Hypertension

Pathophysiology, Diagnosis, and Management

Second Edition

VOLUME ONE

Hypertension
Pathophysiology, Diagnosis, and Management

Second Edition

VOLUME ONE

Editors

John H. Laragh, M.D.
*Director, Cardiovascular Center and
Hypertension Center
Chief, Cardiology Division
Hilda Altschul
Master Professor of Medicine
The New York Hospital-
Cornell Medical Center
New York, New York*

Barry M. Brenner, M.D.
*Director, Renal Division
Department of Medicine
Brigham and Women's Hospital, and
Director, Harvard Center for the Study of Kidney Disease, and
Samuel A. Levine Professor of Medicine
Harvard Medical School
Boston, Massachusetts*

Raven Press ⚚ New York

Raven Press, Ltd., 1185 Avenue of the Americas, New York, New York 10036

Made in the United States of America

Library of Congress Cataloging-in-Publication Data

Hypertension: pathophysiology, diagnosis, and management/editors,
　　John H. Laragh, Barry M. Brenner.—2nd ed.
　　　　p.　cm.
　　Includes bibliographical references and index.
　　ISBN 0-7817-0157-0 (set)
　　1. Hypertension.　I. Laragh, John H., 1924–　.　II. Brenner, Barry M.,
　1937–　.
　　[DNLM: 1. Hypertension.　WG 340 H996354　1995]
　RC685.H8H9144　1995
　616.1′32—dc20
　DNLM/DLC
　for Library of Congress

94-26916
CIP

9　8　7　6　5　4　3　2　1

To my teachers and colleagues who taught me physiology, clinical medicine, and the disciplines of research. In particular my physiology professor, Robert Pitts, a man of penetrating logic, showed me how to design, perform, and analyze an experiment. Harry Goldblatt taught me about experimental hypertension. Homer Smith introduced me to free water clearance and taught me how to tell a good experiment from a bad one. Marcel Goldenberg, who found norepinephrine in adrenal tissue and differentiated its action in humans from that of epinephrine, showed me the excitement of clinical discovery and convinced me anew that cardiology had to involve hormonal signals, chemical transmitters, and cellular mechanisms. This warm, gentle, volatile man died prematurely of malignant hypertension. He asked me to care for him but, sadly, there was little to do. I am especially fortunate to work with my wife, Dr. Jean Sealey, a creative scientist with unique skills that I lack who always gives more than she expects in return.

These scientists, a number of others like them, and my trainees with whom I have worked side by side make every working day a joy. Asking questions and discovering new things to be true has its own rewards.

J.H.L.

To my students and trainees—for they shared heavily in the toil that created and continues to create the richness of new knowledge that has been my lodestar.

B.M.B.

Contents

VOLUME ONE

Section I: Background and Historical Aspects

Section II: Epidemiological Dimensions of Hypertension

Section V: Blood Pressure Regulation in Normal and Hypertensive States

Part A: Arterior Physiology and Pathophysiology

Section V. Part C: Metabolic and Local Humoral Factors in Hypertension

Section V. Part D: Calcium and Magnesium in Blood Pressure Regulation

Section V. Part E: Molecular-Genetic Factors in Hypertension

**Section VI: The Kidneys and the Renin-Angiotensin Aldosterone Axis:
Role in Sodium-Volume Homeostasis and Arterial Tone
in Pathogenesis of Hypertension**

VOLUME TWO

Section VII: Clinical and Laboratory Evaluation of Hypertensive Disorders

Section VIII: Pathophysiology, Diagnosis and Treatment of Specific Forms of Hypertension

Part A: Secondary Forms of Hypertension

1. *Renal Disorders*

2. *Adrenal Disorders*

Section VIII. Part B: Other Endocrine Disorders: Diabetes and Obesity

Section VIII. Part C: Hypertension in Special Situations

Section X. Part C: Future Horizons in Therapy

Contributors

Gyorgy Abraham, M.D., *First Department of Medicine, Albert Szent-Gyorgyi Medical University, Szeged, Hungary H-6701*

Daine Alcorn, M.D., *Department of Anatomy and Cell Biology, University of Melbourne, Parkville 3052, Victoria, Australia*

Michael H. Alderman, M.D., *Department of Epidemiology and Social Medicine, Albert Einstein College of Medicine, 1300 Morris Park Avenue, Bronx, New York 10461*

G. Peter Aldred, M.D., *Department of Medicine, University of Melbourne, Austin Hospital, Heidelberg 3084, Victoria, Australia*

R. Wayne Alexander, M.D., *Department of Medicine, Division of Cardiology, Emory University, Atlanta, Georgia 30322*

Andrew M. Allen, M.D., *Howard Florey Institute of Experimental Physiology and Medicine, University of Melbourne, Parkville 3052, Victoria, Australia*

Bella T. Altura, Ph.D., *Department of Physiology, State University of New York, Health Science Center at Brooklyn, 450 Clarkson Avenue, Brooklyn, New York 11203*

Burton M. Altura, Ph.D., *Departments of Physiology and Medicine, State University of New York, Health Science Center at Brooklyn, 450 Clarkson Avenue, Box 31, Brooklyn, New York 11203*

John Amerena, M.D., *Department of Internal Medicine, Division of Hypertension, University of Michigan Medical Center, 3918 Taubman Center, Ann Arbor, Michigan 48109*

A. Amery, M.D., *Hypertension and Cardiovascular Rehabilitation Unit, Department of Pathophysiology, Faculty of Medicine, University of Leuven, B-3000 Leuven, Belgium*

Richard P. Ames, M.D., *St. Lukes's Roosevelt Hospital, 1000 Tenth Avenue, New York, New York 10019*

Sharon Anderson, M.D., *Division of Nephrology and Hypertension PP262, Oregon Health Sciences University, 3181 Southwest Sam Jackson Park Road, PP Suite 262, Portland, Oregon 97201*

Leonard F. Arnolda, M.D., *Department of Medicine and Centre for Neuroscience, Flinders University, Bedford Park, Adelaide, South Australia 5042, Australia*

Steven A. Atlas, M.D., *Cardiovascular Center, The New York Hospital-Cornell Medical Center, 525 East 68th Street, New York, New York 10021*

Phyllis August, M.D., *Cardiovascular Center, The New York Hospital-Cornell University Medical Center, 525 East 68th Street, New York, New York 10021*

Paul T. Baker, Ph.D., *Department of Anthropology, The Pennsylvania State University, State College, Pennsylvania 16802*

Luciano Barajas, M.D., *Department of Pathology, Harbor-UCLA Medical Center, 1000 West Carson Street, Torrence, California 90509*

William M. Barron, M.D., *Division of General Internal Medicine, Loyola University Medical Center, Building 54, Room 109, 2160 South First Avenue, Maywood, Illinois 60153*

Alfred H. Beil, M.D., *Department of Internal Medicine IV, University of Erlangen-Nürnberg, Kontumazgarten 14-18, 90429, Nürnberg 80, Germany*

Lawrie J. Beilin, M.D., *University Department of Medicine, Royal Perth Hospital, University of Western Australia, 35 Victoria Square, Perth, Western Australia 6000, Australia*

Gordon M. Bell, M.D., *Department of Medicine, Royal Liverpool University Hospital, (6Z-Link Unit), Liverpool L7 8XP, United Kingdom*

Caroline P. Bell-Quilley, M.D., *Department of Pharmacology, New York Medical College, Valhalla, New York 10595*

Marc Bellet, M.D., *Laboratoire Roussel UCLAF, 111 Route de Noisy, 93230 Romainville, France*

Kathleen H. Berecek, M.D., *Department of Physiology and Biophysics, and Vascular Biology and Hypertension Program of the Division of Cardiovascular Disease, Department of Medicine, University of Alabama at Birmingham, UAB Station, Birmingham, Alabama 35294*

Italo Biaggioni, M.D., *Clinical Research Center and Departments of Medicine and Pharmacology, Division of Clinical Pharmacology, AA3228 MCN, Vanderbilt University, Nashville, Tennessee 37232*

Giuseppe Bianchi, M.D., *Division of Nephrology and Hypertension, University of Milan; and Department of Science and Biomedical Technology, San Raffaele Hospital, Via Olgettina 60, 20132 Milan, Italy*

Edward G. Biglieri, M.D. (Retired), *Department of Medicine, General Clinical Research Center, San Francisco General Hospital, 1001 Portrero Avenue, San Francisco, California 94110*

W. H. Birkenhäger, M.D., *Department of Medicine, University Hospital, Maastricht; and Erasmus University, Rotterdam, The Netherlands*

Henry R. Black, M.D., *Professor of Internal Medicine, Chairman, Department of Preventive Medicine, Rush-Presbyterian-St. Luke's Medical Center, Rush University, 1725 West Harrison Street, Suite 117, Chicago, Illinois 60612*

Seymour G. Blank, Ph.D., *Cardiovascular Center, The New York Hospital-Cornell Medical Center, 525 East 68th Street, Starr-4, New York, New York 10021*

M. Donald Blaufox, M.D., Ph.D., *Department of Nuclear Medicine, Albert Einstein College of Medicine and Montefiore Medical Center, 1300 Morris Park Avenue, Bronx, New York 10461*

Jon D. Blumenfeld, M.D., *Cardiovascular Center, New York Hospital-Cornell Medical Center, 525 East 68th Street, New York, New York 10021*

Peter Bolli, M.D., F.A.C.P., *Director, Hypertension Clinic and Hypertension Laboratory, Professor of Medicine, Health Sciences Center, Room GE421, 820 Shrbrook Street, Winnepeg, Manitoba, Canada R3A 1R9*

Gerd Bönner, M.D., *Department II of Internal Medicine, University of Cologne, Merheim Hospital, Ostmerheimer Straße 200, D-51109 Köln, Germany*

Serge Bottari, M.D., *Centre d'Etudes Nucléaires, INSERM U244, B.P. 85X, F-38041 Grenoble, France*

Michael W. Brands, M.D., *Department of Physiology and Biophysics, University of Mississippi Medical Center, 2500 North State Street, Jackson, Mississippi 39216*

Barry M. Brenner, M.D., *The Harvard Center for the Study of Kidney Disease, Harvard Medical School; and Renal Division and Department of Medicine, Brigham and Women's Hospital, 75 Francis Street, Boston, Massachusetts 02115*

Arnold S. Brickman, M.D., *University of California at Los Angeles, San Fernando Valley Program, Sepulveda V.A. Medical Center, 16111 Plummer Street, Mail Code 111, Sepulveda, California 91343*

Josephine P. Briggs, M.D., *Departments of Internal Medicine and Physiology, Division of Nephrology, The University of Michigan Medical School, 1150 West Medical Center Drive, 1560 Medical Science Research Building II, Ann Arbor, Michigan 48109-0679*

Eric Brodde, M.D., *Medizinische Klinik & Poliklinik, Abt Nieren & Hicgdryckkranke, Universitatsklinikum, Hufelandstrasse 55, D-4300 Essen, Germany*

Alexander C. Brownie, M.D., *Department of Biochemistry, State University of New York at Buffalo, School of Medicine, 102 Cary Hall, Buffalo, New York 14214*

P. Bruneval, M.D., *Service d'Anatomopathologie, Hôpital Broussais, 96 rue Didot, 75014 Paris, France*

Tobias A. Bruning, M.D., *Department of Pharmacotherapy, Academic Medical Center, University of Amsterdam, Meibergdreef 15, 1105 AZ Amsterdam, The Netherlands; and Department of Nephrology, University Hospital, Rijnsburgerweg 10, 2333 AA Leiden, The Netherlands*

Hans R. Brunner, M.D., *Division of Nephrology and Hypertension, Centre Hospitalier Universitaire, Chu Vaudois, Départment de Médicine, 1001 Lausanne, Switzerland*

Vardaman M. Buckalew, Jr., M.D., *Department of Internal Medicine, Section on Nephrology, Bowman Gray School of Medicine, Wake Forest University, Medical Center Boulevard, Winston-Salem, North Carolina 27157*

Fritz R. Bühler, M.D., *Department of Pathophysiology and Pharmaceutical Medicine, University of Basel; and Head, International Clinical Research and Development, F. Hoffman La-Roche Limited, 4002 Basel, Switzerland*

Richard D. Bukoski, M.D., *Department of Internal Medicine, University of Texas Medical Branch at Galveston, Galveston, Texas 77555*

Valerie Burke, M.D., F.R.A.C.P., *University Department of Medicine, Royal Perth Hospital, University of Western Australia, 35 Victoria Square, Perth, Western Australia 6000, Australia*

Geoffrey Burnstock, M.D., D.Sc., *Department of Anatomy and Developmental Biology, University College London, Gower Street, London WC1E 6BT, United Kingdom*

Richard L. Byyny, M.D., *Division of Internal Medicine, University of Colorado Health Science Center, Denver, Colorado 80262*

Jean M. Cacciabaudo, M.D., *Cardiovascular Center, The New York Hospital-Cornell Medical Center, 525 East 68th Street, New York, New York 10021*

David A. Calhoun, M.D., *Vascular Biology and Hypertension Program of the Division of Cardiovascular Disease, Department of Medicine, University of Alabama at Birmingham, 1034 Zeigler Research Building, UAB Station, Birmingham, Alabama 35294*

François Cambien, M.D., *INSERM SC7, 17 rue du Fer à Moulin, 75005 Paris, France*

Wallace G. Campbell, Jr., M.D., *Department of Pathology, Cornell University Medical Center, 525 East 68th Street, New York, New York 10021*

Francesco P. Cappuccio, M.B.B.S., M.D., M.Sc., *Environmental Epidemiology Unit, Department of Public Health and Policy, London School of Hygiene and Tropical Medicine, London WC1E 7HT, England*

Ernesto Carafoli, M.D., *Laboratory of Biochemistry, Swiss Federal Institute of Technology (ETH), 8092 Zurich, Switzerland*

Robert M. Carey, M.D., *Division of Endocrinology and Metabolism, Department of Medicine, University of Virginia School of Medicine, University Avenue, Charlottesville, Virginia 22908*

Oscar A. Carretero, M.D., *Department of Medicine, Hypertension and Vascular Research Division, Heart and Vascular Institute, Henry Ford Hospital, 2799 West Grand Boulevard, Detroit, Michigan 48202*

Daniel F. Catanzaro, Ph.D., *Cardiovascular Center, Department of Medicine, and Department of Physiology and Biophysics, The New York Hospital-Cornell Medical Center, 525 East 68th Street, New York, New York 10021*

Anne Chabanel, Ph.D., *Laboratoire Central d'Hématologie, Hopital de l'Hotel Dieu, Paris, France*

Siew Yeen Chai, M.D., *University of Melbourne, Department of Medicine, Austin Hospital, Heidelberg, Victoria 3084, Australia*

J. P. Chalmers, M.D., *Department of Medicine and Centre for Neuroscience, Flinders University, Bedford Park, Adelaide, South Australia 5042, Australia*

Pamela Charney, M.D., *Primary Care Clinic--3N-31, Bronx Municipal Hospital Center, Pelham Parkway South and Eastchester Road, Bronx, New York 10461*

Gilles Chatellier, M.D., *Centre d'Investigations Cliniques, Hôpital Broussais, 96 rue Didot, 75014 Paris, France*

Pei Yen Chen, M.D., *Nephrology Research and Training Center, Departments of Medicine and Physiology, Division of Nephrology, University of Alabama at Birmingham, 1900 University Boulevard, Birmingham, Alabama 35294-0007; and Veterans Affairs Medical Center, Birmingham, Alabama 35294*

Yiu-Fai Chen, Ph.D., *The Vascular Biology and Hypertension Program of the Division of Cardiovascular Disease, Department of Medicine, University of Alabama at Birmingham, 1034 Zeigler Research Building, UAB Station, Birmingham, Alabama 35294*

Glenn M. Chertow, M.D., *Renal Division and Department of Medicine, Brigham and Women's Hospital and Harvard Medical School, Boston, Massachusetts 02115*

Shu Chien, M.D., Ph.D., *Institute for Biomedical Engineering, University of California at San Diego, La Jolla, California 92093*

Michele Chiesi, Ph.D., *Department of Research, Pharmaceuticals Division, Ciba-Geigy Ltd., 4002 Basel, Switzerland*

Aram V. Chobanian, M.D., *Boston University School of Medicine, Boston University Medical Center, 80 East Concord Street, Boston, Massachusetts 02118*

Paul C. Churchill, Ph.D., *Department of Physiology, Wayne State University School of Medicine, 5263 Scott Hall, 540 East Canfield, Detroit, Michigan 48201*

Eric Clauser, M.D., *INSERM U36, Collège de France, 3, rue d'Ulm, 75005 Paris, France*

Ellen Cohen, M.D., *Department of Medicine, Montefiore Medical Center-Centennial 3, 111 East 210 Street, Bronx, New York 10467*

Thomas G. Coleman, Ph.D., *Department of Physiology, University of Mississippi Medical Center, 2500 North State Street, Jackson, Mississippi 39216*

Pierre Corvol, M.D., *INSERM U36, Collège de France, 3, rue d'Ulm, 75005 Paris, France and Service d'Hypertension Artérielle, Hôpital Broussais, 96 rue Didot, 75014 Paris, France*

John Cruickshank, M.D., *Royal Brompton and National Heart and Chest Hospital, London, United Kingdom*

J. J. Curtis, M.D., *Division of Nephrology, University of Alabama at Birmingham, 1900 University Boulevard, University Station, Birmingham, Alabama 35294*

Jeffrey A. Cutler, M.D., M.P.H., *Prevention and Demonstration Research Branch, Division of Epidemiology and Clinical Applications, National Heart, Lung, and Blood Institute, Federal Building, Room 604, 7550 Wisconsin Avenue, Bethesda, Maryland 20892*

Richard C. Dage, M.D., *Marion Merrell Dow Research Institute, 2110 East Galbraith Road, Cincinnati, Ohio 45215*

Robert C. Davidson, M.D., *Department of Medicine, Division of Nephrology, RM-11, Department of Medicine, University of Washington, Seattle, Washington 98195*

Martin Day, M.D., *Centre d'Investigations Cliniques, Hôpital Broussais, 96 rue Didot, 75014 Paris, France*

Jacques de Champlain, M.D., *P.O. Box 6128, Branch A, University of Montreal, Montreal H3C 357, Canada*

Marc de Gasparo, M.D., *Cardiovascular Research K-125 10.15, Ciba-Geigy Ltd., CH4002 Basel, Switzerland*

P. W. de Leeuw, M.D., *Department of Internal Medicine, University Hospital Maastricht, P.O. Box 5800, 6202 AZ Maastricht, The Netherlands; and Erasmus University, Rotterdam, The Netherlands*

Richard B. Devereux, M.D., *Department of Medicine, Cornell University Medical College and Director, Adult Echocardiography Laboratory, Division of Cardiology, The New York Hospital-Cornell Medical Center, 525 East 68th Street, New York, New York 10021*

Gerald F. DiBona, M.D., *Department of Internal Medicine, University of Iowa College of Medicine, Iowa City, Iowa 52242*

Robert G. Dluhy, M.D., *Endocrine-Hypertension Division, Brigham and Women's Hospital, Boston, Massachusetts 02115*

Annette M. Doherty, M.D., *Senior Director, Cardiovascular Cancer/Peptides Chemistry, Parke-Davis Pharmaceutical Research, Warner-Lambert Company, 2800 Plymouth Road, Ann Arbor, Michigan 48105*

Austin E. Doyle, M.D., *(Deceased)*

Raghvendra K. Dubey, M.D., *Department of Medicine, Division of Clinical Pharmacology and Department of Research, Laboratory of Vascular Research, University Hospital, Petersgraben 4, CH-4031 Basel, Switzerland*

Michael J. Dunn, M.D., *Department of Medicine, Case Western Reserve University, School of Medicine and Division of Nephrology, University Hospitals of Cleveland, 2074 Abington Road, Cleveland, Ohio 44106*

Brent M. Egan, M.D., *Department of Pharmacology and Medicine, and Departments of Pharmacology and Medicine, Division of Clinical Pharmacology, Clinical Science Building, 826H, Medical University of South Carolina, 171 Ashley Avenue, Charleston, South Carolina 29426*

Paul Erne, M.D., *Chiles Research Institute, Providence Medical Center and Oregon Health Sciences University, Portland, Oregon 97213*

Joseph W. Eschbach, M.D., *Department of Medicine, Divisions of Hematology and Nephrology, RM-10, University of Washington, Seattle, Washington 98195*

Murray Esler, M.D., *Baker Medical Research Institute, P.O. Box 348, Commercial Road, Prahran 3181, Melbourne, Australia*

Dominique Evéquoz, M.D., *Division of Nephrology and Hypertension, Centre Hospitalier Universitaire, Départment de Médicine, Chu Vaudois, 1001 Lausanne, Switzerland*

R. Fagard, M.D., Ph.D., *Hypertension and Cardiovascular Rehabilitation Unit, Department of Pathophysiology, Faculty of Medicine, University of Leuven, B-3000 Leuven, Belgium*

Ele Ferrannini, M.D., *Metabolism Unit, C.N.R. Institute of Clinical Physiology, University of Pisa, Via Savi, 8, 56100 Pisa, Italy*

Patrizia Ferrari, M.D., *PRASSIS, Sigma Tau Research Institute, Via Forlanini, 3, 20019 Milan, Italy*

Eugene J. Fine, M.D., *Department of Nuclear Medicine, Albert Einstein College of Medicine and Montefiore Medical Center, 1300 Morris Park Avenue, Bronx, New York 10461*

Danilo Fliser, M.D., *Department of Internal Medicine, University of Heidelberg, Bergheimer Straße 56a, 69115, Heidelberg, Germany*

Gary A. Flynn, Ph.D., *Discovery Chemistry, Marion Merrell Dow Research Institute, P.O. Box 156300, 2110 East Galbraith Road, Cincinnati, Ohio 45215*

Björn Folkow, M.D., *Department of Physiology, University of Göteborg, S-400 33 Göteborg, Sweden*

Stanley S. Franklin, M.D., *RMC, 3856 Long Beach Boulevard, Long Beach, California 90807*

Edward D. Freis, M.D., *Hypertensive Research Unit, Department of Veterans Affairs Medical Center, 50 Irving Street, Northwest, Washington D.C. 20422*

John F. French, M.D., *Marion Merrell Dow Research Institute, 2110 East Galbraith Road, Cincinnati, Ohio 45215*

Curt D. Furberg, M.D., Ph.D., *Department of Public Health Sciences, Bowman Gray School of Medicine, Medical Center Boulevard, Winston-Salem, North Carolina 27157-1063*

Fuad Gahnem, D.Sc., *Department of Physiology, Cornell University Medical Center, 525 East 68th Street, New York, New York 10021*

C. A. Gaillard, M.D., *Department of Internal Medicine, University Hospital Maastricht, M/6202 AZ Maastrict, The Netherlands; and Erasmus University, Rotterdam, The Netherlands*

Detlev Ganten, M.D., Ph.D., *Max-Delbrück Center for Molecular Medicine, Robert-Rössle Straße 10, 13125 Berlin-Buch, Germany*

Diego L. Garcia, M.D., *Renal Division, Department of Medicine, Brigham and Women's Hospital, and Harvard Center for the Study of Kidney Disease, Harvard Medical Center, Boston, Massachusetts 02115*

J. M. Gasc, *INSERM U36, Collège de France, 3 rue d'Ulm, 75005 Paris, France*

Robert S. Gaston, M.D., *Nephrology Research and Training Center, Departments of Medicine and Physiology, Division of Nephrology, University of Alabama at Birmingham, 1900 University Boulevard, Birmingham, Alabama 35294-0007 and Veterans Affairs Medical Center, Birmingham, Alabama 35294*

Haralambos Gavras, M.D., *Hypertension and Atherosclerosis Section, Department of Medicine, Boston University School of Medicine, 80 East Concord Street, Boston, Massachusetts 02118*

Irene Gavras, M.D., *Hypertension and Atherosclerosis Section, Department of Medicine, Boston University School of Medicine, 80 East Concord Street, Boston, Massachusetts 02118*

Paolo Gazzotti, Ph.D., *Laboratory of Biochemistry, Swiss Federal Institute of Technology (ETH), 8092 Zurich, Switzerland*

Gerhard H. Giebisch, M.D., *Department of Cellular and Molecular Physiology, Yale University School of Medicine, 333 Cedar Street, P.O. Box 208026, New Haven, Connecticut 06510*

Ray W. Gifford, Jr., M.D., *Department of Clinical Medicine, New York University Medical Center, 324 East 30th Street, New York, New York 10016; and The Cleveland Clinic, Cleveland, Ohio 44195*

James M. Gloor, M.D., *University of Virginia School of Medicine, Charlottesville, Virginia 22908*

Allan Goldberg, M.D., *Cardiovascular Clinical Research, Merck Research Laboratories, 10 Sentry Parkway, BL3-1, Blue Bell, Pennsylvania 19422*

Michael Goldberg, M.D., Ph.D., *Clinical Pharmacology, Merck Research Laboratories, 10 Sentry Parkway, BL3-1, Blue Bell, Pennsylvania 19422*

Peter J. Goldblatt, M.D., *Department of Pathology, Dean, Graduate School, Medical College of Ohio, C.S. 10008, Toledo, Ohio 43699*

R. Ariel Gomez, M.D., *Pediatric Nephrology, Director, Child Health Research Center, Medical Research Building MR4, Room 2001, University of Virginia Health Science Center, Charlottesville, Virginia 22908*

Richard D. Gordon, M.D., Ph.D., F.R.A.C.P., *Endocrine-Hypertension Research Unit, Department of Medicine, University of Queensland, Greenslopes Hospital, Brisbane, 4120, Australia*

Göran Granerus, M.D., *Department of Clinical Physiology, Faculty of Health Sciences, University Hospital, University of Linköping, S-581 85 Linköping, Sweden*

Guido Grassi, M.D., *Cattedra di Medicina Interna, Universitá di Milano, Ospedale S. Gerardo dei Tintori, Monza; Centro Auxologico Italiano, Via F. Sforza 35, Milano 20122, Italy*

Kathy K. Griendling, Ph.D., *Division of Cardiology, Emory University, P.O. Box LL, Atlanta, Georgia 30322*

Clarence E. Grim, M.D., *Hypertensive Research Center, Department of Medicine, Charles R. Drew University of Medicine and Science, 1621 East 120th Street, Los Angeles, California 90059*

Ehud Grossman, M.D., *Hypertension Unit, The Chaim Sheba Medical Center, Tel-Hashomer, 52621, Israel*

Markus G. Grütter, M.D., *Pharmaceuticals Division, Biotechnology Research Department, K-681.545, CIBA-Geigy Ltd., CH 4002 Basel, Switzerland*

Eduardo Guarda, M.D., *Department of Internal Medicine, Division of Cardiology, University of Missouri Health Sciences Center, Columbia, Missouri 65212*

Mark Gunning, M.D., *Department of Medicine, Harvard Medical School, and Renal Division, Department of Medicine, New England Deaconess Hospital and Joslin Diabetes Center, 110 Francis Street-Suite 9D, Boston, Massachusetts 02215*

Jack Guralnik, M.D., Ph.D., *Epidemiology and Demographic Office, National Institute on Aging, Gateway Building, Room 3C309, 7201 Wisconsin Avenue, Bethesda, Maryland 20892*

Arthur C. Guyton, M.D., *Department of Physiology and Biophysics, University of Mississippi Medical Center, 2500 North State Street, Jackson, Mississippi 39216*

Francis J. Haddy, M.D., *Department of Physiology, Uniformed Services University of the Health Sciences, 4301 Junes Bridge Road, Bethesda, Maryland 20814*

John E. Hall, Ph.D., *Department of Physiology and Biophysics, University of Mississippi Medical Center, 2500 North State Street, Jackson, Mississippi 39216*

Jean-Michel Halimi, M.D., *Department of Medicine and Nephrology, Centre Hospitalier Universitaire, Hôpital Lapeyronie, 34059 Montpellier Cedex, France*

Pavel Hamet, M.D., Ph.D., *Laboratory of Molecular Pathophysiology, Centre de Recherche, Hôtel-Dieur de Montréal, Université de Montréal, Marie-de-la-Ferre Pavilion, 3850 St. Urbain Street, Montréal, Quebec H2W 1T8, Canada*

Bruce P. Hamilton, M.D., *Department of Medicine, University of Maryland School of Medicine and V.A. Medical Center, 655 West Baltimore Street, Baltimore, Maryland 21201*

John M. Hamlyn, M.D., *Department of Physiology, University of Maryland School of Medicine, 655 West Baltimore Street, Baltimore, Maryland 21201*

Diane Handy, Ph.D., *Hypertension and Atherosclerosis Section, Department of Medicine, Boston University School of Medicine, 80 East Concord Street, Boston, Massachusetts 02118*

Lennart Hansson, M.D., *Department of Geriatrics, University of Uppsala, P.O. Box 2151 S-75002 Uppsala, Sweden*

Linda C. Harlan, Ph.D., *Division of Cancer Prevention and Control, National Cancer Institute, National Institutes of Health, Bethesda, Maryland 20892*

William R. Harlan, M.D., *Institute of Disease Prevention, National Institutes of Health, Bethesda, Maryland 20892*

Sandra C. Harm, M.S., *Cardiovascular Clinical Research, Merck Research Laboratories, 10 Sentry Parkway, BL3-1, Blue Bell, Pennsylvania 19422*

Raymond C. Harris, M.D., *Departments of Medicine and Biochemistry, Vanderbilt University School of Medicine, 21st Avenue South, Nashville, Tennessee 37232*

Greg S. Hartman, M.D., *Department of Anesthesiology, The New York Hospital-Cornell Medical Center, 525 East 68th Street, New York, NY 10021*

Daniel C. Hatton, M.D., *Department of Medicine, Division of Nephrology and Hypertension, Oregon Health Sciences University, 3314 Southwest US Veterans Hospital Road, Portland, Oregon 97201*

Richard J. Havlik, M.D., M.P.H., *Epidemiology, Demography, and Biometry Program, National Institute on Aging, Gateway Building, Room 3C309, 7201 Wisconsin Avenue, Bethesda, Maryland 20892*

Anthony M. Heagerty, M.D., M.R.C.P., *Department of Medicine, University Hospital of South Manchester, Nell Lane, West Didsbury, Manchester M20 8LR, United Kingdom*

Maarten G. C. Hendriks, M.D., *Department of Pharmacotherapy, Academic Medical Center, Meibergdreef 15, 1105 AZ Amsterdam, The Netherlands*

James P. Henry, M.D., Ph.D., *Department of Research, Division of Nephrology and Hypertension MP II, Charles R. Drew University of Medicine and Science, Hawkins Building, 1621 East 120th Street, Los Angeles, California 90059*

Kent Hermsmeyer, Ph.D., *Oregon Regional Primate Research Center, 505 Northwest 185th Avenue, Beaverton, Oregon 97006*

Brian B. Hoffman, M.D., *Department of Medicine, Stanford University School of Medicine; and Geriatric Research, Education and Clinical Center, Veterans Affairs Medical Center (GRECC/182-B), 3801 Miranda Avenue, Palo Alto, California 94304*

Sigrid Hoffman, Ph.D., *Max-Delbrück Center for Molecular Medicine, Robert Rössle Straße 10, 13125 Berlin-Buch, Germany*

Norman K. Hollenberg, M.D., Ph.D., *Departments of Medicine and Radiology, Harvard Medical School and Brigham and Women's Hospital, 75 Francis Street, Boston, Massachusetts 02115*

Tadashi Inagami, Ph.D., *Departments of Medicine and Biochemistry, Vanderbilt University School of Medicine, 21st Avenue South, Nashville, Tennessee 37232*

Gary D. James, Ph.D., *Departments of Medicine/Physiology and Biophysics, Cardiovascular Center, The New York Hospital-Cornell Medical Center, 525 East 68th Street, New York, New York 10021*

Xavier Jeunemaitre, M.D., *Inserm U 36, Collége de France, 3 rue d'Ulm, 75005 Paris, France; and Service d'Hypertension Arténelle, Hôpital Broussais, 75014 Paris, France*

Colin Ivor Johnston, M.D., *University of Melbourne, Department of Medicine, Austin Hospital, Heidelberg, Victoria 3084, Australia*

Stevo Julius, M.D., Sc.D., *Department of Internal Medicine, Division of Hypertension, University of Michigan, 3918 Taubman Center, Ann Arbor, Michigan 48109-0356*

William B. Kannel, M.D., M.P.H., *Section of Preventive Medicine and Epidemiology, Evans Department of Clinical Research, University Hospital, Boston University Medical Center, 5 Thurber Street, Framingham, Massachusetts 01701*

Michael Kashgarian, M.D., *Department of Pathology, Yale University School of Medicine, 20 Lauder Hall, 310 Cedar Street, P.O. Box 3333, New Haven, Connecticut 06510*

Claudio E. Kater, M.D., *Department of Medicine, Section of Endocrinology, Escola Paulista de Medicina, Sao Paulo, Brasil*

Stephen A. Katz, Ph.D., *Department of Physiology, University of Minnesota School of Medicine, Minneapolis, Minnesota 55455; and Senior Investigator, Division of Nephrology, Hennepin County Medical Center, D-Building, 5th Floor, 914 South 8th Street, Minneapolis, Minnesota 55415*

William F. Keane, M.D., *Department of Medicine, Division of Nephrology, Hennepin County Medical Center, Minnesota Medical School, 701 Park Avenue South, Minneapolis, Minnesota 55415*

Raymond P. Kelly, M.D., *Cardiology Department, St. Vincent's Hospital, Sydney, New South Wales 2010, Australia*

Raouf A. Khalil, M.D., Ph.D., *Department of Physiology in Medicine, Harvard Medical School and Cardiovascular Division, Beth Israel Hospital, 330 Brookline Avenue, Boston, Massachusetts 02215*

Genjiro Kimura, M.D., *Renal Division, Department of Medicine, Brigham and Women's Hospital, 75 Francis Street, Boston, Massachusetts 02115*

Andrew J. King, M.D., *Renal Division, New England Medical Center, Box 390, 750 Washington Street, Boston, Massachusetts 02111; and Brigham and Women's Hospital, 75 Francis Street, Boston, Massachusetts 02115*

Wolfgang Kiowski, M.D., *Division of Cardiology, Department of Medicine, University Hospital, Basel, Switzerland*

Arthur L. Klatsky, M.D., *Division of Cardiology, Department of Medicine, Kaiser Permanente Medical Center, 280 West MacArthur Boulevard, Oakland, California 94611*

Irwin Klein, M.D., *Division of Endocrinology, Department of Medicine, North Shore University Hospital, Cornell University Medical College, 300 Community Drive, Manhasset, New York 11030*

Hollis D. Kleinert, Ph.D., *Pharmaceutical Research and Development, Abbott Laboratories, One Abbott Park Road, Department 48G, Building AP6A, Abbott Park, Illinois 60064*

Shelley A. Klemm, M.D., *Endocrine-Hypertension Research Unit, Department of Medicine, University of Queensland, Greenslopes Hospital, Brisbane, 4120, Australia*

Brian Kobilka, M.D., *Departments of Medicine and Molecular and Cellular Physiology, Stanford University School of Medicine, Stanford, California 94304*

Hermes A. Kontos, M.D., Ph.D., *Department of Medicine, Medical College of Virginia, 11th and Marshall Streets, Richmond, Virginia 23298*

Michael C. Kontos, M.D., *Department of Medicine, Medical College of Virginia, 11th and Marshall Streets, Richmond, Virginia 23298*

Ulla C. Kopp, Ph.D., *Department of Internal Medicine, University of Iowa College of Medicine, Iowa City, Iowa 52242*

Diane R. Krieger, M.D., *Northwestern Memorial Hospital, Wesley Pavilion, Room 296, 250 East Superior Street, Chicago, Illinois 60611*

Lewis Kuller, M.D., *Graduate School of Public Health, University of Pittsburgh, A527 Crabtree Hall, 130 DeSoto Street, Pittsburgh, Pennsylvania 15261*

Theodore W. Kurtz, M.D., *Long Hospital, Room 518, University of California, San Francisco, 505 Parnassus Avenue, Room L-518, San Francisco, California 94143*

Vicente Lahera, Ph.D., *Department of Physiology, Universidad Complutense, Madrid, Spain*

Lewis Landsberg, M.D., *Northwestern Memorial Hospital, Wesley Pavilion, Room 296, 250 East Superior Street, Chicago, Illinois 60611*

John H. Laragh, M.D., *Department of Cardiology, Cardiovascular Center, The New York Hospital-Cornell Medical Center, 525 East 68th Street, New York, New York 10021*

John M. Ledingham, M.D., *University of London, London SW7 IJL, England*

Frans H. H. Leenen, M.D., *Hypertension Unit, Room 4360, University of Ottawa Heart Institute, 1053 Carling Avenue, Ottawa, Ontario K1Y 4E9, Canada*

Kennedy R. Lees, M.D., F.R.C.P., *Department of Medicine and Therapeutics, University of Glasgow, Gardiner Institute, Western Infirmary, Glasgow G11 6NT, Scotland*

Tomas Lenz, M.D., *Department of Nephrology, University of Frankfurt, Frankfurt, Germany*

Bruce B. Lerman, M.D., *Division of Cardiology, Department of Medicine, The New York Hospital-Cornell Medical Center, 525 East 68th Street, Starr 4, New York, New York 10021*

Nigel R. Levens, M.D., *Cardiovascular Research, K 125-10.15, Ciba-Geigy Ltd., CH4002 Basel, Switzerland*

Roberto Levi, M.D., *Department of Pharmacology, The New York Hospital-Cornell Medical Center, Lasdon Center 419, 525 East 68th Street, New York, New York 10021*

John A. Lewicki, M.D., *Scios Nova Incorporated, 2450 Bayshore Parkway, Mountain View, California 94043*

Richard P. Lifton, M.D., *Boyer Center for Molecular Medicine, Section of Nephrology, Yale University School of Medicine, 2073 LMP, 333 Cedar Street, New Haven, Connecticut 06510*

M. Ligueros, M.D., *Department of Clinical Pharmacology, Royal Postgraduate Medical School, Hammersmith Hospital, London, United Kingdom*

Marshall D. Lindheimer, M.D., *Departments of Obstetrics and Gynecology, and Medicine University of Chicago, 5841 South Maryland Avenue, Chicago, Illinois 60637-1470*

Neal Lippman, M.D., *Division of Cardiology, Department of Medicine, The New York Hospital-Cornell University Medical Center, 525 East 68th Street, Starr 4, New York, New York 10021*

Joann Liu, M.D., *Department of Research, Division of Nephrology and Hypertension MPII, Drew University of Medicine and Science Hawkins Building, 1621 East 12th Street, Los Angeles, California 90059*

Li Liu, M.D., *Department of Pathology, Harbor-UCLA Medical Center, 1000 West Carson Street, Torrance, California 90509*

Susanne Ljungman, M.D., *Department of Nephrology, Sahlgrenska Hospital, University of Gothenburg, S-413 45 Gothenburg, Sweden*

Gérard M. London, M.D., *Division of Nephrology, Centre Hospitalier Manhes, Fleury Merogis, France*

Walter M. Lovenberg, Ph.D., *Merrel Dow Research Institute, Strasbourg Center, 16 Rue D'Ankara, Strasbourg 67084, France*

Robert G. Luke, M.D., *University of Cincinnati Medical Center, University of Cincinnati College of Medicine, 231 Bethesda Avenue, ML #0557, Cincinnati, Ohio 45239*

Per Lund-Johansen, M.D., *Department of Heart Disease, University of Bergen, School of Medicine, Bergen, Norway and Department of Heart Disease, Haukeland Hospital, N-5021 Bergen, Norway*

Thomas F. Lüscher, M.D., *Departments of Internal Medicine and Research, Division of Cardiology, University Hospital, Inselspital, CH-3010 Bern, Switzerland*

Thomas Maack, M.D., *Department of Physiology, The New York Hospital-Cornell Medical College, 1300 York Avenue, New York, New York 10021*

Duncan P. MacGregor, M.D., *Department of Medicine, University of Melbourne, Austin Hospital, Heidelberg 3084, Victoria, Australia*

Graham A. MacGregor, M.D., F.R.C.P., *Blood Pressure Unit, Department of Medicine, St. George's Hospital Medical School, Crammer Terrace, London SW17 ORE, United Kingdom*

Harold S. Mackenzie, M.D., Ch.B., M.R.C.P. (UK), *Renal Division, Department of Medicine, Brigham and Women's Hospital, and Harvard Center for the Study of Kidney Disease, Harvard Medical Center, Boston, Massachusetts 02115*

Stephen MacMahon, Ph.D., M.P.H., *Clinical Trials Research Unit, Department of Medicine, Auckland Hospital, Private Bag 92 024, Auckland, New Zealand*

Giuseppe Mancia, M.D., *Cattedra di Medicina Interna, Ospedale S. Gerardo dei Tintori, Monza; Universitá di Milano, Centro Auxologico Italiano, Via F Sforza 35, Milano 20122, Italy*

William M. Manger, M.D., Ph.D., *Department of Clinical Medicine, New York University Medical Center, 324 East 30th Street, New York, New York 10016; and The Cleveland Clinic, Cleveland, Ohio 44195*

Arie J. Man in't Veld, M.D., *Department of Internal Medicine I, Room Ca 327, University Hospital Dijkzigt, Erasmus University Rotterdam, Dr. Molewaterplein 40, 3015 GD Rotterdam, The Netherlands*

Samuel J. Mann, M.D., *Cardiovascular Center The New York Hospital-Cornell University Medical Center, 525 East 68th Street, New York, New York 10021*

R. Davis Manning, Jr., Ph.D., *Department of Physiology, University of Mississippi Medical Center, 2500 North State Street, Jackson, Mississippi 39216*

Franco Mantero, M.D., *Universita-Degli-Studi de Ancona, Cattedra di Endocrinologica, Ospedale Generalo Regionale de Torrette, 06110 Ancona, Italy*

Paolo Manunta, M.D., *Department of Physiology, University of Maryland School of Medicine, 655 West Baltimore Street, Baltimore, Maryland 21201*

Paul R. Marantz, M.D., M.P.H., *Department of Epidemiology and Social Medicine, Albert Einstein College of Medicine, 13 Morris Park Avenue, Bronx, New York 10461*

RoseMerie Marion, R.N., *Cardiovascular Center, The New York Hospital-Cornell Medical Center, 525 East 68th Street, New York, New York 10021*

Allyn L. Mark, M.D., *Cardiovascular Division, Cardiovascular Center, University of Iowa College of Medicine, 200 Hawkins Drive, Iowa City, Iowa 52242; and The Veterans Administration Medical Center, Iowa City, Iowa 52242*

David A. McCarron, M.D., *Department of Medicine, Division of Nephrology and Hypertension, Oregon Health Sciences University, 3314 Southwest U.S. Veterans Hospital Road, PP Suite 262, Portland, Oregon 97201*

John C. McGiff, M.D., *Department of Pharmacology, New York Medical College, Valhalla, New York 10595*

Woerner P. Meehan, Ph.D., *Diabetes/ Medicine Division, University of Southern California, Los Angeles Medical Center, 1010 Mission Road, Los Angeles, California 90031*

Jay I. Meltzer, M.D., *Department of Medicine, Columbia University College of Physicians and Surgeons, New York, New York 10032*

Joël Ménard, M.D., *Centre de Médicine Préventive Cardiovasculaire, Hôpital Broussais, 96 rue Didot, 75014 Paris, France and INSERM U36, 17 rue du Fer à Moulin, 75005 Paris, France*

Frederick A. O. Mendelsohn, M.D., Ph.D., F.R.A.C.P., *Department of Medicine, University of Melbourne, Austin Hospital, Heidelberg 3084, Victoria, Australia*

Chantal Mercure, M.D., *Institut de Recherches Cliniques de Montréal, 110 Pine Avenue West, Montréal, Quebec, Canada H2W 1R7*

P. A. Meredith, M.D., *University Department of Medicine and Therapeutics, Gardiner Institute, Western Infirmary, University of Glasgow, Glasgow G11 6NT, Scotland*

Franz H. Messerli, M.D., *Ochsner Clinic, Department of Hypertension, and Alton Ochsner Medical Foundation, 1514 Jefferson Highway, New Orleans, Louisiana 70121*

Danielle Methot, M.D., *Institut de Recherches Cliniques de Montréal, 110 Pine Avenue West, Montréal, Quebec, Canada H2W 1R7*

Michael L. Middleton, M.D., *Department of Nuclear Medicine, Albert Einstein College of Medicine and Montefiore Medical Center, 1300 Morris Park Avenue, Bronx, New York 10461*

Albert Mimran, M.D., *Department of Medicine and Nephrology, Centre Hospitalier Universitaire, Hôpital Lapeyronie, 34059 Montpellier Cedex, France*

Jane B. Minson, M.D., *Department of Medicine and Centre for Neuroscience, Flinders University, Bedford Park, Adelaide, South Australia 5042, Australia*

Kenneth D. Mitchell, Ph.D., *Department of Physiology SL39, Tulane University School of Medicine, 1430 Tulane Avenue, New Orleans, Louisiana 70112*

Carl Erik Mogensen, M.D., *Department of Endocrinology and Diabetes, Aarhus Kommunehospital, University Hospitals in Aarhus, DK-8000 Aarhus C, Denmark*

R. C. Morris, Jr., M.D., *University of California, San Francisco, General Clinical Research Center, School of Medicine, 1202 Moffitt, Box 0126, San Francisco, California 94143*

Rogelio Mosqueda-Garcia, M.D., Ph.D., *Clinical Research Center and Departments of Medicine and Pharmacology, Division of Clinical Pharmacology, Vanderbilt University, Nashville, Tennessee 37232*

Georges Mourad, M.D., *Department of Medicine and Nephrology, Centre Hospitalier Universitaire, Hôpital Lapeyronie, 34095 Montpellier Cedex, France*

Michael J. Mulvany, Ph.D., D.M.Sc., *Danish Biomembrane Research Centre and Institute of Pharmacology, Aarhus University, Universitetsparken 240, DK-8000 Aarhus C, Denmark*

Hector Myers, Ph.D., *Charles R. Drew University of Medicine and Science, Hypertension Research Center, 1621 East 120th Street, Los Angeles, California 90059*

Elizabeth G. Nabel, M.D., *Cardiovascular Research Center, Departments of Internal Medicine and Biological Chemistry, Howard Hughes Medical Institution, University of Michigan Medical Center, 3560 MSRBII, Box 0688, 1150 West Medical Center Drive, Ann Arbor, Michigan 48109-0688*

Gary J. Nabel, M.D., Ph.D., *Departments of Internal Medicine and Biological Chemistry, Howard Hughes Medical Institution, University of Michigan Medical Center, 3560 MSRBII, Box 0688, 1150 West Medical Center Drive, Ann Arbor, Michigan 48109-0688*

Kazuwa Nakao, M.D., Ph.D., *Second Division, Department of Internal Medicine, Kyoto University Faculty of Medicine, 54 Shogoin Kawahara-cho, Sakyo-ku, Kyoto 606, Japan*

L. Gabriel Navar, Ph.D., *Department of Physiology Tulane University Medical Center, 1430 Tulane Avenue, New Orleans, Louisiana 70112*

James D. Neaton, M.D., *School of Public Health, Division of Biostatistics, University of Minnesota, 2221 University Avenue, Southeast, Suite 200, Minneapolis, Minnesota 55414*

Edward B. Nelson, M.D., *Merck Research Laboratories, 10 Sentry Parkway, BL3-1, Blue Bell, Pennsylvania 19422*

Roger A. Norman, Jr., M.D., *Clinical Research, North Mississippi Medical Center, Tupelo, Mississippi 38801*

Andrew C. Novick, M.D., *Department of Urology, The Cleveland Clinic Foundation, 9500 Euclid Avenue, Cleveland, Ohio 44195*

Michael Nowicki, M.D., *Department of Internal Medicine, University of Heidelberg, 69115 Heidelberg, Germany*

Michael D. Nyby, M.S., *University of California Los Angeles, San Fernando Valley Program, Sepulveda V.A. Medical Center, 16111 Plummer Street, Mail Code 111E, Sepulveda, California 91343*

Michael P. O'Donnell, Ph.D., *Regional Kidney Disease Program, 914 South 8th Street, Minneapolis, Minnesota 55405*

Jürg Nussberger, M.D., *Division of Nephrology and Hypertension, Centre Hospitalier Universitaire, Départment de Médicine, Chu Vaudois, 1011 Lausanne, Switzerland*

Yoshihiro Ogawa, M.D., *Second Division Department of Internal Medicine, Kyoto University Faculty of Medicine, 54 Shogoin Kawahara-cho, Sakyo-ku, Kyoto 606, Japan*

Jacqueline Ohanian, M.D., *Department of Medicine, University Hospital of South Manchester, Nell Lane, West Didsbury, Manchester M20 8LR, United Kingdom*

Kaie Ojamaa, Ph.D., *Division of Endocrinology, Departments of Medicine and Pediatrics, North Shore University Hospital, Cornell University Medical Center, 300 Community Drive, Manhasset, New York 11030*

Per Omvik, M.D., *Department of Heart Disease, University of Bergen, School of Medicine, Bergen, Norway*

Suzanne Oparil, M.D., *Vascular Biology and Hypertension Program of the Division of Cardiovascular Disease, Department of Medicine, University of Alabama at Birmingham, 1034 Ziegler Building, UAB Station, Birmingham, Alabama 35294*

John A. Opsahl, M.D., *School of Medicine, University of Minnesota, Minneapolis, Minnesota 55455 and Division of Nephrology, Hennepin County Medical Center, 914 South 8th Street, Minneapolis, Minnesota 55415*

Sergei N. Orlov, *University of Moscow, Moscow, Russia*

Michael F. O'Rourke, M.D., *Medical Professional Unit, University of New South Wales and Department of Medicine, St. Vincent's Hospital, Sydney, New South Wales 2010, Australia*

Adrian M. Ostfeld, M.D., *Department of Epidemiology and Public Health, Yale University School of Public Health, 60 College Street, Room 404, New Haven, Connecticut 06510*

Martin Paul, M.D., *German Institute for Blood Pressure Research*

Paolo Pauletto, M.D., *Instituto di Medicina Clinica, Universitá di Padova, Via Giustiniani 2, I-35126 Padova, Italy*

Olaf B. Paulson, M.D., *University of Copenhagen, Department of Neurology, Rigshospitalet, 9 Blegdamsvej, DK-2100 Copenhagen, Denmark*

Mark S. Pecker, M.D., *Department of Clinical Medicine, Cardiovascular Center, The New York Hospital-Cornell Medical Center, Hypertension Center, 525 East 68th Street, New York, New York 10021*

Achille C. Pessina, M.D., *Instituto di Medicina Clinica, Universitá di Padova, Via Giustiniani 2, I-35126 Padova, Italy*

Jurij Petrin, M.D., *Bristol-Myers Squibb, Volkarstrasse 83, D-8000 Munich 19, Germany*

Marc A. Pfeffer, M.D., Ph.D., *Department of Medicine, Cardiovascular Division, Brigham and Women's Hospital, 75 Francis Street, Boston, Massachusetts 02115*

Stephen J. Phillips, M.B.B.S., F.R.C.P. (C), *Department of Medicine, Camp Hill Medical Center, Dalhousie University, 5303 Morris Street, Halifax, Nova Scotia, B3J 1B6, Canada*

Thomas G. Pickering, M.D., D.Phil., *Cardiovascular Center, The New York Hospital-Cornell Medical Center, 525 East 68th Street, Starr-4, New York, New York 10021*

Sir George Pickering, M.D., *(Deceased)*

Paul M. Pilowsky, M.D., *Department of Medicine and Centre for Neuroscience, Flinders University, Bedford Park, Adelaide, South Australia 5042, Australia*

F. Pinet, Ph.D., *INSERM U36, Collège de France, 3 rue d'Ulm, 75005 Paris, France*

Gérard E. Plante, M.D., *Departments of Medicine, Physiology, and Pharmacology, University of Sherbrooke, Sherbrooke (Québec) Canada*

P. F. Plouin, M.D., *Service d'Hypertension Artérielle, Hôpital Broussais, 96 rue Didot, 75014 Paris, France*

Anton Y. Postnov, M.D., *Institut de Recherches Cliniques de Montréal, 110 Pine Avenue West, Montréal, Quebec, Canada H2W 1R7*

Kenneth V. Powers, M.S., *Department of Pathology, Harbor-UCLA Medical Center, 1000 West Carson Street, Torrance, California 90509*

B. N. C. Prichard, M.D., *Department of Clinical Pharmacology, University College of London, Gower Street, WC1E 6BT London, England, United Kingdom*

Andrew A. Protter, M.D., *Scios Nova Incorporated, 2450 Bayshore Parkway, Mountain View, California 94043*

Bruce M. Psaty, M.D., Ph.D., *Departments of Medicine, Epidemiology, and Health Services, Cardiovascular Health Research Unit, University of Washington, Metropolitan Park, East Tower, 1730 Minor Avenue, Suite 1360, Seattle, Washington 98101-1488*

I. B. Puddey, M.D., *University Department of Medicine, Royal Perth Hospital, University of Western Australia, 35 Victoria Square, Perth, Western Australia, 6000 Australia*

John Quilley, M.D., *Department of Pharmacology, New York Medical College, Valhalla, New York 10595*

Joseph Rahuel, M.D., *Biotechnology Research Department, Pharmaceuticals Division, Ciba-Geigy Ltd., CH4002 Basel, Switzerland*

Vera Ralevic, M.D., *Department of Anatomy and Developmental Biology, University College London, Gower Street, WC1E 6BT London, United Kingdom*

Jeffrey L. Ram, M.D., *Department of Internal Medicine, Division of Endocrinology, Wayne State University School of Medicine, University Health Center, 4201 St. Antone Avenue, Detroit, MI 48201*

Djamel Ramla, M.D., *Institut de Recherches Cliniques de Montréal, 110 Pine Avenue West, Montréal, Quebec, Canada HRW 1R7*

John P. Rapp, M.D., *Department of Medicine, Medical College of Ohio, Toledo, Ohio 43699*

Alessandro Rappelli, M.D., *Institute of Clinical Medicine, University of Ancona, Ancona, Italy*

John L. Reid, D.M., F.R.C.P., *University Department of Medicine and Therapeutics, Western Infirmary, Glasgow G11 6NT, Scotland*

Donald J. Reis, M.D., *The New York Hospital-Cornell Medical Center, 411 East 69th Street, New York, New York 10021*

Efrain Reisin, M.D., *Department of Medicine, Nephrology Section, Louisiana State University, 1542 Tulane Avenue, Room A319, New Orleans, Louisiana 70112*

Lawrence M. Resnick, M.D., *Division of Endocrinology and Hypertension, Wayne State University Medical Center, 4201 St. Antoine Avenue, Detroit, Michigan 48201*

Timothy L. Reudelhuber, Ph.D., *Institut de Recherches Cliniques de Montréal, 110 Pine Avenue West, Montréal, Quebec, Canada H2W 1R7*

Jean Ribstein, M.D., *Department of Medicine and Nephrology, Centre Hospitalier Universitaire, Hôpital Lapeyronie, 34059 Montpellier Cedex, France*

Eberhard Ritz, M.D., *Department of Internal Medicine, University of Heidelberg, Bergheimer Straße 56A, 69115 Heidelberg, Germany*

David Robertson, M.D., *Professor of Medicine, Pharmacology, and Neurology, Director, Clinical Research Center, Vanderbilt University Medical Center, 1161 21st Avenue South, Nashville, Tennessee 37232-2195*

Mary J. Roman, M.D., *Department of Medicine, The New York Hospital-Cornell Medical Center, Echocardiography Laboratory, 1300 York Avenue, New York, New York 10021*

Juan Carlos Romero, M.D., *Department of Physiology and Biophysics, Mayo School of Medicine, 833 11th Street, Southwest, Rochester, Minnesota 55901*

Gabor M. Rubanyi, M.D., Ph.D., *Berlex Biosciences, Cardiovascular Research, 15049 San Pablo Avenue, Richmond, California 94804*

Speranza Rubattu, M.D., *Il Facolta di Medicina e Chirurgia, Universita di Napoli, Napoli, Italy*

Luis Ruilope, M.D., *Division of Hypertension, Hospital de Octubre, Universidad Complutense, Madrid, Spain*

Marcel Ruzicka, M.D., *Hypertension Unit, Room H360, University of Ottawa Heart Institute, 1053 Carling Avenue, Ottawa, Ontario K1Y 4E9, Canada*

Carolyn Ryan, M.S., R.N., *Cardiovascular Center, The New York Hospital-Cornell Medical Center, 525 East 68th Street, New York, New York 10021*

Michel E. Safar, M.D., *Department of Internal Medicine and INSERM U337, Hôpital Broussais, 96 rue Didot, 75014 Paris, France*

Antonio Saino, M.D., *Cattedra di Medicina Interna, Universitá di Milano, Ospedale S. Gerardo dei Tintori, Monza; Centro Auxologico Italiano, Via F. Sforza 35, Milano 20122, Italy*

Eduardo C. Salido, M.D., *Department of Pathology, Harbor-UCLA Medical Center, 1000 West Carson Street, Torrance, California 90509*

Paul W. Sanders, M.D., *Nephrology Research and Training Center and Division of Nephrology, Departments of Medicine and Physiology, University of Alabama at Birmingham, and VA Medical Center, Birmingham, Alabama 35294*

Saverio Sartore, M.D., *Department of Biomedical Sciences, University of Padova, Via Giustiniani 2, I-35100 Padova, Italy and C.N.R. Unit for Muscle Biology and Physiopathology, Padova, Italy*

Riccardo Sarzani, M.D., *Institute of Clinical Medicine, University of Ancona, Ancona, Italy*

Roland E. Schmeider, M.D., *Department of Internal Medicine IV, University of Erlangen-Nürnberg, Kontumazgarten 14-18, Nürnburg 80, Germany*

Jürgen Schnermann, M.D., *Department of Physiology, The University of Michigan, Ann Arbor, Michigan 48109-0676*

A. Guillermo Scicli, Ph.D., *Hypertension and Vascular Research Division, Department of Medicine, and Heart and Vascular Institute, Henry Ford Hospital, Detroit, Michigan 48202*

Jean E. Sealey, D.Sc., *Cardiovascular Center, The New York Hospital-Cornell Medical Center, 525 East 68th Street, New York, New York 10021*

Anthony Sebastian, M.D., *University of California, San Francisco, General Clinical Research Center, School of Medicine, 1202 Moffitt, San Francisco, California 94143*

Shahnaz Shahinfar, M.D., *Director, Cardiovascular Clinical Research, Merck Research Laboratories, 10 Sentry Parkway, BL3-1, Blue Bell, Pennsylvania 19422*

C. Shakelton, M.D., *British Columbia Transplant Society, East Tower, 4th Floor, 555 West 12th Avenue, University of British Columbia, Vancouver, BC V5Z 3X7, Canada*

Alfonso Siani, M.D., *Institute of Internal Medicine and Metabolic Diseases, University of Naples, "Federico II" Medical School, Via Sergio Pansini, 5-80131 Naples, Italy*

Geza Simon, M.D., Ph.D., *Hypertension Clinic, Veterans Affairs Medical Center, Department of Veterans Affairs, One Veterans Drive, Minneapolis, Minnesota 55417*

F. Olaf Simpson, M.D., *Wellcome Medical Research Institute, University of Otago Medical School, P.O. Box 913, Dunedin 9001, New Zealand*

Alan R. Sinaiko, M.D., *Department of Pediatrics, University of Minnesota Medical School, Box 357 UMHC, 420 Delaware Street Southeast, Minneapolis, Minnesota 55455*

Michael C. Smith, M.D., *Department of Medicine, Case Western Reserve University, School of Medicine and Division of Nephrology, University Hospitals of Cleveland, 2074 Abington Road, Cleveland, Ohio 44106*

Shawna Smith, M.D., *Department of Internal Medicine, Division of Hypertension, University of Michigan, 3918 Taubman Center, Ann Arbor, Michigan 48109*

Sheldon C. Sommers, M.D., *Cardiovascular Center, New York Hospital-Cornell Medical Center, 525 East 68th Street, New York, New York 10021*

R. Ernest Sosa, M.D., *The James Buchanan Brady Foundation, Department of Surgery, Division of Urology, The New York Hospital-Cornell University Medical Center, 525 East 68th Street, New York, New York 10021*

Florent Soubrier, Ph.D., *INSERM U36, 3 rue d'ULM, 75005 Paris, France*

James R. Sowers, M.D., *Department of Medicine and Physiology, Division of Endocrinology, Metabolism, and Hypertension, Wayne State University School of Medicine, University Health Center, 4201 St. Antoine Avenue, Detroit, Michigan 48201*

J. David Spence, M.D., F.R.C.P.C., F.A.C.P., *Department of Clinical Pharmacology and Neurology, University of Western Ontario, London, Ontario N6A 4G5, Canada; and 375 South Street, London, Ontario N6A 4G5, Canada*

Jeremiah Stamler, M.D., *Department of Preventive Medicine, Northwestern University Medical School, Suite 1102, 680 North Lake Shore Drive, Chicago, Illinois 60611-4402*

Paul R. Standley, M.D., *Department of Internal Medicine, Division of Endocrinology, Wayne State University School of Medicine, University Health Center, 4201 St. Antone Avenue, Detroit, MI 48201*

Herman H. Stein, Ph.D., *Abbott Pharmaceutical Laboratories, Research and Development, One Abbott Park Road, Department 48G, Building AP6A, Abbott Park, Illinois 60064*

Kenneth M. Stein, M.D., *Division of Cardiology, Department of Medicine, The New York Hospital-Cornell Medical Center, 525 East 68th Street, Starr-4, New York, New York 10021*

Konrad Stepniakowski, M.D., *Departments of Pharmacology and Medicine, Division of Clinical Pharmacology, Clinical Science Building, 826H, Medical University of South Carolina, 171 Ashley Avenue, Charleston, South Carolina 29426*

Naftali Stern, M.D., *Sourasky-Tel Aviv Medical Center, Tel Aviv University, Tel Aviv, Israel*

Michael Stowasser, M.D., *Endocrine-Hypertension Research Unit, Department of Medicine, University of Queensland, Greenslopes Hospital, Brisbane, 4120, Australia*

Svend Strandgaard, M.D., *Department of Medicine and Nephrology B, Herlev Hospital, DK-2730 Herlev, Copenhagen, Denmark*

Pasquale Strazzullo, M.D., *Institute of Internal Medicine and Metabolic Diseases, University of Naples, "Federico II" Medical School, Via Sergio Pansini, 5-80131 Naples, Italy*

Yao Sun, M.D., Ph.D., *Department of Internal Medicine, Division of Cardiology, University of Missouri Health Sciences Center, Columbia, Missouri 65212*

John D. Swales, M.D., *Department of Medicine, Clinical Sciences Building, Leicester Royal Infirmary, P.O. Box 65, Leicester LE2 7LX, United Kingdom*

Charles S. Sweet, Ph.D., *Cardiovascular Clinical Research, Merck Research Labs., 10 Sentry Parkway, BL3-1, Blue Bell, Pennsylvania 19422*

Deborah M. Swiderski, M.D., *Residency Program in Social Medicine, Montefiore Medical Center, 111 East 210th Street, Bronx, New York 10467*

Stephen J. Thomas, M.D., *Department of Anesthesiology, The New York Hospital-Cornell Medical Center, 525 East 68th Street, New York, New York 10021*

Pieter B. M. W. M. Timmermans, Ph.D., *The DuPont Merck Pharmaceutical Company, Inflammatory Diseases Research Experimental Station, P.O. Box 80400, Wilmington, Delaware 19880-0400*

Louis Tobian, M.D., *University of Minnesota Hospital, Minneapolis, Minnesota 55455*

Johanne Tremblay, M.D., *Centre de Recherche, Hôtel-Dieu de Montréal, Université de Montréal, 3850 St. Urbain Street, Marie-de-la-Ferre Pavilion, Montréal, Quebec H2W 1T8, Canada*

Michael L. Tuck, M.D., *Department of Medicine and Endocrinology Division, UCLA School of Medicine, VA Medical Center, 16111 Plummer Street, Sepulveda, California 91343*

Terry J. Tunny, M. Appl. Sc., *Endocrine-Hypertension Research Unit, Department of Medicine, University of Queensland, Greenslopes Hospital, Brisbane, 4120, Australia*

Stanley Ulick, M.D., *Department of Medicine, Mount Sinai Medical Center, New York, New York; Adrenal Research Laboratory, Bronx VA Hospital, Bronx, New York; Cornell University Medical Center, 525 East 68th Street, New York, New York 10021*

Jason G. Umans, M.D., Ph.D., *Department of Medicine and Clinical Pharmacology, Section of Nephrology, University of Chicago, 5841 South Maryland Avenue, MC-5100, Chicago, Illinois 60637*

Robert J. Unwin, M.R.C.P., Ph.D., *Department of Nephrology, Institute of Urology & Nephrology, University College London Medical School, Gower Street, London WC1E 6BT, United Kingdom*

Hidenori Urata, M.D., *Max-Delbrück Center for Molecular Medicine, Robert Rössle Straße 10, 13125 Berlin-Buch, Germany*

Cornelius van Breemen, M.D., *Department of Pharmacology and Therapeutics, Faculty of Medicine, University of British Columbia, Vancouver, British Columbia V6T 1Z3, Canada*

Anton H. van den Meiracker, M.D., *Department of Internal Medicine I, Room Ca 327, University Hospital Dijkzigt, Erasmus University Rotterdam, Dr. Molewaterplein 40, 3015 GD Rotterdam, The Netherlands*

Peter A. van Zwieten, M.D., Ph.D., *Departments of Pharmacotherapy and Cardiology, Academic Medical Centre, University of Amsterdam, Meibergdreef 15, 1105 AZ Amsterdam, The Netherlands*

E. Darracott Vaughan, Jr., M.D., *The James Buchanan Brady Foundation, Department of Surgery, Division of Urology, The New York Hospital-Cornell Medical Center, 525 East 68th Street, New York, New York 10021*

Ronald G. Victor, M.D., *Department of Internal Medicine, Cardiology Division, University of Texas Southwestern Medical Center, 5323 Harry Hines Boulevard, Dallas, Texas 75235*

Nicola von Lutterotti, M.D., *c/o Alberto Zanchetti, M.D., Clinica e Ipertensione, Universita de Milano, Ospedale Maggiore, Via Francesco Sforza 35, 20122 Milano, Italy*

Bernard Waeber, M.D., *Division of Nephrology and Hypertension, Centre Hospitalier Universitaire, Départment de Médicine, Chu Vaudois, 1011 Lausanne, Switzerland*

Gernot Wagner, Ph.D., *Division of Clinical Research, Cardiovascular Section, E. Merck, Frankfurter Strasse 250, 64271 Darmstadt, Germany*

Jürgen Wagner, M.D., *Max Delbrück Center for Molecular Medicine, Roberte Rössle Straße 10, 13125 Berlin-Buch, Germany*

Ryk Ward, Ph.D., *Department of Human Genetics, University of Utah, 50 North Medical Drive, Salt Lake City, Utah 84132*

David G. Warnock, M.D., *Nephrology Research and Training Center and Division of Nephrology, Departments of Medicine and Physiology, University of Alabama at Birmingham, UAB Station, 1900 University Boulevard, Birmingham, Alabama 35294-0007 and Veterans Affairs Medical Center, Birmingham, Alabama 35294-0007*

Karl T. Weber, M.D., *Department of Internal Medicine, Division of Cardiology, University of Missouri Health Sciences Center, Room MA432 Medical Sciences Building, Columbia, Missouri 65212*

Michael A. Weber, M.D., *Hypertension Center, Veterans Affairs Medical Center, Long Beach, 5901 East 7th Street, Long Beach, California 90822 and University of California at Irvine, Irvine, California 90822*

Myron H. Weinberger, M.D., *Department of Medicine, Hypertension Research Center, Indianapolis University School of Medicine, 541 Clinical Drive, Room 632, Indianapolis, Indiana 46202*

Deborah N. Wentworth, M.P.H., *Division of Biostatistics, School of Public Health, University of Minnesota, 2221 University Avenue, Southeast, Suite 200, Minneapolis, Minnesota 55414*

Mary E. (Polly) Wheat, M.D., *Student Health Services, Barnard College, 3009 Broadway, New York, New York 10027*

Jack P. Whisnant, M.D., *Departments of Health Sciences Research and Neurology, and the Cerebrovascular Research Center, Mayo Clinic, 200 Southwest 1st Street, Rochester, Minnesota 55905*

Perrin C. White, M.D., *Department of Pediatrics, University of Texas Southwestern Medical Center at Dallas, 5323 Harry Hines Boulevard, Dallas, Texas 75235*

C. S. Wilcox, M.D., Ph.D., *Department of Nephrology, Hypertension and Transplantation, University of Florida College of Medicine, Gainesville, Florida 32608-1197*

Gordon H. Williams, M.D., *Departments of Medicine and Radiology, Harvard Medical School and Brigham and Women's Hospital, 75 Francis Street, Boston, Massachusetts 02215*

Peter W. F. Wilson, M.D., *Framingham Heart Study, 5 Thurber Street, Framingham, Massachusetts 01701*

Pancras C. Wong, M.D., *Inflammatory Diseases Research, The DuPont Merck Pharmaceutical Company, Experimental Station, P.O. Box 80400, Wilmington, Delaware 19880-0400*

Jeannette M. Wood, M.D., *Cardiovascular Research, K 125-10.15, Ciba-Geigy Ltd., CH-4002 Basel, Switzerland*

J. Michael Wyss, Ph.D., *Vascular Biology and Hypertension Program of the Division of Cardiovascular Diseases, Department of Medicine and Cell Biology, University of Alabama at Birmingham, Birmingham, Alabama 35294*

Yukio Yamori, M.D., *Department of Pathology, Shimane Medical University, Izumo 693, Japan*

Yue-Ying Liu, M.D., *Charles R. Drew University of Medicine and Science, Division of Nephrology and Hypertension MP 11, 1621 East 120th Street, Los Angeles, California 90059*

David B. Young, Ph.D., *Department of Physiology and Biophysics, University of Mississippi Medical Center, 2500 North State Street, Jackson, Mississippi 39216*

Eric W. Young, M.D., *Nephrology Section, VA Medical Center, Ann Arbor, Michigan 48105*

Alberto Zanchetti, M.D., *Instituto di Clinica Medica e Terapia Medica, Università di Milano, and Centro di Fisiologia Clinica e Ipertensione, Ospedale Maggiore, Via Francesco Sforza 35, 20122 Milano, Italy*

Jialong Zhuo, M.D., *Department of Medicine, University of Melbourne, Austin Hospital, Heidelberg 3084, Victoria, Australia*

Preface to the First Edition

This textbook is the most ambitious yet attempted in the field of hypertension, which has seen a swiftly accelerating interest and knowledge base over the past 25 years. In these two volumes we have assembled 150 generously referenced and indexed chapters written by over 250 internationally recognized authorities and their colleagues. Even so, inevitably, there will be gaps—nobody can fully contain such a fast moving knowledge base. We have given great thought to the choice of authors and subjects, and we hope that our vertical cut into a growing mass, selective as it must be, will provide a valuable source of information for a respectable number of years.

Our aim is that this work will be a useful reference for clinicians, scientists, and related health care professionals who practice their many disciplines in this large, expanding field. These volumes should also appeal to scientists and health planners from academia, industry, and government.

Hypertension is unique as a biomedical discipline. Unlike the fields of cardiology, nephrology, or neurology, it is not organ-oriented. Neither is it identified with a discrete disease process such as cancer or arthritis. Rather, hypertension is a physical sign common to a large group of pathophysiologic disorders that appear to express basic disturbances in integrative physiology. Whatever the origin of the sign, the whole body becomes involved and the involvement is mediated by, or reflected in, demonstrably abnormal endocrine, paracrine, and neural signals. Sooner or later, the heart, brain, and kidney are involved.

That is why there is something in it for everybody. The field of hypertension brings together basic biomedical scientists and clinicians, epidemiologists, and health planners. It is not surprising that this melting pot of disciplines has spawned a rich store of knowledge and created innovative drugs with broad applications in cardiology, nephrology, endocrinology, and general medicine, all with enormous economic and social impact on the health care system.

We felt it appropriate to begin this book with a historical section that reprints a classic treatise by the late Sir George Pickering on the nature of essential hypertension. This is accompanied by an afterword by his son, Dr. Thomas Pickering, a hypertension scholar in his own right. Two following chapters by distinguished contemporary scientists recount other landmark contributions: Dr. Peter Goldblatt reviews and interprets his father's research and Dr. John Ledingham considers anew Byrom's classic work on the vascular fault in hypertension. The historical section concludes with viewpoints from two senior contemporary scientists that provide a historical orientation on the roles of adrenal cortical function and of dietary sodium and potassium as factors in hypertension. This leads naturally into the chapters that review the epidemiologic dimensions of human hypertension.

The remainder of these volumes is organized into sections that address overall circulatory physiology and blood pressure regulation by cardiovascular, neural, and hormonal mechanisms, including what we have lately come to know about the atrial hormone and such local transmitters as endothelin and EDRF. We then consider the role of genetic and metabolic factors in the expression or mediation of these mechanisms in experimental models or humans. This is followed by two renal sections, one on intrarenal hemodynamic mechanisms and the other on renal-endocrine mechanisms as they regulate blood pressure over the long term and contribute to the causation or maintenance of hypertensive states. In these discussions, the reader will find considerable overlap, but this is by design, reflecting an intent to present different lines of evidence and perception in order to provide a diversity of perspectives and interpretations of data on unresolved issues.

In this setting, these volumes then deal comprehensively with the latest concepts of clinical and laboratory diagnosis and the treatment, with and without drugs, of the entire spectrum of human hypertensive disorders. This includes full discussions of presently available classes of drugs as well as agents not yet available for human use but which are of theoretical interest and promise in pre-clinical testing. These volumes conclude with a provocative discussion of changing strategies for drug design, development, and clinical evaluation.

Overall, this was a larger undertaking than we anticipated when we first conceived it during an intermission at a scientific meeting—such breaks often provide more valuable opportunities to exchange information than the formal sessions. We were in solid agreement that the currently enormous hypertension knowledge base needed a new attempt at organization and synthesis. Traditional academic societies and their meetings seem neither inclined nor able to bring together, in one place, all the relevant scientific activity on this topic.

There was a kind of inevitability in this collaboration, for we have known each other a long time. Many years ago we shared an interest in natriuretic hormone research but our concentrations later diverged into different aspects of renal phenomena. However, our research approaches and our dialogue have always been complementary—and this book is a happy outcome of that. But then, we are only the taskmasters. Whatever this book accomplishes, of course, is owed to the authors who toiled only for love of their subject, tolerating our prodding with grace and enthusiasm. To each of them we express our gratitude for their fine contributions and splendid cooperation.

Last, but most of all, we sincerely hope that from these pages readers will conceive novel ideas for great new experiments. Advancement in understanding of hypertension will only come from creative research.

John H. Laragh, M.D.
Barry M. Brenner, M.D.

Preface

The first edition of this book far exceeded our expectations in terms of worldwide sales and favorable reviews. All of this conspired to persuade us to have another go at it.

While only five years have gone by, the task proved more difficult than expected. This is because hypertension research continues to explode, spawning new concepts, revealing new hormones, and creating new products with tremendous impact on patient care, touching on almost every specialty, but especially family medicine, internal medicine, cardiology, nephrology and endocrinology.

The second edition has been enriched by the addition of over 60 brand new chapters and over 150 new contributors and by extensive revision of all other chapters. We have again proceeded from the basic sciences through the spectrum of clinical medicine, diagnostic medicine, therapeutics, and epidemiology. As before we have given great thought to author and topic selection. Even so there will always be gaps in such an ambitious undertaking.

We retain the same format and the same overall goals. We hope this effort will be as successful as the first for communicating new knowledge and enabling creative research. To our colleagues who contributed so effectively we extend our warmest appreciation.

John H. Laragh, M.D.
Barry M. Brenner, M.D.

Acknowledgments

We express our appreciation to many dedicated professionals at Raven Press for their guidance and assistance in matters pertaining to the publication of this work. In particular, we acknowledge the enormous efforts of Mary Rogers, Lisa Berger, and Nicholas Radhuber. It is with pleasure that we also acknowledge several extremely able editorial assistants in our respective offices who not only provided invaluable help in the preparation of this book but also enabled us to delegate many other responsibilities in order to devote extensive time and effort to this project: Barbara Kramer and Dorothy Carmine in New York and Michelle Deraney in Boston.

SECTION I

Background and Historical Aspects

Hypertension: Pathophysiology, Diagnosis, and Management, Second Edition,
edited by J.H. Laragh and B.M. Brenner,
Raven Press, Ltd., New York © 1995.

CHAPTER 1 (Part I)

Hypertension

Definitions, Natural Histories, and Consequences

Sir George Pickering[1]

[This chapter was originally published in *Hypertension Manual: Mechanisms, Methods, Management,* J. H. Laragh, ed., Yorke Medical Books, New York, 1973. The copyright is now owned by Butterworth Publishers, Stoneham, Massachusetts.]

It has been known for over a century that high arterial pressure lessens life expectancy and for half that time that in most patients the raised pressure and its consequences constitute the disease (essential hypertension). Thus the first question the physician asks is "What is hypertension? Beyond what figure do I make the diagnosis?" "For," says the doctor, "until I can make the diagnosis, how can I foretell prognosis and prescribe treatment?" Such reasoning was understandable 25 years ago, when little was known of the behavior of arterial pressure and the relationship between raised pressure and its consequences. We now understand that arterial pressure is a quantity and that its dangerous consequences are related to it quantitatively; the higher the pressure, the worse the prognosis. Moreover, arterial

pressure varies enormously during an average day; the doctor's reading represents its value under the rather special circumstances of the doctor's office. The answer to the physician's question "What is hypertension?" depends on the purpose for which the answer is to be used. We may defer it until the major facts have been displayed.

THE FALLACY OF THE DIVIDING LINE

A great deal of effort has been devoted to the search for a dividing line between "normotension" and "hypertension." Table 1 shows some proposals. It is evident that not all can be correct. In fact, there is no evidence for any. I have challenged every medical audience that I have addressed in the last 25 years to provide such evidence. The challenge has not been accepted because there is no such evidence. When we study the frequency distribution curves of arterial pressure in populations, there is no dividing line. The relationship between arterial pressure and mortality is quantitative; the higher the pressure, the worse the prognosis. So is the relationship

---

[1] Deceased.

TABLE 1. *Some suggested dividing lines between "normotension" and "hypertension"*

Division (pressure, mm Hg)	Source
120/80	Robinson and Brucer 1939 (1)
130/70	Browne until 1947 (2)
140/80	Ayman 1934 (3)
140/90	Perera 1948 (4)
150/90	Thomas 1952 (5)
160/100	Bechgaard 1946 (6)
180/100	Burgess 1948 (7)
180/110	Evans 1956 (8)

between arterial pressure and incidence of coronary heart disease, severity of changes in the renal arteries, size of the heart, frequency of cerebral hemorrhage in Japan, and every other variable so far capable of measurement (9,10). The dividing line is, in fact, nothing more than an artifact.

THE VARIABILITY OF ARTERIAL PRESSURE

It has long been known that arterial pressure is influenced by environmental factors, being raised by anger, fear, pain, cold and exercise, among other things. There was also evidence that it fell during sleep (for review, see Pickering (9)). However, it was convenient for the doctor to assume that the pressure he registered in his office was the pressure which the patient had throughout his normal existence, in the absence of extraneous circumstances, for this enabled him to label his patients "hypertensive" and "normotensive." Sokolow and his colleagues (11) developed a portable recorder in which,

however, the subject had to inflate the cuff. The variations in pressure found in normal subjects during ordinary day-to-day living were much greater than most would have expected.

Automatic Recording of Arterial Pressure

Our first apparatus (12) employed a Gallavardin double cuff which inflated automatically at 5-min intervals, the arterial pressure being estimated by the pulsations recorded from the lower cuff. This showed for the first time the huge fall in arterial pressure during sleep. In Dr. Richardson himself, the systolic pressure varied during the 24 hours from 65 to 134 mm Hg, and the diastolic pressure from 40 to 95 mm Hg. In a 34-year-old patient with episodic forgetfulness, the pressure ranged from 150 to 240 mm Hg systolic and from 96 to 162 mm Hg diastolic. The usefulness of this method was limited by the size and weight of the apparatus.

Dr. Stott designed, and Drs. Honour and Bevan used, a truly automatic portable apparatus (13). It calls for the introduction of a thin nylon catheter into the brachial artery at the elbow by the Seldinger technique. This catheter is perfused continuously with saline solution at a rate of 2 ml/hr and is connected to a pressure transducer through 4 ft of 0.4-mm-bore Teflon tubing. The perfusion pump and transducer are carried on a harness in front of the manubrium sterni. The transducer leads to a galvanometer which records optically on slow-moving paper. The galvanometer and photographic recorder are housed in a small case which can easily fit into a coat or trouser pocket.

Figure 1 shows the results obtained in Dr. Bevan with

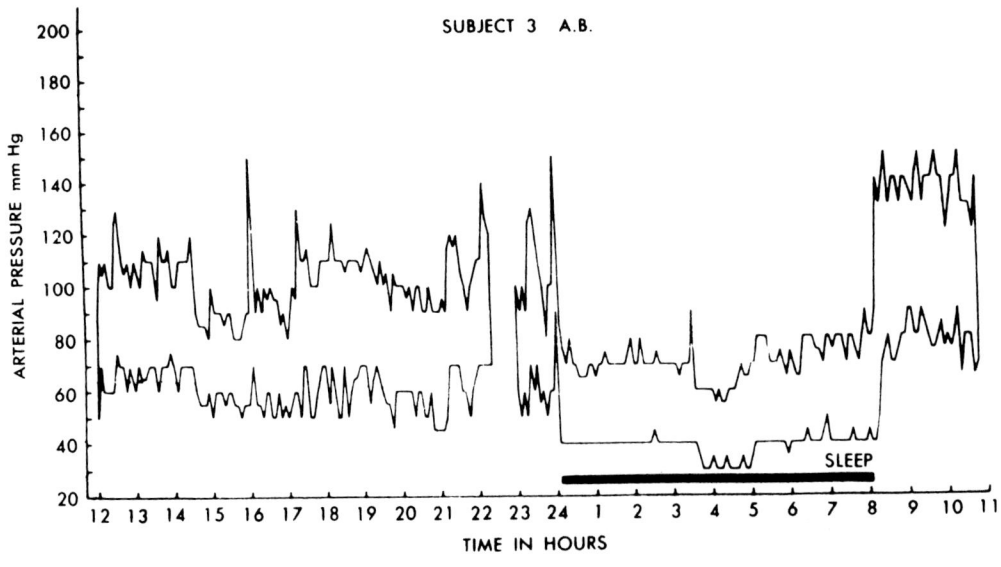

FIG. 1. Arterial pressure plotted at 5-min intervals. The period of sleep is shown by the horizontal bar. The high pressures shown at 16.00 hours and 24.00 hours are due to a painful stimulus and coitus, respectively. (From ref. 13.)

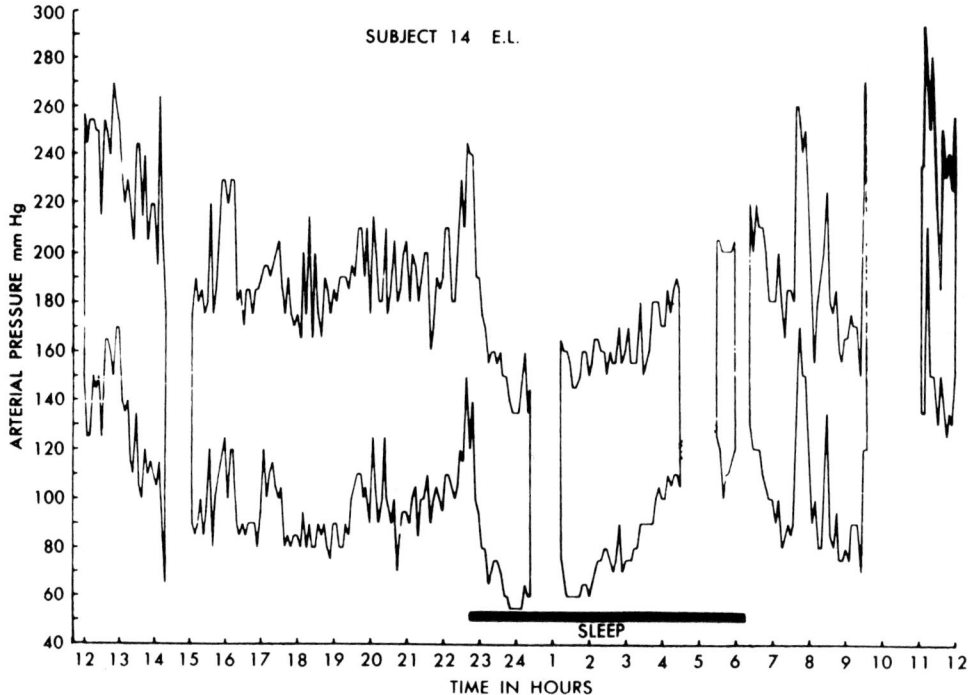

FIG. 2. Arterial pressure plotted at 5-min intervals in a patient with essential hypertension in the benign phase. The period of sleep is shown by the horizontal bar. (From ref. 13.)

this device. Between 15.00 and 16.00 hours he was standing and listening to me conducting a ward round. His arterial pressure was surprisingly low, reaching 80/50 mm Hg. He was clearly bored, perhaps almost asleep. The head nurse stuck a pin into his behind, and his pressure rose abruptly to 150/70 mm Hg. The abrupt rise at 24.00 hours represented the effect of coitus. This was followed by sleep, during which his arterial pressure was

grossly reduced, falling as low as 55/30 mm Hg. The pressure rose to relatively high levels after waking at 8.00 hours during the time that he was helping to get his children off to school. Figure 2 shows a similar record in a 63-year-old patient with essential hypertension. Again there is a huge fall in pressure during sleep. The fluctuations in this patient were enormous. The lowest pressures recorded were 140 mm Hg systolic and 55 mm Hg dia-

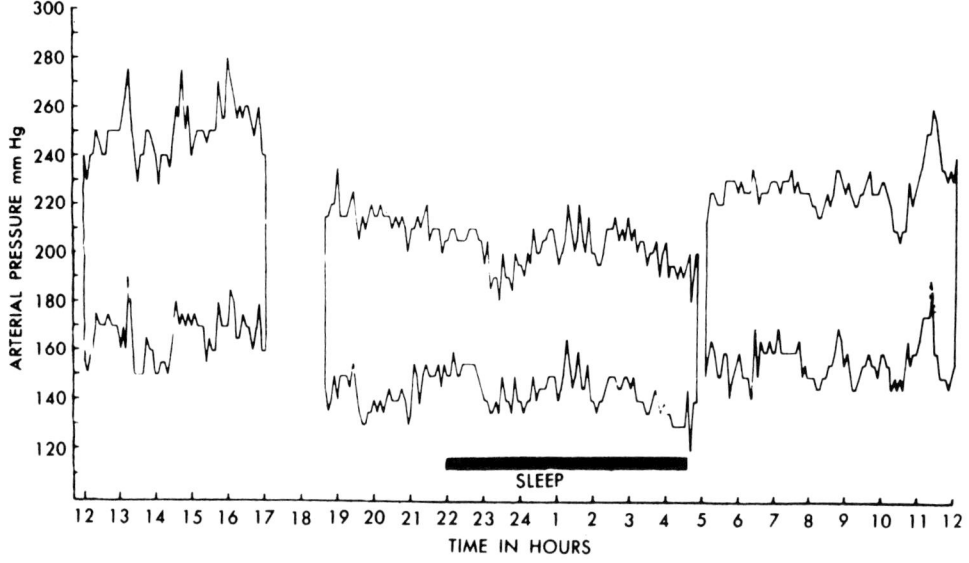

FIG. 3. Arterial pressure plotted at 5-min intervals in a patient with essential hypertension in the malignant phase. The period of sleep is shown by the horizontal bar. (From ref. 13.)

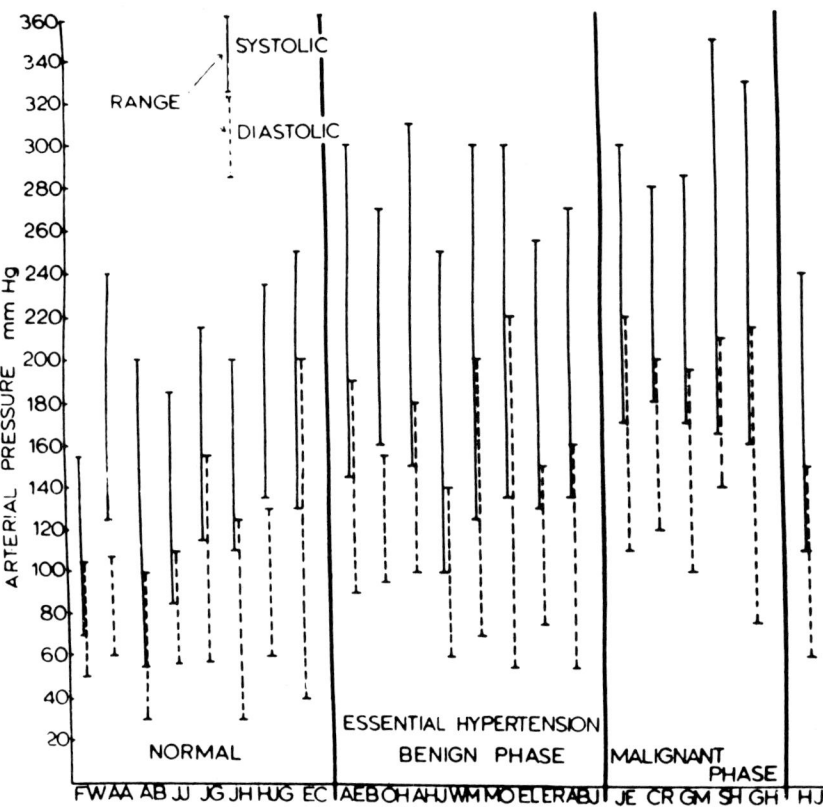

FIG. 4. Extreme range of arterial pressure. (From ref. 13.)

stolic, the highest 300 mm Hg systolic and 170 mm Hg diastolic. Figure 3 shows a similar record in a patient who had essential hypertension in the malignant phase. The fluctuations are smaller. Again pressure is relatively low during sleep. Figure 4 shows the limits in those subjects investigated by this method. The fluctuations in pressure are very large in the subjects classified as normal and in those with essential hypertension in the benign phase and essential hypertension in the malignant phase. It is not possible so far to relate the size of such fluctuations to the age of the patient or to the benign or malignant phase of hypertension. All that can be said is that in every subject investigated the swing is enormous. No doubt had the occupations of the subjects during the day been chosen to represent more extreme forms of behavior, the fluctuations would have been even greater.

ARTERIAL PRESSURE AS MEASURED IN THE OFFICE OR CLINIC

Although the arterial pressure as measured in the office or clinic by no means represents the arterial pressure at other times of the day or night, it is in fact a value which is reasonably replicable, provided that the usual precautions are taken of ensuring that the patient is comfortable, resting, quiet, and at ease. Millions of such measurements have been made, and they constitute nearly all the large-scale data.

However, it should be recognized that the doctor and his surrounding circumstances by no means represent a neutral environment. Pavlov long ago showed the importance in animal behavior of the orienting and defense reflexes, of which a rise in blood pressure, pulse rate, and cardiac output are important components. The extreme form of such a stimulus is provided by the cardiopulmonary laboratory, with men in masks, gowns, and hoods, not unlike the Ku Klux Klan, armed with sharp needles which they plunge into the subject, who is surrounded by forbidding pieces of apparatus. I suspect that what is known as "early hypertension," characterized by an increased cardiac output and a moderately raised pressure, represents a group of subjects who have an unusually large defense reflex.

The first hint that the doctor himself caused a rise in arterial pressure came from Ayman and Goldshine (14), who found that in 30 percent of their patients with essential hypertension, systolic pressure readings were 40 mm Hg lower in the home than in the clinic. Methods of continuously recording arterial pressure have shown how much arterial pressure is related to environmental events.

Pavlov showed that the curiosity and defense reflexes are weakened by repeated exposure to the stimulus when that is not reinforced by an emotive event. Such appears to be the explanation for the facts recorded in Fig. 5 (15), which shows the gradual fall of arterial pressure in a patient who received no treatment and who attended an outpatient clinic at weekly intervals. Initial pressures of 204 mm Hg systolic and 120 mm Hg diastolic fell to 160 mm Hg systolic and 98 mm Hg diastolic during the 12-

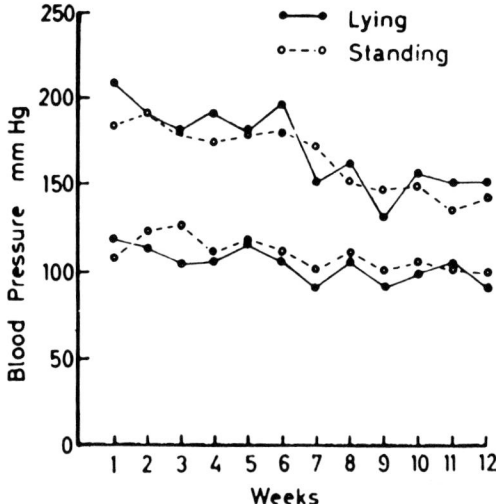

FIG. 5. Arterial pressure measured at weekly intervals in a clinic patient receiving inert tablets. (From ref. 15.)

week period. This fall represents the slow extinction of the defense reflex.

Stewart (16) collected the data on 40 young men with established hypertension. In 12 of these, with an average age of 35 years, the diastolic pressure fell gradually without treatment from an average established level of 105 to 88 mm Hg over 6 to 7 years. Stewart considered that in these 12 men, the hypertension had "lapsed." An alternative and more probable explanation would be that this fall represented the extinction of the defense reflex.

What we can say, then, is that the arterial pressure as measured in the clinic is a useful measurement so long as the doctor does not depend too slavishly upon it or give it greater significance in assessing the patient's condition than it deserves.

COMPLICATIONS OF HYPERTENSION

At least since Janeway's (17) work, it has been known that patients with elevated arterial pressure tend to die prematurely. The most common cause of death in these patients is heart disease; the next most common cause is apoplexy, and uremia is the least common cause. About a third of these patients die of intercurrent disease, that is, diseases unrelated to the arterial pressure.

We are now able to be much more precise about the complications of hypertension that cause disability and death. Thus heart disease includes coronary artery disease, congestive heart failure, and left ventricular failure. Arterial pressure is a substantial factor in the external work of the heart; other things being equal, reduction of a greatly elevated arterial pressure would be expected to alleviate or cure heart failure—and it does. It arrests an attack of acute pulmonary edema due to left ventricular failure. If the pressure is kept low, no further attacks occur. Reduction of a very high arterial pressure will also

abolish congestive cardiac failure, which, again, may not recur if the pressure is kept low. We will consider coronary artery disease later.

Apoplexy is due to cerebral thrombosis (or infarction) and cerebral hemorrhage. These have long been known to have quite different epidemiologic patterns which are now explained because they are due to different types of arterial disease.

Renal failure represents either the effects of the malignant phase caused by fibrinoid arterial necrosis or the progression of some primary renal disease unidentified in the search for a specific cause. Very rarely the kidneys may fail due to other forms of arterial disease, particularly atheroma of the larger vessels and fatty hyaline intimal thickening (arteriolar sclerosis) of the smaller arteries. Arterial disease is the chief complication of hypertension and merits close attention.

ARTERIAL DISEASE IN HYPERTENSION

The terms *arteriosclerosis* and its less happy successor, *atherosclerosis,* have concealed the diversity of arterial disease and their different relationships to raised arterial pressure. Three conditions which may cause disability and death are uncertainly related to raised arterial pressure and therefore will be mentioned only briefly. They are: (i) a congenital medial defect of the arteries of the circle of Willis, causing intracranial aneurysm and its sequel, subarachnoid hemorrhage; (ii) a medial defect of the aorta, causing dissecting aneurysm; and (iii) a medial defect of aorta and large arteries, causing "arteriosclerotic aneurysm."

There are four chief arterial diseases which are known to occur with increased frequency in patients with hypertension, three of which are the chief causes of morbidity and mortality.

Atheroma or Nodular Arteriosclerosis

Nodular arteriosclerosis is the best name for this disease because it is specific and descriptive. Councilman (18) adapted it from Virchow's name. Osler (19) adopted it for his textbook. It is one of the several diseases contained in "atherosclerosis," a name coined by Marchand (20) to combine atheroma and arteriosclerosis.

Nodular arteriosclerosis is a disease of the intima of the larger arteries characterized by the presence of fibrous and fibrofatty plaques on which thrombi may form. The disease is symptomless until a thrombus closes the vessel to produce ischemia or infarction with death of tissue. Disease of the coronary arteries is the most frequent cause of symptoms resulting in angina pectoris, myocardial infarction, and sudden death. Disease of the arteries of the neck and circle of Willis is the next most frequent cause, resulting in various forms of stroke, from

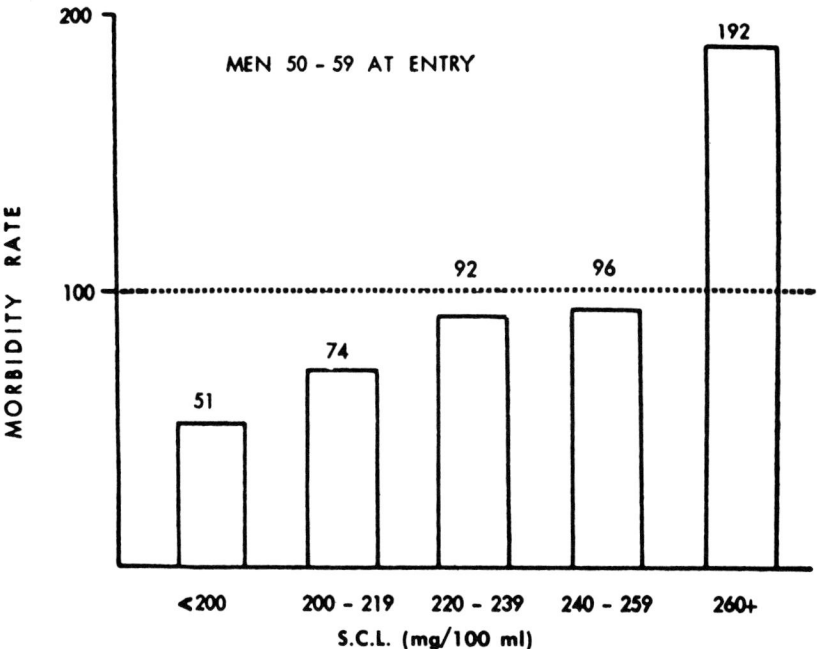

FIG. 6. Risk of developing coronary heart disease in 8 years according to initial serum cholesterol level (Framingham survey). (From ref. 22.)

the transient paralysis due to platelet micro-emboli to the dense hemiplegia of cerebral infarction. Disease of the arteries of the legs results in intermittent claudication and gangrene, as does that of the aortic bifurcation (Leriche syndrome). Disease of the renal arteries may give rise to hypertension and impaired renal function. The arteries of the upper limbs are more rarely affected.

The pathogenesis of the disease is still disputed. Most believe it represents a disturbance of lipid metabolism. A few (of whom I am one) think it more likely to be a thrombotic disease throughout, with the plaques representing previous episodes of mural thrombi that have undergone organization.

Much is known about the factors related to the incidence of coronary heart disease. They are as follows:

1. *Age.* The older the subject, the more widespread and severe the disease.
2. *Sex.* A given severity is recorded about 15 years later in females than in males (21).
3. *Serum cholesterol level.* Figure 6 shows the Framingham figures (22). The higher the cholesterol level the greater the risk of coronary heart disease.
4. *Arterial pressure.* Figure 7 shows the Framingham figures (22). The higher the arterial pressure, the greater the risk of coronary heart disease.

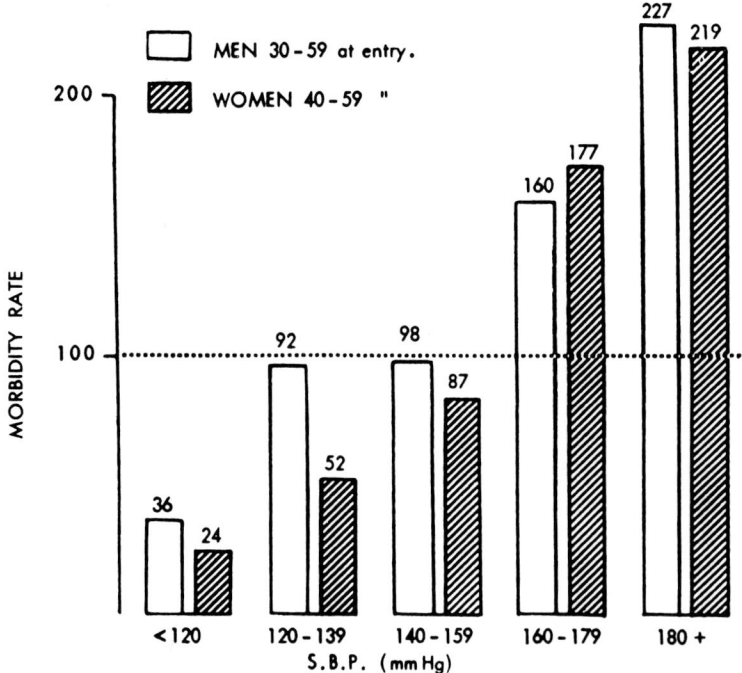

FIG. 7. Risk of developing coronary heart disease in 8 years according to initial systolic blood pressure level (Framingham survey). (From ref. 22.)

5. *Cigarette smoking.* The greater the number of cigarettes smoked in a day, the greater the risk of myocardial infarction (23).

6. *Lack of physical exercise.* Myocardial infarction is more common in bus drivers and in post office clerks than in bus conductors and in postmen who deliver letters (24).

7. *Diet.* Substituting unsaturated for saturated fats in the diet will reduce plasma cholesterol levels. There is some, but not yet conclusive, evidence that this reduces mortality and morbidity.

8. *Inheritance.* Evidence is up to now inconclusive as to whether inheritance influences disposition to this malady.

Much less is known about the factors involved in strokes and in occlusion of the arteries of the lower limbs. It is known that the arterial pressure is sometimes raised, sometimes not, but there is a tendency toward raised pressure. In our series of patients with the Leriche syndrome, arterial pressure averaged 22 mm Hg systolic and 9 mm Hg diastolic above the level found in the population at large when adjusted to age 60 (25). The mean cholesterol level in these patients was 244 mg/100 ml; 12 of 13 were male and all smoked.

From our present standpoint, the outstanding fact is that arterial pressure is only one factor, and perhaps not the most important, in the pathogenesis of myocardial and cerebral infarction. When arterial pressure is reduced by hypotensive drug therapy, coronary artery disease is the least affected and becomes the major cause of death in treated patients.

Charcot-Bouchard Aneurysms

The story of these important lesions is one of the most romantic in the field of medicine. Miliary aneurysms of very small cerebral arteries were described in 1868 by Charcot and Bouchard (26) in 60 elderly subjects dying of cerebral hemorrhage. These investigators recognized that the miliary aneurysms differed considerably in nature and frequency from atheroma. "Miliary aneurysms may be present and are frequently found in considerable numbers independently of any atheromatous lesion of the arteries of the base or of the branches that are distributed to the meninges. The opposite is also true, namely, that quite often the most marked atheromas are encountered and still no single aneurysm is found in the brain." Figure 8 is a drawing by Charcot himself of the aneurysms, one of which is in the middle of a hemorrhage.

Although Charcot was one of the most famous clinicians who ever lived, these lesions were and are forgotten. They are still not mentioned in some current textbooks of medicine in the United States and United Kingdom. They are not mentioned in the latest WHO Report No. 469, Cerebrovascular Diseases: Prevention, Treatment and Rehabilitation, which ascribes cerebral

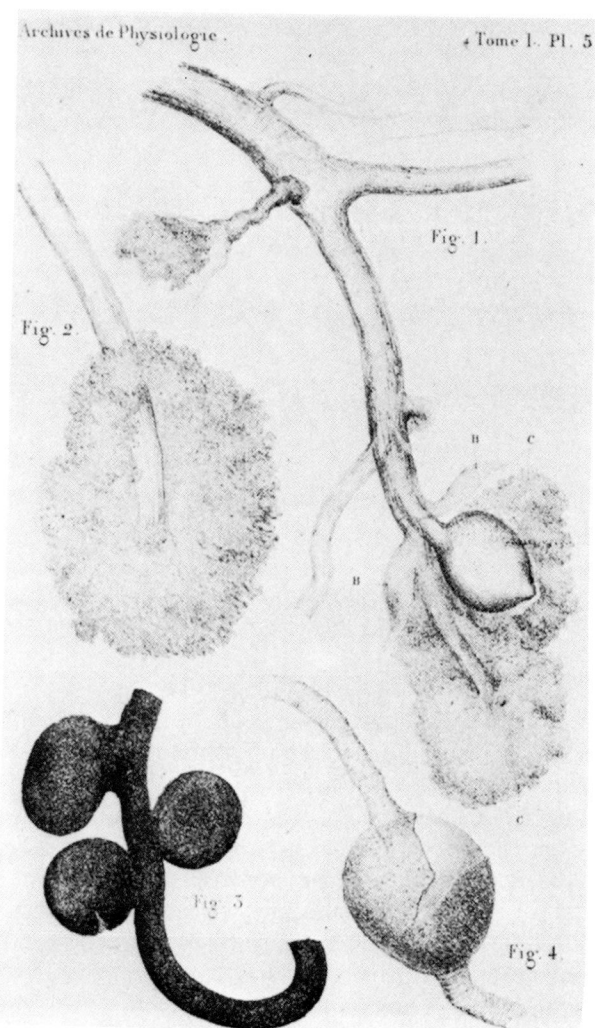

FIG. 8. Charcot's drawings of the microaneurysms. (From ref. 26, courtesy of the New York Academy of Medicine Library.)

hemorrhage to atherosclerosis. Poor Charcot, he must be turning in his grave, muttering "How long, Oh Lord, how long?" These aneurysms were rediscovered in 1963 by Russell (27), whose photographs (Figs. 9 and 10) clearly display their nature. They occur on small perforating arteries of less than 1 mm diameter, especially in the basal ganglia and subcortical regions. The media disappears at the neck of the aneurysm, whose walls consist of intima and adventitia.

The most recent and extensive work on these aneurysms is by Cole and Yates (28). Like Russell, they injected barium sulfate gelatin into the arteries in 100 brains obtained from dead subjects whose diastolic arterial pressure had exceeded 100 mm Hg and whose heart had weighed more than 400 g in males and 350 g in females; they did the same in 100 brains obtained from "normotensive subjects" matched with the "hypertensive subjects" on the sole criteria of sex and age. The patients with raised arterial pressure were a consecutive series of whom 20 had died from massive intracerebral

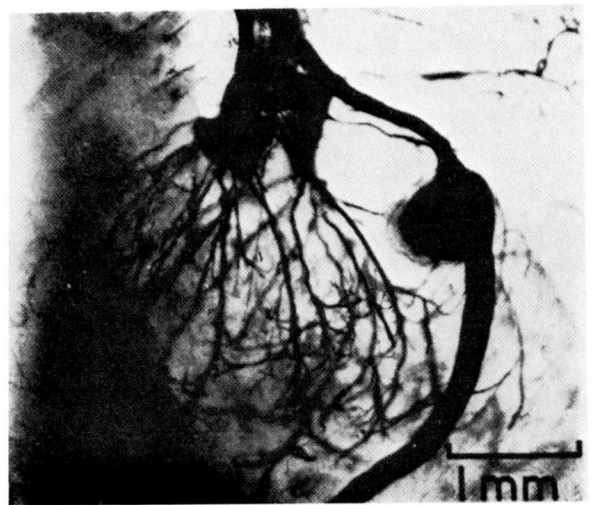

FIG. 9. Aneurysm 0.8 mm in diameter on long penetrating artery from parietal cortex in a 71-year-old man dying of cerebral hemorrhage. Injection mass leaks from aneurysm. (From ref. 27.)

hemorrhage. Microaneurysms of the same structure, size, and distribution were found in 46 of the patients with hypertension, which included the 20 with massive intracerebral hemorrhage. They were also found in seven of the normotensive subjects, none of whom showed cerebral hemorrhage. In the hypertensive group, the youngest patient in whom aneurysms were found was aged 44 years; the frequency increased in each age group up to a maximum of 71 percent in the 70- to 74-year age group. Of the seven normotensive patients with aneurysms, none was younger than 66 years; three were over 75 years of age.

Cerebral hemorrhage is unusually common in Japan. Fukuda (29) measured arterial pressure in 130,000 Japanese railway workers over the age of 40 in 4 successive years. The incidence of cardiovascular episodes was proportional to systolic pressure. The increased incidence was most remarkable in cerebral hemorrhage, followed by undifferentiated apoplexy, and less remarkable in coronary heart attacks.

It now seems almost certain that these microaneurysms are responsible for cerebral hemorrhage in association with high arterial pressures in subjects over the age of 40. They represent, of course, a totally different disease from that causing myocardial and cerebral infarction. Here is the probable clue to the problems that have long puzzled physicians. Why is the relationship between arterial pressure and cerebral hemorrhage so much closer than the relationship between arterial pressure and cerebral infarction? Why do cerebral vascular disease and coronary artery disease behave differently in epidemiologic studies? The answer is delightfully simple. The disease that causes cerebral hemorrhage is quite different from that which causes cerebral thrombosis and

myocardial infarction. The former is a disease of small cerebral arteries in which the media gives way, causing aneurysm and rupture. The latter is a disease of large arteries all over the body in which intimal plaques narrow the lumen, which is ultimately closed by thrombus.

Only two factors are known in the pathogenesis of Charcot-Bouchard aneurysms: age and arterial pressure.

Fibrinoid Necrosis of Small Arteries and Arterioles

Malignant hypertension was first recognized by Volhard and Fahr (30) in 1913. It was characterized by the development of neuroretinopathy (then called albuminuric retinitis), progressive renal failure, and a rapidly downhill course to death, usually within the year, of uremia, cerebral hemorrhage or left ventricular failure. Fahr (31) in 1919 recognized that acute fibrinoid necrosis of small arteries and arterioles was the pathologic basis. Rupture of muscle fibers is followed by an enormous exudation of plasma with or without red cells into the arterial wall, with consequent stenosis or obliteration of lumen. Later there may be an inflammatory reaction involving all coats, especially the adventitia, and fibroblasts invade the exudate. The organs so affected are kidney, pancreas, adrenal, gut, brain, heart, and liver, in approximately that order. Hence the frequency of progressive renal failure.

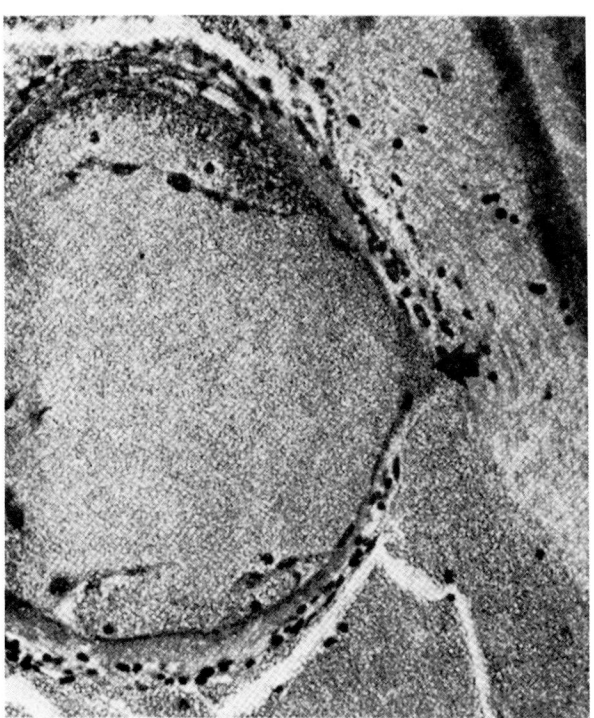

FIG. 10. Aneurysm of lateral striate artery in an elderly subject with hypertension. Injection mass has passed through small break in wall (arrow) into the Virchow-Robin space. (From ref. 27.)

It is now known that the malignant phase may occur in any disease characterized by hypertension, provided the arterial pressure is high enough. It can occur in either sex and at any age from 3 years onwards, although its incidence decreases after the age of 50 years. By far the chief factor in its pathogenesis is the height of the arterial pressure, although the rate of rise and, possibly, such factors as anemia also play a role.

There is now no doubt whatsoever that, provided renal function is intact, the malignant phase can be reversed by reducing the arterial pressure and keeping it down (32–34). The lesion responsible for the raised pressure, or the method used to reduce it (surgical or medical), is quite immaterial. Provided that the pressure is reduced, the retinopathy is reversed, renal function remains intact, and the patient survives. I recently described (35) the follow-up of three patients in whom malignant hypertension had been fully documented, including severe arteriolar necrosis in adrenals and kidneys, and in whom arterial pressure had been reduced by surgery in 1946. In all three, retinopathy had cleared, and renal function remained stable. One, a man of 32, died 9 years later of a cerebral hemorrhage; his arterial pressure had remained between 150 and 170 mm Hg systolic and 100 and 120 mm Hg diastolic. From what we now know, his death was probably due to a Charcot-Bouchard aneurysm. One, a 14-year-old girl, lived for 24 years and then died of a myocardial infarction. The third, an 11-year-old girl, was still alive 25 years later, with a shrunken, scarred kidney but stable renal function. A diagnosis of pyelonephritis had been made in all three on histologic grounds by Heptinstall (36).

Animal experiment has shown that when the arterial pressure is reduced, the exudation is rapidly removed from the arterial wall. The lumen opens again (37). The residue is some fibrosis of muscle fibers and a thickened intima. Harington et al. (32) showed that in a few patients with malignant hypertension, reducing the arterial pressure does not prevent, although it may delay, renal failure. In these patients there is extensive intimal thickening of the interlobular arteries.

TABLE 2. *Mortality ratios[a] for men according to groups of systolic and diastolic (5th phase) blood pressure readings, without minor impairments, all entry ages together[b]*

Systolic reading (mm Hg)	Diastolic reading, 5th phase (mm Hg)				
	64–83	84–88	89–93	94–103	All
118–132	90[c]	91	99	97	92
133–142	99	107	118	134	110
143–152	133	137	141	173	148
153–167	186	178	189	237	210
All	95	100	116	151	106

[a] Actual to expected deaths (expected = 100).
[b] From the Actuarial Society of America and the Association of Life Insurance Medical Directors, 1941 (41).
[c] This included only systolic readings 128 to 132 mm Hg.

TABLE 3. *Deaths from cardiovascular-renal disease, ratios of actual deaths to those expected for this cause in the basic table, all entry ages together[a]*

Systolic reading (mm Hg)	Diastolic reading, 5th phase (mm Hg)		
	54–83	84–93	94–116
108–132	86	101	116
133–142	108	137	171
143–177	175	201	293

[a] From the Actuarial Society of America and the Association of Life Insurance Medical Disorders, 1941 (41).

Arteriolosclerosis

Fatty hyaline thickening of arterioles, particularly of the kidney, has long been known as one of the characteristic lesions of hypertension. Goldblatt (38) saw it as the basic fault in essential hypertension, causing a rise in arterial pressure by, as it were, a myriad of little clamps on the renal arteries. Most regard these lesions as a consequence of the raised arterial pressure. Arteriosclerosis is frequently associated with elastosis of larger vessels. The two, constituting renal vascular disease, were found to be quantitatively related to the arterial pressure by Smithwick and Castleman (39) and Heptinstall (40).

Arteriolosclerosis is usually symptomless, but, along with atheroma and elastosis, it can play a part in producing rare instances of renal failure in benign essential hypertension.

ARTERIAL PRESSURE AND LIFE EXPECTANCY

Insurance companies depend for their profitability on recognizing and measuring factors affecting longevity. A great deal of information has been collected concerning the influence of arterial pressure, and all of it is consistent. The higher the arterial pressure when initially measured, the greater the mortality; this is true from the lowest to the highest pressures. The relationship is quantitative. There is no sudden break. Normotension and hypertension are not merely meaningless concepts, they are wrong.

Table 2 (41) shows an example of the relationship between mortality and pressure. Table 3 (41) shows that deaths from cardiovascular renal disease rise in the same way over the same range of pressure. In Fig. 11, similar data are displayed in a different manner (42). Life expectancy in each age group and in each sex decreases as arterial pressure increases. Note the formidable life expectancy of a 55-year old woman with an arterial pressure of 130/90 mm Hg; she may be expected to live to the age of 82. Yet Robinson and Brucer (1) would have considered this woman to have hypertension! The data from hypertension clinics are less extensive, but they extrapolate the

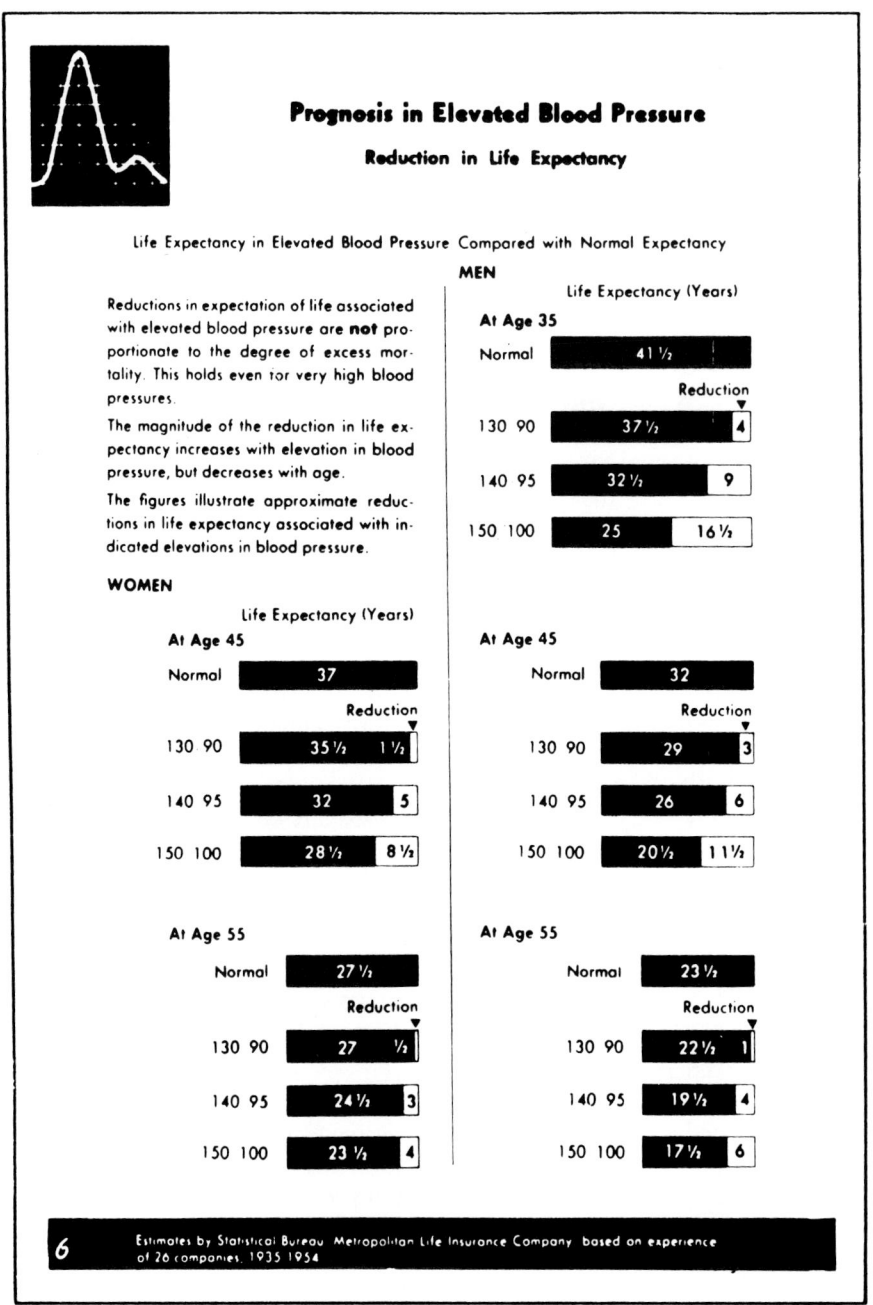

FIG. 11. Life expectancy table. Normal means 120/80 mm Hg or less. (From ref. 42.)

same inverse relationship between arterial pressure and life expectancy, into the higher pressures.

What is true for mortality as a whole is true for its components. Renal artery disease and coronary thrombosis have been specified. In a follow-up study of men employed by the Japanese Railways, Fukuda (29) found that the incidence of death from cerebral hemorrhage was related to the height of the arterial pressure.

All these data are in agreement in showing a quantitative relationship between arterial pressure and its morbid associations. They seem to be consequences since, as Freis (43) shows, reducing arterial pressure reduces the frequency of these morbid events. The quantitative relationship between arterial pressure and its consequences is the chief evidence for the hypothesis that essential hypertension represents a kind of disease hitherto unrecognized by medicine, a disease in which the deviation from the norm is one of degree, not of kind, a quantitative rather than a qualitative disease (44).

CLASSIFICATION OF HYPERTENSION

Hypertension may be classified in two ways, by kind and by degree.

Classification by Kind

Raised arterial pressure is of course a manifestation of some underlying process. It is a symptom of disease, and the diseases causing it are numerous. Investigation of a patient with raised pressures is directed to the detection of any recognizable disease that is present. If no disease is detected, the diagnosis of essential hypertension, hyperpiesia, or hypertension without ascertained cause is made.

The following is a classification of hypertension by kind:

A. Systolic hypertension in which the systolic pressure only is raised
   I. Increased stroke output of the left ventricle (complete heart block, aortic reflux, arteriovenous fistula, patent ductus arteriosus. Paget's disease of bone, thyrotoxicosis, fever, pregnancy).
   II. Increased rigidity of aorta due to degenerative disease of wall.
   III. Decreased capacity of aorta in coarctation.
B. Hypertension in which both systolic and diastolic pressures are raised
   I. Secondary hypertension: hypertension occurring as manifestation of known disease.
     1. Diseases of the kidneys and the urinary tract:
       a. Type I nephritis;[2] in all stages.
       b. Type II nephritis;[2] in the terminal stage.
       c. Chronic pyelonephritis, unilateral or bilateral.
       d. Disease of the renal arteries.
       e. Polycystic kidney.
       f. Other congenital conditions of the kidney. ⎫
       g. Renal stone and other lesions obstructing the urinary tract. ⎬ Probably by predisposing to pyelonephritis.
       h. "Interstitial nephritis" due to analgesics, gout, hypercalcemia, etc.
       i. Diabetes.
       j. Connective tissue diseases, i.e., polyarteritis nodosa, disseminated lupus erythematosus, and systemic sclerosis.
       k. Certain tumors.
       l. Radiation nephritis.
       m. Amyloid contracted kidney.
       n. "Hereditary nephritis."
     2. Coarctation of the aorta.
     3. Pheochromocytoma.
     4. Cushing's syndrome.
     5. Primary aldosteronism.
     6. Pre-eclamptic toxemia of pregnancy.
     7. Post-toxemic hypertension.
     8. Miscellaneous conditions affecting the nervous system.
   II. Essential hypertension.

These several maladies have their own peculiarities and courses superimposed on the effects of hypertension. It is hypertension and its consequences that alone characterize essential hypertension.

Classification by Degree

The Malignant and Benign Phases of Hypertension

Clinical genius Franz Volhard was the first to recognize that an illness in which raised arterial pressure is the outstanding feature may follow two very different courses, which he called the bad and the good, or the malignant and the benign.

The malignant course occurs at any age but is more frequently found in the young than in the old and is characterized by neuroretinopathy and by a rapid decline in renal function. The pressure is usually very high. Unless the arterial pressure is reduced at an early stage, the patient dies after a few months or years either of renal failure, left ventricular failure, or cerebral hemorrhage. Its pathology is fibrinoid arteriolar necrosis.

The benign phase usually occurs in much older subjects in whom the pressures are not as high. The patient's condition remains relatively stable for years, and death, when it occurs, is either due to heart failure, stroke, or intercurrent disease. There is either no retinopathy or, if present, the kind described by Moore (46) as arteriosclerotic retinopathy; papilledema is rare; the exudates are very small and sharply defined and are often confined to one eye. The course of the benign phase is dominated by atheroma and Charcot-Bouchard aneurysms.

Natural Histories

Each of the maladies listed has its own natural history compounded of that of the underlying disease and that of the hypertension and its consequences. Here we are solely concerned with the latter, which exists in its pure form in essential hypertension. The natural history of hypertension itself is thus that of essential hypertension. This has two aspects: the course of the arterial pressure and the course of its consequences.

In the past it has been customary to consider the course of the arterial pressure in terms of a dividing line. This has two fundamental fallacies. First, there is no agreement about the dividing line, which is itself nothing more than an artifact. Second, the measurements of ar-

---

[2] This is the classification of Ellis (45). Many others have been proposed before and since.

terial pressure obtained in the clinic have no great precision and are not in any way representative of what the pressure is at other times. To say that the onset of hypertension was documented in, say, 1956, and to divide the disease into successive stages, prehypertension, intermittent hypertension, labile hypertension, and fixed hypertension, is to put oneself in an intellectual straitjacket, which is entirely meaningless.

The measurements taken in the clinic, despite their lack of precision, are the only data available to show the course of arterial pressure during a lifetime. There is no doubt that arterial pressure tends to rise with age and that the rate of rise is different in some subjects from that in others; some, like me, indeed might fail to show a rise with age, whereas others show varying rates.

Three examples of measurements continued over a number of years are shown in Fig. 12 (47). Figure 12 (middle) is particularly interesting because, rather exceptionally, the relatively high pressure of the patient at 26 years of age did not increase noticeably in the subsequent 18 years. Miall and Lovell (48) found that the higher the pressure at the initial examination, the more rapid the rate of rise, when a large number of subjects is considered.

At present there is little doubt that at any given age the arterial pressure is dependent on polygenic inheritance (49). The higher the pressure of the parents, the higher the pressures of their offspring at a given age, the coefficient of resemblance being about 0.25. The rate of rise in pressure is decreased by physical work and by the number of children in the family and is probably increased by obesity. Acute rises in arterial pressure occur from time to time. There is some evidence, mostly of an anecdotal kind, that these can be precipitated by psychologic factors, such as conflict and anxiety. They are also known to follow a thrombus in a renal artery or one of its branches and to follow the onset of pyelonephritis as a complication of essential hypertension.

In its early stages, essential hypertension is a symptomless disease. The picture changes if the patient becomes frightened by his doctor, his friends, or both, or if a lesion develops in heart, brain, eye, kidney, or, occasionally, other vascular territory.

Iatrogenic disease is extremely common in essential hypertension. The known effects of moderate rises in pressure on the expectation of life over the subsequent 20 years frighten the doctor. His fear is communicated to the patient and is enhanced by articles in the public press, such as "Hypertension No. 1 Killer." Hence, it is the physician himself who, in applying to the patient the grim label of hypertension, produces the patient's symptoms. In Ayman and Pratt's (50) series the chief early complaints of their patients were headache in 72 percent, pain in 67 percent, and nervousness in 67 percent. The frequency of these symptoms was very similar to those found in 50 psychoneurotic subjects with normal blood pressures. Stewart (51) found that of 104 patients who were unaware of having elevated arterial pressure, 87 had no headache; of 96 who had been told they had hypertension, only 27 had not complained of headache, and its onset then corresponded with the telling. In his experience, it was almost impossible for a patient who had been told of having hypertension to remain symptom-free.

The course of the malignant phase has already been referred to. The symptoms that take the patient to his doctor may be: loss of vision due to papilledema, retinal exudate, or hemorrhage; hematuria; fits; or an attack of breathlessness at night. The arterial pressure by that time has reached very high values. In the benign phase, when the pressures are lower, angina pectoris or a myocardial infarction may herald disease of the coronary arteries. A transient or permanent blindness, a transient or permanent paralysis, or symptoms or signs of basilar artery disease may reveal the presence of atheroma of the arteries of the neck and circle of Willis. Should the patient recover from ischemia due to atheroma in one territory, he is at risk from another attack in the same or related

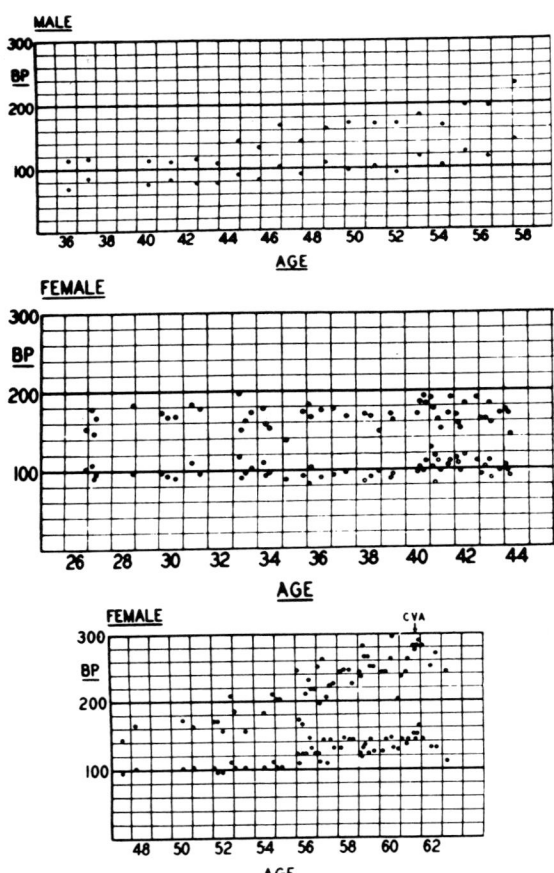

FIG. 12. Three records of arterial pressure over a period of years from Evelyn's analysis of insurance companies' data. (From ref. 47.)

territory. It is not unusual, for example, for a man who has had a myocardial infarct to perish from a stroke and vice versa.

The cerebral hemorrhage that displays the presence of Charcot-Bouchard aneurysms is likewise sudden and unheralded. The further course of these several lesions is beyond our scope.

WHAT IS HYPERTENSION?

The answer to this question depends on the use to which the answer is put. In the past, its purpose has been primarily to appease the physician. He has made a diagnosis; his mind is at rest. But the results in the patients have been catastrophic. Such self-indulgence on the part of the physician has been responsible for the vast amount of iatrogenic psychoneurosis among these patients. Hence, my first rule in treatment: "Never frighten your patient."

If the answer is to be used for insurance purposes, the data are quite clear. There is no division into normotension and hypertension. The higher the pressure, the worse the prognosis. The prognosis is not based on whether "hypertension" is thought to be present, but on the actual pressure recorded.

The question may also be asked from the point of view of diagnosis of the underlying disease. How far am I justified in proceeding to special tests to establish the diagnosis? Every patient should have a full history taken and should undergo a complete physical examination, including microscopic examination of a fresh specimen of urine. He should also have a chest roentgenogram and an electrocardiogram taken. The blood electrolytes, urea, and cholesterol should be measured. These procedures will establish the diagnosis in most patients and will also help in deciding on treatment. If it is decided that the patient's prognosis is sufficiently bad to justify reduction of the arterial pressure, the urinary catecholamines should be determined, and a rapid sequence intravenous pyelogram should be obtained. Procedures which carry a risk to health or life, such as ureteric catheterization and aortography, should be reserved for very special circumstances, such as failure to respond to treatment.

However, the most important question is "At what pressure level should I begin treatment?" Here the data shown in Tables 2 and 3 and Fig. 11 are misleading. The deaths occurred over a period of 20 years from the recording of that arterial pressure. It is extremely probable that death occurred more frequently in those in whom the pressure had risen. From what we know of the effects of therapy (see Dr. Freis's article[3] and ref. 52), patients

whose diastolic arterial pressures exceed 110 mm Hg, after several measurements, fare better and live longer when their arterial pressure is reduced. Because of their special proclivity to atheroma, it is probable that all men with a diastolic pressure of 95 mm Hg and over should be treated. I would suspect that if one were to balance the nuisance value of therapy against its expected benefits, a diastolic pressure of 105 mm Hg would not be far off in women.

Thus the answer to this most important question can be a sterile exercise of great danger to the well-being of the patient, or it may be used constructively to further the patient's own interest. The latter should be the objective of every physician.

SUMMARY

The events provoking disability and death in hypertensive disease are caused by, and related quantitatively to, the high pressure. Left ventricular failure and cardiac failure are usually relieved when a high arterial pressure is reduced. Three types of arterial disease are important: (i) Atheroma or nodular arteriosclerosis, which is a disease of large arteries characterized by fibrous and fibro-fatty plaques and thrombus formation, causes ischemia, notably myocardial, and cerebral infarction; predisposing factors include raised arterial pressure, a metabolic defect associated with a high serum cholesterol level and cigarette smoking. (ii) In Charcot-Bouchard aneurysms of the minute cerebral arteries, whose rupture causes intracerebral hemorrhage, known predisposing factors are age (over 40 years) and arterial pressure (diastolic over 110 mm Hg). (iii) Fibrinoid necrosis of the small arteries and arterioles, the cause of the malignant phase, is due to an extremely high arterial pressure. The role of arterial pressure seems to be greatest in the malignant phase and least in atheroma. Accordingly, when high arterial pressure is reduced by the administration of drugs, atheroma becomes increasingly the common cause of death.

REFERENCES

1. Robinson SC, Brucer M. Range of normal blood pressure. A statistical and clinical study of 11,383 persons. *Arch Intern Med (Chicago)* 1939;64:409.
2. Browne FJ. Chronic hypertension and pregnancy. *Br Med J* 1947;2:283.
3. Ayman D. Heredity in arteriolar (essential) hypertension: a clinical study of the blood pressure of 1,524 members of 277 families. *Arch Intern Med (Chicago)* 1934;53:792.
4. Perera GA. Diagnosis and natural history of hypertensive vascular disease. *Am J Med* 1948;4:416.
5. Thomas CB. The heritage of hypertension. *Am J Med Sci* 1952;224:367.
6. Bechgaard P. Arterial hypertension: a follow-up study of one thousand hypertonics. *Acta Med Scand [Suppl]* 1946:172.
7. Burgess AM. Excessive hypertension of long duration. *N Eng J Med* 1948;239:75.
8. Evans W. *Cardiology,* 2nd edition. London: Butterworth, 1956;386.

---

[3] This refers to a chapter by Dr. Freis in *Hypertension Manual: Mechanisms, Methods, Management,* J. H. Laragh, ed., Yorke Medical Books, New York, 1973, the volume in which the present chapter was originally published.

9. Pickering GW: *High blood pressure,* 2nd edition. London: J & A Churchill, 1968.
10. Pickering GW: *Hypertension, causes, consequences and management.* London: J & A Churchill, 1970.
11. Hinman AT, Engel BT, Bickford AF. Portable blood pressure recorder: accuracy and preliminary use in evaluating intradaily variations in pressure. *Am Heart J* 1962;63:663.
12. Richardson DW, Honour AJ, Fenton GW, Stott FH, Pickering GW. Variation in arterial pressure throughout the day and night. *Clin Sci* 1964;26:445.
13. Bevan AT, Honour AJ, Stott FH. Direct arterial pressure recording in unrestricted man. *Clin Sci* 1969;36:329.
14. Ayman D, Goldshine AD. Blood pressure determinations by patients with essential hypertension. I. The difference between clinic and home readings before treatment. *Am J Med Sci* 1940;200:465.
15. Pickering GW, Cranston WI, Pears MA. *The treatment of hypertension.* Springfield, IL: Charles C Thomas, 1961.
16. Stewart IMG. Long-term observations on high blood-pressure presenting in fit young men. *Lancet* 1971;2:355.
17. Janeway TC. A clinical study of hypertensive cardiovascular disease. *Arch Intern Med (Chicago)* 1913;12:755.
18. Councilman WT. On the relations between arterial disease and tissue changes. *Trans Assoc Am Physicians* 1891;6:179.
19. Osler W. *The principles and practice of medicine,* 9th edition. London: Appleton-Century-Crofts, 1920.
20. Marchand F. Über Arteriosklerose. (Athero-Sklerose). *Verh Kongr Inn Med* 1904;21:23.
21. Mitchell JRA, Schwartz CJ. *Arterial disease.* Oxford: Blackwell Scientific, 1965.
22. Dawber TR, Kannel WB, Revotskie N, Kagan A. The epidemiology of coronary heart disease-the Framingham enquiry. *Proc R Soc Med* 1962;55:265.
23. Doll R, Hill AB. Lung cancer and other causes of death in relation to smoking: a second report on the mortality of British doctors. *Br Med J* 1956;2:1071.
24. Morris JN, Heady JA, Raffle PAB, Roberts CG, Parks JW. Coronary heart-disease and physical activity of work. *Lancet* 1953;2:1053, 1111.
25. Gunning AJ, Hackett MEJ, Mackenzie JR, Oliver DO, Pickering GW, Tibbs DJ. A clinico-pathological study of aorto-iliac thrombosis (the Leriche syndrome). *Q J Med* N.S. 1966;35:475.
26. Charcot JM, Bouchard C. Nouvelles recherches sur la pathogénie de l'hémorrhagie cérébrale. *Arch Physiol* 1868;1:110, 643, 725.
27. Russell RWR. Observations on intracerebral aneurysms. *Brain* 1963;86:425.
28. Cole FM, Yates PO. The occurrence and significance of intracerebral microaneurysms. *J Pathol Bacteriol* 1967;93:393.
29. Fukuda Y. Development of cerebral stroke and coronary heart attack. *Rodoigakukenkyukai* 1970.
30. Volhard F, Fahr T. *Die Brightsche Nierenkrankheit, Klinik, Pathologie und Atlas.* Berlin: Springer-Verlag, 1914.
31. Fahr T. Über Nephrosklerose. *Virchow's Arch Path Anat Physiol* 1919;226:119.
32. Harington M, Kincaid-Smith P, McMichael J. Results of treatment in malignant hypertension: a seven-year experience in 94 cases. *Br Med J* 1959;2:969.
33. Dustan HP, Schneckloth RE, Corcoran AC, Page IH: The effectiveness of long-term treatment of malignant hypertension. *Circulation* 1958;18:644.
34. Perry HM Jr, Schroeder HA, Catanzaro FJ, Moore-Jones D, Camel GH. Studies on the control of hypertension. VIII. Mortality, morbidity, and remissions during twelve years of intensive therapy. *Circulation* 1966;33:958.
35. Pickering GW. Reversibility of malignant hypertension. *Lancet* 1971;1:413.
36. Pickering GW, Wright AD, Heptinstall RH. The reversibility of malignant hypertension. *Lancet* 1952;2:952.
37. Allison PR, Bleehan N, Brown W, Pickering GW, Robb-Smith AHT, Russell RP. The production and resolution of hypertensive vascular lesions in the rabbit. *Clin Sci* 1967;33:39.
38. Goldblatt H. The renal origin of hypertension. *Physiol Rev* 1947;27:120.
39. Smithwick RH, Castleman B. Some observations on renal vascular disease in hypertensive patients based on biopsy material obtained at operation. In: Bell ET, ed. *Hypertension.* Minneapolis: University of Minnesota Press, 1951;199.
40. Heptinstall RH. Renal biopsies in hypertension. *Br Heart J* 1954;16:133.
41. Actuarial Society of America and the Association of Life Insurance Medical Directors. *Supplement to blood pressure study.* New York: Actuarial Society of America and the Association of Life Insurance Medical Directors, 1941.
42. Metropolitan Life Insurance Company. *Blood pressure: insurance experience and its implications.* New York: Metropolitan Life Insurance Co., 1961.
43. Freis ED. Medical treatment of chronic hypertension. *Mod Concepts Cardiovasc Dis* 1971;40:17.
44. Pickering GW. *High blood pressure.* London: J & A Churchill, 1955.
45. Ellis A. Natural history of Bright's disease; clinical, histological and experimental observations. *Lancet* 1942;1:1, 34, 72.
46. Moore RF. The retinitis of arteriosclerosis, and its relation to renal retinitis and to cerebral vascular disease. *Q J Med* 1917;10:29.
47. Evelyn KA. The natural history and prognosis of hypertension. Proceedings of the 42nd Annual Meeting of the Medical Section, American Life Convention, Mackinac Island, MI, June 17–19, 1954.
48. Miall WE, Lovell HG. Relation between change of blood pressure and age. *Br Med J* 1967;2:660.
49. Miall WE, Oldham PD. The hereditary factor in arterial blood pressure. *Br Med J* 1963;1:75.
50. Ayman D, Pratt JH. Nature of the symptoms associated with essential hypertension. *Arch Intern Med (Chicago)* 1931;47:675.
51. Stewart IMG. Headache and hypertension. *Lancet* 1953;1:1261.
52. Freis ED. The treatment of hypertension: why, when and how. *Am J Med* 1972;52:664.

Hypertension: Pathophysiology, Diagnosis, and Management, Second Edition,
edited by J.H. Laragh and B.M. Brenner,
Raven Press, Ltd., New York © 1995.

CHAPTER 1 (Part II)

Modern Definitions and Clinical Expressions of Hypertension

Thomas G. Pickering

As described in the previous chapter, the definition of hypertension was one of my father's favorite scientific topics. His conviction was that blood pressure is distributed continuously in the population, with a skew to the higher end of the curve (a log-gaussian distribution), and that any separation between normotension and hypertension is quite arbitrary (1). Hypertension should thus be defined quantitatively rather than qualitatively on a yes-no or binary basis.

His view has received little, if any, formal challenge since the time that he crossed pens with Sir Robert Platt (2), although a recent analysis from a population survey in Tecumseh, Michigan, concluded that there were indeed two subpopulations with different blood pressures (3). Nevertheless, the distribution curve of blood pressure in this population shows no clearly defined dividing line separating the two, and the populations can only be separated by including variables other than blood pressure.

HYPERTENSION DEFINED AS A TREATMENT THRESHOLD

In spite of this tacit acceptance that there is no absolute separation between normotension and hypertension, the problem has not gone away. The reason for this

T. G. Pickering: Cardiovascular Center, The New York Hospital-Cornell Medical Center, New York, New York 10021.

is not hard to find: at some level of blood pressure we must decide whether or not to prescribe drug treatment or to set a treatment threshold, a decision which is inevitably of a binary nature. In practical terms, hypertension implies ill health and a need for treatment; normotension implies good health and no need for treatment. The debate as to where the dividing line lies has recently been resumed with the demonstration of the efficacy of treating patients with quite mild elevations of blood pressure (4) and the introduction of ambulatory monitoring as a potential clinical tool for defining who needs treatment and who does not (5).

In practice, there are two main reasons to strive for definition of hypertension. One is scientific, the other clinical. Because blood pressure, like many other biological variables, is distributed in a log-gaussian manner, any definition of hypertension is arbitrary, and there is no a priori reason why the same definition should be used for the two purposes. Even if there are indeed two subpopulations with slightly different blood pressures, as suggested by the Tecumseh study, the overlap between them is so great that a single dividing line would not reliably separate them. For scientific purposes it is often appropriate to treat blood pressure quantitatively so that the question of definition need not arise. If a binary classification is to be used, it matters little where the cut is made, as long as it is consistent. The distribution curves of blood pressure are of similar shape in different populations, and it has been shown by Rose and Day (6) that the population mean predicts the number of deviant individuals, however these are defined.

It could be argued that we should define hypertension by the level of blood pressure at which the benefits of treatment outweigh the risks or, in other words, as a treatment threshold. Deciding what this level should be is no easy matter. It entails the assessment of risk without treatment, the reduction of risk conferred by treatment, and the costs and side effects of treatment. Since blood pressure is but one of many risk factors for cardiovascular disease, and since the interactive effects of the various risks tend to be multiplicative rather than additive, it is clear that two individuals with identical levels of blood pressure may have quite different prognoses (Fig. 1). Furthermore, the benefits from treatment are likely to be very different. As shown in Fig. 1, the slope of the line relating risk to blood pressure is much steeper when other risk factors are present than when high blood pressure is the only risk factor (7,8). Lowering blood pressure by a given amount is therefore likely to produce a greater absolute reduction of risk in the "high risk" individual.

While the clinical trials of antihypertensive treatment have proven conclusively that treatment can reduce cardiovascular morbidity (4), they have also introduced a paradox, namely, that treatment benefits the population but not necessarily the patient. This, of course, is because the probability of an individual patient deriving benefit from treatment is very low while the probability of side effects is relatively high, and the majority must bear the costs of treatment for the benefit of the few. Two solutions to this dilemma would be to use safer and cheaper treatment (in which case the low benefit rate would be of less concern) or to stratify patients more accurately according to their levels of risk, so that treatment could be reserved for those who truly need it. There is little hope of achieving the first solution at present without any evidence of greater efficacy in reducing morbidity, especially in the face of new drugs such as the calcium antagonists and angiotensin-converting enzyme (ACE) inhibitors which have added dramatically to the costs of treatment. There is, thus, an urgent need to improve the stratification of risk in mildly hypertensive patients.

All of this presupposes that we actually *can* describe an individual's blood pressure by a single number which we may call the true blood pressure. In earlier times this problem was relatively simple because there was only one way in which blood pressure could be measured routinely, and that was in the clinic. Our knowledge of the risks associated with hypertension and the benefits of treating it were, and to a large extent still are, based on such measurements. Today, the situation is becoming much more complicated. We have three practical methods for measuring blood pressure: in the clinic, by self-monitoring, and by ambulatory monitoring. Each method gives different values of blood pressure.

WILL AMBULATORY BLOOD PRESSURE MONITORING HELP TO DEFINE HYPERTENSION?

The introduction of ambulatory monitoring has provided a new impetus to the attempts to define normotension and hypertension. For ambulatory monitoring to become clinically useful, there is generally thought to be a need to develop some sort of criteria of normality, notwithstanding the problems already discussed with the definition of a normal clinic pressure. The problem here is how the normal range should be established. For a tightly regulated and normally distributed variable such

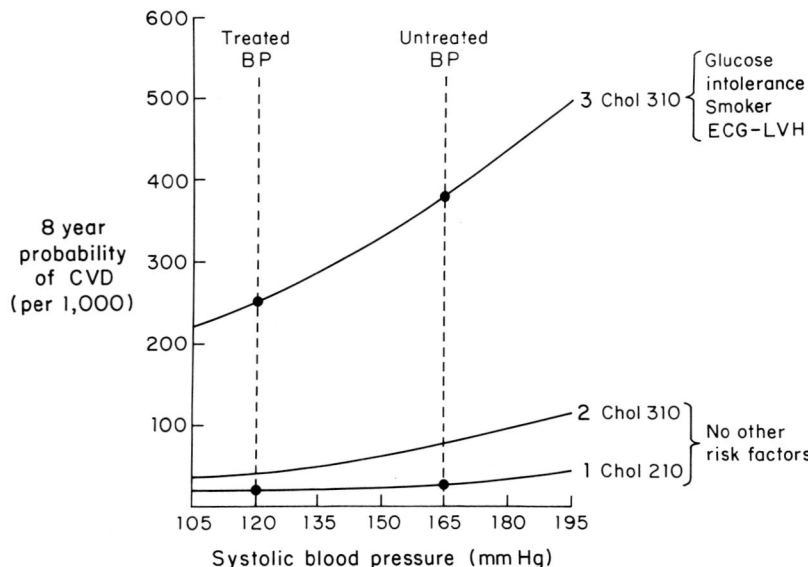

FIG. 1. Relationship between blood pressure (BP) and risk of cardiovascular morbidity (CVD), based on data from the Framingham Study. The lines show how three different hypothetical combinations of risk factors affect the 8-year probability of CVD. Chol, blood cholesterol; ECG-LVH, electrocardiogram-left ventricular hypertrophy. (From refs. 7 and 8, with permission.)

as serum sodium, the solution is relatively simple, and it is generally agreed that the 5th and 95th percentiles are suitable cutoff points (Fig. 2) (8). In the majority of cases where the values lie outside this range, the subject is obviously sick or the deviation is due to measurement error and disappears on repeat testing. In this example, therefore, the equation of normality with health works quite well. Why not do the same for blood pressure? This is indeed what is being presently undertaken in a number of studies, although other methods are also being used. A population or community is evaluated with ambulatory monitoring, and the 95th percentile of the daytime or 24-hour pressure calculated (9). While this is a straightforward approach, it presents a number of problems. Paramount among these is the method used to select the subjects. If a genuinely representative population sample is obtained, it will include many hypertensive individuals, and the 95th percentile might be as high as 175 mm Hg, which is of course far above any acceptable treatment threshold. If, on the other hand, it is decided to exclude the hypertensive individuals, the distribution curve of blood pressure in the population that remains will be determined primarily by the criteria used to exclude the hypertensives. Put another way, to define normotension we must first define hypertension.

Another approach is to define the ambulatory pressure which corresponds to a given level of clinic pressure, such as 140/90 mm Hg (10). This can be done by calculating the regression line between the two variables from a population with a wide range of clinic and ambulatory pressures. One advantage of this is that we do not need to make any a priori blood pressure limit for the reference population and can include normotensive and hypertensive individuals. The disadvantage is that it is still based on the imperfect relationship between clinic pressure and risk.

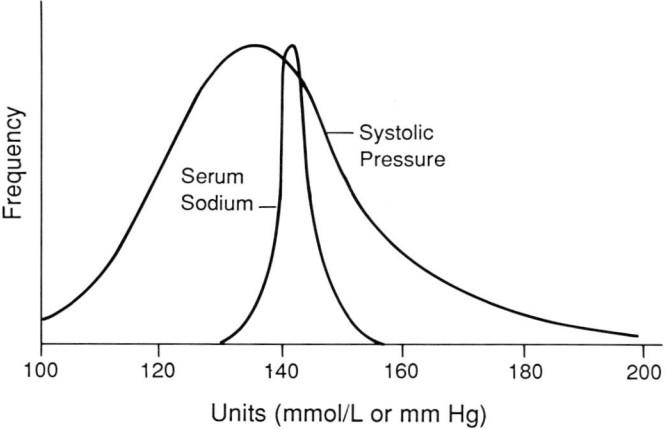

FIG. 2. Comparison of the population distribution of serum sodium and systolic blood pressure. (From ref. 8, with permission.)

Ambulatory monitoring has certainly contributed greatly to our understanding of hypertension. It has demonstrated the enormous variability of blood pressure but at the same time has led to the quite simple concept that hypertension can be regarded as an upward resetting of the set point of blood pressure (the tonic component), with regard to which the short-term changes (the phasic component) occur in approximately the same way as in normotensive individuals. It has also confirmed the unreliability of clinic pressure as a surrogate measure of the true blood pressure. In the majority of hypertensive subjects the clinic pressure is higher than at other times. In a substantial proportion of these patients the pressure outside the clinic may be normal, indicating the phenomenon of *white coat hypertension* (11).

Ambulatory monitoring also appears to give a better estimate of the true blood pressure than clinic measurement. This may be attributed to the greater number of readings that can be obtained and to the fact that they are taken under more representative circumstances than the clinic setting. The validity of this statement is supported both by cross-sectional studies showing that ambulatory pressure gives a closer correlation with target organ damage than does clinic pressure (5) and by much more limited longitudinal data (12).

What it is not likely to do, however, is to give any clearer separation between "normal" and "elevated" blood pressure, since any such separation is quite arbitrary, as my father so clearly enunciated. Given the uncertainties with any definition based solely on blood pressure, it seems clear that what is needed is to relate—either directly and prospectively or indirectly—ambulatory blood pressure to the risk of cardiovascular morbidity by using a surrogate outcome measure such as left ventricular mass. In both cases, the relationship between blood pressure and risk should be stronger for ambulatory than for clinic pressure, offering an easier prospect for deciding the level of blood pressure above which the risk becomes unacceptable. This does not mean to suggest that a dividing line, if one can be agreed upon should become a universal treatment threshold. The decision to start treatment should be based on an assessment of all the major risk factors, not just blood pressure, and on an evaluation of the costs and benefits of treatment. The definition of hypertension should not automatically imply a need for treatment.

CLINICAL EXPRESSIONS OF HYPERTENSION

However it is defined, hypertension can be subdivided in two ways: by its underlying cause and by its severity. While it has been traditional to regard essential hypertension as a single entity, it is likely that an increasing number of distinct phenotypes and genotypes will be identified in the coming years and that the proportion of patients relegated to the diagnosis of essential hypertension will diminish. Some of the terms used to describe the severity or other characteristics of essential hypertension are discussed below.

Although the traditional separation of benign- and malignant-phase hypertension is still methodologically valid, the term *benign hypertension* is now considered to be politically incorrect because it implies an absence of risk. In the past few years there has been increasing emphasis on the need to treat ever-lower levels of blood pressure. The *malignant phase* is defined by the concurrence of very high pressures and papilledema; it has a distinct pathophysiology resulting in a vicious cycle of increasing blood pressure and vascular damage (1).

The term *white coat hypertension (office hypertension)* has become widely used in the past few years as a result of the introduction of ambulatory monitoring and measurements taken outside the clinic. While any definition is arbitrary, it can be generally defined as a persistently elevated clinic pressure with a normal ambulatory pressure. As described above, there is no consensus on what a normal ambulatory pressure should be, but an average daytime value of less than 134/90 mm Hg seems reasonable. It is clinically important because it may define a subgroup at low risk of cardiovascular morbidity, as discussed elsewhere in this volume.

Borderline hypertension is a term which has been used to describe patients with blood pressures between 140/90 and 160/95 mm Hg. *Labile hypertension* and *prehypertension* formerly identified borderline hypertension or "high normal" blood pressure, but these terms are now obsolete.

Most truly hypertensive patients have an elevated blood pressure throughout the day and night. In contrast with white coat hypertension, these patients may be described as having *sustained hypertension.*

In a small proportion of apparently hypertensive patients, the act of inflating a blood pressure cuff may cause a transient elevation of blood pressure (13). This phenomenon, termed *cuff inflation hypertension,* can be identified by continuous blood pressure monitoring (e.g., with a Finapres) during cuff inflation. It appears to be distinct from white coat hypertension.

In most societies systolic blood pressure tends to increase with age to a much greater extent than diastolic pressure. *Isolated systolic hypertension of the elderly* is generally defined as a systolic pressure of more than 160 mm Hg with a diastolic pressure of less than 90 mm Hg. As described elsewhere in this volume, it appears to have a different pathophysiology from essential hypertension, the main factor being an increased stiffness of the arterial wall.

In some elderly patients conventional noninvasive methods of measuring blood pressure may give a falsely

TABLE 1. *Classification of blood pressure*

Category	Systolic (mm Hg)	Diastolic (mm Hg)
Normal	<130	<85
High normal	130–139	85–89
Hypertension		
Stage 1 (mild)	140–159	90–99
Stage 2 (moderate)	160–179	100–109
Stage 3 (severe)	180–209	110–119
Stage 4 (very severe)	≥210	≥120

From ref. 14, with permission.

high estimate of the intraarterial pressure because of incompressibility of the arteries. Since increased arterial stiffness is associated with aging, this is commonly referred to as *pseudohypertension of the elderly.* Physiologically, of course, it is quite distinct from white coat hypertension, but shares with it the discrepancy between an apparently elevated clinic pressure and an absence of target organ damage. It is described elsewhere in this volume.

It should be emphasized that, with the possible exception of the definition for *malignant hypertension,* all the definitions are arbitrary, and conditions may coexist. White coat hypertension, for example, may commonly occur in patients with isolated systolic hypertension. The new classification proposed by the Joint National Committee on Detection, Evaluation, and Treatment of High Blood Pressure (14) is shown in Table 1.

REFERENCES

1. Pickering GW. *High blood pressure.* London: Churchill-Livingstone; 1968.
2. Swales JD. *Platt versus Pickering: an episode in recent medical history.* London: Keynes Press; 1985.
3. Julius S, Krause L, Schork MJ, et al. Hyperkinetic hypertension in Tecumseh, Michigan. *J Hypertens* 1991;9:77–84.
4. Collins R, Peto R, MacMahon S, et al. Blood pressure, stroke, and coronary heart disease. Part 2, short-term reductions in blood pressure: overview of randomized drug trials in their epidemiological context. *Lancet* 1990;335:827–838.
5. Pickering TG. *Ambulatory monitoring and blood pressure variability.* London: Science Press; 1991.
6. Rose G, Day S. The population mean predicts the number of deviant individuals. *Brit Med J* 1990;301:1031–1034.
7. Kannel WB, Gordon T: *The Framingham study: an epidemiological investigation of cardiovascular disease.* Section 31; 1976; DHEW publication no (NIH)76–1083.
8. Pickering TG. The Ninth Sir George Pickering Memorial Lecture: ambulatory monitoring and the definition of hypertension. *J Hypertens* 1992;10:401–409.
9. Staessen JA, Fagard RH, Lignen PJ, Thijs L, van Hoof R, Amery AK. Mean and range of the ambulatory pressure in normotensive subjects from a meta-analysis of 23 studies. *Am J Cardiol* 1991;67:723–727.
10. Baumgart P, Walger P, Jurgens U, Rahn KH. Reference data for ambulatory blood pressure monitoring: what results are equivalent to the established limits of office blood pressure? *Klin Wochenschrift* 1990;68:723–727.
11. Pickering TG, James GD, Boddie C, Harshfield GA, Blank S, Lar-

agh JH. How common is white coat hypertension? *JAMA* 1988;259:225–228.

12. Perloff D, Sokolow M, Cowan R, Juster RP. Diagnostic value of ambulatory blood pressure measurements: further analyses. *J Hypertens* 1989;7[Suppl 3]:S3–S10.

13. Mejia AD, Egan BM, Schork NJ, Sweifler AJ. Artifacts in measurement of blood pressure and lack of target organ involvement in the assessment of patients with treatment-resistant hypertension. *Ann Intern Med* 1990;112:270–277.

14. National Institutes of Health. *The fifth report of the Joint National Committee on Detection, Evaluation, and Treatment of High Blood Pressure,* 1993. NIH publication no 93–1088.

Hypertension: Pathophysiology, Diagnosis, and Management, Second Edition,
edited by J.H. Laragh and B.M. Brenner,
Raven Press, Ltd., New York © 1995.

CHAPTER 2

The Goldblatt Experiment

A Conceptual Paradigm

Peter J. Goldblatt

The primary definition of a paradigm, according to Webster (1), is "an outstandingly clear or typical example, or archetype." The title of this chapter, then, implies that the experiment of Goldblatt and associates, reported in 1932 (2) and published in 1934 (3), represents a clear example of the application of the experimental method to the solution of a problem of human disease. On several occasions, Harry Goldblatt expressed his fervent belief in the experimental method and avowed that he was a "follower of William Harvey," who was among the first to apply it in medicine (4). The question remains, what human disease? From that initial report of the production of persistent hypertension by means of a silver clamp applied to the main renal arteries (2,3), which also demonstrated that narrowing of a single artery resulted in at least transient elevation of the blood pressure in dogs, came the recognition of a human counterpart, known as *Goldblatt hypertension* or *renovascular hypertension*. Although he found this gratifying (see Harry Goldblatt's Perspective of the Paradigm, below), it was clear that the latter was an entirely unanticipated finding. As will be evident from his writings, which are abstracted below, Harry Goldblatt intended to simulate the benign and/or malignant phase of *human essential hypertension*. There is a certain irony in the fact that Goldblatt (renovascular) hypertension is classified as a "secondary" type of hypertension in most texts on the subject. I

will review some of the background that led to the development of the experimental method, and present some abstracts from the initial experiments (2,3,5–9) of the Goldblatt group, which helped to elucidate the mechanism of hypertension in this model. Then, using Harry Goldblatt's own words, as well as my own, I will give an interpretation of these and some more recent investigations, in an attempt to relate this experimental model to *essential* hypertension and its most frequently associated pathologic finding—nephrosclerosis. It was the effects of nephrosclerosis that Harry Goldblatt was trying to simulate when he developed his paradigm.

HISTORICAL PERSPECTIVE

Harry Goldblatt (Fig. 1) graduated from McGill University School of Medicine in 1916. He was selected as the recipient of the final-year prize (10) and took the opportunity at the graduation ceremony to chide the school for resting on its laurels as a great clinical school (Sir William Osler had only recently departed for Johns Hopkins). He suggested that they would slip from prominence unless they embraced the rapidly developing sciences of biochemistry and physiology and became leaders in biomedical research. This admonition from one so new to medicine was hardly received with great favor. According to my aunt (Alta Kahn, *personal communication*), the dean became livid and thanked my father for his remarks, in icy tones, stating that it was "too bad that Goldblatt *wouldn't* be with us, to lead us into

P. J. Goldblatt: Department of Pathology, Medical College of Ohio, Toledo, Ohio 43699.

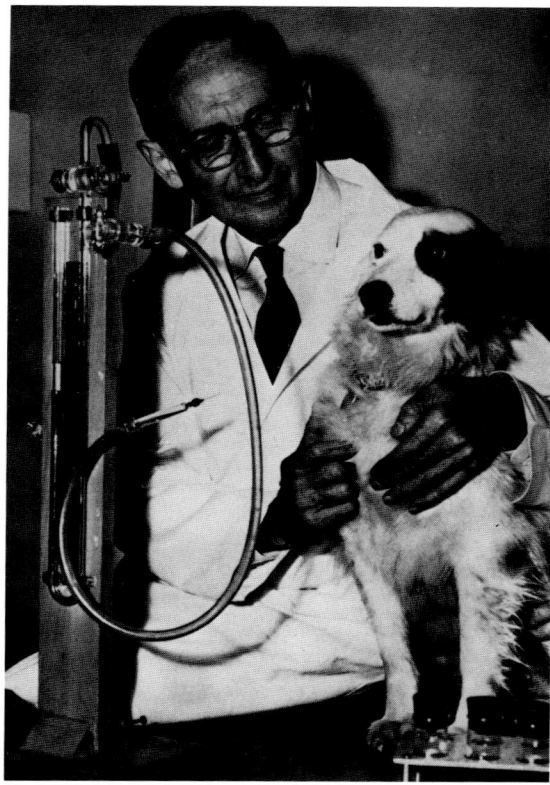

FIG. 1. Harry Goldblatt and "Flossie," research dog hero of the year, about 1955. Dr. Goldblatt was in his sixties, and Flossie was about the same in dog years.

this new era." Indeed, he was with them for one more year, but, perhaps because of these remarks, as a house officer in surgery at the Royal Victoria Hospital rather than in internal medicine, his first choice (Alta Kahn, *personal communication*).

As a student, Goldblatt was exposed to the classical concepts of hypertension and vascular disease which stemmed from the observations of Bright in 1832, who is usually justly given credit for drawing attention to the relationship between scarred kidneys and a large, heavy heart (8,11,12). Harry Goldblatt's medical school notes indicate that he was taught that the vascular disease in the kidneys *resulted* from the hypertension. Like Bright's hypothesis on the "alteration of blood flow," this suggestion—which came from Dr. Mahomed of Guy's Hospital (12)—preceded any reliable clinical means for measuring blood pressure. The latter came with the development of the sphygmomanometer, by Riva Rocci, in 1910 (12). This instrument was available to Harry Goldblatt, and he used it during his surgical house officership to make an observation that he later felt was a significant one in developing his hypothesis (13) (see also Harry Goldblatt's Perspective of the Paradigm, below). A young woman was admitted with a palpable abdominal mass and was taken to surgery. The surgeon pro-

ceeded to resect the mass, only to find that it was an unusual form of horseshoe kidney and that it represented the patient's only functional renal tissue. As reported by my father, he followed her to her death, which took 6 days, and though she became "profoundly uremic, at no time did she develop hypertension." And so he said, "I salted away the idea that, at least, 'No kidneys, no hypertension.'"[1]

Following Harry Goldblatt's first year as a surgeon, in which he rose to the rank of chief resident with 120 surgical beds under his care, because Canada was drafting its physicians into the army, and Goldblatt was a United States citizen, he became a volunteer in pathology while awaiting his call to service. During this time, Volhard and Fahr (11,12) were writing their articles on the classification of hypertension and were debating the origin of the renal vascular disease, particularly the development of the lesion associated with malignant hypertension. Fahr asserted that the extreme pressure was responsible, whereas Volhard felt that biochemical alterations associated with uremia were at least necessary cofactors (12). The debate, which became heated at times, was well known to my father, who corresponded with Volhard, at least, in later years. Nonetheless, again, Harry Goldblatt later asserted that his early experience with multiple autopsies, which continued during his service in the army (although he was a battle surgeon and ended his military career as chief of an evacuation hospital), cemented his and others' conviction that nephrosclerosis almost always accompanied hypertension (11,14). He claimed that it was even at this time that he began to question his early instruction and to formulate the hypothesis that perhaps, "the vascular disease came first, and then, and only then, the hypertension develops."[2] Though the majority view today still favors the reverse, it was this hypothesis that he set out to test when the opportunity presented.

THE GOLDBLATT EXPERIMENT

As mentioned previously, the experiments began in 1928, were presented orally before the Academy of Medicine in Cleveland in 1932 (2), and were finally published in the *Journal of Experimental Medicine* in 1934 (3). As attested in the letter of acceptance (Fig. 2), the editors recognized the significance of the paradigm they had been privileged to receive. "It is a pleasure for us as editors to receive a paper of such large significance, so admirably written," wrote Peyton Rous, whose own investigative work later won him the Nobel Prize. The

---

[1] H. Goldblatt, in "The Agony and Ecstasy of Medical Research," a movie of a talk at the Armed Forces Institute of Pathology, May 1963.
[2] Ibid.

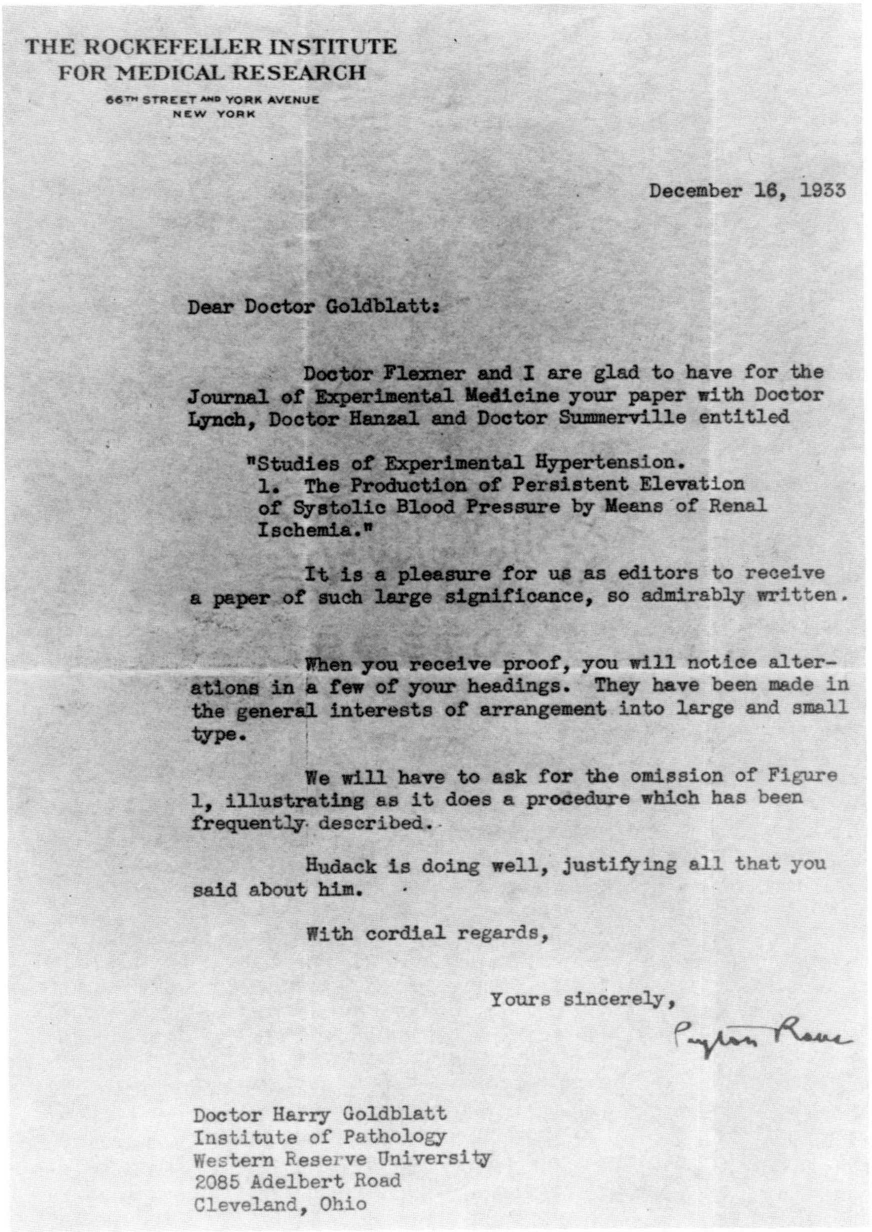

THE ROCKEFELLER INSTITUTE
FOR MEDICAL RESEARCH
66TH STREET AND YORK AVENUE
NEW YORK

December 16, 1933

Dear Doctor Goldblatt:

Doctor Flexner and I are glad to have for the Journal of Experimental Medicine your paper with Doctor Lynch, Doctor Hanzal and Doctor Summerville entitled

"Studies of Experimental Hypertension.
1. The Production of Persistent Elevation of Systolic Blood Pressure by Means of Renal Ischemia."

It is a pleasure for us as editors to receive a paper of such large significance, so admirably written.

When you receive proof, you will notice alterations in a few of your headings. They have been made in the general interests of arrangement into large and small type.

We will have to ask for the omission of Figure 1, illustrating as it does a procedure which has been frequently described.

Hudack is doing well, justifying all that you said about him.

With cordial regards,

Yours sincerely,

Peyton Rous

Doctor Harry Goldblatt
Institute of Pathology
Western Reserve University
2085 Adelbert Road
Cleveland, Ohio

FIG. 2. Letter of acceptance for Harry Goldblatt's first article (3) published in *Journal of Experimental Medicine*. The signature is that of Peyton Rous, later a winner of the Nobel Prize.

"Doctor Flexner" referred to is Simon Flexner, a pathologist and the first director of The Rockefeller Institute, not his brother, Abraham, whose famous report for the Carnegie Foundation is often credited with revolutionizing medical education. Since this first article is one of those most frequently cited in the medical literature and, in Stamey's estimation (15), "stimulated more medical research than any single experiment in medical history," it is excerpted extensively below. Parenthetically, Stamey's assessment appears justified by the enormous additional literature that has accumulated in the 30 plus years since it was made! The following excerpt has been taken from ref. 3:

STUDIES ON EXPERIMENTAL HYPERTENSION
I. The Production of Persistent Elevation of Systolic Blood Pressure by Means of Renal Ischemia[3,4]

Harry Goldblatt, M.D., James Lynch, M.D.,
Ramon F. Hanzal, Ph.D.,
and Ward W. Summerville, M.D.

(From the Institute of Pathology, Western Reserve University, Cleveland, received for publication, December 1, 1933)

[3] Presented before the American Association of Pathologists and Bacteriologists in Washington, D.C., on May 9, 1933.
[4] Aided by a grant from the Committee on Scientific Research of the American Medical Association.

The production of elevated blood pressure in animals has been attempted[5] by various methods involving injury to the kidneys. In the experiments of long duration for the purpose of producing persistent hypertension, the methods used were injection of nephrotoxic substances, irradiation of the kidneys by Roentgen rays, renal venous stasis, and excision of varying amounts of kidney tissue, with or without ligation of some branches of the renal arteries. The elevation of blood pressure, which occurred as a result of some of these methods, did not prove persistent. Cash, one of those who used the method mentioned last, drew attention to the fact that the increase of pressure occurred only when some necrotic kidney tissue was undergoing absorption within the body. He gave as the conditions under which he observed temporary elevation of blood pressure in dogs, that the total kidney substance be reduced at least 50 percent and that, in addition, a portion of kidney which has been deprived of its circulation be allowed to remain *in situ.*

Although it has been suggested (Fahr) that renal ischemia, by itself, may play an important part in the development of the hypertension which is associated with more or less diffuse vascular disease in man, the validity of this contention has not, up to the present time, been investigated experimentally in animals by a study designed to test the effect on blood pressure of renal ischemia alone.

In the investigation here reported, the working hypothesis adopted was that ischemia *limited to the kidneys* may be the initial condition in the pathogenesis of the hypertension that is associated with nephrosclerosis. If this be true, then renal ischemia, no matter how produced, should be followed by elevation of blood pressure. This report deals with the effect on the blood pressure of dogs of experimentally produced ischemia limited to the kidneys. The simplest method for this purpose being obviously constriction of the main renal arteries, this was the method chosen.

METHOD

Animals and Diet

Dogs of various mixed breeds were used. The animals, all females, varied in weight and age. Their exact age was not known, but they were all full grown, seemingly normal dogs. Examination of blood pressure, blood, and urine during a long control period revealed nothing to indicate renal disease. They were kept in individual roomy cubicles and fed throughout the entire experimental period on Purina dog chow, a complete food adequate to maintain adult dogs in good state of nutrition. The amount of water was not limited.

To effect a narrowing of the main renal artery a clamp was devised whereby the degree of constriction of the vessel could be varied and controlled. Various contrivances were devised for this purpose, but the clamp illustrated diagrammatically in Text-Fig. 1 (Fig. 3) was finally found the most satisfactory.

The Clamp

The entire clamp is made of one type of pure silver. The sides and back (B) are 0.75 mm, the compressing plate (C) 0.75 mm, and the removable plate (D) 0.5 mm in thickness. The double acting screw (A) whereby the compressing plate is moved is made of round silver wire measuring 3 mm in diameter. The chamber of the clamp found most suitable for dogs weighing between 10 and 20 kilos measures $3 \times 3 \times 6$ mm.

Instruments for the Application of the Clamp

For the purpose of applying the clamp to the renal artery, which necessitates working at considerable depth, retroperitoneally, special instruments were devised, which are illustrated diagrammatically in Text-Figs. 2, 3, and 4 (see Fig. 3). The instrument for holding the clamp while it is being applied to the vessel is shown in Text-Fig. 2. The device for the insertion of the removable plate (D, Text-Fig. 1) which helps to encase the renal vessel in the clamp is shown in Text-Fig. 3. Text-Fig. 4 is a screwdriver with which to screw down the compressing plate (C) and turn the retaining screw (N) which fixes the clamp in the holder or releases it after application to the vessel.

Application of the Clamp

The clamp, without the removable plate (D), is placed with the head of the double-acting screw (A) pointing downward in the lower part of the clamp holder (Text-Fig. 2, position 1) and held firmly in place by means of the retaining screw (N). The portion of the renal artery dissected out for the purpose is lifted into the upturned clamp and is then encased in the clamp by the insertion of the removable plate (D) into the clamp by means of the special instrument illustrated in Text-Fig. 3. The removable plate is held tightly in the jaws of this instrument while it is being inserted in the clamp. In order to be able to compress the vessel to the desired degree by means of the compressing plate (C), the clamp holder is so fashioned that pressure upon the knob (H) in the handle of the clamp holder (Text-Fig. 2) releases the part that holds the clamp so that it turns over on a hinge and inverts the clamp (Text-Fig. 2, positions 1, 2, and 3). This brings the head of the screw (A) of the clamp uppermost (Text-Fig. 2, position 3) and makes it accessible for the purpose of screwing down the compressing plate (C). When this has been accomplished, the retaining screw (N) is turned back and the clamp, thus released, is easily pushed out of the holder and left on the vessel which it encases and constricts to the desired degree.

The remainder of the article presents details of the initial experiments undertaken using the clamp. By today's standards, the techniques and the experiments themselves may seem rather unsophisticated. It must be remembered that, for instance, heparin was not yet available and that continuous monitoring of blood pressure was impossible because the catheters would become occluded by thrombi. The method of blood pressure esti-

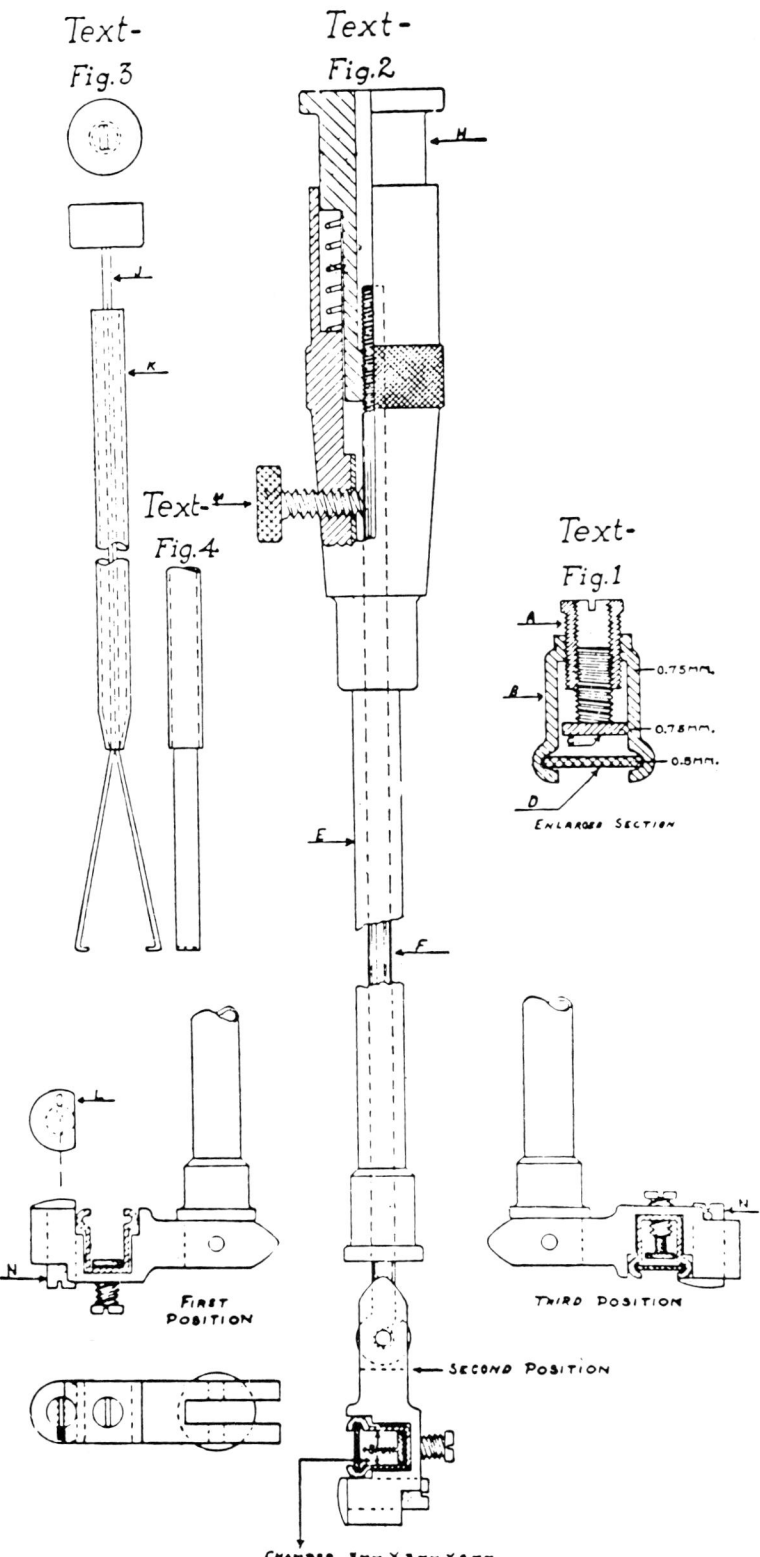

Text-Fig.3

Text-Fig.2

Text-Fig.4

Text-Fig.1

ENLARGED SECTION

FIRST POSITION

THIRD POSITION

SECOND POSITION

CHAMBER 3mm.X3mm.X6mm.

FIG. 3. The clamp and the instrument for insertion (Text-Figs. 1–4, ref. 3). The following are the original explanations of the diagrams. **Text-Fig. 1:** The clamp. A, screw which carries the movable plate; D, removable plate. **Text-Fig. 2:** The clamp holder with clamp inserted. M, a screw, the loosening of which permits the knob H to be pressed down and makes it possible for the part that holds the clamp to assume any one of the three positions illustrated. **Text-Fig. 3:** Holder for removable plate D, Text-Fig. 1. The metal tube K slides down or up and tightens or loosens the grip of the metal jaws on the removable plate. **Text-Fig. 4:** Screw-driver for tightening of screw A (Text-Fig. 1), which carries the movable plate C (Text-Fig. 1).

mation was the carotid loop method of Van Leersum (cited in ref. 3), which gave only systolic values and which Harry Goldblatt himself suspected as being subject to various interpretations. He later abandoned the method in favor of direct femoral arterial puncture, which again yielded *mean* blood pressure rather than both systolic and diastolic pressures, which he considered a crucial element in the diagnosis of hypertension. This led to a series of subsequent investigations that will be commented upon further.

The remainder of the first article dealt with determination of the effect of the degree of constriction of the main renal artery on renal blood flow, variations in the sequence of clamping and/or release, assessment of the effect of clamping on renal function, and an early exploration of mechanism, including removal of one adrenal and destruction of the adrenal medulla on the contralateral side (see ref. 3 for details). Also investigated was the effect of ischemia of *other* organs on blood pressure, as well as of nephrectomy on renal hypertension.

In the discussion, he presented three possible mechanisms (3):

> (a) Afferent impulses from the affected nerve endings in the ischemic kidneys to the sympathetic ganglia or vasomotor center may result in general vasoconstriction and consequent elevation of blood pressure.
> (b) Afferent impulses from the ischemic kidneys may, in some way, bring about increased output of some internal secretion which, by peripheral or central action, may effect general vasoconstriction and thus raise the blood pressure.
> (c) There may be an accumulation or new formation of some substance, or there may occur a disturbance of chemical equilibrium between substances present in the blood which may effect a pressor action like that of a hormone.

These suggested mechanisms were followed by a series of investigations, some of which will be commented upon further, that occupied Goldblatt for nearly 40 more years. In summarizing his initial publication (3), Goldblatt offered the following concluding statements:

> These experiments indicate that, in dogs at least, ischemia localized to the kidneys is a sufficient condition for the production of persistently elevated systolic blood pressure. When the constriction of both main renal arteries is made only moderately severe in the beginning, the elevation of systolic blood pressure is unaccompanied by signs of materially decreased renal function. In this respect the hypertension in these animals resembles the hypertension which is associated with so-called benign nephrosclerosis in man. Subsequent increase of the constriction of the main renal arteries does not materially damage renal function, probably because of adequate development of accessory circulation. More delicate methods of detecting a change may yet prove that some damage does occur. Almost complete constriction of both main renal arteries, from the beginning, results in great elevation of systolic blood pressure which is ac-

companied by severe disturbance of renal function and uremia. This resembles the type of hypertension which is associated with so-called malignant nephrosclerosis, in the sense of Fahr.[6] In several of the animals with persistent elevation of systolic blood pressure, anatomical changes were observed in the glomeruli, vessels, and parenchyma of the kidneys which are probably directly referable to the ischemia.

> It is hoped that these investigations will afford a means of studying the pathogenesis of hypertension that is associated with renal vascular disease.

The articles that followed (5–9) established that it was possible to produce experimental renal hypertension despite extensive splanchnic denervation (5), that *both* systolic and diastolic pressure rose following renal artery constriction in rhesus monkeys (6), and that retinal vascular changes appeared similar to those seen in the malignant phase of essential hypertension when renal ischemia was severe enough to produce uremia (7). Destruction of the anterior spinal nerve roots failed to prevent or abolish renal hypertension (9). In an extensive study of the pathogenesis of experimental hypertension, published in 1937, Harry Goldblatt concluded (8):

> Persistent hypertension has been produced in animals (dog and monkey) by constricting the main renal arteries, which reduces the blood flow to the functioning components of the kidneys (renal ischemia).

> Hypertension without or with disturbance of renal function, resembling in this respect the benign and malignant types, respectively, in man, can be produced by varying the degree of constriction of the renal arteries.

> The results of various experiments indicate that this type of experimental hypertension is due primarily to a humoral and not to a nervous mechanism initiated by the ischemia of the kidneys.

> The nature of the effective substance responsible for inducing the hypertension has not yet been elucidated.

> The present indication is that the adrenal cortical hormone plays a part in conjunction with the hypothetical effective substance of renal origin in the pathogenesis of hypertension due to constriction of the main renal arteries.

Following this, Goldblatt reviewed his own and others' work, which was beginning to fill in the details of the paradigm, in a Harvey Lecture delivered in May 1938 (11). In both of these he extensively reviewed the available literature. He first established the relationship between the adrenal cortex and renal hypertension, and he showed that renal hypertension could be prevented by renal vein ligation and significantly affected by total adrenalectomy. In the Harvey Lecture he reviewed the evidence and, for the first time (that I have found), clearly discussed the relationship of the humoral factor discovered by Tigerstedt and Bergmann (cited in ref. 11) to the model he developed (11):

---

[6] References deleted; see original publication.

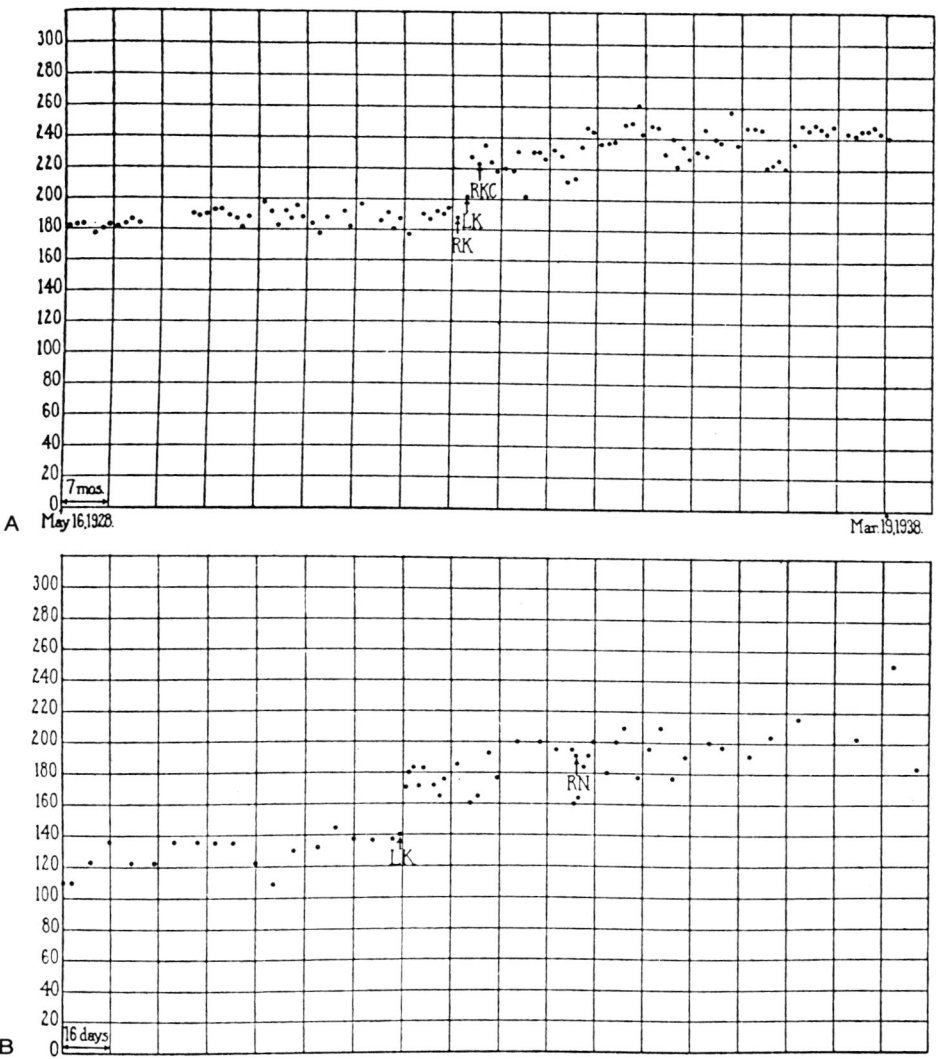

FIG. 4. Illustrative charts from ref. 11, showing **(A)** the effect of bilateral moderate constriction of the renal artery and **(B)** unilateral constriction followed by nephrectomy. **A:** "Blackie," short-haired mongrel, female, age about 1 year, in 1928. Initial weight 21.4 kg. Present weight 21.6 kg. RK, moderate constriction of right main renal artery; LK, moderate constriction of left main renal artery; RKC, occlusion of right main renal artery; ●, systolic blood pressure, mm Hg, van Leersum carotid loop method. The dog was still alive when ref. 11 was published. **B:** Dog 3–14, male, bulldog, young. Initial weight 11 kg. Present weight 11.8 kg. LK, severe constriction of left main renal artery; RN, right nephrectomy; ●, mean blood pressure, mm Hg, direct method, femoral artery.

Since the original investigation by Tigerstedt and Bergmann,[7] who obtained a pressor effect with saline extract of normal rabbits' kidneys when they injected it intravenously into other rabbits, many workers have repeated the experiments with different kinds of extracts, expressed juices, and autolysates of normal kidneys of various animals, with conflicting results. Some confirmed Tigerstedt and Bergmann's finding; others obtained only depressor effects; on the whole, most investigators found both a depressor and pressor effect, the latter usually following the former. Pressor effects have also been ob-

tained with extracts from other organs. The search for the possible chemical substance involved in the humoral mechanism of renal origin in the cause of experimental hypertension due to constriction of renal arteries has resulted in a number of investigations that have dealt with the presence of a pressor principle in normal and ischemic kidneys. Tigerstedt and Bergmann actually suggested that there might be an increase of the pressor substance, *rennin* they called it, in the kidneys of hypertensives. The recent isolation by Landis and collaborators of an extract of normal kidney which elevated blood pressure without diminishing skin temperature and without reducing the amplitude of arterial pulsation is of special interest. A similar extract of ischemic kidney

---

[7] References deleted; see original publication.

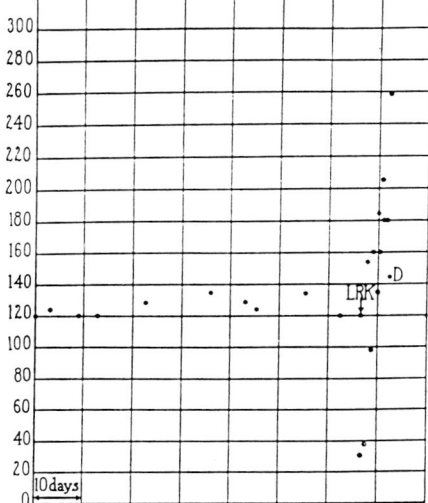

FIG. 5. Severe clamping of the main renal arteries bilaterally with severe hypertension and rising BUN. Such severe constriction produced a picture similar to malignant hypertension with arteriolar necrosis (see Fig. 6) (11). Dog 3–90, female, mixture of collie and airdale, middle-aged. Initial weight 10.9 kg., final weight 12.2 kg. LRK, almost complete constriction of left and right main renal arteries; D, died; ●, mean blood pressure, mm Hg, direct method, femoral artery; ☉, blood urea nitrogen, mg per 100 mL of plasma.

should be made and compared quantitatively with the extract of normal kidney.

In that article he presented graphs (Figs. 4 and 5) illustrating the response to bilateral clamping, unilateral clamping with contralateral nephrectomy (Fig. 4), and bilateral clamping severe enough to result in uremia (Fig. 5). Parenthetically, the dog "Blackie" referred to in the first graph lived to about 14 years of age. Her blood pressure was elevated for at least 12 years, and I remember her well since she was frequently demonstrated to visitors and was more a pet than an experimental animal. This was true of most of his dogs (see "Flossie" in Fig. 1).

Another issue raised in that article (11) that has subsequently been debated and misinterpreted was the pathogenesis of the lesions of *malignant* hypertension that appeared particularly in the intestinal arterioles (but not in the kidneys) (Fig. 6), in which severe clamping resulted in hypertension and uremia (see chart, Fig. 5). As illustrated in Fig. 6, there was fibrinoid necrosis, along with other features closely resembling the lesions in humans. Goldblatt commented (11):

> Nothing is known about the pathogenesis of the arteriolar degeneration and necrosis which are found in many internal organs, but most frequently in the kidneys[8] and gastrointestinal tract in human benign or malignant hy-

---

[8] References deleted; see original publication.

pertension. The degenerative and necrotizing arteriolar lesions of the animals which have been described above are not distinguishable from those found in most cases of malignant hypertension in man except that they are more severe and more widespread than in the latter. This indicates a greater susceptibility of the dog's arterioles to these changes. In human malignant hypertension, skeletal muscles and lungs also rarely show necrosis of arterioles, although hyalinization and other changes may occur in those of the muscles. *The only striking difference between the lesions in man and dog is that in the latter the kidneys do not, while in the former they very frequently do, show arteriolar necrosis* [emphasis added]. This discrepancy is easily explained and actually affords a clue to the pathogenesis of this lesion. In the animals, the intravascular pressure, within the kidney, is low, because the ischemia is due to the constriction of the main renal artery. In man, the intrarenal vascular tension is undoubtedly high, because there is sclerosis and constriction of the preglomerular arterioles. In some of the larger vessels of the human kidney the lumen is also frequently narrowed, due to proliferation of the intima, but it has never been shown that the arterioles belonging to such vessels become necrotic. It may be that only those arterioles become necrotic that are subjected to the high bursting tension as well as to the hypothetical toxic substance or substances in the blood which result from the renal insufficiency. There are some human cases in which necrosis of small renal arterioles is not found. These may be cases in which the renal insufficiency is due to widespread intimal proliferation in the small arteries and large arterioles and not to the reduction in the caliber of the preglomerular arterioles. This may also account for the difference and point to one of the probable factors and necessary conditions in the pathogenesis of arteriolar necrosis and hemorrhage; namely, elevated pressure within these vessels. That the accumulation of chemicals in the blood is not by itself a sufficient condition for the production of the arteriolar lesions is shown by the fact that bilaterally nephrectomized dogs that develop azotemia but no hypertension do not develop the generalized hyalinization and necrosis of arterioles and associated hemorrhages in the organs. That hypertension alone is not sufficient to determine the formation of the necrotizing lesions of the arterioles is shown by the fact that animals that have had severe hypertension for more than five years, without accompanying significant disturbance of renal function, have not developed this lesion. That the lesions of the arterioles are not due to ischemia is shown by the absence of the lesions from the severely ischemic kidneys of the dogs and their presence in organs in which there is no preexistent ischemia. In the dogs, at least, the combination of hypertension and severe disturbance of renal function, with consequent accumulation of chemical substances in the blood, is at least a necessary condition for the manifestation of the arteriolar necrosis and associated hemorrhages in various organs. Since the hypertension is not present within the intrarenal blood vessels of the animals with the main renal arteries, or the aorta above the origin of the renal arteries, constricted, the lesion does not manifest itself there. The same explanation (absence of local hypertension) probably applies to the absence of the lesion in the pulmonary arteries of man as well as of animals. What the nature of the chemical substance or substances is that plays a part in the production of these lesions is not elucidated by these in-

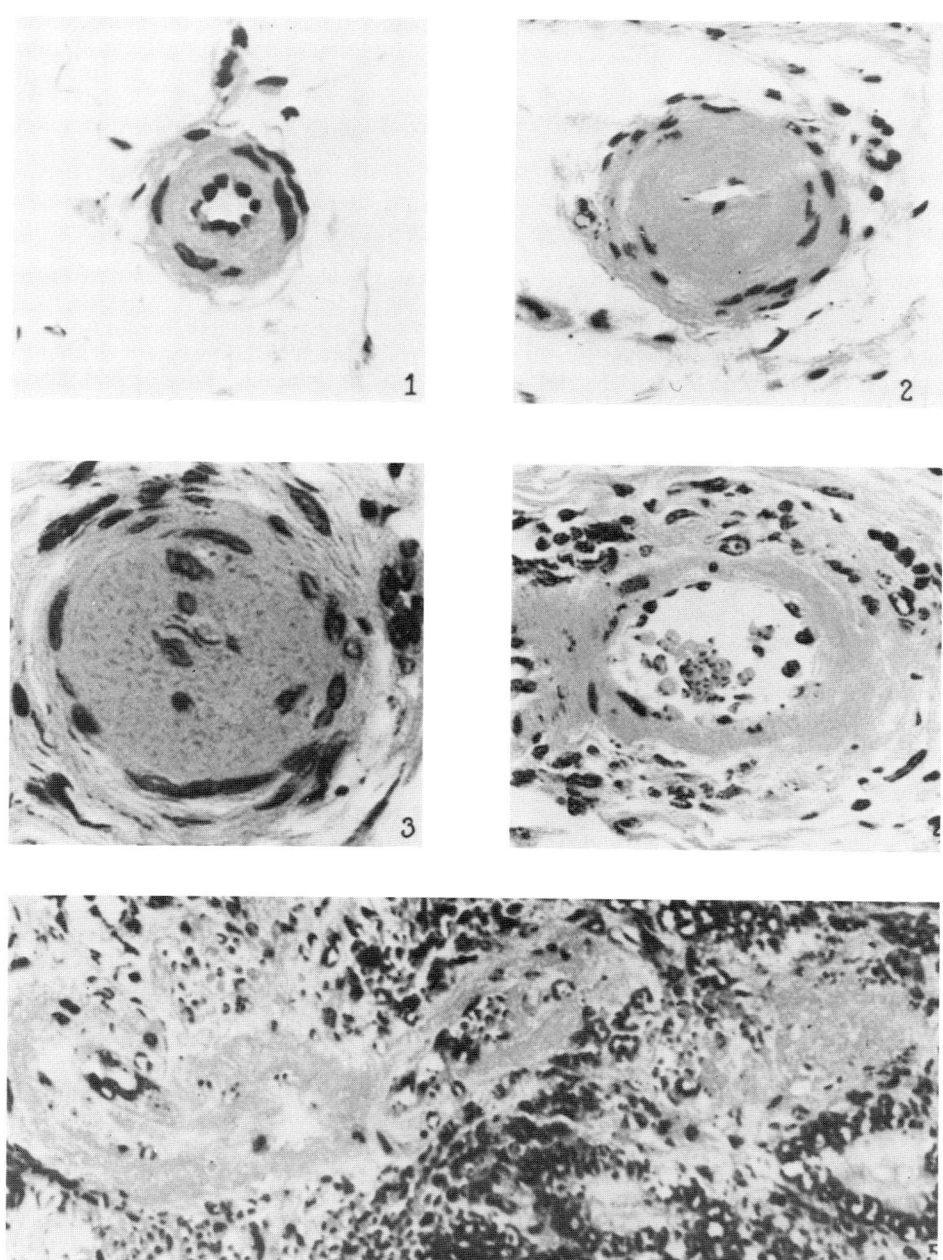

FIG. 6. Illustrations of various arteriolar lesions in the stomach and small intestine in dogs with uremia and severe hypertension (11).

vestigations on experimental hypertension that have been carried out so far but they do show that hypertension, severe disturbance of renal function, and generalized degenerative changes, including severe hyalinization and necrosis, of the arterioles, all indistinguishable from those found in the malignant phase of hypertension in man, can be induced experimentally by severe reduction of the blood supply to the kidneys.

This has been misconstrued as showing that my father believed in the so-called protected kidney in benign (es-

sential!) hypertension resulting from, or accompanied by, unilateral renal artery stenosis. The evidence I have been able to find for the latter is still, 50 years later, not entirely convincing. Obviously, Harry Goldblatt believed that hypertension was a factor in the pathogenesis of particularly the arteriolar lesions in the *malignant* phase of hypertension. The nature of the "toxic principle," which was also postulated by others (3,11,12), has been elusive and still warrants investigation (see below).

A final comment from the early writings indicates

clearly where Harry Goldblatt thought the paradigm was leading (11):

One obvious surgical therapeutic procedure which suggests itself as the result of this work is the possible improvement of blood supply to the functioning components of the kidney by increasing the accessory circulation. In the animals with experimental hypertension induced by renal ischemia, whenever there is a return of the blood pressure to a lower level, it is due to inadequate initial clamping of the renal arteries or to the development of effective accessory circulation by way of ureteral and capsular vessels, which become very prominent. If, before constricting the renal artery, the kidney is decapsulated and adipose tissue or muscle is attached to the denuded cortical surface, the accessory circulation becomes very prominent and interferes with the development of pronounced elevation of blood pressure. Since in the animals the constriction is only of the main renal artery, such accessory circulation can be of functional significance. The fact that animals have survived several years the complete closure of both main renal arteries, when effected gradually by increasing the constriction at intervals, is proof that such accessory circulation can be functionally highly effective. Unfortunately, in human essential hypertension, the vascular disease most frequently involves also the preglomerular arterioles, so that collateral communication with the larger vessels would not improve circulation to glomeruli. Whether improvement of blood supply to some glomeruli, to tubules, and to interstitial tissue would occur and whether it would be effective in lowering blood pressure in human essential hypertension cannot be determined without trying. Although the author has hesitated to recommend it, there is probably more justification on an experimental basis for making this test than there has been for some of the surgical procedures that have already been practiced. The cases in which the production of accessory circulation would be most effective would be those in which the hypertension is due to sclerosis of the main renal arteries alone[9] or their very large branches. The difficulty of making such a diagnosis is obvious, so that unless the method can be applied to essential hypertension associated with renal arteriolar sclerosis the procedure would be of greatly restricted value.

An interesting practical application of this work, which centers upon the renal origin of so-called essential hypertension, has been the finding in children and adults of hypertension associated with unilateral pyelonephritis and vascular disease, and the prompt return of the blood pressure to normal after excision of the diseased kidney. Until 1930, according to Bell and Pedersen, hypertension associated even with bilateral pyelonephritis had not been reported. Since then, several authors have reported this occurrence in some cases and from the meagre studies of the kidneys in these cases it becomes probable that the hypertension associated with unilateral or bilateral pyelonephritis in children and adults occurs only in those cases in which there is associated vascular sclerosis or in which the inflammatory disease produces the same effects on renal circulation as does vascular disease. In cases of unilateral arteriolar nephrosclerosis with hypertension, which have been reported by Moritz and Oldt, if the diagnosis could be made in life, removal of the diseased kidney might result in a return of the blood pressure to normal, as in the cases of unilateral pyelonephritis [see Addendum]. Unfortunately, unless the production of accessory circulation would be effective, *nothing but transplantation of a normal kidney or kidneys, with removal of both diseased kidneys, could be expected to relieve the hypertension and prove the renal origin of the disease in cases of human hypertension associated with bilateral pyelonephritis or arteriolar sclerosis of the kidneys* [emphasis added]. Whether this can ever be accomplished in man, as it can in animals, is for the future to disclose.

Addendum. From the James Buchanan Brady Urological Institute and Department of Medicine of Johns Hopkins Hospital there have been reported two cases of hypertension associated with unilateral renal vascular disease in which the removal of the diseased kidney resulted in a prompt return of the blood pressure to normal. A similar result has been obtained in a third unreported case (Personal Communication, Professor Hugh Young).

HARRY GOLDBLATT'S PERSPECTIVE OF THE PARADIGM

As indicated above, Harry Goldblatt felt that the model was sufficiently similar to human essential hypertension that it would unravel the pathogenesis of that disorder *and* its relationship to the development of widespread vascular disease. As recipient of the Ferdinand C. Valentine Award of the American Urological Society, he said (14):

I am not at all sure that the evidence I have presented in this lecture has convinced you that so-called essential human hypertension is primarily of renal origin. . . .

In any event, I hope you will concede that the category of essential hypertension has dwindled considerably during the past 30 years. Although you may not grant that the experiments have provided unequivocal proof of the renal origin of essential hypertension, I do hope you will agree that the recognition of a clinical entity, renovascular hypertension, admittedly due to renal ischemia, has happened as a result of these experiments. I hope you will also concede that, as in animals, this type of hypertension can be cured by the excision of the ischemic kidney, if the ischemia is due to intrarenal disease and the other kidney is not diseased. If the renal ischemia is due to stenosis or obstruction of the main renal artery of one or both kidneys, the hypertension can be cured by surgical correction of the vascular lesion, provided there is no intrarenal cause of ischemia in either kidney. I hope you will agree that in such cases it would be illogical to expect the blood pressure to fall as a result of the excision of a kidney, or correction of a stenosal lesion of the main renal artery, if, as some believe, the hypertension comes first and causes these lesions. In turn, I am willing to concede that more proof for the renal origin of essential hypertension is highly desirable, and I hope that, in the not too distant future, it will be provided.

Ten years later he wrote an article titled "Reflections" (13), which I have referred to above, but which I think bears repeating as the best example of how he viewed both the origin and the result of his contribution:

---

[9] References deleted; see original publication.

During the 40 years since the publication of my first paper on experimental hypertension [3], I have been asked many times why, in attempting to produce a type of hypertension in animals resembling benign essential hypertension in man, I chose a method which obviously incriminated the kidney as the site of origin of the cause of elevated blood pressure.

As a medical student (1912–1916), I was taught that benign, so-called essential, human hypertension, is best defined as persistently elevated blood pressure, of unknown origin, unaccompanied by significant renal excretory functional disturbance recognizable by clinical and laboratory methods. Although it was known even then that intrarenal arterial and arteriolar sclerosis is a frequent finding at autopsy in human hypertensives, I was taught, and it is still being taught by some, that the elevated blood pressure comes first and that the vascular sclerosis, including that of the kidney, is the result of the persistently elevated blood pressure. It was known then that, in some cases of human hypertension, impairment of renal excretory function eventually does develop and that fatal uremia may occur.

As a resident in surgery, in 1916, I witnessed a tragic event which made me realize, however, that uremia alone is certainly not a sufficient condition for the elevation of the blood pressure. In a middle-aged woman a kidney was removed, presumably for a tumour. It proved to be a congenitally anomalous kidney; there was no tumour and, unfortunately, no other kidney. The patient survived six days and I had the opportunity to follow the fatal course. She died in pronounced uremia, but at no time was there any elevation of blood pressure.

In 1928, after I had been a pathologist for a number of years and had performed autopsies on a large number of hypertensive patients, I began to give serious thought to the problem of the origin of the elevated blood pressure. The striking thing to me was that, no matter what the mode of death (cardiac, cerebral or obviously renal), almost invariably at autopsy some form of disease of the kidney was present—most frequently, by far, obliterative bilateral, intrarenal arterial, and arteriolar sclerosis. In most cases, of course, vascular sclerosis was also present in other parts of the body, so it was hazardous to incriminate the kidneys. I had, however, seen a number of cases of widespread arteriosclerosis with little or no involvement of the kidneys and no history of hypertension, as well as some cases of vascular sclerosis almost exclusively involving the kidneys, with a definite history of persistent hypertension.

Contrary, therefore, to what I had been taught, I began to suspect that the vascular disease comes first and that, when it involves the kidneys, the resultant impairment of the renal circulation probably, in some way, causes elevation of the blood pressure. This condition I assumed to be renal ischemia, an idea which I considered amenable to experimental investigation. I reasoned that if the idea were correct, the production of variable degrees of bilateral renal ischemia, by any means, should result in the development of elevated blood pressure, and, at some degree of ischemia, perhaps, without accompanying impairment of renal excretory function. This would satisfy the definition of benign essential human hypertension.

I did not known then, nor do I know now, how to produce intrarenal, obliterative vascular sclerosis, so I decided to simulate the probable hemodynamic effects of widespread, intrarenal, obliterative vascular sclerosis by producing varying degrees of permanent constriction of the main renal artery of both kidneys in a series of dogs. I must confess that my assumption was that in order to produce elevated blood pressure, both main renal arteries would have to be constricted. Bilateral moderate constriction of both main renal arteries did result in persistent hypertension, without significant disturbance of renal excretory function, in some dogs. All the subsequent experiments by us and many others on animals with this type of persistent hypertension, which have resulted in the elucidation of the humoral (renin-angiotensin) mechanism found to be directly responsible for the elevation of the blood pressure, have been found to apply also to human hypertension associated with renal vascular disease.

One of the earliest, unexpected, experimental findings, however, was that, in the dog at least, constriction of only one renal artery was a sufficient condition for what proved to be a temporary elevation of the blood pressure. This serendipitous finding of hypertension due to unilateral renal ischemia led to the recognition of the existence of unilateral renal disease associated with persistent hypertension in man and in some animals. An important experimental finding was that, in the dog, early release of the single, constricted main renal artery, or the excision of the one ischemic kidney, resulted in the prompt return of the blood pressure to normal, provided the contralateral kidney was normal. This finding led to the recognition of the occurrence, in humans, of hypertension associated with unilateral renal ischemia secondary to critical degrees of partial obstruction or stenosis of any part of the main renal artery.

As in the animal, relief of the ischemia by surgical correction of the stenosis or obstruction, or by excision of the stenotic portion, or by a bypass, or by removal of the ischemic kidney, provided the other kidney is normal, has led to the return of the blood pressure to normal in many humans. As a result, it has been realized that the presence of only a single kidney, provided it is normal, insures a normal blood pressure. This has led directly to the performance of bilateral nephrectomy and transplantation of a single normal kidney, from a living person or a cadaver, for the possible cure of renovascular hypertension and restoration of normal renal excretory function in many humans with severe bilateral renal disease. In such cases, a favourable outcome depends entirely on the survival of the transplanted kidney in a normal state. Unfortunately, frequent rejection of a transplanted kidney is still a stumbling block to progress in this field.

ANOTHER GOLDBLATT PERSPECTIVE

Since the first edition of this compendium, numerous investigators have continued to elucidate the physiological and pathophysiological role of the renin-angiotensin mechanism. Several of the pioneers, like Leonard Skeggs, have left the field, or as in the case of Irvine Page and Erwin Haas, have passed away. Dr. Haas, who died in January 1990, left a large body of data on the enzymology of renin, some of it unpublished, which his family generously donated to the Allen Memorial Library in Cleveland. During the years that he and Harry Goldblatt collaborated, Haas meticulously recorded every detail of their experiments together, and my father never took a note because he had total faith in him. These notebooks may still contain insights that would be fruitful to investigate.

Investigation of the renin-angiotensin system has now clearly entered the era of molecular biology (16). As cited in the review by Menard (16), "the slow pressor effect of the chronic infusion (of angiotensin II) at subpressor doses has shown that a minimal but prolonged stimulation of the renin-angiotensin system may be an etiologic factor in the chronic elevation of blood pressure" (see also Dickinson and Lawrence, ref. 14 cited in ref. 16). This statement underscores the role of the renin-angiotensin system in chronic hypertension and lends further credence to the statements I made in my previous Perspective section, based on the Goldblatt group's studies of acetylated renin (17) and slow infusion of subpressor amounts of renin (18). These studies showed that acetylated renin could induce "anti-renin" and blood pressure lowering in chronically hypertensive dogs (17) and that slow infusion of minute amounts of renin, usually undetectable by the standard dog assay technique, could produce marked elevation of blood pressure (18). It thus appears to me more certain that measurement of "levels" of various components of the renin-angiotensin system may have little or no relevance to their role in chronic hypertension.

The role of extrarenal renin, discussed in this section in the previous edition and elsewhere previously (19,20) remains elusive (see also Lenz and Sealy [21]). What seems to be becoming clearer is the central role of the angiotensin I–converting enzyme (ACE) with its multiple interrelationships to the kinin and other systems (22). The availability of ACE inhibitors too has shown that this enzyme may have a role in cardiac hypertrophy, failure, and the pathogenesis of arterial and arteriolar sclerosis in relationship to hypertension (16,23,24).

There is increasing evidence that the vascular lesions in association with hypertension are not simply the result of the pressure per se. The association of obesity and hyperinsulinemia (or perhaps hyperproinsulinemia, since the early assays did not distinguish proinsulin from insulin) has received increasing attention. The use of various antihypertensive agents with differing pharmacological effects (calcium channel blockers, ACE inhibitors, and others) to lower blood pressure, while yielding somewhat conflicting results, nevertheless has pointed to the presence of factors other than pressure as playing a role in the generation of at least the small vessel disease regularly associated with human hypertension (24,25).

This leads me to a restatement of the conclusions I reached in the previous edition (19). As mentioned there, the Goldblatt experiment has led to the elucidation of the renin-angiotensin system, which certainly plays a role, albeit of undetermined dimensions, in human hyperten-

sion of various types including essential hypertension. It has led directly to the cure of many individuals, most of whom would have been diagnosed as essential hypertensives without the recognition that their raised blood pressure was caused by renal artery stenosis. The model in its various permutations has yielded a reliable and reproducible system with which to explore hypertensive mechanisms. And, again, the usefulness of this model for the exploration of the causes and prevention of vascular diseases in association with hypertension has yet to be fully realized. For these reasons, the paradigm that Harry Goldblatt devised in the early 1930s will continue to be useful well into the twenty-first century.

REFERENCES

1. *Webster's new collegiate dictionary.* Springfield, MA: G & C Merriam Company, 1975;830.
2. Goldblatt H, Lynch J, Hanzal RF, Summerville WW. Experimental hypertension due to renal ischemia. *Bull Acad Med Cleve* 1932;xvi:6. Preliminary report before the experimental section of the Academy of Medicine of Cleveland, November 11, 1932.
3. Goldblatt H, Lynch J, Hanzal RF, Summerville WW. Studies on experimental hypertension. 1. The production of persistent elevation of systolic blood pressure by means of renal ischemia. *J Exp Med* 1934;59:347–379.
4. Goldblatt H. Acceptance Talk, Gold Headed Cane Award. American Association of Pathologists and Bacteriologists. *Am J Pathol* 1966;48:1071–1073.
5. Goldblatt H, Gross J, Hanzal RF. Studies on experimental hypertension. II. The effect of resection of splanchnic nerves on experimental renal hypertension. *J Exp Med* 1937;65:347–379.
6. Goldblatt H. Studies on experimental hypertension. III. The production of persistent hypertension in monkeys (macaque) by renal ischemia. *J Exp Med* 1937;65:671–675.
7. Keyes JEL, Goldblatt H. Experimental hypertension. IV. Clinical and pathologic studies of eyes: preliminary report. *Arch Ophthalmol* 1937;17:1040–1054.
8. Goldblatt H. Studies on experimental hypertension. V. The pathogenesis of experimental hypertension due to renal ischemia. *Ann Intern Med* 1937;11:69–103.
9. Goldblatt H, Wartman WB. Studies on hypertension. VI. The effects of section of the anterior spinal nerve roots on experimental hypertension due to renal ischemia. *J Exp Med* 1937;66:527–534.
10. Goldblatt D. Historical notes: The remarkable case of Dr. X, with notes on George Hoyt Whipple (1878–1976) and Harry Goldblatt (1891–1977). *Semin Neurol* 1985;5:367–373.
11. Goldblatt H. Experimental hypertension induced by renal ischemia. *Harvey Lect* 1938;May 19:237–275.
12. Pickering JW. *High blood pressure.* London: JA Churchill, 1955;122–130.
13. Goldblatt H. Reflections. Reproduced from Joseph J. Kaufman, Guest editor: *The Urologic Clinics of North America.* Symposium on Management of Renovascular Hypertension, vol 2, no 2, 1975;219–221.
14. Goldblatt H. Hypertension due to renal ischemia. The Third Ferdinand C. Valentine Memorial Lecture, delivered before the Section on Urology of the New York Academy of Medicine, March 21, 1964. *Bull NY Acad Med* 1964;40:745–758.
15. Stamey TA. *Renovascular hypertension.* Baltimore: Williams & Wilkins, 1963;15.
16. Menard J. Anthology of the renin-angiotensin system: a one hundred reference approach to angiotensin II antagonists. *J Hypertens* 1993;11(suppl 3):S3–S11.
17. Deodhar SD, Haas E, Goldblatt H. Induced changes in the antigenicity of renin and the production of antirenin to homologous renin and to human renin. *Can Med Assoc J* 1964;90:236–239.
18. Goldblatt H, Haas E, Haas R. Studies on renin II. Continuous in-

fusion of homologous renin at very low rates in intact and nephrectomized dogs. *Circ Res* 1972;31:74–82.

19. Goldblatt PJ. The Goldblatt experiment: a conceptual paradigm. In: Laragh JH, Brenner BM, eds. *Hypertension: pathophysiology, diagnosis and management.* New York: Raven Press, 1990;21–32.

20. Goldblatt PJ. What is the role of extrarenal renin? *Arch Pathol* 1986;110:1128.

21. Lenz T, Sealy JE. Tissue renin systems as a possible factor in hypertension. In: Laragh JH, Brenner BM, eds. *Hypertension: pathophysiology, diagnosis and management.* New York: Raven Press, 1990;1319–1328.

22. Ehlers MRW, Riordan JF. Angiotensin converting enzyme. Biochemistry and molecular biology. In: Laragh JH, Brenner BM, eds. *Hypertension: pathophysiology, diagnosis and management.* New York: Raven Press, 1990;1217–1231.

23. Dzau VJ, Colucci WS, Williams GH, Curfman G, Meggs L, Hollenberg NK. Sustained effectiveness of converting enzyme inhibition in patients with severe congestive heart failure. *N Engl J Med* 1980;302:1373–1379.

24. Powell JS, et al. Inhibitors of angiotensin-converting enzyme prevent myointimal proliferation after vascular injury. *Science* 1989;245:186–188.

25. Anderson S, Rennke HG, Brenner BM. Therapeutic advantages of converting enzyme inhibitors in arresting progressive renal disease associated with systemic hypertension in the rat. *J Clin Invest* 1986;77:1925–1930.

Hypertension: Pathophysiology, Diagnosis, and Management, Second Edition, edited by J.H. Laragh and B.M. Brenner, Raven Press, Ltd., New York © 1995.

CHAPTER 3

The Vascular Fault in Hypertension

Byrom's Work Revisited

John M. Ledingham

Frank Byrom received his medical training at the London Hospital Medical College. After graduation he trained in both pathology and clinical medicine and held appointments in both disciplines—in pathology, under Professor Hubert Turnbull and, in medicine under Professor Arthur Ellis. In 1930 he was granted a Rockefeller Foundation Fellowship to study at the University of Chicago, where he undertook research into water and mineral metabolism in epilepsy (1) under the direction of Professor Russell Wilder. Returning to the London Hospital, he directed his attention to the study of the role of the pituitary antidiuretic hormone in eclampsia and preeclamptic toxemia, but he failed to confirm the pre-

viously reported finding of pressor and antidiuretic activity in ultrafiltrates of plasma in these conditions (2). Despite these negative findings and in the knowledge that the bioassay method in the rat, as used previously, was relatively insensitive, he set out to examine the effects of vasopressin administered to rats, following the report of eclampsia like lesions in the liver and kidneys of guinea pigs injected with this substance. Byrom reported (3) gross lesions in the kidneys, liver, and other organs as well as in the arteries following large injections of vasopressin, and he speculated that the intense vasoconstrictor spasm induced by vasopressin precipitated infarction or ischemic degenerative changes in the tissues, led to increased permeability of the vascular tree beyond the constricted area, and resulted in necrosis of the artery itself. However, he recognized, in light of his

J. M. Ledingham: University of London, London SW7 IJL, England.

earlier work, that the dose of vasopressin administered was grossly in excess of that occurring endogenously in eclampsia. He therefore advanced the hypothesis that, although vascular spasm was likely to be responsible for eclamptic lesions observed clinically, the cause of the spasm was likely to be other than oversecretion of vasopressin. He further speculated that the lesions observed clinically in malignant hypertension and in massive cortical necrosis of the kidney, which closely resembled those following the administration of vasopressin, might also be the direct result of severe vasospasm.

This speculation led Byrom to undertake the study of the nature of the vascular crisis in hypertension, a study that exclusively occupied him for the rest of his working life. At this time and almost simultaneously, Goldblatt (4) and Wilson, working on the Medical Unit of the London Hospital, and Pickering, in the department of Clinical Research at University College Hospital (5), described acute arterial lesions in dogs and rabbits, respectively, made hypertensive by the Goldblatt technique. Byrom joined his younger colleague, Wilson, and together they commenced a study of experimental renal hypertension induced in rats by applying a clip to the renal artery. For the next 3 years they cooperated in seminal studies (6,7), out of which arose the "vicious circle" concept of the pathogenesis of renal hypertension. This concept implied that the hypertension arising through interference with the renal circulation was itself directly responsible for damage to the kidney, resulting in a further exacerbation of the hypertension. The concept has proved to be of the utmost importance to our understanding of the natural history of all forms of hypertension, both clinical and experimental.

Byrom had been supported by a full-time British Medical Research Council grant that was terminated shortly before the outbreak of war. His deep commitment to basic research led him to emigrate to Australia, where for the next 17 years he worked at the Prince Henry and St. Vincent's Hospitals and at the University in Sydney and pursued, single-mindedly, his studies into the vascular consequences of hypertension, being supported by a series of short-term grants; finally, when the grants were used up, he paid for these studies out of his own pocket. During these years he consolidated the concept of the vicious circle in hypertension (8) and advanced evidence for an acute rise in intravascular pressure as being responsible for overdistension and vascular damage in hypertension (9). He developed meticulous techniques for the study of (a) the pathogenesis of acute hypertensive vascular lesions in the cerebral arteries of the rat and (b) the nature of hypertensive encephalopathy (10).

Returning to London in 1957, he was enabled to continue his research at the Bethlem Royal and Maudsley Hospital, being supported by grants from that institution and by the Medical Research Council. The study was extended to observations on the retinal arteries of the hypertensive rat (11) and to the renal vascular damage produced by the administration of angiotensin (12). In his last working years he returned to the laboratories of the Medical Unit of the London Hospital, then under the direction of Professor Clifford Wilson. His lifetime work is described in the monograph he published in 1969 (13); his mature views, written in retirement, are recorded in the Third Volhard Lecture of the International Society of Hypertension in 1976 (14). He died within a year, of acute viral encephalitis.

Byrom was the supreme individualist who steadfastly believed that experimental research was "still a function, not of the team, the Unit, the Department or the Institute, but of the individual, wherever he may work, who wants to find things out—himself" (13). He was a perfectionist, and, rather than accept help from those with less exacting standards, he preferred to pursue his studies uninterruptedly and quietly on his own, although he appreciated the importance of working in a scientific environment. Research was his paramount interest, and he was not to be deflected in any way by extraneous activities. Technical assistance was sporadic, and, at times, he was ably assisted by his wife; even his children were pressed into service on holidays, being rewarded with a sixpenny piece whenever they were required to observe his hypertensive rats and to report at once when hypertensive encephalopathy developed. From time to time he experienced difficulties over personal support and laboratory facilities, and when he was eventually required, at short notice, to leave his laboratory in the medical department of the university, he decided to return to England. Notwithstanding this individualistic attitude in research, Byrom was very ready to communicate with others over mutual research problems, and the writer himself benefited much from long thoughtful handwritten letters discussing such problems. Throughout his scientific life he applied the highest critical standards to his work and only reached a conclusion after the most careful assessment of all the evidence. He was a superb craftsman, and his skill in constructing acrylic windows in the rat skull for the observation of pial vessels is outstanding. In retirement, his technical skill was utilized to the full in the repair of antique clocks, of which he had a remarkable collection.

In some ways, Byrom was the archetypal researcher of an era long departed, when enlightened gentlemen, in the tradition of William Harvey and Stephen Hales, motivated by an intense spirit of inquiry, pursued their solo investigations for the pure intellectual satisfaction of discovery.

THE BASIS FOR THE "VICIOUS CIRCLE" CONCEPT

Goldblatt's discovery in 1934 (15)—that a constriction placed on one or both renal arteries of the dog produced, respectively, transient or permanent hypertension—opened up the study of hypertensive diseases to countless research workers over subsequent years. In 1936, Byrom and Wilson, as clinicians working in Professor Arthur Ellis's department, were deeply involved in attempting to clarify the nature of the unusual form of essential hypertension in which the disease ran a malignant course, ending in death within a few years. This unusual form had been termed *malignant sclerosis* by Fahr (16) to emphasize the severe arterial lesions seen in the kidney and elsewhere. Fahr considered that these lesions were primary, whereas subsequent workers had pointed out that, in the early stages, renal changes were minimal or absent (17,18). The severe changes observed in the late stages of the disease, referred to at this time as *chronic interstitial nephritis,* resembled those seen in the late stages of chronic primary nephritis. Byrom and Wilson recognized that the Goldblatt model of experimental hypertension might provide a means of clarifying the nature of this acute form of hypertension and stated, as their objective (6): "If it could be shown experimentally that this picture of chronic interstitial nephritis may be caused by hypertension alone, the concept of malignant hypertension would be greatly strengthened." In 1938, it had been shown by Wilson and Pickering in rabbits (5) that acute arterial lesions, identical to those seen in clinical malignant hypertension, could be demonstrated in various internal organs but not in the kidneys, strongly suggesting that the lesions elsewhere were due to raised intravascular pressure, whereas the renal vessels were protected by the clamp on the renal artery. At the same time, Goldblatt (4) had made similar observations in dogs but only observed the lesions when the clamp was so tight as to cause a degree of renal excretory failure, which they considered to be an essential factor in the causation of these lesions. In preliminary experiments, Wilson and Byrom had discovered that severe permanent hypertension could be produced in the rat by a constriction placed on one renal artery, leaving the opposite kidney *in situ* and thus exposed to central arterial pressure. They adapted a silver ribbon clip, as previously used in rabbits (19), to rats and developed a plethysmographic technique for the measurement of systolic blood pressure in this animal (20). They performed the experiment in 157 rats, 101 of which developed hypertension (6). The course of the hypertension was variable but was of two broad types. In one, the blood pressure rose gradually and continued for several months at a high level, with the animal continuing in good health. In the other, the course of the blood pressure was irregular with peaks and troughs, accompanied by periodic severe weakness, wasting, coma, and convulsions, often ending in death due to heart failure. The level of blood urea in rats with these symptoms was normal in 22 of the 24 rats examined, indicating that nitrogen retention was not an essential factor in the syndrome. There was a dramatic differ-

ence in the histology of the "clamped" and "opposite" (untouched) kidneys. The clamped kidney either appeared normal macroscopically and microscopically or, more often, showed diffuse tubular atrophy and partial infarction, these changes being found more commonly in the second type of hypertension, although even then the kidney might appear normal. No arterial or glomerular lesions were present. In the opposite kidney, the afferent arterioles showed hyaline or fibrinoid swelling or, more frequently, severe changes with necrosis of the full thickness of the vessel wall, which contained fibrin and red cells, surrounded by an adventitial inflammatory cellular reaction. The lumen was narrowed by intimal swelling and sometimes by cellular intimal proliferation stretching and fragmenting the elastica interna. The glomeruli showed a variety of acute and chronic changes, including focal or total necrosis or hemorrhagic infarction of the tuft with periglomerular fibroblastic proliferation. The tubules were often dilated with hyaline casts or were atrophied and separated by interstitial fibrosis. Similar acute arterial lesions were observed in the pancreas, intestine, stomach, and heart and, more rarely, in the adrenal glands, liver, and testis but not in the brain, eye, or striated muscle, which were, however, only occasionally examined.

In almost every respect the histological changes in the opposite, untouched, kidney could be matched with those occurring in clinical malignant hypertension (Fig. 1).

Wilson and Byrom presented their views on the pathogenesis of the lesions as follows (6):

Since only one kidney is operated on, renal insufficiency is an unlikely factor in the aetiology of the lesions. This conclusion is supported by the absence of nitrogen-retention. The fact that the lesions do not occur in the clamped kidney appears to indicate (1) that they are not due to a circulating toxin, (2) that they are not due to simple ischaemia, and (3) that vasoconstriction due to a circulating pressor substance cannot be solely responsible for them. It is concluded therefore that the production of the lesions is related in some way to the increased intra-arterial tension from which the ischaemic kidney is protected by the clip on the renal artery. We can say with certainty that neither the absolute level of the blood pressure, nor its duration, is an essential factor, since the lesions have been minimal or absent in animals with a blood pressure of over 200 mm Hg persisting for several months. We incline to the belief that the determining factor is probably a sudden strain imposed on the vessel wall by the combination of severe vasoconstriction and the resultant rapid rise in blood pressure. This could presumably produce a vascular necrosis which in the case of a gradually rising pressure might be prevented by the development of compensatory hypertrophy of the arterial wall.

The authors went on to relate their findings to malignant hypertension in humans and stated their belief that the pathogenesis of Fahr's "malignant nephrosclerosis," rather than being the result of inflammation produced

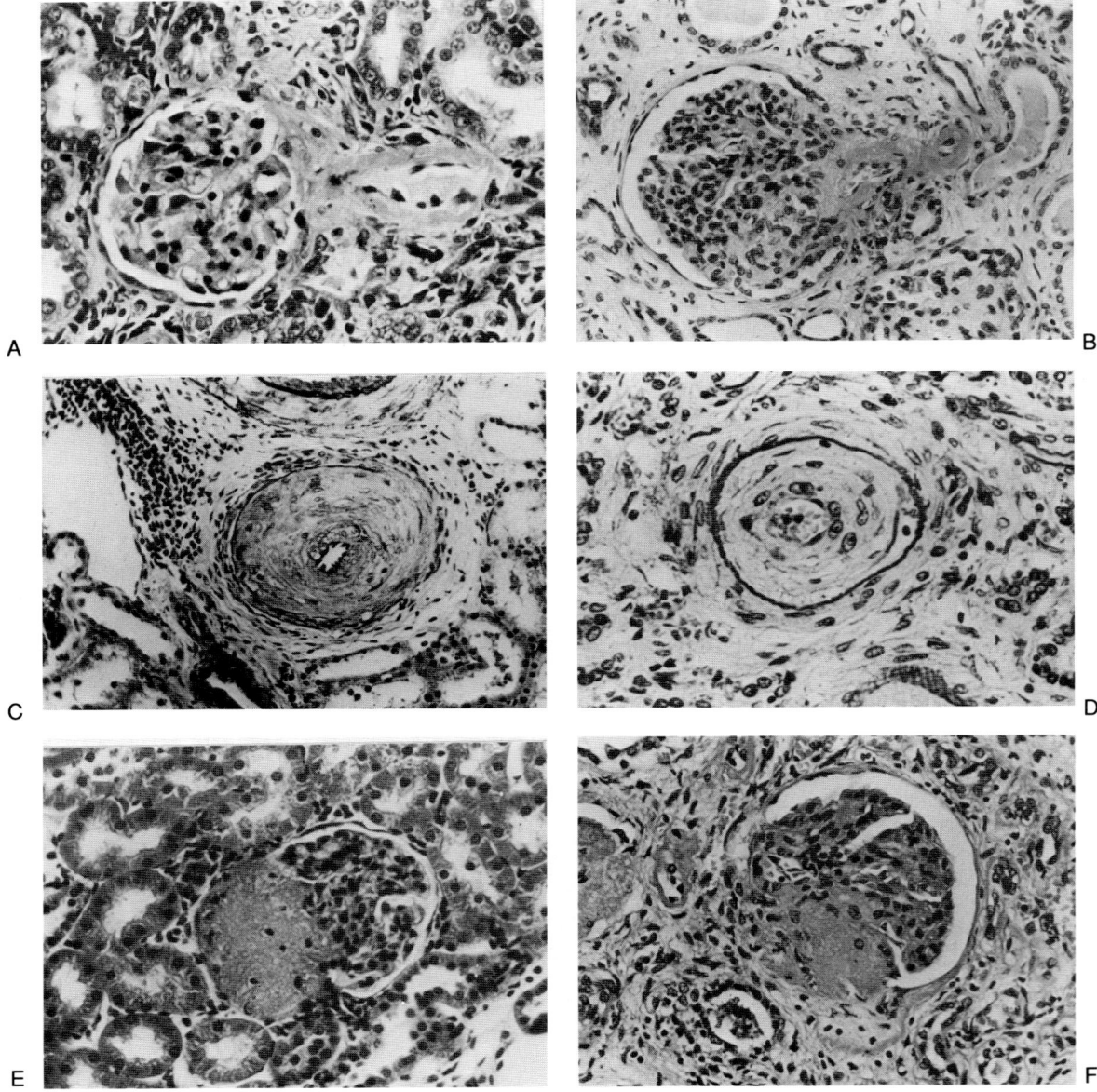

FIG. 1. (A) Untouched (opposite) rat kidney: Acute necrosis of afferent arteriole to glomerulus. **(B)** Human kidney: malignant hypertension showing similar lesion. **(C)** Untouched (opposite) rat kidney: cellular thickening of medium-sized artery ("endarteritis fibrosa"). Elastica interna greatly stretched and fragmented. **(D)** Human kidney: malignant hypertension showing similar lesion in interlobular artery. **(E)** Untouched (opposite) rat kidney: acute focal glomerular necrosis. **(F)** Human kidney: malignant hypertension showing similar lesion in glomerulus. (From ref. 6.)

by a toxic agent ("chronic interstitial nephritis" as it was then called), was the direct consequence of arterial necrosis produced by hypertension. They concluded (6):

> The demonstration that arterial lesions can be produced in the kidney by experimental hypertension also throws light on the clinically malignant course of the human disease; for when vascular lesions occur in malignant hypertension as a result of the high blood pressure, they will presumably give rise to a reduction in renal blood-flow. This may be expected to aggravate the hypertension, and

so a vicious circle will be established in which a rising blood-pressure is associated with progressive renal destruction. Furthermore we have already described . . . the striking and hitherto perplexing similarity, both clinical and histological, that may characterise the terminal stages of chronic nephritis and malignant hypertension. The same manifestations may occasionally be observed in the terminal phase of any form of chronic renal disease with high blood-pressure. It thus appears that not only essential hypertension but also hypertension secondary to renal disease can set in motion the vicious circle which we have envisaged above. This "malignant termination" has therefore no specific character derived from the original disease but is an attribute of the high blood-pressure which is common to all.

The authors concluded their article by enunciating a new interpretation of the clinical condition of hypertensive encephalopathy (6):

> The clinical symptoms in the hypertensive rat also stand in close relation to the human disease. The syndrome we have described of weakness, wasting, coma, and convulsions has been produced by operative interference with one kidney and is not attended by renal insufficiency. In animals moribund from this condition immediate and lasting improvement, with return of the blood-pressure to normal, has been produced by excision of the ischaemic kidney. The syndrome appears to be a close counterpart to hypertensive encephalopathy in man (the pseudouraemia of Volhard).

So important did Wilson and Byrom consider their findings that they proceeded to repeat and expand on their experiment on a much larger scale (7) to obtain further evidence in support of the "vicious circle" concept. In general their findings when one renal artery was clamped (Fig. 2A) confirmed their earlier work, although on this occasion they observed "vascular crises" with severe constitutional disturbances not only at the onset of hypertension but also during the course of chronic persistent hypertension. Evidence was obtained that a relationship existed between the severity of the lesions in the opposite kidney and the degree and duration of hypertension, but with admirable scientific caution they concluded (7):

> The fallacies involved in estimating the extent of the renal lesions . . . are too great to expect any close quantitative relationship, but it is clear on the one hand that extensive lesions in the unclamped kidney are always associated with hypertension of high degree, though not necessarily long sustained; on the other hand it is equally obvious that a marked degree of hypertension may persist for many months without producing significant histological damage in the unclamped kidney. Whether this discrepancy is due to individual differences in the susceptibility of the rat to increased blood-pressure, or due to different rates in the development of the hypertension, is not clear, but the fact emerges that neither the height nor the duration of the hypertension alone determines the production of lesions in the unclamped kidney. . . . Future work must decide what additional factor determines the malignancy of the hypertension; our observations suggest that it may well be sudden development or sudden exacerbation of the high blood-pressure.

Effect of Excision of the Clamped Kidney on the Course of the Hypertension (Fig. 2B)

Shortly before these studies, it had been shown, in dogs (21–23) with hypertension resulting from a clamp either on both renal arteries or on one renal artery with the opposite kidney excised, that release of the clamps or exci-

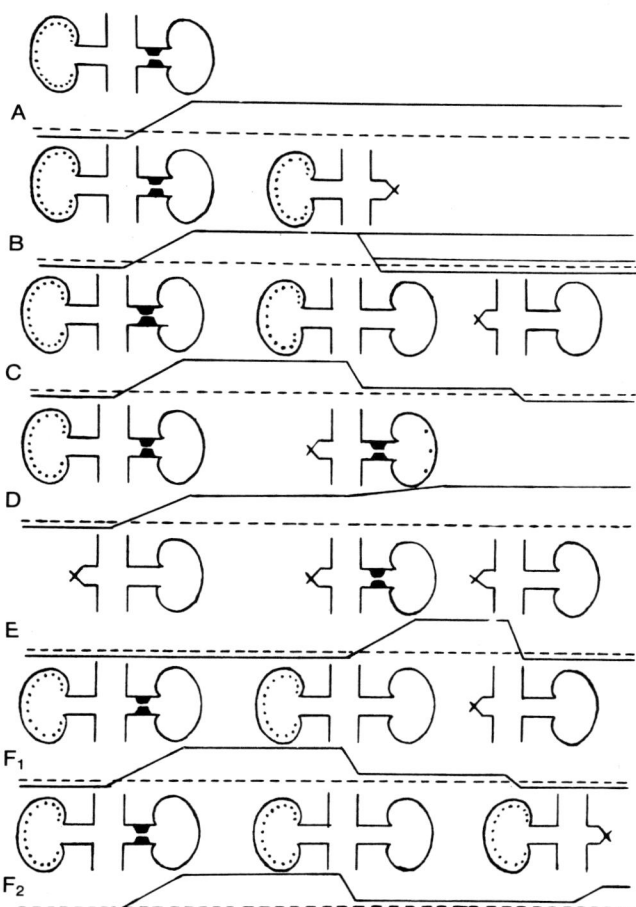

FIG. 2. A–E: Schematic representation of stages in the operative procedures and their consequences in the studies of Wilson and Byrom (6,7). The clip is shown constricting the left renal artery. The *dots* on the right kidney represent the presence of vascular lesions. The systolic blood pressure is shown by the *continuous line,* and the upper limit of normal systolic pressure is shown by the *interrupted line.* **F1** and **F2:** Schematic representation of Floyer's experiment (26). See text for full description.

sion of the single clamped kidney abolished the hypertension. In the experiment of Wilson and Byrom, persistent hypertension was produced by clamping the renal artery to one kidney only; when this kidney was later removed, the influence of the opposite kidney on the future course of the blood pressure could be studied. The clamped kidney was removed in rats with varying degrees of hypertension and at different intervals after constricting the renal artery. The subsequent course of the blood pressure was variable, ranging from persistence of a high level to disappearance of the hypertension. A fairly consistent relationship was found between the degree of residual hypertension and the severity of the lesions in the opposite kidney, particularly in regard to the number of abnormal glomeruli. The authors concluded that the residual hypertension was most likely caused by this damage to the opposite kidney, although they thought it was possible, but unlikely, that arterial lesions in other organs might increase peripheral resistance sufficiently to account for the persistent hypertension. The possibility that the residual hypertension could produce progressive damage to the remaining kidney resulting in eventual renal failure was considered, but experiments had to be terminated by the outbreak of war and the closure of the laboratory. However, several examples of acute fibrinoid necrosis of arteries and arterioles in the kidney and other internal organs were seen in rats that died 2 to 4 months after the clamped kidney was removed.

Effect of Removal of the Clamp from the Renal Artery Followed by Excision of the Untouched (Opposite) Kidney (Fig. 2C)

This procedure was undertaken in four rats. After removal of the clip, the blood pressure fell, but some residual hypertension persisted. In two rats the untouched kidney was then removed with the result that the blood pressure fell further, in one rat to the normal level.

Effect of Removal of the Untouched (Opposite) Kidney After Clamping One Renal Artery (Fig. 2D)

This sequence was performed in 14 rats: in four rats, no hypertension had been present before removing the untouched kidney, and no hypertension developed subsequently; in the other ten rats, earlier hypertension had been present, and the blood pressure rose to a higher level after removing the untouched kidney. At autopsy, the clamped kidney appeared normal in size or slightly atrophied. In half the cases, the kidneys showed slight cortical atrophy, as had been found in previous experiments, but, in the other half, changes similar to those found in the untouched kidney were present, including glomerular adhesions and necroses. These changes were interpreted as resulting from a sudden rise in pressure distal to the clip when the untouched kidney was excised; it was emphasized that such lesions never occurred in the clamped kidney when the opposite kidney was still *in situ*.

As in their earlier article, Wilson and Byrom demonstrated the very striking resemblance of the vascular and parenchymal lesions in the rat kidneys to those occurring in malignant hypertension in humans and also in the terminal stages of chronic Bright's disease and concluded that the acute vascular lesions in these clinical conditions were secondary to hypertension.

The fundamental question of whether malignant hypertension (in humans) is renal in origin or primarily due to some extrarenal factor was considered, and attention was drawn to the presentation of certain patients with papilledema before the occurrence of albuminuria or renal excretory impairment; at autopsy, such patients had been found to show acute fibrinoid necrosis in the kidneys. Wilson and Byrom also pointed out that certain cases of pituitary basophilism developed a malignant type of hypertension (18). They rejected Goldblatt's contention (4) that the acute arterial lesions were due to a combined effect of hypertension and uremia and that clinical malignant hypertension was caused by a primary obstruction to the renal blood flow analogous to the dog experiments. These experiments gave rise to fundamental clarification in the interpretation of the natural history and renal pathology of chronic Bright's disease (7):

> The malignant termination can so dominate both the clinical and histological pictures that it may be impossible in the later stages to recognise the original nature of the disease. We have observed this terminal picture in cases of chronic nephritis, chronic pyelonephritis, hypertensive renal disease following toxaemia of pregnancy, and the chronic hypertension of lead workers.

Classification of Bright's disease was earlier based on the complexities of renal pathology, without recognition of the consequences, if present, of hypertension (7):

> Our work throws no light on the primary cause of essential hypertension or nephritis, but it provides the reason for the unsatisfactory nature of many of the classifications put forward from time to time both by clinicians and pathologists, namely, that the different types of Bright's disease, which in their early stages are quite distinct, tend, as the disease progresses, to lose their separate identities, to pursue a common clinical course, characterized by hypertension and renal failure, and to acquire finally a common histological picture in the kidney. Once the view is accepted that the chronic stages of these diseases are chiefly determined by irreversible hypertension, and that this hypertension may arise either outside the kidney or as a result of primary renal damage, then it becomes evident that an acceptable classification can be derived only from the study of the life history of the disease and of the primary aetiological factors.

Finally, Wilson and Byrom drew attention to cases of hypertension in humans due to unilateral kidney disease that had recently been described and in which removal of the diseased kidney cured the hypertension (24,25) and pointed out that their experiments warned of the possibility that secondary vascular damage in the apparently normal opposite kidney might result, in other circumstances, in persistence or even worsening of the hypertension, a warning that has been amply fulfilled over subsequent years.

Collaboration between Wilson and Byrom came to an end with the outbreak of World War II, and it was left to Byrom to continue his experiments along similar lines some years later in Australia.

These two most important articles, which established (a) the "vicious circle" concept as applied to the hypertensive diseases in humans and (b) the interpretation of the pathological changes in the kidney occurring therein, had a dramatic impact on our understanding of the natural history of hypertension. The work has been confirmed by many other observers who have carried out similar manipulations on the circulation of the kidneys. One such experiment is illustrated in Fig. 2F (26). The results of this experiment clearly confirmed Byrom's predictions, and a remarkable clinical parallel to this experiment has been reported (27). It is now generally accepted that when hypertension results from a known primary cause, removal of this cause may or may not result in the cure of the hypertension. This applies to pheochromocytoma, Cushing's syndrome, aldosteronoma, and unilateral renal disease of many types. Sometimes it has proved possible to predict failure through biopsy of the kidneys (or of the opposite kidney in the case of unilateral renal disease) and through the demonstration of hypertensive vascular damage. However, the clear definition of the precise functional change in the kidney brought about by its exposure to hypertension—and which, in turn, may perpetuate the hypertension—remains uncertain. It is certainly true that the persistence of hypertension after removing the clamped kidney in the experiments of Wilson and Byrom could be broadly correlated with the severity of histological damage to the remaining kidney, but at the present time there is no one combination of tests on the opposite kidney that clearly predicts the outcome. If we accept Guyton et al.'s (28) hypothesis that the level of blood pressure is set by the relationship between renal perfusion pressure and natriuresis, then it becomes a question of defining what precise functional change in the kidney, produced by exposure to hypertension, brings about an alteration in this relationship. There are many candidates for this role, including structural changes in the vessels (29), the reduction of hypotensive medullary lipids (30), the reduction in urinary dopamine (31,32), and many others, all of whose importance in this respect await evaluation. That the severity of the hypertensive structural lesion in the kidney is the determinant of the change in course of the hypertension from the benign to the malignant form has been shown in rats subjected to aortic ligation between the renal arteries (33); both those rats destined to pursue a benign course and those destined to pursue a malignant course developed, within 3 days, acute fibrinoid necrosis in many vascular territories, including the kidneys, but the lesions in the latter were more severe than in the former and were associated with microinfarcts in the right kidney. The vascular and parenchymal damage in the malignant group then progressively developed, whereas in the benign group no further acute lesions occurred and the earlier lesions healed.

BYROM'S SUBSEQUENT WORK ON THE "VICIOUS CIRCLE" CONCEPT

In 1949 Byrom and Dodson provided evidence (8) that established beyond doubt that "human hypertensive disease should be considered potentially reversible except when it derives from, or has itself caused extensive bilateral disorganisation of, the kidneys." In the introduction to this work, the authors stated (8):

> Wilson and Byrom demonstrated a correlation between the extent of the damage in the intact kidney and the occurrence of residual hypertension, but recognised that this did not constitute proof that the two were cause and effect, and they admitted that an unknown factor, independent of the kidney, might have intruded to perpetuate the hypertension. [Thus] it has been widely believed in the past that the generalised increase in arteriolar tone which is the essential abnormality in hypertension leads in time to an irreversible structural narrowing of the arterioles.

A delightfully simple experiment was devised to test the validity of this possibility. The right kidney was excised, and 2 weeks later a clip was applied to the left renal artery (Fig. 2E). After $4\frac{1}{2}$ to 32 weeks, during which time animals developed mild to severe hypertension, successful clip removal was performed and the blood pressure was recorded for a further period ranging from 5 to 19 weeks. In all but one rat, shown at necropsy to have developed perinephritis from cotton wool left *in situ* at operation, clip removal promptly and permanently abolished the hypertension within 24 h. The authors concluded (8):

> Since the present results show that no extra-renal mechanism intrudes in chronic renal hypertension in the rat, it follows that the residual hypertension observed by Wilson and Byrom must have derived from the damaged remaining kidney. Since as we have shown elsewhere [9], the evidence strongly indicates that hypertension is responsible for this damage, the conception of the vicious circle acquires further experimental support.

They summarized their views on the clinical implications of their findings (8):

> From a considerable body of evidence, both clinical and experimental, it is now possible to extract a tentative generalisation, namely that hypertension is an irreversible condition only insofar as it may derive from, or has itself caused extensive irreparable damage involving, both kidneys.

It should be emphasized that, although Byrom's experiment demonstrates the preeminence of the kidney in determining the level of blood pressure, it in no way excludes extrarenal mechanisms, including nonrenal humoral and neurogenic, from contributing to the process but indicates that these other processes must be switched on by damage to the kidney and switched off by restoring a normal kidney to the circulation.

THE PATHOGENESIS OF THE ACUTE VASCULAR LESION AND OF HYPERTENSIVE ENCEPHALOPATHY

Three controversies need to be resolved:

1. Is the acute vascular lesion primarily due to raised intravascular pressure?
2. Is the lesion due to spasm or overdistension?
3. Is hypertensive encephalopathy due to decreased or increased cerebral blood flow?

The Saline Injection Experiment

After proposing the "vicious circle" concept, Byrom directed his attention to the pathogenesis of the acute vascular lesion of malignant hypertension, fibrinoid necrosis of the arterioles. At the time he was aware of three possibilities that were currently held. Byrom and Dodson wrote (9):

> According to one view, necrotising arteritis in the hypertensive animal is due essentially, if not wholly, to increased intravascular tension and the necrotising arteritis and associated parenchymatous renal damage of malignant hypertension are, by inference, likewise the effects of the hypertension. This view is therefore in complete accord with the modern concept of malignant hypertension. On the other hand, other writers believe that hypertension can cause vascular necrosis only in the presence of a second (renal) factor, variously designated as uraemia and toxic absorption from dead or dying kidney tissue.

A remarkably simple, but most revealing, experiment was undertaken in which 2 mL of saline was forcibly and repeatedly injected into the carotid artery of the anesthetized rat (9). The rise in pressure was crudely measured in the lower abdominal aorta by a mercury manometer. In some experiments a loop of thread around the left renal artery was pulled to occlude the vessel and protect the kidney during each injection. The kidneys were exposed and observed throughout (9):

> During each injection the cortex blanched momentarily as the wave of saline swept through. At first the normal colour was immediately regained, but after several injections residual pallor was sometimes observed, usually limited to small irregular areas which slowly changed in shape and size.

The animals recovered rapidly and were then killed 3 days later, and the kidneys were examined histologically (9):

> Typical acute necrotising arteritis [was found] in 10 of 23 rats. The lesions were focal and usually limited to one or two vessels in a complete section. The vessels involved were the arcuate and interlobular arteries and the afferent glomerular arterioles, and the essential lesion was necrosis of the muscle, often involving only a segment of the circumference.

Byrom and Dodson concluded (9):

> It is evident from the present experiment that while occasional renal arteries subjected to mechanical strain undergo necrosis, many more react by a spasmodic contraction intense enough to blanch the adjacent cortex. The lack of necrosis of the renal parenchyma, which is very sensitive to sustained ischaemia, indicates that these contractions are very transient and are probably not, at least in the present circumstances, an essential link in the chain leading to arterial necrosis. The occurrence of spasm is, however, interesting in view of the widespread suspicion that some of the acute symptoms in malignant hypertension, and especially those associated with encephalopathy, may be caused by transient vasospasm.

This experiment clearly demonstrated that an acute rise in intravascular pressure was by itself capable of causing acute necrotizing arteritis and that neither uremia nor preexisting renal damage were necessary associated factors. However, Byrom was aware that, under other circumstances, factors such as these could play a part in the pathogenesis of the lesion, and he initiated some preliminary experiments that will be referred to in the next section. The precise manner in which a rise in intravascular pressure caused the acute lesion, whether in consequence of severe spasm or of excessive stress dilatation, became Byrom's major research interest.

The experiment of forcible injection of saline into the arterial system of rats has been repeated (34,35), with results similar to those of Byrom; experiments have also been performed using the vasodilator aminophylline (35). In the latter study, the acute arterial lesions in the kidneys occurred at a far lower level of imposed pressure than in animals not so pretreated, and the author concluded that these findings supported the concept that vascular lesions occur preferentially in already dilated vessels.

Direct Observation of the Cerebral Vessels

From clinical observations in renal hypertensive rats, Byrom had been greatly impressed by the dramatic occurrence of hypertensive encephalopathy and decided to undertake experiments designed to establish the mechanism of this complication. He had already established that it occurred in rats that were not necessarily in renal failure; indeed, Volhard and Fahr (36) had earlier referred to it as *pseudouremia* to emphasize this point. In the nineteenth century a controversy had arisen as to whether this form of encephalopathy was due to cerebral ischemia from arterial spasm or from overperfusion through dilated arteries. Byrom considered that only by direct observation of the cerebral arteries could this controversy be resolved, and he developed a technique for casting and fitting an individually molded acrylic cranial window into the dorsal surface of the rat's skull in order to overcome the herniation of the brain through a simple craniotomy (10). The technique is described in detail in his monograph (13). Through these windows, under light ether anesthesia, he was able to observe the pial vessels in normal and hypertensive rats, both in the benign phase and in various stages of encephalopathy. The intracranial pressure was also measured through a needle in the cisterna magna; the blood flow in the common carotid was measured by means of a small Ludwig stromuhr, the external carotid being occluded intermittently so that the internal flow could be measured. Rats were made hypertensive by constricting the left renal artery and excising the right kidney. When encephalopathy developed, certain changes were regularly observed (10):

Pallor of the surface of the brain was often obvious on inspection and was almost always demonstrable in serial colour photographs. In the smaller cerebral arteries the typical changes consisted of conspicuous uniform narrowing, which was often intense enough to render the affected branch almost invisible throughout its entire length. This change, though widespread, was usually patchy and some vessels escaped. Not infrequently, sharply localised beads of quite marked dilatation were visible along the course of the constricted vessel or at the origin of a branch. In the larger cerebral arteries similar, though usually less extreme, diffuse contraction was quite common; but as a rule the contraction was more localised, irregular zones of narrowing alternating with regions in which the calibre appeared either normal or somewhat dilated. Uniform dilatation of either large or small arteries was never seen. Spasm showed no tendency to change in position, and, when intense, was only rarely observed to relax—and then usually rather abruptly—on prolonged observation. On the other hand, the calibre of the unaffected regions of the larger arteries sometimes fluctuated appreciably in degree, in company with the blood-pressure, if the level of anaesthesia changed. In a few instances where a larger artery was affected in successive cerebral attacks, focal spasm

tended to reappear at the same points along the affected vessel—a finding possibly related to the uneven distribution of muscle-fibres in the cerebral arteries [Fig. 3A].

When encephalopathy and hypertension were abolished by clip removal, photography 3 days later revealed perfectly normal vessels (Fig. 3B). Similar focal spasm during encephalopathy was observed in the arteries on the surface of the intestine (Fig. 4). In another series of experiments, rats were killed during an attack of encephalopathy, and serial sections of the brain were cut. These revealed a number of organic lesions, including (a) focal arterial necrosis of terminal or medium-sized arteries, (b) recent healing or healed infarcts, and (c) major and minor hemorrhages in a number of rats, but there was no correlation between the severity of the preceding encephalopathy and the presence of organic lesions. Byrom concluded that although acute organic lesions occurred commonly (55% of cases) in encephalopathy, they did not occur in almost half and could not, therefore, be held to explain the symptoms of encephalopathy. Furthermore, the symptoms regularly disappeared within a few hours of clip removal, long before the organic lesion could have healed. In further experiments, a solution of trypan blue, a dye which normally does not cross the blood-brain barrier, was injected intravenously during the course of the encephalopathy. Thirty minutes later the rats were killed, and the cerebral vessels were flushed out with saline to reveal "conspicuous rounded or rosette-shaped blue spots varying from 0.5 to 3.0 mm in diameter on the surface of the brain," indicative of patchy increases in capillary permeability. This finding was supported by the demonstration that the water content of the cerebrum, but not the cerebellum, was significantly increased. Byrom interpreted his observations as follows (10):

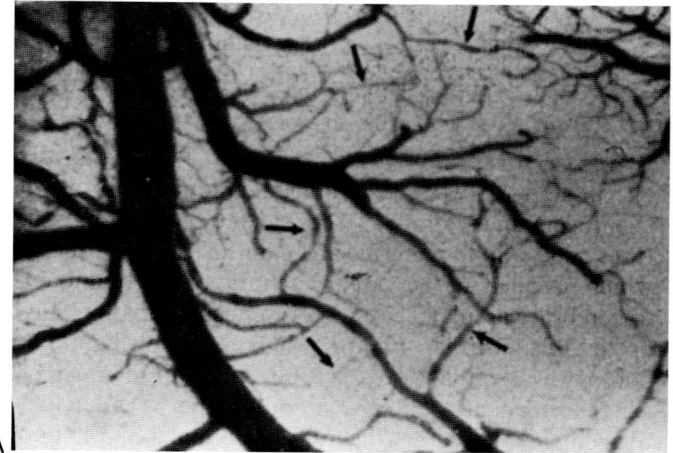
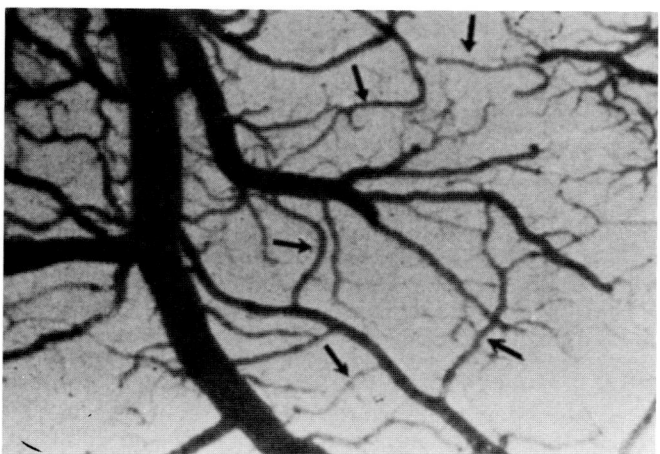

FIG. 3. (A) Pial vessels seen through window in rat's skull in late encephalopathy (blood pressure: 160 mm Hg), with left-sided myoclonic convulsions, showing the following: intense uniform constriction of terminal arteries; slight focal contraction of main artery; and diffuse and focal contraction of medium-sized arteries. **(B)** Same field seen 10 days later after removing renal artery clip. (From ref. 10.)

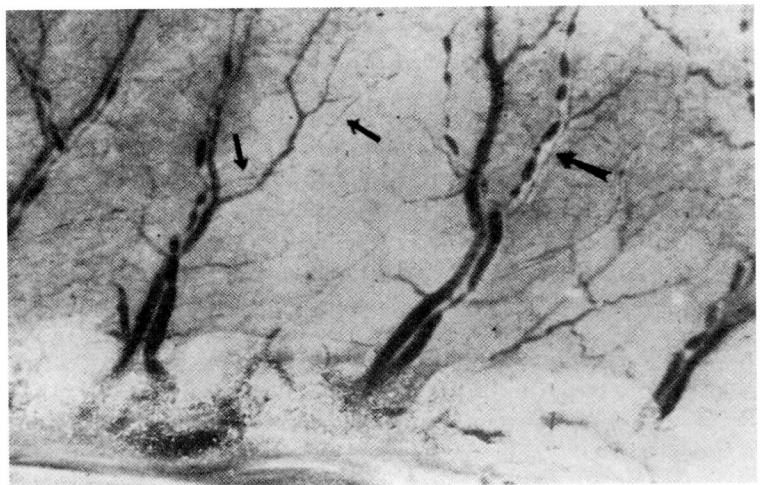

FIG. 4. Vessels on the outer surface of a loop of intestine in a rat with encephalopathy, as seen at laparotomy, showing the following: uniform obliterative spasm of smallest arteries; focal spasm alternating with dilatation of medium-sized arteries; and dilatation predominating in the larger arteries. The veins appear normal. (From ref. 10.)

The evidence . . . indicates that . . . encephalopathy and the focal arterial necrosis which is the essential lesion of malignant hypertension are different expressions of a common local circulatory disturbance which can be . . . related to a simple physiological property of arterial and other plain muscle. The fact that the clamp on the renal artery protects the kidney against arterial necrosis provides strong, if not conclusive, evidence that the local functional disturbance which leads to necrosis is a direct response of the artery to the physical strain of an extremely high blood-pressure. This strain apparently provokes in the affected arteries complex changes in calibre, consisting in intense (often obliterative) spasm of terminal arteries and more focal contraction (sometimes alternating with focal dilatation) of the larger arteries. If the evidence of spasm is accepted there is little room for doubt that the physiological basis for this extreme response to a rise in blood-pressure lies in Bayliss's (1902) long-neglected demonstration that the tension within an artery is a normal and direct stimulus to contraction. And if the intra-arterial tension is both a normal stimulus to contraction and the direct cause of the spasm of encephalopathy and arterial necrosis it is difficult to avoid the inference that it must contribute directly and progressively to the vasoconstriction of the intervening hypertensive state. The nature of this contribution is as yet obscure. It may well be entirely secondary, the rising blood-pressure simply augmenting a vasoconstriction which is initiated by some entirely distinct mechanism. But, it seems at least possible that the initial vasoconstriction may represent the response of abnormally irritable arteries to the physical stimulus of normal blood-pressure. This last is mere speculation: The important point is that in severe hypertension the contribution of the intra-vascular tension, whatever its nature, becomes great enough in degree to play a decisive part in converting orderly diffuse vasoconstriction into uncontrolled focal spasm. The effects of this spasm depend on its intensity, duration and extent. They may be attributed to anoxia, anaemia, or asphyxia (1) of the capillary endothelium, causing increased permeability and focal oedema; (2) of the organ or tissue concerned, causing local or general disturbance of function and, if severe, local infarction; and (3) of the arterial wall causing, if sufficiently intense, focal arterial necrosis, with or without rupture of the wall or occlusion of the lumen.

Although at this time Byrom considered that it was most likely that the intense focal constriction was the mediator of focal necrosis, he did admit that "an alternative explanation of arterial necrosis is that blood trapped between two zones of constriction may be squeezed into the vessel wall." Such caution was wise in light of subsequent research (*vide infra*). In discussing the nature of hypertensive encephalopathy, Byrom says (10):

This form of encephalopathy occurs in severe hypertension of recent origin, such as eclampsia, or during exacerbations of chronic hypertension. It is characterised by generalised or local convulsions, visual disturbances, coma, and sometimes symptoms of raised intracranial tension. It has long been suspected that the condition is in some way related to cerebral oedema; but clinical or gross pathological evidence of cerebral oedema may be absent, even in fatal cases. Opinion on the cause of this oedema is divided. The earlier view, attributed to Traube (1871), was that the thin-walled cerebral arteries dilated under the increased tension and so increased the effective filtration pressure in the capillary bed. Other writers have supported the diametrically opposed view of Volhard (1914), who regarded the oedema as a local result of increased capillary permeability caused by arterial spasm. The present study lends no support to the former hypothesis but, on the contrary, provides direct and detailed confirmation of Volhard's opinion.

Byrom, at this time, was clearly of the opinion that the encephalopathy was due to an acute reduction in blood flow focally in the brain and considered that his observations on flow in the internal and external carotid arteries, which revealed an increase in the ratio of cerebral to extracerebral vascular resistance in encephalopathy, supported this view. He admitted, however, that the methodology was crude and that this speculation must be treated with caution. The later controversy as to whether the cerebral circulatory disturbance in malignant hypertension is one of vasoconstriction (as postulated by Byrom) or of overperfusion will be referred to later. In regard to the general problem of malignant hypertension, Byrom concluded (10):

Turning from cerebral symptoms to the wider problem, the present findings suggest that the dividing line between the benign and malignant phases of hypertension may be defined tentatively as the level of pressure at which the Bayliss reflex gets out of hand and translates diffuse physiological vasoconstriction into uncontrolled focal spasm.

Six years after Byrom's monumental study of the cerebral vessels, his findings were confirmed in the hypertensive cat (37) and monkey (38).

The Retinal Arteries in Hypertension

Byrom expressed concern that the "cerebral arterial spasm observed in oedematous brains through cranial windows could be an artefact" (11), and he commenced a further study in the hypertensive rat of the behavior of the retinal arteries, a study not involving operative interference. He observed that as systolic pressure rose above 170 mm Hg the retinal arteries commenced to show alternating zones of constriction and dilatation, giving rise to a beaded appearance as previously seen in the pial vessels (Fig. 5A). Sometimes there was generalized narrowing and tortuosity. The changes might occur early or late in the course of hypertension. The zones of constriction and dilatation remained fixed in an artery but could be abolished by deepening the level of anesthesia (Fig. 5B), only to reappear in the same sites when anesthesia lightened (Fig. 5C). As hypertension continued, the constricted zones became less responsive to anesthetic changes but were completely abolished by clip removal

and cure of the hypertension, nearly always within a few hours, whereas the zones of dilatation rarely reverted to normal. Focal or diffuse narrowing of the arteries was observed in 74% of rats examined when in acute encephalopathy and in 60% of those not in encephalopathy. In his study of the pial arteries, Byrom had thought that the spasm was an "all or nothing change appearing abruptly at the onset of acute cerebral symptoms." In light of the study of the retinal arteries, he abandoned this concept (11)

in favour of a more or less progressive labile vasoconstriction—irregular perhaps merely because of unevenly distributed muscle fibres, reaching a critical level, at which even a small increment is enough to precipitate a local or general vascular crisis which may resolve, recur or persist. If the overstressed artery does behave in this way . . . the focal oedema and minute infarcts of malignancy may be attributed to simple ischaemia, and the arteriolar necrosis, aneurysms and haemorrhage to simple disruption of muscle fibres under the dual strain and/or extrusion of blood or plasma into the vessel wall.

Writing shortly after this work was published, Byrom remained uncertain in his mind as to whether the focal cerebral edema and structural lesions of malignancy were due to "excessive vasoconstriction (spasm), over dilatation or a combination of the two that is injurious. . . . In renal hypertension, although focal constriction may be very severe, no local reduction in blood flow has yet been demonstrated, and the possibility that the less conspicuous dilatation may cause the damage cannot be excluded" (39). Further light was shortly to be

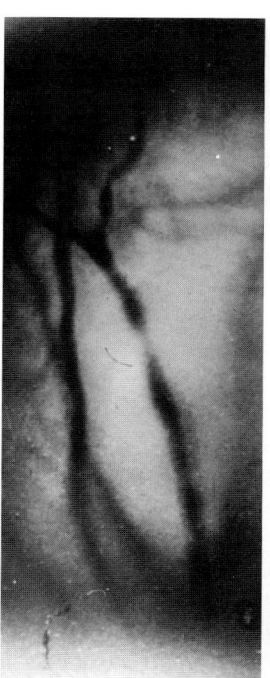 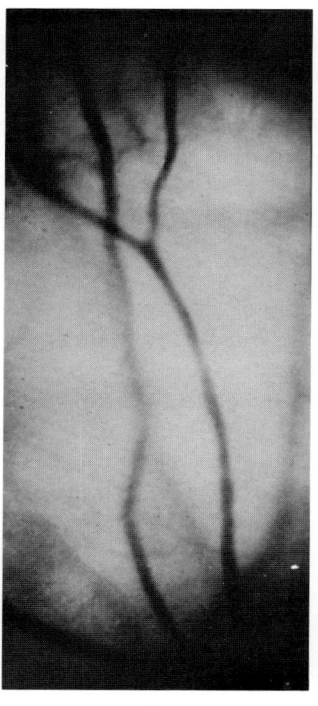 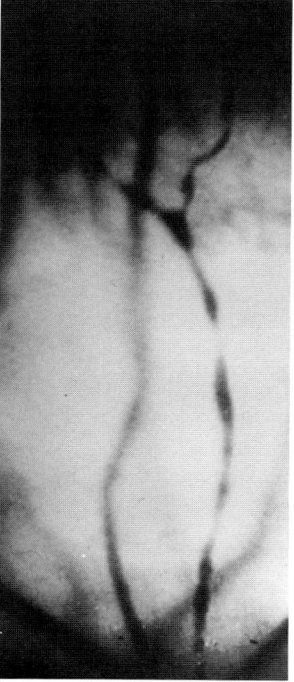

A   B   C

FIG. 5. Retinal vessels in the rat, showing labile nature of the focal arterial narrowing in hypertensive encephalopathy. **(A)** Light ether anesthesia: artery and branches showing alternating constriction and dilatation; veins normal. **(B)** Five minutes later under deep ether anesthesia: the artery is almost normal in caliber. **(C)** Ten minutes later under light anesthesia: constrictions and dilatations have reappeared. (From ref. 11.)

shone on this problem by the work of Giese (40) on vascular reactions as seen in the mesenteric arteries of the rat, occurring during acute hypertension resulting from an infusion of angiotensin. Using an injection of colloidal carbon to detect an increase in vascular permeability, it was clearly demonstrated that when alternating focal spasm and dilatation were visible *in vivo*, carbon particles were found to be present at necropsy only in the walls of the dilated segments. The experiment was repeated with similar findings (41), and it was further demonstrated that the extent of carbon deposition in the vessel wall correlated with the height of the mean blood pressure induced by angiotensin. By electron microscopy it was shown that focal breaks in endothelium, as well as amorphous deposits containing electron-dense material resembling fibrin, were confined to the dilated segments of the arterioles (42). Similar observations have subsequently been made in the mesenteric (43), intestinal submucosal (44), and myocardial (45) arteries of the rat. Although the mode of producing acute hypertension used in these studies differed from that used by Byrom, it is most unlikely that the mechanism responsible for the damage is different, although this possibility has not been disproved. Byrom, writing several years later in his Volhard lecture (16), accepted that the vascular damage in his experiments was due to overdistension and not to intense vascular spasm. He writes (14):

> The vital clue is the irregularity of arterial calibre which heralds an attack of encephalopathy. The change clearly stems directly from the rising pressure which is threatening the reserves of compensatory hypertrophy of the resistance arteries and if it is assumed that these reserves are limited and that muscle fibres are not quite evenly distributed along the course of the vessels a simple explanation of the calibre changes can be observed from first principles. The problems of a small artery derive from the fact that, as a muscular tube containing a high pressure, it becomes progressively weaker when it dilates and stronger when it constricts, because the tension imposed on its fibres by the filling tension of a normal blood pressure varies not only with that pressure, but also with the first power of the diameter of the vessel, according to the law of Laplace. But although the artery has the remarkable ability to contract or relax against a rising or falling blood pressure it is not free to protect itself fully because the flow of blood which it is controlling varies with the fourth power of the calibre, and only small changes in calibre are acceptable. . . . I must emphasize that the choice between over stretching and excessive constriction has not been lightly made. The spectacle of narrow zones in hypertensive cerebral arteries contracting to the full against maximal rises of pressure and maintaining this constriction indefinitely is unforgettable.

Some indirect support for Byrom's concept of vascular spasm as the primary functional disturbance leading to damage of the vessel wall has subsequently been advanced (46,47). On applying L-norepinephrine to the surface of exposed arteries in the rat's leg, it was shown that within a few days the smooth muscle cells herniated widely into each other and occasional necroses occurred in the contracted segments. It was suggested that dilatation in a vessel exposed to raised intravascular pressure might be occurring in segments previously damaged by severe spasm. However, in Byrom's experiments, focal spasm recurred repeatedly at the same sites in the cerebral vessels, and there was no evidence that these sites progressively transformed into dilated segments. On balance, it must be concluded that primary overdistension due to excessive intravascular pressure is the most likely cause of the acute vascular lesion.

The Pathogenesis of Hypertensive Encephalopathy

The role of a change in cerebral blood flow in the pathogenesis of hypertensive encephalopathy was a further recurring problem to Byrom. Accompanying the encephalopathy, he had observed multiple minute areas of focal cerebral edema that he later found to be very closely associated with acute vascular lesions and therefore likely to be arising from increased permeability of the damaged arterial wall. Although cerebral edema arising in this manner was considered to be largely responsible for encephalopathy, Byrom felt that this was not the only mechanism (13):

> The symptoms may stem entirely from this source, but some symptoms appear with dramatic suddenness and disappear with remarkable rapidity with appropriate treatment, while in the brain vasodilatation is overshadowed by widespread constriction and pallor, and localised obliterative constriction has been observed . . . and shown to be labile in innumerable cerebral and other arteries. In view of the profound effect on the circulation of even slight changes in calibre it therefore seems unwise to overlook the possible contribution of the observed overconstriction to the morbid syndrome.

This interpretation was strongly challenged by the work of Strandgaard et al. (48), who showed that the autoregulatory range of cerebral blood flow was shifted upward in hypertensive men as compared with normotensive controls. When the blood pressure was raised with angiotensin there was a "breakthrough" in flow when the upper limit of autoregulation was exceeded with immediate overperfusion, and there was no evidence of vasospasm even transiently reducing flow. The study was confirmed in the baboon (49) using a more reliable technique for blood flow measurement. Byrom remained unconvinced that acute encephalopathy occurring in the course of renal hypertension in humans or rats was due to the breakthrough of autoregulation, and he stressed the different situation of sudden angiotensin-induced hypertension and the very much more gradual rise in pressure occurring in malignant hypertension in his experiments on the rat. In the Volhard lecture he wrote: "But I am not convinced that breakthrough of cerebral autoregulation occurs in spontaneous encephalopathy. . . . It seems that more work is needed before the breakthrough hypothesis of encephalopathy is accepted" (14).

Some support for Byrom's hypothesis comes from the report that when acute hypertension is produced in the rabbit by the infusion of angiotensin, regional cerebral flow, assessed by the [^{14}C]-antipyrine method, was reduced in the watershed areas of the brain at the peak of the induced hypertension and for the following hour, although mean cerebral blood flow was increased for most of this period (50). It is in these areas that permeability increases and leads to focal edema. However, more recent work on hypertensive encephalopathy occurring in stroke-prone spontaneously hypertensive rats revealed that in the early stages of disruption of the blood-brain barrier, the regional flow, measured by the same method, was increased, not decreased, and it was only in the later stages when focal cerebral edema had developed that regional blood flow decreased (51).

This work was undertaken in another form of experimental hypertension from that studied by Byrom and was not designed precisely to explore the possibility that, in the earliest stages of encephalopathy, focal areas of reduced cerebral blood flow were present. Thus, the evidence for and against Byrom's hypothesis must remain evenly balanced until noninvasive techniques become available for monitoring regional cerebral blood flow at the commencement of hypertensive encephalopathy.

THE ROLE OF VASOACTIVE AGENTS, IN ADDITION TO RAISED INTRAVASCULAR PRESSURE, IN THE PATHOGENESIS OF THE ACUTE VASCULAR LESION

Byrom had established in 1948 (9) that mechanical stress alone, in one experimental situation, was a sufficient explanation for acute arterial necrosis. However, he also considered the possibility that, in other situations, both clinically and experimentally, other factors might be involved—in particular, the presence of uremia, a hypothesis advanced by Goldblatt (52).

By 1964 it was generally known that acute fibrinoid necrosis was a feature of hypertension arising in a wide variety of clinical and experimental situations. These included total nephrectomy, renal infarction, renal artery stenosis, primary malignant hypertension, chronic renal failure, pheochromocytoma, Cushing's syndrome, and the experimental administration of a number of agents, including renal extracts (53) and deoxycorticosterone (54). Uncertainty remained as to whether the rapidity of development and the severity of the hypertension in all these situations could, by themselves, account for the acute vascular lesions or whether other factors were implicated. Byrom had demonstrated in 1937 (3) that large doses of vasopressin repeatedly injected subcutaneously into rats caused (a) an acute rise in systolic pressure of 50

mm Hg or more and (b) transient focal areas of pallor on the surface of the kidneys. At sacrifice 24 h later, wedge-shaped anemic infarcts were present in the kidneys, with medial necrosis involving all the renal arteries from the hila to the afferent glomerular arterioles. He compared his findings with identical lesions sometimes observed at the site of injection of epinephrine and ergotamine, and he postulated that spasm was, in some way, responsible. The suggestion was made that "the increased endothelial permeability which follows the spasm induced by vasopressin may allow plasma or blood to escape into the vessel wall" (3).

The Vascular Consequences of Angiotensin Injection

In 1958 Byrom again took up the problem of vasoactive agents as mediators of vessel wall damage and undertook a preliminary study of the effects of synthetic angiotensin II, administered intravenously in various ways, on the renal vessels of the rat. In his later definitive study (12), large doses of angiotensin (up to 10 μg or more) were required to produce visible damage, and in these doses, maximal rises of blood pressure, of 80 mm Hg or more, occurred within 10 to 30 sec:

> During this period the exposed kidney blanched considerably and its main artery, after momentary contraction, became dilated as far as, or slightly beyond, the origin of its primary branches, where dilatation gave way abruptly to marked contraction. These changes disappeared as the blood pressure returned to normal. They recurred, but to a lesser extent after further doses.

At autopsy, 24 h later, medial necrosis, involving part or the whole of the circumference, was found in the larger arteries in the hilum of the kidney and, occasionally, in smaller branches. The glomeruli showed aneurysms and focal necroses. Byrom concluded that "the necrosis appears to be an immediate result, direct or indirect, of the double physical stress imposed on the arteries by overstimulation and excessive filling tension" (12). At the same time as this study, a vascular permeability factor of renal origin was described (55) which, on injection into rats, caused serous effusions and hemoconcentration. This factor was later shown to reside in the cortex and either to be renin or some substance with similar properties (56). The factor was then further purified, and at all stages in its purification the pressor and vascular permeability activities ran parallel and could not be dissociated (57); it was concluded that the factor was indeed renin. Commenting later on this work, Byrom remarked "it must therefore be concluded that the effusions, haemoconcentration and arterial necrosis provoked by renal extracts are caused not by a specific permeability factor but by the rise in blood pressure, or by the unknown changes which cause this rise" (13).

Byrom maintained this view in his Volhard lecture

and did not consider the possibility that when hypertension is brought about by a variety of different mechanisms, all of which can result in acute arterial necrosis, the height of the blood pressure required to produce the lesion might differ according to the particular mechanism promoting the hypertension. Thus it is conceivable that the liability to acute fibrinoid necrosis in various forms of hypertension may depend on the pressure gradient down the arterial tree, and this may differ considerably according to the pathogenesis of the hypertension. In rats with Goldblatt-type hypertension, pressure in small arterioles (30-μm diameter) is normal; however, in rats with deoxycorticosterone (DOC)/salt hypertension, the pressure is above normal in these vessels (58). This may be the explanation of the finding that rats with post-DOC hypertension have significantly fewer arteriolar fibrinoid lesions than rats with ongoing DOC hypertension and the same level of blood pressure (59). The elucidation to this problem poses serious difficulties, because it would necessitate continuous blood pressure measurement throughout the whole course of an experiment and at all levels down the vascular tree. I am not aware of any published studies meeting these stringent requirements. However, evidence of the possibility that renin, in addition to the level of blood pressure, may be involved in causing malignant Goldblatt hypertension in the rat has been advanced (60). Unfortunately, the experiment did not meet the stringent requirements mentioned above. Evidence has also been advanced that an increase in permeability may occur in myocardial and cerebral vessels in the absence of elevated pressure in rats treated with angiotensin (44,61). In a further study (62) the response of the cerebral vessels to systemic angiotensin was examined in both the presence and absence of sympathetic blocking drugs, which diminished the pressor response, and it was claimed that similar lesions occurred in both situations.

Clearly, the possibility that renin/angiotensin is capable of inducing vascular injury by an action on the vessel wall directly in addition to the effects of the elevated blood pressure that it brings about is of great importance both experimentally and clinically (63). Myocardial necrosis results from the administration of angiotensin in large doses to rabbits (64); furthermore, the severity of the lesions has been correlated with the increase of arterial pressure, and these lesions have been found predominantly in the left, rather than the right, ventricle (65). No lesions were observed in the arteries or arterioles, and it was concluded that a hypertensive, rather than vasculotoxic, pathogenesis for the lesions was more likely. Recent work has suggested that angiotensin-induced spasm in the epicardial vessels may produce myocardial necrosis through anoxia but may not be of sufficient severity to damage the vessel wall (44,62). There is no doubt, however, from Byrom's saline injection experiments that mechanical stress alone is capable of producing the lesion. Furthermore, in the presence of reduced or absent renin/angiotensin, as in deoxycorticosterone acetate (DOCA)/salt or renoprival hypertension, the same lesion occurs. The evidence to date for a specific vasculotoxic action of angiotensin, independent of the hypertension it induces, can be said to be no more than suggestive. High concentrations of vasoactive agents injected subcutaneously, including vasopressin (3), epinephrine, and ergotamine, induce local spasm and necrotizing vascular lesions, but whether lesions can arise in this manner and not through the effects simply of the raised blood pressure, when the agent is injected into the bloodstream and is thereby diluted, has not been clearly established. Byrom's view was that spasm, however induced, was capable of causing vascular damage. The possibility of a direct vasculotoxic action of endogenous angiotensin must be regarded as still an open question.

THE VULNERABILITY OF THE VESSEL WALL TO THE EFFECTS OF STRESS

The Role of Vascular Hypertrophy

Byrom commented on the liability to hypertensive encephalopathy at a relatively low level of arterial pressure in eclampsia and acute nephritis (13). He surmised that this could be due to the exposure of nonhypertrophied vessels to the sudden stress of hypertension. This liability to acute vascular damage is also observed following correction of coarctation of the aorta. Byrom observed medial necrosis in the renal artery, as well as glomerular aneurysms and necroses, 24 h after removing the clip from a solitary kidney, during which period the blood pressure had fallen to normal (66). Similarly, arterial necrosis in large and medium-sized renal arteries was seen in the clipped kidney but not in the opposite kidney of the hypertensive rat infused with angiotensin (12); renal vascular hypertrophy was present in the latter but not in the former. The importance of protective structural changes in the vessels developing in the course of hypertension has been subsequently confirmed. Whereas the permeability of the blood-brain barrier, as assessed by radioiodinated serum albumin, is the same in spontaneously hypertensive and normotensive rats, an acute rise in blood pressure induced to an equal degree in the two groups by infusing phenylephrine produced a significantly greater permeability of the barrier in the normotensive group (67). Electron microscopy of the middle cerebral artery in spontaneously hypertensive rats revealed a twofold increase in tight strands at the interendothelial junctions as compared with normotensive controls, suggesting that structural modification in the endothelium may also be of importance in counteracting the stress of hypertension (68).

The Role of Sympathetic Innervation

In early experiments in the hypertensive rat, Byrom found that encephalopathy was neither prevented nor cured by bilateral cervical sympathectomy (10). He did not explore the reverse possibility that the sympathetic might have a beneficial effect in protecting vessels from hypertensive damage. It has now been shown that unilateral superior cervical ganglionectomy attenuates the development of ipsilateral hypertrophy of parenchymal cerebral vessels in the stroke-prone spontaneously hypertensive rat (69) and predisposes to cerebral hemorrhage and to hyalinosis and fibrinoid changes in these vessels (70). Furthermore, permeability of the blood-brain barrier was found to be significantly increased in the sympathetically denervated (as compared with the innervated) hemisphere (71), and it was concluded that sympathetic innervation may protect against encephalopathy, possibly through some trophic action on the hypertrophic response of vessels to chronically raised pressure (72).

The Role of Age

Byrom's experiments were undertaken exclusively in young rats, and the influence of age on hypertensive vascular damage was not studied. It has subsequently been shown in spontaneously hypertensive rats that vascular lesions were more severe in rats averaging 91 weeks of age than in those less than 52 weeks (73); it was concluded that both the level of blood pressure and the age were involved in the pathogenesis of the lesions. It was suggested that the age factor could simply be an indicator of the duration of hypertension, which was really the crucial factor, but it is also possible that aging processes in the vessel walls, analogous to those occurring after x-irradiation (*vide infra*), could be responsible.

The Role of Preexisting Damage to the Vessel Wall

X-Irradiation

When the brain is exposed to a large x-ray dose, fibrinoid necrosis occurs in the cerebral vessels. The exposure of one kidney to a lower dosage leads to the development of hypertension and the appearance of fibrinoid necrosis in both kidneys, the lesions being much more severe in the irradiated kidney (74). This vulnerability of irradiated vessels has also been shown in mesenteric and spinal arteries (75,76). Byrom and Asscher (13) exposed one-half of the brain of rats to a moderate x-ray dose and subsequently made the rats hypertensive. Observation of the pial vessels through bilateral cranial windows revealed that those on the irradiated side became rather more dilated and tortuous and many rats later died of massive intracranial hemorrhage occurring on this side. Byrom concluded that mild to moderate x-irradiation renders vessels more vulnerable to the stress of raised intravascular pressure and that heavy irradiation may render them susceptible to the normal level of blood pressure.

Uremia

Byrom's work proved conclusively that hypertension was capable of causing lesions in the absence of uremia, and Byrom did not consider the problem further. However, the possibility remains as to whether, in the presence of uremia, the vessels are more vulnerable to the stress of hypertension. The study of this problem poses considerable difficulty, because it would require careful comparison of the severity and frequency in two groups of animals developing hypertension at the same rate and to the same degree, one group having reduced and the other having normal renal excretory function. I am not aware of any such study being performed. However, early workers in the field of renoprival hypertension expressed the view that the rise of blood pressure alone was not the main factor in the development of vascular lesions (77). The problem of the role of uremia, per se, in the pathogenesis of acute fibrinoid necrosis remains unresolved.

Steroid Hypertension

Byrom did not study DOC/saline-induced hypertension, but it is of interest that in a microangiographic and histologic study of the pathogenesis of hypertensive vascular and glomerular lesions in this form of hypertension in the rat, the impression was gained that significant lesions could occur with only a mild rise in blood pressure, suggesting that other factors may be involved (78). Furthermore, high-pressure injection of saline into the arterial system of rats pretreated with DOC/saline produced more severe lesions than in normal rats, and it was concluded that the findings supported the concept that vascular lesions were occurring in dilated hyperdistended vessels and in the glomeruli distal to them (35).

Primary Arterial Disease

Byrom was deeply concerned with the clarification of the controversy between Volhard and Fahr (36) over their interpretation of their observations on malignant nephrosclerosis, the condition that would now be termed *primary malignant hypertension* or *essential malignant hypertension.* Fahr maintained that there was primary inflammation of the kidney and secondary hypertension, whereas Volhard maintained that the hypertension was primary and responsible for the structural lesions in the kidney. From his own experiments, Byrom was convinced that Volhard's interpretation was correct, but he conceded that there might be circumstances when the vessels were rendered more vulnerable to the stress of intravascular pressure (14):

> For if a pathologically high blood pressure can cause lesions of malignant nephrosclerosis by overstretching normal (or even hypertrophied) arteries, a normal blood pressure, which is still high, may reasonably be expected to cause identical lesions in an artery weakened by disease or adverse circumstances such as storage for transplantation or, perhaps, rejection.

Byrom refers to diseases including scleroderma, postpartum acute renal failure, and hemolytic uremic syndrome as examples of vessels rendered more vulnerable to the stress of normal blood pressure. The vascular lesion in such patients who have, at least in the early stages, a normal blood pressure, has been extensively studied and has been considered to differ in some respects from those developing in the course of essential malignant hypertension (79).

The last words must be Byrom's (14):

> Only when we perceive that we are all dealing with nothing more obscure than an overstretched artery can we comprehend that the views of Franz Volhard and Theodor Fahr are not contradictory but complementary, appreciate the full significance of their joint contribution to the understanding of Bright's disease, and proceed rationally to build on that contribution.

ACKNOWLEDGMENTS

I wish to acknowledge the publishers of the following journals for permission to reproduce short extracts from the texts of published works: *Lancet; Quarterly Journal of Medicine; Clinical Science; Journal of Pathology; British Journal of Experimental Pathology;* and *American Heart Journal.* I also wish to acknowledge Heinemann Medical Books for permission to reproduce an extract from Byrom's monograph.

REFERENCES

1. Byrom FB. A study of the total exchange of water, sodium, potassium and nitrogen in epilepsy. *Q J Med* 1932;N.S.1:289–304.
2. Byrom FB, Wilson C. The alleged pituitary origin of the eclamptic and pre-eclamptic "toxaemias" of pregnancy. *Q J Med* 1934;N.S.3:361–368.
3. Byrom FB. Morbid effects of vasopressin on the organs and vessels of rats. *J Pathol Bacteriol* 1937;45:1–16.
4. Goldblatt H. Studies on experimental hypertension. VII. The production of the malignant phase of hypertension. *J Exp Med* 1938;67:809–826.
5. Wilson C, Pickering GW. Acute arterial lesions in rabbits with experimental renal hypertension. *Clin Sci* 1938;3:343–351.
6. Wilson C, Byrom FB. Renal changes in malignant hypertension: experimental evidence. *Lancet* 1939;1:136–139.
7. Wilson C, Byrom FB. The vicious circle in chronic Bright's disease: experimental evidence from the hypertensive rat. *Q J Med* 1941;N.S.10:65–93.
8. Byrom FB, Dodson LF. The mechanism of the vicious circle in chronic hypertension. *Clin Sci* 1949;8:1–10.
9. Byrom FB, Dodson LF. The causation of acute arterial necrosis in hypertensive disease. *J Pathol Bacteriol* 1948;60:357–368.
10. Byrom FB. The pathogenesis of hypertensive encephalopathy and its relation to the malignant phase of hypertension: experimental evidence from the hypertensive rat. *Lancet* 1954;2:201–211.
11. Byrom FB. The nature of malignancy in hypertensive disease: evidence from the retina of the rat. *Lancet* 1963;1:516–520.
12. Byrom FB. Angiotensin and renal vascular damage. *Br J Exp Pathol* 1964;45:7–12.
13. Byrom FB. *The hypertensive vascular crisis: an experimental study.* London: William Heinemann, 1969.
14. Byrom FB. Tension and the artery: the experimental elucidation of pseudouraemia and malignant nephrosclerosis. *Clin Sci Molec Med* 1976;51(suppl):3–11.
15. Goldblatt H, Lynch J, Hanzal RF, Summerville WW. Studies on experimental hypertension. VII. The production of the malignant phase of hypertension. *J Exp Med* 1938;67:809–826.
16. Fahr TH. Uber Nephrosclerose. *Virchows Arch* 1919;226:119–178.
17. Kimmelstiel P, Wilson C. Benign and malignant hypertension and nephrosclerosis. *Am J Pathol* 1936;12:45–81.
18. Ellis AWM. Malignant hypertension. *Lancet* 1938;1:977–980.
19. Pickering GW, Prinzmetal M. Experimental hypertension of renal origin in the rabbit. *Clin Sci* 1938;3:357–368.
20. Byrom FB, Wilson C. A plethysmographic method for measuring systolic blood pressure in the intact rat. *J Physiol (Lond)* 1938;93:301–304.
21. Goldblatt H. Studies on experimental hypertension. V. The pathogenesis of experimental hypertension due to renal ischemia. *Ann Intern Med* 1937;11:69–103.
22. Blalock A, Levy SE. Studies on the etiology of renal hypertension. *Ann Surg* 1937;106:826–847.
23. Dicker E. A propos de l'hypertension arterielle consecutive à une entrave de la circulation rénale. *C R Soc Biol* 1937;125:1046–1047.
24. Butler AM. Chronic pyelonephritis and arterial hypertension. *J Clin Invest* 1937;16:889–897.
25. Leadbetter WF, Burkland CE. Hypertension in unilateral renal disease. *J Urol* 1938;39:611–626.
26. Floyer MA. The effect of nephrectomy and adrenalectomy upon the blood pressure in hypertensive and normotensive rats. *Clin Sci* 1951;10:405–421.
27. Thal AP, Grage TB, Vernier RS. Function of the contralateral kidney in renal hypertension due to renal artery stenosis. *Circulation* 1963;27:36–43.
28. Guyton AC, Coleman TG, Cowley AW, Scheel KW, Manning RD, Norman RA. Arterial pressure regulation. Overriding dominance of the kidneys in long-term regulation and in hypertension. *Am J Med* 1972;52:584–594.
29. Folkow B, Gothberg G, Lundin S, Ricksten SE. Structural renal vascular changes in renal hypertensive rats. *Acta Physiol Scand* 1977;101:254–256.
30. Muirhead EE. Renomedullary system of blood pressure control. *Hypertension* 1966;8(suppl 1):38–46.
31. Lee MR. Dopamine and the kidney. *Clin Sci* 1982;62:439–448.
32. Casson IF, Lee MR, Brownjohn AM, Parsons FM, Davidson AM, Will EJ, Clayden AD. Failure of renal dopamine response to salt loading in chronic renal disease. *Br Med J* 1983;286:503–506.
33. Chatelain RE, Dardik BN, Shainoff JR. Acute arterial fibrinoid deposition and ischaemic parenchymal damage of the kidney. Pathogenic factors in the development of malignant hypertension. *J Pathol* 1983;141:125–142.
34. Wolfgarten M, Margarey FR. Vascular fibrinoid necrosis in hypertension. *J Pathol Bacteriol* 1959;77:597–603.
35. Hill GS. Studies on the pathogenesis of hypertensive vascular dis-

ease. Effect of high pressure intra-arterial injections in rats. *Circ Res* 1970;27:657–668.

36. Volhard F, Fahr T. *Die Brightsche Nierenkrankheit.* Berlin: Springer, 1914.

37. Meyer JS, Waltz AG, Gotoh F. Pathogenesis of cerebral vasospasm in hypertensive encephalopathy. II. The nature of increased irritability of smooth muscle of pial arteries in renal hypertension. *Neurology* 1960;10:859–867.

38. Rodda R, Denny-Brown D. The cerebral arterioles in experimental hypertension. *Am J Pathol* 1966;49:53–76.

39. Byrom FB. The caliber of the retinal arteries in hypertension. *Am Heart J* 1963;66:727–730.

40. Giese J. Acute hypertensive vascular disease. 2. Studies on vascular reaction patterns and permeability changes by means of vital microscopy and colloidal tracer technique. *Acta Pathol Microbiol Scand* 1964;62:497–515.

41. Goldby FS, Beilin LJ. Relationship between arterial pressure and the permeability of arterioles to carbon particles in acute hypertension in the rat. *Cardiovasc Res* 1972;6:384–390.

42. Goldby FS, Beilin LJ. How an acute rise in arterial pressure damages arterioles. Electron microscopic changes during angiotensin infusion. *Cardiovasc Res* 1972;6:569–584.

43. Wiener J, Giacomelli F. The cellular pathology of experimental hypertension. VII. Structure and permeability of the mesenteric vasculature in angiotensin-induced hypertension. *Am J Pathol* 1973;72:221–240.

44. Thorball N, Olsen F. Ultrastructural pathological changes in intestinal submucosal arteries in angiotensin-induced acute hypertension in rats. *Acta Pathol Microbiol Scand (A)* 1974;82:703–713.

45. Giacomelli F, Anversa P, Wiener J. Effect of angiotensin-induced hypertension on rat coronary arteries and myocardium. *Am J Pathol* 1976;84:111–138.

46. Joris I, Majno G. Cell-to-cell herniae in the arterial wall. I. Pathogenesis of vacuoles in the normal media. *Am J Pathol* 1977;87:375–398.

47. Joris I, Majno G. Medial changes in arterial spasm induced by L-norepinephrine. *Am J Pathol* 1981;105:212–222.

48. Strandgaard S, Olesen J, Skinhoj E, Lassen NA. Autoregulation of brain circulation in severe arterial hypertension. *Br Med J* 1973;1:507–510.

49. Strandgaard S, MacKenzie ET, Sengupta D, Rowan JO, Lassen NA, Harper AM. Upper limit of autoregulation of cerebral blood flow in the baboon. *Circ Res* 1974;34:435–440.

50. Dinsdale HB, Robertson DM, Haas RA. Cerebral blood flow in acute hypertension. *Arch Neurol* 1974;31:80–87.

51. Tamaki K, Sadoshima S, Baumbach GL, Iadecola C, Reis DJ, Heistad DD. Evidence that disruption of the blood-brain barrier precedes reduction in cerebral blood flow in hypertensive encephalopathy. *Hypertension* 1984;6(suppl 1):75–81.

52. Goldblatt H. The renal origin of hypertension. *Physiol Rev* 1947;27:120–165.

53. Masson GMC, Kashii C, Panisset JC, Yagi S, Page IH. Production of hypertension and vascular disease by kidney extracts. *Circ Res* 1964;14:150–163.

54. Masson GMC, Hazard JB, Corcoran AC, Page IH. Experimental vascular disease due to deoxycorticosterone and anterior pituitary factors. *Arch Pathol Lab Med* 1950;49:641–664.

55. Asscher AW, Anson SG. A vascular permeability factor of renal origin. *Nature* 1963;198:1097–1099.

56. Cuthbert MF, Asscher AW, Jones JH. Characterization of a vascular permeability factor of renal origin. *Clin Sci* 1966;31:325–336.

57. Cuthbert MF, Peart WS. Studies on the identity of a vascular permeability factor of renal origin. *Clin Sci* 1970;38:309–325.

58. Meininger GA, Harris PD, Joshua IG. Distributions of microvascular pressure in skeletal muscle of one-kidney, one clip, two-kidney, one clip, and deoxycorticosterone-salt hypertensive rats. *Hypertension* 1984;6:27–34.

59. Reid R, Lindop G, Brown W, Lever AF, Lucie N, Webb D. Similar blood pressure but different outcome in rats with DOC and post-DOC hypertension. *J Hypertens* 1983;1:303–310.

60. Chatelain RE, DiBello PM, Ferrario CM. Experimental benign and malignant hypertension with malignant nephrosclerosis. *Br J Exp Pathol* 1980;61:401–410.

61. Grammas P, Giacomelli F, Wiener J. Carotid artery constriction in acute hypertension. *Am J Pathol* 1981;103:226–233.

62. Bhan RD, Giacomelli F, Wiener J. Adrenoreceptor blockade in angiotensin-induced hypertension. *Am J Pathol* 1982;108:60–71.

63. Laragh JH. Renin as a predictor of hypertensive complications. *Ann NY Acad Sci* 1978;304:165–177.

64. Gavras H, Kremer D, Brown JJ, et al. Angiotensin and norepinephrine induced myocardial lesions: experimental and clinical studies in man. *Am Heart J* 1975;89:321–332.

65. Kremer D, Lindop G, Brown WCB, Morton JJ, Robertson JIS. Angiotensin-induced myocardial necrosis and renal failure in the rabbit: distributions of lesions and severity in relation to plasma angiotensin II concentration and arterial pressure. *Cardiovasc Res* 1981;15:43–46.

66. Byrom FB. The vascular crisis in hypertension. In: Gross F, ed. *Antihypertensive therapy.* Berlin: Springer-Verlag, 1966;499.

67. Mueller SM, Heistad DD. Effect of chronic hypertension on the blood-brain barrier. *Hypertension* 1980;2:809–812.

68. Majack RA, Bhalla RC. Ultrastructural characteristics of endothelial permeability pathways in chronic hypertension. *Hypertension* 1981;3:586–595.

69. Hart MN, Heistad DD, Brody MJ. Effect of chronic hypertension and sympathetic denervation on wall/lumen ratio of cerebral vessels. *Hypertension* 1980;2:419–423.

70. Sadoshima S, Busija D, Brody M, Heistad D. Sympathetic nerves protect against stroke in stroke-prone hypertensive rats. *Hypertension* 1981;3(suppl 1):124–127.

71. Sadoshima S, Heistad D. Sympathetic nerves protect the blood-brain barrier in stroke-prone spontaneously hypertensive rats. *Hypertension* 1982;4:904–907.

72. Bevan RD. Trophic effects of peripheral adrenergic nerves on vascular structure. *Am J Pathol* 1984;6(suppl III):19–26.

73. Mandal AK, Bell RD, Parker D, Nordquist JA, Lindeman RD. An analysis of the relationship of malignant lesions of the kidney to hypertension. *Microvasc Res* 1977;14:279–292.

74. Wilson C, Ledingham JM, Cohen M. Hypertension following X-irradiation of the kidneys. *Lancet* 1958;1:9–16.

75. Asscher AW, Wilson C, Anson SG. Sensitisation of blood-vessels to hypertensive damage by X-irradiation. *Lancet* 1961;1:580–583.

76. Asscher AW, Anson SG. Arterial hypertension and irradiation damage to the nervous system. *Lancet* 1962;2:1343–1346.

77. Muirhead EE, Turner LB, Grollman A. Hypertensive cardiovascular disease. Nature and pathogenesis of the arteriolar sclerosis induced by bilateral nephrectomy as revealed by a study of its tinctorial characteristics. *Arch Pathol Lab Med* 1951;52:266–279.

78. Hill GS, Heptinstall RH. Steroid-induced hypertension in the rat. *Am J Pathol* 1968;52:1–39.

79. Bohle A, Grund KE, Helmchen U, Meyer D. Primary malignant nephrosclerosis. *Clin Sci Molec Med* 1976;51(suppl):23–25.

SECTION II

Epidemiological Dimensions of Hypertension

Hypertension: Pathophysiology, Diagnosis, and Management, Second Edition, edited by J.H. Laragh and B.M. Brenner, Raven Press, Ltd., New York © 1995.

CHAPTER 4

Does Hypertension Predispose to Coronary Disease?

Conflicting Epidemiological and Experimental Evidence

Austin E. Doyle[1]

There is widespread agreement that the most frequent complications that develop in patients with high blood pressure are those due to myocardial ischemia. These include myocardial infarction, sudden death, and angina pectoris. It is widely assumed that these clinical events are due to atherosclerotic disease of the major coronary arteries, and it is supposed that the elevated blood pressure favors the development of more severe atherosclerosis of the major coronary arteries with consequent myocardial ischemia. Although there is certainly experimental and clinicopathological evidence to support this view, there are other possible explanations that could account for the increased incidence of myocardial ischemia in hypertensive patients. It is, for example, possible that myocardial ischemia could result from cardiac hypertrophy causing relative ischemia, because the metabolic demands of the hypertrophied heart outstrip the available blood supply, even in the absence of coronary atherosclerosis. In such a situation, myocardial ischemia could develop in the absence of atherosclerosis of the coronary arteries, and it would certainly be likely to occur in the presence of relatively modest atherosclerosis.

Other possible relationships between coronary atherosclerosis and hypertension can be envisaged. For exam-

ple, atherosclerosis could conceivably be the primary lesion, with hypertension occurring as a result, rather than as a cause, of the vascular disease. Finally, the two conditions, hypertension and atherosclerosis, might be separate conditions with certain pathogenetic factors in common, in which case they might be expected to coexist frequently, without one being caused by the other.

Resolution of these possibilities is of considerable importance in determining the appropriate therapeutic approach to the problem of myocardial ischemia in hypertensive patients. This chapter reviews some of the conflicting evidence from experimental, epidemiological, and clinicopathological sources.

EXPERIMENTAL HYPERTENSION AND CORONARY ATHEROSCLEROSIS

Few, if any, experimental animal models are suitable for the study of this problem, because most experimental animals such as dogs and rats seldom, if ever, spontaneously develop atheroma. For example, the spontaneously hypertensive rat develops left ventricular hypertrophy (1), thickening of the medial muscular layer in medium and small arteries (2), and fibrinoid necrosis in the same-sized vessels, but no occlusive internal lesions of atherosclerotic type. On the other hand, the combina-

---

[1] Deceased

tion of high-cholesterol diet and hypertension has been shown to induce atheroma in some experimental animals, but not others. In the cynomolgus monkey fed a diet containing 2% cholesterol and 10% butter for 6 months, experimental coarctation of the midthoracic aorta was followed by severe and extensive lesions of the main coronary arteries and their branches, with narrowing of the lumen. In the absence of the coarctation, the same diet induced minor atherosclerotic lesions of the major coronary arteries, with only 12% narrowing of the lumen. Coarctation in monkeys fed a low-cholesterol diet did not induce atherosclerotic lesions, although there was thickening of both the media and the intima, with some narrowing of the lumen of the smaller branches of the coronary arteries (3).

It has been shown that the rise of blood pressure leads to increased arterial wall tension (4), which favors the passage of albumin and lipids into dog aorta (5).

These and other data do provide convincing experimental evidence that hypertension is capable of promoting the development of atheroma in combination with other factors in the experimental animal.

Experimental studies have also given information about the regression of established atherosclerotic lesions. In the rhesus monkey, coronary atherosclerotic lesions induced by a high-cholesterol diet regressed gradually over a prolonged period after the substitution of a low-cholesterol diet (6), whereas in the study on experimental coarctation in the cynomolgus monkey (3) it appeared that control of both the hypertension and the hyperlipidemia was necessary to induce regression of the lesions. These observations may suggest that although hypertension can aggravate the development of atherosclerotic lesions, regression of these lesions may be less dependent on the level of blood pressure.

HYPERTENSION AND CORONARY DISEASE IN HUMANS: CLINICOPATHOLOGICAL STUDIES

There have been several autopsy studies relating the incidence of coronary artery disease to hypertension. Bell and Clawson (7) studied autopsy findings in 420 cases of primary hypertension with the associated clinical findings. This study has some imperfections. *Hypertension* was defined as cases with a systolic blood pressure exceeding 150 mm Hg. However, in only 220 of the 420 cases was the blood pressure known to have been at this level. In 184 cases, the diagnosis of hypertension was based on a heart weight above 500 g in males and 450 g in females. On the basis of the major clinical findings and the autopsy data, cases were subdivided into five types according to cause of death. Of the 420 cases, 187 (44.5 percent) were considered to have died of myocardial insufficiency, 182 of whom had passive hepatic venous

congestion. Death was thought to have been due to coronary disease in 67 cases (16 percent), on the basis of sudden death or death during an attack of anginal pain. An unstated number of patients who died suddenly had chronic congestive heart failure.

The authors also compared the incidence of coronary disease in 151 hypertensive hearts with that in hearts of patients dying of rheumatic valve disease or syphilitic aortitis. They concluded that coronary disease was much more common in the hypertensive hearts than in the control group, but the control group may not have been typical of the general population.

A more convincing study was that by Murphy et al. (8), who studied autopsy material from 375 patients known to have had persistent systolic blood pressures of 160 mm Hg and diastolic blood pressures above 100 mm Hg. Of these, 188 patients died of cardiac causes; 105 of these 188 patients developed paroxysmal nocturnal dyspnea as the first symptom. In the whole series of 375 cases, angina pectoris occurred in 42 patients (11.2 percent). Coronary artery occlusion or severe narrowing was found in 25 percent of cases.

Both of these series emphasize the fact that in untreated hypertension, death from congestive heart failure accounts for over half the deaths, whereas coronary disease caused only 10 to 12 percent of deaths. Flaxman (9) reported that about 65 percent of hypertensive patients died of congestive heart failure, and only 11 percent of coronary occlusion in a series of 189 cases followed clinically and at autopsy.

The question of the relationship between the severity of coronary disease and blood pressure is an important but unresolved issue, since as pointed out by Bell and Clawson (7) the association does not imply a causal relationship between hypertension and coronary atheroma. Davis and Klainer (10) addressed the relationship between blood pressure levels in life and autopsy evidence of coronary atheroma. They found more frequent coronary atherosclerotic lesions in the hypertensive population than in normotensive individuals. However, within the hypertensive population, there was no relationship between the height of the blood pressure in life and the severity of the coronary disease (10), and indeed severe coronary artery disease occurred more commonly in mild hypertension than in the severe type. In a following study (11), these authors examined the extent of coronary atheroma in patients dying of hypertension due to renal disease and reported a greatly reduced incidence of atheroma as compared with that found in essential hypertension. These authors suggested that the association between coronary artery disease and hypertension was unlikely to be the result of the high blood pressure; and they hypothesized, instead, that arterial disease might be a predisposing cause of hypertension.

Harrison and Wood (12) made a careful clinicopathological study of the hearts of patients who first presented to Hammersmith Hospital between 1935 and 1939 suffering from either hypertensive or ischemic heart disease. All the hypertensives had marked elevation of blood pressure and presented with dyspnea and left ventricular failure. About half of those diagnosed as ischemic because of anginal pain or myocardial infarction had some elevation of blood pressure. Postmortem coronary angiography revealed marked coronary irregularities and narrowing in the ischemic group, but none of the hypertensive patients with heart failure had narrow coronary arteries, and the coronary arteries at autopsy were smooth and widely dilated (Fig. 1). This study suggests that hypertensive heart failure, the most common cause of death in untreated hypertensive patients, is not usually associated with evidence of coronary atheroma but is, instead, associated with dilatation of the coronary circulation, presumably as a result of an increased workload and demand for an increased blood supply. It is possible that growth of the left ventricular muscle may protect, in some way, from the atheromatous process.

These studies, while confirming the frequent coexistence of coronary atheroma and hypertension, suggest

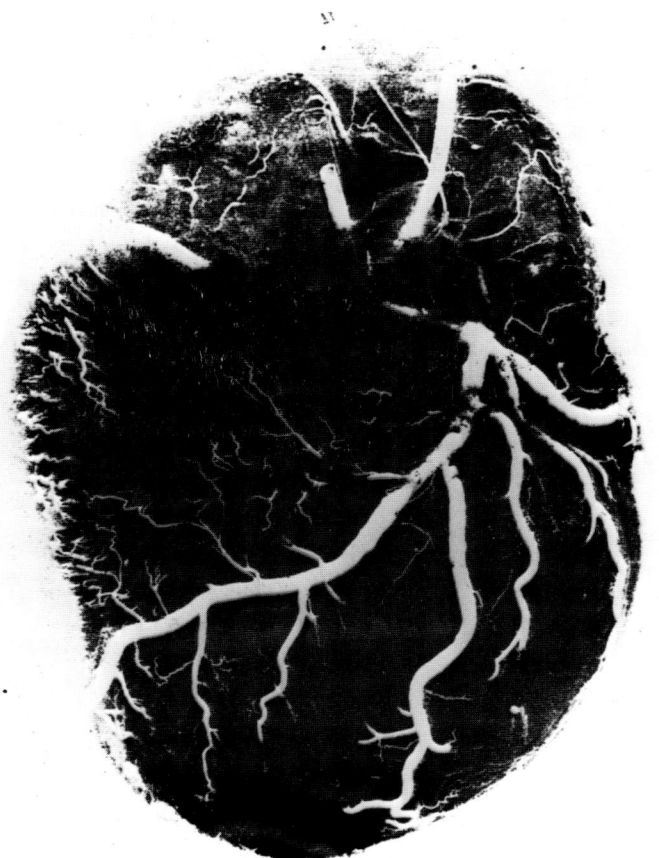

FIG. 1. Postmortem coronary angiogram of a hypertensive heart, weight 545 g. Cleared injected specimen showing dilatation of coronary lumen and smooth outlines, indicating absence of occlusive coronary atheroma. (From ref. 11, with permission.)

that the raised blood pressure itself may not be the direct cause of the coronary disease. Obviously the relationship between the two problems is not a simple one and requires further study. In particular, it would be of interest to know whether independent markers of coronary heart disease can be identified with a view to evaluating the distribution of blood pressure among coronary-prone individuals.

It is a matter of major importance to decide whether or not hypertension per se causes coronary artery disease. If it could be demonstrated that hypertension and coronary disease are independent, but associated, problems, the selection of patients requiring treatment of hypertension would be greatly simplified, because treatment would mainly be needed in the rather small proportion of patients with hypertension severe enough to cause heart failure or stroke. In light of the present evidence, this may be the best policy available.

CORONARY HEART DISEASE IN UNTREATED AND TREATED HYPERTENSIVES

There are few studies from the period before the introduction of antihypertensive drug treatment that indicate with any reliability the precise incidence of coronary disease in untreated hypertensive patients. Diagnostic criteria for myocardial infarction have changed considerably in the last 50 years, and few of the earlier studies refer to the electrocardiogram whereas none refer to more modern criteria such as estimation of cardiac enzymes. Nevertheless, the clinical features of hypertensive heart disease are very clearly described by Flaxman (9) and by Theodore Janeway in his classic paper of 1913 (13). To cite Flaxman:

The symptoms that indicated the onset of hypertensive heart disease were dyspnea, precordial or epigastric pain or both, palpitation, weakness, persistent indigestion, and marked loss in weight. Only 6.6 per cent of the white patients were below 40 years of age at the onset of symptoms, but 16.6 per cent of the colored patients were below that age. The largest incidence among the colored patients occurred in the decade from 41 to 50 years (47.6 per cent); while among the white patients the highest incidence fell in the sixth decade, 51 to 60 years (49.7 per cent).

The symptoms were usually slowly progressive after an insidious onset but the numerous exceptions made attempts to estimate prognoses very difficult. The life-expectancy was short when the symptoms appeared suddenly and were not preceded by any omens of cardiac distress. The average duration of symptoms before the occurrence of heart failure was one year. The main reason for the short interval between the onset of symptoms and the appearance of congestive heart failure appeared to be the sufferers' reluctance to seek medical attention for the relief of symptoms.

A comparison of the duration of the disease after the onset of congestive heart failure in the known deceased and in the living patients indicates approximately similar percentages. Of the deceased white 89.2 per cent and of the deceased colored patients 88.5 per cent had died within one year after the occurrence of congestive heart failure. The percentages of living patients who came under observation within one year after congestive failure occurred were, in the white 88.4 per cent and in the colored patients 88.0 per cent.

As to the age of death in hypertensive heart disease, 30.2 per cent of the white and 65.2 per cent of the colored patients had died before they were 50 years old.

The common cause of death was congestive heart failure (as Table 1 indicates). Uremia was the next most common cause of death; it was more frequent in the colored patients and in males of both races. Coronary thrombosis and cerebral hemorrhage were the causes of death of many patients, especially of those who died within one week after the sudden onset of symptoms. Coronary thrombosis was found to be the third most frequent cause of death.

Janeway described 458 patients, all seen in private practice by himself or his father. Of 212 deaths, 67 were attributed to gradual cardiac failure, 46 to uremia, 29 to apoplexy, and 10 to angina pectoris, with 28 of unknown cause. Janeway further observed that those with angina were older than most other groups. He also commented that the group who died of angina had lower blood pressures, when first seen, than those who died of uremia, apoplexy, or gradual cardiac insufficiency; similarly, the blood pressures of those whose early symptoms were "anginoid" pain were also lower than in the remaining groups.

In their study of the relationship between basal blood pressures and life expectancy, Smirk et al. (14) found a strong positive correlation between the height of the basal blood pressure and congestive heart failure, left ventricular failure, cardiac enlargement, and retinopathy. However, no relationship was found between the height of the basal blood pressure and the extent of coronary disease. In this study, deaths were classified as hypertensive, coronary, unrelated to hypertension, or unknown. In men, those who died of hypertension had higher basal blood pressures than those who died of coronary causes, who, in turn, had higher basal blood pressures than those who died of other causes. In women, those who died of coronary disease had basal pressures that were as high as in those dying of hypertensive causes, with both of these being higher than in those dying of unrelated causes.

It appears from these data that in untreated severe hypertension, the most common cause of death is congestive heart failure, with uremia and stroke also being relatively common. Although all authors note a significant incidence of coronary disease, these accounted for less than 20% of deaths; in those patients, blood pressures appeared to be less elevated.

By contrast, the major cause of death in treated hypertension has consistently been found to be myocardial infarction. Myocardial infarction caused death in 40% of men in Bulpitt's series (15), in 42% of Hodge and Smirk's (16) series, in 41% of Dollery et al.'s series (17), and in 41% from the Glasgow Hypertension Clinic (18) (Table 2).

Taken overall, these data indicate that antihypertensive treatment has greatly reduced the incidence of complications of hypertension that are directly due to the raised blood pressure, most notably congestive heart failure. By contrast, the percentage of deaths due to coronary events has risen since the introduction of antihypertensive drug treatment, leaving it as the major cause of death in treated hypertension. Presumably the removal of other causes of death, along with the lengthened survival time in hypertensive patients, allows the development of coronary artery disease, which is apparently little, if at all, affected by control of blood pressure.

The results of recent clinical trials in mild hyperten-

TABLE 1. *Percentage of causes of death in 189 cases[a,b]*

Causes of death	White				Black			
	M	F	T	%	M	F	T	%
1. Congestive heart failure	63	14	77	64.8	32	13	45	64.3
2. Uremia	13	4	17	14.3	11	3	14	20.1
3. Coronary thrombosis	13	0	13	10.9	2	0	2	2.8
4. Cerebral hemorrhage	3	3	6	5.2	6	1	7	10.0
5. Ruptured dissecting aortic aneurysm	1	0	1	0.8	1	0	1	1.4
6. Spontaneous rupture, ascending aorta	0	0	0	0	1	0	1	1.4
7. Adams-Stokes syndrome	1	0	1	0.8	0	0	0	0
8. Diabetic coma	1	0	1	0.8	0	0	0	0
9. Mesenteric thrombosis	1	0	1	0.8	0	0	0	0
10. Incarcerated inguinal hernia	1	0	1	0.8	0	0	0	0
11. Septicemia	0	1	1	0.8	0	0	0	0
Total:	97	22	119	100.0	53	17	70	100.0

[a] From ref. 9, with permission.
[b] M, male; F, female; T, total.

TABLE 2. *Causes of death in treated hypertension*

	Dollery et al. (17)		Bulpitt et al. (15)		Hodge and Smirk (16)		Isles et al. (18)	
	n	%	*n*	%	*n*	%	*n*	%
Ischemic heart disease	32	41	148	36	72	42	308	41
Stroke	15	19	74	18	39	22	172	23
All vascular	63	80	256	62	139	80	560	75
Nonvascular	16	20	154	37	34	20	190	25
Total:	79		410		173		750	

sion seem to have provided further evidence for a dissociation between hypertension and coronary disease. Placebo-controlled clinical trials of antihypertensive drug treatment, mainly in mild hypertension, have recently been concluded. The results of the British MRC trial (19), the Australian therapeutic trial in mild hypertension (20), and the European trial in the elderly (21) have yielded rather similar results. All three studies demonstrated a small, but significant, reduction in the incidence of stroke in the treated populations as compared with the untreated groups. However, none of the studies revealed any difference in the incidence of coronary events between treated and control groups (Table 3). In all three studies, coronary events were the most frequent cause of both death and morbidity in both the treated and control groups. The numbers of patients involved in these studies are comparatively small, which has led to the suggestion that a real reduction in coronary events may have been missed. Although this possibility cannot be excluded, the trials were large enough to detect differences in the incidence of stroke, which is numerically less common than coronary events, and they were also large enough to demonstrate an increased frequency of coronary events in smokers and men. Thus whereas a protective effect on coronary events in treated mild hypertensives cannot be finally excluded, any effect must be very small compared with the obvious differences noted between hypertensive and nonhypertensive persons in the epidemiological data.

There have been other suggestions advanced for the apparent failure of antihypertensive drug treatment to reduce coronary events. The most popular of these is the suggestion that the use of beta-blocking drugs or diuret-

ics, or both, leads to adverse effects on lipoproteins, which antagonize the protective action of a reduced blood pressure. There is certainly evidence that beta-blockers raise VLDL cholesterol and reduce HDL cholesterol (22), whereas diuretics increase triglyceride levels (23). However, there is also evidence for a protective role of beta-blocking drugs in the secondary prevention of myocardial infarction (24). Whether the adverse effects of beta-blockers on lipoprotein profiles would antagonize any protective effect of their blood pressure-lowering action remains a possibility.

EPIDEMIOLOGICAL DATA

There are few, if any, data available from the era prior to the use of antihypertensive drugs. Moreover, changing diagnostic criteria over the last 40 years make evaluation of the incidence of coronary disease difficult. The concept that hypertension is an important pathogenetic factor in the development of coronary disease is due largely to major prospective epidemiological studies and, in particular, to the Framingham study (25) and the Pooling Project (26). Both of these studies revealed clear evidence that with increasing systolic and diastolic blood pressure levels, the likelihood of coronary events and death from coronary artery disease increased. In addition to blood pressure levels, the data indicate that increasing levels of serum cholesterol, increasing levels of tobacco usage, increasing age, and the male sex were all factors that appeared to predispose to an increased risk of coronary events. Data from the Pooling Project relating levels of blood pressure at various ages to the risk of coronary events are shown in Figs. 2 and 3. These indicate very clearly that the risk of coronary events increases sharply above the age of 50 years in men; at all ages there is an increased risk of coronary events as blood pressure increases, with a particularly steep increase with diastolic blood pressures above 104 mm Hg or systolic pressures above 160 mm Hg. The authors interpreted these data as indicating that the height of blood pressure was an important factor predisposing to the risk of coronary disease, with the implication that increasing levels of blood pressure were a causative factor in the pathogenesis of atherosclerosis of the coronary arteries. Hypertension

TABLE 3. *Comparison of strokes and coronary events in active and treated groups in three clinical trials*

	MRC	EWPHE	Australian trial	Total
Strokes				
Active	60	13	17	90
Placebo	109	24	31	164
Coronary events				
Active	222	42	98	362
Placebo	234	37	109	380

Risk of coronary event

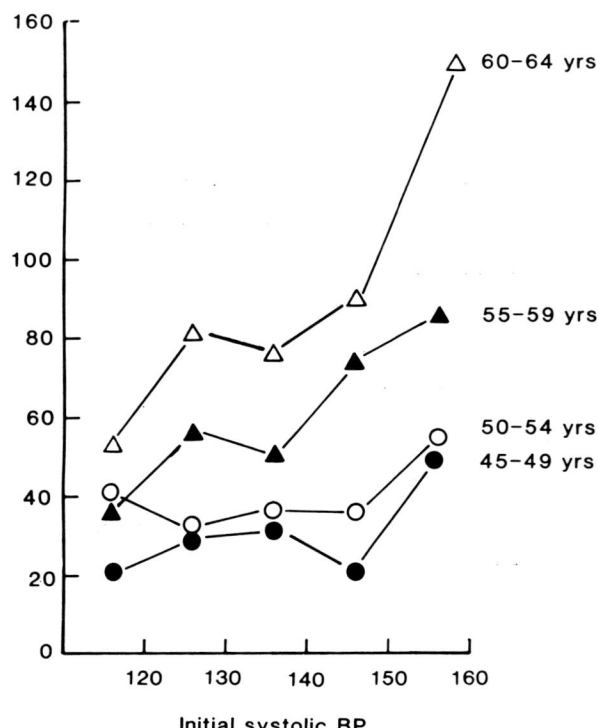

FIG. 2. Risk of coronary events in men, related to age and initial systolic pressure. [Derived from data published by the Pooling Project Research Group (26).]

A major problem in interpretation of these data is the difficulty of distinguishing events due to major epicardial coronary atheroma from those secondary to left ventricular hypertrophy in the absence of coronary disease. Hypertrophy of the left ventricle due to hypertension or aortic valve disease may lead to relative ischemia, because although the coronary arteries dilate, the coronary supply remains inadequate to supply the metabolic needs of the hypertrophied ventricle (29). There is also evidence in experimental left ventricular hypertrophy that the coronary reserve is diminished, particularly in the subendocardial region (30). Pisani et al. (31) have emphasized that hypertension and coronary artery disease may each lead to symptoms that are clinically indistinguishable. This must cast doubt on the concept that hypertension is a risk factor for coronary disease, since the endpoints measured may be due to either hypertension or coronary disease. The situation is further complicated by the fact that coronary disease undoubtedly coexists with hyper-

added to other risk factors such as cigarette smoking, raised cholesterol levels, and the male sex.

The concept that coronary risk increases progressively over the whole range of blood pressure has been challenged by Anderson (27), who reanalyzed data from the Framingham study and concluded that the increased risk of coronary events did not occur with diastolic pressures below 90 mm Hg (Fig. 4).

There has been widespread acceptance of the concept that hypertension is a causative factor in the pathogenesis of coronary atherosclerosis and, hence, of coronary events.

However, the association noted in epidemiological studies may be interpreted in other ways. In a recent analysis of the Framingham data, Harris et al. (28) have demonstrated that systolic blood pressure, both before and after the age of 65 years, is significantly associated with an increased risk of vascular disease. It is, however, possible that elevated systolic pressure is itself a marker of vascular disease and that the higher systolic pressures merely identify those individuals who already have disease of the major arteries. The available data do not allow a clear distinction between this possibility and the idea that hypertension causes atheroma.

Most of the epidemiological data relate death from vascular causes to the degree of blood pressure elevation.

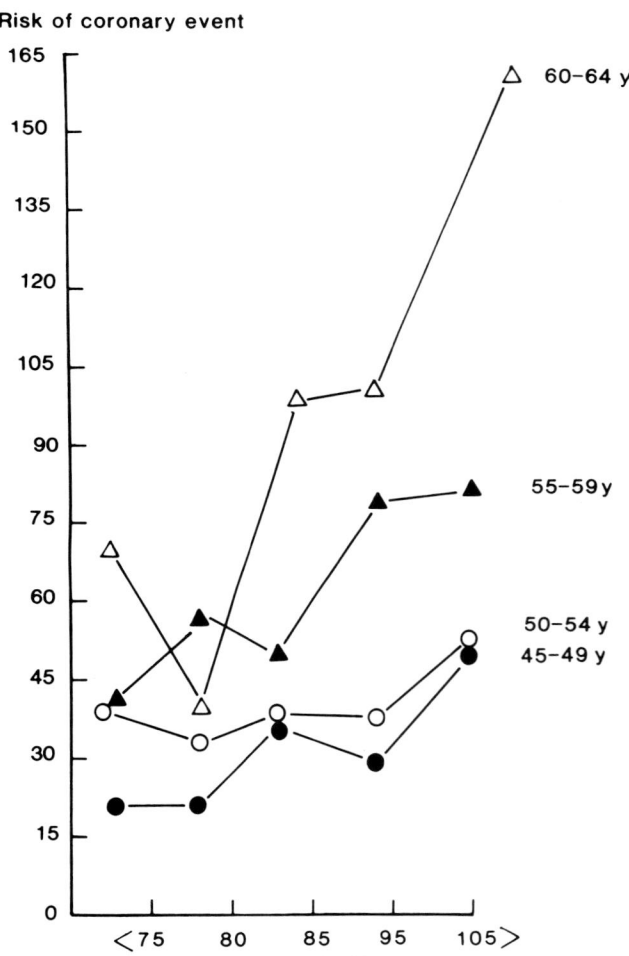

FIG. 3. Risk of coronary events in men, related to age and initial diastolic pressure. [Derived from data published by the Pooling Project Research Group (26).]

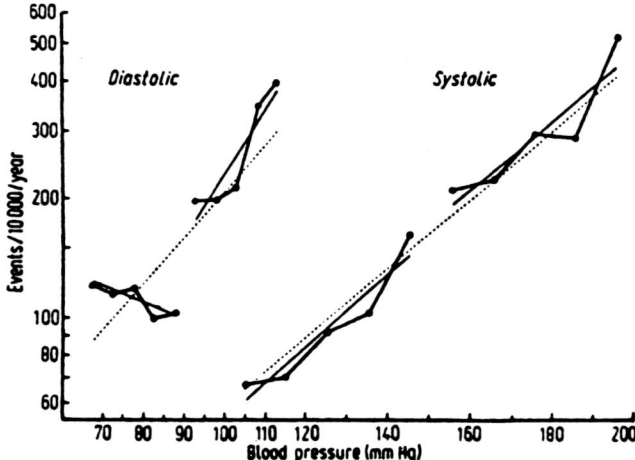

FIG. 4. Annual incidence of cardiovascular events at Framingham over 18 years of follow-up by level of blood pressure, all ages; mean of male and female rates are plotted on logarithmic vertical scale. Logistic curves are shown as dotted lines. Separate regression lines for the upper and lower five points are shown as solid lines. (From ref. 27, with permission.)

tension, in which case minor degrees of coronary narrowing would assume greater pathological significance in the hypertrophied heart. As Frolich (32) has pointed out, there is an urgent need for more precise diagnosis, particularly to establish the presence or absence of coronary disease in the presence of left ventricular hypertrophy.

Finally, there is the disturbing possibility that lowering of blood pressure may, in some instances, actually lead to a fall in cardiac blood flow and may therefore precipitate ischemia or myocardial infarction (33). Although such a mechanism has not been clearly established, it might account for the undoubted fact that myocardial infarction has emerged as the leading cause of death in treated hypertension.

It is clear that the interrelationships between coronary atherosclerosis, hypertension, and left ventricular hypertrophy are complex, and they remain inadequately understood. Recognition of this is a prerequisite for the initiation of further studies designed to clarify these issues.

REFERENCES

1. Sen S, Tarazi RC, Khairallah PA, Bumpus FM. Cardiac hypertrophy in spontaneously hypertensive rats. *Circ Res* 1974;35:775–781.
2. Folkow B, Hallback M, Lundgren G, Weiss L. Structurally based increase of flow resistance in spontaneously hypertensive rats. *Acta Physiol Scand* 1970;79:373–378.
3. Hollander W, Maddoff IM, Paddock J, Kirkpatrick B. Aggravation of coronary and cerebral atherosclerosis by hypertension in a subhuman primate model. *Circulation* 1974;52(Suppl 2):124.
4. Glagov S. Haemodynamic risk factors: mechanical stress, mural architecture, medial nutrition and the vulnerability of arteries to atherosclerosis. In: Wissler RH, Greer JC, eds. *The pathogenesis of atherosclerosis.* Baltimore: Williams & Wilkins, 1972.
5. Duncan LE Jr, Buck K, Lynch A. The effect of pressure and stretching on the passage of labeled albumin into canine aortic wall. *J Atherosclerosis Res* 1965;5:69–79.
6. Armstrong ML, Warner ED, Couner WE. Regression of coronary atheromatosis in rhesus monkeys. *Circ Res* 1970;27:59–67.
7. Bell ET, Clawson BJ. Primary (essential) hypertension. *Arch Pathol* 1928;5:939–1001.
8. Murphy FD, Grill J, Pessin B, Moxon GF. Essential (primary) hypertension: a clinical and morphological study of 375 cases. *Ann Intern Med* 1933;6:31–53.
9. Flaxman N. The course of hypertensive heart disease: 1. Age of onset, development of cardiac insufficiency, duration of life, and cause of death. *Ann Intern Med* 1936;10:748–753.
10. Davis D, Klainer MJ. Studies in hypertensive heart disease. II. The role of hypertension, per se, in the development of coronary sclerosis. *Am Heart J* 1940;19:193–197.
11. Davis D, Klainer MJ. Studies in hypertensive heart disease. I. The incidence of coronary atherosclerosis in cases of essential hypertension. *Am Heart J* 1940;19:185–192.
12. Harrison CV, Wood P. Hypertensive and ischaemic heart disease: a comparative clinical and pathological study. *Br Heart J* 1949;11:205–209.
13. Janeway T. A clinical study of hypertensive cardiovascular disease. *Arch Intern Med* 1913;12:755–798.
14. Smirk FH, Veale AMO, Alstad KS. Basal and supplemental blood pressures in relationship to life expectancy and hypertension symptomatology. *NZ Med J* 1959;58:711–735.
15. Bulpitt CJ, Beevers DG, Butler A, Coles EG, Hunt D, Munro-Faure AD, Newson RB, O'Riordan PW, Petrie JC, Rajagopalan B, Rylance PB, Twallin G, Webster J, Dollery CT. The survival of treated hypertensive patients and their causes of death: a report from the DHSS Hypertensive Care Computing Project (DHCCP). *J Hypertens* 1986;4:93–99.
16. Hodge JV, Smirk FH. The effect of drug treatment of hypertension on the distribution of death from various causes. *Am Heart J* 1967;73:441–452.
17. Dollery CT, Hartlet K, Bulpitt PF, Daymard M, Bulpitt CJ. Fifteen year survival of patients beginning treatment with Methyldopa between 1962 and 1966. *Hypertension* 1984;6(5, Pt II):ii-82–ii-86.
18. Isles CG, Walker LM, Beevers DG, Brown I, Cameron HL, Clarke J, Hawthorne V, Hole D, Lever AF, Robertson JWK, Wapshaw JA. Mortality in patients of the Glasgow Blood Pressure Clinic. *J Hypertens* 1986;4:141–156.
19. Medical Research Council Working Party. MRC Trial of Treatment of Mild Hypertension: principal results. *Br Med J* 1985;291:97–104.
20. Report by the Management Committee. The Australian Therapeutic Trial in Mild Hypertension. *Lancet* 1980;1:1261–1267.
21. Amery A, Brixko P, Clement D, de Schaepdryver A, Fagard R, Forte J, Henry JF, Leonetti G, O'Malley K, Strasser T, Birkenhager W, Bulpitt C, Deruyttere M, Dollery C, Forette F, Hamdy R, Joossens JV, Lund-Johansen P, Petrie J, Tuomilehto J, Williams B. Mortality and morbidity results from the European Working Party on High Blood Pressure in the Elderly Trial. *Lancet* 1985;1:1349–1354.
22. Helgeland A, Hjermann I, Leren P, Enger S, Holme I. High density lipoprotein cholesterol and antihypertensive drugs: the Oslo Study. *Br Med J* 1978;2:403.
23. Helgeland A, Hjermann I, Leren P. Possible metabolic side effects of beta-adrenergic blocking drugs. *Br Med J* 1978;1:828.
24. Norwegian Multicentre Study Group. Timolol-induced reduction in mortality and reinfarction in patients surviving acute myocardial infarction. *N Engl J Med* 1981;304:801–807.
25. Gordon T, Kannell WB. *The Framingham Study,* Section 30 (DHEW publication no NIH74-599). Washington, DC: US Government Printing Office, 1974.
26. Pooling Project Research Group. Relationship of blood pressure, serum cholesterol, smoking habits, relative weight and ECG abnormalities to incidence of major coronary events. Final report of the Pooling Project. *J Chron Dis* 1978;31:201–306.
27. Anderson TW. Re-examination of some of the Framingham blood pressure data. *Lancet* 1978;2:1139–1141.

28. Harris T, Cook EF, Kannel W, Schatzkin A, Goldman L. Blood pressure experience and risk of cardiovascular disease in the elderly. *Hypertension* 1987;7:118–123.

29. Woods JD. Relative ischaemia in the hypertrophied heart. *Lancet* 1961;1:696–698.

30. O'Keefe DD, Hoffman JIE, Cheitlin R, O'Neill MJ, Allard JR, Shapkin E. Coronary blood flow in experimental canine left ventricular hypertrophy. *Circ Res* 1978;43:43–51.

31. Pisani LM, Frank MJ, Carr AA, Von Dohlen TW, Abdullah AM. Editorial: How can we diagnose coronary heart disease in hypertensive patients? *Hypertension* 1987;10:467–472.

32. Frolich ED. Editorial: co-existence of hypertensive and coronary arterial disease. *Hypertension* 1987;10:473–475.

33. Stewart IMcDG. Relation of reduction in pressure to first myocardial infarction in patients receiving treatment for severe hypertension. *Lancet* 1979;1:861–865.

A. E. DOYLE (1923–1993)

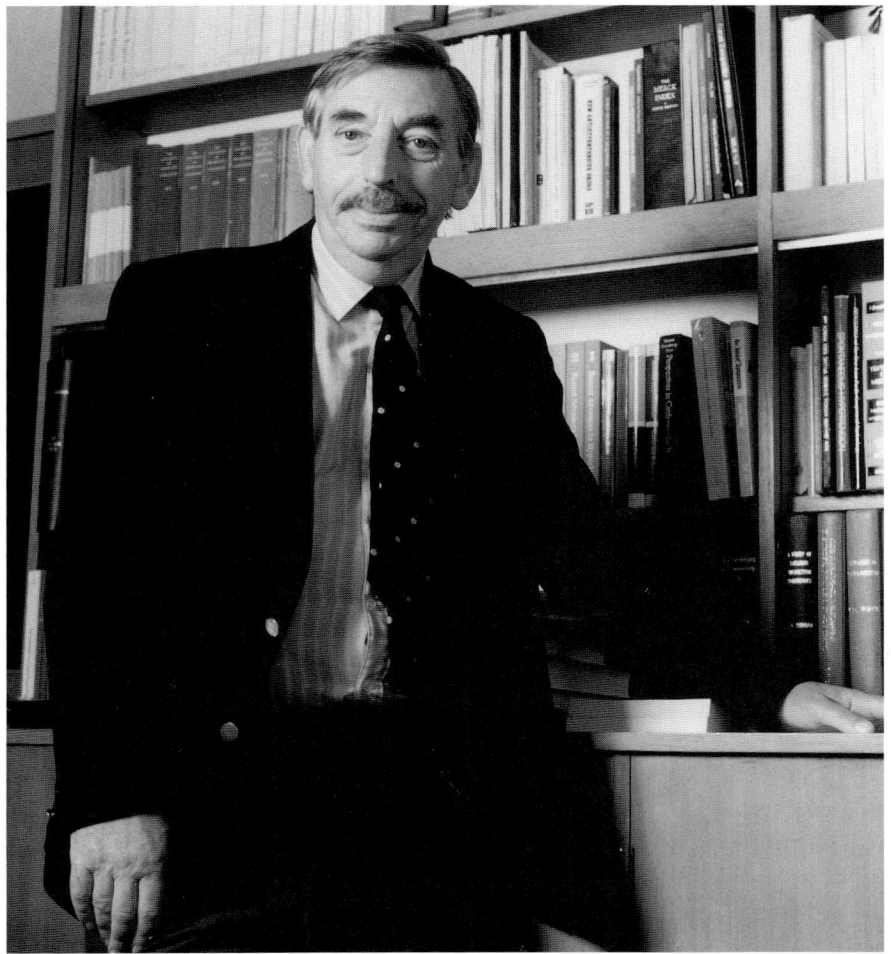

Austin Doyle was a pioneer researcher and clinician in hypertension. He was one of a small group who laid the foundations for the study of hypertension as an important specialty, with widespread public health implications. His life spanned the whole era of studying high blood pressure from seeing patients die within 12 months from malignant hypertension, through all the different classes of antihypertensive agents. Furthermore, because he was active throughout this period, he made significant contributions to many different areas including the pathophysiology and treatment of hypertension, to large scale clinical trials and epidemiology. In these days of intense specialization, this may seem enviable if not impossible, but few could have matched his protean and seminal contributions. In some ways he was iconoclastic and this is seen best in this chapter. He was always sceptical, quizzical, and critical but then again, always open to new ideas and always enthusiastic and positive. He especially questioned dogma and causality deduced from statistically and epidemiological associations. This chapter reflects those qualities and as he rightly points out the evidence directly linking hypertension and ischemic heart disease, although widely accepted, is by no means based on conclusive evidence. Unfortunately he will not be here to see these issues resolved.

Hypertension: Pathophysiology, Diagnosis, and Management, Second Edition, edited by J.H. Laragh and B.M. Brenner, Raven Press, Ltd., New York © 1995.

CHAPTER **5**

Familial Aggregation and Genetic Epidemiology of Blood Pressure

Ryk Ward

There is general agreement that the relatively high prevalence of hypertension (approximately 15 percent) in most developed societies exerts a significant impact on the risk of cardiovascular disease, renal disease, and stroke. Despite the pervasive distribution of this risk factor, the fundamental etiology of essential hypertension remains largely unknown. Since there is considerable evidence that risk of hypertension clusters in families, it becomes important to determine whether this is due to genetic factors and, if so, also to determine the magnitude of the genetic component. Although this issue has been a concern for the past half century, thus far the major advances in this field have revolved around the enhancement of statistical methodology to estimate relative genetic risk, rather than the identification of genetic traits that can be used to characterize the individual.

In large part, this continued emphasis on developing statistical tools reflects the fact that the molecular advances that have revolutionized our understanding of lipid profiles have not yet had a significant impact on the genetic analysis of blood pressure. In the absence of defined molecular markers, the unit of measure remains blood pressure itself, rather than any of the physiological intermediates that interact to yield the final phenotype. Since the basic observations have remained essentially unchanged for decades, a historical perspective of the development of analytic strategies is required in order to understand the contemporary position regarding the genetic etiology of hypertension. Consequently, this chapter will first review the various strategies that have been used to identify the genetic components of blood pressure, before evaluating some of the more recent methodological advances.

BLOOD PRESSURE AND THE NATURE–NURTURE CONTROVERSY

The first intimation that high blood pressure tends to cluster in families was indirect and stemmed from the eighteenth-century observation of Morgagni (1) that the father of a patient who had died of a cerebral hemorrhage had himself died of apoplexy. This gave rise to the speculation that certain families might contain a disproportionate number of individuals whose deaths were due to strokes. Although the connection between high blood pressure and risk of "apoplexy" was imperfectly un-

R. Ward: Department of Human Genetics, University of Utah, Salt Lake City, Utah 84132.

derstood at the time, Morgagni's observations (and those of later physicians) represent the first documented evidence that "hypertension" exhibited a distinct tendency to cluster within families.

Two centuries later, there is now abundant evidence to support the contention that high blood pressure aggregates more in certain families than in others. Building on a series of early population surveys, there is now general agreement that the familial aggregation of blood pressure is a general phenomenon that occurs throughout the entire blood pressure range in virtually all populations that have been studied (2,3). Irrespective of whether the probands are hypotensive, normotensive, or hypertensive, the blood pressures of their family relatives tend to be significantly more similar than expected by chance. There is somewhat less agreement as to whether the fundamental causes that underlie the familial resemblance of blood pressure are predominantly genetic or environmental (4). Furthermore, there is still considerable dispute about the most probable genetic mechanism that leads to the observed familial clustering of blood pressure, particularly with respect to the role played by genetic factors in the distribution of hypertension within and between families.

The heart of the problem revolves around two ineluctable facts: (a) Since family relatives share not only genes but also environments, there are practical difficulties in apportioning the relative contribution of shared environments due to cultural transmission versus genetically inherited backgrounds, and (b). Since blood pressure in general, and hypertension in particular, are complex traits in which the clinically defined phenotype can arise through a wide array of pathophysiological mechanisms (5), identification of the genetic causality of hypertension ideally requires a systematic evaluation of the physiological processes that underlie the clinical endpoint. Hence, the inability to establish experimental contrasts in human families, as well as the imprecision inherent in defining adequate assays for underlying physiological processes, represents a significant impediment with regard to defining causation.

However, the past decade has seen considerable progress on both fronts, so that there is now hope that the next decade will see a considerable resolution of the problem. On the one hand, there has been the development of statistical techniques (6) that, when applied to the analysis of the familial aggregation of blood pressure, allow identification of the relative magnitude of culturally transmitted lifestyle factors and genetic inheritance (7). There have also been significant advances in developing conceptual models that lead to effective strategies in determining the specific kind of genetic mechanism that influences the distribution of hypertension (8). When both of these strategies are then used to examine the distribution of specific physiological processes that are likely to be involved in hypertension, the results in-

dicate that it is now possible to determine the contribution that a single genetic locus makes to the distribution of hypertension in the population (9).

NATURE VERSUS NURTURE: CONTRASTS WITHIN POPULATIONS

Although the familial distribution of environmental factors, or *nurture,* has been touted as a possible explanation for the aggregation of blood pressure within families, there is no instance of a carefully conducted study that has unequivocally concluded that components of the family environment are more important than genetic relationships. In part, the failure to identify a series of culturally transmitted variables that exert a predominant influence on blood pressure clustering within families can be attributed to the lack of experimental control in human families and, hence, to the difficulty in discriminating between the influence of common genes and common environments. As noted below, there are only two study designs—adoption studies and twin studies—that represent a "quasi-experimental" approach to the discrimination of the two confounding factors. Other study designs rely on sophisticated statistical procedures to differentiate between the influence of genes and of family environments. However, the lack of conclusive evidence regarding the influence of the family environment on the familial aggregation of blood pressure also reflects the fact that a few family environmental variables have been identified that unambiguously elevate blood pressure.

Excessive weight, or obesity, is one familial factor that not only exhibits a tendency to aggregate in families but also has a marked influence on blood pressure. For more than 50 years, obesity has been shown to be perhaps the single most important "environmental" variable that influences the population distribution of adult blood pressure (10) and hypertension (11,12). In children, it appears that overall body size and growth rate may represent more important determinants of blood pressure but that after adolescence the most important determinant becomes relative weight. This change in the relationship between blood pressure and obesity may then result in a shift in the characteristic distribution of blood pressure with age, when adults are compared with children (7). Since obesity is also well known to cluster among families, it has been suggested that the familial clustering of blood pressure is merely the secondary consequence of this aggregation.

In this connection, it is relevant that a number of studies, especially those of adopted children, have indicated that the household environment has a marked influence on the distribution of relative weight (13,14). This observation would support the hypothesis that the familial aggregation of blood pressure is influenced by the immediate family environment, mediated by the distribution of relative obesity. However, in evaluating the relationship between the distribution of relative weight and familial aggregation of blood pressure, Kotchen (15) found that the familial aggregation of relative weight was insufficient to account for the familial aggregation of blood pressure. A more detailed study of the relationship between the familial clustering of weight and the aggregation of blood pressure in Muscatine, Iowa, concluded that 30 percent of the correlation of systolic blood pressure between young siblings was due to the aggregation of weight in these households (16). These results suggest that although the familial aggregation of obesity may enhance the aggregation of blood pressure, other factors also operate. Whereas the familial aggregation of obesity is, to some extent, a reflection of culturally transmitted dietary habits, there is increasing evidence that genetic factors also influence the distribution of obesity. In two independent studies of adopted children—one in Scandanavia (17) and one in the American Midwest (18)—the distribution of obesity in children was shown to be a function of the relative level of obesity of their natural parents, rather than of their adoptive parents. A more detailed study of the distribution of weight in a series of Canadian adoptive families also suggested that genetic transmission, in addition to shared family environments, has a significant influence on the distribution of relative weight (13). Hence, a substantial proportion of the familial aggregation of obesity now appears to be due to genetic factors. This, in turn, suggests that the genetic influence on the distribution of blood pressure may operate through a variety of mechanisms. With the recent demonstration that genetic factors may underlie differences in underlying metabolic rates (19,20), a plausible physiological mechanism now exists to suggest that some genes may influence both the familial clustering of obesity and the consequent familial aggregation of blood pressure.

Although a number of other factors that influence blood pressure also show some level of familial clustering, their effect on blood pressure tends to be less substantial than that of obesity. In addition, most of these factors are even less likely than obesity to be the product of culturally transmitted factors. Smoking habits and personality profile may have some influence on blood pressure aggregation within families, but there is little evidence of this. In upper-middle-class U.S. individuals, the amount of routine physical exercise seems to be inversely correlated with blood pressure (21). However, the familial resemblance in the amount of recreational exercise is more likely a reflection of learned values than of biological imperatives. Also, despite the marked influence of exercise on blood pressure levels, the *a priori* family clustering of blood pressure in this population still remains the most important predictor of hypertension (21). Hence, despite the familial aggregation of a large number of lifestyle factors that are potentially important

for the risk of elevated blood pressure (22), there is little evidence that culturally transmitted lifestyle factors are more important than underlying genetic factors in influencing the degree of familial aggregation of blood pressure.

NATURE VERSUS NURTURE: CONTRASTS BETWEEN POPULATIONS

An alternative approach to identifying the relative roles of genetic and environmental factors is to evaluate the distribution of blood pressure between genetically distinct groups. Somewhat paradoxically, the comparison of the distribution of blood pressure between different ethnic groups has tended to provide some of the strongest evidence for the influence of nongenetic, socioculturally derived environmental factors. Early in the first series of epidemiological characterizations of blood pressure within populations, it was realized that, unlike the situation in white populations of Europe or of the United States, essential hypertension was extremely rare in many African societies (23). However, the initial conclusion that these differences between genetically distinct groups were due to differences in genetic background was overturned by a number of subsequent studies of black populations in the United States. These studies indicated that the prevalence of hypertension in U.S. blacks was approximately double that of U.S. whites (24). Despite some claims that the two ethnic groups studied in the United States came from comparable socioeconomic backgrounds, subsequent evidence implicated environmental factors as the root cause of the different prevalence of hypertension between black and white populations. The classic studies of Scotch (25) convincingly demonstrated that for Zulu populations the composite factors that accompanied the change from a traditional lifestyle to the complexities of urban life were responsible for an increase in the prevalence of elevated blood pressure. A number of comprehensive surveys in Africa have indicated not only that there is considerable variation in the prevalence of hypertension throughout the continent (thereby arguing against an ethnically defined distribution of blood pressure), but also that this variability is readily explained by the relative degree of acculturation to a "Westernized" lifestyle. Thus, the prevalence of hypertension is lowest in populations that still retain some of the aspects of a traditional tribal society, whereas it is highest in those that have adopted an urbanized lifestyle with predominantly Western influences (26,27). Studies from many other regions of the world, especially the Pacific (28), have come to the same conclusion (29).

Identification of the specific environmental components that contribute to the difference between traditional societies and more Westernized communities has proved more difficult. An early investigation of the causes underlying the marked differences in the prevalence of hypertension in two Polynesian groups suggested that the different levels of salt intake, which were correlated with the varying levels of "Westernization," was the responsible factor (30). Subsequent studies on other traditional societies substantiated the view that the low salt intake frequently associated with such communities was a primary factor leading to the virtual absence of hypertension in many of these populations (31), with the most dramatic evidence coming from completely unacculturated Yanomama villages, where a virtual absence of dietary sodium is associated with extremely low levels of blood pressure (32).

However, whereas differential levels of salt use may contribute to the diversity of blood pressure levels between ethnically distinct populations, at least three other factors are likely to play an important role (29). They are: the distribution of obesity within the community (4,5,11,12); the relative level of physical activity (21); and the overall degree of psychological stress (25). Overall, it is probable that the characteristic distribution of blood pressure in unacculturated societies, compared with modern Westernized communities, is due to a fairly complex interaction between all four major "environmental factors." As a result, the difference extends not only to lower mean levels of blood pressure but also to the lack of an association of increasing blood pressure with age. As Epstein and Eckoff (33) noted, there is a consistent tendency for blood pressures to rise more steeply with age in those populations in which the average blood pressure levels are high—an observation that is more consistent with the cumulative effects of a series of complex interactions than with the action of a single environmental variable. Hence, the results of the varied studies that have attempted to identify the causes underlying the contrast in blood pressure distribution between distinct ethnic groups have found little evidence to support the hypothesis that the characteristic blood pressure distribution is a result of genetic differences rather than a result of the unique environmental features that characterize distinct ethnic groups (26,29).

An alternative approach to the issue of whether the major genetic differences between ethnic groups result in a different propensity for hypertension is to evaluate the influence of biological ancestry on the distribution of blood pressure in genetically admixed populations. This strategy, which uses genetic ancestry to define the relationship between genetic contrasts and levels of blood pressure, is the counterpart of the epidemiological strategy of studying migrant populations in order to identify the influence of major environmental contrasts. In an early study of this type, the distribution of diastolic blood pressure in 433 adult blacks in Rochester, New York, was evaluated with respect to the degree of an individual's level of African ancestry, estimated by informative genetic markers. After controlling for the effects of age, sex, and relative weight, a statistically significant regression was found between an individual's degree of African ancestry and their diastolic blood pressure. Each 10 percent increase in the proportion of African ancestry was associated with an approximate 2-mm Hg rise in diastolic pressure (34). However, since there was no control for socioeconomic factors, the authors cautioned against a too literal genetic interpretation.

A subsequent study carried out in inner-city Detroit used skin color as a surrogate measure of African ancestry and, in the context of no detectable socioeconomic effect, found a significant association between blood pressure and darker skin color (35,36). However, as noted by Tyroler and James (37), the relationship between skin color, socioeconomic variables, and psychosocial stress in urban North America is so pervasive that it seems unlikely that the Detroit study was able to eliminate these subtle influences. Other studies that attempted to find a relationship between skin color and blood pressure in southern blacks determined that any apparent relationship disappeared once socioeconomic factors were taken into account (38). The most recent study that evaluated the relationship between African ancestry, as determined by genetic markers and blood pressure, found no association in a relatively socially homogeneous Caribbean community (39). Hence, there is little substantive evidence to support the hypothesis that the presence of genetic differences between individuals of predominantly African ancestry and individuals of predominantly Caucasian ancestry has a marked influence on an underlying susceptibility to hypertension. Rather, in parallel with the studies on the contrast in blood pressure between ethnic groups, the studies of genetically admixed populations point to the pervasive effect of the sociocultural environment on the prevalence of hypertension, with little evidence that genetic heterogeneity plays a role.

The balance of data thus indicates that unlike the situation within a population group—where familial factors may account for as much as 20 to 40 percent of the variation in blood pressure (40) and where identifiable mendelian genes may account for up to 20 percent of hypertension (9)—the major differences between populations most probably reflect their characteristic distribution of environmental and lifestyle factors. The predominant factor influencing the characteristic—and sometimes dramatic (32)—differences in blood pressure distribution between ethnic groups appears to be the pervasive relationship between ethnicity and level of adherence to a highly Westernized lifestyle. In general, the transition to such a lifestyle is accompanied by complex changes in all four of the major risk factors (increase in dietary sodium, decrease in physical activity, increase in obesity, and increase in psychosocial stress) and a resulting change in blood pressure. Although one of these factors, obesity, is likely to have a genetic component (17–20), the influence of the other three factors tends to be socio-cultural rather than genetic. Hence, a fuller understanding of the influence of genetic factors on the distribution of hypertension requires a more comprehensive evaluation of the contribution made by genetic factors to the familial aggregation within populations.

EARLY STUDIES: ONE GENE OR MANY?

Despite the initial observations in the seventeenth and eighteenth centuries that the clinical features associated with high blood pressure tended to cluster within families, direct evidence for the familial aggregation of blood pressure was not established until the third and fourth decades of this century. Although the comparative recency of these observations was partly due to an imperfect appreciation of the relationship between elevated blood pressure and risk of significant cardiovascular disease, it was primarily due to the inability to obtain routine and reliable measurements of blood pressure in a noninvasive manner. The development of a succession of instruments for measuring blood pressure in the late nineteenth century was a necessary prerequisite for the establishment of familial aggregation of blood pressure in the twentieth century. Early in this century, the marriage of Riva-Rocci's inflatable pneumatic cuff to von Basch's sphygmomanometer yielded the basic mechanical apparatus for measuring blood pressure. At the same time, Korotkoff's categorization of arterial sounds represented a system for recording blood pressure values in a consistent and reproducible fashion. These developments presaged the survey of blood pressure in relatively large samples of individuals and set the stage for determining the distribution of blood pressure in relatives of individuals, selected either because they had hypertension or because they were representative of the general population.

Shortly after the development of these instruments, the increased clinical interest in blood pressure extended to an interest as to whether related individuals exhibited similar blood pressure values and, if so, whether a genetic explanation was likely. More than 65 years ago, one of the first systematic studies was carried out by Weitz (41). He attempted to identify the etiological factors associated with "hypertension" by evaluating the relatives of patients with high blood pressure and comparing them to age- and sex-matched controls. In a similar vein to Morgagni's observations 160 years previously, he found that the majority of patients with essential hypertension (77 percent of 82 patients) had a family history of excessive deaths due to heart disease or stroke, whereas this was not true for the controls (only 30 percent of 267 normotensive individuals had such a family history).

Weitz also measured blood pressure in 93 adult siblings of 42 hypertensive probands and found that they had elevated blood pressure as compared to 359 controls of similar age. Since he noticed that blood pressure rose with age, he then focused attention on the older siblings of hypertensive patients, under the supposition that older individuals would be more likely to exhibit the consequences of any underlying genetic liability. In this regard, Weitz's work foreshadowed the concept of age-dependent penetrance of genetic liability—now a routine component of modern genetic statistics. By combining information on blood pressure in living relatives with information about cause of death of dead relatives, he determined that approximately 50 percent of a small series of older siblings ($N = 58$) had hypertension (or had died from heart disease or stroke). This apparent 1:1 ratio was interpreted as evidence for the action of a single, dominantly inherited mendelian locus (41). Further support for the hypothesis of single dominant gene was adduced from the distribution of hypertension over three generations in this selected series of families.

Although a number of reports, all based on the clinical evaluation of the members of a single family, continued to be published in support of the concept that hypertension was due to the segregation at a single locus (42), an additional quarter of a century elapsed before the next systematic attempts to determine the genetic etiology of high blood pressure. By the mid-twentieth century it had become apparent that elevated blood pressure was a major risk factor for coronary heart disease and early mortality (43), and the causes of high blood pressure were sought with renewed vigor. In order to define the etiology of essential hypertension, Platt (44) utilized a strategy similar to that previously used by Weitz (41). After first identifying a series of patients with essential hypertension, he then evaluated the distribution of hypertension in their parents as compared to the parents of normotensive control patients. He established that 59 percent of the parents of hypertensive parents appeared to be hypertensive themselves, compared with only 26 percent of the parents of normotensive patients. Since he also found evidence of hypertension transmitted over three generations in a small number of families (4 of 54), he concluded—like Weitz before him—that essential hypertension was caused by the inheritance of a dominant gene (44).

During the same time, Sobye (45) conducted a more extensive study in which 2,023 relatives of 186 hypertensive probands were evaluated. When the distribution of hypertension in these relatives was compared to the distribution of hypertension in a series of age/sex-matched controls, the first-degree relatives of the hypertensive probands were found to exhibit a significant excess of hypertension: 61 percent of their parents and 23 percent of their siblings. Although no formal statistical analyses were performed, Sobye concluded that hypertension was inherited as a mendelian dominant, with a population frequency of 30 to 40 percent (45).

Although these early studies, and others like them, uniformly concluded that essential hypertension was due to a single mendelian gene (usually with dominant inheritance), two aspects of their study design weakened this conclusion. First, such studies focused almost exclusively on the distribution of hypertension among the relatives of highly selected hypertensive individuals. Second, cardiovascular death was frequently used as a surrogate for high blood pressure in the antecedent generations. Both features exacerbate the potential for ascertainment bias, and they lead to exaggerated estimates of the familial clustering of hypertension. Hence, the inference from such study designs is suspect and should be applied to the general population only with extreme caution. An alternative strategy is to evaluate the distribution of *measured* blood pressure within families that are representative of the general population.

An early application of such a strategy was Ayman's 1934 evaluation of the blood pressure distribution among 1,524 individuals belonging to 277 nuclear families (46). After defining hypertension as blood pressure above 140/80, he established that in families in which neither parent was hypertensive, 3.1 percent of the offspring had hypertension, compared to 28.3 percent of the offspring in whom one parent was hypertensive and 45.5 percent in whom both parents were hypertensive. Similarly, whereas 65.3 percent of the siblings of hypertensive probands were hypertensive, so too were 33.1 percent of the siblings of normotensive probands. Since these results were clearly incompatible with the segregation of a single dominant mendelian gene, they represented the first serious challenge to such a hypothesis.

Twenty years later, the research strategy of attempting to understand the inheritance of hypertension by evaluating the distribution of blood pressure within families with a defined relationship to the general population was finally realized in the classic "St. Mary's study" (47–49). This study, conducted by Hamilton, Pickering, and their associates, marked a significant advance in the genetic epidemiology of hypertension in four important respects. First, and perhaps most important, was the insistence on designing the study around the concept that hypertension was merely the quantitatively defined upper tail of a continuous distribution of blood pressure, rather than a qualitatively distinct attribute. Hence, blood pressure itself became the unit of observation, rather than some arbitrarily defined "hypertensive" phenotype. Since this is now the prevailing view, with essentially universal acceptance by clinicians, epidemiologists, and geneticists alike, it is nowadays difficult to comprehend the far-reaching significance of this important conceptual advance. As noted below, the final battle between the "mendelians" (espousing a single gene) and the "galtonians" (espousing many) was essentially decided on this issue.

Second, the investigators took pains to ensure not only that their sample of probands was large but also that their blood pressures could be related to the distribution of blood pressure in the general population. Third, they recognized that concomitant variables, such as age and sex, not only influenced blood pressure but were themselves nonrandomly distributed within families, leading to potential biases in estimation. Accordingly, instead of analyzing "raw blood pressure," they carried out their statistical analysis on values adjusted for the influence of age and sex. Fourth, they adopted the biometrical approach of quantitative genetics in order to define the relationship between the blood pressure of family relatives in standard statistical terms, thereby facilitating explicit hypothesis testing. The first three innovations of the St. Mary's study foreshadowed what has become the accepted practice in obtaining and transforming observations on blood pressure, preparatory to conducting genetic analyses. The fourth innovation, borrowed from the field of quantitative genetics, has also become a regular component of the genetic epidemiologist's armamentarium, albeit with an important difference: The etiological influence of a major mendelian locus is now assessed in conjunction with an assessment of the etiological influence of "polygenes."

Since the St. Mary's study anticipated so many of the subsequent developments in the area of genetic epidemiology, it is perhaps not surprising that their basic conclusions also remain intact. The study involved measuring (a) the blood pressure of 2,031 individuals representative of the population at large in order to define a representative distribution of blood pressure (47), (b) the blood pressure of 376 first-degree relatives of 109 probands whose diastolic pressures were above 100 mm Hg, and (c) the blood pressure of 373 relatives of probands whose diastolic pressures were below 85 mm Hg. The population distribution was used to define age- and sex-specific adjusted scores (48) (equivalent to today's z-scores), and the relationship between blood pressure of first-degree relatives was then evaluated by linear regression of the resulting scores (49). The results showed a uniform level of aggregation of blood pressure within families, defined by a regression coefficient of 0.22 for systolic pressure and 0.18 for diastolic pressure. The significant regressions occurred irrespective of whether the probands were hypertensive or normotensive. More specifically, after combining their data with Sobye's earlier study (45), Hamilton et al. (48,49) determined the overall correlation between siblings to be 0.24 for systolic pressure and 0.22 for diastolic pressure—values identical with those commonly accepted today (see Table 1). Based on these results, Hamilton et al. concluded that what was inherited was not "hypertension" *per se* but, rather, the "average" blood pressure value of an individual. Furthermore, they concluded that the inheritance of blood

TABLE 1. *Familial aggregation of blood pressure in adults: correlations of blood pressure in first-degree relatives (data from selected studies)*

Relationship	Population	Reference	N	Systolic	Diastolic
Mother–child	South Wales, UK	69	319	0.31	0.30
	Tecumseh, USA	70	1464	0.13	0.06
	Framingham, USA	71	1495	0.16	0.14
	Poland	72	183	0.28	0.15
	Taiwan	73	955	0.11	0.18
	Polynesian	7	535	0.14	0.16
Father–child	South Wales, UK	69	273	0.25	0.14
	Tecumseh, USA	70	1464	0.16	0.08
	Framingham, USA	71	1495	0.14	0.15
	Poland	72	183	0.02	0.13
	Taiwan	73	955	0.18	0.23
	Polynesian	7	425	0.21	0.17
Parent–offspring	South Wales, UK	69	538	0.24	0.16
	Tecumseh, USA	70	1066	0.12	0.12
	Evans Co., USA	74	545	0.13	0.14
Siblings	South Wales, UK	69	1088	0.30	0.25
	Tecumseh, USA	70	1232	0.17	0.12
	Framingham, USA	71	953	0.18	0.18
	Evans Co., USA	74	545	0.20	0.17
	Polynesian	7	1082	0.17	0.13

pressure resembled that of a continuously distributed quantitative character, such as height, rather than the inheritance of a discrete mendelian trait (49).

Hard on the heels of this seminal study, which overturned the tenets of the proponents for a single-gene etiology, came two comprehensive, population-based studies. The aim of these studies was to define the statistical relationship between blood pressure measurements within families selected to be representative of a defined community. Each focused on the distribution of blood pressure among all available relatives of randomly selected probands sampled from distinct Welsh communities. The first study, carried out in the mining village of Rhondda Fach (50,51), used a random 1:90 sample of the entire population over 5 years old to identify 250 probands representative of the community. Of the 1,005 relatives of these 250 probands who lived within a 25-mile radius, 978 (97 percent) were then sampled. The resulting distribution of blood pressures was then analyzed by the same strategy that had been employed by the St. Mary's study. Like the St. Mary's study, the regression of age-adjusted blood pressure was found to be (a) statistically significant (with a value of 0.24) and (b) essentially independent of both the proband's blood pressure and sex (50).

The subsequent study, conducted in the rural farming area of the Vale of Glamorgan, used the same strategy to identify 373 representative probands and their 1,267 first-degree relatives (52). Since the data from the Vale of Glamorgan were essentially identical to the data from the Rhondda Fach, the two data sets were combined into a single sample to give greater precision to the statistical estimates. After suitable adjustment, the regression for blood pressure scores of first-degree relatives of the probands was found to be 0.22 for systolic pressures and 0.18 for diastolic pressures. Furthermore, the results of a follow-up study in both communities, 4 years later, served to confirm the original findings and establish the uniformity of the familial aggregation of blood pressure over the entire range of the distribution (53).

In common with later studies, the analysis of the combined longitudinal data set for both communities indicated that siblings had higher correlations than did parent–offspring combinations and that same-sex siblings had higher correlations than unlike-sex siblings. The final overall regression was slightly higher than in the initial surveys, being 0.29 for systolic pressure and 0.22 for diastolic pressure, suggesting that polygenic genetic factors accounted for 33 percent and 22 percent of the population variability in systolic and diastolic pressure, respectively (53). These extensive epidemiological studies of the distribution of blood pressure, within and between families, gave the first conclusive evidence that blood pressure is inherited as a quantitative character in the population at large. Consequently, the familial clustering of hypertension was interpreted as an inevitable consequence of the combined influence of polygenic factors coupled with environmental factors.

In the meantime, the challenge to the mendelian interpretation of the familial clustering of hypertension did not go unnoticed. To counter the claims of Pickering's group, Platt (54) focused attention on hypertensive patients aged 45 to 59 years, to exclude cases of secondary hypertension, and combined his own observations with those of Sobye (45). However, instead of evaluating the distribution of blood pressure (or hypertension) within families, he chose to focus on the shape of the distribution of blood pressure measurements in siblings of the hypertensive probands. The resulting plot of the recorded blood pressure values was suggestive of an "antimode" at 150 mm Hg for systolic values and 90 mm Hg for diastolic values. This apparent partition of the distribution into two components was interpreted to imply that the siblings of the hypertensive probands fell into two distinct groups: a normotensive group with pressure below 150/90 mm Hg and a hypertensive group with pressures above 150/90 mm Hg. Since the two groups were represented in roughly equal proportions, this result was taken as (a) refutation of Pickering's conclusions and (b) confirmation of the segregation of two distinct mendelian traits for blood pressure, with the 1:1 ratio implying dominance of the hypertensive trait.

The resulting controversy simmered for almost a decade, with little modification of their different interpretations by the two chief protagonists—right up to the final, back-to-back publication of their opposing viewpoints (55,56). Unfortunately, since the bulk of the attention was directed toward the shape of the blood pressure distribution in selected groups of relatives, rather than toward a critical examination of the distribution of blood pressure values within families, there was little hope of a definitive test of hypothesis to resolve the issue. In rejoinder to Platt, Oldham et al. (57) pointed out that the apparent bimodal nature of his distribution could be accounted for by failure to adjust for age-related changes in blood pressure, with older siblings falling to the right of the "antimode" and younger sibs falling to the left. The existence of digit preference in recording blood pressures was also felt to be a contributory factor. A further study by Platt (58) complicated the picture because he felt that the distribution of blood pressure in 238 siblings of hypertensive probands now gave evidence for a trimodal distribution—the leftmost mode corresponding to normotensive homozygotes, the middle mode corresponding to heterozygotes with borderline hypertension, and the rightmost mode representing homozygous hypertensives. It was left to Murphy (59) to clarify the situation by using simulated data sets to show conclusively that small samples drawn from a unimodal distribution were inherently likely to display all irregularities and, even more convincingly, that no definitive genetic conclusions could be derived from analyses that were restricted to an evaluation of the population distribution of blood pressure values (60).

Although the controversy slowly yielded to the more genetically oriented analyses of the distribution of blood pressure within families, it is clear that, in many respects, the last word belongs to Pickering (42,61). Despite all attempts to identify discontinuities in the distribution of blood pressure, the evidence is overwhelming that the population distribution of blood pressure is continuous and unimodal. Over the past 60 years, a succession of surveys (10,50–52,62,63) has led to the following general conclusions concerning the population distribution of blood pressure: (a) There is no obvious discontinuity in blood pressure distribution, irrespective of the age or sex of the population under study (47–49,50–53,61); (b) In the majority of populations investigated, there is a marked tendency for blood pressure to rise with age (64)—the only exceptions being a scattering of traditional societies, in which mean blood pressure is remarkably low by Western standards (33); (c) The rate of increase of blood pressure with age tends to follow a characteristic distribution for each sex—being steeper for males in early adulthood until late middle age, when the rise with age becomes steeper for females (42,52,64); (d) The age-related rise of blood pressure in children tends to exhibit a distinct slope compared to that in adults (65), and this difference in slope is especially marked in traditional populations where mean blood pressure is low; furthermore, the rise of adult pressures by age is small (7); (e) As the mean level of blood pressure increases with advancing age, there is also a concomitant increase in the dispersion of blood pressures near the age-specific mean (47–49,63), so that the variance is dependent on the age-specific mean; and (f) The continuous frequency curves for blood pressure deviate (in a subtle, but important, way) from the standard "gaussian" curve by being "tail heavy"—especially the upper tail of the distribution (66).

The importance of the statistical characteristics of blood pressure revealed by these early studies is twofold. First, as a number of workers have emphasized (56,59,61,66), deviations from gaussian expectation cannot be used to infer the mode of inheritance of blood pressure. This is especially true for relatively small samples ($N < 1,000$), where any number of perturbations can arise (59). The misplaced focus on the shape of the blood pressure distribution served to prolong the controversy between Pickering and Platt, because it diverted attention from the essential requirement for testing genetic hypotheses—namely, a statistical evaluation of the distribution of blood pressure *within* families. Not only is it extremely difficult to obtain rigorous statistical evidence to support the contention of multimodality due to an underlying mixture of distributions, but the presence, or lack thereof, of multiple modes does not represent an adequate test of *any* genetic hypothesis.

Second, in order to conduct any meaningful genetic analyses of the familial aggregation of blood pressure, the "raw" blood pressure measurements must first be adjusted to remove the potentially confounding effects of age, sex, obesity, and other concomitants that are likely to be nonrandomly distributed in families. Despite the clear demonstration of the importance of this principle, 35 years ago, by the St. Mary's study (47–49) and the subsequent Welsh studies (50–53), there still remains a surprising lack of appreciation for this essential principle as well as for the means of achieving it. Since the majority of genetic studies deal, perforce, with relatively small numbers of independent individuals, application of regression techniques across the entire sample—as if there were a homogeneous linear relationship—can lead to inappropriate results. A better strategy is to adjust separately for the characteristic means and variances of each major category of the relevant concomitants (7)—which is essentially the strategy initially devised by Fraser Roberts (48).

It should be stressed that both of these caveats apply with equal force to the interpretation of the genetic basis of "intermediate phenotypes" (8). In particular, the misplaced focus on the shape of the population distribution continues to surface in a slightly altered guise to confound the genetic interpretation of the distribution of those physiological processes that are potentially implicated in the pathogenesis of hypertension. Hence, considerable caution should be exercised before interpreting any deviation in the shape of the population frequency distribution from the gaussian standard, as evidence for single gene inheritance. Increased sophistication of statistical models designed to identify mixtures of distributions do not by themselves overcome the inherent pitfalls of inferring genetic causality from the "non-normal" distribution of a complex trait. The problem will only be exacerbated by inadequate sample sizes and by failure to adjust for concomitants. For an adequate test of any hypothesis of genetic etiology—mendelian or nonmendelian—it is mandatory that the distribution of the trait within families be evaluated by the appropriate genetic model. This strategy remains the *sine qua non* for identifying underlying genetic etiology.

EXTENT OF FAMILIAL AGGREGATION OF BLOOD PRESSURE

The increasing acceptance of Pickering's concept that the distribution of blood pressure was both continuous and unimodal, with the physiological state of hypertension being represented by the upper tail of this distribution, sparked an increased interest in establishing the extent of the familial aggregation of blood pressure in a variety of populations. Whereas some of the early surveys merely attempted to replicate aspects of the St. Mary's study (67), others focused on a more critical evaluation of the distribution of familial aggregation. One important issue was whether a completely different ethnic group, examined in a "non-European" environment, would display the same level of familial aggregation of blood pressure that had been observed in the various British studies. An early attempt to address this issue established that the level of familial aggregation among

black Jamaicans was essentially identical to that observed in Great Britain (68). Like the previous studies, this analysis found the regression of blood pressure among first-degree relatives to be 0.19 and 0.18 for systolic and diastolic pressure, respectively (68). Hence, the overall familial resemblance in blood pressure appeared to be consistent across major differences in genetic background and environments—a conclusion that was subsequently verified by a number of other studies (see Table 1).

With the recognition that the average relationship between first-degree relatives could be defined in terms of a regression coefficient of approximately 0.2, and that roughly 20 to 40 percent of the population variability in blood pressure was due to genetic factors, attention turned to an evaluation of the specific distribution of correlations between different types of family relatives. The Welsh study had indicated that siblings tended to resemble each other to a greater extent than children resembled their parents (53,69) and that there appeared to be differences in parent-offspring resemblance, depending on the sex of parent and child. Since there was clearly a substantial environmental component influencing the distribution of blood pressure, these patterns in the distribution of familial correlations were potentially informative in identifying the extent to which shared environments played a role. Accordingly, a substantial emphasis was placed on defining the correlations in blood pressure between different relatives—a feature that would subsequently allow a more specific estimation of the differing contributions of genetic and environmental factors by the method of path analysis (6).

Other issues that required resolution included the following: (a) At what age was the familial resemblance manifested? and (b) Did cohabitation in the same household exert a significant impact on the magnitude of the correlation? Since the number of separate correlations that required estimation increased substantially once the nuclear family was subdivided into all combinations of generation–sex-specific pairwise relationships, the overall sample size also had to increase substantially. For this reason, the initial results concerning the distribution of specific correlations were constrained to the two major community surveys in the United States—Tecumseh (70) and Framingham (71)—plus the early Welsh survey. However, a large number of additional surveys were rapidly initiated, leading to a substantial degree of information regarding the distribution of familial aggregation of blood pressure within the nuclear family in a variety of populations. These results are briefly reviewed below.

Familial Aggregation in Adults

Subsequent to the seminal British studies, the aggregation of blood pressure defined by two large community surveys in the United States (70,71) was found to be somewhat lower, though still statistically significant (Table 1). As data accumulated from other studies in such diverse populations as Poland (72), Taiwan (73), and Tokelau (7), it became clear that the majority of results were consistent with the Framingham and Tecumseh studies, and hence somewhat lower than the estimates from Wales. This was also true for an epidemiological survey carried out in the southern United States (74). Although it is not entirely clear why the majority of studies tend to yield lower correlations than those of the Welsh study, irrespective of ethnic group or environment, a likely possibility relates the partial elimination of temporal variability in the Welsh data. Since temporal variability has been estimated to account for 15 to 40 percent of the population variability in blood pressure (2), the fact that the familial correlations in the Welsh data were based on the average values of longitudinal data would tend to result in higher values as compared to those of the other studies, which were mostly conducted at a single point in time.

One problem in comparing the results from different studies is that the extent of adjustment often varies widely from one study to the next, and this will have a corresponding impact on the variability between studies. As demonstrated in the original British studies (49,52), failure to adjust for age and sex can lead to an appreciable diminution of the resulting correlations. However, the direction of change is quite dependent on the demographic composition of the population (7), whereas addition of other concomitants to the adjustment procedure also exerts a substantial effect (7,13,16). In addition, when the relationship between the concomitants and blood pressure is nonlinear—which is frequently the case (7,48,50,52,65)—use of the "z-score" approach will yield different results than those obtained by the use of linear regression. Hence, given the diversity of adjustment procedures, it is quite remarkable that the values in Table 1 are so similar.

In addition to the consistency of familial aggregation across diverse ethnic groups living in distinct ecosystems, it is also notable that the familial aggregation of blood pressure in adults is remarkably stable over time. Although this point was specifically evaluated in the early Welsh study (53,69), the data from Framingham are striking in that 25 years elapsed between the blood pressure measurement of parent and offspring. Despite that gap, the familial correlations from Framingham are not significantly lower than those from the other studies. Similarly, 609 pairs of adult siblings were followed for 16 years in Framingham, and the correlations remained essentially constant despite the fact they were living in different households and had different spouses, different diets, and different lifestyles (4,71). A similar degree of temporal stability in correlations is also found in other

studies and tends to reinforce the concept that genetic factors are at least partly responsible for the observed levels of familial aggregation.

Last, the pattern of correlations has been examined in some detail to try to identify the action of specific environmental factors. As already noted, with regard to blood pressure values, the resemblance between adult siblings tends to be greater than the resemblance between parent and child. This could reflect a residual aging effect or the fact that parents and offspring never share their environment to the same extent as siblings. Within a sibship, sex appears largely irrelevant, once the appropriate adjustment is made. In the main, this is also true for parent–offspring relationships (Table 1), though some investigators have reported the virtual absence of any correlation between father and offspring and have interpreted this in terms of a maternal effect (75). Overall, there is very little evidence for the existence of a strong maternal effect in adults.

The fact that correlations between spouse pairs is essentially negative (2,7,70,74,76) indicates that the influence of the household environment exerts only a minimal effect on blood pressure variability once adulthood is attained. The same observation extends to other types of unrelated inlaws (2). In addition, apart from a small number of exceptions, the length of time the spouses have cohabited appears not to have a significant influence on the magnitude of their correlation in blood pressure. Collectively, the various observations on the familial aggregation of blood pressure among different types of adult relatives are consistent with the hypothesis that once adulthood is reached, the household environment plays only a minimal role because (a) siblings living apart do not become appreciably dissimilar and (b) spouses living together do not become appreciably more similar. This, in turn, implies that the establishment of familial aggregation occurs relatively early in life and that an analysis of family resemblance in children and infants is likely to give a more detailed perspective on the origins of blood pressure aggregation.

Familial Aggregation in Children

Although there have been only a small number of studies investigating the familial aggregation of blood pressure, this is an important area of research for two reasons. First, since the etiology of hypertension begins several years before its clinical manifestation it is important to identify the factors that are likely to have an early influence on the distribution of blood pressure (77). Second, the temporal stability of familial aggregation of blood pressure that is observed in adults, in conjunction with the observation that the immediate household environment has little influence on the magnitude of the aggregation, indicates that the genesis of resemblance in blood pressure begins early in life. As a corollary, if familial aggregation of blood pressure does begin early in life, this information can be used to identify "high-risk" families in which a high proportion of individuals are predisposed to develop hypertension.

The onset of information about the aggregation of blood pressure in children began with a follow-up study of children born in the Boston City Hospital between 1956 and 1970 (78). The distribution of blood pressure in a total of 721 children belonging to 190 mothers was evaluated and, after adjustment for the influence of age and sex, significant familial aggregation was found in the 12- to 14-year-old children. The sibship correlations, which were 0.34 for systolic pressures and 0.32 for diastolic pressures, were somewhat higher than the correlations reported for adult siblings (Table 2). However, the maternal–offspring regression (0.16 for systolic pressure and 0.19 for diastolic pressure) was exactly equivalent to the majority of results reported for the correlations between mothers and their adult offspring.

This set of families was subsequently followed at intervals of 4 and 8 years, and the correlations between mother and child, and between siblings, were found to be essentially identical to the initial results (77). Hence, familial aggregation appears to be as stable throughout childhood as it is in adulthood. This study also included the additional observation that measurements of urinary kallikrein in children and in their parents also showed significant family aggregation. Thus it is apparent not only that the familial resemblance of blood pressure begins early in childhood but also that the physiological processes associated with high blood pressure tend to exhibit significant familial aggregation at an early age.

Other studies have served to verify this initial result (see Table 2). An evaluation of 491 families in London (79) indicated that children had a sibship correlation of

0.29 for systolic pressure and a mother–child correlation of 0.18. The resemblance between father and child was also significant (correlations ranging from 0.17 to 0.29), lending weight to the concept that genetic factors are likely to underlie the observed correlations. Similarly, an evaluation of the familial resemblance of blood pressure in Tokelau children, living in their traditional atoll environment, indicated significant familial resemblance (80). The Tokelau study also allowed an assessment of whether the familial aggregation of blood pressure in children was demonstrably different from the aggregation in adults belonging to the same population. As comparison of the relevant data in Tables 1 and 2 indicates, the values are virtually identical. Hence, the analysis of blood pressure distribution in this isolated Polynesian community indicates that the joint influence of genes and the "family environment" acts early in childhood— by age 5—to yield significant familial aggregation of blood pressure and is remarkably stable thereafter.

With the demonstration that blood pressure clusters in childhood, it was natural to extend these investigations into infancy. An evaluation of the relationship between the longitudinal blood pressure distribution in children of hypertensive mothers suggested that familial resemblance started early in infancy. A more extensive study evaluated the blood pressure of babies within a few days after delivery, using an ultrasonic device, as well as of their parents (81). Although the mother–infant correlations were low (0.10), they were statistically significant. In a separate study, significant sibship aggregation was found by 1 month of age (82).

A more extensive investigation involved the evaluation of 1,326 newborn infants and their mothers and conclusively demonstrated that the infant's blood pressure is correlated with the mother's blood pressure at birth (83). However, the correlation between father's blood pressure and the infant's blood pressure did not

TABLE 2. *Familial aggregation of blood pressure in children and infants: correlations of blood pressure with mothers and siblings (data from selected studies)*

Relationship	Population	Reference	N	Systolic	Diastolic
		Children (>2 years)			
Mother–child	New England, USA	78	190	0.16	0.19
	London, UK	79	491	0.18	—
	Polynesian	7	410	0.23	0.21
Sibling	New England, USA	78	190	0.34	0.32
	London, UK	79	491	0.29	—
	Polynesian	7	616	0.14	0.16
		Infants (<2 years)			
Mother–child	New England, USA	81	257	0.09	0.13
	New England, USA	82	730	0.14	0.17
Sibling	New England, USA	83	43	0.21	0.17
	New England, USA	82	554	0.17	0.27

become statistically significant until the infant was 1 month old. This suggests that maternal factors predominate in the first few days/weeks of life, with the full impact of genetic factors and the household environment not being manifest until 1 month or later.

Despite a small number of studies that failed to find a significant aggregation of blood pressure between mother and newborn infant (77), it seems clear that the tendency for familial resemblance in blood pressure starts virtually at birth, or soon thereafter, and is then maintained throughout the rest of life. Hence, a full understanding of the physiological interactions leading to hypertension in adulthood, and identifying their genetic and environmental components, is likely to require a more intensive evaluation of blood pressure and its concomitants than has hitherto been the case. Although the extensive evidence for the initiation of familial clustering of blood pressure early in life, as well as for its subsequent stability, suggests the operation of genetic factors, a more extensive statistical analysis is required in order to test this hypothesis. The mere existence of familial correlations is not sufficient to allocate the relative influence of genetic and familial environments. To accomplish this, the statistical procedures outlined in the following section are required.

PARTITIONING THE RELATIVE CONTRIBUTION OF GENES AND ENVIRONMENTS: PATH ANALYSIS

Since the familial aggregation of blood pressure is both ubiquitous (occurs in all ethnic groups in diverse environments) and consistent (stable over space and time), the challenge is to identify the causal factors behind the phenomenon. Genetic factors remain the prime candidates because of the consistency and stability of familial aggregation, but the influence of the culturally transmitted family environment may also play an important role. This is particularly true if familial background results in a significant correlation of relative weight within families because the familial aggregation of weight has been estimated to account for up to a third of the familial aggregation of blood pressure (16). The essence of the problem is to discriminate between these two factors, which are so inextricably confounded in most populations.

One strategy for partitioning out the relative influence of genetic and culturally transmitted factors is to adopt an experimental approach in which genetic contrasts are manipulated independently of contrasts involving family background. Apart from the quasi-experimental design of twin studies or adoption studies as discussed below, the approach is not feasible in our species. An alternative approach is to devise a statistical approach to estimate the relative contribution of genetic and familial factors to blood pressure aggregation by evaluating the

pattern of correlations within a nuclear family, or a similar set of relationships.

Although a number of statistical methods have been developed to achieve this aim, all are predicated on the same concept: Within a cluster of related individuals (such as a nuclear family) and without invoking too many restrictive assumptions, the pattern of genetic correlations has a simple and predictable structure. Significant deviations from the genetically predicted correlational structure can be attributed to the influence of socioculturally transmitted factors, and the pattern of the deviations gives some inference about the type of sociocultural factor (e.g., maternal effect, common sibship effect, etc.). Hence, in order to partition out the relative contribution of genetic factors and sociocultural factors to the familial aggregation of blood pressure, the entire set of correlations for each type of relationship must first be defined. The resulting suite of correlations is then used as the basis for estimating the underlying genetic influences.

Since the estimated correlations themselves form the basis for the next round of estimation, it is important that their values not be distorted by the influence of family structure or of other uncontrolled vagaries of study design. In general, the estimation of familial correlations is complicated by the fact that the correlations between different family members are themselves correlated. In addition, for estimating parent–offspring interclass correlations, the influence of multiple offspring on the estimate has to be considered (84), and the intraclass correlation that defines sibship resemblance has to take account of the parental contribution (85). Since most nuclear families in an epidemiological sample will tend to have a variable number of children in the survey, the resulting unbalanced design can also complicate the issue of testing hypotheses (86). The most effective approach requires the use of an "ensemble" estimate that incorporates a weighing scheme to remove the potential problems caused by different types of family structure (87). Failure to carry out these procedures can result in unstable estimates of the individual familial correlations and a distortion of the true correlational structure. This, in turn, can lead to inappropriate estimates of the relative contribution made by genetic factors.

An early application of the strategy of evaluating the distribution of resemblance among sets of relatives who shared a defined proportion of genes in common was the innovative "family set" approach of Schull et al. (88). In this study design, a linear model approach was used to contrast (a) the resemblance between an individual and two biological relatives (a sibling and a cousin) with (b) the resemblance between the individual and two unrelated individuals (spouse and a random control). The distribution of relationships within and between households allowed estimation of the influence of (a) the immediate-family environment, (b) the "neighborhood" environment, and (c) the underlying genetic factors (88). However, when this approach was carried out in a detailed study of blacks and whites living in high- and low-stress environments of Detroit, the resulting estimates suggested that genetic factors were relatively unimportant (89). Instead, it appeared that blood pressure variability in both populations was primarily influenced by unidentifiable environmental factors. This finding, which was at variance with the accepted role for genetic factors (90), now appears to be due to stratification of the data into subsamples (which precluded rejection of the null hypothesis) rather than to a flaw in the study design. As noted below, a reanalysis of the data yields estimates that are consistent with other studies and reaffirms the general utility of the family set approach.

A somewhat different strategy emphasizes the analysis of the pattern of correlations within a nuclear family (or similar unit) by path analytic procedures (6), as compared to the more explicit contrasts embodied in the family set approach (88). The path analysis procedure developed by Morton and colleagues (6) is based on the concept that the expected value of every observed correlation can be defined in terms of the underlying factors presumed to influence familial resemblance. The relationship is specified as a function of the partial regression coefficients that result when blood pressure is regressed on the underlying factors. The squares of these coefficients then specify the relative contribution of that factor to the population variability of blood pressure. The addition of an "environmental index," defined by the re-

gression of blood pressure on concomitants such as obesity, allows identification of specific sociocultural factors in addition to genetic factors (6).

In path analysis, the first step requires the formulation of the underlying model of causation because this consequently defines the set of functions for the expected correlations. An example of a causal model is displayed in Fig. 1, with the sociocultural influences of parents on their children defined separately by sex (7). In the diagram, the squares represent observed variables, whereas the circles represent the underlying causal factors. Hence, P refers to the observed blood pressure, and I represents the "environmental index"; C and G refer, respectively, to the underlying sociocultural and genetic factors that influence blood pressure. The subscripts F, M, D_1, D_2, S_1, and S_2 refer, respectively, to father, mother, daughters, and sons. The arrows in the diagram refer to the paths of causation that act to influence blood pressure, with the labels referring to the partial regression coefficients that are estimated from the data. The determination of blood pressure is through a genetic component (with coefficients h_P in parents and h_O in offspring) and a sociocultural component (with coefficients c_P in parents and c_O in offspring). The relationships between the underlying causal factors are defined either in terms of correlations represented by double-headed arrows for the sociocultural correlations between spouses (u), brother (v_S), sisters (v_D), and brothers and sisters (w) or in terms of the determining factors. Here f_{FD}, f_{FS}, f_{MD}, and f_{MS} represent the sociocultural transmission of father to daughter, father to son, mother to daughter, and

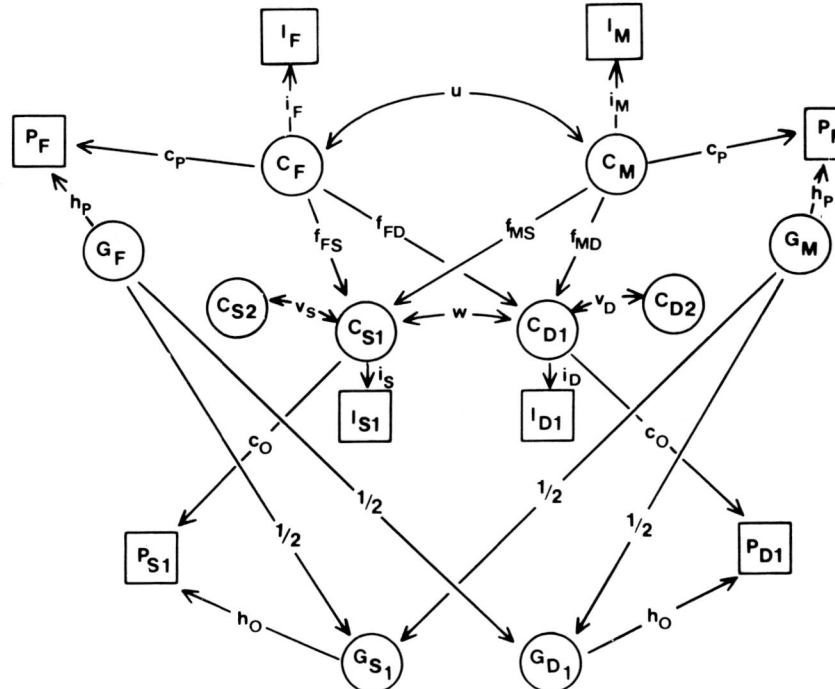

FIG. 1. Path diagram depicting causal factors likely to influence the distribution of blood pressure in nuclear families. P and I refer to blood pressure and the environmental index (obtained by regression on the familially distributed concomitants), respectively—both being directly observable. C and G refer to the underlying, and inherently unobservable, sociocultural and genetic factors that influence blood pressure. The influence of these underlying factors is estimated by the coefficients of determination, c and h—which act as indicated by the arrows in the diagram. The subscripts F, M, D, and S refer, respectively, to father, mother, daughter, and son. For further details see text.

mother to son, respectively; finally, genetic transmission is defined by the $\frac{1}{2}$, as is characteristic of mendelian segregation.

The path diagram can be used to define the expected correlation between any individual in terms of the underlying causal determinants. Thus the expected correlation between the blood pressure of mother and daughter—$r(P_M, P_D)$—is defined to be equal to $h_P \cdot (\frac{1}{2}) \cdot h_O + c_P \cdot r_{MD} \cdot c_O$, where $r_{MD} = f_{MD} + f_{FD} \cdot u$. This strategy results in establishing a set of equations for each of the possible correlations. The simultaneous solution of this equation set then gives the appropriate estimates of the coefficient of determination. Specific hypotheses can then be tested by setting one, or more, of the coefficients equal to a predefined value and comparing the likelihood of the two models. Thus the null hypothesis that the familial aggregation is not caused by genetic factors is tested by setting $h_P = h_O = 0$.

As indicated in Table 3, this strategy has been applied to a variety of populations, with the consistent result that genetic factors are estimated to be of primary importance in influencing the familial aggregation of both systolic and diastolic blood pressure. One of the first such studies differed from the model outlined in Fig. 1 in that the contrast was afforded by evaluating the correlations between half sibs versus full sibs in school children examined during the Bogalusa epidemiological survey (91). In such a study design, no direct estimate of sociocultural transmission is possible, leading to the relatively high composite estimate for genetic heritability shown in Table 3. It should be noted that although the estimates for systolic pressures were identical for blacks and whites, the influence of genetic factors on diastolic pressure appeared to be more important in whites than in blacks.

The successive studies on Japanese-Americans (92) and Brazilians (93) were based on complete nuclear families and thus provided more reliable estimates of sociocultural transmission. As indicated by the data in Table 3, derived from a reanalysis of both studies (94), the genetic heritability of blood pressure in the relatively old Japanese-American sample appears to be less important than in the younger Brazilian families, with a corre-

sponding reversal for sociocultural factors. Hence, the Brazilian data, in conjunction with the Bogalusa data, supported the concept that sociocultural transmission might be relatively unimportant in younger families. A more direct evaluation of the relationship between age of children and importance of sociocultural factors was afforded by the Tokelau study, in which both juvenile families and adult families were studied in the same community (7). That study also offered the opportunity to evaluate families living in two distinct environments—the traditional environment of Tokelau (where blood pressures were low) and the relatively urbanized environment of New Zealand (where blood pressures were higher) (95). As indicated in Table 3, the major change in environments was not associated with a substantial shift in the relative contribution of sociocultural factors to blood pressure variability (96). Also, the estimates of overall influence of sociocultural factors derived from juvenile families were similar to those derived from adult families, though the pattern of transmission was different by family type (96). These results are consistent with the evidence from cross-cultural comparisons that neither major shifts in environmental factors nor differences in genetic background exert a significant influence on the relative contribution of genetic factors to blood pressure variability within populations (29).

As noted above, the initial analysis of the Detroit data by the "family set" method suggested that genetic factors were unimportant. However, a reanalysis of the same data set by maximum likelihood techniques, as well as by the family set procedure, yielded the results shown in Table 3, which are now consistent with other studies (97). The determination of significant estimates for genetic heritability in the Detroit study was largely influenced by the increase in statistical power when the data were agglomerated instead of being stratified into small subsamples. Hence the family set approach will yield valid estimates of the influence of genetic factors, provided that the data sets are reasonably homogeneous. Finally, a reanalysis of the original Tecumseh data (70) using a path analytic approach also gave results consistent with the other studies (98).

TABLE 3. *Estimates of genetic heritability and of the influence of culturally transmitted factors on blood pressure distribution, in a series of populations*

Population	Reference	Genetic heritability		Cultural transmission	
		Systolic	Diastolic	Systolic	Diastolic
Children, USA	91	43.0%	24.0%	0.0%	0.0%
Japanese-American	92	24.4%	14.7%	15.6%	12.8%
Brazilian	93	30.6%	34.6%	4.2%	0.8%
Nonmigrant, Tokelau	96	21.9%	38.7%	22.0%	18.6%
Migrant, Tokelau	96	34.4%	36.4%	23.6%	17.3%
Whites, Detroit	97	32.0%	23.0%	28.6%	32.7%
Blacks, Detroit	97	13.0%	28.5%	5.2%	8.8%
Tecumseh	98	41.7%	30.1%	16.7%	15.2%

Overall, it is clear not only that is there considerable consistency between populations in the degree of familial aggregation of blood pressure (99) but also that a more vigorous analysis of the familial correlations yields remarkably similar estimates of genetic heritability. Although there are a small number of outliers, the overall contribution of genetic factors to the population variability of blood pressure is approximately 30 percent—a value very close to that originally estimated by the early British studies (49–53). By contrast, there is evidence for some variability in the influence of sociocultural factors, which may partly be attributable to differences in study design and statistical analysis. Additional information about the factors influencing blood pressure variability is derived from "quasi-experimental" studies as well as from more focused studies of the physiological components of hypertension (8,9).

QUASI-EXPERIMENTAL DESIGNS: ADOPTION STUDIES AND TWIN STUDIES

As opposed to the indirect strategy of evaluating the distribution of familial aggregation of blood pressure and then using complex statistical procedures to partition out the influence of genetic and culturally transmitted variables, there are two types of family structures—namely, adoptions and twins—that lend themselves to a more direct assessment of the relative role played by genes and environment. In both cases, the specific family structure can be viewed as a single "quasi-experimental" contrast—either genetic or environmental. Studies of adoptive families can be set up to provide an informative environmental contrast in addition to a simple genetic contrast. This requires evaluating both the natural parents and the adoptive parents of the adopted child. Although such a study design has not been accomplished for blood pressure, it has been accomplished for evaluating the relative influence of environmental factors and genetic factors on obesity (17,18). A reduced design is also possible for adoptive families in which the blood pressures of the adopted children are contrasted solely with the distribution of blood pressure in the other members of their adoptive families. As noted below, this reduced design has proved extremely informative as a way of identifying the influence of the common household environment on the distribution of both blood pressure and relative weight (13,14).

Twin studies can be viewed as the converse of adoption studies in that the "quasi-experimental" contrast tends to be genetic rather than environmental. However, the fundamental assumption of the genetic contrast between monozygous twins, who share 100 percent of their genes, and dizygous twins, who share only half their genes, is that the distribution of environmental factors is equivalent for both sets of twins. This assumption is rarely justified. Apart from the fact that the pairs of monozygous twins and dizygous twins are virtually never evaluated when living in the same household, there is considerable evidence to suggest that monozygous twins are exposed to a more uniform family environment than are dizygous twins. Hence, the distribution of genetic correlations tends to be confounded with the distribution of environmental effects. This problem, in conjunction with the concern that twin pairs are not necessarily representative of the general population, suggests that, despite their popularity, twin studies may not be as informative as many other types of family studies. This caveat has even greater force if the twin study is constrained solely to sets of twin pairs, with no evaluation of their parents, siblings, or offspring.

Adoption Studies

Despite the fact that adoption studies represent an extremely useful study design for eliminating some of the confounding influence of common family environments and common genetic relationships, there is little information concerning the blood pressure distribution in adoptive families. The most informative study has been carried out by Biron and colleagues (14,100,101) on a series of adoptive families in Montreal. Their focus on French-Canadian families was designed to eliminate the potentially confounding effect of ethnic heterogeneity within and between adoptive families. Their study was also designed to provide contrasts between (a) families in which all children were adopted, (b) families with a mixture of adopted and natural children, and (c) families with only natural children. They also evaluated the influence of single-parent families as compared to that of families with both parents. The final sample contained information on 756 adopted children, 445 natural children, and 1,176 parents distributed among 606 households. After adjusting the measured blood pressure for the influence of age and sex, they determined that family composition (i.e., number of parents, mixture of adopted and natural children, etc.) had no significant influence on the distribution of blood pressure (102). Hence, they were able to interpret their results in terms of the interaction between genetic influences and the effect of the common household environment.

As depicted in Table 4, the aggregation of blood pressure was strikingly different for the adopted children as compared to the natural children. For both systolic and diastolic blood pressures, the correlation between parents and their natural children was approximately two-fold greater than the correlation between parents and their adopted children. A similar situation was observed for the correlation between siblings. Natural siblings had correlation coefficients approximately twice those observed for the correlations between adopted siblings (i.e.,

TABLE 4. *Aggregation of blood pressure within adoptive households: the Montreal study[a]*

Correlations	Systolic	Diastolic
Between parents (mother–father)	0.15	0.18
Between mother and natural children	0.27	0.26
Between father and natural children	0.24	0.21
Between mother and adoptive children	0.08	0.10
Between father and adoptive children	0.09	0.13
Between natural siblings	0.38	0.53
Between adoptive siblings	0.16	0.29

[a] Data are from refs. 14, 101, and 103.

biologically unrelated children living in the same household). However, it will be noted that the correlations between children within the household are substantially greater than the correlations between parent and child. This implies that the common household environment exerts a significant influence on the distribution of blood pressure in children. Hence, the correlation between the biologically unrelated adopted children is roughly the same as the correlation between parents and their natural children. Additional proof of the important influence of the common household environment on children's blood pressure was given by the observation that the correlation between adopted siblings who had lived in the same household for at least 4 years was substantially higher than that between adopted children who had lived together in the same household for less than 4 years.

In order to estimate the factors contributing to the distribution of blood pressure in this population, the full set of correlations was analyzed to give maximum likelihood estimates of the genetic and common household variance components (101,103). For systolic blood pressure, it was estimated that genetic factors accounted for 34 percent of the population variability, whereas the influence of the common household environment accounted for 11 percent. Random, nonfamilial factors accounted for the remaining 55 percent of the population variability. Based on these estimates, it was concluded that 61 percent of the observed correlations between natural children and their parents, or between natural siblings, was due to shared genes, with the remaining 39 percent being due to the influence of the shared family environment. The situation for diastolic pressure was somewhat more complicated. Genetic factors were estimated to account for 30 percent of the population variability, and the influence of the common household environment (shared by both parents and children) accounted for 11 percent. However, environmental factors common to children accounted for only 20 percent of the diastolic variability in children, whereas the shared environment of parents (or a tendency for assortative mating) accounted for 9 percent of the variability in adult diastolic pressures. As a consequence of the greater influence of the household environment in children, it

was estimated that 67 percent of the sibling correlation in diastolic blood pressure was attributable to the effect of shared environments, whereas only 33 percent was attributable to common genes. By contrast, it was estimated that 58 percent of the correlation between parent and offspring was attributable to shared genes, whereas only 42 percent was attributable to the influence of the household environment.

Overall, the results from this adoptive study, which indicate that genetic factors account for 34 percent of the population variability in systolic pressures and 30 percent of the variability in diastolic pressures, are similar to the estimates displayed in Table 4. However, the study of adoptive families allows a greater resolution of the influence of common household environments on blood pressure. The fact that common household environments exert a greater influence on children's blood pressure than on the blood pressure of adults is consistent with the evidence that blood pressure tracking in children is partly explained by the familial co-aggregation of weight (16). In this context, it is significant that the household environment shared by children has a substantial influence on the distribution of relative weight (13). Hence, this data set provides some support for the hypothesis that the much higher correlations between young siblings, compared to the correlations between parent and offspring, are mediated in part by the co-aggregation of childhood obesity, where the distribution of excess relative weight is partly due to common household factors (13) and partly due to genetic factors (13,17,18).

Twin Studies

In contrast to the paucity of data on adoptive families, the obverse quasi-experimental design afforded by evaluating the distribution of blood pressure in twins has been extensively used for well over half a century. One of the earliest studies, by Stocks (104), was also one of the most informative because he took care to relate the blood pressure distribution in twins to the distribution of blood pressure in matched sets of siblings. The study population was a set of English school children comprising 93 pairs of monozygous twin pairs, 101 pairs of opposite-sex dizygous twins, and 85 pairs of same-sex dizygous twins. In addition, blood pressure was recorded for 248 sets of brothers and sisters and 286 sets of same-sex sibships. After standardizing for the influence of age and sex and analytically removing the influence of temporal variability (calculated by repeatedly measuring blood pressure on five adults for 50 days), the intraclass correlation in systolic pressure was estimated to be 0.81 for monozygous twins, 0.44 for same-sex dizygous twins, and 0.45 for same-sex sibships. Using the conventional statistical procedures for twin studies (105), these values would give a genetic heritability of 60 percent. However, Stocks noted that if these correlations in blood pressure were compared to similar correlations in height (assumed to be completely heritable), then a genetic heritability of 20 to 30 percent would be a more appropriate estimate. That conclusion, along with the actual distribution of correlations between the different types of twins, has scarcely changed during the subsequent half century (105–110).

As indicated in Table 5, the majority of twin studies yield (a) very high correlations between monozygous twins and (b) substantially lower correlations for dizygous twins. With few exceptions, the estimates of genetic heritability derived from twin studies tend to be substantially higher than estimates derived from other types of study design, with the probable cause being the greater extent of shared environments in early childhood (105). However, as is clear from Stocks' early study, the greater environmental covariance of twin pairs is most likely to affect monozygous twins, giving rise to an upwardly biased estimate of genetic heritability (106). If this bias exists, it appears to act at a very early age because the analysis of infant twins gives the same results as does the analysis of adult twins (106). Similarly, estimates of genetic heritability appear elevated if blood pressure is measured in response to a stressor (107), as opposed to casual readings (108–110).

An alternative use of twins is to evaluate the distribution of blood pressure in the families of monozygous twins, using path analytic strategies (or similar procedures) to analyze the resulting pattern of correlations. Although this study design is potentially informative, it has only been used infrequently—with somewhat discordant results. One investigation gave evidence for a strong maternal effect (111), which is at variance with other studies. However, a more extensive evaluation of 341 offspring of 76 monozygous-twin-pair families (112) excluded the existence of a maternal effect and suggested that genetic heritability ranged from 23 percent to 44 percent, depending on whether or not blood pressure was adjusted for relative weight.

Overall, the results from twin studies have to be viewed with some caution, because the resulting estimates appear to be substantially higher than estimates from other types of study design. One consequence of the excessive sharing of sociocultural environments by twin pairs, especially monozygous twin pairs, is that twin studies may be exceptionally sensitive to the set of statistical procedures carried out to obtain adjusted blood pressure. The analysis of lifestyle factors in Utah twins (22) suggests that, compared to other family structures, adjustment for relative weight (and similar variables) may be much more important than adjustment for age and sex. Hence, compared to adoption studies, twin studies appear less reliable and less informative with respect to estimating the factors that underlie familial aggregation. However, twin studies represent an ideal strategy for gaining an initial impression of whether genetic factors are likely to influence specific physiological processes leading to elevated blood pressure, as exemplified by evaluating the probable influence of genetic factors on renal function (113). However, once the initial results from twin studies have been obtained, they should be followed up by more informative study designs. Unfortunately, although a number of twin studies have given suggestive evidence for the genetic heritability of a variety of physiological variables (106), the appropriate follow-up studies have yet to be done.

TOWARD MORE REALISTIC GENETIC MODELS

Thus far, it is clear that familial aggregation of blood pressure is consistently present in the majority of populations evaluated; it is also clear that genetic heritability accounts for approximately 30 percent of the population variability, whereas the familial distribution of sociocultural factors accounts for 20 percent. With respect to the question of whether "nature" or "nurture" is more important, these consistent results indicate that genetic factors are primarily responsible for the observed familial aggregation of blood pressure within populations. Overall, it appears that approximately 60 to 70 percent of familial aggregation is ultimately due to genetic background, with familial transmission of cultural factors being responsible for the remainder. However, it should also be stressed that nonfamilial factors still account for approximately half the population variability in blood pressure, so there is an upper limit to the extent to which the etiology of hypertension can be defined in terms of familial factors.

Although the importance of genetic factors is no longer in doubt, the exact form of the underlying genetic mechanism remains unanswered. This issue represents the major puzzle still to be solved in understanding the genetic basis of hypertension. Although the Platt–Pickering controversy has died down, the conceptual legacy of their disagreement remains: Is hypertension likely to be influenced by the segregation of identifiable mendelian loci, or is genetic liability—like blood pressure it-

TABLE 5. *Comparison of correlations in blood pressure between monozygotic (MZ) and dizygotic (DZ) twins*

Population	Reference	Systolic		Diastolic	
		MZ	DZ	MZ	DZ
Children (N = 279)	104	0.81	0.39	—	—
Children (N = 200)	107	0.85	0.50	0.80	0.54
Children (N = 187)	108	0.54	0.40	0.54	0.27
Adults (N = 514)	110	0.55	0.25	0.58	0.27

self—a completely continuous trait with no possibility of identifying genetically meaningful risk categories within the continuum? Two recent developments in genetic epidemiology suggest that the issue may be resolved more effectively than the previous exhaustive, but fruitless, analysis of the shape of the blood pressure distribution.

One development is conceptual and represents an extension of Pickering's original view (56) that the inheritance of hypertension can be understood only in terms of the inheritance of the constituent physiologic and anatomic traits that combine to result in elevated blood pressure. This concept, also championed by Morton (92), has recently been expanded by Sing and coworkers (8,114), resulting in a series of analytic strategies designed to discriminate effectively between more realistic models. Second, a robust statistical procedure has been developed that facilitates the identification of a segregating major locus that acts against a polygenic background (115). The conjunction of these complementary developments finally promises to resolve some of the critical issues surrounding the origin of the ubiquitous familial aggregation of risk of essential hypertension.

An evaluation of the data suggests that the most appropriate response to the Platt–Pickering controversy requires a two-pronged approach. First, the primary target for genetic analysis should be the physiological processes likely to influence the risk of hypertension, rather than blood pressure itself. Second, the genetic analysis of such "intermediate phenotypes" (8) needs to be formulated in terms of a compromise position between the two extreme viewpoints of Platt and Pickering. Such a compromise holds that whereas the action of specific distinguishable mendelian loci may influence the distribution of an underlying physiologic process, the consequences of such loci will only be discernible against a multifactorial background caused by polygenic factors—in addition to the family environment. Furthermore, each major locus is likely to be specific for a defined physiological process. Hence, genetic risk of hypertension will be conferred by a heterogeneous set of mendelian loci, each acting against a complex multifactorial background. As stressed by Sing and coworkers (8,114), these complex interactions require that we utilize molecular markers in order to define a set of "measured genotypes" that ultimately can be used to categorize the distribution of genetic risk in the population.

As noted previously, factors influencing sodium levels are likely to be critical components of the genetic liability to hypertension (30,31). Consequently, cation transport mechanisms that regulate the cellular flux of sodium are prime candidates for potential "intermediate phenotypes." This is especially true for the Na–Li countertransport system because high rates of Na–Li countertransport are consistently associated with hypertension (116,117). Although a number of studies have investigated the shape of the distribution of Na–Li

countertransport in the population and concluded that an underlying mixture of genotypic proportions is likely (8,114,118), it should be recognized that this argument suffers from the same deficiencies as when applied to blood pressure (59,60). A critical test of genetic hypotheses requires that the distribution of Na–Li countertransport be evaluated *within* families by application of complex segregation analysis (115). This has now been accomplished in a number of samples, with general support for the hypothesis that Na–Li countertransport is influenced by a major gene that acts against a polygenic background (9,118–120). Although the conclusion of some studies was weakened by evidence for nonmendelian segregation (118) or for heterogeneity within pedigrees (119), data from Seattle not only support the existence of a major gene for Na–Li countertransport but also suggest that this locus accounts for a substantial proportion of systolic hypertension (9,120). These results indicate that Na–Li countertransport is an excellent example of an "intermediate phenotype" that is influenced by mendelian segregation at a single locus which, in turn, has a significant impact on the risk of hypertension. Two challenges result. First, molecular markers need to be identified to "measure" the segregating genotypes in the population. Second, many other intermediate phenotypes need to be extensively studied so that we can identify the other distinguishable loci that also influence risk of hypertension.

An important aspect of these more realistic genetic models for hypertension is that they assume that clinical risk of hypertension stems from the joint interaction between susceptible genotypes and deleterious environments. In this regard, the interactions are likely to change during an individual's life span, as the lifestyle of the individual changes. It will therefore become important to determine which components of the temporally changing sociocultural environment are critical for specific ages. In the context of modeling the temporal change in heritability (121), Province and Rao investigated whether the influence of sociocultural factors on blood pressure changed with age (122). Their analysis of blood pressure in the Japanese-American families previously analyzed (92) indicated that sociocultural factors increased in importance during early adulthood, reaching a maximum at age 36 and declining thereafter. Genetic heritability remained constant (122). Although the specific factors involved in the temporal change were not directly identified, the distribution of concomitants suggests that temporal changes in obesity are the most likely cause for the changing influence of the familial environment.

Although this result suggests that genetic factors remain constant throughout life, it is also possible that specific genes may be developmentally regulated such that their influence on blood pressure is only expressed at a certain age (123). Since this hypothesis requires evaluating the distribution of familial correlations over time, it is difficult to test. However, one attempt to test this hypothesis concluded there was no evidence for the sequential expression of genes influencing blood pressure (124). Hence, the evidence to date suggests that the well-defined "tracking" of blood pressure through adolescence (125) is probably due to the consistent expression of genetic factors, in conjunction with relatively stable household environments. This combination is also the probable cause for the concomitant tracking of relative weight and the resulting co-aggregation of weight and blood pressure (16). Even when the transmission pattern of sociocultural factors influencing blood pressure changes drastically, as when populations migrate (126), the pattern of correlations remains quite stable (96). With only a single study reporting a significant temporal change in familial correlations (127), it appears that the genetic components influencing blood pressure are expressed consistently throughout life and that fluctuations in sociocultural factors are generally insufficient to alter the overall level of familial resemblance over time. Changes in lifestyle factors that lead to changing levels of obesity—and, hence, to an altered distribution of blood pressure—are likely to be the only exception. As a consequence, the distribution of genetically mediated intermediate phenotypes is likely to be relatively constant throughout an individual's lifetime. This implies that once the genetic etiology of an intermediate phenotype has been determined, and an assay developed to identify the segregating genotypes, this information can be used to define preclinical risk of hypertension.

PERSONAL VIEWPOINT

The contemporary evidence suggests that in any population, the characteristically continuous distribution of blood pressure results from the combined interaction of a number of genetically influenced intermediate phenotypes, each acting in conjunction with environmental factors. Some of these environmental factors are socioculturally transmitted within family units, while others are randomly dispersed throughout the population. Whereas the mean level of blood pressure fluctuates widely across populations, the shape of the blood pressure distribution appears to be generally similar. Thus far, there is no evidence that changes in mean blood pressure levels across populations are influenced by genetic differences (29) or by differences in the distribution of familially transmitted sociocultural factors (126). Instead the population differences in mean blood pressure appear to be a function of nongenetic factors that have a relatively uniform distribution within the population. Such factors include the overall extent of obesity (11), the average amount of sodium intake (31,128,129), and the level of physical activity (21,29). There is also some

suggestion that the population variability in blood pressure may be proportional to the mean level (32), with the influence of socioculturally transmitted factors being most important in the high-mean, high-slope, extensively acculturated populations (33).

The more important issue relates to the impact of genetic factors on the distribution of hypertension within a population. Here the conceptual approach championed by Sing et al. (8) will be required in order to (a) identify the intermediate phenotypes that have a strong genetic component and (b) apply molecular techniques to identify the measured genotypes. The distribution of the relevant measured, or identified, genotypes within high-risk pedigrees can then be evaluated to determine (a) how they interact and (b) whether they can be used as preclinical markers of liability to hypertension. The process is likely to be time-consuming, because genetic risk of hypertension is undoubtedly influenced by a diverse number of intermediate phenotypes—each influenced, in turn, by a unique locus plus a polygenic background. Thus, the distribution of risk is likely to be due to the combination of relatively rare alleles of moderate effect that segregate at single loci in conjunction with a continuously distributed liability caused by polygenotypes, defined by the simultaneous segregation of multiple loci, each with small effect. This implies that different pedigrees, in which there is a conspicuous aggregation of hypertension, are likely to have a distinct distribution of intermediate phenotypes and correspondingly distinct Mendelian loci. Thus, some pedigrees are likely to show aggregation of hypertension due to the major locus for Na–Li countertransport (9,120), whereas others may have a major locus influencing, say, urinary kallikrein. Still others will exhibit co-aggregation of obesity due to a combination of genetic background (16–18) and sociocultural factors (13), rather than exhibiting an identifiable major gene. Each piece of this complex puzzle will have to be painstakingly identified before the complete picture can emerge.

Overall, the intermediate phenotypes that are likely to be most informative are those that have some bearing on sodium metabolism and renal function. This approach has already proved productive in identifying one Mendelian locus that exerts a significant influence on risk of hypertension (9,118–120). Similar loci undoubtedly exist. A focus on physiologic processes related to sodium metabolism is also likely to determine whether genetic liability due to altered renal function interacts with increased sodium intake to enhance the risk of hypertension (128). Experimental data already exist in support of the concept that an appreciable fraction of hypertensive individuals are "salt-sensitive," whereas the bulk of normotensive individuals are not (129). In particular, hypertensives exhibit a significant correlation between total body sodium and blood pressure, whereas this is not seen in normotensives (130,131). Hypertensives are also more likely than normotensives to experience a rise in blood pressure under a regime of salt loading (132,133).

Overall, it is extremely likely that the hypertensive population is heterogeneous with respect to genetic risk. Hence, whereas some individuals will be at genetic risk for hypertension because of a segregating major gene that influences a specific intermediate phenotype, other individuals will owe their risk to segregation at a completely different locus that influences a different physiological process. Still other individuals will have an increased genetic liability because of the cumulative effect of segregating alleles at many independent loci, none of which has a discernible effect on blood pressure. This "compromise" viewpoint rejects both Platt's concept of a single "monolithic" gene that causes hypertension and Pickering's concept of a completely polygenic distribution of liability, without provision for the action of major genes. Furthermore, the compromise viewpoint predicts that there are an appreciable number of "risk genotypes" for hypertension (i.e., around 10 or more), all of which are potentially measurable at the molecular level. The effect of each gene will be mediated through a specific physiological process, with few individuals (or families) being affected by more than one locus. The next decade is sure to see (a) the identification of a substantial proportion of these major genes and (b) a corresponding understanding of how the physiological processes they regulate contribute to the elevation of blood pressure. Although a number of these major genes are likely to modulate different aspects of renal function, other physiological processes will almost certainly be involved. In the end, the overall diversity of genetic risk factors is likely to rival, if not surpass, the current diversity of environmental risk factors.

REFERENCES

1. Morgagni JB. *De sedibus et causus Morboreum per Anatomen Indagatis,* vol 1. Venice: Remondiana, 1761.
2. Feinlieb M. Genetics and familial aggregation of blood pressure. In: Onesti G, Klimt CR, eds. *Hypertension determinants, complications and intervention.* New York: Grune and Stratton, 1979;35–48.
3. Rapp JP. Genetics of experimental and human hypertension. In: Genest J, Kuchel O, Hamet P, Cantin M, eds. *Hypertension: physiopathology and treatment,* 2nd ed. New York: McGraw-Hill, 1983;582–598.
4. Kannel WB. Host and environmental determinants of hypertension. In: Kesteloot H, Joosens JV, eds. *Epidemiology of arterial blood pressure.* The Hague: Martinus Nijhoff, 1980;265–295.
5. Genest J, Kuchel O, Hamet P, Cantin M, eds. *Hypertension: physiopathology and treatment,* 2nd ed. New York: McGraw-Hill, 1983.
6. Rao DC, Morton NE, Yee S. Resolution of cultural and biological inheritance by path analysis. *Am J Hum Genet* 1976;28:228–242.
7. Ward RH, Chin PG, Prior IAM. Genetic epidemiology of blood pressure in a migrating isolate: Prospectus. In: Sing CF, Skolnick MH, eds. *Genetic analysis of common diseases.* New York: Alan Liss, 1979;675–709.
8. Sing CF, Boerwinkle E, Turner ST. Genetics of primary hypertension. *Clin Exp Hypertens [A]* 1986;A8:623–651.
9. Motulsky AG, Burke W, Billings PR, Ward RH. Hypertension and the genetics of red cell membrane abnormalities. In: Bock G, Collins G, eds. *Molecular approaches to human polygenic disease.* Chichester: Wiley, Ciba Symposium 130, 1987;150–166.
10. Master AM, Dublin LI, Marks HH. The normal blood pressure range and its clinical implications. *JAMA* 1950;143:1464–1473.
11. Whyte HM. Blood pressure and obesity. *Circulation* 1959;19:511–522.
12. Kannel WB, Brand N, Skinner JJ, et al. The relation of adiposity to blood pressure and development of hypertension. *Ann Intern Med* 1967;67:48–59.
13. Annest JL, Sing CF, Biron P, et al. Familial aggregation of blood pressure and weight in adoptive families. III. Analysis of the role of shared genes and shared household environment in explaining family resemblance for height, weight and selected weight/height indices. *Am J Epidemiol* 1983;117:492–506.
14. Mongeau J-G, Biron P, Sing CF. The influence of genetics and household environment on the variability of normal blood pressure: the Montreal adoption study. In: Filer LJ, Lauer RM, eds. *Children's blood pressure.* Columbus, OH: Ross Laboratories, 1985;55–62.
15. Kotchen JM. Effect of relative weight on familial blood pressure aggregations. *Am J Epidemiol* 1977;105:214–222.
16. Hanis CL, Sing CF, Clarke WR, et al. Multivariate models for human genetic analysis: aggregation, co-aggregation and tracking of systolic blood pressure and weight. *Am J Hum Genet* 1983;35:196–210.
17. Stunkard AJ, Sorensen TIA, Hanis C, et al. An adoption study of human obesity. *N Engl J Med* 1986;314:193–198.
18. Price RA, Cadoret RJ, Stunkard AJ, Troughton E. Genetic contributions to human fatness: an adoption study, *Am J Psychiatry* 1987;144:1003–1008.
19. Bogardus C, Lillioja S, Ravussin E, et al. Familial dependence of the resting metabolic rate. *N Engl J Med* 1986;315:96–100.
20. Ravussin E, Lillioja S, Knowler WC, et al. Reduced rate of energy expenditure as a risk factor for body weight gain. *N Engl J Med* 1988;318:467–472.
21. Paffenbarger RS, Wing AL, Hyde RT, Jung DL. Physical activity and incidence of hypertension in college alumni. *Am J Epidemiol* 1983;117:245–257.
22. Slattery ML, Bishop DT, French TK, et al. Lifestyle and blood pressure levels in male twins in Utah. *Genet Epidemiol* 1988;5:277–287.
23. Donnison CP. Blood pressure in the African native: its bearing upon the aetiology of hyperplasia and arteriosclerosis. *Lancet* 1929;i:6–9.
24. Keith KM, Wagener HP, Barker NW. Some different types of essential hypertension—their course and prognosis. *Am J Med Sci* 1939;197:332–339.
25. Scotch NA. Sociocultural factors in the epidemiology of Zulu hypertension. *Am J Public Health* 1963;53:1205–1213.
26. Akinkugbe OO. Epidemiology of hypertension and stroke in Africa. In: Hateno S, ed. *Hypertension and stroke control in the community.* Geneva: World Health Organization, 1976;28–42.
27. Vaughn JP, Miall WE. Cardiovascular measurements in subjects of African origin. *Bull WHO* 1979;57:281–289.
28. Murphy W. Some observations on blood pressure in the humid tropics. *NZ Med J* 1955;54:64–67.
29. Ward RH. Genetic and sociocultural components of high blood pressure. *Am J Phys Anthropol* 1983;62:91–105.
30. Prior IAM, Evans JG, Harvey HPB, et al. Sodium intake and blood pressure in two Polynesian populations. *N Engl J Med* 1968;279:515–520.
31. Page LB. Epidemiologic evidence on the etiology of human hypertension and its possible prevention. *Am Heart J* 1976;91:527–534.
32. Oliver WJ, Cohen EL, Neel JV. Blood pressure, sodium intake and sodium related hormones in the Yanomama Indians, a "no-salt" culture. *Circulation* 1975;52:146–151.
33. Epstein FH, Eckoff RD. The epidemiology of high blood pressure—geographic distribution and etiologic factors. In: Stamler J, Stamler R, Pullman TM, eds. *Epidemiology of hypertension.* New York: Grune and Stratton, 1967;155–166.
34. MacLean CJ, Adams MS, Leyshon WC, et al. Genetic studies on hybrid populations. III. Blood pressure in an American Black community. *Am J Hum Genet* 1974;26:614–626.

35. Harburg E, Gleibermann L, Roeper P. Skin colour, ethnicity and blood pressure: Detroit. I. Blacks. *Am J Public Health* 1978;68:1177–1183.

36. Harburg E, Gleibermann L, Ozgoren F. Skin color, ethnicity and blood pressure: Detroit. II. Whites. *Am J Public Health* 1978;68:1184–1188.

37. Tyroler HA, James SA. Blood pressure and skin colour. *Am J Public Health* 1978;68:1170–1172.

38. Keil J, Tyroler H, Boyle E. Hypertension: effects of social class and racial admixture. *Am J Public Health* 1977;634–639.

39. Hutchinson J. Relationship between African admixture and blood pressure variation in the Caribbean. *Hum Hered* 1986;36:12–18.

40. Feinlieb M, Garrison RJ, Havlik RJ. Environmental and genetic factors affecting the distribution of blood pressure in children. In: Lauer RM, Shekelle RB, eds. *Childhood patterns of atherosclerosis and hypertension.* New York: Raven Press, 1980;271–279.

41. Weitz W. Zur atiologie der genuinen oder vascularen Hypertension. *Z Klin Med* 1923;96:151.

42. Pickering GW. *High blood pressure,* 2nd ed. New York: Grune and Stratton, 1968.

43. Bechgaard P. Arterial hypertension. A follow up study of 1,000 hypertonics. *Acta Med Scand* 1946;172:1–158.

44. Platt R. Heredity in hypertension. *Q J Med* 1947;16:111–132.

45. Sobye P. Heredity in essential hypertension and nephrosclerosis. A genetic-clinical study of 200 propositi suffering from nephrosclerosis. *Hered Hum* 1948;16:1–225.

46. Ayman D. Heredity in arteriolar (essential) hypertension: A clinical study of blood pressure of 1,524 members of 277 families. *Arch Intern Med* 1934;53:792–803.

47. Hamilton M, Pickering GW, Roberts JAF, Sowry GSC. The etiology of essential hypertension. I. The arterial pressure in the general population. *Clin Sci* 1954;13:11–35.

48. Hamilton M, Pickering GW, Roberts JAF, Sowry GSC. The etiology of essential hypertension. 2. Scores for arterial blood pressure adjusted for differences in age and sex. *Clin Sci* 1954;13:37–49.

49. Hamilton M, Pickering GW, Roberts JAF, Sowry GSC. The etiology of essential hypertension. 4. The role of inheritance. *Clin Sci* 1954;13:273–304.

50. Miall WE, Oldham PD. A study of arterial blood pressure and its inheritance in a sample of the general population. *Clin Sci* 1955;14:459–488.

51. Miall WE. Follow up study of arterial pressure in the population of a Welsh mining valley. *Br Med J* 1956;ii:1204–1208.

52. Miall WE, Oldham PD. Factors influencing arterial blood pressure in the general population. *Clin Sci* 1958;17:409–444.

53. Miall WE, Oldham PD. The hereditary factor in arterial blood pressure. *Br Med J* 1963;i:75–80.

54. Platt R. The nature of essential hypertension. *Lancet* 1959;2:55–57.

55. Platt R. The influence of heredity. In: Stamler J, Stamler R, Pullman TN, eds. *The epidemiology of hypertension.* New York: Grune and Stratton, 1967;9–17.

56. Pickering GW. The inheritance of arterial pressure. In: Stamler J, Stamler R, Pullman TN, eds. *The epidemiology of hypertension.* New York: Grune and Stratton, 1967;18–27.

57. Oldham PD, Pickering GW, Roberts JAF, Sowry GSC. The nature of essential hypertension. *Lancet* 1960;i:1085–1093.

58. Platt R. Heredity in hypertension. *Lancet* 1963;i:899–904.

59. Murphy EA. One cause? Many causes? The argument from the bimodal distribution. *J Chronic Dis* 1964;17:301–324.

60. Murphy EA, Thomas CB, Bolling DR. The precursors of hypertension and coronary disease: statistical considerations of distributions in a population of medical students. II. Blood pressure. *Johns Hopkins Med J* 1967;120:1–20.

61. Pickering GW. *The nature of essential hypertension.* New York: Grune and Stratton, 1961.

62. Alvarez WC. Blood pressures in fifteen thousand university freshmen. *Arch Intern Med* 1923;32:17–30.

63. Boe J, Hummerfelt S, Wedervang F. The blood pressure in a population: blood pressure and height and weight determinations in the adult population of the city of Bergen. *Acta Med Scand* [*Suppl*] 1957;321:1–336.

64. Miall WE, Lovell HG. Relation between change of blood pressure and age. *Br Med J* 1967;ii:602–660.

65. Weiss NS, Hammill PVV, Drizd T. *Blood pressure levels of children 6–11 years: relationship to age, sex, race and socioeconomic status.* National Health Survey Series 11, no. 135. Rockville, MD: US Department of HEW, 1973.

66. Karlin S. Non-gaussian phenotypic models of quantitative traits. In: Weir BS, Eisen EJ, Goodman MM, Nankong J, eds. *Proceedings of the 2nd International Conference on Quantitative Genetics.* Sunderland: Sinauer, 1988;123–149.

67. Gearing FR, Clark EG, Perera GA, et al. Hypertension among relatives of hypertensives: progress report of a family study. *Am J Public Health* 1962;52:2058–2061.

68. Miall WE, Kass EH, Ling J, et al. Factors influencing arterial pressure in the general population in Jamaica. *Br Med J* 1962;ii:497–506.

69. Miall WE, Heneage P, Khosal T, Lovell HG, Moore P. Factors influencing the degree of resemblance in arterial pressure of close relatives. *Clin Sci* 1967;33:271–283.

70. Johnson BC, Epstein FH, Kjelsberg MO. Distributions and familial studies of blood pressure and serum cholesterol levels in a total community—Tecumseh, Michigan. *J Chronic Dis* 1965;18:147–160.

71. Havlik RJ, Garrison RJ, Feinleib M, Kannel WB, Castelli WP, McNamara PM. Blood pressure aggregation in families. *Am J Epidemiol* 1979;110:304–312.

72. Wolanski N. An approach to the problem of inheritance of systolic and diastolic arterial blood pressure. *Genet Pol* 1969;10:263–268.

73. Tseng WP. Blood pressure and hypertension in an agricultural and a fishing population in Taiwan. *Am J Epidemiol* 1967;86:513–525.

74. Hayes CG, Tyroler HA, Cassell JC. Family aggregation of blood pressure in Evans County, Georgia. *Arch Intern Med* 1971;128:965–975.

75. Bengtsson B, Thulin T, Schersten B. Familial resemblance in casual blood pressure—a maternal effect? *Clin Sci* 1979;57:2795–2815.

76. Sackett DL, Anderson GD, Milner R, Feinleib M, Kannel WB. Concordance for coronary risk factors among spouses. *Circulation* 1975;52:589–595.

77. Zinner SH, Rosner B, Kass EH, Oh W. Familial aggregation of blood pressure in infants and children. In: Filer LJ, Lauer RM, eds. *Children's blood pressure.* Columbus, OH: Ross Laboratories, 1985;582–598.

78. Zinner SH, Levy PS, Kass EH. Familial aggregation of blood pressure in childhood. *N Engl J Med* 1971;284:401–409.

79. Holland WW, Beresford SAA. Factors influencing blood pressure in children. In: Paul O, ed. *Epidemiology and control of hypertension.* Miami: Symposia Specialists, 1975;375–386.

80. Beaglehole R, Salmond CE, Prior IAM. A family study of blood pressure in Polynesians. *Int J Epidemiol* 1975;4:217–220.

81. Lee YH, Rosner B, Gould JB, Lowe EW, Kass EH. Familial aggregation of blood pressure of newborn infants and their mothers. *Pediatrics* 1976;58:722–730.

82. Hennekens CH, Jesse MJ, Klein BE, Gourley JE, Blumenthal S. Aggregation of blood pressure in infants and their siblings. *Am J Epidemiol* 1976;103:457–467.

83. Zinner SH, Rosner B, Oh W, Kass EH. Significance of blood pressure in infancy: familial aggregation and predictive effect on later blood pressure. *Hypertension* 1985;7:411–416.

84. Rosner B, Donner A, Hennekens CH. Estimation of interclass correlations from familial data. *Appl Stat* 1977;26:179–187.

85. Donner A, Koval JJ. The estimates of intraclass correlations in the analysis of family data. *Biometrics* 1980;36:19–25.

86. Skoukri MM, Ward RH. On the estimation of the intraclass correlation. *Commun Stat Theor Methods* 1984;13:1239–1255.

87. Karlin S, Cameron EC, Williams PT. Sibling and parent offspring correlation estimation with variable family size. *Proc Natl Acad Sci USA* 1981;78:2664–2668.

88. Schull WJ, Harburg E, Erfurt JC, Schork MA, Rice R. A family set method for estimating heredity and stress. II. Preliminary results of the genetic methodology in a pilot survey of Negro blood pressure, Detroit, 1966–67. *J Chronic Dis* 1970;23:83–92.

89. Chakraborty R, Schull WJ, Harburg E, Schork MA, Roeper P.

Heredity, stress and blood pressure, a family set method. V. Heritability estimates. *J Chronic Dis* 1977;30:683–700.

90. Tyroler HA. The Detroit project studies of blood pressure. A prologue and review of related studies and epidemiological issues. *J Chronic Dis* 1977;30:613–624.

91. Weinberg R, Shear CL, Avet LM, et al. Path analysis of environmental and genetic influences on blood pressure. *Am J Epidemiol* 1979;109:588–596.

92. Morton NE, Gulbrandsen Cl, Rao DC, Rhoads CG, Kagan A. Determinants of blood pressure in Japanese-American families. *Hum Genet* 1980;53:261–266.

93. Krieger H, Morton NE, Rao DC, Azevedo E. Familial determinants of blood pressure in northeastern Brazil. *Hum Genet* 1980;53:415–418.

94. Iselius L, Morton NE, Rao DC. Family resemblance for blood pressure. *Hum Hered* 1983;33:277–286.

95. Ward RH, Raspe PD, Ramirez ME, Kirk RL, Prior IAM. Genetic structure and epidemiology: the Tokelau study. In: Eriksson AW, ed. *Population structure and genetic disorders.* London: Academic Press, 1980;301–325.

96. Ward RH, Chin PG, Prior IAM. The effect of migration on the familial aggregation of blood pressure. *Hypertension* 1980;2:143–154.

97. Moll PP, Harburg E, Burns TL, Schork MA, Ozgoren F. Heredity, stress and blood pressure, a family set approach: the Detroit project revisited. *J Chronic Dis* 1983;36:317–328.

98. Longini IM, Higgins MW, Hinton PC, Moll PP, Keller JB. Environmental and genetic sources of familial aggregation of blood pressure in Tecumseh, Michigan. *Am J Epidemiol* 1984;120:131–144.

99. Cruz-Coke R, Donoso H, Barrera R. Genetic ecology of hypertension. *Clin Sci Mol Med* 1973;45:55s–65s.

100. Biron P, Mongeau JG, Bertrand D. Familial aggregation of blood pressure in 558 adopted children. *Can Med Assoc J* 1976;115:773–774.

101. Biron P, Mongeau J-G. Familial aggregation of blood pressure and its components. *Pediatr Clin* 1978;25:29–33.

102. Annest JL, Sing CF, Biron P, Mongeau JG. Familial aggregation of blood pressure and weight in adoptive families. I. Comparisons of blood pressure and weight statistics among families with adopted, natural or both natural and adopted children. *Am J Epidemiol* 1979;110:479–491.

103. Annest JL, Sing CF, Biron P, Mongeau JG. Familial aggregation of blood pressure and weight in adoptive families. II. Estimation of the relative contributions of genetic and common environmental factors to blood pressure correlations between family members. *Am J Epidemiol* 1979;110:492–503.

104. Stocks P. A biometric investigation of twins and their brothers and sisters. *Ann Eugen* 1930;4:49–62.

105. Feinleib M, Garrison R, Borhani N, Rosenman R, Christian J. Studies of hypertension in twins. In: Paul O, ed. *Epidemiology and control of hypertension.* New York: Grune and Stratton, 1975;3–17.

106. Christian JC. Twin studies of blood pressure. In: Filer LJ, Lauer RM, eds. *Children's blood pressure.* Columbus, OH: Ross Laboratories, 1985;51–55.

107. McIhany ML, Shaffer JW, Hines EA. The heritability of blood pressure: an investigation of 200 twin pairs using the cold pressure test. *Johns Hopkins Med J* 1975;136:57–74.

108. Havlik RJ, Garrison RJ, Katz SH, Ellison RC, Feinleib M, Myrianthopoulos NC. Detection of genetic variance in blood pressure of seven-year-old twins. *Am J Epidemiol* 1979;109:512–516.

109. Borhani NO, Feinleib M, Garrison RJ, Christian JC, Rosenman R. Genetic variance in blood pressure. *Acta Genet Med Gemellol (Roma)* 1976;25:137–144.

110. Feinleib M, Garrison RJ, Fabsitz R, et al. The NHLBI twin study of cardiovascular disease risk factors: methodology and summary of results, 1977. *Am J Epidemiol* 1977;106:284–295.

111. Ewell LW, Nance WE, Corey LA, Boughman JA. Blood pressure studies on monzygotic twins and their families. In: Nance WE,

ed. *Twin research: clinical studies.* New York: Alan Liss, 1978;29–38.

112. Rose RJ, Miller JZ, Grim CE, Christian JC. Aggregation of blood pressure in the families of identical twins. *Am J Epidemiol* 1979;109:503–511.

113. Grim CE, Miller JZ, Luft F, Christian JC, Weinberger MH. Genetic influences on renin, aldosterone, and the renal excretion of sodium and potassium following volume expansion and contraction in normal man. *Hypertension* 1979;1:583–590.

114. Sing CF, Boerwinkle E. The genetics of blood pressure variability: an overview. In: Filer LJ, Lauer RM, eds. *Children's blood pressure.* Columbus, OH: Ross Laboratories, 1985;35–43.

115. Lalouel J-M, Rao DC, Morton NE, Elston RC. An unified model for complex segregation analysis. *Am J Hum Genet* 1983;33:816–826.

116. Canessa M, Adragna N, Solomon HS, Connolly TM, Tosteson DC. Increased sodium-lithium countertransport in red cells of patients with essential hypertension. *N Engl J Med* 1980;302:772–776.

117. Canessa M, Brugnara C, Escobales N. The Li$^+$-Na$^+$ exchange and Na$^+$-K$^+$-Cl$^-$ cotransport systems in essential hypertension. *Hypertension* 1987;10:4–10.

118. Boerwinkle E, Turner ST, Weinshilboum R, et al. Analysis of the distribution of erythrocyte sodium-lithium countertransport in a sample representative of the general population. *Genet Epidemiol* 1986;3:365–378.

119. Hasstedt SJ, Wu LL, Ash KO, et al. Hypertension and sodium-lithium countertransport in Utah pedigrees: evidence for major locus inheritance. *Am J Hum Genet* 1988;43:14–22.

120. Ward RH, Billings PR, Burke W, Hornung S, Motulsky AG. A major gene for sodium-lithium countertransport and its influence on hypertension. *N Engl J Med* 1989; submitted for publication.

121. Province MA, Rao DC. Path analysis of family resemblance with temporal trends: applications to height, weight and quetelet index in northeastern Brazil. *Am J Hum Genet* 1985;37:178–192.

122. Province MA, Rao DC. A new model for the resolution of cultural and biological inheritance in the presence of temporal trends: application to systolic blood pressure. *Genet Epidemiol* 1985;2:363–374.

123. Eaves LJ, Long J, Heath AC. A theory of developmental change in quantitative phenotypes applied to cognitive development. *Behav Genet* 1986;16:143–162.

124. Corey LA, Eaves LJ, Mellen BG, et al. Testing for developmental changes in gene expression on resemblance for quantitative traits in kinships of twins: application to height, weight and blood pressure. *Genet Epidemiol* 1986;3:73–83.

125. Clarke WR, Schrott HG, Leaverton PE, Connor WE, Lauer RM. Tracking of blood pressures in school age children. The Muscatine Study. *Circulation* 1978;58:626–634.

126. Ward RH, Prior IAM. Genetic and sociocultural factors in the response of blood pressure to migration of the Tokelau population. *Med Anthropol* 1980;4:339–366.

127. Sims J, Hewitt JK, Kelly KA, Carroll D, Turner JR. Familial and individual influences on blood pressure. *Acta Genet Med Gemellol (Roma)* 1986;35:7–21.

128. Freis ED. Salt, volume and the prevention of hypertension. *Circulation* 1976;53:589–595.

129. Page LB. Dietary sodium and blood pressure: evidence from human studies. In: Lauer RM, Shekelle RB, eds. *Childhood prevention of atherosclerosis and hypertension.* New York: Raven Press, 1980;291–303.

130. Lever AF, Beretta-Piccoli C, Brown JJ, et al. Sodium and potassium in essential hypertension. *Br Med J* 1981;283:463–468.

131. Beretta-Piccoli C, Davies DL, Boddy K, et al. Relation of arterial pressure with body sodium, body potassium and plasma potassium in essential hypertension. *Clin Sci* 1982;63:250–257.

132. Sullivan JM, Ratts TE, Taylor JC, et al. Hemodynamic effects of dietary sodium in man. *Hypertension* 1980;2:506–514.

133. Fujita T, Henry WL, Bartter FC, et al. Factors influencing blood pressure in salt sensitive patients with hypertension. *Am J Med* 1980;69:334–344.

Hypertension: Pathophysiology, Diagnosis, and Management, Second Edition, edited by J.H. Laragh and B.M. Brenner, Raven Press, Ltd., New York © 1995.

CHAPTER **6**

Low Birth Weight as a Risk Factor for Juvenile and Adult Hypertension

Glenn M. Chertow and Barry M. Brenner

Dietary sodium intake and abnormalities in renal sodium handling have been linked to the pathogenesis of hypertension for many years. According to prevailing views (1–3), hypertension is thought to be initiated by the acute expansion of extracellular fluid and plasma volume, followed by an increase in central venous pressures and cardiac output. Blood pressure elevation then leads to increased renal blood flow and natriuresis, attenuating the rise in blood pressure. With time, cardiac output returns to normal, while total peripheral resistance rises. Systemic hypertension thereby evolves from an acute high-cardiac-output form of hypertension to one characterized by increased peripheral resistance. Guyton et al. (3) suggested that hypertension is characterized by an abnormal pressure-natriuresis phenomenon. In the normotensive individual, increased sodium intake is matched by increased sodium excretion, resulting in minimal blood pressure elevation with salt loading. In the hypertensive individual, however, sodium excretion is impaired, and the kidneys require a supranormal perfusion pressure to maintain volume homeostasis.

Sodium intake cannot entirely explain blood pressure variability, however, as individuals and populations vary widely in renal and systemic response to sodium loading

(4,5). It is known that some individuals with hypertension fail to modulate renal blood flow in response to changes in sodium intake (6). Others demonstrate an abnormally small rise in plasma renin activity and aldosterone when salt intake is reduced (7) or when diuretic therapy is instituted (8). There is wide variability in clinical response to sodium restriction (9) and to different classes of antihypertensive agents (10). Although the exact pathogenesis is unclear, an abnormal relationship between blood pressure and natriuresis appears to play a critical role in some cases of essential hypertension, particularly among those considered to be salt-sensitive (11).

AN INVERSE RELATIONSHIP BETWEEN BLOOD PRESSURES AND NEPHRON NUMBER

Brenner et al. (12) postulated that essential hypertension may be initiated by decreased glomerular filtration surface area, due to a reduced number of glomeruli and/or a decrease in filtration surface area per glomerulus. In this model, renal sodium retention initially elevates plasma volume and blood pressure. Systemic hypertension then leads to glomerular capillary hypertension and eventually to glomerulosclerosis, which in turn further decreases filtration surface area, perpetuating a vicious cycle. Inherited deficiencies in filtration surface area may explain the variable rates of progression of renal disease,

G. M. Chertow and B. M. Brenner: Renal Division and Department of Medicine, Brigham and Women's Hospital and Harvard Medical School, Boston, Massachusetts 02115.

as those endowed at birth with a lesser number of nephrons may be less able to sustain renal function after initial injury (12). Just as alterations in renal hemodynamics, reduced ability to excrete sodium, and raised blood pressure characterize the adaptive response to an acquired decrease in the number of functioning nephrons, as from renal ablation or renal disease, inborn deficiencies may also enhance susceptibility to essential hypertension.

This susceptibility appears to be genetically determined. The risk of hypertension increases dramatically when both parents are hypertensive (13); a compelling familial concordance has been noted in baseline blood pressure (14) and in sodium sensitivity of blood pressure among parents and offspring (4). An inherited decrease in nephron number or filtration surface area could constitute an important pathogenetic determinant of salt-sensitive hypertension (11). Inborn deficits in nephron number could contribute to the observed differences in susceptibility to hypertension, irrespective of dietary factors, which characterize distinct population groups. For instance, Japanese individuals (15) and African-Americans (16,17) share an increased incidence of hypertension, and autopsy series reveal their kidneys to be smaller in size than those of Caucasians (12,18). A consistent finding among African-Americans is salt-sensitivity. In a study of normotensive adults, Luft et al. (19) demonstrated that as compared to Caucasians, African-American subjects had higher blood pressures with oral or intravenous salt loading. Hypertensive African-Americans exhibit increased renal vascular resistance (20), impaired natriuretic response to dopamine (21), increased plasma volumes (22), and a form of hypertension which tends to respond to diuretic therapy (23). The salt-sensitive hypertension exhibited by many African-Americans may be due to reduced nephron number or glomerular filtration surface area (11,12). This could partly explain the early development of hypertension and greater risk of renal disease in this population.

Gender may also play a role in susceptibility to hypertension. Women tend to have smaller kidneys than do men (24) and approximately 10–20 percent fewer glomeruli (25,26). Women also exhibit greater age-related increases in blood pressure (27). When gender and race are considered together, African-American women exhibit the steepest rise in blood pressure after saline infusion (28).

Finally, age-related nephron loss may contribute to the increased incidence of hypertension seen among the elderly. The number of intact glomeruli tends to decrease after age 40, as a consequence of aging (29). This gradual loss of nephrons may explain the observation that older individuals are less efficient at excreting an administered or ingested sodium load (30) and typically exhibit the low plasma renin profile and diuretic-responsive type of hypertension shared by younger individuals with reduced nephron number. The incidence and magnitude of age-related hypertension may relate to the congenital complement of nephrons. Those individuals born with a supranormal nephron number may be destined to enjoy normal or low blood pressure throughout life, with a low likelihood of cardiovascular and renal disease. On the other hand, those with congenital "oligonephropathy" may have accelerated nephron loss and risk of early development of renal and cardiovascular disease.

An experimental analogue to this condition is found in the prehypertensive Dahl salt-sensitive rat, a strain with a congenital reduction in nephron number (31). In this strain, renal blood flow and glomerular filtration rates fall to lower levels with graded decrements in perfusion pressure than in salt-resistant strains, demonstrating an abnormal pressure-natriuresis relationship (32). Impaired ability to excrete sodium and failure to increase renal blood flow after sodium loading suggest an underlying renal hemodynamic abnormality reminiscent of human nonmodulators (33). Therefore, inborn differences in nephron number may lead to an altered pressure-natriuresis relationship and essential hypertension and may explain observed differences in arterial pressure responses to dietary sodium intake. Furthermore, the increases in renal vascular pressures that serve initially to restore sodium balance may eventually prove maladaptive and perpetuate the cycle of nephron loss.

VARIABILITY OF NEPHRON NUMBER

Although generally not appreciated, kidneys from normal individuals exhibit considerable variation in weight, cortical volume, and nephron number, depending on the sex, body weight or surface area, and age of the individual. Morphometric data from several studies reveal a wide variation in numbers of glomeruli per kidney (26,34,35). Nyengaard and Bendtsen (26) reported mean glomerular counts per kidney of $0.62 \pm 0.25 \times 10^6$ with a remarkably wide range of 0.33 to 1.1×10^6 (Fig. 1). Direct pathologic studies of nephron number and hypertension in humans are scarce. Hayman et al. (36), in a study of patients with and without renal disease, found systolic blood pressure to be above 150 mm Hg in all individuals with less than 0.7×10^6 glomeruli per kidney (30 percent below the median count).

Experimentally, nephron number, dietary sodium intake, and hypertension are definitively linked. In the rat, removal of 70 percent or more of functional renal mass consistently leads to systemic and glomerular hypertension, characterized by increased plasma volume (37) and low plasma renin activity (38). With this degree of renal ablation, hypertension can be observed in the absence of high sodium intake. With lesser degrees of ablation, (e.g., uninephrectomy), hypertension typically does not develop in rats fed standard chow, but may develop as so-

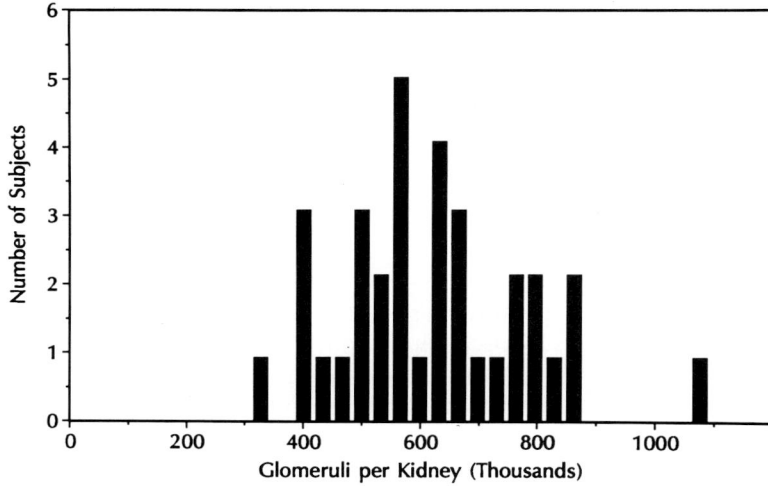

FIG. 1. Frequency distribution of glomerular number per kidney. (From ref. 26, with permission.)

dium intake is increased (39). Koletsky and Goodsitt (40) found that by increasing dietary sodium content, hypertension could be induced in 100 percent of rats with 75 percent nephrectomy after two weeks, in 94 percent of uninephrectomized rats after 4 months, and in 66 percent of rats with two intact kidneys after 8 months (40).

In humans, major congenital or acquired nephron deficits are frequently associated with hypertension and progressive renal injury. For example, in oligomeganephronia (a congenital condition characterized by a marked reduction in nephron number), proteinuria, glomerulosclerosis, hypertension, and renal failure typically ensue before the third decade (41,42). Hypertension is common among individuals with a congenital solitary kidney (43), those who have undergone surgical excision of renal mass due to tumor (44), and those who have undergone uninephrectomy for living-related organ transplantation (45,46). Thus, a 50-percent reduction in nephron number, though insufficient to produce progressive renal failure in most subjects, clearly accelerates the development of systemic hypertension.

Hypertension is also particularly common among renal transplant recipients (47). Several factors may contribute to elevated blood pressure in this group, including glucocorticoid and cyclosporin therapy, renal artery stenosis, rejection, and recurrence of underlying glomerular disease. In addition, transplant recipients have substantially reduced nephron number and filtration surface area secondary to injury induced by organ recovery and preservation, and in many cases, acute rejection or tubular necrosis. Recent review of the North American Transplant Registry at UCLA and the International Transplant Study Registry in Heidelberg suggested that factors associated with an imbalance of nephron supply and demand (e.g., transplantation of pediatric, elderly, female, or African-American kidneys, especially to recipients of large body mass) may seriously jeopardize long-term graft survival (48).

NEPHROGENESIS AND LOW BIRTH WEIGHT

In early fetal development, the kidneys are formed by successive interactions among the pronephros, mesonephros, and metanephros. The renal corpuscles and tubules arise from the metanephric blastema, while the excretory segments, including the collecting ducts, calyces, pelvis, and ureter, derive from the ureteric bud (24). If development is impaired, its manifestations depend upon the stage of organogenesis at which ineffective cell-to-cell communication or frank injury occurs (49).

In the human, an insult occuring within the first weeks of fetal life will likely result in unilateral or bilateral renal agenesis. An insult taking place within the second or third month may induce a congenital malformation such as hypoplasia, or an abnormality of the renal collecting system such as urethral atresia or posterior urethral valves. An insult occurring beyond the fourth month will most likely affect the renal parenchyma rather than the pelvicalyceal system, which is already well-defined at this stage in fetal life (50). It is at this stage that more subtle nephron deficits may originate. In the human, nephrogenesis is completed at a body weight of approximately 2300 g. No nephrogenesis in the human occurs after birth, in contrast to some other animal species (51).

Loss of renal mass during early development is most often the result of a congenital malformation or a perinatal vascular catastrophe (49). While the response of the fetal kidney to injury is variable, compensatory hypertrophy during the postnatal period is well-documented (52). Based on a review of infants born with unilateral multicystic dysplasia, Laufer and Griscom (53) concluded that compensatory renal hypertrophy does not occur in the human fetus. However, by 1 year of age, the volume of the intact kidney in their subjects was equal to that of two normal kidneys.

The magnitude of functional adaptation of remnant nephrons may depend upon the time at which loss of renal mass takes place. In dogs subjected to three-fourths nephrectomy at birth, glomerular filtration rate (GFR) 6 weeks later was equal to that of sham-operated controls, suggesting substantial compensatory hypertrophy (54). In contrast, animals operated upon at 8 weeks of age had a GFR 6 weeks later which was only 45 percent of that of controls (54). In rats, uninephrectomy soon after birth resulted in more rapid development of proteinuria and glomerulosclerosis than when uninephrectomy was performed in the adult animal (55).

Oligonephronia may be induced *in utero* by several experimental approaches. Gilbert and coworkers (56,57) exposed rats to gentamicin from the tenth day of gestation to term (day 21). The number of nephrons present at birth in the offspring of gentamicin-treated mothers was reduced by 20 percent, and at a concentration of gentamicin lower than that measured in the kidney of human fetuses after a single injection of aminoglycosides to pregnant women (58). Premature glomerulosclerosis and proteinuria also developed; unfortunately, blood pressures were not recorded (57). Zeman (59) reported that maternal protein restriction in rats resulted in decreased birth weight in offspring. The liver and kidneys of these young were smaller in proportion to total body weight, suggesting that these organs may have been the most severely affected. Zeman (60) and Merlet-Benichou and co-workers (61) later described specific morphologic effects of maternal protein restriction on the kidneys of newborn rats. Pregnant rats were restricted to a 6-percent-casein diet supplemented with additional carbohydrate, while controls were fed an isocaloric 24-percent-casein chow. Kidneys from newborn rats were removed after birth and showed significant reductions in overall size, glomerular number, and proportion of mature glomeruli in the protein-restricted group. The latter also demonstrated fewer tubular structures, which were replaced with increased connective tissue. The progeny of rats fed the 6-percent-casein diet had markedly lower mean inulin clearance (3.84 ± 1.15 vs. 16.31 ± 5.67 ml/hour/100 g body wt); blood pressures were not measured (62). These studies demonstrate that antenatal nutritional deficiency in the rat may affect nephrogenesis and result in adverse postnatal sequelae.

Merlet-Benichou and co-workers (61) also induced oligonephronia by creating intrauterine growth retardation (IUGR) in rats by partial artery ligation of a single uterine horn on day 17 of gestation. The fetuses in the

TABLE 1. *Relationship between birth weight and number of glomeruli in rats*

	Birth wt (g)	Kidney wt (mg)	Glomeruli (no.)
Control (n = 19)	5.10 ± 0.11	19.2 ± 0.9	4817 ± 291
IUGR (n = 27)	3.65 ± 0.15	12.6 ± 0.1	2858 ± 227

From ref. 61, with permission.

TABLE 2. *Relationship between birth weight and number of glomeruli in human infants*

	Birth wt (g)	Kidney wt (g)	Glomeruli (per optical field)
non-IUGR (n = 14)	3373 ± 253	17.0 ± 2.8	59 ± 10
IUGR (n = 10)	2148 ± 320	12.7 ± 4.6	48 ± 19

From ref. 63, with permission.

contralateral horn served as controls. After delivery of the rats by cesarean section on day 21, a comparison of body weight and kidney weight was performed in IUGR and control pups. Body weights, kidney weights, and nephron number per kidney were significantly reduced in the IUGR group (Table 1). This study suggests that growth retardation per se, rather than a specific nutritional factor, results in an inborn nephron deficit.

A single report also describes kidney size and nephron number in full-term human infants with or without IUGR. Leroy et al. (63) examined kidney cross sections from these infants who died in a neonatal intensive care unit of nonrenal causes. Infants with low birth weight (below the tenth percentile) were compared with controls (infants with usual weight for gestational age). Kidney weights and number of glomeruli were found to be significantly reduced in IUGR infants (Table 2) (63).

Thus, a nephron deficit may predispose an individual to sodium-sensitive hypertension (11). Intrauterine growth retardation appears to result in a congenital nephron deficit, i.e., oligonephropathy. If this is indeed so, the adverse effect of intrauterine growth retardation on nephrogenesis could contribute, at least in part, to an inverse relationship between birth weight and blood pressure.

AN ASSOCIATION OF LOW BIRTH WEIGHT AND ELEVATED BLOOD PRESSURE

Clinical Evidence: Childhood

A number of reports have implicated low birth weight as a predictor of elevated blood pressure in childhood. Simpson and coworkers reported the results of the Dunedin Multidisciplinary Health and Development Study, a cohort of 692 children born in Dunedin, New Zealand, during 1972 and 1973 (64). This study aimed to investigate whether parental, perinatal, nutritional, developmental, or behavioral factors were associated with childhood variations in blood pressure. There were small but significant differences in birth weight among the children in the "high" blood pressure group compared with those in the "medium" group (3.24 ± 0.55 vs. 3.40 ± 0.55 kg, $p < 0.05$) (64). Cater and Gill (65) reported the findings of a 10-year follow-up examination of 143 low-birth-weight infants and 139 controls. The

TABLE 3. *Blood pressures in 143 children[a] of low birth weight and 139 controls*

Birth weight (g)	Blood pressure (mm Hg)	
740–2000	112/74	
2001–2500	113/74	
>2500	107/70	p < 0.05

From ref. 65, with permission.
[a] 10 years of age.

TABLE 5. *Systolic blood pressure related to birth weight: Brompton Study*

Age	Mean SPB difference[a] (mm Hg)
4 days	−1.0
6 weeks	−0.8
6 months	−0.6
1 year	−0.4
2 years	−0.3
3 years	−1.4
4 years	−2.5
5 years	−1.1
6 years	−1.9
7 years	−1.1
8 years	−1.6
9 years	−0.7
10 years	−1.3

From ref. 78, with permission.
[a] Per kg increase in birth weight.
SPB, systolic blood pressure.

mean body weight of the low-birth-weight children was significantly less than that of the control group (28.3 ± 4.8 vs. 30.2 ± 4.7 kg, $p = 0.01$). Despite the lower current body weight, the low-birth-weight group had systolic and diastolic blood pressures which were significantly higher (Table 3). A third and larger study was reported by Whincup et al. (66), in which a cross-sectional survey of 3,591 schoolchildren in 9 British towns aged 5–7.5 years was performed. Univariate analysis showed no significant relationship between birth weight and systolic or diastolic blood pressure. However, when current weight (which was positively correlated with blood pressure) was considered, mean systolic and diastolic blood pressures were inversely related to birth weight within each fifth of the current weight distribution in both boys and girls (Table 4). The investigators also found associations between childhood blood pressure and maternal age, birth rank, and history of hypertension; these later findings were independent of the birth weight effect.

Barker et al. (67) studied 9,921 10-year-old children included in the British births survey of 1970. There was an inverse relationship between systolic blood pressure at age 10 and birth weight in both boys and girls. These findings were confirmed in the Brompton study conducted from 1975–1977 (68). In this study, 1,895 consecutive infants were followed up at 4 days, 6 weeks, 6 months, 1 year, and yearly thereafter until age 10. There was a consistent association between elevated blood

pressure and lower birth weight (Table 5). Moreover, the relationship between systolic blood pressure and birth weight did not depend on shortened gestation, suggesting that elevated blood pressure was initiated by processes associated with reduced growth *in utero*.

Maternal and fetal influences on early childhood blood pressure were studied by Law et al. (69), in which 405 children aged 4 years were visited at home for blood pressure and growth measurements. Data on maternal factors were abstracted from obstetrical records. The relationships between current weight, birth weight, placental weight, and systolic blood pressure at 4 years of age were analyzed by multivariate regression. Systolic blood pressure was directly correlated with weight at age 4 and with placental weight, but inversely correlated with birth weight (Table 6).

The mechanism of the relationship between placental weight and blood pressure is unknown. Anemia, a common complication of pregnancy, may be associated with increased placental size (70). A study of Gambian chil-

TABLE 4. *Mean systolic blood pressures in children[a] in relation to birth weight and current weight*

Boys

Birth wt (g)	SBP (mm Hg) in each qunitile of current weight				
<3000	96.5	100.6	100.8	103.1	108.6
>3800	96.4	98.0	99.7	100.8	104.4

Girls

Birth wt (g)	SBP (mm Hg) in each qunitile of current weight				
<2820	97.7	99.7	102.6	105.3	105.5
>3690	95.6	97.9	98.9	99.5	104.5

From ref. 66, with permission.
[a] 5–7.5 years of age.
SBP, systolic blood pressure.

TABLE 6. *Mean systolic blood pressure in children[a] related to birth weight and placental weight*

Birth weight (g)	Mean difference from reference blood pressure (mm Hg)
<3000	0
3001–3300	−0.8
3301–3600	−0.9
>3600	−2.6

Placental weight (g)

<550	0
551–650	−0.1
651–750	−0.6
>750	−2.6

From ref. 69, with permission.
[a] 4 years of age.

dren noted an association between the failure of mothers to gain weight during the third trimester of pregnancy and elevated blood pressure in offspring at 8–10 years of age (71). Large placentas can be produced in sheep by depriving the ewe of food during pregnancy (72). Based on these observations, Barker (73) and others have postulated that maternal undernutrition may influence blood pressure in offspring. Whether the placental size is simply a marker of maternal nutritional status or of the presence or absence of other factors affecting fetal-placental interchange is unknown.

In a study of 166 twin pairs, Levine and co-workers (74) demonstrated a negative correlation between within-pair differences in birth weight and systolic blood pressure. Among monozygotic twin pairs (n = 67), the lighter twin tended to have higher systolic blood pressure at the age of 1 year. As monozygotic twins are genetically identical, this observation strongly suggests that an intra-uterine influence related to growth and development affects blood pressure during infancy. We have postulated that impaired nephrogenesis induced by IUGR is this "intrauterine influence" which predisposes to higher postnatal blood pressures (75).

Clinical Evidence: Adolescence

In a follow-up to the Dunedin Study, Williams and co-workers (76) reported a small difference in systolic blood pressure between the IUGR groups and normals at age 18; these were limited to IUGR infants of appropriate ponderal index (weight [g] per length^3 [cm]), rather than those of low ponderal index (Table 7) (76). These findings suggest that the pattern of growth retardation, rather than the presence of IUGR alone, may be important in determining the birth-weight–blood-pressure relationship, although these findings contradict those of Law et al. (69) described above.

Finally, a 32,580-subject study in Israel by Seidman et al. (77) showed a significant correlation of birth weight to blood pressure variability at age 17; however, there were no statistically significant increases in systolic or diastolic blood pressure for those with low birth weight

TABLE 7. *Mean change at follow-up^a in systolic blood pressure in children with intrauterine growth retardation and in children large for gestational age compared to controls*

	IUGR-API	IUGR-LPI	LGA	
Age 7	3.2	−1.2	−1.4	(mm Hg)
Age 18	0.8	−1.2	−0.7	(mm Hg)

From ref. 76, with permission.
^{a} 18 years of age.
Ponderal index = weight (g) per length^3 (cm).
IUGR-API, intrauterine growth retardation-appropriate ponderal index; IUGR-LPI, intrauterine growth retardation-low ponderal index; LGA, large for gestational age.

(<2500 g). The authors suggested that major environmental effects on blood pressure were exerted during childhood, rather than *in utero,* and which correlated most closely with changes in weight from childhood to adult life.

It is unclear why the association between low birth weight and elevated blood pressure observed in several studies of children and adults (see below) has not been uniformly observed in adolescents. This may be due to confounding hormonal or other physiologic factors which affect blood pressure in adolescents. It would be expected that the effect of an inborn nephron deficit would be amplified with age-related nephron loss. This may explain why the association between low birth weight and elevated blood pressure appears to be stronger in adults than in children thus far studied (78).

Clinical Evidence: Adulthood

Gennser et al. (79) first reported the inverse association of birth weight and blood pressure in adults. The authors reviewed hospital birth records of 104 randomly selected male Swedish army conscripts whose blood pressures had been measured at 28 years of age. Thirty-two (31 percent) were noted to have a diastolic blood pressure of 90 mm Hg or more. Of the men whose full birth records were available (n = 77), those with resting diastolic blood pressure elevation were more likely to have been below the mean and one standard deviation for birth weight. The calculated odds ratio for subsequent development of diastolic hypertension among men with low birth weight was 3.6 in this study (79). Unfortunately, this study was limited by its small sample size and retrospective case-control design.

The finding of an inverse relationship between height and cardiovascular disease among individuals in Norway (80), Finland (81), and Great Britain (82), and of a correlation between geographic differences in cardiovascular mortality and infant mortality 60 years earlier in England and Wales (83,84) led Barker and co-workers (67) to thoroughly investigate whether an association was present between growth *in utero* and blood pressure in adult life. The 1946 Medical Research Council cohort consisted of 5,362 children included in a national survey of health and development in Great Britain. Of the original 5,362 subjects, 3,259 (61 percent) were available for study as adults. There was a strong, statistically significant inverse relationship between systolic pressure at age 36 and birth weight, which was not associated with gestational age and which was independent of current weight. Among adult men within each body weight group, mean systolic blood pressure fell by 2.57 mm Hg from the lowest to the highest birth weight group. Among women, the effect was 1.83 mm Hg (67).

This group also studied 449 men and women born in Preston, Lancashire, between 1935 and 1943. Data on placental weight, birth weight, and blood pressure at ages 46–54 were available, and demonstrated that mean systolic blood pressure in adult life rose by 13 mm Hg as placental weight increased from <1 lb to >1.5 lb, and fell by 10 mm Hg as birth weight increased from <5.5 lb to >7.5 lb in a graded dose-response nature (Table 8). These relationships were independent, such that the highest blood pressures occured in individuals who had been small infants with large placentas (85). The authors suggested that changes in hemodynamic load related to placental size and function may alter arterial structure, thereby leading to hypertension in later life.

The Hertfordshire survey of 5,654 men born between 1911 and 1930 was also analyzed by Barker and co-workers (86). Its results suggested strongly that death risk due to ischemic heart disease was inversely related to birth weight and weight at 1 year of age. Again, a detailed analysis of this cohort demonstrated an inverse relationship between birth weight and blood pressure at age 64 when current body mass was considered.

In a later report (78), the authors determined that systolic blood pressure at ages 64–71 years decreased 5.2 mm Hg for each kg increase in birth weight. They suggested that the effect linking birth weight and blood pressure was initiated *in utero*. This linkage was evident in infancy and childhood, and became amplified with increasing age. The authors speculated that the initiating process could be related to changes in fetal blood flow or to the increased activity of a trophin or mitogen. Instead, we have proposed that impaired nephrogenesis leading to a deficit in nephron number or glomerular filtration surface area is the event which initiates essential hypertension (Fig. 2) (75).

Microalbuminuria is increasingly recognized as a reliable predictor of overt proteinuria, macrovascular disease, progressive glomerulosclerosis, and end-stage renal failure in diabetics (87–89). Microalbuminuria is also a predictor of serious cardiovascular disease, including hypertension in nondiabetic subjects (90–95). Gould et al.

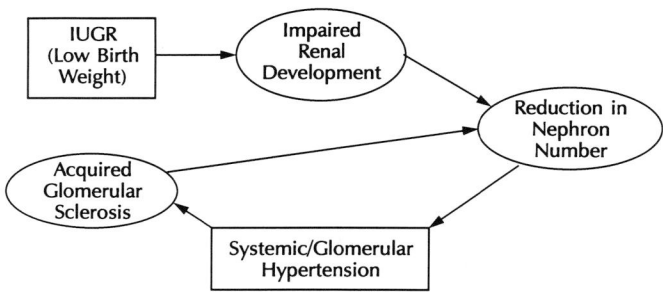

FIG. 2. Hypothesis: Essential hypertension results from an inborn nephron deficit due to intrauterine growth retardation (IUGR).

(96) recently obtained evidence in men for an inverse correlation between microalbuminuria and height, the latter known to vary directly with birth weight (97). An inverse association between height and risk of coronary artery disease has also been reported (82,98), once again presumed to reflect evidence of factors acting *in utero* or in early childhood.

It was Folkow (99) who initially proposed that essential hypertension was determined by mechanisms of initiation and amplification. We have outlined clinical and experimental evidence above related to nephron number and hypertension which fits well into the initiation-amplification model. An infant may be born with mild to moderate growth retardation and a reduced nephron number, perhaps less than 0.5×10^6 per kidney. This abnormality leads to a susceptibility to sodium-sensitive hypertension and a diminished nephron reserve in the face of hypertensive or other renal injury. A cycle of gradual nephron loss ensues with age, exacerbating blood pressure elevation. Ultimately, vascular complications (e.g., stroke, coronary artery disease) may develop, particularly if additional risk factors (e.g., tobacco abuse, hypercholesterolemia) are present.

HYPERTENSION IN AFRICAN-AMERICANS— A CRISIS IN PART RELATED TO LOW-BIRTH-WEIGHT INFANTS?

The risks of stroke, left ventricular hypertrophy, and end-stage renal disease are higher among African-Americans than among Caucasians (100). As outlined above, a trend toward salt-sensitivity and low-renin, diuretic-responsive hypertension may be a manifestation of an underlying nephron deficit in the African-American population at large. Any individual born with an additional nephron deficit related to IUGR might be even more apt to develop systemic hypertension. In this regard, there is marked racial disparity in the incidence of low birth weight (<2500 g) and very low birth weight (<1500 g) in infants, with African-Americans at 2–3 times greater risk for this complication (Table 9) (101).

TABLE 8. *Mean change in systolic blood pressure associated with birth weight and placental weight in adults*[a]

Birth weight (lb)	Mean difference from reference blood pressure (mm Hg)
<5.5	0
5.5–6.5	−4
6.5–7.5	−7
>7.5	−10
Placental weight (g)	
<550	0
551–650	4
651–750	3
>750	13

From ref. 85, with permission.
[a] 46–54 years of age.

TABLE 9. *Frequency of very low birth weight according to race in 3 geographical areas*

Area and race	Live births no.	VLBW no. (%)	Risk ratio (95% CI)
Boston (1980–1985)			
Black	16,977	404 (2.4)	3.1 (2.6–3.7)
White	22,508	172 (0.8)	
St. Louis (1985–1986)			
Black	9,279	297 (3.2)	2.3 (1.8–2.8)
White	6,807	96 (1.4)	
Mississippi (1984–1986)			
Black	7,002	143 (2.0)	2.5 (1.9–3.3)
White	9,245	76 (0.8)	

From ref. 101, with permission.

Those low-birth-weight infants who survive may do so with a persistent nephron deficit and an enhanced susceptibility to hypertension and renal disease in later life. It is critical to learn whether there exist factors, potentially related to nutrition during pregnancy, which may be associated with prematurity and/or intrauterine growth retardation in this racial group.

SUMMARY

Low birth weight has been associated with elevated blood pressure in children and with blood pressure elevation and risk of ischemic heart disease in adults. This association appears to be particularly strong when coupled with increased placental weight. The mechanisms responsible for these associations have yet to be determined. In rats, intrauterine growth retardation is associated with a deficit in nephron number. Abnormal nephrogenesis also occurs when pregnant rats are fed a protein-deficient diet. Could protein deprivation in pregnant women be an important factor contributing to low birth weight and subsequent hypertension in offspring? Which hormone(s), growth factor(s), or cytokine(s) serves as the critical "nephrogenesis factor"? Would protein supplementation during gestation augment intrauterine renal development, possibly endowing a rich supply of nephrons?

Based on the foregoing, we postulate that essential hypertension results from congenital oligonephropathy. The effects of reduced nephron number are amplified with age, by a positive feedback related to glomerular hyperfiltration, glomerular capillary hypertension, and eventually, glomerular sclerosis. African-Americans may be particularly susceptible to the consequences of this inborn nephron deficit. Experimental efforts aimed at defining the determinants of normal and abnormal nephrogenesis and clinical trials aimed at modifying these determinants may ultimately lead to primary prevention of essential hypertension and reduced risk of expression of clinical renal disease.

REFERENCES

1. Ledingham JM, Cohen RD. *Lancet* 1963;2:979–981.
2. Borst JGG, Borst-De Geus A. *Lancet* 1963;1:677–682.
3. Guyton AC, Coleman PJ, Cowley AW Jr. et al. *Circ Res* 1974;35:159–176.
4. Luft FC, Miller JZ, Weinberger MH, et al. *Klin Wochenschr* 1987;65:101–109.
5. Denton D. In: Denton D, ed. *The hunger for salt. An anthropological, physiological and medical analysis.* New York: Springer-Verlag, 1982;542–629.
6. Williams GH, Moore TJ, Hollenberg NK. *Am J Kidney Dis* 1987;10:39–44.
7. Coughlan JP, Doyle AE, Jerums G, Scoggins BA. *Clin Sci* 1972;42:15–23.
8. Matsubara H, Umeda Y, Yamane Y, et al. *Am J Cardiol* 1987;60:708–714.
9. Swales JD. In: Laragh JH, Brenner BM, eds. *Hypertension: pathophysiology, diagnosis and management.* New York: Raven Press, 1990;2001–2019.
10. Muller FB, Laragh JH. In: Laragh JH, Brenner BM, eds. *Hypertension: pathophysiology, diagnosis and management.* New York: Raven Press, 1990;2107–2115.
11. Kimura G, Brenner BM. *Current Opinion Nephrol Hypertens* 1993;2:341–349.
12. Brenner BM, Garcia DL, Anderson S. *Am J Hypertens* 1988;1:335–347.
13. Deutscher S, Epstein FH, Kjelsberg MO. *Circulation* 1966;33:911–924.
14. Miller JZ, Daugherty SA, Weinberger MH, et al. *Hypertension* 1983;5:790–795.
15. Takahashi E, Sasaki N, Takeda J, Ito H. *Hum Biol* 1957;29:139–166.
16. Drizd T, Dannenberg AL, Engel A. *Vital Health Stat* 1986;234:10–18.
17. Jones CA, Agadoa L. *Am J Kid Dis* 1993;21(4),S1:6–9.
18. Tauchi H, Tsuboi K, Okutomi J. *Gerontologia* 1971;17:87–97.
19. Luft FC, Rankin LI, Bloch R, et al. *Circulation* 1979;60:697–706.
20. Frohlich ED, Messerli FH, Dunn FG, et al. *Miner Electrolyte Metab* 1984;10:173–177.
21. Gordon MS, Steunkel CA, Conlin PR, et al. *J Clin Endocrinol Metab* 1989;69:426–432.
22. Lilley JJ, Hsu L, Stone RA. *Ann Intern Med* 1976;84:707–11.
23. Veterans Administration Cooperative Study on Antihypertensive Agents. *JAMA* 1982;248:2004–2011.
24. Tisher CC, Madsden KM. In: Brenner BM, Rector FC Jr, eds. *The kidney.* Philadelphia: WB Saunders, 1991;3–75.
25. McLachlan MSF, Guthrie JC, Anderson CK, Fuller MJ. *J Pathol* 1977;121:65–78.
26. Nyengaard JR, Bendtsen TF. *Anat Record* 1992;232:194–201.
27. Page LB, Danion A, Moellering RC Jr. *Circulation* 1974;49:1132–1146.
28. Luft FC, Fineberg NS, Miller JZ, et al. *Am J Med Sci* 1980;279:15–24.
29. Kappel B, Olsen S. *Virchows Arch (A)* 1980;387:271–277.
30. Luft FC, Weinberger MH, Grim CE. *Am J Med* 1982;72:726–736.
31. Azar S, Iwai J, Weller D. *Kidney Int* 1978;14:691A.
32. Roman RJ. *Am J Physiol* 1986;251:F57–F65.
33. Tuck ML, Williams GH, Dluhy RG, et al. *Circ Res* 1976;39:711–716.
34. Moore RA. *Anat Rec* 1931;48:153–168.
35. Dunnill MS, Halley W. *J Pathol* 1973;110:113–121.
36. Hayman JM Jr., Martin J Jr., Miller M. *Arch Int Med* 1939;64:69–83.
37. Kaysen GA, Watson JB. *Am J Physiol* 1982;343:F372–378.
38. Anderson S, Meyer TW, Rennke HG, Brenner BM. *J Clin Invest* 1985;76:612–619.
39. Koletsky S. *Arch Pathol* 1959;68:11–22.

40. Koletsky S, Goodsitt AM. *Arch Pathol* 1960;69:654–662.
41. Fetterman HG, Habib R. *Am J Clin Pathol* 1969;52:199–207.
42. McGraw M, Poucell S, Sweet J, Bramal R. *Int J Pediatr Nephrol* 1984;5:67–72.
43. Rugiu C, Oldrizzi L, Lupo A, et al. *Nephron* 1986;43:10–15.
44. Novick AC, Gephardt G, Guz B, Steinmuller D, Tubbs RR. *N Engl J Med* 1991;325:1058–1062.
45. Hakim R, Goldszer RC, Brenner BM. *Kidney Int* 1984;25:930–936.
46. Talseth T, Fauchald P, Skrede S, et al. *Kidney Int* 1986;29:1072–1076.
47. Kirkman RL, Strom TB, Weir MR, Tilney NL. *Transplantation* 1982;34(6):347–351.
48. Brenner BM, Cohen RA, Milford EL. *J Am Soc Nephrol* 1992;3(2):162–169.
49. Spitzer A, Chevalier RL. In: Seldin DW, Giebsch G, eds. *The kidney: physiology and pathophysiology.* New York: Raven Press; 1992;829–883.
50. McCrory WW. In: *Pediatric kidney disease.* Edelmann CH, ed. Boston: Little Brown; 1978;3–25.
51. Potter EL, Thierstein ST. *J Pediatr* 1943;22:695–706.
52. Karp R, Brasel JA, Winnik MD. *Am J Physiol* 1971;121:186–188.
53. Laufer I, Griscom NT. *Am J Roentgenol Radium Ther Nucl Med* 1971;113:464–472.
54. Aschinberg LC, Koskimies O, Bernstein J, et al. *Yale J Biol Med* 1978;51:341–45.
55. Celsi G, Bohman SO, Aperia A. *Pediatr Nephrol* 1987;1:290–296.
56. Gilbert T, Lelieve-Pegorier M, Merlet-Benichou C. *Pediatr Nephrol* 1990;4:445–450.
57. Gilbert T, Lelievre-Pegorier M, Merlet-Benichou C. *Pediatr Res* 1991;30:450–456.
58. Bernard B, Garcia-Cazares SJ, Ballard CA, et al. *Antimicrob Agents Chemother* 1977;11:688–694.
59. Zeman FJ. *J Nutrition* 1967;93:167–170.
60. Zeman FJ. *J Nutrition* 1968;94:111–116.
61. Merlet-Benichou C, Lelievre-Pegorier M, Gilbert T, Muffat-Joly M, Leroy B. *J. Am Soc Nephrol* 1992;49P.
62. Hall SM, Zeman FJ. *J Nutrition* 1969;95:49–54.
63. Leroy B, Josset P, Morgan G, Costil J, Merlet-Benichou C. *Pediatr Nephrol* 1991;5:C21.
64. Simpson A, Mortimer JG, Silva PA, Spears G, Williams S. In: Onesti G, Kim KE, eds. *Hypertension in the young and old.* New York: Grune and Stratton, 1981:153–163.
65. Cater J, Gill M. In: Illsley R, Mitchell RG, eds. *Low birth weight, a medical, psychological and social study.* Chichester: John Wiley, 1984:191–205.
66. Whincup PH, Cook DG, Shaper AG. *Br Med J* 1989;299:587–591.
67. Barker DJP, Osmond C, Golding J, Kuh D, Wadsworth MEJ. *B Med J* 1989;298:564–567.
68. deSwiet M, Fayers P, Shinebourne EA. *B Med J* 1992;304:23–26.
69. Law CM, Barker DJP, Bull AR, Osmond C. *Arch Dis Child* 1991;66:1291–1295.
70. Beishcer NA, Sivasamboo R, Vohra S, Silpisornkosal S, Reid S. *Journal of Obstetrics and Gynecology of the British Commonwealth* 1970;77:398–409.
71. Margette B, Rowland MGM, Foord FA, et al. *Int J Epidemiol* 1991;20:938–943.
72. Farchney GJ, White GA. *Aust J Biol Sci* 1987;40:365–377.
73. Barker DJP. *J Hypertens* 1992;10[Suppl 7]:S39–S44.
74. Levine RS, Hennekens CH, Jesse MJ. 1993;*B Med J* 1994 [in press].
75. Brenner BM, Chertow GM. *Current Opinion Nephrol Hyertens* 1993;2:691–695.
76. Williams S, St. George IM, Silva PA. *J Clin Epidemiol* 1992;45(11):1257–1263.
77. Seidman DS, Laor A, Gale R, et al. *B Med J* 1991;302:1235–1237.
78. Law CM, de Swiet M, Osmond C, et al. *B Med J* 1993;306:24–27.
79. Gennser G, Rymark P, Isberg PE. *B Med J* 1988;296:1498–1499.
80. Waaler HT. *Acta Med Scand* 1984;679:1–56.
81. Notkola V. *Living conditions in childhood and coronary heart disease in adulthood.* Helsinki: Finnish Society of Science and Letters, 1985.
82. Marmot MG, Shipley MJ, Rose G. *Lancet* 1984;1:1003–1006.
83. Barker DJP, Osmond C. *Lancet* 1986;1:1077–1081.
84. Barker DJP, Osmond C. *B Med J* 1987;295:83–86.
85. Barker DJP, Bull AR, Osmond C, Simmonds SJ. *B Med J* 1990;301:259–262.
86. Barker DJP, Winter PD, Osmond C, Margetts B, Simmonds SJ. *Lancet* 1989;2:577–580.
87. Viberti GC, Hill RD, Jarrett RJ, et al. *Lancet* 1982;1:1430–1432.
88. Mogensen CE, Christensen CK. *N Engl J Med* 1984;311:89–93.
89. Mattock MB, Keen H, Viberti GC, et al. *Diabetologia* 1988;31:82–87.
90. Kannel WB, Stampfer MJ, Castelli WP, Verter J. *Am Heart J* 1984;108:1347–1352.
91. Yudkin JS, Forest RD, Jackson CA. *Lancet* 1988;2:530–533.
92. Haffner SM, Stern MP, Kozlowski Gruber MK, et al. *Arteriosclerosis* 1990;10:727–731.
93. Liungman S. *Am J Hypertens* 1990;3:956–960.
94. Bianchi S, Bigazzi R, Baldari G, Campese VM. *Am J Hypertens* 1991;4:291–296.
95. Winocour PH, Harland JOE, Millar JP, Laker MR, Alberti KGMM. *Atherosclerosis* 1992;93:71–81.
96. Gould MM, Mohamed-Ali V, Goubet SA, Yudkin JS, Haines AP. *B Med J* 1993;306:240–242.
97. Kuh D, Wadsworth M. *Int J Epidemiol* 1989;18:663–668.
98. Morris JN, Marr JW, Clayton DG. *B Med J* 1977;2:1307–1319.
99. Folkow B. *Clin Sci* 1978;55:3–22S.
100. Hypertension Detection and Follow-up Program Cooperative Group. *JAMA* 1982;247:633–638.
101. Kempe A, Wise PH, Barkan SE, et al. *N Engl J Med* 1992;327:969–973.

Hypertension: Pathophysiology, Diagnosis, and Management, Second Edition,
edited by J.H. Laragh and B.M. Brenner,
Raven Press, Ltd., New York © 1995.

CHAPTER 7

Hypertension, Other Risk Factors, and the Risk of Cardiovascular Disease

Peter W. F. Wilson and William B. Kannel

A persistent and inappropriate elevation of blood pressure is, by any criterion, a direct cause of (a) serious cardiovascular disease and (b) premature mortality from such disease. The high prevalence of hypertension, as well as its large impact and controllability, has justifiably caused this condition to be given a high priority for detection and treatment by physicians and health officials.

While hypertension may be associated with encephalopathy and renal insufficiency, progressive atherosclerosis is the most common sequela. Whereas the fibrinoid arteriolar necrosis and Charcot-Bouchard aneurysms appear to be direct consequences of the high pressure, the atherosclerotic sequelae of hypertension involve a more complex pathogenesis. Hypertension plays a critical and independent role in atherogenesis, but its impact is greatly influenced by coexistent contributors to the occurrence of atherosclerosis, particularly the blood lipids.

P. W. F. Wilson: Framingham Heart Study, Framingham, Massachusetts.

W. B. Kannel: Section of Preventive Medicine and Epidemiology, Evans Department of Clinical Research, University Hospital, Boston University Medical Center, Boston, Massachusetts.

ATHEROSCLEROTIC HAZARDS

Atherosclerotic cardiovascular sequelae (CVD), including stroke, coronary heart disease (CHD), and peripheral arterial disease, all occur with a two- to threefold-increased frequency in hypertensives as compared to normotensives the same age (1–3). The relative risk is greatest for stroke, but because of its much greater incidence, coronary heart disease, particularly myocardial infarction (MI), is the most common sequela of hypertension (Table 1).

The uncertain efficacy of antihypertensive treatment in avoiding coronary heart disease has led some to unjustifiably doubt the atherogenicity of hypertension and its direct causal relationship to CHD. However, the risk of developing initial clinical manifestations of CHD is clearly related to prior blood pressure level. The incidence of every clinical manifestation of CHD is increased in hypertensive persons, and the risk is proportional to the severity of the antecedent hypertension (Table 2).

There is thus strong evidence linking blood pressure to clinical atherosclerotic pathology. In fact, blood pressure appears to be critical to the atherosclerotic process, because lesions seldom occur in low-pressure parts of the

TABLE 1. *Incidence of atherosclerotic cardiovascular events by hypertensive status, 30-year follow-up, Framingham Study*

| Age (years) | Hypertensive status | Age-adjusted annual rate per 1000 | | | | | |
| | | Atherothrombotic brain infarction | | Myocardial infarction | | Peripheral arterial disease | |
		Men[a]	Women[a]	Men[a]	Women[a]	Men	Women
35–64	Normal	0	0	4	1	2[a]	1[a]
	Mild	1	1	8	2	4[a]	1[a]
	Definite	4	2	10	3	5[a]	3[a]
65–94	Normal	3	1	7	4	6[b]	3[b]
	Mild	5	4	17	7	7[b]	3[b]
	Definite	12	9	21	9	9[b]	5[b]

[a] $p < .001$.
[b] Not significant.

TABLE 2. *Clinical manifestations of CHD by hypertensive status, 30-year follow-up, Framingham Study*

| Hypertensive status[a] | Age-adjusted rate per 1000 | | | | | | | |
| | Angina pectoris | | Myocardial infarction | | Sudden death | | Total CHD | |
	Men[b]	Women[b]	Men[b]	Women[b]	Men[b]	Women[b]	Men[b]	Women[b]
Normal	7.6	5.8	8.4	3.0	4.2	1.3	17.4	9.6
Mild	14.7	10.1	16.8	5.8	7.5	2.3	32.2	17.5
Definite	16.1	12.4	12.1	8.0	9.4	2.7	43.5	23.4

[a] Normal, <140/90 mm Hg; mild, 140–159/90–94 mm Hg; definite, 160/95 mm Hg and over.
[b] All trends significant at $p < .001$; subjects 35–94 years of age.

circulation such as the pulmonary arteries or veins, despite their exposure to atherogenic blood lipids. Animal experiments have clearly demonstrated that lipid-induced atherogenesis can be accelerated or retarded by manipulating the blood pressure (4,5).

UNRECOGNIZED MYOCARDIAL INFARCTION

Isolated systolic hypertension predisposes to ischemic infarction of the myocardium in either sex and in the elderly as well as the young (Fig. 1). Some 28 percent of myocardial infarctions in men and 33 percent in women are silent or exhibit atypical symptoms and go unrecognized (6). Hypertension, for reasons which are unclear, appears to predispose particularly to these kinds of occult myocardial infarction. In hypertensive men and women,

respectively, 35 percent and 45 percent of infarctions are unrecognized (Table 3). This is true even if confounding factors such as diabetes, electrocardiogram-left ventricular hypertrophy (ECG-LVH) and antihypertensive treatment are excluded (7). It would appear that the hypertensive person should be periodically monitored by ECG for occurrence of a silent MI. Unrecognized MIs cannot be ignored, because they carry as serious a long-term prognosis as typical symptomatic infarctions (6).

CHARACTER OF HYPERTENSION

It is widely believed that significant hypertension is distinguishable from innocuous blood pressure elevation by the character of the elevated pressure. Diastolic elevations are accorded more importance than systolic in-

TABLE 3. *Proportion of myocardial infarctions unrecognized by hypertensive status excluding possible predisposing conditions*

| Hypertensive status | Percent of myocardial infarctions unrecognized | | | | | |
| | Excluding diabetics[a] | | Excluding anti-HBP Rx[a] | | Excluding LVH[a] | |
	Men	Women	Men	Women	Men	Women
Normal	18.5	30.7	17.8	26.6	19.6	29.0
Mild	28.3	36.1	30.2	35.5	30.1	35.3
Definite	33.2	48.1	34.8	48.5	32.7	50.5

[a] Also excludes persons with coronary heart disease at exam immediately preceding myocardial infarction.
LVH, left ventricular hypertrophy; HBP Rx, high blood pressure medication.

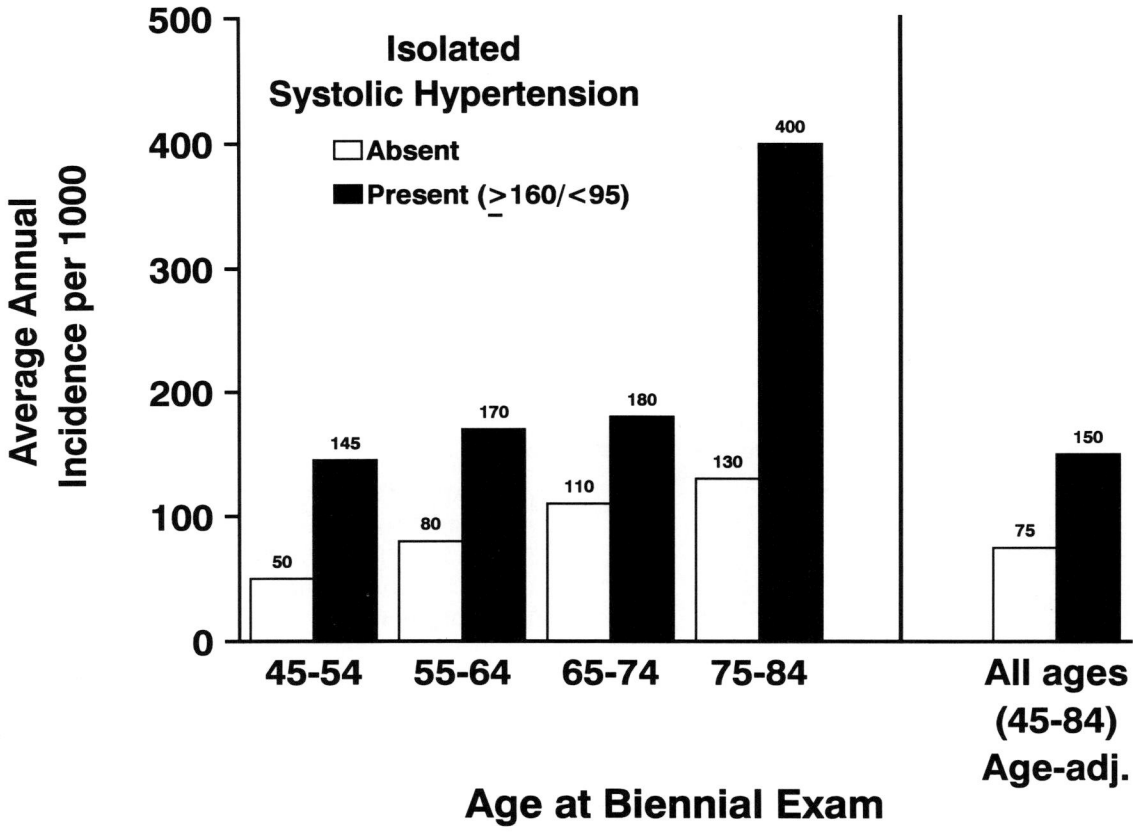

FIG. 1. Risk of myocardial infarction with isolated systolic hypertension (>160/<95 mm Hg), 24-year follow-up, Framingham Study, men aged 45–84 years (*p* < 0.01)

creases. There is, however, no evidence from Framingham (8) or Multiple Risk Factor Intervention Trial (MRFIT) data (9) that major cardiovascular sequelae are more closely linked to the diastolic than the systolic pressure (Table 4). Comparison of regression coefficients for systolic and diastolic pressure in relation to development of cardiovascular disease, suitably standardized to equalize for the different range of values, gives no indication of a greater impact of diastolic pressure. In the elderly,

the diastolic component loses a great deal of its impact, particularly in women.

In the elderly, systolic pressure rises disproportionately as the arteries lose their compliance. This arterial rigidity results in a wide pulse pressure with isolated systolic hypertension (Fig. 2). In the elderly with isolated systolic hypertension, knowledge of the accompanying diastolic pressure is often used to judge the need for treatment. This would appear to be unwise, because risk of

TABLE 4. *Incidence of cardiovascular disease by levels of systolic and diastolic pressure, 30-year follow-up, Framingham Study*

| | Annual age-adjusted rate per 1000 | | | | | | | | |
| | 35–64 | | 65–94 | | Diastolic pressure | 35–64 | | 65–94 | |
Systolic pressure	Men	Women	Men	Women		Men	Women	Men	Women
74–119	10	4	20	14	20–74	12	6	32	25
120–139	12	6	26	23	75–84	12	6	32	23
140–159	21	11	39	25	85–94	19	10	41	33
160–179	31	13	61	27	95–104	25	13	70	23
180–300	40	23	86	48	105–160	39	22	94	44
Standardized regression coefficient:	.406[a]	.442[a]	.463[a]	.282[a]		.351[a]	.368[a]	.300[a]	.122[b]

[a] *p* < .001.
[b] *p* < .05.

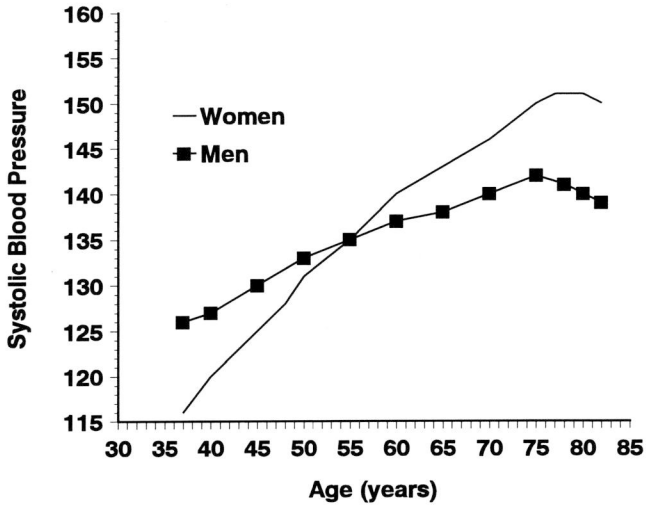

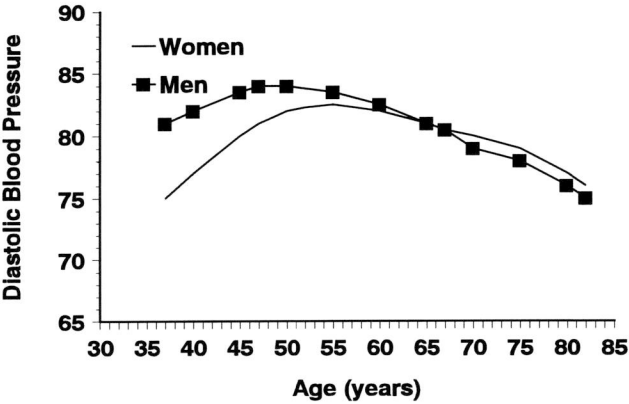

FIG. 2. Top: Cross-sectional age trends in systolic blood pressure levels (mm Hg), Framingham Study, exams 3–16. **Bottom:** Cross-sectional age trends in diastolic blood pressure levels (mm Hg), Framingham Study, exams 3–16.

cardiovascular sequelae in the Framingham Study elderly with systolic hypertension was unrelated to the accompanying diastolic pressure (10). In diastolic hypertensives, on the other hand, accompanying systolic pressure was highly predictive (Fig. 3). Thus, reliance on the diastolic pressure can be misleading. In persons whose diastolic pressures had never exceeded 95 mm Hg over 30 years of follow-up, risk of cardiovascular disease was shown to be related to systolic pressure at all ages, including the elderly (Fig. 4).

Labile blood pressure elevations are considered to be relatively innocuous, and only fixed elevations are thought to be dangerous enough to warrant treatment. However, any designation of labile or fixed hypertension has been shown to be questionable and without prognostic utility (11). Lability of blood pressure increases with age and with the level of the pressure so that, taken alone, lability is associated with *increased* risk. However, multivariate analysis, taking age and the level of pressure into account, indicates that at any given average pressure, risk of cardiovascular disease is unaffected by the variability of the pressure. Dismissing labile elevations of pressure as innocuous is unjustified if the average of a series of office pressures is high. The need for treatment should be based on the *average,* not the lowest pressure recorded on a patient.

ISOLATED SYSTOLIC HYPERTENSION

Owing to a disproportionate rise in systolic blood pressure as age advances, the prevalence of isolated systolic hypertension increases sharply in advanced age (Fig. 5). This variety is the predominant type of hypertension encountered in the elderly (10). This isolated systolic hypertension is not innocuous, and affected persons experience a twofold increase in risk of cardiovascular disease (Table 5) (12). The high systolic pressure appears to be a direct cause of this cardiovascular morbidity and mortality rather than only a sign of the diseased rigid artery. Systolic hypertension is a persistent risk factor when arterial rigidity is taken into account (10).

The chief determinant of systolic hypertension in advanced age is prior elevated blood pressure in middle age (Fig. 6). All components of pressure appear to predispose, particularly the prior systolic pressure. About one-third of isolated systolic pressure appears to evolve from prior diastolic or combined hypertension.

CORRELATES OF HYPERTENSION

Hypertension occurs in association with various atherogenic factors which either promote its occurrence or influence its impact on cardiovascular health. A number of nutritional factors believed to affect blood lipids and atherosclerotic cardiovascular disease also may affect blood pressure, including saturated fat, excess calories, and low calcium and magnesium intake (4,5). Essential hypertension is more common in persons with a family history of hypertension, and when so predisposed there is substantial evidence incriminating high salt and low potassium intake (4).

In the Framingham Study, adiposity, a rapid heart rate, high-normal hematocrit, and elevated blood sugar have all been found to be related to the occurrence of hypertension in one or both sexes. Adiposity is a major controllable contributor to hypertension which also promotes all of the atherogenic cardiovascular risk factors.

In the usual range of hematocrit accepted as within normal limits, there is a threefold variation in the prevalence of hypertension (3). Partially, but not entirely, as a result of this, CHD and stroke incidence are increased in persons with high-normal hematocrit (3). Both hematocrit and hypertension are associated with elevated fibrinogen values (13), and the latter has been

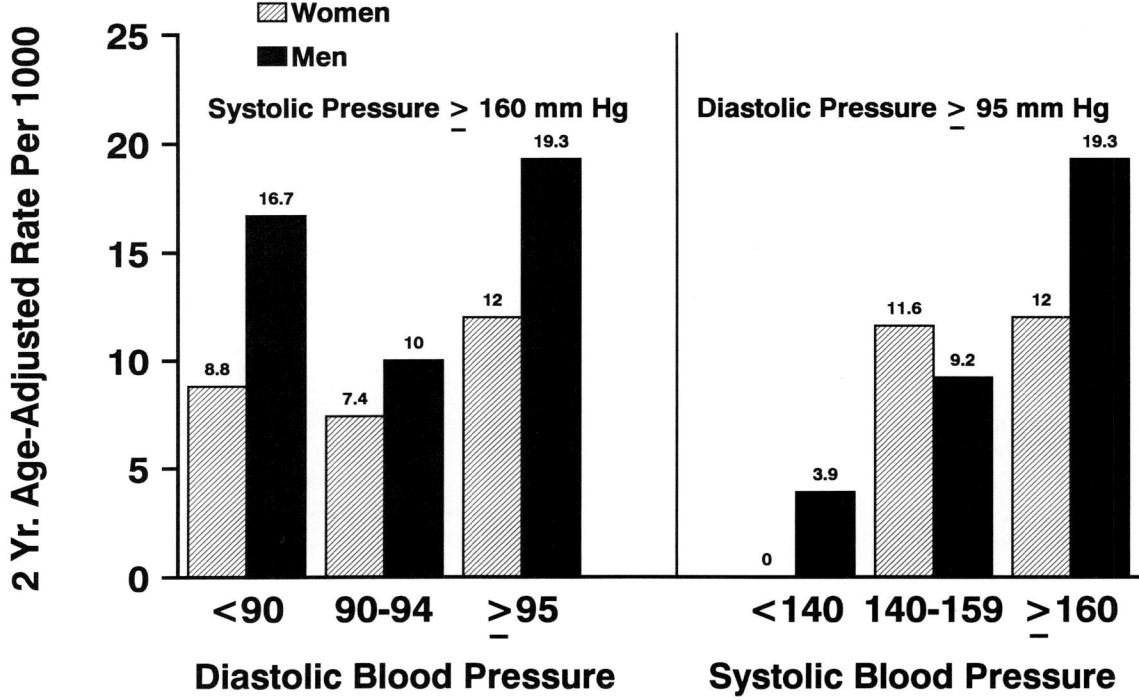

FIG. 3. Risk of stroke according to systolic and diastolic pressures in subjects with systolic or diastolic hypertension, Framingham Study, 26-year follow-up. The subjects were 35–84 years of age.

shown to be associated with an increased risk of CHD and stroke (14,15).

Although the hazards of hypertension and the efficacy of treatment are now well appreciated, the precursors and determinants of most hypertension in the general population are not well understood. Prevention of this powerful and highly prevalent force of morbidity and mortality would appear preferable to early detection and a lifetime of antihypertensive treatment. An understand-

ing of the precursors of hypertension is essential to the development of effective preventive programs.

OBESITY AND HYPERTENSION

Personal attributes found to be related to systolic or diastolic blood pressure at the first examination in the Framingham offspring sample were examined for a re-

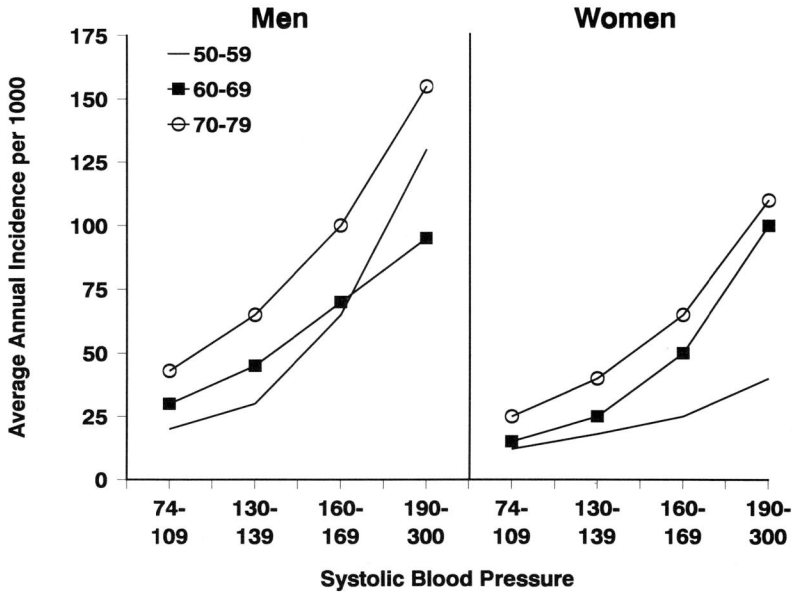

FIG. 4. Risk of cardiovascular disease according to systolic blood pressure, for persons with diastolic blood pressure ≤ 95, Framingham Study, 20-year follow-up. The subjects were men and women, 50–79 years of age.

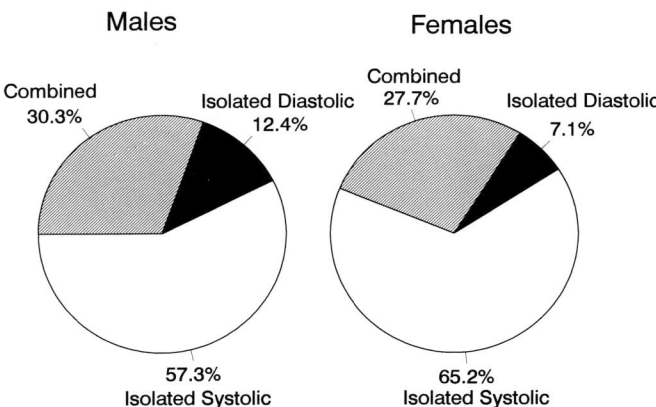

Males

Females

FIG. 5. **Left:** Distribution of hypertensives among Framingham Study elderly males, aged 65–89. **Right:** Distribution of hypertensives among Framingham Study elderly females, aged 65–89.

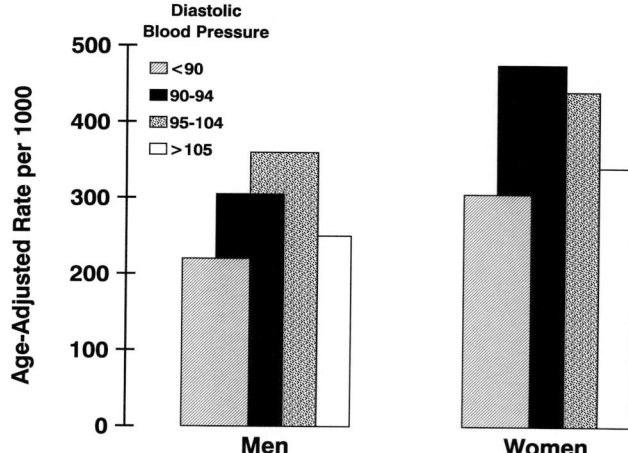

FIG. 6. Risk of developing isolated systolic hypertension by diastolic blood pressure level, 24-year follow-up, Framingham Study.

lations to subsequent development of hypertension over the ensuing 8 years (Table 6). Prominently included among these correlated factors were the various measures of weight or adiposity (16).

Graphic display of hypertension incidence according to the subscapular skinfold thickness indicates a remarkably strong relationship in all but the youngest age group of men (Fig. 7). Hypertension rarely developed in lean men in their fourth and fifth decade. Multivariate analysis indicated a significant and prominent net effect of adiposity, taking other correlated variables into account (see Table 6). Subscapular skinfolds rank high among the independent contributors to hypertension risk, judging from the size of the standardized regression coefficients. Comparison of bivariate coefficients (including only age) with multivariate coefficients (including all cofactors) indicates that only 15 percent of the subscapular skinfold effect is accounted for by other risk factors for hypertension. Future hypertensives tended to evolve from the upper end of the normal blood pressure distribution. Hence, initial blood pressure is actually the best single predictor of future hypertension incidence. However, a fat person is at increased risk of future hypertension, whatever the initial pressure. Baseline blood pressure ex-

plains no more than 20 percent of the hypertension-obesity-incidence relationship.

Further documentation of the close (and probably directly causal) relationship between obesity and hypertension is provided by an examination of the relationship between (a) change in subscapular skinfold thickness and (b) change in recorded systolic and diastolic blood pressure. Even after controlling for baseline blood pressure, changes in body fatness are related to observed changes in systolic and diastolic blood pressure.

Although the efficacy of early detection and treatment is well documented, the treated hypertensive remains at above average risk for cardiovascular disease. A lifetime of antihypertensive treatment is no small matter and includes a substantial penalty in cost, inconvenience, and

TABLE 5. *Risk of cardiovascular events and mortality in subjects with isolated systolic hypertension, 24-year follow-up, Framingham Study*

	Factor of increased risk[a]		Rate per 100	
	Men	Women	Men	Women
Cardiovascular events	2.5	2.4	82.3	42.6
Cardiovascular mortality	2.1	3.1	29.6	11.9
Overall mortality	1.9	1.9	52.6	26.8

[a] Summary odds ratio: ISH/normotensive.
ISH, isolated systolic hypertensive.

TABLE 6. *Independent contributions of specified risk factors for development of hypertension, Framingham Offspring Study*

	Multiple logistic standardized regression coefficients	
Risk factors	Men (1313)	Women (1507)
Subscapular skinfold	.283[a]	.373[a]
Cigarette smoking	.166[b]	−.086[b]
Alcohol	.132[b]	.202[c]
Heart rate	.293[a]	.302[a]
Hematocrit	.071[b]	.247[a]
Glucose	−.149[b]	−.035[b]
Protein	.200[b]	.201[b]
Triglyceride	.179[c]	.091[b]
Phosphorous	.029[b]	.049[b]
Age	.581[d]	.746[d]

[a] $p < .01$.
[b] Not significant.
[c] $p < .05$.
[d] $p < .001$.

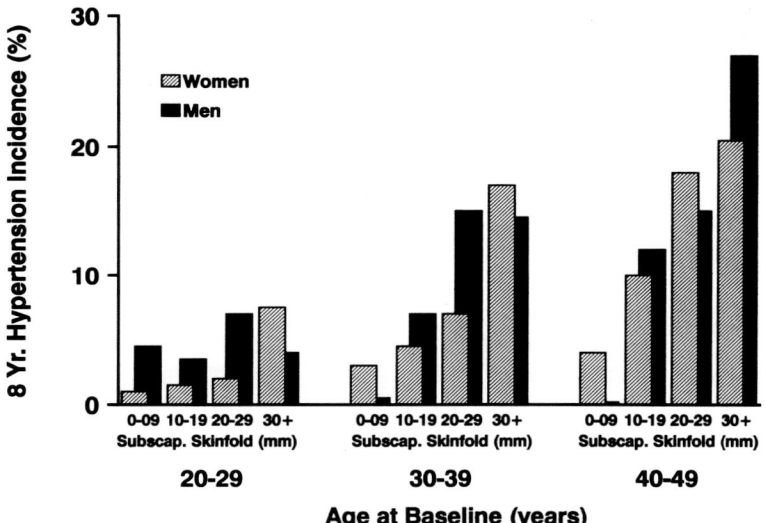

FIG. 7. Incidence of hypertension by subscapular skinfold thickness for three age groups of middle-aged men and women.

side effects. Despite aggressive treatment of hypertension in recent years, there is little evidence that the prevalence of hypertension has declined. Among the modifiable predisposing factors for hypertension, adiposity stands out. Although the hypertension hazard of obesity is well demonstrated in this and other studies, the mechanism is not well understood.

Abnormalities in cell membrane cation transport have been demonstrated in both obesity and hypertension. Hyperinsulinemia is common in obesity, and this can enhance renal tubular sodium reabsorption and retention. Interventions known to improve insulin sensitivity—including weight reduction, exercise, and low-fat, high-fiber diets—do lower blood pressure.

Weight reduction has been shown to reduce blood pressure whether concomitant dietary sodium intake is high or low. The data suggest that obesity is a powerful contributor to hypertension in young adults. The majority of hypertension in women, as well as much of the

early-onset hypertension in men, can be attributed to excess body fat. Attributable risk estimates, using an obesity threshold of 1 cm of subscapular skinfold, suggest that 78 percent of hypertension in men, as opposed to 65 percent in women, is directly attributable to adiposity (16). These data suggest that weight control could have a major impact on the occurrence of hypertension in young and middle-aged adults.

INFLUENCE OF COFACTOR(S)

The propensity of the hypertensive patient to develop cardiovascular sequelae is markedly influenced by coexistent cardiovascular risk factors (3). Judgment as to the need for treatment, particularly in those with mild hypertension, must take into account the presence of other risk factors (Fig. 8) (17). Also, attention to these coexistent risk factors is needed if maximum benefit is to be

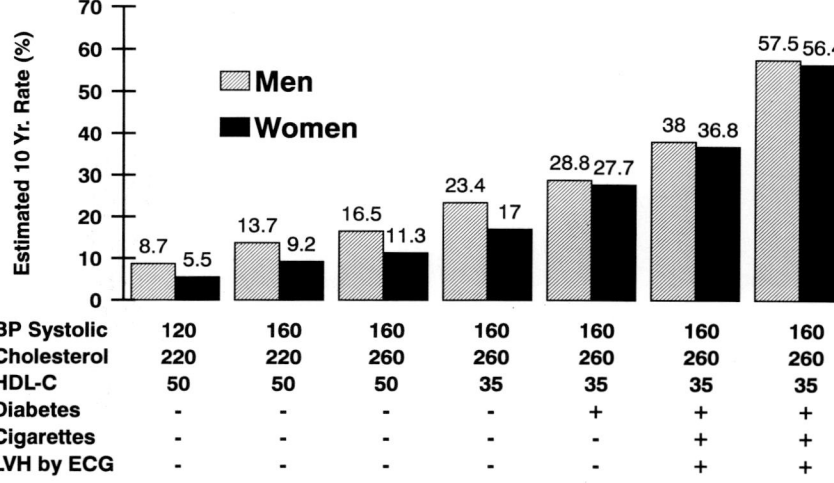

BP Systolic	120	160	160	160	160	160	160
Cholesterol	220	220	260	260	260	260	260
HDL-C	50	50	50	35	35	35	35
Diabetes	-	-	-	-	+	+	+
Cigarettes	-	-	-	-	-	+	+
LVH by ECG	-	-	-	-	-	+	+

FIG. 8. Estimated risk of coronary heart disease over 10 years according to various combinations of risk factor levels for men and women. (From ref. 17, with permission.)

TABLE 7. *Risk of cardiovascular disease[a] in hypertensives by age and sex, 30-year follow-up, Framingham Study*

Age	Risk ratios[b]		Biennial rate per 1000	
	Men	Women	Men	Women
35–44	1.9	1.7	28	10
45–54	1.8	1.7	54	22
55–64	1.8	1.9	88	54
65–74	1.9	1.5	122	62
75–84	2.0	1.3	228	96

[a] Cardiovascular disease: coronary heart disease, stroke, cardiac failure, and occlusive peripheral arterial disease.

[b] Ratio of rate in hypertensive (>160/95 mm Hg) to that in normotensive (<140/90 mm Hg).

achieved. Drugs which lower pressure at the expense of raised low-density lipoprotein (LDL) cholesterol, blood sugar, and uric acid values may not improve the total risk profile. This may explain why the results of antihypertensive treatment trials have been so disappointing for CHD (18). Attention to coronary risk factors through diet, exercise, and weight control may also help control the blood pressure.

AGE AND SEX

Except in some primitive societies, the blood pressure level and the prevalence of hypertension tend to rise with age (19). Whatever the variety of hypertension encountered in the elderly, it is clearly dangerous. Whether judged by the absolute risk, risk ratios, risk gradient, or attributable risks, hypertension is as hazardous in the el-

derly as in the young. However, in the long term the young hypertensive has more to lose, because the chance to reach advanced age is much reduced. Hypertension at any age in either sex is dangerous (Table 7).

INFLUENCE OF BLOOD LIPIDS

The lipoproteins are fundamental to the atherosclerotic process and greatly affect the impact of hypertension on the pace of atherogenesis. An association between the serum total cholesterol and the rate of occurrence of CHD has long been recognized, and this greatly affects the influence of blood pressure on CHD incidence. The established association of the serum total cholesterol with CHD incidence is now recognized as a direct consequence of the atherogenic LDL cholesterol component (20,21). The high-density lipoprotein (HDL) cholesterol fraction also greatly influences the rate of hypertension-induced atherogenesis by augmenting the rate of removal of excess cholesterol from the tissues (20). Thus, the serum total cholesterol actually reflects a two-way traffic of cholesterol in and out of the tissues, and jointly these have a profound effect on the impact of hypertension (Fig. 9).

The very-low-density lipoprotein (VLDL) is a precursor of LDL and is involved in HDL metabolism. It also transports some cholesterol, but it chiefly transports triglyceride (20). However, the VLDL and its cholesterol or triglyceride content make no apparent independent contribution to atherogenesis. The addition of knowledge of triglyceride to a lipid profile comprised of HDL and LDL cholesterol does not improve prediction of the likelihood of developing CHD (22).

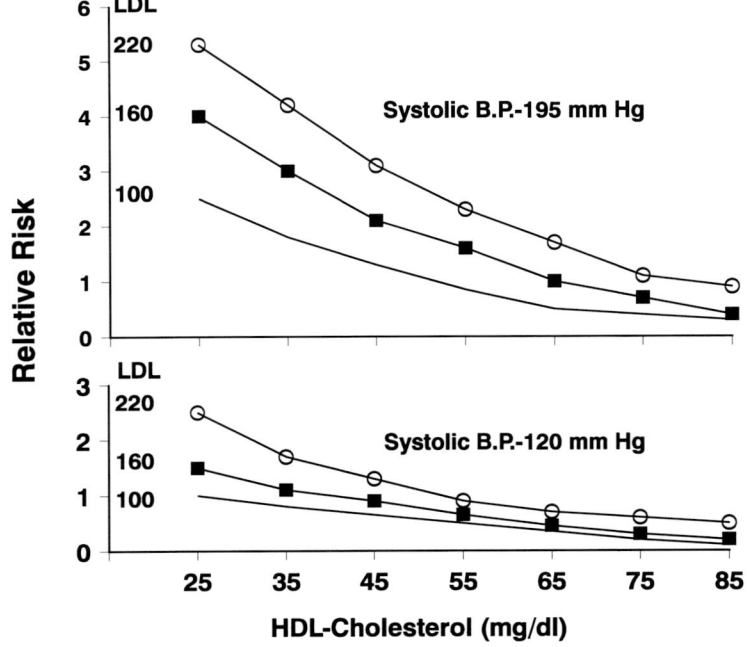

FIG. 9. Relative risk of coronary heart disease according to high-density lipoprotein cholesterol (HDL), low-density lipoprotein cholesterol (LDL), and systolic blood pressure, Framingham Study. The subjects were men, 50–70 years of age.

A practical and efficient means for assessing the combined influence of the atherogenic LDL and protective HDL components of the serum total cholesterol is to form a ratio of LDL (or total) cholesterol to HDL cholesterol. This lipoprotein profile conveniently estimates risk over a wide range at all ages and even beyond age 65, when the serum total cholesterol has less predictive power (2). It also does so within the usual range of serum cholesterol values often not considered to be of high risk (20). It greatly helps to assess the risk among hypertensive persons.

Serum total cholesterol values exceeding 200 mg/dl are, on average, suboptimal for cardiovascular health. A favorable response to antilipemic therapy is to achieve a total-cholesterol-to-HDL-cholesterol ratio below 5.0, the standard risk. An optimal ratio (which corresponds to half the high average CHD rate in the United States) is about 3, which may be required in order to slow or regress accelerated atherogenesis encountered in hypertensive persons. The protective effect of HDL cholesterol is at least as strong as the atherogenic influence of LDL cholesterol. For every 5 mg/dl difference in HDL cholesterol, risk is affected 11 percent in middle-aged adults (23).

Some antihypertensive agents, including widely used thiazide diuretics and beta blockers, may adversely affect the atherogenic lipid profile. Although direct evidence is unavailable, there is no reason to believe that lipid derangements induced by medication have a different significance than those induced by lifestyles. Fortunately, most of the measures recommended for avoiding CHD in general, such as exercise, weight reduction, and avoidance of cigarettes, raise HDL cholesterol (24). Weight control has been shown to control the adverse effects of antihypertensive treatment on blood lipids and glucose tolerance (25,26).

Although the relation of serum cholesterol to occurrence of CHD is clear, its association with the incidence of atherothrombotic brain infarction is weaker (27). Also, epidemiologic studies often show a quadratic relation of overall mortality to serum total cholesterol, with an excess of deaths at both extremes of the cholesterol distribution (28). Reports suggest that this may be due to an excess of cancer mortality and hemorrhagic stroke at low serum cholesterol values and high coronary mortality at elevated cholesterol levels (27). The excess cancer mortality associated with low serum total cholesterol values appears to be largely in the form of colon cancer. It is unlikely that this is a causal relationship. The low serum cholesterol may in fact be a consequence of already existent occult cancer of the colon because the relationship wanes with length of follow-up (28,29). Furthermore, this relationship is not found in women and is not biologically explicable. It is actually paradoxical because high-fat diets commonly associated with elevated cholesterol values have been incriminated in colon cancer (28).

Also countries with low serum cholesterols and low CHD mortality rates have *low,* not high colon cancer rates.

DIET AND SODIUM

The nature of the diet has been incriminated in both hypertension and atherogenesis. International comparisons, migrant studies, secular trends, and experimental studies all indicate powerful environmental influences on the serum total cholesterol, and no environmental factor determines the serum total cholesterol and its atherogenic LDL component more than the nature of the diet (30). Both are raised by excess calories, saturated fats, dietary cholesterol, and possibly animal protein. Fiber, polyunsaturated fat, weight reduction, fiber, and possibly vegetable protein will lower these atherogenic lipids (30). Recent Joint National Committee V recommendations for diet include restriction of alcohol intake to less than 1 oz/day and sodium to less than 100 mmol/day (equivalent to <2.3 g sodium or <6 g sodium chloride). Maintenance of normal calcium, potassium, and magnesium intakes was also suggested (31).

Appropriate dietary modifications can reduce the incidence of hypertension (32), lower the degree of dependence on antihypertensive drugs, and counteract drug-induced lipid derangements, glucose intolerance, hypopotassemia, and magnesium diuresis. Diet must be presumed to be a major determinant of the pace of atherogenesis because of its influence on atherogenic blood lipids, on blood pressure; and, through obesity, on glucose tolerance.

Renin profiling may also bear relationship to CHD risk. A recent prospective study reported that higher-than-normal renin levels for a given daily sodium excretion, independent of smoking and other risk factors (33),

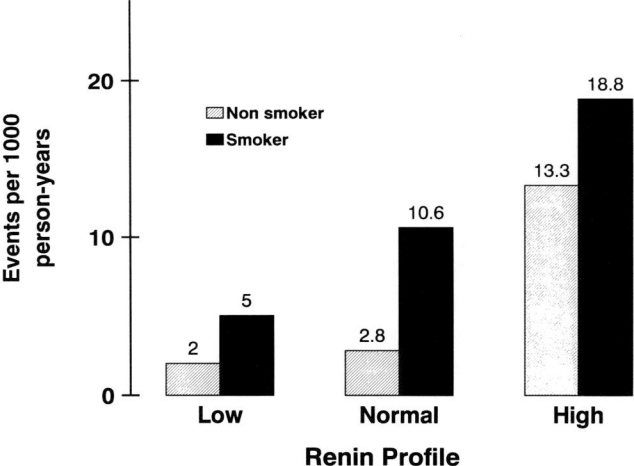

FIG. 10. CHD incidence according to cigarette use and renin profile (From ref. 33, with permission.)

were associated with increased risk of myocardial infarction. This relationship was not found to hold for stroke or noncardiovascular disease (Fig. 10). Measurement of sodium excretion and plasma renin levels holds the greatest promise for coronary risk prediction among individuals at mild-to-moderate risk with little evidence of other risk factors.

GLUCOSE INTOLERANCE

Hypertension is a common problem in the diabetic, and many hypertensive persons have impaired glucose tolerance. Diabetes is often associated with a suboptimal cardiovascular risk profile, including a low HDL cholesterol, obesity, and high blood pressure. The risk of clinical manifestations of CHD in hypertensive persons is greatly worsened by coexistent diabetes (see Fig. 8). The impact of concurrent diabetes is greater in women than in men, making women equally vulnerable to cardiovascular sequelae. Since diabetes may directly damage the myocardium, hypertensive susceptibility to cardiac failure is enhanced. Diuretic-induced hyperglycemia may be a liability in controlling hypertension. This may be controlled by either weight reduction or a shift to other antihypertensive agents when this is a problem.

Some, but not all, of the increased risk of CHD associated with diabetes is a consequence of associated risk factors, and diabetics with a low level of other risk factors fare much better than those burdened with multiple risk factors. Nevertheless, there is some unique atherogenic feature of diabetes which may be a consequence of associated thrombogenic tendencies, such as abnormal factors VII and VIII and increased fibrinogen or platelet aggregation (13).

OBESITY

Approximately 70 percent of newly acquired hypertension in the Framingham Study was attributed to prior obesity (34). Obesity is common in middle-aged Americans, particularly in those who develop hypertension. The obese are at increased risk of coronary disease, stroke, and cardiac failure. Some, but not all, of this increased risk in the obese is attributable to its effect on cardiovascular risk factors.

All of the atherogenic accompaniments of hypertension, as well as the hypertension itself, can be improved by weight reduction (3). The adverse effects of antihypertensive agents employed to control hypertension can often be alleviated by weight reduction (26). It is alleged that obesity of the upper trunk, rather than generalized obesity, is particularly dangerous (35). It is also alleged that hypertension associated with obesity is not as serious as that which occurs in lean persons. Examination of the prognosis of hypertension in relation to degree of

TABLE 8. *Multivariate logistic regression coefficients for HBP for each level of BMI controlled for age and cigarette smoking by sex*[a]

BMI	Men	Women
<21	.823	.722
21	.614	1.532
22	.661	.949
23	.751	.601
24	.217	.915
25	.702	.589
26	1.036	.819
27	.847	.470
28	1.237	.860
29	.680	1.124
30	.805	.777

[a] Eight-year incidence of cardiovascular disease is the outcome variable. This involved cross-sectional pooling using 32-year follow-up baseline exams 1, 5, 9, and 13.
HBP, hypertension; BMI, body mass index.

associated adiposity in the Framingham cohort indicates no less impact in the obese than in the lean (Table 8).

Of particular relevance to the atherosclerosis-prone hypertensive person, obesity promotes rises in serum total cholesterol, LDL cholesterol, triglycerides, blood glucose, and uric acid (36). It also reduces the HDL cholesterol, causing a deterioration in the LDL/HDL cholesterol ratio. Weight control is a major hygienic necessity for the hypertensive candidate for cardiovascular disease.

ORGAN INVOLVEMENT

Most hypertension is, for a long time, an asymptomatic condition; and antihypertensive treatment has side effects, leading many physicians to consider that treatment prior to evidence of organ involvement is meddlesome. However, awaiting indications of organ involvement cannot be justified (37). More than half of all coronary attacks in hypertensive persons will occur before subclinical evidence of organ involvement appears on biennial exam. Too often, the first indication of organ involvement is an unheralded myocardial infarction, a sudden death, or a stroke.

A frequent manifestation of organ involvement in hypertension is ECG-LVH (Fig. 11) (38). It is far from an incidental finding, however, and augurs ill once it appears, particularly if accompanied by repolarization abnormalities (38). Clinical manifestations of CHD occur at about two to three times the rate of the general population. Comparison of ECG-LVH with the occurrence of silent myocardial infarction indicates a similar prognosis, with subsequent rates of clinical coronary events similar to those for ECG-MI (Table 9). The risk of stroke and cardiac failure associated with ECG-LVH is actually

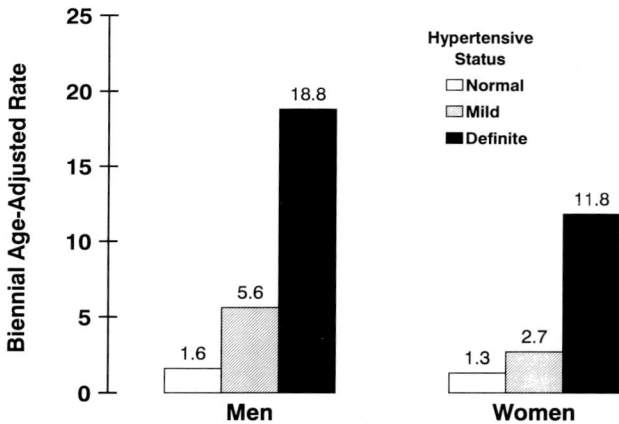

FIG. 11. Development of electrocardiogram-left ventricular hypertrophy (ECG-LVH) by hypertensive status, 30-year follow-up. Framingham Study. The subjects were 35–84 years of age. Trends were significant at $p < 0.001$.

significantly greater than that following appearance of ECG-MI; in women, this risk persists after adjustment for coexistent hypertension. Since ECG-LVH behaves like ECG-MI, it would appear appropriate to treat hypertensive persons with ECG-LVH as if they had already sustained a myocardial infarction. The prevalence of both hypertension and ECG-LVH have declined over the past three decades, and on a population basis antihypertensive treatment can prevent ECG-LVH. Whether treatment after ECG-LVH is established can reduce CVD risk remains to be determined.

An enlarged heart on X-ray also escalates the risk of cardiovascular sequelae in hypertensive persons (38). Hypertrophy on X-ray, however, is not as ominous as ECG-LVH. In the hypertensive candidate for cardiovascular disease, echocardiography is a more sensitive detector of hypertrophy, which has been found to be associated with an increased risk of CHD in prospective analyses (39). Other ECG abnormalities, such as intraventricular conduction disturbance and nonspecific S-T and T-wave abnormalities, are also more commonly found in persons with hypertension; all of the ECG abnormalities are associated with an increased risk of cardiovascular sequelae (38).

HYPERTENSION IN THE ELDERLY

Disease, disability, and death from cardiovascular disease are major and growing problems for the elderly. Hypertension predominates as a predisposing factor because of its high prevalence and continuing impact into advanced age. In the elderly, a greater emphasis on the systolic pressure is needed because there is a disproportionate rise in systolic pressure which continues into advanced age, while diastolic pressure levels off and falls (see Fig. 2). The high frequency of isolated systolic hypertension which ensues is far from an innocuous accompaniment of arterial rigidity, because it carries a two- to threefold excess cardiovascular morbidity and mortality (see Table 5). This contribution to risk is independent of degree of arterial rigidity measured by pulse wave configuration (10).

Whether predominantly systolic or diastolic, labile or fixed, hypertension in the elderly of either sex is clearly dangerous in terms of absolute risk, relative risk, risk gradients, or attributable risk. Some 30 to 60 percent of all cardiovascular disease in the elderly appears to be attributable to either mild or severe hypertension. Cardiovascular mortality in the hypertensive elderly is tripled as compared to that in normotensives the same age.

In the elderly, systolic hypertension is a more reliable predictor of cardiovascular disease than is diastolic pressure, because diastolic pressure is often actually misleading in the elderly with systolic hypertension (see Fig. 3). There is no sign of a diminishing impact of systolic pressure with advancing age. Pressure after age 65 is as strongly related to cardiovascular risk in the elderly as pressure prior to that age (Fig. 12).

The impact of hypertension, as measured by relative risk, is greatest for stroke; but in terms of absolute incidence, coronary disease is the most common sequela under age 65. Although the absolute risk is lower, relative and attributable risks are just as large for women as for men over age 65 (see Table 7). Lability of blood pressure increases with age and blood pressure level; but at a given average pressure, lability has no influence on risk in the older hypertensive patient.

Adiposity, heart rate, alcohol intake, hematocrit, blood sugar, serum cholesterol, and triglyceride are all

TABLE 9. *Ten-year, age-adjusted incidence (rate/100) of coronary heart disease morbidity among subjects with ECG-LVH or ECG-MI*

Event	ECG-LVH	Men, ECG-MI	General rate[a]	ECG-LVH	Women, ECG-MI	General rate
Coronary heart disease	30.1	42.9	19.1	27.8	38.1	12.9
	42/132[b]	34/81	213/2240	37/134	20/53	109/2815
Myocardial infarction	16.1	21.7	10.0	9.8	15.0	5.0
	21/132	17/81	103/2240	13/134	8/53	29/2815

[a] Based on the general Framingham sample.
[b] Number of events/number at risk.
ECG-LVH, electrocardiogram-left ventricular hypertrophy; ECG-MI, electrocardiogram-myocardial infarction.

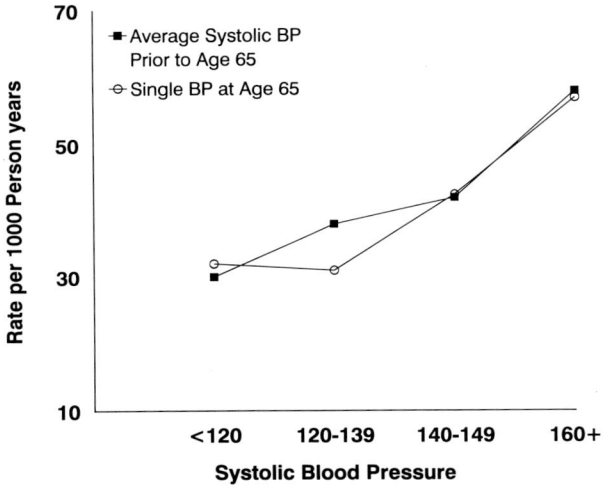

FIG. 12. Systolic blood pressure and risk of cardiovascular disease after age 65 in Framingham Study.

TABLE 10. *Effect of therapy for isolated systolic hypertension on vascular disease risk*

Event	Relative risk	95% Confidence interval for relative risk
Stroke	0.63	0.49–0.82
MI	0.67	0.47–0.96
Severe CHD*	0.75	0.60–0.94
CVD	0.68	0.58–0.79

* Includes myocardial infarction (MI) and coronary heart disease (CHD) death.
From SHEP Cooperative Research Group, ref. 12.

related to occurrence of hypertension in the elderly, and, as in younger hypertensives, cardiovascular risk is markedly affected by coexistent atherogenic cofactors. Hypertension in the elderly is best regarded as a component of a multifactorial cardiovascular risk profile, both for assessment of the hazard it imposes and in implementing optimal therapy. Preventive management should take into account not only the height and character of the blood pressure elevation, but the multivariate risk profile as well.

Awaiting evidence of target organ involvement is also unjustified in the elderly, since half the cardiovascular events precede its appearance. The occurrence of ECG-LVH is particularly ominous, and indicates impending cardiovascular sequelae such as a stroke (Fig. 13). The recently completed Systolic Hypertension in the Elderly

Program (SHEP), a trial of therapy for isolated systolic hypertension, showed that administration of a low-dose thiazide effectively prevents CVD in this age group, reducing incidence of stroke by 37 percent and severe CHD (nonfatal MI plus CHD death) by 25 percent (Table 10) (12).

MORTALITY

Risk of sudden death was increased threefold in hypertensive persons in the Framingham Study; it was increased even more so in terms of relative risk if there was no intervening overt coronary heart disease (Table 11). Men receiving antihypertensive treatment had more than a doubled risk of sudden death whether or not they had prior manifestations of coronary heart disease (Table 12). Approximately 20 percent of men who died suddenly were receiving antihypertensive therapy as compared to 8.4 percent of the population-at-risk of the same age. In those with overt CHD, 34 percent of those dying suddenly were on antihypertensive treatment as compared to 18 percent of those of the same age in the general population.

Population studies such as Framingham do not usually allow an accurate appraisal of the type, amount, and compliance with treatment. However, during the period when most of the sudden deaths occurred, the predominant treatment available consisted of diuretics and reserpine. Other studies have shown an association of diuretic

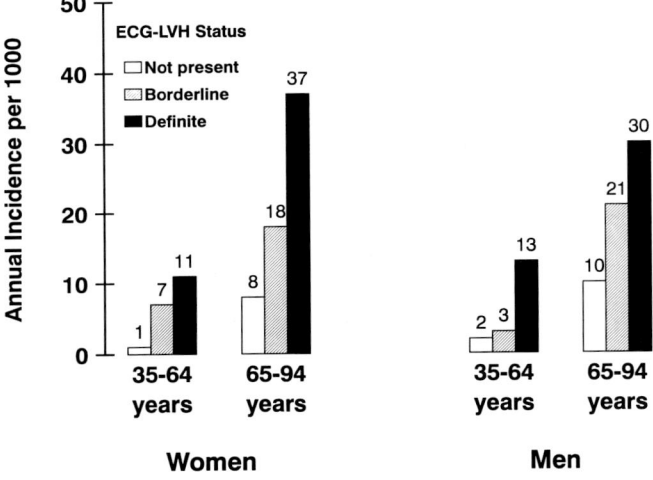

FIG. 13. Average annual rates for stroke and TIA according to ECG-LVH status, Framingham Study, 30-year follow-up.

TABLE 11. *Risk of sudden death by hypertensive status, 30-year follow-up, Framingham Study*

Hypertensive status	Age-adjusted rate per 1000			
	No CHD		Prior CHD	
	Men[b]	Women[b]	Men[c]	Women[b]
Normal	2.1	0.9	24.3	8.0
Mild	4.8	1.6	28.8	11.9
Definite	5.4	1.8	35.1	12.3

[a] Subjects were 35–94 years of age.
[b] p < .0001.
[c] Not significant.
CHD, coronary heart disease.

TABLE 12. *Sudden death incidence in high-risk candidates[a] by ECG and antihypertensive status, 30-year follow-up, Framingham Study[b]*

Anti-HBP treatment	Age-adjusted biennial rate per 1000			
	No abnormal ECG		Abnormal ECG	
	Men	Women	Men	Women
No prior CHD				
Untreated	2.1[d]	1.3[e]	6.0[g]	3.3
Treated	3.7[d]	3.5[e]	11.3[f]	4.4
Prior CHD				
Untreated	5.2[d]	4.5[g]	31.3[g]	12.0
Treated	36.4[e]	5.7[g]	58.5[g]	25.9

[a] High-risk subjects: >20 cigarettes/day; definite HBP glucose intolerance; cholesterol > 20 mg/dl.
[b] Subjects were 35–94 years of age.
[c] Abnormal ECG also includes ECG-MI as well as LVH and NSA.
[d] $p < .001$.
[e] $p < .05$.
[f] $p < .12$.
[g] $p < .07$.

therapy with ventricular arrhythmias (40,41) and, in persons with prior CHD, with sudden death (42). It is not clear whether hypokalemia is responsible for these associations (41).

Since the mid-1960s there has been a major decline in cardiovascular mortality. This reverses an epidemic CHD risk during the previous two decades. During the decade ending in 1990, age-adjusted death rate for CHD has declined over 50 percent. The current rate of decline is 3 to 4 percent per year. For stroke death, the rate of decline since 1972 is 6 percent per year. The improvement included all age groups, both sexes, all races, and all geographic areas in the United States. It was greatest in the educated, in the young, and in blacks. The dramatically reduced mortality is substantial, sustained, and not artifactual.

Whether this dramatic decline is actually a product of improved lifestyle or of better medical care, it is clear that cardiovascular mortality rates can be favorably influenced. The lowered cardiovascular mortality coincided with improvements in risk factors and greater access to more effective medical services. It has been estimated that change in risk-factor-related lifestyle accounts for over half the decline and that medical interventions are responsible for 40 percent. Hypertension treatment and control is considered to be a major factor in the influence of medical intervention. Whatever the reason, the remarkable declines in CHD, stroke, and hypertensive mortality in the United States are a major public health achievement.

The decline in stroke and cardiovascular mortality in the United States and some other countries over the past two decades is, to an extent, very likely a result of the successful detection and treatment of hypertension (43). Although the decline in stroke mortality preceded the widespread introduction of effective drug therapy, it definitely has accelerated in its rate of decrease since the emphasis on therapy. This indicates that hypertension control is, on the whole, beneficial.

ANTIHYPERTENSIVE TREATMENT

Randomized controlled trials indicate the benefit of antihypertensive treatment. These include the Veterans Administration Cooperative Study, United States Public Health Service (USPHS) Hospital Trial, Australian National Blood Pressure Study, Hypertension Detection and Follow-up Program, Oslo Trial, the Medical Research Council (MRC) Mild Hypertension Trial, International Prospective Primary Prevention Study in Hypertension (IPPSH) Trial, and Multiple Risk Factor Intervention Trial (44). On the whole, these trials have provided extensive evidence of the benefit of antihypertensive drug treatment for all grades of hypertension. There are, however, some troublesome aspects such as a lack of proved efficacy in white women and in young hypertensives, as well as a less than expected benefit for the CHD outcome.

As the incidence and mortality from stroke, cardiac failure, and renal failure decline, more emphasis will have to be put on reducing coronary mortality and sudden death. Antihypertensive agents for this purpose may have to be tailored to a profile which is more effective against atherogenesis and less inclined to increase myocardial irritability. Diuretic therapy tends to worsen the lipid profile and to decrease glucose tolerance and serum potassium (18).

The MRC trial of mild hypertension provides an assessment of the value of treatment for stroke, overall mortality, and coronary events and compares diuretic with beta-blocker therapy. Once again, efficacy was demonstrated for stroke, but overall rates of CHD events were unaffected. Also, overall mortality was not improved in women. Stroke risk was better controlled by diuretic therapy. There was some indication that beta blockers might be effective in reducing CHD risk, but only in nonsmokers (45).

The IPPSH Trial failed to demonstrate the efficacy of oxprenolol as an additive to diuretic therapy in reducing CHD risk. The trial did, however, indicate that CHD rates were favorably influenced by the degree of blood pressure reduction with therapy, taking all other risk factors into account, and beta-blocker therapy was particularly beneficial in nonsmoking men (46).

Data from Framingham and MRFIT appear to confirm observations in clinical trials that there may be a subgroup of hypertensive persons in which treatment may actually increase risk of sudden death (26,47).

When patients of the MRFIT special care group were compared with those in the usual care group, an adjusted relative risk indicating a 67-percent excess mortality was noted in the former group (26). The excess coronary mortality among the hypertensive men with ECG abnormalities was attributed chiefly to sudden death. Also, this excess mortality was independent of the baseline blood pressure level. An interaction between ECG abnormality and diuretic treatment was noted. The MRFIT data suggest a 67-percent *excess* mortality in hypertensives treated too vigorously with diuretics in the presence of coexistent ECG abnormality (26). Framingham data suggest an *increased* risk of sudden death in association with antihypertensive treatment, even taking into account blood pressure level, coexistent CHD, ECG abnormality, and cardiac failure. However, the excess risk of sudden death in those treated was not confined to those with ECG abnormalities. Some feature of antihypertensive treatment as practiced in the general population may contribute to sudden coronary death.

Controlled trials indicate that on balance, hypertensive persons who receive treatment live longer than those who do not (48). However, clinical trials indicate that antihypertensive therapy primarily reduces the occurrence of stroke, cardiac failure, renal insufficiency, and aortic aneurysm (49–52). Data indicating benefits for CHD have been less consistent, but summary analyses demonstrate a 14-percent decrease in CHD rates when the experience of several large trials of therapy for diastolic hypertension is summarized (Fig. 14) (48). A controlled trial involving a modest sample of older men has also suggested an adverse effect of antihypertensive treatment with diuretics on coronary mortality (53). National health surveys indicate a substantial improvement in the detection, treatment, and control of hypertension in the United States. Both proportion of hypertensives on treatment and the control rate have improved sharply since 1959. Improvement in control of hypertension preceded the subsequent decline in cardiovascular mortality in the United States and appears to have contributed to it.

However, more detailed information is required in order to better define the indications, contraindications, best drugs, hazards, and side effects of antihypertensive treatment for the avoidance of CHD. Therapy for mild-to-moderate hypertension could well be nonpharmacologic for the coronary candidate. There is growing evidence that nonpharmacologic therapy may be a reasonable alternative to drug therapy. Such therapy includes weight reduction; reduced sodium, fat, and alcohol intake; and consideration of adequate potassium, magnesium, and calcium intake (31,54).

PREVENTIVE IMPLICATIONS

At midcentury, knowledge about hypertension was quite limited and we were unimpressed with its prevalence and could do little about it. Over the past three decades, antihypertensive treatments were developed which could safely and effectively reduce blood pressure. We have come to recognize that hypertension is an insidious and eventually fatal disease. It is now also appreciated that hypertension is a major factor in atherogenesis.

There are now millions of people whose hypertension is controlled, thereby sparing them from needless episodes of stroke, cardiac failure, and premature death. This escalation of detection and treatment of hypertension has fueled the decline in cardiovascular mortality—particularly since 1972, when the National High Blood Pressure Education Program was implemented. There is now enough information, skill, and effective agents and experience to bring hypertension under good control.

However, assessment of hypertension for treatment should include evaluation of other cardiovascular risk factors and tests for evidence of organ involvement. This is particularly important for mild hypertension, where the excess risk is concentrated in those individuals with other risk factors. Optimal preventive management should be multifactorial, including reduction of saturated fat and cholesterol intake to optimize lipids; weight control; restriction of salt and alcohol intake; maintenance of adequate potassium, calcium, and magnesium intake; prudent exercise; and smoking cessation. Inducing the hypertensive cigarette smoker to quit, for example, can promptly reduce CHD risk to half that of those who continue to smoke (31). Awaiting the appearance of organ involvement prior to initiating treatment is imprudent. Within 5 years of the first appearance of cardiac failure or ECG-LVH, more than half will die. Also, most overt cardiovascular sequelae of hypertension, such as sudden death, precede the appearance of laboratory evidence of target organ involvement.

The benefits of therapy for diastolic hypertension (48)

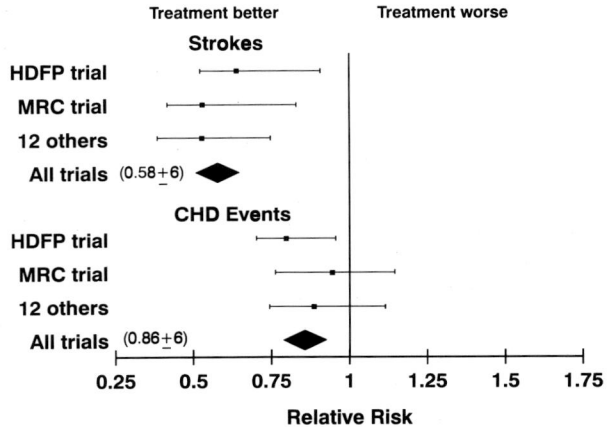

FIG. 14. Estimated relative risk (with confidence intervals) for strokes and coronary heart disease (CHD) events in clinical trials. (From ref. 48, with permission.)

and for low-dose diuretic therapy to treat isolated systolic hypertension in the elderly (12) are now better appreciated. However, as the clinician faces the task of preventing coronary disease and stroke, it is imperative that preventive measures be directed at the entire risk profile. It is not sufficient to treat the blood pressure level alone, and attention must also be focused on underlying vascular disease risk factors such as obesity, diet, diabetes, and smoking.

REFERENCES

1. Stamler J. Epidemiology and treatment of hypertension. In: Carlson RJ, Cunningham R, eds. *Future directions in health care: a new public policy.* Cambridge: Ballinger, 1978.
2. Smith WM. Epidemiology of hypertension. *Med Clin North Am* 1977;61:467–486.
3. Kannel WB, Sorlie P. Hypertension in Framingham. In: Paul O, ed. *Epidemiology and control of hypertension.* Symposia Specialists, 1993.
4. Dustan HP. Role of hypertension and its control—experimental aspects. *Prog Biochem Pharmacol* 1983;19:177–191.
5. Tobian LJ. Interrelationships of sodium volume, CNS and hypertension. *Prog Biochem Pharmacol* 1983;19:208–229.
6. Kannel WB, Abbott RD. Incidence and prognosis of unrecognized myocardial infarction. An update on the Framingham Study. *N Engl J Med* 1984;311:1144–1147.
7. Kannel WB, Dannenberg AL, Abbott RD. Unrecognized myocardial infarction and hypertension: The Framingham Study. *Am Heart J* 1985;109:581–585.
8. Kannel WB, Gordon T, Schwartz MJ. Systolic versus diastolic blood pressure and risk of coronary heart disease: The Framingham Study. *Am J Cardiol* 1971;27:335–345.
9. Stamler J, Stamler R, Neaton JD. Blood pressure, systolic and diastolic, and cardiovascular risks: U.S. population data. *Arch Intern Med* 1993;153:598–615.
10. Kannel WB, Wolf PA, McGee DL, Dawber TR, McNamara PM, Castelli WP. Systolic blood pressure, arterial rigidity and stroke. The Framingham Study. *JAMA* 1981;245:1225–1228.
11. Kannel WB, Sorlie P, Gordon T. Labile hypertension: a faulty concept? The Framingham Study. *Circulation* 1980;61:1183–1187.
12. SHEP Cooperative Research Group. Prevention of stroke by antihypertensive drug treatment in older persons with isolated systolic hypertension: final results of the Systolic Hypertension in the Elderly Program (SHEP). *JAMA* 1991;265:3255–3264.
13. Meade TW, Chakrabarti R, Haines AA, North WRS, Stirling Y. Characteristics affecting fibrinolytic activity and plasma fibrinogen concentrations. *Br Med J* 1979;1:153–156.
14. Ernst E, Resch KL. Fibrinogen as a cardiovascular risk factor: a metanalysis and review of the literature. *Ann Intern Med* 1993;118:956–963.
15. Kannel WB, D'Agostino RB, Wilson PWF, Belanger AJ, Gagnon DR. Diabetes, fibrinogen, and risk of cardiovascular disease: the Framingham experience. *Am Heart J* 1990;120:672–676.
16. Garrison RJ, Kannel WB, Stokes J III, Castelli WP. Incidence and precursors of hypertension in young adults: The Framingham Offspring Study. *Prev Med* 1987;16:234–251.
17. Anderson KM, Wilson PWF, Odell PM, Kannel WB. An updated coronary risk profile. A statement for health professionals. *Circulation* 1991;83:357–363.
18. Weinberger MH. Treatment of hypertension in the 1990s: optimizing the benefit of blood pressure reduction by minimizing risk factors for cardiovascular disease. *Am J Med* 1987;82(suppl 1A):44–49.
19. Intersalt Cooperative Research Group. Intersalt: an international study of electrolyte excretion and blood pressure results for 24 hour urinary sodium and potassium excretion. *Br Med J* 1988;297:319–328.
20. Kannel WB, Castelli WP, Gordon T. Cholesterol in the prediction of atherosclerotic disease. New perspectives based on the Framingham Study. *Ann Intern Med* 1979;90:85–91.
21. Gordon T, Kannel WB, Castelli WP, Dawber TR. Lipoproteins, cardiovascular disease, and death: The Framingham Study. *Arch Intern Med* 1981;141:1123–1131.
22. NIH Consensus Development Panel on Triglyceride High-Density Lipoprotein, and Coronary Heart Disease. Triglyceride, high-density lipoprotein, and coronary heart disease. *JAMA* 1993;269:505–510.
23. Wilson PWF, Anderson KM, Castelli WP, Kannel WB. Twelve-year incidence of coronary heart disease in middle-aged adults during the era of hypertensive therapy: The Framingham Offspring Study. *Am J Med* 1991;90:11–16.
24. Wilson PWF. High-density lipoprotein, low-density lipoprotein and coronary artery disease. *Am J Cardiol* 1990;66(Suppl A):7–10.
25. Kannel WB. High-density lipoproteins: epidemiologic profile and risks of coronary artery disease. *Am J Cardiol* 1983;52:9–12.
26. Multiple Risk Factor Intervention Trial Research Group. Baseline rest ECG abnormalities, antihypertensive treatment and mortality in the MRFIT. *Am J Cardiol* 1985;55:1–15.
27. Iso H, Jacobs DR Jr., Wentworth D, Neaton JD, Cohen JD, for the MRFIT Research Group. Serum cholesterol levels and six-year mortality from stroke in 350,977 men screened for the Multiple Risk Factor Intervention Trial. *N Engl J Med* 1989;320:904–910.
28. Feinleib M. On a possible relationship between serum cholesterol and cancer mortality. *Am J Epidemiol* 1981;114:5–10.
29. Rose G, Shipley MJ. Plasma lipids and mortality: a source of error. *Lancet* 1980;1:523–526.
30. Consensus Development Conference. Lowering blood cholesterol to prevent heart disease. *JAMA* 1985;253:2080–2086.
31. Joint National Committee on Detection Evaluation and Treatment of High Blood Pressure. The fifth report of the Joint National Committee on detection, evaluation, and treatment of high blood pressure (JNC V). *Arch Intern Med* 1993;153:154–183.
32. Stamler R, Stamler J, Gosch FC, et al. Primary prevention of hypertension by nutritional-hygienic means: final report of a randomized, controlled trial. *JAMA* 1989;262:1801–1807.
33. Alderman MH, Madhavan S, Ooi WL, Cohen H, Sealey JE, Laragh JH. Association of the renin-sodium profile with the risk of myocardial infarction in patients with hypertension. *N Engl J Med* 1991;324:1098–1104.
34. Garrison RJ, Kannel WB, Stokes J, Castelli WP. Incidence and precursors of hypertension in young adults: The Framingham Offspring Study. *Prev Med* 1987;16:235–251.
35. Kissebah AH, Vydelingum N, Murray R, et al. Relation of body fat distribution to metabolic complications of obesity. *J Clin Endo Metab* 1982;54:254–260.
36. Wilson PWF, Garrison RJ, Abbott RD, Castelli WP. Factors associated with lipoprotein cholesterol levels: The Framingham Study. *Arteriosclerosis* 1983;3:273–281.
37. Kannel WB, Wolf PA, Verter J. Manifestations of coronary disease predisposing to stroke. The Framingham Study. *JAMA* 1983;250:2942–2946.
38. Kannel WB, Soli WP. Left ventricular hypertrophy in hypertension. Prognostic and pathogenetic implications: The Framingham Study. In: Strauer BE, ed. *The heart in hypertension.* Berlin: Springer-Verlag, 1981:223–242.
39. Levy D, Garrison RJ, Savage DD, Kannel WB, Castelli WP. Prognostic implications of echocardiographically, determined left ventricular mass in the Framingham Heart Study. *N Engl J Med* 1990;322:1561–1566.
40. Holland OB, Nixon JV, Kuhnert L. Diuretic-induced ventricular ectopic activity. *Am J Med* 1981;70:762–768.
41. Medical Research Council Working Party on Mild to Moderate Hypertension. Ventricular extrasystoles during thiazide treatment: substudy of MRC Mild Hypertensive Trial. *Br Med J* 1983;287:1249–1253.
42. Duke M. Thiazide-induced hypokalemia: association with acute myocardial infarction and ventricular fibrillation. *JAMA* 1978;239:43–45.
43. Kannel WB, Thom TJ. Declining cardiovascular mortality. *Circulation* 1984;70:331–336.
44. Thompson MG. An appraisal of the large scale trials of antihypertensive treatment. In: Bulpitt CJ, ed. *Handbook of hypertension*

6: *epidemiology of hypertension.* Amsterdam: Elsevier, 1985:331–343.

45. Medical Research Council (MRC) Working Group. MRC trial of treatment of mild hypertension: principal results. *Br Med J* 1985;291:97–104.

46. The IPPSH Collaborative Group. Carciovascular risk and risk factors in a randomized trial of treatment based on the beta blocker oxprenolol: the International Prospective Primary Prevention Study in Hypertension (IPPPSH). *J Hypertension* 1985;3:379–392.

47. Cutler JA, MacMahon SW, Furberg CD. Controlled clinical trials of drug treatment for hypertension: a review. *Hypertension* 1989;13:I36–I44.

48. Collins R, Peto R, MacMahon S, et al. Blood pressure, stroke, and coronary heart disease. Part 2, short-term reductions in blood pressure: overview of randomised drug trials in their epidemiological context. *Lancet* 1990;335:827–838.

49. Veterans Administration Cooperative Study Group on Antihyper- tensive Agents. Effects of treatment on morbidity in hypertension II. Results in patients with diastolic blood pressure averaging 90 through 114 mm Hg. *JAMA* 1970;213:1143–1152.

50. Report of the Management Committee. The Australian therapeutic trial in mild hypertension. *Lancet* 1980;1:1261–1267.

51. Helgeland A. Treatment of mild hypertension—a 5, year controlled drug trial. The Oslo Study. *Am J Med* 1980;69:625–732.

52. Hypertension Detection and Follow-up Program Cooperative Group. Five, year findings of the Hypertension Detection and Follow-up Program. I. Reduction in mortality of persons with high blood pressure, including mild hypertension. *JAMA* 1979;242:2562–2571.

53. Morgan T, Adam WP, Hodgson M, Gibberd RW. Failure of therapy to improve prognosis in elderly males with hypertension. *Med J Aust* 1980;2:27–31.

54. Final Report of the Subcommittee on Nonpharmacological Therapy. Nonpharmacological approaches to the control of high blood pressure. *Hypertension* 1986;8:444–467.

*Hypertension: Pathophysiology, Diagnosis,
and Management, Second Edition,*
edited by J.H. Laragh and B.M. Brenner,
Raven Press, Ltd., New York © 1995.

CHAPTER 8

Human Population Biology and Blood Pressure: Evolutionary and Ecological Considerations and Interpretations of Population Studies

Gary D. James and Paul T. Baker

Hypertension is generally believed to be a "disease" of modern Western society, afflicting an estimated 15 to 20 percent of the adult population of the United States and other industrialized nations (1–3). One reason for this belief is that many traditional, non-Western, nonindustrialized societies have been reported to have a low prevalence of high blood pressure (3).

Over the past seven decades, many researchers have reported on casual blood pressures in traditional non-Western populations. This work identified a number of groups that exhibited low average blood pressure and

that did not show the age increase in pressure common to modern Western groups (2–9). However, what was often neglected in this research was an assessment of how the genetic and environmental diversity that characterized these traditional groups was related to blood pressure. Specifically, while risk factors such as salt intake (10) or psychosocial stress (11,12) were assessed with regard to their effects on blood pressure, little attention was focused on genetic adaptations or idiosyncratic environmental, cultural, or historic factors peculiar to the groups which may have influenced the risk factor–blood pressure relationships. That is, genetic and ecological mechanisms that might determine how salt, stress, or other factors affect blood pressure were generally neglected in the study of traditional non-Western groups. Therefore, in this chapter, the blood pressure research on tradition-

G. D. James: Cardiovascular Center, The New York Hospital–Cornell Medical Center, New York, New York.
P. T. Baker: Department of Anthropology, The Pennsylvania State University, State College, Pennsylvania.

ally living populations is evaluated from an evolutionary and ecological perspective in which these mechanisms are examined.

EVOLUTIONARY PRINCIPLES

Assumptions and Definitions

A fundamental assumption of the approach used in ecologically oriented studies of humans is that populations adapt to the specific environments they inhabit either through cultural practices or by natural selection (13–15). Because human groups evolve like other populations of organisms, survival depends upon the successful adaptation of individuals to specific environmental stressors. Some of these stressors may be pervasive in the environment, such as the low partial pressure of oxygen at high altitude, but others may be transient, such as nutritional deprivation. These stressors will affect the fitness of the population by either altering gene frequencies through the differential survival of specific genotypes or by modifying the phenotypic expression of the genes in the individual. The population may also adapt by adopting cultural practices that buffer individuals from the environmental insult. A simple example of such a cultural practice is the wearing of furs to warm the body in response to cold temperature.

Other stochastic processes, such as genetic drift through isolation or inbreeding may also modify the gene pool of the population, so that specific genes become fixed. Trait variants defined by these genes may not adversely affect survival in the given environment; but, when that environment changes, survival of the population may be jeopardized because there is less genetic variation on which natural selection can operate.

Finally, how human populations evolve is also likely to be population-specific, depending upon the allelic variation in the population's gene pool and the nature of the population's indigenous cultural practices. Thus, for example, while environmental changes that occur with modernization in lifestyle have been associated with elevating average blood pressure in many populations, the genetic or environmental mechanisms that cause this increase may be completely different from population to population.

Blood Pressure, Genetics, and Adaptation

Blood pressure is a dynamic physiological function that varies with each heartbeat (16). The level of systolic/diastolic pressure at any given heartbeat depends upon several characteristics of the cardiovascular system. These include the lumenal diameter and elasticity of the arteries, the circulating levels of vasoactive hormones and the sensitivity of their receptors, smooth muscle tone, and the contractile strength of the heart (17). From a genetic standpoint, blood pressure is not a quantitative trait in the same sense as stature (18), meaning that the genes involved in producing it do not do so in a strictly additive fashion. Rather, blood pressure is maintained as a dynamic steady state through constant compensation among the structural and hormonal factors noted above. Given the nature of blood pressure as a trait, pathologically high blood pressure can be thought of as a "disease" of adaptation, as articulated by Selye (19,20), Cannon (21), and Hinkle (22), in that it occurs because one or more of the mechanisms, acting through negative feedback to maintain a central value of pressure, fails in its function. If the failure of a particular system is heritable (that is, has some genetic component), the development of high blood pressure will aggregate in families. However, the mechanisms that are inherited in one family may not be the same as those inherited in another. This principle is probably also true of populations. Because human populations have evolved under different circumstances for varying lengths of time, the nature of the interaction between genes that affect pressure and the environment will also likely be different. Thus, the similarities or differences in blood pressure patterns across these groups may occur because of different pressure-maintaining mechanisms.

METHODOLOGICAL CONSIDERATIONS

Research Design in Non-Western Population Studies

Blood pressure in non-Western populations has usually been studied in two ways. The first is an epidemiologic examination that addresses questions about the blood pressure distributions of populations (12). The second approach is one in which the population is studied from a particular problem orientation such as examining the effects of psychosocial factors on blood pressure (11).

These approaches have provided Western medicine with some useful information, such as the fact that blood pressure need not increase with advancing age (2–9). However, mistaken conclusions have also been drawn from these studies. The reason for the mistaken interpretation of results is that in many instances, a hypothesis about a relationship between some single environmental factor and blood pressure is not properly tested. That is, even though the data support the expected relationship, the lack of attention to confounding variables that may affect blood pressure, the specific factor, or both compromises the stated conclusions (23).

Recently, there have been studies in which blood pressure has been examined as one of many variables that describe or influence the health and fitness of the populations assessed (see for example 24,25). These studies do not pursue a single hypothesis about blood pressure. They are an integrated examination of many questions that address how the biology and behavior of a population interact to produce observed patterns of fertility, morbidity, and mortality (23,26). The focus of this research is on how a population evolves and adapts to its environmental circumstance. Blood pressure is thus studied as a biological trait in the context of the population's genetics, natural environment, and behavioral pattern. This approach, while rarely used, allows for firmer conclusions given that many of the variables that confound blood pressure and risk factor relationships are also examined.

Sampling Bias

In nearly all studies of non-Western traditionally living groups, the sample of subjects studied is *not* a random sample of the population. Rather, it is often the case that the people measured are those who agreed to be measured or who happened to be around on the day when the research team was there (10). In addition, such studies usually concentrate on a single or a few villages which are rarely representative of the entire population. Thus, when examining the reported distributions of pressure by age, sex, or other demographic division of the population, it is generally incorrect to assume that the reported values represent the population at large.

Measurement Error

In addition to sampling biases, the studies of traditional, non-Western populations often take place in exotic environments, and collecting data (casual blood pressures) comparable to that gathered in studies of modern Western populations is often impossible (10). Even in Western medicine, research on the validity and reliability of casual blood pressure shows that this method of measurement is confounded by many factors. For example, pressures read by physicians in a clinic setting are consistently higher than those measured at home (27,28). Readings may also be influenced by the relationship between the measurer and subject (29) and even by whether these people are of the same or different sex (30). Accurate readings are further compromised by observer bias such as digit preference (31,32). All of these factors are likely to affect the blood pressure measurements in non-Western groups.

It should also be noted that in many studies of traditional groups, only one measurement per subject is taken. These pressures may not only be influenced by all the above sources of measurement error, but also by other factors such as the emotional state of the subject (33,34). And, while it is recommended that subjects be seated quietly for at least 5 minutes before a reading is taken, it may not be possible to follow this protocol perfectly because of time constraints or other situational factors (7).

Finally, more than one observer usually takes pressures in studies of traditional people as there is often a limited time frame in which to measure the entire group (35). Interobserver biases are thus also part of the measurement error in these studies. Because of these many sources of possible error in measurement, caution should be used in comparing the results of these studies.

LOW BLOOD PRESSURE POPULATIONS

Although there are significant methodological problems, over the years many populations outside the influence of Western culture have been reported to have a low

TABLE 1. *Populations in which blood pressure does not increase with age in either one or both sexes*

Population	Location	Author (ref. no.)
Africa		
Ituri pygmies	Congo (Zaire)	36
Non-Baganda	Uganda	37
Faili	N. Cameroons	6
Kurumba	Upper Volta	38
Kalahari Bushman	South Africa	39
Samburu	Kenya	40
Kikuyu	Kenya	40
Americas		
Eskimo	Greenland	41
Navajo	New Mexico (U.S.)	42
Cuna	Panama	43
Wajana	Surinam	6
Yanomamo	Venezuela	10
Carajas	Brazil	44
Shipibo	Peru	45
Mestizo	Peru	45
Aymara	Chile	46
Asia		
Toda	India	47
"Najafagarh"	India	48
Pacific		
Aborigines	Central Australia	49
Aborigines	Queensland Australia	49
Aborigines	Torres Strait, Australia	49
Chimbu	New Guinea	50
Kikori	New Guinea	50
Chimbu	New Guinea	51
"Delta"	New Guinea	52
"Highland"	New Guinea	52
Tinam-Aigram	New Guinea	53
Ponape	East Carolines	54
Abaiang	Gilbert Islands	55
Fijians	Fiji	56
Fijians (Indians)	Fiji	56
Puka-Pukans	Cook Islands	57
Tokelauans	Tokelau	58
Nasioi	Solomons	60
Nagovisi	Solomons	60
Lau	Solomons	60
Baegu	Solomons	60
Aita	Solomons	60
Kwaio	Solomons	60

Modified from ref. 6.

prevalence of hypertension and little or no blood pressure increase with age. These populations practiced many different customs and modes of subsistence. In addition, they inhabited a variety of environments with differing climates and had different diets. Often, when intragroup comparisons were made, subgroups that had assimilated a number of aspects of Western culture into their lifestyle showed a rising of blood pressure with age, and other changes such as rising serum lipids (3). Table 1 is a list of some populations studied over the past 70 years which showed little or no age increase in blood pressure in either one or both sexes when they were studied. A variety of ethnic groups and natural environments are represented. Although most of the populations retained their traditional societal behavior, several, such as the Fijians and Navaho, were partially associated with Western societies at the time of measurement. However, it is important to recognize that today, most of these groups have neither the same blood pressure profile or traditional societal behavior as when they were first studied. All have had some Western contact.

MODERNIZATION, ADAPTATION, AND BLOOD PRESSURE: CURRENT INTERPRETATIONS AND CRITIQUE

Reviews of cross-cultural blood pressure studies tend to dichotomize populations into two groups: those who practice their traditional culture, and those who have adopted modern lifeways (modernized groups) (see for example 5,8,9). The traditional societies, their cultural practices, and populations are often characterized as well-organized, cohesive, and generally without stress (9). There is also a cultural evolutionary perspective that is generally included in which it is argued that traditionally living populations have evolved an age increase in blood pressure as their social organization has become more complex and similar to modern Western societies (5,8,9).

There are a number of problems with the current interpretations of cross-cultural studies of blood pressure. The first is that all traditional cultures cannot be lumped together. There is a substantial body of evidence in cultural ecology and anthropology which shows that human populations employ both their biological and cultural resources to adapt to their environments (14,61–67). Although there is considerable scientific debate about particular aspects of how specific cultures evolved and continue to change, there is a growing acceptance of the idea that cultural behavior (including technology) develops as part of the adaptive framework of a human population (15). It is recognized by anthropologists that while there are extant cultures with differing levels of technological complexity, these differences relate more to the ecological context of the population, and not to some degree of "primitiveness" (15). Social organizations and cultural practices devised by traditional people likely developed as part of the response to environmental challenges. The correlation of social structure and blood pressure is therefore probably caused by another factor related to both parameters.

A second concern is that the effects of differential mortality of individuals on the average blood pressure of the population are ignored. For example, in many traditional populations, life expectancies are much less than they are in modern Western populations (68). There is a substantial selective mortality in many traditional groups, much of which occurs in infancy (69,70). The people who are measured as adults in blood pressure studies are a select group of all those born. Thus, blood pressures measured among them may be lower in part because, by definition, these survivors are a healthier and heartier group.

It has also been argued from the comparisons of cross-cultural data that genetics plays little or no role in the development of hypertension (3). The reasoning of this position is that if two groups of similar genetic background live in different environments and one has higher average blood pressure (modernized group) than the other (traditional group), the difference is due to environmental factors. The fallacy of the argument is that the modernized group lived traditionally at one time, and any genetic adaptations to the traditional environment may simply be inappropriate or maladaptive in the modernized one. Thus, intragroup differences in blood pressure by modernization status do not exclude genetic contributions to high blood pressure.

Fourthly, modernization is sometimes treated as a monolithic process primarily sociological, cultural, and psychological in nature that stresses the individual (9). As has been described, the process also includes changes in diet (both food and food choices), type of activity, pace of activity, patterns of activity, and the introduction or removal of drugs or stimulants (26,71). It is difficult to disentangle the separate effects of each of these and other factors on blood pressure during the modernization process (8).

A final problem is that there is often overgeneralization in the interpretation of the data. For example, some have advocated that it is the psychosocial stresses of Western life that increase the average blood pressure of modern Western populations over that measured in traditional groups. Specifically, it is hypothesized that the primary cause of increased pressures in now modernized but once traditional populations is the psychological stress due to "dissonance between the social milieu in latter life and expectations based on early experiences" (5,8,9). Others have suggested that the psychological stress of rapid modernization or culture change has very little to do with the increased pressures in Western societies. They suggest that it is either a biological change such as increase in body weight that causes the elevated pressure (72), or that the level of pressure is directly related to the amount of salt consumed (3,73). These latter advocates hypothesize that increased salt consumption is the principal cause of increased blood pressure in modern Western societies. None of these generalizations are entirely correct. Because populations tend to adapt to their specific environments both culturally and biologically and because modernization defines change in many life dimensions, any single explanation of why blood pressure increases as culture changes around the world is, at our present state of knowledge, unwarranted.

In sum, populations with traditional cultures cannot be considered homogeneous. Their similarity in age-specific blood pressure is probably related to selective mortality and population-specific cultural and biological adaptations to the local environments. Changes in blood pressure associated with modernization are probably related to multiple factors, with perhaps different factors affecting different populations.

POPULATION BIOLOGY AND BLOOD PRESSURE

Many of the traditional peoples whose blood pressure has been studied lived in environments far removed from that of the temperate climates of North America and Western Europe. Given their simpler technologies, environmental stressors including high-altitude hypoxia, hot climate, and cold climate have played a significant role in shaping their biology and culture. The adaptations and acclimatizations made to these stressors may have had a significant impact on their blood pressures. The following sections briefly describe some of these adaptations and their possible effect on blood pressure.

Cardiovascular Adaptations to High-altitude Hypoxia in Traditional Populations

The cardiovascular traits of the traditionally living natives at altitudes of some 4,000 meters above sea level are considerably different than those of natives living at sea level. Much of the research of cardiovascular function in high-altitude natives has been conducted on South American Andean populations (74–77). Histologic studies among these natives have shown that after the first months of postnatal development, children born at high altitude develop a thickening of the muscular layer of the pulmonary arteries and arterioles that resembles the development of the fetal pulmonary vascular tree (76,78,79). These changes along with the viscosity accompanying polycythemia contribute to an increased pulmonary arterial pressure in the adult natives (80,81). As a consequence of increased pulmonary resistance, there is also right ventricular hypertrophy (78,82). But, in spite of these pulmonary changes, cardiac output of high-altitude natives during rest and exercise is similar to that attained at sea level (76,81), suggesting that oxygen requirements in these natives are met by more efficient oxygen extraction rather than by greater blood flow, as occurs in low-altitude natives who sojourn at high altitude (67,76).

While pulmonary arterial pressure is greater, casually measured systemic blood pressures in adult high-altitude natives are lower than those reported for sea level populations (see Table 2). The frequency of hypertension and ischemic heart disease is also correspondingly low (76,83). The lower blood pressure at altitude may indicate that chronic hypoxia has a relaxing effect on smooth muscle (84). Exposure to high-altitude hypoxia also results in increased vascularization so that it is possible that the lower pressures in the native traditionally living populations are related in part to a reduction in peripheral resistance to blood flow and not solely to their traditional lifestyle (76). Although modernization effects on blood pressure have been recently studied in high-altitude native populations in the Andes (77), the results may not be generalizable beyond the study population because of the physiological adaptations and acclimatizations peculiar to native Andean groups.

Cardiovascular Adaptations to Heat Stress in Traditional Populations

Adaptation to heat stress requires an increase in the flow of blood from the viscera and body core to the skin

TABLE 2. *Comparisons of the casual blood pressures of matched low (<300 m above sea level) and high (4,000 m+ above sea level) altitude populations from the Andean region of South America*

| | Peru[a] | | Chile[b] | | | |
| | Men | | Men | | Women | |
	Sea level	Altitude	Sea level	Altitude	Sea level	Altitude
N	38	25	53	62	52	77
Age	22 ± 4	21 ± 1	35 ± 12**	45 ± 13	33 ± 12	36 ± 15
Systolic pressure	127 ± 8**	118 ± 9	124 ± 11*	119 ± 12	120 ± 14**	112 ± 13
Diastolic pressure	70 ± 6	73 ± 7	79 ± 8	78 ± 8	74 ± 9	73 ± 9

[a] From ref. 80. Altitude natives reside at 4,540 m; sea level natives reside at 150 m.
[b] From ref. 46. Altitude natives from four villages above 4,070 m; sea level natives from two villages below 300 m.
* High and low altitude different at $p < 0.01$.
** High and low altitude different at $p < 0.001$.

and muscles of the extremities (17,85). This rearrangement of flow is necessary to rid the body of excess heat that is reflected in the rise of core (rectal) temperature (86). Chronic exposure to heat stress may also have a lowering effect on blood pressure (86).

In addition to blood flow and pressure changes, sweating is increased to better facilitate heat loss by water evaporation on the skin. The increase in sweating, however, also causes an increase in the loss of sodium chloride, and there is a relationship such that the greater the sweat output, the greater the loss of sodium (87).

Frisancho (76) has summarized a series of studies of the physiological response to heat stress in a number of traditional populations living in chronically hot environments, including South African Bushmen, Bantu tribesmen (sub-Saharan African blacks), and Australian Aborigines. In comparison to South African whites (both heat-acclimatized and nonacclimatized), the average sweat rates in these groups during work in heat were significantly lower. In addition, nearly all of the men from these groups completed the heat stress tests and maintained a tolerable (<40°C) rectal temperature while, on average, the white comparison groups did not. The implication of these findings is that populations indigenous to hot climates may be able to maintain thermal homeostasis during heat stress with lower body fluid (and concomitant sodium) loss (76). This ability to retain fluid and sodium has a further benefit in that it also helps adapt these populations to the limited availability of salt in their ecosystems (76,88).

Data from traditional populations in the tropics have been used to argue that excessive salt in the diet of Western populations is a major cause of hypertension (3,10). The data from the Bushmen and other studies noted here suggest that traditional populations in chronically hot environments may have low blood pressure along with salt retention mechanisms as part of their adaptive response to heat stress. That is, there may be no specific link between salt intake and low blood pressure in these groups in their traditional environments. This is not to say that salt plays no role in hypertension, but rather that the confounding effects of heat adaptation have not been properly considered in the interpretation of blood pressure data from tropical populations.

Cardiovascular Adaptations to Cold Stress in Traditional Populations

As summarized by Steegman (89), there are substantial interpopulation differences in the response to cold stress; the most relevant to this discussion are those related to extremity cooling in the form of cold pressor tests (usually hand immersion in cold water). As expected, blood pressure is elevated in all groups tested, although the average increase in systolic pressure of Eskimos (a cold-adapted population) is less than that of whites (76,90).

The most clearly different response that occurs with peripheral cooling between populations is the differences found in cold-induced vasodilation (CIVD). Specifically, cooling induces a sympathetically driven immediate constriction of the vessels in the extremities which conserves body heat by cutting down the peripheral flow of blood. CIVD is a relatively rapid and periodic release of this constriction which allows rewarming so that the tissues of the hand are not as subject to frostbite or damage from chronically low tissue temperatures. Adult blacks from a number of populations, when compared with adult male whites of equivalent background and state of cold acclimatization, show a reduced CIVD response (89,91–93). Specifically, blacks generally show more intense peripheral vasoconstriction in response to a cold pressor test with a high frequency of individuals who fail to show any CIVD. This rewarming failure is a clear population contrast in cold physiology which is related to the global distributions of indigenous populations. It has been suggested that since most Subsaharan tropical African populations were rarely exposed to chronically low or freezing temperatures, they did not develop this form of peripheral response to cold through natural selection (89). It may be speculated that this genetically based, sympathetically driven, peripheral vasoconstriction contributes to the greater prevalence of hypertension in U.S. black populations who live in temperate and freezing climates. This is not to say that the average populational difference in cold tolerance is a singular explanation of the greater prevalence of hypertension. Rather, the point being made is that genetic adaptations that evolved under one set of environmental circumstances may be detrimental and contribute to health problems when those environmental circumstances are changed.

SALT AND HYPERTENSION

Excessive dietary salt has long been touted as a primary cause of hypertension (94), but it has also been recognized from clinical studies that there is a considerable variability in the sensitivity of blood pressure to dietary salt in hypertensive patients (95). Nonetheless, when the relationship between salt and hypertension has been examined at the population level, the hypotheses generated and tested have tended to ignore many fundamental aspects of human biological variation. That is, in order to identify salt as the single most important correlate of blood pressure, relevant genetic and ecological factors are overlooked. The following sections evaluate two of these hypotheses from the perspective of human population biology.

The Association of Salt Intake and Blood Pressure: The INTERSALT Study

INTERSALT, a study of the relationship between blood pressure and sodium and potassium intake, included data from 52 ethnically diverse population samples from 32 countries (96). The primary hypothesis (reported prior to the analysis [96]) was that the average blood pressure and prevalence of hypertension of a population was directly and linearly related to the population's average levels of sodium intake, potassium intake (inversely), and the sodium:potassium intake ratio (96,97). That is, the study was designed to test the premise that the differences in blood pressure levels between world populations were directly related to differences in sodium (and potassium) intake. The relationships among sodium, potassium, and blood pressure were examined within as well as between populations (96–99).

The intrapopulational analyses revealed that after adjusting for several relevant covariates (age, sex, body mass index [BMI], level of alcohol consumption, and potassium intake), 8 of the 52 population samples had statistically significant positive associations between the rate of 24-hour urinary sodium excretion and systolic pressure (there were also two groups who showed significant negative associations) and 3 of the 52 had significant positive associations with diastolic pressure (three groups also had significant negative associations) (97). Only two (both from the People's Republic of China) showed statistically significant positive associations between the rate of 24-hour urinary sodium excretion and both systolic and diastolic blood pressure (97). When the relationships between the median rate of 24-hour urinary sodium excretion and the median systolic and diastolic pressure among the 52 populations were examined (again adjusting for sex, age, BMI, and alcohol intake), small positive associations were found. However, this between-group regression analysis was dominated by the median data from four equatorial population samples (Yanomamo and Xingu Indians from the Amazon basin in Brazil, Luo tribesman from the Lake Victoria region of Western Kenya, and people from the Asaro valley in the eastern highlands of Papua New Guinea) which all had extremely low median 24-hour urinary sodium excretion and low median systolic and diastolic pressure (97,99,100). When these groups were omitted from the analysis, there were no associations between the rate of sodium excretion and systolic or diastolic blood pressure among the remaining populations. The only reported consistent association across the groups was between the slopes of systolic and diastolic pressure with age (calculated for each population from the within-population cross-sectional data) and the median rate of sodium excretion of the populations (97,99). From these data, the architects of INTERSALT concluded that "lower average sodium intake might have a favorable influence on blood pressure, on change of blood pressure with age, and hence on cardiovascular mortality" (p. 326) (97).

The findings of INTERSALT have been widely reported and debated (101–103). Most of what has been discussed concerns the public health implications of the data and their utility with regard to guiding patient care. However, no one has really questioned the basic premise of the study. Can one determine an interpopulation relationship between sodium intake and blood pressure given the study design and assumptions of INTERSALT? Were the study assumptions valid?

An implicit assumption in the sampling design of INTERSALT is that there is a uniform probability of survival to a given age in all the populations studied. That is, it is assumed that there are no natural selective processes in any population, related to salt consumption or otherwise, that may affect the age-related distributions of blood pressure or the salt–blood pressure relationship. Furthermore, there also is an assumption that none of the populations studied have adapted genetically or culturally to the availability of dietary salt or any other stressor in their local environments in ways that could affect their blood pressure. From the data and theory reviewed in previous sections of this chapter, it is clear that these assumptions are invalid. There are ample data which show that climatic and other environmental stressors have played an important role in shaping both the biology and culture of human populations, including those sampled in INTERSALT. Therefore, the INTERSALT data can neither refute nor support the central hypothesis of the study that sodium intake is related to blood pressure level on a population basis. However, ironically, the fact that the overwhelming majority of the intrapopulational analyses showed no significant relationship between blood pressure and urinary sodium excretion may provide supportive evidence for the idea that excessive dietary salt is not necessarily a universal health risk.

The Slavery Hypothesis

There are ample data showing that the average level of blood pressure and the prevalence of hypertension are higher among American black populations when compared with American white and African black populations (104,105). Recently, Wilson and Grim (105) have hypothesized that an important contributor to this difference was a natural selection for salt conservation that occurred as a consequence of shipboard conditions experienced by Africans during the slave trade. The conditions included crowding and restricted movement (immobilization stress), acute heat stress, extreme psychological stress, and dramatically increased exposure to communicable diseases, particularly smallpox and dysentery with their enhanced potential for severe electrolyte depletion (106). The basis of the hypothesis is that because the major causes of death among the African captives were salt-depletive infectious diseases, those individuals with an enhanced genetically-based ability to conserve salt had a survival advantage and were therefore more likely to be the progenitors of the current generation of black Americans. The logical consequence of the selection is that American blacks, who inherited the salt-retaining genotype, have a propensity toward greater fluid retention which, in a salt-rich environment, injures the kidneys, causing earlier onset and more severe hypertension and subsequent cardiovascular disease (CVD) morbidity and mortality.

Jackson (106), in evaluating this hypothesis, noted that rather than constricting genetic diversity in the survivors of the slave trade as Wilson and Grim suggest (105), the severe infectious disease-related stresses may have actually enhanced it, by accelerating rates of mutation, genetic recombination, and the presence of mobile genetic elements. She further noted that the survivors of the Middle Passage and the generations of their offspring have also been exposed to new biotic and abiotic selective pressures, enhanced gene flow with other populations, and genetic drift in the American environment which have likely acted to further increase the genotypic diversity of present-day groups as well. She concluded that because many factors have combined to maintain or even increase the genetic variation of American black populations when compared with native African populations, it is highly unlikely that the single historical event of the Middle Passage was a major contributor to the higher average pressures and greater prevalence of hypertension in present-day American black populations.

The slavery hypothesis was developed to provide a framework for testing the genetic basis of salt-sensitive hypertension in American black populations (105). While it has been challenged on theoretical grounds, its basic premise has not been questioned. Is it reasonable to hypothesize that the natural selective response to intense infectious disease stress is the preservation of a genotype that fosters salt retention? In order to determine the validity of the slavery hypothesis, one needs to examine existing empirical data concerning genetic selection to infectious diseases in humans. The key question is whether genotypes are selected to protect against the infection (i.e., the infecting agent) or whether they are selected to alleviate symptoms caused by the infection.

The best documented example of natural selection to infectious disease in humans is the genotypic responses to malarial infection among African and European populations (107). Malaria is a debilitating and potentially lethal infectious disease caused by a plasmodium that attacks red blood cells. Symptoms of the infection include fevers, chills, and dehydration. There are ample data showing that the genotypic changes (of which there are several) that have arisen through natural selection to the malarial infection improve individual survival by altering the reproductive ability of the infecting plasmodium, not by modifying the physiological responses to the infection such as those related to thermoregulation or salt and water retention (107). That is, people with the selected genotypes are protected from the infecting agent itself, not the symptoms it causes.

By the same logic, people who survived the horrendous conditions of the slave trade (from a natural selection standpoint) would be those whose genotype either completely protected them from the infections that caused vomiting, diarrhea, and other electrolyte-depleting symptoms or rendered the infection sufficiently mild so that the debilitating effects of the diseases were not lethal. That is, if natural selection occurred, it would have been for genotypes that protected the individual from infection, not the symptoms of salt depletion that they caused. Therefore, the hypothesis that a salt-retaining genotype arose as a consequence of natural selection to symptoms of salt-depleting diseases is not valid because it is based on an incorrect premise.

ECOLOGICAL STUDIES OF BLOOD PRESSURE: THE SAMOAN EXAMPLE

While the effects of salt on blood pressure remain an important issue in population biological studies of blood pressure, other cardiovascular epidemiologists have concerned themselves with how the changes associated with modernization, acculturation, Westernization, or other processes affect the blood pressure of traditional populations. As previously noted, the changes that occur are multiple and complex and likely differ between the populations studied. Recently, the results of a long-term study of the health of a traditional people in the process of modernizing, the Samoans, have been summarized (24). This population study is a useful illustration of how blood pressure variation can be examined in an ecological context and how stochastic processes specific to a population can affect its biology.

The Samoans are a Polynesian population with significant subpopulations residing in Western Samoa (an independent nation), American Samoa (U.S. Territory), New Zealand, Hawaii, and California. The socioeconomic conditions in these areas range from traditional villages in Western Samoa, which depend primarily on subsistence agriculture and fishing and are traditional in social viewpoint, to almost fully modern as reflected in the lifestyles characteristic of the urban areas of Hawaii, the west coast of the continental U.S., and New Zealand (108). Although these subpopulations live under diverse conditions, they continue to share a common cultural and genetic heritage since the outmigrations to the more modern Western areas occurred only recently (108).

As with most studies of intrapopulation comparisons of blood pressure, the most traditionally living groups show the lowest average levels of pressure, with generally little age increase (59,109). However, a more detailed analysis of the data reveals that the average pressures of those groups with an intermediate contact with Western culture (subpopulations in American Samoa) may have the highest age-specific pressures as well as the steepest pressure increase with age (59,109). This pattern among

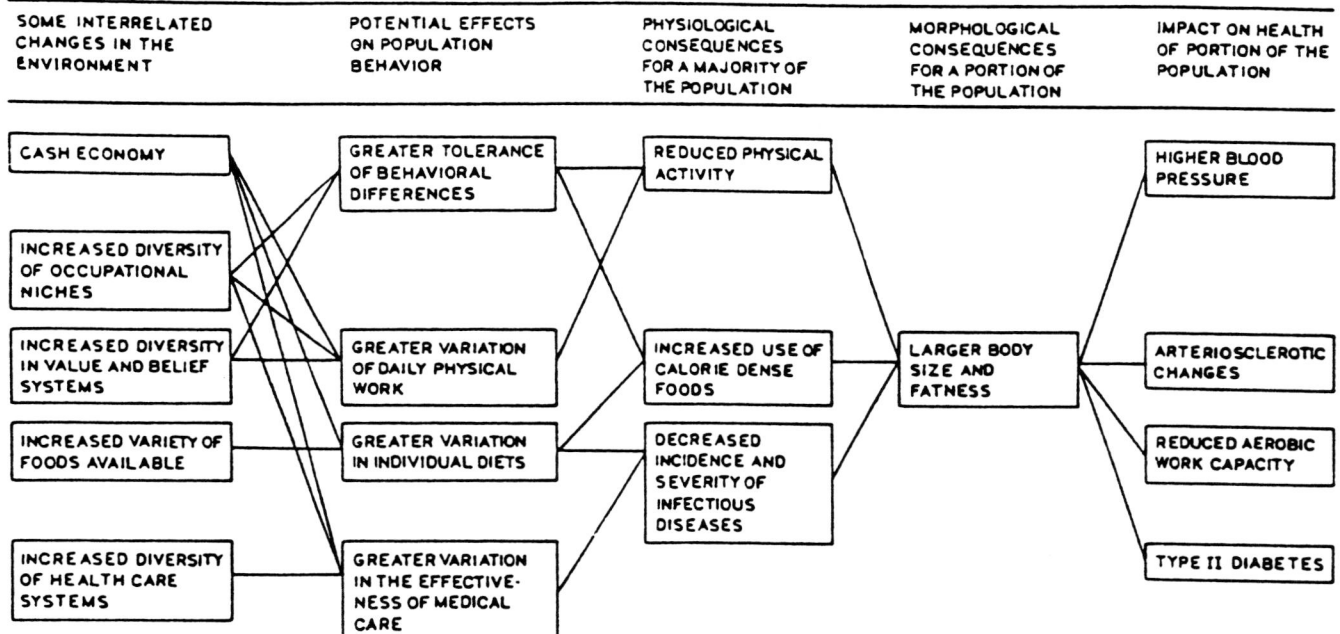

| SOME INTERRELATED CHANGES IN THE ENVIRONMENT | POTENTIAL EFFECTS ON POPULATION BEHAVIOR | PHYSIOLOGICAL CONSEQUENCES FOR A MAJORITY OF THE POPULATION | MORPHOLOGICAL CONSEQUENCES FOR A PORTION OF THE POPULATION | IMPACT ON HEALTH OF PORTION OF THE POPULATION |

FIG. 1. A hypothetical schema of how the socioeconomic changes resulting from modernization may be linked to an increase in average body weight thus affecting health. The presumed links from left to right are generally based on observed associations rather than known mechanisms. (From ref. 26, with permission.)

the Samoans suggests that the stresses of adopting Western lifestyles elevates pressures more than when those lifestyles are fully attained.

The most important correlate of blood pressure among all the Samoan subgroups is weight (fatness), although age (59), diet (110), and psychosocial stress (59,71,111) have all been shown to contribute in some way to the variability in pressure in different subgroups. Why fatness (which also dramatically increases with modernization in a similar pattern with blood pressure, [112]) contributes most to the elevated pressures of the Samoans is probably related to their genetic heritage (109) which was shaped by the founding ancestors of the Samoan islands. These ancestors, who likely endured long sea voyages, may have carried more calories as body fat, which allowed them to better survive bouts of starvation and perhaps cold stress during their ocean-going ordeal (109,113,114). The descendants of these survivors, given a greater diversity of food, a change in activity, and reduced mortality in infancy, probably develop obesity more easily, and with it, elevated rates of diabetes (115) and hypertension (59). Figure 1 shows a hypothetical schema of how sociocultural changes interact with the behavior and biology, leading to the measured health changes of the Samoans.

CONCLUSIONS

Blood pressure studies conducted in traditional populations are often cited to support etiologic arguments in

the studies of hypertension in modern Western populations. While there is substantial data from these populations showing that blood pressure need not increase with age, interpretations relating to why they have low blood pressures in their traditional setting, why pressures increase with modernization, or simply why different populations have different average blood pressure levels are more tenuous. The reasons for this uncertainty are that biological and cultural adaptations as well as the effects of stochastic genetic processes such as drift are often ignored when studying traditional groups or when comparing populations.

In this chapter, we have tried to draw attention to some of these adaptations, as well as to point out that specific genetic and cultural factors may better explain the observed patterns of average pressures in traditional groups. Perhaps the most important conclusion that can be drawn from this brief review is that generalizations about the causes of high blood pressure should not be based solely on evidence from traditional population studies.

It should also be realized that the discussion of stressors such as hypoxia, cold, and heat and their effects on blood pressure has focused on their *singular* effects. Populations (and individuals) actually experience many of these stressors simultaneously, and the measured values of traits such as blood pressure reflect a compromise (or the "best" value) which allows continued survival and reproduction in the face of all of them. Furthermore, other nutritional stresses and adaptations aside from those related to salt and the effects of infectious disease have not been discussed at all, but they also have a profound impact on blood pressure (3,4,7,41,110,116) as well as on the gene pool and culture of many traditional populations (13,15,66,69,76,114,117).

Finally, it is relevant to ask what these studies mean for the treatment of hypertension in Western clinical medicine. The information from these studies points to the fact that there is less constancy in physiological response to stress between groups than is often believed. The data, when considered in an ecological context, strongly support the idea that hypertension has many underlying causes and that these causes may be specific to the genetic and cultural background of the patient. Thus, the data can be interpreted to suggest that treatment for hypertension should be tailored specifically to the biological maladaptations of each individual patient.

REFERENCES

1. *The fifth report of the Joint National Committee on Detection, Evaluation, and Treatment of High Blood Pressure.* Washington, DC: National Institutes of Health; 1993; NIH publication no 93-1088.
2. Epstein FH, Eckhoff RD. The epidemiology of high blood pressure—geographic distributions and etiologic factors. In: Stamler J, Stamler R, Pullman TN, eds. *The epidemiology of hypertension,* New York: Grune and Stratton; 1967:155–166.
3. Page LB. Epidemiologic evidence on the etiology of human hypertension and its possible prevention. *Am Heart J* 1976;91:527–534.
4. Murrill RI. Racial blood pressure studies: a critique of methodology. *Proc Am Phil Soc* 1955;99:277–324.
5. Henry JP, Cassel JC. Psychosocial factors in essential hypertension: recent epidemiologic and animal experimental evidence. *Am J Epidemol* 1969;171–200.
6. Huizinga J. Casual blood pressure in populations. In: Vorester DJM, ed. *Human biology of environmental change.* London: International Biological Programme; 1972:164–169.
7. Akinkuge OO. *High blood pressure in the African.* London: Churchill Livingstone; 1972.
8. Waldron I, Nowotarski M, Freimer M, et al. Cross-cultural variation in blood pressure: a quantitative analysis of the relationships of blood pressure to cultural characteristics, salt consumption and weight. *Soc Sci Med* 1982;16:419–430.
9. Henry JP. Salt, stress, and hypertension. *Soc Sci Med* 1988;26:293–302.
10. Oliver WJ, Cohen EL, Neel JV. Blood pressure, sodium intake, and sodium related hormones in the Yanomamo Indians, a "no-salt" culture. *Circulation* 1975;52:146–151.
11. Scotch NA, Geiger J. The epidemiology of essential hypertension II. *J Chron Dis* 1963;16:1183–1213.
12. Dressler WW, Grell GAC, Gallagher PN, Viteri FE. Blood pressure and social class in a Jamaican community. *AJPH* 1988;78:714–716.
13. Boyden SV, ed. *The impact of civilization on the biology of man.* Toronto: University of Toronto Press; 1970.
14. Baker PT. The adaptive limits of human populations. *Man (NS)* 1984;19:1–14.
15. Boyden S. *Western civilization in biological perspective: patterns in biohistory.* Oxford: Clarendon press; 1987.
16. O'Rourke MF. What is blood pressure? *Am J Hypertens* 1990;3:803–810.
17. Rowell LB. *Human circulation: regulation during physical stress.* New York: Oxford University Press; 1986.
18. Acheson RM, Fowler GB. On the inheritance of stature and blood pressure. *J Chron Dis* 1967;20:731–751.
19. Selye H. The general adaptation syndrome and the diseases of adaptation. *J Clin Endocrinol* 1946;6:117–230.
20. Seyle H. *The stress of life.* New York: McGraw-Hill; 1976.
21. Cannon WB. Stresses and strains of homeostasis. *Am J Med Sci* 1935;189:1–14.
22. Hinkle LE. Stress and disease: the concept after 50 years. *Soc Sci Med* 1987;25:561–566.
23. Baker PT. Problems and strategies. In: Baker PT, ed. *Human population problems in the biosphere: some research strategies and designs.* Paris: UNESCO; 1977: 11–32.
24. Baker PT, Hanna JM, Baker TS, eds. *The changing Samoans: behavior and health in transition.* Oxford: Oxford University Press; 1986.
25. Friedlander JS, ed. *The Solomon Islands Project: A long-term study of health, human biology, and culture change.* Oxford: Clarendon Press; 1987.
26. Baker PT: Rationale and research design. In: Baker PT, Hanna JM, TS Baker, eds. *The changing Samoans: behavior and health in transition.* Oxford: Oxford University Press; 1986:3–18.
27. Ayman D, Goldshine AD. Blood pressure determinations by patients with essential hypertension I. The difference between clinic and home readings before treatment. *Am J Med Sci* 1940;200:465–474.
28. Beckman M, Panfilou V, Silvertsson R, et al. Blood pressure and heart rate recordings at home and at the clinic. *Acta Med Scand* 1981;210:97–102.
29. Shapiro A, Meyers T, Reiser MF. Comparison of blood pressure response to veriloid and to the doctor. *Psychosom Med* 1954;16:478–488.
30. Comstock GW. An epidemiologic study of blood pressure levels in a biracial community in the southern United States. *Am J Hyg* 1957;65:271–315.
31. Rose G. Standardization of observers in blood pressure measurement. *Lancet* 1965;1:673–674.
32. Armitage P, Fox W, Rose GA, Tinker CM. The variability of measurements of casual blood pressure II: survey experience. *Clin Sci* 1966;30:337–344.
33. James GD, Yee LS, Harshfield GA, et al. The influence of happiness, anger, and anxiety on the blood pressure of borderline hypertensives. *Psychosom Med* 1986;48:502–508.
34. Pickering TG, James GD, Boddie C, et al. How common is white coat hypertension? *JAMA* 1988;259:225–228.
35. McGarvey ST, Baker PT. The effects of modernization and migration on Samoan blood pressure. *Human Biol* 1979;51:461–479.
36. Mann GV, Roels OA, Price DL et al. Cardiovascular disease in African Pygmies. *J Chron Dis* 1962;15:341–371.
37. Shaper AG, Saxton GA. Blood pressure and body build in a rural community in Uganda. *E Afr Med J* 1969;46:228–245.
38. Huizinga J: Human biological observations on some African populations of the thorn savanna belt. I.II. *Proc Kon Ned Akad Wetensch, Ser C* 1968;71:356–390.
39. Kaminer B, Lutz WBW. Blood pressure in Bushmen of the Kalahari desert. *Circulation* 1960;22:289–295.
40. Williams AW. Blood pressure differences in Kikuyu and Sanburu communities in Kenya. *E Afr Med J* 1969;46:262–272.
41. Thomas WA. Health of a carnivorous race. *JAMA* 1927; 88:1559–1562.
42. Fulmer HS, Roberts RW. Coronary heart disease among the Navajo Indians. *Ann Int Med* 1963;59:740–764.
43. Kean BH. The blood pressure of the Cuna Indians. *Am J Trop Med* 1944;24:341–343.
44. Lowenstein FW. Blood pressure in relation to age and sex in the tropics and subtropics. A review of the literature and an investigation in two tribes of Brazil Indians. *Lancet* 1961;2:389–392.
45. Tenbrinck MS. Blood pressure comparisons in tropical Africans and Peruvians. *NY State J Med* 1964;Oct:2584–2587.
46. Makela M, Barton SA, Schull WJ, et al. The multi-national Andean genetic and health program—IV. Altitude and the blood pressure of the Aymara. *J Chron Dis* 1973;31:587–603.
47. Kapur YP, Patt AJ. Hearing in Todas of South India. *Arch Otolaryng* 1967;85:400–406.
48. Padmavati S, Gupta S. Blood pressure studies in rural and urban groups in Delhi. *Circulation* 1959;19:395–405.

49. Casley Smith JR. Blood pressure in Australian Aborigines. *Med J Austr* 1959; May 9:627–633.

50. Whyte HM. Body fat and blood pressure of natives in New Guinea: reflections on essential hypertension. *Austr Ann Med* 1958;7:36–46.

51. Maddocks I, Rovin L. A New Guinea population in which blood pressure appears to fall as age advances. *Papua N Guinea Med J* 1965;8:17–21.

52. Maddocks I. Blood pressure in Melanesians. *Med J Austr* 1967;54:1123–1126.

53. Stanhope JM. Blood pressure of Tinam-Aigram people, Madang district, Papua. *N Guinea Med J* 1968;11:60–61.

54. Murrill RI. Blood pressure of natives of Ponape Island. *Human Biol* 1949;21:47–57.

55. Maddocks I. Possible absence of essential hypertension in two complete Pacific island populations. *Lancet* 1961;396–399.

56. Lovell RRH, Maddocks I, Rogerson GW. The casual arterial pressure of Fijians and Indians in Fiji. *Austr Ann Med* 1960;9:4–17.

57. Prior IAM, Evans JG, Harvey HPB, et al. Sodium intake and blood pressure in two Polynesian populations. *New Engl J Med* 1968;279:515–520.

58. Prior IAM. The Tokelau island migrant study: a progress report 1979. In: Fleming C, Prior IAM, eds. *Migration, adaptation, and health in the Pacific.* Wellington, New Zealand: Epidemiology Unit Wellington Hospital; 1981:27–38.

59. McGarvey ST, Schendel DE. Blood pressure of Samoans. In: Baker PT, Hanna JM, Baker TS, eds. *The changing Samoans: behavior and health in transition.* Oxford: Oxford University Press, 1986: 350–393.

60. Page LB, Damon A, Moellering RC. Antecedents of cardiovascular disease in six Solomon Islands societies. *Circulation* 1974;59:1132–1146.

61. Steward J. *Theory of culture change.* Urbana, IL: University of Illinois Press; 1955.

62. Bates M. *The prevalence of people.* New York: Charles Scribner and Sons; 1955.

63. Bresler JB. *Human ecology: collected readings.* Reading, MA: Addison-Wesley; 1966.

64. Rappaport RA. Nature, culture, and ecological anthropology. In: Shapiro HL, ed. *Man, culture, and society.* Oxford: Oxford University Press; 1971:237–267.

65. Vayda AP, ed. *Environment and cultural behavior: ecological studies in cultural anthropology.* American Museum Sourcebooks in Anthropology. Garden City, NY: The Natural History Press; 1969.

66. Moran EF. *Human adaptability: an introduction to ecological anthropology.* Belmont, CA: Duxbury Press; 1979.

67. Little MA, Morren Jr GEB. *Ecology, energetics, and human variability.* Dubuque, IA: Wm. C. Brown Company; 1976.

68. Titlebaum MS. Relevance of demographic transition theory for developing countries. *Science* 1975;188:420–425.

69. Baker PT, Dutt JS. Demographic variables as measures of biological adaptation: a case study of high altitude human populations. In: Harrison GA, Boyce AJ, eds. *The structure of human populations.* Oxford: Clarendon Press; 1972:352–378.

70. Baker PT, Crews DE. Mortality patterns and some biological predictors. In: Baker PT, Hanna JM, Baker TS, eds. *The changing Samoans: behavior and health in transition.* Oxford: Oxford University Press; 1986:93–122.

71. James GD, Baker PT, Jenner DA, Harrison GA. Variation in lifestyle characteristics and catecholamine excretion rates among young Western Samoan men. *Soc Sci Med* 1987;25:981–986.

72. Ostfeld A, D'Atri D. Rapid sociocultural change and high blood pressure. *Adv Psychosom Med* 1977;9:20.

73. Freis ED. Salt, volume, and the prevention of hypertension. *Circulation* 1976;53:589–595.

74. Baker PT, Little MA, eds. *Man in the Andes: a multidisciplinary study of high altitude Quechua.* Stroudsburg, PA: Dowden, Hutchinson and Ross; 1976.

75. Baker PT, ed. *The biology of high altitude peoples.* New York: Cambridge University Press; 1978.

76. Frisancho AR. *Human adaptation: a functional interpretation.* St. Louis: C.V. Mosby; 1979.

77. Cruz-Coke R. Correlation between the prevalence of hypertension and degree of acculturation. *J Hyperten* 1987;5:47–50.

78. Saldana M, Arias-Stella J. Studies on the structure of the pulmonary trunk. Part 2. the evolution of the elastic configuration of the pulmonary trunk in people native to high altitudes. *Circulation* 1963;27:1094–1100.

79. Arias-Stella J, Recavarren S. Right ventricular hypertrophy in native children living at high altitude. *Am J Path* 1962;41:55–59.

80. Penaloza D, Sime F, Banchero N, et al. Pulmonary hypertension in healthy men born and living at high altitudes. *Am J Cardiol* 1963;11:150–157.

81. Banchero N, Sime F, Penaloza D, et al. Pulmonary pressure, cardiac output, and arterial oxygen saturation during exercise at high altitude and at sea level. *Circulation* 1966;33:249–262.

82. Penaloza D, Gamboa R, Dyer J, et al. The influence of high altitudes on the electrical activity of the heart. Electrocardiographic and vectorcardiographic observations in adolescence and adulthood. *Am Heart J* 1961;61:101–107.

83. Marticorena E, Ruiz L, Severino J, et al. Systemic blood pressure in white men born at sea level: changes after long residence at high altitudes. *Am J Cardiol* 1969;23:364–368.

84. Heath D, Williams DR. *Man at high altitude: the pathophysiology of acclimatization and adaptation.* Edinburgh: Churchill Livingstone; 1977.

85. Ladell WSS. The influence of environment in arid regions on the biology of man. *Human and animal ecology, reviews of research.* Paris: UNESCO; 1957.

86. Briggs LC. Environment and human adaptation in the Sahara. In: Damon A, ed. *Physiological anthropology.* New York: Oxford University Press; 1975:93–129.

87. Ladell WSS. Terrestrial animals in humid heat: man. In Dill DB, Adolph EF, Wilber CG, eds. *Handbook of physiology, vol 4, adaptation to the environment.* Baltimore: Williams & Wilkins; 1964:625–659.

88. Gleibermann L. Blood pressure and dietary salt in human populations. *Ecology of Food and Nutr* 1973;2:83–90.

89. Steegman AT. Human adaptation to cold. In: Damon A, ed. *Physiological anthropology.* New York: Oxford University Press; 1975:130–166.

90. LeBlanc J. *Man in the cold.* Springfield, IL: Charles C. Thomas Publisher; 1975.

91. Adams T, Covino BG. Racial variations to a standardized cold stress. *J Appl Physiol* 1958;12:9–12.

92. Rennie DW, Adams T. Comparative thermoregulatory responses of Negroes and white persons to acute cold stress. *J Appl Physiol* 1957;11:201–204.

93. Newman RW. A comparison of Negro and White responses in a 5°C water bath. *Am J Phys Anthropol* 1967;27:249 (abst).

94. Denton D. *The hunger for salt.* Berlin: Springer-Verlag; 1980.

95. Pecker MS, Laragh JH. Dietary salt and blood pressure: a perspective. *Hypertension* 1991;17(Suppl I):I97–I99.

96. The INTERSALT Co-operative Research Group. INTERSALT Study: An international co-operative study on the relation of blood pressure to electrolyte excretion in populations. I. Design and methods. *J Hypertens* 1986;4:781–787.

97. INTERSALT Cooperative Research Group. INTERSALT: An international study of electrolyte excretion and blood pressure. Results for 24 hour urinary sodium and potassium excretion. *Br Med J* 1988;297:319–328.

98. Elliot P, Stamler R. Manual of operations for INTERSALT. *Controlled Clin Trials* 1988;9:1S–118S.

99. Stamler J, Rose G, Elliot P, et al. for the INTERSALT Cooperative Research Group. Findings of the international cooperative INTERSALT study. *Hypertension* 1991;17(Suppl I):I9–I15.

100. Carvalho JJM, Baruzzi RG, Howard PF, et al. Blood pressure in four remote populations in the INTERSALT study. *Hypertension* 1989;14:238–246.

101. Swales JD. Salt saga continued [Editorial]. *Br Med J* 1988;297:307–308.

102. Simpson FO. Salt saga continued [Letter]. *Br Med J* 1988;297:684.

103. Stamler R. Implications of the INTERSALT study. *Hypertension* 1991;17(Suppl I):I16–I20.

104. Anderson ND, Meyers HF, Pickering T, Jackson JS. Hyperten-

sion in blacks: psychosocial and biological perspectives. *J Hypertens* 1989;7:161–172.

105. Wilson TW, Grim CE. Biohistory of slavery and blood pressure differences in blacks today: a hypothesis. *Hypertension* 1991; 17(Suppl I):I22–I28.

106. Jackson FLC. An evolutionary perspective on salt, hypertension, and human genetic variation. *Hypertension* 1991;17(Suppl I): I29–I32.

107. Lefevre-Whitier P. An anthropological perspective on the epidemiology of hemoglobin defects and glucose-6-phosphate dehydrogenase deficiencies in the northern half of the African continent. In: Chakraborty R, Szathmary EJE, eds. *Diseases of complex etiology in small populations: ethnic differences and research approaches.* New York: Alan R. Liss, Inc; 1985:367–397.

108. Baker PT, Hanna JM. Modernization and the biological fitness of Samoans: a progress report on a research program. In: Fleming C, Prior IAM, eds. *Migration, adaptation, and health in the Pacific.* Wellington, New Zealand: Epidemiology Unit, Wellington Hospital; 1981:14–26.

109. Baker PT. Migration, genetics, and the degenerative disease of South Pacific islanders. In: Boyce A, ed. *Migration and mobility.* London: Taylor and Francis, Ltd; 1984:209–239.

110. Hanna JM, Pelletier DL, Brown VJ. The diet and nutrition of contemporary Samoans. In: Baker PT, Hanna JM, Baker TS, eds. *The changing Samoans: behavior and health in transition.* Oxford: Oxford University Press; 1986:275–296.

111. James GD, Jenner DA, Harrison GA, Baker PT. Differences in catecholamine excretion rates, blood pressure, and lifestyle among young Western Samoan men. *Human Biol* 1985;57:635–647.

112. Bindon JR, Baker PT. Modernization, migration, and obesity among Samoan adults. *Annals of Human Biol* 1985;12:67–76.

113. Neel JV. Diabetes mellitus: a thrifty genotype rendered detrimental by "progress"! *Am J Hum Genet* 1962;14:353–362.

114. Prior IAM. The price of civilization. *Nutrition Today* 1971;6:2–11.

115. Crews DE, MacKeen PC. Mortality related to cardiovascular disease and diabetes mellitus in a modernizing population. *Soc Sci Med* 1982;16:175–181.

116. Saunders GM. Blood pressure in Yucatecans. *Am J Med Sci* 1933;185:843–851.

117. Stini WA. Evolutionary implications of changing nutritional patterns in human populations. *Am Anthropologist* 1971;73:1019–1030.

Hypertension: Pathophysiology, Diagnosis, and Management, Second Edition,
edited by J.H. Laragh and B.M. Brenner,
Raven Press, Ltd., New York © 1995.

CHAPTER 9

Impact of Systolic and Diastolic Blood Pressure on Cardiovascular Mortality

James D. Neaton, Lewis Kuller, Jeremiah Stamler, and Deborah N. Wentworth

There is growing recognition of the importance of systolic blood pressure (SBP) as well as diastolic blood pressure (DBP) in assessing a person's risk of cardiovascular disease (CVD) and in making a decision about use of BP lowering treatment. Two recent reviews that discussed the relative importance of SBP and DBP each concluded that both SBP and DBP should be considered in assessing a person's risk of CVD (1,2). Furthermore, the importance of treating persons with an elevated SBP even when their DBP is below usual treatment levels has been affirmed in a recent clinical trial (3). Two other similar clinical trials are ongoing (4,5). As a consequence of a growing body of observational data and the results of the Systolic Hypertension in the Elderly Program (SHEP) (3), the Fifth Report of the Joint National Committee on Detection, Evaluation, and Treatment of High Blood Pressure (JNC-V) defined stages of hypertension based on both SBP and DBP (6). Thus, it is generally accepted that classification of hypertensives by DBP only, and

treatment and monitoring based only on DBP and not SBP, are inappropriate.

In this chapter, relationships between SBP and DBP and death from coronary heart disease (CHD) and stroke are reviewed. To quantify the relative impact of SBP and DBP on risk of specific causes of death, data from the ongoing mortality follow-up of the 361,662 men screened for the Multiple Risk Factor Intervention Trial (MRFIT) are used (7). Reports after 6 and 12 years of follow-up for this cohort established the strong, graded relationship of both SBP and DBP with death from CHD and stroke (8–11), the increased risk of these outcomes associated with isolated systolic hypertension (8,12), the stronger relationship of SBP as compared with DBP with both end points (8,9,12), the declining relative risk and increasing absolute excess risk with age and the presence of diabetes associated with elevated blood pressure (9,13,14), the strong association of SBP and DBP with death from renal disease (15), and the similar association of SBP and DBP with death from CHD, stroke, and renal disease for men in different ethnic groups (7,10,15).

This cohort has now been followed for an average of 16 years. For the group of 347,978 men without a previous myocardial infarction and with both SBP and DBP measurements, on whom most analyses in this chapter are based, 11,149 CHD deaths and 1,233 deaths from stroke have now been identified during the 16-year follow-up. Following a brief description of this large cohort, the chapter is divided into six parts: (a) prevalence of hypertension by JNC-V criteria, (b) SBP and DBP and

J. D. Neaton: Division of Biostatistics, School of Public Health, University of Minnesota, Minneapolis, Minnesota 55414.

L. Kuller: Graduate School of Public Health, University of Pittsburgh, Pittsburgh, Pennsylvania 15261.

J. Stamler: Department of Preventive Medicine, Northwestern University Medical School, Chicago, Illinois 60611.

D. N. Wentworth: Division of Biostatistics, School of Public Health, University of Minnesota, Minneapolis, Minnesota 55414.

risk of death from CHD, (c) SBP and DBP and risk of death from stroke, (d) SBP and DBP and risk of death from any cause, (e) SBP and DBP and risk of death among men with a history of myocardial infarction, and (f) conclusions.

THE MRFIT COHORT

The MRFIT was a randomized, multicenter primary prevention trial to study the effect of an intervention program on blood pressure, serum cholesterol, and cigarette smoking on the incidence of CHD (16,17). Between 1973 and 1975, 361,662 men aged 35 to 57 years from 18 cities in the United States were screened for entry to the MRFIT (18,19). Of those screened, 347,978 had both SBP and DBP measurements and reported that they had not been previously hospitalized for a heart attack.

Race/ethnicity was ascertained at screening. Men are grouped into five categories for this report: white, black, Hispanic, Oriental, and other. Blood pressure was measured by trained observers using a standard mercury sphygmomanometer (20). The first and fifth Korotkoff phases were recorded as SBP and DBP. Three readings were taken of SBP and DBP with a 2-minute rest between readings. The average of the last two readings is used to define SBP and DBP in this report. For the cohort under study, SBP averaged 130.0 (SD = 15.9) and DBP averaged 83.7 (SD = 10.5).

Vital status of all men screened has been ascertained through December 1990 with the National Death Index (1979 to 1990) and the Social Security Administration (1973 through 1986). Methods concerning the collection of vital status information have been described (21). CHD death is defined as International Classification of Diseases, Ninth Revision (ICD-9) codes 410-414 and 429.2 (22). The ICD-9 code 429.2 identifies "cardiovascular disease, unspecified"; most of these certificates would have been coded to the CHD rubric 412.4 under the eighth revision (23). The ICD-9 codes 430 to 438 are used to define death from stroke.

PREVALENCE OF HYPERTENSION BY JNC-V CRITERIA

The JNC-V report identifies six categories of blood pressure for adults age 18 years and older: normal, high normal, stage 1 (mild hypertension), stage 2 (moderate hypertension), stage 3 (severe hypertension), and stage 4 (very severe hypertension) (6). In addition, the JNC-V report notes that among persons with normal blood pressure, optimal levels are SBP < 120 mm Hg and DBP < 80 mm Hg. Thus the "normal" category has been divided into two groups for the purpose of analyses here: (a) optimal, and (b) normal but not optimal. The resulting seven categories are defined in Table 1 in terms of SBP and DBP. Also shown are the percentages of MRFIT men in each category for each of five age groups and overall. The prevalence of hypertension overall (stages 1–4) and for each stage was higher with age. For the youngest age group (35–39 years), 26 percent were hypertensive; for the oldest group (55–57 years), 45 percent were hypertensive. Within each age group the vast majority of hypertensives had stage 1 hypertension (SBP 140–159 mm Hg or DBP 90–99 mm Hg). Overall 74 percent of men aged 35 to 57 years with elevated BP (DBP ≥ 90 or SBP ≥ 140 mm Hg) had stage 1 hypertension. Less than 20 percent of men overall had optimal blood pressure levels.

As a consequence of using both SBP and DBP measurements to define hypertension, prevalence was higher (Table 2). Based on SBP criteria alone, 23.6 percent of MRFIT men were hypertensive; 27.3 percent were hypertensive based on DBP criteria alone. With the JNC-V criteria, which use both SBP and DBP, 35.1 percent of men were hypertensive. The largest absolute effect was for stage 1 hypertension. For this group, the percent of men identified as hypertensive increased from 19 percent or 20 percent using SBP or DBP alone to almost 26 percent with use of both. It is estimated that approximately 50 million Americans have hypertension by JNC-V criteria (6).

TABLE 1. *Age-specific percentage distribution of blood pressure: men screened for MRFIT*

BP category[a]	Systolic BP (mm Hg)		Diastolic BP (mm Hg)	Age in years (N)—percent					
				35–39 (72,566)	40–44 (76,773)	45–49 (82,274)	50–54 (80,544)	55–57 (35,821)	Total (347,978)
Optimal	<120	and	<80	22.5	20.2	17.8	15.0	13.5	18.2
Normal but not optimal	120–129	or	80–84	28.4	26.2	24.1	21.9	19.8	24.5
High normal	130–139	or	85–89	22.8	22.3	22.1	22.0	21.5	22.2
Hypertension									
Stage 1 (mild)	140–159	or	90–99	21.0	23.8	26.3	29.2	31.6	25.9
Stage 2 (moderate)	160–179	or	100–109	4.3	5.9	7.4	9.0	10.3	7.1
Stage 3 (severe)	180–209	or	110–119	0.8	1.3	1.8	2.3	2.7	1.7
Stage 4 (very severe)	≥210	or	≥120	0.2	0.3	0.5	0.6	0.6	0.4
Total				100.0	100.0	100.0	100.0	100.0	100.0

[a] Classification of BP as according to Fifth Joint National Committee Report.

TABLE 2. *Percent classified as hypertensive using systolic BP alone, diastolic BP alone and either systolic or diastolic BP: men screened for MRFIT*

Hypertensive status	Systolic BP alone		Diastolic BP alone		Systolic or diastolic BP[a] criterion met (percent)
	Criterion	Percent	Criterion	Percent	
Stage 1 (mild)	140–159	18.9	90–99	20.1	25.9
Stage 2 (moderate)	160–179	3.8	100–109	5.5	7.1
Stage 3 (severe)	180–209	0.8	110–119	1.3	1.7
Stage 4 (very severe)	≥210	0.1	≥120	0.4	0.4
Total hypertensive		23.6		27.3	35.1

[a] As in Fifth Joint National Committee Report.

The percent with hypertension based on an SBP of 140 or greater was higher for each age group, ranging from 15 percent (35–39 years) to 37 percent (55–57 years) (Fig. 1). The percent of men with a DBP 90 mm Hg or higher was not greater for men age 45 and older. Largely as a consequence of the higher SBP with age, the percent hypertensive based on either SBP or DBP criteria (as per JNC-V) ranged from 26 percent to 45 percent over the age span investigated. The continually higher SBP for persons 50 years of age and older, and the plateau of average DBP after the fifth or sixth decade of life have been reported for several other cohorts (24–26).

Among the 347,978 men without a history of a myocardial infarction 312,993 reported their race as white, 22,471 as black, 4,257 as Oriental, 6,511 as Hispanic, and 1,746 as another race/ethnic group. Prevalence of hypertension based on JNC-V criteria for each ethnic group is shown by age in the upper half of Table 3. The prevalence of hypertension was higher among blacks than the other ethnic groups in each age stratum. Differences within each age group by race are similar to those observed in the National Health and Nutrition Survey conducted at approximately the same time as the screening for MRFIT (24).

Some 5,163 (1.5 percent) men screened reported taking medication for diabetes. Prevalence of hypertension was higher in each age group for men with diabetes compared to those without diabetes (lower half of Table 3). The generally unfavorable cardiovascular risk profile of these men with diabetes is discussed in detail in a recent report (14).

The bivariate percentage distribution of SBP and DBP is given in Table 4. The dotted lines define the seven JNC-V categories of BP for adults. The percentages given in parentheses add to 100 percent within each JNC-V BP category. As noted previously, only 18.2 percent of these middle-aged men had optimal blood pressure levels. Among men with normal, but not optimal, levels, 38.3 percent had above-optimal levels of both SBP and DBP. For those with high normal blood pressure, 76.1 percent had above-optimal levels of both SBP and DBP. Among men with stage 1 hypertension, 32 percent met both SBP and DBP criteria, 27.4 percent met SBP but not DBP criteria, and 40.6 percent met DBP but not SBP criteria. Among those with stage 2 hypertension, 18.3 percent met both SBP and DBP criteria, 25.7 percent met SBP but not DBP criteria, and 56.0 percent met DBP but not SBP criteria. Of men with stage 2 hypertension, 43.9 per-

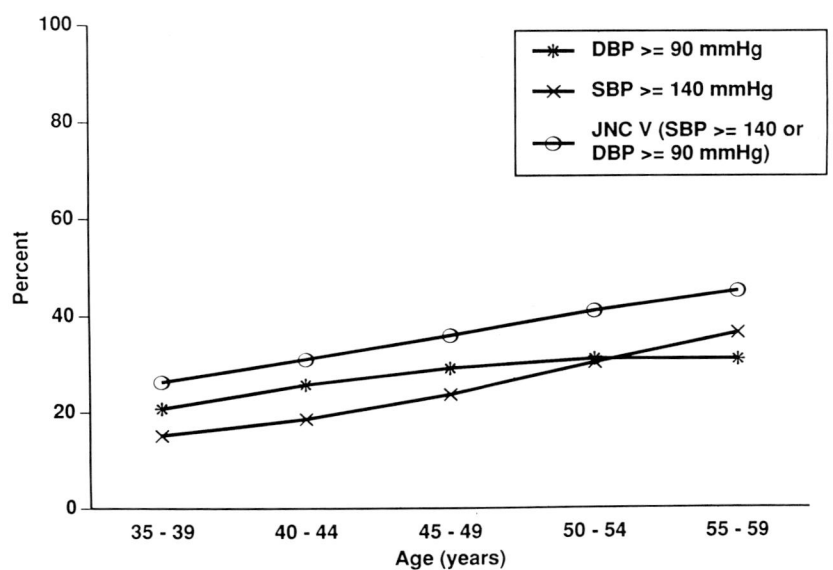

FIG. 1. Percent hypertensive using three criteria by age. Men screened for MRFIT.

TABLE 3. Age-specific prevalence of hypertension[a] by race/ethnicity or diabetes: men screened for MRFIT

	Age (years)					
Ethnicity	35–39	40–44	45–49	50–54	55–57	Total
White	25.6	30.3	35.2	40.3	44.5	34.3
Black	36.8	42.8	47.7	53.5	56.5	46.1
Oriental	23.4	32.8	33.2	39.7	41.5	32.2
Hispanic	25.5	34.0	38.0	43.8	45.9	35.5
Other	26.5	32.2	32.5	41.6	44.8	32.5
Diabetes						
Yes	35.1	42.4	49.4	55.0	57.5	50.8
No	26.3	31.2	35.8	40.8	44.8	34.8

[a] Stage 1 or higher, Fifth Joint National Committee Report.

cent had a DBP of 100 to 109 mm Hg and a SBP 140 to 159 mm Hg. For those with stage 3 hypertension, 14.3 percent met both SBP and DBP criteria, 23.7 percent met SBP but not DBP criteria, and 62.0 percent met DBP but not SBP criteria. Of these middle-aged men with stage 3 hypertension, 34.4 percent had an SBP of 160 to 179 mm Hg and a DBP of 110 to 119 mm Hg. For the 0.4 percent of men with stage 4 hypertension, both SBP and DBP criteria were met for 12 percent, 9.3 percent met SBP but not DBP criteria, and 78.8 percent met DBP but not SBP criteria.

SBP AND DBP AND RISK OF DEATH FROM CHD

Age-adjusted CHD death rates for each of the seven JNC-V blood pressure categories are shown in Table 5.

Age-adjustment is by the direct method (27). Also shown are multivariable adjusted relative risk estimates and the cumulative percent of men dying from CHD 5, 10, and 15 years after blood pressure measurement. Adjusted relative risk estimates were obtained with use of proportional hazards regression (28). The optimal category is used as the reference group and adjustment was for age, race, income, serum cholesterol level, reported cigarettes per day, and use of medication for diabetes. The cumulative percents were estimated using the Kaplan-Meier method (29). With each stage of hypertension, risk of CHD death increases relative to those in the "optimal," "normal," and "high normal" categories. Those with stage 1 hypertension, the vast majority of hypertensives, have CHD death rates more than twice that for men with optimal blood pressure. Furthermore, based on adjusted relative risk estimates, CHD death rates are 31 percent

TABLE 4. Bivariate percentage distribution of SBP and DBP[a]: men screened for MRFIT

	SBP (mm Hg)							
DBP (mm Hg)	<120	120–129	130–139	140–159	160–179	180–209	210+	Total[b]
<80	18.2 (100.0)	10.0 (20.8)	3.9 (17.5)	1.4 (5.5)	0.1 (1.8)	0.0 (1.1)	0.0 (1.1)	33.7
80–84	5.1 (40.9)	9.4 (38.3)	5.5 (24.9)	2.3 (8.8)	0.2 (2.3)	0.0 (1.4)	0.0 (1.0)	22.5
85–89	1.4 (6.4)	5.7 (25.5)	5.7 (25.6)	3.4 (13.1)	0.3 (4.2)	0.0 (1.5)	0.0 (0.6)	16.5
90–99	0.4 (1.5)	3.2 (12.4)	6.9 (26.7)	8.3 (32.0)	1.2 (17.4)	0.1 (6.8)	0.0 (1.3)	20.1
100–109	0.0 (0.1)	0.1 (1.5)	0.7 (10.5)	3.1 (43.9)	1.3 (18.3)	0.2 (12.9)	0.0 (1.7)	5.5
110–119	0.0 (0.1)	0.0 (0.2)	0.0 (1.7)	0.4 (25.6)	0.6 (34.4)	0.2 (14.3)	0.0 (3.6)	1.3
120+	0.0 (0.3)	0.0 (0.1)	0.0 (0.2)	0.0 (5.8)	0.1 (29.4)	0.2 (43.0)	0.5 (12.0)	0.4
Total[b]	25.1	28.4	22.8	18.9	3.8	0.8	0.1	100.0

[a] Percents not in parentheses are of total number of men (347,978). Percents in parentheses are of total number of men in that category of JNC-V BP. The seven categories are defined by the dotted lines beginning in the upper left hand corner: optimal, normal but not optimal, high normal, stage 1, stage 2, stage 3, and stage 4 hypertension.

[b] Some columns do not add to totals due to rounding.

TABLE 5. *Baseline blood pressure and CHD mortality: men screened for MRFIT*

BP category[a]	No. men	No. CHD deaths	Age-adjusted rate per 10,000 person-years[b]	Adjusted relative risk[c]	Cumulative percent dying from CHD[d]		
					5 years	10 years	15 years
Optimal	63,371	942	10.7	1.00	0.3	0.7	1.4
Normal but not optimal	85,273	1,774	14.6	1.31*	0.3	1.0	1.9
High normal	77,248	2,140	18.5	1.61*	0.5	1.4	2.6
Hypertension							
Stage 1 (mild)	90,015	3,934	27.4	2.33*	0.7	2.1	4.1
Stage 2 (moderate)	24,744	1,618	39.9	3.20*	1.2	3.4	6.3
Stage 3 (severe)	5,783	550	57.3	4.64*	1.7	5.1	9.3
Stage 4 (very severe)	1,544	191	83.4	6.88*	2.3	7.3	12.8

[a] Classification of BP is according to Fifth Joint National Committee Report.
[b] Adjusted using the direct method for the age distribution of all men screened.
[c] Estimated using proportional hazards regression model stratified by clinic and adjusted for age, race, income, serum cholesterol level, reported cigarettes per day, and use of medication for diabetes.
[d] Estimated by the Kaplan-Meier method.
* $p < .0001$.

and 61 percent higher for those with normal, but not optimal, and high normal blood pressure compared to those with optimal blood pressure. By 10 years of follow-up, 2.1 percent of men with stage 1 hypertension had died from CHD as compared to 0.7 percent with optimal BP. If, like this cohort, 74 percent of persons in the United States with elevated BP have stage 1 hypertension (approximately 37 million persons), and if the excess risk estimated here is applicable to all persons with stage 1 hypertension, then over 400,000 CHD deaths could possibly be prevented in 10 years by reducing BP to an optimal level.

The strong association of blood pressure and CHD mortality is evident in women as well as in men. Table 6 gives 15-year death rates and relative risk estimates for middle-aged men and women in the Chicago Heart Association Study (10). Like men, few women had optimal blood pressure levels (12 percent in this cohort). With higher SBP and DBP, risk of CHD death increased rapidly. Risk was greatest when both SBP and DBP were elevated. Like men, women who had blood pressures above optimal but not in the hypertensive range also had a higher risk of CHD death than those with optimal levels. Several other observational studies have shown a significant and independent association of blood pressure with CHD in women (30–37).

The association of SBP and DBP with CHD death for men screened for MRFIT is analyzed further in Tables 7 and 8. These tables give age-adjusted CHD death rates and adjusted relative risk estimates (each blood pressure

TABLE 6. *Baseline systolic/diastolic blood pressure (SBP/DBP) and age-adjusted coronary heart disease mortality in the Chicago Heart Association Detection Project in Industry (persons aged 35 to 63 years, mean follow-up)*

SBP/DBP mm Hg	White men (N = 12,035)				White women (N = 9,012)			
	N	Deaths	Rate[e]	RR[b]	N	Deaths	Rate	RR
<120/<80	694	8	7.9	1.00	1130	3	1.8	1.00
<120/80–89	132	3	. . .[c]	. . .	157	0	. . .	. . .
<120/90–99	8	0	. . .	. . .	7	0	. . .	. . .
120–139/<80	1,768	42	19.0	2.40	1766	21	8.8	4.82
120–139/80–89	2,179	74	24.8	3.15	1564	24	12.8	7.05
120–139/90–99	506	31	43.0	5.44	245	2	. . .	. . .
120–139/100+	14	2	. . .	. . .	7	0	. . .	. . .
140–159/<80	471	32	32.1	4.07	379	7	11.0	6.04
140–159/80–89	1,941	102	35.0	4.43	1294	32	14.6	8.02
140–159/90–99	1,730	83	31.8	4.03	893	18	12.2	6.68
140–159/100+	292	18	51.1	6.47	139	5	25.9	14.23
160+/<80	64	1	. . .	. . .	55	2	. . .	. . .
160+/80–89	294	21	40.0	5.07	267	10	18.6	10.24
160+/90–99	867	95	58.7	7.43	573	25	22.1	12.49
160+/100+	1,075	125	73.4	9.30	536	33	36.0	19.79

[a] Age-adjusted rate per 10,000 person-years.
[b] Age-adjusted relative risk.
[c] Numbers too small to estimate.

TABLE 7. *Association of systolic blood pressure and CHD mortality: men screened for MRFIT*

Systolic BP (mm Hg)[a]	No. men	No. CHD deaths	Age-adjusted[b] rate per 10,000 person-years	Adjusted relative risk[c] (95% CI)
<120	87,459	1,412	11.6	1.00 (reference group)
120–129	98,834	2,199	15.5	1.28 (1.19 to 1.36)
130–139	79,308	2,511	20.8	1.66 (1.56 to 1.77)
140–159	65,865	3,487	32.1	2.45 (2.30 to 2.61)
160–179	13,321	1,120	48.4	3.42 (3.16 to 3.71)
180–209	2,863	376	79.6	5.26 (4.68 to 5.90)
≥210	328	44	82.6	6.40 (4.74 to 8.65)
Total	347,978	11,149		

[a] Classification of BP is according to Fifth Joint National Committee Report.
[b] Adjusted using the direct method for the age distribution of all men screened.
[c] Estimated using proportional hazards regression model stratified by clinic and adjusted for age, race, income, serum cholesterol level, reported cigarettes per day, and use of medication for diabetes.

category relative to the lowest one) from a proportional hazards model (28) corresponding to the SBP and DBP levels used in the recent JNC-V recommendations (6). For both SBP (Table 7) and DBP (Table 8) strong graded associations with risk of CHD death are evident. Similar graded relationships have been reported in several other cohorts (38–41).

The importance of SBP as compared to DBP for risk of CHD death is indicated by the data in Tables 7 and 8 and Fig. 2. For example, adjusted relative risk estimates for each of the categories of SBP in Table 7 are higher than the corresponding DBP categories in Table 8, indicating a steeper risk gradient for SBP than DBP with use of these JNC-V cut points. For those with SBP 140 to 159 mm Hg (stage 1 hypertension), the risk of CHD death is 2.45 times greater than the risk of CHD death for those with SBP < 120 mm Hg (optimal). For those with stage 1 BP using DBP (90–99 mm Hg), the corresponding relative risk is 1.84.

Figure 2 gives adjusted relative risk estimates for deciles of SBP and DBP. For each decile relative risks for SBP are higher than for DBP. For SBP the relative risk of CHD death is 3.8 times greater for men in the highest

decile (151 mm Hg or greater) compared with men in the lowest decile (less than 112 mm Hg). For DBP the relative risk for the highest decile (98 mm Hg or higher) compared with the lowest decile (less than 71 mm Hg) is 2.9. These data also clearly demonstrate that there is no evidence for a threshold level below which DBP and SBP are not associated with a lower risk of CHD death. An overview of nine prospective studies, of which MRFIT was one, came to the same conclusion (42). For SBP, risk of CHD death was significantly higher in each decile relative to the lowest. For men with SBP in the second decile (112–117 mm Hg), the adjusted relative risk was 1.19 (95 percent CI: 1.06 to 1.35). For DBP, rates for the lower two deciles (<71 versus 71–75 mm Hg) did not differ significantly (relative risk = 1.03; 95 percent CI: 0.92 to 1.14); however, for men with DBP in the third decile (76–78 mm Hg), the adjusted relative risk was 1.18 (95 percent CI: 1.06 to 1.31). Separate analyses were performed by 5-year age groups (35–39, 40–44, 45–49, and 50–54 years, and for 55–57 years). In no age group was there evidence of a "J-shaped" relationship (data not shown). For men aged 55 to 57 years, a group in which one might expect to see more preexisting coronary dis-

TABLE 8. *Association of diastolic blood pressure and CHD mortality: men screened for MRFIT*

Diastolic BP (mm Hg)[a]	No. men	No. CHD deaths	Age-adjusted[b] rate per 10,000 person-years	Adjusted relative risk[c] (95% CI)
<80	117,278	2,404	14.4	1.00 (reference group)
80–84	78,197	2,056	17.6	1.21 (1.14 to 1.28)
85–89	57,403	1,916	21.9	1.48 (1.39 to 1.57)
90–99	70,067	3,017	27.4	1.84 (1.74 to 1.94)
100–109	19,164	1,207	39.8	2.56 (2.38 to 2.74)
110–119	4,468	381	53.8	3.45 (3.09 to 3.84)
≥120	1,401	168	82.0	5.17 (4.42 to 6.05)
Total	347,978	11,149		

[a] Classification of BP is according to Fifth Joint National Committee Report.
[b] Adjusted using the direct method for the age distribution of all men screened.
[c] Estimated using proportional hazards regression model stratified by clinic and adjusted for age, race, income, serum cholesterol level, reported cigarettes per day, and use of medication for diabetes.

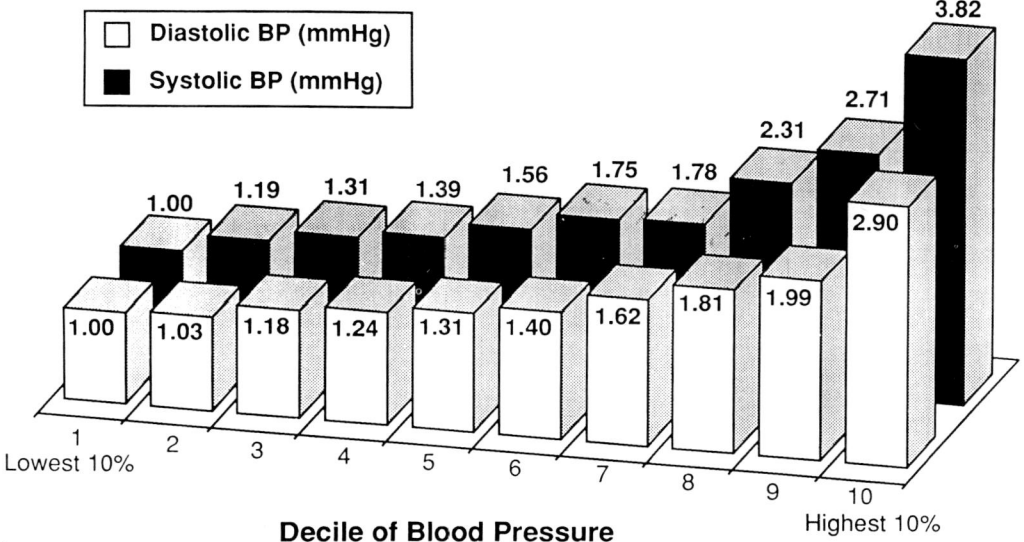

FIG. 2. Relative risk of CHD death for deciles of SBP and DBP. Men screened for MRFIT. SBP deciles are defined by the following cutpoints: <112, 112–117, 118–120, 121–124, 125–128, 129–131, 132–136, 137–141, 142–150, ≥151. DBP deciles are defined by the following: <71, 71–75, 76–78, 78–80, 81–83, 84–85, 86–88, 89–91, ≥98.

ease, risk estimates for the second, third, and fourth deciles relative to the first were 1.12, 1.17, and 1.17 for SBP and 1.06, 1.15, and 1.09 for DBP. None of these estimates differed significantly from 1.

Thus, these data offer minimal support for the "J-shaped" hypothesis (43–45) or for a threshold level for DBP as inferred from some analyses of Framingham data in persons without a history of CVD (46). Whether a threshold level exists for treated blood pressure levels requires further study. Two recent studies do not offer strong experimental support for a threshold level for treated pressure. In SHEP (3), participants were older men and women with isolated systolic hypertension. SBP and DBP averaged 170 and 76 mm Hg at entry. Rates of CHD, stroke, and CVD events were significantly lower with drug treatment as compared with placebo. After 5 years of treatment, those given drug treatment had average SBP and DBP of 144 and 68 mm Hg as compared with 155 and 71 mm Hg for those in the placebo group. In the Treatment of Mild Hypertension Study (TOMHS) (47), CVD incidence was lower in men and women with mild hypertension who were treated with antihypertensive drugs plus nutritional-hygienic intervention compared with those given nutritional-hygienic intervention alone, unless DBP increased to 95 mm Hg or above. Among the participants given drug treatment as well as nutritional advice, SBP and DBP averaged 124 and 78 mm Hg, respectively, after 4 years. Average levels for those initially assigned to nutrition treatment alone were 133 and 82 mm Hg. Thus, aggressive treatment of BP as used in TOMHS and SHEP did not appear to confer harm. Both of these studies ex-

cluded persons with a history or signs of major CVD or other diseases; therefore, the findings may not be generalizable to such persons.

Since the relationship of SBP and DBP varies with age and since previous reports on the men in both this cohort (8–10) and other cohorts (38,48,49) have indicated that the relative importance of SBP and DBP on risk of CHD may vary by age, age-specific summary data are given in Tables 9 and 10. The second column in these tables gives the proportional hazards regression coefficient corresponding to continuous SBP or DBP. With this regression coefficient one can estimate the difference in risk of CHD death associated with a specific difference in SBP or DBP. For example, for men aged 35 to 39 years, the coefficient for SBP is .0232. The relative risk associated with a 10 mm Hg difference in SBP is obtained by multiplying this regression coefficient by 10 and exponentiating the result, e.g., $\exp(.0232 \times 10) = 1.26$. Thus, men in this age-group with a SBP of 150 mm Hg are estimated to have a 26 percent higher risk of CHD death than men with an SBP of 140 mm Hg (150 − 140 = 10 mm Hg difference in SBP). One important assumption of use of this proportional hazards model with a linear term for SBP is that the same difference in risk would be estimated between two persons in this age group with SBPs of 180 and 170 mm Hg (10 mm Hg difference). Another important assumption is that the difference in risk is similar over the entire period of follow-up (16 years); this has been previously examined (9) and appears to be a reasonable assumption.

Even if these assumptions are met (and this appears to be the case with these data), the associations between

TABLE 9. *Association of systolic BP and CHD mortality by age: men screened for MRFIT*

Age (years)	Proportional hazards regression coefficient (SE)[a]	Relative risk[a]—highest to lowest decile (95% CI)	Excess risk: difference (%) in 15-year cumulative CHD mortality[b]—highest decile minus lowest decile (SE)
35–39	.0232 (.0022)	3.44 (2.39 to 4.95)	2.3 (.29)
40–44	.0257 (.0014)	4.74 (3.68 to 6.12)	4.0 (.33)
45–49	.0234 (.0010)	3.79 (3.11 to 4.60)	5.3 (.32)
50–54	.0208 (.0008)	3.86 (3.21 to 4.63)	7.1 (.34)
55–57	.0214 (.0010)	3.40 (2.70 to 4.28)	8.9 (.56)
All ages	.0222 (.0005)	3.82 (3.46 to 4.23)	6.5 (.16)

[a] Estimated using proportional hazards regression model stratified by clinic and adjusted for age, race, income, serum cholesterol level, reported cigarettes per day, and use of medication for diabetes.
[b] Estimated by the Kaplan-Meier method.

SBP and DBP with CHD death are underestimated because of measurement error and temporal variability associated with using BP measurements from only a single visit (42,50). Estimates of the reliability of SBP (0.67) and DBP (0.62) measurements on a subset of this cohort indicate that the regression coefficient for SBP should be multiplied by 1.5 and that for DBP by 1.6 before exponentiating in order to obtain the "true" difference in risk associated with a specific BP difference. Thus, a better estimate of the difference in risk associated with a 10 mm Hg difference in SBP is exp (.0232 × 1.5 × 10) = 1.42, i.e., risk of CHD death is 42 percent higher for a person with 150 as compared with 140 mm Hg.

The third column in Tables 9 and 10 gives the relative risk for the highest decile of BP compared with the lowest, e.g., 151+ versus <112 mm Hg for SBP and 98+ versus <71 mm Hg for DBP. The last column gives excess risk estimates for the highest versus lowest deciles, i.e., the difference in 15-year cumulative CHD mortality from the life table. Regression coefficients and adjusted relative risk estimates (highest to lowest decile) for SBP do not differ very much over this age range. Excess risk increases with age (see Table 9). For DBP, regression coefficients and adjusted relative risk estimates tend to decline with age, while differences in 15-year cumulative CHD mortality increase (Table 10). Relative risk estimates associated with being in the highest decile of BP are greater for SBP than DBP in each age group except the youngest. For men 35 to 39 years, the relative risk (highest vs. lowest decile) is slightly greater for DBP (3.5)

than SBP (3.4). Excess risk estimates are greater for SBP than DBP in each age group. The magnitude of the difference increases with age.

Data from Framingham also suggest a declining relative importance of DBP as compared to SBP with advancing age (38). In that report DBP was a stronger predictor of CHD in persons less than 45 years and SBP was the better predictor in men and women aged 55 and older. Tverdal (48) also found that DBP was more important than SBP in younger men. In a cohort of over 39,000 men he reported that death rates for men 35 to 39 years were greater for those in the upper quintile of DBP as compared to SBP. For men 45 to 49 years, rates were almost identical. Findings were intermediate for those 40 to 44 years. Rosenman et al. (49) reported that SBP was a better predictor of CHD in men 39 to 49 years than DBP and that the two BP measures had similar predictive value in men 50 to 59 years. Each of the above studies had substantially fewer events than the MRFIT cohort.

The joint effect of SBP and DBP on death due to CHD is illustrated in Fig. 3. Men with stage 3 and stage 4 levels of DBP and SBP have been combined because numbers were small. Within each of the JNC-V categories of SBP, differences in age-adjusted CHD rates for DBP categories are modest. A strong risk gradient, however, is evident for SBP within each DBP category. For example, among men with stage 2 hypertension as defined by an elevated SBP (140–159 mm Hg), CHD death rates range from 28.9 to 44.5 per 10,000 person years, rates much higher

TABLE 10. *Association of diastolic BP and CHD mortality by age: men screened for MRFIT*

Age (years)	Proportional hazards regression coefficient (SE)[a]	Relative risk[a]—highest to lowest decile (95% CI)	Excess risk: difference (%) in 15-year cumulative CHD mortality[b]—highest decile minus lowest decile (SE)
35–39	.0355 (.0032)	3.55 (2.57 to 4.90)	2.0 (.25)
40–44	.0394 (.0022)	3.82 (2.99 to 4.87)	3.2 (.28)
45–49	.0311 (.0017)	3.13 (2.57 to 3.82)	4.0 (.30)
50–54	.0283 (.0014)	2.55 (2.19 to 2.97)	5.2 (.37)
55–57	.0263 (.0018)	2.47 (2.03 to 3.00)	6.4 (.64)
All ages	.0308 (.0008)	2.90 (2.65 to 3.18)	4.6 (.15)

[a] Estimated using proportional hazards regression model stratified by clinic and adjusted for age, race, income, serum cholesterol level, reported cigarettes per day, and use of medication for diabetes.
[b] Estimated by the Kaplan-Meier method.

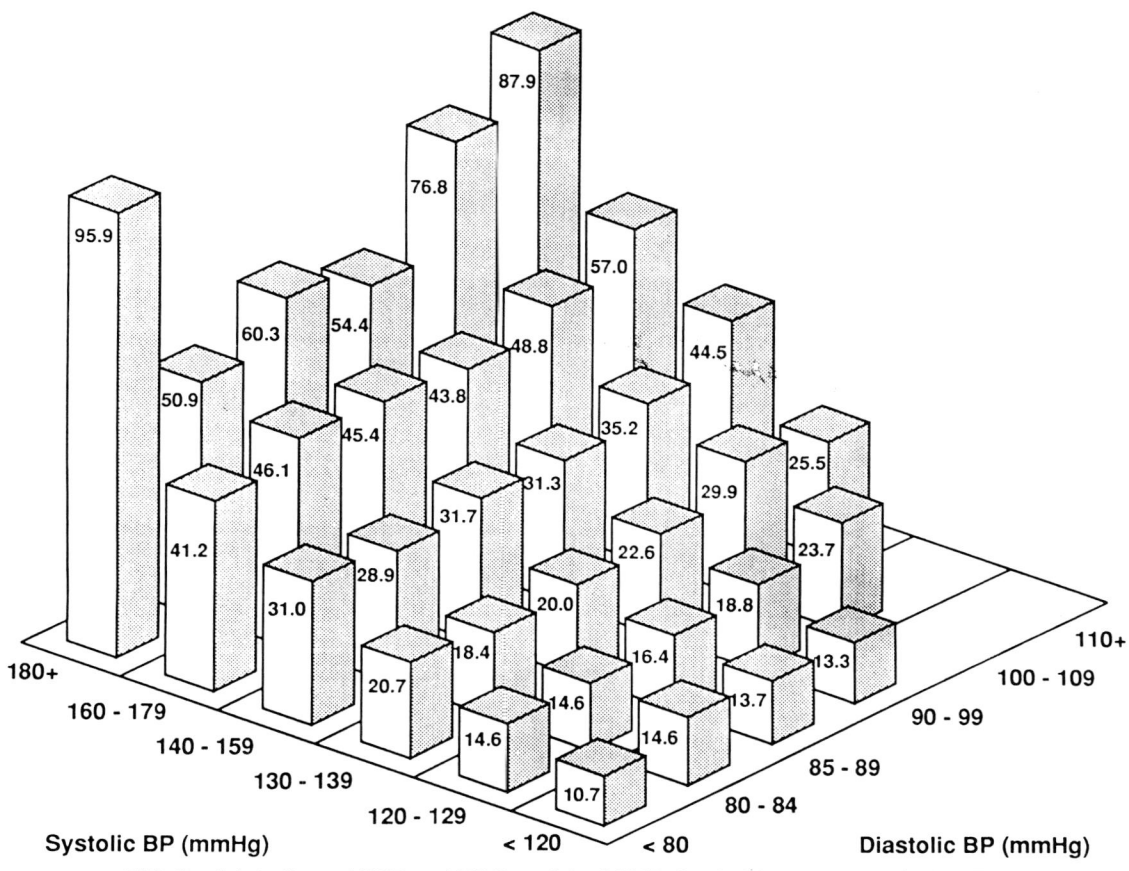

FIG. 3. Joint effect of SBP and DBP on risk of CHD death. Men screened for MRFIT.

than for men with optimal SBP (irrespective of DBP). Similarly, for the subgroup with stage 1 hypertension defined by DBP (90–99 mm Hg), age-adjusted rates for SBP categories range from 13.3 to 54.4 deaths per 10,000 person-years. Those who have stage 1 hypertension defined by SBP have a CHD death rate (31.3) substantially higher than that for those with high normal (22.6), normal but not optimal (18.8), or optimal (13.3) SBP.

If risk were based only on DBP and not on SBP, many participants at high risk of CHD death would not be identified. For example, in the 85 to 89 mm Hg stratum of DBP, each of the four strata of participants defined by SBP 130 mm Hg or above has a CHD death rate higher than the average rate for those in the 90 to 99 mm Hg stratum of DBP and with SBP < 130 mm Hg (18.2) (Fig. 3). The number of men in these strata represent 9.4 percent of those screened (Table 3). In each of the two strata with DBP less than 85 mm Hg there are also four SBP groups with an age-adjusted CHD death rate greater than 18.2 per 10,000 person-years. The number of men in the eight groups with SBP > 130 mm Hg and DBP < 85 mm Hg represent 13.5 percent of those screened (see Table 4).

The increased death rates for men in these two lower strata of DBP (<85 and 85–89 mm Hg) with SBP of 160

mm Hg or higher affirm that isolated systolic hypertension is an important predictor of mortality, as has been previously reported in this (12) and other cohorts (25,48,51–53). These data also indicate that this is not a rare condition, not only in older but also in middle-aged men and women (Tables 4 and 6).

Among men screened for MRFIT the association of SBP and DBP with risk of CHD death was similar for whites, blacks, Orientals, and Hispanics (Table 11). For each of these race/ethnic groups, CHD death rates increased in a graded way with increasing levels of SBP and DBP. Those with optimal BP levels had CHD death rates one-half to one-third of those with stage 1 hypertension, the predominant level of hypertension in each ethnic group. Their CHD death rates were also consistently lower than those for men with high-normal BP.

A strong, significant, graded association of hypertension with risk of CHD death was evident among those with and without diabetes (Table 12). As previously reported (14), risk ratios were smaller for those with diabetes as compared to those without diabetes, but absolute excess risk was greater. For example, the ratio of age-adjusted rates for those with stage 1 hypertension compared to those with optimal BP was 1.72 for men with diabetes and 2.57 for those without diabetes. Excess risk

TABLE 11. *Baseline blood pressure and CHD mortality by race/ethnicity: men screened for MRFIT*

	Race/ethnicity											
	White			Black			Hispanic			Oriental		
BP category[a]	Total	No. CHD deaths	Age-adjusted rate[b]	Total	No. CHD deaths	Age-adjusted rate	Total	No. CHD deaths	Age-adjusted rate	Total	No. CHD deaths	Age-adjusted rate
Optimal	57,833	875	10.7	2,928	43	11.3	1,251	9	6.0	972	9	6.9
Normal but not optimal	77,652	1632	14.6	4,549	102	17.0	1,567	24	11.6	1,049	11	8.1
High normal	70,022	1957	18.5	4,644	132	20.2	1,380	30	16.9	866	11	8.9
Hypertension												
Stage 1	80,412	3582	27.7	6,502	254	26.4	1,688	51	20.9	974	30	23.8
Stage 2	21,287	1455	41.4	2,574	122	31.3	487	22	29.5	300	13	25.7
Stage 3	4,702	464	58.3	883	72	54.3	101	7	49.7	77	4	28.1
Stage 4	1,085	147	88.2	391	41	76.9	37	2	60.2	19	0	0.0
Proportional hazards regression coefficient (SE)[c]												
SBP (mm Hg)	.0223 (.0005)			.0203 (.0016)			.0246 (.0044)			.0220 (.0056)		
DBP (mm Hg)	.0314 (.0009)			.0273 (.0027)			.0255 (.0074)			.0223 (.0101)		

[a] Classification of BP is according to Fifth Joint National Committee Report.
[b] Adjusted using the direct method for the age distribution of all men screened.
[c] Estimated using proportional hazards regression model stratified by clinic and adjusted for age, income, serum cholesterol level, reported cigarettes per day, and use of medication for diabetes; estimates for SBP and DBP are from separate models.

associated with stage 1 hypertension was 38.8 deaths per 10,000 person years for men with diabetes and 16.0 for those without diabetes. The magnitude of excess risk estimates for those with diabetes emphasizes the importance of vigorous risk factor control in these high-risk men.

SBP AND DBP AND RISK OF DEATH FROM STROKE

The presentation of data on the separate and joint association of SBP and DBP with death from stroke paral-

lels that for CHD. For JNC-V BP categories, Table 13 gives age-adjusted rates per 10,000 person years, adjusted relative risk estimates, and life-table estimates of cumulative percent of men dying from stroke. The strong risk gradient evident in Table 13 is also seen when SBP and DBP are considered separately (Tables 14 and 15). These risk gradients were found for both hemorrhagic and nonhemorrhagic stroke (11). These results are consistent with other large bodies of observational data (26,42,54–58). An overview of observational studies indicated that the BP and stroke risk gradient was much steeper than the BP and CHD risk gradient. Since CHD rates are much higher in the United States population,

TABLE 12. *Baseline blood pressure and CHD mortality by diabetes: men screened for MRFIT*

	Diabetes			No diabetes		
BP category[a]	Total	No. CHD deaths	Age-adjusted rate[b]	Total	No. CHD deaths	Age-adjusted rate
Optimal	552	49	53.7	62,819	893	10.2
Normal but not optimal	912	92	62.7	84,361	1,682	14.0
High normal	1,077	108	59.9	76,171	2,032	17.8
Hypertension						
Stage 1	1,673	259	92.5	88,342	3,675	26.2
Stage 2	672	130	122.2	24,072	1,488	37.8
Stage 3	215	48	124.1	5,568	502	54.7
Stage 4	62	13	161.6	1,482	178	80.8
Proportional hazards regression coefficient (SE)[c]						
SBP (mm Hg)	0.0166 (.0018)			.0224 (.0005)		
DBP (mm Hg)	0.0179 (.0032)			.0316 (.0009)		

[a] Classification of BP is according to Fifth Joint National Committee Report.
[b] Adjusted using the direct method for the age distribution of all men screened.
[c] Estimated using proportional hazards regression model stratified by clinic and adjusted for age, race, income, serum cholesterol level, and reported cigarettes per day; estimates for SBP and DBP are from separate models.

TABLE 13. *Baseline blood pressure and stroke mortality: men screened for MRFIT*

BP category[a]	No. men	No. stroke deaths	Age-adjusted rate per 10,000 person-years[b]	Adjusted relative risk[c]	Cumulative percent dying from stroke[d]		
					5 years	10 years	15 years
Optimal	63,371	71	0.8	1.00	.02	.04	.10
Normal but not optimal	85,273	173	1.4	1.73*	.03	.08	.19
High normal	77,248	208	1.8	2.14*	.04	.11	.24
Hypertension							
Stage 1 (mild)	90,015	435	3.0	3.58*	.08	.22	.45
Stage 2 (moderate)	24,744	215	5.3	5.90*	.13	.40	.83
Stage 3 (severe)	5,783	87	9.8	9.66*	.37	.82	1.57
Stage 4 (very severe)	1,544	44	19.0	19.19*	1.06	2.06	3.05

[a] Classification of BP is according to Fifth Joint National Committee Report.
[b] Adjusted using the direct method for the age distribution of all men screened.
[c] Estimated using proportional hazards regression model for stratified by clinic and adjusted for age, race, income, serum cholesterol level, reported cigarettes per day, and use of medication for diabetes.
[d] Estimated by the Kaplan-Meier method.
* $p < .0001$.

TABLE 14. *Association of systolic blood pressure and stroke mortality: men screened for MRFIT*

Systolic BP (mm Hg)[a]	No. men	No. stroke deaths	Age-adjusted[b] rate per 10,000 person-years	Adjusted relative risk[c] (95% CI)
<120	87,459	110	0.9	1.00 (reference group)
120–129	98,834	221	1.6	1.68 (1.34 to 2.11)
130–139	79,308	266	2.2	2.33 (1.87 to 2.92)
140–159	65,865	400	3.7	3.78 (3.05 to 4.69)
160–179	13,321	161	7.2	6.57 (5.13 to 8.41)
180–209	2,863	61	13.2	10.70 (7.77 to 14.72)
≥210	328	14	29.1	24.34 (13.90 to 42.61)
Total	347,978	1,233		

[a] Classification of BP is according to Fifth Joint National Committee Report.
[b] Adjusted using the direct method for the age distribution of all men screened.
[c] Estimated using proportional hazards regression model stratified by clinic and adjusted for age, race, income, serum cholesterol level, reported cigarettes per day, and use of medication for diabetes.

TABLE 15. *Association of diastolic blood pressure and stroke mortality: men screened for MRFIT*

Diastolic BP (mm Hg)[a]	No. men	No. stroke deaths	Age-adjusted[b] rate per 10,000 person-years	Adjusted relative risk[c] (95% CI)
<80	117,278	210	1.3	1.00 (reference group)
80–84	78,197	209	1.8	1.44 (1.19 to 1.75)
85–89	57,403	194	2.2	1.76 (1.45 to 2.15)
90–99	70,067	355	3.2	2.54 (2.14 to 3.02)
100–109	19,164	162	5.3	4.00 (3.25 to 4.93)
110–119	4,468	63	9.3	6.31 (4.74 to 8.39)
≥120	1,401	40	19.2	12.57 (8.91 to 17.74)
Total	347,978	1,233		

[a] Classification of BP is according to Fifth Joint National Committee Report.
[b] Adjusted using the direct method for the age distribution of all men screened.
[c] Estimated using proportional hazards regression model stratified by clinic and adjusted for age, race, income, serum cholesterol level, reported cigarettes per day, and use of medication for diabetes.

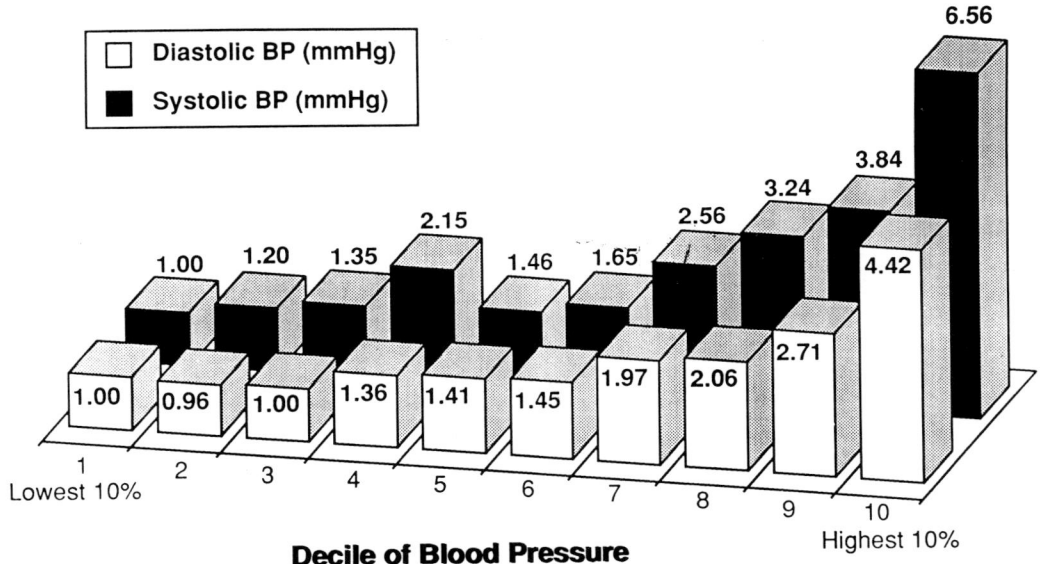

FIG. 4. Relative risk of death from stroke for deciles of SBP and DBP. Men screened for MRFIT. SBP deciles are defined by the following cutpoints: <112, 112–117, 118–120, 121–124, 125–128, 129–131, 132–136, 137–141, 142–150, ≥151. DBP deciles are defined by the following: <71, 71–75, 76–78, 79–80, 81–83, 84–85, 86–88, 89–91, 92–97, ≥98.

absolute excess risk estimates associated with elevated BP are greater for CHD than for stroke.

Like the findings for CHD death, those for death from stroke also indicate a more pronounced risk gradient for SBP than DBP. This is indicated by comparison of relative risk estimates in the last columns of Tables 14 and 15, and by inspection of Fig. 4, which gives relative risk estimates of death from stroke for SBP and DBP deciles. For example, from Fig. 4 the relative risk of death from stroke is 6.6 times greater for men in the highest decile of SBP (151 mm Hg or greater) compared with men in the lowest decile (less than 112 mm Hg). For DBP the relative risk for the highest decile (98 mm Hg or higher) compared with the lowest decile (less than 71 mm Hg) is 4.4.

Also like CHD, age-specific results for death from stroke in Tables 16 and 17 indicate (a) greater differences across age groups in regression coefficients and relative risk estimates for DBP than SBP, (b) higher relative risk estimates for SBP compared with DBP except in the 35 to 39 and 45 to 49 year age groups, and (c) higher absolute excess risk estimates for SBP compared with DBP in all but the youngest age group.

Figure 5 plots the joint effect of SBP and DBP on age-adjusted death rates from stroke. Men with stage 2, 3, or 4 levels of DBP (100–109, 110–119, and 120+ mm Hg) and SBP (160–179, 180–209, and 210+ mm Hg) have been combined since numbers were small. Likewise, men with optimal and with normal but not optimal SBP and DBP have been combined because of the small number of deaths from stroke in these strata. For each category of DBP a strong risk gradient with SBP is evident. Among men with stage 1 hypertension defined by DBP (90–99 mm Hg), age-adjusted death rates from stroke ranged from 1.9 for those with SBP less than 130 mm Hg to 5.6 per 10,000 person-years for those with SBP 160 mm Hg or higher. For those with stage 2 or higher hyper-

TABLE 16. *Association of systolic BP and stroke mortality by age: men screened for MRFIT*

Age (years)	Proportional hazards regression coefficient (SE)[a]	Relative risk[a]—highest to lowest decile (95% CI)	Excess risk: difference (%) in 15-year cumulative stroke mortality[b]—highest decile minus lowest decile (SE)
35–39	.0358 (.0053)	10.5 (2.99 to 36.92)	0.4 (.12)
40–44	.0310 (.0040)	8.20 (3.41 to 19.70)	0.6 (.12)
45–49	.0340 (.0025)	5.59 (3.16 to 9.91)	0.9 (.12)
50–54	.0287 (.0021)	6.20 (3.42 to 11.23)	1.1 (.12)
55–57	.0269 (.0027)	8.65 (3.17 to 23.56)	1.5 (.19)
All ages	.0301 (.0013)	6.56 (4.70 to 9.16)	1.0 (.06)

[a] Estimated using proportional hazards regression model stratified by clinic and adjusted for age, race, income, serum cholesterol level, reported cigarettes per day, and use of medication for diabetes.
[b] Estimated by the Kaplan-Meier method.

TABLE 17. *Association of diastolic BP and stroke mortality by age: men screened for MRFIT*

Age (years)	Proportional hazards regression coefficient (SE)[a]	Relative risk[a]— highest to lowest decile (95% CI)	Excess risk: difference (%) in 15-year cumulative stroke mortality[b]—highest decile minus lowest decile (SE)
35–39	.0580 (.0074)	11.91 (4.07 to 34.84)	0.5 (.11)
40–44	.0473 (.0063)	4.25 (2.03 to 8.89)	0.4 (.09)
45–49	.0503 (.0046)	6.07 (3.12 to 11.80)	0.7 (.11)
50–54	.0460 (.0038)	4.01 (2.48 to 6.48)	0.9 (.13)
55–57	.0361 (.0050)	2.90 (1.64 to 5.13)	0.9 (.24)
All ages	.0458 (.0022)	4.42 (3.33 to 5.87)	0.7 (.06)

[a] Estimated using proportional hazards regression model stratified by clinic and adjusted for age, race, income, serum cholesterol level, reported cigarettes per day, and use of medication for diabetes.
[b] Estimated by the Kaplan-Meier method.

tension based on DBP (100+ mm Hg), death rates from stroke ranged from 2.7 to 10.2 per 10,000 person-years for the four SBP groupings. For specific levels of SBP there were no substantial differences in death rates according to level of DBP.

The association of blood pressure with death from stroke is presented for four ethnic groups in Table 18. The graded association of blood pressure with death from stroke was similar for the four groups. Among whites and blacks, where numbers are larger, death rates from stroke are higher for blacks than whites at each level of blood pressure.

Among men both with and without diabetes, a strong, significant association of blood pressure with death from stroke was observed (Table 19). As for CHD, relative risk

estimates were smaller and excess risk estimates were greater from those with diabetes as compared to those without diabetes.

SBP AND DBP AND RISK OF DEATH FROM ANY CAUSE

Even if blood pressure were unrelated to risk of non-cardiovascular death, a strong association of blood pressure with all-cause mortality among adults in the United States would be expected since a large fraction of deaths are due to cardiovascular causes. Table 20 summarizes the association of blood pressure and all-cause mortality. Men in each blood pressure category above optimal have

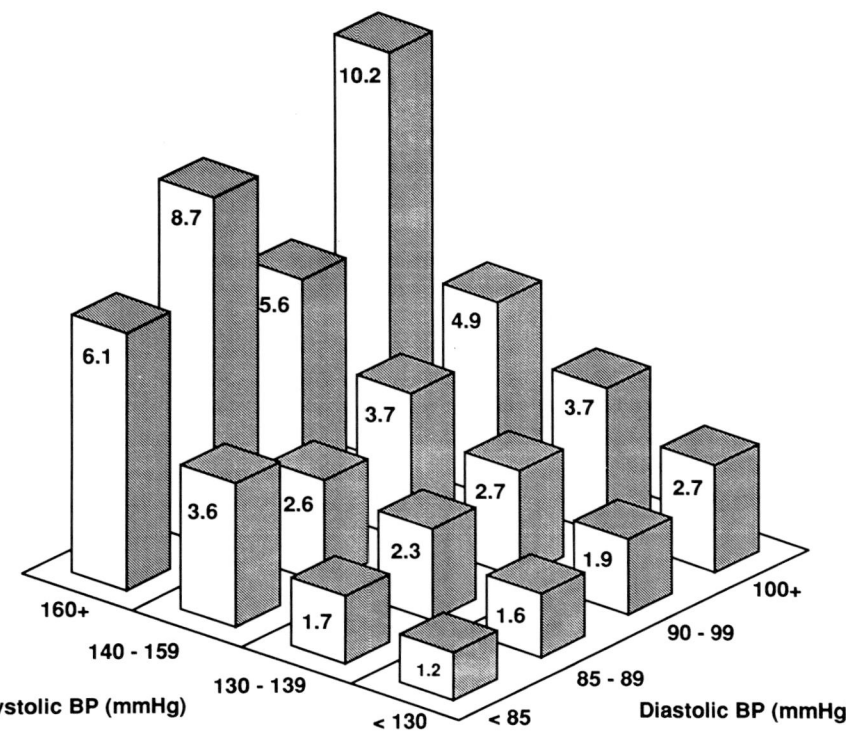

FIG. 5. Joint effect of SBP and DBP on risk of death from stroke. Men screened for MRFIT.

TABLE 18. *Baseline blood pressure and stroke mortality by race/ethnicity: men screened for MRFIT*

	Race/ethnicity											
	White			Black			Hispanic			Oriental		
BP category[a]	Total	No. stroke deaths	Age-adjusted rate[b]	Total	No. stroke deaths	Age-adjusted rate	Total	No. stroke deaths	Age-adjusted rate	Total	No. stroke deaths	Age-adjusted rate
Optimal	57,833	51	0.6	2,928	15	4.2	1,251	2	1.5	972	3	2.9
Normal but not optimal	77,652	150	1.3	4,549	17	2.7	1,567	2	0.9	1,049	3	1.8
High normal	70,022	178	1.7	4,644	23	3.6	1,380	3	1.4	866	3	2.7
Hypertension												
Stage 1	80,412	373	2.9	6,502	42	4.4	1,688	14	5.6	974	5	3.5
Stage 2	21,287	174	4.9	2,574	33	8.6	487	6	7.8	300	1	1.7
Stage 3	4,702	59	7.7	883	24	19.5	101	3	19.0	77	1	6.5
Stage 4	1,085	26	15.4	391	16	29.4	37	1	23.9	19	1	20.0
Proportional hazards regression coefficient (SE)[c]												
SBP (mm Hg)	.0309 (.0014)			.0253 (.0032)			.0398 (.0080)			.0154 (.0126)		
DBP (mm Hg)	.0454 (.0026)			.0428 (.0051)			.0773 (.0129)			.0379 (.0208)		

[a] Classification of BP is according to Fifth Joint National Committee Report.
[b] Adjusted using the direct method for the age distribution of all men screened.
[c] Estimated using proportional hazards regression model stratified by clinic and adjusted for age, income, serum cholesterol level, reported cigarettes per day, and use of medication for diabetes; estimates for SBP and DBP are from separate models.

significantly increased death rates. These rates increase in a graded fashion with higher blood pressure from 49.3 deaths per 10,000 person years for those with optimal blood pressure to 213.7 for those with stage 4 hypertension. Similar findings are available for women (10).

Figure 6 summarizes the joint association of SBP and DBP with death from any cause. The age-adjusted rate for those with SBP < 120 and DBP < 80 mm Hg (optimal levels) was 49.3 per 10,000 person-years; for hypertensive men with both elevated SBP and DBP, rates ranged from 86.2 to 218.7.

SBP AND DBP AND RISK OF DEATH AMONG MEN WITH A HISTORY OF MYOCARDIAL INFARCTION

Preceding analyses were based on the large number of men screened for MRFIT who had not had a prior myocardial infarction at the time of screening. Table 21 describes the association of blood pressure and all-cause mortality for the 5,362 men who reported a history of a myocardial infarction. Approximately 62 percent of all deaths in this cohort were attributed to CHD and 3 per-

TABLE 19. *Baseline blood pressure and stroke mortality by diabetes: men screened for MRFIT*

	Diabetes			No diabetes		
BP category[a]	Total	No. stroke deaths	Age-adjusted rate[b]	Total	No. stroke deaths	Age-adjusted rate
Optimal	552	1	0.9	62,819	70	0.8
Normal but not optimal	912	9	6.0	84,361	164	1.3
High normal	1,077	17	8.1	76,171	191	1.7
Hypertension						
Stage 1	1,673	26	8.8	88,342	409	2.9
Stage 2	672	14	17.0	24,072	201	5.1
Stage 3	215	10	21.2	5,568	77	9.1
Stage 4	62	1	28.9	1,482	43	18.8
Proportional hazards regression coefficient (SE)[c]						
SBP (mm Hg)	0.0246 (.0050)			0.0303 (.0013)		
DBP (mm Hg)	0.0237 (.0094)			0.0471 (.0023)		

[a] Classification of BP is according to Fifth Joint National Committee Report.
[b] Adjusted using the direct method for the age distribution of all men screened.
[c] Estimated using proportional hazards regression model stratified by clinic and adjusted for age, race, income, serum cholesterol level, and reported cigarettes per day; estimates for SBP and DBP are from separate models.

TABLE 20. *Baseline blood pressure and all-cause mortality: men screened for MRFIT*

BP category[a]	No. men	No. deaths	Age-adjusted rate per 10,000 person-years[b]	Adjusted relative risk[c]	Cumulative percent dying[d]		
					5 years	10 years	15 years
Optimal	63,371	4,354	49.3	1.00	1.1	3.0	6.1
Normal but not optimal	85,273	6,822	55.9	1.11*	1.2	3.5	7.2
High normal	77,248	7,281	62.9	1.23*	1.4	4.2	8.4
Hypertension							
Stage 1 (mild)	90,015	11,469	80.1	1.55*	1.9	5.7	11.4
Stage 2 (moderate)	24,744	4,431	108.9	2.04*	2.8	8.3	16.2
Stage 3 (severe)	5,783	1,447	153.0	2.77*	4.3	12.0	22.8
Stage 4 (very severe)	1,544	491	213.7	3.83*	5.7	16.5	29.5

[a] Classification of BP is according to Fifth Joint National Committee Report.
[b] Adjusted using the direct method for age distribution of all men screened.
[c] Estimated using proportional hazards regression model stratified by clinic and adjusted for age, race, income, serum cholesterol level, reported cigarettes per day, and use of medication for diabetes.
[d] Estimated by the Kaplan-Meier method.
* $p < .0001$.

cent were attributed to stroke. Death rates did not differ significantly among the lower three blood pressure categories (optimal, normal but not optimal, and high normal). Rates for those with stage 1 hypertension were approximately 18 percent higher than those with optimal pressure; those with stages 2 to 4 hypertension had rates about 60 percent higher than those with optimal pressure. Although relative risk estimates for this cohort were smaller than for men without a history of myocardial infarction (see Table 20), absolute excess risk estimates were much greater. For example, after 15 years about 45 percent of men with stages 2 to 4 hypertension were

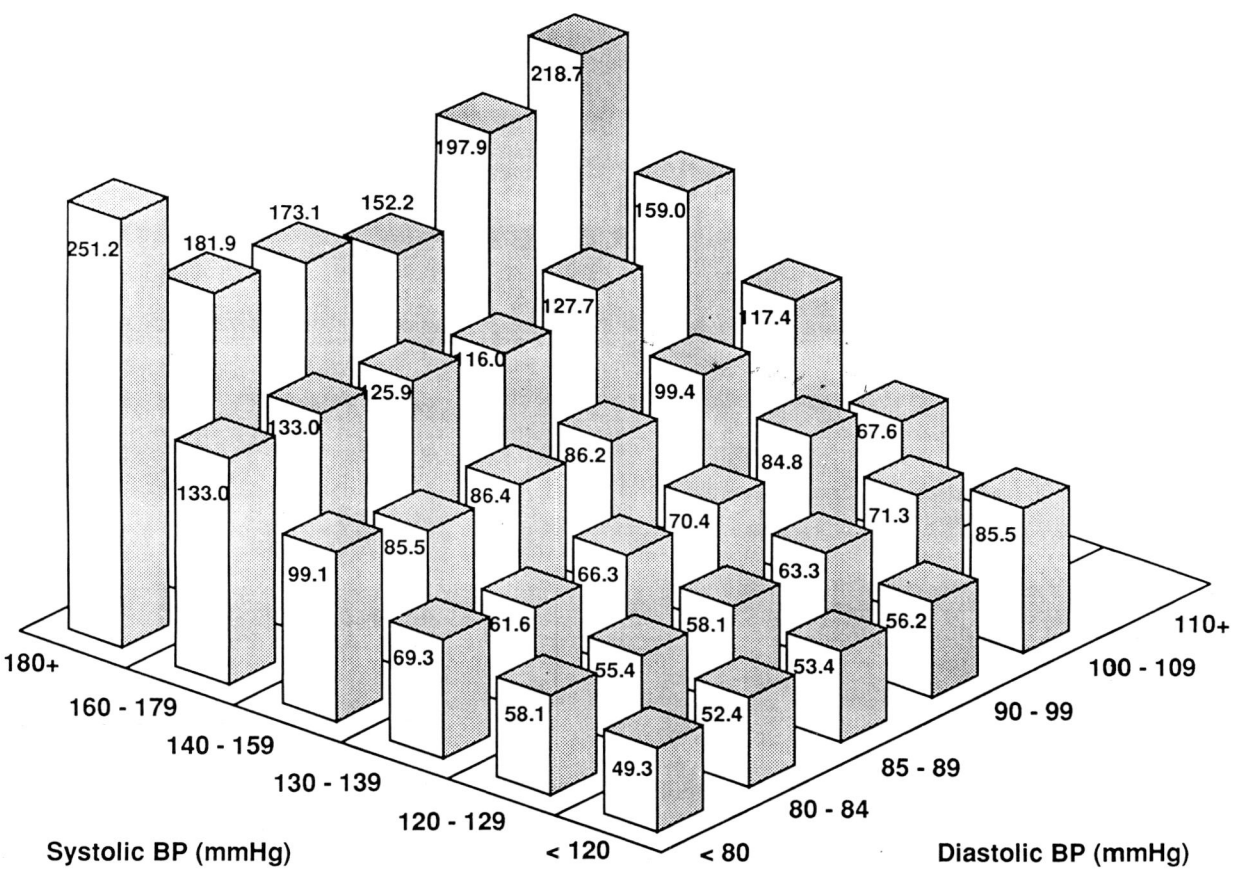

FIG. 6. Joint effect of SBP and DBP on risk of death from any cause. Men screened for MRFIT.

TABLE 21. *Blood pressure and all-cause mortality among men with a history of hospitalization for a myocardial infarction: men screened for MRFIT*

BP category[a]	No. men	No. deaths	Age-adjusted rate per 10,000 person-years[b]	Adjusted relative risk[c]	Cumulative percent dying[d]		
					5 years	10 years	15 years
Optimal	845	277	209.1	1.00	8.5	19.6	31.1
Normal but not optimal	1104	345	203.8	0.92	8.1	18.1	28.9
High normal	1215	423	229.9	1.02	8.4	18.7	32.2
Hypertension							
Stage 1 (mild)	1522	600	267.9	1.18*	9.5	23.0	36.7
Stage 2 (moderate)	505	243	362.7	1.56**	11.9	30.9	46.5
Stage 3 (severe)	133	65	327.2	1.59**	14.3	27.1	46.6
Stage 4 (very severe)	38	17	468.0	1.58	18.4	31.6	44.7
Total	5362	1970					

[a] Classification of BP is according to Fifth Joint National Committee Report.
[b] Adjusted using the direct method for the age distribution of all men screened.
[c] Estimated using proportional hazards regression model stratified by clinic and adjusted for age, race, income, serum cholesterol level, reported cigarettes per day, and use of medication for diabetes.
[d] Estimated by the Kaplan-Meier method.
* $p < .05$.
** $p < .001$.

dead, as compared with 31 percent of those with optimal blood pressure. As noted earlier, further research on the benefit of aggressive blood pressure lowering is needed among persons who have experienced a myocardial infarction. These observational data indicate that the potential for preventing premature deaths is substantial in such persons.

CONCLUSIONS

The data summarized in this chapter indicate:

1. BP elevation is a problem for the majority of middle-aged men and women; a minority have optimal levels.
2. Most persons with hypertension have stage 1 (DBP 90–99 or SBP 140–159 mm Hg).
3. The prevalence of hypertension increases with age in adults largely due to continuing increases in SBP even beyond the age of 50 years.
4. The use of JNC-V criteria, in which both SBP and DBP are considered, results in a higher prevalence of hypertension compared with use of DBP criteria alone.
5. Prevalence of hypertension is higher among blacks than other ethnic groups.
6. Both SBP and DBP are related continuously to risk of death from CHD, stroke, renal disease, and all causes.
7. In all but the youngest age group (35–39 years), SBP is a more important predictor of death from CHD and stroke than DBP.
8. Absolute excess risk of death (predominantly from CHD and stroke) associated with elevated blood pressure is greater among older persons, persons with diabetes, and persons with a history of myocardial infarction.
9. SBP and DBP should be used together to assess a person's risk of CVD since, when used together, a more accurate estimate of risk is obtained than with use of either measure alone.

The heavy burden on society resulting from the high prevalence of high-normal and high BP (hypertension) and their associated morbidity and mortality requires a two-pronged approach to address the problem—an individual-based and a population-based approach (59). With regard to the individual-based or "high-risk" approach, the recent results of TOMHS indicate that low-dose drug treatment, along with vigorous nutritional-hygienic intervention aimed at weight loss, reduced sodium and alcohol intake, and increased physical activity, is an effective strategy for treating stage 1 hypertension (47). Likewise, the results of SHEP (3) and other clinical trials (60) indicate that drug treatment reduces morbidity and mortality from CHD and stroke in persons with isolated systolic hypertension as well as in persons with elevated DBP.

Because the risk of CHD and stroke increases in a continuous manner with SBP and DBP, population-wide efforts to prevent hypertension must accompany efforts to identify and treat hypertensives. This dual approach to "restoration of biological normality" has been advocated by Rose (59) for many diseases. Life-style interventions, e.g., a reduced intake of sodium and alcohol and prevention and control of obesity, to prevent rise of BP with age during adulthood and to lower the mean level of BP in the population may reduce the need for lifelong drug treatment and substantially decrease current morbidity and mortality associated with high BP (61–64).

REFERENCES

1. Rutan GH, McDonald RH, Kuller LH. A historical perspective of elevated systolic vs. diastolic blood pressure from an epidemiological and clinical trial viewpoint. *J Clin Epidemiol* 1989;42:663–673.
2. Bulpitt CJ. Is systolic pressure more important than diastolic pressure? *J Hum Hypertens* 1990;4:471–476.
3. SHEP Cooperative Research Group. Prevention of stroke by antihypertensive drug treatment in older persons with isolated systolic hypertension. Final results of the Systolic Hypertension in the Elderly Program (SHEP). *JAMA* 1991;265:3255–3264.
4. Amery A, Birkenhager W, Bulpitt CJ, et al. (Syst.-Eur.) A multicentre trial on the treatment of isolated systolic hypertension in the elderly: objectives, protocol and organization. *Aging* 1991;3:287–302.
5. Systolic Hypertension in the Elderly's Collaborative Group Coordinating Centre. Systolic hypertension in the elderly: Chinese trial (Syst.-China), interim report (in Chinese with English summary). *Chin J Cardiol* 1992;20:270–275.
6. 1993 Joint National Committee. The 5th Report of the Joint National Committee on the Detection, Evaluation, and Treatment of High Blood Pressure (JNC V). *Arch Intern Med* 1993;153:154–183.
7. Neaton JD, Kuller LH, Wentworth D, Borhani NO. Total and cardiovascular mortality in relation to cigarette smoking, serum cholesterol concentration, and diastolic blood pressure among black and white males follow for up to five years. *Am Heart J* 1984;108:759–770.
8. Stamler J, Neaton JD, Wentworth DN. Blood pressure (systolic and diastolic) and risk of fatal coronary heart disease. *Hypertension* 1989;13(suppl I):2–12.
9. Neaton JD, Wentworth D. Serum cholesterol, blood pressure, cigarette smoking, and death from coronary heart disease. *Arch Intern Med* 1992;152:56–64.
10. Stamler J, Stamler R, Neaton JD. Blood pressure, systolic and diastolic, and cardiovascular risks: U.S. population data. *Arch Intern Med* 1993;153:598–615.
11. Neaton JD, Wentworth DN, Cutler J, Stamler J, Kuller L. Risk factors for death from different types of stroke. *Ann Epidemiol* 1993;3:493–499.
12. Rutan GH, Kuller LN, Neaton JD, Wentworth DN, McDonald RH, Smith WM. Mortality associated with diastolic hypertension and isolated systolic hypertension among men screened for the Multiple Risk Factor Intervention Trial. *Circulation* 1988;77:504–514.
13. Kannel WB, Neaton JD, Wentworth D, Thomas HE, Stamler J, Hulley SB, Kjelsberg MO. Overall and coronary heart disease mortality rates in relation to major risk factors in 325,348 men screened for MRFIT. *Am Heart J* 1986;112:825–836.
14. Stamler J, Vaccaro O, Neaton JD, Wentworth D. Diabetes, other risk factors, and 12-year cardiovascular mortality for men screened in the Multiple Risk Factor Intervention Trial. *Diabetes Care* 1993;16:434–444.
15. Flack JM, Neaton JD, Daniels B, Esunge P. Ethnicity and renal disease: lessons from the Multiple Risk Factor Intervention Trial and the Treatment of Mild Hypertension Study. *Am J Kidney Dis* 1993;21(suppl):31–40.
16. Multiple Risk Factor Intervention Trial Research Group. Statistical design considerations in the NHLI Multiple Risk Factor Intervention Trial. *J Chronic Dis* 1977;30:261–275.
17. Multiple Risk Factor Intervention Trial Research Group: Multiple Risk Factor Intervention Trial risk factor changes and mortality results. *JAMA* 1982;248:1465–1476.
18. Sherwin R, Kaelber CT, Kezdi P, Kjelsberg MO, Thomas HE. The Multiple Risk Factor Intervention Trial (MRFIT) II. The development of the protocol. *Prev Med* 1981;10:402–425.
19. Neaton JD, Grimm RH, Cutler JA. Recruitment of participants for the Multiple Risk Factor Intervention Trial. *Controlled Clin Trials* 1988;8:42S–53S.
20. Dischinger P, DuChene AG. Quality control aspects of blood pressure measurements in the Multiple Risk Factor Intervention Trial. *Controlled Clin Trials* 1986;6:137S–157S.

21. Wentworth DN, Neaton JD, Rasmussen WL. An evaluation of the Social Security Administration MBR file and the National Death Index in the ascertainment of vital status. *Am J Public Health* 1983;73:1270.
22. *International classification of diseases, 9th rev. Vol. I: Clinical modification.* Ann Arbor, MI: Edwards Bros., 1981.
23. Sorlie PD, Gold EB. The effect of physician terminology preference on coronary heart disease mortality: an artifact uncovered by the Ninth Revision ICD. *Am J Public Health* 1987;77:148–152.
24. National Center for Health Statistics. *Blood pressure of persons 6–74 years of age in the United States, 1971–1974.* DHEW Publication No. (HRA) 78-1648. Health Resources Administration, Washington DC: U.S. Government Printing Office, September, 1977.
25. Colandrea MA, Friedman GD, Nichaman MZ, Lynd CN. Systolic hypertension in the elderly. An epidemiologic assessment. *Circulation* 1970;41:239.
26. Kannel WB, Wolf PA, Verter J, McNamara PM. Epidemiologic assessment of the role of blood pressure in stroke. The Framingham Study. *JAMA* 1970;214:301–310.
27. Fleiss JL. *Statistical methods for rates and proportions.* New York: John Wiley, 1973.
28. Cox DR. Regression models and lifetables. *J R Statist Soc B* 1972;24:187–220.
29. Kaplan E, Meier P. Nonparametric estimation from incomplete data. *J Am Stat Assoc* 1958;53:457–481.
30. Kannel WB, Wolf PA, Garrison RF, eds. Section 34: Some risk factors related to the annual incidence of cardiovascular disease and death using pooled repeated biennial measurements. In: *Framingham Heart Study, 30-Year follow-up.* Bethesda, MD: National Institutes of Health; 1987. Publication NIH 87-2703.
31. Wingard DL, Cohn BA. Coronary heart disease mortality among women in Alameda County, 1965 to 1973. In: Eaker ED, Packard B, Wenger N, Clarkson TB, Tyroler HA, eds. *Coronary heart disease in women: proceedings of an NIH workshop.* New York: Haymarket Doyma, 1987;99–105.
32. Stampfer JF, Colditz GA, Willett WC, Rosner B, Speizer FE, Hennekens CH. Coronary heart disease risk factors in women: the Nurses' Health Study experience. In: Eaker ED, Packard B, Wenger NK, Clarkson TB, Tyroler HA, eds. *Coronary heart disease in women: proceedings of an NIH workshop.* New York: Haymarket Doyma, 1987;112–116.
33. Higgins M, Keller JB, Ostrander LD. Risk factors for coronary heart disease in women: Tecumseh Community Health Study, 1959 to 1980. In: Eaker ED, Packard B, Wenger N, Clarkson TB, Tyroler HA, eds. *Coronary heart disease in women: proceedings of an NIH workshop.* New York: Haymarket Doyma, 1987;83–89.
34. Krueger DE, Ellenberg SS, Bloom S, et al. Risk factors for fatal heart attack in young women. *Am J Epidemiol* 1981;113:357–370.
35. Rosenberg L, Miller DR, Kaufman DW, Helmrich SP, Van De Carr S, Stolley PD, Shapiro S. Myocardial infarction in women under 50 years of age. *JAMA* 1983;250:2801–2806.
36. Eaker ED, Packard B, Wenger NK, Clarkson TB, Tyroler HA, eds. *Coronary heart disease in women: proceedings of an NIH workshop.* New York: Haymarket Doyma, 1987.
37. Barrett-Connor E, Khaw KT, Wingard DL. A ten-year prospective study of coronary heart disease mortality among Rancho Bernardo women. In: Eaker ED, Packard B, Wenger NK, Clarkson TB, Tyroler HA, eds. *Coronary heart disease in women: proceedings of an NIH workshop.* New York: Haymarket Doyma, 1987;117–121.
38. Kannel WB, Gordon T, Schwartz MJ. Systolic versus diastolic blood pressure and risk of coronary heart disease. The Framingham Study. *Am J Cardiol* 1971;27:335–346.
39. Lew EA. High blood pressure, other risk factors and longevity: the insurance viewpoint. *Am J Med* 1973;55:281–294.
40. Yano K, McGee D, Reed DM. The impact of elevated blood pressure upon 10-year mortality among Japanese men in Hawaii: The Honolulu Heart Program. *J Chronic Dis* 1983;36:569–579.
41. The Pooling Project Research Group. Relationship of blood pressure, serum cholesterol, smoking habit, relative weight, and ECG abnormalities to incidence of major coronary events: final report of the Pooling Project. *J Chronic Dis* 1978;31:201–306.

42. MacMahon J, Peto R, Cutler J, Collins R, Sorlie P, Neaton JD, Abbott R, Godwin J, Dyer A, Stamler J. Blood pressure, stroke, and coronary heart disease. Part 1, Prolonged differences in blood pressure: prospective observational studies corrected for the regression dilution bias. *Lancet* 1990;335:765–774.

43. Cruickshank JM, Thorp JM, Zacharias FJ. Benefits and potential harm of lowering blood pressure. *Lancet* 1987;1:581–584.

44. Alderman MH, Ooi WL, Madhaven S, Cohen H. Treatment-induced blood pressure reduction and risk of myocardial infarction. *JAMA* 1989;262:920–924.

45. Farnett L, Mulrow CD, Linn WD, Lucey CR, Tuley MR. The J-curve phenomenon and treatment of hypertension: IS there a point beyond which pressure reduction is dangerous? *JAMA* 1991;265:489–495.

46. Anderson TW. Re-examination of some of the Framingham blood pressure data. *Lancet* 1978;2:1139–1141.

47. Neaton JD, Grimm RH, Jr., Prineas RJ, Stamler J, Grandits GA, Elmer PJ, et al. Treatment of Mild Hypertension Study. Final Results. *JAMA* 1993;270:713–724.

48. Tverdal A. Systolic and diastolic blood pressures as predictors of coronary heart disease in middle-aged Norwegian men. *Br Med J* 1987;294:671–673.

49. Rosenman RH, Sholtz RI, Brand RJ. A study of comparative blood pressure measures in predicting risk of coronary heart disease. *Circulation* 1976;54:51–58.

50. Neaton JD, Bartsch GE. Impact of measurement error and temporal variability on the estimation of event probabilities for risk factor intervention trials. *Stat Med* 1992;11:1719–1729.

51. Kannel WB, Dawber TR, McGee DL. Perspectives on systolic hypertension: the Framingham study. *Circulation* 1980;61:1179–1182.

52. Garland C, Barrett-Connor E, Suarez L, Criqui MH. Isolated systolic hypertension and mortality after age 60 years. *Am J Epidemiol* 1983;118:365–376.

53. van den Barr GC, Kampman E, Schouten EG, Kok FJ, van der Heide RM, van der Heide-Wessel C. Isolated systolic hypertension in Dutch middle-aged and all-cause mortality: a 25-year prospective study. *Int J Epidemiol* 1989;18:95–99.

54. Dyken ML, Wolf PA, Barnett HJM, Bergson JJ, et al. Risk factors in stroke: a statement for physicians by the Subcommittee on Risk Factors and Stroke of the Stroke Council. *Stroke* 1984;15:1105–1111.

55. Sacco RL, Wolf PA, Bharucha NE, Meeks SL, et al. Sub-arachnoid and intra-cerebral hemorrhage: natural history, prognosis and precursive factors in the Framingham Study. *Neurology* 1984;34:847–854.

56. Knekt P, Reunanen A, Aho K, et al. Risk factors for sub-arachnoid hemorrhage in a longitudinal population study. *J Clin Epidemiol* 1991;44:933–939.

57. Shaper AG, Phillips AN, Pocock SJ, Walker M, Macfarian PW. Risk factors for stroke in middle-aged British men. *Br Med J* 1991;302:1111–1115.

58. White LR, Losanczy KG, Wolf PA. Cerebrovascular disease. In: Cornani-Huntley JC, Huntley RR, Feldman JJ, eds. *Health status and well-being of the elderly: National Health and Nutrition Examination Survey I—epidemiologic follow-up study.* New York: Oxford University Press, 1990;115–135.

59. Rose G. Sick individuals and sick populations. *Int J Epidemiol* 1985;14:32–38.

60. Collins R, Peto R, MacMahan S, Hebert P, Fiebach NH, Ebeslein KA, Godwin J, Qizilbash N, Taylor JO, Hennekens CH. Blood pressure, stroke, and coronary heart disease. Part 2, short-term reductions in blood pressure: overview of randomized drug trials in their epidemiological context. *Lancet* 1990;335:827–838.

61. INTERSALT Cooperative Research Group. INTERSALT: an international study of electrolyte excretion and blood pressure. Results for 24-hour urinary sodium and potassium excretion. *Br Med J* 1988;297:319–328.

62. Stamler R, Stamler J, Gosch FC, Civinelli J, Fishman J, McKeever P, et al. Primary prevention of hypertension by nutritional-hygienic means. Final report of a randomized controlled trial. *JAMA* 1989;262:1801–1807.

63. Trials of Hypertension Prevention Collaborative Research Group. The effects of nonpharmacologic interventions of blood pressure of persons with high normal levels: results of the Trials of Hypertension Prevention, Phase I. *JAMA* 1992;267:1213–1220.

64. Whelton PK, Adams-Campbell LL, Appel LJ, et al. Report of the National High Blood Pressure Education Program Working Group (PK Whelton, Chair) on the primary prevention of hypertension. *Arch Intern Med* 1993;153:186–208.

Hypertension: Pathophysiology, Diagnosis, and Management, Second Edition, edited by J.H. Laragh and B.M. Brenner, Raven Press, Ltd., New York © 1995.

CHAPTER 10

Epidemiology and Treatment of Hypertension in Older Persons

Adrian M. Ostfeld, Richard J. Havlik, and Jack Guralnik

In most industrialized countries, the proportion of elderly in the population is increasing. In 1950, 8 percent of all persons in the U.S. were aged 65 years or older. By 1990, that proportion had risen to 12.5 percent. By 2040 the percentage is projected to rise to 20 percent with over 75 million persons 65 years and over. This demographic shift toward greater numbers of older individuals has helped to focus attention on the particular problems of hypertension in the elderly (1,2), a segment of the population in which the condition is highly prevalent. This chapter will examine the extent and nature of high blood pressure (BP) at older ages, its significance for survival and health, and the clinical evidence that is available on the efficacy and safety of pharmacologic therapy.

Large population surveys have revealed the extensive problem that exists in the older age groups. Results from the first half of the 1988–1991 National Health and Nutrition Examination Survey (NHANES III) indicate that hypertension, defined as systolic blood pressure (SBP) over 139 mm Hg or diastolic blood pressure (DBP) over 89 mm Hg or requiring antihypertensive medication, is present in about 60 percent of non-Hispanic whites, 71 percent of non-Hispanic blacks, and 61 percent of

Mexican-Americans 60 years and older (2). Previously, the 1976–1980 National Health and Nutrition Examination Survey (3) (NHANES II) generated estimates of hypertension prevalence in the U.S. from a national sample of the civilian, noninstitutionalized population between the ages of 18 and 74. These data show that the prevalence of hypertension, defined in the same way as for NHANES III, increases with age in the overall population, as well as in each race and gender subgroup (Table 1). In each category of persons age 55 and over, hypertension prevalence was estimated to be at least 50 percent. Blacks have higher rates than whites in almost every age group and black women, in particular, are severely affected: over 80 percent of black women aged 65 to 74 years were classified as hypertensive. Although this NHANES study did not include persons aged 75 or older, the prevalence of this condition in this age group has been estimated using data from the screening phase of a large clinical trial of antihypertensive therapy in the elderly (4). Of the 5,566 persons over age 74 who had BPs measured, 75 percent were found to have SBPs above 139 mm Hg and/or DBPs above 89 mm Hg, and/or were receiving treatment.

Cross-sectional observations on BP from the Framingham Heart Disease Study population describe average levels of DBP that rise with age until the mid-fifties for men and the sixties for women (5). Mean SBP, however, does not show the same kind of decline after middle age and continues to increase throughout the seventh decade

---

A. M. Ostfeld: Yale University School of Public Health New Haven, Connecticut 06510

J. Guralnik and R. J. Havlik: Epidemiology, Demography, and Biometry Program, National Institute on Aging, Bethesda, Maryland 20892

TABLE 1. *Hypertension[a] prevalence rates by gender, race and age group in the civilian, noninstitutionalized population, 1976–1980[b]*

Age (year)	Overall (%)	White men (%)	Black men (%)	White women (%)	Black women (%)
18–24	9.2	16.2	10.9	2.3	9.6
25–34	13.7	21.1	23.2	5.7	15.3
35–44	23.7	26.4	44.2	16.6	37.0
45–54	41.3	42.6	55.2	36.3	67.4
55–64	52.6	51.4	66.3	50.0	74.3
65–74	64.3	59.2	67.1	66.2	82.9

[a] Hypertension: average of three single occasion measurements ≥ 140/90/mm Hg or on antihypertensive medication.
[b] From 1976–1980 National Health and Nutrition Examination Survey, with permission.

for both sexes. For women, both SBP and DBP components begin at lower levels and tend to rise more steeply with age, the rate of increase in SBP continuing to be faster than for men throughout the seventies. As the NHANES II data in Table 1 illustrate, these age trends produce hypertension prevalence rates for women that equal male rates by middle age (55–64) and surpass them in the elderly cohort.

The disproportionate increase with age that is observed for SBP relative to DBP presumably reflects changes brought about by the decline in arterial elasticity over time (6,7). Isolated systolic hypertension (ISH), the form of definite hypertension characterized by elevated SBP in the presence of normal DBP, is a condition found almost exclusively among the elderly, particularly among older women. The Evans County, Georgia, study (8) in 1967–1969 showed that ISH (defined as SBP above 160 mm Hg with DBP below 90 mm Hg) was rare before age 40, but rose steadily with increasing age, with a prevalence rate just over 20 percent in those age 70 and above. This pattern of increasing prevalence with age was

also observed in each gender and race subgroup. In a prevalence study limited to those 65 years and older living in central North Carolina (adjusting for various covariables associated with BP such as socioeconomic status, obesity, and diabetes mellitus), untreated ISH was less common in blacks than in whites (9).

Whether or not these observed increases in BP with age are inevitable, it is clear that hypertension, both classically diastolic and disproportionately systolic, is a highly prevalent condition among older individuals. The following section will examine the evidence from epidemiological studies on the prognostic importance of such elevations in BP for the elderly.

SIGNIFICANCE OF HYPERTENSION IN THE ELDERLY: EPIDEMIOLOGICAL OBSERVATIONS

Classical Hypertension

Overall Mortality and Cardiovascular Mortality

Epidemiologic investigations have established a clear association between elevated BP and the risk of certain cardiovascular disease outcomes. The Framingham Heart Disease Study (10), 18 years of follow-up of a general population sample of men and women aged 45 to 74, has shown that overall mortality rates were more than doubled and cardiovascular mortality approximately tripled in persons with definite hypertension when compared with normotensives. (Hypertension in the Framingham Study was defined as SBP above 159 mm Hg or DBP above 94 mm Hg; normotensive as SBP below 140 mm Hg and DBP below 90 mm Hg; and borderline hypertensive as SBP 140–160 and DBP 90–95 mm Hg.) The increase in risk was observed in each sex and at all ages. As Table 2 illustrates, the gradient of risk

TABLE 2. *Total mortality and cardiovascular mortality according to hypertension status by age group Framingham Study: 18 years follow-up*

Average annual incidence rate for death per 10,000 persons at risk at exam

Age	Men			Women		
	Normal	Borderline	Definite	Normal	Borderline	Definite
45–55	64.7	93.1	133.5	37.0	52.4	74.2
55–64	131.5	188.5	268.7	71.4	81.2	92.4
65–74	251.1	352.1	489.4	117.8	173.8	255.1

Average annual incidence rate for death from cardiovascular disease per 10,000 persons at risk at exam

Age	Men			Women		
	Normal	Borderline	Definite	Normal	Borderline	Definite
45–55	26.4	48.3	88.0	7.7	15.8	32.6
55–64	72.2	121.9	204.4	26.7	39.4	58.0
65–74	125.0	190.8	289.1	39.1	90.7	207.4

From ref. 11, with permission.

TABLE 3. *Attributable risk[a] of hypertension for men and women 45–74 years of age: Framingham Study: 20 years follow-up*

Age (yrs)	Overall mortality		Cardiovascular			
			Mortality		Morbidity	
	Men	Women	Men	Women	Men	Women
45–54	17.9	12.0	29.3	28.6	16.4	17.4
55–64	16.1	8.5	21.4	17.5	17.9	26.5
65–74	8.4	14.9	12.9	34.5	18.8	26.9

[a] Attributable risk = (rate for total population − rate for non-hypertensives)/(rate for total population).
From ref. 5, with permission.

from hypertension persists in the elderly as in the younger age groups and is especially impressive for women (11). Framingham data (Table 3) show that after the age of 65, the risk of cardiovascular mortality and morbidity attributable to hypertension is actually greater for women than for men (5).

Data from other communities suggest some of the complexities in understanding BP and mortality risk in the elderly. The Established Populations for Epidemiologic Studies of the Elderly (EPESE) involved the screening of persons 65 years and over residing in East Boston, Massachusetts; New Haven, Connecticut; and Iowa and Washington Counties, Iowa, for BP level and follow-up for cause-specific and total mortality (12). About 10,000 persons were screened and followed. At two years, odds of death from all causes were higher in the lowest third of the SBP distribution (<130 mm Hg) when compared to the middle third (130–159 mm Hg); but by 5 years the cardiovascular deaths increased with increasing SBPs. Similarly, at 2 years cancer deaths were highest in the lowest SBP category; specifically in East Boston all-cause, cardiovascular, and cancer deaths were highest in the lowest DBP group with short-term follow-up. However, when previously collected BPs from some years earlier were utilized in the analysis, these apparent adverse effects with lower BP were no longer evident. The observation suggests that a portion of older persons with lower BP may have chronic disease and disability that both reduces BP and puts that individual at higher risk of short-

term mortality, obscuring the usual relationship of increasing BP with increasing death. There may be some exaggeration of these complexities in the very old. Among men 80 years and older living in a California community, even with control for presence of disease and abnormal blood chemistry values, those with higher DBP had lower all-cause and cardiovascular mortality (13). This was not true for women and for SBP in both genders.

Cardiovascular Morbidity

The risk of congestive heart failure (CHF), in particular, has been strongly linked with hypertension. In the Framingham population, of 5,192 subjects initially free of CHF, 142 experienced definite CHF over a 16-year period of follow-up (14,15). Hypertension was the most common precursor to its development, present in three-quarters of all cases. The risk of developing CHF in hypertensive subjects was six times the risk observed for normotensive persons. Its development was more common with advancing age, but the estimates of relative risk remained high for both men and women in all age groups (Table 4). As with other cardiovascular sequelae there was evidence of a steeper gradient of risk with SBP compared with DBP for both men and women.

Data from the Framingham study have also been used to examine the role of hypertension in the occurrence of cerebrovascular accidents (CVA) (16,17). Such analyses have found no more important factor in the development of CVAs, or atherothrombotic brain infarctions (ABI), in particular, than hypertension. Over 14 years of follow-up, 65 men and 70 women in this population of 5,209 subjects developed stroke (60 percent were ABIs). Although hypertensives (BP above 159/94 mm Hg) when compared with normotensives (BP below 140/90 mm Hg) showed an increased risk for each of the major atherothrombotic diseases (coronary heart disease, intermittent claudication, ABI, and CHF), the relationship of BP to CVA was stronger than for any of the other cardiovascular disease outcomes except CHF. The risk of stroke and of ABI, in particular, was significantly related

TABLE 4. *Relative risk of developing congestive heart failure: hypertensives compared to normotensives according to age and gender*

Age	Men Average annual rate per 10,000 patient years				Women Average annual rate per 10,000 patient years			
	Total	Normal	HTN	RR	Total	Normal	HTN	RR
35–44	4	0	29		4	4	0	
45–54	19	5	68	14.9	6	5	12	2.7
55–64	39	19	93	4.8	27	10	64	6.7
65–74	61	18	124	6.9	39	11	75	6.7

From ref. 15, with permission.
RR, relative risk; CHF, congestive heart failure; HTN, hypertension; PR, relative risk.

to baseline SBP and DBP on a continuous scale. BPs at or above 160/95 mm Hg were associated with more than a tripling of the risk for CVA.

The Chicago Stroke Study (18,19) was a prospective epidemiologic investigation which examined the precursors of stroke in an elderly population. The study cohort consisted of 2,772 subjects aged 65 to 74 years who were initially free of CVA. Hypertension (defined as SBP above 159 mm Hg or DBP above 94 mm Hg) was observed in 42.9 percent of the study group at baseline. As with the Framingham data, this study found that the incidence of stroke was significantly increased in the presence of hypertension. The gradient of risk was observed for both SBP and DBP, with a stronger effect observed for the SBP. The 3-year incidence of stroke among persons with SBP above 179 mm Hg was about three times greater than that observed among persons with SBP below 130 mm Hg. These results held both for the entire cohort as well as for the group with evidence of target organ damage.

Isolated Systolic Hypertension

Overall Mortality and Cardiovascular Mortality

A few studies have focused exclusively on the ISH form of hypertension. In a small study conducted in a retirement community, Colandrea, et al. (20) identified 72 subjects with persistent ISH (SBP above 159 mm Hg and DBP under 90 mm Hg recorded on three separate occasions). The ISH cases were compared to controls matched on gender, age within 5 years, and DBP within 10 mm Hg. All controls had pressures under 140/90 mm Hg. The mean age of subjects was 69 years and the average length of follow-up was approximately 48 months for both cases and controls. Cardiovascular deaths were found to be significantly more frequent in those with ISH than in the controls.

Framingham data have also been used to explore the prognostic importance of ISH. A 20-year follow-up study (21) showed that for men aged 55 to 74 years, all-cause mortality increased by a factor of 2 in subjects with ISH compared with normotensive controls. (ISH was defined as SBP above 159 mm Hg, with DBP under 95 mm Hg.) Compared to normotensives, cardiovascular disease death was 1.8 times greater in men with ISH and 4.7 times greater in women.

Garland (22) followed 2,636 subjects aged 60 and over for an average of 6.4 years. Based on single-day readings of BP, 6.3 percent were classified as having ISH (SBP above 159 mm Hg and diastolic below 90 mm Hg). This study also found an elevated relative risk (adjusted for age and risk factors) for all-cause mortality (1.5) in untreated subjects with ISH compared to normotensive

subjects ($p > 0.10$). Although there was no difference in deaths from ischemic heart disease in men and women with ISH compared with normotensives, men with ISH were found to have more than quadruple the risk factor adjusted relative risk of stroke mortality as normotensives ($p < 0.10$).

Curb, et al. (23) have used data from the Hypertension Detection and Follow-up Program (HDFP) to examine the effects of ISH on all-cause mortality. A random sample of 5,032 subjects with DBP below 90 mm Hg (determined on one occasion) was identified from the HDFP screened population. They were followed for vital status for 8 years and the mortality experience of those with SBP above 160 mm Hg was compared to those with levels below 160 mm Hg. As for all age groups (except the youngest: 30–49 years of age), the sex-race adjusted mortality rate for subjects 60 to 69 years at baseline was higher in the subjects with ISH. Increasing SBP in these subjects was found to be significantly associated with mortality: a 1-mm increase was associated with a 1 percent increase in mortality.

Stroke

The Chicago Stroke Study (18,19) found a 3-year incidence of stroke and class 1 NBI (nonembolic brain infarction) that was 2.5 times higher in elderly subjects with ISH (defined as SBP above 159 mm Hg with DBP below 80 mm Hg.) compared with subjects with SBP below 140 mm Hg. In persons with normal DBP, increasing levels of SBP were associated with an increasing incidence of stroke and class 1 NBI (Table 5).

Twenty-four years of follow-up for stroke incidence in the Framingham cohort has also shown that subjects with antecedent ISH experienced a two- to fourfold increase in strokes compared with normotensives (24). After age adjustment, the risk of stroke increased with the level of SBP in subjects with DBP below 95 mm Hg. This was especially so for men.

Effect of Treatment

The observational studies cited above provide evidence that both diastolic and systolic hypertension put older persons at increased risk. They also suggest that the disproportionate increases in SBP observed in older persons are clinically important and may not be an innocuous accompaniment of aging. However, even with this evidence, questions remained as to whether ISH was an independent and remediable risk factor for cardiovascular disease or merely a marker for atherosclerotic inelastic vessels in the aged (25). This section will report the findings from several observational studies of therapy

TABLE 5. *Three-year incidence of stroke and class 1 NBI by level of systolic blood pressure in persons with diastolic blood pressure less than 80 mm Hg, age 65–74: Chicago Stroke Study*

	Subjects	All stroke			Class 1 NBI		
		No.	Rate/1000	SE	No.	Rate/1000	SE
SBP ≤139	687	12	42	8	14	22	6
SBP 140–159	332	17	55	13	7	26	10
SBP ≥160	204	20	110	27	8	57	23

NBI, nonembolic brain infarction; SBP, systolic blood pressure; DBP, diastolic blood pressure; SE, standard error.

and the results of nine major randomized clinical trials involving older hypertensives.

Observational Studies

An early observational study that suggested beneficial effects of treatment in an elderly population was conducted by Priddle et al. (26). During the period 1963–1967, 183 residents of a Toronto geriatric home with SBP above 179 mm Hg or DBP above 99 mm Hg (on at least two occasions) were identified. Ages ranged from 60 to 96 years, and 86 percent were female. One hundred persons had been treated for hypertension, mostly with thiazide drugs, and 83 were untreated. Although the assignment of treatment group was nonrandom, the two groups did not differ significantly with regard to age, BP at baseline, the incidence of associated diseases, or causes of death. Treatment was effective in reducing BPs by an average of 20 mm SBP and 10 mm DBP. Over the period of follow-up, 78 deaths occurred, with the mortality rate in the treated group about half the rate in the untreated group.

Another observational study examined stroke recurrence in relation to the degree of hypertension control in a group of 162 subjects (27). All patients had recovered from a cerebrovascular episode; all were being treated for hypertension, most with a thiazide diuretic. Forty-seven subjects (29 percent) experienced a second stroke during the average follow-up period of 48 months. The data showed a significant trend of declining recurrence with increasing control of BP levels.

Finally, the issues of treatment as well as control of BP level have been addressed in another study of over 5,000 individuals (28). The National Health and Nutrition Examination Survey (NHANES I) Epidemiologic Follow-up Study assessed vital status over a 9-year period, subsequent to a BP measurement in 1971–1975 among white men and women aged 50 years and older in the U.S. Those at baseline with elevated BP, regardless of history of hypertension or medication intake, had a 27–31 percent increased risk of death. However, among this subgroup with high BP, medication for hypertension was not associated with any substantial excess risk in this population representative of treated but uncontrolled hypertensives.

Randomized Clinical Trials

The Veteran's Administration Cooperative Study

The Veteran's Administration Cooperative Study on Antihypertensive Agents (29–31) was a randomized, double-blind, placebo-controlled clinical trial of the effects of hydrochlorothiazide, reserpine, and hydralazine (Wydase) in the treatment of nonlabile hypertension in males. Begun in April of 1964, the segment of the trial involving patients with moderately severe hypertension at randomization (DBP 115–129 mm Hg) was terminated in May of 1967 when early analyses demonstrated a highly significant effect of treatment (29). The average age was 51 years. The mean baseline BP was 186/121 mm Hg. Although no specific analysis of treatment effects at older ages was performed for subjects with baseline DBP over 115 mm Hg, results were consistent among those over age 59.

For the 380 patients with mild to moderate hypertension (diastolic 90–114 mm Hg at baseline), the VA trial (30) continued until October 1969, resulting in an average follow-up period of approximately 3 years for these subjects. Of these subjects, 43 control and 38 treated subjects were over 59 years of age at entry; 15 in each group were over 69 years (31). As expected, the incidence of severe morbid events increased with age: 63 percent of the untreated and 29 percent of the treated patients over 59 years developed major complications compared with 15 percent and 7 percent of those less than 50 years old. The percentage of reduction in morbid events of treatment was found to be approximately the same in the younger and older age groups: 55 percent in those less than age 50; 68 percent in subjects aged 50–59; and 54 percent in patients over age 59.

The VA study population had a high prevalence of cardiovascular disease at the time of entry into the trial. More than half of the enrolled population showed evidence of cardiovascular or renal abnormalities at baseline, including more than 75 percent of those over 59 years. It should be noted that the 50-percent reduction in outcomes observed in the "no abnormality" group, although not statistically significant, was consistent with the 64-percent reduction found in those with preexisting conditions. Since the VA trial enrolled a relatively small number of patients over age 59 and dealt only with diastolic hypertension in males, it could not provide definitive data on the efficacy of antihypertensive treatment in the elderly.

Hypertension-Stroke Cooperative Study

The Hypertension-Stroke Cooperative Study (32) was a double-blind, randomized trial of the effect of antihypertensive treatment on stroke recurrence in subjects with mild to moderate hypertension. At baseline, SBP was required to be between 140 and 220 mm Hg, with DBP between 90 and 115 mm Hg. Enrollment began September 1966 and ended June 1971. Subjects had to be less than 75 years old and ambulatory at entry, and had to have experienced a stroke (80 percent) or a transient ischemic attack (4 percent), or both (16 percent) in the year prior to enrollment. Treatment consisted of deserpidine (Enduronlyl, Harmonyl, Oreticyl) combined with methylclothiazide.

The mean age of the 452 study subjects was 59 years (44 percent were over 59); 80 percent were black, and 60 percent were male. Among the 156 patients aged 60 to 69 at entry, stroke recurrence affected 18.9 percent of the 74 treated subjects and 22 percent of the 82 untreated patients ($p = 0.79$); cardiovascular endpoints occurred in 8.5 percent and 10.8 percent, respectively ($p = 0.83$); and the combined stroke and cardiovascular event rates were 30.5 percent and 29.7 percent ($p = 0.94$). Of the 44 patients over 70 years of age at entry, 19 were treated and 25 were untreated. Among those on active treatment, only 10.5 percent had a stroke recurrence compared with 36 percent of the placebo group ($p = 0.08$). Cardiovascular endpoints occurred in 5.3 percent of the treated and 12 percent of the placebo patients ($p = 0.62$). Combined stroke recurrence and cardiovascular events affected 15.8 percent and 48 percent of the treated and untreated patients, respectively ($p = 0.06$).

Hypertension Detection and Follow-Up Program

The Hypertension Detection and Follow-Up Program (HDFP) (33–37) was a community-based randomized trial which examined the effect on 5-year mortality of a systematic antihypertensive treatment program (stepped care [SC]) compared to existing community medical therapies for hypertension (regular care [RC]). Screening occurred from February 1973 to May 1974. Baseline

DBP greater than 89 mm Hg was required for enrollment of those up to age 69 years. Treatment consisted of a five-step regimen involving chlorthalidone with reserpine, hydralazine, guanethidine sulfate, and other drugs added as needed to achieve goal diastolic pressure. (Goal pressure was defined as 90 mm Hg or less for those with entry DBP above 99 mm Hg or on antihypertensive medication; or a drop of 10 mm Hg for those with entry DBP between 90 and 99 mm Hg.) Subjects in the SC group did consistently better than those in RC at achieving control over their BP.

To reduce the potential bias from differential endpoint ascertainment for the two treatment groups in this unblinded study, the primary outcome was taken to be death from all causes. Analyses of treatment effect by age group at entry (34) show that benefits accrued primarily to middle-aged and older subjects. A consistent benefit from treatment was demonstrated for the 1,204 SC subjects compared to the 1,172 RC subjects who were 60 to 69 years of age at entry. The percentage reduction in 5-year mortality for the SC group was 16.4 percent for the 60–69 age group. For those subjects with mild hypertension (90–114 mm Hg) at baseline, the reduction was 17.2 percent for the older age group.

Analysis of data for cause of death (37) confirmed that strokes in the elderly could be reduced by an aggressive treatment program. In the overall trial population, strokes accounted for 12.4 percent of deaths in the RC group compared with 8.3 percent in the SC group. Fatal and nonfatal strokes combined were significantly reduced in the SC group compared with the RC subjects (1.9 percent and 2.9 percent, respectively; $p < 0.01$). The greatest reduction in total stroke rate (from 5.5 percent in RC to 3 percent in SC—45.5 percent) was observed in those aged 60 to 69 years at baseline. Total cardiovascular mortality was reduced by 21.8 percent in the 60–69-year-old group (9.6 percent versus 7.5 percent for RC and SC, respectively) (35).

Australian Therapeutic Trial in Mild Hypertension

The Australian Therapeutic Trial in Mild Hypertension (38,39) was a randomized trial designed to assess the effect of treatment of mild, symptomless hypertension. Subjects between the ages of 30 and 69 with no previous treatment for hypertension and with no clinical, biochemical or electrocardiographic evidence of cardiovascular or other major diseases at baseline were eligible. At entry, DBP had to be between 95 and 109 mm Hg, with SBP below 200 mm Hg. Treatment consisted of chlorothiazide (Diuril), with methyldopa, propranolol, or pindolol (Visken) added as second-order drugs. Beginning in 1973, 3,427 subjects were enrolled. Sixty-three percent were male.

Seventeen percent of the trial participants were between the ages of 60 and 69 at entry (293 on active treatment and 289 on placebo). Subgroup analyses of this elderly cohort (39) by intention-to-treat showed that the active group experienced a reduction of 26 percent in the rate of all trial endpoints compared to the placebo group, primarily due to a reduction in nonfatal endpoints (−27 percent). As for the overall population, the differences in total events resulted largely from reductions in IHD and stroke rates.

In the overall population, the beneficial effects of treatment were observed in both genders. However, in the analysis of the older participants the authors reported that the benefits accrued largely to men (who comprised 55 percent of the over-59 age group). It was suggested that such differences could have mitigated the influence of treatment in this age group.

European Working Party on Hypertension in the Elderly

The European Working Party on Hypertension in the Elderly (EWPHE) (40–42) was a randomized, double-blind trial designed to assess the effectiveness of antihypertensive drug therapy in persons over the age of 59. Subjects aged 60 or more with DBP between 90 and 119 mm Hg and SBP between 160 and 239 mm Hg were eligible. Enrollment was begun in 1972. Trial criteria excluded patients with certain complications of hypertension and concurrent diseases such as malignancy and diabetes requiring insulin treatment. Eight hundred forty subjects were randomized to an active treatment of hydrochlorothiazide and triamterene, (with methyldopa added if needed) or placebo. Seventy percent of the subjects were women, and the mean age was 72 years. Average BP at baseline was 183/101 mm Hg. Trial participants were followed on treatment for an average of 3 years; mortality outcomes were ascertained up to July 1984, for a mean overall follow-up of 4.6 years.

Analysis by intention-to-treat, which includes persons in the treatment group regardless of their overall compliance, showed a decline in the observed morality rate of only 8 percent. Cardiovascular mortality, however, declined by 27 percent ($p = 0.037$); the latter decrease was largely due to a fall in cardiac mortality of 38 percent ($p = 0.036$) and a nonsignificant decline in cerebrovascular mortality of 34 percent ($p = 0.16$).

Data on morbidity outcomes (available for the period on treatment) show that study-terminating (defined as those events resulting in removal from the double-blind aspect of the protocol) nonfatal cardiovascular events (cerebral hemorrhage, papilledema, retinal hemorrhage or exudates, CHF not controlled by digitalis) were significantly reduced on active treatment (−60 percent, $p = 0.0064$), mainly due to a 63-percent decline in severe

CHF. Only seven patients (3 placebo, 4 treated) had a nonfatal cerebral hemorrhage. Study-terminating cardiac events, fatal and nonfatal combined, fell 54 percent ($p = 0.0016$). Terminating cerebrovascular events declined 46 percent ($p = 0.058$). The estimated rate of nonfatal MI was actually more frequent in the treated group (14/1000 patient years) than in the untreated (9/1000 patient years). Overall, there was a reduction of 36 percent ($p = 0.0015$) in combined cardiovascular terminating and nonterminating events for subjects on active treatment.

The main benefits identified in this study were a reduction in cardiac mortality (fatal MI, including sudden death) and stroke. There was some indication from these data that the effect of treatment on cardiovascular mortality and on all cardiovascular study-terminating events (fatal events and nonfatal cardiovascular morbid study-terminating events) decreased with age. The investigators concluded that the benefits of treatment could not be established with confidence in those patients over 80 years of age.

Randomized Trial of Elderly Patients in Primary Care (PPC)

This study (43) was a randomized, non-placebo-controlled (but observed subgroup) trial of the effects of atenolol (tenoretic) and bendroflurazide in the treatment of hypertension in an elderly population. Subjects between the ages of 60 and 79 were recruited from practice lists of the National Health Service in Britain during 1978–1981. Blood pressure requirements at entry were SBP above 169 mm Hg or DBP above 104 mm Hg. There were various exclusion criteria. The mean age at entry was 69 years, and 70 percent were female. The mean BP at baseline was 196/99 mm Hg. Blood pressure was lower on active treatment by an average of 18 mm systolic and 11 mm diastolic compared with the control group.

Subjects were followed for an average of 4.4 years. Total mortality was not found to be significantly different between the treatment groups (60 events over 1,845 patient-years in treated group, 69 events over 2,055 patient-years in the observed but untreated group). The rate of fatal stroke among the treated subjects, however, was one-third the level observed among the controls ($p < 0.025$); both fatal and nonfatal strokes combined were significantly reduced by treatment (−42 percent; $p < 0.03$). Overall, there was a nonsignificant decline (−22 percent) in cardiovascular deaths, but the incidence and mortality of myocardial infarction and the incidence of sudden death were unaffected.

Subgroup analyses of patients by age group at entry to the trial and by sex showed a consistent decrease in total stroke for all groups: the rate for those aged 60–69 was for the treated group 14.3 per 1000 compared to 7.5 for the controls (−48 percent); and for those 70–79 the rate was 34.4 compared to 18.7 (−46 percent). For men the reduction was from 31.9 to 16.8 (−47 percent) and for women from 16.5 to 10.7 (−35 percent). Although statistical significance was lost due to the limitations of subgroup sizes, these findings suggested that women as well as men benefited from a decrease in strokes and that the response appeared to be maintained up to age 80.

Systolic Hypertension in the Elderly Program (SHEP)

After the SHEP pilot study (44,45) demonstrated feasibility, a randomized, double-blind, placebo-controlled clinical trial was conducted to assess the safety and efficacy of drug treatment for ISH in persons aged 60 and over (46). Treatment consisted of chlorothalidone (with atenolol available as a Step II drug). Intake into the trial began in 1985. The screening procedure used in this trial involved measurement of BPs on four separate occasions before randomization. The final screening SBP had to fall between 160 and 219 mm Hg, with DBP below 90 mm Hg. Of 447,921 individuals screened in the community in this trial, 4,736 subjects were eventually randomized (2,365 to treatment and 2,371 to placebo): Fifty-seven percent were female, 14 percent were black and 59 percent were over 70 years old.

The primary endpoint was nonfatal and fatal stroke with secondary endpoints being cardiovascular morbidity and mortality and all-cause mortality. The average follow-up for the study was 4.5 years and the average SBP was 155 mm Hg for the placebo group and 143 mm Hg for the active treatment group. Corresponding DBPs were 72 and 68 mm Hg, respectively. These BP differences resulted in a 5-year incidence of total stroke of 5.2 per 100 participants in the treated group and 8.2 per 100 participants in the comparison group. Significant reductions in nonfatal myocardial infarction, in left ventricu-

lar failure, and in all coronary heart disease were also found. The relative risk of treatment versus placebo for nonfatal myocardial infarction and coronary death was 0.73. The 36-percent reduction in total stroke could be translated into an absolute benefit of 30 less events per 100 treated participants. Although SHEP is considered by most as a definitive study, there were not enough events to determine the effect on vascular dementia and certain other endpoints. In Europe a randomized, placebo-controlled, cooperative trial called SYST-EUR has been started to assess the effect of treating ISH on morbidity and mortality in patients over 60 years of age (47). This study will use a calcium antagonist as the primary treatment with an angiotensin-converting enzyme inhibitor or diuretic as secondary therapy. It is projected to be a 5-year study in about 3,000 patients.

Swedish Trial in Old Patients With Hypertension (STOP-Hypertension)

The STOP-Hypertension study addressed the issue of benefits of treatment of either predominantly elevated SBP or DBP in Swedish men and women aged 70–84 years (48). There were 1,627 patients, recruited in health centers, who met screening criteria which included SBP between 180 and 230 mm Hg with a DBP of at least 90 mm Hg, or a DBP between 105 and 120 mm Hg without regard to SBP, on 3 separate occasions over a 1-month period. The mean BP of entrants was 195/102 mm Hg. About 60 percent were eligible mainly by virtue of SBP, although true ISH patients were excluded. Patients were randomized in a prospective double-blind intervention study to compare the effects of antihypertensive therapy to placebo on various fatal and nonfatal cardiovascular end points. The therapy used was a mixture of diuretics and/or beta blockers.

The study lasted 65 months (1985–1990) but the average time in the study was about 2 years. The average SBP

TABLE 6. *Randomized clinical trials of antihypertensive therapy subjects 60 years and older*

Trial	Time period	No. subjects T	No. subjects C	Mean age at entry (range)	Female (%)	Entry BP criteria DBP	Entry BP criteria SBP	Mean entry SBP/DBP	Follow-up mean years
HDFP	73–79	1204	1173	na (60–69)	25%	>89	None	170/101	5
Australia	73–79	293	289	64 (60–69)	45%	95–110 and	<200	165/101	4
EWPHE	72–84	416	424	72 (60–80+)	70%	90–119 and	160–239	182/101	4.6
PPC	75–85	419	465	69 (60–79)	69%	>104 or	>169	196/99	4.4
SHEP	85–91	2365	2371	72 (60–80+)	57%	<90 and	>160	170/77	4.5
STOP-Hyper	85–91	812	815	76 (70–84)	63%	105–120 or	90 + 180–230	195/102	2.1
MRC	82–92	2183	2213	70 (65–74)	58%	<115 and	160–209	185/91	5.8

HDFP, Hypertension Detection and Follow-up Program; EWPHE, European Working Party on Hypertension in the Elderly; PPC, Patients in Primary Care; SHEP, Systolic Hypertension in the Elderly Program; STOP-Hyper, Swedish Trial in Old Patients with Hypertension; MRC, Medical Research Council Trial of Treatment of Hypertension in Older Adults; T, treated; C, control; BP, blood pressure; DBP, diastolic blood pressure; SBP, systolic blood pressure.

difference was 20 mm Hg and DBP 8 mm Hg. There was a significant reduction of 40 percent compared to placebo in the number of primary cardiovascular endpoints (94 vs. 58, $p = 0.003$) as well as a reduction in stroke by 47 percent (53 vs. 29 events, $p = 0.008$). Noteworthy was the significantly reduced number of total deaths (-43 percent) for those on active therapy. This study adds further support for the premise that antihypertensive therapy in the elderly is beneficial. The benefit of treatment was great, with treatment of fourteen elderly patients over 5 years expected to prevent one stroke and one death.

Medical Research Council (MRC) Trial of Treatment of Hypertension in Older Adults

General practices in the UK were sites for a randomized, placebo-controlled, single-blind trial of antihypertensive therapy in 4,396 patients aged 65–74 years (49). A much larger number of patients were screened for persistently elevated BP. The overall mean for SBP had to be 160–209 mm Hg and mean DBP had to be 114 mm Hg or less. Overall, the mean BP of the participating group was 193/91 mm Hg. Two interventions, a beta blocker, or hydrochlorothiazide, and placebo were randomly assigned. Adjustments in treatment were made so that sufficient BP reduction occurred over a 5.8-year period. When compared to the placebo group, the treated group had a 25-percent reduction in strokes, a 1.9-percent reduction in coronary events, and a 3-percent reduction in all deaths. Although BP was reduced for both treatments compared to placebo, after adjusting for baseline characteristics, only the diuretic group had a reduction in risk for stroke 31 percent ($p = 0.04$), coronary events 44 percent ($p = 0.001$) and all deaths 16 percent ($p = 0.13$). The beta-blocker group had similar disease experience to the placebo group. Although some questions have been raised about the substantial rate of dropout and loss to follow-up, especially in the beta-blocker group, it appears that diuretics outperformed the beta-blocker subgroup in this clinical trial.

TABLE 8. *Trial outcomes: cardiovascular mortality*

Trial	Treated (T) No.	%	Control (C) No.	%	Effectiveness (T − C)/C
HDFP	90	7.5	112	9.6	−21.8%
Australia	2	0.7	5	1.7	−60.5%
EWPHE	67	16.1	93	21.9	−26.6%
PPC	35	8.4	50	10.8	−22.3%
SHEP	90	3.8	112	4.7	−20.0%
STOP-Hyper	17	NA	41	NA	NA
MRC	161	12.8	180	14.1	−9.0%

NA, not available.

Summary of Trials

Table 6 presents a summary of the major completed clinical trials initiated in the 1970s and 1980s that have been reviewed. The major results pertaining to mortality and morbidity for subjects over age 59 are shown in Tables 7–9. (All results are in terms of intention to treat.) Overall, mortality rates were consistently lower, although often not significantly reduced, on treatment. The main benefits of antihypertensive therapy are seen in the impressive reductions in cardiovascular mortality (Table 8), especially in the prevention of stroke events in this age group (Table 9). Of the six trials that reported coronary mortality separately (Table 10), EWPHE noted a substantial reduction; the Australian study also showed a reduction, although the number of events was small. Less dramatic reductions were shown by SHEP and MRC, and PPC was negative (detail from STOP-Hypertension was lacking). The incidence of CHF responded well to treatment (EWPHE, PPC, SHEP), but a modest effect on nonfatal MIs was observed in the SHEP, Australia, and PPC studies). After reviewing these studies, a group of British authors concluded that convincing evidence for treatment exists mainly for patients up to 80 years of age and that diuretics rather than beta blockers (based mainly on the MRC results) are the treatment of choice for uncomplicated hypertension (50). More targeted randomized trials in very old patients utilizing clinical endpoints and the newer antihypertensive

TABLE 7. *Trial outcomes: all-cause mortality*

Trial	Treated (%) No.	%	Control (C) No.	%	Effectiveness (T − C)/C
HDFP	153	12.7	178	15.2	−16.4%
Australia	7	2.4	9	3.1	−23.3%
EWPHE	135	32.5	149	35.1	−7.7%
PPC	60	14.3	69	14.8	−3.5%
SHEP	213	9.0	242	10.2	−13.0%
STOP-Hyper	36	2.0	63	3.5	−43.0%
MRC	301	2.4	315	2.5	−3.0%

TABLE 9. *Trial outcomes: all strokes (fatal and nonfatal)*

Trial	Treated (T) No.	%	Control (C) No.	%	Effectiveness (T − C)/C
HDFP	NA	3.0[1]	NA	5.5[1]	−45.5%
Australia	7	2.4	9	3.1	−23.3%
EWPHE	25	6.0	34	8.0	−25.1%
PPC	23	5.5	44	9.5	−42.0%
SHEP	102	5.2	156	8.2	−36.0%
STOP-Hyper	29	1.7	53	3.1	−47.0%
MRC	101	8.1	134	10.8	−25.0%

[1] HDFP, 5-year incidence rate, adjusted for race, sex, entry BP.

TABLE 10. *Other trial outcomes*

Trial	Treated (T)		Control (C)		Effectiveness (T − C)/C
	No.	%	No.	%	
I. Fatal myocardial infarction (inc. sudden death)					
Australia	1	0.3	4	1.4	−75.3%
EWPHE	29	7.0	47	11.1	−37.1%
PPC	25	6.0	28	6.0	−0.9%
SHEP	59	2.5	73	3.1	−20.0%
STOP-Hyper	10	NA	20	NA	NA
MRC	85	6.7	110	8.6	−22.0%
II. Congestive heart failure					
EWPHE	7	1.7	17	4.0	−58.0%
PPC	18	4.3	32	6.9	−37.6%
SHEP	56	2.4	109	4.6	−55.0%
STOP-Hyper	19	NA	39	NA	NA
III. Myocardial infarction					
Australia	6	2.0	5	1.7	18.4%
PPC	10	2.4	10	2.2	11.0%
SHEP	104	4.4	141	5.9	−27.0%
STOP-Hyper	25	1.4	28	1.7	−13.0%
MRC	128	1.0	159	1.3	−19.0%

NA, not available.

drugs would be necessary before more definitive statements could be made.

ADHERENCE TO TREATMENT AMONG ELDERLY SUBJECTS

Long-term adherence to a prescribed medication regimen is necessary for the effective control of hypertension. None of the major clinical trials discussed above found that their elderly participants had major problems complying with medication protocols due to lack of ability or inclination. In the HDFP, no age pattern in the active participation rates after 1 year was found (51). The overall adherence rate for age group 60–69 was 81 percent. Older participants were not only as compliant as younger subjects, they also achieved better control of DBP. After 1 year, 60 percent of the SC and 33.8 percent of RC subjects aged 60–69 were at or below goal compared with 53.4 percent and 30.5 percent, respectively, for those 50–59 at entry. In the EWPHE trial, only 22 of the 416 subjects randomized to active treatment (5 percent), and 30 of the 424 untreated (7 percent) refused to continue their treatment regimen (42). During the pilot phase of the PPC, compliance was tested in the twelve patients in the treated group with a mean decrease of 10 mm Hg or less in systolic pressure; only one patient was found to be noncompliant when serum levels of the treatment drug were examined (43). In the SHEP feasibility study, compliance tests involving pill counts, self-reports, and urine screens found that after 1 year, more than 85 percent of subjects in each treatment group were adhering to their prescribed treatments (44).

SIDE-EFFECTS OF ANTIHYPERTENSIVE THERAPY

The Veterans Administration study of mild to moderate hypertension did not report age-specific data on the incidence of side effects. However, in the overall study population (31), there were 7 reports of depression among the 186 treated, and 5 reports among the 194 untreated. Peptic ulcer developed in six treated and four untreated subjects. This trial employed a multiple drug treatment protocol (hydrochlorothiazide 50/mg plus reserpine 0.1/mg twice daily, and hydralazine 25/mg three times daily) and modifications in the level of drugs were often required.

In the HDFP trial, the 5-year incidence of adverse reactions were actually lower among the older participants (51). The overall rates of side effects were 34.6 percent, 35 percent, and 26.6 percent for subjects aged 40–49, 50–49, and 60–69, respectively. When adverse reactions are restricted to definite or probable effects only, the rates were 9.6 percent, 10.5 percent, and 7.0 percent, respectively. The reports for most specific side effects, including orthostatic hypotension, depression, lethargy, and drowsiness were also lower among the oldest participants in this trial.

In the PPC study (43), 70 percent of the treated subjects were on 100 mg of atenolol per day and 60 percent required the addition of bendroflurazide as the Step II drug in order to achieve a satisfactory BP response. Approximately 25 percent of the treated patients were not able to tolerate atenolol, with the most common reported side effects being general fatigue, muscular weakness, and breathlessness on exertion. This study administered a specially designed questionnaire after the first year in order to ascertain side effects such as headache, breathlessness, fatigue, and depression. Although this was not a placebo-controlled or a blinded trial, no differences in the level of complaint of perceived symptoms were detected among those on drug treatment compared with the observed group.

There was no evidence in the Australian trial that side effects resulted in a disproportionately high number of treatment withdrawals among the elderly participants (39). Thirty-three percent of the active group and 35 percent of the placebo patients over age 59 stopped treatment prematurely, almost identical to the proportions observed in the overall population (34 percent treated and 35 percent untreated). The reason for stopping was rarely given as side effects.

In the SHEP feasibility trial, inquiry was made about 22 specific symptoms at the baseline and at 1 month and

1 year follow-up visits (44). At 1 month, approximately one-third of those on treatment and taking placebo reported one or more troublesome or intolerable symptoms and no symptom was reported significantly more often in the treatment group. At 1 year the groups were still comparable in terms of reported symptoms, although reports of problems in sexual function were more common among the treated men (6 percent compared with zero among the controls; difference not statistically significant). In the SHEP feasibility trial there was no evidence that treatment was related to a diminution of cognitive function or increase in depression (52).

Biochemical changes associated with the use of diuretics are relatively common. Most trials (EWPHE, PPC, Australia, and SHEP feasibility) reported increases in serum uric acid and serum creatinine in patients on active treatment (39,40,43,44). In the PPC and MRC trials, there was an excess of clinical gout reported among the treated subjects (43,49). The combination of thiazide treatment with the use of a potassium-sparing agent (triamterene) in the EWPHE trial prevented a significant change in serum potassium levels on treatment. In the PPC trial of atenolol and bendrofluarzide, the mean serum potassium concentration was also almost unchanged after 1 and 2 years (43). In the SHEP feasibility trial, mean potassium levels fell significantly after 4 weeks on treatment (from 4.5 to 3.9 mEq/L; 21 percent of subjects had levels below 3.5 mEq/L) and after 1 year, potassium supplements had been prescribed for 13 percent of the active treatment group (44). The SHEP study also found a moderate elevation in the mean nonfasting serum glucose level of the treated group ($p = 0.09$); only one case of glucose intolerance requiring treatment was recorded. Other trials have also reported small increases in glucose intolerance in those on active treatment (EWPHE, PPC, MRC) (43,49,53). Biochemical changes with diuretics can be minimized by using the lowest effective dose, equivalent to 12.5–25 mg of hydrochlorothiazide per day (54).

NONPHARMACOLOGIC TREATMENT OF HYPERTENSION

Although adherence to drugs in older persons is generally good and subjective and objective side effects relatively uncommon, support for the use of nonpharmacologic methods in BP control is growing (55,56). Principally, salt restriction and mental relaxation techniques were recommended in the past, but more recently recommendations have been expanded by the World Health Organization (WHO) to include weight loss, aerobic exercise, and increased potassium intake. Such strategies are supported by a randomized trial with BP reduction as the endpoint (55). Participants in this study ranged in age from 60 to 85 years and had a DBP of 85–

100 mm Hg. The experimental arm of the trial was a combination of weight reduction, sodium restriction, and physical activity provided at group and individual sessions over 6 months. Of the 56 randomized participants, 47 completed the study. Weight reduction was successful; there was a 2.1-kg weight loss in treated group and 0.3-kg gain in the control group. There was no significant difference in 24-hour urine sodium. The mean SBP and DBP differences were 4.2 and 4.9 mm Hg respectively. The authors concluded that borderline and mild elevation in DBP could be treated nonpharmacologically. The WHO recommendations suggest that nonpharmacological means may be a method to reduce drug dosage (56).

CONCLUSIONS

The widespread prevalence of hypertension at older ages and the growing ranks of the elderly make the issue of hypertension control one of central importance for the health of this segment of the population. Epidemiologic data have shown that elevations in SBP, as well as DBP, continue to contribute after age 65 to the risk of such disease endpoints as stroke, heart attack, congestive heart failure, aortic aneurysms, and renal failure. The weight of the evidence from clinical drug trials indicates that (a) hypertension can be treated successfully, with good compliance at older ages and with few side effects if dose levels are properly monitored; and (b) successful treatment reduces the incidence of cardiovascular mortality and morbidity in the elderly as it does in those at younger ages.

Recommendations and issues concerning treatment of hypertension in older persons have been discussed in a number of review articles and editorials (54,57,58). However, the recent report of the Joint National Committee on Detection, Evaluation, and Treatment of High Blood Pressure probably represents the current consensus view on hypertension in older patients (2). The committee stated that "the value of treating hypertension in older patients has now been established." Specifically, there is support for the treatment of ISH with reduction of SBPs to less that 160 mm Hg in those with SBPs greater that 180 and to lower BP by 20 mm Hg for those with SBPs between 160 and 179. The goals of therapy for DBP in older persons are very similar to goals for younger persons, except that antihypertensive drug therapy should be carried out with more caution in older patients. Nonpharmacologic treatment could be used as an adjunct to drug therapy. It is important to reiterate, however, because of the presence of multiple comorbidities and other unknown factors, that extrapolation on the basis of current data to treatment effects in those over 80–84 years of age is less substantiated and should be based on individual patient considerations. Further research on appropriate hypertension treatment is needed in this oldest age group.

REFERENCES

1. Gifford R Jr. Geriatric Hypertension: Chairman's Comments on the NIH Working Group Report. *Geriatr* 1987;42(5):45–50.
2. National High Blood Pressure Education Program. The fifth report of the Joint National Committee on detection, evaluation, and treatment of high blood pressure. NIH Publication 93-1088, 1993,35–37.
3. National Health Survey Series 11, No. 234. Blood pressure levels in persons 18–74 years of age in 1976–80, and trends in blood pressure from 1960 to 1980 in the United States. DHHS Publication (PHS) 1986;86–1684.
4. Subcommittee on Definition and Prevalence of the 1984 Joint National Committee. Hypertension prevalence and the status of awareness, treatment, and control in the United States. *Hypertension* 1985;7:457–468.
5. Kannel W. Evaluation of Cardiovascular Risk in the Elderly: the Framingham Study. *Bull NY Acad Med* 1978;54(6):573–591.
6. Fleg J. Alterations in cardiovascular structure and function with advancing age. *Am J Cardiol* 1986;57:33C–44C.
7. Sowers J. Hypertension in the Elderly. *Am J Med* 1987;82[Suppl 1B]:1–8.
8. Wing S., et al. Isolated systolic hypertension in Evans County-I. prevalence and screening considerations. *J Chron Dis* 1982;35:735–742.
9. Svetkey LP, George LK, Burchett BM, Morgan PA, Blazer DG. Black/white differences in hypertension in the elderly: an epidemiologic analysis in central North Carolina. *Am J Epidemiol* 1993;137(1):64–72.
10. Kannel W. Role of blood pressure in cardiovascular disease: the Framingham Study. *Angiology* 1975;26(1):1–14.
11. Shurtleff. Some characteristics related to the incidence of cardiovascular disease and death: Framingham Study 18-year follow-up. DHEW Pub (NIH) 1974;74–599.
12. Taylor JO, Cornoni-Huntley J, Curb JD, Manton KG, Ostfeld AM, Scherr P, Wallace KG. Blood pressure and mortality risk in the elderly. *Am J Epidemiol* 1991;134(5):489–501.
13. Langer RD, Ganiats TG, Barrett-Connor E. Facts associated with paradoxical survival at higher blood pressures in the very old. *Am J Epidemiol* 1991;134(1):29–38.
14. McKee P, et al. The natural history of congestive heart failure: the Framingham Study. *N Engl J Med* 1971;285(26):1441–1446.
15. Kannel W, et al. Role of blood pressure in the development of congestive heart failure: the Framingham Study. *N Engl J Med* 1972;287(16):781–787.
16. Kannel W, et al. Epidemiologic assessment of the role of blood pressure in stroke: the Framingham Study. *JAMA* 1970;214(2):301–310.
17. Kannel W, et al. Components of blood pressure and risk of atherothrombotic brain infarction: the Framingham Study. *Stroke* 1976;7(4):327–331.
18. Ostfeld A, et al. Epidemiology of stroke in an elderly welfare population. *Am J Public Health* 1974;64(5):450–458.
19. Shekelle R, Ostfeld A, Klawans H. Hypertension and risk of stroke in an elderly population. *Stroke* 1974;5:71–75.
20. Colandrea M, et al. Systolic hypertension in the elderly: an epidemiologic assessment. *Circulation* 1970;41:239–245.
21. Kannel W, Dawber T, McGee D. Perspectives on systolic hypertension: the Framingham Study. *Circulation* 1980;61(6):1179–1182.
22. Garland C, et al. Isolated systolic hypertension and mortality after age 60 years. *Am J Epidemiol* 1983;118(3):365–376.
23. Curb J, et al. Isolated systolic hypertension in 14 communities. *Am J Epidemiol* 1985;121(3):362–370.
24. Kannel W, et al. Systolic blood pressure, arterial rigidity, and risk of stroke: the Framingham Study. *JAMA* 1981;245(12):1225–1229.
25. Gifford R. Isolated systolic hypertension in the elderly: some controversial issues. *JAMA* 1982;247(6):781–785.
26. Priddle W, et al. Amelioration of high blood pressure in the elderly. *J Am Geriatr Soc* 1968;16(8):887–892.
27. Beevers D, et al. Antihypertensive treatment and the course of established cerebral vascular disease. *Lancet* 1973;1:1407–1409.
28. Havlik RJ, et al. Antihypertensive drug therapy and survival by treatment status in a national survey. *Hypertension* 1989;13[Suppl I]:I28–I32.
29. Veterans Administration Cooperative Study Group on Antihypertensive Agents. Effects of treatment on morbidity in hypertension: results in patients with diastolic blood pressures averaging 115 through 129 mm Hg. *JAMA* 1967;202(11):116–122.
30. Veterans Administration Cooperative Study Group on Antihypertensive Agents. Effects of treatment on morbidity in hypertension: II. Results in patients with diastolic blood pressure averaging 90 through 114 mm Hg. *JAMA* 1970;213(7):1143–1152.
31. Veterans Administration Cooperative Study Group on Antihypertensive Agents. Effects of treatment on morbidity in hypertension: III. Influence of age, diastolic pressure, and prior cardiovascular disease; further analysis of side effects. *Circulation* 1972;45:991–1004.
32. Hypertension-Stroke Cooperative Study Group. Effect of antihypertensive treatment on stroke recurrence. *JAMA* 1974;229(4):409–418.
33. Hypertension Detection and Follow-Up Program Cooperative Group. Five-year findings of the Hypertension Detection and Follow-Up Program: I. Reduction in mortality of persons with high blood pressure, including mild hypertension. *JAMA* 1979;242(23):2562–2570.
34. Hypertension Detection and Follow-Up Program Cooperative Group. Five-year findings of the Hypertension Detection and Follow-Up Program. II. Mortality by race-sex and age. *JAMA* 1979;242(23):2572–2577.
35. Curb J, et al. Detection and treatment of hypertension in older individuals. *Am J Epidemiol* 1985;121(3):371–376.
36. Hypertension Detection and Follow-Up Program Cooperative Group. The effect of treatment on mortality in "mild" hypertension: results of the Hypertension Detection and Follow-Up Program. *N Engl J Med* 1982;307(16):976–980.
37. Hypertension Detection and Follow-Up Program Cooperative Group. Five-year findings of the Hypertension Detection and Follow-Up Program. III. Reduction in stroke incidence among persons with high blood pressure. *JAMA* 1982;247(5):633–638.
38. Report by the Management Committee. The Australian Therapeutic Trial in mild hypertension. *Lancet* 1980;(1):1261–1267.
39. Report by the Management Committee. Treatment of mild hypertension in the elderly. *Med J Aust* 1981;2:398–402.
40. Amery A, et al. Antihypertensive therapy in elderly patients: pilot trial of the European Working Party on High Blood Pressure in the Elderly Trial. *Gerontology* 1977;23:426–437.
41. Amery A, et al. Efficacy of antihypertensive drug treatment according to age, sex, blood pressure, and previous cardiovascular disease in patients over the age of 60. *Lancet* 1986;2:589–592.
42. Amery A, et al. Mortality and morbidity results from the European Working Party on High Blood Pressure in the Elderly Trial. *Lancet* 1985;1:1349–1354.
43. Coope J, Warrender T. Randomized trial of treatment of hypertension in elderly patients in primary care. *Br Med J* 1986;293:1145–1152.
44. Hulley S, et al. Systolic Hypertension in the Elderly Program (SHEP): antihypertensive efficacy of chlorthalidone. *Am J Cardiol* 1985;56(15):913–920.
45. Hulley S, et al. Systolic Hypertension in the Elderly Program (SHEP): the first three months. *J Am Geriatr Soc* 1986;34(2):101–105.
46. SHEP Cooperative Research Group. Prevention of stroke by antihypertensive drug treatment in older persons with isolated systolic hypertension. *JAMA* 1991;265:(24)3255–3264.

47. Forette F, Boller F. Hypertension and the risk of dementia in the elderly. *Am J Med* 1991;90[Suppl 3A]:3A-14S–3A-19S.
48. Dahlof B, Lindholm LH, Hansson L, Schersten B, Ekbom T, Wester PO. Morbidity and mortality in the Swedish trial in old patients with hypertension (STOP-Hypertension). *Lancet* 1991;338:1281–1285.
49. MRC Working Party. Medical Research Council Trial of treatment of hypertension in older adults: principal results. *Br Med J* 1992;304:405–411.
50. Beard K, Bulpitt C, Taylor HM, O'Malley K, Sever P, Webb S. Management of elderly patients with sustained hypertension. *Br Med J* 1992;304:412–416.
51. Hypertension Detection and Follow-Up Program Cooperative Group. Patient participation in a hypertension control program. *JAMA* 1978;239(15):1507–1514.
52. Gurland BJ, Teresi J, McFate-Smith W, Black D, Hughes G, Edlavitch S. Effects of treatment of isolated systolic hypertension on cognitive status and depression in the elderly. *J Am Geriatr Soc* 1988;36:1015–1022.
53. Amery A, et al. Glucose intolerance during diuretic therapy: results of trial by European Working Party on High Blood Pressure in the Elderly. *Lancet* 1978;1:681–683.
54. Applegate WB, Rutan GH. Advances in management of hypertension in older persons. *JAGS* 1992;40:1164–1174.
55. Applegate WB, Miller ST, Elam JT, Cushman WC, El Derwi D, Brewer A, Graney MJ. Nonpharmacologic intervention to reduce blood pressure in older patients with mild hypertension. *Arch Intern Med* 1992;152:1162–1166.
56. Luft FC. Can nonpharmacological interventions reduce doses of drugs needed for the treatment of hypertension. *Bull WHO* 1992;70(6):685–690.
57. New trials in older hypertensives. *Lancet* 1991;338:1299–1300.
58. Farnsworth TA, Heseltine D. Treatment of elderly hypertensives: some questions remain unanswered. *Age Aging* 1993;22:1–4.

Hypertension: Pathophysiology, Diagnosis, and Management, Second Edition,
edited by J.H. Laragh and B.M. Brenner,
Raven Press, Ltd., New York © 1995.

CHAPTER 11

Hypertension in Women

Ellen Cohen, Mary E. Wheat, Deborah M. Swiderski, and Pamela Charney

In recent years, increasing attention has been focused on the importance of gender in presentation, diagnosis, and management of many common medical conditions. In addition, it has been recognized that frequently women subjects are inadequately represented in clinical research. When women are included, data analysis by gender is infrequently reported (1). Hypertension is the most common chronic medical condition requiring office visits to physicians, and is a major contributing factor to cardiovascular disease. Its importance as a cardiovascular risk factor is at least as significant in women as in men. However, significant questions remain regarding efficacy and safety of antihypertensive therapy in women (2). Before evaluating the impact of gender on management of hypertension, one must reexamine the existing epidemiologic data.

EPIDEMIOLOGY: A GENDER PERSPECTIVE

The current definition of hypertension emphasizes that risk increases with an increasing level of blood pressure. In the United States the threshold for defining hypertension has gradually been lowered. In the Framing-

ham study, hypertension was defined as greater than 160/95, with a borderline category encompassing those with blood pressures between 140/90 and 160/95. Since 1984, however, the Joint National Committee on Detection, Evaluation, and Treatment of High Blood Pressure has defined hypertension as beginning at 140/90 (3). When examining gender trends in the epidemiology of hypertension, it is critical to be aware of differences between studies both in techniques used to assess hypertension (e.g., number of measurements), as well as in its definition.

National surveys based on probability samples of the entire population have examined the epidemiology of hypertension in the United States according to gender and race. The most reliable data pertain to blacks and whites. Some information is available regarding hypertension in Latinos, but no population-based data has been reported for Asian Americans. The National Health and Nutrition Examination Survey II (4) (NHANES II) reported the prevalence of several different categories of hypertension in people 18 to 74 years of age (Fig. 1). When one looks at all hypertensives (defined by systolic blood pressure [BP] >160 or diastolic BP >95 or taking antihypertensive medications), blacks clearly have much higher prevalence rates than whites. Among blacks, women have a higher overall prevalence of hypertension than men. Among whites, women and men have comparable overall rates. In both black and white hypertensives, however, women have a much greater likelihood of having their blood pressure effectively controlled at the time of screening. This observation is sup-

  E. Cohen: Department of Medicine, Montefiore Medical Center, Bronx, New York 10467.
  M. E. Wheat: Student Health Services, Barnard College, New York, NY 10027.
  D. M. Swiderski: Residency Program in Social Medicine, Montefiore Medical Center, Bronx, NY 10467.
  P. Charney: Primary Care Clinic, Bronx Municipal Hospital Center, Bronx, NY 10461.

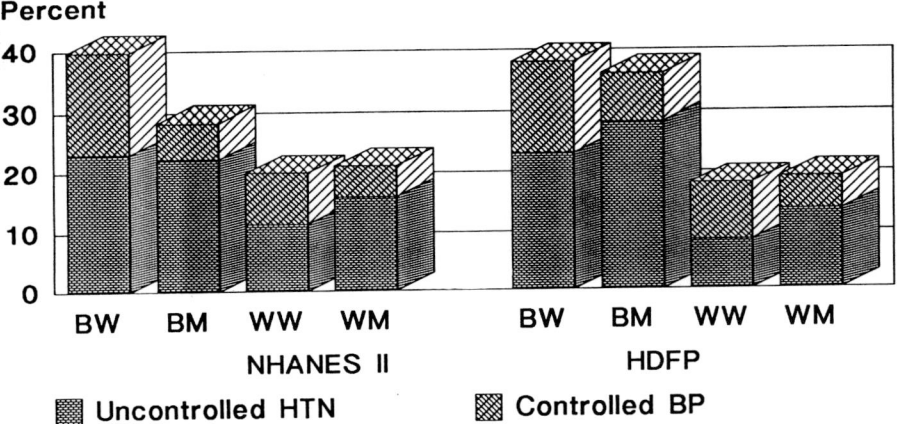

FIG. 1. Race–sex and hypertension, controlled plus uncontrolled HTN.

ported by data from other studies, such as the large, population-based, multicenter Hypertension Detection and Follow-up Program (HDFP) (5). These studies also indicate that women have a greater likelihood than men of knowing that they have high blood pressure, and of taking antihypertensive medications at the time of screening.

NHANES II also reported data for all hypertensives, controlled and uncontrolled, based on a definition of 140/90 (Table 1). Using this definition, the prevalence among all groups except black women rises substantially, particularly among black and white men. White men now have a greater prevalence of hypertension than white women, although black women with hypertension still exceed black men. Prevalence rates among blacks still exceed that for whites by nearly ten percentage points overall.

Information about the prevalence of hypertension in Latina women is based on several recent population surveys, all of which are somewhat problematic in terms of generalization to the diverse Latino population in the United States. Two studies, the Laredo study (6) and the San Antonio Heart study (7), examined prevalence in predominantly Mexican-American populations. The Laredo study found prevalence rates in women that were similar to those observed in white women until age 59, and then were higher at older ages, similar to those found in black women. The San Antonio Heart Study found Mexican-American women to have rates very similar to white non-Latina women in comparable socioeconomic groups.

The only survey that has examined the prevalence of hypertension in different Latino subgroups in this country is the Hispanic Health and Nutrition Examination Survey (HHANES) (8). The population prevalences found in HHANES are lower than those noted previously in blacks or whites, and lower than most other surveys including either Mexican-Americans or Puerto Ricans. Several methodologic problems have been identified that may make this an unreliable estimate of hypertension in Latina women (9). Nonetheless, among older age groups, the prevalence of hypertension in Mexican-American women and men equalled that in whites, but the prevalence in Cuban-Americans and Puerto Ricans continued to be lower (Table 2). As in whites, the prevalence of hypertension in Mexican-American and Cuban-American women exceeded that in men after age 65.

Another way to look at gender differences in hypertension is to examine incidence rates. Data for black and white women and men is provided by the NHANES I Epidemiologic Follow-up Study (NHEFS), which looked at the development of newly detected hypertension a mean of 9.5 years after initial screening for NHANES I (10). According to NHEFS, women and men developed hypertension at similar rates in all age groups, with steadily increasing incidence rates at each 10-year age interval. At all ages black women and men consistently had incidence rates at least twice those of their white counterparts. As the population ages, women and men develop hypertension at similarly increasing rates, while at the same time men are dying at younger ages than women.

TABLE 1. *NHANES II: hypertension prevalence by gender and race for ages 18–74*[a]

Women		Men		All races		Women and men	
Black	White	Black	White	Women	Men	Black	White
38.6	25.3	37.9	32.6	26.8	33.0	38.2	28.8

[a] Figures are percentages. SBP >140 or DBP >90, average of three readings on one occasion, or on antihypertensive medication.

TABLE 2. *Hypertension prevalence by gender and age in latinos, blacks, and whites in HHANES and NHANES II[a]*

Age group	Mexican-American[b]		Cuban-American[b]		Puerto Rican[b]		White[c]		Black[c]	
	Women	Men	Women	Men	Women	Men	Women	Men	Women	Men
18–74	14.1	16.8	15.5	22.8	11.5	15.6	25.3	32.6	38.6	37.9
45–54	24.1	28.5	15.2	37.5	23.7	26.4	36.3	42.6	67.4	55.2
55–64	44.9	47.2	35.6	41.4	47	51.1	50	51.4	74.3	66.3
65–74	66.8	59.6	49.8	46.3	55.2	[d]	66.2	59.2	82.9	67.1

[a] Figures are percentages.
[b] HHANES subjects. SBP >140 or DBP >90, average of two measurements on one occasion, or on antihypertensive medication.
[c] NHANES II subjects. SBP >140 or DBP >90, average of three measurements on one occasion, or on antihypertensive medication.
[d] Sample size too small for reliable estimate.

Thus, by age 65, hypertensive women actually outnumber hypertensive men in the overall population.

The potential sequelae of hypertension include stroke, myocardial infarction, congestive heart failure, and renal insufficiency. Treatment of hypertension is justified by documenting a reduction of such endpoints, hopefully translating into a reduction of overall mortality, when blood pressure is reduced. Because cardiovascular disease is the major cause of morbidity and mortality in women and men over age 60 in the United States, the most clinically relevant way to look at the relative risk of hypertension in women and men is in terms of its contribution to cardiovascular events. Hypertensive men have a higher incidence of cardiovascular endpoints than do hypertensive women at all ages, as demonstrated by 20-year follow-up data from the Framingham study (11). However, the attributable risk percent, that is, the proportion of such events that could theoretically be prevented by removing hypertension as a risk factor ([Ihypertensive − Inormotensive]/Ihypertensive) is similar or higher in women than in men at all ages. Extrapolating Framingham data to the entire white U.S. population shows that the absolute number of cardiovascular events attributable to hypertension is actually greater in women than in men by age 65 to 74 years (Fig. 2). This parallels prevalence data in all racial groups studied which indicate a higher prevalence of hypertension in women than in men by age 65.

These epidemiologic data confirm that hypertension is common in women, that many women are treated for hypertension, and that such treatment, if effective in reducing adverse outcomes, has major public health implications.

TARGET ORGAN ASSESSMENT

Preventing damage to target organs is an important goal of reducing elevated blood pressure. As discussed previously, men have a higher incidence rate of total cardiovascular endpoints than women at all ages. However, when one looks at a specific endpoint such as stroke, which is most associated with hypertension as a risk factor, hypertensive men and women have a similarly increased relative risk of stroke over time (2.3 for women,

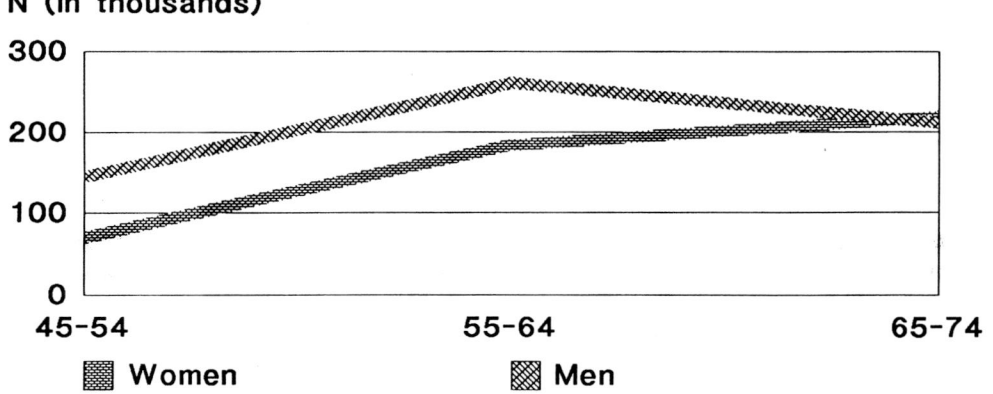

Framingham Data Extrapolated to White U.S. Population

N (in thousands)

FIG. 2. Cardiovascular events attributable to hypertension.

2.7 for men at 18 years follow-up in the Framingham study) (12).

The significance of left ventricular hypertrophy (LVH) as a sequela of hypertension has also been elucidated by the Framingham study. Echocardiographically-proven LVH was independently associated with increased risk of all measured endpoints (13). For cardiovascular disease overall, women and men with LVH had a similarly increased relative risk (women 1.49, men 1.57). For cardiovascular death and death from all causes, women with LVH had a greater increase in relative risk than men (women 2.12 and 2.01 compared with men 1.73 and 1.49). To date there is no adequate data regarding the effect of antihypertensive therapy on LVH in women (14,15).

Several studies have recently examined the contribution of hypertension to the development of renal disease, utilizing serum creatinine determinations in population-based studies (16–18). Women on average have lower serum creatinine values than men, a difference that is not taken into account in some data analyses, making the validity of their gender-specific findings questionable. The one study that did correct for normal gender differences in serum creatinine found that both women and men with higher blood pressure levels in 1974 had an increased risk of hypercreatininemia 15 years later (relative odds 1.56 in women, 2.08 in men) (16).

Overall it appears that women and men suffer similar consequences of hypertension, at fairly comparable rates. Hypertensive women should thus be monitored for the development of cerebrovascular disease and renal insufficiency. Whether or not hypertensive women or men should routinely be evaluated echocardiographically for the presence of LVH remains controversial.

MANAGEMENT OF HYPERTENSION

Evaluation for Secondary Causes

There are multiple secondary causes of elevated blood pressure that occur in women. The most common of these, alcohol use (see section on Nonpharmacological Therapy), oral contraceptives, and noncompliance with treatment, are often overlooked by clinicians.

Oral contraceptives are cited as the most frequent reversible cause of secondary hypertension. Cohort studies of women taking estrogen/progestogen pills indicate an average 5–7 mm Hg increase in systolic blood pressure, with a smaller 1–2 mm Hg rise in diastolic blood pressure. This increase is more likely to occur in women in their mid-30s and older. The risk of developing overt hypertension is increased two- to sixfold, and occurs in about 5 percent of women (19). Some data suggests that these changes differ among races (20–22). Increases in blood pressure seem to be attributable both to the estro-

genic and progestogenic content. Little data is available regarding the risks of hypertension associated with progesterone only methods (e.g., Norplant, mini-pill).

Women using oral contraceptives need periodic monitoring of their blood pressure. If overt hypertension occurs, the medication should be stopped and in most cases blood pressure will normalize within 3 months. For women whose pressure increases to the high normal range and who have high cardiovascular risk profiles, other contraceptive options should be explored, and the risks of an unwanted pregnancy weighed against the risks of an increase in blood pressure.

Renovascular disease, the cause of elevated blood pressure in about 0.5 percent of all hypertensives, is important to diagnose since its treatment may enable the cessation of antihypertensive therapy. Atherosclerosis is responsible for about two-thirds of all renovascular hypertension and occurs twice as frequently in younger men than women with the sex distribution equalizing in the elderly. Fibromuscular dysplasia, on the other hand, is the most common cause of renovascular hypertension under age 40 and occurs predominantly in women (23,24). Findings suggestive of renovascular hypertension include abdominal bruits and lack of response to intensive pharmacotherapy.

Pheochromocytoma is an exceedingly rare cause of hypertension (0.1 percent), but should be thought of in women because it may first appear during pregnancy and, if not identified, be associated with adverse outcomes. Orthostatic hypotension, sweating, pallor, and tachycardia should alert the clinician to the possibility of pheochromocytoma (25). Thyroid disease occurs ten times more frequently in women than men; however, its role as a cause of hypertension remains unclear (26).

Effects on Hypertensive Complications

The major clinical trials have enrolled variable proportions of women subjects, and may or may not analyze data for women separately. In addition, they have examined and combined different clinical endpoints, making comparisons between studies somewhat confusing (Table 3). Three of the major trials (the Veterans Administration trials, the Oslo study, and the Multiple Risk Factor Intervention Trial) included no women subjects. None of the major treatment trials, even those that included women, set out to examine effects of hypertension therapy by gender; thus, such *post hoc* analyses must be viewed with caution (2).

The clinical endpoint for which there is the clearest evidence of benefit from blood pressure reduction in both black and white women, as well as men, is the incidence of stroke. This finding has now been demonstrated clearly in several treatment trials, the earliest of which was HDFP (27). Unlike the other major treatment trials,

TABLE 3. *A quarter century of hypertension treatment studies*

Study (reference)	Number of subjects	Percentage of women	Analysis by gender
Hypertension Detection and Follow-up Program	10,940	46	Decreased mortality in black women and all men Possible increased mortality in white women [Reduced strokes in all groups]
The Australian Therapeutic Trial	3,427	37	36% decrease in adverse outcome in women (p = N.S.) 26% decrease in adverse outcome in men ($p < 0.05$)
Medical Research Council Trial	17,354	48	26% increased mortality in women (p = N.S.) 15% decreased mortality in men ($p < 0.05$) Reduced total cardiovascular events in women and men
European Working Party on Hypertension in the Elderly	840	70	18% reduction in cardiovascular mortality in women (p = N.S.)
Systolic Hypertension in the Elderly Program	4,736	57	Decreased strokes in black and white women and white men Reductions in other cardiovascular events in total population
Medical Research Council Trial in Older Adults	4,396	58	Decreased strokes in women and men
Multiple Risk Factor Intervention Trial	12,866	0	Not applicable
The Oslo Study	785	0	Not applicable
Veterans Administration Cooperative Study	523	0	Not applicable

HDFP was not placebo-controlled, but randomized subjects to either a systematic antihypertensive regimen with free access to health care (stepped care), or their usual source of care in the community (referred care). At 5 years of follow-up the investigators found significant reductions in the secondary endpoints of both fatal and nonfatal stroke in all four race-gender groups (blacks and whites, women and men). More recently, the Systolic Hypertension in the Elderly Program (SHEP) (28) and the Medical Research Council (MRC) trial of treatment of hypertension in older adults (29) both demonstrated reductions in stroke rates in women and men over age 60 by treating either isolated systolic hypertension in the case of SHEP or combined hypertension in the MRC trial.

When looking at effects of antihypertensive therapy on other cardiovascular endpoints in women, studies have shown conflicting results. Given the inadequate numbers of women enrolled and their relatively low rates of cardiovascular events, it is difficult to draw conclusions about the effects of antihypertensive therapy on non-stroke cardiovascular outcomes in women. A met-analysis currently in progress seems to suggest that the cardiovascular benefit in women is similar to that in men (S. Wassertheil-Smoller, M. E. Wheat, D. M. Swiderski, E. Cohen, and P. Charney, 1994).

The summary criterion for the overall efficacy of any therapeutic maneuver is all-cause mortality. In the assessment of antihypertensive therapy in women, mortality analysis yields conflicting results. For example, HDFP showed a reduction in all-cause mortality in the total study population in the Stepped Care group (30). A

post hoc analysis showed the greatest reduction in mortality in black women, and substantially reduced mortality in black and white men in stepped care, but a small, nonsignificant increase in mortality in white women in stepped care (31). Similarly, the MRC trial showed a statistically significant reduction in all-cause mortality in men, but a nonstatistically significant increased mortality in women in the active treatment group (32). In fact, the difference in mortality rates between women and men was statistically significant. Conversely, the Australian Therapeutic Trial found a statistically significant reduction in total events in men, whereas women had a numerically greater reduction that did not achieve statistical significance. However, this study combined all-cause mortality with total cardiovascular morbidity (33). Thus, in *post hoc* analyses of these three major studies, one suggested benefit, one showed no effect, and one suggested increased risk in treated white women.

Overall, these data demonstrate the efficacy of antihypertensive therapy in reducing stroke rates in both women and men, black and white. However, given the small numbers of women studied and differences in data reported, conclusions regarding effects on other cardiovascular events and mortality cannot be drawn.

Blood Pressure Response to Pharmacotherapy

Innumerable small and large trials comparing blood pressure response to a variety of drugs have included variable proportions of women subjects. Few of these studies, however, include gender analysis or offer meaningful information about differences or similarities between women and men in terms of blood pressure response to drugs.

Two small studies suggested that diltiazem might be particularly effective in women (34,35). Applegate et al. (34) compared atenolol, enalapril, and diltiazem in 240 women 65 years of age or older. They found all three drugs to effectively lower blood pressure, but diltiazem lowered it more. A small study in middle-aged, obese black women found a thiazide to be more effective than clonidine in lowering both systolic and diastolic blood pressure (36). Interestingly, hypertensive women have been observed to have lower renin levels than men, which might provide a physiologic explanation for these findings (36a,37).

The MRC trial did report drug withdrawal rates by gender (38). Thirty-three percent of women were withdrawn from diuretic therapy, compared with 40 percent in the beta-blocker and placebo groups. The withdrawal rates in men were 43 percent, 42 percent, and 47 percent, respectively. Thus, women were withdrawn from diuretic therapy less often than men ($p < 0.05$). However, since drug withdrawal occurred both because of lack of efficacy as well as side effects, even this large trial with substantial numbers of women contributes little to our knowledge of gender response to pharmacotherapy.

Nonpharmacologic Therapy

Since all antihypertensive drug therapies have at least some adverse effects, whether biomedical or financial, nonpharmacologic therapy is indicated as primary or adjunctive therapy in all hypertensive persons. Women have been included in most trials of these therapeutic modalities; however, gender analyses of different lifestyle modifications have rarely been performed.

Consistent evidence supports the antihypertensive efficacy of weight reduction. Randomized controlled trials have demonstrated the ability of weight loss to reduce blood pressure in both normotensive and hypertensive persons (39,40), as well as their efficacy in the primary and secondary prevention of hypertension (41–43). Indeed, as noted by Reisin (44), only two groups of investigators failed to note a positive effect of weight loss on reduction of high blood pressure, and these studies were characterized by several design flaws. In three of the larger nonpharmacologic therapy trials, between 30 and 45 percent of the subjects were women, with total subjects ranging from 692 to 2,182 (39,40,43). Nonetheless, none of these studies analyzed their results separately for men and women, although gender was included in linear regression analyses and did not alter results significantly. Given the results of these and other studies (45–47), there seems little reason to question the beneficial blood

pressure effects of weight reduction in overweight women. Since obesity in the United States is significantly more common among middle-aged women than middle-aged men (48), and the benefits of pharmacologic antihypertensive therapy are less well-defined among white women, particularly those under 60 years of age, weight reduction is a particularly important approach to reducing hypertensive complications.

Physical activity is an important component of any weight reduction program; however, its effect on blood pressure has been much less well-studied in women than in men. A recent review of the efficacy of habitual physical activity in lowering blood pressure (49) identified eight randomized, controlled trials published since 1980. Three of these trials included a total of 19 women; one additional trial with 33 participants included men and women, but did not specify numbers. No gender analyses have been performed. An earlier review of the literature identified two additional small controlled trials which included women, the larger of which was an adolescent population (50). Nonetheless, because physical activity has well-documented benefits in women, including reduced risk of osteoporosis (51,52), facilitation of weight control (48), lower rates of diabetes (53), and decreased overall mortality (54), its inclusion as a potentially useful modality to lower blood pressure is justified.

A strong body of literature also supports the efficacy of sodium restriction in reducing blood pressure, in both hypertensive and normotensive persons (55). As with weight reduction, many of these trials have included women, but gender analyses have not been performed. Furthermore, many investigators have noted marked heterogeneity in sodium sensitivity, as well as the interaction of sodium sensitivity with dietary intake of potassium and calcium (56). Weinberger's group also noted that plasma renin activity was significantly lower in sodium-sensitive individuals than in those who were sodium-resistant, although renin activity alone did not predict sodium responsiveness accurately (57). Data from the Trial of Antihypertensive Interventions and Management (TAIM) study also indicated an interaction between plasma renin levels and diastolic blood pressure response to nonpharmacologic therapy (weight reduction, low sodium/high potassium) (58). Since hypertensive women have been observed to have lower renin levels than hypertensive men (37), a possible gender difference in the antihypertensive efficacy of sodium restriction should be specifically examined in future research.

Studies examining other dietary maneuvers such as potassium supplementation, calcium or magnesium supplementation, and reduction of saturated fat have yielded conflicting results (59). The potential interaction of these ions with dietary sodium intake has already been mentioned. Heterogeneity has been noted in both blood pressure response to calcium or magnesium supplementation, and in epidemiologic associations between calcium and magnesium intake and blood pressure levels (60,61). Serum ionized calcium and magnesium levels have been observed to vary with plasma renin activity, although in opposite directions (62). Because of the suggestion of an interaction of gender with plasma renin activity, gender may be an important consideration in delineating groups likely to benefit from particular dietary advice and deserves specific investigation. When considering the potential usefulness of increased potassium intake as a nonpharmacologic therapy for hypertension in women, one must remember that regardless of the inconclusive data to date regarding its antihypertensive efficacy, epidemiologic data from the Rancho Bernardo study suggests a 4.8-fold increase in stroke-associated mortality in women (compared with 2.6 in men) in the lowest tertile of potassium intake when compared with those in the top two tertiles (63).

Alcohol intake has been associated with increased blood pressure in several large cross-sectional and cohort studies which included both substantial numbers of women and gender analyses (64–68). The risk of hypertension appears to follow a j-shaped curve, being lowest in those reporting 1–7 drinks per week, in women as in men. The risk of increased blood pressure increases significantly at intakes greater than 2–3 drinks per day. In addition, elevated blood pressure can be associated with alcohol withdrawal. In the Hypertension Control Program, which enrolled participants from the HDFP trial, alcohol reduction was combined with other nutritional changes (weight loss, sodium restriction) to control blood pressure effectively (47). A post hoc regression analysis, however, did not report alcohol as a significant contributor to the study effect. Furthermore, no gender analyses were performed, although approximately 40 percent of the trial participants were women.

Relaxation techniques have been shown to reduce blood pressure in some studies (69), but not in others (39,70). Again, women have been represented in these studies, but gender analyses have not been performed. Interestingly, Pickering et al. noted that "white-coat" hypertensives are significantly more likely to be women (71). Perloff noted that the increased discrepancy between office blood pressure and ambulatory blood pressure that occurred with increasing age was more pronounced in women (72). This study also found that the difference in the number of adverse events between those with high and low ambulatory blood pressures was significant in women only for systolic blood pressure. In men it was significant both for systolic and diastolic blood pressure. This suggestion of greater blood pressure reactivity among women supports the need for studies to explore the efficacy of relaxation and/or biofeedback approaches to reducing blood pressure in women.

Since questions remain regarding optimal drug therapy in women, particularly those who are white and

younger, gender analyses of women's response to non-pharmacologic therapy would be welcome. Even with post hoc analyses, consistency of effect among the different trials would be important information to support a vigorous approach to nonpharmacologic therapy in women. If, on the other hand, gender analyses of nonpharmacologic maneuvers yield conflicting results, as they have with drug therapy, this would argue that additional studies in women were needed, including research to elucidate separately in women and men pathophysiologic parameters of importance, such as plasma renin activity or blood pressure reactivity.

SIDE EFFECTS OF ANTIHYPERTENSIVE DRUGS

The side effects of antihypertensive drugs are legion. They include serious adverse effects such as metabolic disturbances and financial and quality-of-life issues. Proper selection of indicated antihypertensive drugs minimizes such risk and may even confer benefit (e.g., thiazides and reduced risk of hip fracture) (73).

General Side Effects

Most of the major hypertension treatment trials include information about general side effects of therapy. A gender analysis of side effects, however, is available only from the MRC trial, and, to a limited extent, from HDFP. In the MRC trial, women were less likely than men to be withdrawn from thiazide therapy because of adverse effects (12.8 percent versus 17 percent, $p < 0.05$), while women and men on propranolol had similar withdrawal rates (38). Although women in the placebo group reported higher rates of all side effects than did men, men and women treated with diuretic and propranolol reported new complaints of most specific adverse effects with the same frequency. One exception was the incidence of gout and hyperuricemia, which was increased in men, but not women on thiazides. The HDFP trial also suggested that black and white women were more likely than men to report at least one symptomatic side effect at baseline (74). For new symptoms not reported at baseline, however, men of both races were more likely to list at least one side effect than women (16 percent versus 11 percent for whites; 15 percent versus 12 percent for blacks, $p < 0.05$).

In a large postmarketing surveillance study of captopril, the proportion of patients reporting adverse events did not differ by gender (75). There was no gender analysis of specific adverse events except sexual function (see below). A small randomized controlled trial of captopril suggested that women were more likely than men to develop a cough, although this did not reach statistical significance (76). Finally, Croog et al. examined adverse effects according to gender in black hypertensive women and men randomized to atenolol, captopril, or verapamil-SR (77). There were no differences between drug groups at the end of the trial when examined by gender. Both women and men reported less hand numbness and headache on atenolol. Women also reported less feeling worn out, faint, or depressed. Men on captopril and verapamil-SR reported no improvement for any parameters; however women on captopril were less worn out, less faint, less fatigued, and reported fewer headaches. Only dry mouth was reported less frequently by women taking verapamil-SR.

Quality-of-life Effects

In recent years, clinical studies of antihypertensive drug therapy have focused increasingly on the effects of drug therapy on various measures of quality of life. Many of these studies have included a significant proportion of women subjects, thus making gender analysis possible.

In the Treatment of Mild Hypertension (TOMH) Study, only women reported an improvement in general health associated with weight loss, although both men and women showed a statistically significant improvement in energy/fatigue measures and general function with weight loss (78). Data on older women is also available from Applegate's trial of the efficacy and quality of life effects of atenolol, diltiazem, and enalapril (34). Withdrawal rates were similar for the three drugs, though there was a trend toward less withdrawal from enalapril (46 percent versus 53 percent and 54 percent). There was also a trend toward lower quality of life for participants on atenolol in the areas of general well-being, depression, and digit symbol manipulation; however, many comparisons were made and only one reached statistical significance.

The most detailed quality-of-life data has been reported by Croog in the study mentioned earlier (77). There were no significant intergroup differences between women and men at the conclusion of the trial for any quality-of-life measures. Women reported a significant improvement in general well-being and scored higher on measures of visual-motor coordination on all three drugs. Women on captopril and atenolol reported fewer physical symptoms. Women on captopril also reported less irritability/anger, whereas women on atenolol reported improved sleep.

From the limited data available there is no clear gender trend regarding general side effects or quality-of-life effects of antihypertensive therapy. Women appear to report more symptoms at baseline, but the development of new symptoms while on therapy is comparable between men and women. Future studies should collect and report side effects by gender; accurate data on adverse effects could facilitate appropriate selection of therapy for an individual patient.

Sexual Side Effects

Since sexual side effects are often cited as a common reason for patient dissatisfaction or noncompliance with antihypertensive therapy, it is important to document their impact in women. The sexual response cycle has similar physiologic mechanisms in women and men. It would therefore seem reasonable to hypothesize that medications that cause sexual dysfunction in men may have similar effects in women. Although few of the earlier treatment trials examined sexual side effects in women, more recent studies are reporting this data (79).

The TAIM study showed no statistically significant sexual impairment in women treated with low-dose chlorthalidone or atenolol as compared with placebo (80). Interestingly, sexual function improved in women and men treated with weight loss regardless of concurrent assignment to drug therapy or placebo. Although the SHEP study did not include a separate gender analysis of sexual side effects, 57 percent of subjects were women and there was no statistically significant increase in sexual side effects in the drug-treated participants. Croog provided a more detailed analysis of sexual side effects among black men and women on atenolol, verapamil, and captopril. In men on captopril, sexual function improved significantly. Women demonstrated a numerically larger improvement on the sexual function scale used, but this failed to reach statistical significance since fewer women were randomized to captopril. The TOMH Study reported a 3 percent incidence of problems related to sexual activity in women, as compared with a 10 percent incidence in men. However, there were no statistically significant differences between any of the six drug and placebo treatment groups in women or men. In the postmarketing study of captopril mentioned previously, a statistically significant improvement was noted in sexual quality of life among both women and men. Importantly, there was no placebo control.

Assessment of sexual side effects has been further confounded by study methodology. Many studies have framed their questions about sexual function in terms of male physiology (e.g., erection, ejaculation). One recent study has evaluated the utility of a self-administered diary for assessing sexual function in women (81). Future treatment trials must continue to include such survey instruments.

This preliminary data suggest that women experience sexual dysfunction with antihypertensives analogous to that previously reported in men. Clearly, however, more detailed information is needed about gender-specific sexual side effects of a variety of pharmacologic agents from studies that include adequate numbers of women, and that stratify subjects by gender at randomization.

Serum Lipids

Levels of serum lipids, including total, high-density lipoprotein (HDL), and low-density lipoprotein (LDL) cholesterol have been shown to be related to cardiovascular endpoints in women and men (82). The potential benefits of antihypertensive drug therapy in reducing cardiovascular risk may be compromised by adverse alterations in lipid levels caused by these medications.

Although lipid physiology is known to differ by gender, few studies of antihypertensive therapy have included gender analysis of effects on lipids (83). Clearly such analysis must include menopausal status as a critical confounding variable. The MRC Trial did show an increase in total cholesterol in both women and men treated with bendrofluazide, propranolol, or methyldopa (38). However, neither specific lipoprotein levels nor menopausal status was reported. Boehringer et al. found an increase in LDL and total cholesterol in postmenopausal but not premenopausal women treated with chlorthalidone. Unfortunately, menopausal status was defined by age alone (84). In the TAIM study chlorthalidone raised total cholesterol, whereas nutritional therapy lowered it (40). In a multiple regression analysis of factors related to change in total cholesterol, gender was not a significant predictor.

It is essential that future research on antihypertensive therapies include analysis of lipid effects by gender, as well as defining menopausal status by clinical and laboratory markers.

APPROACH TO THE INDIVIDUAL WOMAN

There is a noticeable scarcity of data regarding the management of hypertension in women. However, the published data suggest that gender, like race (85,86) and age (28,87), influences the natural history, and the response to treatment of hypertension. It is clear that hypertension is quite prevalent in women, that it causes sequelae similar to those experienced by men, and that blood pressure reduction leads to reduction in stroke rates in women.

When a woman has been diagnosed with mild (140–159/90–99) or moderate (160–179/100–109) hypertension, a vigorous 3 to 6-month trial of indicated nonpharmacologic therapy should be pursued. Because of its lower risk profile, nonpharmacologic therapy must always be considered the cornerstone of blood pressure treatment. Its benefit has been demonstrated not only in those labeled hypertensive, but also in those with high-normal blood pressure (SBP 130–139 or DBP 85–89) who are at high risk of developing frank hypertension. If there is evidence of target organ damage (TOD) or of other cardiovascular risk factors, then the prompt addition of pharmacologic treatment is appropriate. Because epidemiologic data suggests more dramatic benefit from

TABLE 4. *Individualizing antihypertensive therapy*

Drug class	Co-morbid conditions	Contraindications or special monitoring required
Initial therapy		
Thiazide diuretics	Osteoporosis; CHF*	Glucose intolerance; hypercholesterolemia; preeclampsia; IHSS**; gout
Loop diuretics	Renal insufficiency; diabetes; gout	
Potassium-sparing diuretics		Renal insufficiency; ACE-inhibitor use
Beta blockers	Angina; IHSS; vascular headaches; post-MI***	CHF*, bronchospasm; heart block; bradycardia; PAD****
ACE-inhibitors	CHF*; diabetes	Pregnancy or planning pregnancy; IHSS**; renal artery stenosis
Calcium antagonists	Angina; diabetes; IHSS**#; vascular headaches	CHF*; bradycardia; heart block
Alpha₁ antagonists	Hypercholesterolemia	IHSS**
Supplemental agents		
Alpha₂ agonists	Pregnancy or planning pregnancy##	Depression; liver disease##
Direct vasodilators	Pregnancy or planning pregnancy (Hydralazine)	Agina; IHSS**; post-MI***
Reserpine		Depression; Peptic Ulcer Disease

* CHF, Congestive heart failure.
** IHSS, Idiopathic hypertrophic sub-aortic stenosis.
*** Post-MI, Post myocardial infarction.
**** PAD, peripheral arterial disease.
#, Diltiazem, Verapamil.
##, Methyldopa.

pharmacologic therapy in black women than white, the treatment threshold may be lower in blacks. Nonpharmacologic therapy should continue to be employed, particularly in view of its favorable impact on side effects such as sexual dysfunction.

Women with mild or moderate hypertension who have not responded to nonpharmacologic therapy should be begun on monotherapy. At this time, unless contraindicated, diuretics or beta blockers should be the initial pharmacotherapy, since these are the only agents demonstrated to decrease stroke, mortality, and probably other cardiovascular endpoints (88). Other authorities contest this recommendation, noting that the relative failure of antihypertensive therapy to have impact on rates of myocardial infarction, as compared with stroke, may be a result of unfavorable effects of these agents on lipid and glucose metabolism (89). Noting that calcium-channel antagonists, angiotensin-converting enzyme inhibitors, and selective α_1-adrenergic blockers are all effective monotherapies for blood pressure reduction, they cite evidence of favorable metabolic and vascular actions of these drugs that could augment their effectiveness in reducing cardiovacsular complications of hypertension. Gender-specific data analysis regarding responses to the newer antihypertensive agents is currently only available in a limited number of short-term studies. In addition, the cost of pharmacotherapy increases with the newer agents which may have a more adverse impact on women, who are more likely to be poor or lack insurance (90).

Black women, who tend to have lower renin levels than whites, may do better with a diuretic or calcium-channel blocker than with a beta blocker or angiotensin-converting enzyme (ACE) inhibitor. Thiazide diuretics may be particularly desirable in women at risk for osteoporosis (e.g., thin, white women). Table 4 outlines advantages and disadvantages of commonly used pharmacologic agents for hypertensive woman.

There is a striking paucity of data regarding side effects of the commonly used antihypertensive agents in women. Clinicians need to be vigilant in monitoring for potential adverse effects. A collaborative working relationship between the woman and her physician will facilitate compliance and accurate reporting of side effects during prolonged treatment of a chronic condition.

REFERENCES

1. Charney P, Morgan C. "Do treatment recommendations reported in the 1990 research literature consider differences between men and women?" 1993. (Submitted for publication).
2. Anastos K, Charney P, Charon RA, et al. *Ann Intern Med* 1991;115:287–293.
3. "The Fifth Report of the Joint National Committee on Detection, Evaluation, and Treatment of High Blood Pressure." *Arch Intern Med* 1993;153:154–183.
4. National Center for Health Statistics, Rowland M, Roberts J. *Advance data from vital and health statistics of the National Center for Health Statistics of the National Center for Health Sciences.* Rockville, MD: Public Health Service; 1982; No. 84:1–12.
5. Hypertension Detection and Follow-up Program Cooperative Group. *JAMA* 1977;237:2385–2391.
6. Stern MP, Gaskill SP, Allen CR, Garza V, Gonzales JL, Waldrop RH. *Am J Epidemiol* 1981;113(5):556–562.
7. Franco LJ, Stern MP, Rosenthal M, Haffner SM, Hazuda HP, Comeaux PJ. *Am J Epidemiol* 1985;121:684–696.
8. Pappas G, Gergen PJ, Carroll M. *Am J Public Health* 1990;80:1431–1436.
9. Geronimus AT, Neidert LJ, Bound J. *Am J Public Health* 1990;80:1437–1442.
10. Cornoni-Huntley J, LaCroix AZ, Havlik RJ. *Arch Intern Med* 1989;149:780–788.
11. Lerner DJ, Kannel WB. *Am Heart J* 1986;111:383–390.
12. Kannel WB, Wolf PA, Verter J, McNamara P. *JAMA* 1970;214:301–310.
13. Levy D, Garrison RJ, Savage DD, Kannel WB, Castelli WP. *N Engl J Med* 1990;322:1561–1566.
14. Schulman SP, Weiss JL, Becker LC, et al. *N Engl J Med* 1990;322:1350–1355.
15. McFate Smith W. *Am J Cardiol* 1985;55:3A–8A.
16. Perneger TV, Nieto FJ, Whelton PK, Klag MJ, Comstock GW, Szklo M. *JAMA* 1993;269:488–493.
17. Perneger TV, Klag MJ, Feldman HI, Whelton PK. *JAMA* 1993;269:1272–1277.
18. Shulman NB, Ford CE, Hall WD, et al. *Hypertension* 1989;13(Suppl I):180–I93.
19. Woods JW. *Hypertension* 1988;11:II11–II15.
20. Khaw K, Peart WS. *Br Med J* 1982;285:402–407.
21. Layde PM, Beral V, Kay CR. *Lancet* 1981;1:541–546.
22. Blumenstein BA, Douglas MB, Hall WD. *Am J Epidemiol* 1980;112:539–552.
23. Mann SJ, Pickering TC. *Ann Intern Med* 1992;117:845–853.
24. Ram C, Venkata S. *Cardiol Clin* 1988;6:483–508.
25. Manger WM, Gifford RW, eds. Laragh JH, Brenner BM, *Hypertension: pathophysiology, diagnosis, and management.* New York: Raven Press Ltd, 1990:1639–1657.
26. Klein I. In: Laragh JH, Brenner BM, eds. *Hypertension: pathophysiology, diagnosis, and management.* New York: Raven Press; 1990:1661–1672.
27. Hypertension Detection and Follow-up Program Cooperative Group. *JAMA* 1982;247:633–638.
28. SHEP Cooperative Research Group. *JAMA* 1991;265:3255–3264.
29. MRC Working Party. *Br Med J* 1992;304:405–412.
30. Hypertension Detection and Follow-up Program Cooperative Group. *JAMA* 1979;242:2572–2577.
31. Schnall PL, Alderman MH, Kern R. *NY State J Med* 1984;84:299–301.
32. Medical Research Council Working Party. *Br Med J* 1985;291:97–104.
33. Report by the Management Committee. *Lancet* 1980;1:1261–1267.
34. Applegate WB, Phillips HL, Schnaper J, et al. *Arch Intern Med* 1991;151:1817–1823.
35. Massie B, MacCarthy EP, Ramanathan KB, et al. *Ann Intern Med* 1987;107:150–157.
36. Reisin E, Weed SG. *J Hypertens* 1992;10:489–493.
36a. Alderman M, Madhavan S, Cohen H, Sealey J, Laragh JH. 1993. (Submitted for publication).
37. Meade TW, Imeson JD, Gordon D, Peart WS. *Clin Science* 1983;64:273–280.
38. Medical Research Council Working Party on Mild to Moderate Hypertension. *Lancet* 1981:539–543.
39. The Trials of Hypertension Prevention Collaborative Research Group. *JAMA* 1992;267:1213–1220.
40. Oberman A, Wassertheil-Smoller S, Langford HG, et al. *Ann Intern Med* 1990;112:89–95.
41. Stamler R, Stamler J, Gosch FC, et al. *JAMA* 1989;262:1801–1807.
42. Langford HG, Blaufox MD, Oberman A, et al. *JAMA* 1985;253:657–664.
43. Hypertension Prevention Trial Research Group. *Arch Intern Med* 1990;150:153–162.

44. Reisin E. In: Laragh JH, Brenner BM, eds. *Hypertension: pathophysiology, diagnosis, and management.* New York: Raven Press; 1990:2025–2033.
45. Schotte DE, Stunkard AJ. *Arch Intern Med* 1990;150:1701–1704.
46. Reisin E, Abel R, Modan M, Silverberg DS, Eliahou HE, Modan B. *N Engl J Med* 1978;298:1–5.
47. Stamler R, Stamler J, Grimm R, et al. *JAMA* 1987;257:1484–1491.
48. Thompson JK, Jarvie JG, Lahey BB, Cureton KJ. *Psychol Bull* 1982;91:55–79.
49. Arroll B, Beaglehole R. *J Clin Epidemiol* 1992;45:439–447.
50. Seals DR, Hagberg JM. *Med Sci Sports Exercise* 1984;16:207–215.
51. Aloia JF, Cohn SH, Ostuni JA, Cane R, Ellis K. *Ann Intern Med* 1978;89:356–358.
52. Michel BA, Bloch DA, Fries JF. *Arch Intern Med* 1989;149:2325–2329.
53. Helmrich SP, Ragland SR, Leung RW, Paffenbarger RS. *N Engl J Med* 1991;325:147–152.
54. Blair SN, Kohl HW, Paffenberger RS, Clark DG, Cooper KH, Gibbons LW. *JAMA* 1989;262:2395–2401.
55. Cutler JA, Follman D, Elliott P, Suh I. *Hypertension* 1991;17:I27–I33.
56. Weinberger MH. In: Laragh JH, Brenner BM, eds. *Hypertension: pathophysiology, diagnosis, and management.* New York: Raven Press; 1990:1999–2007.
57. Weinberger MH, Miller JZ, Luft FC, Grim CE, Fineberg NS. *Hypertension* 1986;8:II127–II34.
58. Blaufox MD, Lee HB, Davis B, Oberman A, Wassertheil-Smoller S, Langford H. *JAMA* 1992;267:1221–1225.
59. Kaplan NM. *Hypertension* 1991;18:I153–I160.
60. Cutler JA, Brittain E. *Am J Hypertens* 1990;3:1375–1465.
61. Whelton PK, Klag MJ. *Am J Cardiol* 1989;63:26G–30G.
62. Resnick LM, Laragh JH, Sealey JE, Alderman MA. *N Engl J Med* 1983;309:888–891.
63. Khaw K, Barrett-Connor E. *N Engl J Med* 1987;316:235–239.
64. Ueshima H, Ozawa H, Baba S, et al. *J Clin Epidemiol* 1992;45:667–673.
65. Witteman JCM, Willette WC, Stampfer MJ, et al. *Am J Cardiol* 1990;65:633–637.
66. Moore RD, Levine DM, Southard J, Entwisle G, Shapiro S. *Am J Hypertens* 1990;3:1–7.
67. Gruchow HW, Sobocinski KA, Barboriak JJ. *JAMA* 1985;253:1567–1570.
68. Klatsky A, Friedman G, Armstrong M. *Circulation* 1986;73:628–636.
69. Patel C, Marmot MG, Terry DJ, Carruthers M, Hunt B, Patel M. *Br Med J* 1985;290:1103–1106.
70. van Montfrans GA, Karemaker JM, Wieling W, Dunning AJ. *Br Med J* 1990;300:1368–1372.
71. Pickering TG, James GD, Boddie C, Harshfield GA, Blank S, Laragh JH. *JAMA* 1988;259:225–228.
72. Perloff D, Sokolow M, Cowan R. *JAMA* 1983;249:2792–2798.
73. LaCroix AZ, Wienpahl J, White LR, et al. *N Engl J Med* 1990;322:286–290.
74. Curb JD, Borhani NO, Blaszkowski TP, Zimbaldi N, Fotiu S, Williams W. *JAMA* 1985;253:3263–3268.
75. Schoenberger JA, Testa M, Ross AD, Brennan WK, Bannon JA. *Arch Intern Med* 1990;150:301–306.
76. Lefebvre J, Poirier L, Lacourciere Y. *Ann Pharmacother* 1992;26:161–164.
77. Croog SH, Kong W, Levine S, et al. *Arch Intern Med* 1990;150:1733–1741.
78. The Treatment of Mild Hypertension Research Group. *Arch Intern Med* 1991;151:1413–1423.
79. *Med Lett Drugs Ther* 1992;34:73–78.
80. Wassertheil-Smoller S, Blaufox MD, Oberman A, et al. *Ann Intern Med* 1991;114:613–620.
81. Hodge RH, Harward MP, West SM, Krongaard-DeMong L, Kowal-Neeley MB. *J Gen Intern Med* 1991;6:290–294.
82. Godsland IF, Wynn V, Crook D, Miller NE. *Am Heart J* 1987;114:1467–1503.
83. Lardinois CK, Neuman SL. *Arch Intern Med* 1988;148:1280–1288.
84. Boehringer K, Weidmann P, Mordasini R, et al. *Ann Intern Med* 1982;97:206–209.
85. Kittner SJ, White LR, Losonczy KG, Wolf PA, Hebel JR. *JAMA* 1990;264:1267–1270.
86. Moser M. *Am J Med* 1990;88(Suppl 3B):24S–31S.
87. Vokonas PS, Kannel WB, Cupples LA. *J Hypertens* 1988;6(Suppl 1):S3–S9.
88. Alderman MH. *JAMA* 1992;267:2786–2787.
89. Weber MA, Laragh JH. *Arch Intern Med* 1993;153:149–152.
90. Horton JA, ed. *The women's health data book: a profile of women's health in the United States.* Washington, DC: Elsevier; 1992.

Hypertension: Pathophysiology, Diagnosis, and Management, Second Edition, edited by J.H. Laragh and B.M. Brenner, Raven Press, Ltd., New York © 1995.

CHAPTER 12

High Blood Pressure in Blacks: Salt, Slavery, Survival, Stress, and Racism

Clarence E. Grim, James P. Henry, and Hector Myers

(Continued on following page)

C. E. Grim, J. P. Henry, and H. Myers: Charles R. Drew University of Medicine and Science, 1621 E. 120th St., Los Angeles, California 90059

---

*It is significant that there are no authentic reports
of low-blood pressure communities of negroid stock
in the Americas or the Caribbean.*
O. O. AKINKUGBEE, 1985

The purpose of this chapter is to review the epidemiology, history, physiology, neuroendocrinology, and sociology of blood pressure variations seen in black populations of sub-Saharan African descent. The terms *blacks* and *whites* are used in this manuscript to denote ethnocultural groups that differ in genetic, cultural, social, and psychological roots.

The prevalence of hypertension in African Americans is the highest in the world, whereas some of the lowest rates are found in sub-Saharan Africans. These epidemiological observations have engendered two major hypotheses:

1. **The evolution of a salt-conserving genotype hypothesis.** For millennia, evolutionary pressures in salt-poor West Africa resulted in the evolution of a salt-conserving genotype. The frequency of this genotype in Western Hemisphere blacks was further increased due to selective survival during the slavery period of history due to selective survival based on the ability to conserve sodium. In a high dietary salt environment, blood pressure increases.

2. **The stress of living in a racist society.** The "stress" experienced by those of African descent living in a historically slave, and currently racist, society such as the US evokes neuroendocrine responses that increase blood pressure.

SELECTIVE SURVIVAL

Helmer first suggested that survival in salt-poor west Africa has, for thousands of years, been selecting those best able to conserve sodium. During the 400 years of the African slave trade to the Americas it is estimated that at least 12 million men, women, and children arrived in the Western Hemisphere. It is likely that at least this number also died in the process of getting there. Upon arrival, these hardy survivors were placed in living and work conditions that continued to result in a mortality rate of 10 percent per year for the next several years. The major causes of death during this experience were diarrhea and febrile illnesses. This high adult mortality, combined with an infant mortality that exceeded 50 percent, again primarily due to diarrhea, required continued massive importation to sustain the work force needed in the agricultural enterprises of sugar, cotton, rice, indigo, and tobacco as well as in mines and other enterprises in which the work conditions were so severe that nonslaves refused to do the work. The transportation and work conditions, due to heat and humidity, placed great strains on the physiological demands of sodium and volume regulation. One of us (CEG) has suggested that selective survival based on those best able to conserve sodium during this process has resulted in a greater prevalence of the salt-sensitive blood pressure genotype in the descendants of the survivors.

RACISM

It is clear that the sociological, cultural, and economic heritage of the slavery period of history, in which whites considered "Africans" as property with no more rights than livestock, has resulted in the racist milieu still rampant in the former slave countries today. The slave trade ruptured virtually all sociological, religious, mythological, and family ties with Africa and prevented, for 400 years, the development of a stable family milieu. In the US, slavery officially ended only six generations ago. This socioeconomic heritage set the stage for the severely disordered family structure still present in many of today's black populations in the Western Hemisphere. In addition, the oppressive economic hardships following the end of slavery, combined with the effectiveness of the racist society in blocking access to educational and economic opportunities, have placed the US African American in a social milieu unlike any other in the world. The stress hypothesis suggests that the neuroendocrine patterns induced by the psychosocial stresses of competing for the desiderata of today's society in this racist environment results in higher blood pressure. Animal studies emphasize the importance of both genetic and sociological stress on the type of neurohumoral and blood pressure response.

If one wishes to use the rationale of the two hypotheses to prevent high blood pressure in African Americans, the time course and feasibility of the solutions are remarkably different. The racism hypothesis suggests that we will be able to prevent high blood pressure only when racism disappears. If this ever happens, it will almost certainly take generations. On the other hand, the survival/salt hypothesis predicts that lowering dietary salt intake below some critical level will lower blood pressure in most African Americans in matter of a few weeks, and a slowing of the rate of development of new hypertensives in those with high normal blood pressure could likely be tested in only 3 years. A major problem in this area is what is the absolute level of sodium restriction that must be achieved in order to reduce blood pressure? Few quantitative studies have been done in hypertensive African Americans. MacGregor et al. (1) studied seven blacks and twelve whites in England with a double-blind crossover design of a 60- to 80-mM sodium diet. Blood pressure was lowered to nearly normal within 2 weeks. It decreased more in blacks than in whites. In the US it seems likely that perhaps 70 percent of the high blood pressure in blacks could be reversed, decreasing sodium intake to a critical level (2) and that even a greater percent could be prevented. The human and public health implications of such a likelihood are enormous. However, to develop adequate evidence for such recommendations, it is necessary to identify African Americans who have or are likely to develop salt-sensitive hypertension and then to test the salt hypothesis. A major impediment to large-scale trials is a simple way to identify salt sensitivity (discussed elsewhere in this volume). In a recent review of the large-scale feasibility trials of hypertension prevention, Kumanyika et al. (3) concluded that it is difficult to reduce sodium intake below 80 mM, and in their experience an average reduction of only 43.9 mM was achieved.

This chapter focuses on the pathophysiology of high blood pressure in African Americans as this is the best studied subpopulation of the African diaspora. The first section presents an overview of epidemiology of high blood pressure, coronary artery disease, and salt-sensitive blood pressure in blacks. The next reviews the survival hypothesis of survival during slavery, the third section reviews the concept that the neuroendocrine responses to social stress in man, as in animals, likely re-

sults in higher blood pressure that is heterogeneous in its pathophysiology.

EPIDEMIOLOGY OF BLOOD PRESSURE IN BLACKS

High Blood Pressure: The Major Health Problem in Populations of Sub-Saharan African Descent

High blood pressure is the major health problem in most black populations in the Western Hemisphere and is emerging as a major problem in many urban areas of Africa (4). It is the major problem because it is so common (33 percent of all black adults in the Western Hemisphere) and because only 20 percent of those with high blood pressure have it under adequate control. Several excellent textbooks have been devoted to many aspects of the problem of high blood pressure in blacks (5–7) and these should be reviewed for more detailed discussions of the epidemiology, the physiology of intracellular ions, the renin-angiotensin-aldosterone system, and for information on lifestyle changes and pharmacological methods to lower blood pressure that need to be considered in populations of African descent.

High Blood Pressure Affects the Health of Blacks from Conception to Old Age

Effects of High Blood Pressure In Utero

High blood pressure begins disproportionately to affect the health of blacks before they are born. This is due to the higher blood pressure of black females of child-bearing age. Higher blood pressure in the mother is associated with vasoconstriction in the placenta, placental ischemia, and smaller fetuses. Because small infants are less likely to survive it seems likely that higher blood pressure in black women may be the major contributor to the high infant mortality in blacks. High blood pressure complications are the major reason for maternal death in pregnant black women worldwide.

Effects of High Blood Pressure in Childhood

During childhood, blood pressure is higher in blacks (8), and the most consistent black-white difference in blood pressure regulatory systems seems to be that blacks have lower levels of renin and aldosterone (9). Manatunga et al. (10) have found that black children have a more rapid rise in blood pressure than do white children. It appears that this higher blood pressure results in more fatty streaks in the large blood vessels in black than in white teenagers (11). Small vessel thickening is also more common at a younger age in kidneys of blacks than whites (12).

Blacks Have the Highest Rate of Renal Failure in the World

In the US, black-white differences in renal failure due to hypertension appear by age 15–19 (13), and by age 40–44 the 1986–89 point prevalence rate of dialysis for renal failure due to hypertension was 20 times greater in blacks. In the US in 1989 about six new black patients began dialysis every day for renal failure due to hypertension. The possibility that the risk of renal failure may be familial in blacks was first suggested by our group (14) and this has now been expanded by studies in North Carolina (15), where 40 percent of blacks on dialysis for high blood pressure and 32 percent of those with diabetes as a cause of renal failure had a first-, second-, or third-degree relative who also had renal failure. Having a first-degree relative with end-stage renal disease (ESRD) increased the risk of ESRD ninefold (OR 9.1; 95 percent Cl, 2.6–31.8). This strongly suggests that renal failure due to high blood pressure is under strong genetic control in blacks.

High Blood Pressure is a Major Contributor to Disability, Unemployment, and Low Educational Achievement in Blacks

Although the sociological effects of African-American history have set the stage for the traditional high rates of unemployment, disability, and low educational achievement, we posit that the higher blood pressure and its complications are also likely to contribute to these problems. For example, most jobs that require a physical examination for employment will not hire anyone who has uncontrolled high blood pressure. Because many blacks have no health insurance, they do not have the resources to get medical care to get their blood pressure under control so they can be employed—a real "Catch 22." The high rates of nonfatal strokes, myocardial infarction, and ESRD result in significant disability so that blacks cannot be employed. Finally, the high rate of dropout of the educational system by US blacks is associated, as expected, with a high unemployment rate. Unexpectedly, those who do not graduate from high school have a systolic blood pressure that is strikingly higher in those blacks with less white admixture, as estimated by skin reflectance (15 mm higher systolic by age 45), compared to those with the darkest skin but who do graduate from high school (16). The major explanation for this observation is the stress of being able to compete in society is increased by lack of education, especially in those with darker skin. It also seems possible that high blood pressure itself may contribute to the high dropout rate of the educational system by US blacks. This possibility comes

from several considerations about the necessary conditions required to complete a high school education: financial resources, family support, and mental ability. High blood pressure and its vascular complications, especially in the inner-city black community, may interfere with some or all of these requirements. We have already mentioned the loss of income that can come from disability or unemployability due to high blood pressure. The family support system in many inner-city blacks hinges on a single mother and/or grandmother. Because of the high prevalence of high blood pressure in black women, especially over the age of 50 (2 of 3 have high blood pressure), many of these families will be severely crippled or disintegrate when disability or death from a high blood pressure complication occurs. Finally, because higher blood pressure in blacks appears early in life, one needs to consider whether this higher blood pressure itself results in subtle progressive vascular changes (such as seen in the kidneys) that may impair neuronal function and the mental abilities required for high school graduation. It is interesting that in the Philippines, where each grade of students is divided into 4 to 5 groups based on "mental ability," there was an inverse relationship between the level of academic rank and the level of blood pressure (17). Wyss et al. (18) have shown that spontaneously hypertensive rats (SHR) do not learn as well as normotensive control rats. Thus, the higher blood pressure seen in blacks who do not graduate from high school may simply be a manifestation that they came from a family with inherited high blood pressure and the effects of this hypertension on the family and the individual may make it less likely that family members will graduate from high school. The high blood pressure at age 45 may be a result of the inherited factors as well as the stresses produced by not graduating from high school.

High Blood Pressure is the Major Risk Factor for Deaths Due to "Major Cardiovascular Diseases" in Blacks

Major cardiovascular diseases are the leading causes of death in the adult black community in the US and are becoming the major problem in any black urban community in the world. The severe consequences of high blood pressure can best be appreciated from the data from Evans County, Georgia, in which it was estimated that between the ages of 40 and 65, 25 percent of all deaths in black males and 50 percent of all deaths in black females are due to hypertension and its complications (19).

Major cardiovascular diseases are the leading causes of death in the adult black community in Los Angeles. Although it had generally been held that coronary artery disease in blacks is an unusual event (or at least much less frequent) compared to whites, recent authors have stressed the fact that this may be untrue, perhaps related to misclassification of cause of death. In a 1980 review of mortality from major cardiovascular disease in Los Angeles (Table 1) (20), it was noted that the overall crude mortality rate for blacks (319.3) was only 60 percent of the rate for whites (530.7).

However, as can be seen in Table 2, when age and sex were adjusted, blacks have in fact a greater mortality rate than whites for these broad groups of major cardiovascular diseases (418 deaths per 100,000 in whites vs. 459 in blacks).

Furthermore, as can be seen in Table 1, black subjects had higher mortality rates for cardiovascular disease at each decade until the age of ≥ 75 years. In women, the black mortality ratio was over two times as great at ages 35–44, 45–54, and 55–64. Thus it appears that, at least in Los Angeles, younger blacks are dying of cardiovascular causes at a significantly higher rate than whites.

The reasons for the greater mortality in Los Angeles from cardiovascular disease in blacks under age 75 are not apparent and not explained by the greater death rates from hypertensive disease and stroke. Three major possibilities come to mind: (a) the biobehavioral stresses and strains of being black and poor may induce physiological alterations leading to increased risk; (b) hypertension, present in 66 percent of blacks over the age of 50 in this community may be inadequately treated, predisposing to coronary artery disease (CAD)—in California only 20 percent of blacks with hypertension are being adequately controlled; (c) current treatment for hypertension may be harmful and increase the risk of CAD; (d) genetic differences in other atherosclerotic risk factors could account for the higher death rate in blacks compared to whites.

High Blood Pressure is a Major Risk Factor for Coronary Artery Atherosclerosis

The high prevalence of hypertension in blacks and the pivotal role of hypertension as a risk factor for CAD suggests that it may play a key role in the development of CAD in African Americans. The increased risk of CAD in hypertension is shown by two important studies. Frank et al. (21) in 1968 reported on prospective data from the Health Insurance Plan of New York. Of 275 men who developed angina over 4 years, 25 percent had hypertension (160/95) and the rate of subsequent myocardial infarction (MI) or death was 2.5 times greater in the hypertensive men over the next 30 months. Men who were hypertensive prior to an MI had a 1-month mortality of 43 percent vs. only 21 percent in the normotensive men. Men who survived the first month but who were hypertensive before MI had a twofold greater likelihood of having a subsequent MI and a fivefold greater chance of dying over the next 4 to 5 years.

In the Rochester, Minnesota, study (22) of white persons who developed angina, 56 percent of men and 73 percent of women had preexisting hypertension. Preexisting hypertension was also present in 53 percent of men and 89 percent of women who developed an MI. Indeed, in women over 60 who developed MI, 94 percent were hypertensive! Patients with angina and normal blood pressure had survival curves that were no different over 10 years than an age-corrected general population. Those with hypertension and MI or angina who were treated for their hypertension had significantly better 10-year survival than those not treated. Even inadequate treatment for hypertension increased survival.

In Framingham (23), left ventricular hypertrophy (LVH) by electrocardiogram (EKG) has been shown to

TABLE 1. Annual mortality rate[a] from major cardiovascular diseases, by sex and race in Los Angeles County, 1980

Sex	Age	White	Black	Black-White Ratio
Male	<35	7.7	12.1	1.57
	35–44	79.7	171.2	2.15
	45–54	326.4	490.8	1.50
	55–64	814.7	1,087.3	1.33
	65–74	2,154.1	2,336.4	1.08
	75–84	5,410.7	5,160.4	.95
	>84	13,831.5	9,822.7	.71
	Total Male	512.3	335.0	.65
Female	<35	5.1	12.0	2.35
	35–44	25.3	62.4	2.47
	45–54	111.9	246.7	2.20
	55–64	317.8	682.2	2.15
	65–74	1,151.5	1,569.6	1.36
	75–84	3,878.2	3,795.9	.98
	>84	12,070.9	9,459.5	.78
	Total female	548.1	305.2	.56
	Total male and female	530.7	319.3	.60

[a] Deaths per 100,000 population.

TABLE 2. *Age- and sex-adjusted mortality rates[a] by ethnic group, Los Angeles County*

Causes of death (ICD code number)	United States: 1980	Los Angeles County (deaths)	White (deaths)	Black (deaths)
All causes	818.8	800.3	850.2	1016.4
		(179,529)	(153,415)	(21,656)
Major cardiovascular diseases (390–448)	401.1	399.2	418.2	459.3
		(89,553)	(78,803)	(8,815)
Diseases of the heart (390–398, 402, 404–429)	308.9	305.9	322.9	347.1
		(68,632)	(60,565)	(6,729)
Ischemic heart disease (IHD) (410–414)	229.2	191.5	205.0	186.3
		(42,952)	(38,668)	(3,477)
Myocardial infarction and acute IHD (410, 411)	123.3	89.8	96.8	85.7
		(20,149)	(18,100)	(1,648)
Chronic IHD (412–414)	105.9	101.7	108.2	100.6
		(22,803)	(20,568)	(1,829)
Hypertensive disease[b] (401–404)	13.3	20.3	18.7	47.7
		(4,550)	(3,472)	(973)
Cerebrovascular disease (strokes) (430–438)	69.0	71.7	73.2	89.6
		(16,075)	(13,911)	(1,659)

[a] Direct method of adjusted rates, with Los Angeles County 1980 population as standard. 1979–81 age- and sex-adjusted mortality rates per 100,000 population.
[b] Includes essential hypertension (401), hypertensive heart disease (402), and hypertensive heart disease either with (404) or without renal disease.

be a significant risk factor for sudden death. Studies by Messerli et al. (24) suggest that this may be related to increased ventricular ectopic activity seen in patients with LVH and hypertension. These studies seemed to exclude this increased activity as being due to increased sympathetic outflow, nor could they account for irritability by hypokalemia.

In the biracial Hypertension Detection Follow-up Program (HDFP) (25), the risk of fatal and nonfatal coronary artery disease was benefited by blood pressure control. When stepped care (SC) was compared to routine care (RC), the following was found: (a) if baseline EKG was normal, new EKG LVH was decreased by 25 percent; (b) if baseline EKG had a prominent R-wave, therapy decreased new LVH by 112 percent; (c) if baseline EKG was normal, there was a 17.6 percent decrease in new MI by EKG; (d) if baseline EKG demonstrated an old MI at baseline, 5-year survival was 70 percent in SC but only 52 percent in RC.

HDFP 5-year mortality also demonstrated a marked effect of social class of a three- to fivefold magnitude. This was more marked in those with LVH in whom the age-adjusted mortality doubled. Tyroler (26) suggests that, based on the limited data available, the importance of any standard risk factor seems to be about equal for blacks or whites, but that the effect of blood pressure on mortality is stronger per unit of blood pressure. He further stresses that blood pressure has a strong monotonic, highly significant association for both ischemic heart disease and all-cause mortality for middle-aged blacks.

The mechanism whereby hypertension predisposes to cardiovascular disease mortality and morbidity is not known in blacks or whites, but may be changing. Before antihypertensive therapy was generally available, the major cause of death was congestive heart failure. Although other vascular complications of hypertension such as strokes and dissecting aortic aneurysms have clearly decreased with antihypertensive therapy, a decrease in deaths due to coronary artery disease or renal failure has been more difficult to demonstrate.

The potential harmful effect of antihypertensive agents on coronary artery disease in blacks has been emphasized by Curry et al. (27). They noted that 50 percent of patients admitted to Howard University Hospital were taking diuretics, presumably for hypertension. Cholesterol was 20 mg/dL higher in patients on diuretics. Considering Lipid Research Clinic (LRC) studies showing a 2 percent decrease in CAD risk with every 1 percent decrease in cholesterol they have raised the question, Are diuretics increasing risk in blacks by increasing cholesterol or other lipid parameters?

African Americans Have Less of a Decline in Blood Pressure at Night

It is intriguing that clinic blood pressure is such a strong predictor of heart disease, given the considerable variation of this measure. This may be especially important in that we have shown blacks living in Los Angeles to have a minimal decline in blood pressure at night (28). This higher 24-hour blood pressure for a given clinic blood pressure (because of the lack of a nocturnal decline) may be an unrecognized risk factor for LVH and CAD, especially in blacks. Similar higher blood pressures at night have been reported in Chicago blacks (29) and in Afro-Caribbeans living in England (30), but the nocturnal decline in blacks in South Africa (29), in Barbados, and in Africans living in the US was more like that seen in whites. Even in childhood, blood pressure is higher at night in blacks in the US (31).

Hypertensive heart disease has been defined traditionally as the presence of both EKG LVH and hypertension. The advent of new sensitive approaches to diagnosis of LVH with substantial prognostic significance (32) has stimulated interest in whether such heart disease could help to explain the apparent paradox of a significant excess of heart disease death in the black population despite studies suggesting less obstructive epicardial coronary artery disease in the blacks (33,34). The electrocardiogram (with or without the chest x-ray) has been used traditionally to assess the presence or absence of LVH in clinical and epidemiological studies of hypertensive subjects. Such studies have shown black hypertensive subjects have a higher prevalence of hypertensive heart disease when compared with white hypertensive subjects. For example, blacks in HDFP were three to four times more likely than whites to have electrocardiographic LVH, with prevalences in the white men and women ranging from 1.7 percent to 3.1 percent and those in black men and women ranging from 7.8 percent to 9 percent (35). This excess of LVH in black hypertensive subjects persisted even after adjustment for age and blood pressure level. The Evans County Study (36) showed similar excess hypertrophy and cardiac enlargement in blacks by EKG and chest x-ray even after adjusting for blood pressure differences. The risk of subsequent morbidity and mortality escalates rapidly with the advent of EKG LVH, which confers a two- to ninefold increased risk of stroke, cardiac failure, overt coronary event, and symptomatic peripheral arterial disease in some populations. Finally, EKG LVH is a marker of advanced hypertension, with 35 percent of men and 20 percent of women dead within 5 years of its appearance in one study (37).

In HDFP, age-adjusted 5-year mortality in the stratum with mild hypertension at baseline (stratum I) was approximately double for (usual care) black males who had electrocardiographic LVH compared to those who did not have such LVH (38). Some subgroups of black subjects had even greater mortality associated with the presence of LVH than did comparable white subjects. For example, age-adjusted analyses of black men with less than a high school education who were not receiving medications at baseline (usual care) indicated a 33.2 percent 5-year mortality in those with EKG LVH. White men with this similar education level who had LVH (and were not receiving medications at baseline) had only a 12.4 percent 5-year mortality.

More sensitive and specific noninvasive diagnostic tools such as M-mode and two-dimensional echocardiography (echo) (39), as well as computerized electrocardiography (40), are being used to investigate prevalence, incidence, characteristics (including reversibility), and prognostic significance of hypertensive heart disease in black and white subjects. Only small studies of black subjects have been published to date, and these show the heterogeneity of heart findings in hypertensive subjects. Echo has demonstrated LVH in 16 percent of blacks with mild hypertension whereas in only 8 percent of whites (41). Other studies have shown greater left ventricular mass (42), greater left ventricular wall thickness (43), or no echo differences in small samples of black hypertensive patients compared with white patients with similar blood pressure levels (44).

Echo LVH is one of the most powerful risk factors for coronary heart disease events (independent of the standard cardiovascular risk factors) in apparently healthy white subjects over age 60 years (45). For example, apparently healthy white men had a 66 percent greater risk of a coronary disease event in 4 years for each additional 50 g of echocardiographic left ventricular mass. This increased risk was independent of the standard cardiovascular disease risk factors, including office blood pressure. No such quantitative risk data are available for black subjects. However, a national sample of black men aged 35 years and older, in the top quintile of left ventricular mass (estimated from computerized electrocardiograms), had a 60 percent 12-year death rate from cardiovascular disease as compared to a less than 25 percent death rate for a similar-aged group of white men also with left ventricular mass in the top quintile (46). This raises the possibility that not only may black men have a greater incidence of hypertensive heart disease but also that such disease may be more "malignant" in black men than in white men. The greater sudden death rate in black athletes (47) is frequently associated with LVH. The role of blood pressure level in this problem urgently needs to be clarified.

Changes of increasing peripheral vascular resistance associated with hypertensive heart disease may start in young black men before office blood pressures reflect elevated blood pressure. Soto et al. (48), in a study of over 500 black and white children from a population sample in Bogalusa, Louisiana, found that black boys between the ages of 12 and 22 years showed, on average, increasing levels of peripheral vascular resistance, whereas white boys and girls, as well as black girls, showed declining peripheral resistance between these ages. Thus, black adolescents and young adults have patterns of increasing peripheral vascular resistance that is seen in middle-aged white men and women and may represent a harbinger of premature CAD and hypertensive heart disease in black men. The increasing blood pressure at night as black adolescents (49) may be a reflection of this same increasing resistance. Prevention of hypertensive heart disease is important, but these early hemodynamic findings in black men and boys suggest that preventive actions may need to occur very early.

Blacks in the Western Hemisphere Have Higher Blood Pressure Than Blacks in Africa

Since the 1930s it has been known that blacks have higher blood pressure than whites and that blacks in the Western Hemisphere have higher blood pressure than blacks in Africa. A metanalysis of the English literature noted that even within Africa there are striking variations in blood pressure between genetic and culturally different black populations (50). Indeed the greatest variation in blood pressure within racial groups was that in blacks reported by Intersalt (51), in which the highest prevalence of high blood pressure in the world was in blacks in Mississippi (35 percent) and one of the lowest (5 percent) was in blacks in Kenya. Most have suggested these differences are due to environmental factors such as psychosocial stress and/or dietary sodium intake between blacks and whites in the west or between American and African blacks. The psychosocial concept does not consider the striking genetic differences within those peoples called black that are reflected in Africa by marked regional and tribal variations in height, weight, body habitus, skin color, frequency of inherited diseases such as sickle cell trait, etc. More widespread variations in genotype are seen in black populations in the US where, in many regions, there is considerable merging of the African, European, and Amerindian gene pool. A pivotal observation was made by Akinkugbe in a 1985 review (52) of the worldwide epidemiology of hypertension in blacks in which he stated "it is significant that there are no authentic reports of low-blood pressure communities of negroid stock in the Americas or the Caribbean." Indeed, this observation was one of the "triggers" that suggested the survival during slavery hypothesis to Grim.

A History of the Evolutionary/Slavery/Survival Hypothesis

Helmer (53) was the first to report that African Americans have a strikingly lower level of renin than white Americans. He was also the first to suggest selective survival for the ability to conserve sodium in a hot, humid tropical environment was related to the present high prevalence of low renin and high blood pressure in African Americans (54). Next, Gleiberman (55) reasoned that low salt availability in Africa was related to the high blood pressure in US Blacks today. Denton posited (56) that western hemisphere blacks were descended from "progenitors . . . representing twenty to forty thousand or more generations of existence in tropical to subtropi-

cal conditions largely in the interior of the continents, and with considerable stress on sodium homeostasis. Greater hedonic liking for salt and less capacity to excrete it could result." After reviewing the history of West African salt availability for his PhD thesis in history, Wilson (57–59) suggested that variations in supplies of salt within ancient West Africa may be important in understanding today's geographical variability of blood pressure in the same areas. He speculated that the ancestors of US blacks may have migrated from the very low salt areas within West Africa and were thus not able to withstand its physiological effects, increased blood pressure. A common concept of these and others (60–63) was related to physical evolution caused by adaptation to heat and salt supplies within Africa.

Interested in the blood pressure differences between US blacks and African blacks, Waldron et al. [at the suggestion of one of us (JH)] in 1982 suggested that the social legacy of slavery in the cultural history of US blacks may be partially responsible for their higher blood pressure (64). In 1983 Blackburn and Prineas (65) emphasized the Atlantic passage during the slavery period was characterized by conditions that may be related to, presumably, a genetic-based salt-sensitive hypertension. In 1988 Grim (66) focused the thinking on the evolution of salt-conservation and salt-sensitive blood pressure in Western Hemisphere blacks by hypothesizing that the conditions of slavery (not just the Atlantic passage) favored those with an enhanced ability to conserve salt. He also introduced the selective potential of salt-depletive diseases like diarrheas and fevers combined with the influence of excessive sweating from heat and work and low salt supplies. He asserted that the descendants of slaves would have a higher prevalence of salt-sensitive blood pressure than the current population of blacks in Africa, and that inheritance played a very important role in these differences. Thus, whereas Helmer, Denton, Gleiberman, Wilson, and others suggested long-term adaptation/evolution of a population adept at conserving salt, Grim suggested an accelerated evolution of salt sensitivity due to possible selective survival only during the past 400 years! Grim and Wilson have detailed the biohistorical (67,68) and physiological basis of the hypothesis (69) elsewhere.

THE HYPOTHESIS OF SURVIVAL DURING SLAVERY

An Overview

Most blacks in the West are descended from survivors of the so-called slavery period of history (1500–1800s), a period of forced migration unlike any other in the recorded history of mankind. During this period, over 12 million black people were transported against their will, under inhumane conditions, to the Western Hemisphere to provide slave labor in the agricultural enterprises of rice, indigo, sugar, tobacco, and in mines. Research by economists and historians over the last 20 years has produced a large amount of qualitative data relative to this period of history. Indeed, the Nobel Prize in Economics was just awarded to Dr. Robert W. Fogel, in part for the monumental work by him and Dr. Stanley Engerman, *Time on the Cross: The Economics of American Negro Slavery* (70). A review of this extensive literature has revealed conditions that must have imposed severe demands on sodium conservation and led to selective survival of those best able to conserve sodium. On-board ship conditions were crowded, access to water and food was limited, food consisted of mostly unsalted products, sea sickness was common and prolonged, and conditions of extreme heat and humidity were characteristic. That high heat below decks may have been a major contributor to death is suggested by the reports that using human-powered ventilators to keep the lower decks cool resulted in a striking reduction of deaths (71). Common illnesses were diarrhea and febrile disorders, both of which may result in severe sodium depletion and were the major causes of death not only on board ship, but also at other stages in the process. Estimated mortality in Africa after capture has averaged 10 percent (range 4–50 percent), on board ship 15 percent (3–80 percent) and was 5 percent (3–30 percent) while awaiting sale in the Americas. After arrival, work conditions were severe and death rates averaged 10 percent/yr (2–50 percent) for the first 2 years and were highest during the hottest parts of the year. It was well known that newly imported Africans were much more likely to die during slavery than those born in the Western Hemisphere, suggesting that the descendants of the survivors were more fit for the slavery environment. Thus, on the average, only about 60 percent ($0.9 \times 0.85 \times 0.95 \times 0.9 \times 0.9$) of those captured survived more than 2 years. In the Brazilian trade perhaps only 28 percent survived the first 4 years of this process (72). If, during this period of high mortality, mortality was not random, the process of selective survival would alter the gene pool of the survivors and their descendants from that of the nontransported African gene pool. Of course, death is never random. Grim has hypothesized that those individuals most efficient at retaining salt (sodium) were better able to maintain sodium and volume homeostasis and thus defend against fatal sodium depletion resulting from the combination of poor dietary sodium intake and excessive losses from sweat and diarrhea. The survivors provided the gene pool for future generations who were likewise forced to slave under severe conditions. Indeed, the mortality was so severe that most areas had to import a continuous supply of people as the death rate of adults and children exceeded the birth rate. The hypothesis predicts an inherited (genetic) increased ability to conserve salt in Western Hemisphere

blacks, which has led to a greater prevalence of salt-sensitive hypertension in present-day blacks of this ancestry compared to present-day black Africans (or Americans) without this ancestry. In the presence of excess dietary salt intake such individuals may develop increases in blood pressure and its health consequences.

What Behavioral Traits Would Have Increased the Likelihood of Survival During Slavery?

The concept that many human behavioral traits are strongly inherited has been emphasized by the recent publication of data in identical white twins raised apart (73). This study suggested that most personality variables, psychological interests, and social attitudes are primarily influenced by inherited factors. Therefore, one must also consider the possibility that genetically determined behavioral traits may have increased the likelihood of survival during the high mortality of slavery and these behavioral traits may be affecting blood pressure today in the US racist society. It seems to us that survival during the slavery process would have been increased in those who were more intelligent; those who could learn special skills valuable to the slave owner including cooking, carpentry, etc.; those who could suppress anger, those who had the ability to behave in a passive manner; and those who could accept and survive the loss of control characteristic of American slavery.

In summary, this theory of selective survival suggests Western Hemisphere slavery was a major evolutionary event in the history of mankind. As a consequence of this short-term, high-mortality selection process, the gene pool of Western hemisphere blacks is different from African blacks with respect to sodium metabolism and perhaps to behavioral characteristics. This gene pool difference will be maintained unless there is selective mortality against these physiological characteristics or there is intermarriage with a population with a less efficient ability to conserve sodium or different biobehavioral/neurohumoral characteristics.

Critiques of the Evolutionary/Slavery/Survival Hypothesis

A number of critiques of this hypothesis are frequently expressed and include: "evolution can't happen this fast," "the changes would have disappeared by now," "a racist hypothesis." Recently, Dr. Phillip Curtin, a prominent historian of this period, has published a detailed critique of this hypothesis (74), and it should be reviewed. Unfortunately, he and others have failed to grasp several key physiological and epidemiological principles underlying the hypothesis. His critique appropriately divides the hypothesis into three separate components, but does not appreciate critical details of each:

1. "The ancestral experience in Africa emphasizes the possible genetic consequences of a low-salt diet over many centuries." Curtin asserts that salt was not scarce in West Africa, yet some of his own publications describe this area as "salt starved." The hypothesis emphasizes both historically low salt availability and high physiological salt needs. The greatest loss was likely that from sweating mandated by the need to prevent fatal hyperthermia or heat stroke. Sodium losses through sweating can reach 25 grams of sodium chloride in only 162 minutes (75). In addition, one continually loses small amounts of sodium in normal stools and may lose fatal amounts during diarrhea (still the leading cause of infant death in this area). The urine likewise is a continual source of sodium loss, which can be dramatically increased by even brief periods of starvation or dehydration. Females are further subjected to the sodium-depleting conditions of pregnancy, parturition, and breast-feeding. Unless these losses are replaced by dietary sources a person will ultimately die.

2. "Genetic changes caused by the trauma of the ocean passage from Africa to America during the slave trade . . . individuals were more likely to survive if they already had an ability to conserve salt." Dr. Curtin and other critics have mistakenly focused on the "middle passage" as the key or only step in the slavery process that likely led to fatal sodium depletion. The original hypothesis emphasized the *cumulative* nature of deaths due to sodium losses that occurred during the entire slavery process. For research purposes historians have divided the slavery process into a number of steps including capture, forced marching to the coast, holding for sale in barracoons, holding on board ship while "slaving the coast," the middle passage, quarantine in the West, transportation to the final work site, and finally the gauntlet of forced labor euphemistically called *seasoning*. Although historians have estimated the mortality at each of these steps, my (CEG) contribution has been to emphasize the pivotal role of the sodium-depleting conditions of the trade and to apply the concept of cumulative mortality at each step to calculate the astounding final mortality figures. I reasoned that each step in the process progressively increased the frequency of the salt-conserving phenotype, who, in today's high salt intake, will have higher blood pressure. Dr. Joseph Miller (76), a professor of history at the University of Virginia, has also recently summarized these figures for the Brazilian trade and calculated that only 28 percent of captives in Africa survived the first 4 years of the Portugese slavery process!

3. "Genetic consequences of life under slavery . . . conditions that caused high death rates and hence genetic changes among the survivors." Curtin concludes this aspect of his critique by summarizing that slavery conditions in the US South were such that the health of blacks under slavery was not worse than the health of poor whites in the South. In other words, he suggests that individual freedom and an intact family milieu are not important to health!

Sodium Conservation and Sodium Loss

The human species has an incredible ability to conserve sodium and, as is true of all biological traits, some individuals are better at this than others. Therefore, under conditions of severe sodium losses (sweat, stool, vomit) and/or inadequate sodium intake to replace losses, it follows that all humans will eventually die because of sodium and volume depletion. Some will die sooner than others. To illustrate the effect of this concept let us assume that we subject a population of humans (or any other animal) to a standardized condition in which the life-threatening, sodium-depleting conditions are exactly the same for all subjects. Under these standardized conditions the time of death of each individual will be dictated by two factors: genetic and environmental.

Genes dictate the physiological systems controlling the rate of sodium conservation and sodium loss in both whites (77) and blacks (78). These genetic factors are a direct result of the evolutionary history of each individual and include the well-known genetic variations in the structure and the function of thermoregulation (especially the sweat gland system), the kidney's ability to conserve and excrete sodium, the renin-angiotensin-aldosterone system, the sympathetic nervous system, and skeletal mass (the major storage site of sodium in the body is bone) as well as other as yet unknown genetic factors that regulate sodium and volume homeostasis.

Environmental supplies of salt interact with the genetic substrate to set the organism's total salt content. These environmental circumstances will be determined by the environmental history superimposed on the genetic substrate of each individual. The environmental factors would include prior access to dietary sodium, water, and calories as well as the environmental conditions of temperature, humidity, and exposure to sodium-depleting illnesses that would affect appetite and/or produce sweating, vomiting, diarrhea, or increased urine output. Obviously, those who had better sodium stores at the start of sodium-depleting stress would live longer. Now, if the fatal progress of the sodium depletion is stopped before all have died, it is clear that those who survived must be different from those who died. The genetic traits that permitted survival would be inherited by their descendants; however, the environmental conditions that affected sodium balance before the stress would not be inherited but would continue to be dictated by one's environment.

Of course, the genetic traits selected by this process will remain forever in the descendant population unless: (a) environmental conditions change such that these previously advantageous, genetic-driven, salt-conserving traits now lead to decreased fertility of these salt-conserving genotypes; and/or (b) there is gene flow of non–salt-conserving genotypes from the original population or from other populations (this clearly has occurred between the black, white, and Amerindian ethnic groups in the US and other parts of the Western Hemisphere); and/or (c) spontaneous mutations occur that change the sodium-conserving genotype.

An Animal Model for the Rapid Evolution of a Salt-Sensitive Genetic Trait

Rapid evolution of salt sensitivity is strongly supported by the observations of Dahl and Shackow's animal model (79). They showed that artifical selection of rats could, in only three generations, produce one strain with extreme salt sensitivity and another with extreme salt resistance. Dahl and colleagues had noted that an unselected population of Sprague-Dawley rats demonstrated striking variation in the effect of a high salt intake on blood pressure. To test if this was related to genetic factors, his group examined the effect of selective breeding on the blood pressure response to salt. First the blood pressure response to high dietary salt intake was determined in an unselected group of rats. Matings were produced between a pair with the lowest change in blood pressure with salt loading, the ancestors of the salt-resistant (SR) strain, and another pair with the greatest increase in blood pressure, the ancestors of the salt-sensitive (SS) strain. The first generation of these selective matings demonstrated a significant difference in the blood pressure–raising effects of high salt intake. This process was continued for two more generations, at which time there was no overlap between SS and SR responses to the blood pressure–raising effects of high dietary salt. Importantly, renin levels were significantly lower in the salt-sensitive rats, and they died rapidly with severe hypertension on a high-salt diet. Recent studies by Rapp et al. (80) have demonstrated that the salt sensitivity is related to alterations in the renin genotype. The genotype that is associated with low levels of renin is the one associated with salt sensitivity. Although this model is accepted as likely being similar to salt-sensitive hypertension in man, it seems likely to us that this may not be the case. This concern is due to the likely differences in how the Dahl SS rat was selected and how human salt-sensitive hypertension likely evolved. As discussed above, the Dahl SS rat was selected only if blood pressure increased on a high-salt diet. The selection that likely produced human salt-sensitive hypertension more likely acted on genes that protect against fatal sodium depletion. The probability that the physiology and genetics of these two selective survival paradigms are the same seems low. Therefore, one should be cautious in translating the animal model to man.

The Importance of Salt Sensitivity on Blood Pressure in African Americans

Hypertension presents an especially challenging problem for physiologists and geneticists because it seems likely that increased blood pressure is the sign of a disturbance of one or more of the several key blood pressure control systems. Whatever this disturbance is, it must alter the renal pressure–natriuresis curve (81), i.e., the renal handling of sodium, in order to increase blood pressure.

Perhaps the most important environmental determinant of the increase in blood pressure with age in a population is dietary salt intake, as recently reported by Intersalt. This study clearly demonstrated that those populations that eat less than 80 mM of sodium per day have no or a minimal increase in blood pressure with age and essentially no hypertension. Intersalt also demonstrated that low sodium intake was associated with a minimal increase in blood pressure with age in populations that are great linguistic and genetic distances apart: Kenyans, Borneo aboriginals, and Amerindians. Although this study suggests that low sodium intake is associated with a low population blood pressure independent of the genetic substrate, the blood pressure–raising effects of a high-sodium diet appear to vary considerably between ethnic groups such as Africans in Tanzania, Afro-Caribbeans in Trinidad-Tobago, African Americans, Amerindians in Mexico, Portuguese in Portugal, and Chinese in China. Thus, it would appear that SS may be present in all populations.

It is of interest that Weinberger and Fineberg (82) have suggested that salt sensitivity of blood pressure itself may be a new method to predict those who will get an increase in blood pressure with aging as Weinberger has recently reported a 10-year follow-up on 31 normotensive and hypertensive subjects determined to be SS using the Saline-Lasix protocol (15 SS and 16 SR). Over the ensuing 10 years the SS group developed an increase in mean arterial pressure (MAP) of 10.2 ± 3.6 mm Hg ($p < .02$), whereas the SR group had a nonsignificant decrease of $-.02 \pm 1.8$ mm Hg for the same period. Thus the SS subjects developed an increase in MAP that averaged 1.42 ± 0.39 mm Hg/year ($p < .001$).

GENETIC STUDIES ON BLOOD PRESSURE IN BLACKS

Blood pressure is clearly influenced by genetic factors in whites and in blacks, and even normotensive blacks are more sensitive to the blood pressure–raising effects of salt than are whites (83). Our own preliminary studies in black twins in Los Angeles and Barbados have shown that the distribution of blood pressure in the population is primarily influenced by genetic factors (84). However, blood pressure is also influenced by environmental factors including diet (calories, alcohol, sodium, potassium, etc.), biosocial factors (psychological stress, job stress, socioeconomic status, education, social interaction, type of society, and social isolation), and by exercise, demonstrating that although genetic factors may be important in "setting" a basic level of blood pressure, variations around this set point are modified by environmental influences.

Because salt sensitivity is present in about 75 percent of all black hypertensives, we are working to identify the gene(s) related to blood pressure and salt sensitivity as an important step toward understanding the etiology of hypertension and in the identification of individuals who are at high genetic risk for salt-sensitive hypertension. We do not believe that the genes for salt sensitivity are likely to be much different in blacks than in whites, but the high frequency makes this group a more efficient group to search for the genes. Our studies conducted over the last 3 years have shed important new light on the physiology and genetics of salt sensitivity of blood pressure in African Americans. We will discuss the physiological factors that we have found to be under genetic control in African Americans as our assumption is that unless a system is under genetic control it is not likely to be involved in high blood pressure in African Americans.

The ultimate goal of medical genetics is to understand the genetic causes of human diseases so that affected or high-risk families may be counseled about diagnosis, prognosis, treatment, and prevention. In the past, medical genetics research followed a classical progression of description of a familial phenotype, segregation analysis to determine mode of inheritance, description of the underlying metabolic disorder, and finally, mapping of the gene. Until recently, the last two steps were rarely successful. However, during the past decade the technology of molecular genetics has made it possible to reverse the investigative process, going from genetic markers directly to mapping and sequencing of genes without prior knowledge of the gene product. This powerful new "reverse genetics" and the availability of numerous DNA markers has made it theoretically possible to map and sequence any segregating human gene. Progress in the area of hypertension has been slow until the recent report (85) of a specific genetic marker and mechanism for familial glucocorticoid remedial hypertension. This syndrome has not yet been reported in blacks. The next major challenge for medical physiologists and geneticists is to identify genes that have major influences on physiological control systems that lead to increases in blood pressure, blood sugar, obesity, and cholesterol, culminating in coronary atherosclerosis. This will likely be a long time in coming because in a recent review of the human genome we identified at least 274 that are likely involved in the hypertensive/atherosclerotic process (86).

In an interesting study (87) on the Caribbean island of Le Desirade, in which most inhabitants are descendants of original French settlers and their slaves, it was found that those with the higher proportion of African genes had higher blood pressures. The proportion of African genes was estimated by both family pedigrees and by detailed genotyping.

The Twin Method for the Study of Genetic Influences on Blood Pressure in African-American Twins

We have used the power of the study of twins to examine the relative contribution of genes and environment to blood pressure variation in blacks in the US (88) and Barbados (89). The efficiency and rationale of the twin method is based on knowledge that monozygotic (MZ) twins share 100 percent of their genes, whereas DZ twins share 50 percent of their genes on the average. Therefore, if MZ twins are significantly more similar than dizygotic (DZ) twins for blood pressure, body-size variables, or biochemical markers for SS (renin, etc.), it may be concluded that the observed variables (phenotype) are influenced by genetic factors, assuming that relevant environmental factors shared by members of the same twin pair are similar in both MZ and DZ twins. Similarly, in multivariate analyses, if the cross-correlations between blood pressure in one twin with body size in the cotwin are found to be greater in MZ twins than in DZ twins, this suggests some correlation among genetic influences important to both phenotypes (90). Recent advances in the multivariate extension of univariate behavioral genetic analysis have been reviewed by Defreis and Fulker (91).

In this, our first detailed analysis of our Los Angeles twin data (92), we have used the multivariate twin design for blood pressure, height, and weight in 52 pairs of black MZ and dizygotic DZ twins to examine genetic and environmental sources of variance underlying observed individual differences in both blood pressure and body size using traditional comparisons of MZ and DZ twin similarity for each variable. In addition, state-of-the-art multivariate genetic analyses provide a new opportunity to determine the genetic and environmental sources of covariation underlying any observed relationship between blood pressure and body size. Through these multivariate biometrical analyses we addressed the following questions: (a) In African Americans, to what extent are individual differences in systolic and diastolic blood pressure, height, and weight explained by genetic and by environmental factors shared by cotwins? and (b) Is the observed relationship between blood pressure and body size in African Americans a function of correlated hereditary factors, correlated environmental factors, or both?

In other words, is there a common, inherited biological predisposition to the underlying individual differences in both blood pressure and body size, or is this known relationship due to other noninherited factors common to both variables, such as diet and exercise?

Means and standard deviations for systolic and diastolic blood pressure, height, weight, and age are presented in Table 3.

Hierarchical multiple regression analyses revealed significant main effects for gender on systolic blood pressure (t = −4.103, p < .001), height (t = −6.55, p < .001), and weight (t = −4.69, p < .001), and a marginally significant gender effect in diastolic blood pressure (t = −1.669, p < .10). Furthermore, there were significant linear effects of age for systolic (t = 4.22, p < .001) and diastolic blood pressure (t = 5.749, p < .001), as well as for weight (t = 5.255, p < .001). Age had a marginally significant (linear) effect on height (t = 1.924, p < .06). There were also some quadratic age effects. The effects of sex and age (both linear and quadratic) were removed by multiple regression and all subsequent analyses presented here are based on age- and sex-adjusted scores: adjusted systolic (ASYS), diastolic (ADIAS), height (AHT), and weight (AWT).

To examine the genetic and environmental etiologies of ADIAS, ASYS, AHT, AWT, and their covariation, multivariate biometrical analyses of the within-pair twin similarities were employed. In addition to providing estimates of proportions of observed variance in these scales due to sources of genetic and environmental influence, the multivariate analyses yield information concerning the factor structures of each class of influences. From these analyses, the extent to which the correlations among twins may be due to shared genetic or shared environmental influences were examined. Maximum-likelihood estimates of the three component matrices were obtainable using the LISREL VI program based on a multiple-group specification that makes full use of the six observed mean-square/cross-product matrices. More exact program specifications can be found in Ho et al. (93).

The resulting data were then transformed into a matrix of genetic correlations (R_g), shared environmental correlations (R_c), and specific environmental correlations (R_s). These are presented in Table 4, along with heritabilities (h^2), common environmentalities (c^2), and specific environmentalities (s^2) for each measure.

As can be seen, relative portions of variance explained by genetic factors (h^2, also called *heritability*) range from 0.16 to 0.80 for the four measures of blood pressure and

TABLE 4. *Maximum-likelihood estimates of genetic and environmental contributions to variations on blood pressure, height, and weight in African Americans*

	Systolic	Diastolic	Height	Weight
		R_G		
ASYS	1.00			
ADIAS	0.55*	1.00		
AHT	−0.28	−0.61*	1.00	
AWT	0.39	0.30	0.59	1.00
h^2	0.64*	0.80*	0.59*	0.16
		R_C		
ASYS	1.00			
ADIAS	0.00	1.00		
AHT	0.00	0.00	1.00	
AWT	0.00	0.00	−0.21	1.00
c^2	0.00	0.00	0.15	0.48*
		R_S		
ASYS	1.00			
ADIAS	0.38*	1.00		
AHT	0.05	0.35*	1.00	
AWT	−0.35*	0.10	0.00	1.00
s^2	0.36*	.20*	0.26*	0.36*

* p < .05. Data are sex- and age-adjusted.

ASYS, adjusted systolic; ADIAS, adjusted diastolic; AHT, adjusted height; AWT, adjusted weight; h^2, heritability; c^2, common environmentality; s^2, specific environmentality; R_G, genetic correlations; R_C, shared environmental correlations; R_S, specific environmental correlations.

body-size characteristics, although genetic variance is nonsignificant for weight. Genetic factors to be considered as influencing blood pressure include blood pressure control systems as well as genetic influences on behavioral traits.

It should be noted that environmental factors shared by twins, c^2, account for little or no variance in blood pressure and height, while contributing more than genetic factors to weight variations. Such factors should include family milieu or education experiences through high school, as all of these twins were raised together. The remaining variance in each measure, s^2, is explained by environmental factors not shared by members of a twin pair, which include the influences of their idiosyncratic experiences and/or errors in measurement. These factors appear to have a significant influence on blood pressure, height, and weight. Thus, factors in the nonshared environment of twin pairs such as differences in diet, alcohol intake, exercise, or psychosocial stress appear to influence blood pressure.

Salt Sensitivity of Blood Pressure is Under Genetic Control in African Americans

We have used the power of the study of twins to test the hypothesis that salt sensitivity of blood pressure (BP)

TABLE 3. *Mean and standard deviations for systolic and diastolic blood pressure, height, and weight*

	Males		Females	
	Mean	SD	Mean	SD
Systolic	125.10	10.03	117.61	11.63
Diastolic	73.03	11.03	70.65	11.08
Height	68.26	5.64	61.42	5.48
Weight	175.10	50.83	141.16	40.54
Age	28.49	11.86	30.26	11.72

is under genetic control in normotensive African Americans (94). Salt sensitivity was tested with the Saline-Lasix protocol developed by Grim and Weinberger of the Indiana group. Blood pressure was measured by trained observers ten times at the end of the saline infusion and at the end of the Na^+ depletion. If systolic BP decreased ($p < .01$) after salt loading, the subject was classified as SS, otherwise as SR. A total of 85 studies were completed in 26 twin pairs (17 MZ) and in 14 unrelated subjects. For SS the decrease in systolic BP was 14 mm Hg and SR only 0.8 mm Hg. The prevalence of SS was 75 percent, repeatability of SS testing was 75 percent (n = 16). Concordance of SS was 82 percent in MZ and 55 percent in DZ. The within-twin pair difference in BP change was 4.8 mm Hg in MZ and 8.5 mm Hg in DZ. As can be seen in Fig. 1, change in systolic blood pressure with sodium depletion is under genetic control.

Although based on a small number of twins, it appears that SS to this protocol is very common in normotensive African Americans, is under strong genetic control, and is likely due to a major gene or at most only a few genes. Now that SS has been shown to be under genetic control in African Americans the next issue is, What other factors are under genetic control or differ between SS blacks and SR blacks?

Plasma Renin is Under Genetic Control in African Americans

Using the power of the study of twins we have recently reported that plasma renin is under genetic control, but renin substrate is not (95).

Blood Pressure is Higher in Normotensive, Salt-Sensitive African Americans

As can be seen in Fig. 2, SS African Americans have higher blood pressure at nearly every point of the Saline-Lasix protocol except the last one, when the pressures have been equalized after sodium depletion with Lasix.

Hypertensive African Americans Have an Impaired Ability to Excrete a Sodium Load

Although documented first by Luft et al. (96), the mechanism has not been clarified. A manifestation of this is that the higher proportion of sodium excretion occurs in African Americans at night. This suggests that during the day they store salt better (see below) and during the night it is excreted to maintain balance. The higher blood pressure at night may be one of the mechanisms whereby sodium excretion is prevented from falling. Another consideration is that in order to maintain sodium balance, they must keep their renal perfusion pressure higher at night. Harshfield (97) has recently shown that African American adolescents who have the higher night blood pressure have lower creatinine clearances.

African Americans Store More Salt on Going From a Low- to a High-Salt Diet

A recent report by Wedler et al. (98) demonstrated that in going from a low- to a high-sodium diet, normotensive blacks took a longer time to come into balance. As sodium intake increased, the $T_{\frac{1}{2}}$ increased. This demonstrates that African Americans are especially good at storing sodium when going from a low-salt to a high-salt situation.

How could these two differences in sodium metabolism protect against death from sodium depletion? In considering the slavery survival hypothesis, Wilson (99) has suggested that the good sodium conserver (more likely to survive) would more rapidly come into balance on a low-sodium diet and, when changed to a high-

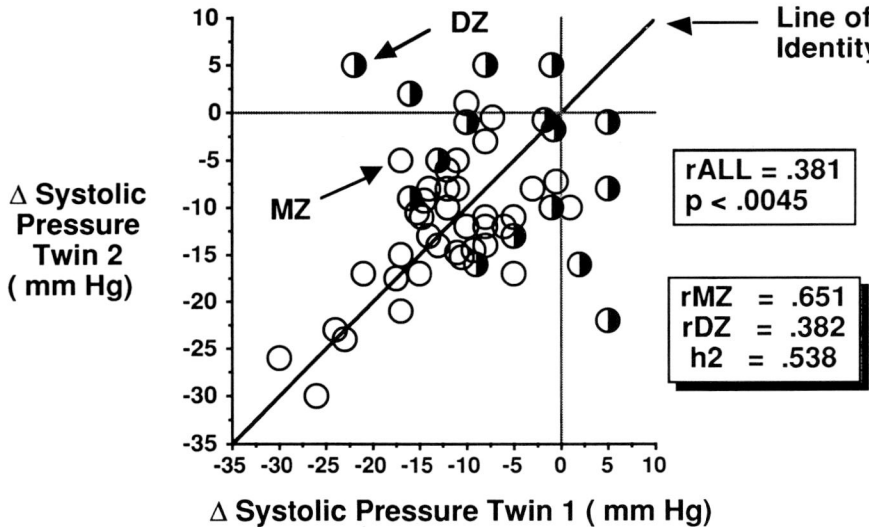

FIG. 1. A graph of the Spearman rank correlation of the change in blood pressure between twin pairs from the post-Saline point to the post-Lasix point. This is highly correlated in the subjects (r = .381, p <.0045). Heritability (h^2) was .538.

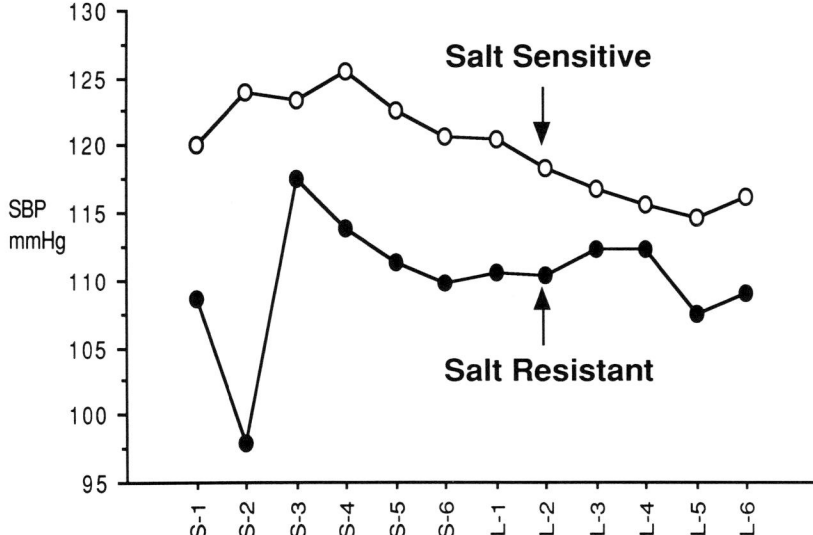

FIG. 2. Blood pressure measured every 4 hours throughout the Saline-Lasix protocol. Systolic pressure was higher in salt-sensitive African Americans. S, saline day; L, Lasix day; 1–6 indicates 4 hour periods starting at 8 am.

sodium diet, they would come into balance slower, thus storing more sodium in preparation for the next potentially fatal sodium-depleting stress. Black-white differences in the $T_{\frac{1}{2}}$ of sodium when going on a low-sodium diet are not different, but the data of Wedler in African Americans is compatible with this suggestion when going from a low- to a high-sodium diet.

Renal Function is Lower in Normotensive, Salt-Sensitive African Americans

As can be seen in Fig. 3, normotensive salt-sensitive African Americans have higher plasma creatinine con-

centrations, suggesting that at this early stage of salt sensitivity, renal function is already lower.

Plasma Norepinephrine Concentration is Higher in Salt-Sensitive African Americans and Appears to be Under Genetic Control

We have recently reported that SS African Americans have a higher level of circulating norepinephrine (NE) than SS (Fig. 4) (100). Our twin studies have also shown that plasma NE is under genetic control (Fig. 5). This suggests that activation of the sympathetic nervous system is present in SS African Americans.

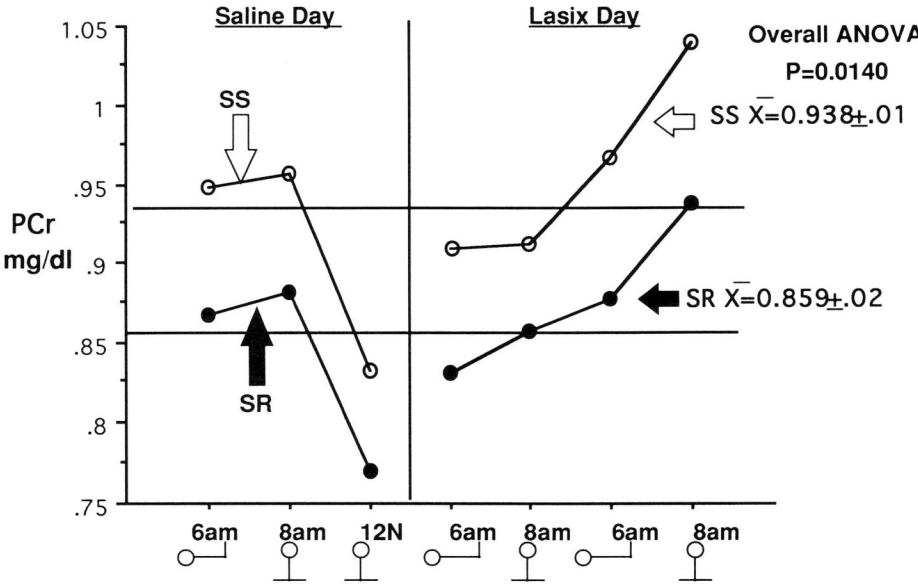

FIG. 3. Serum creatinine measured during the Saline-Lasix protocol. It was always higher in salt-sensitive African Americans.

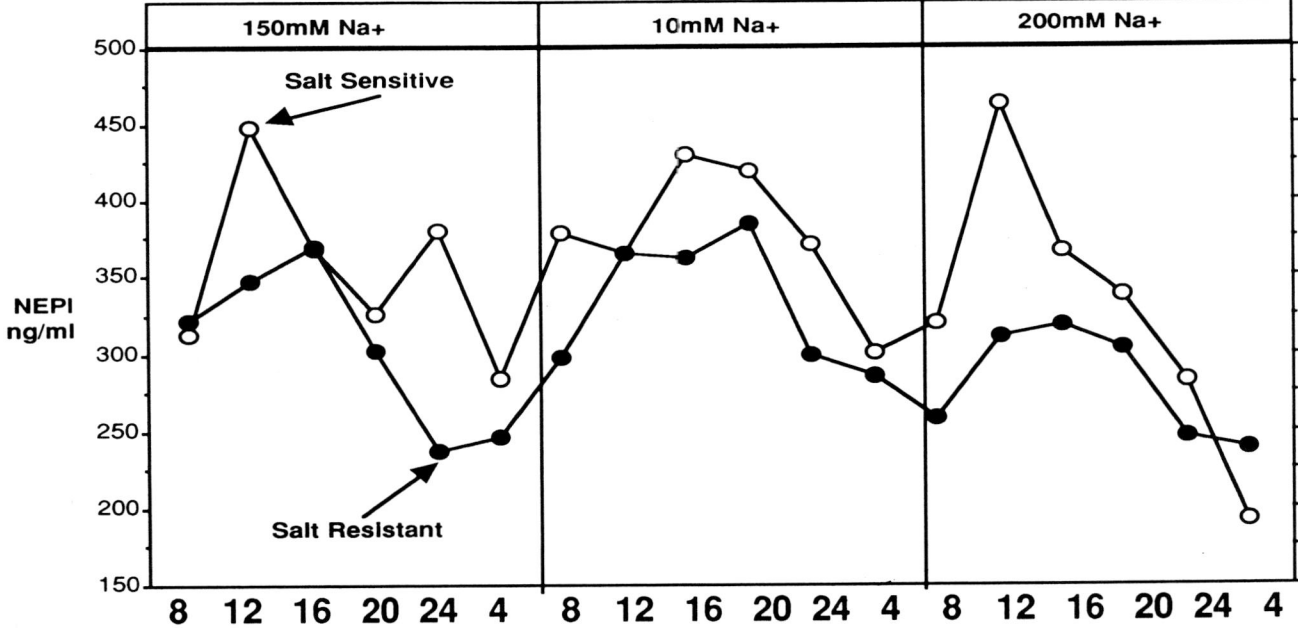

FIG. 4. Plasma norepinephrine (NE) measured every 4 hours on three different diets. Note that the salt-sensitive African Americans had a higher plasma NE.

Insulin Resistance is Probably Not Involved in Salt Sensitivity of Blood Pressure in African Americans

Although hyperinsulinemia has been reported in hypertension since 1966, there has been a recent surge of interest with new observations that one of the metabolic correlates of increased blood pressure is insulin resistance. This has led Reaven and Hoffman (101) to suggest a role for insulin in the hypertensive process as insulin stimulates the Sympathetic Nervous System (SNS), increases renal sodium retention, and may stimulate hypertrophy of vascular smooth muscle and modulate cation transport. A major argument against this hypothesis is that insulin resistance is neither a necessary nor a sufficient condition for increased blood pressure, perhaps best illustrated by observations in Pima Indians who have a high rate of insulin resistance but a low rate of hypertension. One of the earliest reports of the blood pressure–insulin relationship in blacks was that reported by Voors (102) in black children from Bogolusa, Louisiana. A 6-year follow-up study found that insulin levels did not predict rises in blood pressure in black children

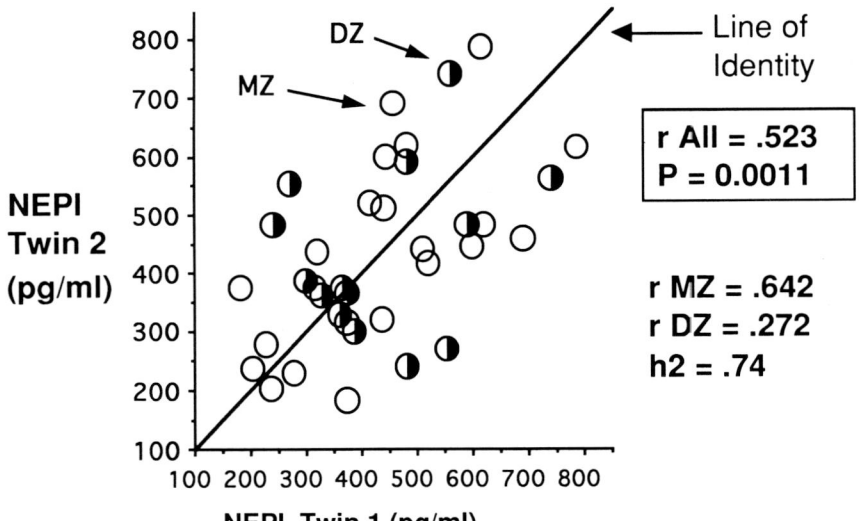

FIG. 5. Spearman correlation of plasma NE in twin pairs. There is a significant correlation in all twins. Monozygotic (MZ) correlations are higher than dizygotic (DZ). $h^2 = .74$.

but was an independent predictor in white children (103). On the other hand, Falkner et al. (104) recently studied insulin resistance and blood pressure in black men and women with normal blood pressure (<135/85) or with borderline hypertension (≥135/95) using the euglycemic hyperinsulinemic clamp technique. Borderline hypertensives had higher fasting insulin levels and greater insulin resistance. A nonobese group (n = 33) had a significant correlation with insulin resistance and sex, BP group, and systolic BP. In striking contrast to Falkner's report in borderline hypertensives, Saad et al. reported no relationship of insulin resistance to blood pressure in adult blacks or in Pima Indians. Mean blood pressure was correlated (r = −.41) with fasting insulin levels in whites but not in blacks (r = −.10) or in Pima Indians (r = −.06). However, if the BP-insulin association is genetic and specific to whites, then blacks showing this association may be admixed with whites, i.e., the white pattern appears in black populations by virtue of admixture with white genes for a BP-insulin correlation. Thus, the small study by Falkner et al. may have included a more admixed population of blacks than was studied by Saad or by Voors. Finally, Akanji et al. (105), in a study of Nigerians in Nigeria, found that a reduced insulin response to glucose loading was blunted and that, as found by Saad, there was no correlation between insulin values and blood pressure.

In our own studies we reasoned that if high insulin levels are important in SS of blood pressure in African Americans, then insulin levels measured around the clock should also be increased. We studied 27 normotensive African-American men with a 12-day protocol of 4 days of a 150-mM Na diet, then 4 days of 10 mM Na and 4 days of 200 mM Na. On day 4 of each diet, 24-hour BP was measured and every 4 hours we measured urinary sodium excretion, plasma insulin, and glucose. Subjects were classified as SS if mean 24-hour BP increased significantly from the 10-mM diet to the diet of 200 mM Na. Others were SR: 7 were SS and 19 SR (Table 5).

Repeated measures ANOVA demonstrated that insulin and glucose levels were significantly lower in SS than in SR (p < .01). There was no effect of diet on insulin or glucose levels. There was no correlation between insulin, 4-hour sodium excretion and 4-hour or 24-hour BP.

TABLE 5. *Insulin and glucose levels in salt-sensitive and salt-resistant African Americans*

Na Diet (Mm)	Insulin (μU/mL)		Glucose (mg%)		ENa (mM/4 hr)	
	SS	SR	SS	SR	SS	SR
150	15	31	95	112	18.0	12.6
10	17	21	98	100	2.7	3.9
200	15	20	94	96	22.0	22.7

SS, salt-sensitive; SR, salt-resistant; ENa, sodium excretion.

These results confirm that a positive insulin-BP relationship is not present in African Americans and indeed that SS have lower 24-hour insulin levels than SR blacks.

A Marker for African-Descent Mitochondria DNA is Associated with CAD Risk Factors in Blacks

Denaro et al. (106) have shown that human mitochondrial DNA (MT-DNA) has six restriction fragment patterns when digested with Hpa I, and that there is a strong correlation between these patterns and maternal ethnic lineage. We have been the first to use this marker, which is inherited only from one's mother, to examine the effect of African descent on cardiovascular risk factors by using white cells saved from our previous studies of twins in Barbados (107). The effect of maternal lineage on systolic pressure (SBP), and 17 plasma assays including aldosterone (PA), angiotensin-converting enzyme (ACE) activity, cholesterol (Chol), and white blood cell count (WBC) was assessed in 40 black normotensive volunteers. DNA was isolated from WBC, digested with endonuclease Hpa 1, electrophoresed in 1 percent agarose gel, and transferred to nytran filters. Blots were hybridized with ^{32}P-labeled MT-DNA probes. Only Denaro's pattern 2 (non-African, n = 18) and 3 (African, n = 22) were found. Classic twin analysis suggested a genetic influence on systolic blood pressure, plasma aldosterone, cholesterol, and triglycerides. There was no effect of MT-DNA type on anthropometric measurements including height, weight, and arm circumference. The major results are tabulated below (Table 6).

ANOVA demonstrated significant influences of maternal lineage on all variables. Thus, blacks (at least in Barbados) with an African maternal lineage are more likely to have the phenotype associated with an increase in blood pressure and cholesterol and a decrease in aldosterone and WBC. The influence of the African MT-DNA pattern on blood pressure and plasma aldosterone is of special interest in light of the report by Pratt (108) that in white MZ twins the twin-twin correlation for urinary aldosterone excretion (sleep) was 0.672 (p = .0002) and in DZ it was 0.103 (p = .309). In addition, they reported that in black families the sib-sib intraclass correlation for urinary aldosterone excretion was 0.510 (p = .0014). These results suggest that, in blacks and whites, aldosterone metabolism may be under strong genetic control. The lower WBC count in blacks with the African MT-DNA is also of great interest and will be a stimulus for further research into the well-known lower WBC count in blacks (or increased WBC in whites). The MT-DNA results suggests a genetic origin for this finding. As it is well known that leukocytes may play a role in atherogenesis, we are intrigued by the possibility that a lower WBC in blacks may be protective against atherosclerosis in blacks.

TABLE 6. *Effect of maternal lineage on systolic pressure, aldosterone, cholesterol, and white blood count in black normotensives*

MT-DNA type (Denaro)	Systolic pressure (mm Hg)	Plasma aldosterone (ng/100 mL)	Plasma cholesterol (mg%)	WBC ($\times 10^3$/mL)
2 (Non-African, n = 18)	114	11.3	181	6.8
3 (African, n = 22)	121	7.0	220	3.9
ANOVA	$p < .05$	$p < .04$	$p < .03$	$p < .0007$

MT-DNA, mitochondrial DNA.

Intracellular Ions and Salt Sensitivity in Blacks

The Williams group (109), in a series of white Utah pedigrees and sibship analyses, suggested a recessive monogenic effect and high total heritability for urinary kallikrein, high fat pattern index, intraerythrocytic sodium, Na-Li countertransport, and ouabain binding sites. Familial correlations more strongly attributable to shared environment than to genetic effects were found for Na/K ATPase, intraerythrocytic magnesium, plasma digoxin-like factor, plasma renin activity, and plasma sodium concentration.

This issue has recently been reviewed in detail by Cooper and Borke (110), who conclude that persons of African descent function at a higher level of intracellular sodium while exhibiting lower rates of ouabain-sensitive and -insensitive membrane transport. The etiology of this difference is not known. There are two major possibilities. Due to another problem most likely residing in the kidney, blacks have increased sodium retention and volume expansion when ingesting today's sodium diet. This stimulates the release of natriuretic volume regulating hormones that increase intracellular sodium by any of a number of ways. This factor(s) is responsible for the epiphenomena of higher intracellular sodium which, by increasing intracellular Ca^{2+} in vascular smooth muscle cells, leads to vasoconstriction. Campese (111) has recently reported that calcium supplementation or pretreatment with slow release infedipine blunted the blood pressure increase with dietary sodium load in African Americans.

PSYCHOSOCIAL STRESS AS A MAJOR CONTRIBUTOR TO THE HIGHER BLOOD PRESSURE IN BLACKS

Animal Studies Suggest that the Neuroendocrine/Blood Pressure Response Will Be Heterogeneous

The following discussion is based on the details of an organism's response to psychosocial stress as discussed in detail in the chapter by Henry. It is clear from the older and recent work of Henry and others that in order for "psychosocial stress" to raise blood pressure in mice or rats, two separate factors must be carefully brought together: a set of genetically determined behavioral traits and a set of environmentally dictated social interactions that result in competition for the desiderata of the caged society—food, territory, and sex. If these two key factors are not precisely matched there will be only one of two outcomes: no competition and no effect on blood pressure or such severe competition that the male rats kill each other. However, when certain genetic endowments are mixed with certain biobehavioral situations, blood pressure increases as does left ventricular mass and small vessel hypertrophy, and premature death results from hypertensive complications.

The greater prevalence and severity of hypertension in blacks in the US has, for years, been suggested to be due to their systematic exposure to a wider array of chronic psychosocial stressors than their white counterparts. It seems likely to us that in man, as in mice and rats, it is the complexity and heterogeneity of both the individual's inherited neuroendocrine and behavioral responses to chronic socioeconomic stress and the intensity of that stress that leads to the higher blood pressure in African Americans. We also will present the argument that the chronic neuroendocrine responses to stress can lead to stimulation, suppression, or no change in the renin-angiotensin system seen in the high, medium, or low range of renin hypertensive variants of African Americans and other ethnic groups. We suggest that in man, as in animals, unexpressed anger induces sympathetic arousal, activation of the renin-angiotensin system, structural vascular changes, and a high-renin state. At the other extreme of the neuroendocrine response to stress, the repeated defeat experienced by some animals (and some humans) results in suppression of the SNS and stimulation of the pituitary adrenal axis, dysplasia of the adrenal glomerulosa-fasciculata complex, and an increased aldosterone/renin ratio.

The different pharmacological responses of these renin subtypes likely reflect their underlying behavioral and neurological heterogeneity. In some neuroendocrine subsets the fight-flight reaction and elevated catecholamines drive the high-renin state and combine to hasten vascular and cardiac hypertrophy and atherosclerosis. These archetypes should respond to relaxation therapy, beta-sympathetic blockade and/or ACE inhibitors. Thus, the low response of blacks to beta blockage and ACE inhibition suggests that African Americans are not demonstrating the fight-flight type of reaction. By contrast, the suppression of emotion and activation of the pituitary-adrenal axis characteristic of defeat should be associated with low-renin hypertension and incomplete suppression of mineralocorticoid activity. This state would resist psychotherapy, but the manifestations of high mineralocorticoid activity should respond to salt restriction, thiazides, calcium-channel blockers, or mineralocorticoid antagonists. In the low-renin state, pathophysiological changes and mortality should be less, perhaps because alexithymic suppression of chronic emotional responses lessens the neuroendocrine changes that accompany the low-renin state. The excellent response to diuretics suggests that this neuroendocrine response to stress is more common in black hypertensives.

High Blood Pressure as a Response to Psychosocial Stressors

The association of controlled anger with high blood pressure was first clearly enunciated by Alexander over 50 years ago (112). His often-cited accurate perception that hypertensives chronically inhibit the expression of the hostile impulses that result from arousal of the fight-flight response is now supported by compelling evidence (113,114). The recent, extensive book-length review by Fray and Douglas (115) of the pathophysiology of hypertension in blacks contends that it is no longer appropriate to speak of essential but of psychosocial hypertension. This is because it is their view, and also that of Anderson and McNally (116), that the critical factor initiating the condition is chronic psychosocial stress. This works through an interplay of constitutional factors, coping resources, and behavioral factors to induce increased sympathetic activity and its pathophysiological consequences. The psychosocial interplay based on the fight-flight response, as originally proposed by Alexander, results in more or less arousal depending on the balance between arousing stress and calming social support, as well as the endogenous set of the neuroendocrine system.

The Severe and Various Stressors in African-American Culture

In common with many others in the field, Fray and Douglas (117) and Johnson (118) focus on an anger of which the individual and others are not fully aware because they avoid self-disclosure, i.e., concealed anger as the activating mechanism of essential hypertension. Our theme is that although this is accurate in some individuals, high blood pressure cannot be solely attributed to suppression of the fight-flight response. They ignore other less well recognized but increasingly understood neuroendocrine mechanisms that result from psychosocial interactions. As Dressler (119) puts it in his presen-

tation of the way in which "social and cultural factors induce hypertension in blacks," there have been profound social changes that, from an evolutionary viewpoint, abruptly moved mankind from the original closely integrated hunter-gatherer bands. It was in such bands during the millenia that man evolved a brain that is not so well suited for modern industrial society with its melange of peoples, cultures, and societies. Dressler describes the changes as an abandonment of tightly knit groups that relied on relationships and a reciprocity of services that permitted little internal competition. Modern society has increased the emphasis on the autonomous individual and on status and power based on appearance and possessions. It is lifestyle that is important now, rather than the attachments of the complex extended family. Western values are widely marketed and individuals strive toward a lifestyle whose attainment is measured in terms of goods such as magazines, radios, stoves, refrigerators, televisions, cars, etc. that the individual uses. Dressler's convincing quantitative data show how those whose lifestyle exceeds their class, rank, and/ or income suppress awareness of the discrepancy as they struggle to maintain their unstable social status. Years of education and type of work are critical determinants both of class and rank. In the US and the Western Hemisphere, skin color is still important in ranking. Yet Dressler's data indicate that a high-status lifestyle that lacks the appropriate network of social support, because class and rank have been outstripped, carries with it an eightfold increased risk of high blood pressure. If education and occupation are low and the skin color is black then, for the young, the social orientation provided by the family loses significance and the extent of non-kin support (i.e., peer or "gang") becomes critical (120,121).

Fray and Douglas (118) have pointed out that lifestyle incongruity due to socioeconomic status is perpetuated in black American society by poor, overcrowded schools, community violence, and unemployment, all the legacy of the slavery history. The John Henryism phenomenon is a further problem. This refers to the fact that young blacks who, despite a lack of the requisite resources, strive by hard work and determination to overcome the disadvantages of limited education in a racist society. The evidence indicates as they struggle with such insuperable obstacles their chronically aroused physiology leads to increases in blood pressure.

Different Psychosocial Mechanisms of High Blood Pressure

Fray and Douglas (118) note that although the general physiological principles underlying higher blood pressure and the importance of psychophysiological stressors in increasing blood pressure are beginning to be more clearly appreciated, there remain some tantalizing gaps in our understanding. For the most part, those describing the condition in psychological terms agree that it is the consequence of an anger that has for long not been disclosed, often because it is not recognized at all. The conditions at home and especially at work provide good reasons that irritation not be displayed. A striking example is the unexpected response of San Francisco bus drivers, most of whom were black, to their stressful experiences. They ranged from difficult passengers to severe traffic problems and restrictive regulations. Yet despite the obvious problems there was a startling inverse relation between the drivers' subjective appraisal of job stress and their blood pressure (122,123). The higher the blood pressure, the less the drivers reported being stressed.

This denial or "repression" seen in these hypertensive bus drivers has long been recognized as a source of misleading information concerning the stressors to which subjects are being exposed. The mechanism of denial has been related to the condition of alexithymia or the failure to express and experience emotion. The 1970s studies of Weinberger et al. (124) on this question of a repressive and defensive coping style superimposed on anxiety and the muffling of its expression have been repeatedly confirmed. They perceive an unexpressed distress as a trigger that leads to increased blood pressure even in those who, like the bus drivers, deny being stressed (124,125). Our point is that there are different neuroendocrine responses according to whether control is being experienced by the person or whether control has been lost. It appears that the repressive alexithymic response that is associated with low renin but higher blood pressure is an expression of a defeated or subordinated hormonal pattern as opposed to the endocrine response of the organism that is still striving for control and experiencing the fight-flight response. In other words, there is not just a single neuroendocrine response to psychosocial challenge and stimulation (stress). There is a spectrum depending on how much control the individual perceives (126) and the neurohumoral response patterns dictated by endogeneous, inherited behavioral patterns (Fig. 6).

Figure 6 summarizes the range of responses. The defense reaction is activated when the organism is challenged but remains in control. When the challenge is severe, a response must be made to the threat as the individual strives to retain a sense of control. There are neuroendocrine changes with the shift from a purely active response to a perception that passive or avoidant behavior may be necessary. There are increases of adrenaline, renin, and fatty acids as the sympathetic adrenal medullary system shifts from an emphasis on fight to flight. A further change occurs as with more severe challenge the sympathetic adrenal medullary system progressively gives way to a sense of defeat and an activation of the pituitary adrenal cortical system (127).

The central amygdalar nuclei are closely associated with the fight-flight cardiovascular response (128) and

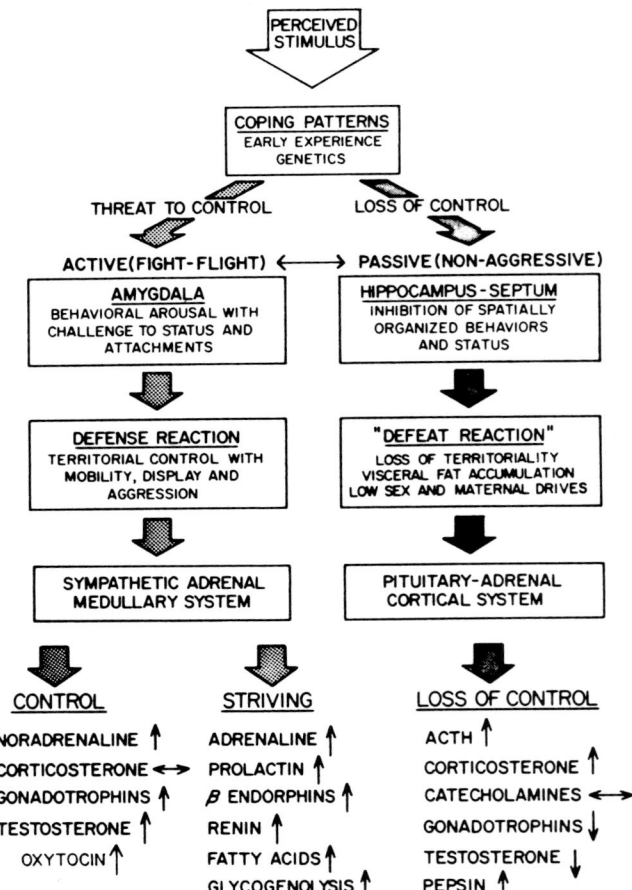

FIG. 6. The defense response involving fight and/or flight activation of the sympathoadrenal system is aroused when the organism is challenged in its control of the environment. With loss of territorial control and failure to meet expectations the adrenocortical system becomes more involved, and a nonaggressive coping response may take over. Hormonal reactions are indicated in the left-hand column in the lower portion of the figure. The physiological consequences of these two response patterns differ as shown. (From ref. 134.)

Folkow (129) has described the contrast between this defense reaction critical for the development of renin-dependent high blood pressure and the defeat reaction. Koolhaas and Bohus et al. (130,131) have emphasized the neuroendocrine as well as the behavioral contrast between the two. They argue that control versus loss of control in the social environment determines the varied pathology that follows social stress: controllability with predictability, loss of control, and threat to control have differing effects because they elicit different neuroendocrine responses and consequently different emotions.

Recently, Bjorntorp and his associates (132), working both with humans and rats, have proposed that with the loss of control in the defeated condition with its diminished sex and maternal drive there is a whole new pattern of disease susceptibility. They point to physical changes including an increased deposition of fat around the waist and a vulnerability to type II diabetes. They suggest that hormonal patterns differ because these people are depressed and defeated rather than hopeful and striving. They suffer from the classic Selyean distressed state with arousal of the hypothalamo-pituitary-adrenal axis with a vulnerability to hyperadrenocorticism, rather than a predominance of Cannon's defense fight-flight catecholamine-driven response. As the following will indicate, the same defeated neuroendocrine response may be the cause of those with low-renin hypertension (133).

Psychological Characteristics of Renin-Dependent and Low-Renin Hypertension

The concepts derived by our and others' examination of the neuroendocrine response to challenge in mice and rats in a social situation can be used to analyze the heterogeneous responses found when types of human hypertension are contrasted. Daunting psychosocial environmental factors are involved in the situations endured by so many blacks where there is low socioeconomic status (i.e., low control and high demand both at work and in the home) (134). As Fig. 7 indicates, there is likely a genetically transferred predisposition to respond with a suppression of emotion and an acceptance of loss of control. This may be made stronger by negative events during childhood.

Inherited traits can readily be exaggerated in infancy by insecure early attachment together with low access to social controls. Our recent work with mice and rats supports this concept (135). In this study it was shown that psychosocial stress can become involved in the induction of chronic hypertension in various strains of rats that would otherwise remain normotensive throughout their lives. Three strains that differ in aggressiveness were chosen. One was the Wistar-Kyoto hyperactive rat (WKHA), developed from the SHR by Hendley's group. Repeated observation confirmed that the males did not fight regardless of provocation. The second strain was the familiar Sprague-Dawley albino. When placed in a communal cage, the males did not bite each other but they did scratch and squabble. Although brief fights broke out, they did not hurt each other. They were regarded as intermediate between the WHKA and the third strain, the Long-Evans rat. This strain of rat has routinely been used as fighters to intimidate other rats because of their "proven level of aggression." In communal cages with females they lived up to their reputation, becoming involved in serious fights with biting (136). On these three distinct behavioral genetic substrates we induced social instability by placing four males with four females in each of four, two-foot square cages. The arousal of the animals in this colony milieu could be made more severe by periodic mixing of the males from different boxes. This social paradigm had no observable effect on the peaceable WKHA, induced some observable effects on the Sprague-Dawley males, and greatly stimulated the Long-Evans males. The different types of psychosocial stress (i.e., mixed or stable populations) and the different

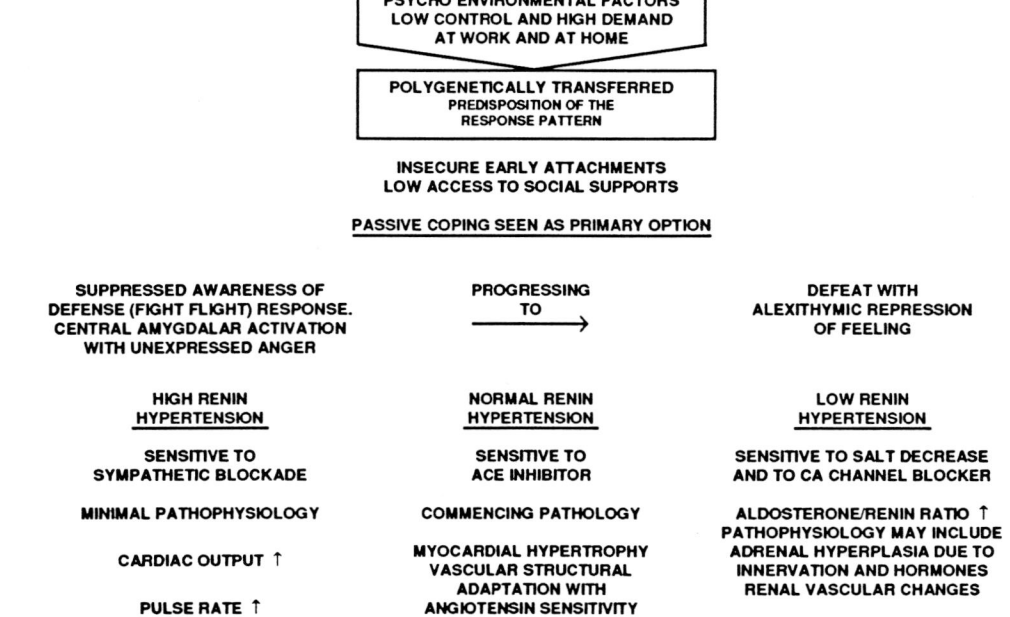

FIG. 7. Modification of Folkow's presentation of the principal pathogenetic elements in primary hypertension with comments on the nature of the psychoemotional factors involved. Changes with time and the critical structural role of the blood vessels are featured. (From ref. 134.)

genetics combined to induce a spectrum of neuroendocrine and blood pressure changes over a period of 6 months. Thus, inherited behavioral traits were clearly exaggerated by the social experience or milieu (137).

As Bouchard et al. (138) have emphasized in their study of human twins raised apart, inherited factors determine personality and temperament as well as intelligence. Parents and culture influence these traits to some extent, but the effects were "not as great as had been imagined." As in the rat, in man there is a strong gene-environment covariance. Thus, heredity likely determines whether the individual traits can readily be exaggerated in infancy by such experiences as insecure early attachment together with low access to social support.

In this context Anderson and McNally (134) point out that the social milieu in which many African Americans exist not only contributes to the experiences of angry feeling but simultaneously punishes their expression. Figure 8 presents the related difference that both Thailer et al. of the Cornell group noted in preliminary work (139) and more recently Perini et al. (140) have noted in a detailed comparison of the behavior of high- and low-renin hypertensives.

Testing of the group to determine which were high-and which low-renin subjects was performed after 5 to 7 days of diet containing only 70 mmol/day. This nor-mally stimulates renin secretion (142). Renin categorization was based on the PRA 24-hour urine sodium nomo-gram of Laragh and Sealey (142).

In the Perini study, comprehensive psychological testing interviews provided measures of the following: the experience and expression of anger, i.e., the State Trait Anger Expression Inventory (STAXI); trait anxiety using the Bendig 20-item short form of the Taylor Manifest Anxiety Scale, and the defensive tendency not to report unfavorable information about oneself, using the Marlowe Crowne Social Desirability (MCSD) scale. Those who scored in the lower third of the Bendig anxiety scale but in the upper quartile of the MCSD defensiveness scale were classified as "responders." The Perini group found that low-renin patients did not experience anger or anxiety. They were defensive "nonresponders" who successfully denied their emotions, a difference that is likely an inherited characteristic. In contrast, the high-renin subjects avoided self-disclosure, thus concealing their anger and anxiety from others (143); they could be discriminated by their positive responses to the STAXI, i.e., the SCL-90 scale of Spielberger. This is the scale used by Perini. This group should respond to psychotherapy and to relaxation therapy. By contrast, the patients with low renin had far lower scores for anxiety, hostility, and emotional distress. Unlike the high-renin group, Perini

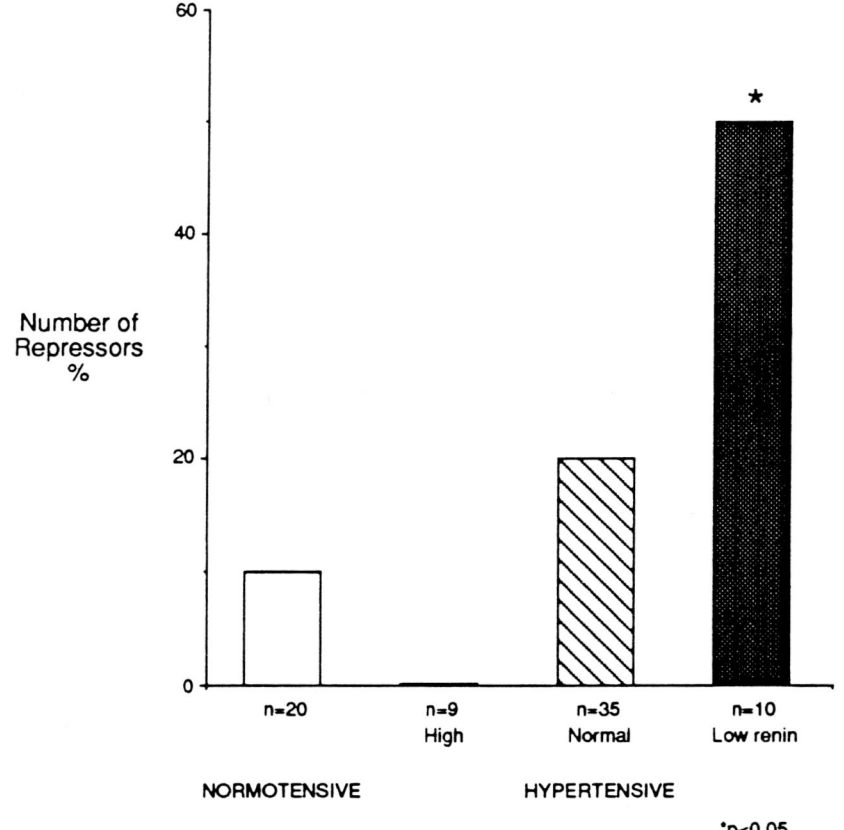

FIG. 8. The number of "repressors" in a normotensive group are contrasted with those in hypertensive patients classified by renin-sodium profiles. $p < .05$ for the low-renin versus the high-renin patients and the normotensive group. From ref. 141.

says they are not just failing to disclose, they simply do not experience, recognize, and verbalize feelings. In addition, they do not respond to relaxation therapy, while giving a convincing impression of well-adjusted poise. The extent to which these differing behavioral traits are genetically determined in man is as yet not known, and similar biobehavioral studies of blacks by renin profile are not available.

It is of interest, as noted above, that 60 percent of the over 1,000 bus drivers studied in San Francisco by Winkleby et al. (122) were black, and a majority suppressed feelings elicited by job stressors. There was a gross underreporting of specific stressful situations. In this group, a majority of whom were probably low-renin, there was a direct inverse relation between the intensity of the stressors they were experiencing and blood pressure. Their "repression" contrasts with the responsiveness of high-renin subjects who are more likely to be angry and anxious.

Pathophysiological and Pharmacotherapeutic Differences Between High- and Low-Renin Hypertension

The different neuroendocrine response patterns between renin types are accompanied by marked pathophysiological differences and their long-term effect. Alderman et al. (144), also of Cornell, have recently reported a decade-long study that involved over 1,700 patients that showed the sharp differences between the high, normal, and low renin profiles. With variations in renin profile came a significant difference in the incidence of myocardial infarction and mortality from all causes. The rate of infarction was 14.7/1,000 in the high-renin group, 5.6/1,000 in the normal-renin group, and only 2.8/1,000 in those with low renin.

Different Stressors Induce Different Neuroendocrine Responses

In brief, it might be said that different genetic substrates respond to the same stimuli with different neuroendocrine patterns. There is growing evidence of the neurophysiological basis for the clear-cut heterogeneity of the types of hypertension. It does not find expression only in behavior, responses to drugs, and pathophysiology. Recent work by Van de Kar et al. (145) has followed up on earlier studies of the close relation of the amygdalar central nuclei with the paraventricular nuclei responsible for corticosterone, vasopressin, and oxytocin release. Different methods of inducing "stress" produced strikingly different neuroendocrine responses. When the stress of immobilization was contrasted with the stress of the conditioned fear of receiving an expected series of shocks, sharply differentiated responses were produced.

In addition, central amygdalar lesions inhibited the corticosterone response to both the immobilization and the conditioned fear. However, the renin response was blocked only in the shock-fear paradigm. The work of Saphier (146) shows the differing responses of the neural mechanisms, including the raphe, which regulate the secretion of oxytocin and vasopressin. Thus, the raphe as well as the central amygdala, the paraventricular nucleus, and the stria terminalis respond in the high-renin fear-anxiety state. It appears that the renin, corticosterone, and prolactin patterns of stimulation differ when the stress-emotion paradigm is fear of loss of control (restraint) as opposed to actual helplessness (repeated shock). Clearly, there are differing routes taken by responses of the amygdalar nuclei to the catecholamine and renin expression of the fight-flight mechanism. However, there are demonstrable differences between this state and the passive acceptance forced by helpless immobilization. The latter is associated with the high ACTH (corticosterone) and prolactin responses of helplessness (i.e., loss of control), a psychological state compatible with the low-renin response.

The Neuroendocrine Response to Psychosocial Stimulation Involves the Adrenal as Well as the Kidney

The evidence for different stressors producing differing neuroendocrine responses is not confined to the central nervous system. Carlsson's work (147) with the direct innervation of the adrenal cortex suggests that steroidogenesis is controlled not only by neuronally regulated blood flow, but also by neurotransmitter effects on the glomerulosa itself to change rates of corticosterone and aldosterone production (148). Furthermore, independent control of stress-induced vasopressin and oxytocin release by the stria terminalis has been demonstrated by Gray et al. (149). Malendowicz et al. have cited evidence that these hormones can serve as mineralocorticoid secretagogues acting directly on the glomerulosa cells (150). Indeed, the extensive work of Ulick's group (151) over the years indicates that salt-saving mineralocorticoid effects can result from corticosterone itself if genetically determined local inactivating mechanisms fail.

Stress and the Hypermineralocorticoid-Adrenal Hyperplasia Syndromes

The low renin levels seen in hypertensive US blacks is compatible with subtle disturbances in the aldosterone/mineralocorticoid production seen in stress-induced adrenal hyperplasia. The greater prevalence of adrenal hyperplasia in blacks was first noted by the Hopkins study (152), and several groups have reported an increased prevalence of the primary aldosteronism in blacks. Screening of hypertensive subjects for primary aldosteronism using the ratio of aldosterone to renin was first reported by Grim et al. in 1979 (153) and was successful in detecting subjects with normokalemic aldosteronism (154). These early reports have been verified by Hiramatsu et al. (155) in screening for aldosterone-producing adenomas and by Gordon et al. (156) who detect primary aldosteronism in its early normokalemic stages, a condition that they report to be far more common than previously thought. In addition, Gordon's extensive previous studies of aldosteronism, including those of Gomez-Sanchez et al. (157), have shown that it is a multiform disorder of the adrenal transitional zone between the glomerulosa and the fasciculata. To Gordon's group the term *aldosteronism* covers a spectrum of conditions that are expressed as hyperplasia as well as outright neoplasia. In fact, even in classic primary aldosteronism due to a solitary benign adrenocortical adenoma, the zona glomerulosa is often found to be hyperplastic, suggesting that the abnormality is not limited to the adenoma cells. These observations have a long background. In 1976, Grim et al. (158) had already demonstrated how commonly adrenal hyperplasia or very small tumors are found in low-renin hypertension. His group and that of Gunnells et al. (159) showed that bilateral adrenalectomy frequently cures such hypertension and that the removed adrenals frequently showed hyperplasia. More recently, Halber et al. (160) have demonstrated that many hypertensive patients have a sustained aldosterone secretion. They fall into Laragh's low-renin group so common in blacks in the US and in whom Gordon et al. have demonstrated a high aldosterone/renin ratio. Approximately one-third of Halber's patients with primary (i.e., essential) hypertension had elevated aldosterone levels similar to those in patients of Grim et al. and Gunnells et al. with surgically confirmed hyperplastic adrenals and characterized by a high aldosterone/renin ratio.

The origins of the hyperplasia that are often found associated with an adenoma and/or microadenomas are by no means clear. Gordon would attribute much to genetics. However, our own data suggest that the psychosocial environment can also lead to hyperplasia. Animal studies show that adrenal hyperplasia often accompanies the hypertrophy that results from chronic psychosocial stimulation. Indeed, Wexler (161) has shown that mixed male and female breeder rats subjected to repeated changes in group composition develop not only hypertension but also enlargement and hyperplasia of the adrenal with increased synthesis of corticosterone as well as catecholamines. As noted above, Henry et al. have reproduced some of these results showing that male and female rat colonies chronically exposed to psychosocial stimulation develop not only high blood pressure and increased heart weight but also adrenal hypertrophy (136). It remains to be seen whether the aldosterone/renin ratio of such socially stressed animals is increased together with the frequency of adrenal hyperplasia.

Stress and High-Renin Hypertension

It is now well established that high-renin hypertension is associated with arousal of the fight-flight response and increased sympathetic activity (162,163). In their 1990 presentation of the psychosocial mechanisms of primary hypertension, Henry and Grim reviewed the evidence that stress and activation of the fight-flight response followed by structural vascular adaptation could account for the phenomenology of renin-dependent hypertension. Henry and Grim presented evidence that the low-renin variant could also be explained by the emotionally driven (i.e., neuroendocrine) changes (see Fig. 6) (134). It was suggested that when an organism is in a situation demanding passive acceptance, as when nonaggressive response is dictated by racial prejudices, there will be a strict control of behavior. This often goes with repression of awareness of the situation. The neuroendocrine picture is one of increasing adrenal cortical stimulation. The hypertrophy of activation will often progress to adrenal hyperplasia (164). It is now evident that adrenal cortical function is directly influenced by the autonomic innervation as well as by trophic effects of hormones. Our own observations in the 1970s of the effects of denervation (165) had suggested that, as Carlsson has recently shown in his work in Folkow's laboratories, the cortex is under autonomic control (148). There is no longer any question that repeated psychosocial stress can lead to sustained and fixed hypertension in mice and rats, nor that this psychosocially induced condition involves heterogeneous responses (i.e., the high and low renin syndromes). The division into two operative mechanisms, as Laragh has said, is "no mere academic exercise." (165) The different components are separated neuroendocrinologically and the mechanisms driving renin secretion can be shown to follow more than one pathway in the brain. The connections are changed from one set of pathways to another when the emotion involved becomes anger as opposed to the depression of loss of control. In short, the heterogeneity of the responses to psychosocial stimuli leads to different neuroendocrine mechanisms of high blood pressure with different treatments and prognoses.

PSYCHOSOCIAL FACTORS IN HYPERTENSION IN BLACKS

Having discussed the theoretical basis of stress-induced increases in blood pressure, we will now turn to specific psychosocial factors that may be related to the higher blood pressure in African Americans (166). As noted by Myers, Anderson, and Strickland (167), the absence of an integrated, multidisciplinary perspective that considers multiple contributors to psychosocial stress is a major obstacle to advancing our understanding of how this disease develops and is maintained in different population groups, especially blacks in a racist society.

We present a multidimensional model that starts with the premise that essential hypertension develops in persons who possess an underlying biological vulnerability for this disease. This biological substrate is acted upon by psychosocial factors, including socioeconomic status, lifestyle factors, psychological attributes, and family dynamics that contribute, either singly or in interaction, to the timing of the onset of the disease, to the disease course, and ultimately to disease morbidity and mortality. This model has been variously referred to as a *diathesis-stress model* or, more recently, as a *biobehavioral* or *biopsychosocial model* (see 168,169 for a more detailed discussion). Here we will discuss the evidence linking four psychosocial factors to the elevation of blood pressure. Two are socioecological factors: socioeconomic status and socioecologic stresses; and two are psychological factors: the predisposition toward active, effortful coping with stress (i.e., John Henryism), and styles of coping with anger and hostility. We also argue that greater attention needs to be paid to the patterns of interpersonal interactions within families as this is the primary setting in which psychosocial factors are mediated and expressed as well as the observation that the black-white difference in blood pressure appears before children leave the home.

Socioeconomic Status is Associated with Blood Pressure in All Ethnic Groups

There is substantial evidence that lower socioeconomic status (SES), whether measured by education, income, occupation, or some combination of these variables, is associated with greater morbidity and mortality from essential hypertension and its sequelae in all ethnic and gender groups (170–176). The Hypertension Detection and Follow-Up Group (177) found that lower education was associated with significantly higher resting blood pressures and a higher prevalence of hypertension. Blacks were twice as likely to be hypertensive as whites, and this racial imbalance was evident in all age groups and in both genders.

There is also historical evidence that lower SES appears to be particularly pathogenic for blacks (i.e., poverty results in greater negative consequences for blacks than for other ethnic groups) (178). It has been argued that in an antiblack, racist society, a lower socioeconomic status exposes blacks to greater social and economic oppression and discrimination than that experienced by whites or other groups due to the confluence of debilitating social context deficits, as well as high-risk behaviors and lifestyles found in poverty-stricken communities. Thus, low-SES blacks are more likely to reside in high socioecologic stress neighborhoods (i.e., high crime, high unemployment, low income, high marital and family instability), to consume diets high in sodium and saturated fats but low in calcium and potassium, to be overweight (especially black women), and to consume excessive amounts of alcohol, tobacco, and illegal drugs. All of these aspects of a poverty-stricken lifestyle interact to substantially enhance the risk for hypertension above and beyond that which is attributable simply to low education or low income.

Socioecologic Stress and Social Disorganization

The psychosocial variable consistently associated with higher blood pressure is living in high socioecologic stress areas. The often-cited studies by Harburg et al. (179,180) showed that for both males and females, black and white, those who lived in communities characterized by high crime, high unemployment, low income, high social instability, and disorganization were significantly more likely to evidence higher resting blood pressures and a higher prevalence of essential hypertension than their ethnic and gender counterparts living in more socioecologically wholesome communities. The highest resting blood pressures were observed in those communities that were both low in SES and high in social instability.

In these socioecologic environments, young black males were 2.5 times more likely to have elevated diastolic blood pressures (i.e., >95 mm Hg) than their cohorts in less socioecologically stressful areas. However, in black men over the age of 40 the living area did not increase the risk of increased blood pressure. Syme (181) has suggested that these results reflect the efforts of younger black men to gain control over difficult and uncontrollable circumstances and the associated greater feelings of anger and frustration. Thus, human environments that are psychologically oppressive because of low economic and social resources, low access to the critical social pathways of opportunity, high threat to personal safety, and/or unstable social structures enhances one's risk for developing hypertension. This risk is enhanced by other high-risk behaviors inherent to these areas: smoking, poor diet, alcoholism, and substance use. Because not everyone in these areas has high blood pressure, what protects those who remain normotensive?

John Henryism

James and colleagues (182) hypothesized that persons with "a strong personality predisposition to cope actively with psychosocial stressors in [their] environment," but with few resources for successful coping (e.g., low education) would be at enhanced risk for hypertension compared to either their counterparts without this predisposition or those similarly disposed but who possess the requisite resources. This coping style has been labeled *John Henryism* (JH) after the legendary black folk hero, John Henry, who epitomized the value of hard work as a means of overcoming overwhelming odds. This hypothesis was first tested in a study of rural black men (182) and later on a community sample of black and white men and women (183). The results of the first study confirmed their hypothesis: black men who were high in JH but with low educational attainment had the highest mean blood pressures. This relationship was further enhanced by perceptions among the more successful blacks that race had interfered with their success. In a more recent study (184), these investigators tested this hypothesis across races and gender groups and found confirmation of greater prevalence of hypertension in high-JH–low-SES black men and women, but not in whites. However, the JH-SES interaction effect was not obtained when mean resting systolic and diastolic blood pressures were tested in each of the ethnic groups. The authors noted that differences in the meaning of SES among blacks may have mitigated against confirming the association between SES, JH, and blood pressure. In whites, the narrow range of SES may have precluded finding any significant association between SES, JH, and blood pressure or any differences in the prevalence of hypertension.

In any event, these studies support the suggestion by Syme (185) that young blacks who are striving to achieve some modicum of social mobility and are predisposed to compensate for their limited educational resources by active, effortful coping (i.e., hard work and determination) run substantially higher risk of becoming hypertensive than other blacks. This evidence may also be congruent with Dressler's social incongruity hypothesis, which posits enhanced risk for hypertension in blacks whose lifestyles exceed their occupational status. However, none of this evidence should be interpreted as suggesting that effortful coping is unhealthy for blacks (e.g., that laziness and giving up the fight is healthier than continuing to struggle). Rather, they underscore the importance of a balance between educational and other resources and one's aspirations on the one hand, and the demands and obstacles one faces in the pursuit of these aspirations on the other. Without the requisite resources, compensating with increased effort or living beyond one's psychological and social means may incur the additional cost of a compromised cardiovascular system.

Coping with Anger and Hostility

As mentioned above, Alexander's (186) hypothesis that hypertensives experience conflict over the expression of hostility, aggression, and other strong emotions has met with failed attempts to identify a specific hypertensive personality (187). Investigators have begun to focus attention on the specific contribution that the experience and expression of anger and hostility might play in this disease. Thus suppressed anger, unexpressed hostility, and inhibited power motivation have been associated with elevated blood pressure (188–191) in both blacks and whites, but especially in younger black males. It is not clear if suppressed anger is part of the core psychodynamics of all hypertensives, only relevant to a subset, or whether suppressed anger operates as a psychological risk enhancer that interacts with other biological vulnerabilities (e.g., a sodium retention trait). If the former is true, we would expect that an anger-suppression style would be evident in a substantial majority of essential hypertensives. On the other hand, if the latter is true then we would expect that this coping style would manifest its effect only in the presence of some other underlying vulnerability.

The accumulating evidence indicates that the risk of higher blood pressure is greater in those with a tendency to suppress anger (192–195). For example, Harburg, Gentry, and associates found that individuals who habitually suppressed anger when provoked had higher resting blood pressures compared to those who expressed their anger when provoked. An anger-suppressing style enhanced the risk for hypertension after adjusting for race, gender, and neighborhood stress in both adolescents and adults (196–202).

Finally, behavioral observations and experimental manipulations suggest that the anger-suppressing style found in many hypertensives may be part of a psychological profile that includes a lack of appropriate assertiveness and a tendency toward greater interpersonal self-consciousness, anxiety, and submissiveness (203, 204). Two recent reports by Cumes-Rayner and Price (205,206) indicated that hypertensives evidenced a greater preference not to self-disclose, but would increase their level of self-disclosure if the situation required. This responsiveness to situational demands was associated with potent dysregulatory effects on their blood pressures. Normotensives were more self-disclosing and showed no associated BP dysregulation (207). In their second study, they investigated the impact of perceived social approval and disapproval on level of self-disclosure and BP reactivity in normotensives and borderlines and found that self-disclosing under conditions of perceived mild social disapproval produced marked BP reactivity only in the borderlines (208), as discussed previously. This evidence was partially confirmed by the results obtained by Winkleby, Ragland, and Syme (209) in San Francisco bus drivers who deny the subjective experience of stress even in high-stress jobs. These findings indicate that there is at least a subset of essential hypertensives who evidence a pattern of hypersensitivity to social exposure/social judgement and have difficulty acknowledging stress and expressing anger and hostility without guilt or conflict (i.e., are likely to be deniers or repressors).

It is also noteworthy that although most published studies report an association between increased blood pressure and inhibited anger, other studies have either failed to find this association (210,211) or have found it only in subgroups, e.g., white men but not black men or women of either race (212). Still others have found the apparently contradictory association between anger directed outward and increased blood pressure (213,214). For example, Harburg et al. (215) found that blacks who reported a tendency to express anger outwardly to an angry boss had higher diastolic blood pressures than those who reported a tendency to suppress anger or to use a more reflective coping style. Some researchers have also observed greater hostility and aggressiveness in hypertensive compared to normotensive subjects (216).

In an effort to account for these apparently contradictory findings, several investigators have suggested that both habitual anger-in and habitual anger-out coping styles, i.e., reflexive rather than reflective anger coping, are associated with elevated blood pressure, and that the relationship between anger-coping style and blood pressure is mediated by a variety of personal and environmental characteristics. For example, Manuck et al. (217) and others explain the apparent contradictory findings by suggesting that lack of "appropriate assertiveness" may be the psychological Achilles heel in a subset of hypertensives. This group of hypertensives may respond to provocation with either inappropriate submissiveness and/or with heightened hostility and aggressiveness. In one study, Manuck et al. (218) subjected borderline hypertensives and normotensives to a challenging role-play task and also asked their significant other to rate their level of social competence. Their results indicated that compared to normotensives, there were at least two distinct subgroups of hypertensives: one subgroup exhibited high levels of hostility and aggressiveness and significant increases in systolic blood pressure and heart rate during the role play whereas a second subgroup that behaved less assertively during the role play were rated as socially less competent by their significant other, and exhibited somewhat higher diastolic blood pressures. Thus, these results suggest that enhanced risk for hypertension may not be associated with one anger-coping style but (a) by how the anger stimulus is perceived and (b) by the degree of arousal and conflict that is experienced in that setting and in response to the provocation. In appropriately assertive persons, both psychological and physiological arousal would be appropriate to the provocation regardless of how the anger was expressed. In less appropriately assertive persons, however, provocation may result in excessive psychological and physiological arousal and a struggle over how to cope with the anger. The resultant neuroendorcrine/behavioral response could be either excessive aggressiveness (high renin) or inappropriate submissiveness (low renin), along with excessive physiological arousal.

Also, although several studies report an association between anger expression and resting blood pressure levels in both hypertensives and normotensives, it is unclear whether the pattern of anger expression and assertiveness mediate cardiovascular stress reactivity only in individuals already diagnosed as hypertensive or who are biologically at risk for the disease. In a study in which black hypertensive and normotensive women were asked to discuss a family conflict while being filmed, McClure (219) found that anger expression style mediated the blood pressure responses only in the hypertensives. Smith and Houston (220) also failed to find a relationship between measures of anger expression and blood pressure responses in normotensive males presented with two challenging tasks.

A recent study by Durel et al. (221) further complicates this picture by reporting gender and race differences in the patterns of association between anger trait, anger expression style, and blood pressure at rest and during active coping stress. These differences may be more evident in response to some types of stresses but not to others. They reported that white women evidenced a strong positive association between State-Trait anger (STAI-T), SBP, and DBP at rest and under active interpersonal conflict stress, whereas black women evidenced strong associations between STAI-T anger, SBP, and DBP at rest, work, and in response to cold pressor stress. On the other hand, among black men, only cognitive anger was associated with DBP at rest, whereas among white men there was a negative association between hostility (Ho scale) and SBP at rest and during a video game task, and a negative association between somatic anger and SBP and DBP reactivity to the cold pressor task.

Clearly, anger coping is a complex issue and the available evidence seems to suggest that one pathway worth further investigation involves whether a reflexive style of coping with anger (i.e., habitual anger-in and/or habitual anger-out) confers additional risk for this disease. It is also worth noting that different measures of anger and different contexts in which anger is elicited and blood pressure is measured may yield different results, and that these differences may be mediated by gender and race.

The Role of Racism and Discrimination in Hypertension in Blacks

A number of scholars have speculated that the disproportionate burden of morbidity and mortality from essential hypertension and related psychosomatic disorders in blacks is, at least in part, attributable to conflicts related to the experience of racism and discrimination (222–228). These investigators have argued that a major developmental task for blacks, and especially for black males, is to develop ways of coping with the ego-deflating experiences and the resulting anger and frustration they are likely to face throughout their lives because of their race. Empirical support for this hypothesis is provided by Gentry (229), who found in the Detroit blood pressure study that blacks evidenced significantly higher interracial hostility than whites, and that those blacks who also possessed the tendency to suppress anger were most likely to evidence the highest mean diastolic blood pressures. In an effort to further explore this question, Harrell (230) proposed six cognitive styles or philosophical perspectives that blacks have developed to cope with racism. They include: (a) an apathetic style characterized by passivity and accommodation to social demands and expectations; (b) a "piece of the action" style in which efforts are continuously made to succeed and to gain socially valued resources despite obstacles; (c) adopting countercultural solutions to racism that transcend the problems of life rather than confront them directly (e.g., developing nonmainstream lifestyles); (d) adopting an activist, black nationalist style with a strong commitment to confront racism in all of its various forms and faces; (e) adopting an authoritarian style in which rules are used to remove ambiguity by prescribing specific ways of responding "appropriately" to racial conflicts; and (f) adopting a style characterized by cognitive flexibility, historical awareness, and open-mindedness. It is clear to us that most of these behavioral traits may have been even more valuable in the struggle to survive the atrocity that was called slavery and that they may even have led to an increased likelihood of survival during slavery.

Efforts by Clark and Harrell (231) to investigate whether a particular racial coping style would be associated with enhanced cardiovascular reactivity to an active coping stressor (i.e., mental arithmetic), however, failed to support their expectations that an apathetic-submissive style would be associated with lower blood pressures. The only coping style that was consistently associated with any pattern of BP reactivity was a cognitively flexible style, which was associated unexpectedly with higher resting SBP and higher recovery DBP. In a subsequent study utilizing more emotionally involving stimuli (i.e., fearful, neutral vs. racist stimuli), Sutherland and Harrell (232) found that black undergraduate females evidenced more reactive heart rates and EMGs to both the racist and fearful imagery. These studies yielded somewhat contradictory results, although only the second study actually tested the impact of exposure to racism on cardiovascular functioning. In a more recent and better-designed study, Armstead et al. (233) tested the hypothesis that exposure to racially provocative stimuli would elicit consistently stronger cardiovascular reactivity in blacks than anger-provoking but nonracist stimuli or neutral stimuli. Their results were consistent with the hypothesis that blacks exhibited higher cardiovascular reactivity to the racist stimuli than to either the anger-provoking/nonracist stimuli or the neutral stimuli. However, self-reported anger arousal (i.e., state anger) was obtained in response to both the racist and the anger-provoking/nonracist stimuli.

This is the first concrete experimental evidence supporting the hypothesis that anger elicited by racist experiences or by racially loaded encounters results in marked cardiovascular reactivity in blacks, above and beyond that which is observed in response to racially neutral anger provocation. However, this evidence does not prove that racially triggered anger is more cardiovascularly pathogenic than anger elicited by any other stimulus, or that this type of anger is more deleterious to blacks than to others. We cannot assume, for example, that whites would not also evidence cardiovascular reactivity to racist stimuli (although the emotional content of that arousal might be different than in blacks) or that women would be any less angry and reactive to sexist stimuli. What this study does show, however, is that by virtue of greater exposure to racist and discriminatory encounters, blacks may run a greater risk than whites of exposure to anger-eliciting stimuli that provoke very strong conflicted emotions with commensurate cardiovascular hyperreactivity. Evidence from the work by James et al. (234,235) would predict that this greater exposure to racially induced stresses should result in even greater risk for hypertension in those blacks who respond with increased effort and determination but lack adequate instrumental resources (i.e., high JH and low education).

Future studies will need to pursue this question about the role of racism-induced anger and reactivity in hypertension and to investigate how individual anger-coping styles might mediate this additional stress burden. We might hypothesize, consistent with previous evidence on anger coping, that greater cardiovascular reactivity and slower recovery should be observed in blacks who are *reflexive* anger responders (i.e., both habitual suppressors and habitual overexpressors), whereas lower reactivity and faster recovery should be observed in those who have developed (or inherited) more *reflective* coping strategies.

Family Factors in Hypertension

Blood pressure and other risk factors cluster in families (236–240), in populations from diverse geographic and cultural backgrounds (241), and in children, adolescents, and adults (242–244). Although the moderate concordance of blood pressures in families (245–248) is compatible with a genetic effect, one also needs to consider a "family psychosomatic" hypothesis of hypertension, i.e., investigating what proportion of attributable familial risk for this disease is due to nongenetic familial processes (249). Some have suggested that the moderate levels of concordance observed between family members and genetically unrelated individuals living together (e.g., married couples) cannot be attributed to genetic factors in the usual sense. However the tendency for nonrandom mating in man, i.e., the tendency for people to marry or adopt persons with similar genetic traits such as skin color, height, or weight and even blood pressure (250) complicates the interpretation of "nongenetic" family environment. Although attributes of the shared environment including diet, nutrition, life stresses, the development of complementary styles of managing stresses, etc. (251,252) may lead to strong nongenetic familial influences on a person's underlying physiology and behavior and influence blood pressure, our studies in black twins provide little evidence for this. In a study involving 233 families, Connor et al. (253) provided evidence of a strong linkage between family dietary habits, familial metabolic aggregation (e.g., familial aggregation for urinary sodium, potassium, and creatinine excretion), and mean familial systolic blood pressure. Familial aggregation of salt sensitivity has been reported in whites, and our twin studies demonstrate a higher concordance in M2 twins.

In the case of blacks, there is ample evidence that their diets are lower in potassium and calcium and have higher sodium/potassium and sodium/calcium ratios than those reported by whites (254–259). Myers et al. (260) argued that these black-white differences in electrolyte intake probably reflect socioeconomic and sociocultural differences, and that these differences are established and maintained through family and community processes. However, the reports of similar lower urinary potassium excretions in blacks in Barbados (261), in Nigeria (262), in South Africa (263), and in Zaire (264) suggest that lower urinary excretion of potassium is a uniform phenomenon in black populations. Any biological differences that may exist between the races such as in sodium metabolism (265,266) could either be exacerbated or minimalized by these environmental influences.

The work by Baer and colleagues (267–269) and others also suggests that models of coping with conflict and anger provided by hypertensive parents may contribute additional risk in offspring above and beyond that which is attributable simply to biological inheritance. Personality characteristics such as denial and an unwillingness to admit to neurotic and aggressive feelings have been reported in a subgroup of young adults with a family history of hypertension (270). Gentry (271) also contends that anger-coping styles are learned and may be related to the psychological attributes of the dominant parent.

Although only a few studies have compared the family relationships and interaction patterns both within hypertensive families and between these families and the families of normotensives, the few that have made these comparisons suggest that negative behaviors (i.e., communication-disrupting behaviors) are associated with increases in blood pressure, and that communication skills training can reduce both hostile communication and the associated physiological reactivity in hypertensives during their interactions with their spouses (272,273).

In a series of studies with family triads, Baer and colleagues (274,275) reported greater gaze aversion in families with a hypertensive parent compared to families with normotensive parents. They suggested that this gaze aversion reflected conflict avoidance (i.e., by reducing information and confrontation), and suggested further that this style of coping with conflict may generate impaired anger management in the children and thereby increase their risk for developing the disorder. In one study, Baer et al. measured blood pressures before and after a family conflict role-play task and found greater SBP reactivity in the offspring of hypertensives along with more parental conflict-avoidant nonverbal behavior. Similar results were noted by McClure and Myers (276) in an unpublished study with black hypertensive and normotensive mother-daughter pairs. These investigators found that the hypertensive mother-daughter dyads exhibited more avoidant behaviors than the normotensive dyads during discussions of conflictual family issues (e.g., dating). The hypertensive family dyads were more likely to avoid eye contact, introduce irrelevant topics, and maintain silence when a response was clearly warranted. They also exhibited higher DBP reactivity during the conflict discussion. This pattern of conflict coping is congruent with the evidence reported by Cumes-Rayner and Price (277,278) that hypertensives evidence a preference for self-concealment, especially in potentially nonsupportive social encounters. In contrast, the normotensive mother-daughter dyads exhibited both more negative verbal behavior (e.g., openly criticized and voiced disagreements) and more positive nonverbal behavior (e.g., more smiling and touching), engaged in more problem solving (e.g., accepted responsibility for their behavior and made compromises), and evidenced lower SBP and DBP reactivity to the conflict discussion task.

Although it is unclear if physiological hyperreactivity is an early marker of the disorder or part of the inherited predisposition to the disorder in the offspring of hypertensives, there is an impressive body of literature that suggests that children of hypertensives do in fact exhibit enhanced physiological responses to a variety of stressors (279). That this is likely an inherited patten, at least in whites, is suggested by the studies of Rose et al. (280) that patterns of cardiovascular reactivity to stresses, at least in white twins, are under strong genetic control (281–283). In blacks, McClure and Myers also reported concordance of BP reactivity in their black mother-daughter dyads. Although we have suggested that at least the results of the McClure and Myers study could also be interpreted as indicating that cardiovascular responses to a conflict stressor may be mediated in part by shared or complementary coping strategies, this concept must be tempered by the recent report on the strong genetic influence on behavioral traits in white identical twin pairs raised apart. Most behavioral and psychological traits, as well as blood pressure, were as alike in twins raised apart as raised together. Twins raised apart and families of identical twins are some of the most efficient ways to tease apart these interactions, but such studies have never been reported in blacks.

THE CASE FOR AN INTERDISCIPLINARY APPROACH

The evidence reviewed here indicates that historical, genetic, and psychosocial factors have been implicated in the excessive morbidity and mortality from essential hypertension suffered by blacks. The evidence is quite substantial that blacks descended from slavery, who now have lower SES backgrounds and live in high socioecologically stressful and socially disorganized communities, have higher resting blood pressures and are at substantially greater risk of developing this disease than both whites and other blacks from less oppressive backgrounds. Evidence is also growing that blacks who cope with life demands by compensating for limited instrumental resources by increasing effort and determination (i.e., high JH) also run additional cardiovascular risks. The evidence is also accumulating that blacks, and especially black men, who characteristically respond to anger provocation with reflexive anger suppression or reflexive anger overreaction/expression, are particularly at risk for this disease. Finally, there is a growing body of evidence that suggests that family context and process variables also contribute to enhanced risk for developing essential hypertension.

Unfortunately, these bodies of research are developing in a haphazard and unintegrative fashion, and we are therefore unable to fully appreciate the degree to which this evidence is potentially complementary. It is important that studies begin incorporating all of these variables into their designs. For example, would black men with both high-risk socioecologic backgrounds and high-risk psychological profiles (i.e., high JH and anger-suppressing or anger-overreacting styles) evidence the highest resting BPs and the greatest cardiovascular reactivity to acute stresses compared to their black peers who possess only some of these risk factors? Is JH inherited? Would sodium metabolism be affected by these traits? in other words, do these psychosocial risk factors confer risk in an additive fashion or do they interact synergistically to increase risk in some nonlinear fashion? How much additional risk is conferred by these factors above and beyond that attributable to other known lifestyle risks such as smoking, sedentary lifestyles, obesity, increased alcohol intake, high-sodium/low-potassium, high-sodium/low-calcium and high-cholesterol diets? Also, does the source of stress and anger provocation

(e.g., racially loaded vs. racially neutral provocation) impact differently on the contribution that the other psychosocial and lifestyle risk factors make to elevated resting BP, to cardiovascular stress reactivity to acute stresses, and to long-term risk for developing stable hypertension in blacks? Do these factors operate differently as a function of SES and/or gender? Finally, as we make more progress in the genetics of blood pressure and behavior, are there specific genetic markers of the blood pressure control systems that predict reactions to the environmental stress imposed on blacks and other ethnic groups?

These and similar questions direly need to be answered and require that investigators approach their studies of the contribution of psychosocial factors in hypertension in blacks from a multidimensional perspective. Such a perspective would include, but not be limited to, the following: (a) careful assessment and consideration of the major known lifestyle risk factors in their analyses; (b) assessment of personal/family SES and of socioecologic stress level of the neighborhoods in which the subjects reside; (c) assessment of coping styles, either in terms of constructs such as JH or the coping styles suggested by Harrell for dealing with racism and/or those suggested by Lazarus and colleagues for dealing with daily hassles; (d) more careful assessment of styles of coping specifically with anger provocation, with consideration of the psychological significance of the provocation (e.g., racial discrimination, ego insult, infringement on personal control, etc.), and the methodology used for measuring the variable (i.e., self-reports vs. ratings of overt behavior); (e) more careful assessment of the neuroendocrine profiles associated with these behavioral profiles; (f) using pharmacological probes to assess the interaction of behavior with blood pressure regulatory systems; and (g) careful studies contrasting the role of culture and genetics in blood pressure variations in Africa and throughout the black diaspora.

ACKNOWLEDGMENTS

This research was supported in part by Research Centers in Minority Institutions (RCMI) award G12RR03026, 7 K04HL01885, T32MHL07655, and RR03026 from the NIH; award 878-F1 from the American Heart Association, Greater Los Angeles Affiliate.

REFERENCES

1. MacGregor GA, Markandu ND, Best FI, Elder DM, Cam JM, Sagnella GA, Squires M. Double-blind randomized crossover trial of moderate sodium restriction in essential hypertension. *Lancet* 1982;1:351–355.
2. Freis ED, Reda DJ, Materson BJ. Volume (weight) loss and blood pressure response following thiazide diuretics. *Hypertension* 1988;12:244–250.

3. Kumanyika SK, Hebert PR, Cutler JA, Lasser VI, et al. Feasibility and efficacy of sodium reduction in the Trials of Hypertension Prevention, phase I. *Hypertension* 1993;22:502–512.

4. World Health Organization. *Arterial hypertension.* 1988; Technical report series N.628.

5. Hall WD, Saunders E, Shulman NB, eds. *Hypertension in blacks: epidemiology, pathophysiology and treatment.* Chicago: Year Book Medical Publishers, 1985.

6. Fray JCS, Douglas JG, eds. *Pathophysiology of hypertension in blacks.* New York: Oxford University Press; 1993.

7. Saunders E, ed. *Hypertension in blacks.* 1991.

8. Voors AW, Foster TA, Frerichs RR, Webber LS, Berenson GS. Studies on blood pressure in children ages 5–14 years in a total biracial community. *Circulation* 1976;54:319–347.

9. Pratt JH, Jones JJ, Miller JZ, et al. Racial differences in aldosterone excretion and plasma aldosterone concentrations in children. *N Engl J Med* 1989;321:1152–7.

10. Manatunga AK, Jones JJ, Pratt JH. Longitudial assessment of blood pressures in black and white children. *Hypertension* 1993;22:84–89.

11. Newman WP III, Freedman DS, Voors AW, Gard PD, Srinivasan SR, Cresanta JL, Williamson GS, Webber LS, Berenson GS. Relation of serum lipoprotein levels and systolic blood pressure to early atheroclerosis: the Bogalusa Heart Study. *N Engl J Med* 1986;3114:1138–144.

12. Tracy RE, Guzaman MA, Oalmann MC, Newman WP, Strong JP. Nephrosclerosis in three cohorts of black and white men born 1925 to 1944, 1934 to 1953 and 1943–1962. *Am J Hypertens* 1993;6:185–192.

13. US Renal Data System, *USRDS 1992 Annual data report.* The National Institutes of Health, National Institute of Diabetes and Digestive and Kidney Diseases, Bethesda, August 1992, B.14.

14. Ferguson R, Grim CE, Opgenorth TJ. A familial risk of chronic renal failure among blacks on dialysis. *J Clin Epidemiol* 1988;41:1189–1196.

15. Freedman BI, Spray BJ, Tuttle AB, Buckalew VM. The familial risk of end-stage renal disease in African Americans. *Am J Kidney Dis* 1993;21:387–93.

16. Klag MJ, Whelton PK, Coresh J, Grim CE, Kuller LH. The association of skin color with blood pressure in US blacks with low socioeconomic status. *JAMA* 1991;265:599–602.

17. Micozzi MS. Childhood hypertension and academic standing in the Phillippines. *Am J Public Health* 1980;70:530–532.

18. Wyss JM, Fisk G, van Groen T. Impaired learning and memory in mature spontaneously hypertensive rats. *Brain Res* 1992;592:135–140.

19. Deubner DC, Tyroler HA, Cassel JC, Hames CG, Becker C. Attributable risk, population attributable risk, and population attributable fraction of death associated with hypertension in a biracial population. *Circulation* 1975;52:901–908.

20. Frerichs FF, Chapman JM, Maes EF. Mortality due to all causes and to cardiovascular diseases among seven race-ethnic populations in Los Angeles County, 1980. *Int J Epidemiol* 1984;13:291–297.

21. Frank CW, Weinblatt E, Shapiro et al. Prognosis of men with coronary heart disease as related to blood pressure. *Circulation* 1969;38:432–438.

22. Connolly DC, Elveback LR, Cxman HA. Coronary heart disease in residents of Rochester, MN. 1950–75. III. Effect of Hypertension and its treatment of survival of patients with coronary artery disease. *Mayo Clin Proc* 1983;58:249–254.

23. Dawber TR. *The Framingham Study.* Cambridge: Harvard University Press, 1980.

24. Messerli FH, Ventura HO, Elizardi DJ, et al. Hypertension and sudden death. Increased ventricular ectopic activity in left ventricular hypertrophy. *Am J Med* 1984;77:18–60.

25. The beneficial effect of the hypertensive detection and follow up program stepped care regime on indices of coronary artery and myocardial disease. *Am J Cardiol* 1982;49:912.

26. Tyroler HA. Overview of risk factors for coronary heart disease in black population. *Am Heart J* 1984;108:658–660.

27. Curry CL, Oliver J, Mumtuz FG. Coronary disease in blacks: risk factors. *Am Heart J* 1984;108:653–657.

28. Harshfield GA, Hwang C, Grim CE. Circadian variation of blood

29. pressure in blacks: influence of age, gender and activity. *J Hum Hypertens* 1990;4:43–47.

29. Fumo MT, Teeger S, Lang RM, Bednarz J, et al. Diurnal blood pressure variation and cardiac mass in American blacks an whites and South African blacks. *Am J Hypertens* 1992;5:111–116.

30. Chaturvei N, McKeigue PM, Marmot MG. Resting and ambulatory blood pressure differences in Afro-Caribbeans and Europeans. *Hypertension* 1993;22:90–96.

31. Harshfield GA, Pulliam DA, Somes GW, Alpert BS. Ambulatory blood pressure patterns in youth. *Am J Hypertens* 1993;6:968–973.

32. Savage DD. Significance of increased left ventricular mass in black and white hypertensive patients. *J Natl Med Assoc* 1988;80[Suppl]:7–11.

33. Carryon P, Mathews MM. Clinical and coronary arteriographic profile of 100 black Americans: focus on subgroup with undiagnosed suspicious chest discomfort. *J Natl Med Assoc* 1987;79:265–71.

34. Maynard D, Fisher LD, Passamani ER. Survival of black persons compared with white persons in the Coronary Artery Surgery Study (CASS). *Am J Cardiol* 1987;60:513–518.

35. Taylor JO, Borhani NO, Entwisle G, Farber M, Hawkins CM on behalf of the HDFP Cooperative Group. Summary of the baseline characteristics of the hypertensive participants. *Hypertension* 1983;5[Supp]:IV-44–IV-50.

36. Beaglehole R, Tyroler HA, Cassel JC, Duebner DC, Bartel A, Hames CG. An epidemiological study of left ventricular hypertrophy in a biracial population of Evans County, Georgia. *J Chron Dis* 1975;28:554–559.

37. Kannel WB, Dannenberg AL. Prevalence and natural history of electrocardiographic left ventricular hypertrophy. In: Messerli F, ed. *The heart and hypertension.* New York: Yorke Medical Books, 1987;53–61.

38. Tyroler HA. Overview of risk factors for coronary heart disease in black populations. *Am Heart J* 1984;108[Suppl]:658–660.

39. Liebsoon PR, Savage DD. Echocardiography in hypertension: a review. I. Left ventricular wall mass, standardization, and ventricular function. *Echocardiography* 1986;3:181–218.

40. Rautaharju PM, et al. Electrocardiographic estimate of left ventricular mass versus radiographic cardiac size and the risk of cardiovascular disease mortality in the epidemiologic follow-up study of the first National Health and Nutrition Examination Survey. *Am J Cardiol* 1988;62:60–66.

41. Hammond IW, Devereux RB, Alderman MH, et al. The prevalence and correlates of echocardiographic left ventricular hypertrophy among employed patients with uncomplicated hypertension. *J Am Coll Cardiol* 1986;7:639–650.

42. Dunn FG, Oigman W, Sungard-Riise K, et al. Racial differences in cardiac adaptation to essential hypertension determined by echocardiographic indexes. *J Am Coll Cardiol* 1983;5(1):1348–1351.

43. Hammond IW, Devereux RB, Alderman MH, et al. Contrast in cardiac anatomy and function between black and white patients with hypertension. *J Natl Med Assoc* 1984;76:247–55.

44. Savage DD, Henry WL, Mitchell JR, et al. Echocardiographic comparison of black and white hypertensive subjects. *J Natl Med Assoc* 1979;71:709–712.

45. Levy D, Garrison RJ, Savage DD, Kannel WB, Castelli WP. Left ventricular mass and incidence of coronary heart disease in an elderly cohort: the Framingham Study. *Ann Intern Med* 1989;110:101–107.

46. Rautaharju PM, et al. Electrocardiographic estimate of left ventricular mass versus radiographic cardiac size and the risk of cardiovascular disease mortality in the epidemiologic follow-up study of the first National Health and Nutrition Examination Survey. *Am J Cardiol* 1988;62:60–66.

47. Mason BJ, Shirani J, Mueller FO, Cantu RC, Roberts WC. *Cardiovascular causes of "Athletic field" deaths: analysis of sudden death in 84 competitive athletes.* AHA Scientific sessions, November 8–11, 1993, Atlanta, Georgia.

48. Soto LF, Kikuchi D, Arcilla RA, Savage DD, Berenson GS. Blood pressure levels and echocardiographic function in children: the Bogalusa Heart Study. *Am J Med Sci* 1989;297:271–279.

49. Harshfield GA, Pulliam DA, Somes GW, Alpert BS. Ambulatory

blood pressure patterns in youth. *Am J Hypertens* 1993;6:968–973.

50. Wilson TW, Holifield LR, Grim CE. Systolic blood pressure levels in black populations in sub-Sahra Africa, the West Indies and the United States: a meta-analysis. *Hypertension* 1991;18[Supp I]:I-87–I-91.

51. Intersalt Cooperative Research Group. Intersalt: an international study of electrolyte excretion and blood pressure. Results for 24 hour urinary sodium and potassium excretion. *Br Med J* 1988;297:319–328.

52. Akinkugbe OO. World epidemiology of hypertension in blacks. In: Hall WD, Saunders E, Shulman NB, eds. *Hypertension in blacks: epidemiology, pathophysiology and treatment.* Chicago: Year Book Medical Publishers, 1985, 11.

53. Helmer OM. Renin-angiotensin system and its relation to hypertension. *Prog Cardiovasc Dis* 1965;8:117–128.

54. Helmer OM. Hormonal and biochemical factors controlling blood pressure. In: Masson et Cie, eds. *Les concepts de Claude Bernard sur le milieu interieur.* Paris: Libraires de l'Académie de Médecine, 1967, 115–128.

55. Gleibermann L. Blood pressure and dietary salt in human populations. *Ecology of Food and Nutrition* 1973;2:143–156.

56. Denton, D. The hunger for salt: an anthropological, physiological and medical analysis. Berlin: Springer-Verlag, 1982, 616.

57. Wilson TW. Africa, Afro-Americans, and hypertension: an hypothesis. In: Kiple KF, ed. *The African exchange: toward a biological history of black people.* Durham: Duke University Press, 1988:257–274.

58. Wilson TW. *Ancient environments and modern disease.* Ann Arbor: University Microfilms, 1988.

59. Wilson TW. History of salt supplies in West Africa and blood pressures today. *Lancet* 1986;i, 784–786.

60. Grollmann A. A conjecture about the prevalence of essential hypertension and its high incidence in the black. *Texas Rep Biol Med* 1978;36:25–32.

61. Williams R, Hopkins PN. Salt, hypertension, and genetic-environmental interactions. *Prog Clin Biol Res* 1979;32:183–194.

62. Lee MR. The kidney fault in essential hypertension may be a failure to mobilize renal dopamine adequately when dietary sodium chloride is increased. *Cardiovasc Rev Rep* 1981;2:785–789.

63. Schachter J, Kuller LH. Blood volume expansion among blacks: an hypothesis. *Medical Hypotheses* 1984;14:1–19.

64. Waldron I, Nowotarski M, Freimer M, Henry JP, Post N, Witten C. Cross-cultural variation in blood pressure: a quantitative analysis of the relationships of blood pressure to cultural characteristics, salt consumption, and body weight. *Soc Sci Med* 1982;16:419–430.

65. Blackburn H, Prineas R. Diet and hypertension: anthropology, epidemiology, and public health implications. *Prog Biochem Pharmacol* 1983;19:31–79.

66. Grim CE. On slavery, salt and the greater prevalence of hypertension in black Americans. *Clin Res* 1988;36:430.

67. Wilson TW, Grim CE. Biohistory of slavery and blood pressure differences in blacks today: a hypothesis. *Hypertension* 1991;17[Suppl I]:I-122–I-128.

68. Wilson TW, Grim CE. The possible relationship between the trans-Atlantic slave trade and blood pressure in blacks today. In: Inkori JE, Engerman SE, eds. *The Atlantic slave trade: gainers and losers.* Durham: Duke University Press, 1992.

69. Grim CE, Wilson TW. Salt, slavery and survival: physiological principles underlying the evolutionary hypothesis of salt sensitive hypertension in western hemisphere blacks. In: Fray JCS, Douglas JG, eds. *The pathophysiology of hypertension in blacks.* New York: Oxford University Press, 1993, 22–48.

70. Fogel RW, Engerman SL. *Time on the cross: the economics of American negro slavery.* Boston: Little, Brown and Company, 1974.

71. Hales S. A treatise on ventilators, wherein an account is given of the happy effects of the several trials that have been made of them, in different ways and for different purposes: which has occasioned their being received with general approbation and applause, on account of their utility for the great benefit of mankind, part second. London: Richard Manby, 1758;82–99.

72. Miller JC. *Way of death: merchant capitalism and the Angolan slave trade, 1730–1830.* Madison, Wisconsin: University of Wisconsin Press, 1988;447–442.

73. Bouchard TJ, Lykken DT, McGue M, Segal NL, Tellegen A. Sources of human psychological differences: the Minnesota Study of Twins Reared Apart. *Science* 1990;250:223–228.

74. Curtin PD. The slavery hypothesis for hypertension among African Americans: the historical evidence. *Am J Public Health* 1992;82:1681–1686.

75. Ladell WSS. The changes in water and chloride distribution during heavy sweating. *J Physiol* 1949;108:440–50.

76. Miller JC. *Way of death: merchant capitalism and the Angolan slave trade, 1730–1830.* Madison, Wisconsin: University of Wisconsin Press, 1988;447–442.

77. Grim CE, Miller JZ, Luft FC, Christian JC, Weinberger MH. Genetic influences on renin, aldosterone, and renal excretion of sodium and potassium following volume expansion and contraction in normal man. *Hypertension* 1979;1:583–590.

78. Grim CE, Li J, Jamgotchian NJ, Eggena PH, Hu MS, Barrett JD, Frodal AM, Lee DBN. Active renin but not prorenin or renin substrate are under genetic control in African Americans. *Am Soc Nephrol* 1993;4:S33.

79. Dahl LK, Shackow E. Effects of chronic excess salt ingestion: experimental hypertension in the rat. *Can Med Assoc J* 1964;90:155–160.

80. Rapp JP, Wang SM, Dene W. A genetic polymorphism in the renin gene of Dahl rats cosegregates with blood pressure. *Science* 1989;243:542–544.

81. Guyton AC. Blood pressure control–special role of the kidneys and body fluids. *Science* 1991;252:1813–1860.

82. Weinberger MH, Fineberg NS. Sodium and volume sensitivity of blood pressure: age and pressure change over time. *Hypertension* 1991;18:67–71.

83. Luft FC, Grim CE, Higgins JT, Weinberger MH. Differences in response to sodium administration in normotensive white and black subjects. *J Lab Clin Med* 1977;90:555–562.

84. Grim CE, Wilson TW. Blood pressure in blacks: twin studies in Barbados. *Hypertension* 1990;15:803–808.

85. Lifton RP, Dluhy RG, Powers M, Rich GM, Cook S, Ulick S, Lalouel JM. A chimeric 11 beta-hydroxylase/aldosterone synthase gene causes glucocorticoid—remedial aldosteronism and human hypertension. *Nature* 1992;255:262–265.

86. Grim CE, Robinson M. Genetics of hypertension in genetic factors in coronary heart disease. Goldbourt U, De Faire U, Berg K, eds. Netherlands: Kluwer Academic Publishers (*in press*).

87. Darlu P, Sagnier PP, Bois E. Genealogical and genetical African admixture estimations, blood pressure and hypertension in a Caribbean community. *Ann Hum Biol* 1990;17:387–397.

88. Grim CE, Harshfield GA, Baker LA, Savage DD, Anderson SJ, Hwang C. Evidence that blood pressure is inherited independently of body weight and left ventricular mass in black twins. *Circulation* 1987;76[II]:IV-9.

89. Grim CE, Wilson TW. Blood pressure in blacks: twin studies in Barbados. *Hypertension* 1990;15:803–808.

90. Plomin R, DeFries JC. Multivariate behavioral genetic analysis of twin data on scholastic abilities. *Behav Genet* 1979;9:505–517.

91. DeFries JC, Fulker DW. Multivariate behavioral genetics and development: an overview. *Behav Genet* 1986;16:1–10.

92. Grim CE, Harshfield GA, Baker LA, Savage DD, Anderson SJ, Hwang C. Evidence that blood pressure is inherited independently of body weight and left ventricular mass in black twins. *Circulation* 1987;76(II):IV-9.

93. Ho H-Z, Baker LA, Decker SN. The genetic and environmental covariation of intelligence and speed-of-information processing. *Behav Genet* 1988;18:247–261.

94. Grim CE, Li J, Gamble F, Abisuga OO. Salt sensitivity of blood pressure is under genetic control in African Americans. *Circulation* 1993;88:I-416.

95. Grim CE, Li J, Jamgotchian NJ, Eggena PH, Hu MS, Barrett JD, Frodal AM, Lee DBN. Active renin but not prorenin or renin

substrate are under genetic control in African Americans. *Am Soc Nephr* 1993;

96. Luft FC, Grim CE, Higgins JT, Weinberger MH. Differences in response to sodium administration in normotensive white and black subjects. *J Lab Clin Med* 1977;90:555–562.

97. Harshfield GA, Pulliam DA, Alpert BS. Ambulatory blood pressure and renal function in healthy children and adolescents. *Am J Hypertens* (in press).

98. Wedler B, Brier ME, Wiersbitzky M, Gruska S, et al. Sodium kinetics in salt-sensitive and salt resistant normotensive and hypertensive subjects. *J Hypertens* 1992;10:663–669.

99. Wilson TW. Salt consumption on British slave ships, 1682–1704: historical evidence on the "slavery hypothesis" of hypertension in blacks. *J Hum Hypertens* 1990;4:790.

100. Grim CE, Mendez GJ, Mohan C. 24 hour norepinephrine levels are higher in salt sensitive African Americans. *Circulation* A1992.

101. Reaven GM, Hoffman BB. A role for insulin in the aetiology and course of hypertension? *Lancet* 1987;2:435–437.

102. Voors AW, Radhakrishamurthy B, Srivinasan SR, Webber LS, Berenson GS. Plasma glucose level related to blood pressure in 272 children, ages 7–15 sampled from a total biracial population. *Am J Epidemiol* 1981;113:347–356.

103. Hwang X, Srinivasan SR, Bao W, Berenson G. Association of fasting insulin with longitudinal changes in blood pressure in children and adolescents. *Am J Hypertens* 1993;6:564–569.

104. Falkner B, Hulman S, Kushner H. Insulin stimulated glucose utilization and borderline hypertension in young adult blacks. *Hypertension* 1993;22:18–25.

105. Akanji AO, Ojule AC, Kladiri S, Osotimehin BO. Plasma glucose loading and insulin responses to oral glucose loading in nonobese Nigerian subjects with essential hypertension. *J Natl Med Assoc* 1993;85:267–272.

106. Denaro M, Blanc H, Johnson MJ, et al. Ethnic variation in Hpa I endonuclease cleavage patterns of human mitochondrial DNA. *Proc Nat Acad Sci* 1981;78:5768–72.

107. Grim CE, Miller RW, Fischel-Ghodsian N, Wilson TW, Ansari A, Fraser HS, Nicholson GD, Hassell TA. *Mitochondrial genotype is related to cardiovascular risk factors in blacks.* Presented at the AHA Council for High Blood Pressure Research, September 1991, Chicago, Illinois.

108. Pratt JH, Manatunga AK. Genetic influences on the urinary excretion of aldosterone in children. *N Engl J Med* 1991;42:192–197.

109. Williams RR, Hasstedt SJ, Hunt SC, Wu LL, Hopkins PL, Berry TD, Stults BM, et al. Genetic traits related to hypertension and electrolyte metabolism. *Hypertension* 1991;17[Suppl I]:I-69–I-73.

110. Cooper RS, Borke JL. Intracellular ions and hypertension in blacks. In: Fray JC, Douglas JG, eds. *Pathophysiology of hypertension in blacks.* New York: Oxford University Press, 1993; Published for the American Physiological Society.

111. Campese V. *Personal communication.*

112. Alexander F. Emotional factors in essential hypertension: *Psychosom Med* 1939;1:172–183.

113. Johnson EH. *The deadly emotions: the role of anger, hostility and aggression in health and emotional well-being.* New York: Praeger, 1990.

114. Sommers-Flanagan J, Greenburg R. Psychosocial variables and hypertension: a new look at an old controversy. *J Nerv Ment Dis* 1989;177:15–24.

115. Fray JC, Douglas JG. *Pathophysiology of hypertension in blacks.* New York: Oxford University Press, 1993; Published for the American Physiological Society.

116. Anderson NB, McNally M. Autonomic reactivity and hypertension in blacks: toward a contextual model. In: Fray JC, Douglas JG, eds. *Pathophysiology of hypertension in blacks:* New York: Oxford University Press, 1993.

117. Fray JC, Douglas JG. *Pathophysiology of hypertension in blacks.* New York: Oxford University Press, 1993; Published for the American Physiological Society.

118. Johnson EH. *The deadly emotions: the role of anger, hostility and aggression in health and emotional well-being.* New York: Praeger, 1990.

119. Dressler WW. Psychosomatic symptoms, stress and modernization: a model. *Cult Med Psychiatry* 1985;9:257–286.

120. Fray JC, Douglas JG. *Pathophysiology of hypertension in blacks.* New York: Oxford University Press, 1993; Published for the American Physiological Society.

121. Dressler WW. Social and cultural dimensions of hypertension in blacks: underlying mechanisms. In: Fray JC, Douglas JG, *Pathophysiology of hypertension in blacks.* New York: Oxford University Press, 1993;69–89a.

122. Winkleby MA, Ragland DR, Syme L. Self-reported stressors and hypertension: evidence of an inverse association. *Am J Epidemiol* 1988;127:124–134.

123. Albright CL, Winkleby MA, Ragland DR, Fish J, Syme L. Job strain and prevalence of hypertension in a biracial population of urban bus drivers. *Am J Public Health* 1992;82:984–989.

124. Weinberger DA, Schwartz GE, Davidson RJ. Low-anxious, high-anxious and repressive coping styles: psychometric patterns and behavioral and physiological responses to stress. *J Abnorm Psychol* 1979;88:369–380.

125. King A, Taylor B, Albright C, Haskell WL. The relationship between repressive and defensive coping styles and blood pressure responses in healthy middle-aged men and women. *J Psychiatr Res* 1990;34:461–71.

126. Albright CL, Winkleby MA, Ragland DR, Fish J, Syme L. Job strain and prevalence of hypertension in a biracial population of urban bus drivers. *Am J Public Health* 1992;82:984–989.

127. Henry JP. Biological basis of the stress response. *NIPS* 1993;8:69–73.

128. Pascoe JP, Kapp BS. Electrophysiological characteristics of amygdaloid central nucleus neurons during Pavlovian fear conditioning in the rabbit. *Behav Brain Res* 1985;16:117–133.

129. Folkow B. Stress and blood pressure in adrenergic blood pressure regulation. In: Birkenhager WH, Folkow B, Strikeer Boucher HAJ, eds. Current Clinic Practice Series. *Excerpta Medica* 1985;87–93.

130. Koolhaas J, Bohus B. Social control in relation to neuroendocrine and immunological responses. In: Steptoe A, Appels A, eds. *Stress personal control and health.* New York: Wiley, 1989.

131. Bohus B, Koolhaas M, de Ruiter AJH, Heijnen. Psycho-social stress: differential alterations in immune system functions and tumor growth. pp 607–621 In: Kvetnansky R, McCarty R, Axelrod J, eds. *Stress: neuroendocrine and molecular approaches,* New York: Gordon and Breach, 1992.

132. Bjorntorp P. The association between obesity adipose tissue distribution and disease. *Acta Med Scand* 1987;723:121–134.

133. Henry JP, Grim CE. Psychosocial mechanisms of primary hypertension. *J Hypertens* 1990;8:783–793.

134. Anderson NB, McNally M. Autonomic reactivity and hypertension in blacks: toward a contextual model, pp 107 In: Fray JC, Douglas JG, eds. *Pathophysiology of hypertension in blacks.* New York: Oxford University Press, 1993.

135. Henry JP, Liu Y, Nadra WE, et al. Psychosocial stress can induce chronic hypertension in normotensive strains of rats. *Hypertension* 1993;21:714–723.

136. Adams N, Blizard DA. Defeat and cardiovascular response. *Psychol Record* 1987;37:349–368.

137. Henry JP, Stephens PM. *Health and the social environment: a sociobiologic approach to medicine.* New York: Springer Verlag, 1977.

138. Bouchard TJ, Lykken DT, McGue M, et al. Sources of human psychological differences: the Minnesota study of twins reared apart. *Science* 1990;250:223–228.

139. Thailer SA, Friedman R, Harshfield GA, et al. Psychologic differences between high-, normal- and low-renin hypertensives. *Psychosom Med* 1985;47:294–298.

140. Perini C, Smith DHG, Neutel JM, Smith AM, Henry JP, et al. A repressive coping style protecting from emotional distress in low renin essential hypertensives, (in press *J Hypertens*).

141. Henry JP, Stephens PM. Psychosocial stress induces high blood

pressure in a population of mammals on a low salt diet. *J Hypertens* 1988;6:139–144.

142. Laragh TH, Seeley JG. Renin-sodium profiling; Why, how and when in clinical practice. In: Laragh JH, ed. *Topics in hypertension.* New York: Yorke Med Publn, 1980;221–243.

143. Cumes-Rayner DP. *Essential hypertension and self disclosure.* Ph.D Dissertation, Department of Psychology New Queensland, 1987.

144. Alderman MH, Madhavan S, Ooi WL, et al. Association of the renin-sodium profile with the risk of myocardial infarction in patients with hypertension. *N Engl J Med* 1991;324:1098–104.

145. Van de Kar LD, Piechowski RA, Rittenhouse PA, Gray TS. Amygdaloid lesions: differential effect on conditioned stress and immobilization-induced increases in corticosterone and renin secretion. *Neuroendocrinology* 1991;54:89–95.

146. Saphier D. Paraventricular nucleus magnocellular neuronal responses following electrical stimulation of the midbrain dorsal raphe. *Exp Brain Res* 1991;85:359–363.

147. Carlsson S. The postganglionic extrinsic innervation of the adrenal gland: a physiological and histological study in the rat. Dissertation, Department of Physiology, University of Goteborg, 1992.

148. Erhart-Bornstein M, Bornstein SR, Scherbaum WA, Pfeiffer EF, Holst JJ. Role of the vasoactive intestinal peptide in a neuroendocrine regulation of the adrenal cortex. *Neuroendocrinology* 1991;54:623–628.

149. Gray TS, Piechowski RA, Yracheta JM, Rittenhouse PA, Bethea CL, Van de Kar LD. Ibotenic acid lesions in the bed nucleus of the stria terminalis attenuate conditioned stress-induced increases in prolactin, ACTH and corticosterone. *Neuroendocrinology* 1993;57:571–524.

150. Malendowicz LK, Nussdorfer GG, Markowaska A, Nowak KW, Torlinski L. Effects of neuromedin-N on the pituitary-adrenocortical axis of dexamethasone-suppressed rats. *Neuropeptides* 1993;24:1–4.

151. Ulick S, Wang JZ, Blumenfeld JD, Pickering TG. Cortisol inactivation overload: a mechanism of mineralocorticoid hypertension in the ectopic adrenocorticotropin syndrome. *Clin Endocrinol Metab* 1992;74:963–967.

152. Russell RR, Masi AT, Richter ED. Adrenal cortical adenomas and hypertension. *Medicine* 1972;51:211–225.

153. Grim CE, Weinberger MH, Luft FC, Pratt JC, Ganguly A. An algorithm for the diagnosis of primary aldosteronism and renovascular hypertension. *Am Heart Assoc* 1979 (*presented*).

154. Weinberger MH, Grim CE, Hollifield JW, Kem DC, Ganguly A, Kramer NJ, Yune HY, Wellman H, Donohue JP. Primary aldosteronism: diagnosis, localization and treatment. *Ann Intern Med* 1979;90:386–395.

155. Hiramatsu K, Yamada T, Yukimura Y, et al. A screening test to identify aldosterone-producing adenoma by measuring plasma renin activity, Results in hypertensive patients. *Arch Intern Med* 1981;141:1589–1593.

156. Gordon RD, Klemm SA, Tunny TJ, et al. Primary aldosteronism: hypertension with a genetic basis. *Lancet* 1992;340:159–161.

157. Gomez-Sanchez CE, Gill JR, Ganguly A, et al. Glucocorticoid-suppressible aldosteronism: a disorder of the adrenal transitional zone. *J Clin Endocrinol Metab* 1988;66:444–448.

158. Grim CE, Keitzer WF, Esterly JA, Longo DL. The inappropriate secretion of aldosterone associated with adrenal hyperplasia. *J Univ Mich Med Center* 1976;42:54–59.

159. Gunnells JC, McGuffin WL Jr, Robinson RR, et al. Hypertension, adrenal abnormalities and alterations in plasma renin activity. *Ann Intern Med* 1970;73:901–911.

160. Halber A, Wambach G, Hummerich W, et al. Evidence for a subgroup of essential hypertensives with non-suppressible excretion of aldosterone during sodium loading. *Klin Wochenschr* 1980;58:439–447.

161. Wexler BC. Correlation of adrenocortical histopathology with anteriosclerosis in breeder rats. *Acta Endocrinol* 1964;46:613–631.

162. Sommers-Flanagan J, Greenburg R. Psychosocial variables and hypertension: a new look at an old controversy. *J Nerv Ment Dis* 1989;177:15–24.

163. Julius S. Hemodynamic, pharmacologic and epidemiologic evidence for behavioral factors in hypertension. In: Julius S, Bassett DR, eds. *Handbook of hypertension,* vol. 9. Amsterdam: Elsevier, 59–84.

164. Henry JP, Kross ME, Stephens PM, et al. Evidence that differing psychosocial stimuli lead to adrenal cortical stimulation by autonomic or endocrine pathways. In: Usdin E, Kvetnansky R, Kopin IJ, eds. *Catecholamines and stress.* New York: Oxford 1976;457–468.

165. Laragh JH. Personal views on the mechanisms of hypertension. In: Genest J, Kuchel O, Hamet, Ganten M, eds. *Hypertension, physiology and treatment,* 2nd ed. New York: McGraw-Hill, 1983.

166. Anderson NB, Myers HF, Pickering T, Jackson JS. Hypertension in blacks: psychosocial and biological perspectives. *Hypertension* 1989;161–172.

167. Myers HF, Anderson NB, Strickland TL. A biobehavioral perspective on stress and hypertension in black adults. In: Jones RL, ed. *Black adult development and aging* Berkeley: Cobb & Henry Publ. 1989;311–349.

168. Anderson NB, Myers HF, Pickering T, Jackson JS. Hypertension in blacks: Psychosocial and biological perspectives. *Hypertension* 1989;161–172.

169. Myers HF, Anderson NB, Strickland TL. A biobehavioral perspective on stress and hypertension in black adults. In: Jones RL, ed. *Black adult development and aging* Berkeley: Cobb & Henry Publ. 1989;311–349.

170. Hypertension Detection and Follow-up Cooperative Group: Race, education, and prevalence of hypertension. *Am J Epidemiol* 1977;106:351–361.

171. Roberts J, Roland M. *Hypertension in adults 25–74 years of age, United States, 1971–1975.* Vital and Health statistics, Series II, data from the National Survey No. 221 (DDHS publication No. (PHS) 81-1671). Hyattsville, MD: Dept. of Health and Human Services, 1981.

172. Rowland M, Roberts J. National Center for Health Statistics. *Blood pressure levels and hypertension in persons ages 6–74 years: United States, 1976–1980.* Vital and Health Statistics, AdvanceData, No. 84, Public Health Service, Washington, U.S. Government Printing Office, 1982;1–11.

173. Prineas RJ, Gillum RF. US Epidemiology of hypertension in blacks. In: Hall WD, Saunders E, Shulman NB, eds. *Hypertension in blacks: epidemiology, pathophysiology and treatment.* Chicago: Yearbook Medical Publishers, 1985;37–48.

174. Akinkugbe OO. *Cardiovascular disease in Africa.* Paper presented at the first All-Africa Cardiovascular Symposium, University of Ibadan, Nigeria, March 15–18, 1976.

175. Anderson N, Jackson JS. Race, ethnicity and health psychology. In: Stone GD, Weiss SM, Matarazzo JD, Miller NE, Rodin J, Schwartz GE, Belar CD, Follick MJ, Singer JE, eds. *Health psychology: a discipline and a profession.* Chicago: University of Chicago Press, 1987;265–283.

176. James SA. Psychosocial and environmental factors in black hypertension. In: Hall WD, Saunders E, Shulman NB, eds. *Hypertension in blacks: epidemiology, pathophysiology and treatment* Chicago: Yearbook Medical Publishers, 1985;132–143.

177. Hypertension Detection and Follow-up Cooperative Group. Race, education, and prevalence of hypertension. *Am J Epidemiol* 1977;106:351–361.

178. Kessler RC, Neighbors HW. A new perspective on the relationships among race, social class and psychological distress. *J Health Soc Behav* 1986;27:107–115.

179. Harburg E, Geibermann L, Roeper P, Schork MA, Schull WJ. Skin color, ethnicity, and blood pressure. I: Detroit blacks. *Am J Public Health* 1978;68:1177–1188.

180. Harburg E, Geibermann L, Roeper P, Schork MA, Schull WJ. Skin color, ethnicity, and blood pressure. II: Detroit whites. *Am J Public Health* 1978;68:1189–1198.

181. Syme SL. Psychosocial determinants of hypertension. In: Onesti E, Klimt C, eds. *Hypertension: determinants, complications and interventions.* New York: Grune & Stratton, 1979;95–99.

182. James SA, LaCroix AZ, Kleinbaum DG, et al. John Henryism

and blood pressure differences among black men II: The role of occupational stressors. *J Behav Med* 1984;7:259–275.

183. James SA, Hartnett SA, Kalsbeek WD. John Henryism and blood pressure differences among black men. *J Behav Med* 1983;6:259–275.

184. James SA, Strogatz DS, Wing SB, Ramsey DL. Socioeconomic status, John Henryism and hypertension in blacks and whites. *Am J Epidemiol* 1987;126:664–673.

185. Syme SL. Psychosocial determinants of hypertension. In: Onesti E, Klimt C, eds. *Hypertension: determinants, complications and interventions.* New York: Grune & Stratton, 1979;95–99.

186. Alexander F. Emotional factors in essential hypertension: presentation of a tentative hypothesis. *Psychosom Med* 1939;1:175–179.

187. Harrell JP. Psychological factors in hypertension: a status report. *Psych Bull* 1980;87:482–501.

188. Diamond EL. The role of anger and hostility in essential hypertension and coronary heart disease. *Psych Bull* 1982;92:410–433.

189. Gentry WD, Chesney AP, Fary HE, Hall RP, Harburg E. Habitual anger-coping styles: effect of mean blood pressure and risk for essential hypertension. *Psychosom Med* 1982;44:195–202.

190. Harburg E, Erfurt JC, Hauenstein L, Chape C, Schull WJ, Schork MA. Socio-ecological stress, suppressed hostility, skin color, and black-white male blood pressure: Detroit. *Psychosom Med* 1973;35:276–296.

191. Harburg E, Blakelock EH, Roeper PJ. Resentful and reflective coping with arbitrary authority and blood pressure: Detroit. *Psychosom Med* 1979;41:189–202.

192. Gentry WD. Relationship of anger-coping styles and blood pressure among black Americans. In: Chesney MA, Rosenman RH, eds. *Anger and hostility cardiovascular and behavioral disorders.* Washington: Hemisphere Publishing Corporation, 1985;139–147.

193. Harburg E, Erfurt JC, Hauenstein L, Chape C, Schull WJ, Schork MA. Socio-ecological stress, suppressed hostility, skin color, and black-white male blood pressure: Detroit. *Psychosom Med* 1973;35:276–296.

194. Harburg E, Julius S, McGinn NF, McLoed J, Hoobler SW. Personality traits and behavioral patterns associated with systolic blood pressure levels in college males. *J Chron Dis* 1964;17:405–414.

195. Gentry WD. Relationship of anger-coping styles and blood pressure among black Americans. In: Chesney MA, Rosenman RH, eds. *Anger and hostility in cardiovascular and behavioral disorders.* Washington: Hemisphere Publishing Corporation, 1985;139–147.

196. Harburg E, Erfurt JC, Hauenstein L, Chape C, Schull WJ, Schork MA. Socio-ecological stress, suppressed hostility, skin color, and black-white male blood pressure: Detroit. *Psychosom Med* 1973;35:276–296.

197. Harburg E, Blakelock EH, Roeper PJ. Resentful and reflective coping with arbitrary authority and blood pressure: Detroit. *Psychosom Med* 1979;41:189–202.

198. Gentry WD. Relationship of anger-coping styles and blood pressure among black Americans. In: Chesney MA, Rosenman RH, eds. *Anger and hostility in cardiovascular and behavioral Disorders.* Washington: Hemisphere Publishing Corporation, 1985;139–147.

199. Cottington EM, Brock BM, House JS, Hawthorne VM. Psychosocial factors and blood pressure in the Michigan Statewide Blood Pressure Survey. *Am J Epidemiol* 1985;121:515–529.

200. Dimsdale JE, Pierce C, Schoenfeld D, Brown A, Zusman R, Graham R. Suppressed anger and blood pressure: the effects of race, sex, social class, obesity, and age. *Psychosom Med* 1986;48:430–436.

201. Johnson EH, Schork NJ, Spielberger CD. Emotional and familial determinants of elevated blood pressure in black and white adolescent females. *J Psychosom Res* 1987a;31:731–741.

202. Johnson EH, Spielberger CD, Worden TJ, Jacobs GA. Emotional and familial determinants of elevated blood pressure in black and white adolescent males. *J Psychosom Res* 1987b;31:287–300.

203. Harris RE, Sokolow M, Carpenter LG, Freedman M, Hunt SP. Response to psychologic stress in persons who are potentially hypertensive. *Circulation* 1953;7:572–578.

204. Pilowski I, Spalding D, Shaw J, Korner PI. Hypertension and personality. *Psychosom Med* 1973;35:50–56.

205. Cumes-Rayner DP, Price J. Understanding hypertensives' behaviour I: Preference not to disclose. *J Psychosom Res* 1989;33:63–74.

206. Cumes-Rayner DP, Price J. Understanding hypertensives' behavior: II: Perceived social approval and blood pressure reactivity. *J Psychosom Res* 1990;34:141–152.

207. Cumes-Rayner DP, Price J. Understanding hypertensives' behaviour I: Preference not to disclose. *J Psychosom Res* 1989;33:63–74.

208. Cumes-Rayner DP, Price J. Understanding hypertensives' behavior: II: Perceived social approval and blood pressure reactivity. *J Psychosom Res* 1990;34:141–152.

209. Winkleby MA, Ragland DR, Syme SL. Self-reported stressors and hypertension: Evidence of an inverse association. *Am J Epidemiol* 1988;127(1):124–134.

210. Julius M, Harburg E, Cottington EM, Johnson E. Anger-coping types, blood pressure, and all-cause mortality: A follow-up in Tecumesh, Michigan (1971–1983). *Am J Epidemiol* 1986;124:220–233.

211. Knight RGG, Paulin JM, Waal-Manning HJ. Self-reported anger intensity and blood pressure. *Br J Clin Psychiatry* 1987;26:65–66.

212. Dimsdale JE, Pierce C, Schoenfeld D, Brown A, Zusman R, Graham R. Suppressed anger and blood pressure: The effects of race, sex, social class, obesity, and age. *Psychosom Med* 1986;48:430–436.

213. Harburg E, Blakelock EH, Roeper PJ. Resentful and reflective coping with arbitrary authority and blood pressure: Detroit. *Psychosom Med* 1979;41:189–202.

214. Siegel JM. Anger and cardiovascular risk in adolescents. *Health Psychol* 1984;3:293–313.

215. Harburg E, Blakelock EH, Roeper PJ. Resentful and reflective coping with arbitrary authority and blood pressure: Detroit. *Psychosom Med* 1979;41:189–202.

216. Schachter J. Pain, fear, and anger in hypertensives and normotensives. *Psychosom Med* 1957;19:17–29.

217. Manuck SB, Morrison RL, Bellack AS, Polefrone JM. Behavioral factors in hypertension: Cardiovascular responsivity, anger, and social competence. In: Chesney MA, Rosenman RH, eds. *Anger and hostility in cardiovascular and behavioral disorders.* New York: Hemisphere/McGraw-Hill, 1985;149–172.

218. Manuck SB, Morrison RL, Bellack AS, Polefrone JM. Behavioral factors in hypertension: cardiovascular responsivity, anger, and social competence. In: Chesney MA, Rosenman RH, eds. *Anger and hostility in cardiovascular and behavioral disorders.* New York: Hemisphere/McGraw-Hill, 1985;149–172.

219. McClure FH. *Cardiovascular stress responses in black hypertensive and normotensive families.* Paper presented at the Meeting of the American Psychological Association, New Orleans, LA, August 1989.

220. Smith MA, Houston BK. Hostility, anger expression, cardiovascular responsivity, and social support. *Bio Psych* 1987;24:39–48.

221. Durel LA, Carver CS, Spitzer SB, Llabre MM, Weintraub JK, Saab PG, Schneiderman N. Associations of blood pressure with self-report measures of anger and hostility among black and white men and women. *Health Psychol* 1989;8:557–575.

222. James SA. Psychosocial and environmental factors in black hypertension. In: Hall WD, Saunders E, Schulman NB, eds. *Hypertension in blacks: epidemiology pathophysiology and treatment* Chicago: Yearbook Medical Publishers, 1985;132–143.

223. Kessler RC, Neighbors HW. A new perspective on the relationships among race, social class and psychological distress. *J Health Soc Behav* 1986;27:107–115.

224. Gentry WD. Relationship of anger-coping styles and blood pressure among black Americans. In: Chesney MA, Rosenman RH, eds. *Anger and hostility in cardiovascular and behavioral disorders.* Washington: Hemisphere Publishing Corporation, 1985;139–147.

225. Harrell JP. Analyzing black coping styles: a supplemental diagnostic system. *J Black Psych* 1979;5:99–108.

226. Myers HF. Stress, ethnicity and social class: a model for research on black populations. In: Jones EE, Korchin S, eds. *Minority mental health* New York: Holt, Rhinehart & Winston, 1982;118–148.

227. Myers HF, (Chair) et al. Summary of workshop III: Working group on socioeconomic and sociocultural influences in coronary heart disease. *Am Heart J* 1984;108(3 part 2):706–710.

228. Anderson N, Jackson JS. Race, ethnicity and health psychology. In: Stone GD, Weiss SM, Matarazzo JD, Miller NE, Rodin J, Schwartz GE, Belar CD, Follick MJ, Singer JE, eds. *Health psychology: a discipline and a profession.* Chicago: University of Chicago Press, 1987;265–283.

229. Gentry WD. Relationship of anger-coping styles and blood pressure among black Americans. In: Chesney MA, Rosenman RH, eds. *Anger and hostility in cardiovascular and behavioral disorders.* Washington: Hemisphere Publishing Corporation, 1985; 139–147.

230. Harrell JP. Analyzing black coping styles: a supplemental diagnostic system. *J Black Psych* 1979;5:99–108.

231. Clark VR, Harrell JP. The relationship among type A behavior, styles used in coping with racism, and blood pressure. *J Black Psych* 1982;8:89–99.

232. Sutherland ME, Harrell JP. Individual differences in physiological responses to fearful, racially noxious, and neutral imagery. *Imag Cog Perso* 1986–1987;6:133–150.

233. Armstead CA, Lawler KA, Gorden G, Cross J, Gibbons J. Relationship of racial stressors to blood pressure responses and anger expression in black college students. *Health Psychol* 1989;8(5): 541–556.

234. James SA, Hartnett SA, Kalsbeek WD. John Henryism and blood pressure differences among black men. *J Behav Med* 1983;6:259–278.

235. James SA, Strogatz DS, Wing SB, Ramsey DL. Socioeconomic status, John Henryism and hypertension in blacks and whites. *Am J Epidemiol* 1987;126:664–673.

236. Grolnick L. A family perspective of psychosomatic factors in illness: a review of the literature. *Fam Proc* 972;11:457–486.

237. Miall WE, Heneage P, Khosla T, Lovell HG, Moore F. Factors influencing the degree of resemblance in arterial pressure of close relatives. *Clin Sci* 1967;33:271–283.

238. Zinner SH, Levy PS, Kass EH. Familial aggregation of blood pressure in childhood. *N Engl J Med* 1971;284:401–404.

239. Zinner SH, Rosner B, Oh W, Kass EH. Significance of blood pressure in infancy: familial aggregation and predictive effect on later blood pressure. *Hypertension* 1985;7:411–416.

240. Speers MA, Kasl SV, Freeman DH, Ostfield AM. Blood pressure concordance between spouses. *Am J Epidemiol* 1986;123:818–829.

241. Tyroler HA. The Detroit project studies of blood pressure: a prologue and review of related studies and epidemiological issues. *J Chron Dis* 1977;30:613–624.

242. Zinner SH, Rosner B, Oh W, Kass EH. Significance of blood pressure in infancy: familial aggregation and predictive effect on later blood pressure. *Hypertension* 1985;7:411–416.

243. Biron P, Mongeau J. Familial aggregation of blood pressure and its components. *Pediatr Clin North Am* 1978;25:1057–1063.

244. Mongeau JG, Biron P. The influence of genetics and of household environment in the transmission of normal blood pressure. *Clin Exp Hypertens* 1982;3(4):593–596.

245. Zinner SH, Levy PS, Kass EH. Familial aggregation of blood pressure in childhood. *N Engl J Med* 1971;284:401–404.

246. Zinner SH, Rosner B, Oh W, Kass EH. Significance of blood pressure in infancy: familial aggregation and predictive effect on later blood pressure. *Hypertension* 1985;7:411–416.

247. Epstein FH. How useful is a family history of hypertension as a predictor of future hypertension? *Ann Clin Res* 1984;20:583–592.

248. Higgins MW, Keller JB, Metzner HL, Moore FE, Ostrander LD. Studies of blood pressure in Tecumesh, Michigan. II. Antecedents in childhood of high blood pressure in young adults. *Hypertension* 1980;2[Suppl. 1]:117–123.

249. Myers HF. *Family contributions in essential hypertension in blacks.* Paper presented at the Meetings of the American Psychological Association, Washington, D.C., August 22–26, 1986.

250. Rose RJ, Fulkes DW, Miller JZ, Grim CE, Christian JC. Heritability of systolic blood pressure: analysis of variance in MZ twin parents and their children. *Acta Genet Med Gemelol* 1980;29: 143–149.

251. Grolnick L. A family perspective of psychosomatic factors in illness: a review of the literature. *Fam Proc* 972;11:457–486.

252. Speers MA, Kasl SV, Freeman DH, Ostfield AM. Blood pressure concordance between spouses. *Am J Epidemiol* 1986;123:818–829.

253. Connor SL, Connor WE, Henry H, Sexton G, Keenan EJ. The effects of familial relationships, age, body weight, and diet on blood pressure and the 24 hour urinary excretion of sodium, potassium, and creatinine in men, women, and children of randomly selected families. *Circulation* 1984;1:76–85.

254. Grim CE, Luft FC, Miller JZ, Brown PL, Cannon MA, Weinberger MH. Effects of sodium loading and depletion in normotensive first-degree relatives of essential hypertensives. *J Lab Clin Med* 1979;94:764–771.

255. Luft FC, Grim CE, Fineberg N, Weinberger MH. Effects of volume contraction in normotensive whites, blacks and subjects of different ages. *Circulation* 1979;59:643–650.

256. Luft FC, Rankin LI, Bloch R, et al. Cardiovascular and humoral responses to extremes of sodium intake in normal white and black men. *Circulation* 1979b;60:697–706.

257. Frisancho AR, Leonard WR, Bolletins L. Blood pressure in blacks and whites and its relationship to dietary sodium and potassium intake. *J Chron Dis* 1984;37:515–519.

258. Langford HG, Langford FPJ, Tyler M. Dietary profile of sodium, potassium, and calcium in U.S. blacks. In: Hall WD, Saunders E, Shulman NB, eds. *Hypertension in blacks: epidemiology pathophysiology and treatment.* Chicago: Yearbook Medical Publishers. 1985;49–57.

259. McCarron DA, Morris DA, Cole C. Dietary calcium in human hypertension. *Science* 1982;217:267–269.

260. Myers HF, (Chair) et al. Summary of workshop III: Working group on socioeconomic and sociocultural influences in coronary heart disease. *Am Heart J* 1984;108(3 part 2):706–710.

261. Grim CE, Wilson TW. Blood pressure in blacks: twin studies in Barbados. *Hypertension* 1990;15:803–808.

262. Wilson TW, Grim CE, Egbunike AC, Wilson D. *Blood pressure does not increase with age in a high sodium intake, rural population in Imo State, Nigeria.* AHA National Meeting, 1990.

263. Barlow RJ, Connell MA, Levendig BJ, Gear JSS, Milne FJ. A comparative study of urinary sodium and potassium excretion in normotensive urban black and white South African males. *S Afr Med J* 1982;62:939–941.

264. Intersalt study.

265. Luft FC, Grim CE, Fineberg N, Weinberger MH. Effects of volume contraction in normotensive whites, blacks and subjects of different ages. *Circulation* 1979;59:643–650.

266. Luft FC, Rankin LI, Bloch R, et al. Cardiovascular and humoral responses to extremes of sodium intake in normal white and black men. *Circulation* 1979b;60:697–706.

267. Baer PE. Conflict management in the family: The impact of paternal hypertension. *Adv Fam Int Assess Theory* 1983;3:161–184. 1:1167–1170.

268. Baer PE, Vincent J, Williams B, Bourianoff GG, Bartlett P. Behavioral response to induced conflict in families with a hypertensive father. *Hypertension* 1980;2:70–77.

269. Baer PE, Reed J, Bartlett PC, Vincent JP, Williams BJ, Bourianoff GG. Studies of gaze during induced conflict in families with a hypertensive father. *Psychosom Med* 1983;45:233–242.

270. Jorgensen RS, Houston BK. Family history of hypertension, personality patterns, and cardiovascular reactivity to stress. *Psy.*

271. Gentry WD. Relationship of anger-coping styles and blood pressure among black Americans. In: Chesney MA, Rosenman RH, eds. *Anger and hostility in cardiovascular and behavioral disorders.* Washington: Hemisphere Publishing Corporation, 1985; 139–147.

272. Ewart CK, Burnett KF, Taylor CB. Communication behaviors

that affect blood pressure: an A-B-A-B analysis of marital interaction. *Behav Med* 1983;7:331–344.

273. Ewart CK, Taylor CB, Kraemer HC, Agras WS. Reducing blood pressure reactivity during interpersonal conflict: effects of marital communication training. *Behav Ther* 1984;15:473–484.

274. Baer PE, Vincent J, Williams B, Bourianoff GG, Bartlett P. Behavioral response to induced conflict in families with a hypertensive father. *Hypertension* 1980;2:70–77.

275. Baer PE, Reed J, Bartlett PC, Vincent JP, Williams BJ, Bourianoff GG. Studies of gaze during induced conflict in families with a hypertensive father. *Psychosom Med* 1983;45:233–242.

276. McClure FH, Myers HF. Blood pressure responses in black hypertensive and normotensive families during conflict (*Unpublished paper*).

277. Cumes-Rayner DP, Price J. Understanding hypertensives' behaviour I: Preference not to disclose. *J Psychosom Res* 1989;33:63–74.

278. Cumes-Rayner DP, Price J. Understanding hypertensives' behavior: II: Perceived social approval and blood pressure reactivity. *J Psychosom Res* 1990;34:141–152.

279. Matthews KA, Rakaczky CJ. *Familial aspects of the Type A behavior pattern and physiologic reactivity to stress.* Paper presented at the Biobehavioral Factors in Heart Disease conference, Winterscheid: Federal Republic of Germany, June 1984.

280. Rose RJ, Grim CE, Miller JZ. Familial influences on cardiovascular stress reactivity. Studies on normotensive twins. *Behav Med Update* 1984;6:21–24.

281. Carmelli D, Chesney MA, Ward MM, Rosenman RH. Twin similarity in cardiovascular stress response. *Health Psychol* 1985;4:413–423.

282. Carroll D, Hewitt JK, Last KA, Turner JR, Sims J. A twin study of cardiac reactivity and its relationship to parental blood pressure. *Phys Behav* 1985;34:103–106.

283. Ditto B. Sibling similarities in cardiovascular reactivity to stress. *Psychophysiology* 1987;24:353–360.

*Hypertension: Pathophysiology, Diagnosis,
and Management, Second Edition,*
edited by J.H. Laragh and B.M. Brenner,
Raven Press, Ltd., New York © 1995.

CHAPTER 13

Childhood Hypertension

Alan R. Sinaiko

The relevance of hypertension to the pediatric population has been generally acknowledged for only a few decades. As a consequence, blood pressure measurement, as an integral component of the pediatric physical examination, dates to the early 1970s. Before that time, high blood pressure was rarely diagnosed in children. Only the most severe cases of hypertension were recognized, and those were almost always associated with some other primary condition, such as renal parenchymal disease, renal artery stenosis, or coarctation of the aorta (1).

Hypertension as a health care concern in children began to surface in the 1960s (2). Shortly thereafter, comprehensive data from large-scale epidemiologic studies established that mild hypertension is more common than previously acknowledged during childhood, particularly in adolescents (3–6). The report of the 1977 National Institutes of Health Task Force on Blood Pressure Control in Children was the initial response to the many questions raised by these studies (7). It established blood pressure measurement as a part of the routine pediatric examination; it incorporated epidemiologic data on the distribution and natural history of blood pressure in children and set accurate standards for normal blood pressure distribution; it defined hypertension as blood pressure greater than the 95th percentile of distribution for age and sex; and it provided guidelines for evaluation and treatment of hypertensive children. A decade later

the Second Task Force on Blood Pressure Control in Children (8) significantly modified and strengthened the first report.

The following generalizations have not changed over the years: (a) Blood pressure is lower in children than adults and increases gradually throughout the first and second decades of life; (b) the diagnosis of hypertension in children is made at levels of blood pressure considerably lower than in adults; and (c) when hypertension at a level sufficiently high enough to require antihypertensive therapy occurs in children, it is usually secondary in nature (i.e., the result of some identifiable cause such as renal disease, renal artery stenosis, etc.). However, there has been a substantial change in the focus of interest in childhood blood pressure. Although the diagnosis and treatment of secondary hypertension continue to be important, equal clinical emphasis is now placed on early recognition of children with essential hypertension, and research efforts have intensified in this age group in an attempt to identify precursors of elevated blood pressure. Although the prevalence of hypertension is much lower in children than adults, persuasive evidence from familial and longitudinal studies strongly suggests that factors influencing the development of hypertension are operative during the childhood years.

Other chapters in this textbook are devoted to specific diseases, physiologic systems, classes of drug, etc., relating to hypertension. Consequently, these topics are addressed in the present chapter only as they relate to childhood issues of blood pressure and hypertension. Normal

A. R. Sinaiko: Department of Pediatrics, University of Minnesota Medical School, Minneapolis, Minnesota 55455

blood pressure and the natural history of blood pressure during childhood and adolescence are discussed. Hypertension is presented according to age, etiology, diagnostic evaluation, and treatment. It is anticipated that the reader will gain an appreciation of the relevance of childhood blood pressure to cardiovascular risk, both during the childhood years and as it relates to adult disease processes.

MEASUREMENT OF BLOOD PRESSURE IN CHILDREN

Blood pressure should be measured in children once each year after the age of 3 years, as recommended by the American Academy of Pediatrics (9) and the Task Force on Blood Pressure Control in Children (8). The basic methodology and instrumentation for blood pressure measurement are not different in children from adults. However, certain factors are unique to the pediatric blood pressure examination.

First, blood pressure measurement by conventional auscultation, although quite reliable in older children, is almost always impractical in children younger than 3 years of age. This is due to the problem of keeping infants and young children quiet and free from anxiety. Infant blood pressure was formerly measured by the "flush" method (10). However, this is an imprecise measurement technique because it is subjective and measures mean blood pressure. Rarely, if ever, is there any indication for its use.

Doppler and oscillometric automatic devices have been widely used in children. The correlation coefficient between Doppler and simultaneously obtained intraarterial measurements is 0.8 for systolic and 0.7 for diastolic blood pressure (11). In contrast, the intraarterial-oscillometric correlation is 0.97 for systolic and 0.9 for diastolic blood pressure (12). The accuracy of oscillometric devices is inversely correlated with infant size, and in general, measurements in premature infants are not as well correlated to intraarterial measurements as those in older children (13).

Second, appropriate blood pressure cuff size is crucial for accurate blood pressure measurements (14,15). The blood pressure cuff (i.e., bladder) should be long enough to encircle the upper arm completely and wide enough to cover at least 75 to 80 percent of the arm between the antecubital fossa and axilla. Currently, manufactured cuffs have been designed so that use of either circumference or width will provide the correct size. Occasionally, the widths of two adjacent-sized cuffs both will be close to the measured width of the arm. In that case, the cuff with the larger width should be used. A small cuff will cause inaccurately high readings, whereas use of a cuff slightly larger than suggested by the upper arm measurement rarely will lower blood pressure enough to prevent the recognition of true hypertension.

TABLE 1. *Distribution of the difference between fourth phase (D4) and fifth phase (D5) diastolic blood pressures for 19,274 fifth- to eighth-grade students in Minneapolis and St. Paul*

Difference between D4 and D5 (mm Hg)	No.	%
0	9,682	500
1–4	2,837	15
5–10	3,908	20
11–77	2,847	15
Total	19,274	100

Third, diastolic blood pressure is recorded differently in children from adults. In children 12 years of age and younger, it is defined as the fourth Korotkoff phase (D4), and in children 13 years of age and older, the fifth Korotkoff phase (D5) is used (8). These recommendations are based on clinical experience recognizing that (a) D5 may not be present in infants and children (i.e., blood pressure sounds heard all the way to 0 mm Hg); and (b) blood pressure measurement in larger children and adolescents is similar to, and should be evaluated in the same context as, that of adults.

The use of D4 or D5 to define diastolic blood pressure has been a source of conflict in pediatrics (16,17). Neither Korotkoff phase represents true intraarterial diastolic blood pressure in children, with D4 tending to be higher and D5 lower (18). An evaluation of diastolic blood pressure from a screening of American school children (Table 1) showed a strong correlation between D4 and D5 but confirmed that there are substantial differences between the two (19). This also has been found in 6- to 18-year-old Finnish children (20). Because standard diastolic reference data published by the 1987 Task Force (see next section) use only D4 or D5, depending on age, the incorrect choice of D4 or D5 for diastolic blood pressure can have a potentially significant effect on the diagnosis of diastolic hypertension.

NATURAL HISTORY OF BLOOD PRESSURE IN CHILDREN

Normal Blood Pressure

Blood pressure in children is directly correlated with age from infancy through the second decade of life, and it appears to be directly correlated with gestational development in the premature newborn. The normal, healthy full-term newborn has a systolic blood pressure of 60 mm Hg and diastolic blood pressure of 40 mm Hg at birth. The adjustment to extrauterine life is characterized by a gradual increase in blood pressure during the first few hours after birth (21).

Data from the 1987 Task Force blood pressure curves, derived from blood pressure measurements in approximately 70,000 children, show that systolic and diastolic blood pressure follow separate patterns during the first year of life (Figs. 1 and 2). Systolic blood pressure increases on a daily basis the first week after birth (22) (Table 2) and then increases more slowly until 2 months of age (23,24). From 2 to 12 months of age, systolic blood pressure remains stable. Diastolic blood pressure increases slightly during the first week of life, then declines steadily to reach a nadir at approximately 2 to 3 months. For the remainder of the first year, it increases slowly but it never exceeds the 1-week level.

Systolic blood pressure increases at a relatively steady rate from 1 year of age through adolescence (Fig. 3). There is very little change in diastolic blood pressure until 5 to 6 years of age when it begins a gradual ascent, in parallel to systolic blood pressure. The reason for this variability between systolic and diastolic blood pressure during development is not known. Similar blood pressure patterns were found in 28,000 4- to 19-year-old European children, although mean values for systolic blood pressure were approximately 6 mm Hg higher than American children for both boys and girls (25).

There are few published data on normal blood pressure in premature infants, primarily because most prematures are treated with volume expansion, pharmacologic agents, and/or respiratory support and are not in a basal physiologic condition. Nevertheless, it is clear that blood pressure in premature infants is even lower than that of full-term infants and is directly related to body weight and gestational age (26–28).

The data base for premature infant blood pressure is derived from direct arterial measurements. Systolic and diastolic blood pressure during the first 12 hours of life are correlated with both birth weight (26,27) and gestational age (26,28). However, body weight appears to be the better standard in small-for-gestational-age infants (26). As in full-term infants, blood pressure increases daily in premature infants (29). Figure 4 represents systolic and diastolic blood pressure at day 7 of life in stable untreated infants of varying gestational age hospitalized in the Neonatal Unit at the University of Minnesota Hospital.

Blood Pressure Tracking in Children

"Tracking" refers to the tendency of children at a given percentile of blood pressure distribution to maintain that percentile relative to their peer group as they grow older. As an example, a child with a systolic blood pressure of 107 mm Hg at age 5 years and 120 mm Hg at age 12 years is tracking at a high normal level of systolic blood pressure.

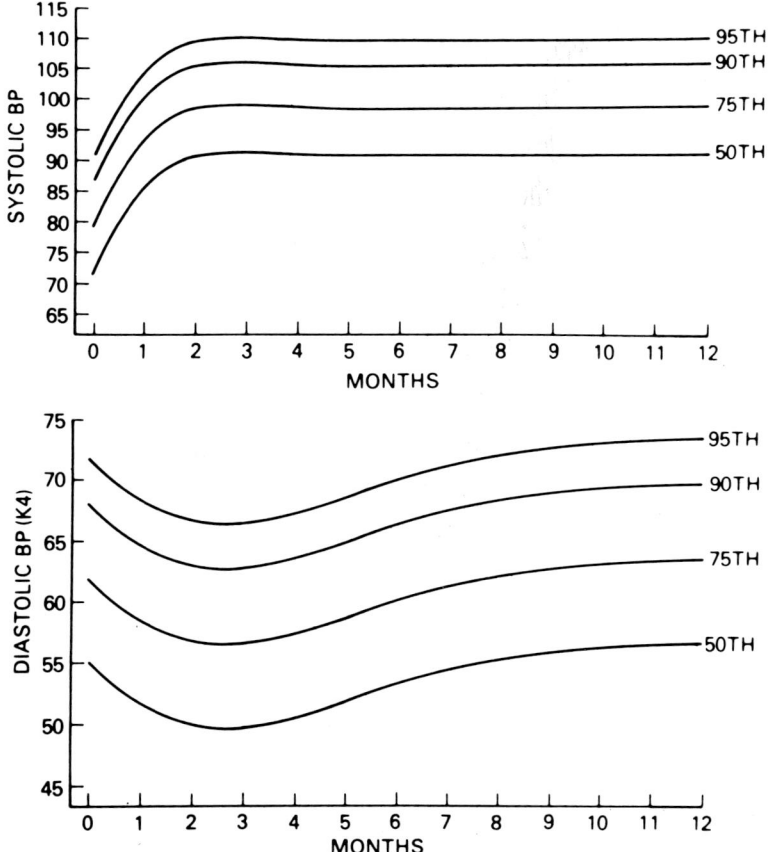

FIG. 1. Age-specific percentiles of blood pressure measurements in boys, birth to 12 months. (From ref. 8, with permission.)

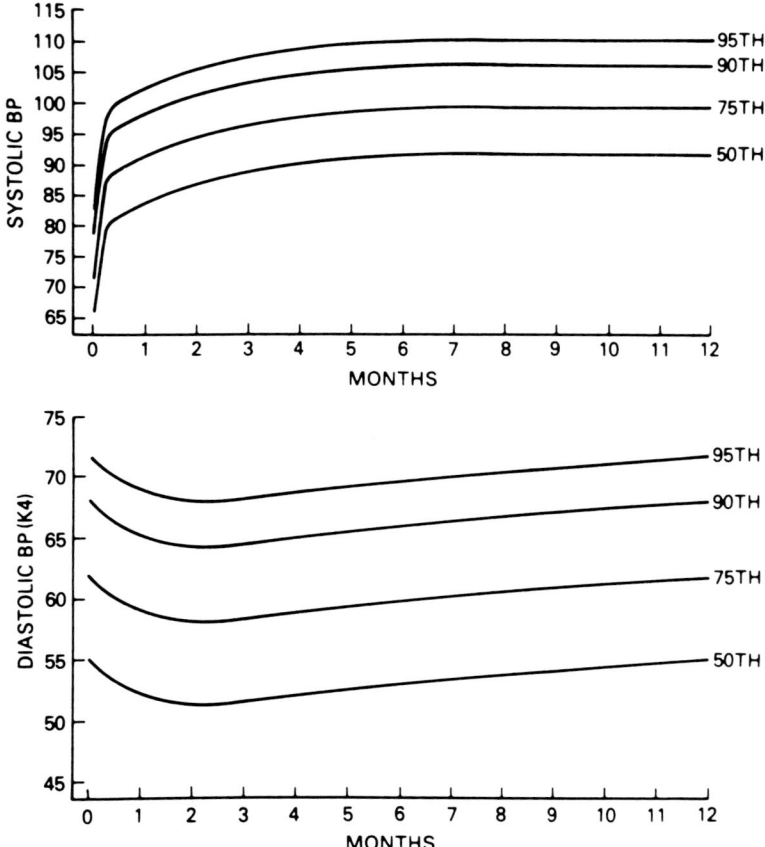

FIG. 2. Age-specific percentiles of blood pressure measurements in girls, birth to 12 months. (From ref. 8, with permission.)

Tracking begins at some point during the first year of life. Newborn blood pressures are not correlated significantly with measurements taken during the first 2 years of life (30). However, beginning at 6 months of age, systolic blood pressure is correlated significantly with blood pressure measured over the ensuing 7 years (24,30,31). Diastolic blood pressure does not show a significant tracking pattern during this stage of development (31).

Several analytic methodologies have been used to evaluate tracking in older children. There is a high degree of variability between studies that may be accounted for

by differences in the precision of blood pressure measurement, differences in sample size, age of the children, and duration of longitudinal blood pressure evaluation. In particular, the frequency of blood pressure measurement over the course of the study is an important factor in improving the tracking analysis (32–34).

Regression analyses between baseline blood pressure and blood pressure at some later age show uniformly positive correlations, ranging from 0.30 to 0.66 for systolic and 0.12 to 0.57 for diastolic blood pressure (as summarized in ref. 32). The correlations are higher for systolic blood pressure, and there is a greater variability for diastolic blood pressure (D4 or D5).

Tracking can be demonstrated by examining changes in quartile or quintile distribution of blood pressure over time. In the U.S. Health Examination Surveys of children 6 to 12 years old (35), 41 percent of children in the lowest blood pressure quintile in 1963 to 1965 remained in the lowest quintile and another 27 percent had increased only to the next highest quintile at the second survey 3 to 4 years later. Conversely, of children in the highest quintile in 1963 to 1965, 45 percent remained in that quintile and 22 percent had fallen only to quintile 4 at the second survey. Almost identical data have come from the Minneapolis Children's Blood Pressure Study (32) in which 55 percent of children in the highest quartile at age 6 to 8 years remained in the top quartile at age

TABLE 2. *Blood pressure (mean ± SD) during the first month of life*

Age	Blood pressure (mm Hg)	
	Systolic	Diastolic
1 day	65 ± 6	48 ± 6
2 days	68 ± 6	50 ± 6
3 days	72 ± 7	53 ± 8
4 days	75 ± 8	56 ± 8
5 days	77 ± 10	55 ± 10
6 days	77 ± 10	55 ± 10
1 week	79 ± 10	55 ± 10
2 weeks	80 ± 10	50 ± 8
1 month	85 ± 10	46 ± 9

Data from author and refs. 18 and 19.

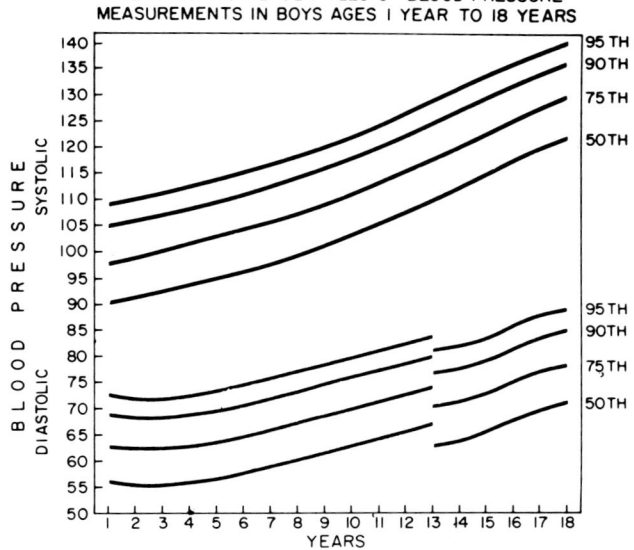

AGE-SPECIFIC PERCENTILES OF BLOOD PRESSURE
MEASUREMENTS IN BOYS AGES 1 YEAR TO 18 YEARS

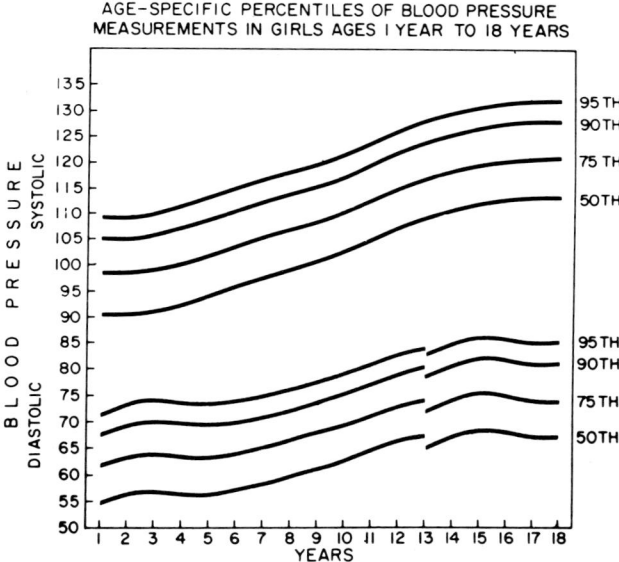

AGE-SPECIFIC PERCENTILES OF BLOOD PRESSURE
MEASUREMENTS IN GIRLS AGES 1 YEAR TO 18 YEARS

FIG. 3. Age-specific percentiles of blood pressure measurements in boys (*top*) and girls (*bottom*) ages 1 year to 18 years. The interruption in the diastolic blood pressure curves at age 13 years is due to the use of the 4th Korotkoff phase (D4) to define diastolic blood in children 12 years and younger and the 5th Korotkoff phase to define diastolic blood pressure in children 13 years and older. (Adapted from ref. 8, with permission.)

pressure measurements (36). As seen in Fig. 5, tracking patterns are similar for the two cohorts. The mean blood pressures parallel one another but remain significantly different at each screening. Similar but even more striking differences were observed in small cohorts of students in the Minneapolis study selected from the upper 1 percentile and lowest 5 percentiles at the first screening (37) and followed for 7 years.

The quintile of systolic blood pressure distribution after 5 years of observation is significantly correlated not only with the initial systolic blood pressure but also with height, weight, pulse rate, and maternal systolic blood pressure (38). In an analysis of tracking, according to the trend of change and variability of blood pressure over time (39), approximately 12 percent of children were found to be tracking toward future high blood pressure, because they had either a high percentile rank of blood pressure distribution at each examination or a persistent upward trend in their percentile distribution. Level and trend of blood pressure also were closely related to level and trend of body size measurements. Thus, blood pres-

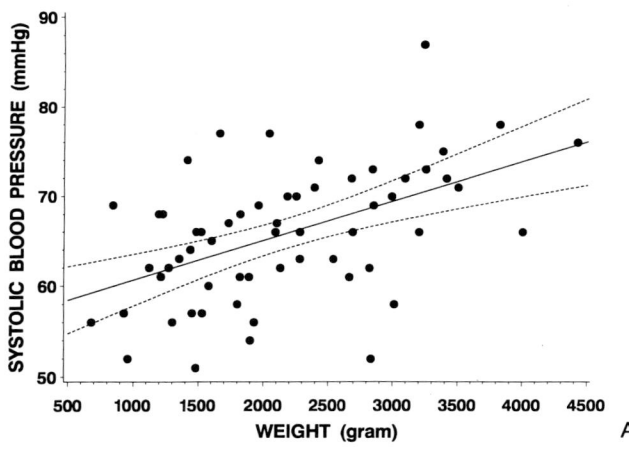

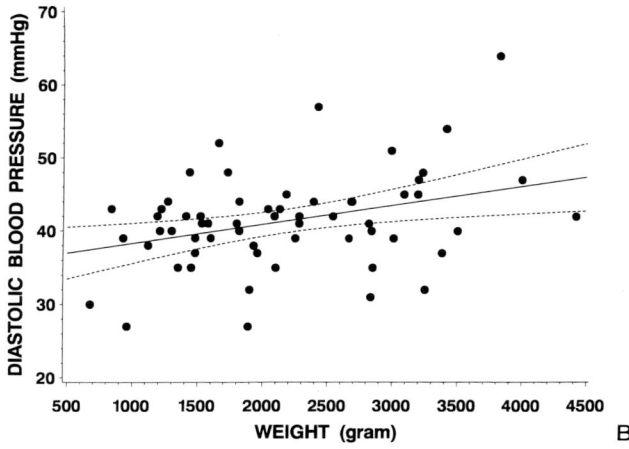

FIG. 4. Linear regression (*solid lines*) and 95 percent confidence limits (*broken lines*) of systolic (**A**) and diastolic (**B**) blood pressures based on weight at day 7 of life. (From M Georgieff, M Mills, O Gomez-Marin, and A Sinaiko, *unpublished data*.)

11 to 13 years (i.e., after 5 years of follow-up) and from the Bogalusa Heart Study (33), in which 68 percent of children with three serial blood pressure measurements in the highest quartile during the 8-year longitudinal evaluation remained in the highest quartile at the end of the study.

Tracking also has been evaluated by dividing children into two cohorts of high and low blood pressure and following their progress longitudinally with a series of blood

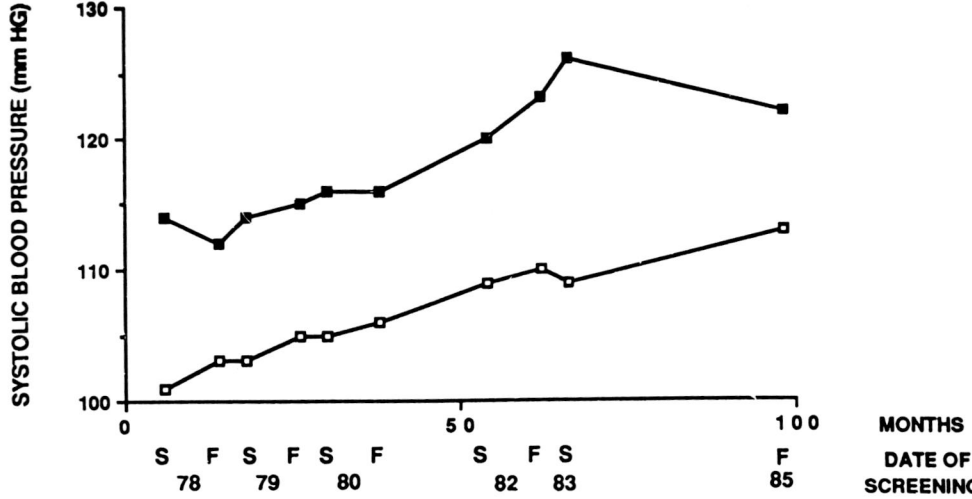

FIG. 5. Blood pressure tracking in two cohorts of children selected on the basis of systolic blood pressure of 120 mm Hg or greater (*solid boxes*) or less than 120 mm Hg (*open boxes*) in spring 1983. Each box represents the group mean at the respective screening. *S,* spring; *F,* fall. The children were in grades one, two, and three at the first screening (spring 1978) and grades eight, nine, and ten at the fifteenth screening (fall 1985). (Adapted from ref. 28, with permission, and RJ Prineas and O Gomez-Marin, *unpublished data.*)

sure tracking is not an isolated phenomenon. It represents the integrated effect of body size, family history, race, and other factors known to influence blood pressure.

Tracking is a well-known phenomenon in adults (40). Data are now available to establish that blood pressure tracking extends from childhood through adolescence and into adult life (41–43). In the Muscatine study, correlations of childhood (7 to 18 years) and adult (20 to 30 years) blood pressures range from 0.21 to 0.39 for systolic and 0.01 to 0.15 for diastolic blood pressure, and the main predictors for development of high blood pressure were childhood blood pressure and change in body size (41). In a study conducted in the San Francisco area childhood blood pressure beginning at age 6 years was a predictor for blood pressure at age 30 years, and blood pressure at age 50 years was best predicted by school-age blood pressures (43). In the Tecumseh study, young adults with borderline hypertension also had higher blood pressure during childhood (42).

Other Factors Influencing Blood Pressure in Children

Race

Differences in blood pressure between blacks and whites are not pronounced during childhood and adolescence. Blood pressure in blacks and whites is the same from birth through the first 2 years of life (30,44), and there is general unanimity that blood pressure does not differ substantially between black and white older children and adolescents (45). In particular, significant racial differences were not noted in the nine studies used to compile the Task Force report (8). However, some small but significant differences have been reported. In the Bogalusa study of children 5 to 14 years old, blacks had significantly higher blood pressure when the analysis was limited to children from the upper 5 percentiles of distribution (5); in a Houston study of children aged 3 to 17 years, whites had low systolic and diastolic blood pressure, even after adjustments were made for body size (46); in Indianapolis school children (mean age, approximately 8.8 years at time of entry into the study), blacks had significantly higher systolic and diastolic blood pressures and a significantly greater rate of rise of blood pressure during 2 to 5 years of evaluation (47); and in the NHLBI growth and health study (48), systolic blood pressure was significantly higher in 9 to 10-year-old black than white girls.

Other ethnic groups have not been studied as thoroughly. Blood pressure in Mexican-American children is similar to whites (45,46). Blood pressure of Southeast Asian children is significantly higher than white and black children, and these differences become more significant when blood pressure is adjusted for body size (49).

Family History

Studies from several countries have shown the strong relation of blood pressure between children and their parents (50–52), and this is intensified in the presence of other risk factors (e.g., obesity) (53). Genetic factors begin to influence blood pressure at birth if not earlier. Both systolic and diastolic blood pressures are correlated significantly between mothers and their newborn infants (24). This relationship, which is not found in father–infant pairs, is maintained through the first 8 years of life (54,55), during which time significant correlations also are found between infant and sibling blood pressures. Familial aggregation of blood pressure has been used to document the genetic influence on blood pressure. In 6- to 18-year-old children from 163 separate families, the variance of blood pressure within families is significantly less than the variance observed when all children are studied together (56).

Data from families with both nonbiologic (or adopted) and biologic children offer the opportunity to investigate genetic influences under controlled environmental conditions. Correlations in these families are many times lower between parents and their adopted children than between the same parents and their biologically related children (57). Similar relationships were observed between parents and children in the Minneapolis study (32).

Children with normal blood pressure but at the upper percentiles of distribution tend to have parents with established hypertension or other forms of cardiovascular disease (33,38). A striking difference in family history was recorded between 8- to 9-year-old children selected from the upper 0.26 percent and lowest 5 percent of blood pressure distribution (58). The high blood pressure group had a history of hypertension, stroke, or heart disease in 40 percent of first-degree family relatives, whereas only 18 percent of the low blood pressure group had a similar family history. In a study from Brazil, 10- to 15-year-old children with blood pressure above the 95th percentile had siblings and mothers with significantly higher blood pressure than children with blood pressure below the 50th percentile (59). Despite the strong correlation between parent and child blood pressure, presence of hypertension in a parent can be used only to identify risk and has not yet proven of value in predicting hypertension in offspring (60).

Body Size

Body size is the main factor accounting for blood pressure variability among children, but this relationship is not firmly established until the early grade-school years. There is a very low correlation between blood pressure and height, weight, body mass index, or body surface area during the first year of life (30). These correlations do not change appreciably during the preschool years, a developmental period when blood pressure plateaus while body growth continues at a steady rate.

The positive relationship between body size and blood pressure is established by age 6 years (32), and the two parallel one another thereafter (8,35,38,39). In Hispanic children, a substantial proportion of the variance in blood pressure can be attributed to body fatness by age 5 to 6 years (61). Not all overweight children will become hypertensive. Nevertheless, as one moves toward the extremes of the blood pressure distribution, the relationship becomes more pronounced. Average weight differences between 8- to 9-year-old children from the upper 0.26 percent and lower 5 percent of the blood pressure distribution have been reported to be 15.6 kg (58); percent overweight in adolescents is correlated significantly with systolic and diastolic blood pressure ($r = .64$ and .41, respectively) (62); and systolic and diastolic blood pressure distributions in obese adolescents are skewed greater than 1 standard deviation to the right when compared with normal blood pressure distributions (63).

It is not clear whether fatness has an independent role in childhood hypertension. A small but significant correlation has been shown between central body fat (determined by subscapular skinfold measurements) and blood pressure (64). Data from the Health Examination Survey (65) suggested that weight–blood pressure relationships are not related to fat but to other components of body mass.

Sex

Blood pressure in boys is virtually identical to girls during childhood (see Fig. 3), and significant differences do not become apparent until the teenage years. Systolic blood pressure is significantly higher in teenage boys (45), and diastolic blood pressure tends to be significantly higher in girls in early adolescence. However, between the ages of 13 to 18 years, diastolic blood pressure also becomes significantly higher in boys. Attempts have been made to correlate degree of sexual development with level of blood pressure (35), but the reliability of this type of analysis is open to question. Although it has been suggested that differences in sexual maturity may help explain the blood pressure differences between black and white girls (66), there is a confounding effect of growth and body size on sexual maturity. Moreover, blood pressure is independent of objective indicators of sexual development, such as serum follicle-stimulating hormone (FSH) or luteinizing hormone (LH) (67).

HYPERTENSION

Definition and Prevalence

Hypertension, with all the clinical and prognostic cardiovascular implications attributable to hypertension in adults, occurs at some upper level of blood pressure distribution. Unlike the situation in adults in which natural history studies and therapeutic clinical trials have established prevalence and risk according to incremental changes in blood pressure, long-term experience on risk and outcome are not available in children. Current definitions of hypertension and recommendations for evaluation and therapy are based on clinical experience and limited published data (7,8). At the present time, the consensus report from the 1987 Task Force (8) is the acknowledged reference source for childhood and adolescent hypertension.

A major contribution of the 1977 Task Force (7) was defining hypertension as blood pressure equal to or greater than the 95th percentile of distribution for sex and age. This definition was reaffirmed in the 1987 report (8), and a new category of "high normal" blood pressure was established to ensure that children with blood pressure at the upper end of the distribution have careful longitudinal evaluation (Table 3). A great deal of controversy continues to surround diagnosis, evaluation, and intervention in mild-to-moderate hypertension. Far less than 5 percent of children will be hypertensive, and less than 1 percent will ultimately require evaluation and treatment.

The diagnosis of hypertension is made only after blood pressure is confirmed to be greater than the 95th percentile at three separate examinations. The average blood pressure from two or more measurements is calculated at each visit, and the percentile distribution is determined from the graphs in Figs. 1 to 3. Despite the use of the 95th percentile on the Task Force curves, less than 5 percent of children will have hypertension when the three-examination protocol is followed. With repeated blood pressure measurements, high blood pressure tends to fall, as a result of accommodation on the part of the child to the measurement procedure and the statistical phenomenon of regression toward the mean. The Task Force distribution curves were constructed from single blood pressure measurements per child. Therefore, only after

TABLE 3. *Definitions of blood pressure categories in children*

Blood pressure category	Definition
Normal	Systolic and diastolic blood pressures less than the 90th percentile for sex and age
High normal	Average systolic and/or diastolic blood pressure between the 90th and 95th percentiles for age and sex
Hypertension	Average systolic and/or diastolic blood pressures equal to or greater than the 95th percentile for age and sex with measurements obtained on at least three occasions

Adapted from ref. 8, with permission.

TABLE 4. *Classification of hypertension by age group*

Age group	Hypertension (mm Hg)	
	Significant	Severe
Newborn		
7 days	SBP ≥ 96	SBP ≥ 106
8–30 days	SBP ≥ 104	SBP ≥ 110
Infant (<2 years)	SBP ≥ 112	SBP ≥ 118
	DBP ≥ 74	DBP ≥ 82
Children (3–5 years)	SBP ≥ 116	SBP ≥ 124
	DBP ≥ 76	DBP ≥ 84
Children (6–9 years)	SBP ≥ 122	SBP ≥ 130
	DBP ≥ 78	DBP ≥ 86
Children (10–12 years)	SBP ≥ 126	SBP ≥ 134
	DBP ≥ 82	DBP ≥ 90
Adolescents (13–15 years)	SBP ≥ 136	SBP ≥ 144
	DBP ≥ 86	DBP ≥ 92
Adolescents (16–18 years)	SBP ≥ 142	SBP ≥ 150
	DBP ≥ 92	DBP ≥ 98

From ref. 8, with permission.
SBP, systolic blood pressure; DBP, diastolic blood pressure.

the initial measurement can the blood pressure of 5 percent of children be expected to be at the 95th percentile or above, and it is expected that the percentage of children with hypertensive levels will decrease with each subsequent visit.

Childhood hypertension is divided into two categories (Table 4). "Significant" hypertension is defined as blood pressure between the 95th and 99th percentiles of distribution, and "severe" hypertension is defined as blood pressure at the 99th percentile or above. A limited amount of information is published about the prevalence of hypertension, but, from all indications, prevalence is low in children. Only 26 of 10,000 6- to 8-year-olds (0.26 percent) in the Minneapolis study (6) had a systolic blood pressure of 130 mm Hg or a diastolic blood pressure of 90 mm Hg (58) at the time of the initial screening. In the Muscatine study of children 5 to 18 years old, the prevalence of blood pressure 140/90 mm Hg or greater was less than 1 percent (68); and in the Dallas screening of eighth- to twelfth-grade students, the prevalence of significant hypertension was only 1.6, 1.7, and 1.9 percent in separate eighth-, tenth-, and twelfth-grade surveys (69). In contrast, a survey from Ireland found that 8 percent of boys and 9 percent of girls had blood pressure greater than the Task Force 95th percentile using the average of two measurements taken at the same examination (70). Using 1987 Task Force curves, data from a screening of 20,000 fifth-, sixth-, seventh-, and eighth-grade students were analyzed (71). After the two examinations, using the average of two measurements at each examination, the prevalence of significant systolic, diastolic, and systolic and/or diastolic hypertension was 0.3, 0.8, and 1.1 percent, respectively.

The low prevalence of hypertension in children should

not detract from current recommendations to monitor blood pressure yearly. The diagnosis of severe hypertension, although uncommon, is most often associated with secondary identifiable causes that may be amenable to specific forms of therapy. Of equal importance is the longitudinal evaluation of blood pressure to detect individuals tracking in the upper ten percentiles of blood pressure distribution.

TABLE 5. *Signs of hypertension in the newborn and infant*

Failure to grow
Irritability
Feeding problems
Vomiting
Cyanosis
Respiratory distress
Cardiac failure
Seizures

Causes of Hypertension

It is generally recognized that the incidence of secondary hypertension (i.e., hypertension resulting from a disease process that is usually identifiable, in contrast to primary or essential hypertension) is directly related to the level of blood pressure and inversely correlated with age. Thus, secondary hypertension is likely to be diagnosed in children with severe hypertension, particularly those of grade-school age and younger, whereas it is far less likely that a secondary cause will be uncovered in an adolescent with blood pressure in the significant, or mildly elevated, range. Many diseases can cause hypertension in children. However, only a few of these occur with any frequency, and these are responsible for most cases.

Causes for hypertension vary according to age. The classifications in the tables are listed in approximate decreasing frequency, and this is discussed in detail in the text. In some cases, the age category for a specific disease is very clear, but for most diseases, there is overlap. For this reason, preschool and grade-school age groups were combined. Despite its low prevalence, the finding of severe hypertension requires a thorough medical evaluation. A clear understanding of probable etiologies is required to formulate a rational, efficient plan for diagnostic investigation.

Neonate and Infant

Hypertension occurs in approximately 1 to 2 percent of all newborns admitted to neonatal intensive care nurseries (72–74). Neonates and infants in the first few months of life commonly present in extreme distress, particularly when hypertension develops after discharge from the hospital. The initial signs of hypertension are usually related to congestive heart failure (Table 5) (i.e., irritability, feeding problems, vomiting, cyanosis, and respiratory distress). This progresses steadily and rapidly to circulatory collapse with severe respiratory distress, oliguria, hypotension, and seizures, followed by cardiac arrest. Although it rarely is possible to distinguish at the initial examination between cardiac failure caused by hypertension and congenital heart disease, blood pressure in hypertensive infants may be in the upper normal range, a finding generally not consistent with overt cardiac failure from other causes. It is not clear why the adverse effect of systemic hypertension is so much more dramatic and precipitous in infants than in older children or adults.

Renal artery thrombosis has become the most common cause of neonatal hypertension (75) (Table 6). Despite recognition of this potential complication and attempts to maintain catheter placement at an aortic level below the renal arteries, the problem continues to be seen. Renal arterial thrombosis is the consequence of embolization of thrombotic plaques formed at the catheter tip, producing small areas of renal infarction. The resultant hypertension is usually mild or moderate in degree but can be severe. In either case, it rarely persists longer than a few weeks or months. The overall prognosis is excellent despite residual severe unilateral renal atrophy (75).

Renal artery stenosis is rare in young infants. Reviews from major teaching hospitals (76,77) include very few cases younger than 1 year of age. At the University of Minnesota Hospital, five young infants, 1 week to 10 months old, have been treated for renal artery stenosis in the past 30 years. Each of these infants presented with severe cardiac failure, and hypertension was not recognized until the cardiac failure was corrected. These patients were managed conservatively with antihypertensive drug therapy until the age of 4 or 5 years, at which time the lesions were treated successfully by surgery.

Other causes are listed in Table 6. Hypertension occurs in 100 percent of infants with autosomal recessive polycystic kidney disease (78) and tends to be more severe in early infancy. It is less frequent in infants with the dominant form of the disease (78). Hypertension can develop in infants with bronchopulmonary dysplasia (74,79,80). The etiology is unknown but may be related to hypoxia-mediated changes in vasoreactivity or angiotensin converting enzyme activity (81). Hypertension has been reported as a frequent complication of extracorporeal membrane oxygenation (ECMO) (82,83), developing in 93 percent of infants and associated with intracranial hemorrhage. Significant risk factors also include prenatal cocaine exposure (84), patent ductus arteriosus, and intraventricular hemorrhage (74).

TABLE 6. *Causes of hypertension in the neonate and infant*

Renal artery thrombosis (after umbilical artery catheterization)
Coarctation of the aorta
Congenital renal structural or parenchymal disease
Renal artery stenosis
Bronchopulmonary dysplasia
Abdominal surgery (85)
Extracorporeal membrane oxygenation (ECMO)
Patent ductus arteriosus
Intraventricular hemorrhage

Children 1 to 10 Years

Hypertension in children after infancy is usually discovered during a routine physical examination, even in patients presenting with the most severe degrees of blood pressure elevation. Certain clinical features are characteristic of hypertension and should draw the clinician's attention to the diagnosis (Table 7). Headache can be a sign of hypertension but may be difficult to evaluate because it is such a common, nonspecific complaint in this age group. Cardiac failure is less common, but cardiac enlargement may be an indication of chronic disease. The initial and only indication of illness may be a stroke. This can vary from transient localized neurologic findings to hemiplegia. In general, the prognosis for ultimate full neurologic recovery is good. An uncommon, but unique, sign of hypertension is facial paralysis or Bell's palsy (86,87). It is believed to be the result of a vascular lesion within the facial canal and is reversible with control of the hypertension. Hypertension has recently been described as a parodoxical complication of hypovolemia (88).

The principal cause of hypertension in preschool and grade-school children is renal disease (Table 8). It is diagnosed in approximately 43 to 84 percent of children with hypertension referred to major medical centers (89–91), and this percentage does not appear to be changing. The presence of hypertension can have important implications for severity and prognosis of the renal disease, and these vary according to the basic disease process (Table 9).

TABLE 7. *Symptoms and signs of hypertension in children and adolescents*

Failure to thrive (i.e., growth retardation)
Nausea and/or vomiting
Lethargy
Irritability
Headache
Visual problems
Cardiac failure
Seizures
Stroke
Facial palsy

TABLE 8. *Causes of hypertension in children and adolescents*

1 Year to 10 Years
　Renal disease
　Coarctation of the aorta
　Renal artery stenosis
　Hypercalcemia
　Neurofibromatosis
　Neurogenic tumors
　Pheochromocytoma
　Mineralocorticoid excess
　　Primary hyperaldosteronism
　　11β-hydroxylase deficiency
　　17α-hydroxylase deficiency
　　Dexamethasone-suppressible hyperaldosteronism
　　Apparent mineralocorticoid excess
　　Liquorice ingestion
　Hyperthyroidism
　Transient hypertension after urologic surgery
　Immobilization (traction)-induced hypertension (124–126)
　Sleep apnea-associated hypertension (127)
　Essential hypertension (rare)
10 Years to Adolescence
　Renal disease
　Essential hypertension
　Diagnoses listed above in 1- to 10-year category

Hypertension is found in 75 to 80 percent of hospitalized patients with acute poststreptococcal glomerulonephritis and is reported to be the most common physical finding in this disease (92,93). It appears to be the consequence of sodium and fluid retention. Analysis of FENa in patients who develop hypertension during hospitalization has shown that blood pressure does not increase to hypertensive levels when the FENa is greater than 0.5, whereas patients with a FENa less than 0.5 develop hypertension (93).

Hypertension is found during the initial examination in 26 percent of children presenting with the nephrotic syndrome (94,95), and the presence of hypertension in this syndrome has important adverse prognostic implications, particularly for older children (94). Although 20 percent of children with minimal change nephrotic

TABLE 9. *Frequency of hypertension in selected renal diseases at time of initial presentation*

Renal disease	% with hypertension
Acute poststreptococcal glomerulonephritis	75–80
Nephrotic syndrome	26
Minimal change	21
Focal segmental glomerulosclerosis	36–50
Membranoproliferative glomerulonephritis	42–51
Membranous nephropathy	6–50
Hemolytic-uremic syndrome	49–73
Chronic pyelonephritis	14–20
Schönlein-Henoch purpura	14
IgA nephropathy	6

syndrome have hypertension, it is usually very mild. In contrast, approximately 50 percent of children with focal segmental glomerulorsclerosis (94,95) and membranoproliferative glomerulonephritis (94,96) will have hypertension. In both diseases, hypertension persists long-term but does not accelerate the disease process. The incidence of hypertension in membranous nephropathy varies widely between referral centers (97,98), and these children seem more likely to progress to chronic renal failure than patients without hypertension.

Hypertension is extremely common in children with hemolytic-uremic syndrome, affecting 50 percent of children developing the disease in their first 3 years of life and approximately 75 percent of older children (99). Persistent hypertension is an ominous sign, indicating active disease or incomplete resolution of the renal lesion. Patients with hemolytic uremic syndrome can have the most severe degrees of hypertension during the active phase of their disease, and some with the atypical form of disease (i.e., non-*Escherichia coli*) have required bilateral nephrectomy to control blood pressure, despite aggressive antihypertensive therapy.

Hypertension occurs in 14 to 35 percent of children with pyelonephritis (89–91) and is closely associated with renal cortical scar formation. Scarring and hypertension may appear months after active infection or after surgical correction of vesicoureteral reflux (VUR). Hypertension is infrequent in patients with Schönlein Henoch purpura nephritis (100) and IgA nephropathy (101).

Renal artery stenosis is seen with a frequency of one to two per year at major referral centers (76,77). The physical examination of these children is usually unremarkable, with the exception of blood pressure. A careful search for abdominal bruits should be conducted, but these will be found in fewer than one-third of patients (76,77). Conventional laboratory tests are also not particularly helpful. Peripheral plasma renin activity (PRA) may be elevated but cannot be relied on to establish the diagnosis. Low serum potassium in the presence of normal PRA may be a clue to a hyperreninemic state (102). Radiographic studies other than arteriogram have been uniformly disappointing (76). Intravenous pyelogram, renal ultrasonography, and isotopic renograms have low sensitivity with an excessive number of false-negative results. Administration of captopril before the renogram increases the reliability of this procedure.

Renovascular hypertension may be the result of other disease processes. Children with abdominal aortic and/or other abdominal artery disease may have had undocumented intrauterine infection (e.g., rubella) (103). Multiple artery involvement may also be seen in Takayasu arteritis (104). Somewhat more common is neurofibromatosis, in which the pathogenesis for renal artery stenosis is a proliferation of Schwann cells within the arterial wall (105), and Williams syndrome, a disorder of calcium metabolism in which hypertension is the clinical expression of hypercalcemia, nephrocalcinosis, or renal artery stenosis (106).

The main nonrenal cause of hypertension in children and infants is coarctation of the aorta. Most children with this disease will be identified before they start school, but the diagnosis is frequently missed and detection may be delayed to later childhood (107). A careful physical examination is the key to diagnosis and characteristically includes hypertension in the arms, a reduction in blood pressure of 20 mm Hg or more in the legs, and reduced or absent femoral pulses. The presence of an abdominal bruit is common and can misdirect the evaluation toward renal artery stenosis. Echocardiography will usually confirm the diagnosis.

The etiology for coarct-induced hypertension continues to be a matter of controversy. It is probably caused in part by mechanical obstruction of aortic blood flow, but the main etiologic relationship appears to be a reduction in renal perfusion pressure, similar to the effect of renal artery stenosis. A prerequisite for coarct hypertension is the presence of renal tissue distal to the arterial constriction (108), suggesting the involvement of a renal pressor agent. Plasma renin activity increases after aortic coarctation is produced but returns to normal within a few weeks (109). Plasma renin activity is not significantly higher in children with coarctation than normal children unless stimulated by volume depletion (110). Plasma renin activity decreases significantly after surgical coarctation repair (111).

Hypertension is also a problem in the immediate postoperative period after coarctation repair (112). In its most exaggerated form, it is associated with a syndrome of mesenteric arteritis, characterized by abdominal pain, rebound tenderness, vomiting, fever, leukocytosis, and ileus (113). On rare occasions, bowel infarction occurs. The hypertension is thought to be related to activation of the sympathetic nervous (114) and renin-angiotensin systems (112). In support of this, administration of propranolol pre- and postoperatively will reduce the postcoarctectomy hypertensive response (114,115). Despite nonrecurrence of the coarctation, hypertension persists in 24 percent of patients (116). Clinical success appears to be related to the patient's age at the time of surgery, with repair after the age of 5 to 6 years associated with a higher incidence of residual hypertension (116).

Other causes of hypertension occur infrequently in this age group. It is found in only 20 percent of children with neurogenic tumors (e.g., neuroblastoma) (117). Pheochromocytoma is an extremely rare tumor in childhood (90,91). Its clinical presentation differs from adults because of the sustained rather than intermittent nature of the hypertension, lower frequency of cardiovascular symptoms, and higher incidence of extraadrenal tumor sites (118).

Mineralocorticoid-induced hypertension also is extremely rare in childhood. A reliable clue is a significant reduction in PRA, whereas other tests (e.g., serum potassium) have a lower sensitivity. Primary hyperaldosteronism has been reported in only 21 children and is usually the result of bilateral adrenal hyperplasia rather than tumor (119). Other etiologies in children are congenital deficiencies of 11 beta-hydroxylase or 17 alpha-hydroxylase (120); dexamethasone-suppressible hyperaldosteronism (121), a rare familial syndrome in which aldosterone secretion is totally suppressible with dexamethasone or other glucocorticoid therapy; and "apparent mineralocorticoid excess" (122), a syndrome with severe hypertension, low renin, and hypokalemia but without an increase in steroid production. These children may be treated successfully with spironolactone. A related uncommon cause of hypertension is liquorice ingestion (123). Liquorice contains glycyrhinic acid, which inhibits 11 beta-dehydrogenase, the enzyme involved in the conversion of cortisol to cortisone.

Early and Late Adolescence

Secondary causes for hypertension become less frequent beginning in late childhood and continuing through adolescence as more children are recognized with early mild essential hypertension. In cases of secondary hypertension, renal-related diseases continue to be the predominant diagnosis (see above). It has become clear that mild-to-moderate elevations in blood pressure are more common than previously recognized, particularly in children of junior high school age and older. Although the evaluation of children in this age range is designed to eliminate secondary causes of hypertension, attention should begin to focus on essential hypertension in the context of general cardiovascular risk.

In contrast to information on the overall prevalence of hypertension in children and adolescents (as noted earlier in this section), there are few data on the specific prevalence of essential hypertension. Reviews from major pediatric centers include, in most cases, only patients with severe hypertension (89–91), thus increasing the prevalence of secondary causes. The consensus reflected in the 1987 Task Force Report (8) and from contemporary clinical experience suggests that the percentage with primary hypertension is substantially increased when children with blood pressure in the significant hypertension range (i.e., 95 to 99 percentiles of distribution) also are considered.

Few attempts had been made until recently to identify factors that are active during childhood in influencing the development of essential hypertension. A study of eight-year-olds with high and low blood pressure (58) showed that plasma norepinephrine levels were not significantly different between the two groups at rest, after 2 hours of upright posture, or after vigorous exercise. Plasma renin activity was significantly lower in the high

blood pressure group under the same sampling conditions (58), and 24-hour urinary kallikrein excretion was significantly lower in the high blood pressure group (128). A role for sympathetic nervous system hyperactivity was suggested by the dramatic response to mental stress exhibited by adolescents with borderline hypertension and a family history of hypertension (129); these individuals also had a higher risk for the eventual development of fixed essential hypertension (130).

Within the past few years, greater attention has been given to potential etiologic mechanisms and documentation of early target-organ effects. Studies suggest that the insulin–blood pressure relation is present before adulthood. Fasting insulin is correlated significantly with blood pressure, even after adjustment for body mass index, as early as 5 years of age (131), and insulin resistance has been demonstrated in young black boys with only borderline hypertension, independent of body mass index (132,133). Obesity also is an important factor in this relation. Significant differences in fasting insulin have been noted in obese children during the first decade of life (134). Obesity, insulin, and blood pressure have been more extensively studied in adolescents (135). In the obese adolescent population, insulin resistance has been associated with chronic sodium retention (136), sodium sensitivity (137), and structural changes in forearm resistance vessels (138), and these are reversible with weight loss and exercise (139).

The bulk of the data on target-organ effects relates to the cardiovascular system. Approximately 40 percent of children and adolescents with blood pressure greater than the 90th percentile have left ventricular hypertrophy, when compared with criteria for normal children (140). In a direct comparison between 9- to 11-year-old children with blood pressure greater than the 95th percentile and children with normal blood pressure, left ventricular mass, corrected for body surface area, was significantly greater in the former group and was associated with other risk factors (141). A longitudinal study in 6- to 11-year-old children concluded that subsequent systolic blood pressure was predicted by baseline left ventricular mass, and subsequent left ventricular mass was predicted by baseline left ventricular mass and exercise diastolic blood pressure (142). Finally, a significant interrelationship between blood pressure and other cardiovascular risk factors early in development is suggested by the positive correlation between blood pressure, serum lipids, and arterial (aortic and coronary) fatty streaks in young subjects dying from noncardiovascular causes (143). A potential early effect on the kidney has been suggested by the finding that offspring (mean age, 9.5 yrs) of essential hypertensive parents are more likely to have a lower renal functional reserve and higher levels of microalbuminuria than offspring of normotensive parents (144).

EVALUATION OF THE HYPERTENSIVE CHILD

There is considerable controversy among pediatricians with regard to which children with hypertension should be investigated with laboratory and other tests and the extent of the investigation. There is a difference in the approach to children with severe and mild hypertension. In the former group, particularly when symptoms are present or there are signs of target-organ involvement, there is general agreement that a complete diagnostic evaluation should be conducted. In the latter group, there is less benefit from an intensive investigation. It is unreasonable to initiate a major investigation in a child suspected of having mild-to-moderate hypertension without confirmation from three separate examinations that the level of blood pressure falls under the definitions listed in Table 4. Investigation is not indicated for children with blood pressure in the high normal range, even those with an occasional reading above the 95th percentile, unless the medical history or physical examination suggests a specific disease entity.

Diagnostic evaluation should be designed to fit the clinical presentation and age of the child (see Tables 6 and 8). When there are not any clues to the etiology, the diagnostic plan should be directed in its early stages toward renal disease. Table 10 lists an outline for evaluation of hypertensive children. It is arranged to begin with general screening tests, proceeding in a stepwise fashion to more complicated procedures required to diagnose the less common causes of hypertension. This list is intended only as a guide. The medical history, family history, or physical examination may provide information enabling the clinician to move more rapidly to investigation of specific disease entities.

The initial evaluation consists of a complete blood count (serum electrolytes, creatinine, urea nitrogen, calcium, uric acid, and cholesterol) and urinalysis. A urine culture is also obtained because of the silent nature of chronic pyelonephritis. Plasma renin activity is obtained primarily to look for suppression of activity, suggesting mineralocorticoid excess. Plasma renin activity is less useful in the diagnosis of renal artery stenosis because of overlap in values between these patients and patients with other forms of hypertension. It is crucial that normal standards for PRA be established by the laboratory performing the test, because PRA values vary according to age in children (145). Serum cholesterol will not aid in the diagnosis but is important for the introduction of the broader concept of cardiovascular risk in the context of hypertension.

Because of the high incidence of renal disease in children with hypertension, a detailed examination of the kidney is indicated. The intravenous pyelogram (IVP) is rarely used today without a specific indication. Kidney size and anatomy are evaluated by renal ultrasound, and renal blood flow is evaluated by the renogram. Unfortunately, the sensitivity of the isotopic renogram in the diagnosis of renal artery stenosis is limited (76,77). This can be circumvented in part by the use of diethylene triamine pentacetic acid (DTPA), which is excreted at the glomerulus and is not excreted or absorbed by the renal tubule. Pretreatment of the patient with captopril before administration of DTPA will enhance flow differences between the affected and normal kidney by further reducing glomerular filtration rate and clearance of DTPA on the stenotic side (146). Even this maneuver cannot be depended on to detect branch arterial stenotic lesions, commonly missed without an arteriogram.

An echocardiogram should be obtained in children with severe hypertension and in any child considered for antihypertensive therapy (147,148). The chest X-ray is not a sensitive enough measure of early cardiac changes. Echocardiographic examination is not indicated for children with mild hypertension, even though early changes in left ventricular geometry have been shown to be present across the normal distribution of childhood blood pressure (149).

Catecholamine production is evaluated by measurement of 24-hour urinary excretion of catecholamines or catechol metabolites (i.e., vanillylmandelic acid [VMA]). In some centers, plasma measurements are also used, but these do not appear to be as sensitive as urinary measurements (150). Measurement of VMA and homovanillic acid (HVA) in randomly collected urine specimens is now used for neuroblastoma detection but has not been tested in patients with pheochromocytoma (151). In the patient with a very low PRA, plasma samples for aldosterone and other steroids should be obtained to eliminate the possibility of mineralocorticoid excess.

In the severely hypertensive child, particularly in the infant and young child, renal arteriography should be performed when other causes for hypertension have been eliminated, even when the isotopic renogram is normal (152). This study should be performed at an in-

TABLE 10. *Diagnostic evaluation of the hypertensive child*

Complete blood count
Serum electrolytes, creatinine, urea nitrogen, calcium, uric acid, cholesterol
Urinalysis
Urine culture
Plasma renin activity
Renal ultrasound
Isotopic renogram
Echocardiogram
Urine collection for catecholamines
Plasma and urinary steroids
Renal arteriography

stitution with the capability for transluminal angioplasty, although care must be taken with regard to patient selection and the angioplastic procedure itself to prevent procedural mishaps. Renal vein renin measurements have traditionally been obtained in children (153), but with mixed results. The test was introduced in adults to assist in distinguishing between renovascular and essential hypertension, but this is not a problem in pediatric patients with hypertension. At the University of Minnesota Hospital, renal vein renin determinations are no longer part of the routine evaluation of renal artery stenosis.

TREATMENT OF CHILDHOOD HYPERTENSION

Antihypertensive therapy clearly is indicated for children with severe hypertension to prevent adverse cardiovascular events (154). It is less clear what approach is best for the child with persistent mild-to-moderate hypertension. The goal of treatment is reduction of blood pressure to a level below the 95th percentile. This may take a period of days or weeks to accomplish. The most important factor is steady progress in blood pressure reduction once treatment has begun, because there is not any evidence that more rapid reduction of blood pressure, except for those patients with extreme hypertension, improves prognosis or well-being.

Nonpharmacologic Therapy

Children with blood pressure in the "significant" hypertension range should be started on a nonpharmacologic regimen, introduced in the context of cardiovascular risk, including family history, lipids, tobacco, overweight, and exercise. Nonpharmacologic therapy includes weight reduction, exercise, and diet adjustment. The effectiveness of each of these is related directly to motivation on the part of the patient and reinforcement on the part of the parents and health care provider. There is general agreement that exercise can be an important addition to antihypertensive control (155). In successful weight loss programs, blood pressure decreases in response to weight reduction (62), and the reduction is greatest in the heaviest children. The reduction in blood pressure is not an isolated finding but occurs in conjunction with other components of cardiovascular risk (156). Aerobic exercise reduces blood pressure in adolescents (63,157,158) and has a beneficial effect on serum lipids (156). Weight training (i.e., static exercise) also reduces blood pressure (159), but is not recommended over aerobic training because of its questionable effect on cardiovascular fitness.

An important issue for the older hypertensive child is strenuous exercise during participation in organized sports. Blood pressure increases significantly with exercise in normal children as well as those with high blood pressure (160), and there is not any evidence to suggest that children with mild hypertension are at increased risk (161). Without evidence of cardiac disease or an abnormality on the electrocardiogram or echocardiogram, participation in sports for these children is not contraindicated, provided blood pressure is carefully monitored with regular examinations (162). The child with severe hypertension is likely to be at greater risk and should not participate in strenuous sports activity. Successful reduction of blood pressure with treatment probably reduces overall exercise risk, but there is not any evidence to support this. Because exercise has a positive effect on blood pressure and cardiovascular risk, it should be unconditionally contraindicated only in those individuals with ongoing severe hypertension.

Dietary intervention has focused on modification of sodium or potassium intake, but few studies have been reported in children or adolescents, and almost all have been of short duration. The effect of low sodium on children has been mixed, with a reduction in blood pressure seen by some (163,164) but not others (165–167). Potassium supplements have not been effective in children (168), but a significant reduction in blood pressure was seen when potassium was combined with sodium restriction (165). When a decrease in blood pressure has been seen, the response has occurred only (166,169,170), or primarily (164), in girls. Significant correlations between urinary sodium and blood pressure have not been found in children under free-living conditions (169–172).

The only long-term intervention study was recently completed in adolescent boys and girls treated with either low-sodium intake or potassium supplementation over 3 years (175). There was not any significant effect noted when the boys and girls were combined and compared with a placebo group. However, when the boys and girls were examined separately, the rates of rise (slopes) of blood pressure of the girls' low-sodium and potassium groups were not significantly different from zero and lower than the slope of the girls' placebo group. Moreover, there was a highly significant difference in slope between the girls' low-sodium and potassium groups and the respective boys' groups.

Intervention studies with calcium have not been reported in children, and the data, in general, on the relation between calcium and blood pressure are conflicting (174–178).

Antihypertensive Drug Therapy

Drug therapy in childhood hypertension is based on the same principles established for adults and has been described in detail elsewhere (179). Drugs are added in a stepwise fashion until blood pressure control is achieved.

When more than one drug is required, drugs acting on the same physiologic system are not used simultaneously.

Severe hypertension in children resulting from primary renal disease frequently requires aggressive therapy with multidrug regimens. These patients may experience a deterioration in renal function coincident with a reduction in blood pressure (180). With ongoing therapy, renal function should return to pretreatment levels.

Acute hypertensive emergencies (Table 11) are usually defined by blood pressure likely to cause some immediate major vascular accident. Patients without neurologic symptoms can be treated with the calcium channel blocker nifedipine (181). Sodium nitroprusside and labetalol are widely used in these children because they are effective and the rate of blood pressure reduction can be controlled (182). Diazoxide is also a very effective drug, but its use is often accompanied by a precipitous fall in blood pressure that is best avoided. Hydralazine is less potent and has a short duration of action. It is useful over the short term but loses its effectiveness when frequent repeated dosing is required.

The availability of newer antihypertensive agents has greatly improved the management of children with chronic hypertension (Table 12). Converting enzyme inhibitors and calcium antagonists are now included with diuretics and beta blockers as options for initial therapy.

Converting enzyme inhibitors have been widely used in children (183) with all degrees of renal function (184). They are particularly useful in newborn infants but should be initiated at 10 percent of the usual children's dose to avoid adverse effects (185,186). Neonatal hypertension can be treated with intravenous enalaprilat (187).

Published experience with calcium antagonists in children has been limited to nifedipine (181) and nitrendipine (188), but the latter is no longer available in the United States.

Diuretics are an important component of antihypertensive therapy in children with renal disease. The thiazides have proved to be exceptionally free from adverse effects. Furosemide is generally reserved for patients with a reduction in renal function to 50 percent of normal or lower. All members of the class of beta-blocking drugs have been used safely in children, as have the remainder of the drugs listed in Table 12.

TABLE 11. *Antihypertensive drug therapy for hypertensive emergencies*

Drug	Dose
Sodium nitroprusside	0.5–8 µg/kg/min intravenous
Labetalol	1–3 mg/kg intravenous
Diazoxide	2–5 mg/kg intravenous
Hydralazine	0.2–0.4 mg/kg intravenous
Nifedipine	0.25–0.5 mg/kg oral
Minoxidil	0.1–0.2 mg/kg oral

TABLE 12. *Antihypertensive drugs for chronic therapy*

Drug	Dose (mg/kg/day) Initial	Maximum
Converting enzyme inhibitors		
Captopril		
Neonates	0.03–0.15	2
Children	1.5	6
Enalapril	0.15	?
Calcium antagonists		
Nifedipine	0.25	3
Diuretics		
Hydrochlorothiazide	1	2–3
Metolazone	0.1	3
Furosemide	1	12
Bumetanide	0.02–0.05	0.3
Spironolactone	1	3
Triamterene	2	3
Beta-adernergic blockers		
Propranolol	1	8
Atenolol	1	8
Alpha blockers		
Prazosin	0.05–0.1	0.5
Vasodilators		
Hydralazine	0.75	7.5
Minoxidil	0.1–0.2	1
Alpha agonists		
Clonidine	0.05–0.1	
MethylDOPA	5	10

REFERENCES

1. Loggie JMH. *J Pediatr* 1969;74:331–355.
2. Londe S. *Pediatrics* 1966;5:71–78.
3. U.S. Department of Health, Education and Welfare: DHEW publication No. (HRA) 74-1617, Vital and Health Statistics-Series 11-135, 1973.
4. Lauer RM, Connor WE, Leaverton PE, Reiter MA, Clarke WR. *J Pediatr* 1975;86:697–706.
5. Voors AW, Foster TA, Frerichs RR, Webber LS, Berenson GS. *Circulation* 1976;54:319–327.
6. Prineas RJ, Gillum RF, Horibe H, Hannan PJ. *Hypertension* 1980;2(suppl I):I18–I28.
7. Report of the Task Force on Blood Pressure Control in Children. *Pediatrics* 1977;59:797–820.
8. Report of the Second Task Force on Blood Pressure Control in Children—1987. *Pediatrics* 1987;79:1–25.
9. American Academy of Pediatrics: Guidelines for health supervision. *News Comment* May 1982.
10. Moss AJ, Liebling W, Austin WO, Adams FH. *Pediatrics* 1957;20:53–62.
11. Reder RF, Dimich I, Cohen ML, Steinfeld L. *Pediatrics* 1978;62:326–330.
12. Park MK, Menard SM. *Pediatrics* 1987;79:907–914.
13. Wareham JA, Haugh LD, Yeager SB, Horbar JD. *Am J Dis Child* 1987;141:1108–1110.
14. Gomez-Marin O, Prineas R, Rastam L. *J Hypertens* 1992;10:1235–1241.
15. Jenner D, Vandongen R, Beilin L. *J Hum Hypertens* 1992;6:367–374.
16. Moss AJ. *Pediatrics* 1983;71:854–855.
17. Londe S. *Pediatrics* 1985;76:460–461.
18. Moss AJ, Adams FH. *Am J Dis Child* 1963;106:747–77.
19. Sinaiko AR, Gomez-Marin OG, Prineas RJ. *Am J Epidemiol* 1990;132:647–655.
20. Uhari M, Nuutinen M, Turtinen J, Pokka T. *Lancet* 1991;338:159–161.
21. Lagler U, Duc G. *Biol Neonate* 1980;37:243–245.

22. Hulman S, Edwards R, Chen Y, Polansky M, Falkner B. *J Perinatol* 1991;XI:231–234.
23. de Swiet M, Fayers P, Shinebourne EA. *Pediatrics* 1980;65:1028–1035.
24. Zinner SH, Rosner B, Oh W, Kass EH. *Hypertension* 1985;7:411–416.
25. de Man S, Andre J, Bachmann H, et al. *J Hypertens* 1991;9:109–114.
26. Versmold HT, Kitterman JA, Phibbs RH, Gregory GH, Tooley WH. *Pediatrics* 1981;67:607–613.
27. Moscoso P, Goldberg RN, Jamieson J, Bancalari E. *J Pediatr* 1983;103:114–117.
28. Adams MA, Pasternak JF, Kupfer BM, Gardner TH. *Pediatrics* 1983;71:23–30.
29. Spinazzola R, Harper R, de Soler M, Lesser M. *J Perinatol* 1991;XI:147–151.
30. Schacter J, Cutler LH, Perfetti C. *Am J Epidemiol* 1982;116:29–41.
31. Burke GL, Voors AW, Shear CL, et al. *Pediatrics* 1987;80 (suppl):784–788.
32. Prineas RJ, Gillum RF, Gomez-Marin O. In: Loggie JMH, Horan MJ, Gruskin AB, Hohn AR, Dunbar JB, Havlik RJ, eds. *NHLBI workshop on juvenile hypertension.* New York: Biomed Infor Serv; 1984:21–35.
33. Shear CL, Burke GL, Freedman DS, Berenson GS. *Pediatrics* 1986;77:862–869.
34. Gillman M, Rosner B, Evans D, et al. *Pediatrics* 1991;87:708–711.
35. Lauer RM, Anderson AR, Beaglehole R, Burns TL. *Hypertension* 1984;6:307–314.
36. Prineas RJ, Gomez-Marin O, Sinaiko AR. *Clin Exp Hypertens (A)* 1986;8:583–604.
37. Sinaiko AR, Bass J, Gomez-Marin O, Prineas RJ. *J Hypertens* 1986;4(suppl 5):S378–S380.
38. Prineas RJ, Gomez-Marin O, Gillum RF. *Ann Behav Med* 1985;7:25–29.
39. Lauer RM, Clarke WR, Beaglehole R. *Circulation* 1984;69:242–249.
40. Leitschuh M, Cupples A, Kannel W, Gagnon D, Chobanian A. *Hypertension* 1991;17:22–27.
41. Mahoney L, Clarke W, Burns T, Lauer R. *Am J Hypertens* 1991;4:608S–610S.
42. Julius S, Jamerson K, Mejia A, Krause L, Schork N, Jones K. *JAMA* 1990;264:354–358.
43. Nelson M, Ragland D, Syme L. *Am J Epidemiol* 1992;136:633–645.
44. Schacter J, Kuller LH, Perkins JM, Radin ME. *Am J Epidemiol* 1979;110:205–218.
45. Baron AE, Freyer B, Fixler DE. *Am J Epidemiol* 1986;123:809–817.
46. Gutgesell M, Terrell G, Labarthe D. *Hypertension* 1981;3:39–47.
47. Manatunga A, Jones J, Pratt H. *Hypertension* 1993;22:84–89.
48. NHLBI growth and health study. *Am J Public Health* 1992;82:1613–1620.
49. Munger R, Gomez-Marin O, Prineas RP, Sinaiko AR. *Am J Epidemiol* 1991;133:1257–1265.
50. Lauer R, Burns T, Clarke W, Mahoney L. *Hypertension* 1991;18(suppl I):1-74–I-81.
51. St. George I, Williams S, Silva P. *Circulation* 1990;82:1675–1680.
52. Hansen H, Rokkedal Nielsen J, Hyldebrandt N, Froberg K. *J Hypertens* 1992;10:677–682.
53. Burns T, Moll P, Lauer R. *Pediatrics* 1992;89:262–268.
54. Wilson D, Klesges L, Klesges R, et al. *J Clin Epidemiol* 1992;45:959–969.
55. Fossali E, Ruzza ML, Codega C, et al. *Acta Paediatr Scand* 1990;79:1213–1218.
56. Zinner SH, Martin LF, Sacks F, Rosner B, Kass EH. *Am J Epidemiol* 1974;100:437–442.
57. Biron P, Morgeau JG. *Pediatr Clin North Am* 1978;25:29–33.
58. Sinaiko AR, Gillum RF, Jacobs DR, Sopko G, Prineas RJ. *Hypertension* 1982;4:299–306.
59. Brandao AP, Brandao AA, Araujo E, Oliveira R. *Hypertension* 1992;19(suppl II):II-214–II-217.
60. Watt G, Foy C, Holton D, Edwards H. *J Hypertens* 1991;9:55–58.
61. Gutin B, Basch C, Shea S, et al. *JAMA* 1990;264:1123–1127.
62. Brownell KD, Kelaran JH, Stunkard AJ. *Pediatrics* 1983;71:515–523.
63. Rocchini AP, Katch V, Anderson J, et al. *Pediatrics* 1988;82:16–23.
64. Shear CL, Freedman DS, Burke GL, Harsha DW, Berenson GS. *Hypertension* 1977;9:236–244.
65. Stallones L, Mueller WH, Christensen BL. *Hypertension* 1982;4:483–486.
66. Kozinetz C. *Am J Dis Child* 1991;145:142–147.
67. Londe S, Johanson A, Kronemer NS, Goldring D. *J Pediatr* 1975;87:896–900.
68. Rames LC, Clarke WR, Connor WE, Recher MA, Lauer RM. *Pediatrics* 1978;61:245–251.
69. Fixler DE, Laird WP. *Pediatrics* 1983;72:459–463.
70. Maguire H, Shelley E. *Ir Med J* 1990;83:90–92.
71. Sinaiko AR, Gomez-Marin O, Prineas RJ. *J Pediatr* 1989;114:664–669.
72. Skalina MEL, Kliegman RM, Fanaroff AA. *Am J Perinatol* 1986;3:235–239.
73. Buchi KF, Siegler RL. *J Hypertens* 1986;4:525–528.
74. Singh H, Hurley R, Myers T. *Am J Hypertens* 1992;5:51–55.
75. Adelman RD. *Pediatr Nephrol* 1987;1:35–41.
76. Daniels SR, Loggie JMH, McEnerny PT, Towbin RB. *Pediatrics* 1987;80:698–704.
77. Watson AR, Balfe JW, Hardy BE. *J Pediatr* 1985;106:366–372.
78. Cole BR, Conley SB, Stapleton FB. *J Pediatr* 1987;111:693–699.
79. Abman SH, Warady BA, Lum GM, Koops BL. *J Pediatr* 1984;104:928–931.
80. Anderson AH, Warady BA, Daily DK, Johnson JA, Thomas MK. *Am J Perinatol* 1993;10:190–193.
81. Mattioli L, Zakheim RM, Mullis K, Molteri A. *J Pediatr* 1978;87:97–101.
82. Sell LL, Cullen ML, Lerner GR, Whittlesey GC, Shanley CJ, Klein MD. *Surgery* 1987;102:724–730.
83. Boedy F, Goldberg A, Howell C, Hulse E, Edwards E, Kanto W. *J Pediatr Surg* 1990;25:258–261.
84. Horn P. *J Pediatr* 1992;121:288–291.
85. Adelman RD, Sherman MP. *J Pediatr* 1980;97:642–644.
86. Lloyd AVC, Jewett DE, Still JDL. *Arch Dis Child* 1968;41:292–294.
87. Siegler R, Brewer E, Corneli H, Thompson J. *Pediatrics* 1991;87:387–389.
88. Bissler J, Welch T, Loggie J. *Pediatr Emer Care* 1991;7:350–352.
89. Dillon MJ. *Pediatr Nephrol* 1987;1:59–68.
90. Uhari M, Kostinies O. *Acta Paediatr Scand* 1979;68:193–198.
91. Loirat C, Pillion G, Blum C. *Adv Nephrol* 1982;11:65–97.
92. Lieberman E, Donnell GN. *Medicine* 1965;109:398–407.
93. Mota-Hernandez F, Feiman R, Gordillo-Paniagua G. *J Pediatr* 1984;104:560–563.
94. International Study of Kidney Disease in Children. *Kidney Int* 1978;13:159–165.
95. Southwest Pediatric Nephrology Study Group. *Kidney Int* 1985;27:442–449.
96. West CD. *Kidney Int* 1986;29:1077–1093.
97. Habib R, Kleinknecht C, Gubler MC. *J Pediatr* 1973;82:754–756.
98. Ramirez F, Brouhard BH, Travis LB, Ellis EN. *J Pediatr* 1982;101:677–681.
99. Habib R, Levy M, Gagnadoux MF, Broyer M. *Adv Nephrol* 1982;11:99–128.
100. Levy M, Broyer M, Arsan A, Levy-Bantolila D, Habib R. *Adv Nephrol* 1976;6:183–228.
101. Southwest Pediatric Nephrology Study Group. *Kidney Int* 1982;22:643–652.
102. Bunchman TE, Sinaiko AR. *Pediatr Nephrol* 1990;4:169–170.
103. Menser MA, Dorman DC, Reye RDK, Reid RR. *Lancet* 1966;1:790–792.
104. Wiggelinkhuizea J, Cremin BS. *Pediatrics* 1978;62:209–217.
105. Hallman R, Roth FJ. *Clin Exp Hypertens* 1986;A8:893–899.
106. Daniels SR, Loggie JMH, Schwartz DC, Strife JL, Kaplan S. *J Pediatr* 1985;106:249–251.

107. Stafford MA, Griffiths SP, Gersony WM. *Pediatrics* 1982;69: 159–163.
108. Scott HW, Collins HA, Langa ASM, Olsen NS. *Surgery* 1954;36: 445–459.
109. Yogi S, Kramsch DM, Madoff IM, Hollander W. *Am J Physiol* 1968;215:605–610.
110. Alpert BS, Baur HH, Balfe JW, Kidd BSL, Olley PM. *Am J Cardiol* 1979;43:828–834.
111. Parker FB, Streeter DHP, Farrell B, Blackman MS, Sondheimer HM, Anderson GH. *Circulation* 1982;66:513–514.
112. Rocchini AP, Rosenthal A, Barger AC, Castaneda AR, Nadas AS. *Circulation* 1976;54:382–387.
113. Ho ECK, Moss AJ. *Pediatrics* 1972;49:40–45.
114. Leenen FHH, Balfe JA, Pelech AN, Barker GA, Balfe JW, Olley PM. *Am Heart J* 1987;5:1164–1173.
115. Gidding SS, Rocchini AP, Beekman R, et al. *N Engl J Med* 1985;312:1224–1228.
116. Nanton MA, Olley PM. *Am J Cardiol* 1976;37:769–772.
117. Weinblatt ME, Heisel MA, Siegel SE. *Pediatrics* 1983;71:947–951.
118. Hodgkinson DJ, Telander RL, Sheps SG, Gilchrist GS, Crowe JK. *Mayo Clin Proc* 1980;55:271–276.
119. Rauh W, Oberfield SE. *Pediatr Adolesc Endocrinol* 1984;13:210–230.
120. White PC, New MI, Dupont B. *N Engl J Med* 1986;8:669–676.
121. Connell JMC, Kenyon CJ, Corrie JET, Fraser R, Watt R, Lever AF. *Hypertension* 1986;8:669–676.
122. Ulick S, Levine LS, Gunezler P, et al. *J Clin Endocrinol Metab* 1979;449:757–764.
123. van der Zwan A. *Clin Neurol Neurosurg* 1993;95:35–37.
124. Linshaw MA, Stapleton FB, Gruskin AB, Baluarte HJ, Harbin GL. *J Pediatr* 1979;95:994–996.
125. Karpati R, Mak R, Lemley K. *Child Nephrol Urol* 1991;11:215–219.
126. Heif HA, Ekkelkamp S, Vos A. *Eur J Pediatr* 1992;151:543–545.
127. Ross RD, Daniels SR, Loggie JMH, Meyer RA, Ballard ET. *J Pediatr* 1987;111:253–255.
128. Sinaiko AR, Glasser RJ, Gillum RF, Prineas RJ. *J Pediatr* 1982;100:938–940.
129. Falkner B, Onesti G, Angelakos ET, Fernandes M, Langman C. *Hypertension* 1979;1:23–30.
130. Falkner B, Kushner H, Onesti G, Angelakos ET. *Hypertension* 1981;3:521–527.
131. Jiang X, Srinivasan S, Bao W, Berenson G. *Arch Intern Med* 1993;153:323–328.
132. Falkner B, Hulman S, Kushner H. *Hypertension* 1993;22:18–25.
133. Falkner B, Hulman S, Tannenbaum J, Kushner H. *Hypertension* 1990;16:706–711.
134. Kanai H, Matsuzawa Y, Tokunaga K, et al. *Int J Obes* 1990;14: 1047–1056.
135. Rocchini A. *Hypertension* 1991;17:837–842.
136. Rocchini A, Katch V, Kveselis D, et al. *Hypertension* 1989;14: 367–374.
137. Rocchini AP, Kee J, Bondie D, et al. *N Engl J Med* 1989;321: 580–585.
138. Rocchini A, Moorehead C, Katch V, Key J, Finta K. *Hypertension* 1992;19:615–620.
139. Rocchini AP, Katch V, Schork A, Kelch RP. *Hypertension* 1987;10:267–273.
140. Daniels S, Meyer R, Loggie J. *Circulation* 1990;82:1243–1248.
141. Hansen H, Rokkedal Nielsen J, Froberg K, Hyldebrandt N. *J Hum Hypertens* 1992;6:41–45.
142. Mahoney L, Schieken R, Clarke W, Lauer R. *Hypertension* 1988;12:206–213.
143. Newman WP, Freedman DS, Voors AW, et al. *N Engl J Med* 1986;314:138–144.
144. Grunfeld B, Perelstein E, Simsolo R, Gimenez M, Romero J. *Hypertension* 1990;15:257–261.
145. Dillon MJ, Ryness JM. *Br Med J* 1975;4:316–319.
146. Sfakianakis GN, Bourgoignie JJ, Jaffe D, Kyriakides G, Perez-Stable E, Duncan RC. *J Nucl Med* 1987;28:1383–1392.
147. Shieken RM, Clarke WR, Lauer RM. *Hypertension* 1981;3:669–675.
148. Culpepper WS, Sodt PC, Messerli FH, Reschhaupt DG, Arcilla RA. *Ann Intern Med* 1983;98:1–7.
149. Burke GL, Arcilla RA, Culpepper WS, Webber LS, Chiang LK, Berenson GS. *Circulation* 1987;75:106–114.
150. Duncan MW, Compton P, Lazarus L, Smythe GA. *N Engl J Med* 1988;319:136–142.
151. Tuchman M, Morris CL, Ramnaraine ML, Bowers LD, Krivit W. *Pediatrics* 1985;75:324–328.
152. Guzzetta PC, Potter BM, Ruley EJ, Majd M, Bock GH. *J Pediatr Surg* 1989;24:1236–1240.
153. Deal JE, Snell MF, Barratt TM, Dillon MJ. *J Pediatr* 1992;121: 378–384.
154. Heyden S, Bartel AG, Hames CG, McDonough JR. *JAMA* 1969;209:1683–1689.
155. Concensus Statement by the World Hypertension League. *J Hypertens* 1991;9:283–287.
156. Becque MD, Katch VL, Rocchini AP, Marks CR, Moorehead C. *Pediatrics* 1988;81:605–612.
157. Hagberg JM, Goldring D, Ehsani AA, et al. *Am J Cardiol* 1983;52:763–768.
158. Hansen HS, Froberg K, Hyldebrandt N, Nielsen JR. *Br Med J* 1991;303:682–685.
159. Hagberg JM, Ehsani AA, Goldring D, Hernandez A, Sinacore DR, Holloszy JO. *J Pediatr* 1984;104:147–151.
160. Wilson SL, Gaffney FA, Laird WP, Fixler DE. *Hypertension* 1985;7:417–422.
161. Fixler DE, Laird WP, Browne R, Fitzgerald V, Wilson S, Vance R. *Pediatrics* 1979;64:579–583.
162. Strong WB. *Pediatrics* 1979;64:693–695.
163. Costa FV, Ambrosioni E, Montepugnoli L, Paccalmi L, Vasconi L, Magnani P. *Clin Sci* 1981;61:215–235.
164. Ellison RC, Capper AL, Stephenson WP, et al. *J Clin Epidemiol* 1989;42:201–208.
165. Grobbe DE, Hofman A, Roelandt JT, Boomsma F, Schalekamp MA, Valkenburg HA. *J Hypertens* 1987;5:115–119.
166. Miller JZ, Weinberger MH, Daughtery SA, Fineberg NS, Christian JC, Grim CE. *Am J Clin Nutr* 1988;47:113–119.
167. Howe PRC, Cobiac L, Smith RM. *J Hypertens* 1991;9:181–186.
168. Miller JZ, Weinberger MH, Christian JC. *Hypertension* 1987;10: 437–442.
169. Geleijuse JM, Grobbee DE, Hofman A. *Br Med J* 1990;300:899–902.
170. Zwianer K, Eberlein G, Widhalm K. *Wien Klin Wochenschr* 1991;103:519–523.
171. Cooper R, Lin K, Trevisan M, Miller W, Stamler J. *Hypertension* 1983;5:135–139.
172. Jenner DA, English DR, Vandongen R, et al. *Am J Clin Nutr* 1988;47:1052–1059.
173. Sinaiko A, Gomez-Marin O, Prineas R. *Hypertension* 1993;21: 989–994.
174. Perlman SA, Prebis JW, Gruskin AB, et al. *Semin Nephrol* 1983;3:149–158.
175. Hunt SC, Williams RR, Quida H. *Am J Hypertens* 1991;4:1–8.
176. Grobbee DE, Hackeng WHL, Birkenhager JC, Hofman H. *Br Med J* 1988;296:814–816.
177. Grobbee DE, Hofman A. *Lancet* 1986;2:703–708.
178. Yamakawa H, Suzuki H, Anakamura M, Onho Y, Saruta T. *Hypertension* 1992;19:528–534.
179. Sinaiko AR. In: Yaffe SJ and Aranda JV, eds. *Pediatric pharmacology, therapeutic principles in practice.* Philadelphia: WB Saunders; 1992:425–436.
180. Green TP, Nevins TE, Hauser MT, Sibley R, Fish AJ, Sinaiko AR. *Pediatrics* 1983;67:850–854.
181. Siegler RL, Brewer ED. *J Hypertens* 1988;112:811–813.
182. Deal JE, Barratt TM, Dillon MJ. *Arch Dis Child* 1992;67:1089–1092.
183. Mirkin BL, Newman TJ. *Pediatrics* 1985;75:1091–1100.
184. Sinaiko AR, Mirkin BL, Hendrick DA, Green TP, O'Dea RF. *J Pediatr* 1983;103:799–805.
185. O'Dea RF, Mirkin BL, Alward CT, Sinaiko AR. *J Pediatr* 1988;113:403–406.
186. Tack ED, Perlman JM. *J Pediatr* 1988;112:805–810.
187. Wells TG, Bunchman TE, Kearns GL. *J Pediatr* 1990;117:664–667.
188. Wells TG, Sinaiko AR. *J Pediatr* 1991;118:638–643.

Hypertension: Pathophysiology, Diagnosis,
and Management, Second Edition,
edited by J.H. Laragh and B.M. Brenner,
Raven Press, Ltd., New York © 1995.

CHAPTER 14

Hypertension in the Elderly

Richard L. Byyny

Large numbers of old people in a population represent a major new phenomenon and change. In the United States, about 5,000 people reach age 65 years daily, resulting in rapid growth of the older population. In the past, most people died by age 65 years, but now it is commonplace to grow old. In 1985, a 65-year-old individual had an average life expectancy of 15.1 additional years for men and 19.5 years for women (1). More startling is the growth of the "old-old" group—those older than 85 years and who represent 2.7 million people—that will increase fivefold to about 16 million in the next 40 years.

R. L. Byyny: Division of Internal Medicine, University of Colorado Health Science Center, Denver, Colorado 80262.

Although the elderly represent 12 percent of the population, they account for one-third of all the U.S. health care dollars spent each year.

The elderly vary widely in physical, behavioral, cognitive, and emotional characteristics, as well as independence, severity of illness, and choices of medical care.

The main health goals for this group are prevention of premature mortality, prevention of disability, and maintenance of function and independence.

It has been said, "A man is only as old as his arteries." This observation is supported by data indicating that cardiovascular disease accounts for most morbidity and mortality in Western cultures. The single most potent, common, and remedial risk factor for cardiovascular disease is hypertension, which greatly increases the risk of death or disability (2). Cardiovascular risk increases independently with increases in either systolic (SBP) or diastolic blood pressure (DBP) (3). The higher the pressure, the greater the risk, but with advancing age, the risk from elevated SBP predominates (4).

Population studies and recent clinical trials provide strong evidence that cardiovascular disease is not an inevitable part of aging. We can prevent cardiovascular disease in the elderly and decrease premature mortality, decrease chronic disability, and improve quality of life.

The following is reviewed in this chapter: the definition of hypertension in the elderly; epidemiology; pathophysiology; etiology; clinical assessment and diagnosis; treatment; and application of the principles in clinical practice. Five recent clinical trials convincingly demonstrate that treatment of hypertension, either systolic or combined systolic and diastolic, decreases cardiovascular morbidity and mortality. These results provide important information about the risk of hypertension, enhance our management strategies, and solidify the beneficial effects of treatment for elderly hypertensive patients. Accumulating evidence indicates that systolic hypertension—which is common, easy to detect, and treatable—is the main risk factor for cardiovascular morbidity and mortality in the elderly (5).

DEFINITIONS

Hypertension

Hypertension can be defined as the arterial pressure above which risk escalates and benefit from treatment exists. Previously, the Framingham study and the World Health Organization defined hypertension as SBP and DBP greater than 160/95 mm Hg, and many epidemiologic studies have used this criteria. However, the fifth report of the Joint National Committee on Detection, Evaluation, and Treatment of High Blood Pressure (JNCHBP) provides a new classification to define stages of blood pressure (6). Table 1 illustrates the blood pressure classification for adults 60 years and older.

Several blood pressure measurements obtained in patients not taking antihypertensive drugs and who are not acutely ill are used for classification. Hypertension is staged by blood pressure ranges. The classification uses the higher category when the SBP and DBP fall into different categories. Isolated systolic hypertension (ISH), defined as SBP of 140 mm Hg or greater and DBP less than 90 mm Hg, is staged by the SBP. Another change in the classification, the designation of the presence or absence of target-organ disease and other risk factors, increases the ability to assess risk and make wise management decisions. In contrast to the recommendations for follow-up of younger adults, I recommend that all individuals over the age of 60 years have their blood pressure rechecked annually, those with stage I hypertension have their blood pressure confirmed within 1 month, and those with higher blood pressure or with target-organ damage be referred and evaluated within 1 week or sooner.

Increments in SBP correlate best with cardiovascular risk, and reduction in elevated SBP decreases cardiovascular events. Patients with combined systolic and diastolic or isolated systolic hypertension (SBP of 160 mm Hg or greater) with or without target-organ damage or multiple risk factors will most often be treated with lifestyle modifications followed by antihypertensive drugs appropriate to their individual risk factors and target-organ damage, with the major goal of reduction in the SBP.

EPIDEMIOLOGY

Figure 1 illustrates the typical rise in SBP and DBP with age in most industrial societies (7). Systolic blood pressure increases to age 70 or 80 years and the DBP to age 50 to 60 years when DBP levels or decreases slightly. Between the third and seventh decade, the rise in SBP is about 1 to 9 mm Hg greater for women than for men, and the DBP increases slightly more in women. In the United States, SBP increases 5 to 10 mm Hg and DBP 5 to 6 mm Hg between ages 40 and 70 years (8). Both SBP and DBP are on average higher in blacks than whites after age 30 years (9). The lower the blood pressures when young, the less the rise with advancing age, and vice versa (10).

The rise in blood pressure with age does not occur in

TABLE 1. *Classification of blood pressure for older adults*

Classification	Blood pressure (mm Hg)		Target organ damage	Other risk factors
	Systolic	Diastolic		
Normal	<130	<85	Absent	None
High normal	130–139	85–89	Present/absent	List
Hypertension				
Stage 1 (mild)	140–159	90–99	Present/absent	List
Stage 2 (moderate)	160–179	100–109	Present/absent	List
Stage 3 (severe)	180–209	110–119	Present/absent	List
Stage 4 (very severe)	≥210	≥120	Present/absent	List

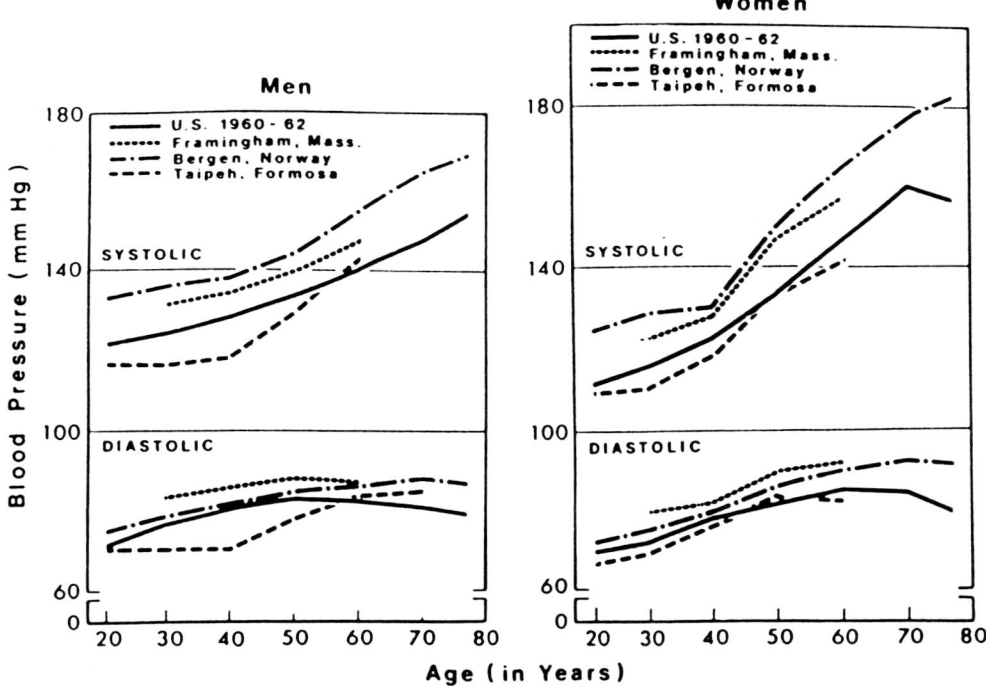

FIG. 1. Rise in systolic and diastolic blood pressure for men and women with increasing age in the United States and in three other countries.

some primitive populations (11–14) and may represent lifestyle differences or other factors. Many elderly individuals in industrialized societies retain normal or low blood pressures and have lower cardiovascular mortality and morbidity rates (15).

Prevalence

The recent National Health and Nutrition Examination Survey (NHANES III) found hypertension prevalence, an average blood pressure of 140/90 mm Hg or greater in those older than age 60 years, to be 60 percent for non-Hispanic whites, 71 percent of non-Hispanic blacks, and 61 percent of Hispanic Americans (6). In the NHANES II survey, the subgroup prevalence of hypertension was black women, 82.9 percent; black men, 67.1 percent; white women, 66.2 percent; and white men, 59.2 percent. The prevalence was 45 percent if a higher blood pressure of greater than 165/95 mm Hg was used.

Sixty-eight percent of those 65 to 74 years old who were screened in the Systolic Hypertension in the Elderly Program (SHEP) were hypertensive (16).

The prevalence of ISH increases with advancing age. The prevalence of ISH, using a SBP of 160 mm Hg or greater and a DBP less than 90 mm Hg after four visits, increases from 7 percent in those ages 60 to 69 years to 25 percent in those older than age 90 years. Isolated systolic hypertension was slightly more common in women than men and in nonwhites than whites (17).

Risk of Hypertension

Cardiac and cerebrovascular disease account for more than half of all mortality in individuals older than age 65 years. Cardiovascular and renal diseases decrease life expectancy by about 10 years. Table 2 summarizes the average annual incidence in rate of cardiovascular events per 1,000 elderly men and women reported by the Fra-

TABLE 2. *Average annual incidence of cardiovascular events in elderly men and women in the Framingham study: 20-year follow-up[a]*

Coronary heart disease		Cerebrovascular disease		Peripheral arterial disease		Congestive heart failure	
Men	Women	Men	Women	Men	Women	Men	Women
20.4	14.5	8.4	8.6	6.3	3.8	8.2	6.8

From ref. 2, with permission.
[a] Rate per 1,000 population.

TABLE 3. *Risk of cardiovascular disease in relation to hypertensive status in the elderly in the Framingham study: 20-year follow-up[a]*

Hypertensive status[b]	Men 65–74 years	Women 65–74 years
Normal	17.1	8.6
Borderline	32.7	22.5
Hypertension	51.0	35.6

From ref. 2, with permission.
[a] Incidence per 1,000 population.
[b] Normal, pressure < 140/90 mm Hg; stage I, pressure of 140–160/90–95 mm Hg; stage II–III, pressure > 160/95 mm Hg (6).

mingham Study. According to these data, about 2 percent of elderly men and 1.5 percent of elderly women will develop coronary heart disease each year, and there is a very high incidence of strokes, peripheral arterial disease, and congestive heart failure. Table 3 illustrates the risk of cardiovascular disease in elderly Framingham study subjects with normal blood pressure (less than 140/90 mm Hg), compared with stage I to III hypertension.

Increases in both SBP and DBP increase risk, but with advancing age, the SBP is the predominant risk factor (18). Figure 2 illustrates the steep increase in probability of cardiovascular disease in low-risk elderly men and women from the Framingham study during 8 years of follow-up related to SBP (19). An increase in SBP from 140 to 185 mm Hg in a 70-year-old nearly doubles the probability of a cardiovascular event.

Table 4, from the Framingham study, shows the significant increase in risk of cardiovascular events related to increased levels of DBP in elderly men and women (20).

Seventy-three percent of men and 81 percent of women who died in the Framingham study were hypertensive (21). Stage I hypertension increases cardiovascular mortality fourfold for men and twofold for women in the age range from 65 to 74 years (2).

Others report a 40 percent prevalence of cardiac disease in those 65 to 74 years of age and more than 50 percent in those older than age 75 years. Electrocardiographic (ECG) abnormalities occur in about half of old people (22,23). Advancing age increases mortality rates from myocardial infarction to 38 percent for ages 60 to 69 years, 43 percent for 70 to 79 years, and 58 percent for 80 to 89 years (24). After a stroke, those older than age 60 years have a 20 percent likelihood of good recovery compared with 30 to 50 percent of younger patients (25). The gender advantage in cardiovascular risk decreases with age. Results from the European Working Party Trial on High Blood Pressure in the Elderly (EWPHE) reported a cardiovascular mortality rate of 47 per 1,000 patient-years, cerebrovascular disease mortality of 16 per 1,000 patient-years, and cardiac mortality of 47 per 1,000 patient-years (26). The Medical Research Council Trial of Treatment of Hypertension in Older

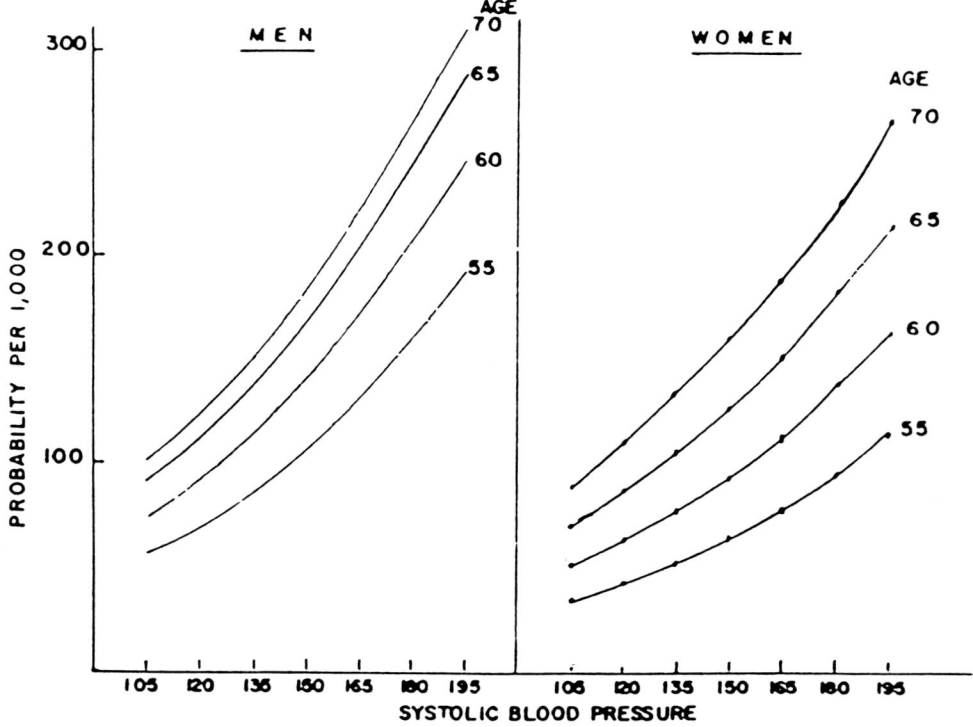

FIG. 2. Probability of cardiovascular disease in low-risk Framingham subjects: a serum cholesterol level of 185 mg per 100 ml, do not smoke, and have no glucose intolerance or left ventricular hypertrophy by electrocardiogram.

TABLE 4. *Risk of cardiovascular events according to diastolic blood pressure in men and women aged 65–74 in the Framingham study: 18-year follow-up[a]*

Diastolic blood pressure (mm Hg), men			Diastolic blood pressure (mm Hg), women		
<90	90–109	≥110	<90	90–109	≥110
24.2	42.9	55.6	17.2	32.4	54.5

From ref. 20, with permission.
[a] Average annual incidence per 1,000 population.

Adults (MRC-THOA) reported, in placebo-treated patients, a stroke mortality rate of 3.3 per 1,000 patient-years, fatal coronary event rate of 8.6 per 1,000 patient-years, and mortality rate for all cardiovascular deaths at 14.1 per 1,000 patient-years. In the MRC-THOA report, men on placebo suffered a cardiovascular mortality rate of 22.1 per 1,000 patient-years compared with 8.6 per 1,000 patient-years in women. Smokers on placebo had higher rates of coronary events and all cardiovascular events but no difference in stroke rates (27). The placebo-treated subjects in the Swedish Trial in Old People with Hypertension (STOP-Hypertension) had 4.5 fatal myocardial infarction deaths per 1,000 patient-years, 8.4 fatal stroke deaths per 1,000 patient-years, 6.8 sudden deaths per 1,000 patient-years, 3.4 other cardiovascular deaths per 1,000 patient-years, and 35.4 total deaths per 1,000 patient-years (28).

In the Framingham study, ISH increased the risk of stroke fourfold in elderly men and more than twofold in elderly women (29). Isolated systolic hypertension increased mortality in the Chicago Blood Pressure Study and increased stroke incidence 2.5-fold in 3 years (4,30). The SHEP reported 9.4 cardiovascular deaths per 1,000 patient-years in those with ISH on placebo (31).

Hypertension in the elderly is responsible for 33 percent of all cardiac disease and 42 percent of strokes in elderly men and 70 percent in elderly women (32).

In the EWPHE study, a 1-mm increase or difference in SBP increases cardiovascular mortality by 1.4 percent, but a rise in DBP did not increase risk. In this study, an SBP of 160 to 169 mm Hg resulted in 32 fatal cardiovascular events per 1,000 patient-years compared with 60 events per 1,000 patient-years when the initial SBP was 180 to 199 mm Hg. Each additional year of age increased cardiovascular mortality 10.4 percent. For those 60 to 64 years old, there were eight fatal cardiovascular events per 1,000 patient-years compared with 64 events per 1,000 patient-years in subjects 75 to 97 years of age. Men had twice the cardiovascular mortality. Cardiovascular complication at entry increased cardiovascular risk by 43.5 percent. Isolated systolic hypertension in the SHEP study nearly doubled the 5-year cumulative stroke rate for those 70 to 79 years old compared with those 60 to 69 years old.

Other risk factors also increase the risk for developing coronary heart disease in elderly patients (2).

Eight to ten percent of elderly individuals have ECG evidence of left ventricular hypertrophy (LVH) (33). Left ventricular hypertrophy by ultrasound criteria occurs in about 60 percent of elderly hypertensive subjects (34). Left ventricular hypertrophy by ECG criteria increases the risk of congestive heart failure, coronary heart disease, and stroke by 3 to 15 percent. In elderly hypertensive patients, LVH demonstrated by ultrasound increases the risk of mortality 14-fold and is the best predictor of cardiovascular events. Left ventricular hypertrophy risk increases with high SBP, long duration of hypertension, congestive heart failure, or arrhythmias. In the elderly, an increase in SBP from 131 to 171 mm Hg increases left ventricular mass index by 20 percent.

Left ventricular hypertrophy increases the risk of left ventricular systolic and diastolic dysfunction. Diastolic dysfunction limits left ventricular filling and is characterized by heart failure symptoms, supranormal ejection fraction, and a prolonged early diastolic filling period (35).

Pathophysiology

A rise in blood pressure is not a normal part of the aging process. Rat models of aging, some aging populations, and many individuals do not demonstrate any increase in blood pressure with increasing age (36–39).

The normal aorta and its branches provide a distensible reservoir that modifies the pulsatile flow from the left ventricle and maintains continuous flow for perfusion (40). The thoracic aorta attenuates pressure in the arterial system and stores approximately 50 percent of the stroke volume during systole. It subsequently propels flow during diastole to maintain mean perfusion pressure (41–43).

The cause of changes in the cardiovascular system with normal aging remains uncertain. Some theorize that genes in fibroblasts, endothelium, and smooth muscle are programmed for senescence and death (44,45). Others hypothesize that somatic mutations or gene errors result in DNA variability with subsequent errors in protein structure and death (46). Age-related changes in collagen, ground substance, extracellular protein matrix, and cross-linkage changes occur (47–49), which alter the anatomy and dynamic mechanical properties of the vasculature. Arterial wall elastin decreases with age, resulting in thin elastic laminae and fragmented, poorly demarcated media. Calcium and lipids accumulate in blood vessel media and calcium binds to the altered elastin. Undifferentiated muscle cells migrate through the elastic laminae to the intima, proliferating, and producing connective tissue with thickening and fibrosis of the intima, which cause arterial wall thickness and stiffness.

The aorta becomes elongated and tortuous with increased diameter and volume. Increased aortic cross-sectional area, vascular stiffness, and pulse-wave velocity begin about age 20 years, and the increase is linear with advancing age (50–53). In young people, the aorta distends dramatically with increases in pressure from 50 to 160 mm Hg and accommodates a proportional increase in aortic volume, but with further increases in pressure, the aorta cannot distend further with increased pressure and cannot accommodate more volume. The volume in the large blood vessels increases with age and, with the rigid vessel walls, results in decreased DBP. The decreased elasticity, increased aortic stiffness, and reduced diastolic recoil increase impedance with aging, and the larger end-diastolic aortic volume diminishes the aorta's contribution to forward blood flow. For the same stroke volume, aortic pressure rises more in the elderly. These changes increase left ventricle work at the onset of systole. A recent study demonstrated increased end-diastolic diameter and cross-sectional area of elastic large central arteries and a decrease or no change in the muscular distal medium-sized arteries (54).

The above changes are associated with the following effects at rest: normal left ventricular end-diastolic pressure; normal heart rate; prolonged left ventricular ejection time; prolonged isovolemic relaxation time; and decreased cardiac output due to a reduced stroke volume. Systolic blood pressure and systemic vascular resistance increase, and with maximal exercise, one observes the following: an exaggerated rise in left ventricular end-diastolic pressure; decreased maximal oxygen consumption; decreased maximal heart rate; and higher arterial blood pressure and vascular resistance (55).

Cardiac output and peripheral resistance determine the level of mean arterial pressure, whereas stroke volume, arterial capacitance, and left ventricular ejection affect the pulse pressure (56). The arterial compliance, or rigidity, is the ratio of pulse pressure-to-stroke volume and can be defined as the slope of the curve relating volume to pressure in the large arteries. Aging decreases compliance and shifts the arterial–pressure curve downward in both normotensive and hypertensive individuals. If mean arterial pressure increases by raising cardiac output or peripheral resistance, pulse pressure also increases. The combination of high SBP, normal cardiac output, and normal DBP increases both total peripheral resistance and work of the heart. For each 10-mm Hg rise in SBP, the DBP must fall 5 mm Hg if peripheral resistance remains normal. However, cardiac work increases whenever SBP is elevated. The expected compensatory decrease in DBP with vascular rigidity does not usually occur, which suggests that other factors are causative in the hypertension associated with aging (57).

Table 5 illustrates the pathophysiologic characteristics of a carefully selected group of elderly to young hypertensive subjects (34). Cardiac output, heart rate, stroke

TABLE 5. *Pathophysiologic differences in hypertensive patients*

Parameter	Elderly	Young	P values
Age (years)	73.0	32.2	
Systolic pressure (mm Hg)	182	153	$<10^{-5}$
Mean arterial pressure (mm Hg)	114	113	
Diastolic pressure (mm Hg)	80.7	93.2	$<10^{-5}$
Heart rate (beats/min)	67.1	72.4	<0.0186
Cardiac output (liters/min)	4.70	6.22	$<10^{-5}$
Cardiac index (liters/min/m^2)	2.60	3.38	$<10^{-5}$
Stroke volume (ml)	70.7	88.3	<0.0009
Mean LV[a] ejection rate (ml/sec)	213	292	$<10^{-5}$
Total peripheral resistance (units)	25.8	18.8	$<10^{-5}$
Ejection time (msec)	332	295	$<10^{-5}$
LV stroke work (units)	161	175	
Central blood volume (liters)	2.36	2.77	<0.0497
Total blood volume (liters)	4.10	4.64	<0.0327
Renal blood flow (ml/min)	674	1110	<0.0006
Renal vascular resistance (units)	1691	1012	$<10^{-5}$
Norepinephrine (pg/ml)	418	331	
Epinephrine (pg/ml)	95	98	
Dopamine (pg/ml)	63	62	
Plasma renin activity (μg/ml/min)	0.454	1.154	<0.047
LV diastolic diameter (mm)	51.4	49.3	
LV systolic diameter (mm)	29.8	33.2	
LV wall thickness (mm)	12.0	9.7	<0.0297
Septal thickness (mm)	11.2	10.5	<0.0444
LV mass (g)	311	222	<0.0340
LV mass index (g/m^2)	169	123	<0.0190
Velocity of circumferential fiber shortening (circ/sec)	123	107	
Radius/posterior wall thickness	224	243	

From ref. 34, with permission.
[a] LV, left ventricular.

volume, intravascular volume, renal blood flow (RBF), and plasma renin activity were significantly lower in elderly than in young hypertensives. Total peripheral resistance and renal vascular resistance, left ventricular posterior wall and septal thicknesses, and left ventricular mass were higher in the elderly hypertensives. Peripheral vascular resistance was inversely related to intravascular volume in both groups. Therefore, hypertension in the elderly is characterized by increased total and peripheral resistance and decreased cardiac output and intravascular volume with concentric cardiac hypertrophy, a slow heart rate, and reduced stroke volume. Renal blood flow is disproportionately reduced (34,58).

Unfortunately, no studies have been published to compare age-matched elderly hypertensives with elderly normotensives.

ETIOLOGY OF HYPERTENSION IN THE ELDERLY

The etiology of hypertension in the elderly is unknown, but important observations relating to possibly etiologic factors have been made.

Vascular Changes

Aging arterials demonstrate hyaline degeneration within the media, which decreases the lumen-to-wall ratio and the overall lumen cross-sectional area. Intimal thickening and duplication of the elastic lamina and changes in the hyaline in the media of vessels result in arteriolar and arterial thickening and a decrease in cross-sectional diameter of the lumen. Large and medium arteries demonstrate atherosclerosis (59). Narrowed vessels result in increased vasoconstrictor-induced resistance (60). These changes, the fracturing and uncoiling of the elastic fibers, and deposition of calcium and collagenous matrix within the vessel walls reduce arterial compliance (56,61). Vascular hypertension further increases arterial stiffening, which further increases SBP more than DBP (62).

Baroreceptor Sensitivity

Baroreceptor reflexes, which normally attenuate sudden increases or decreases in arterial pressure, are blunted in the elderly (63,64). Normally, sudden standing transiently decreases blood pressure, which activates carotid sinus and aortic baroreceptors that transmit afferent signals to the area of the nucleus tractus solitarius, resulting in efferent adrenergic vasoconstrictor stimulation from the medulla plus cholinergic inhibition. This reflex increases peripheral resistance and heart rate, resulting in stabilization of the blood pressure. Conversely, a rise in blood pressure is normally attenuated by baroreceptor reflexes.

Pharmacologically induced tachycardia or bradycardia can be used to determine baroreflex sensitivity. Administration of the alpha-adrenergic vasoconstrictor agonist phenylephrine to elderly normals or to hypertensive subjects produces less bradycardia than in young normotensive subjects. Administration of vasodilators including nitroprusside, calcium channel blockers, and hydralazine produces less tachycardia in elderly normal or hypertensive subjects than in young normotensives (65). Diminished baroreceptor sensitivity results in orthostatic hypotension in elderly normotensive or hypertensive subjects (66). Because plasma norepinephrine response to upright pressure rises steadily with increasing age, the afferent limb of the baroreceptor reflex appears intact. Thus, alteration in the efferent limb is implicated as the cause (67). Atherosclerosis in the carotid body and aorta may be responsible for the impairment of baroreceptor function (68). Alterations in baroreceptor reflex mechanisms may contribute or initiate the rise in blood pressure that occurs in the elderly and probably explain the blood pressure variability (69).

Cellular Sodium Transport

Na-K ATPase activity declines in red blood cells and myocardium with advancing age (70). Although alterations in red blood cell and white blood cell sodium transport have been demonstrated in younger hypertensives and their relatives, erythrocyte Na^+-K^+ cotransport is similar in normotensive and hypertensive elderly subjects (71,72).

Hormonal Changes

Renin-Angiotensin-Aldosterone

Plasma renin levels decrease with increasing age (73–77) and renin responsiveness is blunted at any given level of salt intake (78,79). The suppression of plasma renin is greater in elderly hypertensive than normotensive subjects (76,80). These effects may be caused by age-related decreased juxtaglomerular apparatus responsiveness to normal stimuli due to hyaline degeneration in the afferent arterioles of the kidney with aging and/or a decreased juxtaglomerular beta-adrenergic receptor response (81). The diminished renin response to upright posture may predispose to orthostatic hypotension (82). Basal plasma angiotensin II (AII) levels and AII-receptor affinity do not change with age or blood pressure, and AII receptors in platelets increase with age (83). Plasma aldosterone does not decrease in elderly hypertensive subjects (84). However, a decrease in the sensitivity of the adrenal zona glomerulosa to AII infusion can be demonstrated (85). Plasma aldosterone levels appear to be partially controlled by factors other than renin and angiotensin.

Sympathetic Nervous System

Plasma norepinephrine levels increase with age independently of the age-related increase in obesity. Plasma norepinephrine levels average 410 pg/ml at age 80 years or approximately twice the levels of those age 10 years (86–89). Kinetic studies indicate that the increase in plasma norepinephrine probably represents increased secretion (90). Upright posture and hand-grip isometric exercise increase plasma norepinephrine more in the elderly than in the young (79). Elderly and young subjects demonstrate a similar rise in plasma norepinephrine with exercise, although the heart rate response in the elderly is less (90). The increase in plasma norepinephrine with age is even greater in normotensive than hypertensive subjects (87–91). Plasma norepinephrine, epinephrine, and dopamine from basal or continuous venous sampling are lower in hypertensive compared with age-matched normotensive individuals (92,93).

Beta-adrenoreceptor responses are altered in the elderly. Isoproterenol, a beta$_1$-adrenoreceptor agonist, increases heart rate less in elderly than young subjects (94). Although animal studies demonstrate an age-related reduction in blood vessel relaxation with beta$_2$-adrenergic stimulation, the vasodepressor response to beta$_2$-adrenergic agonists is not altered with aging in humans. Others have demonstrated a greater increase in forearm blood flow caused by intraarterial isoprenaline administration in young subjects compared with older subjects (95). Propranolol, a nonselective beta-adrenoreceptor antagonist, produces less effect in elderly than young subjects despite higher plasma drug levels (95). Because the elderly are not less sensitive to timolol—a nonracemate, nonselective beta-adrenoreceptor antagonist—the age-related effects of propranolol may be caused by differences in the stereoselective metabolism of this racemate molecule (96). Beta-adrenoreceptor number and affinity in myocardial cells, lymphocytes, and pulmonary cells do not change with age, but there is a 30 percent decrease in isoproterenol-stimulated adenylate cyclase activity in myocardial membranes in aged rat myocardium (97). The infusion of salbutamol, a beta$_2$-adrenoreceptor-selective agonist, demonstrates less effect on plasma cyclic adenosine monophosphate (AMP) in elderly than young subjects.

In summary, beta$_1$-cardiac adrenoreceptor responsiveness decreases in the elderly and is probably caused by decreased postreceptor mechanisms. Beta$_2$-adrenoreceptor-mediated vasodilation may be reduced in some vascular beds and in the kidney.

Alpha$_1$-adrenoreceptor response is probably unchanged by aging. Elliott et al. (98) demonstrated that a lower dose of phenylephrine would increase SBP 20 mm Hg in elderly than young volunteers. Blockade of alpha$_1$ adrenoreceptors with prazosin can be overcome with smaller doses of phenylephrine in the elderly, but prazosin results in comparable orthostatic hypotension in the elderly. *In vitro* studies indicate no age-related changes in alpha-adrenoreceptor sensitivity in human blood vessels (99). When phentolamine, an adrenoreceptor antagonist, is infused into normal forearm blood ves-

sels, responses are similar in young and old (100). Simpkins et al. (101) and McAdams et al. (102) demonstrated decreased responsiveness to norepinephrine but not to the alpha$_1$-selective agonist methoxamine in the aorta of old rats. In summary, there is no definite abnormality in alpha$_1$-adrenoreceptor responsiveness with increased age.

A decreased alpha$_2$-adrenoreceptor responsiveness could increase blood pressure. Hyland and Docherty (103) observed that the alpha$_2$ agonist yohimbine had less effect in older rats. However, Featherstone et al. (104) demonstrated similar plasma norepinephrine suppression after orally administered clonidine in old and young subjects. Therefore, alpha$_2$-adrenoreceptor-mediated function appears unchanged in elderly men.

Anticholinergic blockade with atropine results in less tachycardia in aged rats and in older humans (105,106). Both the bradycardia and negative inotropic responses to muscarinic cholinergic agonists are reduced in aged rats (105). Older humans, but not older rats, demonstrate reduced vasodilation with acetylcholine administration (107,108).

In summary, altered adrenergic responsiveness with aging has been most consistent for cardiac beta$_1$ adrenoreceptors, cardiac muscarinic cholinergic receptors, vascular beta adrenoreceptors, and vascular alpha$_2$ adrenoreceptors. The increase in norepinephrine with age does not appear to be related to the increase in blood pressure. A good review of this subject is by Docherty (37).

The Kidney

Glomerular filtration rate (GFR) averages 140 ml/min/1.73 m^2 until age 30 years and then declines linearly by about 8 ml/min/1.73 m^2 per decade (109,110). However, recent studies demonstrate that the decline in GFR with age is not necessarily part of the aging process. If subjects with hypertension, renal, or urinary tract disease or treatment with a diuretic are excluded, the mean decrease in GFR is 0.75 ml/min/year. About one-third demonstrate no decrease in GFR, and a small group actually shows an increase in GFR with advancing age (111). The RBF average is about 350 ml/min through the fourth decade and subsequently declines by about 10 percent per decade (107,112). Decreased RBF response to the vasodilator acetylcholine and to a sodium load occurs with increasing age. Because there is a progressive reduction in RBF per unit of kidney mass, reduction in RBF cannot be caused solely by a reduction in renal mass. Cortical RBF is reduced most with redistribution of flow from the cortex to the medulla, which may account for the demonstrated increase in filtration fraction. These changes are associated with an increase in urinary protein and albumin excretion. With aging, sclerotic glomeruli increase from less than 5 percent at age

40 years to about 40 percent by the eighth decade, resulting in loss of functioning glomeruli and reduced renal weight. Anderson and Brenner (113) suggested these changes are partly accounted for by increased RBF and glomerular pressure from high dietary protein.

Changes in RBF, functioning glomeruli, and tubular function increase the time required to excrete a sodium chloride load in the elderly. In those older than age 60 years, it takes about 31 hours to excrete a sodium load compared with 18 hours for those younger than age 25 years. After 6 days on a high- or low-salt diet, there is no demonstrable difference in sodium balance. Elderly subjects may also have more difficulty conserving sodium when placed on a low-sodium diet (114,115). The elderly demonstrate decreased ability to concentrate and dilute their urine. Increased levels of atrial natriuretic peptide have been demonstrated in aged men, which could be caused by sodium retention, atrial stretch caused by other factors, or decreased peripheral receptor response, but any relation to hypertension in the elderly is unclear (116).

It does not appear that alterations in renal function explain hypertension in the elderly.

Insulin Resistance

Nonobese, nondiabetic hypertensive and normotensive subjects have similar basal plasma insulin and C-peptide levels but significantly enhanced response to oral glucose or a mixed meal. Hypertensives had impaired insulin-stimulated glucose uptake and decreased insulin metabolic clearance rates but no difference in hepatic glucose production. Older hypertensive and especially obese hypertensive subjects manifest insulin resistance when measured in fat cell biopsy specimens by adipocyte 2-deoxyglucose uptake. Both hypertensive and normotensive elderly had increased fat cell intracellular calcium levels. The calcium channel blocker nitrendipine normalized intracellular calcium levels and insulin responsiveness (117). Therefore, alteration in insulin response and/or metabolism may relate to hypertension in the elderly (118).

Impaired Endothelial Function

Endothelial function, measured by normal direct vasodilation and reduced vasodilator response to acetylcholine, an endothelium-dependent vasodilator, has been demonstrated in essential hypertension. However, the role of this endothelial dysfunction is unclear (119).

Obesity

Aging is associated with a decrease in lean body mass and an increase in adipose tissue (120). There is a positive but weak association between increasing body mass index and increasing blood pressure in the elderly (121).

Physical Inactivity

Increasing age decreases the ability to do physical work, and elderly subjects demonstrate an average decreased maximum oxygen consumption (VO$_2$[max]) of 0.9 ml/min/kg per year (122). However, the elderly can be well conditioned, and the average VO$_2$ (max) for elderly athletes is 60 percent higher than that in sedentary elderly and only 15 percent lower than in young athletes. Although peripheral vascular resistance and mean arterial pressure increase with exercise in aged individuals (123), basal SBP decreases an average of 14 mm Hg after an endurance training program in institutionalized geriatric men averaging 71.5 years old (124). Barry et al. (125) demonstrated a decrease in resting SBP with conditioning and DeVries (126) a 12-mm Hg reduction in peak SBP with submaximal exercise after a 6-week training program in 66 elderly subjects. Therefore, deconditioning may well contribute to the increase in blood pressure with age.

Sleep Disorders

Subjects with sleep apnea frequently have hypertension. Sleep apnea and snoring, a reliable clinical correlate, are more common among hypertensive subjects (127–130). Elderly hypertensive subjects may have either nocturnal elevations or reduction in blood pressure with sleep-related breathing disorders (131). The decrease in mean arterial pressure during the episodes was 53 mm Hg and could impair cerebral blood flow (132).

The role of sleep disturbances in hypertension remains unclear.

DIAGNOSIS AND CLINICAL ASSESSMENT

Direct and indirect blood pressure measurements demonstrate a very consistent correlation in the elderly (133–136). Blood pressure measurement in the elderly and young should be the same.

Errors in Diagnosis

There are at least three main causes of misdiagnosis of hypertension in the elderly: labile (or office hypertension), the auscultatory gap, and pseudohypertension. The first is self-explanatory and represents a situation in which automated noninvasive ambulatory blood pressure monitoring (ABPM) or home blood pressure measurement may be useful. Twenty-four-hour ABPM in elderly hypertensive subjects indicates that clinical SBP averages 20 mm Hg higher than ABPM measurements, but the DBP is the same. Those with only high office pressures failed to decrease ABPM on therapy, but office pressure fell significantly. Studies in ISH report variable blood pressure correlation (137–139).

Failure to recognize the auscultatory gap underestimates the SBP. In the elderly, there is often a wide gap between the first Korotkoff sound and subsequent beats. Failure to recognize accurately the first sound will underestimate SBP.

Pseudohypertension or pseudohypotension occur when a sclerotic brachial artery can only be compressed with very high pressures, resulting in a discrepancy of 10 to 100 mm Hg between the auscultated and intraarterial blood pressure. Osler's maneuver for pseudohypertension is positive when the radial artery remains palpable and rigid despite very high cuff pressures. Without measuring intraarterial blood pressure, measurement will frequently over- or underestimate blood pressure (57,140,141).

Clinical Assessment

Clinical assessment and laboratory evaluation are the same as recommended by JNCHBP, plus lying and standing blood pressure to assess orthostatic hypotension.

Secondary Causes of Hypertension

A search for secondary causes of hypertension is not routine, but evaluation for secondary causes is indicated if the patient exhibits the following conditions: onset of a DBP of 105 mm Hg or greater after age 55 years; resistance to an antihypertensive regimen that has previously been effective; a DBP of 100 mm Hg or greater despite a rational triple-drug regimen; or accelerated hypertension, spontaneous hypokalemia, and symptoms or signs suggesting a secondary cause (140). A rise in serum creatinine with an angiotensin-converting-enzyme (ACE) inhibitor suggests the possibility of bilateral renal artery stenosis.

Resistant Hypertension

A complete discussion of resistant hypertension is provided in other chapters.

Resistant hypertension, in compliant elderly patients with ISH on appropriate treatment, is a failure to reduce SBP to less than 170 mm Hg if the initial SBP was greater than 200 mm Hg, or to less than 160 mm Hg and greater than 10 mm Hg if it was initially 160 to 200 mm Hg.

Left Ventricular Hypertrophy

Left ventricular hypertrophy occurs frequently in elderly hypertensive subjects, especially those with the highest SBP, longest duration of hypertension, and arrhythmias or congestive heart failure (141). Left ventricular hypertrophy increases the risk of left ventricular diastolic dysfunction. Left ventricular hypertrophy with a normal ECG can be diagnosed by cardiac ultrasound, which may help identify diastolic dysfunction in symptomatic patients.

Some antihypertensive drugs reverse LVH, but if one chooses drugs that do not reverse LVH, a diagnostic ultrasound should be considered.

TREATMENT

Recent advances in treating hypertension in older patients come from five recent clinical trials. The results convincingly demonstrate that treatment of ISH (SBP of 160 mm Hg or greater) or combined hypertension (SBP of 160 mm Hg or greater and DBP of 90 mm Hg or greater) decreases cardiovascular morbidity. Studies provide important information about the risk and treatment benefits. The next section summarizes, evaluates, and compares the clinical trials.

Earlier Clinical Trials

The Veterans Administration Cooperative Study on Antihypertensive Agents, a classic double-blind placebo-controlled trial, evaluated compliant hypertensive men with an average baseline blood pressure 178/102 mm Hg, and treatment reduced cardiovascular events in those older than 60 years from 62.8 to 28.9 percent, with an overall treatment effectiveness of 54 percent (142).

Subanalysis for hypertension over age 60 years was reported for the single-blind randomized Australian Therapeutic Trial in Mild Hypertension (ATTMH) (143) and the Hypertension Detection and Follow-up Program

TABLE 6. *Effects of therapy in older hypertensive subjects: subanalysis of clinical trial in mild to moderate hypertension*

Study	Australian Therapeutic Trial	Hypertension detection & follow-up
Number of subjects	582	2,374
Subanalysis age range (years)	60–69	60–69
Mean initial BP (mm Hg)	165/101	170/101
Average reduction in risk (%)		
Stroke	−33	−44
Coronary Artery Disease	−18	−15
All cardiovascular disease	−31	−16

(HDFP) study of stepped care to referred care (144), and these are summarized in Table 6.

Several other small controlled trials in the elderly failed to demonstrate the benefit of treatment, or the magnitude of benefit did not reach statistical significance (145–147).

Table 7 summarizes the characteristics of the subjects, blood pressure criteria, treatments, and blood pressure reduction and success from the five recent major clinical trials on hypertension in the elderly. These trials are EWPHE, Coope and Warrender Trial of Hypertension in the Elderly in Primary Care (HEPC), STOP-Hypertension,

TABLE 7. *Summary of randomized clinical trials on hypertension in the elderly*

	EWPHE	HEPC	STOP-Hypertension	MRC-THOA	SHEP
Study Design	Double-blind	Controlled trial No blinding	Double-blind	Single-blind	Double-blind
No. of Patients	840	884	1,627	4,396	4,736
Age Range (yrs)	60–97	60–79	70–84	65–74	60+
Mean Age (yrs)	72		76	70	72
Blood Pressure Criteria (mm Hg)					
SBP	160–239 sitting	190–230 sitting	180–230 or ≤180	160–209 sitting	160–219
DBP	90–119	105–120	90–120 105–120	<115	<90
Mean Baseline (mm Hg)					
SBP	183	197	195	185	170
DBP	101	100	102	91	77
Goal BP					
SBP		<170	<160	<160 if >180 <150 if <180	<160 if >180 >20 mm decrease if 160–179
DBP	<90	<105	<95		
Intervention					
Level 1	HCTZ 25 mg with triamterene 50 mg/day or placebo	Atenolol 100 mg/day	Beta blocker Metoprolol 100 mg/day, pindolol 5 mg/day, or atenolol 50 mg/day; or HCTZ 25 mg/amiloride 2.5 mg/day or placebo	HCTZ 25 mg/amiloride 2.5 mg/day or atenolol 50 mg/day or placebo	Chlorthalidone 12.5 mg/day or placebo
Level 2	HCTZ 50 mg with triamterene 100 mg/day or placebo	Add bendrofluazide 5 mg/day	Add diuretic or β blocker or placebo	HCTZ 50 mg/amiloride 5 mg/day or atenolol 100 mg/day or placebo	Chlorthalidone 25 mg/day or placebo
Level 3	Methyldopa 250–2,000 mg/day	Methyldopa 500 mg/day		Add HCTZ/amiloride to atenolol; add atenolol to HCTZ/amiloride	Add atenolol 25 mg/day or placebo
Level 4		Nifedipine 20 mg b.i.d.		Nifedipine	Add atenolol 50 mg/day or placebo
Placebo	Yes	No	Yes	Yes	Yes
Mean blood pressure on treatment					
Control SBP/DBP	171/95	180/88	186/96	167/85	155/71
Active SBP/DBP	149/85	162/77	167/87	152/79	144/68
Change in BP	−23/−9	−18/−11	−19/−9	−15/−6	−11/−3
% Successes					
SBP			70		
DBP			78		
Overall	>65			>62	72

MRC-THOA, and SHEP (26–28,148,149). Most of the trials evaluated hypertensive patients aged 60 to 75 years, with mean ages of 70 to 72 years, except for the STOP-Hypertension trial, with subjects aged 70 to 84 years and a mean age of 76 years.

The baseline SBP was similar in the EWPHE and MRC-THOA trials. However, in the STOP-Hypertension study, the SBP was 10 to 12 mm Hg higher at 195 mm Hg. The SHEP trial enrolled subjects with ISH with an average SBP of 170 mm Hg, or 13 to 25 mm Hg lower than the other trials, and the initial DBP averaged 77 mm Hg. The MRC-THOA trial enrolled subjects with DBP greater than and less than 90 mm Hg and included predominantly systolic hypertension. The MRC-THOA trial was single-blinded, and the others were double-blind.

The EWPHE goal was based on reduction in DBP, and the others were based on a reduction in SBP.

The average SBP reduction was 11 to 23 mm Hg, depending on drug, dose, and population studied. Goal blood pressure was achieved in 62 to 75 percent of those randomized to drug treatment. The reduction in DBP varied inversely with the level of baseline DBP.

The EWPHE and SHEP trials selected low-dose diuretics as the level 1 intervention, with an increase dose if necessary. Additional drugs, methyldopa in EWPHE or atenolol in SHEP, could be added if needed. Both the STOP-Hypertension and MRC-THOA trials randomized subjects to low-dose diuretics, beta blockers, or placebo for level 1 intervention, and diuretics could be added to the beta blockers or vice versa for level 2 or 3 intervention. The MRC-THOA permitted the addition of nifedipine if needed. All predominantly evaluated white men and women.

Table 8 summarizes the outcomes from these clinical trials and the MRC-THOA diuretic-treated group, including percentage reduction in events and the confidence intervals when they were reported. The diuretic-treated subjects in the MRC-THOA and EWPHE trials demonstrated significant decrease in all cardiovascular mortality of 26 and 27 percent, respectively. Fatal strokes were significantly reduced in HEPC by 70 percent, STOP-Hypertension by 73 percent, and MRC-THOA diuretic-treated group by 24 percent. Similar reductions in stroke mortality were observed in the other trials, but they did not reach statistical significance. Cardiac mortality significantly decreased with treatment in EWPHE by 38 percent and in the MRC-THOA diuretic-treated group by 41 percent, and fatal myocardial infarctions were reduced by 60 percent in EWPHE. Beta-blocker intervention did not decrease cardiac mortality or fatal myocardial infarction.

Diuretic treatment significantly reduced nonfatal strokes by 35 to 52 percent. Nonfatal myocardial infarctions and cardiac death were reduced 30 to 40 percent in SHEP and in the MRC-THOA diuretic-treated group. All nonfatal cardiovascular events were significantly reduced in most studies. In studies that reported outcomes of congestive heart failure and progression to severe hypertension, treatment markedly decreased these morbid conditions.

All studies reported a significant 25 to 49 percent reduction in combined fatal and nonfatal strokes, and SHEP and the MRC-THOA diuretic-treated group demonstrated a 27 to 44 percent reduction in combined cardiac events. In most studies, all cardiovascular mortality was reduced by 32 to 40 percent. Stroke mortality was reduced most in subjects with the highest baseline SBP. Diuretic-treated subjects with combined systolic and diastolic hypertension demonstrated the greatest decrease in cardiac and myocardial infarction mortality. In the EWPHE trial, elderly hypertensives with stage I combined hypertension on entry had comparable results to those with stage II hypertension, suggesting that those with the mildest hypertension benefited from treatment.

In the EWPHE trial, cardiovascular mortality increased as expected with advancing age and also with higher SBP but not with higher DBP. Benefit was evident in both men and women, with and without cardiovascular complications on entry, and at all levels of SBP. Both smokers and nonsmokers benefited, but nonsmokers benefited more. There was no apparent benefit from treatment in those older than age 80 years, and most of the benefit in the age group 70 to 79 years was caused by decrease in cardiovascular terminating events rather than mortality. In the STOP-Hypertension trial, patients benefited up to age 84 years. The average reduction in events for those with combined hypertension were as follows: fatal events—stroke −47 percent, cardiac −17 percent, all cardiovascular −19 percent, total deaths −15 percent, myocardial infarctions −28 percent; nonfatal—stroke −30 percent, myocardial infarctions −13 percent, all cardiac −17 percent, all cardiovascular −37 percent, congestive heart failure −50 percent, progression to severe hypertension −89 percent; and combined events—stroke −41 percent, cardiac −16 percent, and all cardiovascular −29 percent. In comparison, the average reduction in events in isolated systolic hypertension were as follows: fatal—stroke −29 percent, cardiac −20 percent, all cardiovascular −20 percent, total deaths −13 percent; nonfatal—stroke −37 percent, myocardial infarctions −33 percent, all cardiovascular −40 percent, progression to severe hypertension −54 percent; and combined events—stroke −35 percent, cardiac −27 percent, and all cardiovascular −32 percent. Combining average reduction in events from combining all trial results was as follows: fatal—stroke −43 percent, cardiac −21 percent, all cardiovascular −20 percent, total deaths −14 percent; nonfatal—stroke −37 percent, myocardial infarction −18 percent, all cardiac −23 percent, all cardiovascular −37 percent, congestive heart failure −50 percent, severe hypertension −77 percent; and combined events—

TABLE 8. *Clinical trial treatment results (% change) in intention to treat or on randomized treatment*

Outcome	EWPHE	TEPC	STOP-Hypertension	MRC-THOA	SHEP	MRC-THOA Diuretic Group
Fatal events						
Stroke	−32 (−61 to +19)	−70 (−16 to −89)	−73[a] (−16 to −94)	−12 (−44 to +37)	−29 (−69 to +59)	−24[a] (NR)
Cardiac	−38 (−61 to −1)[a]	+1 (−42 to +71)	−25 (−79 to +47)	−22 (−41 to +4)	−20 (−44 to +13)	−41[a] (NR)
All cardiovascular	−27 (−46 to −1)	−22 (−49 to +20)	NR	−9 (−27 to +12)	−20 (−40 to +5)	−26[a] (NR)
All noncardiovascular	+14 (−21 to +64)	NR	NR	+5 (−17 to +33)	+5 (NR)	
Total deaths	−9 (−28 to +15)	−3 (−30 to +42)	−43[a] (−63 to −13)	−3 (−18 to +14)	−13 (−27 to +5)	
Myocardial infarction	−60 (−84 to −4)	0 (−48 to +71)	−25 (−79 to +147)			
Nonfatal Events						
Stroke	−52[a] (−76 to −7)	−29 (NR)	−38[a] (NR)	−30 (NR)	−37[a] (−18 to −51)	−35[a] (NR)
Myocardial infarction	−35 (NR)	+11 (−54 to +68)	−16 (NR)	NR	−33[a] (−4 to −53)	
All cardiac	−9 (NR)	−30 (−59 to +39)	NR	−13 (NR)	−40[a] (NR)	−39[a] (NR)
All cardiovascular[b]	−60[a] (−88 to −19)	−26 (NR)	NR	−26[a] (NR)	−36[a] (NR)	−38[a] (NR)
Congestive heart failure	−63[a] (−85 to −10)	−37 (−65 to +11)	−51 (NR)	NR	−54[a] (−35 to −67)	
Severe hypertension	−90[a] (−98 to −59)	NR	−88[a] (NR)	NR		
Combined Events						
Stroke	−49[a] (NR)	−42[a] (−4 to −65)	−47[a] (−14 to −67)	−25[a] (−3 to −42)	−35[a] (NR)	−31[a] (−3 to −51)
Cardiac	−19 (NR)	−14 NR	−13 (−51 to +56)	−19 (−36 to +2)	−27[a] (−6 to −43)	−44[a] (−21 to −60)
All cardiovascular	−36 (NR)	−24 NR	−40[a] (−15 to −57)	−17 (−2 to −29)	−32[a] (−21 to −42)	−35 (−17 to −49)

[a] P < .05.
[b] Termination event only with nonterminating −35%.
NR, not reported.

stroke −40 percent, cardiac −18 percent, all cardiovascular −30 percent. The results from the predominantly diuretic-treated group were similar to those from all the other studies. In conclusion, all the trials revealed a substantial reduction in most fatal and nonfatal events.

In summary, all trials reveal substantial reduction in most fatal and nonfatal events. Diuretic-only regimens fared as well as combined drug treatment regimens and seemed to decrease cardiac events. Treatment of ISH resulted in a greater reduction in nonfatal and combined cardiac events.

The number of patients needed to be treated to prevent an event provides potentially useful information for making clinical decisions. Over 5 years, one needs to treat only 12 elderly hypertensive patients to prevent one cardiovascular event, 16 to prevent one stroke, and 40 to prevent one cardiac event. Reduction in morbidity as well as mortality remains an important goal. The few elderly hypertensive patients who need to be treated to prevent nonfatal strokes ($n = 34$), cardiac events ($n = 41$), severe congestive heart failure ($n = 29$), and severe hypertension ($n = 14$) provide strong support for treatment. There is a three- to fourfold difference in the effect of other risk factors on the magnitude of treatment benefit. One will need to treat about 30 men and 54 women who are younger lower-risk patients with stage 1 isolated hypertension with diuretics for 5 years to prevent one cardiovascular event compared with 11 older men and 13 older women who are smokers with stage II combined hypertension and abnormal ECGs.

The mortality outcomes in these trials in treatment of hypertension in the elderly were 40 to 50 percent lower than expected, and this difference probably is caused by the enrollment of healthy older individuals. Also, many of the subjects allocated to placebo received active drug treatment. For example, a high percentage of the placebo group received antihypertensive medication: SHEP 44 percent, STOP-Hypertension 20 percent, MRC-THOA 50 percent.

Diuretic-based treatment regimens resulted in high percentage success rates in elderly hypertensives: EWPHE trial, 51 percent on low-dose and 65 percent on high-dose diuretic; STOP-Hypertension 78 percent; MRC-THOA 62 percent; SHEP 46 percent on low-dose and 88 percent on high-dose diuretics. The evidence indicates that diuretic regimens are highly effective as monotherapy, and increasing the dose improves success rates, especially in ISH.

Side Effects

Drug treatment was well tolerated and withdrawals caused by side effects were as follows: MRC-THOA diuretic drugs 15 percent, beta blockers 30 percent, and placebo 4 percent; SHEP, active 13 percent and placebo 7 percent; STOP-Hypertension, active 7 percent and placebo 6 percent; and EWPHE active 2.1 percent and placebo 1.7 percent. Side effects reported were typical of the study drugs. Diuretic drugs produced significantly more gout, muscle cramps, nausea, faintness, loss of consciousness, rapid heart beat, sexual dysfunction, falls, thirst, and rashes than placebo. Beta blockers caused cold hands, swollen ankles, sleep disorder, sexual dysfunction, difficulty with memory, Raynaud's disease, lethargy, and headache. Data from the MRC-THOA trial indicate one withdrawal for side effects in 11 patients treated with diuretic or 5 patients treated with a beta blocker.

Metabolic Effects

Modest metabolic changes were largely associated with diuretic treatment. Serum potassium decreased on average 0.2 to 0.3 mEq/liter with low-dose HCTZ combined with potassium-sparing diuretics or with low-dose chlorthalidone and potassium replacement. Earlier reports from SHEP using high-dose diuretics and clinical trials in younger subjects have reported an average reduction in serum potassium of 0.6 mEq/liter.

The average fasting glucose increased about 5 percent with low-dose diuretic drugs and 35 percent with higher doses, especially if the serum potassium level was low. Postprandial glucose rose more, but significant glucose intolerance developed in only three to four patients in 1,000 patient-years of treatment. Both uric acid and serum creatinine increased slightly with diuretic treatment. Total serum cholesterol levels did not change with low-dose diuretic drugs or beta blockers but increased about 3 percent with higher doses of diuretics.

Compliance

These elderly populations demonstrated excellent treatment compliance, with high success rates. The SHEP trial measured compliance and reported that 76 percent reported compliance with the treatment regimen and 71 percent took 80 percent or more of prescribed medication (which was confirmed by urine testing). Of those still in the trial, 91 percent reported compliance with the treatment regimen, and 88 percent took 80 percent or more of the prescribed drug, which was confirmed in 86 percent (149).

Other Observations from Recent Clinical Trials

"White Coat" Effect

In the STOP-Hypertension trial, the physician-measured blood pressure or "white coat phenomenon" averaged 10/3 mm Hg higher than with trained nurses.

Effect of Smoking

Smoking increased cardiovascular event rates in older hypertensive subjects 1.5- to threefold. In EWPHE, smokers and nonsmokers benefited, but women smokers benefited more than nonsmokers. In the MRC-THOA trial, only male and female nonsmokers demonstrated a reduction in stroke and all cardiovascular events. This beneficial effect was mainly in those taking diuretic drugs. Diuretic-treated smokers demonstrated a 50 percent average decrease in coronary events compared with beta-blocker or placebo treatment. In the HEPC trial, only treated nonsmokers had a reduction in stroke.

Total Mortality

Total mortality was significantly reduced in the STOP-Hypertension trial, which included older, more hypertensive subjects. Most studies reported a slight decrease in all-cause mortality. The studies were designed to detect cardiovascular outcomes in mortality and may have been terminated too soon to detect a true difference.

Abnormal Electrocardiograms, Diuretic Drugs, and Outcomes

Earlier studies raised the question of whether diuretic-treated subjects with baseline ECG abnormalities had worse outcomes with treatment. In the SHEP study, the relative risk of fatal myocardial infarction or coronary death in those with normal baseline ECG with diuretic treatment was 0.83 (confidence interval [CI], 0.53 to 1.29) compared with 0.69 (CI, 0.50 to 0.94) in those with ECG abnormalities. This probably indicates a benefit in those with and without ECG abnormalities.

Beta-Blocker Coronary Prevention

The MRC-THOA trial reported a 35 percent reduction in risk of all cardiovascular events and 29 percent in cardiovascular deaths in diuretic-treated subjects but not in beta-blocker-treated subjects. The rate of coronary events in the diuretic-treated group, 7.6 per 1,000 patient-years, was significantly lower than the 12.8 per 1,000 patient-years in the beta-blocker-treated group. Total deaths were reduced in the diuretic-treated group but not in the beta-blocker-treated group. In the SHEP trial, 32 percent of the active-treated group were taking atenolol. Chlorthalidone alone decreased total mortality, coronary heart disease, and cardiovascular disease, and the addition of atenolol markedly attenuated all these benefits (150). The relative risk for atenolol versus no atenolol for coronary heart disease events was 1.04 (CI, 0.58 to 1.86). Therefore, the treatment benefit appears

to be mostly caused by low-dose chlorthalidone without significant additional benefit attributable to atenolol (150). These differences could be caused by other factors (e.g., more severe hypertension, less treatment response, and longer interval before blood pressure control).

Is There a J-Shaped Mortality Curve in Treatment of Hypertension in The Elderly?

The mortality was highest and rose in those with the highest SBP on and off treatment (151). The mortality curve in treated and untreated subjects was J-shaped. In the EWPHE trial, total mortality increased most for the lowest or middle third of blood pressures. The J-shaped and U-shaped mortality curves do not appear to be a treatment effect.

In the SHEP trial, there was no J-shape relationship in cardiovascular mortality for reduction in either SBP or DBP. An increase in total and mostly noncardiovascular mortality was associated with the greatest reduction in SBP (152). In conclusion, lowering blood pressure to levels achieved in these trials does not increase cardiovascular mortality or morbidity.

Left Ventricular Hypertrophy

Regression of LVH shown by ECG and chest radiography should reduce age-adjusted cardiovascular risk by about 25 percent (153). In the EWPHE trial, there was a significant decrease in LVH by ECG with a diuretic drug plus methyldopa (154). There was no apparent correlation with blood pressure reduction or outcomes.

SYSTOLIC HYPERTENSION IN THE ELDERLY

Systolic hypertension increases the risk of cardiovascular diseases (154). The EWPHE and SHEP trials demonstrated that reduction in SBP predicts nearly all the treatment benefit. The SHEP trial reported a 37 percent reduction in nonfatal strokes, 33 percent reduction in nonfatal myocardial infarction, 40 percent reduction all cardiac events, 36 percent reduction in all cardiovascular events, 54 percent reduction in severe hypertension, 35 percent reduction in combined stroke events, 27 percent reduction in combined cardiac events, and 32 percent reduction in all cardiovascular events. The SHEP 5-year cumulative stroke rates indicated that reduction in stroke rates occurs in all age groups and continues well into the 80s. In SHEP, all age groups and all levels of entry systolic blood pressure benefited from treatment. This clearly establishes the benefit of treatment of ISH in the elderly. Systolic blood pressure increases with age in most populations, and its high prevalence combined with ease of diagnosis and new data demonstrating a clear treatment benefit make it one of the more important and treatable cardiovascular risk factors in the elderly (155).

Both the STOP-Hypertension trial and the MRC-THOA trial provided data on how much better diuretic regimens are for lowering SBP than are beta blockers. In the STOP-Hypertension and MRC-THOA trials, beta blockers and diuretic drugs reduced DBP equally. However, diuretic drugs reduced SBP by 6.2 to 12.3 mm Hg more than beta blockers in STOP-Hypertension and by 8 mm Hg more in MRC-THOA. Combined diuretic and beta-blocker treatment will control blood pressure in 60 to 72 percent of those treated.

Treatment and Clinical Application

An average SBP of 160 mm Hg or greater without other mitigating factors should result in the diagnosis of systolic hypertension, and treatment should be initiated in older men and women up to age 85 years. The goal is to prevent premature mortality and morbidity from strokes and coronary heart disease and to prevent dysfunction secondary to angina and congestive heart failure. The goal blood pressure with treatment should be an SBP of 140 to 150 mm Hg. In selected patients, a lower blood pressure goal may increase the benefit. Treatment of combined systolic and diastolic hypertension should be aimed at reducing the SBP to these levels unless the DBP is greater than 110 mm Hg. With this level of DBP, it is important to reduce effectively both SBP and DBP. If an older patient has another disease worsened by elevated SBP, such as angina or congestive heart failure, therapy should be initiated for an SBP in the range of 140 to 160 mm Hg, and the goal SBP reduction may be greater. In hypertensive patients older than age 80 years who are "biologically young" or who have other risk factors or target-organ damage, treatment should be individualized.

Lifestyle Modifications

Lifestyle factors including obesity, excess alcohol intake, sedentary lifestyle, coffee intake, instability, social isolation, high serum cholesterol, and diabetes are associated with hypertension in the elderly (156). Lifestyle modifications including weight reduction, increased physical activity, moderation of dietary sodium, and decreased alcohol intake, either alone or in combination with drug treatment, may effectively reduce blood pressure in the elderly. In most elderly patients with stage 1 and stage 2 systolic hypertension, lifestyle changes can be prescribed as empiric therapy trial.

Short-term studies of salt restriction in elderly hyper-

tensive subjects indicate variable responses, with some demonstrating decreased blood pressure (157).

Aging is associated with a decrease in lean body mass and an increase in body fat. Exercise and diet-reduced weight loss of 2.1 kg over 6 months in an elderly hypertensive population reduced average SBP/DBP $-4.2/-4.9$ mm Hg compared with the control group (158). A community-based cardiovascular risk reduction program reported that 33 percent of men and 45 percent of women aged 65 to 74 years were able to lose weight when advised to do so (159). Therefore, weight loss in those obese (130 percent or more) elderly hypertensive patients is reasonable.

Exercise conditioning in sedentary elderly subjects decreases blood pressure and should be recommended in the absence of other factors.

Hypertensive subjects who average more than 4 oz of alcohol intake per day should reduce alcohol intake.

Calcium intake is usually low in elderly individuals, and calcium supplementation is being advocated for postmenopausal women. Oral calcium supplementation has been demonstrated to decrease blood pressure in the elderly (160), and if prescribed for other reasons, the antihypertensive effect can be assessed and maintained if there is a good response. Although lifestyle modifications may not reduce blood pressure to the established goal, these interventions may reduce the number and doses of antihypertensive medications needed to manage hypertension (161). Lifestyle modifications are indicated for those with additional cardiovascular risk factors. Intervention to stop cigarette smoking, a major risk factor for cardiovascular disease, must be recommended. Clinical trials indicate that elderly hypertensive smokers benefit from pharmacologic treatment but may not receive the full degree of protection from antihypertensive therapy unless they stop smoking.

Pharmacologic Treatment

Drug treatment should be prescribed for most elderly hypertensive patients not qualifying for or not responding to lifestyle modifications. Treatment should be individualized, because the elderly frequently have other clinical conditions that may benefit from or are worsened by antihypertensive drugs. This can often simplify the regimen for patients, improve compliance, and avoid adverse effects. Important factors to consider in drug selection include congestive heart failure, LVH, obstructive airways disease, diabetes, gout, peripheral vascular disease, angina pectoris, glaucoma, orthostatic hypotension, poor mobility, urinary frequency, memory deficits, depression, urinary incontinence, obstructed urinary flow, and renal dysfunction.

In selecting drugs in the elderly, other issues are important, including the pharmacologic response of the drug in elderly hypertensive subjects; the risk of orthostatic hypotension; the altered physiology with decreased GFR or abnormal hepatic metabolism; coexisting clinical disorders; concurrent drug therapy; and the cost of drugs. Altered pharmacokinetics in drug responses are commonly observed in the elderly. In general, fat stores increase with age while total body water, plasma volume, and lean body mass decrease, resulting in a decrease in volume of distribution of lipid-soluble drugs (162). Elderly hypertensive subjects may have reduced metabolism or excretion of drugs because of alterations in hepatic metabolism or decreased GFR. Dosage reduction in thiazide diuretics, amiloride, verapamil, ACE inhibitors, hydrophilic beta blockers, clonidine, methyldopa, guanfacine, and gunadrel need to be considered due to the decrease in GFR. Calcium channel blockers and guanfacine demonstrate decreased hepatic clearance in the elderly. Pharmacokinetics of alpha-adrenoreceptor blocking drugs and labetalol are not altered by age. Older subjects have reduced beta-receptor sensitivity but unchanged alpha-receptor function (163). Autoregulation of the cerebral and other circulation operates around a higher mean arterial pressure in elderly hypertensive subjects. Although the elderly hypertensive patient can readapt autoregulation with effective antihypertensive therapy, it often takes several days for readaptation to occur. Therefore, the blood pressure should be lowered gradually, with no more than an initial 25 percent decrease, even in situations requiring rapid reduction in blood pressure (164,165).

Diuretic Therapy

When no other clinical condition is present, low-dose HCTZ or chlorthalidone 12.5 to 25 mg/day when combined with a potassium-sparing diuretic (e.g., amiloride 2.5 to 10 mg/day or triamterene 50 to 100 mg/day) is the best first choice based on proven results, cost, convenience, and safety. These drugs decrease cardiovascular mortality and morbidity, including strokes, coronary heart disease, and congestive heart failure, and have a favorable cost-benefit result (166). One can expect 60 to 70 percent responders with diuretic monotherapy. The expected decrease should be about −23/−9 mm Hg in those with combined systolic and diastolic hypertension and about −11/−3 mm Hg in those with ISH. Salt restriction should be an integral part of the diuretic regimen to enhance the blood pressure-lowering effect and to minimize potassium loss. Some will not be able to tolerate the drugs because of impotence, cramps, hypokalemia, or orthostatic hypotension. Diuretics will be particularly useful in patients with coexisting disease, including LVH, congestive heart failure, asthma, angina,

and osteoporosis, but should be avoided in patients with gout and renal failure (167). Because monotherapy with diuretics may increase mortality in diabetics, other drugs or combined therapy is a better choice (168).

Many elderly patients will be taking nonsteroidal antiinflammatory drugs for chronic arthritis, and some of these drugs may attenuate the antihypertensive effects of diuretics and other drugs (169).

Nondiuretic Therapy

Beta-Blocking Drugs

In contrast to younger hypertensive patients, beta-blocking drugs cannot be considered an initial drug for elderly hypertensive subjects. Beta blockers are considerably less effective in lowering blood pressure and decreasing events (170). Beta blockers also reduce cardiac output and increase peripheral resistance. Despite being less effective as monotherapy, beta blockers are indicated to prevent second myocardial infarction and to treat angina pectoris, arrhythmias, migraine headaches, essential or senile tremor, or other disorders. Beta blockers combined with a low-dose diuretic are efficacious (171,172). Beta blockers should be avoided in patients with chronic and reversible airway disease, brittle insulin-dependent diabetes mellitus, allergic rhinitis, congestive heart failure, atrioventricular (AV) conduction abnormalities, bradycardia, and depression. Unfortunately, beta blockers often produce fatigue and exercise intolerance in the elderly, which may decrease functional capacity.

The clearance of water-soluble, long-acting beta blockers (e.g., nadolol or atenolol) may be decreased on the elderly. Those beta blockers metabolized in the liver (e.g., propranolol and metoprolol) have decreased clearance and decreased volume of distribution, resulting in higher plasma levels for a given dose (173,174).

Other Drugs

Other antihypertensive drugs, including adrenergic-depleting drugs, central alpha$_2$-adrenergic agonists, peripheral alpha$_1$-adrenergic antagonists, calcium channel blockers, ACE inhibitors, and direct vasodilators, provide alternative choices to diuretics or beta blockers in some patients. These drugs differ in their ability as monotherapy to decrease SBP in the elderly (175). Clonidine, a central alpha$_2$-adrenergic agonist, is the most effective in decreasing SBP, with an average decrease of 16.2 mm Hg and a 62 percent success rate in lowering SBP to less than 140 mm Hg. Diltiazem, a calcium channel blocker, is nearly as effective with a 13-mm Hg reduction in SBP and a 52 percent success rate. Captopril, an ACE inhibitor, appears to be least effective, and prazosin, an alpha$_1$-adrenergic antagonist, was intermediate. In one study, both diltiazem and HCTZ were similar to clonidine in blood pressure reduction but were better tolerated (175). In a study of diltiazem, enalapril, and atenolol in older women, diltiazem reduced SBP by 14.2 mm Hg compared with 12.7 mm Hg for enalapril and less with atenolol, which lowered quality of life (176). Prazosin and clonidine had the highest and HCTZ the lowest rate of termination caused by side effects. In a study comparing monotherapy in older black and white men, the mean reduction in SBP (in mm Hg) with each drug was as follows: whites—placebo −3, clonidine −17, prazosin −17, HCTZ −13, diltiazem −12, atenolol −12, captopril −11; and for blacks—placebo −3, clonidine −17, HCTZ −16, diltiazem −15, prazosin −13, atenolol −9, captopril −7. Drug effects on DBP were different but effective with all except captopril (177). Almost no data exist for direct-acting vasodilators or reserpine in lowering SBP in the elderly.

Clonidine, a calcium channel blocker, or diltiazem would make a reasonable alternative first choice for treatment of elderly hypertensives unless ACE inhibition or alpha$_1$-adrenergic inhibition would be preferable for other reasons. All the drugs have high success rates when combined with diuretics (178).

Central Alpha$_2$-Adrenergic Agonists

Clonidine has been demonstrated to be effective and well tolerated when used alone or with a diuretic (179). Blood pressure was reduced from an average of 168/102 mm Hg to 132/84 mm Hg with oral clonidine 0.2 to 0.6 mg/day. About 10 percent withdrew due to side effects of dry mouth, drowsiness, and constipation.

The method of administration can improve tolerability and decrease side effects. Renal clearance is decreased, and the drug can often be administered once a day with sustained action. When administered at bedtime, the drug will peak with high concentration while asleep and be active during the highest blood pressures of the day. Clonidine induces sleep and minimizes daytime side effects. The evening dose should usually remain about twice the morning dose when used twice daily.

Transdermal delivery of clonidine is effective in the elderly (180). The lack of drug peaks may decrease sedation and dry mouth. Patches can be administered once a week to improve control and compliance. However, 10 to 30 percent of patients will develop skin reactions, thereby limiting the usefulness of this delivery system in some patients.

Guanabenz, guanfacine, or methyldopa can be used by those most familiar with these central alpha$_2$-adrenergic agonists.

Calcium Channel Blockers

Diltiazem reduces SBP very well with few side effects. Verapamil, nifedipine, nicardipine, felodopine, isradapine, amlodopine, and nitrendipine have demonstrated efficacy in elderly hypertensives (181,182). Peak plasma concentrations and prolonged half-life in the elderly occur with verapamil, diltiazem, nifedipine, and nitrendipine compared with young hypertensive subjects (183–185). Long-acting forms of verapamil and the dihydropyridines may have fewer side effects (186).

Nifedipine (10 mg) acutely decreased average blood pressure from 224/122 to 155/78 mm Hg in a group of elderly subjects undergoing eye surgery. Although they reported no serious side effects, more than 25 percent reduction in mean arterial pressure reduces cerebral blood flow and may cause adverse events (187).

Some calcium channel blockers, verapamil and diltiazem, depress the sinus node and decrease AV conduction. Most of these drugs depress myocardial function and can worsen congestive heart failure in some patients. The main side effects include edema without fluid retention, dizziness, tachycardia, headache, and gastrointestinal side effects. Verapamil causes severe constipation, and preventive measures should be used when initiating therapy. Most of these drugs are expensive, which may limit their use.

Alpha$_1$-Adrenoreceptor Blockers

Prazosin, terazosin, and doxazosin are alpha$_1$-adrenoreceptor blocking drugs with differing half-life. Prazosin is efficacious but has frequent side effects.

In the elderly, peak plasma levels of terazosin were higher and the terminal elimination half-life for terazosin longer. Prazosin kinetics were not effected by age. Supine blood pressure was not affected by either drug in the elderly; peak fall and upright blood pressure were less for the elderly. Doxazosin has longer duration of action. The elderly complain less often of postural dizziness than young subjects (188).

There are few adverse metabolic effects and no central nervous system effects.

Obstructive uropathy caused by benign prostatic hypertrophy and hypertension can be treated with alpha$_1$-adrenoreceptor blockade to improve urine flow (189). Hypotension, which occurs more frequently in patients who are volume-depleted or treated with a diuretic, can exacerbate subclinical cerebrovascular disease, worsen coronary heart disease, cause loss of consciousness, or lead to an injury from a fall. The first-dose hypotension from the short-acting drugs in this class can be minimized by starting or restarting with a small dose at bedtime while supine and then increasing the dose in the same manner. Often a diuretic is required in the elderly for optimal blood pressure control.

Combination Alpha₁- and Beta-Adrenoreceptor Blockers

Labetalol, with or without a diuretic, effectively lowers blood pressure in the elderly (190).

Oral and intravenous labetalol decreases standing blood pressure more in elderly than young subjects due to higher peak plasma concentrations and markedly prolonged half-life (191).

The main adverse effect is orthostatic hypotension. Other side effects include malaise, fatigue, gastrointestinal disturbances, and nightmares.

The same precautions for drug initiation should be used for labetalol as for prazosin and terazosin.

Angiotensin-Converting-Enzyme Inhibitors

Most ACE inhibitors have demonstrated efficacy in treatment of the elderly (192–195). These drugs act as vasodilators and reduce total peripheral resistance without causing a reflex stimulation of heart rate and cardiac output. They do not cause metabolic abnormalities and central nervous system side effects, and they maintain qualify of life (196). They are also effective in managing congestive heart failure and are most effective in reversing LVH (197). Hyperkalemia is a potential problem with these drugs, and they should be used carefully in patients with impaired renal function, should not be combined with potassium salts and potassium-retaining diuretics, and should be used cautiously with nonsteroidal anti-inflammatory drugs (NSAID). The ACE inhibitors in some patients with arterial nephrosclerosis or bilateral renal artery stenosis can result in renal failure. Therefore, when these drugs are administered to older hypertensive subjects, they should be followed closely. All the drugs cause rash, cough, angioedema, taste disturbances, and in some patients, a decrease in renal function.

Direct Vasodilators

Some have advocated traditional vasodilators (hydralazine or minoxidil) because the adrenergic responses should be blunted in the elderly. In my experience, many elderly subjects develop tachycardia, fluid retention, and headaches with hydralazine. These drugs are most effective when used in combination with a diuretic and an antiadrenergic agent. They should probably be reserved for two to three drug combinations in drug-resistant elderly hypertensive subjects.

Reserpine

Reserpine is effective when used in combination with a diuretic (198). Its only two advantages are very low cost and long duration of action. It has not been studied extensively in the elderly. In low doses (0.1 to 0.25 mg/day), side effects are usually low. However, depression, orthostatic hypotension, peptic ulcer disease, nasal congestion, and weight gain occur as important side effects.

Guanethidine and Guanadrel

These adrenergic-depleting drugs should be avoided in the elderly because of orthostatic hypotension and other side effects.

The reader is referred to the chapters on antihypertensive drugs for a more complete discussion of pharmacology and the use of these drugs.

Serotonin Antagonists

Ketanserin, a 5-HT₂-receptor antagonist, has been demonstrated to lower blood pressure more effectively in the elderly than young subjects (199).

Failure of Monotherapy

If monotherapy is unsuccessful, another drug can be substituted or added. The most effective combination in elderly women appears to be an ACE inhibitor and a diuretic drug (200). The ACE inhibitors provide a good choice when a diuretic drug was given first or adding a diuretic when ACE inhibitors were first.

Sequence of Treatment

A proposed treatment algorithm for hypertension in the elderly is summarized in Fig. 3. The diagnosis of hypertension depends on demonstrating an average SBP of 160 mm Hg or greater. If there is another important clinical condition, treatment is individualized, recognizing the relative efficacy and secondary effects of each drug. In the absence of another important clinical condition, a low-dose diuretic drug, usually with a potassium-sparing diuretic, would be prescribed. This would be continued if the SBP decreased to less than 160 mm Hg or decreased by more than 20 mm Hg if the SBP was initially 160 to 170 mm Hg. In patients who have a partial response, addition of an ACE inhibitor is recommended because the combination will decrease blood pressure synergistically. Most would recommend stopping the diuretic for up to 2 weeks before initiation of ACE-inhibitor therapy because of the occasional marked hy-

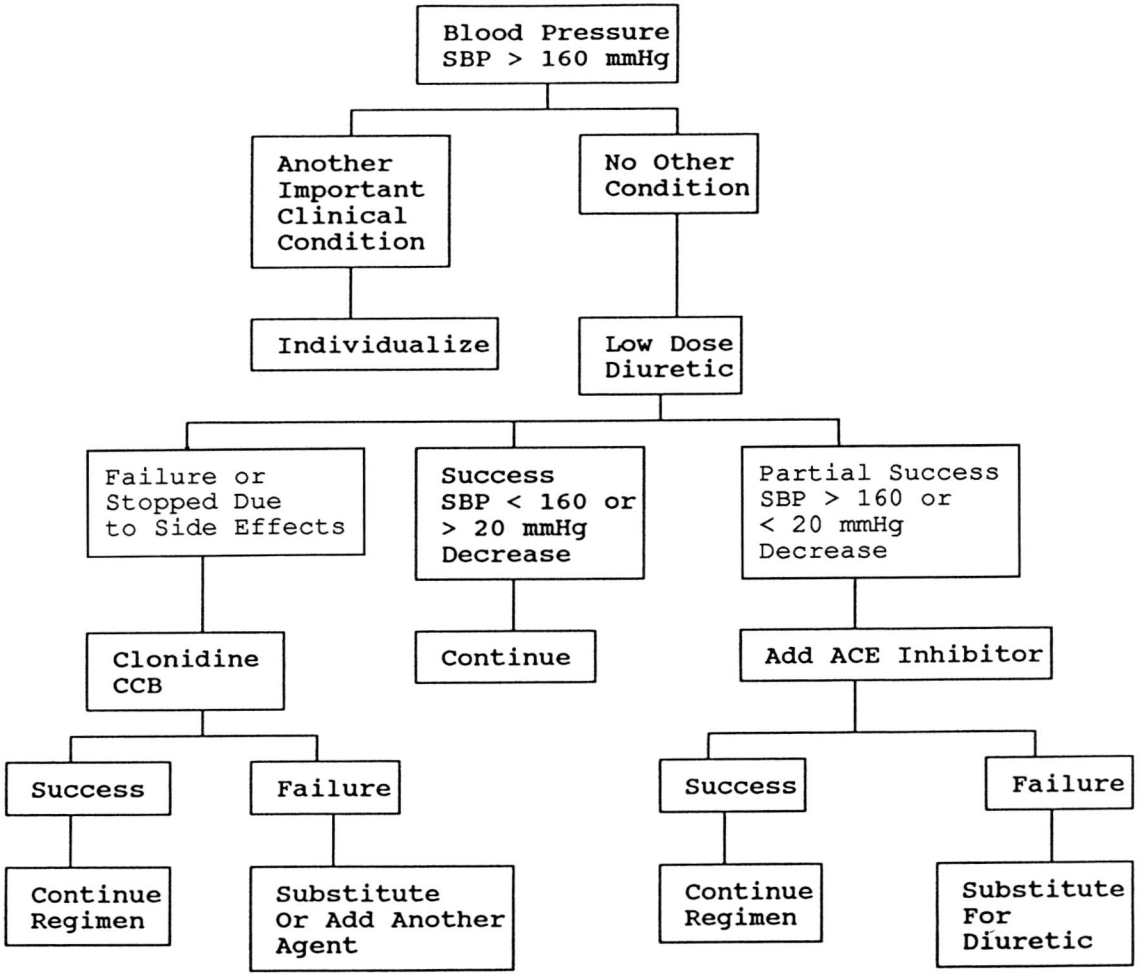

FIG. 3. Algorithm of treatment protocol for hypertension in the elderly. *SBP,* systolic blood pressure; *CCB,* calcium channel blocker; *ACE,* angiotensin-converting enzyme.

potension of this combination. The potassium-sparing diuretic drug would not be restarted. Both the ACE inhibitor and the diuretic doses would be combined and slowly increased with assessment of efficacy. If the patient stopped the diuretic because of side effects or if there was no response to the diuretic, one should probably substitute clonidine or a calcium channel blocker. If the patient cannot tolerate a diuretic drug initially, then the choices are usually clonidine or a calcium channel blocker with the addition of another nondiuretic medication if needed.

Drugs and Isolated Systolic Hypertension

The efficacy of treating ISH in the elderly with low-dose diuretics supports this choice for initial therapy. Clonidine, calcium channel blockers, and ACE inhibitors have demonstrated efficacy in reducing SBP in ISH

and can be used as individualized initial therapy, added to or substituted for a diuretic (201,202).

Compliance

Elderly patients are more motivated to follow their treatment regimens than younger patients. Several studies have demonstrated high compliance rates in elderly hypertensive patients. Average compliance rates of 74 percent for three-drug regimens, 84 percent for two-drug regimens, and 95 percent for one-drug regimens have been reported in the elderly. Diet advice decreased 24-hour sodium excretion from 188 mmol/day to 83 mmol/day (203).

In the HDFP study, the 60 to 69 year old age group was more compliant with their regimens, and 75 percent were at their goal blood pressure as compared with 59 percent of those 30 to 49 years of age (138). In the

SHEP study, 80 to 90 percent of those older than age 60 years were compliant, including those older than age 80 years (204).

Adverse Events

In the HDFP study, those 60 to 69 years old had a lower 5-year incidence of adverse drug reactions requiring discontinuation of drug treatment than did younger subjects, 29.8 percent versus 34 to 38 percent.

In the Australian Trial on Mild Hypertension (ATTMH), 33 percent of the subjects aged 60 to 69 years stopped active treatment prematurely as compared with 35 percent in the placebo-treated group (143). In the more recent trials, withdrawal caused by side effects was noted in 15 percent of the actively treated patients and 2 to 7 percent of the placebo-treated patients. However, the dropout rates from side effects was much greater from beta-blocking drugs than from diuretics. Therefore, antihypertensive drugs appear to be well tolerated in the elderly and result in side effects no more frequently in the elderly than in the young.

Drug Interactions

Because the elderly have many chronic diseases requiring treatment, polypharmacy is often necessary. One must be alert to drug interaction. For example, NSAIDs are frequently prescribed and may block the effect of diuretics, beta blockers, alpha-adrenergic blockers, and ACE inhibitors. The risk appears greatest in the elderly, and the average increase in mean arterial pressure is 10 mm Hg. Some NSAIDs may have less effect on blood pressure (205).

Stepdown Therapy

Between 25 and 41 percent of elderly hypertensive patients receiving antihypertensive drugs have remained normotensive for 10 or more months after withdrawal of the medication (206). Therefore, elderly patients with excellent blood pressure control without cardiovascular complications and without documented severe hypertension in the past can reduce their medications carefully and have it restarted if their hypertension recurs. This will also enable the clinician to restart treatment with drugs that have been demonstrated to be safer and more effective in the elderly.

CONCLUSIONS

Hypertension in the elderly is highly prevalent and increases the risk of cardiovascular complications. Treatment of ISH and combined systolic and diastolic hypertension is safe and effectively reduces cardiovascular morbidity and mortality, including decreased rates of stroke, coronary heart disease, and congestive heart failure. The initial selection of specific antihypertensive drugs is empirical, but individualization of drug choice based on clinical criteria should be used when possible. If there are no specific characteristics to influence drug choice, low-dose diuretic-based regimens have the best evidence for efficacy and tolerability. Systolic blood pressure correlates best with cardiovascular risk and benefit of treatment. Therefore, an increase in SBP to 160 mm Hg or greater should be reduced to less than 160 mm Hg or by greater than 20 mm Hg if it was initially between 160 to 179 mm Hg. With low-dose diuretic regimens, one can expect a 60 percent success rate, good tolerability, and slow reversal of LVH. Therapy should be slowly initiated with low doses of medication and be monitored to effectiveness, failure, or adverse effects, with care to avoid orthostatic hypotension. If monotherapy is unsuccessful, other drugs can be substituted or an ACE inhibitor can be added. Treatment should be aggressive to age 80 years and likely will continue through age 84 years. Treatment should not adversely affect the individual's functional capacity or qualify of life. Compliance is good, and metabolic effects are minimal in this population.

REFERENCES

1. Wenger NK, Marcus FL, O'Rourke RA. Cardiovascular disease in the elderly. *J Am Coll Cardiol* 1987;10:80a–87a.
2. Kannel WB, Gordon T. Evaluation of cardiovascular risk in the elderly: the Framingham Study. *Bull NY Acad Med* 1978;54:573–591.
3. Morton PA. Ordinary insurance: the build and blood pressure study. *Trans Soc Actuaries* 1959;11:987–997.
4. Kannel WB. Some lessons in cardiovascular epidemiology from Framingham. *Am J Cardiol* 1976;37:269–274.
5. Morgenstern N, Byyny RL. Epidemiology of hypertension in the elderly. *Drugs Aging* 1992;2:222–242.
6. The National High Blood Pressure Education Program. National Institutes of Health, National Heart, Lung, and Blood Institute. *The Fifth Report of the Joint National Committee on Detection, Evaluation, and Treatment of High Blood Pressure.* NIH Publication No. 93-1088, 1993, pp. 3–4.
7. Gordon T. *Blood pressure of adults by age and sex, United States 1960–62.* National Center for Health Statistics, PHS Publication 1000, series 11, No. 4, 1964.
8. Miller HW. National Center for Health Statistics. *Plan and operation of the National Health and Nutrition Examination Survey.* United States 1971-1973 Vital and Health Statistics, series 1, Nos. 10a and 10b. US Dept of Health, Education, and Welfare Publication No. 73-1310. Washington, DC: US Government Printing Office; 1973:46.
9. Roberts J, Maurer K. *Blood pressure levels of persons 60–74 years, United States, 1971–1974.* National Center for Health Statistics, 1977;1.
10. Szklo M. Epidemiologic patterns of blood pressure in children. *Epidemiol Rev* 1979;1:143.
11. Lowenstein FW. Blood pressure in relation to age and sex in the tropics and subtropics: a review of the literature and an investigation in two tribes of Brazil Indians. *Lancet* 1961;1:389–392.

12. Maddocks I. Possible absence of essential hypertension in two complete Pacific Island populations. *Lancet* 1961;2:396–399.

13. Prior IAM, Harvey HPB, Naeve MN, Davidson F. *The health of two groups of Cook Island Maoris.* New Zealand Department of Health Special Report, series No. 26. Wellington, New Zealand: Government Press.

14. Sinnett PF, Whyte HM. Epidemiological studies in total highland population, Tukisenta, New Guinea. Cardiovascular disease and relevant clinical, electrocardiographic, radiological, and biochemical findings. *J Chronic Dis* 1973;26:265–290.

15. Kannel WB, Gordon T. Evaluation of cardiovascular risk in the elderly: the Framingham Study. *Bull NY Acad Med* 1978;54:573–591.

16. Hulley SB, Furberg CD, Gurland B, et al. The systolic hypertension in the elderly program (SHEP): antihypertensive efficacy of chlorthalidone. *Am J Cardiol* 1985;56:913–920.

17. Vogt TM, Ireland CC, Black D, Camel G, Hughes G. Recruitment of elderly volunteers for a multicenter clinical trial: the SHEP Pilot Study. *Controlled Clin Trials* 1986;7:118–133.

18. Kannel WB, Dawber TR, McGee DL. Perspectives on systolic hypertension—the Framingham study. *Circulation* 1980;61:1179–1182.

19. Kannel WB. Some lessons in cardiovascular epidemiology. *Am J Cardiol* 1976;37:269–274.

20. Report of the Joint National Committee on Detection. Evaluation and treatment of high blood pressure. *Arch Intern Med* 1984;144:1045–1047.

21. Prior I. Hypertension in the elderly: stages and causes. In: Gross FH, Robertson JIS, eds. *Arterial hypertension.* London: Pitman Medical Publishing Co.; 1979:140–152.

22. Caird FI, Kennedy RD. Epidemiology of heart disease in old age. In: Caird FI, Dall JLC, Kennedy RD, eds. *Cardiology in old age.* New York: Plenum Press; 1976:1–10.

23. Campbell A, Caird FI, Jackson TR. Prevalence of abnormalities of electrocardiogram in old people. *Br Heart J* 1974;36:1005–1011.

24. Ostfeld AM. Elderly hypertensive patient—epidemiologic review. *NY State J Med* 1978;78:1125–1129.

25. Ostfeld AM, Shekelle RB, Klawans H, et al. Epidemiology of stroke in an elderly welfare population. *Am J Public Health* 1974;64:450–462.

26. Amery A, Brixko P, Clement D, et al. Mortality and morbidity results from the European Working Party on High Blood Pressure in the Elderly Trial. *Lancet* 1985;1:1349–1354.

27. Medical Research Council trial of treatment of hypertension in older adults: principal results. *Br Med J* 1992;304:4305–4312.

28. Dahlof B, Lindholm LH, Hansson L, et al. Morbidity and mortality in the Swedish Trial in Old Patients with Hypertension (STOP-Hypertension). *Lancet* 1991;1:1281–1284.

29. Kannel WB, Wolf PA, McGee DL, et al. Systolic blood pressure, arterial rigidity, and risk of stroke. *JAMA* 1981;245:1225–1229.

30. Shekelle RB, Ostfeld AM, Klawans HL. Hypertension and risk of stroke in an elderly population. *Stroke* 1974;5:71–75.

31. Prevention of stroke by antihypertensive drug treatment in older persons with isolated systolic hypertension. Final results of the Systolic Hypertension in the Elderly Program (SHEP). *JAMA* 1991;265:3255–3264.

32. Applegate WB. Hypertension in the elderly. *Generations* 1987;Fall:16–19.

33. Levy D, Garrison RJ, Savage DD, et al. Prognostic implications of echocardiographically determined left ventricular mass in the Framingham Heart Study. *N Engl J Med* 1990;322:1561–1566.

34. Messerli FH, Ventura HO, Glade LB, et al. Essential hypertension in the elderly: hemodynamics, intravascular volume, plasma renin activity and circulating catecholamine levels. *Lancet* 1983;2:983–986.

35. Topol EJ, Thaile JA, Fortuin NJ. Hypertensive hypertrophic cardiomyopathy. *N Engl J Med* 1985;312:277–283.

36. McCarty R. Sympathetic-adrenal medullary and cardiovascular responses to acute cold stress in adult and aged rats. *J Auton Nerv Syst* 1985;12:15–22.

37. Docherty JR. Aging and the cardiovascular system. *J Auton Pharmacol* 1986;6:77–84.

38. Friedman SM, Middleton AG, Friedman CL. Diminished blood pressure lability in aging rats. *Gerontologia* 1958;2:47–54.

39. Lee JC, Karpeles LM, Downing SE. Age-related changes of cardiac performance in male rats. *Am J Physiol* 1972;222:432–438.

40. Hallock P, Benson IC. Studies on the elastic properties of human isolated aorta. *J Clin Invest* 1934;16:595–602.

41. Bader H. Dependence of wall stress in the human thoracic aorta on age and pressure. *Circ Res* 1967;20:354–361.

42. Gerstenblith G, Lakatta EG, Weisfeldt ML. Age changes in myocardial function and exercise response. *Prog Cardiovasc Dis* 1976;19:1–21.

43. Yin FCP. The aging vasculature and its effects on the heart. In: Weisfeldt ML, ed. *The aging heart.* New York: Raven Press; 1980:137–213.

44. Hayflick L. The limited *in vitro* life-time of human diploid cell strains. *Exp Cell Res* 1961;25:585.

45. Roth GS. Age-associated changes in hormone action: the role of receptors. In: Schimke RT, ed. *Biologic mechanisms in aging.* Washington, D.C.: Department of Health and Human Services; 1980:678.

46. Medvedev ZA. Repetition of molecular-genetic information as a possible factor in evolutionary changes in life span. *Exp Gerontol* 1972;7:227.

47. Harmon D. The aging process. *Proc Natl Acad Sci USA* 1981;78:7124.

48. Bjorksten J. The cross-linkage theory of aging. *Finska Kemists Medd* 1971;80:23.

49. Strehler BL. *Time, cells, and aging.* New York: Academic Press; 1977.

50. Yin FCP. The aging vasculature and its effects on the heart. In: Weisfeldt ML, ed. *The aging heart.* New York: Raven Press; 1980:137–213.

51. Gonza ER, Marble AE, Shaw A, Holland JG. Age-related changes in the mechanics of the aorta and pulmonary artery of man. *J Appl Physiol* 1974;36:407–411.

52. Hallock P, Benson IC. Studies on the elastic properties of human isolated aorta. *J Clin Invest* 1937;16:595–602.

53. Lakatta EG. Alterations in the cardiovascular system that occur in advanced age. *Fed Proc* 1979;38:163–167.

54. Boutouyrie P, Laurant S, Benetos A, Girard XJ, Hoeks AP, Safar ME. Opposing effects of aging on distal and proximal large arteries in hypertension. *J Hypertens* 1992;10:589–591.

55. Granath A, Jonsson B, Strandell T. Circulation in healthy old men, studied by right heart catheterization of rest and during exercise in supine and sitting position. *Acta Med Scand* 1964;176:425–446.

56. Koch-Weser J. Correlation of pathophysiology and pharmacology in primary hypertension. *Am J Cardiol* 1973;32:499–508.

57. Franklin SS. Geriatric hypertension. *Med Clin North Am* 1983;67:395–417.

58. Messerli FH. The age factor in hypertension. *Hosp Pract* 1986;21:103–112.

59. Weller RO. Vascular pathology in hypertension. *Age Ageing* 1979;8:99–103.

60. Folkow B, Hallback M, Lundgren Y, Siverston Weiss L. Importance of adaptive changes in vascular design for establishment of primary hypertension studied in man and in spontaneously hypertensive rats. *Circ Res* 1973;32(suppl 1):2.

61. Tarazi RC, Magrini F, Dustan HP. The role of aortic distensibility in hypertension. In: Milliez P, Safer M, eds. *Recent advances in hypertension.* Vol II. Reims, England: Boehringer Ingelheim; 1975:113.

62. Hickler RB. Aging and hypertension. *J Am Geriatr Soc* 1983;3:421–425.

63. Shimada K, Kitazumi T, Sadakane N, Ogura H, Ozawa T. Age-related changes in baroreflex function, plasma norepinephrine, and blood pressure. *Hypertension* 1985;7:113–117.

64. Gribbin B, Pickering LTG, Slight P, Petro R. Effect of age and high blood pressure on baroreflex sensitivity in man. *Circ Res* 1971;29:424.

65. McGarry K, Laher M, Fitzgerald D, Horgan J, O'Brien E, O'Malley K. Baroreflex function in elderly hypertensives. *Hypertension* 1983;5:763–766.

66. Caird FI, Andrews GR, Kenned RD. Effects of posture on blood pressure in the elderly. *Br Heart J* 1973;35:527–530.

67. Sowers JR, Rubenstein LZ, Stern N. Plasma norepinephrine responses to posture and isometric exercise increase with age in the absence of obesity. *J Gerontol* 1983;38:315–317.

68. Appenzeller O, Descarries L. Circulatory reflexes in patients with cerebrovascular disease. *N Engl J Med* 1964;271:820–823.

69. Drayer JIM, Weber MA, DeYoung JL, Wyle FA. Circadian blood pressure patterns in ambulatory hypertensive patients. Effects of age. *Am J Med* 1982;73:493–499.

70. Gambert SR, Duthie EH. Effect of age on red cell membrane sodium-potassium dependent adenosine triphosphate (Na$^+$-K$^+$-ATPase) activity in healthy men. *J Gerontol* 1983;38:23–25.

71. Editorial. Cells, ions, and blood pressure. *Lancet* 1982;2:965–967.

72. Stessman J, Mekler J, Ben-Ishay D. Erythrocyte Na$^+$-K$^+$ cotransport in elderly hypertensive subjects. *Isr J Med Sci* 1985;121:314–316.

73. Crane MG, Harris JJ, Johns VJ. Hyporeninemic hypertension. *Am J Med* 1972;52:457–466.

74. Crane MG, Harris JJ. Effect of aging on renin activity and aldosterone excretion. *J Lab Clin Med* 1976;87:949–959.

75. Noth RH, Lassman MN, Tan SYM, et al. Age and the renin-aldosterone system. *Arch Intern Med* 1977;137:1414–1417.

76. Weidmann P, Beretta-Piccoli C, Ziegler WH, et al. Age versus urinary sodium for judging renin, aldosterone, and catecholamine levels—studies in normal subjects and in patients with essential hypertension. *Kidney Int* 1978;14:619–628.

77. Weidmann P, DeMyttenaere-Bursztein S, Maxwell MH, et al. Effect of aging on plasma renin and aldosterone in normal man. *Kidney Int* 1975;8:325–333.

78. Carey RM, Douglas JG, Schweikert JR, et al. The syndrome of essential hypertension and suppressed plasma renin activity. *Arch Intern Med* 1972;130:849–854.

79. Dunn MJ, Tannen RL. Low-renin hypertension. *Kidney Int* 1974;5:317–325.

80. Tuck ML, Williams GH, Cain JP, et al. Relation of age, diastolic pressure and known duration of hypertension to presence of low renin essential hypertension. *Am J Cardiol* 1973;32:632–637.

81. Osborne JL, DiBona GF, Thames MD. Beta-1 receptor mediation of renin secretion elicited by low frequency renal nerve stimulation. *J Pharmacol Exp Ther* 1981;216:265–270.

82. Stern N, Tuck ML. Homeostatic fragility in the elderly. *Geriatr Cardiol* 1986;4:201–211.

83. Duggan J, Kilfeather S, O'Brien E, O'Malley K, Nussberger J. Effects of aging and hypertension on plasma angiotensin II and platelet angiotensin II receptor density. *Am J Hypertens* 1992;5:687–693.

84. Nowarcynski W, Genest J, Kuchel O, et al. Age- and posture-related changes in plasma protein binding and metabolism of aldosterone in essential and secondary hypertension. *J Lab Clin Med* 1977;90:475–490.

85. Tadeka R, Morimoto S, Uchida K, et al. Effect of age on plasma aldosterone response to exogenous angiotensin II in normotensive subjects. *Acta Endocrinol* 1980;94:553–558.

86. Henry DP, Luft FC, Weinberger MH, et al. Norepinephrine in urine and plasma following provocative maneuvers in normal and hypertensive subjects. *Hypertension* 1980;2:20–28.

87. Lake CR, Ziegler MG, Coleman MD, et al. Age-adjusted plasma norepinephrine levels are similar in normotensive and hypertensive subjects. *N Engl J Med* 1977;296:208–209.

88. Young JB, Rowe JW, Pallotta JA, et al. Enhanced plasma norepinephrine response to upright posture and oral glucose administration in elderly human subjects. *Metabolism* 1980;29:532–535.

89. Sowers JR, Rubenstein LZ, Stern N. Plasma norepinephrine responses to posture and isometric exercise increase with age in the absence of obesity. *J Gerontol* 1983;38(3):315–317.

90. Esler M, Skews H, Leonard P, Jackson G, Bobik A, Korner P. Age-dependence of noradrenaline kinetics in normal subjects. *Clin Sci* 1981;60:217–219.

91. Goldstein DS, Lake CR, Chernew B, et al. Age dependence of the hypertensive-normotensive differences in plasma norepinephrine. *Hypertension* 1983;5:100–107.

92. Gavras SI, Gavras H, Chobanian AV, et al. Hypertension and age: clinical and biochemical correlates. *Clin Exp Hypertens* (A) 1982;4:1097–1106.

93. Stern N, Beahm E, McGinty D, et al. Dissociation of 24-hour catecholamine levels from blood pressure in older men. *Hypertension* 1985;7:1023–1029.

94. Vestal RE, Wood AJJ, Shand DG. Reduced β-adrenoreceptor sensitivity in the elderly. *Clin Pharmacol Ther* 1979;26:186–191.

95. VanBrummelen PV, Buhler FR, Kiowski W, Amann FW. Age related decrease in cardiac and peripheral vascular responsiveness to isoprenaline. *Clin Sci* 1981;60:571–577.

96. Klein C, Gerber JG, Gal J, Nies AS. Beta-adrenergic receptors in the elderly are not less sensitive to timolol. *Clin Pharmacol Ther* 1986;40:161–164.

97. Abrass IB, Davis JL, Scarpace PJ. Isoproterenol responsiveness and myocardial β-adrenergic receptors in young and old rats. *J Gerontol* 1982;37:156–160.

98. Elliott HL, Sumner DJ, McLean K, Reid JL. Effect of age on the responsiveness of vascular alpha-adrenoreceptors in man. *J Cardiovasc Pharmacol* 1982;4:388–392.

99. Scott PJW, Reid JL. The effect of age on the responses of human isolated arteries to noradrenaline. *Br J Clin Pharmacol* 1982;13:237–239.

100. Buhler FR, Kiowski W, VanBrummelen P, Amann FW. Bertal and cardiac, renal and peripheral vascular adrenoreceptor mediated responses indifferent age groups of normal and hypertensive subjects. *Clin Exp Hypertens* 1980;2:409–428.

101. Simpkins JW, Field FP, Ress RJ. Age related decline in adrenergic responsiveness of the kidney, heart and aorta of male rats. *Neurobiol Aging* 1983;4:233–238.

102. McAdams RP, Lattimer N, Rhodes KF, Waterfall JR. The effect of age on activation of pre- and post-synaptic alpha-adrenoreceptors in the rat. *Br J Pharmacol* 1985;86:494.

103. Hyland L, Docherty JR. An investigation of age-related changes in pre- and post-junctional alpha-adrenoreceptors in human saphenous veins. *Eur J Pharmacol* 1985;110:241–246.

104. Featherstone JA, Veith RC, Flatness D, Murburg MM, Villacres EC, Halter JB. Age and alpha-2 adrenergic regulation of plasma norepinephrine kinetics in humans. *J Gerontol* 1987;42:271–276.

105. Kelliher GJ, Conahan ST. Changes in vagal activity and response to muscarinic receptor agonists with age. *J Gerontol* 1980;45:842–849.

106. Dauchot P, Gravenstein JS. Effects of atropine on the electrocardiogram in different age groups. *Clin Pharmacol Ther* 1971;12:274–280.

107. Hollenberg NA, Adams DR, Solomon HS, Rashid A, Abrams HL, Merrill JP. Senescence and the renal vasculature in normal man. *Circ Res* 1974;34:309–316.

108. Fleisch JH. Age related changes in the sensitivity of blood vessels to drugs. *Pharmacol Ther* 1980;8:477–480.

109. Davies DF, Shock NW. Age changes in glomerular filtration rate, effective renal plasma flow and tubular excretory capacity in adult males. *J Clin Invest* 1950;29:496–507.

110. Rowe JW, Andres R, Tobin JD, Norris AH, Shock NW. The effect of age on creatinine clearance in men: a cross sectional and longitudinal study. *J Gerontol* 1976;31:155–163.

111. Lindeman RD, Tobin J, Shock NW. Longitudinal studies on the rate of decline in renal function with age. *J Am Geriatr Soc* 1985;33:178–285.

112. Wesson LG. Renal hemodynamics in physiologic states. In: Wesson LG, ed. *Physiology of the human kidney.* New York: Grune & Stratton; 1969:96–108.

113. Anderson S, Brenner BM. Effects of aging on the renal glomerulus. *Am J Med* 1986;80:435–442.

114. Epstein M, Hollenberg NK. Age as a determinant of renal sodium conservation in normal man. *J Lab Clin Med* 1976;87:411–417.

115. Garcia-Iglesias C, Rollan A. Plasma volume, renin-angiotensin system and sodium balance in healthy elderly men. *Proc Int Congress Gerontol* 1985;13:371.

116. Ohasi M, Fujio N, Nawata H, et al. High plasma concentration of human atrial natriuretic polypeptide in aged men. *J Clin Endocrinol Metab* 1987;64:81–85.

117. Byyny RL, LoVerde M, Lloyd S, Mitchell W, Draznin B. Cyto-

solic calcium and insulin resistance in elderly patients with essential hypertension. *Am J Hypertens* 1992;5:459–464.

118. Giugliano D, Salvatore T, Paolisso G, et al. Impaired glucosemetabolism and reduced insulin clearance in elderly hypertensives. *Am J Hypertens* 1992;57:249–252.

119. Panza JA, Quyyum AA, Callahan TS, Epstein SE. The effect of antihypertensive treatment on endothelium-dependent vascular relaxation in patients with essential hypertension. *J Am Coll Cardiol* 1993;21:1145–1151.

120. Durning FJ, Womerskly J. Body fat assessed from total body density and its estimation from skin fold thickness: measurements on 481 men and women age 16–72 years. *Br J Nutr* 1974;32:77–97.

121. Byyny RL. Analysis of NHANES II data. *Unpublished observations.*

122. Dehn MM, Bruce RA. Longitudinal variation in maximal oxygen intake with age and activity. *J Appl Physiol* 1972;33:805–807.

123. Posner JD, Gorman KM, Klein H, Woldow A. Exercise capacity in the elderly. *Am J Cardiol* 1986;57:52C–59C.

124. Stamford BA. Physiologic effects of training upon institutionalized geriatric men. *J Gerontol* 1972;27:451–455.

125. Barry AJ, Daly JW, Pruett EDR, et al. The effects of physical conditioning on older individuals. *J Gerontol* 1966;21:182–191.

126. DeVries HA. Physiologic effects of an exercise training regimen upon men aged 52–58. *J Gerontol* 1970;25:325–336.

127. Guilleminau HC, Tilkian A, Demment WC. The sleep apnea syndrome. *Annu Rev Med* 1976;27:465–484.

128. Kales A, Bixler EO, Cadieux RJ, et al. Sleep apnea and the hypertensive population. *Lancet* 1983;2:1005–1008.

129. Williams AJ, Houston D, Finberg S, et al. Sleep apnea and essential hypertension. *Am J Cardiol* 1985;55:1019–1022.

130. Lugarisi E, Criginotta E, Coccagano G, et al. Some epidemiologic data on snoring and cardiocirculatory disturbance. *Sleep* 1980;3:221–224.

131. Stern N, Beahm E, McCarty D, et al. Dissociation of 24-hour catecholamine levels from blood pressure in older men. *Hypertension* 1985;7:1023–1029.

132. McGinty D, Beahm E, Stern N, et al. Occult nocturnal hypotension in older men with sleep related breathing disorders. *Sleep Res* 1985;14:190.

133. Editorial. Hypertension in the over 60's. *Lancet* 1980;1:1396.

134. Spence JD, Sibbald WJ, Cape RD. Pseudohypertension in the elderly. *Clin Sci Mol Med* 1978;55:3995–4025.

135. O'Callaghan WG, Fitzgerald DJ, O'Malley K, O'Brien E. Accuracy of indirect blood pressure measurement in the elderly. *Br Med J* 1983;286:1545–1546.

136. Vardan S, Mookherjee S, Warner R, et al. Systolic hypertension. Direct and indirect BP measurements. *Arch Intern Med* 1983;143:935–938.

137. Fatherby MD, Potter JR. Reproducibility of ambuatory and clinic blood pressure measurement in elderly hypertensive subjects. *J Hypertens* 1993;11:573–579.

138. Thijs L, Amery A, Clement D, et al. Ambulatory blood pressure monitoring in elderly patients with isolated systolic hypertension. *J Hypertens* 1992;10:693–699.

139. Rutan GH, McDonald RH, Kuller LH. Comparison of ambulatory and clinic blood pressure and heart rate in older persons with isolated systolic hypertension. *Am J Hypertens* 1992;5:880–886.

140. Bos WJ, van Goudoever J, Wesseling KH, et al. Pseudohypertension in the measurement of blood pressure. *Hypertension* 1992;20:26–31.

141. Oliner CM, Elliott WJ, Gretler DD, Murphy MB. Low predictive value of positive Osler's maneuver for diagnosing psuedohypertension. *J Hum Hypertens* 1993;7:65–70.

142. Veterans Administration Cooperative Study Group on Antihypertensive Agents. Effects of treatment on morbidity in hypertension III. Influence of age, diastolic pressure, and prior cardiovascular disease; further analysis of side effects. *Circulation* 1982;XIV:991–1004.

143. Management Committee. Treatment of hypertension in the elderly. *Med J Aust* 1981;2:398–402.

144. Five-Year Findings of the Hypertension Detection and Follow-up Program. Mortality by race, sex, and age. *JAMA* 1979;141:2572–2577.

145. Kuramota K, Matsushita S, Kuwajima I, Murakami M. Prospective study on the treatment of mild hypertension in the aged. Japanese mild hypertension trial. *Jpn Heart J* 1981;22:75–85.

146. Carter AB. Hypotensive therapy in smoke survivors. *Lancet* 1970;1:485–489.

147. Spackling ME, Mitchell JRA, Short AH, Walt G. Blood pressure reduction in the elderly: a randomized controlled trial of methyldopa. *Br Med J* 1981;283:1151–1153.

148. Coope J, Warrender TS. Randomized trial of treatment of hypertension in elderly patients in primary care. *Br J Med* 1986;293:1145–1151.

149. Hulley SB, Furberg CD, Gurland B, et al. Systolic Hypertension in the Elderly Program (SHEP): antihypertensive efficacy of chlorthalidone. *Am J Cardiol* 1985;56:913–920.

150. Kostis JB. Beta blockers and cardiovascular events in SHEP. *Am J Hypertens* 1992;5:100A.

151. Staessen J, Balpitt C, Clement D, et al. Relation between morality and treated blood pressure in elderly with hypertension: report of the European Working Party on High Blood Pressure in the Elderly. *Br Med J* 1989;298:1552–1556.

152. Davis BR. Is there a J-shaped curve relationship between blood pressure reduction and cardiovascular mortality and morbidity in the Systolic Hypertension in the Elderly Program? Presented at the American Society of Hypertension Meeting 1A:21, 1992.

153. Schulman SD, Weiss JL, Becker LC, et al. The effects of antihypertensive therapy on left ventricular mass in elderly patients. *N Engl J Med* 1990;322:1350–1356.

154. Amery A, Birkenhager W, Brixko R, et al. Efficacy of antihypertensive drug treatment according to age, sex, blood pressure, and previous cardiovascular disease in patients over age 60. *Lancet* 1986;2:499–592.

155. Morgenstern N, Byyny RL. Epidemiology of hypertension in the elderly. *Drugs Aging* 1992;2:222–242.

156. Burke V, Beilin LJ, German R, et al. Association of lifestyle and personality characteristics with blood pressure and hypertension: a cross-sectional study in the elderly. *J Clin Epidemiol* 1992;45:1061–1070.

157. Luft FC, Weinberger HH, Feinberg NS, Mitler JZ, Grim CE. Effects of age on renal sodium homeostasis and its relevance to sodium sensitivity. *Am J Med* 1987;82(1B):9–15.

158. Applegate WB, Miller ST, Elam JT, et al. Nonpharmacologic intervention to reduce blood pressure in older patients with mild hypertension. *Arch Intern Med* 1992;152:1162–1166.

159. Jeffery RW, Folsom AR, Luepker RV, et al. Prevalence of overweight and weight loss behavior in a metropolitan adult population: the Minnesota Heart Survey experience. *Am J Public Health* 1984;74(4):349–352.

160. Tabuchi Y, Ogihara T, Hashizume K, Saito H, Kumahara Y. Hypotensive effect of long term oral calcium supplementation in elderly patients with essential hypertension. *J Clin Hypertens* 1986;3:254–262.

161. Little P, Girling G, Hasler A, Trafford A. A controlled trial of low sodium, low fat, high fibre diet in treated hypertensive patients: effect on antihypertensive drug requirement in clinical practice. *J Hum Hypertens* 1991;5:175–181.

162. Greenblatt DJ, Sellers EM, Shader RI. Drug disposition in old age. *N Engl J Med* 1982;306:1081–1087.

163. Piepho RW, Fendler KJ. Antihypertensive therapy in the aged patient. Clinical pharmacokinetic considerations. *Drugs Aging* 1991;1:194–211.

164. Strandgaard S. Autoregulation of cerebral blood flow in hypertensive patients. The modifying influence of prolonged antihypertensive treatment on the tolerance to acute drug induced hypotension. *Circulation* 1976;53:720–727.

165. Strandgaard S, Oleson J, Skinhoj E, et al. Autoregulation of brain circulation in severe arterial hypertension. *Br Med J* 1973;1:507–510.

166. Hansson L. Future goals for treatment of hypertension in the elderly with reference to STOP-Hypertension, SHEP, and the MRC trial in older adults. *Am J Hypertens* 1993;6:40S–43S.

167. Wasnich R, Davis J, Ross P, Vogel J. Effect of thiazide on rates of bone mineral loss: a longitudinal study. *Br Med J* 1990;301:1303–1305.

168. Warran JH, Laffel LM, Valsania P, Christlieb AR, Kroleski AS.

Excess mortality associated with diuretic therapy in diabetes mellitus. *Arch Intern Med* 1991;151:1350–1356.

169. Anderson RJ, Hart GR, Lee DK. Pitfalls in management of essential hypertension: diuretic therapy. *Prim Cardiol* 1979:63.

170. Niarchos AP, Laragh JH. Hypertension in the elderly. *Mod Concepts Cardiovasc Dis* 1980;XLIX:49–54.

171. Wikstrand J, Westergren G, Berglund G, et al. Antihypertensive treatment with metoprolol or hydrochlorothiazide in patients aged 60–75 years. *JAMA* 1986;255:1304–1310.

172. Down PF, Rao SK, Braverman AM, Poloniecki JD. Treatment of hypertension in the elderly with a low dose combination of beta-adrenoreceptor blocker and a thiazide diuretic: comparison with methyldopa. *Br J Clin Pract* 1983;37:371–374.

173. Castledon CM, George CK. The effect of aging on the hepatic clearance or propranolol. *J Clin Pharmacol* 1979;7:49–54.

174. Kendall MJ, Brown D, Yates RA. Plasma metoprolol concentrations in young and old and hypertensive subjects. *Br J Clin Pharmacol* 1972;4:497–499.

175. Cashman WC, Reda DJ, Materson BJ, et al. Comparison of monotherapy with different classes of drugs on systolic and diastolic blood pressure reduction in hypertension. *Am J Hypertens* 1992;25:7A–8A.

176. Applegate WB, Phillips HL, Schnaper H, et al. A randomized trial of the effects of three antihypertensive agents on blood pressure control and quality of life in older women. *Arch Intern Med* 1991;151:1817–1823.

177. Materson BJ. Veterans Affairs Cooperative Study Group on Antihypertensive Agents. Single drug therapy for hypertension in men. *N Engl J Med* 1993;328:914–921.

178. Materson BJ, Cushman WC, Goldstein G, et al. Treatment of hypertension in the elderly. I. Blood pressure and clinical changes. *Hypertension* 1990;15:348–360.

179. Thananopavarn C, Golub MS, Sambhi MP. Clonidine in the elderly hypertensive: monotherapy and therapy with a diuretic. *Chest* 1983;83:410–411.

180. Jeunemaitre X, Ged E, Ducrocq MB, Alhenc-Gelas F, Corvol P, Menard J. Effects of transdermal clonidine in young and elderly patients with mild hypertension: evaluation by three noninvasive methods of blood pressure measurement. *J Cardiovasc Pharmacol* 1987;10:162–167.

181. Erne P, Bolli P, Bertel O, et al. Factors influencing the hypotensive effects of calcium antagonists. *Hypertension* 1983;5(suppl 2):II-97–II-102.

182. Muller FB, Bolli P, Erne P, Kiowski W, Buhler FR. Use of calcium antagonists as monotherapy in the management of hypertension. *Am J Med* 1984;77(suppl 2B):11–5.

183. Ben-Ishay D, Leibel B, Stessman J. Calcium channel blockers in the management of hypertension in the elderly. *Am J Med* 1986;81(suppl 6A):30–34.

184. Schnapp P, Hermann H, Cernak P, Kahay J. Nifedipine monotherapy in the hypertensive elderly. *Curr Med Res Opin* 1987;10:407–413.

185. Schwartz JB, Abernathy DR. Responses to intravenous oral diltiazem in elderly and younger patients with systemic hypertension. *Am J Cardiol* 1987;59:1111–1117.

186. Abernathy DR, Schwartz JB, Todd EL, Ludie R, Show E. Verapamil pharmacodynamics and disposition in young and elderly hypertensive patients. *Ann Intern Med* 1986;105:329–336.

187. Adler AG, Leahy JJ, Cressman MD. Management of periopera-

tive hypertension using sublingual nifedipine. *Arch Intern Med* 1986;146:1927–1930.

188. McNeil JJ, Drummer OH, Conway EL, Workman BS, Louis WJ. Effect of age on pharmacokinetics of blood pressure responses to prazosin and terazosin. *J Cardiovasc Pharmacol* 1987;10:168–175.

189. Ramsay JWA, Scott GI, Whitfield HN. A double-blind controlled trial of a new alpha-1 blocking drug in the treatment of bladder outflow obstruction. *Br J Urol* 1985;57:657–659.

190. Eisalo A, Virta P. Treatment of hypertension in the elderly with labetalol. *Acta Med Scand* 1984;665S:129–133.

191. Abernathy DR, Schwartz JB, Plachetka JR, Todd EL, Egan JM. Comparison in young and elderly patients of pharmacodynamics and disposition of labetalol in systemic hypertension. *Am J Cardiol* 1987;60:697–702.

192. Jenkins AC, Knill JR, Dreslinski GR. Captopril in the treatment of the elderly hypertensive patient. *Arch Intern Med* 1985;145:2029–2031.

193. Woo JK, Wook S, Kin T, Vallance-Owen J. A single-blind randomized crossover study of angiotensin-converting enzyme inhibitor and triamterene and hydrochlorothiazide in the treatment of mild to moderate hypertension in the elderly. *Arch Intern Med* 1987;147:1386–1388.

194. Ajayi AA, Hockings N, Reid JL. Age and the pharmacodynamics of angiotensin converting enzyme inhibitor enalapril and enalaprilat. *Br J Clin Pharmacol* 1986;21:349–357.

195. Laher MS, Natin D, Rao SK, Jones RW, Carr P. Lisinoprilin elderly patients with hypertension. *J Cardiovasc Pharmacol* 1987;9(suppl 3):569–571.

196. Croog SH, Levine S, Testa MA, et al. The effects of antihypertensive therapy on the quality of life. *N Engl J Med* 1986;314:1657–1664.

197. Dahlof B, Hansson L. Regression of left ventricular hypertrophy in previously untreated essential hypertension: different effect of enalapril and HCTZ. *J Hypertens* 1992;10:1513–1524.

198. Luxenberg J, Feigenbaum LZ. The use of reserpine for elderly hypertensive patients. *J Am Geriatr Soc* 1983;31(9):556–559.

199. Doyle AE. Age-related effects of 5-HT$_2$ antagonists. *J Cardiovasc Pharmacol* 1991;17(suppl 5):S29–34.

200. Perry HM, Hall WD, Due DL, Spiro MA. Atenolol, enalapril, and isradapine for hypertension in elderly women. *Am J Hypertens* 1992;5:7A–7B.

201. Silagy CA, McNeil JJ, McGrath BP. Cross-over comparison of atenolol, enalapril, hydrochlorothiazide, and isradapine for isolated systolic hypertension. *Am J Cardiol* 1992;70:1299–1305.

202. Espinel CH, Bruner DE, Davis JR, Wiliams JC. Analapril and verapamil in the treatment of isolated systolic hypertension in the elderly. *Clin Ther* 1992;14:835–844.

203. Morgan TO, Nowson C, Murphy J, Snowden R. Compliance and the elderly hypertensive. *Drugs* 1986;31(suppl 4):174–183.

204. Black DM, Brand RJ, Greenlick M, et al. Compliance to treatment for hypertension in elderly patients: the SHEP pilot study. *J Gerontol* 1987;42:552–557.

205. Houston MC. Nonsteroidal anti-inflammatory drugs and antihypertensives. *Am J Med* 1991;90:42S–47S.

206. Herman KJ, Eisalo A. Possibility of reduction of antihypertensive therapy in hypertension (abstract). *Proc Sci Meeting Int Soc Hypertens* 1980;7:136.

Hypertension: Pathophysiology, Diagnosis, and Management, Second Edition, edited by J.H. Laragh and B.M. Brenner, Raven Press, Ltd., New York © 1995.

CHAPTER 15

Public Health Issues in Hypertension Control: What Has Been Learned From Clinical Trials

Jeffrey A. Cutler, Bruce M. Psaty, Stephen MacMahon, and Curt D. Furberg

Hypertension is one of the most common chronic conditions. Approximately 50 million Americans have elevated blood pressure or are taking antihypertensive drugs. The public health problem represented by elevated blood pressure lies primarily with its cardiovascular complications. The goal of antihypertensive therapy is to reduce the risk of stroke, acute myocardial infarction (MI), congestive heart failure, and other cardiovascular conditions.

A large number of randomized clinical trials conducted during the past three decades have established

J. A. Cutler: Prevention and Demonstration Research Branch, Division of Epidemiology and Clinical Applications, National Heart, Lung, and Blood Institute, Bethesda, Maryland 20892.

B. M. Psaty: Departments of Medicine, Epidemiology and Health Services, Cardiovascular Health Research Unit, University of Washington, Seattle, Washington 98101.

S. MacMahon: Clinical Trials Research Unit, Department of Medicine, University of Auckland, Auckland, New Zealand.

C. D. Furberg: Department of Public Health Sciences, Bowman Gray School of Medicine, Winston-Salem, North Carolina 27157.

much about the clinical benefit of hypertension control. Research usually triggers more research. So it is of interest to draw attention to the important shifts in research focus during this period. The early landmark trials documented the benefit of controlling severely elevated diastolic blood pressure, and subsequently also of reducing moderate and mild elevations. Recently, based on epidemiologic data showing a strong association between the level of systolic blood pressure and risks of stroke and MI, attention has been directed toward elevations of systolic blood pressure. Clinical trials have now documented the benefit of control of isolated systolic hypertension. The initial trials involved mostly middle-aged hypertensive subjects. Recent trials in elderly persons have shown that this group stands to benefit much more in absolute terms than their younger counterparts.

The high cost of hypertension control with drugs, particularly the more recently introduced calcium-channel blockers and angiotensin-converting enzyme (ACE) inhibitors, as well as the side effects of pharmacologic treatment, have also directed attention and resources toward nonpharmacologic or lifestyle interventions for blood pressure reduction. The role of nonpharmacologic therapies is now clearly specified in treatment guidelines produced both nationally and internationally.

Analyses of the cost-effectiveness of antihypertensive treatment have triggered discussions concerning resource allocation, treatment costs, and related public health issues. What additional health benefits should be expected from new, expensive, and mostly untested antihypertensive agents compared with the older, less expensive ones with proven mortality and morbidity benefits? Should efforts be made to shift the promotion of hypertension control from middle-aged but often low-risk hypertensives to high-risk elderly hypertensives? Conversely, is it timely to place major new emphasis on reducing the incidence of hypertension, both through application of existing knowledge and through further research?

Although remarkable progress has been made in the area of hypertension control, new scientific questions have emerged and need to be explored. The purpose of this review is to examine the data as they relate to the public health benefits of antihypertensive regimens, including those relevant to potential for primary prevention, and to highlight areas for future clinical and public health research.

CLINICAL TRIALS THAT ADDRESS THE QUESTION OF WHETHER LOWERING BLOOD PRESSURE BY ANTIHYPERTENSIVE DRUGS REDUCES CARDIOVASCULAR MORBIDITY AND MORTALITY

By the end of the last decade, available data from randomized controlled trials of antihypertensive treatment demonstrated that a modest blood pressure reduction maintained for a few years reduced the incidence of stroke, coronary heart disease (CHD), and cardiovascular mortality (1). The 14 trials completed at that time involved almost 37,000 patients among whom a 5–6 mm Hg reduction in diastolic blood pressure (DBP) reduced cardiovascular mortality by about a fifth and the incidence of stroke by between a third and a half. (Although underemphasized in reports from these trials, the reductions in DBP were accompanied by approximately two-fold greater reductions in systolic blood pressure [SBP].) The reduction in CHD incidence was less impressive, and the confidence interval (CI) for the combined trial results was consistent with a true effect in the range of a 4 to 22 percent reduction. However, a useful perspective was gained from prospective observational studies; the estimated potential effects of a prolonged DBP difference of 5–6 mm Hg (accompanied by an approximately two-fold greater SBP difference) were reductions in stroke incidence of 35 to 40 percent and in CHD incidence of 20 to 25 percent (2). Hence the trial results indicated that much or all of the long-term potential benefits for stroke

were achieved soon after beginning treatment. For CHD, however, the benefits achieved by a few years of BP reduction appeared to be substantially less than the full long-term potential benefits.

At that time, there was comparatively little evidence available about the effects of antihypertensive treatment in older patients; only two trials, involving a total of 1,724 patients, had recruited older patients exclusively (3,4). One of these studies provided evidence of a conventionally significant reduction in stroke incidence (3), but neither showed a significant reduction in CHD incidence nor in cardiovascular death. While the other 12 studies included about 2,000 patients over the age of 60 years, separate data on outcome in these individuals were not available in most studies. However, as the available data did not indicate any significant heterogeneity between the effects of treatment in older patients and in younger patients, it seemed likely that some benefits of antihypertensive treatment extended to older patients, although the size of such benefits remained uncertain.

In the early 1990s, three new studies of antihypertensive treatment were completed: the U.S. Systolic Hypertension in the Elderly Program (SHEP) (5), the Scandinavian STOP-Hypertension trial (6), and the British Medical Research Council (MRC) trial of the treatment of hypertension in older adults (7). These trials increased by severalfold the available data about effects of antihypertensive treatment in elderly patients; they also increased by about half the total information (clinical events) available from all age groups about the effects of antihypertensive treatment on CHD. Thus, results from these trials, in combination with those of previous trials, now provide an opportunity both to assess directly the effects of BP reduction on stroke and CHD in older patients and to reduce the uncertainty about the size of the reduction in CHD achieved within a few years of BP-lowering.

Overview of Randomized Trials of Antihypertensive Treatment

Study Populations

Data on effects of antihypertensive treatment in younger and older patients are now available from 17 randomized trials involving 47,653 persons. Of these, five studies involving 12,483 subjects were conducted exclusively in persons over 60 years of age (3–7). The characteristics of the study populations of trials in younger and older subjects are summarized in Table 1. Overall, the average age was 57 years, half were male, and the average blood pressure at entry was about 168/96 mm Hg. In the trials conducted exclusively in older individuals, the average age was 21 years greater, and the proportion of female subjects was 30 percent greater, than in the other studies; additionally, the average entry SBP was about 18

TABLE 1. *Characteristics of study populations in 17 randomized trials of antihypertensive treatment*

	All 17 trials	5 trials in older patients	12 trials in younger patients
N patients	47,653	12,483	35,170
Mean age	57	72	51
Percent male	50	40	54
SBP	168[a]	181	163[a]
DBP	96	88	99

[a] Not available from all trials.
SBP, systolic blood pressure; DBP, diastolic blood pressure.

TABLE 2. *Estimates from prospective observational studies of the potential effects of prolonged differences in blood pressure*

Difference in usual		Difference in incidence of	
SBP[a]	DBP[a]	Stroke	CHD
9	5	35%	21%
14	7.5	46%	29%
19	10	56%	37%

From ref. 2, with permission.
[a] mm Hg.
SBP, systolic blood pressure; DBP, diastolic blood pressure; CHD, coronary heart disease.

mm Hg higher and the entry DBP 11 mm Hg lower in the trials in older subjects.

Study Treatments and Blood Pressure Reductions

For three-quarters of all subjects assigned to active treatment in the trials, the initial study drug was a diuretic; for most of the remainder it was a beta blocker. The mean duration of follow-up (weighted by sample size) was 4.9 years, during which average BP differences between study groups was about 6 mm Hg diastolic and about 13 mm Hg systolic. However, since these BP differences were estimated only from subjects who attended study clinics, net differences between all those assigned to study treatment and those assigned to control

are likely to be somewhat less—perhaps about 5–6 mm Hg diastolic and 11–12 mm Hg systolic. In the trials in older subjects the reduction in SBP appeared to be about 2 mm Hg greater than in the other studies, whereas the reduction in DBP was similar in both groups of trials.

Effects on Stroke and Coronary Heart Disease Incidence

From prospective, observational studies (2) it can be calculated that a prolonged BP difference of the magnitude typically achieved in the trials (5–6 mm Hg diastolic and 11–12 mm Hg systolic) should in the long term reduce stroke by about 35 to 40 percent and CHD by 20 to 25 percent (Table 2). In Fig. 1, the effects of several years'

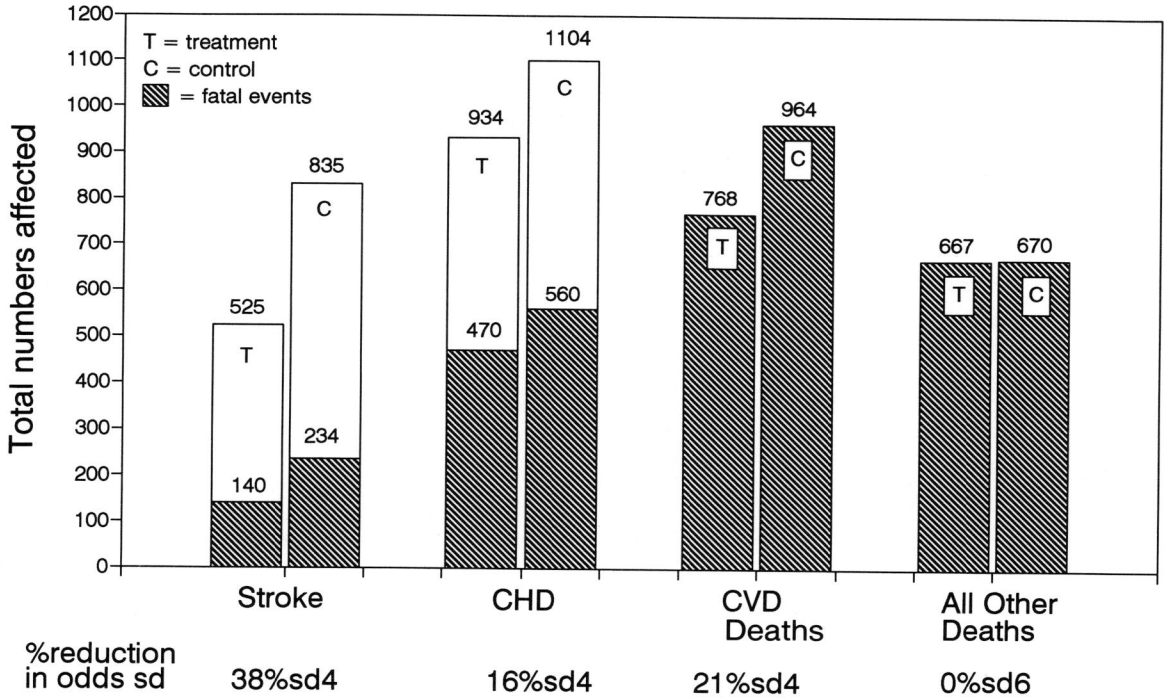

FIG. 1. Effects of antihypertensive treatment on stroke, CHD, total cardiovascular deaths, and total noncardiovascular deaths from the combined results of 17 randomized trials. CHD, coronary heart disease; CVD, cardiovascular disease; sd, standard deviation.

antihypertensive treatment on the incidence of stroke, CHD, total cardiovascular death, and total noncardiovascular death are estimated from the combined results of all 17 randomized trials. Overall, in these trials, among the patients assigned study treatment, stroke incidence was reduced by 38 percent (SD = 4 percent) and CHD incidence was reduced by 16 percent (SD = 4 percent), with similar reductions in fatal and nonfatal events. The 95 percent CI for reduction in stroke was 31 percent to 45 percent, and for reduction in CHD it was 8 percent to 24 percent. Deaths from all cardiovascular causes were reduced by 21 percent (SD = 4 percent) among those assigned active treatment. Because deaths from other causes were not different between active treatment and control groups, total mortality was also reduced, by 12 percent (SD = 3 percent).

These results therefore confirm the previous observation (1) that the reduction in stroke conferred by several years of antihypertensive treatment represents much or all of the expected, long-term potential effect of the BP reduction. They also suggest that about two-thirds of the long-term potential benefit for CHD was achieved. Moreover, the 95 percent Cl for the reduction in CHD indicates that the benefit conferred by several years of treatment is at least a third of the expected long-term benefit, and quite possibly, much or all of the benefit. The proportion of the long-term potential benefit for CHD achieved by BP reduction in these trials was rather similar to that observed in trials of cholesterol lowering,

in which the reduction in CHD with a few years of treatment was about two-thirds of the long-term potential benefit of the achieved cholesterol reduction (8). The accumulated results from these trials of blood pressure reduction now seem to argue against the view that treatment with a diuretic- or beta-blocker-based regimen produces substantially less than the expected benefit for CHD.

Effects in Older and Younger Patients

Results from the five individual trials conducted exclusively in older subjects (3–7), together with combined results from these trials and combined results from trials conducted predominantly in younger subjects, are shown in Figs. 2 and 3. The proportional reduction in stroke incidence in older subjects (34 percent ± 6 percent) was similar to that observed in younger subjects (43 percent ± 6 percent) (Fig. 2), but the absolute reduction in stroke incidence in older subjects (4.9/1,000 person-years) was more than twice as great as that in younger subjects (1.9/1,000 person-years). Incidence of CHD was reduced by 19 percent (±7 percent) in older subjects. Once again, this proportional reduction was similar to that observed in younger subjects (14 percent ± 5 percent) (Fig. 3), yet the absolute reduction in the older subjects (2.7/1,000 person-years) was more than twice as great as that in the younger subjects (1.0/1,000 person-

Trial (or group of trials)	N	% Events Study	Control	Odds Ratio & CL	Reduction ± SD
Older Patients					
SHEP	4,736	4.4%	6.8%		36% ± 10
STOP-H	1,627	3.7%	6.7%		46% ± 17
MRC Older	4,396	4.6%	6.1%		25% ± 12
2 smaller trials	1,724	6.2%	9.8%		39% ± 14
Subtotal:	12,483	4.6%	7.0%		34% ± 6
Younger Patients					
HDFP	10,940	1.9%	2.9%		36% ± 10
MRC Younger	17,354	0.7%	1.3%		45% ± 12
10 smaller trials	6,876	2.2%	3.8%		49% ± 11
Subtotal:	35,170	1.3%	2.3%		43% ± 6
All Patients					
Total stroke	47,653	2.2%	3.5%		38% ± 4
Fatal stroke		0.6%	1.0%		40% ± 8
Nonfatal stroke		1.6%	2.5%		37% ± 5

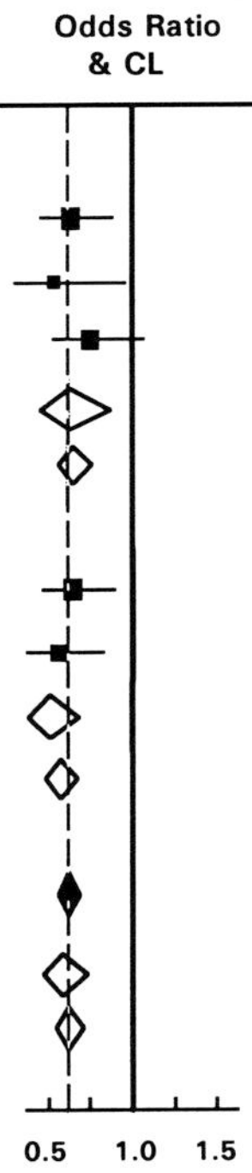

0.5   1.0   1.5

X² test for heterogeneity between age groups: 1.34; P = 0.2; NS
Treatment effect: 2P < 0.0001

FIG. 2. Effects of antihypertensive treatment on stroke incidence in older and younger patients from combined results of 5 and 12 randomized trials, respectively (DBP reduction 5–6 mm Hg, SBP reduction 10–12 mm Hg, follow-up 5 years). N, sample size; CL, confidence limits; SD, standard deviation; DBP, diastolic blood pressure; SBP, systolic blood pressure; SHEP, Systolic Hypertension in the Elderly Program; MRC, Medical Research Council; STOP-H, Swedish Trial of Older Persons-Hypertension; HDFP, Hypertension Detection and Follow-up Program.

Trial (or group of trials)	N	% Events Study	% Events Control	Odds Ratio & CL	Reduction ± SD
Older Patients					
SHEP	4,736	4.4%	6.0%		19% ± 19
STOP-H	1,627	3.8%	3.9%		3% ± 25
MRC Older	4,396	5.9%	7.2%		19% ± 11
2 smaller trials	1,724	9.9%	10.9%		11% ± 15
Subtotal:	12,483	5.6%	6.8%		19% ± 7
Younger Patients					
HDFP	10,940	5.0%	6.3%		21% ± 7
MRC Younger	17,354	2.6%	2.7%		6% ± 9
10 smaller trials	6,876	2.6%	2.8%		8% ± 14
Subtotal:	35,170	3.3%	3.8%		14% ± 5
All Patients					
Total CHD	47,653	3.9%	4.6%		16% ± 4
Fatal CHD		2.0%	2.4%		16% ± 5
Nonfatal MI		1.9%	2.3%		15% ± 6

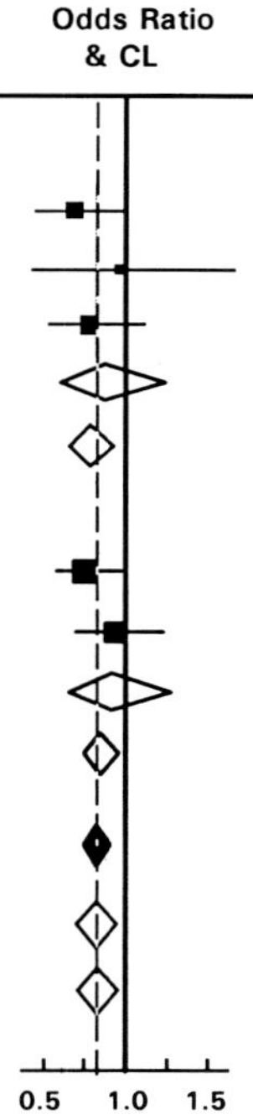

0.5   1.0   1.5

X^2 test for heterogeneity between age groups: 0.46; P = 0.5; NS
Treatment effect: 2P = 0.0001

FIG. 3. Effects of antihypertensive treatment on CHD incidence in older and younger patients from combined results of 5 and 12 randomized trials, respectively (DBP reduction 5–6 mm Hg, SBP reduction 10–12 mm Hg, follow-up 5 years). CHD, coronary heart disease; MI, myocardial infarction; all other abbreviations same as Fig. 2.

years). The proportional reductions in overall cardiovascular mortality were also similar in older and younger subjects (23 percent ± 6 percent and 19 percent ± 6 percent, respectively), and the absolute reduction in older subjects (3.6/1,000 person-years) was more than three times as great as that in younger subjects (1.0/1,000 person-years).

These results clearly establish that there are benefits of treatment for both younger and older persons with hypertension. The proportional reductions in stroke and CHD were quite similar in the trials in older and younger subjects, despite a variety of differences between the study populations (Table 1). However, because the incidence of events increases with age, the absolute differences in outcome were consistently more than twice as great in older subjects than in younger subjects.

Estimation of Effects of Actual Treatment

A proportion of subjects assigned to active treatment in these trials stopped taking treatment during follow-up (drop-outs), and a proportion of those assigned to control began active treatment (drop-ins). Consequently, the results underestimate both the BP-reducing effects of the treatments studied and the potential effects of these treatments on morbidity and mortality. Particularly because of drop-ins, the BP effects of these treatments in compliant patients could well be 15 to 20 percent greater than

the net BP differences observed in these trials. If the relationship between BP level and disease incidence is approximately linear, then the effects on cardiovascular disease would be increased by a similar proportion. In such circumstances, in elderly persons at similar risk of cardiovascular disease to those included in the trials, antihypertensive treatment with diuretic-based treatment should prevent about one major cardiovascular event (a stroke or myocardial infarction) among every 20 patients treated for about 5 years. Among younger patients at similar risk to those included in the trials, one event would be prevented among every 60 patients treated for about 5 years. However, since patients who volunteer to participate in randomized trials typically experience lower mortality and morbidity than do others, and since many of the trials excluded patients at highest risk of cardiovascular events, the use of antihypertensive treatment in usual medical practice may well result in larger absolute benefits than those that are suggested by the results of these randomized trials.

Unresolved Questions About the Effects of Antihypertensive Treatment on Cardiovascular Disease

More or Less Blood Pressure Reduction

The same epidemiologic data indicating continuous relationships between BP and the incidence of stroke and of CHD (2) also suggest that greater reductions in BP should confer greater reductions in cardiovascular death and serious morbidity. However, some uncertainty remains about the effects of greater BP reduction particularly in patients with a history of cardiovascular disease, especially CHD. This uncertainty arises largely as a consequence of reports from nonrandomized observational studies that have suggested that patients who develop the lowest DBP levels have an increased risk of death relative to those with slightly higher levels (9,10); however, an alternative explanation is that more severe coronary (and perhaps also cerebrovascular) disease both lowers BP and independently increases the risk of death (11). From observational studies it is not really possible to determine which of these explanations is correct. However, data from randomized trials, although few, suggest that vigorous BP reduction in hypertensive patients with a history of myocardial infarction or stroke confers a reduced risk of recurrent cerebrovascular or coronary events, rather than an increase in risk.

The combined results of two small trials (12,13) of antihypertensive treatment in patients with preexisting cerebrovascular disease demonstrate a 38 percent ± 16 percent reduction in the risk of recurrent stroke among patients assigned to active treatment. Additionally, the results of the Hypertension Detection and Follow-up Program for patients with a history of self-reported myocardial infarction at baseline indicated a 24 percent ± 13 percent reduction in the risk of recurrent infarction among patients assigned to study treatment. These observations are consistent with the secondary prevention trials: even among "normotensives" with a history of coronary heart disease, drugs such as beta-blockers that lower BP typically reduce rather than increase the risk of recurrent events, and the benefits are undiminished among those with the very lowest initial BP levels (14–16). This failure of randomized studies to demonstrate the increased frequency of recurrent events that would be expected if low BP were itself to confer increased risk has also recently extended to some small studies of BP-lowering drugs in "normotensive" patients with a history of stroke (17, S. Eriksson, *unpublished presentation,* Oslo, 1993).

Several trials have addressed the question of more versus less BP reduction, albeit in subjects free of diagnosed cardiovascular disease. Results from the Treatment of Mild Hypertension Study (18), which compared nondrug treatment alone with nondrug plus drug treatment (see the following section), are consistent with the hypothesis that larger BP reductions, even in patients with very mild hypertension, produce larger cardiovascular benefits. On the other hand, preliminary results from the Swedish Study *Behandla Blodtryck Bättre* (BBB) ("treat blood pressure better") have not shown a clear difference in cardiovascular disease outcomes among patients randomized to more intensive therapy compared with those randomized to less intensive therapy (19). However, the total number of cardiovascular events observed in that study was few (57 in total), and the trial did not have adequate statistical power to detect plausible effects of the modest blood pressure difference (10/7 mm Hg) achieved. A larger trial addressing a similar question is now being conducted by the same investigators (20).

Blood Pressure Reduction in Nonhypertensive Patients

The possibility that BP reduction may confer worthwhile benefits among patients without hypertension but who are for other reasons at high risk of cardiovascular events is suggested both by epidemiologic evidence indicating similar relationships between BP and cardiovascular diseases in hypertensives and normotensives (2), and by the trial results indicating similar proportional effects of BP reduction in patients with mild, moderate, or more severe hypertension, i.e., absence of attenuation of benefit as entry BP decreases (1). Such high-risk "normotensive" patients would include persons with preexisting cerebrovascular disease, CHD, peripheral cardiovascular disease, renal failure, or diabetes. Thus, for example, among patients with a history of transient ischemic attacks (TIAs), the annual risk of completed stroke is about 5 percent (21). If a BP-lowering treatment regimen reduced average BP by just 8/4 mm Hg in such individuals, both the observational and randomized trial data would predict a reduction in stroke risk by about one-fourth within a few years of beginning treatment. Among these normotensive TIA patients the absolute reduction in stroke incidence would be about 12/1,000 person-years. Moreover, since these patients are also at particularly high risk of CHD, such treatment could prevent a few additional CHD events per 1,000 person-years. Absolute benefits of this magnitude in high-risk normotensive patients would be severalfold greater than those that are likely to be achieved in persons with uncomplicated hypertension.

The existence of such benefits remains, however, to be established by large-scale randomized trials. The effects of atenolol in nonhypertensive patients with a history of stroke or TIA have recently been studied in two small trials (21) (S. Eriksson, *unpublished presentation,* Oslo, 1993); however, the BP reductions achieved in those studies were too small (2–3 mm Hg diastolic) to have had measurable effects on stroke incidence, given the study sample sizes (2,193 patients in total). The 95 percent CI for the combined results of these studies includes both a 20 percent increase in stroke and a 30 percent decrease in stroke among patients assigned to atenolol. A trial involving several thousand patients with a history of cerebrovascular disease, and an intervention that lowered BP by at least 4 mm Hg diastolic, would be required to detect reliably a one-quarter reduction in the risk of stroke.

Such an effort is probably warranted, given the large potentially absolute benefits of moderate BP reductions in such high-risk patients.

Newer or Older Antihypertensive Agents

A major area of uncertainty in the treatment of hypertension concerns the effects of newer classes of antihypertensive agents on the incidence of cardiovascular disease. These agents reduce BP by an amount similar to the older agents (17). It seems unlikely that they will have any greater effects on stroke incidence, since a few years of treatment with diuretic-based regimens appears to confer the expected long-term potential effect of the BP reductions achieved, and since none of the newer agents are known to possess any independent cerebroprotective effects. On the other hand, trials of ACE inhibitors after myocardial infarction suggest that these agents may have some independent cardioprotective effects (14,15), while the results of similar trials of dihydropyridine calcium antagonists suggest that these drugs may possess cardiotoxic effects (22,23). Any such relative advantages or disadvantages of the newer agents for CHD risk may be modest rather than large when compared with the effect of diuretics or beta blockers. Consequently, the reliable demonstration of plausible differences in CHD incidence between active treatment regimens will require randomized trials in which a few thousand CHD events are observed. Given that only about 2,000 CHD events were observed in all the previous trials collectively, new trials comparing various agents will need to be very large and focus on high-risk patients such as the elderly or those with prior cardiovascular disease.

CLINICAL TRIALS THAT ADDRESS THE QUESTION OF WHAT TREATMENTS TO CHOOSE FOR REDUCING BLOOD PRESSURE

Epidemiologic studies that show an association between blood pressure (BP) level and incidence of disease do not necessarily prove the existence of a causal relationship. However, the results of clinical trials reviewed in the previous section confirm the role of high BP as a cause of cardiovascular complications and establish the reversibility of the cardiovascular disease (CVD) risk. In this section, we review the available data that compare different treatments, beginning with studies that used major disease endpoints to compare types of drug treatment, followed by comparisons of nonpharmacologic and pharmacologic therapies.

Pharmacologic Therapy and Major Disease Endpoints

The purpose of pharmacologic therapy of hypertension is to reduce the incidence of cardiovascular compli-

cations of untreated hypertension. In addition, quality-of-life differences among antihypertensive agents are important, especially if the particular agents are known to be equally effective in preventing stroke and coronary heart disease. Although a variety of antihypertensive agents, including the newer agents such as calcium-channel blockers and ACE inhibitors, have been evaluated in terms of their effect on BP level and quality of life, only the diuretics and the beta blockers have been evaluated extensively in terms of their effect on major disease endpoints. Here, we discuss first the trials that compared diuretics and beta blockers and, subsequently, effects of each class of agents when compared with control groups in the clinical trials of antihypertensive treatment in the elderly.

In three trials among middle-aged subjects (24–26), beta blockers were directly compared with diuretics. In terms of the outcome of stroke, diuretics were slightly but not significantly better than beta blockers (cumulative incidence of 9.8 versus 10.9 strokes per 1,000 for diuretics and beta blockers, respectively; 11 percent risk reduction in favor of diuretics). In terms of the CHD outcome, beta blockers were slightly but not significantly better than the diuretics (cumulative incidence of 27.2 versus 28.8 coronary events per 1,000 for beta blockers and diuretics, respectively; 6 percent risk reduction in favor of beta blockers). Although the power to detect differences between drugs was relatively small, diuretics and beta blockers were comparable in middle-aged populations.

In the British MRC trial in older adults (7), 4,396 hypertensive men and women 65 to 74 years of age were randomized to placebo, atenolol, or hydrochlorothiazide plus amiloride, and followed for an average of 5.8 years. During the early part of the trial, participants on diuretics had lower levels of BP than those on beta blockers. After two years, the treatment groups had similar levels of both SBP and DBP, although a higher proportion of the participants randomized to beta blockers required supplemental drug therapy (52 percent for beta blockers versus 38 percent for diuretics).

In a direct comparison between the two treatment arms in the MRC trial in older adults, diuretics were significantly better than beta blockers: the cumulative incidences of coronary events were 44.4 per 1,000 for diuretics and 72.6 per 1,000 for beta blockers (risk reduction of 39 percent [95 percent CI, 13 percent to 57 percent] in favor of the diuretics); and the cumulative incidences of stroke were 41.6 per 1,000 for diuretics and 50.8 per 1,000 for beta blockers (risk reduction of 18 percent [95 percent CI = −20 percent to 44 percent] in favor of diuretics). Loss to follow-up in the MRC trial was high, about 25 percent of subjects in the trial. The cumulative percentages of subjects who stopped taking their randomized therapy, including withdrawal of medications and loss to follow-up, were 48 percent of the diuretic group, 63 percent of the beta-blocker group, and 53 percent of the placebo group.

Two of us (B.P., C.F.) recently reviewed the randomized trials of antihypertensive therapy in the elderly (27). The eight clinical trials, which all included a control group, were divided into those that used diuretics or beta blockers as first-line therapy (Fig. 4). Compared with control, diuretics reduced the risk of CHD (risk reduction of 21 percent with 95 percent CI of 10 percent to 31 percent) and stroke (risk reduction of 35 percent with 95 percent CI of 25 percent to 46 percent); beta blockers reduced the risk of stroke (risk reduction of 31 percent with 95 percent CI of 13 percent to 45 percent) but not coronary heart disease (risk reduction 1 percent with 95 percent CI of 19 percent–22 percent). However, the lower confidence limit (19 percent risk reduction) almost overlaps the estimated risk reduction with diuretics. While both diuretics and beta blockers reduced the incidence of congestive heart failure in the elderly, only the diuretics were associated with a statistically significant reduction in total mortality (Fig. 4). Again, it should be noted that the confidence limits for each drug included the point estimate for the other. In general, the recent clinical trials that studied diuretics as first-line therapy in the elderly used diuretics in low doses and sometimes in

combination with potassium-sparing agents; and these low-dose diuretic therapies may be responsible for the beneficial effect of diuretics on CHD in the elderly (28).

In summary, the treatment trials support the recent recommendations from the Joint National Committee: "Because diuretics and beta-blockers are the only classes of drugs that have been used in long-term controlled clinical trials and shown to reduce morbidity and mortality, they are recommended as first-choice agents unless they are contra-indicated or unacceptable, or unless there are special indications for other agents." (29) The other classes of antihypertensive agents, including calcium-channel blockers, ACE inhibitors, and alpha blockers, have not been evaluated in long-term trials with major disease endpoints as the primary outcome, although several such trials are ongoing or being planned (19,30,31).

Trials of Pharmacologic and Nonpharmacologic Therapies

Diuretics and beta blockers have been available as pharmacologic therapies for hypertension since the 1950s and the 1960s, respectively (32). In the last decade, a variety of new agents have been approved for the treatment of hypertension, and the clinical trials that led to

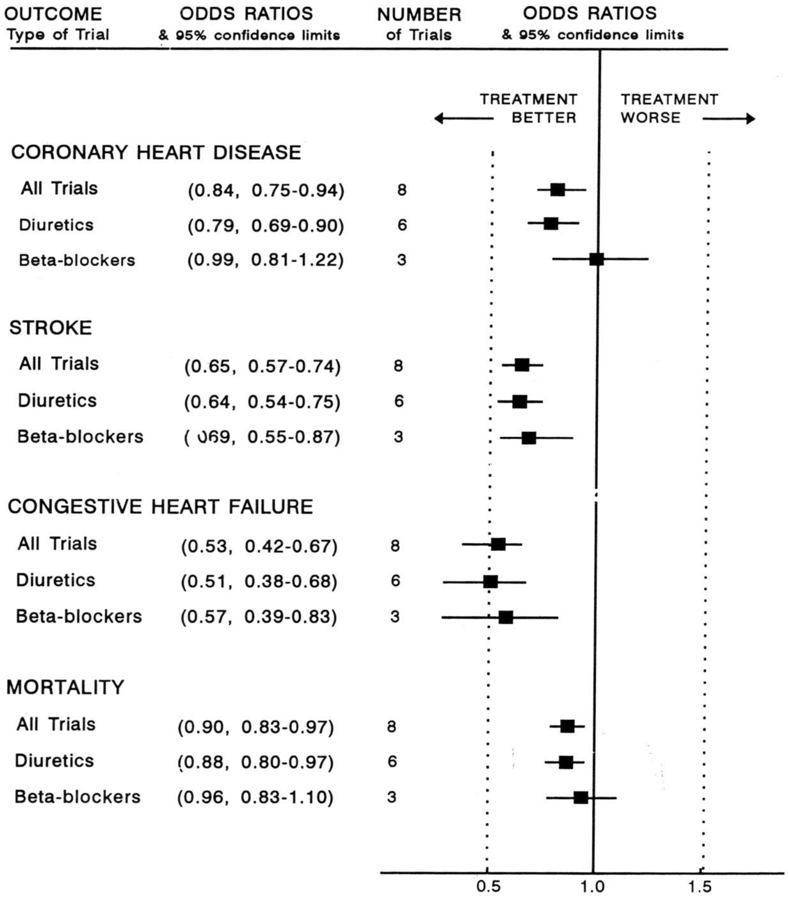

OUTCOME Type of Trial	ODDS RATIOS & 95% confidence limits	NUMBER of Trials	ODDS RATIOS & 95% confidence limits
CORONARY HEART DISEASE			
All Trials	(0.84, 0.75-0.94)	8	
Diuretics	(0.79, 0.69-0.90)	6	
Beta-blockers	(0.99, 0.81-1.22)	3	
STROKE			
All Trials	(0.65, 0.57-0.74)	8	
Diuretics	(0.64, 0.54-0.75)	6	
Beta-blockers	(0.69, 0.55-0.87)	3	
CONGESTIVE HEART FAILURE			
All Trials	(0.53, 0.42-0.67)	8	
Diuretics	(0.51, 0.38-0.68)	6	
Beta-blockers	(0.57, 0.39-0.83)	3	
MORTALITY			
All Trials	(0.90, 0.83-0.97)	8	
Diuretics	(0.88, 0.80-0.97)	6	
Beta-blockers	(0.96, 0.83-1.10)	3	

FIG. 4. Effects of antihypertensive treatment, according to class of first-line drugs, on CHD, stroke, congestive heart failure, and total mortality from the combined results of eight randomized trials in the elderly. (From the American Heart Association, 1993, with permission.)

FDA approval for these new agents generally compared only one new agent to placebo in an effort to demonstrate an effect on BP level. The Treatment of Mild Hypertension Study (TOMHS) included multiple agents within a single study (17). A multicenter randomized placebo-controlled clinical trial of a nutritional-hygienic regimen alone or with one of five drugs as monotherapy, TOMHS focused on a variety of endpoints, including measures of quality of life and subclinical disease such as left ventricular mass.

Men and women 45 to 69 years of age were eligible for TOMHS if their DBP averaged 90–99 mm Hg over three visits; those already on treatment were withdrawn from therapy and were eligible if DBP averaged 85–99 mm Hg. All subjects received nutritional-hygienic intervention that focused on a reduction in weight, sodium intake, and alcohol intake as well as an increase in physical activity. With perhaps the exception of acebutolol, the five study drugs were initially given in low doses.

Table 3 summarizes the primary results of TOMHS after 4 years of follow-up. Compared with placebo, all forms of drug therapy reduced SBP and DBP significantly. The diuretic-reduced systolic pressure the most. Levels of total and low-density lipoprotein (LDL) cholesterol declined and levels of high-density lipoprotein (HDL) increased in all groups over 4 years (Table 3). Doxazosin was associated with the most favorable lipid changes; compared with other agents, acebutolol produced a larger LDL reduction, but a smaller HDL rise. Interestingly, after 1 year of follow-up in TOMHS, chlorthalidone had been associated with a statistically significant adverse effect on total cholesterol and LDL cholesterol compared with the other active therapies; but at 4 years, although the declines in total and LDL cholesterol were smallest among those on chlorthalidone, the difference between chlorthalidone and the other active treatments was no longer significant. While the effects of diuretics and beta blockers on lipids are relatively well-known (33), TOMHS has provided important comparisons of three other classes of drugs within a single study.

Compared with placebo in TOMHS, pharmacologic therapy with any of the five agents (combined for this analysis) was associated with a nonsignificant reduction in major cardiovascular events (relative risk = 0.64 with 95% CI of 0.35–1.18; $p = 0.15$). TOMHS also included measures of subclinical disease (Table 3). Due to a reduction in left ventricular volume, chlorthalidone was associated with the largest decrease in echocardiographic left ventricular mass ($p < 0.01$ compared with enalapril). By echocardiogram, the incidence of left ventricular hypertrophy (LVH) did not differ among treatments; the incidence of LVH by electrocardiogram (ECG) was highest for placebo and acebutolol, and was reduced among those on amlodipine compared with acebutolol. There were no significant differences in the incidence of ST segment depression by ambulatory ECG. The use of technologies such as echocardiogram and ECG to evaluate antihypertensive therapies is an important recent development. Not all new therapies can be evaluated in clinical trials that have as their primary outcomes major disease endpoints. It can be argued that measures of subclinical disease are a better surrogate for the events of interest in trials of antihypertensive therapy than are their effects on BP levels or cardiovascular risk factors such as lipids. In addition to electrocardiography and echocardiography, carotid ultrasound is also being used to assess the effects of antihypertensive therapy on arterial-wall thickness as a measure of atherosclerosis (34).

Table 3 also includes data on the seven quality-of-life measures used in TOMHS. Compared with placebo, acebutolol and chlorthalidone were both associated with significant improvements in the overall test that combined the seven quality-of-life indices ($p < 0.01$). At the doses used in this trial, there were few differences among specific drugs for the seven quality-of-life measures considered individually. For instance, the general health index was better among those on acebutolol compared with amlodipine, enalapril, and placebo ($p < 0.01$); chlorthalidone was associated with increased energy and improved general functioning compared with placebo ($p < 0.01$); the mental health index was significantly improved among those on either chlorthalidone or acebutolol compared with those on placebo ($p < 0.01$); social contacts were reduced among those on chlorthalidone compared with amlodipine ($p < 0.01$); but there were no significant differences among drugs in the index for satisfaction with physical abilities. The comparable effects of these five drug therapies in low doses on measures of quality of life are new and important findings. In the context of some of the industry-sponsored trials (35,36), the beneficial effects of diuretics and beta blockers on quality-of-life measures are perhaps surprising.

In the Trial of Antihypertensive Interventions and Management (TAIM), investigators used a factorial design to study the effect of diet and drug therapies on BP level and quality of life, including sexual function (37,38). Among men on their usual diet, erection-related problems were worse in those taking chlorthalidone compared with either placebo ($p = 0.009$) or atenolol ($p < 0.05$). A weight-reduction diet ameliorated this adverse effect of chlorthalidone. Compared with usual diet or the weight-reduction diet, the low-sodium/high-potassium diet was associated with significantly greater fatigue. The weight-loss diet had the greatest benefit on quality of life: total physical complaints were decreased ($p < 0.001$), and satisfaction with health was increased ($p < 0.001$) (38).

The studies on antihypertensive therapy and quality of life published before 1991 have recently been reviewed (39). This metanalysis included 1,620 subjects from nine trials. For the five constructs—sexual function, sleep,

TABLE 3. *Change from baseline in blood pressure, quality of life, cholesterol, and incidence of selected measures of subclinical disease for participants in Treatment of Mild Hypertension Study by treatment group[a]*

	Acebutolol N = 126	Amlodipine maleate N = 120	Chorthalidone N = 124	Doxazosin mesylate N = 129	Enalapril maleate N = 127	Placebo N = 221
Systolic BP, mm Hg[b]	−17.0	−15.6	−17.7	−12.2	−14.7	−9.1
Diastolic BP, mm Hg[c]	−13.1	−12.9	−12.3	−11.7	−11.5	−8.6
Total cholesterol[d]						
mmol/L	−0.30	−0.17	−0.12	−0.36	−0.21	−0.13
mg/dL	−11.7	−6.7	−4.5	−13.8	−8.0	−5.1
LDL cholesterol[e]						
mmol/L	−0.27	−0.13	−0.09	−0.29	−0.15	−0.09
mg/dL	−10.6	−5.1	−3.6	−11.3	−5.9	−3.6
HDL cholesterol[f]						
mmol/L	0.006	0.05	0.05	0.06	0.07	0.04
mg/dL	0.2	2.0	2.1	2.4	2.6	1.4
General health index[g]	2.2	0.6	1.5	1.2	0.8	1.0
Energy/fatigue index[h]	1.4	0.7	1.4	0.5	0.8	0.7
Mental health index[i]	3.1	2.0	2.7	1.6	1.3	1.4
General functioning index[j]	0.1	0.1	0.1	−0.3	−0.1	−0.3
Satisfaction with physical abilities	0.4	0.5	0.4	0.3	0.4	0.3
Social functioning relative to others[k]	0.2	0.1	0.2	0.0	0.1	−0.1
Social contacts[l]	0.1	0.4	−0.2	0.0	0.1	0.2
ECHO LV mass, grams[m]	−24	−25	−34	−24	−23	−27
ECHO LVH incidence, %[n]	12.6	11.5	11.9	9.3	16.5	13.1
ECG LVH incidence by MC, %[o]	5.4	0.0	1.6	2.3	0.0	4.8
Tall R-waves incidence by ECG, %[p]	15.5	3.4	1.8	6.5	3.4	11.7
ECG VCD incidence, %[q]	17.9	7.6	19.7	8.1	12.4	9.3
ST depression on ambulatory ECG, %	19.6	20.2	26.3	18.4	26.9	19.6

[a] BP, blood pressure; LDL, low-density lipoprotein; HDL, high-density lipoprotein; ECHO, echocardiographic; LV, left-ventricular; LVH, LV hypertrophy; ECG, electrocardiographic; MC, Minnesota code; VCD, ventricular conduction defect. For the measures of quality of life, higher numbers indicate better quality.

[b] $p < 0.01$ for each active drug treatment vs. placebo; acebutolol vs. doxazosin; chlorthalidone vs. doxazosin and enalapril; and all active drug treatments combined vs. placebo based on longitudinal analysis.

[c] $p < 0.01$ for each active drug treatment vs. placebo; and all active drug treatments combined vs. placebo based on longitudinal analysis.

[d] $p < 0.01$ for doxazosin vs. amlodipine, chlorthalidone and placebo; and acebutolol vs. chlorthalidone based on longitudinal analysis.

[e] $p < 0.01$ for doxazosin vs. amlodipine, chlorthalidone and placebo; and acebutolol vs. chlorthalidone and placebo based on longitudinal analysis.

[f] $p < 0.01$ for acebutolol vs. doxazosin and enalapril based on longitudinal analysis.

[g] $p < 0.01$ for amlodipine, enalapril, and placebo vs. acebutolol based on longitudinal analysis.

[h] $p < 0.01$ for placebo vs. chlorthalidone based on longitudinal analysis.

[i] $p < 0.01$ for placebo vs. acebutolol and chlorthalidone; and placebo vs. all active drug treatments based on longitudinal analysis.

[j] $p < 0.01$ for placebo vs. chlorthalidone based on longitudinal analysis.

[k] $p < 0.01$ for placebo vs. acebutolol; and placebo vs. all active drug treatments combined based on longitudinal analysis.

[l] $p < 0.01$ for chlorthalidone vs. amlodipine based on longitudinal analysis.

[m] $p < 0.01$ for chlorthalidone vs. enalapril based on longitudinal analysis.

[n] LV mass index at least 134 g/m^2 for men and at least 110 g/m^2 for women.

[o] $p < 0.01$ for amlodipine vs. acebutolol.

[p] $p < 0.01$ for amlodipine, chlorthalidone, and enalapril vs. acebutolol; amlodipine, chlorthalidone, and enalapril vs. placebo; and all active drug treatments combined vs. placebo.

[q] $p < 0.01$ for amlodipine and placebo vs. chlorthalidone.

psychomotor, general well-being, and mood—Beto and Bansal reported that the various pharmacologic drug groups were associated with either no effect or a small improvement in quality of life. They identified no negative effect of treatment.

In general, dietary modifications to reduce weight or to lower sodium intake result in more modest BP decreases than drug therapy (17,37). These nutritional-hygienic approaches nonetheless remain important adjuncts to pharmacologic therapy. In clinical trials, interventions to decrease weight and sodium intake have reduced the need for or decreased the number of drugs required for

BP control (40) and permitted up to 40% of subjects with mild hypertension to stop pharmacologic therapy for as long as 4 years (41,42).

CLINICAL TRIALS THAT ADDRESS QUESTIONS RELATED TO PREVENTION OF HYPERTENSION

Background

The availability of effective therapy for reducing the morbid complications of hypertension, and for prolonging survival of hypertensive patients, has resulted in widespread and increasing use of antihypertensive drugs (29). Despite the generally acknowledged public health benefits from such treatment, concerns are often raised about prospects of decades-long treatment—usually requiring antihypertensive drugs—for 20 percent or more of the adult population. All drugs have side effects, and costs of medical care are considerable. For these reasons, the primary prevention of hypertension is considered a desirable goal.

Consideration of primary prevention inevitably raises questions of what it is that one wishes to prevent: What is the nature of the hypertensive condition(s)? Conventional definitions of hypertension are arbitrary. The relationship between BP and cardiovascular risks is continuous, as demonstrated most clearly among the approximately 350,000 men without a history of prior myocardial infarction and 35–57 years of age when screened during 1973–1975 for the Multiple Risk Factor Intervention Trial (43). Indeed, these and other long-term cohort studies show that SBP and DBP ". . . have continuous, graded, strong, independent, etiologically significant relationships to the outcome variables. These relationships are documented for young, middle-aged, and older men and for middle-aged and older women of varying socioeconomic backgrounds and ethnicity. Among persons aged 35 years or more, most have SBP/DBP above optimal (>120/>80 mm Hg); hence, they are at increased CVD risk, i.e., the blood pressure problem involves most of the population, not only the substantial minority with clinical HBP. For middle-aged and older persons, SBP related even more strongly to risk than DBP; at every DBP level, higher SBP results in greater CVD risk and curtailment of life expectancy" (43).

This concept of continuous risk has two important implications. First, the goal of preventive strategies should not be confined solely to reducing the incidence of clinically diagnosed hypertension, but should also include avoiding the rise in BP with age beyond that accompanying normal growth. The objective is to shift the entire BP distribution toward lower levels. Secondly, evidence about BP-lowering effects of various interventions derived from clinical trials in hypertensive patients is likely to be generalizable to nonhypertensive individuals. Thus, this review encompasses trials in both kinds of study populations. Trials of lifestyle interventions in hypertensive groups are largely short-term, with follow-up periods of weeks or months, in part because many such subjects eventually require addition of hypertensive drugs. Although many trials in nonhypertensive persons are also short-term, some investigators have conducted long-term studies using *incidence of hypertension* as an outcome measure, and these important trials are described separately. Finally, this review also includes data from observational epidemiologic studies that have generated hypotheses for testing in trials, as well as providing important information in their own right regarding etiologic factors.

Population studies of various designs, as well as clinical and animal experimental research, have clearly shown that the control of BP and the etiology of hypertension are multifactorial. Hence, although scientific understanding is advanced by designs and analytic methods that isolate the effects of individual factors, practical application also requires evidence on whether effects are additive, whether they interact in various ways, and whether they are consistent in various population groups. Despite advances in our understanding of etiology and prevention, it is clear that many of these issues require further study.

Short-term and Single-factor Trials

Weight Control and Physical Activity

Nearly all observational studies, cross-sectional or longitudinal, have found adiposity to be strongly associated with BP and prevalence or incidence of hypertension, both in adults and children (44,45). Adiposity is usually measured indirectly by the body mass index (BMI), which is weight divided by height squared. The associations with BMI have been observed in many ethnic groups and societies and across a wide range of adiposity. Furthermore, it is not merely an artifact of arm and BP cuff size. Most randomized trials of weight loss diets in hypertensive patients have found reductions in DBP and SBP (46). However, only in the past few years have these findings been replicated in nonhypertensive subjects— middle-aged adults with "high-normal" DBP (47,48). With regard to the issue of whether adiposity is simply a marker of excess intake of specific nutrients such as sodium, these recent trials have demonstrated small or no group differences in urinary sodium excretion.

Since physical activity, as part of caloric balance, influences weight, distinguishing a physical-activity effect on BP from that of body weight can be difficult. Nevertheless, a number of observational studies have reported an inverse association between BP/hypertension and physical activity and/or fitness that is at least in part independent of adiposity (49–52). The relationship has been documented in several age and ethnic groups, and may be stronger in women, perhaps because in Western societies their level of activity is lower, a range where the effect may be more pronounced (53–55). Indeed, one of the conclusions stated in Arroll and Beaglehole's review of clinical trials (56) is that lower-intensity/higher-frequency activity is probably as effective as or more effective than higher-intensity exercise, and this finding was confirmed by a subsequent trial in Japanese hypertensive patients (57). That review of 22 studies (13 controlled trials) concludes that although most did not meet high quality standards, an independent BP-lowering effect is likely.

Alcohol Consumption

Nearly all of about 30 cross-sectional epidemiologic studies in diverse populations, reviewed by MacMahon, found a direct association of alcohol intake with BP level or prevalence of hypertension, and many showed an apparent threshold at approximately three drinks (about 40 gm ethanol) per day (58). More recent studies, better controlled for confounding factors such as body mass, physical activity, and sodium intake, have reported similar findings (59–61). Prospective observational studies, including those with information on change in alcohol intake, have found consistent results (62–64). Several randomized trials have been conducted, including two by Australian investigators comparing low- versus normal-alcohol beer in 6-week crossover designs (65,66). In both trials, one in hypertensive subjects and the other in normotensives, significant lowering of SBP and DBP by 3–5 mm Hg was associated with alcohol reductions of about 80 percent, to a level of about three drinks per week. Less extreme change in intake, obtained with individual counseling, has yielded only suggestive evidence of a BP-lowering effect in one small trial (67); a larger, long-term U.S. trial involving a similar intervention is underway (68). A recent trial of the aforementioned crossover design has demonstrated the independence and additive nature of BP reduction with alcohol restriction and weight loss, using a 2 × 2 factorial design (69).

Sodium and Potassium Intake

Observational studies of sodium intake and BP have had to contend with the major challenge of characterizing individuals' usual intakes, which vary a great deal from day to day in most populations (70). In order to capture both discretionary (via the saltshaker) and nondiscretionary intake, measurement needs to employ timed urine collections, usually for 24 hours, a cumbersome method. Significant direct associations between sodium and BP (particularly systolic) have been found by pooling data from many populations, both without (71) and with (72) control for multiple confounding factors. In INTERSALT, a second 24-hour urine was also collected on a subsample to adjust for the underestimation of regression coefficients by imprecisely measuring usual intake (72). Law and colleagues have shown that with this adjustment for so-called regression dilution bias, the strength of the sodium-BP relationship *within* populations is quite consistent with that observed *across* populations (73,74).

Epidemiologic studies have also used the ratio of sodium to potassium urinary concentrations as a predictor of BP levels, for physiologic as well as methodologic reasons. (This simple measure eliminates the need for timed 24-hour urine collections.) This ratio has consistently shown a direct association with BP levels, but so has potassium excretion alone (inversely) (75). Thus, as for all ratios, the individual effects of the components cannot easily be etiologically disentangled.

Clinical trials have established that sodium reduction lowers BP, both in hypertensive and nonhypertensive subjects, and have suggested an effect of increased potassium as well. In pooled analyses that included 22 randomized trials, sodium reduction—typically, by 80–100 mmol/day—lowered SBP and DBP by about 5/3 mm Hg in hypertensives and 2/1 mm Hg in nonhypertensives (76). Five subsequent trials have all shown significant reductions in DBP, about 6 mm Hg in hypertensives, 2–4 mm Hg in nonhypertensives (48,77–80). Two of these were factorial trials in which the other intervention (low-fat/high-fiber diet, fish oil) had no effect (79,80). In the first double-blind, crossover trial of sodium repletion in normotensives (84), the results extended the positive findings seen in similar trials in hypertensives. Finally and perhaps most importantly, the Trials of Hypertension Prevention (TOHP), Phase I, was the largest trial in normotensives to date that achieved long-term net reduction of sodium intake through dietary counseling, and significant BP-lowering was seen (48). Details are described in the next section.

Two metanalyses of potassium supplementation trials have found significant BP-lowering in trials studying hypertensives, of about 5/3 mm Hg (81,82). Of these reviews, only Whelton et al. also separately pooled the results of six randomized trials in normotensives, including the large TOHP sample, and found only a small, nonsignificant trend toward BP reduction. Moreover, almost all of the 22 randomized trials tested potassium salts delivered by pill in large doses (60–120 mmol/day), which are not likely to be achievable by dietary means. Indeed, Siani et al. (83) recently reported a 1-year dietary intervention trial in hypertensives in which they succeeded in raising potassium excretion by only 20–25 mmol/day; this amount was, however, associated with ability to reduce substantially the amount of antihypertensive medication.

Magnesium and Fiber

Because levels of potassium, magnesium, and certain types of dietary fiber are highly correlated in foods, it has been difficult to isolate their respective associations with BP in observational studies (84). In two large prospective studies among health professionals using self-reported BP and incident hypertension as outcome variables, all three dietary components were inversely associated with these endpoints in some analyses. However, after adjustment for the other two dietary variables, results were inconsistent: magnesium was the most robust predictor in women (nurses) and fiber in men (other health professionals) (85,86). Seven randomized trials of magnesium supplementation, six of which studied primarily hypertensive subjects, found no significant BP reduction (48,87,88), except for one trial of thiazide-treated hypertensive patients (89). Subgroup analysis suggested an effect in those with low pretreatment urinary magnesium (88), but this finding was not confirmed in the large TOHP trial (48), in which a significant increase in lower gastrointestinal complaints was also seen. As for fiber, only one of six trials testing an increase in wheat bran, pectin, oat bran, or a fiber mixture (in some cases, combined with reduced fat intake) reported BP reduction (79,90–94).

Several possible explanations have been proposed for the contrast between results of observational studies of magnesium, fiber, and potassium (in normotensives) and findings from clinical trials: (a) each component may individually have a small effect, difficult to detect with the small-to-moderate sample sizes in most trials; (b) they may have additive or even interactive (synergistic) effects, especially when consumed as foods rather than supplements; and/or (c) there may be susceptible subgroups that are not as well represented in trial volunteers as in population-based studies. The notion of combined effects is concordant with observational and intervention studies of vegetarian diets, which have rather consistently shown a relationship with lower BP levels (95).

Macronutrients

The literature on vegetarian diets and BP has fueled investigation into the roles of dietary fat and protein. Observational studies of fat and BP have had mixed results. For example, analyses from the Multiple Risk Factor Intervention Trial, based on averaging 4 to 5 annual 24-hour dietary recalls, have shown significant direct associations of SBP with saturated fatty acids (percent Kcal),

dietary cholesterol (mg/1,000 Kcal), and Key's formula (96). On the other hand, neither of the large health professional cohort studies found associations between BP and total fat or specific types of fatty acids (85,86). Of the randomized trials that reduced total fat and/or saturated fatty acids (SFA) and replaced the calories with carbohydrates, monounsaturates, or polyunsaturated fatty acids (PFA), or simply increased the PFA/SFA ratio with a linoleic acid supplement, only one reported significantly reduced BP (79,92,97–104).

With regard to the small fraction of fat intake consisting of omega-3 (n-3) PFAs (found in higher-fat fish or commercial fish oil), the observational epidemiologic evidence is scant, but nearly 20 randomized trials have been conducted, generally using encapsulated fish oil. A metanalysis including 17 of the trials concluded that the BP effect from the trials in normotensives was small and only marginally significant, while among hypertensives, it was significant and substantial (5.5/3.5 mm Hg, for SBP and DBP, respectively) (105). This seems to represent at least in part a dose-response phenomenon: (a) all but two of the trials in hypertensives used doses of >3 gm/day of n-3 PFAs; (b) one trial found an effect with 15 gm/day but none with 3 gm/day (106); and (c) the TOHP component that also tested 3 gm/day with a large sample size found no effect (48). Moreover, TOHP showed a substantial incidence of unpleasant side effects with fish oil capsules, and increasing n-3 PFA consumption by >3 gm/day through dietary means appears to be impractical.

The studies on vegetarians suggest that a decrease in animal protein or increase in vegetable protein might lower BP. This effect has not been observed in three small controlled trials (107–109). Recently, a series of analyses from large observational studies have added strength to the hypothesis that higher total or vegetable protein intake might decrease BP levels (96,110,111). This hypothesis has probably not been adequately tested in the aforementioned trials.

Calcium Intake

While most of the more than 30 observational studies have found inverse associations between calcium intake, or calcium-rich foods, and BP or prevalence of hypertension, there have been notable exceptions, including most analyses from the U.S. National Health and Nutrition Examination Surveys (112). Of the two large prospective studies in health professionals mentioned previously, an inverse association with hypertension incidence was found in women but not in men (86,87). In both studies, the association tended to be more evident in leaner, younger persons. In keeping with these apparent effect modifiers (age, BMI), a study in 3- to 6-year-old children reported an inverse relationship with systolic (but not diastolic) BP, measured at the end of a 1-year period during which ten dietary records were collected (113).

Of the 25 randomized trials testing increased calcium intake, 12 studied normotensives. Six of these found significant reductions in systolic and/or diastolic BP. However, the largest trial, TOHP, was negative (48), and a pooled analysis of all 12 trials found no significant effects (estimated mean changes of about $-1/-0.5$ mm Hg) (114). All but three of these trials used calcium salts in fairly large doses (1.0–1.5 gm of calcium/day). The others increased calcium consumption from foods, and each observed a fall in either SBP or DBP, but not both (115–117). Even when a pooled analysis included the trials in hypertensives, the effect estimate was small ($-1.5/-0.3$ mm Hg), and was significant only for SBP (114). Just as with the inconsistency between observational and trial findings for other dietary factors (see above), explanations may lie in uncontrolled confounders in the diet or heterogeneity of response among population subgroups.

Stress Management

The well-established relationships between acute stress and BP, along with numerous physiologic and hormonal mediators, have stimulated many epidemiologic studies of chronic stress and BP levels or hypertension (119). One of the most promising formulations of the chronic stress concept has been "job strain," defined as work with high psychological demand and low decision latitude. However, various studies have found both positive and no associations between this measure and hypertension (118–120). Some of the inconsistency may be due to interactions with gender and alcohol consumption (121,122). Other studies have suggested that race (black versus white) may be an important effect modifier (123).

Examination of such potential heterogeneity has not been a prime focus of clinical trials, which have tested such interventions as progressive muscle relaxation, biofeedback, and cognitive coping methods, generally in unselected hypertensive patients. In one review of 25 randomized trials, about half of the trials showed significant BP reduction (124). but in a collaborative metanalysis of 12 trials there was little evidence of an overall BP effect (125). In the only large, long-term (18-month) trial in normotensive subjects, the TOHP found no effect of stress management on BP (48).

Incidence Trials

Three groups of investigators have undertaken long-term trials of lifestyle modification in nonhypertensive subjects with high-normal DBP, and reported on hypertension incidence as a primary or secondary endpoint. The Primary Prevention of Hypertension (PPH) study was a 5-year trial that tested a multifactor intervention

(weight loss, reduction of sodium and alcohol intake, increased physical activity). Hypertension incidence was significantly reduced, by 54 percent (cumulative incidence of 8.8 percent and 19.2 percent, for intervention and control groups, respectively). Correlational analysis implicated weight loss (average of 3 kg) and, to a lesser extent, sodium reduction (average of 20 percent) as the main factors in the BP reduction (126). Subsequently, the Hypertension Prevention Trial tested these two interventions, separately and combined, as well as the combination of sodium reduction and increased dietary potassium, in a 3-year trial with a similar population as the PPH study. Significant reductions in SBP and DBP (about 2 mm Hg) were seen with weight loss, and a trend toward lower incidence of hypertension. The very modest reduction in sodium intake (about 10 percent at end of follow-up) was not associated with significant mean BP reduction, but again a trend toward lower hypertension incidence was seen. The two combined interventions did not produce significant BP effects, due probably to lesser weight loss when the weight intervention was combined with sodium reduction compared with weight reduction alone, and to the limited ability to increase potassium intake by diet (47).

The first phase of the TOHP, alluded to in earlier sections of this chapter, was designed to detect small effects on mean BP of seven interventions, tested individually during a 6-month (dietary supplements) or 18-month (lifestyle change) period. As noted previously, none of the supplements—calcium, magnesium, potassium, fish oil—showed significant effects, nor did stress management. Weight loss (which included an exercise component) and sodium reduction produced significant BP reductions through end of follow-up of 2–3 mm Hg systolic and 1–2 mm Hg diastolic. Furthermore, hypertension incidence was also reduced by 51 percent with weight loss (statistically significant) and 24 percent with sodium reduction (48). Given the modest lifestyle changes achieved (net reductions of 3.7 kg and 44 mmol sodium/24 hr, respectively, at 18 months), these incidence effects are impressive. Phase II of TOHP, a 3-year trial, is further evaluating benefits of sodium reduction and weight loss, singly and in combination, and will provide a more precise estimate of effects on hypertension incidence.

In summary, evidence from clinical trials and observational studies are concordant in supporting the efficacy of weight loss, sodium reduction, moderation of alcohol intake, and increased physical activity for prevention of hypertension (Table 4). The evidence is discordant or lacking in important respects with regard to dietary supplementation with potassium, magnesium, calcium, or fiber; macronutrient alterations; and stress management. Trials of increasing some nutrients also have raised questions of feasibility, as lifestyle changes, or tolerability, as dietary supplements.

TABLE 4. *Trial results on efficacy of interventions for primary prevention of hypertension*

Documented efficacy	
Weight loss	Reduced alcohol consumption
Exercise	Reduced sodium intake

Limited or unproven efficacy	
Potassium supplementation	Macronutrient alteration
Magnesium supplementation	Fish oil supplementation
Fiber supplementation	Calcium supplementation
Stress management	

Adapted from ref. 114.

CONCLUSIONS

Clinical trials completed during the past 25 years have provided a firm knowledge base for controlling hypertension to achieve substantial public health benefits. The effectiveness of pharmacologic treatment of diastolic (or combined) and, now, isolated systolic hypertension in reducing cardiovascular morbidity and mortality, and hence total mortality, is well established. Symptomatic side effects, occasionally troubling to patients, do occur with all agents, but with low doses, with substitution of drugs as necessary, and especially with accompanying lifestyle treatments, quality of life is on average not impaired. Although there is much reassuring evidence to the contrary, some clinicians remain concerned that "excessive" BP reduction may be hazardous to some patients; ongoing or proposed trials should help to resolve this issue.

Because of the very high prevalence of hypertension in most populations, there is justifiable concern about where the limits of treatment should be set, given the aggregate demands on health care resources. Expert groups, reflecting different social milieus for health care decision-making, not surprisingly propose different answers to the question of "whom to treat" (29,127,128). In addition to absolute risk of patients selected for treatments, the cost-effectiveness of treatment depends to a considerable extent on selection of modes of treatment, particularly choice of drugs (129). For the majority of patients, there is no firm basis for choosing more expensive drugs, but results of ongoing trials are needed to inform such judgments further.

Lifestyle counseling is effective for some patients, but if required on an indefinite basis through a traditional clinical setting, may not be more cost-effective than drugs (130). However, from a philosophic viewpoint it is probably not desirable to maintain hundreds of millions of people, worldwide, on decades of drug treatment, if there are safe and inexpensive alternatives. Current knowledge of etiology (including prevention trials), while certainly incomplete, does provide the means for building preventive strategies. To the extent that these are fashioned as community-wide efforts—a population strategy—in addition to high-risk approaches through primary medical care, the control of hypertension through prevention may well be more cost-effective, and has the potential to address above-optimal but nonhypertensive BP levels as well. Convincing evidence that this potential can be realized will also require intervention trials, a challenge to public health researchers at least as great as that successfully met by clinical trials in the past.

ACKNOWLEDGMENTS

Dr. MacMahon is the recipient of a Senior Research Fellowship from the Health Research Council of New Zealand. Dr. Psaty's work was supported in part by Grants HL43201 and AG09556 from the National Institutes of Health. He is also a Merck/SER Clinical Epidemiology Fellow (sponsored by the Merck Co. Foundation, Rahway, NJ, and the Society for Epidemiologic Research, Baltimore, MD). The expert typing and editorial assistance of Ms. Colleen Brown is gratefully acknowledged.

REFERENCES

1. Collins R, Peto R, MacMahon S, et al. Blood pressure, stroke, and coronary heart disease. Part 2, short-term reductions in blood pressure: overview of randomised drug trials in their epidemiological context. *Lancet* 1990;335:827–838.
2. MacMahon S, Peto R, Cutler J, et al. Blood pressure, stroke, and coronary heart disease: Part 1, prolonged differences in blood pressure: prospective observational studies corrected for the regression dilution bias. *Lancet* 1990;335:765–774.
3. Amery A, Brixko P, Clement D, et al. Mortality and morbidity results from the European Working Party on High Blood Pressure in the Elderly Trial. *Lancet* 1985;1:1349–1354.
4. Coope J, Warrender TS. Randomised trial of treatment of hypertension in elderly patients in primary care. *Br Med J* 1986;293:1145–1152.
5. SHEP Cooperative Research Group. Prevention of stroke by antihypertensive drug treatment in older persons with isolated systolic hypertension: final results of the Systolic Hypertension in the Elderly Program (SHEP). *J Am Med Assoc* 1991;265:3255–3264.
6. Dahlof B, Lindeholm LH, Hansson L, Schersten B, Ekbom T, Wester P-O. Morbidity and mortality in the Swedish Trial in Old Patients with Hypertension (STOP-Hypertension). *Lancet* 1991;338:1281–1284.
7. MRC Working Party. Medical Research Council trial of treatment of hypertension in older adults: principal results. *Br Med J* 1992;304:405–412.
8. Peto R, Yusuf S, Collins R. Cholesterol-lowering trial results in their epidemiologic context. *Circulation* 1985;72(Suppl III):451.
9. Cruickshank JM, Thorp JM, Zacharias FJ. Benefits and potential harm of lowering high blood pressure. *Lancet* 1987;1:581–584.
10. Farnett L, Mulrow CD, Linn WD, Lucey CR, Tuley MR. The J-curve phenomenon and the treatment of hypertension. Is there a point beyond which pressure reduction is dangerous? *J Am Med Assoc* 1991;265:489–495.
11. MacMahon S, Sharpe N. The J-curve phenomenon and the treatment of hypertension. *J Am Med Assoc* 1991;266:64–65.
12. Carter AB. Hypotensive therapy in stroke survivors. *Lancet* 1970;1:485–489.

13. Hypertension-Stroke Cooperative Study Group. Effect of antihypertensive treatment on stroke recurrence. *J Am Med Assoc* 1974;229:409–418.

14. Pfeffer MA, Braunwald E, Moye LA, et al. Effect of captopril on mortality and morbidity in patients with left ventricular dysfunction after myocardial infarction: results of the Survival and Ventricular Enlargement Trial. *N Engl J Med* 1992;327:669–677.

15. Yusuf S, Pepine CJ, Garces C, et al. Effect of enalapril on myocardial infarction and unstable angina in patients with low ejection fractions. *Lancet* 1992;340:1173–1178.

16. The Beta-Blocker Pooling Research Group. The Beta-Blocker Pooling Project (BBPP): subgroup findings from randomized trials in post infarction patients. *Eur Heart J* 1988;9:8–16.

17. The TIA Trial Study Group. Trial of secondary prevention with atenolol after transient ischemic attack or non-disabling ischemic stroke. *Stroke* 1993;24:543–548.

18. Neaton JD, Grimm RH Jr, Prineas RJ, et al. Treatment of Mild Hypertension Study (TOMHS): final results. *J Am Med Assoc* 1993;270:713–724.

19. Hansson L, Dahlöf B, Abelin J, for the BBB study group. Cardiovascular morbidity and mortality in BBB Study. *Proceedings of the European Society of Hypertension meeting.* Milan, Italy, 1993.

20. Hansson L, Hedner T, Dahlof B. Prospective Randomized Open Blinded Endpoint (PROBE) Study: a novel design for intervention trials. *Blood Pressure* 1992;1:113–119.

21. Dennis M, Bamford J, Sandercock P, Warlow C. Prognosis of transient ischemic attacks in the Oxfordshire Community Stroke Project. *Stroke* 1990;21:848–853.

22. Held PH, Yusuf S, Furberg CD. Calcium channel blockers in acute myocardial infarction and unstable angina: an overview. *Br Med J* 1989;299:1187–1992.

23. Yusuf S, Held P, Furberg C. Update of effects of calcium antagonists in myocardial infarction or angina in light of the second Danish Verapamil Infarction Trial (DAVIT-II) and other recent studies. *Am J Cardiol* 1991;67:1295–1297.

24. Medical Research Council Working Party. MRC trial of treatment of mild hypertension: principal results. *Br Med J* 1985;291:97–104.

25. The IPPPSH Collaborative Group. Cardiovascular risk and risk factors in a randomized trial of treatment based on the beta-blocker oxprenolol: the International Prospective Primary Prevention Study in Hypertension (IPPPSH). *J Hypertens* 1985;3:379–392.

26. Wilhelmsen L, Berglund G, Elmfeldt D, et al. Beta-blockers versus diuretics in hypertensive men: main results from the HAPPHY trial. *J Hypertens* 1987;5:561–572.

27. Psaty BM, Furberg CD. Treatment trials: morbidity and mortality. *Hypertension Primer: The Essentials of High Blood Pressure,* eds Izzo JL Jr, Black HR, Taubert KA. Dallas, TX: American Heart Association, 1993:197–201.

28. Siscovick DS, Raghunathan TF, Psaty BM, et al. Diuretic therapy for hypertension and primary cardiac arrest. (Submitted for publication).

29. Joint National Committee on Detection, Evaluation, and Treatment of High Blood Pressure. The fifth report of the Joint National Committee on Detection, Evaluation, and Treatment of High Blood Pressure (JNC V). *Arch Intern Med* 1993;153:154–183.

30. Oparil S. Antihypertensive therapy—efficacy and quality of life. *N Engl J Med* 1993;328:959–961.

31. Amery A, Birkenhager W, Bulpitt CJ, et al. A multicentre trial on the treatment of isolated systolic hypertension in the elderly: objectives, protocol, and organization. *Aging* 1991;3:287–302.

32. Gross TP, Wise RP, Knapp DE. Antihypertensive drug use: trends in the United States from 1973 to 1985. *Hypertension* 1989;13(Suppl I):I113–I118.

33. Rohlfing JJ, Brunzell JD. The effects of diuretics and adrenergic-blocking agents on plasma lipids. *West J Med* 1986;145:210–218.

34. Furberg CD, Byington RP, Borhani NA, for the MIDAS Research Group. Multicenter Isradipine Diuretic Atherosclerosis Study (MIDAS): design features. *Am J Med* 1989;86(suppl):37–39.

35. Croog SH, Levine S, Testa M, et al. The effects of antihypertensive therapy on the quality of life. *N Engl J Med* 1986;314:1657–1664.

36. Croog SH, Levine S, Sudilovsky A, Baume RM, Clive J. Sexual symptoms in hypertensive patients: a clinical trial of antihypertensive medications. *Arch Intern Med* 1988;148:788–794.

37. Langford HG, Davis BR, Blaufox D, et al. Effect of drug and diet treatment of mild hypertension on diastolic blood pressure. *Hypertension* 1991;17:210–217.

38. Wassertheil-Smoller S, Blaufox MD, Oberman A, et al. Effect of antihypertensives on sexual function and quality of life: the TAIM study. *Ann Intern Med* 1991;114:613–620.

39. Beto JA, Bansal VK. Quality of life in the treatment of hypertension: a meta-analysis of clinical trials. *Am J Hypertens* 1992;5:125–133.

40. Beard TC, Cooke HM, Bray WR, Barge R. Randomized controlled trial of a no-added-salt diet for mild hypertension. *Lancet* 1982;2:455–458.

41. Langford HG, Blaufox D, Oberman A, et al. Dietary therapy slows the return of hypertension after stopping prolonged medication. *J Am Med Assoc* 1985;253:657–664.

42. Stamler R, Stamler J, Grimm R, et al. Nutritional therapy for high blood pressure: final report of a four-year randomized controlled trial—the Hypertension Control Program. *J Am Med Assoc* 1987;257:1484–1492.

43. Stamler J, Stamler R, Neaton JD. Blood pressure, systolic and diastolic, and cardiovascular disease: U.S. population data. *Arch Intern Med* 1993;153:598–615.

44. Stamler J. Epidemiologic findings on body mass and blood pressure in adults. *Ann Epidemiol* 1991;1:347–362.

45. Labarthe DR, Mueller WH, Eissa M. Blood pressure and obesity in childhood and adolescence: epidemiologic aspects. *Ann Epidemiol* 1991;1:337–345.

46. MacMahon S, Cutler J, Brittain E, Higgins M. Obesity and hypertension: epidemiological and clinical issues. *Eur Heart J* 1987;8:57–70.

47. Hypertension Prevention Trial Research Group. The Hypertension Prevention Trial: three-year effects of dietary changes on blood pressure. *Arch Intern Med* 1990;150:153–162.

48. The Trials of Hypertension Prevention Collaborative Research Group. The effects of nonpharmacologic interventions on blood pressure of persons with high normal levels: results of the Trials of Hypertension Prevention. *J Am Med Assoc* 1992;267:1213–1220.

49. Folsom AR, Caspersen CJ, Taylor HL, et al. Leisure time physical activity and its relationship to coronary risk factors in a population-based sample. *Am J Epidemiol* 1985;121:570–579.

50. Tuomilehto J, Marti B, Salonen JT, Virtala E, Lahti T, Puska P. Leisure-time physical activity is inversely related to risk factors for coronary heart disease in middle-aged Finnish men. *Eur Heart J* 1987;8:1047–1055.

51. Caspersen CJ, Bloemberg BPM, Saris WHM, Merritt RK, Kromhout D. The prevalence of selected physical activities and their relation with coronary heart disease risk factors in elderly men: the Zutphen Study. *Am J Epidemiol* 1991;133:1078–1092.

52. Paffenbarger RS, Jung DL, Leung RW, Hyde RT. Physical activity and hypertension: an epidemiological view. *Ann Med* 1991;23:319–327.

53. Blair SN, Goodyear NN, Gibbons LW, Cooper KH. Physical fitness and incidence of hypertension in healthy normotensive men and women. *J Am Med Assoc* 1984;252:487–490.

54. Ainsworth BE, Keenan NL, Strogatz DS, Garrett JM, James SA. Physical activity and hypertension in black adults: the Pitt County Study. *Am J Public Health* 1991;81:1477–1479.

55. Reaven PD, Barrett-Connor E, Edelstein S. Relation between leisure-time physical activity and blood pressure in older women. *Circulation* 1991;83:559–565.

56. Arroll B, Beaglehole R. Does physical activity lower blood pressure: a critical review of the clinical trials. *J Clin Epidemiol* 1992;45:439–447.

57. Matsusaki M, Ikeda M, Tashiro E, et al. Influence of work load on the antihypertensive effect of exercise. *Clin Exp Pharmacol Physiol* 1992;19:471–479.

58. MacMahon S. Alcohol consumption and hypertension. *Hypertension* 1987;9:111–121.

59. Kono S, Shinghi K, Ikeda N, Yanai F, Imanishi K, Handa K. Lifestyles, glucose tolerance and blood pressure in male self-

defense officials in northern Kyushu, Japan. *J Hum Hypertens* 1992;6:101–105.

60. Miyao M, Furuta M, Sakakibara H, et al. Analysis of factors related to hypertension in Japanese middle-aged male workers. *J Hum Hypertens* 1992;6:193–197.

61. Salvaggio A, Periti M, Miano L, Tavanelli M, Marzorati D. Analysis of the relation between blood pressure and both self-reported and biochemically inferred alcohol consumption. *J Hypertens* 1991;9:S276–S277.

62. Gordon T, Kannel WB. Drinking and its relation to smoking, BP, blood lipids and uric acid. *Arch Intern Med* 1983;143:1366–1374.

63. Kromhout D, Bosschieter EB, Coulander C de L. Potassium, calcium, alcohol intake and blood pressure: the Zutphen Study. *Am J Clin Nutr* 1985;41:1299–1304.

64. Gordon T, Doyle JT. Alcohol consumption and its relationship to smoking, weight, blood pressure and blood lipids: the Albany Study. *Arch Int Med* 1986;146:262–265.

65. Puddey IB, Beilin LJ, Vandongen R, Rouse IL, Rogers P. Evidence for a direct effect of alcohol consumption on blood pressure in normotensive men: a randomized controlled trial. *Hypertension* 1985;7:707–713.

66. Puddey IB, Beilin LJ, Vandongen R. Regular alcohol use raises blood pressure in treated hypertensive subjects. *Lancet* 1987;1:647–651.

67. Maheswaran R, Beevers M, Beevers DG. Effectiveness of advice to reduce alcohol consumption in hypertension patients. *Hypertension* 1991;19:79–84.

68. Cushman WC, Bingham SF, Cutler JA, Harford TC, Collins JF for the PATHS Group. Prevention and Treatment of Hypertension Study (PATHS): effect of alcohol reduction on blood pressure. Design and baseline characteristics. *Am J Hypertens* 1991;4:109A.

69. Puddey IB, Parker M, Beilin LJ, VanDongen R, Masarei JRL. Effects of alcohol and caloric restrictions on blood pressure and serum lipids in overweight men. *Hypertension* 1992;20:533–541.

70. Liu K, Cooper R, McKeever J, et al. Assessment of the association between habitual salt intake and high blood pressure: methodological problems. *Am J Epidemiol* 1979;110:219–226.

71. Elliott P. Observational studies of salt and blood pressure. *Hypertension* 1991;17(Suppl I):I3–I8.

72. Intersalt Cooperative Research Group. Intersalt: an international study of electrolyte excretion and blood pressure. Results for 24 hour urinary sodium and potassium excretion. *Br Med J* 1988;297:319–328.

73. Law MR, Frost CD, Wald NJ. By how much does dietary salt reduction lower blood pressure? I—analysis of observational data among populations. *Br Med J* 1991;302:811–815.

74. Frost CD, Law MR, Wald NJ. By how much does dietary salt reduction lower blood pressure? II—analysis of observational data within populations. *Br Med J* 1991;302:815–818.

75. Bruce NG, Cook DG, Shaper AG, Ratcliffe JG, Thomson AG. Casual urine concentrations of sodium and potassium and geographic blood pressure variations in Great Britain. *J Hum Hypertens* 1992;6:157–164.

76. Cutler JA, Follmann D, Elliott P, Suh I. An overview of randomized trials of sodium reduction and blood pressure. *Hypertension* 1991;17(Suppl I):I27–I33.

77. Mascioli S, Grimm R Jr, Launer C, et al. Sodium chloride raises blood pressure in normotensive subjects. The study of sodium and blood pressure. *Hypertension* 1991;17(Suppl I):I21–I26.

78. Benetos A, Xiao YY, Cuche JL, Hannaert P, Safar M. Arterial effects of salt restriction in hypertensive patients: a 9-week, randomized, double-blind, crossover study. *J Hypertens* 1992;10:355–360.

79. Sciarrone SEG, Beilin LJ, Rouse IL, Rogers PB. A factorial study of salt restriction and a low-fat/high-fibre diet in hypertensive subjects. *J Hypertens* 1992;10:287–298.

80. Cobiac L, Nestel PJ, Wing LMH, Howe PRC. A low-sodium diet supplemented with fish oil lowers blood pressure in the elderly. *J Hypertens* 1992;10:87–92.

81. Cappuccio FP, MacGregor GA. Does potassium supplementation lower blood pressure? A meta-analysis of published trials. *J Hypertens* 1991;9:465–473.

82. Whelton PK, Appel LA, Seidler AJ, Thaker CK, Klag MJ. Potassium supplementation in the treatment and prevention of hypertension. *J Hypertens* 1992;10(Suppl 4):S108.

83. Siani A, Strazzullo P, Giacco A, Pacioni D, Celentano E, Mancini M. Increasing the dietary potassium intake reduces the need for antihypertensive medication. *Ann Intern Med* 1991;115:753–759.

84. Reed D, McGee D, Yano K, Hankin J. Diet, blood pressure, and multicollinearity. *Hypertension* 1985;7:405–410.

85. Witteman JCM, Willett WC, Stampfer MJ, et al. A prospective study of nutritional factors and hypertension among US women. *Circulation* 1989;80:1320–1327.

86. Ascherio A, Rimm EB, Giovannucci EL, et al. A prospective study of nutritional factors and hypertension among U.S. men. *Circulation* 1992;86:1651–1653.

87. Whelton PK, Klag MJ. Magnesium and blood pressure: review of the epidemiologic and clinical trial experience. *Am J Cardiol* 1989;63:26G–30G.

88. Lind L, Lithell H, Pollare T, Ljunghall S. Blood pressure response during long-term treatment with magnesium is dependent on magnesium status: a double-blind, placebo-controlled study in essential hypertension and in subjects with high-normal blood pressure. *Am J Hypertens* 1991;4:674–679.

89. Paolisso G, De Maro G, Cozzolino D. Chronic magnesium administration enhances oxidative glucose metabolism in thiazide treated hypertensive patients. *Am J Hypertens* 1992;5:581–586.

90. Wright A, Burstyn PG, Gibney MJ. Dietary fibre and blood pressure. *Br Med J* 1979;2:1541–1543.

91. Kelsay JL, Behall KM, Prather ES. Effect of fiber from fruits and vegetables on metabolic responses of human subjects. I. Bowel transit time, number of defecations, fecal weight, urinary excretions of energy and nitrogen and apparent digestibilities of energy, nitrogen, and fat. *Am J Clin Nutr* 1978;31:1149–1153.

92. Brussard JH, van Raaij JMA, Stasse-Wolthuis M, Katan MB, Hautvast JGAJ. Blood pressure and diet in normotensive volunteers: absence of an effect of dietary fiber, protein, or fat. *Am J Clin Nutr* 1981;34:2023–2029.

93. Margetts BM, Beilin LJ, Vandongen R, Armstrong BK. A randomized controlled trial of the effect of dietary fibre on blood pressure. *Clin Sci* 1987;72:343–350.

94. Swain JF, Rouse IL, Curley CB, Sacks FM. Comparison of the effects of oat bran and low-fiber wheat on serum lipoprotein levels and blood pressure. *N Engl J Med* 1990;322:147–152.

95. Sacks FM, Kass EH. Low blood pressure in vegetarians: effects of specific foods and nutrients. *Am J Clin Nutr* 1988;48:795–800.

96. Stamler J, Caggiula A, Grandits A. Relationships of dietary variables to blood pressure (BP): findings of the Multiple Risk Factor Intervention Trial (MRFIT). *Circulation* 1992;85:867.

97. National Diet-Heart Study Research Group. The National Diet-Heart Study final report. *Circulation* 1968;37(Suppl I):I1–I419.

98. Medical Research Council. Controlled trial of soya-bean oil in myocardial infarction. *Lancet* 1968;2:693–700.

99. Iacono JM, Judd FT, Marshall MW, et al. The role of dietary essential fatty acids and prostaglandins in reducing blood pressure. *Prog Lipid Res* 1981;20:349–364.

100. Puska P, Iacono JM, Nissinen A, et al. Controlled, randomised trial of the effect of dietary fat on blood pressure. *Lancet* 1983;1:1–5.

101. Margetts BM, Beilin LJ, Armstrong BK, et al. Blood pressure and dietary polyunsaturated and saturated fats: a controlled trial. *Clin Sci* 1985;69:165–175.

102. Sacks FM, Rouse IL, Stampfer MJ, Bishop LM, Lenherr CF, Walther RJ. Effect of dietary fat and carbohydrate on blood pressure of mildly hypertensive patients. *Hypertension* 1987;10:452–460.

103. Sacks FM, Stampfer MJ, Munoz A, McManus K, Canessa M, Kass EH. Effect of linoleic and oleic acids on blood pressure, blood viscosity, and erythrocyte cation transport. *J Am Coll Nutr* 1987;6:179–185.

104. Mensink RP, Janssen M-C, Katan MB. Effect on blood pressure of two diets differing in total fat but not in saturated and polyunsaturated fatty acids in healthy volunteers. *Am J Clin Nutr* 1988;47:976–980.

105. Appel LJ, Miller ER, Seidler AJ, Whelton PK. Does supplementation of diet with fish oil reduce blood pressure? A meta-analysis

of controlled clinical trials. *Arch Intern Med* 1993;153:1429–1438.

106. Knapp HR, FitzGerald GA. The antihypertensive effects of fish oil: a controlled study of polyunsaturated fatty acid supplements in essential hypertension. *N Engl J Med* 1989;320:1037–1043.

107. Prescott SL, Jenner DA, Beilin LJ, Margetts BM, Vandongen R. Controlled study of the effects of dietary protein on blood pressure in normotensive humans. *Clin Exp Pharmacol Physiol* 1987;14:159–162.

108. Sacks FM, Breslow JL, Wood PG, Kass EH. Lack of an effect of dairy protein (casein) and soy protein on plasma cholesterol of strict vegetarians. An experiment and a critical review. *J Lipid Res* 1983;24:1012–1020.

109. Sacks FM, Wood PG, Kass EH. Stability of blood pressure in vegetarians receiving dietary protein supplements. *Hypertension* 1984;6:199–201.

110. Elliott P, Kesteloot H, Dyer A, et al. 24-hour urinary nitrogen excretion and blood pressure: INTERSALT findings. *Circulation* 1991;84(Suppl 2):II-698 (abst).

111. Liu K, Ruth KJ, Shekelle RB, Stamler J. Macronutrients and long-term change in systolic blood pressure. *Circulation* 1993;87:679 (abst).

112. Cutler JA, Brittain E. Calcium and blood pressure: an epidemiologic perspective. *Am J Hypertens* 1990;3:137S–146S.

113. Gilman MW, Oliveria SA, Moore LL, Ellison RC. Inverse association of dietary calcium with systolic blood pressure in young children. *J Am Med Assoc* 1992;267:2340–2343.

114. National High Blood Pressure Education Program. *Working Group Report on primary prevention of hypertension.* U.S. Department of Health and Human Service 1993; NIH publication no 93-2669.

115. Bierenbaum ML, Wolf E, Bisgeier G, Maginnis WP. Dietary calcium: a method of lowering blood pressure. *Am J Hypertens* 1988;1:1495–1525.

116. van Beresteijn ECH, van Schaik M, Schaafsma G. Milk: does it affect blood pressure? A controlled intervention study. *J Intern Med* 1990;228:477–482.

117. Vinson JA, Mazur T, Bose P. Comparison of different forms of calcium on blood pressure of normotensive young males. *Nutr Rep Int* 1987;36:497–505.

118. Johnson JV, Hall EM. Job strain, workplace social support, and cardiovascular disease: a cross-sectional study of a random sample of the Swedish working population. *Am J Public Health* 1988;78:1336–1342.

119. Schnall PL, Pieper C, Schwartz JE, et al. The relationship between job strain, workplace diastolic blood pressure, and left ventricular mass. *J Am Med Assoc* 1990;263:1929–1935.

120. Albright CL, Winkleby MA, Ragland DR, Fisher J, Syme SL. Job strain and prevalence of hypertension in a biracial population of urban bus drivers. *Am J Public Health* 1992;82:984–989.

121. Light KC, Turner JR, Hinderliter AL. Job strain and ambulatory work blood pressure in healthy young men and women. *Hypertension* 1992;20:214–218.

122. Schnall PL, Schwartz JE, Landsbergis PA, Warren K, Pickering TG. Relation between job strain, alcohol, and ambulatory blood pressure. *Hypertension* 1992;19:488–494.

123. Murphy JK, Alpert BS, Walker SS. Ethnicity, pressor reactivity and children's blood pressure: five years of observations. *Hypertension* 1992;20:327–332.

124. Johnston DW. The behavioral control of high blood pressure. *Curr Psychol Res Rev* 1987;6:99–114.

125. Kaufmann PG, Jacob RG, Ewart CK, et al. Hypertension Intervention Pooling Project. *Health Psychol* 1988;7(Suppl):209–224.

126. Stamler R, Stamler J, Gosch FC, et al. Primary prevention of hypertension by nutritional-hygienic means: final report of a randomized, controlled trial. *J Am Med Assoc* 1989;262:1801–1807.

127. Sever P, Beevers G, Bulpitt C, et al. Management guidelines in essential hypertension: report of the second working party of the British Hypertension Society. *Br Med J* 1993;306:983–987.

128. Jackson R, Barham P, Bills J, et al. Management of raised blood pressure in New Zealand: a discussion document. *Br Med J* 1993;307:107–110.

129. Edelson JT, Weinstein MC, Tosteson ANA, Williams L, Lee TH, Goldman L. Long-term cost-effectiveness of various initial monotherapies for mild to moderate hypertension. *J Am Med Assoc* 1990;263:408–413.

130. Johannesson M, Aberg H, Agreus L, Borgquist L, Jonsson B. Cost-benefit analysis of non-pharmacological treatment of hypertension. *J Intern Med* 1991;230:307–312.

SECTION III

Diet and Hypertension

Hypertension: Pathophysiology, Diagnosis, and Management, Second Edition,
edited by J.H. Laragh and B.M. Brenner,
Raven Press, Ltd., New York © 1995.

CHAPTER **16**

Blood Pressure and Sodium Intake

F. Olaf Simpson

SPECIAL POSITION OF SALT IN HYPERTENSION

It is not difficult to marshal evidence that salt intake has some connection with hypertension (1–8). It is also not difficult to demonstrate flaws and deficiencies in the evidence (9–14), though in most cases the criticism is not that the link between salt intake and hypertension is demonstrably fallacious but rather that it has not been proved sufficiently to warrant a massive change in salt intake by whole populations.

Salt intake holds a unique position among the environmental factors that are known to affect blood pressure (BP): it is possible that if salt intake were sufficiently low, there would be no essential hypertension. None of the other known or possible factors (low intake of calcium, potassium, or fiber; overweight; excess alcohol; high intake of saturated fat; too little exercise; stress) appears capable of a similar role. The implication is that these other factors would be largely or wholly inoperative if life-long salt intake was low. Very conceivably, however, these other factors can modify the effect of a given level of salt intake; thus a population with none of the other risk factors for hypertension might be able to take more salt and yet have a lower BP than another population that takes less salt but has many of the other risk factors for hypertension.

This chapter will review evidence relating the development of hypertension to a high or medium salt intake and will consider possible mechanisms. For reasons of space, studies in humans have been given preference over studies in hypertensive rats, fascinating though the latter are.

There is, unfortunately, no easy way to measure salt intake accurately. Self-assessment can be grossly misleading, dietary questionnaires fail in the case of sodium, and duplicate diets are cumbersome and expensive. Urinary sodium excretion is the best guide to sodium intake, at least to that part of sodium intake that is surplus to what is lost through the skin (which can be considerable in hot climates or hot occupations) and by the bowel (which is normally a very small amount). Unfortunately, 24-hour collections of urine are needed; overnight samples are not reliable in that the day/night ratio of sodium excretion varies and may be affected by the presence of the high BP itself (15). Thus overnight or single casual urine specimens should be used only to monitor the adherence of an individual or group to a salt-reduced diet, and not to provide data for epidemiological work.

It should be noted that much of the work on salt in the context of hypertension has concerned the sodium ion rather than chloride. This is reflected also in the present chapter although the anion aspect should not be neglected.

F. O. Simpson: Wellcome Medical Research Institute, University of Otago Medical School, Dunedin, New Zealand.

EPIDEMIOLOGICAL DATA ON SALT AND HYPERTENSION

Until 1988, interpopulation analyses of the relationship between salt intake and hypertension depended on data obtained in various populations by individual research groups. These analyses were usually based on data for people aged 50–59 years, an age at which hypertension has often already developed but complications are just starting. Such analyses (4,16–18) show a highly significant linear regression of BP on sodium intake, with a slope equivalent to an increase of about 0.9–1.1 mm Hg systolic and 0.5–0.7 mm Hg diastolic for every 10 mmol increase in sodium intake. The data were collected by various techniques and protocols, so that the basis for the analyses was inevitably a little shaky. Two international studies (Intersalt and WHO-CARDIAC) were therefore set up.

Intersalt (19) gathered data on BP and 24-hour urinary sodium and potassium excretion for over 10,000 men and women aged 20–59 years in 52 centers throughout the world. Blood pressure did not rise with age in four communities living in traditional ways and having sodium excretions of 60 mmol/24h or less. Overall, BP was significantly related to sodium intake (as measured by sodium excretion) but the slope of the relationship amounted to only 0.22 mm Hg systolic per 10 mmol of sodium after body mass index and alcohol intake were allowed for. This has been taken (20) to mean that salt intake has little importance for hypertension. However, the study also showed that for every 10 mmol rise in a population's sodium intake there was an increase of 0.9 mm Hg systolic and 0.45 mm Hg diastolic in the population's mean rise in BP from age 25 to age 55, again after allowing for body mass index and alcohol intake. This was clearly a result of at least equal importance.

The other large international study, WHO-CARDIAC (21), has also given somewhat equivocal results. This study, which looked at various other dietary factors in addition to sodium and potassium excretion, was based on about 10,000 people aged 48–56 years in 46 communities around the world. Significantly, BP was positively related to sodium excretion in the men but not in the women.

In general, then, the *inter*population data give support to the notion that the level of salt intake is related to the rise in BP in the second half of life, but they give some ammunition also to the skeptics. *Intra*population data are also difficult to interpret. A highly significant regression of BP on sodium excretion has been found in Japanese (22), Koreans (23), Chinese (24,25), Kashmiris (26), and Kenyans (27) but generally not in Western populations (e.g., 28–32). However, even in Western populations, any relationship that is found between BP and some parameter of salt intake is usually positive.

Various explanations have been put forward for the rather indeterminate showing of sodium intake as an important contributor to hypertension:

1. *Noise in the data.* Many of the studies are based on a single 24-hour collection of urine for each individual. These are reliable for giving the mean or median value for a community, but the day-to-day variation in the individual is very considerable and several 24-hour specimens are needed to give a reliable estimate of a person's sodium consumption habits (33). When noise in the sodium data is allowed for, the relationship of BP to sodium intake (measured as excretion) can be shown to become stronger (34).
2. *Too little variation in salt intake* in a single population. The range is in fact quite wide in most populations, but there is no doubt that the bulk of a population occupies a fairly narrow part of the range.
3. *Genetic variability.*
4. *A threshold level* at about 60–70 mmol/day, above which the amount taken may not matter (2).
5. *The long time frame* for the development of hypertension. Current salt intake may, in some way, be less important than overall past intake.
6. *Other nutritional factors* (such as other cations, type of fat, alcohol, and overweight) may affect or obscure the relationship between BP and salt intake.

INTERRELATIONSHIPS BETWEEN SODIUM INTAKE AND OTHER NUTRIENTS

Chloride

Sodium chloride has a greater effect on BP than other salts of sodium (35,36). In this connection, it is curious that so much continues to be written and spoken about "grams per day" of salt intake. It is usually impossible to measure salt intake as such, and the grams-per-day figure is nearly always an estimate based on the supposition that all the sodium in the urine is present as sodium chloride. This is not so, as has been shown in a study of the sodium and chlorine content of daily diets by neutron activation analysis (37); the "salt content" was 40–50 percent higher when calculated from the sodium content than when calculated from the chlorine content. The discrepancy was presumably due to the presence of sodium salts other than the chloride; the proportions of such salts in the diet will vary in different populations and in different individuals.

Potassium

Blood pressure usually has a negative relationship to 24-hour potassium excretion in epidemiological studies (19,38); thus, Na/K ratio may be an important factor, in addition to the absolute levels of intake of these electrolytes. However, the effect of potassium is very minor when sodium intake is low (39).

Calcium

The relationship of calcium intake to sodium handling and BP is extremely complicated but also of great interest (40). Epidemiological studies show a tendency to an inverse relationship between calcium intake and BP (17) and some BP-lowering effect of calcium administration has been demonstrated in clinical trials (41–43), the effect being seen particularly in connection with a high salt intake and in salt-sensitive rather than in salt-resistant subjects. A further link between salt and calcium is to be found in their handling by the kidney: the more salt that is consumed (and thus the more sodium that is excreted), the more calcium is excreted by the kidneys (44,45). Further, a dietary calcium supplement can have a natriuretic effect (46). This link between sodium and calcium excretion appears to be due to a local renal tubular mechanism; it must inevitably affect calcium balance and calcium-regulating hormones and thus, potentially, intracellular calcium levels and vascular reactivity. Thus the interplay between sodium and calcium at hormonal, renal, and cellular levels is probably highly relevant to the link between salt intake and hypertension.

Fatty acids

A combination of fish oil and a low-salt diet lowers BP in elderly people more than a combination of fish oil and a normal salt diet or sunflower oil and a low-salt diet (47). Thus there may be some interaction between the type of fat eaten and the degree of salt sensitivity; this could perhaps be relevant to the fact that the relationship between salt intake and BP is more readily found in populations whose fat intake tends to be low.

This interrelatedness of the effects on BP of salt and other nutrients raises the question (48,49) of whether the prevention of hypertension could be obtained equally well by attention to better potassium and calcium intake, better exercise habits, and avoidance of overweight and excessive alcohol. It would certainly be foolish to neglect these other factors. Their relative importance compared to salt will vary according to the eating habits of each population and the type of change in diet that the population is willing to make. Perhaps the least painful way for people to achieve lifetime normotension is to make moderate adjustments to their lifestyle in all these areas, rather than a very drastic change in any one of them. It is likely, nevertheless, that salt occupies a central position and that without some general reduction in salt intake, hypertension will continue to be a prevalent and damaging nuisance in the second half of life.

SALT RESTRICTION IN ESTABLISHED HYPERTENSION

Salt restriction undoubtedly can lead to a reduction in the required dose of many antihypertensive drugs (50,51) such as thiazides, beta blockers, and angiotensin-converting enzyme inhibitors (but not calcium antagonists).

The results of moderate salt restriction used alone (i.e., without drugs) are somewhat conflicting. Interpretation of the results has been equally diverse. For instance, Morgan and Nowson (52), reviewing a large number of published studies of manipulation of salt intake, found the evidence convincing that BP does change with change in sodium intake, to the extent of about 1 mm Hg for every 10 mmol of sodium intake; the fall in BP was greatest in people with more severe hypertension and was scarcely detectable below about 130/90 mm Hg. Grobbee and Hofman (53), on the other hand, reviewing 13 randomized studies of salt restriction, found the hypotensive effect to be small and to involve mainly systolic pressure; however, five of these studies were done in people averaging 25 years of age or less and having group mean diastolic pressures of 61–73 mm Hg. It is difficult to see how any reduction in BP can be expected in such subjects.

An extensive metanalysis of published trials by Law et al. (54) showed a highly significant effect of salt restriction on BP in hypertension, though this analysis has been criticized (55) for including uncontrolled trials.

Recent individual studies of salt restriction and supplementation have strengthened the case for salt playing a significant role (56,57). Salt restriction greatly increases the likelihood of hypertensives being able to stay off drug therapy when this is stopped (58,59). The large US trial of Hypertension Prevention (60) showed that an average reduction in sodium intake of 44 mmol/day led to a small but significant fall in BP (1.7/0.9 mm Hg) in people with "high normal" pressures. Portuguese investigators (61) succeeded in reducing salt intake in one of two rural communities with enormous salt intakes (averaging about 360 mmol/day with a 30-percent prevalence of hypertension); BP fell by an average of 5/5 mm Hg in this community after 2 years, while rising slightly in the control community.

Salt-loading studies in population groups with low salt intakes have shown a definite tendency for the BP to rise, even in the short term (62–64).

SALT SENSITIVITY

When hypertensives restrict their sodium intake, the group mean BP response is usually a small fall, as outlined above, but the individual response may be a fall or no change, occasionally even a small rise (65). The concept of "salt sensitivity" therefore developed (66–70), though its etiological significance has been challenged (71). It has been estimated (67) that 50–60 percent of clinical hypertensives are sensitive to sodium intake. The precise definition of this is not yet settled; in many studies it is based on short-term (3–7 days) and very drastic reductions in sodium intake (e.g., to 10 mmol/day), even supplemented in some cases with furosemide to speed up the negative sodium balance. This sort of test is unlikely to be a good model for the response to years of moderate reduction of sodium intake, e.g., to 70–90 mmol/day.

Factors influencing the response of the BP to reduction of salt intake include the following:

1. *The severity of the hypertension.* Salt restriction appears to be more effective in severe hypertension (52–54). While this is probably at least partly true (in that normotensives show little BP response to salt restriction), it should be noted that the same pattern of response is seen also in trials of antihypertensive therapy, and its validity has been questioned (72) on the grounds that the change in BP is mathematically not independent of the baseline BP.
2. *Age.* The BP of older people is more sensitive than that of younger ones to changes in sodium intake (73–76).
3. *Race.* Salt sensitivity is more common in African-Americans than in Caucasians (75,77).
4. *A genetic or familial factor.* The BP response to salt restriction has been found to show significant mother-offspring, sibling-sibling and twin-twin resemblance (78).
5. *Renal abnormalities.*
   a. *Azotemia.* In renal failure, blood volume and extracellular fluid volume become more sensitive to the load of sodium chloride that has to be excreted (76).
   b. *Bilateral renal artery stenosis or stenosis of the artery to a sole kidney.*
6. *Certain abnormalities of the renin-angiotensin-aldosterone system (67):*
   a. *Primary aldosteronism.* BP is sensitive to salt intake in this condition (79,80), for reasons that are not clear. A very low sodium intake is clearly physiologically more suited to the high circulating aldosterone levels.
   b. *Low renin states (other than primary aldosteronism).* These states may be of various origins. Where mineralocorticoid secretion is inappropriately high, or in people taking licorice as a sweetmeat (81,82) or chewing tobacco (83), the mechanism is presumably akin to that seen in primary aldosteronism. In others, however, it is not clear just why plasma renin is low. Plasma renin gradually falls with increasing age (84), and there may be a link here with the tendency for the BP of the elderly to be relatively salt-sensitive.
   c. *States where the reaction of the renin-angiotensin-aldosterone system to sodium restriction is sluggish* (85). The body will be less able to protect itself against sodium loss. This will lead to a relatively great contraction of fluid volume when salt intake is reduced and there will be a tendency for the BP to fall, especially in the standing position. Again,

this becomes increasingly common in the elderly but is not confined to this age group.
   d. *Normal-renin "non-modulators."* Hollenberg and Williams (67) believe that most salt-sensitive hypertensives fall into this category. These people have normal plasma renin levels but do not adequately adjust their renovascular and adrenal responsiveness to angiotensin II when salt intake is changed.

ADAPTATION TO LOW SALT INTAKE

Fears are sometimes voiced that salt restriction could adversely affect health. Some of the fears are probably based on the effects of severe salt restriction (e.g., daily sodium intakes of 20 mmol) but clearly the adaptations to a reduced salt intake need to be examined for deleterious side effects.

1. *Extracellular fluid volume (ECFV), plasma volume, and cardiac output.* These fall when salt intake is reduced. Tiredness, postural faintness, and circulatory collapse are all theoretically possible and no doubt can and do occur if salt restriction is sudden and over-enthusiastic, especially in the elderly or in people treated with diuretics or angiotensin-converting enzyme (ACE) inhibitors (76). The incidence of such events is uncertain and probably not high but it certainly has to be remembered that sudden reduction of salt intake is quite a major change and that the dosage of most antihypertensive drugs will need to be adjusted. Salt restriction should be (and, fortunately, usually is) a gradual process. It is not clear whether people having a moderately low salt intake get into special difficulty if they develop diarrhea or vomiting or if they holiday in a hot climate. Sodium loss in sweat is lower when salt intake is low (86) and exercise tolerance in hot laboratory conditions has been shown to be unaffected by a low salt intake (86).
2. *Hematocrit, hemoglobin, and plasma albumen.* These all rise when sodium intake is abruptly reduced (87), probably due mainly to a fall in plasma volume. This will lead to increased blood viscosity.
3. *Renin, angiotensin and aldosterone.* The secretion and plasma levels of these hormones increase when salt intake is reduced. A renin level that is high in relation to salt intake has been shown to have bad prognostic significance for vascular complications in hypertensives (88,89), but there is no evidence that raising the plasma renin by reducing salt intake has a similar prognostic significance. A high aldosterone level will stimulate sodium-for-potassium exchange in the distal nephron but this does not cause potassium depletion as long as the amount of sodium reaching the distal nephron is small.
4. *Norepinephrine, insulin, uric acid, total cholesterol*

and *LDL cholesterol* rise significantly when sodium intake is suddenly reduced to low levels (87,90–92).

5. *Creatinine* tends to rise when salt intake is drastically reduced (90), probably partly due to reduction in plasma volume. However, renal blood flow and glomerular filtration rate will also fall; when renal function is marginal, this could lead to a more serious rise in plasma creatinine (76).

6. *Platelet function* is reported to be activated by salt restriction (93).

More data are required on whether these undesired effects are of real importance in the context of moderate salt restriction. They are, to some extent at least, counterbalanced by the fact that salt restriction has some desirable effects in addition to what it may do to the BP:

1. *Calcium excretion* is reduced when sodium excretion is reduced (44,45). Thus salt restriction may reduce the prevalence of osteoporosis in the elderly.

2. *Arterial compliance* improves significantly when salt intake is reduced (94–96). This is probably a particularly valuable feature in view of the importance that is now being assigned to raised systolic pressure (97); there is, in fact, evidence that isolated systolic hypertension responds well to salt restriction (98).

3. *Left ventricular mass* is lower when salt intake (measured as sodium excretion) is lower, not only in adults (99–101), but also in adolescents (102).

4. *Stroke* may be related to salt intake, independently of the effect on BP (103).

5. *Stomach cancer* appears to be related to salt intake (104).

ADAPTATION TO HIGH SALT INTAKE

The healthy human body copes astonishingly well, in the short term, with a huge range of daily sodium intake, up to 500 mmol or more, but it has to make big adaptations and we must consider not only short- and medium-term adaptations, but also adaptations over 60 years or more.

Known adaptations to a high salt intake include: expansion of extracellular fluid volume (ECFV) (105); rise in cardiac output (106,107) and renal blood flow (42); fall in plasma epinephrine, norepinephrine, and dopamine (108–110); fall in PRA, angiotensin II and aldosterone (111–113); rise in plasma ANP (113,114); and rise in plasma (ouabainlike) natriuretic hormone which may affect arteriolar smooth muscle and thus be a link in the chain of events that link salt intake to hypertension (115,116).

The purpose of these adjustments is presumably to make sodium output equal to intake, to keep body sodium and body fluid volumes as near as possible to a standard norm, and perhaps to minimize the disturbance to organ blood flow. There is a lay impression that body sodium is kept virtually constant in spite of large changes in salt intake. However, body sodium is higher on a high salt intake than on a low one (117), and there is ample evidence that when there is a step change downward in sodium intake, there is a net loss of sodium over the next 3–6 days.

The exact location of the additional sodium in the body when salt intake is high is not entirely clear. Some of it may be in cells (118–120) and some is undoubtedly in the plasma and ECFV (105). Some of it must be in the gut, where it may influence cardiovascular and renal function via gut hormones such as vasoactive intestinal peptide (121).

A high sodium excretion leads, as mentioned earlier, to a high calcium excretion (44–45). This must inevitably affect calcium balance and calcium-regulating hormones and thus, potentially, intracellular calcium and vascular reactivity.

The question of long-term adaptations to high salt intake over several decades is potentially of great interest. Changes in the walls of arteries, hypertrophy of the left ventricle, and changes in the endocrine control of sodium homeostasis may be examples of such adaptations.

PATTERNS OF ESSENTIAL HYPERTENSION IN RELATION TO SALT INTAKE

Hypertensives on an "average" sodium intake (120–200 mmol/day) can have high, medium, or low PRA and high, medium, or low aldosterone in various permutations (122–125); on average, PRA is lower than in normotensives. Plasma ANP (which is high in primary aldosteronism (126) seems to vary in essential hypertension, being high in some studies (127,129) and normal in others (126,130). Body sodium of hypertensives has been found to range from −20 percent to +40 percent of normal (131); in hypertensives there is reported to be a significant correlation between body sodium and BP (132), although (unlike the situation in primary aldosteronism) the mean value for body sodium in essential hypertensives is not increased.

Some hypertensives, mainly those with a low PRA, have an abnormally small rise in PRA or aldosterone when salt intake is drastically reduced (122,124) or when furosemide (Lasix) is given (133). Some fail to lower their aldosterone production as much as normal subjects do when sodium intake is increased (134,135) or are slow to suppress PRA when a saline load is given (136). Some fail to adjust (modulate) their renal blood flow in response to change in sodium intake (137), even though their PRA is normal; in the same subjects, aldosterone production by the adrenal cortex responds only sluggishly and poorly to angiotensin (137), thus exaggerating a tendency that is found in the normal elderly (138). Some hypertensives have, as reviewed earlier, a BP that is sensitive to short- or medium-term reduction in salt intake, whereas others do not.

There is a strong theory (81,115,116) that a starting point for hypertension is a reduced ability of the kidneys to excrete sodium. It is not at present clear whether this applies to all hypertensives, and it seems likely that the defect is not necessarily the same in all hypertensives. Some salt-sensitive patients (68,106) retain a great deal of sodium when placed on a high-salt diet. However, many hypertensives excrete an intravenous (i.v.) saline load faster than normotensives do (139–143) and it is difficult to imagine that this characteristic does not apply in some way also to salt taken by mouth. The phenomenon is much more marked in those with low plasma renin and/or a renin that is unresponsive to sodium restriction or furosemide (133,142,143). Such people have a particularly large rise in plasma ANP when given an intravenous saline load (133), and this may be of relevance. The most extreme example of a low and nonresponding PRA is, of course, primary aldosteronism; in this condition, plasma ANP levels are high (126), and a saline load is very rapidly excreted (144,145). There are some difficulties, then, in the renal defect in sodium excretion.

Some of the above-mentioned phenomena and abnormalities are known (or thought) to be linked, while others may be independent of each other. Their interrelationships are not clear and it is at present not easy to gather all the various threads together into a coherent scheme. It is, however, of intense interest to the subject of salt intake and hypertension that hypertensives have so often some deviation from normal in matters relating to the endocrine and renal control of sodium. Are these deviations from normal the cause of the rise in BP? or are they secondary to the hypertension? Do they arise directly from some inborn defect? or do they develop (perhaps because of an inborn defect) as a response to years of "average" or high salt intake? If the latter, they seem to follow different patterns in different individuals and this diversity is of great interest. After all, if a life-long low-salt diet would abolish essential hypertension, it would presumably abolish most of the above-mentioned patterns. It is not too surprising that physiological processes might become either worn out or less sensitive in some way if subjected to a lifetime of either excessive or suboptimal stimulation. Perhaps it is also not too surprising that human beings may vary in their response to this situation.

BODY SODIUM AND SODIUM INTAKE: THE STRAUSS CONCEPT

In this difficult area of salt intake and human hypertension, there is unfortunately a large central hole in our knowledge: body sodium. Apart from a very small number of studies (e.g., 82,117,131,132,146), this remains something of a black box due to the technical and ethical difficulties involved in its measurement in man. It is necessary, therefore, to make up for the lack of hard data by examining the theoretical aspects of the relationship between salt intake and body sodium. For this, the concept originally put forward by Strauss et al. (147) is a useful start.

Strauss (147) pointed out that when sodium intake is reduced to a level just sufficient to cover obligatory (skin and fecal) losses, sodium excretion falls exponentially over a few days, virtually to zero. He also showed that when a small amount of sodium chloride is then infused intravenously, it will be excreted; thus there is in these circumstances no true deficit. However, when a diuretic is given along with the low sodium diet, a saline load does not lead to the appearance of sodium in the urine until the deficit has been made up. He therefore postulated that on a very low sodium intake alone (i.e., without a diuretic), the individual does not have a true sodium deficit but is in a special state of "neither surfeit or deficit." This state was subsequently termed the *set-point for sodium* by Hollenberg (148), but for various reasons *basal body sodium* seems preferable (149–151).

Thus we can develop the concept of body sodium being composed, as it were, of two fractions: (a) *basal body sodium,* i.e., the level at which sodium excretion becomes virtually zero, provided that the kidneys are functioning reasonably normally, and at which the amount of sodium presented to the distal nephron must exactly equal the amount of sodium reabsorbed in the distal nephron (151); (b) *extra body sodium,* i.e., sodium in the body over and above the basal level and available to be excreted. It follows that two people with the same sodium intake and the same total body sodium could have achieved this in different ways. For instance, one person could have a fairly high basal body sodium and a very small amount of extra sodium. The other could have a relatively low basal body sodium and a larger amount of extra sodium. Possibly this is why the measurements of total body sodium in hypertension have been difficult to interpret.

The level of *basal body sodium* appears to be determined mainly by aldosterone (or mineralocorticoid activity in general). This can be deduced from the fact that people with primary aldosteronism on an average salt intake have a high total body sodium (16 percent above normal [146]). As such, people very rapidly shut off their sodium excretion when placed on a low sodium diet (152), their extra body sodium must be very low and therefore their basal body sodium must be even more than 16 percent above normal (149,150). In the opposite situation, people with adrenocortical insufficiency, body sodium falls to extremely low levels when a low sodium diet is given (117); thus the basal body sodium of such people must be very low indeed.

The amount of *extra sodium* in the body depends on sodium intake and on the half-time of the exponential decay in sodium excretion, in the same way (148) that the amount of a drug in the body depends on the dosage and on the half-time of the drug's metabolism and/or excretion. The half-time of the exponential decay in sodium excretion can be calculated from the 24-hour urinary sodium excretion pattern following a sudden switch to a low sodium intake. It has been shown to be about 18 hours in normal young people, 23 hours in normal adults, and 31 hours in the elderly (153). The data of Uchida et al. (152), when interpreted in the same way, indicate that people with primary aldosteronism have an abnormally short half-time for the excretion of extra sodium. At the opposite end of the scale, people with adrenal insufficiency have an abnormally long half-time (154). Thus it is evident that aldosterone does not slow down the excretion of extra sodium. Rather, it seems that extra sodium is excreted very quickly by people whose aldosterone activity is fixed and high, and very slowly by people whose aldosterone activity is fixed and low. The half-time of the decay in sodium excretion depends presumably on factors such as hemodynamics, ANP, natriuretic hormone, dopamine, prostaglandins, etc.

Overall, it would appear that the amount of extra sodium in the body is very low in primary aldosteronism, low in normal young people, "average" in normal adults, higher in the elderly, and very high in adrenocortical insufficiency. Exactly where essential hypertensives lie on this scale is not clear: some must hold very little extra sodium, because they lose very little sodium when put on a low sodium diet (152) while others, including at least some salt-sensitives (66,106), retain a lot of sodium when placed on a high salt intake. What then are the principles involved?

SALT INTAKE, BODY SODIUM, AND SALT SENSITIVITY

It should be noted that basal body sodium is not in any sense an ideal state. Rather, it represents a critical level and a concept that can help us to obtain some insight into the different patterns of abnormality that can affect sodium homeostasis in relation to BP. Applied to salt sensitivity, the concept suggests that there may be three broad categories of salt-sensitive hypertensives:

1. *Those whose problem is too high a high basal body sodium,* due to excessive mineralocorticoid activity. A low salt intake will be physiologically more suited to the high mineralocorticoid and should reduce extra sodium and total body sodium a little. This should lead to less natriuretic hormone secretion and a lower BP. Even on a low salt intake, however, the total body sodium of such people will remain somewhat high.

2. *Those whose problem is some defect (perhaps in-* volving renal tubules, prostaglandins, dopamine, vasoactive intestinal peptide, etc.) in the excretion of sodium, leading to too high an extra sodium, and whose basal body sodium is normal. A low salt intake will greatly reduce the high extra sodium and the expanded fluid volumes, and BP will become more normal. Total body sodium should become normal. Thus the salt restriction will compensate more fully for the defect.

3. *Those whose hypertension is due to some other mechanism but whose renin-angiotensin-aldosterone (R-A-A) system is hyporesponsive to salt restriction.* In this theoretical situation, total body sodium should be normal but will be made up of a low basal body sodium and a rather high extra sodium. Salt restriction will result in a big drop in extra and total body sodium and a gratifying fall in BP but total body sodium may become subnormal. In such people, salt restriction might not be correcting a defect but rather might be making use of the impairment in the R-A-A defense mechanism to achieve a large fall in fluid volumes and BP.

Proof of the difference between groups 2 and 3 would require accurate measurement of body sodium on "normal" and low-sodium diets. This will probably never be easy on a large scale and it is to be hoped that the problem can be elucidated by indirect means.

CONCLUSIONS

1. There is a positive correlation between BP and sodium intake in interpopulation studies. Hypertension scarcely exists in populations where sodium intake is 60 mmol/day or less.
2. A similar but weaker correlation is found within some populations but usually not in Western ones.
3. While clearly there are other environmental factors involved, it is possible that a relatively high salt intake is the basic essential factor without which the other factors would not be able to cause hypertension.
4. Salt restriction reduces the dosage requirements of antihypertensive drugs other than the calcium antagonists.
5. Short-term salt restriction lowers BP in about 50–60 percent of hypertensives ("salt-sensitive") but not in others ("salt-resistant"). Salt-sensitivity seems to be related to various forms of lack of sensitivity of the renin-angiotensin-aldosterone system, though these are not necessarily the primary abnormality. It is not clear whether these abnormalities of sodium homeostasis are inevitable consequences of aging or, more probably, secondary to years of high salt intake and therefore preventable.
6. Body sodium may hold clues to the problem of salt sensitivity but is an inadequately researched field. The concept of *basal body sodium* (which is attained when sodium intake is very low and just sufficient to cover

obligatory losses) and *extra sodium* (which is proportional to sodium intake and is excreted exponentially with different rate constants in different people) may be useful in separating different syndromes.

7. The ideal sodium intake has not yet been established. It will depend on circumstances but may well be the amount that leads to a urinary sodium excretion of about 70–100 mmol/day.

REFERENCES

1. Meneely GR, Dahl LK. *Med Clin N Amer* 1961;45:273–283.
2. Freis ED. *Circulation* 1976;53:589–595.
3. Joossens JV, Geboers J. *Prev Med* 1983;12:53–59.
4. Simpson FO. In: Bulpitt CJ, ed. *Handbook of hypertension: epidemiology of hypertension,* vol 6. Amsterdam: Elsevier, 1985;175–190.
5. Weinberger MH. *N Eng J Med* 1987;317:1084–1086.
6. Elliott P. *Klin Wochenschr* 1991;69[Suppl 25]:3–10.
7. Cappucio FP, Markandu ND, MacGregor GA. *Klin Wochenschr* 1991;69[suppl 25]:17–25.
8. Beilin LJ. *Kidney Int* 1992;41[Suppl 37]:S90–S96.
9. Simpson FO. *Clin Sci* 1979;57:463S–480S.
10. Laragh JH, Pecker MS. *Ann Intern Med* 1983;98:735–743.
11. Brown JJ, Lever AF, Robertson JIS, Semple PF. *Q J Med* 1984;53:427–437.
12. Nicholls MG. *Hypertension* 1984;6:795–801.
13. Swales JD. *Am J Hypertens* 1990;3:645–649.
14. Heagerty AM. *Klin Wochenschr* 1991;69[Suppl 25]:26–29.
15. Staessen J, Broughton PM, Fletcher AE, et al. *J Hypertens* 1991;9:1035–40.
16. Gleibermann L. *Ecol Food Nutr* 1973;2:143–156.
17. McCarron DA, Henry HJ, Morris CD. *Hypertension* 1982;4[Suppl III]:III-2–III-13.
18. Law MR, Frost CD, Wald N. *BMJ* 1991;302:811–815.
19. Intersalt Cooperative Research Group. *Br Med J* 1988;297:319–328.
20. Swales JD. *Br Med J* 1988;297:307–308.
21. Yamori Y. *Clin Exp Hypertens* 1989;A11:957–972.
22. Kihara M, Fujikawa J, Ohtaka M, et al. *Hypertension* 1984;6:736–742.
23. Kesteloot H, Park BC, Lee CS, Brems-Heyns E, Joosens JV. In: Kesteloot H, Joossens JV, eds. *Epidemiology of arterial blood pressure.* The Hague; Martinus Nijhoff, 1980;453–470.
24. Nara Y, Zhao GS, Huang ZD, et al. *J Cardiovasc Pharmacol* 1990;16[Suppl. 8]:S40–S42.
25. He J, Tell GS, Tang Y-C, Mo P-S, He G-Q. *Hypertension* 1991;17:378–385.
26. Mir MA, Newcombe R. *J Hum Hypertens* 1988;2:241–246.
27. Poulter N, Khaw KT, Hopwood BEC, Mugambi M, Peart WS, Sever PS. *J Cardiovasc Pharmacol* 1984;6:S197–S203.
28. Staessen J, Fagard R, Lijnen P, Amery A, Bulpitt C, Joossens JV. *J Epidem Community Health* 1981;35:256–261.
29. Simpson FO, Waal-Manning HJ, Bolli P, Phelan EL, Spears GFS. *Clin Sci Mol Med* 1978;55:373s–375s.
30. Smith WCS, Crombie IK, Tavendale RT, Gulland SK, Tunstall-Pedoe HD. *BMJ* 1988;297:329–330.
31. Karvonen MJ, Punsar S. *Acta Med Scand* 1977;202:501–507.
32. Ljungman S, Aurell M, Hartford M, Wikstrand J, Wilhelmsen L, Berglund G. *Hypertension* 1981;3:318–326.
33. Liu K, Cooper R, McKeever J, et al. *Am J Epidemiol* 1979;110:219–226.
34. Frost CD, Law MR, Wald NJ. *BMJ* 1991;302:815–818.
35. Shore AC, Markandu ND, MacGregor GA. *J Hypertens* 1988;6:613–617.
36. Boegehold MA, Kotchen TA. *Hypertension* 1991;17[Suppl I]:I.158–I.161.
37. Teramoto K, Horiguchi S, Wakitani F, et al. *Osaka City Med J* 1990;36:175–180.
38. Bulpitt CJ, Broughton PMG, Markowe HLJ, et al. *J Chronic Dis* 1986;39:211–219.
39. Grimm RH, Neaton JD, Elmer PJ, et al. *N Engl J Med* 1990;322:569–574.
40. Resnick LM. *Am J Med* 1992;93[Suppl 2A]:11S–20S.
41. Saito K, Sano H, Furuta Y, Fukuzaki H. *Hypertension* 1989;13:219–226.
42. Rich GM, McCullough M, Olmedo A, Moore TJ. *Am J Hypertens* 1991;4:642S–645S.
43. Sowers JR, Zemel MB, Zemel PC, Standley PR. *Am J Hypertens* 1991;4:557–563.
44. Goulding A, McFarland BE. *J Cardiovasc Pharmacol* 1990;16[Suppl 7]:S47–S49.
45. Zemel MB, Gualdoni SM, Walsh MF, et al. *J Hypertens* 1986;4[Suppl 5]:S364–S366.
46. He J, Tell GS, Tang Y-C, Mo P-S, He G-Q. *J Hypertens* 1992;10:671–676.
47. Cobiac L, Nestel PJ, Wing LMH, Howe PRC. *J Hypertens* 1992;10:87–92.
48. McCarron DA. *Hypertension* 1991;17[Suppl I]:I-170–I-172.
49. Hense H-W. *Klin Wochenschr* 1991;69[Suppl 25]:11–16.
50. Luft FC, Weinberger MH. *Hypertension* 1988;11[Suppl I]:I.229–I.232.
51. Singer DRJ, Markandu ND, Sugden AI, Miller MA, MacGregor GA. *Hypertension* 1991;17:798–803.
52. Morgan T, Nowson C. *Can J Physiol Pharmacol* 1986;64:786–792.
53. Grobbee DE, Hofman A. *Brit Med J* 1986;293:27–29.
54. Law MR, Frost CD, Wald NJ. *BMJ* 1991;302:819–824.
55. Swales JD. *J Hypertens* 1991;9[Suppl 6]:S42–S46.
56. MacGregor GA, Markandu ND, Sagnella GA, Singer DRJ, Cappucio FP. *Lancet* 1989;2:1244–1247.
57. Australian National Health & Medical Research Council Dietary Salt Study Management Committee. *Lancet* 1989;1:399–402.
58. Langford HG, Blaufox D, Oberman A, et al. *JAMA* 1985;253:657–664.
59. Morgan T, Anderson A. *Can J Physiol Pharmacol* 1987;65:1752–1755.
60. The Trials of Hypertension Prevention Collaborative Research Group. *JAMA* 1992;267:1213–1220.
61. Forte JG, Pereira Miguel JM, Pereira Miguel MJ, de Padua F, Rose G. *J Hum Hypertens* 1989;3:179–184.
62. Rikimaru T, Fujita Y, Okuda T, Kajiwara N, Miyatani S, Alpers MP, Koishi H. *Am J Clin Nutr* 1988;47:502–508.
63. Mtabaji JP, Nara Y, Yamori Y. *J Hum Hypertens* 1990;4:80–81.
64. Mufunda J, Chimoskey JE, Matenga J, Musabayane C, Sparks HV Jr. *J Hypertens* 1992;10:279–285.
65. Longworth DL, Drayer JIM, Weber MA, Laragh JH. *Clin Pharmacol Ther* 1980;27:544–546.
66. Kawasaki T, Delea CS, Bartter FC, Smith H. *Am J Med* 1978;64:193–198.
67. Hollenberg NK, Williams GH. *Am J Hypertens* 1989;2:809–815.
68. Dustan HP, Valdes G, Bravo EL, Tarazi RC. *Am J Med Sci* 1986;292:67–74.
69. Weinberger MH. *Am J Hypertens* 1991;4:615S–616S.
70. Wedler B, Wiersbitzki M, Wolf E, Luft FC. *Clin Exp Hypertens A* 1992;14:1037–1049.
71. Watt GCM. *Klin Wochenschr* 1991;69[Suppl 25]:30–35.
72. Gill JS, Zezulka AV, Beevers DG, Davies P. *Lancet* 1985;1:567–569.
73. Myers J, Morgan T. *Clin Exp Hypertens Theory & Practice* 1983;A5:99–118.
74. Zemel MB, Sowers JR. *Am J Cardiol* 1988;61:7H–12H.
75. Luft FC, Miller JZ, Grim CE, Fineberg NS, Christian JC, Daugherty SA, Weinberger MH. *Hypertension* 1991;17[Suppl 1]:I.102–I.108.
76. Mimran A, Ribstein J, Jover B. *Kidney Int* 1992;37[Suppl]:S107–S113.
77. Sullivan JM, Prewitt RL, Ratts TE. *Am J Med Sci* 1988;295:370–377.
78. Miller JZ, Weinberger MH, Christian JC, Daugherty SA. *Am J Epidemiol* 1987;126:822–830.
79. Bravo E, Tarazi RC, Dustan HP, Fouad FM. *Hypertension* 1985;7:90–96.

80. Pedrinelli R, Clerico A, Panarace G, et al. *J Hypertens* 1991;9: 457–463.
81. Borst JGG, Borst-de Guis A. *Lancet* 1963;1:677–682.
82. Beretta-Piccoli C, Salvade G, Crivelli PL, Weidmann P. *J Hypertens* 1985;3:19–23.
83. Westman EC, Guthrie GP. *New Eng J Med* 1990;322:850.
84. Weidmann P, de Myttenaere-Burstein S, Maxwell MH, de Lima J. *Kidney Int* 1975;8:325–333.
85. Borghi C, Borghi S, Costa FV, Ambrosioni E. *Clin Exp Hypertens A* 1992;14:837–851.
86. Hargreaves M, Morgan TO, Snow R, Guerin M. *Clin Sci* 1989;76:553–557.
87. Weder AB, Egan BM. *Klin Wochenschr* 1991;69[Suppl 25]:45–50.
88. Laragh JH, Sealey JE. *Clin Chem* 1991;37:1820–1827.
89. Alderman MH, Madhavan S, Wee LO, Cohen H, Sealey JE, Laragh JH. *N Eng J Med* 1991;324:1098–1104.
90. Egan BM, Weder AB, Petrin J, Hoffman RG. *Am J Hypertens* 1991;4:416–421.
91. Ruppert M, Diehl J, Kolloch R, Overlack A, Kraft K, Gobel B, Hittel N, Stumpe KO. *Klin Wochenschr* 1991;69[Suppl 25]:51–57.
92. Masugi F, Ogihara T, Hashizume K, Hasegawa T, Sakaguchi K, Kumahara Y. *J Hum Hypertens* 1988;1:293–298.
93. Ikeda T, Gomi T, Sakurai J, Toya Y, Fujinami K, Yuhara M, Ikegami F. *Jpn Heart J* 1989;30:365–373.
94. Avolio AP, Clyde CM, Beard TC, Cooke HM, Ho KKL, O'Rourke MF. *Arteriosclerosis* 1986;6:166–169.
95. Safar M, Laurent S, Safavian A, Pannier B, Asmar R. *Am J Med* 84[Suppl 1B]15–19.
96. Benetos A, Xiao YY, Cuche JL, Hannaert P, Safar M. *J Hypertens* 1992;10:355–360.
97. SHEP Cooperative Research Group. *JAMA* 1991;265:3255–3264.
98. Niarchos AP, Weinstein DL, Laragh JH. *Am J Med* 1984;77: 1061–1068.
99. Schmieder RE, Messerli FH, Garavaglia GE, Nunez BD. *Circulation* 1988;78:951–956.
100. Blake J, Devereux RB, Borer JS, Szulc M, Pappas TW, Laragh JH. *Am J Med* 1990;88:477–485.
101. du Cailar G, Gallay P, Ribstein J, Daures JP, Grolleau R, Mimran A. *Arch Mal Coeur* 1990;83:2045–2049.
102. Martell N, Rodrigo JL, Fernandez-Pernilla C, et al. *J Hypertens* 1991;9[Suppl 6]:S258–S259.
103. Perry IJ, Beevers DG. *J Hum Hypertens* 1992;6:23–25.
104. Joossens JV, Geboers J. In: Levin B, Riddell RH, eds. *Frontiers of gastrointestinal cancer.* New York: Elsevier, 1984;167–183.
105. Seely JF, Levy M. In: Brenner BM, Rector FC, eds. *The kidney,* vol 1. Philadelphia: WB Saunders, 1981;371–407.
106. Fujita T, Henry WL, Bartter FC, Lake CR, Delea CS. *Am J Med* 1980;69:334–344.
107. Sullivan JM, Ratts TE. *Hypertension* 1983;5:814–820.
108. Romoff MS, Keusch G, Campese VM, et al. *J Clin Endocrinol Metab* 1979;48:26–31.
109. Kuchel OG, Kuchel GA. *Hypertension* 1991;18:709–721.
110. Williams GH, Gordon MS, Stuenkel CA, Conlin PR, Hollenberg NK. *Am J Hypertens* 1990;3:112S–115S.
111. Brown JJ, Fraser R, Lever AF, Love DR, Morton JJ, Robertson JIS. *Lancet* 1972;2:1106–1107.
112. Sealey JE, Laragh JH. *Kidney Int* 1974;6:281–290.
113. Sagnella GA, Markandu MD, Buckley MG, Miller MA, Singer DR, Cappucio FP, MacGregor GA. *Can J Physiol Pharmacol* 1991;69:1592–1600.
114. Kohno M, Yasunari K, Murakawa K, Kanayama K, Matsuura T, Takeda T. *Am J Cardiol* 1987;59:1212–1215.
115. Blaustein MP, Hamlyn JH. *Hypertension* 1991;18[Suppl III]:III.184–III.195.
116. de Wardener HE. *Hypertension* 1991;17:830–836.
117. Brown WJ, Brown FK, Krishan I. *Circulation* 1971;43:508–519.
118. Trevisan M, Cooper R, Ostrow D, et al. *Clin Sci* 1981;61[Suppl 1]:29s–32s.
119. Ambrosioni E, Costa FV, Borghi C, et al. *Clin Sci* 1982;63:231s–234s.
120. Lijnen P, M'Buyama-Kabangu JR, Fiocchi R, et al. *Postgrad Med J* 1986;62[Suppl 1]:3–12.
121. Duggan KA, Macdonald GJ. *Clin Sci* 1987;72:195–200.
122. Laragh JH, Sealey JE, Brunner HR. *Am J Med* 1972;53:649–663.
123. Buhler FR, Laragh JH, Sealey JE, Brunner HR. *Am J Cardiol* 1973;32:554–561.
124. Coghlan JP, Doyle AE, Jerums G, Scoggins BA. *Clin Sci* 1972;42: 15–23.
125. Agabitei Rosei E, Brown JJ, Cumming AMM, et al. *Clin Endocrinol* 1978;8:141–147.
126. Yamaji T, Ishibashi M, Sekihara H, Takaku F, Nakaoka H, Fujii J. *J Clin Endocrinol Metab* 1986;63:815–818.
127. Sagnella GA, Markandu ND, Shore AC, MacGregor GA. *Lancet* 1986;1:179–181.
128. Iimura O, Shimamoto K, Ando T, et al. *Can J Physiol Pharmacol* 1987;65:1701–1705.
129. Kohno M, Yasunari K, Matsuura T, Murakawa K, Takeda T. *Am Heart J* 1987;113:1160–1163.
130. Larochelle P, Cusson JR, Gutkowska J, et al. *Br Med J* 1987;294: 1249–1252.
131. Davies DL, Schalekamp MA, Beevers DG, et al. *Lancet* 1973;1: 683–686.
132. Beretta-Piccoli C, Davies DL, Boddy K, et al. *Clin Sci* 1982;63: 257–270.
133. Matsubara H, Umeda Y, Yamane Y, Nishikawa M, Taniguchi T, Inada M. *Am J Cardiol* 1987;60:708–714.
134. Collins RD, Weinberger MH, Dowdy AJ, Nokes GW, Gonzales CM, Luetscher JA. *J Clin Invest* 1970;49:1415–1426.
135. Kloppenborg PWC, Drayer JIM, Smals AGH, Benraad ThJ. *Clin Exper Hypert* 1982;A4:1881–1893.
136. Tuck ML, Williams GH, Dluhy RG, Greenfield M, Moore TJ. *Circ Res* 1976;39:711–717.
137. Hollenberg NK, Moore T, Shoback D, Redgrave J, Rabinowe S, Williams GH. *Am J Med* 1986;81:412–418.
138. Takeda R, Morimoto S, Uchida K, Miyamori I, Hashiba T. *Acta Endocrinol* 1980;94:552–558.
139. Birchall R, Tuthill SW, Jacobs WS, Trautman WJ, Findley T. *Circulation* 1953;7:258–267.
140. Baldwin DS, Biggs AW, Goldring W, Hulet WH, Chasis H. *Am J Med* 1958;24:893–902.
141. Buckalew VM, Puschett JB, Kintzel JE, Goldberg M. *J Clin Invest* 1969;48:1007–1016.
142. Krakoff LR, Goodwin FJ, Baer L, Torres M, Laragh JH. *Circulation* 1970;42:335–345.
143. Schalekamp MADH, Krauss XH, Schalekamp-Kuyken MPA, Kolsters G, Birkenhager WH. *Clin Sci* 1971;41:219–231.
144. Rovner DR, Conn JW, Knopf RF, Cohen EL, Hsueh MT-Y. *J Clin Endocrinol* 1965;25:53–64.
145. Biglieri EG, McIlroy MB. *Circulation* 1966;33:73–86.
146. Beretta-Piccoli C, Davies DL, Brown JJ, et al. *J Hypertens* 1983;1:197–205.
147. Strauss MB, Lamdin E, Smith WP, Bleifer DJ. *Arch Int Med* 1958;102:527–536.
148. Hollenberg NK. *Kidney Int* 1980;17:423–429.
149. Simpson FO. In: Puschett JB, Greenberg A, eds. *Diuretics II: chemistry, pharmacology, and clinical applications.* New York: Elsevier, 1987;569–576.
150. Simpson FO. *Lancet* 1988;2:25–29.
151. Simpson FO, Ledingham JM. *Nephron* 1990;54:61–69.
152. Uchida K, Morimoto S, Takeda R, Murakami M. *Jpn Circ J* 1972;36:1301–1311.
153. Epstein M, Hollenberg NK. *J Lab Clin Med* 1976;87:411–417.
154. Lipsett MB, Pearson OH. *J Clin Invest* 1958;37:1394–1402.

Hypertension: Pathophysiology, Diagnosis, and Management, Second Edition, edited by J.H. Laragh and B.M. Brenner, Raven Press, Ltd., New York © 1995.

CHAPTER 17

Dietary Sodium Restriction in Hypertension

John D. Swales

Dietary salt restriction is included in all national and international guidelines for treating hypertension as part of a nonpharmacological strategy (1). In addition, salt restriction is recommended by some groups as a population measure for a reduction in the mortality and morbidity associated with hypertension (2). Although much of the rationale for such recommendations is based upon the hypothesis that excessive salt intake plays a pathogenetic role in hypertension, the scientific justification for advocating salt restriction rests upon a number of assumptions. Lowering salt intake should reduce blood pressure in hypertensive patients and prevent blood pressure elevation in those at risk. In addition, the adverse effects of salt restriction should be outweighed by the blood pressure lowering effect (3). Most scientific studies in this field have concentrated on blood pressure lowering efficacy in hypertensive and normotensive individuals. The large, long-term trials required to demonstrate prevention and to assess possible adverse effects have not been attempted and indeed are unlikely to be set up. As a result, any overview of the value of salt restriction is limited to assessment of trials of efficacy and extrapolation from clinical and experimental data on the effects of salt restriction.

J. D. Swales: Department of Medicine, Leicester Royal Infirmary, Leicester, England.

SODIUM AS A CAUSE OF HYPERTENSION

It has been argued that a high salt intake is a fairly recent aberration in the evolution of the human species and that hypertension is therefore a consequence of inappropriate dietary habits (4). Such evolutionary arguments should carry little weight in determining the advice to be given to individual hypertensive patients. Indeed, the invocation of Darwinian natural selection would not seem relevant to the needs of Western man, since in other fields the health practices of our antecedents have not been accepted in any sense as a desirable model.

The sodium hypothesis was originally based upon an apparent association between dietary salt intake and the prevalence of hypertension in cross-cultural studies (5). These studies have now been superceded in both rigor and magnitude by the Intersalt Study (6). Fifty-two centers in 32 countries each recruited 200 subjects in whom sodium intake was estimated from 24-hour urinary sodium excretion. After adjustment for age and sex, sodium excretion and systolic blood pressure were significantly and positively correlated in 15 centers and negatively in 2. The number of centers for diastolic blood pressure were 4 and 1, respectively. However, since this relationship could be due to other dietary factors, multiple regression analysis was carried out after adjustment for body mass index, alcohol consumption, and urinary potassium. This indicated that confounding factors did indeed account for some of the observed association since the number of significant positive associations fell to 8 for systolic blood pressure and to 3 for diastolic blood pressure. Significant negative associations remained at 2 and 3, respectively. Pooling of the regression coefficients over all 52 centers yielded a significant overall regression coefficient for systolic but not diastolic blood pressure. The magnitude of the correlation was, however, extremely small. After adjustment, the rise in systolic blood pressure for 100-mmol increase in sodium excretion was 2.2 mm Hg and for diastolic blood pressure 0.1 mm Hg. The four centers with very low sodium excretions were found to influence the cross-center analysis. When these were excluded there was no relationship between the prevalence of blood pressure and sodium excretion or between median blood pressure and sodium excretion. Perhaps the most important aspect of this part of the Intersalt Study is the demonstration that some of the association is attributable to confounding factors which were not completely assessed in the smaller, older investigations. A second, more positive finding from the Intersalt Study was the demonstration of a significant relationship between the slope of blood pressure with age and both systolic and diastolic blood pressure. It is difficult to decide if this is an artifact of retrospective subgroup analysis of a cross-sectional study or whether it has physiological meaning. It is possible that there is a growing importance of salt intake with aging; there is some evidence of this from the Intervention Studies (see below). In addition, exchangeable sodium rises with age and is correlated with blood pressure only in older hypertensives; it is reduced in younger hypertensives (7).

The Intersalt Study provides relevant negative and positive data on the salt/blood pressure relationship. The largest epidemiologic investigation of the association between sodium intake and blood pressure in a single population provides remarkably concordant results. Blood pressure and 24-hour urinary sodium excretion were measured in a random sample of 7,354 Scottish subjects (8). A weakly positive correlation between blood pressure and sodium excretion disappeared when adjusted for body mass index, alcohol consumption, and urinary potassium. The data in this study are greater than pooled data from previous small investigations which are of limited value by reason of low statistical power and unrecognized, possibly confounding factors.

Taken in isolation, such population-based associations do not provide an adequate basis for therapeutic or public health interventions. Taken in conjunction with intervention studies, however, they provide valuable information on the possible role of sodium intake in determining blood pressure levels in the population.

INTERVENTION STUDIES IN SECONDARY HYPERTENSION

Sodium retention produces high blood pressure in the majority of patients with advanced renal failure managed by intermittent dialysis (9–11). Not only is it possible to demonstrate a relationship between exchangeable sodium and blood pressure in these patients, but removal of sodium lowers blood pressure (10,11). On the other hand, in a minority of patients on chronic dialysis, severe hypertension persists despite dialytic sodium depletion (10,11).

In some respects such patients physiologically resemble patients with renovascular hypertension due to unilateral renal artery stenosis (12) and some patients with severe malignant hypertension (13,14) where very high blood pressure levels may give rise to negative sodium balance, presumably through perfusion pressure natriuresis. Isolated case reports suggest that saline infusion may produce clinical improvement in such cases (14,15). Data from experimental study in rats with Goldblatt hypertension have confirmed the validity of such clinical observations. Acute dialytic sodium removal (16) or dietary sodium depletion (17,18) fails to lower blood pressure in animals with unilateral renal ischemia and a normal opposite kidney (Goldblatt 1 clip 2 kidney hypertension). Bilateral nephrectomy, however, produces sodium-responsive blood pressure (16). Renal mechanisms (which include the renin-angiotensin system and probably the renomedullary vasodepressor system) clearly override sodium-dependent blood pressure changes.

Among patients with essential hypertension there is no evidence for sodium retention unless cardiac failure has supervened or in the absence of sodium-retaining antihypertensive drugs. Exchangeable sodium and extracellular fluid measured isotopically in milder hypertensive and younger hypertensive subjects are indeed slightly reduced (19,20). One study has described a positive correlation between body sodium and blood pressure in older subjects only, resulting in sodium retention (7). This was interpreted as reflecting secondary renal changes. Excluding the patients with advanced renal failure or with mineralocorticoid hypertension and perhaps some elderly individuals, dietary salt restriction cannot be advocated on the grounds that it corrects a pathophysiological abnormality. In such patients its justification lies in claims that reducing salt intake lowers blood pressure.

INTERVENTION STUDIES IN ESSENTIAL HYPERTENSION

The observation that sodium restriction lowers blood pressure dates from the early years of this century

TABLE 1. *Trials of sodium restriction in subjects selected for high blood pressures*

Trial (ref.)	No.	Design	Duration (months)	Achieved U Na (mmol/24 h)	Change U Na (mmol/24 h)	BP Change (mm Hg) SBP	DBP	Initial BP (mm Hg) SBP	DBP
Parijs et al. (27)	15	CX	1	93	−98	−6.7	+3.2	175	112
Morgan et al. (28)	31/31	PG	24	157	−34	−1.5	−6.9	160	97
Macgregor et al. (29)	19	DBCX	1	80	−76	−10	−5.0	156	98
Watt et al. (30)	18	DBCX	1	87	−56	−0.5	−0.3	136	82
Puska et al. (31)	15/19	PG	1.5	77	−115	+1.3	+0.9	148	96
Silman et al. (32)	21/16	PG	12	117	−53	−8.7	−6.3	163	99
Richards et al. (33)	12	CX	1	80	−105	−5.2	−1.8	150	92
Erwtemann et al. (34)	44/50	PG	1	72	−58	−1.9	−1.5	143	95
Chalmers et al. (35)	48/52	PG	3	86	−54	−5.1	−4.2	156	97
Logan (36)	42/43	PG	6	121	−43	−1.1	−0.2	"Mild"	"Mild"
Grobbee et al. (37)	40	DBCX	1.5	57	−72	−0.8	−0.8	143	78
MacGregor et al. (38)	20	DBCX	1	49	−59	−8.0	−5.0	155	95
ANHMRC (39)	88	DBCX	2	90	−67	−3.6	−2.1	153	95
ANHMRC (40)	50/53	PG	2	90	−71	−5.5	−2.8	155	95
TOHP (41)	327/417	PG	18	111	−44	−1.7	−0.9	125	84
Sinaiko et al. (42)	35/34 (m)	PG	36	162	+20	+1.8	−4.	114	63
	35/35 (f)	PG	36	119	−14	−5.7	−5.1	114	63
Fotherby et al. (43)	17	DBCX	1.2	95	−79	−5.0 (Ambulatory)	−2.0	150	87
						−8.0 (Clinic)	−1.0	171	96

Treatment group data placed first in parallel group studies.

PG, parallel group; CX, crossover; DB, double blind; SBP, systolic blood pressure; DBP, diastolic blood pressure.

(21,22). Kempner's rice-fruit diet was shown to lower blood pressure effectively in severely hypertensive patients (23–25). This diet reduced sodium intake to approximately 5 mmols a day and also radically altered other dietary components: most relevant perhaps is the fact that the Kempner rice-fruit diet is particularly rich in potassium. The Medical Research Council (MRC) Study, however, provided evidence that the reduction in sodium was at least partially responsible for the fall in blood pressure because the addition of only modest amounts of sodium chloride to the diet restored blood pressure to baseline levels (24). The unpleasantness of

the Kempner rice-fruit diet combined with the grave social disadvantages attendant upon it led to poor compliance, although its efficacy cannot be questioned. As a result, relatively few clinicians were persuaded to incorporate it into clinical practice. In addition, the development of effective antihypertensive drugs shortly thereafter removed some of the clinical need for dietary methods of blood pressure lowering. In the 1970s, however, salt restriction and other nonpharmacological methods of lowering blood pressure began to be reassessed. This followed from the appreciation that blood pressure reduction, even in patients with mild to moder-

TABLE 2. *Trials of sodium restriction in normotensive subjects*

	No.	Design	Duration (months)	Achieved U Na (mmol/24 h)	Change U Na (mmol/24 h)	BP change (mm Hg) SBP	DBP	Initial BP (mm Hg) SBP	DBP
Skrabal et al. (44)	20	CX	0.5	40	−170	−2.7	−3.0	125	76
Puska et al. (31)	19/19	PG	0.5	77	−117	−0.5	−0.4	131	81
Cooper et al. (45)	113	CX	0.8	45	−69	−0.6	−1.4	109	61
Watt (HH) et al. (46)	35	DBCX	1	56	−74	−1.4	+1.2	114	63
Watt (LL) et al. (46)	31	DBCX	1	68	−60	−0.5	+1.4	111	64
El-Ashry et al. (47)	26	CX	0.5	37	−81	−0.0	−2.5	129	70
Myers (48)	172	CX	0.5	71	−130	−3.5	−1.9	121	77
HPTRG (49)	174/177	PG	36	155	−16	+0.1	+0.2	124	83
Howe et al. (50)	90	CX	2	98	−81	−1.0	−0.4	115	60

PG, parallel group; CX, crossover; DB, double blind; SBP, systolic blood pressure; DBP, diastolic blood pressure; HH, offspring of two parents with high blood pressure; LL, offspring of two parents with low blood pressure.

ate hypertension, carries significant benefit. The need to treat increasingly large numbers of patients for the duration of their lives created new economic and social pressures to find alternatives to pharmacological therapy (26). Although severe salt restriction to 10 mmol/day or less sodium was unacceptable to the majority of active hypertensive patients, more moderate degrees of salt restriction (i.e., reducing the intake to below 100 mmol/day) are feasible, although with some social difficulty.

Accordingly, over the last two decades a series of dietary intervention trials has been carried out to assess the effect of such moderate salt restriction on blood pressure (27–43) (Table 1). Other workers have recruited normotensive volunteers (Table 2) (44–50). The interpretation of these studies has given rise to considerable debate, although a much broader consensus is now emerging. Table 1 includes studies which were interpreted by those carrying them out as both positive and negative. The apparent conflict of results is attributable to at least three factors. These are: design of studies, number of patients included in each study (statistical power), and differences in initial blood pressure of patients recruited.

DESIGN OF STUDIES

Sustained reduction in sodium intake is not easy to achieve in Western societies. In addition to refraining from adding salt to food at the table, it is necessary to abstain from salt in cooking and to avoid high salt-containing (usually processed) foods. The difficulties are well exemplified by the final achieved 24-hour urinary sodiums (used as measures of sodium intake) in clinical trials (see Tables 1 and 2). Only modest falls in urinary sodium were obtained in longer term trials. Further, better compliance was achieved in experimental studies in well-motivated normotensive volunteers (see Table 2) (44–50) compared with hypertensive subjects (see Table 1) (27–43).

The nature of the control group or period is critical in view of the need to detect a small effect upon blood pressure in the presence of a marked placebo effect when blood pressure is repeatedly measured. Thus, in the trial reported by Silman et al. (32), blood pressures in the control group (whose members continued to attend for a year) fell from 159/98 to 139/87 mm Hg. In the intervention group, blood pressure fell from 167/99 to 139/81 mm Hg. Although the difference between the two was not statistically significant, the fall in blood pressure in the control group was considerably greater than that recorded in intervention groups in most of the other studies. In another study, a significant fall in blood pressure from baseline to intervention periods was observed in both salt-restricted and control groups, although there was no significant increase in blood pressure in either group during the final washout phase (31). The fall in

blood pressure in the control group is also evident in the parallel group design trial reported by Morgan et al. (28). Without proper controls, therefore, nonspecific falls in blood pressure due to habituation and (in the hypertensive group) due to regression to the mean as well will lead to spurious effects. It is therefore essential if specific salt-related effects are to be identified to use proper randomization employing either a parallel group or crossover design so that nonspecific time-related changes in blood pressure are excluded.

There is another difficulty in the design of trials of salt restriction. When patients are placed on a low-salt diet, potentially relevant factors other than sodium are altered: these include lipids, fiber, and dietary protein. The potential importance of this confounding factor became evident during the earlier Australian National Health and Medical Research Council trials (35). Two hundred and twelve subjects were randomized to normal diet, high-potassium diet, reduced-sodium diet, or high-potassium/low-sodium diet. Systolic and diastolic blood pressure fell by 3.8/1.6 mm Hg in the normal diet group and by 8.9/5.8 mm Hg in the low-sodium group. However, when patients were rerandomized to placebo or sodium chloride supplements, blood pressure was not elevated significantly by restoring sodium intake. The authors could not therefore exclude the possibility that factors other than changes in sodium or potassium intake contributed to the fall in blood pressure during the diet phase of their study. The possible confounding effect of changes in other dietary components is eliminated in the most sophisticated approach to this problem, the double-blind design. All patients are stabilized on a low-salt diet and then randomly allocated in a double-blind fashion to placebo or salt supplement (29,30,37–39,43). It is essential in any overview of clinical trials that due account is paid to trial design if fallacious conclusions are to be avoided.

STATISTICAL POWER

The statistical power of some studies has been severely restrained by their relatively small size making the detection of small change in blood pressure difficult. Thus, in some cases apparently appreciable and clinically significant falls in blood pressure are documented which do not reach statistical significance (32,33). Duration of intervention is another potentially important feature. The maneuver proposed, i.e., dietary salt restriction, is intended for lifelong application. Possible long-term changes in compliance and in physiological adaptation to a low-salt diet require evaluation. In diuretic-treated patients, for instance, progressive rise in plasma renin activity has been recorded over a two-year period (51). Whether a similar phenomena occurs with dietary salt restriction is unknown. Conversely, it is possible that reversal of longstanding vascular hypertrophy might result in amplification of any blood pressure lowering effect (52,53).

DIFFERENCES IN INITIAL BLOOD PRESSURE OF RECRUITED PATIENTS

One of the most important explanations for discordance in published reports lies in the differences in initial blood pressures of the patients recruited. There is a necessary mathematical relationship between the degree of change in a variable and the initial value of that variable, since each shares a common component (54). It would therefore be predicted that studies in normotensive subjects will observe less blood pressure lowering than studies in hypertensives.

There is another physiological explanation for the lesser efficacy of salt restriction in the lower blood pressure ranges. One of the mechanisms by which the circulation is protected against volume depletion is the renin-angiotensin system. The activity of this system is inversely related to the height of blood pressure in unselected populations of normal subjects and patients with essential hypertension (55). Inhibition of the system may therefore be associated with a blood pressure response to salt depletion which is not observed in patients with a normally responding renin-angiotensin system. Two reported studies have in this context shown a close relationship between the blood pressure response to salt restriction on the one hand, and the initial plasma renin and the response of plasma renin to stimuli such as sodium depletion on the other (33,56). The lower plasma renins observed in elderly subjects may explain an apparent greater efficacy of salt restriction in the elderly which emerge from one pooled analysis (57).

METANALYSES OF SALT RESTRICTION

The technique of metanalysis has been widely employed to assess the efficacy of therapeutic maneuvers. Its value depends upon the ability to recognize possible pitfalls. Pooling of data may amplify statistical power by increasing group size, but it will also amplify any systematic bias. The possible systematic bias inherent in poorly controlled and nonrandomized studies of antihypertensive therapy has already been discussed. Placebo effects and regression to the mean may wrongly be attributed to sodium restriction. Publication bias in favor of positive results has been demonstrated elsewhere (58,59) and it is impossible to exclude when examining the effects of such a widely employed maneuver as salt restriction. This is particularly likely to be a factor where studies are selected independently of size, since small negative studies are less likely to be published than small positive studies. Lastly, pooling of data depends upon the assumption of

homogeneity at least as far as the relevant effect is concerned (60,61). Nevertheless, studies of salt restriction clearly differ in such important variables as baseline blood pressures, trial design, compliance with sodium restriction, and patient age. Conclusions derived from pooling of different studies cannot necessarily be extrapolated to each clinical and experimental situation included in the overall analysis.

It is not perhaps surprising under the circumstances that two recent metanalyses have produced radically different conclusions. Law et al. analysed the results of 78 trials of dietary salt restriction (62). Their conclusions were age-stratified, but they calculated that in subjects 50–59 years old a reduction in daily sodium intake of 100/mmol would lower systolic blood pressure by 14 mm Hg in hypertensive subjects and 10 mm Hg in normotensive subjects if sustained for 5 weeks or more. Diastolic blood pressure would be lowered by about half as much. As a result, they concluded that even more modest reductions in sodium intake would have a major impact upon strokes and heart attacks in the general population. One important point emphasized in their analysis was that trials lasting 4 weeks or less had a lesser effect upon blood pressure than more lengthy trials. This metanalysis was based upon only 10 randomized controlled trials and 68 nonrandomized trials. Although all trials employed a control period in the strict sense of the term, this was in the majority of cases part of a fixed sequence (e.g., a baseline period was followed by sodium restriction). Indeed, the earliest study included antedates the era of the modern clinical trial (63). Comparison of the results from adequately controlled trials in this metanalysis with poorly controlled studies indicates that most of the late fall in blood pressure calculated was attributable to the impact of poor controls (64). Indeed, in properly controlled studies smaller effects were observed with longer durations than with shorter duration of salt restriction (64). In view of the poor quality of most of the underlying data, it is surprising that the conclusions of the Law metanalysis have been so widely cited.

Cutler et al. (65) adopted a more rigorous approach and accepted only properly controlled randomized trials not apparently confounded by other effects (65). Twenty-three such studies were identified. Overall moderate salt restriction produced a lowering of 4.9/2.6 mm Hg in hypertensive subjects and 1.7/1.0 mm Hg in normotensive subjects. For 100-mmol/day reduction in sodium they calculated that blood pressure would be reduced by 2.2/1.3 mm Hg in normotensive subjects and 5.7/2.7 mm Hg in hypertensive subjects. These substantially more conservative conclusions reflect the greater rigor with which trials were selected.

The metanalysis by Cutler et al. omits several large studies which reported subsequent to the analysis being carried out. The inclusion of trials in which patients were receiving antihypertensive therapy or other nonpharma-

TABLE 3. *Mean changes in blood pressure (weighted by group size)*

| | No. | Hypertensive BP change | | No. | Normotensive BP change | |
		SBP	DBP		SBP	DBP
Overall	18	−2.80	−2.11	9	−1.28	−0.78
<100 mmol Na/d achieved	9	−2.30	−2.37	8	−1.73	−0.82
Double-blind trials	6	−3.92	−2.23	2	−0.98	+1.29
Open trials	12	−2.46	−1.56	7	−1.31	−1.00

BP, blood pressure; SBP, systolic blood pressure; DBP, systolic blood pressure.

cological antihypertensive measures may also have contributed to the result. Accordingly, a further metanalysis has been carried out on studies published between 1973 and 1993 (see Tables 1 and 2). Inclusion criteria were that trials should be randomized, compliance assessed by urinary sodium excretion, systolic and diastolic blood pressure independently provided, and no other dietary maneuver carried out. In addition, only trials of 2 or more weeks duration were included and more than ten patients in each study had to be subjected to dietary sodium restriction. The latter was included as a criterion since the risks of publication bias in favor of positive studies is more likely with smaller trials. Eighteen trials were identified in patients selected for high blood pressure and nine in normotensive subjects (see Tables 1 and 2). The large majority of trials in both groups show reductions in systolic and diastolic pressure, although in most cases these were fairly small. Thus, weighting trials by group size, an overall mean blood pressure fall of 2.80/2.11 mm Hg was observed in hypertensive subjects and 1.28/0.78 mm Hg in normotensive subjects. Adjusted to 100-mmol/day sodium reduction (Table 4), these values are slightly lower than those reported by Cutler et al. (65) for normotensive subjects, but of similar order for hypertensive subjects.

Some trials obtained only a disappointing reduction in sodium intake. In one case sodium intake actually rose (42). It could be argued on an "intention-to-treat" basis that these should not be excluded. However, failure to achieve the goal of less than 100 mmol/day does not materially affect the above conclusions (Tables 3, 4). Previous metanalyses have not considered the possibility that trial design may produce confounding effects through changes in components of diet other than sodium. This possibility is avoided in the double-blind design in which only sodium chloride intake is altered. Analyzing double-blind and open studies separately indicates, however, that this concern is not justified, at least in hypertensives (see Table 3 and 4). Since only two trials (both carried out by the same group) in normotensive subjects used the double-blind design, conclusions have to be guarded for these subjects.

After much controversy, the reporting of properly constructed trials of salt restriction is now leading to a reasonable consensus. Modest blood pressure lowering is achieved in hypertensive subjects, though this is only a fraction of what would be anticipated from antihypertensive drugs or dietary weight reduction (see Table 3). This is related to blood pressure level and longer duration trials indicate substantial drop in compliance. Only very small blood pressure falls are observed in normotensive subjects (Figs. 1,2). Properly constructed studies provide no evidence for greater efficacy with prolonged sodium restriction and, disappointingly, the effects of sodium restriction on blood pressure become less impressive, with lower baseline blood pressures indicating more limited value when sodium restriction is used as a preventive measure for patients with high normal pressures.

It is interesting to observe that the extent of blood pressure lowering in normotensive subjects (see Table 4) is of a similar order of magnitude to the change in blood pressure which would be anticipated from the Intersalt observational study when other dietary factors had been adjusted for. The concordance in observational and intervention studies in demonstrating weak effects supports the validity of this type of analysis.

TABLE 4. *Mean weighted reductions in blood pressure expressed per 100 mmol Na reduction*

| | No. | Hypertensive BP change | | No. | Normotensive BP change | |
		SBP	DBP		SBP	DBP
Overall	18	−5.44	−4.10	9	−1.48	−0.94
<100 mmol Na/d achieved	9	−3.30	−3.40	8	−1.63	−0.77
Double-blind trials	6	−5.76	−3.27	2	−1.45	+1.94
Open trials	12	−5.31	−3.36	7	−1.55	−1.19

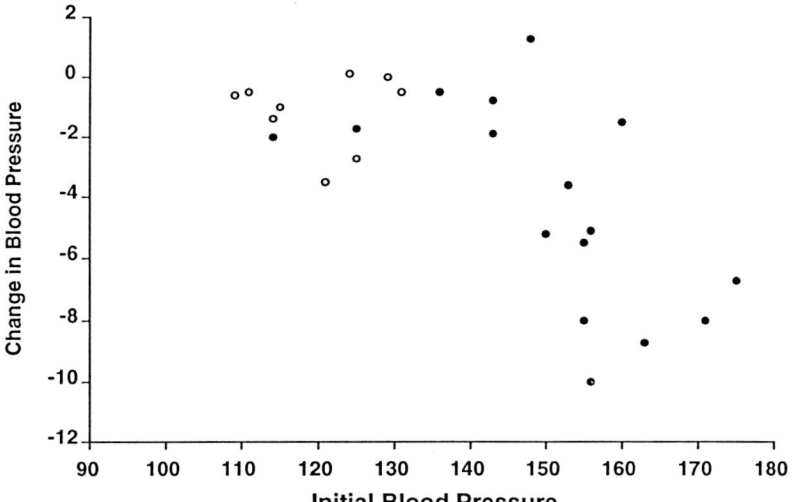

FIG. 1. Change in blood pressure in trials of salt restriction in relation to initial systolic blood pressure. Normotensive volunteers (*open circles*), subjects selected for blood pressure elevation (*closed circles*).

COSTS AND ADVERSE EFFECTS

In any assessment of drug treatment both the risks and costs of treatment as well as benefits have to be evaluated. The economic cost of dietary salt restriction has not been formally evaluated. One of its major attractions as both a therapeutic and a preventive measure is its economy, compared, for instance, to drug treatment. This, however, is more apparent than real. The advantage to providers of health care is that much of the cost of dietary modification is provided by others. These costs may fall upon the patients. Food costs may increase as selection is made from a narrower range of more expensive foods, and an increased burden may also fall upon manufacturers who have to change their processing. The expenditure of health care providers is largely limited to dietary advice and reinforcement. Even public health campaigns are not usually funded by the direct providers of health

care. These costs have to be set against efficacy of the maneuver. Blood-pressure-lowering efficacy can now be predicted with a reasonable degree of precision (see Tables 3,4). The efficacy of individual and population advice in reducing sodium intake is more uncertain. While one New Zealand community study using a short, intensive training program produced falls in sodium intake of 70 and 47 mmol/day in men and women, respectively (66), a larger program in two Belgian towns reduced sodium intake by 25 mmol in women and failed to influence it significantly in men: no effect upon blood pressure was observed in either sex (67). Although probably less intensive than the New Zealand trial, the Belgian study employed a media campaign and individual advice from doctors. It was concluded that reduction in salt intake is difficult to achieve at the population level. The disappointing reduction in sodium intake observed in some of the intervention trials underlines this problem

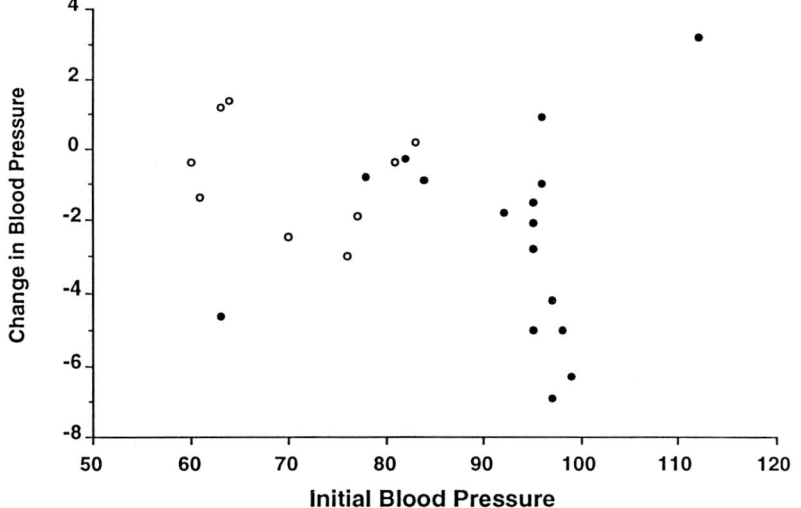

FIG. 2. Change in blood pressure in trials of salt restriction in relation to initial diastolic blood pressure. Normotensive volunteers (*open circles*), subjects selected for blood pressure elevation (*closed circles*).

(42,49). On the other hand, the use of sodium restriction as part of a general program of "hygienic measures" carried out by other groups has resulted in a sustained reduction in sodium intake (68). At an individual level, few attempts have been made to calculate the cost of sodium restriction. In the most detailed study, a program of nonpharmacological treatment (dietary weight reduction, alcohol restriction, and sodium restriction) was employed in a group of obese patients with mild hypertension for a period of 1 year (69). This regime was compared with drug treatment. Outcome was assessed on different assumptions based upon observed changes in cardiovascular risk factors such as hypertension and lipids. The cost of life-years gained varied substantially, of course, with different assumptions, but in general nonpharmacological treatment was much more costly in relation to benefits than was drug treatment. No assessment of quality of life was included in this analysis and the uncertainties led the authors to conclude that it was impossible to draw any definitive conclusions. Nevertheless, this important study does emphasize the major labor costs involved in nonpharmacological management which are often ignored.

There are few data on the incidence of adverse reactions to salt restriction in man, though this is of central importance when recommendations are made to large populations. The only systematic attempt at comparing the impact of sodium reduction and drug therapy upon quality of life was carried out by the Trail of Antihypertensive Interventions and Management (TAIM) investigators (70). Patients were randomized to one of three agents (placebo, chlorthalidone or atenolol) or one of three diets (usual, low-sodium–high-potassium, and weight loss). Low sodium intake in this study was associated with a higher incidence of fatigability and problems with erection in men and, in combination with drugs, a greater incidence of sleep disturbances in patients receiving drugs (an approximate doubling of incidence in each case). By contrast, weight reduction was associated with improvement in most measures of quality of life. Experimental studies have in general used severe salt depletion and the results cannot necessarily, therefore, be extrapolated to more moderate degrees of salt restriction, although if the physiological responses are linear, modest effects which may be of importance in large populations may still occur. Folkow and Ely have, in particular, emphasized the need for critical examination of the consequences of salt restriction (71). Both low and high salt intakes can compromise the circulation in experimental studies. Thus, severe salt restriction impairs the cardiovascular responses to such challenges as blood loss; furthermore, hypertensive animals are particularly susceptible in this regard, at least in the the case of the rat. Folkow has argued that, given free choice, animals select a salt intake approximately midway in the range of salt intakes, at the extremes of which adverse effects on the

circulation and growth were evident (72). Extrapolation to man after adjustment for differences in weight and basic metabolic rate indicates an equivalent sodium intake of 250 mmol/day. At this level, protective cardiovascular responses to physiological stress are optimal. It should be emphasized, however, that in Folkow's experimental studies the responses in changes to dietary sodium were nonlinear (i.e., only observed at each extreme of sodium intake) and it cannot therefore be assumed that intakes of sodium below the calculated optimal level are harmful.

One of the important factors in this context seems to be reduced noradrenaline response per nerve impulse, causing an animal to maintain a higher level of sympathetic activity and higher renin secretion in order to maintain blood pressure (71). This may in turn reduce the potential neuroendocrine support which can be called upon in the face of an emergency. This impairment of a normal physiological response may account for the greater operative mortality when salt-depleted animals undergo surgical procedures (73). It seems likely that sodium depletion has similar adverse consequences when major surgery is carried out in humans, although there are no controlled data in this area (74). The predisposition of salt-depleted animals to acute tubular necrosis may reflect the same physiological effect (75,76).

The effect of moderate degrees of salt restriction has not been systematically studied from this viewpoint, either in the laboratory animal or in humans. Moderate salt restriction may be free of these problems, or the incidence of adverse sequelae may be merely reduced, depending upon assumptions of linearity. In addition, patients may not be homogeneous. The elderly, for instance, are particularly at risk from diuretic-induced sodium and water depletion and may also be exposed to greater risks when consuming a low-salt diet. Whether hypertensive patients (like hypertensive rats) are at increased risk is also unknown.

HOW FAR SHOULD SALT INTAKE BE RESTRICTED?

Earlier studies of salt restriction showed substantial blood pressure lowering in severely hypertensive patients when salt intake was reduced to levels below 10 mmol/day. Murray et al. (77) attempted to define a dose-response relationship in normal subjects exposed to changes in salt intake ranging between 10 and 1500 mmols/day. Although the resultant graph showed a clear reduction in blood pressure at the extreme lower ends of salt intake (10 mmol/day), there was little relationship with blood pressure over the physiological range of sodium intake encountered in Western society. Freis (78) has postulated that efficacy of dietary salt restriction requires extracellular fluid and plasma volume contraction, which occur only when salt intake is reduced to below 3 g (50 mmol/day sodium). The only systematic approach to testing this hypothesis was undertaken by MacGregor et al. (38). Twenty hypertensive patients were randomized in double-blind fashion to sodium intakes of 50, 100 and 200 mmol/day each for 1 month. The resulting blood pressures suggested a linear response with values, respectively, of 147/91, 155/95, and 163/100 mm Hg. Pooled data from trials in hypertensive patients (see Table 1) provide little evidence for linearity when change in either urinary sodium or attained urinary sodium are examined in relation to the blood pressure response. The reduction in urinary sodium overall in the trials shown in Table 1 was 51.4 mmol/day per recruited patient. The heterogeneity of these trials, however, both in terms of basal blood pressure level and in duration and design, makes an attempt to construct a dose-response relationship hazardous. The available evidence does, however, indicate that even a reduction in sodium intake of 50 mmol/day in hypertensive subjects produces the modest blood pressure response recorded in Table 3. The degree of sodium restriction achieved in normotensive subjects was much greater (mean reduction 82.7 mmol/day), and the achieved sodium intake was much lower in normotensive compared with hypertensive patients (see Table 2). This is consistent with the particular population recruited for these studies, i.e., healthy volunteers in whom compliance is likely to be good. Patients in Table 2 are more homeogeneous, at least in terms of baseline blood pressures, compared with hypertensive patients in Table 1 and the available data suggests in some studies that the very low intakes of sodium achieved (i.e., less than 50 mmol/day) achieved a greater blood pressure fall.

SALT RESTRICTION COMBINED WITH OTHER NON-PHARMACOLOGICAL MEASURES

Salt restriction, combined with other nonpharmacological measures such as dietary weight reduction and alcohol restriction, produces useful blood-pressure-lowering effects and reduces the need of patients for an-

tihypertensive medication (68). How far the value of such regimes depends upon the sodium restriction component rather than the other components has not been examined.

The relationship between urinary sodium/potassium ratio and blood pressure in the Intersalt Study was in general stronger than the relationship between sodium intake and blood pressure (6). This and other observational studies reporting similar data (79) have led to attempts to lower blood pressure by combining sodium restriction with potassium supplementation (Table 5). The results indicate no greater fall in blood pressure than was observed in trials of sodium restriction. Where sodium restriction was formally compared with reduction in dietary sodium/potassium ratio, this conclusion was reinforced in all but one case where reduced urinary sodium/potassium produced a greater impact on blood pressure than sodium restriction alone (37). The net effect was, however, small. Smith et al. (80) formally compared the putative benefits of the two approaches by sodium restricting hypertensive subjects and then supplementing their diet with potassium in a double-blind fashion. The addition of potassium to the sodium restriction regime produced no significant further lowering in blood pressure. In summary, therefore, the available evidence does not support the view that combining potassium supplementation with sodium restriction adds to the blood-pressure-lowering effects of sodium restriction alone. This raises the interesting question of why the epidemiological association between blood pressure and urinary sodium/potassium ratio is stronger than that between blood pressure and sodium. The explanation would seem to be that the urinary sodium/potassium ratio is acting as a marker for other dietary components or lifestyle influences, rather than indicating a direct impact of these cations on blood pressure.

A number of studies have examined the impact of combining dietary weight reduction and sodium restriction on blood pressure following the original suggestion that the effect of weight reduction was mediated through altered salt intake (81,82). Some studies have shown that dietary weight reduction lowers blood pressure independent

TABLE 5. *Trials in which dietary sodium/potassium ratio was decreased*

	No.	Design	Duration	Urinary Na/K		BP change (mm Hg)		Initial BP (mm Hg)	
				Initial	Final	SBP	DBP	SBP	DBP
ANHMRC (39)	53/55	PG	3	2.21	0.95	−4.0	−2.6	153	95
Skrabal et al. (44)	20	CX	0.5	2.95	0.16	−2.3	−3.5	125	73
Smith[a] et al. (80)	20	DBCX	1	0.94	0.68	−2.0	0.0	163	103
Grobbee et al. (37)	40	DBCX	1.5	1.68	0.53	−1.8	−3.3	137	74
HPTRG (49)	195/196	PG	36	2.8	2.3	+0.1	+0.2	124	82
Langford et al. (81)	79/90	PG	6	2.36	1.41	+1.7	−0.7	145	75

[a] Patients sodium-restricted initially.

BP, blood pressure; SBP, systolic blood pressure; DBP, diastolic blood pressure; PG, parallel group; CX, crossover; DB, double blind.

dently of sodium intake (83,84). Tuck et al. (85) tested the proposition more formally by examining the influence of major weight reduction in obese subjects on two different dietary sodium intakes (120 mmols or 40 mmol/day). Blood pressure reduction was achieved in both groups of patients independently of salt intake. On the other hand, Andersson et al. (86) compared the blood pressure response in obese subjects to two regimens: in one, energy intake only was restricted and in the other, energy intake and sodium intake were restricted, the latter by 91 mmol/day. Significant falls in blood pressure were only achieved when energy and sodium restriction were combined. However, the data reported indicate a fall in blood pressure in the group subject only to calorie restriction, although this was not significant statistically (5.7/4.9 mm Hg, compared with 13.1/9.6 mm Hg). These observations are therefore still consistent with additive effects of the two maneuvers. Rocchini et al. (87) obtained rather different conclusions in a group of adolescent subjects. A major reduction in urinary sodium (from 220 to 35 mmol/day) achieved a significant fall in mean arterial pressure. Patients were then subjected to a weight loss program and, among those who lost more than 1 kg in weight, blood pressure sensitivity to changes in dietary sodium disappeared. The explanation of this phenomenon is uncertain but the authors suggest that it may be attributable to either hyperinsulinemia, hyperaldosteronism, or increased nervous system activity in the obese with the correction of these abnormalities by dietary weight reduction. Although there are significant differences in design and interpretation in all these studies, it seems probable that the effects of dietary salt restriction and dietary weight reduction are additive, although not all studies have had the statistical power to detect such effects.

There have been few formal studies of additive effects of sodium restriction with other nonpharmacological maneuvers. Parker et al. (88) used a factorial design to study blood pressure lowering effects of alcohol reduction in treated hypertensive heavy drinkers and sodium restriction (less than 60 mmols/day). Sodium restriction in this group of subjects failed to have any additional effects on the blood pressure lowering achieved by alcohol restriction. The confidence limits for the effects of sodium restriction were, however, wide and the study is perfectly consistent with sodium restriction achieving the degree of blood pressure fall recorded in Table 1. There is less evidence on the combination of sodium restriction with other nonpharmacological maneuvers. Using a factorial design, Sciarrone et al. (89) investigated the additive and independent effects of sodium restriction and diet (low in fat, high in polysaturated-to-saturated fatty acid, and high in fiber) in hypertensive patients, most of whom were receiving drug treatment. Sodium restriction significantly lowered blood pressure while the low-fat, high-fiber diet not only influenced

blood pressure but favorably influenced cholesterol levels. It was concluded that the combined effect on blood pressure and lipids carried additive benefits. Cobiac et al. (90) examined the interaction between dietary fish oil supplementation and sodium restriction in elderly normotensive subjects using a double-blind parallel group design. Sodium restriction alone produced a modest fall in systolic blood pressure (−4.2 mm Hg) but no change in diastolic blood pressure. While the fish oil supplementation produced no significant fall in blood pressure as a sole maneuver, in combination with salt restriction a useful blood pressure fall was observed (−6.7/5.2 mm Hg). Analysis of variance, adjusting for such variables as weight reduction, showed an additive effect of the two maneuvers on systolic blood pressure and a positive interaction on diastolic blood pressure.

SALT RESTRICTION AND ANTIHYPERTENSIVE MEDICATION

Dietary advice in multifactorial intervention trials has been associated with a reduction in the amount of antihypertensive medication required to control blood pressure (68). A more specific study of the interaction between dietary salt restriction and antihypertensive medication was carried out by Beard et al. (91). Ninety patients receiving medication were randomly allocated to a fairly severe salt restriction regime (37 mmol/day) or to a control group. Members of the salt-restricted group were able to halve their medication, and one patient in three was able to discontinue medication entirely. Two-thirds of the control group remained on the same dose of medication, and only 9 percent discontinued drugs. The protocol selectively resulted in diuretics being withdrawn from the diet-treated group, since diuretics were discontinued (and other agents substituted) if urinary sodium fell below 50 mmol/day. Despite this, however, the consumption of beta blockers and other antihypertensives was reduced in the diet group, suggesting that the interaction between diet and therapy was indeed a real one. The duration of the trial was 12 weeks. Therefore, it is uncertain how sustained the reduction in medication was. Other studies provide only limited information. In the TAIM trial, 878 mildly hypertensive subjects were randomly assigned to chlorthalidone, atenolol, or placebo, together with either weight loss or a low-sodium, high-potassium diet, or usual diet (81). The low-sodium, high-potassium diet did not add significantly to the antihypertensive effect of either drug. However, the decrease in urinary sodium (27.4 mmol/day) was only small. In the Treatment of Mild Hypertension Study (TOHMS) trial, 221 patients were randomly allocated to placebo or treatment with one of each major classes of antihypertensive agent (92). In addition, patients were placed on a nutritional hygienic regimen which included weight loss, sodium restriction, alcohol restriction and physical activity. The fall in blood pressure on the latter alone was 10.6/8.1 mm Hg while the fall in the combined drug and nutritional hygienic regime ranged from 16–22 mm Hg systolic blood pressure and 12–14 mm Hg diastolic blood pressure. In the absence of a control usual diet regime, however, it is not possible to determine how far blood pressure falls were attributable to the nutritional hygienic regime.

These studies do not, therefore, help to define adjuvant effects of dietary salt restriction as a sole maneuver on specific forms of antihypertensive medication. Several investigators have addressed this problem.

Diuretics

The extent to which the diuresis induced by diuretics accounts for their blood-pressure-lowering action is still controversial. There is, however, evidence that dietary salt intake influences the efficacy of diuretics as antihypertensive agents. In one study, ingestion of 20 g of sodium chloride daily for a week abolished the antihypertensive response to thiazide diuretics (93). In other investigations, raising salt intake from 50 to 100 mmol/day (94,95) and from 4.25 to 11.25 g/day virtually inhibited the blood-pressure-lowering efficacy of diuretics. Finnerty et al. replaced urinary sodium losses induced by thiazides or frusemide with saline infusion and found that blood pressure was restored to baseline levels (96). Interestingly, plasma volume expansion with dextran had no such effect. In another study, the blood pressure rise produced by the cessation of diuretic therapy was prevented by severe salt restriction (97). Other controlled studies using less extreme changes in sodium intake have been less encouraging. One crossover trial reported a small additive effect when salt restriction was combined with diuretic therapy (27), whereas two other groups reported no effect (34,98). Although this may reflect inadequate power, it is notable that one of these studies was able to detect an additive effect of sodium restriction on beta-blocker treatment (34).

Sodium depletion increases salt appetite and it is therefore possible that diuretic-treated patients may voluntarily increase sodium intake. It has been postulated that this phenomenon may explain "secondary escape" from the antihypertensive action of diuretics in some cases. Thus, Langford et al. (99) reported significantly higher urinary sodium excretion in patients on antihypertensive therapy as compared with untreated women. However, these patients were known to be taking a variety of drugs. In the previously cited crossover trial, Parijs et al. (27) reported increased urinary sodium excretion in diuretic-treated hypertensives. However, Bing et al. (51), in a longitudinal study, followed up thirty-two hypertensive patients treated with bendrofluazide (5 mg/day) as sole medication for 2 years. No change in mean 24-hour urinary sodium excretion occurred over this period and individual patients who had an increase in urinary sodium showed no preferential tendency for blood pressure to increase. Interestingly, a progressive rise in plasma renin activity (PRA) suggested that renin-angiotensin activation was a more likely mechanism for secondary escape.

Other Antihypertensive Drugs

Much less work has been carried out on the interaction between dietary salt restriction and other antihypertensive drugs. There is, however, good physiological and clinical support for the belief that the antihypertensive potency of converting enzyme inhibitors is potentiated by sodium depletion (100). Erwteman et al. (34) carried out a double-blind crossover study of beta blockade, diuretics, and moderate sodium restriction (sodium intake reduced from 130 to 70 mmol/day). They observed a useful additive effect when salt restriction was combined with the selective beta blocker metoprolol.

There is no evidence for any useful interaction between sodium restriction and calcium channel blockers. Thus, sodium restriction has not potentiated the antihypertensive action of nitrendipine (101,102), verapamil hydrochloride (103,104) or nifedipine (Adalat, Procardia) (105–107) in controlled trials. Indeed, in one brief report there was a slight pressor effect when nifedipine-treated patients were salt restricted (105). Although some of these reports are only brief and only a small fall in sodium excretion was observed in one case (102), it does seem that sodium restriction has little to add to the management of patients on calcium antagonists (105). With this exception, sodium restriction probably has small additive effects to most classes of antihypertensive agents and this may contribute to the reduction in dosage of antihypertensive medication when nutritional hygienic measures are used. The long-term difficulty in securing substantial reductions in sodium intake and possible adverse effects on quality of life may limit the usefulness of this maneuver.

SALT SENSITIVITY AND HYPERTENSION

The heterogeneity of hypertension has provided a tantalizing prospect to numerous research workers since the original debate between Platt and Pickering on the modality of blood pressure distribution curves (108). Although distinct subgroups are not evident on population distribution curves for blood pressure, it is still probable that the hypertensive population includes distinct subgroups in which multiple factors play varying roles (109). As was pointed out by one of the contributors to the Platt-Pickering debate, a unimodal distribution of, for instance, intelligence quotients or hemoglobin, conceals discrete, genetically determined disorders such as phenylketonuria or sickle-cell anemia (110).

Dahl's development of an inbred strain of rat which develops sustained hypertension after being fed a high-salt diet led naturally to the search for analogous forms of hypertension in humans (111). Kawasaki et al. (112) changed salt intake from 9 to 249 mmols of sodium per day in nineteen patients with essential hypertension, allowing a week for equilibration on each diet (112). Patients were classified into salt-sensitive and non-salt-sensitive groups, depending on whether they showed an increase in mean blood pressure of more than 10 percent. The procedures used to demonstrate "salt sensitivity" have varied widely since this pioneering study. Fujita et al. (113) used 25 mg mefruside daily instead of a period of low-salt diet and then supplemented subjects salt intake to a level of approximately 390 mmol/day. Other groups have employed intravenous saline for the salt-loading maneuver and severe sodium depletion coupled with a loop diuretic to induce sodium depletion (114). The prevalence of "sodium sensitivity" in hypertensive subjects increases with age and is higher in black subjects (115). In addition, differences between sensitive and nonsensitive subjects have been reported in a variety of relevant features, including activity of the renin-angiotensin-aldosterone system, kallikrein, circulating catecholamines, urinary dopamine, response to stress, salt taste, forearm vascular resistance, baroreflex sensitivity, intracellular electrolytes, cellular transmembrane ion fluxes, concomitant intake of chloride, potassium and calcium, oral contraceptive use, and a positive family history of hypertension (116).

Such associations may be secondary or attributable to confounding factors which may influence both the variable being assessed and the blood pressure response to changes in sodium intake. One of the key questions is how far salt sensitivity is genetically determined or how far it is a secondary effect. The apparent increase in the prevalence of salt sensitivity with age would suggest the latter. There is, however, evidence for genetic factors as well. Thus, an association has been reported between the haptoglobin phenotype Hp-1 and sodium sensitivity, although there was considerable overlap between salt-sensitive and salt-resistant individuals in this respect (117). This report awaits confirmation with more detailed family linkage studies.

Other reports have suggested that sodium sensitivity is more common in subjects with a family history of hypertension (44,118). Such family histories are notoriously unreliable, however. In the most carefully documented study, Watt et al. (46) examined the effect of changed dietary sodium in subjects whose parents both belonged to the upper part of the blood pressure distribution and those whose parents belonged to the lower part (46). No difference in responsiveness was observed, although the changes in dietary sodium were in general less than those used in other studies of salt sensitivity. Nevertheless, as an investigation of blood pressure responsiveness to a range of diets encountered in Western civilization, this study suggests that those who inherit a predisposition to hypertension have no greater incidence of sodium sensitivity. This is not the case, however, in hypertensive individuals in whom sensitivity to changes in sodium intake is clearly greater (see Tables 1, 2).

The issue of sodium sensitivity is of prime importance in both the management of individual patients and population advice. If subjects can be be identified who show a particularly favorable response to sodium restriction, this clearly has importance for treatment. Additionally, if genetically determined sodium sensitivity leads to the development of hypertension in individuals exposed to a Western intake of salt, sodium restriction may offer an important preventative strategy. In this context it has been reported that sodium-sensitive subjects show an increase in blood pressure with age. Weinberger and Fineberg examined 31 subjects (18 normotensive, 13 hypertensive) who had, 10 or more years previously, been classified according to sodium sensitivity (119). Over this period, the sodium-resistant subjects showed little or no change in blood pressure while the salt-sensitive patients showed a highly significant increase (1.42 mm Hg systolic blood pressure per year). However, the salt-sensitive subjects in this study were both older and had a higher initial blood pressure. Both of these characteristics may have influenced the subsequent blood pressure change.

VALUE OF THE CONCEPT OF SALT SENSITIVITY

The role of genetic factors in salt sensitivity is controversial. Even if their importance were established, it still could not be concluded that salt sensitivity is pathogenetically important. It might develop as a consequence of elevated blood pressure in which, of course, genetic factors are important. One possible explanation, for instance, is that hypertension impairs the mechanisms by which blood pressure is buffered against changes in sodium intake. Notably, baseline renin levels and renin responsiveness to salt depletion appear to be greater in salt-resistant normotensive and hypertensive subjects. This is consistent with the observation that salt sensitivity is more frequent in blacks and in the elderly (115). There is, therefore, a strong possibility of secondary impairment of renin responsiveness or perhaps biological variability in renin secretion as one factor in salt sensitivity. The renin-angiotensin system helps maintain blood pressure in the face of sodium depletion, and inhibition of the renin response exacerbates the fall in blood pressure produced by salt depletion (100). Interestingly, PRA is slightly elevated in first-degree relatives of hypertensive patients (120), suggesting that impairment of renin secretion is a secondary change. There is no evidence to support the original contention by Kawasaki et al. (112) that there is a subgroup of hypertensive subjects with genetically determined abnormality of sodium excretion. Although Luft et al. (120) reported reduced capacity to excrete a sodium load in first-degree relatives of hypertensives over a 24-hour period after saline infusion, other protocols have suggested that in such individuals the immediate response to saline infusion is an accelerated sodium excretion, perhaps related to slightly elevated 24-hour blood pressure levels (121).

The most important deficiency in most reports on salt sensitivity, however, is the absence of data on specificity and reproducibility. Genetically predisposed subjects may show an abnormally great pressor response to several stressful stimuli. This was the case with the Dahl salt-sensitive rat, for instance (122). The presence in some studies of indices of sympathetic adrenergic activation emphasizes the need for studies of specificity (123) before a specific role can be attributed to sodium in "salt-sensitive hypertension."

Most studies on salt sensitivity present no data on reproducibility. Blood pressure variability will lead to apparent changes in blood pressure being attributed to changes in sodium balance. The smaller the changes in blood pressure selected as a criterion for salt sensitivity, the more likely classification is to be confounded by blood pressure variability. If variability is increased in some populations, apparent salt sensitivity will also be increased. In some studies, for instance, greater spontaneous blood pressure variability has been observed in blacks compared with whites (124). Recognizing the need for a robust and reproducible set of criteria, Flack et al. (125) have shown that where a change in diastolic blood pressure of more than 2 mm Hg is used as a criterion on changing either from or to a low-salt diet, the chance probability of diagnosing sensitivity is as high as 0.49 (125). Where both an increase of this magnitude on salt loading and a decrease on salt restriction is required, the probability falls to 0.07. Where a change in diastolic blood pressure of more than 8 mm Hg is required, the relevant figures are 0.124 and 0.01. The increase in specificity is, of course, obtained at the cost of a loss of sensitivity. The problem would be made easier if there had been sufficient reports of reproducibility using different maneuvers. Sharma et al. (126) used a dietary regime to define salt sensitivity in fifteen normotensive subjects. *Salt sensitivity* was defined as a fall in mean arterial pressure greater than 3 mm Hg calculated as the difference between the average of 30 readings during the high and low period. There was near-perfect agreement between classification on the two occasions, although there was little correlation between the blood pressure change using the two maneuvers. Weinberger and Fineberg (119) used a more vigorous regime employing intravenous saline to produce sodium loading and a combination of diuretics and severe sodium restriction to produce sodium depletion. Twenty-eight normotensive and hypertensive individuals were studied: four changed categories on restudy and six subjects changed to the indeterminate category on restudy, after initial classification as salt-sensitive and salt-resistant. A decrease in mean arterial pressure of 10 mm Hg or greater was required as a criterion for sodium sensitivity and a change in blood pressure of 5 mm or less as a criterion for sodium resistance. Although the authors conclude that classification was reproducible, the correlation between changes in blood pressure on the two occasions was small (r = 0.56), indicating that only one-third of the variance of blood pressure change was reproducible. Changes in classification in this study, despite the extremely robust criterion required for the definition of salt sensitivity, suggest that where less stringent criteria are used reproducibility must be low. In summary, while it seems likely that there is heterogeneity in the response of hypertensive patients to salt restriction, there are no biochemical or physiological markers which are currently of value to the clinician in treating the individual patient, although population associations are of scientific interest. The phenomenon has not been adequately characterized in terms of reproducibility, specificity, or basic mechanisms and, in particular, even where salt sensitivity can be demonstrated it still remains uncertain whether it is of primary importance or a secondary effect of elevated blood pressure or aging.

REFERENCES

1. Swales JD. Guidelines on guidelines. *J Hypertens* 1993;11:[in press].
2. National High Blood Pressure Education Program Working Group. Report on Primary Prevention of Hypertension. *Arch Int Med* 1993;153:186–208.
3. Swales JD. Studies of salt intake in hypertension: what can epidemiology teach us. *Am J Hypertens* 1990;3:645–649.
4. Denton D. Hypertension a malady of civilisation? In Sambhi MP, ed. *Systemic effects of antihypertensive agents.* New York: Grune & Stratton, 1976;577–583.
5. Dahl LK. Salt and hypertension. *Am J Clin Nutr* 1972;25:231–244.
6. Intersalt Cooperative Research Group. Intersalt: an international study of electrolyte excretion and blood pressure. Results of 24 hour urinary sodium and potassium excretion. *Br Med J* 1988;297:319–328.
7. Beretta-Piccoli C, Davies DL, Boddy K, Brown JJ, Cumming AMM, East BW, Fraser R, Levert AF, Padfield PL, Semple PF, Robertson JIS, Weidmann P, Williams ED. Relation of arterial pressure with body sodium, body potassium and plasma potassium in essential hypertension. *Clin Sci* 1982;62:257–270.
8. Smith WCS, Crombie IK, Tavendale RT. Urinary electrolyte excretion, alcohol consumption and blood pressure in the Scottish Heart Health Study. *Br Med J* 1988;297:329–330.
9. Merrill JP, Schupak E. Mechanisms of hypertension in renoprival man. *Canad Med Assoc J* 1964;90:326.
10. Vertes V, Cangiano JL, Berman LB, Gould A. Hypertension in end-stage renal disease. *N Engl J Med* 1969;280:978–981.
11. Wilkinson R, Scott DF, Uldall PR, Kerr DNS. Plasma renin and

exchangeable sodium in the hypertension of chronic renal failure. *QJ Med* 1970;39:377–394.

12. McAreavey D, Brown JJ, Cumming AMM, Davies DL, Fraser R, Lever AF, MacKay A, Morton JJ, Robertson JIS. Inverse relation of exchangeable sodium and blood pressure in hypertensive patients with renal artery stenosis. *J Hypertens* 1981;1:297–302.

13. Barraclough MA. Sodium and water depletion with acute malignant hypertension. *Am J Med* 1966;40:265–272.

14. Kaneda H, Yamauchi T, Murata R, Matsumoto J, Haruyama T. Treatment of malignant hypertension with infusion of sodium chloride; a case report and a review. *Tohoku J Exper Med* 1980;132:179–186.

15. Thomas RD, Lee MR. Sodium repletion and beta-adrenergic blockade in treatment of salt depletion with accelerated hypertension. *Br Med J* 1976;2:1425–1426.

16. Swales JD, Tange JD. The influence of acute sodium depletion on experimental hypertension in the rat. *J Lab Clin Med* 1971;78:369–379.

17. Thurston H, Swales JD. Influence of sodium restriction upon two models of renal hypertension. *Clin Sci Mol Med* 1976;51:275–279.

18. Munoz-Ramirez H, Schatelain RE, Bumpus FM, Khairallah PA. Development of two kidney Goldblatt hypertension in rats under dietary sodium restriction. *Am J Physiol* 1980;238:G889–G894.

19. Bing RF, Smith AJ. Plasma and interstitial volumes in essential hypertension: relationship to blood pressure. *Clin Sci* 1981;61:287–293.

20. Bauer JH, Brooks CS. Body-fluid composition in normal and hypertensive man. *Clin Sci* 1982;62:43–49.

21. Ambard L, Beaujard E. Causes de l'hypertension arterelle. *Arch Gen Med* 1904;1:520–533.

22. Allen FM, Sherrill JW. The treatment of arterial hypertension. *J Metab Res* 1922;2:429–545.

23. Dole VP, Dahl LK, Cotzias GC, Eder HA, Krebs ME. Dietary treatment of hypertension: clinical and metabolic studies of patients on the rice-fruit diet. *J Clin Invest* 1950;29:1189–1206.

24. Medical Research Council. The rice diet in the treatment of hypertension. *Lancet* 1950;2:509–513.

25. Corcoran AC, Taylor RD, Page IH. Controlled observations on the effect of low sodium diet therapy in essential hypertension. *Circulation* 1951;3:1–16.

26. Joint National Committee on Detection, Evaluation and Treatment of High Blood Pressure. Non-pharmacological approaches to the control of high blood pressure. *Hypertension* 1986;8:444–467.

27. Parijs J, Joossens JV, Van der Linden L, Verstreken G, Amery AKPC. Moderate sodium restriction and diuretics in the treatment of hypertension. *Am Heart J* 1973;8:22–34.

28. Morgan T, Gillies A, Morgan G, Adam W, Wilson M, Carney S. Hypertension treated by salt restriction. *Lancet* 1978;1:227–233.

29. MacGregor GA, Markandu N, Best F, Elder D, Cam J, Squires M. Double-blind randomised crossover trial of moderate sodium restriction in essential hypertension. *Lancet* 1982;1:351–354.

30. Watt GCM, Edwards C, Hart JJ, Hart M, Walton P, Foy CJW. Dietary sodium restriction for mild hypertension in general practice. *Br Med J* 1983;286:432–436.

31. Puska P, Iacono JM, Nissinen NA, Korhonen HJ, Vartianen E, Pietenen P, Dougherty R, Leino U, Mutanen M, Moisio S, Huttimen J. Controlled randomised trial of the effect of dietary fat on blood pressure. *Lancet* 1983;1:1–5.

32. Silman AJ, Locke C, Mitchell P, Humpherson P. Evaluation of the effectiveness of a low sodium diet in the treatment of mild to moderate hypertension. *Lancet* 1983;1:1179–1182.

33. Richards AM, Espiner EA, Mashofwski AH, Nicholls MG, Ikram H, Hamilton EJ, Walls JE. Blood pressure response to moderate sodium restriction and to potassium supplementation in mild essential hypertension. *Lancet* 1984;1:757–761.

34. Erwteman RM, Nagelkerke N, Lubsen J, Koster M, Dunning AJ. B-blockage, diuretics and salt restriction for the management of mild hypertension: a randomised double-blind trial. *Br Med J* 1984;289:406–409.

35. Chalmers J, Morgan T, Doyle A, Dickson B, Hopper J, Matthews G, Moulds R, Myers J, Nowson C, Scoggins B, Stebbing M. *Australian National Health and Medical Research Council* 1986;4[Suppl 6]:S629–637.

36. Logan AG. Sodium manipulation in the management of hypertension. The view against its general use. *Can J Physiol Pharmacol* 1986;64:793–801.

37. Grobbee DE, Hofman A, Roelandt JT, Boomsma F, Schalekamp MA, Valkenburg HA. Sodium restriction and potassium supplementation in young people with mildly elevated blood pressure. *J Hypertens* 1987;5:115–119.

38. MacGregor GA, Markandu ND, Sagnella GA, Singer DR, Cappuccio FP. Double-blind study of three sodium intakes and long-term effects of sodium restriction in essential hypertension. *Lancet* 1989;2:1244–1247.

39. Australian National Health and Medical Research Council Dietary Salt Study Management Committee. Effects of replacement sodium intake in subjects on a low sodium diet: a crossover study. *Clin Exp Hypertens*(A) 1989;11:1011–1024.

40. Australian National Health and Medical Research Council Dietary Salt Study Management Committee. Fall in blood pressure with modest reduction in dietary salt intake in mild hypertension. *Lancet* 1989;1:399–402.

41. The Trials of Hypertension Collaborative Research Group. The effects of non-pharmacologic interventions on blood pressure of persons with high normal levels. Results of the Trials of Hypertension Prevention Phase I. *JAMA* 1992;267:1213–1220.

42. Sinaiko AR, Gomez-Marin O, Prineas RJ. Effect of low sodium diet or potassium supplementation on adolescent blood pressure. *Hypertension* 1993;21:989–994.

43. Fotherby MD, Potter JF. Effects of moderate sodium restriction on clinic and 24 hour ambulatory blood pressure in elderly hypertensive subjects. *J Hypertens* 1993;11:657–663.

44. Skrabal F, Auback J, Hortnagl H. Low sodium/high potassium diet for prevention of hypertension: probable mechanism of action. *Lancet* 1981;2:895–900.

45. Cooper R, Van Horn L, Liu K, Trevisan M, Nanas S, Ueshima H, Larbi E, Yu CS, Sempos C, Le Grady D, Stamler J. A randomised trial on the effect of decreased dietary sodium intake on blood pressure in adolescents. *J Hypertens* 1984;2:361–366.

46. Watt GCM, Foy CJW, Hart JT, Bingham G, Edwards C, Hart M, Thomas E, Walton P. Dietary sodium and arterial blood pressure evidence against genetic susceptibility. *Br Med J* 1985;291:1525–1528.

47. El-Ashry A, Heagerty AM, Alton SM, Bing RF, Swales J, Thurston H. Effects of manipulation of sodium balance on erythrocyte sodium transport. *J Hum Hypertens* 1987;1:105–111.

48. Myers JB. Reduced sodium chloride intake normalises blood pressure distribution. *J Hum Hypertens* 1989;3:97–104.

49. Hypertension Prevention Trial Research Group. The Hypertension Prevention Trial: three year effects of dietary changes on blood pressure. *Arch Intern Med* 1990;150:153–162.

50. Howe PRC, Cobiac L, Smith RM. Lack of effect of short-term changes in sodium intake on blood pressure in adolescent children. *J Hypertens* 1991;9:181–186.

51. Bing RF, Thurston HG, Swales JD. Salt intake and diuretic treatment of hypertension. *Lancet* 1979;2:121–123.

52. Lever AF. Slow pressor mechanisms in hypertension: a role for hypertrophy of resistance vessels? *J Hypertens* 1986;4:515–524.

53. Korner P. Causal and homeostatic factors in hypertension. *Clin Sci* 1982;63:5s–26s.

54. Oldham PD. A note of the analysis of repeated measurements of the same subjects. *J Chronic Dis* 1962;15:967–977.

55. Meade TW, Imeson JD, Gordon D, Peart WS. The epidemiology of plasma renin. *Clin Sci* 1983;64:273–280.

56. Cappuccio FP, Markandu ND, Sagnella GA, MacGregor GA. Sodium restriction lowers high blood pressure through a decreased response of the renin system. Direct evidence using saralasin. *J Hypertens* 1985;3:243–247.

57. Grobbee DE, Hofman A. Does sodium restriction lower blood pressure. *Br Med J* 1986;293:27–29.

58. Easterbrook PJ, Berlin JA, Gopalan R, Mathews DR. Publication bias in clinical research. *Lancet* 1991;337:867–872.

59. Stewart LA & Parmar MKB. Meta-analysis of the literature or of individual patient data: is there a difference. *Lancet* 1993;341:418–422.

60. Thompson SG, Pocock SJ. Can meta-analysis be trusted? *Lancet* 1991;338:1127–1130.

61. Swales JD. Meta-analysis as a guide to clinical practice. *J Hypertens* 1993;11[Suppl] [in press].

62. Law MR, Frost CD, Wald NJ. By how much does dietary salt reduction lower blood pressure? 3-analysis of data from trials of salt reduction. *Br Med J* 1991;302:819–824.

63. Perera GA & Blood DW. Relation of sodium chloride to hypertension. *J Clin Invest* 1947;26:1109–1118.

64. Swales JD. Dietary salt and blood pressure: the role of meta-analyses. *J Hypertens* 1991;9[Suppl 6]:S42–S46.

65. Cutler JA, Follmann D, Elliott P, Suh I. An overview of randomised trials of sodium reduction and blood pressure. *Hypertension* 1991;17[Suppl 1]:1-27–1-33.

66. Thaler BI, Paulin JM, Phelan EL. A pilot study to test the feasibility of salt restriction in the community. *N Z Med J* 1982;95: 839–842.

67. Staessen J, Bulpitt CJ, Fagard R, Joosens JV, Lijnen P, Amery A. Salt intake and blood pressure in the general population. A controlled intervention trial in two towns. *J Hypertens* 1986;6: 965–973.

68. Stamler R, Grimm R, Gisch FC, Elmer P, Dyer A, Berman R, Fishman J, Van Heel IV, Civinelli J, McDonald A, Stamler J. Control of high blood pressure by nutritional therapy: final report of a four-year randomised controlled trial—the Hypertension Control Program. *JAMA* 1987;257:1484–1491.

69. Johannesson M, Fagerberg B. Health economic comparison of diet and drug treatment in obese men with mild hypertension. *J Hypertens* 1992;10:1063–1070.

70. Wassertheil-Smoller S, Blaufox MD, Oberman A, Davis BR, Swencionis C, Knerr MO'C, Hawkins CM, Langford HG. Effect of antihypertensives on sexual function and quality of life. The TAIM study. *Ann Int Med* 1991;114:613–620.

71. Folkow B, Ely DL. Dietary sodium effects on cardiovascular and sympathetic neuroeffector function as studied in various rat models. *J Hypertens* 1987;5:383–395.

72. Folkow B. Critical review of studies on salt and hypertension. *Clin Exp Hypertens* (A) 1992;14:1–14.

73. Webb DJ, Clark SA, Brown WB, Fraser R, Lever AF, Murray GD, Robertson JIS. Dietary sodium deprivation raises blood pressure in the rat but does not produce irreversible hyperaldosteronism. *J Hypertens* 1987;5:525–532.

74. Thompson JE, Vollman RW, Austin DJ, Kartchner MM. Prevention of hypotensive and renal complications of aortic surgery using balanced salt solutions. *Ann Surg* 1968;167:767–776.

75. McDonald FD, Thiel G, Wilson DR, Di Bona GF, Oken DR. The prevention of acute renal failure in the rat by long term saline loading: a possible role of the renin-angiotensin axis. *Proc Soc Exp Biol Med* 1969;131:610–614.

76. Di Bona GF, Sawin LL. The renin-angiotensin system in acute renal failure in the rat. *Lab Invest* 1971;25:528–532.

77. Murray RH, Luft FC, Bloch R, Weyman E. Blood pressure response to extremes of sodium intake in normal man. *Proc Soc Exp Biol Med* 1978;159:432–436.

78. Freis ED. Does moderate salt restriction lower blood pressure? *Hypertension* 1986;8:265–266.

79. Swales JD. Dietary sodium potassium and blood pressure. In: Bursztyn P, ed. *Nutrition and blood pressure.* London: John Libby, 1987;85–109.

80. Smith SJ, Markandu ND, Sagnella GA, MacGregor GA. Moderate potassium chloride in essential hypertension: is it additive to moderate sodium restriction? *Br Med J* 1985;290:110–113.

81. Langford HG, Davis BR, Blaufox D, Oberman A, Wassertheil-Smoller S, Hawkins M, Ziembaldi N. Effect of drug and diet treatment of mild hypertension on diastolic blood pressure. *Hypertension* 1991;17:210–217.

82. Dahl LK, Silver L, Christie RW. Role of salt in the fall of blood pressure accompanying reduction of obesity. *New Engl J Med* 1958;258:1186–1192.

83. Reisin E, Abel R, Modan M, Silverberg DS, Eliahou HE, Moden B. Effect of weight loss without salt restriction on the reduction of blood pressure in overweight hypertensive patients. *New Engl J Med* 1978;298:1–6.

84. Maxwell MH, Kushiro T, Dornfield LP, Tuck ML, Waks AU. Blood pressure changes in obese hypertensive subjects during rapid weight loss: comparison of restrictive versus unchanged salt intake. *Arch Int Med* 1984;144:1581–1584.

85. Tuck ML, Sowers J, Dornfeld L, Kledzik G, Maxwell M. The effect of weight reduction on blood pressure, plasma renin activity and plasma aldosterone levels in obese patients. *New Engl J Med* 1981;304:930–933.

86. Andersson OK, Fagerberg B, Hedner T. Importance of dietary salt in the haemodynamic adjustement to weight reduction in obese hypertensive men. *Hypertension* 1984;6:814–819.

87. Rocchini AP, Key J, Bondie D, Chuo R, Moorehead C, Katel V, Martin M. The effect of weight loss on the sensitivity of blood pressure to sodium in obese adolescents. *New Engl J Med* 1989;321:580–585.

88. Parker M, Puddey IB, Beilin LJ, Vandongen R. Two-way factorial study of alcohol and salt restriction in treated hypertensive men. *Hypertension* 1990;16:398–406.

89. Sciarrone SEG, Beilin LJ, Rouse IL, Rogers PB. A factorial study of salt restriction and a low fat/high fibre diet in hypertensive subjects. *J Hypertens* 1992;10:287–298.

90. Cobiac L, Nestel PJ, Wing LMH, Howe PRC. A low sodium diet supplemented with fish oil lowers blood pressure in the elderly. *J Hypertens* 1992;10:87–92.

91. Beard TC, Gray WR, Cooke HM, Barge R. Randomised controlled trial of a no-added-sodium diet for mild hypertension. *Lancet* 1982;2:455–463.

92. Treatment of Mild Hypertension Research Group (TOHMS Study) The treatment of mild hypertension study: a randomised placebo controlled trial of a nutritional hygienic regimen along with drug monotherapies. *Arch Int Med* 1991;151:1413–1423.

93. Winer N. The antihypertensive mechanisms of salt depletion induced by hydrochlorothiazide. *Circulation* 1961;24:788–796.

94. Johnson OD, Ruchelman H, Ford RV. Diuretics and hypertension: effect of sodium balance. *N Engl J Med* 1962;267:336–338.

95. Fries ED, Wanko A, Wilson IM. Treatment of essential hypertension with chlorothiazide (Diuril). Its use and combined with other antihypertensive agents. *JAMA* 1958;166:137–139.

96. Finnerty FA, Davidov M, Kakavdiatos IVC. Relation of sodium balance to arterial pressure during drug-induced saluresis. *Circulation* 1968;37:175–183.

97. Hollander W, Chobaniasn AV, Wilkins RW. Relationship between diuretic and antihypertensive effects of chlorothiazide and mercurial diuretics. *Circulation* 1959;19:827–838.

98. Van Brummelen P, Schalekamp M, de Graeff J. Influence of sodium intake on hydrochlorothiazide-induced changes in blood pressure, serum electrolytes, renin and aldosterone in essential hypertension. *Acta Med Scand* 1978;204:151–157.

99. Langford HG, Watson RL, Gavras J. Increased salt appetite in the treated hypertensive. *Clin Res* 1975;23:55A.

100. MacGregor GA, Markandu ND, Singer DRJ, Cappuccio FP, Shore AC, Sagnella G. Moderate sodium restriction with angiotensin converting enzyme in essential hypertension: a double-blind study. *Br Med J* 1987;294:531–534.

101. Nicholson JP, Resnick LM, Di Fibio B, James HD, Jennis R, Laragh JH. Sodium restriction and the antihypertensive effect of nitrendipine. *Clin Res* 1986;34:404A (abst).

102. Salvetti A, Arzilli F, Innocenti P, Ponzalelli F, Cagianelli A, Saba P. The antihypertensive effect of nitrendipine and its interaction with sodium intake: a multicentre crossover trial. *J Hypertens* 1991;9[Suppl 6]:S364–S365.

103. Nicholson JP, Resnick LM, Laragh JH. The antihypertensive effect of verapamril at extremes of dietary sodium intake. *Ann Intern Med* 1987;107:329–334.

104. Redon-Mas J, Abellan-Aleman J, Aranda-Lara P, Figuera-von Wichmann M, de la, Luque-Otro M, Rodicio-Diaz JL, Ruilope-Urioste LM, Velasco-Quintna J. For the VERSAL study group. Hypertensive activity of verapamil: impact of dietary sodium. *J Hypertens* 1993;11:665–671.

105. Morgan T, Anderson A, Wilson D, Myers J, Murphy J, Nowson C. Parodoxical effect of sodium restriction on blood pressure in people on slow channel calcium blocking drugs. *Lancet* 1986;1: 793.

106. Cappuccio FP, Markandu ND, MacGregor GA. Calcium antagonists and sodium balance: effect of changes in sodium intake and of the addition of a thiazide diuretic on the blood pressure lowering effect of nifedipine. *J Cardio Pharmacol* 1987;10[Suppl 10]:S57–S60.

107. Luque-Otero M, Fernandez-Pinilla C, Catalan P, Nartell-Claros

N, Fernandez-Cruz A, Martinez-Gomez ME. Acute antihypertensive effect of nifedipine on high and low salt diet. *J of Cardio Pharmacol* 1987;10[Suppl 10]:S147–S148.

108. Swales JD. *Platt versus Pickering: an Episode in Recent Medical History.* London: The Keynes Press, British Medical Association, 1985;155.

109. McManus IC. Bimodality of blood pressure levels. *Stat Med* 1983;2:253–258.

110. Pickering GW. Logic and hypertension. *Lancet* 1962;1:1349.

111. Dahl LK, Heine M, Tassinari L. Effects of chronic excess salt ingestion: evidence that genetic factors play an important role in susceptibility to experimental hypertension. *J Exp Med* 1962;115:1173–1190.

112. Kawasaki T, Delea CS, Bartter FC, Smith H. The effect of high-sodium and low-sodium intakes on blood pressure and other related variables in human subjects with idiopathic hypertension. *Am J Med* 1978;64:193–198.

113. Fujita T, Henry WL, Bartter FC, Lake CR. Factors influencing blood pressure in salt-sensitive patients with hypertension. *Am J Med* 1980;69:334–344.

114. Weinberger MH, Miller JZ, Luft FC, Grim CE, Fineberg NS. Definitions and characteristics of sodium sensitivity and blood pressure resistance. *Hypertension* 1986;8[Suppl II]:II-127–II-134.

115. Luft FC, Miller JZ, Grim CE, Fineberg NS, Christian JC, Daugherty SA, Weinberger MH. Salt sensitivity of blood pressure: age and race as factors in physiological responses. *Hypertension* 1991;17[Suppl 1]:I-102–I-108.

116. Grobbee DE. Methodology of sodium sensitivity assessment: the example of age and sex. *Hypertension* 1991;17[Suppl 1]:I-109–I-114.

117. Weinberger MH, Miller JZ, Fineberg NS, Luft FC, Grim CE, Christian JC. Association of haptoglobin with sodium sensitivity and resistance of blood pressure. *Hypertension* 1987;10:443–446.

118. Oshima T, Matsuura H, Ishibashi K, Kainouchi M, Ishida T, Ozono R, Fujii T, Kajiyama G. Familial influence upon NaCl sensitivity in patients with essential hypertension. *J Hypertens* 1992;10:1089–1094.

119. Weinberger MH, Fineberg NS. Sodium and volume sensitivity of blood pressure: age and pressure change over time. *Hypertension* 1991;18:67–71.

120. Luft FC, Weinberger MH, Grim CE. Sodium sensitivity and resistance in normotensive humans. *Am J Med* 1982;72:726–736.

121. Wiggins RC, Basar I, Slater IDH. Effect of arterial pressure and inheritance on the sodium excretory capacity of normal young men. *Clin Sci Mol Med* 1978;54:639–647.

122. Dahl LK, Heine M, Thompson K. Genetic influence of the kidneys on blood pressure: evidence from chronic renal homografts in rats with opposite predispositions to hypertension. *Circ Res* 1974;34:94–101.

123. Skrabal F, Hergholz H, Neumayr M, Hamberger L, Ledochowski M, Sporer H, Hortnagl H, Schwarz, Schoritzer D. Salt sensitivity in humans is linked to enhanced sympathetic responsiveness and enhanced proximal tubular sodium reabsorption. *Hypertension* 1984;6:152–158.

124. Grim CE, Luft FC, Miller JZ, Meneely GR, Battarbee HD, Hames CG, Dahl LK. Racial differences in blood pressure in Evans County, Georgia: relationship to sodium and potassium intake and plasma renin activity. *J Chron Dis* 1980;33:87–94.

125. Flack JM, Ensrud KE, Mascioli S, Launer CA, Svendsen K, Elmer PJ, Grimm RH. Racial and ethnic modifers of the salt-blood pressure response. *Hypertension* 1991;17[Suppl 1]:I-115–I-121.

126. Sharma AM, Schattenfroh S, Kribben A, Distler A. Reliability of salt sensitivity testing in normotensive subjects. *Kllinische Wochenschrift* 1989;67:632–634.

Hypertension: Pathophysiology, Diagnosis, and Management, Second Edition,
edited by J.H. Laragh and B.M. Brenner,
Raven Press, Ltd., New York © 1995.

CHAPTER 18

The Protective Effects of High-Potassium Diets in Hypertension, and the Mechanisms by Which High-NaCl Diets Produce Hypertension—A Personal View

Louis Tobian

Evidence that potassium (K) is a very important element in human nutrition has been growing steadily for the last four decades. When considering the subject of K in the diet, one should realize that prehistoric humans and hominids (living from 3.5 million to around 10,000 years ago) lived as pure hunter-gatherers and ate only the natural food that could be obtained from hunting or collecting vegetable materials such as roots, fruits, tubers, nuts, grains, and seeds. This native food contains not only a very low amount of sodium (Na) but also a very high amount of K (1,2). The few colonies of humans living as hunter-gatherers today take in between 200 and 285 mEq of K per day (1,2). On the other hand, urban whites in the United States eat about 65 mEq/day (3), and certain population groups such as blacks in the southeastern United States average 25 to 30 mEq/day (4,5).

There is wide diversity among peoples concerning the habitual daily intake of K. All modern-day people, how-

ever, take in less than one-fourth the amount of K eaten by their prehistoric hunter-gatherer forebears. During those 3 million years of human and hominid existence, evolutionary forces were at work, and, according to Darwinian principles, it is reasonable to expect that human beings became exceedingly well adapted to this very-high-K diet (6). Such a diet could be considered the "natural" diet of humans and is in great contrast to modern-day diets. This contrast could lead to the suspicion that the modern low-K diet could have some sort of adverse physiological effect.

It may be a coincidence, but groups of people habitually on low-K diets appear to have increased cardiovascular complications. For instance, blacks in the southeastern part of the United States eat such a diet and also seem to have a higher stroke rate than any other U.S. geographic or ethnic group (5). These same blacks also have an inordinately high incidence of the type of end-stage renal disease caused by hypertension, an incidence 18 times higher than that in whites (7).

The people of Scotland are also on a relatively low-K diet, averaging about 46 mEq/day. It is well documented

L. Tobian: University of Minnesota Hospital, Minneapolis, Minnesota 55455.

that they have a considerably greater incidence of cardiovascular disease than the people of southern England, France, or Italy, regions where higher levels of K are consumed. The people of Tibet eat a very-low-K diet, about 20 mEq/day, and have an exceedingly high incidence of strokes, far more than are found in other areas of China or in Japan. The stroke rate in China and Japan, however, is also very much higher than that in certain Western countries, and stroke has long been considered the leading cause of death in those two countries. Coincidence or not, recent surveys indicate that the people in China and Japan average about 45 mEq of K per day, a level that could be considered on the low side, compared with the K intake of average American or European Caucasians. Sasaki et al. (8) described two adjoining prefectures in northern Japan (Akita and Aamori) that have contrasting diets. Farmers living in the Aamori district eat 8 to 10 apples per day, whereas those in the Akita prefecture do not, but they eat more rice instead. The consumption of this quantity of apples would provide a greater K intake and possibly a lower Na intake as well, and it is clear that the people of the apple-eating district have a significantly lower stroke rate than those in the rice-eating district.

POTASSIUM INTAKE AND BLOOD PRESSURE IN VARIOUS POPULATIONS

Primitive peoples worldwide eat very low amounts of Na and very high amounts of K and have literally no hypertension (1). Several studies suggest that K intake may indeed have an effect upon blood pressure (BP). For instance, Langford (5) collected 24-hr urines for 6 consecutive days in 101 young black women of about 20 years of age. BP was measured three times daily for 8 days. In this group, with its mixture of those genetically susceptible and those not susceptible to hypertension, there was actually no significant correlation between BP and level of Na excretion. There was, however, a positive correlation between the urinary Na/K ratio and the diastolic BP ($r = 0.37$, $p < 0.02$).

Walker et al. (9) studied a large group of people in Baltimore and could find no significant correlation between BP and Na intake, but he did find a highly significant negative correlation between K excretion and recumbent diastolic BP ($r = -0.23$, $p < 0.0001$).

Page et al. (10) found that among men of the Qash'qai tribe of northern Iran there was a correlation between BP and Na intake. The women of that tribe did not show a significant correlation between BP and Na excretion, but they did exhibit a positive correlation between BP and the Na/K ratio in the urine.

A recent report from Norway (5) showed an almost perfect correlation between mean urinary Na/K ratios and mean diastolic BP in three different areas whose populations have different BPs and K excretions.

Recent studies in Rancho Bernardo, California (11), on the island of St. Lucia in the Caribbean (12), and in Honolulu (13) found a significant positive correlation between BP and the Na/K ratio in the diet and found a negative correlation between the K/creatinine ratio in the urine and K in the diet. Similarly, in Zutphen in the Netherlands, K intake was inversely correlated with BP (14).

At least six studies in the United States indicate that blacks consume less K than whites. Watson et al. (15) studied black and white females averaging 20 years of age. The 24-hr K excretion was 28 mEq in black females and 36 mEq in white females, a significant difference.

In Evans County, Georgia, Grim et al. (4) reported an estimated K intake of 23 mEq/day in black men versus 54 mEq/day in white men, a highly significant difference. Black men had an average urinary K excretion of 24 mEq/day, compared with 40 mEq/day for white men, once again a significant difference. Similar differences were found in women of the area. A study by Zinner et al. (16) showed that black youths between the ages of 5 and 18 were likely to have a lower urinary K concentration than white youths.

In a study at five Veterans Administration Hospitals, Cushman and Langford (17) reported that the average 24-hr K excretion among blacks was 40 mEq, whereas among whites it was 70 mEq ($p < 0.001$). Voors et al. (18) found that black children excreted only two-thirds as much K per day as white children. Langford (19) found similar results in Holmes County, Mississippi, with blacks eating significantly less K than whites. Walker et al. (9), in a study in Baltimore, also confirmed that blacks take in considerably less K than do whites. Dai et al. (20) found the same pattern of K intake in three U.S. cities. These differences in K intake may have important implications for the previously mentioned hypertension in blacks, with its resultant strokes and renal disease.

Many studies show a decrease in the BP of hypertensive patients resulting from dietary K supplementation. The earliest studies were those by Addison (21) and Priddle (22). Iimura et al. (23) in Japan found a marked hypotensive effect of a high-K diet in patients with essential hypertension. MacGregor et al. (24) in England, in a very well-controlled study, noted that K supplementation brought about a decrease in BP of about 6 mm Hg systolic and 4 mm Hg diastolic in patients with essential hypertension. Morino et al. (25) found that K supplements will reduce the BP of hypertensive patients, and Svetkey et al. (26) found a reduction in BP averaging 7 mm Hg systolic and 4 mm Hg diastolic with K supplementation in patients with essential hypertension. Kaplan et al. (27) had a number of patients with essential hypertension on treatment with small doses of thiazide diuretics; these patients were given K supplements for one treatment period and not given the supplements for a contrasting period. The average BP was significantly lower by 7 mm Hg systolic and 4 mm Hg diastolic when the supplements were given.

THE EFFECT OF DIETARY POTASSIUM ON DEATHS RELATED TO STROKES

Khaw and Barrett-Connor (3) analyzed the relationship of K intake to the stroke-related death rate in a group of individuals over 50 years of age in Rancho Bernardo, California. The quantity of foods taken in was assessed with the use of food models, and this 24-hr dietary recall was carefully analyzed according to the University of Minnesota Nutrition Coordinating Center data base. The incidence of stroke-related deaths over the succeeding 12 years was ascertained and showed a very significant negative correlation with the daily intake of K. For instance, among women who took in less than 49 mEq of K per day, the stroke death rate was 5.3 per 100. When the K intake was between 49 and 66 mEq/day, the stroke death incidence was 2.1 per 100. Most striking, if the K intake was greater than 67 mEq/day, there were no stroke-related deaths at all. Each of these three groups represents tertiles of K intake, with 168 individuals in each of the tertiles. A similar relationship showed among the men in the study. When the correlation between K and the death rate was corrected for age, calorie intake, and systolic or diastolic BP, or for the fiber, magnesium, or calcium content of the food, the results still held up. Using these corrected data, it could be deduced that a 10-mEq/day increase of K intake would bring about a 40 percent decrease in the incidence of stroke-related death over 12 years. This amounts to only one full extra helping of fruits, citrus fruit juices, vegetables, or potatoes per day, which emphasizes the fact that relatively small daily increases of K intake are associated with very marked decreases of stroke-related deaths. In this study the same strong relationship could be seen if the influence of BP was totally factored out. A similar relationship of K to coronary artery events was not found.

Clearly the reduction of stroke-related deaths was related only in a minor way to a reduction of BP, whereas the protective effect of added dietary K appeared to be exerted without any change in BP. This was precisely what had been found by Tobian et al. (28) in rats with high BP. Most variations of K in the diet could be accounted for by differences in the intake of fruits and vegetables. This could be the basis for strong advice to individuals to increase somewhat their intake of fruits and vegetables, particularly since such advice would appear to be a perfectly safe alternative and one that might have a salutary effect on cancer (29,30) as well as on cardiovascular disease (31,32).

PROTECTIVE EFFECTS OF POTASSIUM IN ANIMALS

Renal Lesions

In Dahl S rats that have a genetically conditioned salt-induced high BP, one finds a gradual, progressive injury to the kidney with "normal" levels of K in the diet. Photomicrographs will show large dilated tubules filled with "casts" in the renal cortex, renal outer medulla, and renal papilla of Dahl S rats eating 4 percent NaCl and a normal amount of K. Table 1 shows what happened when a group of Dahl S rats on 4 percent NaCl was fed the same diet with 1.36 percent K added to achieve a final K concentration of 2.1 percent. (This is about the same percentage of K in the dry diet as one would find in the diet of a prehistoric human hunter-gatherer eating only natural foods.) Despite no lowering of BP, the Dahl S rats on the high-K diet had a 51 percent improvement in lesions in the renal cortex, a 32 percent improvement in lesions of the renal outer medulla, and a 43 percent improvement in lesions of the renal papilla (33).

This same protective effect can be seen in a different way. In another set of Dahl S rats fed a 4 percent NaCl diet for 24 weeks, there was uniformly severe hypertension both in rats on diets with no added K salts and in rats receiving K supplements up to a final concentration of 2.1 percent K. Figure 1 shows, however, that after 24 weeks on the usual K intake the plasma flow to the renal papilla had gone down to 13.5, which is 18 percent lower than the papillary plasma flow one finds in an S rat on a low-NaCl diet. This 18 percent reduction in plasma flow to the renal papilla in the severely hypertensive S rat was

TABLE 1. *Renal tubular dilation scores and glomerular lesion scores in Dahl S rats on diets containing varying amounts of Na and K*

Diet	BP (mm Hg)	Renal tubular dilation scores			Glomerular lesion scores
		Cortex	Outer medulla	Papilla	
4% NaCl; no K added (*n* = 18)	171	41	79	49	29
4% NaCl; 1.36% K added (*n* = 20)	174	20; −51% ($p < 0.001$)	54; −32% ($p < 0.001$)	28; −43% ($p < 0.001$)	24; −19% ($p < 0.005$)

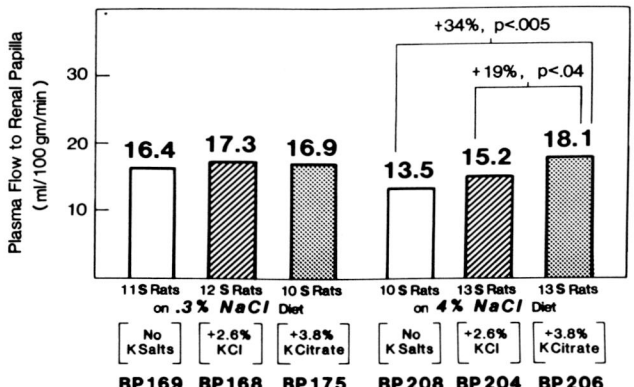

FIG. 1. Renal papillary plasma flow and mean blood pressure (BP, mm Hg) in Dahl S rats fed for 24 weeks on either low (0.3 percent)-NaCl or high (4 percent)-NaCl diets containing various potassium (K) supplements.

probably due to advancing renal lesions, including nephrosclerosis of the glomeruli and dilation of the tubules. In the Dahl S rats fed a supplement of 3.8 percent K citrate (2.1 percent total K in the diet), however, the flow to the renal papilla was not reduced at all and actually increased by 7.1 percent. The addition of 3.8 percent K citrate to S rats on a 4 percent NaCl diet actually increased the plasma flow to the renal papilla by 34 percent, compared to the S rats on the same 4 percent NaCl diet that had no added K in their diet (34). Seemingly the addition of K citrate prevented nephron loss and thereby prevented the reduction in papillary plasma flow that usually accompanies nephron loss.

Twenty-one Dahl S rats were fed a diet with 2 percent NaCl for 40 weeks to imitate the typical 2 percent NaCl diet of the United States. Ten of these S rats were fed a normal-K diet, and their isolated kidneys showed a decrease of 81 percent in the "intrinsic" glomerular filtration capacity when perfused with blood at a 125 mm Hg inflow pressure, when compared to other S rats on a low-NaCl diet. Eleven other S rats were on a similar 2 percent NaCl diet for 40 weeks, but with enough K citrate added to achieve a final K concentration of 2.1 percent. In these high-K rats, the "intrinsic" glomerular filtration rate (GFR) decreased only 52 percent even though the BP was just as high as with the normal-K diet. Thus after 40 weeks on 2 percent NaCl, the Dahl S rats on the high-K diet had an "intrinsic" GFR that was 2.6 times greater than that of the S rats on the normal-K diet ($p < 0.05$). Both these groups had almost identical *in vivo* plasma creatinine levels, indicating that the normal-K Dahl S rats were employing considerable hemodynamic adaptations in order to have the same plasma creatinine level as the high-K Dahl S rats. It appears that the high-K diet preserves glomerular function as well as tubular function in S rats on a high-NaCl diet.

Microscopic kidney slides in the Dahl S rats and in control Dahl R rats that are highly resistant to NaCl-induced hypertension were studied for arteriolar dimensions. As seen in Fig. 2, if a 4 percent NaCl diet is fed to an S rat, the rat develops hypertension, and the wall thickness of the renal arterioles increases by 38 percent. This is a well-known effect described by Volhard 73 years ago. When 1.36 percent K was added to the 4 percent NaCl diet (2.1 percent total K concentration), the Dahl S rats still became as hypertensive as ever, yet the average thickness of their renal arterioles was no thicker than the walls of the R rats that had no hypertension. Thus the added K salts greatly diminished the expected thickening of the arteriolar walls, even though the BP was not reduced (33).

These studies showed that it was possible to have high BP and no thickening of the arteriolar wall. It was as if the extra K in the diet permitted the arteriole to resist the usual effects of the high BP. The stretching effect of the hypertension was there, but additional dietary K seemed to allow the artery to be unaffected by it. This amounted to prevention of a type of arteriolar lesion in the kidney that usually results from long-standing hypertension.

Cerebral Lesions

The fact that dietary K supplements could prevent kidney arteriolar lesions led to similar studies in other parts of the body. Strokes often result from common types of arterial disease in the brain. Hypertension, which is a frequent forerunner of such strokes, causes damage primarily through a chronic overstretching of the walls of the cerebral arteries. This leads to a thickening of the artery wall with possible eventual total closure of the artery lumen, leading to a brain infarct. Thrombo-

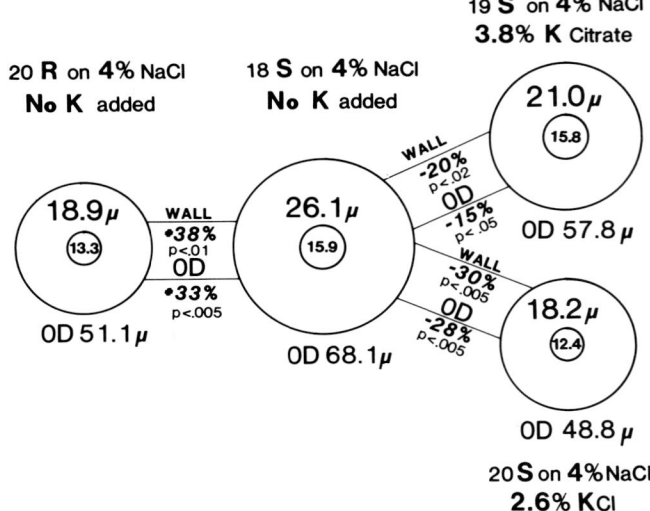

FIG. 2. Measurement of renal arteries. Average outer diameter (OD), wall thickness, and lumen size in arteries from Dahl S and R rats fed diets containing varying amounts of Na and K.

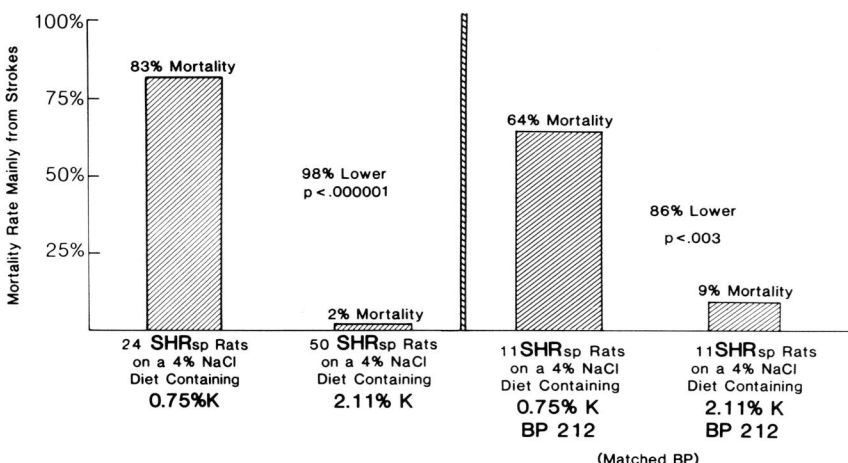

FIG. 3. The *left-hand panel* indicates the remarkable lowering of mortality rate when SHRsp eat a high-K diet (2.1 percent K) versus a normal-K diet (0.75 percent K). The *right-hand panel* shows that even when blood pressure (BP) is exactly equal in the groups being compared, the SHRsp on the high-K diet had an 86 percent lower mortality rate than the SHRsp on the normal-K diet.

sis on the diseased artery walls may hasten the total closure of the cerebral artery. On the other hand, overstretching of the cerebral arteries can also cause (a) local thinning of the wall and (b) Charcot-Bouchard microaneurysms of these arteries. Such microaneurysms have a high wall tension brought about by high intraarterial pressure and the larger radius. When stretched by the high arterial pressure, the thin-walled microaneurysm often bursts, resulting in a cerebral hemorrhage. This is another important category of strokes that result from high BP. Both types of strokes could possibly be prevented with a high-K diet.

It has been demonstrated many times that when stroke-prone spontaneously hypertensive rats (SHRsp) are fed a Japanese-style diet with 4 percent NaCl, the incidence of stroke increases, compared to an American-style diet. After 17 weeks of feeding two Japanese-type diets, each containing 4 percent NaCl, 20 of the 24 SHRsp in the diet group with no added K (0.75 percent total K) had died, an 83 percent mortality rate (Fig. 3, left side). During this same period, 49 of the 50 rats on the same diet, but with the addition of 1.36 percent K

(2.11 percent total K), were still alive and showed no evidence of a nonfatal stroke. One rat had died in the final week, giving a 2 percent mortality rate to the K-supplemented group ($p < 0.000001$) (28). The K supplements significantly reduced BP in the SHRsp, which is undoubtedly a partial explanation for the remarkable protective effect of the K supplements. However, the K supplements also appeared to reduce the death rate for a given level of hypertension. With two groups of SHRsp having virtually equal average BPs of 212 mm Hg, the group of 11 K-supplemented rats had only one death (9 percent mortality rate), whereas the group of 11 rats without K supplements had seven deaths (64 percent mortality rate). In these two groups, very closely matched for BP, the 86 percent decrease in mortality rate was significant (Fig. 3, right side). This difference indicates that K supplementation in SHRsp is very effective for preventing death even though BP is almost identical in the two groups being compared.

In another study (Fig. 4), after 10 weeks of high-NaCl diets, 18 of 33 Dahl S rats on the diet with no K supplement (0.75 percent total K) had died (55 percent mortal-

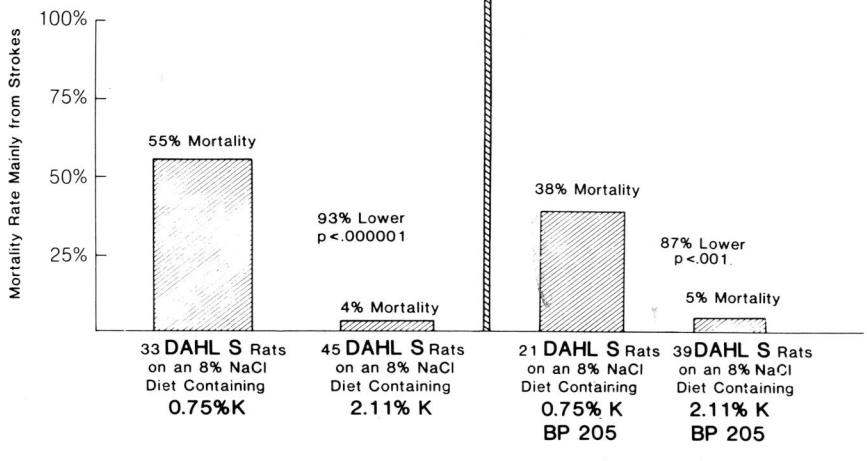

FIG. 4. The *left-hand panel* indicates the remarkable lowering of the mortality rate when Dahl S rats eat a high-K diet (2.1 percent K) versus a normal-K diet (0.75 percent K). The *right-hand panel* shows that even when blood pressure (BP) is exactly equal in the groups being compared, the Dahl S rats on the high-K diet had an 87 percent lower mortality rate than the Dahl S rats on the normal-K diet.

ity rate), whereas only two of 45 Dahl S rats on the diets with 1.36 percent K supplements (2.11 percent total K) had died (4 percent mortality rate). This 93 percent reduction in mortality rate was highly significant ($p < 10^{-6}$) (28). K supplementation did effect a modest reduction in BP in the Dahl S rats on an 8 percent NaCl diet, but again it was possible to remove the effect of this reduction of BP and still be able to analyze the influence of K supplements on mortality rate. In two groups of Dahl S rats with very closely matched BPs, the mortality rate was 38 percent (eight of 21) in the group with no K supplement, as compared to 5 percent (two of 39) in the groups with K supplementation. This 87 percent reduction in mortality rate was significant ($p < 0.001$).

In a second study of SHRsp, after 22 weeks of the diets, 18 of 28 rats had died in the group with no added K, a 64 percent mortality rate. In contrast, among the SHRsp receiving a K supplement, only two of 36 had died, a 5.6 percent mortality rate. This represents a 91 percent reduction in mortality ($p < 10^{-6}$) (28). Among the survivors in this second batch of SHRsp, each brain was examined for spots of hemorrhage. In the group of 10 survivors not receiving K supplements, four of 10 brains had spots of cerebral hemorrhage, a 40 percent incidence. Among the 34 survivors in the SHRsp that did receive K supplements, not a single brain had any spot of cerebral hemorrhage. Thus K supplementation was associated with a striking reduction in the incidence of cerebral hemorrhage ($p < 0.0001$). Survival in these three studies was greatly improved by the high-K diets (Fig. 5).

The relatively small lowerings of BP brought about by the high-K diet probably had only a minor effect in reducing the death rate. Nevertheless, it is clear that anything that lowers the BP in a hypertensive rat should have at least some small effect in reducing the death rate from strokes. So an additional study using more precise methods of taking BP was done. Male SHRsp were fed a Japanese-style diet containing 4 percent NaCl. At the end of this study, 69 percent of the SHRsp on the normal (0.75 percent)-K diet had died (40 of 58), most of them of a stroke (Fig. 5). In the group receiving K supplementation (2.11 percent K), only two of 95 rats had died, a 2 percent mortality rate ($p < 0.000001$). During the 10th week, each rat was tested for intra-arterial BP in the femoral artery under light ether anesthesia both during the day and at night. These two pressures were averaged to obtain a mean BP representative for that given rat. The feeding of a high-K diet reduced the mean BP by 17 mm Hg, with the rats on the normal-K diet having a mean BP of 187, whereas the rats on the high-K diet had a mean BP of 170 mm Hg ($p < 0.001$). With these data it was possible to obtain two perfectly matching groups of rats with equal mean BP by discarding some rats on the normal-K diet with the highest BPs and also discarding some of the rats on the high-K diet with the lowest BPs. Thus a group of 47 SHRsp on a normal-K diet with a

mean BP of 182 mm Hg were compared with 35 other SHRsp on the high-K diet that also had a mean BP of 182 mm Hg. The mortality rate in the group of SHRsp on a normal-K diet was 64 percent, whereas the mortality rate of the SHRsp on the high-K diet was 6 percent (-91 percent, $p < 0.001$) (Fig. 6). Thus it appears even more certain that the ability of the high-K diet to prevent death from strokes does not depend on a lowering of the arterial pressure.

In another study, multiple sagittal sections of the brain were obtained at 0.5-mm intervals and were examined "blindly" for the presence of brain infarcts. Among the surviving SHRsp on a normal (0.75 percent)-K diet, 13 of the 36 slides (36 percent) showed evidence of a brain infarct. In contrast, among the 11 surviving SHRsp on a 2.11 percent high-K diet, only one of 44 slides had evidence of a brain infarct, a 2 percent incidence. This was a 94.5 percent reduction of infarcts ($p < 0.0001$). This study gave clear indications that the high-K diet prevents brain infarcts in the SHRsp.

In another series of SHRsp, 25 rats fed the normal (0.75 percent)-K diet for an 8-week period had a 72 percent incidence of cerebral hemorrhage, whereas the 36 SHRsp on the high-K diet had only a 5.5 percent incidence of brain hemorrhage, a 92 percent reduction. The rats in this study were killed after 8 weeks on the diet before any of them had died of a stroke. In this period of time there was a strikingly high (72 percent) incidence of cerebral bleeding in the rats on the regular-K diet and a very low (5.5 percent) incidence in the rats on the high-K diet.

In still another group of SHRsp, it was investigated whether a high-K diet would protect against lethal strokes after there had been a bilateral carotid ligation. A number of these SHRsp were placed either on a normal- or high-K diet. After 8 weeks the BPs of each rat were taken intra-arterially under light ether anesthesia, and two groups of rats were selected with precisely matching mean BPs of 168 mm Hg. The rats underwent a bilateral carotid ligation under inactin anesthesia and were observed for the next 3 hr. Within that 3-hr interval, 48 percent of the rats on the normal-K diet had died, whereas only 23 percent of the rats on the high-K diet had died. This is a 52 percent reduction in mortality rate ($p < 0.05$). Most normal rats easily survive a bilateral carotid ligation. Among hypertensive rats there are a number of deaths after bilateral carotid ligation because the collateral arterial vessels of hypertensive rats do not dilate in a normal fashion after ligation of some of the main arteries supplying the brain. Apparently a high-K diet enables these collateral arterial channels to dilate with a much greater degree of efficiency, thereby reducing the amount of ischemia and death from brain infarcts.

In another study of hypertensive arterial hypertrophy, male SHRsp (5 weeks old) were fed 6 percent NaCl diets containing either normal (0.75 percent) K ($n = 25$) or

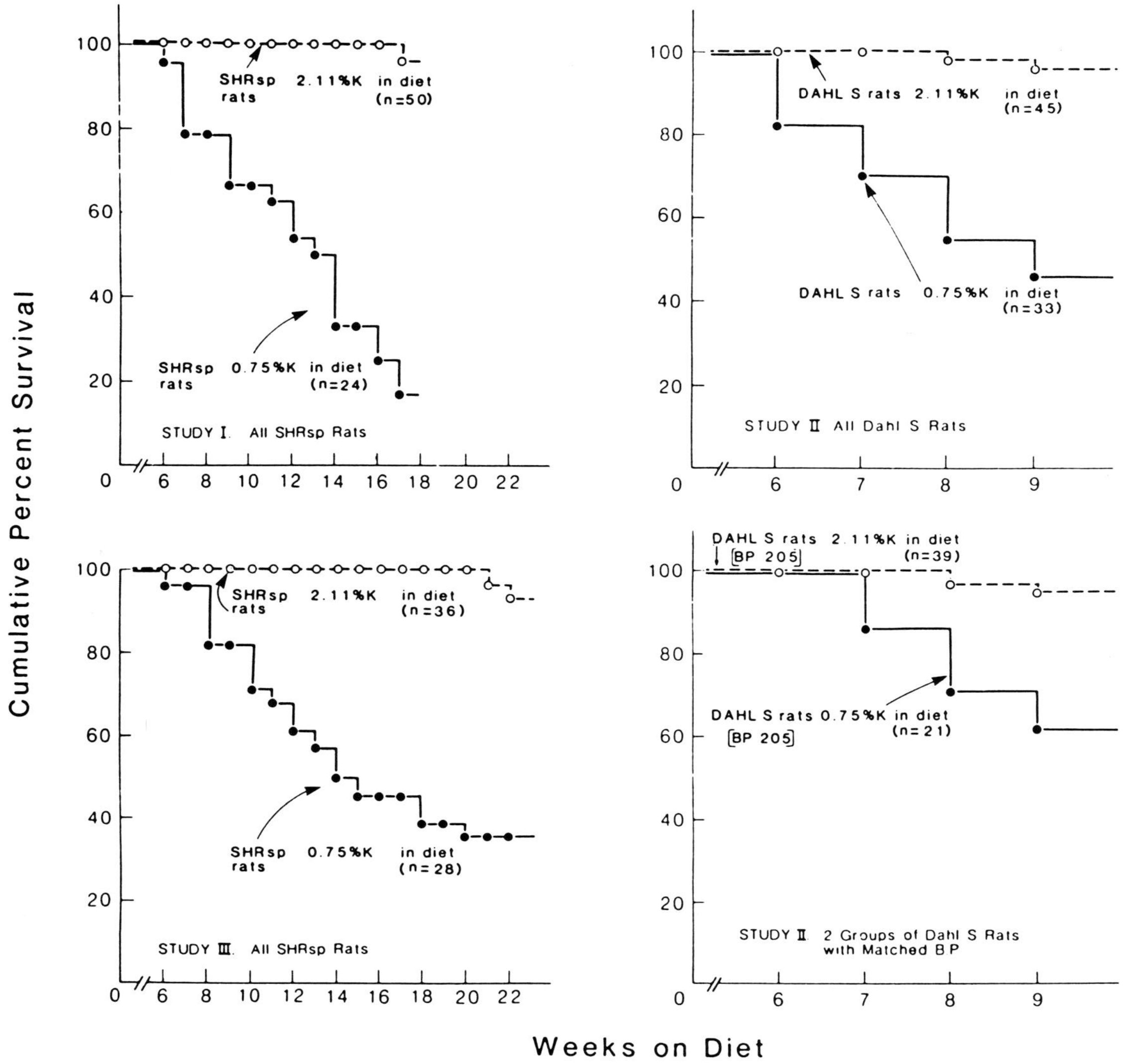

FIG. 5. These graphs plot the cumulative percentage survival rates in several studies. The *upper left-hand panel* plots the survival data of SHRsp. The two *right-hand panels* plot the survival data of Dahl S rats. The *lower left-hand panel* plots the survival rate in a second group of SHRsp. In this second group there was a 64 percent mortality among SHRsp on the 0.75 percent normal-K diet, as compared to a 5 percent mortality rate among SHRsp on the 2.1 percent high-K diet ($p < 0.000001$).

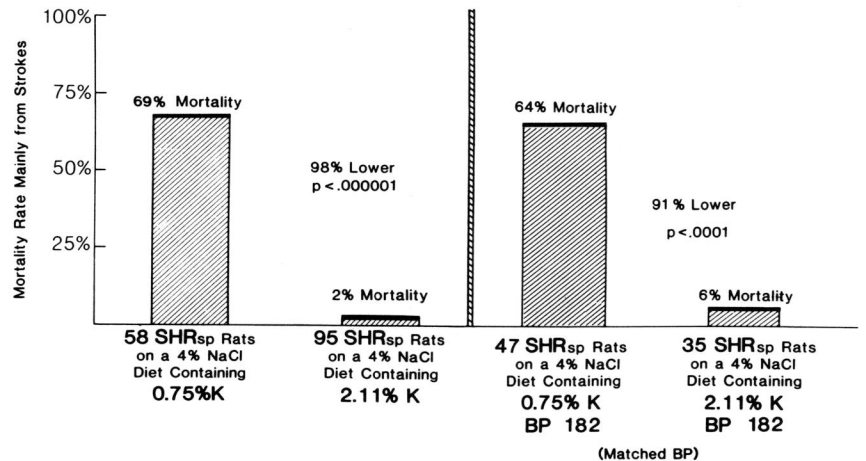

FIG. 6. Results of a study involving very accurately matched blood pressures in SHRsp. In the matched groups there was a 64 percent mortality rate among the SHRsp eating the 0.75 percent normal-K diet, in sharp contrast to the 6 percent mortality rate among SHRsp eating the 2.1 percent high-K diet.

high (2.1 percent) K ($n = 47$) for 8 weeks. Age-matched Wistar-Kyoto (WKY) rats ($n = 15$) were fed a 6 percent NaCl diet with normal K (BP 138). BPs under inactin anesthesia in these SHRsp were not different: normal K = 207 mm Hg; high K = 208 mm Hg. After perfusion fixation, average medial thicknesses (μm), normal K versus high K, were: aorta, 123 versus 94 (-24 percent); mesenteric, 72 versus 58 (-19 percent); carotid, 65 versus 56 (-14 percent); basilar, 31 versus 25 (-20 percent) ($p < 0.001$ for each). Thus all four arteries were less hypertrophied in high-K rats, with aorta and mesenterics no thicker than in normotensive WKY rats.

In these same rats, average "blind" intimal injury scores, normal K versus high K, were: aorta, 28 versus 13 (-54 percent); mesenteric, 18 versus 10 (-44 percent); carotid, 29 versus 19 (-35 percent) ($p < 0.001$ for each). In aorta and mesenterics, average intimal injury scores in high-K SHRsp were similar to scores in normotensive WKY rats. Thus high-K diets have a highly protective effect against hypertensive arterial injury in SHRsp, including prevention of intimal lesions and medial hypertrophy, even though BPs were equally high in the normal- and high-K groups. A protective effect of high-K diets against endothelial cell injury could partially explain both intimal and medial protection, since release of endothelium and macrophage-derived growth factors would be diminished with a healthier endothelium. This would reduce the medial hypertrophy and the intimal hypercellularity that results when medial smooth muscle cells migrate into the intimal layer in response to the chemoattraction of these growth factors. Reduced intimal lesions in the high-K group indicate, in all likelihood, less endothelial cell injury. With less damage to endothelium, fewer macrophages would migrate into the intima, and the release of growth factors from macrophages and damaged endothelium would be diminished, thereby causing less medial smooth muscle cell hypertrophy and less migration of smooth muscle cells from media to intima and less hyperplasia of these migrated intimal smooth muscle cells. Heart weight (gram dry weight) to body weight (kg) ratios averaged 0.98 on 0.75 percent K versus 0.85 on 2.1 percent K, 13 percent less on high K, $p < 0.001$, even though blood pressures were the same in the two groups. It thus can no longer be considered a certainty that hypertension will invariably lead to a significant thickening in the walls of arteries and arterioles. The high-K diet, even in the face of severe hypertension, can bring about a substantial reduction in wall thickening in both large and small arteries of SHRsp.

ENDOTHELIAL CELL STUDIES

Recent evidence by Tobian et al. (35) provides a strong link between high-K feeding and preservation of the integrity of arterial endothelial cells. It has been known for a decade that endothelial cells secrete a relaxing factor that acts on the smooth muscle cell of arteries. Certain vasodilating substances act directly on the smooth muscle cell, whereas others cause release, from endothelial cells, of what has been termed *endothelium-derived relaxing factors* (EDRF). These may include nitric oxide. Our investigations revealed that severe hypertension in SHRsp on a high-NaCl diet induces injury to the endothelial cells, which causes them to release much lower quantities of EDRF when stimulated with the vasodilator acetylcholine. However, when other SHRsp with equally high BP and on a high-NaCl diet are given dietary supplements of K citrate, the endothelial cell's capacity for releasing EDRF was completely preserved (35). It has also been recently reported that EDRF released from endothelial cells inhibits platelet adhesion to endothelial cells and also inhibits platelet aggregation (36–38). Thus a deficiency of EDRF release, such as would be found in hypertensive arteries, would encourage platelet adhesion to endothelial cells as well as platelet aggregation in the vicinity of the adhering platelets. This would strongly increase the likelihood of thrombosis on artery walls. Many infarct-type strokes in hypertensive people and rats are the result of thrombus formation in cerebral arteries. High-K diets greatly reduce brain infarcts in SHRsp (39) and, at the same time, protect the endothelium from hypertensive dysfunction. This preservation of EDRF release could be an important factor in reducing these thrombotic infarcts. These findings (35–39), using two separate approaches, provide strong evidence that the arterial endothelial cells are protected from hypertensive injury by the high-K diet.

Tissue Content of Potassium

To explain the protective effect of high-K diets in still another way, measurements of total exchangeable Na and total exchangeable K in Dahl S rats and in SHRsp after 23 days on either a normal- or a high-K diet were examined. Neither of the high-K diets significantly increased total exchangeable K in the Dahl S rats or in the SHRsp. Moreover, in the SHRsp, the total exchangeable Na was not altered significantly by a high-K diet. Among Dahl S rats a high-K diet resulting from the addition of KCl did not significantly alter total exchangeable Na (even though this diet provided a strong degree of protection against death from strokes as well as against hypertensive hypertrophy of arteries), but when the high-K diet was achieved by the addition of K citrate, there was a 6.5 percent reduction of body Na ($p < 0.0001$). Both KCl and K citrate, however, provided great protection against stroke deaths in Dahl S rats, even though KCl was associated with an unchanged total body Na while K citrate resulted in a reduced body Na. It is thus apparent that a reduction in total exchangeable Na is not a requisite for a marked prevention of death from hypertensive strokes.

It was also considered that high-K diets might increase the K content of skeletal muscle or the wall of the aorta, but studies in both SHRsp and Dahl S rats showed no changes in skeletal muscle or aortic wall K. The remarkable protective effect of the high-K diet can be achieved without any changes in total body K, muscle K, aortic wall K, bone K, or plasma K.

EFFECTS OF POTASSIUM

In our experiments, the mortality rate in Dahl S rats on 8 percent NaCl exceeded 50 percent. Werber et al. (40) observed a similarly high mortality rate in Dahl S rats; all 37 of his Dahl S rats were dead after 18 weeks of eating a Japanese-style chow containing 8 percent NaCl. Seventy-eight percent of his Dahl S rats had sustained a stroke after the 18 weeks of feeding, with a 35 percent incidence of cerebral hemorrhage and a 68 percent incidence of cerebral infarction. Meneely and Ball (41) reported a significantly reduced death rate in 5.6 percent NaCl-fed Sprague-Dawley rats after the addition of 1.2 percent K to the control diet. In this study, the KCl supplementation prolonged life even though the BP was not reduced below control levels. Gordon and Drury (42) produced renal hypertension in rabbits, which caused a mesenteric vascular disease with many tiny hemorrhages. Supplements of K in these rabbits did not reduce the BP but did greatly reduce the number of small hemorrhages, suggesting a partial prevention of mesenteric vascular lesions.

The precise mechanism by which extra dietary K reduces stroke deaths is, at present, elusive. Moderately severe hypertension can cause stretching in a tense arterial endothelial layer, which could cause endothelial cell dysfunction and increase the permeability of the endothelial lining (43). Such endothelial injury in cerebral arteries could ultimately produce strokes. Our data indicate that the high-K diet preserves the integrity of endothelial cells even when they are under great tension from the high BP, thereby preventing artery wall lesions with subsequent cerebral hemorrhage and infarcts.

Thus a return toward the high-K levels of prehistoric cuisine might very well diminish the high attack rates of stroke and hypertensive renal failure. As these studies indicate, the added dietary K appears to retard the development of lesions in cerebral arteries exposed to high arterial pressure.

SODIUM CHLORIDE AND HYPERTENSION

I still believe that essential hypertension in humans has a strong NaCl relationship. Several points of evidence lead to this conclusion. First, relatively primitive peoples all over the world with a lifelong low-NaCl diet (less than 60 mEq daily) have virtually no hypertension and no rise of blood pressure with advancing age. When equally primitive peoples take in generous amounts of NaCl, they develop their share of hypertension. Page et al. (44) described a group in the Solomon Islands that cooks its food in sea water. Even though quite primitive, this particular group had a sizeable incidence of hypertension. Shaper (45) describes Samburu herdsmen that were quite normotensive as they ate their native low-NaCl diet (50 mEq/day) but developed a higher incidence of hypertension when they began eating 308 mEq of NaCl daily as draftees in the army of Kenya.

The second point is that very-high-NaCl diets will raise the blood pressure in almost any human being if the NaCl intake is high enough (46). Moreover, specific groups of people such as those in the Akita Prefecture of northern Japan (47) and in Newfoundland (48) both have a very-high-NaCl diet as well as a high prevalence of hypertension.

The third point is that diets with less than 10 mEq of daily NaCl will lower the blood pressure of most hypertensive patients. The reduction may not be all the way to normotensive levels, but there is usually a significant drop of blood pressure (49).

The fourth point of evidence is that thiazide diuretics will lower the blood pressure somewhat in most hypertensive patients. This effect is NaCl-related, since it can be prevented when the thiazide diuretic is combined with a very-high-NaCl diet (50).

The fifth point of evidence is that high-NaCl diets also induce hypertension in a variety of animal species, but genetic susceptibility plays a very definite role here with various genetic strains of rats having marked differences in susceptibility to NaCl-induced hypertension. Human beings have a marked genetic variation in their susceptibility to NaCl-induced essential hypertension. One likely explanation is that those with the genetic susceptibility to hypertension have kidneys that are unable to excrete a sodium load rapidly. Possibly one of every five people is in this category. When such a person is on a lifelong low-NaCl diet, there is no tendency for a buildup of body sodium and hence no stimulus for a rise in BP. However, when such an individual eats a high-NaCl diet there is a tendency for NaCl retention, and this can gradually bring about a rise in BP. Those with a genetic resistance to hypertension probably have kidneys that excrete a sodium load in a very rapid, efficient fashion. When such people eat high-NaCl diets they will have no tendency for buildup of body Na and will remain normotensive. Grim et al. (51) found that normotensive relatives of hypertensive individuals have an abnormally slow rate of excretion of a NaCl load, providing some support for this concept. The Dahl S rat is a classic example of a rat with a strong genetic susceptibility to NaCl-induced hypertension. Several studies indicate that the kidneys of these

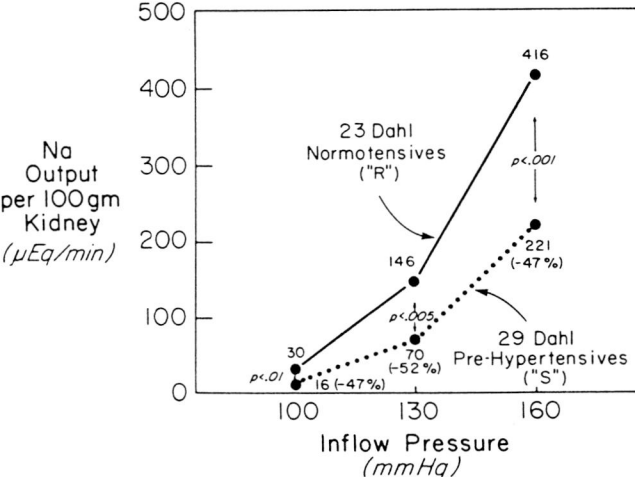

FIG. 7. Sodium excretion of isolated kidneys from S and R rats at varying inflow pressures. The distance between the large black dot (the mean value) and the tip of the arrowhead represents the standard error of the mean.

Dahl S rats have a slow rate of sodium excretion for a given arterial inflow pressure, even when they are normotensive while eating a low-NaCl diet (52) (Fig. 7). When sodium excretion by the kidney is facilitated with the addition of a thiazide diuretic, these Dahl S rats remain normotensive while consuming a high-NaCl diet (53).

When one considers a NaCl-related type of hypertension such as essential hypertension in humans or in the Dahl S rat, it is usually the combination of a high-NaCl diet plus a kidney with slow Na excretion that brings about the rise of BP. Either one of these items alone will generally not cause hypertension. In prehistoric times, when most people were living in a low-NaCl world, it was a great biological advantage to have a kidney with a capacity for avidly retaining Na. With such a kidney there was no likelihood of any buildup of body Na because the natural diet was so low in NaCl. However, this same characteristic, when carried into modern times, can be quite disadvantageous because NaCl is cheap and readily obtainable and, with such a kidney, can readily lead to hypertension.

MECHANISMS FAVORING SODIUM RETENTION IN DAHL S RATS

In the prehypertensive Dahl S rat there are several demonstrated abnormalities that could lead to an increased tendency for Na retention. We have recently shown that in this prehypertensive state the Dahl S rat shows no increase in GFR after an infusion of amino acids, indicating that there is no reserve capacity for increasing glomerular filtration (54). With this defect in glomerular filtration, maximum hemodynamic adapta-

tions are required in order to barely achieve a normal GFR. On the other hand, the Dahl R rat increased its GFR by 81 percent after the amino acid infusion, indicating that it has a great reserve capacity for increasing GFR. The isolated kidneys from prehypertensive Dahl S rats have a 33 percent reduction in GFR compared to those from Dahl R rats when both types of kidneys are perfused with blood at 100 mm Hg inflow pressure (52). Lithium clearance is also diminished in the Dahl S rat, suggesting a reduced rate of Na reabsorption from the proximal convoluted tubule. Prostaglandin E_2 levels are diminished in the cortex and in the outer and inner medullas of quick-frozen kidneys from prehypertensive Dahl S rats. This reduction in prostaglandin E_2 would lead to excessive Na reabsorption from the ascending thick limb of Henle's loop as well as from the cortical collecting tubule and the inner medullary collecting duct (55,56). Moreover, in the quick-frozen outer medulla the Dahl S rat has about a 33 percent reduction in the concentrations of prostaglandins E_2, I_2, and D_2, all of which are vasodilator prostaglandins, and a 50 percent increase in the concentration of thromboxane, which is a vasoconstrictor prostaglandin (56). The deficit in vasodilator prostaglandins and the excess of a vasoconstrictor prostaglandin would tend to cause vasoconstriction in the descending vasa recta, which should lead to a diminished papillary plasma flow. In fact, in the prehypertensive Dahl S rat on a low-NaCl diet we have measured a 25 percent reduction in plasma flow to the renal papilla (57). The vasoconstriction of the descending vasa recta along with the diminished papillary plasma flow would encourage Na retention. There is also evidence that the Dahl S rat has humoral agents that reduce Na excretion in isolated kidneys (53). It is not clear how many of these renal alterations occur in human beings genetically susceptible to essential hypertension. However, they do have reduced lithium clearance similar to that in Dahl S rats (58).

When a Dahl S rat begins eating a 4 percent high-NaCl diet, a change occurs in the kidney that further compromises GFR. As seen in isolated kidneys perfused with blood at normotensive pressures, 20 days of a high-NaCl diet will reduce the "intrinsic" GFR by 42 percent, whereas only 5 days of the high-NaCl diet causes almost no reduction (59). These changes brought about by 20 days of a high-NaCl diet in a susceptible species could be partially irreversible, with the kidney and the BP never completely recovering even when a very-low-NaCl diet is reinstituted (60).

HOW IS THE SODIUM CHLORIDE SIGNAL TRANSMITTED?

When the combination of a high-NaCl diet plus a kidney with sluggish Na excretion brings on hypertension in a susceptible human or rat, it is still a mystery as to how the NaCl signal is perceived. In certain people this NaCl signal may not be perceived at all. We see signs of this in individuals who gradually go into renal failure with no hypertension whatsoever and in whom a large expansion of extracellular fluid volume for 4 weeks under dialysis conditions leads to no rise of BP (61). This lack of reception of the NaCl signal may be present in as many as 20 percent of people. One possible NaCl receptor would be the juxtaglomerular cells in the walls of the renal afferent arterioles. An increased extracellular volume, as well as an increased concentration of NaCl in plasma, diminishes renin secretion (62,63). It is also possible that the signal for excess NaCl could be perceived in the central nervous system (CNS). Various lesions in the CNS of the Dahl S rat can greatly attenuate NaCl-induced hypertension. 6-Hydroxy dopamine injected into the lateral brain ventricle destroys many catecholamine-containing neurons and reduces NaCl hypertension by 50 percent (64). Bilateral lesions of the paraventricular nuclei will also reduce NaCl hypertension by 50 percent (65). A thermal lesion at the anterior end of the third brain ventricle (AV3V area) will reduce NaCl hypertension by 60 percent (66). Moreover, a bilateral lesion of the suprachiasmatic nuclei, which are at the bottom of the third brain ventricle, will actually increase NaCl hypertension by 15 mm Hg and will also increase heart-weight/body-weight ratios by 15 percent (64). Thus, it is essential to have certain CNS systems intact in order to get the full expression of NaCl-induced hypertension. This could indicate the possibility that the NaCl signal is somehow received in the brain.

If such is the case it would be helpful to know just how the NaCl signal is received. It is well known that hypertonic NaCl introduced into the lateral brain ventricle will induce a pressor response, and such pressor responses are greatly exaggerated in the prehypertensive Dahl S rat (67). When an excessive amount of NaCl is incorporated in food, it would transiently increase the NaCl concentration and tonicity of extracellular fluid, and the signal could be perceived in this way. In order to investigate this, we have recently prepared a high-NaCl liquid diet to be fed to Dahl S rats for 12 weeks with no additional water offered. These liquid diets contain 8 g of NaCl per 100 g of soluble nutrients. These components were dissolved in a minimal amount of water to produce a hypertonic liquid diet (1.4 percent NaCl), and these same components were also dissolved in a much greater volume of water to produce a hypotonic (0.45 percent NaCl) diet. Eleven Dahl S rats ate the hypertonic 1.4 percent NaCl diet, and 12 other Dahl S rats ate the hypotonic 0.45 percent NaCl diet. At the end of 12 weeks on either of the diets, the average intra-arterial mean BP was 195 mm Hg for both the hypertonic and the hypotonic groups. Since just as much of a rise of blood pressure occurred when the NaCl was introduced in a hypotonic fashion, it is quite unlikely that a high NaCl concentration is the signal that brings about a rise in BP. If a rise in NaCl concentration is not the signal, the most likely alternate signal would be a rise in extracellular fluid volume in some specialized receptor area. It is a common experience that a week at an international scientific conference with all the attendant high-NaCl food leads to some puffiness of hands and feet with difficulty in removing wedding rings. Many control systems involving body water are located in nuclei surrounding the third brain ventricle, which is a vertical, slit-like structure (see Fig. 8). It is conceivable that a high-NaCl diet could bring on some "puffiness" (excessive extracellular fluid volume) in the local tissues on either side of the slit that consti-

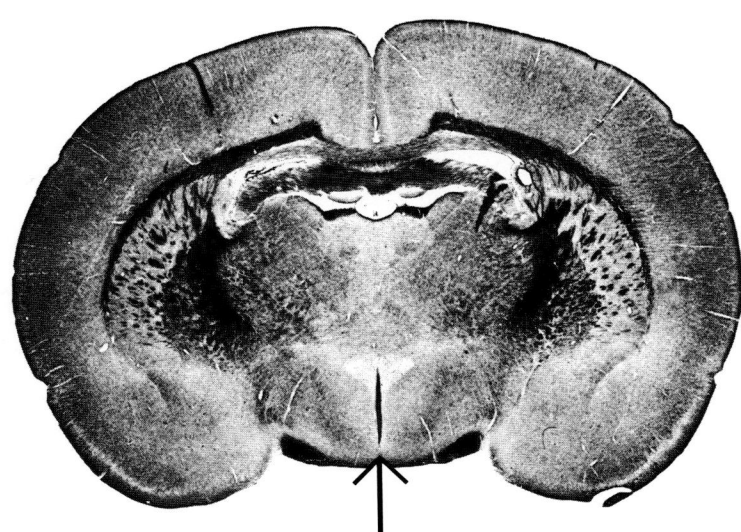

THIRD VENTRICLE

FIG. 8. Photomicrograph of the third brain ventricle. Notice that it is in the shape of a slit.

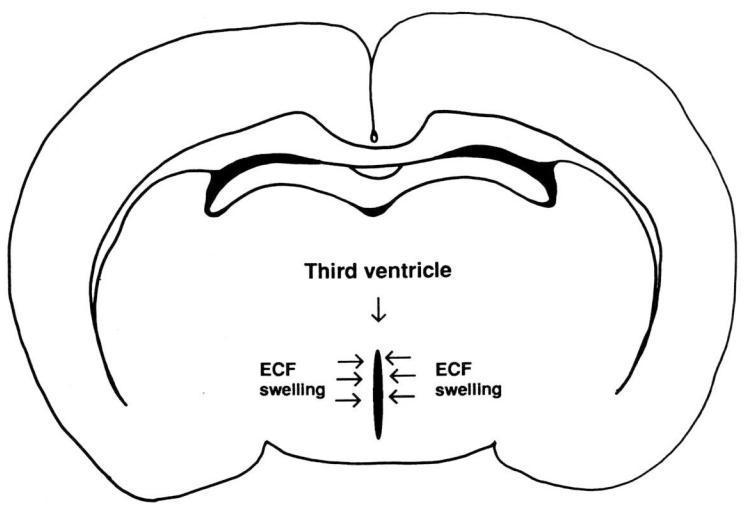

Third ventricle

↓

ECF → | ← ECF
swelling → | ← swelling
→ | ←

FIG. 9. High-NaCl diets could produce ECF swelling of tissue on either side of the third ventricle. This could close parts of the slit of the third ventricle, allowing ependymal cells and nerve fibers to touch, which could give off a signal indicating an increased ECF volume.

tutes the third brain ventricle (see Fig. 9). This localized extracellular fluid (ECF) swelling of tissue on either side of the slit could cause the ependymal cells and nerve fibers in the walls of the slit to touch one another, which could give off a neurogenic or humoral signal indicating an increased ECF volume (see Fig. 9). We decided to test this hypothesis by blocking the aqueduct of Sylvius stereotaxically with an inert silicone material in various Dahl S rats. Such a block brings on some hydrocephalus of the third brain ventricle, thereby preventing ependymal cells or nerve fibers from touching one another in response to a high-NaCl diet. Twenty Dahl S rats on a 0.23 percent low-NaCl diet had a verified block of the aqueduct as described above, while 26 other Dahl S rats on the same low-NaCl diet had a sham aqueduct block. After 6 weeks on these diets, both groups had an average intra-arterial mean BP of 130 mm Hg. Thus, the block of the aqueduct had no influence on the BP of Dahl S rats as long as they were on a very-low-NaCl diet. Thirty-four other Dahl S rats underwent a sham aqueduct block and then began eating a 6 percent high-NaCl diet. After 6 weeks the intra-arterial mean BP of these rats averaged

177 mm Hg, indicating a 47 mm Hg rise in blood pressure as a result of the high-NaCl diet. In contrast to this, 17 other Dahl S rats underwent a subsequently verified true aqueduct block and then began eating the 6 percent high-NaCl diet. After 6 weeks, the average BP of this group was 149 mm Hg, indicating a 19 mm Hg increase in BP as a result of the high-NaCl diet. Thus the true aqueduct block abolished 60 percent of the NaCl-induced rise in BP ($p < 0.001$). These results appeared to support the hypothesis that the touching of ependymal and nerve cells lining the third ventricle produces the signal that ultimately raises the BP in a susceptible species. After 12 weeks on the 6 percent high-NaCl diet, the mortality rate for the 34 Dahl S rats with the sham aqueduct block was 64 percent, whereas the mortality rate for the 17 Dahl S rats with the true aqueduct block was only 6 percent. Thus the block of the aqueduct resulted in a 90 percent reduction in mortality rate ($p < 0.001$). There were no deaths among either group of Dahl S rats on the 0.23 percent low-NaCl diet. Cumulative survival curves in Fig. 10 indicate the striking increase in survival among the S rats with the verified true aqueduct block. At the

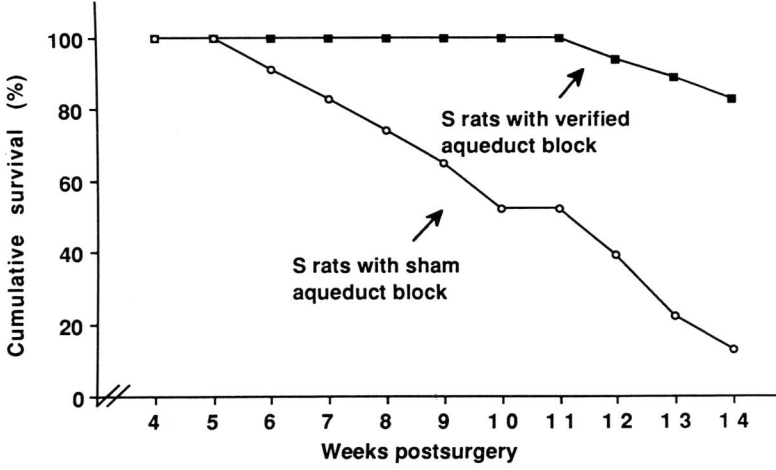

FIG. 10. Cumulative survival in Dahl S rats on a 6 percent NaCl diet that have either a verified true aqueduct block ($n = 17$) or a sham aqueduct block ($n = 34$).

11th week after surgery, none of the high-NaCl rats with the true aqueduct block had died, whereas 50 percent of those with the sham aqueduct block had already perished. The albumin in the 24-hr urine was also reduced 54 percent in the high-NaCl S rats with the true aqueduct block, compared to those with the sham aqueduct block ($p < 0.001$). When the aqueduct is blocked with silicone, it is quite possible that some of the periaqueductal fibers of passage and nuclei might be destroyed by the pressure of the silicone, and this possible periaqueductal lesion could bring about the large reduction of BP and mortality rate in the S rats on the high-NaCl diet. To examine this possibility, we made discrete thermal lesions stereotaxically in the periaqueductal structures of other S rats just before they began eating the 6 percent high-NaCl diet for 6 weeks. These rats were compared with another group of S rats on the same diet, who underwent sham thermal lesions. At this point, 25 rats with the true thermal lesion and 13 rats with the sham thermal lesion have been examined, and their respective average mean intra-arterial BPs are 176 and 166. The BP was actually higher with the thermal lesion than with the sham lesion, but there is one chance in six ($p < 0.16$) that this difference is due to chance. Thus a thermal lesion of periaqueductal fibers of passage certainly did not reduce the degree of NaCl-induced hypertension in the Dahl S rats, which strengthens the notion that it is the hydrocephalus of the third brain ventricle that is reducing the hypertension and mortality in these NaCl-fed S rats. In summary, these preliminary studies give a fairly strong indication that a signal for excess body NaCl could be a localized increase of ECF volume in the tissues surrounding the slit-like third ventricle. The local pressure from this ECF swelling could narrow the slit of the third ventricle, thereby causing ependymal cells and nerve fibers to come in contact with one another. This contact could set off a signal indicating increased ECF volume, which could ultimately cause a rise in BP with its attendant increase in mortality rate.

REFERENCES

1. Denton D. *Hunger for salt, an anthropological, physiological and medical analysis.* New York: Springer-Verlag, 1982;573–575.
2. Eaton SB, Konner M. Paleolithic nutrition. A consideration of its nature and current implications. *N Engl J Med* 1985;312:283–289.
3. Khaw KT, Barrett-Connor E. Dietary potassium and stroke-associated mortality: a 12-year prospective population study. *N Engl J Med* 1987;316:235–240.
4. Grim CE, Luft FC, Miller JZ, et al. Racial differences in blood pressure in Evans County, Georgia: relationships to sodium and potassium intake and plasma renin activity. *J Chronic Dis* 1980;33:87–94.
5. Langford HG. Dietary potassium and hypertension: epidemiologic data. *Ann Intern Med* 1983;98(Suppl):770–772.
6. Darwin C. *On the origin of species.* Cambridge: Harvard University Press, 1984.
7. Rostand SG, Kirk KA, Rutsky EA, Pate BA. Racial differences in the incidence of treatment for end-stage renal disease. *N Engl J Med* 1982;306:1276–1279.
8. Sasaki N, Mitsuhashi T, Fukushi S. Effects of the ingestion of large amounts of apples on blood pressure in farmers in Akita prefecture. *Igaku Seibutsugaku* 1959;51:103–105.
9. Walker WG, Whelton PK, Saito H, et al. Relation between blood pressure and renin, renin substrate, angiotensin II, aldosterone and urinary sodium and potassium in 574 ambulatory subjects. *Hypertension* 1979;1:287–291.
10. Page LB, Vandevert DE, Nader K, et al. Blood pressure of Qash'qai pastoral nomads in Iran in relation to culture, diet and body form. *Am J Clin Nutr* 1981;34:527–538.
11. Khaw KT, Barrett-Connor E. Dietary potassium and blood pressure in a population. *Am J Clin Nutr* 1984;39:963–968.
12. Khaw KT, Rose G. Population study of blood pressure and associated factors in St. Lucia, West Indies. *Int J Epidemiol* 1982;11:372–377.
13. Reed D, McGee D, Yano K, Hankin J. Diet, blood pressure, and multicollinearity. *Hypertension* 1985;7:405–410.
14. Kromhout D, Bosschieter EB, Coulander CDL. Potassium, calcium, alcohol intake and blood pressure: the Zutphen Study. *Am J Clin Nutr* 1985;41:1299–1304.
15. Watson RL, Langford HG, Abernethy J, et al. Urinary electrolytes, body weight, and blood pressure: pooled cross-sectional results among four groups of adolescent females. *Hypertension* 1980;2(Suppl 2):I-93–I-98.
16. Zinner SH, Margolius HS, Rosner B, et al. Familial aggregation of urinary kallikrein concentration in childhood: relation to blood pressure, race and urinary electrolytes. *Am J Epidemiol* 1976;104:124–132.
17. Cushman WC, Langford HG, for Veterans Administration Cooperative Study Group on Antihypertensive Agents. Urinary electrolyte differences in black and white hypertensives. *Clin Res* 1983;31:843A (abst).
18. Voors AW, Dalferes ER Jr, Frank GC, et al. Relation between ingested potassium and sodium balance in young blacks and whites. *Am J Clin Nutr* 1983;37:583–594.
19. Langford HG. In: Horan MJ, Blaustein M, Dunbar JB, et al, eds. *Potassium and hypertension. Proceedings of NIH workshop on nutrition and hypertension.* New York: Biomedical Information Corp, 1985;147–153.
20. Dai WS, Kuller LH, Miller G. Arterial BP and urinary electrolytes. *J Chronic Dis* 1984;37:75–84.
21. Addison W. The uses of sodium chloride, potassium chloride, sodium bromide and potassium bromide in cases of arterial hypertension which are amenable to potassium chloride. *Can Med Assoc J* 1928;18:281–285.
22. Priddle WW. Observations on the management of hypertension. *Can Med Assoc J* 1931;25:5–8.
23. Iimura O, Kijima T, Kikuchi K, Miyama A, Ando T, Nakao T, Takigami Y. Studies on the hypotensive effect of high potassium intake in patients with essential hypertension. *Clin Sci* 1981;61(Suppl):77–80.
24. MacGregor GA, Smith SJ, Markandu ND, Banks RA, Sagnella GA. Moderate potassium supplementation in essential hypertension. *Lancet* 1982;Sept 11:567–570.
25. Morino T, McCaa R, Langford HG. Effect of potassium on blood pressure, sodium excretion and plasma renin activity in hypertensive patients. *Clin Res* 1978;26:805a (abst).
26. Svetkey LP, Yarger WE, Feussner JR, DeLong E, Klotman PE. Placebo-controlled trial of oral potassium in the treatment of mild hypertension. *Clin Res* 1986;34:487A (abst).
27. Kaplan NM, Carnegie A, Raskin P, Heller JA, Simmons M. K supplementation in hypertensive patients with diuretic-induced hypokalemia. *N Engl J Med* 1985;312:746–749.
28. Tobian L, Lange J, Ulm K, Wold L, Iwai J. Potassium reduces cerebral hemorrhage and death in hypertensive rats even when BP is not lowered. *Hypertension* 1985;7(Suppl 2):I-110–I-114.
29. Colditz GA, Branch LG, Lipnick RJ, et al. Increased green and yellow vegetable intake and lowered cancer deaths in an elderly population. *Am J Clin Nutr* 1985;41:32–36.
30. Hirayama T. Diet and cancer. *Nutr Cancer* 1979;1:67–81.
31. Kushi LH, Lew RA, Stare FJ, et al. Diet and 20-year mortality from coronary heart disease: the Ireland-Boston Diet-Heart Study. *N Engl J Med* 1985;312:811–818.

32. Acheson RM, Williams DRR. Does consumption of fruit and vegetables protect against stroke? *Lancet* 1983;1:1191–1193.

33. Tobian L, MacNeill D, Johnson MA, Ganguli MC, Iwai J. Potassium protection against lesions of the renal tubules, arteries and glomeruli and nephron loss in salt-loaded hypertensive Dahl S rats. *Hypertension* 1984;6(Suppl 1):170–176.

34. Ganguli MC, Tobian L, Iwai J, Johnson MA. Potassium citrate feeding protects against nephron loss in severe NaCl hypertension in rats. *Clin Sci* 1981;61(Suppl):73–75.

35. Tobian L, Sugimoto T, Johnson MA, Hanlon S. High K diets protect against endothelial injury in stroke-prone SHR rats. *J Hypertens* 1987;5(Suppl 5):263–265.

36. Radomski MW, Palmer RMJ, Moncada S. Comparative pharmacology of endothelium-derived relaxing factor, nitric oxide and prostacyclin in platelets. *Br J Pharmacol* 1987;92:181–187.

37. Radomski MW, Palmer RMJ, Moncada S. Endogenous nitric oxide inhibits human platelet adhesion to vascular endothelium. *Lancet* 1987;ii:1057–1058.

38. Radomski MW, Palmer RMJ, Moncada S. The role of nitric oxide and cGMP in platelet adhesion to vascular endothelium. *Biochem Biophys Res Commun* 1987;148:1482–1489.

39. Sugimoto T, Tobian L, Ganguli MC. High K diets protect against dysfunction of endothelial cells in stroke-prone SHR. *Hypertension* 1988;in press.

40. Werber AH, Baumbach GL, Wagner DV, Mark AL, Heistad DD. Factors that influence stroke in Dahl salt-sensitive rats. *Hypertension* 1985;7:59–64.

41. Meneely GR, Ball COT. Experimental epidemiology of chronic NaCl toxicity and the protective effects of potassium chloride. *Am J Med* 1958;25:713–725.

42. Gordon DB, Drury DR. The effect of potassium on the occurrence of petechial hemorrhages in renal hypertensive rabbits. *Circ Res* 1956;4:167–172.

43. Goldby FS, Beilin LJ. Relationship between arterial pressure and the permeability of arterioles to carbon particles in acute hypertension in the rat. *Cardiovasc Res* 1972;6:384–390.

44. Page LB, Danion A, Moellering RC Jr. Antecedents of cardiovascular disease in six Solomon Islands societies. *Circulation* 1974;49:1132–1146.

45. Shaper AG. Cardiovascular disease in the tropics: III. Blood pressure and hypertension. *Br Med J* 1972;3:805–807.

46. Murray RH, Luft FC, Block R, Weyman AE. Blood pressure responses to extremes of sodium intake in normal man. *Proc Soc Exp Biol Med* 1978;159:432–436.

47. Takahashi E, Sasaki N, Takeda J, Ito H. The geographic distribution of cerebral hemorrhage and hypertension in Japan. *Hum Biol* 1957;29:139–160.

48. Fodor JG, Abbott EC, Rusted IE. An epidemiologic study of hypertension in Newfoundland. *Can Med Assoc J* 1973;108:1365–1380.

49. Watkin DM, Froeb HF, Hatch FT, Gutman AB. Effects of diet in essential hypertension: II. Results with unmodified Kempner rice diet in fifty hospitalized patients. *Am J Med* 1950;9:441–499.

50. Winer BH. The antihypertensive actions of benzothiadiazines. *Circulation* 1961;23:211–218.

51. Grim CE, Luft FC, Miller JZ, Brown PL, Gannon MA, Weinberger MH. Effects of sodium loading and depletion in normotensive first-degree relatives of essential hypertensives. *J Lab Clin Med* 1979;94:764–771.

52. Tobian L, Lange J, Azar S, Iwai J, Koop D, Coffee K, Johnson MA. Reduction of natriuretic capacity and renin release in isolated, blood-perfused kidneys of Dahl hypertension-prone rats. *Circ Res* 1978;43(Suppl):92–98.

53. Tobian L, Lange J, Iwai J, Hiller K, Johnson MA, Goossens P. Prevention with thiazide of NaCl-induced hypertension in Dahl "S" rats: evidence for a Na-retaining humoral factor in "S" rats. *Hypertension* 1979;1:316–323.

54. Tobian L, Johnson MA, Hanlon S, Bartemes K. Prehypertensive Dahl S rats show no rise in GFR after amino acid infusion. *FASEB J* 1988;2:A1280.

55. Tobian L, Ganguli M, Johnson MA, Iwai J. Influence of renal prostaglandins and dietary linoleate on hypertension in Dahl S rats. *Hypertension* 1982;4(Suppl II):149–153.

56. Tobian L, Uehara Y, Iwai J. Prostaglandin alterations in barely hypertensive Dahl S rats. *Trans Assoc Am Phys* 1985;XCVIII:378–383.

57. Ganguli M, Tobian L, Dahl L. Low renal papillary plasma flow in both Dahl and Kyoto rats with spontaneous hypertension. *Circ Res* 1976;39:337–341.

58. Weder AB. Red-cell lithium-sodium countertransport and renal lithium clearance in hypertension. *N Engl J Med* 1986;314:198–201.

59. Tobian L, Lange J, Ulm K, Wold L, Iwai J. NaCl feeding in Dahl S rats markedly reduces GFR and RBF in isolated kidneys perfused at normotensive inflow pressures. *J Hypertens* 1986;4(Suppl 6):S370–S372.

60. Tobian L, Johnson MA, Lange J, Magraw S. Effect of varying perfusion pressures on the output of sodium and the vascular resistance in kidneys of rats with "post-salt" hypertension and Kyoto spontaneous hypertension. *Circ Res* 1975;36(Suppl 1):162–170.

61. Onesti G, Kim KE, Greco JA, Del Guercio ET, Fernandes M, Swartz C. Blood pressure regulation in end-stage renal disease and anephric man. *Circ Res* 1975;36(Suppl 1):145–152.

62. Tobian L. The interrelationship of electrolytes, juxtaglomerular cells and hypertension. *Phys Rev* 1960;40:280–312.

63. Tobian L. Some aspects of the relationship of salt and hypertension. *Trans Am Clin Climatol Assoc* 1966;78:153–160.

64. Tobian L, Ganguli M, Goto A, Ikeda T, Johnson MA, Iwai J. The influence of renal prostaglandins, central nervous system and NaCl on hypertension of Dahl S rats. *Clin Exp Pharmacol Physiol* 1982;9:341–353.

65. Goto A, Ikeda T, Tobian L, Iwai J, Johnson MA. Brain lesions in the paraventricular nuclei and catecholaminergic neurons minimize salt hypertension in Dahl salt-sensitive rats. *Clin Sci* 1981;61:53s–55s.

66. Goto A, Ganguli M, Tobian L, Johnson MA, Iwai J. Effect of an anteroventral third ventricle lesion on NaCl hypertension in Dahl salt-sensitive rats. *Am J Physiol* 1982;243:H614–H618.

67. Ikeda T, Tobian L, Iwai J, Goossens P. Central nervous system pressor responses in rats susceptible and resistant to sodium chloride hypertension. *Clin Sci Mol Med* 1978;55:225s–227s.

Hypertension: Pathophysiology, Diagnosis, and Management, Second Edition,
edited by J.H. Laragh and B.M. Brenner,
Raven Press, Ltd., New York © 1995.

CHAPTER 19

The Role of Dietary Protein in Hypertensive Disease

Walter M. Lovenberg and Yukio Yamori

Traditionally, the finding and consumption of food has been thought of as a basic need for survival. Increasingly, it is recognized that components of food may have subtle beneficial or deleterious effects on the health of humans. This seems to be particularly true with regard to cardiovascular disease. These subtle effects of food constituents are particularly difficult to study because they often take years to be expressed in humans and because their significance is profoundly affected by the genetic makeup of the individual. If one uses the example of dietary lipids and cholesterol, it is likely that 20 or more years will pass before the effects of a nonoptimal diet are apparent. Because there are very significant genetic differences in humans with regard to how the dietary lipids are handled, it is clear that a diet that may be harmful to one individual may not be harmful for another. However, a significant portion of a person's lifetime may pass before the damaging effects of an inappropriate diet are recognized. Thus, there is clearly an interaction of genetic, environmental, and behavioral factors which accounts for the eventual atherosclerosis. An analogous analysis could be made for sodium intake. Clearly, excessive sodium intake can lead to hypertensive diseases in certain individuals and not in others. There is also fragmentary evidence that subtle changes in the quantity or quality of

dietary protein affect the development of hypertension and the subsequent hypertensive diseases that it spawns. However, our knowledge of the relationship between dietary protein and hypertensive diseases is far less advanced than is the case for dietary lipids and sodium. In both atherosclerosis and sodium-dependent hypertension, significant advances in our understanding of the disease process have been made because we have had useful animal models. In the 1970s, Watanabe and his colleagues in Japan developed a strain of hyperlipidemic rabbits [1] which were later found to be defective in the low-density lipoprotein (LDL) receptor [2]. This animal model, which develops atherosclerosis similar to that seen in humans with familial hypercholesterolemia, has been found to have essentially the same genetic defect. This is an apparent loss of the LDL receptor which is essential for the uptake and metabolism of LDL. Consequently, individuals with a genetic LDL-receptor deficiency are much more likely to develop atherosclerosis when consuming a diet rich in cholesterol or cholesterol-producing constituents.

The role of sodium as a pathogenic factor in hypertension is less well defined on a molecular basis. The classic observation of Lewis Dahl and his co-workers [3] relating to the sensitivity and resistance of rats to excessive sodium intake has provided clues to the possible role of sodium in human hypertension. Based on these observations, they [4] developed outbred strains of rats that were both sensitive and resistant to excessive sodium in the diet. More recently [5], inbred strains of salt-sensitive

W. Lovenberg: Merrel Dow Research Institute, Strasbourg Center, Strasbourg 67084, France.

Y. Yamori: Department of Pathology, Shimane Medical University, Izumo 693, Japan.

and salt-resistant rats have been developed from the original outbred colonies. It would appear that the basic differences in the handling of sodium lie in the kidney (6), although the molecular or cellular basis for the difference is not known. Since many strains of rats show at least modest increases in blood pressure when exposed to a high-sodium diet, the sodium-resistant strain may be the most interesting to study. However, once again, it appears that it is the interaction of environmental, behavioral, and genetic factors that leads to sodium-dependent hypertension.

Aside from gross malnutrition arising from diets deficient in protein or containing proteins which do not provide sufficient quantities of the essential amino acids, little is known about the subtle effects of proteins on cardiovascular disease.

In this chapter, we will summarize the existing evidence for a role of dietary protein in the development of hypertensive disease.

ANIMAL MODELS FOR HYPERTENSIVE DISEASE

In 1963, Okamoto and Aoki (7) separated a new strain of genetically hypertensive rats. This strain and substrains derived from them were destined to become some of the most widely used animal models in research. Subsequently, a number of other hypertensive rat strains have been derived, but none has attained the distribution and use in research that the spontaneously hypertensive rat (SHR) has obtained. A summary of the characteristics of these various rat strains can be found in a recent review (8). An attractive feature of the SHR was that these animals manifested much of the pathology normally seen in human hypertensive disease (9). In 1974, Okamoto et al. (10) reported a substrain of the SHR which exhibited a very high incidence of stroke during its first year of life. These stroke-prone SHRs (SHR-SPs) exhibit significantly higher blood pressures than do normal SHRs; and when they develop cerebral lesions, many of the lesions correspond to the types of lesions seen in human stroke (11). It would appear that genetic factors other than those simply associated with severe hypertension may be involved in the pathogenesis of the cerebral lesions. In certain experimental conditions, the incidence of apparent stroke is less in spite of maintenance of extremely high blood pressures. Ogata et al. (12–14) have also studied the pathology of SHR-SPs, and their findings suggested that lesions seen in the brain and other tissues are much more similar to those occurring with malignant hypertension. These workers report that the occurrence of a major infarction or hemorrhage in the brains of these rats is infrequent and that the cerebral damage more closely resembles the generalized tissue damage seen with severe high blood pressure.

More recent studies, however, suggest that the initiat-

ing events in the degenerative process may have many features in common with the human disease. It now appears that the initiating event in this disease process may be medial necrosis in vascular tissue (15,16) that is caused in part by the well-established decrease in cerebral blood flow (17) when the rats are allowed to develop severe hypertension. There is some evidence to suggest that medial smooth muscle cells from the SHR-SPs may also be more sensitive to deprivation of oxygen and nutrients (18). Thus in the SHR-SP a combination of factors may come into play. The reduction in cerebral blood flow leads to a partial loss of oxygen and nutrients in the outer medial cells which, in turn, because of their increased sensitivity, start the necrotic process. This eventually leads to the loss of the blood-brain barrier in discrete locations, as demonstrated recently by Fredriksson et al. (19). These, then, are the precursor lesions for the more obvious hemorrhages and infarctions that occur in the latter stages of the disease.

While the relevance of the cerebral lesions in SHR-SPs to those seen in humans following a stroke remains to be completely resolved, it is clear that the SHR-SP represents a good model for examining the effects of very severe hypertension on the brain. The reproducibility and the frequency of cerebral lesions allow one to modify nutritional or environmental elements to determine the interplay of these factors with hypertension.

THE EFFECT OF DIET ON CEREBRAL LESIONS IN ANIMAL MODELS

In 1975, we initiated studies with this new strain of hypertensive rat (SHR-SP). The initial focus of this research was simply to utilize these rats as animal models of hypertension (20,21). By 1978, it became apparent that the SHR-SPs maintained at the National Institutes of Health (NIH) in Bethesda, Maryland, were much less susceptible to stroke than the original reports from Japan had indicated. A study was then undertaken to attempt to understand the difference in the frequency of cerebral lesions in the rats maintained in the U.S. At this time, Yamori et al. (22) had already realized that dietary factors could influence the incidence of cerebral lesions. It was therefore decided to undertake a series of joint experiments between the laboratories at the NIH and those in Japan to determine whether dietary or genetic changes led to the lower incidence of stroke observed in SHR-SPs in the U.S. laboratories. The breeding pairs of SHR-SPs were returned to Japan along with a sufficient quantity of the rat food normally used at the NIH. In the experiment, groups of rats derived from these breeding pairs were fed either the NIH open formula diet (Ralston Purina) or the Funahashi-SP diet (Funahashi Farm). Likewise, groups of rats derived from the strain of SHR-SP maintained in Japan were fed the same diets. Rats were fed these diets from 10 weeks of age until 10 months of

TABLE 1. *Comparison of the incidence of stroke in stroke-prone rats receiving different diets*

Physiologic or pathologic response	Group 1 Japanese diet (n = 28)	Group 2 American diet (n = 34)
Blood pressure (mm Hg)		
3 months of age	225 ± 5	230 ± 4
9 months of age	211 ± 3	233 ± 9
Body weight (g)	305 ± 5	306 ± 10
Incidence (%) of cerebral	28 of 32	10 of 34
lesion	(88%)	(30%)[a]
Pathology		
Infarction	20/28	8/10
Hemorrhage	3/28	—
Combined	5/28	2/10
Location		
Occipital lobe	12/28	6/10
Anteromedial cortex	10/28	4/10
Basal ganglia	7/28	3/10
Temporal cortex	9/28	2/10
Neurological symptoms		
Grade 0		
(no symptoms)	5/32	26/34
Grade I (irritable)	20/32	8/34
Grade II (lethargy)	5/32	0
Grade III (akinetic)	2/32	0

From ref. 24.
[a] Significant difference from Group 1 ($p < 0.0001$).

age. The results of this experiment (23) were rather dramatic in that 56 percent of the rats receiving the Japanese diet either died or exhibited the symptoms of stroke, whereas none of the animals receiving the NIH diet appeared to have suffered severe cerebral lesions. Of interest was the fact that the body weight gain and development of hypertension were similar in all groups of animals. This would suggest that there are subtle differences in these two diets that affect the consequences of severe hypertension. One could conclude that while hypertension is a necessary element in the development of stroke or cerebral lesions, other factors can influence the expression of the pathological event. In this study, the major difference in the two diets appeared to be in the protein content of the food, as determined by amino acid analysis of the hydrolyzed food. The total amino acids represented 17 percent of the Japanese diet and 24 percent of the NIH diet. Clearly, while these differences in protein content had no effect on growth or the development of hypertension, they may have been responsible for the differences in cerebral lesions.

Subsequently, a similar experiment was carried out at the NIH (24). The design of this experiment was somewhat different in that only stroke-prone rats that had been bred at the NIH were used to compare the two diets. Groups of animals were maintained on either of the two diets with tap water for drinking, and the progression of blood pressure and body weight was determined from 6 weeks of age until 9 months. At the end of 9 months, the surviving animals were killed, and their brains were examined for the presence of cerebral lesions. As can be seen in Table 1, upon pathological examination, only 30 percent of the animals receiving the American diet had detectable lesions in the brain, whereas 88 percent of those receiving the Japanese diet had significant lesions.

TABLE 2. *Comparison of American and Japanese laboratory stock diets*

Nutrient	Japanese diet (Funahashi-SP)	American diet (NIH)	Ratio A/J
Crude protein (%)	19.7	25.3	1.3
Crude fat (%)	4.8	5.3	1.1
Crude fiber (%)	3.4	3.5	1.0
Ash (%)	6.2	6.6	1.1
Minerals			
Calcium (%)	1.20	1.0	0.9
Phosphorus (%)	0.96	0.94	1.0
Cobalt (ppm)	0.36	0.40	1.1
Copper (ppm)	16.2	16.1	1.0
Iron (ppm)	214.0	255.0	1.2
Manganese (ppm)	52.6	61.1	1.2
Magnesium (%)	0.26	0.19	0.7
Zinc (ppm)	56.1	52.3	0.9
Iodine (ppm)	1.7	1.9	1.1
Selenium (ppm)	0.37	0.33	0.9
Vitamins			
Choline (%)	0.24	0.22	0.9
Niacin (ppm)	110	110	1.0
Pantothenic acid (ppm)	38.1	30.9	0.8
Pyridoxine (ppm)	12	10	0.8
Riboflavin (ppm)	10	8	0.8
Thiamine (ppm)	13	15	1.2
α-Tocopherol (ppm)	70	70	1.0
Vitamin K_3 (ppm)	0.5	0.5	1.0

From ref. 24.
A/J, American/Japanese; NIH, National Institutes of Health.

In these studies (24) the analyses of the diets were carried out in detail. Nutrient, mineral, and vitamin analyses (Table 2) revealed once again that while other minor differences in the composition of the food were present, the major difference was that the American diet contained significantly more protein. Not only was the total content different, but significant relative differences in the amino acid composition were observed. The only essential amino acid that was disproportionately higher in the American diet was methionine. Several of the minor amino acids such as taurine, hydroxyproline, ornithine, and methyl histidine were greatly enriched in the American diet, probably reflecting the greater use of animal sources for the protein of the rat food from the U.S. From the above studies, it was clear that subtle changes in diet could have unexpected and significant impacts on the expression of cardiovascular disease. The major outstanding questions are: What is the mechanism of this protective effect of protein? and Does this finding relate to human cardiovascular disease?

POSSIBLE MECHANISMS FOR THE EFFECT OF DIETARY PROTEIN ON CARDIOVASCULAR DISEASE

The mechanism underlying the ability of dietary protein to limit the cerebral pathology caused by severe hypertension in the SHR-SP is unknown. There are several hypothetical explanations that can be put forth, but all remain to be proved. One such hypothesis is that the increased availability of amino acids from the diet permits vascular hypertrophy to occur during the development of hypertension. There are several studies in the literature which show that vascular hypertrophy normally occurs in the SHR and SHR-SP. While such hypertrophy is often thought of as a negative consequence of hypertension, in the case of stroke it may be viewed as a protective adaptation. Folkow et al. (25) have studied in detail the adaptive changes that take place as the walls of the small blood vessels hypertrophy are related to this phenomenon. The observation that the sympathetic nervous system may regulate the expression of this hypertrophic process has been made in several laboratories.

In 1974 (26) it was found that lysine was incorporated more rapidly into the protein of small blood vessels from SHRs than into the corresponding vessels from normotensive control animals. This increased incorporation of an amino acid into protein of blood vessels was not solely due to the response to the increased pressure, since it occurred in young SHRs before they experienced a significant rise in blood pressure. Later experiments (27) provided evidence that this increased amino acid incorporation was controlled by the sympathetic nervous system. The rate of lysine incorporation into small blood vessels of the SHRs and SHR-SPs is about twice that observed in normotensive controls. Denervation of the vessels or ganglionic blockade has little effect on lysine incorporation in normotensive animals but reduces the rate of incorporation in hypertensive animals to approximately control levels. In other studies, Bevan (28) found that denervation of rabbit ear arteries slows the rate of amino acid incorporation into proteins of the vessel. Further evidence for the role of innervation on hypertrophy of vessels was the finding of Sadoshima et al. (29) that the wall-to-lumen ratio of cerebral blood vessels of hypertensive rats was reduced following denervation of the vessels.

The apparent increased sympathetic nerve activity often associated with hypertension may also serve a protective role by permitting the hypertrophy and strengthening of the blood vessels. This concept was further strengthened by the work of Sadoshima et al. (29,30), who found that when unilateral superior cervical ganglionectomy was carried out in stroke-prone rats, the majority of subsequent strokes or cerebral lesions occurred in the denervated half of the brain. It is interesting to note that in the above studies (29,30) the differential incidence of cerebral lesions could be seen only in rats receiving the low-protein Japanese rat diet. That an increased level of circulating amino acids might be a requirement for the expression of the trophic effects is a subject that should be explored. More direct experiments on the effects of dietary protein on vascular strength and responsiveness have been reported (23). Aortas from SHR-SPs fed a high-protein diet (50 percent soybean) have significantly greater ductile strength than the aortas from similar rats fed a normal-protein diet. Furthermore, SHR-SPs on a low-protein diet show a marked reduction in cerebral blood flow and chemical cerebrovascular reactivity compared to normotensive control animals. These measures of cerebrovascular performance can be largely normalized by maintaining the rats on a high-protein diet. In the above experiments the severity of the hypertension was not affected by increasing the protein in the diet of the SHR-SPs. From these studies it was concluded that dietary protein can have a significant effect on the strength and reactivity of the blood vessels.

An alternate possibility for the protective effect of dietary protein is that one or more amino acids and/or their metabolites directly affect the disease process. With this in mind we examined the effects of supplementing the diets of stroke-prone rats with either methionine or taurine. The American rat diet was relatively high in these two amino acids.

Preliminary studies suggested that methionine supplementation had only a small effect on blood pressure but did reduce the incidence of cerebral lesions in stroke-prone rats receiving a Japanese-type rat diet (31). In somewhat more complete studies with taurine (32), it was found that the levels of taurine in the liver and plasma of SHR-SPs were substantially below those found in SHRs and normotensive control animals. Treatment for 3 months with 3 percent taurine in the drinking water led to a significant reduction in blood pressure in the SHR-SPs, a slight reduction in the blood pressure in the SHRs, and no change in blood pressure in the normotensive animals. Chronic treatment with taurine did not lead to a sustained rise in tissue taurine. The tissue taurine had returned to pretreatment levels 1 day after the conclusion of the 3-month study.

The mechanism by which taurine exerts its effect on blood pressure is unknown, although it possibly occurs by a neural mechanism. It can be demonstrated that intraventricular administration of taurine causes a significant fall in blood pressure in hypertensive animals (31).

An area which has yet to be studied in detail but which deserves further investigation is the effect of excess protein intake on the excretion of sodium. It is possible that intake of protein in excess of the requirements for growth and maintenance of the animal produces a natriuretic and diuretic effect in the rat. In the dietary studies cited above (24), the sodium content of the Japanese diet was slightly higher (3.7 mg/g) than that of the American diet (2.7 mg/g). This small increase in the sodium content of the diet in itself should not be deleterious. However, if the increased protein in the diet produced metabolites that were natriuretic, coupled with the lower sodium content, it might make a significant difference in the sodium balance. In the absence of solid experimentation, such a conjecture must be considered speculative. However, of interest is a recent study which showed that SHRs maintained on 1 percent NaCl had significantly lower blood pressures when fed a high-protein diet. Furthermore, the animals receiving the high-protein diet had nearly a doubling of renal sodium clearance (33).

The fact that urea formed from the protein may be responsible for this increased sodium excretion is suggested by the work of Wang et al. (34). In this study the inclusion of 13.5 percent urea in a normal-protein diet of hypertensive rats fed 1 percent NaCl led to a marked increase in sodium and water excretion with a concomitant reduction in the severity of the hypertension and in the incidence of cerebral lesions.

A preliminary study done in human volunteers (35) also suggests that dietary protein may have an effect on the response of certain salt-sensitive individuals to increased sodium intake. In these experiments, Yamori et al. divided a group of young male volunteers into two groups, depending on whether they had a positive family history of hypertension. The group with a family history of hypertension had slightly higher control blood pressures when maintained on a diet containing 6 g of NaCl and 40 g of protein per day. When NaCl intake was increased to 25 g/day there was no change in blood pressure of the group without a positive family history, whereas the group with a positive history showed a sig-

nificant rise in mean arterial pressure. This rise in arterial pressure could be prevented if the level of animal protein in the diet was increased from 40 to 110 g/day. It therefore appears that in this specific group of subjects, increased protein intake could reduce the effects of increased sodium on blood pressure.

DIETARY PROTEIN AND RENOVASCULAR DISEASE

In contrast to the apparent beneficial effects of dietary protein in ameliorating cerebrovascular complications of hypertension, it would appear that restriction of dietary protein is beneficial when renovascular disease is the cause of or associated with hypertension. Nath et al. (36), investigating a remnant kidney model in the rat, found that reducing dietary protein from 20 percent to 6 percent led to a greater preservation of the renal function. Both glomerular filtration rate and renal clearances were improved. It was necessary to impose the dietary restriction prior to the renal injury. In a very different model, fawn-hooded rats are genetically susceptible to renal failure and significant increases in blood pressure when maintained on a normal-protein diet. DeKeijzer and Provoost (37) studied lifelong feeding on a low (12 percent) protein diet versus a high (36 percent) protein diet. The low-protein diet resulted in prolonged life span and an increased period of stable renal function with limited proteinemia. It is interesting to note that hypertension was somewhat reduced in group receiving the high-protein diet. In this regard, it is also interesting to note that another group (38) has developed a model of hypertension in the rat using chronic salt loading together with a low-protein diet. These studies are consistent with protein having a protective effect on the development of hypertension even though it may be deleterious to the kidney when other causes of renal damage are present. In man, a study has been done with eleven patients with insulin-dependent diabetes (39). This study indicated that restriction of dietary protein had a sustained beneficial effect on the course of diabetic nephropathy. Taken as a whole, these studies would suggest that adequate or increased amounts of dietary protein may be beneficial for hypertension or cerebrovascular disease; a low-protein diet may be more appropriate with renal vascular disease.

DIETARY PROTEIN AND HYPERTENSIVE DISEASE IN HUMANS

The establishment of dietary factors (such as protein intake) as subtle contributory factors to hypertensive diseases is difficult. The length of time involved, the individual variation, and the changing lifestyles of individuals and populations represent parts of the problem.

Adequately controlled, prospective studies are essentially impossible because of the time required and the complexity of human behavior. We must therefore attempt to uncover clues from epidemiologic studies. These approaches have been valuable in discerning the role of saturated lipids and salt in the development of hypertensive diseases. With the exception of gross malnutrition, few indices of quantity and quality of protein in the diet have been established, and few have been correlated with epidemiologic data on the occurrence of hypertensive diseases. Perhaps the best-measured index of quantitative protein intake is urinary urea or the urea: creatinine ratio because approximately 85 percent of the excreted nitrogen arising from protein metabolism is found as urinary urea. This index, however, gives no indication of the quality of the protein with regard to the distribution of amino acids which it contains. Other approaches such as dietary recall are also useful in estimating both quantity and quality of dietary protein either in an individual or among a cohort of individuals.

Although no study has unequivocally demonstrated a relationship between protein intake and hypertensive diseases in humans, there are several studies which could be considered to be suggestive of such a relationship. The traditional Japanese culture appears to present a natural experimental setting for evaluating factors such as dietary sodium and protein as they relate to cardiovascular disease.

Traditionally, the people in rural Japan consumed relatively high quantities of salt and rather low amounts of protein in their diets. Komachi (40) has recently analyzed data from nutrition surveys done on Japanese diets in the period from 1945 to 1955. In general, there were high intakes of salt and carbohydrate and a relatively low intake of protein, particularly as compared to Western diets. Salt intake in some of the rural provinces reached 25 g/day. At this time, ischemic heart disease in Japan was very rare, while the incidence of stroke was extremely high. In the succeeding 30 years, significant changes have taken place in the Japanese diet. Diets today contain considerably more animal protein and fat and proportionally less carbohydrate and salt. In Japan, there has been a dramatic reduction in the incidence of stroke and a significant increase in ischemic heart disease. While these major shifts in the distribution of cardiovascular disease correlate well with dietary changes, it should be remembered that the quality of health care in Japan has greatly improved over the years, particularly in the treatment of hypertension.

Although few epidemiologic studies have been directed primarily at the question of the role of dietary protein in the frequency of hypertensive diseases, there are other data which support a negative correlation between blood pressure and dietary protein. Reed and co-workers (41–43) have attempted to correlate dietary habits with blood pressure in a large number (8,000) of men of Japanese origin living in Hawaii. While several correlations of dietary components with blood pressures were observed, two of the most significant were a positive correlation with alcohol intake and a negative correlation with dietary protein. In any study such as this there are so many variables that cause and effect cannot be easily discerned, but it is interesting that such correlations are apparent. It will be interesting to follow this Honolulu Heart Study to completion, at which time it may be possible to correlate (a) adverse events associated with cardiovascular disease with (b) individual dietary components. A more recent study from this group examined a subset of this cohort (43). In this subset, 615 men were investigated in detail with regard to their diets. Once again a strong negative correlation between consumption of protein and blood pressure was observed. In this case, the strongest correlation was between vegetable protein and blood pressure. This observation provides an example of how difficult it is to interpret such studies since the vegetable content of the diet may contain other beneficial factors such as potassium or fiber.

Yamori et al. (44) have also undertaken a number of studies in an attempt to unravel the role of diet in hypertensive diseases. These workers attempted to establish simple measurements that could be made on samples collected in the field. Through the use of experiments with normal volunteers on diets containing high or low salt and high or low protein, they suggested that Na/creatinine, urea/creatinine, and sulfate/creatinine ratios measured in evening-deposit urine provided reasonable indices of sodium, total protein, and animal protein intake, respectively. They then went on to compare these parameters in a farming village and in a fishing village in the Shimane prefecture of Japan. These villages were selected because previous demographic studies had indicated that the death rate from stroke was approximately twice as high in the farming village as in the fishing village. Mean blood pressures were slightly higher in the farming village. There appeared to be no differences in total salt intake (about 16 g/day) or in the total protein intake (urea/creatinine). There was, however, a significantly reduced sulfate/creatinine ratio in the farming village, probably reflecting the larger amount of animal protein (fish) consumed in the fishing village. It was concluded that in the presence of a high-salt diet, the type of protein consumed may be very important in determining the pathologic sequelae of hypertension. Clearly, more complete studies are needed, particularly in cohorts other than the Japanese.

A major effort is underway to attempt to take advantage of remaining cultural differences in the world with regard to dietary habits. This is a World Health Organization (WHO)-sponsored study which has been given the acronym CARDIAC. In this WHO-CARDIAC program, 23 nations involving 54 research centers have taken part under the coordination of Dr. Yukio Yamori.

Several reports arising from this massive undertaking have appeared (45–48), although the final report is not yet finished. In each of the participating centers, 100 men and 100 women were randomly selected from the population. Blood pressures were measured with uniform methodology and 24-hour urine collections were done with a standardized procedure. Samples from all centers were analyzed at the WHO Collaborating Center for Research on Primary Prevention of Cardiovascular Disease in Izumo, Japan. This study has resulted in a number of important findings. However, the relationship between an index for dietary protein and blood pressure is most relevant to this chapter. The amino acid methyl histidine is found primarily in animal proteins and its urinary excretion is considered an index of animal protein intake. There appears to be a consistent negative correlation between blood pressure, both systolic and diastolic, and urinary methyl histidine. This relationship can be seen in Fig. 1, which summarizes the data from a number of centers in People's Republic of China. As one might expect, these studies also revealed a positive correlation of Na^+ excretion with blood pressure. In the Chinese centers, a negative correlation of taurine excretion and blood pressures was observed.

While it is impossible to draw unquestioned conclusions from these types of data, there is a strong suggestion that adequate dietary protein with reduced sodium intake would minimize the severity of hypertension. Clearly, there are many possible contributing factors such as the presence of polyunsaturated fatty acids in fish-containing diets.

CONCLUSIONS

A number of studies with animal models have led to a hypothesis that the level of protein in the diet can have a subtle but profound effect on the manner in which a mammalian organism responds to the potentially damaging effects of sustained high blood pressure. One possible explanation for this phenomenon is that the increased protein consumption and metabolism promotes the excretion of sodium, which may be one of the causative factors in the development of cerebral lesions as a result of high blood pressure.

Another explanation is that dietary protein has an effect on vascular structure; however, a role for dietary protein in the incidence of stroke in humans is remote.

Nevertheless, there is an increasing number of epidemiologic studies which are at least consistent with such a hypothesis and which correlate quite well with the animal model experiments.

Because of the magnitude of the pathologic conditions such as stroke that result from hypertension in the world today, nonpharmacologic approaches such as diet modifications are attractive. It is therefore imperative that further understanding of the role of diet and dietary proteins in the suppression of hypertensive diseases be pursued.

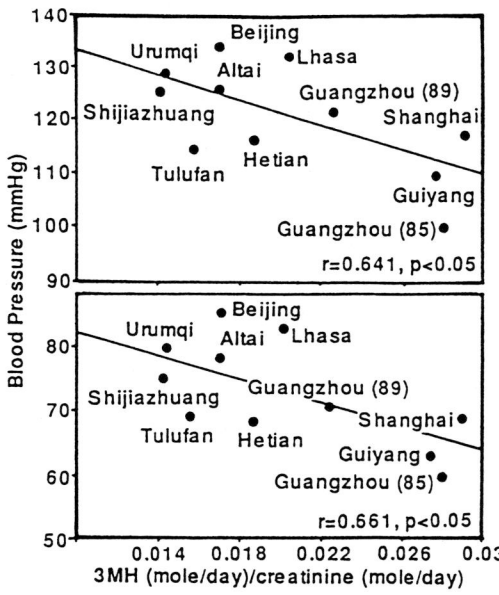

FIG. 1. Relationship between systolic blood pressure (SBP) and diastolic blood pressure (DBP), and urinary 3-methyl histidine (3MH) excretion divided by creatinine. From ref. 46.

SBP: y=-1151.1x + 144.0
DBP: y=-937.2x + 91.7

REFERENCES

1. Watanabe Y. Serial inbreeding of rabbits with heritable hyperlipidemia (WHHL-rabbit): incidence and development of atherosclerosis and xanthoma. *Atherosclerosis* 1980;36:261–268.
2. Kita T, Brown MS, Watanabe Y, Goldstein JL. Deficiency of LDL receptor in liver and adrenal gland of the WHHL rabbit, an animal model of familial hypercholesterolemia. *Proc Natl Acad Sci USA* 1981;78:2268–2272.
3. Dahl LK, Heine M, Tassinari L. Role of genetic factors in susceptibility to experimental hypertension due to chronic excess salt ingestion. *Nature* 1962;194:431–456.
4. Knudsen KD, Dahl LK, Thompson K, Iwai J, Heine M, Leitl C. Effects of chronic excess salt ingestion: inheritance of hypertension in the rat. *J Exp Med* 1970;132:976–1000.
5. Rapp JP, Dene H. Development and characteristics of inbred strains of Dahl salt-sensitive and salt-resistant rats. *Hypertension* 1985;7:340–349.
6. Dahl LK, Heine M. Primary role of renal homografts in setting chronic blood pressure in rats. *Circ Res* 1975;36:692–696.
7. Okamoto K, Aoki K. Development of a strain of spontaneously hypertensive rats. *Jpn Circ J* 1963;27:282–293.
8. Lovenberg W. Animal models for hypertension research. *Prog Clin Biol Res* 1987;229:225–240.
9. Okamoto K. Spontaneous hypertension in rats. In: Richter GW, Epstein MA, eds. *International review of experimental pathology*, vol. 7. New York: Academic Press, 1969;227–270.
10. Okamoto K, Yamori Y, Nagaoka A. Establishment of a strain of stroke-prone SHR. *Circ Res* 1974;34/35(1):143–153.
11. Yamori Y, Horie R, Akiguchi I, Kihara M, Nara Y, Lovenberg W. Symptomatological classification in the development of stroke in stroke-prone spontaneously hypertensive rats. *Jpn Circ J* 1982;46:274–282.

12. Ogata J, Fujishima M, Tamaki K, Nakatomi Y, Ishitsuka T, Omae T. Stroke-prone spontaneously hypertensive rats as an experimental model of malignant hypertension. *Acta Neuropathol* 1980;51:179–184.

13. Ogata J, Fujishima M, Tamaki K, Nakatomi Y, Ishitsuka T, Omae T. Vascular changes underlying cerebral lesions in stroke-prone spontaneously hypertensive rats. *Acta Neuropathol* 1981;54:183–188.

14. Ogata J, Fujishima M, Tamaki K, Nakatomi Y, Ishitsuka T, Omae T. Stroke-prone spontaneously hypertensive rats as an experimental model of malignant hypertension. *Virchows Arch* 82;394:185–194.

15. Tagami M, Nara Y, Kubota A, et al. Ultrastructural characteristics of occluded perforating arteries in stroke-prone spontaneously hypertensive rats. *Stroke* 1987;18:733–740.

16. Tagami M, Kubota A, Kitamura J, Nara Y, Yamori Y. Electron microscopic studies of ruptured and occluded arteries in stroke-prone spontaneously hypertensive rats. *Hypertension* 1986;4:S413–S415.

17. Yamori Y, Horie R. Developmental course of hypertension and regional cerebral blood flow in stroke-prone spontaneously hypertensive rats. *Stroke* 1987;8:456–461.

18. Yamori Y, Horie R, Nara Y, et al. Pathogenesis and dietary prevention of cerebrovascular diseases in animal models and epidemiological evidence for the applicability in man. In: Yamori Y, Lenfant C, eds. *Prevention of cardiovascular diseases: an approach to active long life.* Amsterdam: Elsevier, 1987;22:163–177.

19. Fredriksson K, Nordborg C, Kalimo H, Olsson Y, Johansson BB. Cerebral microangiopathy in stroke-prone spontaneously hypertensive rats: an immunohistochemical and ultrastructural study. *Acta Neuropathol* 1988;75:241–252.

20. Nagaoka A, Lovenberg W. Plasma norepinephrine and dopamine-β-hydroxylase in genetic hypertensive rats. *Life Sci* 1976;19:29–34.

21. Nagaoka A, Lovenberg W. Regional changes in the activities of aminergic biosynthetic enzymes in the brains of hypertensive rats. *Eur J Pharmacol* 1977;43:297–306.

22. Yamori Y, Horie R, Akiguchi I, Ohtaka M, Nara Y, Fukase M. New models of spontaneously hypertensive rat (SHR) for studies on stroke and atherogenesis. *Clin Exp Pharmacol Physiol* 1976;3:199–203.

23. Yamori Y, Horie R, Ikeda K, Nara Y, Lovenberg W. Prophylactic effect of dietary protein on stroke and its mechanisms. In: Yamori Y, Lovenberg W, Fries E, eds. *Perspectives in cardiovascular research, vol 4: prophylactic approach to hypertensive diseases* (Katz AM, series ed.). New York: Raven Press, 1979;497–504.

24. Yamori Y, Horie R, Tanase H, Fujiwara K, Nara Y, Lovenberg W. Possible role of nutritional factors and the incidence of cerebral lesions in stroke-prone spontaneously hypertensive rats. *Hypertension* 1984;6:49–53.

25. Folkow B, Hallbäck M, Lundgren Y, Sivertsson R, Weiss L. Importance of adaptive changes in vascular design for establishment of primary hypertension, studied in man and in spontaneously hypertensive rats. *Circ Res* 1973;2(Suppl I):32–33.

26. Yamabe H, Lovenberg W. Increased incorporation of 3144C lysine into vascular proteins of the spontaneously hypertensive rat. *Eur J Pharmacol* 1974;29:109–116.

27. Yamori Y, Nakada T, Lovenberg W. Effect of antihypertensive therapy on lysine incorporation into vascular protein of the spontaneously hypertensive rat. *Eur J Pharmacol* 1976;38:349–355.

28. Bevan RD. Effect of sympathetic denervation on smooth muscle cell proliferation in the growing rabbit ear artery. *Circ Res* 1975;97:14–19.

29. Sadoshima S, Busija D, Brody M, Heistad D. Sympathetic nerves protect against stroke in stroke-prone hypertensive rats. A preliminary report. *Hypertension* 1981;3:I-124–I-127.

30. Sadoshima S, Heistad D. Sympathetic nerves protect the blood-brain barrier in stroke-prone spontaneously hypertensive rats. *Hypertension* 1982;4(6):904–907.

31. Yamori Y, Nara Y, Horie R, Ooshima A, Lovenberg W. Pathophysiological role of taurine in blood pressure regulation in stroke-prone spontaneously hypertensive rats (SHR). In: Shaffer S, Baskin S, eds. *The action of taurine on excitable tissue.* New York: Spectrum Press, 1981;391–403.

32. Nara Y, Yamori Y, Lovenberg W. Effect of dietary taurine on blood pressure in spontaneously hypertensive rats. *Biochem Pharmacol* 1978;27:2689–2692.

33. Kanamaru T, Nakanishi N, Igarashi N, Kato M, Kato S, Sugino N. Effect of dietary protein on blood pressure and renal function in spontaneously hypertensive and control rats. *Hypertension* 1986;4:S457–S458.

34. Wang H, Ikeda K, Kihara M, et al. Effect of dietary urea on blood pressure in spontaneously hypertensive rats. *Clin Exp Pharmacol Physiol* 1984;11:555–561.

35. Yamori Y, Horie R, Nara Y, et al. Nutritional causation and prevention of cardiovascular diseases: experimental evidence in animal models and man. In: Lovenberg W, Yamori Y, eds. *Nutritional prevention of cardiovascular disease.* Orlando, FL: Academic Press, 1984;37–51.

36. Nath KA, Kren SM, Hostetter TH. Dietary protein restriction in established renal injury in the rat. *J Clin Invest* 1986;78:1199–1205.

37. DeKeijzer MH, Provoost AP. Effects of dietary protein on the progression of renal failure in the fawn-hooded rat. *Nephron* 1990;55:203–209.

38. Strekalova VV, Khachirov DG, Dedonkov AN, Suvorov II, Shvatsabaia IK. Modeling of experimental hypertension by chronic salt loading combined with a low-protein diet in Wistar rats. *Biull Usesoiuznogo Kardiol Nauchn Tsentra* 1989;12:48–51.

39. Evanoff G, Thompson C, Brown J, Weinman E. Prolonged dietary protein restriction in diabetic nephropathy. *Arch Intern Med* 1989;149:1129–1133.

40. Komachi Y. Japanese dietary life and diseases. *Asian Med J* 1987;30:317–323.

41. Reed D, McGee D, Yano K. Biological and social correlates of blood pressure among Japanese men in Hawaii. *Hypertension* 1982;4:406–414.

42. Reed D, McGee D, Yano K, Hankin J. Diet, blood pressure and multicollinearity. *Hypertension* 1985;7:405–410.

43. Joffres M, Reed D, Yano K. Relationship of magnesium intake and other dietary factors to blood pressure: the Honolulu Heart Study. *Am J Clin Nutr* 1987;45:469–475.

44. Yamori Y, Tsunematsu T, Note S, Ishikawa S, Fukase M. Nutritional improvement for stroke prevention. In: Yamori Y, Lovenberg W, Fries E, eds. *Perspectives in cardiovascular research, vol 4: prophylactic approach to hypertensive diseases.* New York: Raven Press, 1979;587–593.

45. Yamori Y, Nara Y, Mizushima S, Mano M, Sawamura M, Kihara M, Horie R. International cooperative study on the relationship between dietary factors and blood pressure: A report from the cardiovascular diseases and alimentary comparison (CARDIAC) study. *J Cardiovasc Pharmacol* 1990;16(8):S43–S47.

46. Nara Y, Zhao GS, Huang ZD, Li YH, Mizushima S, Mano M, Zhang HX, Sun SF, Sato T, Horie R, Zhang MX, He BS, Mori C, Hatano S, Liu LS, Yamori Y. Relationship between dietary factors and blood pressure in China. *J Cardiovasc Pharmacol* 1990;16(8):S40–S42.

47. Yamori Y, Nara Y, Mizushima S, Murakami S, Ikeda K, Sawamura M, Nabika T, Horie R. Gene-environment interaction in hypertension, stroke and atherosclerosis in experimental models and supportive findings from a world-wide cross-sectional epidemiological survey: A WHO-CARDIAC study. *Clin Exp Pharmacol Physiol* 1992;19(20):43–52.

48. Yamori Y. Predictive and preventive pathology of cardiovascular diseases. *Acta Pathol Jpn* 1989;39(11):683–705.

SECTION IV

Circulatory and Target Organ Pathophysiology of Hypertensive Disease

Hypertension: Pathophysiology, Diagnosis, and Management, Second Edition, edited by J.H. Laragh and B.M. Brenner, Raven Press, Ltd., New York © 1995.

CHAPTER **20**

Hemodynamic Patterns of Untreated Hypertensive Disease

Per Lund-Johansen and Per Omvik

Hypertension may be defined as a hemodynamic disease—a disturbance in the ratio between the cardiac output (CO) and total peripheral resistance (TPR), the two most important factors determining the blood pressure (BP) in the systemic circulation. Total peripheral resistance is calculated as the ratio between mean arterial pressure (MAP) and the CO:

$$MAP = CO \times TPR \text{ or } TPR = MAP/CO.$$

Strictly, this equation is valid only for laminar flow in straight rigid tubes (1). Total peripheral resistance is mainly determined by the diameter of the arterioles and their total number, but flow resistance is also influenced by the blood viscosity (2,3), as a relatively small increase in viscous resistance may increase BP (4).

  P. Lund-Johansen: Department of Heart Disease, University of Bergen, School of Medicine, Bergen, Norway.
  P. Omvik: Department of Heart Disease, University of Bergen, School of Medicine, Bergen, Norway.

The hemodynamic pattern behind an increased BP may vary considerably and is influenced by the age of the subject as well as by the severity of the hypertensive disease (5–14 for review).

Although there is general agreement on the hemodynamic pattern in severe hypertension of long duration, it is still unclear why, how, and when the hemodynamic alterations leading to permanent hypertension really start.

HEMODYNAMIC METHODS

The Blood Pressure

The BP is recorded most accurately by a pressure transducer via a thin polyethylene catheter introduced into the brachial or the radial artery. Beat-to-beat changes may then be studied and, when the catheter is first in place, the BP may be recorded continuously without disturbing the patient. For the measurements of all types of rapid changes in the BP, this method has to be used. Although the classic conventional Riva Rocci method is surprisingly accurate in resting subjects with a normal arm circumference and a suitable cuff (12), cuff methods are inaccurate during physical exercise because of muscular tension or noise problems. Intraarterial recordings are then mandatory (15).

During the last decade many automatic and semiautomatic noninvasive recording systems have been developed. Their use during muscular exercise is still a matter of controversy, but it is obvious that the number of erroneous readings then will be substantial (16–18).

The Cardiac Output

The most accurate methods are the Fick method (19), the dye dilution method (20) (preferably by Cardiogreen), and the thermodilution method (21). However, the methods record mean flow over a 15- to 60-second period—or even more for the Fick method. The carbon dioxide rebreathing method also seems to be quite reliable (22). Less accurate are impedance cardiography and echocardiography (without Doppler).

The combination of echo and Doppler measures the diameter of the aorta by echo, and the blood velocity by the Doppler and allows determination of stroke volume beat-by-beat (23,24). The mean of several stroke volumes are multiplied by the heart rate to get CO. Although some investigators have found the method useful also during exercise, others have found poor agreement between the echo-Doppler results and those obtained by dilution methods or by the classic Fick principle. The method seems most useful for recording relative changes in CO during resting situations over short time periods.

The thermodilution method is based on the Swan Ganz catheter and allows serial determination of CO (21) and the pressures in the pulmonary circulation. The isotope dilution technique based on 99-TC is also used, but seems to overestimate CO by approximately 30 percent (25).

Body Size Correction

In order to facilitate comparison between small and large individuals, correction for body surface area (BSA) is often useful. This should always be included in papers on hemodynamics, making calculation of the index (I) parameters (CI = CO/BSA, TPRI = MAP/CI) possible and thus allowing comparison of results between different laboratories (12).

The Experimental Situation

Observations on 24-hour BP recorded intraarterially—or intraarterial recordings from various laboratory situations—have shown that the BP is very labile in most subjects and may easily be influenced by several external stimuli.

In a relaxed subject with intraarterial BP being recorded, just the mere sight of a Riva Rocci apparatus to be used for comparison of the two methods (12) may sometimes increase the BP 10 mm Hg or more.

Also, just the sight of a physician during a hospital round may increase resting BP by 10–20 mm Hg or more (26). Conversation about "neutral" topics may also sometimes increase BP 10 mm Hg or more (12,27).

The Awareness Problem

The subject's awareness of his BP may be a crucial factor for the blood pressure level and possibly also for the hemodynamic situation (28). Studies based on military recruits drawn from mass screening and later drawn in for studies of the BP show that those who had gotten a letter telling them that they had high BP had a higher pressure than those who had a letter with a different text not mentioning the BP problem, but pretending that this was a "general health check." In recruits with the same BP level, those who had the letter mentioning high BP had the highest pressures at the restudy (29,30).

When a full-day study is undertaken, food intake causes problems, as a meal increases metabolism, CO and heart rate (HR), and reduces TPR (12,31). If a subject falls asleep, this will obviously influence the hemodynamic pattern (32).

It follows from these observations that standardization of the experimental situation is extremely important in order to arrive at meaningful results.

CENTRAL HEMODYNAMICS IN NORMALS

Studies During Rest

Age influences central hemodynamics. There is general agreement that in nearly all human populations there is an increase in resting BP with aging. The increase is greatest for the systolic BP. The diastolic BP also increases from childhood up to the age of 60, but during the last period of life a fall in diastolic BP has been reported (33–37). The picture is less clear with respect to CO.

In several studies from 1965 to recent years—where CO was measured by the Fick method or by the dye dilution or thermodilution methods—the general finding was that the CO during rest supine declined with aging about 1 percent per year (38–40). However, if only small groups of subjects covering a short span of life were studied, this finding was not always present (12,37,41,42).

Since there is a fall in CO and an increase in BP, it follows that calculated TPR increases with aging (12).

In contrast, observations from Baltimore in healthy, selected subjects 30–80 years studied by gated radionuclide angiography suggested that there was no reduction in resting CO with increasing age. The reduction in HR with aging was compensated by increase in stroke volume (43–45).

Exercise Studies

Many studies based on invasive methods have shown a reduction in CO during exercise with aging due to decrease in stroke volume (12,33,39,40). The maximal HR during very strenuous exercise is lower in older than in younger subjects. The filling pressures of both right and left heart ventricle increase with aging, particularly during exercise (46).

In the Baltimore study no reduction in CO during exercise was seen with aging. Exercise HR decreased, but was compensated by increase in the stroke volume (45). Most studies seem to agree that the BP and TPR increases with aging, also during exercise (12,33,47).

The decrease in exercise HR with advancing age could be due to decrease in beta-adrenergic responsiveness (48,49). The greater increase in systolic BP during exercise with aging is usually explained by a combination of loss of elasticity in the aorta (50,51) and less sensitive baroreflexes at higher age (52).

The reduction in exercise CO and stroke volume with aging (observed in most of the invasive studies) is probably due to a reduction in compliance of the left ventricle and reduced diastolic filling. With aging, left ventricular filling time is increased (53–56) and as heart rate increases during exercise, stroke volume becomes subnormal.

CENTRAL HEMODYNAMICS IN HYPERTENSIVE DISEASE: BORDERLINE AND MILD HYPERTENSION (THE STARTING PHASE)

It is obviously very difficult to find subjects definitely in the starting phase of essential hypertension. In most earlier studies the approach was to invasively study subjects in their twenties to forties with borderline or mild hypertension and to compare them with age-matched normotensive controls. Recently, large groups of "hypertensive" children and adolescents have been studied, but with less accurate noninvasive methods.

Studies During Rest

Invasive Studies in Young Adults

In young adults (18–40 years) with borderline (some readings above and some readings below 140/90 mm Hg) or with mild hypertension (diastolic blood pressure 90–105 mm Hg), the characteristic hemodynamic disturbance is a high CI, a high HR and a numerically "normal" calculated TPR. This has been shown in numerous studies from different parts of the world from 1967 until today, all based on the most accurate available methods (CO measured by dye dilution technique and blood pressure recorded intraarterially) (57–64).

In most of these studies the mean BP has been about

TABLE 1. *Mean values for mean arterial pressure (MAP), cardiac index (CI), total peripheral resistance index (TPRI), heart rate (HR), and stroke index (SI) in young subjects (aged 20–40 years) with borderline or mild essential hypertension in the supine position at rest*[a]

References	n	MAP (mm Hg)	CI (L min^{-1} m^{-2})	TPRI (dyn sec cm^{-5} m^2)	HR (beats min^{-1})	SI (ml stroke^{-1} m^{-2})
Bello et al. (60)	11	108 (91)	4.10 (3.39)	2110 (2210)	81 (74)	51 (44)
Lund-Johansen (13)	25	102 (84)	4.14 (3.45)	1970 (1950)	75 (63)	56 (55)
Frohlich et al. (62)	9	106 (93)	3.53 (3.05)	2400 (2440)	77 (68)	46 (45)
Safar et al. (63)	23	105 (86)	4.09 (3.15)	2100 (2220)	80 (72)	51 (44)
Julius et al. (64)	77	100 (83)	3.79 (3.31)	2220 (2090)	76 (67)	50 (50)

[a] Mean values for control groups are in parentheses.

15 percent higher than in the normotensive controls, with a similar relative increase in CI and in HR, but individual variations have been great (12,65).

A survey of typical studies from the 1960s in hypertensives and normotensive age-matched controls is found in Table 1. More recent invasive studies have supported these older findings (66–68).

Although calculated TPR was numerically not significantly different from controls in these studies and usually called "normal," it should be stressed that the TPR was increased when related to the blood flow.

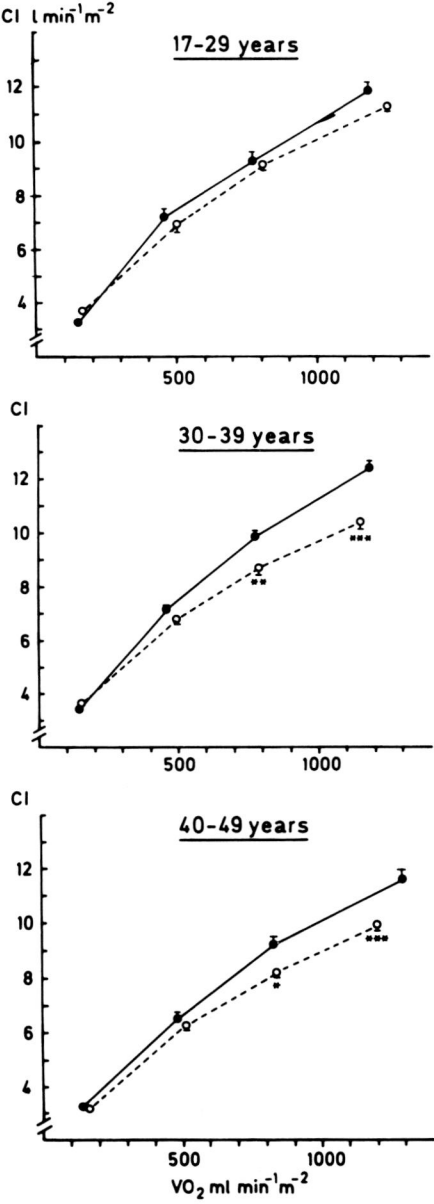

FIG. 1. Cardiac index (CI) at rest (sitting) and during bicycle exercise (sitting) at 50, 100, and 150 W in hypertensives (---) and in age-matched normotensives (—) in different age groups. Mean values and SEM. VO$_2$, oxygen consumption. *$p < 0.05$; **$p < 0.01$; ***$p < 0.001$. (Adapted from ref. 12.)

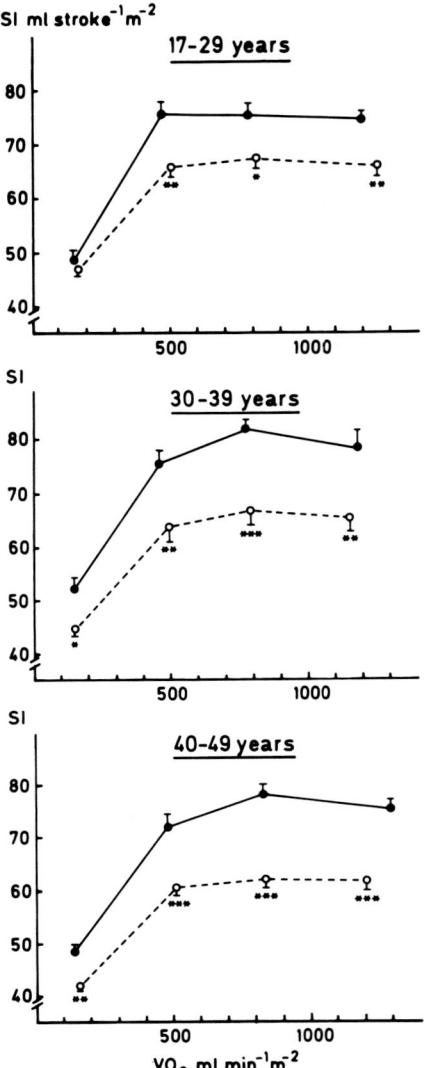

FIG. 2. Stroke index (SI) at rest (sitting) and during bicycle exercise (sitting) in hypertensives (---) and in age-matched controls (—). Mean values and SEM. VO$_2$, oxygen consumption. *$p < 0.05$; **$p < 0.001$; ***$p < 0.001$. (Adapted from ref. 12.)

When borderline hypertension exists in older subjects (above 40 years of age), CI is no longer increased, but similar to that seen in age-matched normotensive controls (69). Exceptions are rare (70).

Children and Adolescents

In the Muscatine screening program 264 children (9–18 years) were studied by the automatic Arteriosonde cuff method for BP and by echocardiography for CI (71). Cardiac index at rest supine ranged from 1.5 to 5.5 L/min/m^2. When the subjects were stratified according to the BP in three categories (low, about 100/50 mm Hg, middle, and high 112/55 mm Hg), those with the highest

BP had slightly higher HR and CI than those who had the lowest BP.

In a similar study from Baltimore (age 8–19 years), slightly higher CI values were found in those with "mild hypertension" (BP 141/94 mm Hg) versus the controls (BP 114/68 mm Hg) (72).

Thus the Muscatine as well as the Baltimore study showed a slight trend toward higher CI values in the children with the highest BP, but the differences between "hypertensives" and controls were less than in the invasive studies in 20- to 30-year-old men. The most dramatic changes, however, were seen in left ventricular mass, which was much greater in the highest BP group.

In contrast to the trend seen in these studies, Hofmann et al. (73,74) found no increase in CI in "hypertensive" children and adolescents (10–19 years) unaware of their BP level (recruited by screening programs) and suggest

that the changes in BP over time are caused by a gradual increase in TPRI—beginning early in life—possibly due to high levels of circulating catecholamines.

Offspring of Hypertensive Parents

Central hemodynamics have been studied invasively in offspring from hypertensive parents who at the time of the hemodynamic study had BP averaging only 137/84 mm Hg (75). Still, this BP was higher than in controls. There was, however, no difference between CI in the two groups; TPRI was slightly increased in the offspring group.

Falkner (76) has found that children from hypertensive parents have higher baseline HR and react more strongly to stress stimuli than age-matched controls.

At present time it is difficult to explain why the nonin-

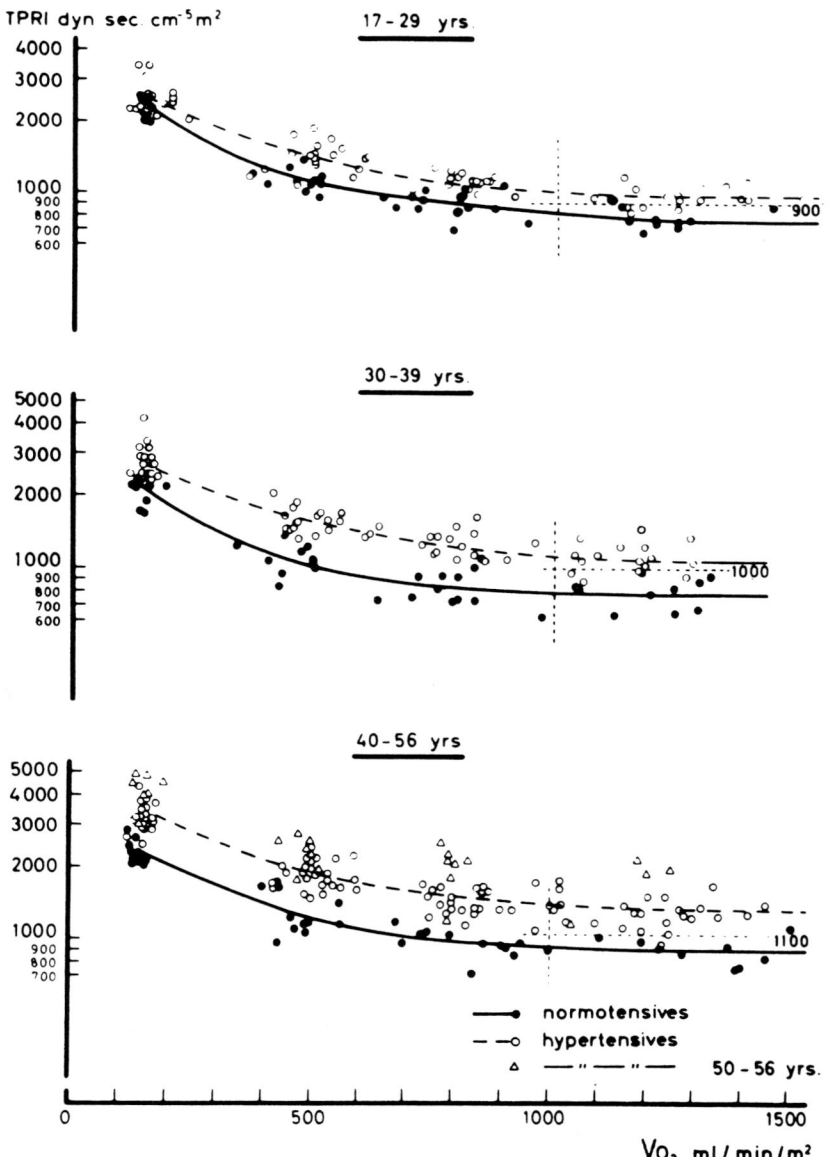

FIG. 3. Total peripheral resistance index (TPRI) at rest (sitting) and during bicycle exercise (sitting) in hypertensives (---) and in age-matched normotensives (—). Individual and mean values. VO$_2$, oxygen consumption. (From ref. 12.)

vasive studies in children and adolescents have not indicated a typical hyperkinetic circulatory state as the dominating pattern. But since so far no long-term observations are available in these children—who often have very mildly increased BP—it is difficult to know whether they represent the starting phase of essential hypertension. Furthermore, the CO has been obtained by rather inaccurate methods (echocardiography). In a recent study from our laboratory in offspring from hypertensive and normotensive parents (based on 27 years of BP observations), hypertensive offspring had higher 24-hour BP, but not HR when corrections were made for smoking habits (77).

A Truly Hyperkinetic Phase—a Myth?

The original observation from studies in experimental renal hypertension in rats that the initial increase in blood pressure was caused by increase in CO (again due to fluid retention and increase in plasma volume) in the presence of normal TPR (78–80), induced a large series of studies on central hemodynamics in young subjects with essential hypertension. As already discussed, most of these invasive studies showed a higher CI in hypertensives than in controls. Theoretically, the increased CO could lead to an overperfusion of blood in the different tissues, and this in turn could induce vasoconstriction and a reduction in blood flow. The increase in TPR would maintain the increased BP (81).

However, four independent studies in young hypertensive males all showed that in addition to the 15-percent increase in CO, there was a similar increase in oxygen consumption and the arteriovenous oxygen difference was normal (12,82–84). Thus the "whole body autoregulation theory" (81) did not fit.

In this context it is interesting that Gorlin in 1962 (85)

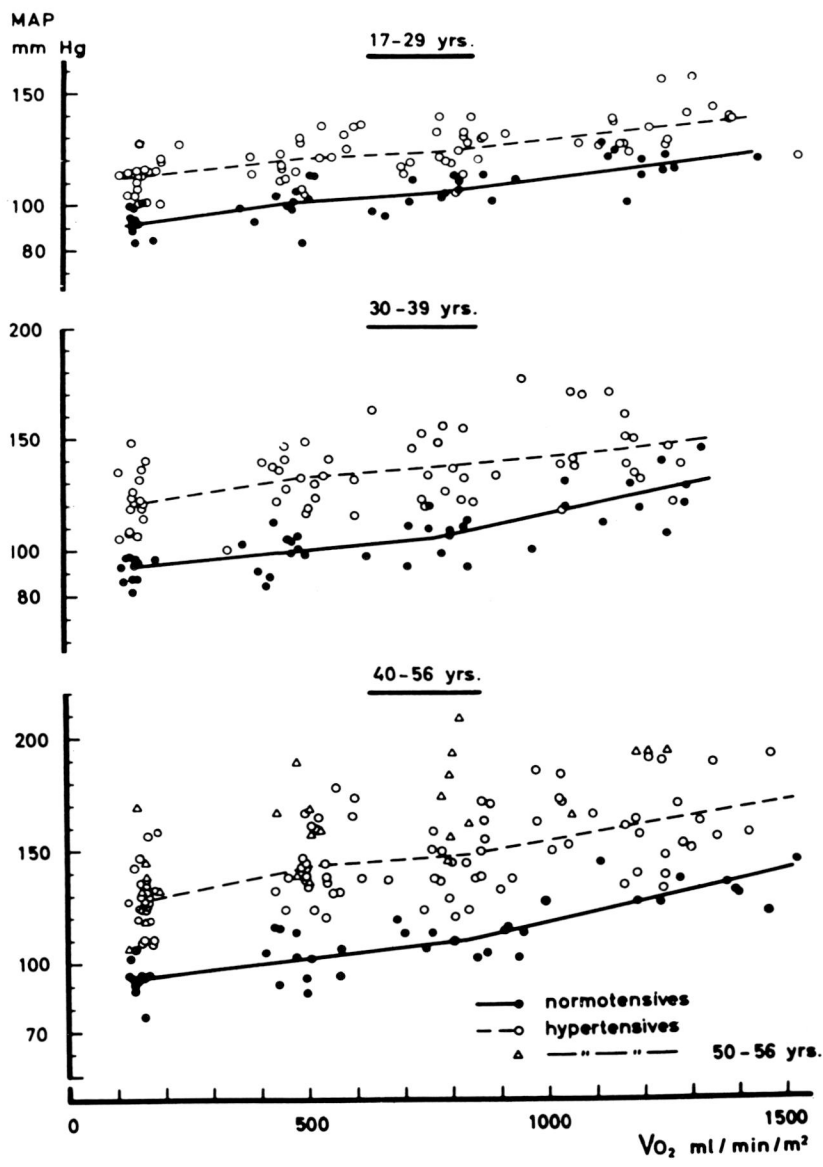

FIG. 4. Mean arterial blood pressure (MAP) recorded intra-arterially at rest (sitting) and during bicycle exercise (sitting) in hypertensives (---) and in age-matched normotensives (—). Individual and mean values. VO₂, oxygen consumption. (From ref. 12.)

described a so-called idiopathic hyperkinetic heart syndrome, characterized by tachycardia and cardiac awareness and extremely high CI (5.7 L/min/m^2), or 38 percent higher than in controls. Arteriovenous oxygen difference was abnormally low (only 2.9 versus 4.0 mL oxygen per 100 blood in normals). These were truly hyperkinetic subjects, but very few had developed hypertension at the follow-up 10–15 years later (86). A few exceptions to these major results in early hypertension have been described (87).

Studies During Exercise

When the circulatory system is really challenged, such as during heavy muscular exercise, the hemodynamic pattern in mild and borderline hypertension is not hyperkinetic by any meaning of the word (12,88). In contrast, CI is usually subnormal (Fig. 1) due to an insufficient increase in stroke index (Fig. 2) and the arteriovenous oxygen difference is slightly on the higher side.

The abnormally low exercise stroke volume is probably due to reduced compliance in the left ventricular wall. This has been demonstrated by echocardiography and by the gated blood pool method (89,90).

Invasive data on exercise hemodynamics in children are lacking, but in a study in adolescents (mean age 16 years) the BP rise during treadmill exercise was similar to that seen in normotensive age-matched controls (91). This finding is in agreement with the BP response during exercise seen in mildly hypertensive males between 20 and 40 years (12,92).

An important finding in the exercise studies is that the apparently normal TPR during rest situation in subjects with mild hypertension is no longer present during exercise, as TPRI does not fall to the same low levels as in normotensive age-matched controls but is abnormal at an early stage (Fig. 3) (12). The systolic arterial pressure (SAP), diastolic arterial pressure, and MAP (intraarterially recorded) increase parallel to what is seen in normals (Fig. 4) (12,82,92). Most laboratories have agreed on these results, but a few exceptions have been published (93).

ESTABLISHED HYPERTENSION

Studies During Rest

In adults with moderately severe essential hypertension (BP 180–160/115–100 mm Hg) of several years duration, the dominating hemodynamic disturbance is an increase in TPR, while CO is usually lower than in normotensive controls and lower than in younger hypertensive stage I subjects. The HR, however, is usually higher than in controls and the stroke volume is normal or low (94–102).

Left ventricular wall thickness is increased and left ventricular filling rate and compliance are reduced. The ejection fraction is usually normal but may be slightly reduced (14,103,104).

Studies During Exercise

In subjects with moderately severe essential hypertension, TPR during exercise is clearly higher than in normotensive age-matched controls and also higher than in younger hypertensive subjects with borderline mild hypertension (12,92). Exercise CO is abnormally low due to insufficient increase in stroke volume. Blood pressure increases parallel to what is seen in normals when related to work load or to oxygen uptake. When related to blood flow or CO, the rise is steeper (12).

This abnormally low heart-pump function during exercise is most probably due to reduced compliance of left ventricle as the ejection fraction during rest is usually normal (14,90,104).

SEVERE HYPERTENSION

With increasing severity of hypertension and complications (WHO stage III) the circulatory system is characterized by a pronounced increase in TPR and often a substantial decrease in CO, particularly if coronary heart disease coexists. Stroke volume is reduced. In subjects with very severe hypertension refractory to triple treatment, very high resistance values have been seen (105,106). A few exceptions to this pattern (severe hypertension and a high CI) have been reported (107).

HYPERTENSION AND HEART FAILURE—THE END-STAGE

The pioneer studies on hemodynamics in hypertension were performed by heart catheterization in subjects with severe hypertension and heart failure. The studies showed a marked increase in TPR and a very low CO (108–110). Left ventricular filling pressures as well as the pressures in the pulmonary circulation were increased. Later it has been shown that left ventricular ejection fraction and maximal circumferential fiber shortening is reduced (111).

In *malignant* hypertension of long duration, left ventricular wall thickness is increased and ejection fraction reduced. When the duration of hypertension is short, wall thickness may be normal, but the diastolic filling rate is reduced quite early (112).

LONG-TERM CHANGES IN CENTRAL HEMODYNAMICS

Only longitudinal studies can tell what will really happen with the hemodynamic patterns in hypertension.

Over the years several long-term studies (mostly 2–5 years follow-up) have been published (113–119). A review of these studies is given in Table 2. The selection of patients and the situation at the follow-up examination vary considerably. In general, all these studies show a decrease in CI and an increase in TPRI and usually only minor changes in blood pressure during the follow-up period.

Andersson et al. (118) studied 33 borderline hypertensives and 22 normotensive controls (initial age 18–21 years). After 5 years, central hemodynamics was completely unchanged in the normotensive controls. In contrast, there was a fall in CI and a slight increase in TPRI in the entire borderline group. As in many similar studies, BP was unchanged (138/75 mm Hg at study 1 and 136/74 mm Hg at study 2). In a hyperkinetic subgroup the reduction in CI was impressive (from 4.51 to 3.30 L/min/m^2) and associated with increase in TPRI.

The Bergen Long-Term Study on Central Hemodynamics in Essential Hypertension

In our laboratory our hypertensive subjects were followed for 20 years, and to our knowledge this is the only study which includes exercise hemodynamics. The series includes 77 male patients with mild to moderate essential hypertension, recruited from the Bergen population survey (12). All subjects had blood pressure above 140/90 mm Hg at the screening in 1965 and at two follow-up examinations over a period of 6 months. All patients below the age of 60 were in WHO stages I or II. For comparison 33 normotensive males, aged 17–49 years, were studied.

Central hemodynamics were studied invasively at rest sitting and during exercise at 50, 100 and 150 W on bicycle ergometer. Heart rate was recorded by ECG, CO (in duplicate) by the Cardiogreen method, and BP by a catheter in the brachial artery. The methods and the initial results have been described in detail elsewhere (12).

Ten Years Follow-Up

At the initial hemodynamic study, most of the hypertensives under age 40 were found to have mild hypertension not considered to need drug treatment, while nearly all patients over 40 were advised to have drug treatment. By conventional clinical methods at yearly intervals, no complications could be disclosed in the two youngest age groups (less than 40 years) during this period (119).

At the 10-year follow-up all available untreated subjects in age groups I (n = 16) and II (n = 13), and 5 untreated subjects in group III were studied by exactly the same methods as during the first study. Details about the material have been published elsewhere (12,119).

The oxygen consumption at rest had decreased in age group I but was almost unchanged in group II, and during exercise there were only small changes in both age groups.

The blood pressure showed remarkably small changes. During rest there were no significant changes in SAP, DAP, or MAP. During 150-W exercise there was a significant increase in MAP from 133 mm Hg to 141 mm Hg in age group I and from 141 mm Hg to 147 mm Hg in group II. The pressure changes at rest and during exercise in age group I are seen in Fig. 5.

Cardiac index had decreased significantly in both age groups at rest as well as during exercise. At rest the CI had decreased in all but two in age group I and in all but one in age group II. In age group I the mean value decreased from 3.81 to 3.22 L/min/m^2 at rest, and in group II from 3.64 to 2.81 L/min/m^2. During the 150-W exercise the mean value decreased from 11.1 to 9.4 L/min/m^2 in group I and from 10.4 to 8.96 L/min/m^2 in group II. The changes in CI at rest and during exercise in

TABLE 2. *Hemodynamic follow-up studies in essential hypertension showing change in cardiac output (CO) and total peripheral resistance (TPR)*

References	No. of patients		Therapy	Experimental condition of study 1 and study 2	Follow-up time (years)	Hemodynamic changes in study 2
	Study 1	Study 2				
Eich et al. (83)	68	41	In some	Different; rest only	~4	CO↓ TPR↑
Eliasch et al. (113)	83	20	Sympathectomy in some	Different	8–17	CO↓ TPR↑ BP↔
Birkenhäger et al. (114)	15	15	In all (intermittent)	Same; rest only	1–4	CO↓ TPR↑
Weiss et al. (115)	37	37	0	Same; rest only	~4	CO↓ TPR↑ SAP↑ DAP↔
Lund-Johansen (120)	34	33	0	Same; rest and exercise	9–10	CO↓ TPR↑ BP↔
Julius et al. (64)	24	24	In 9	Same; rest only	5–6	CO↓ TPR↑ BP↔
Andersson et al. (118)						
HT subjects	44	33	0	Same; rest only	5	CO↓ TPR↑ BP↔
NT controls	29	22	0			No change
Birkenhäger, de Leeuw (117)	17	17	0	Same; rest only	2	CO↓ TPR↑ BP↔

↑, increased; ↓, reduced; ↔, unchanged.

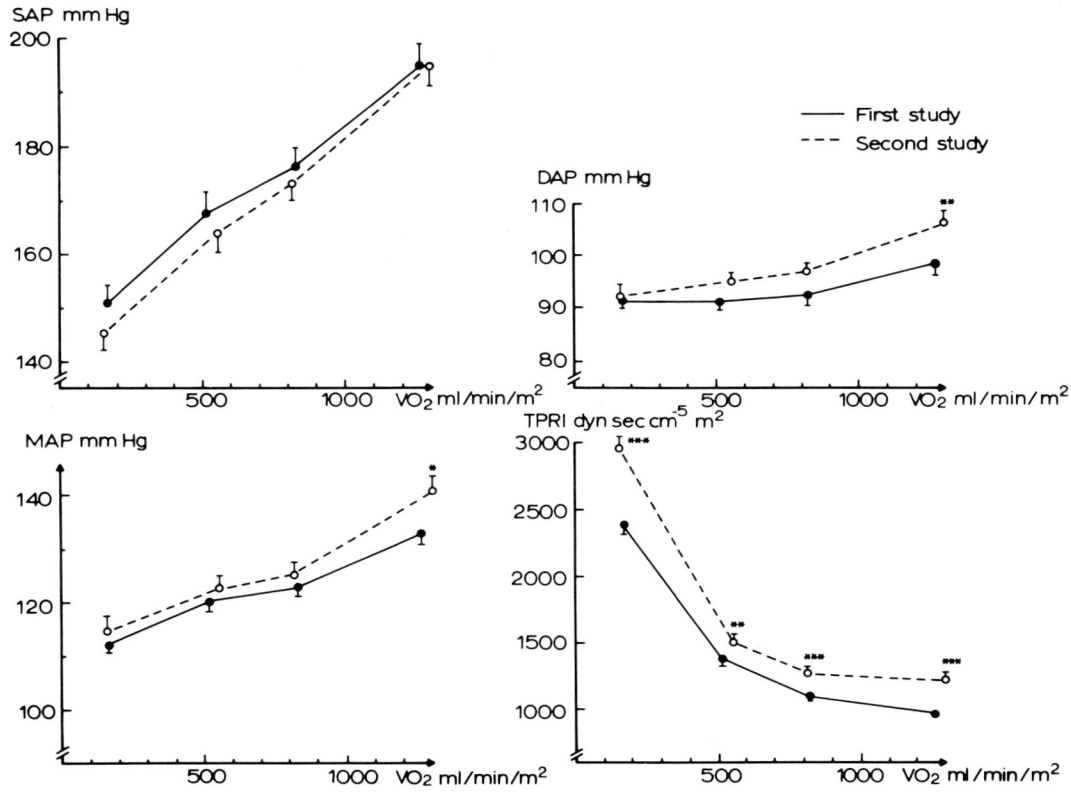

FIG. 5. Systolic (SAP), diastolic (DAP), and mean (MAP) arterial pressure, as well as total peripheral resistance index (TPRI), at initial study and at 10-year follow-up in age group I (17–29 years at first study). VO_2, oxygen consumption. *$p < 0.05$; **$p < 0.01$; ***$p < 0.001$.

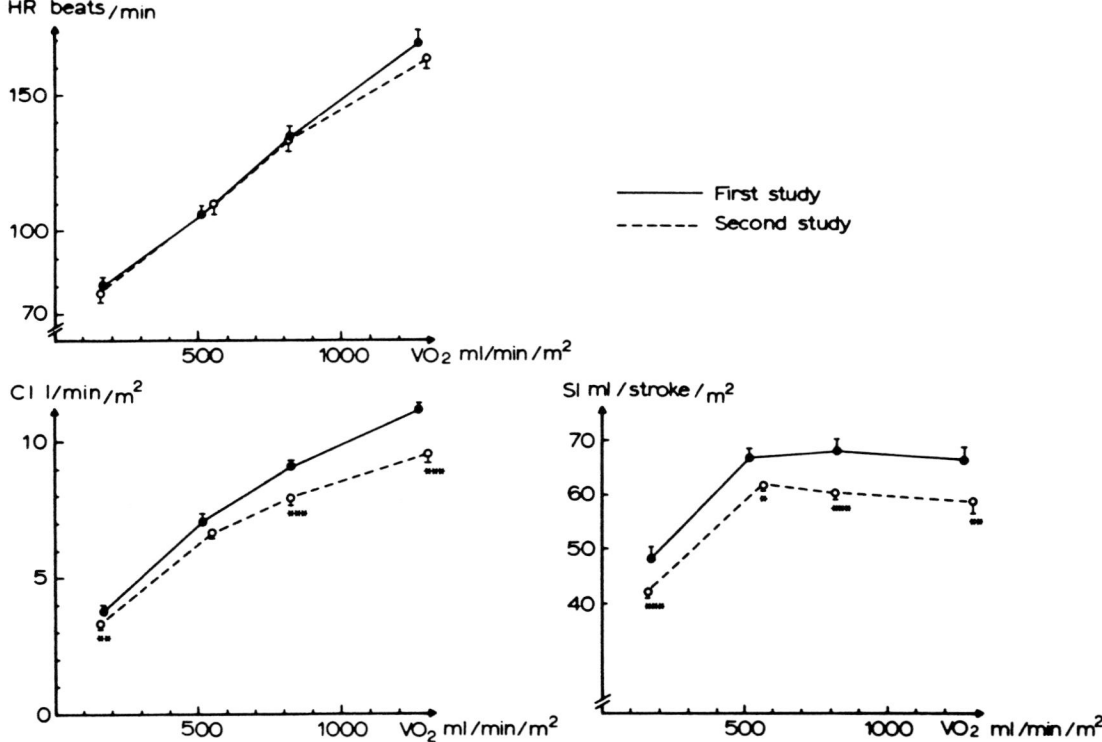

FIG. 6. Central hemodynamics at rest and during exercise at initial study (—) and 10 years later (---) in 15 males with untreated essential hypertension in age group I (17–29 years at first study). Mean values and SEM. HR, heart rate; CI, cardiac index; SI, stroke index; VO_2, oxygen consumption. *$p < 0.05$; **$p < 0.01$; ***$p < 0.001$.

group I are seen in Fig. 6. The changes in group II were very similar.

In both age groups reduction in CI was associated with a significant decrease in SI at rest as well as during exercise. At rest SI decreased from 48.0 to 41.7 mL/stroke/m² in group I and from 45.6 to 39.9 mL/stroke/m² in group II. During exercise the stroke index (SI) had decreased about 6–8 mL/stroke/m² in both age groups.

In age group I the HR at rest and during exercise showed only small and insignificant changes. In group II there was a significant decrease in the resting value. During exercise there were no significant changes.

Total peripheral resistance index increased significantly at rest as well as during exercise in both age groups. During rest situation TPRI had increased in all but two in age group I and in all but one in age group II.

A subgroup analysis in patients who initially had high CI values and "normal" TPRI—versus those who initially had low or normal CI and high TPRI values—showed that the latter group had increased their BP values more over the 10 years and they were found to need treatment after the 10-year follow-up study. In contrast,

in the initially hyperkinetic group very few (only 3 of 10) clearly increased BP to values indicating need for hypertensive treatment (guidelines DAP > 100 mm Hg).

The fall in CI over the 10 years was mainly caused by reduction in SI at rest as well as during exercise.

Thus these long-term observations indicate a reduction in the heart pump function and in the ability to dilate the resistance vessels during exercise over the years.

In age group III (40–49 years, only five untreated), there was also an increase in BP at rest as well as during exercise, a marked increase in TPRI, and a decrease in CO. In this small group the deterioration of the heart pump function and the changes in the resistance vessels seemed to be greater than in those over 40 years of age.

Twenty-Years Follow-Up

After the 10-year follow-up, nearly all patients were seen by the investigator (P.L-J) with yearly intervals (a few were controlled by their general practitioners). From a scientific point of view it would have been most interesting to have also followed these subjects untreated over

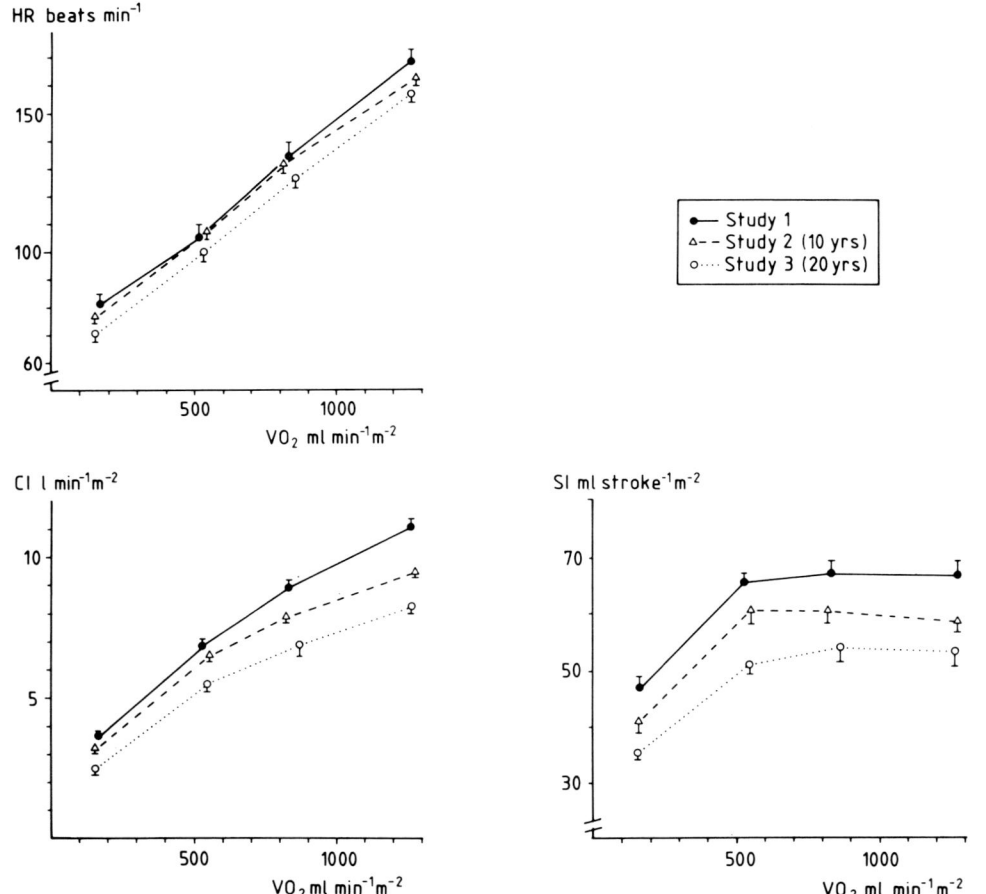

FIG. 7. Central hemodynamics at rest and during exercise in age group I (17–29 years) at initial study and at 10- and 20-year follow-ups. Mean values (n = 14) and SEM. HR, heart rate; CI, cardiac index; SI, stroke index; VO₂, oxygen consumption. *$p < 0.05$; **$p < 0.01$; ***$p < 0.001$. See text for details.

the next decade. For ethical reasons this was not feasible. When DAP rose to 100 mm Hg or more (recorded several times over at least a 3-month period), antihypertensive treatment was started (generally by diuretics, beta blockers, or a combination of the two).

Nevertheless, the clinical status and hemodynamic situation in these subjects after 20 years was thought to be of interest. Since most of the patients (over 40 years of age) had only mild to moderately severe hypertension, it was found ethically justifiable to withdraw drug treatment (under clinical control) for 2 months before a third hemodynamic study (at 20 years follow-up).

Since the patients in age group 40–49 years initially had somewhat more severe hypertension, treatment was therefore withdrawn only for approximately 2 weeks in these subjects. The clinical outcome has been published elsewhere (120).

The invasive hemodynamic studies showed that in the two youngest age groups there was a further reduction in CI of approximately the same magnitude as the reductions seen during the first decade of follow-up. The SI had declined further and there was a marked increase in TPRI.

Figures 7 and 8 show the most important hemodynamic changes in age group I over the 20 years. Mean values are shown at the initial study, at the 10-year and at the 20-year follow-up. It is seen that CI continued to fall during the next decade of follow-up, mainly due to further decrease in SI. The reduction in HR was small. Compared to the first study, HR during 150-W exercise was reduced only by 7 percent in group I and by 6 percent in group II.

Since a large fraction of these patients had been treated between the 10- and 20-year follow-up (but had been without drugs the last 2 months before the third hemodynamic study), they do not represent a completely untreated group during the last decade. However, the results were very similar to those seen in eight completely untreated subjects (initially below 40 years of age) followed over 17 years.

Twenty-Years Follow-Up in Age Group III (Treated Group)

All but two of these patients had been treated during the last 10 years before the 20-year restudy (mainly by

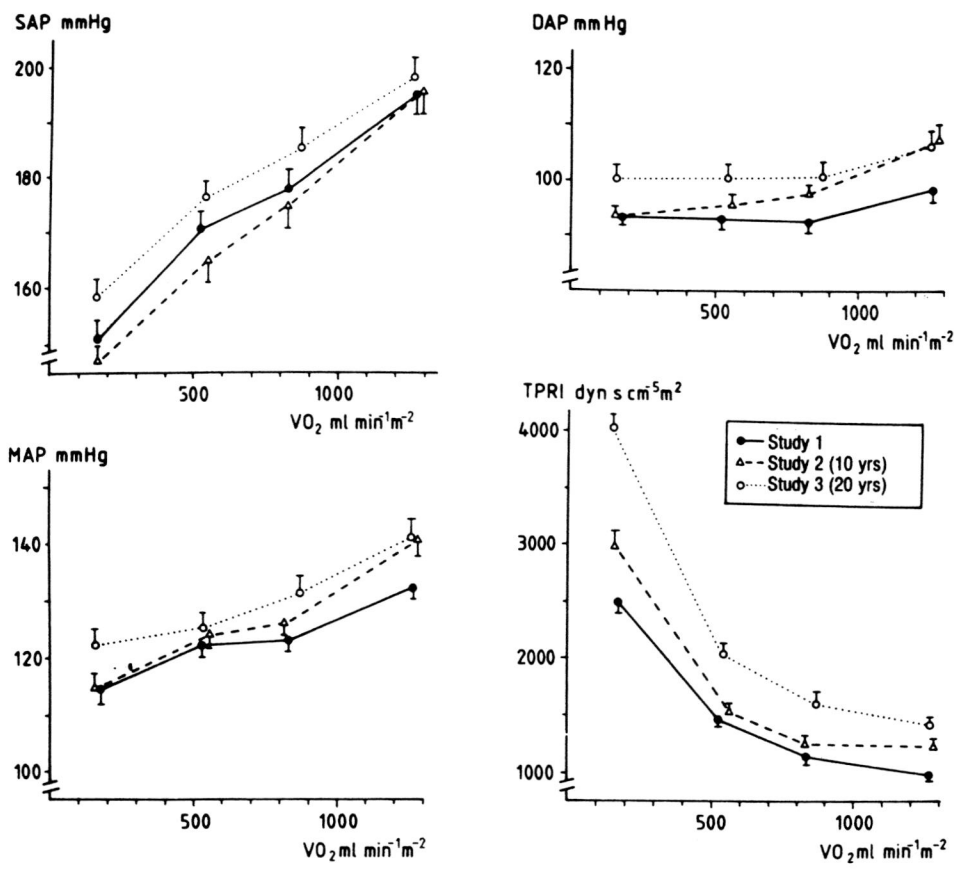

FIG. 8. Central hemodynamics (pressures and total peripheral resistance index [TPRI]) at rest and during exercise in age group I (17–29 years) at initial study and at 10- and 20-year follow-ups. SAP, systolic arterial pressure; DAP, diastolic arterial pressure; MAP, mean arterial pressure; VO₂, oxygen consumption. See text for details.

diuretics, beta blockers, or combination of the two, aiming at a DAP < 90 mm Hg without side effects). To exclude the immediate drug effects, treatment was withdrawn about 1–2 weeks before the 20-year follow-up (no complications or dramatic changes in the BP were seen).

At the restudy, DAP had been reduced significantly from 102.4 ± 11.5 mm Hg to 86.0 ± 4.4 mm Hg (16 percent) at rest and from 108.7 to 89.5 mm Hg (18 percent) during 150-W exercise (compared to the initial values 20 years earlier). The reduction in MAP was slightly less. Somewhat surprisingly, the effect on SAP had been very modest, from 167.9 to 162.8 mm Hg (3 percent, not significant) at rest sitting, and 7 percent, 8 percent, and 8 percent during 50-, 100-, and 150-W exercise, respectively.

In spite of clinically satisfactory diastolic BP control over all these years, there had been a dramatic increase in TPRI: 28 percent at rest and 19 percent, 34 percent, and 65 percent during exercise. Cardiac index was reduced by 31 percent at rest and by 25–40 percent during exercise, mainly due to fall in SI, but there was also a

significant reduction in HR, 17 percent at rest and approximately 12 percent during exercise.

Comparison of the Hemodynamic Pattern in the Young and in the Old

If we compare the mean values of the hemodynamic parameters at the first study in the youngest age group (17–29 years) with those seen after 20 years of hypertension (although treated) in the oldest group (60–69 years at the restudy) marked contrasts are seen (Figs. 9,10). Incidently, the two groups had almost the same MAP at rest sitting, 114 mm Hg. However, in the oldest group the SAP was higher and the DAP lower than in the youngest group. The increase in BP during exercise was much steeper in the older than in the younger group. The TPRI was about twice as high. Cardiac index during 150-W exercise was 11.1 L/min/m^2 in group I at the first study and approximately half of this value (5.94 L/min/m^2) in the oldest group. Although the two groups had the same

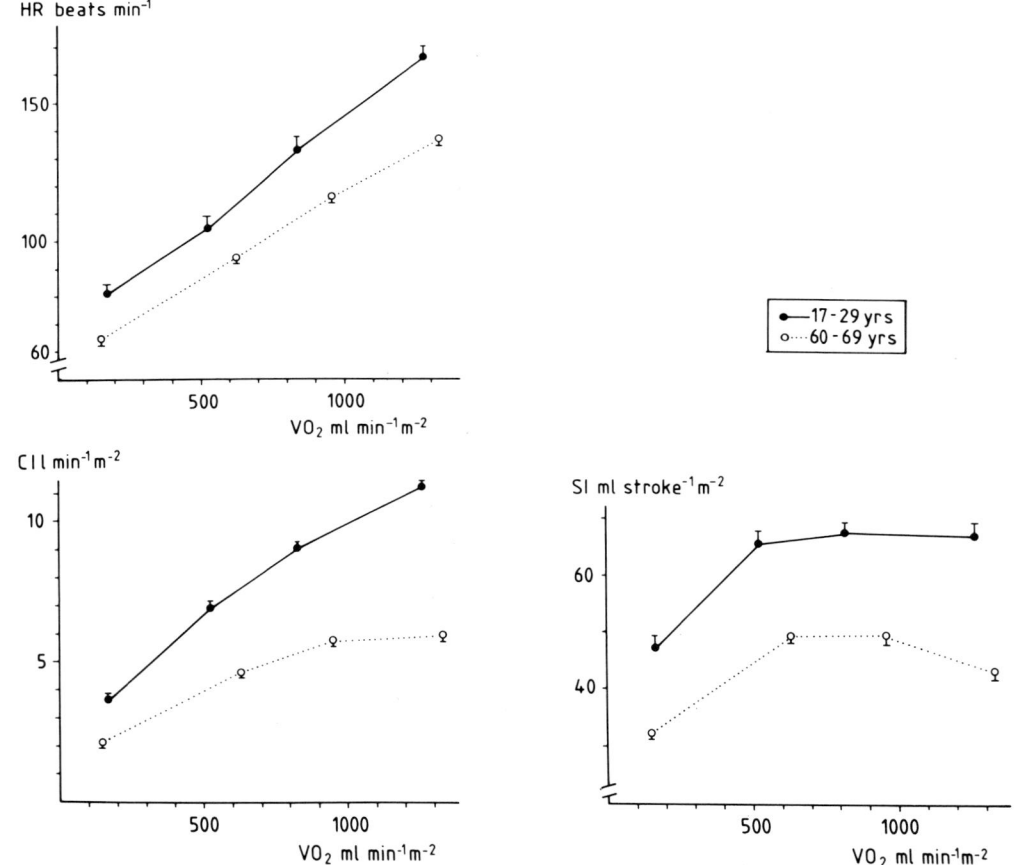

FIG. 9. Contrasting hemodynamic patterns at rest and during exercise in age group 17–29 years (n = 14) at initial study versus subjects aged 60–69 years (n = 19). Note that stroke index (SI) declines with increasing load in the oldest group. Mean values and SEM. HR, heart rate; CI, cardiac index; VO$_2$, oxygen consumption.

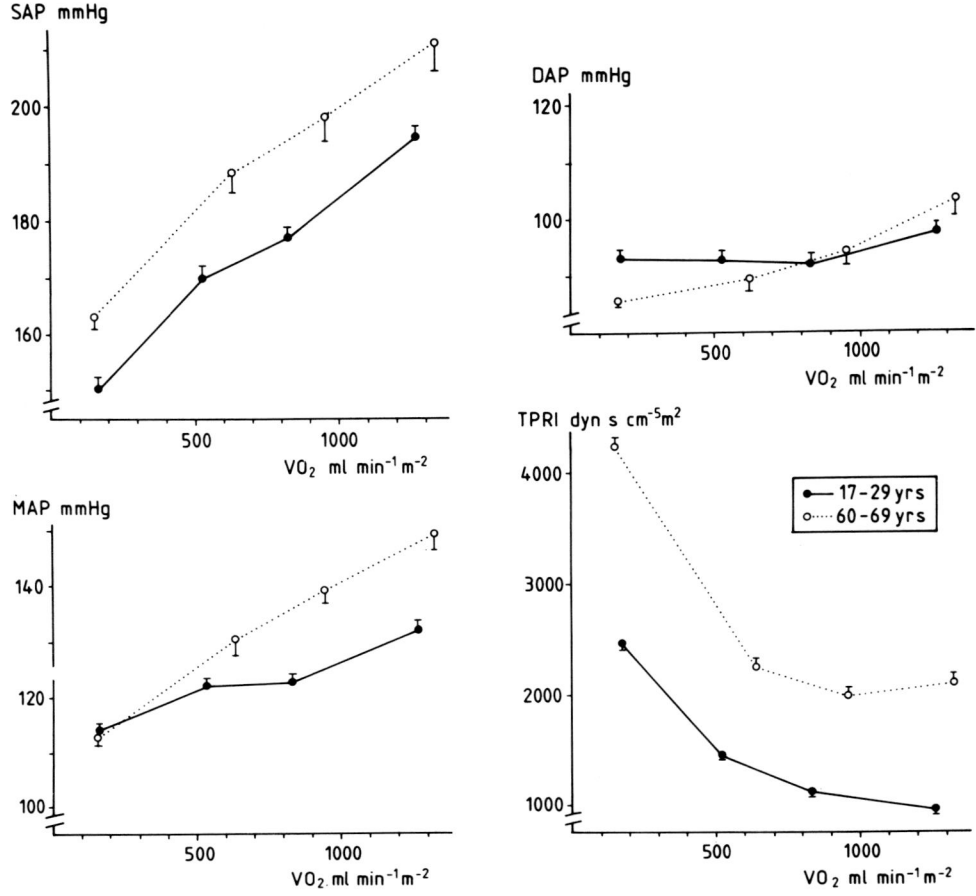

FIG. 10. Contrasting hemodynamic patterns at rest and during exercise in subjects aged 17–29 years (n = 14) at initial study versus subjects aged 60–69 years (n = 19). Mean values and SEM. Note that mean arterial pressure (MAP) is similar during rest, but increases are steeper in the oldest age group during exercise. Also note that total peripheral resistance index (TPRI) is almost twice as high in the older group as compared with the younger. SAP, systolic arterial pressure; DAP, diastolic arterial pressure; VO$_2$, oxygen consumption.

MAP at rest, central hemodynamics at rest as well as during exercise were widely different in these groups—representing the early phase and the late phase of essential hypertension. In the late phase, systolic hypertension was very marked (in spite of previous drug therapy).

CENTRAL HEMODYNAMICS IN VERY OLD HYPERTENSIVE SUBJECTS

There are relatively few studies on very old patients (over 70 years of age). In a study from Japan (121), CI and SI were much lower in the old hypertensives than in the young normotensives; TPRI was markedly increased in the oldest group.

In another Japanese study (122) including 126 patients aged 60 to above 80 years, low values for CI and SI were found. In fourteen men above 80 years of age, CI was 2.55 L/min/m^2 versus 3.03 in age group 60–69 years. Low values for CI and SI agree well with the findings in

our own series (age group 60–69 years). Exceptions to this hemodynamic pattern in elderly hypertensives have been described (123).

REGIONAL CIRCULATION

The regional circulation is more difficult to study than central hemodynamics. Furthermore, it is very difficult to establish where in the macro- and microvasculature of a given organ the resistance is disturbed. In the spontaneously hypertensive rats, the vascular resistance is increased in every organ system (124). However, microvascular pressure measurements in the kidney, in the skeletal muscles, in the small intestine, and in the cerebral cortex have shown that pressures are increased in the arteries and in the arterioles, but are normal in the precapillary arterioles, capillaries, and venules.

In subjects with essential hypertension in different stages, the disturbances in the pressure flow ratio (or in the calculated TPR) are not shared to the same extent in the various parts of the body (125).

Renal Circulation

It seems well accepted that in established hypertension the renal blood flow is usually reduced and the renal vascular resistance is increased—like in the rest of the body (126). London et al. (127) measured renal blood flow by [132]I-labeled hippuran in young patients with blood pressure 183/100 (versus 133/73 mm Hg in the controls). Cardiac index was not significantly different in the two groups, but TPRI was higher in the hypertensives than in the controls (2,923 vs. 1,997 dyn sec cm^{-5}m^2). Renal blood flow was reduced in the hypertensives (735 vs. 853 mL/min/m^2). The renal fraction of the cardiac output was 20.8 percent in the hypertensives versus 23.1 percent in the controls.

In 200 patients with uncomplicated essential hypertension studied under standardized conditions, a considerable increase in renal vascular resistance and reduction in renal blood flow were seen (126), and also a fall in renal plasma flow as the mean blood pressure increased from 110 to 140 mm Hg (126). The nature and the site of the increased renal vascular resistance are still poorly understood, but it is likely to occur mainly in the outer cortical zone in the preglomerular vessels.

In borderline hypertensives, findings have been more controversial. An increased renal blood flow (correlated to cardiac output) has been reported (65,128), while others have found renal blood flow to be within normal limits, even in subjects with increased cardiac output (129).

Bianchi et al. (130) reported increased renal plasma flow in offspring from hypertensive parents (with mean age of 25 years, BP about 124/80 mm Hg) and normal CO.

Splanchnic Circulation

The splanchnic circulation may be estimated by dye dilution method (usually Cardiogreen). In subjects with borderline hypertension with increased CO, the hepatic blood flow was found to be normal (129). In established hypertension the resistance was increased as in the rest of the body (131).

Skeletal Muscles

The blood flow in the skeletal muscles (forearm or leg) is usually studied by isotope methods or by plethysmography (with the latter method the skin blood flow will also be included) (132–136).

In summary, for patients with borderline hypertension and increased CO, an increase in muscle blood flow seems to be typical. When the hypertension becomes fixed, the resistance increases and the blood flow falls. Minimal resistance (during artificial vasodilatation) may be abnormal already in normotensive subjects with positive family history of hypertension (137–139).

Coronary Circulation

All methods for measurement of myocardial blood flow require rather invasive procedures, and for this reason the picture about the coronary hemodynamics in hypertensive heart disease in different ages and stages is quite incomplete (140,141).

No systematic studies are available in children and adolescents. Strauer (111) studied the coronary reserve after vasodilation with dipyridamole in a few patients in the early stage of hypertension (with normal ECG). Already at this stage he could demonstrate a reduction in the coronary reserve. With more severe hypertension the reduction in the coronary reserve was greater. Maximal coronary blood flow per gram of myocardial tissue is reduced when left ventricular hypertrophy is present (142,143). Since increase in left ventricular mass is seen in children with very mild hypertension, one may wonder whether coronary blood flow could already be affected at this stage.

Pulmonary Circulation

Hypertension also seem to affect—or involve—the lesser circulation. It has been shown that even in patients with mild and moderately severe hypertension (without any clinical signs of heart failure) there is often an increase in the pulmonary artery pressure (144,145). Probably as a consequence of this, there is also an involvement of the right ventricle with reduced ejection fraction, and thus functional disturbances in both the left and the right side of the heart (46).

The cause of the increased pulmonary artery pressure in subjects with mild hypertension is not known. A redistribution of the blood flow from the systemic circulation to the central circulation is possible, perhaps caused by an overreactive neural stimulation, not only on the systemic, but also on the pulmonary vessels.

INTRACARDIAC HEMODYNAMICS

Although the first studies on hemodynamics in hypertension were performed by right heart catheterization—and demonstrated increased filling pressures of left ventricle in patients with severe hypertension—most of our knowledge about the details in intracardiac hemodynamics in hypertension derives from more recent echo-Doppler studies.

The heart responds to the increased afterload by a concentric left ventricular hypertrophy (14). The increased systolic wall stress leads to replication of sarcomers, an increase in cell width, and an increase in, and remodeling of, the collagen network (146). Studies of the diastolic filling rate have shown that this is reduced at an early stage in essential hypertension (147–150) and it seems likely that this is a consequence of the remodeling of the left ventricular wall which becomes stiffer (146).

The transport of blood from the left atrium to the left ventricle involves two phases: first the rapid early filling phase (the E-phase) and then the atrial contraction (the A-phase). With increasing stiffness of the left ventricular wall, the atrial phase becomes more important for the filling of the ventricle and the A-phase increases. The ratio between these two (the E/A-ratio) is often used as an indication of the diastolic function. It appears that this ratio might be one of the most sensitive indexes of an early functional disturbance in the hypertensive heart. In hypertensive hearts this ratio may range from about 1.7 to 0.6, depending on the age and severity of hypertension (151).

It is also well known that physical training induces increased left ventricular mass, but in contrast to hypertension it is not associated with diastolic dysfunction (152,153). The concentric left ventricular hypertrophy (LVH) seen in established essential hypertension is related to the increased TPR (154), but several nonhemodynamic factors also seem to influence the development of LVH and affect the E/A-ratio (14), and the cause of decreased ventricular relaxation is often unclear.

At least initially, LVH involves an adaptive benefit. It permits distribution of the pressure overload to a greater cross-section of the myocardium, and fiber shortening and stroke volume remain close to normal—at least during rest. However, as demonstrated 25 years ago in our own hemodynamic studies, exercise testing unveils subnormal stroke volume already in the early phase of essential hypertension (12), and this has also been shown later by others with different methods (155). Today it appears likely that the reduced systolic function of the heart during exercise is a consequence of the pathologic diastolic function of the left ventricle (156).

Due to the risk involved in left heart catheterization, systematic studies of intracardiac pressures by this method have not been performed in early essential hypertensives. Most of the catheterization studies have been undertaken in patients with chest pain, when coronary heart disease has been suspected. When hypertension has been untreated for many years, heart failure may develop, associated with increased left ventricular end-diastolic pressure and reduced ejection fraction and stroke volume. However, the mechanisms whereby hypertension leads to cardiac failure are not fully defined. The transition from hypertensive LVH with normal ejection fraction to definite congestive heart failure may depend on several factors such as structural changes, biochemical or humoral abnormalities, compensatory mechanisms, or myocardial ischemia (12).

WHAT CAUSES THE HEMODYNAMIC DISTURBANCES IN ESSENTIAL HYPERTENSION?

What are the most important factors responsible for the increased pressure and the hemodynamic disturbances in the various phases of essential hypertension? This is a very complex field and since many of the most important factors involved (in the starting phase as well as in chronic fixed hypertension) will be discussed in separate chapters in this book, studies dealing mainly with both central hemodynamics and regulating mechanisms will be discussed briefly.

The Sympathetic Nervous System

It is generally believed that the increased CO, HR, and oxygen consumption seen in many patients with early essential hypertension—at least during testing situation—is due to an "overactivity" in the sympathetic nervous system, but this has been difficult to prove. There is disagreement about how an "overactivity" in the sympathetic nervous system should be expressed (157–159).

Measurements of just plasma noradrenaline concentration or 24-hour excretion of catecholamines in the urine could be misleading because the most important information needed concerns what happens at the nerve terminal. Esler et al. (157,158) have suggested that the noradrenaline spillover rate—preferably from individual organ systems—would be the best index.

Plasma noradrenaline recorded during rest is strongly influenced by age. In a review of about 80 studies on catecholamines in essential hypertension, it was concluded that only a minority of younger subjects with essential hypertension had elevated norepinephrine values during rest (159). Younger patients with essential hypertension had increased renal noradrenaline spillover rates and elevated 24-hour norepinephrine levels.

In patients with borderline hypertension, Messerli et al. (160) found an age-dependent increase in norepinephrine level and a decrease in epinephrine level. Several investigators have reported a positive correlation between plasma noradrenaline and TPR or CI or HR in mildly hypertensive patients (161,162).

When the sympathetic nervous system is blocked by propranolol and the parasympathetic system by atropine, an imbalance between the sympathetic and parasympathetic nervous system in a large proportion of patients with mild borderline hypertension have been demonstrated (163). Julius (163,164) considers that the hemodynamic abnormalities during rest seen in early essential hypertension are most easily described through neurogenic mechanism.

Many investigators have tried to demonstrate that children or adolescents with hypertensive parents are "hyperreactors" to various stress stimuli. Such tests have been used trying to identify young subjects who later develop hypertension (165). Falkner (76) has shown a greater BP and HR response to stress in young subjects who later developed hypertension, and regarded these findings consistent with a dysregulatory neurogenic component in the pathogenesis of essential hypertension.

It is often claimed that the stress of everyday life in industrialized societies is responsible for the increase in BP seen over years. In this context it is interesting that in nuns from a secluded order, who had a very quiet life with no contact with the rest of the world, there was practically no change in the BP over a 20-year period, in contrast to a similar group of women living in the neighborhood under normal conditions (166).

In recent years it has been shown that the effect of the catecholamines seem to be dependent on the sodium ion. Sodium-sensitive hypertensives have been found most sensitive to neurogenic stimuli (167). Thus, this whole field on "hyperreactivity"—what causes it and whether it induces hypertension over time—is very complex.

Blood Volume and the Capacitance Vessels

In order to obtain an increased or normal CO in the presence of an increased afterload, an enhanced filling of the heart is important. Many studies have shown that there is an increase in cardiopulmonary blood volume in hypertension (168–173). Total blood volume, however, is usually normal in mild hypertension and tends to be decreased in more severe forms. The blood volume is usually inversely correlated with the BP (174). A positive correlation between cardiopulmonary blood volume and CO has been demonstrated (65).

A reduced distensibility (compliance) of the venous system could partly contribute to a redistribution of the blood volume and increase in left ventricular filling pressure. More than 20 years ago it was noted that a rapid infusion of dextran caused a greater increase in the central venous pressure in hypertensive subjects than in normotensives (12,175–178). This was interpreted as a reduced compliance of the venous system. In recent years, studies based on other methods (e.g., plethysmography) have also suggested a reduction in the venous compliance as a typical phenomenon in essential hypertension (179,180). This seems to occur very early in the process of hypertension (181), even in normotensive offspring from hypertensive families (182).

Structural Changes in the Left Ventricle and in the Resistance Vessels

In the spontaneously hypertensive rats, hypertrophy and reduced compliance of the left ventricle occur at a very early stage, sometimes after only a few weeks (183–185).

In man it is well established that a reduction in the left ventricular compliance and filling rate are seen very early in the process of essential hypertension, even before there is an increase in the wall thickness (147,186). It seems reasonable to explain the subnormal stroke volume during exercise as a consequence of the increased filling time of the left ventricle.

During the last 15 years there has also been a large number of echo studies of the heart in children with slight elevation in the BP (71,72,148–150). These studies have all shown an increase in left ventricular mass with increase in BP.

Hopefully, with improvement of the technique, the echo-Doppler method should be able to give useful information, not only on the structure of the heart and on blood velocity, but also on the cardiac dynamics and on the heart pump function—measured as stroke volume and CO during exercise. Then a complete correlation between structure and function should be possible.

Structural changes in the resistance vessels have been demonstrated at a very early stage in the spontaneously hypertensive rats (170). In humans with borderline or

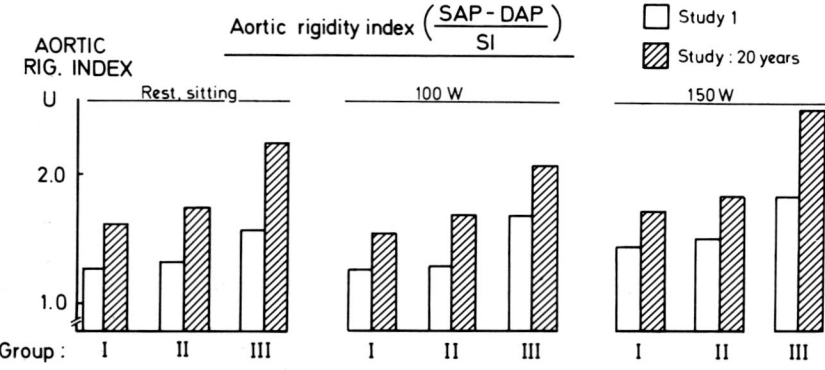

FIG. 11. Aortic rigidity index [(SAP − DAP)/SI] in units (U) at first study (open bars) and at restudy 20 years later (hatched bars) in age groups I, II, and III at rest (sitting) and at 100 and 150 W exercise. Mean values. Note increase in the aortic rigidity index decade by decade and by aging over 20 years.

mild hypertension it has been shown that TPR does not fall to normal levels during exercise (12) or after autonomic blockade (164) or after heating and exercise when maximal vasodilatation is assumed to be present (136). This "residual" increase in TPR is usually explained on the basis of increase in the wall-to-lumen ratio in the arterioles, similar to what has been demonstrated in the spontaneously hypertensive rats (181–185).

An increase in aortic rigidity index (SAP-DAP/SI) was seen in all age groups in our 20-year follow-up study (Fig. 11).

HEMODYNAMIC ALTERATIONS— THERAPEUTIC CONSIDERATIONS

This review has demonstrated that the hemodynamic patterns and mechanisms behind increased BP differ greatly in the various stages of hypertensive disease. From a hemodynamic point of view, treatment of hypertension should aim at normalization of central as well as peripheral hemodynamic abnormalities—at rest and during exercise. Deterioration of the heart pump function and increase in arteriolar resistance should be prevented.

The various classes of antihypertensive agents act quite differently on central hemodynamics at rest and during exercise. This has recently been reviewed quite extensively (187). The purpose of this brief discussion is to emphasize that, at least in subgroups of hypertensive patients, it is important to use a hemodynamically correct drug.

The immediate effects on central hemodynamics induced by a special type of an antihypertensive agent may differ quite markedly from the long-term effects. Initially, counter-regulatory mechanisms (such as baroreflex-triggered increase in HR) may try to reduce the BP fall induced by the pharmacological effect of the drug. During long-term use, some of these counter-regulatory reactions may disappear (188). Also, gradual regression of structural changes in the heart and in the resistance vessels may contribute to normalization of the hemodynamic situation. Thus, it is not only the pharmacological effect of a drug which determines how the hemodynamic disturbances are affected over time.

Antihypertensive agents like thiazide diuretics, alpha-receptor blockers (like prazosin or doxazosin), calcium antagonists and angiotensin-converting enzyme (ACE) inhibitors all lower BP through reduction in TPRI (187). The reduction in TPR is, of course, achieved through very different mechanisms (i.e., effect on receptors, on angiotensin, on calcium transport). Extensive studies in humans with mild to moderate essential hypertension— at rest and during exercise—indicate that all these classes of drugs during chronic treatment tend to normalize central hemodynamics more or less. Since they do not cause

any reduction in heart pump function at rest and during exercise, these compounds do not seem to reduce exercise tolerance. Peripheral as well as renal blood flow is maintained or may be increased.

The beta blockers are different (189). When the beta blockers were introduced in treatment of hypertension many years ago, they were referred to as a "paradoxic" way of treating hypertension. The paradox implied that, in established essential hypertension, pretreatment CO was generally subnormal and the beta blockers induced a further reduction in CO in most patients, while TPR did not seem to be reduced. During rest there are important differences with respect to beta blockers with or without intrinsic sympathicomimetic activity (ISA), but during physical exercise all commonly used beta blockers reduce CO in subjects with uncomplicated hypertension. The oxygen delivery to the tissues is achieved through an increase in the arteriovenous oxygen difference. For this reason, most subjects are able to tolerate a 20- to 25-percent reduction in exercise CO without serious symptoms as long as the exercise load is not too severe and does not last too long.

However, during endurance exercise it is well established that beta blockers reduce the performance (13,190). For this reason, beta blockers are not the drug of first choice in physically very active subjects. Then other alternatives would seem to be preferable.

The beta blockers are usually contraindicated in hypertensives with heart failure when CO is very low. In patients with heart failure the ACE inhibitors have been shown to be extremely effective (in hypertensives as well as in normotensive subjects). The ACE inhibitors have a strong effect on preload as well as an afterload, and they seem to be the drug of first choice in hypertensive patients with heart failure (187).

Since most beta blockers (without ISA) reduce BP as well as HR, they may induce a substantial reduction in the workload on the heart (the pressure × heart rate product). Partly for this reason, the beta blockers are generally very useful in hypertensive patients with angina pectoris and, if contraindications are not present, the beta blockers belong to the first line of drugs in this type of hypertensive subject. When contraindicated, the calcium antagonists—also improving coronary blood flow—would seem to be the best choice. Further comprehensive discussions on the proper choice of antihypertensive agents are available to the the reader (187).

CONCLUSIONS

What have we learned from the hemodynamic studies over the three last decades? There is still no agreement on how to define subjects definitely representing the "starting phase" of essential hypertension. In our opinion, observations from mildly hypertensive children, adolescents, and young adults indicate that there is probably no uniform starting phase from a hemodynamic point of view. High CO, HR, and oxygen consumption have been demonstrated in a large fraction of such subjects who were permanently hypertensive (at least initially) during some months before the initial hemodynamic investigation and who remained hypertensive during the following 20 years, with some increase in BP over time. Thus, the subjects were undoubtedly hypertensive at the time of the first study. However, it also seems reasonable that the high CO phase is not present in all subjects and that essential hypertension may start by an increase in TPR as well. The high CO phase usually disappears over a 5- to 10-year period, and TPR increases. It is exceptional to find high CO in elderly hypertensives, but it has been reported.

Very recently the Dutch Hypertension and Offspring Study has reported that offspring from normotensive and hypertensive parents did have the same oxygen consumption during rest and almost the same CI values (191). The BP in the hypertensive offspring (age 22.8 years) was 126.9/78.7 mm Hg versus 116.4/71.0 mm Hg in the normotensive offspring (age 19.5 years). The studies were noninvasive, and the CI values were surprisingly low—only about 1.8 L/min/m^2 in all offspring groups. It remains to be seen how many in the different groups will develop definite hypertension (BP > 140/90 mm Hg). As in many similar studies, left ventricular mass index was slightly higher in the hypertensive offspring than in the normotensive offspring.

Increased activity in sympathetic nervous system—or an imbalance between the sympathetic or vagal tone—may at least partially be responsible for the hemodynamic alterations in the early phase.

Studies of heart pump function during exercise, together with echo-Doppler studies (mainly during rest), have unveiled changes in the study of pump function and of cardiac dynamics early in the process of hypertension. In particular, disturbances in the diastolic function—reduction in the elasticity of the left ventricle with increase in filling time—seem to be present very early, even before wall thickness is increased. The systolic function is affected much later. The triggering mechanism of the hemodynamics in essential hypertension is yet far from understood, and there are also many unsolved questions about why hemodynamic patterns may develop differently in different groups of patients over the years. It seems likely that this is due to inherited as well as external factors.

During the last two decades there has been a tendency to oversimplification of the treatment of hypertension. There has been too much concern about BP level and relatively little interest in the hemodynamic mechanisms behind the increased pressure and how this could be best corrected by the different types of antihypertensive agents (192).

It is hoped that this review has shown that the hemodynamic mechanisms behind the same BP levels in young and in elderly subjects may be widely different. The various classes of antihypertensive agents affect the hemodynamic disturbances quite differently. Proper use of antihypertensive agents—also based on hemodynamic effects and effects on other physiological regulating systems—should lead to a more physiological approach to treatment of hypertension (193) and should also be better tolerated and induce better long-term results than the older drugs seem to do.

ACKNOWLEDGMENTS

This work has been supported by the Norwegian Council on Cardiovascular Diseases. The authors also wish to thank Janicke Bjørke for excellent assistance in preparation of the manuscript.

REFERENCES

1. Peterson LH. In: Brest AN, Moyer JH, eds. *Hypertension. Recent advances.* Philadelphia: Lea and Febriger, 1961;45–52.
2. Pickering ThG. *Am J Cardiol* 1986;58:12D–15D.
3. Letcher RL, Chien S, Pickering ThG, et al. *Hypertension* 1983;5:757–762.
4. Smith WCSS, Lowe GDO, Lee AJ, et al. *J Hypertens* 1992;10:467–472.
5. Freis ED. *Physiol Rev* 1960;40:27–54.
6. Birkenhäger WH, de Leeuw PW, Schalekamp MADH. *Control Mechanisms in Essential Hypertension.* Amsterdam, New York, Oxford: Elsevier Biomedical Press, 1982.
7. Lund-Johansen P. State of the art review. *Clin Sci* 1980;59:343s–354s.
8. Folkow B. *Physiol Rev* 1982;62:347–504.
9. Conway FJ, Lund-Johansen P, Hansson L, et al. *Acta Med Scand* 1982;212:253–260.
10. Lund-Johansen P. In: Robertson JIS, ed. *Handbook of hypertension,* vol 1, *Clinical aspects of essential hypertension.* Amsterdam: Elsevier Science Publishers BV, 1983;151–173.
11. Conway J. *Physiol Rev* 1984;64:617–660.
12. Lund-Johansen P. *Acta Med Scand* 1967;181[Suppl 482]:1–101.
13. Lund-Johansen P. *Am J Cardiol* 1987;59:98A–107A.
14. Frohlich ED, Apstein C, Chobanian AV, et al. *N Engl J Med* 1992;998–1008.
15. Karlefors T, Nielsen R, Westling H. *Acta Med Scand* 1966;180[Suppl 449]:91–98.
16. Ellestad MH. *Am J Cardiol* 1989;983–985.
17. West JNW, Townend JN, Davies P, et al. *Hypertension* 1991;18:593–597.
18. White WB, Lund-Johansen P, Omvik P. *Am J Cardiol* 1990;65:60–66.
19. Fagard R, Conway J. *Eur Heart J* 1990;11[Suppl 1]:S1–S5.
20. Lund-Johansen P. *Eur Heart J* 1990;11[Suppl 1]:S6–S12.
21. Conway J, Lund-Johansen P. *Eur Heart J* 1990;11[Suppl 1]:S17–S20.
22. Reybrouck T, Fagard R. *Eur Heart J* 1990;11[Suppl 1]:S21–S25.
23. Wallerson DC, Ganau A, Roman MJ, et al. *Eur Heart J* 1990;11[Suppl 1]:S67–S78.
24. Lacolley PJ, Pannier BM, Levy BI, et al. *Eur Heart J* 1990;11[Suppl 1]:S62–S66.
25. Fouad-Tarazi FM, MacIntyre WJ. *Eur Heart J* 1990;11[Suppl 1]:S33–S40.
26. Mancia G, Bertineri G, Grassi G, et al. *Lancet* 1983;2:695–698.
27. Silverberg DS, Rosenfeld JB. *Isr J Med Sci* 1980;16:41–43.
28. Birkenhäger WH. *J Hypertens* 1991;[Suppl 6]:S2–S9.

29. Rostrup M, Kjeldsen SE, Eide IK. *Am J Hypertens* 1990;3:912–917.
30. Rostrup M, Mundal HH, Westheim A, et al. *J Hypertens* 1991;9:159–166.
31. Fagan TC, Conrad KA, Mar JH, et al. *Clin Pharmacol Ther* 1986;39:255–260.
32. Bristow JD, Honour AJ, Pickering TG, et al. *Cardiovasc Res* 1969;3:476–485.
33. Amery A, Wasir H, Bulpitt C, et al. *Acta Cardiol* 1978;6:443–467.
34. Kannel WB, Dawber TR, McGee DL. *Circulation* 1980;61:1179–1184.
35. Landahl S, Bengtsson C, Sigurdsson JA, et al. *Hypertension* 1986;8:1044–1053.
36. Schoenberger JA. *Am J Cardiol* 1986;57:45C–51C.
37. Shannon RP, Maher KA, Santinga JT, Royal HD, Wei JY. *Am J Cardiol* 1991;67:1110–1116.
38. Brandfonbrener M, Landowne M, Shock NW. *Circulation* 1955;12:557–566.
39. Granath A, Johnsson B, Strandell T. *Acta Med Scand* 1964;176:425–432.
40. Strandell T. In: Caird FI, ed. *Cardiology in old age.* Plenum Press, 1976;81–100.
41. Hanson JS, Tabakin BS, Levy AM. *Circulation* 1968;37:345–360.
42. Julius S, Amery A, Whitlock LS. *Circulation* 1967;36:222–230.
43. Fleg JL. *Am J Cardiol* 1986;57:33C–43C.
44. Rodeheffer RJ, Gerstenblith G, Becker LC, et al. *Circulation* 1984;69:203–213.
45. Lakatta EG. *Eur Heart J* 1990;11[Suppl C]:S22–S29.
46. Guazzi MD, De Cesare N, Fiorentini C, et al. *Circulation* 1987;75[Suppl I]:I-56–I-62.
47. Levy AM, Tabakin BS, Hanson JS. *Circulation* 1967;35:1063–1072.
48. Conway J, Wheeler R, Sannerstedt R. *Cardiovasc Res* 1971;5:577–584.
49. Frohlich ED, Tarazi RC, Dustan HP. *Am J Med Sci* 1969;257:9–23.
50. Lowenthal DT, Kim KE, Affrime MB, et al. *Chest* 1983;2[Suppl]:408–409.
51. Smulyan H, Csermely TJ, Mookherjee S, et al. *Arteriosclerosis* 1983;3:199–205.
52. McGarry K, Laher M, Fitzgerald D, et al. *Hypertension* 1983;5:763–771.
53. Iskandrian AS, Hakki A-H. *Am Heart J* 1986;112:75–84.
54. Wei JY. *N Engl J Med* 1992;327:1735–1739.
55. Manvari DE, Patterson Ch, Johnson D, et al. *J Am Geriatr Soc* 1985;33:758–767.
56. Templeton GH, Platt MR, Willerson JT, et al. *Circ Res* 1979;44:189–197.
57. Widimsky J, Fejfarova MH, Fejfar Z. *Cardiologia* 1957;31:381–389.
58. Fejfar MH, Widimsky J. In: Cort JH, Fencl V, Hejl Z, Jirka J, eds. *The pathogenesis of essential hypertension.* Prague: State Medical Publishing House, 1961;33–39.
59. Eich RH, Peters RJ, Cuddy RP, et al. *Am Heart J* 1962;63:188–195.
60. Bello CT, Sevy RW, Harakal C. *Am J Med Sci* 1967;253:194–208.
61. Kuramoto K, Murata K, Yazaki Y, et al. *Jpn Circ* 1968;32:981–998.
62. Frohlich ED, Kozyl VJ, Tarazi RC, et al. *Circ Res* 1970;25[Suppl I]:55–69.
63. Safar M, Fendler J-P, Weil B, et al. *La Press Medicale* 1970;78:111–114.
64. Julius S, Pascual AV, Sannerstedt R, et al. *Circulation* 1971;43:382–390.
65. Messerli FH, DeCarvalho JGR, Christie B, et al. *Circulation* 1978;58:441–448.
66. Jern S. *Acta Med Scand* 1982;[Suppl 662]:1–54.
67. Fujita T, Noda H. *Jpn Circ J* 1983;47:795–801.
68. Sato T. *Jpn Circ J* 1983;47:221–229.
69. Messerli FH, Frohlich ED, Suarez H, et al. *Circulation* 1981;64:760–764.
70. Kuwajima I. *Nippon Ronen Igakkai Zasshi* 1979;16:29–37.
71. Schieken RM, Clarke WR, Lauer RM. *Hypertension* 1981;3:669–675.
72. Zahka KG, Neill CA, Langford H, et al. *Hypertension* 1981;3:664–668.
73. Hofmann A, Roelandt JTRC, Boomsa F, et al. *Clin Sci* 1981;61:169–174.
74. Hofmann A, Ellison RC, Newburger J, et al. *Br Heart J* 1982;48:377–380.
75. Ohlsson O. *Haemodynamic studies of relatives to hypertensive parents.* Malmö: Malmö University Press, 1981;1–29.
76. Falkner B. *J Cardiovasc Pharmacol* 1986;8[Suppl 5]:S44–S47.
77. Mo R, Lund-Johansen P, Omvik P. *Blood Pressure* 1993;2:197–204.
78. Ledingham JM, Cohen RD. *Lancet* 1963;2:979–981.
79. Guyton AC, Coleman TG, Cowley AW Jr, et al. In: Onesti G, Kim KE, Moyer JH, eds. *Hypertension: mechanisms and management.* New York: Grune & Stratton, 1983;25–36.
80. Liard JF. In: Guyton AC, Young DHB, eds. *Cardiovascular physiology.* Baltimore: University Park Press, 1979;317–355.
81. Cowley AW. *Am J Med* 1980;68:906–916.
82. Sannerstedt R. *Acta Med Scand* 1966;458[Suppl 180]:1–83.
83. Eich RH, Cuddy RP, Smulyan H, et al. *Circulation* 1966;34:299–307.
84. Julius S, Conway J. *Circulation* 1968;38:282–288.
85. Gorlin R. *JAMA* 1962;182:823–829.
86. Gillum RF, Teichholz LE, Herman MV, et al. *Am Heart J* 1981;102:728–734.
87. Widimsky J, Jandova R, Ressle J. *Eur Heart J* 1981;2:307–315.
88. Levy AM, Tabakin BS, Hanson JS. *Circulation* 1967;35:1063–1072.
89. Fouad FM, Tarazi RC, Dustan HP, et al. *Am Heart J* 1978;96:646–654.
90. Fouad FM. *Circulation* 1987;75[Suppl I]:I-48–I-55.
91. Klein AA, McCrory WW, Engle MA, et al. *JACC* 1984;3:381–386.
92. Amery A, Julius S, Whitlock LS, et al. *Circulation* 1967;36:231–237.
93. Widimsky J. *Cor Vasa* 1984;26:147–154.
94. Glazer GA. *Cor Vasa* 1963;5:165–176.
95. Bello CT, Sevy RW, Harakal C. *Am J Med Sci* 1967;253:194–208.
96. Amery A. *Malattie Cardiovasc* 1969;10:227–245.
97. Frohlich ED, Pfeffer MA. *Clin Sci Mol Med* 1975;48[Suppl 2]:225s–238s.
98. Chau N-P, Safar ME, Weiss YA, et al. *Contrib Nephrol* 1977;8:109–115.
99. de Leeuw PW, Kho TL, Falke HE, et al. *Acta Med Scand* 1978;[Suppl 622]:1–15.
100. Lund-Johansen P. In: Onesti G, Kim KE, eds. *Hypertension in the young and the old.* New York: Grune & Stratton, 1980;236–249.
101. Aoki, Sato K. *Jpn Heart J* 1986;27:467–474.
102. Fagard R, Staessen J. *Am J Cardiol* 1991;67:585–589.
103. Devereux RB, Savage DD, Sachs I, et al. *Am J Cardiol* 1983;51:171–176.
104. Wikstrand J. *Clin Physiol* 1986;6:115–127.
105. Anderson O, Hansson L, Sivertsson R. *Circulation* 1978;58:615.
106. Omvik P, Lund-Johansen P. *J Hypertens* 1984;2:73–79.
107. Ibrahim MM, Tarazi RC, Dustan HP, et al. *Am J Cardiol* 1975;35:667–674.
108. Werkö L, Lagerlöf H. *Acta Med Scand* 1949;133:427.
109. Varnauskas E. *Scand J Clin Lab Invest* 1955;7[Suppl 17]:1–117.
110. Taylor SH, Donald KW, Bishop JM. *Clin Sci* 1957;16:351–376.
111. Strauer B-E. *Am J Cardiol* 1979;44:999–1006.
112. Shapiro LM, Mackinnon K, Beevers DG. *Br Heart J* 1981;46:374–379.
113. Eliasch H, Varnauskas E, Werkö L. In: Hansson L, ed. *Hypertoni och arterioscklerosfrågor.* Göteborg, Lindgren, 1971;17–19.
114. Birkenhäger WH, Schalekamp MADH, Krauss XH, et al. *Lancet* 1972;1:560–564.
115. Weiss YA, Safar ME, London GM, et al. *Am J Med* 1978;64:382–387.

116. Julius S, Quadir H, Gajendragadkar S. In: Gross F, Strasser T, eds. *Mild hypertension: natural history and management.* Proceedings of the Joint WHO/ISH meeting, Susono, Japan. Bath: Pitman Medical, 1979;116–126.
117. Birkenhäger WH, de Leeuw PW. *J Hypertens* 1984;2:121–125.
118. Andersson OKI, Sannerstedt R, Beckman M, et al. *J Hypertens* 1983;1[Suppl 2]:91–93.
119. Lund-Johansen P. In: Onesti G, Klimt CR, eds. *Hypertension—determinants, complications, and intervention.* New York: Grune & Stratton, 1979;201–218.
120. Lund-Johansen P. *Hypertension* 1991;18[Suppl III]:III-54–III-61.
121. Terasawa F, Kuramoto K, Ying LH, et al. *Acta Gerontol Jap* 1972;56:47–56.
122. Sato I, Tazumi K, Kato K, et al. *Jpn J Geriatr* 1977;14:99–109.
123. Kuwajima I. *Nippon Ronen Igakkai Zasshi* 1979;16:29–35.
124. Bohlen HG. *Hypertension* 1986;8:181–183.
125. Brod J, Fencl V, Hejl Z, et al. *Clin Sci* 1962;23:339–349.
126. de Leeuw PW, Birkenhäger WH. *J Hypertens* 1983;1:321–331.
127. London GM, Safar ME, Bouthier JL, et al. *Clin Sci* 1984;67:313–319.
128. Hollenberg NK, Adams DF. *Am J Med Sci* 1971;261:232–239.
129. Temmar MM, Safar ME, Levenson JA, et al. *Clin Sci* 1981;60:653–658.
130. Bianchi G, Gatti M, Ferrari P, et al. *Lancet* 1979;1:173–177.
131. Messerli FH, Genest J, Nowaczynski W, et al. *Circulation* 1975;51:114–119.
132. Conway J. *Circulation* 1963;27:520–529.
133. Amery A, Bossaert H, Verstracle M. *Am Heart J* 1969;78:211–216.
134. Romanovska I, Prerovsky I, Jandova R, et al. *Cor Vasa* 1980;20:33–40.
135. Fantini F, Nuzzaci G, Padeletti P, et al. *Angiology* 1977;28:549–554.
136. Sivertsson R, Sannerstedt R, Lundgren Y. *Clin Sci Mol Med* 1976;51[Suppl 3]:65s–71s.
137. Berglund G, Ljungman S, Hartford M, et al. *J Hypertens* 1983;1[Suppl 2]:286–288.
138. Gudmundsson O, Andersson OK, Aurell M, et al. *J Hypertens* 1984;2:291–296.
139. Takeshita A, Mark AL. *Jpn Circ J* 1983;47:256–257.
140. Marcus ML, Wilson RF, White CW. *Circulation* 1987;76:245–253.
141. Collins P. *Br Heart J* 1993;69:279–281.
142. Nichols AB, Sciacca RR, Weiss MB, et al. *Circulation* 1980;62:329–340.
143. Strauer BE, Schwartzkopff B, Motz W, et al. *J Cardiovasc Pharmacol* 1991;18[Suppl 3]:S20–S27.
144. Ferlinz J. *Circulation* 1980;61:61:156–162.
145. Widimsky J, Jandova R, Ressle J. *Cor Vasa* 1980;22:156–167.
146. Weber KT, Brilla CG. *Circulation* 1991;83:1849–1865.
147. Inouye I, Massie B, Loge D, et al. *Am J Cardiol* 1984;53:120–126.
148. Johnson GL, Kotchen JM, McKean HE, et al. *Am Heart J* 1983;105:113–118.
149. Labovitz AJ, Pearson AC. *Am Heart J* 1987;114:836–851.
150. Snider AR, Gidding SS, Rocchini AP, et al. *Am J Cardiol* 1985;56:921–926.
151. Shahi M, Thom S, Poulter N, Sever PS, Foale RA. *Eur Heart J* 1991;12:974–979.
152. Granger CB, Karimeddini MK, Smith VE, Shapiro HR, Katz AM, Riba AL. *J Am Coll Cardiol* 1985;5:862–868.
153. Smith VE, Schulman P, Karimeddini MK, White WB, Meeran MK, Katz AM. *J Am Coll Cardiol* 1985;5:869–874.
154. Blake J, Devereux RB, Herrold EM, et al. *Am J Cardiol* 1988;62:246–252.
155. Wasserman AG, Katz RJ, Varghese PJ, et al. *N Engl J Med* 1984;311:1276–1280.
156. Cuocolo A, Sax FL, Brush JE, Maron BJ, Bacharach SL, Bonow RO. *Circulation* 1990;81:978–986.
157. Esler MD, Hasking GJ, Willett IR, et al. *J Hypertens* 1985;3:117–129.
158. Ferrier C, Esler MD, Eisenhofer G, et al. *Hypertension* 1992;19:62–69.
159. Tuck ML. *Am Heart J* 1986;112:877–886.
160. Messerli FH, Frohlich ED, Suarez H, et al. *Circulation* 1981;64:760–764.
161. Miura Y, Kobayashi K, Sakuma H, et al. *Clin Sci Mol Med* 1978;55[Suppl 4]:69s–71s.
162. Muisan G, Agabiti-Rosei E, Alicandri C, et al. In: Albertini A, Da Prada A, Peska BA, eds. *Radioimmunoassay of drugs and hormones in cardiovascular medicine.* New York: Elsevier, 1979;123–132.
163. Julius S. *Schweiz Med Wochensctr* 1976;106:1698–1705.
164. Julius S. *Am J Cardiol* 1991;67:3B–7B.
165. Parker FC, Croft JB, Cresanta JL, et al. *Am Heart J* 1987;113:1174–1179.
166. Timio M, Verdecchia P, Ronconi M, et al. *J Hypertens* 1985;3[Suppl 3]:S387–S388.
167. Koolen MI, van Brummelen P. *Hypertension* 1984;6:820–825.
168. Safar ME, Weiss YA, London GM, et al. *Postgrad Med J* 1977;3:35–39.
169. Dustan HP, Tarazi RC. *Annu Rev Med* 1978;29:485–493.
170. Brod J. *Contrib Nephrol* 1981;25:36–43.
171. Julius S, Pascual AV, Reilly K, et al. *Arch Int Med* 1971;127:116–119.
172. Dustan HP, Tarazi RC, Bravo EL. *Am J Med* 1972;52:610–622.
173. Tarazi RC. *Circ Res* 1976;38[Suppl II]:II-73–II-83.
174. Bing RF, Smith AJ. *Clin Sci* 1981;61:287–293.
175. Ulrych M, Hofman J, Hejl Z. *Am Heart J* 1964;68:193–203.
176. London GM, Safar ME, Simon AC, et al. *Circulation* 1978;57:995–1000.
177. Safar ME, London GM, Levenson JA, et al. *Hypertension* 1979;1:615–623.
178. Ulrych M. *Angiology* 1979;30:104–116.
179. Safar ME, London GM. *Hypertension* 1987;10:133–139.
180. Safar ME, London GM. *Clin Sci* 1985;69:497–504.
181. Takeshita A, Imaizumi T, Ashihara T, et al. *Circ Res* 1982;50:671–677.
182. Widgren BR, Berglund G, Wikstrand J, et al. *J Hypertens* 1992;10:459–465.
183. Folkow B. *Hypertension* 1990;16:89–101.
184. Yamori Y, Mori C, Nishio T, et al. *Am J Cardiol* 1979;44:964–969.
185. Lundin SA, Hallbäck-Nordlander M. *Cardiovasc Res* 1980;14:561–567.
186. Culpepper WS III, Sodt PC, Messerli FH, et al. *Ann Int Med* 1983;98:1–7.
187. Lund-Johansen P. In: Doyle AE, ed. *Handbook of hypertension,* vol 5: *Clinical pharmacology of antihypertensive drugs.* Amsterdam: Elsevier, 1988;41–72.
188. Lund-Johansen P. *Med Clin N Am* 1987;71:947–957.
189. Omvik P, Lund-Johansen P. *Cardiovasc Drugs Ther* 1993;7:193–206.
190. Lund-Johansen P. *Eur Heart J* 1983;4[Suppl D]:1–12.
191. van Hooft IMS, Grobbee DE, Waal-Manning HJ, Hofman A. *Circulation* 1993;87:1100–1106.
192. The Fifth Report of the Joint National Committee on Detection, Evaluation, and Treatment of High Blood Pressure (JNC V). *Arch Intern Med* 1993;153:154–208.
193. Weber MA, Laragh JH. Hypertension: Steps forward and steps backward (The Fifth Report of the Joint National Committee). *Arch Intern Med* 1993;153:149–152.

Hypertension: Pathophysiology, Diagnosis, and Management, Second Edition,
edited by J.H. Laragh and B.M. Brenner,
Raven Press, Ltd., New York © 1995.

CHAPTER **21**

Evaluation of Arterial Wave Forms in Hypertension and Normotension

Raymond P. Kelly and Michael F. O'Rourke

HISTORY

Use of the arterial pulse in the clinical evaluation of disease states has a long history dating back to antiquity. Examination of the arterial pulse is recorded by historians as being an essential part of ancient Chinese, Indian, and Greek medicine (1). Palpation of the pulse, however, was very much a part of the "art" of medicine with a bewildering array of terminologies being passed down by oral tradition, and in the voluminous Galenic tomes. The first accurate recording of the arterial pulse in man was performed by Etienne Jules Marey (2) last century. Marey developed a series of mechanical devices used to record the radial pulse in humans for physiological and clinical studies (Fig. 1). Marey was a physician with an interest in recording movement graphically, and by rapid-sequence photography. His device for the recording the peripheral arterial pulse, the *sphygmogram,* was soon taken up by leading clinicians of the day, particularly in England. Articles written by Mahomed (3), Broadbent (4), and Mackenzie (5) document the importance which these clinicians placed on the contour of the arterial pressure wave recorded by sphygmography as a

means for diagnosing clinical hypertension. Following the work by Bright (6) on the effects of renal disease on arterial pressure, cardiac hypertrophy, and stroke, interest developed in detecting the onset of hypertension in asymptomatic individuals before the development of target organ damage. The principal means of doing this in the late nineteenth century was using a variety of types of sphygmographs to record the arterial pulse in a wide range of asymptomatic individuals. Hence, for the first time the range of contours of the human arterial pulse was recorded and interpreted. Mahomed sought to quantify and illustrate the "hardness of the pulse" which had been emphasized by Bright. Mahomed described essential hypertension (interpreting it as the "pre-albuminuric stage of Bright's disease") in 1874 (7), and documented the course of hypertension on the basis of his recordings and interpretation of the peripheral arterial pulse (Fig. 2).

> These persons appear to pass on through life pretty much as others do and generally do not suffer from their high blood pressure except in their petty ailments upon which it imprints itself. . . . as age advances the enemy gains accession of strength . . . the individual has now passed forty years, perhaps fifty years of age, his lungs begin to degenerate, he has a cough in the Winter time, *but by his pulse you will know him. . . .* Alternatively, headache, vertigo, epistaxis, a passing paralysis, a more severe apoplectic seizure, and then the final blow.

In discussing the etiology of hypertension and its relationship to renal disease, Mahomed wrote:

R. P. Kelly: Cardiology Department, St Vincent's Hospital, New South Wales 2010, Australia.

M. F. O'Rourke: Medical Professorial Unit, University of New South Wales, St Vincent's Hospital, New South Wales 2010, Australia.

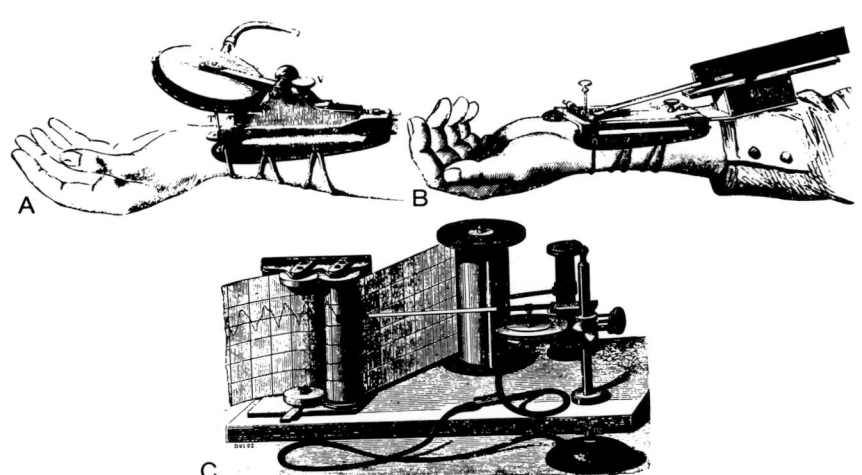

FIG. 1. Sphygmograms developed by E Marey. **A.** Air-filled system with base plate overlying artery connected to transducer. **B.** Mechanical sphygmogram without air-filled tubing which writes directly onto smoked paper, moved by a clockwork mechanism. **C:** Kymograph with cup-shaped sensor in foreground. (From ref. 86, with permission.)

What has been the cause in one case may be the result in another; thus general disorder may cause high arterial pressure and this in turn kidney changes; while on the other hand kidney changes may be primary and acute, they may in their turn produce impurity of blood and this general pressure. But whether we read the tale backward or forward, it is the same tale in the end.

All of this brilliant clinic work was done with the aid of the sphygmogram, and through interpretation of pulse tracings—and decades before introduction of the sphygmomanometer cuff. It is of historical interest that at the time of the first diagnosis of hypertension based on arterial pressure wave forms, the role of the kidney in its etiology was discussed much as we still do today. The points raised by Mahomed regarding the kidneys in the pathogenesis of essential hypertension are still addressed today (8).

Although the role of the kidneys in essential hypertension continues to be debated, a more consensual approach to the treatment of hypertension has been reached. This view is based entirely on sphygmomanometric measurement of systolic and diastolic pressure. The view initially emphasized diastolic brachial sphygmomanometric pressure in diagnosis and as a goal of treatment, but the equal importance of systolic arterial pressure as a risk for target organ damage is now more fully appreciated (9,10). Consideration of reversal of target organ damage influences the choice of drug therapy for hypertension. The effects of various pharmacologic agents on left ventricular hypertrophy (11,12), renal function (especially diabetic proteinuria) (13), properties of large arteries (14,15), and on coexistent risk factors (16), are important factors in deciding appropriate treatment of hypertension. This current situation was foretold by Mahomed as quoted above. Our treatment approach to hypertension a century after Mahomed's writings is dictated by the target organ damage described by Gull and Sutton (1) and alluded to by Mahomed. As will be discussed later, the contour of the arterial pulse

in normotension and hypertension provides important information regarding the pathogenesis of hypertension and its response to treatment.

By the turn of the century, examination of the peripheral pulse using the sphygmogram was a refined clinical procedure, and various types of pulses were recorded and

3. *On the sphygmographic evidence of arterio-capillary fibrosis.*

By F. A. MAHOMED, M.D.

FIGS. 5 and 6 are tracings obtained from a male, aged about 35, and a female, æt. 45; they illustrate a form of pulse frequently met with in apparently healthy persons, but who, not uncommonly, are subjects of the gouty diathesis, dyspeptics,

WOODCUT 5.

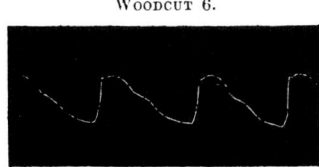

alcoholists, or who possess one or other of the predisposing causes to chronic Bright's disease. They do not, however, present any other symptoms; their urine is normal, and the character of the pulse alone affords an indication of their condition. The pulse presents the signs usually recognised as those of high tension; the most

WOODCUT 6.

FIG. 2. Reproduction of the first page of an 1877 article illustrating the radial artery pressure wave form in two relatively young patients with what would now be regarded as essential hypertension. Pressure waves show a secondary or "tidal" wave in late systole whose amplitude is close to or greater than the initial peak (or percussion wave), and absent or small diastolic wave. (From ref. 7, with permission.)

classified. Three major textbooks were written during this period, all of which gave prominence to the interpretation of the recorded peripheral arterial pulse in clinical evaluation. The first was written by Marey himself in 1881 (2), the second was written by Broadbent in 1890, encompassing much of what Mahomed had published before his untimely death (4), and the third by Sir James Mackenzie in 1902 (5). This last book described Mackenzie's experience with the sphygmograph which represented recordings from a large number of patients seen frequently over long periods of time in Mackenzie's general practice. Mackenzie subsequently utilized this data on human pulse wave forms in normal aging and in patients with hypertension as part of his consultant physician practice in London. Both Broadbent and Mackenzie were among the most prominent physicians in London at the turn of the century. Their books, which record the contour of the human arterial pulse in hypertension and normotension, over a wide variety of ages, and in different disease states, provided the first objective graphic recording used to supplement the clinical examination in evaluation of patients. At this time neither the electrocardiogram nor X-ray nor sphygmomanometer had been introduced into clinical practice. The sphygmograph represented the standard investigative procedure in assessing not only disease states but the response to therapy. Indeed, the first description of the favorable effects of nitroglycerine in angina pectoris by Murrell (17) included sphygmomanographic tracings of the radial pulse before and after drug administration (Fig. 3). It is of interest that recordings of arterial wave forms following administration of nitroglycerine are still today providing us with insights into the mechanisms of action and therapeutic applications of this drug (1,14).

Introduction of the sphygmograph into clinical practice marked an important advance in clinical medicine. It provided for the first time objective recordings of pulse contour in disease states and following treatment. It heralded the dramatic advances made in the twentieth century in supplementing clinical patient assessment with objectively recorded data. There were, however, limitations to the accuracy of the sphygmograph. Most sphygmographs were quite cumbersome devices (see Fig. 1), dependent on a system of levers to transform the diameter fluctuations of the peripheral radial artery into a recorded wave form. They were quite dependent on the skill of the operator using the instrument. The sphygmomanometer, introduced at this time following the work of Riva-Rocci (1896) and Korotkov (1905), was much simpler to use and allowed the clinician to base diagnosis and treatment on two numbers, the systolic and diastolic pressures, rather than requiring the rigors of wave form interpretation. Thus the sphygmomanometer was rapidly introduced into clinical practice, coming to replace the sphygmogram and wave form interpretation as part of the evaluation of hypertension. This reliance on the

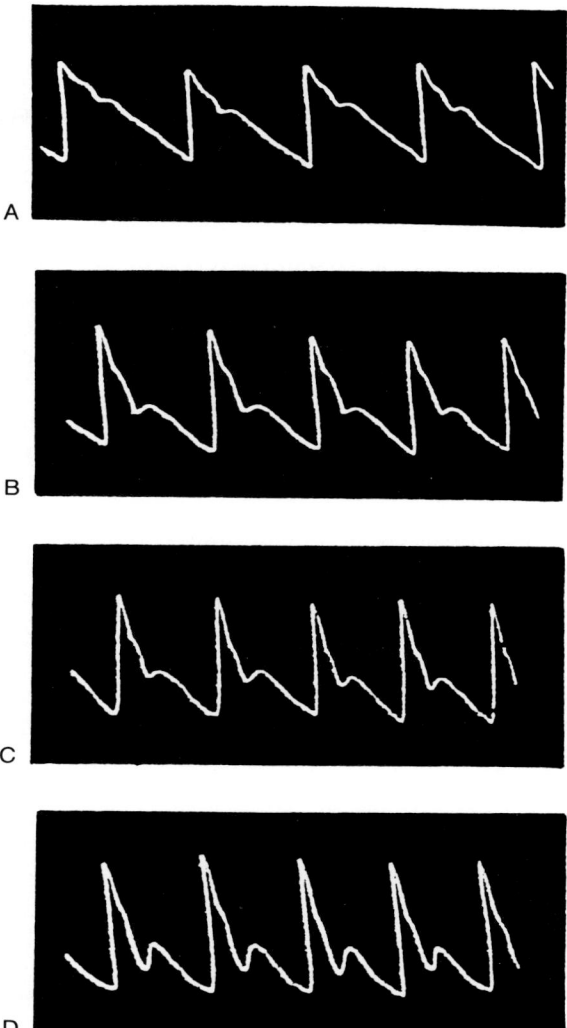

FIG. 3. Radial artery sphygmograph published by Murrell and showing in detail the effects of nitroglycerine as causing progressive reduction in the last systolic shoulder of the pulse. **A:** Before dose; **B:** 2 minutes after dose; **C:** 8 minutes after dose; **D:** 9 minutes after dose. (From ref. 17, with permission.)

maximum and minimum values of arterial pressure, with the abandonment of interpretation within these two limits, occurred just at the time when the interpretation of electrocardiographic wave forms as an important part of clinical assessment was increasing in popularity.

In the early twentieth century, major advances were made in the study of arterial hemodynamics in research physiology laboratories through the development of accurate optical manometers by Otto Frank in Germany (18). Frank's basic studies on the heart formed the foundation of Starling's description of the *Law of the Heart* in 1914. Frank (18,36) recorded the arterial pulse in different arteries of experimental animals under different conditions and produced a theory for the interpretation of pressure wave contour. Frank interpreted the pressure wave form as having a basic filling and emptying curve or "Grundform" upon which was superimposed the effects of wave "reflections" from peripheral beds. Frank also described the means by which the arterial pressure pulse could be described in the frequency domain by a Fourier series of harmonics. Frank's work on the pressure pulse contour was continued by Carl Wiggers, who had traveled to Germany from the United States to gain experience in Frank's laboratory. Wiggers (19) recorded the pulse directly in experimental animals and also performed indirect recordings from the peripheral arteries in man. His findings were later extended by Hamilton and colleagues (20,21), who further emphasized the change in pressure pulse contour as a result of its transmission from the aorta to peripheral sites. These accurate manometers introduced by Wiggers, together with the introduction of venous and arterial catheterization, allowed pressure waves in human subjects to be recorded with great accuracy. However, the recording of these wave forms remained in the realm of physiologic research. Further technical developments resulted in the introduction of diagnostic cardiac catheterization in man in 1944 and the golden era of cardiac hemodynamics, as well as coronary arteriography.

Despite these advances, the application of arterial pressure wave analysis to clinical hypertension languished until the 1980s. The development of the electromagnetic flow meter for the registration of blood flow both by a cuff applied to an exposed vessel, or through a catheter inserted through a peripheral vessel, had allowed recordings of arterial impedance to be made in normotensive and hypertensive states (22–25). Impedance measurement remains largely a research procedure, and has not been utilized in the routine clinical evaluation of patients with hypertension, but it has provided a sound physiologic basis on which the pulse may be interpreted. Landmark recordings were made in the cardiac catheter laboratory by Murgo et al. in 1980 (26) and Takazawa et al. in 1985 (27). These studies were able to provide a detailed interpretation of the ascending aortic pressure wave in individuals at varying ages and levels of blood pressure, drawing upon impedance measurement to give a lucid explanation for the variety of contours found. Such studies have led to a reawakening of interest in pressure wave contour analysis in essential hypertension (1). Until this recent reemergence of interest in wave contours, pressure data obtained invasively, either in the cardiac catheter laboratory or from intraarterial monitoring lines, was still largely interpreted in terms of the systolic and diastolic pressures between which the pressure wave fluctuated. Oftentimes, intraarterial wave forms are extensively filtered and smoothed to produce a wave form on a bedside monitor which is given little attention or interpretation apart from its maximum and minimum numerical values.

There have, however, been some instances during this century where the pressure wave contour has been utilized in the clinical evaluation of patients. Both Framingham (28) and Japanese (29) epidemiological studies have employed pressure contour analysis. In the Framingham Study, plethysmographic volume wave forms were recorded noninvasively, using a cuff placed around the finger. In this study in over 1,000 individuals, the investigators focused their attention on the diastolic wave following the dicrotic notch. They showed that with increasing age there was a decreasing prevalence of the diastolic wave with a less clearly defined dicrotic notch than seen in youth (Fig. 4). This finding has been confirmed by more recent invasive data (26) and explained by alteration in timing of reflected waves due to vascular stiffening, as detailed in the following section. In addition to an age relationship, the investigators also noted a correlation between wave contour and the clinical incidence of coronary heart disease. We now know that the aging changes in the arterial waveform are due to the degenerative effects of arteriosclerosis. Widespread arterial degeneration in the Western world is, of course, associated with obstructive coronary disease, although the use of peripheral wave forms in predicting the severity of coronary artery disease has limited application. Recent studies by Japanese researchers (30) have rediscovered that patients with obstructive coronary disease and myocardial infarction indeed have evidence of widespread

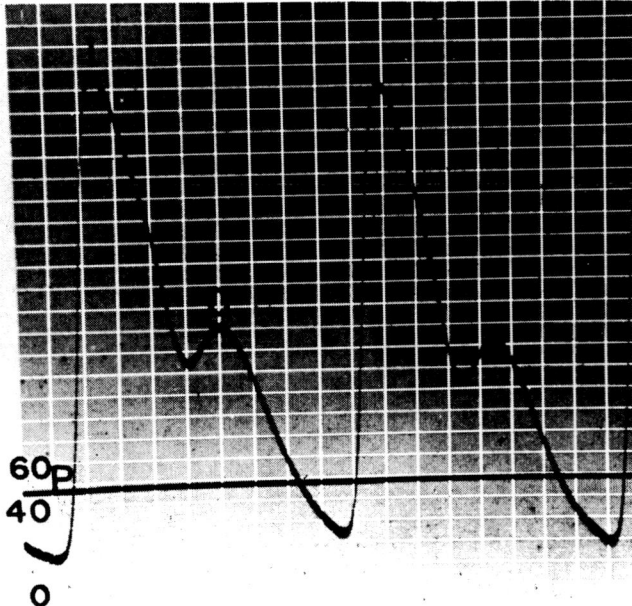

FIG. 4. Normal arterial pulse waves recorded from the third digit of a healthy 25-year old man. The vertical lines are time signals 0.1 second apart and the horizontal lines represent pressure increments of 10 mm Hg in the cuff applied about the finger. The cuff pressure (*P*) is recorded simultaneously but independently of the components of the pulse wave. Note initial wave (*I*) and well-defined dicrotic wave (*D*). (From ref. 87, with permission.)

vascular degeneration and arterial stiffening. Japanese epidemiologic studies have looked at analysis of wave forms also derived from a finger plethysmogram. In these studies (29), the second derivative of such wave forms has been used to highlight fluctuations in the pressure wave and quantify them. They have shown that features of the peripheral wave contour are strongly indicative of the degree of vascular degeneration associated with age. They have also shown that these fluctuations can be altered by pharmacologic intervention with angiotensin or nitroglycerine administration.

The modern interpretation of wave form changes associated with aging and arterial degeneration associated with hypertension, diabetes, and atherosclerotic disease draws heavily upon the findings of measurements of vascular impedance performed in the middle of this century following the development of accurate instruments to record simultaneous pressure and flow wave contours. We now interpret these wave forms based both on large vessel compliance and also the timing and intensity of wave reflection from peripheral beds (31–33). Such interpretations extend the earlier work of Frank, Wiggers, and Hamilton. They have also a solid foundation in studies which show the relationship between precise measures of vascular impedance in the frequency domain and wave contour analysis in the time domain (see Fig. 5).

Throughout the history of assessment of arterial pressure wave forms in interpreting cardiovascular function, it has often been assumed that the pressure recorded at any one site in the vasculature represents the pressure throughout the rest of the arterial tree. However, there are clearly differences in pressure at different parts of the arterial tree recorded in any individual at any particular time (1,34,35). This difference in pressure wave contour was a feature noticed in the earliest studies of hemodynamics, particularly those performed by Wiggers (19) (see Fig. 6) and Hamilton (29). The fact that the arterial pressure wave changes as it travels along the arterial tree from the heart to the periphery has important implications in terms of the way we model the arterial system and the assumptions which we make in clinical practice. The arterial tree has often been described as a *Windkessel* with respect to its elastic properties (36). However the limitation of the Windkessel model is that it assumes that the response to injection of a volume into the arterial tree is the same and occurs simultaneously in all parts of the vasculature. The Windkessel model fails to take into account the effects of linear transmission of arterial wave forms along the vasculature and cannot explain differences in pressure amplitude or wave contour in different arteries. Measurements of vascular impedance in the middle of the twentieth century gave clear explanations for the change in both pressure and flow wave contours based on the physical properties of the systemic vasculature. Such findings have important clinical implications. The most important and relevant is that we cannot assume that pressure recorded at the brachial site by sphygmomanometry represents the pressure at the aortic root with which the heart interacts. These concepts are pursued in detail later in this chapter. Use of peripherally recorded wave forms to enhance our evaluation and treatment in hypertension has come full circle in recent years with the development of a "transfer function" to allow prediction of the ascending aortic root pressure contour from a wave form recorded at a peripheral site (37). There are several groups around the world who are now utilizing such technology to enhance the brachial sphygmomanometric measurement of arterial pressure so as to fully utilize the information contained in the pressure wave form as it fluctuates between its maximum and minimum values. We are now at the stage where quantitative assessment of pressure by cuff sphygmomanometer can be combined with precise evaluation of pressure wave contour as was used by physicians over 100 years ago when hypertension was first diagnosed and treated.

PRESSURE FLOW RELATIONSHIPS IN THE ASCENDING AORTA AND IN PERIPHERAL ARTERIES

The arterial pulse is generated by flow input from the heart into the system vasculature (1,38). The function of the systemic circulation is to provide adequate perfusion to vital organs in order to supply nutrients to, and remove waste products from, body tissues. At the organ level, these functions are achieved through continuous, nonpulsatile flow through a large capillary network. The energy for such flow is imparted to the circulation by the contraction of the left ventricle as it ejects blood at high velocity into the ascending aorta. Blood is distributed from the ascending aorta to the capillary bed by the branching arterial tree and arteriolar beds. In addition to this distributive function, the arteries and arterioles have a second important function, which is to cushion the large flow fluctuations that result from intermittent ventricular ejection and to smooth it so that capillary flow is continuous and hence most efficient (33,39,40). Arterial pulsation occurs as a result of this intermittent cardiac contraction. The shape of the arterial pulse is determined by both the pattern of ventricular contraction and the properties of the arterial system and arterioles (1,38). More specifically, when arterial pressure is measured at any particular site in the body, its contour is the result of the pattern of flow input into the system from the cardiac source and both the local properties of the arteries at the recording site, together with the influence of transmission properties of the branching systemic vasculature throughout the body. In other words, the arterial system is not a simple elastic chamber within which events occur simultaneously at all sites in response to flow input from the heart. The Windkessel model of the circulation helps describe the simple elastic properties of the arterial system but cannot explain the details of the contour of the human arterial pulse. This simple elastic chamber model fails to account for the spatially distributed, complex branching nature of the human arterial tree (41,42). The most obvious consequence of the complex spatial distribution of the systemic vasculature interposed between the heart and the peripheral organs is the fact that the arterial pressure pulse recorded at any site in the body has secondary fluctuations (see Figs. 2–6) despite the fact that the heart beats only once every cardiac cycle. These secondary fluctuations are due to wave travel and reflection within the arterial tree. The pressure pulse contour changes as one progresses from the aortic root to the peripheral parts of the circulation, because of effects of finite linear wave travel velocity [as first described by Thomas Young (43)] and the superimposed effects of wave reflection. We will now consider in more detail the pressure flow relationships in the ascending aorta and the way these are altered by transmission through the sys-

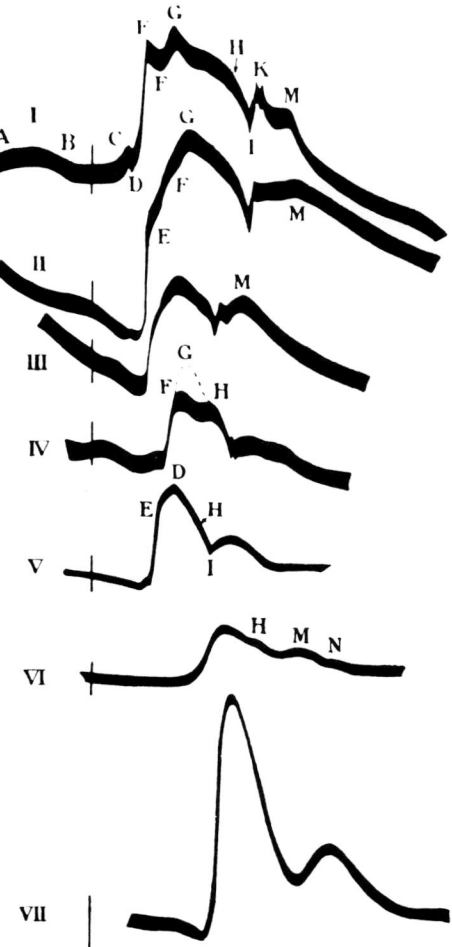

FIG. 6. Pressure waves recorded noninvasively in human subjects: Subclavian pulses (*I and II*); carotid pulses (*III and IV*); brachial pulse (*V*); radial pulse (*VI*); femoral pulse (*VII*). (From ref. 19, with permission.)

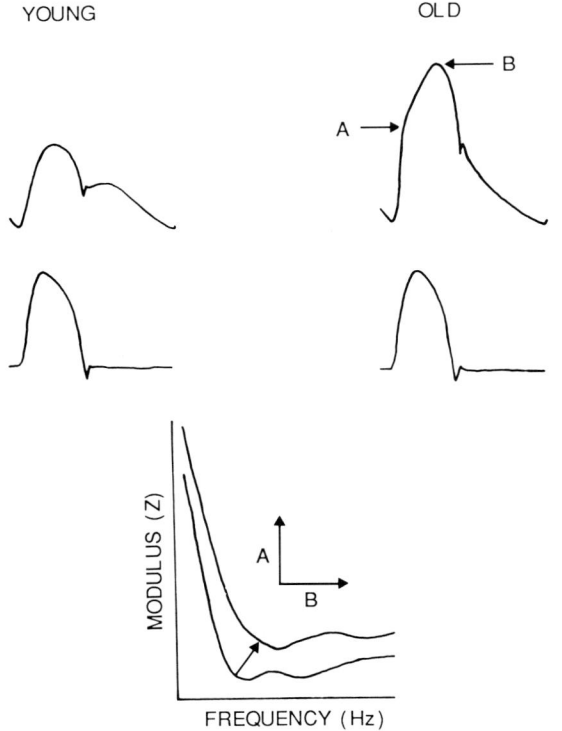

FIG. 5. Below: Impedance modulus plotted against frequency under normal conditions (*lower curve*) and in hypertension (*upper curve*). Above: The pressure wave resynthesized from impedance curves using the same ventricular ejection flow wave (*center*). Changes in impedance and in pressure waves are attributable to (1) increased peripheral resistance leading to increased mean pressure, (2) increased aortic stiffness leading directly to increased characteristic impedance and to the first shoulder on the pressure wave and (3) early wave reflection causing rightward shift of the impedance curve and to the late systolic peak of pressure. (From ref. 57, with permission.)

temic vasculature under normotensive conditions and in hypertension.

In the ascending aorta, once left ventricular pressure rises above aortic diastolic pressure, the aortic valve opens and an arterial pressure pulse is generated by flow from the heart into the aortic root. In the early part of systolic ejection, the aortic pressure is created by the interaction of ventricular flow and the local elastic properties of the ascending aorta. Beyond the initial part of systolic ejection, secondary influences determine the shape of the aortic pulse, in addition to the local elastic properties of the ascending aorta. These influences include the effects of wave reflection from the peripheral arterial beds. Thus, to understand the determinants of the arterial pulse and particularly its secondary fluctuations, it is necessary to be clear about the timing of events in the systemic circulation.

When the left ventricle contracts, it ejects blood into the aorta at a speed which rises quickly to a peak of ap-

| MAN | SHEEP | DOG | RABBIT | GUINEA PIG |

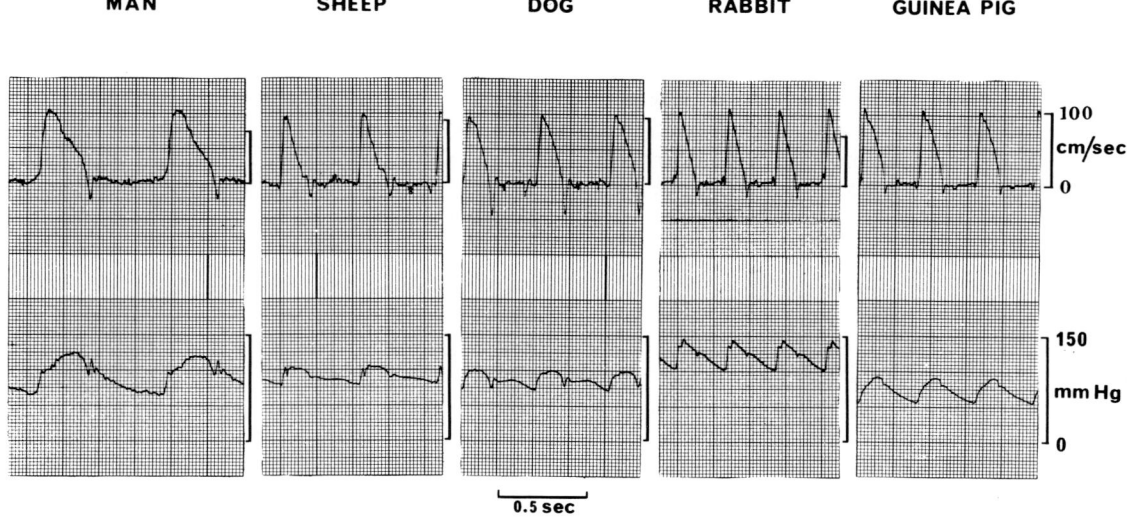

FIG. 7. Flow (*above*) and pressure (*below*) waves in the ascending aorta of five different mammals. Flow calibration (100 cm/sec in each case) is different for each animal. Pressure calibration (0–150 mm Hg) and time scale are the same for all. (From ref. 33, with permission.)

proximately 80–120 cm/sec, some 80 msec after the opening of the aortic valve. After a rapid rise to this peak, aortic flow velocity falls more slowly in the latter part of systole back to zero at the time of aortic valve closure. After a small amount of backflow as the aortic valve shuts, there is no flow into the ascending aorta throughout diastole. The pattern of ventricular ejection and the resulting flow velocity profile recorded in the ascending aorta is remarkably similar in man and in all large animal species that have been studied (Fig. 7). There is some difference in duration of systole between animals in that larger animals tend to have a slower heart rate and a longer systolic ejection period, but the flow velocity contour and maximum velocity of flow are virtually identical in all animal species under normal conditions (44–46). Ejection of blood into the aorta dilates the aorta and

generates a pressure wave in the aortic root. The energy so transmitted to the systemic vasculature generates a pulse wave, the effects of which may be measured at any particular site by the detection of blood flow or the resultant pressure wave created by the interaction of flow and properties of the arterial wall. This impulse of energy is transmitted quickly along the systemic vasculature, along the walls of the arteries and arterioles. The speed at which the pulse travels down the arterial tree varies with age (Fig. 8), but is in the order of 5–12 m/sec (47–50). This figure is crucial to our understanding of the contour of the arterial pulse. It is much faster than the local velocity of flow of red blood cells recorded in the ascending aorta or at any other sites. It is also very fast with respect to the length of the arterial tree. Given that the average human height is <2 meters, it is clear that the pulse can

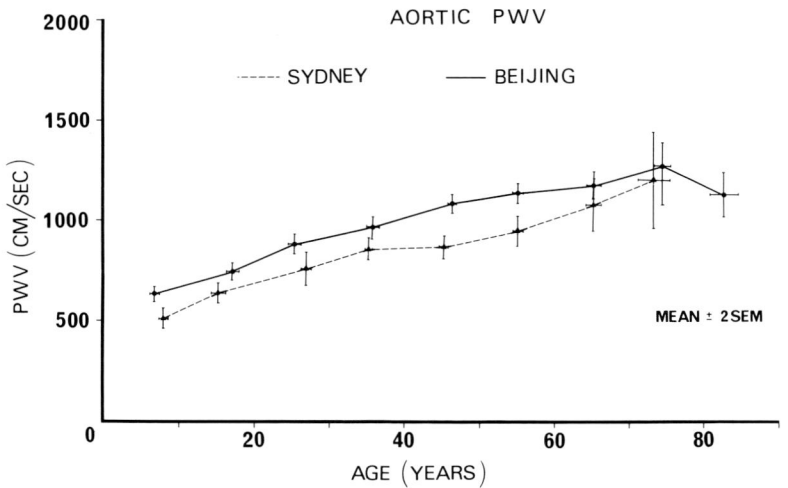

FIG. 8. Comparison of age-related changes in pulse wave velocity measured in normal subjects of Beijing (O ------- O), Sydney (Δ ——— Δ), and Guangzhou (O – – – – O). After the first decade, pulse wave velocity of rural Guangzhou subjects is significantly lower than that of Beijing and Sydney subjects. Serum cholesterol levels were similar in Beijing and Guangzhou subjects. Urinary sodium excretion, however, was significantly higher in Beijing subjects. Pulse wave velocities in Sydney subjects were similar to those measured in subjects with high and low serum cholesterol levels. These data indicate that arterial pulse wave velocity (and stiffness) increases with age and that sodium (not cholesterol) influences an increase in pulse wave velocity at a given age.

be transmitted to the periphery and return well within the duration of one cardiac cycle (0.8–1.0 sec). The pressure wave contour at any particular site is a composite of a forward-traveling "incident" wave and a wave which is the net result of peripheral wave reflections (1,41, 42,46). The pressure wave can indeed be decomposed into forward-traveling and backward-traveling components (46).

The contour of the ascending aortic pressure and flow waves in humans has been systematically studied by Murgo et al. (26). Normal subjects of a wide variety of ages were studied at cardiac catheterization, and aortic pressure flow relationships were determined both in the time domain as wave forms and in the frequency domain as impedance. Three different patterns of ascending aortic pressure were described (Fig. 9). In the first, designated type A, the pressure wave rose from its diastolic level to a systolic shoulder and then further to a late systolic peak. The second type of pressure wave, designated type C, was characterized by a pressure wave which rose from diastole to an early systolic peak with no late systolic rise, but rather a slight decline in pressure throughout systolic ejection to the incisura, which was followed by a prominent diastolic wave. The third pattern, designated type B, was intermediate between types A and C. Pattern A was so-called because it was most commonly seen in adult subjects, while C was the pattern found in subjects in their late teenage years or early twenties.

These three types of pressure waves relate to the patterns of flow which have been described in the central part of the vasculature from recordings of brachiocephalic flow in humans (51). Brachiocephalic flow can be classified into three basic forms, again dependent on the patient's age (Fig. 10). Both the aortic pressure and brachiocephalic flow wave patterns are explicable on the basis of simultaneous impedance measurements. These latter data provide evidence for altered timing and intensity of wave reflection as humans age and their vasculature becomes stiffer and less compliant. The type A pressure wave (as described by Murgo [26]) corresponds to the Type I flow wave (as described by Mills [51]) (Fig. 11); both occur in older subjects and have their contour influenced by reflections from peripheral beds returning to the central part of the vasculature in late systole (Fig. 12). The influence of wave reflections was further demonstrated by Murgo, who also reported the effect of the Valsalva maneuver on the aortic pressure and flow contours (Fig. 13). These studies and others have demonstrated that, as humans age, degenerative changes in the systemic vasculature result not only in a mild elevation in peripheral vascular resistance, but also in a stiffening of the arterial bed upstream from the arterioles with an earlier return of wave reflection. This accounts for the disappearance of the diastolic wave following the incisura and the increase in the late systolic wave. This increase in late systolic wave accounts not only for a rise in systolic pressure with age (which in its extreme form produces isolated systolic hypertension) (52,53), but also

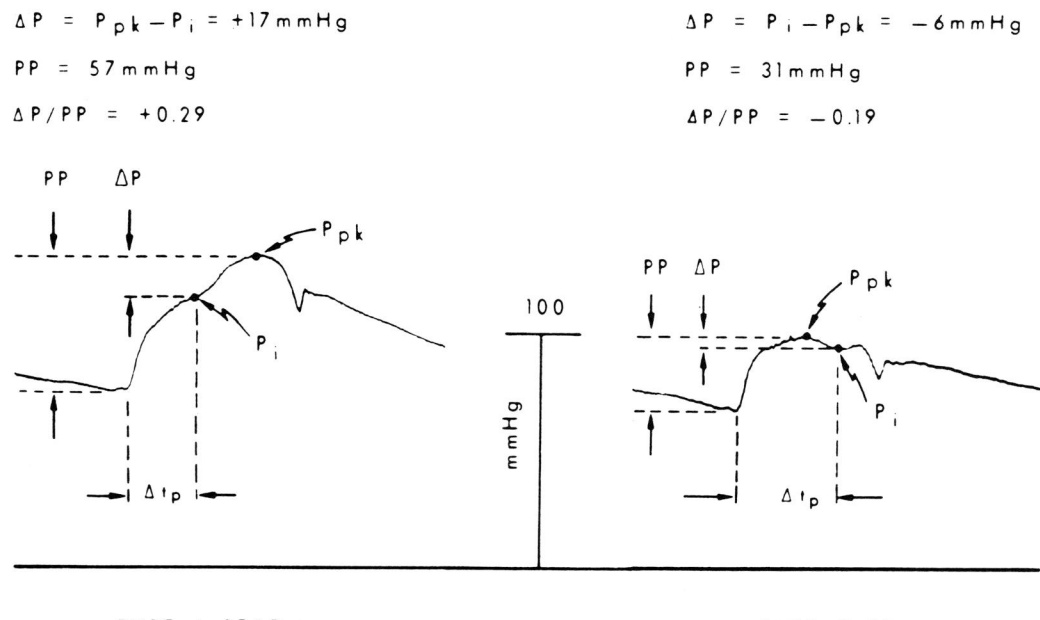

FIG. 9. Pressure wave form classification and an example of how the two different wave forms were evaluated. P1, inflection point; Ppk, peak pressure. P = Ppk − P1. PP, total pulse pressure; Δ to change in time.

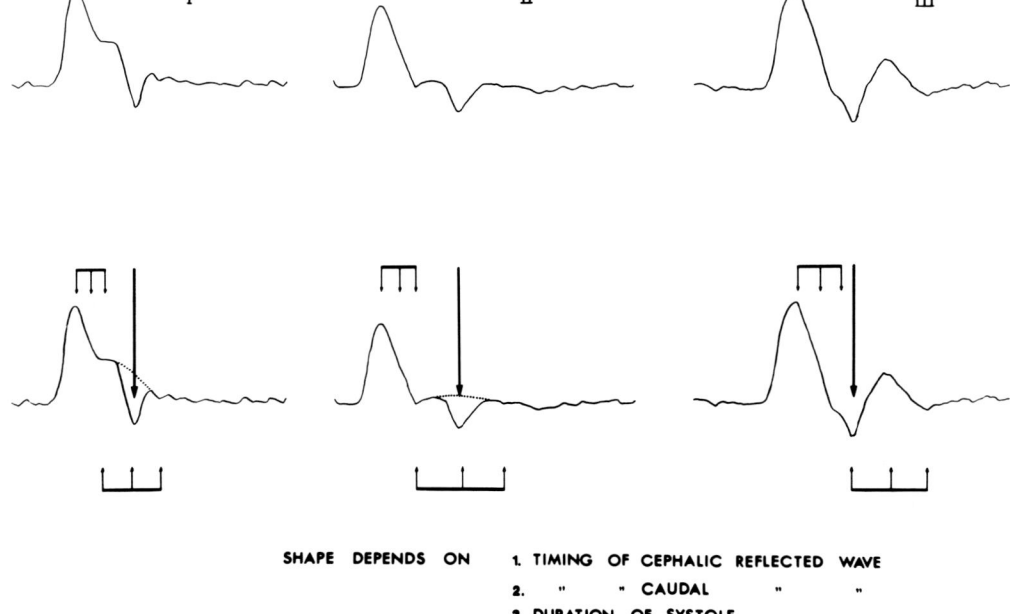

SHAPE DEPENDS ON
1. TIMING OF CEPHALIC REFLECTED WAVE
2. " " CAUDAL " "
3. DURATION OF SYSTOLE

FIG. 10. Flow waves recorded in the brachiocephalic artery of an older (*left*), intermediate (*center*) and young (*right*) human. These waves are explained (*below*) on the basis of earliest wave reflection from the upper body (*arrows above*) decelerating flow, and later wave velocity from the lower body (*arrows below*) accelerating flow into the brachiocephalic artery. The incisura is caused by aortic valve closure (*single arrow and dotted line*). The difference between young (*right*) and older (*left*) pattern is explicable on the basis of earlier wave reflection from the lower body in the older subject. (From ref. 51, with permission.) O'Rourke, Avolio (88).

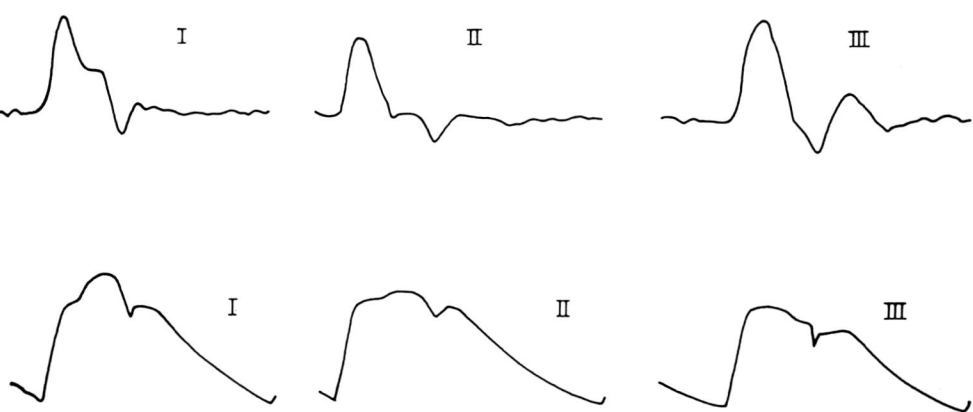

FIG. 11. Comparison of types I, II, and III brachiocephalic flow waves (*top*) with corresponding ascending aortic pressure waves (*bottom*). Explanations are identical. The different flow and pressure patterns are attributable to differences in timing of wave reflection from the lower parts of the body, with the reflected wave returning before aortic valve closure in type I (and A), during valve closure in type II (and B), and after valve closure in type III (and C). (From refs. 26, 33, and 51, with permission.)

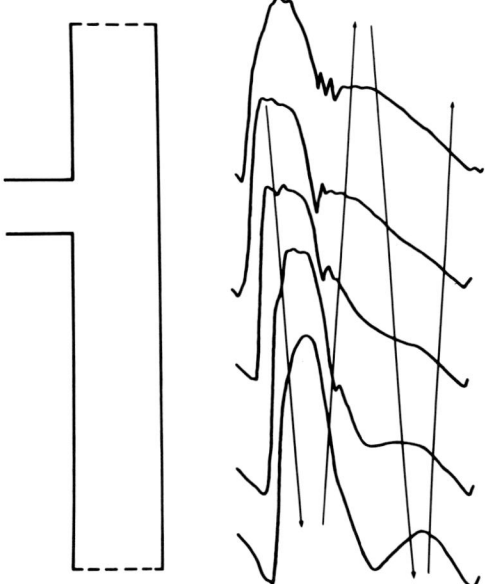

FIG. 12. The asymmetric T model of the systemic arterial system. Pressure waves in a dog (*left*) and in an old human subject with arterial degeneration and stiffened arteries (*right*) are recorded in the aortic arch (*top*), iliac artery (*below*), and intermediate points. A line is drawn parallel to the wave foot to indicate wave travel and reflection at arterial terminations in the lower and upper parts of the body. In both cases, wave contour in all arteries can be explained on the basis of reflection and rereflection of the initial impulse generated by ventricular ejection. Differences between the dog (left) and older human (right) are readily explained on the basis of more rapid wave travel in the human's stiffened arteries, with earlier return of wave reflection. (From ref. 89, with permission.)

means that the time of peak aortic and left ventricular pressure is shifted from early to late systole. Hence, peak pressure occurs in the aorta and the left ventricle at a time when ventricular volume is reaching its nadir just prior to closure of the aortic valve. This combination of peak pressure and minimal volume results in increased left ventricular wall stress, and has important implications for myocardial oxygen consumption and ventricular efficiency. These findings show that increased pulsatile load per se, independent of mean resistance, can influence left ventricular function. This has been confirmed in animal studies (54,55) and has important implications for the treatment of hypertension and regression of target organ damage.

Murgo's grouping of aortic pressure-flow relations in man into three discrete types has been confirmed and extended by Nichols et al. (39), who assembled data from different studies to demonstrate a continuum of changes in ascending aortic pressure wave contour and impedance with age and their implications for ventriculovascular interaction. Nichols showed that aging was as-

sociated with a progressive change in the ascending aortic pattern from C in young people through B to A in adults, but with little change in the ascending aortic flow pattern. The age-related changes in pressure and flow waves result in a pattern of impedance that produces greatest opposition to flow from the heart where flow components, expressed in the frequency domain, are maximal (Fig. 14). Hence, with human aging there is a "detuning" of the optimal ventriculo-vascular coupling which is found in children and in other mammalian species which do not attain the longevity of adult humans (39,40). As discussed below, hypertension accelerates the age-related degenerative changes found in normotensive humans and exacerbates the detuning of ventriculovascular coupling that occurs with age.

The contour of pressure and flow waves in the ascending aorta and central part of the vasculature differ from the contour of waves recorded in peripheral vessels. This was demonstrated by the classical investigations of Hamilton and Dow (20,21), Remington (34) and others (35,36). As shown in Fig. 15, the contour of the pressure and flow waves change dramatically as the pulse is transmitted from the central part of the vasculature to the periphery. The factors contributing to this change in contour, as originally put forward by Wiggers and later modified by McDonald (23) are: (a) the attenuation of the pressure wave during its travel from the aortic root to the peripheral site because of the viscoelastic properties of the arterial wall and the viscosity of the blood contained within; (b) dispersion of the pressure wave created by different velocities at which different frequency components of the wave traveled; (c) the effect of waves reflected from peripheral sites causing summation with the forward-propagating wave and so producing amplification of the pulse wave as it traveled from a central site to the periphery; (d) the occurrence of natural vibrations or "resonance" in various parts of the arterial tree; and (e) amplification of the pulse in peripheral arteries because of the greater stiffness of the arterial walls at peripheral sites compared to the properties of the proximal aorta.

To summarize, the pressure pulse contour increases in amplitude and changes in contour as it is transmitted to the periphery due to increasing stiffness of the arterial walls and the different timing of wave reflections at different sites. The flow wave contour is also strongly influenced by timing of wave reflections and also changes as volume is distributed to various organ beds along the route of transmission.

Knowledge of physiologic determinants of pressure wave contour has been greatly enhanced by studies assessing the effects of vasoactive drugs on pressure-flow relationships. Animal studies (22) have shown that altering mean arterial pressure produces dramatic changes in the central pressure pulse contour (Fig. 16). By increas-

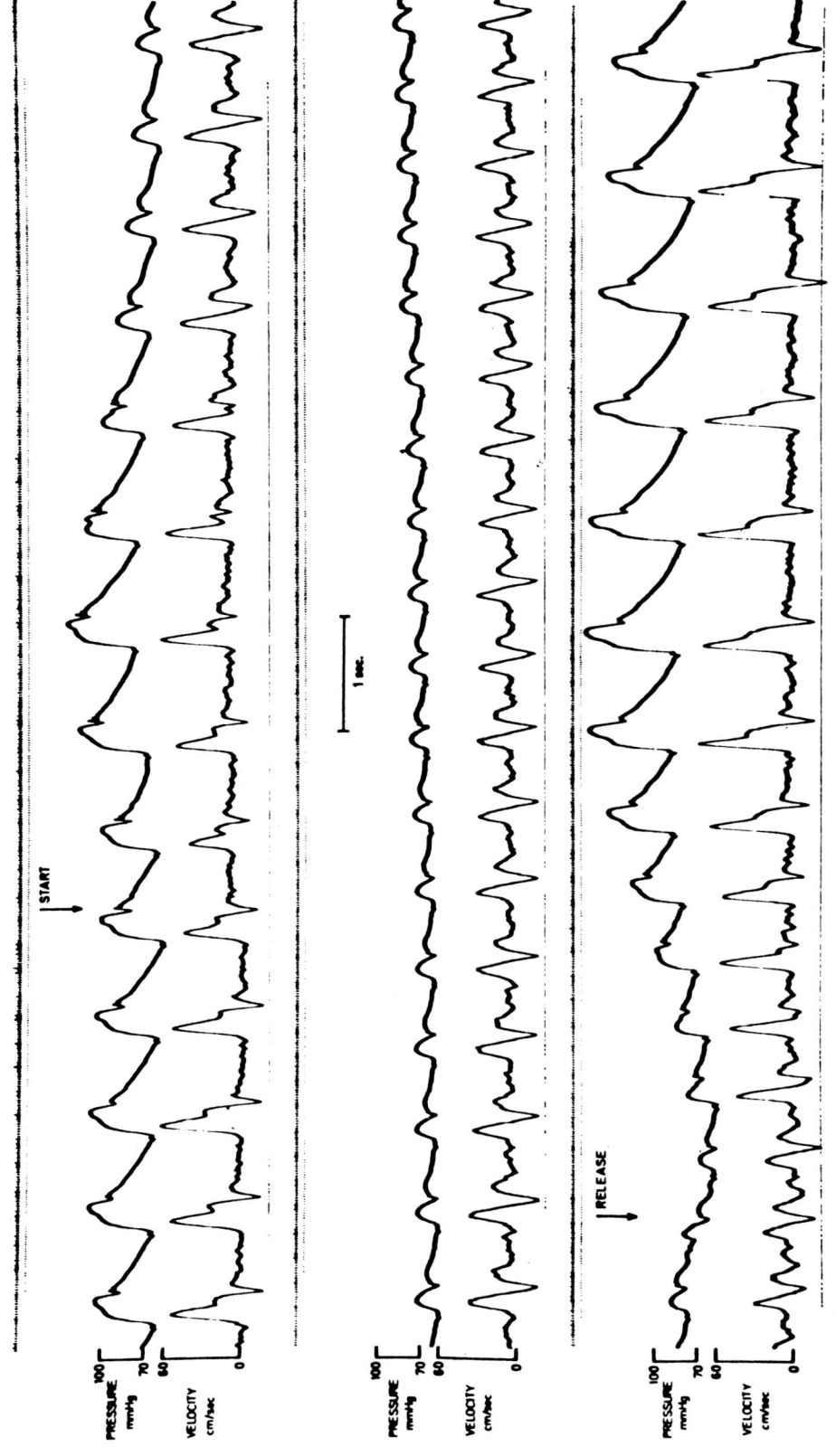

FIG. 13. Continuous recording of brachiocephalic pressure (above) and flow (below) in a human subject before, during and after Valsalva maneuver. (From ref. 51, with permission.)

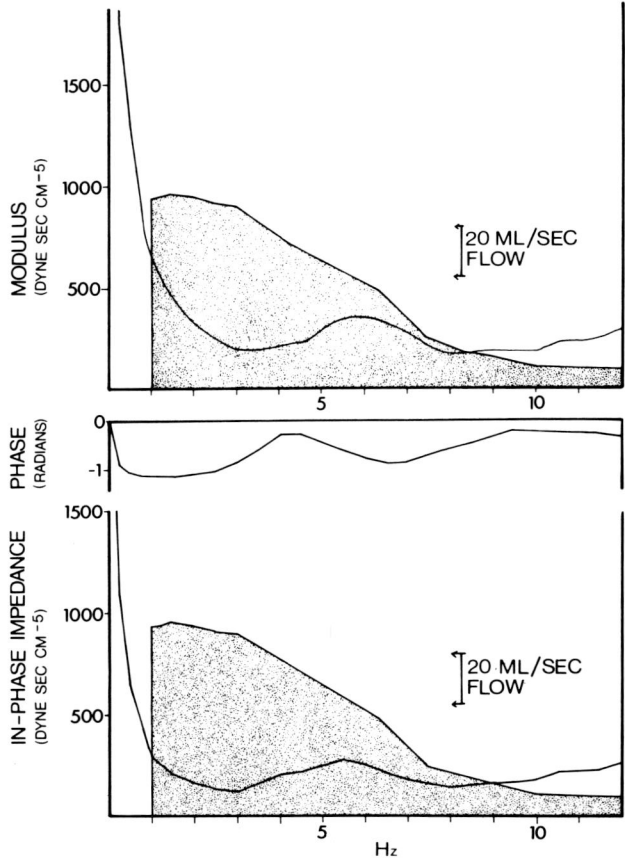

FIG. 14. Relationship between harmonic content of the left ventricular ejection wave (shaded area) and (above) modulus of ascending aortic impedance and (below) in-phase impedance in a dog. (From ref. 90, with permission.)

ing mean arterial pressure, epinephrine infusion changes the carotid artery pressure wave in rabbits from a wave similar to a human aortic type C wave to type A—one which has a prominent notch on the upstroke with a subsequent late systolic peak and loss of diastolic wave (Fig. 17). It is interesting to note that the pressure wave contours in all animal species generally show a "young" waveform by human standards (type C). Even studies performed in "aged" animals under control conditions are unable to reproduce the hemodynamic conditions found in adult humans with vascular degeneration; this appears to be a species-specific phenomenon and related to relative longevity in humans (Fig. 18). It is only by pharmacologically raising mean arterial pressure or artificially "stiffening" the aorta (54) in animals that human adult wave forms can be reproduced. Reduction in mean arterial pressure, for example by pilocarpine infusion, produces a carotid pressure wave which has an early peak, no notch on the upstroke, and a prominent diastolic wave. These effects of epinephrine and pilocarpine are interpreted in terms of the nonlinear elastic proper-

ties of the vasculature. As arteriolar tone is increased, mean pressure rises and more of the hydraulic load is taken up by the collagenous components of the arterial walls than can be accommodated by the elastin fibers. This "stiffening" of the arterial vasculature results in a faster pulse-transmission time and so earlier return of reflected waves from the arteriolar terminations. This "shifts" the effect of wave reflection from diastole into late systole, producing the "late-peaking" aortic pressure wave.

Such pharmacologically-induced changes in arterial pressure contour are not solely determined by mean arterial pressure. It is possible to dilate selectively a regional vascular bed and to reduce the intensity of reflection, while maintaining mean pressure in the systemic vasculature. Regional vascular dilation results in a change in pressure wave form which is explicable from simultaneous impedance measurements as being due to improved compliance and reduced wave reflection (20,21,24,25).

These animal studies show that aging effects in humans on the contour of the pulse can be reproduced in animals by producing hypertension. Indeed, subsequent studies in humans have shown that hypertension of any cause simulates the effects of aging on pulse contour (1,33,34–41,57–60) (Fig. 19). Compared to the effects of normal age-related arterial degeneration on the aortic pressure wave contour, hypertension results in (a) higher mean pressure; (b) a higher pressure shoulder or notch on its upstroke due to reduced aortic compliance; and (c) a more prominent late systolic peak due to increased wave reflections.

All these effects are the same as occur with aging, but they occur earlier, and to a greater extent in hypertensive subjects. Hypertension increases pulsatile arterial load (items [b] and [c] above), both directly through damage to the architecture of arterial walls and indirectly through elevation of mean arterial pressure (41,46). Elevation of mean pressure increases pulsatile load because more of the hydraulic load is borne by the collagen than by the elastin fibers in the media of its wall. Collagen is stiffer than elastin, which bears most of the hydraulic load at lower levels of mean pressure.

Recent studies have shown that antihypertensive drugs differ in their ability to affect mean and/or pulsatile load in hypertension. The effects of vasoactive drugs on the arterial pressure wave form in human subjects have been most extensively investigated with nitroglycerin (17,27,62–65). In low dose, nitroglycerin reduces the late systolic peak of both the aortic and left ventricular pressure waveforms (27,62–65) due to a reduction in pulsatile load, and quite independently of any change in mean arterial pressure. Angiotensin infusion (27) increases the late systolic pressure peak (Fig. 20).

The study of effects of pharmacologic therapy on pres-

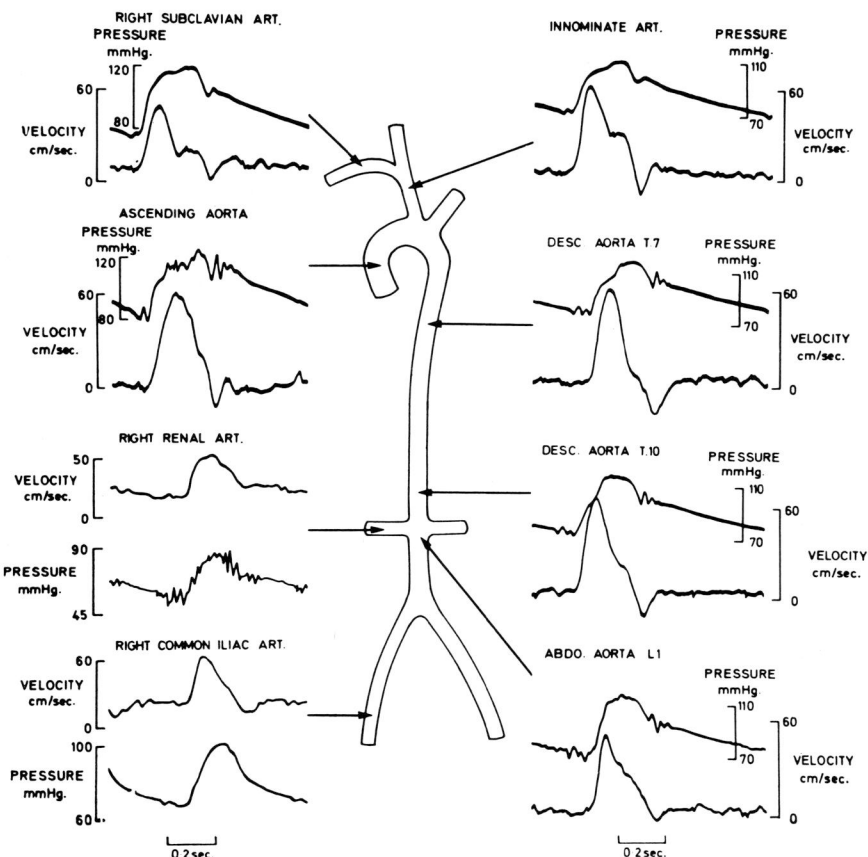

FIG. 15. Simultaneously recorded pressure and flow waves in human arteries. Data recorded at diagnostic cardiac catheterization. (From ref. 51, with permission.)

sure flow relationships in the ascending aorta have been greatly extended by the ability to record the "central" pressure pulse noninvasively at the carotid site. The noninvasive determination of arterial pressure and flow waves in states of normotension and hypertension is discussed below. Several studies have shown that the noninvasively recorded carotid pulse serves as an adequate guide to events in the ascending aorta. That is, the carotid pulse in its contour is more akin to the ascending aortic pulse than to the peripheral radial, brachial, or femoral pulse. Studies by Kelly et al. (66–68) and Fuji et al. (69) have both shown that the carotid pulse alters with age and hypertension in similar fashion to the ascending aortic pressure pulse. Similarly, drugs such as nitroglycerine reduce the late systolic pressure wave in the carotid pulse, as they do in the ascending aortic pulse. Kelly et al. (64) have noted that this effect can dissociate drug effects in different parts of the vasculature. In a series of noninvasive studies, with pressure recorded at carotid and radial sites, it was shown that a drug such as nitroglycerine may reduce the late systolic pressure peak by up to 20 mm Hg, but with little reduction in brachial or radial systolic pressure (64). However, the contour of the brachial pulse did change significantly, and in the way first described by Murrell (17) (Fig. 21). The difference in effect on systolic pressure at the central and peripheral sites is due to the fact that differential timing of wave reflection causes the carotid peak systolic pressure to be determined by the reflected wave, whereas this was not the case for the brachial wave. As discussed above, the pressure pulse contour recorded at "peripheral" sites differs from that recorded at "central" sites, and in consequence of transmission properties of the arterial vasculature between the two sites. The ability to predict the

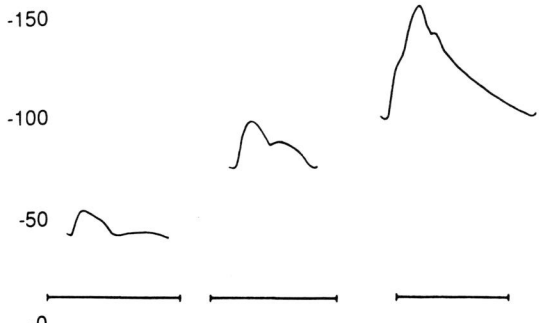

FIG. 16. Effects of increasing pressure on contour of pressure waves in the ascending aorta of a rabbit. (From refs. 22 and 89, with permission.)

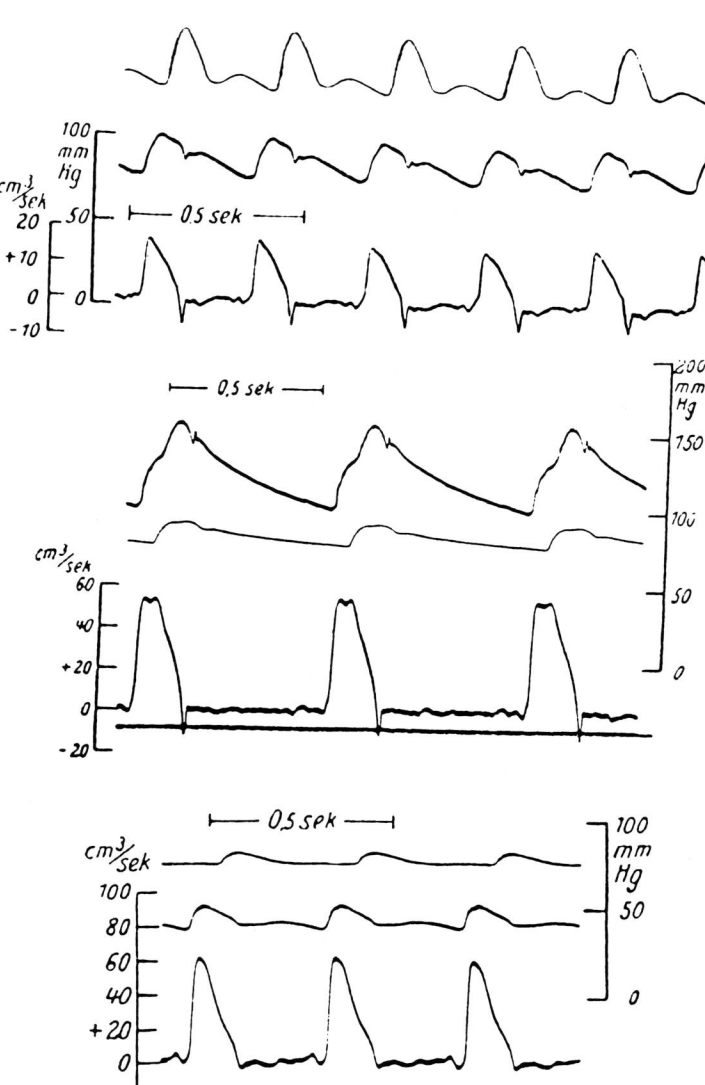

FIG. 17. Flow and pressure waves with induced hypotension in a rabbit. **Top:** Femoral artery pressure, carotid pressure, and ascending aortic flow under control conditions. **Center:** Carotid artery pressure, femoral artery pressure, and ascending aortic flow following injection of epinephrine. **Bottom:** Femoral artery pressure, carotid artery pressure, and ascending aortic flow after injection of pilocarpine. (From ref. 22, with permission.)

ascending aortic pressure pulse from a recorded pulse at the radial or brachial site depends on the ability to characterize the properties of the vasculature between these two sites. Based on knowledge of values for pulse wave velocity and invasively recorded data, it is possible to for-

mulate a "transfer function" which models the effect of pulse transmission along this part of the systemic vasculature (70) (Fig. 22). Remarkably, studies thus far have shown that this transfer function for human subjects between the aortic and brachial sites is relatively constant across various age groups and under different physiologic conditions (70). This gives rise to the possibility of synthesizing an aortic pressure pulse contour from a pressure wave recorded at a peripheral brachial or radial site utilizing a generalized transfer function.

NONINVASIVE DETERMINATION OF ARTERIAL PRESSURE AND FLOW WAVES

The arterial pressure wave form has been recorded noninvasively by several techniques. In the 1960s, Freis et al. (71) reported on the contour of the carotid wave

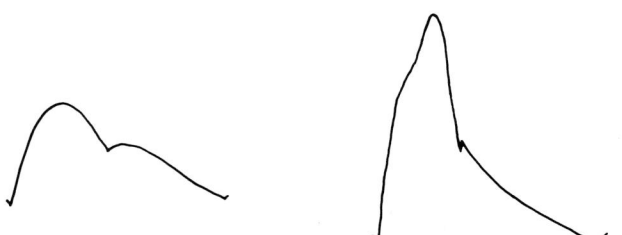

FIG. 18. Pressure wave pattern as seen in young human adults and in experimental animals (*left*) contrasted to pressure wave pattern as seen in mature human adults (*right*).

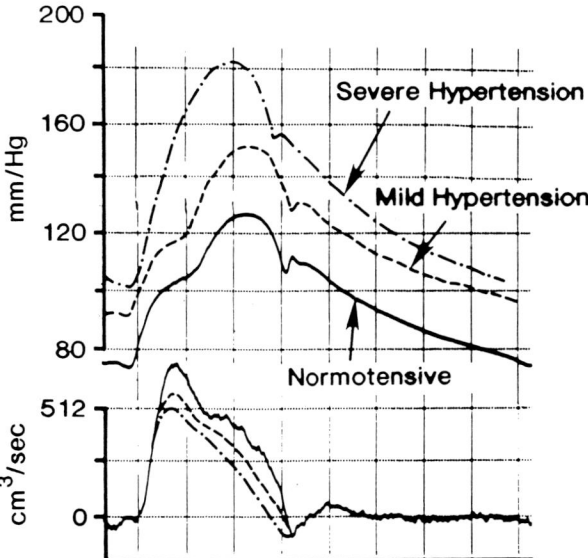

FIG. 19. Pressure and flow waves recorded in one normotensive and two hypertensive subjects of approximately the same age. As mean arterial pressure increases, the late secondary rise in systolic pressure is augmented and Δ tp decreases until, in severe hypertension, there is no inflection point and the pressure wave changes from a Type A to a Type D beat. With increasing severity of hypertension, systolic pressure increases 65 mm Hg while diastolic pressure increases 26 mm Hg.

recorded noninvasively by a suction cap device. This air-filled chamber was affixed to the skin overlying the carotid pulse. Underlying diameter fluctuations of the carotid pulse resulted in compression of the air contained within the chamber and was converted to an electrical signal by a charged membrane within the capsule. This recording device produced wave forms comparable to invasively recorded wave forms, but was limited both by the damping effects of the recording system and by movement artifact. In the 1980s, development of micromanometer technology was applied to a noninvasive instrument which was also used to record pressure pulses. Drawing on previous experience in ocular tonometry in ophthalmological practice, a device was developed which would accurately record noninvasive intraarterial pressure wave forms when applied against a superficial pulse point (72,73). By flattening the surface of a curved pressure-containing structure, circumferential forces inherent in the wall were normalized to the direction of pressure recordings so that there was little distortion of the intraarterial pressure pulse. This tonometric device allowed wave forms to be recorded at superficial pulse sites in large numbers of subjects and on repeated occasions (Figs. 23, 24). Perhaps the greatest contribution of tonometry was its use in defining effects of antihypertensive drugs. In a series of studies Kelly et al. (14) showed that the late systolic peak of the carotid pressure pulse

was able to be abolished by the administration of a small dose of sublingual nitroglycerine. This was associated with a simultaneous change in contour in the brachial or radial pulse recorded noninvasively, although there was not always a significant change in systolic pressure at the peripheral site. These findings were confirmed in the cardiac catheterization laboratory (64) in a series of fourteen subjects where ascending aortic and brachial artery pressure waves were recorded by micromanometer techniques in patients undergoing brachial artery catheterization. These studies confirmed that the administration of a small dose of sublingual nitroglycerine was able to reduce the late systolic peak in the aortic wave form with a marked reduction in systolic pressure and often in the presence of little change in systolic pressure recorded at the brachial site. Such findings have important implications for antihypertensive drug medication (Fig. 25). It is known that antihypertensive agents are not equally efficacious in reducing pulsatile vascular load. Angiotensin-converting enzyme inhibitors (1,14,74,75) and calcium channel blockers (1,14,74) reduce pulsatile load while beta blockers may increase it (76). Initial studies (11,74–76) indicate that antihypertensive drugs which reduce pulsatile load (arterial stiffness and wave reflection), as well as reducing mean resistance, are more effective in producing regression of hypertensive left ventricular hypertrophy. The use of noninvasive pressure pulse recording may provide additional important information on the mechanism of action of different antihypertensive drugs despite a similar effect on brachial sphygmomanometric values (77).

Noninvasive pressure recordings have also been popularized by the use of the photoplethysmographic noninvasive blood pressure device (Finapres). Whereas the tonometer requires calibration with a sphygmomanometric brachial pressure, the Finapres device is a self-contained unit which records digital artery systolic and diastolic pressures as well as the wave contour in between these two extremes. The Finapres device works on the principle of a vascular-unloading technique whereby intraarterial pressure fluctuations are counterbalanced by an external inflated cuff which equalizes pressure across the arterial wall (78).

Arterial flow waves have been recorded noninvasively using Doppler ultrasound techniques. Such techniques provide ready access to flow velocity profiles in both the ascending aorta and peripheral vessels. It has been observed for many years now that aging is associated with a reduction in peak velocity in the ascending aorta as well as a reduction in the acceleration of flow (68,79). These changes are exaggerated in states of cardiac failure (80). More recently, attention has been directed to the contour of the flow velocity profile on the downstroke of the wave beyond the initial systolic peak. Indices of pulsatile loading conditions such as the effect of wave reflection have been developed from these noninvasively-recorded flow

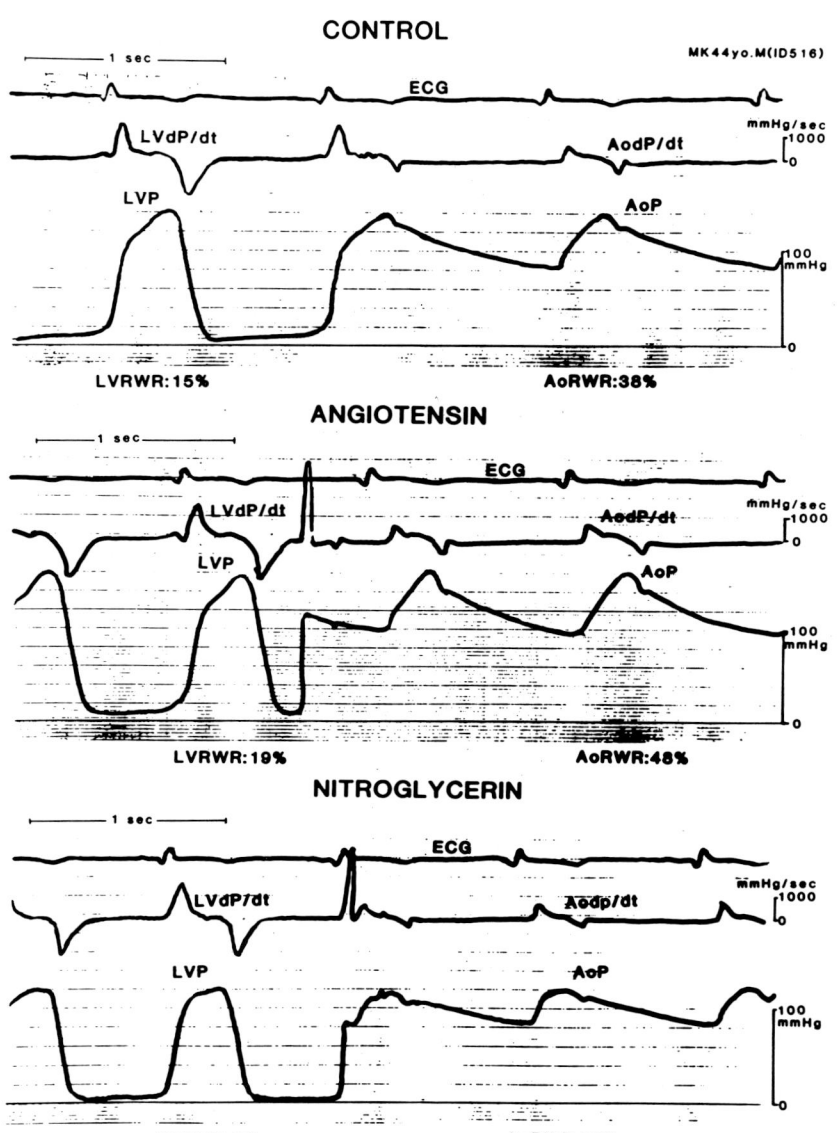

FIG. 20. Pressure recorded in the left ventricle (*left*) with a micromanometer catheter system and (*right*) after withdrawal into the ascending aorta of a patient studied at diagnostic cardiac catheterization under control conditions (*top*), during infusion of angiotensin (*center*), and after sublingual nitroglycerin 0.6 mg (*bottom*). (From ref. 91, with permission.)

waves (81). Such flow-wave indices may enhance our ability to assess vascular loading conditions in normotensive and hypertensive subjects undergoing routine Doppler ultrasound studies.

DETERMINATION OF CENTRAL FROM PERIPHERAL PRESSURE

As discussed above, blood pressure is not the same in all arteries in any individual and, furthermore, the specific physiologic factors which determine peak systolic pressure differ at various sites. These determinants also vary according to the age of the patient. Hence, in the central part of the vasculature, ascending aortic and ca-

rotid artery systolic pressure in middle-aged to older humans is determined by a late systolic pressure wave. This late systolic peak is the net effect of wave reflection from multiple sites, particularly in the lower part of the body. This "reflected wave" can also be seen in the contour of the pressure pulse at peripheral sites such as the brachial and radial, but it does not determine peak systolic pressure at these sites. In the periphery, wave reflection is an important determinant of wave contour, and effects of drugs on wave reflection can be inferred from changes in the peripheral pulse contour. Since our aim in treating hypertension is to reduce cardiovascular morbidity and mortality and reduce target organ effects, the ability to measure pressure at the sites of these organ effects would seem logical. It is the ascending aortic pressure with

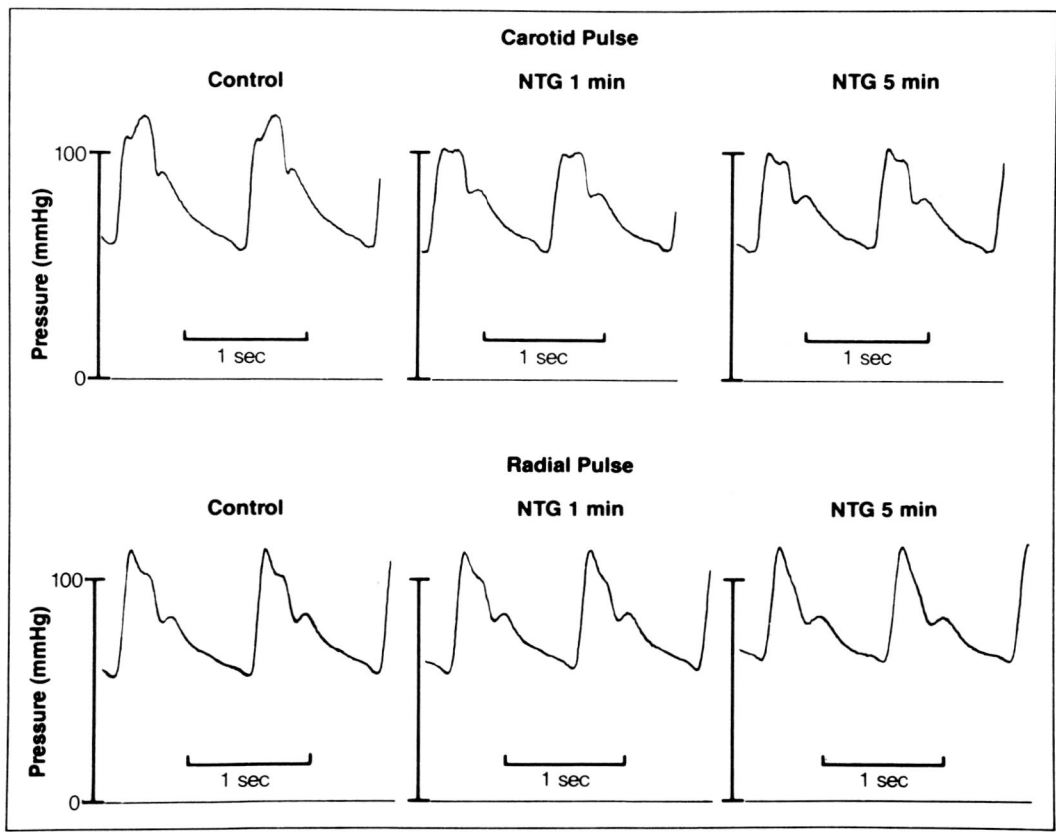

FIG. 21. Tonometric, noninvasively recorded carotid (*above*) and radial artery (*below*) pressure waves in a 50-year-old man under control conditions (*left*) and 1 minute (*center*) and 5 minutes (*right*) after administration of nitroglycerin 0.3 mg sublingually. Calibrations refer to sphygmomanometric measurement of brachial artery pressure. (From ref. 14, with permission.)

which the heart interacts, and it is the cerebral pressure in the carotid artery and its branches to which the brain is exposed. Yet our current treatment approach to hypertension still relies on a single measurement of pressure taken at the brachial site.

Similarly, the differential effects of antihypertensive medications on pulsatile versus mean pressure load and on target organ effects indicates that a full assessment of the patient with hypertension in the future will require more than just brachial sphygmomanometric measurements. One approach to this is to try to directly measure the target-organ effects noninvasively as part of clinical assessment. The role of echocardiography in the workup of the hypertensive patient is currently debated and has important cost-effectiveness implications.

Such considerations have led investigators, including ourselves, to develop a method whereby the central arterial pressure can be evaluated at the bedside from simple measurements of blood pressure and pulse contour at a peripheral site. Although some noninvasive methods such as tonometry allow direct recording of the carotid

pulse (67,82), there are methodologic problems with this which limit its widespread implication in routine clinical management. Carotid tonometry is operator-dependent and requires care to be taken with regard to correct placement of the instrument over the carotid vessel with the patient in a recumbent position. A simpler approach is to record the radial pulse contour, calibrating it with brachial sphygmomanometric systolic and diastolic levels, and thence to synthesize the corresponding ascending aortic pressure contour as based on known transmission line properties between the aortic and radial sites. In this way a generalized "transfer function" can be applied to obtain a calibrated ascending aortic pressure wave as part of the routine bedside evaluation in patients with hypertension (1,41). Experience thus far has indicated that the transfer function from the ascending aorta along the upper limb to the radial site is surprisingly constant across varying age groups and under widely different physiologic conditions (70). Application of this method allows a bedside report to be generated, displaying not only brachial sphygmomanometric and radial pressure contours,

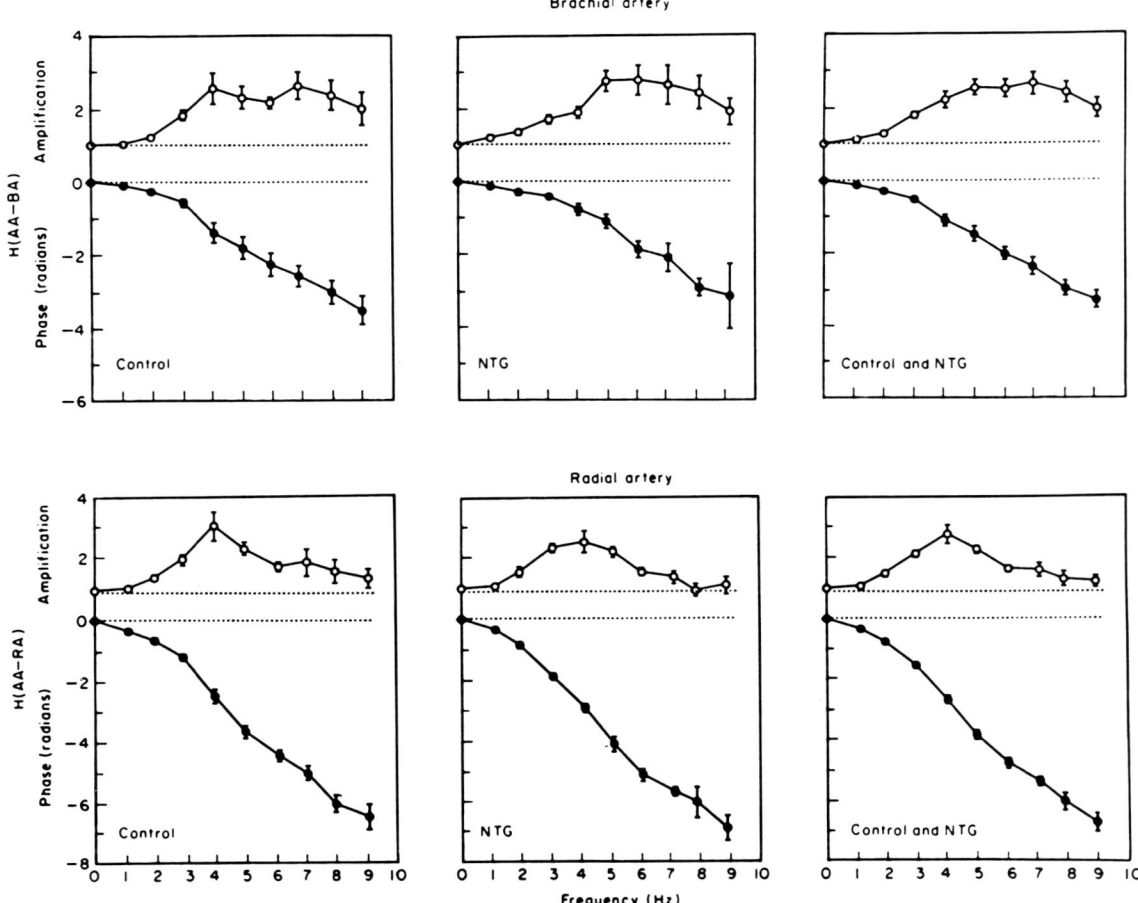

FIG. 22. Calculated transfer function and its change with age in man between ascending aorta (*AA*) and brachial artery (*BA*).

but also the ascending aortic pressure contour (Fig. 26). From these recordings, a number of physiologic indices can be determined directly or indirectly which may assist in the therapeutic approach to patients with hypertension. Indices of ventricular-vascular interaction include systolic and diastolic time intervals, a subendocardial viability index (83) based on such intervals, an augmentation index to determine effects of wave reflection (68,1) and end-systolic pressure to stroke volume ratio (55,84). One such application is to derive a subendocardial viability index based on the relative durations of systole and diastole (81,82).

Such an approach is not the only means available of obtaining more accurate hemodynamic information from peripheral recordings. There are alternative ways of estimating central aortic pressure from upper limb (84) or carotid (82) recordings. Furthermore, measurement of arterial diameter by ultrasound techniques provides important data on the distensibility of large arteries in states of normotension and treated hypertension (85).

These techniques (1,81,82,84,85) may allow us in the future to more accurately assess the hemodynamic status of any individual with hypertension, to more precisely select an appropriate drug to offset the hemodynamic derangement so found, and to follow up the patient response to this therapy with repeated noninvasive measurements in the office or clinic. These devices also open many opportunities for future research into the coupling of cardiac function with vascular properties. The combination of noninvasive aortic pressure measurement and Doppler-derived aortic flow contours may provide a powerful tool in the future for assessing ventriculoarterial coupling, not only in aging and hypertension but also in other disease states such as cardiac failure. Such clinical and research advances in the future in assessing afterload properties will depend on progressing beyond the brachial sphygmomanometer to more informative means of assessing arterial pressure. They constitute a return to our heritage of obtaining as much information as possible from the arterial pulse.

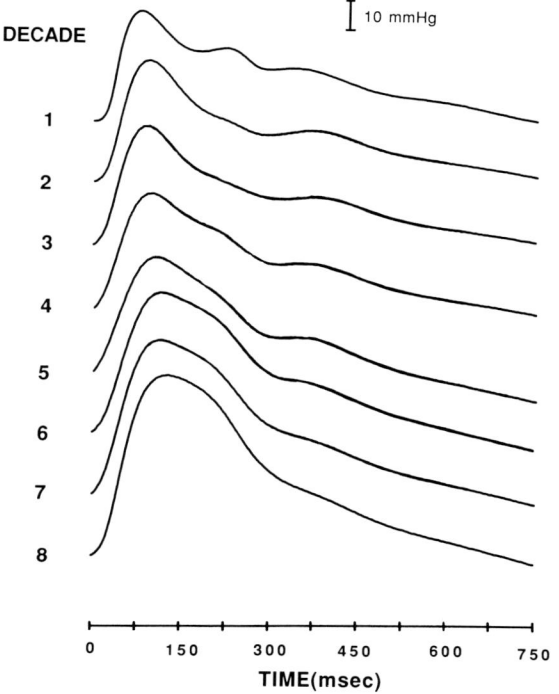

FIG. 23. Change in contour and amplitude of the human radial artery pressure wave with age. (From ref. 68, with permission.)

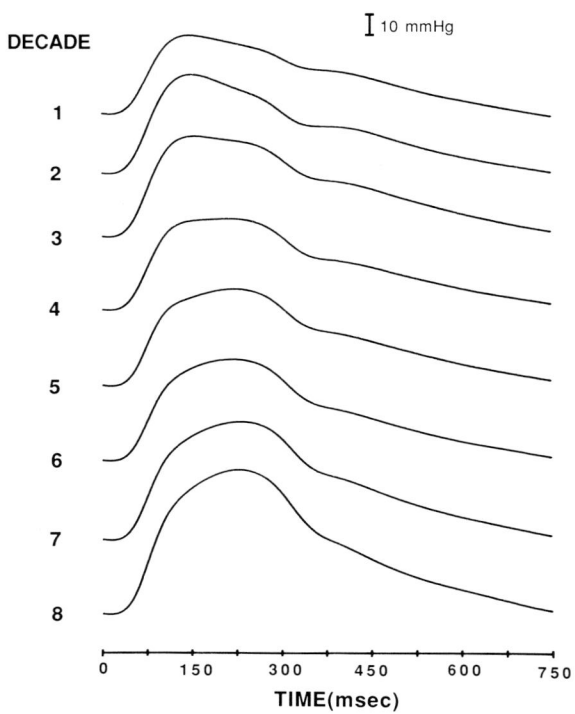

FIG. 24. Change in contour and amplitude of the human carotid artery pressure wave with age. (From ref. 68, with permission.)

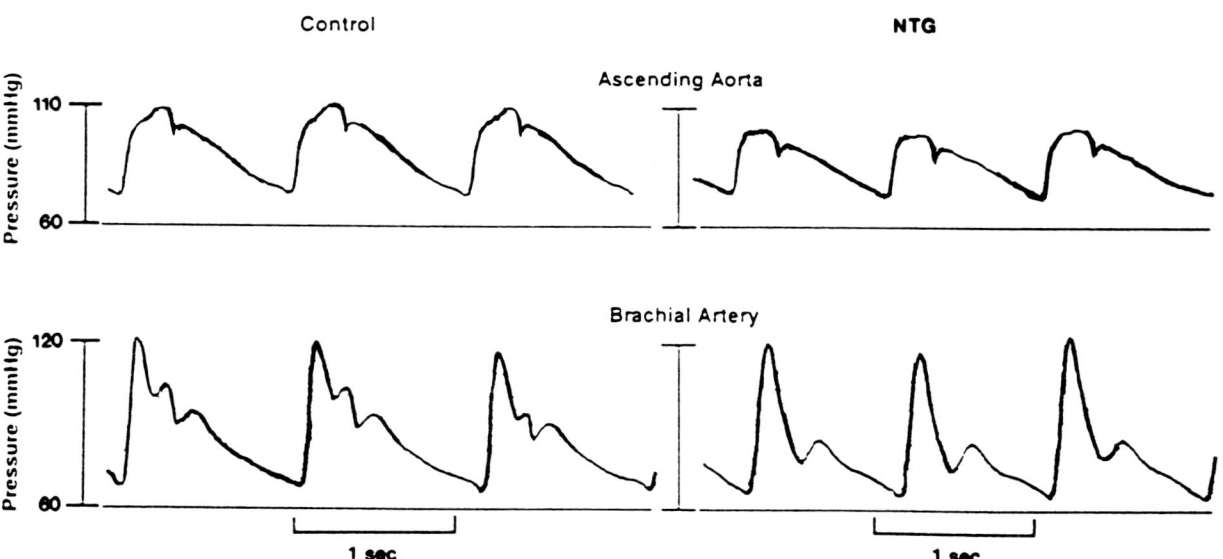

FIG. 25. Pressure waves recorded directly with a micromanometer in the ascending aorta (*above*) and brachial artery (*below*) in a middle-aged man before (*left*) and after (*right*) administration of 0.3 mg nitroglycerin sublingually. (From ref. 64, with permission.)

Patient ID =   Operator ID =   8
Patient Name= GISELLE ERT
Sex = F   Age = 77
Address   = D/153 BAYSWATER RD, RUSHCUTTERS BAY 2011
Current Medication =RENITEC, CARTIA

Date Of Inspection = TUE 13/JUL/1993 10:34

Heart Rate =71 Bpm Ejection Duration =310 mSec Reference Age =58

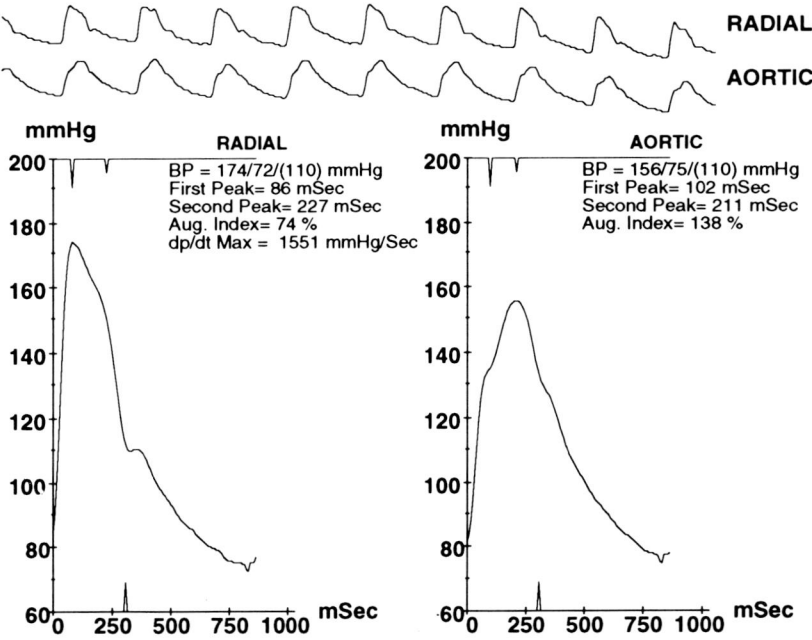

Central Pressure Indices

Augmented pressure	= 21	**mmHg**
Tension Time Index	= 2947	**mmHg.Sec/min**
Diastolic Time Index	= 3682	**mmHg.Sec/min**
Subendocardial Viability	= 125	**%**
Mean Systolic Pressure	= 136	**mmHg**
Mean Diastolic Pressure	= 96	**mmHg**
End Systolic Pressure	= 133	**mmHg**

FIG. 26. Sample report of arterial pressure wave form analysis in 50-year-old patient with history of essential hypertension.

REFERENCES

1. O'Rourke MF, Avolio AP, Kelly RP. *The Arterial Pulse.* Baltimore: Lea & Febiger; 1991.
2. Marey EJ. *La circulation du sang a l'etat physiologique et dans les maladies.* Paris: Masson; 1881.
3. Mahomed FA. The physiology and clinical use of the sphygmograph. *Medical Times and Gazette* 1872;1:62–64, 128–130, 220–222.
4. Broadbent W. *The pulse.* Philadelphia: Lea; 1890.
5. Mackenzie J. *The study of the pulse.* London: Pentland; 1902.
6. Bright R. *Select reports of medical cases.* London: Longmans; 1827.
7. Mahomed F. The aetiology of Bright's Disease and the prealbumenuric stage. *Med Chir Trans* 1874;57:197–228.
8. Luke RG. Essential hypertension: A renal disease? *Hypertension* 1993;21:380–390.
9. Kannel WB, Wolf PA, McGee DL, Dawber TR, McNamara P, Castelli WP. Systolic blood pressure, arterial rigidity and risk of stroke. The Framingham Study. *JAMA* 1981;245:1225–1229.
10. Rutan GH, Kuller LH, Neaton JD, Wentworth DN, McDonald RH, McFate-Smith W. Mortality associated with diastolic hypertension and isolated systolic hypertension among men screened for Multiple Risk Factor Intervention Trial. *Circulation* 1988;77:504–514.
11. Schulman SP, Weiss JL, Becker LC, et al. The effects of antihypertensive therapy on left ventricular mass in elderly patients. *New Engl J Med* 1990;322:1350–1356.
12. Pfeffer MA, Pfeffer JM. Reversing cardiac hypertrophy in hypertension. *New Engl J Med* 1990;322:1388–1390.
13. Pettinger WA, Lie HC, Reisch J, Mitchell HC. Long-term improvement in renal function after short-term strict blood pressure control in hypertensive nephrosclerosis. *Hypertension* 1989;13:766–772.
14. O'Rourke MF, Kelly RP, Avolio AP, Hayward CS. Effects of arterial dilator agents on central aortic systolic pressure and on left ventricular hydraulic load. *Am J Cardiol* 1989;63:38I–44I.
15. O'Rourke MF, Safar ME, eds. Functional and structural properties of large arteries. *J Hypertens* 1992;10[Suppl 6]:S1–S146.
16. Kannel WB. In: Kaplan NM, Stamler J, eds. *Prevention of coronary heart disease.* Philadelphia: WB Saunders; 1983.

17. Murrell W. Nitroglycerine as a remedy for angina pectoris. *Lancet* 1879;1:80–81, 151–152, 225–227.

18. Frank O. Der Puls in den Arterien. *Zeitschrift fur Biologie* 1905;46:441–553.

19. Wiggers CJ. *The pressure pulse in the cardiovascular system.* London: Longmans; 1928.

20. Hamilton WF, Dow P. An experimental study of the standing waves in the pulse propagated through the aorta. *Am J Physiol* 1939;125:48–59.

21. Hamilton WF. The patterns of the arterial pressure pulse. *Am J Physiol* 1944;141:235–241.

22. Wetterer E. Flow and pressure in the arterial system, their hemodynamic relationship and the principles of their measurement. *Minnesota Med* 1954;37:77–86.

23. McDonald DA. *McDonald's blood flow in arteries.* London: Arnold; 1960.

24. O'Rourke MF, Taylor MG. Vascular impedance of the femoral bed. *Circ Res* 1966;18:126–39.

25. O'Rourke MF, Taylor MG. Input impedance of the systemic circulation. *Circ Res* 1967;20:365–380.

26. Murgo JP, Westerhof N, Giolma JP, Altobelli SA. Manipulation of ascending aortic pressure and flow wave reflections with the Valsalva manoeuvre: relationship to pressure wave forms. *Circulation* 1981;62:122–132.

27. Takazawa K. A clinical study of the second component of left ventricular systolic pressure. *J Tokyo Med Coll* 1987;45:256–270.

28. Dawber TR, Thomas HE, McNamara PM. Characteristics of the dicrotic notch of the arterial pulse wave in coronary heart disease.

29. Takazawa K, Fujita M, Yabe K, Sakai T, Kobayashi T, Maeda K, et al. Clinical usefulness of the second derivative of plethysmogram. *Japanese Cardiac J* [in press].

30. Hirai T, Sasayama S, Kawasaki T, Yagi S. Stiffness of systemic arteries in patients with myocardial infarction. *Circulation* 1989;80:78–86.

31. O'Rourke MF. Pressure and flow waves in systemic arteries and the anatomical design of the arterial system. *J Appl Physiol* 1967;23:139–149.

32. O'Rourke MF, Blazek JV, Morreels CL, Krovetz LJ. Pressure wave transmission along the human aorta. *Circ Res* 1968;23:567–579.

33. O'Rourke MF. *Arterial function in health and disease.* Edinburgh: Churchill Livingstone; 1982.

34. Remington JW, Wood EH. Formation of peripheral pulse contour in man. *J Appl Physiol* 1956;9:433–442.

35. Rowell LB, Brengelmann GL, Blackmon JR et al. Disparities between aortic and peripheral pulse pressures induced by upright exercise and vasomotor changes in man. *Circulation* 1968;37:954–964.

36. Frank O. Schatzung des Schlagvolummens des menschlichen Herzens auf grund der wellenund Windkessel Theorie. *Zeitschrift fur Biologie* 1930;90:405–409.

37. Karamanoglu M, O'Rourke MF, Avolio AP, Kelly RP. An analysis of the relationship between central aortic and peripheral upper limb pressure waves in man. *Eur Heart J* 1993;14:160–167.

38. O'Rourke MF. Influence of ventricular ejection on the relationship between central aortic and brachial pressure pulse in man. *Cardiovasc Res* 1970;4:291–300.

39. Nichols WW, O'Rourke MF, Avolio AP, Yaginuma T, Murgo JP, Pepine CJ, Conti CR. Effects of age on ventricular/vascular coupling. *Am J Cardiol* 1985;55:1179–1184.

40. O'Rourke MF, Avolio AP, Nichols WW. Left ventricular systemic arterial coupling in man and strategies to improve coupling in disease states. In: Yin FCP, ed. *Vascular ventricular coupling.* New York: Springer-Verlag; 1985;1–19.

41. O'Rourke MF, Kelly RP. Wave reflection in the systemic circulation and its implication in ventricular function in man. *J Hypertens* 1993;11:327–337.

42. Latham RD, Westerhof N, Sipkema P, Rubal B, Reuderink P. Regional wave travel and reflections along the human aorta: a study with six simultaneous micromanometric pressures. *Circulation* 1985;72:1257–1269.

43. Young T. Hydraulic investigations subservient to an intended Croonian lecture on the motion of the blood. *Phil Trans Roy Soc* (London) 1808;98:164–186.

44. Milnor WR. Aortic wavelength as a determinant of the relationship between heart rate and body size in mammals. *Am J Physiol* 1979;237:R3–R6.

45. O'Rourke MF. Commentary on aortic wave length as a determinant of the relationship between heart rate and body size in mammals. *Am J Physiol* 1981;240:R393–395.

46. Nichols WW, O'Rourke MF. *McDonald's blood flow in arteries,* 3rd ed. London: Arnold; 1990.

47. Bramwell JC, Hill AV. Velocity of transmission of the pulse wave and elasticity of arteries. *Lancet* 1922;1:891–892.

48. Ho K. *Effects of aging on arterial distensibility and left ventricular load in an Australian community* [Thesis] Sydney: University of NSW, 1982.

49. Avolio AP, Chen S-G, Wang R-P, Zhang C-L, Li M-F, O'Rourke MF. Effects of aging on changing arterial compliance and left ventricular load in a northern Chinese urban community. *Circulation* 1983;68:50–58.

50. Avolio AP, Deng FQ, Li W, et al. Effects of aging on arterial distensibility in populations with high and low prevalence of hypertension: comparisons between urban and rural communities in China. *Circulation* 1985;71:202–210.

51. Mills CJ, Gabe IT, Gault JH, et al. Pressure-flow relationships and vascular impedance in man. *Cardiovasc Res* 1970;4:405–417.

52. O'Rourke MF. Arterial stiffness, systolic blood pressure, and logical treatment of arterial hypertension. *Hypertension* 1990;15:339–347.

53. O'Rourke MF. What is blood pressure? *Am J Hypertens* 1990;3:803–810.

54. O'Rourke MF. Steady and pulsatile energy losses in the systemic circulation under normal conditions and in simulated arterial disease. *Cardiovasc Res* 1967;1:313–326.

55. Kelly R, Tunin R, Kass D. Effect of reduced aortic compliance on left ventricular contractile function and energetics in vivo. *Circ Res* 1992;71:490–502.

56. Kroeker EJ, Wood EH. Beat-to-beat alterations in the relationship of simultaneously-recorded central and peripheral arterial pressure pulses during Valsalva manoeuvre and prolonged expiration in man. *J Appl Physiol* 1956;8:483–494.

57. O'Rourke MF. Pulsatile arterial haemodynamics in hypertension. *Aust NZ J Med* 1976;16[Suppl 2]:40–48.

58. Merillon JP, Fontenier G, Chastre J, Lerallut JF, Jaffrin MY, Gourgon R. Etude du spectre d'impédance chez l'homme normal et hypertendie. Effects de l'accroissement de frequence cardiaque et des croques vasomotrics. *Arch Mal Couer* 1980;73:83–90.

59. Merillon JP, Motte G, Masquet C, Azancot I, Guiomard A, Gourgon R. Relationship between physical properties of the arterial system and left ventricular performance in the course of aging and arterial hypertension. *Eur Heart J* 1982;3[Suppl A]:95–101.

60. Ting CT, Brin KP, Lin SJ, Wang SP, Chang MS, Chiang BN, Yin FCP. Arterial hemodynamics in human hypertension. *J Clin Invest* 1986;78:1462–1471.

61. Ting CT, Chang MS, Wang SP, Chiang BN, Yin FCP. Regional pulse wave velocities in hypertensive and normotensive humans. *Cardiovasc Res* 1990;24:865–872.

62. Yaginuma T, Avolio AP, O'Rourke MF, Nichols WW, et al. Effects of glyceryl trinitrate on peripheral arteries alters left ventricular hydraulic load in man. *Cardiovasc Res* 1986;20:153–160.

63. Latson TW, Hunter WC, Ketoh N, Sagawa K. Effect of nitroglycerin on aortic impedance diameter and pulse wave velocity. *Circ Res* 1988;62:884–890.

64. Kelly RP, Gibbs H, O'Rourke MF, Daley JE, Mang K, Morgan JJ, Avolio AP. Nitroglycerin has more favorable effects on the left ventricular afterload than apparent from measurement of pressure in a peripheral artery. *Eur Heart J* 1990;11:138–144.

65. Fitchett DH, Simkus GJ, Beaudry JP, Marpole DG. Reflected pressure wave in the ascending aorta: effect of glyceryl trinitrate. *Cardiovasc Res* 1988;22:494–500.

66. Kelly RP, Hayward CS, Ganis J, Daley JM, Avolio AP, O'Rourke MF. Non-invasive registration of the arterial pressure pulse waveform using high-fidelity applanation tonometry. *J Vasc Med Biol* 1989;1:142–149.

67. Kelly RP, Karamanoglu M, Gibbs H, Avolio AP, O'Rourke MF. Non-invasive carotid pressure registration as an indication of ascending aortic pressure. *J Vasc Med Biol* 1989;1:241–247.

68. Kelly RP, Hayward CS, Avolio AP, O'Rourke MF. Non-invasive

determination of age-related changes in the human arterial pulse. *Circulation* 1989;80:1652–1659.

69. Fujii M, Yaginuma T, Takazawa K, et al. Non-invasive detection of reflection wave in the arterial system. *Automedica.* New York: Gordon & Breach; 1987:9, 49.

70. Karamanoglu M, O'Rourke MF, Avolio AP, Kelly RP. An analysis of the relationship between central aortic and peripheral upper limb pressure waves in man. *Eur Heart J* 1993;14:160–167.

71. Freis ED, Kyle MC. Computer analysis of carotid and brachial pulse waves. Effects of age in normal subjects. *Am J Cardiol* 1968;22:691–695.

72. Pressman GL, Newgard PM. A transducer for the continuous external measurement of arterial blood pressure. *IEEE Trans Biomed Elect* 1963;(BME-10):73–81.

73. Drzewiecki GM, Melbin J, Noordergraaf A. Arterial tonometry: review and analysis. *J Biomed* 1983;16(2):141–153.

74. Safar ME, Toto-Moukouo JJ, Bouthier JA, Asmar RE, Levenson JA, Simon ACh, London GM. Arterial dynamics, cardiac hypertrophy and anti-hypertensive treatment. *Circulation* 1987; 75[Suppl 1]:156–161.

75. Asmar RG, Pannier B, Santoni JP, et al. Reversion of cardiac hypertrophy and reduced arterial compliance after converting enzyme inhibition in essential hypertension. *Circulation* 1988;78: 941–950.

76. Zusman RM, Christensen DM, Federman EB, et al. Nifedipine but not propranolol improves left ventricular systolic and diastolic function in patients with hypertension. *Am J Cardiol* 1989;64: 51F–61F.

76. Ting CT, Chou CY, Chang MS, Wang SP, Chiang BN, Yin FCP. Arterial hemodynamics in human hypertension: effects of adrenergic blockade. *Circulation* 1991;84:1049–1057.

77. Kelly RP, Daley J, Avolio A, O'Rourke M. Arterial dilation and reduced wave reflection: benefit of dilevalol in hypertension. *Hypertension* 1989;14:14–21.

78. Wesseling KH, de Wit B, Settels Jj, Klawer WH. On indirect registration of blood pressure after Penaz. *Funkt Biol Med* 1982;1:245–250.

79. Gardin JM, Burn CS, Childs WJ, Henry WL. Evaluation of blood flow velocity in the ascending aorta and main pulmonary artery of normal subjects by Doppler echocardiography. *Am Heart J* 1984;107:310–319.

80. Gardin JM, Isei LT, Elkayan U, et al. Evaluation of dilated cardiomyopathy by pulsed Doppler echography. *Am Heart J* 1983;106: 1057–1065.

81. Miyashita H, Ikeda U, Tsuruya Y, Sekiguchi H, Shimoda K, Yaginuma T. Non invasive evaluation of the influence of aortic valve reflection on left ventricular ejection during auxotomic contraction. *Heart and Vessels* 1993 [in press].

82. Roman M, Saba PS, Pini R, Spitzer M, Ganau A, Devereux RB. Parallel and vascular adaptation in hypertension. *Circulation* 1992;86:1909–1918.

83. Buckberg GD, Fisher DE, Archie JP, Hoffman JIE. Experimental subendocardial ischemia in dogs with normal coronary arteries. *Circ Res* 1972;30:67–81.

84. Sharir T, Marma A, Ting CT, Chen JW, Liu CP, Chang MS, et al. Validation of a method for noninvasive measurement of central arterial pressure. *Hypertension* 1993;21:74–82.

85. Safar M, Peronneau J, Levenson J, Simon A. Pulsed Doppler: diameter, velocity and flow of brachial artery in sustained essential hypertension. *Circulation* 1981;63(II):393–400.

86. Snellen, HA. *EJ Marey and Cardiology.* Rotterdam: Kookyer; 1980.

87. *Circulation* 1958; Vol XVIII.

88. O'Rourke MF, Avolio AP. Pulsatile flow and pressure in human systemic arteries; studies in man and in a multi-branched model of the systemic arterial tree. *Circ Res* 1980;44:363–372.

89. O'Rourke MF. The arterial pulse in health and disease. *Am Heart J* 1971;82:687–702.

90. O'Rourke MF. Vascular impedance in studies of arterial cardiac function. *Physiol Rev* 1982;62:570–623.

91. Takazawa K. A clinical study of the second component of left ventricular systolic pressure. *J Tokyo Med Coll* 1987;45:256–270.

Hypertension: Pathophysiology, Diagnosis,
and Management, Second Edition,
edited by J.H. Laragh and B.M. Brenner,
Raven Press, Ltd., New York © 1995.

CHAPTER **22**

Blood Viscosity as a Factor in Human Hypertension

Anne Chabanel and Shu Chien

Increased systemic flow resistance is a hemodynamic feature of established essential hypertension (EH). The resistance to flow is a function of (a) the geometric features of the vasculature, and (b) the flow properties of blood. Although blood viscosity has usually been ignored as a determinant of vascular resistance, there has been a recent increase in interest in monitoring blood viscosity changes in several hematological and cardiovascular disorders. Improved methodology for the measurement of factors determining blood viscosity has demonstrated that high blood viscosity occurs in several forms of cardiovascular diseases (1,2). High rates of cardiovascular morbidity have been reported in patients with hypertension and blood hyperviscosity (3). Furthermore, evidence is accumulating which shows that an improvement in blood fluidity is associated with clinical benefits.

In this review on blood viscosity factors in relation to hypertension, we begin with a general discussion of the relationship between blood viscosity and blood pressure and with a description of blood rheology and the determinants of blood viscosity. Next, we review the clinical observations linking blood viscosity changes to hypertension. Finally, the effects of antihypertensive treatments on blood viscosity are presented.

RELATIONSHIP BETWEEN BLOOD PRESSURE AND BLOOD VISCOSITY

The mean arterial pressure (MAP) varies directly with the cardiac output (CO) and the resistance to flow (R):

$$MAP = CO \times R$$

A. Chabanel: Laboratoire Central d'Hématologie, Hopital de l'Hotel Dieu, Paris, France.
S. Chien: Institute for Biomedical Engineering, University of California, San Diego, La Jolla, California 92093.

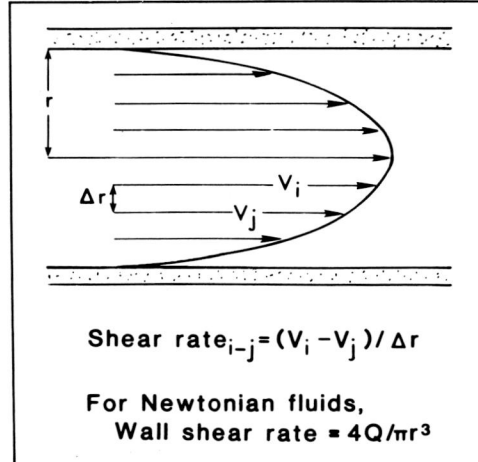

$$\text{Shear rate}_{i-j} = (V_i - V_j)/\Delta r$$

For Newtonian fluids,
Wall shear rate = $4Q/\pi r^3$

FIG. 1. Cross-section of a cylindrical tube showing the velocity profile in laminar flow. The shear rate is the difference in velocity of adjacent layers of flowing fluid per unit distance between the layers. For example, the shear rate between the layers with velocities of v_i and v_j separated by a distance Δr is $(v_i - v_j)/\Delta r$. The velocity profile is such that the shear rate is near zero in the tube center and increased to a maximum next to the wall.

The resistance, in turn, is the product of blood viscosity and vascular hindrance (Z), which represents the contribution of vascular geometry to the resistance (4). An elevation of Z usually results from vasoconstriction. Therefore, blood viscosity and the degree of arteriolar constriction together determine the total peripheral resistance. The elevation of arterial pressure must then be analyzed in terms of not only the CO and vascular hindrance, but also the blood viscosity. Cardiac output is elevated in the early phase of hypertension, but generally is normal in established hypertension (5,6). Until recently, the rise of BP in hypertension has usually been explained solely by an increase in vascular hindrance due to contraction of arteriolar smooth muscle cells (7). However, a significant correlation between blood viscosity and BP has been demonstrated in patients with EH (8,9). Moreover, blood viscosity is increased in patients with EH even in the early phase of borderline elevation of arterial pressure (1,10) or in normotensive relatives of EH patients (11). In apparently normal adults, several epidemiological studies have revealed statistically significant correlations between arterial blood pressure and blood viscosity or its determinants (12–20).

RHEOLOGICAL BEHAVIOR OF BLOOD

Rheology is the study of the relations between stresses applied to a material and the resulting deformation and flow. Blood rheology, or hemorheology, is the science which examines the deformation and flow of blood.

A fluid flowing in a tube exhibits a velocity gradient (shear rate): the velocity is zero near the wall and increases progressively to the center of the tube (Fig. 1). Viscosity is defined as a ratio of the shear stress, which is the shear force acting tangentially on a unit area, to the shear rate.

Non-Newtonian Behavior of Blood

Blood is a very complex fluid. The most remarkable aspect of blood viscosity is that blood remains fluid even at hematocrit values as high as 95–98 percent. In contrast to blood, suspensions of rigid particles achieve the consistency of a brick at concentrations as low as 60 percent (21). This unique property of blood is due to the deformability of its cellular elements (22). The viscosity of blood rises with decreasing shear rate (Fig. 2). Although whole blood might exhibit viscosities in the order of 100-

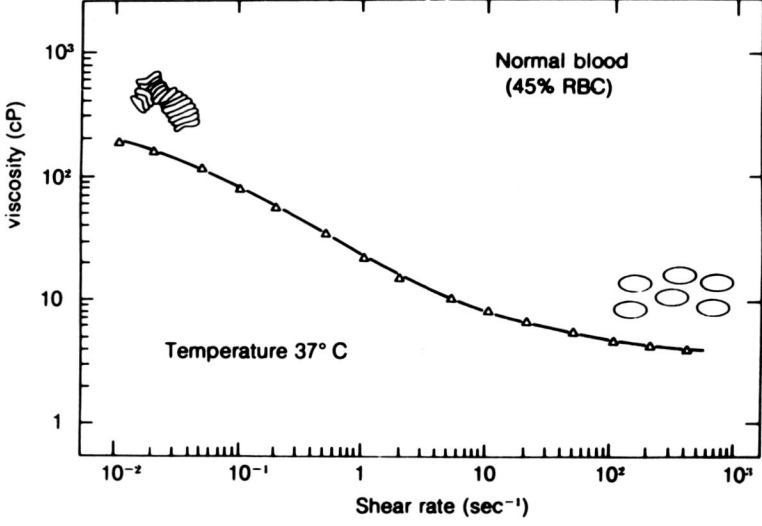

FIG. 2. Logarithmic plot showing the relationship between the apparent viscosity of normal human blood and the shear rate. The inset sketches show the aggregation of red blood cells at low shear rates and their disaggregation and deformation at high shear rates (123).

fold higher than water at near-zero shear rates, at high shear rates it shows a viscosity of only about four times that of water. This shear-dependent behavior characterizes blood as a non-Newtonian fluid (4). The elevation of blood viscosity at low shear rates reflects the aggregation of red blood cells (RBCs), whereas the diminution at high shear rates is due to disaggregation, deformation, and orientation of the cells (22).

In vivo, depending on local shear rates, the viscosity of blood varies greatly in different segments of the circulation. The highest shear rates are encountered in the arterioles and precapillary vessels, while the lowest shear rates are found in postcapillary venules (4). Under normal conditions, the shear rates in most parts of the circulatory system are sufficiently high to ensure disaggregation and deformation of RBCs, thus maintaining blood viscosity at a low level; the only parts of the circulation which might have shear rates low enough to favor RBC aggregation are the postcapillary venules, where wall shear rates could be less than 20 sec^{-1} (23). In pathologic situations, shear rates can increase (at stenosis) or decrease (poststenotic region) beyond physiologic ranges, thereby causing perturbations to blood flow. It is worthy to note that since the shear rate approaches zero at the center of axial flow, RBC aggregates might persist in the center of vessels in spite of high shear rates at the wall.

Factors Determining Blood Viscosity

Blood viscosity at a given temperature depends on the plasma viscosity, cell concentration, cell aggregation, and cell deformability, with the last two factors being shear-dependent.

Plasma behaves as a Newtonian fluid, i.e., its viscosity does not vary with shear rate. At a given temperature, plasma viscosity is strongly dependent on the concentration of plasma proteins, especially proteins with molecular asymmetry, such as fibrinogen and some of the globulin fractions. Plasma viscosity can be measured by capillary (24) Couette (25), or other types of viscosimeters.

Blood viscosity varies nonlinearly with the hematocrit value (4). Elevation of systemic hematocrit or local hemoconcentration due to increased vascular permeability can exert undesirable hemodynamic effects (12).

Normal RBCs are deformable in response to shear stress. Red blood cell deformability is a function of cell geometry (especially the surface-area/cell-volume ratio), internal viscosity, and membrane viscoelastic properties (26). These factors influencing RBC deformability can be assessed by several techniques (27). Measurements of the viscosity of RBC suspensions in Ringer-albumin solution over a range of shear rates lead to the estimation of RBC deformability. In the rheoscope, an deformation of individual RBCs under shear flow in a rotational de-

vice can be measured directly under microscopic observation (28). In the ektacytometer, the laser diffraction pattern gives information on the deformability of a population of cells (29); by monitoring the cell elongation as a function of the osmolarity of the medium, one can evaluate changes in the different determinants governing RBC deformability (30). Red blood cell deformability can also be studied by determining the pressure-flow relationship of RBC suspensions passed through polycarbonate filters with pore diameters ≥ 3 microns under a constant pressure (31) or a constant flow (32). Red blood cell passage is dominated by cell geometry for a pore diameter of 3 microns and by internal and membrane viscosities for a pore diameter of 7 microns (33). Polycarbonate sieves with pore diameters less than 1 micron have also been used to determine RBC membrane elasticity. The length of the protrusions induced by a small aspiration pressure on the cell surface is measured by scanning electron microscopic examination (34). Aspiration of a small segment of the RBC membrane into a micropipette can be used to investigate the viscoelastic properties of the membrane (35–37).

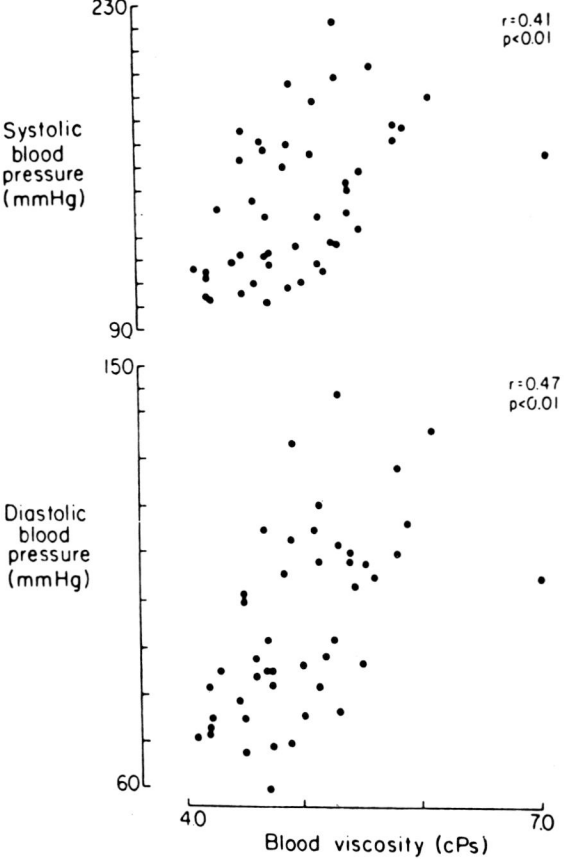

FIG. 3. Correlation between blood pressure and blood viscosity (shear rate = 0.52 sec^{-1}) in normal controls and patients with essential hypertension. At higher shear rates (52 sec^{-1}), blood viscosity is correlated with systolic and diastolic arterial pressures (n = 48) (9).

As mentioned earlier, RBC aggregation is a major determinant of blood viscosity at low shear rates. Aggregates of blood cells can cause an increase in the resistance to flow, thereby leading to microvascular occlusion. Red blood cell aggregation depends on the cell surface properties and on the composition and concentration of plasma proteins (38,39). Instruments based on optical methods have been designed to study the kinetics of RBC aggregation and the shear resistance of aggregates (40–42).

In most of the commercially available instruments, there are on-line computational facilities and automated devices.

BLOOD VISCOSITY IN HUMAN HYPERTENSION

In 1930, Harris and McLoughlin (43) reported that blood viscosity was abnormally elevated in untreated hypertensive patients. Since this early observation, several groups have reported an increase in blood viscosity for EH patients when compared to sex- and age-matched normotensive subjects (3,8,9,11,44–54). The correlation between blood viscosity and blood pressure is illustrated in Fig. 3 (9), and this has been confirmed by Zannad et al. (47). High blood viscosity can be due to an elevation of any one of the blood viscosity determinants or their

TABLE 1. *Blood rheology in hypertension*

References	Year of publication	No. studied Patients	No. studied Controls	Blood viscosity (shear rates sec⁻¹)	Plasma Viscosity	Plasma Fibrinogen	Hematocrit	RBC aggregation	RBC rigidity (method)
Tibblin et al. (8)	1966	14	11	+ (23–230)	+		+		
Chien (44)	1977	32	31	+ (0.5, 2.08)	+				+ (viscometry)
Dintenfass and Girolami (67)	1978	71	71						+ (viscometry)
Letcher et al. (9)	1981	49	49	+ (0.1–208)	+	+	+		
Palareti et al. (58)	1981	28	30	0 (23); + (230)		+	0		+ (filtration)
Freitas et al. (46)	1983						0		+ (filtration)
Letcher et al. (10)ᵇ	1983	25	25	+ (0.1–208)	+	+	+	+	
Devereux et al. (56)	1984	24	13	0 (0.5); + (140)		+	+		
Petralito et al. (65)	1985	68	30					+	
Fallo et al. (48)	1986			+	0	0			
Naftilan et al. (70)	1986								+ (filtration)
Chien (1)	1986			+	+	+	+		
Longhini et al. (11)	1986	25	20	+ (11.5–230)	+		−	+	
Leschke et al. (62)	1987	43	34	+	+	+		+	
Cherubini et al. (71)	1987	20	20						+ (filtration)
Torricelli et al. (107)	1987	15	11	0 (0.2, 94.5)					
Lorient-Roudaut et al. (49)	1987	20	20	+	0	0	0		
Levenson et al. (51)	1987	81	33	+ (0.2–240)	+		+		
Puniyani et al. (52)	1987	12	35	+ (45–225)	+		0	+	+
Zannad et al. (47)	1988	52	70	+ (0.2–128)	+	+	0	+	0 (filtration)
Chabanel et al. (60)	1991	49	35		+		0	+	
Puniyani et al. (53)	1991	37	37	+	+			+	
Razavia et al. (64)	1992	21	17	+ (240)	+	+		+	
Vaya et al. (54)	1992	21	60	+ (23–230)	+		0	+	+ (filtration)

ᵇ Borderline hypertension.
RBC, red blood cell; +, increased; −, decreased; 0, no significant difference.

combinations. We will review the abnormalities in the various blood factors which may be involved in the increased blood viscosity in human hypertension (Table 1).

Variation of Hematocrit in Hypertension

In epidemiological studies on relatively large population samples (12,16,18–20,55), it has been found that a high diastolic pressure can be correlated with elevated hematocrit or hemoglobin levels. The Framingham Study showed that subjects with a blood hemoglobin concentration over 15 g/dl for women and 16 g/dl for men subsequently developed a diastolic pressure above 90 mm Hg approximately twice as often as subjects with hemoglobin concentrations below these levels (12). An elevated hematocrit in the subjects with high blood pressure was found by several groups of investigators (see, e.g., refs. 1,8,9,51,55–57), but not by others (see, e.g., 11,46,47,49,52,53,58–60).

Some of the variabilities in results might be due to differences in the subclasses of hypertensive patients studied. When EH patients were subgrouped according to plasma renin activity in relation to the 24-hour urinary Na excretion, Chien (44) reported that, while hematocrit was elevated in high-renin patients, the low-renin patients had a decreased hematocrit, which may compensate for the elevation of plasma viscosity, resulting in an essentially normal blood viscosity. Moreover, hypertensive patients with renal failure are anemic (16), and the low hematocrit compensates for their high fibrinogen and serum globulin levels.

In twenty-five patients with borderline hypertension, the hematocrit was increased as compared to twenty-five control subjects (10). Heilman et al. (61) described a correlation between blood pressure and RBC concentration in the hypertension of preeclampsia (61).

Leakage of plasma fluid into the extravascular space under increased arterial pressure has been proposed as the main reason for the hemoconcentration in hypertension (8).

Variation of Plasma Composition and Viscosity in Hypertension

When blood viscosity was measured at constant hematocrit, hypertensive patients still had significantly higher blood viscosity than normotensive controls (9,62), indicating the participation of the other determinants of blood viscosity in its increase in hypertension.

After an extensive study of 973 men born in 1913, Tibblin et al. (8) reported an elevated total plasma protein concentration in subjects with diastolic blood pressure higher than 100 mm Hg. There was no single fraction of plasma protein which was more responsible for the elevation than any other. They also observed a significantly decreased plasma volume and increased plasma viscosity at rest in the hypertensive group, as compared to the normotensive. Exercise exacerbated the increase in plasma protein level and the decrease of plasma volume in the hypertensive group.

In subjects with established EH, plasma viscosity was significantly higher than that of controls (9,11,44,47,50–53,62–64). In ten newly diagnosed hypertensives, plasma viscosity was also increased when compared to normal subjects (52). Only two groups did not find any difference in plasma viscosity between EH patients and controls, although they did find an increased blood viscosity in hypertensives (48,49).

Letcher et al. (9) attributed the increase in plasma viscosity to the rise in fibrinogen levels (+36 percent) and also partially to an increased globulin concentration (+7 percent). A higher plasma fibrinogen level in EH patients than in normotensive controls was reported by a number of investigators (50,57,58,60,64), as well as higher total plasma protein concentrations (51,64).

In borderline hypertensive patients, plasma viscosity and fibrinogen concentration were significantly increased above the normal levels; the increases were not solely explained by hemoconcentration, since not all plasma protein concentrations were raised to the same degree (10).

Variation of Red Cell Aggregability in Hypertension

Early evaluations of RBC aggregability were deduced from viscosimetric measurements. In EH, the increase in blood viscosity was inversely related to shear rate (9,51), suggesting the involvement of RBC aggregation in the rise of blood viscosity. At low shear rates, the increase in blood viscosity ranged between 20 and 28 percent when compared with normal subjects (9,51).

By measuring erythrocyte aggregation directly, several groups confirmed the elevation in RBC aggregability in EH patients (11,47,50,60,62,64,65). Chien (44) noticed an increased tendency of RBC aggregation for the blood of hypertensive patients with high renin activity level. In twenty-one newly diagnosed hypertensives, RBC aggregability was increased when compared to normal subjects (54). In patients with borderline hypertension, RBC aggregation was enhanced (10). Petralito et al. (65) found that the degree of RBC aggregation increased progressively with the evolution of the disease. Systolic, diastolic, and mean arterial blood pressures were positively correlated with the aggregation index (47). In addition to the increased rate and extent of aggregation, the shear resistance of RBC aggregates was found to be increased in EH (60,64). These findings are of considerable interest in view of the observation that in certain areas of the circulation, *in vivo* shear stresses are lower in EH patients than in normotensive subjects (66).

Variation of RBC Deformability in Hypertension

In twenty-four EH patients with high plasma renin activity, the increase in blood viscosity was attributed, in part, to a reduced RBC deformability assessed by measuring the viscosity of suspensions of 45 percent RBCs in Ringer-albumin solution (44).

Using blood viscosity measurement, Dintenfass and Girolami (67) also deduced a decreased RBC deformability in seventy-one hypertensive patients as compared to seventy-one normotensive subjects. They explained the decrease in RBC deformability by an increased internal cellular viscosity.

By examining RBC filtration, several laboratories also concluded that there was a decreased deformability for the RBCs of the hypertensive patients (11,46,47, 49,54,57,58,68–71). In twenty-one newly diagnosed hypertensives, RBC filterability was decreased when compared to normal subjects (54).

In fifty-three patients with borderline hypertension, Hossman et al. observed a significant impairment of erythrocyte filterability (72).

Essential hypertension has been associated with various functional abnormalities of RBCs in humans and animals. Calcium binding (73,74) and lipid fluidity are altered in human hypertensive patients (73). As a result of alterations in cellular sodium transport systems (11,75), the sodium content is elevated in RBCs (76), promoting calcium entry (77) and resulting in elevated free-calcium concentration (78) in patients with EH. In hypertensive patients, high cytosolic calcium concentration values were associated with a reduced RBC deformability (78). Huai-yong et al. (79) found that erythrocyte membrane Ca^{2+}-Mg^{2+}-adenosinetriphosphatase (ATPase) activity was lower in children with a family history of EH compared with children with no such family history. These perturbations might change the physical state and mechanical properties of the RBC membrane, thereby affecting RBC deformability (11) and aggregation.

Hemorheological Profile in Malignant Hypertension and in Diseases Associated With Hypertension

Isles et al. (80) addressed the question whether the hemorheological disturbances reported in hypertension were amplified in malignant hypertension. They compared two groups of eighteen subjects with either malignant or nonmalignant hypertension and a group of eighteen matched healthy subjects. They concluded that blood rheological abnormalities in malignant hypertensive patients were not different from nonmalignant hypertensives having similar levels of blood pressure. However, when EH was associated with a cardiovascular disorder such as coronary artery disease, higher levels of plasma viscosity and fibrinogen were found than in patients with EH and normal coronary arteries (62).

The hemorrheological disturbances observed in various diseases are enhanced in the presence of hypertension. This situation has been observed in diabetes (60,81), obesity (82), hypertriglyceridemia (83), and cerebrovascular disorders (60).

Blood Viscosity and Plasma Renin Profile

Patients with EH can be classified according to their plasma renin activity normalized for 24-hour urinary Na excretion. A high plasma renin activity is associated with a higher risk for vascular injury (84). Chien (1,44) reported that, in EH, the increases in blood viscosity and in the components of blood viscosity were greatest for the patients with the highest plasma renin activity. The dependency on the renin profile is already seen in the borderline hypertensive patients before the full establishment of hypertension.

VASCULAR RESPONSE TO INCREASED BLOOD VISCOSITY

According to Folkow (7), there is a functional autoregulatory vasoconstriction as the first and immediate line of defense for keeping flow normal in spite of a rise in blood pressure. *In vitro* blood viscosity measurements can be correlated with *in vivo* measurements of circulatory dynamics (85) and body fluid volumes (86). The determination of the pressure-flow relationship *in vivo* allows the calculation of flow resistance which will, in turn, give information on vascular hindrance (resistance/blood viscosity) if blood viscosity is measured.

Chien (1) studied *in vivo* hemodynamic functions in two groups of EH patients with different degrees of severity. The first group of patients had a relatively mild hypertension (average mean arterial pressure 105 mm Hg). The blood viscosity in these patients was elevated and the vascular hindrance was approximately 10 percent lower than controls. Their cardiac index (stroke volume index × heart rate) increased in proportion to the arterial pressure. Therefore, the elevation in blood pressure in these patients was associated with increases in CO and blood viscosity, whereas the total peripheral resistance decreased. It was proposed that in these mild hypertensive subjects, a compensatory vasodilation prevents the pressure from going higher (1). In the second group, the

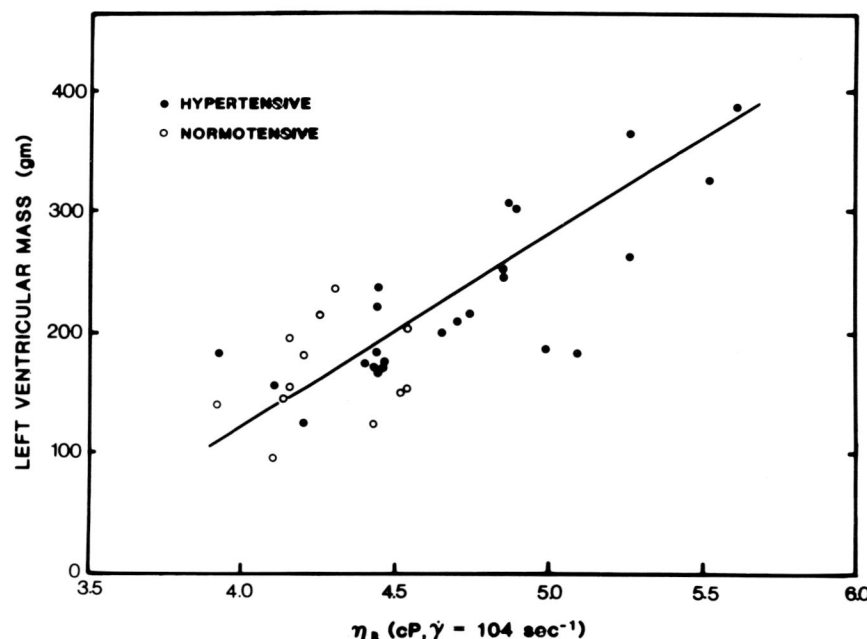

FIG. 4. Correlation between left ventricular mass and blood viscosity (h_b) at a shear rate of 104 sec^{-1} in 24 hypertensive patients (*dots*) and 13 normotensive subjects (*open circles*). The coefficient of correlation is 0.80. (Modified from ref. 56.)

patients had a higher level of hypertension (mean arterial pressure 122 mm Hg). Blood viscosity increased in parallel to total peripheral resistance, indicating that the systemic vascular hindrance was not altered in these patients with moderate (rather than mild) hypertension. These findings suggest that, as the severity of hypertension progresses from being mild to moderate, the patients lose the ability for compensatory vasodilation.

BLOOD VISCOSITY AND COMPLICATIONS OF HYPERTENSION

Attempts to correlate the left ventricular mass with various hemodynamic parameters such as arterial pressure, CO, and cardiac work, have yielded coefficients of correlation less than 0.6 (56). In twenty-four patients with EH, Devereux et al. (56) found a strong correlation between blood viscosity and left ventricular mass (r = 0.80, $p < 0.001$) (Fig. 4). Furthermore, hypertensive patients with normal blood viscosity had normal left ventricular mass despite having elevated blood pressure. The correlation between blood viscosity and left ventricular mass was confirmed by another laboratory in addition to a significant correlation with the RBC aggregation index (47). In another study, however, left ventricular hypertrophy was best correlated with plasma viscosity (50).

In hypertensive patients without coronary artery disease, those with a low coronary reserve had a significantly elevated hematocrit and plasma viscosity when compared to normotensive controls, whereas those with a higher coronary reserve did not manifest any rheological alternation. Moreover, there was a clear correlation

between the reduction of coronary reserve and the amount of rheological abnormalities in hypertensive patients (63). The possible involvement of blood rheology alternations in the reduction of the capacity of coronary regulation is supported by the clinical finding that plasmapheresis in patients with multiple myeloma improved coronary reserve in parallel to the reduction in plasma viscosity (67).

Although one cannot draw conclusions on causal relationship from correlation, these results suggest the possibility that high blood viscosity in hypertension may constitute a potentiating factor for ventricular hypertrophy and/or reduction of coronary vascular reserve.

BLOOD RHEOLOGY IN ANIMAL MODELS OF ESSENTIAL HYPERTENSION

The spontaneously hypertensive rat (SHR) is hemodynamically similar, in many respects, to the human essential hypertensive patients, and SHR has become the animal model of choice (88,89). Similar abnormalities in RBC membrane calcium binding and in lipid fluidity are shared by human essential hypertensives and SHRs (74,90–92). In rats with hypertension induced by deoxycorticosterone or renal factors, there was no alteration of RBC membrane structure or function (91).

Two groups have shown that SHRs suffer from blood hyperviscosity (93,94). It appeared that the elevated hematocrit value was not the only cause for the high blood viscosity (93).

With the use of the micropipette technique, Chabanel et al. (95) found a significant increase of RBC membrane rigidity in young SHRs during the developmental phase of hypertension (3–5 weeks). After the establishment of the hypertension (7–8 weeks), however, the deformability of the RBC membrane of SHRs improved and became comparable to that of the Wistar-Kyoto (WKY) controls. An abnormal RBC membrane deformability, by contributing to an increase in flow resistance, could be a cause of the initial increase in blood pressure. The later recovery of RBC membrane elasticity after 7 weeks of age might reflect an adaptive process.

Animal models of EH have been used to examine the effects of therapy. The decrease in blood viscosity resulting from isovolemic hemodilution was associated with a significant reduction of high blood pressure in SHRs (94). De Clerck et al. (96) showed a drop in blood pressure correlated with a parallel fall in whole blood viscosity in hypertensive dogs treated with ketanserin. In hypertensive rats, heparin was shown to lower blood pressure and to decrease the hematocrit (97). The possibility exists that heparin decreased blood pressure by reducing blood viscosity (97).

EXPERIMENTAL MANIPULATIONS OF BLOOD RHEOLOGY AND THEIR EFFECTS ON BLOOD PRESSURE

Experiments have been performed on SHRs to study the hemodynamic effects of manipulating blood viscosity (98). The hematocrit was chronically reduced by bleeding or by heparin injection, and the blood pressure was shown to fall in parallel to the hematocrit. When the heparin-treated SHRs were subjected to a transfusion of packed RBCs, the decreases in hematocrit and in blood pressure were both prevented. These experiments suggest that a drop in blood viscosity, as a consequence of a decreased hematocrit, leads to a reduction in arterial pressure. In conscious sheep, the elevation of blood viscosity, induced by RBC transfusion, caused the development of left ventricular hypertrophy (99).

Studies on dogs have shown that elevations of hematocrit or colloid concentrations can stimulate renin release (100,101). Simchon et al. (102) studied the effect of alteration in apparent blood viscosity on renal hemodynamics in anesthetized dogs. Blood viscosity was isovolemically altered either by transfusion of RBCs or by dextran administration. The hyperviscosity of blood was associated with a decrease of renal vascular hindrance. Thus, a compensatory renal vasodilation occurred as a result of increased blood viscosity. Moreover, plasma renin activity increased and was strongly correlated with renal hindrance. These results have been interpreted to suggest that the increase in plasma renin activity associated with experimental hyperviscosity (due to moderate hemoconcentration and dextran administration) is a response to the autoregulatory renal vasodilation.

MEDICATION IN HYPERTENSION: EFFECTS ON BLOOD VISCOSITY

Hypertensive patients with impaired renal function have been successfully treated by plasmapheresis. The decrease in plasma renin activity and the improvement in renal function have been interpreted as the result of improved microcirculation due to a reduced blood viscosity (103). On the other hand, acute hypervolemic hemodilution produced by saline infusion did not reduce high blood pressure in thirteen men with primary hypertension. Reduction in hematocrit, and hence improved blood rheology, did not affect calculated vascular resistance, indicating that vasoconstriction might have counteracted the possibly beneficial effect of change in viscosity (104).

In patients with EH, treatment with the alpha blocker prazosin induced a reduction in blood viscosity (105). The decrease in blood viscosity showed a significant correlation with the diminution of blood pressure. The hematocrit was found to change in parallel to the blood viscosity. Frohlich et al. (106) reviewed the hemodynamic effect of alpha-adrenergic receptor agonist compounds. The reduction in arterial pressure elicited by these drugs was reported to be accompanied by an expansion in plasma volume that was associated with a decreased blood viscosity and hematocrit.

Several beta blockers have been tested for their effect on hemorrheological parameters. In vivo, atenolol has been shown to improve blood viscosity at low and high shear rates without modifying the levels of hematocrit and fibrinogen in EH patients, while chlorthalidone had no such effects (107). An in vivo study of alprenolol indicated that it reduces blood viscosity in hypertensive patients (108). Timolol maleate also induced a significant decrease in blood viscosity (108a). Carvedilol, a beta blocker with a vasodilating action, improved RBC deformability and aggregability, decreased plasma viscosity, but did not change the hematocrit value, after 4 and 8 weeks of treatment (109). On the other hand, oxprenolol hydrochloride, which does lower the blood pressure, does not cause a decrease in blood viscosity (121).

Ketanserin, a serotonin antagonist, has been shown to lower blood pressure in hypertensive patients (110). This effect was assumed to be the consequence of the vasodilator properties of ketanserin. However, acute administration of ketanserin has been shown to decrease whole blood viscosity at high and low shear rates (111) and to improve RBC filterability in hypertensive subjects (112,113), indicating that the drug might also act through a beneficial effect on blood rheology. Waal-Manning et al. (114) tested the chronic effect of the drug and confirmed its beneficial effect on blood cell deformability. The ouabain-induced deterioration of RBC deformability was prevented by a single dose of 60 mg of ketanserin. This finding has led De Cree et al. (115) to propose that the beneficial effect of ketanserin in hypertension might be related to a regulation of the sodium content of RBCs.

The effect of calcium antagonists on blood viscosity has been studied by several groups. For twenty-one untreated patients with EH, the intravenous injection of nicardipine resulted in the lowering of plasma and blood viscosities (116). In an open study including forty patients, the effects of nifedipine (Adalat, Procardia), verapamil hydrochloride, and diltiazem hydrochloride (Cardizem) on RBC deformability were tested. There was no significant change in the RBC filtration time for any of these drugs when compared to the group taking no drug (117). Felodipine did not improve blood rheology over a 2-week treatment period (118). Isradipine, administered for 6 to 12 weeks, caused an improvement in the hemodynamics without a reduction in blood viscosity or modification of hematocrit, fibrinogen (57,59), or plasma viscosity (59), but with a restoration of whole blood filterability (57).

Ernst and Matrai (119) found an increased mortality in hypertensives treated with diuretics. Palareti et al. (58) and Koenig et al. (118) noted that diuretics induced a worsening of rheological parameters and that this was prevented by beta blockers (58).

Two groups showed that, in polycythemic patients with EH, treatment with alpha-methyldopa induced a plasma volume expansion which, in turn, led to decreases in hematocrit, plasma protein concentration, and blood viscosity (3,120).

Among the various types of antihypertensive drugs, those with an action to concurrently improve blood rheological parameters (e.g., alpha blockers, beta blockers, ketanserin) might be more suitable than those which simultaneously increase blood viscosity (e.g., diuretics).

CONCLUSIONS

The general consensus is that blood viscosity is elevated in human EH and that there is a direct correlation between blood pressure and blood viscosity. Elevated hematocrit and plasma viscosity seem to be responsible for the increased blood viscosity at high shear rates, whereas enhanced cell aggregation, increased plasma viscosity, and elevated hematocrit are the basis for the increased blood viscosity at low shear rates (1). An increased RBC rigidity could also be an initiating factor for the rise of blood pressure (11,72,95,121).

Some of these rheological changes might be the consequences of hypertension: for example, leakage of plasma fluid into the extravascular space under increased arterial pressure may be the main reason for the hemoconcentration. Elevated catecholamine and other humoral changes in hypertension could result in a chronic phase

protein reaction with raised fibrinogen level, leading to increased plasma viscosity and RBC aggregation.

On the other hand, the high blood viscosity may represent an etiologic pathway and a risk factor in hypertensive disorders. Elevated blood viscosity can promote and aggravate arterial hypertension due to an increase of peripheral resistance (1,122). During the development phase, before the full establishment of hypertension, there is already an increase in blood viscosity (10,11) which can be correlated with systolic and diastolic pressures (10). The hyperviscosity state in EH is associated with an unfavorable prognosis since it is correlated with the severity of the disease, as well as its complications, including left ventricular hypertrophy (47,50,56) and reduction of coronary reserve (63).

Evidence is accumulating that rheological factors play a role in the pathogenesis of hypertension and there lies the possibility that therapeutic procedures to decrease blood viscosity may be beneficial to the course of the disease.

REFERENCES

1. Chien S. Blood rheology in myocardial infarction and hypertension. *Biorheology* 1986;23:633–653.
2. Dintenfass L. *Blood viscosity, hyperviscosity and hyperviscosaemia.* Lancaster, Pennsylvania: MTP Press, 1985.
3. Chrysant SG, Frohlich ED, Adampoulos PN, et al. Pathophysiologic significance of stress or relative polycythemia in essential hypertension. *Am J Cardiol* 1976;37:1069–1072.
4. Chien S. Biophysical behavior of red cells in suspensions. In: Surgenor DM, ed. *The red blood cell,* vol 2, 2nd ed. New York: Academic Press, 1975;1031–1133.
5. Lund-Johansen P. The hemodynamics of essential hypertension. Vol 1. Clinical aspects of essential hypertension. In: Robertson JIS, ed. *Handbook of hypertension.* Amsterdam: Elsiever, 1983;151–173.
6. Frohlich ED. Hemodynamic consideration in clinical hypertension. *Med Clin North Am* 1987;71:803–812.
7. Folkow B. Cardiovascular structural adaptation, its role in the initiation and maintenance of primary hypertension. *Clin Sci* 1978;55:3s–22s.
8. Tibblin G, Bergentz SE, Bjure J, Wilhelmsen L. Hematocrit, plasma protein, plasma volume and viscosity in early hypertensive disease. *Am Heart J* 1966;72:165–176.
9. Letcher RL, Chien S, Pickering TG, Sealey JE, Laragh JH. Direct relationship between blood pressure and blood viscosity in normal and hypertensive subjects: role of fibrinogen and concentration. *Am J Med* 1981;70:1195–1202.
10. Letcher RL, Chien S, Pickering TG, Laragh JH. Elevated blood viscosity in patients with borderline essential hypertension. *Hypertension* 1983;5:757–762.
11. Longhini E, Agosti R, Cherubini P, et al. Haemorheology in hypertension. *Clin Hemorheol* 1986;6:567–576.
12. Kannel WB, Gordon R, Wolf PA, McNamara P. Haemoglobin and the risk of cerebral infarction; The Framingham Study. *Stroke* 1972;3:409–420.
13. Sorlie PD, Garcia-Palmieri MR, Costas R, Havlik RJ. Hematocrit and risk of coronary heart disease. The Puerto Rico Heart Health Program. *Am Heart J* 1981;101:456–461.
14. Carter G, McGee D, Reed D, et al. Hematocrit and the risk of coronary heart disease: the Honolulu Heart Program. *Am Heart J* 1983;105:674–679.
15. Wilhelmsen L, Svardsudd K, Korsan-Bengsten K, et al. Fibrino-

gen as a risk factor for stroke and myocardial infarction. *N Engl J Med* 1984;311:501–505.

16. Lowe GDO, Robertson J, Dunn FG, et al. Haematocrit in patients attending a hypertension clinic. *Scott Med* 1985;30:168–172.

17. De Simone G, Devereux RB, Chien S, et al. Relation of blood viscosity to demographic and physiologic variables and to cardiovascular risk factors in apparently normal adults. *Circulation* 1990;81:107–117.

18. Göbel BO, Schulte-Göbel A, Weisser B, et al. Arterial blood pressure. Correlation with erythrocyte count, hematocrit and hemoglobin concentration. *Am J Hypertens* 1991;4:14–19.

19. Smith WCS, Lowe GDO, Lee AJ, Tunstall-Pedoe H. Rheological determinants of blood pressure in a Scottish adult population. *J Hypertens* 1992;10:467–472.

20. Cirillo M, Laurenzi M, Trevisan M. Hematocrit, blood pressure and hypertension. The Gubbio population study. *Hypertension* 1992;20:319–326.

21. Chien S, Usami S, Dellenback RJ, Gregersen MI. Blood viscosity: influence of erythrocyte deformation. *Science* 1967;157:827–829.

22. Chien S. Shear dependence of effective cell volume as a determinant of blood viscosity. *Science* 1970;168:977–978.

23. Chien S. Rheology in the microcirculation in normal and low flow states. *Adv Shock Res* 1982;8:71–80.

24. Harkness J. A new instrument for the measurement of plasma viscosity. *Lancet* 1963;2:280–284.

25. Chien S, Usami S, Dellenback RJ, Bryant CA. Comparative hemorheology. Hematological implications of species differences in blood viscosity. *Biorheology* 1971;8:35–57.

26. Chien S. Principles and techniques for assessing erythrocyte deformability. *Blood Cells* 1977;3:71–99.

27. Chien S. Red cell deformability and its relevance to blood flow. *Ann Rev Physiol* 1987;49:177–192.

28. Schmid-Schönbein H, Gaehtgens P, Fisher T, Stohr LM. Biology of red cells: non-nucleated erythrocytes as fluid drop-like cell fragments. *Int J Microcirc Clin Exp* 1984;3:161–196.

29. Bessis M, Mohandas N. A diffractometric method for the measurement of cellular deformability. *Blood Cells* 1975;1:307–313.

30. Féo CJ, Noscal M, Jones E, Bessis M. Une nouvelle technique d'étude de la physiologie des globules róuges. La mesure de leur déformabilité en fonction de l'osmolarité. Résultats obtenus par un ektacytometre automatisé sur du sang normal et dans différentes anémies hémolytiques. *CR Acad Sci Paris* 1982; 295:687–691.

31. Hanss M. Erythrocyte deformability measurement by the initial flow rate method. *Biorheology* 1983;20:199–211.

32. Schmalzer EA, Skalak R, Usami S, et al. Influence of red cell concentration on filtration of blood cell suspensions. *Biorheology* 1982;20:29–40.

33. Reinhart WH, Chien S. Roles of cell geometry and cytoplasmic viscosity in red cell passage through narrow pores. *Am J Physiol* 1985;C473–C479.

34. Baker RF. Membrane deformability of metabolically depleted human red cells. *Blood Cells* 1987;7:551–556.

35. LaCelle PL, Weed RI. The contribution of normal and pathologic erythrocytes to red cell rheology. *Progr Hematol* 1971;7:1–31.

36. Evans EA, Hochmuth RM. Membrane viscoelasticity. *Biophys J* 1976;16:1–11.

37. Chien S, Sung KLP, Skalak R, et al. Theoretical and experimental studies on viscoelastic properties of red cell membrane. *Biophys J* 1978;24:463–488.

38. Goldstone J, Schmid-Schönbein H, Wells R. The rheology of red blood cell aggregates. *Microvasc Res* 1970;2:273–286.

39. Chien S, Sung LA, Simchon S, et al. Energy balance in red cell interactions. *Ann New York Acad Sci* 1983;190–206.

40. Usami S, Chien S. Optical reflectometry of red cell aggregation under shear flow. *Bibl Anat* 1973;11:91–97.

41. Schmid-Schönbein H, Volger E, Teitel P, Kiesewetter H, Daver V, Heilmann L. New hemorheological techniques for the routine laboratory. *Clin Hemorheol* 1982;2:93–105.

42. Snabre P, Bitbol M, Mills P. Cell disaggregation behavior in shear flow. *Biophys J* 1987;51:795–807.

43. Harris I, McLoughlin G. The viscosity of blood in high blood pressure. *Q J Med* 1930;23:451–464.

44. Chien S. Blood rheology in hypertension and cardiovascular diseases. *Cardiovasc Med* 1977;2:356–360.

45. Dintenfass L. *Hyperviscosity in hypertension.* New York: Pergamon Press, 1981.

46. Freitas J, Braz-Nogueira J, Nogueira da Costa J, Martins e Silva J. Whole blood filterability and blood oxygen transport in human hypertension. *Clin Hemorheol* 1983;3:367–373.

47. Zannad F, Voisin Ph, Brunotte F, et al. Haemorheological abnormalities in arterial hypertension and their relation to cardiac hyptertrophy. *J Hypertens* 1988;6:293–297.

48. Fallo F, Procidano M, de Angelis V, et al. Erythrocyte Na^+-Li^+ countertransport and blood viscosity in arterial hypertension. *Res Exp Med (Berl)* 1986;186:71–77.

49. Lorient-Roudaut MF, Roudaut R, Freyburger G, et al. Hemorheological abnormalities in essential hypertension. *Clin Hemorheol* 1987;7:537.

50. Leschke M, Motz W, Blanke H, Strauer BE. Blood rheology as a determinant of left ventricular hypertrophy in hypertension. *Clin Hemorheol* 1987;7:400.

51. Levenson J, Simon AC, Cambien A, Beretti C. Cigarette smoking and hypertension. Factors independently associated with blood hyperviscosity and arterial rigidity. *Arteriosclerosis* 1987;7:572–577.

52. Puniyani RR, Annapurna V, Chaturani P, Kale PA. Haemorheological profile in cases of hypertension. *Clin Hemorheol* 1987;7:767–772.

53. Puniyani RR, Ajmani R, Kale PA. Risk factors evaluation in some cardiovascular diseases. *J Biomed Eng* 1991;13:441–443.

54. Vaya A, Martinez M, Garcia J, Aznar J. Hemorrheological alterations in mild essential hypertension. *Thromb Res* 1992;66:223–229.

55. McDonough JR, Hames CG, Garrison GE, et al. The relationship of hematocrit to cardiovascular states of health in the negro and white population of Evans County, Georgia. *J Chron Dis* 1965;18:243–257.

56. Devereux RB, Drayer JIM, Chien S, et al. Whole blood viscosity as a determinant of cardiac hypertrophy in systemic hypertension. *Am J Cardiol* 1984;54:592–595.

57. Slonim A, Paran E, Cristal N. Effect of isradipine on factors affecting blood viscosity. *Am J Hypertens* 1991;4:172S–174S.

58. Palareti G, De Fabritiis A, Poggi M, et al. Haemorheological parameters in essential hypertension and early changes during antihypertensive treatments. *Clin Hemorrheol* 1981;1:495.

59. Wysocki M, Persson B, Bagge U, Anderson OK. Flow resistance and its components in hypertensive men treated with the calcium antagonist isradipine. *Eur J Clin Pharmacol* 1992;43:463–468.

60. Chabanel A, Slama G, Samama M. Evaluation of a technique to assess red blood cell aggregation: clinical applications and influence of hypertension. In: Stoltz JF, Donner M, Copley AL, ed. *Hémorrhéologie et agrégation érythrocytaire*, vol 3. Paris: EM Internationales, 1991;238–249.

61. Heilmann L, Siekmann U, Schmid-Schönbein H, Ludwig H. Hemoconcentration and pre-eclampsia. *Arch Gynecol* 1981;231:7–21.

62. Leschke M, Motz W, Blanke H, Strauer BE. Blood rheology in hypertension and hypertensive heart disease. *J Cardiovasc Pharmacol* 1987;10[Suppl 6]:S103–S110.

63. Leschke M, Vogt M, Motz W, Strauer BE. Blood rheology as a contributing factor in reduced coronary reserve in systemic hypertension. *Am J Cardiol* 1990;65:56G–59G.

64. Razavia SM, Del Pino M, Simon A, Levenson J. Increase in erythrocyte disaggregation shear stress in hypertension. *Hypertension* 1992;20:247–252.

65. Petralito A, Malatino LS, Fione CE. Erythrocyte aggregation in different stages of arterial hypertension. *Thromb Haemost* 1985;54:555.

66. Simon AC, Levenson J, Flaud P. Pulsatile flow and oscillating wall shear stress in the brachial artery of normotensive and hypertensive subjects. *Cardiovasc Res* 1990;24:129–136.

67. Dintenfass L, Girolami A. Rigidity of red cells in essential hypertension. *Haemostatis* 1978;7:298–302.

68. Isles C, Lowe GDO, Drummond MM, et al. Blood rheology in malignant phase hypertension. *Scand J Clin Lab Invest* 1981;41[Suppl 156]:175–176.

69. Ranieri MG, Provera FP, Bottoni P, et al. Valutazione della deformabilita eritrocitaria in sogetti con ipertensione arteriosa essentiale. *La Ricerca Clin Lab* 1983;13:401–404.

70. Naftilan AJ, Dzau VJ, Loscalzo J. Preliminary observations on abnormalities of membrane structure and function in essential hypertension. *Hypertension* 1986;8[Suppl II]; II.174–II.179.

71. Cherubini P, Bozzoni M, Agosti R, et al. Red blood cell filterability in essential hypertension: role of transmembranary ions fluxes. *Clin Hemorheol* 1990;9:89–101.

72. Hossmann V, Bönner G, Wambach G, et al. Blood viscosity: a pathogenetic factor in the development of essential hypertension? *Clin Exper Ther Pract* 1986;A8:673–680.

73. Orlov SN, Postnov YV. Calcium binding and membrane fluidity in essential and renal hypertension. *Clin Sciences* 1982;63:281–284.

74. Cirillo M, Trevisan M, Laurenzi M. Calcium binding capacity of erythrocyte membrane in human hypertension. *Hypertension* 1989;14:152–155.

75. Garay RP, Dagher G, Pernollet M-G, et al. Inherited defect in a $Na^+ K^+$-co-transport system in erythrocytes from essential hypertensive patients. *Nature* 1980;284:281–283.

76. Weder AB, Fitzpatrick MA, Toretti BA, et al. Red blood cell Li^+-Na^+ counter transport, Na^+-K^+ co-transport and the hemodynamics of hypertension. *Hypertension* 1987;9:459–466.

77. Caimi G, Serra A, Presti RL, et al. Red cell Ca^{2+} content (total and cytosolic) and erythrocyte membrane fluidity in several clinical conditions. *Clin Hemorheol* 1993;13:227–235.

78. David-Dufilho M, Astarie C, Pernollet M-G, et al. Control of the erythrocyte free Ca^{2+} concentration in essential hypertension. *Hypertension* 1992;19:167–174.

79. Huai-yong C, Li-sheng L, De-yu Z. Comparison of erythrocyte membrane Ca^{2+}-Mg^{2+}-ATPase activity in children with and without family history of essential hypertension. *J Human Hypertens* 1990;4:147–148.

80. Isles C, Lowe GD, Rankin BM, et al. Abnormal haemostasis and blood viscosity in malignant hypertension. *Thromb Haemost* 1984;52:253–255.

81. Rampling MW, Feher MD, Elkeles RS, Sever P. Haemorheological disturbances in type II diabetes are enhanced in the presence of hypertension. *Clin Hemorheol* 1987;7:518.

82. Fioravanti M, Solerte SB, Ferrari E. Arterial hypertension in essential obesity: role of blood hyperviscosity and reduced erythrocyte deformability. *Clin Hemorheol* 1987;7:494.

83. Gerlach A, Spurk P, Angelkort B. Qualitative analysis of the effects of arteriosclerosis risk factors on blood fluidity. *Clin Hemorheol* 1987;7:439.

84. Laragh JH, Baer L, Brunner HR, et al. Renin, angiotensin and aldosterone system in pathogenesis and management of hypertensive vascular disease. *Am J Med* 1972;52:633–652.

85. Frohlich ED. Clinical significances of hemodynamic findings in hypertension. *Chest* 1973;64:94–99.

86. Dustan HP, Tarazi RC, Bravo EL, Dart RA. Plasma and extracellular fluid volumes in hypertension. *Circ Res* 1973;12/13:173–183.

87. Strauer BE, Fatah-Moghadam A, Kment A, et al. Use of plasmapheresis and of immunosuppresive therapy in coronary microangiopathies. *Bibl Haematol* 1981;47:213–227.

88. Okamoto K, Aoki K. Development of a strain of spontaneously hypertensive rats. *Jpn Circ J* 1963;27:282–293.

89. Trippodo NC, Frohlich ED. Similarities of genetic (spontaneous) hypertension. Man and rat. *Circ Res* 1981;48:309–319.

90. Daveloose D, Viret J, Molle D, Leterrier F. Mise en évidence par marquage de spin d'une modification structurale de la membrane érythrocytaire du rat génétiquement hypertendu. *C R Acad Sci Paris* 1980;240[Série D]:85–88.

91. Orlov SN, Gulak PV, Litinov IS, Postnov YV. Evidence of altered structure of the erythrocyte membrane in spontaneously hypertensive rats. *Clin Sci* 1982;63:43–45.

92. Devynck MA, Pernollet M-G, Nunez A-M, Aragon I, Montenay-Garestier T, Helene C, Meyer P. Diffuse structural alterations in cell membranes of spontaneously hypertensive rats. *Proc Natl Acad Sci USA* 1982;79:5057–5060.

93. De Clerck F, Beerens M, Van Gorp L, Zhonneux R. Blood hyperviscosity in spontaneously hypertensive rats. *Thrombos Res* 1980;18:291–295.

94. Seiffge D. Hemodilution in spontaneously hypertensive rats: its effect on blood pressure and blood rheology. *Bibl Haematol* 1981;47:70–76.

95. Chabanel A, Schachter D, Chien S. Increased red cell membrane rigidity in young spontaneously hypertensive rats. *Hypertension* 1987;10:603–607.

96. De Clerck F, Jagenau A, Dom J. Haemorheological effects of ketanserin, a selective 5-hydroxytryptamine-2 receptor antagonist in aged, spontaneously hypertensive dogs. *Arch Int Pharmacodyn Ther* 1982;258:100–115.

97. Susic D, Mandal AK, Kentera D. Heparin lowers the blood pressure in hypertensive rats. *Hypertension* 1982;4:681–685.

98. Susic D, Mandall AK, Kentera D. Hemodynamic effects of chronic alternation in hematocrit in spontaneously hypertensive rat. *Hypertension* 1984;6:262–266.

99. Sakai A, Ueda G, Kobayashi T, et al. Effects of elevated-hematocrit levels on pulmonary circulation in conscious sheep. *Jpn J Physiol* 1984;34:871–884.

100. McDonald KM. Effects of hematocrit and colloid-induced changes in blood viscosity on renal hemodynamics and renin release in the dog. *Circ Res* 1974;34:112–122.

101. Hall JE, Guyton AC. Changes in renal hemodynamics and renin release caused by increased plasma oncotic pressure. *Am J Physiol* 1976;231:1550–1556.

102. Simchon S, Chen YZ, Carlin RD, et al. Effects of blood viscosity on plasma renin activity and renal hemodynamics. *Am J Physiol* 1986;250:F40–F46.

103. Glasson P. Traitement de l'hypertension artérielle par plasmaphérèse. *Schweiz med Wschr* 1983;113:189–191.

104. Wysocki M, Persson B, Aurell M, et al. Haemodynamic and haemorheological effects of hypervolaemic haemodilution in men with primary hypertension. *J Hypertens* 1987;5:185–189.

105. Letcher RL, Chien S, Laragh JH. Changes in blood viscosity accompanying the response to prazosin in patients with essential hypertension. *J Cardiovasc Pharmacol* 1979;1[Suppl]:S8–S20.

106. Frohlich ED, Messerli FH, Pegram BL, Kardon MB. Hemodynamic and cardiac effects of centrally acting antihypertensive drugs. *Hypertension* 1984;6:1176–1181.

107. Torricelli P, Palareti G, Marchetta F, et al. Atenolol, but not chlorthalidone improves haemorheology in patients with essential hypertension. *Clin Hemorheol* 1987;7:485.

108. Dintenfass L, Lake B. Beta blockers and blood viscosity. *Lancet* 1976;1:1026.

108a. Caimi G, Catania A, Frazetta F, et al. Essential hypertension: the behaviour of the haemorheological determinants and their trends during beta-blocker treatment. *Jpn Heart J* 1983;24:723–729.

109. Nagakawa Y, Akedo Y, Kaku S, Orimo H. Effects of carvedilol on common carotid arterial flow, peripheral hemodynamics, and hemorheologic variables in hypertension. *Eur J Clin Pharmacol* 1990;38:S115–S119.

110. Hedner T, Person B, Berglund G. Ketanserin: a novel 5-hydroxytryptamine antagonist: monotherapy in essential hypertension. *Br J Clin Pharmacol* 1983;16:121–125.

111. Konishi M, Sakakura M, Tsushima N. Effects of ketanserin on microhemodynamics and hemorheology in patients with essential hypertension. *Cardiovasc Drugs Ther* 1990;4:101–104.

112. Ernst E, Matrai A. Ketanserin treatment in essential hypertension. *Brit Heart J* 1984;52:359–360.

113. Zannad F, Voisin P, Pointel JP, et al. Effects of ketanserin on platelet function and red cell filterability in hypertension and peripheral disease. *J Cardiovasc Pharmacol* 1985;7:S32–S34.

114. Waal-Manning HJ, Brown SA, Spears GF, Simpson FO. Clinical studies with ketanserin in hypertension. *J Cardiovasc Pharmacol* 1985;7:S154–S158.

115. De Cree J, Leempoels J, Demoven B, Verhaegen H. Ketanserin and RBC sodium content in hypertension. *J Cardiovasc Pharmacol* 1985;7:S41–S43.

116. Zannad F, Voisin P, Sadoul N, et al. Effets de la nicardipine intraveineuse sur la pression artérielle, 'hémorhéologie et les fonctions plaquettaires dans l'hypertension artérielle. Relations dose-effet. *Arch Mal Coeur* 1987;80:844–850.

117. Lin M-S, Huang C-S, Leen D-Y. Lack of effects of calcium antagonists on red blood cell deformability in hypertension. *Int J Clin Pharmac Ther Tox* 1988;26:585–587.

118. Koenig W, Sund M, Ernst E, et al. Effects of felodipine ER and hydrochlorothiazide on blood rheology in essential hypertension. A randomized, double-blind, crossover study. *J Int Med* 1991;229:533–538.

119. Ernst E, Matrai A. Increased mortality in hypertensives treated with diuretics. A hemorheological problem? *Clin Hemorheol* 1984;4:589–590.

120. Emery AC, Whitcomb WH, Frohlich ED. Stress polycythemia and hypertension. *JAMA* 1974;229:159–162.

121. Dintenfass L. Internal viscosity of the red cell: problems associated with defibrination of plasma viscosity and effective volume of red cells in the blood viscosity equation. *Biorheology* 1975;12:253–256.

122. Chien S. Hemorheology: normal physiology and pathological changes in blood viscosity and blood flow. Pharmacological approach to the treatment of limb ischaemia. *Symp Frontiers Pharmacol* 1983;3:15–33.

Hypertension: Pathophysiology, Diagnosis, and Management, Second Edition, edited by J.H. Laragh and B.M. Brenner, Raven Press, Ltd., New York © 1995.

CHAPTER **23**

Vascular Compliance and Blood Volume in Essential Hypertension

Michel E. Safar, Gérard E. Plante, and Gérard M. London

Adequacy of the circulation is strictly dependent on the filling pressure of the vascular compartment, in particular on the filling pressure of the heart (1,2). Looking at the overall vascular system, a well-defined relationship has been documented between changes in blood volume and changes in circulatory filling pressure (1). The slope of the relationship between vascular volume and pressure defines compliance, which represents the inherent elasticity of the vascular system (1,2). Changes in vascular compliance are of critical importance in the control of cardiovascular function and extracellular fluid volume (1–3), which include the vascular space and the interstitial fluid compartment, a strategic zone of heterogeneous composition and physicochemical characteristics (4,5), in close contact with the microcirculation on one side and the cellular mass on the other.

In arterial hypertension, a number of hemodynamic abnormalities, including changes in several cardiovascular and fluid volume control mechanisms, have been described (6–10), the end result of which is a decrease in total vascular compliance, mainly that of the venous compartment (11–14). While a relatively large number of studies on the venous system have been performed in experimental models of arterial hypertension (15–17), almost no research has been done in hypertensive human subjects.

The purpose of this review is to examine the critical importance of alterations in the venous system and their hemodynamic correlates with body fluid compartments in human hypertensive subjects. We will only consider systemic capacitance function of the peripheral circulation. Data obtained on local segments of the venous system (forearm studies) will be used only when measurements of the total peripheral venous compartment is unavailable. This review will include information obtained in a large number of untreated, uncomplicated essential hypertensive patients in which the following hemodynamic parameters were obtained: cardiac output; total and cardiopulmonary blood volumes; and filling pressure of the heart. The methods used have been previously described and validated in our laboratory (11,18). Finally, reference will be made to the relationships between venous pathophysiology, interstitial fluid volume alteration, and cardiac and kidney dysfunction in arterial hypertension.

M. E. Safar: Department of Internal Medicine and INSERM U337, Hôpital Broussais, Paris, France.

G. E. Plante: Departments of Medicine, Physiology, and Pharmacology, University of Sherbrooke, Sherbrooke (Québec), Canada.

G. M. London: Division of Nephrology, Centre Hospitalier Manhes, Fleury Merogis, France.

PRESSURE-VOLUME RELATIONSHIP IN ARTERIES AND VEINS

The elastic structural component and the perivascular smooth muscle give these organs unique characteristics—resistance to stretching forces and the ability to return to original resting length after stretching—as defined by Hooke's law:

$$T = E \times \Delta L/L$$

where T is the tension developed by stretching an elastic element by a given force (F), expressed per cross-sectional area (S), giving $T = F/S$; L and ΔL represent the initial and the stretch-induced change in length; finally the term E, called Young's modulus, defines the elasticity of the stretched structure. Hooke's law has been developed to describe phenomena in longitudinal elements, and is therefore difficult to apply to anatomical structures, which resemble either pouches (lungs) or cylinders (blood vessels). For this reason, physiologists have proposed to quantify the elastic properties of anatomical structures by measuring the volume changes which result from changes in pressure capable of distending those structures (19). The distending pressure is considered to be the transmural pressure.

The slope of the curve which describes volume (abcissa) and pressure (ordinate) is called *elastance* (E'). This term is equivalent to Young's modulus, used in Hooke's law:

$$E' = \Delta P/\Delta V$$

where ΔP and ΔV represent the changes in pressure and volume, respectively. Therefore, E' is a reliable quantitative evaluation of anatomical structure elasticity. Nevertheless, most physiologists define the elastic behavior of tissues in terms of compliance (C), which is the reciprocal of elastance:

$$C = \Delta V/\Delta P$$

However, in most anatomical structures, the pressure-volume relationship cannot be extrapolated to zero, and the intercept of that curve (assuming a linear model) must be defined as:

$$C = (V - V0)/(P - 0)$$

where $V0$ is the unstressed volume, [e.g., the volume contained within the compliant structure when the transmural pressure (P) is zero (0)] and V is the volume contained in the vascular structure when the transmural pressure is P. All units for measuring compliance are expressed in mL/mm Hg or in mL/kg/mm Hg. Under such conditions, it is clear that compliance expresses the inherent elasticity of the anatomical structures studied.

TOTAL VASCULAR COMPLIANCE IN EXPERIMENTAL STUDIES

In cardiovascular physiology, compliance is defined as the relationship between changes in the vascular volume and blood pressure. Over a wide range of values, this relationship is nonlinear. However, for a limited range of volume and pressure measurements, a linear curve can be approximated to define compliance (20). In a closed model of the circulation, what is being measured represents total vascular compliance, and includes the sum of individual compliance values of all segments of the circulation, from the large arteries to the central veins (19,20). In experimental animals, total vascular compliance is obtained from the determination of the curve relating mean circulatory filling pressure ($MCFP$) to blood volume (V). MCFP refers to the pressure level that would develop over the entire circulation, should the heart be stopped suddenly, and the vascular volume redistributed within the vascular compartment according to the capacity of blood vessels (2,21). Total vascular compliance (TVC) can therefore be calculated from the change in blood pressure and the change in MCFP, as follows:

$$TVC = (V - V0)/(MCFP - 0) \quad \text{or} \quad TVC = \Delta V/\Delta MCFP$$

where V is the blood volume and $V0$ is the unstressed blood volume, defined as V contained in the vascular system when $MCFP$ is equal to zero.

According to this definition, it becomes clear that the functional capacity of the circulatory system is determined by vascular compliance and unstressed volume. It is important to recognize these two distinct parameters. When a given change in blood volume passively dilates or shrinks the vascular system, the resulting alteration in pressure is determined only by compliance. When the vascular tone is modified, the pressure resulting from the change in volume depends upon both unstressed volume and compliance. Classical estimation of MCFP requires that the systemic flow is stopped. To obviate this methodological constraint, different methods have been developed to measure vascular compliance. Instead of measuring MCFP, determination of the central venous pressure (CVP) has been proposed (11,20,22,23). Under such conditions, it has been well established that CVP gives values that are very close to MCFP.

Compliance of the smallest body fluid volume, the vascular compartment, has been examined, and includes both the arterial and the venous components. Studies performed in dogs revealed compliance values ranging between 1.4 and 4.2 mL/kg/mm Hg, with an average of 2.57 mL/kg/mm Hg (2,19,20,23–25) for the venous system, whereas for the arterial component of the circulation, compliance values averaged 0.067 mL/kg/mm Hg (19), which represents a very small portion (1–3 percent) of the total vascular compliance. Therefore, it is reasonable to use the total vascular compliance as a reliable index of that critical parameter, the venous system. The total vascular compliance is then taken as the summation of values obtained in both the peripheral and the cardiopulmonary veins. In the latter system, compliance values are much lower than in the peripheral venous system, in the order of 0.213–0.627 mL/kg/mm Hg (26,27). Since veins are able to hold relatively large volumes of fluid for small changes in pressure, they are currently called *capacitance vessels,* and considered as a blood reservoir connected in series with the heart. Consequently, MCFP, the characteristic pressure in this reservoir, represents the upstream pressure for venous return, which depends essentially upon the two dominant characteristics of capacitance vessels: the compliance and the vascular volume.

EFFECTIVE VASCULAR COMPLIANCE IN NORMAL HUMANS

In human subjects, MCFP cannot readily be measured, therefore another hemodynamic parameter has to be chosen and utilized. Studies in experimental animals and in humans revealed that blood volume changes and pressure values, measured in different segments of the venous circulation, are well correlated under conditions of free flow. Pressure values are usually obtained from the central veins or from the right atrium. The slope of the correlation between CVP and V ($\Delta V/\Delta CVP$) under these circumstances is equivalent to compliance (mL/mm Hg). In order to differentiate the $\Delta V/\Delta CVP$ from that obtained using MCFP, the former parameter is identified as the *effective* total vascular compliance.

This distinction is important and necessary, since CVP is not exclusively dependent upon blood volume and elastic properties of the vascular bed. In fact, the right atrial pressure is not only determined by the venous flow, but also by the pumping ability of the heart itself (2). Therefore, CVP becomes a valid measure of blood volume, or compliance, only if the heart dynamics are normal. Changes in cardiac output induced by acute volume expansion, for instance, exert only minimal effect on the right atrial pressure and compliance measurements unless cardiac output is associated with neurohumoral effects on the venous tone (20,22). In addition, to avoid any time-dependent variations in compliance and to minimize extravasation from the vascular volume to the interstitial space of the marker utilized to measure plasma volume (28), all samples and parameter measures must be performed very quickly—within 3 minutes (22). Even under these ideal conditions, CVP is not exactly equivalent to MCFP. Nevertheless, the latter parameter can be computed from the CVP and the flow-related pressure drop along the veins. During blood volume changes, the pressure along the venous system varies in parallel (20,23), but it appears that the gradient for venous return to the heart changes simultaneously (23,25). Appropriate corrections for CVP must be done, therefore, for changes in pressure drop (16). Finally, CVP alterations activate various neural reflex mechanisms which, in turn, may influence mechanical properties of the blood vessels, and likely the appropriate evaluation of compliance (22,23). For all the above-mentioned reasons, it becomes evident that only the *effective* compliance is available for measurement in human subjects.

Total effective vascular compliance has easily been determined in normal human subjects by recording the changes in right atrial pressure (CVP) induced by acute blood retransfusion (11,23). Several studies revealed that the effective total vascular compliance under these circumstances ranges between 2.1–2.7 mL/kg, and behaves as a genuine biological constant (11,23,26,27,29). As stated above for the dog, total effective vascular compliance is the arithmetic sum of the arterial, which is very low in man (0.034 mL/kg/mm Hg, or 1–3 percent) (30), and the venous compliance value, which accounts for 97–98 percent of the total compliance. More direct evaluation of the intrathoracic compliance gave a value of 0.45 mL/kg/mm Hg (31), i.e., approximately 20 percent of the total compliance. These data obtained in human subjects are close to those reported in animal studies (26,27).

COMPLIANCE OF EXTRAVASCULAR FLUID COMPARTMENTS

The concept of vascular compliance, which so well suits peripheral hemodynamics physiology, has not been extended to the behavior of the other two body fluid compartments, the interstitium and the intracellular volume, quantitatively much more important than the vascular, since they together represent approximately 55 percent of the total body weight (32). Similarly, the role of endothelial permeability which plays a critical role (33), in association with capillary Starling physical forces (34) in determining the net transfer of fluid and solutes in the interstitium, has not been extensively examined either. Finally, the contribution of plasma membrane of the cellular mass (specific for each organ), which controls the passage of fluid and solutes between the interstitium and the intracellular milieu (35), has not received more attention since the sprint given in that direction by deWardener and his group (36).

A brief discussion on that matter is necessary at this point to understand the main subject of this paper, since changes in interstitial and/or cellular volume compliance may be associated with alterations in the volume and compliance of the venous reservoir. First, regional capillary permeability is determined by two physiological parameters, modulated by a large number of autacoids and hormones: pre- and postcapillary resistances (37), and endothelial cell permeability (an active process which requires activation of the cytoskeleton and dysfunction of cell-cell attachments) (38). Second, voloregulation of the cell mass is under the control of several pump and channel systems (39), including the sodium-potassium adenosine triphosphatase (ATPase) (40), the sodium-calcium (41) and the sodium-hydrogen (42) exchangers, and the sodium-potassium-chloride cotransporter (43), also under the control of several endogenous autacoids and hormones (44). Taking into consideration the number and interactions of the control systems involved in the regional microcirculation, as well as the voloregulation of the cell mass and the critical role these two important fluid compartments have on the vascular system, it becomes evident that the venous volume and compliance characteristics, under normal conditions, are the result of complex and delicate physiological interactions.

VASCULAR VOLUME AND COMPLIANCE IN HYPERTENSION

In patients with uncomplicated essential hypertension, total effective vascular compliance is reduced by approximately 30 percent, when compared to normal subjects of similar age and sex, as shown in Table 1 (11,18). For a given rise in extracellular volume, the elevation in CVP is higher in the patients when compared to matched controls. This reduction in compliance is due to a decrease in systemic vessel capacitance, not to a defect in the thoracic vascular bed (31). As shown in experimental animal studies (45,46), the findings reported in the hypertensive subjects are related to a reduced distensibility of the extrathoracic venous compartment (12).

Since the capacitance system holds approximately 80 percent of the vascular volume (17,23), measurement of the latter represents a reasonable estimate of that amount of fluid contained in the reservoir vessels. Moreover, since this blood volume is mainly distributed between two major areas, the thoracic and the extrathoracic, adequate estimation of the former is a prerequisite for understanding the complex relationship between vascular compliance and volume in hypertensive patients.

Values of total blood volume obtained in hypertensive individuals are compared to those of normal matched controls and shown in Table 2. The controversy existing about the question of total blood and plasma volumes being increased, normal, or decreased, in patients with essential hypertension, is critical and must be discussed at this point. In fact, even if most investigators have reported that the blood volume of such patients is reduced (47), we feel that a critical point of methodology is to be clarified. First, the dilution technique utilized in most reported studies, using either radioactive albumin or Evans blue dye, overestimates the blood volume (47) because hypertension is associated with a uniform extravasation of plasma from the vascular space to the interstitium (48,49). Second, the frame of reference to express blood volume measurements is inadequate. The best reference parameter to report blood volume is the body surface area, according to a new mathematical approach described by Chau and co-workers (50). When expressed in terms of body height, blood volume can also be overestimated (47) because most hypertensive patients are overweight, while underestimation may occur if blood volume is expressed in terms of body weight. Nevertheless, these limitations being considered, it appears that the vascular volume is significantly reduced in patients with uncomplicated essential hypertension, even in those with obesity: in 150 hypertensive patients compared to 50 age-matched controls, blood volume was found to be reduced by approximately 25 percent (2,274 vs. 2,953 mL/m^2 body surface area, respectively), as shown in Table 2 and Fig. 1.

Interestingly, despite the significant reduction observed in the total blood volume of hypertensive patients, the arterial component of the vascular system is increased: the diameter of the thoracic aorta and that of

TABLE 1. *Different values of compliance in controls and hypertensive men*[a]

Compliance	Controls	Sustained essential hypertensive patients	Reference
Total effective vascular compliance (mL/mm Hg/kg)	2.08 ± 0.09	1.49 ± 0.06***	11,12,13,18,68
Cardiopulmonary effective vascular compliance (mL/mm Hg/kg)	0.45 ± 0.03	0.45 ± 0.06	31,54
Arterial compliance (mL/mm Hg/kg)	0.044 ± 0.004	0.025 ± 0.0019***	30
Left ventricular compliance (mL/mm Hg.10)	0.07 ± 0.16	0.014 ± 0.10***	51,68

[a] Normalization of left ventricular compliance could not be obtained in the literature.

TABLE 2. *Fluid volumes in healthy and hypertensive men*

	Healthy		Hypertensive	
EFV (mL/m²)	5528	± 102	5603	± 79
PV (mL/m²)	1628	± 23	1524	± 20**
PV/IF (%)	40.7 ±	1.2	36.0 ±	0.7**
TBV (mL/m²)	3039	± 45	2784	± 42**
CPBV (mL/m²)	668	± 17	655	± 21
CPBV/TBV (%)	22.1 ±	0.5	23.6 ±	0.8

From refs. 6,7,47,50,59,60,84.
Values are mean ± standard error of the mean.
** *p* < 0.01.
EFV, extracellular fluid volume; PV, plasma volume; PV/IF, plasma volume on interstitial fluid volume ratio; TBV, total blood volume; CPBV, cardiopulmonary blood volume.

several peripheral arteries is significantly augmented (51). On the other hand, the cardiopulmonary blood volume (CPBV) being strictly normal in hypertensive patients, as shown in Table 3, it becomes evident that the reduction in the total blood volume measured in those patients is entirely accounted for by a marked reduction in the extrathoracic venous compartment. These findings further indicate that the ratio between intrathoracic and total blood volumes (CPBV/V) is increased in essential hypertension (11,52,53). This pathophysiological situation should trigger, and/or perhaps downregulate, the cardiopulmonary mechanoreceptor system under baseline conditions, as well as during volume expansion. In fact, during the latter situation, CPBV increases more in hypertensive than in normal subjects (54), resulting in a higher stretch of cardiac mechanoreceptors. As a consequence of the latter pathophysiological phenomenon, increased secretion of the atrial natriuretic peptide could well develop (55). In addition to its vasodilatory properties (56) and its diuretic and natriuretic effects (57), this peptide increases capillary permeability and promotes plasma extravasation into the interstitium (58). The latter vascular effect could therefore further aggravate the reduction in the extrathoracic venous volume, potentially affecting the compliance of the interstitial space, and creating a mostly vicious circle.

Control mechanisms of the vascular volume are not oriented toward the maintenance of a rigid fixed volume. On the contrary, the net effect resulting from activation of these mechanisms is the control of blood volume relative to the holding capacity of the vascular space. For a long time, the finding of an inverse correlation between blood or plasma volumes and blood pressure (or total peripheral resistance), was taken as an argument to support the view that the blood volume is rigidly maintained by a primary disturbance of volume regulation in essential hypertension. In addition, this view was used to classify essential hypertensive patients into hypovolemic or hypervolemic artificial subgroups (7,14,59,60). From a pathophysiological point of view, the blood volume–peripheral resistance correlation cannot provide an acceptable basis for the evaluation of circulatory "fullness," or in other words, the control of blood volume relative to the holding capacity of the vascular space. Arterial pressure and peripheral resistance are hemodynamic parameters entirely related to the high pressure system whose function is almost uniquely "resistive." The compliance of this portion of the vascular system is quite low and its capacitance role very limited (2,19,23). It is the low-pressure, post-capillary extrathoracic venous system that plays the role of the circulatory reservoir function (2,17,21). A more appropriate way to classify essential hypertensive patients should be based on the relationship between blood volume and the mechanical properties of the capacitance low-pressure system. Thus, blood volume should be examined as a function of the total vascular compliance. In normal individuals, a positive correlation is obtained between vascular volume and total vascular compliance. Those with a high vascular compliance value have a tendency to show a higher blood volume, and vice versa (12,53). This trend also applies to hypertensive patients, but in a more attenuated fashion. However, when the entire population of control and hypertensive subjects is examined together, the correlation obtained is dramatic, as illustrated in Fig. 2: blood volume and total vascular compliance are positively correlated to a single regression curve, and the hy-

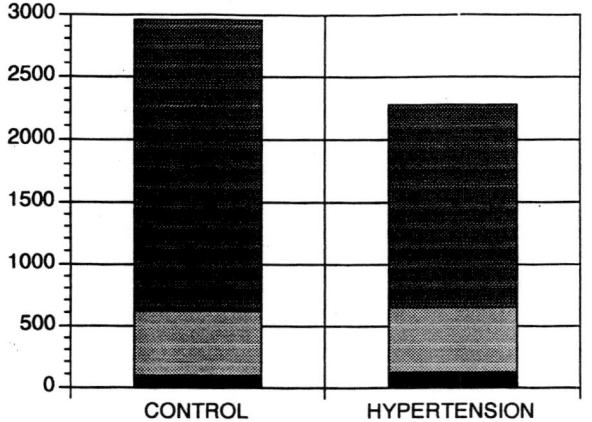

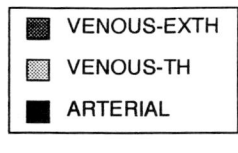

Values in ml/m2

Safar et al. Personal Data

FIG. 1. Intravascular volumes (mL/m² of body surface area) obtained in control and hypertensive subjects: arterial, venous extrathoracic (venous-exth) and thoracic (venous-th).

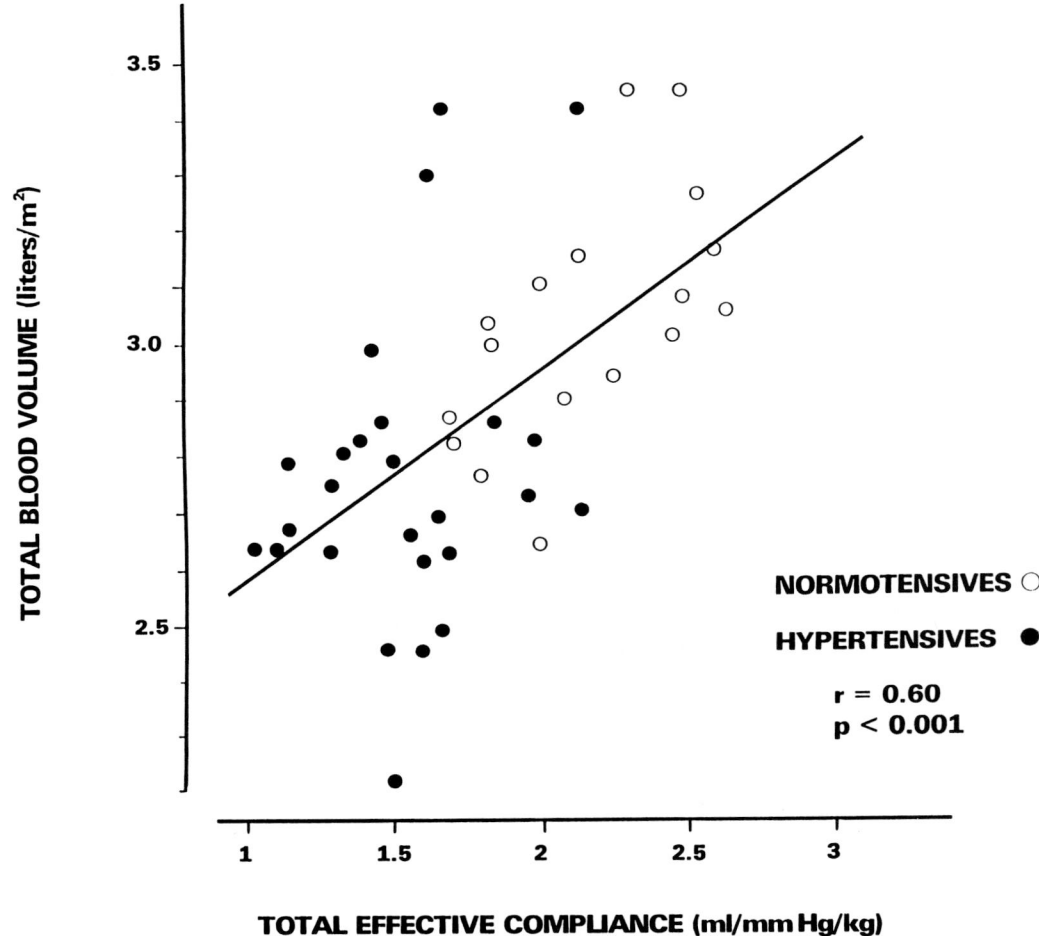

FIG. 2. Relationship between total effective compliance and total blood volume in normotensive and hypertensive subjects.

pertensive population is then neither hypovolemic nor hypervolemic. Intravascular volume is reduced in patients with essential hypertension. However, from a hemodynamic point of view, the circulatory fullness is normal, or even increased, as will be discussed in further details below.

EXTRAVASCULAR COMPLIANCE IN HYPERTENSION

The reduction in absolute blood volume and the decrement in extrathoracic venous compliance, well documented in the essential hypertensive patient (11,18,47), could be explained by either a structural and/or a functional defect in the capacity of the large extrathoracic venous reservoir to dilate, or by increased external pressure on this venous system due to primary extravasation of fluid and solutes (in particular macromolecules such as albumin) in the interstitial space—which is, in itself, of

limited compliance, as is the cellular volume (39), especially in organs tightly enveloped by serosa (such as the skeletal muscle) or capsules (such as the kidney, liver, and spleen) (61). Extravasation of fluid in the interstitium of such organs, with limited capacity to expand and which contain a significant fraction of total body fluid (32), would then be associated with increased interstitial hydrostatic pressure (62). As a consequence, it is likely that all surrounding structures would be affected by such compressive forces, including the low-pressure venous compartment of the circulation.

The notion of increased capillary permeability leading to plasma leakage into the interstitium in hypertension is not a new finding. In fact, it has been documented previously but attributed in these studies to the nonspecific effect of high blood pressure per se (48,49). In contrast, the possibility of a primary dysfunction of capillary permeability in essential hypertension, leading to abnormal distribution of body fluid volumes, alteration of venous compliance, and finally, arterial hypertension, appears more attractive and is supported in fact by the following observation. In the spontaneously hypertensive rat model, we documented a selective enhanced extravasation of albumin in the kidney before the appearance of hypertension, ruling out the nonspecific effect of elevated pressure on capillary permeability (63). Complementary data obtained from these studies revealed that this permeability defect could be reversed by B2 bradykinin receptor blockade (64). The suggestion that the kidney might be the site of a primary dysfunction leading to hypertension is a renal physiologist's dream which originated with the pioneer work of Guyton and co-workers (2,21), and has been revigorated from time to time (as a pertinent example, see the interesting paper by Lucas and Floyer (65). In a model of renoprival hypertension, these authors have demonstrated that the vascular/interstitial volume ratio was diminished, suggesting a net transfer of fluid toward the interstitium. They attributed this defect to the absence of renal tissue, suggesting that a humoral factor produced by the kidney might have been responsible for this unique finding.

CARDIAC OUTPUT, FILLING PRESSURE, VENOUS COMPLIANCE

In human studies, the right atrial pressure (CVP) represents the most accurate estimation of circulatory filling. There is a concensus in the literature supporting the fact that right atrial pressure is slightly but consistently elevated in patients with sustained essential hypertension, even in the absence of congestive heart failure (53,54,66). In parallel to this finding, increased pulmonary arterial and wedge pressures were also reported (54,66). The pressure gradient across the pulmonary circulation is identical in hypertensive and control subjects, as is the total pulmonary resistance. Furthermore, arterial, right atrial, pulmonary, and wedge pressure values are all correlated with each other (54,66). The right atrial pressure is influenced by parameters which regulate both the venous return and the pumping ability of the right ventricle (2). Theoretically, elevation of the CVP in hypertension could result from three possibilities: a reduction in the pump function, a decreased vascular compliance, or a majorated blood volume.

The adjustment of stroke volume to blood inflow is described as the Frank-Starling "law of the heart." It is expressed in terms of cardiac function curves by plotting stroke volume against right atrial pressure (2). In patients with essential hypertension, right cardiac function curves exhibit a rightward shift, of otherwise normally shaped curves (12,31). The pump operates normally but at a higher basic pressure level. The increased basic pressure level might theoretically be a passive consequence of heart hypertrophy, and result from a backward effect of elevated arterial pressure (66). However, such a passive phenomenon is unlikely to be the main factor responsible for elevation of venous pressure in hypertension. Cardiopulmonary and thoracic low-pressure systems are compliant and, as such, increase their volume whenever exposed to increased pressure. Nevertheless, an elevation of CVP is observed in patients with essential hypertension, yet cardiopulmonary and total blood volumes are normal and decreased, respectively. Therefore, only a decrement in venous compliance would satisfactorily explain the change in right atrial pressure. Several findings obtained from clinical studies support this interpretation. In hypertensive as well as in normal subjects, a negative correlation is obtained between CVP and blood volume, and also between CVP and total vascular compliance (53). In other words, in essential hypertension, the slight elevation of CVP results from a reduction of total vascular compliance, and this phenomenon is observed in the presence of a blood volume decrement.

In patients with essential hypertension, the contribution of vascular capacitance to the regulation of cardiac output is particularly important, in view of the three following hemodynamic characteristics of the heart: normal cardiac output, decreased vascular volume, and cardiac hypertrophy in the absence of congestive failure. Indeed, it is now well accepted that the normal cardiac output, in the presence of increased afterload, is achieved through cardiac hypertrophy which causes a loss in left ventricular compliance (9,10,14). Under such conditions, the presence of established cardiac hypertrophy would lead to a reduction in stroke volume without adequate compensation. The latter could take the picture of increased cardiac filling pressure of left and right ventricles. In patients with essential hypertension, a slight elevation in capillary wedge pressure is observed, suggesting a rise in left atrial pressure (54,66). Since the right atrial pressure is also elevated (54,66), for the hypertrophied heart to receive an adequate driving pressure, a reduction in venous compliance appears essential. Using the isotonic saline load maneuver, Ulrych and colleagues (67) have demonstrated that the rise in cardiac output obtained under these conditions was enhanced in hypertensive subjects. They suggested that a reduction in the peripheral vascular capacity was responsible for this finding. A more direct evidence is provided by the following observation: a negative correlation is obtained between cardiac output (or stroke volume) and effective vascular compliance in patients with essential hypertension. In other words, the higher cardiac output is associated with the more reduced compliance (11). Thus, despite cardiac hypertrophy and decreased vascular volume, the normal cardiac output observed in sustained essential hypertension is achieved by a reduction in the extrathoracic venous compliance, a finding confirmed by the study of mathematical models of the circulation (6).

EXTRAVASCULAR VOLUMES AND THE KIDNEY

Despite past controversies and disputes over the subject, it is now relatively well accepted that the external sodium and fluid balance in experimental and human essential hypertension is normal. Since the total extracellular fluid volume is within the limits of normalcy while total blood volume is reduced, a significant reduction in the plasma to interstitial fluid volume ratio (PV/IT) obtains in uncomplicated essential hypertension. These findings suggest that forces regulating fluid and solutes movements across capillaries (14,47) and/or changes in endothelial permeability per se (48,64,68) and/or inadequate removal of filtered albumin by lymphatic drainage (69) are responsible for this abnormal profile of body fluid distribution. With respect to a potential abnormality in lymphatic drainage, it is of interest that endothelial nitric oxide production, which appears to be diminished in hypertensive states (70), plays a critical role in the pulsative function of lymphatic vessels (71). An increased capillary filtration rate (extrarenal hyperfiltration) has been clearly documented in hypertensive patients: the transcapillary escape rate of radioactive albumin was shown to be directly correlated with mean arterial pressure (48,67). Such findings could be explained by at least three independent and/or combined physiological disturbances: (a) inappropriate tonus of the precapillary resistance (relative dilatation); (b) increased postcapillary resistance (relative constriction) because of the reduction in venous and/or interstitial compliance; (c) alteration in endothelial cell permeability of selected networks (64) or of the entire microcirculation (48,67). It is important at this point to recall that increased permeability to albumin absolutely requires humoral-induced endothelial cell dysjunction (72,73), and cannot be the mere consequence of increased capillary hydrostatic pressure (72). The decrease in PV/IT observed in hypertensive patients is negatively correlated with CVP, and positively with total vascular compliance, independently of the level of arterial pressure and vascular resistance values (12,53). These findings could therefore be taken as a strong argument in favor of the capacitance system failure to regulate body fluid volume partition in essential hypertension (68).

The maintenance of a normal external sodium and fluid balance, which characterizes the essential hypertensive patient, occurs in the presence of paradoxical subtle renal hemodynamic and tubular dysfunctions that should, on the contrary, predispose to sodium and fluid retention (2,3,13). Renal plasma flow is significantly reduced while glomerular filtration remains unchanged.

As a consequence, filtration fraction rises and the peritubular protein concentration and oncotic pressure is also expected to increase (13). Under such circumstances, passive proximal tubular reabsorption of sodium and fluid should rise (74), leading to positive external balance. Maintenance of sodium and fluid balance despite enhanced proximal tubule net reabsorption is not entirely incompatible, since several extrarenal and intrarenal adaptive mechanisms are already existing in the hypertensive patient and/or can be induced (36).

1. Peripheral blood atrial natriuretic peptide, not measured in the reported studies, was probably elevated because of the rise in CVP documented in the hypertensive patients, a known potent stimulus for the synthesis and release of this peptide (55).
2. Ouabain, another important natriuretic compound (36), the release of which appears to be more influenced by expansion of the interstitial than of the vascular compartment (75), could also be involved in the adaptative process described above. This endogenous natriuretic compound inhibits the sodium-potassium ATPase, including that of the thick ascending limb of Henle, the putative site of its renal action (76).
3. Another natriuretic substance, bradykinin (77), could also participate in the renal adaptation. The interstitial cells of the renal medulla represent an important source of kinins (78), the synthesis and release of which are triggered, at least in part, by elevation of intrarenal hydrostatic pressure (79).
4. Simple elevation of intrarenal pressure was shown to enhance natriuresis (pressure natriuresis), apparently without any need for humoral intervention (62).

Finally, we assume of course, that the observed decrement in renal plasma flow, on which all the above discussion is based, represents a reliable measurement. In fact, since the radio-hippuran clearance method was used to measure renal plasma flow, and since the renal extraction of this marker could not be performed in the human studies reported (13,53), it is possible that the reduction in the radio-hippuran clearance was overestimated, due to the fact that intrarenal blood flow redistributed to the deep nephrons which do not secrete hippuran (80). Since positive sodium and fluid balance fails to develop in uncomplicated essential hypertension, this possibility appears remote because such redistribution of flow and filtrate would be expected to produce avid sodium retention, this population of nephrons being reputed for its high capacity to reabsorb this cation (81).

A number of arguments support the relationship between the body fluid changes observed and the renal functional disturbances measured in essential hypertensive patients. Changes in the venous capacity could be at least partly responsible for the maintenance of sodium balance. Lowenstein and co-workers (82) have found that renal venous pressure was higher than normal in patients with essential hypertension, and increased further during volume loading. Such modifications could well account for the adjusted natriuresis (protection against enhanced proximal passive reabsorption), and could explain, as well, the exaggerated natriuresis obtained in hypertensive patients after volume loading (82). It is likely, therefore, that increased hydrostatic force in the low-pressure system compensates for the small elevation of the calculated peritubular oncotic pressure in the hypertensive kidney (13,83). In fact, the renal filtration fraction is negatively correlated to vascular capacitance in normotensive and hypertensive subjects. Similarly, a negative correlation is obtained between peritubular oncotic pressure and vascular compliance. Conversely, a positive relationship is observed between CVP and postglomerular oncotic pressure (13). Thus, the elevation of filling pressure in the low-pressure system, secondary to decreased systemic capacitance, may underlie the extrarenal hyperfiltration responsible for the decreased vascular/interstitial fluid volume ratio. The same rise in hydrostatic pressure, neutralizing the elevation of oncotic pressure and described for the peritubular capillary network (3,83), could well obtain in other microcirculation beds. Two arguments support this hypothesis: (a) the difference in peritubular oncotic pressure (−3 mm Hg) between normal and hypertensive subjects is almost equal to the difference (+2 mm Hg) measured in the CVP; (b) a highly significant correlation between filtration fraction and the vascular/interstitial volume ratio is observed in the hypertensive patients (84). Suffice it to recall again that the possibility of a primary capillary permeability dysfunction in a putative hypertension genetic trait, leading to extravasation of plasma from the vascular to the interstitial compartment (64,65) and giving rise to most of the hemodynamic abnormalities reported above, has not yet been ruled out and remains a challenging hypothesis to further examine. If ever demonstrated in human hypertension, it would fit nicely with the results obtained in the spontaneously hypertensive rat before the appearance of hypertension (64).

VENOUS COMPLIANCE: STRUCTURAL OR FUNCTIONAL DEFECT?

The venous wall contains elastin and collagen fibers, ground substance including proteoglycans (85), and smooth muscle cells. Therefore, the tonus of this organ can be influenced either by alteration in function or by structural changes: elastin/collagen/proteoglycan ratio (2,3,15). Unlike the resistance vessels which adjust their shape in response to local metabolic changes, the capacitance vessels are regulated by the sympathetic nervous system and also by a variety of autacoids and hormones such as histamine (17), prostagandins (86), endothelins (87), and endothelium-derived relaxing factor (88). In essential hypertension, the venous function can be altered by structural and/or functional changes as well. Venous wall hypertrophy and alteration in tissue water and electrolyte contents have been suggested as possible structural abnormalities in different models of experimental hypertension. These changes were considered for a long time as occurring in a venous system where pressure remains normal (86,89). Recently, the dynamic aspects of the interstitial space, which occupies the subendothelial portion of blood vessels, was revitalized by a series of observations suggesting that the proteoglycans of the ground substance were interacting with sodium and calcium, two critical ions involved in the vascular smooth muscle contraction (90–92). Under conditions where the composition of the interstitium is expected to be altered, such as arterial hypertension in which increased endothelial permeability to fluid and solutes has been documented (48,49,64) or—even more critical—following pharmacological treatment of hypertension itself (93), it is likely that the functional behavior of the venous system will also be modified. As shown in patients with hypertension, venous pressure is slightly elevated, so that the Laplace law should be operating (94). On the other hand, increased neurogenic tone and/or enhanced contractile response to vasoactive autacoids have been suggested to explain the functional alterations described. Increased plasma catecholamines or sympathetic nervous system activity could influence vascular compliance, as suggested by the finding of a negative correlation between total effective vascular compliance and serum dopamine beta-hydroxylase activity in normal and hypertensive subjects (15).

Finally, the role of physiological senescence per se must be taken into consideration when evaluating the structural and functional aspects of decreased venous compliance. Clinical studies have shown that, as arterial blood pressure and peripheral resistance rise with age, venous compliance also decreases, but in a steeper fashion in hypertension (18). In other words, there is a serious possibility that the functional alterations of the venous system described in hypertension project a similar influence on the functional and structural alterations of the arterial system during the course of the disease. Clearly, these important questions, as well as the recently proposed hypothesis suggesting nephron heterogeneity with discordant renin secretion (95), remain to be solved, among many others raised over the past decade by the discovery of a myriad of potent vasoactive autacoids likely involved in the pathophysiology of hypertension.

REFERENCES

1. Gauer OH, Henry JP. Neurohumoral control of plasma volume. In: Guyton AC, Cowley AW, eds. *International review of cardiovascular physiology II*, vol. 9. Baltimore: University Park Press, 1976;145–190.

2. Guyton AC, Coleman TG, Granger HJ. Circulation: overall regulation. *Ann Rev Physiol* 1982;34:13–44.

3. Seely JG, Levy M. Control of extracellular fluid volume. In: Brenner BM, Rector FC, eds. *The kidney.* Philadelphia: Saunders, 1981;371–407.

4. Aukland K, Nicolaysen G. Interstitial fluid volume: local regulatory mechanisms. *Physiol Rev* 1981;61:556–673.

5. Jackson RL, Busch SJ, Cardin AD. Glycosaminoglycans: molecular properties, protein interactions, and role in physiological processes. *Physiol Rev* 1991;71:481–601.

6. Chau NP, Coleman TG, London GM, Safar ME. Meaning of the cardiac output-blood volume relationship in essential hypertension. *Am J Physiol* 1982;243:R318–R328.

7. Safar ME, Chau NP, Weiss YA, London GM, Simon AC, Milliez PL. The pressure-volume relationship in normotensive and permanent essential hypertensive patients. *Clin Sci Mol Med* 1976;50: 207–212.

8. Tarazi RC, Dustan HP, Frohlich ED. Plasma volume in men with essential hypertension. *N Engl J Med* 1968;762:278–284.

9. Tarazi RC, Dustan HP, Frohlich ED. Relation of plasma to interstitial fluid volume in essential hypertension. *Circulation* 1969;40: 357–364.

10. Ulrych M, Frohlich ED, Tarazi RC, Dustan HP, Page IH. Cardiac output and distribution of blood volume in central and peripheral circulations in hypertensive and normotensive man. *Br Heart J* 1969;570:31–42.

11. London GM, Safar ME, Weiss YA, Simon AC. Total effective compliance of the vascular bed in essential hypertension. *Am Heart J* 1978;95:325–330.

12. London GM, Safar ME, Simon AC, Alexandre JM, Levenson JA, Weiss YA. Total effective compliance, cardiac output and fluid volumes in essential hypertension. *Circulation* 1978;57:995–1000.

13. London GM, Safar ME, Levenson JA, Simon AC, Temmar MA. Renal filtration fraction, effective vascular compliance and partition of fluid volumes in sustained essential hypertension. *Kidney Int* 1981;20:97–103.

14. Tarazi RC. Hemodynamic role of extracellular fluid in hypertension. *Circ Res* 1976;73[Suppl II]:38–47.

15. Cooper KE. Functional aspects of the venous system. In: Schwartz CJ, Werthessen NT, Wolf S, eds. *Structure and function of the circulation*, vol 2. New York: Plenum, 1981;457–485.

16. Rothe CF. The venous System. The physiology of the capacitance vessels. In: Shepherd JT, Abboud FM, eds. *Handbook of physiology. The cardiovascular system. Peripheral circulation and organ blood flow*, vol III, Sect 2. Bethesda: Am Physiol Soc, 1983;397–452.

17. Shepherd JT, Van Houtte PM. *Veins and their control*, vol 1. Philadelphia: Saunders, 1975;269–287.

18. London GM, Safar ME, Safar AL, Simon AC. Blood pressure in the low-pressure system and cardiac performance in essential hypertension. *J Hypertens* 1985;3:337–342.

19. Green JF. *Mechanical concepts in cardiovascular and pulmonary physiology*. Philadelphia: Lea & Fiberger, 1977;166–213.

20. Shoukas AA, Sagawa K. Total systemic vascular compliance measured as incremental volume-pressure ratio. *Circ Res* 1971;277: 28–37.

21. Guyton AC. Mean circulatory pressure, mean systemic pressure and mean pulmonary pressure and their effect on venous return. In: *Circulation physiology. Cardiac output and its regulation.* Philadelphia: Saunders, 1963;193–208.

22. Shoukas AA, Sagawa K. Control of total systemic vascular capacity by the carotid sinus baroreceptor reflex. *Circ Res* 1973;32:33–39.

23. Hecht M, Duweling J, Gauer OH, Lange L. Effective compliance of the total vascular bed and the intrathoracic compartment derived from changes in central venous pressure induced by volume changes in man. *Circ Res* 1974;34:61–72.

24. Drees JA, Rothe CF. Reflex venoconstriction and capacity vessels pressure-volume relationships in dog. *Circ Res* 1967;360:213–219.

25. Harlan JC, Smith EE, Richardson TQ. Pressure-volume curves of systemic and pulmonary circuit. *Am J Physiol* 1967;499:213–219.

26. Engelberg J, Dubois AB. Mechanisms of pulmonary circulation in isolated rabbit lungs. *Am J Physiol* 1959;401:196–208.

27. Maseri A, Caldini P, Horward P, Josmi RC, Permutt S, Zierler KL. Determinants of pulmonary vascular volume recruitment versus distensibility. *Circ Res* 1972;218:31–38.

28. Venkatachalam MA, Karnovsky MJ. Extravascular protein in the kidney: an ultrastructural study of its relation to renal peritubular capillary permeability using protein tracers. *Lab Invest* 1972;27: 435–441.

29. Gauer OH. Mechanoreceptors in the intrathoracic circulation and plasma volume control. In: Epstein M, ed. *The kidney in liver disease*, vol. 1. New York: Elsevier, 1978;3–17.

30. Simon AC, Safar ME, Levenson JA, London GM, Levy BI, Chau NP. An evaluation of large arteries compliance in man. *Am J Physiol* 1979;235:H550–H554.

31. London GM, Safar ME, Payen DM, Gitelman RC, Guerin AM. Total peripheral and intrathoracic effective compliances of the vascular bed in normotensive and hypertensive patients. In: Brod J, ed. *Contribution to nephrology*. Basel: Karger, 1982;144–153.

32. Edelman IS, Liebman J. Anatomy of body water and electrolytes. *Am J Med* 1959;27:256–266.

33. Simionescu N. Cellular aspects of transcapillary exchange. *Physiol Rev* 1983;63:1536–1617.

34. Earley LE, Schrier RW. Intrarenal control of sodium excretion by hemodynamic and physical factors. In: Orloff J, Berliner RW, eds. *Handbook of physiology: renal physiology.* Washington: Am Physiol Soc, 1973;721–762.

35. Robinson JR. Metabolism of intracellular water. *Physiol Rev* 1960;40:112–187.

36. DeWardener HE, Clarkson EM. Concept of natriuretic hormone. *Physiol Rev* 1985;65:658–759.

37. Dworkin LD, Ichikawa I, Brenner BM. Hormonal regulation of glomerular function. *Am J Physiol* 1983;244:F95–F104.

38. Sirois MG, Plante GE, Braquet P, Sirois P. Role of eicosanoids in PAF-induced increases of vascular permeabilities in rat airways. *Br J Pharmacol* 1990;101:896–900.

39. Seifter JL, Aronson PS. Properties and physiological roles of the plasma membrane sodium-hydrogen exchanger. *J Clin Invest* 1986;78:859–864.

40. Tuck ML, Corry DB, Maxwell M, Stern N. Kinetic analysis of erythrocyte Na-K pump and cotransport in essential hypertension. *Hypertension* 1987;10:204–211.

41. VanBreemen C, Aaronson P, Loutzenhiser R. Na-Ca interaction in mammalian smooth muscle. *Pharmacol Rev* 1979;30:606–718.

42. Grinstein S, Rothstein A. Mechanisms of regulation of the Na/H exchanger. *J Membr Biol* 1986;10:1–12.

43. Brugnara C, Canessa M, Cusi D, Tosteson DC. Furosemide-sensitive Na and K fluxes in human red cells: net uphill Na extrusion and equilibrium properties. *J Gen Physiol* 1986;87:91–112.

44. Owen NE. Regulation of Na-K-Cl cotransport in vascular smooth muscle cells. *Biochem Biophys Res Commun* 1984;125:500–508.

45. Ricksen SE, Yao T, Thoren P. Peripheral and central vascular compliances in conscious normotensive and spontaneously hypertensive rats. *Acta Physiol Scand* 1981;112:167–169.

46. Trippodo NC, Yamamoto J, Frohlich ED. Whole-body venous capacity and effective total tissue compliance in SHR. *Hypertension* 1981;3:104–111.

47. Safar ME, London GM, Simon AC, Chau NP. Volume factors, total exchangeable sodium and potassium in hypertension disease. In: Genest J, Kuchel O, Hamet P, Cantin M, eds. *Hypertension: physiopathology and treatment.* New York: McGraw-Hill, 1983;42–54.

48. Parving MH, Gyntelberg F. Transcapillary escape rate of albumin and plasma volume in essential hypertension. *Circ Res* 1973;643: 32–39.

49. Ulrych M. Plasma volume decrease and elevated Evans blue disappearance rate in essential hypertension. *Clin Sci Mol Med* 1973;173:45–52.

50. Chau NP, Tarazi RC, Fouad FM, Safar ME, Birkenhager WH, DeLeeuw PW. Index for normalization of blood volume. *Clin Sci Mol Med* 1982;63:375s–377s.

51. Isnard RN, Pannier BM, Laurent S, London GM, Diebold B, Safar ME. Pulsatile diameter and elastic modulus of the aortic arch in essential hypertension: a noninvasive study. *J Am Coll Cardiol* 1989;13:399–405.

52. Julius S, Pascual AV, Reilly K, London GM. Abnormalities of plasma volume in borderline hypertension. *Arch Int Med* 1971;127:116–119.

53. London GM, Levenson JA, London AM, Simon AC, Safar ME.

Systemic compliance, renal hemodynamics and sodium excretion in hypertension. *Kidney Int* 1984;16:342–350.

54. London GM, Levenson JA, Safar ME, Simon AC, Guerin AP, Payen D. Hemodynamic effects of head-down tilt in normal subjects and sustained hypertensive patients. *Am J Physiol* 1983;245:H194–H202.

55. Morris M, Alexander N. Baroreceptor influences on plasma atrial natriuretic peptide (ANP): sinoaortic denervation reduces basal levels and the response to an osmotic challenge. *Endocrinology* 1988;122:373–375.

56. Currie MG, Geller DM, Cole BR, Boylan JG, YuSheng W, Holmberg SW, Needleman P. Bioactive cardiac substances: potent vasorelaxant activity in mammalia atria. *Science* 1983;221:71–73.

57. Camargo MJF, Atlas SA, Maack T. Role of increased glomerular filtration rate in atrial natriuretic factor-induced natriuresis in the rat. *Life Sci* 1986;38:2397–2404.

58. Almeida FA, Suzuki M, Maack T. Atrial natriuretic factor increases hematocrit and decreases plasma volume in nephrectomized rats. *Life Sci* 1986;39:1193–1199.

59. London GM, Safar ME, Weiss YA, Corvol PL, Lehner JP, Menard JM, Simon AC, Milliez PL. Volume-dependent parameters in essential hypertension. *Kidney Int* 1977;11:204–208.

60. Safar ME, London GM, Weiss YA, Milliez PL. Altered blood volume regulation in sustained essential hypertension. A hemodynamic study. *Kidney Int* 1975;8:42–47.

61. Koch KM, Aynedhan HS, Bank N. Effect of acute hypertension on sodium reabsorption by the proximal tubule. *J Clin Invest* 1968;47:1696–1709.

62. Hall JE, Granger JP, Hester RL, Montani JP. Mechanisms of sodium balance in hypertension: role of pressure natriuresis. *J Hypertens* 1986;4[Suppl 4]:S57–S65.

63. Bissonnette M, Sirois MG, Sirois P, Regoli D, Plante GE. Anomalies de la microcirculation rénale chez le rat spontanément hypertendu. *Médecine Sciences* 1989;12[Suppl 3]:42A.

64. Plante GE, Bissonnette M, Sirois MG, Regoli D, Sirois P. Renal permeability alteration precedes hypertension and involves bradykinin in the spontaneously hypertensive rat. *J Clin Invest* 1992;89:2030–2034.

65. Lucas L, Floyer MA. Changes in body fluid distribution and interstitial tissue compliance during the development and reversal of experimental hypertension in the rat. *Clin Sci Mol Med* 1974;47:1–10.

66. Ferlinz J. Right ventricular performance in essential hypertension. *Circulation* 1980;61:156–162.

67. Ulrych M, Hofman J, Hejl Z. Cardiac and renal hyperresponsiveness to acute plasma volume expansion in hypertension. *Am Heart J* 1964;68:193–199.

68. Safar ME, London GM, Levenson JA, Simon AC, Chau NP. Rapid dextran infusion in essential hypertension. *Hypertension* 1979;1:615–623.

69. Aukland K, Reed RK. Interstitial-lymphatic mechanisms in the control of extracellular fluid volume. *Physiol Rev* 1993;73:1–78.

70. Arnal JF, Warin L, Michel JB. Determinants of chronic cyclic guanosine monophosphate in hypertension induced by chronic inhibition of nitric oxide synthase. *J Clin Invest* 1992;90:647–652.

71. Elias RM, Eissnhoffer J, Johnston MG. Role of endothelial cells in regulating hemoglobin-induced changes in lymphatic pumping. *Am J Physiol* 1992;263:H1880–1887.

72. Sirois MG, Jancar S, Braquet P, Plante GE, Sirois P. PAF increases vascular permeability in selected tissues: effect of BN-52021, and L-655,240. *Prostaglandins* 1988;36:631–637.

73. Wysolmerski RB, Lagunoff D. Involvement of myosin light-chain kinase in endothelial cell retraction. *Proc Nat Acad Sci* 1990;87:16–19.

74. Brenner BM, Falchuk KH, Keimowitz JD, Berliner RW. The relationship between peritubular capillary protein concentration and fluid reabsorption by the renal proximal tubule. *J Clin Invest* 1969;48:1519–1529.

75. Plante GE, Hebert RL. Platelet activating factor in renal physiology and pathophysiology. Interest of the gingkolides. In: Braquet P, ed. Gingkolides: chemistry, biology, pharmacology and clinical perspectives. Barcelona: Prous Science Publishers, 1988;575–602.

76. Plante GE, Prevost C, Chainey A, Braquet P, Sirois P. Diuretic and natriuretic properties of prestegane B, a mammalian lignan. *Am J Physiol* 1987;253:R375–R378.

77. Lortie M, Regoli D, Rhaleb NE, Plante GE. Dissociation of hemodynamic and tubular effects of intrarenal bradykinin infusion. *Am J Physiol* 1992;262:R72–R77.

78. Scicli AG, Gandolfi R, Carretero OA. Site of formation of kinins in the dog nephron. *Am J Physiol* 1978;234:F36–F42.

79. Roman RJ, Kaldunski ML, Scicli AG, Carretero OA. Influence of kinins and angiotensin II on the regulation of papillary blood flow. *Am J Physiol* 1988;255:F690–F696.

80. Burg MB, Orloff JP. Aminohippurate uptake and exchange by separated renal tubules. *Am J Physiol* 1969;217:1064–1068.

81. Horster M, Thurau K. Micropuncture studies on the filtration rate of single superficial and juxtamedullary glomeruli in the rat kidney. *Eur J Physiol* 1968;301:162–181.

82. Lowenstein J, Beranbaum ER, Chasis H, Baldwin DS. Intrarenal pressure and exaggerated natriuresis in essential hypertension. *Clin Sci Mol Med* 1970;38:359–375.

83. Jobin J, Hemmings R, Plante GE. Effect of renal vein pressure on urinary sodium and hydrogen excretion. *Can J Physiol Pharmacol* 1978;56:166–174.

84. Simon ACH, Safar ME, Levenson JA, Aboras NE, Alexandre JM, Pauleau NI. Extracellular fluid volume and renal indices in essential hypertension. *Clin Exp Hypertens* 1979;1:557–561.

85. Bevan JA, Siegel G. Blood vessel wall matrix flow sensor: evidence and speculation. *Blood Vessels* 1991;28:552–556.

86. London GM, Hornych A, Safar ME, Levenson JA, Simon AC. Plasma prostaglandin E2 and I2a, total effective vascular compliance and renal plasma flow in essential hypertension. *Nephron* 1982;32:118–124.

87. Miller WL, Redfield MM, Burnett JC. Integrated cardiac, renal, and endocrine actions of endothelin. *J Clin Invest* 1989;83:317–323.

88. Brenner BM, Troy JL, Ballermann BJ. Endothelium-dependent vascular responses. Mediators and mechanisms. *J Clin Invest* 1989;84:1373–1380.

89. Pamnami MB, Overbeck HW. Abnormal ion and water composition of veins and normotensive arteries in coarctation hypertension in rats. *Circ Res* 1976;38:375–378.

90. Bevan JA, Wellmann GC, Joyce EH. Flow-induced constriction of rabbit resistance artery is sodium-dependent. *Blood Vessels* 1990;27:369–372.

91. Bevan JA, Joyce EH. Flow-induced relaxation in a resistance artery is associated with an amiloride-sensitive sodium-dependent mechanism in vascular smooth muscle. *J Vasc Med Biol* 1991;2:281–288.

92. Bevan JA, Joyce EH. Saline infusion into lumen of resistance artery and small vein causes contraction. *Am J Physiol* 1990;259:H23–H28.

93. Lehoux S, Sirois MG, Chakir M, Sirois P, Plante GE. Diuretics alter vascular permeability in selected organs. In: Puschett JB, Greenberg JD, eds. *Diuretics IV: chemistry, pharmacology and clinical applications.* New York: Elsevier, 1993;[in press].

94. Folkow B. Physiological aspects of primary hypertension. *Physiol Rev* 1982;62:347–504.

95. Laragh JH. On the renal basis for essential hypertension: nephron heterogeneity with discordant renin secretion and sodium excretion causing a hypertensive vasoconstriction-volume relationship. *J Hypertens* 1988;6:763–777.

Hypertension: Pathophysiology, Diagnosis, and Management, Second Edition,
edited by J.H. Laragh and B.M. Brenner,
Raven Press, Ltd., New York © 1995.

CHAPTER 24

Red Blood Cell Mass/Erythropoietin and Blood Pressure: Lessons from Patients with Renal Disease

Joseph W. Eschbach and Robert C. Davidson

Chronic renal failure (CRF), regardless of the cause, is often associated with a hypoproliferative anemia. This anemia may develop at any time that the serum creatinine rises to greater than 2 mg/dL, but usually is not symptomatic until the hematocrit decreases to below 30. By the time dialysis therapy is required, which usually corresponds to an endogenous creatinine clearance of 5–7 mL/min, most patients with CRF are anemic. In the past there was no effective treatment for this anemia, and most patients whose lives were maintained with repetitive dialysis functioned at a suboptimal level because of this anemia.

In December 1985, the first clinical trial with recombinant human erythropoietin (epoetin), a new biotechnology product, was begun in anemic, hemodialysis patients (1). Subsequent experience indicated that this hormone, which is essentially identical to natural human erythropoietin (2), increased the hematocrit or red cell mass in a dose-dependent manner and resulted in marked clinical benefits for patients with CRF suffering with hematocrit levels of 15–30, many of whom previously required repeated red cell transfusions in order to relieve symptoms of moderate to marked anemia. However, an increase in blood pressure (≥ 10 mm Hg in mean arterial pressure [MAP]) was noted in up to 33 percent of hemodialysis patients treated with epoetin in most clinical trials. The hypertension that may develop in patients responding to epoetin often requires an increase in either diuretics or dialysis ultrafiltration and antihypertensive drugs, occasionally may be difficult to control, and rarely seizures may occur. Since there are over 500,000 dialysis patients in the world, of whom approximately 300,000 are receiving epoetin to treat the hypoproliferative anemia of CRF, this hypertensive complication is of much potential significance. This chapter will explore the relationship between red cell mass and blood pressure, and whether epoetin, per se, is a direct or indirect vasopressor agent. Since epoetin is not usually associated with a hypertensive response in anemic subjects with normal renal function (3), the underlying hypertension of CRF is therefore an important

J. W. Eschbach: Department of Medicine, Divisions of Hematology and Nephrology, University of Washington, Seattle, Washington 98195.

Robert C. Davidson: Department of Medicine, Division of Nephrology, University of Washington, Seattle, Washington 98195.

prerequisite for the epoetin-related hypertension. Markedly elevated levels of serum erythropoietin, present in patients with hemolytic disorders, are not associated with an increased incidence of hypertension.

ERYTHROPOIETIN AND CHRONIC RENAL FAILURE

Erythropoietin is produced primarily from the peritubular capillary endothelial cells of the kidney and is secreted in response to hypoxia or anemia, so that with increasing anemia there is increased production of erythropoietin. In CRF, the kidney is unable to respond adequately to the anemic stimulus, resulting in plasma erythropoietin levels that are "normal," but are inappropriately low for the degree of anemia (4). The hypoproliferative anemia of CRF used to be considered multifactorial in its etiology, with the major causes being erythropoietin deficiency, shortened red cell survival, retention of uremic inhibitors of erythropoiesis, and bleeding secondary to the qualitative uremic platelet defect (4). However, since infusions of equal amounts of erythropoietin into normal and uremic sheep or normal and uremic humans produces similar erythropoietic responses, it now is apparent that the anemia of CRF is primarily due to relative erythropoietin deficiency (4,5), and is not an anemia due to uremia.

HYPERTENSION IN RENAL DISEASE

Overview

Hypertension usually develops as the glomerular filtration rate decreases. By the time so-called end-stage renal disease occurs, i.e., dialysis or renal transplantation is required to maintain life, 75–90 percent of patients are hypertensive and/or are requiring antihypertensive medication(s) (6). Most forms of renal disease can be associated with hypertension, with variable incidence, but glomular and vascular diseases of the kidney are the most common forms. Once dialysis is begun, hypertension can usually be controlled through a combination of

plasma volume control via dialysis ultrafiltration and/or antihypertensive drugs. It is also likely that the anemia of CRF, through anemic, hypoxic vasodilatation, will moderate the hypertension.

Pathophysiology

This has been reviewed in the chapter by Smith and Dunn. There are two and possibly three major factors contributing to the elevated blood pressure, and most patients may have a mixture of these elements. An expanded plasma volume is the first factor. Reducing excessive plasma volume by strict control of sodium balance through diet and dialysis ultrafiltration will normalize blood pressure in the majority of dialysis patients (7). A second factor is increased systemic vascular resistance due to increased vasoconstriction. A significant minority of dialysis patients will have a vasoconstrictor-related form of hypertension requiring antihypertensive medication, in addition to dialysis ultrafiltration, to maintain a normal blood pressure. Increased vasoconstrictor activity is implied because of several observations: peripheral renin activity (PRA) may be increased in 30 percent of dialysis patients; there is an inappropriate secretion of renin in relation to the plasma volume; and angiotensin-converting enzyme inhibition of arterial wall angiotensin II is effective in lowering blood pressure even if the PRA is low (6). The autonomic nervous system is the third factor which may be involved. Baroreflex sensitivity is diminished in CRF so that adrenergic outflow continues even at higher blood pressures.

Hemodynamic Parameters

The hemodynamic changes that occur with CRF and hypertension have been well studied. In comparison to normal subjects, cardiac output or index, heart rate, and MAP are increased, whereas stroke volume and peripheral resistance (the mean for all CRF patients) are unchanged (8). However, anemia has a major role in these hemodynamic changes. Normotensive and hypertensive CRF patients with the same hematocrit—23—have sim-

TABLE 1. *Hemodynamic studies in normotensive and hypertensive hemodialysis patients and normal subjects*

	Normotensive	Hypertensive	Normal
Numbers of patients	23	52	42
Hematocrit (%)	23	23	43
Cardiac index (L/min/m^2)	4.55 ± 0.15	4.39 ± 0.14	3.39 ± 0.08
Heart rate (beats/min)	89 ± 2.0	91.1 ± 1.4	66 ± 1.2
Stroke index (mL/stroke/m^2)	51 ± 1.6	49 ± 1.6	52 ± 1.4
Arterial pressure (mm Hg)	93 ± 1.8	139 ± 2.9	91 ± 1.6
Mean TPRI (dynes sec/cm^5)	1670 ± 61	2703 ± 120	2187 ± 59

From Kim et al., ref. 8.
TPRI, total peripheral resistance index.

ilar cardiac indices and heart rates (although still higher than normal subjects); but total peripheral resistance index (TPRI) in the normotensive CRF patients is lower than in normal subjects. In the hypertensive CRF patients the TPRI is much higher than normal (8). Therefore, increased peripheral vascular resistance rather than increased cardiac output is responsible for the hypertension of CRF. However, anemia through hypoxic vasodilation contributes to maintaining a normal MAP in some patients (Table 1). This is even more obvious when the anemia is reversed. When the hematocrit was increased from 20 to 30 and then to 40 by red cell transfusions in six hemodialysis patients, cardiac output decreased toward normal with the normalization in red cell mass, while TPRI increased from normal or below normal values to elevated values, which then led to a marked increase in diastolic blood pressure (9).

RED CELL MASS, BLOOD PRESSURE AND HEMODYNAMICS

Since anemia is associated with reduced TPRI in CRF, particularly in the absence of hypertension, it is important to evaluate the effect of red cell mass on blood pressure in subjects with normal renal function. When the blood pressure was measured in forty patients with various hematological diseases (three of whom had polycythemia vera), there was a positive correlation between systolic and diastolic pressures and the hemoglobin or hematocrit levels (10). The hemoglobin ranged from 3.1 to 19.7 g/dL (corresponding to a hematocrit range of 09 to 62). The MAP was 79.1 ± 10.9 in the 21 patients with hemoglobin levels < 10.0 g/dL, but 89.9 ± 13.4 in the 19 patients with hemoglobin levels > 10.0 g/dL (p < 0.01) (Fig. 1). Even though cardiac output decreased as the hemoglobin increased, TPRI continued to increase, accounting for the rise in blood pressure in the polycythemic state. These authors stated (in 1986) that "such a strong relation between hemoglobin concentration and both systolic and diastolic blood pressure has not been noted before."

However, in one large study, the incidence of hypertension in polycythemia vera was only 32 percent (11), and there was no hypertension in three patients with hematocrit values of 77, 66, and 81 (12). "Stress" polycythemia is associated with a high incidence of hypertension, but red cell volume is not increased in these patients and antihypertensive therapy often lowers the hematocrit (13). Animal (dog) models of exchange transfusion have also failed to show a consistent relationship between an elevated hematocrit and hypertension (14,15), whereas marked polycythemia in the rat (hematocrit 72 ± 3), induced by epoetin, led to a rise in MAP from 107 to 126 (16). Milder polycythemia (hematocrit 59 ± 2) failed to induce hypertension, presumably be-

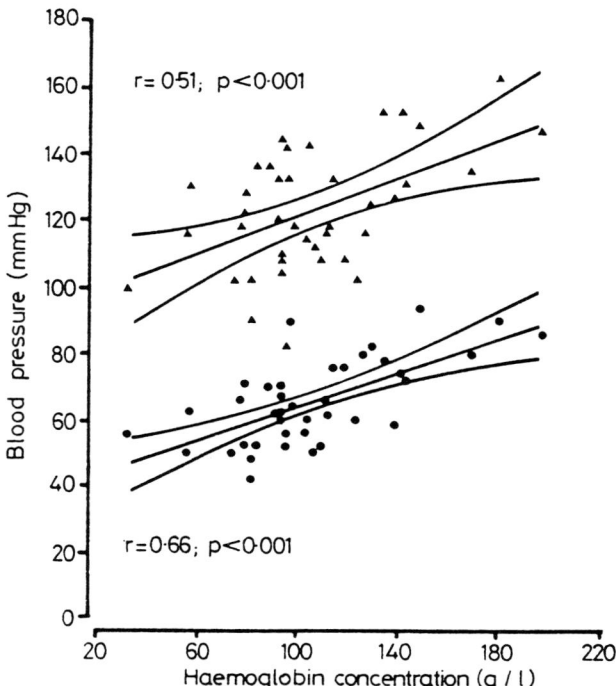

FIG. 1. The relationship between hemoglobin concentration and systolic and diastolic blood pressure in forty patients with various forms of nonrenal anemias. From Daniel et al. (10).

cause of autoregulatory factors such as increased nitric oxide release from endothelial cells (16). However, the spontaneously hypertensive rat will experience an increase in blood pressure in association with a rise in hematocrit (17).

In contrast to the inconsistent relationship between hypertension and polycythemia in humans, anemia from various causes generally lowers blood pressure (18–21). The effect of anemia in animals is variable: anemia lowers blood pressure in the rat (15), but not in the dog (22,23).

When anemia is corrected (i.e., by iron, folic acid, vitamin B12, antihelminthic therapy or red cells, depending on the etiology of the anemia), there may be significant blood pressure and/or hemodynamic changes. Most patients reported (some more than 50 years ago) were very anemic prior to therapy (hemoglobin levels of 8–57 percent of normal, n = 47 [18]; hemoglobin 1.5–6.5 g/ dL, n = 51 [19]; hemoglobin 1.9–3.8 g/dL, n = 7 [20]; hematocrit 20.3 ± 4.8, n = 15 [21]; hemoglobin 4.4 ± 1.5 g/dL, n = 18 [24]). When anemia was corrected in the patients in these studies, selected follow-up found that 14 of 23 patients had a >10-mm Hg rise in diastolic pressure, with one patient's BP changing from 125/60 to 190/115 (18); the MAP increased by 24.2 ± 13.4 mm Hg in six of eleven patients (19); diastolic pressure increased from 61 ± 22 to 74 ± 23 (p < 0.05) in seven patients (20); MAP increased from 88 to 103 in fifteen patients when the hematocrit increased from 20 to 36 (21); and dia-

TABLE 2. *Blood pressure changes following treatment of nutritional or blood loss anemias*

Study	Baseline Hgb (g/dL)	Baseline Hct	Treated Hgb	Treated Hct	DBP or MAP ≥ 10-mm Hg rise
Ellis et al. (18)	1.2–8.6		"normal"		14/23 patients
Roy et al. (19)	3.5 ± 1.6		10.8 ± 1.1		6/11
Cropp (20)	3.3 ± 0.7		13.0 ± 1.6		4/7
Duke et al. (21)		20.3 ± 4.8		36.1 ± 2.7	13/15
Porter (24)	4.6 ± 1.3		10.7 ± 1.1		10/15
Total					47/71 (66%)

DBP, diastolic blood pressure; MAP, mean arterial pressure; Hgb, hemoglobin; Hct, hematocrit.

stolic pressure increased by 10.9 ± 8.0 in fifteen patients (six of whom had a rise of >10 mm) when the hemoglobin increased from 4.6 to 10.7, two of whom had rises in blood pressure from 118/65 to 146/118 and 130/80 to 165/105 (24). These studies are summarized in Table 2. Note that 47 of 71 patients (66 percent) had a ≥10-mm Hg rise in diastolic or MAP when their hemoglobin or hematocrit increased to greater than 10 g/dL or 30, respectively. Therefore, a rise in blood pressure is common in normotensive subjects with normal renal function as severe anemia is corrected. But the development of hypertension is uncommon, probably because the rise in MAP essentially reverses the lower MAP that occurred as a consequence of the anemic state, and it is conceivable that the more reactive subjects may have had hypertension prior to becoming anemic.

ERYTHROPOIETIN-RELATED HYPERTENSION

Clinical Significance

During the initial clinical trials with epoetin in 1986, the sudden development or accentuation of hypertension was observed. Unfortunately, in a few cases hypertensive encephalopathy developed (1,25). As more dialysis patients were treated with epoetin in various clinical trials, almost all published series (most of which were uncontrolled) indicated a significant incidence of increasing hypertension following an erythropoietic response to epoetin therapy. Of 15 clinical trials in hemodialysis patients reported between 1986 to 1991, 273 of 999 patients (27 percent) developed hypertension or became more hypertensive (usually defined as an increase of at least 10 mm Hg in MAP or diastolic blood pressure) (1,25–39). In addition, the largest clinical trial, occurring in the US, noted these blood pressure changes in 88 of 251 patients (35 percent) (40). Placebo-controlled studies noted an increased need for antihypertensive medications in 28 percent (28 of 99) of patients receiving epoetin and a 9 percent (3 of 32) incidence in placebo-treated patients (38). In another study, 58 percent of 151

epoetin-treated and 37 percent of 78 placebo-treated dialysis patients became more hypertensive (39). Extrapolating from the placebo-controlled studies, the corrected frequency for the development or worsening of hypertension in dialysis patients treated with epoetin is 21 percent.

The development or aggravation of hypertension was also noted when epoetin was used to treat the anemia of patients with renal insufficiency not yet requiring dialysis. Using the same criteria as mentioned above, 43 of 123 patients (35 percent) had a significant rise in blood pressure during the induction phase of epoetin therapy (41–51). However, in a multicenter trial using epoetin intravenously, which included six of the above reported individual studies, there was no difference in the incidence of hypertensive responses between 86 placebo- and epoetin-treated patients (52). This discrepancy remains unexplained. Despite these findings, the aggravation of hypertension during the induction phase of epoetin therapy in patients with progressive renal insufficiency does occur, whether given intravenously or subcutaneously, and blood pressure must be monitored frequently. Hypertensive encephalopathy with seizures has been a rare, but disturbing complication of the epoetin-related hypertension (53).

Pathophysiology

The pathophysiology of the pressor response to epoetin is incompletely understood. Some studies suggest that epoetin exerts a direct pressor effect, whereas most investigators believe that the response is indirectly due to an increase in red cell mass associated with an incomplete reversal in hemodynamic parameters.

Is Epoetin a Direct Pressor Agent?

There are several observations that suggest that epoetin may have a direct pressor effect in the patient with CRF: (a) the pressor response may occur prior to a change in hematocrit (54); (b) the perfusion of epoetin into rat renal and mesenteric arteries results in vasoconstriction of vascular smooth muscle (55); (c) when a specific erythropoietin receptor on the endothelial cell is stimulated with epoetin, this results in the proliferation of endothelial cell growth *in vitro* (56); (d) epoetin results in increased platelet intracellular uptake of calcium (and therefore possibly of endothelial cells) (57); (e) and endothelin-1 production and blood pressure is increased by epoetin (58–60).

On the other hand, these observations must be put in perspective by the following findings:

1. Only patients with CRF develop a pressor response to epoetin, and then in only about 20 percent of the patients. The blood pressure in hypertensive dialysis patients on antihypertensive medication often fluctuates unrelated to epoetin therapy, and even patients receiving placebo instead of epoetin may become more hypertensive (38,39).

2. The amount of epoetin that resulted in vasoconstriction of rat arteries (55) exceeded by five- to tenfold the amount of erythropoietin that circulates in severe hemolytic anemia (1000–2000 mU/mL, usually the highest circulating levels of erythropoietin), and by 10–20 times the level observed after standard epoetin therapy for the anemia of CRF. In contrast to this study, two studies have failed to show any epoetin-induced vasoconstriction of either human subcutaneous arterioles *in vitro* (61) or of isolated perfused Sprague-Dawley rat kidney infused with 1000 mU/mL of epoetin (62).

3. There has yet to be confirmation by other investigators that there is an endothelial cell erythropoietin receptor. Even if there is an erythropoietin receptor on the endothelial cell, the amount of epoetin required to significantly stimulate endothelial growth *in vitro* was in concentrations greater than 2000 mU/mL (56). These concentrations are rarely achieved with standard doses of epoetin. Intravenous injections of 50 U/kg result in a transient (1–2 hours) rise in plasma epoetin levels to 800–1000 mU/mL, whereas subcutaneous injection of the same dose rarely achieves a plasma level greater than 100 mU/mL (63).

4. Epoetin increases the intracellular concentration of calcium in the erythroid precursor cells (64), as well as in the platelets (57). However, there are no data as yet to indicate that the endothelial cell concentration of calcium is greater in those patients who have a pressor response from epoetin.

5. Endothelin-1, a potent vasoconstrictor peptide derived from endothelial cells, has been shown to increase from endothelial cells in culture (58,59), and also in the plasma following epoetin administration (60). However, nonphysiological amounts of epoetin were used in the *in vitro* studies [800–6,600 mU/mL (58) and 200,000 mU/mL (59)]. What role, if any, endothelin-1 plays in the pressor-response is unclear since the levels of endothelin-1 were similar in the pressor-responsive and pressor-nonresponsive dialysis patients receiving epoetin (59), only two of ten pressor-responsive epoetin-treated patients in another study had significantly elevated endothelin-1 levels (65), and no patients in a third study had a pressor response despite a rise in endothelin-1 levels (66).

6. Hormones associated with hypertension and/or vasoconstriction, such as aldosterone, catecholamines, angiotensin, vasopressin (67,68), atrial natriuretic factor (69), and endalin activity (endogenous digitalislike substances) (70) generally are not elevated following epoetin therapy.

Therefore, based upon the above observations, there is insufficient evidence that epoetin, in physiological and clinical doses, exerts a direct vasopressor effect upon the endothelium of vascular smooth muscle. Furthermore, there is no evidence that epoetin raises the levels of known circulating vasoconstrictors.

HEMODYNAMIC EFFECTS OF AN INCREASING RED CELL MASS

As discussed above, anemia, or its correction, result in significant hemodynamic changes affecting cardiac output and peripheral resistance. In addition, the viscosity of blood also may play a role in these hemodynamic changes. Whole blood viscosity is higher in hypertensive than normotensive subjects, and higher in hypertensive patients with higher hematocrit values, which is associated with higher fibrinogen levels (71). A rise in blood viscosity has been thought by some to be a factor in the rise in epoetin-associated hypertension (72,73), but this increase is proportional to the rise in hematocrit (50), and is similar in pressor responders and nonresponders.

Many hemodynamic studies, using either invasive or noninvasive techniques, have been performed. The majority of these studies confirm that the anemic CRF patient has an elevated cardiac output/index and a decreased TPRI. Following an epoetin-induced rise in hematocrit there is a decrease toward normal in the elevated cardiac output, with a compensatory increase in TPRI into the normal range (74–77). These are changes similar to that induced by red-cell transfusion when the hematocrit was increased from 20 to 30, and then from 30 to 40 (9). These hemodynamic changes occur regardless of whether there is a significant increase in MAP. The TPRI does not rise to levels greater than normal in the epoetin-treated patients, in contrast to what was observed in dialysis patients whose hematocrit was increased with red-cell transfusions (9) or in anemic hypertensive patients as seen in Table 2. Cardiac output/index decreases, but does not always return to normal levels. This incomplete correction in cardiac output, without an elevation to greater-than-normal levels of TPRI, has been claimed to contribute to the epoetin-associated rise in blood pressure (68,77). However, since the hematocrit was not returned to normal, the incomplete correction of cardiac output may also have been due to the persistence of mild anemia. Another possible explanation for the slightly elevated cardiac output after partial correction of anemia with epoetin is the effect of the arteriovenous fistula or graft that is present in all hemodialysis patients (78). However, hemodynamic studies done in anemic dialysis patients have failed to demonstrate any change before and after creation of such arteriovenous shunts (79). Of interest is that despite the rise in peripheral resistance, cardiac output is reduced enough so that the pressor effect, if it does develop, may moderate, resulting in a return to baseline BP levels (Fig. 2), (80,81).

Vascular reactivity may be increased in those patients who derive a pressor effect from epoetin. The loss of anemic, hypoxic vasodilation may contribute to the epoetin-induced hypertension, but other factors may also contribute. Those patients who develop the pressor response are more likely to develop forearm vascular resistance to an increase in pO_2 as induced by breathing 60 percent oxygen (82). Angiotensin II infusion increases epinephrine and norepinephrine levels, but in epoetin-treated patients the amount of angiotensin II necessary to increase the MAP by 20 mm Hg actually decreased after 6 weeks and 3 months of epoetin therapy as the hematocrit was rising (83). However, none of these patients developed a pressor response. In the Wistar rat, epoetin induces a pressor response which is blocked by the simultaneous administration of an angiotensin-converting enzyme inhibitor (84). However, in our experience, the epoetin-related pressor response in patients with CRF is not uniformly helped with angiotensin-converting enzyme inhibitors. Autonomic nervous system dysfunction is not a factor in this pressor response (85).

There are two perplexing questions. Why don't all patients with CRF become hypertensive when their red-cell mass increases following epoetin therapy? Why don't some severely anemic patients with normal renal function not become hypertensive following epoetin therapy? A genetic predisposition to hypertension may increase the likelihood of a pressor response related to epoetin therapy (86). This observation needs confirmation. Another possible explanation is suppression of the renin-

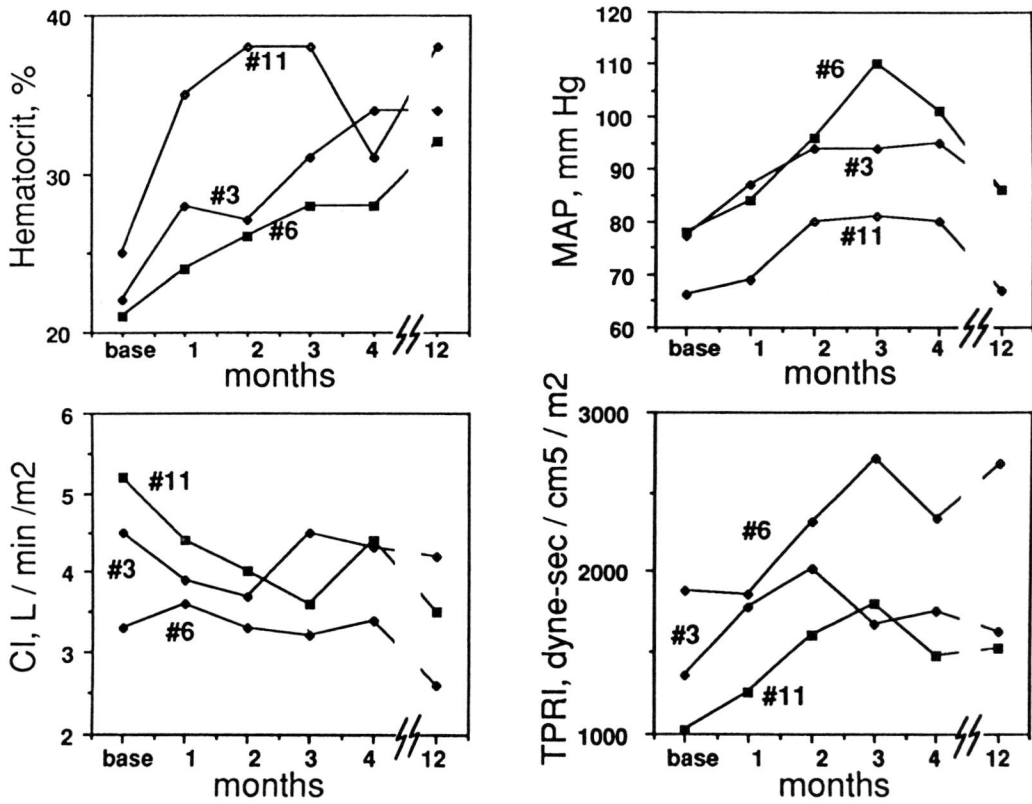

FIG. 2. Hematocrit, mean arterial pressure, cardiac index, and total peripheral vascular resistance index followed serially for up to 1 year in three normotensive (on no antihypertensive medication), anemic hemodialysis patients treated with epoetin, IV, three times a week, either 50 U/kg (patients 3 and 6) or 150 U/kg (patient 11). Patient 6 required an angiotensin-converting enzyme inhibitor drug temporarily between months 3 and 4 of epoetin therapy. Note the return in MAP to near-baseline levels at 1 year despite persistence of a near-normal hematocrit and an elevated-but-normal TPRI. (From ref. 81, with permission.)

angiotensin-aldosterone axis by epoetin in those patients who remain normotensive (87). Plasma renin and aldosterone levels actually decreased in nine dialysis patients treated with epoetin, none of whom had an increase in blood pressure when their hematocrit increased from 19.1 ± 0.8 to 24.5 ± 1.1. However, no patients who developed a pressor response to epoetin were studied. A better explanation for the irregularity of the pressor response and eventual autoregulation, if a pressor response does occur, may be that there is modulation of the production of the vasodilator nitric oxide by endothelial cells in the presence of an epoetin-enhanced red-cell mass (16). As more patients with nonrenal anemias are treated with epoetin, subjects with preexisting hypertension may be less likely to autoregulate, and hypertension will probably be reported to occasionally occur (88).

Clinical Example

The following patient history illustrates various aspects in the presentation, hemodynamics, significance, and management of the hypertensive consequences of epoetin therapy in the anemia of CRF.

This 32-year-old female was diagnosed with a nonhereditary interstitial renal disease at the age of 6 years. She was very anemic and normotensive for many years prior to the onset of hemodialysis in November, 1982. The hematocrit remained below 20 until epoetin was begun in February 1987 as part of a clinical study (150 units/kg, intravenously, three times a week) (40). Blood pressure (BP) was normal at 140/80 at the onset of therapy when the hematocrit was 17. For the next 10 weeks as the hematocrit rose, the BP remained approximately 140/80. Occipital and frontal headaches then developed, associated with a BP of 136/100 and a hematocrit of 34. Metoprolol (Lopressor) 50 mg twice daily was begun. The next day two grand mal seizures occurred when the BP was 164/104. Neurological workup was normal, consisting of normal optic fundi, CT scan, and EEG. Phenytoin and nifedipine (Adalat, Procardia) were prescribed. Because the hematocrit was now 38, 250 ml of blood was removed by phlebotomy. Epoetin was continued at 75 U/kg, three times a week. Although the hematocrit remained approximately 30, hypertension persisted and was associated with bitemporal headaches and vomiting after almost every meal. Five weeks after the initial seizures, there was another seizure. Epoetin was discontinued and the hematocrit dropped to 18 within 3 weeks, but the BP remained elevated at 158/100–180/110. There was now weakness in the left arm and leg and blurred vision in the right eye. An MRI showed a left intracerebral hemorrhage, and hemorrhagic exudates were observed in the right retina. Minoxidil was added to the metoprolol therapy which controlled the BP. All antihypertensive medications were discontinued approximately 6 months later, after there was complete neurological recovery. Antiepileptic medication was discontinued several years later.

The hematocrit remained between 18 and 22 from mid-1987 to February 1992, when epoetin was resumed at the patient's request. Figure 3 details the hematocrit

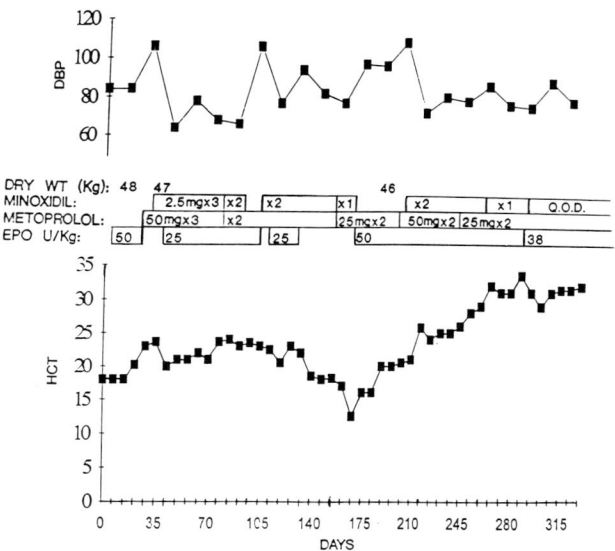

FIG. 3. Diastolic pressure changes related to epoetin-induced hematocrit changes in a previously normotensive, anemic hemodialysis patient who 5 years earlier developed hypertensive encephalopathy related to epoetin therapy (see text for details). The patient subsequently was able to taper off and discontinue both antihypertensive medications.

and BP responses to 25, 50, and 37.5 U/kg of epoetin. Contrary to the initial experience when the BP didn't increase until the hematocrit reached 34, the diastolic pressure increased abruptly with minimal increase in hematocrit (from 18 to 23). By reducing dry weight through dialysis ultrafiltration and prompt resumption of minoxidil and metoprolol antihypertensive therapy, it was possible to safely increase the hematocrit to 34. During the subsequent 18 months, antihypertensive medication has been tapered and eventually discontinued. The blood pressure is now 124/84 with a hematocrit of 34, maintained with 37.5 U/kg of epoetin IV, three times a week.

Noninvasive hemodynamic studies (75) indicated a reversal in the baseline (anemic) elevated cardiac index and low TPVRI (Table 3).

Although this patient's pressor response was more severe than most, it illustrates a number of important clinical points. The pressor response:

1. May occur even in patients without a history of hypertension.

2. Is not related to the dose of epoetin.

3. May occur suddenly and result in hypertensive encephalopathy with or without seizures.

4. If not controlled, can lead to intracerebral bleeding.

5. May not be controlled unless epoetin is discontinued and/or phlebotomy lowers the red-cell mass.

6. May occur at any hematocrit (although usually it occurs when the hematocrit has increased by more than 6–8 percentage points).

7. May require potent vasodilatory drugs to control.

8. May be modified by maintaining good ultrafiltration control (as the red-cell mass increases, plasma vol-

TABLE 3. *Hemodynamics before and during epoetin therapy*

Date	2/13/1987	7/30/1992	9/9/1993
Hematocrit	17	25	32
Epoetin dose, U/kg, T.I.W.	none	50	37.5
Blood pressure	140/80	172/97	128/84
BP medicines	none	minoxidil 50 mg b.i.d. metoprolol 50 mg b.i.d.	none
Cardiac index (L/min/m^2)	5.2	5.0	3.1
Heart rate (beats/min)	73	63	89
Stroke volume (mL/stroke)	97	114	52
TPRI (dynes sec/cm^5)	1707	1952	2489

TPRI, total peripheral resistance index; b.i.d., twice daily; T.I.W., three times a week.

ume should decrease, but it may not– there then may be an increase in volume that contributes to the rise in blood pressure).

9. Eventually, moderates as autoregulation may occur, resulting in the elimination of antihypertensive medication.

While the rate of rise in the hematocrit is not a factor in the incidence of epoetin-associated hypertension (75), it is conceivable that the initial rate of rise in hematocrit for this patient, who had adjusted to severe anemia for many years, was greater than compensatory factors could achieve, resulting in the sudden onset of hypertensive encephalopathy. When lower doses of epoetin were employed 5 years later, the sudden rise in diastolic pressure recurred, although at a lower hematocrit. Closer clinical monitoring detected an expanded plasma volume and prompt vasodilator therapy and dialysis ultrafiltration controlled the blood pressure, allowing for epoetin to be continued to achieve the target hematocrit.

Management

In general, there may be an increase of 10 mm Hg in diastolic pressure as the hematocrit increases from 20 to 30 (9). Therefore, prior to initiating epoetin therapy, blood pressure must be controlled and the patient should be "dry" of excessive extracellular fluid. Controlling plasma volume is crucial to controlling blood pressure in the dialysis patient (89) and equally important in controlling the blood pressure once the epoetin therapy is begun in patients with CRF (90).

There is no evidence that the dose of epoetin is a determinant of a possible pressor response (39,75,91,92). Epoetin therapy is usually initiated with 50 U/kg intravenously three times a week, or 4000 Units subcutaneously two to three times a week, with adjustments every 2–4 weeks if necessary. During this initiation phase, i.e., until the target hematocrit level is attained, BP should be monitored with each dialysis, or every 2 weeks in the predialysis outpatient. The hematocrit should be mea-

sured during this phase at least every other week. If the BP increases to hypertensive levels and/or symptoms of hypertensive encephalopathy develop, epoetin should be discontinued and vasodilator antihypertensive medication prescribed to reduce peripheral resistance. Drugs such as alpha-adrenergic blockers, direct vasodilators, calcium channel blockers, and angiotensin-converting enzyme inhibitors may be effective. However, beta-blocker drugs may also be helpful, considering that cardiac output may remain inappropriately elevated. If the hematocrit increases to levels higher than anticipated, phlebotomy may be necessary to control the BP (93), or a lowering of the hematocrit by reducing epoetin dosage may be sufficient (80). Readjustment downward in the patient's "dry" weight also may be necessary.

As noted in the case example (see Fig. 3), it is possible to attain a target hematocrit in a patient who has marked vascular reactivity to an increasing red cell mass by using vasodilating drugs and dialysis ultrafiltration. Once the target hematocrit is achieved, autoregulatory factors may ensue during the next 6–18 months to allow for a reduction or elimination of antihypertensive drugs (80,92). If autoregulation does not occur, the hypertension usually is not difficult to control. In a follow-up of 55 hemodialysis patients treated with epoetin for 3–5 years, 15 initially became more hypertensive, but their blood pressures were easily controlled and similar to their pressures prior to epoetin therapy (94). Once the target hematocrit has been achieved, epoetin does not need to be discontinued because of transient elevations of BP (which are common in the dialysis patient—even prior to epoetin therapy). It is important to maintain epoetin therapy to maximize saturation of the erythroid progenitor receptors.

CONCLUSIONS

Blood pressure is influenced by the red-cell mass. Anemia results in an increase in cardiac output with a compensatory decrease in peripheral vascular resistance, which is often associated with a lowering in MAP. Polycythemia is occasionally associated with a rise in blood pressure. Severe anemias, whether due to iron, B12, folate, or erythropoietin deficiencies, when partially or completely corrected by appropriate replacement therapy, may be associated with a significant rise in MAP. In CRF there is a high incidence of hypertension, and partial correction of the associated hypoproliferative anemia with recombinant human erythropoietin may result in elevations in MAP of ≥ 10 mm Hg in 20 percent of the patients. It is presently difficult to identify the patient at risk who might develop the epoetin-associated pressor response, although the higher the baseline MAP, the greater the development of significant hypertension. Rarely, hypertensive encephalopathy may result as a consequence of this hemodynamic change.

While a mild elevation in MAP is expected in any patient whose anemia improves from appropriate therapy, the patient with CRF has an increased vascular reactivity that exaggerates this pressor response when initially receiving epoetin. A vasodilatory effect from endothelial-cell-generated nitric oxide may be blunted due to binding of nitric oxide by hemoglobin as the red-cell mass expands, and may also contribute to the epoetin-associated hypertension. Despite this exaggerated pressor response from epoetin in a minority of patients with CRF, blood pressure can usually be well controlled with a combination of antihypertensive medications and maintaining normal plasma volume. Autoregulation may occur in some patients, allowing for the eventual discontinuation or reduction of antihypertensive medicines.

REFERENCES

1. Eschbach JW, Egrie JC, Downing MR, Browne JK, Adamson JW. *N Engl J Med* 1987;316:73–78.
2. Egrie JC, Strickland TW, Lane J, et al. *Immunobiology* 1986;72:213–224.
3. Erslev AJ. *N Engl J Med* 1991;324:1339–1344.
4. Eschbach JW. *Kidney Int* 1989;35:134–148.
5. Eschbach JW, Haley NR, Egrie JC, Adamson JW. *Kidney Int* 1992;43:407–416.
6. Acosta JH. *Kidney Int* 1982;22:702–712.
7. Charra B, Calemard E, Ruffet M, Chazot C, Terrat J, Vanel T, Laurent G. *Kidney Int* 1992;41:1286–1291.
8. Kim KE, Onesti G, Schwartz AB, Chinitz JL, Swartz C. *Circulation* 1972;46:456–464.
9. Neff MS, Kim KE, Persoff M, Onesti G, Swartz C. *Circulation* 1971;43:876–883.
10. Daniel MK, Bennet B, Dawson AA, Rawles JM. *Br Med J* 1986;292:923–926.
11. Berlin NI. *Semin Hematol* 1975;12:339–351.
12. DeWardener HE, McSwiney RR, Miles BD. *Lancet* 1951;2:204–206.
13. Emery AC, Whitcomb WA, Frohlich ED. *JAMA* 1974;229:159–162.
14. Richardson TQ, Guyton AC. *Am J Physiol* 1959;197:1167–1170.
15. Myers BD, Deen WM, Robertson CR, Brenner BM. *Circulation Res* 1975;36:425–435.
16. Wilcox CS, Deng X, Doll AH, Snellen H, Welch WJ. *Kidney Int* 1993;44:430–435.
17. Susic D, Mandal AK, Jovovic D, Veljkovic V, Panajotovic V, Bell RD, Kentera D. *Am J Hypertens* 1992;5:713–718.
18. Ellis LB, Faulkner JM. *N Engl J Med* 1939;220:943–952.
19. Roy SB, Bhatia ML, Mathur VS, Virmani S. *Circulation* 1963;28:346–356.
20. Chopp GJA. *Circulation* 1969;39:775–784.
21. Duke MD, Abelmann WH. *Circulation* 1969;39:503–515.
22. Vatner SF, Higgins CB, Franklin D. *Circulation Res* 1972;30:731–740.
23. Schrier RW, Earley LE. *J of Clin Inves* 1970;49:1656–1667.
24. Porter WB. *Am Heart J* 1937;13:550–579.
25. Winearls G, Oliver D, Pippar M, et al. *Lancet* 1986;2:1175–1178.
26. Casati S, Passerini P, Campise M, et al. *Br Med J* 1987;295:1017–1020.
27. Bommer J, Kugel M, Schoeppe W, et al. *Contrib Nephrol* 1988;66:85–93.
28. Urabe A, Takaku F, Mizoguchi H, et al. *Int J Cell Cloning* 1988;6:179–191.
29. Samtleben W, Baldamus CA, Bommer J, et al. *Contrib Nephrol* 1988;66:114–122.
30. Besarab A, Gaughan W, Medina F. *Kidney Int* 1989;35:240.
31. Sundal E. *Nephrol Dial Transplant* 1989;4:979–987.
32. Schaefer R, Buerner B, Zech M, et al. *Int J Artif Organs* 1988;11:249–254.
33. Kreis H, Zins B, Naret C, et al. *Transpl Proc* 1989;21:55–61.
34. Nielsen OJ, Thaysen. *J Int Med* 1989;226:89–94.
35. Sundal E, Businger J, Kappeler A. *Nephrol Dial Transplant* 1991;6:955–965.
36. Suzuki M, Hirasawa Y, Hirashima K, et al. *Contrib Nephrol* 1989;76:166–178.
37. Duff MD, Golper TA, Sloan RS, Brier ME, Aronoff GR. *Am J Kidney Dis* 1991;18:60–64.
38. Canadian Erythopoietin Study Group. *Am J Nephrol* 1991;11:23–26.
39. Abraham PA, Macres MG. *J Am Soc Nephrology* 1991;2:927–936.
40. Eschbach JW, Abdulhadi MII, Browne JK, et al. *J Ann Int Med* 1989;1111:992–1000.
41. Lim VS, DeGowin RL, Zavala D, Kirchner PT, Abels R, Perry P, Fangman. *J Ann Int Med* 1989;110:108–114.
42. Stone WJ, Graber SE, Krantz SB. *Am J Med Sci* 1988;296:171–179.
43. Eschbach JW, Kelly MR, Haley NR, Abels RI, Adamson JW. *N Engl J Med* 1989;321:158–163.
44. Kleinman KS, Schweitzer SU, Perdue ST, Bleifer KH, Abels RI. *Am J Kidney Dis* 1989;14:486–495.
45. Teehan BP, Sigler MH, Brown JM, et al. *Transpl Proc* 1989;21:63–66.
46. Onoyama K, Kumagai H, Takeda K, Shimamatsu K, Fujishima M. *Nephrol Dial Transplant* 1989;4:966–960.
47. Frenken LAM, Verberckmoes R, Michielsen P, Koene RAP. *Nephrol Dial Transplant* 1989;4:782–786.
48. Abraham PA, Opsahl JA, Rachael KM, Asinger R, Halstenson CE. *Am J Nephrol* 1990;10:128–136.
49. Schwartz AB, Kelch B, Terzian L, Prior J, Kim KE, Pequinot E, Kahn SB. *ASAIO Trans* 1990;36:691–696.
50. Brown CD, Friedman EA. *Am J Nephrol* 1990;10:29–33.
51. Frenken LAM, Wetzels JFM, Sluiter HE, Koene RAP. *Kidney Int* 1992;41:384–387.
52. The US Recombinant Human Erythropoietin Predialysis Study Group. *Am J Kidney Dis* 1991;18:50–59.
53. Edmunds ME, Walls J. *Semin Dialysis* 1991;4:163–167.
54. Baskin S, Lasker N. *N Engl J Med* 1990;323:999–1000.
55. Heidenrich S, Rahn K, Zidek W. *Kidney Int* 1991;39:259–265.
56. Anagnostou A, Lee ES, Kessimian N, Levinson R, Steiner M. *Proc Natl Acad Sci* 1990;87:5978–5982.
57. Van Geet C, Van Damme-Lombaerts R, Vanrusselt M, de Mol A, Proesmans W, Vermylen J. *Thromb Haemostasis* 1990;64:7–10.
58. Carlini RG, Dusso AS, Obialo CI, Alvarez UM, Rothstein M. *Kidney Int* 1993;43:1010–1014.
59. Bode-Böger SM, Böger RH, Kuhn M, Radermacher J, Frölich J. *J Cardiovasc Pharmacol* 1992;20(Suppl 12):S25–S28.

60. Carlini R, Obialo CI, Rothstein M. *AJH* 1993;6:1–5.
61. Bund SJ, Heagerty A, Edmunds M, Walls J. *Nephron* 1989;53:173.
62. Pagel H, Jelkmann W, Weiss C. *Horm Metabol Res* 1989;21:224.
63. Brockmöller J, Köchling J, Weber W, Looby M, Roots I, Neumayer H. *Br J Clin Pharmac* 1992;34:499–508.
64. Miller BA, Scaduto RC Jr, Tillotson DL, Botti JJ, Cheung JY. *J Clin Invest* 1988;82:309–315.
65. Takahashi K, Totsune K, Imai Y, et al. *Clin Sci* 1993;84:47–50.
66. Takayama K, Nagai T, Kinugasa E, Akizawa T, Koshikawa S. *Trans Am Sc Artif Intern Organs* 1991;37:M187–M188.
67. Paganini E, Thomas T, Fouad F, Garcia J, Bravo E. *Kidney Int* 1988;33:204.
68. Hori K, Onoyama K, Iseki K, Fujimi S, Fujishima M. *Clinical Nephrology* 1990;6:293–298.
69. Nonnast-Daniel B, Frei U, Brabant EG, Talartschik J, Schaeffer J, Daniel WG, Koch KM. *Nephrol Dial Transplant* 1989;29:478.
70. Epstein D, Valeri A, Neusy A-J, Lowenstein J. *JASN* 1991;2:376.
71. Letcher RL, Chien SC, Pickering TG, Sealey JE, Laragh JH. *AJM* 1981;70:1195–1202.
72. Rainer AEG. *Lancet* 1988;97–99.
73. Schaefer RM, Leschke M, Strauer BE, Heidland A. *Am J Nephrol* 1988;8:449–453.
74. Nonnast-Daniel B, Creutzig A, Kühn K, et al. *Contr Nephrol* 1988;66:185–194.
75. Buckner FS, Eschbach JW, Haley NR, Davidson RC, Adamson JW. *Am J Hypertens* 1990;3:947–955.
76. London GM, Zins B, Pannier B, et al. *Kidney Int* 1989;36:878–882.
77. Mayer G, Cada EM, Watzinger U, Barnas U, Graf H. *Am J Kidney Dis* 1991;42:286–289.
78. Dongradi G, Rocha P, Baron B. *Clin Nephrol* 1981;15:75–79.
79. Munclinger M, Nemecek K, Serf B, et al. *Nephron* 1987;46:105–106.
80. Nonnast-Daniel B, Deschodt G, Brunkhorst R, Cruetzig A, Bahlmann J, Shaldon S, Koch KM. *Nephrol Dial Transplant* 1990;5:444–448.
81. Davidson RC, Haley NR, Easterling TR, Ahmad S, Adamson JW, Eschbach JW. *Kidney Int* 1990;37:237(A).
82. Roger SD, Grasty MS, Baker LRI, Raine AEG. *Kidney Int* 1992;42:975–980.
83. Jandeleit K, Heintz B, Gross-Heitfeld E, Kindler J, Sieberth HG, Kirsten R, Nelson K. *Nephron* 1990;56:220–221.
84. Eggena P, Willsey P, Jamgotchian N. *Am J Physiol* 1991;261:E642–E646.
85. Roger SD, Baker LRI, Raine AEG. *Clin Nephrol* 1993;39:103–110.
86. Ishimitsu T, Tsukada H, Ogawa Y, Numabe A, Yagi S. *AJM* 1993;94:401–406.
87. Yaqoob M, Morris K, Bell GM, Ahmad R. *Nephrol Dial Transplant* 1992;7:125–128.
88. Abels RI. *Sem in Oncology* 1992;19:29–35.
89. Kim KE, Onesti G, DelGuercio ET, Greco J, Fernandes M, Eidelson B, Swartz B. *Hypertension* 1980;2:102–110.
90. Anastassiades E, Howarth D, Howarth J, et al. *Nephrol Dial Transplant* 1993;8:621–625.
91. Spinowitz B. *Am J Nephrol* 1990;10[Suppl 2]:24–28.
92. van de Borne P, Tielemans C, Vanherweghem J-L, Degaute J-P. *Nephrol Dial Transplant* 1992;7:45–49.
93. Fahal IH, Yaqoob M, Ahmad R. *Nephron* 1992;61:214–216.
94. Eschbach JW, Aquiling T, Haley NR, Fan MH, Blagg CR. *Clin Nephrol* 1992;38[Suppl 1]:S98–S103.

Hypertension: Pathophysiology, Diagnosis, and Management, Second Edition,
edited by J.H. Laragh and B.M. Brenner,
Raven Press, Ltd., New York © 1995.

CHAPTER **25**

Interactions Between the Sympathetic Nervous System and the Renin Angiotensin System

Giuseppe Mancia, Antonio Saino, and Guido Grassi

A large body of evidence indicates that the sympathetic nervous system and the renin-angiotensin system are both majorly involved in the modulation of the circulation (1,2). More recently, it has also become clear that these two systems do not operate independently but interact with each other in accomplishing their cardiovascular regulation. This interaction has been shown both in experimental animal species and in man with and without cardiovascular disease.

This chapter will focus on the interactions between the sympathetic nervous system and the renin-angiotensin system based on the evidence collected in humans by our group and by other laboratories. Emphasis will be given to the implications of these interactions for the cardiovascular function in hypertension, congestive heart failure, and ischemic heart disease.

SYMPATHETIC INFLUENCES ON THE RENIN-ANGIOTENSIN SYSTEM

Animal Background

In several animal species electrical stimulation of renal sympathetic nerves is associated with the renal release of renin (3,4). The increase in renin release accompanying

renal nerve stimulation can be seen also when the concomitant reduction in renal blood flow is prevented by blockade of alpha-adrenergic receptors by phenoxybenzamine (Dibenzyline) (5,6). It can be seen even when the electrical stimulus is performed at a frequency so low as to be unable to cause any detectable renal vasoconstriction (7). The renin release increase can, on the other hand, be abolished by blockade of beta-adrenergic receptors via propranolol (Inderal) without affecting the renal vasoconstriction (5,6). Thus, the sympathetic nervous system has a large influence on the renin secretory process occurring in the kidney. This influence is exerted not only through alterations in renal hemodynamics but also through a direct influence on the secretion which takes place in the juxtaglomerular apparatus. This is presumably effected by the sympathetic fibers which innervate beta-adrenergic receptors in the juxtaglomerular cells.

Electrical stimulation is an artificial means to activate sympathetic influences. However, a large body of animal evidence shows that these influences also operate under stimuli elicited more physiologically via the brain. For example, Richardson et al. (8,9) have shown that in anesthetized cats electrical stimulation of several areas in the hindbrain was associated with a large increase in renin release in an innervated kidney but not in the contralateral denervated one. The increase persisted when the concomitant renal vasoconstriction was prevented by phenoxybenzamine and abolished following administration of propranolol (10). Furthermore, Ueda et al. (11) and Passo et al. (12) have shown that marked increases

G. Mancia, A. Saino, and G. Grassi: Cattedra di Medicina Interna, Università di Milano, Ospedale S. Gerardo dei Tintori, Monza; Centro Auxologico Italiano, Milano, Italy.

in renin release also followed electrical stimulation of the hypothalamus and other sites of the forebrain. Finally, an increase in renin release has been repeatedly shown under circumstances in which animals' behavior was altered to cause central sympathetic stimulation, i.e., during exercise, defense reaction, etc. (13–15).

Animal data further document that renin release can be significantly modulated via reflex alterations in sympathetic drive. Although several reflexogenic areas are involved, a most important contribution to reflex renin control originates from volume receptors in the cardiopulmonary region. In dogs and cats activation of these receptors by atrial stretching is associated with an inhibition of renin release via a reflex reduction in renal sympathetic nerve traffic (16,17). Conversely, a deactivation of these receptors by vagal nerve cooling (which reversibly blocks afferent nerve conduction) is associated with a reflex increase in sympathetic nerve traffic and renin release (18). A substantial increase in renin release can be obtained also when (a) concomitant changes in renal hemodynamics are prevented and (b) the cardiopulmonary receptor deactivation is produced not by blockade of afferent nerve signal but by a reduction in central blood volume by hemorrhage or tilting (19,20).

Thus, sympathetic modulation of renin release is under the continuous restraint of reflex influences originating from volume receptors in the intrathoracic areas. This represents a feedback mechanism for blood volume control.

Evidence in Normal Humans

In normal human beings renin release undergoes an increase during mental stress and dynamic exercise, suggesting that in our species central activation of the sympathetic nervous system has a stimulating effect (21,22). Human evidence about central influences on renin release is limited, however, because behavioral stimuli are often too short-lasting to substantially affect renin release. Furthermore, in conditions such as sleep a central sympathetic deactivation is associated with a marked blood pressure fall which results in a direct baroreceptor stimulation of renin secretion, preventing observation of the sympathetic-dependent reduction (23,24).

On the other hand, substantial evidence exists as to the importance of reflex control of renin release in man. This was observed by Kiowski and Egan and co-workers in normotensive subjects in whom a moderate reduction in venous return to the heart and central blood volume were obtained by inflation of cuffs positioned around the tights (25,26). This maneuver resulted in an increase in plasma renin activity in most individuals. The increase was abolished by previous administration of propranolol and not at all evident in few subjects with renal denervation from kidney transplantation, suggesting a reflex

control of renin release from modulation of renal sympathetic nerve activity by volume cardiopulmonary receptors, similar to the one shown in animal studies.

Our group has recently examined in more detail the reflex control of renin release exerted by cardiopulmonary receptors in healthy humans (27,28). Central venous pressure and left ventricular volume (echocardiography) were increased by passive leg raising and reduced by application of a mild negative pressure to the lower body. The increase and reduction were maintained for 20–30 minutes and obtained with only minimal alterations of blood pressure and heart rate. The increase in central venous pressure and cardiac volume caused a reduction in plasma norepinephrine and a forearm vasodilatation, indicating reflex sympathetic inhibition. The reduction in central venous pressure and cardiac volume caused an increase in plasma norepinephrine and a forearm vasoconstriction, indicating reflex sympathetic stimulation. The sympathetic inhibition and stimulation

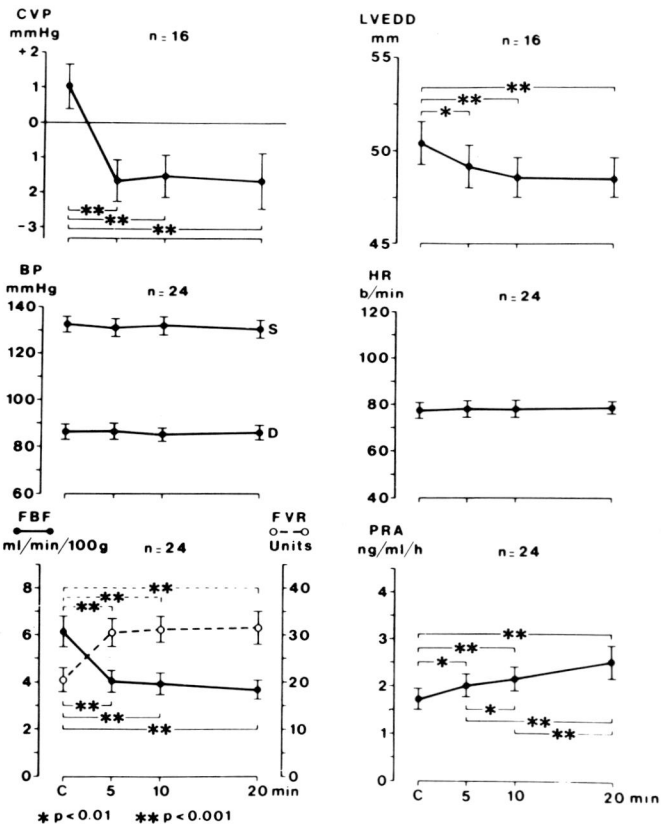

FIG. 1. Effects of 20 minutes nonhypotensive lower-body negative pressure (−14.8 ± 1.6 mm Hg) on central venous pressure (CVP), left ventricular end-diastolic diameter (LVEDD), systolic (S) and diastolic (D) blood pressure (BP), heart rate (HR), forearm blood flow (FBF), forearm vascular resistance (FVR) and plasma renin activity (PRA). Values are shown as means ± SE from 24 subjects (n = 16 for CVP and LVEDD). Asterisks refer to statistical significance between different values. C, control. From ref. 28, with permission.

were accompanied by a reduction and an increase, respectively, of plasma renin levels. The changes in plasma renin activity increased with the increasing duration of the reflexogenic stimuli and at the thirtieth minute modified baseline plasma renin activity by 92 ± 15 percent. Thus, in normal man renin secretion is restrained by cardiopulmonary receptors. This restraint is such as to substantially modify plasma renin levels in both directions over a relatively short time.

A debated question is whether and to what extent other reflexogenic areas participate in reflex control of renin release in man. In six healthy volunteers Mark et al. (29) reported that a reduction in venous return caused an increase in plasma renin activity only when so marked as to induce a blood pressure fall, suggesting that reflexogenic control of renin release needs arterial baroreceptor involvement. However, the bulk of the remaining evidence rather suggests a predominant role of cardiopulmonary receptors with little arterial baroreceptor contribution. Firstly, in the study of Kiowski et al. (25), the increase in plasma renin activity induced by cuff inflation at the tights was obtained with no apparent blood pressure alteration. This was clearly the case in our studies with lower-body negative pressure even when blood pressure was more precisely measured by intraarterial monitoring (Fig. 1) (27,28). Secondly, in a subsequent study of our group, the increase in plasma renin activity induced by lower-body negative pressure was abolished

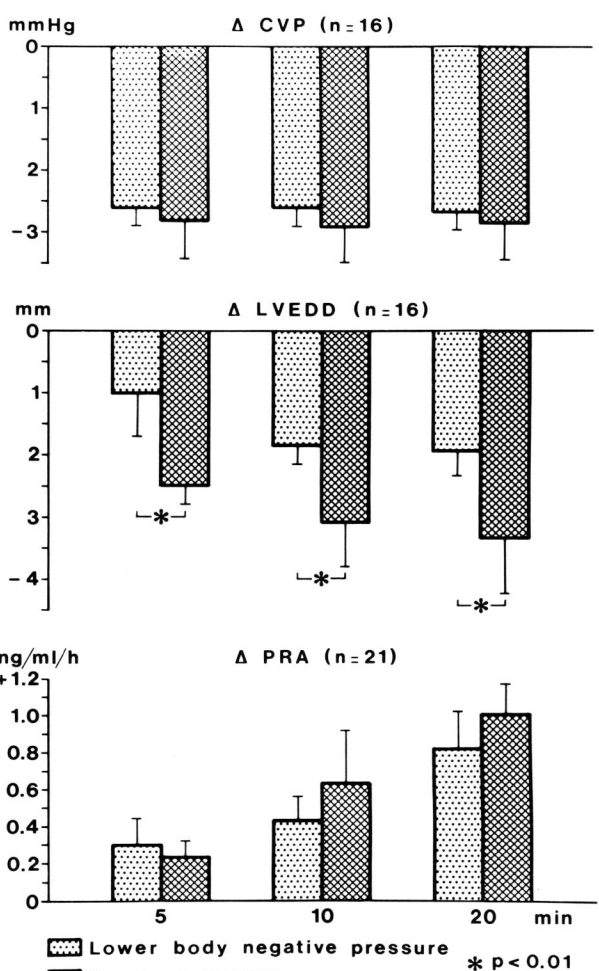

FIG. 3. Mean (±SE) changes in central venous pressure (CVP), left ventricular end-diastolic diameter (LVEDD), and plasma renin activity (PRA) induced by nonhypotensive lower-body negative pressure and head-up tilting. From ref. 28, with permission.

in patients with a recent heart transplantation, even when the negative pressure was so marked as to cause hypotension and thus engage the arterial baroreflex (Fig. 2) (30). Three, the increase in plasma renin activity induced by head-up tilting, i.e., a maneuver which deactivates not only cardiopulmonary receptors (reduction in central venous pressure) but also carotid baroreceptors (displacement of the carotid sinuses above the heart), was entirely reproduced by an identical reduction in central venous pressure through nonhypotensive lower-body negative pressure (Fig. 3) (28).

Thus, in normal humans, cardiopulmonary receptors can modulate renin release even in absence of an arterial baroreceptor involvement; indeed, heart transplantation data suggest this to be a role played by receptors located in the heart. This modulation is largely responsible for the changes in plasma renin activity occurring during alterations in posture.

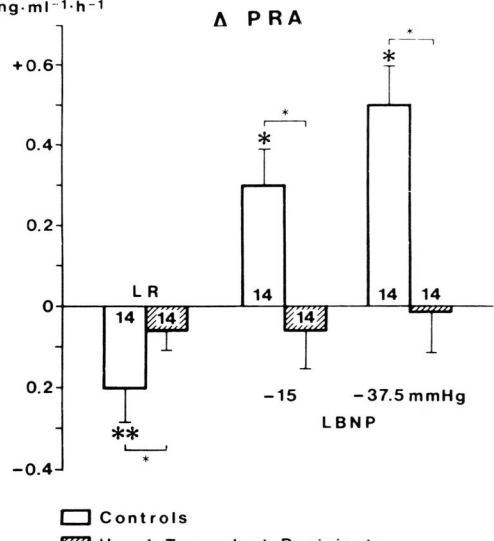

FIG. 2. Mean (±SE) changes in plasma renin activity (PRA) induced by leg raising (LR) and lower-body negative pressure (LBNP) at −15 and −37.5 mm Hg in 14 controls and 14 age-matched cardiac-transplant subjects. Large asterisks on each histogram refer to the statistical significance of the changes from baseline values. Small asterisks refer to the statistical significance of the difference between controls and cardiac-transplant subjects. *p < 0.05 **p < 0.01. From ref. 30, with permission.

Hypertension and Congestive Heart Failure

In twelve patients with an untreated mild hypertension, plasma renin activity was measured before and during an increase and a reduction in central venous pressure caused by passive leg raising and nonhypotensive lower-body negative pressure, respectively (28). Plasma renin activity was reduced during leg raising and increased during lower-body negative pressure. The changes were similar to those seen in age-matched controls, suggesting no impairment of cardiopulmonary reflex modulation of renin release in uncomplicated essential hypertension.

Preservation of cardiopulmonary receptor control of renin release does not apply to more advanced hypertension stages, however. In twelve patients with hypertension and marked left ventricular hypertrophy, the changes in plasma renin activity induced by cardiopulmonary receptor deactivation and stimulation via nonhypotensive lower-body negative pressure and leg raising were markedly reduced as compared to those seen in normotensive controls and hypertensives with no left ventricular hypertrophy (Fig. 4) (31). The reduction was paralleled by a reduction in other sympathetically mediated reflex responses (e.g., plasma norepinephrine and forearm vascular resistance). It was accompanied, however, by an unchanged plasma renin response to other neural stimuli, indicating that an impaired responsiveness of the juxtaglomerular cells to renin-secreting stimuli was not involved. Thus, reflex sympathetic modulation of renin release is unaltered in early hypertension but impaired in hypertensive conditions in which structural cardiovascular changes have occurred. This implies less tonic restraint of renin release and a tendency for this humoral substance to increase. Such increase may favor a progression of the hypertensive condition. It may also favor the adverse effects of an excessive production of angiotensin II on the cardiovascular system (cardiac hypertrophy, vascular hypertrophy and hyperplasia, etc.).

Several studies have shown that reflex control of the circulation is impaired in congestive heart failure and that the impairment involves the cardiac and vascular modulation exerted by both arterial baroreceptors and cardiopulmonary receptors (32–36). Little evidence exists, however, as to whether the reflex impairment includes modulation of renin release. Preliminary data from our group suggest that this is indeed the case because in subjects with congestive heart failure the changes in plasma renin activity induced by leg raising and nonhypotensive lower-body negative pressure were about 70 percent less than those seen in age-matched controls (37). The impairment was evident not only in patients belonging to class III and IV of the New York Heart Association (NYHA) classification but also in those belonging to class NYHA II. The impairment of the cardiopulmonary reflex control of renin release occurring in congestive heart failure may contribute to the activation of the renin-angiotensin system typical of this

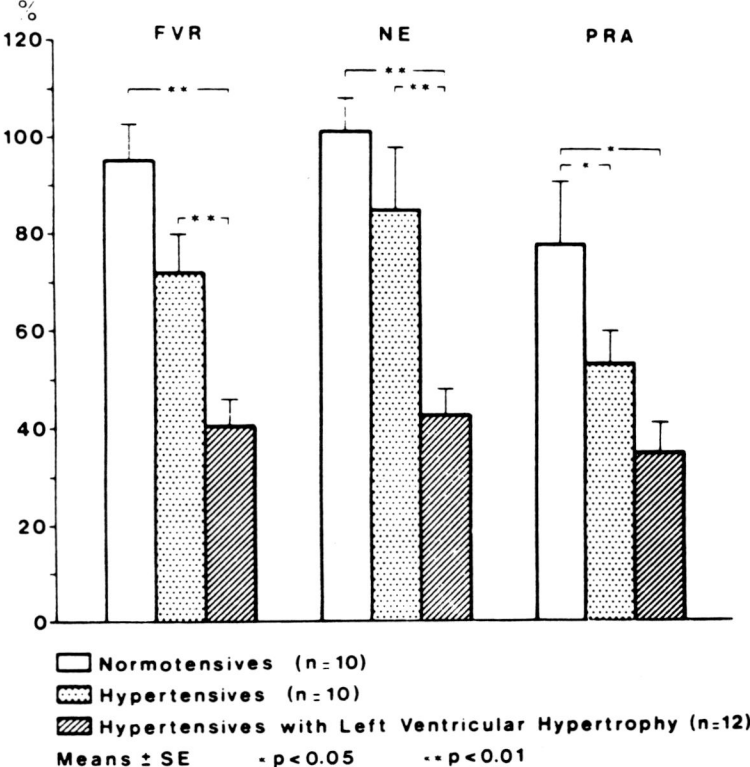

FIG. 4. Mean (±SE) percent changes in forearm vascular resistance (FVR), plasma renin activity (PRA), and plasma norepinephrine (NE) induced by leg raising and nonhypotensive lower-body negative pressure in normotensive subjects and in hypertensives without and with cardiac hypertrophy. Changes induced by leg raising and lower-body negative pressure are added to evaluate the overall responses. From ref. 31, with permission.

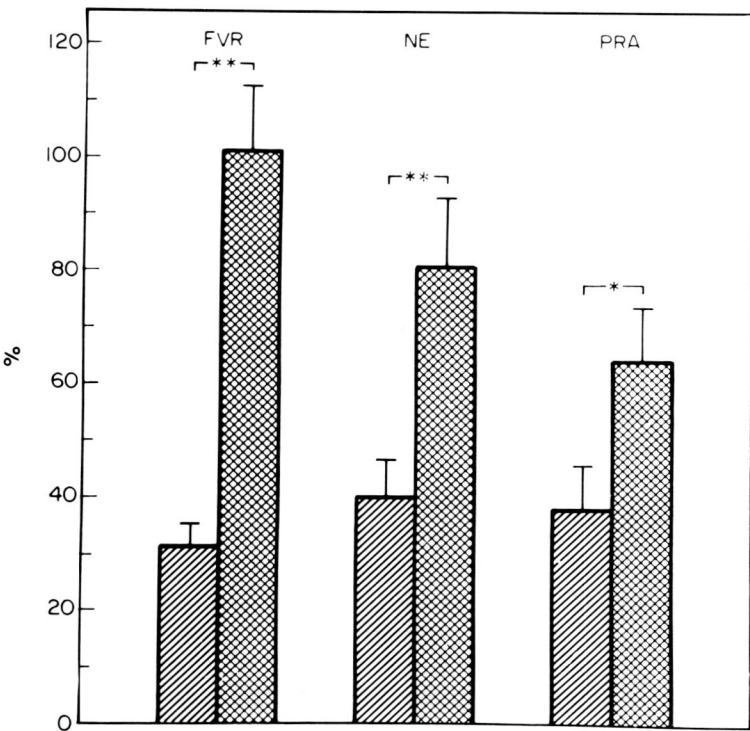

FIG. 5. Mean (±SE) percent changes in forearm vascular resistance (FVR), plasma norepinephrine (NE), and plasma renin activity (PRA) induced by leg raising and nonhypotensive lower-body negative pressure in seven hypertensives before (▨) and after (▦) therapeutic regression of left ventricular hypertrophy. Changes induced by leg raising and lower-body negative pressure are added to evaluate the overall responses. *$p < 0.05$; **$p < 0.01$.

condition. It may also enhance the concomitant sympathetic activation because of the facilitating effect of angiotensin II on sympathetic neural drive (see below) (34,36).

Does treatment reverse the impaired reflex control of renin release occurring in cardiovascular disease? At present, evidence is limited to hypertension and refers to subjects in whom the elevated blood pressure values were effectively reduced for 1 year, achieving a regression of the left ventricular hypertrophy diagnosed before treatment (31). As shown in Fig. 5, 2 weeks after withdrawal of antihypertensive treatment (to avoid direct effects of antihypertensive drugs on the reflex responses), leg raising and nonhypotensive lower-body negative pressure were accompanied by changes in plasma renin activity much greater than those seen before treatment. Thus, the impaired reflex control of renin release occurring in hypertension is reversible, provided that the structural alterations induced by hypertension are reversed.

RENIN-ANGIOTENSIN INFLUENCES ON THE SYMPATHETIC NERVOUS SYSTEM

Animal Background

A large number of animal studies documents that angiotensin II facilitates sympathetic influences on the heart and the systemic blood vessels. Because injection of angiotensin II into blood vessels perfusing the brain (or topical brain application of this substance) was followed by a sympathetically mediated increase in blood pressure and vascular resistance (38–44), this facilitation can be produced through a central mechanism. However, peripheral mechanisms also play a role because angiotensin II has a stimulating influence on neural transmission across sympathetic ganglia (45,46). Furthermore, release of norepinephrine from sympathetic nerve terminals is increased by angiotensin II due to stimulation of presynaptic angiotensinergic receptors (47–50) or other complex synaptic mechanisms (51,52). Finally, in pithed rats, angiotensin II has been shown to amplify the local vascular effects of catecholamine infusion (53), thereby increasing the responsiveness of adrenergic receptors to their physiological stimuli. Thus, multifold mechanisms are involved in the enhancing effects of angiotensin II on sympathetic circulatory control in animals. These effects establish a reciprocal reinforcement which favors a progressive activation of the renin-angiotensin system and the sympathetic nervous system regardless which is initially stimulated. This reinforcement may be further promoted by the fact that, as shown in several animal species, arterial baroreflex sensitivity is attenuated by angiotensin II (54–56), reducing an important restraint to cardiac and vascular sympathetic drive.

Human Data

Forearm Circulation

More than 20 years ago Abboud (57) showed that in healthy normotensive volunteers, intravenous administration of angiotensin II was accompanied by an increase in forearm vasoconstriction induced reflexly by deactivating cardiopulmonary receptors through lower-body negative pressure. This was confirmed by other investigators who made use also of subpressor intravenous doses of angiotensin II (58) or of doses of angiotensin II infused directly into the brachial artery (59,60). There is therefore little doubt that the enhancing effect of this substance on sympathetic vascular influences also takes place in normal man. This can be further inferred from the results obtained by a more indirect approach, i.e., blockade of angiotensin II formation through administration of an angiotensin-converting enzyme (ACE) inhibitor. In subjects with mild or moderate essential hypertension we observed that the sympathetic constriction of the forearm arterioles reflexly induced by cardiopulmonary receptor deactivation via lower-body negative pressure was attenuated following an oral dose of captopril (Capoten) capable of markedly reducing plasma angiotensin II levels (61). Similar results were obtained after (a) administration of benazepril (Zinadril) (62) and (b) administration of the ACE inhibitors for several weeks (61,62). Thus, although ACE inhibitors alter the tissue and plasma concentrations of several other vasoactive substances (63), sympathetic vascular influences are probably blunted by the acute removal of angiotensin II with little recovery when the removal is more chronically maintained.

Coronary Circulation

An important question is whether in man the facilitating effect of angiotensin II on sympathetic influences involves areas other than forearm resistance vessels, which mainly reflect skeletal muscle circulation. In this context, Benjamin et al. (64) have shown that in healthy, normal volunteers the reflex venoconstriction caused by deep breathing is augmented by intravenous administration of angiotensin II. Furthermore, Seidelin and Struthers (65) have shown that intravenous subpressor doses of angiotensin II enhance the inotropic response of the normal human heart to adrenergic stimulation by isoproterenol (Norisodrine). Finally, Jakobsen et al. (66)

have demonstrated that the reflex tachycardia induced by administration of vasodilators in hypertensive patients is blunted by concomitant ACE inhibition. Thus, the facilitating effect of angiotensin II on sympathetic influences extends beyond skeletal muscle resistance vessels and involves the heart.

Our group has recently shown that the enhancing effect of angiotensin II on sympathetic influences is particularly evident in human coronary circulation. The study made use of diving (67), i.e., a stimulus which causes a mild sympathetic coronary vasoconstriction in the presence of mild coronary artery disease and a marked sympathetic coronary vasoconstriction in the presence of severe coronary artery lesions (68). In a first series of seven subjects with mild coronary artery disease (angiographic examination) a 30-second diving increased arterial blood pressure (arterial catheter) and coronary blood flow (coronary sinus thermodilution) with little change in coronary vascular resistance. During an intracoronary infusion (left coronary artery) of a dose of angiotensin II (1.27 ± 0.16 ng/min, mean $\pm$ SE) devoid of any systemic or coronary hemodynamic effect, however, diving increased blood pressure to a similar extent but it reduced coronary blood flow, thereby markedly increasing coronary vascular resistance (Table 1). Conversely, in a second series of nine subjects with severe coronary artery disease, diving increased blood pressure markedly and reduced coronary blood flow with a marked increase in coronary vascular resistance. Following an oral dose of 25 mg of captopril the pressor response was unchanged but the reduction in coronary blood flow was replaced by an increase with a marked attenuation of the coronary vasoconstriction (Fig. 6) (69).

Two further questions are (a) the mechanisms responsible for the facilitating effect of angiotensin II on sympathetic activity in man and (b) the relationship of this effect to the plasma renin and angiotensin II levels.

Concerning the first question in mild or moderate essential hypertensive patients, Taddei et al. (60) have shown that the increased reflex forearm vasoconstriction associated with brachial artery infusion of angiotensin II was accompanied by an increased release of norepinephrine from the forearm tissues. However, intraarterial infusion of angiotensin II may lead to nonphysiological

TABLE 1. *Changes in coronary and systemic hemodynamics induced by diving during the intracoronary infusion of saline and angiotensin II*

	Baseline	Saline (%)	Angiotensin II (%)	p^a
Systolic blood pressure	127.5 ± 3.9	$+21 \pm 3$	$+21 \pm 2$	NS
Diastolic blood pressure	74.7 ± 2.3	$+18 \pm 6$	$+27 \pm 5$	NS
Mean arterial pressure	92.2 ± 2.5	$+19 \pm 4$	$+24 \pm 3$	NS
Heart rate	63.2 ± 4.2	-9 ± 1	-12 ± 1	NS
Coronary blood flow	104.8 ± 10.2	$+14 \pm 4$	-16 ± 5	<0.01
Coronary vascular resistance	0.92 ± 0.1	$+7 \pm 6$	$+52 \pm 9$	<0.01

[a] Statistical significance of the difference between changes induced by saline and angiotensin II.

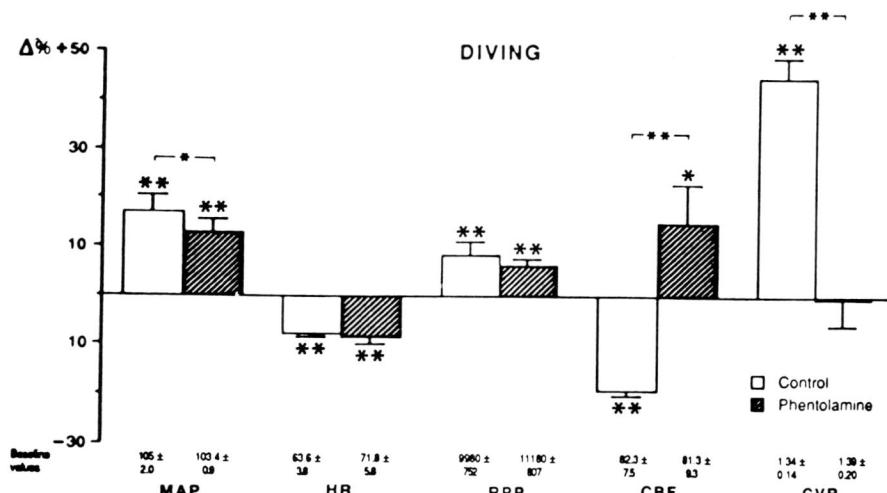

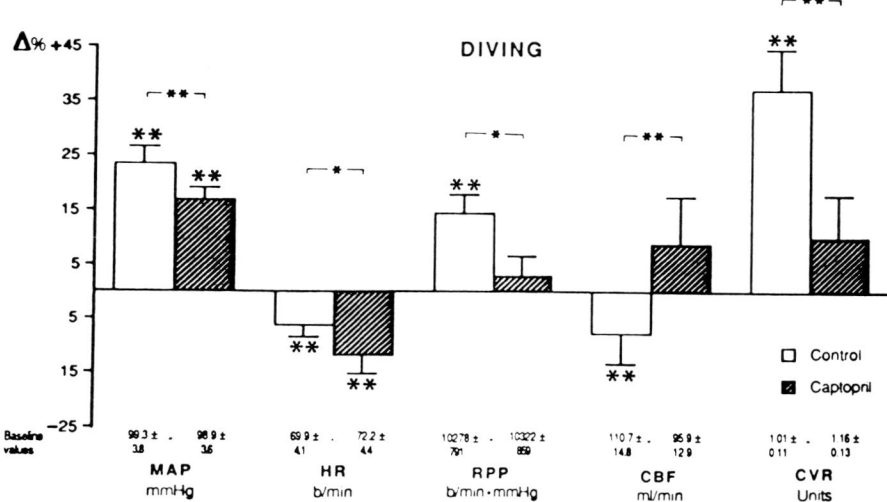

FIG. 6. Effects of intravenous phentolamine infusion (*top panel,* n = 5) and oral captopril administration (*bottom panel,* n = 9) on systemic and coronary hemodynamic responses to diving. Data are expressed as mean (±SE) percent changes from baseline values (*bottom, each panel*). Large asterisks refer to statistical significance of the responses whereas small asterisks to statistical significance of the difference between changes observed in control condition (*open bars*) and after administration of phentolamine or captopril (*hatched bars*). MAP, mean arterial pressure; HR, heart rate; RPP, rate-pressure product; CBF, coronary blood flow; CVR, coronary vascular resistance. *p < 0.05; **p < 0.01. From ref. 69, with permission.

concentration and distribution of this substance, and other studies have reported that during intravenous infusion of angiotensin II the enhanced sympathetic vasoconstriction is not accompanied by an overflow of norepinephrine (70). Furthermore, in our hypertensive subjects the attenuation of the reflex forearm vasoconstriction that followed ACE inhibition was not paralleled by any attenuation in the plasma norepinephrine response (61). Finally, as mentioned above, evidence has been produced that in man the inotropic responses to isoproterenol are enhanced by angiotensin II (65). Thus, a postsynaptic mechanism is likely to be involved in the angiotensin II enhancement of sympathetic cardiovascular influences in man (71). Whether this is caused by circulating angiotensin II or by production of this substance at tissue level is unknown.

As to the second question, sympathetic influences are clearly enhanced when plasma levels of angiotensin II are increased by exogenous infusion. However, even the low plasma angiotensin II levels characterizing a large proportion of subjects have been shown to have a sympathofacilitating effect (61,69). Thus, it appears that in man the renin-angiotensin system interacts with the sympathetic nervous system, even at low degrees of activation.

Clinical Implications

The interactions between the renin-angiotensin and the sympathetic nervous systems may have complex effects on blood pressure homeostasis.

Blood pressure homeostasis may be improved by the

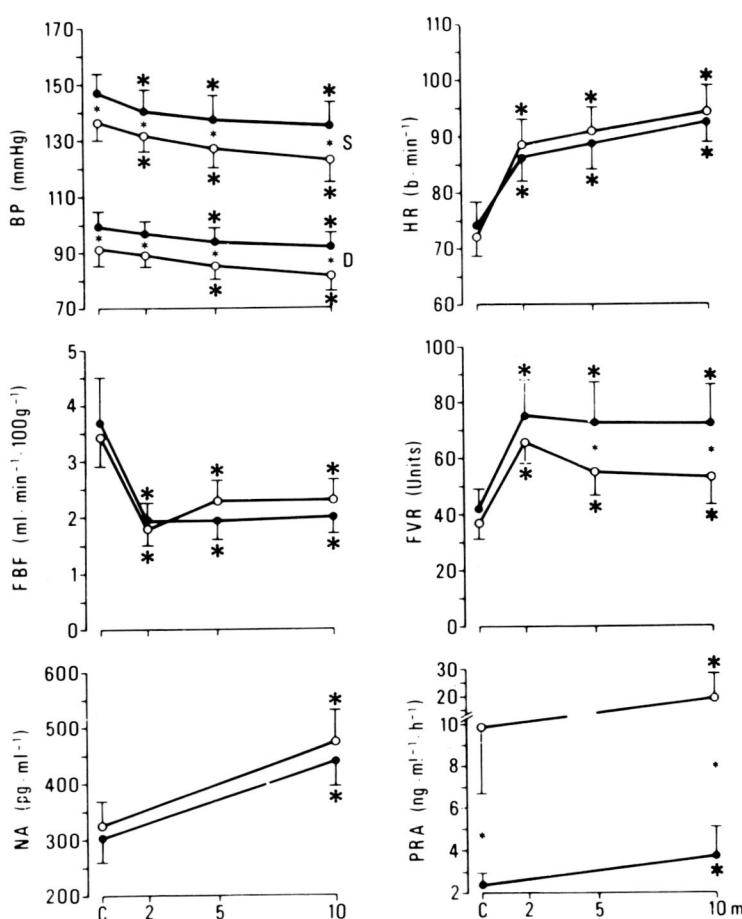

FIG. 7. Effects of hypotensive lower body negative pressure (−37.5 ± 0.5 mm Hg) on systolic (S) and diastolic (D) blood pressure (BP), heart rate (HR), forearm blood flow (FBF), forearm vascular resistance (FVR), plasma norepinephrine (NA), and plasma renin activity (PRA) before (*closed circles*) and after (*open circles*) chronic angiotensin-converting enzyme inhibition in nine hypertensive patients. Data are shown as mean ± SEM; *$p < 0.05$. From ref. 61, with permission.

angiotensin-II-dependent increase in cardiac and vascular sympathetic influences. It may also be worsened, however, by the baroreflex impairment caused by angiotensin II (72). It is likely that, in acute conditions, the improvement prevails because in our study acute removal of plasma angiotensin II by ACE inhibition was followed by a greater hypotensive effect of marked lower-body negative pressure (73) (Fig. 7), indicating a less effective blood pressure adjustment to orthostaticlike challenges (74–76). Furthermore, in conditions in which the renin-angiotensin system is activated (e.g., congestive heart failure), acute ACE inhibition may not too infrequently be accompanied by a profound hypotension despite an increase in baroreflex sensitivity (77–80).

On the other hand, chronic administration of ACE inhibitors is only exceptionally followed by hypotensive phenomena during orthostasis and exercise, suggesting that later compensatory factors may allow recovery of neural cardiovascular adjustments (81). It is also possible, however, that this recovery is due to partial escape of angiotensin II production from ACE inhibition (82).

Regardless the effects on blood pressure homeostasis, the reciprocal reinforcement of the renin-angiotensin and the sympathetic nervous systems may have clear ad-

verse effects in several cardiovascular disorders. For example, this reinforcement may increase the neurohumoral activation occurring in congestive heart failure; i.e., it may modify in an unfavorable fashion a variable with an adverse impact on patients' prognoses (83,84). Furthermore, it may increase neurohumoral activation occurring immediately after an acute myocardial infarction (85), also with adverse consequences on prognosis. Finally, because of this interaction, the trophic effects of angiotensin II and catecholamines may be increased with a greater tendency to develop cardiac and vascular hypertrophy and thus to have structural alterations of clinical relevance in hypertension. All this may account for the beneficial effects of ACE inhibition in the diseases mentioned above.

REFERENCES

1. Mancia G, Ferrari AU, Zanchetti A. In: Zanchetti A, Tarazi R, eds. *Handbook of hypertension,* vol 8. Amsterdam: Elsevier, 1986;47–68.
2. Sealey JE, Laragh JH. In: Laragh JH, Brenner BM, eds. *Hypertension: pathophysiology, diagnosis and management.* New York: Raven Press, 1990;1287–1318.
3. Vander AJ. *Am J Physiol* 1965;209:659–662.

4. Johnson JA, Davis JO, Witty RT. *Circ Res* 1971;29:646–653.
5. Loeffler JR, Stockigt JR, Ganong WF. *Neuroendocrinol* 1972;10: 129–138.
6. Coote JH, Johns EJ, Macleod VM, Singer B. *J Physiol* 1972;226: 15–36.
7. Lagrange RG, Sloop CH, Schmid HE. *Circ Res* 1973;33:704–712.
8. Richardson D, Stella A, Leonetti G, Bartorelli A, Zanchetti A. *Clin Sci Mol Med* 1973;45(Suppl 1):243–246.
9. Richardson D, Stella A, Leonetti G, Bartorelli A, Zanchetti A. *Circ Res* 1974;34:425–434.
10. Zanchetti A, Stella A. *Clin Sci Mol Med* 1975;48(Suppl 2):215–223.
11. Ueda H, Yasuda H, Takabatake Y, et al. *Jpn Heart J* 1967;8:498–506.
12. Passo SS, Assaykeen TA, Otsuka K, Wise BL, Goldfein A, Ganong WF. *Neuroendocrinol* 1971;7:1–10.
13. Tsukiyama H, Otsuka K, Kyuwo S, Fujishima S, Kijima F. *Jpn Circ J* 1973;37:1265–1271.
14. Clamage DN, Sanford CS, Vander AJ, Mouw DR. *Am J Physiol* 1976;231:1290–1297.
15. Bing J, Povlsen K. *Acta Physiol Scand* 1979;107:251–256.
16. Zehr JE, Hasbergen JA, Kurz KD. *Circ Res* 1976;38:232–239.
17. Thames MC. *Am J Physiol* 1977;233:H181–H184.
18. Mancia G, Romero JC, Shepherd JT. *Circ Res* 1974;36:529–535.
19. Stella A, Zanchetti A. *Am J Physiol* 1977;232:H500–H507.
20. Stella A, Dampney RAL, Golin R, Zanchetti A. *Circ Res* 1978;43(Suppl 1):I107–I111.
21. Hotchen TA, Hartley LH, Rice TW, Mougey EH, Jones LG, Masow JW. *J Appl Physiol* 1971;31:178–184.
22. Galbo H. *Hormonal and metabolic adaptation to exercise.* New York: Thieme-Stratton, 1983.
23. Vagnucci AH, McDonald RH, Drash AL, Wrong AKC. *J Clin Endocrinol Metab* 1974;38:761–776.
24. Mancia G, Zanchetti A. In: Orem J, Barnes CD, eds. *Physiology in sleep.* New York: Academic Press, 1980;1–55.
25. Kiowski W, Julius S. *J Clin Invest* 1978;62:656–663.
26. Egan BM, Julius S, Cottier C, Osterziel KJ, Ibsen H. *Hypertension* 1983;5:779–786.
27. Grassi G, Giannattasio C, Cuspidi C, et al. *Am J Med* 1988;84(Suppl 3A):97–104.
28. Grassi G, Giannattasio C, Saino A, et al. *Hypertension* 1988;11: 92–99.
29. Mark AL, Abboud FM, Fitz AE. *Am J Physiol* 1983;235:H29–H33.
30. Giannattasio C, Del Bo M, Cattaneo BM, et al. *Hypertension* 1993;21:461–469.
31. Grassi G, Giannattasio C, Cleroux J, et al. *Hypertension* 1988;12: 227–237.
32. Mancia G. *Eur Heart J* 1990;11(Suppl A):3–11.
33. Creager MA. *Am J Cardiol* 1992;69:10G–16G.
34. Mancia G, Seravalle G, Giannattasio C, et al. *Am J Cardiol* 1992;69:17G–23G.
35. Ferguson DA. *Circulation* 1993;87(Suppl VII):68–75.
36. Seravalle G, Cattaneo BM, Giannattasio C, et al. *J Human Hypertens* 1993;7(Suppl 2):S13–S18.
37. Osculati G, Giannattasio C, De Ceglia S, et al. *Eur Heart J* 1993;14:9(Abstr).
38. Reid IA. *Am J Physiol* 1984;246:F533–F543.
39. Buckley JP. *Fed Proc* 1972;31:1332–1337.
40. Sweet CS, Kadowitz PJ, Brody MJ. *Am J Physiol* 1971;221:1640–1644.
41. Scroop GC, Katic F, Joy MD, Lowe RD. *Brit Med J* 1971;1:324–326.
42. Ferrario CM, Gildenberg PL, McCubbin JW. *Circ Res* 1972;30: 257–262.
43. Andreatta SH, Averill DB, Santos RAS, Ferrario CM. *Hypertension* 1988;11(Suppl I):I163–I166.
44. Ueda H, Katayama S, Kato R. *Adv Exp Biol Med* 1972;17:109–116.
45. Reit E. *Fed Proc* 1972;31:1338–1343.
46. Farr WC, Grupp G. *J Pharmacol Exp Ther* 1971;177:48–55.
47. Zimmerman BG, Gomer SK, Liao JC. *Fed Proc* 1972;31:1344–1350.
48. Szabo B, Hedler L, Schurr C, Starke K. *J Cardiovasc Pharmacol* 1990;15:968–975.
49. Majewski H, Hedler L, Schurr C, Starke K. *J Cardiovasc Pharmacol* 1984;6:888–896.
50. Johnson EM, Marshall GR, Needleman P. *Brit J Pharmacol* 1974;51:541–547.
51. Roth RH. *Fed Proc* 1972;31:1358–1364.
52. Khairallah PA. *Fed Proc* 1972;31:1351–1357.
53. Clough DP, Collis MG, Conway J, Hatton R, Keddie JR. *Am J Cardiol* 1982;49:1410–1414.
54. Lee WB, Ismay MJ, Lumbers ER. *Circ Res* 1980;47:286–292.
55. Hatton R, Clough DP, Adigun SA, Conway J. *Clin Sci* 1982;62: 51–56.
56. Guo GB, Abboud FM. *Am J Physiol* 1984;246:H80–H89.
57. Abboud FM. *Fed Proc* 1974;33:143–149.
58. Seidelin PH, Coutie WJR, McFarlane L, Struthers AD. *Brit J Clin Pharmacol* 1990;29:144–145.
59. Webb DJ, Seidelin PH, Benjamin N, Collier JG, Struthers AD. *J Hypertens* 1988;6(Suppl 4):S542–S543.
60. Taddei S, Favilla S, Duranti P, Simonini N, Salvetti A. *Hypertension* 1991;18:266–277.
61. Morganti A, Grassi G, Giannattasio C, et al. *J Hypertens* 1989;7: 825–835.
62. Giannattasio C, Cattaneo BM, Omboni S, et al. *J Hypertens* 1992;10:373–378.
63. Dollery CT. In: Sonnenblick EH, Laragh J, Lesch M, eds. *New frontiers in cardiovascular therapy.* Amsterdam: Excerpta Medica, 1989;47–54.
64. Benjamin N, Collier JG, Webb DJ. *Clin Sci* 1988;75:337–340.
65. Seidelin PH, Struthers AD. *Clin Sci* 1989;76(Suppl 20):47.
66. Jakobsen J, Glaus L, Graf P, et al. *J Hypertens* 1992;10:1045–1052.
67. Brick I. *J Appl Physiol* 1966;21:33–36.
68. Saino A, Perondi R, Alessio P, et al. *Eur Heart J* 1992;13:299–303.
69. Perondi R, Saino A, Tio RA, et al. *Circulation* 1992;85:2004–2013.
70. Seidelin PH, Coutie WJR, Struthers AD. *Brit J Clin Pharmacol* 1987;24:699–704.
71. Seidelin PH, Coutie WJR, Sudah Pai M, Morton J, Struthers AD. *J Hypertens* 1987;5(Suppl 5):S121–S124.
72. Matsukawa T, Gotoh E, Miyajima E, et al. *J Hypertens* 1988;6(Suppl 4):S501–S504.
73. Mancia G, Giannattasio C, Grassi G, Morganti A, Zanchetti A. *J Hypertens* 1988;6(Suppl 3):S45–S49.
74. Ibsen H, Egan B, Osterziel K, Vander A, Julius S. *Hypertension* 1983;5(Suppl 1):184–191.
75. Morganti A, Pickering TG, Lopez-Ovejero JA, Laragh JH. *J Clin Endocrinol Metab* 1980;50:748–754.
76. Rasmussen S, Hesse B, Bonde-Petersen F, et al. *Scand J Clin Lab Invest* 1986;46:81–88.
77. Ibsen H, Egan B, Julius S. *J Hypertens* 1983;1(Suppl 2):222–224.
78. Ebert TJ. *Hypertension* 1985;7:602–606.
79. Mancia G, Parati G, Pomidossi G. *Am J Cardiol* 1982;49:1415–1419.
80. Clementi WA, Durst NL, McNay JL, Keeton TK. *Hypertension* 1986;8:229–237.
81. Semple PF, Thoren P, Lever AF. *J Hypertens* 1988;6:601–606.
82. Unger T, Yukimura T, Marine-Grez M, Lang RE, Rascher W, Ganten D. *Eur J Pharmacol* 1982;78(4):411–420.
83. Mancia G. *Eur Heart J* 1990;11(Suppl A):3–11.
84. Packer M, Lee WH, Kessler PD, Gottlieb SS, Bernstein JL, Kukin ML. *Circulation* 1987;75(Suppl IV):80–92.
85. Karlsberg RP, Cryer PE, Roberts R. *Am Heart J* 1981;102:24–29.

Hypertension: Pathophysiology, Diagnosis,
and Management, Second Edition,
edited by J.H. Laragh and B.M. Brenner,
Raven Press, Ltd., New York © 1995.

CHAPTER 26

Hypertensive Cardiac Hypertrophy: Pathophysiologic and Clinical Characteristics

Richard B. Devereux and Mary J. Roman

Since the mid-1970s, accurate measurements of left ventricular (LV) mass by echocardiography or by other techniques have been used to show that left ventricular hypertrophy (LVH) is more prevalent, more heterogeneous in its anatomic and pathophysiologic patterns, and more important as a determinant of prognosis in hypertensive patients than previously revealed by electrocardiogram (ECG) or chest radiogram (1–6). In this chapter, the expanding knowledge of cardiac adaptation to hypertension will be reviewed as follows: (a) prevalence of LVH in human hypertension; (b) determinants of hypertensive cardiac hypertrophy and geometric remodeling; (c) relations between cardiac and vascular changes in hypertension; (d) clinical consequences of hypertensive cardiac hypertrophy; (e) reversibility of hypertensive

cardiac involvement; and (f) the role of cardiovascular hypertrophy in the evolution of hypertensive cardiovascular disease.

PREVALENCE OF LEFT VENTRICULAR HYPERTROPHY IN HUMAN HYPERTENSION

The normal left ventricle grows continuously from infancy until adulthood (7–9), with cellular enlargement (hypertrophy) accounting for most of the increase in size (10). Further increases, or at times decreases, in LV muscle mass may occur due to physiologic or pathologic alterations in the hemodynamic load imposed on this chamber (11–15). While LV mass thus ranges from subnormal to markedly increased values, it is at times convenient for clinical decision-making to identify LVH as a categorical abnormality. Accurate assessment of LV anatomy identifies the cardiac response to the various hemodynamic and nonhemodynamic stimuli to myocardial growth.

R. B. Devereux: Cornell University Medical College, Echocardiography Laboratory, New York Hospital, New York, New York 10021.

M. J. Roman: Department of Medicine, Cornell University Medical College, New York, New York 10021.

Normal Left Ventricular Size

The LV was shown in initial autopsy studies to weigh ≤175 g in normal adults of average size and ≤215 g in those of large build or physical activity (16). More recent studies have used anatomically validated echocardiographic methods (17–21) to clarify the factors that should be incorporated in clinically useful normal limits of LV anatomic measurements. The closest correlate of LV mass is a measure of body size in both normal children (7,8,22–24) and adults (12,25–32). Body size has traditionally been taken into account by indexing LV mass for body surface area, with similar upper normal limits for LV mass index reported from Cornell (26,32) and Framingham (28) in adult men (134 g/m^2 and 131 g/m^2, respectively) and women (109 g/m^2 and 100 g/m^2).

This method of LV mass indexation is useful to detect LVH due to hypertension, but may misclassify obesity-induced LVH as normal (12,29,31,33,34). A physiologic approach to the problem imposed by obesity is to index LV mass for lean body mass (12,26), but this is impractical for routine purposes. Alternatively, body height may be used as an indirect measure of normal body size to index LV mass (29,34). However, use of LV mass/body height does not take into account the curvilinear relation between LV mass and height in normal children and adults (31) (Fig. 1). Recent research indicates that LV mass in different normal populations is proportional to between height^2 and height$^{2.7}$ (31,35,36); linear dimensions such as LV diameter and wall thicknesses are best indexed for body height (31,37).

Indexation of echocardiographic LV measurements by appropriate measures of body size eliminates gender differences in primary LV dimensions, but not in LV mass/body surface area or height$^{2.7}$, which are 10–20 percent greater in normal men than women (26,30,31,38). This gender difference parallels the sex difference in lean body mass and may reflect genetic, hormonal, or exercise effects that influence both skeletal and heart muscle (12,26,39,40). Relations between age and LV dimensions or mass have been either absent or weakly positive—especially in women—in normal adults (12,26,38, 41,42). Thus, body size and gender need to be taken into account for LV mass upper normal limits, while age in women and systolic blood pressure in the normal range contribute little to multivariate predictive models (12,28,41,42).

Prevalence of Left Ventricular Hypertrophy in Hypertensive Patients

In contrast to the 3–8 percent of patients with mild to moderate essential hypertension who have ECG LVH (5,6), echocardiographic LV mass is increased in from 12 to 30 percent of relatively unselected hypertensive adults (27,34,43–45), and in 20–60 percent of patients with uncomplicated hypertension seen in referral centers (6,13,46,47). This difference reflects selection bias, as patients with both higher blood pressure and more target organ damage are disproportionately referred to secondary or tertiary care centers (43). Consideration of the LV wall thickness/chamber radius ratio (relative wall thickness [48,49]) in addition to LV mass identified increased relative wall thickness but normal LV mass in an additional 15 percent of uncomplicated hypertensive patients in four studies (50–53). We have coined the term *concentric remodeling* to describe this previously unrecognized LV geometric pattern (50).

Prevalences of LVH may exceed 90 percent among patients with sustained severe or malignant hypertension (33,54), but LVH has been found in as few as 10 percent of patients with new-onset malignant hypertension or preeclampsia (54,55). Fundoscopic changes or other target organ abnormalities used to classify patients as having stage 2 essential hypertension under the World Health Organization schema (56) identified patients with a high prevalence of echocardiographic LVH in one series of hypertensive inpatients (43), but not in another group of asymptomatic hypertensive outpatients (57). The prevalence of LVH among patients with renovascular hypertension (58) or pheochromocytoma (59,60) is similar to that in essential hypertension of similar severity.

The prevalence of LVH among hypertensive patients is influenced by gender, obesity, and possibly by age. Sex-

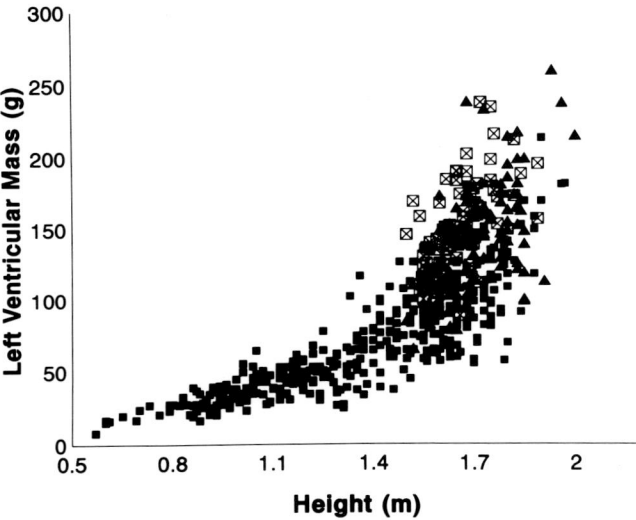

FIG. 1. Relation between left ventricular mass and height in 611 normotensive, normal-weight subjects ranging in age from 4 months to 72 years. It may be seen that this relationship is curvilinear, with the "allometric" (growth) power of the relationship (LV mass-height$^{2.7}$) approximating that expected between one-dimensional height and three-dimensional myocardial volume, and precluding use of the simple LV mass/height ratio to normalize LV mass for body size in individuals of different heights. (From ref. 31, with permission.)

specific criteria for LV mass index identify LVH in more women than men with systemic hypertension, both among employed adults (26), clinical patients (13,46), and subjects with systolic blood pressure of $\geq$140 mm Hg in the Framingham population sample (34). The reasons for this sex difference include (a) selective elimination of hypertensive men with LVH from asymptomatic populations due to accelerated complications of coronary artery disease and (b) the greater increase in arterial pressure from lower levels in normal young women that is needed to meet diagnostic criteria for hypertension. The prevalence of hypertensive LVH is increased 1.5- to 2-fold by coexisting obesity (12,34,61,62), whereas the effect of advancing age reflects mostly age-related increases in blood pressure (12).

DETERMINANTS OF HYPERTENSIVE CARDIAC HYPERTROPHY AND REMODELING

Although one might expect that elevated arterial pressure would consistently induce LVH, the data reviewed above indicate this is not the case. Numerous studies have been undertaken to resolve this apparent discrepancy by examining the role of hemodynamic and nonhemodynamic stimuli in hypertensive LVH.

Hemodynamic Stimuli to Hypertensive Left Ventricular Hypertrophy

Although the initial report of Evans (1) indicated that LV mass was closely related to clinical blood pressure, this has not been true in subsequent studies (6,12, 13,33,45–47,63–65). However, the importance of hemodynamic factors in determining LV mass in hypertensive patients has been understated for two reasons: (a) clinical blood pressure measurements are frequently unrepresentative of the pressure load imposed by hypertension (66) and (b) the hemodynamic load imposed on the heart is due not only to the level of blood pressure but also to concomitant hemodynamic volume load, arterial stiffness, and other factors (14,67,68).

Ambulatory Blood Pressure

Understanding of the impact of blood pressure on the heart has been advanced by use of well-validated methods for ambulatory blood pressure monitoring (69,70). Left ventricular muscle mass or wall thicknesses are more closely related to 24-hour than to casual blood pressures (13,71–75). Among the components of 24-hour blood pressure, daytime pressures usually predict LV anatomic measurements better than those during sleep (13,66,71,72), although this may not be the case

among African-American patients (76,77). Left ventricular muscle mass is usually more closely related to systolic blood pressure, whether it is measured at rest (14,46) or during activity (13,66,71,72). Conversely, LV wall thicknesses or relative wall thickness correlate more closely with diastolic blood pressure (13,46). This difference parallels the known relation between diastolic blood pressure and peripheral resistance (i.e., "pure" pressure load, which induces an increase in LV wall thicknesses) and the added impact of stroke volume on pulse pressure and hence systolic pressure (i.e., mixed pressure and volume load, in which chamber enlargement due to increased stroke volume multiplies the effect of LV wall thickness on LV mass [14,67,78]).

The relations between ambulatory blood pressure and LV anatomy may be illustrated by detailed consideration of studies from our laboratory (13,52,79). In one group of 100 subjects, the weak correlation between LV mass and casual systolic pressure (r = 0.24, $p < 0.05$) rose only to 0.38 ($p < 0.001$) for 24-hour pressure, largely because of a poor relation with sleep pressures (r = 0.10, p = NS). A greater improvement was observed, however, in the 60 subjects in whom ambulatory systolic pressure was measured during occupational work (r = 0.50 with LV mass index, $p < 0.001$). In parallel, LV mass index and ambulatory systolic blood pressure measured at home were most strongly related (r = 0.48, $p < 0.001$) in subjects who went to work the day of recording (13). In all 100 subjects, LV relative wall thickness was most closely related to work diastolic pressure (r = 0.59, $p < 0.001$) (13).

The results of this study suggest a special impact on the heart of blood pressure responses to regularly recurring stress at work, with possible "spillover" of this effect to home blood pressure on working days (13). Further study in an employed population revealed that both ambulatory blood pressure and LV mass were higher in those in jobs characterized by high "job strain" (i.e., high psychological job demands and low decision-making latitude) (79). Job strain is in turn related to increased risk of cardiovascular morbidity (80,81). In a study of 191 normotensive or hypertensive adults (52), the patients with concentric LV hypertrophy (increased LV mass and relative wall thickness) had the highest daytime and work systolic and diastolic pressures, while those with eccentric hypertrophy (a geometric pattern associated with increased cardiac output [50]) had significantly lower ambulatory than clinical pressures (52).

Exercise Blood Pressure

Because physical exercise increases arterial pressure and stroke volume, blood pressure responses to physical activity might, analogous to the hypertrophy induced by vigorous exercise (82), contribute to determining LV structure in hypertensive as well as normotensive adults.

Left ventricular mass index in hypertensive patients is more closely correlated with systolic blood pressure at the end of maximal (83,84) or submaximal exercise (85) than with resting systolic pressure (r = 0.53–0.65 versus r = 0.16–0.46). As a result, LV hypertrophy is more prevalent among subjects with the highest exercise blood pressures, whether they are classified as hypertensive (84) or normotensive (86) by casual pressure measurements.

Hemodynamic Volume Load

Left ventricular volume load, as measured by cardiac output or stroke volume, is usually normal in hypertension. However, supranormal cardiac output is well documented in children with high normal blood pressures (87) and in adults with mild (27,88,89) or more severe essential (57,90,91) and/or renovascular (58,92–95) hypertension. Conversely, low normal or subnormal cardiac output and stroke volume may occur with markedly elevated peripheral resistance in patients with relatively severe hypertension (88,96) or in mildly hypertensive patients with concentric LV remodeling (50).

These alterations in LV stroke volume influence end-diastolic chamber size, and hence the volume encircled by the myocardium. Chamber enlargement without increased myocardial mass increases cavity radius and decreases wall thicknesses (as the myocardium is stretched over a larger surface), both of which increase LV wall stress (by the LaPlace relationship, tension = [pressure × radius]/wall thickness). Since increased wall stress is the principal mechanical stimulus to LV hypertrophy (51,97,98), wall thickness then increases to normalize

relative wall thickness, resulting in eccentric LV hypertrophy (Fig. 2). Eccentric LV hypertrophy occurs commonly in both essential (28,50,52,62,99) and renovascular (58) hypertension.

Conversely, reduced LV stroke volume and resultant diminished LV chamber size in some hypertensives with low cardiac output allow wall thicknesses and relative wall thickness to increase while LV mass remains normal, producing the geometric pattern of concentric LV remodeling (50) (see Fig. 2). The important role of volume load in the pathogenesis of hypertensive LVH is underscored by the fact that LV chamber size and stroke volume are more closely related than systolic pressure to LV mass in normotensive and mildly hypertensive humans (14), as well as normal or hypertensive rats (95,100).

Two factors in the pathogenesis of essential hypertension—obesity (101–103) and high sodium intake (104,105)—exert their effects at least partially by increasing cardiac output. In our studies (12,62,99) and those of Messerli et al. (33), obesity was associated with increased cardiac output and eccentric LVH at all levels of blood pressure. In keeping with these observations, MacMahon et al. (106) reported that LV mass and wall thicknesses decreased in young, overweight hypertensive patients who lost weight. Dietary sodium intake is positively related to LV mass in both cross-sectional (12,107) and longitudinal (108) studies. High sodium intake has been associated with eccentric LV hypertrophy in hypertension in clinical (99) and experimental (100) studies. Expansion of plasma volume in hypertensive patients with eccentric LV hypertrophy, and reduction of it

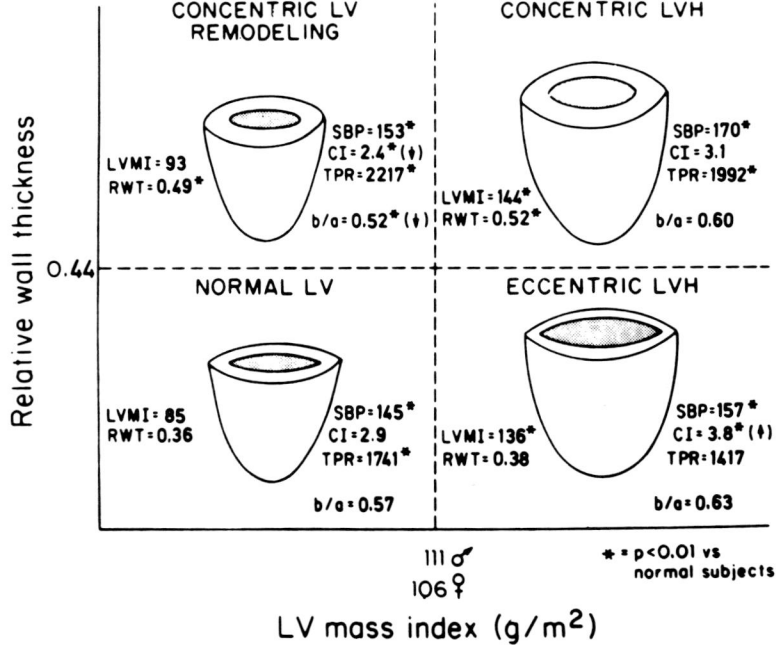

FIG. 2. Hemodynamic and geometric profiles in hypertensive patients with the four patterns of left ventricular (LV) geometry. The short-axis/long-axis ratio (b/a) was derived by two-dimensional echocardiography. CI, cardiac index; LVH, left ventricular hypertrophy; LVMI, left ventricular mass index; RWT, relative wall thickness; SBP, systolic blood pressure; TPR, total peripheral resistance. (From ref. 50, with permission.)

in those with concentric remodeling (109), may mediate the dietary sodium effects.

Arterial Structure and Resistance

Closely related to LV anatomic adaptations to hypertension, arterial structure and resistance are discussed more fully below.

Blood Viscosity

Although vascular resistance is usually considered to be determined by vascular structure and tone, the Poiseuille-Hagan relation reveals that resistance to flow of a fluid is also directly proportional to the fluid's viscosity. Whole blood viscosity or components thereof have been shown in numerous studies to be elevated in patients with hypertension (110–114). We have shown (42,65), and others have confirmed (115), that LV wall thicknesses and mass are directly related to whole blood viscosity, extending Strandell's previous documentation (116) that heart volume is related to total hemoglobin.

Nonhemodynamic Stimuli to Hypertensive Left Ventricular Hypertrophy

Considerable attention has been devoted to the possible contribution of nonhemodynamic factors to hypertensive LV hypertrophy (117). Research has focused on: (a) the sympathetic nervous system; (b) circulating and intracellular renin-angiotensin systems; and (c) genetic and other intracellular signals.

Sympathetic Nervous System

The concept that cardiac adrenergic activity modulates myocardial hypertrophy is based on studies in which catecholamine administration induced LVH that appeared out of proportion to hemodynamic changes (118,119), or in which sympatholytic interventions diminished the myocardial hypertrophy response to exercise (120), anemia (121), and hypertension (122,123). Parallelisms also exist between sympathetic activity and myocardial hypertrophy under some experimental (124,125) or clinical (126) conditions, while α-1 adrenergic agonists stimulate hypertrophy of fetal cardiac myocytes (127–129).

However, other evidence suggests only a limited independent role for adrenergic activity in *in vivo* hypertensive cardiac hypertrophy. First, hemodynamic pressure or volume load responses to adrenergic stimulation or blockade have generally not been well characterized. Second, chemical or surgical sympathectomy do not prevent LV hypertrophy in response to experimental interventions (130–135). Third, catecholamines do not induce hypertrophy of cultured adult cardiac myocytes (136). Finally, patients with pheochromocytoma, the prototypic state of hyperadrenergic hypertension, have LVH that is proportionate to their level of blood pressure (59,60). Thus, doubt has been cast on the "catecholamine hypothesis" of hypertensive cardiac hypertrophy.

Renin-Angiotensin System

Extensive research has established the fundamental physiological role of the circulating renin-angiotensin-aldosterone system, while recent studies have demonstrated expression of genes for angiotensinogen and angiotensin-converting enzyme in the heart and other organs (137–140). In addition to its effects on cardiac hemodynamic load, angiotensin has a positive inotropic effect (141,142) but also increases coronary vascular resistance (143). Angiotensin II has stimulated steps in myocardial protein synthesis after brief infusion in some (144,145) but not all (146) studies. Striking decreases in LV mass have also occurred in patients who received angiotensin-converting enzyme inhibitors (see below). Finally, it has been suggested that locally produced angiotensin II may stimulate vascular smooth muscle hypertrophy (147), indirectly affecting cardiac structure.

However, an independent role of circulating or intracellular renin-angiotensin systems in hypertensive LVH remains unproven because of conflicting observations (148). Thus, angiotensin II infusion increased heart weight in pressor but not in subpressor doses (149), and reduction of LV mass by angiotensin-converting enzyme inhibition has depended on arterial pressure lowering in some (150) but not all (151) studies. Several investigators have failed to find physiologically meaningful concentrations of renin messenger ribonucleic acid (mRNA), the *sine qua non* of a functioning local renin-angiotensin system, in normal or hypertrophied myocardium, using polymerase chain reaction or other sensitive techniques (152–157). In clinical studies, we found no difference in LV mass among patients with high-, normal- or low-renin forms of essential hypertension (158), or between patients with renovascular hypertension, the prototype of high-renin hypertension, and matched patients with essential hypertension (58). Finally, we performed an experiment in rats (159) to stimulate the circulating renin-angiotensin system either in the presence of pressure overload (by renal artery clipping) or in its absence (by dietary salt deprivation) and assess the responses of both heart weight and the molecular isoforms of myosin heavy chain, quantitatively the most important myocardial protein. As may be seen in Fig. 3, both interventions markedly stimulated plasma renin activity, although blood pressure increased only in clipped animals on normal or high-salt diets (159). In Fig. 4 it can be seen that

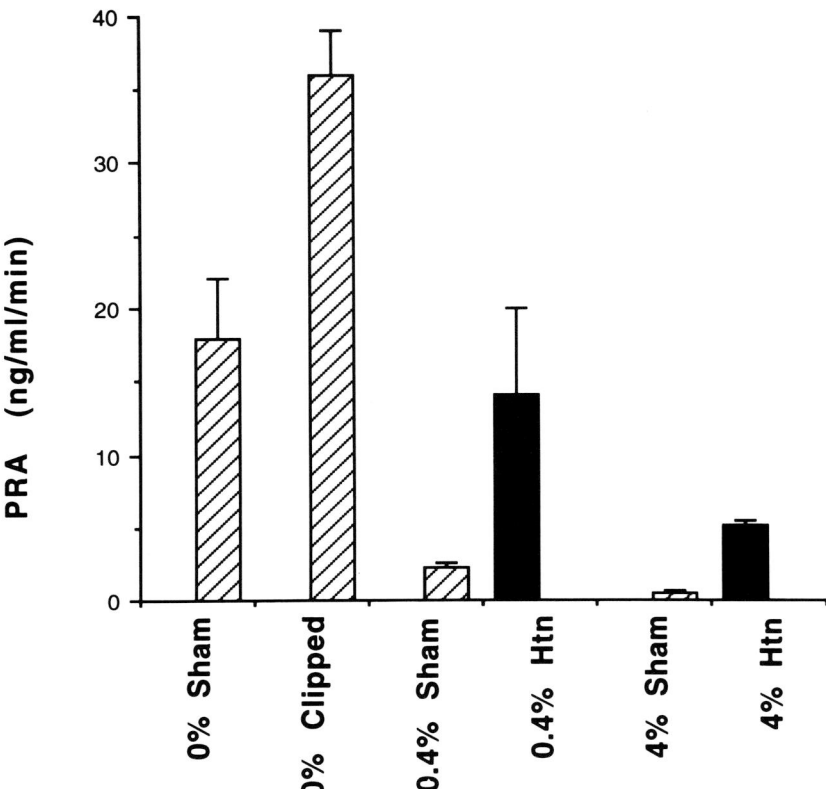

FIG. 3. Plasma renin activity in two-kidney, one-clip Goldblatt hypertensive rats and sham-operated controls on 0.0035 percent, 0.4 percent, and 4.0 percent NaCl diets. Plasma renin activity is stimulated to an even greater extent by severe salt restriction than by renal artery clipping on a normal salt diet. Blood pressure elevation was produced by renal artery clipping only in the animals on 0.4 percent or 4 percent NaCl diets (*filled bars*). (From data in ref. 159, with permission.)

heart weight increased and the ratio of alpha to beta myosin heavy chain decreased only in hypertensive animals. In fact, both Goldblatt and sham-operated animals on the salt-deprived diet had increased alpha/beta myosin ratios (159), a molecular transformation directionally opposite to that seen with myocardial hypertrophy.

These data suggest that the renin-angiotensin system does not contribute directly to the pathogenesis of hypertensive LV hypertrophy (148). Other data suggest that renin system activity may adversely affect cardiac function (58,158). This may be due to pathologic transformations of myocardial connective tissue in response to aldosterone (160–162).

Intracellular and Genetic Factors

The stimuli discussed above must be transduced intracellularly to induce protein synthesis and cause cell growth. Factors that stimulate myocardial protein synthesis have been isolated from hearts with established or developing hypertrophy and partially characterized (163,164). A promising avenue of research concerns the role of growth factors and protooncogenes, the expression of which may induce cardiac cell growth or division (165–167). Acute induction of hypertension was found by Izumo et al. (166) to lead within 1 hour to ventricular

expression of mRNA for the *c-myc* and *c-fos* protooncogene, followed within 2 days by ventricular expression of mRNA for fetal isoforms of contractile proteins and for atrial natriuretic factor. Of greatest interest, supranormal expression of the *myc* gene, caused by insertion of extra gene copies, substantially increased heart weight due to *in utero* cardiac myocyte hyperplasia in a murine model (167). In this experiment, perinatal death occurred in nearly 50 percent of animals with *myc*-gene-induced cardiac enlargement (167), paralleling increased morbidity in patients with LVH.

Although intracellular effectors of LV hypertrophy in humans have not yet been clarified, indirect evidence from phenotypic studies documents genetic influences. Normotensive offspring of hypertensive parents have greater than normal LV mass (75,168), but this may be related to higher 24-hour blood pressure levels (75). Twin studies show an influence of heredity on LV mass that is decreased but remains significant after blood pressure, body size, and physical activity are taken into account (39,40,169). Similarly, greater cardiac hypertrophy in black as opposed to white hypertensives (170–172) parallels the greater frequency and severity of hypertension in blacks (173) and may reflect genetic influences, although many nongenetic factors affect comparisons between racial groups (174).

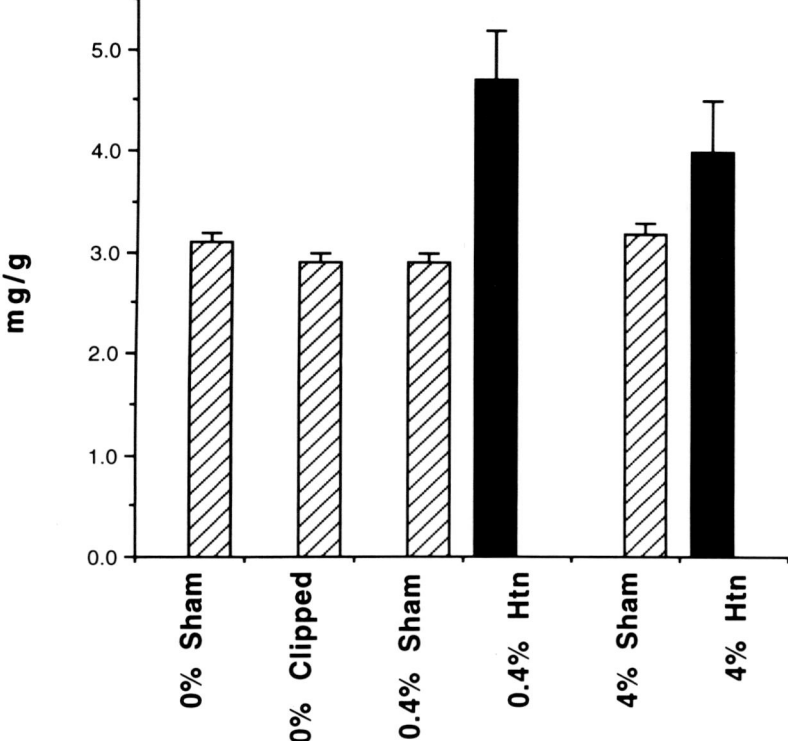

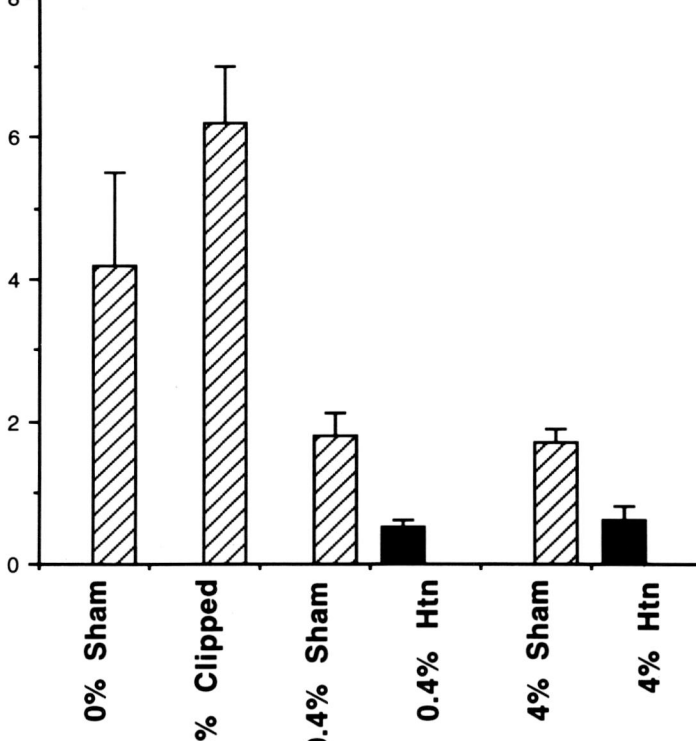

FIG. 4. Top: Heart weight/body weight ratio in two-kidney, one-clip (2K1C) Goldblatt hypertensive rats and sham-operated controls on 0.0035 percent, 0.4 percent, and 4.0 percent NaCl diets. Animals with mildly elevated plasma renin activity and blood pressure due to renal artery clipping on normal or high-sodium diets (*filled bars*) had increased heart weight, whereas heart weight was normal in the animals with more striking hyperreninemia due to salt deprivation. **Bottom:** Ratio of alpha to beta myosin mRNA. Animals with elevated plasma renin activity (Fig. 3) due to salt restriction have elevated alpha/beta myosin ratios, as opposed to the decrease in this ratio in 2K1C animals on normal or elevated NaCl diets that had hypertension and increased heart weight (*filled bars*). (From ref. 159, with permission.)

Increased Left Ventricular Mass as a Precursor of Hypertension

The possibility that LVH might not only be a consequence of hypertension, but could also precede it was first raised by the observation that baseline LV mass in children and adults contribute independently to predicting their blood pressure 4 years later (24). To assess whether this also occurred in adults, we compared baseline findings in 117 normal subjects who remained normotensive and disease-free 5 years later to those in 15 individuals from the same population who developed borderline hypertension (175). The strongest predictor of subsequent hypertension was initial LV mass (Fig. 5) with additional independent prediction by the 24-hour urinary sodium/potassium excretion ratio (175). Subsequent studies (176,177) have confirmed the ability of high baseline values of LV mass to predict subsequent increases in blood pressure independently of standard risk factors for hypertension. These results raise the possibility that LV mass is more closely linked than is blood pressure to the etiology of hypertension, or conversely, that some individuals may have elevated ambulatory blood pressures but normal clinic pressures, a phenomenon that might be termed *white coat normotension.*

Synthesis: Extracellular Stimuli and Intracellular Effectors of Hypertensive Left Ventricular Hypertrophy

Available evidence suggests that hypertensive cardiac hypertrophy is principally determined by mechanical stimuli (Fig. 6). Increases in LV mass are stimulated by higher blood pressure or stroke volume, as well as by

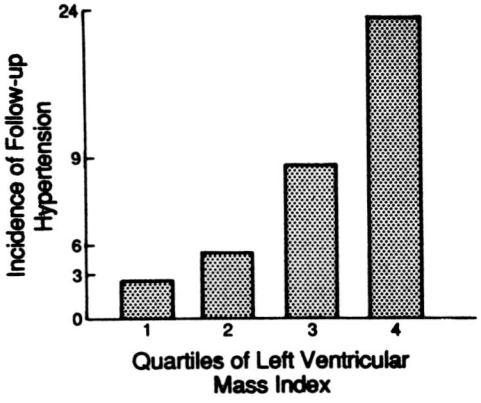

FIG. 5. Incidence of arterial hypertension during 4-year follow-up in relation to quartiles of initial left ventricular mass index. The relation is exponential (*p* < 0.001). Upper cutoff points for left ventricular mass index in men and women, respectively, for each quartile are as follows: first quartile, 70.2 g/m² and 57.2 g/m²; second quartile, 84.3 g/m² and 70.0 g/m²; third quartile, 96.1 g/m² and 81.9 g/m². (From ref. 175, with permission.)

impaired myocardial contractile performance (14,50,51, 97,98). Fig. 7 represents a three-dimensional diagram in which one can move from a surface representing average normal LV mass to higher LV mass due to increases in blood pressure or stroke volume or decreases in contractile efficiency (14). This conceptual schema explains why LV mass does not decrease when blood pressure is reduced by vasodilator drugs that increase stroke volume (67,178) or by isotonic exercise training (179), and why it remains normal in hypertensive patients with supranormal LV performance (180–182). Although LV mass is better predicted by these three mechanical stimuli in multivariate analysis than by blood pressure alone (R^2 = 0.66 vs. 0.20) (14), significant residual variability remains. In part, this may reflect variations in the arterial pressure wave form due to wave reflections or other alterations in arterial function, which place a load on the heart that is not measured by the levels of systolic and diastolic blood pressure (183–184).

The search for understanding of the scatter in the relationship between blood pressure and LV mass has led to extensive exploration of nonhemodynamic stimuli to myocardial hypertrophy (185). Clinical and experimental studies indicate that the adrenergic and renin-angiotensin systems are not the primary determinants of myocardial growth. Progress in identifying the role of intracellular protooncogenes and other growth factors in cardiac myocyte growth holds out the prospect of elucidating the basic mechanisms of hypertensive cardiac hypertrophy, but measurements of hemodynamic pressure and volume load and myocardial inotropic state are needed in studies of genetic interventions or assessment of molecular phenotypes. Clarification of the mechanisms by which myocardial wall stress, considered to be the trigger of hypertrophy at the organ level (97,98), is transduced intracellularly should facilitate separation at the molecular level of the influences of mechanical and nonhemodynamic stimuli to hypertensive LVH.

RELATIONS BETWEEN CARDIAC AND VASCULAR CHANGES IN HYPERTENSION

Functional (186–193) and structural (194–197) alterations in resistance vessels have been studied in human and experimental hypertension, as is extensively reviewed in the chapters by Folkow and Mulvany.

Increased vascular resistance and vascular hypertrophy (an increase in wall thickness relative to radius) have been related to LV adaptive changes in some but not all human studies. In one study (187), minimum calf vascular resistance was related to echocardiographic LV mass and posterior wall thickness when hypertensive and control subjects were pooled, but not when the groups were analyzed separately. Geri et al. (188) found a weak but significant relation (r = 0.33, *p* < 0.05) between calf minimum vascular resistance and LV mass in 52 patients

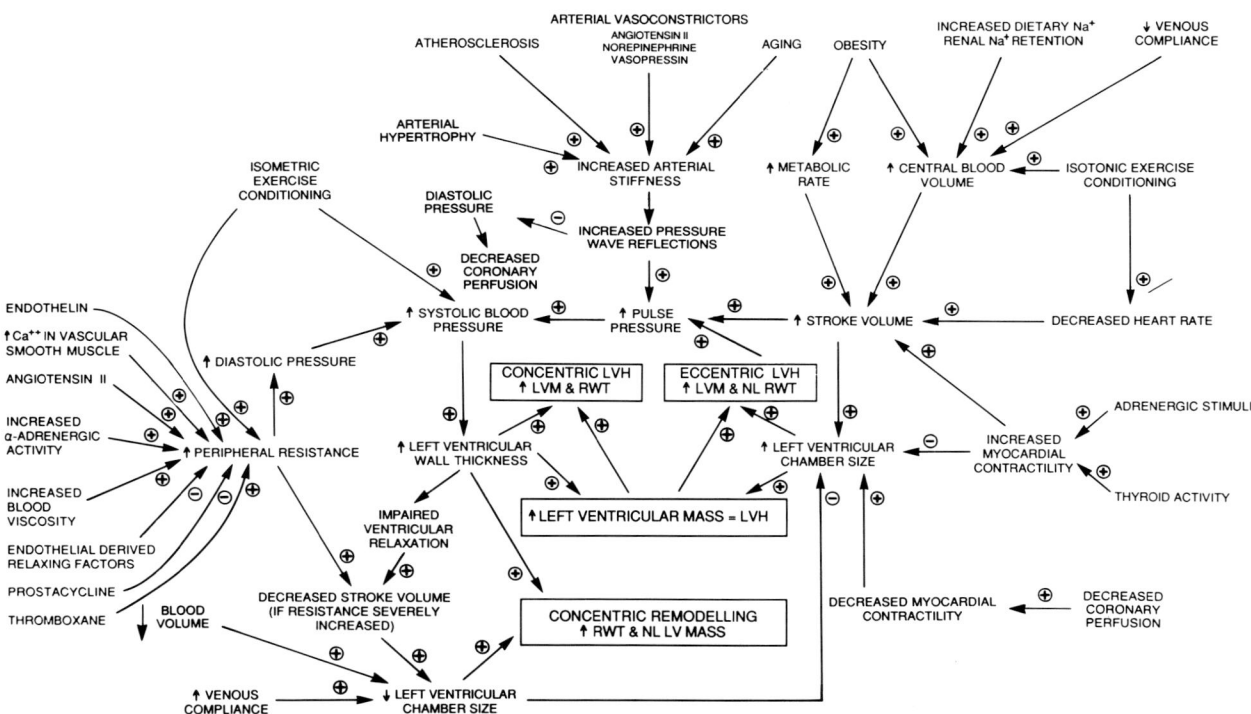

FIG. 6. Postulated relationships between hemodynamic stimuli and hypertensive cardiac hypertrophy. Depending on the combination of stimuli, the cardiac geometric response may be characterized by increases in both left ventricular (LV) mass and relative wall thickness (concentric LV hypertrophy), increased LV mass with increased chamber volume (eccentric LV hypertrophy), or increased relative wall thickness (RWT) with (N) LV mass (concentric LV remodeling). (Adapted from ref. 371, with permission.)

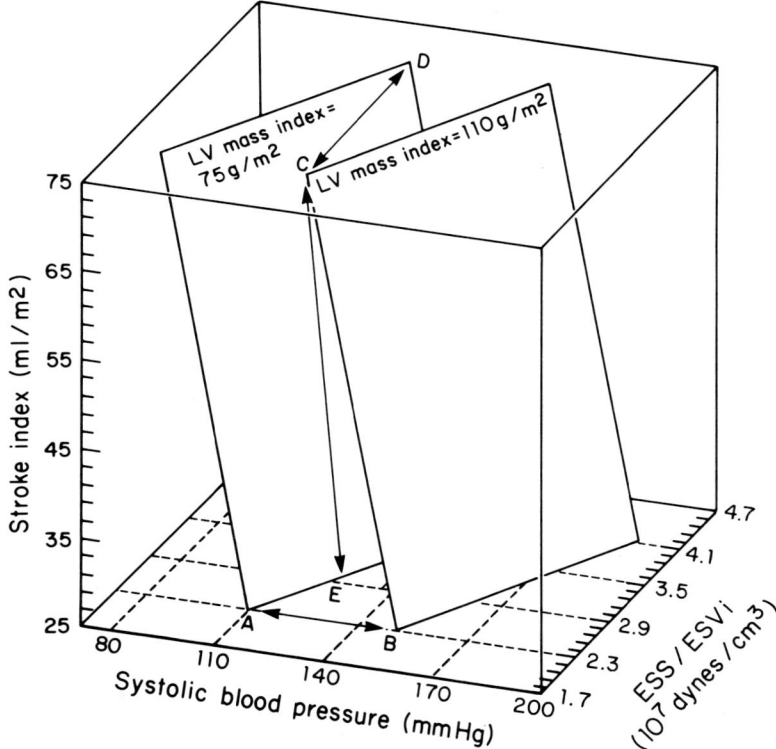

FIG. 7. Three-dimensional plot of the interrelations revealed by multivariate analysis among left ventricular (LV) mass index, systolic blood pressure, stroke index, and the ratio of end-systolic stress (ESS) to end-systolic volume index (ESVi) as a simple measure of LV contractile performance. The two planes depicted correspond to different levels of LV mass index (75 and 110 g/m², respectively). Each plane describes the possible interactions between systolic pressure, stroke index, and ESS/ESVi responsible for a given level of LV mass index. Displacements between planes due to changes in blood pressure (A, B), contractility (C, D), or stroke volume (C–E) are indicated. (From ref. 14, with permission.)

with essential hypertension but noted a higher prevalence of LVH in patients with normal than with elevated vascular resistance (50 percent vs. 27 percent), suggesting that LVH precedes alterations in vascular structure. No relation was found between minimum forearm vascular resistance and LV mass in 29 patients with essential hypertension (192), and regression of LVH did not correlate with forearm vascular resistance in another study (198). In contrast, Schulte et al. (193) found a significant relation between forearm vascular resistance and LV mass in hypertensive patients ($r = 0.32$, $p < 0.01$). In part, variability of results may relate to the extent to which elevated blood pressure is sustained primarily by increased cardiac output rather than increased peripheral resistance, with the latter group more likely to demonstrate concentric LV hypertrophy or remodeling and the former eccentric hypertrophy (50,52,96,199). Alternatively, the reliance on functional (minimal vascular resistance or total peripheral resistance) rather than structural (absolute or relative wall thickness) vascular characterization may underestimate relations between vascular and ventricular structure. Furthermore, elevated "minimal" forearm resistance during induced ischemia and localized heating in hypertensive patients may be lowered further by drugs (190).

Structural (68,200–202) and functional (203–208) alterations of the larger conduit arteries have likewise been documented in human hypertension. However, structural differences have not been consistently noted (208,209) and the independence of decreased vascular compliance from distending pressure has been questioned (183,202,210).

The availability of accurate noninvasive, ultrasound imaging of large arteries and the heart (17,211) has recently allowed *in vivo* comparison of human cardiac and vascular structure (68) and of the impact of altered vascular properties on ventricular adaptation (184,212–216). Pulse wave velocity, an index of vascular stiffness, and brachial artery compliance have been related to the LV mass-volume ratio (212–214). In addition, the pulsatile component of blood pressure, assessed either by pulse pressure (215) or the augmentation index (186), appears to influence LV adaptation independent of mean arterial pressure.

Direct ultrasound measurement of LV and carotid artery anatomy in untreated, asymptomatic hypertensive patients demonstrates greater absolute (0.89 ± 0.21 vs. 0.71 ± 0.15 mm, $p < 0.00005$) and relative (0.30 ± 0.07 vs. 0.26 ± 0.06, $p < 0.005$) wall thicknesses than in matched controls (68). A significant univariate relation between carotid and LV wall thicknesses ($r = 0.40$, $p < 0.005$) remained independent in multivariate analyses, taking age and blood pressure into account. Vascular hypertrophy was more common than LV hypertrophy (28 percent vs. 14 percent) among the hypertensive patients, suggesting that vascular hypertrophy may precede or be

a more sensitive marker of end-organ damage in hypertension (68). Significant increases have also been found in intimal-medial thickness of carotid and femoral (200) arteries in hypertensive patients.

CLINICAL CONSEQUENCES OF HYPERTENSIVE CARDIAC HYPERTROPHY

Myocardial hypertrophy affects both prognosis and cardiac function in hypertension.

Prognostic Implications of Hypertensive Cardiac Hypertrophy

Electrocardiographic LV hypertrophy is well-known to predict morbidity and mortality in patients with hypertension (2–3,217) in the general population (4,218) and in catheterized patients with or without coronary artery obstruction (219), but it was uncertain whether these patterns derived their significance from cardiac hypertrophy or from ECG manifestations of myocardial ischemia. This uncertainty has been resolved by the demonstration that increased LV mass is a potent predictor of cardiovascular morbidity and mortality, independent of blood pressure or other risk factors (51,57,220–230).

In the first of these studies (220), we followed 140 men with initially uncomplicated essential hypertension for 5 years to determine the incidence of "hard" cardiovascular morbid events (cardiac death, myocardial infarction, stroke, or angina pectoris requiring coronary bypass surgery). The 29 or 20 percent of the patients in whom baseline LV mass exceeded 125 g/m^2, a partition value for LVH chosen on the basis of previous findings in employed adults (27), had a roughly fourfold higher rate of morbid events (7 of 29 or 24 percent) than the men without LVH (7 of 111 or 6 percent, $p < 0.01$) (220).

We subsequently extended this study to follow-up of more than 10 years of 280 women and men with initially uncomplicated essential hypertension (51). Left ventricular mass index > 125 g/m^2 strongly predicted all-cause mortality (Fig. 8) and cardiac death, as well as myocardial infarction or need for coronary revascularization (51). Considered as a continuous variable, LV mass index eliminated all conventional risk factors except age from multivariate models; after age adjustment LV mass remained a strong predictor of adverse cardiovascular events. Subdivision of patients into groups with the four LV geometric patterns shown in Fig. 2 revealed that those with concentric LV hypertrophy (increased LV mass and relative wall thickness) had the highest rates of all-cause mortality (Fig. 9, upper panel) and cardiovascular morbid events (Fig. 9, lower panel), while patients with eccentric hypertrophy (increased LV mass alone) or concentric remodeling (increased relative wall thickness alone) had rates of morbidity that fell between those of

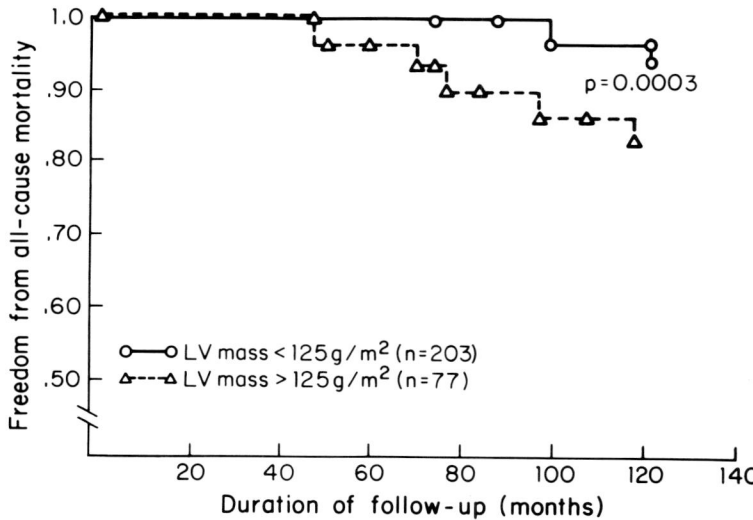

FIG. 8. A 10-year longitudinal study of 280 women and men with initially uncomplicated essential hypertension. The incidence of all-cause mortality was approximately fourfold higher in those with, than those without, echocardiographic left ventricular mass > 125 g/m². (From ref. 51, with permission.)

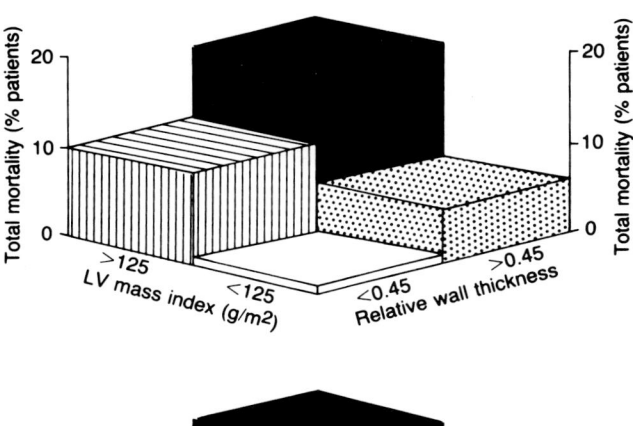

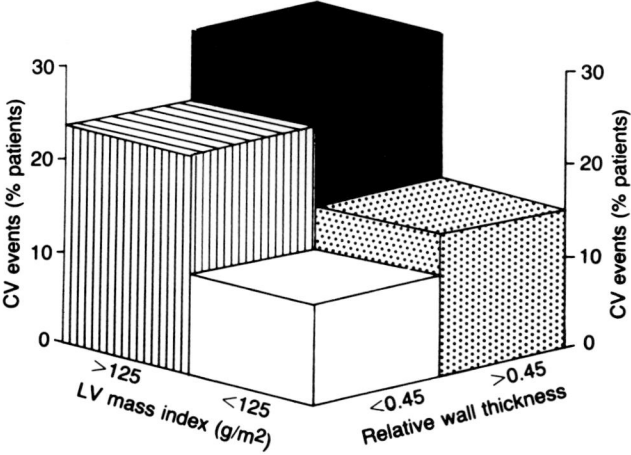

FIG. 9. The relation of total mortality (*top*) and cardiovascular (CV) events (*bottom*) to patterns of left ventricular (LV) geometry in 253 patients with essential hypertension. Mortality and event rates are highest in patients with concentric hypertrophy (*solid column*), lower in patients with normal ventricular geometry (*open column*), and intermediate in patients with eccentric hypertrophy (*lined column*) and concentric remodeling (*stippled column*) ($p < 0.001$ for total mortality and $p = 0.03$ for CV events by analysis of variance). (From ref. 51, with permission.)

patients with concentric hypertrophy and the low-risk group with normal LV geometry (51). Further analyses during up to 15 years follow-up revealed an especially adverse prognosis in patients with LV mass index > 175 g/m² (57).

Other studies have confirmed and extended these findings by demonstrating that LV mass is a strong predictor, independent of blood pressure or other risk factors, of cardiac and cerebrovascular morbidity and mortality among middle-aged and elderly women and men in the general population (222,225,229), in patients with diverse forms of heart disease including hypertension (223,224,226–228), and in catheterized patients with and without coronary artery disease (230). A report from the Framingham Heart Study documented that LV mass strongly predicted all-cause and cardiac death and coronary heart disease events in adults over age 40, and noted that "only LV mass index and age were strong and consistent predictors of all three outcome events in all age and sex subgroups" in analyses that included conventional risk factors (229). Of note, the same level of indexed LV mass (140 g/m of height) identified high-risk status in both women and men (229), similar to our finding that LV mass > 125 g/m² predicted death or morbid events equally in both genders (51). In another important study, Ghali et al. (230) documented that increased, as opposed to normal, LV mass predicted subsequent mortality more strongly (odds ratio 3.7) in catheterized patients without obstructive coronary artery disease than in those with stenosis of large coronary arteries (odds ratio 1.9) (Fig. 10).

These results suggest that echocardiographic LV mass summarizes the integrated adverse effects on the heart of increased hemodynamic load and vascular damage and, when elevated, predisposes directly to complications. One mechanism of such predisposition is enhancement

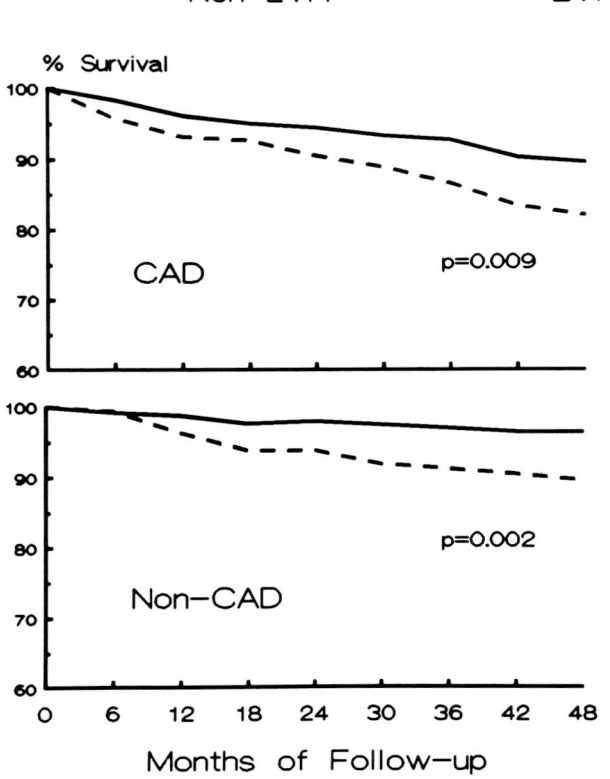

FIG. 10. Cumulative survival in patients with (– – –) and without (——) left ventricular hypertrophy in the presence and absence of coronary artery disease. CAD, coronary artery disease; LVH, left ventricular hypertrophy. (From ref. 230, with permission.)

by hypertensive LV hypertrophy of the extent (231) and rapidity of development (232) of myocardial infarction, and risk of sudden death following infarction (233). Increase in total myocardial oxygen demand by the combination of increased pressure load and increased myocardial mass may contribute to adverse effects of hypertensive LVH (234). Reduced coronary flow reserve secondary to increased basal demand and/or altered microvascular function has been documented in patients with hypertensive LVH (235,236), whereas flow reserve may be reduced on a microvascular basis in some patients without LVH (237). Conversely, LV hypertrophy can also be stimulated by repeated brief coronary artery occlusions (238) and may occur in normotensive patients with coronary artery disease who have not suffered myocardial infarction (239,240).

A second mechanism by which LVH may predispose to cardiac morbidity is by induction of electrophysiologic abnormalities (241–243) and consequently of arrhythmias (244). Left ventricular mass is strongly associated with both simple and complex ventricular arrhythmias in hypertensive patients (245,246) and unselected adults (247). Electrocardiographic LVH independently predicts morbid events in hypertensive patients (244), but the contribution of hypertensive LVH to the approximately 400,000 sudden cardiac deaths per year in the U.S. (248) and the ability of diuretic-induced hypokalemia or other drug effects to exacerbate arrhythmias associated with hypertension and LV hypertrophy (249–252) remain uncertain (253).

Evidence that hypertensive LVH is associated with systemic vascular hypertrophy and atherosclerosis (68,254) and that it amplifies the morbid consequences of coronary artery obstruction (51,230–234,255) may help resolve the persisting controversy concerning the strength of association between hypertension and coronary atherosclerosis (256). This controversy arises from the discordance between epidemiologic evidence of a strong association between elevated blood pressure and coronary heart disease (248,257,258) and pathologic demonstration of only a weak association between hypertension and coronary atherosclerosis, with epicardial coronary arteries tending to be normal or even enlarged in severely hypertensive patients who died of heart failure (259–261). Effective antihypertensive treatment has dramatically reduced stroke or heart failure mortality in hypertensive patients (262–265) but has had variably significant (266–270) or insignificant (271–275) effects on coronary disease morbidity in controlled trials. These disparate observations could be reconciled if coronary atherosclerosis were largely independent of hypertension, but its morbid consequences were exacerbated by hypertensive LVH or by activity of the renin-angiotensin system (276) and were not effectively reversed by the blood pressure reduction or the medication by which it was achieved in most therapeutic trials.

Performance of the Hypertrophied Left Ventricle

Echocardiography and radionuclide angiography make it possible to assess LV functional characteristics in unselected hypertensive patients. In most mildly to moderately hypertensive patients, LV systolic performance at rest is normal or mildly increased (6,46,47,63, 96,99,180–182,277–280). Supernormal LV ejection fraction or fractional shortening in patients or experimental animals with mild hypertension and little or no LVH has been interpreted as reflecting enhanced myocardial contractility (180–182), whereas marked concentric LVH in severely hypertensive patients facilitates LV contraction by reducing wall stress (96,277,281). However, a conceptual mismatch exists in analyses relating chamber size or shortening at the endocardium to the mean level of end-systolic wall stress, which is applied approximately at the LV midwall (282). When midwall shortening-end-systolic stress relations were analyzed in relatively unselected hypertensive patients, patients with concentric LVH had decreased myocardial contractility, and no significant hypercontractility was observed in patients without LVH (283,284).

Many hypertensive patients have normal resting LV function but abnormal ejection fraction responses to exercise (99,278,285,286). We have found that abnormal exercise responses of both LV ejection fraction (99) and pulmonary capillary wedge pressure (287) were associated with eccentric LV hypertrophy and with obesity, a cause of LV volume overload.

In contrast to the general normality of systolic LV performance in uncomplicated hypertension, LV diastolic filling is abnormal in many adults (288–296) and even children with hypertension (297). Characteristically, early diastolic LV filling is impaired with normal or enhanced filling during atrial systole, identifying subnormal LV relaxation but not compliance (298–300). Markedly impaired LV diastolic relaxation occurs in patients in whom extreme LVH with preserved systolic function is complicated by heart failure (281), and reduced early diastolic LV filling is strongly related to LV mass in cross-sectional (290,292) and longitudinal studies (295). However, diastolic LV filling may be abnormal in hypertensive patients with normal LV anatomy and is usually normal in athletes with hypertrophy (301–302).

Patterns of Hypertrophy and Cardiovascular Function in Hypertension

Evidence for heterogeneity of cardiac pathophysiologic patterns in hypertension (50,303,304) comes from clinical and experimental study of two questions: What are the clinical and functional correlates of the previously described patterns of cardiac geometric adaptation? and, What are the relations between LV and arterial geometry and function?

As may be seen in Table 1, blood pressure in hypertensive patients with concentric LVH is principally elevated by increased peripheral resistance with slightly above-average normal cardiac output (50). The concentrically hypertrophied heart derives the increased work capacity needed to sustain moderately elevated blood pressure from increased LV mass and the mechanical advantage bestowed by high relative wall thickness, despite decreased myocardial contractility (50,52,283). In patients with eccentric hypertrophy, increased cardiac output with minimal or no elevation of peripheral resistance supports blood pressure elevation that is milder during normal activity than in the clinic (50,52). Increased LV mass with normal relative wall thicknesses and roughly normal contractility, but increased preload due to plasma volume expansion, sustains LV ejection phase performance that is normal at rest but may be subnormal during exercise (50,52,99,109,283). Patients with concentric LV remodeling have relatively mild hypertension, despite markedly elevated peripheral resistance, because cardiac output is subnormal (50). The mechanical advantage associated with high relative wall thickness sustains the pressure load at rest and during activity, despite normal LV mass and reduced preload due to diminished plasma volume (52,109). Patients with normal LV geometry tend to have mild hypertension with above-average normal peripheral resistances and/or cardiac outputs (50). The mild overload is offset by slightly above-average normal LV mass with normal contractility (50,52,53,283).

Analogous relations among LV geometric pattern, LV function, and systemic hemodynamics have been observed by other investigators in adults with hypertensive (181,182,280,281) and athletic (305) LVH. Colan et al. (305) reported that power lifters with concentric LVH and relative wall thickness out of proportion to arterial pressure had supranormal resting LV fractional shortening, whereas runners with eccentric LVH had reduced chamber function. Thus, pure pressure or volume loads, whether "physiologic" or "pathologic," are similarly matched to patterns of ventricular geometry and function.

TABLE 1. *Clinical and hemodynamic correlates of patterns of left ventricular geometric adaptation to hypertension in hypertensive patients[a]*

Characteristic	Reference	Normal geometry	Concentric remodeling	Eccentric hypertrophy	Concentric hypertrophy
Age	50, 53	+	++	++	++
Gender (Female/Male)	50, 53	=	=	+ Female	+ Female
Body Mass Index	50, 53	+	+	++	++
Cardiac Index	50	=	−−	+++	+
Peripheral Resistance	50	+	+++	=	++
Awake Ambulatory Blood Pressure	52	+	++	+	+++
Plasma Volume	109	=	−−	++	=
Left Ventricular Mass	50, 52, 53	= to +	= to +	++	+++
Relative Wall Thickness	50, 52, 53	=	++	=	+++
Midwall Shortening	283	=	−	=	−

[a] Data based on quantitative comparison with concurrently studied normotensive subjects expressed from much greater (+++) to much less (−−−), or similar (=).

REVERSAL OF HYPERTENSIVE CARDIAC HYPERTROPHY AND ITS POTENTIAL CLINICAL BENEFIT

The adverse effects of hypertensive LVH on prognosis and cardiac function have made the reversibility of this abnormality a central problem in hypertension research. As reviewed elsewhere (306–311), numerous studies over nearly four decades have established that blood pressure reduction may reverse hypertensive LVH, but leave unresolved the questions of how this is best achieved and whether it leads to improved prognosis and cardiac performance.

Do Hypertensive Treatments Differ in Their Effect on Cardiac Hypertrophy?

Interest in this topic has been stimulated by the suggestion that regression of LVH may be produced by some but not other classes of antihypertensive drugs (312,313). This possibility was first raised by the experimental observations that LVH was prevented by agents with sympatholytic or anti-renin-angiotensin system activity but not by other classes of drug that lowered blood pressure, most notably direct-acting vasodilators (122,123,314–319). However, this claim of pharmacologic specificity with regard to LVH regression has been tempered by the subsequent recognition that vasodilators cause a substitution of volume for pressure load on the heart (14,67,178) and by documentation that long-term hydralazine (Wydase) therapy begun early in life reduces ventricular weight in spontaneously hypertensive rats (320–322).

Numerous echocardiographic studies have documented reduction of LV mass during effective antihypertensive treatment with drugs (308–311), weight reduction (106), or salt depletion (108). Available evidence indicates that regression of LVH can be induced by most antihypertensive drugs if blood pressure is reduced substantially (323) and for a prolonged period (324). Statistically significant but relatively weak relations (r = ≤0.54) exist between the reduction in mean blood pressure and the induced change in echocardiographic LV mass in various published reviews or metanalyses (308–311,325) of clinical trials of antihypertensive treatment.

The possibility that different pharmacologic classes of antihypertensive drugs might have different capacities to reverse LVH is examined in Fig. 11, derived from the metanalysis of Cruickshank et al. (311). In this figure, data are displayed separately for trials using converting enzyme inhibitors (326–332), beta-adrenergic blockers (126,328,333–340), diuretics (333,335,341–345), vasodilators (344–346), alpha-methyldopa (342,343,347), dihydropyridine calcium blockers (345), nondihydropyridine calcium blockers (348), and other types of drugs or

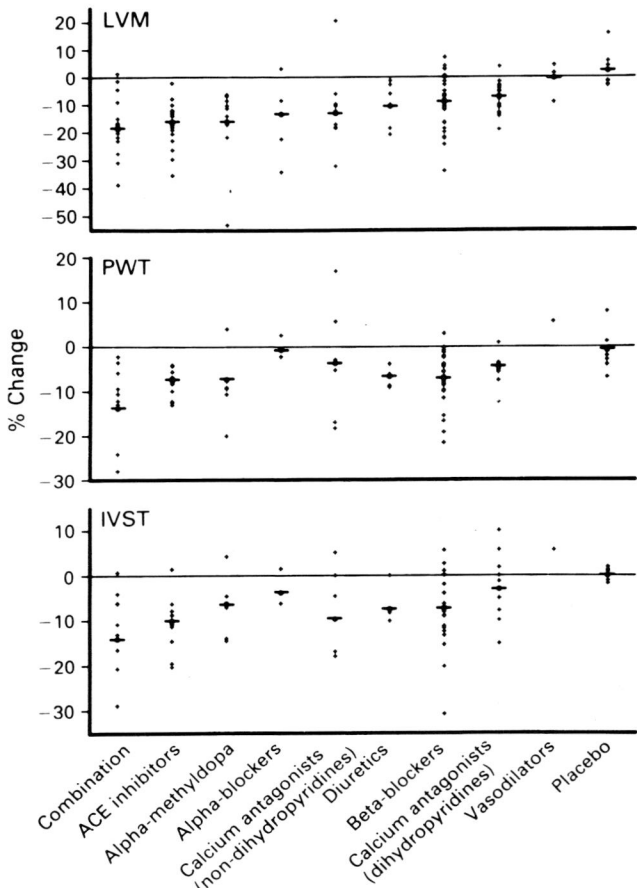

FIG. 11. Effect of different classes of antihypertensive therapy upon left ventricular mass (index) [LVM (I)]. PWT, posterior wall thickness; IVST, intraventricular septal thickness; %, percentage change. Weighted means shown. (From ref. 311, with permission.)

drug combinations (340,342–344,347,349–352). The most striking result in these and other published studies (353–356) is that significant LV mass reduction was produced in none of the studies using direct-acting vasodilators and in a minority of trials using diuretic therapy, as compared to virtually all trials using converting enzyme inhibitors, a majority of those using beta- and/or alpha-adrenoceptor blockers, and most studies using other drugs or drug combinations.

Thus, currently available human data tend to support, but not prove, the hypothesis that antihypertensive drugs that inhibit the renin-angiotensin or, to a lesser extent, the adrenergic system reverse LVH more consistently than agents that do not affect or may even stimulate these systems, but with sufficient overlap to suggest that any difference is quantitative, not absolute. However, these data are not definitive because of serious limitations of most available studies (332,357). The problems with many existing studies include small size and disparate selection of patient populations; lack of blinding to drug usage or study sequence of echocardiogram interpretation; small blood pressure effects in the "negative" arms of some studies of LV hypertrophy regression (341,343,348,358–359); lack of information on blood pressure during normal activity or induced changes (if any) in hemodynamic volume load; short study durations (often 3 months or less); possible admixture of subjects with white coat hypertension (360,361); and study of drug effects in subjects who had been rendered normotensive with normal LV mass by nutritional-hygienic therapy (359). Further research with improved study design is needed to test definitively the hypothesis, suggested by available data, that control of blood pressure by agents that interrupt renin system activity is more likely to induce regression of LVH than other drug treatments of hypertension.

Left Ventricular Mass Change and Prognosis in Treated Hypertensive Patients

Although it has long been presumed that regression of hypertensive LV hypertrophy would be clinically beneficial, only recently have data become available to support this hypothesis. Among 166 patients with initially uncomplicated essential hypertension who remained free of morbid events for approximately 5 years between a baseline and follow-up echocardiogram, we found a higher risk of subsequent cardiovascular events in those in whom LV hypertrophy persisted or developed despite treatment than in those in whom LV mass remained normal or fell (362,363). In a cooperative study from eastern Europe, Yurenev et al. (364) found that failure to decrease LV mass from baseline to the end of study or to the last annual echocardiogram before complications occurred was strongly associated with the occurrence of morbid events.

THE ROLE OF CARDIOVASCULAR HYPERTROPHY IN THE EVOLUTION OF HYPERTENSIVE DISEASE

Hypertension and other risk factors, especially elevated cholesterol and glucose levels and cigarette smoking, help predict premature mortality and nonfatal morbid events, and their control variably reduces the incidence of events. However, the ability to predict risk and to reduce it by control of hypertension or other risk factors are both imperfect. These limitations occur in part because the progression from risk factor exposure to morbid events depends on the variable likelihood that individuals exposed to the same risk factors will progress through two stages (schematically depicted in Fig. 12): (a) the development of asymptomatic or "preclinical" anatomic and functional cardiovascular disease in response to standard risk factors and other variables, and (b) the precipitation of morbid events by progression of preclinical disease or by the action of additional "triggering" mechanisms in the presence of preclinical disease (365,366). Advances in diagnostic methodology now allow noninvasive detection in many asymptomatic individuals of LVH or other manifestations of preclinical disease such as carotid atherosclerosis or renal dysfunction. As shown in Table 2, detection of different measures of preclinical disease identifies patients at substantially increased risk (51,220,225,229,230,367–370). Progress in elucidating stimuli to LVH and in defining its independent prognostic significance demonstrates that focusing separately on these two stages of disease

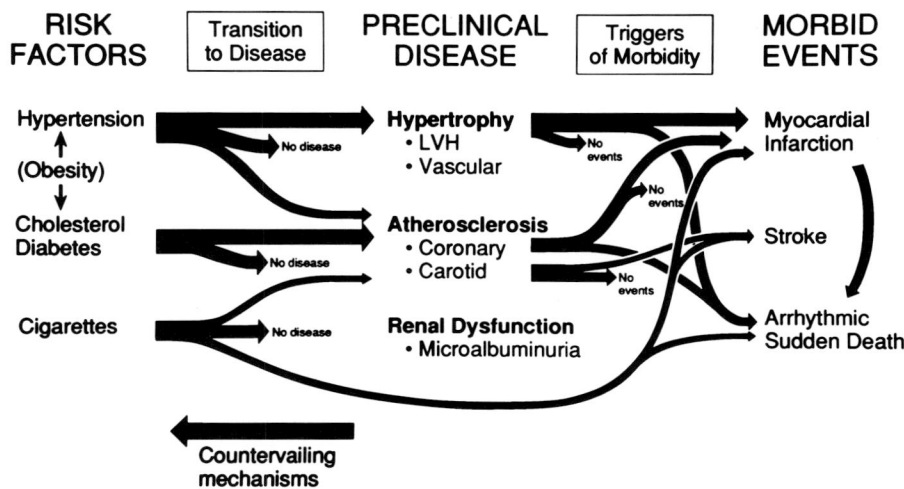

FIG. 12. Schematic representation of the pathways from risk-factor exposure to preclinical disease and ultimate development of clinical morbid events. Note that at each step some individuals do not make the next transition. (From ref. 365, with permission.)

TABLE 2. *Incidence[a] of morbid events in subjects with and without different forms of cardiovascular disease*

Reference	Method of measurement	Preclinical disease	End-point	With preclinical disease	Without preclinical disease
Cohn et al. (367)	Angiography	Coronary stenosis ≥75% narrowing	Death	2.7	—
Kent et al. (368)	Angiography	Coronary stenosis ≥50% narrowing	Death	3.0	—
Casale et al. (220)	Echocardiography	LV mass >125 g/m²	Death, MI, CVA, severe angina	4.6	1.2
Levy et al. (225)	Echocardiography	LV mass >150 g/m	Angina	2.8[b]	0.6[b]
			CHD other than angina	3.2[b]	0.7[b]
Levy et al. (229)	Echocardiography	LV mass >140 g/m (>116 g/m²)	All-cause mortality	2.0[b]	0.8[b]
			All cardiovascular events	3.3[b]	1.4[b]
Koren et al. (51)	Echocardiography	LV mass >125 g/m²	Cardiovascular death	1.4	0.1
			All cardiovascular events	6.3	2.2
Salonen et al. (369)	Carotid ultrasonography	Intimal-medial thickening or plaque	Myocardial infarction	2.8[c]	0.8[c]
Yudkin et al. (370)		Microalbuminuria >20 ug/min	All-cause mortality	9.3	0.6
Ghali et al. (230)	Echocardiography	LV mass >131 g/m² (men), LV mass >100 g/m² (women)	Death:		
			Patients with CAD	5.3	2.9
			Patients without CAD	2.9	0.8

From ref. 343, with permission.
[a] Incidence of morbid events per 100 patient years.
[b] Age-adjusted rate.
[c] Percent of subjects with events over 1- to 30-month follow-up period.
CAD, angiographic coronary artery disease; CHD, coronary heart disease; CVA, cerebrovascular accident; LV, left ventricular; MI, myocardial infarction.

evolution is a fruitful research strategy and may also be valuable in guiding clinical care. The closer relation of measures of preclinical disease than risk factors to the subsequent risk of complications indicates that their detection improves clinical risk stratification. However, whether clinical outcome is improved or treatment cost is lowered by basing antihypertensive or antihyperlipidemic treatment decisions in part on the presence of LVH or other measures of preclinical cardiovascular disease needs to be tested before this strategy becomes the standard of care.

ACKNOWLEDGMENTS

We thank Virginia Burns for her assistance in preparation of this manuscript and Dr. Peter Buttrick for his provision of Figs. 3 and 4.

REFERENCES

1. Evans G. A contribution to the study of arteriosclerosis, with special reference to its relation to chronic disease. *Q J Med* 1921;14:215–282.
2. Sokolow M, Perloff D. The prognosis of essential hypertension treated conservatively. *Circulation* 1961;23:697–713.
3. Breslin DJ, Gifford RW Jr, Fairbairn JF II. Essential hypertension: a twenty-year follow-up study. *Circulation* 1966;33:87–97.
4. Kannel WB, Castelli WP, McNamara PM, McKee PA, Feinleib M. Role of blood pressure in the development of congestive heart failure: the Framingham study. *N Engl J Med* 1972;287:781–787.
5. Hypertensive Detection and Follow-up Program Cooperative Group: Five year findings of the Hypertension Detection and Follow-up Program: reduction of mortality of persons with high blood pressure, including mild hypertension. *JAMA* 1979;242:2562–2571.
6. Savage DD, Drayer JIM, Henry WL, et al. Echocardiographic assessment of cardiac anatomy and function in hypertensive subjects. *Circulation* 1979;59:623–632.
7. Henry WL, Ware J, Gardin JM, Hepner SI, McKay J, Weiner M. Echocardiographic measurements in normal subjects: growth-related changes that occur between infancy and early adulthood. *Circulation* 1978;57:278–285.
8. Roge CLL, Silverman NH, Hart PA, Ray RM. Cardiac structure growth pattern determined by echocardiography. *Circulation* 1978;57:285–290.
9. de Simone G, Devereux RB, Daniels SR, Meyer RA. The role of puberty in development of gender differences in left ventricular mass. *Am J Cardiol (submitted).*
10. Linzbach AJ. Hypertrophy, hyperplasia and structural dilatation of the human heart. *Adv Cardiol* 1976;18:1–13.
11. Milliken MC, Stray-Gundersen J, Peshock RM, Katz J, Mitchell JH. Left ventricular mass as determined by magnetic resonance imaging in male endurance athletes. *Am J Cardiol* 1988;62:301–305.
12. Hammond IW, Devereux RB, Alderman MH, Laragh JH. Relation of blood pressure and body build to left ventricular mass in normotensive and hypertensive employed adults. *J Am Coll Cardiol* 1988;12:996–1004.
13. Devereux RB, Pickering TG, Harshfield GA, et al. Left ventricular hypertrophy in patients with hypertension: importance of blood pressure responses to regularly recurring stress. *Circulation* 1983;68:470–476.
14. Ganau A, Devereux RB, Pickering TG, et al: Relation of left ventricular hemodynamic load and contractile performance to left ventricular mass in hypertension. *Circulation* 1990;81:25–36.
15. St. John Sutton MG, Plappert T, Crosby L, Douglas P, Mullen J, Reichek N. Effects of reduced left ventricular mass on chamber architecture, load, and function: a study of anorexia nervosa. *Circulation* 1985;72:991–1000.

16. Bove KE, Rowland DT, Scott RC. Observations on the assessment of cardiac hypertrophy using a chamber partition technique. *Circulation* 1966;33:558–568.

17. Devereux RB, Reichek N. Echocardiographic determination of left ventricular mass in man. Anatomic validation of the method. *Circulation* 1977;55:613–618.

18. Reichek N, Helak J, Plappert T, St John Sutton M, Weber KT. Anatomic validation of left ventricular mass estimates from clinical two-dimensional echocardiography: initial results. *Circulation* 1983;67:348–352.

19. Woythaler N, Singer SL, Kwan OL, et al. Accuracy of echocardiography versus electrocardiography in detecting left ventricular hypertrophy: comparisons with post-mortem mass measurements. *J Am Coll Cardiol* 1983;2:305–311.

20. Devereux RB, Alonso DR, Lutas EM, et al. Echocardiographic assessment of left ventricular hypertrophy: comparison to necropsy findings. *Am J Cardiol* 1986;57:450–458.

21. Byrd BF III, Finkbeiner W, Bouchard A, Silverman MH, Schiller NB. Accuracy and reproducibility of clinically acquired two-dimensional echocardiographic mass measurements. *Am Heart J* 1989;118:133–137.

22. Burke GL, Arcilla RA, Culpepper WS, Webber LS, Chiang Y-K, Berenson GS. Blood pressure and echocardiographic measures in children: the Bogalusa Heart Study. *Circulation* 1987;75:106–114.

23. Daniels SR, Meyer RA, Liang Y, Bove KE. Echocardiographically determined left ventricular mass index in normal children, adolescents and young adults. *J Am Coll Cardiol* 1988;12:703–708.

24. Mahoney CT, Schieken RM, Clarke WR, Lauer RM. Left ventricular mass and exercise responses predict future blood pressure: the Muscatine study. *Hypertension* 1988;12:206–213.

25. Henry WL, Gardin JM, Ware JH. Echocardiographic measurements in normal subjects from infancy to old age. *Circulation* 1980;62:1054–1061.

26. Devereux RB, Lutas EM, Casale PN, et al. Standardization of M-mode echocardiographic left ventricular anatomic measurements. *J Am Coll Cardiol* 1984;4:1222–1230.

27. Hammond IW, Devereux RB, Alderman MH, et al. The prevalence and correlates of echocardiographic left ventricular hypertrophy among employed patients with uncomplicated hypertension. *J Am Coll Cardiol* 1986;7:639–650.

28. Savage DD, Garrison RJ, Kannel WB, et al. The spectrum of left ventricular hypertrophy in a general population sample: the Framingham study. *Circulation* 1987;75(suppl I):I-26–I-33.

29. Levy D, Savage DD, Garrison RJ, Anderson KM, Kannel WB, Castelli WP. Echocardiographic criteria for left ventricular hypertrophy: the Framingham study. *Am J Cardiol* 1987;59:956–960.

30. Byrd BF III, Wahr D, Wang YS, Bouchard A, Schiller NB. Left ventricular mass and volume/mass ratio determined by two-dimensional echocardiography in normal adults. *J Am Coll Cardiol* 1985;6:1021–1025.

31. de Simone G, Daniels SR, Devereux RB, et al. Left ventricular mass and body size in normotensive children and adults: assessment of allometric relations and of the impact of overweight. *J Am Coll Cardiol* 1992;20:1251–1260.

32. Devereux RB, Casale PN, Kligfield P, et al. Performance of primary and derived M-mode echocardiographic measurements for detection of left ventricular hypertrophy in necropsied subjects and in patients with systemic hypertension, mitral regurgitation and dilated cardiomyopathy. *Am J Cardiol* 1986;57:1388–1393.

33. Messerli FH, Sundgaard-Riise K, Reisen ED, et al. Dimorphic cardiac adaptation to obesity and arterial hypertension. *Ann Intern Med* 1983;99:757–761.

34. Levy D, Anderson KM, Savage DD, Kannel WB, Christiansen JC, Castelli WP. Echocardiographically detected left ventricular hypertrophy: prevalence and risk factors. *Ann Intern Med* 1988;108:7–13.

35. Lauer MS, Anderson KM, Larson MG, Levy D. A new method for indexing left ventricular mass for differences in body size. *Am J Cardiol* 1994 (in press).

36. de Simone G, Devereux RB, Daniels SR, Meyer RA. Left ventricular mass in children and adults: Differences in the allometric relations with body size. *Clin Res* 1993;41:620A.

37. Gutgesell HP, Rembold CM. Growth of the human heart relative to body surface area. *Am J Cardiol* 1990;65:662–668.

38. Valdez RS, Motta JA, London E, et al. Evaluation of the echocardiogram as an epidemiologic tool in an symptomatic population. *Circulation* 1979;60:921–929.

39. Harshfield GA, Grim CE, Hwang C, Savage DD, Anderson SJ. Genetic and environmental influences on echocardiographically determined left ventricular mass in black twins. *Am J Hypertens* 1990;3:538–543.

40. Verhaaren HA, Schieken RM, Mosteller M, Hewitt JK, Eaves LJ, Nance WE. Bivariate genetic analysis of left ventricular mass and weight in pubertal twins (the Medical College of Virginia Twin Study). *Am J Cardiol* 1991;68:661–668.

41. Dannenberg AL, Levy D, Garrison RJ. Impact of age on echocardiographic left ventricular mass in a healthy population (The Framingham Study). *Am J Cardiol* 1989;64:1066–1068.

42. de Simone G, Devereux RB, Roman MJ, et al. Gender differences in left ventricular anatomy, blood viscosity and volume regulatory hormones in normal adults. *Am J Cardiol* 1991;68:1704–1708.

43. Devereux RB, Casale PN, Hammond IW, et al. Echocardiographic detection of pressure-overload left ventricular hypertrophy: effect of criteria and patient population. *J Clin Hypertens* 1987;3:66–78.

44. Laufer E, Jennings GL, Korner PI, Dewar E. Prevalence of cardiac structural and functional abnormalities in untreated primary hypertension. *Hypertension* 1989;13:151–162.

45. Liebson PR, Grandits G, Prineas R, et al. Echocardiographic correlates of left ventricular structure among 844 mildly hypertensive men and women in the Treatment of Mild hypertension Study (TOMHS). *Circulation* 1993;87:476–486.

46. Devereux RB, Savage DD, Sachs I, Laragh JH. Relation of hemodynamic load to left ventricular hypertrophy and performance in hypertension. *Am J Cardiol* 1983;51:171–176.

47. Abi-Samra F, Fouad RM, Tarazi RC. Determinants of left ventricular hypertrophy and function in hypertensive patients. *Am J Med* 1983;75(suppl 3A):26–33.

48. Ford LE. Heart size. *Circ Research* 1976;39:297–303.

49. Reichek N, Devereux RB. Reliable estimation of peak left ventricular pressure by M-mode echographic determined end-diastolic relative wall thickness: identification of severe valvular aortic stenosis in adult patients. *Am Heart J* 1982;103:202–209.

50. Ganau A, Devereux RB, Roman MJ, et al. Patterns of left ventricular hypertrophy and geometric remodeling in essential hypertension. *J Am Coll Cardiol* 1992;19:1550–1558.

51. Koren MJ, Devereux RB, Casale PN, Savage DD, Laragh JH. Relation of left ventricular mass and geometry to morbidity and mortality in men and women with essential hypertension. *Ann Intern Med* 1991;114:345–352.

52. Devereux RB, James GD, Pickering TG. What is normal blood pressure? comparison of ambulatory pressure level and variability in patients with normal or abnormal left ventricular geometry. *Am J Hypertens* 1993;6:211s–215s.

53. Roman MJ, Alderman MH, de Simone G, Schwartz J, Laragh JH, Devereux RB. Echocardiography in hypertensive and normotensive employed adults. *Proceedings of the NIH Workshop on Echocardiography in Hypertension*

54. Shapiro LM, MacKinnon J, Beevers DG. Echocardiographic features of malignant hypertension. *Br Heart J* 1981;46:374–379.

55. Thompson JA, Hays PM, Sagar KB, Cruikshank DP. Echocardiographic left ventricular mass to differentiate chronic hypertension from pre-eclampsia during pregnancy. *Am J Obstet Gynecol* 1986;155:994–999.

56. World Health Organization Expert Committee: Arterial hypertension. Geneva: World Health Organization: 1978:8–10.

57. Mensah GA, Pappas TW, Koren MJ, Ulin RJ, Laragh JH, Devereux RB. Comparison of classification of hypertension severity by blood pressure level and World Health Organization criteria for prediction of concurrent cardiac abnormalities and subsequent complications in essential hypertension. *J Hypertension* 1993 (in press).

58. Vensel LA, Devereux RB, Pickering TG, Herrold EMcM, Borer JS, Laragh JH: Cardiac anatomy and function in renovascular hypertension produced by unilateral and bilateral renal artery stenosis. *Am J Cardiol* 1986;58:575–582.

59. Shub C, Cueto-Garcia L, Sheps SG, Ilstrup DM, Tajik AJ. Echocardiographic findings in pheochromocytoma. *Am J Cardiol* 1986;57:971–975.

60. Fouad-Tarazi FM, Imamura M, Bravo EL, et al. Differences in left ventricular structural and functional changes between pheochromocytoma and essential hypertension. *Am J Hypertension* 1992;5:134–140.

61. Lauer M, Anderson KM, Kannel WB, Levy D. The impact of obesity on left ventricular mass and geometry. *JAMA* 1991;266:231–236.

62. de Simone G, Devereux RB, Roman MJ, Alderman MH, Laragh JH. Relation of obesity and gender to left ventricular hypertrophy in normotensive and hypertensive adults. *Hypertension* 1994 (*in press*).

63. Dunn FG, Chandraratna PN, de Carvalho JGR, Basta LL, Frohlich ED. Pathophysiologic assessment of hypertensive heart disease with echocardiography. *Am J Cardiol* 1977;39:789–795.

64. Kleinert HD, Harshfield GA, Pickering TG, et al. What is the value of home blood pressure measurement in patients with mild hypertension? *Hypertension* 1984;6:574–578.

65. Devereux RB, Drayer JIM, Chien S, et al. Whole blood viscosity as a determinant of cardiac hypertrophy in systemic hypertension. *Am J Cardiol* 1984;54:592–595.

66. Devereux RB, Pickering TG. Ambulatory blood pressure in assessing the cardiac impact and prognosis of hypertension. In: O'Brien E, O'Malley K, eds. *Handbook of hypertension, vol. 14: blood pressure measurement.* Amsterdam: Elsevier, 1991;261–285.

67. Leenen FH, Tsoporis J. Cardiac volume load as a determinant of the response of cardiac mass to antihypertensive therapy. *Eur Heart J* 1990;11(suppl G):s100–s106.

68. Roman MJ, Saba PS, Pini R, et al. Parallel cardiac and vascular adaptation in hypertension. *Circulation* 1992;86:1909–1918.

69. Bevan AT, Hanan AJ, Stott FD. Direct arterial pressure recording in unrestricted man. *Clin Sci* 1969;36:329–344.

70. Harshfield GA, Pickering TG, Blank S, Lindahl C, Strand L, Laragh JH. A validation study of the Del Mar Avionics ambulatory blood pressure system. *Ambulatory Electrocardiography* 1979;1:7–12.

71. Rowlands DB, Glover DR, Ireland MA, et al. Assessment of left ventricular mass and its response to antihypertensive treatment. *Lancet* 1982;1:467–470.

72. Drayer JIM, Weber MA, deJong JL. Blood pressure as a determinant of cardiac left ventricular muscle mass. *Arch Intern Med* 1983;143:90–92.

73. Prisant LM, Carr AA. Ambulatory blood pressure monitoring and echocardiographic left ventricular wall thickness and man. *Am J Hypertension* 1990;3:81–89.

74. Verdecchia P, Schillaci G, Guerrieri M, et al. Circadian blood pressure changes and left ventricular hypertrophy in essential hypertension. *Circulation* 1990;81:528–536.

75. Ravogli A, Trazzi S, Villani A, et al. Early 24-hour blood pressure elevation in normotensive subjects with parental hypertension. *Hypertension* 1990;16:491–497.

76. Harshfield GA, Hwang C, Grim CE. Circadian variation of blood pressure in blacks: influence of age, gender and activity. *J Human Hypertens* 1990;4:43–47.

77. Fumo MT, Teeger S, Lang RM, et al. Diurnal blood pressure variation and cardiac mass in American blacks and whites and South African blacks. *Am J Hypertension* 1992;5:111–116.

78. Safar ME, St Laurent S, Safarian AL, Pannier BM, London GM. Pulse pressure in sustained essential hypertension: a haemodynamic study. *J Hypertension* 1987;5:213–218.

79. Schnall PL, Schwartz JE, Landsbergis PA, Warren K, Pickering TG. Relation between job strain, alcohol and ambulatory blood pressure. *Hypertension* 1992;19:488–494.

80. Karasek RA, Baker D, Marxer F, Ahlbom A, Theorell T. Job decision latitude, job demands, and cardiovascular disease: a prospective study of Swedish men. *Am J Public Health* 1981;71:694–706.

81. Karasek RA, Theorell T, Schwartz JE, Schnall PL, Pieper CF, Michela JL. Job characteristics in relation to the prevalence of myocardial infarction in the US Health Examination Survey (HES) and Health and nutrition examination survey (HANES). *Am J Public Health* 1988;78:1–9.

82. Washburn RA, Savage DD, Dearwater SR, et al. Echocardiographic left ventricular mass and physical activity: quantification of the relations in spinal cord injured and apparently health active men. *Am J Cardiol* 1986;58:1248–1253.

83. Gosse P, Campello G, Aouizerate E, Roudant R, Broustet J-P, Dallochio M. Left ventricular hypertrophy in hypertension: correlation with rest, exercise and ambulatory systolic blood pressure. *J Hypertension* 1986;4(suppl 5):s297–s299.

84. Ren J-F, Hakki A-H, Kotler MN, Iskandrian A. Exercise systolic blood pressure: a powerful determinant of increased left ventricular mass in patients with hypertension. *J Am Coll Cardiol* 1985;5:1224–1231.

85. Nathwani D, Reeves RA, Marquez-Julio A, Leenen FHH. Left ventricular hypertrophy in mild hypertension: correlation with exercise blood pressure. *Am Heart J* 1985;109:386–387.

86. Gottdiener J, Brown J, Zoltick J, Fletcher R. Left ventricular hypertrophy in men with normal blood pressure: relation to exaggerated blood pressure response to exercise. *Ann Intern Med* 1990;112:161–166.

87. Schieken RM, Lauer RM, Clarke WR. Hemodynamics in childhood hypertension. *Clin Exp Hypertension* 1986;8:703–720.

88. Lund-Johansen P. Haemodynamics in essential hypertension. *Clin Sci* 1980;59:343s–354s.

89. Varnauskas E. Studies in hypertensive cardiovascular disease, with special reference to cardiac function. *Scand J Clin Lab Invest* 1955;7(suppl 17):1–117.

90. Ibrahim MM, Tarazi RC, Dustan JP, Bravo El, Gifford RW Jr. Hyperkinetic heart in severe hypertension: a separate clinical hemodynamic entity. *Am J Cardiol* 1975;35:667–674.

91. Finkelmen S, Worcel M, Agest A. Hemodynamic patterns in essential hypertension. *Circulation* 1965;31:356–368.

92. Tarazi RC, Frohlich ED, Dustan HP. Contribution of cardiac output to renovascular hypertension in men: relation to surgical treatment. *Am J Cardiol* 1973;31:600–605.

93. Ledingham JM, Cohen RD. Changes in the extracellular fluid volume and cardiac output during the development of experimental renal hypertension. *Canad Med Assoc J* 1964;90:292–294.

94. Bianchi G, Tilde Tenconi L, Lucca R. Effect in the conscious dog of constriction of the renal artery to a sole remaining kidney on haemodynamics, sodium balance, body fluid volumes, plasma renin concentration and pressor responsiveness to angiotensin. *Clin Sci* 1970;38:741–766.

95. de Simone G, Devereux RB, Camargo MJF, et al. In vivo left ventricular anatomy in rats with 2-kidney, 1-clip and 1-kidney, 1-clip renovascular hypertension. *J Hypertension* 1992;10:725–732.

96. Blake J, Devereux RB, Herrold EMcM, et al. Relation of concentric left ventricular hypertrophy and extracardiac target organ damage to supranormal left ventricular performance in established essential hypertension. *Am J Cardiol* 1988;62:246–252.

97. Grant C, Green DG, Bunnell IL. Left ventricular enlargement and hypertrophy. *Am J Med* 1965;39:895–904.

98. Grossman W, Jones D, McLaurin LD. Wall stress and patterns of hypertrophy in the human left ventricle. *J Clin Invest* 1975;56:56–64.

99. Blake J, Devereux RB, Borer JS, Szulc M, Pappas TW, Laragh JH. Relation of obesity, high sodium intake and eccentric left ventricular hypertrophy to left ventricular exercise dysfunction in essential hypertension. *Am J Med* 1990;88:477–485.

100. de Simone G, Devereux RB, Camargo MJF, Wallerson DC, Laragh JH. Influence of sodium intake on in vivo left ventricular anatomy in one-kidney one-clip and two-kidney one-clip Goldblatt rats. *Am J Physiol* 1993;264:H2103–H2120.

101. Dustan HP. Mechanisms of hypertension associated with obesity. *Ann Intern Med* 1983;98:860–864.

102. White FMM, Pereira LH, Garner JB. Body mass index and hypertension in women. *Canad Med Assoc J* 1986;135:1070–1072.

103. Rocchini AP, Moorehead C, Wentz E, Deremier S. Obesity-induced hypertension in the dog. *Hypertension* 1987;9(suppl III):III-64–III-68.

104. Khaw KT, Barrett-Connor E. The association between blood pressure, age, and dietary sodium and potassium: a population study. *Circulation* 1988;77:53–61.

105. Omirk P, Lund-Johansen P. Is sodium restriction effective treat-

ment of borderline and mild essential hypertension? A long-term haemodynamic study at rest and during exercise. *J Hypertension* 1986;4:535–541.

106. MacMahon SW, Wilcken DEL, Macdonald GJ. The effect of weight reduction on left ventricular mass: a randomized controlled trial in young, overweight hypertensive patients. *N Engl J Med* 1986;314:334–339.

107. Schmeider RE, Messerli FH, Garavaglia GE, Nunez BE. Dietary salt intake: a determinant of cardiac involvement in essential hypertension. *Circulation* 1988;78:951–956.

108. Ferrara LA, de Simone G, Pasanisi F, Mancini M, Mancini M. Left ventricular mass reduction during salt depletion in arterial hypertension. *Hypertension* 1984;6:755–759.

109. Ganau A, Arru A, Saba PS, et al. Stroke volume and left heart anatomy in relation to plasma volume in essential hypertension. *J Hypertension* 1991;9(suppl 6):s150–s151.

110. Tibblin G, Bergentz SE, Bjure J, Wilhelmsen L. Hematocrit, plasma protein, plasma volume and viscosity in early hypertensive disease. *Am Heart J* 1966;72:165–176.

111. Chrysant SG, Frohlich ED, Adamopoulos PN, et al. Pathophysiological significance of "stress" or relative polycythemia in essential hypertension. *Am J Cardiol* 1976;37:1069–1072.

112. Letcher RL, Chien S, Pickering TG, Sealey JE, Laragh JH. Direct relationship between blood pressure and blood viscosity in normal and hypertensive subjects. *Am J Med* 1981;70:1195–1202.

113. Letcher RL, Chien S, Pickering TG, Laragh JH. Elevated blood viscosity in patients with borderline essential hypertension. *Hypertension* 1983;5:757–762.

114. Fowkes FGR, Lowe GDO, Rumley A, Lennie SE, Smith FB, Connan PT. The relationship between blood viscosity and blood pressure in a random sample of the population aged 55 to 74 years. *Eur Heart J* 1993;14:597–601.

115. Zannod F, Voisin P, Brunette F, et al. Hemorheological abnormalities in arterial hypertension and their relation to cardiac hypertrophy. *J Hypertension* 1988;6:293–297.

116. Strandell T. Total haemoglobin, blood volume and haemoglobin concentration at rest and circulatory adaptation during exercise in relation to some anthropometric data in old men compared with young men. *Acta Med Scand* 1964;176:219–232.

117. Frohlich ED, Tarazi RC. Is arterial pressure the sole factor responsible for hypertensive cardiac hypertrophy. *Am J Cardiol* 1979;44:959–963.

118. Alderman EL, Harrison DC. Myocardial hypertrophy resulting from low dose isoproterenol administration in rats. *Proc Soc Exp Biol Med* 1970;136:268–270.

119. Laks MM, Morady F, Swan HJC. Myocardial hypertrophy produced by chronic infusion of subhypertensive doses of norepinephrine in the dog. *Chest* 1973;64:75–78.

120. Ostman-Smith I. Prevention of exercise-induced cardiac hypertrophy in rats by chemical sympathectomy (guanethidine treatment). *Neuroscience* 1976;1:497–507.

121. Rossi MA, Carillo SV. Pathogenesis of cardiac hypertrophy in iron deficiency anemia: The role of noradrenaline. *Br J Exp Pathol* 1982;63:269–277.

122. Sen S, Tarazi RC, Khairallah PA, Bumpus FM. Cardiac hypertrophy in spontaneously hypertensive rats. *Circ Res* 1974;35:775–781.

123. Fernandes M, Onesti G, Fiorentini T, Kim KE, Swartz C. Effect of chronic administration of propranolol on the blood pressure and heart weight in experimental renal hypertension. *Life Sci* 1976;18:967–970.

124. Ostman-Smith I. Cardiac sympathetic nerves as the final common pathway in the initiation of adaptive cardiac hypertrophy. *Clin Sci* 1981;61:265–272.

125. Lindpointer K, Sen S. Role of sodium in hypertensive cardiac hypertrophy. *Circ Res* 1985;57:610–617.

126. Corea L, Bentivoglio M, Verdecchia P. Echocardiographic left ventricular hypertrophy as related to arterial pressure and plasma norepinephrine concentration in arterial hypertension: reversal by atenolol treatment. *Hypertension* 1983;5:837–843.

127. Simpson P. Norepinephrine-stimulated hypertrophy of cultured rat myocardial cells is an alpha$_1$-adrenergic response. *J Clin Invest* 1983;72:732–738.

128. Simpson P. Stimulation of hypertrophy of cultured neonatal rat heart cells through an α_1-adrenergic receptor and induction of

beating through α_1 and β_1-adrenergic receptor interaction. *Circ Res* 1985;56:884–894.

129. Simpson P, Bishoprick N, Couglin S, et al. Dual trophic effects of the alpha-1-adrenergic receptor in cultured neonatal rat heart muscle cells. *J Mol Cell Cardiol* 1986;18(suppl):45–58.

130. Cohen J. Role of endocrine factors in the pathogenesis of cardiac hypertrophy. *Circ Res* 1974;34(suppl II):II-49–II-57.

131. Cutilletta AF, Erinoff L, Hellar A, Low J, Oparil S. Development of left ventricular hypertrophy in young spontaneously hypertensive rats after peripheral sympathectomy. *Circ Res* 1977;40:428–434.

132. Page E, Oparil S. Effect of peripheral sympathectomy on left ventricular ultrastructure in young spontaneously hypertensive rats. *J Mol Cell Cardiol* 1978;10:301–305.

133. Tomanek RJ, Bhatnagar RK, Schmid P, Brody MJ. Role of catecholamine in myocardial cell hypertrophy in hypertensive rats. *Am J Physiol* 1982;242:H1015–H1021.

134. Vaughan-Williams EM. The absence of effect of chemical sympathectomy on ventricular hypertrophy induced by hypoxia in young rabbits. *Cardiovasc Res* 1983;17:379–389.

135. Tomanek RJ, Carlson DW, Palmer PJ, Bhatnager RK. Role of sympathetic nerves during developing cardiac hypertrophy in Grollman hypertensive rats. *Am J Physiol* 1987;253:H818–H825.

136. Mann DL, Kent RL, Parsons B, Cooper G IV. Adrenergic effects on the biology of the adult mammalian cardiocyte. *Circulation* 1992;85:790–804.

137. Campbell DJ, Habener JF. Angiotensinogen gene is expressed and differentially regulated in multiple tissues of the rat. *J Clin Invest* 1986;78:31–39.

138. Fabris B, Jackson B, Kohzuki M, Perich R, Johnston CI. Increased cardiac angiotensin-converting enzyme in rats with chronic heart failure. *Clin Exp Pharmacol Physiol* 1990;17:309–314.

139. Yamada H, Fabris B, Allen AM, Jackson B, Johnston CI, Mendelsohn FAO. Localization of angiotensin converting enzyme in rat heart. *Circ Res* 1991;68:141–149.

140. Fabris B, Yamada H, Cubela B, Jackson B, Mendelsohn FAO, Johnston CI. Characterization of cardiac angiotensin converting enzyme (ACE) and *in vivo* inhibition following oral quinipril to rats. *Br J Pharmacol* 1990;100:651–653.

141. Freer RJ, Pappano AJ, Peach MJ, et al. Mechanism for the positive inotropic effect of angiotensin II on isolated cardiac muscle. *Circ Res* 1976;39:178–183.

142. Hirakata H, Fouad-Tarazi FM, Bumpus FM, et al. Angiotensin and the failing heart. Enhanced positive inotropic response to angiotensin I in cardiomyopathic hamster heart in the presence of captopril. *Circ Res* 1990;66:891–899.

143. Faxon DP, Creager MA, Halperin JL, Sussman HA, Gavras H, Ryan TJ. The effect of angiotensin converting enzyme inhibition on coronary blood flow and hemodynamics in patients without coronary artery disease. *Int J Cardiol* 1982;2:251–262.

144. Roth RH, Hughes J. Acceleration of protein biosynthesis by angiotensin: correlation with angiotensin's effect on catecholamine biosynthesis. *Biochem Pharmacol* 1972;21:3182–3187.

145. Boodle-Biber MC, Hughes J, Roth RH. Acceleration of catecholamine biosynthesis in sympathetically innervated tissues by angiotensin II-amide. *Br J Pharmacol* 1972;46:289–299.

146. Hill RN, Severs WB, Lin DK. Inability of angiotensin to stimulate RNA synthesis in isolated rat atria. *Proc Soc Exp Biol* 1975;148:418–419.

147. Owens GK. Influence of blood pressure on development of aortic medial smooth muscle hypertrophy in spontaneously hypertensive rats. *Hypertension* 1987;9:178–187.

148. von Lutteroti N, Catanzaro DF, Sealey JE, Laragh JH. Renin is not synthesized by cardiac and extrarenal vascular tissue: a review of experimental evidence. *Circulation* 1994;89:458–470.

149. Khairallah PA, Kanabus J. Angiotensin and myocardial protein synthesis. In: Tarazi RC, Dunbar JB, eds. *Perspectives in Cardiovascular Research,* Vol 8. New York: Raven Press, 1983;337–347.

150. Unger T, Mattveldt T, Lamberly V, et al. Effect of early onset angiotensin converting enzyme inhibition in myocardial capillaries. *Hypertension* 1992;20:478–482.

151. Linz W, Scholkens BA, Ganten D. Converting enzyme inhibition

specifically prevents the development of cardiac hypertrophy in rats. *Clin and Exper Hypertension* 1989;11:1325–1350.

152. Ekker M, Tronik D, Rougeon F. Extra-renal transcription of the renin gene in multiple tissues of mice and rats. *Proc Natl Acad Sci (USA)* 1989;86:5155–5158.

153. Sigmund CD, Jones CA, Fabian JR, et al. Tissue and cell-specific expression of a renin promoter-reporter gene construct in transgenic mice. *Biochem Biophys Res Commun* 1990;170:344–350.

154. Tada M, Fukamizu A, Seo MS, Takahashi S, Murakami K. Renin expression in the kidney and brain is reciprocally controlled by captopril. *Biochem Biophys Res Comm* 1989;158:1065–1071.

155. Lou Y, Smith DL, Robinson BG, Morris BJ. Renin gene expression in various tissues determined by single-step polymerase chain reaction. *Clin Exp Pharmacol Physiol* 1991;18:357–362.

156. Okura T, Kitami Y, Iwata T, Howada K. Quantitative measurement of extra-renal mRNA by polymerase chain reaction. *Biochem Biophys Res Comm* 1991;179:25–31.

157. Quinones M, Do YS, Kurabayashi M, et al. Analysis of the human intracardiac renin angiotensin system (Abstr) *Hypertension* 1992;20:415.

158. Devereux RB, Savage DD, Drayer JIM, Laragh JH. Left ventricular hypertrophy and function in high-, normal-, and low-renin forms of essential hypertension. *Hypertension* 1982;4:524–531.

159. Buttrick P, Kaplan M, Camargo MJF, et al: The influence of dietary salt and plasma renin activity on myosin heavy chain gene expression in rat hearts. *Am J Hypertension* 1993;6:579–585.

160. Brilla CG, Pick R, Tan LB, Janicki JS, Weber KT. Remodelling of the rat right and left ventricle in experimental hypertension. *Circ Res* 1990;67:1355–1364.

161. Brilla CG, Janicki JS, Weber KT. Impaired diastolic function and coronary reserve in genetic hypertension: role of interstitial fibrosis and medial thickening of intramyocardial coronary arteries. *Circ Res* 1991;69:107–115.

162. Brilla CG, Weber KT. Mineralocorticoid excess, dietary sodium, and myocardial fibrosin. *J Lab Clin Med* 1992;120:893–901.

163. Hammond GL, Lai YK, Markert CL. The molecules that initiate cardiac hypertrophy are not species-specific. *Science* 1982;216:529–531.

164. Sil P, Misono K, Sen S. Myotrophin in human cardiomyopathic heart. *Circ Res* 1993;73:98–108.

165. Starksen NF, Simpson PC, Bishopric N, et al. Cardiac myocyte hypertrophy is associated with c-myc proto-oncogene expression. *Proc Natl Acad Sci USA* 1986;83:8348–8350.

166. Izumo S, Nadal-Ginard B, Mahdavi V. Proto-oncogene induction and reprogramming of cardiac gene expression produced by pressure overload. *Proc Natl Acad Sci* 1988;85:339–343.

167. Jackson T, Allard MF, Sreenan CM, Dos LK, Bishop SP, Swain JL. The c-myc proto-oncogene regulates cardiac development in transgenic mice. *Mol Cell Biol* 1990;10:3709–3716.

168. Radice M, Alli C, Avanzini F, et al. Left ventricular structure and function in normotensive adolescents with a genetic predisposition to hypertension. *Am Heart J* 1986;111:115–120.

169. Fagard R, Van der Brocke C, Bielen E, Amery A. Maximum oxygen uptake and cardiac size and function in twins. *Am J Cardiol* 1987;60:1362–1367.

170. Dunn FG, Oigman W, Sungaard-Riise K, et al. Racial differences in cardiac adaptation to essential hypertension determined by echocardiographic indexes. *J Am Coll Cardiol* 1983;1:1348–1351.

171. Hammond IW, Alderman MH, Devereux RB, Lutas EM, Laragh JH. Contrast in cardiac anatomy and function between black and white patients with hypertension. *J Natl Med Assoc* 1984;76:247–255.

172. Koren MJ, Mensah GA, Blake J, Laragh JH, Devereux RB. Comparison of left ventricular mass and geometry in black and white patients with essential hypertension. *Am J Hypertension* 1993;6:815–823.

173. Persky V, Pan WH, Stamler J, Dyer A, Levy P. Time trends in the US racial difference in hypertension. *Am J Epidemiol* 1986;124:724–737.

174. Cooper R. A note on the biologic concept of race and its application in epidemiologic research. *Am Heart J* 1984;108:715–723.

175. de Simone G, Devereux RB, Roman MJ, Schlussel Y, Alderman MH, Laragh JH. Echocardiographic left ventricular mass and electrolyte intake predict subsequent arterial hypertension in initially normotensive adults. *Ann Intern Med* 1991;114:202–209.

176. Iso H, Kiyama M, Doi M, et al. Left ventricular mass and subsequent blood pressure changes among middle-aged men in rural and urban Japanese populations. *Circulation* 1994 (*in press*).

177. Post WS, Larson MG, Levy D. Cardiac structural precursors of hypertension. *Circulation* 1993;88(suppl I):I-614.

178. Tsoporis J, Leenen FHH. Effects of arterial vasodilators on cardiac hypertrophy and sympathetic activity in rats. *Hypertension* 1988;11:376–386.

179. Jennings GL, Laufer E, Esler MD, Korner PI. Long term effects of exercise on blood pressure, sympathetic activity, and left ventricular hypertrophy in essential hypertension. *Hypertension* 1987;10:371.

180. Lutas EM, Devereux RB, Reis G, et al. Increased cardiac performance in mild essential hypertension: left ventricular mechanics. *Hypertension* 1985;7:979–988.

181. Hartford M, Wikstrand JCM, Wallentin I, Ljungman SMG, Berglund GL. Left ventricular wall stress and systolic function in untreated primary hypertension. *Hypertension* 1985;7:97–104.

182. de Simone G, DiLorenzo L, Costantino G, Moccia D, Buonissimo S, de Vitiis O. Supernormal contractility in primary hypertension without left ventricular hypertrophy. *Hypertension* 1988;11:457–463.

183. Roman MJ, Pini R, Pickering TG, Devereux RB. Non-invasive measurements of arterial compliance in hypertensive compared with normotensive adults. *J Hypertens* 1992;10(suppl 6):S115–S118.

184. Saba PS, Roman MJ, Pini R, Ganau A, Devereux RB. Relation of arterial pressure waveforms to left ventricular and carotid anatomy in normotensive subjects. *J Am Coll Cardiol* 1993;22:1873–1880.

185. Morgan H, Baker KM. Cardiac hypertrophy, mechanical, neural, and endocrine dependence. *Circulation* 1991;83(1):13–25.

186. Folkow B, Grimby G, Thulesius O. Adaptive structural changes of the vascular walls in hypertension and their relation to control of the peripheral resistance. *Acta Physiol Scand* 1958;44:255–272.

187. Shkhvatsabaya IK, Usubaliyen NN, Yurenev AP, Panfilov VV. The interrelations of cardiac and vascular wall hypertrophy in arterial hypertension. *Cardiovasc Rev Rep* 1981;2:1145–1149.

188. Geri A, Agabiti-Rosei E, Muiesan ML, Romanelli G, Platto L, Muiesan G. Interrelations of cardiac and arterial vascular wall hypertrophy in essential hypertension. *J Hypertens* 1985;3(suppl 3):s335–s337.

189. Hartling OJ. In vivo studies of peripheral vascular structure in hypertensive patients. *J Clin Hypertens* 1987;3:349–354.

190. Schulte K-L, Braun J, Meyer-Sabellek W, Wegscheider K, Gotzen R, Distler A. Functional versus structural changes of forearm vascular resistance in hypertension. *Hypertension* 1988;11:320–325.

191. Egan B, Schork N, Panis R, Hinderliter A. Vascular structure enhances regional resistance responses in mild essential hypertension. *J Hypertens* 1988;6:41–48.

192. Lucarini AR, Spessot M, Picano E, et al. Lack of correlation between cardiac mass and arteriolar structural changes in mild-to-moderate hypertension. *J Hypertens* 1991;9:1187–1191.

193. Schulte K-L, Liederwald K, Meyer-Sabellek W, van Gemmeren D, Lenz T, Gotzen R. Relationships between ambulatory blood pressure, forearm vascular resistance, and left ventricular mass in hypertensive and normotensive subjects. *Am J Hypertens* 1993;6:786–793.

194. Mulvany MJ. The structure of the resistance vasculature in essential hypertension. *J Hypertens* 1987;5:129–136.

195. Mulvany MJ, Hansen PK, Aalkjaer C. Direct evidence that the greater contractility of resistance vessels in spontaneously hypertensive rats is associated with a narrowed lumen, a thickened media, and an increased number of smooth muscle cell layers. *Circ Res* 1978;43:854–864.

196. Aalkjaer C, Eiskjaer H, Mulvany MJ, et al. Abnormal structure and function of isolated subcutaneous resistance vessels from essential hypertensive patients despite antihypertensive treatment. *J Hypertens* 1989;7:305–310.

197. Heagerty AM, Aalkjaer C, Bund SJ, Korsgaard N, Mulvany MJ. Small artery structure in hypertension. Dual processes of remodeling and growth. *Hypertension* 1993;21:391–397.

198. Cifkova R, Niederle P, Romanovska L, et al. Heart and vessel hypertrophy in hypertension: possibilities of regression. *J Hypertens* 1987;5(suppl 5):S407–S410.

199. Devereux RB, Savage DD, Sachs I, Laragh JH. Relation of hemodynamic load to left ventricular hypertrophy and performance in hypertension. *Am J Cardiol* 1983;51:171–176.

200. Gariepy J, Massonneau M, Levenson J, Heudes D, Simon A. Evidence for in vivo carotid and femoral wall thickening in human hypertension. *Hypertension* 1993;22:111–118.

201. Arcaro G, Laurent S, Jondeau G, Hoeks AP, Safar ME. Stiffness of the common carotid artery in treated hypertensive patients. *J Hypertens* 1991;9:947–954.

202. Laurent S, Hayoz D, Trazzi S, et al. Isobaric compliance of the radial artery is increased in patients with essential hypertension. *J Hypertens* 1993;11:89–98.

203. Megnien JL, Simon A, Valensi P, Flaud P, Merli I, Levenson J. Comparative effects of diabetes mellitus on physical properties of human large arteries. *J Am Coll Cardiol* 1992;20:1562–1568.

204. Simon AC, Safar ME, Levenson JA, London GM, Levy BI, Chau NP. An evaluation of large arteries compliance in man. *Am J Physiol* 1979;237:H550–H554.

205. Avolio AP, Deng FQ, Li WQ, et al. Effects of aging on arterial distensibility in populations with high and low prevalence of hypertension: comparison between urban and rural communities in China. *Circulation* 1985;71:202–210.

206. Nichols WW, O'Rourke MF, Avolio AP, Yaginuma T, Pepine CJ, Conti CR. Ventricular/vascular interaction in patients with mild systemic hypertension and normal peripheral resistance. *Circulation* 1986;74:455–462.

207. Ting CT, Brink P, Lin SJ, et al. Arterial hemodynamics in human hypertension. *J Clin Invest* 1986;78:1462–1471.

208. Bouthier J, Benetos A, Simon A, Levenson J, Safar M. Pulsed Doppler evaluation of diameter, blood velocity and blood flow of common carotid artery in sustained hypertension. *J Cardiovasc Pharmacol* 1985;7(suppl 2):S99–S104.

209. Salonen JT, Salonen R. Association of serum low density lipoprotein cholesterol, smoking and hypertension with different manifestations of atherosclerosis. *Int J Epidemiol* 1990;19:911–917.

210. Gribben B, Pickering TG, Sleight P. Arterial distensibility in normal and hypertensive man. *Clin Sci* 1979;56:413–417.

211. Pignoli P, Tremoli E, Poli A, Oreste P, Paoletti R. Intimal plus medial thickness of the arterial wall. A direct measurement with ultrasound imaging. *Circulation* 1986;74:1399–1406.

212. Bouthier JD, De Luca N, Safar ME, Simon AC. Cardiac hypertrophy and arterial distensibility in essential hypertension. *Am Heart J* 1985;109:1345–1352.

213. Safar ME, Toto-Moukouo JJ, Bouthier JA, et al. Arterial dynamics, cardiac hypertrophy, and antihypertensive treatment. *Circulation* 1987;75(suppl I):I-156–I-161.

214. Asmar RG, Pannier B, Santoni JP, et al. Reversion of cardiac hypertrophy and reduced arterial compliance after converting enzyme inhibition in essential hypertension. *Circulation* 1988;88:941–950.

215. Pannier B, Brunel P, El Aroussy W, Lacolley P, Safar ME. Pulse pressure and echocardiographic findings in essential hypertension. *J Hypertens* 1989;7:127–132.

216. O'Rourke MF, Kelly RP. Wave reflection in the systemic circulation and its implications in ventricular function. *J Hypertens* 1993;11:327–337.

217. Isles CG, Walker LV, Beevers DG, et al. Mortality in the Glasgow blood pressure clinic. *J Hypertens* 1987;4:141–156.

218. Kannel WB, Abbott RD. A prognostic comparison of asymptomatic left ventricular hypertrophy and unrecognized myocardial infarction: The Framingham Study. *Am Heart J* 1986;111:391–397.

219. Sullivan JM, Vander Zwaag R, El-Zeky F, Ramanathan KB, Mirvis DM. Left ventricular hypertrophy: Effect on survival. *J Am Coll Cardiol* 1993;22:508–513.

220. Casale PN, Devereux RB, Milner M, et al. Value of echocardiographic measurement of left ventricular mass in predicting cardiovascular morbid events in hypertensive men. *Ann Intern Med* 1986;105:173–178.

221. Nestrova AL, Novikov ID, Yurenev AP. Prognostic significance of blood pressure and left ventricular hypertrophy in systematic and nonsystematic treatment of essential hypertension. *Kardiologia* 1986;8:89–91.

222. Levy D, Plehn JF, Wolf PA, et al. Left ventricular mass and risk of stroke in men (abst) *Circulation* 1987;76(suppl IV):IV-143.

223. Aronow WS, Epstein S, Koenigsberg M, Schwartz KS. Usefulness of echocardiographic left ventricular hypertrophy, ventricular tachycardia and complex ventricular arrhythmias in predicting ventricular fibrillation or sudden death in elderly patients. *Am J Cardiol* 1988;62:1124–1125.

224. Wofford JL, Wasilauskas CH, Byington RP, et al. Left ventricular mass index as a predictor of mortality (abstr) *Circulation* 1988;78(suppl II):II-63.

225. Levy D, Garrison RJ, Savage DD, Kannel WB, Castelli WP. Left ventricular mass and incidence of coronary heart disease in an elderly cohort: The Framingham Study. *Ann Intern Med* 1989;110:101–108.

226. Cooper RS, Castaner A, Simmons B, Suntanan V, Chali JL, Mar M. Left ventricular hypertrophy is associated with worse survival independent of ventricular function and number of coronary arteries severely narrowed. *Am J Cardiol* 1990;65:441–445.

227. Parfrey PS, Harnett JD, Griffiths SM, et al. The clinical course of left ventricular hypertrophy in dialysis patients. *Nephron* 1990;55:114–120.

228. Silberberg JS, Barre PE, Prichard SS, Sniderman AD. Impact of left ventricular hypertrophy on survival in end-stage renal disease. *Kidney Int* 1989;36:286–290.

229. Levy D, Garrison RJ, Savage DD, Kannel WB, Castelli WP. Prognostic implications of echocardiographically determined left ventricular mass in the Framingham Heart Study. *N Engl J Med* 1990;322:1561–1566.

230. Ghali JK, Liao Y, Simmons B, Castaner A, Cao G, Cooper RS. The prognostic role of left ventricular hypertrophy in patients with or without coronary artery disease. *Ann Intern Med* 1992;117:831–836.

231. Koyanagi S, Eastham CL, Harrison DG, Marcus ML. Increased size of myocardial infarction in dogs with chronic hypertension and left ventricular hypertrophy. *Circ Res* 1982;50:55–62.

232. Dellsperger KC, Clothier JL, Hartnett JA, Hann LM, Marcus ML. Acceleration of the wavefront of myocardial necrosis by chronic hypertension and left ventricular hypertrophy in dogs. *Circ Res* 1988;63:87–96.

233. Koyanagi S, Eastham CL, Marcus ML. Effects of chronic hypertension and left ventricular hypertrophy on the incidence of sudden cardiac death after coronary artery occlusion in conscious dogs. *Circulation* 1982;65:1192–1197.

234. Inou T, Lambeth WC Jr, Koyanagi S, Harrison DG, Eastham CL, Marcus ML. Relative importance of hypertension after coronary occlusion in chronic hypertensive dogs with LVH. *Am J Physiol* 1987;253:H1148–H1158.

235. Houghton JL, Frank MJ, Carr AA, von Dohlen TW, Prisant LM. Relations among impaired coronary flow reserve, left ventricular hypertrophy and thallium perfusion defects in hypertensive patients without obstructive coronary artery disease. *J Am Coll Cardiol* 1990;15:43–51.

236. Polese A, DeCesare N, Montorsi P, et al. Upward shift of the lower range of coronary flow autoregulation in hypertensive patients with hypertrophy of the left ventricle. *Circulation* 1991;83:845–853.

237. Antony I, Nitenberg A, Foult J-M, Aptecar E. Coronary vasodilator reserve in untreated and treated hypertensive patients with and without left ventricular hypertrophy. *J Am Coll Cardiol* 1993;22:514–520.

238. Fujita M, Mikuniya A, McKown DP, McKown MD, Franklin D. Regional myocardial volume alterations induced by brief repeated coronary occlusion in conscious dogs. *J Am Coll Cardiol* 1988;12:1048–1053.

239. Pech HJ, Witte R, Romaniuk R, Parsi RA, Porstmann W. Left ventricular mass in coronary artery disease without hypertension. *Br Heart J* 1974;36:362–367.

240. Gould KL, Lipscomb K, Hamilton GW, Kennedy JW. Relation

of left ventricular shape, function and wall stress in man. *Am J Cardiol* 1974;34:627–634.

241. Versailles JT, Verscheure Y, LeKim A, Pourrias B. Comparison between the ventricular fibrillation thresholds of spontaneously hypertensive and normotensive rats—investigation of antidysrhythmic drugs. *J Cardiovasc Pharmacol* 1982;4:430–435.

242. Aronson RS. After potentials and triggered activity in hypertrophied myocardium from rats with renal hypertension. *Circ Res* 1981;48:720–727.

243. Martins JB, Kim W, Marcus ML. Chronic hypertension and left ventricular hypertrophy facilitate induction of sustained ventricular tachycardia in dogs 3 hours after left circumflex coronary artery occlusion. *J Am Coll Cardiol* 1989;14:1365–1373.

244. Zehender M, Meinertz T, Hohnloser S, et al. Prevalence of circadian variations and spontaneous variability of cardiac disorders and ECG changes suggestive of myocardial ischemia in systemic arterial hypertension. *Circulation* 1992;85:1808–1815.

245. Messerli FH, Ventura HO, Wlizardi DJ, Dunn FG, Frohlich ED. Hypertension and sudden death: increased ventricular ectopic activity in left ventricular hypertrophy. *Am J Med* 1984;77:18–22.

246. McLenachan JM, Henderson E, Morris KI, Dargie HG. Ventricular arrhythmias in patients with hypertensive left ventricular hypertrophy. *N Engl J Med* 1987;317:787–792.

247. Levy D, Anderson KM, Plehn J, Savage DD, Christiansen JC, Castelli WP. Echocardiographically determined left ventricular structural and functional correlates of complex or frequent ventricular arrhythmias on one-hour ambulatory electrocardiographic monitoring. *Am J Cardiol* 1987;159:836–840.

248. Kannel WB, Thom TJ. Incidence, prevalence, and mortality of cardiovascular diseases. In Hurst JW, Schlant RC, Rackly CE, Sonnnenblick EH, Wenger NK, eds. *The Heart, Arteries and Veins*, 7th ed. New York: McGraw-Hill, 1990;627–638.

249. Holland OB, Nixon JV, Kuhnert L. Diuretic-induced ventricular ectopic activity. *Am J Med* 1981;70:762–768.

250. Multiple Risk Factor Intervention Trial Research Group: Baseline rest electrocardiographic abnormalities, antihypertensive treatment, and mortality in the Multiple Risk Factor Intervention Trial. *Am J Cardiol* 1985;55:1–15.

251. Papademetriou V, Fletcher R, Katri IM, Freis ED. Diuretic-induced hypokalemia in uncomplicated systemic hypertension: effect of plasma potassium correction on cardiac arrhythmias. *Am J Cardiol* 1983;52:1017–1022.

252. Bause GS, Fleg JL, Lakatta EG. Exercise-induced arrhythmias in diuretic-treated patients with uncomplicated systemic hypertension. *Am J Cardiol* 1987;59:847–877.

253. Devereux RB. 'Silent ischemia,' ventricular arrhythmias, and complications of hypertension. *Circulation* 1992;85:1948–1950.

254. Roman MJ, Spitzer M, Pini R, Pickering T, Devereux RB. The association of carotid atherosclerosis and increased left ventricular mass in hypertension. *J Am Coll Cardiol* 1992;19:86A.

255. Rabkin SW, Mathewson FAL, Tate RB. Prognosis after acute myocardial infarction: relation to blood pressure values before infarction in a prospective cardiovascular study. *Am J Cardiol* 1977;40:604–610.

256. Doyle AE. Hypertension and vascular disease. *Am J Hypertension* 1991;4:s103–s106.

257. Kannel WB, Sorlie P. Hypertension in Framingham. In: Paul O, ed. *Epidemiology and Control of Hypertension*. New York: Stratton Intercontinental, 1975;553–590.

258. Pooling Project Research Group: Relationship of blood pressure, serum cholesterol, smoking habits, relative weight and ECG abnormalities to incidence of major coronary events. Final report of the pooling project. *J Chronic Dis* 1978;31:201–306.

259. Davis D, Kloiner MJ. Studies in hypertensive heart disease. I. The incidence of coronary atherosclerosis in cases of essential hypertension. *Am Heart J* 1940;19:185–192.

260. Davis D, Kloiner MJ. Studies in hypertensive heart disease. II. The role of hypertension, per se, in the development of coronary sclerosis. *Am Heart J* 1940;19:193–197.

261. Harrison CV, Wood P. Hypertensive and ischaemic heart disease: a comparative clinical and pathological study. *Brit Heart J* 1949;11:205–209.

262. Bell ET, Clawson BJ. Primary (essential) hypertension. A study of four hundred and twenty cases. *Arch Pathol* 1928;5:939–1001.

263. Goldring W, Chasis H. *Hypertension and Hypertensive Disease.* New York: Commonwealth Fund, 1945.

264. Hodge JV, Smirk FH. The effect of drug treatment of hypertension on the distribution of death from various causes. *Am Heart J* 1967;73:441–452.

265. Collins R, Peto R, MacMahon S, et al. Blood pressure, stroke and coronary heart disease. Part 2, short-term reductions in blood pressure: Overview of randomized drug trials in their epidemiological context. *Lancet* 1990;335:827–839.

266. Hypertension Detection and Follow-Up Program cooperative Study: Five-year findings of the HDFP, 1: reduction in mortality of persons with high blood pressure, 2: mortality by race, sex and age. *JAMA* 1979;242:2562–2579.

267. Wikstrand J, Warnold I, Olsson G, et al. Primary prevention with metoprolol in patients with hypertension. Mortality results from the MAPHY study. *JAMA* 1988;259:1976–1982.

268. SHEP Cooperative Research Group. Prevention of stroke by antihypertensive drug treatment in older persons with isolated systolic hypertension. Final results of the Systolic Hypertension in the Elderly Program. *JAMA* 1991;265:3255–3264.

269. MRC Working Party. Medical Research Council trial of treatment of hypertension in old adults: principal results. *BMJ* 1992;304:405–412.

270. Dahlof B, Lindholm LH, Hansson L, Schersten B, Ekbom T, Wester P-O. Morbidity and mortality in the Swedish Trial in Old Patients with Hypertension. (STOP-Hypertension). *Lancet* 1991;338:1281–1285.

271. Medical Research Council Working Party: MRC Trial of treatment of mild hypertension: principal results. *Brit Med J* 1985;291:97–104.

272. Report by the Management Committee: The Australian therapeutic trial in mild hypertension. *Lancet* 1980;1:1261–1269.

273. Amery A, Brixko P, Clement D, et al. Mortality and morbidity results from the European working party on high blood pressure in the elderly trail. *Lancet* 1985;1:1349–1354.

274. Hegeland A. Treatment of mild hypertension: a five-year controlled drug trial: the Oslo Study. *Am J Med* 1980;69:725–732.

275. Multiple Risk Factor Intervention Trail Research Group: Baseline rest electrocardiographic abnormalities, antihypertensive treatment and mortality in the Multiple Risk Factor Intervention Trial. *Am J Cardiol* 1985;55:1–15.

276. Alderman MH, Madhavan S, Ooi WL, Cohen H, Sealey JE, Laragh JH. Association of the renin-sodium profile with the risk of myocardial infarction in patients with hypertension. *N Engl J Med* 1991;234:1098–1104.

277. Takahashi M, Sasayama S, Kawai C, Kotoura H. Contractile performance of the hypertrophied left ventricle in patients with systemic hypertension. *Circulation* 1980;62:116–126.

278. Borer JS, Jason M, Devereux RB, Pickering T, Erle S, Laragh JH. Left ventricular performance in the hypertensive patient: Exercise-mediated non-invasive separation of loading influences from intrinsic muscle dysfunction. *Chest* 1983;2:29–34.

279. Boudoulas H, Manzouratos D, Sahn YH, Weissler AM. Left ventricular mass and systolic performance in chronic systemic hypertension. *Am J Cardiol* 1986;57:232–237.

280. de Simone G, DiLorenzo L, Moccia D, Costantino G, Buonissimo S, deDivitiis O. Hemodynamic hypertrophied ventricular patterns in systemic hypertension. *Am J Cardiol* 1987;60:1317–1321.

281. Topol EJ, Traill TA, Fortuin NJ. Hypertensive hypertrophic cardiomyopathy of the elderly. *N Eng J Med* 1985;312:277–283.

282. Shimuzu G, Hirota Y, Kita Y, Kawamura K, Saito T, Gaasch WH. Left ventricular midwall mechanics in systemic arterial hypertension. Myocardial function is depressed in pressure-overload hypertrophy. *Circulation* 1991;83:1676–1684.

283. de Simone G, Devereux RB, Roman MJ, et al. Assessment of left ventricular function by the mid-wall fractional shortening-end-systolic stress relation in human hypertension. *J Am Coll Cardiol* 1994 (*in press*).

284. Porchellati C, Verdecchia P, Schillaci G, et al. Low mid-wall fractional shortening identifies a subgroup of hypertensive patients with increased left ventricular mass and ambulatory blood pressure. *J Hypertens* (in press).

285. Wasserman AG, Katz RJ, Varghese PJ, et al. Exercise radionu-

clide ventriculographic responses in hypertensive patients with chest pain. *N Engl J Med* 1984;311:1276–1280.

286. Miller DD, Ruddy TD, Zusman RM, et al. Left ventricular ejection fraction response during exercise in asymptomatic systemic hypertension. *Am J Cardiol* 1987;59:409–413.

287. Cody RJ, Kubo SH, Devereux RB, Shaknovich A, Ryman KS, Laragh JH. Adverse influence of eccentric hypertrophy and obesity on exercise cardiac performance in hypertension. *Proceedings of the Second Annual Meeting of the American Society of Hypertension* 1987:70.

288. Fouad FM, Tarazi RV, Gallagher JH, MacIntyre WJ, Cook SA. Abnormal left ventricular relaxation in hypertensive patients. *Clin Sci* 1980;59:411s–414s.

289. Gibson DG, Traill TA, Hall RJC, Brown DJ. Echocardiographic features of secondary left ventricular hypertrophy. *Br Heart J* 1979;41:54–59.

290. Fouad FM, Slominski JM, Tarazi RC. Left ventricular diastolic function in hypertension: relation to left ventricular mass and systolic function. *J Am Coll Cardiol* 1984;3:1500–1506.

291. Inouye I, Massie B, Loge D, et al. Abnormal left ventricular filling: an early finding in mild to moderate systemic hypertension. *Am J Cardiol* 1984;53:120–126.

292. Smith V-E, Schulman P, Karimeddini M, White WB, Meeran MK, Katz AM. Rapid left ventricular filling in left ventricular hypertrophy: II. Pathologic hypertrophy. *J Am Coll Cardiol* 1985;5:869–874.

293. Papademitriou V, Gottdiener JS, Fletcher RD, Freis ED. Echocardiographic assessment by computer-assisted analysis of diastolic left ventricular function and hypertrophy in borderline or mild hypertension. *Am J Cardiol* 1985;56:546–550.

294. Gardin JM, Drayer JI, Rohan MK, et al. Doppler evaluation of left ventricular filling in mild and severe hypertension. *J Am Coll Cardiol* 1986;7:185–192.

295. Smith V-E, White WB, Meeran MK, Karimeddini MK. Improved left ventricular filling accompanies reduced left ventricular mass during therapy of essential hypertension. *J Am Coll Cardiol* 1986;8:1449–1454.

296. Pearson AC, Labovitz AJ, Mrosek D, Williams GA, Kennedy HL. Assessment of diastolic function in normal and hypertrophied hearts: comparison of Doppler echocardiography and M-mode echocardiography. *Am Heart J* 1987;113:1417–1425.

297. Snider AR, Gidding SS, Rocchini AP, et al. Doppler evaluation of left ventricular diastolic filling in children with systemic hypertension. *Am J Cardiol* 1985;56:921–926.

298. Glantz SA, Parmley WW. Factors which affect the diastolic pressure-volume curve. *Circ Res* 1978;42:171–180.

299. Stoddard MF, Pearson AC, Kern MJ, Ratcliff J, Mrosek DG, Labovitz AJ. Left ventricular diastolic function: Comparison of Doppler echocardiographic and hemodynamic indexes in subjects with and without coronary artery disease. *J Am Coll Cardiol* 1989;13:327–336.

300. Devereux RB. Left ventricular diastolic dysfunction: early diastolic relaxation and late diastolic compliance. *J Am Coll Cardiol* 1989;13:337–339.

301. Granger CB, Karimeddini MK, Smith V-E, Shapiro HR, Katz AM, Riba AL. Rapid ventricular filling in left ventricular filling in left ventricular hypertrophy. I. Physiologic hypertrophy. *J Am Coll Cardiol* 1985;5:862–868.

302. Pearson AC, Schiff M, Mrosek D, Labovitz AJ, Williams GA. Left ventricular diastolic function in weight lifters. *Am J Cardiol* 1986;58:1254–1259.

303. Laragh JH. Cardiac pathophysiology and its heterogeneity in patients with established hypertensive disease. The first Robert C. Tarazi lecture. *Am J Med* 1988;84(suppl 3):3–11.

304. Devereux RB. Echocardiographic insights into the pathophysiology and prognostic significance of hypertensive cardiac hypertrophy. *Am J Hypertension* 1989;2:186s–195s.

305. Colan SD, Sanders SP, Borow KM. Physiologic hypertrophy: effects on left ventricular systolic mechanics in athletes. *J Am Coll Cardiol* 1987;9:776–783.

306. Hall O, Hall CE, Ogden E. Cardiac hypertrophy in experimental hypertension and its regression following reestablishment of normal blood pressure. *Am J Physiol* 1953;174:175–178.

307. Beznak M, Korecky B, Thomas G. Regression of cardiac hyper-

trophies of various origins. *Canad J Physiol Pharmacol* 1969;7:579–586.

308. Liebson PR, Savage DD. Echocardiography in hypertension: a review. II. Echocardiographic studies of the effects of antihypertensive agents on left ventricular wall mass and function. *Echocardiography* 1987;4:215–249.

309. Liebson PR. Clinical studies of drug reversal of hypertensive left ventricular hypertrophy. *Am J Hypertens* 1990;3:512–517.

310. Dahlof B, Pennert K, Hansson L. Reversal of left ventricular hypertrophy in hypertensive patients: A metaanalysis of 109 treatment studies. *Am J Hypertens* 1992;5:95–110.

311. Cruickshank J, Lewis J, Moore V, Dodd C. Reversibility of left ventricular hypertrophy by differing types of antihypertensive therapy. *J Hum Hypertens* 1992;6:85–90.

312. Tarazi RC. Cardiovascular hypertrophy in hypertension. Arthur C. Corcoran Memorial Lecture. *Hypertension* 1986;8(suppl II):II-187–II-190.

313. Tarazi RC. Reversal of cardiac hypertrophy by medical treatment. *Ann Rev Med* 1985;36:407–414.

314. Sen S, Tarazi RC, Bumpus FM. Cardiac hypertrophy and antihypertensive therapy. *Cardiovasc Res* 1977;11:427–433.

315. Sen S, Tarazi RC, Bumpus FM. Effect of convertin enzyme inhibitor (SQ 14225) on myocardial hypertrophy in spontaneously hypertensive rats. *Hypertension* 1980;2:169–176.

316. Sen S, Tarazi RC, Bumpus FM. Reversal of cardiac hypertrophy in renal hypertensive rats: medical vs surgical therapy. *Am J Physiol* 1981;240:H408–H412.

317. Sen S, Tarazi RC. Regression of cardiac hypertrophy: experimental animal model. *Am J Physiol* 1983;244:H97–H101.

318. Pegram BL, Ishise S, Frohlich ED. Effect of methyldopa, clonidine and hydralazine on cardiac mass and hemodynamics in Wistar-Kyoto and spontaneously hypertensive rats. *Cardiovasc Res* 1982;16:40–46.

319. Oparil S, Erinoff L, Cutilletta A. Catecholamines, blood pressure, renin, and myocardial infarction in the spontaneously hypertensive rat. *Clin Sci Mol Med* 1976;51:455s–459s.

320. Weiss L, Lundgren Y. Left ventricular hypertrophy and its reversibility in young spontaneously hypertensive rats. *Cardiovasc Res* 1978;12:635–638.

321. Jespersen LT, Nyberg NCB, Pedersen OL, Mikkelsen EO, Mulvany MJ. Cardiac mass and peripheral vascular structure in hydralazine-treated spontaneously hypertensive rats. *Hypertension* 1985;7:734–741.

322. Narayan S, Janicki JS, Shroff SG, Pick R, Weber KT. Myocardial collagen and mechanics after preventing hypertrophy in hypertensive rats. *Am J Hypertens* 1989;2:675–682.

323. Drayer JIM, Gardin JM, Weber MA. Echocardiographic left ventricular hypertrophy in hypertension. *Chest* 1983;84:217–221.

324. Sau F, Cherchi A, Seguro C. Reversal of left ventricular hypertrophy after treatment of hypertension by atenolol for one year. *Clin Sci* 1982;63:367s–369s.

325. Devereux RB, Pickering TG, Cody RJ, Laragh JH. Relation of renin-angiotensin system activity to left ventricular hypertrophy and function in experimental and human hypertension. *J Clin Hypertens* 1987;3(1):87–103.

326. Dunn FG, Oigman W, Ventura HO, Messerli FH, Kobrin I, Frohlich ED. Enalapril improves systemic and regional hemodynamics and allows regression of left ventricular mass in essential hypertension. *Am J Cardiol* 1984;53:105–108.

327. Ventura HO, Frohlich ED, Messerli FH, Kobrin I, Kardon MB. Cardiovascular effects and regional blood flow distribution associated with angiotensin converting enzyme inhibition (captopril) in essential hypertension. *Am J Cardiol* 1985;55:1023–1026.

328. Lombardo M, Zaini G, Pastori F, Fusco M, Pacini S, Foppoli C. Left ventricular mass and function before and after antihypertensive treatment. *J Hypertens* 1983;1:215–219.

329. Nakashima Y, Fouad F, Tarazi RC. Regression of left ventricular hypertrophy from systemic hypertension by enalopril. *Am J Cardiol* 1984;53:1044–1049.

330. Shahi M, Thom S, Poulter N, et al. Regression of hypertensive left ventricular hypertrophy and left ventricular diastolic function. *Lancet* 1990;336:458–461.

331. Julien J, Dufloux M-A, Prasquier R, et al. Effects of captopril and minoxidil on left ventricular hypertrophy in resistant hyperten-

sive patients: a 6 month double-blind comparison. *J Am Coll Cardiol* 1990;16:137–142.

332. Devereux RB. Angiotensin converting enzyme inhibition and regression of hypertensive left ventricular hypertrophy. In: *Current Advances in ACE Inhibition-2.* London: Churchill Livingston, 1991;43–52.

333. Ibrahim MM, Madkour MA, Mossallam R. Factors influencing cardiac hypertrophy in hypertensive patients. *Clin Sci* 1981;61:105s–108s.

334. Rowlands DB, Glover DR, Stallard TJ, Littler WA. Control of blood pressure and reduction of echocardiographically assessed left ventricular mass with once-daily timolol. *Br J Clin Pharmacol* 1982;14:89–95.

335. Arora R, Nair M, Gupta GD, Gupta MP. Assessment of left ventricular changes in systemic hypertension—before and after therapy. *Indian Heart J* 1984;36:155–160.

336. Kane U, Mohan JC, Bhatia ML. Effects of labetalol on left ventricular mass and function in hypertension—an assessment by serial echocardiography. *Int J Cardiol* 1984;5:461–469.

337. Plotnick GD, Fisher ML, Wohl B, Hamilton JH, Hamilton BP. Improvement in depressed cardiac function in hypertensive patients during pindolol treatment. *Am J Med* 1984;76:25–30.

338. Trimarco B, Ricciardelli B, deLuca N, et al. Effect of acebutalol on left ventricular hemodynamics and anatomy in systemic hypertension. *Am J Cardiol* 1984;53:791–796.

339. Weinberg P, Berezow J, Charlap S, et al. Inability of oral labetalol to reverse left ventricular hypertrophy in hypertensive patients: a noninvasive assessment (abstr) *Clin Res* 1984;32:341A.

340. Russell GI, Pohl JEF, Baldwin J, et al. Treatment of essential hypertension: changes in blood pressure, echocardiography and electrocardiography on three regimens. *Eur J Clin Pharmacol* 1985;28:119–124.

341. Drayer JIM, Gardin JM, Weber MA, Aronow WS. Changes in ventricular septal thickness during diuretic therapy. *Clin Pharmacol Therap* 1982;32:283–288.

342. Reichek N, Franklin BB, Chandler T, Muhammed A, Plappert T, St. John Sutton M. Reversal of left ventricular hypertrophy by antihypertensive therapy. *Eur Heart J* 1982;3(suppl A):165–169.

343. Drayer JIM, Weber MA, Gardin JM, Lipson JL. Effect of long-term antihypertensive therapy on cardiac anatomy in patients with essential hypertension. *Am J Med* 1983;75(suppl 3A):116–120.

344. Wollam GL, Hall WD, Porter VD, et al. Time course of regression of left ventricular hypertrophy in treated hypertensive patients. *Am J Med* 1983;75(suppl 3A):100–110.

345. Ferrara LA, de Simone G, Mancini M, Fasano ML, Pasanisi F, Vallone G. Changes in left ventricular mass during a double-blind study with chlorthalidone and slow-release nifedipine. *Eur J Clin Pharmacol* 1984;27:525–528.

346. Drayer JIM, Gardin JM, Weber MA, Aronow WS. Cardiac muscle mass during vasodilation therapy of hypertension. *Clin Pharmacol Ther* 1983;33:727–733.

347. Fouad FM, Nakashima Y, Tarazi RC, Salcedo EE. Reversal of left ventricular hypertrophy in hypertensive patients treated with methyldopa. *Am J Cardiol* 1982;49:795–801.

348. Schulman SP, Weiss JL, Becker LC, et al. The effects of antihypertensive therapy on left ventricular mass in elderly patients. *N Engl J Med* 1990;322:1350–1356.

349. Schlant RC, Felner JM, Heymsfield SB, et al. Echocardiographic studies of left ventricular anatomy and function in essential hypertension. *Cardiovasc Med* 1977;2:477–491.

350. Dunn FG, Bastian B, Lawrie TDV, Lorimer AR. Effect of blood pressure control on left ventricular hypertrophy in patients with essential hypertension. *Clin Sci* 1980;59:441s–443s.

351. Rowlands DB, Glover DR, Ireland MA, et al. Assessment of left ventricular mass and its response to antihypertensive treatment. *Lancet* 1982;1:467–470.

352. Devereux RB, Pickering TG, Cody RJ, Laragh JH. Relation of renin-angiotensin system activity to left ventricular hypertrophy and function in experimental and human hypertension. *J Clin Hypertens* 1987;3:87–103.

353. Mace PJE, Littler WA, Glover DR, et al. Regression of left ventricular hypertrophy in hypertension: comparative effects of three different drugs. *J Cardiovasc Pharmacol* 1985;7:s52.

354. Drayer JIM, Hall WD, Smith V-E, Weber MA, Wollam GL, White WB. Effect of the calcium channel blocker nitrendipine on left ventricular mass in patients with hypertension. *Clin Pharmacol Ther* 1986;40:679–685.

355. Dunn FG, Ventura HO, Messerli FH, Kobrin I, Frohlich ED. Time course of regression of left ventricular hypertrophy in hypertensive patients treated with atenolol. *Circulation* 1987;76:254–258.

356. Leenen FHH, Smith DL, Farkas RM, Reeves RA, Marquez-Julio A. Vasodilators and regression of left ventricular hypertrophy: hydralazine versus prazosin in hypertensive humans. *Am J Med* 1987;86:969–978.

357. Devereux RB, Laragh JH. Angiotensin converting enzyme inhibition of renin system activity induces reversal of hypertensive target organ changes: Do these effects predict a reduction in long-term morbidity? *Am J Hypertens* 1992;5:923–926.

358. Dahlof B, Herlitz H, Aurell M, Hansson L. Reversal of cardiovascular structural changes when treating essential hypertension. The importance of the renin-angiotensin-aldosterone system. *Am J Hypertens* 1992;5:900–911.

359. Neaton JD, Grimm RHJ Jr, Prineas RJ, et al. Treatment of Mild Hypertension Study: Final results. *JAMA* 1993;270:713–724.

360. Mancia G, Parati G, Pomidossi G, Grassi G, Casadel R, Zanchetti A. Alerting reaction and rise in blood pressure during measurement by physician and nurse. *Hypertension* 1987;9:209–215.

361. Pickering TG, James GD, Boddie C, Harshfield GA, Blank S, Laragh JH. How common is white coat hypertension? *JAMA* 1988;259:225–228.

362. Koren MJ, Savage DD, Casale PN, Laragh JH, Devereux RB. Changes in left ventricular mass predict risk in essential hypertension. *Circulation* 1990;82(suppl III):III-29.

363. Koren MJ, Ulin RJ, Laragh JH, Devereux RB. Reduction of left ventricular mass during treatment of essential hypertension is associated with improved prognosis. *Am J Hypertens* 1991;4:1A.

364. Yurenev AP, Dyakonova HG, Novikov ID, et al. Management of essential hypertension in patients with different degrees of left ventricular hypertrophy: Multicenter trial. *Am J Hypertens* 1992;5:182s–189s.

365. Devereux RB, Alderman MH. Role of preclinical cardiovascular disease in the evolution from risk factor exposure to clinical morbid events. *Circulation* 1993 (in press).

366. Muller JE, Abela GS, Nesto RW, Tofler GH. Triggers, acute risk factors, and vulnerable plaques: The lexicon of a new frontier. *J Am Coll Cardiol* 1994 (in press).

367. Cohn PF, Harris P, Barry WH, Rosati RA, Rosenbaum P, Waternaux C. Prognostic importance of anginal symptoms in angiographically defined coronary artery disease. *Am J Cardiol* 1981;47:233–237.

368. Kent KM, Rosing DR, Ewels CJ, Lipson L, Bonow R, Epstein SE. Prognosis of asymptomatic or mildly symptomatic patients with coronary artery disease. *Am J Cardiol* 1982;49:1823–1831.

369. Salonen JT, Salonen R. Ultrasound B-mode imaging in observational studies of atherosclerotic progression. *Circulation* 1993;87(suppl II):II-56–II-65.

370. Yudkin JS, Forrest RD, Jackson CA. Microalbuminuria as a predictor of vascular disease in non-diabetic subjects. Islington diabetes survey. *Lancet* 1988;2:530–533.

371. Devereux RB. Hypertensive cardiac hypertrophy: pathophysiologic and clinical characteristics. In: Laragh JH, Brenner BM, eds. *Hypertension: pathophysiology, diagnosis and management.* New York: Raven Press, 1990;359–377.

Hypertension: Pathophysiology, Diagnosis, and Management, Second Edition,
edited by J.H. Laragh and B.M. Brenner,
Raven Press, Ltd., New York © 1995.

CHAPTER **27**

Hypertensive Disease and Kidney Structure

Michael Kashgarian

The number of patients developing end stage renal disease secondary to hypertension, associated nephrosclerosis is increasing and accounts for 25 percent of new dialysis patients in the US. The mechanisms involved in the sclerotic process are not only a sequelae of hypertension but also contribute to its pathogenesis.

The role that the renal vessels play in the pathogenesis and progression of essential hypertension has been debated for many years, and a historical perspective will help to set a framework for our understanding of the consequences of hypertension on the kidney. The interplay between the kidney and the cardiovascular systems was recognized as far back as 1868 in Johnson's report on Bright's disease (1). He associated the thickening of the walls of the arterioles of the granular kidney of Bright's disease with cardiac hypertrophy. Shortly thereafter, Gull and Sutton (2) described a generalized small-vessel disease which they called "arterio-capillary fibrosis," and they suggested that the vascular disease was a primary pathologic change responsible for hypertension. The description of two types of contracted kidneys—inflammatory and arteriosclerotic—by Jores in 1904 (3) provided an anatomic basis for differentiating secondary hypertension associated with renal disease from primary essential hypertension.

By the early twentieth century, three apparently divergent theories began to emerge. One postulated that renal disease was primary and that associated vascular disease and hypertension were its results. The second suggested that renal disease was part of a primary diffuse vascular disease and that progressive vascular sclerosis increased peripheral resistance, resulting in systemic hypertension. The third maintained that essential hypertension itself was a primary disease and that the vascular diseases seen in all organs were a result rather than a cause. Even from the simplistic analysis of the formula which relates mean arterial pressure to a product of the cardiac output and the total peripheral resistance, it can be seen that the structure of the small vessels is an important determinant in the pathogenesis of systemic hypertension.

The unique importance of the small vessels of the kidney was emphasized by Fishberg (4). He described a pattern of vascular damage in patients with chronic hypertension, and recently, morphometric studies by Tracy (10) have confirmed that the renal arteriolar lesions are related to the severity and length of hypertension, while Bohle and co-workers (11,12) have begun to separate out the effects of hypertension on preglomerular and postglomerular vasculature in an attempt to distinguish the direct effects of increased pressure from changes due to ischemia. The relationship between the vascular disease and the endocrine role of the kidney vis-à-vis the renin-angiotensin system, the effects of antidiuretic hormone, the prostaglandin system, and other vasoactive or ion-transport-related systems further complicates and enhances the role of the kidney in hypertension.

Aside from the virtues of any of these theories relative to the primary or secondary nature of the renal vascular lesions, it is clear that the vasculopathy of hypertension is a distinct, and perhaps unique, lesion which involves the kidney preferentially. Furthermore, the structural vascular changes play an integral role in the development, maintenance and progression of the disease. It is,

M. Kashgarian: Department of Pathology, Yale University School of Medicine, New Haven, Connecticut 06510.

therefore, of importance to understand the anatomic and biochemical nature of the arteriolar changes seen in hypertension.

MICROVASCULAR DISEASE OF THE KIDNEY IN HYPERTENSION

The vessels most susceptible to pathologic change in hypertension are the small arteries and arterioles. This has been repeatedly observed in humans (13,14) and has recently been quantified in the hypertensive rat model (15,16). The preglomerular vessels tend to be more prominently affected than the postglomerular arterioles. Small arteries measuring 50–150 μm in diameter are characterized by one to three layers of vascular smooth muscle in the media. The endothelium is separated from the media by a fenestrated internal elastic lamina. The endothelium or intima consists of a single layer of endothelial cells on an opposed basement membrane. The arterioles are vessels which have outer diameters measuring 50 μm or less with only a single layer of smooth muscle and no elastic lamina. The endothelial cells of both small arteries and arterioles are joined by incomplete tight junctions. The cytoplasm contains the usual complement of cytoplasmic organelles, including coated pits and pinocytotic vesicles. The incomplete tight junctions and pinocytotic vesicles may represent an anatomic correlate of a double system of pores for transendothelial transport of low- and high-molecular-weight substances.

The vascular pathology of the small arteries and arterioles of the kidney falls into three general categories: hyaline arteriolar sclerosis; myointimal hypertrophy and hyperplasia; and fibrinoid necrosis. Hyaline arteriolar sclerosis is seen in all forms of hypertension, whereas hyperplastic vasculopathy and necrotizing arteriolitis have been considered hallmarks of malignant hypertension.

HYALINE ARTERIOSCLEROSIS

Perhaps the most interesting microvascular pathology is the lesion of hyaline arteriosclerosis (17). Indeed, the lesion has been described by Zollinger (18) as playing the role of the great sphinx of renal pathology. Hyaline is derived from the Greek *hyalos*, meaning "glass." It has been given this description since the walls of the vessels are thickened by the deposition of homogeneous glassy material which is eosinophilic (Fig. 1). Ultrastructurally (Fig. 2), the deposition of hyaline is associated with (a) atrophy of the smooth muscle cells, (b) irregular thickening of the basement membrane and collagen, and (c) the presence of a homogeneous dense material which, by immunofluorescence studies, contains plasma proteins such as immunoglobulins and complement. Although mild hyaline arteriosclerosis is often encountered in aged

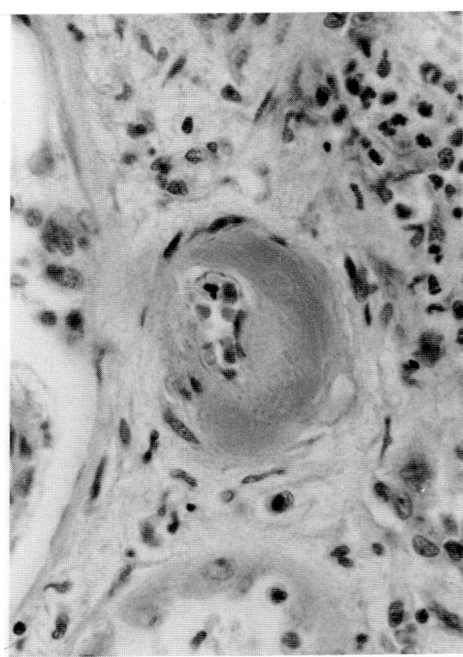

FIG. 1. Photomicrograph of a glomerular arteriole with striking hyaline arteriosclerosis. The vessel wall is thickened by the deposition of a homogeneous, amorphous "glassy" material. There is evidence of atrophy of the cells of the arteriolar wall and narrowing of the lumen. ×600.

patients having moderate systolic hypertension, it is most prominently seen in patients with hypertension or diabetes. The changes associated with aging are usually minimal and focal and are generally not associated with elevations of diastolic pressure. The lesion in patients with hypertension is usually more dramatic. Its presence is unrelated to age and has been shown to have a relationship to both severity and duration of the hypertension (19). Although occasional patients with essential hypertension show minimal changes, this is related either to duration, lability, or lack of severity of the hypertension.

The exact biochemical nature and origin of hyaline is still not completely understood. It appears to be composed largely of glycoproteins mixed with collagenous matrix. Histochemically, it avidly takes the periodic acid-Schiff stain and has positive Millon and sulfhydryl reactions. Lipid is also present, diffusely mixed with the glycoprotein and collagenous matrix. Rokitansky (20) was the first to propose that this material might be derived from substances filtered from the bloodstream. Hueck (9) later described an insudative lesion derived from plasma constituents that had leaked across injured endothelium into the arteriolar wall (21,22). Cuenoud et al. (23) have shown that a chronic nonspecific irritation to the endothelium of arterioles may result in focal infiltration of the vessel wall with blood components and fibrin, and they have postulated that endogenous media-

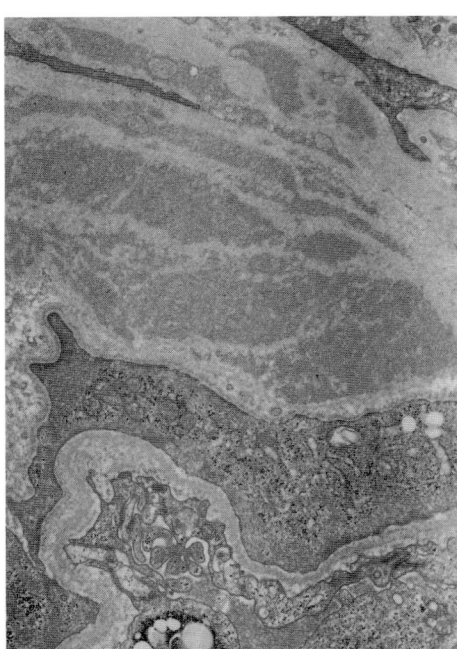

FIG. 2. Electron micrograph of the wall of an arteriole involved with hyaline arteriosclerosis. There is splitting and lamination of the basement membrane by deposition of an electron-dense material which composes the hyaline. Smooth muscle cells cannot be easily identified, and the pericytes are flattened and elongated. ×13,000.

tors are involved in the pathogenesis. Some have felt that hyaline originates from the degeneration or necrosis of smooth muscle cells and medial collagen with release of degenerative components into the media of the vessel (24). Others have suggested that hyaline deposits may be formed by the coalescence of increased amounts of basement membrane material synthesized by endothelial and smooth muscle cells (24,25). Remodeling of the vascular wall by a rearrangement of normal matrix and cell components by subjection to high pressure may precede permanent changes and may comprise a reversible component of nephrosclerosis (26).

Since there is some evidence to support each of these concepts, it is likely to be a combination of all. The end result is a thicker and less compliant small vessel which results in a more or less fixed vascular lumen leading to (a) an elevation of peripheral vascular resistance and (b) relative ischemia of the regions supplied by the vessel. Peripheral ischemia also results in arteriolar rarefaction or the disappearance of microvessels and may compromise a significant component of the increase in peripheral vascular resistance and may limit the reversibility of the structural lesions (27,28).

The interplay between the extracellular matrix and the cellular components of the vessel wall undoubtedly are important in the pathogenesis of hyaline arteriolosclero-

sis. At the present time, at least ten separate types of collagenous proteins have been identified. Of these, at least seven types have been found in the extracellular matrix of vessels or are known to be synthesized by endothelial cells or vascular smooth muscle cells. Types I, III, and VI collagens are found as organized fibrillar collagens in the interstitial connective tissue regions of the vessel wall and adjacent tissues. The basement-membrane collagens IV and V are found in the basal lamina which (a) underlie the endothelium and (b) surround the vascular smooth muscle cells and pericytes. Type VIII collagen and a heparan-inducible 60-kilodalton collagenous protein are synthesized by bovine endothelial cells and vascular smooth muscle cells in culture. In addition, there are a number of matrix-associated proteins (such as the attachment proteins laminin and fibronectin) as well as a variety of glycoproteins (such as glycosaminoglycans). One of these, heparan sulfate proteoglycan, has been demonstrated to be important in regulating the permeability of basement membranes by limiting the penetration of charged macromolecules. The matrix components are synthesized by the various cellular elements of the vessel wall. Unfortunately, except for a few isolated studies, little is known about the alterations in collagen synthesis and structure seen in hypertensive states. The histochemical and morphologic studies of hyaline arteriosclerosis suggest that matrix components comprise at least a part of the material which is deposited (29). Whether this occurs as a result of increased synthesis, increased incorporation of plasma constituents, or decreased degradation, or a combination of these, is presently unclear. Transforming growth factor-beta (TGF-β) has been demonstrated to stimulate synthesis and inhibit degradation of matrix molecules by several cell types in addition to its other activities in tissue repair (30). These findings suggest that it may play a role in the endothelial-mediated responses to blood flow and stretch (31,32).

Biochemical analysis of the composition of the vascular wall in hypertension has demonstrated a number of interesting changes which relate to the structural abnormalities which have been observed. Sodium, calcium, and water content of the vessel walls is increased, and studies on sodium exchange have suggested that the increased sodium is located in the extracellular matrix (33). Glycosaminoglycans, the matrix-associated proteins that are potent binders of cations, have also been shown to be increased in experimental hypertension (34) and may provide the binding sites for these cations. Similarly, increased absolute amounts of collagen and elastin have been found (35). Increased incorporation of [^{14}C]-lysine into collagenous proteins of the vessel walls of animals with experimental hypertension has indicated that stimulated collagen synthesis is of importance. Of particular interest in the experiments of Udenfruend et al. (36) is one in which the potent inhibitor of collagen crosslinking, β-aminopropriononitryl, was given to a strain of spontaneously hypertensive rats. It blocked the increase in lysine incorporation into collagen and was associated with amelioration of the systemic hypertension. These experiments tend to suggest that even if vascular collagenosis and sclerosis is not a primary initiating factor in the pathogenesis of hypertension, its presence influences its persistence and, perhaps, its severity.

The connective tissue components of the vessel wall are synthesized by the various cellular elements, and there is an increasing body of evidence that alterations of cytoskeletal structure can stimulate or modulate synthetic activities. Experiments of the effect of vasoactive amines on vascular smooth muscle demonstrate stimulation of metabolism, with increases in oxygen consumption, cytochrome oxidase activity, and utilization of glucose (37). While increased workload imposed by contraction of the smooth muscle cells may partially account for these effects, increased protein synthesis can also account for this observation. Similar effects have also been identified in endothelial and pericytic cells. On the basis of these experiments, one can postulate that, when vasoactive amines induce persistent or intense contraction of medial smooth muscle cells, alterations in the cytoskeleton have a stimulatory effect on protein synthesis, perhaps mediated by growth factors which lead to hyaline sclerosis. The amines may also be direct mediators of protein synthesis. Thus, in the early phases of hypertension, removal of the stimulus that induces contraction and protein synthesis would allow return of the vessel to its normal tone and structure, whereas persistence of the chemical mediation of hypertension may result in increased deposition of hyaline within the vessel wall, with the structural changes yielding a vessel with fixed compliance—resulting in persistence of hypertension.

Conversely, there is additional evidence that growth and differentiation of cells is influenced directly by the composition of the extracellular matrix. Endothelial cells that have been cultured on an extracellular matrix secreted and deposited by other endothelial cells have a different response to growth factors and vasoactive amines than cells grown on artificial substrates (38). Similarly, epithelial cell differentiation has been shown to be influenced by the matrix upon which cultured cells are grown (39). Proper orientation, cellular differentiation, and the rate of cell growth have been shown to differ relative to the composition and configuration of the extracellular matrix (40) and, more recently, of TGF-β (30). If one accepts the possibility that at least a portion of the hyaline deposits are derived from plasma macromolecules, alterations induced in the matrix by accumulation of these macromolecules may stimulate medial smooth muscle cells to produce additional matrix, thereby contributing to the progression of the arteriosclerosis.

This system would be analogous to those arguments which have been advanced to explain the development of glomerulosclerosis. Changes in glomerular hemodynamics or increased transglomerular traffic of plasma proteins with accumulation in the mesangium have been implicated as possibly serving as the stimulus to the proliferation of mesangial cells and matrix, eventually resulting in glomerulosclerosis (41).

Evidence for transudation of plasma proteins into the vessel wall in hyaline arteriosclerosis associated with hypertension is the finding that IgM and early and late classic complement-pathway components can also be identified within the vessel wall (42). A recent study (43) demonstrates that iC3b is bound via an ester linkage to hydroxyl groups on the repeating disaccharide units of hyaluronic acid, one of the major components of the glycosaminoglycans present in hyaline arteriolosclerosis. Slow, spontaneous activation of either the classical or alternative complement pathway may occur, providing a stimulus to matrix synthesis and deposition.

Hyaline arteriosclerosis is also accelerated in patients with diabetes. Recent studies have demonstrated a reduced synthesis of basement-membrane heparan sulfate proteoglycans at the same time that proline incorporation into laminin and collagenous protein was increased (44). These findings suggest a possible model to account for the glomerular sclerosis of diabetes. Decreased proteoglycan levels would be expected to make the basement membrane more permeable to anionic proteins, and this change could induce the compensatory synthesis of basement-membrane components in an attempt to rectify the increased porosity. The resulting unbalanced synthesis would lead to increased deposition of basement membrane and sclerosis. In other studies, altered microcirculatory dynamics have been demonstrated to influence the rate of development of diabetic glomerular lesions (45). In unclipped normotensive rats, characteristic glomerular lesions developed fully in both kidneys. However, when hypertension is experimentally induced using the two-kidney, one-clip hypertensive model, a distinct asymmetry in the development of lesions is found. In the unclipped kidney exposed to elevated systemic pressure, more severe diabetic glomerular changes are present when compared with normotensive diabetic rats, whereas in the clipped or protected kidney of the hypertensive diabetic rat, there is a lesser degree of glomerulosclerosis when compared to the normotensive diabetic control. These studies suggest that local hemodynamic changes can influence the metabolic alterations and further emphasize the interrelationships among cell, matrix, and hemodynamic and biochemical changes.

MYOINTIMAL HYPERPLASIA

The second morphologic abnormality of small arteries and arterioles which can be attributed to elevated systemic pressures is a hyperplastic lesion involving the smooth muscle and intima of these vessels. Hyperplastic arteriolosclerosis is generally associated with acute or persistent severe elevations of blood pressure and therefore is seen more frequently in malignant hypertension than in benign hypertension. Indeed, Muirhead and Pitcock have found that this lesion was the dominant finding in 41 patients with severe hypertension and renal failure (46). Hyperplastic lesions are not unique to the arterioles and occur in small and large arteries as well.

Tracy et al. (47,48) have drawn greater attention to the contribution of the cortical arteries to the development of nephrosclerosis and have demonstrated a relationship to hypertension. Using morphometric techniques, they have demonstrated progressive intimal thickening of renal cortical arteries with age and increasing blood pressure. The severity of the lesions was also related to differences in sex, race, and ethnic origin. In the small vessels, the uniform concentric thickening of the vessel has led to its description as "onion-skinning" (Figs. 3 and 4). The hyperplasia causes marked narrowing of the lumen.

Although originally described as intimal thickening, suggesting endothelial proliferation, recent studies have identified the cells involved in the hyperplastic thickening to be modified smooth muscle cells or myointimal cells that originate in the media of the vessel (Fig. 5) and

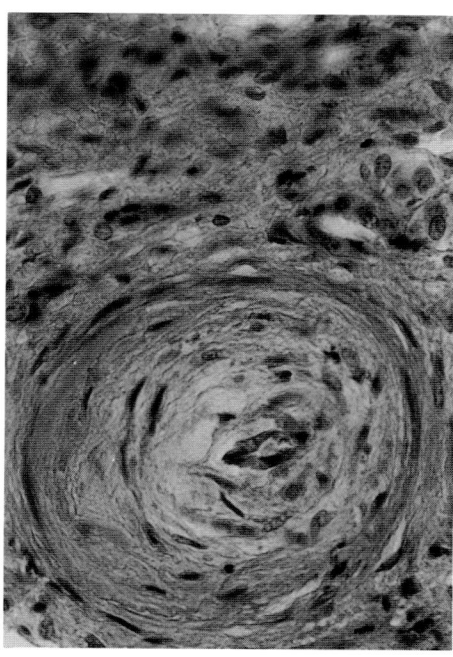

FIG. 4. Photomicrograph of an intralobular artery demonstrating "onion-skinning." The "onion-skinning" is similar to the myointimal proliferation seen in the arterioles, but the nuclei are more elongated and the proliferating myointimal cells are more spindled in their configuration. ×600.

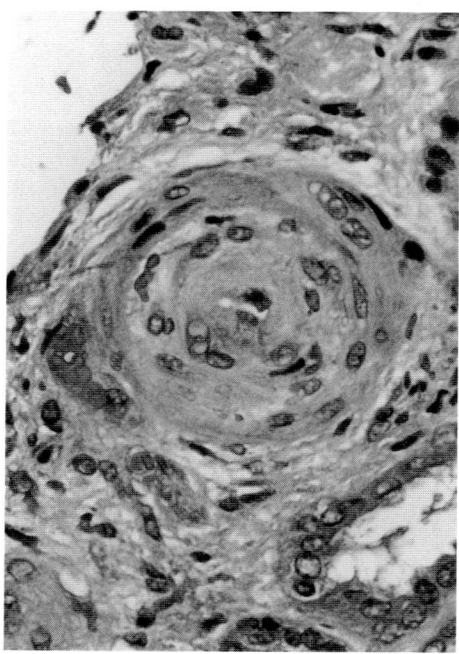

FIG. 3. Photomicrograph of an arteriole with striking myointimal hyperplasia. There is marked narrowing of the lumen by a hyperplasia of the medial cells, as can be seen by the increased numbers of nuclei. In addition, there appears to be an increase of homogeneous matrix material between the cells. ×600.

migrate into the intima through the fenestrations of the incomplete internal elastic lamina (49). The vascular smooth muscle in hypertension has been extensively studied. The changes are hypertrophic as well as hyperplastic. In one study, Friedman et al. (50) have reported that in deoxycorticosterone-induced hypertension in the rat, surface area, and volume of individual smooth muscle cells were increased, demonstrating cellular hypertrophy. The hypertrophy is primarily radial in character (51). Thymidine incorporation is increased, indicating the presence of cell multiplication and hyperplasia. Recent studies (52,53) have shown that hypertension alters DNA synthesis in arterial smooth muscle cells. DNA duplication occurs without karyokinesis or cytokinesis, resulting in smooth muscle polyploidy in large vessels. In small vessels, however, hypertension results in an increase of diploid cells (true hyperplasia).

The molecular mechanisms by which hypertension induces changes in the structure of arterial and arteriolar walls have not yet been identified. The present evidence, however, indicates that changes in cell cycle and activation of gene encoding for proteins relating to growth and secretion of matrix are involved. The remodeling of vessels in nephrosclerosis is the combination of the cellular changes and the mechanical effects of pressure per se. The importance of cell cycle in the pathogenesis of the vascular lesions of hypertension has been demonstrated, in that smooth muscle cells from spontaneously hyper-

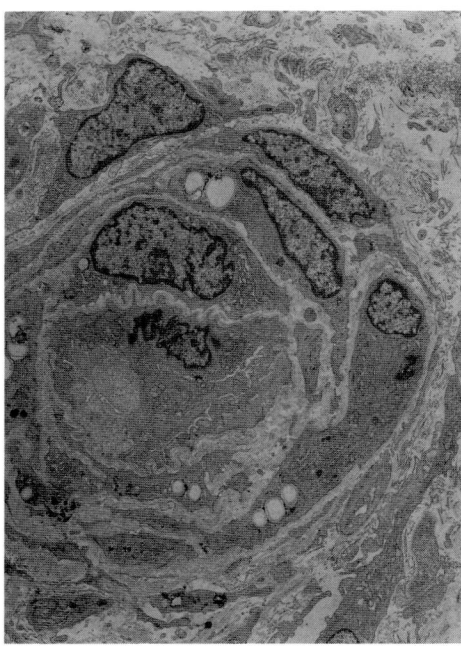

FIG. 5. Electron micrograph of an arteriole with myointimal hyperplasia. The lumen is markedly compromised by the proliferation of cells and by the reduplication of the basement membranes and matrix. The cells are elongated, contain lipid and sparse organelles, and have features of both smooth muscle cells and endothelial cells. ×4500.

tensive rats have an exaggerated response to mitogens, which is the result of a more rapid entry into the S phase (54). The mediation of the change in cell cycle is likely due to activation of growth factor genes. Sarzani et al. (55) have focused attention on TGF-β and it has been suggested that autocrine secretion of TGF-β may mediate this response by acting synergistically with other growth factors (56) such as epidermal growth factor. Genetic factors also affect growth-factor responsiveness since TGF-β inhibits EGF-stimulated mitogenesis in normal fibroblasts while stimulating EGF response in fibroblasts derived from keloids (57). Dunstan (58) has hypothesized that the differential response to growth factors of cells *in vitro* and in genetic hypertension of experimental animals may explain the differences in severity of hypertension and renal disease seen in different racial groups.

One interesting mechanism which combines these molecular mechanisms with mechanical effects of vasoconstriction has been postulated to explain the vascular lesions (59). At critical levels the action of vasoactive amines such as angiotensin II, adrenaline, and vasopressin results in an intermittent vascular contraction, producing a "sausage-string" appearance. In the nonconstricted zones there is an increase in the permeability of the vessel wall to plasma proteins (60). The turbulence produced in such vessels results in endothelial damage

and platelet activation. Platelet factors, including thromboxane and platelet-derived growth factor, are released and enhance the intermittent contraction of the vessel and stimulate proliferation and migration of the myointimal cells.

FIBRINOID ARTERIOLAR NECROSIS

The third, and perhaps the most dramatic, lesion is necrotizing arteriolitis. Fibrinoid necrosis of the arterioles is considered by some to be the hallmark of malignant or accelerated hypertension. The lesion is generally superimposed upon existing hyperplastic or hyaline lesions, but it is also occasionally seen as a first event in children and adolescents acutely presenting with severe acute malignant hypertension. Indeed, Linton (61) has hypothesized that a primary arteriolitis resulting in insudation of fibrin into the vascular walls may account for hypertension in such cases. The presence of immunoglobulins within the vessel wall has also led Paronetto (42) to postulate an immunologic mechanism. The lesion consists of obliteration of the normal medial architecture by necrosis, accompanied by the deposition of a deep eosinophilic, granular, fibrinlike material (Fig. 6). Ultrastructural examination reveals the fibrillar material embedded in hyaline to have a periodicity considered to be characteristic of fibrin or fibrinogen.

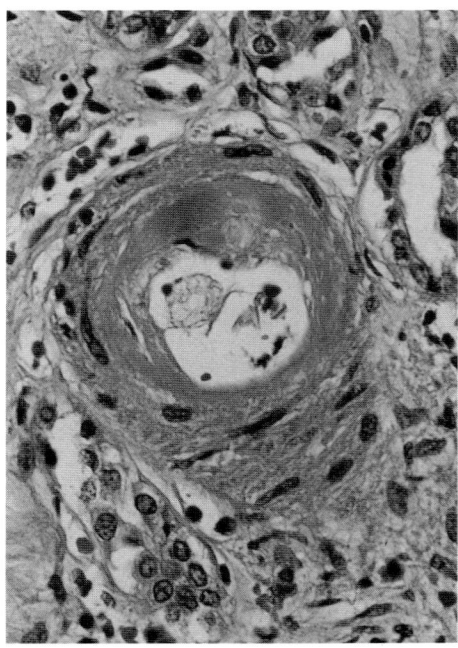

FIG. 6. Photomicrograph of an arteriole with fibrinoid necrosis of the vessel wall. The architecture of the wall is obliterated and destroyed by necrosis, which is accompanied by the deposition of material which stains positively for fibrin. The arteriole in the center shows a concentric deposition of fibrin, whereas the adjacent arteriole contains fibrin in only one portion of the wall. ×600.

Immunofluorescence studies have also confirmed the presence of fibrin in the walls (62). It seems likely that the intramural fibrin comes from the transudation of plasma proteins into the vessel wall secondary to endothelial damage associated with an increased transmural pressor gradient (29,63). The fibrin is sometimes accompanied by extravasation of red blood cells and intraluminal thrombosis. Occasionally, leukocytes may also be present within the walls, suggesting an inflammatory arteriolitis. Intravascular thrombosis may be superimposed on the necrotic vessel wall lesion. Hemorrhage in the adjacent interstitium may be seen when the necrosis is transmural. As the lesions resolve, the fibrin and necrotic tissue are replaced with collagen, leaving a vessel with a narrowed lumen and an acellular collagenous vascular wall (64).

RENAL CONSEQUENCES OF MICROVASCULAR DISEASE

The sequelae of arterial narrowing can be related to the degree and rate at which the narrowing occurs. Acute complete obstruction is associated with infarction, whereas gradual or incomplete obstruction is associated with a decrease in function and subsequent atrophy. Truly mild forms of ischemia may have little or no sequelae. Since the vascular lesions of hypertension primarily affect the small arteries in the preglomerular arterioles, the glomeruli and postglomerular structures are subject to the ischemic changes.

In mild or early hypertension, many glomeruli are normal and there is little evidence of tubular atrophy or interstitial fibrosis. As the hypertension progresses in severity or duration, the same structures begin to demonstrate direct hypertensive injury (65,66) as well as ischemic changes. The glomerular capillary tufts begin to collapse and show wrinkling, and the capillary walls appear thickened by light microscopy (Fig. 7). The tuft gradually undergoes a degree of collapse to the point where the glomeruli appear solid and the nuclei are concentrated, giving a hypercellular appearance. The condensation is followed by glomerulosclerosis, which initially is segmental but gradually becomes global. Ultrastructurally, the changes initially show (a) collapse of the capillary loop with wrinkling of the basement membrane in the paramesangial region and (b) coalescence of the collapsed basement membrane with the mesangial matrix (Fig. 8). There is a gradual increase of mesangial matrix, accompanied by obliteration of the glomerular capillary lumina, loss of endothelial cells, and increase in basement-membrane-like material. Dramatic changes also occur in Bowman's capsule, where there is thickening by the deposition of collagenous material which appears to extend into the urinary space, particularly in the hilar region. Eventually, both the glo-

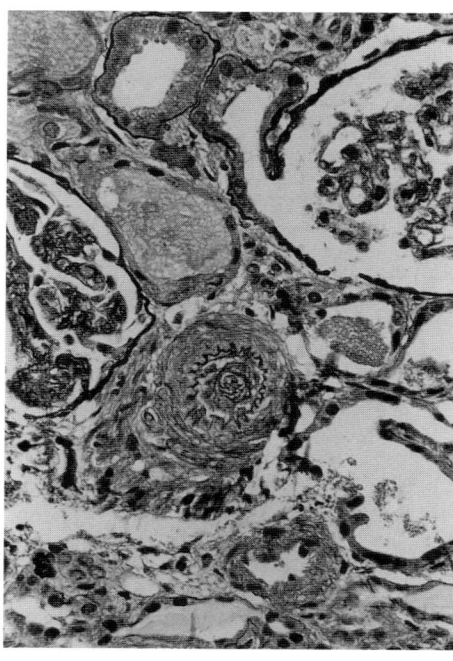

FIG. 7. Photomicrograph of a needle biopsy of a patient with hypertensive nephropathy. The inner lobular artery in the center shows myointimal hyperplasia and reduplication of the elastic lamina. Portions of two glomeruli are present, one of which shows ischemic glomerular capillary collapse with wrinkling of the capillary loops, while the other shows condensation and hyalinization of the glomerular tufts. ×150.

merular capillary shrinkage and hyaline sclerosis of Bowman's capsule coalesce, resulting in the global sclerosis of the glomerulus.

The tubules are also affected by ischemia and gradually become atrophic. There is thickening of the tubular basement membrane with either collapse of the tubules and loss of tubular epithelium or dilatation of the tubules with accumulation of hyaline casts in the lumen. The atrophy of the tubules is accompanied by an increase in interstitial collagen, which occasionally is accompanied by a lymphoplasmacytic infiltrate. The reason for the presence of chronic inflammatory cells in ischemic atrophy is not clear.

In 1925, in his treatise on nephrosclerosis, Fahr (5) described changes which differed from both the ischemic alterations of benign nephrosclerosis and the more active necrotic and proliferative lesions associated with malignant nephrosclerosis. He described these changes as being characteristic of what he termed "decompensated benign nephrosclerosis." The glomerular alterations which are present include glomerular cell proliferation, focal capillary loop necrosis, and hyaline change of the glomerular epithelial cell. This lesion has largely been ignored until recently, when Meyer et al. (12) and Bohle and Ratschek (11) rekindled interest with their descriptions of primary hypertensive glomerulopathy and mor-

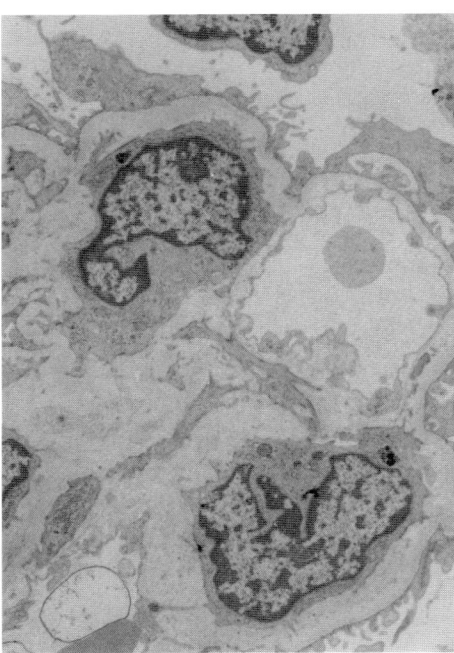

FIG. 8. Electron micrograph of a glomerulus showing glomerular capillary collapse, thickening of the basement membranes, and an increase in mesangial matrix. There is an apparent increase in mesangial cellularity as a result of the mesangial sclerosis. ×8000.

phometric studies of the sclerotic kidney. In the early stage of what they term "hypertensive glomerulopathy," they describe a thickening of the basement membrane of the glomerular capillaries, along with an irregular increase in mesangial matrix as well as hyaline droplet change in the visceral podocytes. As the lesion progresses, there is an increase in cellularity, accompanied by adhesion of the glomerular capillaries to each other and to Bowman's capsule, associated with swelling of the endothelial cells and epithelial cells, which appear as apparent epithelial cell proliferation or even crescent formation. The lesion progresses into periodic acid–Schiff-positive scarring and what has been described as "pseudo-tubule" formation in Bowman's capsule, and then finally to glomerular hyalinosis. Since this lesion appears more prominently in glomeruli supplied by larger arteries, the authors postulate that the lesion is the result of a direct effect of greatly elevated blood pressure on the glomeruli. They further emphasize that the lesion is seen most commonly in patients who develop secondary malignant hypertension superimposed on long-standing benign essential hypertension.

Thus, in benign hypertension, glomerular damage occurs either as a result of ischemia secondary to narrowing of the preglomerular vessels by arteriosclerosis or as a result of direct damage to the glomerular capillaries by increased pressure resulting from an inability of the preglomerular vessels to respond and regulate in a normal

fashion (65). Both forms of glomerular injury could easily correlate with the degree of proteinuria seen in various stages of the course of hypertension, but the direct hypertensive glomerular capillary lesion is more likely to account for the higher levels of proteinuria. Furthermore, it is of interest that recent studies of the Dahl salt-sensitive hypertensive rat (67) have demonstrated that a glomerular lesion can precede the development of hypertension in this model. These results suggest that the glomeruli may play a more important role in the genesis and progression of hypertension than has been previously suggested. In most patients, renal insufficiency is usually mild, but end-stage renal disease does occur and there is increasing evidence that the scarred kidney may continue to play a central role in the perpetuation of hypertension (68).

The glomeruli in malignant nephrosclerosis showed changes in addition to those described for benign and decompensated nephrosclerosis. The fibrinoid necrosis of the afferent arterioles sometimes extends into the glomerulus, and focal necrosis of the glomerular tuft can also be seen (Fig. 9). Thrombosis of the capillaries and proliferation of the capillary tuft cells can accompany these changes (Fig. 10). Occasionally, well-formed crescents can be found associated with adhesions of the necrotic tuft to Bowman's capsule. These changes can be attributed either to intense ischemia of the glomeruli with subsequent endothelial damage or to a direct action of increased transmural pressure of the glomerular capil-

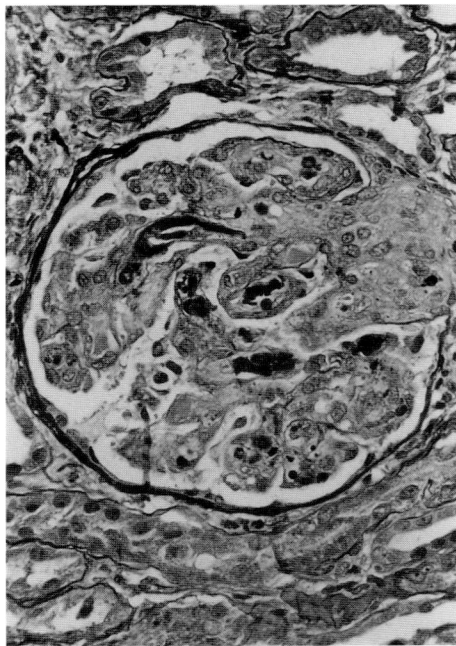

FIG. 9. Photomicrograph of a glomerulus from a patient with malignant hypertension. There is necrosis of the vascular pole and collapse of the capillaries. Thrombosis of some of the capillary loops is present. ×600.

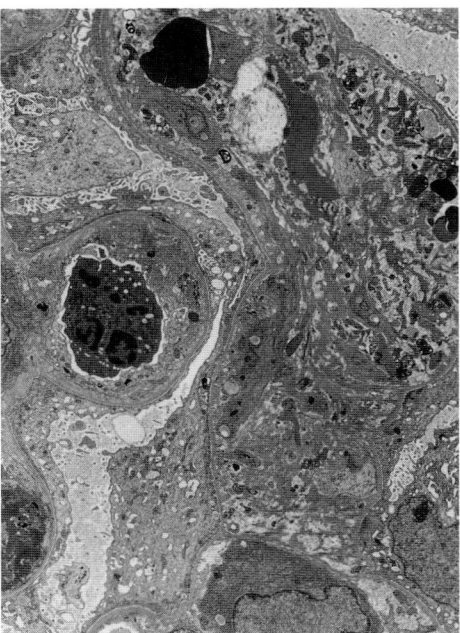

FIG. 10. Electron micrograph of a capillary loop of a glomerulus from a patient with malignant hypertension. Thrombosis of the capillary is present, along with fibrin, red cell fragments, and cellular debris filling the capillary lumen. ×8000.

lary wall. The juxtaglomerular apparatus is frequently enlarged, and there appears to be hyperplasia of the juxtaglomerular cells associated with an increase in granulation.

RENAL ARTERIAL DISEASE

Although small-blood-vessel disease in the kidney is probably the most important vascular complication from a functional viewpoint, the larger renal arteries also are subject to pathologic change. Atheromatous disease of the major renal arteries is accelerated in patients with hypertension and can perpetuate the disease by creating renal artery stenosis. In addition, the major renal arteries may also be the source of atheromatous emboli, contributing to distal renal parenchymal infarction with its consequent loss of functional renal parenchyma. Arteries down to the arcuate size can show arteriosclerotic changes, but the smaller vessels are more commonly involved in an intimal thickening of the fibroelastic type similar to that seen in the small arteries.

Disease of the major renal arteries becomes of particular importance when it is unilateral; it causes significant stenosis of the renal artery, resulting in secondary hypertension. The lesions can be generally broken down into three major categories: (a) atherosclerosis; (b) dysplastic diseases of the fibromuscular vessels; and (c) a miscellaneous group which includes congenital anomalies, Takayasu's aortitis, and radiation injury. The most common cause of renal artery stenosis is obstruction by an atheromatous plaque involving the orifice of the main renal artery. It is usually associated with severe atheromatous disease of the aorta and, as such, is seen more frequently in males and patients with diabetes mellitus. The incidence increases with increasing age. The lesion is frequently associated with (a) aneurysmal dilatation of the aorta distal to the renal arteries and (b) mural thrombosis.

The second group of lesions leading to stenosis are the so-called dysplastic lesions of the renal artery (69) (Table 1). The dysplastic lesions can involve other systemic vessels, suggesting that it may be a genetic disease; but they become clinically important when they cause obstruction of the major renal artery, initiating severe hypertension by creating a Goldblatt kidney. The lesions can be subdivided into six separate groups: intimal fibroplasia, medial fibroplasia, medial hyperplasia, perimedial fibroplasia, medial dissection, and periarterial fibroplasia. The term *fibromuscular dysplasia* has been used to encompass several of these separate categories, but it appears useful to subclassify them because they may affect different patient populations.

In intimal fibroplasia, the lesion involves only the intima of the vessel, with the elastica and media maintaining a normal architecture. There is hyperplasia of the intima, which is essentially indistinguishable from the

TABLE 1. Dysplastic lesions of the renal artery

	Age (years) and sex incidence	Relative frequency[a] (%)	Lesion
Intimal fibroplasia	1–50 M = F	1–2	Narrowing by intimal proliferation without lipid
Medial fibroplasia with aneurysms	30–60 F > M	60–70	"String of beads"; alternating stenosis and mural thinning
Medial hyperplasia	30–60 F > M	5–15	Smooth muscle hyperplasia and thickening
Perimedial fibroplasia	30–60 F > M	15–24	Fibrosis of outer media; occasionally aneurysms
Medial dissection	30–60 F > M	5–15	Fibrosis of media with dissecting aneurysms
Periarterial fibroplasia	15–50 F > M	1	Perivascular fibrosis and inflammation

M, male; F, female. [a]Relative to all forms of dysplastic lesions, ie. medialfibroplasia is the most common form of renal arterial dysplasia.

proliferative stage of atherosclerosis but is not associated with an increased deposition of lipids. The proliferation can be of such severity as to cause significant narrowing of the lumen. The lesion has been reported in individuals as young as 1 year of age but is most commonly seen in the third and fourth decades. The most common of the medial lesions is medial fibroplasia. This usually results in a multifocal stenotic lesion alternating with microaneurysms, producing a characteristic "string of beads" appearance by renal arteriography (70). Histopathologically, there is atrophy of the muscle and fibrosis of the wall in the region of the small aneurysms alternating with the stenotic lesions, where there is medial muscular hypertrophy with an increase of interstitial collagen. The second most frequently encountered variation of fibromuscular hyperplasia is perimedial fibroplasia. In contrast to medial fibroplasia, segmental aneurysmal dilatation is not present but focal aneurysms occasionally occur. The lesion consists of thickening of the outer half of the media by an increase in fibrous tissue. The muscle is disoriented and there is a generalized thickening of the wall, although the elastica and intima, as well as the inner portion of the media, retain a relatively normal architecture. Less commonly seen is medial hyperplasia. Here, there is hyperplasia of the muscle which results in a uniform thickening of the vessel wall and resultant generalized narrowing of the lumen. Periarterial fibroplasia is a rare lesion in which fibrosis of the adventitia extends into the surrounding adipose and connective tissue—resulting in constriction of the vessel from without, rather than from within, the vessel wall. The fibrosis is frequently accompanied by an infiltrate of chronic inflammatory cells.

Of the miscellaneous causes of renal artery stenosis, radiation injury probably deserves some discussion. Chronic radiation injury results in loss of the muscle cells and an intense fibrosis of all layers of the vessel wall. It occurs as a distinct event after radiation exposure, usually in the form of radiation therapy for a malignant lesion. Takayasu's aortitis, or pulseless disease, is a chronic sclerosing aortitis of unknown etiology which can cause renal artery stenosis due to osteal narrowing. An inflammatory infiltrate is seen in addition to the fibrotic lesion, suggesting a possible immunologic mechanism for the aortitis.

In unilateral renal arterial disease the ischemic kidney generally is smaller than the contralateral kidney and shows diffuse ischemic atrophy. The glomeruli appear small, and the tubules are collapsed. Interstitial fibrosis is associated with more marked tubular atrophy if the stenosis is longstanding. The juxtaglomerular apparatus is hyperplastic, and there is increased granulation seen with special stains. The small vessels are protected from the hypertension, in contrast to the contralateral kidney where hypertensive microvasculature is prominent.

In summary, the microangiopathic changes of hypertension have long been recognized to be associated with systemic hypertension. It now seems clear that these changes—in particular, hyaline arteriosclerosis—probably play an important pathologic role in the progression of the disease. This occurs as a result of fixing peripheral resistance through loss of compliance of the small vessels and through its ischemic effects on the renal parenchyma served by those vessels. Macrovascular disease of the kidney, on the other hand, is of importance in the initiation and perpetuation of renal vascular hypertension by producing a Goldblatt kidney. Both arterial sclerotic and dysplastic lesions of renal artery can result in stenosis, which may be amenable to surgical or intraluminal intervention.

REFERENCES

1. Johnson GI. On certain points in the anatomy and pathology of Bright's disease. *Trans Med Chir Soc* 1868;51:57–78.
2. Gull WW, Sutton HG. On the pathology of the morbid state commonly called chronic Bright's disease with contracted kidney (arterio-capillary fibrosis). *Trans Med Chir Soc* 1872;55:273–329.
3. Jores L. Uber die arteriosklerose der kleinen organ arterien. *Virchows Arch* 1904;178:367–406.
4. Fishberg AM. Anatomic findings in essential hypertension. *Arch Intern Med* 1925;35:650–668.
5. Fahr T. Pathologishe Anatomie des Morbus Brightii. In: *Handbuch der Speziellen Pathologishen Anatomie und Histologie*. Berlin: Springer-Verlag; 368ff.
6. Moritz AR, Oldt MR. Arteriolar sclerosis in hypertensive and nonhypertensive individuals. *Am J Pathol* 1937;13:679–728.
7. Goldblatt H, Lynch J, Hanzal RF, et al. Studies on experimental hypertension. I. The production of persistent elevation of systolic blood pressure by means of renal ischemia. *J Exp Med* 1934;59:347–379.
8. Goldblatt H. The renal origin of hypertension. *Physiol Rev* 1947;27:120–165.
9. Hueck W. Anatomishes zur fruge nach wesen and ursache der arteriosclerose. *Munch Med Wochenschr* 1920;67:835–837.
10. Tracy RE. Hypertension and arteriolar sclerosis of the kidney, pancreas, adrenal gland and liver. *Virchows Arch* 1981;391:91–106.
11. Bohle A, Ratschek M. The compensated and decompensated form of benign nephrosclerosis. *Pathol Res Pract* 1982;174:357–367.
12. Meyer D, Helmchen U, Bohle A. Hypertensive glomerulare. *Schaden Verh Dtsch Ges Pathol* 1973;57:392–393.
13. Fishberg G, Ditscherlein G. Renal histopathology in hypertensive diabetic patients. *Hypertension* 1985;7:II-29–II-32.
14. Tracy RE, Mercante DE, Mondada A, Berenson G. Quantitation of hypertension nephrosclerosis on an objective rational scale of measure in adults and children. *Am J Clin Pathol* 1986;85:312–318.
15. Miller BC, Connors BA, Bohlen HG, Evan AP. Cell and wall morphology of intestinal arterioles from 4 to 6 and 17 to 19 week old Wistar-Kyoto and spontaneously hypertensive rats. *Hypertension* 1987;9:59–68.
16. Khan NA, Hampton JA, Lacher DA, Rapp JP, Cohara AF, Goldblatt PJ. Morphometric evaluation of the renal arterial system of Dahl salt sensitive and salt resistant rats on high salt. *Lab Invest* 1987;57(6):714–723.
17. Dustin P Jr. Arteriolar hyalinosis. *Int Rev Exp Pathol* 1962;1:73–138.
18. Zollinger HV. Niere und Ableitende Harnwege. In: Doerr W, Uehlinger E, eds. *Spezielle Pathogishe Anatomie Band 3*. Berlin: Springer-Verlag, 1966;577.
19. Sommers SC, Melamed J. Renal pathology of essential hypertension. *Am J Hypertens* 1990;3:583–587.
20. Rokitansky C. Uber einige der wichtigsten Kranicheiten der arterien. *Denkschrift Konigl Akad Nis* 1852;4:49.

21. Fisher ER, Perez SE, Pardo V. Ultrastructural studies in hypertension. *Lab Invest* 1966;15:1409–1433.

22. Schloss G. Die Histogenese und pathogenese der gefassverenderungen beim experimentellen renalen Drosselung-Schochdruck der Ratte. *Schweiz Z Allg Pathol* 1948;11:109–113.

23. Cuenoud HF, Joris I, Langer RS, Majno G. Focal arteriolar insudation. *Am J Pathol* 1987;127:592–604.

24. McGee WF, Ashworth CT. Fine structure of chronic hypertensive arteriopathy in the human kidney. *Am J Pathol* 1963;43:273–299.

25. Wiener J, Spiro D, Lattes RG. The cellular pathology of experimental hypertension. II. *Am J Pathol* 1963;47:457–485.

26. Mulvaney MJ. The development and regression of vascular hypertrophy. *J Cardio Pharm* 1992;19:522–527.

27. Boegehold MA, Johnson MD, Overbeck HN. Pressure independent arteriolar rarefaction in hypertension. *Am J Physiol* 1991;261:H83–H87.

28. Greene AS, Tonelato PJ, Lui J, Lombard JH, Cowley AW. Microvascular rarefaction and tissue vascular resistance in hypertension. *Am J Physiol* 1989;256:H126–H131.

29. Wiener J, Lattes RG, Meltzer BG, et al. The cellular pathology of experimental hypertension. *Am J Pathol* 1969;54:187–207.

30. Sporn MB, Roberts AB, Wakefield LM, deCrombrugge B. Some recent advances in the chemistry and biology of transforming growth factor-beta. *J Cell Biol* 1987;105:1039–1046.

31. Langille BL, O'Donnell F. Reductions in arterial diameter produced by decreases in blood flow are endothelium dependent. *Science* 1986;231:405–407.

32. Furchgott RF. Role of endothelium in responses of vascular smooth muscle. *Circ Res* 1983;53:557–573.

33. Tobian L, Olson R, Chesley G. Water content of arteriolar wall in renovascular hypertension. *Am J Physiol* 1969;216:22–24.

34. Pamnani MB, Overbeck HW. Vascular wall composition in renal hypertension [Abstract]. *Fed Proc* 75;34:282.

35. Woliasky H. Longterm effects of hypertension on the rat aortic wall. *Circ Res* 1972;30:301–309.

36. Udenfruend S, Cardinale G, Spector S. Hypertension induced vascular fibrosis and its reversal by antihypertensive drugs. In: Laragh JH, Buhler FR, Seldin DW, eds. *Frontiers in hypertension research.* New York: Springer, 1981;404–411.

37. Amer MS, Comoll AW, Perhach JL. Aberrations of cyclic-nucleotide metabolism in the hearts and vessels of hypertensive rats. *Proc Natl Acad Sci USA* 1974;71:4930–4934.

38. Kleinman HK, Klebe RJ, Martin GR. The role of collagenous matrices in the addition and growth of cells. *J Cell Biol* 1981;88:473–479.

39. Gospadorowicz D, Cheng J, Livette M. Bovine brain and pituitary growth factors: comparison of their abilities to support the proliferation of human bovine vascular endothelial cells. *J Cell Biol* 1983;97:1677–1685.

40. Hall HD, Farson DA, Bissell MJ. Lumen formation by epithelial cell lines in response to collagen overlay. *Proc Natl Acad Sci USA* 1982;79:4672–4676.

41. Olsen JL, Hostetter TH, Rennke HG, et al. Altered charge and size selective properties of the glomerular wall: a response to reduced renal mass. *Kidney Int* 1982;22:112–118.

42. Paronetto F. Immunocytochemical observations on the vascular necrosis and renal glomerular lesions of malignant nephrosclerosis. *Am J Pathol* 1965;46:901.

43. Gamble CN. The pathogenesis of hyaline arteriosclerosis. *Am J Pathol* 1986;122:410–420.

44. Rohrbach DH, Wagner CW, Star VL, et al. Reduced synthesis of basement membrane heparan sulphate proteoglycan in streptazotocin-induced diabetic mice. *J Biol Chem* 1983;258:11672–11677.

45. Mauer SM, Steftes MW, Azar S, et al. The effects of Goldblatt hypertension on the development of the glomerular lesions of diabetes mellitus in the rat. *Diabetes* 1978;27:738–744.

46. Muirhead EE, Pitcock JA. Histopathology of severe renal vascular hypertension in blacks. *Clin Cardiology* 1989;12:IV58–IV65.

47. Tracy RE, Berenson GS, Cuoto-Garcia L, Wattigney WA, Barrett TJ. Nephrosclerosis and aortic atherosclerosis from age 6 to 70 in the United States and Mexico. *Virchows Arch A* 1992;420:479–488.

48. Tracy RE, Bhandura SY, Oalmann MC, Guzman MA, Newman WP. Blood pressure and nephrosclerosis in black and white men and women aged 25 to 54. *Modern Path* 1991;4:602–609.

49. Buck RC. Intimal thickening after ligature of arteries. *Circ Res* 1961;9:418–426.

50. Friedman SM, Nakashima M, Mar MA. Morphologic assessment of vasoconstriction and vascular hypertrophy in sustained hypertension of the rat. *Microvasc Res* 1971;3:416.

51. Miller BC, Connors BA, Bohlen HG, Evan AP. Cell and wall morphology of intestinal arterioles from 4 to 6 and 17 to 19 week old Wistar Kyoto and spontaneously hypertensive rats. *Hypertension* 1987;9:59–68.

52. Schwartz SM, Campbell GR, Campbell JH. Replication of smooth muscle in vascular disease. *Circ Res* 1986;58:427–444.

53. Gordon D, Schwartz SM. Replication of smooth muscle cells in hypertension and atherosclerosis. *Am J Cardiol* 1987;59:44A–48A.

54. Hadrava V, Tremblay J, Sekaly RP, Hamet P. Accelerated entry of aortic smooth muscle cells from spontaneously hypertensive rats into the S phase of cell cycle. *Biochem Cell Biol* 1992;70:599–604.

55. Sarzani R, Brecher P, Chobanion AV. Growth factor expression in aorta of normotensive and hypertensive rats. *J Clin Invest* 1989;83:1404–1408.

56. Saltis J, Agrotis A, Bobik A. TGFβ1 potentiates growth factor stimulated proliferation of smooth muscle cells in genetic hypertension. *Am J Physiol* 1992;263:C420–C428.

57. Russell SB, Trupin KM, Rodrigues-Eaton S, Russell JD, Trupin JS. Reduced growth factor requirement of keloid derived fibroblasts may account for tumor growth. *Proc Natl Acad Sci USA* 1988;85:587–591.

58. Dunstan HP. Growth factors and racial differences in severity of hypertension and renal disease. *Lancet* 1992;339:1339–1340.

59. Kincaid-Smith P. Malignant hypertension: mechanisms and management. *Pharmacol Ther* 1980;9:245–269.

60. Wilson SK, Heptinstall RH. Effects of acute angiotensin-induced hypertension on intra-renal arteries in the rat. *Kidney Int* 1984;25:492–501.

61. Linton AL. Microangiopathic hemolytic anemia and the pathogenesis of malignant hypertension. *Lancet* 1969;1:1277.

62. Valenzuela R, Gogate PA, Deodar SD, Gifford RW. Hyaline arteriolonephrosclerosis. Immunofluorescent findings in vascular lesions. *Lab Invest* 1980;43:530–534.

63. Jones DB. Arterial and glomerular lesions associated with severe hypertension. *Lab Invest* 1974;31:303–313.

64. Harrington M, Kincaid-Smith P, McMichael J. Results of treatment of malignant hypertension. A seven-year experience in 94 cases. *Br Med J* 1959;2:969.

65. Anderson S, Meyer TW, Rennke HG, Brenner BM. Control of glomerular hypertension limits glomerular injury in rats with reduced renal mass. *J Clin Invest* 1985;76:612–619.

66. Dworkin LD, Feiner HO. Glomerular injury in uninephrectomized spontaneously hypertensive rats. *J Clin Invest* 1986;77:797–809.

67. Sterzel RB, Gao Y, Kriz W, Waldherr R, Briggs J, Schnermann J. Renal disease precedes hypertension in salt sensitive Dahl rats. *Kidney Int* 1986;29:259.

68. Curtis JJ, Luke RG, Dustan HP, et al. Remission of essential hypertension after renal transplantation. *N Engl J Med* 1983;309:1009–1015.

69. Harrison EG, McCormack LJ. Pathologic classification of renal arterial disease in renovascular hypertension. *Mayo Clin Proc* 1971;46:161–166.

70. McCormack LJ, Poutasse EF, Meaney TF, Noto TJ, Dustan HP. Arteriographic correlation of renal artery disease. *Am Heart J* 1966;72:188–198.

Hypertension: Pathophysiology, Diagnosis, and Management, Second Edition, edited by J.H. Laragh and B.M. Brenner, Raven Press, Ltd., New York © 1995.

CHAPTER 28

Hypertensive Disease and Cerebral Circulation

Olaf B. Paulson and Svend Strandgaard

Hypertension profoundly influences the cerebral circulation by causing structural and functional hemodynamic changes in the resistance vessels. Hypertension is also a major risk factor for stroke, both ischemic and hemorrhagic, and one of the major benefits afforded by modern antihypertensive treatment is stroke prevention. Occasionally, however, clinical blood pressure lowering may escape control and precipitate the very cerebral ischemia that it aimed to prevent. These and related problems are reviewed in the present chapter.

PHYSIOLOGY OF THE CEREBRAL CIRCULATION

The cerebral circulation supplies the brain with nutrients, clears it for waste products, and is meticulously adjusted to meet the metabolic demands of the tissue. The local capillary density in the brain is closely adjusted to the metabolism and flow in the local area (1). In normal man, average cerebral blood flow (CBF) in the resting condition is slightly below 50 mL/100 g/min, and the oxygen saturation in the venous outflow from the brain is 60–70 percent (2–5). The blood-brain barrier, located in the vascular endothelium, is impermeable for most hydrophilic substances, glucose being a notable exception (6). The cerebral circulation and the blood-brain barrier play key roles in maintaining a constant chemical

 O. B. Paulson: Department of Neurology, University of Copenhagen, Rigshospitalet, DK-2100 Copenhagen, Denmark.
 S. Strandgaard: Department of Medicine and Nephrology B, Herlev Hospital, DK-2730 Herlev, Copenhagen, Denmark.

microenvironment in the brain. It is not surprising, therefore, that there are several mechanisms regulating or influencing CBF.

Mechanisms Regulating Cerebral Blood Flow

The three most important mechanisms regulating CBF are autoregulation, chemical regulation, and metabolic regulation; CBF is also adjusted to changes in hemoglobin concentration.

Autoregulation ensures that CBF is kept constant despite rather wide fluctuations of blood pressure. Autoregulation is of major importance for the understanding of the cerebral circulation in hypertension and will be discussed in detail later in the present chapter.

A major factor in *chemical regulation* is the arterial CO_2 tension. Hypercapnia causes cerebral vasodilation with a CBF increase; it causes cerebral vasoconstriction with a CBF decrease (7,8). It is not the CO_2 tension per se that is responsible for the flow changes, but the accompanying shift in periarteriolar pH (9). Since the blood-brain barrier is impermeable to H^+ and HCO_3^- and freely permeable to the lipophilic gas CO_2, the periarteriolar pH will be determined by the HCO_3^- concentration in the periarteriolar tissue and the CO_2 tension in the arterial blood flowing through the arterioles. The impermeability of the blood-brain barrier to H^+ and HCO_3^- also means that systemic metabolic acid base changes are not reflected by similar cerebral periarteriolar changes and thus essentially are not accompanied by CBF changes (10). If a shift of the arterial CO_2 tension is maintained for a longer period, adaptation occurs, resetting both the cerebral pH and the CBF to normal levels within 6–24 hours (11,12).

Potassium is another chemical factor regulating CBF. Within the physiological range an increase of the periarteriolar K^+ concentration dilates the arterioles and increases CBF (13). Changes in periarteriolar K^+ concentration may be of major significance for the metabolic regulation of CBF. A special transport system via the astrocytes seems to secure an immediate periarteriolar concentration change in response to potassium release from the neurones (14).

Nitric oxide (NO) is an *endothelial-derived* relaxing factor with strong vasodilatory properties and of considerable interest for blood flow regulation in most organs. Inhibition of NO by nitro-l-arginine does not modify autoregulation of CBF and NO seems thus not to be of significance for this important mechanism of cerebral flow regulation (15). In contrast, blocking of NO results in an attenuation of the normal CBF increase during hypercapnia (16–18), an effect that is also seen following indomethacin administration (19).

The term *metabolic regulation* denotes that there normally is a close coupling between CBF, cerebral metabolism, and cerebral function (20–22).

CBF is adjusted to changes in the blood *hemoglobin concentration*. Thus, in anemia with low oxygen binding capacity of the blood CBF is high, and in polycytemia CBF is low. The cerebral circulation thus tends to keep on constant oxygen tension in the cerebral venous blood. The oxygen-binding capacity of the blood as well as the oxyhemoglobin dissociation curve—and to some extent, the blood viscosity—seem to be involved in this regulation (23,24).

Autoregulation

Autoregulation of blood flow ensures that the flow through an organ or a vascular bed is maintained fairly constant despite changes in the arterial blood pressure. The vessels dilate in response to blood pressure decreases and constrict in response to blood pressure increases. Autoregulation is present in most organs but is particularly well developed in the brain (Fig. 1). The concept of cerebral autoregulation has recently been extensively reviewed by us (25).

Autoregulation of CBF is effective over a wide range of arterial blood pressures, but has a lower as well as an upper pressure limit. Under normal conditions these limits are about mean blood pressures of 60 and 150 mm Hg, respectively (26–28). When the blood pressure falls below the lower limit, CBF decreases as vasodilation becomes inadequate. The resistance vessels reach only submaximal dilation in the autoregulatory response, and can be further dilated pharmacologically (29–31). If systemic blood pressure drops moderately below the lower limit of autoregulation (less than around 50 percent with a CBF decrease of 30 percent or less), then the oxygen uptake of the brain is maintained at its normal level by an increase of the oxygen extraction from the blood in proportion to the fall in CBF. At this stage clinical symp-

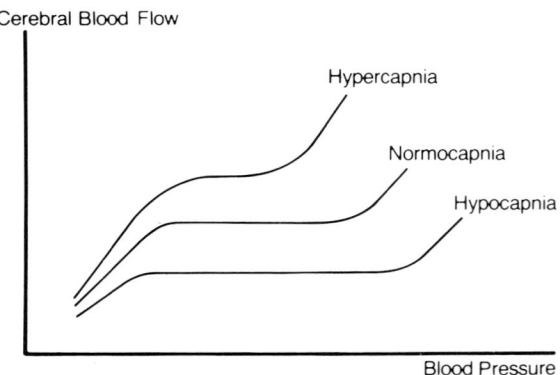

FIG. 1. Autoregulation of cerebral blood flow (CBF). The diagram shows the autoregulatory plateau and its lower and upper limits. During hypercapnia, the cerebral resistance vessels are dilated, CBF is increased, and the autoregulatory plateau is shortened. Conversely, during hypocapnia, cerebral vasoconstriction causes a decrease in CBF and a widening of the autoregulatory plateau.

toms are insignificant. If pressure drops further, symptoms of incipient fainting develop with dizziness, pallor, sweating, yawning, etc. With further pressure reduction, consciousness is lost and finally ischemic brain damage occurs, first reversible and then irreversible. At these stages, with blood pressure markedly below the lower limit of autoregulation, the increase in oxygen extraction from the blood can no longer counterbalance the decrease in CBF and there is a decrease in the cerebral uptake of oxygen, i.e., in the cerebral metabolic rate of oxygen.

Above the upper limit of autoregulation, constriction of cerebral resistance vessels gives way to the high pressure and CBF increases (32–34). The intraluminal pressure rise in the arterioles and capillaries may result in forceful dilation of segments of the arterioles leading to caliber variations and blood-brain barrier damage (35–37). If the high pressure is maintained, brain edema may develop with a possible secondary flow decrease. Such a sequence of events is probably of major pathogenetic significance for the development of the clinical condition of hypertensive encephalopathy, as discussed later in this chapter.

Cerebral blood flow autoregulation responds not only to blood pressure changes but also to changes in intracranial pressure (29,38). It is, in fact, the perfusion pressure (arterial blood pressure minus intracranial pressure) that is determining for the limits of autoregulation. However, in the normal situation and in diseases without changes in intracranial pressure, the variations in perfusion pressure are essentially identical to those in arterial blood pressure.

Two possible mechanisms have been suggested to explain the nature of autoregulation. One is a *myogenic mechanism* in which the arterioles and small arteries constrict or dilate in response to an increase or decrease in the transmural pressure gradient. The other is a *metabolic mechanism* in which changes in the metabolic microenvironment are thought to be responsible for the vasomotor response. The fact that CBF is very well maintained at its resting level when perfusion pressure changes has been interpreted to speak against the metabolic hypothesis, since one would assume that some flow change would be needed in order to trigger the metabolic changes.

The rapidity of the autoregulatory response, which is initiated within a few seconds after a change in transmural pressure of the resistance vessels (39–43), and largely completed within 15–30 sec or less, favors a myogenic response. The myogenic properties have been measured directly *in vitro* in isolated branches from the posterior cerebral artery from normotensive and spontaneously hypertensive rats. Responses of autoregulatory nature following changes in transmural pressure were observed (44). This study indicates that purely myogenic responses can account for at least a portion of the adjust-

ment in cerebral arterial and arteriolar caliber required for CBF autoregulation.

Physiological Modulation of Cerebral Autoregulation

Both the sympathetic nervous system and the renin-angiotensin system have a physiological modulating influence on CBF autoregulation. Activation of the sympathetic nervous system thus shifts the lower and upper limits of autoregulation toward higher pressures, and blocking of the renin-angiotensin system shifts the limits toward lower pressures. The limits of autoregulation will furthermore be shifted during increase or decrease of CBF as induced by hyper- or hypocapnia, with a narrowing of the autoregulatory plateau at high CBF levels. The limits of autoregulation in an individual are thus not completely fixed but influenced by other physiological mechanisms.

Changes in the activity of the *sympathetic nervous system* does not influence the CBF within the autoregulatory range or influences it only very transiently (45–47). Activation of the alpha-adrenergic sympathetic nerves, however, shifts the limits of autoregulation toward higher pressures, and acute denervation shifts the limits of autoregulation toward lower pressure (Fig. 2) (48–53). Chronic sympathetic denervation does not shift the limits of autoregulation (53). Spontaneous increases of the systemic blood pressure always involve enhanced sympathetic activity. Thus, the shift of the upper limit of cerebral autoregulation toward higher pressure during sympathetic activation must be considered as a physiological widening of the autoregulatory range protecting

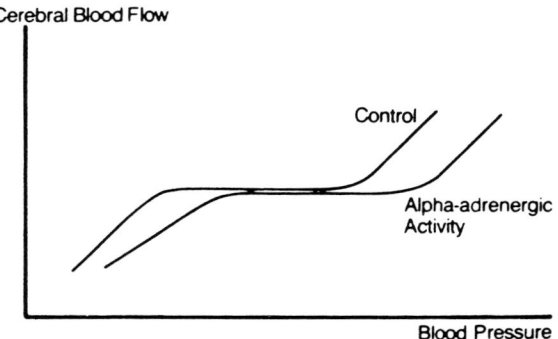

FIG. 2. Effect of stimulation of the alpha-adrenergic perivascular sympathetic nerves on autoregulation of cerebral blood flow (CBF). In the autoregulatory range, sympathetic constriction of the larger "inflow tract" cerebral arteries is compensated by autoregulatory dilatation of the smaller resistance vessels further downstream. As the lower limit is approached, this autoregulatory compensation becomes inadequate, with the net result of a shift of the lower limit toward higher pressure. This is the situation occurring in hemorrhagic shock. Conversely, during endogenous pressure peaks, sympathetic vasoconstriction assists autoregulatory constriction, resulting in a shift of the upper limit toward higher pressure.

the brain against the high blood pressure. Sympathetic stimulation thus attenuates the blood-brain barrier damage occurring when blood pressure is increased above the normal upper level of cerebral autoregulation (49,54).

Physiological falls in blood pressure are often associated with a low sympathetic tone and here the shift toward low pressure of the CBF autoregulation also acts as a physiological widening of the autoregulatory plateau protecting the brain against the reduced blood pressure. However, sympathetic tone is not always low at low blood pressures, but may in some instances be high, e.g., during hemorrhagic hypotension. Here a resulting upward shift of the lower limit of autoregulation is not per se advantageous for the brain, but rather is part of the general regulatory mechanisms of the body to a shock condition with a balance between mechanisms trying to keep up the blood pressure and the mechanism trying to avoid ischemia of vital organs.

The alpha-adrenergic sympathetic nervous system predominantly exerts its vasomotor function in the larger cerebral resistance vessels (the "inflow tract"), whereas autoregulation is predominantly a function of the smaller resistance vessels (45,55–59). During sympathetic activation with constriction of the larger resistance vessels, the smaller resistance vessels further downstream will dilate as an autoregulatory response to keep CBF constant as long as blood pressure is within the autoregulatory range. The opposite takes place if the sympathetic tone is reduced. Only at the limits of autoregulation may the vasomotor function of the larger resistance vessels affect CBF, because the smaller resistance vessels no longer have the full autoregulatory capacity. Thus if the larger resistance vessels have constricted and the smaller have dilated in an autoregulatory response to hypotension, then less capacity is left for further autoregulatory dilation of the smaller vessels (60). If systemic blood pressure is now lowered, the lower limit of autoregulation will be reached at a higher pressure than if the larger resistance vessels had not constricted. Further, the combination of constricted large resistance vessels and dilated small resistance vessels may lead to inhomogeneous perfusion with patchy tissue ischemia (60). At the upper limit of autoregulation a sympathetic constriction of the larger resistance vessels will add to the vasoconstrictor capacity of the smaller resistance vessel, resulting in a shift of the upper limit of autoregulation toward higher pressures (61).

The *renin-angiotensin* system also modulates cerebral autoregulation. The angiotensin-converting enzyme inhibitor captopril (Capoten, Capozide), as well as fosinopril and ceranapril, thus shift both the lower and upper limits of autoregulation to lower blood pressure levels when administered to rats (Fig. 3) (62–64). The renin-angiotensin system must therefore have some tonus in the cerebral resistance vessels. When captopril was given directly in the cerebral ventricles, it did not influence autoregulation (65). Thus, the converting enzyme inhibitor

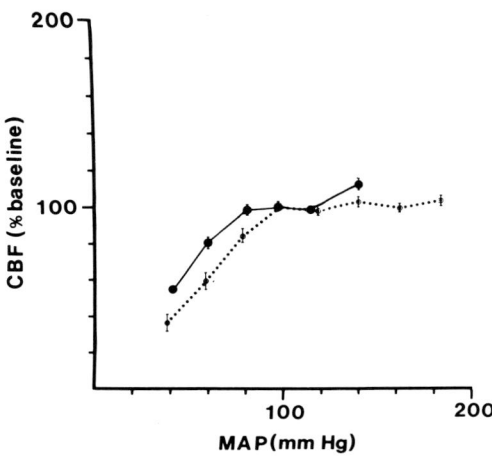

FIG. 3. Captopril, given acutely intravenously, shifts the lower limit of autoregulation of cerebral blood flow (CBF) toward lower blood pressure. Captopril caused the blood pressure to fall below the lower limit of autoregulation with no change in CBF. The blood pressure was lowered further by controlled hemorrhage. When the blood pressure in another group of animals following captopril was raised with intravenous norepinephrine, the upper limit of autoregulation was found to be shifted toward lower pressure, with a shortening of the autoregulatory plateau. MAP, mean arterial pressure. (From ref. 62, with permission.)

appeared to influence the vessel wall renin system rather than the brain renin system. The renin-angiotensin system presumably influences mainly the larger cerebral resistance vessels, and converting enzyme inhibition causes dilation of these vessels. Therefore the limits for cerebral autoregulation are shifted to lower pressure levels for reasons quite similar to those discussed above for the sympathetic nervous system. The response of the cerebral circulation to converting enzyme inhibitors appears also to depend on whether the drugs are given orally or parenterally. This will be discussed further below in the section on pharmacological influence on cerebral autoregulation; here we shall deal only with the physiological aspects.

An interaction can be shown between the renin-angiotensin system and the sympathetic nervous system. Thus the downward shift of the upper limit of autoregulation is attenuated by simultaneous stimulation of the superior cervical sympathetic ganglion in the rat (Fig. 4) (66). This observation is obviously of major interest for the treatment of hypertensive patients with converting enzyme inhibitors because spontaneous increases of the systemic blood pressure always involve enhanced sympathetic activity. The effect of captopril on the limits of autoregulation in the rat is still present following chronic sympathetic denervation (67). This demonstrates that the renin-angiotensin system influences CBF flow autoregulation independently of the sympathetic nervous system.

In awake man, the effect of converting enzyme inhibition with captopril is less pronounced than in the anes-

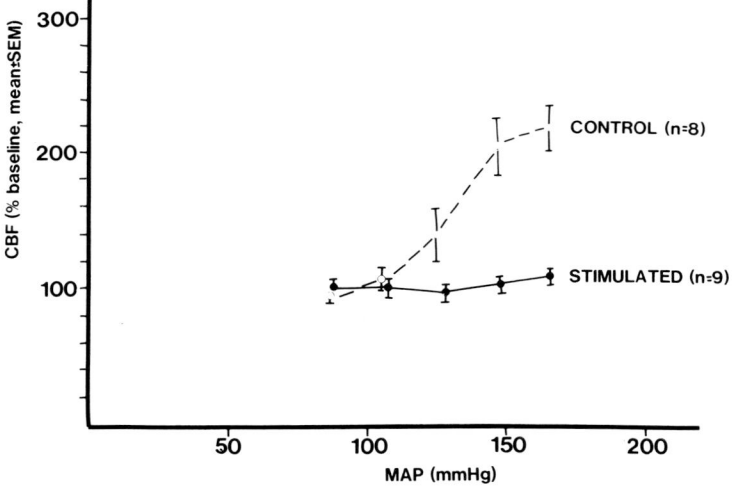

FIG. 4. Electric stimulation of the cervical sympathetic trunk abolishes the effect of captopril (given acutely intravenously) on the upper limit of autoregulation of cerebral blood flow (CBF) in spontaneously hypertensive rats. Following captopril, the upper limit of autoregulation was lowered, and intravenous norepinephrine caused a marked rise in CBF (upper curve). This was completely prevented by concomitant sympathetic stimulation. MAP, mean arterial pressure (lower curve). (From ref. 66, with permission.)

thetized rat, possibly because of a lower activity of the sympathetic nervous system in anesthetized animals. In patients with heart failure, captopril caused a marked fall in blood pressure with no changes in CBF, suggestive of a shift in autoregulation toward low pressure (68). In one study in normotensive and hypertensive individuals, the observations suggest some downward shift of the lower limit of autoregulation but statistically only at the limits of significance (69); however, in another study by the same group a significant reduction was reached in patients with normal-pressure hydrocephalus (70). The upper limit of autoregulation was not reached by moderate blood pressure increase in either of the studies.

The *level of CBF* influences the autoregulation as the autoregulatory plateau is shortened at high CBF and widened at low CBF. This is best illustrated by CBF changes induced by arterial PCO_2 changes (see Fig. 1) (29,71,72). It has not been studied for flow changes due to metabolic regulation. At high CBF the resistance vessels are dilated and do not have enough dilatory capacity to keep CBF constant down to the normal lower limit of autoregulation. At the upper limit of autoregulation the dilated resistance vessels will be more vulnerable and resist the increased intravascular pressure less well. Thus the upper limit of autoregulation will be shifted downward at high flow levels.

STRUCTURAL VASCULAR CHANGES IN THE BRAIN IN HYPERTENSION

Chronic hypertension is associated with adaptive and degenerative structural changes in the cerebral resistance vessels. In the larger conduit arteries, including the circle of Willis and its branches, hypertension accelerates atherosclerosis and contributes to the development and rupture of saccular aneurysms, thereby increasing the risk of major cerebral infarcts and subarachnoid hemorrhage, respectively. In the smaller arteries and arterioles, which play the main role in regulating CBF, hypertension causes structural remodeling with wall thickening and luminal narrowing. In longstanding hypertension, degenerative changes in the form of "lipohyalinosis" may prevail, sometimes associated with a tendency to develop Charcot-Bouchard microaneurysms (73). These various degenerative changes may be the source of small "lacunar" cerebral infarcts and cerebral hemorrhage (74). Binswanger's encephalopathy, also known as *leukoaraiosis* or *subcortical arteriosclerotic demyelinization with progressive dementia,* is also associated with hypertension (75) and is sometimes misleadingly called "chronic hypertensive encephalopathy."

HYPERTENSIVE ADAPTATION OF AUTOREGULATION OF CEREBRAL BLOOD FLOW

The absolute value of CBF is the same in hypertensive and normotensive man without neurological deficit (3). Thus, in hypertension, vascular resistance is elevated in the brain as elsewhere in the body. This state of permanently elevated vascular resistance is associated with the structural changes described above in the small arteries and arterioles. Correspondingly, the flow velocity is unchanged in hypertension in the larger cerebral arteries, as determined by intracranial Doppler technique (76). In hypertensive rats, the sympathetic perivascular nerves appear to play a role in the development of this cerebrovascular adaptation (77). Once established, however, arteriolar narrowing and wall thickening is of a structural nature and impairs the vessel's capacity for maximal vasodilation. Hence, the hypertensive individual's tolerance to blood pressure lowering is impaired, as manifested by a shift of autoregulation of CBF toward higher levels on the blood-pressure axis.

Interestingly, endothelium-dependent dilatation of cerebral arterioles has been found to be impaired in stroke-prone SHR, whereas endothelium-independent dilatation was intact (78).

In an early study by Finnerty and coworkers (79), it was shown that during controlled hypotension in hypertensive and normotensive individuals, consciousness was lost when global CBF was approximately halved. This happened at blood pressures reduced proportionately to the individual's habitual pressure (Fig. 5). In 1965, Gottstein (80) published data from the literature of CBF measurement during controlled hypotension and suggested a shift of the lower end of the autoregulation curve in hypertension. This shift had been predicted in Lassen's classical review from 1959 (4). Finally, hypertensive adaptation of the lower end of the CBF autoregulation curve was shown in individual hypertensive patients in the early 1970s (Fig. 6) (26,28), and later in baboons with renovascular hypertension (81) and in rats with spontaneous and renal hypertension (82,83).

In a study in baboons with renovascular hypertension, it was further shown that the upper limit of autoregulation was shifted toward higher pressure (84). Thus, the hypertensive vascular changes that impair the tolerance to hypotension concomitantly improve the tolerance to hypertension. Actually, in spontaneously hypertensive rats, the upper limit of autoregulation has been found to be shifted more toward higher pressure than the lower limit, with a consequent widening of the autoregulatory plateau (Fig. 7) (85). Thus, it is understandable that hypertensive patients can tolerate for prolonged periods blood pressures that would soon precipitate a hypertensive crisis in an otherwise normotensive individual.

The cerebrovascular response to hypocapnia and hypercapnia is unaltered in hypertension (Fig. 8) (8). This

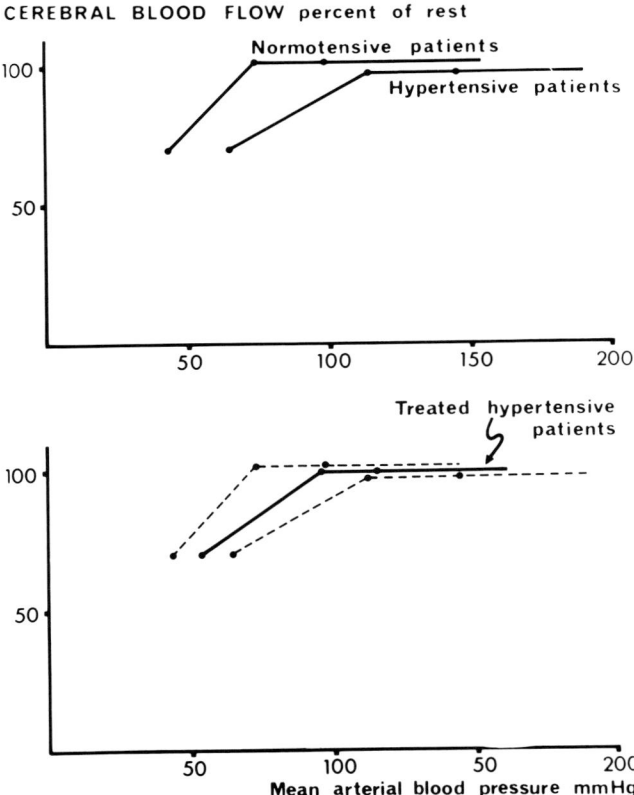

FIG. 6. Mean autoregulation curves from normotensive, untreated and uncontrolled hypertensive, and effectively treated hypertensive patients. Blood pressure was lowered gradually by trimethaphan infusion combined with head-up tilt. On each curve is marked the resting blood pressure, the lower limit of autoregulation, and the lowest tolerated blood pressure where mild symptoms of cerebral hypoperfusion were encountered. (From ref. 28, with permission of the American Heart Association, Inc.)

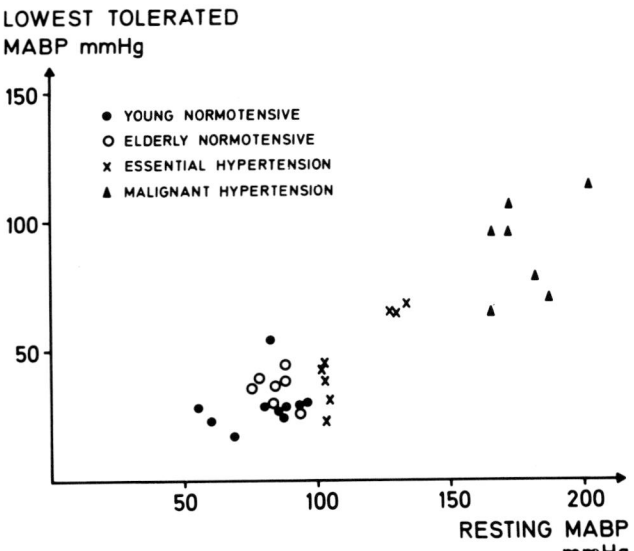

FIG. 5. Relation between mean arterial blood pressure at rest and during controlled hypotension at the level where transient symptoms of cerebral ischemia developed. (Drawn from data from ref. 79.)

actually is a result of structural vascular adaptation, since in a normotensive individual the combination of hypercapnia and induced hypertension would expectedly cause an extreme rise in CBF. In chronic hypertension the hypercapnic CBF response must be understood to be restricted by the adaptive resistance vessel wall changes.

The cerebrovascular reactivity is also influenced by aging. Thus, the flow increase in response to hypercapnia decreases and the lower limit of autoregulation is shifted to higher blood pressure during maturation and aging (86). This may, at least to some extent, be a consequence of an increase of the blood pressure with advancing age.

Readaptation of Autoregulation of Cerebral Blood Flow During Long-Term Antihypertensive Treatment

Despite the structural adaptation of cerebral resistance vessels to high blood pressure and the consequent shift of autoregulation, antihypertensive treatment does not in the great majority of patients carry any risk of inducing

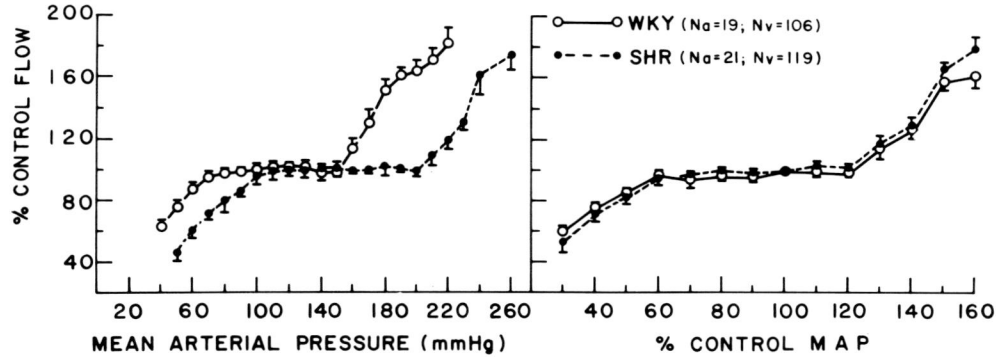

FIG. 7. Autoregulation of cerebral blood flow in normotensive Wistar-Kyoto rats and spontaneously hypertensive rats. The shift of the upper limit toward high pressure is more marked than the shift of the absolute lower limit, but the relative shift is the same. (From ref. 85, with permission.)

cerebral ischemia. This paradox will be discussed in some detail in a later section; one contributing factor, however, may be that during antihypertensive treatment, structural changes in cerebral resistance vessels and, consequently, autoregulation, may readapt toward normal. In a study of the lower limit of CBF autoregulation in man, effectively treated hypertensive patients were found to have autoregulation curves that on the average were intermediate between severely untreated or uncontrolled patients and normotensives, overlapping both of these groups. This suggested that the effectively treated patients had in some, but not all, instances readapted their cerebral resistance vessels toward normal during treatment (28).

In some patients readaptation could be demonstrated following approximately 1 year of effective treatment. In

others, no such readaptation was apparent (28). Studies of the vascular bed in the forearm of patients with long-standing hypertension point to an only partial readaptation of structural hypertensive changes during treatment (87).

In rats with renal hypertension of 2 months' duration, the lower limit of CBF autoregulation was found to be shifted around 20 mm Hg toward higher blood pressure. By a further 2 months of effective antihypertensive treatment with hydrochlorothiazide, apresoline, and reserpine, the lower limit was shifted completely back to normal, whereas in a control group that remained hypertensive for 4 months, an additional shift of autoregulation of the order of 20 mm Hg was seen (Fig. 9) (88). A similar shift of autoregulation back to normal in rats with renovascular hypertension was seen during chronic treatment with the converting enzyme inhibitor perindopril (89). These studies in rats may reasonably be taken to be predictive of the response of CBF autoregulation to hypertension and antihypertensive treatment in younger patients. In elderly patients or patients with longstanding hypertension, degenerative changes and connective tissue proliferation may prevail in the arteriolar walls, and none or limited readaptation of CBF autoregulation should be expected.

CEREBROVASCULAR DISEASES IN HYPERTENSION

Stroke

Several epidemiological studies indicate that the frequency of stroke in hypertension is increased considerably as compared with normotensive subjects (90–95). In the Framingham Study, a linear correlation was found between blood pressure, both systolic and diastolic, and the incidence of stroke (90,92). In contrast, other studies have demonstrated that there is not a relation between blood pressure and stroke incidence at low pressure lev-

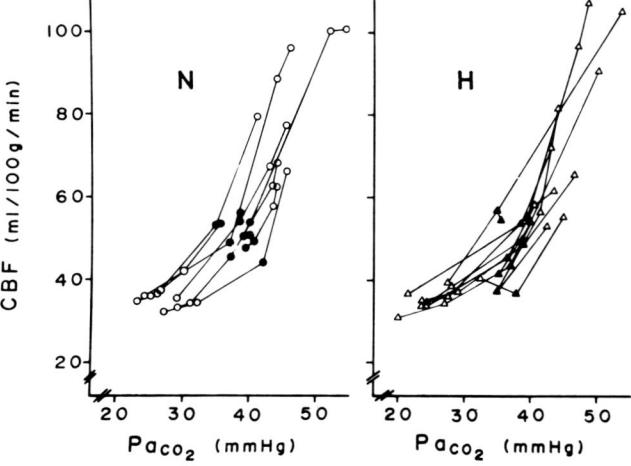

FIG. 8. Cerebrovascular CO_2 reactivity in normotensive and hypertensive man. In each subject, cerebral blood flow (CBF) was measured by the intracarotid ^{133}Xe injection method at normocapnia (*filled circles and triangles*), during CO_2 inhalation, and during hyperventilation. No differences in response were found between normotensive and hypertensive subjects (From ref. 8, with permission of the American Heart Association, Inc.)

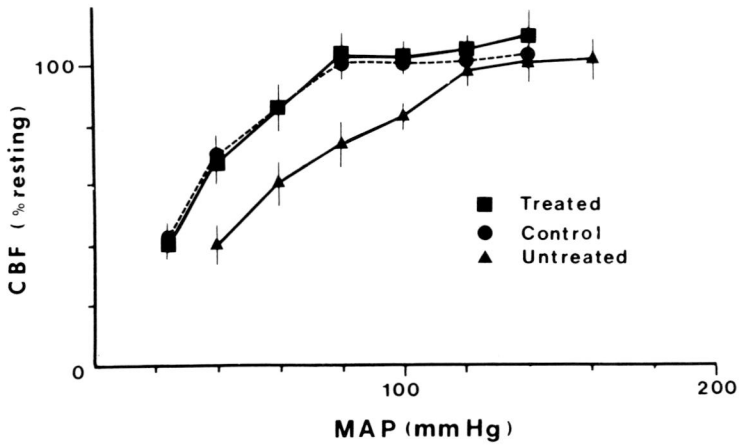

FIG. 9. Effect of renal hypertension and chronic anti-hypertensive treatment on autoregulation of cerebral blood flow (CBF) in rats. At approximately 1 month of age, Wistar-Kyoto rats were subjected to unilateral renal infarction and contralateral nephrectomy. This was followed by the development of hypertension, and after 2 months, half the animals were placed on antihypertensive treatment with hydrochlorothiazide, reserpine, and dihydralazine in the drinking water. After a further 2 months of normotension, CBF autoregulation was studied by controlled hemorrhage using the intracarotid ^{133}Xe method. Chronic hypertension caused a marked shift of the lower limit of the autoregulation curves toward higher pressure, and this was completely reversed by the antihypertensive treatment. (From ref. 88, with permission of the American Heart Association, Inc.)

els, but an exponential increase of stroke at high pressure levels (94). About half of patients developing stroke have preexisting hypertension (96–98). In the acute phase of a stroke, hypertension is even more common and blood pressure at or above 170/110 mm Hg has been reported to be present in about 70 percent of the patients because of the acute brain damage (99).

Stroke in hypertension may be large-vessel disease (atherothrombotic) or small-vessel disease, resulting in lacunar lesions or an intracerebral hemorrhage. The atherothrombotic ischemic strokes are caused by arteriosclerosis and a sudden thromboembolic occlusion of an artery supplying the brain. Occasionally a hemodynamic mechanism may operate when the blood pressure is lowered in the presence of a severe stenosis on a cerebral end artery. The lacunar strokes are due to degenerative changes in penetrating small arteries causing small, sometimes multiple lesions, and often located deep in the white matter of the hemispheres (100). They can probably have several causes: small ischemic lesions, small hemorrhages that have been resorbed, or localized hypertensive damage due to hypertensive episodes with disturbed blood-brain barrier function. The intracerebral hemorrhages may be spontaneous but have often been assumed to arise from a Charcot-Bouchard microaneurysm on a small intracerebral artery or, less commonly, from a larger vascular malformation. It should be noted that these microaneurysms are quite different from the saccular aneurysms on the larger cerebral arteries, which are discussed below in the section on subarachnoid hemorrhage.

One of the main benefits of modern antihypertensive treatment is stroke prevention (101–105). It has been debated whether antihypertensive treatment prevents all three types of strokes (74,106,107). It might be assumed that especially the incidence of lacunar infarction and intracerebral hemorrhage would decrease with antihypertensive treatment because hypertension is closely associated with vascular lipohyalinosis and microaneurysm formation. If antihypertensive treatment prevents

the progression of arteriosclerosis in the larger arteries, a decrease of the incidence of thromboembolic strokes might also be expected in the long term. Actually, the observation that the entire excess risk of stroke in hypertension is eliminated by antihypertensive treatment (105) suggests prevention of both lacunar, hemorrhagic, and ischemic stroke.

At present there are few epidemiological studies in which it has been possible to differentiate between the different stroke types using more extensive evaluation, including computed tomography (CT) scan and/or autopsy. In a Finnish study the mortality of stroke in 1972–1973 and 1978–1980 was compared. A decline in the incidence of hemorrhages but not of ischemic lesions was observed, and this difference was attributed to improved care of hypertension (108). In an unpublished study quoted by Spence (107), the incidence of patients hospitalized with stroke decreased from 1977 to 1984, a period when CT scan had been routine and the proportion of strokes due to hypertensive hemorrhage and hypertensive lacunar infarction had decreased from 50 percent to 10 percent of the patients. This has not, however, been confirmed in larger series and it is still generally accepted that about 10 percent of all strokes are intracerebral hemorrhage and 30 percent are lacunes. Therefore, further epidemiological investigation is definitely warranted before more firm conclusions can be drawn.

Subarachnoid Hemorrhage

These are hemorrhages that occur directly into the subarachnoidal space. There will be some overlap to the intracerebral hemorrhages discussed above. The cause of the subarachnoidal hemorrhage is in about 70 percent a ruptured saccular arterial aneurysm at the bifurcation of the larger cerebral arteries, in 10 percent a bleeding from an arteriovenous malformation, and in the remaining 20 percent a rupture of a seemingly normal vessel. The subarachnoid hemorrhage in most instances occurs in situations with episodes of physiological increase of the blood pressure such as coitus, isometric exercise, etc. It should be noted that the saccular arterial aneurysms and the vascular malformations are not protected by cerebral autoregulation against episodes of increased blood pressure because they most often arise from the larger resistance vessels.

It would be expected that chronic arterial hypertension would also increase the risk of subarachnoidal hemorrhage and of the formation of the saccular intracranial aneurysms. Epidemiological studies support this assumption. A clear correlation between rupture of intracranial aneurysms and hypertension was observed in the Framingham Study (109), and the risk of subarachnoidal hemorrhage was found increased in hypertensive patients in a case-control population study (110).

Acute Hypertensive Encephalopathy

Acute hypertensive encephalopathy in the strict sense is a vascular cerebral crisis of acute onset and storming course. The patient develops an intense headache, nausea and vomiting, convulsions, focal neurological signs and symptoms, and a decreasing level of consciousness. The blood pressure is high, but especially in young children and pregnant women may be only moderately elevated. If untreated, the syndrome leads to the patient's death in coma; with proper treatment, patients may recover cerebrally to a surprising extent.

The intense headache experienced by some patients with very high blood pressure and fundoscopic changes signifying malignant hypertension may be a mild analogue of the full-blown syndrome of acute hypertensive encephalopathy. Indeed, patients with malignant hypertension often have a raised cerebrospinal fluid pressure (111).

The term *acute hypertensive encephalopathy* was suggested in 1928 by Oppenheimer and Fishberg (112) in replacement of the earlier "eclamptic uremia" or "pseudouremia" (113). The syndrome should not be confused with lacunar brain infarction or Binswanger's encephalopathy, briefly mentioned in an earlier paragraph. Clinicians probably tend to overuse the diagnosis of hypertensive encephalopathy (114). True acute hypertensive encephalopathy is a rare condition, most likely as a result of the widespread use of antihypertensive treatment.

The pathogenesis of acute hypertensive encephalopathy has been under discussion for more than a century, with the earliest concepts curiously resembling the current ones. Basically the discussion has focused on rather simple hemodynamic mechanisms of opposite nature: some authors have claimed that the syndrome is due to cerebral vasospasm with ischemia, whereas others have favored forced cerebral vasodilation with hyperemia as the key initiating event.

The vasospasm hypothesis was prevailing in the literature for decades, dating back to the observation of Kussmaul and Tenner in 1857 (115) that carotid ligation in a rabbit caused epileptiform convulsions. Hypertensive retinal changes have been conventionally interpreted in terms of vasospasm (116), and the vasospasm concept found support in Byrom's (117) early interpretation of the so-called sausage-string pattern of alternating constrictions and dilations seen in the small arteries or on the surface of the rat brain in severe hypertension.

The vasospasm hypothesis was, however, severely questioned by Giese's (118) observation in the rat mesentery that during acute hypertension, leaking of plasma protein (or colloidal carbon as a marker) invariably took place in the dilated and never in the constricted segments of the sausage-string pattern. These observations prompted Byrom to revise his concepts, and in his book from 1969 (119) he came out clearly in favor of forced vasodilation as the key event in acute hypertensive encephalopathy.

A later study in cats has demonstrated that the narrow segments of the sausage-string phenomenon are indeed the remnants of autoregulatory constriction, and that the segmental vasodilation may develop into a state of general vasodilation with a massive rise in CBF (34,120). Studies of CBF during acutely induced hypertension have repeatedly demonstrated an upper limit of autoregulation beyond which CBF increases (32,33,84), whereas cerebral ischemia, consequent of hypertensive vasospasm, has never been found in such studies. Acute hypertension may also cause blood-barrier dysfunction with protein extravasation, along with CBF increase (35–37).

The forced vasodilation hypothesis may be formulated as follows (121,122): high blood pressure, either rising acutely or sustained at very high levels, or both, causes localized and later possibly global cerebral vasodilation and a high CBF; this is associated with vascular leakage of plasma protein causing brain edema that is initially focal and later becomes generalized. This brain edema causes the clinical symptoms. As brain edema continues to develop and the patient lapses into coma, CBF decreases to low levels. It will be understood that a clear proof of this hypothesis has not been presented; it is nonetheless rather solidly founded on experimental evidence, and some clinical consequences can be drawn from the current state of knowledge. Thus, based on the vasospasm hypothesis it was once advocated to treat these patients with CO_2 inhalation; this should be regarded as extremely dangerous as it would add a further increase to CBF and cause a further rise in intracranial pressure and acceleration of the development of brain edema. On the contrary, apart from controlling the patient's blood pressure, it is extremely important to avoid hypercapnia and hypoxia; opiates should not be used for sedation, and the patient should be placed on artificial ventilation if necessary. Extreme care should be taken to avoid precipitous blood pressure falls in the initial phase of treatment, where the aim should be a moderate reduction and not an immediate normalization of blood pressure. This is discussed in detail later in the present chapter.

EFFECTS OF ANTIHYPERTENSIVE TREATMENT OF THE CEREBRAL CIRCULATION

The Cerebrovascular Pharmacology of Antihypertensive Drugs

With *acute* pharmacological blood pressure lowering, two types of effects can be anticipated in the cerebral circulation. First, the CBF response will depend on how much the pressure falls. With a moderate blood pressure reduction, autoregulation will operate to keep CBF constant; with a more marked fall in pressure to below the lower limit of autoregulation, CBF will fall. Second, specific pharmacological actions of antihypertensive drugs in the cerebral vessels may modify this response; a vasodilating drug such as dihydralazine may increase CBF along with lowering of the blood pressure, and both vasodilators and converting enzyme inhibitors may sustain a normal CBF well below the lower limit of autoregulation.

With *chronic* antihypertensive treatment, the possibility arises that CBF autoregulation may readapt itself partly or completely to normal; this can be expected in young patients and would allow a gradual normalization of even the most severely elevated pressures. The time factor in this readaptation has not been studied in man, but based on animal studies it would be expected to be rather short: young rats with renal hypertension normalized their CBF autoregulation in the course of a few weeks or months of antihypertensive treatment (88,89). Studies in the peripheral circulation of hypertensive rats suggest that the time factor required for structural vascular readaptation may be even shorter, on the order of 2–3 weeks (123). On the other hand, in the human forearm, functional signs of structural hypertensive changes were still present after 5 years of effective pressure lowering (87). Thus, an irreversible element of hypertensive vascular remodeling and degenerative changes in the vessel walls may prevail no matter how long the pressure is kept down.

A Classification of Drugs Used for Emergency Antihypertensive Treatment

Based on their effect on the cerebral circulation, drugs used for acute blood pressure reduction can be classified in at least five different groups:

Drugs with No Pharmacological Action in the Cerebral Vessels

Diazoxide is the most extensively studied drug in this group. When a small dose of diazoxide is given intravenously, blood pressure falls moderately, and CBF is unaltered. When the once-clinically-favored "bolus dose" of 5 mg/kg body weight was given to rats with spontaneous or renal hypertension, blood pressure was approximately halved in less than 30 sec and CBF fell on the average to 70 percent of the resting level. Comparison with autoregulation curves in the rats obtained by controlled bleeding showed that CBF after diazoxide had fallen to the level expected when the pressure fell below the lower limit of autoregulation (124). If a pressor drug is given after diazoxide-induced hypertension, CBF is restored and autoregulation is intact (125). In man, a moderate dose of diazoxide caused no changes in CBF, whereas higher doses induced a fall in CBF as the pressure went below the anticipated lower limit of autoregulation (126). Diazoxide has been incriminated in many of the published studies of cerebral ischemia caused by antihypertensive treatment, as discussed in a later section. It has been learned that the steep, massive fall in pressure caused by the "bolus dose" treatment with diazoxide is unnecessarily risky; in repetitive moderate doses, e.g., 1.5 mg/kg or by intravenous infusion, the drug appears to be quite safe (127).

Cerebral Vasodilators

Dihydralazine given intravenously increases CBF in normal and hypertensive patients (128,129). In neurosurgical patients, dihydralazine was found to increase CBF and cause a marked rise in an already elevated intracranial pressure (130). In normal cats, dihydralazine caused a modest rise in intracranial pressure associated with pial arteriolar dilation; the pial venules were not dilated by the drug (131). In rats with spontaneous or renal hypertension, incremental doses of dihydralazine caused a gradual fall in blood pressure with an unchanged CBF even below the lower limit of autoregulation; at the lowest pressure, CBF tended to rise (Fig. 10) (132). When a pressor drug was given after dihydralazine-induced hypotension, CBF rose massively, showing a paralyzed autoregulation (125). Intracranial pressure was not measured in these rat studies.

Sodium nitroprusside at low blood pressure dilates cerebral resistance vessels, at least in anesthetized patients (133). The drug increases intracranial pressure, but this tends to wear off as hypotension becomes more profound (134). When pressor drugs are given under sodium-nitroprusside-induced hypotension, CBF autoregulation is shown to be paralyzed (135). In awake man, sodium-nitroprusside-induced hypotension paradoxically causes

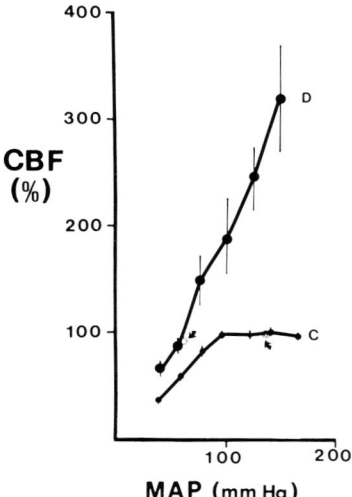

FIG. 10. Effect of dihydralazine on cerebral blood flow (CBF) and its autoregulation in spontaneously hypertensive rats. Following repetitive incremental doses of intravenous dihydralazine, blood pressure fell to below the lower limit of autoregulation with no fall in CBF. When the blood pressure was subsequently raised by norepinephrine infusion, CBF rose massively, showing that autoregulation was paralyzed. (From ref. 125, with permission of S. Karger Publishers.)

a decrease in CBF because of hyperventilation and alpha-adrenergic activation (136).

Cerebral vasodilators should not be given to patients with acute cerebral lesions or to patients in whom a raised intracranial pressure for other reasons might be suspected. This includes patients with fundoscopic signs of malignant hypertension (111) and acute stroke patients. Focal cerebral ischemia may actually be worsened by cerebral vasodilators, which may increase perfusion only in the healthy tissue causing a "steal" from the ischemic tissue (blood flow reduction). On the other hand, the risk associated with the undesired effects of the drugs are restricted to these limited groups of patients, and should not preclude their use in other groups. Thus, sodium nitroprusside is an effective agent for induction of hypotension during anesthesia.

Calcium Antagonists

Calcium antagonists may cause some intracerebral vasodilatation. When nifedipine (Adalat, Procardia) was given orally to severely hypertensive patients, blood pressure fell markedly but CBF was unchanged; a comparable fall in blood pressure induced with clonidine was associated with a fall in CBF (137). In spontaneously hypertensive rats (SHR), nifedipine caused a fall in blood pressure and a marked rise in CBF (138). Nitrendipine in hypertensive patients caused a fall in blood pressure with no change in CBF (137). Nimodipine (Nimotop) in patients with normal-pressure hydrocephalus caused no

change in CBF but a rise in intracranial pressure (139). In animal studies, nimodipine has been found to impair CBF autoregulation (140–142). At least one calcium antagonist has been found to cause a steal of blood away from an ischemic lesion in acute stroke (143).

Alpha-Adrenergic Blockers and Ganglionic Blockers

These drugs tend to improve autoregulation at low pressure by counteracting the weak alpha-adrenergic constrictor effect on the larger "inflow tract" cerebral resistance vessels. This has been shown in baboons with the alpha-blocker phenoxybenzamine (48), which is seldom used clinically. The ganglionic blocker trimethaphan is recommended for moderate blood pressure lowering in neurosurgical patients because it does not raise intracranial pressure (134). Alpha-blockers such as chlorpromazine (Thorazine) and labetalol (Normodyne, Trandate) are used clinically for emergency pressure lowering. Labetalol does not influence intracranial pressure in dogs, irrespective of the presence or absence of preexisting intracranial hypertension (144). Contrary to this, chlorpromazine has been found to cause an additional increase in the already increased intracranial pressure in neurosurgical patients (145).

Converting Enzyme Inhibitors

The effect of captopril on CBF has been extensively studied in rat and man. In the rat, captopril given intravenously shifted the lower limit of autoregulation toward lower pressure, as mentioned above under modulation of autoregulation (62). In patients with heart failure, captopril caused a marked fall in blood pressure with no change in CBF, suggestive of an acute shift in autoregulation toward low pressure (68). It has been proposed that these effects are mediated by a release in angiotensin-II-dependent tone of the larger resistance vessels. Intravenous administration of captopril in spontaneously hypertensive rats shifted not only the lower but also the upper limit of autoregulation toward low pressure (see Fig. 3) (62). A similar effect was seen with fosinopril and ceranapril (63,64). Autoregulation was not paralyzed, but the autoregulatory plateau was considerably shortened. In a later study in rats in which captopril was given orally, the shift of the lower limit was still present, whereas the shift of the upper limit was largely attenuated (146). In normotensive and hypertensive man, acutely given captopril caused a slight, barely significant downward shift of the lower end of the autoregulation curve as tested by lower body suction (147). Studies with moderate degrees of controlled hypertension in man have shown that the upper limit of autoregulation is not easily reached following oral captopril (147). Possible reasons for these differences between rat and man are discussed in an earlier section of this chapter. Captopril did not influence intracranial pressure in a study in patients with normal-pressure hydrocephalus (70). In patients with moderate hypertension, acute and short-term (12-week) treatment with fosinopril produced a significant reduction in blood pressure, but CBF was left unchanged (148).

Cardiac Output and Cerebral Blood Flow During Induced Hypotension

Drugs used for emergency blood pressure lowering are sometimes classified by those that lower cardiac output, such as the ganglionic blockers, and those that raise it, such as dihydralazine or diazoxide. Whereas this classification is important from the point of view of the circulation as a whole, it is of no relevance for the cerebral circulation. The cerebral circulation does not participate in the overall regulation of the circulatory system, and cardiac output only influences the cerebral circulation by way of its effect on the blood pressure. If the blood pressure is reduced acutely below the lower limit of autoregulation, CBF will decrease whether cardiac output is high or low.

Which Drug Should be Preferred for Emergency Blood Pressure Lowering?

It is easier to say what should be avoided than what should be preferred when selecting a drug for emergency blood pressure lowering. First, it should be understood that in many clinical situations, even very high blood pressures should not be lowered acutely by drugs given intravenously. If a patient is asymptomatic and a very high blood pressure is found incidentally (e.g., by routine medical checkup), a period of observation and blood pressure measurement is almost always warranted, and if it is decided that the blood pressure must be lowered, it is generally preferable to do it with conventional antihypertensive drugs given orally in moderate initial doses.

If on the other hand a hypertensive emergency is present, some advice can be given as to what should *not* be done. Cerebral vasodilators, dihydralazine (Wydase) in particular, should be given only with extreme care when a raised intracranial pressure may be present, e.g., in malignant hypertension or in acute stroke. In particular, if a patient's blood pressure is refractory to one of these drugs, dosage should not be increased indiscriminately because the combination of a paralyzed CBF autoregulation and a persistently very high blood pressure is potentially disastrous. Further, precipitous drops in blood pressure such as may be caused by "bolus dose" diazoxide should be avoided as the risk of therapy-induced

cerebral ischemia is unacceptably high. On balance, of the drugs listed above, the alpha-blockers and the converting enzyme inhibitors have the most favorable hemodynamic profile in the cerebral circulation. Angiotensin-converting enzyme (ACE) inhibitors, on the other hand, may cause unexpected drastic pressure falls in patients whose renin system is activated because of dehydration or unrecognized renovascular hypertension. Good studies in patients or animals of the effect on CBF of alpha-blockers such as labetalol are, unfortunately, not available.

Pharmacological Effects of Chronic Antihypertensive Treatment on the Cerebral Circulation

As mentioned above, chronic antihypertensive treatment may induce regression of structural vascular hypertensive changes and hence readaptation of CBF autoregulation toward normal. Whether this process is facilitated by some antihypertensive drugs more than by others is not known. As mentioned previously, readaptation has been found both with a combination of hydralazine, reserpine, and hydrochlorothiazide (88), and with the ACE-inhibitor perindopril (89). Readaptation would tend to obscure any chronic pharmacological effects of antihypertensive drugs on CBF and its regulation. Further, in SHR, it appears that during chronic treatment captopril retains its beneficial effect on the lower limit of autoregulation while the potentially harmful effect on the upper limit disappears (146). Chronic treatment with another ACE-inhibitor, cilazapril, was found in hypertensive rats to normalize cerebral vascular "reserve," i.e., the maximal attainable level of CBF (149).

The ACE-inhibitor enalapril given to chronically hypertensive patients was found to cause no change in CBF with little change in blood pressure (150). The influence of long-term treatment with the converting enzyme inhibitor captopril has been studied in two series of patients with severe congestive heart failure. In one series no changes of CBF were observed (68), whereas a 20-percent increase of CBF was observed in the other series (151).

In elderly patients, the postsynaptic alpha-1 blocker prazosin combined with hydrochlorothiazide caused an approximate 10-mm Hg fall in mean blood pressure with no change in CBF (152). Similar observations have been made with clonidine (153), the vasodilating beta-blocker carvedilol (154), and the calcium antagonists nifedipine and nitrendipine (137).

The headache sometimes seen during treatment with hydralazine or calcium antagonists would suggest a state of chronic cerebral vasodilatation, possibly with a somewhat raised intracranial pressure; this, however, has not been studied.

In What Clinical Settings Is There a Real Risk of Overtreating Hypertension and Causing Cerebral Ischemia?

Despite hypertensive adaptation of CBF autoregulation, clinical blood pressure lowering very seldom causes cerebral ischemia. On the contrary, the brain is the one organ that has benefited most from modern antihypertensive treatment. There are at least three factors contributing to explain this paradox. First, despite hypertensive adaptation of CBF autoregulation, there is in most hypertensive patients considerable scope for pressure lowering before cerebral perfusion is impaired. Thus, in an acute study in man (28), blood pressure could be reduced by about 25 percent before the lower limit of autoregulation was reached, and by about 50 percent before mild symptoms of cerebral hypoperfusion were encountered. Second, when the blood pressure falls below the lower limit of autoregulation, the brain can extract more oxygen from the blood, thereby maintaining a normal metabolism with a reduced CBF. This oxygen reserve in the blood is not available in the heart, as discussed in the final section of the present chapter. And third, as discussed earlier, CBF autoregulation may readapt itself toward normal during long-term antihypertensive treatment.

Despite these factors, overzealous antihypertensive treatment may occasionally cause cerebral ischemia. This occurs mainly in a few characteristic clinical settings, some of which should be easily recognizable.

Initial or Intensified Treatment of Severe Hypertension

A number of reports have described how overzealous blood pressure lowering in patients with very high blood pressure causes cerebral ischemia with, for example, blindness, paresis, or even death (155–159). Many different drug regimens have been given to the patients in these reports, but the "pulse dose" diazoxide appears relatively frequently. Blindness has been caused by infarction of the optic nerves (156) or occipital cortex (159). Occasionally, the cerebral lesions have the form of "border-zone" infarcts in the watershed areas between the major brain arteries (155,160,161). Stenosis of cerebral arteries may be revealed during treatment-induced hypotension as focal neurologic symptoms are provoked (162). The lesson to be learned from these reports is that reduction of blood pressure in severely hypertensive patients should be gradual and that precipitous pressure falls should be fought actively and immediately. With time, allowing for vascular readaptation to occur, patients with the most severe malignant hypertension may tolerate surprisingly low or even normal pressures.

Hypertension in the Elderly

Recent controlled trials have demonstrated a marked beneficial effect of antihypertensive treatment in elderly hypertensive patients, with large-scale prevention of stroke and heart disease (163–166). Surprisingly, even treatment of isolated systolic hypertension in the elderly results in prevention of strokes (163). These studies in fit elderly hypertensive patients, however, should not be applied uncritically in the more frail elderly, in whom the risk of overtreatment of hypertension is real. Reports on this are of an anecdotal nature (167–169), but suggest that in particular preexisting postural hypotension is a risk factor.

Patients with Transient Cerebral Ischemic Attacks of Hemodynamic Origin

The majority of transient cerebral ischemic attacks are of thromboembolic origin and are unrelated to changes in blood pressure. Occasional patients, however, have transient cerebral ischemic episodes of hemodynamic origin that are precipitated by drops in blood pressure, mostly orthostatic episodes. Here a significant stenotic lesion of an artery in the neck or of an intracranial artery feeding the brain results in a "low-pressure area" without sufficient vasodilator reserve capacity, and a blood pressure drop may cause focal ischemic symptoms (170). Antihypertensive treatment may be dangerous in such patients, and vascular surgery, including extra-intracranial bypass, is often indicated (171,172).

Hypotensive Anesthesia in Treated Hypertensive Patients

A risk of cerebral ischemia may be present when treated hypertensive patients are subjected to hypotensive anesthesia. This would apply to those patients who do not readapt their CBF autoregulation toward normal during antihypertensive treatment. At least one such case has been reported (159).

Patients with Acute Stroke and High Blood Pressure

About 50 percent of stroke patients have a history of hypertension; but in the acute phase of stroke, about 70 percent of the patients have an elevated blood pressure (99). Recommendations vary considerably as to how high blood pressure should be handled in the acute stroke patient. Hemodynamically, a fresh cerebral infarct with very low perfusion is in the early phase often surrounded by a "penumbral" zone of underperfused but viable tissue; this infarct may be surrounded by zones of hyperemia because of lactic acidosis or reperfusion of the more proximal parts of the infarction following thrombolysis (173,174). Zones of cerebral hypo- and hyperperfusion may, in fact, change within a few hours. A cerebral hemorrhage, once bleeding has stopped, may also be surrounded by ischemic and hyperemic tissue. The most severe stroke cases, both large hematomas and massive infarcts with secondary edema formation, may be accompanied by a rise in intracranial pressure. This may, in itself, threaten the cerebral circulation and its autoregulation. Cerebral perfusion pressure in such patients may be considerably lower than the blood pressure, and the patients will therefore not tolerate a blood pressure reduction otherwise judged to be desirable. Even in less severe stroke cases, acute blood pressure lowering may jeopardize perfusion in the borderline ischemic areas described above; conversely, hypertensive overperfusion of the hyperemic parts of the tissue may lead to brain edema. Very high blood pressure would also carry a risk of repeated cerebral hemorrhage or the transforming of an ischemic into a hemorrhagic infarct in case thrombolysis has occurred. It is thus not possible, on the basis of pathophysiological knowledge, to decide which blood pressure is optimal for the individual stroke patient.

There is little doubt that marked acute lowering of blood pressure in the acute stroke patient can be harmful, by worsening the symptoms and contributing to the patient's demise (99,175). This applies in particular if the patient's hypertension is transient and a consequence, rather than a cause, of the stroke. Some authors recommend moderate reduction of pressure in stroke patients (176,177), whereas others recommend a conservative approach, delaying antihypertensive treatment until the convalescent phase, when physical rehabilitation has started (178,179). The Joint Committee for Stroke Facilities of the American Heart Association (180) gives no unequivocal advice but recommends treatment of severely elevated blood pressure. It is the policy of the present authors to give antihypertensive treatment to patients with acute stroke in whom diastolic blood pressure remains at or above 130–135 mm Hg for more than a few hours after admission. If possible, antihypertensive agents are given orally. Diuretics are avoided in dehydrated patients. Otherwise, conventional antihypertensive drugs are used. Possibly, converting enzyme inhibitors are advantageous because they shift the lower limit of autoregulation toward lower pressures. If parenteral treatment is necessary, cerebral vasodilators such as dihydralazine or sodium nitroprusside should be avoided, because they may raise intracranial pressure and cause "steal" of blood away from diseased tissue. Small refractory intravenous doses of diazoxide or alpha-adrenoceptor blockers such as labetalol are recommended.

WHY DOES ANTIHYPERTENSIVE TREATMENT PREVENT STROKE BUT NOT MYOCARDIAL INFARCTION?

Although modern antihypertensive treatment effectively prevents stroke and heart failure, it has failed to influence the increased incidence of myocardial infarction associated with hypertension. It has been proposed that myocardial infarction is more directly related to atherosclerosis than to stroke and that atherosclerosis, which is accelerated by high blood pressure, is not remediable by therapeutic blood pressure lowering (181). It is, however, hard to understand why atherothrombotic infarction in the heart should have a different natural history than the same disease in the brain. For this hypothesis to be tenable it would be a prerequisite that antihypertensive treatment in particular should reduce the incidence of lacunar cerebral infarction and cerebral hemorrhage, both related to the development of hypertensive degenerative vascular changes in the brain (74,182). Whether this is the case remains uncertain, as discussed previously.

Alternatively, an explanation might be sought with regard to differences in autoregulatory capacity and blood oxygen extraction reserve in the heart and brain. It will be recalled from an earlier section of this chapter that oxygen saturation in the jugular venous blood at rest is 60–70 percent. Below the lower limit of autoregulation, cerebral oxygen metabolism can be maintained at an unchanged rate by increasing oxygen extraction from the blood until CBF is reduced by about 30 percent of the autoregulatory resting level (28). By contrast, in the coronary sinus, oxygen saturation is on the order of 30 percent (183); and if the blood pressure falls, myocardial oxidative metabolism cannot be maintained by an increased oxygen extraction from the blood. Further, in the heart, part of the vasodilatory capacity is used to counterbalance the myocardial compressive tissue pressure. This pressure is particularly high in the subendocardium, where it may reach intracavitary pressure.

Therefore, in the subendocardial myocardium, the lower end of the autoregulatory curve is shifted toward higher pressure, as compared with the subepicardium (184). In hypertension, it is possible that the shift is even more marked, since coronary vasodilatory reserve is known to be restricted even in young hypertensive patients without atherosclerosis on coronary angiography (185). Hence, the hypertensive subendocardium must be expected to be especially prone to develop ischemia when the blood pressure is lowered by drug treatment, even though pressure lowering causes a decrease in myocardial oxygen consumption. This vulnerability would be further enhanced by atherosclerotic stenoses of larger branches of the coronary arteries. On this background, it has been hypothesized that in the heart, benefit and harm of the blood pressure lowering cancel each other, whereas the brain, with its oxygen reserve in the blood, is better suited to exploit the benefit of blood pressure lowering (186).

REFERENCES

1. Kuschinsky W, Paulson OB. Capillary circulation in the brain. *Cerebrovasc Brain Metab Rev* 1992;4:261–286.
2. Kety SS, Schmidt CF. The determination of cerebral blood flow in man by the use of nitrous oxide in low concentration. *Am J Physiol* 1945;143:53–66.
3. Kety SS, Hafkenschiel JH, Jeffers WA, Leopold IH, Shenkin HA. The blood flow, vascular resistance, and oxygen consumption of the brain in essential hypertension. *J Clin Invest* 1948;27:511–514.
4. Lassen NA. Cerebral blood flow and oxygen consumption in man. *Physiol Rev* 1959;39:183–238.
5. Madsen PL, Holm S, Herning M, Lassen NA. Average blood flow and oxygen uptake in the human brain during resting wakefulness: a critical appraisal of the Kety-Schmidt technique. *J Cereb Blood Flow Metab* 1993;13:646–655.
6. Knudsen GM. Application of a double-indicator technique for measurement of blood-brain barrier permeability in humans. *Cerebrovasc Brain Metab Rev* 1994;6:1–13.
7. Olesen J, Paulson OB, Lassen NA. Regional cerebral blood flow in man determined by the initial slope of the clearance of intra-arterially injected 133Xe. Theory of the method, normal values, error of measurement, correction for remaining radioactivity, relation to other flow parameters, and response to PaCO$_2$ changes. *Stroke* 1971;2:519–540.
8. Tominaga S, Strandgaard S, Uemura K, Ito K, Kutsuzawa T, Lassen NA, et al. Cerebrovascular CO$_2$ reactivity in normotensive and hypotensive man. *Stroke* 1976;7:507–510.
9. Wahl M, Deetjen P, Thurau K, Ingvar DH, Lassen NA. Micropuncture evaluation of the importance of perivascular pH for the arteriolar diameter on the brain surface. *Pfluegers Arch Ges Physiol* 1970;316:152–163.
10. Fencl V, Vale JR, Broch JA. Respiration and cerebral blood flow in metabolic acidosis and alkalosis in humans. *J Appl Physiol* 1969;27:67–76.
11. Severinghaus JW, Chiodi H, Eger EI, Brandstater B, Hornbein TF. Cerebral blood flow in man at high altitude. Role of cerebrospinal fluid pH in normalization of low in chronic hypocapnia. *Circ Res* 1966;19:274–282.
12. Christensen MS, Brodersen P, Olesen J, Paulson OB. Cerebral apoplexy (stroke) treated with or without prolonged artificial hyperventilation: II. Cerebrospinal fluid acid-base balance and intracranial pressure. *Stroke* 1973;4:620–631.
13. Kuschinsky W, Wahl M, Bosse O, Thurau K. Perivascular potassium and pH as determinants of local pial arterial diameter in cats. A microapplication study. *Circ Res* 1972;31:240–247.
14. Paulson OB, Newman EA. Does the release of potassium from astrocyte endfeet regulate cerebral blood flow? *Science* 1987;237:896–898.
15. Wang Q, Paulson OB, Lassen NA. Is autoregulation of cerebral blood flow in rats influenced by nitro-1-arginine, a blocker of the synthesis of nitric oxide? *Acta Physiol Scand* 1992;145:297–298.
16. Iadecola C. Does nitric oxide mediate the cerebrovasodilation elicited by hypercapnia? *Proc Natl Acad Sci USA* 1992;89:3913–3916.
17. Wang Q, Paulson OB, Lassen NA. Effect of nitric oxide blockade by NG-nitro-1-arginine on cerebral blood flow response to changes in carbon dioxide tension. *J Cereb Blood Flow Metab* 1992;12:947–953.
18. Pelligrino DA, Koenig H, Albrecht RF. Nitric oxide synthesis and regional cerebral blood flow responses to hypercapnia and hypoxia in the rat. *J Cereb Blood Flow Metab* 1993;13:80–87.
19. Wang Q, Paulson OB, Lassen NA. Indomethacin abolishes cerebral blood flow increase in response to acetazolamide-induced ex-

tracellular acidosis: a mechanism for its effect on hypercapnia? *J Cereb Blood Flow Metab* 1993;13:724–727.
20. Henriksen L, Paulson OB, Lassen NA. Visual cortex activation recorded by dynamic emission computed tomography of inhaled Xenon-133. *Eur J Nucl Med* 1981;6:487–489.
21. Petersen SE, Fox PT, Snyder AZ, Raichle ME. Activation of extrastriate and frontal cortical areas by visual words and work-like stimuli. *Science* 1990;33:1041–1044.
22. Zeki S, Watson JDG, Luech CJ, Friston KJ, Kennard C, Frackowiak RSJ. A direct demonstration of functional specialization in human visual cortex. *J Neurosci* 1991;11:641–649.
23. Paulson OB, Parving HH, Olesen J, Skinhøj E. Influence of carbon monoxide and of hemodilution on cerebral blood flow and blood gases in man. *J Appl Physiol* 1973;35:111–116.
24. Henricksen L, Paulson OB, Smith RJ. Cerebral blood flow following normorolemic hemodilution in patients with high hemocrit. *Ann Neurol* 1981;9:454–457.
25. Paulson OB, Strandgaard S, Edvinsson L. Cerebral autoregulation. *Cerebrovasc Brain Metab Rev* 1990;2:161–192.
26. Strandgaard S, Olesen J, Skinhøj E, Lassen NA. Autoregulation of brain circulation in severe arterial hypertension. *Br Med J* 1973;1:507–510.
27. McHenry JLC, West JW, Cooper ES, Goldberg HI, Jaffe ME. Cerebral autoregulation in man. *Stroke* 1974;5:695–705.
28. Strandgaard S. Autoregulation of cerebral blood flow in hypertensive patients. The modifying influence of prolonged antihypertensive treatment on the tolerance to acute, drug-induced hypotension. *Circulation* 1976;53:720–727.
29. Häggendal E, Johansson B. Effects of arterial carbon dioxide tension and oxygen saturation on cerebral blood flow autoregulation in dogs. *Acta Physiol Scand* 1965;66[Suppl258]:27–53.
30. MacKenzie ET, Farrar JK, Fitch W, Graham DI, Gregory PC, Harper AM. Effects of hemorrhagic hypotension on the cerebral circulation. I: Cerebral blood flow and pial arteriolar caliber. *Stroke* 1979;10:711–718.
31. Postiglione A, Bobkiewicz T, Vinholdt-Pedersen E, Lassen NA, Paulson OB, Barry DI. Cerebrovascular effects of angiotensin converting enzyme inhibition involve large artery dilatation in rats. *Stroke* 1991;22:1362–1368.
32. Skinhøj E, Strandgaard S. Pathogenesis of hypertensive encephalopathy. *Lancet* 1973;1:461–462.
33. Strandgaard S, MacKenzie ET, Sengupta D, Rowan JO, Lassen NA, Harper AM. Upper limit for autoregulation of cerebral blood flow in the baboon with experimental renovascular hypertension. *Circ Res* 1974;34:435–440.
34. MacKenzie ET, Strandgaard S, Graham DI, Jones JV, Harper AM, Farrar JK. Effect of acutely induced hypertension in cats on pial arteriolar caliber, local cerebral blood flow and the blood-brain barrier. *Circ Res* 1976;39:33–41.
35. Westergaard E, van Deurs B, Brøndsted H. Increased vesicular transfer of horseradish peroxydase across cerebral endothelium, evoked by acute hypertension. *Acta Neuropath (Berl)* 1977;37:141–152.
36. Johansson BB. Hypertension and the blood-brain barrier. In: Neuwelt E. *Implications of the blood-brain barrier and its manipulation,* vol. 2. New York: Plenum Press, 1989:389–410.
37. Sokrad TED, Kalimo H, Olsson Y, Johansson BB. Transient hypertensive opening of the blood-brain barrier can lead to brain damage. *Acta Neuropath (Berl)* 1988;75:557–565.
38. Sadoshima S, Thames M, Heistad D. Cerebral blood flow during elevation of intracranial pressure: role of sympathetic nerves. *Am J Physiol* 1981;241[Heart Circ Physiol 10]:H78–H84.
39. Symon L, Held K, Dorsch NWC. A study of regional autoregulation in the cerebral circulation to increased perfusion pressure in normocapnia and hypercapnia. *Stroke* 1973;4:139–147.
40. Kontos HA, Wei EP, Navari RM, Levasseur JE, Rosenblum WI, Patterson JL. Responses of cerebral arteries and arterioles to acute hypotension and hypertension. *Am J Physiol* 1978;234[Heart Circ Physiol 3]:H371–383.
41. Johansson BB, Nilsson B. Cerebral vasomotor reactivity in normotensive and spontaneously hypertensive rats. *Stroke* 1979;10:572–576.
42. Aaslid R, Newell DW, Stooss R, Sorteberg W, Lindegaard KF.

43. Florence G, Seylaz J. Rapid autoregulation of cerebral blood flow: a laser-Doppler flowmetry study. *J Cereb Blood Flow Metab* 1992;12:674–680.

44. Osol G, Halpern W. Myogenic properties of cerebral blood vessels from normotensive and hypertensive rats. *Am J Physiol* 1985;249[Heart Circ Physiol 18]:H914–H921.

45. Harper AM, Deshmukh VD, Rowan JO, Jennett WB. The influence of sympathetic nervous activity on cerebral blood flow. *Arch Neurol* 1972;27:1–6.

46. Sercombe R, LaCombe P, Aubineau P, Mamo H, Pinard E, Reyneir-Rebuffel AM, et al. Is there an active mechanism limiting the influence of the sympathetic system on the cerebral vascular bed? Evidence for vasomotor escape from sympathetic stimulation in the rabbit. *Brain Res* 1979;164:81–102.

47. Busija DW, Heistad DD, Marcus ML. Effects of sympathetic nerves on cerebral vessels during acute, moderate increases in arterial pressure in dogs and cats. *Circ Res* 1980;46:696–702.

48. Fitch W, MacKenzie ET, Harper AM. Effects of decreasing arterial blood pressure on cerebral blood flow in the baboon. *Circ Res* 1975;37:550–557.

49. Bill A, Linder J. Sympathetic control of cerebral blood flow in acute arterial hypertension. *Acta Physiol Scand* 1976;96:114–121.

50. Edvinsson L, Owman C, Siesjö B. Physiological role of cerebrovascular sympathetic nerves in the autoregulation of cerebral blood flow. *Brain Res* 1976;117:518–523.

51. Gross PM, Heistad DD, Strait MR, Marcus ML, Brody MJ. Cerebral vascular responses to physiological stimulation of sympathetic pathways in cats. *Circ Res* 1979;44:288–294.

52. MacKenzie ET, McGeorge AP, Graham DI, Fitch W, Edvinsson L, Harper AM. Effects of increasing arterial pressure on cerebral blood flow in the baboon: influence of the sympathetic nervous system. *Pfluegers Arch* 1979;378:189–195.

53. Sadoshima S, Fujishima M, Yoshida F, Ibayashi S, Shiokawa O, Omae T. Cerebral autoregulation in young spontaneously hypertensive rats. Effect of sympathetic denervation. *Hypertension* 1985;7:392–397.

54. Heistad DD, Marcus ML. Effect of sympathetic stimulation on permeability of the blood-brain barrier to albumin during acute hypertension in cats. *Circ Res* 1979;45:331–338.

55. Olesen J. The effect of intracarotid epinephrine, norepinephrine and angiotensin on the regional cerebral blood flow in man. *Neurology (Minn)* 1972;22:978–987.

56. Stromberg DD, Fox JR. Pressures in the pial arterial microcirculation of the cat during changes in systemic arterial blood pressure. *Circ Res* 1972;31:229–239.

57. Baumbach GL, Heistad DD. Effects of sympathetic stimulation and changes in arterial pressure on segmental resistance of cerebral vessels in rabbits and cats. *Circ Res* 1983;52:527–533.

58. Auer LM, Ishiyama N. Pial vascular behavior during bilateral and contralateral cervical sympathetic stimulation. *J Cereb Blood Flow Metab* 1986;6:298–304.

59. Gotoh F, Fukuuchi Y, Amano T, Tanaka K, Uematsu D, Suzuki N, et al. Comparison between pial and intraparenchymal vascular responses to cervical sympathetic stimulation in cats. Part 1. Under normal resting conditions. *J Cereb Blood Flow Metab* 1986;6:342–347.

60. Hamar J, Kovach ABG, Reivich M, Nyary I, Durity F. Effect of phenoxybenzamine on cerebral blood flow and metabolism in the baboon during haemorrhagic shock. *Stroke* 1979;10:401–407.

61. Beausang-Linder M, Bill A. Cerebral circulation in acute arterial hypertension—protective effects of sympathetic nervous activity. *Acta Physiol Scand* 1981;111:193–193.

62. Barry DI, Jarden JO, Paulson OB, Graham DI, Strandgaard S. Cerebrovascular effects of converting enzyme inhibition. I: effects of intravenous captopril in spontaneously hypertensive and normotensive rats. *J Hypertens* 1984;2:589–597.

63. Waldemar G, Pedersen EV, Barry DI. Cerebral blood flow autoregulation during angiotensin converting enzyme inhibition. *J Cereb Blood Flow Metabol* 1987;7[Suppl 1]:S283.

64. Torup M, Waldemar G, Paulson OB. Ceranapril and cerebral blood flow autoregulation. *J Hypertens* 1993;11:399–405.

65. Jarden JO, Barry DI, Juhler M, Graham DI, Strandgaard S, Paulson OB. Cerebrovascular aspects of converting enzyme inhibition. II. Blood-brain barrier permeability and effect of intracerebroventricular administration of captopril. *J Hypertens* 1984;2:599–604.

66. Waldemar G, Paulson OB, Barry DI, Knudsen GM. Angiotensin converting enzyme inhibition and the upper limit of cerebral blood flow autoregulation: effect of sympathetic stimulation. *Circ Res* 1989;64:1197–1204.

67. Waldemar G. Acute sympathetic denervation does not eliminate the effect of angiotensin converting enzyme inhibition on CBF autoregulation in spontaneously hypertensive rats. *J Cereb Blood Flow Metab* 1990;10:43–47.

68. Paulson OB, Jarden JO, Vorstrup S, Holm S, Godtfredsen J. Effect of captopril on the cerebral circulation in chronic heart failure. *Eur J Clin Invest* 1986;16:124–132.

69. Waldemar G, Schmidt JF, Andersen AR, Vorstrup S, Paulson OB. Angiotensin converting enzyme inhibition and cerebral blood flow autoregulation in normotensive and hypertensive man. *J Hypertens* 1989;7:229–235.

70. Schmidt JF, Andersen AR, Paulson OB, Gjerris F. Angiotensin converting enzyme inhibition, CBF autoregulation and ICP in patients with normal-pressure hydrocephalus. *Acta Neurochirurg* 1990;106:9–12.

71. Ekstrøm-Jodal B, Häggendal E, Linder LE, Nilsson NJ. Cerebral blood flow autoregulation at high arterial pressures and different levels of carbon dioxide tension. *Eur Neurol* 1971;6:6–10.

72. Paulson OB, Olesen J, Christensen MS. Restoration of autoregulation of cerebral blood flow by hypocapnia. *Neurology (Minn)* 1972;22:286–293.

73. Charcot JM, Bouchard CH. Nouvelles recherches sur la pathogénie de l'hémorragie cérébrale. *Arch Phys (Norm Pathol)* 1868;1:110–127,643–665,725–735.

74. Russell RW. Pathological changes in small cerebral arteries causing occlusion and haemorrhage. *J Cardiovasc Pharmacol* 1984;6:S691–S695.

75. Hachinski VC, Potter P, Mershey H. Leuko-araiosis. *Arch Neurol* 1987;44:21–23.

76. Malatino LS, Bellofiore S, Costa MP, Lo Manto G, Finocchiaro F, Di Maria GU. Cerebral blood flow velocity after hyperventilation-induced vasoconstriction in hypertensive patients. *Stroke* 1992;23:1728–1732.

77. Hart MN, Heistad DD, Brody MJ. Effect of chronic hypertension and sympathetic denervation on wall/lumen ratio of cerebral vessels. *Hypertension* 1980;2:419–423.

78. Yang ST, Mayhan WG, Faraci FM, Heistad DD. Endothelium-dependent responses of cerebral blood vessels during chronic hypertension. *Hypertension* 1991;17:612–618.

79. Finnerty FAJ, Witkin L, Fazekas JF. Cerebral hemodynamics during cerebral ischemia induced by acute hypotension. *J Clin Invest* 1954;33:1227–1232.

80. Gottstein U. Physiologie und Pathophysiologie des Hirnkreislaufs. *Med Welt* 1965;15:715–726.

81. Jones JV, Fitch W, MacKenzie ET, Strandgaard S, Harper AM. Lower limit of cerebral blood flow autoregulation in the baboon. *Circ Res* 1976;39:555–557.

82. Fujishima M, Omae T. Lower limit of cerebral autoregulation in normotensive and spontaneously hypertensive rats. *Experientia* 1976;32:1019–1021.

83. Barry DI, Strandgaard S, Graham DI, Brændstrup O, Svendsen UG, Vorstrup S, et al. Cerebral blood flow in rats with renal and spontaneous hypertension: resetting of the lower limit of autoregulation. *J Cereb Blood Flow Metab* 1982;2:347–353.

84. Strandgaard S, Jones JV, MacKenzie ET, Harper AM. Upper limit of cerebral blood flow autoregulation in the baboon with experimental renovascular hypotension. *Circ Res* 1975;37:164–167.

85. Harper SL, Bohlen HG. Microvascular adaptation in the cerebral cortex of adult spontaneously hypertensive rats. *Hypertension* 1984;6:408–419.

86. Lartaud I, Bray-des-Boses L, Chillon JM, Atkinson J, Capdeville-

Atkinson C. In vivo cerebrovascular reactivity in Wistar and Fischer 344 rat strains during aging. *Am J Physiol* [Heart Circ Physiol 3 Pt 2] 1993;264:H851–H858.

87. Sivertsson R. The hemodynamic importance of structural vascular changes in essential hypotension. *Acta Physiol Scand* 1970;[Suppl 343]:1–56.

88. Vorstrup S, Barry DI, Jarden JO, Svendsen UG, Brændstrup O, Graham DI, et al. Chronic antihypertensive treatment in the rat reverses hypertension-induced changes in cerebral blood flow autoregulation. *Stroke* 1984;15:312–318.

89. Muller F, Lartaud I, Bray L, Atkinson J, Janian P, Burlet C, et al. Chronic treatment with the angiotensin I converting enzyme inhibitor, perindopril, restores the lower limit of autoregulation of cerebral blood flow in the awake renovascular hypertensive rat. *J Hypertens* 1990;8:1037–1042.

90. Shurtleff D. Some characteristics related to the incidence of cardiovascular disease and death: the Framingham Study. 18 year follow-up. *The Framingham study, an epidemiologic investigation of cardiovascular disease.* Washington: US Dept. of Health (NIH), 1974:74–559.

91. Herman B, Schmitz PIM, Leyten AC M, van Luijk JH, Frenken CW, GM, de Coul AA, WO, et al. Multivariate logistic analysis of risk factors for stroke in Tilburg, The Netherlands. *Am J Epidemiol* 1983;118:514–525.

92. Wolf PA, Kannel WB, Verter J. Current status of risk factors for stroke. *Neurol Clin* 1983;1:317–343.

93. Davis PH, Dambrosia JM, Schoenberg BS, Schoenberg DG, Pritchard DA, Lilienfeld AM, et al. Risk factors for ischemic stroke: a prospective study in Rochester, Minnesota. *Ann Neurol* 1987;22:319–327.

94. Boysen G, Nyboe J, Appleyard M, Sørensen PS, Boas J, Somnier F, et al. Stroke incidence and risk factors for stroke in Copenhagen, Denmark. *Stroke* 1988;19:1345–1353.

95. MacMahon S, Peto R, Cutler J, Collins R, Sorlie P, Neaton J, et al. Blood pressure, stroke and coronary heart disease. part 1, prolonged differences in blood pressure: prospective observational studies corrected for the regression dilution bias. *Lancet* 1990;335:765–774.

96. Brott T, Thalinger K, Hertzberg V. Hypertension as a risk factor for spontaneous intracerebral hemorrhage. *Stroke* 1986;17:1078–1083.

97. Schulte BP, Leyten AC, Herman B. Pre-stroke and immediate post-stroke hypertension: neuroepidemiological data. *Br J Clin Pract* [Symp Suppl] 1985;39:31–33.

98. Roberts WC. Frequency of systemic hypertension in various cardiovascular diseases. *Am J Cardiol* 1987;60:1E–8E.

99. Britton M, Carlsson A, de Faire U. Blood pressure course in patients with acute stroke and matched controls. *Stroke* 1986;17:861–864.

100. Fisher CM. The arterial lesions underlying lacunes. *Acta Neuropathol* (*Berl*) 1969;12:1–15.

101. Veterans Administration Cooperative Study Group on Antihypertensive agents. Effects of treatment on morbidity in hypertension. Results in patients with diastolic blood pressures averaging 115 through 129 mm Hg. *JAMA* 1967;202:1028–1034.

102. Veterans Administration Cooperative Study Group on Antihypertensive agents. Effects of treatment on morbidity in hypertension. II: Results in patients with diastolic blood pressure averaging 90 through 114 mm Hg. *JAMA* 1970;213:1143–1152.

103. Management Committee of the Australian Hypertension Trial. The Australian therapeutic trial in mild hypertension. *Lancet* 1980;1:1261–1267.

104. Medical Research Council Working Party. MRC trial of treatment of mild hypertension: principal results. *Br Med J* 1985;291:97–104.

105. Collins R, Peto R, MacMahon S, Hebert P, Fiebach NH, Eberlein KA, et al. Blood pressure, stroke and coronary heart disease, part 2, short-term reduction in blood pressure: overview of randomised drug trials in their epidemiological context. *Lancet* 1990;335:827–838.

106. Russell RWR. How does blood-pressure cause stroke? *Lancet* 1975;2:1283–1285.

107. Spence JD. Antihypertensive drugs and prevention of atherosclerotic stroke. *Stroke* 1986;17:808–810.

108. Kotila M. Declining incidence and mortality of stroke? *Stroke* 1984;15:255–259.

109. Sacco RL, Wolf PA, Bharucha NE, Meeks SL, Kannel WB, Charette LJ, et al. Subarachnoid and intracerebral hemorrhage: natural history, prognosis, and precursor factors in the Framingham Study. *Neurology* 1984;34:847–854.

110. Bonita R. Cigarette smoking, hypertension and the risk of subarachnoid hemorrhage: a population-based case-control study. *Stroke* 1986;17:831–835.

111. Kincaid-Smith P, McMichael J, Murphy EA. The clinical course and pathology of hypertension with papilloedema (malignant hypertension). *Q J Med New Series* 1958;27:117–153.

112. Oppenheimer BS, Fishberg AM. Hypertensive encephalopathy. *Arch Intern Med* 1928;41:264–278.

113. Volhart F, Fahr T. *Die Brightsche Nierenkrankheit.* Berlin: Julius Springer, 1914.

114. Ziegler DK, Zosa A, Zileli T. Hypertensive encephalopathy. *Arch Neurol* 1965;12:472–478.

115. Kussmaul A, Tenner A. Untersuchungen über der Ursprung und Wesen der fallsuchtartigen Zuckungen bei der Verblutung. *Untersuchungen zur Naturlehre der Menschen und der Tiere.* Frankfurt am Main: Meidinger, 1857:1–124.

116. Keith NM, Wagner HP, Barker NW. Some different types of essential hypertension. Their course and prognosis. *J Am Med Sci* 1939;197:332–334.

117. Byrom FB. The pathogenesis of hypertensive encephalopathy and its relation to the malignant phase of hypertension. Experimental evidence from the hypertensive rat. *Lancet* 1954;2:201–211.

118. Giese J. Acute hypertensive vascular disease. 2: studies on vascular reaction patterns and permeability changes by means of vital microscopy and colloidal tracer technique. *Acta Pathol Microbiol Scand* 1964;62:497–515.

119. Byrom FB. *The hypertensive vascular crisis. An experimental study.* London: Heinemann, 1969.

120. Farrar JK, Jones JV, Graham DI, Strandgaard S, MacKenzie ET. Evidence against cerebral vasospasm during acutely induced hypertension. *Brain Res* 1976;104:176–180.

121. Lassen NA, Agnoli A. The upper limit of autoregulation of cerebral blood flow—on the pathogenesis of hypertensive encephalopathy. *Scand J Clin Lab Invest* 1973;30:113–116.

122. Strandgaard S. Autoregulation of cerebral circulation in hypertension. *Acta Neurol Scand* 1978;57[Suppl 66]:1–82.

123. Lundgren Y. Adaptive changes of cardiovascular design in spontaneous and renal hypertension (thesis). *Acta Physiol Scand* 1974;[Suppl 408]:1–62.

124. Barry I, Strandgaard S, Graham DI, Brændstrup O, Svendsen UG, Bolwig TG. Effect of diaxozide induced hypotension on cerebral blood flow in hypertensive rats. *Eur J Clin Invest* 1983;13:201–207.

125. Barry DI, Strandgaard S. Acute effects of antihypertensive drugs on autoregulation of cerebral blood flow in spontaneously hypertensive rats. *Progr Appl Microcirc* 1985;8:206–212.

126. Goldberg HI, Codario RA, Banka RS, Reivich M. Patterns of cerebral dysautoregulation in severe hypertension to blood pressure reduction with diazoxide. *Acta Neurol Scand* 1977;56[Suppl 64]:64–65.

127. Vidt DG. Current concept in treatment of hypertension emergencies. *Am Heart J* 1986;111:220–225.

128. Schroeder T, Sillesen H. Dihydralazine induces marked cerebral vasodilatation in man. *Eur J Clin Invest* 1987;17:214–217.

129. Rowe GG, Maxwell GM, Crumpton CW. The cerebral haemodynamic response to administration of hydralazine. *Circulation* 1962;25:970–972.

130. Overgaard J, Skinhøj E. A paradoxical cerebral haemodynamic effect of hydralazine. *Stroke* 1975;6:402–404.

131. Johansson BB, Auer LM, Trummer UG. Pial vascular reaction to intravenous dihydralazine in the cat. *Stroke* 1980;11:369–371.

132. Barry DI, Strandgaard S, Graham DI, Svendsen UG, Brændstrup O, Paulson OB. Cerebral blood flow response to intravenous di-

hydralazine in renal and spontaneously hypertensive rats. *Stroke* 1984;15:102–107.

133. Henriksen L, Thorshauge C, Harmsen A, Christensen P, Sørensen M, Lester J, et al. Controlled hypotension with sodium nitroprusside: effects of cerebral blood flow and cerebral venous blood gases in patients operated for cerebral aneurysms. *Acta Anaesthesiol Scand* 1983;27:62–67.

134. Turner JM, Powell D, Gibson RM, McDowall DG. Intracranial pressure changes in neurosurgical patients during hypotension induced with sodium nitroprusside or trimethaphan. *Br J Anaesthesiol* 1977;49:419–420.

135. Keaney NP, McDowall DG, Turner JM, Lang JR, Okuda Y, Pickerodt VW, et al. Cerebral blood flow autoregulation, cerebrospinal fluid acid-base parameters and profound hypotension induced by sodium nitroprusside and deep halothane anaesthesia. In: Langfitt TW, McHenry LC, Reivich M, Wollman H. *Cerebral circulation and metabolism.* Heidelberg: Springer, 1975:21–23.

136. Henriksen L, Paulson OB. The effects of sodium nitroprusside on cerebral blood flow and cerebral venous blood gases. II. Observations in awake man during successive blood pressure reduction. *Eur J Clin Invest* 1982;12:389–393.

137. Conen D, Rüttmann S, Noll G, Schneider K, Müller J. Short- and long-term cerebrovascular effects of nitrendipine in hypertensive patients. *J Cardiovasc Pharmacol* 1988;12[Suppl 14]:S64–S68.

138. Ooboshi H, Sadoshima S, Fujii K, Yao H, Ibayashi S, Fujishima M. Acute effects of antihypertensive agents on cerebral blood flow in hypertensive rats. *Eur J Pharmacol* 1990;179:253–261.

139. Schmidt JF, Albeck M, Gjerris F. The effect of nimodipine on intracranial pressure and cerebral blood flow in patients with normal-pressure hydrocephalus. *Acta Neurochirurg* 1990;102:11–13.

140. Harris RJ, Branston NM, Symon L, Bayhan M, Watson A. The effects of a calcium antagonist, nimodipine, upon physiological responses of the cerebral vasculature and its possible influence upon focal cerebral ischaemia. *Stroke* 1982;13:759–766.

141. Gaab MR, Höllerhage HG, Zumkeller M, Trost HA. The effect of the Ca-antagonist nimodipine on cerebral blood flow autoregulation. *J Cereb Blood Flow Metab* 1987;7[Suppl 1]:S170.

142. van den Kerckhoff W, Kazda S. The autoregulation of cerebral blood flow is influenced by calcium antagonists. *J Cereb Blood Flow Metab* 1987;7[Suppl 1]:S169.

143. Vorstrup S, Andersen A, Blegvad N, Paulson OB. Calcium antagonist (PY 108-068) treatment may further decrease flow in ischemic areas in acute stroke. *J Cereb Blood Flow Metab* 1986;6:222–229.

144. van Aken H, Puchstein C, Schweppe ML, Heinecke A. Effect of labetalol on intracranial pressure in dogs with and without intracranial hypertension. *Acta Anaesth Scand* 1982;26:615–619.

145. Hirose S, Handa Y, Kobayashi H, Kawano H, Nozaki J, Hayashi M. Effects of antihypertensive drugs on intracranial hypertension. *Zentralbl Neurochirurg* 1991;52:69–75.

146. Pedersen EV, Bobkiewicz-Kozlowska T, Barry DI. Cerebrovascular effects of chronic antihypertensive treatment with captopril in spontaneously hypertensive rats. *Eur J Clin Invest* 1987;17:A38.

147. Andersen AR, Vorstrup S, Ibsen H, Schmidt J, Paulson OB, Waldemar G. Converting enzyme inhibition and the autoregulation of cerebral circulation in hypertension and stroke. *Eur J Clin Invest* 1987;17:A19.

148. Waldemar G, Ibsen H, Strandgaard S, Paulson OB, Andersen AR, Rasmussen S. The effect of fosinopril sodium on cerebral blood flow in moderate essential hypertension. *Am J Hypertens* 1990;3:464–470.

149. Clozel J-P, Kuhn H, Helfi F. Effects of cilazapril on the cerebral circulation in spontaneously hypertensive rats. *Hypertension* 1989;14:645–651.

150. Frei A, Müller-Brand J. Cerebral blood flow and antihypertensive treatment with enalapril. *J Hypertens* 1986;4:365–367.

151. Rajagopalan B, Raine AEG, Cooper R, Ledingham JGG. Changes in cerebral blood flow in patients with severe congestive cardiac failure before and after captopril treatment. *Am J Med* 1984;76(5B):86–90.

152. Ram CVS, Meese R, Kaplan NM, Devous MD, Bonte FJ, Cutler

RE. Antihypertensive therapy in the elderly. Effects on blood pressure and cerebral blood flow. *Am J Med* 1987;82[Suppl 1A]:53–57.

153. Guell A, Le Traon AP, Chatellier G, Bes A. Effects of clonidine on cerebral blood flow in hypertensive patients. *Curr Ther Res* 1991;49:801–806.

154. Kuriyama Y, Nakamura M, Kyougoku I, Sawada T. Effects of carvedilol on cerebral blood flow and its autoregulation in previous stroke patients with hypertension. *Eur J Clin Pharmacol* 1990;38:S120–S121.

155. Graham DI, McGeorge A, Fitch W, Jones JV, MacKenzie ET. Ischaemic brain damage induced by rapid lowering of arterial pressure in hypertension. *J Hypertens* 1984;2:297–304.

156. Cove BH, Seddom M, Fletcher RF, Dukes DC. Blindness after treatment for malignant hypertension. *Br Med J* 1979;2:245–246.

157. Ledingham JGG, Rajagopalan B. Cerebral complications in the treatment of accelerated hypertension. *Q J Med New Series* 1979;48:25–41.

158. Hulse JA, Taylor DSI, Dillon MJ. Blindness and paraplegia in severe childhood hypertension. *Lancet* 1979;2:553–556.

159. Strandgaard S, Andersen GS, Ahlgreen P, Nielsen PE. Visual disturbances and occipital brain infarct following acute, transient hypotension in hypertensive patients. *Acta Med Scand* 1984;216:417–422.

160. Graham DI. Ischaemic brain damage of cerebral perfusion failure type after treatment of severe hypertension. *Br Med J* 1975;4:739.

161. Brierley JB, Brown AW, Excell BJ, Meldrum BS. Brain damage in the rhesus monkey resulting from profound arterial hypotension. I. Its nature, distribution and general physiological correlates. *Brain Res* 1969;13:68–100.

162. Jensen H, Ring-Larsen H, Garsdal P, Fruergaard P. Carotid artery stenosis exposed by an adverse effect of captopril. *Br Med J* 1986;293:1073–1074.

163. SHEP, Cooperative Research Group. Prevention of stroke by antihypertensive drug treatment in older persons with isolated systolic hypertension. Final results of the systolic hypertension in the elderly program. *JAMA* 1991;265:3255–3264.

164. MRC Working Party. Medical Research Council trial of treatment of hypertension in older adults: principal results. *Br Med J* 1992;304:405–412.

165. Dahlöf B, Lindholm LH, Hansson L, Scherstén B, Ekbom T, Wester PO. Morbidity and mortality in the Swedish trial in old patients with hypertension (STOP-hypertension). *Lancet* 1991;338:1281–1285.

166. Amery A, Brixko P, Clement D, et al. Mortality and morbidity results from the European Working Party on High Blood Pressure in the Elderly. *Lancet* 1985;1:1349–1354.

167. Hankey GJ, Gubbay SS. Focal cerebral ischaemia and infarction due to antihypertensive therapy. *Med J Austr* 1987;146:412–414.

168. Jackson G, Pierscianowski TA, Mahon W, Condon J. Inappropriate antihypertensive therapy in the elderly. *Lancet* 1976;2:1317–1318.

169. Jansen PAF, Gribnau FWJ, Schultz BPM, Poels EFJ. Contribution of inappropriate treatment for hypertension to pathogenesis of stroke in the elderly. *Br Med J* 1986;293:914–917.

170. Ruff RL, Talman WT, Petito F. Transient ischemic attacks associated with hypotension in hypertensive patients with carotid artery stenosis. *Stroke* 1981;12:353–355.

171. Vorstrup SV, Lassen NA, Henriksen L, Haase J, Lindewald H, Boysen G, et al. CBF before and after extracranial-intracranial bypass surgery in patients with ischemic cerebrovascular disease studied with 133Xe-inhalation tomography. *Stroke* 1985;16:616–626.

172. Vorstrup S. Tomographic cerebral blood flow measurements in patients with ischemic cerebrovascular disease and evaluation of the vasodilatory capacity by the acetazolamide test. *Acta Neurol Scand* 1988;77[Suppl 114]:1–47.

173. Paulson OB. Cerebral apoplexy (stroke). Pathogenesis, pathophysiology and therapy as illustrated by regional blood flow measurements in the brain. *Stroke* 1971;2:327–360.

174. Olsen TS. Regional cerebral blood flow after occlusion of the middle cerebral artery. *Acta Neurol Scand* 1986;73:321–337.

175. Lavin P. Management of hypertension in patients with acute stroke. *Arch Intern Med* 1986;146:66–68.
176. Gottstein U, Seel AW. Antihypertensive therapy in stroke patients. *Acta Neurol Scand* 1977;56[Suppl 64]:174–175.
177. Spence JD, del Maestro RF. Hypertension in acute ischemic stroke. Treat. *Arch Neurol* 1985;42:1000–1002.
178. Bannan LT, Beevers DG, Jackson SD, Wright N. ABC of blood pressure reduction. Special problems. *Br Med J* 1980;281:1200–1202.
179. Yatsu FM, Zivin J. Hypertension in acute ischemic strokes. Not to treat. *Arch Neurol* 1985;42:999–1000.
180. American Heart Association. Report of the Joint Committee for Stroke Facilities. VII. Medical and surgical management of stroke. *Stroke* 1973;4:270–309.
181. Oliver MF. What are we trying to prevent by controlling hypertension? *Am Heart J* 1987;114:1011–1013.
182. Russell RWR. Observations on intracranial aneurysms. *Brain* 1963;86:425–442.
183. Klocke FJ, Mates RE, Copley DP, Orlick AE. Physiology of the coronary circulation in health and coronary artery disease. *Symposium on coronary circulation.* Philadelphia: Lea & Febiger, 1976;7:1.
184. Haunsø S. Lower limits of blood flow autoregulation in different myocardial layers of the left ventricular free wall of dogs. *Acta Physiol Scand* 1981;112:349–350.
185. Strauer BE. Structural and functional adaptation of the chronically overloaded heart in arterial hypertension. *Am Heart J* 1987;114:948–957.
186. Strandgaard S, Haunsø S. Why does antihypertensive treatment prevent stroke but not myocardial infarction? *Lancet* 1987;2:658–661.

Hypertension: Pathophysiology, Diagnosis, and Management, Second Edition, edited by J.H. Laragh and B.M. Brenner, Raven Press, Ltd., New York © 1995.

CHAPTER **29**

Hypertension and Stroke

Stephen J. Phillips and Jack P. Whisnant

Stroke is the most devastating complication of hypertension. This chapter reviews the evidence implicating hypertension as a risk factor for stroke, examines the role of hypertension in the pathogenesis of stroke, and discusses antihypertensive therapy with regard to the primary prevention of stroke, blood pressure management during the acute phase of stroke, and the prevention of stroke recurrence.

HYPERTENSION AS A RISK FACTOR FOR STROKE

Epidemiologic Evidence

The Framingham Heart Disease Epidemiology Study (1)—the first and longest-running prospective population-based study of the determinants of cardiovascular and cerebrovascular morbidity and mortality—has provided much of the epidemiologic evidence incriminating hypertension as the most important modifiable risk factor for stroke. The Framingham Study cohort comprises a random sample (and some volunteers) of the adults who were resident in the town in 1948 and who were free of cardiovascular disease (including stroke) when examined in 1950. These 5,127 men and women aged 30–62 have since received a standardized biennial cardiovascular evaluation that includes a history, three blood pressure readings, a physical examination, and several ancillary investigations.

Stroke data have been reported for 14 (2), 18 (3), 24 (4), 26 (5), and 30 (6) years of follow-up. Diagnosis of stroke type has been largely based on findings from clinical examination, lumbar puncture, and autopsy. Cerebral angiography was performed on some patients—especially those with suspected intracranial hemorrhage—and computerized tomographic (CT) brain scanning has been performed on patients in recent years (5,6). The investigators defined five categories of stroke: atherothrombotic brain infarction; intracerebral hemorrhage; subarachnoid hemorrhage; (cardiogenic) cerebral embolism; and transient ischemic attack (1).

After 24 years, 85 percent of the Framingham cohort had taken each exam and 3 percent had been lost to follow-up (4). A total of 345 strokes had occurred, 60 percent of them categorized as atherothrombotic brain infarction. The risk of brain infarction was positively associated with blood pressure throughout its range, there being no evidence of a critical pressure below which stroke did not occur (Figs. 1, 2). At 18 years of follow-up (3), definite hypertension (blood pressure ≥ 160/95 mm Hg) was associated with a relative risk of stroke of 2.7 for

S. J. Phillips: Department of Medicine, Dalhousie University, Halifax, Nova Scotia, Canada.

J. P. Whisnant: Departments of Health Sciences Research and Neurology and the Cerebrovascular Research Center, Mayo Clinic, Rochester, Minnesota 55905.

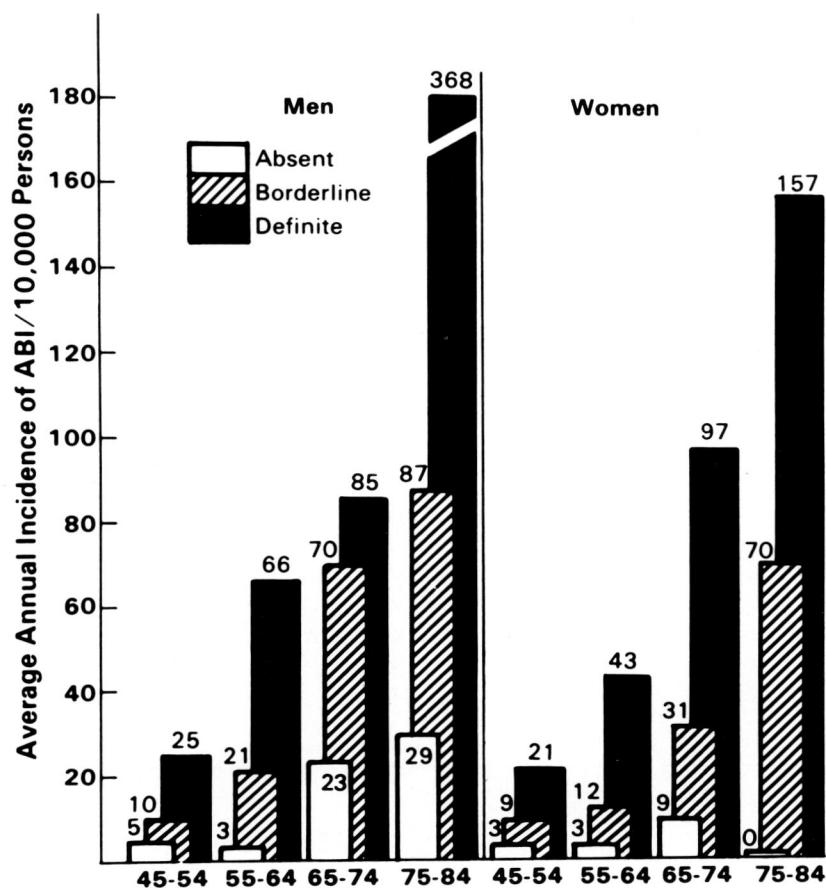

FIG. 1. Hypertension and risk of athero-thrombotic brain infarction (ABI) in men and women participating in the Framingham Study (24 years of follow-up). Definite hypertension refers to systolic pressure ≥ 160 and/or diastolic ≥ 95 mm Hg; absent hypertension refers to blood pressure < 140/90 mm Hg; borderline hypertension refers to all intermediary values. (From ref. 4, with permission.)

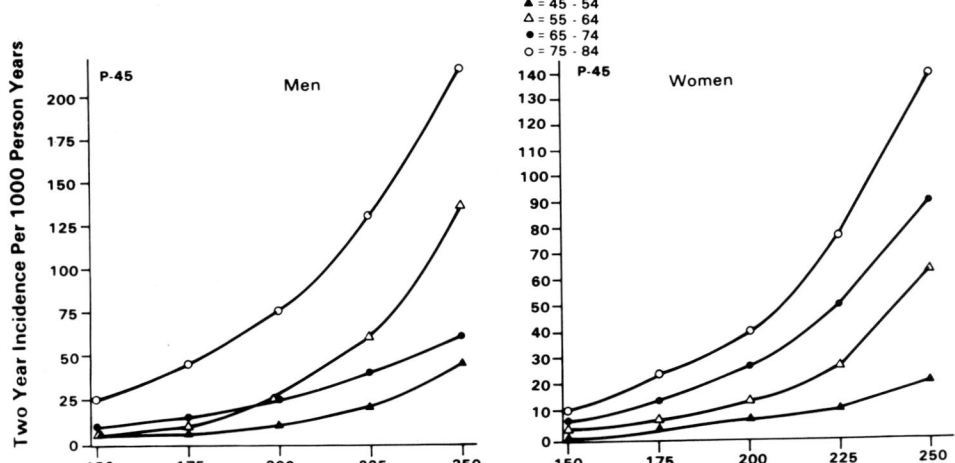

FIG. 2. Incidence of atherothrombotic brain infarction, according to systolic blood pressure (mm Hg) (*abscissa*) and age, in men and women participating in the Framingham Study (24-years follow-up). (From ref. 4, with permission.)

men and 2.3 for women, after multivariate adjustment for age, serum cholesterol, cigarette smoking, left ventricular hypertrophy, and glucose intolerance. Systolic pressure was more closely linked to the incidence of atherothrombotic brain infarction than other components of blood pressure such as diastolic pressure, pulse pressure, and mean arterial pressure (4,7,8). Among subjects aged 65–84 years, isolated systolic hypertension (systolic pressure ≥ 160 and diastolic < 95 mm Hg) was associated with at least a twofold increased risk of brain infarction (4).

Several other population-based case-control studies and cohort studies conducted in different parts of the world have confirmed that hypertension is the most important modifiable risk factor for stroke (9–20). A statistical overview (21) of nine major prospective observational studies showed that prolonged decreases in usual diastolic blood pressure of 5, 7.5 and 10 mm Hg were respectively associated with at least 34 percent, 46 percent, and 56 percent less stroke. Comparisons of Japanese men living in Japan with those living in Hawaii (19), and of black and white Americans living in the same region (22–24), suggest that genetic, dietary, or other factors may modify the deleterious cerebrovascular effects of chronically elevated blood pressure.

Study of the population of Rochester, Minnesota, has provided a different perspective of the association between hypertension and stroke. Medical care for residents of Rochester and the surrounding area has been centered at the Mayo Clinic since the beginning of this century. Each patient's medical record contains a master sheet that lists all diagnoses for that patient, whether made in a hospital, in an outpatient clinic, at a home visit, or at autopsy (25). These diagnoses are coded and entered into a computer file which allows retrieval of all cases of stroke or stroke-related disorder in the popula-

tion. This medical records and records-linkage system has provided the only available data concerning temporal trends for the incidence of stroke in North America (26). Cerebral thrombosis and embolism (collectively, cerebral infarction), intracerebral hemorrhage, subarachnoid hemorrhage, and stroke of unknown type have been defined according to clinical criteria, findings at lumbar puncture, and findings at autopsy (27).

The incidence of stroke of all types, in both sexes, was relatively constant between 1935 and 1954 (28). After 1954, incidence rates among women gradually declined, but among men there was little change until 1969 when rates began to decline sharply (28). There was a 46 percent decline in incidence rates for both sexes through the 1970s (29,30), and a 17 percent increase in the early 1980s (31). Study of population-based controls, matched to cases who had their first stroke during the period 1950 through 1979, showed that the prevalence of diastolic pressure greater than or equal to 105 mm Hg fell 26 percent in men and 70 percent in women from 1950 to 1959 and 1970 to 1979 (32). Prevalence of diastolic pressures in the range of 95–104 mm Hg decreased 5 percent in men and 58 percent in women. The incidence of stroke was four times higher among hypertensive individuals (systolic pressure ≥ 160 or diastolic pressure ≥ 95 mm Hg on at least one occasion) than among normotensives (33). Increasing control of hypertension had an almost inverse linear relationship with the decreasing incidence of stroke in women, but the incidence of stroke in men did not decrease until 10 years after the improvement in blood pressure control began (Fig. 3). The data suggest that improvements in the detection and control of hypertension contributed to the decline of stroke in Rochester, but the cause of the delay in the fall of incidence rates for men is unknown. The cause of the recent increase in the incidence of stroke has not been fully ex-

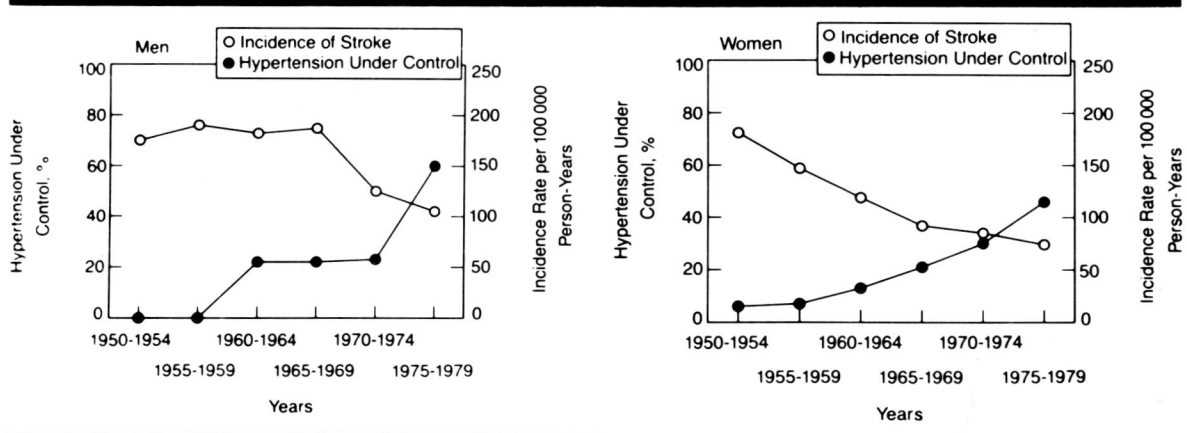

FIG. 3. Average annual incidence rates (adjusted for age to 1950 US white population) for stroke in Rochester, Minnesota, and percentage of men (*left*) and women (*right*) with hypertension under control (diastolic blood pressure < 95 mm Hg) in consecutive 5-year periods, 1950–1979. (From ref. 32, with permission.)

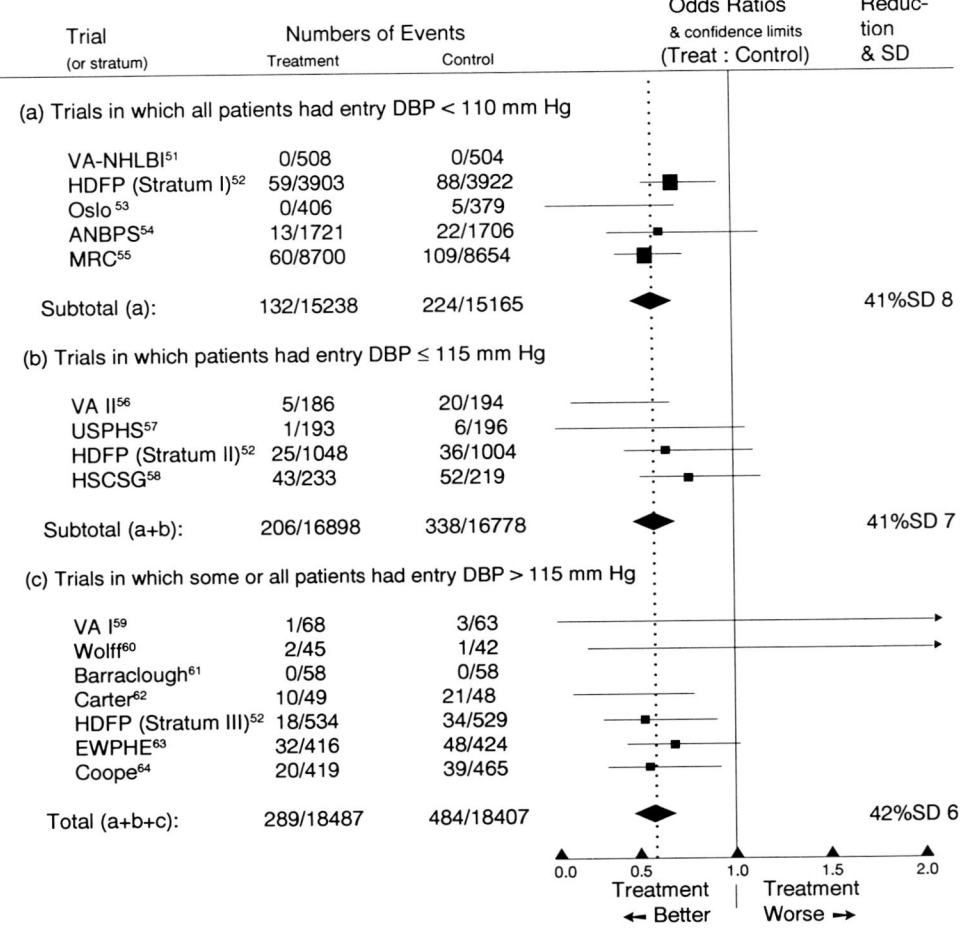

Trial (or stratum)	Numbers of Events		Odds Ratios & confidence limits (Treat : Control)	Reduction & SD
	Treatment	Control		

(a) Trials in which all patients had entry DBP < 110 mm Hg

VA-NHLBI[51]	0/508	0/504		
HDFP (Stratum I)[52]	59/3903	88/3922		
Oslo[53]	0/406	5/379		
ANBPS[54]	13/1721	22/1706		
MRC[55]	60/8700	109/8654		
Subtotal (a):	132/15238	224/15165		41%SD 8

(b) Trials in which patients had entry DBP ≤ 115 mm Hg

VA II[56]	5/186	20/194		
USPHS[57]	1/193	6/196		
HDFP (Stratum II)[52]	25/1048	36/1004		
HSCSG[58]	43/233	52/219		
Subtotal (a+b):	206/16898	338/16778		41%SD 7

(c) Trials in which some or all patients had entry DBP > 115 mm Hg

VA I[59]	1/68	3/63		
Wolff[60]	2/45	1/42		
Barraclough[61]	0/58	0/58		
Carter[62]	10/49	21/48		
HDFP (Stratum III)[52]	18/534	34/529		
EWPHE[63]	32/416	48/424		
Coope[64]	20/419	39/465		
Total (a+b+c):	289/18487	484/18407		42%SD 6

0.0 0.5 1.0 1.5 2.0

Treatment ← Better | Treatment Worse →

FIG. 4. Effects on stroke in the unconfounded randomized trials of antihypertensive drug treatment. Solid squares represent the odds ratios (treatment:control) in each trial, and the sizes of the squares are proportional to amount of information contributed by that study; 99 percent confidence intervals (for individual trials) (*lines*) and 95 percent intervals (for overviews of trials) are denoted by diamonds. (From ref. 50, with permission.)

plained either, although increased case-ascertainment due to CT scanning may have contributed (31). The increase in incidence occurred despite improvement in blood-pressure control in the population (34), indicating that the effect of hypertension control on stroke incidence has limitations, and that other (unknown) factors have contributed (35,36). Similarly, studies of temporal trends in stroke *mortality* (37) suggest that improvement in blood pressure control is responsible for only a small proportion of the reduction in rates observed in the US (38) and other westernized countries in recent decades (39).

Epidemiologic data concerning stroke subtypes are more difficult to ascertain than information about stroke in general. Hypertension was identified as an important precursor of primary intracerebral hemorrhage in the Framingham cohort (5) and in the population of Rochester (40). Temporal trends in the incidence of primary intracerebral hemorrhage in Rochester have mirrored those for all stroke. For spontaneous subarachnoid hem-

orrhage (which is usually due to rupture of an intracranial aneurysm), the status of hypertension as a risk factor remains uncertain because of conflicting evidence from epidemiological, clinical, and laboratory studies (41–48). Some of the discrepancy may be due to the difficulties in distinguishing the effects of factors that induce aneurysm formation from those that cause rupture. In the population of Rochester, the incidence of subarachnoid hemorrhage has remained stable (49) in the face of substantial declines in the incidence of all stroke and the prevalence of hypertension.

Evidence from Antihypertensive Treatment Trials

An overview analysis of 14 randomized trials of antihypertensive pharmacotherapy was reported recently (50). The analysis pooled data from 37,000 individuals who were treated (chiefly with thiazide diuretics or beta blockers) for an average of 5 years. Diastolic blood pressure differed by an average of 5–6 mm Hg between the treated and untreated groups. Stroke was reduced by 42 percent (95 percent confidence interval, 33–50 percent) (Fig. 4). Since this overview analysis was published, three more large randomized placebo-controlled trials have been reported (65–67). All three studied only older hypertensive adults (each trial used a slightly different definition of "old" and "hypertension"), and showed that active treatment (thiazide diuretic and/or a beta blocker) reduced the occurrence of stroke by 25–47 percent.

ROLE OF HYPERTENSION IN THE PATHOGENESIS OF STROKE

The brain receives its blood supply via two arterial systems that arise from the anterior cerebral, middle cerebral, posterior cerebral, and basilar arteries: (a) small-diameter end-arteries that supply the phylogenetically older, medial and basal portions of the brain and brainstem (the "vascular centrencephalon") (68); and (b) larger circumferential arteries supplying the newer structures. Strokes that occur in the territories of these two systems have different but overlapping clinical and pathologic features. At least some of this heterogeneity may be due to the different effects that hypertension has on large and small cerebral arteries. In this section we discuss these effects and their role in the pathogenesis of cerebral infarction and intracerebral hemorrhage. The experimental evidence implicating hypertension in the development, growth, and rupture of intracranial saccular (berry) aneurysms has been reviewed recently (47), and will not be further discussed. Binswanger's disease is considered separately.

Large-Vessel Disease

Atherosclerosis, a noninflammatory, multifocal disease of unknown cause that affects large and medium-sized arteries, is commonly found in the cervical and cerebral arteries of persons who have had a stroke, and tends to be more frequent and more severe in hypertensives than in normotensives (69). The typical atherosclerotic lesion, or plaque, consists of an accumulation of intimal, lipid-laden smooth-muscle cells, surrounded by lipid, collagen, elastic fibers, and proteoglycans. Together, the cells and extracellular matrix components form a fibrous cap that covers a large, deeper deposit of free extracellular lipid intermixed with cell debris. Plaques tend to occur at sites of arterial branching or tortuosity. In the cerebral circulation, the sites of predilection are the bifurcations of the common carotid arteries, the carotid siphons, the origins of the vertebral arteries, the basilar artery, the circle of Willis and the proximal parts of the cerebral arteries (70). Lesions in the aorta, proximal to the origins of the great vessels, also cause

cerebral ischemia in some patients (71). Atherosclerotic plaques develop over many years. They usually produce symptoms only when they become complicated by necrosis, calcification, thrombosis, or hemorrhage. Cerebral ischemia may be caused by partial or complete occlusion of an artery by such a plaque, or by embolization of atherothrombotic debris from a plaque. Infarction produced by these mechanisms (atherothromboembolism) characteristically involves the cerebral or cerebellar cortex (Fig. 5A). The deeper structures of the vascular centrencephalon may be involved as well if the infarct is large, or if a penetrating branch vessel is blocked by an embolus, or if a penetrating vessel is occluded at its origin by a plaque in the wall of the parent artery. This latter scenario may be especially likely to occur in the pons, which is supplied by small penetrating vessels that arise directly from the atherosclerosis-prone basilar artery (72,73). The precise frequency of stroke due to atherothromboembolism is unknown because: (a) the clinical and pathological features of this form of cerebral infarction are nonspecific; (b) patients often harbor more than one condition with the potential to cause stroke; and (c) our means of delineating the pathophysiologic events that occur at the time of a stroke are rather limited.

Epidemiologic evidence indicates that hypertension is associated with an increased frequency of complications of atherosclerosis (74,75). The relationship between hypertension and atherosclerosis has been studied in experimental animals, but in none has it been possible to exactly replicate the pattern and severity of the cerebral artery involvement seen in man (76). According to the response-to-injury hypothesis of atherogenesis, sustained endothelial damage results in plaque formation by promoting a complex series of interactions between the exposed subendothelial connective tissue and circulating low-density lipoprotein particles, platelets, and monocytes (77). Elevated blood pressure is thought to contribute to this process by damaging the arterial endothelium (78,79). However, there is disagreement regarding the exact mechanisms by which this occurs. Hypertension also induces medial hypertrophy and other alterations in the walls of large and medium-sized arteries (76,80,81). These changes protect the cerebral microcirculation from the deleterious effects of high blood pressure by increasing cerebral vascular resistance (82). Paradoxically, they may also predispose to focal cerebral ischemia by impairing the response of cerebral blood vessels to vasodilator stimuli (83).

Prospective, randomized antihypertensive treatment trials have shown a rather modest 14 percent (95 percent confidence interval, 4–22 percent) reduction in the occurrence of atherosclerotic coronary heart disease (50). This contrasts sharply with the substantial reduction in stroke (50) (see Fig. 4) which occurred within just a few years of blood pressure lowering, even among chronically hypertensive elderly subjects (65–67) who would be

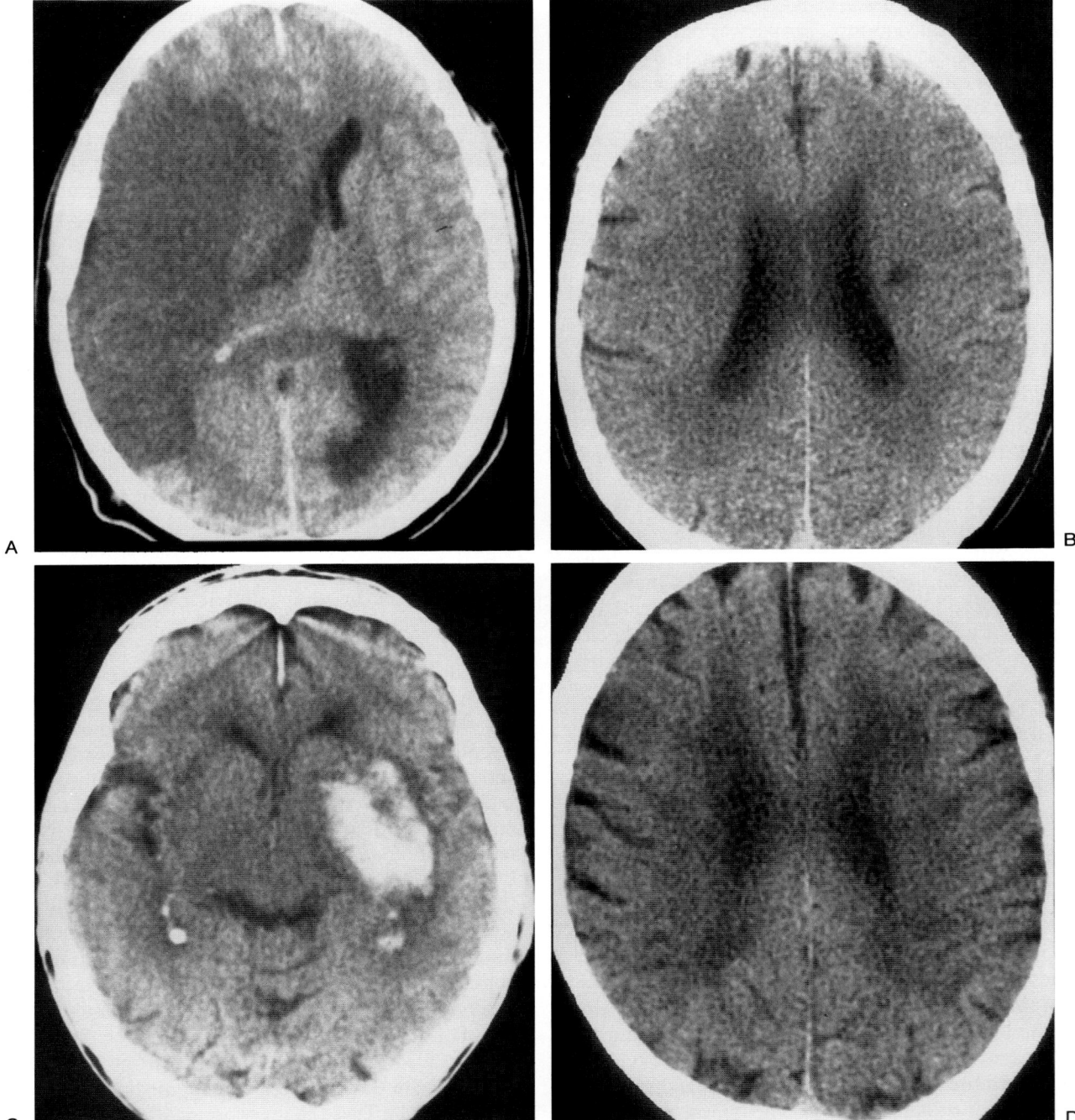

FIG. 5. Computed tomographic images of brain lesions caused by hypertension-associated cerebral vascular disease: **A:** large, middle cerebral artery territory infarct caused by atherothrombotic occlusion of the proximal internal carotid artery; **B:** small, deep (lacunar) infarct in the corona radiata caused by occlusion of a penetrating end-artery; **C:** basal ganglia hemorrhage caused by rupture of a penetrating end-artery; and **D:** diffuse periventricular white matter rarefaction (leuko-araiosis) associated with arteriolosclerosis of the penetrating end-arteries.

expected to have advanced irreversible structural arterial disease. These observations suggest that the impact of antihypertensive therapy on stroke was not mediated solely through an effect on atherothromboembolic mechanisms. The disparate effects of antihypertensive treatment on stroke and coronary heart disease may be better explained by differences in the physiologic regulatory mechanisms of the cerebral and myocardial circulations and their dynamic adaptation to changes in perfusion pressure (84).

Small-Vessel Disease

Disease of the penetrating cerebral end-arteries is the principal cause of small, deep infarcts (lacunes) (Fig. 5B) (69,85,86), and an important cause of primary intracerebral hemorrhage (Fig. 5C) (87). Population-based studies indicate that lacunar infarction accounts for 10–20 percent of first strokes, and intracerebral hemorrhage for about 10 percent (31,88–90).

The association of hypertension with primary intracerebral hemorrhage has long been known. A large-scale autopsy study carried out at the Office of the Chief Medical Examiner of the state of Maryland during the years 1951 to 1967 showed that hypertension-associated hemorrhages occurred at the following sites (listed in descending order of frequency): basal ganglia, pons, thalamus, cerebellum, and deep hemispheric white matter (91). Lacunar infarcts are similarly distributed and are frequently observed in the brains of patients who die from primary intracerebral hemorrhage (69). Clinically, small hemorrhages and lacunar infarcts may be indistinguishable (90,92). A study of intracerebral hemorrhage in Greater Cincinnati in 1988 (93), showed that 60 percent of all (fatal and nonfatal) hemorrhages occurred in the basal ganglia, thalamus, pons, and cerebellum. The remaining 40 percent were located more superficially in the cerebral hemispheres (lobar hemorrhages). The prevalence of prestroke hypertension was about the same among the cases of lobar hemorrhage as among the cases of deep hemorrhages.

Although the small-diameter penetrating end-arteries that supply the vascular centrencephalon would seem to be particularly vulnerable to the deleterious effects of elevated blood pressure since they arise directly from main arterial trunks (94)—an arrangement that is unique to the cerebral circulation—the existence of a unique cerebrovascular lesion attributable to hypertension remains in question (95). Furthermore, we understand little about the mechanisms by which hypertension-accelerated cerebral small-vessel damage occurs or the factors that influence whether hemorrhage or infarction occurs in the territory of a diseased vessel.

Charcot and Bouchard (96), on the basis of observations made in autopsy material at L'Hopital de la Salpe-

trière in 1886, first proposed that microaneurysm rupture leads to intracerebral hemorrhage. Studies by Ross Russell (97), Cole and Yates (98), and Fisher (87) later provided more evidence to support this hypothesis. Ross Russell (97) postulated that: (a) massive hemorrhage is most likely to result if a microaneurysm ruptures early in its development; (b) if rupture does not occur when the elastic lamina of the parent vessel is breached, the aneurysm wall becomes stretched and thickened, and the lumen occluded by thrombus; (c) involvement of the parent vessel by the thrombotic process may result in a small area of softening (infarction) in the distribution of the aneurysmal artery. Other investigators have since provided evidence that this latter mechanism is a cause of lacunar infarction (99,100).

However, a recent report (101) disputes the significance and prevalence of microaneurysms, suggesting that these lesions were artifacts of the injection technique used to demonstrate them. Challa et al. (101) used a histochemical stain that labeled endothelial cells with a radiodense precipitate. Microradiographs of sections from brains of 35 hypertensive and 20 normotensive patients showed no aneurysms; instead, the vessels contained many tight coils and twists. If the lumen of such a coil is filled with contrast medium, an X-ray of the overlapping loop could be misinterpreted as showing a solid structure that would be called an aneurysm. Further studies will be required to resolve this controversy.

Fisher coined the terms *lipohyalinosis* and *microatheroma* to describe other pathological changes in the small penetrating cerebral arteries of patients with hypertension and stroke (87,99,102,103). Lipohyalinosis was first recognized by European investigators who gave it a confusing variety of names: fibrinoid necrosis, hyaline arterionecrosis, atherosclerosis of small arteries, hyaline fatty change, plasmatic vascular destruction, hyalinosis, angionecrosis, fibrinoid arteritis, and—in its chronic healed stage—segmental arterial disorganization (87, 99). Lipohyalinosis affects arteries less than 200 microns in diameter and is characterized by loss of the normal arterial architecture, subintimal hyaline deposition, infiltration by fatty macrophages or foam cells, and perivascular accumulation of monocytes (99). Microatheroma affects arteries 400–900 microns in diameter and is characterized by focal plaques of macrophages or foam cells (103). Although histologically distinct from the fibrolipid plaques of classic atherosclerosis, these "tiny beads of atheroma" (103) have been postulated to be the small-vessel equivalent of the plaques found in large and medium-sized arteries. Lipohyalinosis is thought to be the arteriopathy underlying small (often asymptomatic) lacunes, whereas microatheroma causes larger symptomatic lacunar infarcts (103).

It should be noted that Fisher's postulates were based on observations made in a few cases, and that similar vascular lesions are seen in normotensives. Lipohyalinosis is probably a close cousin of the hypertensive lesions seen elsewhere in the body, rather than a hypertensive lesion unique to the brain (95). Epidemiologic data indicate that prestroke hypertension is no more prevalent among patients with lacunar infarcts (small-vessel territory stroke) than it is among those with large-vessel territory stroke caused by presumed atherothromboembolic mechanisms (104).

Hypertension, then, may best be regarded as having an aggravating and accelerating, but nonspecific, influence on degenerative cerebrovascular disease. The apparent vulnerability of the cerebral circulation to the deleterious effects of elevated blood pressure is most likely due to pathophysiologic as well as pathoanatomic factors.

Binswanger's Disease

The nosological status of "subcortical arteriosclerotic encephalopathy," or Binswanger's disease (105), is controversial. Traditionally considered a complication of elevated blood pressure, Binswanger's disease is being diagnosed with increased frequency (106) despite the decline in the prevalence of hypertension (107).

The confusion stems from Binswanger's original description, in 1894, of a disease which he named "encephalitis subcorticalis chronica progressiva" (108). (This article was translated and critically reviewed by Olszewski in 1962 [109]). In eight patients he observed a slowly progressive dementing illness accompanied by focal neurologic symptoms and signs—a rather nonspecific clinical picture. The one patient he described in detail had a history of syphilis. Macroscopic examination of this patient's brain showed enlargement of the temporal and parietooccipital horns of the lateral ventricles, with corresponding loss of white matter, and preservation of the cerebral cortex. No histological examination was reported. Comments regarding the cerebral vasculature were confined to the arteries at the base of the brain which showed "only insignificant, isolated whitish plaques." Eight years later, in a review of various clinical and pathologic forms of cerebral arteriosclerosis, Alzheimer stated that Binswanger's encephalitis subcorticalis chronica progressiva was "caused by a particularly severe arteriosclerosis of the long vessels of the deep white matter with intense atrophy of the white matter of the cerebral hemispheres" (109,110). In a report of a single case published in 1920, Nissl (109,111) gave the first histological description of the arteriosclerotic lesions. The features were those of hypertensive arteriolosclerosis. Affected vessels were found both in the foci of white matter degeneration and in normal white matter.

Based on the opinions of the majority of the early authors, and without attempting to define the disease in clinical terms, Olszewski (109) proposed that the term *subcortical arteriosclerotic encephalopathy* (Bin-

swanger's type) be used to describe a form of cerebral arteriosclerosis that predominantly affects the vessels of the white matter and subcortical gray substance. More recently, the emphasis on the pathological changes in the blood vessels has shifted to the white matter. Symmetrical involvement of the white matter of the occipital lobes and periventricular regions has been reported most frequently (105,112). The lesions are multifocal, have irregular edges, are interspersed with normal-looking white matter, and consistently spare the subcortical U-fibers (105,112). Various microscopic changes have been described: swollen myelin sheaths; loss of myelin and oligodendroglia with relative preservation of axons; and cystic change resulting from destruction of both axons and myelin (105,112). Astrocytic gliosis is almost invariably present and may be quite prominent (105,112). The pathogenesis of these lesions is uncertain. It has been postulated that they result from chronic ischemia caused by arteriolosclerosis of the long perforating arteries to the white matter (113–115). Others have argued that if this were so, the subcortical U-fibers would be expected to bear the brunt of the insult rather than being spared (116).

The clinical features of Binswanger's disease have not been clearly defined. Dementia and the subacute accumulation of focal, usually bilateral, neurologic symptoms and signs (particularly motor signs and pseudobulbar palsy) over a period of weeks to months have been considered characteristic (113). However, this clinical picture could be produced by the multiple lacunar infarctions which frequently coexist with the white matter changes (105,109,112,113,116). "Characteristic" pathologic changes have been described in a patient without any clinical evidence of a neurologic or psychiatric disorder (114), and in a patient with documented normotension (117), but such cases are exceptional.

The term *leuko-araiosis* (106) (Greek for "white-matter rarefaction") was coined to describe the appearance of diffuse white-matter changes on CT (Fig. 5D) and nuclear magnetic resonance imaging scans. The prevalence of leuko-araiosis increases with age (118,119). In the Dutch TIA trial (120), which involved patients with transient ischemic attacks or minor strokes, those who had leuko-araiosis on CT scan were 7 years older, more often had hypertension, and had a higher risk of subsequent stroke than patients with normal white matter. The neuropsychologic correlates of leuko-araiosis are of particular interest currently because of the resurgence of interest in vascular dementia (121). Some investigators have found that white matter changes are associated with cognitive impairment (122–124), while others have not (114,125–127). Such discrepancies are probably explicable on the basis of selection bias, different definitions of cognitive impairment, interobserver variation in the definition of the white matter changes, and the heterogeneity of the underlying histopathological changes.

Hypertension has been postulated to play a pathogenetic role in the development of periventricular white matter lesions by promoting arteriolosclerosis, which in turn impairs cerebral blood flow autoregulation, thereby rendering the periventricular white matter vulnerable to ischemia, particularly during periods of relative hypotension (113,114,128). Then, if chronic low-grade white-matter ischemia, or zones of "incomplete infarction" (128), were to interrupt a sufficient number of association pathways in the periventricular regions, a detectable change in cognition would be expected (129). However, it should be pointed out that these theories have not been substantiated. In fact, in the Systolic Hypertension in the Elderly Program (65), in which patients under active treatment experienced an average reduction in systolic blood pressure of nearly 26 mm Hg and in diastolic blood pressure of more than 9 mm Hg, the incidence of dementia in the active treatment and placebo groups was not significantly different.

ANTIHYPERTENSIVE THERAPY AND STROKE

Primary Prevention

The evidence implicating hypertension as a major modifiable risk factor for stroke is incontrovertible (130). Antihypertensive treatment is beneficial to men and women of all ethnic groups, and to patients with isolated systolic hypertension, as well as those with diastolic hypertension. The challenge is in getting the treatment to the people. Rose (131,132) conceptualized a "high-risk" strategy (treatment of hypertensive individuals), and a mass strategy aimed at reducing the population mean blood pressure. These complementary but different approaches to the patient and to the population have been reviewed recently by the National High Blood Pressure Education Program (133,134). In the past, interventions have been targeted mainly at young and middle-aged adults, yet the prevalence of hypertension (107) and the incidence of stroke (31) are greatest in the elderly. Recent studies indicating the efficacy of antihypertensive treatment in older adults highlight the need for a specific approach to the management of hypertension in this segment of society (65–67,135–137).

Management of Hypertension during the Acute Phase of Stroke

Cerebral Infarction

In a recent report (138), the Emergency Cardiac Care Committee and Subcommittees of the American Heart Association recommended that antihypertensive drugs be used "rarely and cautiously" in acute ischemic stroke

(139). The vagueness of this recommendation stems from the fact that there has been only one very small prospective randomized trial of antihypertensive treatment in this setting (140). Consequently, we do not know the relative risks and benefits of antihypertensive treatment in patients who present with an acute ischemic stroke, or whether one antihypertensive agent is better than another.

Severe hypertension during acute ischemic stroke is an indicator of poor prognosis (141), but there is no convincing evidence that rapid lowering of elevated blood pressure is beneficial in this situation. On the contrary, there are several published reports of patients in whom neurological deterioration was associated with precipitous falls in blood pressure induced by emergency antihypertensive treatment (142,143). Although cerebral blood flow was not measured in these patients, it is generally assumed that neurological deterioration occurred because blood pressure dropped below the lower limit of cerebral blood-flow autoregulation and caused more widespread cerebral hypoperfusion. The frequency of this occurrence in clinical practice has not been established.

The risk of causing harm, together with the lack of evidence of benefit, and knowledge that elevated blood pressure settles spontaneously in a few days (144), suggest that rapid lowering of blood pressure is best avoided during the acute phase of an uncomplicated ischemic stroke (145,146). However, given the quality of the evidence, the absence of proof of benefit does not mean that antihypertensive therapy is of no value. Some clinical investigators (147–149) have argued persuasively in favor of aggressive blood pressure management (particularly if the diastolic pressure is in excess of 120 mm Hg) to attenuate edema formation and reduce the risk of hemorrhage into ischemic brain. In addition, there may be co-morbid conditions present, such as aortic dissection or acute myocardial ischemia, that would require antihypertensive treatment in their own right.

The clinician who elects to treat a hypertensive stroke patient next has to decide which drug to use and how far to lower the blood pressure. Two recent reviews (150,151) of the management of hypertensive urgencies and emergencies recommended sodium nitroprusside as the drug of first choice, and labetalol (Normodyne, Trandate), diazoxide, or nifedipine (Adalat, Procardia) as alternatives. Most authorities (147,150,151) agree that mean arterial blood pressure (calculated as diastolic pressure plus one-third of the pulse pressure) should be reduced by about 20–25 percent over 24 hours. This recommendation is largely based on the results of a study (152) of global cerebral blood flow in 22 hypertensive patients and 10 normotensive controls which showed that mean arterial blood pressure could be reduced by about 25 percent before the lower limit of autoregulation was reached, and by about 50 percent before symptoms of cerebral hypoperfusion occurred. The 24-hour time frame is somewhat arbitrary; positron emission tomography has shown that cerebral blood flow is unstable for the first few days after stroke onset (153).

Intracerebral Hemorrhage

Again, there are inadequate data, and controversy reigns (154–156). Acute intracerebral hemorrhage is frequently accompanied by very severe systemic hypertension and elevated intracranial pressure. Sodium nitroprusside may increase intracranial pressure by causing cerebral vasodilation. Therefore, labetalol is the preferred antihypertensive agent in this situation. Monitoring intracranial pressure helps ensure that adequate cerebral perfusion pressure is maintained when the blood pressure is lowered. Head-positioning, hyperventilation, mannitol, furosemide (Lasix), and ventricular drainage may be used to control intracranial pressure. Surgical evacuation of the hematoma may be performed in some cases. However, superiority of one form of treatment over another has not been convincingly demonstrated (157), and optimal management remains controversial. Patients with small, uncomplicated intracerebral hemorrhages probably do not require emergency hypotensive therapy.

Subarachnoid Hemorrhage

The Cooperative Aneurysm Study (158,159) showed that elevated blood pressure was associated with an increased rate of rebleeding during the 30-day period after the initial rupture. However, induced hypotension may predispose to vasospasm and secondary ischemic brain damage. Hypertension may increase the risk of rebleeding if the aneurysm has not been repaired, but reduce the risk of vasospasm postrepair (160). The competing risks of rebleeding and vasospasm influence many facets of the management of the patient with a recent aneurysmal subarachnoid hemorrhage; decisions regarding the treatment of blood pressure are no exception (161). Nimodipine, a cerebroselective dihydropyridine calcium antagonist, improves outcome after subarachnoid hemorrhage, but this effect is probably not mediated through an effect on systemic blood pressure (162).

Prevention of Stroke Recurrence

There are conflicting data concerning the relationship between stroke recurrence rates and the presence and management of hypertension. In summary, antihypertensive therapy appears to be more effective in the primary prevention of stroke than in the prevention of stroke recurrence. This is probably because blood pressure was not normalized in a substantial proportion of the patients in the published studies.

In the Framingham Study (163), the cumulative 5-year recurrence rate for atherothrombotic brain infarction was 42 percent for men and 24 percent for women. Rates were reduced by excluding from the analyses patients who—before their first stroke—were hypertensive (blood pressure ≥ 160/95 mm Hg on two separate examinations), and who had combined hypertension and coronary heart disease and/or congestive heart failure.

In Rochester, Minnesota (164), stroke recurrence rates remained stable at around 5 percent per year between 1950 and 1979, in contrast to the decline in initial stroke incidence rates during this time (30). Neither level of blood pressure in the year before the first stroke, nor management of hypertension in the year afterward, had any apparent effect on stroke recurrence rates throughout the period of follow-up.

Data from the hospital-based Lehigh Valley Stroke Register suggest that hypertension ranks below transient ischemic attack (TIA), coronary heart disease, and diabetes as a risk factor for stroke recurrence (165).

Two randomized controlled trials have examined the efficacy of poststroke antihypertensive therapy (58,62). In the British study reported in 1970 by Barham Carter (62), 99 patients with either diastolic (≥110 mm Hg) or systolic (≥160 mm Hg) hypertension and probable cerebral infarction were randomly assigned to drug therapy or to no treatment. After 2–6 years of follow-up, the stroke recurrence rate in the treated group was approximately 50 percent lower than that in the untreated group (10 vs. 21 strokes). Actuarial methods were not used to analyze the data. The other trial (58), performed in the US, was placebo-controlled and involved 452 patients with diastolic hypertension (90–115 mm Hg) and a recent history of stroke or TIA. The net reduction in diastolic pressure in the active treatment group was 12 mm Hg. After an average of 3 years of follow-up, there was a nonsignificant (probably because of the small sample size) difference in the number of strokes and TIAs in the active treatment and placebo groups (37 vs. 42). However, congestive heart failure was significantly less frequent in the active treatment group.

CONCLUSIONS

Hypertension is a major risk factor for cerebral infarction and intracerebral hemorrhage. Treatment of even mild hypertension substantially lowers the probability of stroke occurrence, but the best means of optimizing blood-pressure control in the general population are not yet clear. Elevated blood pressure appears to predispose to stroke through effects on the small-diameter penetrating cerebral arteries and by aggravating atherosclerosis. The factors that precipitate stroke in the territory of a vessel damaged by hypertension have not been fully elucidated. Further understanding of these mechanisms may lead to a much-needed expansion of our prophylactic armamentarium—"prevention is still the key to an important impact on stroke incidence, morbidity and mortality" (166).

ACKNOWLEDGMENT

Doctor Phillips receives support from the W. Garfield Weston Foundation, Toronto, Ontario, Canada.

REFERENCES

1. Dawber TR. *The Framingham Study: the epidemiology of atherosclerotic disease.* Cambridge: Harvard University Press, 1980.
2. Kannel WB, Wolf PA, Verter J, McNamara PM. Epidemiologic assessment of the role of blood pressure in stroke: the Framingham Study. *JAMA* 1970;214:301–310.
3. Shurtleff D. Some characteristics related to the incidence of cardiovascular disease and death: the Framingham Study. 18 year follow-up. In: Kannel WB, Gordon T, eds. *The Framingham Study, an epidemiological investigation of cardiovascular disease,* Publication (NIH) 74-599. Washington, DC: US Dept. of Health, Education, and Welfare, 1974;Section 30.
4. Wolf PA, Kannel WB, Verter J. Current status of risk factors for stroke. *Neurol Clin* 1983;1:317–343.
5. Sacco RL, Wolf PA, Bharucha NE, et al. Subarachnoid and intracerebral hemorrhage: natural history, prognosis, and precursive factors in the Framingham Study. *Neurology* 1984;34:847–854.
6. Wolf PA, Kannel WB, Cupples LA, D'Agostino RB. Risk factor interaction in cardiovascular and cerebrovascular disease. In: Furlan AJ, ed. *The heart and stroke: exploring mutual cerebrovascular and cardiovascular issues.* Berlin: Springer-Verlag, 1987; 331–355.
7. Kannel WB, Dawber TR, McGee DL. Perspectives on systolic hypertension: the Framingham Study. *Circulation* 1980;61: 1179–1182.
8. Kannel WB, Wolf PA, McGee DL, Dawber TR, McNamara P, Castelli WP. Systolic blood pressure, arterial rigidity, and the risk of stroke: the Framingham Study. *JAMA* 1981;245:1225–1229.
9. Herman B, Leyten AC, van Luijk JH, Frenken CW, Op de Coul AA, Schulte BP. An evaluation of risk factors for stroke in a Dutch community. *Stroke* 1982;13:334–339.
10. Salonen JT, Puska P, Tuomilehto J, Homan K. Relation of blood pressure, serum lipids, and smoking to the risk of cerebral stroke: a longitudinal study in eastern Finland. *Stroke* 1982;13:327–333.
11. Welin L, Svardsudd K, Wilhelmsen L, Larsson B, Tibblin G. Analysis of risk factors for stroke in a cohort of men born in 1913. *N Engl J Med* 1987;317:521–526.
12. Okada H, Horibe H, Ohno Y, Hayakawa N, Aoki N. A prospective study of cerebrovascular disease in Japanese rural communities, Akabane and Asahi. Part I. Evaluation of risk factors in the occurrence of cerebral hemorrhage and thrombosis. *Stroke* 1976;7:599–607.
13. Ueshima H, Iida M, Shimamoto T, et al. Multivariate analysis of risk factors for stroke. Eight-year follow-up study of farming villages in Akita, Japan. *Preventive Med* 1980;9:722–740.
14. Tanaka H, Ueda Y, Hayashi M, et al. Risk factors for cerebral hemorrhage and cerebral infarction in a Japanese rural community. *Stroke* 1982;13:62–73.
15. Tanaka H, Hayashi M, Date C, et al. Epidemiologic studies of stroke in Shibata, a Japanese provincial city: preliminary report on risk factors for cerebral infarction. *Stroke* 1985;16:773–780.
16. Kagan A, Popper JS, Rhoads GG. Factors related to stroke incidence in Hawaiian Japanese men: the Honolulu Heart Study. *Stroke* 1980;11:14–21.
17. Stemmerman GN, Hayashi T, Resch JA, Chung CS, Reed DM, Rhoads GG. Risk factors related to ischemic and hemorrhagic cerebrovascular disease at autopsy: the Honolulu Heart Study. *Stroke* 1984;15:23–28.
18. Kagan A, Popper JS, Rhoads GG, Yano K. Dietary and other risk factors for stroke in Hawaiian Japanese men. *Stroke* 1985;16: 390–396.
19. Takeya Y, Popper JS, Shimizu Y, Kato H, Rhoads GG, Kagan A. Epidemiologic studies of coronary heart disease and stroke in Japanese men living in Japan, Hawaii and California: incidence of stroke in Japan and Hawaii. *Stroke* 1984;15:15–23.
20. Boysen G, Nyboe J, Appleyard M, et al. Stroke incidence and risk factors for stroke in Copenhagen, Denmark. *Stroke* 1988;19: 1345–1353.
21. MacMahon S, Peto R, Cutler J, et al. Blood pressure, stroke, and coronary artery disease. Part 1, prolonged differences in blood pressure: prospective observational studies corrected for the regression dilution bias. *Lancet* 1990;335:765–774.
22. Ostfeld AM, Shekelle RB, Klawans H, Tufo HM. Epidemiology of stroke in an elderly welfare population. *Am J Public Health* 1974;64:450–458.
23. Heyman A, Karp HR, Heyden S, et al. Cerebrovascular disease in the biracial population of Evans County, Georgia. *Arch Intern Med* 1971;128:949–955.
24. Gross CR, Kase CS, Mohr JP, Cunningham SC, Baker WE. Stroke in South Alabama: Incidence and diagnostic features—a population based study. *Stroke* 1984;15:249–255.
25. Kurland LT, Molgaard CA. The patient record in epidemiology. *Sci Am* 1981;245:54–63.
26. Malmgren R, Warlow C, Bamford J, Sandercock P. Geographical and secular trends in stroke incidence. *Lancet* 1987;2:1196–1200.
27. Matsumoto N, Whisnant JP, Kurland LT, Okazaki H. Natural history of stroke in Rochester, Minnesota, 1955 through 1969: an extension of a previous study, 1945 through 1954. *Stroke* 1973;4: 20–29.
28. Homer D, Whisnant JP, Schoenberg BS. Trends in the incidence rates of stroke in Rochester, Minnesota, since 1935. *Ann Neurol* 1987;22:245–251.
29. Garraway WM, Whisnant JP, Furlan AJ, Phillips LH II, Kurland LT, O'Fallon WM. The declining incidence of stroke. *N Engl J Med* 1979;300:449–452.
30. Garraway WM, Whisnant JP, Drury I. The continuing decline in the incidence of stroke. *Mayo Clin Proc* 1983;58:520–523.
31. Broderick JP, Phillips SJ, Whisnant JP, O'Fallon WM, Bergstrahl EJ. Incidence rates of stroke in the eighties: the end of the decline in stroke? *Stroke* 1989;20:577–582.
32. Garraway WM, Whisnant JP. The changing pattern of hypertension and the declining incidence of stroke. *JAMA* 1987;258:214–217.
33. Davis PH, Dambrosia JM, Schoenberg BS, et al. Risk factors for ischemic stroke: a prospective study in Rochester, Minnesota. *Ann Neurol* 1987;22:319–327.
34. Phillips SJ, Whisnant JP, O'Fallon WM, Hickman RD. A community blood pressure survey: Rochester, Minnesota, 1986. *Mayo Clin Proc* 1988;63:691–699.
35. Ebrahim S. *Clinical epidemiology of stroke.* New York: Oxford University Press, 1990.
36. Bonita R. Epidemiology of stroke. *Lancet* 1992;339:342–344.
37. Bonita R, Beaglehole R. Cerebrovascular disease. Explaining stroke mortality trends. *Lancet* 1993;341:1510–1511.
38. Klag MJ, Whelton PK, Seidler AJ. Decline in US stroke mortality. Demographic trends and antihypertensive treatment. *Stroke* 1989;20:14–21.
39. Bonita R, Stewart AW. International trends in stroke mortality: 1970–1985. *Stroke* 1990;21:989–992.
40. Furlan AJ, Whisnant JP, Elveback LR. The decreasing incidence of primary intracerebral hemorrhage: a population study. *Ann Neurol* 1979;5:367–373.
41. McCormick WF, Schmalstieg EJ. The relationship of arterial hypertension to intracranial aneurysms. *Arch Neurol* 1977;34:285–287.
42. Wiebers DO, Whisnant JP, O'Fallon WM. The natural history of

unruptured intracranial aneurysms. *N Engl J Med* 1981;304:696–698.

43. de la Monte S, Moore GW, Monk MA, Hutchins GM. Risk factors for the development and rupture of intracranial berry aneurysms. *Am J Med* 1985;78:957–964.

44. Longstreth WT, Koepsell TD, Yerby MS, van Belle G. Risk factors for subarachnoid hemorrhage. *Stroke* 1985;16:377–385.

45. Bonita R. Cigarette smoking, hypertension and the risk of subarachnoid hemorrhage: A population-based case-control study. *Stroke* 1986;17:831–835.

46. Wiebers DO, Whisnant JP, Sundt TM Jr, O'Fallon WM. The significance of unruptured intracranial saccular aneurysms. *J Neurosurg* 1987;66:23–29.

47. Stehbens WE. Etiology of intracranial berry aneurysms. *J Neurosurg* 1989;70:823–831.

48. Knekt P, Reunanen A, Aho K, et al. Risk factors for subarachnoid hemorrhage in a longitudinal population study. *J Clin Epidemiol* 1991;44:933–939.

49. Ingall TJ, Whisnant JP, Wiebers DO, O'Fallon WM. Has there been a decline in subarachnoid hemorrhage mortality? *Stroke* 1989;20:718–724.

50. Collins R, Peto R, MacMahon S, et al. Blood pressure, stroke, and coronary heart disease. Part 2, short-term reductions in blood pressure: overview of randomised drug trials in their epidemiological context. *Lancet* 1990;335:827–838.

51. Perry HM, Goldman AI, Lavin MA, et al. Evaluation of drug treatment in mild hypertension: VA-NHLBI feasibility trial. *Ann NY Acad Sci* 1978;304:267–292.

52. Daugherty SA, Berman R, Entwhisle G, Haerer AF. Cerebrovascular events in the Hypertension Detection and Follow-up Program. *Prog Cardiovasc Dis* 1986;29(3 Suppl 1):63–72.

53. Helgeland A. Treatment of mild hypertension: a five year controlled drug trial. The Oslo study. *Am J Med* 1980;69:725–732.

54. Report by the Management Committee. The Australian therapeutic trial in mild hypertension. *Lancet* 1980;1:1261–1267.

55. Medical Research Council Working Party. MRC trial of treatment of mild hypertension: principal results. *Br Med J* 1985;291:97–104.

56. Veterans Administration Cooperative Study Group on Antihypertensive Agents. Effects of treatment on morbidity in hypertension II. Results in patients with diastolic blood pressure averaging 90 through 114 mm Hg. *JAMA* 1970;213:1143–1152.

57. US Public Health Service Hospitals Cooperative Study Group, Smith WM. Treatment of mild hypertension: results of a ten-year intervention trial. *Circ Res* 1977;40(Supp I):I-98–I-105.

58. Hypertension-Stroke Cooperative Study Group. Effect of antihypertensive treatment on stroke recurrence. *JAMA* 1974;229:409–418.

59. Veterans Administration Cooperative Study Group on Antihypertensive Agents. Effects of treatment on morbidity in hypertension: results in patients with diastolic blood pressures averaging 115 through 129 mm Hg. *JAMA* 1967;202:116–122.

60. Wolff FW, Lineman RD. Effects of treatment in hypertension: results of a controlled study. *J Chron Dis* 1966;19:227–240.

61. Barraclough M, Bainton D, Cochranee AL, et al. Control of moderately raised blood pressure: report of a co-operative randomised controlled trial. *Br Med J* 1973;3:434–436.

62. Barham Carter A. Hypotensive therapy in stroke survivors. *Lancet* 1973;1:1407–1409.

63. Amery A, Birkenhager W, Brixko P, et al. Mortality and morbidity results from the European Working Party on High Blood Pressure in the Elderly trial. *Lancet* 1985;1:1349–1354.

64. Coope J, Warrender TS. Randomised trial of treatment of hypertension in the elderly in primary care. *Br Med J* 1986;293:1145–1151.

65. SHEP Cooperative Research Group. Prevention of stroke by antihypertensive drug treatment in older persons with isolated systolic hypertension: final results of the Systolic Hypertension the Elderly Program (SHEP). *JAMA* 1991;265:3255–3264.

66. Dahlöf B, Lindholm LH, Scherstén B, Ekbom T, Wester P-O. Morbidity and mortality in the Swedish Trial in Old Patients with Hypertension. *Lancet* 1991;338:1281–1285.

67. MRC Working Party. Medical Research Council trial of treatment of hypertension in older adults: principal results. *Br Med J* 1992;304:405–412.

68. Hachinski V, Norris JW. *The acute stroke.* Philadelphia: Davis, 1985;27–40.

69. Fisher CM. Lacunes: small, deep cerebral infarcts. *Neurology* 1965;15:774–784.

70. Lie JT. Pathology of occlusive disease of the extracranial arteries. In: Sundt TM Jr, ed. *Occlusive cerebrovascular disease: diagnosis and surgical management.* Philadelphia: Saunders, 1987;19–37.

71. Karalis DG, Chandrasekaran K, Victor MF, Ross JJ Jr, Mintz GS. Recognition and embolic potential of intra-aortic atherosclerotic debris. *J Am Coll Cardiol* 1991;17:73–78.

72. Fisher CM, Caplan LR. Basilar artery branch occlusion: a cause of pontine infarction. *Neurology* 1971;21:900–905.

73. Fisher CM. Bilateral occlusion of basilar artery branches. *J Neurol Neurosurg Psychiat* 1977;40:1182–1189.

74. Kannel WB, Sorlie P. Hypertension in Framingham. In: Paul O, ed. *Epidemiology and control of hypertension.* New York: Stratton, 1975;553–592.

75. Robertson WB, Strong JP. Atherosclerosis in persons with hypertension and diabetes mellitus. *Lab Invest* 1968;18:538–551.

76. Graham DI. Hypoxia and vascular disorders. In: Hume Adams J, Corsellis JAN, Duchen LW, eds. *Greenfield's neuropathology,* 5th edition. New York: Oxford University Press, 1992;153–268.

77. Ross R. The pathogenesis of atherosclerosis—an update. *N Engl J Med* 1986;314:488–498.

78. Chobanian AV. The influence of hypertension and other hemodynamic factors in atherogenesis. *Prog Cardiovasc Dis* 1983;26:177–196.

79. Grady PA. Pathophysiology of extracranial cerebral arterial stenosis—a critical review. *Stroke* 1984;15:224–236.

80. Chobanian AV. Hypertension, antihypertensive drugs, and atherogenesis: mechanisms and clinical implications. *J Clin Hypertens* 1986;3:148S–157S.

81. Baumbach GL, Heistad DD. Remodeling of cerebral arterioles in chronic hypertension. *Hypertension* 1989;13:968–972.

82. Baumbach GL, Heistad DD. Cerebral circulation in chronic arterial hypertension. *Hypertension* 1988;12:89–95.

83. Faraci FM, Heistad DD. Regulation of large cerebral arteries and cerebral microvascular pressure. *Circ Res* 1990;66:8–17.

84. Strandgaard S, Paulson OB. Hypertensive disease and the cerebral circulation. In: Laragh JH, Brenner BM, eds. *Hypertension: pathophysiology, diagnosis, and management.* New York: Raven Press, 1990;399–416.

85. Fisher CM. Lacunar strokes and infarcts: a review. *Neurology* 1982;32:871–876.

86. Pullicino PM. Pathogenesis of lacunar infarcts and small deep infarcts. In: Pullicino PM, Caplan LR, Hommel M, eds. *Advances in Neurology,* Vol. 62. New York: Raven Press, 1993;125–140.

87. Fisher CM. Pathological observations in hypertensive cerebral hemorrhage. *J Neuropathol Exp Neurol* 1971;30:536–550.

88. Sacco SE, Whisnant JP, Broderick JP, Phillips SJ, O'Fallon WM. Epidemiologic characteristics of lacunar infarcts in a population. *Stroke* 1991;22:1236–1241.

89. Bamford J, Sandercock P, Dennis M, et al. A prospective study of acute cerebrovascular disease in the community: The Oxfordshire Community Stroke Project 1981–1986. *J Neurol Neurosurg Psychiatry* 1988;51:1373–1380.

90. Bamford J, Sandercock P, Jones L, Warlow C. The natural history of lacunar infarction: the Oxfordshire Community Stroke Project. *Stroke* 1987;18:545–551.

91. Freytag E. Fatal hypertensive intracerebral hematomas: a survey of the pathological anatomy of 393 cases. *J Neurol Neurosurg Psychiatry* 1968;31:616–620.

92. Mori E, Tabuchi M, Yamadori A. Lacunar syndrome due to intracerebral hemorrhage. *Stroke* 1985;16:454–459.

93. Broderick JP, Brott T, Tomsick T, Leach A. Lobar hemorrhage in the elderly. The undiminishing importance of hypertension. *Stroke* 1993;24:49–51.

94. Hughes W. The origin of lacunes. *Lancet* 1965;2:19–21.

95. Ostrow PT, Miller LL. Pathology of small artery disease. In: Pullicino PM, Caplan LR, Hommel M, eds. *Advances in Neurology,* Vol. 62. New York: Raven Press, 1993;93–123.

96. Charcot JM, Bouchard C. Nouvelles recherches sur la pathogenie

de l'hemorrhagie cerebrale. *Arch Physiol Norm Pathol* 1868;1: 110–127, 643–665, 725–734.

97. Ross Russell RW. Observations on intracerebral aneurysms. *Brain* 1963;86:425–442.

98. Cole FM, Yates PO. The occurrence and significance of intracerebral micro-aneurysms. *J Path Bact* 1967;93:393–411.

99. Fisher CM. The arterial lesions underlying lacunes. *Acta Neuropathol (Berl)* 1969;12:1–15.

100. Benhaiem-Sigaux N, Gherardi R, Salama J, Gray F, Amouroux J, Poirier J. Thrombosis of a saccular microaneurysm causing cerebral (pontine) lacunae. *Acta Neuropathol (Berl)* 1986;69:332–336.

101. Challa VR, Moody DM, Bell MA. The Charcot-Bouchard aneurysm controversy: impact of a new histopathologic technique. *J Neuropathol Exp Neurol* 1992;51:264–271.

102. Fisher CM. Cerebral miliary aneurysms in hypertension. *Am J Pathol* 1972;66:313–324.

103. Fisher CM. Capsular infarcts: the underlying vascular lesions. *Arch Neurol* 1979;36:65–73.

104. Lodder J, Boiten J. Incidence, natural history, and risk factors in lacunar infarction. In: Pullicino PM, Caplan LR, Hommel M, eds. *Advances in Neurology,* Vol. 62. New York: Raven Press, 1993;213–227.

105. van Swieten JC, Caplan LR. Binswanger's disease. In: Pullicino PM, Caplan LR, Hommel M, eds. *Advances in Neurology,* Vol. 62. New York: Raven Press, 1993;193–211.

106. Hachinski VC, Potter P, Merskey H. Leuko-araiosis. *Arch Neurol* 1987;44:21–23.

107. National Center for Health Statistics, Drizd T, Dannenberg AL, Engel A. Blood pressure levels in persons 18–74 years of age in 1976–80, and trends in blood pressure from 1960 to 1980 in the United States. *Vital and health statistics,* Series 11, no. 234. DHHS publication no (PHS)86-1684. Public Health Service. Washington, DC: US Government Printing Office, July 1986.

108. Binswanger O. Die Abgrenzung der allgemeinen progressiven Paralyse. (Referate erstattet auf der Jahresversammlung des Vereins Deutscher Irrenarzte zu Dresden am 20 September, 1894.) *Berl Klin Wochschr* 1894;31:1103–1105; 1137–1139; 1180–1186.

109. Olszewski J. Subcortical arteriosclerotic encephalopathy: review of the literature on the so-called Binswanger's disease and presentation of two cases. *World Neurol* 1962;3:359–375.

110. Alzheimer A. Die Seelenstorungen auf arteriosklerotischer Grundlage. *Z Psychol* 1902;59:695–711.

111. Nissl F. Zur Kasuistik der Arteriosklerotischen Demenz. (Ein Fall von sog. "Encephalitis subcorticalis"). *Z Neurol Psychol* 1920;19: 438–453.

112. Babikian V, Ropper AH. Binswanger's disease: a review. *Stroke* 1987;18:2–12.

113. Caplan LR, Schoene WC. Clinical features of subcortical arteriosclerotic encephalopathy (Binswanger disease). *Neurology* 1978; 28:1206–1215.

114. De Reuck J, Crevits L, De Coster W, Sieben G, Eecken HV. Pathogenesis of Binswanger chronic progressive subcortical encephalopathy. *Neurology* 1980;30:920–928.

115. Loizou LA, Kendall BE, Marshall J. Subcortical arteriosclerotic encephalopathy: a clinical and radiological investigation. *J Neurol Neurosurg Psychiatry* 1981;44:294–304.

116. Huang K, Wu L, Luo Y. Binswanger's disease: Progressive subcortical encephalopathy or multi-infarct dementia? *Can J Neurol Sci* 1985;12:88–94.

117. Loizou LA, Jefferson JM, Smith WT. Subcortical arteriosclerotic encephalopathy (Binswanger's type) and cortical infarcts in a young normotensive patient. *J Neurol Neurosurg Psychiatry* 1982;45:409–417.

118. George AE, de Leon MJ, Gentes CI, et al. Leukoencephalopathy in normal and pathologic aging: 1. CT of brain lucencies. *AJNR* 1986;7:561–566.

119. George AE, de Leon MJ, Kalnin A, Rosner L, Goodgold A, Chase N. Leukoencephalopathy in normal and pathologic aging: 2. MRI of brain lucencies. *AJNR* 1986;7:567–570.

120. van Swieten JC, Kappelle LJ, Algra A, van Latum JC, Koudstaal PJ, van Gijn J. Hypodensity of the cerebral white matter on CT in patients with TIA or minor stroke: influence on the rate of subsequent stroke. *Ann Neurol* 1992;32:177–183.

121. Hachinski V. The decline and resurgence of vascular dementia. *Can Med Assoc J* 1990;142:107–111.

122. Kinkel WR, Jacobs L, Polachini I, Bates V, Heffner RR Jr. Subcortical arteriosclerotic encephalopathy (Binswanger's disease): computed tomographic, nuclear magnetic resonance, and clinical correlations. *Arch Neurol* 1985;42:951–959.

123. Steingart A, Hachinski VC, Lau C, et al. Cognitive and neurologic findings in subjects with diffuse white matter lucencies on computed tomographic scan (leuko-araiosis). *Arch Neurol* 1987;44: 32–35.

124. Kertesz A, Polk M, Carr T. Cognition and white matter changes on magnetic resonance imaging in dementia. *Arch Neurol* 1990;47:387–391.

125. Rao SM, Mittenberg W, Bernardin L, Haughton V, Leo GJ. Neuropsychological test findings in subjects with leukoaraiosis. *Arch Neurol* 1989;46:40–4.

126. Hunt AL, Orrison WW, Yeo RA, et al. Clinical significance of MRI white matter lesions in the elderly. *Neurology* 1989;39: 1470–4.

127. Tupler LA, Coffey E, Logue PE, Djang WT, Fagan SM. Neuropsychological importance of subcortical white matter hyperintensity. *Arch Neurol* 1992;49:1248–1252.

128. Brun A, Englund E. A white matter disorder in dementia of the Alzheimer type: a pathoanatomical study. *Ann Neurol* 1986;19: 253–262.

129. Tatemichi TK. How acute brain failure becomes chronic: a view of the mechanisms of dementia related to stroke. *Neurology* 1990;40:1652–1659.

130. Stamler J, Stamler R, Neaton JD. Blood pressure, systolic and diastolic, and cardiovascular risk. US population data. *Arch Intern Med* 1993;153:598–615.

131. Rose G. Strategy of prevention: lessons from cardiovascular disease. *Br Med J* 1981;282:1847–1851.

132. Rose G. Sick individuals and sick populations. *Int J Epidemiol* 1985;14:32–38.

133. The fifth report of the Joint National Committee on the Detection, Evaluation, and Treatment of High Blood Pressure (JNC V). *Arch Intern Med* 1993;153:154–183.

134. National High Blood Pressure Education Program Working Group Report on primary prevention of hypertension. *Arch Intern Med* 1993;153:186–208.

135. Applegate WB, Miller ST, Elam JT, et al. Nonpharmacologic intervention to reduce blood pressure in older patients with mild hypertension. *Arch Intern Med* 1992;152:1162–1166.

136. Applegate WB, Rutan GH. Advances in management of hypertension in older persons. *JAGS* 1992;40:1164–1174.

137. The Systolic Hypertension in the Elderly Program Cooperative Research Group. Implications of the Systolic Hypertension in the Elderly Program. *Hypertension* 1993;21:335–343.

138. Emergency Cardiac Care Committee and Subcommittees, American Heart Association. Guidelines for cardiopulmonary resuscitation and emergency cardiac care. Part IV—Special resuscitation situations: stroke. *JAMA* 1992;268:2242–2244.

139. Powers WJ. Acute hypertension after stroke: the scientific basis for treatment decisions. *Neurology* 1993;43:461–467.

140. Lisk DR, Grotta JC, Lamki LM, et al. Should hypertension be treated after acute stroke? A randomized controlled trial using single photon emission computed tomography. *Arch Neurol* 1993;50:855–862.

141. Dávalos A, Cendra E, Teruel J, Martinez M, Genís D. Deteriorating ischemic stroke: risk factors and prognosis. *Neurology* 1990;40:1865–1869.

142. Jansen PA, Schulte BP, Gribnau FW. Cerebral ischaemia and stroke as side effects of antihypertensive treatment; special danger in the elderly. A review of the cases reported in the literature. *Neth J Med* 1987;30:193–201.

143. Barry DI. Cerebrovascular aspects of antihypertensive treatment. *Am J Cardiol* 1989;63:14C–18C.

144. Carlberg B, Asplund K, Hägg E. Course of blood pressure in different subsets of patients after acute stroke. *Cerebrovasc Dis* 1991;1:281–287.

145. Yatsu FM, Zivin J. Hypertension in acute ischemic strokes: not to treat. *Arch Neurol* 1985;42:999–1000.
146. Lavin P. Management of hypertension in patients with acute stroke. *Arch Intern Med* 1986;146:66–68.
147. Brott T, MacCarthy EP. Antihypertensive therapy in stroke. In: Fisher M, ed. *Medical therapy of acute stroke.* New York: Marcel Dekker, Inc., 1989;117–141.
148. Brott T, Reed RL. Intensive care for acute stroke in the community hospital setting: the first 24 hours. *Stroke* 1989;20:694–697.
149. Spence JD, Del Maestro RF. Hypertension in acute ischemic strokes: treat. *Arch Neurol* 1985;42:1000–1002.
150. Calhoun DA, Oparil S. Treatment of hypertensive crisis. *N Engl J Med* 1990;323:1177–1183.
151. Gifford RW Jr. Management of hypertensive crises. *JAMA* 1991;266:829–835.
152. Strandgaard S: Autoregulation of cerebral blood flow in hypertensive patients. The modifying influence of prolonged antihypertensive treatment on the tolerance to acute, drug-induced hypotension. *Circulation* 1976;53:720–727.
153. Baron JC. Pathophysiology of acute cerebral ischemia: PET studies in humans. *Cerebrovasc Dis* 1991;1(suppl 1):22–31.
154. Meyer JS, Bauer RB. Medical treatment of spontaneous intracranial hemorrhage by the use of hypotensive drugs. *Neurology* 1962;12:36–47.
155. Ram CV. Hypertension associated with intracranial hemorrhage. *Curr Probl Cardiol* 1982;7:23–25.
156. Wood DH. Managing the hypertensive patient with cerebrovascular disease. *J Natl Med Assoc* 1984;76(suppl):16–23.
157. Batjer HH, Reisch JS, Allen BC, Plaizier LJ, Su CJ. Failure of surgery to improve outcome in hypertensive putaminal hemorrhage: a prospective randomized trial. *Arch Neurol* 1990;47:1103–1106.
158. Nibbelink DW, Torner JC, Henderson WG. Randomized treatment study. Drug-induced hypotension. In: Sahs AL, Nibbelink DW, Torner JC, eds. *Aneurysmal subarachnoid hemorrhage: report of the cooperative study.* Baltimore: Urban & Schwarzenberg, 1981;77–106.
159. Torner JC, Henderson WG, Nibbelink DW. Randomized treatment study. Drug-induced hypotension: statistical evaluation. In: Sahs AL, Nibbelink DW, Torner JC, eds. *Aneurysmal subarachnoid hemorrhage: report of the cooperative study.* Baltimore: Urban & Schwarzenberg, 1981;107–143.
160. Kassell NF, Peerless SJ, Durward QJ, Beck DW, Drake CG, Adams HP. Treatment of ischemic deficits from vasospasm with intravascular volume expansion and induced arterial hypertension. *Neurosurgery* 1982;11:337–343.
161. Biller J, Godersky JC, Adams HP Jr. Management of aneurysmal subarachnoid hemorrhage. *Stroke* 1988;19:1300–1305.
162. Langley MS, Sorkin EM. Nimodipine: a review of its pharmacodynamic and pharmacokinetic properties, and therapeutic potential in cerebrovascular disease. *Drugs* 1989;37:669–699.
163. Sacco RL, Wolf PA, Kannel WB, McNamara PM. Survival and recurrence following stroke: the Framingham Study. *Stroke* 1982;13:290–295.
164. Meissner I, Whisnant JP, Garraway WM. Hypertension management and stroke recurrence in a community (Rochester, Minnesota, 1950–1979). *Stroke* 1988;19:459–463.
165. Alter M, Sobel E, McCoy RL, et al. Stroke in the Lehigh Valley: risk factors for recurrent stroke. *Neurology* 1987;37:503–507.
166. Goldstein M. Cerebrovascular research: the opportunity has never been better. *Stroke* 1986;17:1067–1068.

Blood Pressure Regulation in Normal and Hypertensive States

Part A: Arterior Physiology and Pathophysiology

Hypertension: Pathophysiology, Diagnosis,
and Management, Second Edition,
edited by J.H. Laragh and B.M. Brenner,
Raven Press, Ltd., New York © 1995.

CHAPTER 30

The Structural Factor in Hypertension with Special Emphasis on the Altered Geometric Design of the Systemic Resistance Arteries

Björn Folkow

The *structural factor* is often assumed to be a relative newcomer in hypertension research, but the first *morphological* data were, in fact, at hand long before blood pressure was first measured in man in the 1880s. Thus, in 1836 Richard Bright described left ventricular and aortic wall thickening in Bright's disease, and in 1868 George Johnson observed wall thickening also in arterioles, but hardly in veins (1). However, the *functional-hemodynamic* consequences were largely overlooked for almost a century, partly because little was known about associated luminal changes or about microvascular biophysics, and partly because the wall thickening was assumed to represent late, sclerotic complications—with one notable exception: on confirming Johnson's observations in 1877, Ewald in Germany suggested that they might rather reflect true muscle hypertrophy in response to "*der übermässigen Spannung in Gefäss-system.*"

Ewald even hinted at possible functional consequences, though his fairly vague considerations were apparently not understood and hence left little trace (1).

I became interested in these problems in the early 1950s during studies of the interactions between passive wall distension and myogenic "autoregulatory" reactions in cat resistance vessels and how superimposed nervous influences affected these local events (2). These results, in turn, raised questions about what the hemodynamic outcome would be if resistance vascular walls became thicker, as had for so long been known to be the case in hypertension. This led to plethysmographic-hemodynamic analyses in normotensive and hypertensive forearm vascular beds in 1955–1956 (3,4), revealing also that when hypertensive resistance vessels are completely relaxed their lumina are structurally narrowed when compared with normotensive controls, and to such an extent that minimal resistance (R_{min}) was increased almost as much as was mean arterial pressure (MAP). Particularly when combined with the known wall

---

B. Folkow: Department of Physiology, University of Göteborg, Göteborg, Sweden.

thickening, such a structural luminal narrowing could in biophysical-mathematical analyses be shown to have most important hemodynamic consequences: if present in all systemic resistance vessels, they were, in fact, of such an extent that the raised systemic resistance in hypertensive subjects could for geometric-physical reasons be maintained at largely *normal* levels of smooth muscle activity. There appeared, in other words, to be "no room left" for the generally assumed presence of a continuous increase of vascular smooth muscle activity, an opinion which at that time "bordered on heresy." It was further suggested (4) that the observed structural adaptation of systemic resistance vessels might per se be genetically endowed in essential (primary) hypertension (i.e., via facilitation of some key link(s) in the involved growth processes). If so, even ordinary daily pressor stimuli could be enough to start a slow upward climb of the pressure-resistance balance.

Though these hemodynamic results were within a few years confirmed and extended by Conway (5) (at the same time as Short and Thomson [6] and Furuyama [7]), showing with ingenious morphometric techniques that the lumina and wall/lumen ratios of small resistance arteries in hypertensive subjects were indeed structurally altered as outlined above, it took about another two decades before the physically inevitable consequences of such vascular geometric alterations were generally recognized. This curious delay was mainly due to the prevailing, almost dogmatic assumption that resistance vascular smooth muscle activity must be increased in hypertension, where Harry Goldblatt's classical 1934 experiments on renal hypertension had created an enthusiastic "eureka" atmosphere. This attitude was reinforced by the elegant unraveling of the renin-angiotensin system by Irvine Page and Eduardo Braun-Menendez and their groups in the early 1940s (1), whereby research on essential (primary) hypertension mainly attracted expertise in endocrinology, nephrology, and autonomic nervous function.

It was, in any case, for quite a long time largely overlooked—and sometimes is so even today—that the *hemodynamic* behavior of the resistance microvessels is not dependent on only one factor such as (a) their smooth muscle activity, but is about as much dependent on three additional factors: (b) their geometric design; (c) wall distensibility; and (d) their transmural pressure (8,9). Moreover, these four factors steadily interact during *in vivo* conditions in ways which imply that function and structure continuously adapt to each other, whereby (b) often accomplishes what (a) is assumed to do, which is thoroughly discussed in some recent reviews (8,10) and is also the main theme in this chapter. As the literature on structural cardiovascular changes and their importance in hypertension is by now enormous, reference is made mainly to recent reviews covering various aspects of the topic.

BIOPHYSICAL ASPECTS

To understand the principles of cardiovascular design and its relation to function, the laws of Laplace and Poiseuille are essential, where Laplace's law states:

$$T = P \times r/w$$

where T represents tension per unit wall layer (wall stress), P transmural pressure, r tube radius, and w wall thickness. Thus, if P increases, T remains constant only if w/r_i is proportionally increased, whether by w increase and/or by r decrease—and vice versa upon P reduction. A glance at normal arterial and venous designs or at those of the left and right ventricles indicate how, indeed, the local levels of P determine the regional w/r_i levels: somehow the local pressure load serves to adjust both the direction and the extent of local growth-promoting processes along the Laplace principles, which by no means denies that "remote," neurohormonally conveyed trophic agents often also superimpose modulatory influences (1,11,12), as further dealt with later in this chapter.

Nature here provides a particularly drastic example in the 6-meters-tall giraffe, where MAP at heart level must be kept at 250–300 mm Hg to allow for brain perfusion. For hydrostatic reasons cranial arteries in the erect position are then exposed to only 80–100 mm Hg in transmural pressure, and they show w/r_i values similar to those of human cranial arteries. However, the feet arteries, ordinarily exposed to 400–500 mm Hg, have some 4–5 times higher w/r_i values (1,8,13). The systemic venous "low-pressure side" in man also illustrates these principles well, though at a more humble level. In small children w/r_i ratios in arm and leg veins are quite low and largely the same, but once the erect position intermittently adds a substantial transmural pressure elevation along leg veins, their w/r_i ratios increase proportionally (1,14,15).

However, vascular design also adjusts readily to differences in tissue bulk and/or in metabolic demands, where Poiseuille's law also comes in, according to which flow increases with the *fourth* power of the inner radius (r_i). This principle is drastically exemplified by the profound expansion of the uterine vasculature during pregnancy or by the differences in maximal flow capacity and capillary density in myocardium as compared with skeletal muscle (400–500 ml $\times$ 100 g^{-1} $\times$ mm^{-1} and 3000–4000 capillaries per mm^3 versus 70–120 ml and 300–600 capillaries per mm^3, respectively). Therefore, the problems of structural cardiovascular adaptation may be reduced to three main questions:

1. What happens with r_i, w and w/r_i—particularly in resistance vessels but also in heart, large arteries and venous capacitance vessels—at increased (decreased) P, though at unchanged tissue mass and metabolism?

2. What happens with resistance and capillary vessels when, instead, tissue mass and/or metabolism increase (decrease) but *P* remains unchanged?
3. What happens if (1) and (2) occur *simultaneously,* as for coronary vessels along with hypertensive left ventricular hypertrophy?

Obviously, structural cardiovascular adaptation—whether it occurs "upward" as in hypertension or "downward" as in hypotension—is in the final end of relevance because of the *hemodynamic* consequences, not only concerning pressure, cardiac output, overall resistance, and capacitance functions, but also concerning regional blood supply and blood content, capillary exchange, and barostat functions. It should further be emphasized that even quite small changes in r_i, w and w/r_i can importantly influence resistance and cardiac and capacitance functions for the following reasons:

1. Concerning *resistance vessel function,* maximal flow capacity (and hence R_{min}) varies directly (R_{min} inversely) with the *fourth* power of an average structural r_i change (Poiseuille's law). Furthermore, "vascular reactivity" (i.e. the extent to which a given smooth muscle activation increases resistance) is for geometric reasons strongly influenced by the ratio between w and $r_i (w/r_i)$, as are wall stress, strength of vascular contraction, and wall distensibility (Laplace's law).

2. Concerning *cardiac ventricular function,* the r_i and w dimensions set the upper limit for diastolic filling (as dependent on the "preload") as well as for stroke volume capacity, and here volume changes with the *third* power of r_i. Further, w/r_i determines wall stress and wall distensibility as well as the strength with which the left ventricle can cope with MAP and endsystolic arterial pressure ("afterload").

3. *Venous capacitance function,* all-important for cardiac priming, varies with the *second* power of the average venous r_i. While w/r_i in veins is normally so low that it hardly has any geometric amplifying significance, structural increases of venous w/r_i are nevertheless important, as they reduce venous compliance and also increase contractile strength whenever the media layer is thicker.

The biophysical consequences of changes in r, w and w/r_i will now be discussed in more detail concerning these three major functions.

Systemic Resistance Vessels

It should be remembered that *P* within the dominating precapillary resistance section is also fairly high in normotension, with an *average* w/r_i at full relaxation and distension around 0.15 or so in this section (1). For geometric reasons the relatively large wall mass here acts as an "amplifying lever" which correspondingly exagger-

ates the luminal narrowing, since media contractions ordinarily set out from the outer muscle layer, where the tonically active vasoconstrictor fibers exert their action. As, moreover, resistance varies inversely with the *fourth* power of r_i, even small smooth muscle adjustments can powerfully affect precapillary resistance: actually, a 30- to 35-percent shortening of the outermost muscle layer would almost close the lumina (1), where the increasing tendency of intimal crenation further accentuates the resistance increase for rheological reasons (16). From this follows that even minor structural alterations of average r_i, w and w/r_i in the precapillary resistance section are of greatest relevance in hypertension for three main reasons:

1. A structural r_i narrowing resets upward the very "baseline" for active smooth muscle adjustments because now R_{min} is also elevated (1–10). Note that only a 5-percent *average* r_i reduction means about 20-percent R_{min} increase (Poiseuille's law).

2. A structural w/r_i increase adds, as mentioned, a corresponding amplification of the r_i reduction at any given smooth muscle shortening, which further accentuates the resistance increase, again because of Poiseuille's law (1,3,4,8–10). Therefore, even modest decreases of r_i—and particularly so when associated with relative increases of w and hence of w/r_i—can remarkably elevate resistance also at entirely *normal* levels of smooth muscle activity, as is schematically illustrated in Fig. 1. Thus, generalized to all systemic circuits it will also correspondingly elevate MAP at entirely normal levels of cardiac output and vascular smooth muscle activity.

3. In the long run perhaps even more important in hypertension: Any adaptive-structural vascular change in the mentioned directions invites to a *positive feedback interaction* with functional pressor influences, at least when sustained or often repeated. The reason is that the two tend to mutually reinforce each other (1,8). Whenever generalized, the *structural amplifier* (to use Korner's expressive term [10]), will for any given smooth muscle activation result in accentuated pressure elevations which, in turn, will invite further structural adaptation and so on, along with time (also schematically illustrated in Fig. 1). These biophysical consequences of the characteristic hypertensive changes of resistance vascular geometry (1,8) were recently dealt with in particular detail by Korner and Angus (10), both from a theoretical-mathematical point of view, and toward the background of the various experimental approaches now available.

Because of this per se normal structural adaptation of precapillary resistance vessels and its interactions with smooth muscle function in these vessels, it is in a way more surprising that most people *remain* normotensive throughout life than the fact that resistance and MAP gradually increase in some, the more so as the same process also resets the important "long-term barostat func-

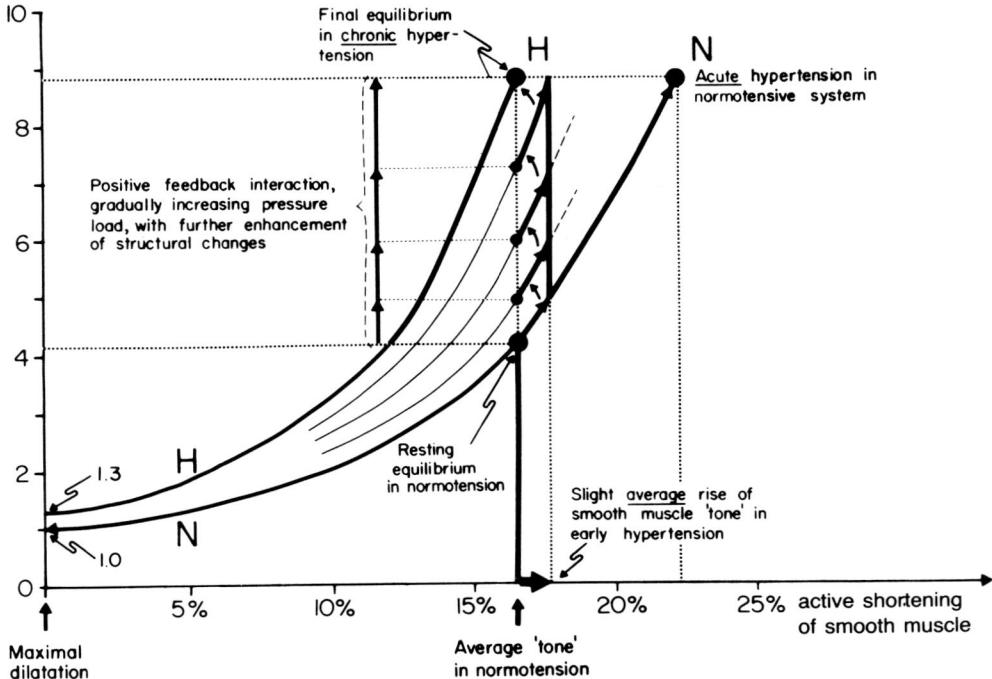

Systemic resistance;
≈Mean arterial pressure,
at unchanged cardiac output

FIG. 1. Principles of the changed relationship between degree of smooth muscle shortening and resulting increase of systemic flow resistance, when a reduction of inner radius (r_i) associated with a relative wall (w) thickening in the precapillary resistance section appear as local responses to an increased average pressure load ("structural autoregulation"). Resistance curve N represents a normotensive precapillary resistance vessel, with w/r_i around 0.2 at complete relaxation; curve H represents a fully "structurally autoregulated" vessel in established hypertension, with average r_i reduced 7 percent and w increased 30–40 percent. Note how the "triggering" pressure elevation (caused by slight, perhaps even transient, though repeated, increases in average smooth muscle tone and/or in cardiac output) needs to be only marginal because of positive-feedback interaction between this functional excitatory influence and the "structural autoregulation." Both reinforce each other with respect to the pressor effects, causing a transfer toward gradually steeper resistance curves as the extent of structural adaptation grows, to which also "trophic" influences (e.g., of neurohormonal origin) may contribute. (From ref. 92, with permission.)

tion" of the kidneys (discussed later in this chapter). A physiologist easily becomes more interested in the evidently durable (but poorly understood so far) negative feedbacks which allow for this, than in the many excitatory influences that may chronically raise pressure. There is much to indicate that the Muirhead "medullipin depressor system" (long-overlooked but increasingly actual) is of particular importance for maintaining normotension (17,18).

Heart

As recently reviewed (19), early "hyperkinetic" primary hypertension is often associated with mild left ventricular *eccentric hypertrophy* (i.e., an increased r_i in response to elevated "preload," with secondary w

thickening to offset increases of both r_i and P ("afterload")). The structurally increased r_i implies that a given myocyte shortening results in a greater stroke volume (in relation to r_i^3), or that a normal stroke volume can be maintained at reduced average myocyte shortening. When *concentric hypertrophy* becomes the dominating cardiac structural change in established or advanced primary hypertension, the increased w/r_i serves not only to balance the raised systolic afterload (19), but adds also a systolic "geometric amplifier" for reducing r_i during blood expulsion (20). Thus, the geometric design is again highly important for cardiac functional performance, though in somewhat different ways than in the resistance vessels. Cardiac function is, moreover, greatly influenced also by the aortic-large artery changes, and will be discussed further in this chapter.

Veins

Concerning *venous resistance and capacitance functions, w/r_i* is normally so low on the venous side ($1/20$–$1/30$) that geometric amplifier influences can be neglected even though some wall thickening and stiffening occurs in hypertension. Therefore, even a 30- to 35 percent smooth muscle shortening would increase postcapillary resistance only 4–5 times, compared with far greater resistance increases on the precapillary side (1,8). Concerning venous capacitance function, the mentioned maximum of media shortening would, on the other hand, expel as much as some 50 percent of venous contents toward the heart, i.e., in proportion to r_i^2. Thus, as human systemic veins contain about 70 percent of blood volume but the heart only about 10 percent, even minor shifts of venous smooth muscle activity or reduced compliance can powerfully influence cardiac filling, as will be further discussed.

METHODOLOGICAL ASPECTS

The apparently straightforward "morphometric" measurements of altered design in vessels and heart, as first used by Johnson in 1868 concerning arterioles, offer considerable problems. First, usually both w and r_i are altered in hypertension and, as already mentioned, often in different directions (1,8,9). Second, if shifts in muscle activity and/or distending pressure occur during fixation or measurement, they invite great errors since w and r_i then change in *opposite* directions where, moreover, resistance changes inversely to the *fourth* power of r_i. Third, concerning the resistance microvessels, regional differences between consecutive sections and in branching characteristics make it difficult to "sample" them in a representative way.

However, thanks to new techniques for standardizing the r_i dimensions, introduced by Short and Thomson (6) and Furuyama (7) almost 100 years after Johnson's pioneering study, fairly precise measurements of r_i, and hence of w and w/r_i in microvessels, may now be performed both *in vitro* and *in vivo* (18,21–25). Here the variant developed by Mulvany, Halpern, and Aalkjaer (21,22) has the added virtue that small artery dimensions can also be related to media contractile strength, while *in situ* estimations of microvascular geometric design (23,24), or on isolated whole microarteries where also length changes are considered (25), add other advantages. Such approaches also provide knowledge about various wall layers (21–24) and, for consecutive microsections *in vivo,* about their contraction characteristics and relative contributions to resistance (21–25).

Thus, already Short and Thomson (6) and Furuyama (7) showed in human hypertension that the structurally reduced r_i and increased w/r_i seemed to be mainly confined to the proximal 50–60 percent of the hypertensive precapillary resistance section, and later shown also in secondary (26) as well as in primary rat hypertension (24). These changes rapidly taper off in "downstream" microvessels, according to Furuyama (7), mainly because they are protected from pressure elevation by the "upstream" structural adaptation. *In vivo* morphometric analyses further indicate that the smallest precapillary arborizations may display some "rarefaction," at least in spontaneously hypertensive rats (SHR) (27,28), though this hardly adds much to overall resistance. Thus, modern morphometric analyses have many advantages, but the mentioned "sampling" difficulties largely remain, as does the "sensitivity problem" inherent in the fact that R_{min} relates inversely to the *fourth* power of r_i. For example, a 5-percent average r_i reduction is not easy to measure directly, but it implies a 20-percent R_{min} increase which is of great hemodynamic relevance.

For such reasons, complementary approaches are indispensable, like the mentioned hemodynamic analyses of average r_i via R_{min} measurements (1–5,8–11). They imply a biological application of the principles used in engineering when the dimensions of complex tube systems or electrical circuits are estimated by use of the Poiseuille and Ohm laws, respectively: as pressures and flows can be precisely measured (e.g., in human limbs) and regional maximal dilatation induced *in vivo* if due precautions are taken (1–4,8–10,29), exact calculations of local R_{min} can be made also in man. Further, as consecutive vascular sections are here exposed to their appropriate transmural pressures, *in vivo* R_{min} closely reflects the "*average*" r_i for the resistance vessels as long as blood viscosity is normal, or when Newtonian fluids are used (e.g., in rat perfusion experiments) (1,8–10).

If R_{min} is then related to *resting* resistance (R_r), which is easily made in plethysmographic forearm or hand studies in man, the R_r/R_{min} ratio reflects the average regional level of resistance in smooth muscle "tone" during "rest" (1,4,5,29). Further, additional smooth muscle activations can be induced regionally by hormonal or neurogenic stimuli and, when these resistance elevations are related to R_{min} and R_r in normotensive and hypertensive subjects, characteristic "resistance curves" can be obtained both in well-established (29) and in mild human primary hypertension (30). For natural reasons, such comparisons can become even more precise and complete in, e.g., *in vitro* paired constant-flow perfusions of normotensive and hypertensive vascular beds in rats (1,8–11), as shown in Fig. 2. Here the differences in maximal "pressor responses" reflect differences in relative media thickness, and the different curve slopes reflect how average w/r_i design has become altered and by its geometric effects affects "*vascular reactivity*" (i.e., the extent of resistance increase for a given smooth muscle

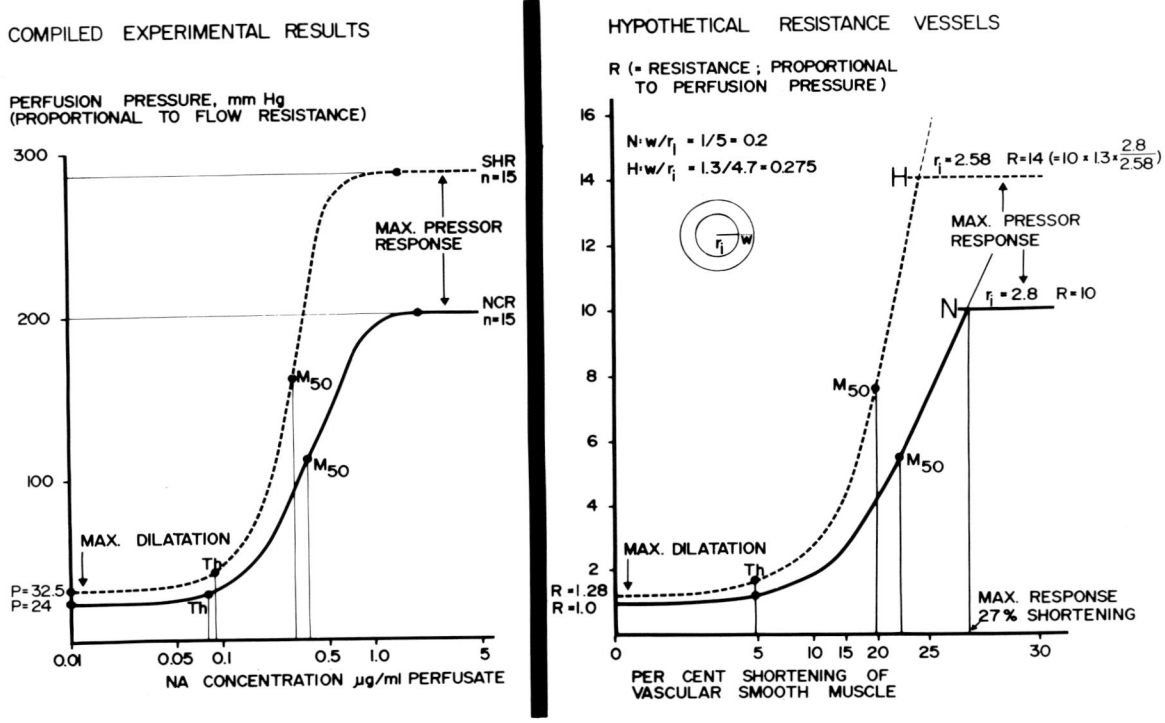

FIG. 2. Left: Average "resistance curves" for pair-perfused hindquarter vascular beds from SHR and normotensive control rats (NCR), based on 15 experiments during constant-flow perfusion. Graded vasoconstriction responses induced by intraarterial norepinephrine infusion at concentrations up to supramaximal levels. **Right:** Mathematically deduced "resistance curves" for two hypothetical resistance vessels, H and N, where H differs from N only by a 30 percent increase of media thickness associated with a 7 percent lumen reduction present already at complete smooth muscle relaxation. Note the striking similarities between the two sets of "resistance curves" with respect to: resistance at maximal relaxation (R_{min}); "threshold" (Th; reflecting smooth muscle sensitivity); steepness of the curves; 50 percent of the maximal pressor (resistance) response (M_{50}); and maximal pressor (resistance) response. (From ref. 93, with permission.)

activation). Selective increases (decreases) of *smooth muscle sensitivity,* on the other hand, show up as parallel left-hand (right-hand) shifts of otherwise identically shaped curves.

While such maximal "pressor responses" cannot be measured in human primary hypertension (Fig. 3), Sivertsson's experiment (29) shows that, besides the raised R_{min}, the entire slope of the resistance curve is much steeper in established human primary hypertension and largely in proportion to the raised pressure, recently confirmed in mild variants of primary hypertension by Egan et al. (30). This means that a given smooth muscle shortening is able to produce the *same* reduction of flow in hypertensive and normotensive subjects despite considerable elevations of both perfusion and transmural pressures in the former. In other words, the extent of structural, upward resetting in human primary hypertension largely matches the raised pressure level, as must be the case also in giraffes. Figure 2 shows the same relationships concerning SHR hypertension, but it also illustrates the increased maximal contractile strength,

while related data to those shown in Figs. 2 and 3 indicate that vascular smooth muscle *sensitivity* is largely unchanged in both human primary hypertension (29,30) and in SHR (8,9).

This hemodynamic test principle of resistance vascular design and function has several advantages besides the fact that changes in smooth muscle length are amplified to the fourth power, or even more so as the high w/r_i adds a "geometric amplifying" effect on r_i. Thus, it automatically provides the *averaged* responses of the entire microvascular network during circumstances when the consecutive sections are appropriately distended. In addition, in normotensive and hypertensive rats paired *in vitro*, comparisons can be made of virtually all systemic circuits (1,8–10), and its consecutive sections can be separately analyzed by pressure recordings along the circuit. For example, "isogravimetric" estimations of mean capillary pressure reveal that the structural resistance increase is largely confined to the *pre*capillary vascular section (1,8). Finally, the noninvasive plethysmographic hemodynamic approach in human primary hyperten-

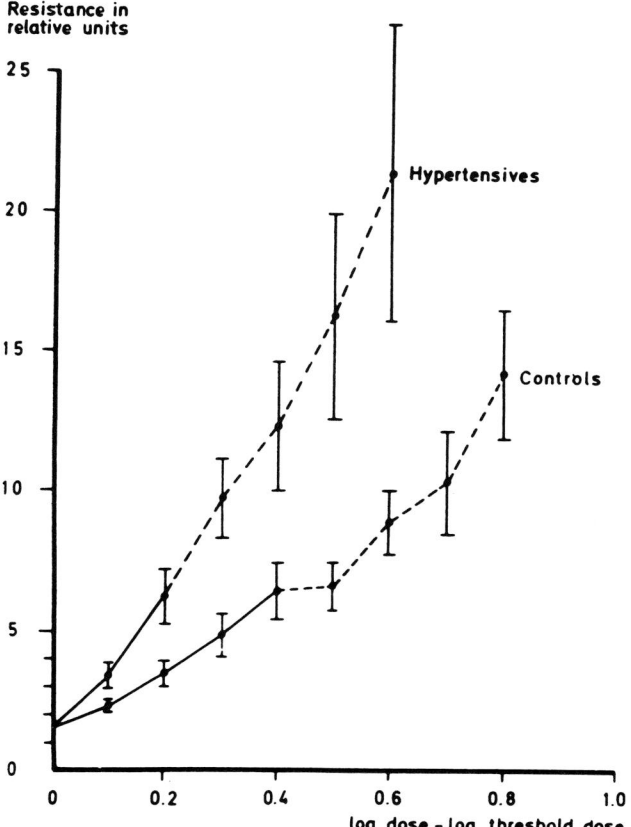

FIG. 3. Dose-resistance response curves to intraarterial nor-epinephrine (NE) infusion to hand vascular beds in subjects with primary hypertension (*H*; n = 16) and matched normo-tensive controls (*C*; n = 16). The abscissa gives the logarithm for the norepinephrine dose (μL $\times$ 100 mL^{-1} $\times$ min^{-1}) minus the log threshold dose, whereas the ordinate gives the resistance as a multiple of the "basal" resistance, which was 60 percent higher, and R_{min} 50 percent higher in H than in C. Even though mean arterial distending and perfusion pressures were 40 percent higher in H than in C, the H resistance vessels display much steeper norepinephrine responses, implying that their w/r_i is structurally increased ("vascular hyper-reactivity"). However, the threshold responses to nor-epinephrine did not differ significantly in H and C, suggesting a largely normal smooth muscle sensitivity to norepinephrine in H. (From ref. 29, with permission.)

sion can be used for repeated analyses of, e.g., forearm and/or hand vascular beds, thus revealing changes in R_{min} (r_i) and vascular reactivity (w/r_i), along with anti-hypertensive treatment (8).

Concerning *the heart,* noninvasive echocardiography provides good estimations of myocardial mass, and also to some extent of left ventricular r_i, w and w/r_i in man (19), even though diastolic distending pressures, which are needed for correct w/r_i estimations, are less accessible. Thus, myocardial mass alone, though easy to measure in animal experiments simply by weighing, tells nothing about the functionally decisive differences in r_i, w and w/r_i in eccentric and concentric hypertrophy.

However, these parameters can be deduced with considerable accuracy if left ventricular diastolic pressure-volume characteristics are also measured in isolated perfused rat hearts (8,19). Finally, concerning *the systemic veins,* changes in volume, wall compliance, and contractile responses can be estimated regionally in man and, concerning rats, for the entire low-pressure system as well (1,8,31,32).

THE STRUCTURAL FACTOR AS RELATED TO OTHER CAUSATIVE ELEMENTS IN PRIMARY HYPERTENSION

General Aspects

To get the right perspective on how the structural factor contributes to hypertension in general, how it depends on both pressure and trophic influences (11,12), and how it in primary hypertension may even be genetically reinforced, the principal etiological elements behind this disorder of regulation will first be outlined (1,8).

Polygenetically linked predisposition is the *sine qua non* of primary hypertension, where genetic profiles in man are more or less randomized, while they are uniform within each of the 5–6 hypertensive rat strains, thanks to inbreeding, though differing between strains. It need not be the consequences of genetic "abnormalities" or "lesions," but rather a matter of specific *constellations* of per se ordinary genetic variants.

Environmental factors include: (a) psychosocial, neurohormonally conveyed excitatory influences; (b) level of salt intake; and (c) other less well-defined electrolyte and nutritional influences, like those of potassium, calcium, excess caloric intake, alcohol, etc. Here the relative impacts of environmental factors to a great extent depend on whether the predisposing genetic elements make the organism more sensitive to any of them.

Structural cardiovascular adaptation is a normal and rapid, sometimes even genetically reinforced tissue response to pressure elevation, which soon dominates hemodynamics to the extent that it may even be difficult to trace polygenetically linked predisposition or environmental factors. The structural factor, which also depends on trophic, growth-promoting influences, serves to reset upward the heart, most barostat mechanisms, the venous capacitance side, and (particularly important) the systemic resistance, not the least because here it introduces the mentioned positive feedback interaction with functional pressor influences.

This scheme also illustrates the complexity of primary hypertension as it ensues from variable interactions between three major elements which are all, in turn, multifactorial. Further, these interactions may vary not only between individuals and species, as discussed elsewhere (1,8,11,33), but also between different stages of primary hypertension, though the structural factor soon seems to dominate hemodynamics in all variants and furthermore invites escalation. In a way, such a physiologically based attitude to primary hypertension owes much to Sir George Pickering's by-now-classical concept (33) that human primary hypertension is likely to represent the right-hand part of the normal Gaussian curve for pressure distribution, rather than being a specific disorder in the usual sense of the word. However, because in most species prolonged elevations of arterial pressure accelerate cardiovascular aging (34) and therefore invite cardiovascular deterioration, true disorder is gradually superimposed in the form of organ lesions. Also, in secondary hypertension structural cardiovascular adaptation soon tends to dominate hemodynamics (1,8,10), but here the functional trigger mechanisms and associated trophic influences are usually more distinct than in primary hypertension, even though they also vary with the type of secondary hypertension. However, the structural factor is here not genetically endowed, except accidentally if secondary hypertension happens to be superimposed on primary hypertension.

As is further dealt with in the next section, the structural factor is sometimes genetically reinforced in primary hypertension, as must also be the case in the fascinating variant of "natural" hypertension present in giraffes, though for different reasons. Because the head is here placed some 3 meters above heart level, the excessive high-pressure state (250–300 mm Hg at heart level) is needed for perfusion of the brain (1,8,13). As briefly mentioned previously, this calls for a profound-though-differentiated structural adaptation of heart and vasculature because it must be closely tailored to the marked regional differences in transmural pressures in this up-to-6-meters tall creature. In this way regional wall stress may be largely the same as in other species, whereby functional adjustments of cardiac output, resistance, and regional flows can be accomplished by similar levels of myocyte activity and range of neurohormonal adjustments. However, it should be noted that cardiovascular tissues in giraffes must also be genetically designed to cope with such extreme pressures because they seem to reach similar ages as other large herbivores, at least when kept protected from predators in zoological gardens. Had man been blessed with the same "genetic protection" against cardiovascular deterioration, primary hypertension may well have been considered a harmless physical variant, like body length, size of ears, etc. Perhaps man sometimes exhibits similar variants of "genetic protection," though more humble in extent, explaining why some individuals seem to endure raised arterial pressure for decades while others rapidly show lesions.

The molecular and cellular processes involved in cardiovascular structural adaptation, as well as their potential relations to the genetic predisposing elements in primary hypertension, have in recent years been intensely studied. This is true not only for membrane characteristics (35), but also for cell responsiveness to pressure, stretch, and to trophic agents of local and remote origins (11,12,36,37), as well as how the various intracellular links involved in growth are affected by, and possibly genetically sensitive to, such stimuli (38–40). However, these biochemical-molecular events are still in many respects poorly understood, where the reader is referred to the mentioned recent reviews for details (35–40). In general, protooncogenes seem to be of key importance for overall control of cellular growth, and thus also for the cardiovascular system, whether heart and vessels are exposed to mechanical stimuli in terms of increases of stretch or work load, or when growth is promoted by local or neurohormonally conveyed trophic agents. These different types of growth-promoting influences are separately outlined below, as they seem to have different roles in the process of structural adaptation.

Pressure- and Flow-Related Stimuli

Because the interest is at present so strongly focused on chemical-trophic agents in general, it is easily overlooked that local changes in pressure and/or in tissue nutritional demands are, indeed, crucial for determining the direction and extent of the geometric changes (i.e., exactly how r_i, w and w/r_i of heart and vessels are tailored to fit the given hemodynamic situation) (compare to earlier section). Certainly agents like catecholamines or angiotensin can stimulate wall growth in both heart and vessels (36–40), but it is equally obvious that the *hemodynamic* consequences are widely different whether a given increase of wall mass surrounds a narrowed or an expanded lumen.

In other words, what finally matters for cardiovascular function and pressure are the dimensions and, in particular, the geometric relationships of r_i and w/r_i, and they seem to be directly related to local pressures as well as to tissue mass and/or metabolic demands (8,41). Thus, as earlier outlined in this chapter, w becomes increased in relation to r_i in all cardiovascular sections exposed to raised transmural pressures, while systemic resistance vessels exhibit a structural increase of R_{min} that is almost proportional to the MAP elevation. The importance of pressure per se is here evident from the fact that the reverse structural changes of r_i and w/r_i occur when regional hypotension is induced in SHR by low aortic obstruction, even though these "low-pressure" vessels are exposed to the same neurohormonal trophic agents as elsewhere (1,8,41).

Alternatively, if, at unchanged pressure, tissue mass and/or metabolism is increased, this initiates a luminal growth in the resistance vessels with a secondary w/r_i adaptation according to Laplace's law, and vice versa at reduced metabolism (8,41). It is therefore likely that the structural r_i decrease of the resistance vessels in hypertension at least in part depends on flow-related local signals, serving to keep maximal flow capacity unchanged despite the increase of perfusion pressure (Poiseuille's law), rather than being only a consequence of increased transmural pressure. For example, the coronary resistance vessels in hypertension, exposed to increases of both pressure and nutritional demands due to cardiac hypertrophy, so adjust R_{min} as to fit not only the raised perfusion pressure but also the increased tissue mass (8,19,41). Furthermore, the aorta-large arteries which, like the resistance vessels, are exposed to increased pressure but are not involved in the control of nutritional flow, show the expected increases of w but here usually in association with *increases* of r_i as studied, e.g., by Safar (42) (discussed later in this chapter).

Alterations in the geometric design of the heart further illustrate how local pressure and flow conditions must be the key signals for directing growth in specialized directions. When, for example, cardiac walls during diastole "sense" increased filling (preload), as in connection with sustained elevations of overall nutritional demands during hyperkinetic circulatory states, a structurally based luminal widening occurs, with a secondary w adaptation to keep w/r_i balanced to the increased r_i (eccentric hypertrophy) (19). Evidently, the myocytes respond to such

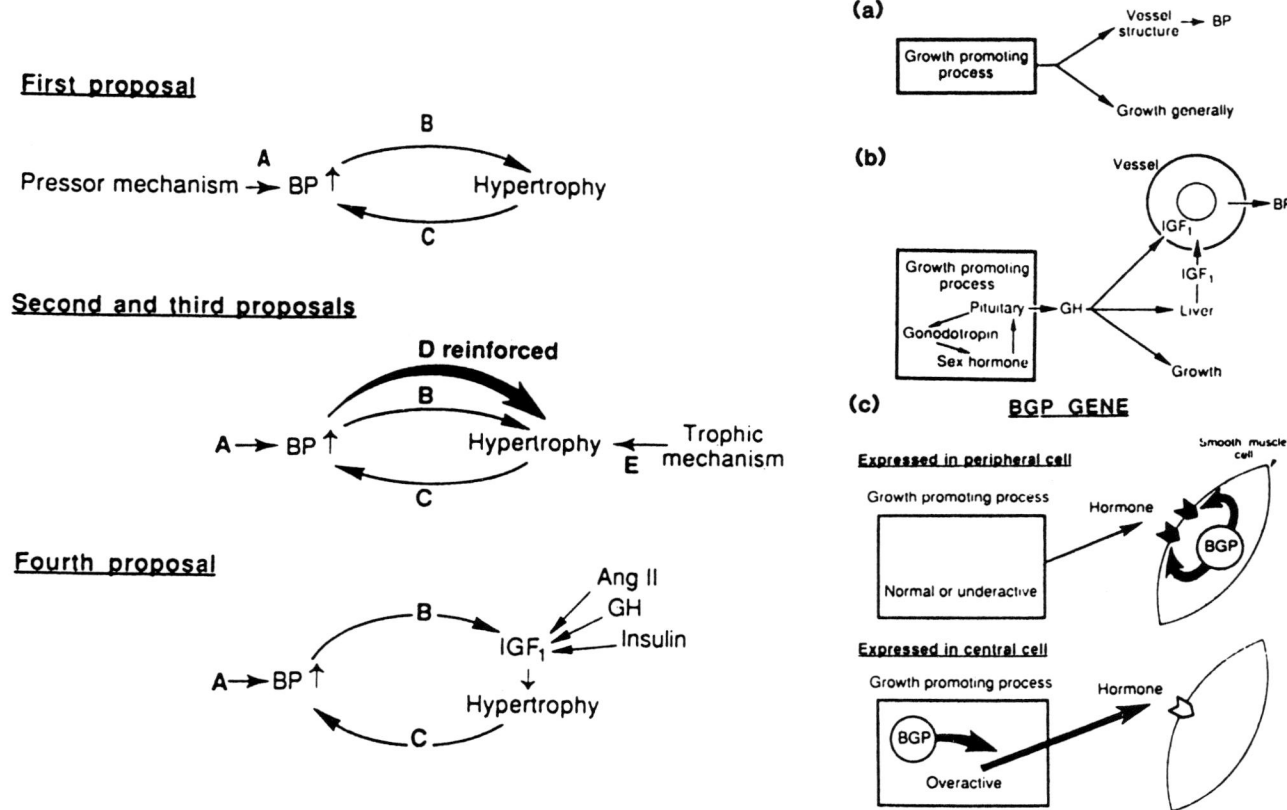

FIG. 4. Left: Four variants of feedback mechanism relating pressure (BP) and vascular structure. According to Lever and Harrap *"First proposal"*: Increased pressure (*A*) causes vascular structural adaptation (*B*) which increases pressure further (*C*). This feedback mechanism might, according to Folkow et al., (4) be genetically reinforced in primary hypertension, as in (*D*), and/or according to Lever, be stimulated by trophic agents, as in (*E*) of *"Second and third proposal."* *"Fourth proposal:"* Agents like growth hormone, angiotensin II, and insulin act in combination with increases of pressure, insulin-like growth factor serving as "final common pathway." **Right:** Schematic illustration by Lever and Harrap of **A:** processes controlling normal growth and maturation of the cardiovascular system which thereby raises systemic resistance and MAP. **B:** detail of one growth-promoting process and of its action on, e.g., a blood vessel. Growth hormone and insulin-like growth factor are here considered to be stimulated by sex hormones which, in turn, are stimulated by gonadotrophins. **C:** the gene(s) controlling "basal growth potential" (BGP) is expressed in vascular smooth muscle cells where it increases receptors for trophic agent(s). Normal concentrations of, e.g., growth hormone then accentuate vascular growth processes. In the lower part of **C** the BGP gene(s) is instead expressed in, e.g., the pituitary gland so that increased growth hormone secretion accentuates vascular growth. (Modified from refs. 4,12, and 36, with permission.)

increases of diastolic stretch by increasing their length and this seems to occur by adding more sarco-meres (43). By contrast, when the ventricles during end-contraction are exposed to an increased afterload, the myocytes instead respond mainly by adding more of parallel acto-myosin filaments to each sarcomere, making them thicker and stronger, but not longer (concentric hypertrophy). Thus, as is the case with the resistance vessels, these examples illustrate how entirely different growth processes are involved, depending on differences in mechanical and/or flow-related signals, which latter evidently operate by means of partly different growth-mod-

ulating factors. Superimposed on these local events, a variety of "extrinsic" trophic factors serve as modulators and, like growth hormone, are likely to exert "permissive-trophic" effects that are necessary for making the local growth-modulating mechanisms fully efficient.

Nature of Trophic Agents

The current intense interest for trophic influences on cardiovascular structural adaptation was, in a way, initiated by Bevan's observation (44) some 20 years ago that

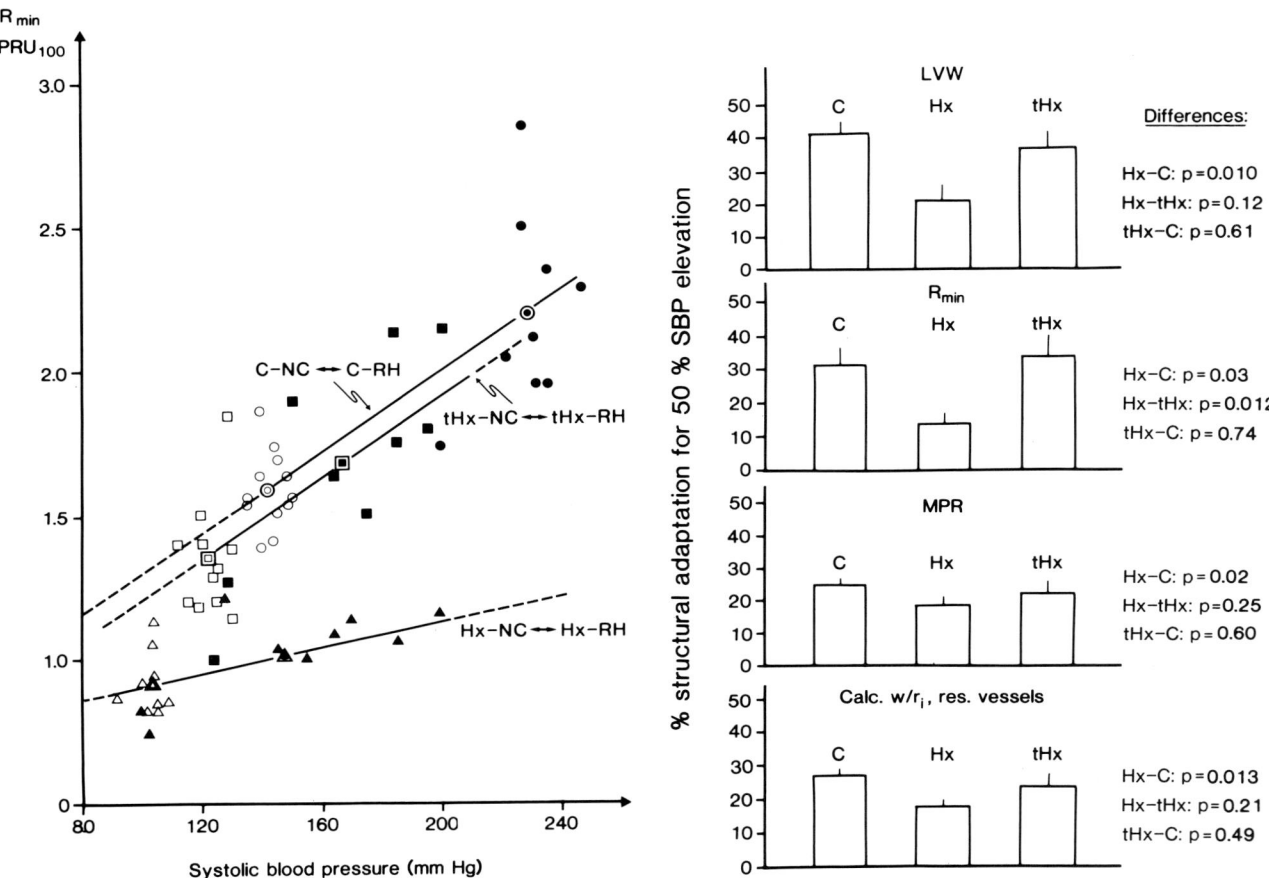

FIG. 5. Left: Relation between systolic blood pressure and R_{min} in individual rats in six groups of animals: normal control rats (C-NC, *open circles*), renal clip hypertension in control rats (C-RH, *closed circles*), hypophysectomized otherwise intact controls (Hx-NC, *open triangles*), hypophysectomized renal clip hypertensive rats (Hx-RH *closed triangles*), hypophysectomized but growth-hormone-thyroxine substituted controls (gt-Hx-NC, *open squares*) and renal clip hypertension-induced in hypophysectomized but substituted rats (gt-Hx-RH, *closed squares*). Mean values for the six groups are given as double symbols. Note how the structural narrowing of r_i is greatly reduced in hypophysectomized, renal hypertensive rats, but is almost the same as in ordinary renal hypertensive rats when substitution with growth hormone and thyroxine is given to Hx-rats. **Right:** Percentage structural adaptation of left ventricular weight (LVW), minimal resistance to flow (R_{min}), maximal pressor response (MPR, reflecting relative w) and w/r_i (calculated from the R_{min} and MPR data), as related to a 50 percent chronic elevation of systolic blood pressure (SBP). Each of the three renal hypertensive groups of rats are here compared with their respective unclipped control groups. Note the marked attenuation of both cardiac and vascular structural adaptation in response to chronic renal clip hypertension in hypophysectomized rats, even though their plasma concentration of "trophic" angiotensin II was particularly high, while growth hormone-thyroxine substitution almost normalized structural cardiovascular adaptation. (From ref. 45, with permission.)

adrenergic transmitters appear to also serve as stimuli for vascular growth. These problems are extensively discussed in recent reviews by Lever (12), Lever and Harrap (36), Schelling et al. (37), and by Jackson and Schwartz (40), which provide good insight into the rapidly growing literature. Apart from their other cardiovascular effects, both catecholamines and angiotensin II exert important trophic influences on heart and vessels, also present during *in vitro* conditions as on tissue cultures. The same is also true for insulin, and it is likely that insulin-like growth factor (IGF-1) serves as a final common pathway for several of these effects, as illustrated in Fig. 4 (36).

Further, it was recently shown in experimental renal hypertension that growth hormone (GH) and thyroxine (t) for heart, vessels, and kidneys serve as important "permissive-trophic" hormones, so denoted because their growth-promoting effects do not alone induce pressure elevation (45). When, however, renal clamping induces angiotensin-II-dependent pressure increases in normal, in hypophysectomized, and in hypophysectomized-but-GH-t-substituted rats, these permissive-trophic influences become fully evident. For any given pressure elevation, the extent of cardiac, vascular, and renal structural adaptation was greatly attenuated in the hypophysectomized group, even though a particularly marked and long-lasting increase of angiotensin release occurred in this group. The differences between the three groups are shown in the left panel of Fig. 5 concerning R_{min} increase in relation to pressure elevation, and in the right panel concerning the relative extents of left ventricular hypertrophy, R_{min}, maximal pressure response and estimated w/r_i increase for a 50-percent increase of pressure (45). These results probably explain the observation by Okamoto (46) that early hypophysectomy largely abolished SHR hypertension. The mentioned study (45) further suggests that GH-t are crucial for the normal remodeling and maturation of the cardiovascular system which occurs around puberty and which in both man and rats is associated with elevation of MAP 10–20 mm Hg. On the basis of these and other recent findings concerning growth-promoting factors, Lever and Harrap (36) discuss how they may control cardiac and vascular growth processes along with the time axis of life in normotensive organisms and in primary hypertension, as further discussed later in this chapter (see Fig. 4).

It should, however, be stressed that several biogenic vasodilator agents like nitric oxide (NO), atrio-natriuretic peptide (ANP), and perhaps also the Muirhead medullipin system (17,18), exert growth-*inhibitory* effects (39), which may be equally important as those of growth-promoting factors. For example, deficiencies of growth-inhibitory actions might facilitate cardiovascular growth almost as efficiently as excess release of growth-promoting factors, which opens up new alternatives for the important control of structural cardiovascular adaptation in high-pressure states.

GENETIC REINFORCEMENT OF THE STRUCTURAL FACTOR

It was long generally assumed that the particular genetic constellations, or macromolecular alterations, behind the predisposition to primary hypertension should express themselves as *functional* deviations from the norm. However, such assumptions are by no means justified because the involved macromolecules, perhaps serving as enzymes, carriers, membrane components, signal or growth-promoting substances, etc., may as well affect some structural characteristics of cells and tissues. This possibility was discussed already in the 1956–58 hemodynamic study of altered resistance vessel design in primary hypertension (4), tentatively involving intrinsic links promoting growth and/or "extrinsic," neurohormonally conveyed trophic influences (1,8,11). If so, "ordinary" pressor stimuli might also be enough to initiate a gradual structural "upward resetting" and hence start the ball rolling (4). Though this proposal was at the time considered by some to be "far-fetched" (8), the interest for a genetic facilitation of the structural factor in primary hypertension has increased greatly in recent years, as evident from a number of reviews (11,12,36–39) covering various aspects of this problem.

During the 70s, several studies of SHR hypertension had already pointed in this general direction (1), and by now the evidence of such a genetic reinforcement of the structural factor is strong (8,11,12,36–39,43). For example, Kanbe et al. (47) observed that tissue culture growth of vascular smooth muscle is more rapid in SHR than in Wistar-Kyoto rats (WKY), pointing to a genetic reinforcement within the myocytes themselves. Moreover, addition of catecholamines further increases this growth (47) at the same time that SHR show a "primary" accentuation of central neurohormonal influences on the cardiovascular system (1,8,11,46). Thus, both local-intrinsic and remote-extrinsic growth-promoting mechanisms seem to be genetically enhanced in SHR. For example, even before birth SHR show structural cardiovascular changes compared with WKY, as studied and reviewed by Gray (48), and at the resistance level these changes even seem to be "in excess" of the pressure rise in the early "borderline" phase (8,9,11).

The presence of such genetic reinforcements of the structural cardiovascular adaptation in primary hypertension should not, after all, come as a surprise. As a parallel, the structural design of another major system, that of skeletal muscle, is also genetically influenced as is obvious from the inherited differences between "athletic" and "leptosomic" body builds (which no-one would ascribe to "abnormal" or "lesioned" genes—not uncommon in primary hypertension). The skeletal muscle system also strikingly illustrates the importance of trophic agents by the abuses of anabolic steroids in modern athletics. Lever and Harrap (36) discuss different ways by which genetic factors may facilitate structural cardiovascular adaptation in primary hypertension, as indicated by the thick arrows in Fig. 4, where alternative "D" best coincides with the 1958 proposal by Folkow et al. (4). Figure 4 also illustrates different ways by which trophic influences may contribute to genetic facilitation of the structural factor in primary hypertension. Thus, the release of trophic agents, or cardiovascular sensitivity to such agents or to pressure elevation, may be enhanced. Here the mentioned permissive-trophic actions of hormones like GH on structural cardiovascular adaptation is of particular interest (45), as it may explain Okamoto's observation (46) that early hypophysectomy largely abolished SHR primary hypertension.

The potential importance of "antitrophic" growth-inhibitory agents should, however, not be forgotten, as their release may be reduced in primary hypertension, and/or cardiovascular sensitivity to them may be attenuated. For example, it was recently shown that the pressure-flow-related release of the Muirhead renomedullary depressor agents (medullipins) is greatly attenuated in SHR (49), implying that the vasodilator, sympatho-inhibitory, and natriuretic actions of these powerful agents (17,18), as well as their possible growth-inhibitory actions, are here almost absent. It is not known whether this is due to genetic or to early-secondary influences; then perhaps consequences of the locally suppressing influence by the sympathetic and renin-angiotensin systems on the medullipin system (17,18,49). In any case, this marked attenuation of the medullipin system in SHR is likely to contribute to the fact that kidney cross-transplantation between SHR and normotensive rats invites to hypertension in the latter.

The question arises: To what extent is the structural factor genetically reinforced in human variants of primary hypertension, where similarities to the SHR model are often close? (1,8,11,36,37) As summarized in recent reviews (36,50), studies of children from families with strong predisposition for primary hypertension suggest that also in man the structural factor may be involved quite early in life. For example, MAP levels tend to aggregate in the upper-normal age range, and this is often associated with increased body weight and not seldom with marginal increases in myocardial mass. Furthermore, adolescents from hypertensive families usually show intensified and prolonged neurohormonal pressor responses to psychosocial stimuli (51) which, as in SHR, may facilitate the gradual development of the structural factor, both via repeated pressor episodes and by means of trophic influences mediated by catecholamines, angiotensin II, etc. (52,53). In general, therefore, much may be gained by early studies of children from hypertensive families, concerning not only functional but also structural expressions of the genetic predisposition, as has been of great value in analyses of juvenile SHR.

LOCATION, EXTENT AND RATE OF RESISTANCE VASCULAR CHANGES

General Aspects

As outlined in previous sections, all pressure-exposed cardiovascular sections in primary hypertension show early, sometimes even genetically-endowed changes of their geometric design, though in different ways depending on their functional role. However, those occurring in systemic precapillary resistance vessels are of particular importance, for the following reasons: (a) they are the major cause of the elevated MAP in chronic high-pressure states; (b) their combination of structurally narrowed lumina with increased wall/lumen ratios is unique; (c) they invite to an aggravating interaction with functional pressor influences; and (d) their renal presence serves to reset upward the "long-term barostat function" of the kidneys as well, which according to Guyton and co-workers (54,55) is a prerequisite for chronic high pressure states. For these reasons the present section will discuss in more detail these microvascular alterations, the more so because they have during recent decades attracted intense interest, where recent reviews cover the by-now-abundant literature (1,8,10–12,20,22,24,27, 36–40).

Thus, the presence of a reduced r_i as combined with an increased w/r_i has been confirmed and quantified by a variety of experimental approaches, both in man and in rat models of primary and secondary hypertension. Further, these geometric changes have been observed in all systemic circuits so far explored (in rats, e.g., in the hindquarter, gastrointestinal, renal, coronary, and cerebral circuits, in which they are essentially confined to the *pre*capillary resistance vessels [1,8]). The Mulvany-Halpern technique (21,22) reveals that the relative media thickening is associated with a proportional increase of contractile strength, while vascular smooth muscle sensitivity is largely unchanged, both in human and rat primary hypertension (1,8,10,22). In addition, hypertensive resistance vessels are not only stronger and, for geometric reasons, hyperreactive (see Figs. 2 and 3), but their walls are also stiffer over the whole range of media contraction (9), as expected when more of coupled actomyosin filaments offer resistance to stretch (8,10).

These geometric, biophysical, and physiological characteristics are all important for the ability of hypertensive precapillary resistance vessels to maintain an increased systemic resistance at normal levels of tonic smooth muscle activity and to allow for a normal range of flow changes, even though they are exposed to often marked elevations of both perfusion and transmural pressures (1,8–10): the vascular system is simply rebuilt to operate at a higher pressure equilibrium and still maintain a normal range of blood flow adjustments. When instead expressed in terms of resistance, the resistance vessels therefore exhibit steeper "resistance curves" because both the baseline (R_{min}) and the w/r_i relationships are re-set upward (see Figs. 1–3), as must also be the case in the "physiological" high-pressure state present in giraffes. These precapillary structural changes which, despite pressure elevation, keep regional flow and capillary pressure largely constant, represent a long-term analogue to functional autoregulation and therefore deserve to be called *structural autoregulation* (2). Both are essentially local responses to upward or downward changes of MAP, though on an acute-functional versus delayed-structural basis. Further, both are entirely adequate for the individual circuit and tissue, as they serve to protect the sensitive capillary exchange section from undue pressure changes, and in the kidneys to keep glomerular filtration pressure constant.

When, however, all systemic circuits are structurally autoregulated upward and cardiac output at the same time remains adjusted to current metabolic needs, MAP inevitably becomes raised also when vascular smooth muscle activity is normal. Furthermore, as structural and functional interactions invite to the previously mentioned positive feedback interaction, MAP may continue to rise in a vicious circle fashion as, indeed, occurs in malignant hypertension. The fact that this does not occur more often in primary hypertension—and evidently not at all in the "physiological" high-pressure state of giraffes—suggests that the cardiovascular system has some durable and potentially powerful *negative* feedbacks which are still poorly understood.

Location and Extent

It may be asked whether these structural changes are evenly distributed along the precapillary resistance section or mainly concentrated to proximal or distal consecutive parts. Indeed, the early human studies by Short and Thomson (6) and Furuyama (7), mentioned in the first section of this chapter, already strongly indicated that they are mainly confined to *proximal* resistance arteries. Thus, a distinct r_i reduction in combination with an increased w/r_i was observed only in arterial vessels with diameters above some 100 μm, with a gradual tapering off toward the capillary level which, according to Furuyama (7), was due to a protective influence of the upstream structural changes. The same is in general true for rat primary and secondary hypertension, as reviewed by Zweifach (27), and recently explored in detail concerning SHR cerebral resistance vessels (24).

Such a concentration of hypertensive structural changes to what corresponds to the proximal 50–60 percent of the precapillary resistance function (22) has, because of the Poiseuille and Laplace laws, interesting consequences concerning r_i, w/r_i and total wall area (w_a): For example, a 35-percent R_{min} increase at 45-percent MAP elevation—as observed in the "established" phases of human (4) and SHR hypertension (9)—would be at a *generalized* luminal narrowing call for only 7 to 8 percent r_i reduction. Such an extent of structural adaptation seems, as mentioned, to be so closely matched to the MAP elevation that there is no need to assume any maintained accentuation of smooth muscle activity (1,8,10), as can also be deduced from Figs. 2 and 3. Even in secondary renal hypertension in rats the extent of structural vascular change is within 3–5 weeks so marked as to alone explain 80–90 percent of the resistance and pressure elevation (45).

If the structural narrowing is concentrated to the proximal 50–60 percent of the precapillary resistance section, the mentioned 35 percent R_{min} increase necessitates a twice-greater r_i reduction in this proximal section, i.e., by some 15 percent, at the same time as w/r_i still needs to be increased by 45 percent to balance off the mentioned 45 percent MAP rise. It can then be calculated from the formula:

$$w_a = \pi(r_e^2 - r_i^2)$$

that such a 45-percent w/r_i increase can be accomplished with no or only minor change of w_a, simply because r_i is so much reduced. This was in essence what Short and Thomson (6) noted in pioneering morphometric comparisons of human hypertensive and normotensive resistance arteries, observed also by Friedman et al. (26) in subsequent measurements in rat secondary hypertension, as reviewed elsewhere (1). Thus, terms like *media hypertrophy* for such hypertensive vascular changes may be justified to emphasize the important w/r_i increase, and was so used by Furuyama (7) as she always related w and w_a to the r_i value. However, if primarily comparing w_a between equivalent hypertensive and normotensive small arteries, morphologists would justly conclude that a largely unchanged w_a in the former is not "hypertrophic," even though wrapped as a thicker sheath around a narrowed lumen. In a way, it boils down to a semantic problem, which here results from the fact that findings of the same type have been arrived at by different experimental approaches and are therefore seen from either a biophysical-hemodynamic or a morphological angle.

Baumbach and Heistad (24), who in SHR have confirmed and extended Short's and Friedman's finding, have overcome such semantic problems by introducing the term *vascular remodeling* to denote the special situation where the r_i reduction is so marked that little or no w_a increase is needed to allow for a pressure-proportional w/r_i increase. However, such processes still call for extensive changes of both cellular and matrix arrangements, where undoubtedly trophic agents as well as pressure changes are involved. Thus, in the absence of GH and thyroxin the structural r_i reduction in response to pressure elevation was almost abolished (as shown in Fig. 5) even though high concentrations of trophically active angiotensin II were at hand (45). While the mentioned hypertensive changes of r_i and w/r_i taper off in distal parts of the precapillary resistance compartment, these microvessels may in return show some "rarefaction," at least in some vascular beds in rat hypertensive models (24,27,28). However, these changes seem to be of late, secondary nature and probably add only little to the overall resistance increase, particularly as the remaining arborizations appear to be slightly widened according to some observations. Due to the inverse relationship between resistance and the fourth power of r_i (Poiseuille), only 10 percent average r_i widening would be enough to offset 30–35 percent reduction of the number of microbranches.

Rate of Development and Regression

To explore the speed at which structural cardiovascular adaptation can occur, renal hypertension in rats has been predominantly used (56,57), as particularly rapid and extensive changes of MAP can here be accomplished by renal clipping and declipping, respectively. When adjusted to the rate of pressure change, it was found that hemodynamically significant changes were noted within 2–3 days (56) and a largely completed "upward structural resetting" of vessels and heart could be accomplished in 10–14 days (1,8,45,56,57). Though the metabolic rate in man is 5–6 times slower than in rats, which should correspondingly influence also structural cardiovascular adaptation, this process seems to be largely completed in 1–2 months in man, if the triggering pressure elevation is rapid. Thus, Aalkjaer et al. (58) noted, in small mesenteric resistance arteries excised in preeclampsia patients undergoing cesarean section, that they showed largely proportional structural changes of r_i, w and w/r_i to the raised pressure level, which in these cases could hardly have been of more than a few months' duration.

It follows that structural cardiovascular adaptation is neither in rats nor in humans the rate-limiting step in the usually slow development of multifactorial primary hypertension: The "structural amplifier" is already of hemodynamic importance in the earliest stages (1,8,13) and may, as mentioned, serve also as a "primary mover" when it is genetically reinforced, as in SHR. In fact, the first biochemical signs of initiated structural adaptation can be traced within an hour after raising the pressure load, as reflected by an increased active uptake and protein incorporation of amino acids in isolated perfused rat hearts exposed to ramplike elevations of afterload (8,59). More recent studies dealing with the early biochemical and cellular growth processes, induced by in-

creases of pressure load and/or by trophic agents, are reviewed by Krieger and Dzau (39) and by Jackson and Schwartz (40).

Provided that the period of pressure elevation is not too long (3–5 weeks in the 2K1C rat model), the regression of these cardiovascular structural changes upon renal declipping is about as rapid as their development (1,8,57). However, at prolonged pressure increases, cardiac and vascular myocytes, besides developing hypertrophy and w/r_i changes, also participate with fibrocytes in the slower process of "interstitial endowment" by producing collagen and other interstitial material (8,60–62). Such a "second line of structural defense" (1,8) not only adds to wall thickening and stiffening, but unfortunately it also reduces and delays structural regression when antihypertensive therapy is induced (61). This seems to be the case not only along with aging in SHR primary hypertension (62) but also if the pressure elevation in secondary rat hypertension has lasted 3–5 months or more (63). Such findings per se argue for early or even preventive antihypertensive treatment to facilitate regression in primary hypertension because the structural cardiovascular changes here seem to dominate hemodynamics already from early stages.

STRUCTURAL CHANGES IN PARTICULARLY IMPORTANT SYSTEMIC CIRCUITS

The renal vascular bed is in this context of particular interest due to its important role in the "long-term barostat function" of the kidneys, as extensively studied by Guyton et al. (54,55). Their computer simulations show that the most efficient way to induce an upward resetting of renal barostat function is to increase the ratio between the pre- and postglomerular resistances, as this to an even greater extent reduces glomerular filtration and hence renal excretory functions.

It is here important to stress that the preglomerular resistance vessels are the equivalents of proximal resistance arteries in other systemic circuits, and already for such reasons they would be expected to show the same early upward structural autoregulation as other systemic circuits in primary hypertension. This is, indeed, also the case (64–67), as illustrated in Fig. 6 concerning pairperfused, age-matched, and maximally vasodilated kidneys from SHR and WKY during recordings of perfusion pressure, perfusate flow, and glomerular filtration rate (GFR).

With perfusion pressure along the abscissa and GFR along the ordinate, a displacement of the pressureGFR relationship to the right will for biophysical reasons indicate an increase of the structurally set prepostglomerular resistance ratio, while a less steep slope of this relationship reflects reduced glomerular filtration capacity. Further, a reduced perfusate flow for a given

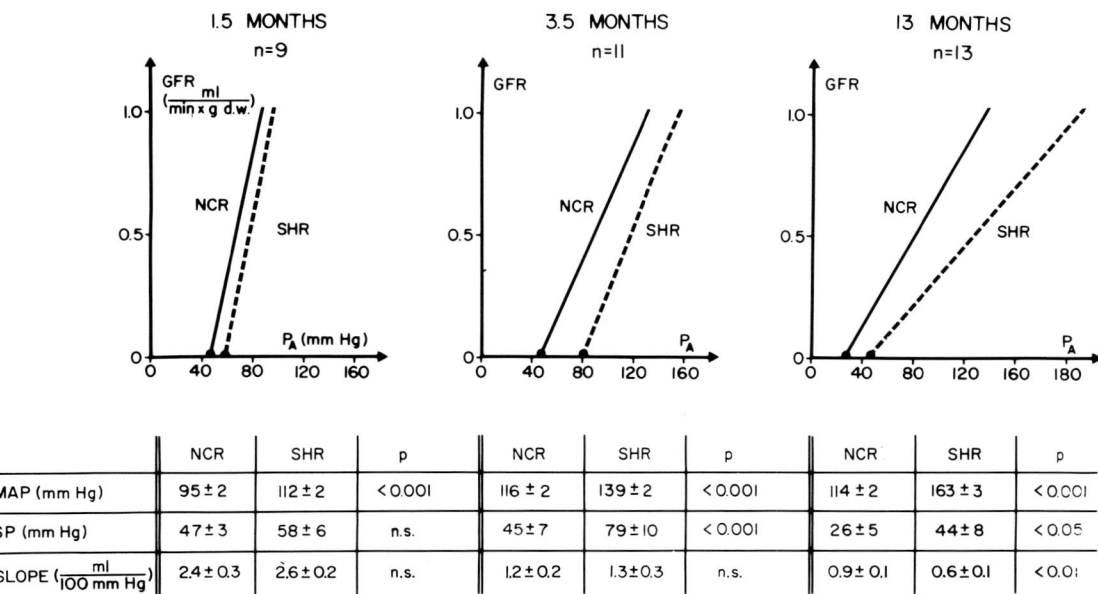

	NCR	SHR	p	NCR	SHR	p	NCR	SHR	p
MAP (mm Hg)	95±2	112±2	<0.001	116±2	139±2	<0.001	114±2	163±3	<0.001
SP (mm Hg)	47±3	58±6	n.s.	45±7	79±10	<0.001	26±5	44±8	<0.05
SLOPE ($\frac{ml}{100\,mm\,Hg}$)	2.4±0.3	2.6±0.2	n.s.	1.2±0.2	1.3±0.3	n.s.	0.9±0.1	0.6±0.1	<0.01

FIG. 6. A diagrammatic comparison between isolated pair-perfused (2 percent Dextran-Tyrode solution) kidneys from "young" (1.5 months), "adult" (3.5 months), and "old" (13 months) spontaneously hypertensive rats (SHR) and matched normotensive Wistar control rats (NCR). The different SHR groups represent the "borderline," "early established," and "long-standing" phases of primary hypertension. Besides showing the differences between SHR and NCR kidneys, the comparisons also illustrate the "ordinary" age-dependent structural alterations of renal hemodynamics in normotensive rats. **Top:** Diagrams showing the relationships between perfusion pressure (P_A) and glomerular filtration rate (GFR), as represented by the "average slopes" and by the "starting points" (SP), respectively; SP (i.e., the intercept of the slope with the pressure axis) reflects the preglomerular/postglomerular resistance ratio, and the slope reflects the glomerular filtration capacity. **Bottom:** Chart showing the average values (±SEM) for SP and slope of the P_A-GFR relationships, as well as for mean arterial pressures (MAP) of the awake rats. (From ref. 65, with permission.)

pressure reflects an increased R_{min} for the whole set of renal resistance vessels, while an increased maximal pressor response to, for example, noradrenaline (66), reflects an increased w/r_i, as for the hindquarter resistance vessels in Fig. 2.

The data based on this experimental approach, as in part presented in Fig. 6 (64–67), reveal the following structural alterations of the SHR renal vascular bed: Already in the early "borderline" phase of primary hypertension (age 6 weeks), when MAP is raised only 10–15 percent and average w/r_i shows a largely proportional increase (66), there is a marginal elevation of the pre- to postglomerular resistance ratio, though GFR is still normal. In "early established" SHR hypertension (age 3.5 months), when both MAP and w/r_i of the renal resistance vessels are raised 25–30 percent, the increase of the pre- to postglomerular resistance ratio is, if anything, even more marked (see center panel, Fig. 6), though GFR is still about the same as in age-matched normotensive controls. In aging SHR (13 months old), with 45-percent MAP elevation and a proportional w/r_i increase to judge from the maximal pressor responses (66), GFR is much more reduced than in age-matched normotensive controls. However, now the increase of the pre- to postglo-

merular resistance ratio in SHR is *less* pronounced than at the 3.5 months of age but, in return, R_{min} for the entire renal circuit is about 30 percent *more* increased. These findings reveal that aging per se has added a substantial structural narrowing of the postglomerular resistance vessels as well, perhaps a compensatory adjustment to offset the declining filtration capacity by instead increasing glomerular filtration pressure. In fact, the normotensive renal vascular bed shows structural alterations along with aging in the same general direction as in SHR, though to a much milder degree. Therefore, these perfusion analyses of the renal vascular bed also illustrate how high blood pressure accelerates the "ordinary" age-related structural deterioration of the cardiovascular system.

Modern morphometric analyses of r_i, w, and w/r_i dimensions have been successfully applied to the renal resistance vessels as well, e.g., by Gattone et al. (68) and by Smeda et al. (69). Gattone et al., who fixated the renal vessels at about their ordinary distending pressures, noted clear reductions of average preglomerular r_i already in young "borderline" SHR, a difference that was still more obvious in "established" SHR hypertension, in agreement with the mentioned "hemodynamic" analyses of the SHR renal resistance vessels. Lee's group (69) did not observe such differences but they evidently used fixation pressures far too low to fully distend the renal vessels, when also hemodynamic R_{min} analyses may fail to reveal R_{min} differences between resistance vessels from SHR and controls (66,67). In return, Lee et al. provided strong evidence of early and marked w/r_i increases in SHR preglomerular vessels, both with morphometric and hemodynamic techniques. Therefore, their conclusions were in general agreement with those arrived at in the mentioned hemodynamic (64–67) and morphometric (68) analyses. Hemodynamic analyses in man strongly indicate that essentially the same structural renovascular changes occur in human primary hypertension (70,71).

To summarize, an early, probably even genetically facilitated structural upward resetting occurs in the SHR preglomerular resistance vessels, evidently of the same nature as in proximal arterial resistance vessels of other systemic circuits. However, the renovascular structural adaptation is of particular importance as it implies an upward resetting of the renal "long-term barostat function," almost as if microclips had been applied to all preglomerular arterioles to increase their resistance in proportion to the MAP elevation. It is, then, not surprising that transplantation of an SHR kidney (or that of other hypertensive strains) to an acutely nephrectomized normotensive rat invites to hypertension, because GFR of the reset hypertensive kidney then becomes reduced while their renin-angiotensin system becomes activated and their renomedullary depressor systems inhibited. Enthusiasts for a genetically-based *renal origin* of primary hypertension often take such experiments as proof of their theory, but it may as well represent one among many consequences of a widespread cardiovascular structural adaptation, which may per se be genetically facilitated by quite different mechanisms. For example, if a giraffe kidney designed for a 250–300 mm Hg MAP level could be transplanted to a normotensive cow, it would surely make this creature hypertensive. However, this by no means proves that giraffe hypertension is renal in origin, as it evidently depends on the fact that the brain is placed 3 meters above the heart (72). Actually, the renovascular changes in SHR (and perhaps in several other hypertensive rat strains and in man as well) might as well ensue from genetic elements which enhance central neurohormonal pressor and trophic stimuli and/or make cardiovascular cells more sensitive to such stimuli and/or, via them, suppress the renomedullary depressor system (49). If so, the kidneys are just one (though no doubt particularly important) "victim" where assumptions about "what comes first, the chicken or the egg," usually depend on initial preferences and interests.

The cerebral vascular bed is, at least in most people, the most important circuit of all due to the organ subserved, and, in addition, a common victim in hypertension. The cerebrovascular structural changes were recently reviewed by Baumbach and Heistad (24), where they (as mentioned) used the expression "vascular remodeling" to denote how the structural r_i narrowing in cerebral proximal resistance vessels in SHR could be so marked that no wall area (w_a) expansion was needed to increase w/r_i in proportion to the raised MAP.

The moment-to-moment control of cerebral blood supply is based on a pronounced precapillary myogenic tone which is precisely adjusted to current metabolic needs by local-chemical feedback influences (73). This highly efficient functional autoregulation also serves to keep flow and—particularly important—the sensitive capillary exchange vessels largely constant at even marked acute changes in pressure, over the range 60–160 mm Hg or so. However, as long-term pressure increases, the cerebral precapillary resistance vessels show the same pressure-related structural autoregulation as in other circuits, which implies a corresponding upward resetting of the pressure range over which functional autoregulation can keep cerebral blood flow and capillary pressure constant (74–76). This naturally provides a better protection against dangerous increases of capillary pressure which occur when accidental pressure bouts overcome the autoregulatory capacity (74,75), but it also implies an upward resetting of the lower end of the autoregulatory range (76). Consequently, accidental pressure falls in hypertensive subjects, of ortostatic nature, or caused by too-rapid pressure reductions during antihypertensive therapy, can induce relative cerebral hypoxia at pressure levels which normotensive subjects readily balance off by functional autoregulation.

The coronary vascular bed, as mentioned earlier, is an important circuit that faces two challenges in hypertension: the resistance vessels must adapt their design both to the increased pressure and to the pressure-related increase of myocardial mass and hence of metabolic demands. Perfusion analyses of the coronary circuit in SHR and WKY hearts indicate that both these demands are, indeed, coped with: Per unit myocardial mass R_{min} and maximal pressor responses, which reflect average r_i and w/r_i, respectively, exhibit the same MAP-related increases as in other systemic circuits. However, R_{min}, and hence maximal coronary flow capacity, also becomes adjusted to the increase of myocardial tissue (19,77,78).

This illustrates particularly well how microvascular design is generally governed both by local transmural pressure and by nutritional and/or flow signals derived from the supplied tissues (8,41). As, however, myocardial metabolic demands are about as imperative and acute as those of the brain, this upward resetting implies that the coronary "blood flow reserve" is correspondingly reduced if MAP is so rapidly lowered (e.g., by antihypertensive therapy) that structural vascular regression cannot keep pace. However, during controlled pressure lowering the coronary vascular bed efficiently down-

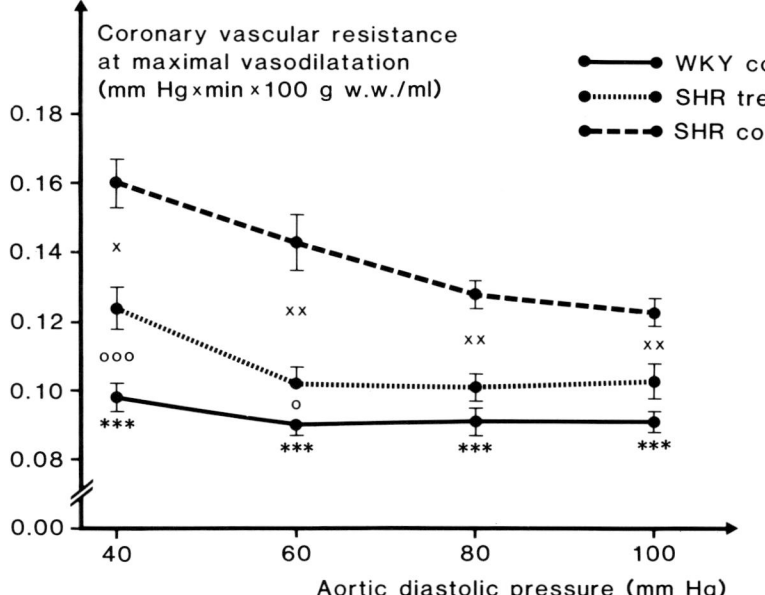

FIG. 7. Minimal coronary vascular resistance (R_{min}) per 100 g of myocardial tissue at four different aortic diastolic pressures in untreated spontaneously hypertensive rats (SHR), in Wistar-Kyoto rats (WKY), and in SHR treated with a β_1-receptor blocker combined with a vasoselective Ca^{2+}-entry blocker (metoprolol and felodipine). Note the 30- to 40 percent higher R_{min} in SHR versus WKY, and note how antihypertensive therapy has almost normalized R_{min} in treated SHR. Means $\pm$ SEM; $***p < 0.001$ between untreated SHR and WKY; $^x p < 0.05$; $^{xx} p < 0.01$ between untreated and treated SHR; $^o p < 0.05$, $^{ooo} p < 0.001$ between WKY and treated SHR. (From ref. 79, with permission.)

regulates its geometric design, as shown in Fig. 7, which compares coronary R_{min} at various perfusion pressures in untreated and treated SHR as well as in WKY (79).

HEMODYNAMIC EFFECTS OF STRUCTURAL CHANGES IN HEART, LARGE ARTERIES, AND VEINS

Though this article for good reasons mainly deals with the nature, extent, and hemodynamic consequences of the structural adaptation of systemic resistance vessels in hypertension, it is justified to briefly summarize major functional consequences of the related structural changes in heart, large arteries, and veins.

Heart

Both early SHR and human borderline primary hypertension commonly exhibit mild eccentric hypertrophy associated with, or perhaps rather a consequence of, a more or less "hyperkinetic" circulatory state (19,80). As myocytes are then elongated by addition of more sarcomeres (43), diastolic volume is increased in proportion to r_i^3 at the same time as a given stroke volume can be expelled at a correspondingly reduced myocardial contraction. This type of cardiac structural adaptation is particularly evident in endurance athletes and explains their increased stroke volume capacity, which can also be traced in hearts of young SHR when myocardial contractile ability is not yet reduced (19).

The gradual shift to concentric hypertrophy, when both systemic resistance and MAP are increased while the mainly rate-dependent increase of cardiac output is

normalized (80), implies a per se appropriate increase of left ventricular w/r_i to cope with the raised afterload. As for the resistance vessels, this w/r_i increase adds a geometric amplifying effect (10,20) which also implies that a given stroke volume can be expelled at reduced average shortening of individual myocytes. A particularly pronounced "concentric" hypertrophy is, for natural reasons, seen in giraffes (13). Thus, at the *local* level both eccentric and concentric hypertrophy appear as adequate structural adaptations to cope with increases of preload and afterload, respectively, at least as long as they are not complicated, e.g., by reduced coronary flow capacity or deteriorating myocyte contractility. Cardiac wall thickening has, however, other obvious consequences, such as increased wall stiffening, which calls for some elevation of diastolic filling pressure, at the same time as it contributes to the upward resetting of cardiac "volume" receptors (81).

In the clinical literature it is often stressed that cardiac hypertrophy is a major risk factor in human hypertension. However, to be strict, this is hardly due to hypertrophy per se, but rather because increased myocardial mass is a particularly obvious "marker" of the widespread structural cardiovascular changes present in chronic high-pressure state. By means of echocardiography the cardiac changes are more accessible than the concomitant microvascular structural changes in man, but these latter changes are probably far more serious for health than cardiac hypertrophy per se. For example, they interfere with cerebral and coronary blood supply, and hence with myocardial function, as well as with renal function, and are thereby the major causes of organ deterioration and lesions in hypertension in association with partly pressure-dependent atherosclerosis. Experimental evidence from hypertensive rat models indicates that cardiac and microvascular structural changes follow each other closely, both in rate and extent (1,8,19). By analogy, echocardiographic estimations of cardiac design in human hypertension are likely to be fairly reliable indicators of prevailing resistance vascular changes, and are probably, for *that* reason mainly, a reliable predictor of risks.

Large Arteries

The aorta and proximal conduit arteries are in this context of considerable hemodynamic importance, and for two reasons: first, their "Windkessel" function serves to transform the rhythmic cardiac output into a more even peripheral flow, at the same time that their distensibility damps the pulsatile pressure oscillations and hence the endsystolic load for the left ventricle, as reviewed by O'Rourke (82). Second, they are the site for the various sets of arterial baroreceptors, and any change of wall distensibility affects baroreceptor function as well.

In hypertension, as in ordinary aging, these vessels exhibit thickened and stiffer walls, though usually associated with *increases* of luminal dimensions (42), in contrast to downstream small resistance arteries. As a result, the pulse amplitude increases, which further adds to left ventricular endsystolic afterload for two reasons, as outlined by O'Rourke (82): An "elastance component" is, of course, added by the wall stiffening per se. However, as wall stiffening also causes up to threefold increases of pulse wave transmission; this wave may after peripheral reflection return to the aortic root even before systole is ended. Therefore, this may add a "reflected wave component" of up to 15–20 mm Hg to left ventricular afterload. As these reflected waves are hardly transferred out along the branchial arteries, they are little noticeable in forearm systolic pressure measurements, but the left ventricle must certainly always face them. The many negative consequences of these aortic-large-artery changes and nutritional supply may be serious indeed, as outlined elsewhere (34).

In addition, the stiffened aortic and carotid walls imply that higher pressures are needed to activate the baroreceptors as these in reality are stretch receptors. Independent of functional adaptive mechanisms, it adds a structural resetting influence whereby these receptors rather serve to maintain than to counteract the high-pressure state (83). It seems, however, as if receptors with unmyelinated afferents are *less* readily reset, perhaps because their nerve endings infiltrate the muscle layers. They therefore serve as if they were partly "series-coupled" receptors, whereby they may also sense wall *tension*. By contrast, the baroreceptors with medullated afferents serve as "parallel-coupled" receptors because

they respond only to circumferential stretch due to their adventitial location (84).

Veins

As earlier mentioned, venous structural design is ordinarily adapted to fairly low transmural pressures and shows additional increases of w to the modest elevations in average venous pressure that are often present already early in hypertension (1). However, to judge from a largely unchanged venous resistance to flow, venous average r_i remains virtually unchanged (1,8,31,32). Nevertheless, even modest venous wall thickening is hemodynamically quite important by reducing overall venous compliance, which tends to centralize blood volume in primary hypertension. This becomes of particular relevance when associated cardiac structural changes decrease diastolic compliance and therefore call for some increase of filling pressure (31,32).

THERAPEUTIC CONSIDERATIONS

As outlined in previous sections, the structural upward resetting dominates the systemic resistance elevation early in primary hypertension and also affects heart, veins, and most barostat functions. Though these adaptive processes are from a *local* point of view appropriate, they invite to the mentioned positive feedback interaction with functional pressor influences when generalized to all systemic circuits. Therefore, the major long-term goal of antihypertensive therapy should be to *reverse* this structural process and, if possible, to facilitate this regression, the more so as high-pressure states in man as in most species accelerate cardiovascular aging and hence invite to deterioration, organ lesions, and true disorder. Here the situation seems to be quite different in the "physiological" high-pressure state of giraffes where heart and vessels evidently are genetically designed to cope with the increased load, and much might be learned by analyzing the underlying cause.

This is not the place for extensive discussions of the many problems inherent in antihypertensive treatment, but a few items related to the present topic should be briefly outlined. Because the pressure elevation per se, as combined with increased cardiovascular muscle activity, serves as the "directing" local stimuli for structural adaptation, though more or less reinforced by trophic factors, therapy should accordingly aim at: (a) reducing the pressure load; (b) reducing cardiovascular muscle activity; (c) concentrating such effects to key sites of hemodynamic disturbance; and (d) reducing reinforcing influences of trophic factors (85,86). It is, indeed, remarkable that already in the 1740s Samuel Schaarschmidt in Berlin intuitively treated patients with *spastische Kontrak-*

tionen der Arterien along with these principles, as outlined elsewhere! (1)

On a more long-range scale, increased knowledge about the genetic-molecular and cellular growth processes may soon allow for more selective, perhaps even preventive, interferences whereby the coupling between "ordinary" pressor influences and the adaptive structural processes may be interrupted or at least attenuated, hopefully with minor side effects. Presently many exploratory studies of such events are going on in rat models of human primary hypertension and with promising results, partly discussed in earlier mentioned reviews (36,37,39,40), though much certainly remains to be done. So far it is clear that several antihypertensive drug principles, among which some also counteract trophic mechanisms, can (in, e.g., SHR) greatly attenuate the early development of hypertension and structural changes, and/or cause their regression, as illustrated in Fig. 7 for coronary vessels.

Unfortunately, it is in man, for sociopsychological reasons, seldom possible to start treatment already in early "borderline" phases except by using nonpharmacological approaches such as increased physical activity, weight reduction, etc., though still mainly on a pilot study basis. As a result, the gradual addition of interstitial endowment complicates the situation once pharmacological therapy must start, because structural regression is then more sluggish and incomplete. Furthermore, it is in man usually not possible to give enough drugs to rapidly normalize pressure due to disturbing side effects, not the least because the upward resetting of the entire system and its barostat mechanisms tends to oppose such an interference. Nevertheless, by means of quantitative estimations of, e.g., forearm R_{min} and, particularly, by the far-more-easily-performed echocardiographic analysis of cardiac dimensions and design (87–89), it seems clear that well-controlled and aggressive treatment can achieve structural regression toward a nearly normalized situation, if started early enough. It should, however, be remembered that the genetic predisposition remains in primary hypertension and that it is often difficult to eliminate the involved environmental pressor influences as well, which may again start the ball rolling. Future model therapeutic studies in hypertensive rat strains may here provide new avenues and principles, clarifying problems of the following type (85,86):

1. How early, intense and prolonged should therapy be to optimize structural regression?
2. Is it possible to design drugs so as to specifically counteract genetic and trophic reinforcements of the structural factor?
3. Do different genetic profiles call for different therapeutic designs to counteract the structural endowment?

4. Can new treatment principles set out from *physiological* depressor mechanisms, like that inherent in the medullipin system of Muirhead (17,18,49), and/or do some of the drugs used partly act by activating this system? (72)
5. Are the involved functional mechanisms in primary hypertension usually so relatively mild that, if structural adaptation can be blocked or fully regressed, the tendency of pressure elevation is usually so modest that it may be balanced off by revisions of living style and of psychosocial environment? There are, in fact, interesting indications that this may be the case also in man, e.g., in the important follow-up study by Timio et al. (90) concerning quite different blood pressure levels in groups of Italian women as related to their different psychosocial life styles.

CONCLUSIONS

Cardiovascular structural adaptation, being the most important quantitative component behind the elevated pressure and systemic resistance in established primary hypertension, and probably often involved also as a "primary" element, is by now fairly well known concerning principal origin, location, extent, rate of development, and hemodynamic effects. Much work is presently concentrated on the involved molecular and cellular mechanisms, how they are initiated and controlled by mechanical and trophic factors, and how they may be genetically endowed, where progress may be rapid.

Considering *hemodynamic* effects, this "normal" process of structural adaptation is potentially so efficient, particularly at the systemic resistance level that it is, in a way, more remarkable that the majority of people *remain* normotensive than that a minority becomes hypertensive. After all, the renal barostat function, as well as most cardiovascular baroreceptors and volume receptors, are rapidly reset upward to operate at a raised MAP level and, to a large extent, by way of the same structural process that raises systemic resistance. Hence these barostat mechanisms soon serve to *maintain*, rather than to offset, the high-pressure state, which invites the question as to where the evidently powerful and durable negative feedbacks are located which manage to maintain *normotension*, and which also may hinder primary hypertension to escalate toward a malignant development (72). Actually, far less is known about this problem than about the various mechanisms which may lead to hypertension, though this appears to be seldom realized. After all, it might be via reinforcements of such normal depressor mechanisms that a more efficient therapy, and perhaps even prevention, can be achieved in the future (72). Strong candidates for such powerful and durable negative-feedback influences may be endothelial depressor mechanisms, in terms of nitric oxide Endothelium-Derived Relaxing Factor (EDRF) release, pioneered by Furchgott (91), and Muirhead's humoral renomedullary depressor system (17,18). In addition, the unmyelinated baroafferents may partly serve similar purposes, as they seem to be far less reset in hypertension than the better known myelinated ones (84).

On balance, it almost appears as if experimental hypertension research has provided more knowledge to the *physiology* of circulatory control than to the apparent enigma of primary hypertension. Perhaps the main reason for this is that primary hypertension may, indeed, represent a "quantitative variant of normality," almost like different types of per se normal body builds, i.e., being the right-hand part of the Gaussean curve for "normal" blood pressure distribution, as originally proposed by Sir George Pickering, rather than being a true disorder in the ordinary sense of this word. Unfortunately, however, medical and pharmacological interventions are usually necessary as raised pressure *invites* to disorder by accelerating cardiovascular aging and deterioration in most species, except perhaps in giraffes which, because of their body build, are genetically designed for very high pressures.

REFERENCES

1. Folkow B. Physiological aspects of primary hypertension. *Physiol Rev* 1982;62:347–504.
2. Folkow B. Functional and structural "autoregulation"—some personal considerations concerning the century-old development of these microvascular concepts: the Benjamin W. Zweifach Award Lecture. *Microvasc Res* 1989;37:243–255.
3. Folkow B. Structural, myogenic, humoral and nervous factors controlling peripheral resistance. In: Harrington M, ed. *Hypotensive drugs.* London: Pergamon, 1956;163–174.
4. Folkow B, Grimby G, Thulesius O. Adaptive structural changes of the vascular walls in hypertension and their relation to the control of the peripheral resistance. *Acta Physiol Scand* 1958;44:255–272.
5. Conway J. A vascular abnormality in hypertension. A study of blood flow in the forearm. *Circulation* 1963;27:520–529.
6. Short DS, Thomson AD. The arteries of the small intestine in systemic hypertension. *J Pathol Bacteriol* 1959;78:321–334.
7. Furuyama M. Histometrical investigations of arteries in reference to arterial hypertension. *Tohoku J Exp Med* 1962;76:388–414.
8. Folkow B. "Structural factor" in primary and secondary hypertension. *Hypertension* 1990;16:89–101.
9. Folkow B, Karlström G. Age- and pressure-dependent changes of systemic resistance vessels concerning the relationships between geometric design, wall distensibility, vascular reactivity and smooth muscle sensitivity. *Acta Physiol Scand* 1984;122:17–33.
10. Korner PJ, Angus JA. Structural determinants of vascular resistance properties in hypertension. *J Vasc Res* 1992;29:293–312.
11. Folkow B. The structural cardiovascular factor in primary hypertension—pressure dependence and genetic reinforcement. *J Hypertens* 1986;4(Suppl 3):S51–S56.
12. Lever AF. Slow pressor mechanisms in hypertension: a role for hypertrophy of resistance vessels? [Editorial]. *J Hypertens* 1986;4:515–524.
13. Goetz RH, Keen EN. Some aspects of the cardiovascular system in the giraffe. *Angiology* 1957;8:542–564.
14. Kügelgen A Von. Über das Verhältnis von Ringmuskulatur und Innendruck in Menschlichen grossen Venen. *Z Zellforsch Mikrosk Anat* 1955;43:168–183.
15. Svejcar J, Prerovsky I, Linhart J, Kruml J. Content of collagen, elastin and water in walls of the internal saphenous vein in man. *Circ Res* 1962;11:296–300.
16. Sleek GE, Duling BR. Coordination of mural elements and myofilaments during arteriolar constriction. *Circ Res* 1986;59:620–627.
17. Muirhead EE. Medullipin system of blood pressure control. *News Physiol Sci* 1990;5:241–244.
18. Karlström G, Folkow B, Göthberg G. The humoral renal antihypertensive system: nervous and hemodynamic effects in normotensive and unclipped renal hypertensive rats. *Am J Med Sci* 1988;295(4):258–262.
19. Friberg P, Nordlander M. Influence of left ventricular and coronary vascular hypertrophy on cardiac performance. (Edit rev). *J Hypertens* 1990;8:879–889.
20. Korner PJ, Angus JA, Bobik A, Jennings GA. Amplifyer function of resistance vessels and the left ventricle in hypertension. *J Hypertens* 1991;9[Suppl 2]:S31–S41.
21. Mulvany MJ, Halpern W. Contractile properties of small arterial vessels in spontaneously hypertensive and normotensive rats. *Circ Res* 1977;41:19–26.
22. Mulvany MJ, Aalkjaer C. Structure and function of small arteries. *Physiol Rev* 1990;70:921–961.
23. Lee RMKW, Garfield RE, Forrest JB, Daniel EE. Morphometric study of structural changes in the mesenteric blood vessels of spontaneously hypertensive rats. *Blood Vessels* 1983;20:57–71.
24. Baumbach GL, Heistad DD. Adaptive changes in cerebral blood vessels during chronic hypertension. (Edit rev). *J Hypertens* 1991;9:987–991.
25. Lew MJ, Angus JA. Wall thickness to lumen diameter ratios of arteries from SHR and WKY. Comparison of pressurized and wire-mounted preparations. *J Vasc Res* 1992;29:435–442.
26. Friedman SM, Nakashima M, Mar MA. Morphological assessment of vasoconstriction and vascular hypertrophy in sustained hypertension in the rat. *Microvasc Res* 1971;3:416–425.
27. Zweifach BW. The microcirculation in experimental hypaertension [state-of-the-art rev]. *Hypertension* 1983;5(Suppl I):I10–I16.
28. Bohlen HG. The microcirculation in hypertension. *J Hypertens* 1989;7(Suppl 4):S117–S124.
29. Sivertsson R. The hemodynamic importance of structural vascular changes in essential hypertension. *Acta Physiol Scand* 1970[Suppl 343]:1–56.
30. Egan B, Schork N, Panis R, Hinderliter A. Vascular structure enhances regional resistance responses in mild essential hypertension. *J Hypertens* 1988;6:41–48.
31. Ricksten S-E, Yao T, Thorén P. Peripheral and central vascular compliance in conscious normotensive and spontaneously hypertensive rats. *Acta Physiol Scand* 1980;112:169–177.
32. Haraldsson B, Nilsson H, Folkow B. Structurally reduced distensibility of cardiovascular "low-pressure" compartments in primary hypertension, as studied in spontaneously hypertensive rats (SHR). *Acta Physiol Scand* 1981;112:473–480.
33. Pickering GW. High Blood Pressure, 2nd ed. London: Churchill, 1968.
34. Folkow B, Svanborg A. Physiology of cardiovascular aging. *Physiol Rev* 1993;73:725–764.
35. Postnov YV. Cell membrane alteration in primary hypertension: an approach to its explanation. *Acta Physiol Scand* 1988;133[Suppl 571]:175–180.
36. Lever AF, Harrap SB. Essential hypertension: a disorder of growth with origins in childhood? (Edit rev). *J Hypertens* 1992;10:101–120.
37. Schelling P, Fischer H, Ganten D. Angiotensin and cell growth: a link to cardiovascular hypertrophy. (Edit rev). *J Hypertens* 1991;9:3–15.
38. Neyses L, Vetter H. Molecular biology of ontogenes and cardiovascular hypertrophy. (Edit rev). *J Hypertens* 1992;10:1447–1452.
39. Krieger JE, Dzau VJ. Molecular biology of hypertension. *Hypertension* 1991;18[Suppl I]:I3–I17.
40. Jackson CL, Schwartz SM. Pharmacology of smooth muscle cell replication. (Edit rev). *Hypertension* 1992;20:713–736.
41. Folkow B. Extrinsic mechanisms of vascular growth. *J Clin Hypertens* 1987;3:328–336.

42. Safar ME, ed. *Arterial and venous systems in essential hypertension.* Dordrecht, The Netherlands: M Nijhoff, 1987.

43. Franticelli A, Josephson R, Danzinger R, Lakatta E, Spurgeon H. Morphologic and contractile characteristics of individual myocytes of rats from maturation to senescence. *Am J Physiol* 1989;257:H259–H265.

44. Bevan RD. Effects of sympathetic denervation on smooth muscle proliferation in the growing rabbit ear artery. *Circ Res* 1975;37:14–19.

45. Folkow B, Isaksson OGP, Karlström G, Lever AF, Nordlander M. Trophic effects of hypophyseal hormones on resistance vessels and the heart in normotensive and renal hypertensive rats. *Acta Physiol Scand* 1992;144:291–306.

46. Okamoto K. Spontaneous hypertension in rats. *Int Rev Exp Pathol* 1969;7:227–270.

47. Kanbe T, Nara Y, Tagami M, Yamori Y. Studies of hypertension-induced vascular hypertrophy in cultured smooth muscle cells from spontaneously hypertensive rats. *Hypertension* 1983;5:887–892.

48. Gray SD. Spontaneous hypertension in the neonatal rat. *Clin Exp Hypertens* (A) 1984;A6(4):755–781.

49. Karlström G, Bergström G, Folkow B, Rudenstam J, Göthberg G. Is the humoral renal antihypertensive activity of the spontaneously hypertensive rat (SHR) reset to the high blood pressure? *Acta Physiol Scand* 1991;141:517–530.

50. Hofman A, Grobbee DE, Schalekamp MADH, eds. The early pathogenesis of primary hypertension. Amsterdam: Exerpta Medica, 1987.

51. Falkner B. Reactivity to mental stress in hypertension and prehypertension. In: Julius S, Basset DR, eds. *Handbook of hypertension, vol 9: Behavioral factors in hypertension.* Amsterdam: Elsevier, 1987;95–103.

52. Folkow B. Psychosocial and central nervous influences in primary hypertension. *Circulation* 1987;76(Suppl I):1–10.

53. Henry JM, Grim CE. Psychosocial mechanisms of primary hypertension (Edit rev). *J Hypertens* 1990;8:783–793.

54. Guyton AC, Coleman TG, Cowley AW Jr, Manning RD Jr, Norman RA Jr, Ferguson JD. A systems analysis approach to understanding long-range arterial blood pressure control and hypertension. *Circ Res* 1974;35:159–176.

55. Guyton AC, Hall JE, Montani J-P. Kidney function and hypertension. *Acta Physiol Scand* 1988;133(Suppl 571):163–173.

56. Lundgren Y, Hallbäck M, Weiss L, Folkow B. Rate and extent of adaptive cardiovascular changes in rats during experimental renal hypertension. *Acta Physiol Scand* 1974;91:103–115.

57. Lundgren Y. Adaptive changes of cardiovascular design in spontaneous and renal hypertension. *Acta Physiol Scand* 1974;91(Suppl 408):1–62.

58. Aalkjaer C, Danielsen H, Johannesen P, Pedersen EB, Rasmussen A, Mulvany MJ. Abnormal vascular function and morphology in preeclampsia: a study of isolated resistance vessels. *Clin Sci* 1985;69:477–482.

59. Hjalmarsson Å, Isaksson OGP. In vitro work load and rat heart metabolism: Effect on protein synthesis. *Acta Physiol Scand* 1972;86:126–144.

60. Udenfriend S, Ooshima A, Cardinale G, Fuller GC, Spector S. Increased formation of collagen in the blood vessels of hypertensive rats. *Ann NY Acad Sci* 1976;275:101–103.

61. Wolinsky H. Long-term effects of hypertension on the rat aortic wall and their relation to concurrent aging changes. *Circ Res* 1972;30:301–309.

62. Weiss L. Aspects of the relation between functional and structural cardiovascular factors in primary hypertension. *Acta Physiol Scand* 1974;91(Suppl 409):1–58.

63. Lundgren Y, Weiss L. Cardiovascular design after 'reversal' of longstanding renal hypertension. *Clin Sci* 1979;57:19s–21s.

64. Göthberg G, Lundin S, Ricksten S-E, Folkow B. Apparent and true vascular resistances to flow in SHR and NCR kidneys as related to the pre/postglomerular resistance ratio. *Acta Physiol Scand* 1979;105:282–294.

65. Göthberg G, Folkow B. Age-dependent alterations in the structurally determined vascular resistance, pre- to postglomerular resistance ratio and glomerular filtration capacity in kidneys, as studied in aging normotensive rats and spontaneously hypertensive rats. *Acta Physiol Scand* 1983;117:547–555.

66. Göthberg G, Hallbäck-Nordlander M, Karlström G, Ricksten S-E, Folkow B. Structurally based changes of renal vascular reactivity in spontaneously hypertensive and two-kidney, one-clip renal hypertensive rats, as compared with kidneys from uninephrectomized and intact normotensive rats. *Acta Physiol Scand* 1983;118:61–67.

67. Göthberg G, Folkow B. "Structural autoregulation" of blood flow and GFR in the two renal vascular beds from two-kidney, one-clip renal hypertensive rats, as compared with kidneys from uninephrectomized and intact normotensive rats. *Acta Physiol Scand* 1983;118:141–148.

68. Gattone VH, Evan AP, Willis LR, Luft FC. Renal afferent arteriole in the spontaneously hypertensive rat. *Hypertension* 1983;5:8–16.

69. Smeda JS, Lee RMKW, Forrest JB. Structural and reactivity alterations of the renal vasculature of spontaneously hypertensive rats prior to and during established hypertension. *Circ Res* 1988;63:518–533.

70. Hollenberg NK, Adams DF. The renal circulation in hypertensive disease. *Am J Med* 1976;60:773–784.

71. Hollenberg NK, Borucki LJ, Adams DF. The renal vasculature in early essential hypertension. Evidence for a pathogenetic role. *Medicine* 1978;57:167–176.

72. Folkow B. Some reflections on today's hypertension research. *Blood Pressure* 1992;1:5–8.

73. Folkow B, Hansson L, Johansson B, eds. Myogenic mechanisms in the control of systemic resistance. *J Hypertens* 1989;7(Suppl 4):S1–S171.

74. Johansson BB. Cerebral vascular bed in hypertension and consequences for the brain. *Hypertension* 1984;6(Suppl III):III-81–III-86.

75. Johansson BB, Strandgaard S, Lassen N. The hypertensive "breakthrough" of autoregulation of cerebral blood flow with forced vasodilatation, flow increase and blood-drain damage. *Circ Res* 1974;34(Suppl I):167–171.

76. Jones JV, Fitch W, MacKenzie ET, Strandgaard S, Harper AM. Lower limit of cerebral blood flow autoregulation in experimental renovascular hypertension in the baboon. *Circ Res* 1976;39:555–557.

77. Noresson E, Hallbäck M, Hjalmarsson Å. Structural "resetting" of the coronary vascular bed in spontaneously hypertensive rats. *Acta Physiol Scand* 1977;101:363–365.

78. Strauer BE. The coronary circulation in hypertensive heart disease. *Hypertension* 1984;6(Suppl III):III-74–III-80.

79. Friberg P, Wåhlander H, Nordlander M. Structural and functional adaptations within the myocardium and coronary vessels after antihypertensive therapy in spontaneously hypertensive rats. *J Hypertens* 1986;4(Suppl 3):S519–S521.

80. Conway J. Hemodynamic aspects of essential hypertension in humans. *Physiol Rev* 1984;64:617–660.

81. Thorén P. Cardiac reflexes in hypertension. In: Zanchetti A, Tarazi RC, eds. *Handbook of hypertension, vol 7: Pathophysiology of hypertension—cardiovascular aspects.* Amsterdam: Elsevier, 1986;102–116.

82. O'Rourke M. Arterial stiffness, systolic blood pressure, and logical treatment of hypertension. (Edit rev). *Hypertension* 1990;15:339–347.

83. Mark AL, Mancia G. Cardiopulmonary baroreflex in humans. In: Shepherd JT, Abboud FM, eds. *Handbook of physiology—the cardiovascular system.* Bethesda: Am Physiol Soc 1983;vol III:795–813.

84. Thorén P, Ricksten S-E. Cardiac C-fiber endings in cardiovascular control under normal and pathophysiological conditions. In: Disturbances in neurogenic control of the circulation. *Am Physiol Soc* 1981;17–31.

85. Folkow B. Physiological approach to future developments in therapy. *J Cardiovasc Pharmacol* 1987;10(Suppl 2):S128–S134.

86. Folkow B. The structural factor in primary hypertension: its relevance for future principles of treatment. *J Hypertens* 1987;5[Suppl 5]:S611–S613.

87. Sivertsson R, Hansson L. Effects of blood pressure reduction on

the structural vascular abnormality in skin and muscle vascular beds in human essential hypertension. *Clin Sci* 1976;51:77s–79s.

88. Korner PI, Jennings GL, Esler MD, Bobik A, Adams M. The role of cardiovascular hypertrophy in hypertension: basis for a new therapeutic strategy. *J Cardiovasc Pharmacol* 1987;10[Suppl 5]:S72–S78.

89. Dahlöf B, Pennert K, Hansson L. Reversal of left ventricular hypertrophy in hypertensive patients. A metaanalysis of 109 treated studies. *Am J Hypertens* 1992;5:95–110.

90. Timio M, Verdecchia P, Venanzi S, Gentili S, Ronconi M, Francucci B, Montanari M, Bichisao E. Age and blood pressure changes. A 20-year follow-up study in nuns in a secluded order. *Hypertension* 1988;12:457–461.

91. Furchgott RF. The 1989 Ulf von Euler Lecture. Studies on endothelium-dependent vasodilatation and the endothelium-derived relaxing factor. *Acta Physiol Scand* 1989;139:257–270.

92. Folkow B. Cardiovascular structural adaptation; its role in the initiation and maintenance of primary hypertension. The Fourth Volhard Lecture. *Clin Sci* 1978;55:3s–22s.

93. Folkow B, et al. Background of increased flow resistance and vascular reactivity in spontaneously hypertensive rats. *Acta Physiol Scand* 1970;80:93–106.

Hypertension: Pathophysiology, Diagnosis, and Management, Second Edition,
edited by J.H. Laragh and B.M. Brenner,
Raven Press, Ltd., New York © 1995.

CHAPTER **31**

Structural Changes in the Resistance Vessels in Human Hypertension

Michael J. Mulvany

It is well established that essential hypertension is associated with increased peripheral resistance (see e.g., ref. 1). Furthermore, since capillary pressure is approximately normal in essential hypertension (2), the main increase in resistance must lie in the *resistance vessels,* that is, those precapillary vessels that contribute to, and control, the peripheral resistance. This increase in resistance can be explained in terms of either a narrowing of the resistance vessels or a decrease in the number of parallel-connected vessels, a process known as rarefaction (3). Although the distribution of the resistance in essential hypertension is not known, evidence from animal models suggests that the precapillary resistance resides in both the *arterioles* (arteries with not more than one layer of smooth muscle cells) and in the more proximal *small arteries* (prearteriolar arteries with lumen diameters less

than approximately 300 μm (4). Recent work concerning abnormalities of resistance vessels in hypertension has therefore been directed toward understanding the abnormalities of both the arterioles and the small arteries. In particular, interest has focused on whether the abnormalities are due to alterations in the vascular smooth muscle (structure or excitation-contraction properties), in the neuromuscular junction, or in the endothelium (5–7).

At present, most information about resistance vessels and hypertension is based on the many animal models, and these have demonstrated a bewildering variety of structural and functional abnormalities apparently associated with hypertension (8). However, the relevance of these data to the human situation is not clear, and recent work has been directed at investigating resistance vessels in essential hypertensive patients. This question has been addressed in a number of ways: hemodynamic studies, direct visualization of vessels, histologic examination of biopsy and autopsy material, and examination of the

M. J. Mulvany: Danish Biomembrane Research Centre and Institute of Pharmacology, Aarhus University, Aarhus, Denmark.

vessels *in vitro*. This chapter discusses the evidence obtained with these different techniques as regards essential hypertension. The reader is referred to Mulvany (8) for a fuller discussion of these results in the context of experimental hypertension.

LOCATION OF PERIPHERAL RESISTANCE

In animal models, the contribution of the various segments of vasculature to the peripheral resistance can be determined from measurement of the intravascular pressure in vessels from the aorta through to the capillaries to the veins. Such investigations (4,8–11) indicate that, under anesthetized conditions, a substantial portion of the systemic pressure is dissipated in the prearteriolar small arteries (as defined above), and that these vessels participate in the control of the peripheral resistance. Furthermore, such vessels also contribute to the increased peripheral resistance of spontaneously hypertensive rats (SHR) (12–15) and renal hypertensive rats (16,17). These findings from anesthetized animals have recently been confirmed in conscious animals (18,19).

In man, such findings are confined to measurements of capillary pressure, which is shown to be about 13 mm Hg, about 14 percent of systemic pressure (2). Moreover, in patients with essential hypertension, the capillary pressure of essential hypertensive patients is about 17 percent of systemic pressure (2), similar to that in normotensive controls. This indicates that the main increase in resistance lies proximal to the capillaries, i.e., in the resistance vessels. The available evidence suggests therefore that studies of the causes of the increased peripheral resistance associated with essential hypertension should be concerned with the precapillary vessels, and the animal data indicate that both the arterioles and the small arteries should be investigated.

METHODS

The past decade has seen great improvements in the means for studying these small vessels, in particular as regards small arteries, both *in vivo* and *in vitro* (20,21), thus enabling previous hypotheses concerning the role of resistance vessels in the pathogenesis of hypertension to be tested. These methods for studying the structure and function of small arteries will be briefly discussed.

Structure

What is the "structure" of a blood vessel? Given the elastic nature of the vascular wall, the dimensions of a vessel depend on the conditions under which they are measured. The structure of a blood vessel must therefore be determined under clearly defined mechanical conditions, e.g., a particular intravascular pressure, such that its intrinsic dimensions (lumen diameter, wall thickness) will then be a function of the amount of material in the wall, the manner in which it is arranged and the elastic moduli of the various wall components. However, the dimensions will also be a function of the degree of smooth muscle activation in the vessel wall, and the magnitude of the intravascular pressure. Meaningful measurements of vascular structure therefore require that the intravascular pressure and state of activation be defined, and for comparative purposes it is usual for structure to be measured with the smooth muscle completely relaxed and, as far as possible, with a specific intravascular pressure, often 100 mm Hg (13.3 kPa). The figure of 100 mm Hg is used both because it is a round number, and because the elastic characteristics of the vascular wall give a logarithmic lumen-intravascular pressure relation such that above 100 mm Hg there is little increase in lumen diameter (22).

It is frequently discussed whether the structure of a vessel should not be determined with the intravascular pressure that it has experienced *in vivo*. However, the purpose of comparing vessels under identical experimental conditions is to compare their intrinsic properties, not their properties *in vivo*. Clearly, extrapolation of results obtained under standardized conditions to the *in vivo* situation must be made with caution.

Another difficulty in measuring structure is the question of which vessels should be compared; should this be on the basis of branching pattern, or on the basis of location (4)? Thus different sampling techniques can give different results. For measurements of wall thickness to lumen diameter ratio (wall/lumen ratio), or smooth muscle cell volume, this is not so serious, for this parameter is less dependent on the precise location (23). However, lumen diameter, wall cross-sectional area (wall volume per unit length), and number of smooth muscle cells per unit length are strongly dependent on the position in the vascular tree. Therefore, for these parameters, slight differences in the architecture of hypertensive and normotensive vasculatures can give erroneous results; conclusions in particular concerning growth or lack of growth in the resistance vasculature of hypertensive individuals need to be treated with caution (24), and more sophisticated sampling techniques are called for (25,26).

Measurement of Vascular Structure

Hemodynamic Studies

An indication of the structural characteristics of resistance vessels *in vivo* can be obtained from hemodynamic studies in which the resistance of a vascular bed is measured with the bed completely relaxed, for example, following reactive hyperemia (27). This provides information about the integrated resistance of the resistance vessels. However, it cannot show whether, for example, an increase in resistance is due to a reduction in average lumen diameter or to a decrease in the number of parallel connected vessels (rarefaction). Nor does this technique allow for the differences in the systemic pressure.

Histological Studies

Information about individual vessels can be obtained from histological studies of postmortem material. To fulfill the conditions indicated above, the material has to be perfusion fixed (25), where the perfusion pressure has a given value, e.g., 100 mm Hg. However, unless precautions are taken (28), the intravascular pressure in the vessels to be examined at the time of fixation is unknown.

Direct Observation In Vivo

For visible vessels, direct observation of their structure is an alternative. In humans, this at present is confined to the eye (29), and nail fold (30), although the techniques do not seem able to provide quantitative information about vascular dimensions. In animal models, other vascular beds can be exposed under anesthesia (e.g., ref. 13). In the future, noninvasive ultrasonic echo techniques may be possible, given the rapid progress in this field (31).

In Vitro Studies

For proximal resistance vessels, in vitro experiments offer the possibility for precise determinations of structure under clearly defined conditions (for review see ref. 4), in which isolated vessels are mounted on a pressure myograph, where vessel segments are cannulated at each end and the relation between lumen diameter and intravascular pressure is determined (32,33), or a wire myograph, where segments are threaded onto two fine wires (Fig. 1) that are then connected to a force transducer and micrometer, respectively, allowing force-internal circumference relations to be determined under closely controlled conditions (34). The utility of these techniques as regards essential hypertension has been substantially increased by the introduction of a human gluteal skin biopsy, taken under local anesthesia, from which subcutaneous small arteries can be dissected (35). For preparations examined on a pressure myograph, structure can easily be measured with the vessels relaxed and under a known intravascular pressure, although here it is important also to standardize the amount of longitudinal stretch (22).

For vessels mounted on a wire myograph, the standardization has to be done indirectly using the Laplace equation to determine the extension corresponding to the given intravascular transmural pressure (36). A direct evaluation of the two methods indicates that they give qualitatively similar results for comparing vessels from hypertensive individuals relative to those from normotensive individuals (22). For more distal resistance ves-

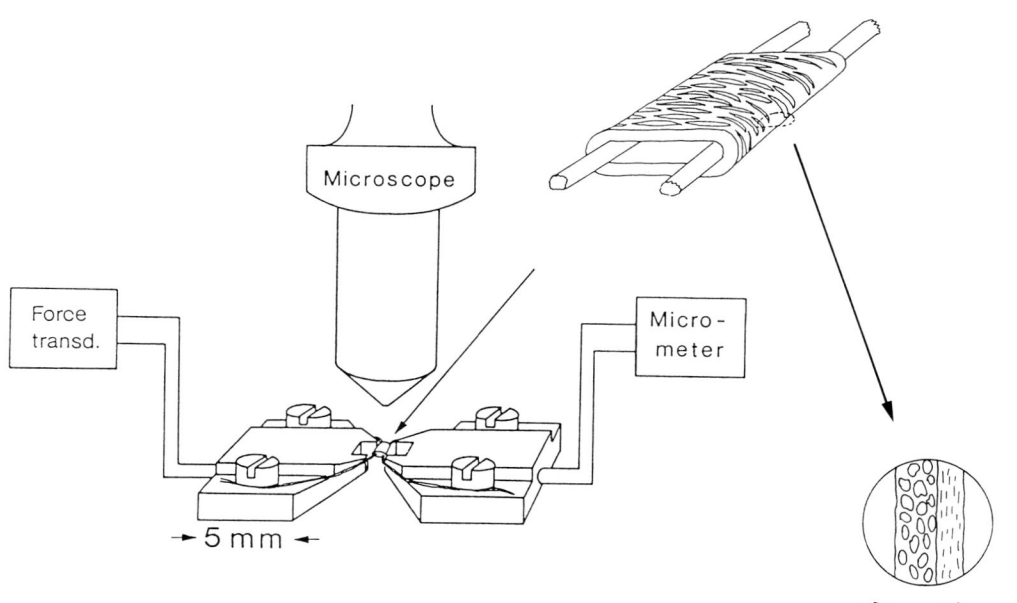

FIG. 1. Wire myograph used to investigate the structural and functional properties of human small arteries (34,77).

sels, present *in vitro* techniques do not allow quantitative examination of isolated human vessels.

Measurement of Excitation-Contraction Coupling Characteristics

Many of the techniques described above can also be used for measurement of resistance vessel function. Thus, measurement of forearm blood flow resistance provides information about the integrated response of the vasculature to infused vasoactive agents (37). Examination of isolated small arteries on wire or pressure myographs can be used for investigation of the contractile responses of the vessels. Pressure myographs are particularly suited for measurement of endothelial function and myogenic responses, while wire myographs are probably best suited for determination of the pharmacology of the receptors as well as of the mechanisms linking receptor activation to contraction (for review see ref. 38). The sophistication of the latter studies has been increased with the ability to measure many other parameters in wire myographs, including membrane potential (39), cytoplasmic calcium (40) and proton (41) activity, transmembrane fluxes (42), and phosophoinositide metabolism (43).

HEMODYNAMIC STUDIES

Structure

Evidence for structural alteration in the resistance vasculature of patients with essential hypertension is obtained from measurements of the resistance of the relaxed hypertensive forearm vasculature ("minimum vascular resistance"), determined during reactive hyperemia; this is found to be increased roughly in proportion to the increase in mean blood pressure (MBP) (27, 44–46). The conclusion that this is a measure of vascular structure, rather than any change in excitation-contraction coupling properties, rests on the belief that the vasculature is indeed fully relaxed (47), and this has been questioned (48). However, further *in vivo* evidence for structural change in the vasculature of essential hypertensive patients comes from clinical determinations of vascular wall stiffness in the forearm (49) and finger (50), using plethysmography, and in the lower leg (51), using a ^{133}Xe-washout technique. Moreover, indirect evidence that the structure of the resistance vasculature of hypertensive subjects is altered comes from the increased pressor response to infused agonists seen in essential hypertensive patients (44,46,52,53), since this is most easily explained in terms of an increased wall/lumen ratio of the resistance vessels (54). The available hemodynamic evidence thus provides strong support for altered resistance vessel structure in essential hypertension.

Excitation-Contraction Coupling

Evidence concerning the threshold sensitivity of the vasculature of essential hypertensive patients (i.e., the minimum dose that will give a response) is sparse. The forearm (44) and the hand (55) show no abnormality concerning noradrenaline sensitivity. However, Robinson et al. (56) and Hulthen et al. (57) found that the ratio between the sensitivity of the forearm vasculature of essential hypertensives to calcium antagonists and to nitroprusside was increased, suggesting some functional abnormality. Also, in the renal vasculature, Ljungman et al. (53) reported a slight increase in the sensitivity to venous infusion of angiotensin II, although some central mechanism could have been involved. However, apart from the evidence described below concerning endothelial-mediated responses, the hemodynamic evidence for substantial altered function in resistance vessels of essential hypertensive subjects is not strong.

In contrast to these negative results concerning agonist responses, following the original report of a reduced endothelial-dependent vasodilator effect of acetylcholine in SHR aorta (58), this phenomenon has been investigated in essential hypertension. Here it has been found that the decrease in forearm vascular resistance in response to acetylcholine is blunted compared to normotensive controls, such blunting not being observed with respect to nitroprusside (59,60). The response to acetylcholine appears to be mediated through activation of nitric oxide synthase (61).

Conclusions

Taken together, these hemodynamic studies provide good evidence that the increased total peripheral resistance seen in essential hypertension is associated with abnormalities in the structure of the precapillary resistance vessels, for the increased resistance seen in fully dilated vascular beds can only be explained in terms of the physical properties of the vasculature. However, the nature of the abnormality cannot be determined from these experiments. The increased minimum vascular resistance could be due either to the vessels being narrower or to rarefaction. Therefore, although the experiments provide rather good evidence for the vasculature being changed in hypertension, their interpretation in terms of specific abnormalities is difficult. Such specific information must be obtained by direct examination of the vessels involved.

HISTOLOGICAL STUDIES

Vascular Morphology

Autopsy studies in the last century (62,63) indicated that the small arteries of patients with hypertension (then

Bright's disease) had abnormally high wall/lumen ratios. However, it was not clear if this was due to a structural change or to the vessels having contracted more strongly during the fixation process. Later, Furuyama (64) and Suwa and Takahashi (65) attempted to circumvent this problem by estimating vascular diameter from the total length of the internal elastic lamina (which corrugates during vascular contraction), and also found an increased wall/lumen ratio of vessels in autopsy material from essential hypertensives. The validity of the method, however, is dependent on the assumption that the internal elastic lamina becomes smooth at the same pressure in hypertensive and control subjects, an assumption that has been questioned (66). Short (25) fixed autopsy samples of mesenteric vasculature while these were being perfused under pressure, and also showed that wall/lumen ratios were increased in essential hypertensives. However, it should be pointed out that even this elegant study had the weakness that the actual pressure in vessels at the moment of fixation could not be controlled, nor was the possibility excluded that the fixative caused contraction of the vessels. Further histological evidence for structural change in resistance vessels comes from a recent investigation of autopsied hearts (67), which indicated that, for a given diameter, the wall of coronary arterioles was thickened in hypertension.

Cell Morphology

An important question, which so far can only be addressed by histological methods, is whether any alteration in vessel structure is associated with a change in the volume of the cells. In essential hypertension, cell volume is normal in subcutaneous small arteries (68). This is also the case for mesenteric small arteries in SHR (69), as in a hypertensive transgenic rat (70). Taken together, the evidence points strongly in favor of smooth muscle cell volume being normal in genetic hypertension. In this respect, genetic hypertension appears to differ from induced hypertension, e.g., in Goldblatt renal hypertension in rats, where smooth muscle cell volume is found to be increased (71).

Conclusions

The histologic data support the hemodynamic evidence that the media/lumen ratios of small arteries is increased in essential hypertension, and suggest further that this is not associated with any increase in smooth muscle cell size.

IN VIVO VISUALIZATION

In man, the vascular beds most suited to direct observation are in the eye and in the nail fold. However, little information has been obtained by this means as regards essential hypertension. A recent study showed that vascular damage in the retina increases with the degree of hypertension, and that this is reduced by antihypertensive treatment (29). Moreover, observations of the conjunctiva of essential hypertensive subjects show a rarefaction of the vasculature (72), and similar findings are reported concerning the capillaries of the nail fold (30). Thus, as in SHR (72–74), available evidence supports the possibility that rarefaction is one of the causes of the increased peripheral resistance in essential hypertension, although more work is needed to validate this (75). It should also be pointed out that a recent theoretical analysis (76) has suggested that rarefaction can only account for a minor proportion of the increased resistance.

IN VITRO EXAMINATION

Structure

Until recently, there had been few investigations of isolated small arteries in essential hypertension. However, the development of the gluteal skin biopsy mentioned above, taken under local anesthesia, from which it is possible to dissect out small arteries for mounting on wire myographs (77), has allowed prospective investigations of small arteries in essential hypertensives. In several investigations (35,68,78,79), small arteries have been isolated from subjects with untreated moderate to severe essential hypertension and from age- and sex-matched controls and mounted on a wire myograph (Fig. 2). In all cases, the small arteries from the essential hypertensive subjects were found to have significantly larger media/lumen ratios than those taken from the controls and smaller lumens (significant in two of the investigations). The maximum response of the vessels from the essential hypertensives to all agonists tested was increased, but the increase corresponded exactly to the increased media thickness; the force production per unit of smooth muscle cross section ("active media stress") was normal (Fig. 3). The experiments thus provide strong support for essential hypertension being associated with abnormal structure of small arteries.

Of particular interest is the question indicated in Fig. 4, as to whether the increased media/lumen ratio of small arteries is associated with growth of these vessels, or whether they can be explained in terms of "remodeling" (80,81), i.e., a rearrangement of the same amount of material around a smaller lumen (24). In favor of remodeling being the primary process is the fact that, as shown in Fig. 5, in none of the four investigations mentioned above was the increased media/lumen ratio associated with any significant increase in the media cross-sectional area (equal to media volume per unit length). There are, however, many caveats (24) to this conclu-

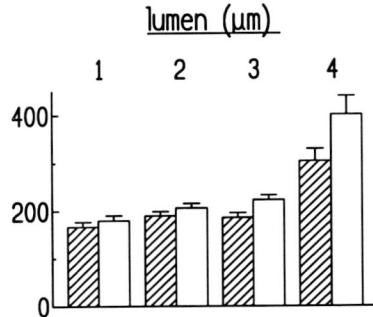
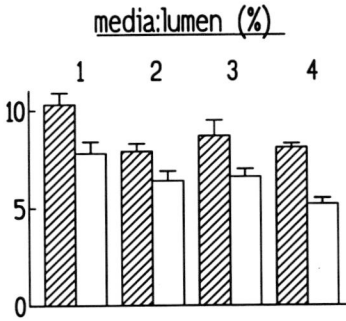

FIG. 2. Lumen diameter and media/lumen ratio of resistance arteries from essential hypertensive patients compared to resistance arteries from age- and sex-matched control subjects. Summary of results from four investigations: 1, ref. 35; 2, ref. 111; 3, ref. 68; 4, ref. 79 (*open columns, left hatch, right hatch,* and *cross hatch,* respectively). Error bars show SE; 8 to 16 subjects in each group.

sion: (a) the work refers only to subcutaneous small arteries; (b) there is statistical room in the data for a small amount of growth (say 15 percent); (c) there is the possibility of a sampling error; (d) the relation of the *in vitro* measurements to the *in vivo* situation is not clear, in particular the relation of the length of the preparations *in vitro* to the *in vivo* situation. Further work is required to determine the importance of the remodeling process, and thereby whether growth factors play a role.

To some extent, the concept that remodeling should be more important than growth processes in the resistance vasculature is in contrast to the more generally accepted view that the structural changes seen in resistance vessels are due to an encroachment of the media into the lumen. However, a consideration of the basic tenets of the Folkow (27) hypothesis shows that remodeling is actually an inherent part of his concept. As shown in Fig. 6, reduction of lumen (according to the Poiseuille fourth power relation) to account for the increased peripheral

resistance, and increase in media/lumen ratio to allow vessels to contract against a higher pressure, actually predict that the altered structure will be due mainly to remodeling, and only in part to growth. The experimental findings (Figs. 2 and 5) therefore agree well with the Folkow hypothesis (27).

Excitation-Contraction Coupling in Smooth Muscle

Although, there is substantial evidence that resistance vessels from SHR are hypersensitive to a variety of agonists, there is no evidence for this in resistance vessels from essential hypertensive subjects (Fig. 3). Thus, sensitivity to noradrenaline, serotonin, and vasopressin is normal in subcutaneous small arteries (35,79). Other functional parameters found to be normal in small arteries from essential hypertensive subjects include the intracellular pH, both under resting and activated conditions,

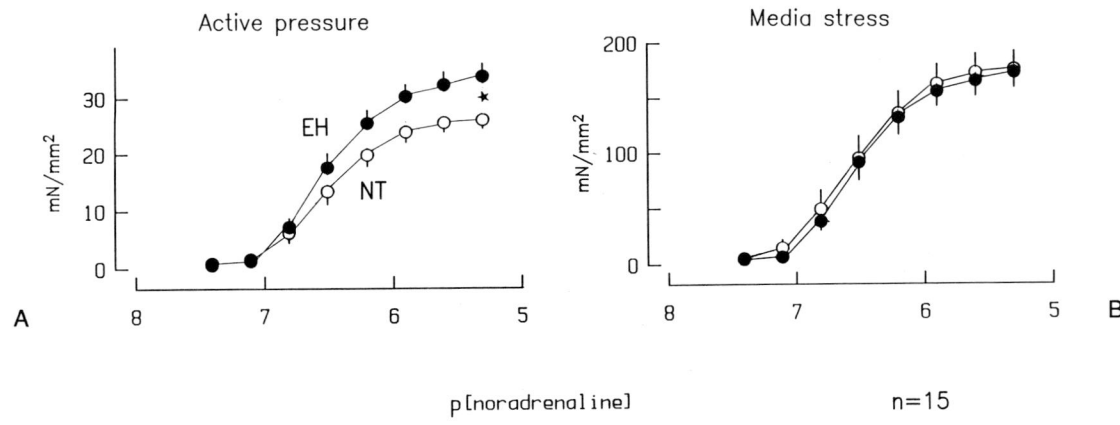

FIG. 3. Noradrenaline concentration-response curves of isolated subcutaneous small arteries from essential hypertensive subjects (*filled symbols*) and from controls (*open symbols*). Noradrenaline doses are given as p (noradrenaline) = −log (noradrenaline concentration [M]), and responses are expressed as effective active pressure (pressure against which vessel could contract, on the basis of the Laplace relation (36) (**A**) and media stress (**B**). *$p < .05$. Error bars show SE; 15 subjects in each group. (From ref. 35, with permission.)

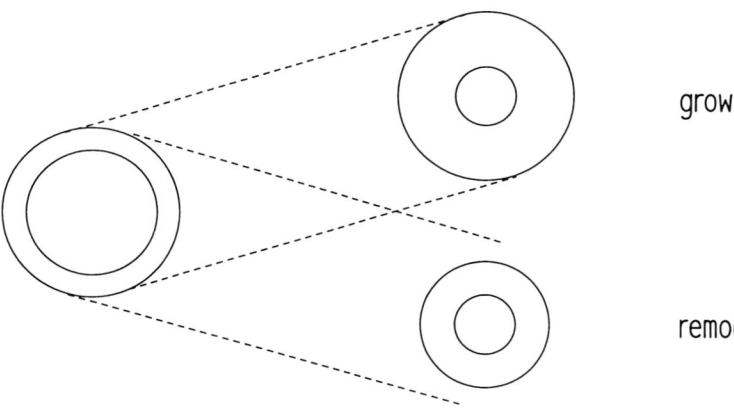

growth

remodelling

FIG. 4. Hypothetical cross sections of vessels in the normotensive situation (*left*) and in the hypertensive situation (*right*) showing how the reduction in the lumen might have arisen: (*top*) by a growth of the wall into the lumen, or (*bottom*) without growth but by a rearrangement of the same amount of material around the smaller lumen—the phenomenon known as vascular "remodeling" (80,81), where the cross-sectional areas of the normotensive and hypertensive vessels are the same. Note that vascular remodeling leading to an increased media/lumen ratio necessarily involves a decrease in both the internal and the external diameter (80,81).

suggesting lack of abnormality in the activity of transsarcolemmal Na,H-exchange (78). An exception to this is the response to endothelin, which is reduced in subcutaneous small arteries from patients with essential hypertension (79), as also is found in SHR and renal hypertensive rats (82,83). It has been suggested that this blunted response is due to endothelin causing increased release of endothelial-derived relaxing factor in hypertension (84).

Conclusions

These *in vitro* data confirm and extend the hemodynamic and histological data as regards the presence of structural abnormalities of the resistance vasculature in essential hypertension. The data suggest that the increased pressor response seen in essential hypertensives is due mainly to changes in structure, rather than excitation-contraction coupling properties. The structural abnormality appears to be an increased media/lumen ratio due mainly to remodeling rather than growth, although, as indicated above, caution needs to be exercised in drawing this conclusion.

RESISTANCE VESSELS AND THE ETIOLOGY OF HYPERTENSION

The evidence reviewed above suggests that essential hypertension is associated with abnormalities of the resistance vessels. The abnormality appears to be mainly structural, such that the media/lumen (or wall/lumen) ratio of the small arteries is increased, and with a decrease in endothelial-dependent relaxation. By contrast, as discussed above, the evidence for functional alterations of the smooth muscle is weaker, for smooth muscle sensitivity appears normal (or perhaps reduced, e.g., endothelin) in essential hypertension. Therefore, on the basis that the dominant resistance vessel abnormality in essential hypertension is structural, this raises the question as to whether these structural abnormalities are involved in causing the raised pressure, or whether they are merely a consequence of the hypertension. According to the original Folkow (27) hypothesis, small increases in blood pressure would cause small structural changes, which would then maintain the increased pressure. In this way, a vicious circle would be created, leading ultimately to substantial increases in blood pressure.

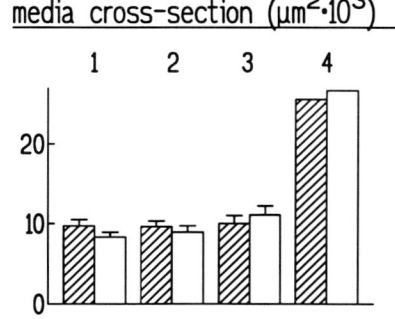

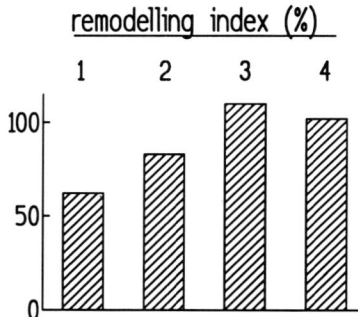

FIG. 5. Growth and remodeling in the resistance arteries from hypertensive individuals compared with resistance arteries from age- and sex-matched controls, shown in Fig. 2, from four investigations: 1, ref. 35; 2, ref. 111; 3, ref. 68; 4, ref. 79 (*open columns, left hatch, right hatch,* and *cross hatch,* respectively). Media cross-sectional area, equal to media volume per vessel segment length, is taken as a measure of growth. Remodeling index is the percentage of the reduction in the lumen that can be explained by a rearrangement of material (80) (see Fig. 4). Error bars show SE; 8 to 16 subjects in each group.

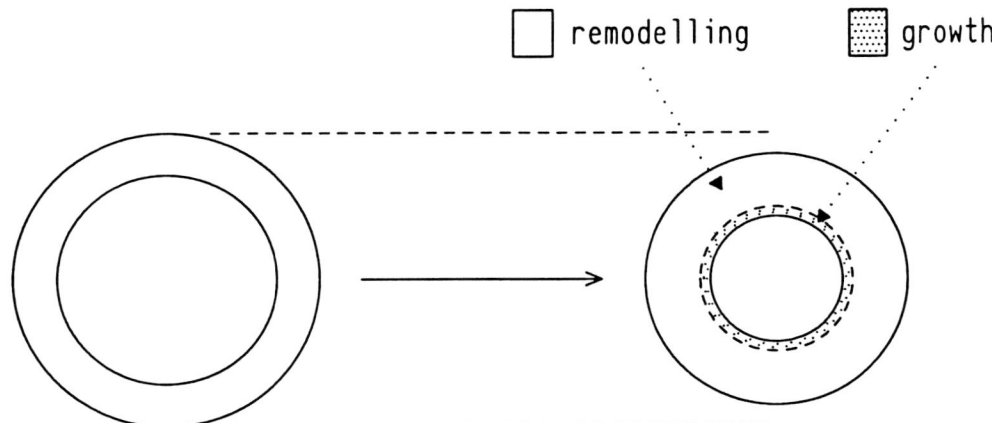

☐ remodelling   ▦ growth

FIG. 6. Predicted growth and remodeling in hypertension. Based on the hypothesis of Folkow (54), a 30 percent increase in blood pressure would be associated with (a) a 30 percent increase in minimum vascular resistance, and hence a 6 percent decrease in resistance vessel lumen diameter; and (b) a 30 percent increase in the resistance vessel media thickness/lumen diameter ratio. Given that the media/lumen ratio of small arteries of normotensive controls is about 0.05 (see Fig. 2), the Folkow hypothesis predicts that the external diameter would decrease by 4 percent, and that the cross-sectional area of the vessels from the hypertensive individual would be 16 percent greater (*shaded area*) than that of normotensive controls; 72 percent of the reduction in lumen can be accounted for by remodeling (a rearrangement of material (80,81). The cartoon illustrates this process, where the radial dimensions have been exaggerated for clarity.

As discussed previously (4), the hallmark of essential hypertension is the increased peripheral resistance, indicating that the resistance vessels must play a key role in the disease. Moreover, the structural abnormalities described above can in themselves explain this increased resistance, without the need for increased levels of neurohumoral activation or alterations in the excitation-contraction coupling properties of the vessels. In this sense, therefore, the structural abnormalities are the cause of hypertension. However, as further discussed (4), it is possible that hypertension is the result of some part of the cardiovascular control system requiring a high blood pressure (85,86), and the resistance vessels are responding to this requirement by providing the increased resistance. Seen in this perspective, the structural changes in the resistance vessels are an adaptation, allowing the resistance vessels to provide this increased resistance most efficiently (7). Which of these two possibilities is correct is still not clear, and the following subsection will point to some of the evidence for each. The importance of deciding between them lies in the strategy that should be used for antihypertensive therapy: Should this be aimed specifically at the resistance vessels, or are there other mechanisms that should be targeted?

Resistance Vessel Structural Abnormalities and Blood Pressure

Untreated Individuals

In adult individuals, as indicated above, there is overwhelming evidence that resistance vessel structure, ex-pressed as media/lumen ratio, is closely and positively correlated with blood pressure, especially as regards small arteries. Furthermore, studies of vascular structure in children of hypertensive parents (87) showed that the structure was altered in proportion to the small increase in blood pressure that was already present. However, this correlation may not always hold, for evidence of pressure-independent structural change in resistance vessels comes from the work of Takeshita et al. (88), who showed that forearm resistance in children of hypertensive parents was increased compared to children matched for blood pressure, and without a family history of hypertension. Thus, the conclusions from the evidence concerning the relation between resistance vessel structure and blood pressure in untreated individuals are not clear-cut.

As regards the impaired endothelial-dependent relaxation seen in hypertensive individuals, evidence from SHR indicates that this develops with age (89). Evidence concerning offspring of essential hypertensive patients is not at present available; thus, as for vascular structure, it is not clear whether this abnormality is a cause or an effect of the hypertension.

Treatment

Further evidence of a possible pressure-independent effect on vascular structure comes from antihypertensive treatment experiments. As reviewed recently (90), it has been a common finding that in essential hypertensive subjects (91–93), as in the SHR (94–102), it is easier to obtain normalization of blood pressure than to obtain normalization of vascular structure. Indeed, up to 6 years of antihypertensive treatment may be required for full normalization of forearm resistance in essential hypertensive patients (103).

Does Resistance Vessel Structure Influence Blood Pressure?

From a theoretical point of view, it is clear that altered resistance vessel structure is functionally equivalent to an alteration in the level of activation (54). It has, however, proved to be surprisingly difficult to obtain evidence that this is indeed the case.

One experimental strategy has been to determine if the rate of rise of blood pressure when treatment is withdrawn is correlated with resistance artery structure (104). The results, however, have not supported this possibility. In a study of 49 essential hypertensive patients who had been on one of five antihypertensive therapies, it was found that the rate of rise of blood pressure when treatment was withdrawn was positively correlated to cardiac output (CO), but negatively correlated to total peripheral resistance (TPR). That is, a low rate of recovery of blood pressure was associated with a low CO and a high TPR. In two animal studies, where rats were treated with a variety of antihypertensive drugs, including angiotensin-converting enzyme inhibitors (ACEIs) in different doses, the rate of rise of blood pressure when therapy was withdrawn did not correlate with resistance artery structure during treatment (101,105).

The conclusion of these studies is that it has not been possible to show a clear relation between resistance artery structure and blood pressure development, but this does not exclude the possibility that other experimental approaches would be able to demonstrate this elusive relation. For example, it has recently been possible to demonstrate that a reduced diameter of renal afferent arterioles in 7-week-old F_2-hypertensive/normotensive rats is a predictor for the development of high blood pressure at age 24 weeks (106). Thus, at least in the kidney, resistance vessel structure may indeed be an important determinant of blood pressure. Definitive evidence, however, is still lacking.

Does Normalization of Resistance Artery Structure Matter?

Given the difficulty of proving that resistance vessel structure has a primary effect on blood pressure, it may be asked whether it is important for antihypertensive therapy to attempt to normalize this structure. At present, there is no direct evidence, but it has been demonstrated (107,108) that the structural changes in the myocardium of hypertensive individuals are associated with a reduced coronary reserve, and that antihypertensive treatment can fail to normalize the coronary reserve.

Furthermore, in mature SHR, decreased reserve in a variety of muscular vascular beds is associated with a decreased capillary filtration coefficient (109). It is therefore possible that the relatively disappointing ability of antihypertensive treatment to reduce myocardial infarction (110) is in part due to failure to obtain complete regression of vascular structure. As indicated above, the ability to achieve full regression of resistance vessel structure appears to depend on the length of the antihypertensive treatment, and possibly the type of therapy. This important hypothesis requires further investigation.

CONCLUSIONS

Although the high blood pressure associated with essential hypertension is caused by an increased peripheral resistance in the face of a normal cardiac output, the role of the resistance vessels in the etiology of the disease remains uncertain. As described in this chapter, certain abnormalities are apparent in the resistance vessels of patients with essential hypertension, including an increased media/lumen ratio, a decreased lumen, and a decreased endothelial-dependent relaxation. Whether the altered structure is due to vascular growth or remodeling (a rearrangement of material) is not certain. Furthermore, although the structural and endothelial abnormalities described could in themselves account for the increased peripheral resistance, it is by no means certain that the abnormalities are primary. The hypertension could be a response to a requirement for some other part of the cardiovascular system for a high blood pressure, in which case the changes in the resistance vessels should be seen as enabling them to provide the needed increase in resistance most conveniently. Nevertheless, regardless of whether the abnormalities are primary or secondary, there are grounds for supposing that failure to obtain complete regression of resistance artery structure with antihypertensive treatment could prevent normalization of coronary reserve, and thus have a deleterious effect on the prognosis. More work is therefore needed to determine means for obtaining rapid normalization of resistance vessel structure and endothelial function.

ACKNOWLEDGMENTS

This chapter was written while the author was receiving support from the Danish Medical Research Council and the Danish Heart Foundation. The review includes work done by the European Working Party on Resistance Artery Disease (EURAD).

REFERENCES

1. Lund-Johansson P. *Clin Sci* 1980;59:343–354.
2. Williams SA, Boolell M, MacGregor GA, Smaje LH, Wasserman SM, Tooke JE. *Clin Sci* 1990;79:5–8.

3. Hutchins PM, Darnell AE. *Circ Res* 1974;34,35(suppl 1):I-161–I-165.
4. Mulvany MJ, Aalkjær C. *Physiol Rev* 1990;70:921–961.
5. Mulvany MJ. *Blood Vessels* 1983;20:1–22.
6. Mulvany MJ. *J Hypertens* 1987;5:129–136.
7. Mulvany MJ. *Hypertension* 1991;18(Suppl 1):I-52–I-57.
8. Mulvany MJ. In: Swales J, ed. *Textbook of hypertension.* Oxford: Blackwell, 1993;in press.
9. Faraci FM, Heistad DD. *Circ Res* 1990;66:8–17.
10. Kanatsuka H, Lamping KG, Eastham CL, Marcus ML. *Circ Res* 1990;66:389–396.
11. Chilian WM, Layne SM. *Circ Res* 1990;66:1227–1238.
12. Zweifach BW, Kovalcheck S, DeLano F, Chen P. *Hypertension* 1981;3:601–614.
13. Bohlen HG. *Hypertension* 1983;5:739–745.
14. Harper SL, Bohlen HG. *Hypertension* 1984;6:408–419.
15. DeLano FA, Schmid Schonbein GW, Skalak TC, Zweifach BW. *Microvasc Res* 1991;41:92–110.
16. Meininger GA, Harris PD, Joshua IG. *Hypertension* 1984;6:27–34.
17. Joyner WL, Davis MJ, Gilmore JP. *Microvasc Res* 1981;22:190–198.
18. Christensen KL, Mulvany MJ. *J Vasc Res* 1993;30:73–79.
19. Christensen KL, Mulvany MJ. *J Hypertens* 1993;11(Suppl 5):s462 (abstract).
20. Mulvany MJ, Aalkjær C, Heagerty AM, Nyborg NCB, Strandgaard S, eds. *Resistance arteries: structure and function.* Amsterdam: Elsevier, 1991.
21. Bevan JA, Halpern W, Mulvany MJ, eds. *The resistance vasculature.* Totowa, NJ: Humana, 1993.
22. Lew MJ, Angus JA. *J Vasc Res* 1992;29:435–442.
23. Korsgaard N, Mulvany MJ. *Proc Int Union Physiol Sci* 1989;17:169.
24. Heagerty AM, Aalkjær C, Bund SJ, Korsgaard N, Mulvany MJ. *Hypertension* 1993;21:391–397.
25. Short D. *Lancet* 1966;1:1302–1304.
26. Gundersen HJG, Bagger P, Bendtsen TF, Evans SM, Korbo L, Marcussen N, Møller A, Nielsen K, Nyengaard fR, Pakkenberg B, et al. *APMIS* 1988;96:857–881.
27. Folkow B. In: Harington M, ed. *Hypotensive drugs.* London: Pergamon, 1956;163–174.
28. Skov K, Mulvany MJ, Korsgaard N. *Hypertension* 1992;20:821–827.
29. Dahlöf B. *Blood Pressure* 1992;1:35–44.
30. Gasser P, Buhler FR. *J Hypertens* 1992;10:83–86.
31. Hayoz D, Rutschmann B, Perret F, Niederberger M, Tardy Y, Mooser V, Nussberger J, Waeber B, Brunner HR. *Hypertension* 1992;20:1–6.
32. Duling BR, Gore RW, Dacey RG, Damon DN. *Am J Physiol* 1981;241:H108–H116.
33. Halpern W, Osol G. *Prog Appl Microcirc* 1985;8:32–39.
34. Mulvany MJ, Halpern W. *Nature* 1976;260:617–619.
35. Aalkjær C, Heagerty AM, Petersen KK, Swales JD, Mulvany MJ. *Circ Res* 1987;61:181–186.
36. Mulvany MJ, Halpern W. *Circ Res* 1977;41:19–26.
37. Seidelin PH, Collier JG, Struthers AD, Webb DJ. *Clin Sci* 1991;81:261–266.
38. Halpern W, Kelley M. *Blood Vessels* 1991;28:245–251.
39. Mulvany MJ, Nilsson H, Flatman JA. *J Physiol* 1982;332:363–373.
40. Jensen PE, Mulvany MJ, Aalkjær C. *Pflugers Arch* 1992;420:536–543.
41. Aalkjær C, Cragoe EJ. *J Physiol* 1988;402:391–410.
42. Aalkjær C, Mulvany MJ. *J Physiol* 1983;343:105–116.
43. Durkin H, Ollerenshaw JD, Heagerty AM. *J Hypertens* 1990;8:557–563.
44. Folkow B, Grimby G, Thulesius O. *Acta Physiol Scand* 1958;44:255–272.
45. Conway J. *Circulation* 1963;27:520.
46. Egan BM, Schork N, Panis R, Hinderliter A. *J Hypertens* 1988;6:41–48.
47. Folkow B. *Hypertension* 1988;12:635–637.
48. Schulte KL, Braun J, Meyer-Sabellek W, Wegscheider K, Gotzen R, Distler A. *Hypertension* 1988;11:320–325.
49. Takeshita A, Mark AL. *Hypertension* 1980;2:610–616.
50. Zweifler AJ, Nicholls MG, Arbor A. *Am Heart J* 1982;104:812–815.
51. Henriksen O, Skagen K, Amtorp O, Hartling O. *Acta Physiol Scand* 1981;112:323–329.
52. Doyle AE, Black H. *Circ Res* 1955;12:974–980.
53. Ljungman S, Aurell M, Hartford M, Wikstrand J, Berglund G. *Hypertension* 1983;5:368–374.
54. Folkow B. *Physiol Rev* 1982;62:347–504.
55. Sivertsson R. *Acta Physiol Scand* 1970;suppl 343:1–56.
56. Robinson BF, Dobbs RJ, Bayley S. *Clin Sci* 1982;63:33–42.
57. Hulthen UL, Bolli P, Kiowski W, Bühler FR. *Gen Pharmacol* 1983;14:193–196.
58. Lüscher TF, Vanhoutte PM. *Hypertension* 1986;8:344–348.
59. Panza JA, Quyyumi AA, Brush JEJ, Epstein SE. *N Engl J Med* 1990;323:22–27.
60. Linder L, Kiowski W, Bühler FR, Lüscher TF. *Circulation* 1990;81:1762–1767.
61. Imaizumi T, Hirooka Y, Masaki H, Harada S, Momohara M, Tagawa T, Takeshita A. *Hypertension* 1992;20:511–517.
62. Johnson G. *Trans R Med Chir Soc* 1868;51:57–58.
63. Gull WW, Sutton HG. *Med Chir Trans* 1872;55:273–326.
64. Furuyama M. *Tohoku J Exp Med* 1962;76:388–414.
65. Suwa N, Takahashi T. *Morphological and morphometric analysis of circulation in hypertension and ischaemic kidney.* Munich: Urban & Schwarzenberg, 1971.
66. Lee RMKW, Forrest JB, Garfield RE, Daniel EE. *Blood Vessels* 1983;20:245–254.
67. Schwartzkopff B, Frenzel H, Dieckerhoff J, Betz P, Flasshove M, Schulte HD, Mundhenke M, Motz W, Strauer BE. *Eur Heart J* 1992;13(Suppl D):17–23.
68. Korsgaard N, Heagerty AM, Aalkjær C, Bund SJ, Mulvany MJ. *Hypertension* 1993;22:523–526.
69. Mulvany MJ, Baandrup U, Gundersen HJG. *Circ Res* 1985;57:794–800.
70. Thybo NK, Korsgaard N, Mulvany MJ. *J Hypertens* 1992;10:1191–1196.
71. Korsgaard N, Mulvany MJ. *Hypertension* 1988;12:162–167.
72. Harper RN, Moore MA, Marr MC, Watts LE, Hutchins PM. *Microvasc Res* 1978;16:369–372.
73. Sokolova IA, Manukhina EB, Blinkov SM, Koshelev VB, Pinelis VG, Rodionov IM. *Microvasc Res* 1985;30:1–9.
74. le Noble JL, Tangelder GJ, Slaaf DW, Van Essen H, Reneman RS, Struyker Boudier HA. *J Hypertens* 1990;8:741–748.
75. Engelson ET, Schmid-Schonbein GW, Zweifach BW. *Microvasc Res* 1986;31:356–374.
76. Korner PI, Angus JA. *J Vasc Res* 1992;29:293–312.
77. Aalkjær C, Pedersen EB, Danielsen H, Fjeldborg O, Jespersen B, Kjaer T, Soerensen SS, Mulvany MJ. *Clin Sci* 1986;71:657–663.
78. Izzard AS, MacIver DH, Cragoe EJ, Heagerty AM. *Clin Sci* 1991;81:65–72.
79. Schiffrin EL, Deng LY, Larochelle P. *J Hypertens* 1992;10:437–444.
80. Baumbach GL, Heistad DD. *Hypertension* 1989;13:968–972.
81. Baumbach GL, Heistad DD. *J Hypertens* 1991;9:987–991.
82. Deng LY, Schiffrin EL. *Am J Hypertens* 1992;5:817–822.
83. Deng LY, Schiffrin EL. *Am J Physiol* 1991;261:H1171–H1177.
84. Dohi Y, Luscher TF. *Hypertension* 1991;18:543–549.
85. Julius S. *J Hypertens* 1988;6:177–185.
86. Julius S. *Diabetes Care* 1991;14:249–259.
87. Aalkjær C, Heagerty AM, Bailey I, Mulvany MJ, Swales JD. *Hypertension* 1987;9(Suppl III):III-155–III-158.
88. Takeshita A, Imaizumi T, Ashihara T, Yamamoto K, Hoka S, Nakamura M. *Circ Res* 1982;50:671–677.
89. Watt PAC, Thurston H. *J Hypertens* 1989;7:661–666.
90. Schachter M. *Am Heart J* 1991;122:316–323.
91. Hansson L. *J Hypertens* 1987;5(Suppl 4):S71–S74.
92. Aalkjær C, Eiskjaer H, Mulvany MJ, Jespersen B, Kjaer T, Soerensen SS, Pedersen EB. *J Hypertens* 1989;7:305–310.
93. Novo S, Abrignani MG, Sapienza ND, Barbagallo M, Pinto A, Di Maria GU, Mistretta A, Strano A. *Int Angiol* 1992;11:137–141.
94. Warshaw DM, Root DT, Halpern W. *Blood Vessels* 1980;17:257–270.
95. Weiss L, Lundgren Y. *Cardiovasc Res* 1978;12:744–751.

96. Scott TM, Pang SC. *Acta Stereologica* 1983;2:127–133.
97. Nyborg NCB, Mulvany MJ. *J Cardiovasc Pharmacol* 1984;6:499–505.
98. Jespersen LT, Nyborg NCB, Pedersen OL, Mikkelsen EO, Mulvany MJ. *Hypertension* 1985;7:734–741.
99. Harper SL. *Circ Res* 1987;60:229–237.
100. Smeda JS, Lee RMKW, Forrest JB. *Circ Res* 1988;63:534–542.
101. Christensen KL, Jespersen LT, Mulvany MJ. *J Hypertens* 1989;7:83–90.
102. Smeda JS, Lee RMKW. *Hypertension* 1991;17:526–533.
103. Hartford M, Wendelhag I, Berglund G, Wallentin I, Ljungman S, Wikstrand J. *JAMA* 1988;259:2553–2557.
104. Korner PI, Bobik A, Jennings GL, Angus JA, Anderson WP. *J Cardiovasc Pharmacol* 1991;17(Suppl 2):S25–S32.
105. Thybo NK, Eriksen S, Christensen KL, Mulvany MJ. *Acta Physiol Scand* 1993;146(Suppl 608):143(abstract).
106. Nørrelund H, Korsgaard N, Christensen KL, Samani NJ, Mulvany MJ. *J Hypertens* 1993;11(Suppl 5):s462 (abstract).
107. Strauer BE, Schwartzkopff B, Motz W, Vogt M. *J Cardiovasc Pharmacol* 1992;18(Suppl 3):s20–s27.
108. Brilla CG, Janicki JS, Weber KT. *Circ Res* 1991;69:107–115.
109. Sexton WL, Korthuis RJ, Laughlin MH. *J Appl Physiol* 1990;69:1073–1079.
110. Collins R, Peto R, MacMahon S, Hebert P, Fiebach NH, Eberlein KA, Godwin J, Qizilbash N, Taylor JO, Hennekens CH. *Lancet* 1990;335:827–838.
111. Izzard AS, Cragoe EJ, Heagerty AM. *Hypertension* 1991;17:780–786.

Hypertension: Pathophysiology, Diagnosis, and Management, Second Edition,
edited by J.H. Laragh and B.M. Brenner,
Raven Press, Ltd., New York © 1995.

CHAPTER 32

Hypertension, Growth Factors, and Their Relevance to Atherosclerotic Vascular Disease

Aram V. Chobanian

Hypertension is a potent promoter of atherosclerosis (1). Although the exact mechanisms have not been elucidated as yet, hypertension may influence several characteristic features of atherosclerotic plaque development including the accumulation of smooth muscle cells (SMC), macrophages, and lymphocytes; intimal deposition of lipid, particularly free cholesterol and cholesterol esters; and accumulation of connective tissue matrix. Such changes are induced experimentally by hypercholesterolemia and are generally consistent with inflammatory responses to arterial injury. The lipid deposition in plaques may be intracellular, particularly in macrophages, causing formation of foam cells and fatty streak lesions. Advanced plaques typically are rich in connective tissue and extracellular lipid as well as in cellular components.

Cells in atherosclerotic lesions proliferate and such proliferation may play an important role in the genesis and growth of the plaque. Cellular growth factors and cytokines appear to be involved in the cellular proliferation and thereby influence plaque enlargement. Hypertension also causes vascular cell growth along with thickening of the arterial intima and media and increase in cellular mass and connective tissue content. A summary of the changes occurring in both intima and media as a result of hypertension is provided in Fig. 1.

This chapter reviews the role of hypertension in mediating cellular growth, the importance of growth factors in the development of vascular changes, and the role of growth inhibitors and of antihypertensive drugs in the responses to arterial injury and in atherogenesis.

CELLULAR ORIGIN OF GROWTH FACTORS

Arterial endothelial cells, smooth muscle cells, macrophages, and T-lymphocytes not only respond to growth factors but also are potential rich sources of these substances. Endothelial cell growth factors include platelet-derived growth factor (PDGF), basic fibroblast growth factor (bFGF), insulin growth factor-1 (IGF-1), interleukin-1 (IL-1), transforming growth factor-beta (TGF-β), tumor necrosis factor (TNF-α), and monocyte colony-stimulating factor (M-CSF) (2). Growth inhibitors which can be made by endothelial cells include nitric oxide, bradykinin, and prostacyclin.

Smooth muscle cells are capable of producing PDGF, IL-1, bFGF, IGF-1, TGF-β, TNF-α, M-CSF, and epidermal growth factor (EGF) (2). Macrophages are a particularly rich source of such growth promoters and inhibitors, as are T-lymphocytes. Thus, several cell types in the vasculature may participate in the regulation of vascular

A. V. Chobanian: Boston University School of Medicine, Boston, Massachusetts 02118.

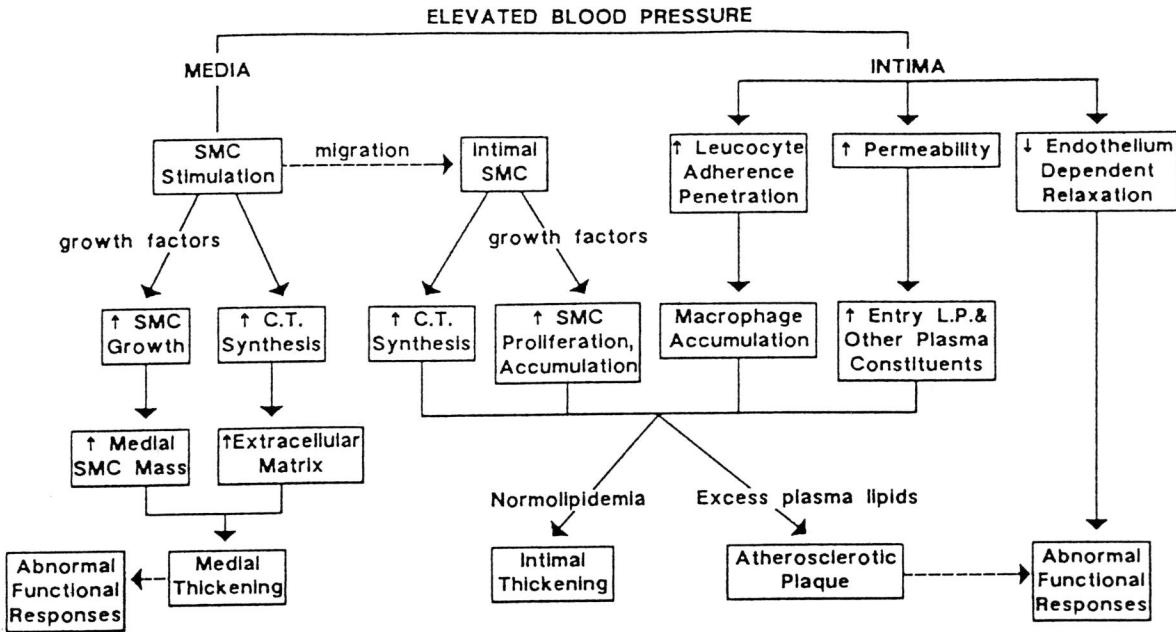

FIG. 1. Diagrammatic representation of the effects of hypertension on the arterial wall. SMC, smooth muscle cell; C.T., connective tissue; L.P., lipoprotein. (From ref. 76, with permission.)

cell growth. Their actions may be targeted to adjacent cells in the vessel wall or to the cells themselves producing these substances.

Experimental studies have demonstrated that the early stages of arterial injury associated with either hypercholesterolemia or hypertension involve damage to the endothelium with resultant changes in endothelial cell function. Very early changes in the endothelium caused by hypercholesterolemia include the rapid induction of adhesive glycoproteins or endothelial leukocyte adherence molecules (ELAMs) and later adherence of leukocytes to the endothelial surface (3). Increased adherence of leukocytes to the endothelium has also been observed with experimental hypertension (4), although no studies of changes in ELAMs with hypertension have been reported as yet.

Other evidence for endothelial cell injury by hypertension includes changes in size and shape of endothelial cells and their nuclei (4). Blood levels of von Willebrand factor, a glycoprotein synthesized by endothelial cells, have been reported to increase in patients with hypertension (5) or with hypercholesterolemia (6), suggesting increased leakage of this glycoprotein from endothelial cells to the circulating blood in these conditions.

HYPERTENSION AND ARTERIAL GROWTH FACTORS

Hypertension appears to induce the growth and/or the proliferation of a subpopulation of arterial cells. In the spontaneously hypertensive rat (SHR), increased thymidine synthesis has been observed in both aortic endothelial cells and SMC (7,8), although at a given time, only a small fraction of such cells (e.g., 1 percent) appear to participate in the process. The rate of proliferation of aortic SMC in aortic explants taken from SHR and DOCA-salt hypertensive rats is also increased as compared with controls (9,10). In addition, cultured SMC from SHR have shown an increased rate of incorporation of ^{3}H-thymidine into DNA in response to PDGF or EGF (11).

In chronic rat models of hypertension such as the SHR, elevated blood pressure causes aortic SMC hypertrophy, which is associated with increased DNA replication and increased nuclear polyploidy (12–14). In contrast, in mesenteric resistance vessels of the SHR, hypertension stimulates SMC hyperplasia rather than hypertrophy (15). Aortic coarctation with acute rise in blood pressure has been reported to cause SMC hyperplasia in rabbit and rat aorta (16,17).

We have been interested in the effects of hypertension on arterial growth factor expression *in vivo*. We have observed that DOCA-salt hypertension increases steady-state messenger ribonucleic acid (mRNA) levels of TGF-β1 in rat aorta but does not appear to influence expression of such growth factors as EGF, acidic and basic FGF, IGFs, and both A and B chains of PDGF (18). Increased aortic expression of TGF-β1 also has been observed in the SHR as a result of both hypertension and increasing age (19). Cellular localization of the TGF-β1 expression in aorta has been studied recently by *in situ* hybridization. In normal aorta, we have observed the TGF-β1 message to be distributed diffusely between the aortic intima, media, and adventitia. With DOCA-salt hypertension, increased message is prominent in the periadventitia, although some increase in the region of the endothelium and in SMC is also apparent (20). The concentration of the TGF-β1 message in the adventitia is of interest, although the role of the adventitia in the regulation of cellular growth is unknown.

In both DOCA-salt hypertensive rats and in SHR, increased aortic expression of the PDGF-beta (PDGF-β) receptor which binds the PDGF-B chain is present (21), but the PDGF ligands themselves are unaffected. Increases in aortic expression of PDGF-β receptor are also apparent with advancing age in the SHR and in both Wistar and Wistar-Kyoto (WKY) normotensive controls (20).

Recent data have suggested that integrin-cell receptors and extracellular proteins may alter growth of cultured cells (22). We therefore have examined the relationship between the changes in arterial extracellular matrix to those in cellular growth as a result of hypertension. The studies have focused on the large protein, fibronectin, which is known to alter endothelial cell function after arterial balloon injury (23) and which can cause phenotypic changes in cultured SMC (24). Several forms of hypertension can induce rapid increases in aortic fibronectin expression, synthesis, and accumulation (25). Such increases may occur within 1 day in the angiotensin II (AngII) infusion model, although it is as yet unclear whether these early changes in fibronectin precede or are a consequence of enhanced cellular growth.

Transforming growth factor-beta appears to be an important regulator of fibronectin and other extracellular proteins (26). The changes in TGF-β and fibronectin in the arterial wall in response to hypertension are associated with overall increase in fibrous tissue and remodeling of the extracellular matrix. Increased expression of TGF-β has also been demonstrated in other forms of tissue injury such as in experimental glomerulonephritis of rats in which marked accumulation of extracellular matrix is associated with renal failure (27). Interestingly, decorin, a natural inhibitor of TGF-β, has been shown to reduce renal scarring and improve renal function, suggesting an important role of TGF-β in this model of renal injury (28). No studies are as yet available regarding the role of TGF-β or of fibronectin on the arterial changes induced by hypertension.

ANGIOTENSIN II AND CELLULAR GROWTH

Abundant evidence now exists to indicate that Ang II can act as a vascular growth factor. Angiotensin II causes hypertrophy of cultured SMC in serum-free medium (29), although it may induce hyperplasia in serum-rich medium (30). The mechanism of the Ang II effect may involve the stimulation of the protooncogenes, c-*myc*, c-*fos*, and c-*jun*, and of TGF-β1 and PDGF-A chain (31). Antisense oligonucleotides of PDGF-A mRNA have been shown to inhibit the SMC growth induced by Ang II, indicating an important role of PDGF-A in the process (32). The changes in TGF-β1 expression caused by Ang II could act to modulate the PDGF-A action on growth (33), although direct evidence for such modulation is lacking as yet. Atrial natriuretic peptide has been observed to reduce the hypertrophic effect of Ang II on arterial SMC without apparently inhibiting expression of protooncogenes, suggesting that other pathways may also be involved (34). Angiotensin II has been reported to induce expression of endothelin-a, a known growth factor for SMC, thus suggesting an additional potential mechanism for Ang II action on growth (35).

Ang II also has been reported to stimulate the migration of SMC *in vitro* in a Boydens Chamber preparation (36). This action is inhibited by sodium nitroprusside and 8-bromo-cyclic guanosine monophosphate (cGMP), suggesting that nitric oxide may counteract the Ang II effect.

We recently have assessed the role of blood pressure in mediating the *in vivo* changes in aortic fibronectin that occur in response to angiotensin administration in the rat (37). Following Ang II infusion for 3 days, there were significant increases in aortic fibronectin expression and content which were inhibited by losartan, indicating the importance of AT-1 receptors in this process. Treatment with prazosin, hydralazine (Apresoline) or I-arginine in doses sufficient to normalize blood pressure did not attenuate the increase in fibronectin response, suggesting that the action of angiotensin on fibronectin is caused, at least in part, by pressure-independent mechanisms.

Non-pressor-related effects of Ang II are also thought to be important with respect to the heart where marked fibrosis has been observed even after brief periods of Ang II infusion (38). It has been proposed that the Ang II effects may be mediated through aldosterone stimulation (38). We have observed very rapid induction of fibrosis in the heart by 3–7 days of Ang II administration which was associated with marked increases in fibronectin expression and total quantity of fibronectin (39). The effects were inhibited by losartan but not by antihypertensive agents that did not inhibit angiotensin. The fibrosis occurred in perivascular areas of both right and left ventricles and appeared to be associated with injury of small arteries and arterioles. By *in situ* hybridization, the fibronectin expression was localized to nonmyocytic cells of the heart in the periadventitial and interstitial fibroblasts. Changes in expression of atrial natriuretic factor, a marker for phenotypic change in the myocyte associated with hypertrophy, appeared to follow slightly those occurring in the fibroblasts. The latter findings suggest that some of the effects of Ang II administration on the cardiac myocyte may be secondary to vascular injury and connective tissue reactions to such injury.

Recent data would suggest that Ang II is a mediator of the responses of cardiac myocytes to stretch (40). Subjecting cultured myocytes to stretch induced marked increases in expression of c-*fos* and atrial natriuretic factor, which were blocked by losartan. Angiotensin II release from the cells was also enhanced. These findings suggest a potentially important role of the local renin-angiotensin system in the heart to hemodynamic alterations. Although data are not available for the arterial wall, it is tempting to speculate that a similar autocrine role for the renin-angiotensin system may be present there as well.

ENDOTHELIN

Endothelin production can be stimulated by Ang II (41). Endothelin is a very potent vasoconstrictor which has been shown to induce the proliferation of vascular SMC (42) and the expression of PDGF-A chain, c-*myc* and c-*fos* (43). Hypertension has been reported to be associated with elevated circulating levels of endothelin in experimental animals (44). Increased levels have also been suggested in markedly hypertensive human subjects (45,46). The role of endothelin in atherogenesis and in the vascular complications of hypertension has not been delineated as yet, but the recent availability of endothelin-1 receptor antagonists provides an excellent opportunity for studying the participation of endothelin in these processes.

NITRIC OXIDE AND ATHEROGENESIS

Recent evidence would indicate that nitric oxide may be involved in protection against atherosclerosis. This potent vasodilator, which is produced by the endothelium, inhibits the growth and proliferation of vascular SMC (47). It also can inhibit leukocyte adherence to endothelium (48,49). Both hypercholesterolemia and hypertension have been shown to impair endothelium-dependent relaxation in experimental animals and man (50–52), suggesting reduced production or release of nitric oxide. Stimulation of nitric oxide production by prolonged dietary administration of its precursor, L-arginine, has been shown to reduce the extent of atherosclerosis and to improve endothelium-dependent arterial relaxation in cholesterol-fed rabbits (53,54). In addition, administration of the nitric oxide synthase inhibitor, L-nitro-arginine methyl ester, has been reported recently to accelerate aortic atherosclerosis in cholesterol-fed rabbits (55). Inhibition of nitric oxide synthase also can increase monocyte adherence to cytokine-activated endothelium (49).

ANTIHYPERTENSIVE DRUGS, VASCULAR CELL GROWTH, AND VASCULAR PROTECTION

Certain antihypertensive drugs have been reported to inhibit the development of arterial disease caused by balloon injury or by hypercholesterolemia. Some of these vasculoprotective effects may be related to inhibitory effects of the drugs on cellular growth.

Balloon Injury

The model of balloon injury with removal of arterial endothelium provides an *in vivo* system for examining the growth-inhibiting properties of antihypertensive drugs. Following endothelial denudation, the lesion which develops is highly proliferative in nature. Intravenous administration of antibodies to PDGF reduces the size of the plaque developing in rat carotid artery following balloon injury (56). Calcium antagonists also may reduce plaque size caused by balloon injury of the rat carotid artery (57). A reduction in intracellular calcium caused by such drugs might be responsible for this action by inhibiting cellular migration and proliferation.

Several angiotensin-converting enzyme (ACE) inhibitors have been reported to inhibit plaque formation in the rat carotid artery model (58). Angiotensin-converting enzyme inhibitors reduce Ang II levels and thereby could influence cellular growth. The bradykinin elevation resulting from ACE inhibition also may play a role to reduce proliferative activity. A recent study has indicated that treatment with losartan is not as effective as that with the ACE inhibitor ramipril in reducing plaque development following balloon injury of rat carotid artery (59). In these studies, combination of ramipril (Altase) with a bradykinin receptor antagonist reduced the effect of ramipril on plaque formation. Although a beneficial action of ACE inhibition following balloon injury has been apparent in the rat, no effect of the ACE inhibitor cilazapril on intimal hyperplasia was demonstrable in the baboon (60). The clinical implications are as yet unknown, but clinical studies are currently in progress to determine the effects of ACE inhibition in patients who have undergone balloon angioplasty of their coronary arteries. In the first completed study of this type, the MERCATOR Study (61), cilazapril (Caposten) failed to inhibit coronary restenosis following angioplasty.

Atherosclerosis

Beta-adrenergic blockers, calcium antagonists, and ACE inhibitors have been reported to reduce the development of atherosclerosis in hypercholesterolemic normotensive animals. One feature common to all of these drugs is their ability to lower blood pressure. Such lowering could contribute to a protective effect of the drug on the vasculature, even in normotensive animals, by altering hemodynamic stresses on the arterial wall. Another common property is their potential to reduce cellular growth either by reducing sympathetic activity (beta blockers and ACE inhibitors), Ang II levels (beta blockers and ACE inhibitors), or cellular calcium content (calcium antagonists).

With calcium antagonists and beta blockers, antiatherosclerotic effects were observed in cholesterol-fed animals (62–65), but no inhibition was apparent in the Watanabe heritable hyperlipidemic (WHHL) rabbit with a deficit in the cellular receptor for low-density lipoproteins (66,67).

Angiotensin-converting enzyme inhibitors reduce atherosclerosis in several species including the WHHL rabbit (68,69), the cholesterol-fed cynomolgus monkey (70) and the cholesterol-fed minipig (71). This action appears to be a class effect since several ACE inhibitors have shown a favorable antiatherosclerotic action. Our studies have demonstrated that ACE inhibitors cause decreases in cellularity of aortic atherosclerotic lesions in the WHHL rabbit (68), although it is unknown whether this action is related directly to a growth-inhibitory effect by reducing Ang II or increasing bradykinin. Several other mechanisms have been proposed (Table 1) including improvement in endothelial function (72), inhibition of monocyte adherence to endothelium and monocyte migration into the media (73), and prevention of oxidation of low-density lipoproteins (74).

The effects of ACE inhibitors on atherosclerosis in man have not been studied as yet. In the recently completed Survival and Ventricular Enlargement Trial (SAVE) Study (75), patients with left ventricular dysfunction treated with captopril following an acute myocardial infarction had a decreased rate of recurrence of myocardial infarction, but whether this effect was related to any action on atherosclerosis is unclear. Clinical trials have recently been initiated to determine whether the course of coronary artery disease, as determined by angi-

ography, is affected by ACE inhibitors. Until the results of these and other studies become available, the clinical implications of the data obtained in hypercholesterolemic animals remain uncertain.

CONCLUSIONS

The responses to arterial injury induced by hypertension and hypercholesterolemia include the stimulation of growth and the proliferation and accumulation of SMC. Several growth factors produced by the vascular cells appear to be involved in these responses and may act together to promote cell proliferation. Hypertension may also be associated with phenotypic changes in the SMC that enhance their proliferative potential and their responses to growth factors.

Angiotensin II can act as a vascular growth factor whose effects may be mediated by protooncogenes and PDGF-A chain. Stimulation of nitric oxide or of cGMP production can counter the growth-promoting effects of Ang II. The effects of Ang II on vascular growth appear to be partially independent of blood pressure and may involve direct stimulation of arterial cells.

Studies in experimental animals indicate that ACE inhibitors, as a class, reduce the development of atherosclerosis induced by hypercholesterolemia and improve endothelium-dependent relaxation. Several mechanisms may be involved in the antiatherogenic action of these drugs, but the inhibition of cellular growth appears to play a prominent role in this protection. A potentially valuable new approach to reducing atherosclerosis in man is therefore suggested by these studies.

REFERENCES

1. Chobanian AV, Lichtenstein AH, Nilakhe V, Haudenschild CC, Drago R, Nickerson C. Influence of hypertension on aortic atherosclerosis in the Watanabe rabbit. *Hypertension* 1989;14:203–209.
2. Schwartz SMdd, Heimark RL, Majesky MW. Developmental mechanisms underlying pathology of arteries. *Physiol Rev* 1990;70:1177–1209.
3. Li H, Cybulsky MI, Gimbrone MA Jr, Libby P. An atherogenic diet rapidly induces CAM-1, a cytokine-regulatable mononuclear leukocyte adhesion molecule, in rabbit aortic endothelium. *Arterioscler Thromb* 1993;13:197–204.
4. Haudenschild C, Prescott MF, and Chobanian AV. Effects of hypertension and its reversal on aortic intimal lesions of the rat. *Hypertension* 1980;2:33–44.
5. Blann AD, Naqvi T, Waite M, McCollum CN. Von Willebrand factor and endothelial damage in essential hypertension. *J Human Hyp* 1993;7:107–111.
6. Duffy A, Blann AD, Anderson J, Miller P, Gowland E, McCollum CN. Increased von Willebrand factor antigen in familial hypercholesterolemia. *Atherosclerosis* 1991;90:226–230.
7. Schwartz SM, Benditt EP. Aortic endothelial cell replication. I. Effects of age and hypertension in the rat. *Circ Res* 1977;41:248–255.
8. Schwartz SM, Campbell GR, Campbell JH. Replication of smooth muscle cells in vascular disease. *Circ Res* 1986;41:248–255.
9. Haudenschild CC, Grunwald J, Chobanian AV. Effects of hyper-

TABLE 1. *ACE inhibitors and potential vasculoprotective mechanisms*

Hemodynamic—reduction of blood pressure
Inhibition of cellular growth and/or migration
   Reduction of angiotensin II
   Reduction of sympathetic activity
   Enhancement of bradykinin
Action on nitric oxide and/or cGMP
   Restoration of endothelial function
   Inhibition of cellular growth
   Reduction of monocyte adherence and migration
Inhibition of foam cell formation
Inhibition of oxidation of low-density lipoproteins

tension on migration and proliferation of smooth muscle in culture. *Hypertension* 1985;7:I-101–I-104.

10. Grunwald J, Chobanian AV, Haudenschild CC. Smooth muscle cell migration and proliferation: atherogenic mechanisms in hypertension. *Atherosclerosis* 1987;67:215–222.

11. Hadrava V, Tremblay J, Hamet P. Abnormalities in growth characteristics of aortic smooth muscle cells in spontaneously hypertensive rats. *Hypertension* 1989;13:589–597.

12. Owens GK, and Schwartz SM. Alterations in vascular smooth muscle mass in the spontaneous hypertensive rat. Role in cellular hypertrophy, hyperploidy and hyperplasia. *Circ Res* 1982;51:280–289.

13. Lichtenstein AH, Brecher P, and Chobanian AV. Effects of deoxycorticosterone-salt hypertension on cell ploidy in the rat aorta. *Hypertension* 1986;8:II-50–II-54.

14. Owens GK. Control of hypertrophic versus hyperplastic growth of vascular smooth muscle cells. *Am J Physiol* 1989;26:H1755–H1765.

15. Mulvany M, Baandrup U, Gundersen H. Evidence for hyperplasia in mesenteric resistance vessels of spontaneously hypertensive rats using a three-dimensional dissector. *Circ Res* 1985;57:794–800.

16. Bevan R, Marthens E, and Bevan J. Hyperplasia of vascular smooth muscle in experimental hypertension in the rabbit. *Circ Res* 1976;38:II-58–II-62.

17. Owens G, and Reidy M. Hyperplastic growth response of vascular smooth muscle cells following induction of acute hypertension in rats by aortic coarctation. *Circ Res* 1985;57:695–705.

18. Sarzani R, Brecher P, Chobanian AV. Growth factor expression in aorta of normotensive and hypertensive rats. *J Clin Invest* 1989;83:1404–1408.

19. Sarzani R, Arnaldi G, Takasaki I, Brecher P, Chobanian AV. Effects of hypertension and aging on PDGF and PDGF receptor expression in rat aorta and heart. *Hypertension* 1991;18:III-93–III-99.

20. Nickerson C, Pavlova A, Chobanian AV, Brecher P. TGFβ and fibronectin expression in cardiac and vascular lesions of hypertensive rats. *Submitted, 1994*.

21. Sarzani R, Arnaldi G, and Chobanian AV. Hypertension-induced changes of platelet-derived growth factor receptor expression in rat aorta and heart. *Hypertension* 1991;17:888–895.

22. Ingber DE. Fibronectin controls capillary endothelial cell growth by modulating cell shape. *Proc Natl Acad Sci* 1990;87:3579–3583.

23. Madri JA, Pratt BM, Tucker AM. Endothelial cell behavior after denudation injury is modulated by transforming growth factor-β1 and fibronectin. *Lab Invest* 1989;60:755–765.

24. Hedin U, Bottger BA, Forsberg E, Johansson S, Thyberg J. Diverse effects of fibronectin and laminin on phenotypic properties of cultured arterial smooth muscle cells. *J Cell Biol* 1988;107:307–319.

25. Takasaki I, Chobanian AV, Sarzani R, Brecher P. Effect of hypertension on fibronectin expression in the rat aorta. *J Biol Chem* 1990;265:21935–21939.

26. Ignotz RA, Endo T, Massague J. Regulation of fibronectin and type I collagen on RNA levels by transforming growth factor-β. *J Biol Chem* 1987;262:6443–6446.

27. Okuda S, Languino LR, Ruoslahti E, Border WA. Elevated expression of transforming growth factor-β and proteoglycan production in experimental glomerulonephritis. *J Clin Invest* 1990;86:453–462.

28. Border WA, Noble NA, Yamamoto T, Harper JR, Yamaguchi Y, Pierschbacher MD, Ruoslahti E. Natural inhibitors of transforming growth factor-β protect against scarring in experimental kidney disease. *Nature* 1992;360:361–364.

29. Geisterfer AA, Owens GK. Arginine vasopressin induced hypertrophy of cultured rat aortic smooth muscle cells. *Hypertension* 1989;14:413–420.

30. Campbell-Boswell M, Robertson A. Effects of angiotensin II and vasopressin on human smooth muscle cells in vitro. *Exp Molec Path* 1981;35:265–276.

31. Naftilan A, Pratt R, Dzau V. Induction of c-fos, c-myc and PDGF A-chain gene expressions by angiotensin II in cultured vascular smooth muscle cells. *J Clin Invest* 1989;83:1419–1424.

32. Itoh H, Pratt RE, Dzau V. Antisense oligonucleotides complementary to PDGF mRNA attenuate angiotensin II-induced vascular hypertrophy. *Hypertension* 1990;16:325 (Abst).

33. Dzau VJ, Gibbons GH. Endothelium and growth factors in vascular remodelling of hypertension. *Hypertension* 1991;18(suppl):III-115–III-121.

34. Itoh H, Pratt RE, Dzau VJ. Interaction of atrial natriuretic polypeptide and angiotensin II on protooncogene expression and vascular cell growth. *Biochem Biophys Res Comm* 1991;176:1601–1609.

35. Oohi Y, Hahn AWA, Boulanger CM, Bühler FR, Luscher TF. Endothelin stimulated by angiotensin II augments contractility of spontaneously hypertensive rat resistance arteries. *Hypertension* 1992;19:131–137.

36. Dubey RK, Ganten D, Lüscher TF. Enhanced migration of smooth muscle cells from ren-2 transgenic rats in response to angiotensin II: Inhibition by nitric oxide. *Hypertension* 1993;22:412–418.

37. Himeno H, Crawford DH, Hosoi M, Chobanian AV, Brecher P. Angiotensin II alters fibronectin independent of hypertension. *Hypertension (in press)* 1994.

38. Weber KT, Brilla CG. Pathologic hypertrophy and cardiac interstitium fibrosis and the renin-angiotensin-aldosterone system. *Circulation* 1991;893:1849–1865.

39. Crawford D, Chobanian AV, Brecher P. Angiotensin II induces fibronectin expression associated with cardiac fibrosis in the rat. *Circ Res* 1994;74:727–739.

40. Sadoshima J, Yuhui X, Slayter HS, Izumo S. Autocrine release of angiotensin II mediates stretch-induced hypertrophy of cardiac myocytes in vitro. *Cell* 1993;75:977–984.

41. Emory T, Hirata Y, Ohta K, Shichiri M, Marumo F. Secretory mechanism of immunoreactive endothelin in cultured bovine endothelial cells. *Biochem Biophys Res Comm* 1989;160:93–100.

42. Simonson MS, Wann S, Meng P, Dubyank GR, Kester M, Nakazato Y, Sedor VR, Dunn MJ. Endothelium stimulates phospholipase C, Na⁺/H⁺ exchange, c-fos expression, and mitogenes in rat mesangial cells. *J Clin Invest* 1989;83:708–712.

43. Dubin D, Pratt RE, Cooke JP, Dzau VJ. Endothelin, a potent vasoconstrictor, is a vascular smooth muscle mitogen. *J Vasc Med Biol* 1989;1:150–154.

44. Saito Y, Makao K, Mukoyama M, Shizakami G, Itoh H, Yamada T, Azai H, Hozoda K, Suga S, Joukazak M, Ogawa Y, Makajiama S, Ueda M, Imura H. Application of monoclonal antibodies for endothelin to hypertension research. *Hypertension* 1990;15:493–496.

45. Schikiri M, Hirata Y, Ando K, Emori T, Ohta K, Kimoto S, Ogura M, Inone A, M-arumo F. Plasma endothelin levels in hypertension and chronic renal failure. *Hypertension* 1990;15:493–496.

46. Wolinsky J, Horki K, Dvorakova J. Plasma endothelin 1,2 levels in mild and severe hypertension. *J Hypertens* 1991;9(suppl 6):S194–S195.

47. Garg, Hassid A. Nitric oxide-generating vasodilators and 8-bromocyclic guanosine monophosphate inhibit mitogenesis and proliferation of cultured rat vascular smooth muscle cells. *J Clin Invest* 1989;83:1774–1777.

48. Kubes PM, Suzuki M, Granger DN. Nitric oxide: An endogenous modulator of leukocyte adhesion. *Proc Natl Acad Sci* 1991;88:4651–4655.

49. Cayatte AJ, Faller DV, Cohen RA. Nitric oxide inhibits monocyte adhesion to cytokine-activated endothelium (Abst). *Circulation* 1993;88:I-565.

50. Cohen RA, Zitnay KM, Haudenschild CC, Cunningham LD. Loss of selective endothelial cell vasoactive functions in pig coronary arteries during hypercholesterolemia. *Circ Res* 1988;63:903–910.

51. Lüscher T, Vanhoutte PM. Endothelium-dependent contractions to acetycholine in the aorta of the spontaneously hypertensive rat. *Hypertension* 1986;8:344–348.

52. Panza JA, Quyyumi AA, Brush JE, Epstein SE. Abnormal endothelium-dependent vascular reactions in patients with essential hypertension. *N Engl J Med* 1990;323:22–27.

53. Cook JP, Singer AH, Tsao P, Zera P, Rowan RA, Billingham ME. Antiatherogenic effects of L-arginine in the hypercholesterolemic rabbit. *J Clin Invest* 1992;90:1168–1172.

54. Girerd XJ, Hirsch AT, Cooke JP, Dzau VJ, Creager MA. L-arginine augments endothelium-dependent vasodilation in cholesterol-fed rabbits. *Circ Res* 1990;67:1301–1308.

55. Cayatte AJ, Palacino JJ, Horten K, Cohen RA. Chronic inhibition

of nitric oxide accelerates neointima foam cell accumulation and impairs endothelial function in hypercholesterolemic rabbits. *Arterioscler Thromb* 1994; In press.

56. Ferns GA, Raines EW, Sprugel KW, Motani AS, Reidy MA, Ross R. Inhibition of neointimal smooth muscle accumulation after angioplasty by an antibody to PDGF. *Science* 1991;253:1129–1132.

57. Handley DA, VanValen RG, Melden MK, Saunders RN. Suppression of rat carotid lesion development by the calcium channel blocker PN 200-100. *Am J Path* 1986;124:88–93.

58. Powell JS, Clozel J-P, Muller RKM, Kuhn H, Hefti F, Hosang M, and Baumgartner HR. Inhibitors of angiotensin-converting enzyme prevent myointimal proliferation after vascular injury. *Science* 1989;245:186–188.

59. Farhy RD, Carretero OA, Ho K, Scili AG. Role of kinins and nitric oxide in the effects of angiotensin converting enzyme inhibitors on neointima formation. *Circ Res* 1993;72:1202–1210.

60. Hanson SR, Powell JS, Dodson T, Lumsden A, Kelly AB, Anderson JS, Clowes AW, Harker LA. Effects of angiotensin converting enzyme inhibition with cilazapril on intimal hyperplasia in injured arteries and vascular grafts in the baboon. *Hypertension* 1993;18: II-70–II-76.

61. The Multicenter European Trial with Cilazapril after Angioplasty to Prevent Transluminal Coronary Obstruction and Restenosis (MERCATOR) Study Group. Does the new angiotensin converting enzyme inhibitor cilazapril prevent restenosis after percutaneous transluminal coronary angioplasty? *Circulation* 1992;86:100–110.

62. Chobanian AV, Brecher P, Chan C. Effects of propranolol on atherogenesis in the cholesterol-fed rabbit. *Circ Res* 1985;56:755–762.

63. Kaplan JR, Manuck SB, Adams MR, Weingand KW, Clarkson TB. Inhibition of coronary atherosclerosis by propranolol in behaviorally predisposed monkeys fed on atherogenic diet. *Circulation* 1987;76:1364–1372.

64. Henry PD, Bentley KI. Suppression of atherosclerosis in cholesterol-fed rabbits treated with nifedipine. *J Clin Invest* 1981;68: 1366–1369.

65. Rouleau J-L, Parmley WW, Stevens J, Wilkman-Cofflet JW, Mahley RW, Havel RJ. Verapamil suppresses atherosclerosis in cholesterol-fed rabbits. *J Am Coll Cardiol* 1983;1:1453–1460.

66. Lichtenstein AH, Drago R, Nickerson C, Prescott MF, Lee SQ, Chobanian AV. The effect of propranolol on atherogenesis in the Watanabe heritable hyperlipidemic rabbit. *J Vasc Med Biol* 1989;1:248–254.

67. Van Niekerk JLM, Hendriks Th, DeBoer HHM, Van't Laar A. Does nifedipine suppress atherogenesis in WHHL rabbits? *Atherosclerosis* 1984;53:91–98.

68. Chobanian AV, Haudenschild CC, Nickerson C, and Drago R. Antiatherogenic effect of captopril in the Watanabe heritable hyperlipidemic rabbit. *Hypertension* 1992;15:327–331.

69. Chobanian AV, Haudenschild CC, Nickerson C, Hope S. Trandolapril inhibits atherosclerosis in the Watanabe Heritable Hyperlipidemic Rabbit. *Hypertension* 1992;20:473–477.

70. Aberg G, Ferrer P. Effects of captopril on atherosclerosis in cynomolgus monkeys. *J Cardiovasc Pharmacol* 1990;15:S-65–S-72.

71. Charpio. Perindopril effects on atherogenesis-induced styructural and functional changes in minipig arteries. *Arterioscler Thromb* 1993;13:1126–

72. Becker RHA, Wiener G, Linz W. Preservation of endothelial function by ramipril in rabbits on a long-term atherogenic diet. *J Cardiovasc Pharmacol* 1991;18:S11.

73. Clozel M, Kühn H, Hefti F, Baumgartner HR. Endothelial dysfunction and subendothelial monocyte macrophages in hypertension. *Hypertension* 1991;18:132–141.

74. Chopra M, Beswick H, Clappeston M, Dargie JH, Smith WE, McMurray J. Anti-oxidant effects of angiotensin-converting enzyme (ACE) inhibitors: free radical and oxidant scavenging are sulfhydryl dependent, but lipid peroxidation is inhibited by both sulfhydryl- and nonsulfhydryl-containing ACE inhibitors. *J Cardiovasc Pharmacol* 1992;19:330–340.

75. Pfeffer MA, Braunwald E, Moye LA, Basta L, Brown EJ, Cuddy TE, Davis BR, Geltman EM, Goldman S, Flaker GC, Klein M, Lamas GA, Packer M, Rouleau J, Rouleau JL, Rutherford J, Wertheimer JH, Hawkins CM. Effect of captopril on mortality and morbidity in patients with left ventricular dysfunction after myocardial infarction. *N Engl J Med* 1992;327:669–677.

76. Chobanian AV. Coronary artery disease and the hypertension-atherosclerosis connection. *Am J Cardiol* (*in press*).

Hypertension: Pathophysiology, Diagnosis, and Management, Second Edition, edited by J.H. Laragh and B.M. Brenner, Raven Press, Ltd., New York © 1995.

CHAPTER 33

Mechanisms of Calcium Mobilization and Homeostasis in Vascular Smooth Muscle and Their Relevance to Hypertension

Raouf A. Khalil and Cornelius van Breemen

The last two decades have witnessed great advances in our understanding of the molecular mechanisms underlying vascular smooth muscle tone. Several mechanisms have been proposed, but the intracellular free Ca^{2+} concentration ($[Ca^{2+}]_i$) is still widely accepted as a major determinant of vascular smooth muscle contraction. In resting smooth muscle cells, $[Ca^{2+}]_i$ is maintained constant by a balance between a variety of Ca^{2+} mobilizing and Ca^{2+} homeostatic mechanisms generally mediated by Ca^{2+} channels and Ca^{2+} pumps located in the plasma membrane and intracellular organelles (Fig. 1). Activation of most types of smooth muscle cells by different external stimuli disturbs the balance between Ca^{2+} mobilization and Ca^{2+} homeostasis with a resultant increase in $[Ca^{2+}]_i$ and smooth muscle contraction. Smooth mus-

cle cells are electrically connected to one another via nexuses and thus can be activated by membrane depolarization. The primary result of membrane depolarization is that Ca^{2+} entry is enhanced by the opening of voltage-gated Ca^{2+} channels. Smooth muscle cells are also covered by a multitude of receptors that interact with a variety of excitatory agonists. The agonist-receptor interaction activates a transducing guanosine triphosphate–binding protein that, in turn, stimulates plasma membrane–associated enzymes, in particular phospholipase C, to generate cascades of second messengers and modulators such as 1,4,5-inositol trisphosphate. Inositol trisphosphate and Ca^{2+} activate separate Ca^{2+} channels in the sarcoplasmic reticulum membrane. The agonist-receptor interaction is also coupled to the opening of receptor-operated Ca^{2+} channels in the plasma membrane. Since both the sarcoplasmic reticulum and the extracellular space contain Ca^{2+} at concentrations 10,000-fold greater than in the cytoplasm, Ca^{2+} is rapidly delivered through various Ca^{2+} channels into the cytoplasm, where it reaches concentrations sufficient to cause

R. A. Khalil: Cardiovascular Division, Beth Israel Hospital, Harvard Medical School, Boston, Massachusetts 02215.

C. van Breemen: Department of Pharmacology and Therapeutics, Faculty of Medicine, University of British Columbia, Vancouver, British Columbia V6T 1Z3, Canada.

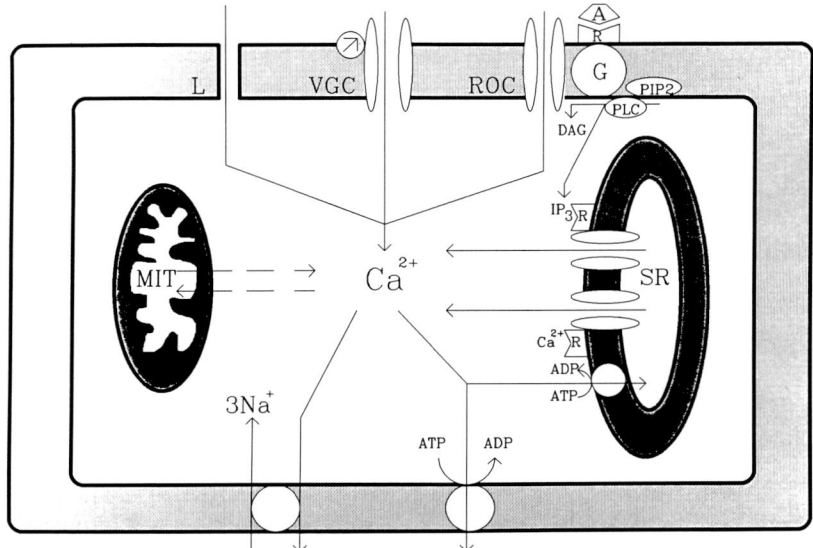

FIG. 1. Schematic representation of the Ca^{2+} mobilizing and Ca^{2+} homeostatic mechanisms in vascular smooth muscle. Extracellular Ca^{2+} enters the cell through the passive Ca^{2+} leak (L), receptor-operated Ca^{2+} channels (ROC), and voltage-gated Ca^{2+} channels (VGC). Intracellular Ca^{2+} stores in the sarcoplasmic reticulum (SR) are released in response to 1,4,5-inositol trisphosphate (IP_3) or to Ca^{2+}. The increased intracellular Ca^{2+} is taken up by the sarcoplasmic reticulum Ca^{2+} pump or extruded by the plasmalemmal Ca^{2+} pump. At high concentrations of Ca^{2+}, the Na^+-Ca^{2+} exchanger and the mitochondria (MIT) may play a role in Ca^{2+} homeostasis. A, agonist; R, receptor; G, guanosine triphosphate-binding protein; PIP_2, phosphatidylinositol 4,5-bisphosphate; PLC, phospholipase C.

smooth muscle contraction. The elevated cytosolic Ca^{2+} simultaneously stimulates Ca^{2+} removal by Ca^{2+} pumps located in the plasma membrane and the sarcoplasmic reticulum membrane that, together, may constitute an integrated buffer barrier against Ca^{2+} entry. At high concentrations of cytosolic Ca^{2+}, the Na^+-Ca^{2+} exchanger may also contribute to Ca^{2+} removal. At extremely high and probably pathological Ca^{2+} concentrations, mitochondrial Ca^{2+} accumulation comes into play. In the following sections the various Ca^{2+} mobilizing and Ca^{2+} homeostatic mechanisms involved in the regulation of vascular smooth muscle function are reviewed. The modification of these mechanisms by different agonists, their heterogeneity in the arterial tree, and their possible alteration in hypertension are also discussed.

MECHANISMS OF CALCIUM MOBILIZATION

Calcium mobilization occurs through Ca^{2+} channels located at the surface membrane and in some intracellular organelles. The Ca^{2+} concentration in the extracellular space and the intracellular organelles is severalfold higher than that in the cytosol. Thus the opening of surface membrane Ca^{2+} channels will allow Ca^{2+} to enter from the extracellular space into the cytosol. On the other hand, the opening of Ca^{2+} channels in the organelle membrane will release Ca^{2+} from the intracellular organelles to the cytosol.

CALCIUM ENTRY FROM EXTRACELLULAR SPACE

Four major Ca^{2+} entry pathways have been identified or suggested in vascular smooth muscle cells: the Ca^{2+} leak, the voltage-gated Ca^{2+} channels, the receptor-operated Ca^{2+} channels, and the stretch-activated Ca^{2+} channels.

Calcium Leak

Ca^{2+} leak is defined as the Ca^{2+} entry pathway through which Ca^{2+} passes down its electrochemical gradient into the resting cell. This Ca^{2+} entry pathway is probably lined with both phosphate and carboxyl groups because it is partially blocked by increasing the hydrogen ion concentration. Also, inorganic trivalent cations such as lanthanum and divalent cations such as cobalt have been shown to block the Ca^{2+} leak by approximately 66 percent (1).

It has generally been assumed that the Ca^{2+} leak pathway represents Ca^{2+} movements that do not require the actual opening of specific Ca^{2+} channels. However, Benham and Tsien (2) have recently described a divalent cation-selective channel that displays occasional spontaneous openings and may contribute to the Ca^{2+} leak. This channel opens at holding potentials below the threshold for activation of voltage-gated Ca^{2+} channel and has a higher conductance than the adenosine triphosphate (ATP)-sensitive Ca^{2+} channel (one type of receptor-operated Ca^{2+} channel); thus, it has been identified as a separate type of channel.

The magnitude of the Ca^{2+} leak in smooth muscle cells has been determined by $^{45}Ca^{2+}$ flux measurements. In the resting rabbit aorta, $^{45}Ca^{2+}$ influx is ~ 14 $\mu mol/Kg/min$ (3). This large Ca^{2+} leak does not cause contraction because it is constantly balanced by Ca^{2+} homeostatic mechanisms such as Ca^{2+} uptake by the sarcoplasmic reticulum and Ca^{2+} extrusion to the extracellular space. However, if these Ca^{2+} homeostatic mechanisms are compromised or the myofilaments force sensitivity to

Ca^{2+} is increased, the Ca^{2+} leak pathway is expected to contribute to smooth muscle contraction.

Voltage-Gated Calcium Channels

The presence of extracellular Ca^{2+} is essential for contraction of certain types of vascular smooth muscle in response to certain stimuli (1). In rabbit aorta, force development in response to membrane depolarization by high K^+ is abolished in the absence of extracellular Ca^{2+}. Also, the maintained norepinephrine-induced contraction in rabbit aorta is significantly inhibited in Ca^{2+}-free medium. The magnitude of Ca^{2+} movement into the cell during activation by various agonists has been determined by measuring the $^{45}Ca^{2+}$ influx (4) and, more recently, the current associated with Ca^{2+} movement (5–8). $^{45}Ca^{2+}$ influx measurements have shown that the Ca^{2+} entry pathway activated by high K^+ depolarization is sensitive to various organic Ca^{2+} antagonists, particularly the dihydropyridines (9). A strong correlation has been found between the Ca^{2+} antagonist-induced blockade of $^{45}Ca^{2+}$ influx and the associated inhibition of force (1). On the other hand, Bay K8644, a Ca^{2+} channel agonist, has been shown to stimulate Ca^{2+} influx and to induce force, thus establishing a causal link between both parameters. These observations suggest that a distinct Ca^{2+} entry pathway exists in the plasma membrane. This pathway is activated by membrane depolarization and has thus been termed a voltage-gated Ca^{2+} channel (10–12).

The advent of the voltage-clamp and patch-clamp techniques has provided further characterization of the voltage-gated Ca^{2+} channels in a variety of vascular smooth muscle cells. Most of these studies have provided evidence for two components of voltage-activated Ca^{2+} current, one of which is activated by relatively large depolarizations and inactivates relatively slowly, while the other is activated by relatively small depolarizations and inactivates relatively rapidly. These two components have been referred to as L and T current, respectively (7).

Both components of the Ca^{2+} current are blocked by lanthanum (5), cadmium (8,13), and cobalt (6,8). However, the two current components can be distinguished by their sensitivity to dihydropyridines. The L current is blocked by dihydropyridines such as nisoldipine, nimodipine, nifedipine, and nitrendipine and is augmented by Bay K8644 and Bay R5417. In contrast, the T current is not significantly affected by these dihydropyridines (5–8).

The question of whether the voltage-gated Ca^{2+} channels are modulated by physiological agonists is still unresolved. Reports on the effects of norepinephrine on voltage-activated Ca^{2+} current in vascular smooth muscle are variable. Some studies have shown that norepinephrine has no effect on the voltage-activated Ca^{2+} current (5,8). However, in the rabbit ear artery, Benham and Tsien (14) have reported that norepinephrine, acting through non-α non-β receptors, stimulates the L type current but not the T type current. Also, in rabbit mesenteric artery, Nelson and co-workers (12) have shown that norepinephrine can activate and increase the open probability of voltage-gated Ca^{2+} channels.

Receptor-Operated Calcium Channels

In contrast to high K^+ depolarization, the increase in Ca^{2+} influx and force induced by physiological agonists such as norepinephrine appears to be refractory to organic Ca^{2+} antagonists. Nevertheless, these agonists still require extracellular Ca^{2+} in order to induce maximal and maintained force. In rabbit aorta, it has been observed that (a) norepinephrine causes further increase in tension after maximal depolarization of the tissue by high K^+; (b) the $^{45}Ca^{2+}$ influx stimulated by simultaneous application of maximal concentrations of norepinephrine and high K^+ depolarizing solution is equal to the sum of that stimulated by each one alone, i.e., an additive effect is demonstrated; and (c) the $^{45}Ca^{2+}$ influx stimulated by Ca^{2+} channel agonists such as Bay K8644 is additive to that induced by maximal concentrations of norepinephrine but not to that stimulated by high K^+-induced depolarization (1,15). These observations suggest that physiological agonists activate Ca^{2+} channels different from those activated by membrane depolarization. These Ca^{2+} channels have been termed receptor-operated Ca^{2+} channels (10,11).

Electrophysiological studies have provided more direct evidence for the receptor-operated Ca^{2+} channels. Benham and Tsien (2) have reported that ATP activates a distinct Ca^{2+} current in the rabbit ear artery. The receptor-operated Ca^{2+} channel activated by ATP displays a 3:1 selectivity for Ca^{2+} over Na^+ at near-physiological ionic conditions. It can be distinguished from the voltage-gated Ca^{2+} channel by its insensitivity to blockade by nifedipine and cadmium, its opening at high negative potentials, and its unitary conductance of ~ 5 pS in 110 mM Ca^{2+} or Ba^{2+}. Since the channel is not activated when ATP is added outside the cell-attached patch pipette, it appears to be directly coupled to receptor activation by ATP rather than through an ATP-induced generation of a freely diffusible messenger (16).

Stretch-Activated Calcium Channels

Since the discovery of the phenomenon of "autoregulation" of peripheral blood flow (17), it has been recognized that stretch of the vascular wall or elevation of the intravascular pressure can produce a maintained increase in vascular smooth muscle tone. It has also been found that the stretch-stimulated vascular tone is highly dependent on extracellular Ca^{2+}, suggesting the activation of a Ca^{2+} channel by stretch (18). Bevan and co-workers have provided evidence that the stretch activated Ca^{2+} channels differ from the voltage-gated Ca^{2+} channels and the receptor-operated Ca^{2+} channels in their sensitivity to Ca^{2+} antagonists, being more sensitive to diltiazem but insensitive to dihydropyridines. In support of this hypothesis, it has recently been found that stretch stimulates $^{45}Ca^{2+}$ influx and opens nonspecific cation channels in smooth muscle membranes (19). The mechanism of activation of the stretch-sensitive Ca^{2+} channels is not clear at present. Recent evidence suggests an intermediary role of the endothelium in the arterial smooth muscle response to stretch (20,21).

CALCIUM RELEASE FROM INTRACELLULAR STORES

Stimulation of smooth muscle by various physiological agonists has been shown to produce a transient contractile response in the absence of extracellular Ca^{2+}. Also, inhibition of Ca^{2+} influx by Ca^{2+} antagonists inhibits the maintained agonist-induced contraction but does not interfere with the transient agonist-induced contraction (9). In addition, agonists stimulate $^{45}Ca^{2+}$ efflux from $^{45}Ca^{2+}$-loaded smooth muscle, particularly in a Ca^{2+}-free medium (22). These observations have suggested that Ca^{2+} release from an intracellular Ca^{2+} storage site may contribute to the agonist-induced smooth muscle contraction.

Ultrastructure studies in smooth muscle have revealed structures consistent with the sarcoplasmic reticulum and electron probe X-ray microanalysis has shown that this organelle can accumulate Ca^{2+} from solutions containing micromolar concentrations of Ca^{2+} (23). The sarcoplasmic reticulum is an intracellular membrane system of tubules (24) and, in some species, flattened cisternae (23). It occupies from 1.5 percent to 7.5 percent of the smooth muscle cell volume (25). The largest volumes of the sarcoplasmic reticulum are encountered in large elastic arteries, such as the rabbit main pulmonary artery, which also show the greatest persistence of contraction in the absence of extracellular Ca^{2+}. In contrast, phasic smooth muscle such as the guinea pig taenia coli and the rabbit mesenteric vein contain relatively small volumes (1.5 percent to 2.5 percent) of sarcoplasmic reticulum and lose their responsiveness more readily in Ca^{2+}-free solutions. However, even this small 2 percent volume of sarcoplasmic reticulum can store sufficient Ca^{2+} for activating a near maximal contraction when released (26).

The sarcoplasmic reticulum has recently been isolated as a microsomal fraction using advanced biochemical techniques. Isolated smooth muscle microsomes have been shown to accumulate $^{45}Ca^{2+}$ and to release it in re-

sponse to Ca^{2+} releasing agents such as caffeine. In addition, the Ca^{2+} release channel in sarcoplasmic reticulum vesicles of smooth muscle has recently been characterized in planar lipid bilayer (27). The problem of losing some essential cellular components during isolation and purification of the sarcoplasmic reticulum vesicles has been circumvented by chemical skinning of smooth muscle using saponin (24,28) or α-toxin (29–31). Chemical skinning has enabled the investigators to study the Ca^{2+} release mechanism under conditions not very far from being physiological. Studies on skinned fibers have shown that Ca^{2+} release from the sarcoplasmic reticulum is triggered by two intracellular second messengers, namely 1,4,5-inositol trisphosphate (IP_3) and Ca^{2+}.

Inositol Trisphosphate–Mediated Calcium Release

One of the earliest biochemical events that follows the agonist-receptor interaction is stimulation of the membrane-associated phospholipase C, which stimulates the breakdown of the plasma membrane phospholipid phosphatidylinositol 4,5-bisphosphate into 1,2-diacylglycerol and IP_3 (32). Diacylglycerol is a lipophilic compound and thus remains in the plasma membrane where it binds to and activates protein kinase C (33). On the other hand, IP_3 is a water-soluble compound that diffuses in the cytosol and stimulates Ca^{2+} release from the sarcoplasmic reticulum (34–37). Studies in smooth muscle cells chemically skinned with saponin have shown that the IP_3-induced Ca^{2+} release is sufficiently large and rapid. The half-maximal effective concentration of IP_3 (~ 1 μM) is low enough to account for the observed transient smooth muscle contraction (34,36,38). Also, a specific phosphatase, which rapidly inactivates IP_3, in accordance with the requirements for its function as a second messenger, has been identified in smooth muscle (39). IP_3 binds to a specific receptor on the surface of the sarcoplasmic reticulum and thereby activates an IP_3-sensitive Ca^{2+} release channel. Heparin, probably because of its electronegative charge, may compete with IP_3 for its receptor and thus inhibit IP_3-induced Ca^{2+} release from the sarcoplasmic reticulum (40).

Calcium-Induced Calcium Release

The observation that small concentrations of Ca^{2+} can induce further Ca^{2+} release from the sarcoplasmic reticulum was first shown in skinned skeletal (24,41) and cardiac muscle (42). Thereafter, Ca^{2+}-induced Ca^{2+} release was demonstrated in chemically-skinned vascular smooth muscle (28). Ca^{2+}-induced Ca^{2+} release is a regenerative process that can be facilitated by Ca^{2+} releasing agents such as caffeine (24). The process is triggered when the concentration of Ca^{2+} in the vicinity of the sarcoplasmic reticulum exceeds a threshold of 3×10^{-6} M.

The threshold Ca^{2+} concentration that stimulates Ca^{2+} release is increased in the presence of Mg^{2+}. Ca^{2+}-induced Ca^{2+} release is enhanced by adenosine 3',5'-cyclic monophosphate (cyclic AMP) and inhibited by procaine (28).

In contrast to skeletal and cardiac muscle, an influx of extracellular Ca^{2+} is not necessary to stimulate Ca^{2+}-induced Ca^{2+} release from smooth muscle sarcoplasmic reticulum. However, an increase in Ca^{2+} concentration in the vicinity of the sarcoplasmic reticulum is essential for this regenerative process to take place. It has been suggested that an initial IP_3-induced Ca^{2+} release from the sarcoplasmic reticulum through a subset of Ca^{2+} release channels may raise $[Ca^{2+}]$ near the sarcoplasmic reticulum above the threshold of 3×10^{-6} M, which in turn stimulates more Ca^{2+} release from the sarcoplasmic reticulum through a second subset of Ca^{2+} release channels (43). Another component of the signal amplification system is suggested by the observation that Ca^{2+} enhances the IP_3-induced Ca^{2+} release from the sarcoplasmic reticulum in skinned smooth muscle preparations (38).

MECHANISMS OF CALCIUM HOMEOSTASIS

In addition to their role in Ca^{2+} mobilization, the smooth muscle plasma membrane and intracellular organelles also play a role in maintaining cellular Ca^{2+} homeostasis. The plasmalemmal Ca^{2+}–adenosine triphosphatase (ATPase) plays the predominant role in maintaining $[Ca^{2+}]_i$ close to the basal levels, while the Na^+-Ca^{2+} exchanger contributes to removal of excess cytosolic Ca^{2+}. In addition to the events occurring at the plasma membrane level, two intracellular organelles determine the cytosolic Ca^{2+} concentration; these are the sarcoplasmic reticulum and the mitochondria. These organelles have pump-leak systems oriented so that there is an active uptake of Ca^{2+} from the cytosol and a passive leak of Ca^{2+} back to the cytosol.

PLASMALEMMAL CALCIUM ATPase

Metabolic inhibition of the smooth muscle of guinea pig tenia coli using iodoacetic acid or 2,4-dinitrophenol has been shown to cause an initial net Ca^{2+} uptake that is similar in magnitude to the passive Ca^{2+} leak (44, 45). These observations have suggested that an ATP-dependent Ca^{2+} extrusion pump contributes to cellular Ca^{2+} homeostasis (46) and that inhibition of the Ca^{2+} pump will cause accumulation of Ca^{2+} inside the cell. The smooth muscle plasmalemmal Ca^{2+} pump is probably similar to the better-studied Ca^{2+} pumps in the squid axon and red blood cells (47). It has a molecular weight of 130 kDa. It is stimulated by calmodulin and inhibited by vanadate. The observation that vanadate causes max-

imal contraction of vascular smooth muscle suggests that the plasmalemmal Ca^{2+} pump plays a major role in the regulation of $[Ca^{2+}]_i$ and thereby vascular tone (48). Also, certain agonists such as oxytocin and prostaglandins have been shown to enhance their contractile response by inhibiting the plasmalemmal Ca^{2+} extrusion pump (49,50).

The plasmalemmal Ca^{2+}-ATPase can be distinguished from other ATPases in the plasmalemma and endoplasmic reticulum by its insensitivity to ouabain (distinction from Na^+,K^+-ATPase), high sensitivity to inhibition by vanadate (more sensitive than endoplasmic reticulum ATPase), sensitivity to K^+ (less sensitive than endoplasmic reticulum ATPase), and sensitivity to calmodulin antagonists (49).

Recent molecular biology studies have reported the molecular cloning, expression, purification, and amino acid sequencing of the plasmalemmal Ca^{2+} pump from several cell types (51,52) including smooth muscle (53).

THE SODIUM-CALCIUM EXCHANGER

The Na^+-Ca^{2+} exchange provides an alternative mechanism in the plasma membrane through which excess intracellular Ca^{2+} is removed to the extracellular space against a large $[Ca^{2+}]$ gradient. The contribution of Na^+-Ca^{2+} exchange to Ca^{2+} homeostasis has been suggested in many cell types including smooth muscle (16,54,55). Studies on membrane vesicles have shown that a Na^+-Ca^{2+} exchange activity co-purifies with plasma membrane markers and thus represents a plasmalemmal activity. The plasmalemmal Na^+-Ca^{2+} exchange has been distinguished from the mitochondrial Na^+-Ca^{2+} exchanger by its significantly different specificity and stoichiometry (56). Also, several studies have reported the isolation and functional reconstitution of the plasmalemmal Na^+-Ca^{2+} exchanger (57,58).

The fundamental questions about the exact nature of the plasmalemmal Na^+-Ca^{2+} exchange, its stoichiometry, its direction, and its physiologic and pathologic significance have been resolved. The process is driven by the transmembrane Na^+ and Ca^{2+} ionic gradients and the membrane potential. The energy derived from either Na^+ or Ca^{2+}, moving down its electrochemical gradient, is balanced by an antiport movement of the coupled ion. The process is electrogenic (59) and has a stoichiometry of $3Na^+$:Ca^{2+} (60).

In vascular smooth muscle, Na^+-Ca^{2+} exchange may contribute to Ca^{2+} extrusion, but the magnitude of its contribution is not well-defined and appears to vary from one tissue to another (61,62). Although often assumed to be mainly a Ca^{2+} efflux pathway, it is now clear that depending upon the membrane potential, the transmembrane ionic gradients of Na^+ and Ca^{2+} and the relative importance of intracellular Ca^{2+}, the Na^+-Ca^{2+} exchanger can contribute to either Ca^{2+} extrusion or Ca^{2+} influx. The significance of Na^+-Ca^{2+} exchange as a source of intracellular Ca^{2+} may be increased in pathological states of the cardiovascular system particularly hypertension (63).

SARCOPLASMIC RETICULUM CALCIUM ATPase

The contribution of the sarcoplasmic reticulum Ca^{2+}-ATPase to Ca^{2+} homeostasis has long been established in skeletal and cardiac muscle. The Ca^{2+}-ATPase of skeletal and cardiac sarcoplasmic reticulum has very high density and therefore is very well characterized (64). It has a molecular weight of 100 kDa. Substantial information is also available on its mechanism of action, its reversibility, the 2:1 stoichiometry between Ca^{2+} transport and ATP hydrolysis, as well as its phosphorylation by various kinases. The ability of sarcoplasmic reticulum to accumulate Ca^{2+} is most marked in skeletal and cardiac muscle and is significantly less in other systems, including smooth muscle (65). However, microsomal sarcoplasmic reticulum preparations showing energy-dependent Ca^{2+} uptake have been isolated from smooth muscle. Also, Ca^{2+} electron probe X-ray microanalysis of saponin-permeabilized smooth muscle has shown the operation of an ATP-dependent nonmitochondrial Ca^{2+}-pump that is blocked by vanadate (23). The affinity of the sarcoplasmic reticulum pump for Ca^{2+} ($K_m = 0.2$ to $0.6 \ \mu M$) is high enough to take up Ca^{2+} and thereby cause relaxation. Also, the high-capacity, low-affinity Ca^{2+}-binding protein calsequestrin, which increases the Ca^{2+} storage capacity, has been demonstrated in isolated preparations from skeletal (66) and smooth muscle (67) sarcoplasmic reticulum. However, the capacity of the sarcoplasmic reticulum to accumulate Ca^{2+} is limited, so that with successive and excessive Ca^{2+} loads the mitochondria may become the major Ca^{2+} pool (68).

MITOCHONDRIA

Although mitochondria occupy approximately 5 percent of the total smooth muscle cell volume (23), questions regarding their role in regulation of intracellular Ca^{2+} under both physiological and pathological conditions are still unresolved. Also, the concentration of free Ca^{2+} in the mitochondrial matrix space is unclear. There are separate Ca^{2+} influx and Ca^{2+} efflux pathways across the mitochondrial membrane (56,69,70). The influx pathway operates as a Ca^{2+} uniporter driven by the large mitochondrial membrane potential (150 mV, inside negative), and the efflux pathway operates as a Ca^{2+}:$2H^+$ or Ca^{2+}:$2Na^+$ antiporter (71,72). The Ca^{2+} efflux pathway is of lower capacity than the Ca^{2+} influx pathway (69). Under physiological conditions the major cytosolic anion is phosphate. When Ca^{2+} is taken up by mitochondria, HPO_4^{2-} is also taken up via HPO_4^{2-}:$2OH^-$ exchange and calcium phosphates are formed. According to Mitchell's (73) hypothesis of mitochondrial energy transfer, the primary event is the development of an electrochemical proton gradient across the mitochondrial membrane with the pH gradient in mitochondria greater than cytoplasm (70). In an alkaline environment the solubility of calcium phosphates is extremely low. Thus, the major determinants of the free $[Ca^{2+}]$ within the mitochondrial matrix space are the extra- and intramitochondrial phosphate concentration, the intramitochondrial pH, and the K_m and V_{max} of the efflux pathway (71).

The role of mitochondria in cellular Ca^{2+} homeostasis can be easily understood by considering the rate of Ca^{2+} uptake into mitochondria as a function of the cytosolic Ca^{2+} concentration. The rate of mitochondrial Ca^{2+} uptake increases dramatically as the cytosolic Ca^{2+} rises to abnormally high levels. Since the Ca^{2+} efflux pathway out of the mitochondria is saturable (69), the rate of mitochondrial Ca^{2+} uptake will exceed the Ca^{2+} efflux rate and a net accumulation of Ca^{2+} by the mitochondria occurs (71). The accumulated Ca^{2+} then deposits into a nonionic calcium pool of calcium phosphate. Thus, the mitochondria function as a sink for Ca^{2+} during Ca^{2+} overload. The mitochondrial free Ca^{2+}, however, is in equilibrium with the large nonionic calcium pool. This arrangement means that the cytosolic free Ca^{2+} is coupled to the nonionic calcium pool in the mitochondria. Consequently, when the cytosolic free Ca^{2+} is lower than the mitochondrial free Ca^{2+}, the nonionic calcium pool is released in order to stabilize the cytosolic free Ca^{2+}. On the other hand, when the cytosolic Ca^{2+} is within the normal basal level ($\sim 0.1 \ \mu M$), the mitochondrial free Ca^{2+} will have a similar value and the plasma membrane and the sarcoplasmic reticulum will be largely responsible for maintaining the cellular Ca^{2+} homeostasis. Also, because the capacity of the mitochondria, although large, is finite, it may be presumed that they slowly release their stored calcium during periods of cellular quiescence when it can be handled by the plasmalemmal and the sarcoplasmic reticulum Ca^{2+} pumps.

The evidence is now overwhelming that the sarcoplasmic reticulum plays the major physiological role as the Ca^{2+} storage site, and that the mitochondria accumulate Ca^{2+} only when cytosolic Ca^{2+} is abnormally high, exceeding 5 μM (23,74). The apparent K_m of mitochondria for Ca^{2+} uptake is approximately 10 to 17 μM, which is higher than that of the sarcoplasmic reticulum ($K_m \sim 1$ μM). Therefore, smooth muscle mitochondria are minimally loaded with Ca^{2+} under physiological conditions (23,74). Thus the mitochondrial large Ca^{2+} buffering capacity plays a role in the regulation of cytoplasmic Ca^{2+} only under pathological conditions when "Ca^{2+} overload" occurs, i.e., when cell death is threatened by massive Ca^{2+} influx. The high Ca^{2+} content of mitochondria isolated from atherosclerotic blood vessels may reflect vascular smooth muscle damage, and such cells containing calcium-loaded mitochondria may become the initial sites of vascular calcification (23).

INTRACELLULAR FREE CALCIUM CONCENTRATION

The level of $[Ca^{2+}]_i$ is regulated by a balance between the Ca^{2+}-mobilizing mechanisms that increase $[Ca^{2+}]_i$, i.e., Ca^{2+} release from the sarcoplasmic reticulum and Ca^{2+} influx from extracellular space, and the Ca^{2+} homeostatic mechanisms that decrease $[Ca^{2+}]_i$, i.e., the plasmalemmal and sarcoplasmic reticulum Ca^{2+}-ATPases, the Na^+-Ca^{2+} exchange and the mitochondria.

$[Ca^{2+}]_i$ has been measured by several techniques. Measurement of $[Ca^{2+}]_i$ often requires loading a Ca^{2+} indicator into the cells. In cells large enough to permit microinjection of suitable metallochromic dyes such as arsenazo III and antipyralzo III (75), microinjection of bioluminescent proteins such as aequorin (76,77), or impalement of the cell with Ca^{2+}-sensitive microelectrodes (78), adequate measurements of $[Ca^{2+}]_i$ have been made. On the other hand, small cells such as smooth muscle are not amenable to microinjection or impalement. This problem was first circumvented by loading smooth muscle with aequorin using a transient cell permeabilization method (79). Thereafter, a group of fluorescent Ca^{2+} indicators has been developed and used for measuring $[Ca^{2+}]_i$ in many cell types, including smooth muscle (80,81). Fluorescent Ca^{2+} indicators are available in both the free acid form and the acetoxymethyl ester form. The nonpolar acetoxymethyl ester, being relatively lipophilic, diffuses freely across the plasma membrane into the cell where it is hydrolyzed by intracellular esterases into the free acid form, acetic acid, and methyl alcohol. The free acid form is too hydrophilic to cross the plasma membrane and therefore accumulates inside the cell. This group of fluorescent Ca^{2+} indicators includes quin-2 (80,82,83), fura-2 (55,81), and indo-1 (84). Regardless of the technique employed, there is a general agreement between all methods that the physiological $[Ca^{2+}]_i$ is in the range between 0.1 and 1 μM.

HETEROGENEITY IN AGONIST-INDUCED RESPONSE

According to the thick-filament regulation hypothesis of smooth muscle contraction, Ca^{2+} binds calmodulin to form a Ca^{2+}-calmodulin complex, which activates myosin light chain kinase (85). Activation of myosin light chain kinase results in the phosphorylation of the 20-

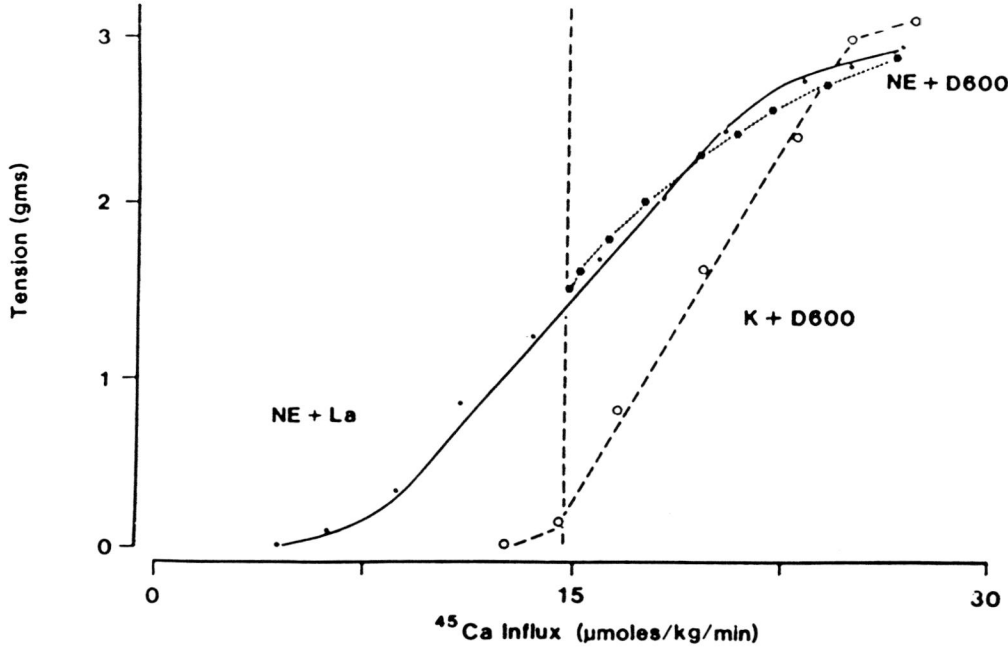

FIG. 2. Ca^{2+} influx-force relationship in rabbit aorta. Maximum high K^+-induced Ca^{2+} influx and force were measured in rabbit aortic rings. The Ca^{2+} channel antagonist D600 was added at increasing concentrations and the gradual inhibition of high K^+-induced Ca^{2+} influx and force was recorded. In parallel experiments, maximum norepinephrine-induced Ca^{2+} influx and force were recorded. Higher concentrations of D600 were needed to block the norepinephrine-induced Ca^{2+} influx but did not inhibit the norepinephrine-induced force completely. To inhibit the norepinephrine-induced force completely, increasing concentrations of La^{3+} were needed to block the Ca^{2+} leak.

kDa light chain subunit of myosin, and the stimulation of actin-activated Mg^{2+}-ATPase of smooth muscle myosin and initiation of actin-myosin interaction (86). At low levels of intracellular Ca^{2+}, a myosin light-chain phosphatase terminates actomyosin interaction and causes smooth muscle relaxation (87).

The thick-filament regulation hypothesis predicts a steady elevation of $[Ca^{2+}]_i$ during maintained agonist-induced smooth muscle contraction. Measurements of isometric tension and $^{45}Ca^{2+}$ influx have provided indirect evidence for an increase in $[Ca^{2+}]_i$ during maintained smooth muscle contraction. In rabbit aorta bathed in Ca^{2+}-free medium supplemented with 2 mM ethyleneglycoltetraacetic acid (EGTA), the phenylephrine-induced tone is significantly inhibited and the high K^+ response is abolished. Also, in rabbit aorta bathed in physiological saline solution, phenylephrine and high K^+ significantly increase $^{45}Ca^{2+}$ influx above basal levels (3,88).

However, the relationships between Ca^{2+} influx and the developed tension during activation of rabbit aorta by high K^+ and norepinephrine are not similar (88). As shown in Fig. 2, increasing concentrations of the Ca^{2+} channel antagonist D600 cause significant inhibition of the high K^+-induced Ca^{2+} influx and tension. In contrast, higher concentrations of D600 are needed to block the norepinephrine-stimulated Ca^{2+} influx but still do not inhibit the norepinephrine-induced contraction completely. To inhibit the norepinephrine-induced contraction completely, increasing concentrations of La^{3+} are needed to block the Ca^{2+} leak. Figure 2 also shows that for the same level of Ca^{2+} influx, norepinephrine causes a greater increase in tension than that induced by high K^+, i.e., there is a shift to the left in the norepinephrine Ca^{2+} influx–force curve as compared to that of high K^+.

Also, measurements of $[Ca^{2+}]_i$ during agonist-induced contraction, using the bioluminescent protein aequorin, have shown a $[Ca^{2+}]_i$ spike during force development that falls to values close to the basal values during force maintenance (79,89). Similarly, simultaneous recordings of force and $[Ca^{2+}]_i$ in rabbit inferior vena cava loaded with fura-2 (90) have shown that norepinephrine initially increases $[Ca^{2+}]_i$ to 264 nM during force development, which drops to a smaller level but still significantly higher than the basal values during maintenance of force (Fig. 3). The transient increase and subsequent decrease in $[Ca^{2+}]_i$ have suggested that a maintained increase in $[Ca^{2+}]_i$ may not be the sole mechanism of smooth muscle contraction.

One way to test the hypothesis is to compare the agonist-induced response with that of an agent that exclusively increases $[Ca^{2+}]_i$. Both Bay K8644 and high K^+ are known to stimulate Ca^{2+} entry specifically through voltage-gated Ca^{2+} channels (1,91). In rabbit inferior vena cava, the Ca^{2+} channel agonist Bay K8644 and

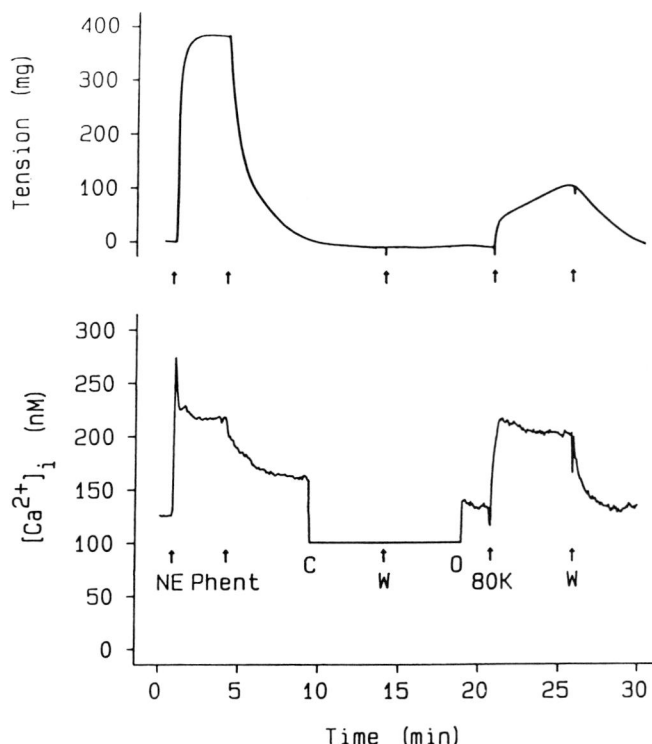

FIG. 3. Effect of norepinephrine and high K^+ on rabbit inferior vena cava. Rabbit inferior vena cava loaded with fura-2 was equilibrated in physiological saline solution for 45 min. The tissue was stimulated by norepinephrine (10 μM), treated with 10 μM phentolamine (Phent), washed with PSS (W) and then activated by high K^+ (80 mM). The changes in tension (*upper panel*) were recorded simultaneously with the changes in $[Ca^{2+}]_i$ (*lower panel*). C, shutter closed; O, shutter open.

membrane depolarization by 80 mM K^+ solution cause a smaller contractile response than norepinephrine but approximately the same steady-state increase in $[Ca^{2+}]_i$ as that induced by norepinephrine (Fig. 3).

$[Ca^{2+}]_i$-force curves have been constructed by measuring the steady-state norepinephrine- and high K^+-stimulated force and $[Ca^{2+}]_i$ at different concentrations of extracellular Ca^{2+}. As shown in Fig. 4A, at 100 μM extracellular Ca^{2+}, the norepinephrine-induced force is very small and that induced by high K^+ is abolished. The steady-state norepinephrine-induced force increases with the increases in extracellular Ca^{2+}, reaches a maximum at 1 to 2 mM extracellular Ca^{2+}, and then starts to decline. On the other hand, the high K^+-induced force increases monotonically with the increases in extracellular Ca^{2+} and does not reach a maximum even at 10 mM extracellular Ca^{2+}.

Changing the extracellular Ca^{2+} concentration also changes the steady-state norepinephrine- and high K^+-induced increase in $[Ca^{2+}]_i$ (Fig. 4B). At 100 μM extracellular Ca^{2+}, the estimated $[Ca^{2+}]_i$ is 124 nM during activation by norepinephrine and 120 nM during activation by high K^+. Increasing the extracellular Ca^{2+} con-

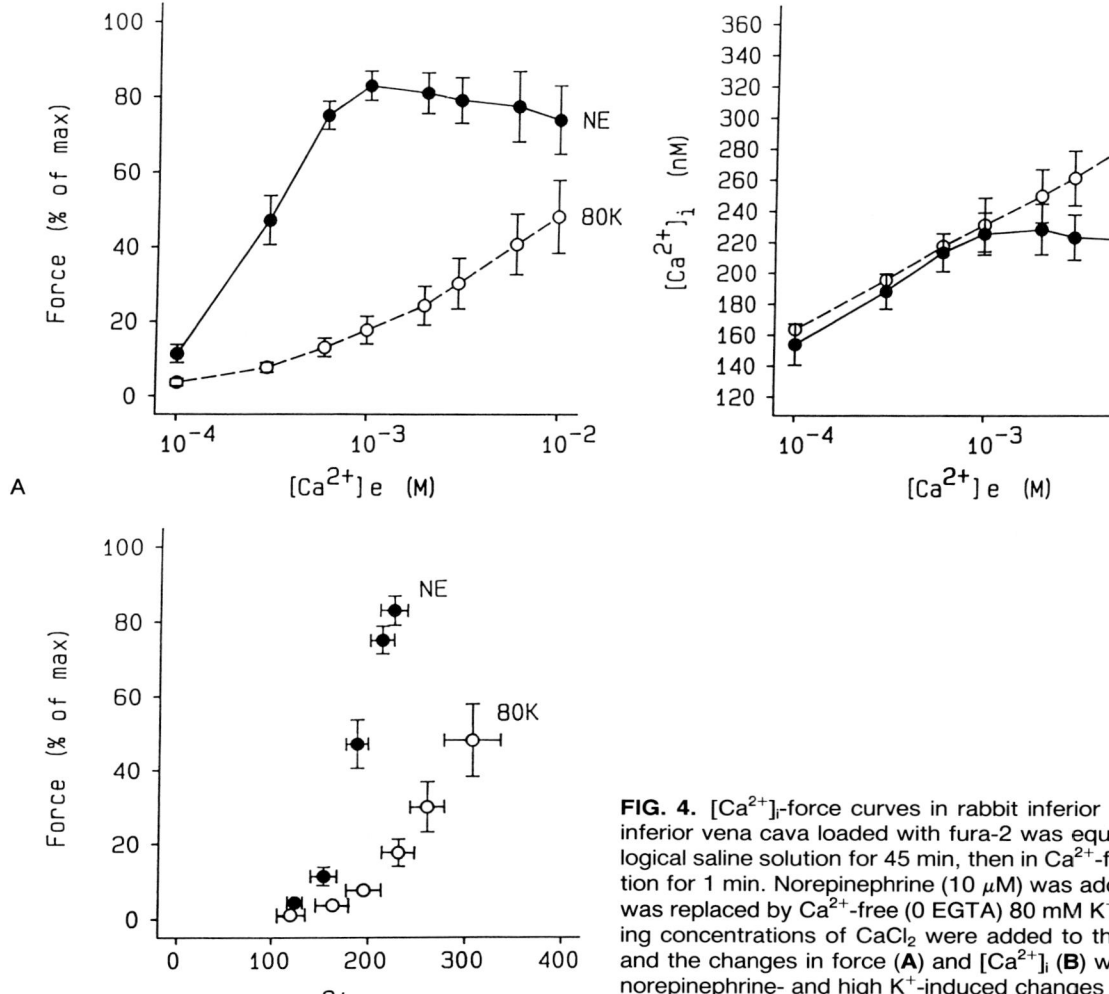

FIG. 4. $[Ca^{2+}]_i$-force curves in rabbit inferior vena cava. Rabbit inferior vena cava loaded with fura-2 was equilibrated in physiological saline solution for 45 min, then in Ca^{2+}-free (0 EGTA) solution for 1 min. Norepinephrine (10 μM) was added or the solution was replaced by Ca^{2+}-free (0 EGTA) 80 mM K^+ solution. Increasing concentrations of $CaCl_2$ were added to the bathing solution and the changes in force (**A**) and $[Ca^{2+}]_i$ (**B**) were recorded. The norepinephrine- and high K^+-induced changes in force were plotted as a function of the simultaneously recorded $[Ca^{2+}]_i$ (**C**).

centration causes a graded increase in the steady-state norepinephrine-stimulated $[Ca^{2+}]_i$, which reaches a maximum of 228 nM at 2 mM extracellular Ca^{2+} and then starts to decline. In contrast, the high K^+-stimulated $[Ca^{2+}]_i$ increases monotonically with the increase in extracellular Ca^{2+} concentration and does not reach a maximum even at 10 mM extracellular Ca^{2+}.

In $[Ca^{2+}]$ versus force curves, the norepinephrine curve is shifted to the left of that of high K^+ (Fig. 4). These results are in accordance with other studies in the ferret aorta and portal vein using the photoprotein aequorin (89). Assuming the high K^+ $[Ca^{2+}]_i$-force curve as control, it has been suggested that physiological agonists increase the myofilament sensitivity to Ca^{2+} by activating a second regulatory pathway other than Ca^{2+}. One of the possible regulatory pathways is activation of protein kinase C (92).

Several studies have shown that phorbol esters can activate protein kinase C (93) and cause smooth muscle contraction (3,94,95) with no detectable increase in $[Ca^{2+}]_i$ (96,97). These observations provide evidence

that activation of protein kinase C increases the myofilament force sensitivity to Ca^{2+} and thus can explain the shift to the left in the $[Ca^{2+}]_i$-force curve during activation by physiological agonists. However, the agonist-induced shift in the $[Ca^{2+}]_i$-force relationship has also been explained by agonist-induced changes in the spatial distribution of $[Ca^{2+}]_i$, as described below.

INTEGRATION OF CALCIUM MOBILIZING AND CALCIUM HOMEOSTATIC MECHANISMS

It seems reasonable to assume, as a working hypothesis, that the difference between the agonist and the high K^+ responses is, in part, due to a difference in the spatial distribution of $[Ca^{2+}]_i$ (Fig. 5). Under resting conditions, Ca^{2+} moves down its electrochemical gradient into the smooth muscle cell through the passive leak pathway. The Ca^{2+} leak is constantly balanced by Ca^{2+} extrusion through the plasmalemmal Ca^{2+}-ATPase and Ca^{2+} up-

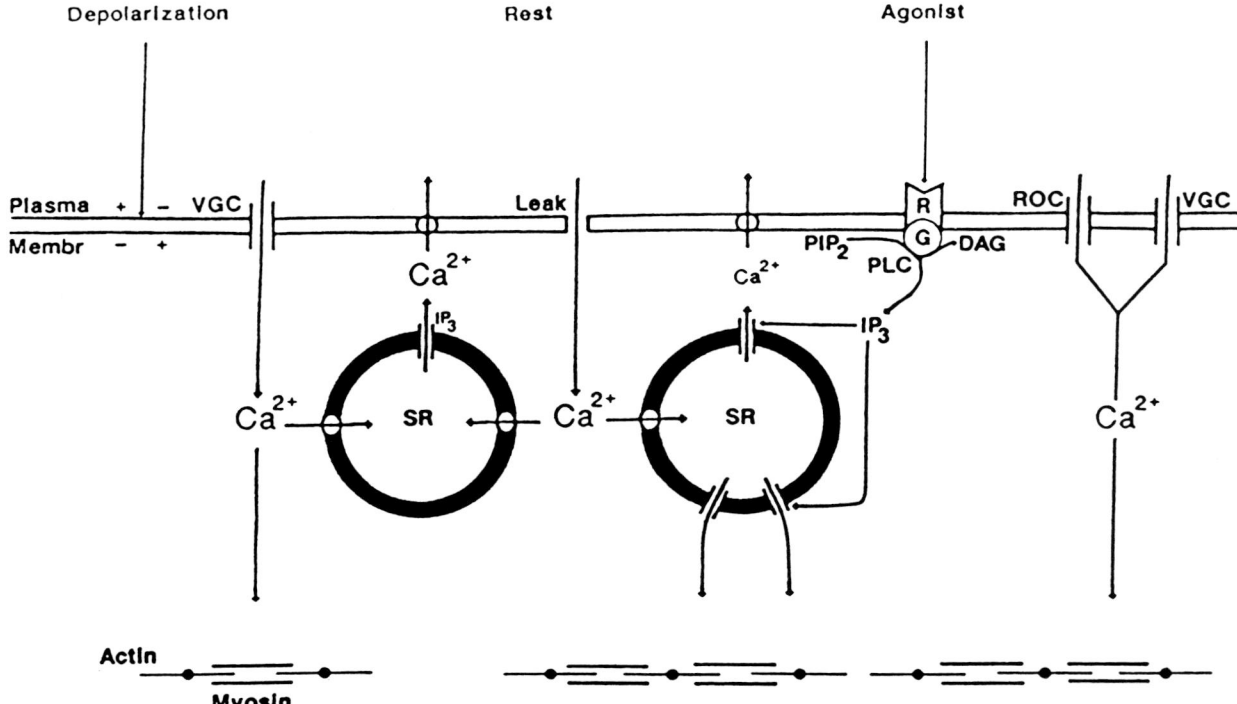

FIG. 5. The superficial buffer barrier in vascular smooth muscle. Under resting conditions, Ca^{2+} moves down its electrochemical gradient into the smooth muscle cell through the Ca^{2+} leak pathway. The Ca^{2+} leak is constantly balanced by Ca^{2+} extrusion through the plasmalemmal Ca^{2+}-ATPase and Ca^{2+} uptake by the sarcoplasmic reticulum Ca^{2+} pump, which, together, may constitute an integrated Ca^{2+} buffering system involving Ca^{2+} uptake by the sarcoplasmic reticulum, Ca^{2+} release toward the plasmalemma, followed by Ca^{2+} extrusion to the extracellular space. Membrane depolarization by high K^+ stimulates Ca^{2+} influx through voltage-gated Ca^{2+} channels (VGC). When the depolarization-induced Ca^{2+} influx exceeds a certain threshold it can bypass the superficial buffer barrier, reach the deep myoplasm, and activate the myofilaments. The agonist-induced response involves cascades of biochemical events that lead to stimulation of Ca^{2+} influx through voltage-gated (VGC) and/or receptor-operated (ROC) Ca^{2+} channels and Ca^{2+} release from the sarcoplasmic reticulum. The agonist-induced Ca^{2+} release keeps the sarcoplasmic reticulum in a state of enhanced permeability and prevents it from accumulating Ca^{2+}, and thus Ca^{2+} entering the smooth muscle cell through the leak pathway and the excitable Ca^{2+} channels will reach the deep myoplasm and activate the myofilaments.

take by the sarcoplasmic reticulum Ca^{2+} pump, which, together, may constitute an integrated Ca^{2+} buffering system involving Ca^{2+} uptake by the sarcoplasmic reticulum, Ca^{2+} release toward the plasmalemma, and ultimately Ca^{2+} extrusion to the extracellular space. Therefore, under steady-state resting conditions, the amount of Ca^{2+} that reaches the deep myoplasm is too small to activate the myofilaments. Membrane depolarization by high K^+ solution stimulates Ca^{2+} influx through voltage-gated Ca^{2+} channels. When the depolarization-induced Ca^{2+} influx is slow, a great proportion of Ca^{2+} entry will be shunted through the sarcoplasmic reticulum to the extracellular space. On the other hand, when the depolarization-induced Ca^{2+} influx exceeds a certain threshold, it can bypass the sarcoplasmic reticulum, reach the deep myoplasm, and activate the myofilaments. As illustrated in Fig. 5, during depolarization by

high K^+, the stimulated Ca^{2+} influx is presumably taken up by a superficially-located sarcoplasmic reticulum and then shunted to the extracellular space via the plasmalemmal Ca^{2+} extrusion pump or the Na^+-Ca^{2+} exchanger. Thus, the level of $[Ca^{2+}]_i$ will be high in the subplasmalemmal space and gradually decreases as one proceeds deeper in the myoplasm. On the other hand, during activation by norepinephrine, the continuous Ca^{2+} release interferes with the buffering capacity of the sarcoplasmic reticulum. Thus, Ca^{2+} entry from the extracellular space will be taken up by the sarcoplasmic reticulum but constantly released toward the deep myoplasm and induce contraction (Fig. 5). Thus when fura-2 is used to measure the average changes in $[Ca^{2+}]_i$ in the whole cytosol of a population of cells, it may give similar $[Ca^{2+}]_i$ levels during activation by high K^+ and norepinephrine (Fig. 6). In other words, the estimated

Depolarization

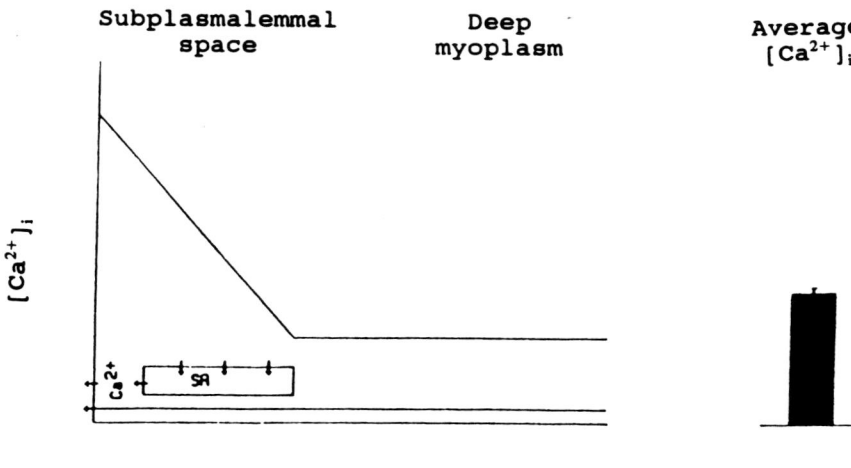

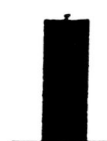

Norepinephrine

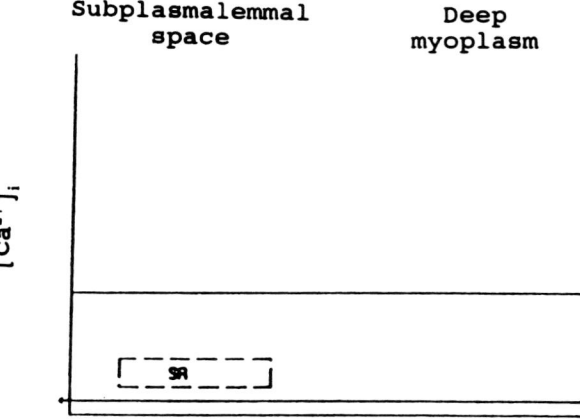

FIG. 6. Predicted steady-state distribution of $[Ca^{2+}]_i$ in smooth muscle during activation by depolarization or norepinephrine. During membrane depolarization by high K^+, the stimulated Ca^{2+} influx is presumably buffered by a superficially-located sarcoplasmic reticulum. Thus, $[Ca^{2+}]$ will be high in the subplasmalemmal space and gradually decrease as it proceeds deeper in the myoplasm. On the other hand, during activation by norepinephrine, the continuous Ca^{2+} release interferes with the buffering capacity of the sarcoplasmic reticulum. Thus, Ca^{2+} entry from the extracellular space will be shunted through the sarcoplasmic reticulum and constantly released toward the deep myoplasm and induce tension. Since fura-2 measures the average changes in $[Ca^{2+}]_i$ in the whole cytosol of a population of cells, it may give similar $[Ca^{2+}]_i$ during activation by high K^+ and norepinephrine.

levels of $[Ca^{2+}]_i$ may not reflect the spatial distribution of $[Ca^{2+}]_i$ with respect to localized gradients or availability to the myofilaments.

THE SUPERFICIAL BUFFER BARRIER

The superficial buffer barrier model assumes that a peripherally located subset of sarcoplasmic reticulum takes up Ca^{2+} as it enters the smooth muscle cell and then releases it preferentially toward the plasmalemma to be extruded to the extracellular space (Fig. 5). This model pre-

dicts that (a) the proportion of Ca^{2+} entering across the plasma membrane and taken up by the superficial sarcoplasmic reticulum is crucial in determining the threshold Ca^{2+} influx that activates tension, (b) the state of the sarcoplasmic reticulum with respect to its permeability to Ca^{2+} and its rate of Ca^{2+}-ATPase activity partly determines the steady state $[Ca^{2+}]_i$, and (c) a variable, outwardly-directed Ca^{2+} gradient exists in a narrow region (in the order of tens of nanometers) just underneath the plasmalemma. The small basal IP_3 production may be sufficient to open Ca^{2+} channels in the junctional surface of the sarcoplasmic reticulum membrane. The localized Ca^{2+} release near the inner surface of the plasma membrane may trigger further vectorial Ca^{2+} release (Ca^{2+}-induced Ca^{2+} release) toward the plasmalemma (1). The resulting high $[Ca^{2+}]$ near the inner surface of the plasma membrane would stimulate Ca^{2+} extrusion via the plasmalemmal Ca^{2+}-ATPase and probably the Na^+-Ca^{2+} exchanger.

A growing body of evidence has provided support to the superficial buffer-barrier model. Measurements of tension and $^{45}Ca^{2+}$ influx in arterial smooth muscle during depolarization by high K^+ have shown that the magnitude of smooth muscle contraction is dependent on the rate rather than the magnitude of net cellular Ca^{2+} gain (4). These observations can be explained by the possibility that a fraction of the high K^+-stimulated Ca^{2+} influx is taken up by the sarcoplasmic reticulum before it reaches the myofilaments. The net Ca^{2+} uptake by the sarcoplasmic reticulum is expected to depend on the rate of Ca^{2+} diffusion inside the cell so that, when the rate of Ca^{2+} diffusion is slower, the sarcoplasmic reticulum will be able to remove a larger proportion of the cytoplasmic Ca^{2+} leading to less myofilament activation (4). These studies have been supported by the observation that depletion of the sarcoplasmic reticulum Ca^{2+} by exposing aortic rings bathed in Ca^{2+}-free solution repeatedly to maximal concentrations of norepinephrine diminishes the ability of subsequent high K^+-stimulated Ca^{2+} influx to activate tension. It has been found that high K^+ depolarization could induce tension only if the norepinephrine-releasable Ca^{2+} store in the sarcoplasmic reticulum is refilled to near its physiological capacity (98).

Ultrastructural studies have shown that a significant portion of the sarcoplasmic reticulum in smooth muscle cells is located close to the inner surface of the sarcolemma and has been termed *peripheral sarcoplasmic reticulum* (23,25,99). In the subplasmalemmal regions where the sarcoplasmic reticulum tubules approach the surface membrane, quasi-periodic bridging structures span the 12 to 18 nm subplasmalemmal space (23). These structures resemble the junctional feet of the skeletal muscle triads (100) and may represent sites for functional integration between the sarcoplasmic reticulum and the plasma membrane.

Several studies have suggested the presence of a Ca^{2+} gradient underneath the plasmalemma. For instance, the Ca^{2+}-sensitive K^+ channels of smooth muscle plasmalemma may show spontaneous opening in the absence of cell contraction (101). Also, α-adrenergic stimulation of intestinal smooth muscle simultaneously increases the quin-2 fluorescence and decreases the contractile response (102). This could be interpreted by localized increase in $[Ca^{2+}]$ near the plasmalemmal Ca^{2+}-activated K^+ channels leading to hyperpolarization of the membrane and inhibition of Ca^{2+} entry through voltage-gated

Ca^{2+} channels and consequently a decrease in myoplasmic $[Ca^{2+}]$. In addition, Rembold (103) has observed that Ca^{2+} depletion of the sarcoplasmic reticulum by repetitive agonist applications in Ca^{2+}-free solution causes temporal dissociation of Ca^{2+}-induced aequorin luminescence from myosin light chain phosphorylation and smooth muscle contraction when Ca^{2+} influx is stimulated by addition of Ca^{2+}.

Since agonist activation may involve many Ca^{2+} regulatory mechanisms, a more direct way to test the superficial buffer barrier hypothesis is to test an agent that exclusively releases Ca^{2+} from the sarcoplasmic reticulum. The plant alkaloid ryanodine has been used in a variety of preparations to study Ca^{2+} release from the sarcoplasmic reticulum (104–107). In smooth muscle of rat aorta and bovine tail artery, pretreatment with ryanodine blocks the caffeine-induced contraction and attenuates the norepinephrine-induced contraction (108). In rabbit aorta, ryanodine stimulates a small but prolonged $^{45}Ca^{2+}$ efflux and reduces the norepinephrine-induced $^{45}Ca^{2+}$ efflux (109). Also, pretreatment of mesenteric resistance vessels with ryanodine significantly enhances their contractile response to high K^+ (110). These observations have suggested that ryanodine stimulates Ca^{2+} release and thus interferes with the sarcoplasmic reticulum Ca^{2+} buffering and allows a greater proportion of the depolarization-induced Ca^{2+} influx to reach the deep myoplasm and induce contraction.

The ryanodine-induced fluctuations in $[Ca^{2+}]_i$ have been monitored in intact rabbit inferior vena cava loaded with fura-2. As shown in Fig. 7, ryanodine causes an initial rise in $[Ca^{2+}]_i$ that is maintained at a steady level for more than 30 min. The ryanodine-induced increase in $[Ca^{2+}]_i$ is in part due to Ca^{2+} entry from the extracellular space because it is inhibited in the absence of external Ca^{2+} and completely abolished by La^{3+}. It is unlikely, however, that the ryanodine response is due to Ca^{2+} influx through activated Ca^{2+} channels because (a) it is not inhibited by the Ca^{2+} channel antagonist diltiazem at a concentration known to block Ca^{2+} entry through voltage-gated channels and to reduce Ca^{2+} entry through receptor-operated channels (15), and (b) ryanodine does not enhance the basal or the high K^+-stimulated Ca^{2+} influx. It is also unlikely that the ryanodine response is solely due to slow and prolonged Ca^{2+} release from the sarcoplasmic reticulum. The time course of the ryanodine-induced increase in $[Ca^{2+}]_i$ is faster in onset and longer in duration than the ryanodine-induced depletion of the Ca^{2+} stores. Thus Ca^{2+} entry from the extracellular space can maintain an increase in $[Ca^{2+}]_i$ initiated by Ca^{2+} release from the sarcoplasmic reticulum. These studies provide evidence for functional integration between the plasma membrane and the sarcoplasmic reticulum—the so-called superficial buffer barrier.

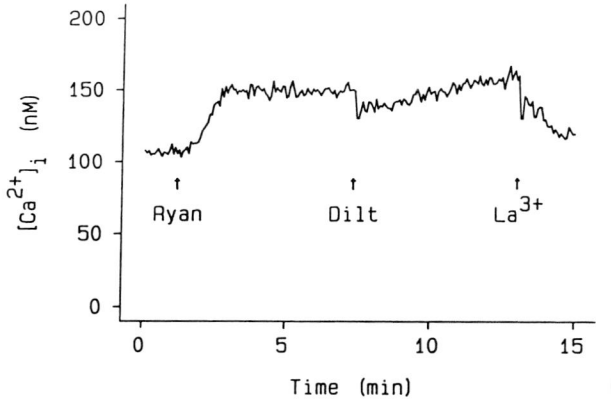

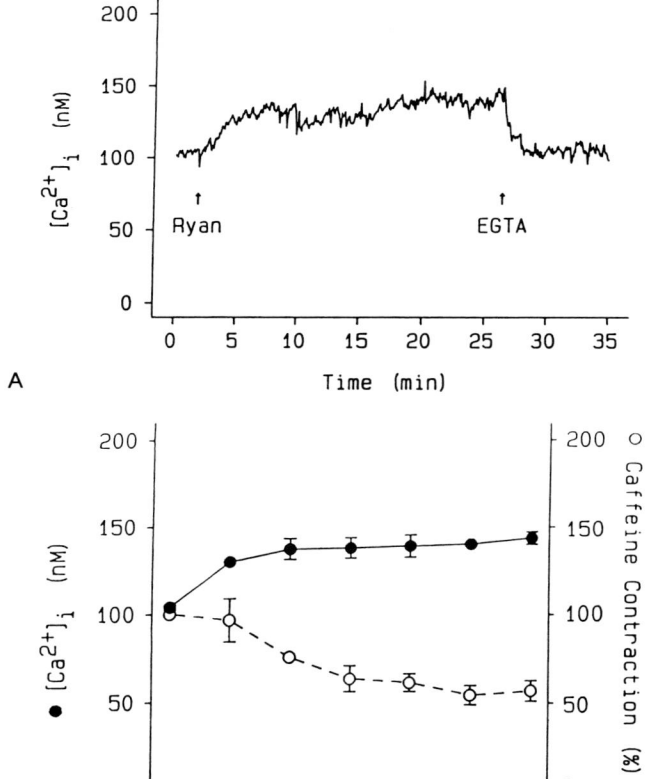

FIG. 7. Effect of ryanodine on $[Ca^{2+}]_i$ in rabbit inferior vena cava. Rabbit inferior vena cava loaded with fura-2 was equilibrated in physiological saline solution (PSS) for 45 min. Ryanodine (30 μM) was added and the changes in $[Ca^{2+}]_i$ were recorded. **A:** Effect of Ca^{2+}-free (2 mM EGTA) solution. **B:** Effect of diltiazem (10 μM) and La^{3+} (1 mM). **C:** Rabbit inferior vena cava loaded with fura-2 was equilibrated in PSS, ryanodine was added, and the changes in $[Ca^{2+}]_i$ were observed (*closed circles*). Rings of rabbit inferior vena cava were equilibrated in PSS for 45 min. After a 25-mM caffeine-control contraction, the tissue was washed in PSS for 1 h in order to replenish the Ca^{2+} stores and allow the tissue to recover from the effects of caffeine. The tissue was preincubated with ryanodine for the specified period of time and then challenged with a mixture of caffeine and ryanodine. The remaining caffeine contractile response was measured as percent of the caffeine control contraction (*open circles*).

HETEROGENEITY ALONG THE ARTERIAL TREE

Blood vessels show great difference in their response to physiological, pharmacological, and electrical stimuli. Larger vessels such as the aorta or the superior mesenteric artery are more sensitive to physiological agonists than smaller arterial branches such as the mesenteric resistance arteries. The norepinephrine concentration-force curve and the norepinephrine concentration–Ca^{2+} influx relationship are steeper in the rabbit mesenteric resistance vessels (fifth branch) than in rabbit aorta. Also, a significant portion of the norepinephrine-induced contraction of the aorta remains in the absence of extracellular Ca^{2+}. On the other hand, the mesenteric vessels are more dependent on extracellular Ca^{2+} and show very small norepinephrine response in a Ca^{2+}-free medium (111). When the superior mesenteric artery and its branches 1 through 4 are compared, the norepinephrine-induced contractile response in a Ca^{2+}-free medium decreases gradually and is significantly reduced in the fourth branch (112). Agonist-induced Ca^{2+} efflux in a Ca^{2+}-free medium can also be used as a measure

of the contribution of the intracellular Ca^{2+} stores to the agonist-induced response. The norepinephrine-stimulated Ca^{2+} efflux in the mesenteric arterial tree is the highest in the superior mesenteric artery and decreases gradually in the branches 1 through 4. These observations suggest that in larger arteries, norepinephrine causes significant Ca^{2+} release from the sarcoplasmic reticulum, which accounts for the rapid initial contraction in these vessels. A simultaneous norepinephrine-stimulated Ca^{2+} influx from the extracellular space will maintain the norepinephrine contractile response in the large arteries. On the other hand, in the smaller diameter resistance vessels, there is less contribution of Ca^{2+} release from the sarcoplasmic reticulum to the norepinephrine-induced contraction, and the vessels are more dependent on Ca^{2+} influx from the extracellular space for contraction (113). These observations may explain the difference between vessels in their sensitivity to Ca^{2+} antagonists. The inhibition of high K^+-induced contractions by diltiazem is similar in all vessels. The IC_{50} for diltiazem-induced inhibition of high K^+ contraction is 6×10^{-7} in the aorta, 3×10^{-7} in the superior mesenteric artery, and 7×10^{-7} in the small resistance vessels. The sensitivity of the high K^+-induced Ca^{2+} influx to diltiazem is also similar in these vessels. In contrast, the sensitivity of norepinephrine-induced contraction to inhibition by diltiazem increases as one moves downward along the arterial tree (112). The concentration that inhibits 50 percent (IC_{50}) for diltiazem is 3×10^{-4} in the aorta, 5×10^{-7} in the superior mesenteric artery, and 2×10^{-8} in the mesenteric resistance vessels (fifth branch). Similarly, diltiazem inhibits the maximal norepinephrine-induced Ca^{2+} influx by 11 percent in the aorta, 66 percent in the superior mesenteric artery, and 87 percent in the mesenteric resistance vessels. Thus the contribution of Ca^{2+} release or Ca^{2+} influx to the norepinephrine-induced contraction is dependent on the diameter of the vessel. The larger the vessel diameter, the greater the contribution of Ca^{2+} release. The opposite is seen in smaller vessels, i.e., the smaller the vessel the less the contribution of the intracellular stores and the greater the contribution of Ca^{2+} influx to norepinephrine-induced contraction.

Blood vessels are also different in their resting membrane potential and their electrical response to external stimuli. The average physiological membrane potential in most blood vessels, with the exception of certain cerebral arteries (114), is between -45 and -60 mV (115). The relationship between membrane potential and active tension is steep, i.e., small changes in membrane potential cause a significant increase in force (116). In the presence of high K^+, the relationship between membrane potential and active tension in the aorta and the small mesenteric resistance vessels is similar. In contrast, norepinephrine activates large arteries such as the aorta with no significant membrane depolarization (117). However, in smaller vessels, norepinephrine produces significant and maximal membrane depolarization to 14 to 20 mV (114,115). Voltage-tension relationship in mesenteric resistance vessels have shown that the norepinephrine-induced depolarization that increases tension from 20 percent to 100 percent of maximum is 14 mV, which is similar to that observed with high K^+. These observations suggest that norepinephrine activates the rabbit aorta mainly through pharmacomechanical coupling, while it activates the mesenteric resistance vessels mainly through electromechanical coupling (117). The changes in membrane potential induced by norepinephrine or high K^+ in other resistance vessels are similar to those observed in the mesenteric vessels. However, in the cerebral arteries the changes are even larger (114). The difference in the electrical properties between large and small arteries can be explained by alteration in the receptor-operated Ca^{2+} channels as one proceeds down the arterial tree. Alternatively, as has been suggested by recent electrophysiological studies, norepinephrine may modify the gating or the conductance of voltage-gated Ca^{2+} channels in resistance vessels (7,12,118,119).

ALTERATIONS IN EXPERIMENTAL HYPERTENSION

Essential hypertension is characterized by normal cardiac output and increased peripheral resistance. Several factors have been suggested as possible causes of increased peripheral vascular resistance. These factors include abnormalities in the vascular wall or the ultrastructure of smooth muscle, augmented vasoconstriction in response to increased vessel sensitivity to sympathetic stimulation and norepinephrine, and impaired Ca^{2+} metabolism in smooth muscle.

An impaired Ca^{2+} metabolism can be caused directly by an increased plasma membrane permeability to Ca^{2+}, decreased Ca^{2+}-ATPase activity in the plasma membrane and the sarcoplasmic reticulum, or decreased activity of the Na^+-Ca^{2+} exchanger. The Ca^{2+} metabolism can be impaired indirectly by increased membrane permeability to Na^+ or decreased activity of the Na^+,K^+-ATPase in the plasma membrane with net accumulation of Na^+. The accumulated Na^+ then leads to accumulation of Ca^{2+} through the Na^+-Ca^{2+} exchanger.

Animal models of hypertension have been used extensively in hypertension research. The most widely-used animal model is the spontaneously hypertensive rat (SHR), which is usually compared with the normotensive Wistar-Kyoto rat (WKY). It has been demonstrated that the sensitivity to norepinephrine in denervated or cocaine-treated mesenteric resistance vessels of the SHR is greater than that of the WKY (120). Also, the dependence of contraction on extracellular Ca^{2+} is greater in norepinephrine-activated but not in depolarized mesenteric resistance vessels of the SHR as compared to that of the WKY (111,120). Although the median effective concentration (EC_{50}) for norepinephrine is not different in the two strains, both the rate of tension development and the maximal tension induced by norepinephrine are greater in the SHR vessels than in the WKY vessels (111).

The difference between the SHR and the WKY in their sensitivity to norepinephrine can be explained either by an enhancement of the Ca^{2+} mobilization mechanisms, due to an increase in Ca^{2+} release from the sarcoplasmic reticulum or an increase in Ca^{2+} influx from the extracellular space, or by a decrease in the Ca^{2+} homeostasis mechanisms. A change in the myofilament sensitivity to Ca^{2+} can be ruled out by the observation that the high K^+-induced contraction is not significantly different in the SHR and the WKY.

Maximal concentrations of norepinephrine have been shown to stimulate Ca^{2+} efflux to the same extent in the SHR and the WKY, suggesting that the difference between the two strains is not due to a difference in Ca^{2+} release (111). Also, measurements of Ca^{2+} influx have shown no significant difference in the basal or in the high K^+-induced Ca^{2+} influx between the SHR and the WKY. In contrast, the norepinephrine-stimulated Ca^{2+} influx is significantly higher in the SHR than in the WKY. These observations suggest an increase in the membrane permeability to Ca^{2+} in the SHR vessels. This is supported by the difference between the SHR and the WKY in their sensitivity to Ca^{2+} antagonists. For instance, the norepinephrine-induced tension and Ca^{2+} influx are less sensitive to nisoldipine or PN 200/110 in the SHR than in the WKY. In contrast, the sensitivity of the high K^+-induced tension and Ca^{2+} influx to nisoldipine or PN 200/110 are similar in the SHR and the WKY. These observations suggest that there may be a difference between the SHR and the WKY in the agonist-stimulated Ca^{2+} influx pathway. Other studies have suggested that the Ca^{2+} homeostasis mechanisms may be compromised in hypertensive animal models. For example, isolated plasma membrane fractions from small arteries and veins of the SHR have shown decreased ATP-dependent Ca^{2+} accumulation as compared to the WKY (121). An increase in Ca^{2+} mobilization and/or a decrease in Ca^{2+} homeostasis is expected to increase $[Ca^{2+}]_i$. Measurement of $[Ca^{2+}]_i$ in smooth muscle cells loaded with quin-2 have shown that arginine-vasopressin produces a greater increase in $[Ca^{2+}]_i$ in the SHR as compared to the WKY (122). Also, measurements of $[Ca^{2+}]_i$ in freshly isolated aortic smooth muscle cells using fura-2 (84) or Ca^{2+}-sensitive microelectrodes (123) have shown that the resting $[Ca^{2+}]_i$ is higher in hypertensive rats as compared to the normotensive rat.

An important question is how the results in animal models of hypertension relate to the clinical cases of hypertension. The available clinical data are not always consistent with the experimental data. Verapamil has been found to be more effective in dilating the forearm vessels of hypertensive patients than in normotensive controls, suggesting that contraction of vessels of hypertensive patients is more dependent on extracellular Ca^{2+} (124,125). However, a decreased dependence on extracellular Ca^{2+} has been demonstrated in norepinephrine-activated subcutaneous vessels isolated from hypertensive patients (126). The discrepancies between the clinical findings and the experimental data obtained from isolated tissues impose caution in extrapolating the data from SHR mesenteric vessels to clinical hypertension. However, studies on various human vascular beds such as the mesenteric, skeletal, and renal resistance vessels have shown similarities to those of the WKY rat. For instance, it has been reported that the norepinephrine-induced contraction of human renal resistance vessels is dependent on extracellular Ca^{2+}. This observation is similar to what has been found in the WKY renal resistance vessels. Also, it has been found that human mesen-

teric vessels respond to atriopeptin III in the same fashion as the WKY mesenteric vessels.

CONCLUSIONS

Ca^{2+} is a major determinant of vascular smooth muscle functions. The intracellular free Ca^{2+} concentration $[Ca^{2+}]_i$ is controlled by two opposing Ca^{2+} handling mechanisms composed of Ca^{2+} channels and Ca^{2+} pumps in the plasma membrane and intracellular organelles. Ca^{2+}-mobilizing mechanisms tend to increase $[Ca^{2+}]_i$, while the Ca^{2+} homeostatic mechanisms have the opposite effect. The balance between the Ca^{2+}-mobilizing and the Ca^{2+} homeostatic mechanisms maintains resting $[Ca^{2+}]_i$ constant. In the presence of a physiological agonist or in pathological states such as hypertension, the balance between the Ca^{2+} mobilizing and the Ca^{2+} homeostatic mechanisms may be compromised with a resulting increase in $[Ca^{2+}]_i$ and vascular smooth muscle contractility.

REFERENCES

1. van Breemen C, Hwang K, Loutzenhiser R, Lukeman S, Yamamoto H. In: Fleckenstein A, van Breemen C, Gross R, Hoffmeister F, eds. *Cardiovascular effects of dihydropyridine-type calcium antagonists and agonists.* New York: Springer-Verlag, 1985;58–71.
2. Benham CD, Tsien RW. *Nature* 1987;328:275–278.
3. Khalil RA, van Breemen C. *J Pharmacol Exp Ther* 1988;244:537–541.
4. van Breemen C. *J Physiol* 1977;272:317–329.
5. Bean BP, Sturek M, Puga A, Hermsmeyer K. *Circ Res* 1986;59:229–235.
6. Loirand G, Pacaud P, Mironneau C, Mironneau J. *Pflugers Arch* 1986;407:566–568.
7. Benham CD, Hess P, Tsien RW. *Circ Res* 1987;61(suppl I):I10–I16.
8. Yatani A, Seidel CL, Allen J, Brown AM. *Circ Res* 1987;60:523–533.
9. Cauvin C, Loutzenhiser R, van Breemen C. *Annu Rev Pharmacol Toxicol* 1983;23:373–396.
10. Bolton TB. *Physiol Rev* 1979;59:606–718.
11. van Breemen C, Aaronson P, Loutzenhiser R. *Pharmacol Rev* 1979;30:167–208.
12. Nelson MT, Standen NB, Brayden JE, Worley III JF. *Nature* 1988;336:382–385.
13. Sturek M, Hermsmeyer K. *Science* 1986;233:475–478.
14. Benham CD, Tsien RW. *J Physiol* 1987;390:98P.
15. Meisheri K, Hwang O, van Breemen C. *J Membr Biol* 1981;59:19–25.
16. Reuter H. *NIPS* 1987;2:168–171.
17. Bayliss WM. *J Physiol* 1902;23:220–231.
18. Bohr DF, Webb RC. *Am J Med* 1984;77:3–17.
19. Kirber MT, Singer JJ, Walsh JV. *Pflugers Arch* 1988;412:339–345.
20. Katusic ZS, Shepherd JT, Vanhoutte PM. *Fed Proc* 1986;45:289.
21. Harder DR. *Circ Res* 1987;60:102–107.
22. Deth R, van Breemen C. *J Membr Biol* 1977;30:363–380.
23. Somlyo AP, Somlyo AV. In Fozzard HA, et al., eds. *Smooth muscle structure and function.* New York: Raven Press, 1986;845–864.

24. Endo M. *Physiol Rev* 1977;57:71–108.
25. Devine CE, Somlyo AV, Somlyo AP. *Philos Trans R Soc Lond* 1973;B265:17–23.
26. Bond M, Kitazawa T, Somlyo AP, Somlyo AV. *J Physiol* 1984;355:677–695.
27. Ehrlich BE, Watras J. *Nature* 1988;336:583–586.
28. Saida K, van Breemen C. *J Gen Physiol* 1984;84:307–318.
29. Cassidy P, Hoar PE, Kerrick WGL. *J Biol Chem* 1979;254:11148–11153.
30. Nishimura J, Kolber M, van Breemen C. *Biochem Biophys Res Commun* 1988;157:677–683.
31. Kitazawa T, Kobayashi S, Horiuti K, Somlyo AV, Somlyo AP. *J Biol Chem* 1989;264:5339–5342.
32. Berridge MJ, Irvine RF. *Nature* 1984;312:315–321.
33. Nishizuka Y. *Science* 1992;258:607–614.
34. Suematsu E, Hirata M, Hashimoto T, Kuriyama H. *Biochem Biophys Res Commun* 1984;120:481–485.
35. Somlyo AV, Bond M, Somlyo AP, Scarpa A. *Proc Natl Acad Sci USA* 1985;82:5231–5235.
36. Yamamoto H, van Breemen C. *Biochem Biophys Res Commun* 1985;130:270–274.
37. Saida K, van Breemen C. *Biochem Biophys Res Commun* 1987;144:1313–1316.
38. Iino M. *Biochem Biophys Res Commun* 1987;142:47–52.
39. Walker JW, Somlyo AV, Goldman YE, Somlyo AP, Trentham DR. *Nature* 1987;327:249–252.
40. Kobayashi S, Somlyo AP, Somlyo AV. *Biochem Biophys Res Commun* 1988;153:625–631.
41. Ford LE, Podolsky RJ. *Science* 1970;107:58–59.
42. Fabiato A, Fabiato F. *Circ Res* 1972;31:293–301.
43. van Breemen C, Saida K. *Annu Rev Physiol* 1989;51:315–329.
44. van Breemen C, Daniel EE. *J Gen Physiol* 1966;49:1299–1317.
45. Somlyo AP, Somlyo AV. *Pharmacol Rev* 1970;22:249–353.
46. Casteels R, van Breemen C. *Pflugers Arch* 1975;359:197–207.
47. Raeymaekers L, Wuytack F, Casteels R. *Biochim Biophys Acta* 1985;815:441–454.
48. Rapp JP. *J Hypertens* 1981;3(suppl I):1168–1172.
49. Popescu LM, Panoiu C, Toescu EC, Nutu O. In: Braquet P, et al., eds. *Prostaglandins and membrane ion transport.* New York: Raven Press, 1984;217–222.
50. Eggermont JA, Vrolix M, Raeymaekers L, Wuytack F, Casteels R. *Circ Res* 1988;62:266–278.
51. Heim R, Iwata T, Zvaritch E, Adamo HP, Rutishauser B, Strehler EE, Guerini D, Carafoli E. *J Biol Chem* 1992;267:24476–24484.
52. Kumar R, Haugen JD, Penniston JT. *J Bone Miner Res* 1993;8:505–513.
53. De Jaegere S, Wuytack F, Eggermont JA, Verboomen H, Casteels R. *Biochem J* 1990;271:655–660.
54. Grover AK, Kwan CY, Rangachari PK, Daniel EE. *Am J Physiol* 1983;244:C158–C165.
55. Pritchard K, Ashley CC. *Pflugers Arch* 1987;410:401–407.
56. Carafoli E, Crompton M. *Ann NY Acad Sci* 1978;307:269–284.
57. Barzilai A, Spanier R, Rahaminoff H. *Proc Natl Acad Sci USA* 1984;81:6521–5625.
58. Matlib MA, Reeves JP. *Biochim Biophys Acta* 1987;904:145–148.
59. Reeves JP, Sutko JL. *Science* 1980;208:1461–1464.
60. Reeves JP, Hale CC. *J Biol Chem* 1984;259:7733–7739.
61. Mulvany MJ, Aalkjaer C, Peterson TT. *Circ Res* 1984;54:740–749.
62. Ashida T, Blaustein MP. *J Physiol* 1987;392:617–635.
63. Blaustein MP, Hamlyn JM. *Am J Med* 1984;77:45–59.
64. Inesi G. *Annu Rev Physiol* 1985;47:573–601.
65. Borlé AB. *Rev Physiol Biochem Pharmacol* 1981;90:13–153.
66. Maclennan DH, Wong PTS. *Proc Natl Acad Sci USA* 1971;68:1231–1235.
67. Wuytack F, Raeymaekers L, Verbist J, Jones LR, Casteels R. *Biochim Biophys Acta* 1987;899:151–158.
68. Waisman DM, Gimble J, Goodman DBP, Rasmussen H. *J Biol Chem* 1981;256:409–414.
69. Puskin JS, Gunter TE, Gunter KK, Russell PR. *Biochemistry* 1976;15:3834–3842.
70. Nicholls DG. In: *Bioenergetics. The interaction of bioenergetic organelles with their environment.* London: Academic Press, 1982;167–179.
71. Rasmussen H, Barrett PG. *Physiol Rev* 1984;64:938–984.
72. Carafoli E. *Annu Rev Biochem* 1987;56:395–433.
73. Mitchell P. *Nature* 1961;191:144–148.
74. Yamamoto H, van Breemen C. *J Gen Physiol* 1986;87:369–389.
75. Scarpa A, Brinley FJ, Tiffert T, Dubyak G. *Ann NY Acad Sci* 1978;307:86–112.
76. Ashley CC. *Ann NY Acad Sci* 1978;307:308–329.
77. Blinks JR, Wier WG, Hess P, Prendergast FG. *Prog Biophys Mol Biol* 1982;40:1–114.
78. Brown HM, Pemberton JP, Owen JD. *Anal Chim Acta* 1976;85:261–276.
79. Morgan JP, Morgan KG. *J Physiol* 1984;351:155–167.
80. Tsien RY. *Annu Rev Biophys Bioeng* 1983;12:91–116.
81. Grynkiewicz G, Poenie M, Tsien RY. *J Biol Chem* 1985;260:3440–3450.
82. Kobayashi S, Kanaide H, Nakamura M. *Science* 1985;229:553–556.
83. Himpens B, Casteels R. *Pflugers Arch* 1987;408:32–37.
84. Sugiyama T, Yoshizumi M, Takaku F, Urabe H, Tsukakoshi M, Kasuya T, Yazaki Y. *Biochem Biophys Res Commun* 1986;141:340–345.
85. Dabrowska R, Aromatorio D, Sherry JMF, Hartshorne DJ. *Biochem Biophys Res Commun* 1977;78:1263–1272.
86. Adelstein RS, Eisenberg E. *Annu Rev Biochem* 1980;49:921–956.
87. Kerrick WGL, Hoar PE, Cassidy PS, Bolles L. *J Gen Physiol* 1981;77:177–190.
88. Lukeman S, van Breemen C. In: Lichtlen PR, eds. *Recent aspects in calcium antagonism.* Stuttgart: Schattauer, 1985;49–65.
89. DeFeo TT, Morgan KG. *J Physiol* 1985;369:269–282.
90. Khalil RA, van Breemen C. *Pflugers Arch* 1990;416:727–734.
91. Schramm M, Thomas G, Towart R, Franchowiak G. *Nature* 1983;303:535–537.
92. Khalil RA, Morgan KG. *NIPS* 1992;7:10–15.
93. Castagna M, Takai Y, Kaibuchi K, Sano K, Kikkawa U, Nishizuka Y. *J Biol Chem* 1982;257:7847–7851.
94. Danthaluri NR, Deth RC. *Biochem Biophys Res Commun* 1984;125:1103–1109.
95. Rasmussen H, Forder J, Kojima I, Scriabine A. *Biochem Biophys Res Commun* 1984;122:776–784.
96. Jiang MJ, Morgan KG. *Am J Physiol* 1987;253:H1365–H1371.
97. Nishimura J, Khalil RA, Drenth JP, van Breemen C. *Am J Physiol* 1990;259:H2–H8.
98. Loutzenhiser R, van Breemen C. *Circ Res* 1983;52:I97–I103.
99. Gabella G. *J Cell Sci* 1971;8:601–609.
100. Cadwell JJS, Caswell AH. *J Cell Biol* 1982;93:543–550.
101. Benham CD, Bolton TB. *J Physiol* 1986;381:385–406.
102. Nelemans A, den Hertog A. *Eur J Pharmacol* 1987;140:39–46.
103. Rembold CM. *J Physiol* 1989;416:273–290.
104. Besch HR, Jr. *Fed Proc* 1985;44:2950–2963.
105. Sutko JL, Ito K, Kenyon JL. *Fed Proc* 1985;44:2984–2988.
106. Rousseau E, Smith JS, Meissner G. *Am J Physiol* 1987;253:C364–368.
107. Lai FA, Erickson HP, Rousseau E, Liu Q, Meissner G. *Nature* 1988;331:315–319.
108. Ashida T, Schaeffer J, Goldman WF, Wade JB, Blaustein MP. *Circ Res* 1988;62:854–863.
109. Hwang KS, van Breemen C. *Pflugers Arch* 1987;408:343–350.
110. Julou-Schaeffer G, Freslon JL. *Br J Pharmacol* 1988;95:605–613.
111. Cauvin C, van Breemen C. *J Cardiovasc Pharmacol* 1985;7(suppl 4):S4–S10.
112. Cauvin C, Saida K, van Breemen C. *Blood Vessels* 1984;21:23–31.
113. Yang S, Bevan RD. *Fed Proc* 1981;40:659.
114. Harder DR. In: Crass MF, Barnes CD, eds. *Vascular smooth muscle: metabolic, ionic and contractile mechanisms.* New York: Academic Press, 1982;71–97.
115. Hermsmeyer K. *Fed Proc* 1983;43:269–270.
116. Hermsmeyer K, Trapani A, Abel P. In: Vanhoutte P, Leusen I, eds. *Vasodilation.* New York: Raven Press, 1981;273–284.
117. Cauvin C, Lukeman S, Cameron J, Hwang O, van Breemen C. *Circ Res* 1985;56:822–828.

118. Droogmans G, Declerck I, Casteels R. *Pflugers Arch* 1987;409:9–12.
119. Pacaud P, Loirand G, Mironneau C, Mironneau J. *Pflugers Arch* 1987;410:557–559.
120. Mulvany MJ, Nyborg N. *Br J Pharmacol* 1980;71:585–596.
121. Kwan CY, Daniel EE. *Eur J Pharmacol* 1981;75:321–324.
122. Nabika T, Velletri PA, Beaven MA, Endo J, Lovenberg W. *Life Sci* 1985;37:579–584.
123. Losse H, Zidek W, Vetter H. *J Cardiovasc Pharmacol* 1984;6:S32–S37.
124. Buhler FR, Bolli P, Erne P, Kiowski W, Muller B, Hulthen UL, Ji BH. *J Cardiovasc Pharmacol* 1985;7(suppl 4):S21–S27.
125. Robinson BF. *Am J Cardiol* 1985;55:24B–29B.
126. Aalkjaer C, Haegerty AM, Petersen KK, Swales JD, Mulvany MJ. *Circ Res* 1987;61:181–186.

Hypertension: Pathophysiology, Diagnosis, and Management, Second Edition, edited by J.H. Laragh and B.M. Brenner, Raven Press, Ltd., New York © 1995.

CHAPTER 34

Angiotensin, Other Pressors, and the Transduction of Vascular Smooth Muscle Contraction

Kathy K. Griendling and R. Wayne Alexander

Vascular smooth muscle contracts in response to neurotransmitters and a variety of circulating hormones. These vasoactive agonists bind to specific cell surface receptors and generate a multitude of intracellular biochemical signals, which ultimately result in vasoconstriction. Vascular smooth muscle contraction generally involves both an initial and a sustained phase, and these two phases utilize different biochemical pathways.

K. K. Griendling and R. W. Alexander: Division of Cardiology, Emory University, Atlanta, Georgia 30322.

PRESSOR AGENTS AND THEIR RECEPTORS

Among the most potent vasoconstrictors are the catecholamines norepinephrine (NE) and epinephrine and the peptides angiotensin II (Ang II), vasopressin, and endothelin (ET). Other circulating agents, such as prostaglandins, adenosine triphosphate (ATP), thrombin, and serotonin, also cause vascular smooth muscle contraction, but may play a smaller role under normal conditions *in vivo*.

Over the past several years, most of the cellular receptors for the major contractile agents have been cloned.

All belong to the G protein–coupled superfamily of receptors (1–4). These receptors have seven transmembrane domains, three intracellular and three extracellular loops, and a carboxyterminal tail of varying length that projects into the cytoplasm (Fig. 1). Extent of glycosylation, agonist binding sites, and G protein–coupling differs among the different classes of receptors. Salient features of each group are discussed in more detail in the following sections, and are summarized in Table 1.

α-Adrenergic Receptors

α-Adrenergic agonists, such as NE and epinephrine, bind to two major subtypes of receptors in the vessel wall, namely, α_1 and α_2 (17–20). Although all α-subtypes mediate contraction, the intracellular signals that they generate appear to differ markedly (21,22) (see below). These receptors also differ in their affinity for agonists and antagonists. The α_1-receptors have an agonist potency series of epinephrine > NE > phenylephrine > clonidine (23), whereas the α_2-receptors exhibit a po-

tency series of epinephrine > clonidine > NE > phenylephrine (24). The α_1-receptors are preferentially blocked by prazosin, and the α_2-receptors are blocked by yohimbine (25). These two major subtypes couple to different intracellular effectors: α_1-receptors couple positively to phospholipase C (PLC), while α_2-receptors couple negatively to adenylate cyclase.

Pharmacological data support the existence of at least two subtypes of α_1-receptors, based on a differential sensitivity to chlorethylclonidine and a differential affinity for WB4101, an adrenergic antagonist (21,26). Cloning techniques have identified three α_1-subtypes and four α_2-subtypes that share limited sequence homology (1,6,9). Specific features of these clones are given in Table 1.

Angiotensin (AT) Receptors

The recent development of non–peptidic pharmacological antagonists has provided definitive evidence for two major subtypes of angiotensin receptors, now denoted AT_1 and AT_2. AT_1 receptors are selectively

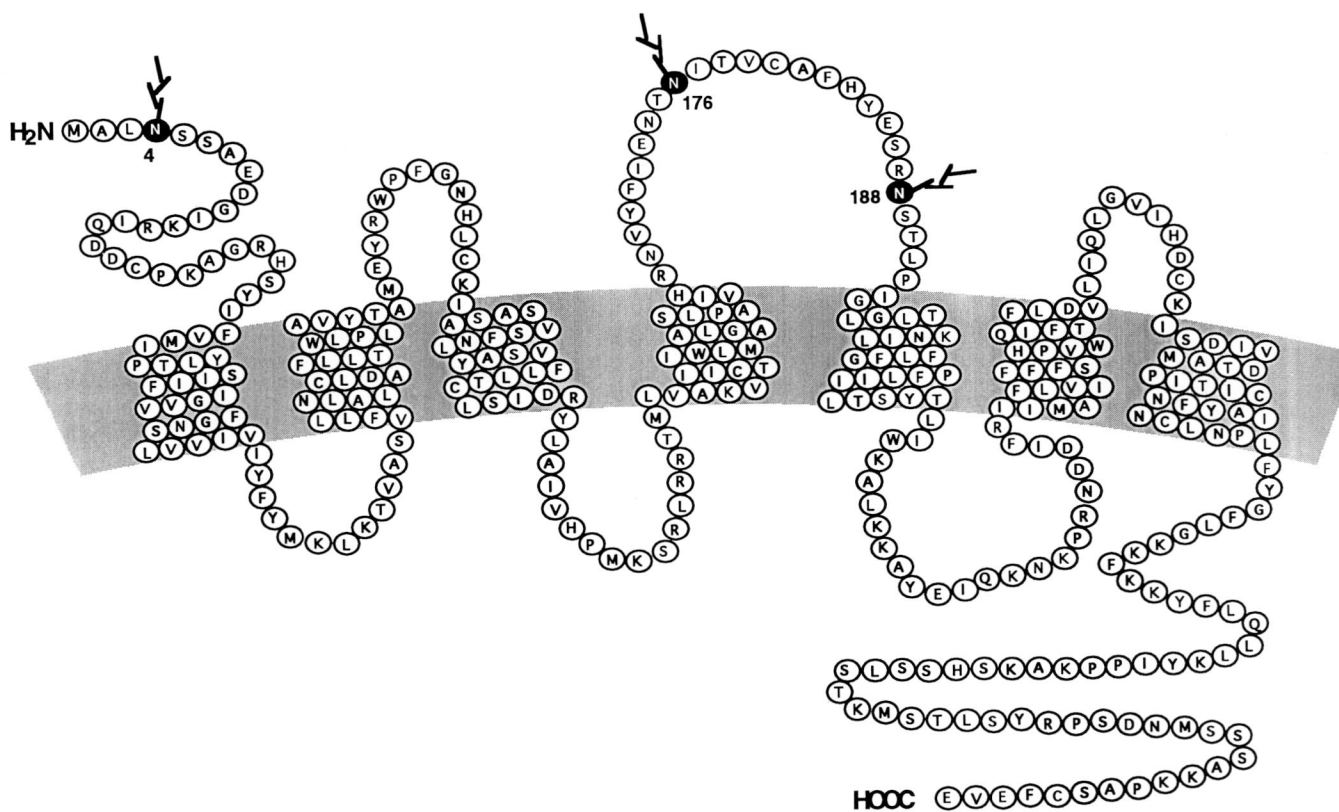

FIG. 1. Structure of G-protein coupled receptors. The sequence shown here is for the AT_1 receptor, but is characteristic of the G-protein superfamily of receptors. These receptors have seven membrane-spanning domains, three extracellular loops, and three intracellular loops. The length of these loops as well as the N-terminus and C-terminus varies among receptors (see Table 1). Often there are glycosylation sites on the extracellular loops and consensus sequences for phosphorylation by protein kinases on the intracellular, cytoplasmic portion of the protein. (From ref. 5, with permission.)

TABLE 1. *Molecular features of vasoconstrictor, G protein–coupled receptors*

Receptor	Cloned	Amino acids (#)	Special features	Glycosylated (# sites)	Potential phosphorylation sites	Effector	Reference
α 1a	Y	560	Long COOH terminus	2	2nd/3rd IC loops, COOH terminus	↑ PLC	6
1b	Y	515	Long COOH terminus	4	2nd/3rd IC loops	↑ PLC	1
2c₁₀	Y	450	Long 3rd IC loop, short COOH terminus	2	2nd/3rd IC loops		7
2c₄	Y	450		2	2nd/3rd IC loops, COOH terminus	↓ Adenylate cyclase	8
2c₂	Y	450	Short NH₂ terminus	0			9
AT 1a	Y	359	Short NH₂ terminus, short 3rd IC loop	3	COOH terminus	↑ PLC	10
1b	Y	359		3	COOH terminus	↑ PLC	11
2	N	N.D.	N.D.	N.D.	N.D.	N.D.	
ET A	Y	427	N terminal signal sequence, long NH₂ terminus	2	COOH terminus	↑ PLC	12,13
B	Y	441		2	3rd IC loop, COOH terminus	↑ PLC	14
C	N	N.D.	N.D.	N.D.	N.D.	N.D.	
V 1a	Y	394		2	3rd IC loop, COOH terminus	↑ PLC	15
1b	N	N.D.	N.D.	N.D.	N.D.	N.D.	
2	Y	370		1	COOH terminus	↑ Adenylate cyclase	16

IC, intracellular; N.D., not determined.

blocked by biphenylimidazoles such as Losartan (Dup753), while AT₂ binding sites are blocked by tetrahydroimidazopyridines typified by PD123177 (27). AT₁ receptors (previously AII-1, AII-B, AIIα) are more responsive to Ang II than Ang III, are positively coupled to PLC, and may be negatively coupled to adenylate cyclase (27). AT₂ binding sites (previously AII-2, AII-A, AIIβ) bind Ang II and Ang III equally well, and may be involved in modulation of the intracellular content of cyclic guanosine monophosphate (cGMP) (28). Most known specific responses to Ang II have been shown to be mediated by AT₁ receptors, including vascular contraction, pressor and tachycardiac responses, aldosterone secretion, Ang II–induced water drinking, and hypertension in renal artery stenosis (29). However, the abundance of AT₂ binding sites in fetal and neonatal rat tissues raises the possibility that they may have a role in development (30).

The cloning of the vascular and adrenal AT₁ receptor confirmed its identity as a member of the G protein–coupled superfamily of receptors. Two subtypes of the AT₁ receptor, termed AT₁ₐ and AT₁ᵦ, have now been cloned, and show a greater than 90 percent sequence homology. The functional significance of these receptor subtypes is unknown, but they do have distinct tissue distributions (31).

ET Receptors

In the past several years, molecular biological techniques have been particularly fruitful in the ET field. Three types of ET have been cloned that are highly homologous but have different biological activities (32). In terms of vasoconstrictor activity, ET-1 and ET-2 are equipotent, while ET-3 is less potent. In addition, two subtypes of ET receptors have been cloned and a third has been identified pharmacologically. The ET₁ₐ receptor is the vascular smooth muscle receptor that binds ET-1 and ET-2 with greater affinity than ET-3 (4). The ET₁ᵦ receptor is found on vascular endothelium, and has approximately equal affinities for ET-1, ET-2, and ET-3. The ET₁c receptor has a high affinity for ET-3 and relatively low affinities for ET-1 and ET-2, and is found in anterior pituitary cells. ET receptors are coupled positively to PLC and to L-type calcium channels (33).

Vasopressin Receptors

Vasopressin also interacts with three subtypes of receptors, termed V1a, V1b, and V2 (34). These receptors have been distinguished by the physiological response to which they are coupled (34), by selective pharmacological agents (35), and more recently by cloning techniques (2). Selective ligands include the V1 receptor antagonist (1-[β-mercapto-β,β-cyclopentamethylenepropionic acid],2-(O-methyl)tyrosine,8-arginine]vasopressin) and the V2 receptor agonist dDAVP ([1-desamino,8-D-arginine]vasopressin). V1a receptors, the subtype present on vascular smooth muscle (36), mediate vasoconstriction. This receptor has been cloned, and has been shown to be a seven membrane–spanning domain receptor that couples to PLC. The V2 receptor has also been cloned (16). It is mainly located in the kidney, and appears to be positively coupled to adenylate cyclase (37).

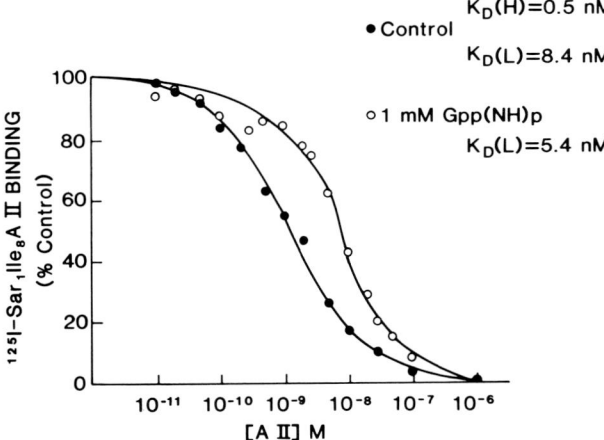

FIG. 2. Effect of guanine nucleotides on the displacement of ^{125}I-Sar^1-Ile^8 angiotensin II binding by unlabeled angiotensin II (AII). K_D(H) is the calculated K_D for the high-affinity state of the receptor; K_D(L) is the calculated K_D for the low-affinity state of the receptor. Gpp(NH)p, a nonhydrolyzable analogue of GTP, converts the high-affinity state into the low-affinity state of the receptor. (Courtesy of Dr. Tommy Brock.)

REGULATION AND MEASUREMENT OF HORMONE-RECEPTOR INTERACTIONS

The first step in transduction of an external stimulus to contraction is binding of the hormone to the receptor. Binding of agonists to receptors has been characterized using radioligand binding techniques. Specificity of binding of a radiolabeled ligand to a given receptor is determined by four criteria: the binding must be saturable, reversible, proportionate to protein concentration, and displaceable by ligands in an order of potency that parallels that of the physiological response (38).

Potency series characteristic for a given receptor subtype can be obtained from displacement experiments. The receptor is radiolabeled with ligand, and the tissue is then incubated with a variety of unlabeled ligands that compete for the receptor sites and displace radiolabeled material. When receptors are radiolabeled with antagonists, displacement curves by agonists are often shallow. This indicates the presence of more than one subtype or "affinity state" of the receptor. An example of angiotensin II displacement of ^{125}I-Sar^1-Ile^8-Ang II (a potent Ang II antagonist) is shown in Fig. 2. The shallowness of the curve suggests that there are heterogeneous binding states for agonist, but not for antagonist, binding. These affinity states have been shown to be interconvertible by guanine nucleotides (35,39–47). Thus, in the presence of nonhydrolyzable analogues of guanosine triphosphate (GTP), Ang II receptors are converted from a high-affinity state to a low-affinity state (Fig. 2). The exact mechanism of this effect is unknown, but this shift in agonist affinity states is thought to represent involvement of a guanine nucleotide regulatory protein (G protein) in receptor activation. Similar results have been obtained for α_1, α_2, ET, and V1 receptors in a variety of tissues (Table 2).

Also shown in Table 2 is the effect of cations on the affinity of the receptor for an agonist. These effects tend to be more variable than those of the guanine nucleotides. Na$^+$, for example, increases the affinity of the Ang II receptor for Ang II in rat mesenteric vascular smooth muscle (39), but decreases the affinity of adrenergic agonists for α_1- and α_2-receptors in rat myocardium (45), rat renal cortex (42), and bovine brain (43). The mechanism of Na$^+$ regulation of agonist binding is unknown, but these observations imply the existence of a monovalent cation-sensitive site that is involved in receptor activation. Additionally, divalent cations uniformly increase the affinity of Ang II, ET, and adrenergic agonists for their respective receptors (39,43,48). Although these observations are incompletely understood, the effect of magnesium, at least, appears to occur at the level of a guanine nucleotide–binding protein (49). Thus, binding

TABLE 2. *Effect of cations and guanine nucleotides on binding affinity of receptors*

Receptor	GTP analogues	Na$^+$	Divalent cations	Tissue (ref.)
Ang II	−	+	++	Rat mesentery (39)
α_1	−	−		Rat renal cortex (42)
	−			Rat liver (40,44)
	−			Rat mesentery (45)
	−	−		Rat myocardium (45)
α_2	−	−		Rat renal cortex (42)
	−	−	+	Bovine brain (43)
	−			Human platelets (41)
	−	−		Rabbit platelets (47)
	−			Rabbit uterus (41)
V$_1$	−			Cultured VSMC (35,36)
	−			Rat liver (35,46)
ET		+		Rat myocardium (48)

(−) indicates decrease in affinity.
(+) indicates increase in affinity.
VSMC, vascular smooth muscle cells.

of a hormone to its receptor appears to be regulated by guanine nucleotides, sodium, and divalent cations. Consequently, these compounds can all affect the initial biochemical signal generated by hormone-receptor interaction, but their effects can be modified by the myriad of subsequent intracellular signaling events.

GENERATION OF SECOND MESSENGERS

Binding of a hormone to a receptor initiates a characteristic series of biochemical events. Ang II, ET, vasopressin, and α-adrenergic agonists all belong to the class of hormones that mobilize intracellular Ca^{2+} as an integral step in causing contraction. Understanding of the biochemical signals generated by these Ca^{2+}-mobilizing hormones has expanded considerably in recent years, primarily because of the identification and characterization of two important second messengers, inositol trisphosphate (IP_3) and diacylglycerol (DG). These two intracellular signals result from agonist-stimulated metabolism of membrane phospholipids that are present in all mammalian cells (for reviews, see refs. 50–55).

The plasma membrane contains many types of phospholipids, but to date only two classes have been identified conclusively as participating in signal transduction: the phosphoinositides and phosphatidylcholine (PC). There are a few reports that phosphatidylethanol is also hydrolyzed in an agonist-dependent manner, but this pathway is only now beginning to be investigated (56). Three major types of phospholipases (A_2, C, and D) act

upon membrane phospholipids, yielding specific second messengers (Fig. 3). Each signaling molecule then initiates a cascade of events, ultimately leading to contraction or growth.

Phospholipase C and Inositol Phospholipid Hydrolysis

There are three major phosphoinositides in the plasma membrane of eukaryotic cells: phosphatidylinositol (PI), phosphatidylinositol 4-phosphate (PIP), and phosphatidylinositol 4,5-bisphosphate (PIP_2), present in a ratio of about 7:1:0.4 (54). These compounds exist in a dynamic equilibrium through the actions of phosphatases and kinases. Stimulation of the cell by Ca^{2+}-mobilizing vasopressors dramatically alters this equilibrium by activating PLC, an enzyme that cleaves the phosphodiester bond between the inositol head group and the glycerol backbone of the lipid substrate, resulting in formation of the inositol phosphates and DG (Fig. 3). Each of these compounds undergoes further metabolism, ultimately resulting in resynthesis of the inositol phospholipids.

The major effect of agonists on this pathway is the stimulation of PIP_2 hydrolysis to form IP_3 and DG. These two molecules have definitive roles as intracellular messengers (see below). Their metabolic products, IP_4 and arachidonic acid, have also been proposed to have physiological functions. IP_4 has been implicated in Ca^{2+} influx (58), and arachidonic acid acts as a precursor for eicosanoids, which also cause secondary cellular activation (54). However, as discussed below, hydrolysis of the

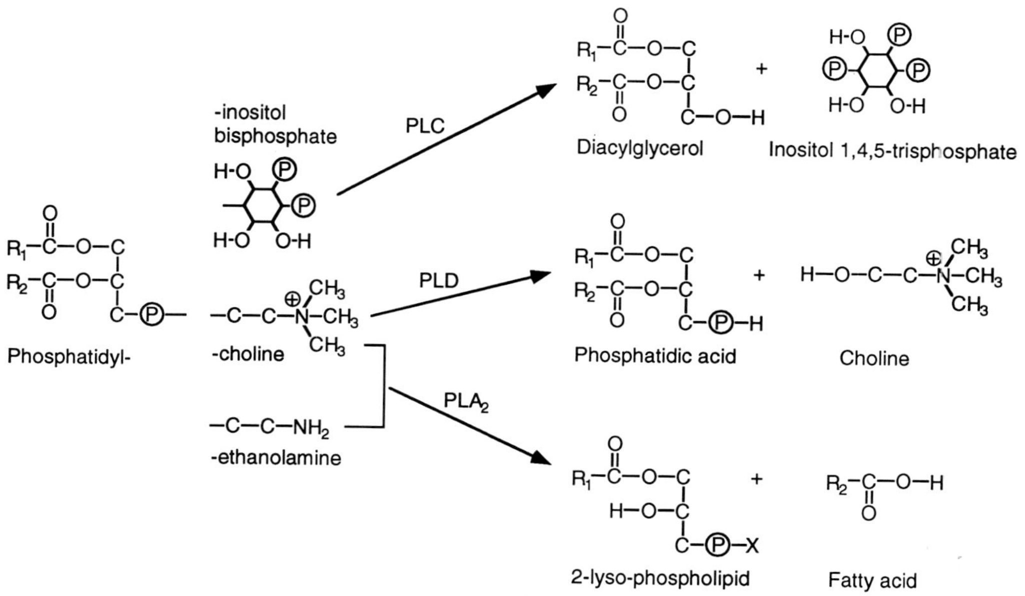

FIG. 3. Phospholipases coupled to vasoconstrictor receptors in vascular smooth muscle. AT_1 receptors are coupled positively to phospholipases A_2, C, and D. As described in the text, phospholipases hydrolyze membrane phospholipids at different positions on the glycerol backbone, releasing diacylglycerol [phospholipase C (PLC)], phosphatidic acid [phospholipase D (PLD)], or 2-lysophospholipid [phospholipase A_2 (PLA$_2$)] and the corresponding head group or fatty acid. (Modified from ref. 57.)

inositol phospholipids by PLC is not the major source of DG in vascular smooth muscle, so that by far the most important signals resulting from PLC activation are IP_3 and increased intracellular Ca^{2+} concentration.

Consequences of PLC Activation: Inositol Trisphosphate Production and Ca^{2+} Mobilization

As noted above, one of the earliest measurable events resulting from Ang II activation of vascular smooth muscle is PLC-mediated hydrolysis of the triphosphorylated form of phosphatidylinositol, PIP_2, to yield IP_3 (59,60) and DG (61). IP_3 formation is transient, peaking at 15 sec and returning to near baseline by 2 min (Fig. 4). In permeabilized porcine coronary artery (63) and cultured vascular smooth muscle cells (64), IP_3 has been shown to cause release of Ca^{2+} from nonmitochondrial intracellular sites, presumably endoplasmic reticulum. In intact cells, the Ang II–induced IP_3 transient slightly precedes a rapid, transient increase in intracellular free Ca^{2+} (Fig. 4), which is, in part, independent of Ca^{2+} influx (65,66). Similar observations have been made in cells exposed to vasopressin and ET (66–68). The effect of α-adrenergic agonists on IP_3 formation and Ca^{2+} mobilization appears to be more complicated than the scenario described above. Although several groups have reported increased turnover of the phosphoinositides following incubation of vascular smooth muscle with NE (69–71), IP_3 forma-

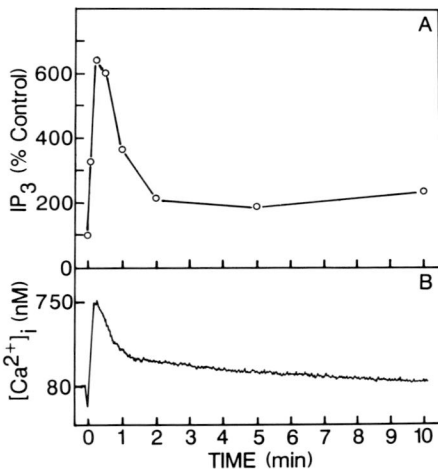

FIG. 4. Time course of IP_3 and Ca^{2+} generation in angiotensin II–stimulated vascular smooth muscle. One of the earliest events stimulated by angiotensin II in vascular smooth muscle is PLC-mediated PIP_2 hydrolysis. This results in a transient generation of IP_3 **(A)**. To measure IP_3, cells were prelabeled with [³H]myoinositol and were exposed to Ang II (100 nM) for the indicated times. IP_3 releases Ca^{2+} from intracellular stores, leading to a sharp increase in cytosolic free Ca^{2+} concentration **(B)**, as measured by the fluorescent dye fura-2. Ca^{2+} levels decline toward baseline, but remain slightly elevated for the duration of the stimulus, due to the stimulated influx of extracellular Ca^{2+}. (From ref. 62, with permission.)

tion has been difficult to measure. One explanation of this difficulty may lie in the observation that the two subtypes of α_1-receptors in rat vas deferens appear to be coupled to different signaling pathways (21). Analysis of the NE-stimulated IP_3 formation in vas deferens showed that only the low-affinity (α_{1b}) subtype of receptor is coupled to IP_3 formation, whereas the higher affinity α_{1a} subtype is coupled directly to Ca^{2+} influx (see below). Regardless of the mechanism and source, the transient nature of the Ca^{2+} signal induced by α-adrenergic agonists in vascular smooth muscle is similar to that induced by Ang II, vasopressin, and endothelin (72).

PLC Isozymes and Regulation of Activity

PLC exists as several isoforms, many of which have been cloned and sequenced (for review, see ref. 73). The PLC-β family of enzymes has been shown to be activated by G proteins, while the PLC-γ family is activated by tyrosine phosphorylation (74). In general, agonists that cause a rapid increase in intracellular Ca^{2+}, including Ang II and ET, couple to PLC via a G protein. Agonists that increase intracellular Ca^{2+} following a perceptible lag, such as growth factors, activate PLC-γ by phosphorylating specific tyrosine residues. With the exception of α_1-adrenergic receptors (see below), none of the receptors for the agonists discussed in this chapter have been proven to couple selectively to one or the other type of PLC, but, based on data from other systems, all are likely to couple to PLC through G proteins.

G proteins are a family of heterotrimeric proteins consisting of α, β, and γ subunits (75). The α-subunits (25–52 kDa) have variable functions, and are the subunits to which guanine nucleotides bind. The $\beta\gamma$ complex serves as a regulatory subunit. G proteins cycle between an inactive guanosine diphosphate (GDP)-binding state and an active GTP-binding state. When GDP is bound, the molecule exists as an $\alpha\beta\gamma$ heterotrimer. When GTP is bound, the α-subunit dissociates from the $\beta\gamma$ chains. Under resting conditions, the conversion from the GDP form to the GTP form is slow. However, upon stimulation of the cell by a hormone whose receptor is coupled to the G protein, the rate of exchange of GTP for GDP is markedly enhanced. The G protein is then said to be "activated," and the GTP-α subunit alters the activity of its target enzyme, such as adenylate cyclase or PLC. Activation is terminated by the guanosine triphosphatase (GTPase) activity of the α chain, and the heterotrimer re-forms. Under continual hormonal stimulation, this cycle continues at an accelerated rate, with some desensitization over time. Nonhydrolyzable analogues of GTP, such as GTPγS or Gpp(NH)p, can irreversibly activate G proteins by binding to the α-subunit since they are resistant to GTPase activity.

Evidence for a role for G proteins in vasoconstrictor-induced PLC activation in vascular smooth muscle has been presented by several laboratories. Numerous studies in permeabilized cells (76) and isolated membranes (77,78) have demonstrated that Gpp(NH)p or GTPγS stimulate PLC-mediated PIP_2 breakdown and IP_3 formation. In some cases, this response is sensitive to pertussis toxin, suggesting that a member of the G_i subfamily of G proteins is the coupling protein. Pertussis toxin has been reported to inhibit or have no effect on ET-, NE- and Ang II–induced PLC activation (68,79–82). In pertussis toxin–insensitive cells, PLC activation still apparently occurs through a G protein, since GTPγS acts synergistically with the agonist (81).

The identity of the pertussis toxin–insensitive G protein coupled to PLC has been investigated using reconstitution and immunochemical experiments. These data showed that members of the G_q class of G protein α-subunits activate PLC-β (74). In particular, the α-subunits of G_q, G_{11}, G_{14}, and G_{16} all activate PLC-β1, while $G\alpha_{16}$ is most effective in activating PLC-β2 (83). Gα subunits also appear to be able to discriminate between subtypes of receptors. The three $α_1$-adrenergic receptors couple to PLC-β1 equally well with $G\alpha_q$ and $G\alpha_{11}$, but $G\alpha_{14}$ and $G\alpha_{16}$ showed differences in specificity for the receptor subtypes (84).

In addition to activation by G proteins, experiments on intact cells have identified other regulators of PLC activity, the most important and ubiquitous of which is protein kinase C (PKC, see below for detailed discussion). In many cell types, including vascular smooth muscle, phorbol esters and synthetic DG (which are potent activators of PKC) have been shown to inhibit polyphosphoinositide hydrolysis (85–90), suggesting a possible role for PKC in attenuating the early phosphoinositide response. In Ang II–stimulated cultured vascular smooth muscle cells, phorbol 12,13-myristic acid (PMA) inhibits IP_3 formation and PIP_2 hydrolysis, as well as Ca^{2+} mobilization (61,85). Similar results have been found with ET (82) and vasopressin (91). Thus, activation of PKC appears to act as a negative feedback mechanism to terminate PLC activation.

In vitro experiments have also implicated Ca^{2+} and pH as potential regulators of PLC. In purified enzyme systems, hydrolysis of PI has been shown to require millimolar concentrations of Ca^{2+}, whereas hydrolysis of PIP_2 occurs at micromolar Ca^{2+} concentrations (92–94). These observations have led to the suggestion that the increase in cytoplasmic Ca^{2+} resulting from hormonal stimulation might serve to shift the dominant substrate for PLC activity from the polyphosphoinositides to PI (93). Although Ca^{2+} may play a modulatory role, it does not appear to be required for PLC activation in intact cells (61). The intracellular hydrogen ion concentration has also been postulated to be important to the function of enzymes involved in the phosphoinositide pathway. The pH optimum for PLC *in vitro* ranges from 5.5

(92,95) to 7.0 (95,96), and depends on the Ca^{2+} concentration of the buffer (97). Extrapolation of these results to intact cells is difficult, since cytosolic pH rarely falls below 6.8 following hormonal stimulation (98,99).

Calcium Influx

There appears to be a component of the Ca^{2+} response to vasoactive agonists that is independent of IP_3 and is dependent on extracellular Ca^{2+}. Several studies have demonstrated hormone-stimulated Ca^{2+} influx, both directly (100–102) and indirectly (65,103). Removal of extracellular Ca^{2+} from cultured vascular smooth muscle cells reduces the magnitude of the increase in cytoplasmic free-Ca^{2+} concentration in response to Ang II and abolishes the small, but measurable, plateau phase (65,67). Vasopressin-mediated increases in cytoplasmic free Ca^{2+} concentration seem to be even more dependent on extracellular Ca^{2+} than those mediated by Ang II, since addition of EGTA nearly abolishes the subsequent vasopressin-stimulated cytoplasmic Ca^{2+} peak (67). The increase in cytoplasmic free Ca^{2+} following activation of $α_{1a}$-receptors in smooth muscle (21) and $α_2$-receptors in blood vessels (104) is totally dependent on extracellular Ca^{2+}. ET appears to increase both the release of Ca^{2+} from intracellular stores (68) and the influx of Ca^{2+} through voltage-dependent calcium channels (105) (see below).

Influx of extracellular Ca^{2+} can be mediated by either voltage-dependent, dihydropyridine-sensitive channels or ligand-operated channels. Vascular smooth muscle appears to contain both types of channels (106), but their relative contribution to hormone-stimulated Ca^{2+} influx remains uncertain. Both Ang II and NE depolarize vascular smooth muscle (107–109), but it is not known whether this change in membrane potential activates voltage-dependent Ca^{2+} influx. Studies with the Ca^{2+} channel blocker D600 suggest that NE-mediated Ca^{2+} influx can be dissociated from that induced by depolarizing concentrations of potassium (110). Vasopressin actually inhibits voltage-dependent Ca^{2+} channel activity in A7r5 cells (111), as does DG, one of the products of PLC-mediated hydrolysis of the phosphoinositides (111). These observations suggest that the Ca^{2+} influx that accompanies receptor activation of vascular smooth muscle occurs mainly via ligand-operated channels. One exception to this conclusion may be ET, although the type of channel activated by this agonist remains controversial (105,112).

Phospholipase D and Phosphatidylcholine Hydrolysis

Although the increase in IP_3 formation in response to agonist stimulation is transient, in most cases the accumulation of DG is not (61,113–115). For example, in

Ang II–stimulated vascular smooth muscle cells, DG formation is sustained for as long as 20 min (61) (Fig. 5). This suggests that not only do IP₃ and DG have different physiological functions, but they also derive from different sources. Over the past several years, evidence has accumulated that most vascular PLC-coupled hormones are also coupled to the enzyme phospholipase D (PLD) (116–120).

PLD cleaves the distal ester bond of the phosphate group at the third position of the glycerol backbone of membrane phospholipids, releasing phosphatidic acid (PA) and a free, water-soluble head group (Fig. 3). In vascular smooth muscle, the major phospholipid hydrolyzed by PLD is PC. The PA formed in this reaction most likely has direct second messenger functions, but in addition, it is acted upon by phosphatidic acid phosphohydrolase to form DG. This pathway thus accounts for 75 to 90 percent of the DG formed in vascular smooth muscle (117).

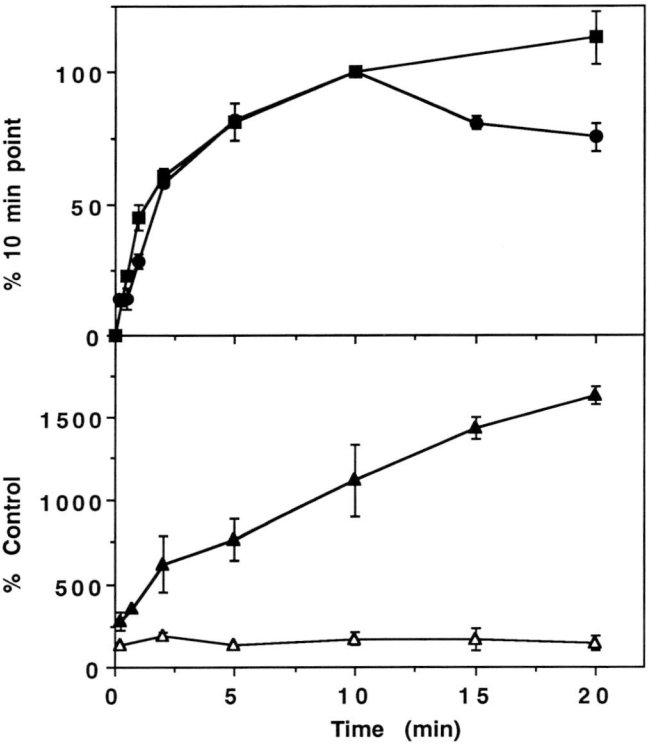

FIG. 5. Angiotensin II stimulation of vascular smooth muscle PLD. Ang II induces PLD-mediated PC hydrolysis, resulting in the formation of PA, and subsequent to the action of PA phosphohydrolase, DG (**top panel**). PLD activity can be measured by following the formation of phosphatidylethanol (PEt) (**bottom panel**), which is formed in a unique transphosphatidylation reaction when PLD is activated in the presence of ethanol. PEt is not further metabolized by the cell, so that its accumulation can be readily measured and is a good indicator of PLD activity. ● – ●, DG; ■ – ■, PA; ▲ – ▲, PEt in presence of ethanol; △ – △, PEt in absence of ethanol. (Courtesy of Dr. Bernard Lassègue.)

Ang II, ET, vasopressin, and NE have all been shown to activate PLD in smooth muscle (116–120). Ang II–induced stimulation of PLD is delayed and sustained, compared with IP₃ generation, and parallels the second phase of DG formation (Fig. 5). Fatty acid analysis of this DG shows that the majority has a fatty acid composition similar to that found in PC (117). A role for PC hydrolysis is supported by the fact that choline release is also sustained in these cells (116). The time course of norepinephrine-stimulated PLD activation is similar to that for Ang II, while ET- and vasopressin-induced stimulation of PLD is more transient (119,121). In all cases, however, both PA and DG accumulate for the duration of the stimulus (117,119–121).

Consequences of PLD Activation: Diacylglycerol and Stimulation of PKC

The massive formation of DG induced by vasoconstrictors has important consequences for cellular activation. DG has been shown to activate PKC, an 80-kDa, Ca²⁺- and phospholipid-dependent serine/threonine kinase present in eukaryotic cells (50,51). DG increases the affinity of PKC for Ca²⁺ and phosphatidylserine, thereby allowing enzyme activation at resting Ca²⁺ levels (50). PKC is an amphitropic protein that, upon activation, translocates from the cytosol to the membrane (122). The translocated enzyme binds tightly to the phospholipid bilayer (51), presumably until dissociation of DG from the complex following attenuation of the transmembrane signal.

PKC represents a group of at least nine isoforms of structurally homologous proteins that have the enzymatic activity described above (123). Several of the PKC isoenzymes isolated by cloning are Ca²⁺-independent, in contrast to the conventional PKCs described above. These isoforms appear to have different activation requirements and substrate specificities. The principal PKC isoforms in vascular smooth muscle are PKC-α and -β (124), which belong to the classic PKCs whose activation is Ca²⁺-dependent.

PKCs phosphorylate numerous cellular proteins, few of which have been identified. Recently, Tsuda et al. (125) have shown that Ang II and ET increase the phosphorylation of an identical group of cellular proteins in cultured vascular smooth muscle cells, a subset of which appears to be PKC-dependent. In general, Ang II–stimulated phosphorylations that are mediated by PKC appear to be sustained (125). Of these, only the lamins (126), caldesmon (127), and an 80-kDa protein with a pI of 4.5 to 5.0 (designated MARCKS for myristoylated alanine-rich C kinase substrate) have been identified (125). This latter substrate is also phosphorylated by vasopressin in cultured Swiss 3T3 fibroblasts (128). Adrenergic-mediated activation of PKC has apparently unique regulatory effects, since phorbol esters have been shown to phosphorylate the α_1-receptor and thereby alter further agonist binding (129) and subsequent signal generation.

PKC activation has been implicated in the downstream stimulation of several other kinases, as well as in the regulation of gene transcription (123). Among the most prominent of the kinase cascades initiated by PKC activation is activation of the MAP/S6 kinases. When simultaneously phosphorylated on tyrosine, MAP kinase in turn phosphorylates pp90[rsk], a cytosolic protein kinase (S6 kinase) that phosphorylates the ribosomal S6 protein (130). Phosphorylated S6 has been proposed to be involved in the transition from G0 to G1, the first step in the mitogenic response. PKC also activates AP-1, a transcription element that controls the transcription of numerous genes, including the early response genes c-*myc* and c-*fos* (131). Thus, in addition to being involved in the signaling cascade leading to contraction, PKC is, perhaps more importantly, implicated in the growth-related signaling pathways of smooth muscle.

Finally, activation of PKC has been shown to stimulate Na^+-H^+ exchange and to cause cytoplasmic alkalinization in a variety of cell types, including vascular smooth muscle (98). This suggests that PKC may function to regulate agonist-mediated induction of Na^+-H^+ exchange, thus affecting the activity of numerous metabolic pathways (see below).

Consequences of PLD Activation: Accumulation of Phosphatidic Acid

The role of PA as a second messenger remains controversial. Early studies implicated PA in the regulation of Ca^{2+} influx (132). The PA/PLD pathway has been suggested to be involved in the sustained Ca^{2+} influx seen during contraction (119). More recently, it has been suggested that PA has a role in mitogenesis (133,134). Finally, PA has been shown conclusively to stimulate reduced nicotinamide-adenine dinucleotide phosphate (NADPH) oxidase activity in neutrophils (135) and vascular smooth muscle cells (136). Although some of these signals may be involved in the transduction of contraction, definitive evidence remains to be determined.

PLD Subtypes and Regulation of Activity

Evidence exists that there are multiple PLD activities, although there has yet to be successful purification or cloning of a mammalian PLD. Both membrane-bound and cytosolic PLDs have been characterized, but neither has been proven to be receptor-coupled (137). PLD activities that are more active against phosphatidylethanolamine than PC have been described, and it has been suggested that this enzyme is important in growth (56).

PLD can be activated by G-protein coupling (138), tyrosine phosphorylation (139), or PKC stimulation (55). It is not known whether these pathways activate specific PLD subtypes or, alternatively, act in combination on a single subtype. Although PKC activators are capable of stimulating PLD, PKC does not appear to be involved in Ang II, ET-, or NE-induced PLD activation (117,118, 140). Stimulation of PLD by these agonists, is, however, at least partially Ca^{2+}-dependent (117), even though PLD is not activated by Ca^{2+} per se. Although it is likely that vasoconstrictors couple to PLD via G proteins, Ang II–induced PLD activation is strongly attenuated by tyrosine kinase inhibitors (unpublished observations), suggesting that tyrosine phosphorylation may be involved in agonist-stimulation of PLD activity in vascular smooth muscle. Unraveling these complicated pathways must await development of the appropriate molecular biological probes.

An additional regulator of PLD activity, at least in Ang II–treated cells, is cellular processing of the receptor-agonist complex. Binding of Ang II to its receptor initiates internalization of the receptor-ligand complex, first within the plane of the membrane, and subsequently into coated pits and vesicles, endosomes, and lysosomes (141). Thus, the activated receptor complex occupies several different cellular domains during the course of signal generation. Movement of the agonist-receptor complex through these domains may be essential for development of the normal sequence of intracellular signals. Interfering with internalization does indeed alter signal generation (142,143). Agents that attenuate receptor internalization inhibit the sustained phase of Ang II–stimulated DG formation and PLD activity (116,142). The precise processing event essential to maintaining DG accumulation probably occurs at the level of the plasma membrane (142). It is interesting that the "processed" Ang II–receptor complex retains its ability to signal (142). These types of observations have not yet been made for other vasoconstrictor agonists, but they do suggest that the physical state and location of the agonist-receptor complex may have a bearing on the regulation of PLD activity and subsequent signal generation.

Intracellular concentration of hydrogen ion also appears to affect PLD activity. Ang II stimulates a biphasic change in intracellular pH that temporally correlates with DG formation (61,98). Alkalinization, such as that which occurs during the sustained phase of hormonal stimulation, enhances Ang II–induced sustained DG accumulation in vascular smooth muscle while having no effect on early DG formation (144). Dimethylamiloride or incubation in Na^+-free buffer, either of which inhibits Na^+-H^+ exchange, also inhibits Ang II–induced sustained DG formation (144). Thus, in Ang II–stimulated vascular smooth muscle cells, DG accumulation, and, by inference, PLD activity appear to be regulated by an intracellular alkalinization that is dependent on Na^+-H^+ exchange.

Phospholipase A₂

A third phospholipase activated by vasoconstrictor hormones is phospholipase A₂ (PLA₂). PLA₂ cleaves the ester bond in position 2 of glycerophospholipids such as PC and phosphatidylethanolamine, releasing a free fatty acid and the lyso- form of the phospholipid (Fig. 3). The composition of mammalian plasma membrane phospholipids is such that arachidonic acid is one of the major fatty acids produced by this reaction. Arachidonic acid is the rate-limiting precursor for the generation of eicosanoids, molecules that themselves have numerous signaling properties. If acted upon by cyclooxygenase, arachidonic acid is converted into the prostaglandins and thromboxanes, which cause either vasodilation or vasoconstriction, depending upon the exact nature of the product. Lipoxygenase action on arachidonic acid results in the formation of hydroperoxyeicosatetraenoate (HPETE) and the leukotrienes, which function in vascular growth (145) and permeability. Cytochrome P-450 monooxygenase converts arachidonic acid to the epoxides, potent vasodilators (146). It should be noted that arachidonic acid can also be generated by the hydrolysis of DG by diacylglycerol lipase, and thus can result indirectly from activation of PLC. Although Ang II and ET have been demonstrated to be directly coupled to PLA₂ (147,148), most studies of vasopressin-stimulated prostaglandin formation do not address the question of direct receptor-PLA₂ interaction (149).

Consequences of PLA₂ Activation: Arachidonic Acid and its Metabolites

Arachidonic acid and the eicosanoids serve both second messenger and paracrine functions in the circulation. Prostacyclin (PGI₂) and prostaglandin E (PGE) relax vascular smooth muscle, while prostaglandin F₂α contracts it. Both Ang II and vasopressin stimulate cultured smooth muscle cells to produce PGI₂ and PGE (149,150), while NE is ineffective, at least for PGE (150). A full discussion of the interaction of eicosanoids with the vasculature can be found in Chapter 57.

Arachidonic acid has also been shown to stimulate the βII, γ, and ε isozymes of PKC in a Ca²⁺-independent fashion, and PKC-α in a Ca²⁺-dependent fashion (123). In addition, fatty acids may activate PKC in different cellular compartments than does DG, since soluble PKC appears to be more sensitive than membrane-bound PKC to these molecules (151). Thus, arachidonic acid may participate in regulating the intracellular signals modulated by PKC.

PLA₂ Subtypes and Activation Requirements

There are at least three types of PLA₂ activities in vascular smooth muscle: secreted, and Ca²⁺-dependent

and -independent intracellular forms (152,153). The secreted PLA₂ has a neutral pH optimum and is critically dependent on ambient Ca²⁺ concentration (152). Release of this enzyme is stimulated by agents that activate adenylate cyclase, but is unaffected by Ang II (153). The Ca²⁺-independent PLA₂ is activated by adenine nucleotides, but there is at present no evidence that it is regulated by receptor activation (152). The intracellular, Ca²⁺-dependent subtype (termed cPLA₂) may be most relevant to intracellular signaling in vascular smooth muscle. This 110-kDa protein is activated by phosphorylation on serine, and is translocated to the membrane upon activation (154). It has been shown unequivocally to be receptor-linked (154). Recent evidence indicates that this protein is stimulated by Ang II in cultured vascular smooth muscle cells (G. Rao, *personal communication*).

Prior to identification of PLA₂ subtypes, numerous investigators showed that receptor-stimulated arachidonic acid release was sensitive to pertussis toxin, or was synergistically enhanced by co-incubation with GTPγS (74). The difficulty with interpreting these results has been that PLC is also coupled to a G protein, so that these effects might be attributed to the interaction of the G protein with PLC, leading to a secondary activation of PLA₂. In some cases, PLC and PLA₂ activation can be temporally separated, or show differential sensitivity to inhibitors (74), simplifying data interpretation. However, direct evidence for G protein–PLA₂ receptor interaction is lacking, particularly in smooth muscle.

The intracellular forms of PLA₂ have been shown to be phosphorylated on serine in a PKC-dependent manner, presumably by activation of mitogen-activated protein (MAP) kinase (154,155). Whether or not this phosphorylation correlates with increased activity is controversial (74). A possible explanation for these disparate results lies in the observation that PKC-induced activation of PLA₂ may require elevation of intracellular Ca²⁺ (149,156). Although Ca²⁺ alone may not be sufficient to activate PLA₂, it has been implicated in mediating translocation of PLA₂ from the cytosol to the membrane (157).

Temporal Pattern of Signal Generation in Vascular Smooth Muscle

From the previous discussion, it is clear that interaction of a vasoconstrictor hormone with its receptor on the surface of a vascular smooth muscle cell results in the activation of numerous enzyme systems and the generation of myriad intracellular second messengers. Order may be brought out of chaos by examining the temporal relationship of these signaling events. Interaction of these effects has been most fully characterized in Ang II–stimulated cultured vascular smooth muscle cells (Fig. 6). When these cells are exposed to Ang II, there is an

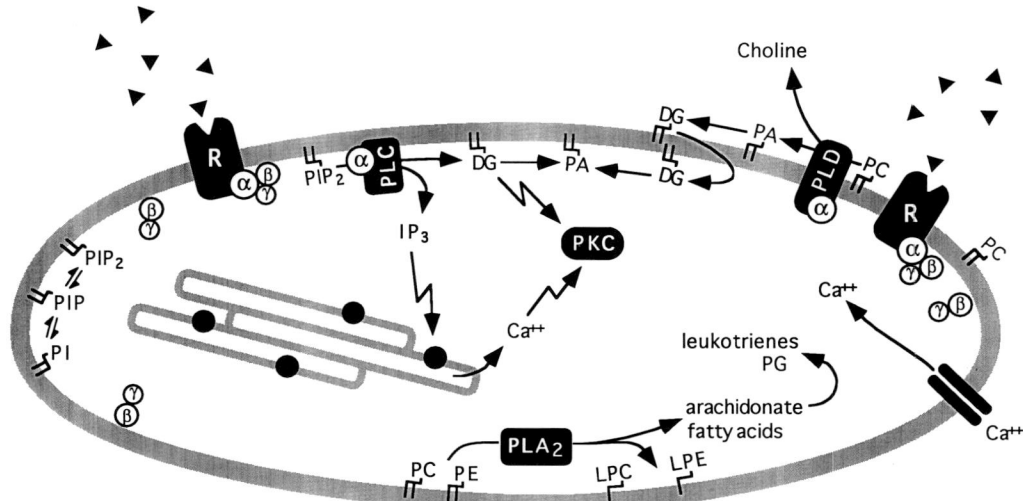

FIG. 6. Hormonal activation of vascular smooth muscle. Ang II and other vasoconstrictors activate PLA$_2$, PLC, and PLD. The second messengers produced (fatty acids, IP$_3$, DG, PA) then activate numerous signaling pathways within the cell. IP$_3$ releases Ca^{2+} from intracellular stores, DG (in the presence of Ca^{2+}) activates PKC, and the fatty acid arachidonic acid is converted into the prostaglandins and leukotrienes. For details of the interaction between these pathways, see text. (Modified from ref. 158.)

initial, rapid hydrolysis of PIP$_2$ to form IP$_3$ and DG. This reaction is mediated by a G protein, possibly of the G$_q$ subfamily. IP$_3$ stimulates the release of Ca^{2+} from intracellular stores, resulting in the activation of Ca^{2+}-calmodulin–dependent protein kinases. The Ang II–receptor complex becomes sequestered in the membrane, allowing initiation of PLD-mediated PC hydrolysis as an additional source of DG. In the presence of elevated intracellular Ca^{2+}, DG activates PKC, resulting in termination of PIP$_2$ hydrolysis, stimulation of Na$^+$-H$^+$ exchange, and possibly stimulation of PLA$_2$. The arachidonic acid released by PLA$_2$ may be metabolized to eicosanoids, or may act to enhance the activity of cellular enzymes, including certain forms of PKC. In addition, PKC phosphorylates numerous cellular proteins and activates other kinases, in particular the MAP kinase cascade. During the sustained phase of the response, ongoing Ca^{2+} influx occurs, maintaining a low, but elevated level of cytoplasmic free Ca^{2+}, which plays a permissive role in many more distal enzymatic reactions. Thus, activation of phospholipases C, D, and A$_2$ acts in concert to generate interdependent second messengers.

CONTRACTION

The second messengers generated by hormonal activation of vascular smooth muscle, in turn, activate enzymes leading to contraction. The transduction of these signals into contraction and force generation has been elucidated in general, but the regulation and interactions of the various enzymes and proteins remain under investigation.

Hormone-Stimulated Contraction

Ang II, ET, NE, and vasopressin all cause vascular smooth muscle contraction, but the profile of force generation varies with the hormone and the vessel. Ang II causes a phasic contraction of rat and rabbit aortae (159,160) and most small arteries and resistance vessels (161), but causes a sustained contraction of dog aorta (160). α-Adrenergic agonists cause a sustained contraction of most vessels studied (160,161), with the exception of canine aorta (162). In rabbit ear artery, NE causes a distinct biphasic contraction: a rapid initial phase followed by a slower, sustained force generation (163). Vasopressin also causes a sustained contraction of both aorta and resistance vessels (161,162), but some arteries, such as canine pulmonary resistance vessels, remain unresponsive to this hormone (161). ET induces a sustained contraction in nearly all vessels studied (105). The magnitude and maintenance of force generation are also dependent on dose. Higher doses of agonist not only cause a greater initial force generation, but also often increase the rate of relaxation of the sustained component (159). The reasons behind the different patterns of contraction induced by these agonists are unknown. It is possible that certain phasic agonists, such as Ang II, stimulate a delayed release of vasorelaxants (e.g., PLA$_2$ metabolites) that attenuate sustained contraction (150). Phasic contraction might also result from rapid desensitization of the receptors.

The initial phase of force development has been studied most extensively. Force generation and contraction of smooth muscle are postulated to depend on formation of actin-myosin cross-bridges. The molecular mechanism underlying the sustained phase of contraction is unclear, but has been termed the latch-state to describe low-level cycling of cross-bridges. These models will be discussed separately below.

Phasic Contraction of Vascular Smooth Muscle

Muscle contraction is dependent upon the interaction of actin and myosin. In skeletal muscle, a "sliding filament" model—a model based on stimulus-induced variation in the amount of overlap between alternating regular arrays of actin and myosin filaments—was proposed to account for muscle shortening (164). According to this model, force generation is accomplished by attachment of the myosin heads (or cross-bridges) to F-actin filaments. This attachment occurs only in stimulated muscle, and it catalyzes ATP hydrolysis to generate tension. Contraction of smooth muscle is also assumed to be regulated by a sliding-filament mechanism, but regulation of actin-myosin interaction is quite different. Smooth muscle has a relatively greater content of actin and tropomyosin, and a lower content of myosin, than does skeletal muscle (165). Tropomyosin does not appear to be important in regulation of actin-myosin interaction (165); its function in smooth muscle is unknown but may involve stabilization of F-actin (166). Indeed, in contrast to skeletal muscle where the major site of Ca^{2+} regulation resides on the actin filament, Ca^{2+} regulation of smooth muscle actomyosin resides with the myosin molecule (165). Smooth muscle myosin consists of two large subunits, each with a molecular weight of 200 kDa, and two small subunits known as the *myosin light chains*. One light chain has a molecular weight of 16 to 17 kDa, and the other has a molecular weight of 20 kDa (167). The 20-kDa myosin light chain appears to be the regulatory subunit (167). The major mechanism of regulation is phosphorylation/dephosphorylation of this subunit. Purified smooth muscle myosin cannot be activated by actin unless the 20-kDa light chain is phosphorylated. Once phosphorylation occurs, actin-activated Mg^{2+}-ATPase activity is stimulated, resulting in cross-bridge cycling.

Smooth muscle actin-myosin interaction is Ca^{2+} dependent, but the Ca^{2+} requirement exists early in the contraction cascade. Myosin light chain phosphorylation is mediated by an enzyme known as *myosin light chain kinase* (MLCK). MLCK has a molecular weight of 130 to 150 kDa and is able to associate with calmodulin, a Ca^{2+}-binding protein (molecular weight 16.7 kDa) required for activation of a number of cytoplasmic enzymes (168). The current theory of phasic contraction rests on a "contraction cascade" initiated by an increase in intracellular free Ca^{2+} (169) (Fig. 7). When Ca^{2+} increases following hormonal stimulation, four molecules of Ca^{2+} bind to calmodulin, which then binds to MLCK. Binding of Ca^{2+}-calmodulin converts MLCK from an inactive to an active form. MLCK then phosphorylates the myosin light chain, permitting actin activation of the Mg^{2+}-ATPase and resulting in cross-bridge formation. When intracellular Ca^{2+} drops below 10^{-7} M, Ca^{2+} dissociates from calmodulin, calmodulin dissociates from MLCK, and MLCK becomes inactive. Myosin light chain phosphatase activity, which is insensitive to Ca^{2+}, then predominates, and myosin is dephosphorylated. The theory predicts that relaxation would then ensue; in fact, smooth muscle often remains contracted (170). Thus, it appears that myosin phosphorylation correlates

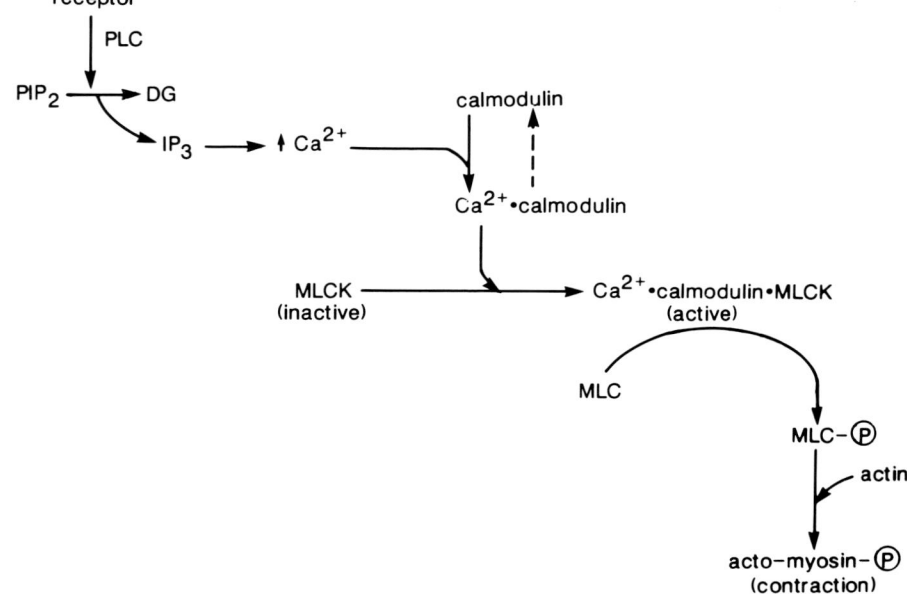

FIG. 7. Cascade of enzymatic reactions leading to contraction in vascular smooth muscle stimulated with calcium-mobilizing hormones. As described in the text, the initial increase in intracellular Ca^{2+} initiates a cascade of kinase activation, ultimately resulting in actin-myosin interaction and contraction. MLC, myosin light chain; MLCK, MLC kinase. (Modified from ref. 167.)

with cross-bridge cycling but not necessarily with tension. This has led to the postulate that a "latch-bridge," a cross-bridge that forms but either does not recycle or recycles only slowly, maintains tension in smooth muscle (171) (see below).

Two additional actin-binding proteins have recently been identified and proposed as possible regulatory molecules. Calponin (MW 34,000) binds to both actin and tropomyosin, inhibiting actomyosin ATPase activity. This inhibition can be released by Ca^{2+}-calmodulin or phosphorylation by PKC (172). Caldesmon (MW 145,000) also alters actomyosin interactions (173). In the absence of Ca^{2+}-calmodulin, caldesmon inhibits cross-bridge formation between actin and phosphorylated myosin, presumably by binding to actin and tropomyosin (173). When intracellular Ca^{2+} increases upon stimulation, the interaction between caldesmon, actin, and tropomyosin changes, permitting cross-bridge formation. Caldesmon is phosphorylated *in vitro* by several protein kinases (172). Recent evidence suggests that phosphorylated caldesmon, acting through actin and tropomyosin, may slow cross-bridge detachment, thus contributing to the formation of latch-bridges (172).

Tonic Contraction of Smooth Muscle

In order for MLCK-mediated actin-myosin interaction to account for sustained contraction, two assumptions must hold: (a) intracellular free Ca^{2+} must remain elevated for the duration of contraction; and (b) the myosin light chain must remain phosphorylated, supporting continued cross-bridge cycling. As noted previously, both of these events are transient in smooth muscle (65,170). Furthermore, energy consumption, as reflected by depletion of ATP, decreases markedly from a high level during initial contraction to a low level during the sustained phase (174). These observations suggest that increased cross-bridge cycling does not occur during sustained contraction. To explain the continued generation of force, Dillon et al. (175) suggested that once the myosin light chain is dephosphorylated, a shift in the properties of the cross-bridges occurs such that a long-lasting cross-bridge between actin and myosin is formed. This new "latch-bridge" is purported to be more sensitive to Ca^{2+} than is the initial activation. No definitive molecular identification of this "latch-bridge" structure has been made.

Activation of PKC has been implicated in sustained contraction of vascular smooth muscle, since phorbol esters, exogenous activators of PKC, cause a slow, sustained contraction of rat and rabbit aortae (176,177). This contraction is not accompanied by phosphorylation of the myosin light chain but is instead accompanied by phosphorylation of several intermediate filament- or actin-binding proteins (127). It has, however, been

difficult to conclusively demonstrate a role for PKC in agonist-stimulated contraction. If it is involved, it appears to have a modulatory role: it may alter the Ca^{2+}-sensitivity of the myofilaments (178) or affect the function of actin-binding proteins such as caldesmon (179).

Ca^{2+} influx may play a much more important role than does PKC in tonic contraction. The sustained phase of contraction is dependent on sustained Ca^{2+} influx, since it is completely inhibited in Ca^{2+}-free medium (127). To account for this Ca^{2+} dependency in the face of the transience of the initial increase in cytosolic free Ca^{2+} concentration, Rasmussen et al. (180) have suggested that hormone-stimulated Ca^{2+} influx, which has been demonstrated to be prolonged in vascular smooth muscle (100–103), results in an increase in the concentration of Ca^{2+} only in the immediate vicinity of the plasma membrane, since Ca^{2+} extrusion mechanisms remain activated by hormonal stimulation. It is also possible that the initial rise in intracellular Ca^{2+} determines the amount of PKC associated with the membrane (180), leading to prolonged activation of this enzyme and modulation of contraction.

Intracellular pH may also serve a modulatory function in the regulation of tonic contraction. Acidosis has been shown to decrease tension development in cardiac and skeletal muscles (181), and intracellular alkalinization by ammonium chloride administration contracts vascular smooth muscle (N. R. Danthuluri, *personal communication*). The mechanism by which pH alters contraction is unknown. It has been suggested that pH alters sarcolemmal binding of Ca^{2+} (182) and that pH modulates calmodulin activity (183). Tkachuk and Men'shikov (183) demonstrated that increasing pH from 6.5 to 7.5 causes an order of magnitude decrease in the K_D of calmodulin for Ca^{2+}, suggesting that alkalinization could increase the degree of activation of calmodulin at resting Ca^{2+} levels, thus prolonging its effects. Additionally, it has been shown that pH can alter actomyosin ATPase activity and may affect the sensitivity of the myofibrils to Ca^{2+} (184). Finally, there is some evidence for an interaction between Ca^{2+} and H^+ in terms of transmembrane fluxes and competition at intracellular binding sites (184). Thus, although the mechanism of pH modulation has not been conclusively demonstrated, in all cases pH appears to alter the stimulatory effects of Ca^{2+} at various levels of the contraction cascade.

ALTERATION OF SIGNAL TRANSDUCTION IN HYPERTENSION

It is clear that any pathological condition that alters receptor binding, phospholipase activity, Ca^{2+} flux, intracellular pH, PKC activity, or the contractile apparatus could have a profound effect on agonist-stimulated or tonic contraction of vascular smooth muscle. In tissue from spontaneously hypertensive rats (SHRs) or from patients with essential hypertension, changes in nearly all of these areas have been documented.

Vascular smooth muscle from hypertensive subjects has been shown to be hyperreactive to agonist stimulation (185). Although some of this increase in contractility can be attributed to an increase in vessel wall mass (185), there remains within a single vessel a differential sensitivity to certain agonists. In the renal vasculature of the hypertensive rat, the contractile response to Ang II is enhanced more than that to NE (186). Some studies have demonstrated an increase in Ang II or α-adrenergic receptor numbers in tissues from SHRs (187,188), but this change appears to depend on the particular tissue and receptor investigated.

Studies on the biochemical signaling pathways in hypertensive versus normotensive rats have documented major changes in the activity of the enzymes and second messengers involved in these pathways. However, alterations in enzymatic activity often depend on the agonist used to stimulate the cells. Ang II, but not vasopressin or ET, causes an increased PLC activity in mesenteric artery smooth muscle cells from SHRs, as compared with normotensive controls (189). Ang II–stimulated Na^+-H^+ exchange is also increased in smooth muscle cells from SHRs, as is activation of S6 kinase (190). Ca^{2+} influx through voltage-dependent Ca^{2+} channels is increased in carotids (191) and mesenteric arteries (192) in SHRs as compared with that in normotensive rats. The DG-PKC pathway is also altered in SHRs in some cell types (193,194), but not apparently in smooth muscle (190).

Increased vascular distending pressure also causes changes in the amounts of contractile proteins. Berner et al. (195) demonstrated that in rabbit portal anterior mesenteric veins that had been exposed to elevated pressures for 2 weeks, the number of actin filaments increased in proportion to cell volume, whereas the number of myosin filaments remained unchanged. These observations suggest that a change in the contractile proteins may be partially responsible for vascular hyperreactivity.

Each of the steps in the transduction of agonist stimulation into contractile activity thus may be altered in hypertension. The final contractile response of the vessel depends on integration of all these parameters. The identification of the biochemical or cytologic lesion(s) responsible for hyperreactivity of isolated vessels from hypertensive subjects may be complicated by the interrelationships of a variety of secondary signals.

ACKNOWLEDGMENTS

This work was supported by National Institutes of Health grants HL38206 and HL47557. We appreciate the editorial assistance of Barbara Merchant and thank Dr. Bernard Lassègue for his help with the illustrations.

REFERENCES

1. Cotecchia S, Schwinn DA, Randall RR, Lefkowitz RJ, Caron MG, Kobilka BK. *Proc Natl Acad Sci USA* 1988;85:7159–7163.
2. Morel A, O'Carroll A, Brownstein MJ, Lolait SJ. *Nature* 1992;356:523–526.
3. Murphy TJ, Alexander RW, Griendling KK, Runge MS, Bernstein KE. *Nature* 1991;351:233–236.
4. Lin HY, Kaji EH, Winkel GK, Ives HE, Lodish HF. *Proc Natl Acad Sci USA* 1991;88:3185–3189.
5. Griendling KK, Murphy TJ, Alexander RW. *Circulation* 1993;87:1816–1828.
6. Lomasney JW, Cotecchia S, Lorenz W, et al. *J Biol Chem* 1991;266:6365–6369.
7. Kobilka BK, Matsui H, Kobilka TS, et al. *Science* 1987;238:650–656.
8. Regan JW, Kobilka TS, Yang-Feng TL, Caron MG, Lefkowitz RJ, Kobilka BK. *Proc Natl Acad Sci USA* 1988;85:6301–6305.
9. Lomasney JW, Lorenz W, Allen LF, et al. *Proc Natl Acad Sci USA* 1990;87:5094–5098.
10. Murphy TJ, Alexander RW, Griendling KK, Runge MS, Bernstein KE. *Nature* 1991;351:233–236.
11. Iwai N, Inagami T. *FEBS Lett* 1992;298:257–260.
12. Arai H, Hori S, Aramori I, Ohkubo H, Nakanishi S. *Nature* 1990;348:730–732.
13. Lin HY, Kaji EH, Winkel GK, Ives HE, Lodish HF. *Proc Natl Acad Sci USA* 1991;88:3185–3189.
14. Sakurai T, Yanagisawa M, Takuwa Y, Miyazaki H, Kimura S, Goto K, Masaki T. *Nature* 1990;348:732–735.
15. Morel A, O'Carroll A-M, Brownstein MJ, Lolait SJ. *Nature* 1992;356:523–526.
16. Lolait SJ, O'Carroll A-M, McBride OW, Konig M, Morel A, Brownstein MJ. *Nature* 1992;357:336–339.
17. DeMey J, Vanhoutte PM. *Circ Res* 1981;48:875–884.
18. McGrath JC. *Biochem Pharmacol* 1982;31:467–484.
19. Drew GM, Whiting SB. *Br J Pharmacol* 1979;67:207–215.
20. Ruffolo RR Jr, Waddell JE, Yaden EL. *J Pharmacol Exp Ther* 1982;221:309–314.
21. Han C, Abel PW, Minneman KP. *Nature* 1987;329:333–335.
22. Erne P, Mittelholzer E, Burgisser E, Fluckiger R, Buhler FR. *J Recept Res* 1984;4:587–604.
23. Wikberg JES. *Nature* 1978;273:164–166.
24. Berthelsen S, Pettinger WA. *Life Sci* 1977;21:595–606.
25. Hoffman BB, Lefkowitz RJ. *N Engl J Med* 1980;302:1390–1396.
26. Johnson RD, Minneman KP. *Mol Pharmacol* 1987;31:239–246.
27. Bumpus FM, Catt KJ, Shiu AT, et al. *Hypertension* 1991;17:720–721.
28. Sumners C, Tang W, Zelezna B, Raizada MK. *Proc Natl Acad Sci USA* 1991;88:7567–7571.
29. Bernstein KE, Alexander RW. *Endocr Rev* 1992;13:381–386.
30. Milan MA, Carvallo P, Izumi S-I, et al. *Science* 1989;244:1340–1342.
31. Kakar SS, Sellers JC, Devor DC, Musgrove LC, Neill JD. *Biochem Biophys Res Commun* 1992;183:1090–1096.
32. Masaki T, Kimura S, Yanagisawa M, Goto K. *Circulation* 1991;84:1457–1468.
33. Simonson MS, Dunn MJ. *FASEB J* 1990;4:2989–3000.
34. Michell RH, Kirk CJ, Billah MM. *Biochem Soc Trans* 1979;7:861–865.
35. Stassen FL, Heckman G, Schmidt D, et al. *Mol Pharmacol* 1987;31:267–272.
36. Stassen FL, Heckman G, Schmidt D, Aiyar N, Nambi P, Crooke ST. *Mol Pharmacol* 1987;31:259–266.
37. Roy C, Hall D, Ausiello DA. *J Biol Chem* 1981;256:3423–3427.
38. Wright GB, Alexander RW, Gimbrone MA Jr. In: Haft JL, Karliner JS, eds. *Receptor Science in Cardiology*. New York: Futura, 1984;163–203.
39. Wright GB, Alexander RW, Ekstein LS, Gimbrone MA Jr. *Circ Res* 1982;50:462–469.
40. Geynet P, Ferry N, Borsodi A, Hanoune J. *Biochem Pharmacol* 1981;30:1665–1675.
41. Hoffman BB, Mullikin-Kilpatrick D, Lefkowitz RJ. *J Biol Chem* 1980;255:4645–4652.
42. Snavely MD, Insel PA. *Mol Pharmacol* 1983;22:532–546.

43. U'Prichard DC, Snyder SH. *J Neurochem* 1980;34:385–394.
44. Goodhardt M, Ferry N, Geynet P, Hanoune J. *J Biol Chem* 1982;257:11577–11583.
45. Colucci WS, Gimbrone MA Jr, Alexander RW. *Circ Res* 1984;55:78–88.
46. Bojanic D, Fain JN. *Biochem J* 1986;240:361–365.
47. Michel T, Hoffman BB, Lefkowitz RJ. *Nature* 1980;288:709–711.
48. Gu XH, Casley D, Nayler W. *Eur J Pharmacol* 1989;167:281–290.
49. Gilman AG. *Annu Rev Biochem* 1987;56:615–649.
50. Nishizuka Y. *Nature* 1984;308:693–698.
51. Bell RM. *Cell* 1986;45:631–632.
52. Williamson JR, Cooper RH, Joseph SK, Thomas AP. *Am J Physiol* 1985;248:C208–C216.
53. Hokin LE. *Annu Rev Biochem* 1985;54:205–235.
54. Majerus PW, Neufeld EJ, Wilson DB. *Cell* 1986;37:701–703.
55. Billah MM, Anthes JC. *Biochem J* 1990;269:281–291.
56. Kiss Z. *Biochem J* 1992;285:229–233.
57. Griendling KK, Lassegue B, Alexander RW. In: August JT, Anders MW, Murad F. *Advances in Pharmacology.* New York: Academic Press, in press.
58. Irvine RF, Letcher AJ, Heslop JP, Berridge MJ. *Nature* 1986;320:631–634.
59. Alexander RW, Brock TA, Gimbrone MA Jr, Rittenhouse SE. *Hypertension* 1985;7:447–451.
60. Smith JB, Smith L, Brown RE, et al. *Proc Natl Acad Sci USA* 1984;81:7812–7816.
61. Griendling KK, Rittenhouse SE, Brock TA, Ekstein LS, Gimbrone MA Jr, Alexander RW. *J Biol Chem* 1986;261:5901–5906.
62. Griendling KK, Berk BC, Socorro L, Tsuda T, Delafontaine P, Alexander RW. *Clin Exp Pharmacol Physiol* 1988;15:105–112.
63. Yamamoto H, van Breeman C. *Biochem Biophys Res Commun* 1985;130:270–274.
64. Smith JB, Smith L, Higgins BL. *J Biol Chem* 1985;260:14413–14416.
65. Brock TA, Alexander RW, Ekstein LS, Atkinson WJ, Gimbrone MA Jr. *Hypertension* 1985;7(suppl 1):105–109.
66. Capponi AM, Lew PD, Vallotton MB. *J Biol Chem* 1985;260:7836–7842.
67. Nabika T, Velletri PA, Lovenberg W, Beaven MA. *J Biol Chem* 1985;260:4661–4670.
68. Muldoon LL, Rodland KD, Forsythe ML, Magun BE. *J Biol Chem* 1989;264:8529–8536.
69. Fox AW, Abel PW, Minneman KP. *Eur J Pharmacol* 1985;116:145–152.
70. Villalobos-Molina R, Ue M, Hong E, Garcio-Sainz JA. *J Pharmacol Exp Ther* 1982;222:258–261.
71. Campbell MD, Deth RC, Payne RA, Honeyman TW. *Eur J Pharmacol* 1985;116:129–136.
72. Morgan KG. *Am J Cardiol* 1987;59:24A–28A.
73. Cockcroft S, Thomas GMH. *Biochem J* 1992;288:1–14.
74. Lambeth JD. In: Kuo JF, ed. *Protein Kinase C.* New York: Oxford University Press, 1993.
75. Stryer L, Bourne HR. *Annu Rev Cell Biol* 1986;2:391–419.
76. Haslam RJ, Davidson MML. *J Recept Res* 1984;4:605–629.
77. Cockcroft S, Gomperts BD. *Nature* 1985;314:534–536.
78. Litosch I. *Biochem J* 1987;244:35–40.
79. Bruns C, Marme D. *FEBS Lett* 1987;212:40–44.
80. Kanaide H, Matsumoto T, Nakamura M. *Biochem Biophys Res Commun* 1986;140:195–203.
81. Socorro L, Alexander RW. *FASEB J* 1988;2:A787.
82. Reynolds EE, Mok LL, Kurokawa S. *Biochem Biophys Res Commun* 1989;160:868–873.
83. Lee CH, Park D, Wu D, Rhee SG, Simon MI. *J Biol Chem* 1992;267:16044–16047.
84. Wu H, Katz A, Lee CH, Simon MI. *J Biol Chem* 1926;7:25798–25802.
85. Brock TA, Rittenhouse SE, Powers CW, Ekstein LS, Gimbrone MA Jr, Alexander RW. *J Biol Chem* 1985;260:14158–14162.
86. Orellana SA, Solski PA, Brown JH. *J Biol Chem* 1985;260:5236–5239.
87. Brown KD, Blakely DM, Hamon MH, Laurie MS, Corps AN. *Biochem J* 1987;245:631–639.
88. MacIntyre DE, McNicol A, Drummond AH. *FEBS Lett* 1985;180:160–164.
89. Corvera S, Schwartz KR, Graham RM, Garcia-Sainz JA. *J Biol Chem* 1986;261:520–526.
90. Cooper RH, Coll KE, Williamson JR. *J Biol Chem* 1985;260:3281–3288.
91. Chardonnens D, Lang U, Rossier MF, Capponi AM, Vallotton MB. *J Biol Chem* 1990;265:10451–10457.
92. Manne V, Kung H. *Biochem J* 1987;243:763–771.
93. Wilson DB, Bross TE, Hofmann SL, Majerus PW. *J Biol Chem* 1984;259:11718–11724.
94. Bennett CF, Crooke ST. *J Biol Chem* 1987;262:13789–13797.
95. Carter HR, Smith AD. *Biochem J* 1987;244:639–645.
96. Chau L, Tai H. *Biochim Biophys Acta* 1982;713:344–351.
97. Griendling KK, Taubman MB, Akers M, Mendlowitz M, Alexander RW. *J Biol Chem* 1991;266:15498–15504.
98. Berk BC, Aronow MS, Brock TA, Cragoe E Jr, Gimbrone MA Jr, Alexander RW. *J Biol Chem* 1987;262:5057–5064.
99. Berk BC, Brock TA, Gimbrone MA Jr, Alexander RW. *J Biol Chem* 1987;262:5065–5072.
100. Benham CD, Tsien RW. *Nature* 1987;328:275–278.
101. Cauvin C, Malik S. *J Pharmacol Exp Ther* 1984;230:413–418.
102. Godfraind T. In: Weiss GB, ed. *Perspectives on calcium antagonists.* Bethesda MD: American Physiological Society, 1981;95–107.
103. Reynolds EE, Dubyak GR. *Biochem Biophys Res Commun* 1985;130:627–632.
104. VanMeel JCA, DeJonge A, Kalkman HO, Wiffert B, Timmermans PBMWM, van Zwieten PA. *Eur J Pharmacol* 1981;69:205–208.
105. Yanagisawa M, Kurihara H, Kimura S, et al. *Nature* 1988;332:411–418.
106. Bolton TB. *Physiol Rev* 1979;59:606–718.
107. Zelcer E, Sperelakis N. *Blood Vessels* 1981;18:263–279.
108. Casteels R, Kitamura K, Kuriyama H, Suzuki H. *J Physiol* 1977;271:41–61.
109. Hermsmeyer K. *Life Sci* 1971;10:223–234.
110. Meisheri KD, Hwang O, van Breeman C. *J Membrane Biol* 1981;59:19–25.
111. Galizzi J, Qar J, Fosset M, Van Renterghem C, Lazdunski M. *J Biol Chem* 1987;262:6947–6950.
112. Mitsuhashi T, Morris RC, Ives HE. *J Clin Invest* 1989;84:635–639.
113. Bocckino SB, Blackmore PF, Exton JH. *J Biol Chem* 1985;260:14201–14207.
114. Thomas AP, Marks JS, Coll KE, Williamson JR. *J Biol Chem* 1983;258:5716–5725.
115. Griendling KK, Tsuda T, Alexander RW. *J Biol Chem* 1989;264:10620–10624.
116. Lassègue B, Alexander RW, Clark M, Griendling KK. *Biochem J* 1991;276:19–25.
117. Lassègue B, Alexander RW, Clark M, Akers MA, Griendling KK. *Biochem J* 1993;292:509–517.
118. Liu Y, Geisbuhler B, Jones AW. *Am J Physiol* 1992;262:C941–C949.
119. Jones AW, Shulka SD, Geisbuhler BB. *Am J Physiol* 1993;264:C609–C616.
120. Welsh CJ, Schmeichel K, Cao H, Chabbott H. *Lipids* 1990;25:675–684.
121. Friedlaender MM, Jain D, Ahmed Z, Hart D, Barnett RL, Nord EP. *Am J Physiol* 1993;264:F845–F853.
122. Wolf M, LeVine H III, May WS Jr, Cuatrecasas P, Sahyoun N. *Nature* 1985;317:546–549.
123. Hug H, Sarre TF. *Biochem J* 1993;291:329–343.
124. Singer HA, Schworer CM, Sweeley C, Benscoter H. *Arch Biochem Biophys* 1992;299:320–329.
125. Tsuda T, Griendling KK, Ollerenshaw JD, Lassègue B, Alexander RW. *J Vas Res* 1993;30:241–249.
126. Tsuda T, Alexander RW. *J Biol Chem* 1990;265:1165–1170.
127. Park S, Rasmussen H. *J Biol Chem* 1986;261:15734–15739.
128. Rodriguez PA, Rozengurt E. *J Cell Physiol* 1986;129:124–130.
129. Leeb-Lundberg LMF, Cotecchia S, Lomasney JW, DeBernardis JF, Lefkowitz RJ, Caron MG. *Proc Natl Acad Sci USA* 1985;82:5651–5655.

130. Tsuda T, Kawahara Y, Ishida Y, Koide M, Shii K, Yokoyama M. *Circ Res* 1992;71:620–630.
131. Naftilan AJ. *J Cardiovasc Pharmacol* 1992;20:S37–40.
132. Putney JW, Weiss SJ, Van De Walle CM, Haddas RA. *Nature* 1980;284:345–347.
133. Moolenaar WH, Kruijer W, Tilly BC, Verlaan I, Bierman AJ, de Laat SW. *Nature* 1986;323:171–173.
134. Yu C, Tsai M, Stacey DW. *Cell* 1988;52:63–71.
135. Agwu DE, McPhail LC, Sozzani S, Bass DA, McCall CE. *J Clin Invest* 1991;88:531–539.
136. Griendling KK, Ollerenshaw JD, Minieri C, Alexander RW. *FASEB* 1993;7:A1.
137. Wang P, Anthes JC, Siegel MI, Egan RW, Billah MM. *J Biol Chem* 1991;266:14877–14880.
138. Bocckino SB, Blackmore PF, Wilson PB, Exton JH. *J Biol Chem* 1987;262:15309–15315.
139. Uings IJ, Thompson NT, Randall RW, et al. *Biochem J* 1992;281:597–600.
140. Gu H, Trajkovic S, LaBelle EF. *Am J Physiol* 1992;262:C1376–C1383.
141. Anderson KM, Murahashi T, Dostal DE, Peach MJ. *Am J Physiol* 1993;264:C179–C188.
142. Griendling KK, Delafontaine P, Rittenhouse SE, Gimbrone MA Jr, Alexander RW. *J Biol Chem* 1987;262:14555–14562.
143. Hunyady L, Merelli F, Baukal AJ, Balla T, Catt KJ. *J Biol Chem* 1991;266:2783–2788.
144. Griendling KK, Berk BC, Alexander RW. *J Biol Chem* 1988;263:10620–10624.
145. Rao GN, Lassègue B, Griendling KK, Alexander RW, Berk BC. *Nucleic Acids Res* 1993;21:1259–1263.
146. Schwartzman M, Ferreri NR, Carroll MA, Songu-Mize E, McFiff JC. *Nature* 1985;314:620–622.
147. Resink TJ, Scott-Burden T, Buhler FR. *Biochem Biophys Res Commun* 1989;158:279–286.
148. Schlondorff D, DeCandido S, Satriano JA. *Am J Physiol* 1987;253:C113–C120.
149. Lang U, Vallotton MB. *Biochem J* 1989;259:477–484.
150. Alexander RW, Gimbrone MA Jr. *Proc Natl Acad Sci USA* 1976;73:1617–1620.
151. Khan WA, Blobe GC, Hannun YA. *J Biol Chem* 1992;267:3605–3612.
152. Miyake R, Gross RW. *Biochim Biophys Acta* 1992;1165:167–176.
153. Pfeilschifter J, Pignat W, Marki F, Wiesenberg I. *Eur J Biochem* 1989;181:237–242.
154. Lin L, Lin AY, Knopf JL. *Proc Natl Acad Sci USA* 1992;89:6147–6151.
155. Lin L, Wartmann M, Lin AY, Knopf JL, Seth A, Davis RJ. *Cell* 1993;72:268–278.
156. Jeremy JY, Dandona P. *Eur J Pharmacol* 1987;136:311–316.
157. Channon JY, Leslie CC. *J Biol Chem* 1990;265:5409–5413.
158. Griendling KK, Lassègue B, Alexander RW. *Thromb Haemost* 1993;70:188–192.
159. Berk BC, Alexander RW, Brock TA, Gimbrone MA Jr, Webb RC. *Science* 1986;232:87–90.
160. Bohr DF, Uchida E. *Circ Res* 1967;20,21(suppl 11):II-135–II-145.
161. Bohr DF, Goulet PL, Jaquini AC Jr. *Angiology* 1961;12:478–485.
162. Somlyo AV, Sandberg RL, Somlyo AP. *J Pharmacol Exp Ther* 1965;149:106–112.
163. McCalden TA, Bevan JA. *Am J Physiol* 1980;238:H618–H624.
164. Huxley AF, Niedergerke R. *Nature* 1954;173:971–973.
165. Hartshorne DJ, Gorecka A. In: Bohr DF, Somlyo AP, Sparks HV Jr, eds. *Handbook of physiology: the cardiovascular system*. Bethesda, MD: American Physiological Society, 1980;4:93–120.
166. Bennett J, Weeds A. *Br Med Bull* 1986;42:385–390.
167. Adelstein RS. In: Genest J, Kuchel O, Hamet P, Cantin M, eds. *Hypertension: physiopathology and treatment*. New York: McGraw Hill, 1983;524.
168. Klee CB, Crouch TH, Richman PG. *Annu Rev Biochem* 1980;49:489–515.
169. Adelstein RS, Eisenberg E. *Annu Rev Biochem* 1980;49:921–956.
170. Aksoy MO, Mras S, Kamm KE, Murphy RA. *Am J Physiol* 1983;245:C255–270.
171. Murphy RA, Aksoy MO, Dillon PF, Gerthoffer WT, Kamm KE. *Fed Proc* 1983;42:51–56.
172. Hathaway DR, March KL, Lash JA, Adam LP, Wilensky RL. *Circulation* 1991;83:382–390.
173. Smith CWJ, Pritchard K, Marston SB. *J Biol Chem* 1987;262:116–122.
174. Gluck E, Paul R. *Pflugers Arch* 1977;370:9–18.
175. Dillon PF, Aksoy MO, Driska SP, Murphy RA. *Science* 1981;211:495–497.
176. Danthuluri NR, Deth RC. *Biochem Biophys Res Commun* 1984;125:1103–1109.
177. Rasmussen H, Forder J, Kojima I, Scriabine A. *Biochem Biophys Res Commun* 1984;122:776–784.
178. Nishimura J, Khalil RA, Drenth JP, Van Breeman C. *Am J Physiol* 1990;259:H2–H8.
179. Ngai PK, Walsh MP. *Biochem J* 1987;244:417–425.
180. Rasmussen H, Takuwa Y, Park S. *FASEB J* 1987;1:177–185.
181. Fabiato A, Fabiato F. *J Physiol* 1978;276:233–255.
182. Langer GA. *Circ Res* 1985;57:374–382.
183. Tkachuk VA, Men'shikov MY. *Biokhimia* 1981;46:963–973.
184. Wray S. *Am J Physiol* 1988;254:C213–C225.
185. Friedman SM. In: Genest J, Kuchel O, Hamet P, Cantin M, eds. *Hypertension: physiopathology and treatment*. New York: McGraw-Hill, 1983;457–473.
186. Berecek KH, Schwertschlag V, Gross F. *Am J Physiol* 1980;238:H287–H293.
187. Bradshaw B, Moore TJ. *Hypertension* 1988;11:49–54.
188. Dawson R Jr, Oparil S. *Pharmacology* 1987;34:131–142.
189. Osani T, Dunn MJ. *Hypertension* 1992;19:446–455.
190. Resink TJ, Scott-Burden T, Baur U, Burgin M, Buhler FR. *Hypertension* 1989;14:293–303.
191. Thompson LP, Bruner CA, Lamb FS, King CM, Webb RC. *Am J Cardiol* 1987;59:29A–34A.
192. Cheung DW, MacKay MJ. *Biochem Biophys Res Commun* 1987;145:1105–1111.
193. Takaori K, Itoh S, Kanayama Y, Takeda T. *Biochem Biophys Res Commun* 1986;141:769–773.
194. Turla MB, Webb RC. *Hypertension* 1987;9(suppl III):III-150–III-154.
195. Berner PF, Somlyo AV, Somlyo AP. *J Cell Biol* 1981;88:96–101.

Hypertension: Pathophysiology, Diagnosis, and Management, Second Edition,
edited by J.H. Laragh and B.M. Brenner,
Raven Press, Ltd., New York © 1995.

CHAPTER 35

The Phosphoinositide Signaling System and the Pathogenesis of Hypertension

Jacqueline Ohanian and Anthony M. Heagerty

The fact that essential hypertension represents the upper echelons of a normal distribution curve implies that a cause is unlikely to be discovered that is present in patients placed above limits defined by risk and sets them apart from subjects falling below such levels. Even allowing for environmental interactions, the contribution from the genetic background of an individual is complex. Research endeavors are currently focusing on studies aimed at defining the genes that may control blood pressure, and the genes and cellular processes that control the adaptive structural changes observed in hypertensive patients and that have been shown to be prognostically important. It has to be conceded from the outset that some of the difficulty in trying to solve the puzzle of why some people have higher blood pressure than others resides in the need to examine cellular and subcellular processes, and the technology required has been developed only comparatively recently. Among these discoveries, the functional description of a relatively minor fraction of phospholipids, the phosphoinositides, located in the cell plasma membrane, has excited researchers in many disciplines. Recently, the key role of these lipids in signal transduction has been established and the major effectors of the signaling pathway described. In addition, evidence has accumulated that derangements of the phosphoinositide signaling system may occur in hypertension. This chapter summarizes the current state of knowledge about this system and examines its possible role in the genesis of hypertension.

PHOSPHOINOSITIDE LIPIDS

The inositol lipids are ubiquitously distributed, being predominantly located in the inner lamella of the plasma membrane (1) and more recently having been reported to be functionally active in the nuclear membrane (see below). The largest fraction comprises phosphatidylinositol (PtdIns), with small contributions from at least two others, namely, phosphatidylinositol 4-phosphate (PtdIns 4-P) and phosphatidylinositol 4,5-bisphosphate (PtdIns 4,5-P_2). Their synthesis occurs in the endoplasmic reticulum, and transport proteins then transfer them

J. Ohanian: Department of Medicine, University Hospital of South Manchester, West Didsbury, Manchester, M20 8LR, United Kingdom.
A. M. Heagerty: Department of Medicine, University Hospital of South Manchester, West Didsbury, Manchester, M20 8LR, United Kingdom.

to the plasma membrane (1). Specific membrane kinases can phosphorylate PtdIns in the 4-position to produce PtdIns 4-P, and then in the 5-position to yield PtdIns 4,5-P_2 (2). The activities of these enzymes are stimulated by Mg^{2+} and inhibited by Ca^{2+}. Monoesterases can dephosphorylate the polyphosphoinositides so that even when unstimulated the inositol lipids are constantly turning over in a futile cycle (3). There is little doubt that other similar lipids exist and as yet remain to be characterized. For example, the importance of the 3-phosphorylated polyphosphoinositol lipids has been recognized recently (4). These lipids are produced by PtdIns 3-kinases, which have been found in a variety of cell types (5,6). They have been implicated in mitogenesis (7) and signal transduction (5,6). The PtdIns 3-Ps are not substrates for PtdIns phospholipase C (PI-PLC), leading to speculation that they are signaling molecules in their own right (7). Little is known about the cellular targets of their action, although it has been shown recently that the ζ isoform of protein kinase C (PKC) is activated *in vitro* by PtdIns 3,4,5-P_3 (8).

Signaling Through the Hydrolysis of Phosphoinositol Lipids

Some G protein–linked receptors and tyrosine kinase receptors are coupled to these lipids; stimulation of such receptors results in the hydrolysis of PtdIns 4,5-P_2 by PI-PLC to produce two second messengers—inositol 1,4,5-trisphosphate (Ins 1,4,5-P_3) and 1,2-diacylglycerol (1,2-DAG). Inositol 1,4,5-trisphosphate is an effector of this system itself because it acts upon a specific receptor to release calcium from intracellular stores, which is the signal for many cellular responses such as secretion, cell proliferation, and the initiation of smooth muscle contraction (9). 1,2-diacylglycerol activates protein kinase C (PKC), which is implicated in many sustained responses such as proliferation (10). The individual components of these signaling systems are now known (Fig. 1). However, not shown in this figure is the diversity of each component; for instance, individual agonists act upon separate receptors, there are multiple G proteins (11) and large families of PLC (12), and inositol trisphosphate re-

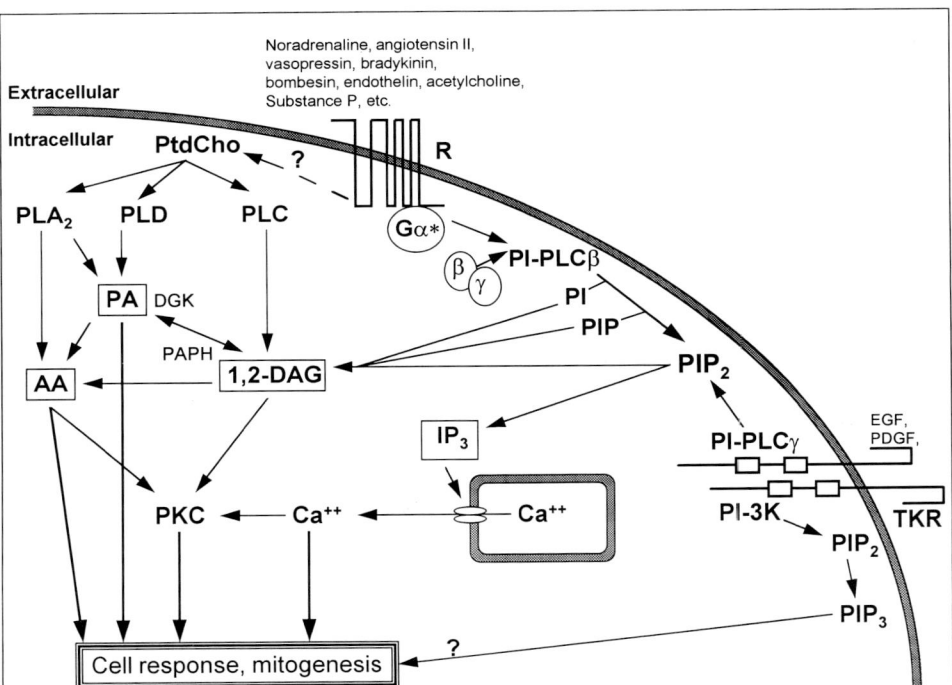

FIG. 1. Diagram summarizing the major receptor activated pathways for the formation of inositol 1,4,5-trisphosphate (IP_3) and 1,2-diacylglycerol (1,2–DAG). The binding of an agonist to a seven-membrane spanning receptor (R) results in the activation of PI-PLC-β, whereas the stimulation of tyrosine kinase receptors (TKR) by polypeptide growth factors will activate PI-PLC-γ. Both pathways result in the hydrolysis of PtdIns 4,5-P_2 (PIP_2) and the formation of IP_3 and 1,2-DAG. In addition, agonists that act on seven-membrane spanning receptors may stimulate phosphatidylcholine (PtdCho) hydrolysis, and activation of tyrosine kinase receptors will stimulate the production of PtdIns 3,4,5-P_3 (PIP_3). DGK, diacylglycerol kinase; PAPH, phosphatidic acid phosphohydrolase; Gα*, activated G protein α subunit (also for βγ subunits); PLD, phospholipase D; PLC, phospholipase C; PKC, protein kinase C; PI-3K, phosphatidylinositol 3-kinase; PI, phosphatidylinositol; PIP, phosphatidylinositol 4-phosphate; EGF, epidermal growth factor; PDGF, platelet-derived growth factor; PLA₂, phospholipase A₂; AA, arachidonic acid.

ceptor (9) and protein kinase C (13) exist. The significance of such diversity is not clear but may reflect modification of the basic signaling system to satisfy the unique needs of individual cells.

G Protein–Linked Receptors

The hormone receptors linked to the activation of PI-PLC belong to the family of seven-transmembrane-segment receptors that have no known enzymatic activity (14). Previous work on the adenylate cyclase signaling system has shown that receptors in this family act through a G protein linking the receptor to its effector, adenylate cyclase (15).

The G proteins involved in the regulation of PI-PLC are heterotrimeric guanosine triphosphate (GTP)-binding proteins composed of α, β, and γ subunits (16, 17). In response to receptor stimulation, the α subunit, which has guanosine triphosphatase (GTPase) activity, dissociates from the membrane-attached $\beta\gamma$ complex and activates the enzymes that generate second messengers (16). Such a system allows amplification of the agonist response, because a single ligand-bound receptor can interact with more than one G protein. Multiple families of G proteins have been identified; the greatest diversity has been found among the α subunits, which have been classified into four families: G_s, G_i/G_o, G_q, and G_{12} (11). Initially it was thought that the α subunits were responsible for activation of the effector, while the $\beta\gamma$ subunits played only a regulatory role (16). However, recent evidence has shown that the $\beta\gamma$ subunits can activate individual adenylyl cyclase isotypes differentially, and that specific $\beta\gamma$ subunits link to different receptor types (18). This has led to speculation that other effectors, such as phospholipases, are regulated by $\beta\gamma$ subunits (19). Indeed, it has been reported recently that PLC-β may be activated by $\beta\gamma$ subunits from transducin (20).

Evidence that G proteins are involved in the regulation of PI-PLC has come from many different types of experiments. Recently, Im and Graham (21) have purified the α_1-adrenergic receptor from rat liver and shown that it is linked to a 75-kDa G protein. However, the most convincing evidence has come from reconstitution studies showing that purified Gαq, Gα_{11}, Gα_{14}, Gα_{15}, and Gα_{16} will activate the PLC-β_1 isoform (22), and most of them activate the PLC-β_2 isoform (23). In addition, free $\beta\gamma$ subunits activate PLC-β_2 but not PLC-β_1 in both cotransfection and cell free assays (24,25), and recently it has been shown that interleukin-8 receptors couple preferentially with Gαq or Gα_{11} subunits, indicating specificity of receptors for G proteins (26).

Tyrosine Kinase Receptors

Polypeptide growth factors transmit signals through tyrosine kinase receptors, resulting in the production of Ins 1,4,5-P$_3$ and 1,2-DAG. Receptor tyrosine kinases contain four major domains: (a) an extracellular domain for the binding of ligand, (b) a tyrosine kinase domain mediating the biological response, (c) a transmembrane domain that spans the membrane a single time, and (d) one or more regulatory domains containing autophosphorylation sites. The fundamental response of growth factor receptors is mediated by their tyrosine kinase activity. Mutations that eliminate this activity abolish the biological function of the receptor (27). The other receptor domains serve to regulate the tyrosine kinase activity (28). Growth factors activate their corresponding receptors by inducing receptor dimerization and subsequent transphosphorylation at specific tyrosine residues (29). Such ligand-bound receptors associate physically with and phosphorylate a set of cytoplasmic proteins implicated in intracellular signal transduction pathways, including PI-PLC-γ_1 and phosphatidylinositol 3-kinase (30) (Fig. 1). PI 3-kinase phosphorylates the inositol ring of PtdIns at the D3 position, generating polyphosphoinositides that are resistant to PI-PLC hydrolysis (7). This enzyme is activated by adding platelet-derived growth factor (PDGF) or epidermal growth factor (EGF) to cells (30). However, little is known about the role of 3'-inositol phosphates in signaling. Growth factor stimulation results in the rapid activation of PI-PLC-γ_1 *in vivo* (31). Tyrosine phosphorylation of PLC appears to be essential but not sufficient for activation (32,33). Delivery of PLC to its substrate at the membrane may be one explanation for increased *in vivo* activity. PtdIns 4- and PtdIns 5-kinases also associate with the EGF receptor (34); these enzymes catalyze PtdIns 4,5-P$_2$ formation. Therefore, enzyme and substrate are assembled together to allow efficient production of the second messengers Ins 1,4,5-P$_3$ and 1,2-DAG.

Phosphoinositol Phospholipase C

The release of Ins 1,4,5-P$_3$ from PtdIns 4,5-P$_2$ is achieved by the activation of PLC. Several distinct PI-PLC enzymes have been purified from a variety of mammalian tissues (the reader is referred to three recent reviews—12,35,36).

There are at least three families of genes in the PI-PLC superfamily designated β, γ, and δ, and each type contains more than one subtype (12,35). The β, γ, and δ isotypes contain two limited regions of sequence homology, named regions X and Y (35). PLC-β and -δ contain short sequences of 50 to 70 amino acids separating the X and Y regions. PLC-γ has a long sequence of approximately 400 amino acids between these regions, which contains Src homology domains (termed SH2 and SH3). These are considered necessary for binding to tyrosine kinase receptors (37). Also, single polypeptide PLCs with molecular masses of 62 to 68 kDa have been purified (35), with an area of weak homology (32–35 percent) to region X (38). These smaller enzymes were named PLC-α. However, Srivastava et al. (39) have shown that the putative PLC-α cDNA actually encodes a thiol:protein-disulfide oxidoreductase that carries no PLC activity. It is believed now that the 62- to 68-kDa enzymes may be proteolytic fragments derived from PLC-β, -γ and -δ isotypes (12). Deletion mutagenesis showed that both regions X and Y were necessary for catalytic activity (40) and presumably represent the active site. The profound structural differences between the isotypes suggest that individual isotypes may (a) play distinctive cellular roles, (b) have different cellular locations, or (c) differ in the regulation of their activity. All the isotypes are known to be phosphoproteins (41–43) and serve as substrates for protein kinases *in vivo* (38,42,44). No alteration of enzyme activity as a result of phosphorylation has been detected *in vitro,* suggesting phosphorylation may affect interaction of the enzyme with activator(s) or substrates (45). PI-PLC-γ_1 is involved in the hydrolysis of phosphoinositides following growth factor stimulation of receptor tyrosine kinases (31). The PLC-βs mediate the effects of agonists that act through G protein–linked receptors (46). Neither the receptors nor the transducer that are coupled to any of the PLC-δs are known. The functional roles of these distinctive isotypes are not understood.

The three major classes of PI-PLC—β, γ, and δ—require inositol lipids as substrates specifically (35). They hydrolyze PtdIns, PtdIns 4-P and PtdIns 4,5-P_2, although PtdIns 4-P and PtdIns 4,5-P_2 are the preferred substrates. The selectivity for PtdIns 4,5-P_2 over PtdIns decreases in the order PLC-β_1 > PLC-δ_1 > PLC-γ_1 (12). The catalytic activities of all three classes of PI-PLC are dependent on calcium. In addition, the substrate preference of the isotypes is affected by pH such that at low pH, PtdIns hydrolysis predominates, changing at neutral pH when PI-PLC-β_1 hydrolysis of PtdIns 4,5-P_2 is favored (35). These differences may provide a mechanism by which cells regulate the isotypes activated and the substrates hydrolyzed. It is not known if such conditions are found *in vivo.*

Recently, the PI-PLC isoenzymes present in smooth muscle have been purified and characterized. Kato et al. (47) have identified PI-PLC-γ_1 and -δ_1 in the aorta of Wistar-Kyoto (WKY) rats. The catalytic fragment PI-PLC-α and a second, different molecular weight protein with PLC activity were demonstrated in rat aortic smooth muscle cells (48). Bovine iris sphincter smooth muscle has been shown to contain PI-PLC-γ_1, -β_1, and -δ_1 (49). Indeed, it has been proposed that sequential activation of different PI-PLC enzymes could occur during agonist stimulation (48). These conclusions are based on measurements of intracellular pH (pH$_i$) and calcium changes in cultured vascular smooth muscle cells in response to angiotensin II, where an initial acidification ac-

companied by elevated calcium was followed by a prolonged alkalinization while calcium levels returned to baseline (50–52). However, care must be taken when extrapolating these results to intact smooth muscle preparations, as Izzard and Heagerty (53) have shown acidification of small artery pH$_i$ during agonist stimulation, which is maintained throughout the response. These conditions may favor different PI-PLC isotypes in the intact tissue. PI-PLC isotypes have predominantly been isolated from cytosolic preparations, although membrane-bound enzymes PI-PLC-β_1, -γ, and -α have been detected (35,38,54). The abundance of cytosolic enzyme raises the possibility that PLC must translocate to the membrane in order to act upon its substrate. The mechanisms for translocation are unknown, but may represent a way of regulating PLC-dependent second messenger generation.

Inositol Phosphates

The activation of phospholipase C and hydrolysis of PtdIns 4,5-P_2 produces Ins 1,4,5-P_3. This compound is water soluble and diffuses into the cytoplasm where it acts on a specific receptor to release calcium from intracellular stores (9). In smooth muscle, this is the early signal, providing sufficient calcium to initiate contraction (55); in other tissues, liberation of calcium in this way is the primary step in evoking physiologic responses. The metabolism of inositol phosphates is extremely complex. For instance, including the cyclic inositol phosphates, the upper limit for the possible number of these compounds is currently considered to be 66 (56). Here, we confine ourselves to the immediate metabolism of Ins 1,4,5-P_3.

There are two alternate routes for the metabolism of Ins 1,4,5-P_3, both of which result in complete dephosphorylation. One of these is the removal of the 5-phosphate by a phosphomonoesterase (5-phosphatase) to produce Ins 1,4-P_2. The other route is the so-called tris-tetrakis pathway, which involves sequential phosphorylation and dephosphorylation to Ins 1,3,4-P_3 via the intermediary inositol 1,3,4,5-tetrakisphosphate (Ins 1,3,4,5-P_4). Effectively, both pathways terminate Ins 1,4,5-P_3 activity because the Ins 1,3,4-P_3 isomer has low affinity for the Ins 1,4,5-P_3 receptor (57). The proposal that Ins 1,3,4,5-P_4 may act in concert with Ins 1,4,5-P_3 to maintain elevated intracellular calcium levels during agonist stimulation (58) led to considerable research into the enzymes 5-phosphatase and 3-kinase. However, whether Ins 1,3,4,5-P_4 has a physiologic role in calcium regulation *in vivo* is currently under debate (59).

Both 5-phosphatase and 3-kinase are widely distributed (60). There is some evidence that 5-phosphatase is stimulated by protein kinase C, but this effect is so far limited to platelets, possibly due to a specific isoform (61). Various groups have shown that 3-kinase is activated by elevated calcium through an interaction with calmodulin and is subject to proteolysis by calpain (60). In addition, it is phosphorylated by protein kinase C, leading to deactivation (62). The relative contribution of these two enzymes to the metabolism of Ins 1,4,5-P$_3$ *in vivo* has not been resolved satisfactorily. In fact, it is difficult to determine which pathway is favored in intact cells because the extremely rapid flux in inositol phosphates makes it necessary to use unphysiologically high doses of agonists in order to amplify the response, so that significant changes in Ins 1,4,5-P$_3$ can be measured. Obviously, under these conditions the levels of inositol phosphates will be higher than the levels the cell normally achieves *in vivo,* and this will alter the normal pattern of metabolism in itself.

There are two principal intracellular calcium channels responsible for mobilizing stored calcium, the Ins P$_3$ and ryanodine receptors, which have considerable structural and functional homology (63,64). The cloning of the Ins P$_3$ receptor has resulted in the identification of a family of receptors that arise from alternative splicing (65,66) and as separate gene products (67). The amino terminal end of the receptor contains the Ins 1,4,5-P$_3$ binding site, and the carboxyl terminal end is responsible for tetramerization and presumably calcium channel formation (68,69). These receptors are mainly located on portions of the endoplasmic reticulum, presumably at the sites of calcium stores (70). The binding of Ins 1,4,5-P$_3$ induces a conformational change in the receptor that may be related to the coupling process leading to channel opening (68). The mechanisms involved in Ins P$_3$–induced calcium release are complex and beyond the scope of this chapter. The reader is referred to two recent reviews for further discussion of this topic (9,59).

1,2-Diacylglycerol

The lipid product of phospholipase C–mediated hydrolysis of any inositol lipid is 1,2-sn-diacylglycerol. Functionally, it is recognized to be the physiological activator of protein kinase C (PKC), an 80-kDa, Ca^{2+}, and phospholipid-dependent serine-threonine kinase present in eukaryotic cells. 1,2-Diacylglycerol increases the affinity of PKC for Ca^{2+} and phosphatidylserine, thereby allowing enzyme activation. The efficiency of 1,2-DAG in terms of PKC activation is dependent on the degree of unsaturation of the fatty acids in the 1 and 2 positions on the glycerol backbone. Those species derived from inositol lipids are enriched with arachidonate and 16 or 18 carbon-chain fatty acids and are particularly useful in this context. It is of interest currently that 1,2-DAG can

be produced from other phospholipids, for instance phosphatidylcholine (PtdCho), by agonist-stimulated PLC or phospholipase D (PLD) activation. PtdCho contains more diverse fatty acids than PtdIns, in particular less arachidonate and more oleate, linoleate, and palmitate (71). Therefore, the 1,2-DAG species released will differ, depending on the phospholipid hydrolyzed. The significance of this is not certain, and it is not known if the diglycerides released by PtdCho can activate PKC.

Leach et al. (72) demonstrated that hydrolysis of PtdCho and increased 1,2-DAG derived from this lipid did not activate PKC in fibroblasts. However, as discussed in the section on PKC, specific PKC isotypes may be activated by 1,2-DAG in the absence of elevated calcium; therefore, extrapolation of these data in fibroblasts to other cell types expressing different and/or additional PKCs may not be valid. Also, it must be borne in mind that PKC may not be the sole or prime determinant of an agonist-induced cellular function, and, furthermore, the assumption that 1,2-DAG levels are increased during inositol lipid hydrolysis may not be valid. Rembold and Weaver (73) found no measurable sustained histamine- or endothelin-induced increase in DAG mass in swine arterial smooth muscle, and we have shown no accumulation of inositol-derived 1,2-DAG species in intact rat small arteries stimulated with vasopressin or noradrenaline (74). However, others have found an increased DAG mass in stimulated vascular smooth muscle (75,76).

There are two major routes for the breakdown of phosphoinositol-derived 1,2-DAG: diacylglycerol kinase, which converts 1,2-DAG to phosphatidic acid, and deacylation by di- and monoglyceride lipases, which leads to a variety of arachidonic acid metabolites. The predominant pathway is tissue-specific (although in many cell lines diacylglycerol kinase appears to be more important [77]) and contributes to the deactivation of PKC, supplies precursors for inositol lipid resynthesis, and produces phosphatidic acid, which has cellular functions of its own (60,78). Diacylglycerol-kinase activity is found in both cytosolic and membrane fractions of cell extracts, and the enzyme is translocated to the membrane in response to increasing levels of substrate. In addition, it is a target for phosphorylation by adenosine 3′,5′-cyclic monophosphate (cyclic AMP)–dependent kinase, Ca^{2+}-calmodulin–dependent kinase, and PKC (79).

The pattern of 1,2-DAG metabolism appears to be agonist-specific (74). For example, angiotensin II causes accumulation of 1,2-DAG and subsequent PKC activation, whereas norepinephrine produces stimulation of diacylglycerol kinase and the accumulation of phosphatidic acid (74). In this context, there has been much interest in angiotensin II being a pressure-independent trophic factor, which is able to promote hypertrophy by increasing membrane levels of 1,2-DAG or PKC activation (80). Again, it is clear that isoforms of diacylglycerol kinase exist. A membrane-associated arachidonoyl-specific DAG kinase has recently been identified (81) that may play a role in metabolism of inositol-derived 1,2-DAG.

Phosphatidic Acid

Phosphatidic acid (PA) is essential for the formation of all phospholipids, and yet is present in minor quantities in nonstimulated cells (82). Accumulation of this lipid has been shown in many cells and intact tissues following agonist stimulation (74,83). Recent studies have demonstrated that the production of PA during receptor-induced inositol lipid hydrolysis is agonist specific; for instance, norepinephrine or phenylephrine stimulate large increases in this lipid, whereas angiotensin II does not in vascular smooth muscle (74,83).

Many roles have been ascribed to PA. When added extracellularly it stimulates PLC and induces DNA synthesis in cultured cells (78), although some of these effects have been ascribed to lyso-phosphatidic acid contamination (84). It increases intracellular calcium and may be involved in vascular smooth muscle contraction (85). Phosphatidic acid produced within the inner membrane leaflet may also have a biological function. Recently, two types of ras-regulatory proteins, GTPase-activating protein (GAP) and a GTPase-inhibiting protein (GIP), have been shown in vitro to be sensitive to PA (86,87). The ras genes were first discovered as retroviral oncogenes and have subsequently been found to be activated in some 30 percent of human tumors. The proteins that they encode are key regulators of cellular growth: 21-kDa guanine nucleotide–binding proteins, which cycle between the active, growth promoting, GTP-bound state, and the inactive, guanosine diphosphate (GDP)-bound form (88). This cycle is regulated by a number of proteins: GAPs, which stimulate the hydrolysis of GTP on ras and speed up its inactivation, counterbalanced by GIPs, which promote the loss of bound GDP and uptake of fresh GTP from the cytosol, so reactivating ras. Stearate-arachidonate–containing species of PA inhibit GAP activity (86), while stearate-arachidonate-PA and 1,2-DAG (dilinolein) activate GIP activity in vitro (87), the net result being that receptor-coupled production of 1,2-DAG and PA, preferentially derived from inositol lipids, would alter the equilibrium of the ras-GAP-GIP system, biasing it toward GIP dominance. The in vivo consequences of this effect are not known, but these data provide evidence for a link between hormone-stimulated inositol lipid hydrolysis and the cellular ras proteins that may be critical in the control of proliferation.

Phosphatidic acid influences enzymes in the inositol lipid cycle. Phospholipase C is stimulated by PA (89,90), and it is a specific activator of phosphatidylinositol-4-phosphate kinase promoting the formation of PtdIns 4,5-P_2 (91). These data suggest that hormone-stimulated elevations of membrane PA may initiate a synergistic activation of PtdIns P kinase and PI-PLC, providing a powerful positive feedback signal for the amplification of cellular responses.

Yet another role for PA has been suggested following the observation that PA-dependent protein phosphorylation occurs in soluble extracts from rat liver, brain, lung, and testis (92). The phosphorylation pattern promoted by PA was distinct from that observed with 1,2-DAG and phosphatidylserine, indicating involvement of a kinase other than PKC. Furthermore, phosphorylation was stimulated by free calcium in the range 360 to 800 nM, which is within the levels of intracellular calcium attained during agonist stimulation (93). The identity of the PA-dependent kinase is unknown, and activity has yet to be shown in intact preparations.

Arachidonic Acid

Inositol phospholipids are highly enriched with arachidonic acid at the Sn-2 position on the glycerol backbone. This eicosanoid is the precursor of cyclooxygenase- and lipoxygenase-derived prostaglandins and leukotrienes, and an increase in the release of arachidonic acid and in the production of prostaglandins has been demonstrated following agonist-evoked breakdown of polyphosphoinositides.

Two major routes for the production of arachidonic acid from phospholipids have been proposed: (a) PI-PLC hydrolysis of inositol lipids releasing arachidonate enriched 1,2-DAG, followed by sequential deacylation by DAG-lipases; and (b) phospholipase A_2 (PLA$_2$) hydrolysis of phospholipids to release arachidonate directly. The main evidence for the former has come from studies in platelets (94). However, recently this pathway has been shown unequivocally to mediate bradykinin-induced release of arachidonate in dorsal root ganglion neurons in primary culture (95). A high-molecular-weight (85.2 kDa) cytosolic PLA$_2$, which selectively hydrolyzes arachidonate-containing phospholipids, has been purified from several sources and a full-length cDNA clone that encodes it has been purified and sequenced (96,97). Cytosolic PLA$_2$ is activated by free Ca^{2+} (0.1–1 μmol), which is within the concentration achieved during agonist stimulation (98,99). Elevated cytosolic calcium concentration also causes translocation of the enzyme from the cytosol to its active site at the membrane (98). Phospholipase A_2 is activated in cells by EGF and PDGF (100). In addition, phorbol esters and membrane-permeant diacylglycerols provoke arachidonic acid release, suggesting PKC may be involved in PLA$_2$ activation (101).

Both free arachidonic acid and its metabolites have been implicated in many cellular processes. Recent reports support the involvement of lipoxygenase metabolites of arachidonic acid in the activation of K^+ channels in a variety of cells ranging from mollusc neurons to mammalian platelets (102–104). Stimulation of mitogenesis by growth factors is accompanied by marked changes in lipid turnover, including release and metabolism of arachidonic acid. A primary response gene, TIS10, which can be superinduced by mitogenic stimuli, encodes an active cyclooxygenase (prostaglandin G/H synthase), suggesting an involvement of prostaglandins in mitogenic control (105). Noncyclooxygenase metabolites of arachidonic acid may also play a role in modulating proliferation induced by various factors, including EGF in Syrian hamster embryo cells and rat mesangial cells (106,107), and angiotensin II in bovine adrenocortical cells (108). In addition, free arachidonic acid has been implicated in smooth muscle contraction, possibly by increasing the sensitivity of the contractile apparatus to calcium (109), although the mechanisms involved are not known.

The Protein Kinase C Family

Protein kinase C, an enzyme widely regarded as a key regulator of cellular homeostasis, was discovered by Nishizuka and co-workers in 1977 (110). The activation of PKC by various hormones, growth factors, neurotransmitters, and phorbol esters is associated with cell signaling events (10,111). Upon receptor-stimulation the enzyme translocates from the cytosol to the membrane, where it is activated by calcium and phospholipid (112). It is known now that there is a gene family coding for several closely related, yet unique enzymes that constitute the PKCs. The reason(s) for PKC heterogeneity are not yet understood. Protein kinase C activation by 1,2-DAG, generated by agonist-stimulated phosphoinositide hydrolysis, is well established. The potential for isoenzyme-specific activation by 1,2-DAG and free fatty acids generated from other phospholipid sources during receptor-activation is currently being investigated (113,114).

Ten subspecies of PKC have been identified in mammalian tissues. These isotypes have been classified into three groups according to differences in their mode of activation (115 and references therein). Group A consists of the classic PKCs (cPKC): α, βI and βII, and γ. Group B consists of the new PKCs (nPKC): δ, ϵ, Γ (L), and θ. Group C consists of two atypical PKCs (aPKC): ζ and λ. The group A PKC enzymes have four conserved (C_1–C_4) and five variable (V_1–V_5) regions. The functions of the conserved regions have now been identified: C_1 is a putative membrane binding site (116), C_2 is related to the calcium sensitivity, C_3 contains the catalytic site, and C_4 appears to be necessary for substrate recognition (115).

These enzymes are activated by calcium, phosphatidylserine, 1,2-DAG, and phorbol esters. In addition, cis-unsaturated acids (e.g., arachidonate) potentiate their activation. The group B enzymes lack the C_2 region and do not require calcium for activation. These enzymes are activated by phosphatidylserine, 1,2-DAG, and phorbol esters (114,117,118). Differences within the group in the susceptibility to cis-unsaturated fatty acids have been shown such that ϵ is, but δ is not, activated by these lipids (118,119). The group B enzymes have been implicated in regulation of nuclear events stimulated by growth factors (120). The group C enzymes have only one cysteine-rich zinc-finger-like region in the C_1 domain and are activated by phosphatidylserine, but not 1,2-DAG, phorbol esters, or calcium. The signaling system to which these enzymes are linked is not known. These differences suggest that co-expressed PKC isotypes would act in parallel rather than interchangeably. Agonist-stimulated hydrolysis of PtdIns 4,5-P_2 will produce different molecular species of 1,2-DAG to those formed from PtdCho breakdown. In addition, the former will elevate intracellular calcium levels. In these circumstances different PKC isotypes may be activated depending on the phospholipid hydrolyzed. Also, it is possible to speculate that the target proteins phosphorylated would change during the response as the initial calcium burst decayed and intracellular calcium levels returned toward the baseline. Through these interactions the cellular response to activation of PKC could be tailored to a specific agonist.

Our knowledge of specific functions of the individual PKC isotypes is still limited. There is evidence to suggest that some members of the PKC family, in particular δ, may function in the regulation of the cell cycle (121). In the membrane, PKCs have been implicated in downregulation of receptors, modulation of ion channels, release of hormones and neurotransmitters, and exocytosis (10). Recently, diacylglycerol kinase has been identified as a substrate for PKC-ϵ, suggesting this enzyme may modulate the PtdIns cycle (122). A role for PKC in sustained vascular smooth muscle contraction has also been proposed (75), although conclusive evidence for this remains elusive.

Smooth Muscle Contraction

Once a vasoconstrictor agonist occupies its receptor, Ins 1,4,5-P_3 is released into the cytoplasm and stimulates the release of calcium from the sarcoplasmic reticulum of smooth muscle. The resulting increase in intracellular calcium concentration may be potentiated by the release of calcium bound to the inside of the plasma membrane, another function influenced by phosphoinositide metabolism (123). Inositol 1,4,5-trisphosphate–stimulated calcium release is detectable within seconds of receptor activation (124) and is of sufficient magnitude to initiate tension development via calcium-calmodulin–mediated activation of myosin light chain kinase (125,126). The exact site of calcium release from sarcoplasmic reticulum may vary, depending upon the length of agonist stimulation (127). Similarly, the exact mechanism by which a contraction is maintained is unclear; activation of the phosphoinositide signaling system is not the only way smooth muscle can be made to contract (128,129). Indeed, membrane depolarization and stretch are two other activating stimuli.

Nevertheless, it appears that neurotransmitters and other pressor stimuli act through Ins 1,4,5-P$_3$ and both functional and kinetic studies have demonstrated that Ins 1,4,5-P$_3$–induced calcium release is rapid enough to account for initiation of smooth muscle contraction (130). The mechanisms sustaining contraction are less clearly defined. Phorbol ester irreversible activators, and cell-permeant diglyceride physiological activators of PKC cause sustained smooth muscle contraction (131,132). However, whether PKC is involved in physiological smooth muscle contraction remains controversial. Both calcium-dependent (group A) and calcium-independent (group B) isotypes have been identified in rat uterus and ferret aorta (133,134), and it has been suggested that the α_1-adrenergic agonist phenylephrine activates a calcium-independent PKC to induce sustained contraction (135). Phorbol ester–induced contractions of rabbit thoracic aorta and porcine carotid artery were accompanied by an increase in cytosolic calcium (136,137). In other vascular smooth muscle preparations, cytosolic calcium was unchanged during phorbol ester–induced contraction (138). Protein kinase C does not appear to regulate contraction through an effect on myosin light chain 20 phosphorylation (134). Indeed, it is uncertain if PKC is activated during physiological contraction in intact preparations. In porcine coronary arteries histamine and endothelin do not increase 1,2-DAG mass (139), and in rat subcutaneous arteries vasopressin decreases arachidonate-containing DAG levels during sustained contraction (74), although others have found increased DAG levels in smooth muscle during agonist stimulation (140).

Recently it has been shown that agonists that act through the hydrolysis of phosphoinositides can increase force in a calcium-independent manner (141). This effect is G protein–linked, and arachidonic acid has been proposed as a mediator of the response (109,142). The origin of the arachidonate has not been shown, although, as previously discussed, agonists that stimulate PtdIns 4,5-P$_2$ breakdown also may increase arachidonate release, providing evidence for sustained contraction through this mechanism.

Nuclear Phosphoinositides

In addition to the plasma membrane, the nucleus contains an autonomous phosphoinositol signaling system. It contains the kinases necessary to phosphorylate PtdIns

and PtdIns 4-P, PLC-β, and DAG kinase (143–146). Insulin-like growth factor-1 stimulates inositol lipid hydrolysis resulting in increased Ins 1,4,5-P$_3$ and DAG within the nucleus in Swiss 3T3 cells (144). Recently, Martelli and co-workers (147) demonstrated that this effect was due to activation of nuclear PLC-β. The purpose of this signaling system within the nucleus is not known. Increased PKC has been found in the nucleus of insulin-like growth factor-1–stimulated Swiss 3T3 cells with a time course similar to the appearance of 1,2-DAG (144). This suggests that nuclear PtdIns hydrolysis could be involved in the control of the phosphorylation of intranuclear proteins, such as components of chromatin, the nuclear lamina, or gene regulatory elements, making this one of the most intriguing areas of phosphoinositol research.

Cell Growth and Proliferation

Within a fully-developed multicellular organism most cells are nondividing, but they may return to the cell cycle when challenged by mitogens. When cells divide, an ordered process is followed that results in DNA synthesis and mitosis (148,149). However, mitosis is not an immediate cellular response following the application of a mitogen. There is a prolonged phase, G$_1$, before the inception of DNA replication at the outset of the S phase. During G$_1$, there is a rapid increase in mRNA activity that occurs very early after mitogenic stimulation (150), with a consequent rise in protein synthesis; at the same time there is phosphorylation of ribosomal proteins (149). Both of these events seem to be important, because blocking them leads to an attenuation of the growth process. However, progression through the cell cycle to cell division is not inevitable following mitogen stimulation. Growth factors must be present throughout the G$_1$ phase and some cells, for instance cardiac myocytes, are unable to divide, and so hypertrophy occurs rather than proliferation.

The events leading to cell growth (hypertrophy and proliferation) can be divided into three phases: extracellular stimuli and receptors, intracellular signal transduction pathways and activation of nuclear transcription factors leading to activation or repression of target genes. Mitogenic stimuli can be divided into two groups: the polypeptide growth factors such as PDGF, EGF, and basic fibroblast growth factor, which act upon receptors with intrinsic tyrosine kinase activity; and factors such as α_1-adrenergic agonists, angiotensin II, endothelin, bombesin, and bradykinin, which act on G protein–coupled receptors (151,152). Despite the remarkable diversity in these mitogens and their signal transduction systems, there is remarkable similarity in the response such that virtually all mitogens lead to the rapid and transient activation of one or a pair of 42- to 44-kDa mitogen-activated protein (MAP) kinase family members (153–155). Recently, major advances have been made in understanding the links in the signaling system leading from tyrosine kinase receptor activation to nuclear events and DNA synthesis (156). A detailed discussion of this kinase cascade is outside the scope of this chapter but the interested reader is referred elsewhere (155–157).

The phosphoinositol-derived signals Ins 1,4,5-P$_3$ and 1,2-DAG are common to both mitogen-activated pathways, but there is conflicting evidence concerning their role in promoting cell growth. In some cells increased PtdIns turnover is not sufficient stimulus to induce mitogenesis; for instance, Chinese hamster lung fibroblasts transfected with M$_1$-muscarinic receptors responded to carbachol with an increase in inositol phosphate release and *fos* and *myc* induction, but there was no DNA synthesis (157). In contrast, the same M$_1$ receptors was mitogenic in CHO cells (158). Antibodies directed against PLC inhibited fibroblast proliferation (159), whereas injection of PLC-β or PLC-γ stimulated DNA synthesis (160).

Phorbol esters are potent mitogens (148,149), suggesting that the 1,2-DAG/PKC pathway is involved in proliferation. Indeed, prolonged treatment with cell-permeable diglyceride and ionophore to mimic Ins 1,4,5-P$_3$–induced calcium release will activate lymphocytes (9). Down-regulation of PKC inhibits the activation of MAP kinase in response to agents that stimulate the M$_1$-muscarinic receptor but not to growth factors, implying that PKC is involved in the mitogenic response to G protein but not tyrosine kinase receptor stimulation (161). α_1-Agonists induce cardiac hypertrophy *in vivo* (162) and *in vitro* (163). In neonatal cardiomyocytes they induce expression of the β isoform of the myosin heavy chain (164), overexpression of PKC-β, but not -α also induced β-MHC expression (165), implying that at least one isoform of PKC is involved in cardiac hypertrophy.

Further evidence for the involvement of the PtdIns system in cell growth comes from measurement of cytosolic calcium during mitogenic stimulation. In fertilized eggs and lymphocytes, persistent repetitive calcium oscillations are observed lasting for several hours (166) in which Ins 1,4,5-P$_3$ plays a central role (9). Calcium is important for mitogenesis as shown by inhibition of cell growth by calcium channel blockers (167) or low extracellular calcium (166). Among other roles it is involved in the activation of certain isoforms of PKC and activated MAP kinase (168). In addition, there is evidence that nuclear calcium increases dramatically following mitogenic stimuli (169). However, there is no evidence as yet for Ins P$_3$ receptors on the inner nuclear membrane; therefore, whether Ins 1,4,5-P$_3$ is involved in the elevation of nuclear calcium levels is unknown.

Phosphoinositide Metabolism and Hypertension

Abnormalities in phosphoinositide signaling lipids could be responsible for the triggering mechanism that generates raised pressure (if present in the central nervous system, for example) or for an exaggerated adaptive-growth response in genetically hypertension-prone individuals or animals.

Much of the early work on this system centered around the measurement of membrane inositol phospholipid content and the rate of ^{32}P incorporation into the phosphoinositides. Abnormalities were found in red blood cell membranes from hypertensive patients, the phosphoinositide lipid content was low (170), and the rate of ^{32}P incorporation into PtdIns 4,5-P$_2$ was raised, implying enhanced turnover (170,171). This effect may be dependent on the stage of the disease, as Riozzi et al. (172) showed enhanced turnover of phosphoinositides in the normotensive offspring of hypertensive subjects, which was slightly reduced when the blood pressure was established. In spontaneously hypertensive rats (SHRs), Kiselev et al. (173) reported an increase in PtdIns 4-P content at 4 weeks and a lower ^{32}P incorporation rate into polyphosphoinositides. In older rats, similar findings are also recorded (174–176), although results do appear to be age-dependent (173). More recent studies have concentrated on measurement of inositol phosphate production in order to determine whether hyperactivity of the system occurs in hypertension. Radiolabeling of tissues or cells with ^{3}H-myoinositol has resulted in detailed studies of both total inositol phosphates and separation into Ins 4-P, Ins 1,4-P$_2$, and Ins 1,4,5-P$_3$. The data obtained from these studies with respect to basal inositol phosphate production are conflicting. In the SHR two studies have reported no difference in basal inositol phosphates in cultured fibroblasts (177) or cultured mesangial and mesenteric myocytes (178). However, in erythrocytes and aorta there were higher levels of Ins 1,4,5-P$_3$ in SHRs compared to WKY rats (47,179), but this was not seen in mesenteric arteries from SHRs (180) at either 5 weeks or 12 weeks of age. Coarctation of the aorta in the rat resulted in a sustained elevation of inositol phosphates in the aorta proximal to the ligature but not in mesenteric arteries also exposed to elevated pressure (181). Furthermore, in a perinephritic model of hypertension, basal inositol phosphates in the aorta were not changed throughout the development of hypertension (182). The reasons for these differences are unclear. However, a consensus does emerge following agonist challenge in hypertensive tissues. Certainly the accumulation of inositol phosphates in response to norepinephrine and angiotensin II is elevated in SHR (177,178,180) compared with WKY and to norepinephrine in perinephritic hypertension (182), suggesting hyperactivity of PLC.

Indeed, there are a number of reports of abnormalities of PLC in hypertension. In SHR it has been demonstrated that there is a restriction fragment-length polymorphism in PLC genes when compared with those from normotensive WKY rats (183). The same group has shown that the restriction fragment length polymorphism band is present in the PLC-δ genomic locus of SHR and stroke-prone SHR (SHR-SP) but not in Sprague-Dawley, Donryu, and WKY normotensive animals (184). DNA sequencing of PLC-δ complementary DNA cloned from an aortic complementary DNA library of SHR revealed three SHR-specific point mutations, two of which result in amino acid substitutions (184). The significance of these findings remains to be established. The authors contend that the amino acid substitutions may explain the enhanced PLC activity in hypertension reported by others (185–187). Certainly it is of interest that the PLC isoform studied by Yagisawa et al. (184) was classified as the δ_1 subtype. Recently, Kato et al. (47) reported hyperactivity of this PLC isoform in the aorta of SHR from 7 to 12 weeks of age, when blood pressure is beginning to rise and becoming established. Furthermore, these authors report that SHR PLC-δ_1 is activated at lower calcium concentrations than that of the WKY enzyme (47). Others have reported that SHR PLC has a different pH dependency (187). Measurements of PLC activity as assessed by hydrolysis of PtdIns 4,5-P$_2$ have been less clear. Makita and Yasuda (188) found no differences in the myocardium at 4 weeks and found depressed hydrolysis at 20 weeks. The latter time period is consistent with some form of pressure-induced down-regulation of inositol lipid breakdown, which has been suggested by data from other groups investigating SHR vascular tissues (180,189,190). In other, pressure-independent tissues, overactive inositol breakdown continues to be observed (191), although this may be dependent on the agonist applied (178).

A number of studies have shown that smooth muscle cells from SHRs cultured in the presence of fetal calf serum proliferate more rapidly and are more numerous at confluency than cells from normotensive WKY rats (192–194). Several reactive pathways are implicated in the onset of proliferation (see above), including tyrosine kinase activation and the hydrolysis of inositol lipids. It has been suggested that hyperactive PLC may be involved in the enhanced proliferative response. However, recently two studies have failed to demonstrate that increased PLC activity is linked to enhanced serum-induced proliferation (195,196), and this trait has not been shown to co-segregate with blood pressure in recent breeding studies (197).

Interest has also developed in the second arm of the phosphoinositide signaling system: the 1,2-DAG/PKC pathway. The development of a sensitive assay for the quantitation of 1,2-DAG (198) has facilitated accurate measurements of this lipid in many tissues. Currently, it is of great interest that 1,2-DAG be produced from other phospholipids such as PtdCho by the agonist-stimulated activation of PLC or PLD (113). In SHR or SHR-SP platelets, the metabolism of PtdCho has been reported to increase even at a prehypertensive stage (199). However, there seems little doubt that inositol-derived diacyl-glycerol is the predominant lipid. Indeed, during the development of left ventricular hypertrophy in SHR myocardium, no evidence of increased PtdCho or phosphatidylethanolamine hydrolysis has been reported. However, in the early stages of left ventricular hypertrophy, mass levels of 1,2-DAG are increased, suggesting a possible pathogenic role of inositol lipid metabolism in this process (200,201). In addition, the diacylglycerol content of the myocardium has been observed to increase in the early stages of diabetic cardiomyopathy and BIO 14.4 myopathic hamsters (202,203). The phospholipid source of 1,2-DAG was not determined in any of these studies. Two studies have been reported from the SHR thoracic aorta (47,204). No significant difference was found in phosphatidylethanolamine or PtdCho (204). Again, at an early prehypertensive point (4 weeks), the 1,2-DAG content of the SHR aorta was significantly increased. This difference had disappeared at 20 weeks of age (204). Again, the parent lipid source was not determined. In the second study, 1,2-DAG levels were increased at 12 weeks but not at 7 weeks (47), implying cyclic changes during the development of hypertension. An increase in 1,2-DAG has also been reported in SHR platelets (203).

There is some evidence for increased production of 1,2-DAG in the SHR during agonist stimulation. Kondo et al. (205) showed enhanced 1,2-DAG levels in the aorta of SHR compared with WKY controls during norepinephrine stimulation. In SHR platelets there is evidence that DAG-kinase activity is significantly reduced by thrombin compared with the fall in activity seen in WKY rat platelets, leading to a greater accumulation of 1,2-DAG (206), although another study using platelets from stroke-prone SHR did not show enhanced 1,2-DAG or PA in response to thrombin (177). The implication of this finding is that not only is more 1,2-DAG produced in hypertension, but that the principal route of metabolism is impaired. This is supported by the observation that 1,2-DAG accumulation in SHR aorta was more than would be expected from the PtdIns 4,5-P$_2$ levels (47). In transformed cells, the translocation of DAG kinase from cytosol to membrane was impaired, leading to increased 1,2-DAG levels and PKC activation (207). Further, in endothelial cells, 15-hydroxyeicosatetraenoic acid, a lipoxygenase metabolite of arachidonate, inhibited DAG-kinase activity and led to mitogenesis (208). These data show that alteration of the function of this kinase can have profound cellular effects.

For the most part, studies of PKC in hypertension have been carried out using phorbol esters or inhibitors of PKC. Both methods are prone to difficulty in interpretation because phorbol esters have other effects on cell metabolism besides irreversibly binding and activating PKC, and few PKC inhibitors can be regarded as truly specific for PKC alone. Sauro and Fitzpatrick (209) reported that SHR aorta had significantly greater basal and phorbol ester–stimulated PKC activity than that in WKY rat aorta. Kravtsov et al. (210) found PKC activity to be raised 1.6- to 2-fold in the lysate of erythrocytes of patients with essential hypertension and in SHR. Tsuda and Masuyama (211) investigated the effects of the PKC inhibitor 1-(5-isoquinolysulfonyl)-2-methyl-piperazine (H-7) on vascular adrenergic transmission in the mesenteric vasculature. Endogenous norepinephrine release during periarterial nerve stimulation was inhibited by H-7 in a dose-dependent manner. H-7 had a greater effect in SHR vessels than those from WKY rats, and the authors contend that PKC overactivity contributes to the enhanced vascular sympathetic nervous activity seen in SHR. Studies with phorbol esters have also been carried out in thoracic aortic strips from rats with coarctation and in the perfused hind limb of the SHR. The SHR aorta and the aorta from rats with coarctation were more responsive to phorbol ester stimulation (212,213) but *in vivo* this was not confirmed in SHR (213). It should be emphasized that although it has been demonstrated repeatedly that phorbol esters can produce contraction in vascular tissues, this does not prove that PKC is causing the response, which may be due to the other effects of the drug. Makita and Yasuda measured PKC activity in the SHR heart of both hypertensive and control rat strains (188). There was no difference at 4 weeks of age; however, it was increased at 20 weeks but only in the control. In contrast, Sauro and Hadden (214) reported an abnormal distribution of PKC activity in the spleen, thymus, and aorta of 6- to 10-week-old SHRs such that particulate activity was higher and cytosolic lower than in WKY controls. In addition, nuclear PKC activity was elevated in the SHRs (214). Increased phorbol ester binding sites have been reported in SHR fibroblasts, implying the presence of increased PKC (215).

An indirect assay of PKC activity was carried out by Koutouzov et al. (216) by measuring a target protein phosphorylated by PKC. Basal levels were not different in SHRs when compared with WKY rats, but thrombin caused greater phosphorylation in SHR platelets, suggesting augmented PKC activity in stimulated cells from genetically hypertension-prone rats. Similar results have been found in isolated glomeruli from SHR (217). Recently, using platelets from hypertensive patients, Haller et al. (218) have shown increased protein phosphorylation in response to thrombin and phorbol ester, suggesting increased activity of PKC in essential hypertension.

In terms of downstream functional activity of PKC, there was great excitement that the activation of Na^+ and H^+ exchange would prove to be the route by which growth might be influenced, because of the demonstration of alkaline pH changes seen in cultured cell lines. An increase in intracellular pH is seen when fibroblasts are activated by various vasoactive peptides before mitosis is observed (219). In such cases this alkalinization is brought about by increased Na^+/H^+ exchange. However,

recent studies in HCO_3-containing medium have led to a reassessment of cytoplasmic alkalinization in cell growth (220). The initial assumptions about cell regulation of pH were too simple. Nevertheless, in SHR resistance vessels, Na^+/H^+ exchange is increased and intracellular pH is more alkaline (221,222). In hypertensive humans, intracellular pH has been shown to be no different when increased and decreased (223–225), and there are a number of reports that the activity of the Na^+/H^+ exchanger appears to be overactive in platelets, erythrocytes, and leukocytes (224,226,227). However, a recent report on human resistance arteries found intracellular pH was similar in vessels from hypertensives when compared with those from control subjects, and Na^+/H^+ exchange was not increased (228). Finally, studies regarding changes in intracellular pH occurring during the development of vascular hypertrophy have shown singularly negative results (229).

CONCLUSIONS

Over the last few years enormous progress has been made in our understanding of the phosphoinositide signal transduction system. Two classes of external stimuli—the "calcium mobilizing hormones" and polypeptide growth factors—have been shown to activate PtdIns $4,5-P_2$ hydrolysis. The receptors used by these stimuli have marked differences, yet the second messengers Ins $1,4,5-P_3$ and 1,2-DAG are common to both. The discovery of the Ins P_3 receptor established that Ins $1,4,5-P_3$ was responsible for the elevation of intracellular calcium following receptor stimulation. The Ins $1,4,5-P_3$–calcium signaling pathway has been shown to be involved in fertilization and development. In differentiated cells the system is adapted to control many functions, for instance smooth muscle contraction, liver metabolism, and secretion.

The role of the phosphoinositide system in cell growth is less clear. Mitogenic stimuli cause PtdIns $4,5-P_2$ hydrolysis, and calcium and 1,2-DAG/PKC have been implicated in proliferation and hypertrophy; however, increased PtdIns turnover does not always lead to mitogenesis.

Also, it has become clear that it is no longer possible to study the phosphoinositide system in isolation, as agents that stimulate PtdIns $4,5-P_2$ hydrolysis frequently stimulate PtdCho breakdown and arachidonate release through activation of PLD and PLA_2. The role played by the different lipid second messengers generated may underlie the different cellular response produced.

With regard to hypertension, abnormalities of PLC and PKC genes have been reported, implying that the system could be involved in the pathogenesis of the disease. However, most of the experiments have used SHR and WKY animals and the relevance of this model to hypertension has been questioned recently (230,231).

The demonstration of changes in inositol phosphates, phosphatidic acid, and early response genes in experimental models of hypertension and cardiac hypertrophy also implicates the phosphoinositide system in adaptive circulatory changes secondary to hypertension. Future work must now build on these studies to try and determine whether changes in the phosphoinositide system would be causative in triggering the disease or merely assume a secondary adaptive role in the circulation. Either way, the search is on for specific inhibitors in the phosphoinositide signaling cascade that may lead to agents that could reverse the pressure-mediated consequences observed throughout the circulation, which are known to be so prognostically important.

ACKNOWLEDGMENTS

Dr. Ohanian is a British Heart Foundation Intermediate Research Fellow. We are grateful to the British Heart Foundation for supporting our studies. We also extend our gratitude to Mrs. M Williamson and Mrs. T Bent for typing this manuscript.

REFERENCES

1. Van Meer G. Transport and sorting of membrane lipids. *Curr Opin Cell Biol* 1993;5:661–673.
2. Paulus H, Kennedy EP. The enzymic synthesis of inositol monophosphatide. *J Biol Chem* 1960;235:1303–1311.
3. Berridge MJ, Irvine RF. Inositol trisphosphate, a novel second messenger in cellular signal transduction. *Nature* 1984;312:315–321.
4. Traynor Kaplan AE, Harris AL, Thompson BL, Taylor P, Skiar LA. An inositol tetrakis phosphate-containing phospholipid in activated neutrophils. *Nature* 1988;334:353–356.
5. Carpenter CL, Cantley LC. Phosphoinositide kinases. *Biochemistry* 1990;29:11147–11156.
6. Downes CP, Carter AN. Phosphoinositide 3-kinase: a new effector in signal transduction. *Cell Signalling* 1991;3:501–513.
7. Lips DL, Marjerus PW, Gorga FR, Young AT, Benjamin TL. Phosphatidylinositol-3-phosphate is present in normal and transformed fibroblasts and is resistant to hydrolysis by bovine brain phospholipase C11. *J Biol Chem* 1989;364:8759–8763.
8. Nakanishi H, Brewer KA, Exton JH. Activation of the isozyme of protein kinase C by phosphatidylinositol 3,4,5-trisphosphate. *J Biol Chem* 1993;268:13–15.
9. Berridge MJ. Inositol trisphosphate and calcium signalling. *Nature* 1993;361:315–325.
10. Nishizuka Y. Studies and perspectives of protein kinase C. *Science* 1986;233:305–312.
11. Simon MI, Strathmann MP, Gautman N. Diversity of G proteins in signal transduction. *Science* 1991;252:802–808.
12. Rhee SG, Choi KD. Regulation of inositol phospholipid-specific phospholipase C isozymes. *J Biol Chem* 1992;267:12393–12396.
13. Parker PJ, Kour G, Marais RM, Mitchell F, Pear SC, Schaap D, Stabel S, Webster C. Protein kinase C—a family affair. *Mol Cell Endocrinol* 1989;65:1–11.
14. Dohlman HG, Thorner J, Caron MG, Lefkowitz RJ. Model systems for the study of seven-transmembrane segment receptors. *Annu Rev Biochem* 1991;60:653–688.
15. Rodbell M. The role of hormone receptors and GTP-regulatory proteins in membrane transduction. *Nature* 1980;284:17–22.
16. Gilman AG. G proteins: transducers of receptor-generated signals. *Annu Rev Biochem* 1987;56:615–649.
17. Linder ME, Gilman AG. G proteins. *Sci Am* 1992;267:36–43.
18. Kleuss C, Scherubl H, Hescheler J, Schultz G, Wittig B. Different beta-subunits determine G-protein interaction with transmembrane receptors. *Nature* 1992;358:424–426.
19. Lefkowitz RJ. The subunit story thickens. *Nature* 1992;358:372.
20. Carozzi A, Camps M, Gierschik P, Parker PJ. Activation of phosphatidylinositol lipid-specific phospholipase C-β_3 by G protein $\beta\gamma$ subunits. *FEBS Lett* 1993;315:340–342.
21. Im M-J, Graham RM. A novel guanine nucleotide-binding protein coupled to the alpha$_1$-adrenergic receptor. *J Biol Chem* 1990;265:18944–18951.
22. Wu D, Katz A, Lee C-H, Simon MI. Activation of phospholipase C by α_1-adrenergic receptors is mediated by the α subunits of Gq family. *J Biol Chem* 1992;267:25798–25802.
23. Lee CH, Park D, Wu D, Rhee SG, Simon MI. Members of the Gq α subunit gene family activate phospholipase C$_\beta$ isozymes. *J Biol Chem* 1992;267:16044–16047.
24. Katz A, Wu D, Simon MI. Subunits $\beta\gamma$ of heterotrimeric G protein activate $\beta 2$ isoform of phospholipase C. *Nature* 1992;360:686–689.
25. Camps M, Carozzi A, Schnabel P, Scheer A, Parker PJ, Gierschik P. Isozyme-selective stimulation of phospholipase C-β_2 by G protein $\beta\gamma$-subunits. *Nature* 1992;360:684–689.
26. Wu D, LaRosa GJ, Simon MI. G protein-coupled signal transduction pathways for interleukin-8. *Science* 1993;261:101–103.
27. Gill GN. Growth factors and their receptors. In: Weinberg RA, ed. *Oncogenes and the molecular origins of cancer.* New York: Cold Spring Harbor Laboratory Press, 1989;67–76.
28. Cadena DL, Gill GN. Receptor tyrosine kinases. *FASEB J* 1992;6:2332–2337.
29. Rozengurt E. Growth factors and cell proliferation. *Curr Opin Cell Biol* 1992;4:161–165.
30. Cantley L, Auger KR, Carpenter C, Duckworth B, Graziani A, Kapeller R, Soltoff S. Oncogenes and signal transduction. *Cell* 1991;64:281–302.
31. Wahl MI, Daniel TO, Carpenter G. Antiphosphotyrosine recovery of phospholipase C activity after EGF treatment of A-431 cells. *Science* 1988;241:968–970.
32. Kim HK, Kim JW, Zilberstein A, Margolis B, Kim JG, Schlessinger J, Rhee SG. PDGF stimulation of inositol phospholipid hydrolysis regulates PLCα, phosphorylation at tyrosine residues 783 and 1254. *Cell* 1991;65:453–461.
33. Vega QC, Cochet C, Filhol O, Chang EP, Rhee SG, Gill GN. A site for tyrosine phosphorylation in the C$_1$ terminus of the EGF receptor is required to activate phospholipase C. *Mol Cell Biol* 1992;12:128–135.
34. Cochet C, Filhol O, Payrastre B, Hunter T, Gill GN. Interaction between the epidermal growth factor receptor and phosphoinositol kinases. *J Biol Chem* 1991;266:637–644.
35. Rhee SG, Suh PG, Lee SY. Studies of inositol phospholipid-specific phospholipase C. *Science* 1989;244:546–550.
36. Cockcroft S, Thomas GMH. Inositol-lipid-specific phospholipase C isoenzymes and their differential regulation by receptors. *Biochem J* 1992;288:1–14.
37. Koch CA, Anderson D, Moran MF, Ellis C, Pawson T. SH2 and SH3 domains: elements that control interactions of cytoplasmic signalling proteins. *Science* 1991;252:668–674.
38. Crooke ST, Bennett CF. Mammalian phosphoinositide-specific phospholipase C isoenzymes. *Cell Calcium* 1989;10:309–323.
39. Srivastava SP, Chen NQ, Liu YX, Holtzman JL. Purification and characterisation of a new isozyme of thiol: protein-disulfide oxidoreductase from rat hepatic microsomes. *J Biol Chem* 1991;266:20337–20344.
40. Bristol A, Hall SM, Kriz RW, Stahl ML, Fan YS, Byers MG, Eddy RL, Shows TB, Knopf JL. Phospholipase C-148: chromosomal location and deletion mapping of functional domains. *Cold Spring Harb Symp Quant Biol* 1988;L111:915–920.
41. Bennett CF, Crooke ST. Purification and characterisation of a phosphoinositide-specific phospholipase C from guinea pig. *J Biol Chem* 1987;262:13789–13797.
42. Kim U-H, Kim JW, Rhee SG. Phosphorylation of phospholipase C by cAMP-dependent protein kinase. *J Biol Chem* 1989;264:20167–20170.
43. Meisenhelder J, Suh PG, Rhee SG, Hunter T. Phospholipase C is

a substrate for the PDGF and EGF receptor protein tyrosine kinases in vivo and in vitro. *Cell* 1989;57:1109–1122.

44. Nishibe S, Wahl MI, Rhee SG, Carpenter G. Tyrosine phosphorylation of phospholipase C-11 in vitro by the epidermal growth factor receptor. *J Biol Chem* 1989;264:10335–10338.

45. Ryu SH, Suh PG, Cho KS, Lee KY, Rhee SG. Bovine brain cytosol contains three immunologically distinct forms of inositolphospholipid-specific phospholipase C. *Proc Natl Acad Sci USA* 1987;84:6649–6652.

46. Martin TFJ. Receptor regulation of phosphoinositidase C. *Pharmacol Ther* 1991;49:329–345.

47. Kato H, Fukani K, Shibasaki F, Homma Y, Takenawa T. Enhancement of phospholipase Cδ, activity in the aortas of spontaneously hypertensive rats. *J Biol Chem* 1992;267:6483–6487.

48. Griendling KK, Taubman MB, Akers M, Mendlowitz H, Alexander RW. Characterisation of phosphatidylinositol-specific phospholipase C from cultured vascular smooth muscle cells. *J Biol Chem* 1991;266:15498–15504.

49. Zhou C-J, Akhtar AA, Abdel Latif AA. Purification and characterisation of phosphoinositol-specific phospholipase C from bovine iris sphincter muscle. *Biochem J* 1993;289:401–409.

50. Brock TA, Rittenhouse SE, Powers CW, Elstein LS, Gimbrone MA Jr, Alexander RW. Phorbolester and 1-oleoyl-2-acetylglycerol inhibit angiotensin activation of phospholipase C in cultured vascular smooth muscle cells. *J Biol Chem* 1985;260:14158–14162.

51. Griendling KK, Delafontaine P, Rittenhouse SE, Gimbrone MA, Alexander RW. Correlation of receptor sequestration with sustained diacylglycerol accumulation in angiotensin II-stimulated cultured vascular smooth muscle cells. *J Biol Chem* 1987;262:14555–14562.

52. Berk BC, Aronow MS, Brock TA, Cragoe E, Gimbrone MA, Alexander RW. Angiotensin II stimulated Na$^+$/H$^+$ exchange in cultured vascular smooth muscle cells. *J Biol Chem* 1987;262:5057–5064.

53. Izzard AS, Heagerty AM. The measurement of internal pH in resistance arterioles: evidence that intracellular pH is more alkaline in SHR and WKY animals. *J Hypertens* 1989;7:173–180.

54. Lee K-Y, Ryu SH, Suh P-G, Choi WC, Rhee SG. Phospholipase C associated with particulate fractions of bovine brain. *Proc Natl Acad Sci USA* 1987;84:5540–5544.

55. Somlyo AV, Bond M, Somlyo AP, Scarpa A. Inositol trisphosphate-induced calcium release and contraction in vascular smooth muscle. *Proc Natl Acad Sci USA* 1985;82:5231–5235.

56. Majerus PW, Connolly TM, Bansal VS, Inhorn RC, Ross TS, Lips DL. Inositol phosphates: synthesis and degradation. *J Biol Chem* 1988;263:3051–3054.

57. Nahorski SR. Inositol polyphosphates and neuronal calcium homeostasis. *Trends Neurosci* 1988;11:444–448.

58. Morris AP, Gallagher DV, Irvine RF, Petersen OH. Synergism of inositol trisphosphate and tetrakisphosphate in activating Ca^{2+}-dependent K$^+$ channels. *Nature* 1987;330:653–655.

59. Irvine RF. Inositol lipids in cell signalling. *Curr Opin Cell Biol* 1992;4:212–219.

60. Shears SB. Regulation of the metabolism of 1,2 diacylglycerols and inositol phosphates that respond to receptor activations. *Pharmacol Ther* 1991;49:79–104.

61. King WG, Rittenhouse SE. Inhibition of protein kinase C by staurosporine promotes elevated accumulations of inositol trisphosphates and tetrakisphosphates in human platelets exposed to thrombin. *J Biol Chem* 1989;264:6070–6074.

62. Sim SS, Kim JW, Rhee SG. Regulation of D-Myo-inositol 1,4,5-trisphosphate 3-kinase by cAMP dependent protein kinase and protein kinase C. *J Biol Chem* 1990;265:10367–10372.

63. Henzi V, MacDermott A. Neuronal inositol trisphosphate receptors. *Neuroscience* 1992;46:251–273.

64. Tsien RW, Tsien RY. Calcium channels, stores, and oscillations. *Annu Rev Cell Biol* 1990;6:715–760.

65. Danop SK, Ferris CD, Donath C, Fischer GA, Munerutsu S, Ullrich A, Snyder SH, Ross CA. Inositol-1,4,5-trisphosphate receptors: District neuronal and non neuronal forms derived by alterative splicing differ in phosphorylation. *Proc Natl Acad Sci USA* 1991;88:2951–2955.

66. Nakagawa T, Okano H, Furuichi T, Aruga J, Mikoshiba K. The

subtypes of the mouse inositol 1,4,5-trisphosphate receptor are expressed in a tissue-specific and developmentally-specific manner. *Proc Natl Acad Sci USA* 1991;88:6244–6248.

67. Sudhof TC, Newton CL, Archer BT III, Ushkaryov TA, Mignery GA. Structure of a novel InsP3 receptor. *EMBO J* 1991;10:3199–3206.

68. Mignery GA, Sudhof TC. The ligand binding site and transduction mechanism in the inositol-1,4,5-trisphosphate receptor. *EMBO J* 1990;9:3893–3898.

69. Miyawaki M, Furuichi T, Ryon Y, Yoshikawa S, Nakagawa T, Saitoh T, Mikoshiba K. Structure function relationships of the mouse inositol 1,4,5-trisphosphate receptor. *Proc Natl Acad Sci USA* 1991;88:4911–4915.

70. Meldolesi J, Madeddu L, Pozzar T. Intracellular Ca^{2+} storage organelles in non-muscle cells: heterogeneity and functional assignment. *Biochim Biophys Acta* 1990;1055:130–140.

71. Mueller HW, O'Flaherty JT, Greene DG, Samuel MP, Wyckle RL. 1-0-alkyl-linked glycerophospholipids of human neutrophils distribution of arachidonate and other acyl residues in the ester-linked and diacyl species. *J Lipid Res* 1984;25:383–388.

72. Leach KL, Ruff VA, Wright TM, Pessin MS, Raben DM. Dissociation of protein kinase C activation and Sn-1,2-diacylglycerol formation. *J Biol Chem* 1991;266:3215–3221.

73. Rembold CM, Weaver BA. [Ca2+], not diacylglycerol, is the primary regulator of sustained swine arterial smooth muscle contraction. *Hypertension* 1990;15:692–698.

74. Ohanian J, Ollerenshaw J, Collins P, Heagerty A. Agonist-induced production of 1,2 diacylglycerol and phosphatidic acid in intact resistance arteries: evidence that accumulation of diacylglycerol is not a prerequisite for contraction. *J Biol Chem* 1990;265:8921–8928.

75. Rasmussen H, Takuwa Y, Park S. Protein kinase C in the regulation of smooth muscle contraction. *FASEB J* 1987;1:177–185.

76. Clark AH, Garland CJ. 5-Hydroxytryptamine-stimulated accumulation of 1,2 diacylglycerol in the rabbit basilar artery: a role for protein kinase C in smooth muscle contraction. *Br J Pharmacol* 1991;102:415–421.

77. Hee-Cheong M, Fletcher T, Kryski SK, Severson DL. Diacylglycerol lipase and kinase activities in rat brain microvessels. *Biochim Biophys Acta* 1985;833:59–68.

78. Knauss TC, Jaffer FE, Abboud HE. Phosphatidic acid modulates DNA synthesis phospholipase C and platelet-derived growth factor mRNAs in cultured mesangial cells: role of protein kinase C. *J Biol Chem* 1990;265:14457–14463.

79. Kanoh H, Yamada K, Sakane F, Imaizumi T. Phosphorylation of diacylglycerol kinase in vitro by protein kinase C. *Biochem J* 1989;358:455–462.

80. Heagerty AM. Angiotensin II-vasoconstrictor or growth factor. *J Cardiovasc Pharmacol* 1991;18(suppl 2):14–19.

81. Lemaitre RN, King WC, MacDonald ML, Glomset JA. Distribution of distinct arachidonoyl-specific and non-specific isoenzymes of diacylglycerol kinase in baboon (Papiocynocephalus) tissues. *Biochem J* 1990;266:291–299.

82. Fukaru K, Takenawa T. Phosphatidic acid that accumulated in platelet-derived growth factor stimulated Balb/C 3T3 cells is a potential mitogenic factor. *J Biol Chem* 1992;267:10988–10993.

83. Danthuluri NR, Deth RC. Acute desensitization to angiotensin II: evidence for a requirement of agonist-induced diacylglycerol production during tonic contraction of rat aorta. *Eur J Pharmacol* 1986;126:135–139.

84. van Corven EJ, Groenink A, Jalink K, Eicholtz T, Moolenaar WH. Lysophosphatidate-induced cell proliferation: identification and dissection of signalling pathway mediated by G proteins. *Cell* 1989;59:45–54.

85. Salmon DM, Honeyman TW. Proposed mechanism of cholinergic action in smooth muscle. *Nature* 1980;284:344–347.

86. Tsai M-H, Yu C-L, Wei F-S, Stacey DW. The effect of GTPase activating protein upon Ras is inhibited by mitogenically responsive lipids. *Science* 1989;243:522–526.

87. Tsai M-H, Yu C-L, Stacey DW. A cytoplasmic protein inhibits the GTPase activity of H-Ras in a phospholipid dependent manner. *Science* 1990;250:982–985.

88. Downward J. Signal transduction: Ras regulation: putting back the GTP. *Curr Biol* 1992;2:329–332.

89. Jackowski S, Rock CO. Stimulation of phosphatidyl inositol 4,5-bisphosphate phospholipase C activity by phosphatidic acid. *Arch Biochem Biophys* 1989;268:516–524.

90. Qian Z, Drewes LR. Cross-talk between receptor-regulated phospholipase D and phospholipase C in brain. *FASEB J* 1991;5:315–319.

91. Moritz A, De Graan PNE, Gispen WH, Wirtz KWA. Phosphatidic acid is a specific activator of phosphatidylinositol-4-phosphate kinase. *J Biol Chem* 1992;267:7207–7210.

92. Bocckino BB, Blackmore PF, Wilson PB, Exton JH. Phosphatidate accumulation in hormone-treated hepatocytes via a phospholipase D mechanism. *J Biol Chem* 1987;262:15309–15315.

93. Roe MW, Hepler JR, Harden K, Herman B. Platelet-derived growth factor and angiotensin II cause increases in cytosolic free calcium by different mechanisms in vascular smooth muscle cells. *J Cell Physiol* 1989;139:100–108.

94. Prescott SM, Majerus PW. Characterisation of 1,2-diacylglycerol hydrolysis in human platelets. Demonstration of an arachidonyl-monoacylglycerol intermediate. *J Biol Chem* 1983;258:764–769.

95. Allen AC, Gammon CM, Ousley AH, McCarthy KD, Morrell P. Bradykinin stimulates arachidonic acid release through the sequential actions of sn-1-diacylglycerol lipase and a monoacyl glycerol lipase. *J Neurochem* 1992;58:1130–1139.

96. Gronich JH, Bonventre JV, Nemenoff RA. Purification of a high molecular-mass form of phospholipase A$_2$ from rat kidney activated at physiological calcium concentrations. *Biochem J* 1990;271:37–43.

97. Piomelli D. Arachidonic acid in cell signalling. *Curr Opin Cell Biol* 1993;5:274–280.

98. Clark JD, Lin L-L, Kriz RW, Ramesha CS, Sultzman LA, Lin AY, Milona N, Knopf JL. A novel arachidonic acid-selective cytosolic phospholipase A$_2$ contains a Ca^{2+} dependent translocation domain with homology to PKC and GAP. *Cell* 1991;65:1043–1051.

99. Channon JY, Leslie CC. A calcium-dependent mechanism for associating a soluble arachidonoyl-hydrolyzing phospholipase A$_2$ in the macrophage cell line RAW 264.7. *J Biol Chem* 1990;265:5409–5413.

100. Lin LL, Lin Ay, Knopf JL. Cytosolic phospholipase A$_2$ is coupled to hormonally regulated release of arachidonic acid. *Proc Natl Acad Sci USA* 1992;89:6147–6151.

101. Felder CC, Williams HL, Axelrod J. A transduction pathway associated with receptors coupled to the inhibitory guanine nucleotide binding protein Gi that amplifies ATP mediated arachidonic acid release. *Proc Natl Acad Sci USA* 1991;88:6477–6480.

102. Bahls FH, Richmond JE, Smith WL, Haydon PG. A lipoxygenase pathway of arachidonic acid metabolism mediates FMRFamide activation of a potassium current in an identified neuron of helisoma. *Neurosci Lett* 1992;138:165–168.

103. Nakajima T, Sugimoto T, Kurachi Y. Platelet-activating factor activates cardiac G$_k$ via arachidonic acid metabolites. *FEBS Lett* 1991;289:239–243.

104. Margalit A, Livine AA. Lipoxygenase product controls the regulatory volume decrease of human platelets. *Platelets* 1991;2:207–214.

105. Kujubu DA, Fletcher BS, Varnum BC, Lim RW, Herschman HR. TIS10, a phorbol ester tumor promoter-inducible mRNA from Swiss 3T3 cells, encodes a novel prostaglandin synthase/cyclo-oxygenase homologue. *J Biol Chem* 1991;266:12866–12872.

106. Glasgow WC, Afshari CA, Barrett JC, Eling TE. Modulation of the epidermal growth factor mitogenic response by metabolites of linoleic and arachidonic acid in Syrian hamster embryo fibroblasts. *J Biol Chem* 1992;267:10771–10779.

107. Sellmayer A, Uedelhoven WH, Weber PC, Bonventre JV. Endogenous non cyclo-oxygenase metabolism of arachidonic acid modulates growth and mRNA levels of immediate-early response genes in rat mesengial cells. *J Biol Chem* 1991;266:3800–3807.

108. Natarajan R, Gonzales N, Hornsby PJ, Nadler J. Mechanism of angiotensin II-induced proliferation in bovine adrenocortical cells. *Endocrinology* 1992;131:1174–1180.

109. Gong MC, Fuglsang A, Alessi D, Kobayashi S, Cohen P, Somlyo AV, Somlyo AP. Arachidonic acid inhibits myosin light chain phosphatase and sensitizes smooth muscle to calcium. *J Biol Chem* 1992;267:21492–21498.

110. Inoue M, Kishimoto A, Takai Y, Nishizuka Y. Studies on cyclic nucleotide-independent protein kinase and its proenzyme in mammalian tissues. *J Biol Chem* 1977;252:7610–7616.

111. Nishizuka Y. The role of protein kinase C in cell surface signal transduction and tumour promotion. *Nature* 1984;308:693–698.

112. Takai Y, Kiskimoto A, Iwasa Y, Kawahari Y, Mori T, Nishizuka Y. Calcium-dependent activation of a multifunctional protein kinase by membrane phospholipids. *J Biol Chem* 1979;254:3692–3695.

113. Exton JH. Signalling through phosphatidylcholine breakdown. *J Biol Chem* 1990;265:1–4.

114. Bell RM, Burns DJ. Lipid activation of protein kinase C. *J Biol Chem* 1991;266:4661–4664.

115. Nishizuka Y. Intracellular signalling by hydrolysis of phospholipids and activation of protein kinase C. *Science* 1992;258:607–614.

116. Ono Y, Fujii T, Igarashi K, Kuno T, Tanaka C, Kikkawa U, Nishizuka Y. Phorbol ester binding to protein kinase C requires a cysteine-rich zinc-finger-like sequence. *Proc Natl Acad Sci USA* 1989;86:4868–4871.

117. Leibersperger H, Gschwendt M, Marks F. Purification and characterization of a calcium unresponsive phorbol ester/phospholipid-activated protein kinase from porcine spleen. *J Biol Chem* 1990;265:16108–16115.

118. Ogita K, Miyamoto S, Yamaguchi K, Koide H, Fujisawa N, Kikkawa U, Sahara S, Fukami Y, Nishizuka Y. Isolation and characterization of δ-subspecies of protein kinase C from rat brain. *Proc Natl Acad Sci USA* 1992;89:1592–1596.

119. Koide H, Ogita K, Kikkawa U, Nishizuka Y. Isolation and characterization of the ε subspecies of protein kinase C from rat brain. *Proc Natl Acad Sci USA* 1992;89:1149–1153.

120. Gomez N, Cohen P. Dissection of the protein kinase cascade by which nerve growth factor activates MAP kinases. *Nature* 1991;353:170.

121. Watanabe T, Ono Y, Taniyama Y, Hazama K, Igarashi K, Ogita K, Kikkawa U, Nishizuka Y. Cell division arrest induced by phorbol ester in CHO cells overexpressing protein kinase C-δ subspecies. *Proc Natl Acad Sci USA* 1992;89:10159–10163.

122. Schaap D, van der Wal J, Blitterswijk WJ, van der Bend RL, Ploegh HL. Diacylglycerol kinase is phosphorylated in vivo upon stimulation of the epidermal growth factor receptor and serine/threonine kinases, including protein kinase C-ε. *Biochem J* 1993;289:875–881.

123. Allan D, Mitchell RH. A calcium-activated polyphosphoinositide phosphodiesterase in the plasma membrane of human and rabbit erythrocytes. *Biochem Biophys Acta* 1978;508:277–286.

124. Burgess GM, Irvine RF, Berridge MJ, McKinney JS, Putney JW. Actions of inositol phosphates in Ca^{2+} pools in guinea pig hepatocytes. *Biochem J* 1984;224:741–746.

125. Suematsu E, Hirata M, Hashimoto T, Kuriyama H. Inositol 1,4,5-trisphosphate releases Ca^{2+} from intracellular store sites in skinned single cells of porcine coronary artery. *Biochem Biophys Res Commun* 1984;120:481–485.

126. Van Breemen C, Leijten P, Yamamoto H, Aaronson P, Cauvin C. Calcium activation of vascular smooth muscle. State of the art lecture. *Hypertension* 1986;8(suppl 2):89–95.

127. Leijten P, van Breemen C. The relationship between noradrenaline-induced contraction and ^{45}Ca efflux stimulation in rabbit mesenteric artery. *Br J Pharmacol* 1986;89:739–747.

128. Karaki H, Weiss GB. Calcium release in smooth muscle. *Life Sci* 1988;42:111–122.

129. Khalil R, Lodge N, Saida K, van Breemen C. Mechanism of calcium activation in vascular smooth muscle. *J Hypertens* 1987;5(suppl 4):5–15.

130. Somlyo AP, Walker JW, Godman YF, Trentham DR, Kobayashi S, Kitazawa T, Somlyo AV. Inositol trisphosphate, calcium and muscle contraction. *Philos Trans R Soc Lond [Biol]* 1988;320:399–414.

131. Danthuluri NR, Deth RC. Phorbol-ester-induced contractions of arterial smooth muscle and inhibition of α-adrenergic response. *Biochim Biophys Res Commun* 1984;125:1103–1109.

132. Ohanian J, Izzard A, Littlewood M, Heagerty AM. Regulation of diacylglycerol metabolism by vasoconstrictor hormones in intact small arteries. *Circ Res* 1993;72:1163–1171.

133. Karibe H, Oishi K, Uchida MK. Involvement of protein kinase C in Ca^{2+}-independent contraction of rat uterine smooth muscle. *Biochem Biophys Res Commun* 1991;179:487–494.

134. Andrea JE, Walsh MP. Protein kinase C of smooth muscle. *Hypertension* 1992;20:585–595.

135. Collins EM, Walsh MP, Morgan KG. Contraction of single vascular smooth muscle cells by phenylephrine at constant $[Ca^{2+}]$. *Am J Physiol* 1992;262:H754–H762.

136. Gleason MM, Flaim SF. Phorbol ester contracts rabbit thoracic aorta by increasing intracellular calcium and by activating calcium influx. *Biochem Biophys Res Commun* 1986;138:1362–1369.

137. Rembold CM, Murphy RA. $[Ca^{2+}]$-dependent myosin phosphorylation in phorbol diester stimulated smooth muscle contraction. *Am J Physiol* 1988;255:C719–C723.

138. Itoh H, Lederis K. Contraction of rat thoracic aorta strips induced by phorbol 12-myristate 13-acetate. *Am J Physiol* 1987;252:C244–C247.

139. Rembold CM, Weaver BA. $[Ca^{2+}]$, not diacylglycerol, is the primary regulator of sustained arterial smooth muscle contraction. *Hypertension* 1990;15:692–698.

140. Clark AH, Garland CJ. 5-Hydroxytryptamine-stimulated accumulation of 1,2-diacylglycerol in the rabbit basilar artery. *Br J Pharmacol* 1991;102:415–421.

141. Nishimura J, Kolber M, van Breeman C. Norepinephrine and $GTP\gamma s$ increases myofilament Ca^{2+} sensitivity in α-toxin permeabilised arterial smooth muscle. *Biochem Biophys Res Commun* 1988;157:677–683.

142. Kitazawa T, Kobayashi S, Horiuti K, Somlyo AV, Somlyo AP. Receptor-coupled permeabilised smooth muscle. Role of the phosphatidylinositol cascade, G proteins and modulation of the contractile response to Ca^{2+}. *J Biol Chem* 1989;264:5339–5342.

143. Irvine RF, Divecha N. Phospholipids in the nucleus-metabolism and possible functions. *Semin Cell Biol* 1992;3:225–235.

144. Divecha N, Banfic H, Irvine RF. The polyphosphoinositide cycle exists in the nuclei of Swiss 3T3 cells under the control of a receptor (for IGF-1) in the plasma membrane and stimulation of the cycle increases nuclear diacylglycerol and apparently induces translocation of protein kinase C to the nucleus. *EMBO J* 1991;10:3207–3214.

145. Smith CD, Wells WW. Phosphorylation of rat liver envelopes, characterization of in vitro phosphorylation. *J Biol Chem* 1983;258:9368–9373.

146. Payrastre B, Nievers M, Boonstra J, Breton M, Verleij AJ, van Bergen EN, Henegouwen PMP. A differential location of phosphoinositide kinases, diacylglycerol kinase, and phospholipase C in the nuclear matrix. *J Biol Chem* 1992;267:5078–5084.

147. Martelli AM, Gilmour RS, Bertagnolo V, Neri LM, Manzoli L, Cocco L. Nuclear localization and signaling activity of phosphoinositidase $C\beta$ in Swiss 3T3 cells. *Nature* 1992;358:242–245.

148. Berridge MJ. Inositol lipids and cell proliferation. *Philos Trans R Soc Lond* [*Biol*] 1987;317:525–536.

149. Berridge MJ. Inositol lipids and cell proliferation. *Biochim Biophys Acta* 1987;907:33–45.

150. Pardee AB, Dubrow R, Hamlin JL, Ketzien RF. Animal cell cycle. *Annu Rev Biochem* 1978;47:715–750.

151. Neyses L, Vetter H. Molecular biology of oncogenes and cardiovascular hypertrophy. *J Hypertens* 1992;10:1447–1452.

152. Rozengurt E. Growth factors and cell proliferation. *Curr Opin Cell Biol* 1992;4:161–165.

153. Cobb M, Boulton TG, Robbins DJ. Extracellular signal-related kinases. ERKs in Progress. *Mol Biol Cell* 1991;2:965–978.

154. Pelech SL, Sanghera JS. MAP kinases: charting the regulatory pathways. *Science* 1992;257:1355–1356.

155. Posada J, Cooper JA. Molecular signal integration. Interplay between serine threonine and tyrosine phosphorylation. *Mol Cell Biol* 1992;3:583–592.

156. Marx J. Forging a path to the nucleus. *Science* 1993;260:1588–1590.

157. Poussegur J, Seuwen K. Transmembrane receptors and intracellular pathways that control cell proliferation. *Annu Rev Physiol* 1992;54:195–210.

158. Ashkenazi A, Ramachandran J, Capon DJ. Acetylcholine analogue stimulates DNA synthesis in brain-derived cells via specific muscarinic receptor subtypes. *Nature* 1989;340:146–150.

159. Smith MR, Liu Y-L, Kim H, Rhee S-G, Kung H-F. Inhibition of serum- and Ras-stimulated DNA synthesis by antibodies to phospholipase C. *Science* 1990;247:1074–1077.

160. Smith MR, Ryu S-H, Suk P-G, Rhee S-G, Kung H-F. S-phase induction and transformation of quiescent NIH 3T3 cells by microinjection of phospholipase C. *Proc Natl Acad Sci USA* 1989;86:3659–3663.

161. de Vries-Smits AMM, Burgering BMT, Leevers SJ, Marshall CJ, Bos JC. Involvement of p21 Ras in activation of extracellular signal-regulated kinase 2. *Nature* 1992;357:602–604.

162. Zierhut W, Zimmer HG. Significance of myocardial α- and β-adrenoreceptors in catecholamine-induced cardiac hypertrophy. *Circ Res* 1989;65:1417–1425.

163. Simpson P. Norepinephrine-stimulated hypertrophy of cultured rat myocardial cells is an α_1-adrenergic response. *J Clin Invest* 1983;22:732–735.

164. Waspe LE, Ordahl CP, Simpson PC. The cardiac myosin heavy chain isogene is induced selectively in α_1-adrenergic receptor-stimulated hypertrophy of cultured rat heart myocytes. *J Clin Invest* 1990;85:1206–1214.

165. Kariya KI, Karns LR, Simpson PC. Expression of a constitutively activated mutant of the β-isozyme of protein kinase C in cardiac myocytes stimulates the promoter of the β-myosin heavy chain isogene. *J Biol Chem* 1990;266:10023–10026.

166. Magni M, Meldolesi J, Pandiella A. Ionic events induced by epidermal growth factor. *J Biol Chem* 1991;266:6329–6335.

167. Takuwa N, Iwamoto A, Kumada M, Yamashita K, Takuwa Y. Role of Ca^{2+} influx in bombesin-induced mitogenesis in Swiss 3T3 fibroblasts. *J Biol Chem* 1991;266:1403–1409.

168. Chao T-S O, Byron KL, Lee K-M, Villereal M, Rosner MR. Activation of MAP kinases by calcium-dependent and calcium-independent pathways. *J Biol Chem* 1992;267:19876–19883.

169. Yamacha H, Mizuguchi J, Nakinishi M. Antigen receptor-mediated calcium signals in B cells as revealed by confocal fluorescence microscopy. *FEBS Lett* 1991;284:249–251.

170. Minenko A, Hajdu I, Oehme P. ^{32}P-einbau in polyphosphoinositide von erythrozyten essentieller hypertoniker. *Acta Biol Med Germ* 1981;40:341–344.

171. Marche P, Koutouzov S, Girard A, Elghozi J-L, Meyer P, Ben-Ishay D. Phosphoinositide turnover in erythrocyte membranes in human and experimental hypertension. *J Hypertens* 1985;3:25–30.

172. Riozzi A, Heagerty AM, Ollerenshaw JD, Swales JD. Erythrocyte phosphoinositide metabolism in essential hypertensive patients and their normotensive offspring. *Clin Sci* 1987;73:29–32.

173. Kiselev G, Minenko A, Moritz V, Oeheme P. Polyphosphoinositide metabolism in erythrocytes of spontaneously hypertensive rats. *Biochem Pharmacol* 1981;30:833–837.

174. Koutouzov S, Marche P, Girard A, Meyer P. Altered turnover of polyphosphoinositides in the erythrocyte membrane of the spontaneously hypertensive rat. *Hypertension* 1983;5:409–414.

175. Boriskina GM, Gulak PV, Postnov YuV. Phosphoinositide content in the erythrocyte membrane of rats with spontaneous and renal hypertension. *Experientia* 1978;34:744.

176. Koutouzov S, Marche P, Cloix JF, Meyer PF. Phospholipid phosphorylation in erythrocytes of spontaneously hypertensive rats. *Am J Physiol* 1982;243:H590.

177. Kawaguchi H, Shoki M, Sano H, Kudo T, Sawa H, Mochizuki N, Okamoto H, Endo Y, Kitabatake A. Polyphosphoinositide metabolism in hypertrophic rat heart. *J Mol Cell Cardiol* 1992;24:1003–1010.

178. Osanai T, Dunn MJ. Phospholipase C responses in cells from spontaneously hypertensive rats. *Hypertension* 1992;19:446–455.

179. Tremblay J, Cherkaoui L, Skuhersta R, Amer V, Hamet P. Increased inositol trisphosphate in erythrocytes of spontaneously hypertensive rats. *J Hypertens* 1990;8:115–120.

180. Durkin H, Ollerenshaw JD, Heagerty AM. Resistance artery

phosphoinositide metabolism in genetic hypertension. *J Hypertens* 1990;8:557–563.

181. Ollerenshaw JD, Heagerty AM, West K, Swales JD. The effects of coarctation hypertension upon vascular inositol phospholipid hydrolysis in Wistar rats. *J Hypertens* 1988;6:733–738.

182. Nixon GF, Hamilton CA, Wadsworth RM, Reid JL. Inositol phosphate formation in arterial smooth muscle from rabbits with perinephritis hypertension. *J Hypertens* 1990;8:1155–1160.

183. Yagisawa H, Emori Y, Nojima H. Phospholipase C genes display restriction fragment length polymorphisms between the genomes of normotensive and hypertensive rats. *J Hypertens* 1991;9:303–307.

184. Yagisawa H, Tanase H, Nojima H. Phospholipase C-δ gene of the spontaneously hypertensive rat harbours point mutations causing amino acid substitutions in a catalytic domain. *J Hypertens* 1991;9:997–1004.

185. Baudouin-Legros M, Meyer P. Hypertension and atherosclerosis. *J Cardiovasc Pharmacol* 1990;15(suppl 1):51–56.

186. Kawaguchi H, Okamoto H, Saito H, Yasuda H. Renal phospholipase C and diglyceride lipase activity in spontaneously hypertensive rats. *Hypertension* 1987;10:100–106.

187. Uehara Y, Ishii M, Ishimitu T, Sugimoto T. Enhanced phospholipase C activity in the vascular wall of spontaneously hypertensive rats. *Hypertension* 1988;11:28–33.

188. Makita N, Yasuda H. Alterations in phosphoinositide-specific phospholipase C and protein kinase C in the myocardium of spontaneously hypertensive rats. *Basic Res Cardiol* 1990;85:435–443.

189. Ollerenshaw JD, Heagerty AM, Swales JD. Abnormal vascular phosphoinositide hydrolysis in the spontaneously hypertensive rat. *Br J Pharmacol* 1986;89:803–807.

190. Ex TP, Campbell MD, Deth RC. Reduction of norepinephrine-induced tonic contraction and phosphoinositide turnover in arteries of spontaneously hypertensive rats. *Am J Hypertens* 1989;2:40–45.

191. Laitinen JT, Torda T, Saavedra JM. Enhanced phosphoinositide hydrolysis in the pineal gland of spontaneously hypertensive rats. *Am J Hypertens* 1990;3:496–498.

192. Kanbe T, Nara Y, Tagami M, Yamori Y. Studies of hypertension-induced vascular hypertrophy in cultured smooth muscle cells from spontaneously hypertensive rat. *Hypertension* 1983;5:887–892.

193. Ishimusu T, Uehara Y, Ishii M, Ikeda T, Matsuoka H, Sugimoto T. Thromboxane and vascular smooth muscle cell growth in genetically hypertensive rats. *Hypertension* 1988;12:46–51.

194. Berk BC, Vallega G, Muslin AJ, Gordon HM, Canessa H, Alexander RW. Spontaneously hypertensive rat vascular smooth muscle cells in culture exhibit increased growth and Na$^+$/H$^+$ exchange. *J Clin Invest* 1989;83:822–829.

195. Paquet J-L, Baudounin-Legros M, Brunelle G, Meyer P. Hyperactivation of phospholipase C does not support the enhanced proliferation of aortic smooth muscle cells from spontaneously hypertensive rats. *Am J Hypertens* 1991;4:651–660.

196. Guicheney P, Wauquier I, Paquet J-L, Meyer P. Enhanced response to growth factors and to angiotensin II of spontaneously hypertensive rat skin fibroblasts in culture. *J Hypertens* 1991;9:23–27.

197. Guicheney P, Soussan K, Dausse E, Rota R. Dissociation of hypertension and genetically enhanced growth capacity in skin fibroblasts of F$_2$-hybrid SHR/WKY rats. *Am J Hypertens* 1992;5:556–565.

198. Preiss J, Loomis CR, Bishop WR, Stein R, Niedel JE, Bell RM. Quantitative measurement of sn-1,2-diacylglycerols present in platelets, hepatocytes and Ras- and sis-transformed normal rat kidney cells. *J Biol Chem* 1986;261:8597–8600.

199. Marche P, Limon I, Blanc J, Girard A. Platelet phosphatidylcholine turnover in experimental hypertension. *Hypertension* 1990;16:190–193.

200. Okumura K, Kondo J, Yoshino M, Ishikawa K, Asano H, Hashimoto H, Ito T. Enalapril reduces the enhanced 1,2-diacylglycerol content and RNA synthesis in spontaneously hypertensive rat hearts before established hypertension. *Mol Cell Biochem* 1992;112:15–21.

201. Okumura K, Kondo J, Shimizu K, Yoshino M, Toki Y, Hashimoto H, Ito T. Changes in ventricular 1,2-diacylglycerol content in rats following monocrotaline treatment. *Cardiovasc Res* 1992;26:626–630.

202. Okumura K, Akiyama N, Hashimoto H, Ogawa K, Sutake T. Alteration of 1,2-diacylglycerol content in myocardium from diabetic rats. *Diabetes* 1988;37:1168–1172.

203. Okumura K, Yamada Y, Kondo J, Ishida A, Hashimoto H, Ito T, Ogana K, Kitoh J. Increased 1,2-diacylglycerol content in myopathic hamster hearts at a prenecrotic stage. *Life Sci* 1988;43:1371–1377.

204. Okumura K, Kondo J, Shirai Y, Muramatsu M, Yamada Y, Hashimoto H, Ito T. 1,2 diacylglycerol content in thoracic aorta of spontaneously hypertensive rats. *Hypertension* 1990;16:43–48.

205. Kondo J, Yamada Y, Okumura K, Hashimoto H, Ito T, Satake T. 1,2-diacylglycerol content in myocardium from spontaneously hypertensive rats during the development of hypertension. *Basic Res Cardiol* 1990;85:435–460.

206. Kato H, Takenawa T. Phospholipase C activation and diacylglycerol kinase inactivation lead to an increase in diacylglycerol content in spontaneously hypertensive rat. *Biochem Biophys Res Commun* 1987;146:1419–1424.

207. Kato M, Kawai S, Takenawa T. Disappearance of diacylglycerol kinase translocation in ras-transformed cells. *Biochem Biophys Res Commun* 1988:154:959–966.

208. Setty BNY, Graeber JE, Short MJ. The mitogenic effect of 15- and 12-hydroxyeicosatetraenoic acid on endothelial cells may be mediated via diacylglycerol kinase inhibition. *J Biol Chem* 1987;262:17613–17622.

209. Sauro MD, Fitzpatrick DF. Atrial peptides inhibit protein kinase C-mediated contraction in rat aorta. *Eur J Pharmacol* 1990;180:373–376.

210. Kravtsov GM, Dulin NO, Postnov IYUV, Orlov SN, Pokudin NI, Kotelevtsev YUV, Postnov YUV. Protein kinase C activity in erythrocytes in primary hypertension regulation of cell shape and cation transport. *Physiol Bohemoslov* 1990;39:27–36.

211. Tsuda K, Masuyama Y. Effects of a protein kinase C inhibitor (H-7) on norepinephrine release from vascular adrenergic neurones in spontaneously hypertensive rats. *Clin Exp Hypertens* 1990;12:581–596.

212. Turla MB, Park SM, Webb RC. Vascular responsiveness to phorbol esters in coarctation-hypertensive rats. *J Hypertens* 1990;8:191–196.

213. Bilder GE, Kasiewski CJ, Perrone MH. Phorbol-12, 13-dibutyrate induced vasoconstriction in vivo: characterization of response in genetic hypertension. *J Pharmacol Exp Ther* 1990;252:526–530.

214. Sauro MD, Hadden JW. Gamma-interferon corrects aberrant protein kinase C levels and immunosuppression in the spontaneously hypertensive rat. *Int J Immunopharmacol* 1992;14:1421–1427.

215. Zhu DL, Herembert T, Marche P. Protein kinase C and cell proliferation in spontaneously hypertensive rats. *Clin Exp Hypertens* [A] 1992;A14:875–887.

216. Koutouzov S, Limon I, Marche P. Receptor-dependent and -independent protein phosphorylation in platelets of spontaneously hypertensive rats. *Thromb Res* 1990;59:475–487.

217. Hano T, Shotani M, Baba A, Ura M, Nakamura Y, Tomobuchi Y, Nishio I, Masuyama Y. Contribution of calmodulin and protein kinase C to renin release in spontaneously hypertensive rats. *Am J Hypertens* 1990;3:206S–209S.

218. Haller H, Lindschau C, Quass P, Distler A. Protein phosphorylation and intracellular free calcium in platelets of patients with essential hypertension. *Am J Hypertens* 1992;5:117–124.

219. Moolenaar WH, Yarden T, De Laat SW, Schlessinger J. Epidermal growth factor induced electrically silent Na$^+$ influx in human fibroblasts. *J Biol Chem* 1982;257:8502–8506.

220. Ganz MB, Boyarsky G, Bern Sterzel R, Boron WF. Arginine vasopressin enhances pH: regulation in the presence of HCO$_3$ by stimulating three acid-base transport systems. *Nature* 1989;337:648–651.

221. Izzard AS, Heagerty AM. The measurement of internal pH in

resistance arteries evidence that intracellular pH is more alkaline in SHR than WKY animals. *J Hypertens* 1989;7:173–180.

222. Izzard AS, Heagerty AM. Resting intracellular pH in mesenteric arteries from spontaneously hypertensive and Wistar-Kyoto rats: effects of amiloride and 4,4′diisothiocyanotostilbene-2 2′-disulphonic acid. *J Hypertens* 1989;7(suppl 6):128–129.

223. Weder AB, Bahadosingh SE, Neagos GR. Platelet intracellular pH in essential hypertensives and normotensives. *J Hypertens* 1987;7(suppl 6):S152–S153.

224. Ng LL, Dudley C, Bomford J, Hawley D. Leucocyte intracellular pH and Na$^+$/H$^+$ antiport activity in human hypertension. *J Hypertens* 1989;7:471–475.

225. Resnick LM, Gupta RK, Sosa RE, Corbett ML, Laragh JH. Intracellular pH in human and experimental hypertension. *Proc Natl Acad Sci USA* 1987;84:7663–7667.

226. Live A, Vitch R, Grinstein S, Balfe JW, Marques-Julio A, Rothstein A. Increased platelet Na$^+$-H$^+$ exchange rates in essential hypertension: application of a novel test. *Lancet* 1987;1:533–536.

227. Orlov SN, Postnov IY, Pokudin NI, Kukharenko VY, Postnov YUV. Na$^+$-H$^+$ exchange and other ion-transport systems in erythrocytes of essential hypertensives and spontaneously hypertensive rats: a comparable analysis. *J Hypertens* 1989;7:781–788.

228. Izzard AS, Cragoe EJ, Heagerty AM. Intracellular pH in human resistance arteries in essential hypertension. *Hypertension* 1991;17:780–786.

229. Izzard AS, MacIver DH, Cragoe EJ, Heagerty AM. Intracellular pH in rat resistance arteries during the development of experimental hypertension. *Clin Sci* 1991;81:65–71.

230. St Lezin E, Simonet L, Pravenec M, Kurtz TW. Hypertensive strains and normotensive "control" strains: How closely are they related? *Hypertension* 1992;19:419–424.

231. Johnson ML, Ely DL, Turner ME. Genetic divergence between the Wistar-Kyoto rat and the spontaneously hypertensive rat. *Hypertension* 1992;19:425–427.

Hypertension: Pathophysiology, Diagnosis, and Management, Second Edition,
edited by J.H. Laragh and B.M. Brenner,
Raven Press, Ltd., New York © 1995.

CHAPTER 36

Intracellular Signaling Mechanisms in Hypertension

Pavel Hamet, Sergei N. Orlov, Johanne Tremblay

CYCLIC NUCLEOTIDES AND ION TRANSPORT PATHWAYS AS COMPONENTS OF INTRACELLULAR SIGNALING

In the last two decades, major progress has been achieved in our understanding of the mechanisms of cellular activation by extracellular stimuli. It has been established that signal transduction and amplification are mediated by transitory increases of intracellular second messengers: cyclic nucleotides (cyclic adenosine monophosphate [cAMP] and cyclic guanosine monophosphate [cGMP]), polyphosphoinositide metabolism intermediates (inositol-1,4,5-trisphosphate [InsP$_3$], inositol-1,3,4,5-tetrakisphosphate [InsP$_4$], diacylglycerol [DAG], phosphatidylinositol-3,4,5-triphosphate [PIP$_3$]) and intracellular calcium ([Ca^{2+}]$_i$). The first section of this chapter briefly reviews our current knowledge of the systems involved in intracellular signaling, paying particular attention to cAMP, cGMP, [Ca^{2+}]$_i$ and monovalent cations. The second section describes the main mechanisms and the potential implications of intracellular signaling in blood pressure regulation. Data on abnormalities of the cyclic nucleotide system and ion transport pathways in hypertension are summarized in the third and fourth sections. The fifth and last section discusses putative mechanisms of abnormalities of intracellular signaling involved in the development and maintenance of hypertension as well as in the expression of disease complications. For a more detailed analysis of the polyphosphoinositide signaling system and its alteration in essential hypertension, the reader is referred to other reviews (1–3).

Cyclic AMP

Figure 1 is a schematic representation of the intracellular signaling pathway involving cyclic nucleotides as

P. Hamet: Centre de Recherche Hôtel-Dieu de Montréal, Université de Montréal, Montréal, Quebec H2W 1T8, Canada.
S. N. Orlov: University of Moscow, Moscow, Russia.
J. Tremblay: Centre de Recherche Hôtel-Dieu de Montréal, Université de Montréal, Montréal, Quebec H2W 1T8, Canada.

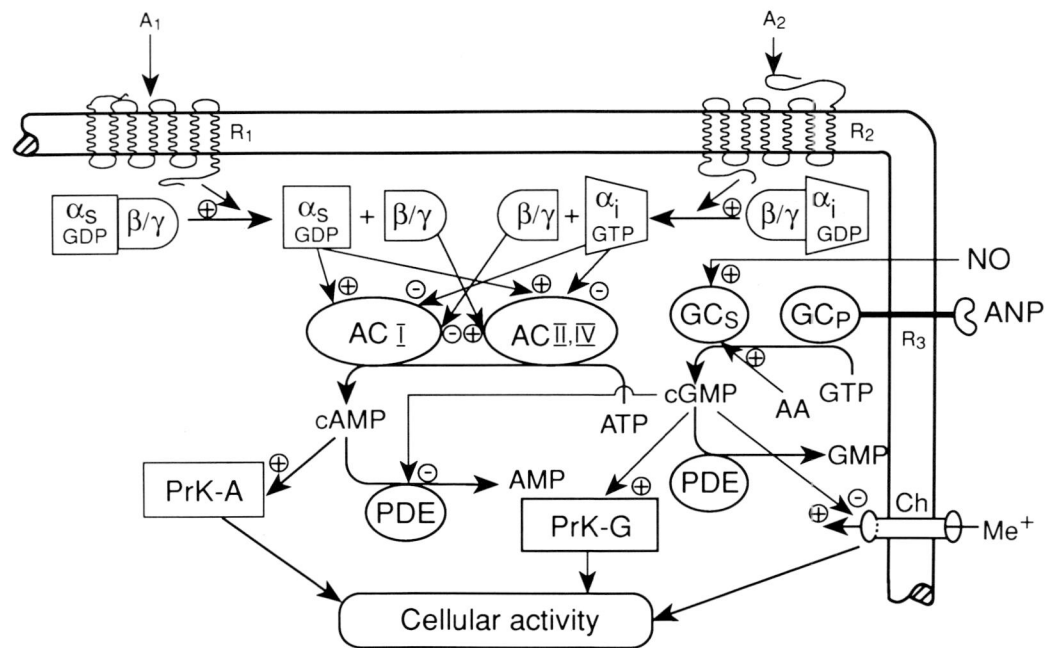

FIG. 1. Cyclic nucleotide-mediated intracellular signaling system. Agonists (A₁, A₂) activate the 7-membrane-spanning receptors (R₁, R₂) coupled with GTP-binding proteins of Gₛ and Gᵢ families, respectively. This interaction results in GDP/GTP exchange and dissociation of the α and β/γ subunits of Gp. Alphaₛ-GTP subunit activates (+) whereas αᵢ-GTP subunit inhibits (−) adenylate cyclase. In the presence of αₛ-GTP β/γ subunits inhibit type I but activate type II and type IV isoforms of adenylate cyclase (AC). Cyclic GMP is generated by soluble guanylate cyclase (GCₛ) or particulate guanylate (GCp) covalently bound with ANP receptors (R₃). Soluble guanylate cyclase is activated by nitric oxide (NO) and arachidonic acid (AA). PDE, phosphodiesterase, PrK-A and PrK-G, cAMP- and cGMP-dependent protein kinases, respectively. In rod outer segment cGMP activates whereas in epithelial cells it inhibits nonselective cation (Me⁺) channels (Ch). For other details, see text.

second messengers. Discovered over 30 years ago by Sutherland and Rall (4), this system led to the establishment of the second messenger concept. Cyclic AMP is generated by several isoforms of a membrane-bound enzyme (adenylate cyclase) via a cyclasing reaction of α-phosphate and pyrophosphate release from the substrate adenosine triphosphate (ATP) in the presence of the magnesium ion. The stimulation of cAMP synthesis in response to hormones is a complex cascade of events which is now almost fully understood. The specificity of this reaction resides in recognition of the ligand hormone by its 7-membrane-spanning receptor at the outer site of the plasma membrane. The ligand-receptor interaction creates an increased affinity of guanosine triphosphate (GTP)-binding protein (Gp) for GTP. Our knowledge of the Gp-mediated cascade of intracellular signaling, gained mostly through the work of Birnbaumer and coworkers (5), was summarized recently (6–12). The Gp involved in the regulation of adenylate cyclase activity is a member of the ubiquitous superfamily of heterotrimer proteins. Up to now, about 20 α-subunits (Mr 40–50 kDa), 4 β-subunits (Mr ~ 35 kDa) and 3 γ-subunits (Mr ~ 10–12kDa) of Gp have been cloned, using the polymerase chain reaction. The Gp heterotrimer interaction with activated receptors increases the affinity of α-

subunits for GTP, induces guanosine diphosphate (GDP)/GTP exchange and dissociates α-GTP from the βγ dimer. The GDP/GTP exchange in αᵢ, αₒ-, and αₜ-subunits of Gᵢ proteins is inhibited by their adenosine diphosphate (ADP)-ribosylation catalyzed by pertussis toxin. Interaction of the α-subunits with target proteins results in increased intrinsic GTPase activity and inactivation of the signaling pathway via the formation of an αβγ complex. The GTPase activity of αₛ- and αₒₗf-subunits is blocked by cholera toxin-induced ribosylation, irreversibly activating the Gₛ-mediated signaling pathway. Neither αz- nor α-subunits of Gq and G₁₂ families are sensitive to bacterial toxins.

The *orthodox* view of Gp signaling pointed to αₛ (αₒₗf) and αᵢ as the only subunits responsible for activation and inhibition of adenylate cyclase, respectively, whereas the βγ dimer regulates the levels of active, free α-subunits and the inactive heterotrimer. Six isoforms of adenylate cyclase (types I to VI) have been cloned in the last few years (13). In accordance with the orthodox view, addition of the βγ dimer decreases the activation of adenylate cyclase by αₛ-GTP in membranes from Sf9 cells infected with the type I isoform of this enzyme. In contrast, type II and IV isoforms were found to be drastically activated by the βγ dimer in the presence of αₛ-GTP (14–16).

These data gave ground to the assumption that the $\beta\gamma$-subunits of Gp, usually coupled to other target proteins (phospholipase C, ionic channels, etc.), may also be involved in the regulation of adenylate cyclase activity. This *heterodox* point of view is supported by data on the activation of cAMP production by α_2-adrenoceptor agonists in HEK-293 and COS-7 cells transfected with type II adenylate cyclase (17) and by findings of increased β-adrenergic-induced cAMP production in vascular smooth muscle cells (VSMC) by angiotensin II, a powerful activator of polyphosphoinositide breakdown (18).

Table 1 summarizes data on the interaction of G-protein subunits with adenylate cyclase and other target proteins observed in the last few years in reconstituted systems and transfected cells (6,14–16,19–32). In addition to Gp-dependent stimulation of adenylate cyclase, the catalytic subunit of the enzyme can be directly activated by forskolin, an alkaloid extract of *Coleus forskolii.* This is an old Indian medicinal herb used for cardiovascular purposes. It is a useful tool to explore the catalytic subunits of adenylate cyclase, since it can stimulate the enzyme both in the absence or presence of Gp (33).

The degradation of cyclic nucleotides is mediated by enzymes called cyclic nucleotide phosphodiesterases. These enzymes degrade cyclic nucleotides by cleavage of the 3'-bond in the presence of a divalent metal, usually magnesium, leading to the formation of 5'-AMP, a compound devoid of the specific activity of cyclic nucleotides. Although most phosphodiesterases are able to hydrolyze both cAMP and cGMP, at least one type of phosphodiesterase specifically hydrolyzes cAMP (34). Other phosphodiesterases include: (a) a calmodulin-stimulated enzyme abundant in brain and cardiac tissues; and (b) a cGMP-stimulating phosphodiesterase originally discovered in the heart (35,36). This particular molecule is an enzyme whose cAMP hydrolytic activity is inhibited by micromolar concentrations of cGMP, constituting one of the levels of interaction of the two cyclic nucleotides. This phosphodiesterase isoform, cGMP-inhibited cAMP-phosphodiesterase (CGI-PDE), has been found in human platelets (37) and in the rat aorta (38).

Protein kinases are enzymes responsible for the posttranslational modification of specific substrates by amino-acid phosphorylation from the γ-phosphate of ATP, leading to functional changes (usually an increase) of the substrates of cellular events of interest (39). Cyclic AMP-dependent protein kinase, discovered by Walsh et al. (40), is one of the best characterized target enzymes of cAMP, translating the cAMP message into specific cellular functions. Cyclic AMP-dependent protein kinase is composed of two regulatory and two catalytic subunits. Upon cAMP binding by the regulatory subunits, the catalytic subunits can dissociate and become active to phosphorylate specific substrates. Particular interchain rearrangement of the catalytic and regulatory subunits is the basis of classification of this enzyme as type I or II (39).

Rapid phosphorylation of G-protein-coupled receptors accompanies agonist-driven (homologous) desensitization. Both second messenger-activated kinases and the more recently discovered G-protein-coupled receptor kinases are involved in this modification. Beta-adrenergic receptor kinase 1 (βARK1) and rhodopsin kinase, the best studied members of this new protein kinase family, probably participate in phosphorylation of several Ser/Thr residues of the carboxyl tail of G-protein-coupled receptors via their interaction with the $\beta\gamma$ dimer. Unlike second messenger-activated protein kinases, βARK1 and rhodopsin kinase have the unique feature of phosphorylating receptors only when they are in an active conformation. This phosphorylation is followed by binding of arrestin and interdicting signal transduction (41).

TABLE 1. *Target proteins coupled to GTP-binding protein subunits*

Subunits	Target-proteins	Activation (↑) or inhibition (↓)	References
α_s	Adenylate cyclase	↑	6
	Ca^{2+} channels	↑	19,20
	Ca^{2+}-activated K$^+$ channels	↑	21
α_i	Adenylate cyclase	↓	6
	Ca^{2+} channels	↓	22
α_{i3}	K$^+$ channels	↑	23,24
α_t	cGMP specific phosphodiesterase	↑	90
α_q, α_{14}, α_{16}, α_{11}	Phospholipase C (β_1 isoform)	↑	25–27
α_0	Ca channels (mod)	↓	29,280
$\beta\gamma$	Phospholipase A$_2$	↑	30
	Phospholipase C (β_2 isoform)	↑	31
$\beta\gamma^*$	Adenylate cyclase type I	↓	15
	Adenylate cyclase type II, IV	↑	14–16
β_1	Ca channels	↓	32
β_3	Ca channels	↓	32

* These experiments were performed in the presence of the α_2 subunit.

Cyclic GMP

In addition to cAMP, cGMP is the only other cyclic nucleotide widely distributed in nature. Although discovered by Price et al. (42) merely a decade after cAMP, its importance in cellular regulation took longer to be established. Two major forms of guanylate cyclase are encountered in most tissues. Soluble guanylate cyclase is a heme-protein heterodimer of 150-kDa molecular weight. It is composed of two unequal subunits of 70 and 80 kDa molecular weight (43,44). Interaction with the heme moiety is essential for the activation of soluble guanylate cyclase by nitrosodilators such as endothelium-derived nitrous oxide (NO) and sodium nitroprusside. Purification of this enzyme has demonstrated that its stimulability is completely lost when the heme moiety is separated from the protein (45–47). In addition to alteration of the heme-protein interaction by nitroso compounds, this enzyme can be modulated by several thiol agents (48) and fatty acids (49). It is also subject to oxygen-dependent activation (50). Many other activators of guanylate cyclase are free radicals which, like NO, bind to the heme moiety and change its interaction with the protein (48). Ascorbate is another potent activator (51,52), which must be kept in mind when it is used as a preservative for such agonists as catecholamines. In addition to a series of activators, soluble guanylate cyclase also has its inhibitors. They include hemoglobin (53) and methylene blue (54,55), largely employed as tools to differentiate soluble from particulate guanylate cyclase.

Particulate guanylate cyclase is found in most animal species, including monocellular organisms (52–56). Most tissues possess both soluble and particulate guanylate cyclase, and the distribution of the two enzymes is equal in such tissues as VSMC (57). Tissues rich in particulate, but with very little soluble guanylate cyclase, include intestinal epithelial cells and glomeruli. This is in contrast to cell types such as platelets, which mainly possess soluble guanylate cyclase (58). The first endogenous hormone found to directly activate particulate guanylate cyclase was atrial natriuretic peptide (ANP), the first peptide identified in the newly-uncovered natriuretic peptide family.

The natriuretic peptide family at present consists of at least three members: ANP (59,60), brain natriuretic peptide (BNP) (61,62) and C-type natriuretic peptide (CNP) (63,64). Three types of receptors of this natriuretic peptide family have recently been identified and cloned. Natriuretic peptide receptor-C (NPR-C) is considered to have mainly a clearance function (65,66), while the other two, natriuretic peptide receptor-A (NPR-A) and natriuretic peptide receptor-B (NPR-B), also known as guanylate cyclase-A (GC-A) and guanylate cyclase-B (GC-B), respectively (67–69), are believed to be biologically active binding sites possessing intrinsic particulate guanylate cyclase activity. These two proteins closely resemble each other in both sequence identity and overall structure, with three distinct domains of homology in addition to a single putative transmembrane domain. Radiation inactivation has been used to characterize the functional domains of GC-A. Radiation-inactivation sizes of about 30 kDa for the cyclase function, 20 kDa for the ANP-binding function and 90 kDa for the inhibitory function have been calculated (70). These studies suggest that GC-A behaves as a multidomain protein and that an intramolecular inhibitory domain represses the guanylate cyclase catalytic domain. Atrial natriuretic peptide binding to the extracellular binding domain activates the cyclase function, probably via modulation of the intramolecular inhibitory function.

It is noteworthy that, in addition to the two functional domains of ligand binding and catalysis, sequence analysis demonstrated a third domain in the intracellular region of the protein with high sequence homology to protein kinases (71). Deletion mutagenesis showed that this kinaselike domain represses guanylate cyclase activity and that this repression is removed after ANP binding.

Guanylate cyclase-A and GC-B can be viewed as an evolutionary intersection among three different and nonoverlapping groups of proteins. They define a large and disparate protein superfamily, including natriuretic peptide receptors, protein kinases and cyclases (72). Chromosomal localization of genes encoding the three human natriuretic peptide receptors NPR-C, GC-A, and GC-B assigned the GC-A gene to 1q21 → q22, GC-B to 9p12 → p21 and NPR-C to 5p13 → p14, illustrating the dispersal of this gene family in the human genome (72).

Several studies have shown that GC-A and GC-B have different ligand selectivity. Guanylate cyclase-A mainly binds ANP and BNP, whereas GC-B mainly binds CNP (67,73,74). This selectivity differential suggests that they play distinct physiological roles. Suga et al. (75) recently reported that GC-B is highly expressed in vascular smooth muscles and that CNP is synthesized in and secreted from endothelial cells in response to various secretagogues, including $TGF\beta_1$. They postulated the existence of a "vascular natriuretic system." In the aorta, we found that GC-B mRNA levels are about 10 times higher than those of GC-A, and this dominance is further amplified (more than 500-fold) in cultured aortic smooth muscle cells (ASMC) (Fujio et al., *submitted for publication*). Interestingly, it has been demonstrated that the CNP effects on natriuresis, diuresis, and vasodilation are only about 1 percent of those of ANP (63). This suggests that the biological activity of GC-B is much weaker than that of GC-A or that the two receptors mediate different functions. Our results on cultured ASMC show that although GC-B messenger ribonucleic acid (mRNA) levels are much higher than those of GC-A, the CNP-induced production of cGMP is similar to that generated by ANP, at least in spontaneously hypertensive rat (SHR) cells

(Tremblay et al., *submitted for publication*). This points to a lower activity of GC-B compared to GC-A, as observed *in vivo*, but also suggests that the selective endogenous agonist of GC-B still remains to be uncovered.

Cyclic GMP-hydrolyzing enzymes have been divided by Beavo et al. (34) according to their ability to bind cGMP and their hydrolytic activity. Cyclic GMP-binding phosphodiesterases are subdivided into three categories: the first is a cGMP-stimulated type, the second occurs specifically in the retina and is regulated by GTP-binding protein, while the third is found in platelets and lung (76). In addition, cGMP can be hydrolyzed by a calcium-calmodulin-sensitive phosphodiesterase (which is, however, also able to hydrolyze cAMP) and by a specific, high-affinity cGMP-phosphodiesterase. As with cAMP-specific phosphodiesterase, cGMP hydrolysis can be modified from the exterior of cells by active cardiovascular agents such as methylxanthines. Chiu et al. (77) explored the effects of vinpocetine and 8-bromo-cGMP derivatives on vasorelaxation. Vinpocetine compound is a specific inhibitor of calmodulin-dependent phosphodiesterase, having an IC_{50} of 19 μM. It produces significant cGMP but not cAMP accumulation in aortic tissue. Thus, besides the specific inhibitor of cGMP-phosphodiesterase, this compound represents another tool known for a long time as M & B-22948, which has also been demonstrated to potentiate the vasodilatory effects of nitrovasodilators (78).

Most mammalian tissues contain cGMP-dependent protein kinase (79), an enzyme distinct from the cAMP-dependent enzyme. It is only a dimer, compared to the tetrameric structure of the cAMP-dependent enzyme (80). Cyclic GMP-binding and catalytic sites reside in two different domains, probably on the same polypeptide chain (81). Specific endogenous substrates for this enzyme have been found in rabbit aortic tissue and cultured ASMC (82).

Cyclic GMP can also interfere with ionic fluxes without the involvement of phosphorylation, via binding of the cGMP molecule to the channel. Ten years ago, this type of cGMP function was shown to be expressed in very specialized tissues of the retina, controlling the permeability of sodium channels and transmission of the light signal (83). It was suggested that such an exquisitely rapid action of cGMP in modifying ionic fluxes may occur in other tissues, including the endothelium, where massive and quick cGMP fluxes are induced by hormonal stimulation with ANP (84). Recently, this theory was confirmed for the amiloride-sensitive sodium channels of epithelial cells (see below).

Polyphosphoinositides and Calcium

Forty years ago, Hokin and Hokin (85,86) demonstrated that treatment of pancreatic slices with acetyl-choline increased the ^{32}P-labeling of phospholipids, eventually identified as polyphosphoinositides. The involvement of polyphosphoinositide metabolism in receptor-induced intracellular signaling was proposed by Michell (87) in 1975, and the role of DAG as well as $InsP_3$ as second messengers was recognized in the mid-1980s in elegant experiments performed by M. Berridge, R. Irvine, and their co-workers. A number of reviews have been published describing this signaling pathway (2,88,89).

Polyphosphoinositide Metabolism Intermediators

Many agonists interacting with 7-membrane-spanning receptors activate two isoforms of phosphatidylinositol-4,5-diphosphate (PIP_2): specific phospholipase C: (PLC)β_1 and β_2. Coupling of these receptors to PLCβ_1 is mediated by the α-subunit of G_{14}-, G_{16}-, G_{11}-, and Gq-proteins (Fig. 2) (see Table 1) (6,14–16,18,19,21–32,90). There is growing evidence that $\beta\gamma$ subunits play a key role in the activation of PLCβ_2 (31) and modulate the efficiency of α-subunits coupling with other isoforms of PLC (91). Breakdown of PIP_2 by PLC results in increased intracellular DAG and $InsP_3$ content. Nishizuka and co-workers (92) demonstrated that DAG is an endogenous activator of (Ca^{2+}-phospholipid)-dependent protein kinase (protein kinase C). $InsP_3$ activates receptors localized on the cytoplasmic surface of the endoplasmic reticulum coupled with Ca^{2+} channels, triggering a rise in $[Ca^{2+}]_i$ (93). Activation of $InsP_3$-kinase results in the formation of $InsP_4$. It has been suggested that this compound increases $[Ca^{2+}]_i$ via the direct activation of plasma membrane Ca^{2+} channels (94). Indeed, $InsP_4$ specifically enhances the activity of Ca^{2+}-permeable channels when added to the intracellular surface of endothelial cell inside-out membrane patches (95). The other activation pathway of polyphosphoinositide metabolism is triggered by antigen, insulin, and growth factors interacting with single membrane-spanning tyrosine kinase receptors. Agonist-induced autophosphorylation of these receptors favors their cross-linking and interaction with the γ_1-isoform of PLC, resulting in phosphorylation of at least three tyrosine residues of this enzyme (tyr 771, 783, and 1,254) that are important for its activation. Tyrosine kinase receptors are also capable of activating other effectors such as phosphotidylinositol 3-OH kinase, which generates PIP_3 and GTPase-activating protein (GAP), triggering the ras → raf 1–MAP-2 kinase cascade of intracellular signaling. There is evidence for the involvement of PIP_3 in activation of the ξ-isoform of protein kinase C (96) and in regulation of the cytoskeleton assembly and GAP/ras interaction (97). The role of the GAP/ras interaction in the regulation of cellular activity has been reviewed (11,98). There is also indirect evidence for the involvement of GAP and ras p21 in reg-

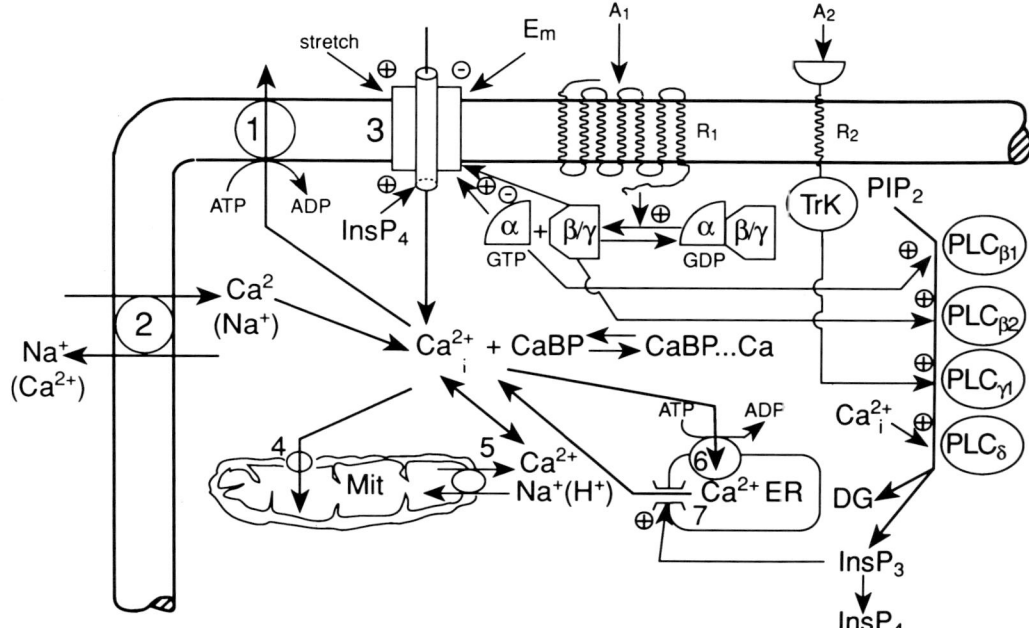

FIG. 2. Systems involved in the regulation of intracellular free calcium $[Ca^{2-}]_i$ concentration. 1, plasma membrane Ca^{2+} pump; 2, Na^+/Ca^{2+} exchanger; 3, Ca^{2+} channels; 4 and 5, Ca^{2+} uniporter and Ca^{2+}/Na^+ (or Ca^{2+}/H^+) exchanger of mitochondria (Mit); 6 and 7, Ca^{2+} pump and Ca^{2+} channels of endoplasmic reticulum (ER). A_1 and A_2, agonists interacting with 7-membrane-spanning receptors (R_1) and tyrosine kinase (TrK)-coupled receptors (R_2); α, β, γ, subunits of G-proteins; PIP_2, phosphatidylinositol-4,5-diphosphate; $InsP_3$, inositol-1,4,5-trisphosphate; DG, diacylglycerol; $PLC\beta_1$, $PLC\beta_2$, $PLC\gamma_1$ and $PLC\delta$, members of phospholipase C family; Em, electrical potential of plasma membrane; CaBP, calcium-binding proteins; + and −, stimulatory and inhibitory pathways of regulation.

ulation of the GTPase activity of G-protein coupling of muscarinic receptors to atrial K^+ channels (99).

Intracellular Calcium

Two peculiarities of $[Ca^{2+}]_i$ as a second messenger should be taken into consideration in the role of this cation in regulating cellular activity.

Diversity of Transport Systems Involved in $[Ca^{2+}]_i$ Regulation

Concentration of cyclic nucleotides and polyphosphoinositide-derived second messengers is under the control of only two key enzymes catalyzing their synthesis and degradation (e.g., adenylate cyclase and phosphodiesterase for cAMP). Figure 2 illustrates the diversity of the ionic transport systems involved in regulating $[Ca^{2+}]_i$ levels. Long-term maintenance of extremely low $[Ca^{2+}]_i$ under basal conditions is mainly provided by the Ca^{2+} pump and Na^+/Ca^{2+} exchanger localized in plasma membranes. The Ca^{2+} pump operates via Mg^{2+}-dependent, Ca^{2+}-activated adenosine triphosphatase (Ca^{2+}-ATPase), coupling hydrolysis of the ATP molecule with

efflux of the calcium ion against its electrochemical gradient (100). An electroneutral operation mode of this pump is probably supported by the countertransport of two protons. The Ca^{2+} efflux via Na^+/Ca^{2+} exchange is supported by an inward electrochemical sodium gradient. The stoichiometry of this exchange varies between $2Na^+:1Ca^{2+}$ (electroneutral mode) and $4Na^+:1Ca^{2+}$ (electrogenic mode) (100,101). To date, there is no known specific inhibitor of the plasmalemmal Ca^{2+} pump. Data on amiloride derivatives and bepridil as Na^+/Ca^{2+} exchange blockers have been summarized by Kaczorowski et al. (102).

A set of channels is involved in inward Ca^{2+} movement. Under basal conditions, most of these channels are quenched and the rate of Ca^{2+} influx is extremely low. Under membrane depolarization conditions, the rate of Ca^{2+} influx increases drastically due to the opening of potential-operated channels (POC). These POC (L- and P-type channels), activated and inactivated at a high membrane potential (Em), are the best characterized calcium-entry pathways, primarily because of the existence of highly selective organic compounds and neurotoxins which inhibit their conductance. No specific ligands are presently available to characterize low-voltage-activated T-type POC (103,104). In several tissues, L-type POC activity is under the control of α_s-,α_1-, α_o-, and β-subunits (see Fig. 2 and Table 1). There are a variety of electrical silent cells including platelets, mast cells, lymphocytes, and neutrophils, in which Ca^{2+} influx involves nonselective channels. These channels are permeable to Ca^{2+}, Na^+, and Mn^{2+}, lack a voltage-dependent gating mechanism, and can be opened by receptor agonists (receptor-operated channels [ROC]), cGMP, $InsP_4$, and stretch (95,105–108).

The other pathway for increased $[Ca^{2+}]_i$ during cell excitation is mediated by calcium release from the endoplasmic reticulum via channels containing high-affinity binding sites for $InsP_3$ ($InsP_3$-activated channels) or ryanodine (Ca^{2+}-activated channels) (2). A special isoform of Ca^{2+}-ATPase is involved in calcium refilling of the endoplasmic reticulum, supporting the short-term regulation of $[Ca^{2+}]_i$ during electrical or pharmacological excitation. It has been postulated that under conditions of intracellular calcium overloading, an electrogenic Ca^{2+} uniporter of the inner mitochondrial membrane takes part in $[Ca^{2+}]_i$ regulation. Normalization of $[Ca^{2+}]_i$ homeostasis is accompanied by its release from mitochondria via Ca^{2+}/Na^+ or Ca^{2+}/H^+ exchange (101).

Diversity of $[Ca^{2+}]_i$ Receptors

Protein kinases are the only receptors of cAMP and DAG that are involved in the regulation of cellular activity. Protein kinases and nonselective ion channels have been described as intracellular cGMP receptors (see Fig. 1). Unlike these second messengers, a set of target proteins containing high-affinity Ca^{2+}-binding sites (the so-called "EF" motif) mediate signaling pathways induced by increments of $[Ca^{2+}]_i$. Calmodulin, troponin C, parvalbumin, calbindin, calpain, gelsolin, $cPLA_2$ and PLCδ are the most widely distributed Ca^{2+}-binding proteins of this superfamily. Some of them are highly specialized. For example, troponin C regulates actomyosin ATPase activity of skeletal and cardiac muscle cells whereas gelsolin mediates Ca^{2+}-dependent regulation of actin polymerization and cytoskeleton assembly. Ca^{2+}-dependent phospholipases ($cPLA_2$, PLCδ) and proteases (calpain) are involved in the catabolism of phospholipids and proteins, as well as in the generation of PIP_2-derived second messengers. Unlike the Ca^{2+}-binding proteins mentioned above, Ca^{2+}-induced conformational calmodulin transition is accompanied by the altered activity of several purified soluble or membrane-bound enzymes, e.g., Ca^{2+}-calmodulin-dependent protein kinases, phosphoproteinphosphatase (calcineurin), phosphodiesterase, type I adenylate cyclase, plasma membrane Ca^{2+}-ATPase, myosin light-chain kinase, etc., indicating the possible involvement of calmodulin in the regulation of these enzymes *in vivo*. The role of some Ca^{2+}-binding proteins (e.g., parvalbumin) is still unclear. It must be

mentioned that the list of intracellular Ca^{2+} receptors is not yet complete. There are no data on the nature of an intracellular calcium sensor responsible for the opening of Ca^{2+}-dependent K^+ channels. For more details, consult recent publications (109–114).

Monovalent Cation Transport Pathways

As mentioned in the previous subsection, monovalent ions are involved in the regulation of $[Ca^{2+}]_i$ via at least two transport pathways, i.e., potential-operated Ca^{2+} channels and the Na^+/Ca^{2+} exchanger. The transport pathways of monovalent ions are also involved in regulating cellular activity and the secretion of hormones, as well as neuromediators via the control of salt and water reabsorption by kidney tubular epithelial cells and adjustment of cellular volume, pH_i and the $[Na^+]_i/[K^+]_i$ ratio. The last three parameters play a key role in the homeostasis of cell growth and proliferation. Collective viewing of these facts indicates that monovalent cation metabolism is an important component of intracellular signaling, showing several points of its involvement in the long-term maintenance of high blood pressure. Here, we will briefly summarize data on the transport systems participating in the regulation of intracellular levels of monovalent cations, cell volume, and the Em of plasma membranes (Fig. 3). Detailed information has been published (104,115–124).

The Na^+,K^+ pump (Mg^{2+}-dependent Na^+,K^+-activated ATPase) operates as a primary active transport system, coupling the energy of ATP hydrolysis with outward Na^+ and inward K^+ fluxes. This pump is a main controller of the equilibrium distribution of monovalent cations between the cytoplasm and extracellular fluids as well as of transcellular salt movement. Due to its stoechiometry ($3Na_i^+:2K_o^+$), the Na^+,K^+ pump is also involved in regulating the Em of cells with relatively high plasma membrane electrical resistance. Its activity is inhibited by cardiac glycosides (ouabain).

Several electroneutral ion carriers ($Na^+,K^+,2Cl^-$ cotransport, K^+,Cl^- cotransport, Na^+/H^+ exchange, anion exchange) operate as secondary active transport systems. Transport mediated by these carriers can occur against an electrochemical gradient but in contrast to primary active transport it is not directly coupled to ATP consumption. Rather, energy is provided by the chemical gradient of one or more co- or countertransporting ions. $Na^+,K^+,2Cl^-$ cotransport is inhibited by diuretics, e.g., furosemide or bumetanide. Depending on the transmembrane ionic gradient, net fluxes of Na^+,K^+ and Cl^- with a stoechiometry of 1:1:2 can occur in either direction. In human and rat erythrocytes, bumetanide inhibits about 5–15 percent of outward and inward Na^+ and K^+ fluxes. On the other hand, in electrically excitable tissue, $Na^+,K^+,2Cl^-$ cotransport mediates up to 80 percent

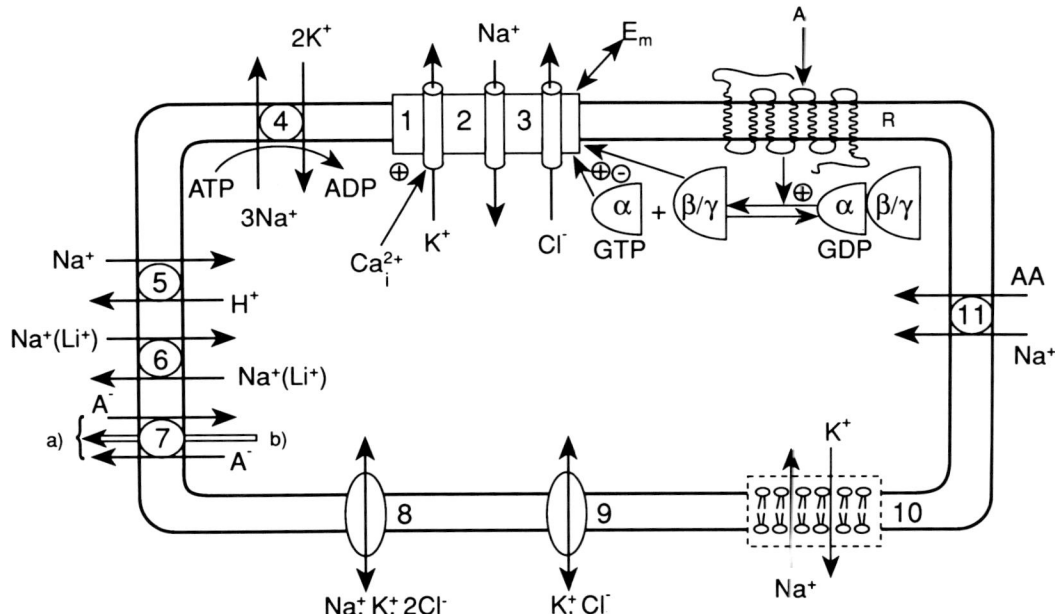

FIG. 3. Systems involved in regulating the intracellular concentration of monovalent ions and plasma membrane electrical potentials (Em). 1, 2, 3, potential- and receptor-operated K^+, Cl^-, and Na^+ channels (K^+ channels may be also activated by $[Ca^{2+}]_i$); 4, Na^+,K^+ pump; 5, Na^+/H^+ exchange; 6, Na^+/Na^+ (Na^+/Li^+) countertransport; 7, anion transport: a) electroneutral mode (anion exchange), b) electrogenic mode (unidirectoral transport); 8, Na^+,K^+,$2Cl^-$ cotransport; 9, K^+,Cl^- cotransport; 10, passive diffusion (leakage); 11, symport of sodium with organic compounds (amino acids, glucose, neurotransmitters, etc.); A, agonist; R, 7-membrane-spanning receptor; α, β, γ, subunits of G-proteins; $+$ and $-$, stimulatory and inhibitory pathways of regulation.

of total potassium influx. In epithelial cells lining the thick ascending limb of Henle's loop, this carrier also plays a key role in NaCl and water reabsorption (see below). Equimolar sodium and proton countertransport (exchange) in all types of vertebrate cells is very much under investigation. Under physiological conditions, this carrier, operating as Na_o^+/H_i^+ countertransport, is inhibited by amiloride derivatives (ethylisopropyl amiloride [EIPA], dimethyl amiloride [DMA], etc.). In erythrocytes, as well as in most nonexcitable cells, Na^+/H^+ exchange is quenched under resting conditions and needs intracellular acidification for its activation. In VSMC, this carrier is the main pathway of Na^+ influx and plays a key role in the regulation of $[Na^+]_i$ (see below).

The highest values of the phloretin-inhibited component of Na^+ (Li^+) fluxes, transactivated by Li^+ (Na^+) and called *Na^+/Na^+* or *Na^+/Li^+ countertransport*, have been found in human, cow, and rabbit erythrocytes. The physiological significance of this electroneutral and equimolar exchanger is still unknown. It has been suggested that Na^+/Li^+ countertransport represents the mode of operation of the Na^+/H^+ exchanger. However, comparative analysis of Na^+/H^+ and Na^+/Li^+ countertransport values in erythrocytes of different species, as well as in *Xenopus laevis* oocytes, does not support this suggestion (125,126).

The Em of resting cells is determined by chemical gradients of monovalent ions and their relative conductance. Ion conductance is dependent on the activity of electrogenic transport pathways, mainly mediated by monovalent ions passing through regulated water pores formed in the lipid bilayer by members of an extended family of ion-channel proteins. As mentioned above, electrogenic ion pumps (e.g., Na^+,K^+-ATPase) and carriers (e.g., anion transporter operated in an unidirectional mode) may also be involved in the regulation of membrane potential. For the majority of monovalent ion channels, their opening and closing are under feedback control of membrane potential (potential-operated channels). Bungarotoxin-sensitive Na^+ channels of postsynaptic membranes are directly coupled with n-cholinergic receptors, triggering the action potential. Tetrodotoxin-sensitive fast Na^+ channels and L-type Ca^{2+} channels are involved in propagation of the action potential in skeletal and smooth muscle cells, respectively. Resting potential and the efficiency of membrane polarization after propagation of the action potential are mainly dependent on the activity of potential-operated K^+ channels. The feedback regulation of membrane potential is increased via a Ca^{2+}-dependent mechanism opening K^+ channels (Ca^{2+}-activated K^+ channels). Ionic channel regulation by G-protein-coupled receptors may be obligatory for opening (e.g., muscarinic atrial K^+

channels) or it may be modulatory with some other stimulus such as membrane depolarization or increased $[Ca^{2+}]_i$ concentration (Ca^{2+}-activated K^+ channels of smooth muscles) (see Table 1).

INTRACELLULAR SIGNALING SYSTEMS IN BLOOD PRESSURE REGULATION

This section outlines the specific roles of the intracellular signaling systems in blood pressure control mentioned above. In accordance with Guyton's concept (127), more attention will be devoted to mechanisms which may be involved in the *long-term* maintenance of elevated (>140 mm Hg) blood pressure. Data on cyclic nucleotide involvement in the regulation of heart rate, renin secretion, ACTH action on the adrenal cortex, and neurotransmitter release have been summarized previously (128), as well as elsewhere in other chapters of this volume.

Vascular Contractility

Observations on endothelium-derived relaxing factors (EDRF), identified as NO and PGI_2, endothelium-derived contractile factor (EDCF), identified as a 21-amino-acid peptide termed *endothelin*, as well as on the mechanism of regulation of VSMC contraction and relaxation, have been reviewed recently (129–132). This section reports only new results obtained during the last 5 years and formulates some unresolved problems.

The Endothelium as a Primary Target of Circulating Vasoactive Substances

It has been shown that acetylcholine, bradykinin, histamine, serotonin, ATP, ADP and substance P enhance the production of vasodilators (PGI_2 and NO) by endothelial cells. All these hormones and neuromediators, designated as Group I compounds, activate polyphosphoinositide/Ca^{2+} signaling systems. Nitrous oxide and PGI_2 synthesis is probably mediated via the activation of Ca^{2+}-dependent phospholipase A_2 and (Ca^{2+}-calmodulin)-dependent NO synthase, respectively (133). Group II compounds (thrombin, α-agonists, TGF$_\beta$) are known as activators of the polyphosphoinositide/Ca^{2+} signaling system. However, unlike Group I, Group II compounds induce endothelin synthesis via protein kinase C-activated domains (two octanucleotide sequences) on the 5' flanking region of the preproendothelin gene (130). The mechanism of predominant activation of Ca^{2+}-dependent and protein kinase C-dependent pathways by Group I and Group II compounds, respectively, is still unknown.

Pulmonary endothelial cells are the major depot of

angiotensin-converting enzyme; angiotensin I is completely converted into angiotensin II within a single passage of blood (134). These observations raise questions about the mechanism of regulation of angiotensin II production by endothelial cells and the relative roles of circulatory as well as endothelium-derived angiotensin in controlling VSMC contractility.

Vascular endothelial cells possess a $Na^+,K^+,2Cl^-$ cotransport system that mediates a major portion of total K^+ influx. This carrier is activated by vasopressin, bradykinin and angiotensin II and is inhibited by compounds which activate cAMP (β-adrenoceptor)- and cGMP (ANP)-mediated signaling pathways (135,136). The mechanism of hormonal regulation of Na^+,K^+ cotransport and the physiological implications of this regulatory pathway are still unclear. It may be suggested that $Na^+,K^+,2Cl^-$ cotransport and other monovalent ion transport systems involved in cell volume regulation via the control of intracellular inorganic osmolytes (Na^+/H^+ exchanger, stretch-activated ion channels) support the integrity of the endothelium monolayer, protecting smooth muscle cells from the direct action of circulating vasoactive compounds and arteriosclerotic damage. Indeed, factors that cause cell shrinkage or retraction are known to increase permeability of the endothelial monolayer for protein molecules (137).

Regulation of Vascular Smooth Muscle Contraction

Intracellular calcium is viewed as a main trigger of VSMC contraction: Ca^{2+} binds to calmodulin, and the Ca-calmodulin complex removes myosin light chain kinase autoinhibition, phosphorylating the serine 19 residue of myosin light chains and facilitating actin-myosin interaction (138). Potential-operated L-type Ca^{2+} channels and $InsP_3$-activated Ca^{2+} channels of the sarcoplasmic reticulum are the main transport pathways, providing an increase of $[Ca^{2+}]_i$ during electrical and pharmacological excitation-contraction coupling, respectively (Fig. 4a). Benham and Tsien (139) and Den Hertog and co-workers (140) presented data on the induction in smooth muscle cells by P_2-purinergic and β_1-adrenergic agonists of an electrogenic L-type channel blocker-insensitive Ca transport pathway referred to as receptor-operated Ca^{2+} channels. However, the lack of selective inhibitors complicates the estimation of the role of these channels in vascular smooth muscle contraction.

As discussed above (see Table 1), potential-operated Ca^{2+} channels in skeletal muscle, atria and GH_3 cells are under the modulatory, activatory, and inhibitory control of G_s and G_o proteins, respectively (19,20,24,32). This pharmacologically important pathway of $[Ca^{2+}]_i$ regulation has not been studied in VSMC.

Contractile agonists such as histamine, endothelin,

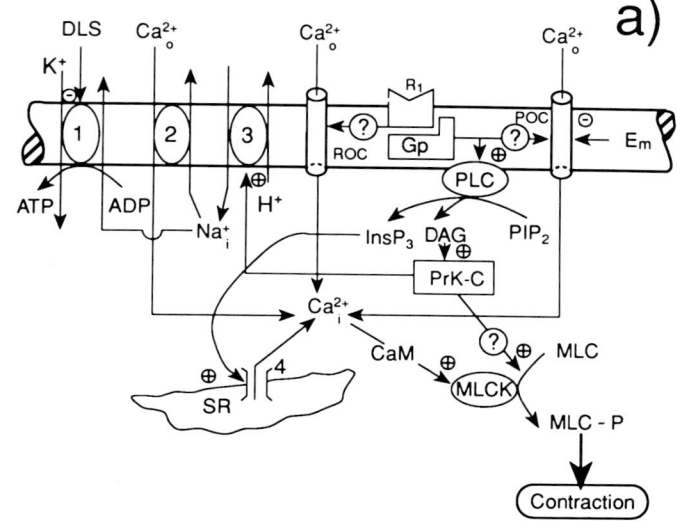

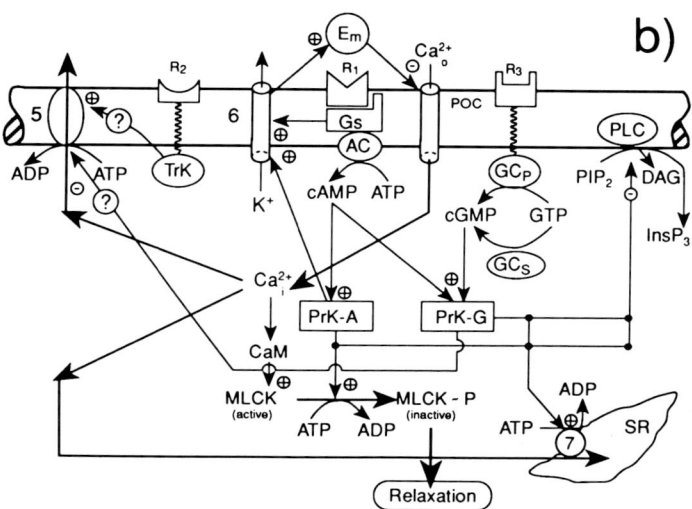

FIG. 4. Cross-talking of signaling pathways involved in vascular smooth muscle contraction a) and relaxation b) 1, Na^+,K^+ pump; 2, Na^+/Ca^{2+} exchanger; 3, Na^+/H^+ exchanger; 4, $InsP_3$-, and Ca^{2+}-operated channels of sarcoplasmic reticulum (SR); 5, Ca^{2+} pump of plasma membrane; 6, Ca^{2+}-activated K^+ channels; 7, Ca^{2+} pumps of sarcoplasmic reticulum; R_1, 7-membrane-spanning receptors coupled with Gp; R_2, receptors coupled with tyrosine kinase (TrK); R_3, ANP receptors coupled with guanylate cyclase (GC); ROC and POC, receptor- and potential-operated Ca^{2+} channels, respectively; Em, plasma membrane electrical potential; DLS, digitalis-like substance(s) or natriuretic hormone; PLC, phospholipase C; AC, adenylate cyclase; PIP_2, phosphatidylinositol-4,5-diphosphate; $InsP_3$, inositol-1,4,5-triphosphate; DAG, diacylglycerol; PrK-C, protein kinase C; PrK-A and PrK-G, cAMP- and cGMP-dependent protein kinases, respectively; MLC, myosin light chains; MLCK, myosin light chain kinase; CaM, calmodulin; + and −, stimulatory and inhibitory pathways of regulation, respectively; −, unidentified mechanisms of regulation.

and phenylephrine induce a greater sensitivity of myosin light chain phosphorylation for $[Ca^{2+}]_i$ than L-type channel or Na_i^+/Ca_o^{2+} exchange activators (131). Moreover, using aequorin-loaded VSMCs, it has been shown that histamine evokes myosin light chain phosphorylation and contractile responses in Ca^{2+}-free medium without any increment of $[Ca^{2+}]_i$. Pharmacomechanical coupling is accompanied by PLC-mediated DAG production, indicating the possible involvement of protein kinase C in the drastic increase of contractile protein affinity for $[Ca^{2+}]_i$ (see Fig. 4a). Indeed, it has been reported that phorbol diesters, exogenous activators of protein kinase C, induce contraction of the swine carotid with resting levels of $[Ca^{2+}]_i$ (141). The mechanism of $[Ca^{2+}]_i$-independent protein kinase C-activated muscle contraction is still unknown. It may be assumed that this

type of contraction is partly caused by the activation of G_i-proteins, leading to decreased cAMP content.

It is known that the Na_i^+/Ca_o^{2+} mode of operation of the Na^+/Ca^{2+} exchanger is increased drastically under membrane depolarization and the influence of factors augmenting intracellular sodium content (101). The Na^+,K^+ pump and Na^+/H^+ exchange as main pathways of Na^+ efflux and influx, respectively, play key roles in the regulation of $[Na^+]_i$ in VSMC (142,143). Fifteen years ago, it was proposed that sarcolemmal Na^+/Ca^{2+} exchange mediates the increase in $[Ca^{2+}]_i$ and vasoconstriction in several forms of arterial hypertension induced by enhanced salt intake (144,145). Up to now, this hypothesis has been supported by data on heightened levels of circulating Na^+,K^+-ATPase inhibitors (the so-called natriuretic hormone or digitalis-like substance

[DLS]) found in hypertensive patients and experimental animals with volume-expanded hypertension (see 146 for review), as well as by numerous reports on increased Na^+/H^+ exchange in essential hypertensives and SHR (see below).

Regulation of Vascular Smooth Muscle Relaxation

Reversible phosphorylation of turkey-gizzard smooth muscle myosin light chain kinase by cAMP-dependent protein kinase A has been demonstrated by Adelstein and co-workers (147). This observation has also been recently confirmed for tracheal smooth muscle cells (148). These data suggest that protein kinase A-mediated myosin light chain kinase inactivation is a main mechanism of cAMP signaling involved in the relaxation of blood vessels. However, to the best of our knowledge, there is no direct evidence positively correlating cAMP-induced phosphorylation of myosin light chain kinase and relaxation of vascular smooth muscle in vivo. On the contrary, it has been shown that forskolin-induced relaxation of carotid arteries is not associated with an altered Ca^{2+} sensitivity of myosin light chain phosphorylation (149). Data on myosin light chain kinase-independent mechanisms of smooth muscle cell relaxation, summarized in Fig. 4b, will be briefly discussed below.

In cardiac muscle cells, β-adrenergic-induced phosphorylation of phospholamban, a 22-kDa protein, is accompanied by a several-fold activation of the sarcoplasmic reticulum Ca^{2+} pump (150). In VSMC, phospholamban phosphorylation occurs at the same site as in cardiac cells but is predominantly mediated by cGMP-dependent protein kinase (151–153). To date, however, there is no direct evidence of cAMP- or cGMP-dependent activation of the Ca^{2+} pump in the vascular smooth muscle sarcoplasmic reticulum. Ten years ago, it was reported that prior activation of platelet protein kinase A, C, or G inhibits calcium mobilization via PLC-coupled receptors (for review see 154). Recently, this negative regulatory pathway mediated by the inhibition of phosphatidylinositol hydrolysis was also revealed in vascular smooth muscle (155,156). It was also suggested that the cGMP signaling system may be involved in VSMC relaxation via protein kinase G-dependent inactivation of $InsP_3$-sensitive Ca^{2+} channels of the sarcoplasmic reticulum, inhibition of cAMP hydrolysis by phosphodiesterase or via activation of K^+ channels and membrane polarization (38,132). These attractive hypotheses should be examined in forthcoming experiments.

Yoshida and co-workers (157) have reported that the maximal activity of plasma membrane Ca^{2+} ATPase, partially purified from the porcine aorta by calmodulin-affinity chromatography, is increased twofold with the addition of cGMP-dependent protein kinase. These results suggest that cGMP-induced vascular smooth muscle relaxation may be mediated via activation of the plasma membrane Ca^{2+} pump. Plasmalemmal Ca^{2+} pump activation is probably also involved in the enhanced efficiency of spontaneous relaxation in vascular smooth muscles pretreated with insulin. Insulin stimulates the Na_o^+-independent component of ^{45}Ca efflux in aortic strips and the rate of $[Ca^{2+}]_i$ recovery to baseline in cultured VSMC after their exposure to PLC activators. Insulin's effect on vascular smooth muscle relaxation and ^{45}Ca efflux in aortic strips is abolished by orthovanadate, the nonselective inhibitor of E_1-E_2 ATPase (158,159).

As mentioned above, potassium efflux through the electrogenic pathway (K^+ channels) is critical for membrane potential regulation in vascular smooth muscles. Beta-adrenergic stimulation of VSMC is accompanied by membrane hyperpolarization (160) and by inhibition of nicardipine-sensitive ^{45}Ca-influx in low- but not in high-potassium medium (161). In tracheal smooth muscle, evidence of direct (membrane-limited G_s-protein-mediated) and indirect (protein kinase A-mediated) coupling of β-adrenoceptor with Ca^{2+}-activated K^+ channels was obtained by the patch-clamp technique (21). These results suggest that β-adrenergic activation of vascular smooth muscle channels is a trigger for membrane polarization, closing L-type Ca^{2+} channels and inducing relaxation.

Vascular Smooth Muscle Growth and Remodeling

In 1970, Folkow et al. (162) demonstrated that an equal vasoconstrictor stimulus produced greater narrowing of the vessels with an increased wall/lumen ratio. These findings, as well as data on blood vessel wall hypertrophy in clinical and experimental hypertension, indicate that the altered geometry of blood vessels is one of the major mechanisms of long-term maintenance of high blood pressure (163). During the last decade, it has been shown that enhanced cell growth, proliferation and so-called remodeling (rearranging existing material without the need to evoke a growth response) are involved in increasing the wall/lumen ratio in primary hypertension (164,165). More rapid proliferation of aortic and mesenteric smooth muscles from SHR, compared with normotensive rats, has also been demonstrated in vitro (166–174). It should be mentioned that the increased growth of VSMC from hypertensive animals appears to be tightly linked with apoptosis, i.e., programmed cell death (175). Numerous data on the hormonal regulation of VSMC replication have been summarized recently in an excellent review (164), as well as elsewhere in this volume. This section merely focuses on the control of

VSMC growth and proliferation by cyclic nucleotide signaling systems and intracellular cations.

Cellular growth regulation, specifically of the cell cycle by modulation of cyclic nucleotide levels as well as of the calcium signal, has long been recognized. Initial studies by Boynton and Whitfield (176) pinpointed the intervention of cyclic nucleotides early in the cell cycle, in the regulated component of G_0-G_1 transition prior to DNA synthesis. Our investigations (177) indicate that cAMP is also involved in regulating the growth potential of VSMC. Thus, the ability of cells to grow in culture correlates directly with adenylate cyclase activity in different lines of VSMC. Adenylate cyclase activity increases after the addition of growth stimuli, and this event appears to precede the rise in [^{3}H]-thymidine incorporation (177). A few years ago, it was shown that the transcriptional stimulation of a number of eukaryotic genes in response to factors increasing intracellular cAMP and/or [Ca^{2+}]$_i$ occurs through a conserved promoter element (178). Several proteins named activating transcription factor, possessing the capacity of cAMP- and Ca-dependent activation of this promoter, have recently been found (179–181). A member of this family, CREB, has been shown to mediate similar levels of Ca^{2+} and cAMP responses. Studies on cAMP-response element binding protein (CREB) indicate that its Ser 133 residue and flanking amino acids constitute a phosphorylation site for cAMP-dependent and Ca^{2+}-calmodulin-dependent protein kinases (179,180).

Several lines of evidence listed below suggest that, in sea urchin eggs, fibroblasts, osteoblast-like cells, and macrophages, activation of Na^+/H^+ exchange is involved in the onset and/or maintenance of the proliferative cascade (182,183):

- growth-promoting agents induce acute activation of the Na^+/H^+ exchanger;
- the proliferative cascade in these cells may be triggered by cytoplasmic alkalinization;
- the mitogen-induced proliferative response of these cells is diminished in a Na^+-free medium;
- Na^+/H^+ exchange blockers inhibit the proliferative response as well as proliferation of these cells under basal conditions;
- upon differentiation of granulocytic HL-60 cells, mRNA and protein expression of the NHE$_1$ isoform of the Na^+/H^+ exchanger is increased by tenfold.

This hypothesis is also supported by data obtained for fibroblasts transfected with the yeast gene of plasma membrane H^+-ATPase (184) and for the Na^+/H^+ antiporter-deficient mutant line of Chinese hamster lung fibroblasts (185). It should be stressed, however, that unlike cAMP and Ca^{2+} signaling systems, the intracellular target(s) mediating pH$_i$-dependent regulation of the cell cycle are still unknown.

Recently, Bobik and co-workers (186) reported that 5-(N-ethyl-N-isopropyl)-amiloride (EIPA), 5-(N,N-dimethyl)-amiloride (DMA), and amiloride attenuated the replication rate of VSMC from the rat aorta. The order of potency of these inhibitors was similar to their suppression of the Na^+/H^+ exchanger (186). Because of the lack of any effect of the reduced Na^+/H^+ exchange activity on the early phases of growth factor-stimulated protein synthesis, these authors speculated that decreased reductions in Na^+/H^+ exchange may convert a normal proliferative response of vascular smooth muscle to growth factors to one in which the cells hypertrophy without replication. In other words, Na^+/H^+ exchange not only regulates the replication rate of VSMC, but also influences the type of vascular hypertrophy. Data on the enhanced activity of this exchanger in primary hypertension will be analyzed in a later section.

Salt and Water Reabsorption by the Renal Tubular Epithelium

According to Guyton's concept, the right shift of the renal function curve (so-called resetting) is a major mechanism of long-term, elevated blood pressure maintenance (187). Figure 5 displays the ion transport systems of renal tubular epithelium cells involved in controlling extracellular fluid volume via the regulation of salt and water reabsorption. Sodium-organic solute (glucose, amino acids) cotransport, Na^+/H^+ exchange, and the anion transporter localized in apical membranes mediate the main part of salt reabsorption in proximal tubular cells. Transcellular salt movement is also under control of the Na^+/K^+ pump and Cl^- channels localized in basal membranes. Passive transport processes dominate in the thin limbs of Henle's loop, whereas Na^+,K^+ 2Cl^- cotransport and Na^+/H^+ exchange mediate salt reabsorption in the thick ascending limb of Henle's loop. Smaller fractions of sodium ions are reabsorbed in the distal tubule and collecting ducts via Na^+, Cl^- cotransport and Na^+ channels (120,188–190).

In the last few years, several isoforms of the Na^+/H^+ exchanger possessing different regulatory properties and different sensitivities to inhibitors have been cloned and transfected in Na^+/H^+ antiporter-deficient cell lines. The ubiquitous Na^+/H^+ exchanger, now referred to as NHE$_1$, is expressed in the basolateral membranes of polarized epithelial cells and in all types of nonepithelial cells studied so far (191). The gene encoding for NHE$_1$ is located on the short arm of human chromosome 1. Its structure has recently been determined (192). The second isoform of the human Na^-/H^+ exchanger (NHE$_2$) is mainly expressed on the apical membrane of epithelial cells (193): The NHE$_3$ isoform is highly expressed in the rabbit colon, small intestine and kidney cortex, whereas NHE$_4$ is found in the rat stomach (193,194). Special NHE$_\beta$ isoforms are expressed in nucleated fish erythrocytes (195).

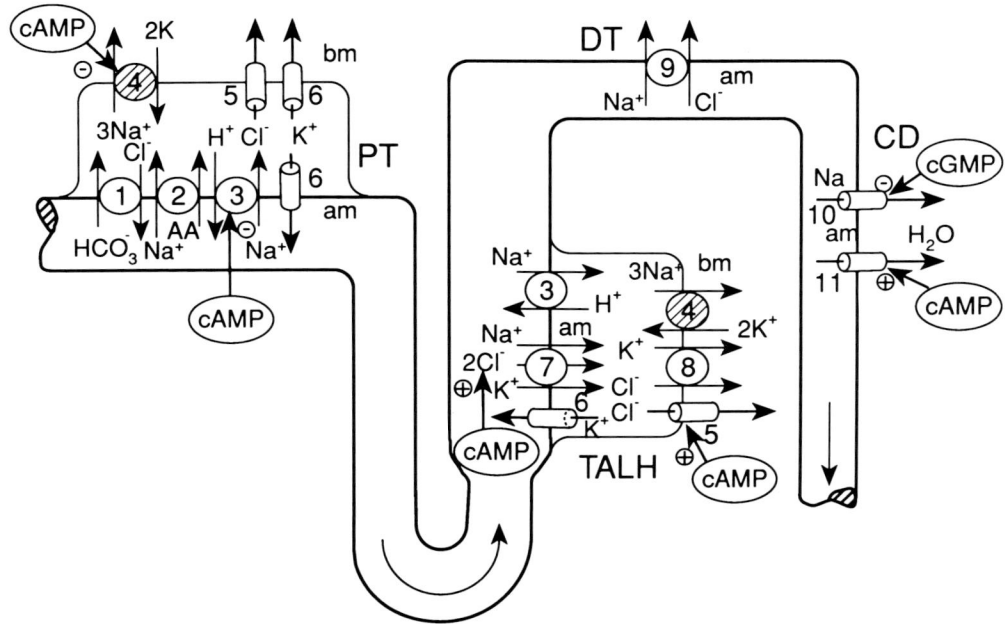

FIG. 5. The main pathways of salt and water reabsorption in kidney tubular epithelium. PT, proximal tubule; DT, distal tubule; TALH, thick ascending limb of Henle's loop; CD, collecting duct; am, apical membrane; bm, basolateral membrane; 1, anion exchanger; 2, (sodium + glucose/amino acid)-cotransport; 3, Na^+/H^+ exchanger (NHE_2 or/and NHE_3 isoforms); 4, Na^+,K^+ pump; 5, chloride channels; 6, potassium channels; 7, $Na^+,K^+,2Cl^-$ cotransport; 8, K^+,Cl^- cotransport; 9, Na^+,Cl^- cotransport; 10, amiloride-sensitive cation channels. Unlike other nephron segments, an apical membrane of epithelial cells of collecting duct is impermeable to water and contains specialized water channels activated by vasopressin via the V_2-receptor-adenylate cyclase-protein kinase A-mediated pathway. See text for other details. (From ref. 11, with permission.)

Data on pharmacological regulation of the Na^+/H^+ exchanger have been obtained for NHE_1, NHE_2 and NHE_β isoforms. The inhibitory constant (K_i) for amiloride derivatives of NHE_2 is about one order of magnitude higher than with NHE_1 (10–150 vs. 1–7 μM, respectively). The NHE_1 isoform is probably more sensitive to activation by protein kinase C- and tyrosine kinase-mediated signaling than NHE_2 or NHE_β (122,196). Beta-adrenergic activation is accompanied by a drastic increase of NHE_β activity via the cAMP-protein kinase A-mediated pathway (195). In canine enteric endocrine cells and in mouse L cells, the β-adrenergic receptor also stimulates NHE_1 activity by two- to threefold. However, neither cholera toxin-sensitive G-proteins nor protein kinase A is involved in this regulation (197). Unlike NHE_1 and NHE_β, the NHE_2 (and/or NHE_3) isoform of the Na^+/H^+ exchanger in rabbit-kidney brush border membranes is under the negative control of protein kinase A (198). Dopamine (DA), the main intrarenal hormone formed in proximal tubular cells, probably contributes to the natriuretic response to high-salt diets via DA_1 receptor-mediated cAMP production and inhibition of the NHE_2 isoform of the Na^+/H^+ exchanger (199) and Na^+K^+ pump (178).

Recently, it was also shown that in rat-kidney brush border membrane vesicles, both AlF_4^- and GTPγS in-

hibit Na^+/H^+ exchange without any alteration of adenylate cyclase activity, indicating a direct regulatory coupling of the carrier with Gp. Peculiarities in the hormonal regulation of different isoforms of the Na^+/H^+ exchanger are thought to be caused by a divergence in structural organization of the cytoplasmic C-terminal domain, which is involved in the protein kinase- and cytoskeleton-mediated control of affinity of 10- to 12-membrane-spanning N-terminal transport domains for intracellular protons (185,195).

Unlike the Na^+/H^+ exchanger, $Na^+,K^+,2Cl^-$ cotransport has not yet been cloned. The protein responsible for $Na^+,K^+,2Cl^-$ cotransport in the shark rectal gland has been characterized by affinity chromatography with immobilized bumetanide (Bumex) and a panel of monoclonal antibodies (200,201). These studies have revealed that this cotransporter is a heavily glycosylated protein with an apparent mass of 195 kDa, of which the polypeptide comprises about 135 kDa. Activation of protein kinase A increases rectal gland $Na^+,K^+,2Cl^-$ cotransport by five- to tenfold and this stimulation is accompanied by phosphorylation of the cotransport protein at serine and threonine residues. In kidney epithelial cells, $Na^+,K^+,2Cl^-$ cotransport is also under positive control of cAMP systems activated by vasopressin via V_2-receptors (189,202). It is accompanied by phosphorylation of a 150-kDa protein (203). In collecting ducts, these receptors are also involved in protein kinase A-mediated activation of water channels (see Fig. 5).

Recently, cDNA encoding a bumetanide-insensitive, thiazide-inhibited electroneutral Na⁺,Cl⁻ cotransporter was isolated from the winter flounder urinary bladder, using an expression cloning strategy (204). Nucleotide sequencing predicted a protein of 1,023 amino acids (112 kDa) with 12-membrane-spanning domains, a long hydrophilic C-terminus of ∼450 amino acid residues and several potential N-linked glycosylation sites between putative transmembrane segments S7 and S8. The intracellular signaling systems involved in regulating the activity of this carrier, localized on apical membranes of renal distal tubular epithelial cells (see Fig. 5), are still unknown.

In the apical membranes of A6 cells (a renal cell line derived from the *Xenopus laevis* kidney), three types of amiloride-blockable channels have been found at the single-channel level. One is a highly Na⁺-selective channel (Na⁺,K⁺ permeability ratio > 30:1) with a low conductance (4–5 pS); another is a less selective channel (Na: K ∼ 4:1) with single-channel conductance of 8–9 pS; the third is a nonselective, highly permeable (20–30 pS) cation channel. Using inside-out patches, it was shown that inactivation and deactivation of G-proteins by the application of GTPγS and GDPβS at the cytosolic surface, respectively, produced a tenfold decrease and five- to sevenfold increase of activity of the highly selective low conductance channel. The effect of GDPβS was mimicked by pertussis toxin, indicating the involvement of G_i proteins in the regulation of this type of amiloride-sensitive channel (205). The apical membranes of collecting duct cells contain amiloride-sensitive nonselective channels whose activity is inhibited by cGMP (206). These channels have been partially cloned, using oligonucleotide probes for the cGMP-binding domain of the rod outer segment of nonselective cGMP-activated channels (207). By employing the polymerase chain reaction, Ahmad and co-workers (208) isolated three cDNA from mouse collecting duct cells and a rat kidney library which differed by 1, 2, and 20 bases from the 426-base coding region of the photoreceptor channel.

In kidney epithelial cells, ANP-induced cGMP production is one to two orders of magnitude less than in glomeruli (57,209) or cultured VSMC and endothelial cells (84). On the basis of these results, it was assumed that ANP receptor-coupled guanylate cyclase of vascular tissue is a major source of plasma and urinary cGMP (210), probably due to the presence of a highly efficient transport system providing cGMP efflux from these cells (84). These data suggest that the nonselective cation channels of renal tubular epithelium cells inhibited by vascular tissue-derived cGMP are the main system mediating ANP-induced natriuresis.

ABNORMALITIES OF THE CYCLIC NUCLEOTIDE SYSTEM IN HYPERTENSION

Cyclic nucleotide studies in hypertension have, from the beginning, generated controversial data. The cyclic nucleotide-synthesizing enzymes adenylate and guanylate cyclases, cyclic nucleotide levels, cyclic nucleotide phosphodiesterases, as well as target protein phosphorylation, have all been reported to be either increased, normal, or decreased in hypertension (for review, see 211–245 and Tables 2–4). We suggest that these discrepancies are analogous to many others in hypertension (normal, high, or low renin levels, for example), and may be due to the use of different models having different mechanisms of pathogenesis, but they can be attributed principally to the heterogeneity of the disease itself and evaluation of its different stages. Descriptions of signaling system abnormalities in hypertension must clearly define at which point the disease is being explored. At least three levels of observation have to be distinguished: (a) the recognition of *primary,* genetically determined events which serve as promoting steps in the initiation of hypertension; (b) the definition of events *maintaining* hypertension chronically—these events start later and evolve with hypertension; and (c) the study of the *consequences* of hypertension at target organs. Genetic and environmental events may and do intervene at all three levels, not only as a primary momentum of hypertension, but also as a means of maintenance and susceptibility to specific complications in target organs. In attempting to propose a unifying hypothesis which can be tested on our data and those of other investigators, we suggested in 1990 that "an abnormality of negative vasodilatory pathways can be implicated in the pathogenesis of high blood pressure" (215). We believe that in the last 3 years, this hypothesis has received further support, some of which will be reviewed in the present section.

Extracellular Cyclic Nucleotides

Over the years, extracellular cyclic nucleotide levels appeared to be a very informative marker of the status of second messenger systems. Cyclic nucleotide levels in plasma reflect hormonal actions. From the first glucagon injection given by Broadus et al. (246) over two decades ago, to the huge cGMP increases seen after ANP infusions (58,247–250), cAMP and cGMP in plasma seemed to be valuable tools. Cyclic nucleotides are intracellular messengers, but their intracellular elevation is almost immediately followed by their egression into the extracellular environment. This egression is the result of an active transport system apparently shared by both cAMP and cGMP (84). Since the extracellular signal continues to accumulate in the extracellular environment, it be-

TABLE 2. Agonist-induced cAMP production in intact cells in primary hypertension

Model of hypertension (age)	Tissue	Agonist	cAMP production[a]	References
SHR vs WKY (6–20 weeks)	Platelets	PGE$_1$	↑	216
SHR vs WKY (6–20 weeks)	Platelets	epinephrine	↑	211
EH vs NP	Platelets	PGE$_1$	↑	217
EH vs NP	Platelets	PGI$_2$ analogue	=	218
SHR vs WKY (5 weeks)	Heart slices	Isoproterenol	=	219
SHR vs WKY (6 weeks) (37 weeks)	Heart slices	Isoproterenol	↓ =	220
SHR vs WKY (10 weeks)	Adipocytes	Adrenaline ACTH	= ↑	221
SHR vs WKY (13 weeks)	Endothelium depleted strips from femoral arteries	Forskolin Norepinephrine	= ↓	222
SHR vs WKY (12–14 weeks)	Primary cultured VSMC	Isoproterenol	=	223
SHR vs WKY (12–16 weeks)	Primary cultured VSMC	Adenosine	=	224
SHR vs WKY (6–8 weeks) (24–28 weeks)	Skeletal muscle	Isoproterenol	= ↓	225
SHR vs WKY (3–20 weeks)	Proximal convoluted tubules	Dopamine analogue Forskolin Gpp(NH)p	↓ = =	226–228
Dahl SS vs SHR (7–8 weeks)	Medullary and cortical tubule cells	Dopamine analogue Forskolin	↓ =	229
SHR vs WKY (12–20 weeks)	Cortical collecting ducts	Dopamine analogue	=	230

[a] Agonist-induced cAMP production in hypertension was reported to be increased (↑), decreased (↓), or not altered (=), respectively.

comes an amplified marker that is readily available for exploration.

Extracellular cyclic nucleotide levels in plasma and urine are under hormonal control, but the short half-life of cAMP and cGMP in plasma (about 3 minutes) is, to a large extent, dependent on renal status. Both cyclic nucleotides are excreted in urine by glomerular filtration, to which cAMP is added in tubules under the effect of parathyroid hormone, and cGMP is enriched by the glomerular and tubular actions of ANP. Urinary cAMP is therefore a sum of glomerular filtration and parathyroid action for its nephrogenous part, while urinary cGMP reflects ANP-dependent plasma levels, glomerular production and the effect of NO on the kidney (250). Impairment of renal function results in elevated cGMP and cAMP plasma levels, which is also the case with many of their peptide agonists. Thus, correction of renal function, as determined by creatinine clearance, is required, but in the case of significant renal impairment even this normalization is inadequate. Indeed, as shown previously, cyclic nucleotides are extremely elevated in the plasma of uremic subjects, both in the presence and absence of the kidneys. The injection of ^{3}H-labeled cAMP

in plasma allows the determination of its half-life, which is significantly prolonged in uremic subjects (251). While no significant differences in creatinine clearance, serum calcium levels, or sodium excretion exist between normotensive and hypertensive subjects, hypertensives have a higher cAMP excretion rate and a higher serum PTH concentration (252).

Several years ago, we presented evidence that infusion of isoproterenol induced a stronger increment of plasma cAMP levels in young subjects with labile hypertension than in age-matched controls. We compared this exaggerated responsiveness to β-adrenergic stimulation with the diminished reaction observed in older subjects with low plasma renin activity (Fig. 6) (253,254). As isoproterenol could not be safely infused in the older population, we used insulin-induced hypoglycemia as a β-adrenergic stimulus. As demonstrated by our group and since confirmed by others, insulin-induced hypoglycemia is indeed under the influence of β-adrenergic stimulation, as it is absent in adrenalectomized subjects and can be entirely abolished by concomitant propranolol infusion (255). Figure 6 shows that plasma cAMP can be utilized to distinguish exaggerated from decreased β-

TABLE 3. *Agonist-induced adenylate cyclase activity in cell-free systems in primary hypertension*

Model of hypertension (age)	Tissue	Agonist	Adenylate cyclase activity[a]	References
SHR vs WKY (8–16 weeks)	Aorta	β-agonists	↓	231–234
SHR vs WKY (10–11 weeks)	Mesenteric arteries	Forskolin	=	235
		β-agonists	↓	
		NaF	↓	
		PGE$_1$	↓	
SHR vs WKY (12 weeks)	Platelets	PGE$_1$	↑	216
SHR vs WKY (54 weeks)	Platelets	PGE$_1$	↓	236
SHR vs WKY (3 weeks)	Myocardium	Isoproterenol	=	237
		Gpp(NH)p	=	
		NaF	=	
(36 weeks)		Isoproterenol	↓	
		Gpp(NH)p	↓	
		NaF	↓	
SHR vs WKY (10–13 weeks)	Myocardium	Isoproterenol	↓	238
		Forskolin	=	
		NaF	=	
		Gpp(NH)p	=	
SHR vs WKY (10–12 weeks)	Myocardium	Gpp(NH)p	=	239
		Isoprenaline	=	
		Forskolin	=	
SHR vs WKY (11–13 weeks)	Myocardium	Isoproterenol	↑	240
		NaF	↑	
		Forskolin	↑	
NP ($^+$FH) vs NP ($^-$FH)	Lymphocytes	Forskolin	↑	241
SHR vs WKY (10–12 weeks)	Lung	Isoproterenol	↑	242
SHR vs WKY (12 weeks)	Kidneys	PGE$_2$	↓	243
		NaF	↓	
		Forskolin	=	
SHR vs WKY (3, 8, and 20 weeks)	Striatum	Dopamine analogue	=	230

[a] Adenylate cyclase activity in hypertension was reported to be increased (↑), decreased (↓), or not altered (=), respectively.

NP ($^+$FH) and ($^-$FH), normotensive subjects with and without a family history of hypertension.

TABLE 4. *G-protein content in spontaneous hypertension*

Model of hypertension (age)	Tissue	Gp subunits	Study	Change[a]	References
SHR vs WKY (10–12 weeks)	Aorta, myocardium	α_i	mRNA expression	↑	244
SHR vs WKY (10–12 weeks)	Myocardium	α_i	Immunoblotting	↑	239
SHR vs WKY (10–11 weeks)	Mesenteric arteries	$\alpha_s, \alpha_{i2}, \alpha_{i3}, \beta_1$	Western blotting	=	235
SHR vs WKY (14–16 weeks)	Long-term cultured VSMC from aorta	α_i, β	ADP-ribosylation, immunoblotting	=	245

[a] The content of Gp subunits in SHR was reported to be increased (↑) or not altered (=), respectively.

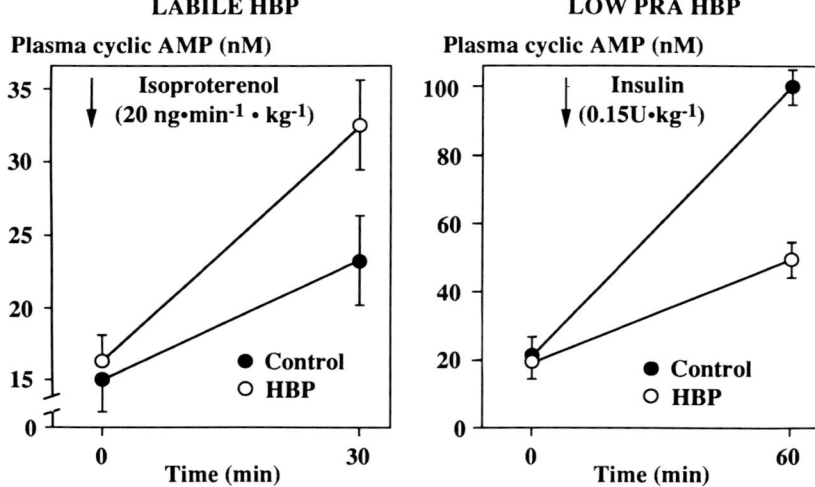

FIG. 6. Increases of plasma cAMP levels after exogenous β-adrenergic stimulation by isoproterenol in labile hypertensive subjects (*left panel*) and in response to endogenous β-adrenergic stimulation induced by insulin hypoglycemia in patients with low plasma renin activity (*right panel*). (From refs. 253 and 254, with permission.)

adrenergic responsiveness. In younger subjects with higher β-adrenergic responses, plasma cAMP levels are actually even significantly correlated (r = 0.633, p < 0.001) with heart rate after isoproterenol infusion (254).

Increased β-adrenergic responses of the cyclic nucleotide system in hypertension, initially demonstrated by us (256) and other investigators (240), have even been reported in neonatal spontaneously hypertensive animals (240). We view β-adrenergic hyperresponsiveness and its modification with age to be in accordance with the evolution of total peripheral resistance and cardiac output. Several decades ago, Widimsky and co-workers (257) observed increased cardiac output in young subjects with labile hypertension and proposed that it was an initial pattern of hypertension presentation evolving to lower cardiac output with a progressive elevation of total peripheral vascular resistance. These observations have been confirmed in experimental hypertension models and extended in different studies of human subjects (258–260). Increased cardiac output may reflect an early

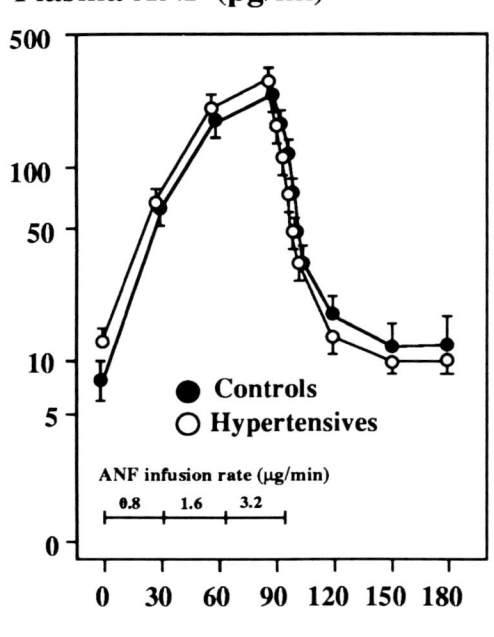

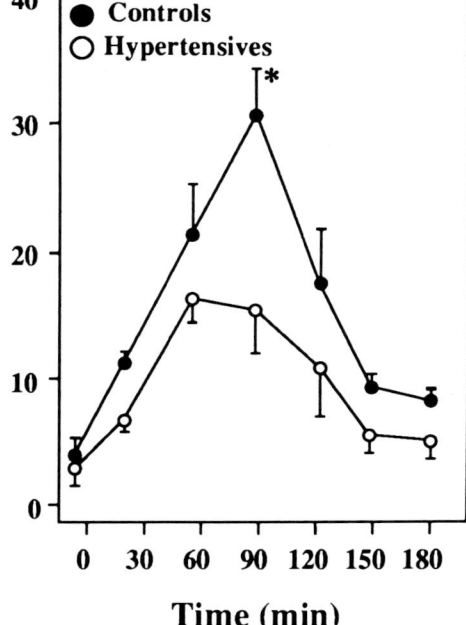

FIG. 7. Plasma atrial natriuretic peptide (ANF) concentration and cGMP levels following infusion of ANF in patients with essential hypertension and control subjects. (From ref. 261, with permission.)

augmented responsiveness of the β-adrenergic system and could thus be one of the initial events in the pathogenesis of hypertension.

Several years ago, we noted that ANP infusion elevated plasma cGMP levels in human hypertensives (Fig. 7) (261). This enhanced cGMP production was accompanied by exaggerated natriuresis and diuresis in these subjects. Analogous findings have been made in SHR and hypertensive monkeys (262). The possible mechanisms of this phenomenon as we see it now will be discussed below.

Cyclic AMP Signaling

Intact Cells and Cell-Free Systems

Data on agonist-induced cAMP production in whole organs, tissue slices, freshly isolated and primary cultured cells are summarized in Table 2. Tables 3 and 4 enumerate data on adenylate cyclase activity and G-protein content in primary hypertension in cell-free systems (tissue homogenates and isolated membrane fractions).

In humans, only circulating cells such as lymphocytes and platelets are readily accessible and present an advantage by studying single-cell types with concomitant observation of cyclic nucleotide or other messenger systems. An inherent problem is that these blood cells may modify their own signaling behavior, as we have demonstrated in platelets (263). However, this system has the advantage of prospective follow-up on the effects of antihypertensive therapy. Biopsies and organ cultures are rarely used. Most studies being performed on cell cultures have many advantages in the characterization of intracellular signaling systems. Problematically, however, a phenomenon persisting in cell culture is usually considered to be independent of blood pressure. The weakness of this paradigm is that cell cultures may reflect a phenomenon induced *in vivo* in hypertensive animals or humans and then perpetuated as a permanent *ex vivo* phenotype. Moreover, the state of cell differentiation or proliferation, the effect of culture media, etc., may also dramatically influence the regulation and behavior of such systems. On the other hand, their strength resides in the possibility of longitudinally studying virtually all intracellular signaling pathways in well-defined situations.

As mentioned above, data obtained on cAMP signaling in hypertension are rather contradictory. Several points should be considered when analyzing these results:

1. The activity of the cAMP system depends on the stage of development of hypertension (see Tables 2, 3). Age-dependent differences between SHR and Wistar-Kyoto (WKY) rats have been revealed by studies of pro-tein kinase A activity. It has been shown that the activity of this enzyme is decreased in the heart of 5-week-old SHR compared with age-matched WKY, without any differences between 18-week-old animals. On the other hand, protein kinase A activity is unaltered in the aorta of 5-week-old SHR but is decreased in 18-week-olds of these species (219).

2. Some cAMP signaling features in primary hypertension are tissue-specific and cannot be viewed as manifestations of widespread abnormalities. Thus, it has been shown that the DA-induced cAMP response is quenched in epithelial cells from medullary and cortical tubules in SHR and Dahl salt-sensitive rats as compared with WKY and Dahl salt-resistant animals, respectively. However, no differences between normotensive and hypertensive rats have been observed in collecting duct epithelial cells (see Table 2). According to the data presented in Table 4, G-protein α_i-subunit content is increased in the aorta and myocardium but not in the mesenteric artery and in long-term cultured VSMC from SHR.

3. At least a part of the abnormalities of cAMP signaling systems occurring in SHR has also been demonstrated in experimental models of secondary hypertension. Thus, as in SHR (Table 4), the hearts of DOCA-salt and one-kidney, one-clip hypertensive rats exhibit an increased expression of the G_i-protein α-subunit (264,265). The features of cAMP signaling in these models also depend on the stage of hypertension. In the early stage of DOCA-salt hypertension, basal adenylate cyclase activity in the heart is increased, whereas isoproterenol- and forskolin-induced increments are unaltered. In contrast, in established secondary hypertension, basal adenylate cyclase activity is unchanged, whereas isoproterenol- and forskolin-induced increments are decreased (238,266). In two-kidney, one-clip hypertension, when the clipped kidney is removed, these alterations return toward normal, like blood pressure and heart weight (238).

4. In some cases, differences apparent in experimental hypertension have not been confirmed in essential hypertension. Thus, decreased blood pressure and natriuretic responses, as well as increased nephrogenous cAMP induced by intravenous DA administration, were drastically augmented in some patients with essential hypertension (267), which contradicted results obtained in isolated tubular segments from SHR and Dahl salt-sensitive rats (see Table 2).

5. The data on cAMP signaling in intact cells and cell-free systems are essentially different. The level of hormonal stimulation of adenylate cyclase in isolated membrane fractions of VSMC is one to two orders of magnitude lower than agonist-induced cAMP responses in cultured cells (235,268). The maximal capacity of β-adrenoceptors in cultured VSMC is 20-fold higher, whereas their affinities are five- to sevenfold lower than

the same parameters in isolated membrane fractions (223,268). These data probably reflect the physical disruption of linkage between receptors, Gp and adenylate cyclase in cell-free systems with broken cytoskeleton networks lacking endogenous cytoplasmic regulators.

Features of Long-Term VSMC Cultures

To ascertain whether or not differences in β-adrenergic responsiveness are present between long-term cultures (6–17 passages) of VSMC from normotensive and hypertensive animals, we undertook the following studies: Basal cAMP levels and those stimulated by forskolin as well as by isoproterenol in cultured VSMC from the aortae of WKY and Brown-Norway (BN.lx) normotensive strains were compared to those in SHR substrains from Taconic Farms (SHRt), Charles River (SHRcr) and Prague (SHRp). The specific reasons for studying BN.lx and SHRp were that these strains have been used as progenitors of newly developed recombinant inbred rats, which enable us to analyze the genetic cosegregation of various hypertension phenotypes (269). These data are summarized in Fig. 8. Although basal adenylate cyclase activity was lower in cells of hypertensive origin (i.e., in all three SHR strains), there was no difference between SHR and WKY or BN.lx in response to forskolin. However, major disparities appeared following exposure to isoproterenol, with an excessive fivefold increase being observed in hypertensives. This excessive cAMP response to isoproterenol was not due to augmented binding affinity or receptor density, as demonstrated by [³H]-dihydroalprenolol (DHA) binding, which was not distinguishable between BN.lx and SHR cells (270).

In attempting to find possible explanations for the huge difference between unaffected forskolin stimulation

(i.e., forskolin's main action being directly on the catalytic subunit of adenylate cyclase) and the increased effectiveness of isoproterenol despite unaltered β-receptor binding subunits, we evaluated Gp/adenylate cyclase interaction in this system. Vascular smooth muscle cell pretreatment with cholera toxin, an activator of G_s-protein, elevated basal activity in both normotensive and hypertensive cells, yet its efficiency was fivefold higher in SHR, while the isoproterenol-induced increment of cAMP following this intervention was significantly decreased in both normotensive and hypertensive cells. These data suggest an enhanced efficiency of signal transduction between G_s-protein and adenylate cyclase. However, viewing the augmented efficiency of this pathway as the only source of heightened β-adrenergic cAMP production in SHR indicates that the same differences may be observed under activation of different types of G_s-protein-coupled receptors. Unlike β-adrenoceptors, cAMP generation under A_2-adenosine receptor activation was decreased by three- to fivefold in SHR compared with normotensive rats (268). These results indicate that increased isoproterenol-induced cAMP production in SHR VSMC is probably caused by the enhanced efficiency of signal transduction between β-adrenoceptors and G_s-proteins. Recently, it was shown that this coupling is under the control of β-arrestin and highly specific β-adrenergic receptor kinase (185). The hypothesis on reduced activity of this feedback regulatory pathway in VSMC in spontaneous hypertension is open to direct evaluation. Forthcoming experiments should clarify the mechanism of this abnormality in long-term cultured cells.

Cyclic GMP Signaling

We have already mentioned that plasma cGMP levels reflect ANP activity, while cGMP in urine indicates ANP's impact on particulate guanylate cyclase as well as the NO pathway effect on soluble guanylate cyclase. We have demonstrated that comparable vasodilatory doses of sodium nitroprusside and ANP increase urinary cGMP, but only ANP elevates both plasma and urinary levels of the nucleotide (250). This dichotomy is probably due to the fact that endothelial cells, although rich in particulate guanylate cyclase and thus responding to ANP, are very poor in soluble guanylate cyclase. Therefore, although both sodium nitroprusside or nitrates and ANP can vasodilate, only the ANP action is mirrored by plasma cGMP levels (271).

The role of ANP in hypertension is still unclear. Overexpression of the ANP gene in transgenic animals results in low blood pressure, while the administration of ANP antibodies increases blood pressure, (272). Accordingly, chronic inhibition of NO synthase leads to hypertension (273).

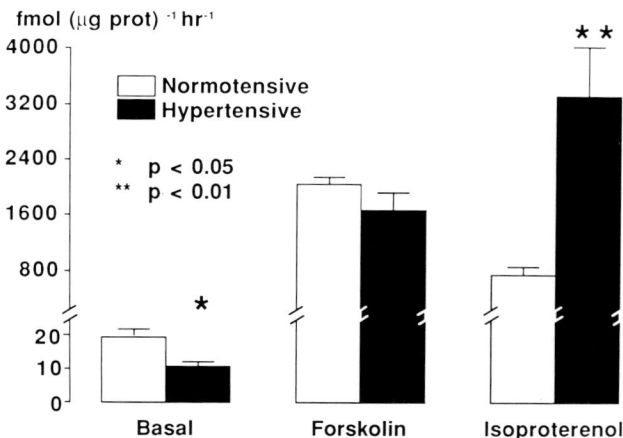

FIG. 8. Cyclic AMP production by quiescent long-term cultured VSMC from normotensive (WKY and BN.lx) and hypertensive (SHRcr, SHRt, and SHRp) rats under basal conditions and in the presence of forskolin (10^{-5} M) and isoproterenol (10^{-5} M) (From ref. 268, with permission.)

As mentioned earlier, ANP infusion elevates exaggerated plasma cGMP levels in human hypertensives, SHR, and hypertensive monkeys. We therefore considered the possible increased responsiveness of the ANP/cGMP system at the onset of hypertension, similar to our suggestion of hyperresponsiveness of the cAMP system. Indeed, we recently established that cGMP production is amplified in glomeruli isolated from SHR compared to several control strains and that this rise is not dependent upon high blood pressure, since the difference is not modified by effective antihypertensive therapy. As glomerular particulate guanylate cyclase is the target en-zyme of ANP in the kidney (57), we directly measured its activity in glomeruli from normotensive and hypertensive rats. We demonstrated that basal particulate guanylate cyclase activity was increased in SHR and remained high after ANP stimulation or solubilization with Triton X-100 (274). This phenotype appeared early in life with a less striking difference at an older age (274).

We also reported a similar exaggerated pattern of cGMP production in long-term cultures (cells between 6 to 15 passages) of VSMC derived from 10-week-old SHR, as compared to age-matched normotensive WKY controls (270). These results are in contrast to earlier

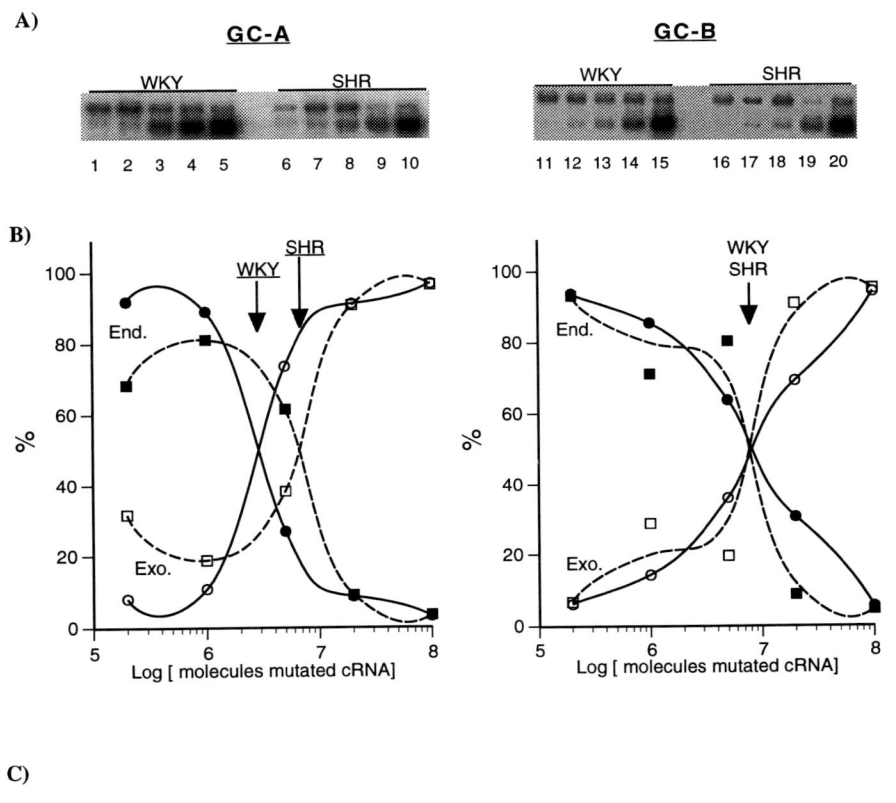

FIG. 9. A: Typical PCR transcript titration assay of GC-A and GC-B mRNA in tissues of WKY and SHR. **B:** Titration curves of GC-A and GC-B mRNA using increasing concentrations of mutated GC-A and GC-B cRNA. **C:** Histogram of GC-A and GC-B mRNA levels of lung tissues in WKY and SHR. (From ref. 274, with permission.)

findings, demonstrating an impaired cGMP response to ANP in SHR VSMC (275). On the other hand, previous studies have reported an exaggerated vasodilatory reaction to ANP in young SHR, but with a similar response in 20-week-old adults (276). This would explain in part the apparent discrepancy in our results, since earlier investigations of cultured VSMC were performed in 20- to 25-week-old animals and on early (between 3 to 6) cell passages where *in vivo* conditions of high circulating ANP levels may still prevail. In fact, we reported that the exaggerated response to ANP in the aorta of 4-week-old SHR is accompanied by an enhanced cGMP reaction to ANP with an evolution from increased to normal cGMP production and blood vessel relaxation in older SHR compared to age-matched normotensive controls (277). This led us to speculate that the high response of the cGMP system to ANP could be a primary event in the pathogenesis of hypertension.

It is therefore interesting to ascertain which receptor subtype (GC-A or GC-B) is exaggeratedly expressed in SHR organs. Since the mRNA levels of these genes are particularly low and thus do not allow their quantitation by northern blot, we have developed a quantitative polymerase chain reaction titration assay. With this assay, we have been able to evaluate the differential expression of GC-A and GC-B, and it actually appears that the GC-B receptor subtype is the predominant specie in glomeruli, renal papillae, lung, and aorta. Only in the adrenal cortex is the GC-A type predominant (278). Titration curves have demonstrated that the GC-A subtype is expressed more selectively in SHR (274) (Fig. 9). Deng and Rapp (279) recently suggested that a locus containing guanylate cyclase A cosegregates with hypertension by using microsatellites in the first intron of the guanylate cyclase A gene. We have obtained very similar results in recombinant inbred strains, demonstrating that a polymorphism (of GC-A) is associated with 6 mm Hg of systolic blood pressure. Our preliminary data suggest that a polymorphism present in the promoter region of this gene is also associated with hypertension in recombinant inbred strains (280).

ION TRANSPORT ABNORMALITIES IN HYPERTENSION

Monovalent Cations

The first direct evidence of increased plasma membrane permeability in primary hypertension was obtained in kinetic studies of isotope ($^{22}Na^+$, $^{42}K^+$, $^{36}Cl^-$) equilibrium in aortic strips from SHR by Jones (281), as well as in erythrocytes from SHR and patients with essential hypertension by Postnov and co-workers (282–284). Later, these findings were confirmed by several research groups (see 285–289 for review). This section focuses on the particulate ion transport pathways involved in these abnormalities.

$Na^+/Na^+(Na^+/Li^+)$ Exchange

In 1980, Canessa and co-workers (290) reported an increased rate of Na^+/Na^+ exchange in erythrocytes from patients with essential hypertension, determined as a maximal rate of Na_o^+/Li_i^+ countertransport (290). This result was reproduced in several studies with the exception of two carried out in black hypertensives (for more details see 287,289,291 for review.) Na^+/Li^+ countertransport in rat erythrocytes is extremely low (125). Data on activity of this carrier in spontaneously hypertensive rodents are absent. There are no systematic studies on Na^+/Na^+ countertransport in other tissues just as there are no data on the physiological implications of electroneutral and equimolar exchangers. However, the findings listed below show that estimation of erythrocyte Na^+/Li^+ countertransport is a useful tool, predicting the probability of essential hypertension and differentiating combined cases of primary and secondary hypertension.

1. The rate of Na^+/Li^+ countertransport is unaltered in patients with secondary hypertension (renovascular hypertension, glomerulonephritis, chronic pyelonephritis) (290,292,293).

2. In patients with secondary hypertension and low Na^+/Li^+ countertransport, blood pressure drops after surgical treatment of the kidney, renal vessels or adrenals. Surgical interventions in patients with combined renovascular and essential hypertension, as well as high rates of Na^+/Li^+ countertransport, have been reported to be function failures (293). The usefulness of Na^+/Li^+ countertransport as a predictor of clinical outcome after reconstruction of renal artery stenosis deserves further evaluation.

3. In both Caucasians and Chinese, Na^+/Li^+ countertransport is increased in young normotensive offspring of patients with essential hypertension (294,295).

4. A cross-sectional association between the rate of Na^+/Li^+ countertransport and hypertension has been found in the general Caucasian population by several research groups (296–299).

5. By comparing Na^+/Li^+ countertransport values in essential hypertensives, it has been shown that the enhanced activity of the carrier is associated with elevated peripheral resistance (300), increased renal sodium reabsorption (301,302), left ventricular hypertrophy (302), and insulin resistance (303). The last finding is in accordance with the three- to fourfold decrease in the Na^+/Li^+ exchange rate in human erythrocytes after 3 hours of preincubation in medium containing 50 mU/L insulin (304). This is an important observation that awaits con-

firmation by other investigators with an explanation of its mechanism.

Na+/H+ Exchange

In 1986 to 1988, an increased rate of Na^+/H^+ exchange in blood cells of essential hypertensive patients and SHR was demonstrated independently by several research teams (305–307). Later, these results were confirmed by other investigators with a few exceptions. As seen in Table 5 (125,173,305–335), increased Na^+/H^+ exchange was also found in cultured VSMC from SHR and in skeletal muscle cells from SHR and patients with essential hypertension *in vivo,* supporting the hypothesis of widespread abnormalities in the plasma membrane-ion transport system in hypertension (286,336). Data on the activity of the Na^+/H^+ exchanger in hypertension were recently discussed in detail by Rosskopf et al. (337). Several conclusions listed below may be drawn from analysis of these results.

1. Based on the tissue-specific expression of NHE_2, NHE_3, and NHE_4 isoforms of the Na^+/H^+ exchanger (see below), it may be supposed that data on enhanced Na^+/H^+ antiporter activity (see Table 5) refer mainly to the ubiquitous NHE_1 isoform. There are two reports of an increased rate of amiloride-inhibited ^{22}Na influx in kidney tubular (254,330) and jejunal (255,331) epithelial cells from SHR. It should be mentioned, however, that these experiments cannot be viewed as strong evidence of enhanced NHE_2 or NHE_3 activity of the exchanger due to the presence of amiloride-sensitive nonselective cation channels in these cells (discussed further below).

2. There are no indications of an altered apparent affinity of platelet, leukocyte, and erythrocyte Na^+/H^+ for extracellular sodium and intracellular protons in essential hypertension (309,313–315,317,318). Hill's co-efficients of the Na^+/H^+ exchanger are unaltered in platelets and leukocytes (317,318) and slightly decreased in erythrocytes (309) of patients with essential hypertension. These results suggest that enhanced Na^+/H^+ antiporter activity in primary hypertension is caused by an increased expression of the NHE_1 isoform or by an augmented rate of carrier turnover due to its posttranslational modification or altered membrane environment. The last suggestion is supported by data on an elevated Na^+/H^+ exchange in immortalized lymphoblasts from essential hypertensive patients without an increment of steady-state NHE_1 mRNA transcript levels (338). Analysis of 93 hypertensive sibling pairs demonstrated that mutations at the NHE_1 gene locus rarely, if ever, contribute to the pathogenesis of hypertension (339).

3. A unimodal distribution of maximal Na^+/H^+ exchange was noted in erythrocytes of normotensive patients with mean values of about 50 mmol (L cells × hr). In hypertensives, distribution was bimodal with mean left and right gauss curves of 40 and 80 mmol (L cells × hr) respectively (309). According to the results of this study, only 40–50 percent of patients with essential hypertension possess enhanced Na^+/H^+ exchanger activity. Increased Na^+/H^+ exchanger activity was observed in SHR (see Table 5) and Dahl salt-sensitive hypertensive rats (319), but not in hypertensive rats of the Milan strain (MHS) (see Table 5). An elevated Na^+/H^+ exchange was found in erythrocytes of normotensive BN.1x rats (340) and in VSMC of normotensive Wistar rats (327) as compared with WKY controls. Erythrocyte Na^+/H^+ exchanger activation of three- to fourfold was noted in normotensive patients with acute, deep venous thrombosis (341).

On the one hand, these results may be interpreted as evidence against Na^+/H^+ exchange as a major contribution to the pathogenesis of hypertension. On the other

TABLE 5. *Na+/H+ Exchange in primary hypertension*

Cells	EH vs NP[a] (ref.)	SHR vs WKY[a] (ref.)
Erythrocytes	↑ (125,307–309,335)	↑ (125)
	= (334)	= (319)
Platelets	↑ (310–314)	↑ (320–322)
	= (315)	
Leukocytes	↑ (306,316–318,424)	ND
Neutrophils	ND	↑ (305)
Lymphocytes	ND	↑ (323)
		= (324)
Mesenteric artery strips	ND	↑ (325)
Cultured vascular smooth muscle cells	ND	↑ (173,326–329)
Kidney tubular epithelium	ND	↑ (330)
Jejunal epithelium	ND	↑ (331)
Cultured mesangial cells	ND	↑ (332)
Skeletal muscle *in vivo*	↑ (318)	↑ (333)

[a] increased (↑) or unaltered (=) Na^+/H^+ exchanger in hypertension, respectively.
ND, activity of the Na^+/H^+ exchanger in primary hypertension was not determined in this type of cell. EH, essential hypertension; NP, normotensive patients.

hand, they underscore the inadequacy of WKY rats as the so-called controls for SHR. Clear evidence of the crucial impact of genetic interaction is furnished by observation of the Na^+/H^+ exchanger in F_2 hybrids of SHR and WKY crosses (340). Since F_2 hybrids have higher values than both parental strains, these data indicate that the measured phenotype is indeed a result of complex interaction of the transporter itself with the specific genetic background of the parental strains. Further studies in genetically defined strains and their crosses are needed for an understanding of contributing phenotypes and their interaction with other genes in the pathogenesis of abnormal ionic transport in hypertension.

$Na^+, K^+, 2Cl^-$ Cotransport

Unlike in smooth muscle cells, Na^+/H^+ exchange in human and rat erythrocytes is quenched under basal conditions. In other words, this carrier cannot be viewed as a cause of the increased ouabain-insensitive ^{22}Na efflux in erythrocytes of SHR and essential hypertension patients seen under steady-state conditions (283,284). In essential hypertension, an increased rate of ^{22}Na efflux may be caused by Na^+/Na^+ exchange. However, in rat erythrocytes, this ion transport pathway is also quenched. Abnormal kinetic characteristics of erythrocyte $Na^+, K^+, 2Cl^-$ cotransport in essential hypertension patients and SHR were reported in 1980 by Garay and co-workers (342) as well as by De Mendonca et al. (343). However, these studies were carried out in SH-reagent-

or mistatin-treated cells with an inverted transmembrane sodium and potassium gradient ($[Na^+]_i \sim 100$ mM/$[K^+]_i = 10$ mM) (see 287,289,344 for details). Data on $Na^+, K^+, 2Cl^-$ cotransport in primary hypertension in intact cells with a physiological $[Na^+]_i/[K^+]_i$ ratio are summarized in Table 6 (125,330,332,340,345–357). Several conclusions could be drawn from an analysis of these investigations.

1. The outward mode of $Na^+, K^+, 2Cl^-$ cotransport, determined as the furosemide (bumetanide)-inhibited component of ^{86}Rb or ^{22}Na (^{23}Na) efflux, was increased in erythrocytes of MHS and SHR by 40–70 percent and 30–50 percent, respectively, in comparison to corresponding normotensive strains (125,345,347), with the exception of one negative report (348). It should be mentioned, however, that the rate constant of the bumetanide-inhibited component of ^{22}Na efflux in this paper was presented without any correction of the different specific radioactivity of intracellular ^{22}Na (see 285 for more methodological details). This difference arises due to the increased intracellular sodium in SHR erythrocytes first reported by Losse and co-workers (358) and confirmed by Yokomatsu et al. (348). This comment has special importance because of possible alterations in the kinetic properties of $Na_i^+, K_i^+, 2Cl_i^-$ cotransport. Indeed, the affinity of the $Na^+, K^+, 2Cl^-$ cotransporter for intracellular Na^+ in MHS erythrocytes was twofold higher, whereas its maximal activity was decreased by 15 percent compared with Milan Normotensive Strain (MNS) (359).

TABLE 6. $Na^+, K^+, 2Cl^-$ Cotransport in primary hypertension

Cells/model of hypertension	Mode of operation of carrier [methods of measurement]	Alterations in hypertension (ref.)
Erythrocytes/MHS vs MNS	Outward [1]	↑ (345)
	Outward [2]	(346)
Erythrocytes/SHR vs WKY	Outward [2]	↑ (346,347)
	Outward [3]	= (348)
	Inward [4]	↑ (125)
Erythrocytes/PHR vs PNR	Inward [4]	↑ (349)
	Inward [5]	= (349)
Erythrocytes/SHR vs BN.1x	Inward [5]	= (340)
Erythrocytes/HP vs NP	Outward [2]	↑ (347)
	Inward [4]	↑ (350,351) = (125)
Quiescent VSMC/SHR vs WKY	Outward [3]	↑ (352)
	Inward [5]	↑ (353,354)
Growing VSMC/SHR vs WKY	Inward [5]	↓ (355)
Quiescent VSMC/MHS vs MNS	Inward [5]	↑ (356)
Mesangial cells/SHR vs WKY	Outward [6]	↑ (332)
Kidney tubular epithelial cells/SHR vs WKY	Inward [4]	= (330)
Kidney tubular epithelial cells/MHS vs MNS	Inward [4]	↑ (330)
Membranes from kidney tubular epithelial cells/MHS vs MNS	Inward [5]	↑ (357)

SHR, MHS, PHR, different strains of spontaneously hypertensive rats; WKY, MNS, PNR, BN.1x, different strains of normotensive rats; HP, NP, hypertensive and normotensive patients; ↑, ↓, =, increased, decreased, unaltered activity of $Na^+, K^+, 2Cl^-$ cotransport; [1], bumetanide-inhibited net Na efflux in Na-free medium; [2], furosemide-inhibited ^{22}Na efflux; [3], bumetanide-inhibited ^{22}Na efflux; [4], furosemide-inhibited ^{86}Rb influx; [5], bumetanide-inhibited ^{86}Rb influx; [6], bumetanide-inhibited ^{86}Rb efflux.

2. The inward mode of $Na^+,K^+,2Cl^-$ cotransport, measured as furosemide-inhibited ^{86}Rb influx was slightly increased (by 15–25 percent) in SHR and Prague hypertensive strain (PHS) erythrocytes as compared with normotensive controls (125,349). Bumetanide-inhibited ^{86}Rb influx was found to be unaltered in PHS (349) and SHR erythrocytes vis-à-vis BN.1x rats (340). The discrepancy may have been caused by furosemide-induced inhibition of Na^+-independent K^+,Cl^- cotransport. Preliminary data on the enhanced activity of this ion transport pathway in SHR erythrocytes were reported by Garay and co-workers (360). Their results await confirmation by other investigators.

3. The data on outward and inward $Na^+,K^+,2Cl^-$ cotransport in erythrocytes of patients with essential hypertension are contradictory (see Table 6), probably because of alteration of this ion transport system in some subjects. Indeed, Cusi and co-workers (361) reported a normal (unimodal) and bimodal distribution of outward $Na^+,K^+,2Cl^-$ cotransport in normotensive Caucasian subjects with no family history of hypertension and in patients with essential hypertension, respectively. The essential hypertensives with higher $Na^+,K^+,2Cl^-$ cotransport values also had increased Na^+/Li^+ countertransport and passive permeability (leakage) of the erythrocyte membrane for sodium.

4. Outward and inward $Na^+,K^+,2Cl^-$ cotransport was augmented in quiescent SHR VSMC as compared with WKY (352–354). Similar results were obtained for inward $Na^+,K^+,2Cl^-$ cotransport in quiescent VSMC from MHS aortae (356). In contrast, O'Donnell and Owen (355) reported decreased inward $Na^+,K^+,2Cl^-$ cotransport in growing SHR VSMC (362). Recently, it was shown that these contradictory results may be partly caused by dependence of the inward mode of $Na^+,K^+,2Cl^-$ cotransport of VSMC on intracellular sodium concentration (268).

5. Table 6 presents data on increased inward $Na^+,K^+,2Cl^-$ cotransport in MHS renal tubular epithelial cells. In MHS rats, faster erythrocyte $Na^+,K^+,2Cl^-$ cotransport is also associated with enhanced tubular reabsorption measured in isolated perfused kidneys (363). Compared with normotensives and normal cotransport hypertensives, high-cotransport hypertensives present lower fractional uric secretion and plasma renin activity with an increased natriuretic response to furosemide (364). These studies, as well as data on the positive correlation of erythrocyte $Na^+,K^+,2Cl^-$ cotransport and blood pressure in F_2 hybrids of MHS and MNS (345), and in SHR and WKY (346), support the hypothesis of the involvement of this carrier in the pathogenesis of primary hypertension. It should be mentioned, however, that to date there is no direct evidence for the biochemical identity of the $Na^+,K^+,2Cl^-$ cotransporter expressed in erythrocytes, VSMC, and renal epithelial cells.

Ca^{2+}-Activated K^+ Channels

Studies performed on erythrocytes and aortic strips from patients with essential hypertension and SHR show that the enhanced rate of univalent ion turnover persists at 2–4 degrees Centigrade (see 287 for details). Keeping in mind the high Q10 values of ion pumps and carriers, the results of these investigations may be viewed as indirect evidence of increased cation diffusion along their electrochemical gradient through the lipid bilayer or/and through specialized ion channels. It has been found that A23187 and propranolol-induced $[Ca^{2+}]_i$-mediated potassium efflux (365,366), as well as membrane hyperpolarization (125), are increased in erythrocytes of SHR compared to WKY rats. The same peculiarities have also been noted in some patients with essential hypertension but not in MHS (125). The differences between SHR and WKY were eliminated at saturating intracellular free calcium concentrations (125,365), demonstrating the enhanced sensitivity of K^+ channels to intracellular Ca^{2+}. Recently, direct evidence in support of this hypothesis was obtained with the patch-clamp technique. Shoemaker and Worrell (367) recorded an increased Ca^{2+} sensitivity of 55-pS K^+ channels in inside-out patches of cultured smooth muscle cells from the aorta of SHR compared to WKY. In cell-attached patches of freshly isolated aortic myocytes, high-conductance (225 pS) Ca^{2+}-dependent channels showed a fivefold higher open-state probability with greater $[Ca^{2+}]_i$ sensitivity in SHR versus WKY (368). It may be assumed that the enhanced Ca^{2+} sensitivity of K^+ channels provides a feedback mechanism limiting augmented vasculature contraction in hypertension. Indeed, it is evident that a pharmacological block of resting K^+ current unmasks enhanced blood vessel contraction in SHR and rats with renal hypertension (369,370).

Calcium

The early studies of $[Ca^{2+}]_i$ handling in SHR and essential hypertension have been summarized elsewhere (287,289,371–373). Table 7 presents data on the intracellular free calcium concentration in SHR and patients with essential hypertension documented by the use of fluorescent Ca^{2+} chelators in the last 10 years. This table shows that the majority of research groups investigating this problem detected an increase of $[Ca^{2+}]_i$ in erythrocytes, platelets, peripheral lymphocytes, and VSMC in primary hypertension. There are single reports of elevated $[Ca^{2+}]_i$ in synaptosomes (374) and cardiac muscle cells (375) of SHR and in erythrocytes (376) and VSMC (377) of MHS. Oshima and co-workers (378) noted that the $[Ca^{2+}]_i$ increase in SHR platelets persists in the prehypertensive stage, suggesting the involvement of this

TABLE 7. *Intracellular free calcium concentration in primary hypertension*

Cells	EH vs NP (ref.)	SHR vs WKY (ref.)
Erythrocytes	↑ (388)	↑ (376,401)
Platelets	↑ (389–395)	↑ (378,390,393,402)
	= (396,397)	
Peripheral lymphocytes	↑ (403–405)	↑ (398,399)
Spleen lymphocytes	ND	= (405)
Neutrophils	= (400)	ND
Brain synaptosomes	ND	↑ (374)
Vascular smooth muscle cells	ND	↑ (406–410)
		= (411)
Cardiac myocytes	ND	↑ (375)

↑, =, increased or unaltered intracellular free calcium concentration in hypertension, respectively. EH, essential hypertension; NP, normotensive patients.

abnormality in the pathogenesis of primary hypertension as a trigger of high blood pressure. This makes it reasonable to consider the possible mechanisms of sustained cellular calcium overloading in primary hypertension.

Ca²⁺ Efflux

Ca^{2+}-ATPase (Ca^{2+} pump) and the Na^+/Ca^{2+} exchanger are major plasma membrane Ca^{2+} transport pathways, providing long-term maintenance of low $[Ca^{2+}]_i$ in resting cells. To the best of our knowledge, there is no direct evidence of Na^+/Ca^{2+} exchanger expression in blood cells or data on the altered activity of this carrier in SHR myocytes. The erythrocyte Ca^{2+} pump from SHR and patients with essential hypertension has been found to be unchanged (379–383) or slightly decreased (384) in comparison to normotensive controls. Using unresealed fragments or inside-out vesicles of erythrocyte membranes, it has been shown that the calmodulin-induced increment of Ca^{2+}-ATPase activity is attenuated in SHR (379,384), MHS (381), and patients with essential hypertension (380,382). The blunted regulation of Ca^{2+}-ATPase activity stimulated by calmodulin was also observed in platelet membrane fractions from patients with essential hypertension (385). No significant difference in Ca^{2+}-ATPase activity was noted between hypertensive and normotensive patients (386) or between SHR and WKY (384) after detergent solubilization of the enzyme. These results reveal that the number of Ca^{2+}-ATPase molecules is the same in primary hypertension and that the reduced activation of this enzyme by calmodulin in inside-out vesicles and erythrocyte ghosts is due to an altered pump environment persisting in intact erythrocytes or induced by erythrocyte ghost and inside-out vesicle procedures.

The last assumption is in accordance with data obtained on saponin-treated erythrocytes. This model allows us to vary the intracellular calcium and ATP concentration without altering cytoplasmic protein content. It has more in common with intact erythrocytes than cytoskeleton-depleted inside-out vesicles. Unlike in inside-out vesicles, neither exogenous calmodulin nor the powerful calmodulin antagonist (R24571) regulates Ca^{2+}-ATPase activity in saponin-treated erythrocytes (387). These data suggest that calmodulin is not involved in the regulation of the Ca^{2+} pump in intact erythrocytes. The Ca^{2+}-ATPase activity of saponin-treated erythrocytes in SHR and MHS is not altered as compared with normotensive WKY and MNS strains (125). Decreased maximal activity of Ca^{2+}-ATPase in saponin-treated erythrocytes of SHR was noted in a study using the BN.1x strain as a normotensive control (340).

Ca²⁺ Influx

Data presented in the previous section indicate that the systems involved in Ca^{2+} transport against its electrochemical gradient are probably unaltered in primary hypertension. Based on these results, it may be assumed that the increment of $[Ca^{2+}]_i$ in primary hypertension (Table 7) (374–376,378,388–411) is caused by activation of the transport pathways mediating Ca^{2+} influx. The mechanism of Ca^{2+} entry through plasma membranes in blood cells is poorly understood. Unlike excitable tissues, neither human nor rat erythrocytes contain Na^+/Ca^+ exchanger (154). Using erythrocytes resealed with Ca-EGTA buffer, it was shown that the rate of ^{45}Ca influx is drastically increased under replacement of intracellular Na^+ and K^+ by choline. On the basis of these data, it was postulated that the major part of the inward calcium flux in these cells is mediated via nonselective $[Ca^{2+}]_o/[Na^+]_i/[K^+]_i$ exchange (143). The activity of this pathway is slightly enhanced (by 15–25 percent) in quin 2-loaded SHR erythrocytes compared with WKY (376). There are no differences between normotensive subjects and patients with essential hypertension in the rate of ^{45}Ca influx in intact erythrocytes (388).

As discussed above, ion channels play a key role in the increment of $[Ca^{2+}]_i$ under cellular excitation. Direct comparison of vascular smooth muscle from SHR and WKY by means of the patch-clamp technique has shown an enhanced calcium current passing through long-lasting L-type channels in spontaneous hypertension (412). Intracellular EGTA enhances the peak amplitude of L-type channels by 60–80 percent in SHR VSMC but does not modify them significantly in WKY (413). The same differences between SHR and WKY are seen in the veins of newborn rats (372). These results are in accordance with data on the increased calcium antagonist-sensitive component of ^{45}Ca influx in cultured smooth muscle cells from the SHR aorta (414).

Calmodulin and Other Ca^{2+}-Binding Proteins

Numerous data obtained in cell-free systems and briefly summarized earlier suggest a key role of Ca^{2+}-binding proteins in signal transduction as intracellular $[Ca^{2+}]_i$ sensors. Calmodulin is the most extensively investigated member of this family in hypertension. Using direct radioimmunoassay (RIA), it has been reported that calmodulin content in the brain, heart, aorta, and kidney of SHR is decreased by 18, 30, 45 and 16 percent, respectively, compared with WKY (415). The same patterns of alteration were observed in the brain, heart, and kidney (but not in the aorta) of rats with secondary (DOCA) hypertension (415). Decreased and unchanged levels of RIA-detectable calmodulin in the aorta of SHR and DOCA-salt hypertensive rats, respectively, were reported by Baba and co-workers (416). When calmodulin content was measured by the ability of tissue samples to activate calmodulin-dependent phosphodiesterase, an increase was recorded in the kidney, aorta, and heart of SHR and in the kidney and heart of spontaneously hypertensive mice (SHM) (417). The same approach did not reveal any alteration of calmodulin content in the SHR brain and liver (417,418) as well as in erythrocytes from SHR and patients with essential hypertension (380). The Ca-binding properties of calmodulin, purified from the SHR brain by affinity chromatography with phenyl-sepharose, were also unaltered in comparison to WKY (418). Enhanced Ca^{2+}-dependent activation of phosphodiesterase by kidney and heart homogenates from SHR and SHM and by homogenates of cultured SHR vascular smooth muscle is probably caused by the presence of calmodulin activator (419). The calmodulin activator is a hydrophobic, heat, acid, and base-stable compound sensitive to proteases. It is optimally extracted by the chloroform/methanol Folch method, and interacts with phosphodiesterase by increasing its apparent affinity for calmodulin. Preliminary identification indicates that it is a low-molecular-weight lipopeptide (420). In SHR, the antihypertensive effect of a high-calcium diet is accompanied by a decreased level of the calmodulin activator in the heart and kidney (420). Further experiments must clarify the involvement of this substance and of PHF, another factor of lipopeptide origin derived from parathyroid glands (421), in the antihypertensive effect of high-calcium diet.

MECHANISMS OF INTRACELLULAR SIGNALING INVOLVED IN THE PATHOGENESIS OF HYPERTENSION

Figure 10 summarizes our present understanding of the possible pathways of intracellular signaling involved in primary hypertension examined in earlier sections on the activation of servomechanisms for long-term maintenance of elevated blood pressure.

Increased $Na^+,K^+,2Cl^-$ cotransport and Na^+/H^+ exchange in the renal tubular epithelium result in the enhanced reabsorption of salt and osmotically obliged water, leading to augmented extracellular fluid volume (EFV), cardiac output, and blood pressure (Pathway #1). The cAMP system may also be involved in augmenting cardiac output via a β-adrenergic-induced positive inotropic effect. Activation of the cAMP signaling system in proximal tubules decreases EFV via inhibition of the Na^+/H^+ exchanger and Na^+,K^+ pump. Unlike in proximal tubules, activation of cAMP signaling in the thick ascending limb of Henle's loop and in collecting ducts increases EFV via activation of $Na^+,K^+,2Cl^-$ cotransport and water channels, respectively. In collecting ducts, cGMP decreases salt reabsorption via inhibition of amiloride-sensitive ion channels (see Fig. 5).

Enhanced Na^+/H^+ exchange in VSMC leads to increased peripheral blood resistance via $[Na^+]_i$-mediated activation of the Na^+/Ca^{2+} exchanger and elevated intracellular free calcium concentration (Pathway #2). As discussed earlier, increased peripheral resistance may also be caused by hyperactivity of the polyphosphoinositide signaling system and activation of protein kinase C. Data on abnormal signaling via this pathway in hypertension are summarized elsewhere in this volume. Cyclic AMP and cGMP involvement in vascular smooth muscle relaxation is discussed in an earlier section.

Both the Na^+/H^+ exchange and cAMP systems are positively involved in VSMC growth and proliferation. As shown earlier, vascular wall hypertrophy (an increased wall/lumen ratio) leads to heightened responsiveness to vasoconstrictors and enhanced total peripheral vascular resistance (Pathway #3). Data on activation of the Na^+/H^+ exchanger in primary hypertension have been mainly obtained for the NHE$_1$ isoform of this carrier, which is expressed in all tissues studied so far. From this point of view, it is noteworthy that data on enhanced

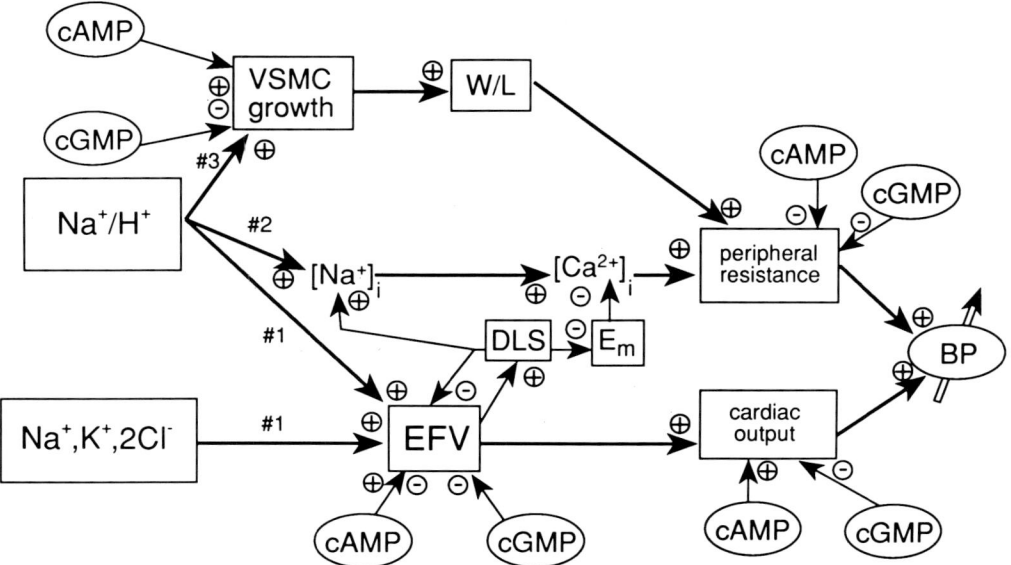

FIG. 10. Mechanisms of the involvement of intracellular signaling systems in the pathogenesis of hypertension. Na^+/H^+, Na^+/H^+ exchanger; $Na^+,K^+,2Cl^-$, $Na^+,K^+,2Cl^-$ cotransport; VSMC, vascular smooth muscle cell; W/L, wall/lumen ratio; EFV, extracellular fluid volume; DLS, digitalis-like substance(s); E_m, plasma membrane electrical potentials; BP, blood pressure. For more details, see text.

growth and proliferation in primary hypertension are not limited to vascular smooth muscles only. Normotensive children of hypertensive parents have an enlarged mass of the left heart ventricle (422). These findings suggest that cardiac hypertrophy precedes the increase in blood pressure. Renal hypertrophy is also reported to coincide with essential hypertension (302).

There are several points of interrelation of these pathways in the maintenance of elevated blood pressure. Thus, EFV expansion increases the production of low- and high-molecular-weight digitalis-like substance(s) (DLS) (146,423). These compounds try to normalize EFV via inhibition of the Na^+,K^+ pump in the renal tubular epithelium. However, the affinity of the kidney Na^+,K^+-ATPase isoform for ouabain and probably for DLS is one order of magnitude less than with the Na^+,K^+ pump in smooth muscle cells and nerve terminals. Acting predominantly on these cells, DLS increases their intracellular sodium concentration and decreases the plasma membrane potential due to electrogenity of the Na^+,K^+ pump (424). Both $[Na^+]_i$-induced activation of the $[Na^+]_i/[Ca^{2+}]_o$ exchanger and opening of POCs lead to elevated $[Ca^{2+}]_i$ in VSMC and nerve terminals, neurotransmitter release, and enhanced total peripheral resistance.

Regulatory pathways of the cAMP and cGMP systems are probably overactive early in hypertension and therefore represent potential primary events characterized by increased cardiac output and vasodilation. As shown in an earlier section, particulate guanylate cyclase is a candidate gene for a potential primary event in hypertension. In chronically established hypertension, the vasoconstrictory pathways related to protein kinase C, phosphoinositol turnover, calcium and monovalent ion transport predominate and are accompanied by decreases of cAMP and cGMP, culminating in increased total peripheral vascular resistance. Alterations in these signaling systems are probably also involved in kidney resetting and hypertrophy of blood vessels. However, to date, the genetic and cellular components of ion transport abnormalities in primary hypertension are still unknown. Our hypothesis of the vasodilatory pathway as a primary event in hypertension is reminiscent of William Osler's *Principles and Practice of Medicine,* a 100-year-old description of the course of cardiac hypertrophy which could be divided into three stages. In the first stage, Osler postulates that there is period of development which varies with the nature of the primary lesion. In the second stage, there is full compensation, a latent state during which the heart meets the requirements of the circulation. Finally, there is a period of "broken compensation." With the signal transduction hypothesis, we propose that in the period of development, vasodilatory systems are overactive, and only their failure and the prevalence of vasoconstrictory systems lead to sustained hypertension.

ACKNOWLEDGMENTS

We gratefully acknowledge the help of Mrs. Josée Bédard-Baker, Mr. Ovid Da Silva, Mr. Pierre Dumas, and Mr. Bruno Lachance in preparing the manuscript. The work was supported by grants from the Medical Research Council of Canada (Grant MT-10802, MT-10803, and MT-11463), from the Heart and Stroke Foundation, and from the Dairy Bureau of Canada to Pavel Hamet and Johanne Tremblay. Sergei N. Orlov is the recipient of a visiting professorship from Pfizer Pharmaceutical Company.

REFERENCES

1. Heagerty AM, Ollerenshaw JD: The phosphoinositide signaling system and the pathogenesis of hypertension. In: Laragh JH, Brenner BM, eds. *Hypertension: pathophysiology, diagnosis, and management,* ed 1. New York: Raven Press, 1990;601–615.
2. Berridge MJ. *Nature* 1993;361:315–325.
3. Touyz RM, Schiffrin EL. *Curr Opin Nephrol Hypertens* 1993;2: 5–16.
4. Sutherland EW, Rall TW. *Pharmacol Rev* 1960;12:265–299.
5. Birnbaumer L, Pohl SL, Krans MJ, Rodbell M. The actions of hormones on the adenyl cyclase system. In: Greengard P, Costa E, eds. *Role of cyclic AMP in cell function,* vol. 3: New York: Raven Press, 1970;185–208.
6. Gilman AG *Annu Rev Biochem* 1987;56:615–649.
7. Birnbaumer L, Abramowitz J, Brown AM. *Biochim Biophys Acta* 1990;1031:185–224.
8. Birnbaumer L. *Cell* 1992;71:1069–1072.
9. Simon MI, Strathmann MP, Gautam N. *Science* 1991;252:802–808.
10. Taylor CW. *Biochem J* 1990;272:1–13.
11. Bourne HR, Sanders DA, McCormick F. *Nature* 1990;348:125–132.
12. Port FD, Malbon CC. *Trends Cardiovasc Med* 1993;3:85–92.
13. Tang WJ, Gilman AG. *Cell* 1992;70:869–872.
14. Gao B, Gilman AG. *Proc Natl Acad Sci USA* 1991;88:10178–10182.
15. Tang WJ, Gilman AG. *Science* 1991;254:1500–1503.
16. Taussig R, Quarmby LM, Gilman AG. *J Biol Chem* 1993;268:9–12.
17. Federman AD, Comklin BR, Schrader KA, Reed RR, Bourne HR. *Nature* 1992;356:159–161.
18. Kubalak SW, Webb JG. *Am J Physiol* 1993;264:H86–H96.
19. Yatani A, Godina J, Imoto Y, Reeves JP. *Science* 1987;288: 1288–1292.
20. Yatani A, Hamm HE, Codina J, Mazzoni MD, Birnbaumer L, Brown AM. *Science* 1988;241:828–831.
21. Kume H, Graziano MP, Kotlikoff MI. *Proc Natl Acad Sci USA* 1992;89:11051–11055.
22. Hescheler J, Rosenthal W, Hinsch KD, Wulfern M, Trautwein W, Schultz G. *EMBO J* 1988;7:619–624.
23. Codina J, Yatani A, Grenet D, Brown AM, Birnbaumer L. *Science* 1987;236:442–444.
24. Yatani A, Codina J, Brown AM, Birnbaumer L. *Science* 1987;235:207–211.
25. Smrcka AV, Hepler JR, Brown KO, Sternweis PC. *Science* 1991;251:804–807.
26. Aragay HM, Katz A, Simon MI. *J Biol Chem* 1992;267:24983–24988.
27. Wu D, Katz A, Lee CH, Simon MI. *J Biol Chem* 1992;267: 25798–25802.
28. Hescheler J, Rosenthal W, Trautwein W, Schultz G. *Nature* 1987;325:445–447.
29. Kleuss C, Hescheler J, Ewel C, Rosenthal W, Schultz G, Wittig B. *Nature* 1991;353:43–48.
30. Jelsema CL, Axelrod J. *Proc Natl Acad Sci USA* 1987;84:3623–3627.
31. Kats A, Wu D, Simon MI. *Nature* 1992;360:686–689.
32. Kleuss C, Scherubl H, Hescheler J, Schultz G, Wittig B. *Nature* 1992;358:424–426.
33. Miller WH, Laughlin SB. *Biophys Struct Mechan* 1983;9:269–276.
34. Beavo JA, Hansen RS, Harrison SA, Hurwitz RL, Martins TJ, Mumby MC. *Mol Cell Endocrinol* 1982;28:387–410.
35. Beavo JA, Hardman JG, Sutherland EW. *J Biol Chem* 1970;245: 5649–5655.
36. Franks DJ, MacManus JP. *Biochem Biophys Res Commun* 1971;42:844–849.
37. Maurice DH, Haslam RJ. *Mol Pharmacol* 1990;37:671–681.
38. Maurice DH, Haslam RJ. *Eur J Pharmacol* 1990;191:471–475.
39. Beebe SJ, Blackmore PF, Chrisman TD, Corbin JD. Use of synergistic pairs of site-selective cAMP analogs in intact cells. In: Corbin JD, Johnson RA, eds. *Methods in enzymology,* vol. 159. New York: Academic Press, 1988;118–139.
40. Walsh DA, Perkins JP, Krebs EG. *J Biol Chem* 1968;243:3763–3774.
41. Lefkowitz RJ. *Cell* 1993;74:409–412.
42. Price TD, Ashman DF, Melicow MM. *Biochim Biophys Acta* 1967;138:452–465.
43. Garbers DL. *J Biol Chem* 1979;254:240–243.
44. Kamisaki Y, Saheki S, Nakane M, Palmieri JA, Kuno T, Chang BY, Waldman SA, Murad F. *J Biol Chem* 1986;261:7236–7241.
45. Ignarro LJ, Degnan JN, Baricos WH, Kadowitz PJ, Wolin MS. *Biochem Biophys Acta* 1982;718:49–59.
46. Gerzer R, Hofmann F, Bohme E, Ivanova K, Spies C, Schultz G. Purification of soluble guanylate cyclase without loss of stimulation by sodium nitroprusside. In: Robison GA, ed. *Advances in cyclic nucleotide research,* vol. 14. New York: Raven Press, 1981;255–261.
47. Gerzer R, Hofmann F, Schultz G. *Eur J Biochem* 1981;116:479–486.
48. Bohme E, Grossman G, Herz J, Mulsch A, Spies C, Schultz G. Regulation of cyclic GMP formation by soluble guanylate cyclase: stimulation by NO-containing compounds. In: Nicosia S, ed. *Advances in cyclic nucleotide and protein phosphorylation research,* vol. 17. New York: Raven Press, 1984;259–266.
49. Glass DB, Frey W, II, Carr DW, Goldberg ND. *J Biol Chem* 1977;252:1279–1285.
50. White AA, Karr DB, Patt CS. *Biochem J* 1982;204:383–392.
51. Clyman RI, Blacksin AS, Manganiello VC, Vaughan M. *Proc Natl Acad Sci USA* 1975;72:3883–3887.
52. Goldberg ND, Haddox MK. *Annu Rev Biochem* 1977;46:823–896.
53. Martin W, Villani GM, Jothianandan D, Furchgott RF. *J Pharmacol Exp Ther* 1985;233(3):679–685.
54. Gruetter CA, Barry BK, McNamara DB, Gruetter DY, Kadowitz PJ, Ignarro LJ. *J Cyclic Nucleotide Res* 1979;5(3):211–224.
55. Ignarro LJ, Harbison RG, Wood KS, Kadowitz PJ. *J Pharmacol Exp Ther* 1986;236:30–36.
56. Hardman JG, Sutherland EW. *J Biol Chem* 1969;244:6363–6370.
57. Tremblay J, Gerzer R, Vinay P, Pang SC, Beliveau R, Hamet P. *FEBS Lett* 1985;181:17–22.
58. Tremblay J, Gerzer R, Hamet P. Cyclic GMP in cell function. In: Greengard P, Robison GA, eds. *Advances in second messenger and phosphoprotein research,* vol. 22. New York: Raven Press, 1988;319–383.
59. Flynn TG, De Bold ML, De Bold AJ. *Biochem Biophys Res Commun* 1983;117:859–865.
60. Kangawa K, Matsuo H. *Biochem Biophys Res Commun* 1984;118:131–139.
61. Sudoh T, Kangawa K, Minamino N, Matsuo H. *Nature* 1988;332:78–81.
62. Minamino N, Kangawa K, Matsuo H. *Biochem Biophys Res Commun* 1988;157:402–409.
63. Sudoh T, Minamino N, Kangawa K, Matsuo H. *Biochem Biophys Res Commun* 1990;168:863–870.
64. Kojima M, Minamino N, Kangawa K, Matsuo H. *FEBS Lett* 1990;276:209–213.
65. Schenk DB, Phelps MN, Porter JG, Scarborough RM, McEnroe GA, Lewicki JA. *J Biol Chem* 1985;260:14887–14890.
66. Fuller F, Porter JG, Arfsten AE, Miller J, Schilling JW, Scarborough RM, Lewicki JA, Schenk DB. *J Biol Chem* 1988;263:9395–9401.

67. Lowe DG, Chang MS, Hellmiss R, Chen E, Singh S, Garbers DL, Goeddel DV. *EMBO J* 1989;8:1377–1384.
68. Chinkers M, Garbers DL, Chang MS, Lowe DG, Chin H, Goeddel DV, Schulz S. *Nature* 1989;338:78–83.
69. Schulz S, Singh S, Bellet RA, Singh G, Tubb DJ, Chin H, Garbers DL. *Cell* 1989;58:1155–1162.
70. Tremblay J, Huot C, Koch C, Potier M. *J Biol Chem* 1991;266:8171–8175.
71. Schulz S, Chinkers M, Garbers DL. *FASEB J* 1989;3:2026–2035.
72. Lowe DG, Klisak I, Sparkes RS, Mohandas T, Goeddel DV. *Genomics* 1990;8:304–312.
73. Koller KJ, Lowe DG, Bennett GL, Minamino N, Kangawa K, Matsuo H, Goeddel DV. *Science* 1991;252:120–123.
74. Komatsu Y, Nakao K, Suga S, Ogawa Y, Mukoyama M, Arai H, Shirakami G, Hosoda K, Nakagawa O, Hama N, Kishimoto I, Imura H. *Endocrinology* 1991;129:1104–1106.
75. Suga S, Nakao K, Kishimoto I, Hosoda K, Mukoyama M, Arai H, Shirakami G, Ogawa Y, Komatsu Y, Nakagawa O, Hama N, Imura H. *Circ Res* 1992;71:34–39.
76. Hamet P, Tremblay J: Platelet cyclic GMP-binding phosphodiesterase. In: Corbin JD, Johnson RA, eds. *Methods in enzymology*, vol. 159. New York: Academic Press, 1988;710–722.
77. Chiu PJS, Tetzloff G, Ahn HS, Sybertz EJ. *Am J Hypertens* 1988;1:262–268.
78. Kukovetz WR, Holzmann S. *Eur J Pharmacol* 1986;122:103–109.
79. Kuo JF. *Proc Natl Acad Sci USA* 1974;71:4037–4040.
80. Takai Y, Nakaya S, Inoue M, Kishimoto A, Nishiyama K, Yamamura H, Nishizuka Y. *J Biol Chem* 1976;251:1481–1487.
81. Inoue M, Kishimoto A, Takai Y, Nishizuka Y. *J Biol Chem* 1976;251:4476–4478.
82. Casnellie JE, Greengard P. *Proc Natl Acad Sci USA* 1974;71:1891–1895.
83. Fesenko EE, Kolesnikov SS, Lyubarsky AL. *Nature* 1985;313:310–313.
84. Hamet P, Pang SC, Tremblay J. *J Biol Chem* 1989;264:12364–12369.
85. Hokin MR, Hokin LE. *J Biol Chem* 1953;203:267–277.
86. Hokin LE, Hokin MR. *Biochim Biophys Acta* 1955;18:102–110.
87. Michell RH. *Biochim Biophys Acta* 1975;45:81–147.
88. Berridge MJ. *Annu Rev Biochem* 1987;56:159–193.
89. Majerus PW, Ross TS, Cunningham TW, Caldwell KK, Jefferson AB, Bansal VS. *Cell* 1990;63:459–465.
90. Stryer L. *Gold Spring Harbor Symp Quant Biol* 1988;53:282–294.
91. Boyer JL, Waldo GL, Harden TK. *J Biol Chem* 1992;267:25451–25456.
92. Nishizuka Y. *Science* 1986;233:305–312.
93. Berridge MJ, Irvine RF. *Nature* 1984;312:315–321.
94. Peterson OH. *Cell Calcium* 1989;10:375–383.
95. Luckhoff A, Clapham DE. *Nature* 1992;355:356–358.
96. Nakanishi H, Brewer KA, Exton JH. *J Biol Chem* 1993;268:13–16.
97. Pike LJ. *Endocr Rev* 1993;268:13–16.
98. Barbacid M. *Annu Rev Biochem* 1987;56:776–827.
99. Yatani A, Okabe K, Polakis P, Helenbeck R, McCormick F, Brown AM. *Cell* 1990;61:769–776.
100. Carafoli E. *Physiol Rev* 1991;71:129–153.
101. Carafoli E. *Annu Rev Biochem* 1987;56:395–433.
102. Kaczorowski GJ, Slaughter RS, King VF, Garcia ML. *Biochim Biophys Acta* 1989;988:287–302.
103. Hullin RE, Biel M, Flockerzi V, Hoffman F. *Trends Cardiovasc Med* 1993;3:48–53.
104. Katz AM. *N Engl J Med* 1993;328:1244–1251.
105. Putney JW. *Trends Pharmacol Sci* 1987;8:481–486.
106. Kirber MT, Walsh TV, Singer TT. *Pflugers Arch* 1988;412:339–345.
107. Cook NJ, Hanke W, Kaupp UB. *Proc Natl Acad Sci USA* 1987;84:585–589.
108. Fasoloto C, Hoth M, Matthew C, Penner R. *Proc Natl Acad Sci USA* 1993;20:3068–3072.
109. Klee CB, Vanaman TC. *Calmodulin Adv Protein Chem* 1993;35:213–321.
110. Dollard TD. *Annu Rev Biochem* 1986;55:987–1035.
111. Burgoyne RD, Geisow MJ. *Cell Calcium* 1989;10:1–10.
112. Heizmann CW, Hunziker W. *Trends Biochem Sci* 1991;16:98–103.
113. Glaser KB, Mobilio D, Chang JY, Senko N. *Trends Biol Sci* 1993;14:92–98.
114. Davis TN. *Cell* 1992;71:557–564.
115. Bernhardt I, Hall AC, Ellory JC. *Studia Biophysica* 1988;126:5–21.
116. Duhm J. Na+ and K+ transport in human and rat erythrocytes: features complicating the interpretation of data. In: Rettig R, Ganten D, Luft FC, eds. *Salt and hypertension. Dietary minerals, volume homeostasis and cardiovascular regulation.* Berlin: Springer Verlag, 1989;35–51.
117. Chipperfield AR. *Clin Sci* 1986;71:465–476.
118. McManus TJ. *Fed Proc* 1987;46:2378–2383.
119. Knauf U: An ion transport in erythrocytes. In: Andreoli TE, Hoffman JF, Fanestich DD, Schulz SG, eds., New York: Plenum Press, 1993;191–230.
120. Lang F. NaCl transport in the kidney. In Gregor R, ed. *Advances in comparative and environmental physiology.* New York: Springer-Verlag, 1988;153–188.
121. Brown AM, Birnbaumer L. *Annu Rev Physiol* 1990;52:197–213.
122. Clark JD, Limbird LE. *Am J Physiol* 1991;261:C945–C953.
123. Counillon L, Pouyssegur J. *Curr Opin Nephrol Hypertens* 1993;2:708–714.
124. McDonough HA, Farley RA. *Curr Opin Nephrol Hypertens* 1993;2:725–734.
125. Orlov SN, Postnov IY, Pokudin NI, Kukharenko VY, Postnov YV. *J Hypertens* 1989;7:781–788.
126. Busch S, Siffert W. *Pflugers Arch* 1992;420:R17.
127. Guyton AC. *Circulatory physiology III: Arterial pressure and regulation.* London-Toronto: Saunders, 1980.
128. Hamet P, Tremblay J. Cyclic nucleotides in the pathogenesis of hypertension. In: Laragh JH, Brenner BM, eds. *Hypertension: pathophysiology, diagnosis, and management.* New York: Raven Press, 1990;617–635.
129. Luscher TF, Diederich D, Buhler FR, Van Houtte PM. Interactions between platelets and the vessel wall. Role of endothelium-derived vasoactive substances. In: Laragh JH, Brenner BM, eds. *Hypertension: pathophysiology, diagnosis, and management.* New York: Raven Press, 1990;637–648.
130. King AJ, Marsden PA, Brenner BM. Endothelin. A potent vasoactive peptide of endothelial origin. In: Laragh JH, Brenner BN, eds. *Hypertension: pathophysiology, diagnosis, and management.* New York: Raven Press, 1990;649–660.
131. Rembold CM. *Hypertension* 1992;20:129–137.
132. Lincoln TM, Cornwell TL. *FASEB J* 1993;7:328–338.
133. Moncada S, Palmer RMJ, Higgs EA. *Pharmacol Rev* 1991;43:109–142.
134. Dzau VJ. *Hypertension* 1986;8:553–559.
135. Brock TA, Brugnara C, Canessa M, Gimbrone MA. *Am J Physiol* 1986;250:C888–C895.
136. O'Donnell ME. *Am J Physiol* 1989;257:C36–C44.
137. Shepard JM, Goderic SK, Brzyski N, Del Vecchio PJ, Malik AB, Kimelberg HK. *J Cell Physiol* 1987;133:389–394.
138. Hartshorne DJ, Kawamura T. *News Physiol Sci* 1992;7:59–64.
139. Benham CD, Tsien RW. *Nature* 1987;328:275–278.
140. Den Hertog A, Nelmans SA, Mollelman A, Hoiting BH, Van den Akker J, Duin M. Regulation of inositol phosphates, intracellular calcium and membrane current via P_2-purinoceptors and alpha-1-adrenoceptors In: Sperilakis N, Wood JW, eds. *Frontiers in smooth muscle research.* New York: Alan R. Liss Inc., 1990;183–192.
141. Cole BR, Kuhnline MA, Needleman P. *J Clin Invest* 1985;76:2413–2415.
142. Little PJ, Cragoe EJ, Bobik A. *Am J Physiol* 1986;251:C707–C712.
143. Orlov SN, Resink TJ, Bernhardt J, Buhler FR. *J Membr Biol* 1992;129:199–210.
144. Blaustein MP. *Am J Physiol* 1977;232:C165–C173.
145. Blaustein MP, Hamllyn JM. *Am J Med* 1993;77:45–59.
146. Buckalew V, Haddy FJ: Circulating natriuretic factors in hypertension. In: Laragh JH, Brenner BM, eds. *Hypertension: patho-*

physiology, diagnosis, and management. New York: Raven Press, 1990;939–954.

147. Adelstein RS, Conti MA, Hathaway DR. *J Biol Chem* 1978;253: 8347–8850.

148. Stull JT, Hsu LC, Tansey MG, Kamm KE. *J Biol Chem* 1990;265:16683–16690.

149. McDaniel NL, Rembold CM, Richard HM, Murphy RA. *J Physiol* 1991;439:147–160.

150. Lindemann JP, Jones LR, Hathaway DR, Henry BG, Watanabe AM. *J Biol Chem* 1993;258:464–471.

151. Raeymaekers L, Hoffmann F, Casteels R. *Biochem J* 1988;252: 269–273.

152. Sarcevic B, Brookes V, Martin TJ, Kemp BE, Robinson PJ. *J Biol Chem* 1989;264:20648–20654.

153. Cornwell TL, Pryzwansky KB, Wyalt TA, Lincoln TM. *Mol Pharmacol* 1991;40:923–931.

154. Scharff O, Foder B. *Physiol Rev* 1993;73:547–582.

155. Chen XL, Rembold CM. *Am J Physiol* 1992;263:C468–C473.

156. Ahn HY, Kang SE, Chang KC, Karakitt PA. *J Pharmacol* 1992;59:263–265.

157. Yoshida Y, Sun HT, Cai TQ, Imai S. *J Biol Chem* 1991;266: 19819–19825.

158. Zemel MB, Johnson BA, Ambrozy SA. *Am J Hypertens* 1992;5: 637–641.

159. Kim YC, Zemel MB. *Hypertension* 1993;22:74.

160. Stekiel WJ, Contney SJ, Rusch NJ. *Hypertension* 1993;21:1005–1009.

161. Orlov SN, Hamet P. β-adrenergic regulation of Ca influx in vascular smooth muscle cells (VSMC) from normotensive rats (BN.1x) and SHR (Abstr.). In: *15th Scientific Meeting of the International Society of Hypertension, Melbourne, March 20–24 1994.*

162. Folkow B, Hallback M, Lundgren Y, Weiss L. *Acta Physiol Scand* 1970;80:93–106.

163. Folkow B. *Physiol Rev* 1982;62:347–503.

164. Jackson CL, Schwartz SM. *Hypertension* 1992;20:713–736.

165. Heagerty AM, Aalkjaer C, Bund SJ, Korsgaard N, Mulvany MJ. *Hypertension* 1993;21:391–397.

166. Yamori Y, Igawa T, Kanbe T, Kihara M, Nara Y, Horie R. *Clin Sci* 1981;61(Suppl.):121S–123S.

167. Hamet P, Hadrava V, Kruppa U, Tremblay J. *J Hypertens* 1988;6(Suppl. 4):S36–S39.

168. Blennerhassett MG, Kannan MS, Garfield RE. *Am J Physiol* 1989;256:C644–C651.

169. Hadrava V, Tremblay J, Hamet P. *Hypertension* 1989;13:589–597.

170. Scott-Burden T, Resink TJ, Baur U, Burgin M, Buhler FR. *Hypertension* 1989;13:295–304.

171. Paquet JL, Baudouin-Legros M, Marche P, Meyer P. *Am J Hypertens* 1989;2:108–110.

172. Hamada M, Harris EL, Millar JA, Simpson FO. *J Vasc Med Biol* 1990;2:136–141.

173. Berk BC, Vallega G, Muslin AJ, Gordon HM, Canessa M, Alexander RW. *J Clin Invest* 1989;83:822–829.

174. Saltis J, Bobik A. *J Hypertens* 1992;60:635–644.

175. Richard L, Dam TV, Teiger E, Tremblay J, Gossard F, Hamet P. Apoptosis in target organs of hypertension (Abstr.). In: *15th Scientific Meeting of the International Society of Hypertension, Melbourne, March 20–24 1994.*

176. Boynton AL, Whitfield JF. The role of cyclic AMP in cell proliferation: a critical assessment of the evidence. In: Greengard P, Robison GA, eds. *Advances in cyclic nucleotide research,* vol. 15. New York: Raven Press, 1983;193–294.

177. Franks DJ, Plamondon J, Hamet P. *J Cell Physiol* 1984;119:41–45.

178. Silver BJ, Bokar JA, Virgin JB, Vallen EA, Milsted A, Nilson JH. *Proc Natl Acad Sci USA* 1987;83:6682–6686.

179. Yamamoto KK, Gonzalez GA, Briggs WHIII, Montininy MR. *Nature* 1988;334:494–498.

180. Sheng M, Thompson MA, Greenberg ME. *Science* 1991;252: 1427–1430.

181. Liu F, Thompson MA, Wagner S, Greenberg ME, Green MR. *J Biol Chem* 1993;268:6714–6720.

182. Grinstein S, Rotin D, Mason MJ. *Biochim Biophys Acta* 1989;988:73–97.

183. Rao G, Sardet C, Pouyssegur J, Berk BC. *Am J Physiol* 1993;264: C1278–C1284.

184. Perara R, Serrano R. *Nature* 1988;334:439–440.

185. Wakabayashi S, Fafournoux P, Sardet C, Pouyssegur J: *Proc Natl Acad Sci USA* 1992;89:2424–2428.

186. Bobik A, Grooms A, Little PJ, Cragoe EJ, Grinpukel S. *Am J Physiol* 1991;260:C581–C588.

187. Guyton A, Hall JE, Coleman TG, Manning RD. The dominant role of the kidney in the long-term regulation of arterial pressure in normal and hypertensive states. In: Laragh JH, Brenner BM, eds. *Hypertension: Pathophysiology, Diagnosis, and Management.* New York: Raven Press, 1990;1029–1052.

188. Gregor G. *Physiol Rev* 1985;65:760–797.

189. Molony DA, Reeves WB, Adreoli TE. *Kidney Int* 1989;36:418–426.

190. Giebisch G: Single nephron studies on the action of furosemide. In *Lasix. Proceeding of the symposium held at Hoechst AG, Frankfurt am Main,* 1993; 17–30.

191. Sardet C, Franchi A, Pouyssegur J. *Cell* 1989;56:271–280.

192. Miller RT, Counillon L, Pages G, Lifton RP, Sardet C, Pouyssegur J. *J Biol Chem* 1991;268:10813–10819.

193. Tse CM, Brant SR, Walker MS, Pouyssegur J, Donowitz M. *J Biol Chem* 1992;267:9340–9346.

194. Orlowski J, Kandasamy RA, Shull CE. *J Biol Chem* 1992;267: 9331–9339.

195. Borgese F, Sardet C, Cappadoro M, Pouyssegur J, Motais R. *Proc Natl Acad Sci USA* 1992;89:6765–6769.

196. Orlov SN, Skryabin GA. *J Comp Physiol* 1993;163:413–420.

197. Barber DL, Ganz MB. *J Biol Chem* 1992;267:20607–20612.

198. Weinmann EJ, Shenolikar S, Kahn AM. *Am J Physiol* 1987;252: 19–25.

199. Felder CC, Cambell T, Albrecht F, Jose PA. *Am J Physiol* 1990;259:F297–F303.

200. Lytle C, Xu JC, Biemesderfer P, Haas M, Forbush B III. *J Biol Chem* 1992;267:25428–25737.

201. Lytle C, Forbush B III. *J Biol Chem* 1992;267:25438–25443.

202. Sun A, Grossman EB, Lombardi M, Hebert SC. *J Membr Biol* 1991;120:83–94.

203. Haas M, Dunham PB, Forbush BIII. *Am J Physiol* 1991;260: C791–C804.

204. Gamba G, Saltzberg SN, Lombardi M, Miyanoshita A, Lytton J, Hediger MA, Brenner BM, Hebert SC. *Proc Natl Acad Sci USA* 1993;90:2749–2753.

205. Ohara A, Matsunaga H, Eaton DC. *Am J Physiol* 1993;264: C352–C360.

206. Light DB, Corbin JD, Stanton BA. *Nature* 1990;344:336–339.

207. Stanton BA, Karlson K. *FASEB J* 1992;6:A1808.

208. Ahmad I, Korbmacher C, Segal AS, Cheung P, Boulpaep EL, Barnstable CJ. *Proc Natl Acad Sci USA* 1992;89:10262–10266.

209. Willenbrock RC, Tremblay J, Garcia R, Hamet P. *J Clin Invest* 1989;83:482–489.

210. Hamet P, Tremblay J, Pang SC, Skuherska R, Schiffrin EL, Garcia R, Cantin M, Genest J, Palmour R, Ervin FR, Martin S, Goldwater R. *J Hypertens* 1986;4(Suppl. 2):S49–S56.

211. Hamet P, Tremblay J, Pang SC: Cyclic nucleotides in pathology. In: Nicosia S, ed. *Advances in cyclic nucleotide and protein phosphorylation research,* vol. 17. New York: Raven Press, 1984;651–659.

212. Hamet P, Coquil JF, Bousseau-Lafortune S, Franks DJ, Tremblay J. Cyclic GMP binding and phosphodiesterase: implication for platelet function. In: Strada SJ, Thompson WJ, eds. *Advances in cyclic nucleotides and protein phosphorylation research,* vol. 16. New York: Raven Press, 1984;119–136.

213. Hamet P, Sands H. Concluding remarks: comments on pathophysiological studies and cyclic nucleotides. In: Hamet P, Sands H, eds. *Advances in cyclic nucleotide research,* vol. 12. New York: Raven Press, 1980;411–412.

214. Hamet P, Franks DJ, Adnot S, Coquil JF. Cyclic nucleotides in hypertension. In: Hamet P, Sands H, eds. *Advances in cyclic nucleotide research,* vol. 12. New York: Raven Press; 1980;11–23.

215. Hamet P, Tremblay J: Cyclic nucleotides in the pathogenesis of

hypertension. In: Laragh JH, Brenner BM, eds. *Hypertension: pathophysiology, diagnosis, and management.* New York: Raven Press, 1990;617–635.

216. Hamet P, Fraysse J, Franks DJ. *Circ Res* 1978;43:583–591.
217. Resink TJ, Burgisser E, Buhler FR. *Hypertension* 1986;8:662–668.
218. Hoffmann G, Gobel BO, Harbrecht U, Vetter H, Dusing R. *Am J Hypertens* 1992;5:847–850.
219. Coquil JF, Hamet P. *Proc Soc Exp Biol Med* 1980;164:569–575.
220. Matsumori Y, Ohyanagi M, Kawamoto H, Shibata R, Iwasaki T. *Jpn Circ J* 1989;53:113–120.
221. Postnov YV, Orlov SN, Reznikova MB, Pokudin NI. *Pflugers Arch* 1980;384:183–188.
222. Asano M, Masuzawa K, Matsuda T, Asano T. *J Pharm Exp Ther* 1988;246(2):709–718.
223. Jazayeri A, Meyer III WJ. *J Hypertens* 1989;7:895–900.
224. Benze J, Griffith VJ, Yang HY, Rosendorff G. *J Hypertens* 1992;10:539–544.
225. Atrakchi A. *Hypertension* 1989;14:54–60.
226. Kinoshita S, Sidhu A, Telder RA. *J Clin Invest* 1989;84:1849–1856.
227. Gesek FA, Schoolwerth AC. *Am J Physiol* 1991;2G1:F526–F536.
228. Felder RA, Konoshita S, Ohbu K, Mouradian MM, Sibley DR, Monsma FJ, Minowa T, Minowa MT, Canessa LM, Jose PA. *Am J Physiol* 1993;2G4:R726–R732.
229. Nishi A, Eklof AS, Bertorello AM, Aperia A. *Hypertension* 1993;761–771.
230. Ohbu K, Felder RA. *Am J Physiol* 1993;2G4:F274–F279.
231. Amer MS, Gomoll AW, Perhach JL, Ferguson HC, McKinney GR. *Proc Natl Acad Sci USA* 1974;71:4930–4934.
232. Triner L, Vulliemoz Y, Verosky M, Marger WN. *Biochem Pharmacol* 1975;24:743–745.
233. Bhalla RC, Sharma RV. *Blood Vessels* 1982;19:109–116.
234. Anand-Srivastava MB. *Biochem Pharmacol* 1988;37:3017–3022.
235. Clark CJ, Milligan G, McLellan AR, Connell JMC. *Hypertension* 1993;21:204–209.
236. Hamet P, Tremblay J: Abnormalities of second messenger systems in hypertension. In: Meyer P, Marche P, eds. *Blood cells and arteries in hypertension and atherosclerosis: the Argenteuil Symposia series,* vol. 12. New York: Raven Press, 1989;171–187.
237. Bhalla RC, Sharma RV, Ramanathan S. *Biochim Biophys Acta* 1980;632:497–506.
238. Kumano K, Upsher ME, Khaizallah PA. *Hypertension* 1983;5(Suppl I):I-175–I-183.
239. Bohem M, Gierschik P, Knorr A, Larish K, Weismann K, Erdmann E. *J Hypertens* 1992;10:1115–1128.
240. Ohsuzu F, Katsushika S, Maie SI, Akanuma M, Yanagida S, Sakata H, Ishida H, Aosaki N, Nakamura H. *Jpn Circ J* 1992;56:301–309.
241. Schultz KD, Fritschka E, Pauliks LB, Philipp T, Distler A. *J Hypertens* 1993;7(Suppl 6):S142–S143.
242. Kamibayashi C, Ramanathan S. *Life Sci* 1989;45:2115–2125.
243. Yoshikawa H, Fukuda K, Baba A, Nishio H, Ueyama T, Yoshikawa A, Kuchii M, Nishio I, Masuyama Y. *Am J Hypertens* 1993;3:230–233.
244. Anand-Srivastava MB, Picard S, Thibault C. *Am J Hypertens* 1991;4:840–843.
245. Resink TJ, Rybin V, Bernhardt J, Orlov S, Buhler FR, Tkachuk VA. *J Vasc Res* 1993;30:169–180.
246. Broadus AE, Kaminsky NI, Northcutt RC, Hardman JG, Sutherland EW, Liddle GW. *J Clin Invest* 1970;49:2237–2245.
247. Gerzer R, Witzgall H, Tremblay J, Gutkowska J, Hamet P. *J Clin Endocrinol Metab* 1985;61:1217–1219.
248. Weil J, Gerzer R, Strom T, Lang RE, Dohlemann C, Knorr D, Bidlingmaier F. *Pediatrics* 1987;80:545–548.
249. Heim JM, Gottmann K, Weil J, Strom TM, Gerzer R. *Eur J Clin Invest* 1989;19:265–271.
250. Roy LF, Ogilvie RI, Larochelle P, Hamet P, Leenen FHH. *Circulation* 1989;79:383–392.
251. Hamet P, Stouder DA, Ginn HE, Hardman JG, Liddle GW. *J Clin Invest* 1975;56:339–345.
252. Papagalanis ND, Skopelitis P, Kourti A, Kostogianni G, Kara-

253. Lowder SC, Hamet P, Liddle GW. *Circ Res* 1976;38:105–108.
254. Messerli FH, Kuchel O, Hamet P, Tolis G, Guthrie GP Jr, Fraysse J, Nowaczynski W, Genest J. *Circ Res* 1976;38(Suppl 2):II42–II47.
255. Hamet P, Lowder SC, Hardman JG, Liddle GW. *Metabolism* 1975;24:1139–1144.
256. Messerli FH, Kuchel O, Tolis G, Hamet P, Fraysse J, Genest J. *Int J Clin Pharmacol* 1976;14:189–194.
257. Widimsky J, Fejfarova MH, Feifar Z. *Cardiology* 1957;31:381–389.
258. Julius S, Conway J. *Circulation* 1968;38:282–288.
259. Frohlich ED, Kozul VJ, Tarazi RC, Dustan HP. *Circ Res* 1970;26–27(Suppl I):55–63.
260. Watanabe K, Nishio T, Mori C, Kihara M, Yamori Y. *Jpn Circ J* 1985;49:446–450.
261. Cusson JR, Hamet P, Gutkowska J, Kuchel O, Genest J, Cantin M, Larochelle P. *J Hypertens* 1987;5:435–443.
262. Hamet P, Testaert E, Palmour R, Larochelle P, Cantin M, Martin S, Ervin F, Tremblay J. *Am J Hypertens* 1989;2:690–695.
263. Hamet P, Skuherska R, Pang SC, Tremblay J. *Hypertension* 1985;7(Suppl II):II135–II142.
264. Anand-Srivastava M, et al. *Am J Hypertens* 1993;6:72–75.
265. Bohm M et al. *Hypertension* 1992;20:103–112.
266. Fukuda N, Honda M, Minato M, Soma M, Izumi Y, Hatano M. *Jpn Circ J* 1990;54:82–88.
267. Schoors DF, Dupont AG. *Am J Hypertens* 1991;4:494–499.
268. Orlov SN, Tremblay J, Hamet P: Impaired β-adrenergic regulation of cAMP production and Na, K cotransport in SHR vascular smooth muscle cells (VSMC) (Abstr). In: *15th Scientific Meeting of the International Society of Hypertension, Melbourne, March 20–24, 1994.*
269. Pravenec M, Klir P, Kren V, Zicha J, Kunes J. *J Hypertens* 1989;7:217–222.
270. Orlov SN, Kunes J, Tremblay J, Hamet P. *Hypertension* 1993;*Submitted.*
271. Tremblay J, Willenbrock R, Cusson JR, Larochelle P, Schiller PW, Leenen FHH, Palmour R, Ervin F, Testaert E, Hamet P: Role of action of particulate guanylate cyclase in the expression of biological actions of ANF. In Needleman P, ed. *Biological and molecular aspects of atrial factors,* vol. 81. New York: Alan R. Liss, Inc., 1988;97–108.
272. Steinhelper ME, Cochrane KL, Field LJ. *Hypertension* 1990;16:301–307.
273. Arnal JF, Warin L, Michel JB. *J Clin Invest* 1992;90:647–652.
274. Tremblay J, Huot C, Willenbrock RC, Bayard F, Gossard F, Fujio N, Koch C, Kuchel O, Debinski W, Hamet P. *J Clin Invest* 1993;92:2499–2508.
275. Resink TJ, Scott-Burden T, Jones CR, Baur U, Bühler FR. *Am J Hypertens* 1989;2:32–39.
276. Mulvany MJ. *Clin Exp Hypertens (A)* 1987;9:1789–1801.
277. Schiffrin EL, Parent A, St-Louis J, Tremblay J, Garcia R, Thibault G. *Cardiovasc Res* 1992;26:857–864.
278. Fujio N, Bayard F, Gossard F, Hamet P, Tremblay J. *J Biol Chem* 1993;*Submitted.*
279. Deng Y, Rapp JP. *Nature Gen* 1992;1:267–272.
280. Tremblay J, Gossard F, Sun YL, Pravenec M, Kren V, Hamet P. A polymorphism in the promoter of natriuretic peptide receptor-A gene is associated with hypertension (Abstr). In: *15th Scientific Meeting of the International Society of Hypertension, Melbourne, March 20–24, 1994.*
281. Jones AW. *Circ Res* 1973;33:563–572.
282. Postnov YV, Orlov SN, Shevchenko AS. *Kardiologiia* 1975;15 (no. 10):88–92.
283. Postnov YV, Orlov SN, Gulak PV, Shevchenko AS. *Pflugers Arch* 1976;365:257–263.
284. Postnov YV, Orlov SN, Shevchenko AS, Adler AM. *Pflugers Arch* 1977;371:263–270.
285. Postnov YV, Orlov SN: Alteration of cell membranes in primary hypertension. In: Genest J, Kuchel O, Hamet P, Cantin M, eds. *Hypertension: physiopathology and treatment,* ed 2. New York: McGraw-Hill, 1983;95–108.

batsos A, Gennadiou M, Thomas S, Samartzis M, Mountokalakis T. *Nephron* 1991;59:226–231.

286. Postnov YV, Orlov SN. *J Hypertens* 1984;2:1–6.
287. Postnov YV, Orlov SN. *Physiological Rev* 1985;65(4):904–945.
288. Hilton PJ. *N Engl J Med* 1986;314:222–229.
289. Aviv A, Lasker N: Proposed defects in membrane transport and intracellular ions as pathogenic factors in essential hypertension. In: Laragh JH, Brenner BM, eds. *Hypertension: pathophysiology, diagnosis and treatment*. New York: Raven Press, 1990;923–937.
290. Canessa M, Adragna N, Solomon HS, Connolly TM, Tosleson DC. *N Engl J Med* 1980;302:772–776.
291. Huot SJ, Aronson PS. *Diabetes Care* 1991;14:521–535.
292. Lyusov VA, Orlov SN, Postnov IY, Ryazhski GG. *Kardiologiia* 1983;23(No. 3):76–80.
293. Petrov VV, Arabidze GG, Levitskii DO, Grishenkov EA, Kaikov MI, Khailov IE. *Teraperticheskki Archiv (Moscow)* 1990;66(6):124–129.
294. Carr SJ, Thomas TH, Laker MF, Wilkinson R. *J Hypertens* 1990;8:139–146.
295. Lau YT, Wu D, Liang HC, Chen WC. *Clin Exp Hypertens (A)* 1992;14:489–503.
296. Laurenzi M, Cirillo M, Trevisan M. *Clin Exp Hypertens (A)* 1992;14:261–269.
297. Britov AN, Kobal AM, Orlov SN, Pokudin NI, Sapozhnikov II, Grishenkov EA. *Kardiologiia* 1991;31(8):54–58.
298. Turner ST, Michels VV. *Hypertension* 1991;18:183–190.
299. Turner ST, Rebbeck TR, Sing CF. *Hypertension* 1992;20:841–850.
300. Weder AB, Fitzpatrick MA, Torretti BA, Hinder-Liter AL, Eggn BM, Tulius S. *Hypertension* 1987;9:459–465.
301. Weder AB. *N Engl J Med* 1986;314:198–201.
302. Nosadini R, Semplicini P, Fioretto P, Lusiani L, Trevisan R, Donadon V, Zanette G, Nicolosi GL, Dall'Aglio V, Zanuttini D, Viberti G. *Hypertension* 1991;18:191–198.
303. Doria A, Fioretto P, Avogaro A, Cararo A, Morocutti A, Trevisan R, Frigato F, Crepadi G, Viberti G, Nosadini R. *Am J Physiol* 1991;261:E684–E691.
304. Foyle WJ, Drury PL. *J Hypertens* 1991;9:713–717.
305. Feig PU, D'Occhio MA, Boylan JW. *J Hypertens* 1986;4(Suppl 5):S224–S226.
306. Ng LL, Harker M, Abel MD. *Clin Sci* 1988;75:521–526.
307. Orlov SN, Postnov IY, Pokudin NI, Kukharenko VY, Postnov YV. *Bull Exp Biol Med (Moscow)* 1988;106:286–289.
308. Semplicini A, Canessa M, Mozzato MG, Cesloto G, Marzola M, Buzzaccarini F, Casolino P, Pessina AC. *Am J Hypertens* 1989;2:903–908.
309. Canessa M, Morgan K, Goldszer R, Moore TJ, Spalvins A. *Hypertension* 1991;17:340–348.
310. Livne A, Veitch R, Grinstein S, Balfe JW, Marquez-Julio A, Rothstein A. *Lancet* 1987;1:533–536.
311. Livne AA, Aharonovitz O, Paran E. *J Hypertens* 1991;9:1013–1019.
312. Weder AB, Schmouder RL, Torretti BA. *J Hypertens* 1990;8:1132–1142.
313. Rosskopf D, Siffert G, Osswald U, Witte K, Dusing R, Akermann TWN, Siffert W. *J Hypertens* 1992;10:839–847.
314. Tokutome G, Tomanari H, Gardner JP, Aladjem M, Fine BR, Lasker N, Gutkin M, Byrd LH, Aviv A. *Hypertension* 1990;16:180–189.
315. Doctor HS, Benjamin N, Todd SD, Ritter JM. *J Human Hypertens* 1991;5:161–165.
316. Ng LL, Dudley C, Bomford J, Hawley D. *J Hypertens* 1989;7:471–475.
317. Ng LL, Fennell DA, Dudley C. *J Hypertens* 1990;8:533–537.
318. Dudley CRK, Taylor DJ, Ng LL, Kemp IJ, Ratcliffe PJ, Radda GK, Ledingham JGG. *Clin Sci* 1990;79:491–497.
319. Pontremoli R, Spalvins A, Menachery A, Torrelli L, Canessa M. *Kidney Int* 1992;42:1355–1362.
320. Feig PU. *Kidney Int* 1987;31:296.
321. Feig PU. *Am J Hypertens* 1990;3:927–932.
322. Markov KHM, Pinelis VG, Kudinov UV, Borin ML, Azizova OA. *Bull Exp Biol Med* 1989;107:188–190.
323. Feig PU, D'Occhio MA, Boylan JW. *Hypertension* 1987;9:287–288.
324. Saleh AM, Battle DC, Gutterman C. *J Clin Invest* 1990;85:1734–1739.
325. Ellstrom DR, Foster CD, Honeyman TW, Scheid CR. *Am J Hypertens* 1993;6:21–27.
326. Ek TD, Deth RC. *Hypertension* 1988;12:331–332.
327. Alexander D, Gerdner JP, Tomonari H, Fine BP, Aviv A. *J Hypertens* 1990;8:867–871.
328. Orlov SN, Resink TJ, Bernhardt J, Buhler FR. Sodium fluoride as a potent activator of Ca^{2+} influx and NA^+/H^+ exchange in cultured vascular smooth muscle cells from WKY and SHR. In: *14th Scientific Meeting of International Society of Hypertension*, Madrid, June 14–18, 1992, p. 294.
329. Inariba H, Kanayama Y, Takaori K, Negoro N, Inoe T, Takeda T. *Clin Exp Pharmacol Physiol* 1992;19:171–176.
330. Orlov SN, Pokudin NI, Postnov YV. *J Hypertens* 1991;9(Suppl):S290–S291.
331. Acra S, Ghishan FK. *Gastroenterology* 1991;101:430–436.
332. Kuriyama S, Nakamura K, Kaguchi Y, Tomonari H, Tokutome G, Hashimoto T, Sakai O. *Nephron* 1992;60:448–452.
333. Sume PP, Aronvon JK, Thompson CH, Williams EM, Green Y, Radda GK. *Clin Sci* 1991;81:743–750.
334. Delva P, Pastori C, Provoli E, Degan M, Arosio E, Montesi G, Steele A, Lechi A. *J Hypertens* 1993;11:823–830.
335. Alonso A, Arrazola A, Garciandia A, Esparza N, Gomez-Alamillo C, Diez J. *Hypertension* 1993;22:348–356.
336. Postnov YV. *Kardiologiia* 1975;15(6):19–23.
337. Rosskopf D, Dusing R, Siffert W. *Hypertension* 1993;21:607–617.
338. Rosskopf D, Fromter E, Siffert W. *J Clin Invest* 1993;92:2553–2559.
339. Lifton RR, Hunt SC, Williams RR, Pouyssegur J, Lalouel JM. *Hypertension* 1991;17:8–14.
340. Orlov SN, Petrunyaka VV, Pokudin NI, Kotelevtsev YV, Postnov YV, Kunes J, Zicha J. *J Hypertens* 1991;9:977–982.
341. Polykarpov SA, Orlov SN. *Experientia* 1992;42:489–491.
342. Garay RP, Dagher G, Pernollet MG, Devynck MA, Meyer P. *Nature* 1980;284:281–283.
343. De Mendonca M, Grichois ML, Garay RP, Sassard J, Ben-Ishay D, Meyer P. *Proc Natl Acad Sci USA* 1980;77:4283–4286.
344. Meyer P, Garay R, De Mendonca M: Ion transport system in hypertension. In: Genest J, Kuchel O, Hamet P, Cantin M, eds. *Hypertension, physiopathology and treatment*. New York: McGraw-Hill, 1983;108–116.
345. Bianchi G, Ferrari P, Trizio D, Ferrandi M, Torielli L, Barber BR, Polli E. *Hypertension* 1985;7:319–325.
346. Orlov SN, Pokudin NI, Kotelevtsev YV, Postnov YV. *Kardiologiia* 1988;28(No. 1):57–63.
347. Feig PU, Mitchell PP, Boylan JW. *Hypertension* 1985;7:423–429.
348. Yokomatsu M, Fujito K, Numahata H, Koide H. *Scand J Clin Lab Invest* 1992;52:497–506.
349. Duhm J, Heller J, Zicha J. *Clin Exp Hypertens (A)* 1990;12:1203–1222.
350. Bin Talib HK, Chipperfield AR, Semple PF. *J Hypertens* 1984;2:405–409.
351. Postnov YV, Kravtsov GM, Orlov SN, Pokudin NJ, Postnov IY, Kotelevtsev YV. *Hypertension* 1988;12:267–273.
352. Tokushige A, Kino M, Tamura H, Hopp L, Searle BM, Aviv A. *Hypertension* 1986;8:379–385.
353. Kuriyama S, Denny TN, Aviv A. *J Cardiovasc Pharmacol* 1988;11:722–729.
354. Orlov SN, Resink TJ, Bernhardt J, Buhler FR. *J Hypertens* 1992;10:733–740.
355. O'Donnell ME, Owen NE. *Am J Physiol* 1988;24:C169–C180.
356. Vallega G, Atkinson W, Tsai E, Torielli L, Canessa M. *FASEB J* 1989;3:A1187.
357. Ferrandi M, Salardi S, Parenti P, Ferrari P, Bianchi G, Brawn R, Karlish SJD. *Biochim Biophys Acta* 1990;1021:13–20.
358. Losse H, Wehmeyer H, Zumkley H: The behaviour of the intracellular electrolytes in arterial hypertension. In: Bajusz E, ed. *Electrolytes and cardiovascular diseases*, ed 2. Karger: Basel, 1966;174–197.
359. Ferrari P, Torielli L, Cirillo M, Salardi S, Bianchi G. *J Hypertens* 1991;9:703–711.
360. Garay RP, Azazola A, Nazaret C, Rota R, Diaz AS, Hannaert P, Beaurand Y, Cragol EJ. Depression of K^+, Cl^- cotransportation

erythrocytes and thymocytes from spontaneously hypertensive rats. In: *Abst. 6th International Symposium on SHR,* Iowa, May 22–24, 1989, p. 2.

361. Cusi D, Fossali E, Piazza A, Tripodi G, Barlassina C, Dozzoli E, Vezzoli G, Stella P, Soldati L, Bianchi G. *Am J Hypertens* 1991;4:725–754.

362. Murphy MB, Kohner E, Lewis PJ, Schumer B, Dollery CT. *Lancet* 1982;2:1293–1295.

363. Salvati P, Pingiroli GP, Bianchi G. *J Hypertens* 1987;5:31–38.

364. Cusi D, Niutta E, Barlassina C, Bollini P, Cesano B, Stella P, Robba C, Nerati G, Bianchi G. *J Hypertens* 1993;11:805–813.

365. Orlov SN, Rjazhsky GG, Kravtsov GM, Postnov YV. *Kardiologiia* 1984;24(3):87–94.

366. Gusev GP, Shulski IA, Khrustaleva RS. *Proc Acad Sci USSR* 1987;297:244–247.

367. Shoemaker RL, Worrell RT. *Proc Soc Exp Biol Med* 1991;196:325–332.

368. England SC, Wooldridge TA, Stekiel WJ, Rusch NJ. *Am J Physiol* 1993;264:H1337–H1345.

369. Rusch NJ, De Lucena RW, Wooldridge TA, England SC, Cowley AW Jr. *Hypertension* 1992;19:301–307.

370. Thompson LP, Bruner CA, Lamb FS, King CM, Webb RC. *Am J Cardiol* 1987;59:29A–34A.

371. Khalil RA, Lodge NJ, Saida K, Gelband CH, Van Breeman C: Calcium mobilization in vascular smooth muscle and its relevance to the etiology of hypertension. In: Laragh JH, Brenner BM, eds. *Hypertension: pathophysiology, diagnosis, and management.* New York: Raven Press, 1990;545–564.

372. Hermsmeyer K, Erne P: Vascular muscle electrophysiology and platelet calcium in hypertension. In: Laragh JH, Brenner BM, eds. *Hypertension: pathophysiology, diagnosis, and management.* New York: Raven Press, 1990;661–666.

373. Fleckenstein-Grun G, Frey M, Thimm F, Hofgarther W, Fleckenstein A. *Drugs* 1992;49(Supp 1):23–30.

374. Orlov SN, Pokudin NI, Kravtsov GN, Postnov YV, Okun IM, Shukanova NA, Rakovich AA, Aksentsev SL, Konev SV. *Bull Exp Biol Med (Moscow)* 1987;103:538–540.

375. Kawaguchi H, Sands H, Iizuka K, Okado H, Kudo T, Kageyema K, Muramoto S, Murakami T, Okamoto H, Mochizuki N. *Circ Res* 1993;75:966–972.

376. Orlov SN, Pokudin NI, Postnov YV. *J Hypertens* 1988;6:829–837.

377. Socorro L, Vallega G, Nunn A, Moore TJ, Canessa M. *Hypertension* 1990;83:822–829.

378. Oshima T, Young EW, McCarron DA. *Hypertension* 1991;18:111–115.

379. Orlov SN, Pokudin NI, Postnov YV. *Pflugers Arch* 1983;397:54–56.

380. Postnov YV, Orlov SN, Reznikova MB, Rjazhsky GG, Pokudin NI. *Clin Sci* 1984;66:459–463.

381. Vezzoli G, Elli AA, Tripodi G, Bianchi G, Carafoli E. *J Hypertens* 1985;3:645–648.

382. Olorunsogo DO, Okudolo BE, Lawal SOA, Falase AO. *Biosci Rep* 1985;5:525–531.

383. Spieker C, Pan N, Schluter H, Zidek W. *Clin Exp Hypertens (A)* 1993;15:143–152.

384. Adeoya AS, Norman RI, Bing RF. *Clin Sci* 1989;77:395–400.

385. Resink TJ, Tkachuk VA, Erne P, Buhler FR. *Hypertension* 1986;8:159–166.

386. Pokudin NI, Orlov SN, Postnov YV. *Kardiologiia* 1986;26(4):68–75.

387. Petrunyaka VV, Panyushkina EA, Severina EP, Orlov SN. *Biochim Biophys Acta* 1990;1030:279–288.

388. David-Dufilho M, Astarie C, Pernollet MG, Del Pino M, Levenson J, Simon A, Devynck MA. *Hypertension* 1992;19:167–174.

389. Erne P, Bolli P, Burgisser E, Buhler FR. *N Engl J Med* 1984;310:1084–1088.

390. Orlov SN, Pokudin NI, Postnov YV. *Kardiologiia* 1984;24(10):93–98.

391. Lechi A, Lechi C, Bonadonna G, Sinigaglia D, Corradini P, Polignano R, Arosio E, Covi G, de Togni P, McCarron DA. *Hypertension* 1987;9:230–235.

392. Astarie C, Levenson J, Simon A, Meyer P, Devynch MA. *J Hypertens* 1988;7:455–491.

393. Bruschi G, Bruschi ME, Caroppo M, Orlandini G, Spaggiari M, Cavatorta A. *Clin Sci* 1985;68:179–184.

394. Shkhvatsabaya IK, Kravchenko AN, Avclonin PV, Men'Shikov MY, Nekrasova AA. *Kardiologiia* 1988;28(6):72–77.

395. Tepel M, Wischniowski H, Zidek W. *Life Sci* 1992;51:161–167.

396. Dominiczak AF, Morton JJ, Murray G, Semple PF. *Clin Sci* 1988;77:183.

397. Tepel M, Wischniowski H, Neusser M, Spieker C, Zidek W. *Am J Hypertens* 1993;6:660–666.

398. Oshima T, Matsuura H, Kido K, Matsumoto K, Fujii H, Masaoka S, Okamoto M, Tsuchioka Y, Kajiyama G, Tsubokura T. *Hypertension* 1988;12:26–31.

399. Alexiewicz JM, Gaciong Z, Parise M, Karaubian F, Massry SG, Campese VM. *Am J Hypertens* 1992;5:536–541.

400. Lew PD, Farre L, Walvoge FA, Vallotton M. *Clin Sci* 1985;69:227–230.

401. Morris MJ, Dufilho MD, Devynch MA. *Am J Hypertens* 1992;5:887–891.

402. Baba A, Fukuda K, Hano T, Shiotani M, Yoshikawa H, Ura M, Nakamura Y, Kuchii M, Nishio I, Masuyama Y. *Am J Hypertens* 1990;3:224S–226S.

403. Bruschi G, Bruschi ME, Caroppo M, Orlandi G, Pavarini G, Cavatorta A. *Life Sci* 1984;35:535–542.

404. Furspan PB, Bohr DF. *Hypertension* 1986;8(Suppl II):II123–II126.

405. Battle DC, Tanss G, LaPointe MC, Libre J, Saleh A. *Am J Hypertens* 1990;3:343–348.

406. Sugiyama T, Yoshizumi M, Takaku F, Yazaki Y. *J Hypertens* 1990;8:369–375.

407. Sugiyama T, Yoshizumi M, Takaku F, Urabe H, Tsukakoshi M, Kasuya T, Yazaki Y. *Biochem Biophys Res Commun* 1986;141:340–345.

408. Erne P, Hermsmeyer K. *Hypertension* 1989;14:145–151.

409. Bendhack LM, Sharma RV, Bhalla RC. *Hypertension* 1992;19(Suppl 2):II142–II148.

410. Bruschi G, Bruschi ME, Regolisti G, Borghetti A. *Blood Pressure* 1992;1:231–238.

411. Nabika T, Velletri PA, Beaven MA, Endo J, Lovenberg W. *Life Sci* 1985;37:579–584.

412. Rusch NJ, Hermsmeyer K. *Circ Res* 1988;63:997–1002.

413. Hermsmeyer K, Rusch NJ. *Hypertension* 1989;14:453–456.

414. Orlov S, Resink TJ, Bernhardt J, Ferracin F, Buhler FR. *Hypertension* 1993;21:195–203.

415. Higaki J, Oginara T, Kumahara Y, Bravo EL. *Clin Sci* 1985;68:407–410.

416. Baba A, Fukuda K, Kuchii M, Ura M, Yoshikawa H, Hamada M, Hano T, Nishio I, Masuyama Y. *Jpn Circ J* 1987;51:1216–1222.

417. Hamet P, Tremblay J, Pang SC, Walter SV, Wen YI. *Can J Physiol Pharmacol* 1985;63:380–386.

418. Pokudin NJ, Orlov SN, Ryazhshi GC, Men'shikov M, Tkachuk VA, Postnov YV. *Kardiologiia* 1985;25(1):72–77.

419. Huang SL, Wen YI, Kupranycz DB, Pang SC, Schlager G, Hamet P, Tremblay J. *J Clin Invest* 1988;82:276–281.

420. Chang E, Tremblay J, Hamet P. *J Cardiovasc Pharmacol* 1994;23(Suppl 3):S42–S49.

421. Benishin C, Labedz T, Guo DD, Lewanczuk RZ, Pang PK. *Am J Hypertens* 1993;6:134–140.

422. Hansen HS, Nielsen JR, Hyldebrandt N, Froberg K. *J Hypertens* 1992;10:677–682.

423. Gonick HC, Weiler EWJ, Khalil-Manish F, Weber MA. *Am J Hypertens* 1993;6:680–687.

424. Goldsmith DJA, Tribe RM, Poston L, Cappuccio FP, Markandu ND, MacGregor GA, Hilton PJ. *J Hypertens* 1990;9:645–653.

Hypertension: Pathophysiology, Diagnosis, and Management, Second Edition, edited by J.H. Laragh and B.M. Brenner, Raven Press, Ltd., New York © 1995.

CHAPTER 37

Endothelium and Platelet-Derived Vasoactive Substances: Role in the Regulation of Vascular Tone and Growth

Thomas F. Lüscher and Raghvendra K. Dubey

In the circulation, the endothelium plays a pivotal functional role in maintaining homeostasis in a normal vessel by generating several substances that modulate vascular smooth muscle tone, as well as growth and coagulation and platelet function. Furthermore, the endothelium also acts as a target organ in hypertension and atherosclerosis.

Functional roles of the endothelium in the circulation include (a) prevention of the adherence and activation of circulating blood cells to the vessel wall; (b) production of factors involved in coagulation (e.g., von Willebrand factor VIII, plasminogen activators and inhibitors, i.e., heparan sulfate); (c) capillary transport; (d) modulation of vascular tone by releasing both vasorelaxants (i.e., nitric oxide, prostacyclins, a putative hyperpolarizing factor) and vasoconstrictors (endothelin, angiotensin II, platelet-derived growth factors, epidermal growth factor, histamine); (e) release of growth regulatory substances that can inhibit growth (i.e., heparin, prostacyclins, nitric oxide) or promote growth (i.e., platelet-derived growth factors, epidermal growth factor, endothelin, angiotensin II); and (f) activation (i.e., angiotensin I) and inactivation (i.e., norepinephrine, serotonin, bradykinin, and adenosine diphosphate) of circulating and local hormones.

T. F. Lüscher: Division of Cardiology, Cardiovascular Research, University Hospital, Inselspital, Bern, Switzerland.

R. K. Dubey: Department of Medicine, Division of Clinical Pharmacology and Department of Research, Laboratory of Vascular Research, University Hospital, Basel, Switzerland.

In addition to the endothelium, several cells such as vascular smooth muscle cells as well as blood-borne cells such as platelets, leukocytes, and monocytes are able to form and release local vasoactive substances and vascular mediators (1).

This chapter focuses on the role of endothelium-derived vasoactive substances in the regulation of vascular tone and growth under physiological conditions as well as in hypertension and atherosclerosis.

ENDOTHELIUM-DERIVED VASOACTIVE SUBSTANCES

Endothelial cells can produce and release a variety of vasoactive substances (Fig. 1) (1,2): (a) endothelium-derived relaxing factors (EDRFs), such as nitric oxide (NO), endothelium-derived hyperpolarizing factor, and prostacyclin, as well as other prostaglandins; and (b) endothelium-derived contracting factors (EDCF), in-cluding cyclooxygenase-derived contracting factors, endothelins, and possibly also angiotensin II either produced locally or taken up from the circulation.

Endothelium-Derived Relaxing Substances

Endothelium-Derived Nitric Oxide

Furchgott and Zawadzki (2) demonstrated that in the presence of endothelium, acetylcholine-induced relaxations cannot be prevented by inhibitors of cyclooxygenase, which block the production of prostacyclin, and suggested that a new endothelium-vasodilator substance other than the prostanoid must be involved. Endothelium-dependent relaxations have been demonstrated in large (conduit) arteries and in resistance vessels of most mammalian species including humans (3). EDRF release can occur both *in vitro* and *in vivo* (1–6). The release of EDRF can be demonstrated under basal condi-

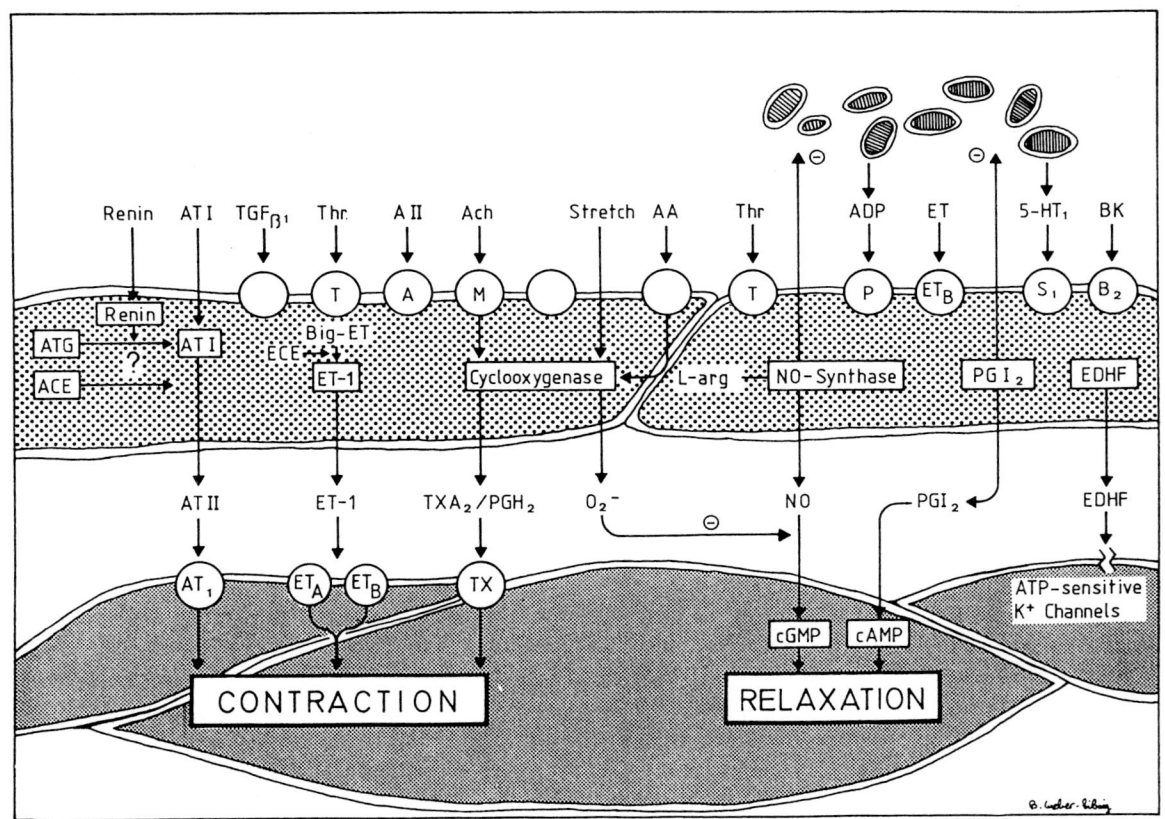

FIG. 1. Endothelium-derived vasoactive substances. The endothelium releases relaxing factors (*right*) and contracting factors (*left*). The relaxing factors include nitric oxide (NO), prostacyclin (PGI₂), and endothelium-derived hyperpolarizing factor (EDHF). NO and PGI₂ not only cause relaxation but also inhibition (Θ) of platelet function. The contracting factors include the local vascular renin-angiotensin (AT) system, endothelin (ET), and cyclooxygenase-derived contracting factor such as thromboxane A₂ (TXA₂) and prostaglandin H₂ (PGH₂). In addition, the cyclooxygenase pathway is a source of oxygen-derived free radicals (O₂⁻). A, angiotensin receptor; AA, arachidonic acid; ADP, adenosine diphosphate; ATG, angiotensinogen; ACE, angiotensin-converting enzyme; Ach, acetylcholine; cAMP, cyclic 3′,5′-adenosine monophosphate; cGMP, cyclic 3′,5′-guanosine monophosphate. (Modified from ref. 1, with permission.)

tions; in response to mechanical forces such as shear stress [exerted by the circulating blood (7,8)]; and after activation of receptor operated mechanisms by acetylcholine, neurotransmitters, various local and circulating hormones, and substances derived from platelets and the coagulation system (see Vascular Effects of Platelet-Derived Products) (Fig. 2) (1–6). EDRF is a diffusible substance with a half-life of a few seconds (2,9), and has now been identified as NO (10–12). Antioxidants such as ascorbic acid, catecholamines, and phenidone inactivate EDRF or NO, demonstrating that the factor is an oxidized substance and that its oxidized state is essential for its biological activity. Bradykinin releases NO from cultured endothelial cells and the relaxations induced by exogenous nitric oxide are indistinguishable from those evoked by EDRF (11). Endothelium-derived nitric oxide (EDNO) has the same chemical characteristics as EDRF (i.e., inactivated by superoxide anions and hemoglobin, and protected by superoxide dismutase, a free radical

scavenger) and is liberated in amounts sufficient to account for the vascular action of EDRF (11).

Vasodilator effects of NO are associated with an increase in intracellular cyclic 3′,5′-guanosine monophosphate (cGMP) in vascular smooth muscle (Fig. 2) (12). The inhibitor of soluble guanylyl cyclase, methylene blue, prevents the production of cGMP and inhibits endothelium-dependent relaxations (13,14). Thus, EDNO causes relaxations by stimulating the enzyme and in turn the formation of cGMP. Soluble guanylyl cyclase is also present in platelets and activated by EDNO (Fig. 2) (15–17). Increased levels of cGMP in platelets are associated with a reduced adhesion and aggregation. Therefore, EDNO causes both vasodilation and platelet deactivation and thereby represents an important antispastic and antithrombotic feature of the endothelium.

EDNO is formed from L-arginine by oxidation of the guanidine-nitrogen terminal of L-arginine (Fig. 2) (14). NO synthase has recently been cloned (18); it is primarily

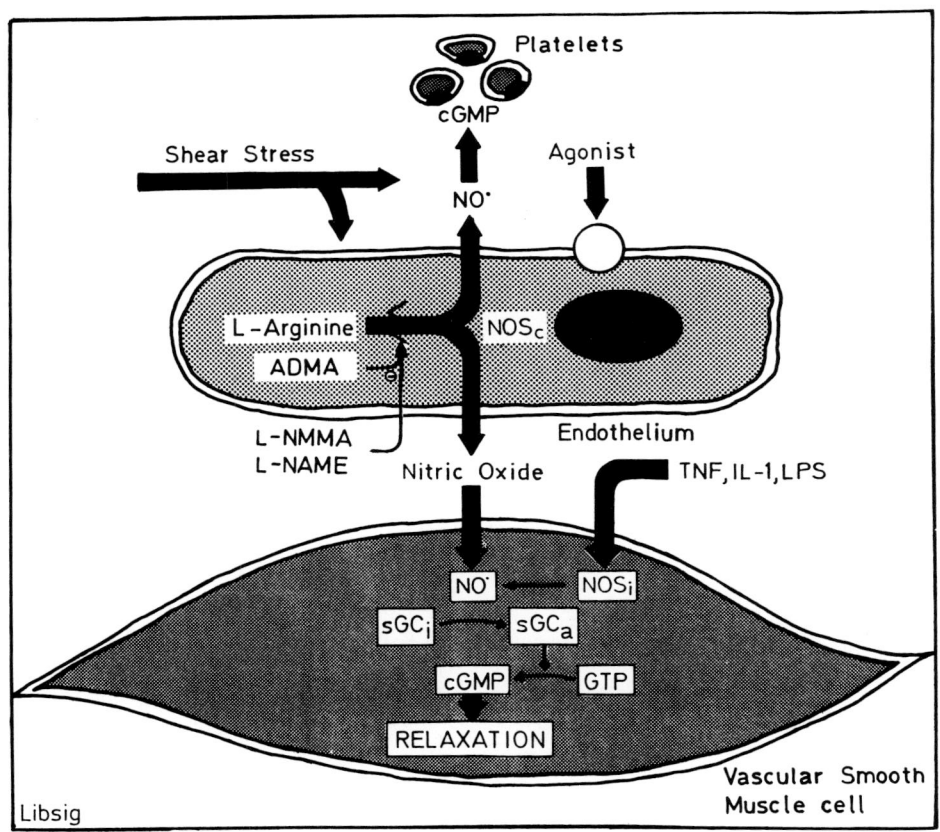

FIG. 2. The L-arginine pathway in the blood vessel wall. Endothelial cells form nitric oxide (NO) from L-arginine via the activity of the constitutive nitric oxide synthase (NOS$_c$), which can be inhibited by analogues of the amino acid such as isometrical dymethyl arginine (ADMA), L-N^G-monomethyl arginine (L-NMMA), or L-nitroarginine methylester (L-NAME). Nitric oxide activates soluble guanylyl cyclase (sGC) in vascular smooth muscle and platelets, and it causes increases in cyclic 3′,5′-guanosine monophosphate (cGMP), which mediates relaxation and platelet inhibition, respectively. Shear stress and receptor-operated agonists stimulate the release of NO. In addition, vascular smooth muscle cells can form NO via the activity of an inducible [by tumor necrosis factor (TNF), interleukin-1 (IL-1), and lipopolysaccharide (LPS)] form of nitric oxide synthase (NOS$_i$). (Modified from ref. 140, with permission.)

a cytosolic enzyme requiring calmodulin, Ca^{2+}, and β-nicotinamide adenine dinucleotide hydrogen phosphate (NADPH) and has similarities with cytochrome P-450 enzymes. Several isoforms of the enzyme occur not only in endothelial cells, but also in platelets (19), macrophages (20), vascular smooth muscle cells (21–23), and the brain (24).

In porcine coronary arteries, endothelium-dependent relaxations to serotonin are inhibited by analogues of L-arginine such as L-N^G-monomethyl arginine (L-NMMA) and are restored by L-arginine, but not D-arginine (25). In quiescent arteries, L-NMMA causes endothelium-dependent contractions (26,27). In intact organs such as the perfused porcine eye, L-nitro arginine methylester (L-NAME) markedly decreases local blood flow (Fig. 3) (28). When infused in rabbits, L-NMMA induces long-lasting increases in blood pressure that are reversed by L-arginine (Fig. 4) (29). This demonstrates that the vasculature is in a constant state of vasodilation because of the continuous basal release of NO from the endothelium. Of particular physiological and pathophysiological interest is the more recent discovery of an endogenous inhibitor of the L-arginine nitric oxide pathway, i.e., asymmetrical dimethyl-arginine (ADMA) (30). This indicates that endogenously produced substances can regulate the activity of this pathway both locally and systematically as it is also detected in plasma. Hence, an increased production and/or elimination of this endogenous inhibitor can profoundly affect the function of the cardiovascular system, for instance in patients with renal failure (30).

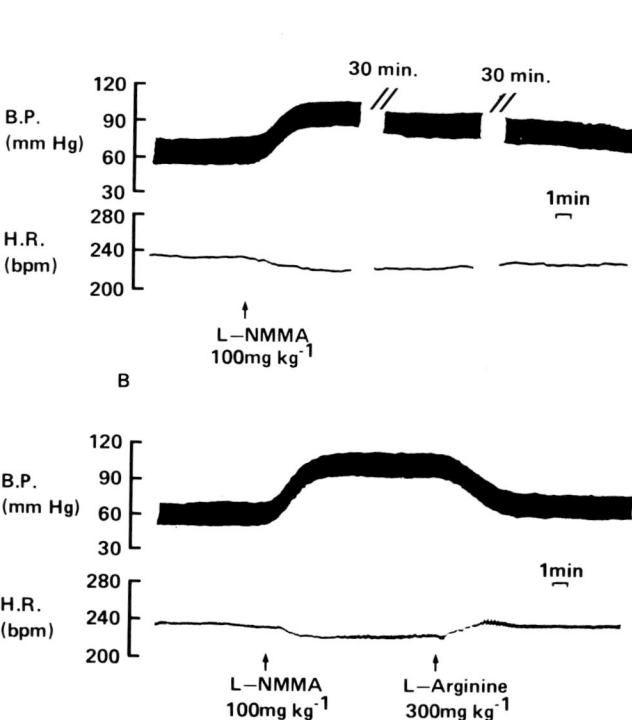

FIG. 4. Effects of intravenous infusion of L-N^G-monomethyl arginine (L-NMMA) on blood pressure (BP) and heart rate (HR) in the intact rabbit. Infusion of L-NMMA causes a marked increase in systolic and diastolic blood pressure and a decrease in heart rate (**A**). This effect can be reversed by high dosages of L-arginine, which competes with L-NAME for the enzyme (**B**). (From ref. 29, with permission.)

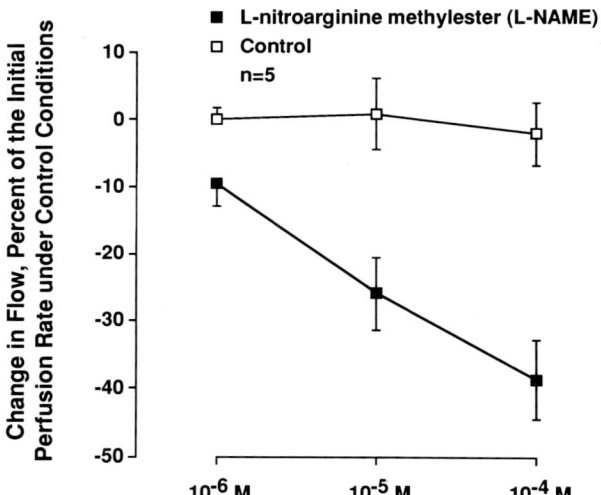

FIG. 3. Effects of the inhibitor of NO production L-nitro arginine methylester (L-NAME) on ophthalmic flow in the intact perfused porcine eye. While flow in the time control remains constant, L-NAME causes a concentration-dependent potent inhibition of ophthalmic flow indicating that the ophthalmic circulation is in a constant state of vasodilation due to the basal formation of NO. (From ref. 28, with permission.)

Endothelium-Derived Hyperpolarizing Factors

In the porcine coronary circulation, L-NMMA inhibits the relaxations to serotonin, but only slightly those to bradykinin (25). As similar effects are obtained by other inhibitors of the action of EDNO such as hemoglobin and methylene blue, endothelial cells appear to release a relaxing factor distinct from NO (31). Since prostacyclin is a weak vasodilator of porcine coronary arteries and indomethacin does not affect the response to bradykinin (25), prostacyclin can be excluded.

Acetylcholine causes not only an endothelium-dependent relaxation, but also an endothelium-dependent hyperpolarization of vascular smooth muscle (32). Whereas the relaxation to the muscarinic agonist is sustained, the hyperpolarization is transient. An endothelium-derived hyperpolarizing factor (EDHF) (Fig. 1) distinct from NO could explain these responses, although the latter was shown to have hyperpolarizing properties under certain conditions (33). The EDHF appears to activate adenosine triphosphate (ATP)-sensitive K^+ channels (34) and/or Na^+, K^+–adenosine triphosphatase (ATPase) in smooth muscle (32). Several candidates for these non–NO-mediated endothelium-dependent responses have been proposed including a putative hyperpolarizing factor (EDHF), products of lipooxygenase, or the cytochrome P-450 pathway.

Prostacyclin

Prostacyclin is the major product of vascular cyclooxygenase pathway in the blood vessel wall, whereas that of platelets is thromboxane A_2 (Fig. 1) (35). Although endothelial cells are an important source of prostacyclin, it is primarily formed in the intima, but also in the media and adventitia in response to shear stress, hypoxia, and several mediators leading also to the formation of EDNO. However, in most blood vessels, the contribution of prostacyclin to endothelium-dependent relaxations is negligible (25,27). Prostacyclin causes relaxation by increasing cyclic 3',5'-adenosine monophosphate (cAMP) in smooth muscle and platelets (35), where it also inhibits platelet aggregation. In human

platelets EDNO and prostacyclin synergistically inhibit platelet aggregation (15).

Most substances evoking endothelium-dependent relaxation, such as acetylcholine, calcium ionophore A23187, thrombin, and histamine, also release prostacyclin and other prostanoids from endothelial cells (1).

Endothelium-Derived Contracting Substances

Cyclooxygenase-Dependent Endothelium-Derived Contracting Factor (EDCF)

Exogenous arachidonic acid can evoke endothelium-dependent contractions prevented by indomethacin (an inhibitor of cyclooxygenase) (36,37). In the human saphenous vein, acetylcholine and histamine evoke endothelium-dependent contractions; in the presence of indomethacin, however, endothelium-dependent relaxations are unmasked (27). The products of cyclooxygenase mediating the contractions are thromboxane A_2, in the case of acetylcholine, and endoperoxides (prostaglan-

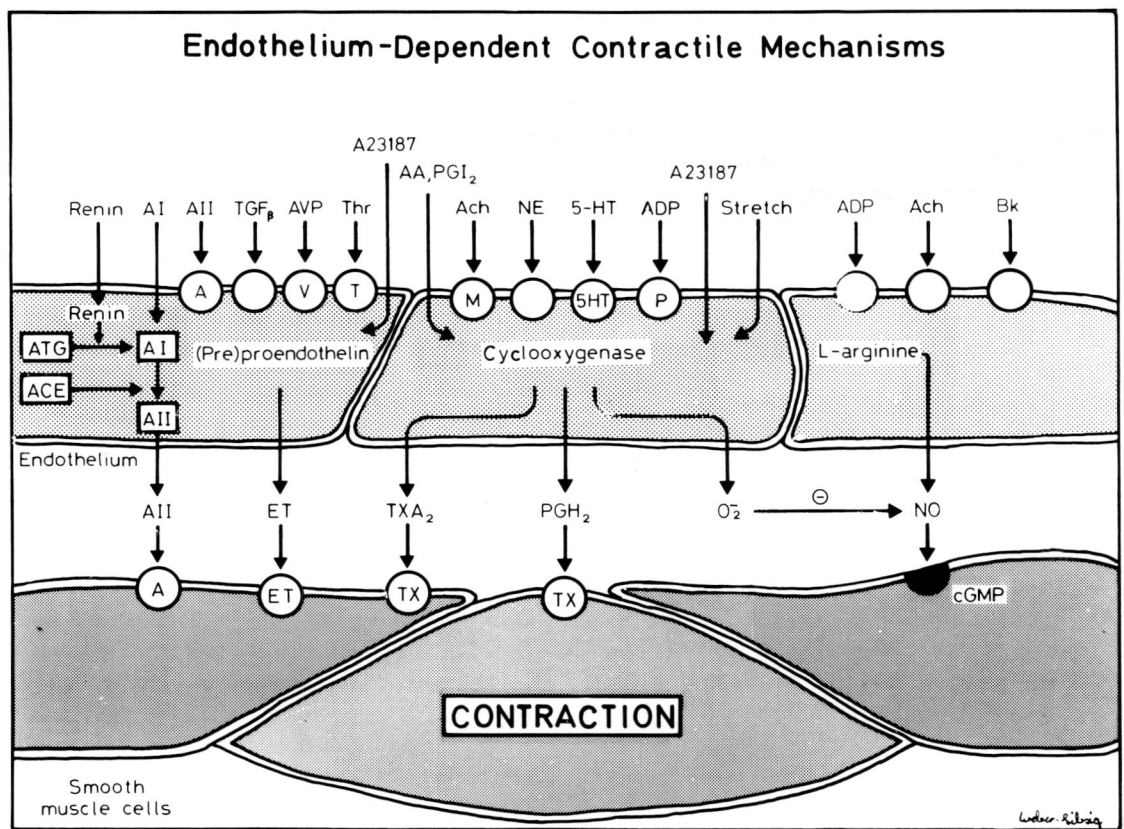

FIG. 5. Endothelium-derived contracting factors. Endothelial cells are a source of numerous substances causing contraction of the underlying smooth muscle. AII, angiotensin II; ATG, angiotensinogen; ACE, angiotensin-converting enzyme; ET, endothelin; NO, nitric oxide; TXA$_2$, thromboxane A$_2$; PGH$_2$ prostaglandin H$_2$; O$_2^-$, superoxide. *Open symbols* represent receptors. (From ref. 41, with permission of the American Heart Association.)

din H$_2$) in that of histamine (27). Thromboxane A$_2$ and endoperoxide activate both vascular smooth muscle and platelets and hence counteract the protective effects of NO and prostacyclin in the blood vessel wall.

Furthermore, the cyclooxygenase pathway is a source of superoxide anions, which can mediate endothelium-dependent contractions either by the breakdown of NO or direct effects on vascular smooth muscle (38,39). Thus, the cyclooxygenase pathway produces a variety of endothelium-derived contracting factors; their release appears particularly prominent in veins and in the cerebral and ophthalmic circulation (Fig. 5) (1).

Endothelin

Endothelial cells produce the 21 amino acid peptide endothelin (Fig. 5) (40,41). Among the three peptides (endothelin-1, endothelin-2, and endothelin-3), endothelial cells appear to produce exclusively endothelin-1.

Translation of messenger RNA generates prepro endothelin, which is converted to big endothelin; its conversion to endothelin-1 by the endothelin-converting enzyme is necessary for the development of full vascular activity (40,41). The expression of messenger RNA and the release of the peptide is stimulated by thrombin, transforming growth factor-β, interleukin-1, epinephrine, angiotensin II, arginine vasopressin, calcium ionophore, and phorbolester (Fig. 6) (40–44). In addition, hypoxia has been shown to stimulate the release of endothelin in isolated vessels (45), as well as in healthy mountaineers at high altitude (46).

Endothelin-1 is a potent vasoconstrictor both *in vitro* and *in vivo* (40,47–50). In the coronary and ophthalmic circulation and the human forearm endothelin causes vasodilation at lower and marked contractions at higher concentrations (28,50,51), which in the heart eventually leads to ischemia, arrhythmias, and death. Also, in human arterial and venous coronary bypass vessels, endothelin causes marked contractions (47).

However, the circulating levels of endothelin-1 are very low, suggesting that little of the peptide is formed under physiological conditions because of the absence of stimuli and/or the presence of potent inhibitory mechanisms or that it is released preferentially toward smooth muscle cells (Fig. 7) (41,52,53). Indeed, three inhibitory mechanisms regulating endothelin production have been delineated: (a) cGMP-dependent inhibition (42,54), (b) cAMP-dependent inhibition (55), and (c) an inhibitory factor produced by vascular smooth muscle cells (53). The cGMP-dependent mechanism can be activated by EDNO, nitroglycerine, 3-morpholino sydnominine (SIN-1) (42,43), and atrial natriuretic peptide, which activates particulate guanylyl cyclase (1,54). Thus, after inhibition of the endothelial L-arginine pathway, the

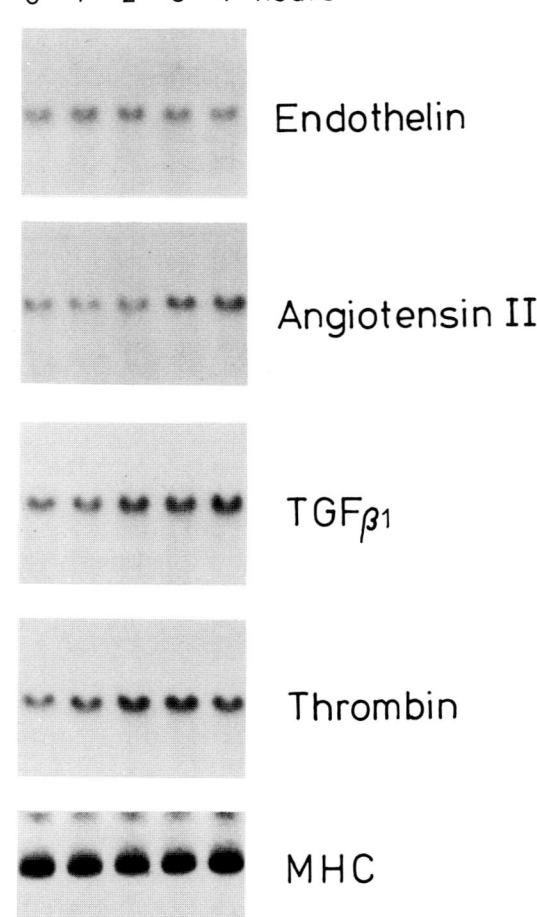

0 1 2 3 4 hours

Endothelin

Angiotensin II

TGFβ1

Thrombin

MHC

FIG. 6. Endothelin gene expression in porcine aortic endothelial cells in culture. While endothelin itself does not increase prepro–messenger RNA (as assessed by cDNA probe), angiotensin II, transforming growth factor β-1, endothelin-1, as well as thrombin, all increase endothelin expression after 1 to 4 hours of stimulation. MHC, control experiments using major histocompatibility complex. (Modified from ref. 44, with permission of the American Heart Association.)

thrombin-induced production of endothelin is augmented (42); on the other hand, SIN-1 prevents the thrombin-induced endothelin release via a cGMP-dependent mechanism (43). Endothelin can also release NO and prostacyclin from endothelial cells, which may represent a negative feedback mechanism (48,56). EDNO also interacts with the effects of endothelin at the level of vascular smooth muscle. Indeed, the contractions to the peptide are enhanced after endothelial removal, indicating that basal production of EDNO reduces its response (47). Stimulation of the formation of EDNO by acetylcholine reverses endothelin-induced contractions in most blood vessels, although this mechanism appears to be less potent in veins (47,57).

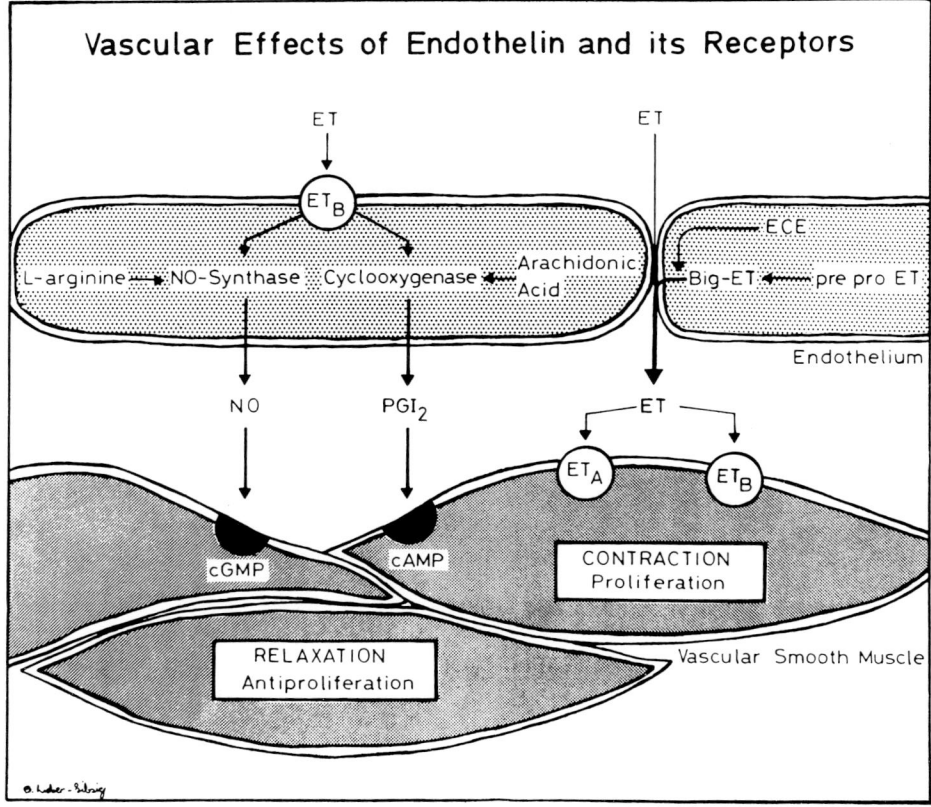

FIG 7. Vascular effects of endothelin and its receptors. Endothelin (ET) is produced from preproendothelin, big endothelin, via the activity of endothelin-converting enzyme (ECE) to its final product, the 21–amino acid peptide ET. Endothelin is mainly released abluminally toward vascular smooth muscle where it interacts with ET_A- and ET_B-receptors mediating contractions and proliferation. In addition, endothelin can interact with endothelial receptors (ET_B-receptors) linked to the formation of nitric oxide (NO) and prostacyclin (PGI$_2$). The latter substances cause relaxation and antiproliferation via cGMP and cAMP, respectively.

Two distinct endothelin receptors have been cloned, the ET_A- and ET_B-receptor (Fig. 7) (58–60). Endothelial cells express ET_B-receptors linked to the formation of NO and prostacyclin, which may explain the transient vasodilator effects of endothelin when infused in intact organs or organisms. In vascular smooth muscle ET_A- and in part ET_B-receptors are mediating contraction and proliferation. ET_B-receptors equally bind endothelin-1 and endothelin-3, whereas ET_A-receptors preferentially bind endothelin-1. Several endothelin receptor antagonists have been developed. Most substances are specific ET_A-receptor antagonists, whereas more recently developed molecules also possess combined ET_A- and ET_B-receptor antagonism (28,61–63). In various vascular preparations, the vasoconstrictor effects of endothelin can be potently inhibited by these newly developed molecules. Furthermore, the fact that these antagonists do lower blood pressure under certain conditions suggests that endothelin may contribute to blood pressure regulation (64,65).

Angiotensin

Angiotensin II is a vasoactive octapeptide formed from its inactive decapeptide precursor, angiotensin I, by the action of a dipeptidyl carboxypeptidase known as angiotensin-converting enzyme (ACE), which is also present in the vascular endothelial cells (Fig. 1) (66,67). Angiotensin I is derived from the cleavage of angiotensinogen by renin and all major components required for the synthesis of angiotensin II are present in vascular tissue (66–68). A local angiotensin II synthesis in the vascular wall is of special interest in view of the multiple vascular actions of angiotensin II. Angiotensin II not only exerts a direct vasoconstrictor effect but also enhances sympathetic noradrenergic transmission (69) and exhibits mitogenic and trophic actions in the vasculature (70,71). Angiotensin is now also known to induce the synthesis of endothelin (72). The observations that infusion of angiotensin II raises blood pressure (73) and angiotensin receptor density increases at sites of intimal thickening (74), together with the finding that inhibitors of ACE can prevent both the rise in blood pressure (71) as well as the hyperplastic growth of the vascular smooth muscle, suggest that vascular or endothelial ACE activity may play an important role in regulating normal vascular function.

Histamine

Rat blood cells can synthesize histamine, and this synthesis increases with increasing shear stress or blood pressure (1). Bovine aortic endothelial cells contain histidine decarboxylase. *In vitro*, the capacity of these cells to form histamine is much greater than that of the media. Locally synthesized histamine, by activating H_2-histaminergic receptors, may cause direct vasoconstriction or induce endothelium-dependent relaxations by activating H_1-histaminergic receptors on the endothelium. In some blood vessels, H_2-histaminergic receptors on vascular

smooth muscle cells can also mediate relaxation. The vascular distribution of inhibitory and excitatory histaminergic receptors determines the physiological response.

VASCULAR EFFECTS OF PLATELET-DERIVED PRODUCTS

Platelets

The most important blood cells releasing vasoactive substances are platelets. Platelets release a variety of substances such as adenine nucleotides (ATP/ADP), serotonin, and thromboxane A_2, and are also able to form nitric oxide (Fig. 8) (3,5,19,75). Once released, platelet-derived substances can interact with the endothelium and vascular smooth muscle cells of the blood vessel wall. At the level of the endothelium, ATP/ADP and, at least in certain arteries, serotonin can activate P_2-

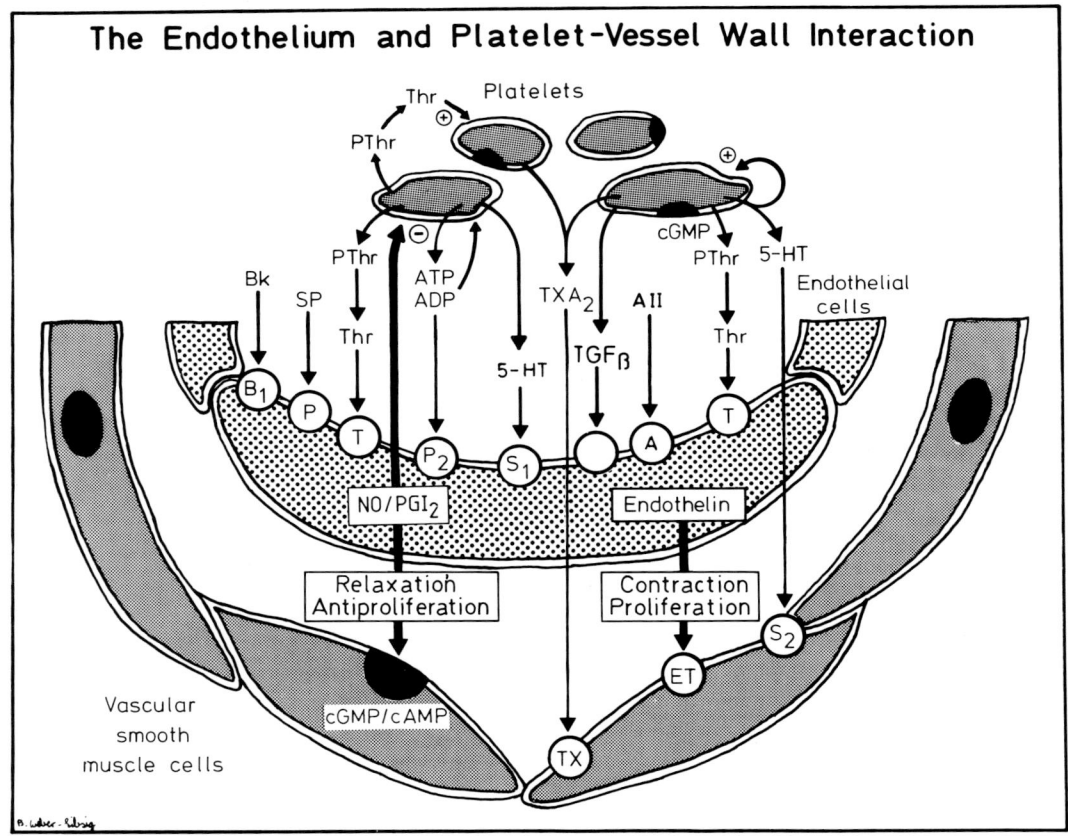

FIG. 8. Endothelium-dependent effects of platelet-derived products. Activated or aggregating platelets may release the following: adenosine diphosphate (ADP) or adenosine triphosphate (ATP), serotonin (5-HT), platelet-activating factor (PAF), or vasopressin (VP). At sites where platelets are activated, thrombin (Thr) is also formed. All these substances may activate specific receptors on endothelial cells, thereby releasing endothelium-derived nitric oxide and prostacyclin (PGI_2). NO and PGI_2 both cause vascular relaxation and inhibition of platelet aggregation ($\ominus$). The effects of NO are mediated by cGMP, and those of PGI_2 are mediated by cAMP. At sites of a dysfunctional or absent endothelial layer, platelet-derived substances may cause contraction.

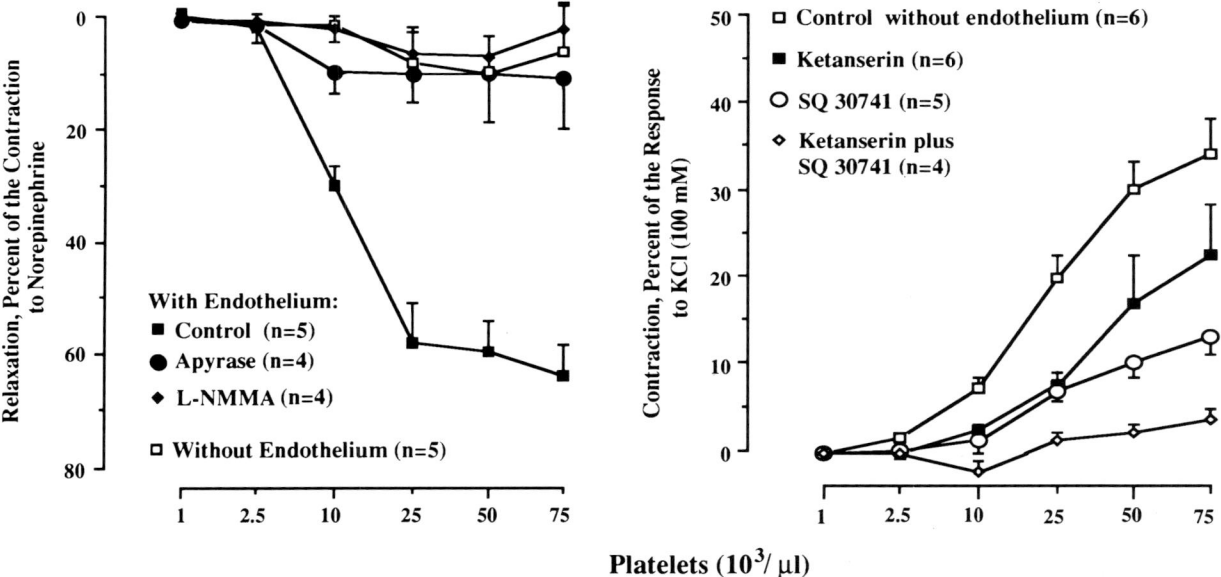

FIG. 9. Effects of aggregating platelets on norepinephrine-induced contraction of isolated human internal mammary artery with or without endothelium. In rings contracted with norepinephrine, aggregating platelets cause endothelium-dependent relaxations prevented by L-N^G-monomethyl arginine (L-NMMA, to inhibit NO formation) or apyrase (to break down ATP and ADP; *left panel*). In quiescent rings without endothelium, platelets cause contractions that are reduced by the 5-HT$_2$-serotonergic antagonist ketanserin and the thromboxane receptor antagonist SQ30741 (*right panel*). Only the combination of both receptor antagonists prevents platelet-induced vasoconstriction. (Modified from ref. 5, with permission.)

purinergic and 5-HT$_1$-serotonergic receptors, respectively. Both receptors, if present, are linked to the release of nitric oxide. Hence, in intact blood vessels aggregating platelets cause endothelium-dependent relaxations (Fig. 9) (3,5,75) even though they release potent vasoconstrictors such as thromboxane A$_2$ and serotonin. On the other hand, in the absence of functional endothelial cells, aggregating platelets can cause profound vasoconstriction, which is mediated through activation of thromboxane and 5-HT$_2$-serotonergic receptors on vascular smooth muscle (Fig. 9) (5). Additionally, platelets have been shown to stimulate the release of endothelin from cultured porcine endothelial cells; in contrast, the release of endothelin from intact aorta is decreased in response to platelets, presumably due to the release of an inhibitory factor from vascular smooth muscle (76).

Thrombin

Thrombin can act as a vasoactive factor both directly or by modulating the effects of other vasoactive factors, particularly those released from platelets (Fig. 8). In isolated vessels with intact endothelium, thrombin induces vasorelaxation through the generation of both NO and prostacyclin; this in turn also prevents platelet activation. On the other hand, in vessels denuded of endothelium thrombin induces profound platelet activation, and in turn the release of thromboxane A$_2$, which causes

marked contraction and further platelet activation (Figs. 8 and 9) (77).

White Blood Cells

Several white blood cells such as leukocytes and monocytes/macrophages are able to produce NO, particularly if stimulated with cytokines and other substances as they express the inducible form of NO synthase (16,78,79). The capacity of these cells to produce large amounts of NO if appropriately stimulated may contribute to local inflammatory responses of the microcirculation (in particular to the increased local tissue blood flow) as well as exerting a toxic effect important for immune responses.

ENDOTHELIUM-DEPENDENT RESPONSES IN HYPERTENSION

Hypertension is associated with morphological and functional alterations of the endothelium (1). In hypertensive blood vessels, endothelial cells have an increased volume and bulge into the lumen, and the subintimal space exhibits structural changes with increased fibrin and cell disposition. Furthermore, the interaction of platelets and monocytes with the endothelium is increased as compared with normotensive controls.

Endothelium-Dependent Relaxations

Endothelium-dependent relaxations to acetylcholine are reduced in the aorta and in the cerebral and peripheral microcirculation of hypertensive rats (80–86). Similarly, the vasodilator effects of acetylcholine in the human forearm of hypertensive subjects is blunted (Fig. 10) (87–90). On the other hand, not all the patients with hypertension appear to have endothelium dysfunction, at least not in the forearm circulation (91). In the coronary circulation, impaired vasodilator responses occur both in epicardial and microvessels of hypertensive patients, in particular in the presence of left ventricular hypertrophy (92–94).

In experimental animals, the degree of impairment of endothelium-dependent responses is positively correlated with the level of blood pressure and seems to become more pronounced as hypertension develops and with increased duration of hypertension (95). This suggests that most if not all of the dysfunction of the endothelium occurring in hypertension is a consequence rather than a cause of hypertension. This could also explain why the degree of activation differs in different studies, or may even be absent in early and/or mild hypertension. More recent data, however, demonstrated that even in pedigrees of hypertensive parents, endothelium-dependent vasodilation in the human forearm circulation may be impaired in the presence of normal blood pressure (96). Because under most circumstances the response to the direct vasodilator sodium nitroprusside remains preserved, impaired responses to acetylcholine must be related to alterations in endothelial function.

Possible Mechanisms of Impaired Endothelium-Dependent Responses in Hypertension

Endothelium-dependent responses of hypertensive arteries could be impaired as a result of (a) a decreased release of EDNO, (b) a decreased release of other endothelium-derived vasodilator substances such as EDHF or prostacyclin, (c) an impaired diffusion of these substances from the endothelium to the vascular smooth muscle cells, (d) a decreased responsiveness of the vascular smooth muscle cells to vasodilator substances, and/or (e) an augmented release of endothelium-derived contracting factors (Fig. 11).

Formation of Nitric Oxide

The basal formation of NO (as assessed by the contractile effects of inhibitors of NO production) is reduced in established but not early hypertension of spontaneously hypertensive rats (SHR), renovascular hypertensive rats, and ren-2 transgenic rats (97–99). Indeed, in the mesenteric resistance circulation, L-NMMA increases vasoconstrictor responses to norepinephrine more in Wistar-Kyoto (WKY) rats than in the SHR (97). In ren-2 transgenic rats, endothelium-dependent contractions to L-NAME become markedly blunted as duration of hypertension increases (99). Similarly, in patients with essential hypertension, infusion of L-NMMA into the brachial artery causes less vasoconstriction (or decreases in forearm blood flow) in hypertensives as compared with normotensives, although the response to phenylephrine is comparable (100). This suggests that the basal forma-

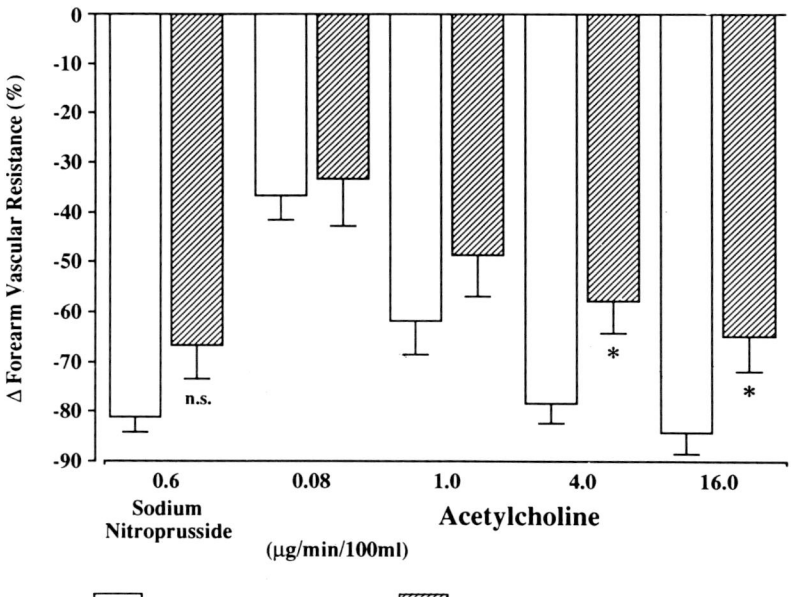

FIG. 10. Endothelium-dependent vasodilation to acetylcholine in the forearm circulation of normotensive and hypertensive subjects. The vasodilator effects of acetylcholine are significantly blunted in hypertensives. (Modified from ref. 87, with permission of the American Heart Association.)

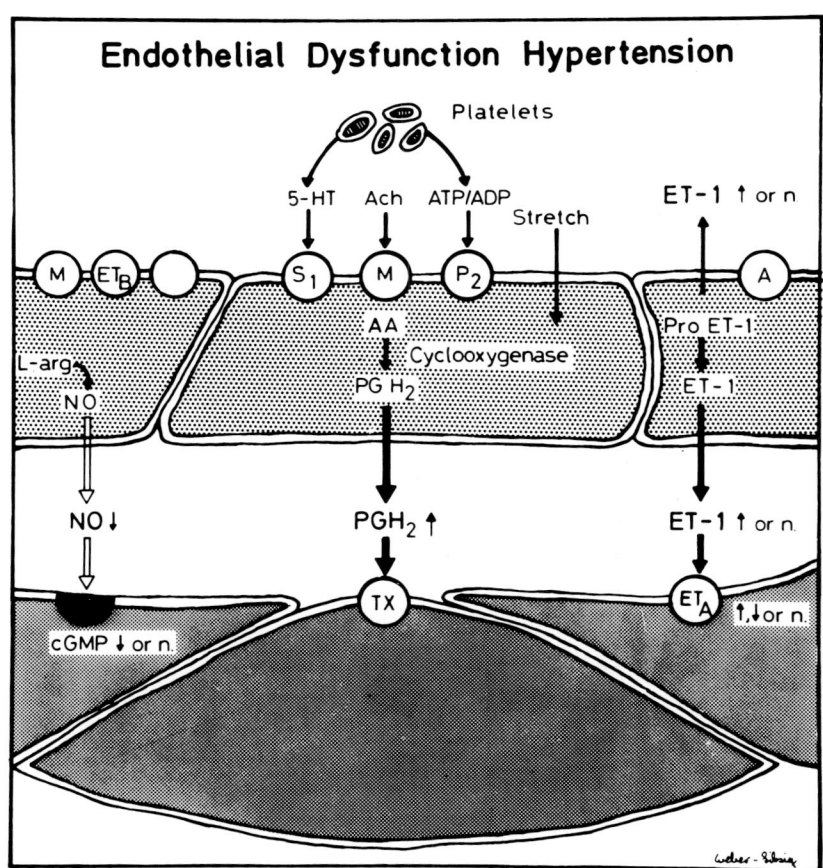

FIG. 11. Endothelial dysfunction in hypertension. In hypertension, the basal formation of NO appears to be reduced under most conditions, whereas the stimulated formation of NO appears to be impaired in more advanced hypertension. In addition, the hypertensive endothelium can form cyclooxygenase-derived contracting factor [prostaglandin H₂ (PGH₂)]. The effects of endothelin (ET-1) in hypertension are controversial. Increased, but mostly normal, circulating levels have been reported. The vascular responsiveness to endothelin can be reduced, normal, or increased. The concomitant reduced formation and responsiveness of vascular smooth muscle to endothelium-derived nitric oxide (NO) leads to an imbalance between NO and endothelium-derived contracting factors (EDCF), which may contribute to the increased peripheral vascular resistance and complications of hypertension. 5-HT, serotonin; Ach, acetylcholine; L-arg, L-arginine; AA, arachidonic acid. (From ref. 41, with permission of the American Heart Association.)

tion of NO is also reduced in patients with essential hypertension.

In an attempt to restore reduced endothelium-dependent vasodilation in patients with essential hypertension, Panza et al. (101) infused L-arginine, which augmented the vasodilation response to acetylcholine in normal subjects, whereas the responses to acetylcholine remained unchanged in subjects with essential hypertension. Ineffectiveness of L-arginine in improving endothelium-dependent vasodilation in hypertensive subjects could involve (a) reduced expression of muscarinic receptors (and possibly other endothelial receptors linked to the L-arginine/NO pathway), (b) impaired signal transduction, (c) an altered uptake mechanism of L-arginine into the endothelium, and/or (d) impaired activity of NO synthase. The possibility of a reduced responsiveness of hypertensive vascular smooth muscle to NO can be excluded, because the response to sodium nitroprusside was identical in normotensive and hypertensive subjects (101). Quite a different explanation may also involve the possibility that an endothelium-derived contracting factor is formed in hypertensive patients as suggested by experimental work (41,83; see Endothelin, below). This has recently also been observed in hypertensive patients in whom acute treatment with a cyclooxygenase inhibitor

such as indomethacin improved endothelium-dependent vasodilation to acetylcholine (90) (see below). However, since inhibition of cyclooxygenase-derived contracting factor (most likely prostaglandin H₂) does not normalize endothelium-dependent vasodilation in hypertensive subjects, this strongly suggests an additional defect, which may in fact involve the L-arginine pathway as discussed above.

In perfused mesenteric resistance arteries of the SHR, endothelium-dependent relaxations are reduced upon intraluminal but not extraluminal application of acetylcholine (97). This suggests that the intraluminal side of the endothelium, which is most exposed to blood pressure, is particularly prone to develop endothelial dysfunction.

However, not all hypertensive blood vessels and not all forms of hypertension are exhibiting alterations of the L-arginine/NO pathway. Indeed, in the coronary circulation of the SHR, very little endothelial dysfunction can be observed except in very old rats (102). Similarly, in the aorta of these animals, endothelium-dependent relaxations are normal in the presence of indomethacin (83) to prevent the formation of vasoconstrictor cyclooxygenase products (35). Also, bioassay experiments using the perfused SHR aorta revealed comparable amounts of biologically active NO (103). Bioassay experiments indicate that at least in SHR luminal release of EDRF and prostacyclin induced by acetylcholine and histamine is normal or slightly increased (103, 104). Hence, under certain conditions, the pathway may be augmented, presumably as a counterregulatory mechanism.

Endothelin

Commonly the circulating levels of endothelin are not increased in experimental or human hypertension (41). This suggests that at least the abluminal release of the peptide into the circulation is unaltered except in the presence of vascular disease, atherosclerosis, or renal failure. However, as more than twice as much endothelin is released abluminally (52) by endothelial cells rather than luminally, measurement of circulating endothelin-levels may not be appropriate to determine local vascular endothelin production. Indeed, in deoxycorticosterone acetate (DOCA)-salt hypertensive rats, an increased production of endothelin in mesenteric resistance arteries can be demonstrated even in the presence of normal circulating levels of the peptide (105). In contrast, in the same preparations obtained from SHR no increased endothelin production can be seen (105).

The vascular responses to endothelin differ depending on the experimental conditions, the model of hypertension studied, and the vascular bed utilized for the experiments (41). Increased, normal, and reduced pressor responses have been reported. No data are available so far as to the responses to endothelin in hypertensive patients.

However, it remains questionable whether pharmacological experiments studying the responses to endothelin at rather high concentrations have any physiological or pathophysiological meaning. Indeed, in most of these experiments, concentrations of the peptide are much higher than those found in plasma under most conditions. Hence, the indirect amplifying effects of endothelin occurring at very low concentrations might be more important. It is therefore of interest that, in contrast to the direct responses to endothelin, the potentiating properties of low and threshold concentrations of endothelin are increased with aging and hypertension (44,106–108), indicating that this indirect amplifying effect of endothelin may contribute to an increased vascular contractility as pressure rises and the blood vessel wall ages. This aspect may be of particular importance, as the circulating levels of endothelin remain quite low in hypertension (for review, see ref. 41), indicating a low production rate of the peptide in the blood vessel wall.

Endothelium-Dependent Contractions

Although it is commonly assumed that impaired endothelium-dependent relaxations or vasodilations, respectively, are primarily related to a reduced formation or release of NO, at least under certain conditions this may also be caused by an increased production of endothelium-derived contracting factors (Fig. 12) (41). Indeed, in the SHR the reduced response to acetylcholine in the aorta is related to the production of a cyclooxygenase-dependent endothelium-derived contracting factor (i.e., prostaglandin H_2) (83,84). Indeed, blockade of endothelium-dependent contractions by inhibitors to

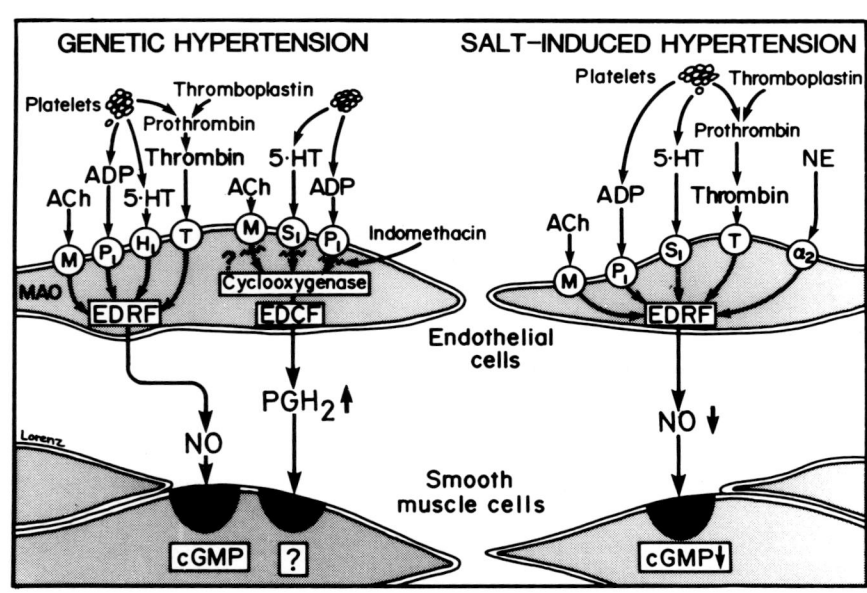

FIG. 12. Proposed mechanisms of altered endothelium-dependent relaxations in genetic (spontaneous) and salt-induced hypertension of the rat. In spontaneously hypertensive rats (left), endothelium-dependent relaxations are decreased because of a concomitant release of endothelium-derived nitric oxide and constricting factors (i.e. prostaglandin H_2, PGH_2). In salt-induced hypertension (right), a reduced vascular responsiveness to NO—and possibly decreased transit of NO—appears to be involved. (From ref. 1, with permission.)

cyclooxygenase or antagonist of the thromboxane receptor normalize endothelium-dependent relaxations to acetylcholine in these animals (83). Similar results were obtained in the cerebral and coronary microcirculation of the SHR with ADP/ATP or serotonin as agonists (85,86,109). Interestingly, also in the human forearm circulation, the impaired vasodilation to acetylcholine is improved (although not normalized) by pretreatment with indomethacin (a cyclooxygenase inhibitor) in patients with essential hypertension (90). This suggests that an increased production of prostaglandin H_2 or another cyclooxygenase-derived contracting factor also contributes to impaired endothelium-dependent vascular regulation in human hypertension. The fact that, at least in the rat, platelets and platelet-derived products (i.e., ADP/ATP, serotonin) are able to stimulate the formation of this contracting factor (84) strongly suggests that this form of endothelial dysfunction may contribute not only to the increased peripheral vascular resistance, but also to the complications of hypertension.

Impaired Response of Vascular Smooth Muscle Cell to Nitric Oxide

In contrast to the SHR, the Dahl rat aorta does not release a cyclooxygenase-dependent EDCF in response to acetylcholine, since indomethacin has no effect on the response to the muscarinic agonist (Figs. 11 and 12) (110). Thus, it is likely that in this model, as in the aorta of DOCA-salt and renal hypertensive rats, a reduced responsiveness of the vascular smooth muscle to NO and possibly also an impaired diffusion of the factor from the endothelium to the vascular smooth muscle cells (due to extensive subendothelial thickening) is responsible for the blunted endothelium-dependent relaxations (1) (Fig. 12).

To judge from experiments with sodium nitroprusside, which also induces relaxations by increasing cGMP (111), the responsiveness of vascular smooth muscle cells to NO is normal in small mesenteric arteries of the SHR, but is slightly impaired in the aorta of these rats (81,82). Van de Voorde and Leusen (104) found normal relaxations to sodium nitroprusside in the aorta of DOCA-salt and renal hypertensive rats. This contrasts with findings of others in these forms of hypertension and in hypertensive Dahl rats where the relaxations to nitrovasodilators were found to be impaired (81,110). However, the relaxations were much less impaired than those to acetylcholine, and the maximal relaxation was not decreased. This would suggest that reduced responsiveness of hypertensive arteries to NO may not fully explain the blunted relaxations to acetylcholine. The different results published in the literature may be related to the duration of hypertension, as it appears that the response to NO be-

comes impaired as the hypertensive vascular changes become more pronounced.

ENDOTHELIUM-DEPENDENT RESPONSES IN ATHEROSCLEROTIC BLOOD VESSELS

Hyperlipidemia

Morphologically, the endothelium remains intact in this pre-stage of atherogenesis (112). Functionally, however, pronounced alterations occur, both as far as endothelium-dependent relaxations as well as the production of contracting factors are concerned. Particularly, oxidized low-density lipoproteins (OX-LDL) are present in human atherosclerotic lesions (113).

Endothelium-Dependent Relaxations

In isolated porcine coronary artery, OX-LDL inhibits endothelium-dependent relaxations to platelets, serotonin, and thrombin (Fig. 13) (114,115). In contrast, relaxations to the NO-donor linsidomine are well maintained, excluding a reduced responsiveness of vascular smooth muscle to EDNO. In the porcine coronary circulation, this inhibition is specific for OX-LDL, as it is not induced by comparable concentrations of native LDL (114). In the rabbit aorta the effect of OX-LDL is mimicked by lysolecithin (a characteristic component of OX-LDL) (116). OX-LDL appears to activate an endothelial receptor distinct from the LDL receptor such as the scavenger receptor (Fig. 14) (114); indeed, dextran sulfate, a competitive antagonist of modified LDL at this receptor (114), prevents the endothelial effects of OX-LDL. The inhibitor of NO production L-NMMA exerts a similar inhibitory effect on endothelium-dependent relaxations as the modified lipoproteins, suggesting that OX-LDL specifically interferes with the L-arginine pathway. The activity of NO synthase, however, appears to remain unaffected as L-arginine evokes a full relaxation in vessels treated with OX-LDL. Pretreatment with L-arginine restores the response to serotonin in vessels treated with OX-LDL. Furthermore, pretreatment of isolated vessels with L-arginine improves or restores the inhibited endothelium-dependent responses to serotonin. Thus, OX-LDL may interact with the intracellular signal transduction mechanisms (for instance, the function of Gi proteins; 117) and/or the availability of L-arginine (Fig. 14). This mechanism may also occur in vivo, as in hypercholesterolemic pigs; a similar inhibition of endothelium-dependent relaxation to serotonin occurs in coronary arteries exposed to OX-LDL (118,119). In humans with hypercholesterolemia, L-arginine infusion augments the blunted increase in local blood flow in re-

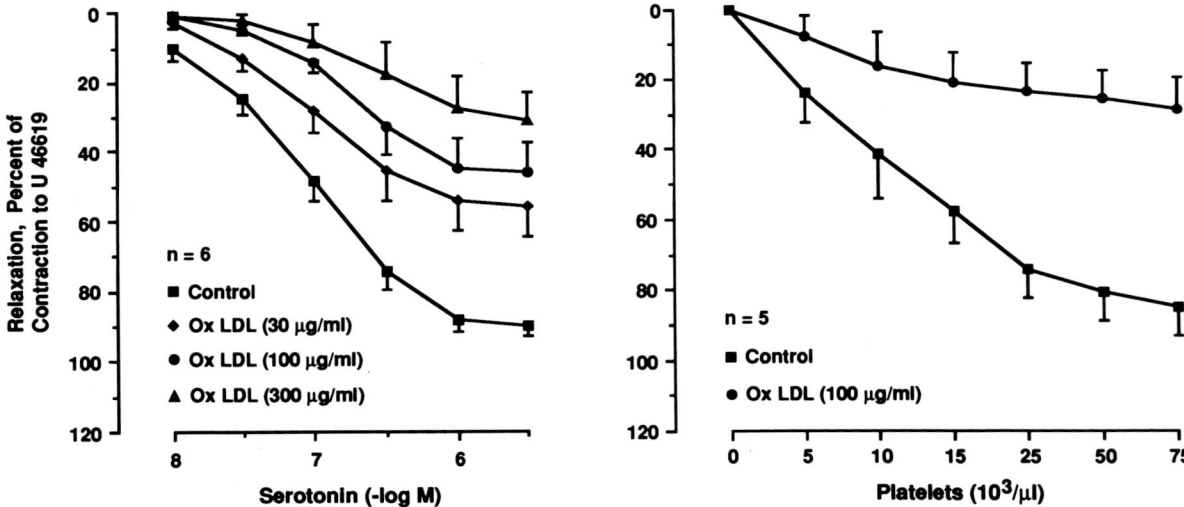

FIG. 13. Effects of oxidized low-density lipoproteins (OX-LDL) on endothelium-dependent relaxations induced by platelets (*right*) and serotonin (*left*) in porcine coronary artery. OX-LDLs markedly reduce the response to aggregating platelets and to serotonin occurring in the presence of ketanserin to inhibit direct contractile effects of the monoamine on vascular smooth muscle. (Modified from ref. 114, with permission of the American Heart Association.)

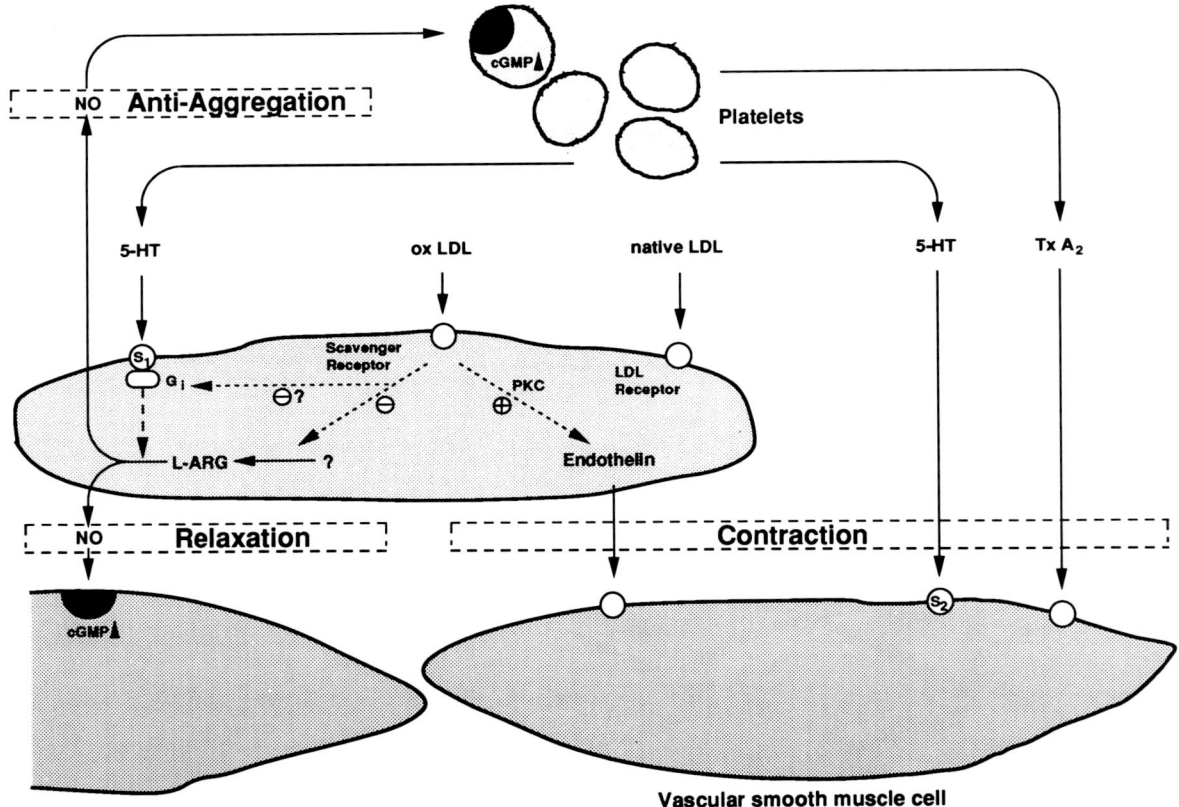

FIG. 14. Schematic representation of the effects of low-density lipoproteins in the blood vessel wall. Most likely, oxidation of LDL is an important step in the dysfunction of the endothelium in hyperlipidemia and atherosclerosis. Oxidized low-density lipoproteins (OX-LDL) may interact with the intracellular availability of L-arginine (L-ARG), the G protein of the serotonergic receptor (S_1), and they may also inactivate NO. In addition, OX-LDL can increase the endothelial production of endothelin-1 via protein kinase C (PKC). Serotonin = 5-HT. (From ref. 140, with permission.)

sponse to acetylcholine (120–122); in contrast, the loss of endothelium-dependent vasodilation to acetylcholine in epicardial coronary arteries is unaffected by the amino acid, possibly because of the presence of fully developed atherosclerosis (121).

In addition to their effect on the L-arginine pathway, both native and OX-LDL inactivate NO and cause endothelium-dependent (115) as well as endothelium-independent contraction (123).

Endothelin

OX-LDL also induces the expression of messenger RNA for endothelin in cultured aortic endothelial cells as well as the release of the peptide from the intact porcine aorta (Fig. 15) (124). In this context it is of interest that threshold and low concentrations of endothelin, which by themselves evoke no appreciable vascular effect, potentiate contractions induced by serotonin in the human coronary artery and to norepinephrine and serotonin in the human internal mammary artery (see above) (108). Thus, OX-LDL inhibits endothelium-dependent relaxations and promotes endothelium-dependent as well as endothelium-independent contractions; the consequences are alterations in vascular tone leading to vasospasm and thrombus formation, both common events in patients with coronary artery disease.

Atherosclerosis

In contrast to hyperlipidemia, atherosclerosis is associated with more or less severe morphological changes of the intima of large arteries (i.e., intimal thickening and accumulation of proliferation of smooth muscle cells and lipid-containing macrophages) (112). Except at late stages, however, endothelial denudation does not occur.

Endothelium-Dependent Relaxations

In porcine coronary arteries, established atherosclerosis severely impairs endothelium-dependent relaxations to serotonin and also reduces endothelium-dependent relaxations to bradykinin, which are maintained in hypercholesterolemia (119). However, endothelium-independent relaxations to nitrovasodilators remain preserved except in severely atherosclerotic arteries. Similarly, in atherosclerotic human coronary arteries, endothelium-dependent relaxations to substance P, bradykinin, aggregating platelets, and calcium ionophore are attenuated (125) and in vivo acetylcholine as well as serotonin cause paradoxical vasoconstriction (126,127).

Mechanism of Impaired Endothelium-Dependent Relaxation

Controversy exists as to the mechanism responsible for the marked impairment or loss of endothelium-dependent relaxations in atherosclerosis. Thus, bioassayable EDRF release in porcine coronary artery with hypercholesterolemia and atherosclerosis clearly is reduced (119). Direct measurements of NO in the rabbit aorta, however, suggest an increased formation of NO with a concomitant massive breakdown of the endogenous nitrovasodilator (to the biologically inactive molecule nitrite, nitrate) (128). The latter observation would suggest an increased formation of superoxide radicals in the endothelium and other products inactivating NO and/or a decreased activity of superoxide dismutase in the blood vessel wall in atherosclerosis. It is conceivable that atherosclerosis in the more developed stages with marked invasion of monocytes and other blood cells induces NO synthase in the subintimal space and vascular smooth muscle cells. However, it is unknown whether similar alterations occur in human coronary arteries as in the rabbit aorta.

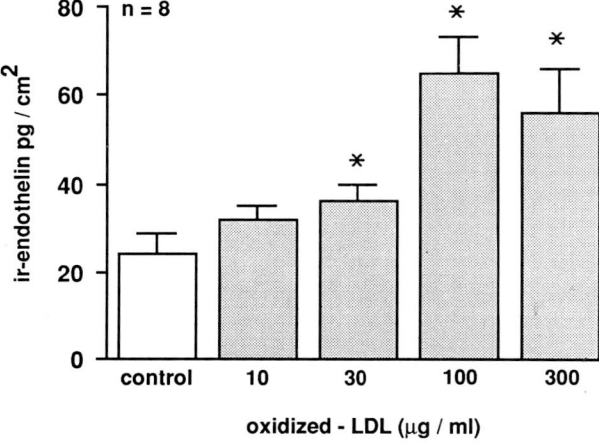

FIG. 15. Stimulating effects of oxidized low-density lipoproteins (OX-LDL) on endothelin production in the intact porcine aorta. Increasing concentrations of OX-LDL augment the amount of immunoreactive (ir) endothelin detected in the supernatant (*top*), a phenomenon that is reduced by dextran sulfate (not shown). *p <.05 vs control; §p <.05 vs OX-LDL. (Data from ref. 124, with permission of the American Heart Association.)

Endothelin

As in most other forms of vascular disease, human atherosclerosis is associated with increased circulating levels of endothelin (129). Interestingly, the circulating endothelin levels are positively correlated with the degree of atherosclerotic disease and the number of involved vascular beds (129). Histological examination of the human aorta suggests that the increased endothelium production is derived not only from endothelial cells of atherosclerotic blood vessels but also from vascular smooth muscle cells migrating into the intima. Indeed, vascular smooth muscle cells in culture produce significant amounts of endothelin, particularly if stimulated with vasoconstrictor hormones, growth factors, or coagulation products (130). Increased local levels of endothelin may contribute to the known increased vasoconstrictor responses of atherosclerotic blood vessels and, because of the proliferative properties of endothelin (131,132), also to the atherosclerotic process itself.

PLATELET FUNCTION AND HYPERTENSION

Increased platelet activity in hypertension, together with an altered endothelial and vascular responsiveness to platelet-derived products, could contribute to the occurrence of vascular complications and/or to the increased peripheral vascular resistance associated with the disease process.

Platelet Adhesion

The adherence of circulating blood cells to the endothelial cell layer is increased in hypertension. The adhering cells are mainly granulocytes, monocytes, and lymphocytes, but—at least in the rat aorta—not platelets (1,133). In cerebral arteries of the SHR, however, adhesion of platelets to the endothelium does occur (134). In human essential hypertension, the adhesiveness of platelets is increased (135).

In atherosclerotic blood vessels, monocytes adhere to endothelial cells early in the disease process (136). The attached monocytes are particularly prominent in junctional areas and between endothelial cells, from where they may migrate into the subendothelial space, accumulate fat, and become foam cells that form the ubiquitous fatty streaks, the earliest lesion in atherosclerosis. Later in the disease process, the endothelial cell layer begins to separate, particularly at branching sites, and the subendothelial space may be exposed to the circulating blood. At these sites, platelets adhere and can release vasoactive substances (e.g., thromboxane A_2, serotonin, adenosine nucleotides) as well as growth factors (e.g., platelet-derived endothelial cell growth factor, transforming growth factor-α, epidermal growth factor, transforming growth factor-β).

Platelet Function

β-Thromboglobulin, a marker of platelet activation, is increased in essential hypertension, whereas the life span of platelets is shortened (135,137). The platelet uptake and endogenous content of serotonin are decreased in patients with essential hypertension, whereas the release

of the monoamine is increased (1,138). The thrombin-induced release of serotonin from platelets of SHR is also enhanced (139). Similar changes occur in patients with essential hypertension (135,139).

Measurements of platelet aggregation in hypertensive patients revealed contradictory results. Whereas some authors found an increased platelet aggregation induced by adenosine diphosphate in hypertensives and in humans with a family history of hypertension, others were unable to demonstrate marked differences between normotensive and hypertensive patients (135,137). Similarly, no conclusive differences in the aggregatory response of normotensive and hypertensive platelets to epinephrine were found. In contrast, aggregatory responses to serotonin increase with age in patients with essential hypertension, particularly in men (138). Thus, a progressive increase in aggregatory response to serotonin, together with a diminished uptake and enhanced release of the monoamine, may provide high local concentrations of serotonin at the blood vessel wall, where serotonergic receptors are located.

ENDOTHELIUM-DEPENDENT REGULATION OF VASCULAR GROWTH

Normal Vessels

The endothelium also produces several factors that regulate growth of underlying smooth muscle cells. In normal vessels, the endothelium appears to synthesize primarily substances like heparan sulfate, NO, and prostaglandins that inhibit growth of smooth muscle cells. This may explain why vascular structure normally remains the same over prolonged periods of time (Fig. 16, left panel). However, under certain conditions the endothelium can generate substances like platelet-derived growth factor (PDGF), basic fibroblast growth factor (bFGF), insulin-like growth factor-1, colony stimulating factor-1, modified LDL, endothelin-1, and transforming growth factor-β or interleukin-1 and tumor necrosis factor-α, which can induce proliferation by themselves and/or stimulate secondary gene expression of growth factors in smooth muscle cells.

Mechanical removal and/or dysfunction of endothelial cells normally results in migration and proliferation of smooth muscle cells (Fig. 16, right panel) (71,74,140, 141), suggesting that the endothelium normally has indeed a net inhibitory influence on these responses.

Hypertensive Vessels

Structural abnormalities of the media of large conduit and resistance arteries is importantly involved in the pathophysiology of hypertension. In large conduit arteries, intimal thickening and atherosclerosis are important

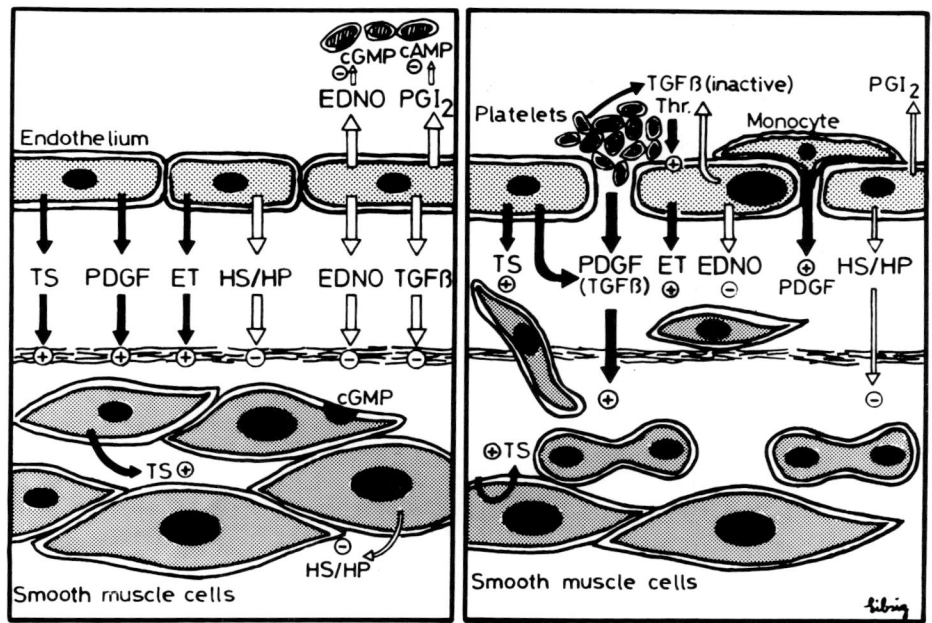

FIG. 16. Endothelium-derived vasoactive factors and vascular growth. The endothelium produces growth inhibitors such as heparin (HP), heparan sulfate (HS), transforming growth factor-beta (TGF-β), and also nitric oxide (EDNO). On the other hand, it releases growth promoters, such as platelet-derived growth factor (PDGF), thrombospondin (TS), and endothelin (ET). At sites of damaged endothelium the production of EDNO and prostacyclin (PGI₂) is diminished, favoring platelet adhesion and aggregation. PDGF is released by aggregating platelets and leads to proliferation as well as migration of vascular smooth muscle cells into the intima. The endothelium most probably takes part in these structural changes of the vascular wall, at least indirectly, by inhibiting platelet aggregation and with that the release of growth-stimulating factors. (From ref. 140, with permission.)

consequences of hypertension and responsible for most of the vascular complications of the disease process. Resistance arteries exhibit increased media/lumen ratios, which primarily involve migration and rearrangement of vascular smooth muscle cells within the media (71,141). The latter changes contribute importantly to the increase in peripheral vascular resistance in hypertension.

Since endothelium-dependent responses are altered in hypertension, an imbalance/alteration in the production of endogenous smooth muscle cell–migration inhibitors or promoters by endothelial cells could result in enhanced smooth muscle cell migration and contribute to the vascular remodeling observed in hypertensive resistance arteries. Nitric oxide derived from nitrovasodilators and cytokine-stimulated smooth muscle cells inhibits fetal calf serum, PDGF, bFGF, epidermal growth factor (EGF), and angiotensin II–induced growth of aortic and arteriolar smooth muscle cells (140–146). Furthermore, NO also inhibits mitogen-induced smooth muscle cell migration (140–146). Prostaglandins have also been evaluated as potential endothelium-derived growth-affecting factors. Prostacyclin, and to a lesser extent, prostaglandin E_1 and E_2, inhibit DNA synthesis and proliferation in cultured aortic smooth muscle cells (71,112,140). Furthermore, prostaglandins may contrib-

ute to a negative feedback regulation of mitogenesis stimulated by peptidergic growth factors (71,112,140, 141). Taken together the findings suggest that decreased production of endothelium-derived relaxing factor or prostaglandins could tilt the balance toward enhanced effects of endothelium-derived growth inducers and result in the abnormal growth of the smooth muscle.

Endothelin induces growth of cultured smooth muscle cells (131,132) and its mitogenic effects are augmented in the presence of other potent vasoactive factors such as angiotensin II. Furthermore, endothelin itself can potentiate the mitogenic effects of vasoactive substances like angiotensin II. On the other hand, angiotensin II, transforming growth factor-β, interleukin-1, epinephrine, arginine, and vasopressin have been shown to induce expression of endothelin messenger RNA in cultured endothelial cells (40–44,72). Although the role of endothelin in hypertension remains controversial (65) (see above), it does have the potential to regulate not only tone but also proliferation of smooth muscle cells.

In addition, properties of the vascular smooth muscle cells themselves are important. Aortic smooth muscle cells from ren-2 transgenic rats show enhanced migration in response to angiotensin II as compared with their age-matched control Sprague-Dawleys (142), suggesting that receptor operated mechanisms may also participate in this process. Indeed, angiotensin II induces expression of proto-oncogenes and causes vascular smooth muscle growth (hyperplastic and hypertrophic) both *in vitro* and *in vivo*. Furthermore, angiotensin II increases the synthesis of platelet-derived growth factor, a smooth muscle mitogen that may act as an autocrine to stimulate the proliferation of these cells (71,112,140,141). Angiotensin II also increases the synthesis and secretion of transforming growth factor-β by vascular smooth muscle cells (SMCs), and transforming growth factor-β increases deposition of extracellular matrix, a characteristic finding in hypertensive arteries. Angiotensin itself may also contribute to these events as it is capable of synthesizing extracellular matrices like collagen and fibronectin (71,112,140,141). Inhibitors of ACE, on the other hand, prevent myointimal proliferation after vascular injury (71,112,140,141).

Atherosclerosis

Endothelium-derived factors play a crucial role in the genesis of atherosclerotic lesions because of their effects on local blood flow, platelet function, and migration and proliferation (112). Although endothelium denudation does not occur except at late stages of atherosclerosis, information gathered from balloon angioplasty studies suggest an important antiproliferative effect of the endothelium. Indeed, denudation of endothelial cells is followed by platelet adhesion and aggregation, probably resulting in release of PDGF as well as other growth factors and invariably leading to intimal hyperplasia. PDGF and bFGF are mitogenic and chemotactic and induce vasoconstriction in smooth muscle cells (71,112,139,140, 148) and it is thought therefore that SMCs stimulated by PDGF or some other growth factors undergo migration and proliferation into the intima resulting in intimal hyperplasia.

Although macrophages do not adhere much to the blood vessel wall, they do so in the early stages of atherosclerosis. In the intima they are able to generate PDGF and bFGF and to induce migration of SMCs from the media into the intima followed by proliferation and plaque formation at the site of endothelial dysfunction/injury. Interaction of the endothelium with macrophages, platelets, and smooth muscle, as well as T lymphocytes, is regulated by endothelial mediators. Nitric oxide, prostacyclin, and heparan sulfate produced by the endothelium are antithrombotic; furthermore, the endothelium can bind specifically to factors like thrombin and factor Xa. Additionally, the endothelium is a source of fibrinolytic systems (e.g., plasminogen activator and urokinase). In atherosclerotic lesions, the formation of plasminogen activator inhibitor (PAI-1) could shift this balance to a prothrombotic state, which be could be particularly deleterious in the later stages of the disease.

The plasma contains factors such as angiotensin II, EGF, insulin-like growth factor, and PDGF. Platelets release at least five mitogens for SMCs (71,112,140,148), including serotonin, thrombospondin, and the three dimeric forms of PDGFs (i.e., -AA, -AB, -BB), and transforming growth factors-β_1, which can stimulate and inhibit SMC migration and proliferation depending on the cell culture conditions (71,112,139,140,147,148). Hence, activation of platelets at a damaged endothelial surface can lead to high local concentrations of growth factors.

In addition, another intriguing molecule that binds to endothelium is lipoprotein-a, which has a structural homology to LDL apolipoprotein B-100. Lipoprotein-a immunoreactivity has been described in the intima of atherosclerotic vessels as well as in the neointima of saphenous vein bypass grafts but not in normal vessels (148). Hence, increased expression of lipoprotein-a at sites of vascular damage may diminish the intrinsic fibrinolytic capacity of the vessel and thereby promote thrombosis in patients with atherosclerosis.

Apart from synthesizing several growth regulatory vasoactive factors (see above), endothelial cells represent the first potential site of oxidation of LDL as they transport LDL into the artery wall. OX-LDL alters endothelial function (see above) and this could lead to increased adherence of platelets, monocytes/macrophages, and T lymphocytes. OX-LDL is a key component in endothelial injury. Once formed by the endothelium, OX-LDL can directly injure the endothelium (toxic effects), change the release of endothelial mediators, and together with other vasoactive substances associated with atherogenesis participate in activation of monocytes into macrophages. Uptake of the OX-LDL by the macrophages leads to foam cell formation and alters gene expression of many growth-regulatory molecules and cytokines. OX-LDL can also form as a result of the action of NO (which is a free radical) or the enzyme responsible for leukotriene formation lipooxygenase (149).

Monocytes/macrophages within the circulation are also a source of growth-regulatory molecules and cytokines. Macrophage is the principal inflammatory mediator of cells in the atheromatous plaque microenvironment. It internalizes OX-LDL and can oxidize LDL through several pathways including lipooxygenase enzymes (71,112,139,140,148). Macrophages also play an important role in the fibroproliferative process because of its capacity to form numerous growth factors like vascular endothelial growth factor, basic fibroblast growth factor, epidermal growth factor, transforming growth factor α and β, interleukin-1, tumor necrosis factor-α (TNF-α), and PGE. In atherosclerosis associated with cardiac transplant rejection, large numbers of macrophages and T lymphocytes occur at the site of lesion, suggesting that localized immune response may have exacerbated macrophage/T-cell interactions and macrophage/smooth muscle cell interactions leading to pronounced proliferation of all these cells, and a similar role for macrophage also can occur in common atherosclerosis and hypertension.

SUMMARY: IMPORTANCE OF PLATELET–VESSEL–WALL INTERACTIONS IN HYPERTENSION

The endothelium plays an important protective role in the circulation by releasing NO and prostacyclin as well as inhibitors of coagulation; these substances cause vasodilation, have antiproliferative properties, and inhibit platelet adhesion and aggregation. Substances released from aggregating platelets can evoke the release of NO and prostacyclin, coagulation, and growth. Thus, if platelets are activated in a blood vessel with intact endothelial cells, vasodilation and inhibition of platelet function occur. This would disaggregate and flush away an evolving clot. In hypertension, endothelium-dependent relaxations are impaired under most conditions; in addition, the release of platelet-derived products, in particular serotonin, is enhanced. This may contribute to vascular complications and/or the increased peripheral resistance in hypertension. If, in hypertensive arteries, atherosclerotic vascular changes are superimposed, endothelium dysfunction becomes further reduced, an event that importantly contributes to the occurrence of myocardial infarction and stroke.

REFERENCES

1. Lüscher TF, Vanhoutte PM. *The endothelium: modulator of cardiovascular function.* Boca Raton: CRC Press, 1990;1–215.
2. Furchgott RF, Zawadzki JV. The obligatory role of endothelial cells in the relaxation of arterial smooth muscle by acetylcholine. *Nature* 1980;299:373–376.
3. Cohen RA, Shepherd JT, Vanhoutte PM. Inhibitory role of the endothelium in the response of isolated coronary arteries to platelets. *Science* 1983;221:273–274.
4. Vanhoutte PM, Lüscher TF. Peripheral mechanisms in cardiovascular regulation: transmitters, receptors and the endothelium. In: Tarazi RC, Zanchetti A, eds. *Handbook of hypertension, vol 8, physiology and pathophysiology of hypertension—regulatory mechanisms.* Amsterdam: Elsevier, 1986;96–123.
5. Yang Z, Stulz P, von Segesser L, Bauer E, Turina M, Lüscher TF. Different interactions of platelets with arterial and venous coronary bypass vessels. *Lancet* 1991;337:939–943.
6. Lüscher TF, Diederich D, Siebenmann R, Lehmann K, Stulz P, von Segesser L, Yang Z, Turina M, Grädel E, Weber E, Bühler FR. Difference between endothelium-dependent relaxations in arterial and in venous coronary bypass grafts. *N Engl J Med* 1988;319:462–467.
7. Rubanyi GM, Romero JC, Vanhoutte PM. Flow-induced release of endothelium-derived relaxing factor. *Am J Physiol* 1986;250: H1145–H1149.
8. Pohl U, Holtz J, Busse R, Bassenge E. Crucial role of endothelium in the vasodilator response to increased flow in vivo. *Hypertension* 1986;8:37–44.
9. Rubanyi GM, Vanhoutte PM. Superoxide anions and hyperoxia inactivate endothelium-derived relaxing factor. *Am J Physiol* 1986;250:H822–H827.
10. Furchgott RF. Studies on relaxation of rabbit aorta by sodium nitrite: the basis for the proposal that acid-activatable inhibitory factor from bovine retractor penis is inorganic nitrite and the endothelium-derived relaxing factor is nitric oxide. In: Vanhoutte PM, ed. *Vasodilation: vascular smooth muscle, peptides, autonomic nerves and endothelium.* New York: Raven Press, 1988;401–414.
11. Palmer RMJ, Ferrige AG, Moncada S. Nitric oxide release accounts for the biological activity of endothelium-derived relaxing factor. *Nature* 1987;327:524–526.
12. Ignarro LJ, Byrns RE, Buga GM, Chaudhuri G, Wood KS. Pharmacological evidence that endothelium-derived relaxing factor is nitric oxide: use of pyrogallol and superoxide dismutase to study endothelium-dependent and nitric oxide-elicited vascular smooth muscle relaxation. *J Pharmacol Exp Ther* 1988;244: 181–189.
13. Rapoport RM, Draznin MB, Murad F. Endothelium-dependent relaxation in rat aorta may be mediated through cyclic GMP-dependent protein phosphorylation. *Nature* 1983;306:174–176.
14. Palmer RMJ, Ashton DS, Moncada S. Vascular endothelial cells synthesize nitric oxide from L-arginine. *Nature* 1988;333:664–666.
15. Radomski MW, Palmer RMJ, Moncada S. Comparative pharmacology of endothelium-derived relaxing factor, nitric oxide and prostacyclin in platelets. *Br J Pharmacol* 1987;92:181–187.
16. Radomski MW, Palmer RMJ, Moncada S. Endogenous nitric oxide inhibits human platelet adhesion to vascular endothelium. *Lancet* 1987;2:1057–1068.
17. Busse R, Lückhoff A, Bassenge E. Endothelium-derived relaxant factor inhibits platelet activation. *Naunyn-Schmiedebergs Arch Pharmacol* 1987;336:566–571.
18. Bredt DS, Hwang PM, Glatt CE, Lowenstein C, Reed RR, Snyder SH. Cloned and expressed nitric oxide synthase structurally resembles cytochrome P-450 reductase. *Nature* 1991;351:714–718.
19. Radomski MW, Palmer RMJ, Moncada S. An L-arginine/nitric oxide pathway present in human platelets regulates aggregation. *Proc Natl Acad Sci USA* 1990;87:5193–5197.
20. Hibbs JB, Taintor RR, Vavrin Z, Rachlin EM. Nitric oxide: a cytotoxic activated macrophage effector molecule. *Biochem Biophys Res Commun* 1988;157:87–94.
21. Bernhardt J, Tschudi MR, Dohi Y, Gut I, Urwyler B, Bühler FR, Lüscher TF. Release of nitric oxide from human vascular smooth muscle cells. *Biochem Biophys Res Commun* 1991;180:907–912.
22. Julou-Schaeffer G, Gray GA, Fleming I, Schott C, Parratt JR, Stoclet J-C. Loss of vascular responsiveness induced by endotoxin involves L-arginine pathway. *Am J Physiol* 1990;259:H1038–H1043.
23. Wright CE, Rees DD, Moncada S. Protective and pathological roles of nitric oxide in endotoxin shock. *Cardiovasc Res* 1992;26: 48–57.
24. Knowles RG, Palacios M, Palmer RMJ, Moncada S. Formation of nitric oxide from L-arginine in the central nervous system: a transduction mechanism for stimulation of the soluble guanylate cyclase. *Proc Natl Acad Sci USA* 1989;86:1–4.
25. Richard V, Tschudi MR, Lüscher TF. Differential activation of the endothelial L-arginine pathway by bradykinin, serotonin and clonidine in porcine coronary arteries. *Am J Physiol* 1990;259: H1433–H1439.
26. Tschudi M, Richard V, Bühler FR, Lüscher TF. Importance of endothelium-derived nitric oxide in intramyocardial porcine coronary arteries. *Am J Physiol* 1990;260:H13–H20.
27. Yang Z, von Segesser L, Bauer E, Stulz P, Tschudi M, Lüscher TF. Differential activation of the endothelial L-arginine and cyclooxygenase pathway in the human internal mammary artery and saphenous vein. *Circ Res* 1991;68:52–60.
28. Meyer P, Flammer J, Lüscher TF. Endothelium-dependent regulation of the ophthalmic microcirculation in the perfused porcine eye. Role of nitric oxide and endothelins. *Invest Ophthalmol Vis Sci* 1993;in press.
29. Rees DD, Palmer RMJ, Moncada S. The role of endothelium-derived nitric oxide in the regulation of blood pressure. *Proc Natl Acad Sci USA* 1989;86:3375–3378.
30. Vallance P, Leeve A, Calver A, Collier J, Moncoda S. Accumulation of an endogenous inhibitor of nitric oxide synthesis in chronic renal failure. *Lancet* 1992;339:573–575.

31. Vanhoutte PM. The end of the quest? *Nature* 1987;327:459–460.
32. Feletou M, Vanhoutte PM. Endothelium-dependent hyperpolarization of canine coronary smooth muscle. *Br J Pharmacol* 1988;93:515–524.
33. Tare M, Parkington HC, Coleman HA, Neild TO, Dusting GJ. Hyperpolarization and relaxation of arterial smooth muscle caused by NO derived from the endothelium. *Nature* 1990;346:69–71.
34. Standen NB, Quayle JM, Davies NW, Brayden JE, Huang Y, Nelson MT. Hyperpolarizing vasodilators activate ATP-sensitive K+-channels in arterial smooth muscle. *Science* 1989;245:177–180.
35. Moncada S, Vane JR. Pharmacology and endogenous roles of prostaglandin endoperoxides, thromboxane A_2 and prostacyclin. *Pharmacol Rev* 1979;30:293–331.
36. De Mey JG, Claeys M, Vanhoutte PM. Endothelium-dependent inhibitory effects of acetylcholine, adenosine diphosphate, thrombin and arachidonic acid in the canine femoral artery. *J Pharmacol Exp Ther* 1982;222:166–173.
37. Miller VM, Vanhoutte PM. Endothelium-dependent contractions to arachidonic acid are mediated by products of cyclooxygenase in canine veins. *Am J Physiol* 1985;248:H432–H437.
38. Vanhoutte PM, Katusic ZS. Endothelium-derived contracting factor: endothelin and/or superoxide anion? *Trends Pharmacol Sci* 1988;9:229–230.
39. Katusic ZS, Vanhoutte PM. Superoxide anion is an endothelium-derived contracting factor. *Am J Physiol* 1989;257:H33–H37.
40. Yanagisawa M, Kurihara H, Kimura S, Mitsui Y, Kobayashi M, Watanabe TX, Masaki T. A novel potent vasoconstrictor peptide produced by vascular endothelial cells. *Nature* 1988;332:411–415.
41. Lüscher TF, Boulanger CM, Dohi Y, Yang Z. Endothelium-derived contracting factors (brief review). *Hypertension* 1992;19:117–130.
42. Boulanger C, Lüscher TF. Release of endothelin from the porcine aorta: inhibition by endothelium-derived nitric oxide. *J Clin Invest* 1990;85:587–590.
43. Boulanger C, Lüscher TF. Hirudin and nitric oxide donors inhibit the thrombin-induced release of endothelin from the intact porcine aorta. *Circ Res* 1990;68:1768–1772.
44. Dohi Y, Hahn AWA, Boulanger CM, Bühler FR, Lüscher TF. Endothelin stimulated by angiotensin II augments vascular contractility of hypertensive resistance arteries. *Hypertension* 1992;19:131–137.
45. Kourembanas S, Marsden PA, McQullan LP, Faller DV. Hypoxia induces endothelin gene expression and secretion in cultured human endothelium. *J Clin Invest* 1991;88:1054–1057.
46. Goerre S, Wenk M, Bärtsch P, Lüscher TF, Niroomand E, Oelz O, Reinhart WH. Endothelin-1 in pulmonary hypertension associated with high altitude exposure. *Circulation* 1994;submitted.
47. Lüscher TF, Yang Z, Tschudi M, von Segesser L, Stulz P, Boulanger C, Siebenmann R, Turina M, Bühler FR. Interaction between endothelin-1 and endothelium-derived relaxing factor in human arteries and veins. *Circ Res* 1990;66:1088–1094.
48. Dohi Y, Lüscher TF. Endothelin-1 in hypertensive resistance arteries: Intraluminal and extraluminal dysfunction. *Hypertension* 1991;18:543–549.
49. Clarke JG, Larkin SW, Benjamin N, Keogh BE, Chester A, Davies GJ, Maseri A, Taylor KM. Endothelin-1 is a potent long-lasting vasoconstrictor in dog peripheral vasculature in vivo. *J Cardiovasc Pharmacol* 1989;13(suppl 5):218–219.
50. Kiowski W, Lüscher TF, Linder L, Bühler FR. Endothelin-1-induced vasoconstriction in man: reversal by calcium channel blockade but not by nitrovasodilators or endothelium-derived relaxing factor. *Circulation* 1991;83:469–475.
51. Neubauer S, Ertl G, Haas U, Pulzer F, Kochsiek K. Effects of endothelin-1 in isolated perfused rat heart. *J Cardiovasc Pharmacol* 1990;16:1–8.
52. Wagner O, Christ G, Wojta J, Vierhapper H, Parzer S, Nowotny P, Schneider B, Waldhäusl W, Binder BR. Polar secretion of endothelin-1 by cultured endothelial cells. *J Biomed Chem* 1992;267:16066–16068.
53. Stewart DJ, Langleben D, Cernacek P, Cianflone K. Endothelin release is inhibited by coculture of endothelial cells with cells of vascular media. *Am J Physiol* 1990;259:H1928–H1932.
54. Saijonmaa O, Ristimäki A, Fyhrquist F. Atrial natriuretic peptide, nitroglycerine, and nitroprusside reduce basal and stimulated endothelin production from cultured endothelial cells. *Biochem Biophys Res Commun* 1990;173:514–520.
55. Yokokawa K, Kohno M, Yasunari K, Murakawa K, Horio T, Takeda T. Endothelin-3 regulates endothelin-1 production in cultured human endothelial cells. *Hypertension* 1991;18:304–315.
56. Warner TD, Mitchell JA, de Nucci G, Vane JR. Endothelin-1 and endothelin-3 release EDRF from isolated perfused arterial vessels of the rat and rabbit. *J Cardiovasc Pharmacol* 1989;13(suppl 5):85–88.
57. Miller VM, Komori K, Burnett JC, Vanhoutte PM. Differential sensitivity to endothelin in canine arteries and veins. *Am J Physiol* 1989;257:H1127–H1131.
58. Arai H, Hori S, Aramori I, Ohkubo H, Nakanishi S. Cloning and expression of a cDNA encoding and endothelin receptor. *Nature* 1990;348:730–732.
59. Sakurai T, Yanagisawa M, Takuwa Y, et al. Cloning of a cDNA encoding a non-isopeptide-selective subtype of the endothelin receptor. *Nature* 1990;348:732–735.
60. Vane J. Endothelins come home to roost. *Nature* 1990;348:673–675.
61. Bazil MK, Lappe RW, Webb RL. Pharmacologic characterization of an endothelin$_A$ (ET$_A$) receptor antagonist in conscious rats. *J Cardiovasc Pharmacol* 1992;20:940–948.
62. Breu V, Clozel M, Löffler B. Binding characterization of Ro-46-2005 a novel nonpeptidic endothelin receptor antagonist. Abstract 3rd International Conference on Endothelin, Houston, Texas, 1993.
63. Seo B-G, Oemas BS, Subermann R, Von Segesse L, Lüscher TF. Both ET$_A$ and ET$_B$ contraction to endothelin-1 in human blood vessels. *Circulation* 1994;89:1203–1208.
64. Nishikibe M, Ikada M, Tsuchida S, Fukuroda T, Shimamoto K, Kobayashi M, Ishikawa K, Yano M, Ikemoto F. Antihypertensive effect of a newly synthesized endothelin antagonist, BQ-123, in genetic hypertension model. *J Hypertens* 1992;10(suppl 4):P53.
65. Lüscher TF, Seo B-G, Bühler FR. Potential role of endothelin in hypertension. Controversy on endothelin in hypertension. *Hypertension* 1993;21:752–757.
66. Erdös EG. Angiotensin I converting enzyme. *Circ Res* 1975;36:247–255.
67. Shai S-Y, Fishel RS, Martin BM, Berk BC, Bernstein KE. Bovine angiotensin converting enzyme cDNA cloning and regulation. Increased expression during endothelial cell growth arrest. *Circ Res* 1992;70:1274–1281.
68. Lilly LS, Pratt RE, Alexander RW, Larson DM, Ellison KE, Gimbrone MA Jr, Dzau VJ. Renin expression by vascular endothelial cells in culture. *Circ Res* 1985;57:312–318.
69. Severs WB, Daniels-Severs AE. Effects of angiotensin on the central nervous system. *Pharmacol Rev* 1973;25:415–449.
70. Dubey RK, Roy A, Overbeck HW. Culture of renal arteriolar smooth muscle cells: mitogenic responses to Ang II. *Circ Res* 1992;71:1143–1152.
71. Jackson CL, Schwartz SM. Pharmacology of smooth muscle cell replication. *Hypertension* 1992;20:713–736.
72. Lüscher TF. Angiotensin, ACE-inhibitors and endothelial control of vasomotor tone. In: Grobecker H, Hensch G, Stranes BG, eds. *Angiotensin and the heart.* Darmstadt: Steinkopff Verlag 1993;15–24.
73. Mistry M, Muierhead EE, Yamaguchi Y, Nasjletti A. Renal function in rats with angiotensin II-salt induced hypertension: effects of thromboxane synthesis inhibition and receptor blockade. *J Hypertens* 1990;8:75–83.
74. Viswanathan M, Strömberg C, Seltzer A, Saavedra JM. Balloon angioplasty enhances the expression of angiotensin II AT$_1$ receptors in meointima of rat aorta. *J Clin Invest* 1992;90:1707–1712.
75. Förstermann U, Mügge A, Bode SM, Frölich JC. Response of human coronary arteries to aggregating platelets: importance of endothelium-derived relaxing factor and prostanoids. *Circ Res* 1988;63:306–312.
76. Beà ML, Oemar BS, Boulanger CM, Lüscher TF. Platelets stimulate endothelin release in cultured endothelial cells but inhibit it in intact blood vessels. *J Vasc Res* 1992;29:82.

77. Yang Z, Arnet U, Bauer E, Van Segessar L, Turina M, Lüscher TF. Thrombin induces endothelium dependent inhibition and direct activation of platelet vessel wall contraction: role of nitric oxide, prostacyclin and thromboxane A_2. *J Vasc Res* 1992;29:228.

78. Rimele TJ, Sturm RJ, Adams LM, Henry DE, Heaslip RJ, Weichman BM, Grimes D. Interaction of neutrophils with vascular smooth muscle: identification as a neutrophil-derived relaxing factor. *J Pharmacol Exp Ther* 1988;245:102–111.

79. Hibbs JB Jr, Vavrin Z, Taintor RR. L-arginine is required for expression of the activated macrophage effector mechanism causing selective metabolic inhibition in target cells. *J Immunol* 1987;138:550–565.

80. Konishi M, Su C. Role of endothelium in dilator responses of spontaneously hypertensive rat arteries. *Hypertension* 1983;5:881–886.

81. Winquist RJ, Bunting PB, Baskin EP, Wallace AA. Decreased endothelium-dependent relaxation in New Zealand genetic hypertensive rats. *J Hypertens* 1984;2:536–541.

82. De Mey JG, Gray SD. Endothelium-dependent reactivity in resistance vessels. *Prog Appl Microcirc* 1985;88:181–187.

83. Lüscher TF, Vanhoutte PM. Endothelium-dependent contractions to acetylcholine in the aorta of the spontaneously hypertensive rat. *Hypertension* 1986;8:344–348.

84. Lüscher TF, Vanhoutte PM. Endothelium-dependent responses to aggregating platelets and serotonin in spontaneously hypertensive rats. *Hypertension* 1986;8(suppl II):55–60.

85. Mayhan WG, Faraci FM, Heistad DD. Impairment of endothelium-dependent responses of cerebral arterioles in chronic hypertension. *Am J Physiol* 1987;253:H1435–H1440.

86. Mayhan WG, Faraci FM, Heistad DD. Responses of cerebral arterioles to adenosine diphosphate, serotonin and the thromboxane analoque U-46619 during chronic hypertension. *Hypertension* 1989;12(suppl 6):556–561.

87. Linder L, Kiowski W, Bühler FR, Lüscher TF. Indirect evidence for release of endothelium-derived relaxing factor in human forearm circulation in vivo: blunted response in essential hypertension. *Circulation* 1990;81:1762–1767.

88. Panza JA, Quyyumi AA, Brush JE Jr, Epstein SE. Abnormal vascular endothelium-dependent vascular relaxation in patients with essential hypertension. *N Engl J Med* 1990;323:22–27.

89. Creager MA, Roddy M-A, Coleman SM, Dzau VJ. The effect of ACE inhibition on endothelium-dependent vasodilation in hypertension. *J Vasc Res* 1992;29:97.

90. Taddei S, Virdis A, Mattei P, Salvetti A. Vasodilation to acetylcholine in primary and secondary forms of human hypertension. *Hypertension* 1993;21:929–933.

91. Cockroft JR, Chewenczyk PJ, Benjamin N, Riller JM. Preserved endothelium-dependent vasodilation in patients with essential hypertension. *N Engl J Med* 1994 (in press).

92. Treasure CB, Manoukian SV, Klein JL, Vita JA, Nabel EG, Renwick GH, Selwyn AP, Alexander RW, Ganz P. Epicardial coronary artery responses to acetylcholine are impaired in hypertensive patients. *Circ Res* 1992;71:776–781.

93. Treasure CB, Klein JL, Vita JA, Selwyn AP, Alexander RW, Ganz P. Left ventricular hypertrophy secondary to hypertension is associated with impaired endothelium-mediated relaxation in the coronary microvessels. *J Am Coll Cardiol* 1991;17:127A.

94. Zeiher AM, Drexler H, Saurbier B, Just H. Endothelium-mediated coronary blood flow modulation in humans. Effects of age, atherosclerosis, hypercholesterolemia and hypertension. *J Clin Invest* 1993;92:652–662.

95. Lüscher TF, Vanhoutte PM, Raij L. Antihypertensive therapy normalizes endothelium-dependent relaxations in salt-induced hypertension of the rat. *Hypertension* 1987;9(suppl III):193–197.

96. Taddei S, Virdis A, Mattei P, Arzilli F, Salvetti. Endothelium-dependent forarm vasodilation is reduced in normotensive with familial history of hypertension. *J Vasc Res* 1992;29:389.

97. Dohi Y, Thiel M, Bühler FR, Lüscher TF. Activation of the endothelial L-arginine pathway in pressurized mesenteric resistance arteries: effect of age and hypertension. *Hypertension* 1990;15:170–175.

98. Dohi Y, Criscione L, Lüscher TF. Renovascular hypertension impairs formation of endothelium-derived relaxing factors and

99. Tschudi MR, Noll G, Arnet U, Novosel D, Ganten D, Lüscher TF. Specific reduction of basal formation of nitric oxide in coronary arteries of hypertensive Ren-2 transgenic rats. *Circulation* 1994;in press.

100. Vallance P, Collier J, Moncada S. Effects of endothelium-derived nitric oxide on peripheral arteriolar tone in man. *Lancet* 1989;2:997–1004.

101. Panza JA, Casino PR, Badar DM, Quyyumi AA. Effect of increased availability of endothelium-derived nitric oxide on endothelium-dependent vascular relaxation in normals and in patients with essential hypertension. *Circulation* 1993;87:1475–1481.

102. Tschudi MR, Criscione L, Lüscher TF. Effect of aging and hypertension on endothelial function of rat coronary arteries. *J Hypertens* 1991;9(suppl 6):164–165.

103. Lüscher TF, Romero JC, Vanhoutte PM. Bioassay of endothelium-derived vasoactive substances in the aorta of normotensive and spontaneously hypertensive rats. *J Hypertens* 1986;4(suppl 6):81–83.

104. Van de Voorde J, Leusen I. Endothelium-dependent and independent relaxation of aortic rings from hypertensive rats. *Am J Physiol* 1986;250:H711–H717.

105. Larivière R, Thibault G, Schiffrin EL. Increased endothelin-1 contents in blood vessels of deoxycorticosterone acetate-salt hypertensive rats but not in spontaneously hypertensive rats. *Hypertension* 1993;21:294–300.

106. Tabuchi Y, Nakamaru M, Rakugi H, Nagano M, Ogihara T. Endothelin enhances adrenergic vasoconstriction in perfused rat mesenteric arteries. *Biochem Biophys Res Commun* 1989;159:1304–1308.

107. Dohi Y, Lüscher T. Aging differentially affects direct and indirect actions of endothelin-1 in perfused mesenteric arteries of the rat. *Br J Pharmacol* 1990;100:889–893.

108. Yang Z, Richard V, von Segesser L, Bauer E, Stulz P, Turina M, Lüscher TF. Threshold concentrations of endothelin-1 potentiate contractions to norepinephrine and serotonin in human arteries: a new mechanism of vasospasm? *Circulation* 1990;82:188–195.

109. Lüscher TF, Rubanyi GM, Aarhus LL, Vanhoutte PM. Serotonin reduces coronary flow in isolated hearts of the spontaneously hypertensive rat. *J Hypertens* 1986;4(suppl 5):148–150.

110. Lüscher TF, Raij L, Vanhoutte PM. Endothelium-dependent responses in normotensive and hypertensive Dahl rats. *Hypertension* 1987;9:157–163.

111. Lüscher TF, Vanhoutte PM, Raij L. Antihypertensive therapy normalizes endothelium-dependent relaxations in salt-induced hypertension of the rat. *Hypertension* 1987;9(suppl III):193–197.

112. Ross R. The pathogenesis of atherosclerosis—an update. *N Engl J Med* 1986;314:488–500.

113. Ylä-Herttuala S, Palinski W, Rosenfeld ME, et al. Evidence for the presence of oxidatively modified low-density lipoproteins in atherosclerotic lesions of rabbit and man. *J Clin Invest* 1989;84:1086–1095.

114. Tanner FC, Noll G, Boulanger CM, Lüscher TF. Oxidized low-density lipoproteins inhibit relaxations of porcine coronary arteries: role of scavenger receptor and endothelium-derived nitric oxide. *Circulation* 1991;83:2012–2020.

115. Simon BC, Cunningham LD, Cohen RA. Oxidized low density lipoproteins cause contraction and inhibit endothelium-dependent relaxation in the pig coronary artery. *J Clin Invest* 1990;86:75–79.

116. Kugiyama K, Kerns SA, Morrisett JD, Roberts R, Henry PD. Impairment of endothelium-dependent arterial relaxation by lysolecithin in modified low-density lipoproteins. *Nature* 1990;344:160–162.

117. Flavahan NA. Atherosclerosis or lipoprotein-induced endothelial dysfunction: potential mechanisms underlying reduction in dysfunction in EDRF/nitric oxide activity. *Circulation* 1992;85:1927–1938.

118. Shimokawa H, Vanhoutte PM. Hypercholesterolemia causes generalized impairment of endothelium-dependent relaxation to aggregating platelets in porcine arteries. *J Am Coll Cardiol* 1989;13:1402–1408.

119. Shimokawa H, Vanhoutte PM. Impaired endothelium-dependent relaxation to aggregating platelets and related vasoactive substances in porcine coronary arteries in hypercholesterolemia and in atherosclerosis. *Circ Res* 1989;64:900–914.

120. Creager MA, Cooke JP, Mendelsohn ME, Gallagher SJ, Coleman SM, Loscalzo J, Dzau VJ. Impaired vasodilation of forearm resistance vessels in hypercholesterolemic humans. *J Clin Invest* 1990;86:228–234.

121. Drexler H, Zeiher AM, Meinzer K, Just H. Correction of endothelial dysfunction in coronary microcirculation of hypercholesterolemic patients by L-arginine. *Lancet* 1991;338:1546–1550.

122. Creager MA, Gallagher SH, Girerd XJ, Coleman S, Dzau VJ, Cooke JP. L-arginine improves endothelium-dependent vasodilation in hypercholesterolemic humans. *J Clin Invest* 1992;90:1248–1253.

123. Galle J, Bassenge E, Busse R. Oxidized low-density lipoproteins potentiate vasoconstrictions to various agonists by direct interaction with vascular smooth muscle. *Circ Res* 1990;66:1287–1293.

124. Boulanger CM, Tanner FC, Hahn AWA, Werner A, Lüscher TF. Oxidized low-density lipoproteins induce mRNA expression and release of endothelin from human and porcine endothelium. *Circ Res* 1992;70:1191–1197.

125. Förstermann U, Mügge A, Alheid U, Haverich A, Frölich JC. Selective attenuation of endothelium-mediated vasodilation in atherosclerotic human coronary arteries. *Circ Res* 1988;62:185–190.

126. Ludmer PL, Selwyn AP, Shook TL, Wayne RR, Mudge GH, Alexander RW, Ganz P. Paradoxical vasoconstriction induced by acetylcholine in atherosclerotic coronary arteries. *N Engl J Med* 1986;315:1046–1051.

127. Golino P, et al. Divergent effects of serotonin on coronary-artery dimensions and blood flow in patients with coronary atherosclerosis and control patients. *N Engl J Med* 1991;324:641–648.

128. Minor RL, Myers RR Jr, Guerra R Jr, Bates JN, Harrison DG. Diet-induced atherosclerosis increases the release of nitrogen oxides from rabbit aorta. *J Clin Invest* 1990;86:2109–2116.

129. Lerman A, Edwards BS, Hallett JW, Heublein DM, Sondberg SM, Burnett JC Jr. Circulating and tissue endothelin immunoreactivity in advanced atherosclerosis. *N Engl J Med* 1991;325:997–1001.

130. Hahn AWA, Resink TJ, Scott-Burden T, Powell J, Roni Y, Bühler FR. Stimulation of endothelin mRNA and secretion in rat vascular smooth muscle cells: a novel function. *Cell Regulation* 1990;1:649–659.

131. Hirata Y, Takagi Y, Fukuda Y, Marumo F. Endothelin is a potent mitogen for rat vascular smooth muscle cells. *Atherosclerosis* 1989;78:225–228.

132. Dubin D, Pratt RE, Cooke JP, Dzau VJ. Endothelin, a potent vasoconstrictor, is a vascular smooth muscle mitogen. *J Vasc Med Biol* 1989;1:13–17.

133. Chobanian AV, Brecher PI, Haudenschild CC. Effects of hypertension and of antihypertensive therapy on atherosclerosis. *Hypertension* 1986;8(suppl I):15–21.

134. Hazaman F, Ozaki T, Amano S. Scanning electron microscopic study of endothelial cells of cerebral arteries from spontaneously hypertensive rats. *Stroke* 1979;10:245–252.

135. Amstein R, Tetovska N, Lüscher TF, Kiowski W, Bühler FR. Age and the platelet serotonin vasoconstrictor axis in essential hypertension. *J Cardiovasc Pharmacol* 1988;11(suppl 1):35–40.

136. De Clerk F. Blood platelets in human essential hypertension. *Agents Actions* 1986;18:563–580.

137. Kamal LA, Quain-bui KHL, Meyer P. Decreased uptake of H₃-serotonin and endogenous content of serotonin in blood platelets of hypertensive patients. *Hypertension* 1984;6:568–573.

138. Baudouin-Legros M, Dard B, Guicheney P. Hyperreactivity of platelets from spontaneously hypertensive rats. *Hypertension* 1986;8:694–699.

139. Casscells W. Migration of smooth muscle and endothelial cells: critical events in restenosis. *Circulation* 1992;86:723–729.

140. Lüscher TF, Tanner FC. Endothelial regulation of vascular tone and growth. *Am J Hypertens* 1993;6:283S–293S.

141. Dzau VJ, Gibbons GH. Vascular remodelling: mechanisms and implications. *J Cardiovasc Pharmacol* 1993;21(suppl I):S1–S5.

142. Dubey RK, Ganten D, Lüscher TF. Enhanced migration of smooth muscle cells from Ren-2 Transgenic rats in response to angiotensin II: inhibition by nitric oxide. *Hypertension* 1993;22:412.

143. Dubey RK, Overbeck HW. Culture of mesenteric arteriolar SMCs: effect of PDGF. AII, and NO on growth. *Cell Tissue Res* 1994;275:133–141.

144. Dubey RK. Effect of nitric oxide synthesizing compounds and 8-bromo-cGMP on the growth of arteriolar smooth muscle cells. *J Vasc Res* 1992;29:107.

145. Garg UC, Hassid A. Nitric-oxide generating vasodilators and 8-bromo-cyclic guanosine monophosphate inhibit mitogenesis and proliferation of cultured rat vascular SMCs. *J Clin Invest* 1989;83:1774–1777.

146. Scott-Burden T, Schini VB, Elizondo E, Junquero DC, Vanhoutte. Platelet-derived growth factor suppresses and fibroblast growth factor enhances cytokine-induced production of NO by cultured aortic SMCs. Effects on cell proliferation. *Circ Res* 1992;71:1088–1100.

147. Ware JA, Heistad DD. Platelet-endothelium interactions. *N Engl J Med* 1993;328:628–635.

148. Scanu AM, Lawn RM, Berg K. Lipoprotein(a) and atherosclerosis. *Ann Intern Med* 1991;87:6959–6963.

149. Yla-Herttuala S, Rosenfeld ME, Parthasarathy S, Glass CK, Sigal E, Witztum JL, Sternberg D. Colocalization of 15-lipoxygenase mRNA and protein with epitopes of oxidized low density lipoprotein in macrophage rich areas of atherosclerotic lesions. *Proc Natl Acad Sci USA* 1990;87:6959–6963.

Hypertension: Pathophysiology, Diagnosis, and Management, Second Edition, edited by J.H. Laragh and B.M. Brenner, Raven Press, Ltd., New York © 1995.

CHAPTER 38

Endothelins: Multifunctional Peptides with Potent Vasoactive Properties

Andrew J. King

Systemic hypertension is a disease characterized by an increase in systemic vascular resistance, frequently associated with structural remodeling of the vessel wall. A circulating factor leading to increased vascular tone, such as catecholamines or angiotensin II (Ang II) can be identified only in a minority of patients. Over the past decade the endothelium has been appreciated to be a lo-

cal modulator of vascular smooth muscle tone by its ability to elicit both vasorelaxant and vasoconstrictor substances (1–5). This has led to the possibility of a dysfunctional endothelium causing systemic hypertension by producing excessive vasoconstrictors and/or deficient vasodilators. In addition, the location of endothelial monolayer at the interface of the vascular lumen and the vascular smooth muscle might render it particularly susceptible to the long-term damaging effects of sustained elevation of systemic blood pressure. One of the endothelium-derived vasoconstrictors, endothelin (now

A. J. King: New England Medical Center, Boston, Massachusetts 02111.

termed *ET-1*), was first described in 1988 by Yanigisawa et al. (6). This 21-amino-acid peptide is a member of a family of three peptides and is the most potent endogenous vasoconstrictor yet identified (7). When infused intravenously, endothelin induces transient hypotension followed by a sustained hypertensive response. However, its role in normal human physiology and in the pathogenesis of human systemic hypertension have not been elucidated. The peptide circulates in normals and is elevated in a variety of pathological conditions associated with altered renal and systemic hemodynamics (8). The tremendous investigation efforts thus far have identified many actions of the peptide other than its pressor effects with potential importance to the hypertension. Most importantly, the peptide has mitogenic properties which might be involved in vascular wall remodeling. This chapter will focus on several aspects of endothelin biology: (a) structural characteristics and gene expression; (b) cellular actions; (c) systemic and renal physiology; (d) potential role in renal pathophysiology; and (e) potential role in human and experimental hypertension.

STRUCTURAL CHARACTERISTICS AND GENE EXPRESSION

Historical Perspectives

The first evidence of an endothelium-derived vasoconstrictor was a report by Hickey et al. (9) of prolonged vasoconstriction of isolated rings of canine, bovine, and porcine arteries that were exposed to medium conditioned by cultured bovine aortic endothelial cells. This response was abrogated by protease pretreatment, indicating that the vasoconstrictor(s) was a peptide. The presence of protease-sensitive and -insensitive endothelium-derived vasoconstrictors was also reported by several other groups (10–12). In 1988, Yanagisawa et al. (6) isolated a 21-amino-acid peptide, endothelin, from the supernatant of serum-free, cultured porcine aortic endothelial cells. Using anion exchange and reverse-phase HPLC, the vasoconstrictor was purified. An oligonucleotide probe was synthesized for amino acids 7–20 and preproendothelin cDNA was then isolated, using a cDNA library constructed from poly(A) messenger ribonucleic acid (mRNA) extracted from porcine aortic endothelial cells. The cDNA sequence and deduced amino acid sequence are depicted in Fig. 1. Screening of a rat genomic library with the same probe revealed a region with 76 percent homology with porcine aortic preproendothelin (13). The deduced amino acid sequence of the mature peptide revealed six amino acid substitutions and was termed *rat endothelin*. However, subsequent screening of multiple species under less stringent conditions indicate that each species has multiple genes cross-

reacting with the endothelin probe. To date, the endothelin family of peptides consists of three isoforms, now called *ET-1, ET-2,* and *ET-3* (see below, Fig. 2) (6,7,13–15). These peptides have since been identified to have wide-ranging biological effects in addition to their vasoconstrictor response.

Structural Characteristics

Mature endothelin molecules are 21-amino-acid peptides characterized by two intrachain disulfide rings, leading to a hairpin loop configuration (see Fig. 2). This configuration is atypical for mammalian peptides but is present in a variety of submammalian venoms. Endothelin has significant regional homologies with alpha scorpion venoms, and in particular with the snake venom sarafotoxin (see Fig. 2) (16–19). The hydrophobic carboxy-terminus portion of the molecule is the most conserved region of the peptide, with variability occurring within the charged hairpin at residues 4–7 (6,7,13,15). Both the carboxy-terminus and the hairpin configuration are necessary for bioactivity of the peptide. Removal of the tryptophan at the end of the hydrophobic tail or reduction of the disulfide bonds leads to approximately 1000-fold reduction in bioactivity of the peptide (20). These studies also indicate that the outer bridge (Cys^1-Cys^{15}) is more important to potency than the inner disulfide bond (Cys^3-Cys^{11}). In-depth analysis of structure-activity relationships has been reviewed (21).

Predictions regarding the three-dimensional structure of the peptide have been made using circular dichroism, nuclear magnetic resonance, and molecular dynamics simulation (21–25). The molecule is believed to be 30–35 percent helical in the region of the hairpin between residues Lys^9 and Cys^{15}. The helical character is lost when the disulfide bonds are broken [ET-1(1,3,11,15-Ala)]. This helical pattern is similar to that observed with apamin and mast-cell-degranulating peptide (22,25,26). The position of the carboxy-terminus portion remains unclear, though for ET-3 it is believed to be in apposition with the helical region (26).

Gene Characteristics

As discussed above, preproendothelin-1 was first isolated and sequenced using a probe encoding for amino acids 7–20 of mature ET-1 (6). Subsequent southern blot analysis using conditions of low stringency identified three independent genes which were present in multiple species (7). The mature peptides of these genes have been termed *ET-1, ET-2,* and *ET-3* (formerly rat endothelin). A fourth isoform expressed exclusively in the intestine, termed *beta-endothelin* or *vasoactive intestinal constrict-*

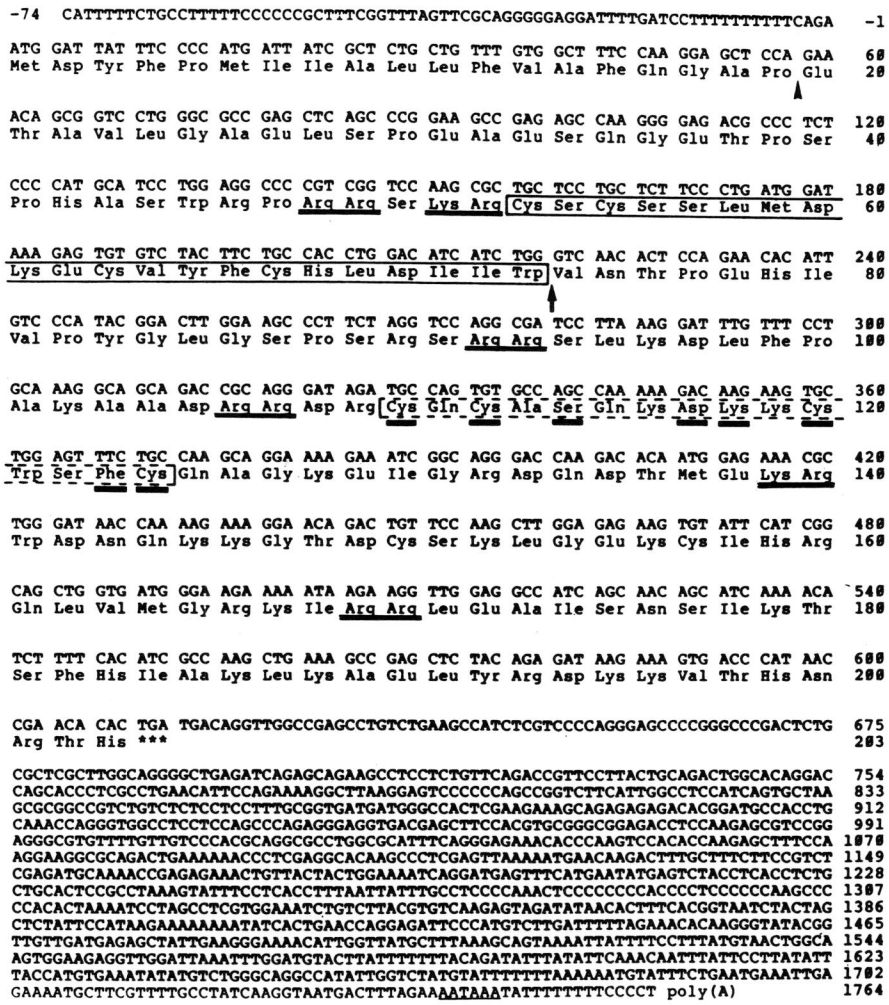

FIG. 1. Nucleotide sequence of preproendothelin-1 cDNA, along with deduced amino acid sequence. Arrowhead represents cleavage site for putative signal sequence. Double underlines indicate paired basic amino acid sequences. Solid lines enclose sequence of mature endothelin peptide; broken lines enclose endothelin-like peptide. The arrow signifies the site of cleavage of the unusual proteolytic processing enzyme (From ref. 6, with permission.)

ing peptide, was cloned and sequenced in both the mouse and rat (27). However, subsequent analysis suggests that this represents an isoform of the ET-2 gene (28).

It is believed that the three isoforms of endothelin arose by gene duplication of a common ancestral gene (29,30). The close resemblance of the mature ET peptides to the submammalian snake venom sarafotoxin is intriguing, and the preserved structure suggests that the gene has biological importance (17–19). The ET-1, ET-2, and ET-3 genes have been localized to chromosomes 6, 1, and 20, respectively (29,31,32). Human genomic clones of ET-1 and -3 demonstrate five exons and four intervening sequences with the mature peptide encoded on the second exon (14,29,32). The third exon contains a 15-amino-acid, endothelin-like peptide, the significance of which is unknown. Several features of the preproendothelin gene suggest possible regulatory mechanisms (33,34). The gene has an initiation site typical for eukaryotic cells (6). There are 5'-Cis-acting sequences which are believed to mediate induction under several conditions, including phorbol ester stimulation, acute physiologic stress, and hormone stimulation (14,32,35). In particular, there is a 10-base pair section in the first exon which is identical to the core of a transforming growth factor-beta (TGF-β)-responsive element which binds nuclear factor 1 (32). This TGF-β has been shown to induce endothelin transcription (36–40). In addition, the 3'-noncoding region contains a highly conserved 250-base pair region with AU-repeat sequences believed to be involved in mRNA destabilization (32). These data

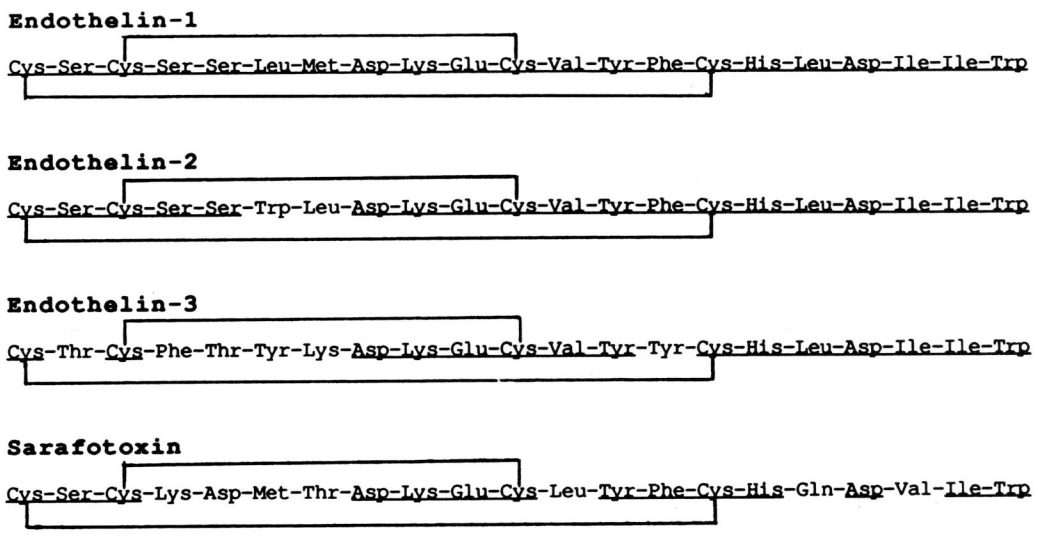

Endothelin-1

Cys-Ser-Cys-Ser-Ser-Leu-Met-Asp-Lys-Glu-Cys-Val-Tyr-Phe-Cys-His-Leu-Asp-Ile-Ile-Trp

Endothelin-2

Cys-Ser-Cys-Ser-Ser-Trp-Leu-Asp-Lys-Glu-Cys-Val-Tyr-Phe-Cys-His-Leu-Asp-Ile-Ile-Trp

Endothelin-3

Cys-Thr-Cys-Phe-Thr-Tyr-Lys-Asp-Lys-Glu-Cys-Val-Tyr-Tyr-Cys-His-Leu-Asp-Ile-Ile-Trp

Sarafotoxin

Cys-Ser-Cys-Lys-Asp-Met-Thr-Asp-Lys-Glu-Cys-Leu-Tyr-Phe-Cys-His-Gln-Asp-Val-Ile-Trp

FIG. 2. Amino acid sequences of endothelin-1, endothelin-2, endothelin-3, and sarafotoxin S6. Bars represent disulfide bridges, and underlined amino acids indicate homologies to endothelin-1.

suggest that cellular endothelin mRNA might be regulated at the level of transcription and mRNA stability. The reader is referred to several excellent reviews of the molecular biology of the endothelin family of genes (33,34,41,42).

Gene Induction and Posttranscription Processing

The proposed biosynthetic pathway of endothelin is depicted in Fig. 3. Amino acids 1–20 of preproendothelin are characteristic of an eukaryotic secretory signal

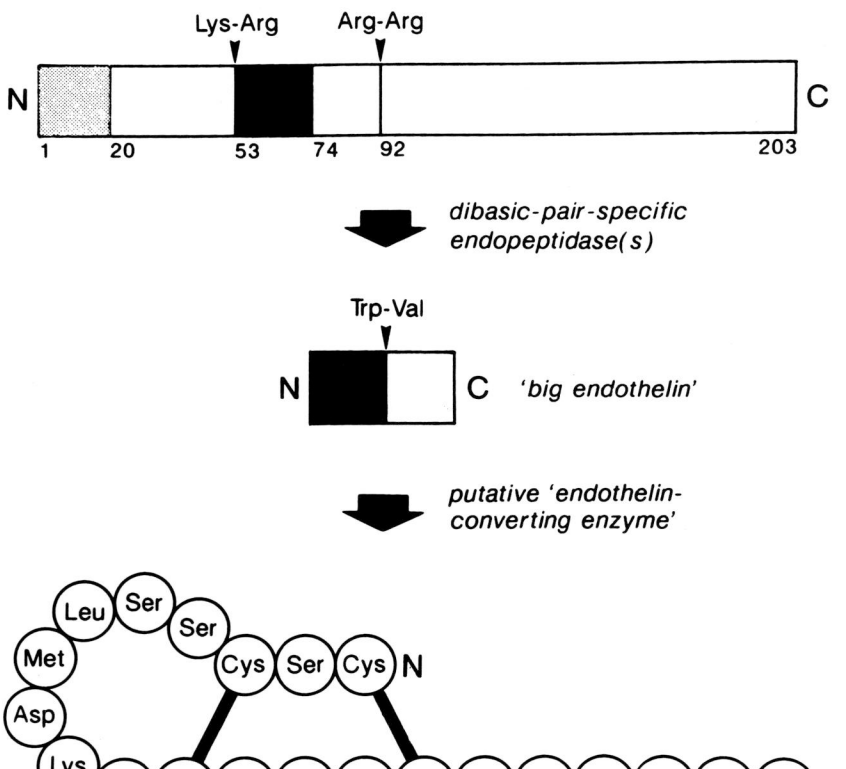

FIG. 3. Proposed biosynthetic pathway of endothelin. Light-shaded box represents putative signal sequence; dark-shaded box signifies mature endothelin sequence. Open boxes indicate the remainder of preproendothelin. (From ref. 6, with permission.)

sequence (6). Mature endothelin is preceded by a dibasic pair (Lys 51-Arg 52), which is a common recognition sequence for processing endopeptidases. Cleavage at this site yields a 39-amino-acid peptide termed *big endothelin,* a molecule with little or no intrinsic vasoconstrictor properties when placed on vascular smooth muscle preparation (43,44). By contrast, the C-terminus of the mature peptide is flanked by Trp 73 and Val 74, which is unusual, leading Yanagisawa et al. (6) to propose a novel "endothelin-converting enzyme" (ECE) with chymotrypsin-like activity (see 21,41,45,46 for review). *In vitro,* chymotrypsin can cleave big endothelin and yield vasoactive byproducts; however, the importance of this *in vivo* has not been established (47,48). Endothelin-converting enzyme activity has also been associated with aspartic proteases and neutral endopeptidases. Endothelin-converting enzyme activity with pH optimum 4.0 is seen in extract of porcine aortic endothelial cells and is completely blocked by pepstatin-A, an inhibitor of aspartic proteases (49). Subsequently, membrane- and cytosol-associated aspartic protease ECE activity has been identified in several cell types (50–53). Although the exact nature of this enzyme(s) has not been determined, it has been suggested that this might represent a cathepsin (48,50,54,55). However, the low pH optimum of these enzymes raises questions regarding the importance of these reactions *in vivo.* Endothelin-converting enzyme activity at neutral pH was first described in a homogenate of bovine endothelial cells (56). This enzyme(s) is a metal-dependent endopeptidase similar to, though different from, neutral endopeptidase 24:11, as it can be inhibited by phosphoramidon or metal chelating agents, but not thiorphan or kelatorphan (46,53,57–62). Whether this enzyme represents a specific protease has not been determined; however, in bovine carotid artery endothelial cells, a cytosolic enzyme has been identified which converts big ET-1 to mature ET-1, but not big ET-3 (57,60,61). Several lines of evidence suggest that ECE is likely to be the metal-dependent neutral endopeptidase. First, release of ET-1 from cultured endothelial cells can be inhibited by phosphoramidon (63,64). Second, the systemic vasoconstrictive effects of intravenous big ET-1, but not ET-1, are markedly inhibited by pretreatment with phosphoramidon (57,58,65–68). These results also suggest that this ECE is accessible to the circulation. By contrast, big ET-3 has much less systemic effect than ET-3, suggesting that a specific ET-3 ECE is not accessible to the circulation (69). Clearly, specific inhibitors of this enzyme would help provide insight into the physiologic effects of endogenous endothelin. For greater depth regarding ECE, the reader is referred to a recent review of ECEs (46).

In the original report, Yanagisawa et al. (6) observed linear release of endothelin from cultured porcine endothelial cells, suggesting that production of endothelin is constitutive. In endothelial cells there are no endothelin-containing secretory granules. However, endothelin-containing vesicles have been identified in the posterior pituitary of the rat and might play a role in the setting of water depletion and/or severe volume depletion (see below) (70,71). A recent report that endothelin secretion by endothelial cells is vectorial has important implications regarding the role of endothelin as a paracrine mediator (see below) (72). In these studies approximately 80 percent of secreted endothelin was released on the basolateral side, a finding that raises concerns regarding the interpretation of circulating levels of endothelin as an indicator of endothelin activity. Preproendothelin mRNA levels and/or endothelin secretion increase in response to a variety of hormonal and mechanical stimuli (Table 1). Note that the potential stimuli and inhibitors for endothelin release include many of the known modulators of systemic and renal hemodynamics as well as volume

TABLE 1. *Factors that stimulate and inhibit endothelin transcription and/or secretion* in vitro

Stimulators	Inhibitors
Hormonal	
Angiotensin II	Atrial natriuretic peptide
Arginine vasopressin	Brain natriuretic peptide
Bradykinin	Bradykinin
Endothelin-1	
Epinephrine	
Insulin	
Glucocorticoids	
Prolactin	
Inflammatory mediators	
Endotoxin	
Interleukin-1	
Tumor necrosis factor	
Interferon-β	
Growth factors	
Epidermal growth factor	
Insulin-like growth factor	
Transforming growth factor-β	
Coagulation factors	
Thrombin	Heparin
Thromboxane A$_2$	Prostacyclin
Tissue plasminogen activating factor	
Other	
Ca^{2+} ionophores	Protein kinase A activators
Hypoxia	Nitric oxide
Mechanical shear stress	ACE inhibitors
Oxidized low-density lipoproteins	
Phorbol esters	
L-NMMA/methylene blue	

homeostasis (see discussion below). However, the multifunctional potential of this family of peptides is highlighted by the stimulation observed with inflammatory mediators, coagulation factors, and growth factors.

It is now clear that a large variety of cells are capable of producing endothelins in a tissue-specific manner (see 41,45,73 for review). Endothelin-1, but not ET-2 or ET-3 mRNA levels have been detected in cultured endothelial cells from various vessels (6,14,29, and others). Cultured vascular smooth muscle cells (39,74) and mesangial cells (40,75–79) secrete endothelin in a linear fashion. Endothelin release has been reported in a number of cultured nonvascular cells, including (but not limited to) renal epithelial cells (37,80–82), glial cells (83), several cancer cell lines (84–86), leukocytes (87,88), endometrial epithelial cells (89), tracheal epithelial cells (90), and Hep G-2 cells (84). By contrast, ET-2 and ET-3 production in cultured cells has been observed only in a few select cell lines. Several investigators have examined the tissue distribution of the isoforms of endothelin using *in situ* hybridization and northern analysis, and have identified ET-1 in a large variety of organs, including (but not exclusively) the lung, central nervous system, heart, kidney, gastrointestinal tract, placenta (see 41,73 for review). Using northern analysis and *in situ* hybridization, there has been considerable variation in the tissue distribution of the isopeptides, at least in part due to the insensitivity of the techniques and species variation. Many organs also have detectable ET-3, but in far lower concentrations. Notable exceptions include the central nervous system, pituitary, gut, and inner medulla of the kidney where ET-3 appears more prominently (28,91,92). To date, ET-2 has been detected almost exclusively in the large and small intestine, with trace levels in muscle and heart (27,92). In summary, a wide variety of cell types express ET-1 and ET-3; however, the endothelium produces exclusively ET-1. Although ET-1 and to a lesser extent ET-3 are detectable in a wide variety of organs and cell types, the physiologic relevance remains to be determined.

CELLULAR ACTIONS OF ENDOTHELIN

Endothelin induces potent dose-dependent contraction in isolated vascular muscle preparations from a variety of species (6,93). The vasoconstrictor effects have been observed in both arteries and veins, irrespective of the vascular source. However, veins appear to be more sensitive than arteries (94). The contractile responses are (a) slow in onset, (b) sustained, and (c) difficult to reverse with a perfusate wash (Fig. 4) (6,13,94–96). In the original report, Yanagisawa et al. (6) observed that constriction was not abrogated by indomethacin, phentolamine, nordihydroguaiaretic acid, atropine, methysergide, or diphenhydramine. The half-maximal constriction concen-

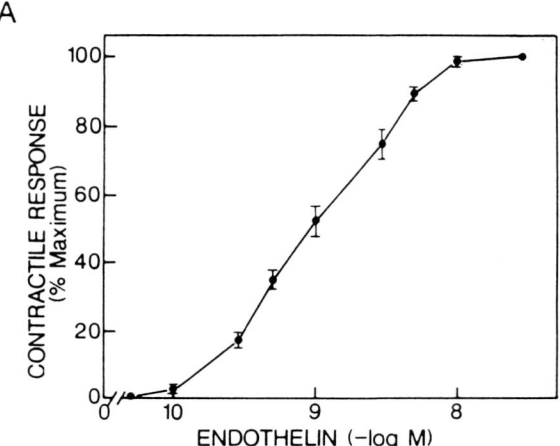

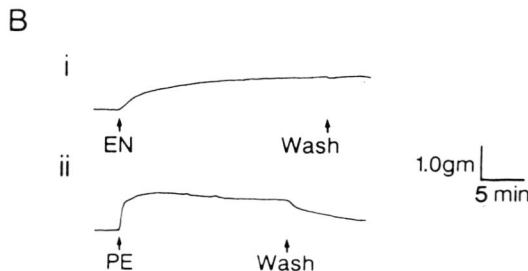

FIG. 4. Endothelin-stimulated contractile responses of rabbit aortic rings. **A:** Cumulative dose-response curve for endothelin-induced aortic contractile response (mean ± SEM). **B:** Contractile response of rabbit aortic rings to (i) 20 nM endothelin (EN) and (ii) 2 μm phenylephrine (PE) (From ref. 95, with permission.)

tration (EC_{50}) for the contractile response ranges from 0.2 to 5.0 nM, depending on the species and tissue source, making endothelin the most potent vasoconstrictor yet identified. The constrictor response is not limited to vascular smooth muscle and has been observed in several smooth muscle preparations. This portion of the chapter will analyze receptor characteristics and signal transduction pathways of endothelin.

Endothelin Receptors

Soon after the description of endothelin, numerous investigators demonstrated high-affinity endothelin binding in a wide variety of tissues and cell types. Binding is rapid, specific, and saturable, with K_d values (0.1–10.0 nM) in the range of the EC_{50} for the biological effects of endothelin (41,97,98). However, an unusual feature of this binding was the slow dissociation rate of the ligand-receptor complex, which is postulated to account, at least in part, for the long-acting nature of the peptide (93). Intravenous infusion of ^{125}I-endothelin identified enrichment of the isotope within the vasculature, as well as to nonvascular organs such as the kidney, brain, adrenal glands, intestine, and lung (41,99,100). In their original report, Yanagisawa et al. (6) speculated that endothelin might be a direct activator of voltage-dependent Ca^{2+} channels. However, labeled endothelin was not displaced by a variety of Ca^{2+} channel blockers, nor was it displaced by other vasoconstrictors such as norepinephrine, Ang II, or arginine vasopressin (AVP) (43,95,101–104). The presence of these binding sites, which were subsequently identified to be specific receptors on both vascular and nonvascular tissues, lends credence to the hypothesis that the endothelin family of peptides might serve multifunctional roles.

Several lines of evidence indicate that many vascular and nonvascular cells manifest multiple-receptor subtypes (see 41,97 for review). Specifically, a variety of cells express different affinity characteristics for the isoforms of endothelin (104–110). Cross-linking studies in brain membranes and mesangial cells identified multiple receptors on individual cells (111,112). In addition, several groups have subsequently cloned endothelin receptor subtype cDNAs from libraries prepared from rat and bovine lung mRNA (113,114), A10 vascular smooth muscle cells (115), and human liver (116) and placenta (117–119). These clones have suggested at least two distinct receptor subtypes, ET_A and ET_B; ET_A binds ET-1 > ET-2 > sarafotoxin $\gg$ ET-3, whereas the ET_B receptor binds all isoforms with equal affinity (114). When expressed in COS-7 cells, ET_A and ET_B have K_d values of 0.18 nM and 2 nM for ET-1, respectively (113,114). In transfected COS-7 cells, both endothelin and sarafotoxin binding increased inositol phosphate production and induced a transient increase in $[Ca^{2+}]_i$ (intracellular calcium) (113). The sequences of these proteins are similar to other G-protein-coupled receptors, with seven stretches of hydrophobic regions which are likely transmembrane-spanning regions, an extracellular N-terminus, and a cytoplasmic C-terminus (113) (Fig. 5). Northern blot analyses indicate that both receptors are widely expressed in vivo with considerable crossover, including brain, lung, kidney, heart, adrenal gland, intestine, and placenta (113,114,120–122). Two important exceptions include cultured human endothelial cells and human aortic smooth muscle cells. Human endothelial cells express ET_B, but not ET_A mRNA, suggesting that endothelin-induced stimulation of nitric oxide and prostacyclin production is mediated by ET_B receptors (120,121). By contrast, aortic smooth muscles express ET_A receptors with little or no detectable ET_B mRNA, suggesting that ET_A is the receptor most likely to modulate vascular smooth muscle tone (113). These findings are supported by in situ hybridization revealing ET_A is largely expressed in vascular smooth muscle, bronchial smooth muscle, myocardium, liver, and in the pituitary gland (122). Endothelin receptor subtype ET_B was not expressed in vascular smooth muscle, though it was

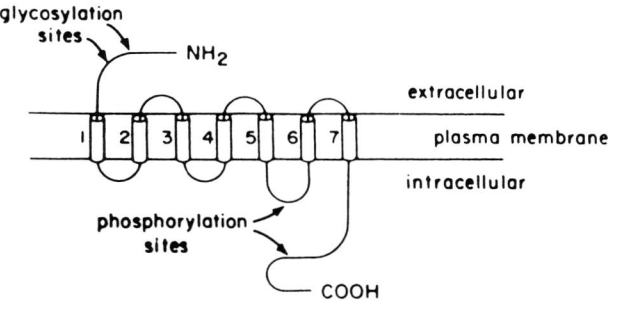

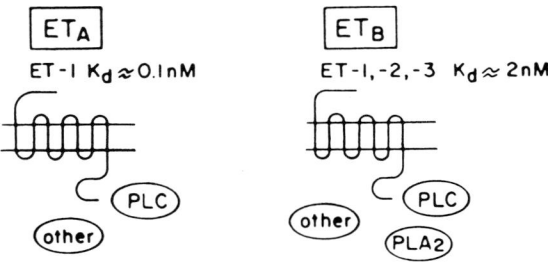

FIG. 5. Illustration of G-protein-coupled receptors. Note that there are 7 α-helical hydrophobic regions which are likely transmembrane-spanning domains similar. Receptor molecules are potentially coupled to various G-proteins, resulting in an array of cellular responses. ET_A, endothelin A receptor; ET_E, endothelin B receptor; PLC, phospholipase C; PLA_2, phospholipase A_2. (From ref. 41, with permission.)

prominently expressed in glial cells, choroid plexus, ependymal cells lining ventricles, atrial and ventricular myocardium, adrenal gland, kidney (see below), and colon (122). The similarity of the endothelin receptors to other G-protein-coupled receptors prompts the idea that the biological response to endothelin in a given cell relates to the interaction of the specific endothelin receptor subtype with various G-proteins, thereby stimulating an array of cell-specific signal transduction pathways (41). Indeed, there is evidence that endothelin receptors are linked to pertussis-toxin-sensitive and -insensitive G-proteins (41). In summary, there are at least two receptors for endothelin that are widely expressed in a tissue-specific fashion. Notably, vascular smooth muscle and endothelial cells express ET_A and ET_B receptors, respectively.

Signal Transduction Pathways

Endothelin-1 induces a rapid contractile response followed by a more sustained tonic phase in a variety of isolated arteries and veins. The response is slower in onset, more sustained, and more difficult to wash out than that induced by other vasoconstrictors (6,13,94–96). Despite these differences, binding of endothelin to its specific receptor initiates an array of cellular events which have many similarities to other vasoactive hormones such as Ang II, norepinephrine, and vasopressin (6,41,123). The receptors for endothelin and these vasoactive agents utilize various G-proteins to trigger a cellular response, the nature of which depends on the specific G-protein(s) and its effector protein (see Fig. 5). One such effector protein which is critical to inducing vascular smooth muscle contraction is phosphoinositide-specific phospholipase C (PLC), the activation of which ultimately leads to an increase in $[Ca^{2+}]_i$. Endothelin induces a dose-dependent, rapid increase in $[Ca^{2+}]_i$ followed by a sustained elevation in $[Ca^{2+}]_i$ in a variety of vascular smooth muscle preparations (Fig. 6) (6,95, 96,124–131). The magnitude of the rise in $[Ca^{2+}]_i$ and the time to peak elevation is concentration-dependent (95); Ca^{2+} signaling induced by endothelin is also observed in nonvascular smooth muscle cells, including endothelial cells (132), heart (133), mesangial cells (134–137), neural cells (138,139), anterior pituitary cells (140), epithelial cells (110), myometrium (141), and other peripheral muscle cells (142). It is now firmly established that endothelin leads to the mobilization of $[Ca^{2+}]_i$ stores

and to transmembrane flux of Ca^{2+} from the extracellular space (see 41,123 for review). Similar to Ang II, norepinephrine, and AVP, endothelin receptor occupation activates PLC, leading to the formation of water-soluble Ins 1,4,5-trisphosphate (1,4,5-P_3) and *sn* 1,2-diacylglycerol (DAG) (Fig. 7). In turn, Ins 1,4,5-P_3 binds to a high-affinity receptor on intracellular storage sites for Ca^{2+}, endoplasmic (or sarcoplasmic) reticulum leading to an increase in $[Ca^{2+}]_i$ (143,144). Indeed, the rapid, dose-dependent, and transient rise in vascular smooth muscle 1,4,5-P_3 is temporally related to the early changes in $[Ca^{2+}]_i$.

The sustained phase of increased $[Ca^{2+}]_i$ is longest for ET-1 and ET-2 and is believed to account, at least in part, for the prolonged actions of the peptides (135,145). With depletion of extracellular calcium, the initial spike in $[Ca^{2+}]_i$ persists; however, the return to baseline $[Ca^{2+}]_i$ is much more rapid (see Fig. 7). It is believed that this influx of calcium occurs through both voltage-sensitive and receptor-gated calcium channels. Evidence that more than one type of calcium channel is involved is

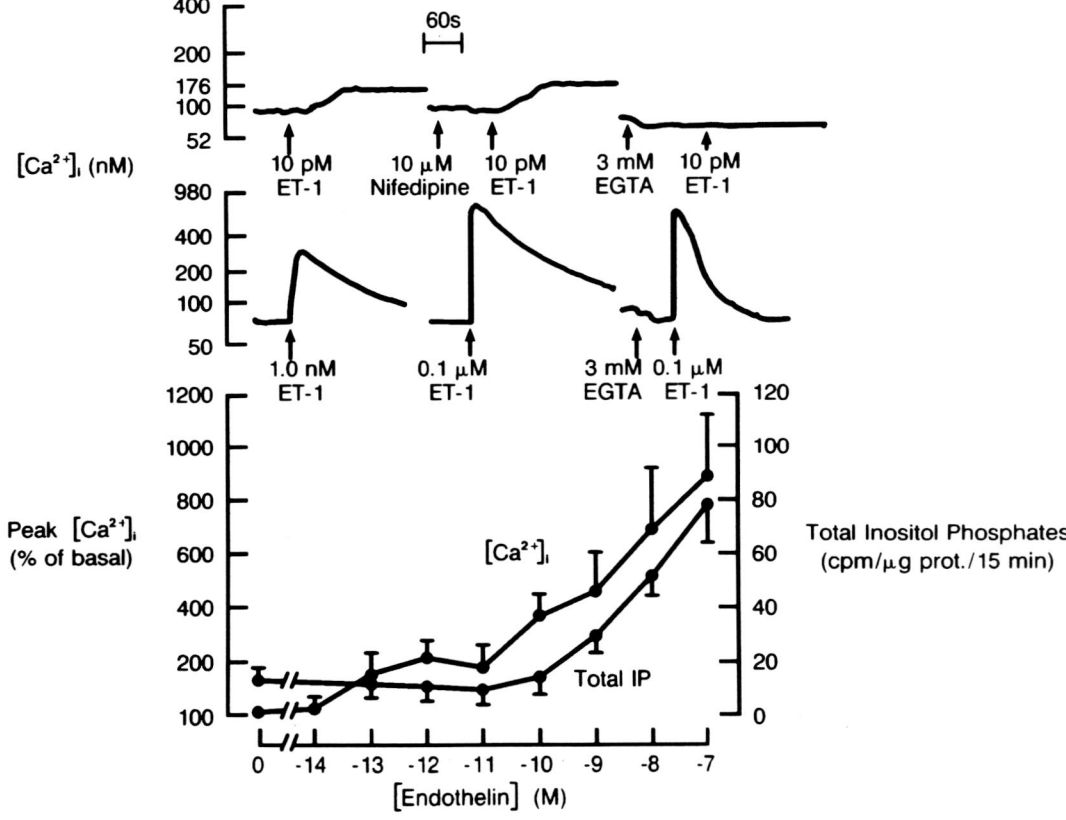

FIG. 6. Effects of ET-1 on cytosolic free Ca^{2+} and inositol phosphate (IP) turnover in mesangial cells. **A:** slow but sustained increase in Ca^{2+} at 10-pM ET-1. **B:** effect of 10-μM nifedipine. **C:** effect of 3.0-mM EGTA pretreatment in Ca^{2+}-free buffer at 10-pM ET-1. **D, E:** transient increase in Ca^{2+} observed at ≥1.0-nM ET-1. Ca^{2+} returned to baseline after 10–12 min. **F:** effect of 3.0-mM EGTA pretreatment at 0.1-μM ET-1. Ca^{2+} returned to baseline after 3.5–4.0 min. Bottom: dose dependence of peak Ca^{2+} and turnover of total inosital phosphates. Data are means ± SEM. $[Ca^{2+}]_i$, intracellular calcium concentration. (From ref. 137, with permission.)

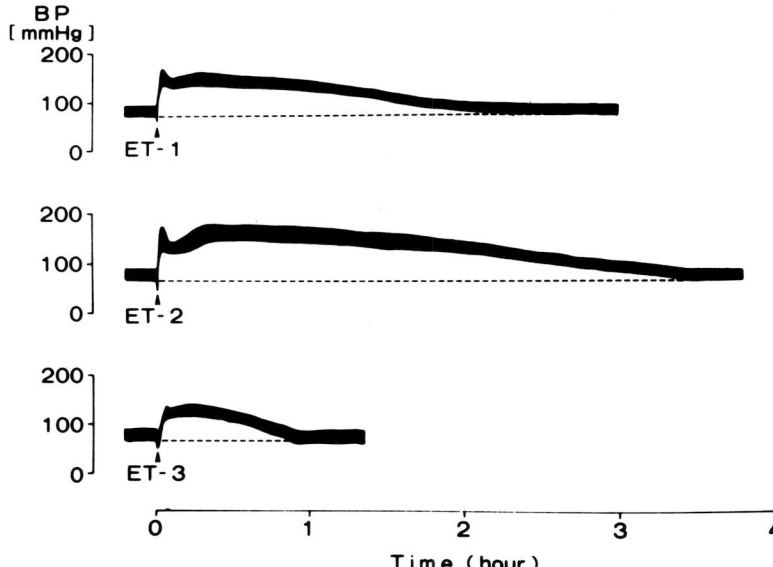

FIG. 7. Tracings of the systemic response to bolus endothelin isopeptides in anesthetized, chemically denervated rats. ET-1, endothelin-1; ET-2, endothelin-2; ET-3, endothelin-3; BP, blood pressure. (From ref. 7, with permission.)

partly derived from the effect of dihydropyridine or phenylalkylamine Ca^{2+} channel blockers, agents that block voltage-sensitive channels on endothelin-induced vasoconstriction and increases in $[Ca^{2+}]_i$. Depending on the experimental conditions, these agents either blunt or have no effect on the calcium influx and vasoconstriction induced by endothelin (see 41,123 for review). The inability of these agents to abrogate the influx provides indirect evidence that receptor-gated calcium channels are involved. Influx is also reduced by a specific inhibitor of this type of channel in NG108-15 cells (146). Stimulation of voltage-sensitive calcium channels most likely occurs by an indirect mechanism involving second messengers and membrane depolarization. Ca^{2+} channel ligands do not interfere with ^{125}I-endothelin binding to vascular smooth muscle, nor does endothelin modulate the binding of radiolabeled calcium-channel blockers (95,101,102,104,147,148). In addition, several patch-clamp studies indicate that endothelin increases Ca^{2+} channel activity of vascular smooth muscle cells in the cell-attached mode, providing evidence that signal transduction via second messengers is involved (125,149,150). In vascular smooth muscle cells, endothelin induces transient membrane hyperpolarization, followed by sustained depolarization, a known signal to open voltage-sensitive Ca^{2+} channels (101). In summary, the influx of calcium is due to opening of multiple channels, including receptor-gated and voltage-sensitive calcium channels and is only partially blocked by Ca^{2+} channel blockers. The reader is referred to several reviews for an in-depth analysis of the effects of endothelin on cellular calcium homeostasis (41,123).

Another potentially important cellular event induced by endothelin is the activation of protein kinase C. Endothelin-triggered hydrolysis of phosphatidylinositol

biphosphate (PIP_2) by PLC leads to biphasic increase of membrane-bound DAG, which in the presence of Ca^{2+} and neutral phospholipid activates protein kinase C (151). Endothelin increases in phosphorylation of protein kinase C in rat aortic vascular smooth muscle cells (152). Furthermore, endothelin leads to translocation of protein kinase C from the cytosol to the plasma membrane in bovine aortic vascular smooth muscle cells (153). Activation of protein kinase C might have several effects pertinent to the biological response to endothelin, including contributing to the sustained vasoconstriction, providing negative feedback for PLC activity, activating Na^{2+}-H^+ exchange, and contributing to the mitogenic effects. Phorbol esters, known stimulators of protein kinase C, induce sustained vasoconstriction of blood vessels similar to endothelin (154–156). The magnitude and duration of endothelin-induced vasoconstriction of rat and rabbit aortic rings are reduced by pretreatment with either staurosporine or H-7, selective inhibitors of protein kinase C (130,131,154,157). Furthermore, downregulation of protein kinase C by pretreating with phorbol 12,13-dibutyrate significantly attenuates the vasoconstriction induced by either endothelin or phorbol esters (152). These findings strongly suggest that protein kinase C activation plays an important role in the vasoconstrictor effects of endothelin. It is noteworthy that treatment of vascular smooth muscle cells with either Ang II or phorbol esters downregulates endothelin binding as well as decreases PLC activity and Ca^{2+} signaling (158,159). Thus, stimulation of protein kinase C might act as a negative feedback mechanism for endothelin. Protein kinase C activation by phorbol esters, endothelin, and a variety of other vasoconstrictors also activates Na^+-H^+ exchange, leading to cytosolic alkalinization in vascular smooth muscle cells (160–164). Alkalinization can be completely blocked by pretreatment with staurosporine, removal of external Na^{2+}, or treatment with an inhibitor of Na^+-H^+ antiport (5-N-ethylisopropyl-amiloride) (124). Finally, the mitogenic effects of endothelin have been postulated to be linked to protein kinase C activation (165,166).

Other potentially important cellular events include stimulation of phospholipase A_2 (PLA_2) and phospholipase D. Numerous studies have demonstrated an increase in phospholipase D activity in vascular smooth muscle cells treated with endothelin (167–170). The significance of this response is unclear; however, it might provide an alternate source of DAG by increasing phosphatidic acid (123,153,167). By contrast, stimulation PLA_2 leads to increased production of vasodilatory prostaglandins and thromboxane, the balance of which might alter the vasoactive properties of endothelin (145,170–176). The mechanism of PLA_2 stimulation has not been fully delineated. However, in transfected Chinese hamster ovary cells, both ET_A and ET_B receptors can activate this phospholipase (177). The relative production of vasodilatory and vasoconstrictor prostanoids is likely tissue-specific. ET-1-stimulated PLA_2 activity increased arachidonate release from mesangial cells as well as release of PGE_2 > PGI_2 > TXA_2 (145,176); whereas, in the rat aorta there is evidence that TXA_2 contributes to the vasoconstriction (178). For more information regarding the signal transduction pathways of endothelin the reader is referred to several excellent reviews.

Mitogenic Actions of Endothelin

Endothelin stimulates growth and proliferation in a variety of cell types, including vascular smooth muscle cells (179,180), endothelial cells (181,182), fibroblasts (166,183,184), glial cells (83), and mesangial cells (137,185). This property suggests a possible role of the peptide in vascular wall remodeling, wound healing, and proliferative glomerular diseases. With incorporation of ^{3}H-thymidine into quiescent cultures, vascular smooth muscle cells, as well as cell number, are increased in a dose-dependent fashion (179). However, stimulation of DNA synthesis is not potent as 10 percent fetal calf serum (179). Similar to Ang II, endothelin increases expression of several protooncogenes which have been implicated in the regulation of DNA transcription, including c-*myc*, c-*fos*, and c-*jun* (137,166,179,180,184, 186–188). It is noteworthy that there is differential expression of c-*fos* and c-*jun*, depending on either the stimulating endothelin isopeptide or the receptor subtype (188). For angiotensin II, this effect is believed to be related, at least in part, to the stimulation of autocrine growth factors, including platelet-derived growth factor (PDGF) and TGF-β (189). In human mesangial cells, endothelin stimulates PDGF A and B chains; thus, the mitogenic effects of endothelin might in part relate to release of other endogenous growth factors (185). It is intriguing that PDGF and TGF-β are both known stimuli for endothelin expression. The cellular mechanism by which endothelin induces these proliferative effects remains unclear, though several possibilities have been suggested (190,191).

ENDOTHELIN: LOCAL MEDIATOR OR CIRCULATING HORMONE?

Despite the tremendous volume of investigation, the question of whether endothelin functions as a circulating mediator or is predominantly an autocrine/paracrine factor in the control of vascular smooth muscle tone has not been resolved. A paracrine role for endothelin is strongly supported by the observation that in cultured human umbilical-vein endothelial cells, approximately 80 percent of endothelin production is secreted toward the basolateral side (192). Whether such polar secretion occurs in all vascular beds has not been established. Similar polarity is seen in cultured inner medullary collecting duct cells (193). Nevertheless, circulating endothelin could potentially be a marker of endothelial production, if not smooth-muscle-derived peptide. Several factors argue against a role for circulating endothelin as a modulator of vasomotor tone under normal circumstances. First, although numerous investigators have identified circulating levels of ET-1 of approximately 3 pg/mL in normal humans and other mammalian species, these levels are unlikely to elicit a physiologic response, as they are well below the estimated K_d for endothelin receptors (see 8 for review of plasma levels in health and disease). Levels of ET-3 are roughly one-third that of ET-1 and circulating ET-2 has not been detected. In addition, confluent human umbilical-vein endothelial cell monolayers grown on acellular amniotic membranes substantially impede the diffusion of mature endothelin, suggesting that circulating peptide may not have ready access to the underlying vascular smooth muscle (72). An important barrier effect is also supported by studies of isolated rabbit femoral artery and vein segments (194). Endothelin applied to the luminal and adventitial surface induced similar vasoconstriction when the endothelium was removed, whereas the vasoconstrictor effects of luminal-applied endothelin were abrogated by an intact endothelium (194). Although this suggests that the peptide had restricted access to the underlying vascular smooth muscle, endothelin might alternatively have triggered the endothelium to produce vasodilators that offset the vasoconstrictor effect (see below). Indeed, endothelin can trigger production of endothelium-derived relaxing factor (EDRF) (94).

Clearly, this barrier effect can be overcome *in vivo*, as intravenous infusion of pharmacologic doses of endothelin induces profound hypertension in a variety of species (195). However, lower doses sufficient to double circulating levels in dogs still lead to significant systemic and renal vasoconstriction in the absence of hypertension (196). In humans, exogenous ET-1 infusion had a mild pressor effect (approximately 3–5 mm Hg) at doses that increased circulating endothelin from 1.2 ± 0.3 pmol/L to 9.9 ± 7.6 pmol/L (197). Levels in this range have been observed in humans with congestive heart failure or acute renal failure, suggesting that under some circumstances circulating levels might have important hemodynamic effects. Although these infusion studies resulted in circulating levels in the range of those found in pathological conditions, one must consider the metabolic fate of infused endothelin. Using isotopic endothelin, the half-life of circulating peptide is brief (approximately 0.66–7 minutes) despite the prolonged pressor effects (198–200). Endothelin is removed from the circulation primarily by the lung > kidney > liver ≫ several other tissues (198–200). Further, degradation products of exogenous radiolabeled endothelin were not present up to 60 minutes following ^{125}I-ET-1 injection, suggesting that removal was mediated by receptor binding (198). Indeed, 93 percent of labeled ET-1 infused into isolated guinea pig lungs was associated with membranes and intracellular organelles (199). Removal of the peptide by passage through the pulmonary vasculature has been documented in humans and other species (85,94,199,201,202). Although it appears that receptor binding is a major source of removal of circulating endothelin, several enzymes have been identified which can metabolize the peptide. Similar to other peptides such as atrial natriuretic peptide (ANP), neutral endopeptidases (NEPs) such as NEP24.11 can metabolize endothelin (203). Due to the avid binding of infused endothelin to

its receptors and the prolonged physiologic response, infusion studies are unlikely to be useful models of *in vivo* pathological states despite achieving similar circulating levels.

IN VIVO ACTIONS OF EXOGENOUS ENDOTHELIN: SYSTEMIC RESPONSE

To date, knowledge of the physiologic effects of endothelin are based largely on studies that infuse the peptide into study animals or human subjects. Most of these studies use pharmacologic doses infused over a short period of time. As outlined above, it is likely that the peptide is secreted in a vectorial manner and the local concentration of endothelin remains unknown. Only recently have effective receptor antagonists become available. Thus, one must interpret infusion studies with caution. Nevertheless, these data help to define the range of potential biological effects.

Systemic Vasodilatory Response

Bolus intravenous infusion of subnanomolar quantities of ET-1 induces transient hypotension, followed by a sustained hypertensive response in a wide variety of species (Fig. 8) (6,7,13,94,204–219). *In vivo*, the depressor effects of ET-3 are more prominent than for ET-1 (7). In the anesthetized rat, the fall in blood pressure is due to a dose-dependent peripheral vasodilatory effect, since cardiac index (CI) does not decrease during this period (205). Anesthetized cats and dogs show a similar peripheral vasodilation, although cardiac output rises significantly in this early phase (206,215). In conscious rats, the hypotensive response triggers an appropriate baroreflex

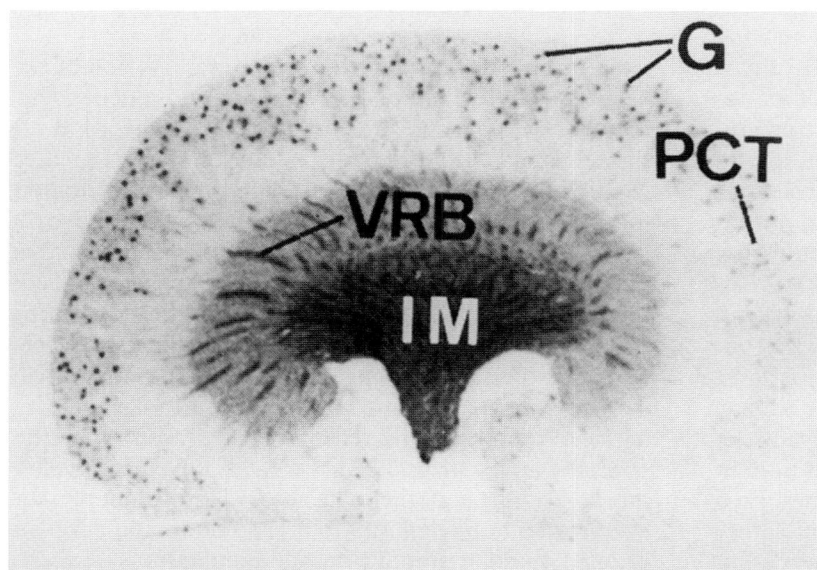

FIG. 8. Autoradiograph of ^{125}I endothelin-1 binding in the rat kidney. G, glomeruli; PCT, proximal convoluted tubules; VRB, *vasa recta* bundles; IM, inner medulla. (From ref. 241, with permission.)

response consisting of an increase in efferent sympathetic nerve activity, tachycardia, and an increase in cardiac output (210,215,218). Autonomic blockade with atenolol and methscopolamine abrogates the reflex tachycardia, though a mild increase in cardiac output persists, suggesting a positive inotropic effect (see below) (218). There are significant regional differences in the vasodilatory response. Endothelin consistently decreases vascular resistance in the hindlimb of both conscious and anesthetized animals (208,210,215,218,220–222). In anesthetized pigs and cats, carotid and bronchial blood flow are increased in the early phase (208,210,217, 221). In the renal and mesenteric vascular beds, the vasodilatory responses are much less apparent with most *in vivo* infusion studies finding immediate vasoconstriction (210,218,220,221). Nevertheless, a biphasic response of renal blood flow has been reported by several groups (216,223,224).

Several factors are likely to contribute to this vasodilatory response and regional variation. Endothelin induces vasorelaxation of isolated perfused mesenteric arteries when applied to the luminal, but not the extraluminal, surface (225). Endothelin stimulates dose-dependent release of the vasodilator, EDRF, from isolated perfused rat mesentery and luminally perfused rabbit aorta; an effect which is obliterated by removal of endothelial cells or concurrent infusion of oxyhemoglobin (94). A role for EDRF production is further supported by studies using analogues of L-Arg that competitively antagonize the conversion of L-Arg to nitric oxide. With EDRF synthesis blockade, the hypotensive effects of endothelin infusion were markedly attenuated (226). These agents also inhibited the vasodilatory effect of ET-3 in isolated perfused mesentery (227). Endothelin-1 and ET-3 both induce vasodilation in isolated perfused mesentery preconstricted with methoxamine, at doses 100-fold less than those required for vasoconstriction (228). With increasing doses the vasodilating effects persist for ET-3, whereas ET-1 induces only vasoconstriction. Thus, the hemodynamic effect of endogenous endothelin in a particular vascular bed might relate to several factors, including the specific isopeptide produced and the magnitude of production. In addition, the distribution of endothelin receptor subtypes is likely to play a role. Endothelial cells, a major source of both EDRF and prostacyclin (PGI_2), express exclusively the ET_B receptors that have equal affinity to ET-1 and ET-3 (see above). Endothelial cells produce only ET-1, suggesting a possible autocrine feedback loop that might attenuate the vasoconstrictive effects of the peptide. Under certain conditions, endothelium production of EDRF might modulate the hemodynamic effects of vascular smooth-muscle-derived endothelin production in a paracrine fashion. In tissues that express ET-3 in substantial quantities, such as the gut, brain, and inner medulla, the vasodilatory effects may predominate, as ET-3 has much lower affinity for ET_A receptors on vascular smooth muscle cells. Finally, as discussed above, inhibition of EDRF production by analogues of L-Arg or inhibition of soluble guanylyl cyclase augment thrombin-stimulated endothelin production in porcine aorta, but not basal production (229). In these studies, 8-bromo cyclic guanosine monophosphate (cGMP), a nonhydrolyzable analogue of cGMP, also reduced thrombin-induced endothelin production, supporting a role for this second messenger in the feedback response.

As discussed above, endothelin leads to activation of PLA_2, and thus increases intracellular arachidonate, the substrate for prostanoid production (99,171–176,178). In isolated perfused rat lungs, ET-1 induced a sustained release of $PGI_2 \gg TXA_2$, whereas production was similar in guinea pigs (94). A similar predominance of vasodilatory prostanoid production was observed in isolated perfused rabbit kidney and spleen (230). In these studies, perfusion pressures in the isolated organs were increased by cyclooxygenase inhibitors supporting prostanoid production that resulted in a net vasodilatory response. In untreated dogs, endothelin infusion led to an increase in plasma 6-keto PGF_{1a} (231). In these studies, the hypotensive response to exogenous ET-1 was markedly reduced by pretreatment with acetylsalicylic acid. Blunting of the hypotensive effects by cyclooxygenase inhibitors has also been observed in the spontaneously hypertensive rat (SHR) (232). Most investigators have noted a persistent hypotensive response despite inhibition of prostanoid production, supporting a role for other factors such as EDRF (94,207). Nevertheless, pretreatment with indomethacin and piroxicam (Feldene) potentiates the pressor response, suggesting that like EDRF, vasodilatory prostanoids might modulate the hemodynamic actions of endothelin *in vivo* (94,207).

Systemic Vasoconstrictor Response

Following the vasodepressor response, infusion of exogenous endothelin induces a sustained, dose-dependent pressor response in a variety of species (see Fig. 8). Both the hypotensive and hypertensive responses are greater when the peptide is infused intraarterially as compared to intravenously (94). Isolated perfused lungs remove 60 percent of the peptide in a single pass, suggesting that this differential effect is due to pulmonary clearance. Indeed, the half-life of circulating endothelin is brief (1–7 minutes), suggesting that the prolonged effects are due to persistent binding and activation of vascular smooth muscle cells (see above). In general, the relative molar potency of the isopeptides *in vivo* reflects that observed in porcine coronary artery strips, ET-1 > ET-2 ≫ ET-3 (7). The 39-amino-acid big endothelin has nearly equivalent pressor effects despite having 100-fold less contractile effect in isolated vascular smooth muscle preparations, suggesting that there is substantial intravascular conversion of this precursor peptide (44). A variety of endopeptidases including chymotrypsin, aspartic proteases, and neutral endopeptidases are capable of converting the precursor peptide (see above). In the anesthetized rat, the hypertensive response to a bolus dose lasts up to 60–90 minutes with an LD_{50} of approximately 450 pmol (6,7,204). As with the magnitude of the pressor response, the duration of response is markedly less with ET-3 than ET-1 or ET-2 (see Fig. 8) (7). Endothelin induces hypertension primarily by increasing peripheral vascular resistance, an effect which has been confirmed in numerous species including in the forearm of humans (205,209,211,233). Indeed, with pharmacologic doses, the pressor effect persists despite a reduction in cardiac output indicative of extreme peripheral vasoconstriction. Mild bradycardia is commonly observed with systemic endothelin infusion (205,210,212,220,234).

The pressor effects are slightly less potent than that observed with Ang II, and yet endothelin has similar regional selectivity in its vasoconstrictor effects (125,205, 211). The renal, mesenteric, and peripheral muscle vascular beds account for the majority of the increase in vascular resistance, whereas the pulmonary bed is less sensitive (224,235). In one study using labeled microspheres, intravenous ET-1 led to pulmonary vasodilation despite peripheral vasoconstriction, an effect not blocked by indomethacin, suggesting a role for EDRF in this response (235). Indeed, endothelin-induced production of EDRF in the pulmonary vasculature has been documented in isolated perfused lung preparations (94).

The potency of endothelin in conscious rats can be enhanced by pretreatment with chlorisondamine, methscopolamine, captopril (Capoten), and $d(CH_2)_5$-Tyr(Me)AVP, suggesting that endothelin triggers a neurohumoral response (214). However, the interaction of endothelin and other neurohumoral systems such as the sympathetic nervous system remains unclear. In conscious dogs, the pressor response to endothelin is blunted by ganglionic blockade (hexamethonium and atropine), an effect not seen in the conscious rats (pentolinium and atropine) (206,211,215). In the conscious rats, the bradycardia induced by endothelin is similar to that induced by equipressor doses of norepinephrine and is attenuated by simultaneous cholinergic and ganglionic blockade (215). Whereas in chloralose-anesthetized rats, a robust pressor response ($+53 \pm 5.4$ mm Hg) is associated with a fall in renal nerve sympathetic nerve activity (-46.4 ± 12.7 percent) (215). Taken together, these data suggest that the baroreflexes remain grossly intact in the endothelin-treated rat. Nevertheless, a potentially important interaction of endothelin and the sympathetic nervous system is suggested by the dose-dependent pressor response to intracerebroventricular injections of endothelin observed in conscious rats (236). The response is blunted by pretreatment with phenoxybenzamine and is associated with increased plasma levels of epinephrine and norepinephrine. Clearly the central nervous system has abundant endothelin receptors and endothelin-producing cells, suggesting that this stimulation of sympathetic outflow might have physiologic significance (see below). This possibility is supported by increased plasma endothelin levels in conditions known to have increased sympathetic tone, such as congestive heart failure or hepatorenal syndrome (8).

Binding of endothelin to its receptor triggers a rapid increase in cytosolic Ca^{2+}, followed by a slow influx of extracellular calcium. The prolonged contraction is dependent on this influx and is thus blunted when extracellular Ca^{2+} is low (see above). Dihydropyridine Ca^{2+} channel antagonists have minimal effects on the rapid phase of the pressor response, though markedly lessen the prolonged phase of vasoconstriction (207,222,237). Similarly, verapamil and manganese blunt the pressor response (238). These studies suggest that in vivo vasoconstriction is, at least in part, due to influx of Ca^{2+} through voltage-dependent dihydropyridine-sensitive Ca^{2+} channels.

ENDOTHELIN AND THE KIDNEY

Since the discovery of endothelin there has been intense investigation of its role in the modulation of renal hemodynamics, sodium, and water handling. This vascular bed is distinguished by the unusual interposition of the glomerular capillary bed between two resistance vessels, the afferent and efferent arterioles (239). Adjustments of the relative resistance of the pre- and postglomerular resistance allows the kidney to modulate glomerular capillary hydraulic pressure and glomerular capillary plasma flow rate and thus maintain filtration over a wide range of renal perfusion pressures. The arterioles and tubules are highly sensitive to a variety of circulating mediators such as Ang II, norepinephrine, and ANP (240). In addition, many of the glomerular cells are capable of synthesizing several of these mediators as well as others and may thus alter renal function in the absence of changes in systemic hemodynamics. Endothelin shares many of the characteristics associated with known endogenous modulators of renal function. The kidney is one of the richest sources of both ET_A and ET_B receptors that reside primarily in the glomeruli and inner medulla. Second, glomerular endothelial cells, mesangial cells, and several renal epithelial cells are capable of synthesizing the peptide. Third, endothelin triggers a robust physiologic effect in the arterioles, mesangial cells, and epithelial cells. Finally, the kidney is a rich source of neutral endopeptidases and might thus serve as an important organ for metabolism of either big endothelin or mature endothelin.

Renal Endothelin Receptors

Autoradiographic studies of a variety of species including humans reveal intense binding of ^{125}I-endothelin in the region of the glomeruli, the vasa recta bundles, and the inner medulla, with lesser binding over proximal tubules (Fig. 9) (97,241–245). As discussed above, this binding is highly specific and nearly irreversible (<10 percent bound ^{125}I displaced by excess unlabeled ET-1 at 24 hours) (243). Saturation binding isotherms of both rat and human sections indicate K_d values (0.4–0.7 nM) in the range where renal physiologic effects are observed (241). Although the pattern of staining is similar to Ang II and ANP, labeled endothelin is not displaced by these peptides, arginine vasopressin, or norepinephrine (241). Similar to vascular smooth muscle cells, binding is also not blocked by L-type voltage-dependent Ca^{2+} channel blockers (241). The pattern of binding sites is similar for the three isopeptides, suggesting that there are both ET_A and ET_B receptors (246).

The presence of multiple receptors in glomerular and renal epithelial cells is supported by equilibrium binding studies, as well as northern analysis for ET_A and ET_B mRNA. Binding studies have been performed using crude membranes derived from kidney glomeruli and papillae (247), epithelial cell lines derived from renal epithelium (248), and most extensively with mesangial cells (112,249,250). Scatchard analyses of endothelin binding to mesangial cell membranes were not uniformly linear, suggesting two receptors with different affinities (112,249). Using displacement studies, two distinct receptors were identified with apparent molecular masses of 60 and 73 kDa (112). Affinity labeling of the 73-kDa receptor by ^{125}I-ET-1 was inhibited by ET-1 but not ET-3, whereas labeling of the 60-kDa receptor was inhibited competitively by all three isopeptides. Indeed, northern blot analysis of rat renal cortex indicates steady state mRNA levels for both ET_A and ET_B receptors (113–115,122). Localization of receptor subtypes by *in situ* hybridization reveal ET_A mRNA in the renal vasculature, including the large vessels and more prominently in the afferent and efferent arterioles (122). By contrast, ET_B was expressed primarily in glomerular endothelial cells, vasa recta bundles, and epithelial cells of thin segments of the Henle's loop, with little or no hybridization signal over epithelial cells of the collecting duct. Using a sensitive technique that couples polymerase chain reaction to reverse transcription on single microdissected renal tubules, ET_A receptor was detected in glomeruli, vasa recta, and arcuate arteries, whereas none was detected in the tubules (251). By contrast, ET_B was widely detected in glomeruli and terminal inner medullary collecting duct (IMCD) > initial IMCD > outer MCD > medullary thick ascending limb (251). Notably, there was no significant ET_A or ET_B amplification products detected in the proximal tubule, a finding which is corroborated by only modest levels of binding by autoradiography (241,245,251). These studies also do not detect substantial receptor expression in mesangial cells, despite the well-characterized binding sites and the robust increase in intracellular free calcium in response to endothelin.

Overall, these studies indicate that the kidney has abundant ET_A and ET_B receptors and is thus likely to be an important target organ for both ET-1 and ET-3. The distribution of the ET_A receptors predominantly on the pre- and postglomerular resistance vessels suggest that the renal vasoconstriction induced by exogenous endothelin is likely secondary to ET_A receptor occupancy. However, the prominent ET_B receptors located on the glomerular endothelial cells raise the possibility that the predominant effect of locally produced endothelin (within the glomerulus) might be production of EDRF or PGI_2. Indeed, intact rat glomeruli treated with endothelin isopeptides increase glomerular cGMP, an effect that is inhibited by an L-arginine analogue N^W-nitro-L-arginine (252). This response strongly suggests ET_B activation as it occurs with both ET-1 and ET-3 and is not inhibitable by BQ-123, a specific ET_A antagonist. Renal

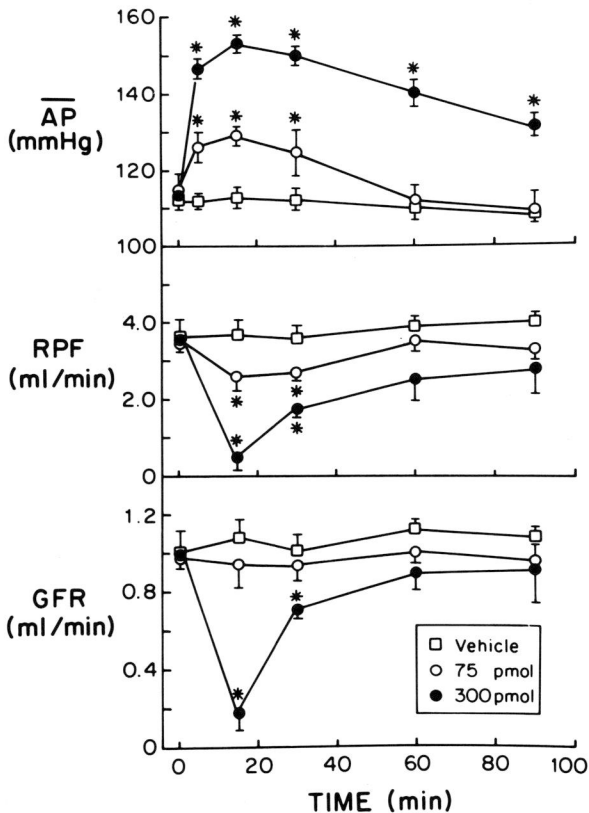

FIG. 9. Time course of mean arterial pressure (AP), renal plasma flow rate (RPF), and glomerular filtration rate (GFR) after a single bolus of ET-1. Note that maximal effect occurs within 15–20 min and that duration of response is sustained. Values are means ± SEM. *$p < 0.05$ vs. baseline; n = 4–5 per dose. (From ref. 204, with permission.)

epithelial cells express exclusively ET_B and, thus, the tubular effects might be mediated by either ET-1 or ET-3.

Renal Production of Endothelin Isopeptides

Several lines of evidence indicate that the kidney is likely to be a prominent source of endogenous endothelin production. First, using northern analysis and polymerase chain reaction, mRNA for ET-1 and ET-3 have been detected in the kidneys of rats and pigs (92,244,253–255). Endothelin-3 is more abundantly expressed than ET-1, and ET-2 is not expressed (92). *In situ* hybridization indicates localization to small blood vessels (arcuate and interlobular arteries) with no apparent hybridization in the capillaries or renal tubules (253). Using the reverse transcription and PCR technique in dissected rat nephron segments, ET-1 is found in glomeruli and IMCD with little or no PCR product observed in proximal tubules or thick ascending limbs (255). Mature ET-1 production by these segments followed the same pattern and was significantly stimulated by fetal calf serum and TGF-β. Studies using immunostaining techniques do not provide the exact cellular source of endothelin, and yet it provides some insight into the distribution of the peptide within the kidney. In normal rat kidneys, endothelin-like immunoreactivity was identified in the renal cortex, medulla, and papilla: the highest density localized primarily to vasa recta (256). In general, staining was restricted to the vascular components including the glomerular capillary. Only focal staining was observed in collecting duct cells and early proximal tubule brush border (256).

Endothelin is expressed and produced *in vitro* in several cultured renal cell models. Each of the primary cells within the glomerular capsule is capable of synthesizing endothelin. Cultured bovine glomerular endothelial cells express a 2.3-kb preproendothelin-1 mRNA which is enhanced by co-incubation with agonists known to increase glomerular endothelial cytosolic free calcium such as bradykinin, thrombin, adenosine triphosphate (ATP), and platelet-activating factor (257). Under basal conditions glomerular endothelial cells were shown to release ET-1 in a time-dependent fashion, a response which was enhanced markedly by co-incubation with bradykinin (257). Several investigators have observed low-level constitutive expression, synthesis, and release of ET-1 from cultured mesangial cells (40,75,77,78). Of note, this expression can be stimulated by a variety of factors potentially important to the pathogenesis of acute glomerulonephritis, including thrombin, TGF-β, and a thromboxane A_2 analogue (U-46619) (40). Other factors that stimulate mesangial production include AVP, fetal bovine serum, PDGF, and phorbol ester; notably, interleukin-1β does not (75,77). By contrast, maneuvers that increase mesangial intracellular cyclic adenosine

monophosphate (cAMP) inhibit serum-stimulated ET-1 production, including isoproterenol, forskolin, or 8-bromo-cyclic AMP (78). Most recently, production of ET-1 has been observed in cultured rat glomerular epithelial cells, the magnitude of which exceeds that of cultured mesangial cells (258). Similar to the mesangial cells, there was stimulation by TGF-β, complement C5b-9, thrombin, and phorbol esters. Thus, each of the major cell types comprising the glomerular tuft is capable of synthesizing endothelin in cell culture, particularly when exposed to inflammatory mediators, growth factors, or thrombin.

Renal epithelial cell lines derived from several species including MDCK, $LLCPK_1$, RK_{13}, BHK-21, COS-7, and NRK-52E have also been shown to release ET-1 in a time-dependent fashion (37,80–82). Cultures of renal epithelial cells derived from each segment of the nephron release ET-3 $\gg$ ET-1 (259). For ET-3 the relative production is IMCD > MTAL = PT = CCT: for ET-1, IMCD > MTAL > CCT $\gg$ PT. It is noteworthy that cultured IMCD cells exhibit polarized secretion of endothelin toward the basolateral side having potential effects on the juxtaposed vasa recta or autocrine effects (193). In addition, endothelin receptors on these cells are primarily located on the basolateral side, suggesting possible autocrine regulation of IMCD function by endothelin. Several inflammatory mediators including tumor necrosis factor, and interleukin-1β, as well as thrombin and TGF-β, stimulate LLCPK cells to produce ET-1, which suggests a possible role for local endothelin production in interstitial nephritis (37). Techniques assessing mRNA levels in normal animals do not indicate substantial epithelial cell transcription. Thus, it is unclear whether under normal conditions these cells produce endothelin *in vivo*. Potentially, the conditions required to maintain cell viability in culture such as fetal serum and/or growth factors also stimulate the cells to produce endothelin *in vitro*.

Finally, the high concentration of endothelin in the urine, and under certain circumstances in the renal vein, suggest that the kidney is capable of substantial synthesis. Urinary concentrations of endothelin in normals are roughly 6–7 times that observed in plasma (86,260). Second only to the lung, the kidney is an important organ for clearance of infused endothelin (94,199,261). It is unclear to which this is due to receptor binding or degradation by neutral endopeptidases. However, the presence of abundant neutral endopeptidases in the proximal tubule make it less likely that urinary endothelin is derived exclusively from the plasma. Under normal circumstances there is little or no increase in endothelin concentrations in the renal vein, suggesting that the kidney is not generating substantial quantities of circulating endothelin. However, in cyclosporine-treated rats there is a substantial step-up of endothelin production across the renal vascular bed (see below) (262).

In summary, the synthetic capacity of the renal vasculature, the cells comprising the glomerulus, and the renal epithelium suggest that the kidney is potentially a rich source of endothelin. Many of these cells have abundant endothelin receptors which induce a physiologic response when occupied. Taken together, these findings suggest that locally generated endothelin might have important autocrine and paracrine effects on renal hemodynamics and tubular function.

Effects of Endothelin on Whole-Kidney Hemodynamic Response

The renal vasculature is exquisitely sensitive to the infusion of exogenous endothelin. Although several investigators have noted a transient renal vasodilatory response *in vivo,* this vasodilation is more brief and less profound than that observed in other vascular beds (208,216,238,263–265). This may be due to the relatively high permeability of renal vascular endothelium, allowing for better access of the peptide to the VSM. Transient renal hyperemia is observed in dogs with intrarenal artery infusion of ET-1 in the absence of systemic effects, supporting local production of vasodilators (266,267). Indomethacin pretreatment abrogated the vasodilatory response and enhanced the subsequent vasoconstriction, supporting a role for vasodilatory prostaglandins. By contrast, ET-3 infusion induces mild renal vasodilation at low doses and at high dose is much less potent a renal vasoconstrictor (268).

As with the systemic response, exogenous ET-1 induces profound renal vasoconstriction in a variety of species (204,233,249,263,266,269–275). In the anesthetized rat, ET-1 intravenous infusion leads to dose-dependent, long-lasting reductions in renal plasma-flow (RPF) rate (Fig. 10) (204). In isolated perfused rabbit kidneys, the renal vasoconstriction is much longer-lasting, and nearly 30 and 500 times more potent than Ang II and norepinephrine, respectively (273). In awake rats, intravenous ET-1 was less potent a renal vasoconstrictor than Ang II, and yet the duration of effect is substantially longer (276). Most of the intravenous studies have utilized pharmacologic doses of endothelin, leading to changes in systemic hemodynamics; doses that also trigger several neurohormonal systems with known renal vasoactive effects including the renin-angiotensin axis, the sympathetic nervous system, and ANP release (212,233,264). However, in dogs, intravenous infusion of ET-1 sufficient to double circulating concentrations leads to a reduction in renal blood flow rate without a change in glomerular filtration rate (GFR), plasma renin activity, or ANP levels (196). An important local vasoconstrictor effect is confirmed in rats and dogs by intrarenal artery infusion studies (without systemic effects) (265,272,277–279) and in isolated perfused kidney preparations (270,273,280–282). In anesthetized dogs, intrarenal infusion of ET-1 led to a proportionately greater reduction in cortical blood flow than medullary blood flow rate, suggesting differences in regional sensitivity within the kidney (263).

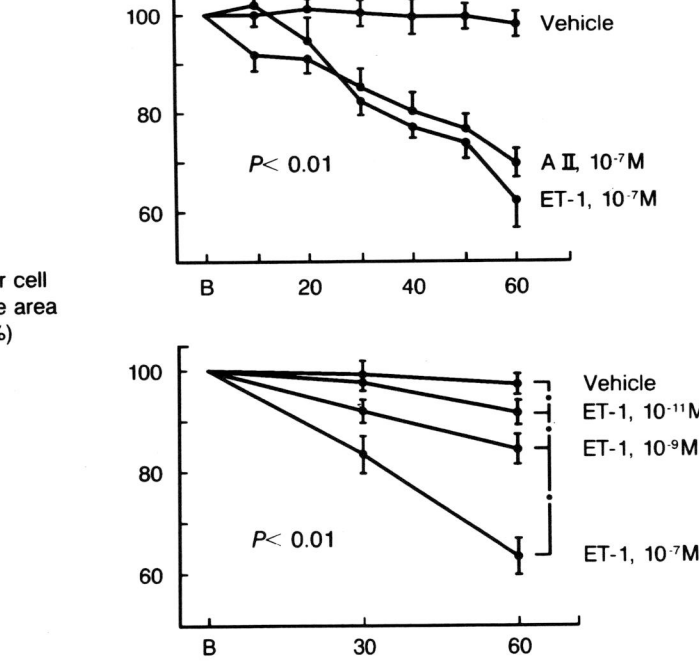

FIG. 10. **Top:** time course of changes in mesangial cell planar cell surface area in response to endothelin-1 (ET-1), angiotensin II (AII), or vehicle. **Bottom:** dose-dependent studies of endothelin-1-induced mesangial contraction. (Adapted from ref. 298.)

Exogenous endothelin also leads to dose-dependent reduction in GFR in dogs, rats, pigs, and rabbits. In the anesthetized rat, lower bolus doses of ET-1 (75 pmol) lead to a proportionately greater decline in RPF rate than GFR; thus, filtration fraction increases (see Fig. 10) (204). Higher doses lead to parallel declines in RPF and GFR. Other studies in dogs and rats that infused ET-1 into the renal artery *in vivo* and into isolated kidney preparations note parallel effects on RPF and GFR (265,266,270,272). The discrepancy is likely related to the magnitude of hypertension and the extent to which other renal vasoactive systems are activated. Indeed, the reduction in RPF and GFR following intravenous ET-1 are partially offset by the rise in renal perfusion pressure (204).

The response to exogenous endothelin can be modified by several maneuvers. As discussed above, pretreatment with either aspirin or indomethacin potentiates the vasoconstriction in anesthetized dogs, suggesting that, like Ang II, endothelin triggers the production of vasodilatory prostanoids that partially offset the vasoactive effects (266,283,284). Intrarenal infusion of ET-1 in dogs markedly increases renal 6-ketoprostaglandin F_{1a} production without stimulating renal renin release or norepinephrine output (266). In the isolated perfused rabbit kidney, perfusion pressure was increased by endothelin infusion concurrent with an increase in effluent PGI_2 > PGE_2, whereas TXA_2 production did not change (230). Taken together, these findings suggest direct stimulation of renal vasodilation which offset the vasoactive effects of endothelin. Others have failed to observe this potentiating effect in rats pretreated with either indomethacin or meclofenamate (285). The reason for this discrepancy is unclear, though it might relate to species differences. In the isolated perfused rabbit kidney, co-infusion with methylene blue or oxyhemaglobin only slightly enhanced the vasoconstrictor effects of endothelin, suggesting minimal stimulation of EDRF release (273). This occurred despite the presence of abundant ET_B receptors within the glomerulus (see above). Indeed, evidence of stimulation of glomerular ET_B receptors is observed in intact glomeruli where cGMP production markedly increases when stimulated by all three isopeptides (286). This effect was totally inhibited by L^W-nitro-L-arginine, but not by BQ-123 (an ET_A receptor antagonist). In summary, inhibition of renal prostanoid and, to a lesser extent, EDRF production can potentiate the renal hemodynamic actions of endothelin.

By contrast, several maneuvers can attenuate the renal hemodynamic effects of endothelin. In keeping with the finding that L-type voltage-dependent Ca^{2+} channels are responsible, at least in part, for the sustained contractile response in vascular smooth muscle preparations, several investigators have noted that Ca^{2+} channel blockers blunt the renal vasoconstriction of exogenous endothelin (276). Co-infusion of a dihydropyridine, nicardipine,

with endothelin into rat renal arteries substantially lessened the reduction in RPF rate and GFR (272). Similar findings have been noted with nifedipine in the awake rat (intravenous infusion) and in isolated perfused rat kidneys (271,276). By contrast, in anesthetized dogs and rats, verapamil and manganese blocked ET-1-induced hypertension, but failed to blunt the renal vasoconstriction (238). Co-infusion of pharmacologic doses of ANP also blunts the systemic and renal effects of endothelin (269,272). Although ET-1 is a potent secretagogue of ANP (68,287,288), it is unclear whether ANP exerts a counter-regulatory influence *in vivo* (212,233,264,272). Finally, there is one report that inhibitors of platelet-activating factor inhibit ET-induced renal hemodynamic effects and mesangial contraction (289).

In summary, several endogenous factors appear to modulate the renal effects of endothelin, and yet a role for endothelin in the regulation of renal hemodynamics has yet to be established. Of note, infusion of antiendothelin antibody or specific endothelin-receptor antagonists into normal animals fails to alter either blood pressure, GFR, or RPF rate, suggesting basal endothelin is not a modulator of systemic or renal hemodynamics under normal physiologic conditions (290–293).

Effects of Endothelin on Glomerular Hemodynamics

As predicted from the whole kidney responses, endothelin has striking effects on the primary determinants of glomerular filtration. Several techniques have been employed to examine the potential effects of endothelin on the individual determinants of single-nephron GFR (SNGFR). Micropuncture studies in Munich Wistar rats indicate that both the pre- and postglomerular resistance vessels contract in response to intravenous and intrarenal artery infusion of ET-1 (134,204,294,295). Continuous intravenous infusion of mildly pressor doses of endothelin lead to a proportionately greater constriction of the efferent arteriole as compared to vehicle-infused rats and, thus, glomerular capillary hydraulic pressure (P_{GC}) is higher (204). Offsetting this profiltration force, the glomerular capillary ultrafiltration coefficient (K_f) is lowered and, thus, SNGFR is similar to vehicle. An increase in P_{GC} has been noted by other laboratories that was abrogated by pretreatment with ibuprofen, raising the possibility that glomerular prostanoid production might play a role in the efferent vasoconstriction (295). In response to high-dose endothelin, isolated glomeruli produce PGF_{2a} and PGF_2 in a 3:2 ratio (295). With bolus intravenous infusions of higher doses, afferent and efferent arteriolar resistances increase roughly proportionately with no change in P_{GC} (134). These studies demonstrate a significant reduction in SNGFR due to a fall in single-nephron plasma flow rate (Q_A) and a marked reduction in K_f. Whether the effect on K_f represents a reduction in glomerular capillary surface area or a reduction in the hydraulic permeability remains unknown (see below). Finally, infusion directly into the renal artery reduces SNGFR by lowering both Q_A and P_{GC} without affecting K_f (294). The relative sensitivity of the afferent and efferent arterioles to endothelin differed among these studies, as reflected by differences in the measured P_{GC}. These discrepancies likely reflect differing doses and modes of delivery, the magnitude of systemic effects, and the variable stimulation of other renal modulators. Indeed, a dose-dependent effect on P_{GC} was noted with intrarenal infusion in dogs with no change at low doses, despite a 23 percent reduction in renal blood flow rate and a significant reduction in P_{GC} at higher doses (279).

Studies of isolated perfused rat renal arterioles indicate the EC_{50} of ET-1 was significantly less for efferent arterioles than afferent arterioles (295,296). These effects are not altered by captopril or saralasin, arguing against a role for locally produced Ang II (296). In isolated rabbit arterioles, relative constrictive effect on the arterioles is ET-1 = ET-2 ≫ ET-3 with similar EC_{50} for constriction of afferent and efferent arterioles (286). However, these studies indicate that the EC_{50} for afferent arteriolar constriction was substantially increased in the presence of nicardipine or verapamil, whereas the sensitivity of the efferent arteriole was unchanged by either. This finding suggests that the vasoconstrictive effects on the afferent arteriole are dependent, at least in part, on the influx of extracellular calcium through voltage-dependent channels, whereas efferent constriction depends either on $[Ca^{2+}]_i$ stores or an alternative channel. This discrepancy in the relative effects of dihydropyridines is also evident in the isolated perfused hydronephrotic rat kidney where endothelin induced predominant afferent arteriolar constriction (271).

These studies must be interpreted with caution as the doses employed are likely to be pharmacologic. In general, the physiologic effects of exogenous endothelin are in keeping with the distribution of endothelin receptors. Specifically, both arterioles vasoconstrict with variable effects on P_{GC} and K_f, depending on the dose and route of administration. Thus, the renal response might differ substantially in the setting of increased circulating levels as compared to increased intraglomerular production, with the latter potentially having little or no effect on the preglomerular resistance. Despite the absence of changes in whole-kidney hemodynamics by endothelin receptor antagonists, micropuncture studies should be performed to assess the possibility of offsetting effects of endogenous endothelin on the individual determinants of glomerular filtration.

Effects of Endothelin on Mesangial Cells

The role of the mesangial cell in the modulation of glomerular filtration or in the pathogenesis of acute or chronic renal disease remains unclear. The majority of these cells exhibit smooth-muscle-like features and are able to constrict *in vitro* when exposed to vasoactive modulators of renal hemodynamics, including Ang II, norepinephrine, and arginine vasopressin (297). It is believed that mesangial cell contraction might alter K_f by reducing the glomerular capillary surface area and/or the hydraulic permeability. A large body of data using primarily cultured mesangial cells has been amassed, suggesting that this cell may be a potential source, as well as a target, for endothelin. As discussed above, these cells have constitutive expression of endothelin which is responsive to a variety of stimuli, and they possess both ET_A and ET_B receptors.

A contractile response of cultured mesangial cells to endothelin has been recognized by several groups (134,145,289,298,299). Endothelin-1 exposure induces a reduction in mesangial planar surface area which is comparable to Ang II (Fig. 11) (298). Endothelin also triggers rearrangements of F-actin filaments indicative of the transition from a stationary cell to a motile cell (145). In addition, the cross-sectional area of isolated glomeruli is also reduced by ET-1, supporting a possible effect on glomerular capillary surface area (289). As with vascular smooth muscle cells, ET-1 induces a rapid rise in intra-

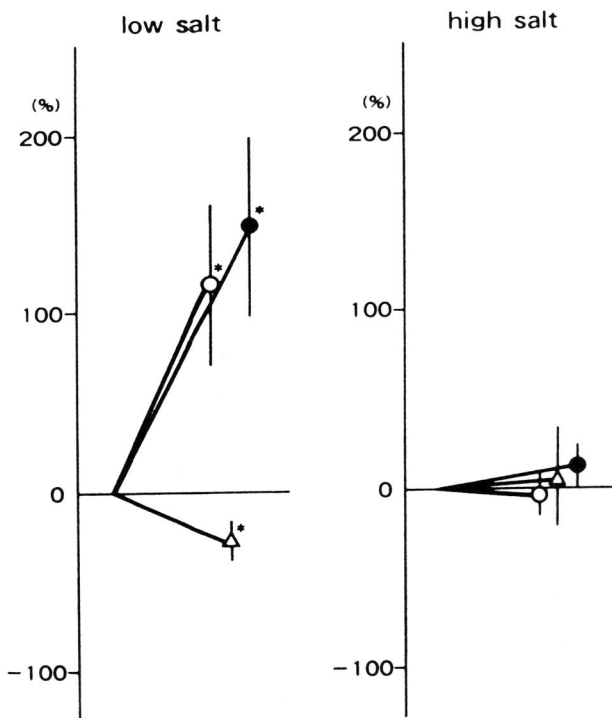

FIG. 11. Percent change of urinary sodium excretion rate ($U_{Na}V$, *open circles*), fractional excretion of sodium (FE_{Na}, *closed circles*), and plasma renin (*open triangles*) in rats receiving antiendothelin antibodies relative to rats infused with nonimmune serum; rats were fed either a low- or high-salt diet. (From ref. 290, with permission.)

cellular free Ca^{2+} due to release of intracellular stores, followed by a sustained increase in cytosolic Ca^{2+} which is dependent upon the influx of extracellular calcium (137). These findings are paralleled by an increase in inositol phospholipid turnover, indicating activation of phospholipase C (134,137).

Similar to vascular smooth muscle, endothelin stimulates PLA_2 activity in mesangial cells, and thus leads to release of arachidonate as well as $PGE_2 > PGI_2 > TXA_2$ (99,134,176). This might attenuate the mesangial contractile response as well as modulate arteriolar tone. Indeed, in vitro PGE_2 significantly reduces the contractile response of ET-1 in these cells (299). A potentially important paracrine effect of endothelin within the glomerulus is also suggested by a sustained increase in PGE_2 production by mesangial cells cocultured with glomerular endothelial cells, an effect which was abrogated by ET-1 antiserum (300). Despite persistently increased basal PGE_2 production, cocultured mesangial cells became desensitized to acute ET-1 exposure due, at least in part, to a marked reduction in mesangial endothelin receptors. These results suggest a potentially important feedback mechanism within the glomerulus. In support of this possibility, downregulation (or less likely prior occupation) of endothelin receptors by autocrine production of endothelin has been observed in human umbilical vein cells, rat aortic endothelial cells, and rat mesangial cells (301).

Finally, several investigators have identified a potent mitogenic effect of endothelin in quiescent cultured mesangial cells with an EC_{50} of 0.9 nM (134,137,185). The exact intracellular mechanism of this mitogenic response remains unclear. As in vascular smooth muscle cells, endothelin stimulates expression of the protooncogenes (see above) (137,188). In addition, endothelin stimulates mitogen-activated protein kinases, a process that involves activation of both protein kinase C and a tyrosine kinase (302). Endothelin also stimulates mesangial cell release of PDGF, which could potentially stimulate glomerular endothelin production. Finally, endothelin activates Na^+/H^+ exchange, leading to intracellular alkalinization, another potential signal for cell proliferation (137).

Whether glomerular endothelial or mesangial cell production of endothelin modulates glomerular hemodynamics under normal physiologic conditions remains unclear. Several inflammatory mediators and coagulation products stimulate endothelin production in the three cell types comprising the glomerulus, the mesangial, endothelial, and epithelial cells. Endothelin has a potent mitogenic and contractile effect on mesangial cells. Taken together, these responses raise the possibility of a role for this mediator in the pathogenesis of the mesangial proliferation and reduced GFR, which are commonly observed in several forms of acute glomerulonephritis.

Effects of Endothelin on Sodium Excretion

There is substantial evidence that renal retention of sodium leading to expansion of extracellular fluid volume plays a prominent role in the pathogenesis of hypertension (303). For this reason there has been intense interest in the effects of endogenous and exogenous endothelin on sodium balance. Depending on the dose and route of delivery, endothelin affects nearly all of the hemodynamic, hormonal, and tubular functions involved in renal sodium handling. However, the net effect of endogenous endothelin on sodium balance remains unclear, as the peptide stimulates both pro- and antinatriuretic processes. Discerning a role for endogenous endothelin on sodium handling in vivo will be fostered greatly by the studies infusing specific endothelin-receptor antagonists and/or ECE inhibitors. This section will examine the effects of exogenous endothelin on whole-kidney sodium handling, as well as on specific hormone systems and renal epithelial proteins of particular importance to salt balance.

Whole Kidney Response/Pressure-Natriuresis

Pharmacologic doses of endothelin induce dose-dependent, long-lasting pressor responses and reductions in GFR. These effects could alter renal sodium handling by inducing a pressor natriuresis and/or a reduction in filtered load of sodium. High-dose intravenous infusions of ET-1 associated with marked reductions in GFR, and thus filtered load of sodium, lead to profound falls in sodium excretion rate (204,212,233, 238,278). By contrast, in the anesthetized rat, endothelin leads to moderate natriuresis when infused in pressor doses that do not substantially impair GFR (204,304–307). The natriuresis is proportional to the rise in blood pressure and is eliminated when renal perfusion pressure is maintained constant, using an aortic snare or with removal of the renal capsule (204,304,305). Most studies using subpressor doses in dogs and rats have noted, little or no change in sodium excretion rates (196,305), whereas others have observed an increase (266). One infusion study in dogs that doubled circulating levels of endothelin (subpressor dose) suggested a mild antinatriuretic response as compared to vehicle-infused animals (196). With intrarenal artery infusion in doses that do not affect systemic blood pressure or GFR, ET-1 has no significant effect on the fractional excretion of sodium in most studies (265,272,278), with one study observing an increase (266). Similar to the intravenous studies, higher intrarenal artery doses lead to parallel reductions in GFR and sodium excretion rate (265,272,277,278). In the isolated perfused kidney, a natriuretic effect is noted, despite substantial reductions in GFR (282,306). In one study of salt-deprived rats, intravenous antiendothelin antibodies increased urinary sodium excretion, increased fractional excretion of sodium, and decreased plasma renin activity in the absence of changes in renal hemodynamics (Fig. 12) (290). However, rats on a high-salt diet had no natriuretic response. This finding suggests a potentially important interaction of the renin-angiotensin axis and endothelin in the renal reply to volume contraction (see below). Overall, the effects of exogenous endothelin on renal sodium handling are highly dose-dependent and are closely related to changes in renal perfusion pressure and GFR.

Atrial Natriuretic Peptide

Pretreatment with pharmacologic doses of ANP markedly attenuates the renal and systemic hemodynamic effects of endothelin and has thus been postulated to be an endogenous modulator of endothelin action. In cultured rat atrial myocytes, neonatal rat atrial and ventricular myocytes, and perfused rat heart, endothelin is a potent secretagogue for ANP (287,288,308). Indeed, several investigators have noted increased plasma levels of ANP with intravenous endothelin infusion (212,233, 307). In one study, coinfusion of anti-ANP antibodies lessened the natriuresis induced by moderately pressor

doses of ET-1 in anesthetized rats (307). However, these increases in ANP are generally modest and achieve levels unlikely to alter the hemodynamic effects of the endothelin. Several studies in rats and dogs using relatively high pressor doses of endothelin do not have significant increases in ANP (264,272,306). In addition, doses sufficient to double circulating ET-1 in dogs failed to increase ANP (196). This is corroborated in humans where intravenous infusion of ET-1, achieving approximately 50-fold increase in circulating concentrations, did not change plasma ANP levels (renal hemodynamics and sodium excretion rates were not measured) (197). By contrast, ET-1 infusion abrogated the systemic and renal effects of intravenous ANP in dogs (309). Overall, the data for regarding the possible interaction of ET and ANP *in vivo* are not sufficient to determine the physiologic significance of their offsetting pharmacological actions.

Arachidonate Biproducts

Several mechanisms other than pressure-natriuresis and ANP have been examined to account for the observed natriuresis, including prostanoids and lipoxygenase products. The natriuretic effects of intravenous ET-1

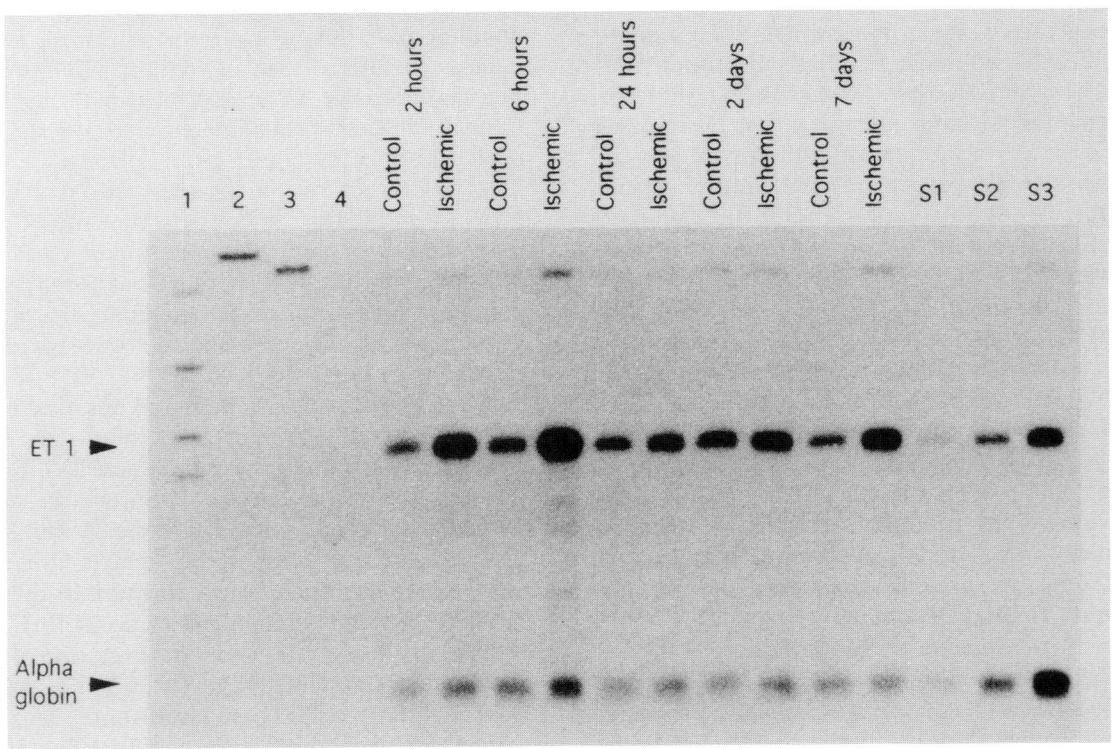

FIG. 12. Time course of expression of ET-1 mRNA in rat kidneys following a 45-minute period of unilateral ischemia, comparing the ischemic and contralateral kidney (control). The autoradiograph was obtained following 16 hours of exposure using a RNAase protection assay of ET-1 mRNA. **Lane 1:** marker, HpaII digest of pBR322. **Lane 2:** ET-1 probe. **Lane 3:** α globin probe. Lane 4: hybridization without RNA. S1–S3: standards containing 50, 100, and 200 μg of pooled rat kidney RNA and 0.5, 1, and 2 μg of K562, a fragment unprotected by the probe. (From ref. 92, with permission.)

in rats are inhibited in rats by pretreatment with either L-651,392, a specific 5-lipoxygenase inhibitor, or an LTC_4/LTD_4 receptor antagonist (306). However these agents also prevent the pressor response to endothelin and, thus, would lessen pressure-induced natriuresis (306). In another intravenous infusion study, meclofenamate failed to alter the natriuretic response to a pressor dose of ET-1, arguing against a role for prostanoids in this process (305). This is supported by the finding that indomethacin or ibuprofen do not alter the response to ET-1 in the isolated perfused kidney model (282). With intrarenal artery infusion of ET-1, indomethacin does not attenuate the increase in fractional excretion of sodium seen in one study, despite obliterating the increase in renal arterial and venous 6-keto-PGF_{2a} (266).

Direct Effects of Endothelin on Renal Tubular Epithelium

There is growing evidence that endothelin might have important effects on several renal tubular epithelial cell proteins pertinent to sodium transport. Tubular effects are suggested by the relative abundance of ET_B (but not ET_A) receptors on tubular epithelial cells, IMCD > medullary thick ascending limb, and the ability of cultured renal epithelial cells to produce both ET-1 and ET-3 (see above). There are very few data regarding the effects of exogenous endothelin on sodium reabsorption in various segments of the nephron *in vivo*. However, lithium clearance is substantially increased in rats given bolus intravenous ET-1 (pressor doses) despite a reduction in GFR, suggesting a reduction in absolute proximal reabsorption of sodium (306). Others have corroborated an ET-induced increase in end-proximal fluid delivery with natriuresis in anesthetized rats (310). It is yet unclear whether this represents altered peritubular capillary hemodynamics or a direct proximal tubular effect. However, only modest quantities of endothelin-like immunoreactivity are identified in early proximal brush-border membranes, and binding of radiolabeled endothelin is substantially less than that observed in the glomerulus and inner medulla (241,256).

Studies of isolated perfused tubules, cortical and inner medullary cell suspensions, and cortical membrane vesicle preparations have yielded conflicting results. In isolated rat proximal straight tubule preparations, endothelin (10^{-9} M) reduces both fluid adsorption rate and bicarbonate absorption, an effect associated with a 20 percent reduction in Na^{2+}/K^+ ATPase activity (311). By contrast, ouabain-sensitive oxygen consumption is unchanged by ET-1 in suspensions of rabbit cortical proximal tubule cells, casting doubt on endothelin modulation of Na^+/K^+ ATPase activity in these cells (312). Oxygen consumption is inhibited in rabbit inner medullary collecting duct cell suspensions treated with ET-1 (EC_{50} 50 pM) (312). This was associated with a reduction

in the initial rate of ouabain-sensitive ^{86}Rb uptake in the IMCD cells, suggesting a reduction in Na^+/K^+ ATPase activity similar to that induced by PGE_2 (312,313). Indeed, this response is likely mediated by prostanoids, as endothelin induces PGE_2 release in these cells, and the effects on oxygen consumption are blocked by ibuprofen (312). Further studies are needed to determine the extent to which endothelin, directly or indirectly, alters Na^+/K^+ ATPase activity in the renal epithelial cells. In rabbit aorta, Na^+/K^+ ATPase activity is increased by endothelin by receptor-mediated activation of protein kinase C and Na^+/H^+ exchange (314).

Vesicle membranes prepared from rabbit renal cortex indicate direct dose-dependent (10^{-8} to 10^{-11} M) stimulation (25 percent) of the apical Na^+/H^+ exchanger and the basolateral Na^+/HCO_3^- cotransporter (315). For both proteins, this effect represented an increase in the V_{max}, with no effect on the K_m, and was blocked by anti-ET antibody. Similar stimulation of Na^+/H^+ exchange has been observed in brush-border membrane vesicles prepared from rat proximal tubule slices (316). The vesicle studies indicate that the effects on the Na^+/H^+ exchanger and the basolateral Na^+/HCO_3^- cotransporter occur independent of intracellular events. Thus, the discrepant results might reflect offsetting cellular effects, in addition to species and/or methodologic differences. Use of specific receptor antagonists and/or ECE inhibitors will help determine the importance of endogenous endothelin in this segment of the nephron.

Interaction of Endothelin and the Renin-Angiotensin-Aldosterone System

The renin-angiotensin-aldosterone system is well recognized as a key modulator of renal hemodynamics and sodium balance. A wide variety of circulating and local factors has been identified which can modulate renal renin secretion. The proximity of the renin-producing juxtaglomerular cells to the afferent arteriolar endothelial cells raises the possibility of an important regulatory effect of the endothelium on renin secretion (317). Several lines of evidence suggest that endothelin might modulate this system and, thus, have an important effect on extracellular fluid volume. Infusion of antiendothelin antibodies leads to a natriuresis and a reduction of plasma renin concentration in salt-deprived rats, suggesting that stimulation of renin release in volume depletion might be directly or indirectly mediated, in part, by endothelin (290). Pressor doses of endothelin in dogs and rats increase plasma renin activity and circulating aldosterone levels (212,233,264,318), whereas lower doses either have no effect or decrease plasma renin activity and aldosterone (196,318,319).

Intrarenal artery infusion of ET-1 in anesthetized rats does not alter plasma renin activity or renin secretory rate in doses that have no (1 ng/kg/min) or only modest effects (2 ng/kg/min) on renal hemodynamics (277). Others note a significant inhibitory effect on renin release in a canine nonfiltering kidney with high and low doses of endothelin (279). These studies block the macula densa mechanism of renin release and, thus, suggest a direct effect of endothelin on renin secretion by the juxtaglomerular cells. Indeed, *in vitro* renin secretion is reduced by endothelin in dispersed juxtaglomerular cells, renal cortical slices, and isolated rat glomeruli (320–324). Endothelin also significantly attenuates cAMP and isoproterenol-stimulated renin release in both cortical slices and isolated juxtaglomerular cells (321,322,325). Isoproterenol-induced renin release is blunted *in vivo* when the agonist is infused into the renal artery of anesthetized rats (277). In humans, exogenous endothelin infusion did not change either plasma concentrations of renin or aldosterone, despite increasing endothelin plasma concentrations by 50-fold and inducing a mild pressor response (197). Endothelin might have effects on aldosterone production independent of renin. Receptors for endothelin have been identified in zona glomerulosa cells, and endothelin induces dose-dependent production of aldosterone, although less potently than Ang II (106). Subthreshold concentrations of endothelin also significantly potentiate the stimulatory effect of adrenocorticotropic hormone in adrenal glomerulosa cells (326,327). The effect on Ang II-stimulated aldosterone production was less clear, with one study showing stimulation (326) and the other showing no effect (327).

Taken together, endothelin might interact with the renin-angiotensin-aldosterone system on several levels. The direct effect of the peptide on aldosterone production suggests a possible antinatriuretic effect independent of renin. Due to its profound systemic and renal hemodynamic effects, endothelin potentially modulates many of the primary determinants of renin synthesis, including baroreceptor function, the macula densa, and/or the sympathetic nervous system (see below). It is clear from the studies outlined above that some of these effects are offsetting. However, studies achieving mild to moderate increases in circulating endothelin levels in the range of those observed under pathological conditions have failed to alter plasma renin activity. In the original report, Yanagisawa et al. (6) indicate that Ang II stimulates endothelin production by endothelial cells, raising the possibility of a negative feedback mechanism for renin production by the juxtaglomerular cells. It is noteworthy that endothelin infusion induces a marked natriuresis in sodium-avid cirrhotic rats with ascites, despite a substantial reduction in the filtered load of sodium (328). Concurrently, ANP and aldosterone levels increased despite suppression of plasma renin activity.

Effects of Endothelin on Water Balance

Pharmacologic doses of endothelin increase levels of circulating AVP) in conjunction with marked changes in systemic hemodynamics (212,233). However, a consistent finding of studies infusing ET-1 *in vivo* is a prominent diuresis, which can occur even when GFR is reduced (204). Concurrently, there is a decrease in urine osmolality, suggesting a direct effect on water reabsorption (212,302,329). Similar effects have been observed for ET-3, suggesting that ET_B receptors are involved (329). ET-3-induced diuresis was not affected by a cyclooxygenase inhibitor, arguing against a role for prostaglandins in this response. In other studies ET-1 significantly reduces urine osmolality without changing circulating AVP levels, suggesting that the increase in free-water clearance is due to the inhibition of AVP action, not release (302). Inhibition at the collecting duct is also supported by studies in the Brattleboro rat, where ET-1 inhibited the antidiuresis of exogenous AVP infusion (329). Arginine vasopressin-induced cAMP accumulation is inhibited in microdissected cortical collecting ducts, and outer and inner medullary collecting ducts (330). In isolated microperfused rat IMCD segments, endothelin (10^{-8}-10^{-10} M) inhibits AVP-stimulated water permeability by roughly 20 percent, but not stimulation by dibutyryl cAMP (331). These findings have been confirmed by others who note rapid desensitization of these segments to the inhibitory effects of ET-1 (332). Furthermore, the reduction in AVP-stimulated water permeability is not altered by indomethacin, though it is abrogated by either pertussis toxin or the protein kinase C inhibitor calphostin (330,332). Similar to IMCD segments, ET-1 inhibits AVP-induced water and Cl absorption in rat cortical collecting ducts (333).

Evidence of a possible autocrine and/or paracrine role for endothelin in the regulation of renal concentrating ability is rapidly accumulating. The inner medulla of the kidney is one of the richest sources of endothelin receptors in the body, with abundant receptors on IMCD cells, medullary interstitial cells, and the vasa recta. Several investigators have demonstrated constitutive synthesis of ET-1 by rat and human IMCD cells, raising the possibility of an autocrine function for the peptide (259,334–336). By contrast, ET-3 production was minimal in human and rabbit IMCD cells (259,335,337). An autocrine effect is supported by the polar expression of endothelin receptors and directional secretion of endothelin in IMCD (193). Specifically, radiolabeled ET-1 binds primarily on the basolateral surface of IMCD cells grown to confluence on semipermeable membranes. Likewise, secretion of ET-1 was predominantly toward the basolateral side (193). In addition, endothelin stimulation of IMCD PGE_2 production and the inhibition of AVP-induced water flux are observed primarily with basolateral exposure to ET-1 (193,331). Preincubation of cultured IMCD cells with anti-ET-1 antibodies not only enhances AVP-dependent cAMP accumulation, it also leads to a sixfold increase in radiolabeled ET-1 binding, suggesting a possible feedback mechanism (335). In addition to possible autocrine effects, a paracrine function on vasa recta tone or medullary interstitial cells is possible. Indeed, cultured rat medullary interstitial cells specifically bind endothelin in a pattern consistent with ET_A receptors and respond to exogenous endothelin by inducing phospholipid turnover, increased $[Ca^{2+}]_i$ and PGE_2 synthesis (110).

Unlike endothelial cells and other cell types, vasopressin, thrombin, bradykinin, and epinephrine failed to alter ET-1 release by rat IMCD (334). There are conflicting data regarding the effects of osmolality on endothelin synthesis by IMCD cells. In tubule suspensions from the inner medulla of rats and rabbits, endothelin transcription and release are stimulated by hyperosmolality induced by NaCl, decreased by urea, and unchanged by mannitol (336). By contrast, increasing osmolality from 300 to 450 mosmol in cultured rat IMCD cells using NaCl or mannitol leads to a time-dependent reduction in ET-1 transcription and release, whereas urea had no effect (338). The reason for these discrepant findings is unclear; however, inhibition of endothelin release by hypertonicity is supported by the finding of significantly reduced urinary ET-1 excretion and inner medullary ET-1 mRNA in water-depleted rats. Although the findings outlined above are strongly suggestive of a role for endothelin in water balance, the importance of these effects *in vivo* remains unclear. It is noteworthy that in the rat, secretory vesicles containing endothelin are located in AVP-producing posterior pituitary cells (70,71). In water-deprived rats these secretory vesicles are absent. Whether secretion of the two mediators is independently regulated remains unclear.

ENDOTHELIN AND RENAL PATHOPHYSIOLOGY

The ability of many renal cells to produce endothelin and the abundance of renal endothelin receptors raises the possibility that the kidney is an important source and target organ for endothelin under pathological conditions. Endothelin has been implicated in several disorders associated with dysfunctional renal endothelium, including cyclosporine (CyA) toxicity, vascular rejection of the transplanted, and acute ischemic renal failure. Most recently, endothelin has been proposed as a pathogenic factor in the hepatorenal syndrome (295). These disorders share the findings of severe renal vasoconstriction and reductions in GFR. Endothelin has also been implicated in the pathogenesis of the progression of renal disease, a condition associated with single-nephron hyperperfusion and hyperfiltration. The divergent nature of the renal hemodynamics in these conditions suggests that the dominant effects might relate to several factors such as peptide concentration, cellular source, and receptor density.

Cyclosporine Nephrotoxicity

Nephrotoxicity is one of the dose-limiting factors for the use of CyA in solid organ transplantation and is a major source of morbidity. In humans and animals CyA therapy leads to renal vasoconstriction with a reduction in GFR, and is commonly associated with systemic hypertension (339). The severity of this response varies considerably among individuals and is dose-related. There is increasing evidence that CyA is toxic to the endothelium, leading to cell lysis and detachment and, thus, might alter both the vasoactive and nonthrombogenic properties of this monolayer of cells (340–344). In one individual who inadvertently received very high dose of CyA immediately following placement of a cadaveric renal allograft, there was an acute cessation of renal function with diffuse sloughing of the endothelial cell layer and extensive necrosis of the glomeruli and tubules; no rejection was evident (345). Endothelin levels were 43-fold higher than normal and 3–4 times higher than dialysis patients. In one study, plasma endothelin levels did not increase in uncomplicated renal transplantation (346). By contrast, a threefold increase was observed in patients with vascular rejection, a condition marked by endovasculitis, infiltration of the intima by mononuclear cells, and fibrinoid necrosis (346). Others find increased circulating levels of endothelin in renal allograft recipients (347), as well as in patients receiving CyA without intrinsic renal disease such as uveitis and liver transplantation (348,349). In liver transplant patients, circulating endothelin levels increase two- to threefold in the first-week posttransplant in association with a rise in blood pressure (349), whereas no significant elevation of endothelin is noted with chronic CyA therapy in cardiac allograft recipients as compared to normals, nor did endothelin levels correlate with blood pressure or creatinine levels (350). In rats treated chronically with CyA (30 days postoperative), urinary excretion of endothelin is elevated as compared to vehicle with no significant difference in plasma levels (351). Urinary endothelin secretion, but not plasma endothelin, was strongly correlated with plasma creatinine in these animals. These results suggest that urinary excretion rates might be a more sensitive indicator of renal endothelin production.

There is increasing experimental evidence that CyA stimulates endothelin production, which subsequently alters renal hemodynamics. Endothelin secretion from human umbilical-vein endothelial cells is increased by CyA in a dose-dependent fashion, an effect which is inhibited by cycloheximide (352). Similar stimulation is seen in LLC-PK1 cells, a renal epithelial cell line (82). In addition, conditioned media from CyA-treated endothelial cells induces proliferation of human smooth muscle cells (352). This mitogenic effect is inhibited by coincubation with antiendothelin antibodies, nifedipine, or verapamil. *In vivo,* endothelin levels are markedly higher in rats receiving acute intravenous CyA therapy (40 pg/mL) than vehicle-treated animals (<2 pg/mL) (262). In these studies CyA induced proportionately greater afferent than efferent arteriolar vasoconstriction with a reduction in SNGFR, effects that were largely prevented by co-infusion of antiendothelin antibodies into the renal artery (262). Antiendothelin antibodies also prevent CyA effects in the isolated perfused kidney model (292). A protective effect related specifically to endothelin has been confirmed using a specific ET_A receptor antagonist, BQ-123 (293). When infused intravenously, antiendothelin antibodies only partially prevent renal vasoconstriction induced by acute CyA, and BQ-123 does not (292,293). Studies of isolated rat renal arteries verify that the afferent arteriole is more sensitive to CyA than the efferent, and note that vasoconstriction of the afferent, but not the efferent, arteriole is blocked by a specific ET_A receptor antagonist (353). These studies also imply that CyA triggers release of endothelin from the afferent arteriole, presumably the endothelium. It is noteworthy that ET_A receptor antagonist also attenuates CyA-induced myosin light chain phosphorylation in cultured mesangial cells and, thus, might help maintain GFR by altering glomerular capillary surface area (354). Finally, 4 days of CyA therapy in rats increases renal endothelin receptor number, urinary excretion rate of endothelin, and plasma creatinine levels (decreased creatinine clearance), effects that were not present in rats cotreated with nifedipine (355,356). Cyclosporine also increases the density of binding sites in cardiac cell membranes (357). Thus, CyA might also enhance the kidney as a potential target organ for endothelin.

In summary, there is substantial evidence of increased production of endothelin in humans and animals in response to CyA. In addition, the renal hemodynamic effects are markedly attenuated by specific inhibitors related to endothelin. Considering the effects of endothelin on voltage-dependent Ca^{2+} channels, it is not surprising that calcium-channel blockers reduce the both arteriolar constrictive effects of CyA and the mesangial constriction. The availability of receptor antagonists raises the exciting possibility of preventing CyA nephrotoxicity in the future.

Acute Renal Failure

In humans and rats, acute ischemic renal failure is manifested by a reduction in RPF rate and a disproportionate fall in GFR (358,359). It has been proposed that the renal hemodynamic effects are due, at least in part, to dysfunctional endothelium resulting in deficient endothelium-derived vasodilator production and/or excessive vasoconstrictor production. Several groups have noted impaired endothelium-dependent vasodilation in rat models of acute renal failure (360,361). In humans, acute renal failure is associated with an increase in circulating endothelin levels which normalize with recovery (362). By contrast, circulating endothelin levels in renal allograft recipients with postoperative acute tubular necrosis (determined by biopsy) were near normal (346). In patients with chronic renal insufficiency, ET-1 levels do not correlate with residual renal function (363). In hemodialyzed patients increased plasma levels of ET-1 are noted by some (364,365), but not all, investigators (363).

A role for endothelin in acute renal failure was first suggested in a rat model of ischemia (25 minutes) where antiendothelin antibodies infused into a branch of the renal artery attenuated the glomerular hypoperfusion and hypofiltration in distribution of that artery 48 hours after the insult (294). In another study of bilateral renal ischemia (45 minutes), antiendothelin antibody rendered a functional and histologic protective effect in rats (366). These studies reveal an increase in renal parenchymal endothelin concentration and in circulating levels. By contrast, in dogs, pretreatment with a specific ET_A receptor antagonist (BQ-123) lessened postischemic (1-hour aortic cross-clamping) renal vasoconstriction without ameliorating the reduction in GFR (291). Hypoxia might be a key component in this response as low oxygen tension increases expression of endothelin from endothelial cells (367). Indeed, ET-1 expression is increased after 25 or 45 minutes of renal ischemia, as compared to the normal contralateral kidney (Fig. 13) (92). The increased mRNA is significant only at 2 hours for 25 minutes ischemia, whereas with 45 minutes it is maximal at 6 hours (>fourfold increase) and persists throughout a 7-day postischemic period. By contrast, ET-3 expression decreased postischemia and ET-2 remained undetectable (92). The significance of reduced ET-3 production is unknown. ET-1 binding-site density of rat cardiac membranes is markedly increased by global ischemia (20–90 minutes), which is further enhanced by reperfusion (368). However, in rats with unilateral renal ischemia (60 minutes), the density and affinity of endothelin receptors was similar in the ischemic and contralateral normal kidney at 2 and 24 hours (369). Indeed, infusion of endothelin in normal animals downregulates renal endothelin receptors, an effect which is preserved in postischemic kidneys (369).

A common cause of acute tubular necrosis in hospitalized patients is bacterial sepsis. The renal vasoconstriction in this setting is believed to be related to endotoxemia. In rats, endotoxin infusion induces renal vasoconstriction and acute renal failure (370,371). A role for endothelin in this vasoconstriction is suggested by marked increases in circulating levels noted in rats, pigs, and sheep infused with endotoxin (372–374). In addition, endotoxin stimulates endothelin production in cultured endothelial cells (372). Endotoxin also induces nitric oxide production from vascular smooth muscle cells which may, in part, counterbalance the effects of ET-1

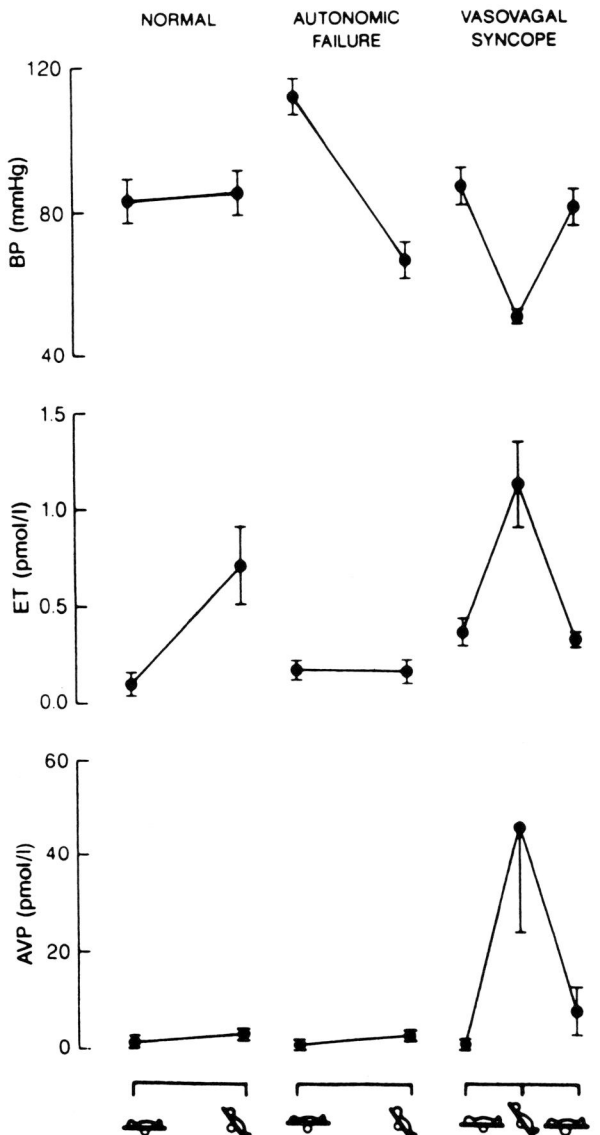

FIG. 13. Effect of tilt on blood pressure (BP), plasma concentrations of endothelin (ET), and arginine vasopressin (AVP) in normal subjects, patients with autonomic failure, and patients with vasovagal syncope. (From ref. 393, with permission.)

(375). In summary, both acute ischemic renal failure and endotoxin-induced renal failure are conditions associated with increased production of endothelin. Potentially, maneuvers that decrease endothelin synthesis or action might offer useful therapy for these disorders, heretofore untreatable.

Progression of Renal Disease

Patients with renal insufficiency typically undergo progressive loss of residual renal function, even in the absence of the original disease. In experimental animals the slow decline in total GFR is accompanied by hyperperfusion, hyperfiltration, and hypertrophy of the residual nephrons with progressive loss of the barrier function of the glomerulus membrane and glomerular scarring. Micropuncture studies have identified systemic and glomerular hypertension as major risk factors for progression in the ablation model of renal insufficiency (376). Several lines of evidence suggest a possible role for endothelin in this model. In two separate studies, 6–7 weeks after 5/6 renal ablation, urinary excretion rate of endothelin is significantly greater in nephrectomized rats than sham operated rats, despite no difference in plasma levels (377,378). Urinary endothelin excretion rate correlates with systolic blood pressure, proteinuria, and percent sclerotic glomeruli (378,379). In addition, renal cortical tissue from ablated rats produced more ET-1 than sham animals. Furthermore, isolated glomeruli from the ablated rats, but not sham animals, increased endothelin production in response to thrombin (377). Preproendothelin-1 mRNA of ablated rat renal tissue increased progressively 30 and 60 days following surgery, whereas transcription in sham rats was unchanged (379). The stimulus and primary source of preproendothelin is unclear. Potentially, the increase in single-nephron renal blood flow increases shear stress on the endothelium, a known stimulus for endothelin expression (380,381). Alternatively, glomerular endothelial cells or mesangial cells might increase endothelin expression in response to inflammatory or coagulation mediators, both of which have been implicated in this model. It is noteworthy that chronic treatment of ablated rats with a specific ET_A receptor antagonist (FR139317) substantially reduces proteinuria and structural injury as compared to untreated rats (382). However, the receptor antagonist also reduced systemic hypertension and, thus, a specific renal protective effect of blocking endothelin must be confirmed. Further studies are also required to discern the impact of endothelin antagonism on glomerular hemodynamics, P_{GC} in particular.

POTENTIAL ROLE OF ENDOTHELIN IN BASAL HEMODYNAMICS AND SHOCK

It is now well established that the endothelium has sensor and effector properties necessary for the transduction of intravascular signals into appropriate changes in vascular smooth muscle tone. The endothelium has specific receptors for a variety of vasoactive hormones, as well as membrane ion channels that are responsive to changes in flow and pressure (1,3,383). The cells can alter vascular smooth muscle tone by eliciting both vasoconstrictive and vasodilatory soluble mediators, or by direct cell-cell contact through gap junctions (384). One of the unique features of endothelin is its long-lasting vasoconstrictive effects which are noted both *in vitro* and *in vivo*. Regulation of endothelin occurs at the level of transcription and, thus, increased production by endothelial cells in response to various signals requires time for transcription, processing, and release. Taken together, these characteristics suggest that endothelin might regulate vascular tone over longer periods of time rather than moment to moment. This section will examine the role of endogenous endothelin in the regulation of blood pressure in the basal state as well as in conditions of threatened systemic hemodynamics.

Role of Endogenous Endothelin in the Regulation of Basal Hemodynamics

Circulating levels of endothelin in normals are well below either the K_d for endothelin binding to its receptor or the EC_{50} for inducing contraction of vascular smooth muscle cells (see section). For several reasons this finding does not necessarily preclude a role for endothelin in the control of vascular tone under normal circumstances. First, the polar secretion of endothelin by endothelial cells raises the possibility that circulating levels underestimate local concentrations in the resistance vessels. In addition, endothelin potentiates the vasoconstrictor effects of other known modulators of systemic vascular resistance such as norepinephrine and, thus, low concentrations of endothelin might indirectly modulate blood pressure (385,386). However, no hypotensive effect is observed in several studies that infuse either antiendothelin antibodies or specific endothelin receptor antagonists into normal animals, despite using doses that inhibit the pressor effects of pharmacologic doses of exogenous endothelin (387–390). These findings cast serious doubt on a major role for peripheral endothelium-derived endothelin in control of basal hemodynamics.

The aforementioned findings do not exclude possible central effects of endothelin on systemic vascular resistance. As discussed above, the central nervous system has both abundant receptors and the ability to produce ET-1 and ET-3. Furthermore, acute or chronic intracerebroventricular administration of endothelin in rats triggers a pressor response and tachycardia (236,391, 392). This response is largely blocked by pretreatment with phenoxybenzamine, and plasma epinephrine and norepinephrine levels increase substantially, lending support to the premise that the peripheral effects are due to stimulation of the sympathetic outflow (236). The pressor response is also inhibited by prazosin, but not a V1 ADH receptor blocker (392). An interaction with sympathetic nervous system-mediated control of blood pressure is also suggested by abrupt increases in plasma endothelin concentrations, which are observed in normals with change in posture from supine to upright position (Fig. 14) (363,393,394). This rise is not observed in patients with autonomic failure, strongly supporting a

role for the baroreflex in this response (393). Several lines of evidence suggest that this is due to release of endothelin from the neurohypophysis and not due to an effect on peripheral endothelin production. First, the rapid rise indicates release of preformed endothelin, and the posterior pituitary has the only endothelin-containing vesicles identified to date (71,395). Second, with tilt plasma, endothelin and AVP increase in parallel (393). Third, the acute rise persists in patients with vasovagal syncope, a condition characterized by a normal afferent limb of the reflex with impaired sympathetic outflow (see Fig. 14) (393). Finally, patients with diabetes insipidus failed to increase endothelin with tilt and had a fall in blood pressure (393). In another study, rapid (5 minutes) postural changes in plasma-immunoreactive endothelin precede the increase in other vasoconstrictor mediators (394). These data suggest that conditions triggering baroreflexes might also lead to release of central vesicles containing endothelin. It is noteworthy that volume infusion does not alter cerebrospinal fluid or plasma endothelin levels in rats, but both decrease with phenylephrine infusion, an effect that was abrogated by sinoaortic denervation (396). Microinjection of endothelin into different regions of the brain has various effects on blood pressure and sympathetic nerve activity, depending on location. In summary, under normal circumstances (including tilt) circulating levels of endothelin are well below that required to trigger cellular responses. There are indications that endothelin release in the brain might be linked to baroreceptor function. Finally, blocking endothelin receptors fails to cause hypotension, casting doubt on the importance of circulating endothelin in the maintenance of basal hemodynamics.

Role of Endogenous Endothelin in Shock and Other Conditions of Disturbed Hemodynamics

Increased levels of circulating endothelin have been identified in several conditions associated with disturbed hemodynamics including congestive heart failure, acute myocardial infarction, shock, anaphylaxis, surgery, and the hepatorenal syndrome (8). Potentially, the high levels might help maintain vascular tone and thus contribute to a compensatory response. The rise in endothelin must reflect an increase in production and/or a decrease in metabolism of the peptide. The pulmonary and renal vascular beds account for the majority of clearance of exogenous endothelin, whereas little is known of the metabolism of endothelin *in vivo*. It is noteworthy that to varying degrees, many of the conditions listed above are associated with impairment of renal and/or pulmonary function. Indeed, renal dysfunction from a variety of causes is associated with increased levels. The cellular source and stimulus for release of endothelin in conditions of disturbed hemodynamics remains unclear. To

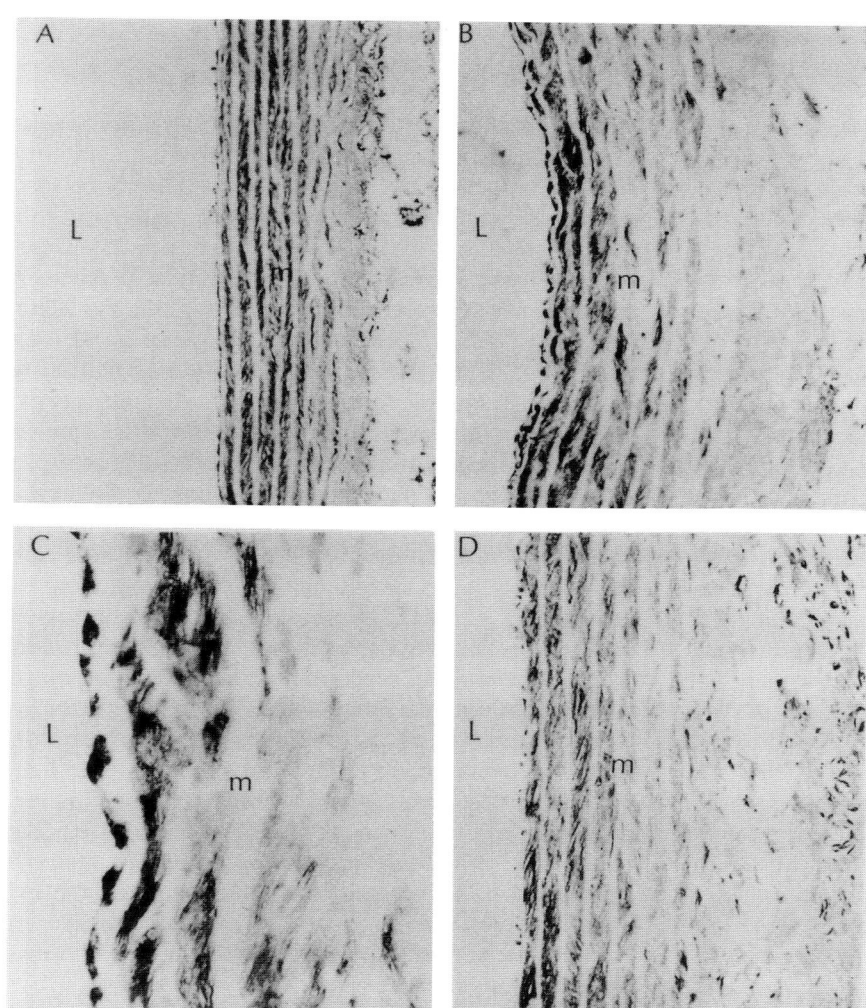

FIG. 14. Immunohistochemical localization of immunoreactive endothelin in the thoracic aorta of uninephrectomized rats (*panel A*) and DOCA-salt hypertensive rats (*panels B, C*). Note the increase in staining in the endothelial monolayer of the hypertensive rats, which was nearly abolished by addition of excess endothelin-1 (*panel D*). L, lumen; m, media. (From ref. 418, with permission.)

varying degrees, these conditions are also associated with parallel increases in several neurohumoral mediators including Ang II, norepinephrine, and AVP; factors that also increase expression of preproendothelin-1 in endothelial cells *in vitro,* raising the possibility of direct stimulation (see Table 1). Evidence against this hypothesis is the finding that acute infusion of AMP, dDAVP, and norepinephrine in normal humans fails to increase circulating endothelin levels (397). Similarly, in rats, acute infusion of either Ang II or phenylephrine fails to increase endothelin levels despite severe hypertension (398). Nevertheless, threshold concentrations of endothelin (10^{-9} M) potentiate norepinephrine and seretonin-induced contractions of human internal mammary and coronary arteries, rabbit aorta, and rat mesenteric arteries, suggesting a potentially important interaction (385,386,399–401).

A central source of the endothelin must also be considered, given the finding of orthostatic increases in endothelin (discussed above). The posterior pituitary ap-

pears to release endothelin concurrently with AVP in response to changes in osmolality (71). Specifically, the neurohypophyseal nerve endings of rats deprived of water have significantly less endothelin and AVP content than controls (71). As outlined in the previous section, stimulation of baroreflexes might also trigger release of neurohypophyseal endothelin and AVP. In general, release of AVP in response to changes in hemodynamics reflects a profound circulatory disturbance. This might explain in part why increased endothelin levels are observed in patients with cardiogenic shock and not in those with mild heart failure (118,402–404). However, factors other than hypotension must be involved as infusion of high-dose nitroprusside fails to increase endothelin levels, nor does severe hypotension due to hemorrhage in the pig and guinea pig (405). Neither of these maneuvers alters osmolality but cause marked stimulation of the sympathetic nervous system and renin-angiotensin system.

Several forms of shock other than cardiogenic have

been associated with increased endothelin levels including anaphylactic, endotoxic, hemorrhagic, and hypoxic (8). Potentially, endothelin might be a factor involved in the early phase of shock where peripheral vasoconstriction is a prominent finding. As discussed above, renal ischemia is associated with a substantial increase in circulating endothelin levels in rats. Shock is characterized by tissue hypoperfusion leading to hypoxia. Calf coronary artery endothelial cells exposed to 2 percent oxygen increase endothelin expression in a time-dependent fashion (406). In addition, increases in endothelin occur in several rat models of acute pulmonary hypoxia (407,408) and in the fetal blood of asphyxiated infants (409,410) and pigs (405). Furthermore, moderate hypoventilation in the anesthetized rat leads to a doubling of the vasoconstrictor potency of endothelin in the mesentery (411). Potentially, tissue hypoxia might be the requisite factor increasing endothelin levels in severe congestive heart failure, which is absent in patients with milder disease. However, prolonged and severe hypoxia (1 hour of 5 percent oxygen) was required in rats to increase endothelin levels, raising questions about the importance of this stimulus *in vivo* (408).

In a variety of species including humans, endotoxin-induced shock has been associated with increased circulating levels of endothelin. Endotoxin infusion in several species also leads to an increase in pulmonary and renal vascular resistance (372–374), the latter of which has been attenuated in rats by co-infusion of antiendothelin antibodies (412). These data suggest a possible role for endothelin in the regional vasoconstriction which occurs with endotoxemia. Cultured bovine aortic endothelial cells and calf pulmonary artery endothelial cells exposed to endotoxin increase release of endothelin (372). In addition, several inflammatory mediators believed to be involved in endotoxemic shock, including TNF_a and interleukin-1, stimulate endothelin expression in endothelial cells (see Table 1) (36,37); TNF_a infusion in rats also increases circulating levels of ET-1 and to a lesser extent ET-3. Another potential cellular source of endothelin in acute infection is the macrophage, a cell that increases endothelin secretion by up to 10 times when treated with endotoxin (87). Notably, in rats, pretreatment with indomethacin substantially lessened the increase in circulating endothelin induced by endotoxin without altering the hypotensive effects (413). These studies suggest a possible role for prostanoids as the stimulus for endothelin release. In summary, increased circulating levels of endothelin are seen in shock associated with several disease states. It is yet unclear whether this increased production represents an epiphenomena or if it is an important component of the compensatory response to impending circulatory collapse. This determination will require further study using specific inhibitors of endothelin.

POTENTIAL ROLE OF ENDOTHELIN IN SYSTEMIC HYPERTENSION

The endothelial cell modulates vascular smooth muscle tone in response to chemical and mechanical intravascular signals by eliciting either vasodilatory or vasoconstrictive factors. Potentially, disruption of either the sensor or effector capabilities of these cells could result in systemic hypertension due to disproportionate release of vasoconstrictive as compared to vasodilatory factors (414,415). When first described, the potent and long-lasting vasoconstrictor properties of endothelin suggested a possible role for the peptide in the pathogenesis of idiopathic hypertension. In addition to direct effects on systemic vascular resistance, endothelin might promote hypertension by altering renal hemodynamics and the pressure-natriuresis relationship, leading to volume expansion. Finally, endothelin might interact with other known modulators of vascular resistance including the sympathetic nervous system. Determining whether endothelin mediates hypertension in humans and experimental models has proved difficult and remains controversial. To invoke endothelin as a mediator of hypertension, one or more of the following aberrations must occur: endothelin production increases, endothelin metabolism decreases, or sensitivity to endothelin is enhanced. Little is known of the metabolism of endogenous endothelin in normals or how it might be altered in hypertension. This section will thus examine the evidence for increased production of endothelin and enhanced vascular sensitivity to endothelin in experimental and human hypertension.

Endothelin Production in Experimental and Human Hypertension

Continuous infusion of endothelin in rats over a 7-day period induces sustained hypertension in rats without any overt change in sodium balance (234). However, plasma endothelin levels in several experimental models fail to show an overt increase in endogenous endothelin production. Indeed, levels are similar or decreased as compared to appropriate controls in the DOCA-salt model (416–418), the spontaneously hypertensive rat (SHR) (398,413,417–420), the SHR stroke-prone rat (417), and the two-kidney, one-clip model (398). One notable exception occurs in rats with malignant range hypertension (280 ± 9 mm Hg systolic) induced by treating SHR rats with DOCA, where levels were twice as high as untreated SHR with systolic blood pressures of 207 ± 8 mm Hg (398). Spontaneously hypertensive rats and SHR stroke-prone rats have lower levels of both big ET-1 and ET-1 than age-matched Wistar-Kyoto (WKY) rats, suggesting that there is reduced transcription and not a reduction in ECE activity (417). This observation is corroborated by evidence of lower endothelin levels in the inner and outer renal medulla and urine of hypertensive SHR rats as compared to WKY, findings not present in prehypertensive SHR rats (91,419,420). Given the ability of endothelin to inhibit Na^+/K^+ ATPase activity and water transport in IMCD cells, it is possible that loss of tonic inhibition leads to sodium retention.

As discussed above, the vectorial secretion of endothelin toward the basolateral side suggests that plasma levels might not accurately reflect vascular production of endothelin (72). Indeed, despite similar plasma levels, segments of thoracic aorta (sixfold) and mesenteric artery (twofold) from DOCA-salt hypertensive rats have significantly more immunoreactive ET-1 than uninephrectomized controls (418). Immunostaining for ET-1 localized the increase in vessel wall endothelin to the endothelium and not the media (Fig. 15) (418). In addition, preproendothelin-1 mRNA levels in these vessels are four- to fivefold higher in DOCA-salt rats than uninephrectomized controls (421). By contrast, aortic ET-1 content was mildly reduced in 16-week hypertensive SHR rats as compared to age-matched WKY rats, whereas immunostaining for ET-1 was similar (418). Mesenteric artery ET-1 content was similar in SHR and WKY rats. Others observe increased release of endothelin from the mesenteric artery of SHR rats as compared to WKY rats. Thus, localized overproduction of endothelin occurs in the DOCA-salt rat, but not the SHR rat. Further studies using receptor antagonists are required to assess the physiologic importance of this enhanced production.

Perhaps the most compelling evidence that endothelin can induce hypertension in humans relates to several patients with hemangioendotheliomas, a rare tumor of the blood vessel that can be associated with severe hypertension and increased circulating levels of endothelin (see Fig. 15) (422,422a). Excision of the tumor leads to a parallel reduction in plasma ET-1 and mean arterial blood pressure. It is noteworthy that the circulating levels are approximately 10–15 times normal, an increase that is substantially greater than other human disease states associated with increased circulating levels (8). Cyclosporine-induced hypertension is another form of secondary hypertension which might be related to endothelin. As discussed above, endothelin levels are increased in some (349,423), but not all, studies (350) of patients treated with cyclosporine. Early after orthotopic liver transplantation, endothelin levels correlate with elevations in blood pressure (349). However, long-term cardiac transplant recipients (average 22 months posttransplant) treated with cyclosporine had no increase in endothelin levels as compared to patients not on cyclosporine, despite a markedly higher incidence of hypertension and higher creatinine levels (350).

Plasma endothelin levels have been measured in a large number of patients with essential hypertension. In general, studies of patients with borderline hypertension or early disease have little or no (0.9- to 1.5-fold) increase in mean plasma endothelin levels with considerable overlap with normotensive controls (363,424–431). Levels are slightly higher in patients with more advanced disease, but generally remain approximately twofold or less (424,425,427). Most studies fail to correlate endothelin levels with either systolic or diastolic blood pressure or heart rate (349,425,427,429,430). Some (424), but not all (349,432), observe a correlation of endothelin levels and serum creatinine levels in patients with essential hypertension, suggesting that renal dysfunction might be an important factor. In one study of patients with atherosclerotic disease, endothelin levels correlated with the number of sites involved, but failed to correlate with age, serum creatinine, or mean arterial blood pressure (433). In summary, endothelin levels in essential hypertension are either modestly elevated or unchanged unless there is advanced end organ disease. No study of patients with essential hypertension has found levels in the range of the rare patient with a hemangioendothelioma. Thus, to the extent that circulating endothelin levels reflect peripheral production of endothelin, there is little evidence that overproduction of the peptide plays a role in essential hypertension.

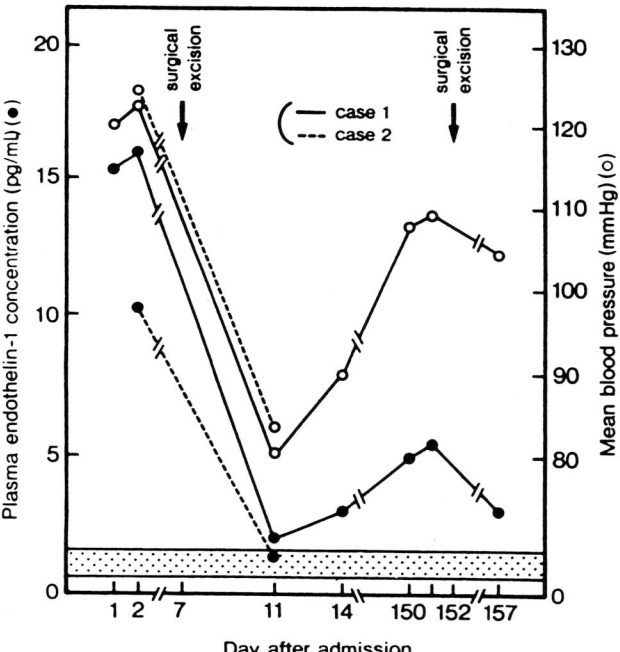

FIG. 15. Plasma endothelin-1 levels (*closed circles*) and mean arterial blood pressure (*open circles*) over time in two patients with malignant hemangioendotheliomas. Shaded area represents normal range. (From ref. 422a, with permission.)

Vascular Responsiveness to Endothelin in Experimental and Human Hypertension

Heightened sensitivity of vascular smooth muscle to endothelin might induce hypertension or amplify the effects of modest increases in endothelin production. Evidence for such an effect in experimental models of hypertension remains controversial. Exogenous endothelin infusion in hypertensive SHR induces a systemic effect similar to WKY rats, i.e., transient hypotension followed by sustained hypertension (207,208,269,434–436). In these studies the magnitude of the vasodepressor response is equivalent or slightly enhanced as compared to control rats, with only minor differences identified in the pressor effects. These experiments in the intact SHR animal do not distinguish the relative effects of endothelin on the endothelium versus the vascular smooth muscle. In perfused mesenteric arteries the sensitivity to extraluminal exposure to endothelin was less in SHR compared to WKY rats, though maximal contraction did not differ (225). With intraluminal dosing of ET-1 or acetylcholine in intact arteries (with endothelium), vasodilation is reduced in the SHR versus the WKY rat, indicating dysfunctional endothelium (225). Others have noted an enhanced contractile response of SHR mesenteric and renal arteries, a discrepancy for which there is no clear answer (207,223). In aortas of SHR and SHR stroke-prone rats, endothelium-dependent vasodilation in response to ET-1 and ET-3 persists, though is impaired compared to WKY rats (437,438). It is noteworthy that endothelin-induced ANP release from atria of SHR is increased compared to WKY rats. However, it is unlikely that this contributes to the early vasodilatory response (434). There is a divergence of findings in aortas from SHR with some noting increased (103,223,413), decreased (439,440), or normal sensitivity to ET-1 (441,442). However, a reduction in the maximal constrictor response is found by several groups (441,442). Potentially, the reduced sensitivity of the vascular smooth muscle might reflect decreased endothelin receptors. Indeed, the density of endothelin binding sites in SHR aortic smooth muscle cells in culture is roughly half that in WKY rats with no difference in the K_d (103). Taken together, the normal circulating levels of endothelin, the reduced endothelin binding sites, and the reduced sensitivity and maximal constriction of most isolated vascular smooth muscle preparations do not point to a primary role for endothelin in the pathogenesis of hypertension in the SHR model.

However, possible interaction of endothelin with other vasoregulatory systems in the SHR is suggested by evidence that threshold concentrations of exogenous ET-1 potentiate contractions induced by norepinephrine in perfused SHR, but not WKY mesentery (399,400). Perfusion of mesentery with high-dose Ang II (10^{-7} M) also potentiates norepinephrine-induced vasoconstriction, an effect likely due to endogenous endothelin as preproendothelin mRNA is increased, and the effect is inhibited by either phosphoramidon or antiendothelin antibodies (399). Augmentation of norepinephrine- and serotonin-induced vasoconstriction by endothelin is also observed in normal human mammary and coronary artery rings and rabbit aorta, an effect that is prevented by a calcium antagonist (385,386). In rats, synergistic pressor effects occur with chronic infusion of exogenous endothelin and Ang II (443). Taken together, these data suggest a possible amplifying effect of the peptide on the renin-angiotensin system. In this regard, the sensitivity to endothelin of mesenteric arterioles in situ in Goldblatt hypertensive rats (one-clip, two-kidney) is increased compared to normotensive controls, whereas the sensitivity and maximal response of isolated aortas to endothelin (with and without endothelium) is similar to control (444). Others find a decrease in sensitivity of the mesenteric artery of rats with renovascular hypertension (445). Thus, large vessels and small vessels might differ significantly in their response to endothelin. It is noteworthy that in Goldblatt hypertensive rats, treatment of blood pressure using an angiotensin-converting enzyme inhibitor, but not a beta blocker or hydralazine, normalized the blunted dose-response curves to ET-1 (446).

As described above in the DOCA-salt model of hypertension, there is an increase in endothelin content in the endothelium of the thoracic aorta and mesenteric artery despite normal circulating levels (418). The pathogenesis of this model of hypertension is believed to be, at least in part, related to volume expansion. However, this evidence suggests that the vasoactive effects of endothelin might also contribute. In isolated thoracic aortas and mesenteric arteries from hypertensive DOCA-salt rats (without endothelium), the maximal vasoconstrictor response is substantially less than uninephrectomized controls (66 percent and 33 percent, respectively) (416). In mesenteric arteries of these animals, the density of binding sites for endothelin is reduced with no change in the K_d, which is mirrored by a decrease in the accumulation of inositol 1,4,5-trisphosphate in response to ET-1 (416). These findings occur in the absence of endothelium and are thus likely to represent receptor downregulation, although given the binding characteristics of endothelin, prior occupancy cannot be ruled out even in isolated preparations. Downregulation of receptors is noted in cultured vascular smooth muscle cells after as little as 30 minutes of treatment with endothelin (447). An increase in endothelin receptors is also seen in rat mesangial cells (ET$_A$), human umbilical-vein endothelial cells (ET$_B$), and rat aortic endothelial cells (ET$_B$) treated with phosphoramidon, suggesting an autocrine effect of endothelin on its receptor (301). Others have noted no change (444) or augmentation (413) of the dose-response of isolated aortas. In support of an augmented response there is potentiation of endothelin-induced phosphoinositide hydrolysis in atria and mesenteric arteries of DOCA-salt rats (448). In the microvasculature, the sensitivity of rat mesenteric arterioles to endothelin was also similar to uninephrectomized controls (444). The divergence of findings might relate to specific experimental conditions, vessel size, or duration of hypertension, which was 2 weeks in the studies showing decreased responsiveness and longer in those showing no change or augmentation. In the Dahl salt-sensitive rat, another model of "volume-related" hypertension, there is an increase in vasoconstriction of isolated aortas prior to inducing hypertension with salt, which normalizes with the onset of hypertension (449).

In summary, controversy persists regarding the responsiveness of vascular smooth muscle in hypertension to exogenous and endogenous endothelin. In the SHR, DOCA-salt model, and Goldblatt models of hypertension, most find a decrease in the sensitivity of large and small vessels to endothelin. In human essential hypertension there is a decrease in sensitivity of subcutaneous resistance arteries to endothelin; otherwise little is known (450). In the SHR and DOCA-salt model the binding capacity of the vessel wall is also decreased, suggesting downregulation of endothelin receptors. In the SHR and Goldblatt hypertension models, exogenous endothelin and Ang II-induced endogenous endothelin can alter the responsiveness of the vessel to norepinephrine, suggesting significant interaction of the renin-angiotensin and sympathetic nervous system with endothelin. In the DOCA-salt model these findings are coupled to a significant increase in endothelial-cell endothelin content. These experimental models of hypertension and human hypertension are also associated with dysfunctional production of nitric oxide. This impairment worsens as hypertension progresses and is ameliorated by antihypertensive agents. It is likely that several factors will be altered by duration and magnitude of hypertension, including endothelium production of endothelin, vascular smooth muscle receptors, and responsiveness to endothelin.

Effect of Specific Blockade of Endothelin on Blood Pressure

The belief that endothelin is directly related to the hypertension in patients with rare hemangioendotheliomas is based on the abrupt parallel reduction of circulating endothelin and blood pressure with excision of the tumor. (Fig. 15). A role for endothelin in the pathogenesis of systemic hypertension would be strongly supported by specific inhibition of endothelin production or binding to its receptor. To date, there are no specific inhibitors of endothelin production. However, phosphoramidon, a nonspecific inhibitor of ECE, lowers blood pressure in the SHR (58). As discussed above, selective ET_A receptor

antagonists and antiendothelin antibodies do not alter blood pressure in normals (387–390). There is a paucity of data regarding the effects of the receptor antagonists on blood pressure in hypertensive animals. In rats with 5/6 nephrectomy, blood pressure rises over a 2- to 4-week period to hypertensive levels and is associated with progressive loss of renal mass. Five-sixths nephrectomized rats treated for 60 days with FR139317, a selective ET_A receptor antagonist, had significantly lower blood pressures than untreated rats, though still higher than sham rats (382). This effect was noted within 30 days of surgery and, thus, is less likely to be related solely to preservation of renal function. A selective ET_A receptor antagonist, BQ-123 has a hypotensive effect in stroke-prone SHR, the magnitude of which depends on the pretreatment blood pressure (451,452). In hypertensive SHR (18 and 40 weeks old) and normotensive WKY rat controls, this agent failed to lower blood pressure (451). Using antiendothelin antibodies, some have observed an antihypertensive effect in the SHR (453), whereas others have not (454). Other preliminary results note lower blood pressure in SHR acutely infused with either BQ-123 (138 ± 4 mm Hg) or another ET_A receptor antagonist, BMS-182874 (123 ± 4 mm Hg), as compared to vehicle (162 ± 5 mm Hg) (388). These changes were accompanied by a reduction in renal blood flow and, with BQ-123, a significant reduction in GFR. Using these highly selective receptor antagonists should help to clarify the role of endothelin in systemic hypertension; however, the present data are insufficient to draw conclusions.

In summary, in essential hypertension, endothelin production is modestly increased as judged by circulating levels. Production in experimental hypertension varies depending on the model studied. It is worth emphasizing that vessel wall endothelin content in the DOCA-salt model is increased despite unchanged circulating endothelin, highlighting the potential insensitivity of plasma endothelin levels. Experimental models indicate that vascular sensitivity to endothelin is altered in hypertension in both large and small vessels, an effect which is, at least in part, related to changes in receptor density. Preliminary results indicate that specific blockade of endothelin has a hypotensive effect. Finally, there is rapidly accumulating evidence of an interaction of endothelin with the renin-angiotensin system and the sympathetic nervous system.

CONCLUSIONS

In the past 5 years there has been an explosion of investigation of the endothelin peptides. The highly preserved structure, abundant cellular sources, and wide distribution of receptors suggest a role for this system in normal physiology. To date, however, that role has not been clearly defined. Regional specificity might be conferred by the relative ability of specific tissues to respond to endothelin-inducing stimuli, the abundance and specificity of ECE, and the density of receptor subtypes. Although many cells are able to produce endothelin, the vascular endothelium and brain are the most prominent sources. Circulating levels of endothelin in normals and in a wide range of disease states fall well below the K_d for receptor binding and the EC_{50} for cellular responses. However, polar secretion of the peptide by endothelial cells suggests that endothelin is more likely a paracrine and/or autocrine mediator than a circulating hormone. Thus, local concentrations within the vessel wall might be sufficient to trigger a cellular response. There are accumulating data to suggest that low concentrations of endothelin also might potentiate other known modulators of systemic and regional hemodynamics such as the renin-angiotensin and sympathetic nervous systems. To date, studies using specific endothelin-receptor antagonists do not support a role for endothelin in the maintenance of basal hemodynamics. Although there is little doubt that exogenous endothelin can lead to hypertension in humans, there are insufficient data to ascribe a role for this potent vasoconstrictor in essential hypertension. Given the pleiotropic nature of the actions of endothelin, the next 5 years will likely define a variety of functions for this peptide in normal and pathophysiologic states.

REFERENCES

1. Brenner BM, Troy JL, Ballermann BJ. Endothelium-dependent vascular responses. *J Clin Invest* 1989;84:1373–1378.
2. Furchgott RF, Zawadzki JV. The obligatory role of endothelial cells in the relaxation of arterial smooth muscle by acetylcholine. *Nature* 1980;288:373–376.
3. Furchgott RF. The role of endothelium in the responses of vascular smooth muscle to drugs. *Ann Rev Pharmacol Toxicol* 1984;24:175–197.
4. Vanhoutte PM. The endothelium—modulator of vascular smooth muscle tone. *N Engl J Med* 1988;318:512–513.
5. Vanhoutte PM. Endothelium-derived relaxing and contracting factors. *Adv Nephrol* 1990;19:3–16.
6. Yanagisawa M, Kurihara H, Kimura S, Tomobe Y, Kobayashi M, Mitsui Y, Yazaki Y, Goto K, Masaki T. A novel potent vasoconstrictor peptide produced by vascular endothelial cells. *Nature* 1988;332:411–415.
7. Inoue A, Yanagisawa M, Kimura S, Kasuya Y, Miyauchi T, Goto K, Masaki T. The human endothelin family: three structurally and pharmacologically distinct isopeptides predicted by three separate genes. *Proc Natl Acad Sci USA* 1989;86:2863–2867.
8. Battistini B, D'Orleans-Juste P, Sirois P. Endothelins: circulating plasma levels and presence in other biologic fluids. *Lab Invest* 1993;68:600–628.
9. Hickey KA, Rubanyi G, Paul RJ, Highsmith RF. Characterization of a coronary vasoconstrictor produced by cultured endothelial cells. *Am J Physiol* 1985;248 (Cell Physiol 17):C550–C556.
10. O'Brien RF, Robbins RJ, McMurtry IF. Endothelial cells in culture produce a vasoconstrictor substance. *J Cell Physiol* 1987;132:263–270.
11. Gillespie MN, Owasoyo JO, McMurtry IF, O'Brien RF. Sustained coronary vasoconstriction provoked by a peptidergic substance released from endothelial cells in culture. *J Pharmacol Exp Ther* 1986;236:339–343.
12. Rubanyi G. Endothelium-dependent pressure-induced contraction of isolated canine carotid arteries. *Am J Physiol* 1988;255 (Heart Circ Physiol 24):H783–H788.
13. Yanagisawa M, Inoue A, Ishikawa T, Kasuya Y, Kimura S, Kumagaye SI, Nakajima K, Watanabe TX, Sakakibara S, Goto K, Masaki T. Primary structure, synthesis, and biological activity of rat endothelin, an endothelium-derived vasoconstrictor peptide. *Proc Natl Acad Sci USA* 1988;85:6964–6967.
14. Inoue A, Yanagisawa M, Takuwa Y, Mitsui Y, Kobayashi M, Masaki T. The human preproendothelin-1 gene. *J Biol Chem* 1989;264:14954–14959.
15. Itoh Y, Yangisawa M, Ohkubo S, Kimura C, Goto K, Masaki T. Cloning and sequence analysis of cDNA encoding the precursor of a human endothelium-derived vasconstrictor peptide, endothelin: identity of human and porcine endothelin. *FEBS* Lett. 1988;231:440–444.
16. Takasaki C, Tamiya N, Bdolah A, Wollberg Z, Kochva E. Sarafotoxins S6: several isotoxins from *Attractaspis engaddensis* (burrowing asp): venon that affect the heart. *Toxicon* 1988;26:543–548.
17. Wollberg Z, Shabo-Shina R, Intrator N, Bdolah A, Kochva E, Shavit G, Oron Y, Vidne BA, Gitter S. A novel cardiotoxic polypeptide from the venom of *Attractaspis engaddensis* (burrowing asp): cardiac effects in mice and isolated rat and human heart preparations. *Toxicon* 1988;26:525–534.
18. Kopeyan C, Martinez G, Rochat H. Primary structure of toxin IV of *Leiurus quinquestriatus:* characterization of a new group of scorpion toxins. *FEBS* Lett. 1985;181:211–217.
19. Kloog Y, Ambar I, Sokolvsky M, Kochva E, Wollberg A, Bdolah A. Sarafotoxin, a novel vasoconstrictor peptide: phosphoinositide peptide: phosphoinositide hydrolysis in rat heart and brain. *Science* 1988;242:268–270.
20. Kimura S, Kasuya Y, Sawamura T, Shinmi O, Sugita Y, Yanagisawa M, Goto K, Masaki T. Structure-activity relationships of endothelin: importance of the C-terminal moiety. *Biochem Biophys Res Commun* 1988;156:1182–1186.
21. Doherty AM. Endothelin: a new challenge. *J Med Chem* 1992;35:1494–1507.
22. Perkins TD, Hider RC, Barlow DJ. Proposed solution structure of endothelin. *Int J Peptide Protein Res* 1990;36:128–133.
23. Saudek V, Hoflack J, Pelton JT. 1H-NMR study of endothelin, sequence-specific assignment of the spectrum and a solution structure. *FEBS* Lett. 1989;257:145–148.
24. Endo S, Inooka H, Ishibashi Y, Kitada C, Mizuta E, Fujino M. Solution conformation of endothelin determined by nuclear magnetic resonance and distance geometry. *FEBS* Lett. 1989;257:149–154.
25. Reily MD, Dunbar JB. The conformation of endothelin-1 in aqueous solution: NMR-derived constraints combined with distance geometry and molecular dynamics calculations. *Biochem Biophys Res Commun* 1992;178:570–577.
26. Mills RG, O'Donoghue SI, Smith R, King GF. Solution structure of endothelin-3 determined using NMR spectroscopy. *Biochemistry* 1992;31:5640–5645.
27. Saida K, Mitsui Y, Ishida N. A novel peptide, vasoactive intestinal constrictor, of a new (endothelin) peptide family. *J Biol Chem* 1989;264:14613–14616.
28. Bloch KD, Hong CC, Eddy RL, Shows TB, Quertermous T. cDNA cloning and chromosomal assignment of the endothelin 2 gene: vasoactive intestinal contractor peptide is rat endothelin 2. *Genomics* 1991;10:236–242.
29. Bloch KD, Eddy RL, Shows TB, Quertermous T. cDNA cloning and chromosomal assignment of the gene encoding endothelin 3. *J Biol Chem* 1989;264:18156–18161.
30. Landan G, Bdolah A, Wollberg Z, Kochva E, Graur D. Evolution of the sarafotoxin/endothelin superfamily of proteins. *Toxicon* 1991;29:237–244.
31. Arinami T, Ishikawa M, Inoue A, Yanagisawa M, Masaki T, Yoshida MC, Hamaguchi H. Chromosomal assignments of the human endothelin family genes: the endothelin-1 gene (EDN1) to 6p23-p24, the endothelin-2 gene (EDN2) to 1p34 and the endothelin-3 gene (EDN3) to 20q13.2-q13.3. *Am J Hum Genet* 1991;48:990–996.
32. Bloch KD, Friedrich SP, Lee M-E, Eddy RL, Shows TB, Querter-

mous T. Structural organization and chromosomal assignment of the gene encoding endothelin. *J Biol Chem* 1989;264:108521–10857.

33. Hilkert RJ, Lee M-E, Quertermous T. Genetic regulation of endothelin-1 in vascular endothelial cells. *Trends Cardiovasc Med* 1992;2:129–133.

34. Phillips PE, Cade C, Parker Botelho LH, Rubanyi GM. Molecular biology of endothelins. In: Rubanyi GM, ed. *Endothelin*. New York: Oxford, 1992;31–40.

35. Lee M-E, Dhadly MS, Temizer DH, Clifford JA, Yoshizumi M, Quertermous T. Regulation of endothelin-1 gene expression by fos and jun. *J Biol Chem* 1991;266:19034–19039.

36. Kanse SM, Takahashi K, Lam HC, Rees A, Warren JB, Porta M, Molinatti P, Ghatei M, Bloom SR. Cytokine stimulated endothelin release from endothelial cells. *Life Sci* 1991;48:1379–1384.

37. Ohta K, Hirata Y, Imai T, Kanno K, Emori T, Shichiri M, Marumo F. Cytokine-induced release of endothelin-1 from porcine renal epithelial cell line. *Biochem Biophys Res Commun* 1990;169:578–584.

38. Kurihara MK, Yoshizuma M, Sugiyama T, Takaku F, Yanagisawa M, Masaki T, Hamaoki H, Kato H, Yazaki Y. Transforming growth factor-β stimulates the expression of endothelin mRNA by vascular endothelial cells. *Biochem Biophys Res Commun* 1989;159:1435–1440.

39. Resink TJ, Hahn AW, Scott-Burden T, Powell J, Weber E, Buhler FR. Inducible endothelin mRNA expression and peptide secretion in cultured human vascular smooth muscle cells. *Biochem Biophys Res Commun* 1990;168:1303–1310.

40. Zoja CS, Orisio S, Perico N, Benigni A, Morigi M, Benatti L, Rambaldi A, Remuzzi G. Constitutive expression of endothelin gene in cultured human mesangial cells and its modulation by transforming growth factor β, thrombi, and a thromboxane A₂ analogue. *Lab Invest* 1991;64:16–25.

41. Simonson MS. Endothelins: multifuntional renal peptides. *Physiol Rev* 1993;73:375–411.

42. Masaki T, Kimura S, Yanagisawa M, Goto K. Molecular and cellular mechanism of endothelin regulation. *Circulation* 1991;84:1457–1468.

43. Kimura S, Kaysuya Y, Sawamura T, Shinmi O, Sugita Y, Yanagisawa M, Goto K, Masaki T. Conversion of big endothelin-1 to 21-residue endothelin-1 is essential for expression of full vasoconstrictor activity: structure-activity relationships of big endothelin-1. *J Cardiovasc Pharmacol* 1989;13:S5–S7.

44. Kashiwabara T, Inagaki Y, Ohta H, Iwamatsu A, Nomizu M, Morita A, Nishikori K. Putative precursors of endothelin have less vasoconstrictor activity in vitro but a potent effect in vivo. *FEBS* Lett. 1989;247:73–76.

45. Rubanyi GM, Parker Botelho LH. Endothelins. *FASEB J.* 1991;5:2713–2720.

46. Opgenorth TJ, Wu-Wong JR, Shiosaki K. Endothelin-converting enzymes. *FASEB J.* 1992;6:2653–2659.

47. McMahon EG, Palomo MA, Mehta P, Olins GM. Depressor and natriuretic effects of M&B 22,948, a guanosine cyclic 3′,5′-monophosphate-selective phosphodiesterase inhibitor. *J Pharmacol Exp Ther* 1989;251:1000–1005.

48. Takaoka M, Hukumori Y, Shiragami R, Ikegawa R, Matsumura Y, Morimoto S. Proteolytic processing of porcine big endothelin-1 catalyzed by cathepsin D. *Biochem Biophys Res Commun* 1990;173:1218–1223.

49. Matsumura Y, Ikegawa R, Takaoka M, Morimoto S. Conversion of porcine big endothelin to endothelin by an extract from the porcine aortic endothelial cells. *Biochem Biophys Res Commun* 1990;167:203–210.

50. Sawamura T, Kimura S, Shinmi O, Sugita Y, Yanagisawa M, Goto K, Masaki T. Purification and characterization of putative endothelin converting enzyme in bovine adrenal medulla: evidence for a cathepsin D-like enzyme. *Biochem Biophys Res Commun* 1990;168:1230–1236.

51. Sawamura T, Kimura S, Shinmi O, Sugita Y, Kobayashi M, Mitsui Y, Yanagisawa M, Goto K, Masaki T. Characterization of endothelin converting enzyme activities in soluble fraction of bovine cultured endothelial cells. *Biochem Biophys Res Commun* 1990;169:1138–1144.

52. Wu-Wong JR, Budzik GP, Devine EM, Opgenorth TJ. Charac-

terization of endothelin converting enzyme in rat lung. *Biochem Biophys Res Commun* 1990;169:1291–1296.

53. Wu-Wong JR, Devine EM, Budzik GP, Opgenorth TJ. Characterization and partial purification of endothelin-converting enzyme in rat lung. *J Cardiovasc Pharmacol* 1991;17:520–525.

54. Sawamura T, Shinmi O, Kishi N, Sugita Y, Yanagisawa M, Goto K, Masaki T, Kimura S. Analysis of big endothelin-1 digestion by cathepsin D. *Biochem Biophys Res Commun* 1990;170:883–889.

55. Lees WE, Kalinka S, Meech J, Capper SJ, Cook ND, Kay J. Generation of human endothelin by cathepsin E. *FEBS* Lett. 1990;273:99–102.

56. Ohnaka K, Takayanagi R, Yamauchi T, Okazaki H, Ohashi M, Umeda F, Nawata H. Identification and characterization of endothelin converting enzyme activity in cultured bovine endothelial cells. *Biochem Biophys Res Commun* 1990;168:1128–1136.

57. Fukuroda T, Noguchi K, Tsuchida S, Nishikibe M, Ikemoto F, Okada K, Yano M. Inhibitions of biological actions of big endothelin-1 by phosphoramidon. *Biochem Biophys Res Commun* 1990;172:390–395.

58. McMahon EG, Palomo MA, Moore WM, McDonald JF, Stern MK. Phosphoramidon blocks the pressor activity of porcine big-endothelin-1 (1-39) in vivo and conversion of big endothelin-1-(1-39) to endothelin-1-(1-21) in vitro. *Proc Natl Acad Sci USA* 1991;88:703–707.

59. Sawamura T, Kasuya Y, Matsushita Y, Suzuki N, Shinmi O, Kishi N, Sugita Y, Yanagisawa M, Goto K, Masaki T, Kimura S. Phosphoramidone inhibits the intracellular conversion of big endothelin-1 to endothelin-1 in cultured endothelial cells. *Biochem Biophys Res Commun* 1991;174:779–784.

60. Matsumura Y, Ikegawa R, Tsukahara Y, Takaoka M, Morimoto S. Conversion of big-endothelin-1 to endothelin-1 by two types of metalloproteinases derived from porcine aortic endothelial cells. *FEBS* Lett. 1990;272:166–170.

61. Takada J, Okada K, Ikenaga T, Matsuyama K, Yano M. Phosphoramidon-sensitive endothelin-converting enzyme in the cytosol of cultured bovine endothelial cells. *Biochem Biophys Res Commun* 1991;176:860–865.

62. Hioki Y, Okada K, Ito H, Matsuyama K, Yano M. Endothelin converting enzyme of bovine carotid artery smooth muscles. *Biochem Biophys Res Commun* 1991;174:446–451.

63. Ikegawa R, Matsumura Y, Tsukahara Y, Takaoka M, Morimoto S. Phosphoramidon, a metalloproteinase inhibitor, suppresses the secretion of endothelin-1 from cultured endothelial cells by inhibiting a big endothelin-1 converting enzyme. *Biochem Biophys Res Commun* 1990;171:669–675.

64. Sawamura T, Kasuya Y, Matsushita Y, Suzuki N, Shinmi O, Kishi N, Sugita Y, Yanagisawa M, Goto K, Masaki T, Kimura S. Phosphoramidon inhibits the intracellular conversion of big endothelin-1 in cultured endothelial cells. *Biochem Biophys Res Commun* 1990;174:779–784.

65. Matsumura Y, Hisaki K, Takaoka M, Morimoto S. Phosphoramidon, a metalloproteinase inhibitor, suppresses the hypertensive effect of big-endothelin-1. *Eur J Pharmacol* 1990;185:103–106.

66. Pollock DM, Opgenorth TJ. Evidence for metalloprotease involvement in the in vivo effects of big endothelin 1. *Am J Physiol* 1991;261:R257–R263.

67. Le Monnier de Gouville A-C, Cavero I. Cross tachyphylaxis to endothelin isopeptide-induced hypotension: a phenomenon not seen with proendothelin. *Br J Pharmacol* 1991;104.

68. Gardiner SM, Compton AM, Kemp PA, Bennett T. The effects of phophoramidon on the regional haemodynamic responses to human proendothelin [1-38] in conscious rats. *Br J Pharmacol* 1991;103:2009–2015.

69. D'Orleans-Juste P, Telemaque S, Claing A. Different pharmacological profiles of big endothelin-3 and big endothelin-1 in vivo and in vitro. *Br J Pharmacol* 1991;104:441–444.

70. Yoshizawa T, Shinmi O, Giaid A, Yanagisawa M, Gibson SJ, Kimura S, Uchiyama Y, Polak JM, Masaki T, Kanazawa I. Endothelin: a novel peptide in the posterior pituitary system. *Science Wash* 1990;247:462–464.

71. Ritz MF, Stuenkel EL, Dayanithi G, Jones R, Nordmann JJ. Endothelin regulation of neuropeptide release from nerve endings of

the posterior pituitary. *Proc Natl Acad Sci USA* 1992;89:8371–8375.

72. Wagner OF, Christ G, Wojta J, Vierhapper H, Parzer S, Nowotny PJ, Schneider B, Waldhausl W, Binder BR. Polar secretion of endothelin-1 by cultured endothelial cells. *J Biol Chem* 1992; 267:16066–16068.

73. Parker Botelho LH, Cade C, Phillips PE, Rubanyi GM. Tissue specificity of endothelin synthesis and binding. In: Rubanyi GM, ed. *Endothelin*. New York: Oxford, 1992;73–102.

74. Kanse SM, Takahashi K, Warren JB, Ghatei M, Bloom SR. Glucocorticoids induce endothelin release from vascular smooth muscle cells but not endothelial cells. *Eur J Pharmacol* 1991;199: 99–101.

75. Sakamoto H, Sasaki S, Hirata Y, Imai T, Ando K, Ida T, Sukurai T, Yanagisawa M, Masaki T, Marumo F. Production of endothelin-1 by rat cultured mesangial cells. *Biochem Biophys Res Commun* 1990;169:462–468.

76. Kohan DE. Production of endothelin-1 by rat cultured mesangial cells: regulation by tumor necrosis factor. *J Lab Clin Med* 1992;119:477–484.

77. Bakris GL, Fairbanks R, Traish AM, Akerstrom V, Kern S. Arginine vasopressin stimulates human mesangial cell production of endothelin. *J Clin Invest* 1991;87:1158–1164.

78. Sakamoto H, Sasaki S, Nakamura Y, Fushimi K, Marumo F. Regulation of endothelin-1 production in cultured rat mesangial cells. *Kidney Int* 1992;41:350–355.

79. Marsden PA, Brenner BM. Transcriptional regulation of the endothelin-1 gene by TNF-alpha. 1992.

80. Shichiri M, Hirata Y, Emori T, Ohta K, Nakajima T, Sato K, Sato A, Marumo F. Secretion of endothelin and related peptides from renal epithelial cell lines. *FEBS* Lett. 1989;253:203–206.

81. Kosaka T, Suzuki N, Matsumoto H, Itoh Y, Yasuhara T, Onda H, Fujino M. Synthesis of the vasoconstrictor peptide endothelin in kidney cells. *FEBS* Lett. 1989;249:42–46.

82. Nakahama H. Stimulatory effect of cyclosporine A on endothelin secretion by a cultured renal epithelial cell line, LLC-PK1 cells. *Eur J Pharmacol* 1990;180:191–192.

83. Maccumber MW, Ross CA, Synder SH. Endothelin in brain: receptors, mitogenesis and biosynthesis in glial cells. *Proc Natl Acad Sci USA* 1990;86:7285–7289.

84. Suzuki N, Matsumoto H, Kitada C, Kimura S, Fujino M. Production of endothelin-1 and big endothelin-1 by tumor cells with endotheliallike morphology. *J Biochem* 1989;106:736–741.

85. Kushuhara M, Yamaguchi K, Nagasaki Y, Hayashi C, Suzaki A, Hori S, Handa S, Nakamura Y, Abe K. Production of endothelin in human cancer cell lines. *Cancer Res* 1990;50:3257–3261.

86. Shichiri M, Hirata Y, Nakajima T, Ando K, Imai T, Yanagisawa M, Masaki T, Marumo F. Endothelin-1 is an autocrine/paracrine growth factor for human cancer cell lines. *J Clin Invest* 1991;87: 1867–1871.

87. Ehrenreich H, Anderson RW, Fox CH, Rieckmann P, Hoffman GS, Travis WD, Coligan JE, Kehrl JH, Fauci AS. Endothelins, peptides with potent vasoactive properties, are produced by human macrophages. *J Exp Med* 1990;172:1741–1748.

88. Ehrenreich H, Burd PR, Rottem M, Hultner L, Hylton JB, Garfield M, Coligan JE, Metcalfe DD, Fauci AS. Endothelins belong to the assortment of mast cell-derived and mast cell-bound cytokines. *New Biol* 1992;4:147–156.

89. Orlando CM, Brandi ML, Peri A, Giannini G, Fantoni G, Calabresi E, Serio M, Maggi M. Neurohypophyseal hormone regulation of endothelin secretion from rabbit endometrial cells in primary culture. *Endocrinology* 1990;126:1780–1782.

90. Black PN, Ghatei MA, Takahashi K, Bretherton-Watt D, Krausz CT, Dollery CT, Bloom SR. Formation of endothelin by cultured airway epithelial cells. *FEBS* Lett. 1989;255:129–132.

91. Kitamura K, Tanaka T, Kato J, Ogawa T, Eto T, Tanaka K. Immunoreactive endothelin in rat kidney inner medulla: marked decrease in spontaneously hypertensive rats. *Biochem Biophys Res Commun* 1989;162:38–44.

92. Firth JD, Ratcliffe PJ. Organ distribution of the three rat endothelin messenger RNAs and the effects of ischemia on renal gene expression. *J Clin Invest* 1992;90:1023–1031.

93. Yanagisawa M, Masaki T. Endothelin, a novel endothelium-derived peptide. *Biochem Pharmacol* 1989;38:1877–1883.

94. De Nucci GD, Thomas R, D'Orleans-Juste P, Antunes E, Walder C, Warner TD, Vane JR. Pressor effects of circulating endothelin are limited by its removal in the pulmonary circulation and by the release of prostacyclin and endothelium-derived relaxing factor. *Proc Natl Acad Sci USA* 1988;85:9797–9800.

95. Marsden PA, Danthuluri NR, Brenner BM, Ballermann BJ, Brock TA. Endothelin action on vascular smooth muscle involves inositol trisphosphate and calcium mobilization. *Biochem Biophys Res Commun* 1989;158:86–93.

96. Auguet M, Delaflotte S, Chabrier PE, Pirotzky E, Clostre F, Braquet P. Endothelin and Ca^{++} agonist Bay K 8644: different vasoconstrictive properties. *Biochem Biophys Res Commun* 1988; 156:186–192.

97. Nayler WG. Endothelin: isoforms, binding sites, and possible implications in pathology. *Trends Pharmacol Sci* 1990;11:96–99.

98. Miyazaki H, Kondoh M, Masuda Y, Watanabe H, Murakami K. Endothelin receptors and receptor subtypes. In: Rubanyi GM, ed. *Endothelin*. New York: Oxford, 1992;58–71.

99. Simonson MS, Dunn MJ. Cellular signaling by peptides of the endothelin gene family. *FASEB J* 1990;4:2989–3000.

100. Vane JR, Botting R, Masaki T. Endothelin. *J Cardiovasc Pharmacol* 1989;13(suppl):S1–S231.

101. Vanrenterghem C, Vigne P, Barhanin J, Schmid-Alliana A, Frelin C, Lazdunski M. Molecular mechanism of action of the vasoconstrictor peptide endothelin. *Biochem Biophys Res Commun* 1988;157:977–985.

102. Gu XH, Liu JJ, Dillon JS, Nayler WG. The failure of endothelin to displace bound, radioactively-labelled, calcium antagonists (PN 200/110, D88 and diltiazem). *Br J Pharmacol* 1989;96:262–264.

103. Clozel M. Endothelin sensitivity and receptor binding in the aorta of spontaneously hypertensive rats. *J Hypertension* 1989;7:913–917.

104. Hirata Y, Yoshimi H, Takaichi S, Yanagisawa M, Masaki T. Binding and receptor down-regulation of a novel vasoconstrictor endothelin in cultured rat vascular smooth muscle cells. *FEBS* Lett. 1988;239:13–17.

105. Clozel M, Fischli W, Guilly C. Specific binding of endothelin on human vascular smooth muscle cells in culture. *J Clin Invest* 1990;83:1758–1761.

106. Cozza EN, Gomez-Sanchez CE, Foecking MF, Chiou S. Endothelin binding to cultured calf adrenal zona glomerulosa cells and stimulation of aldosterone secretion. *J Clin Invest* 1989;84:1032–1035.

107. Emori T, Hirata Y, Marumo F. Specific receptors for endothelin-3 in cultured bovine endothelial cells and its mechanisms of action. *FEBS* Lett. 1990;263:261–264.

108. Fugitani M, Oda K, Takimoto M, Inui T, Okada T, Urade Y. Autocrine receptors for endothelins in the primary culture of endothelial cells of human umbilical vein. *FEBS* Lett. 1992;298: 79–83.

109. Kishino J, Hanasaki K, Kato T, Arita H. Endothelin-induced intracellular Ca^{++} mobilization through its specific receptors in murine peritoneal macrophages. *FEBS* Lett. 1991;280:103–106.

110. Wilkes BM, Ruston AS, Mento P, Girardi E, Hart D, Molen MV, Barnett R, Nord EP. Characterization of endothelin 1 receptor and signal transduction mechanisms in rat medullary interstitial cells. *Am J Physiol* 1991;260 (Renal, Fluid, Electrolyte Physiol 29):F579–F589.

111. Ambar I, Kloog Y, Sokolovsky M. Cross-linking of endothelin-1 and endothelin-3 to rat brain membranes—identification of the putative receptor. *Biochemistry* 1990;29:6415–6418.

112. Martin ER, Brenner BM, Ballermann BJ. Heterogeneity of cell surface endothelin receptors. *J Biol Chem* 1990;265(23):14044–14049.

113. Sakurai T, Yanagisawa M, Takuwa Y, Miyazaki H, Kimura S, Goto K, Masaki T. Cloning of a cDNA encoding a non-isopeptide-selective subtype of the endothelin receptor. *Nature* 1990;348:732–735.

114. Arai H, Hori S, Aramori I, Ohkubo H, Nakanishi S. Cloning and expression of a cDNA encoding an endothelin receptor. *Nature* 1990;348:730–732.

115. Lin H-Y, Kaji EH, Winkel GK, Ives HE, Lodish HF. Cloning and

functional expression of a vascular smooth muscle endothelin-1 receptor. *Proc Natl Acad Sci USA* 1991;88:3185–3189.

116. Nakamuta M, Takayanagi R, Sakai Y, Sakamoto S, Hagiwara H, Mizuno T, Saito Y, Hirose S, Yamamoto M, Nawata H. Cloning and sequence analysis of a cDNA encoding human non-selective type of endothelin receptor. *Biochem Biophys Res Commun* 1991;177:34–39.

117. Nakao K, Arai H, Hosoda K, Ogawa Y, Nakagawa O, Suga S-I, Nakanishi S, Imura H. Molecular cloning of two subtypes of human endothelin receptor. *J Vasc Med Biol* 1991;3:303–307.

118. Ito H, Hirata Y, Hiroe M, Tsujino M, Adachi S, Takamoto T, Nitta M, Taniguchi K, Marumo F. Endothelin-1 induces hypertrophy with enhanced expression of muscle-specific genes in cultured neonatal rat cardiomyocytes. *Circ Res* 1991;69:209–215.

119. Cyr C, Heubner K, Druck T, Kris R. Cloning and chromosomal localization of a human endothelin ETA receptor. *Biochem Biophys Res Commun* 1991;181:184–190.

120. Ogawa Y, Nakao K, Arai H, Nakagawa O, Hosoda K, Suga S, Nakanishi S, Imura H. Molecular cloning of a non-isopeptide-selective human endothelin receptor. *Biochem Biophys Res Commun* 1991;178:248–255.

121. Hosada K, Nakao K, Tamura N, Arai H, Ogawa Y, Suga S, Nakanishi S, Imura H. Organization, structure, chromosomal assignment, and expression of the gene encoding the human endothelin-A receptor. *J Biol Chem* 1992;267:18797–18804.

122. Hori S, Komatsu Y, Shigemoto R, Mizuno N, Nakanishi S. Distinct tissue distribution and cellular localization of two messenger ribonucleic acids encoding different subtypes of rat endothelin receptors. *Endocrinology* 1992;130:1885–1895.

123. Brock TA, Danthuluri NR. Cellular actions of endothelin in vascular smooth muscle. In: Rubanyi GM, ed. *Endothelin.* New York: Oxford, 1992;103–124.

124. Danthuluri NR, Brock TA. Endothelin receptor coupling mechanisms in vascular smooth muscle: a role for protein kinase C. *J Pharmacol Exp Ther* 1990;254:393–399.

125. Goto K, Kasuya Y, Matsuki N, Takuwa Y, Kurihara H, Ishikawa T, Kimura S, Yanagisawa M, Masaki T. Endothelin activates the dihydropyridine-sensitive, voltage-dependent Ca⁺⁺ channel in vascular smooth muscle. *Proc Natl Acad Sci USA* 1989;86:3915–3918.

126. Kai H, Kanaide H, Nakamura M. Endothelin-sensitive intracellular Ca⁺⁺ store overlaps with a caffeine-sensitive one in rat aortic smooth muscle cells in primary culture. *Biochem Biophys Res Commun* 1989;158:235–243.

127. Kasuya Y, Takuwa Y, Yanagisawa M, Kimura S, Goto K, Masaki T. Endothelin-1 induces vasoconstriction through two functionally distinct pathways in porcine artery-contribution of phosphoinositide turnover. *Biochem Biophys Res Commun* 1989;161:1049–1055.

128. Kodama I, Kanaide H, Abe S, Hirano K, Kai H, Nakamura M. Endothelin-induced Ca-independent contraction of the porcine coronary artery. *Biochem Biophys Res Commun* 1989;160:1302–1308.

129. Mitsuhasi T, Morris RC, Ives HE. Endothelin-induced increases in vascular smooth muscle Ca²⁺ do not depend on dihydropyridine-sensitive Ca²⁺ channels. *J Clin Invest* 1989;84:635–639.

130. Ohlstein EH, Horohonich S, Hay DWP. Cellular mechanisms of endothelin in rabbit aorta. *J Pharmacol Exp Ther* 1989;250:548–555.

131. Sugiura M, Inagami T, Hare GMT, Johns JA. Endothelin action: inhibition by a protein kinase C inhibitor and involvement of phosphoinositols. *Biochem Biophys Res Commun* 1989;158:170–176.

132. Yokokawa K, Kohno M, Murakawa K, Yasunari K, Takeda T. Effect of endothelin-1 on cytosolic calcium ions in cultured human endothelial cells. *J Hypertens* 1990;8:843–849.

133. Vigne P, Breittmayer JP, Marsault R, Frelin C. Endothelin mobilizes Ca²⁺ from a caffeine-insensitive and ryanodine-insensitive intracellular pool in rat atrial cells. *J Biol Chem* 1990;265:5925–5928.

134. Badr KF, Murray JJ, Breyer MD, Takahashi K, Inagami T, Harris RC. Mesangial cell, glomerular and renal vascular responses to endothelin in the rat kidney. *J Clin Invest* 1989;83:336–342.

135. Simonson MS, Dunn MJ. Ca⁺⁺ signaling by distinct endothelin peptides in glomerular mesangial cells. *Exp Cell Res* 1991;192:148–156.

136. Simonson MS, Osanai T, Dunn MJ. Endothelin isopeptides evoke Ca²⁺ signaling and oscillations of cytosolic free [Ca⁺⁺] in human mesangial cells. *Biochem Biophys Res Commun* 1990;1055:63–68.

137. Simonson MS, Wann S, Mene P, Dubyak GR, Kester M, Nakazato Y, Sedor JR, Dunn MJ. Endothelin stimulates phospholipase C, Na/H exchange, c-fos expression, and mitogenesis in rat mesangial cells. *J Clin Invest* 1989;83:708–712.

138. Marsault R, Vigne P, Frelin C. Astrocytes are target cells for endothelins and sarafotoxin. *J Neurochem* 1990;54:2142–2144.

139. Yue TL, Gleason MM, Lysko PG, Feuerstein G. Effect of endothelins on cytosolic free calcium concentration in neuroblastoma NG108-15 and NCB-20 cells. *Neuropeptides* 1990;17:7–12.

140. Stojilkovic SS, Merelli F, Ilda T, Krsmanovic LZ, Catt KJ. Endothelin stimulation of cytosolic calcium and gonadotropin secretion in anterior pituitary cells. *Science* 1990;248:1663–1666.

141. Word RA, Kamm KE, Stull JT, Caey ML. Endothelin increases cytoplasmic calcium and myosin phosphorylation in human myometrium. *Am J Obstet Gynecol* 1990;162:1103–1108.

142. Korbmacher CH, Helbing H, Haller H, Erickson-Lamy K, Wiederholt M. Endothelin depolarized membrane voltage and increases intracellular calcium concentration in human ciliary muscle cells. *Biochem Biophys Res Commun* 1989;164:1031–1039.

143. Berridge MJ, Irvine RF. Inositol phosphates and cell signaling. *Nature* 1990;341:197–205.

144. Exton JH. Mechanisms of action of calcium-mobilizing agonists: some variations on a young theme. *FASEB J* 1988;2670–2676.

145. Simonson MS, Dunn MJ. Endothelin-1 stimulates contraction of rat glomerular mesangial cells and potentiates β-adrenergic-mediated cyclic adenosine monophosphate accumulation. *J Clin Invest* 1990;85:790–797.

146. Chan J, Greenburg DA. SK&F 96365, a receptor-mediated calcium entry inhibitor, inhibits calcium responses to endothelin-1 in NG108-15 cells. *Biochem Biophys Res Commun* 1991;177:1141–1146.

147. Clozel M, Fischli W, Guilly C. Specific binding of endothelin on human vascular smooth muscle cells in culture. *J Clin Invest* 1989;83:1758–1761.

148. Kayusa YT, Takuwa T, Yanagisawa M, Kimura S, Goto K, Masaki T. Endothelin-1 induces vasoconstriction through two functionally distinct pathways in porcine coronary artery; contribution of phosphoinositide turnover. *Biochem Biophys Res Commun* 1989;161:1049–1055.

149. Silberberg SD, Poder TC, Lacerda AE. Endothelin increases single-channel calcium currents in coronary arterial smooth muscle cells. *FEBS* Lett. 247;247:68–72.

150. Inoue Y, Oike M, Kitamura K, Kuriyama H. Endothelin augments unitary calcium channel currents on the smooth muscle cell membrane of guinea-pig portal vein. *J Physiol Lond* 1990;423:171–191.

151. Nishizuka Y. Studies and perspectives of the protein kinase C family for cellular regulation. *Cancer* 1989;63:1892–1903.

152. Griendling KK, Tsuda T, Alexander RW. Endothelin stimulates diacylglycerol accumulation and activates protein kinase C in cultured vascular smooth muscle cells. *J Biol Chem* 1989;264:8237–8240.

153. Lee T-E, Chao T, Hu K, King GL. Endothelin stimulates a sustained 1,2-diacylglycerol increase and protein kinase C activation in bovine aortic smooth muscle cells. *Biochem Biophys Res Commun* 1989;162:381–386.

154. Auget M, Delaflotte S, Chabrier PE, Braquet P. Comparative effects of endothelin and phorbol 12,13-dibutyrate in rat aorta. *Life Sci* 1989;45:2051–2059.

155. Danthuluri NR, Deth RC. Phorbol ester-induced contraction of arterial smooth muscle and inhibition of α-adrenergic response. *Biochem Biophys Res Commun* 1984;125:1103–1109.

156. Itoh H, Lederis K. Contraction of rat thoracic aorta strips induced by phorbol 12-myristate 13-acetate. *Am J Physiol* 1987;252:C244–C247.

157. Danthuluri NR, Brock TA. Endothelin receptor coupling mechanisms in vascular smooth muscle: a role for protein kinase C. *J Pharmacol Exp Ther* 1990;254:393–399.

158. Resink TJ, Scott-Burden T, Weber E, Buhler FR. Phorbol ester promotes a sustained down-regulation of endothelin receptors and cellular responses to endothelin in human vascular smooth muscle cells. *Biochem Biophys Res Commun* 1990;166:1213–1219.

159. Roubert P, Gillard V, Plas P, Guillon JM, Chabrier PE, Braquet P. Angiotensin II and phobol esters potently down-regulate endothelin (endothelin-1) binding sites in vascular smooth muscle cells. *Biochem Biophys Res Commun* 1989;164:809–815.

160. Berk B, Brock TA, Gimbrone MA, Alexander RW. Early agonist-mediated ionic events in cultured vascular smooth muscle cells: calcium mobilization is associated with intracellular acidification. *J Biol Chem* 1987;262:5065–5072.

161. Danthuluri NR, Berk BC, Brock TA, Cragoe EJJ, Deth RC. Protein kinase C-mediated intracellular alkalinization in rat and rabbit aortic smooth muscle cells. *Eur J Pharmacol* 1987;141:503–506.

162. Grinstein S, Rothstein A. Mechanism of regulation of the Na^+/H^+ exchanger. *J Membr Biol* 1986;90:1–12.

163. Hatori N, Fine BP, Nakamura A, Cragoe EJ, Aviv A. Angiotensin II effect on cytosolic pH in cultured rat vascular smooth muscle cells. *J Biol Chem* 1987;262:5073–5078.

164. Owen NE. Effect of catecholamines on Na/H exchange in vascular smooth muscle cells. *J Cell Biol* 1986;103:2053–2060.

165. Simonson MS, Herman WH. Protein kinase C and protein tyrosine kinase activity contribute to mitogenic signaling by endothelin-1: cross talk between G protein-coupled receptors and pp60^{c-src}. *J Biol Chem* 1993.

166. Muldoon LL, Pribnow D, Roland KD, Magun BE. Endothelin-1 stimulates DNA synthesis and anchorage-independent growth of rat-1 fibroblasts through a protein kinase C-dependent mechanism. *Cee Regul* 1990;1:379–390.

167. Kester M, Simonson MS, McDermott RG, Baldi E, Dunn MJ. Endothelin stimulates phosphotidic acid formation in cultured mesangial cells: role of a protein kinase C-dependent phospholipase D. *J Cell Physiol* 1992;150:578–585.

168. MacNulty EE, Plevin R, Wakelam MJ. Stimulation of the hydrolysis of phosphotidyinositol 4,5-bisphosphate and phosphatidylcholine by endothelin, a complete mitogen for Rat-1 fibroblasts. *Biochem J* 1990;272:761–766.

169. Pai J-K, Dobek EA, Bishop NR. Endothelin-1 activates phospholipase D and thymidine incorporation in fibroblasts overexpressing protein kinase C beta 1. *Cell Regul* 1991;2:897–903.

170. Resink TJ, Scott-Burden T, Buhler FR. Activation of multiple signal transduction pathways by endothelin in cultured vascular smooth muscle cells. *Eur J Biochem* 1990;189:415–421.

171. Battistini B, Sirois P, Braquet P, Filep JG. Endothelin-induced constriction of guinea pig airways: role of platelet-activating factor. *Eur J Pharmacol* 1990;186:307–310.

172. Resink TJ, Scott-Burden T, Buhler FR. Activation of phospholipase A by endothelin in cultured vascular smooth muscle cells. *Biochem Biophys Res Commun* 1989;158:279–286.

173. Reynolds EE, Mok LL, Kurokawa S. Phorbol ester dissociates endothelin-stimulated phosphoinositide hydrolysis and arachidonic acid release in vascular smooth muscle cells. *Biochem Biophys Res Commun* 1989;160:868–873.

174. Schumacher WA, Steinbacher TE, Allen GT, Ogletree ML. Role of thromboxane receptor activation in the bronchospastic response to endothelin. *Prostaglandins* 1990;40:71–79.

175. Takayasu Okishio M, Terashita Z, Kondo K. Endothelin-1 and platelet activating factor stimulate thromboxane A_2 biosynthesis in rat vascular smooth muscle cells. *Biochem Pharmacol* 1990;40:2713–2717.

176. Zoja C, Benigni A, Renzi D, Piccinelli A, Perico N, Remuzzi G. Endothelin and eicosanoid synthesis in cultured mesangial cells. *Kidney Int* 1990;37:927–933.

177. Aramori I, Nakanishi S. Coupling of two endothelin receptor subtypes to differing signal transduction in transfected Chinese hamster ovary cells. *J Biol Chem* 1992;267:12468–12474.

178. Reynolds EE, Mok LL. Role of thromboxane A_2/prostaglandin H_2 receptor in the vasoconstrictor response of rat aorta to endothelin. *J Pharmacol Exp Ther* 1990;252:915–921.

179. Dubin D, Pratt RE, Cooke JP, Dzau VJ. Endothelin, a potent vasoconstrictor, is a vascular smooth muscle mitogen. *J Vasc Med Biol* 1989;1:150–154.

180. Komuro I, Kurihara H, Sugiyama T, Yoshizumi M, Takaku F, Yazaki Y. Endothelin stimulates c-fos and c-myc expression and proliferation of vascular smooth muscle cells. *FEBS* Lett. 1988;238:249–252.

181. Takagi N, Fukase M, Takata S, Yoshimi H, Tokunaga O, Fujita T. Autocrine effect of endothelin on DNA synthesis in human vascular endothelial cells. *Biochem Biophys Res Commun* 1990;168:537–543.

182. Vigne P, Marsault R, Breittmayer JP, Frelin C. Endothelin stimulates phosphatidylinositol hydrolysis and DNA synthesis in brain capillary endothelial cells. *Biochem J* 1990;266:415–420.

183. Brown KD, Littlewood CJ. Endothelin stimulates DNA synthesis in Swiss 3T3 cells. Synergy with polypeptide growth factors. *Biochem J* 1989;263:977–980.

184. Takuwa Y, Kasuya Y, Takuwa N, Kudo M, Yanagisawa M, Masaki T. Novel vasoactive peptide endothelin stimulates mitogenesis through inositol lipid turnover in Swiss 3T3 fibroblasts. *J Biol Chem* 1989;264:7856–7861.

185. Jaffer FE, Knauss TC, Poptic E, Aboudd HE. Endothelin stimulates PDGF secretion in cultured human mesangial cells. *Kidney Int* 1990;38:1193–1198.

186. Muldoon L, Rodland KD, Forsythe ML, Magun BE. Stimulation of phosphatidylinositol hydrolysis, diacylglycerol release, and gene expression in response to endothelin, a potent new agonist for fibroblasts and smooth muscle cells. *J Biol Chem* 1989;264:8529–8536.

187. Rodland KD, Muldoon LL, Lenormand P, Magun BE. Modulation of RNA expression by intracellular calcium. *J Biol Chem* 1990;265:11000–11007.

188. Simonson MS, Jones JM, Dunn MJ. Differential regulation of *fos* and *jun* gene expression and AP-1 *cis*-element activity by endothelin isopeptides: possible implications for mitogenic signaling by endothelin. *J Biol Chem* 1992;267:8643–8649.

189. Nafitilan AJ, Pratt RE, Dzau VJ. Induction of PDGF A-chain and c-*myc*-gene expressions by angiotensin II in cultured rat vascular smooth muscle cells. *J Clin Invest* 1989;83:1419–1424.

190. Simonson MS, Jones JM, Dunn MJ. Cytosolic and nuclear signaling by endothelin peptides: implications for the mesangial response to glomerular injury. *Kidney Int* 1992;41:542–545.

191. Simonson MS, Wang Y, Dunn MJ. Cellular signaling by endothelin peptides: pathways to the nucleus. *J Am Soc Nephrol* 1992;2:S116–S125.

192. Wagner OF, Christ G, Wojta J, Vierhapper H, Parzer S, Nowotnu PJ, Schneider B, Waldhausl W, Binder BR. Polar secretion of endothelin-1 by cultured endothelial cells. *Proc Natl Acad Sci USA* 1992;267:16066–16068.

193. Kohan DE, Padilla E. Endothelin-1 is an autocrine factor in rat inner medullary collecting ducts. *Am J Physiol* 1992;261 (Renal, Fluid, Electrolyte Physiol 32):F607–F612.

194. Pohl U, Busse R. Differential vascular sensitivity to luminally and adventitially applied endothelin-1. *J Cardiovasc Pharmacol* 1989;13(suppl 5):S188–S190.

195. King AJ, Brenner BM. Renal and systemic hemodynamic actions of endothelin. In: Rubanyi GM, ed. *Endothelin.* New York: Oxford, 1992;158–178.

196. Lerman A, Hildebrand FL, Aarhus LL, Burnett JC. Endothelin has biological actions at pathophysiologic concentrations. *Circulation* 1991;83:1808–1814.

197. Vierhapper H, Wagner O, Nowotny P, Waldhausl W. Effect of endothelin-1 in man. *Circulation* 1990;81:1415–1418.

198. Shiba R, Yanagisawa M, Miyauchi T, Ishii Y, Kimura S, Uchiyama Y, Masaki T, Goto K. Elimination of intravenously injected endothelin-1 from the circulation of the rat. *J Cardiovasc Pharmacol* 1989;6(suppl 4):S98–S101.

199. Anggard E, Galton S, Rae G, Thomas R, McLoughlin L, de Nucci G, Vane JR. The fate of radioiodinatated endothelin-1 and endothelin-3 in the rat. *J Cardiovasc Pharmacol* 1989;6(suppl 4):S46–S49.

200. Sirvio M, Metsarinne K, Saijonmaa O, Fyhrquist F. Tissue distribution and half-life of 125-I endothelin in the rat: importance of pulmonary clearance. *Biochem Biophys Res Commun* 1990;167:1191–1195.

201. Stewart DJ, Levy RD, Cernacek P, Langleben D. Increased plasma endothelin-1 in pulmonary hypertension: marker or mediator of disease? *Ann Intern Med* 1991;114:464–469.

202. Westcott JY, Henson J, McMurtry IF, O'Brien RF. Uptake and metabolism of endothelin in the isolated perfused rat lung. *Exp Lung Res* 1990;16:521–532.

203. Vijayaraghavan J, Scicli AG, Carretero OA, Slaughter C, Moomaw C, Hersh LB. The hydrolysis of endothelins by neutral endopeptidase 24.11 (enkephalinase). *J Biol Chem* 1990;265: 14150–14155.

204. King AJ, Brenner BM, Anderson S. Endothelin: a potent renal and systemic vasoconstrictor peptide. *Am J Physiol* 1989;256 (Renal Fluid Electrolyte Physiol 25):F1051–F1058.

205. King AJ, Pfeffer JM, Pfeffer MA, Brenner BM. Systemic hemodynamic effects of endothelin in the rat. *Am J Physiol* 1990;258 (Heart Circ Physiol 23):H787–H792.

206. Kitayoshi T, Watanabe T, Shimamoto N. Cardiovascular effects of endothelin in dogs: positive inotropic action in vivo. *Eur J Pharmacol* 1989;166:519–522.

207. Miyauchi T, Ishikawa T, Tomobe Y, Yanagisawa M, Kimura S, Sugishita Y, Ito I, Goto K, Masaki T. Characteristics of pressor response to endothelin in spontaneously hypertensive and Wistar-Kyoto rats. *Hypertension* 1989;14:427–434.

208. Wright CE, Fozard JR. Regional vasodilation is a prominent feature of the haemodynamic response to endothelin in anaesthetized, spontaneously hypertensive rats. *Eur J Pharmacol* 1988;155:201–203.

209. Clarke JG, Benjamin N, Larkin SW, Webb DJ, Davies GJ, Maseri A. Endothelin is a potent long-lasting vasoconstrictor in men. *Am J Physiol* 1989;257 (Heart Circ Physiol 26):H2033–H2035.

210. Gardiner SM, Compton AM, Bennett T. Regional hemodynamic effects of endothelin-1 in conscious, unrestrained, Wistar rats. *J Cardiovasc Pharmacol* 1989;6(suppl 4):S202–S204.

211. Given MB, Lowe RF, Lippton H, Hyman AL, Sander GE, Giles TD. Hemodynamic actions of endothelin in conscious and anesthetized dogs. *Peptides* 1989;10:41–44.

212. Goetz KL, Wang BC, Madwed JB, Zhu JL, Leadley RJ. Cardiovascular, renal, and endocrine responses to intravenous endothelin in conscious dogs. *Am J Physiol* 1988;255 (Regulatory Integrative Comp Physiol 24):R1064–R1068.

213. Han SP, Trapani AJ, Fok KF, Westfall TC, Kneupfer MM. Effects of endothelin on regional hemodynamics in conscious rats. *Eur J Pharmacol* 1989;159:303–305.

214. Hinojosa-Laborde C, Osborn JW, Cowley AW. Hemodynamic effects of endothelin in conscious rats. *Am J Physiol* 1989;256 (Heart Circ Physiol 25):H1742–H1746.

215. Kneupfer MM, Han SP, Trapani AJ, Fok KF, Westfall TC. Regional hemodynamic and baroreflex effects of endothelin in rats. *Am J Physiol* 1989;257 (Heart Circ Physiol 26):H918–H926.

216. Lippton H, Goff J, Hyman A. Effects of endothelin in the systemic and renal vascular beds in vivo. *Eur J Pharm* 1988;155: 197–199.

217. Pernow J, Franco-Cereceda A, Matran R, Lundberg JM. Effect of endothelin-1 on regional vascular resistances in the pig. *J Cardiovasc Pharmacol* 1989;6(suppl 4):S205–S206.

218. Rohmeiss P, Photiadis J, Rohmeiss S, Unger T. Hemodynamic actions of intravenous endothelin in the rats: comparison with sodium nitroprusside and methoxamine. *Am J Physiol* 1990;258 (Heart Circ Physiol 27):H337–H346.

219. Scoggins BA, Spence CD, Parkes DG, McDonald M, Wade JD, Coghlan JP. Cardiovascular actions of human endothelin in conscious sheep. *Clin Exp Pharmacol Physiol* 1989;16:235–238.

220. Clozel M, Clozel JP. Effects of endothelin on regional blood flows in squirrel monkeys. *J Pharmacol Exp Ther* 1989;250:1125–1131.

221. Hoffman A, Grossman E, Ohman KP, Marks E, Keiser HR. Endothelin induces an initial increase in cardiac output associated with selective in rats. *Life Sci* 1989;45:249–255.

222. Minkes RK, MacMillan LA, Bellan JA, Kerstein MD, McNamara DB, Kadowitz PJ. Analysis of regional responses to endothelin in hindquarters vascular bed of cats. *Am J Physiol* 1989;256 (Heart Circ Physiol 25):H598–H602.

223. Tomobe Y, Miyauchi T, Saito A, Yanagisawa M, Kimura S, Goto K, Masaki T. Effects of endothelin on the renal artery from spontaneously hypertensive and Wistar-Kyoto rats. *Eur J Pharmacol* 1988;152:373–374.

224. Walder CE, Thomas GR, Thiemermann C, Vane JR. The hemodynamic effects of endothelin-1 in the rat. *J Cardiovasc Pharmacol* 1989;6(suppl 4):S93–S97.

225. Dohi Y, Luscher TF. Endothelin-1 in hypertensive mesenteric resistance arteries. Different intra- and extra-luminal dysfunction. *Hypertension* 1991.

226. Whittle BJR, Lopez-Belmonte J, Rees DD. Modulation of the vasodepressor actions of acetylcholine, bradykinin, substance P and endothelin in the rat by a specific inhibitor of nitric oxide formation. *Br J Pharmacol* 1989;98:646–652.

227. Fukuda N, Izumi Y, Soma M, Watanabe Y, Wantanabe M, Hatano M, Sakuma I, Yasuda H. L-NG-monomethyl arginine inhibits the vasodilating effects of low dose of endothelin-3 on rat mesenteric arteries. *Biochem Biophys Res Commun* 1990;167: 739–745.

228. Warner TD, de Nucci GD, Vane JR. Rat endothelin is a vasodilator in the perfused mesentery of the rat. *Eur J Pharmacol* 1989;159:325–326.

229. Boulanger C, Luscher TF. Release of endothelin from the porcine aorta. *J Clin Invest* 1990;85:587–590.

230. Rae GA, Trybulec M, de Nucci G, Vane JR. Endothelin-1 releases eicosanoids from rabbit isolated perfused kidney and spleen. *J Cardiovasc Pharmacol* 1989;6(suppl 4):S89–S92.

231. Herman F, Magyar K, Chabrier PE, Braquet P, Filep J. Prostacyclin mediates antiaggregatory and hypopotensive actions of endothelin in anaesthetized beagle dogs. *Br J Pharmacol* 1989;98: 38–40.

232. Hom GJ, Touhey B, Rubanyi GM. Potential mechanisms of endothelin-induced transient decreases in arterial pressure in spontaneously hypertensive rats. In: Rubanyi GM, Vanhoutte PM, eds. *Endothelium-derived contracting factors.* Basel: Varger, 1990;98–103.

233. Miller WL, Redfield MM, Burnett JC. Integrated cardiac, renal and endocrine actions of endothelin. *J Clin Invest* 1989;83:317–320.

234. Mortensen LH, Fink GD. Hemodynamic effect of human and rat endothelin administration into conscious rats. *Am J Physiol* 1990;258 (Heart Circ Physiol 27):H362–H368.

235. Lippton HL, Hauth TA, Summer WR, Hyman AL. Endothelin produces pulmonary vasoconstriction and systemic vasodilation. *J Appl Physiol* 1989;66(2):1008–1012.

236. Ouchi Y, Kim S, Souza AC, Iijima S, Hattori A, Orimo H, Yoshizumi M, Kurihara H, Yazaki Y. Central effect of endothelin on blood pressure in conscious rats. *Am J Physiol* 1989;256 (Heart Circ Physiol 25):H1747–H1751.

237. Pernow J. Characterization of the cardiovascular actions of endothelin in vivo: comparisons with neuropeptide Y and angiotensin II. *Acta Physiol Scand* 1989;137:421–426.

238. Cao L, Banks RO. Cardiovascular and renal actions of endothelin: effects of calcium-channel blockers. *Am J Physiol* 1990;258 (Renal Fluid Electrolyte Physiol 27):F254–F258.

239. Maddox DA, Brenner BM. Glomerular ultrafiltration. In: Brenner BM, Rector FC, eds. *The kidney.* Philadelphia: W. B. Saunders, 1991;205–244.

240. Dworkin LD, Hostetter TH, Rennke HG, Brenner BM. Hemodynamic basis for glomerular injury in rats with desoxycorticosterone-salt hypertension. *J Clin Invest* 1984;73:1448–1461.

241. Kohzuki M, Johnston CI, Chai SY, Casley DJ, Mendelsohn FAO. Localization of endothelin receptors in rat kidney. *Eur J Pharmacol* 1989;160:193–194.

242. Koseki C, Imai M, Hirata Y, Yanagisawa M, Masaki T. Autoradiographic distribution in rat tissues of binding sites for endothelin: a neuropeptide? *Am J Physiol* 1989;256:R858–R866.

243. Jones CR, Hiley CR, Pelton JT, Miller RC. Autoradiographic localization on endothelin binding sites in kidney. *Eur J Pharmacol* 1989;163:379–382.

244. Maccumber MW, Ross CA, Glaser BM, Snyder SH. Endothelin: visualization of mRNAs by in situ hybridization provides evidence for local action. *Proc Natl Acad Sci USA* 1989;87:2359–2363.

245. Waeber OF, Hoyer D, Palacios J-M. Similar distribution of [^{125}I]-

sarafotoxin-6b and [^{125}I] endothelin 1,2,3 binding sites in the human kidney. *Eur J Pharmacol* 1990;176:233–236.

246. Nambi P, Wu HL, Pullen M, Aiyar N, Bryan H, Elliot J. Identification of endothelin receptor subtypes in rat kidney cortex using subtype-selective ligands. *Mol Pharmacol* 1992;42:336–339.

247. Martin ER, Marsden PA, Brenner BM, Ballermann BJ. Identification and characterization of endothelin binding sites in rat renal papillary and glomerular membranes. *Biochem Biophys Res Commun* 1989;162:130–137.

248. Neuser D, Zaiss S, Stasch J-P. Endothelin receptors in cultured vascular smooth muscle cells. *Eur J Pharmacol* 1990;176:241–243.

249. Badr KF, Munger KA, Sugiura M, Snajdar RM, Schwartzberg M, Inagami T. High and low affinity binding sites for endothelin on cultured rat glomerular mesangial cells. *Biochem Biophys Res Commun* 1989;161:776–781.

250. Baldi E, Dunn MJ. Endothelin binding and receptor downregulation in rat glomerular mesangial cells. *J Pharmacol Exp Ther* 1991;256:581–586.

251. Terada Y, Tomita K, Nonogughi H, Marumo F. Different localization of two types of endothelin receptor mRNA in microdissected rat nephron segments using reverse transcription and polymerase chain reaction. *J Clin Invest* 1992;90:107–112.

252. Edwards RM, Pullen M, Nambi P. Activation of endothelin ET receptors increases glomerular cGMP via an L-arginine-dependent pathway. *Am J Physiol* 1992;263 (Renal Fluid Electrolyte Physiol 32):F1020–F1025.

253. Nunez DJ, Taylor EA, Oh VM, Schofield JP, Brown MJ. Endothelin-1 mRNA is widely expressed in porcine and human tissue. *Biochem J* 1991;275:1537–1541.

254. Sakurai T, Yanagisawa M, Inoue A, Ryan US, Kimura S, Mitsui Y, Goto K, Masaki T. cDNA cloning, sequence analysis and tissue distribution of rat preproendothelin-1 mRNA. *Biochem Biophys Res Commun* 1991;175:44–47.

255. Ujiie K, Terada Y, Nonoguchi H, Shinohara M, Tomita K, Marumo F. Messenger RNA expression and synthesis of endothelin-1 along rat nephron segments. *J Clin Invest* 1992;90:1043–1048.

256. Wilkes BM, Susin M, Mento PF, Macica CM, Girardi EP, Boss E, Nord EP. Localization of endothelinlike immunoreactivity in rat kidneys. *Am J Physiol* 1991;260 (Renal Fluid Electrolyte Physiol 29):F913–F920.

257. Marsden P. *Am J Hypertens* 1989.

258. Cybulski AV, Stewart DJ, Cybulsky MI. Glomerular epithelial cells produce endothelin-1. *J Am Soc Nephrol* 1993;3:1398–1404.

259. Kohan DE. Endothelin synthesis by rabbit renal tubule cells. *Am J Physiol* 1991;261 (Renal Fluid Electrolyte Physiol 30):F221–F226.

260. Berbinschi A, Ketelslegers JM. Endothelin in urine. *Lancet* 1989;2:46.

261. Pernow J, Hemsen A, Jundberg JM. Tissue specific distribution, clearance, and vascular effects of endothelin in the pig. *Biochem Biophys Res Commun* 1989;161:647–653.

262. Kon V, Sugiura M, Inagami T, Hoover RL, Fogo A, Harvie BR, Ichikawa I. Cyclosporine causes endothelin-dependent caute renal failure (Abst). *Kidney Int* 1990;37:486.

263. Tsuchiya K, Naruse M, Sanaka T, Naruse K, Nitta K, Demura H, Sugino N. Effects of endothelin on renal regional blood flow in dogs. *Eur J Pharm* 1989;166:541–543.

264. Nakamoto H, Suzuki H, Murakami M, Kageyama Y, Ohishi A, Fukuda K, Hori S, Saruta T. Effects of endothelin on systemic and renal haemodynamics and neuroendocrine hormones in conscious dogs. *Clin Sci* 1989;77:567–572.

265. Stacy DL, Scott JW, Granger JP. Control of renal function during intrarenal infusion of endothelin. *Am J Physiol* 1990;258 (Renal Fluid Electrolyte Physiol 27):F1232–F1236.

266. Chou SY, Dahhan A, Porush JG. Renal actions of endothelin: interaction with prostacyclin. *Am J Physiol* 1990;259 (Renal Fluid Electrolyte Physiol 28):F645–F652.

267. Gardiner SM, Compton AM, Bennett T, Palmer RMJ, Moncada S. Control of regional blood flow by endothelium-derived nitric oxide. *Hypertension* 1990;15:486–492.

268. Yamashita Y, Yukimura T, Miura K, Okumura M, Yamamoto K. Effects of endothelin-3 on renal functions. *J Pharmacol Exp Ther* 1991;259:1256–1260.

269. Hirata Y, Matsuoka H, Kimura K, Fukui K, Hayakawa H, Suzuki E, Sugimoto T, Sugimoto T, Yanagisawa M, Masaki T. Renal vasoconstriction by the endothelial cell-derived peptide endothelin in spontaneously hypertensive rats. *Circ Res* 1989;65:1370–1379.

270. Firth JD, Ratcliffe PJ, Raine AEG, Ledingham JGG. Endothelin: an important factor in acute renal failure. *Lancet* 1988;2:1179–1181.

271. Loutzenhiser R, Epstein M, Hayashi K, Horton C. Direct visualization of effects of endothelin on the renal microvasculature. *Am J Physiol* 1990;258 (Renal Fluid Electrolyte Physiol 27):F61–F68.

272. Katoh T, Chang H, Uchida S, Okuda T, Kurakawa K. Direct effects of endothelin in the rat kidney. *Am J Physiol* 1990;258 (Renal Fluid Electrolyte Physiol 27):F397–F402.

273. Cairns HS, Rogerson ME, Fairbanks LD, Neild GH, Westwick J. Endothelin induces an increase in renal vascular resistance and a fall in glomerular filtration rate in the rabbit isolated perfused kidney. *Br J Pharmacol* 1989;98:155–160.

274. Yokokawa K, Kohno M, Murakawa K, Yasunari K, Horio T, Inoue T, Takeda T. Acute effects of endothelin on renal hemodynamics and blood pressure in anesthetized rats. *Am J Hypertens* 1989;2:715–717.

275. Pernow J, Bouttier JF, Franco-Cereceda A, Lacroix JS, Natran R, Lundberg JM. Potent selective vasoconstrictor effects of endothelin in the pig kidney in vivo. *Acta Physiol Scand* 1988;134:573–574.

276. Madeddu P, Yang X, Anania V, Troffa C, Pazzola A, Soro A, Manunta P, Tonolo G, Demontis M, Varoni M, Melis M, Glorioso N. Efficacy of nifedipine to prevent systemic and renal vasoconstrictor effects of endothelin. *Am J Physiol* 1990;259 (Renal Fluid Electrolyte Physiol 28):F304–F311.

277. Matsumura Y, Hisaki K, Okyama T, Hayashi K, Morimoto S. Effects of endothelin on renal function and renin secretion in anesthetized rats. *Eur J Pharmacol* 1989;166:577–580.

278. Banks RO. Effects of endothelin on renal function in dogs and rats. *Am J Physiol* 1990;258 (Renal Fluid Electrolyte Physiol 27):F775–F780.

279. Lin H, Sangmal M, Smith MJ, Young DB. Effect of endothelin-1 on glomerular hydraulic pressure and renin release in dogs. *Hypertension* 1993;21:845–851.

280. Ferrario RG, Foulkes R, Salvati P, Patrono C. Hemodynamic and tubular effects of endothelin and thromboxane in the isolated perfused rat kidney. *Eur J Pharmacol* 1989;171:127–134.

281. Nitta K, Naruse M, Sanaka T, Tsuchiya K, Naruse K, Zeng Z, Demura H, Sugino N. Natriuretic and diuretic effects of endothelin in isolated perfused rat kidney. *Endocrinol Jpn* 1990;36:887–890.

282. Perico N, Dadan J, Gabanelli M, Remuzzi G. Cyclooxygenase products and atrial natriuretic peptide modulate renal response to endothelin. *J Pharmacol Exp Ther* 1990;252:177–178.

283. Gardiner SM, Compton AM, Bennett T. Effects of indomethacin on the regional hemodynamic responses to low doses of endothelins and sarafotoxin. *Br J Pharmacol* 1990;100:158–162.

284. Miura K, Yukimura T, Yamashita Y, Shimmen T, Okumura M, Yamanaka S, Imanishi M, Yamamoto K. Renal and femoral vascular responses to endothelin-1 in dogs: role of prostaglandins. *Am J Hypertens* 1991;3:632–634.

285. Cao L, Banks RO. Cardiorenal actions of endothelin. II. Effects of cycolooxygenase inhibitors. *Life Sci* 1990;46:585–590.

286. Edwards RM, Trizna WT, Ohlstein EH. Renal microvascular effects of endothelin. *Am J Physiol* 1990;259 (Renal Fluid Electrolyte Physiol 28):F217–F221.

287. Mantymaa P, Leppaluoto J, Ruskoaho H. Endothelin stimulates basal and stretch-induced atrial natriuretic peptide secretion from the perfused rat heart. *Endocrinology* 1990;126:587–595.

288. Fukada Y, Hirata Y, Yoshimi H, Kojima T, Kobayashi Y, Yanagisawa M, Masaki T. Endothelin is a potent secretagogue for atrial natriuretic peptide in cultured rat atrial myocytes. *Biochem Biophys Res Commun* 1988;155:167–172.

289. Lopez-Farre A, Gomez-Garre D, Bernabeau F, Montanes I, Mil-

las I, Lopez-Novoa JM. Renal effects and mesangial cell contraction induced by endothelin are mediated by PAF. *Kidney Int* 1991;39:624–630.

290. Yamada K, Yoshida S. Role of endogenous endothelin on renal function in rats. *Am J Physiol* 1991;260 (Renal Fluid Electrolyte Physiol 29):F34–F38.

291. Stingo AJ, Clavell AL, Aarhus LL, Burnett JC. Biological role for the endothelin-A receptor in aortic cross-clamping. *Hypertension* 1993;22:62–66.

292. Perico N, Dadan J, Remuzzi G. Endothelin mediates the renal vasoconstriction induced by cyclosporine in the rat. *J Am Soc Nephrol* 1990;1:76–83.

293. Fogo A, Hellings S, Inagami T, Kon V. Endothelin receptor antagonism is protective in in vivo acute cyclosporine toxicity. *Kidney Int* 1992;42:770–774.

294. Kon V, Yoshioka T, Fogo A, Ichikawa I. Glomerular actions of endothelin in vivo. *J Clin Invest* 1989;83:1762–1767.

295. Munger KA, Takahashi K, Awazu M, Frazer M, Falk SA, Conger JD, Badr KF. Maintenance of endothelin-induced renal arteriolar constriction in rats is cyclooxygenase dependent. *Am J Physiol* 1993;264:F637–F644.

296. Lanese DM, Yuan BH, McMurtry IF, Conger JD. Comparative sensitivities of isolated rat renal arterioles to endothelin. *Am J Physiol* 1992;263:F894–F899.

297. Ausiello DA, Kreisberg JL, Roy C, Karnovsky JM. Contraction of cultured rat glomerular cells of apparent mesangial origin after stimulation with angiotensin and arginine-vasopressin. *J Clin Invest* 1980;65:754–760.

298. Culebras M, Montanes I, Lopez-Farre A, Millas I, Lopez-Novoa JM. Effect of endothelin on renal function and on the contraction of cultured rat mesangial cells. *Med Sci Res* 1989;17:245–246.

299. Dunlop ME, Larkins RG. Insulin-dependent contractility of glomerular mesangial cells in response to angiotensin-II, platelet activating factor and endothelin is attenuated by prostaglandin E2. *Biochem J* 1990;272:561–568.

300. Uchida K, Ballermann BJ. Sustained activation of PGE$_2$ synthesis in mesangial cells cocultured with glomerular endothelial cells. *Am J Physiol* 1992;263 (Cell Physiol 32):C200–C209.

301. Clozel M, Loffler BM, Breu V, Hilfiger L, Maire JP, Butscha B. Downregulation of endothelin receptors by autocrine production of endothelin-1. *Am J Physiol* 1993;265 (Cell Physiol):C188–C192.

302. Goetz K, Wang BC, Leadley R, Zhu JL, Madwed J, Bie P. Endothelin and sarafatoxin produce dissimilar effects on renal blood flow, but both block the antidiuretic effects of vasopressin. *Proc Soc Exp Biol Med* 1989;191:425–427.

303. Guyton AC. Blood pressure control-special role of the kidneys and body fluids. *Science* 1991;252:1813–1816.

304. Uzuner K, Banks RO. Endothelin-induced natriuresis and diuresis are pressure-dependent events in the rat. *Am J Physiol* 1993;265:R90–R96.

305. Takabatake T, Ise T, Ohta K, Kobayashi K. Effects of endothelin on renal hemodynamics and tubuloglomerular feedback. *Am J Physiol* 1992;263 (Renal Fluid Electrolyte Physiol):F103–F108.

306. Perico N, Cornejo RP, Benigni A, Malanchini B, Ladny JR, Remuzzi G. Endothelin induces diuresis and natriuresis in the rat by acting on proximal tubular cells through a mechanism mediated by lipoxygenase products. *J Am Soc Nephrol* 1991;2:57–69.

307. Munger KA, Sugiura M, Takahashi K, Inagami T, Badr KF. A role for atrial natriuretic peptide in endothelin-induced natriuresis. *J Am Soc Nephrol* 1991;1:1278–1283.

308. Gardner DG, Newman ED, Nakamura KK, Nguyen KPT. Endothelin increases the synthesis and secretion of atrial natriuretic peptide in neonatal rat cardiocytes. *Am J Physiol* 1991;261:E177–E182.

309. Ota K, Kimura T, Shoji M, Inoue M, Sato K, Ohta M, Yamamoto T, Tsunoda K, Abe K, Yoshinaga K. Interaction of ANP with endothelin on cardiovascular, renal, and endocrine function. *Am J Physiol* 1992;262 (Endocrinol Metab 25):E135–E141.

310. Harris PJ, Zhou J, Mendelsohn FAO, Skinner SL. Haemodynamic and renal tubular effects of low doses of endothelin in anesthetized rats. *J Physiol* 1991;433:25–39.

311. Garvin J, Sanders K. Endothelin inhibits fluid and bicarbonate

312. Zeidel ML, Brady HR, Kone BC, Gullans SR, Brenner BM. Endothelin, a peptide inhibitor of Na$^+$/K$^+$ ATPase in intact renal tubular epithelial cells. *Am J Physiol* 1989;257 (Cell Physiol): C1101–C1107.

313. Jabs K, Zeidel ML, Silva P. Prostaglandin E inhibits Na/K ATPase activity in the inner medullary collect duct. *Am J Physiol* 1989;257:F424–F430.

314. Gupta S, Ruderman NB, Cragoe EJ, Sussman I. Endothelin stimulates Na-K-ATPase activity by a protein kinase C-dependent pathway in rabbit aorta. *Am J Physiol* 1991;261:H38–H45.

315. Eiam-Ong S, Hilden SA, King AJ, Johns CA, Madias NE. Endothelin-1 stimulates Na$^+$/H$^+$ and Na$^+$/HCO$_3^-$ transporters in rabbit renal cortex. *Kidney Int* 1992;42:18–24.

316. Guntupalli J, Phelps R, Dubose TD. Effect(s) of endothelin-1 on Na-Pi cotransport and Na$^+$-H$^+$ exchange in rat renal brush border membranes (Abst). *J Am Soc Nephrol* 1991;2:402.

317. Campbell WB, Henrich WL. Endothelial factors in the regulation of renin release. *Kidney Int* 1990;38:612–617.

318. Otsuka A, Mikami H, Katahira K, Tsunetoshi T, Minamitani K, Ogihara T. Changes in plasma renin activity and aldosterone concentration in response to endothelin injection in dogs. *Acta Endocrinologica* 1989;121:361–364.

319. Cavero PG, Miller WL, Heublein DM, Margulies KB, Burnett JC. Endothelin in experimental congestive heart failure in the anesthetized dog. *Am J Physiol* 1990;259 (Renal Fluid Electrolyte Physiol 28):F312–F317.

320. Takagi M, Matsuoka H, Atarashi K, S. Y. Endothelin: a new inhibitor of renin release. *Biochem Biophys Res Commun* 1988;157:1164–1168.

321. Takagi M, Tsukada H, Matsuoka H, Yagi S. Inhibitory effect of endothelin on renin release in vitro. *Am J Physiol* 1989;257 (Endocrinol Metab 20):E833–E838.

322. Moe O, Tejedor A, Campbell WB, Alpern RJ, Henrich WL. Effects of endothelin on in vitro renin secretion. *Am J Physiol* 1991;260 (Endocrinol Metab 23):E521–E525.

323. Rakugi H, Nakamaru M, Saito H, Higaki J, Ogihara T. Endothelin inhibits renin release from isolated rat glomeruli. *Biochem Biophys Res Commun* 1988;155:1244–1247.

324. Matsumura Y, Kakase K, Ikegawa R, Haysahi K, Ohyama T, Morimoto S. The endothelium derived vasoconstrictor endothelin inhibits renin release in vitro. *Life Sci* 1989;44:149–157.

325. Kurtz A, Kaissling B, Busse R, Baier W. Endothelial cells modulate renin secretion from isolated mouse juxtaglomerular cells. *J Clin Invest* 1991;88:1147–1154.

326. Cozza EN, Chiou S, Gomez-Sanchez CE. Endothelin-1 potentiation of angiotensin II stimulation of aldosterone production. *Am J Physiol* 1992;262 (Regulatory Integrative Comp Physiol 31): R85–R89.

327. Rosolowsky LJ, Campbell WB. Endothelin enhances adrenocorticotropin-stimulated aldosterone release from cultured bovine adrenal cells. *Endocrinology* 1990;126:1860–1866.

328. Claria J, Jimenez W, Arroyo V, Castro A, Asbert M, Ros J, Rivera F, Rodes J. Doses of endothelin have natriuretic effects in conscious rats with cirrhosis and ascites. *Kidney Int* 1991;40:182–187.

329. Schnermann J, Lorenz JN, Briggs JP, Keiser JA. Induction of water diuresis by endothelin in rats. *Am J Physiol* 1992;263: F516–F526.

330. Tomita K, Nonoguchi H, Marumo F. Effects of endothelin on peptide-dependent cyclic adenosine monophosphate accumulation along the nephron segments of the rat. *J Clin Invest* 1990;85: 2014–2018.

331. Oishi R, Nonoguchi H, Tomita K, Marumo F. Endothelin-1 inhibits AVP-stimulated osmotic water permeability in rat inner medullary collecting duct. *Am J Physiol* 1991;261 (Renal Fluid Electrolyte Physiol 30):F951–F956.

332. Nadler SP, Zimpelmann JA, RLH. Endothelin inhibits vasopressin-stimulated water permeability in rat terminal inner medullary collecting duct. *J Clin Invest* 1992;90:1458–1466.

333. Tomita K, Nonoguchi H, Terada Y, Marumo F. Effects of ET-1 on water and chloride transport in cortical collecting ducts of the

rat. *Am J Physiol* 1993;264 (Renal Fluid Electrolyte Physiol 33): F690–F696.

334. Kohan DE, Fiedorek FT. Endothelin synthesis by rat inner medullary collecting duct cells. *J Am Soc Nephrol* 1991;2:150–155.

335. Kohan DE, Hughes AK. Autocrine role of endothelin in rat IMCD: inhibition of AVP-induced cAMP accumulation. *Am J Physiol* 1993;265 (Renal Fluid Electrolyte Physiol 34):F126–F129.

336. Yang T, Terada Y, Nonoguchi H, Ujiie K, Tomita K, Marumo F. Effect of hyperosmolality on production and mRNA expression of ET-1 in inner medullary collecting duct. *Am J Physiol* 1993;264 (Renal Fluid Electrolyte Physiol 33):F684–F689.

337. Kohan DE. Endothelin production by human inner medullary collecting duct cells. *J Am Soc Nephrol* 1993;3:1719–1721.

338. Kohan DE, Padilla E. Osmolar regulation of endothelin-1 production by rat inner medullary collecting duct. *J Clin Invest* 1993;91:1235–1240.

339. Myers B. Cyclosporine nephrotoxicity. *Kidney Int* 1986;30:964–974.

340. Lau DCW, Wong KL. Cyclosporine toxicity on cultured rat microvascular endothelial cells. *Kidney Int* 1989;35:604–613.

341. Zoja C, Furci L, Ghilardi F, Zilio P, Benigni A, Remuzzi G. Cyclosporin-induced endothelial cell injury. *Lab Invest* 1986;55:455–462.

342. Bossaller C, Forstermann U, Hertel R, Olbricht C, Reschke V, Fleck E. Cyclosporin A inhibits endothelium-dependent vasodilatation and vascular prostacyclin production. *Eur J Pharmacol* 1989;165:165–169.

343. Gerkins JF. Cyclosporine treatment of normal rats produces a rise in blood pressure and decreased renal vascular responses to nerve stimulation, vasoconstrictors and endothelium-dependent dilators. *J Pharmacol Exp Ther* 1989;250:1105–1112.

344. Shulman H, Striker G, Deeg HJ, Kennedy M, Storb R, Thomas ED. Nephrotoxicity of cyclosporin A after allogenic marrow transplantation. *N Engl J Med* 1981;305:1392–1395.

345. Fogo A, Hakim RC, Sugiura M, Inagami T, Kon V. Severe endothelial injury in a renal transplant patient receiving cyclosporine. *Transplantation* 1990;49:1190–1192.

346. Watschinger B, Vychytil A, Schuller M, Hartter E, Traindl O, Pohanka E, Ulrich W, Kovarik J. The pathophysiologic role of endothelin in acute vascular rejection after renal transplantation. *Transplantation* 1991;52:743–746.

347. Grieff M, Al Shoheib S, Loertscher R, Stewart DJ. Cyclosporine A (CSA) induces elevation in circulating endothelin-1 (ET-1) following transplantation (Abst). *Transplantation*.

348. Deray G, Carayon A, Le Hoang P. Increased endothelin level after cyclosporine therapy. *Ann Int Med* 1991;114:809.

349. Lerman A, Click RL, Narr BJ, Wiesner RH, Krom RAF, Textor SC, J.C. B. Elevation of plasma endothelin associated with systemic hypertension in humans following orthotopic liver transplantation. *Transplantation* 1991;51:646–650.

350. Edwards BS, Hunt SA, Fowler MB, Valantine HA, Anderson LM, Lerman A. Effect of cyclosporine on plasma endothelin levels in human after cardiac transplantation. *Am J Cardiol* 1991;67:782–794.

351. Benigni A, Perico N, Ladny JR, Imberti O, Bellizzi L, Remuzzi G. Increased urinary excretion of endothelin-1 and its precursor, big-endothelin-1, in rats chronically treated with cyclosporine. *Transplantation* 1991;52:175–177.

352. Bunchman TE, Brookshire CA. Cyclosporine-induced synthesis of endothelin by cultured human endothelial cells. *J Clin Invest* 1991;88:310–314.

353. Lanese DM, Conger JD. Effects of endothelin receptor antagonist on cyclosporine-induced vasoconstriction in isolated rat renal arterioles. *J Clin Invest* 1993;91:2144–2149.

354. Takeda M, Breyer MD, Noland TD, Homma T, Hoover RL, Inagami T, Kon V. Endothelin-1 receptor antagonist: effects on endothelin- and cyclosporine-treated mesangial cells. *Kidney Int* 1992;42:1713–1719.

355. Brooks DP, Ohlstein EH, Contino LC, Storer B, Pullen M, Caltabiano M, Nambi P. Effect of nifedipine on cyclosporine A-induced nephrotoxicity, urinary endothelin excretion and renal endothelin receptor number. *Eur J Pharmacol* 1991;194:115–117.

356. Nambi P, Pullen M, Contino LC, Brooks DP. Upregulation of renal endothelin receptors in rats with cyclosporine A-induced nephrotoxicity. *Eur J Pharmacol* 1990;187:113–116.

357. Nayler WG, Gu XH, Casley DJ, Panagiotopoulos S, Liu J, Mottram PL. Cyclosporine increases endothelin-1 binding site density in cardiac membranes. *Biochem Biophys Res Commun* 1989;163:1270–1274.

358. Frega NS, DiBona DR, Guertler B, Leaf A. Ischemic renal injury. *Kidney Int* 1976;10(suppl):S17–S25.

359. Levinsky NG. Pathophysiology of acute renal failure. *N Engl J Med* 1977;296:1453–1458.

360. Conger JD, Robinette JB, Schrier RW. Smooth muscle calcium and endothelium-derived relaxing factor in the abnormal vascular responses of acute renal failure. *J Clin Invest* 1988;82:532–537.

361. Lieberthal W, Wolf EF, Rennke HG, Valeri CR, Levinsky NG. Renal ischemia and reperfusion impair endothelium-dependent vascular relaxation. *Am J Physiol* 1989;256 (Renal Fluid Electrolyte Physiol 25):F894–F900.

362. Tomita K, Ujiie K, Nakanishi T, Tomura S, Matsuda O, Ando K, Shichiri M, Hirata Y, Marumo F. Plasma endothelin levels in patients with acute renal failure (letter). *N Eng J Med* 1990;321:1127.

363. Shichiri M, Hirata Y, Ando K, Emori T, Ohta K, Kimoto S, Ogura M, Inoue A, Marumo F. Plasma endothelin levels in hypertension and chronic renal failure. *Hypertension* 1990;15:493–496.

364. Koyama H, Nishizawa Y, Morii EH, Tabata T, Inoue T, Yamaji T. Plasma endothelin levels in patients with uremia. *Lancet* 1989;1:991–992.

365. Totsune K, Mouri T, Takahashi K, Ohneda M, Sone M, Saito T, Yoshinaga K. Detection of immunoreactive endothelin in plasma of hemodialysis patients. *FEBS* Lett. 1989;249[2]:239–242.

366. Shibouta Y, Suzuki N, Shino A, Matsumoto H, Terashita Z-I, Kondo K, Nishikawa K. Pathophysiological role of endothelin in acute renal failure. *Life Sci* 1990;46:1611–1618.

367. Kourembanas S, Marsden P, McQuillen LP, Faller DV. Hypoxia induces endothelin gene expression and secretion in cultured human endothelium. *J Clin Invest* 1991;88:1054–1057.

368. Liu J, Chen R, Casley DJ, Nayler WG. Ischemia and reperfusion increase I-labeled endothelin-1 binding in rat cardiac membranes. *Am J Physiol* 1990;258 (Heart Circ Physiol 27):H829–H835.

369. Wilkes BM, Pearl AR, Mento PF, Maita ME, Macica CM, Girardi EP. Glomerular endothelin receptors during initiation and maintenance of ischemic acute renal failure in rats. *Am J Physiol* 1991;260:F110–F118.

370. Badr KF, Kelley VE, Rennke HG, Brenner BM. Roles for thromboxane A and leukotrienes in endotoxin-induced acute renal failure. *Kidney Int* 1986;30:474–480.

371. Kikeri D, Pennell JP, Hwang KH, Jacob AI, Richman AV, Bourgoignie JJ. Endotoxemic acute renal failure in awake rats. *Am J Physiol* 1986;250 (Renal Fluid Electrol Physiol 19):F1098–F1106.

372. Sugiura M, Inagami T, Kon V. Endotoxin stimulates endothelin-release in vivo and in vitro as determined by radioimmunoassay. *Biochem Biophys Res Commun* 1989;161:1220–1227.

373. Morel DR, Lacroix JS, Hemsen A, Steinig DA, Pittet JF, Lundberg JM. Increased plasma and pulmonary lymph levels of endothelin during endotoxin shock. *Eur J Pharmacol* 1989;167:427–428.

374. Pernow J, Hemsen A, Lundberg JM. Increased plasma levels of endothelinlike immunoreactivity during endotoxin administration in the pig. *Acta Physiol Scand* 1989;137:317–318.

375. Beasley D, Schwartz JH, Brenner BM. Interleukin 1 induces prolonged L-arginine-dependent cyclic guanosine monophosphate and nitrile production in rat vascular smooth muscle cells. *J Clin Invest* 1991;87:602–608.

376. Anderson S, Meyer TW, Rennke HG, Brenner BM. Control of glomerular hypertension limits glomerular injury in rats with reduced renal mass. *J Clin Invest* 1985;76:612–619.

377. Benigni A, Perico N, Gaspari F, Zoja C, Bellizzi L, Gabanelli M, Remuzzi G. Increased renal endothelin production in rats with reduced renal mass. *Am J Physiol* 1991;260:F331–F339.

378. Brooks DP, Contino LC, Storer B, Ohlstein EH. Increased endothelin excretion in rats with renal failure induced by partial nephrectomy. *Br J Pharmacol* 1991;104:987–989.

379. Orisio S, Benigni A, Bruzzi I, Corna D, Perico N, Zoja C, Benatti L, Remuzzi G. Renal endothelin gene expression is increased in remnant kidney and correlates with disease progression. *Kidney Int* 1993;43:354–358.

380. Milner P, Bodin P, Loesch A, Burnstock G. Rapid release of endothelin and ATP from isolated aortic endothelial cells exposed to increase flow. *Biochem Biophys Res Commun* 1990;170:649–656.

381. Yoshizumi M, Kurihara H, Sugiyama T, Takaku F, Yanagisawa M, Masaki T, Yazaki Y. Hemodynamic shear stress stimulates endothelin production by cultured endothelial cells. *Biochem Biophys Res Commun* 1989;161:859–864.

382. Benigni A, Zoja C, Corna D, Orisio S, Longaretti L, Bertani T, Remuzzi G. A specific endothelin subtype A receptor antagonist protects against injury in renal disease progression. *Kidney Int* 1993;44:440–444.

383. Vanhoutte PM. Endothelium and control of vascular function. *Hypertension* 1989;13:658–667.

384. Davies PF, Oleson SP, Clapham DE, Morrel EM, Schoen FJ. Endothelial communication. State of the art lecture. *Hypertension Dallas* 1988;11:563–572.

385. Yang ZH, Richard V, Vonsegesser L, Bauer E, Stulz P, Turina M, Lusher TF. Threshold concentrations of endothelin-1 potentiate contractions to norepinephrine and serotonin in human arteries-a newer mechanism of vasospasm. *Circulation* 1990;82:188–195.

386. Henrion D, Laher I. Potentiation of norepinephrine-induced contractions by endothelin-1 in the rabbit aorta. *Hypertension* 1993;22:78–83.

387. Ihara M, Saeki T, Fukuroda T, Kimura S, Ozaki S, Patel AC, Yano M. A novel radioligand [125I]BQ-3020 selective for endothelin (ETB) receptors. *Life Sci* 1992;51:PL47–PL52.

388. Bird JE, Asaad MM, Giancarli MR, Dorso CR, Chao C-C, Webb ML. Role of endothelin (ET) in regulation of renal function and blood pressure in spontaneously hypertensive rats (Abst). *J Am Soc Nephrol* 1993;4:445.

389. Fujihara CK, De Nucci G, Zatz R. Effect of FR139317, a novel endothelin inhibitor, on glomerular microcirculation and systemic hemodynamics in the rat (Abst). *J Am Soc Nephrol* 1993;4:549.

390. Fogo A, Hellings SE, Inagami T, Kon V. Endothelin receptor antagonism is protective in in vivo acute cyclosporine toxicity. *Kidney Int* 1992;42:770–774.

391. Macrae IM, McAulley MA, Robinson MJ, Reid JL, McCulloch J. Endothelin-1-induced hypertension: a consequence of medullary ischemia? *J Cardiovasc Pharmacol* 1991;17:S496–S499.

392. Yamamoto T, Kimura T, Ota K, Shoji M, Inoue M, Sato K, Ohta M, Yoshinaga K. Central effects of endothelin-1 on vasopressin release, blood pressure, and renal solute excretion. *Am J Physiol* 1992;262:E856–E862.

393. Kaufman H, Oribe E, Oliver JA. Plasma endothelin during upright tilt: relevance for orthostatic hypotension? *Lancet* 1991;338:1542–1545.

394. Stewart DJ, Cernacek P, Costello KB, Rouleau JL. Elevated endothelin-1 in heart failure and loss of normal response to postural change. *Circulation* 1992;85:510–517.

395. Yoshizawa T, Shinmi O, Glaid A, Yanagisawa M, Gibson SJ, Kimura S, Uchiyama Y, Polak JM, Masaki T, Kanazawa I. Endothelin: a novel peptide in the posterior pituitary system. *Science* 1990;247:462–464.

396. Mosqueda-Garcia R, Inagami T, Appalsamy M, Sugiura M, Robertson RM. Endothelin as a neuropeptide. Cardiovascular effects in the brainstem of normotensive rats. *Circ Res* 1993;72:20–35.

397. Wagner OF, Nowotny P, Vierhapper H. Unchanged plasma levels of endothelin-1 in healthy men during short-term infusions of AMP, dDAVP and of norepinephrine. *Horm Metab Res* 1991;23:191–192.

398. Kohno M, Murakawa K, Horio T, Yokokawa K, Yasunari K, Fukui T, Takeda T. Plasma immunoreactive endothelin-1 in experimental malignant hypertension. *Hypertension* 1991;19:93–100.

399. Dohi Y, Hahn AWA, Boulanger CM, Buhler FR, Luscher TF. Endothelin stimulated by angiotensin II augments contractility of spontaneously hypertensive rat resistance arteries. *Hypertension* 1992;19:131–137.

400. Tabuchi Y, Nakamaru M, Rakugi H, Nagano M, Ogihara T. Endothelin enhances adrenergic vasoconstriction in perfused rat mesenteric arteries. *Biochem Biophys Res Commun* 1989;159:1304–1308.

401. Dohi Y, Luscher TF. Aging differentially affects direct and indirect actions of endothelin-1 in perfused mesenteric arteries of the rat. *Br J Pharmacol* 1990;100:889–893.

402. Cody WL, Doherty AM, He JX, Depue PL, Rapundalo ST, Hingorani GA, Major TC, Panek RL, Dudley DT, Haleen SJ, Ladouceur D, Hill KE, Flynn MA, Reynolds EE. Design of a functional hexapeptide antagonist of endothelin. *J Med Chem* 1992;83:3301–3303.

403. Margulies KB, Hildebrand FL, Lerman A, Perrella MA, Burnett JC. Increased endothelin in experimental heart failure. 1990;82:2226–2230.

404. Cernacek P, Stewart DJ. Immunoreactive endothelin in human plasma: marked elevations in patients in cardiogenic shock. *Biochem Biophys Res Commun* 1989;161:562–567.

405. Pernow J, Hemsen A, Lundberg JM. Increased plasma levels of endothelinlike immunoreactivity during endotoxin administration in the pig. *Acta Physiol Scand* 1990;137:317–318.

406. Hieda HS, Gomez-Sanchez CE. Hypoxia increases endothelin release in bovine endothelial cells in culture, but epinephrine, serotonin, histamine and angiotensin II do not. *Life Sci* 1990;47:247–251.

407. Horio T, Kohno M, Yokokawa K, Murakawa K, Yasunari K, Fujiwara H, et al. Effect of hypoxia on plasma immunoreactive endothelin-1 concentration in anesthetized rats. *Metabolism* 1991;40:999–1001.

408. Shirakami G, Nakao K, Saito Y, Magaribuchi T, Jougasaki M, Mukoyana M, et al. Acute pulmonary alveolar hypoxia increases lung and plasma endothelin-1 levels in conscious rats. *Life Sci* 1991;47:969–976.

409. Isaoki-Fukuda Y, Kojima T, Hirata Y, Ono A, Sawaragi S, Sawaeagi I. Plasma immuno reactive endothelin-1 concentration in human fetal blood: its relation to asphyxia. *Ped Res* 1991;30:244–247.

410. Hashiguchi K, Takagi K, Nakabayashi M, Takeda Y, Sakamoto S, Naruse M, et al. Relationship between fetal hypoxia and endothelin-1 in fetal circulation. *J Cardiovasc Pharmacol* 1991;(suppl)17:S509–S510.

411. MacLean MR, Randall MD, Hiley CR. Effects of moderate hypoxia, hypercapnia and acidosis on haemodynamic changes induced by endothelin-1 in the pithed rat. *Br J Pharmacol* 1989;98:1055–1065.

412. Kon V, Badr KF. Biological actions and pathophysiologic significance of endothelin in the kidney. *Kidney Int* 1991;40:1–12.

413. Vemulapalli S, Chiu PJS, Rivelli M, Fostre CJ, Syberts EJ. Modulation of circulating endothelin levels in hypertension and endotoxemia in rats. *J Cardiovasc Pharmacol* 1991;18:895–903.

414. Vanhoutte PM. Is endothelin involved in the pathogenesis of hypertension. *Hypertension* 1993;21:747–751.

415. Luscher TF, Seo B-G, Buhler FR. Potential role of endothelin in hypertension. *Hypertension* 1993;21:752–757.

416. Nguyen PV, A. P, Deng LY, Fluckiger J, Thibault G, Schiffrin EL. Endothelin vascular receptors and responses in deoxycorticosterone acetate-salt hypertensive rats. *Hypertension* 1992;19(suppl II):II-98–II-104.

417. Suzuki N, Miyauchi T, Tomobe Y, Matsumoto H, Goto K, Masaki T, Fujino M. Plasma concentrations of endothelin-1 in spontaneously hypertensive rats and DOCA-salt hypertensive rats. *Biochem Biophys Res Commun* 1990;167:941–947.

418. Lariviere R, Thibault G, Schiffrin EL. Increased endothelin-1 content in blood vessels of deoxycorticosterone acetate-salt hypertensive but not in spontaneously hypertensive rats. *Hypertension* 1993;21:294–300.

419. Hughes AK, Cline RC, Kohan DE. Alterations in renal endothelin-1 production in spontaneously hypertensive rats. *Hypertension* 1992;20:666–673.

420. Bolger GT, Liard F, Jodoin A, Jaramilla J. Vascular reactivity, tissue levels, and binding sites for endothelin: a comparison in the

spontaneously hypertensive and Wistar-Kyoto rats. *Can J Physiol Pharmacol* 1991;69:406–413.

421. Lariviere R, Day R, Schiffrin EL. Increased expression of endothelin-1 gene in blood vessels of deoxycorticosterone acetate-salt hypertensive rats. *Hypertension* 1993;21:916–920.

422. Yokokawa K, Tahara H, Kohno M, Murakawa K, Yasunari K, Nakagawa K, Hamadat, Otani S, Yanagisawa M, Takeda T. Endothelin-secreting tumor. *J Cardiovasc Pharmacol* 1991; 17:S398–S401.

422a. Yokokawa K, Tahara H, Kohno M, Murakawa K, Yasunari K, Nakagawa K, Hamada T, Otani S, Yanagisawa M, Takeda T. Hypertension associated with endothelin-secreting malignant hemangioendothelioma. *Ann Intern Med* 1991;114:213–215.

423. Yamakado M, Hirata Y, Matsuoka H, Sugimoto T. Pathophysiological role of endothelin in renal transplantation. *J Cardiovasc Pharmacol Suppl* 1991;17:S477–S499.

424. Kohno M, Yasunari K, Murakawa KI. Plasma immunoreactivity endothelin in essential hypertension. *Am J Med* 1990;88:614.

425. Saito Y, Nakao K, Mukoyama M, Imura H. Increased plasma endothelin level in patients with essential hypertension (Letter). *N Engl J Med* 1990;322[3]:205.

426. Kamoi K, Sudo N, Ishibashi M, Yamaji T. Plasma endothelin-1 levels in patients with pregnancy-induced hypertension. *N Engl J Med* 1990;323:1486–1488.

427. Naruse K, Naruse M, Watanabe Y, Yoshihara I, Ohsumi K, Horiuchi J, et al. Molecular forms of immunoreactive endothelin in plasma and urine of normal subjects and patients with various disease states. *J Cardiovasc Pharmacol* 1991;17:S506–S508.

428. Haak T, Jungmann E, Felber A, Hillmann U, Usadel KH. Increased plasma levels of endothelin in diabetic patients with hypertension. *Am J Hypertens* 1992;5:161–166.

429. Davenport AP, Ashby MJ, Easton P, Ella S, Bedford J, Dickerson C, Nunez DJ, Capper SJ, Brown MJ. A sensitive radioimmunoassay measuring endothelinlike immunoreactivity in human plasma: comparison of levels in patients with essential hypertension and normotensive control subjects. *Clin Sci* 1990;78:261–264.

430. Predel H-G, Meyer-Lehnert H, Backer A, Stelkens H, Kramer HJ. Plasma concentrations of endothelin in patients with abnormal vascular reactivity. *Life Sci* 1990;47:1837–1843.

431. Schiffrin EL, Thibault G. Plasma endothelin in human essential hypertension. *Am J Hypertens* 1991;4:303–308.

432. Saito Y, Nakao K, Mukoyama M, Shirakami G, Itoh H, Yamada T, Arai H, Hosoda K, Suga A, Jougasaki M, Ogawa Y, Nakajima S, Ueda M, Imura H. Application of monoclonal antibodies for endothelin to hypertensive research. *Hypertension* 1990;15:734–738.

433. Lerman A, Edwards BS, Hallett JW, Heublein DM, Sandberg SM, Burnett JC. Circulating and tissue endothelin immunoreactivity in advanced atherosclerosis. *N Engl J Med* 1991;325:997–1001.

434. Winquist RJ, Scott AL, Vlasuk GP. Enhanced release of atrial natriuretic factor by endothelin in atria from hypertensive rats. *Hypertension* 1989;14:111–114.

435. Kitazumi K, Shiba T, Nishiki K, Furukawa Y, Takasaki C, Tasaka K. Vasodilator effects of sarafotoxins and endothelin-1 in spontaneously hypertensive rats and rat isolated perfused mesentery. *Biochem Pharmacol* 1990;40:1843–1847.

436. Fozard JR, Part ML. No major role for atrial natriuretic peptide in the vasodilator response to endothelin-1 in the spontaneously hypertensive rat. *Eur J Pharmacol* 1990;180:153–159.

437. Schini VB, Kim ND, Vanhoutte PM. The basal and stimulated release of EDRF inhibits the contractions evoked by endothelin-1 and endothelin-3 in aortae of normotensive and spontaneously hypertensive rats. *J Cardiovasc Pharmacol* 1991;17:S266–S270.

438. Wu C, Bohr D. Role of endothelium in the response to endothelin in hypertension. *Hypertension* 1990;16:677–681.

439. Ashida T, Kawano Y, Yoshimi H, Akabane S, Kuramochi M, Omae T. Effects of ouabain and verapamil on endothelin-1-induced contraction of mesenteric artery in young spontaneously hypertensive rats. *J Cardiovasc Pharmacol* 1991;17:S174–S176.

440. Dohi Y, Luscher TF. Endothelin in hypertensive resistance arteries. *Hypertension* 1991;18:543–549.

441. Criscione L, Nellis P, Riniker B, Thomann H, Burdet R. Reactivity and sensitivity of mesenteric vascular beds and aortic rings of SHR to endothelin. *Br J Pharmacol* 1990;100:31–36.

442. Auch-Schwelk W, Vanhoutte PM. Contractions to endothelin in normotensive spontaneously hypertensive rats: role of endothelium and prostaglandins. *Blood Pressure* 1992;1:45–49.

443. Yoshida K, Yasujima M, Kohzuki M, Tsunoda K, Kudo K, Kanazawa M, et al. Chronic synergistic effect of endothelin-1 and angiotensin II on blood pressure in conscious rats. *J Cardiovasc Pharmacol Suppl* 1991;17:S514–S516.

444. Catelli de Carvalho MH, Nigro D, Scivoletto R, Barbeiro HV, Aparecida de Oliveira M, de Nucci G, Fortes ZB. Comparison of the effect of endothelin on microvessels and macrovessels in Goldblatt II and deoxycorticosterone acetate-salt hypertensive rats. *Hypertension* 1990;15(suppl I):I-68–I-71.

445. Dohi Y, Criscione L, Luscher TF. Renovascular hypertension impairs formation of endothelium-derived relaxing factors and sensitivity to endothelin-1 in resistance arteries. *Br J Pharmacol* 1991;104:349–354.

446. Deng LY, Schiffrin EL. Effect of antihypertensive treatment on response to endothelin of resistance arteries of hypertensive rats. *J Cardiovasc Pharmacol* 1993;21:725–731.

447. Roubert P, Gillard V, Plas P, Chabrier PE, Braquet P. Down-regulation of endothelin binding sites in rat vascular smooth muscle cells. *Am J Hypertens* 1990;3:310–312.

448. de Champlain J, Eid HP D. Potentiated endothelin-1-induced phosphoinositide hydrolysis in atria and mesenteric artery of DOCA-salt hypertensive rats. *J Hypertens* 1989;7:S136–S137.

449. Goligorsky MS, Iijima K, Morgan M, Yanagisawa M, Masaki T, Lin L, Nasjletta A, Kaskel F, Frazer M, Badr KF. Role of endothelin in the development of Dahl hypertension. *J Cardiovasc Pharmacol* 1991;17:S484–S491.

450. Schiffrin EL, Deng LY, Larochelle P. Blunted effects of endothelin upon small subcutaneous resistance arteries of mild essential hypertensive patients. *J Hypertens* 1992;10:437–444.

451. Nishikibe M, Tsuchiba S, Okada M, Fukuroda T, Shimamoto K, Yano M, Ishikawa K, Ikemoto F. Antihypertensive effect of a newly synthesized endothelin antagonist, BQ-123, in a genetic hypertensive model. *Life Sci* 1993;52:717–724.

452. Nishikibe M, Ikada M, Tsuchida S, Fukuroda T, Shimamoto K, Kobayashi M, Ishikawa K, Yano M, Ikemoto F. Antihypertensive effect of a newly synthesized endothelin antagonist BQ-123 in genetic hypertension models. *J Hypertens* 1992;10(suppl 4): P53.

453. Ohno A, Naruse M, Kato S, Hosaka M, Naruse K, Demura H, et al. Endothelin specific antibodies decrease blood pressure and increase glomerular filtration rate and renal plasma flow in SHR. *J Hypertens* 1992;10:781–785.

454. Kinoshita O, Kawano Y, Yoshimi H, Ashida T, Yoshida K, et al. Acute and chronic effects of anti-endothelin-1 antibody on blood pressure in SHR. *J Cardiovasc Pharmacol* 1991;17:S511–S513.

Hypertension: Pathophysiology, Diagnosis, and Management, Second Edition, edited by J.H. Laragh and B.M. Brenner, Raven Press, Ltd., New York © 1995.

CHAPTER 39

Vascular Muscle Ion Channels and Cellular Calcium Regulation in Hypertension

Kent Hermsmeyer and Paul Erne

Membrane signal events that regulate the state of contractile activity in the vascular wall are multiple and interactive, and have repeatedly been suggested as likely contributors to hypertension (1–3). The result of excitation in vascular muscle is via ion channels, resulting in the release of intracellular Ca^{2+} and, consequently, triggering of contraction. The topic that this chapter discusses follows the reasoning that membrane signaling could grow sufficiently aberrant to contribute to the etiology of hypertension. Ca^{2+} changes in circulating blood cells will also be explored as an indicator of altered Ca^{2+} signaling in vascular muscle.

MEMBRANE EXCITATION IN VASCULAR MUSCLE

The fundamental alteration of vascular muscle in hypertension does not appear to be the relationship between tension and membrane potential. Numerous studies have shown the strong correlation between membrane potential and tension in vascular muscle (reviewed in refs. 2–11). Studies comparing arteries from both hypertensive and normotensive animals have consistently demonstrated that there is no difference in the relation-

ship between membrane potential and tension in hypertension (4,8,12–15). The most intriguing evidence that changes in membrane potential might occur in hypertension was provided from *in situ* recordings in mesenteric veins by Stekiel and co-workers (15–17). These investigators showed that vascular muscle cells of the mesenteric vein *in situ* were more depolarized as a result of the greater depolarization by a neurotransmitter, the release of which could be blocked by tetrodotoxin. With nerve endings eliminated or blocked, the membrane potentials were the same in hypertensive and normotensive animals. Summaries of the observations on membrane potential of vascular muscle in hypertension have concluded that there is no evidence for altered membrane potential of the vascular muscle cells in hypertension when the neural and humoral depolarizing influences are removed (7,15,18). The vascular muscle cell per se appears to have normal membrane potential.

However, the origin of the membrane potential is altered in the genetic form of hypertension, i.e., in the spontaneously hypertensive rat (SHR) developed by Okamoto and Aoki in 1963. The ionic mechanisms producing membrane potential (electrogenesis) are more dependent upon the electrogenic transport of Na^+ ions out of the cell in SHR than in genetically matched Wistar-Kyoto (WKY) normotensive rats (4,8,12,13,19). This increased dependence of membrane potential on the electrogenic Na^+ pump is associated with increased responses to norepinephrine, and is the hallmark mem-

K. Hermsmeyer and P. Erne: Chiles Research Institute, Providence Medical Center and Oregon Health Sciences University, Portland, Oregon 97213.

brane property change in SHR/WKY hypertension. This characteristic difference between SHR and WKY follows an apparent trophic influence of sympathetic innervation, revealed in cross-transplantation experiments, where these hallmark membrane properties of SHR and WKY were interconverted (20).

The increased dependence on the electrogenic Na^+ pump contributes to hyperactivity under the influence of norepinephrine, in response to which there is increased influx of Na^+ and K^+ in such magnitude that it becomes the dominant influence on membrane potential (eclipsing the much smaller currents of the Na^+ pump), resulting in increased contraction (21). These alterations are best demonstrated by the K^+ return experiment, in which there is transient stimulation of the electrogenic Na^+ pump associated with transient hyperpolarization after incubation in zero K^+ (4,8,12,19–21). Together with evidence from tracer fluxes, which also supports enhanced dependence of membrane potential on the Na^+ pump in SHR (10,21,22), membrane potential and contractile data strongly implicate the altered Na^+ pump in hypertension, and suggest the need for further study of ionic regulatory mechanisms. It is likely that altered ionic mechanisms due to abnormal membrane function are compensated for by other Ca^{2+} regulatory systems that may themselves contribute to abnormally increased blood pressure. Such observations as decreased Mg^{2+} uptake suggest that a comprehensive ion model may be needed to link Ca^{2+} and Na^+ abnormalities (23).

ION CHANNELS OF VASCULAR MUSCLE

The importance of membrane potential for vascular muscle has been increasingly appreciated as more data from single-cell voltage clamp studies have emerged. Detailed mechanisms of ion channel responses to membrane potential show the reason for close correlations. As a large body of evidence has developed on vascular muscle ion channels, the central importance of Ca^{2+} channels in the excitation process has been increasingly apparent. The explanation for the steep dependence of vascular muscle excitation on membrane potential is based primarily on the voltage sensitivity of vascular muscle Ca^{2+} channels (24,25). Detailed studies of Ca^{2+} channels in vascular muscle, stimulation by norepinephrine, and inhibition by Ca^{2+} antagonists have revealed a strong correlation between the membrane potential dependence of excitation and the voltage gating of Ca^{2+} channels (26). Numerous molecular details have been revealed about the Ca^{2+} channel and have allowed identification of individual Ca^{2+} antagonist binding sites (27). It is to be determined if changes in the Ca^{2+} channel protein directly contribute to hypertension. There promises to be many more developments that explain both the cel-

lular and molecular basis for vascular muscle changes in hypertension and for development of medical management of hypertension from Ca^{2+} channel investigation (28).

Considerable evidence has already implicated Ca^{2+} channels in the abnormal voltage-dependent Ca^{2+} influx reported by multiple laboratories that study the basis for genetic hypertension (29–31). While there is evidence for increased Ca^{2+} influx that can be abolished by Ca^{2+} channel blockers (32), these studies also suggest increased Ca^{2+} sensitivity due to increased activity of protein kinase C (PKC) and mechanisms stimulated as a result of phospholipase C activation (33–35). There is increasing evidence for abnormal function due to increased Ca^{2+} channel opening that may be inherent or due to modulation by PKC. Several functional correlates of increased Ca^{2+} entry through voltage-dependent Ca^{2+} channels have been reported in multiple examples of genetic hypertension, particularly in blood vessels from SHR (36–39). Arterial muscle from SHR is consistently more permeable to Ca^{2+} under basal conditions, even in 6-week-old animals in whom hypertension is still developing (36). Ca^{2+} channel opening is known to be enhanced under depolarizing conditions by the dihydropyridine Ca^{2+} agonist, Bay K8644, which consequently contracted arteries from SHR more than from controls (38,39,40). Altered responsiveness of Ca^{2+} channels to dihydropyridine Ca^{2+} agonists and more vigorous responses to Ca^{2+} antagonists have often been reported (37,39,41–47). Thus, studies of Ca^{2+} channels have provided a particularly strong correlation with hypertension, possibly due to being a pathway for increased responsiveness and inappropriately maintained contraction of vascular muscle cells.

Several biochemical investigations of the vascular muscle membrane have revealed alterations that support the Ca^{2+} channel hypothesis of hypertension (28). Related hypotheses have emerged for specific alterations in vascular muscle cell membranes based on phospholipid composition (48–51). A similar hypothesis suggests altered excitation-contraction coupling based on a changed phospholipid environment of ion channels (52). More evidence for the Ca^{2+} channel hypothesis comes from testing the hypothesis by determining whether further increases in Ca^{2+} channel current are found in rats with more severe hypertension. More exaggerated increases in Ca^{2+} channel current were found in SHRs that are stroke-prone (due to more elevated blood pressures) than in non–stroke-prone SHRs (28). This correlation is consistent with a primary role for increased Ca^{2+} channel currents. Additional evidence for altered function, possibly involving decreased cellular Mg^{2+}, may provide a link between Na^+ and Ca^{2+} and warrants further investigation (23). When sufficient studies are reported to allow ion interactions to be understood, the Ca^{2+} hypothesis of hypertension that was first formulated and advocated by Aoki (53) will likely be an important component.

In any analysis, ion channels will play a central role in accounting for alterations of vascular muscle function in hypertension. Notably, changes in Ca^{2+} channels were reported in veins of newborn rats, suggesting that they are a cause, rather than a result, of increased blood pressure (29). Furthermore, Ca^{2+} channel changes persist even after several days in culture, which would rule out humoral or nerve release factors in the Ca^{2+} channel alteration. Because the development of tension is so closely related to activation of Ca^{2+} channels in vascular muscle (4,21,24–26), it is very likely that these increased Ca^{2+} currents translate into increased contraction.

Ca^{2+} INFLUX AND RELEASE IN VASCULAR MUSCLE

Alterations in Ca^{2+} channels would be expected to produce corresponding increases in intracellular Ca^{2+} in arterial muscle cells. Independent tests of the Ca^{2+} channel hypothesis have been explored with imaging technology at high resolution. Studies of localized variations in ionized free-Ca^{2+} concentration, or technically Ca^{2+} activity, have been carried out using several intracellular fluorescence or absorbance Ca^{2+} indicators (24,54). Comparisons of SHR versus WKY intracellular Ca^{2+} activities in various laboratories have revealed all three possible outcomes, i.e., increased intracellular Ca^{2+}, no change in intracellular Ca^{2+}, and decreased intracellular Ca^{2+} in vascular muscle from SHR. These studies have been carried out on different blood vessels and cells, under widely differing conditions and by significantly different techniques, which might explain different results. Detailed studies of single cells have shown localized Ca^{2+} increases in SHR vascular muscle (55,56). However, in studies on segments of artery (where the Ca^{2+} signal is averaged from several hundred cells and without optical definition of the source of Ca^{2+}), measurements actually showed a decrease in Ca^{2+} in SHR under basal conditions (56).

No change in Ca^{2+} concentration was found in basal levels or moderately to maximally norepinephrine-stimulated SHR versus WKY mesenteric arteries or primary cell cultures (57). However, when the area near the surface membrane was separately quantitated, evidence for an increase in Ca^{2+} activity in SHR was evident (54). Furthermore, this increase in intracellular Ca^{2+} near the surface membrane was enhanced by exposure of the cells to Ca^{2+} antagonists (54). These findings suggest alterations of the intracellular mechanisms regulating Ca^{2+}. Differences in Ca^{2+} activity occurring at the subsarcolemmal region, where modulation of both Ca^{2+} and K^+ channels would importantly influence membrane poten-

tial and Ca^{2+} entry, could explain consistent observations suggesting defective intracellular Ca^{2+} signaling (58–60).

Ca^{2+} fluxes through specific cation channels of the cellular membrane are linked to subcellular signals. Targets of hormonal signal transduction are PKC stimulation and formation of inositol 1,4,5-trisphosphate ($InsP_3$). The latter induces Ca^{2+} release from sarcoplasmic reticulum (SR). Since alterations of cellular membrane cation channels and altered cellular responses to various hormones have been described in hypertension, a direct investigation of SR and Ca^{2+} metabolism might give more insight. There is a protein other than calmodulin that sensitizes the contractile proteins to Ca^{2+} (61). Earlier studies had also suggested areas of high regional Ca^{2+} concentrations at submembranous SR localizations (55,56).

Release of Ca^{2+} from intracellular stores is an important component of the conversion of a hormonal signal into cellular responses. Endoplasmic and sarcoplasmic reticula are Ca^{2+} stores of low capacity but rapid release and uptake. SR is able to take up Ca^{2+} through a Ca^{2+}-ATPase–driven pump. This enzyme is regulated by the adenosine 3′,5′-cyclic monophosphate (cAMP)-dependent phospholamban (62). Ca^{2+} release from SR takes place in response to $InsP_3$, disulfide reagents, Ca^{2+}, and a spontaneous leak. $InsP_3$-induced Ca^{2+} release in permeabilized platelets has recently been coupled to hydrolysis of $InsP_3$ to inositol 1,4-biphosphate; there was rapid recovery of the sensitivity of the $InsP_3$-sensitive Ca^{2+} stores after successive additions of $InsP_3$ (increment detection), which appears to be associated with hydrolysis of $InsP_3$ (63). This points to the important role of SR for repetitive stimuli signaling.

It might be assumed that Ca^{2+} release from SR might depend most importantly on $InsP_3$ generation and cytosolic Ca^{2+} activities. Ca^{2+} release from SR results from exposure to and binding of four $InsP_3$ molecules to its receptor in a pattern that is consistent with noncooperative binding of the receptor. However, Ca^{2+} release from SR does not depend on cytosolic Ca^{2+} concentration in the physiologic range, although an elevation of Ca^{2+} in SR (intraluminal Ca^{2+}) does importantly stimulate Ca^{2+} release; at high concentrations of intraluminal Ca^{2+}, increased sensitivities of $InsP_3$-sensitive Ca^{2+} stores to $InsP_3$ are observed. These mechanisms might allow for variable Ca^{2+} transients as well as guarantee conversion of vital stimuli to cellular responses (64). However, the role and putative alteration in hypertension of the different Ca^{2+} release and uptake mechanisms have not been studied in detail. Preliminary studies on adenosine triphosphatase (ATPase)-driven Ca^{2+} transport by SR in platelets did not provide evidence for a close correlation with blood pressure (P. Erne, personal communication), which, taking into account the localized high Ca^{2+} concentrations close to subsarcolemmal SR, could instead suggest alterations of release mechanisms in hypertension.

Alternatively, hormone signal coupling might be altered in hypertension through alterations of the PKC system. Hormonal stimulation involves the activation of phospholipase C and the subsequent generation of second messengers $InsP_3$ and diacylglycerol, which respectively result in an increase of intracellular Ca^{2+} and activation of PKC, the major receptor for tumor-inducing phorbol esters (65). The role of PKC in sustained responses and secretion is generally established. In addition, PKC can act in synergy with Ca^{2+} mobilization. It has been suggested that PKC might play two distinct roles in regulating smooth muscle contractility (66). Stimuli producing a translocation of PKC from the cytosol to the membrane and sarcolemma induce a phosphorylation of protein and slow contraction. Prolonged association of the kinase with the membrane may lead to proteolysis and release into the cytosol of protein kinase M (which induces relaxation of permeabilized muscle fibers), resulting in myosin phosphorylation and relaxation. PKC suppressed the proto-oncogene c-*fos* in rat hearts, consistent with a role in regulation of protein expression (68). Although translocation of PKC upon stimulation as part of its action has been established for several years, the physiologically important protein substrates of PKC have not been identified. Various studies have investigated a putative involvement of PKC in hypertension with variable results (35,48,50,53, 59,66). PKC-depleted cells showed an exaggerated increase in thymidine uptake in response to platelet-derived growth factor (PDGF) stimulation in SHR versus WKY vascular muscle cells (68). Increased PKC activity was found in platelets of SHR (69). Comparison of basal PKC activity distribution between cytosolic and membrane fractions of SHR and WKY aortas and mesenteric arteries revealed no significant difference, although vessels from SHR produced a more sensitive contraction to phorbol esters. This might be due to a more sensitive stimulation of PKC by phorbol ester activation in SHR when compared with WKY (70).

The variability of results observed by use of different models and agonists might be due to the heterogeneity of PKC enzymes (66,71). PKC occurs in at least four Ca^{2+}-dependent (alpha, beta I, beta II, and gamma) and four Ca^{2+}-independent (delta, epsilon, zeta, eta) isoforms (65). In human platelets we have identified three distinct isoforms (alpha, beta, and zeta) that translocate distinctly upon exposure to phorbol esters (72) and physiologic agonists (73). In contrast to platelets, vascular muscle cells, and cardiac myocytes, only the alpha, beta, epsilon, and zeta isoforms have been identified (66). Thus, there is an obvious need for more detailed studies to characterize the role of PKC isoforms in hypertension.

Ca^{2+}-binding proteins, the target of Ca^{2+} signaling, were thought to be altered in hypertension, either by pre- or post-transcriptional changes. In a number of earlier reports, it was suggested that calmodulin, a ubiquitous Ca^{2+}-binding protein, might be involved in cellular adaptation to pressure overload, although results from different studies varied. In the last few years, a number of other Ca^{2+}-binding proteins were identified in vessels and the heart, among which are those of the S100 protein family (74,75). This preferential location and large Ca^{2+}-binding capacity might be important for our further understanding of contraction.

CIRCULATING BLOOD CELLS AND HYPERTENSION

Many studies have been carried out in human and animals on circulating blood cells, which have the virtue of being more readily accessible than vascular muscle cells. Clinical investigators have often studied patients with established essential hypertension, but these data do not allow conclusions with regard to the pathogenic causality. The blood cell results also cannot be directly extrapolated to human vascular muscle cells without verification. However, based on studies in human blood cells, important new information has accumulated, particularly in studies designed to investigate biochemical or functional similarities between blood cells and vascular muscle cells. If these limitations are taken into account, some of the different results between studies can be explained. These discrepancies are partially due to differences between the various blood cells; for example, while data on Na^+ content in primary hypertension are contradictory, white blood cell findings may eventually facilitate drawing a conclusion (76–78). Certainly, differences due to altered pH regulation, such as excessive sensitivity to extracellular acidosis, need to be accounted for in all ion measurements (79).

Other differences might be explained by different patient subpopulations and by inhomogeneities within groups of blood cells, particularly among lymphocytes. Furthermore, studies on animal and human blood cells can lead to different results that are explained by species differences, e.g., differences in functional receptors or different control by intracellular messengers, particularly of the adenylate cyclase system. Therefore, the rest of this chapter concentrates on studies in human blood cells, with special attention to human platelets, exploring cellular Ca^{2+} handling abnormalities related to findings from hypertensive animal models.

CALCIUM CONCENTRATIONS IN CIRCULATING BLOOD CELLS

An elevated content of total Ca^{2+} has been reported in erythrocytes of patients with essential hypertension (80).

By measurement of ion activities with cation-specific electrodes, elevated Ca^{2+} activities were demonstrated in hypertensives (81), which could be normalized by antihypertensive treatments. This group also extended their findings to vascular muscle cells from SHR (82). The lack of functional Ca^{2+} channels in erythrocytes has required alternative explanations involving Ca^{2+}-binding and transport for these changes in Ca^{2+} activities in hypertensives. McCarron et al. (83,84) have provided a model demonstrating that changes in cellular Ca^{2+} activities might be linked to a more general defect in Ca^{2+} metabolism, associated with decreased Ca^{2+} serum levels and elevated urinary Ca^{2+} excretion. The link between altered serum Ca^{2+} concentration and hypertension has been strengthened by observations in patients with low renin hypertension, with implications for additional calciotropic and Mg^{2+}-regulating hormones (85).

There is growing evidence in human and animal studies that disturbed Ca^{2+} metabolism is a major contributing factor in the pathogenesis of essential hypertension. Studies of circulating blood cells and platelets, as well as of vascular muscle cells, reveal altered Ca^{2+} metabolism that has been formulated as an etiologic hypothesis (53). Ca^{2+}-regulating factors, such as parathyroid hormone (PTH) and 1,25-dihydroxyvitamin D3 (1,25-[OH]$_2$D$_3$), have been implicated in interactions with blood pressure regulation. Evidence that PTH increases Ca^{2+} influx in heart cells (86), in osteoblasts (87), and in vascular muscle cells (88) has led to increased recognition of calciotropic hormone participation in the etiology of hypertension. The increased urinary Ca^{2+} excretion observed in hypertensive patients suggests enhanced parathyroid function, and what is perhaps an appropriate response to the increased urinary leak of Ca^{2+} (89). Manipulation of dietary Ca^{2+} and Na^+ has shown that there is a major influence of these important ions on development of hypertension in genetically hypertensive rats (90), and has led to a Ca^{2+} deficiency hypothesis in hypertension (91).

Correlations of Ca^{2+} regulatory hormones with hypertension have been made by several laboratories (92–94). Calciotropic hormones are among the factors that correlate highly with the development of increased blood pressure in hypertension (95), and thus warrant further study. In a recent study of normotensive offspring of either hypertensive or normotensive parents under defined dietary conditions, exposure to a high-salt (NaCl) diet increased blood pressure and platelet Ca^{2+}, associated with an increase in 1,25-(OH)$_2$D$_3$, showing predictive diagnostic value of platelet Ca^{2+} for future development of hypertension (96). The commonly observed increase in urinary Ca^{2+} excretion was confirmed with this study. These and other clinical and *in vitro* evidence suggest a role for the Ca^{2+} regulating hormone 1,25-(OH)$_2$D$_3$ in human and experimental hypertension. This interaction has recently been addressed by patch-clamp and fluorescence spectroscopic techniques, which showed an increase of Ca^{2+} channel current and an intracellular Ca^{2+} transient in rat vascular muscle cells upon exposure to 1,25-(OH)$_2$D$_3$ (97).

This inverse relationship between serum Ca^{2+} and Mg^{2+}, and its possible effects on intracellular cation activities, needs further exploration; in contrast to the decrease in Ca^{2+} activity, elevated intracellular free Mg^{2+} concentrations were reported in erythrocytes from hypertensive patients (98) and from SHR (99). Target structures at which Ca^{2+} and Mg^{2+} might compete for the same binding site include surface membrane, intracellular membranes, and proteins. An enhanced capacity to bind Ca^{2+} has been shown in erythrocyte membranes from hypertensives (100,101), and reduced Mg^{2+}-binding may allow excess Ca^{2+} uptake in rabbit vascular muscle (23). Furthermore, a decreased content of a transmembrane Ca^{2+}-binding protein has been observed in various tissues and erythrocytes, as well as in other cells from hypertensive rats. Such observations are consistent with a decreased transmembranous Ca^{2+} efflux in hypertension (102).

Among human blood cells, erythrocytes are certainly most reactive to the altered shearing forces in established essential hypertension. Information on altered cation concentrations in other circulating cells is also needed. However, studies on human mononuclear leukocytes (103), neutrophils (104), or lymphocytes (105,106) failed to demonstrate a difference in intracellular Ca^{2+} activities between normotensives and hypertensives. In contrast, elevated Ca^{2+} activities in platelets from patients with essential hypertension have been demonstrated (105,107). In various studies, direct correlations between intraplatelet Ca^{2+} activities and blood pressures have been reported in humans (106–112) and in rats (113), and elevated Ca^{2+} activity could be normalized by antihypertensive treatment (107). An abnormally high Na^+ leak and clonidine insensitivity were found in erythrocytes of 25 patients with essential hypertension, suggesting altered ion transport (114).

Subsequently, alterations of other Ca^{2+}-dependent functions (such as an enhanced shape-change reaction and aggregation response), as well as Ca^{2+} release reactions to a variety of hormones (such as adenosine diphosphate (ADP), epinephrine, and thrombin), were found (112,115). The stimulation of platelets by agents acting through Ca^{2+} influx as well as through phosphoinositide breakdown was increased. An increased cAMP sensitivity, greater Ca^{2+}-dependent myosin light chain phosphorylation, and an elevated Ca^{2+}-Mg^{2+}–ATPase activity and blunted responsiveness to calmodulin addition have been observed in calmodulin-deficient platelet membranes from patients with essential hypertension (110,116,117).

Human platelet studies increasingly show utility in diagnosing and adjusting treatment of hypertension, e.g., parallel reduction of Ca^{2+} influx–dependent vasoconstriction and platelet Ca^{2+} activity in patients treated with Ca^{2+} entry and β-adrenoceptor blockade (118). Besides abnormal Ca^{2+} handling in platelets of hypertensives, other ion regulatory alterations have been described in hypertension, e.g., increased Na^+-H^+ exchange (119), increased α_2-receptor number (120), resistance to desensitization (121), indications of altered membrane composition for phosphoinositide breakdown to more readily accessible components (117,122), increased norepinephrine (123) and thromboglobulin secretion (124), and altered serotonin metabolism (125).

The regulation of Ca^{2+} activity in platelets has been addressed in many subsequent studies. Increased intraplatelet Ca^{2+} concentrations have been identified as the common hallmark in certain defined situations, such as in hypertensives with early and end-stage kidney disease (126,127), in hypertensive and diabetic patients (128), in obese patients, with normalization upon weight reduction (129), and in preeclamptic females (130), in which this has been shown to predict increased peripheral resistance (131). This indicates that elevated free Ca^{2+} concentrations in platelets is a rather common phenomenon related to elevated blood pressure and other conditions associated with increased platelet Ca^{2+} activities. There is a growing need for these disorders to be studied further and correlated with post-Ca^{2+} levels.

However, platelet studies have important limitations. For instance, it seems very unlikely that altered functions in platelets from hypertensives are mediated through voltage-gated Ca^{2+} channels, since such channels could not be demonstrated in receptor binding studies (108), although there is some indirect evidence for the presence of a voltage-gated Ca^{2+} channel, which seems to have a minor functional importance for platelets (132,133). On the other hand, dihydropyridine Ca^{2+} agonists can stimulate platelets (134); conversely, various Ca^{2+} antagonists inhibit platelet function both *in vitro* and *in vivo* (135–138). However, evidence has been provided for a ligand-gated Ca^{2+} channel in human platelets (132,133), which could partially explain these discrepancies.

PLATELETS AS INDICATORS OF HYPERTENSION MECHANISMS

The relevance of platelet studies to hypertension is a compelling reason for consideration as a clinical diagnostic tool, namely as an accessible indicator of muscle cell function. Common features include Ca^{2+}-dependent contraction processes and functionally similar receptors for adrenaline, serotonin, vasopressin, etc. (115). The necessity for further investigations of platelets and their interactions with the vessel wall can also be appreciated, based on the increased risk of thromboembolic complications and mortality in hypertensive patients (139). As the main task of platelets, in combination with plasma

coagulation factors, is to protect the body from blood loss, platelets adhere, change shape, take up and release factors and hormones, and aggregate (for a review, see ref. 140). Major stimuli for activation of platelets *in vivo* are thought to be secretion products from endothelial lesions, thrombin, and shearing forces (141,142).

Further evidence for a central role for Ca^{2+} in human essential hypertension has recently been provided in a recent Dutch study (143). The suggestion that PTH levels are higher in the prehypertensive phase was further supported by significantly lower levels of plasma Mg^{2+} and phosphate in prehypertensive offspring of hypertensive parents. The higher urinary Ca^{2+} excretion that seems to increasingly be regarded as a hallmark of genetic hypertension was also increased in the prehypertensive offspring of hypertensive parents. The authors concluded that changes in Ca^{2+} metabolism appear in the early pathogenesis of primary hypertension, and suggested that a reduced renal sensitivity to PTH may be a significant variable (143). Evidence that the signal transduction pathway involving Ca^{2+} is altered in hypertension was provided in SHR/WKY experiments (33). These studies suggest that, at least in rats, the Ca^{2+} influx in response to angiotensin II and PDGF are enhanced in hypertension.

It may well be that increased shearing forces contribute, together with more responsive platelets, to the increased risk of thromboembolic events in hypertension. However, this hypothesis is still speculative, since the primary regulators of physiologic coagulation and anticoagulation *in vivo* are circulating plasma factors. Secretion products of endothelium and platelets, synthesis of activators and inhibitors by vascular muscle cells, and the sensitivity of appropriate receptors in all three cell types are involved in the regulation and maintenance of physiologic vascular integrity, coagulation, and blood viscosity (144–150). Whether any of these factors plays a role in the elevated thromboembolic incidence rates in hypertension is not yet known.

To interpret results from platelet studies, it should be noted that platelets are released from megakaryocytes into circulation as a family of subpopulations of platelets differing in size and function (151–153). In an earlier report, it had been suggested that hypertension is associated with different platelet subpopulations (154). However, this could not be confirmed by others (112). Because platelets are so reactive and possibly hold important clues for both pathophysiologic mechanism and diagnostic utility, much additional research will be needed.

CONCLUSIONS

In conclusion, identified changes in vascular muscle cells involving regulation of Ca^{2+} by the surface and intracellular membranes have been identified and linked to mechanisms that appear to contribute to genetic hypertension. Altered regulation of ions may suggest that there are membrane changes that affect multiple ion channels and ion transport, resulting in the compromised regulation of intracellular Ca^{2+} and sometimes adverse changes in compensatory mechanisms. Although additional mechanisms such as suppressed vasodilator function (155) might also be important to explain excessively constricted blood vessels in hypertensives, the indicators point increasingly to Ca^{2+} regulation. Ca^{2+} channels have been specifically identified as abnormal in SHR, implying that this highly conserved (Ca^{2+} channel) protein may be a site of genetic alteration causing hypertension. In addition, alterations in modulation by PKC and other intracellular signal messengers or membrane phospholipids may be involved, either as a primary hypertension mechanism or as a compensation for altered Ca^{2+} channel function. Much more cell and molecular research is needed to differentiate cause and effect in multiple identified abnormal mechanisms. A Ca^{2+} hypothesis for hypertension, which was originally formulated by Aoki and co-workers (47,53), has been followed and further explored by others (48,58,60,82,92,95, 96,105,107,131,156,158). Additionally, Ca^{2+} influx and release are altered in genetic hypertension, as shown with increasing levels of spatial and temporal resolution. However, to detect these subtle differences, it is apparently necessary to measure Ca^{2+} in localized regions, e.g., the subplasma-membrane space, with resolution of less than 1 second. Under such conditions, increased levels of subsarcolemmal Ca^{2+} have been detected both as a consequence of increased Ca^{2+} release and decreased Ca^{2+} uptake in SHR.

Intracellular sensitizing proteins other than calmodulin apparently result in increased Ca^{2+} sensitivity of the contractile proteins (61), and other proteins need to be investigated. With each of these intracellular regulatory proteins, levels of complexity need to be explored before the definitive pattern is likely to emerge. For example, in the case of PKC, different isoforms with different patterns of regulation, translocation, and function have been identified. Additionally, Ca^{2+}-binding proteins, especially those of the S100 protein family, may be important alterations occurring in hypertension. A very useful diagnostic tool for both recognition of prehypertensives and monitoring treatment effectiveness is Ca^{2+} levels in circulating blood cells, which provide an important window on the function of the cardiovascular system in hypertension. Studies of Ca^{2+} in platelets have revealed abnormally high Ca^{2+} levels, responsiveness to vasopressin, and responses to calciotropic hormones. Increased platelet Ca^{2+} in response to stimulation by PTH and 1,25-$(OH_2)D_3$ in hypertension suggests the diagnostic utility of Ca^{2+} measurements in platelets under a variety of conditions. Examples are early and end-stage kidney disease,

hypertension along with diabetes, obesity, and preeclampsia, all of which have shown the predictive value of platelet Ca^{2+} measurements. Recent evidence that PTH levels are higher in the prehypertensive phase, and that interactions of such stimulants as vasopressin, thrombin, and serotonin might interact with calciotropic hormones, appear to be productive areas for future investigation. There is clearly an underlying reason for the growing evidence in both vascular muscle and circulating blood cells that Ca^{2+} is altered. Such observations of aberrant regulation, because of the importance of the Ca^{2+} signal, warrant further attention.

ACKNOWLEDGMENTS

Research of the authors cited in this chapter was supported by NIH grants HL 38537 and HL 38645. Paul Erne was supported by the Swiss National Fund No. 32-029-975.90.

REFERENCES

1. Abboud FM. The sympathetic system in hypertension. State-of-art review. *Hypertension* 1982;4(suppl 11):200–225.
2. Hermsmeyer K. Calcium antagonist effects on vascular muscle membrane potentials and intracellular Ca^{2+}. In: Rubin RP, Weiss G, Putney IW Jr, eds. *Calcium in biological systems.* New York: Plenum Press, 1985;423–430.
3. Hermsmeyer K. Altered membrane potential control of contraction in arterial muscle in hypertension. *Klin Worchenschr* 1985;63(suppl III):61–62.
4. Hermsmeyer K. Electrogenic ion pumps and other determinants of membrane potential in vascular muscle. *Physiologist* 1982;25:454–465.
5. Nelson MT, Standen NB, Brayden JE, Worley JF III. Noradrenaline contracts arteries by activating voltage-dependent calcium channels. *Nature* 1988;336:382–385.
6. Hermsmeyer K, Mason R. Norepinephrine sensitivity and desensitization of cultured single vascular muscle cells. *Circ Res* 1982;50:627–632.
7. Hermsmeyer K. Vascular muscle membrane cation mechanisms and total peripheral resistance. *Hypertension* 1987;10(suppl I):1-20-1-22.
8. Hermsmeyer K, Harder D. Membrane ATPase mechanism of the K^+ return relaxation in stroke-prone SHR and WKY arterial muscles. *Am J Physiol* 1986;250(*Cell Physiol* 19):C557–C562.
9. Haeusler C. Contraction, membrane potential, and calcium fluxes in rabbit pulmonary artery muscle. *Fed Proc* 1983;42:240–252.
10. Jones AW. Content and fluxes of electrolytes. In: Bohr DF, Somlyo AP, Sparks HV, eds. *Handbook of physiology. The cardiovascular system.* Washington, DC: American Physiological Society, 1980.
11. Siegel C, Walter A, Rettig W, Kampe CH, Ebeling BJ, Bertsche O. Sodium compartments in the arterial wall. In: Zumkley H, Losse H, eds. *Intracellular electrolytes and arterial hypertension.* International Symposium, Munster. Stuttgart: Georg Thieme Verlag, 1980;30–50.
12. Hermsmeyer K. Electrogenesis of increased norepinephrine sensitivity of arterial vascular muscle in hypertension. *Circ Res* 1976;38:362–367.
13. Hermsmeyer K. Cellular basis for increased sensitivity of vascular smooth muscle in spontaneously hypertensive rats. *Circ Res* 1976;38(suppl II):53–57.
14. Mulvany MJ, Aalkjer C, Christensen J. Changes in noradrenaline sensitivity and morphology of arterial resistance vessels during

development of high blood pressure in spontaneously hypertensive rats. *Hypertension* 1980;2:4–71.

15. Stekiel WJ. Electrophysiological mechanisms of force development by vascular smooth muscle membrane in hypertension. In: Lee EMKW, ed. *Blood vessel changes in hypertension: structure and function.* Boca Raton, FL: CRC Press, 1989;127–170.

16. Stekiel WJ, Contney SJ, Lombard JH, Harder DR. Response of venous membrane potential to calcium blockade in spontaneous hypertension. *Hypertension* 1983;5(suppl I):164–169.

17. Lombard JH, Burke MJ, Contney SJ, Willems WJ, Stekiel WJ. Effect of tetrodotoxin on membrane potentials and active tone in vascular smooth muscle. *Am J Physiol* 1982;242:H967–H972.

18. Rusch NJ, Stekiel WJ. Ionic channels of vascular smooth muscle in hypertension. In: Cox RH, ed. *Cellular and molecular mechanisms of hypertension.* New York: Plenum Press, 1991;1–7.

19. Hermsmeyer K. Altered arterial muscle ion transport mechanism in the spontaneously hypertensive rat. *J Cardiovasc Pharmacol* 1984;6:S10–S15.

20. Abel PW, Hermsmeyer K. Sympathetic cross-innervation of SHR and genetic controls suggests a trophic influence on vascular muscle membranes. *Circ Res* 1981;49:1311–1318.

21. Hermsmeyer K. Sodium pump hyperpolarization-relaxation in rat caudal artery. *Fed Proc* 1983;42:246–252.

22. Magliola L, McMahon EG, Jones W. Alterations in active Na-K transport during hypertension. *Am J Physiol* 1986;250:C540–C546.

23. Shetty SS, Weiss GB. Decreasing cellular Mg^{2+} by increasing extracellular Na^+ increases the bound Ca^{2+} fraction mobilized by agonists in vascular smooth muscle. *J Vasc Med Biol* 1991;3:229–234.

24. Hermsmeyer K, Sturek M. Membrane potential, Ca^{2+} influx, and Ca^{2+} release in single vascular muscle cells. *J Cardiovasc Pharmacol* 1986;8(suppl 8):S38–S41.

25. Sturek M, Hermsmeyer K. Calcium and sodium channels in spontaneously contracting vascular muscle cells. *Science* 1986;233:475–478.

26. Bean BP, Sturek M, Puga A, Hermsmeyer K. Calcium channels in vascular muscle cells isolated from rat mesenteric arteries: modulation by dihydropyridine drugs. *Circ Res* 1986;59:229–235.

27. Triggle D. Calcium channel drugs: structure-function relations and selectivity of action. *J Cardiovasc Pharmacol* 1991;18(suppl 10):S1–S6.

28. Hermsmeyer K, Bian K. Calcium channel hypothesis in hypertension. *J Vasc Med Biol* 1991;3:219–222.

29. Rusch NJ, Hermsmeyer K. Calcium currents are altered in the vascular muscle cell membrane of spontaneously hypertensive rats. *Circ Res* 1988;63:997–1002.

30. Rusch NJ, Hermsmeyer K. Vascular muscle calcium channels in hypertension. In: Coca A, ed. *Handbook on ionic transport in hypertension: new perspectives.* Boca Raton, FL: CRC Press, 1993.

31. Bruner CA, Webb RC, Bohr DF. Vascular reactivity and membrane stabilizing effect of calcium in spontaneously hypertensive rats. In: Aoki K, Frohlich ED, eds. *Calcium in essential hypertension.* Tokyo: Academic Press, 1989;275–306.

32. Tomobe Y, Ishikawa T, Yanagisawa M, et al. Mechanisms of altered sensitivity to endothelin 1 between aortic smooth muscle of spontaneously hypertensive and Wistar-Kyoto rats. *J Pharmacol Exp Ther* 1991;257:555–561.

33. Bendhack LM, Sharma RV, Bhalla R. Altered signal transduction in vascular smooth muscle cells of spontaneously hypertensive rats. *Hypertension* 1992;19(suppl II):II-142–II-148.

34. Kishi K, Inoue T. Possible mechanisms of abnormal norepinephrine sensitivity and reactivity of resistance vessels and the development of hypertension in spontaneously hypertensive rats. A hypothesis. *Am J Hypertens* 1990;3:202S–205S.

35. Marche P. Membrane phosphoinositide metabolism in hypertension. *NIPS* 1989;4:230–233.

36. Okamoto K, Aoki K. Development of a strain of spontaneously hypertensive rats. *Jpn Circ J* 1963;27:282–293.

37. Aoki K, Asano M. Effects of Bay K 8644 and nifedipine on femoral arteries of spontaneously hypertensive rats. *Br J Pharmacol* 1986;88:221–230.

38. Aoki K, Asano M. Increased responsiveness to calcium agonist BAY k 8644 and calcium antagonist nifedipine in femoral arteries of spontaneously hypertensive rats. *J Cardiovasc Pharmacol* 1987;10:S62–S64.

39. Hermsmeyer K, Sturek M, Rusch NJ. Calcium channel modulation by dihydropyridines in vascular muscle. *Ann NY Acad Sci* 1988;522:25–31.

40. Storm DS, Turla MB, Todd KM, Webb RC. Calcium and contractile responses to phorbol esters and the calcium channel agonist, Bay K 8644, in arteries from hypertensive rats. *Am J Hypertens* 1990;3:245S–248S.

41. Noon JP, Rice PJ, Baldessarini RJ. Calcium leakage as a cause of high resting tension in vascular smooth muscle from the spontaneously hypertensive rat. *Proc Natl Acad Sci USA* 1978;75:1605–1607.

42. Pederson OL, Mikkelsen E, Andersson KE. Effects of extracellular calcium on potassium and noradrenaline induced contractions in the aorta of spontaneously hypertensive rats—increased sensitivity to nifedipine. *Acta Pharmacol Toxicol* 1978;43:137–144.

43. Robinson BF, Dobbs RJ, Bayley S. Response of forearm resistance vessels to verapamil and sodium nitroprusside in normotensive and hypertensive men: evidence for a functional abnormality of vascular smooth muscle in primary hypertension. *Clin Sci* 1982;63:33–42.

44. Hulthen UL, Bolli P, Amann FW, et al. Enhanced vasodilatation in essential hypertension by calcium channel blockade with verapamil. *Hypertension* 1982;4:26–31.

45. Garthoff S. Calcium antagonist nifedipine normalizes high blood pressure and prevents mortality in salt-loaded DS substrain of DAHL rats. *Eur J Pharmacol* 1981;74:111–112.

46. Takata Y, Hutchinson JS. Exaggerated hypotensive responses to calcium antagonists in spontaneously hypertensive rats. *Clin Exp Hypertens* 1983;A5:827–847.

47. Aoki K, Kawaguchi Y, Sato K, et al. Clinical and pharmacological properties of calcium antagonists in essential hypertension in humans and spontaneously hypertensive rats. *J Cardiovasc Pharmacol* 1982;4:S298–S302.

48. Dominiczak AF, Webb RC, Bohr DF. Calcium and the malfunction of the plasma membrane in hypertension. *J Vasc Med Biol* 1991;3:178–180.

49. Bohr DF. Cell membrane in hypertension. *News Physiol Sci* 1989;4:85–88.

50. Postnov YV, Orlov N. Cell membrane alterations as a source of primary hypertension. *J Hypertens* 1984;2:1–6.

51. Gleason MM, Medow MS, Tulenko TN. Excess membrane cholesterol alters calcium movements, cytosolic calcium levels, and membrane fluidity in arterial smooth muscle cells. *Circ Res* 1991;69:216–227.

52. Cox RH, Tulenko TN. Altered excitation-contraction coupling in hypertension: role of plasma membrane phospholipids and ion channels. In: Moreland RS, ed. *Regulation of smooth muscle contraction.* New York: Plenum Press, 1991;272–290.

53. Aoki K. Development of the calcium-membrane theory of hypertension. In: Kwan CY, ed. *Membrane abnormalities in hypertension.* Boca Raton, FL: CRC Press, 1989;79–114.

54. Erne P, Hermsmeyer K. Intracellular vascular muscle Ca^{2+} modulation in genetic hypertension. *Hypertension* 1989;14:145–151.

55. Hermsmeyer K, Land R, Erne P. Subsarcolemmal increase in intracellular calcium in vascular muscle cells from spontaneously hypertensive rats. *J Vasc Med Biol* 1991;3:261–267.

56. Xue H, McCarron DA, Bukoski RD. 1,25 $(OH)_2$ vitamin D_3-induced 45CA uptake in vascular myocytes cultured from spontaneously hypertensive and normotensive rats. *Life Sci* 1991;49(9):651–659.

57. Bukoski RD. Intracellular Ca^{2+} metabolism of isolated resistance arteries and cultured vascular myocytes of spontaneously hypertensive and Wistar-Kyoto normotensive rats. *J Hypertens* 1990;8(1):37–43.

58. Kwan CY. Dysfunction of calcium handling by smooth muscle in hypertension. *Can J Physiol Pharmacol* 1985;63:366–374.

59. Kwan CY, Belbeck L, Daniel EE. Abnormal biochemistry of vascular smooth muscle plasma membrane as an important factor

in the initiation and maintenance of hypertension in rats. *Blood Vessels* 1979;16:259–268.

60. Lau K, Eby B. The role of calcium in genetic hypertension. *Hypertension* 1985;7:657–667.

61. Bruschi G, Bruschi ME, Borghetti A. Changes in Ca^{2+} sensitivity by release-restitution of cytosoluble proteins in perforated arterial smooth muscle cells. *J Vasc Med Biol* 1991;3:174–177.

62. James P, Inui M, Tada M, Chiesi M, Carafoli E. Nature and sites of phospholamban regulation of the Ca^{2+} pump of sarcoplasmic reticulum. *Nature* 1989;342:90–92.

63. Eberhard M, Erne P. Inositol 1,4,5-trisphosphate-induced calcium release in permeabilized platelets is coupled to hydrolysis of inositol 1,4,5-trisphosphate to inositol 1,4-bisphosphate. *Biochem Biophys Res Commun* 1993;195:19–24.

64. Eberhard M, Erne P. Role of cytosolic and intraluminal Ca^{2+} in inositol 1,4,5-triphosphate-induced Ca^{2+} release in human platelets. (submitted).

65. Nishizuka Y. The molecular heterogeneity of protein kinase C and its implications for cellular regulation. *Nature* 1988;334:661–665.

66. Andrea JE, Walsh MP. Protein kinase C of smooth muscle. *Hypertension* 1992;20:585–595.

67. Yazaki Y, Komuro I. Molecular analysis of stretch-induced proto-oncogene expression in cardiac myocytes. *J Vasc Med Biol* 1991;3:290–296.

68. Bhalla RC, Sharma RV. Increased growth-factor-stimulated DNA synthesis in SHR VSM cells is independent of protein kinase C activity. *J Vasc Med Biol* 1991;3:308–313.

69. Takaori K, Itoh S, Kanayama Y, Takeda T. Protein kinase C activity in platelets from spontaneously hypertensive rats (SHR) and normotensive Wistar Kyoto rats (WKY). *Biochem Biophys Res Commun* 1986;141:769–773.

70. Bazan E, Campbell AK, Rapoport RM. Protein kinase C activity in blood vessels from normotensive and spontaneously hypertensive rats. *Eur J Pharmacol* 1992;227:343–348.

71. Erne P, Crabos M, Woodtli T, Imber R, Fabbro D, Yamakado T, Heizmann CW, Bühler FR. Intraplatelet tropomyosin and protein kinase C isoforms: putative abnormalities in hypertensive platelets. *J Vasc Med Biol* 1991;3:277–284.

72. Crabos M, Imber R, Woodtli TH, Fabbro D, Erne P. Different translocation of three distinct PKC isoforms with tumor-promoting phorbol ester in human platelets. *Biochem Biophys Res Commun* 1991;178:878–883.

73. Crabos M, Fabbro D, Stabel S, Erne P. Effect of tumor-promoting phorbol ester, thrombin, and vasopressin on translocation of three distinct protein kinase C isoforms in human platelets and regulation by calcium. *Biochem J* 1992;288:891–896.

74. Engelkamp D, Schäfer BS, Erne P, Heizmann CW. S100α, CAPL, and CACY: molecular cloning and expression analysis of three calcium-binding proteins from human heart. *Biochemistry* 1992;31:10258–10264.

75. Engelkamp D, Schäfer BW, Mattei MG, Erne P, Heizmann CW. Six S100 genes are clustered on human chromosome 1q21: identification of two genes coding for the two previously identified calcium-binding proteins S100D and S100E. *Proc Natl Acad Sci USA* 1993;90:6547–6551.

76. Friedman SM. Cellular ionic pertubations in hypertension. *J Hypertens* 1983;1:109–114.

77. Postnov YV, Orlov SN. Ion transport across membrane in primary hypertension. *Physiol Rev* 1985;65:904–945.

78. Hilton PJ. Cellular sodium transport in essential hypertension. *N Engl J Med* 1986;314:222–229.

79. Patel P, Sharma S, Bose R. Intracellular calcium, pH, and aggregation changes in spontaneously hypertensive rat platelets in response to extracellular acidosis. *J Vasc Med Biol* 1991;3:314–319.

80. Losse H, Wehmeyer H, Wessels F. Der Wasser-und Elektrolythaushalt von Erythrocyten bei arterieller Hypertonie. *Klin Wochenschr* 1960;38:393–402.

81. Zidek W, Losse H, Dorst K, Zumkley H, Vetter H. Intracellular sodium and calcium in essential hypertension. *Klin Wochenschr* 1982;60:859–862.

82. Losse H, Zidek W, Vetter H. Intracellular sodium and calcium in

vascular muscle of spontaneously hypertensive rats. *J Cardiovasc Pharmacol* 1984;6:532–534.

83. McCarron D, Pingree PA, Rubin RJ, Gaucher SM, Molitch M, Krutzik S. Enhanced parathyroid function in essential hypertension: a homeostatic response to a urinary calcium leak. *Hypertension* 1978;2:162–168.

84. McCarron DA. Low serum concentrations of ionized calcium in patients with hypertension. *N Engl J Med* 1982;307:226–228.

85. Resnick LM, Laragh JH, Sealey JE, Alderman MA. Divalent ions in essential hypertension. Relations between serum ionized calcium, magnesium and plasma renin activity. *N Engl J Med* 1983;309:888–891.

86. Bogin E, Massry SG, Harary I. Effect of parathyroid hormone on rat heart cells. *J Clin Invest* 1981;67:1215–1227.

87. Reid IR, Civitelli R, Halstead LR, Avioli LV, Hruska KA. Parathyroid hormone acutely elevates intracellular calcium in osteoblastic cells. *Am J Physiol* 1987;253(*Endocrinol Metab* 16):E45–E51.

88. Bukoski RD, Wang D, Wagman W. Injection of 1,25 $(OH)_2$ $VitD_3$ enhances resistance artery contractile properties. *Hypertension* 1990;16:523–531.

89. McCarron DA, Pingree PA, Rubin RJ, Gaucher SM, Molitch ME, Krutzik S. Enhanced parathyroid function in essential hypertension: a homeostatic response to a urinary calcium leak. *Hypertension* 1980;2:162–168.

90. McCarron DA, Lucas PA, Schneidman RJ, LaCour B, Drüeke T. Blood pressure development of the spontaneously hypertensive rat after concurrent manipulations of dietary Ca^{2+} and Na^+. *J Clin Invest* 1985;76:1147–1149.

91. McCarron DA, Morris CD. The calcium deficiency hypothesis of hypertension. *Ann Intern Med* 1987;107:919–922.

92. Sowers JR, Zemel MB, Standley PR, Zemel PC. Calcium and hypertension. *J Lab Clin Med* 1989;114:338–348.

93. Resnick LM, Müller FB, Laragh JH. Calcium-regulating hormones in essential hypertension: relation to plasma renin activity and sodium metabolism. *Ann Intern Med* 1986;105:649–654.

94. Hvarfner A, Bergström R, Morlin C, Wide L, Ljunghall S. Relationships between calcium metabolic indices and blood pressure in patients with essential hypertension as compared with a healthy population. *J Hypertens* 1987;5:451–456.

95. Brickman AS, Nyby M, von Hungen K, Eggena P, Tuck L. Calcitropic hormones, platelet calcium, and blood pressure in essential hypertension. *Hypertension* 1990;16:515–522.

96. Yamakawa H, Suzuki H, Nakamura M, Ohno Y, Saruta T. Disturbed calcium metabolism in offspring of hypertensive parents. *Hypertension* 1992;19:528–534.

97. Shan J, Resnick LM, Lewanczuk RZ, Karpinski E, Pang PKT. 1,25 dihydroxy-vitamin D as a cardiovascular hormone: effects on calcium current and cytosolic free calcium in vascular smooth muscle cells. *Am J Hypertens* 1993;6:983–988.

98. Resnick LJ, Gupta RK, Laragh JH. Intracellular free magnesium in erythrocytes of essential hypertension: relation to blood pressure and serum divalent cations. *Proc Natl Acad Sci USA* 1985;81:6511–6515.

99. Matuura T, Kanayama Y, Yasunari K, Murakawa K, Takeda T, Ishimora K, Morishima I, Yonezawa T. Decreased intracellular free magnesium in erythrocytes of spontaneously hypertensive rats. *Biochem Biophys Res Commun* 1987;143:1012–1017.

100. Orlov SN, Postnov YV. Ca^{2+}-binding and membrane fluidity in essential and renal hypertension. *Clin Sci* 1982;63:281–284.

101. Postnov YV, Orlov SN, Reznikova MB, Rjazhsky GC. Calmodulin distribution and Ca^{2+} transport in the erythrocyte of patients with essential hypertension. *Clin Sci* 1984;66:459–463.

102. Kowarski S, Cowen LA, Schachter D. Decreased content of integral membrane calcium-binding protein (IMCAL) in tissues of the spontaneously hypertensive rat. *Proc Natl Acad Sci USA* 1986;93:1097–1100.

103. Shore AC, Beynon GW, Jones JC, Markandu ND, Sagnella GA, MacGregor GA. Mononuclear leucocyte intracellular free calcium—Does it correlate with blood pressure? *J Hypertens* 1985;3:183–187.

104. Favre L, Lew PD, Valloton MB. Cytosolic free calcium and intracellular stores are normal in neutrophils from patients with essential hypertension. *J Hypertens* 1985;2(suppl 3):493–494.

105. Bruschi G, Bruschi ME, Caroppo M, Orlandini G, Spaggiari M, Cavatorta A. Cytoplasmic free Ca²⁺ is in platelets of spontaneously hypertensive rats and essential hypertensive patients. *Clin Sci* 1985;66:179–184.

106. Ashley CC, Castell LM, Ledingham JGG, Osborn C, Pritchard K, Raine AEG, Sommers VK. Relationship between lymphocyte and platelet intracellular free calcium concentrations, plasma ionized calcium, and blood pressure in essential hypertension. *J Physiol (Lond)* 1986;372:81P.

107. Erne P, Bolli P, Burgisser E, Buhler FR. Correlation of platelet calcium with blood pressure: effect of antihypertensive therapy. *N Engl J Med* 1984;310:1084–1088.

108. Erne P, Burgisser E, Buhler FR, Dubach B, Kuhnis H, Meier M, Rogg H. Enhancement of calcium influx in human platelets by CGP 28392, a novel dihydropyridine. *Biochem Biophys Res Commun* 1984;118:842–847.

109. Le Quang Sang KH, Montenay-Garestier T, Devynck MA. Platelet cytosolic free calcium concentration in essential hypertension. *Nouv Rev Fr Hematol* 1985;27:279–283.

110. Erne P, Conen D, Kiowski W, Bolli P, Mueller FB, Buehler FR. Calcium antagonist induced vasodilation in peripheral, coronary and cerebral vasculature as important factors in the treatment of elderly hypertensives. *Eur Heart J* 1987;8(suppl K):49–56.

111. Lindner A, Kenny M, Meadam AJ. Effects of a circulating factor in patients with essential hypertension on intracellular free calcium in normal platelets. *N Engl J Med* 1987;316:509–513.

112. Taylor MA, Ayers CR, Gear ARL. Platelet calcium and quenched-flow aggregation kinetics in essential hypertension. *Hypertension* 1989;13:558–566.

113. Vasdev S, Thompson P, Triggle C, Fernandez P, Bolli P, Ananthanarayanan VS. Fura-2 used as a probe to show elevated intracellular free calcium in platelets of Dahl-sensitive rats fed a high salt diet. *Biochem Biophys Res Commun* 1988;154:380–386.

114. Senn N, Hajem S, Frohly P, Ollivier J-P, Garay RP. Clonidine sensitivity in patients with essential hypertension as a function of red cell ion transport. *J Vasc Med Biol* 1991;3:285–289.

115. Erne P, Resink TJ, Burgisser E, Buhler FR. Platelets and hypertension. *J Cardiovasc Pharmacol* 1985;7(suppl 6):103–108.

116. Resink TJ, Tkachuk VA, Erne P, Buhler FR. Platelet membrane calmodulin-stimulated calcium-adenosine triphosphatase. Altered activity in essential hypertension. *Hypertension* 1986;8:156–166.

117. Resink TJ, Dimitrov D, Zschauer A, Erne P, Tkachuk VA, Buhler FR. Platelet calcium linked abnormalities in essential hypertension. *Ann NY Acad Sci* 1987;488:252–259.

118. Bolli P, Erne P, Hulthen UL, Ritz R, Kiowksi W, Ji BH, Buhler FR. Parallel reduction of calcium-influx-dependent vasoconstriction and platelet free calcium concentration with calcium entry and beta-adrenoceptor blockade. *J Cardiovasc Pharmacol* 1984;6(suppl 7):996–1001.

119. Livne A, Balfe JW, Veitch R, Marquez-Julio A, Grinstein S, Rothstein A. Increased platelet Na⁺-H⁺ exchange rates in essential hypertension: application of a novel test. *Lancet* 1987;1:533–536.

120. Brodde OE, Daul E, O'Hara N, Khalifa AM. Properties of alpha- and beta-adrenoceptors in circulating blood cells of patients with essential hypertension. *J Cardiovasc Pharmacol* 1985;7(suppl 6):162–167.

121. Hollister AS, Onrot J, Lonce S, Nadeau JHJ, Robertson D. Plasma catecholamine modulation of alpha-2-adrenoceptor agonist affinity and sensitivity in normotensive and hypertensive human platelet. *J Clin Invest* 1986;77:1416–1421.

122. Naftilan AJ, Dzau VJ, Loscalzo J. Preliminary observation on abnormalities of membrane structure and function in essential hypertension. *Hypertension* 1986;8:174–179.

123. Mattiason I, Hood B. Efflux of noradrenaline from platelets in normotensive and hypertensive families. *Clin Sci* 1982;62:151–155.

124. Kjieldsen SE, Gjesdal K, Eide I, Aakesson I, Amundson R, Foss OP, Leren P. Increased beta-thromboglobulin in essential hypertension: interaction between arterial adrenaline, platelet function and blood lipids. *Acta Med Scand* 1983;213:369–373.

125. Kamal LA, LeQuan-Bui KH, Meyer P. Decreased uptake of ³H-serotonin and endogenous content of serotonin in blood platelets in hypertensive platelets. *Hypertension* 1984;6:568–573.

126. Schiffl H. Platelet cytosolic free-calcium concentration in hypertension associated with early-stage kidney disease. *Klin Wochenschr* 1989;67:676–681.

127. Schiffl H. Correlation of blood pressure in end-stage renal disease with platelet cytosolic free-calcium concentration. *Klin Wochenschr* 1990;68:718–722.

128. Ishii H, Umeda F, Hashimoto H, Nawata H. Increased intracellular calcium mobilization in platelets from patients with type 2 (non-insulin-dependent) diabetes mellitus. *Diabetologia* 1991;34:332–336.

129. Scherrer U, Nussberger J, Torriani S, Waeber B, Darioli R, Hofstetter JR, Brunner HR. Effect of weight reduction in moderately overweight patients on recorded ambulatory blood pressure and free cytosolic platelet calcium. *Circulation* 1991;83(2):552–558.

130. Haller T, Oeney T, Hauck U, Distler A, Philipp T. Increased intracellular free calcium and sensitivity to angiotensin II in platelets of preeclamptic women. *Am J Hypertens* 1989;2:238–243.

131. Zemel MB, Zemel PC, Berry S, Norman G, Kowalczyk C, Sokol RJ, Standley PR, Walsh MF, Sowers JR. Altered platelet calcium metabolism as an early predictor of increased peripheral vascular resistance and preeclampsia in urban black women. *N Engl J Med* 1990;323:434–438.

132. Zschauer A, van Breemen C, Bühler FR, Nelson MT. Calcium channels in thrombin-activated human platelet membranes. *Nature* 1988;334(6184):703–705.

133. Zschauer A, Resink TJ, Buhler FR. Evidence for a voltage gated calcium channel in human platelets. (Submitted).

134. Resink TJ, Erne P, Buhler FR. The influence of CGP 28392, 1,4-dihydropyridine on human platelet calcium and cyclic AMP metabolism. *Eur J Pharmacol* 1985;113:383–393.

135. MacIntyre DE, Shaw AM, Bushfield M, MacMillan LJ, McNicol A, Pollock WK. Endogenous and pharmacological mechanisms for the regulation of human platelet cytosolic free Ca²⁺. *Nouv Rev Fr Hematol* 1985;27:285–292.

136. Erne P, Mittelholzer E, Resink TJ, Rogg H, Buhler FR. Vasodilating agents and platelet function: intracellular free calcium concentration, cyclic nucleotides and shape-change response. *J Cardiovasc Pharmacol* 1986;8(suppl 8):102–106.

137. Johnson GJ, Leis LA, Francis GS. Disparate effects of the calcium-channel blockers, nifedipine and verapamil, on alpha-2-adrenergic receptors and thromboxane A₂-induced aggregation of human platelets. *Circulation* 1986;73:847–854.

138. Mehta J, Mehta P. Platelet function in hypertension and effect of therapy. *Am J Cardiol* 1981;47:331–334.

139. Kannel WB. Some lessons in cardiovascular epidemiology from Framingham. *Am J Cardiol* 1976;37:269.

140. Weiss HJ. *Platelets, pathophysiology and antiplatelet drug therapy.* New York: Alan R. Liss, 1982.

141. Tschopp TB, Baumgartner HR, Silberbauer K, Sinzinger H. Platelet adhesion and platelet thrombus formation on subendothelium of human arteries and veins exposed to flowing blood *in vitro*. *Haemostasis* 1980;8:19–29.

142. Weiss HJ, Turitto VT, Baumgartner HR. Platelet adhesion and thrombus formation on subendothelium in platelets deficient in glycoproteins IIb-IIIa, Ib, and storage granules. *Blood* 1986;67:322–330.

143. van Hooft IMS, Grobbee DE, Frölich M, Pols HAP, Hofman A. Alterations in calcium metabolism in young people at risk for primary hypertension. The Dutch hypertension and offspring study. *Hypertension* 1993;21:267–272.

144. Collen D. On the regulation and control of fibrinolysis. *Thromb Haemost* 1980;43:77–89.

145. Schwarz HP, Heeb MJ, Griffin JG. Human platelet protein S. *Thromb Haemost* 1985;54:57A.

146. Fair DS, Marlar RA, Levin EG. Human endothelial cells synthesize protein S. *Blood* 1986;67:1168–1171.

147. Kruithof EKO, Tran-Thang C, Bachmann F. Studies on the release of a plasminogen activator inhibitor by human platelets. *Thromb Haemost* 1986;55:201–205.

148. Lane DA, Pejler G, Flynn AM, Thompson EA, Lindhal U. Neutralization of heparin-related saccharides by histidine-rich glycoprotein and platelet factor 4. *J Biol Chem* 1986;261:3980–3986.

149. Leeksma OC, Zandbergen J, Giltai JC, van Mourik JA. Cultured human endothelial cells synthesize a plasma membrane protein complex immunologically related to the platelet glycoprotein IIb/IIIa complex. *Blood* 1986;67:1176–1180.

150. Levin EG. Quantitation and properties of the active and latent plasminogen activator inhibitors in cultures of human endothelial cells. *Blood* 1986;67:1309–1313.

151. Pennington DE, Strattfield K. Heterogeneity of megakaryocytes and platelets. *Semin Hematol* 1975;8:1–48.

152. Thompson C, Eaton KA, Princiotta SM. Kushkin CA, Valeri CR. Size-dependent platelet subpopulations: relationship of platelet volume to ultrastructure, enzymatic activity and function. *Br J Haematol* 1982;50:509–519.

153. Erne P, Wardle J, Sanders K, Lewis SM, Maseri A. Mean platelet volume and size distribution and their sensitivity to agonists in patients with coronary artery disease and congestive heart failure. *Thromb Haemost* 1988;59:259–263.

154. Lande K, Os I, Kjieldsen E, Westheim A, Hjermann I, Eide I, Gjesdal K. Increased platelet size and release reaction in essential hypertension. *J Hypertens* 1987;5:401–406.

155. Toda N, Kitamura Y, Okamura T. New idea on the mechanism of hypertension: suppression of nitroxidergic vasodilator nerve function. *J Vasc Med Biol* 1991;3:235–241.

156. Kwan CY. Abnormalities of vascular muscle membranes with special reference to calcium handling. In: Kwan CY, ed. *Membrane abnormalities in hypertension.* Boca Raton, FL: CRC Press, 1989;115–144.

157. McCarron DA. Is calcium more important than sodium in the pathogenesis of essential hypertension? *Hypertension* 1985;7:607–627.

158. Kamouchi M, Akata T, Xiong Z, Inoue R, Kitamura K, Kuriyama H. Cellular and subcellular clues to hypertension: assessment from calcium mobilization data. *J Vasc Med Biol* 1991;3:205–218.

Hypertension: Pathophysiology, Diagnosis, and Management, Second Edition, edited by J.H. Laragh and B.M. Brenner, Raven Press, Ltd., New York © 1995.

CHAPTER **40**

Role of Products of Univalent Reduction of Oxygen in Hypertensive Vascular Injury

Hermes A. Kontos and Michael C. Kontos

Substantial evidence has accumulated in the past few years that the products of univalent reduction of oxygen, including superoxide anion radical ($\cdot O_2^-$), hydrogen peroxide (H_2O_2), and hydroxyl radical ($\cdot OH$), are mediators of vascular injury in a variety of diverse conditions, including acute hypertension (1), ischemia reperfusion (2,3), and traumatic injury (4). This development has excited considerable interest because of the possibility that therapies directed against these reactive products of oxygen may be helpful in minimizing tissue injury.

This chapter reviews the evidence implicating products of univalent reduction of oxygen in vascular injury from hypertension.

CHEMISTRY OF OXYGEN RADICALS

A molecule with one or more unpaired electrons in its molecular orbitals is termed a free radical (5). The presence of the unpaired electron usually imparts high reactivity to the molecule and renders it unstable and short-lived. However, some free radicals are surprisingly unreactive and may be relatively stable under ordinary conditions.

Free oxygen radicals (also called oxygen radicals or oxyradicals) are particularly interesting because of the abundance of oxygen in biological systems. Oxygen is a biradical because it contains, in each of its two outer molecular orbitals, an unpaired electron; the spin of each of these unpaired electrons is in the same direction (6). Molecules interact by the pairing of electrons that have opposite spin; since quantum mechanical rules forbid the simultaneous introduction of two electrons with the same spin in a molecule and since most organic molecules with which oxygen might react have paired electrons, the structure of oxygen renders it relatively unreactive and favors its univalent reaction.

The univalent reduction of oxygen yields superoxide anion radical (or simply superoxide), hydrogen peroxide, hydroxyl radical, and water (7,8), according to the following sequence:

$$O_2 \xrightarrow{e^-} \cdot O_2^- \xrightarrow{e^-} H_2O_2 \xrightarrow{e^-} \cdot OH \xrightarrow{e^-} H_2O$$

Superoxide is the anion of hydroperoxyl acid ($HO_2\cdot$). The pK_α for the dissociation of the latter is 4.8 (9); hence,

H. A. Kontos and M. C. Kontos: Department of Medicine, Medical College of Virginia, Richmond, Virginia 23298.

at physiological pH, superoxide is the predominant species. At low pH, the concentration of hydroperoxyl acid rises. This is significant because hydroperoxyl acid is more lipid-soluble and is a stronger oxidizing agent than superoxide (10–12). Superoxide is water-soluble and can act either as an oxidizing agent or as a reducing agent. It is less reactive in aqueous media than in aprotic media. In aqueous solution at neutral pH, its preferred reaction is the dismutation reaction, which yields hydrogen peroxide. Superoxide can cross cell membranes via the anion channel. Its passage through this channel is inhibited by blockers of this channel in red-cell membranes (13) and in cerebral vessel *in vivo* (14).

Hydrogen peroxide is not a true radical. It is stable under conditions prevailing in biological materials. It is a moderately strong oxidizing agent. Since it is lipid-soluble it can cross cell membranes with ease (15).

Hydroxyl radical is a powerful oxidant. It is extremely reactive; it reacts very rapidly with a large array of compounds (16). Because of its very high reactivity, it is very short-lived and does not travel more than a few molecular diameters from its site of formation.

Oxygen can also give rise to another reactive product, called singlet oxygen (17,18). Under certain conditions, one of the unpaired electrons of oxygen absorbs sufficient energy and inverts its spin. This changes the molecular structure of oxygen from a triplet state, denoted as $^3O_2$, to the singlet state, or $^1O_2$. Singlet oxygen is lipid-soluble, reactive, and very short-lived in biological systems.

Superoxide reacts rapidly with nitric oxide to generate peroxynitrite (19). The decomposition of peroxynitrite yields a strong oxidant that is very similar in reactivity to hydroxyl radical (19).

CELLULAR SOURCES OF REACTIVE PRODUCTS OF OXYGEN

The cellular sources and mechanism of formation of superoxide, hydrogen peroxide, hydroxyl radical, singlet oxygen, and peroxynitrite are considered in the following subsections.

Superoxide

Superoxide can be produced from a variety of sources. Table 1 lists those sources that are relevant to vascular injury.

Normally, a small portion of the oxygen consumption in mitochondria is accounted for by univalent reduction of oxygen, which produces superoxide (7,20). This results primarily from autoxidation of reduced components of the electron transport chain. Most of mitochondrial superoxide production takes place via autoxidation of ubisemiquinone (21–23). Reduced nicotinamide ade-

TABLE 1. *Sources of oxygen radicals*

Mitochondrial autoxidations
Autoxidations of small molecules
Hemoglobin and myoglobin
Oxidative enzymes
Enzymatic oxidation of unsaturated fatty acids
Metabolism of xenobiotics
Phagocytic cells

nine dinucleotide (NADH) dehydrogenase (21) and dihydroorotic dehydrogenase (24) also produce a small portion of mitochondrial superoxide.

Superoxide production from mitochondria would be expected to increase under hypoxic conditions (when the concentration of reduced components of the electron transport chain is high) (25) or during hyperoxia (when the concentration of oxygen is high) (25).

A variety of small molecules that are normal cellular constituents—such as flavins (26), thiols (27,28), and catecholamines (29)—undergo autoxidation (either spontaneous or catalyzed via transition metals, such as iron or copper) to yield superoxide.

Superoxide is also produced by hemoproteins such as hemoglobin or myoglobin during autoxidation to yield methemoglobin and metmyoglobin (30).

A number of oxidative enzymes reduce oxygen by a univalent pathway and produce superoxide (7,20). The best studied such enzyme is xanthine oxidase, which oxidizes xanthine and hypoxanthine to uric acid (31). Xanthine oxidase is present in different organs in varying concentrations, which also depend on the species. It seems to be concentrated primarily in the endothelium of blood vessels (32). Xanthine oxidase is present in tissues in the dehydrogenase form, which transfers electrons from its substrate to nicotinamide adenine dinucleotide (NAD) (32–34). This form of the enzyme does not produce superoxide. Under conditions of ischemia or severe hypoxia, or in the course of isolating the enzyme from tissues, xanthine dehydrogenase is converted to the oxidase form, probably by proteolytic action (2,3). This form of the enzyme transfers electrons directly to oxygen to produce superoxide. The enzyme also produces hydrogen peroxide via divalent reduction of oxygen (31). The transformation of xanthine dehydrogenase to oxidase requires widely varying times of ischemia in different tissues.

Arachidonate and other unsaturated fatty acids are metabolized in tissues by three pathways: via cyclooxygenase-prostaglandin hydroperoxidase (PGH synthase), via lipoxygenase, and via cytochrome P-450 oxygenases. All three pathways are capable of producing superoxide.

PGH synthase is an iron-containing protein with two activities; the cyclooxygenase activity is responsible for the oxygenation of arachidonate to the endoperoxide prostaglandin G_2 (PGG$_2$), which is a hydroperoxy acid (35). The peroxidase activity of the enzyme converts

PGG$_2$ to another endoperoxide, prostaglandin H$_2$ (PGH$_2$), which is a hydroxy acid. Superoxide is produced in the conversion of PGG$_2$ to PGH$_2$. During the peroxidase action, the enzyme molecule is converted to an intermediate form analogous to compound I of catalase, which is a radical form of the enzyme with the unpaired electron either on or near the iron (36). This intermediate is capable of reacting with reducing agents, such as NADH or reduced nicotinamide adenine dinucleotide phosphate, (NADPH), to convert them to the radical form of NAD or NADP (37). These radicals then react rapidly with oxygen to produce superoxide (38). Thus, superoxide is not a direct product of PGH synthase but is, instead, a product from a side chain (39). Under optimum conditions of cofactor concentrations, the yield of superoxide from this pathway is 1 mole per 10 moles of arachidonate metabolized (39).

The production of superoxide from PGH synthase has several important characteristics (39): It occurs in burst-like fashion with a high initial rate of production, which rapidly subsides to a fraction of its initial rate within a few seconds. This is due to self-inactivation of the enzyme. The rate of production is dependent on the concentration of NADH or NADPH. Although the concentrations of these in cells appear to be adequate to support maximum rates of production, it is not known what their concentrations are in the vicinity of the enzyme. The rate of production of superoxide is relatively insensitive to variations in the concentration of arachidonate. Linoleic acid or PGG$_2$, substituted for arachidonate as substrates, also generate superoxide; however, substitution of PGH$_2$ does not give rise to superoxide.

Certain polypeptides, like bradykinin, are capable of generating superoxide by activating phospholipases, thereby releasing arachidonate and accelerating its metabolism via PGH synthase (14,40). This mechanism accounts for the release of superoxide from human endothelial cells by bradykinin (41).

Soybean lipoxygenase also produces superoxide in the presence of NADH or NADPH but not in their absence. Either linoleic or arachidonic acid can be used as substrates. The yield of superoxide from this pathway is much less than that from PGH synthase (39).

The membrane-bound oxygenases associated with cytochrome P-450 or cytochrome b are also capable of metabolizing arachidonate and produce superoxide in the process (42,43).

Nitric oxide synthase, the enzyme that generates nitric oxide from L-arginine in a wide variety of tissues, is also capable of producing superoxide (44) and hydrogen peroxide (45). Presumably, the latter is generated by the dismutation of superoxide. Nitric oxide synthase has close homology with cytochrome P-450 reductase. The simultaneous production of superoxide and nitric oxide by the same enzyme is important because it may afford the opportunity for the generation of peroxynitrite. N^G-monomethyl-L-arginine (L-NMMA), which inhibits the production of nitric oxide from arginine, does not inhibit the production of superoxide from this enzyme (44). On the other hand, N^G-nitro-L-arginine methylester (L-NAME), which also inhibits nitric oxide production by nitric oxide synthase, also inhibits superoxide production by this enzyme. The differential effects of L-NMMA may account for the reported apparent production of oxygen radicals under the influence of this agent (46).

An NADH oxidase capable of producing superoxide accounts for the production of superoxide when lactate concentration is high in pulmonary arteries (47). Evidently, the same enzyme is widely distributed, not only in vascular tissue but also in parenchymal tissues, and may be an important source of superoxide (M. S. Wolin, personal communication).

Certain drugs or foreign substances introduced in tissues can undergo metabolism via a univalent pathway that converts them to radicals (48). These radical forms can then react with oxygen to produce superoxide. The best-studied such reaction is that of the herbicide methyl viologen (paraquat), which is converted to a radical form via a diaphorase. The production of superoxide from paraquat accounts for its toxicity (49). Hepatic microsomes transfer electrons from NADPH to the quinone moiety of the antimetabolite drug Adriamycin. The resultant anthracycline semiquinone then donates unpaired electrons to molecular oxygen forming superoxide anion (50). The addition of Adriamycin to submitochondrial particles isolated from the bovine heart has been shown to generate superoxide anion (51). Menadione, another quinone, is metabolized in cells by a univalent pathway to a semiquinone, which then reacts with oxygen to generate superoxide (52).

A variety of photosensitizing dyes autoxidize to generate superoxide (53). The best known of these is methylene blue, which, in addition to autoxidation, can undergo enzymatic univalent oxidation in tissues to generate superoxide. This agent inhibits guanylate cyclase in vascular smooth muscle by generating oxygen radicals (54–56). Another agent, 6-anilino-5′8′quinolinedione (LY83583), which is also an inhibitor of guanylate cyclase, generates oxygen radicals by the same mechanism (55,56).

Activated polymorphonuclear leukocytes and macrophages generate superoxide from NADPH oxidase (57). Superoxide is secreted in the extracellular space by these cells and is used in bactericidal action.

Hydrogen Peroxide

The main source of hydrogen peroxide in tissues is the dismutation of superoxide (20):

$$2 \cdot O_2^- + 2H^+ \rightarrow H_2O_2 + O_2$$

This reaction can be spontaneous, or it can be catalyzed by superoxide dismutase (SOD). The spontaneous dismutation is pH sensitive; its rate constant at pH 7.4 is $2 \times 10^5 \, M^{-1} \, sec^{-1}$ (7–9). The pH dependence of the dismutation of superoxide is explained by the rate constants of the following reactions (58):

$$2HO_2 \cdot \rightarrow H_2O_2 + O_2 \quad 7.6 \times 10^5 \, M^{-1} \, sec^{-1}$$

$$HO_2 \cdot + \cdot O_2^- + H^+ \rightarrow H_2O_2 + O_2 \quad 8.5 \times 10^7 \, M^{-1} \, sec^{-1}$$

$$2 \cdot O_2^- + 2H^+ \rightarrow H_2O_2 + O_2 \quad <100 \, M^{-1} \, sec^{-1}$$

Thus at high pH, superoxide predominates over hydroperoxyl acid and is relatively long-lived in the absence of SOD. Half-lives as long as 70 sec have been observed under such conditions (59). The SOD-catalyzed dismutation is much faster, with a rate constant of $2 \times 10^9 \, M^{-1} \, sec^{-1}$, and it is pH insensitive (7–9). The SOD-catalyzed dismutation is favored when the concentration of superoxide is low and when the concentration of SOD is high. These conditions prevail in cells under normal conditions.

Hydrogen peroxide is also produced by divalent reduction of oxygen by a variety of oxidative enzymes such as xanthine oxidase (20).

Hydroxyl Radical

Hydroxyl radical can be produced directly from water via the action of ionizing radiation. Of greater importance is the production of hydroxyl radical in tissues from superoxide and hydrogen peroxide via the iron-catalyzed Haber-Weiss reaction (60). The uncatalyzed Haber-Weiss reaction does not proceed with sufficient speed to produce hydroxyl radicals at significant rates. However, in the presence of catalytic transition metal, usually iron or copper, this reaction can produce hydroxyl radical at significant rates (61). Hydroxyl radical is produced in this sequence via decomposition of hydrogen peroxide through the action of ferrous iron:

$$H_2O_2 + Fe^{2+} \rightarrow \cdot OH + OH^- + Fe^{3+}$$

Superoxide reduces the ferric iron produced by this reaction and makes the repetition of the cycle possible:

$$Fe^{3+} + \cdot O_2^- \rightarrow Fe^{2+} + O_2$$

The toxicity of superoxide is frequently ascribed to the formation of hydroxyl radical. Because of this radical's high reactivity, along with its correspondingly very short range, both of which make effects at large distances unlikely, controversy has arisen as to whether this radical is truly the mediator of superoxide toxicity. Several hypotheses have been proposed to answer criticisms concerning this issue. The first involves site specificity (62). According to this hypothesis, the damage occurs at sites where the catalytic iron for the catalyzed Haber-Weiss

reaction resides (62). The second hypothesis is that the responses ascribed to the hydroxyl radical are not the result of generation of this radical but are, instead, due to the formation of an unidentified ferryl radical whose rate of generation depends on the state of oxidation of the iron (63). Since superoxide reduces iron and hydrogen peroxide oxidizes it, the concentration of these two agents determines the formation of the injurious ferryl radical. Finally, the formation of peroxynitrite from superoxide and nitric oxide may be another explanation (19). It should be noted that peroxynitrite reacts very rapidly with iron chelators, such as deferoxamine (19). Therefore, the inhibition of responses ascribed to hydroxyl radical generation via the Haber-Weiss reaction by deferoxamine, need not be definitive evidence that hydroxyl radical from the Haber-Weiss reaction is involved.

The concentration of iron is limiting in the Haber-Weiss reaction. Iron is stored in cells in the ferric form in combination with ferritin (64). Little is known about the mechanisms of its mobilization or its exact state in the catalysis of the Haber-Weiss reaction. Reduction seems essential for its mobilization (65). Superoxide can release iron from ferritin *in vitro* (60). Also, flavins can achieve the same result very effectively (66). Chelation of iron can render it more effective in the catalysis of the Haber-Weiss reaction. For example, iron chelates with ethylenediaminetetraacetic acid (EDTA) are very efficient catalysts of the Haber-Weiss reaction (61).

It is important to recognize the significance of the formation of the highly destructive hydroxyl radical from its two less-reactive precursors, superoxide and hydrogen peroxide. The latter two, if they escape and enter the extracellular fluid, are more likely to travel some distance from their site of formation and form hydroxyl radical at the site of the catalytic iron, thereby inducing local damage. This mechanism makes remote effects possible.

Peroxynitrite

Peroxynitrite is formed by a diffusion-limited, high-yield reaction between superoxide and nitric oxide as follows:

$$\cdot O_2^- + NO \cdot \rightarrow ONOO^-$$

Peroxynitrite is stable at high pH. However, at lower pH it becomes protonated to peroxynitrous acid, which decomposes spontaneously to yield hydroxyl radical as follows:

$$ONOO^- + H^+ \rightarrow ONOOH \rightarrow HO \cdot + NO_2 \cdot$$

At pH 7.4 the half-life of the decomposition of peroxynitrous acid is 1.9 sec (19). The decomposition is even faster in bicarbonate containing physiological fluids. More recent evidence suggests that the decomposition of peroxynitrite does not yield free hydroxyl radical but rather leads to a vibrationally excited state that has reactivity equivalent to that of hydroxyl radicals (67).

Irrespective of the nature of the oxidant produced by decomposition of peroxynitrite, it is clear that a wide variety of chemicals can be oxidized. These include deoxyribose, dimethyl sulfoxide (DMSO) (19), lipids (68), and sulfhydryl-containing compounds such as cysteine or proteins (69). The oxidation of sulfhydryl compounds can also be accomplished by direct interaction with peroxynitrite (69). This latter direct oxidation of sulfhydryl compounds by peroxynitrite is likely to be more selective than the indiscriminate oxidation due to the powerful oxidant generated by its decomposition and may, therefore, be more important in explaining the toxicity of peroxynitrite.

Singlet Oxygen

Singlet oxygen can be generated in tissues by photochemical reactions (17,18). Singlet oxygen can also be produced by myeloperoxidase in activated leukocytes as follows:

$$H_2O_2 + H^+ + Cl^- \rightarrow H_2O + HOCl$$

$$H_2O_2 + HOCl \rightarrow H_2O + H^+ + Cl^- + {}^1O_2$$

Singlet oxygen has been indirectly shown to be produced by phagocytosing neutrophils (70).

CELLULAR DEFENSES AGAINST RADICALS

Mammalian cells possess enzymatic and nonenzymatic defenses against radicals. Superoxide is eliminated by superoxide dismutases, which greatly accelerate the dismutation of this radical (71). A manganese-containing superoxide dismutase is present in mitochondria. A cytosolic enzyme containing copper and zinc is also present in all mammalian cells. The extracellular fluid contains a high molecular-weight superoxide dismutase, which is a glycoprotein and contains copper and zinc. This is referred to as EC-SOD (72). This enzyme is bound to endothelial cells, from which it can be released by heparin (73). The concentration of superoxide dismutase in the extracellular fluid is much less than in intracellular fluid. For this reason, superoxide can survive longer and travel further once it gains access to extracellular fluid.

Hydrogen peroxide is destroyed by glutathione peroxidase and by catalase (20). The former enzyme utilizes reduced glutathione to convert hydrogen peroxide to water; in the process, glutathione is oxidized. This enzyme is more important in eliminating hydrogen peroxide when the concentration of hydrogen peroxide is low (20). Catalase converts hydrogen peroxide to water without requiring any cofactors (20). It is more important when hydrogen peroxide concentration is higher.

Because of its extremely high reactivity, there are no specific scavengers of hydroxyl radical. A large number of cellular constituents, however, scavenge not only hydroxyl radical but also other radicals, and these constituents act as nonspecific antioxidants. Through this action, they protect more essential cellular components from oxidant attack. Such compounds include vitamin E and ascorbic acid.

CELLULAR EFFECTS OF OXYGEN RADICALS

Oxygen radicals can damage a variety of essential cellular components (Table 2). One or more of these effects can kill the cell.

Oxygen radicals attack the double bonds of unsaturated fatty acids in membrane phospholipids and cause lipid peroxidation. This process is complex (74,75). The radicals can extract hydrogen from the lipid and form a lipid radical. The latter can undergo oxidation in the presence of transition metals to produce a hydroperoxyl radical that then propagates the process by attacking new lipid through a chain reaction. The resultant altered membrane structure is associated with abnormal permeability and consequent effects on function. Thus, ionic permeability of the cell membrane may be affected. The function of cellular organelles whose membranes are altered by oxidant attack cannot proceed normally. Mitochondrial function, for example, may be altered, along with loss of oxidative metabolic capability and reduced energy availability (76).

Oxygen radicals can damage proteins in a variety of ways. Amino acids that contain sulfhydryl groups are vulnerable to oxidation (69,77). Similarly, hydroxyl radical can cause hydroxylation of certain amino acids (78–81). The damaged proteins may undergo cross-linking, with resultant alteration in their physicochemical properties (82).

The alteration in protein structure caused by oxygen radicals inactivates many enzymes. For example, glyceraldehyde-3-phosphate dehydrogenase is inactivated by oxygen radicals, thereby interfering with glycolysis (83). Creatine phosphokinase is inactivated by su-

TABLE 2. *Cellular effects of products of univalent reduction of oxygen*

Lipid peroxidation
Protein denaturation
Inactivation of enzymes
Nucleic acid and DNA damage
Release of calcium ions from intracellular stores
Damage to cytoskeleton
Damage to tissue structural components
Chemotaxis

peroxide and its derivatives (84). Superoxide inactivates catalase (85) and glutathione peroxidase (86), while hydrogen peroxide inactivates superoxide dismutase (87). Na^+,K^+-ATPase is inactivated by oxygen radicals, with resultant alterations in active membrane ionic transport (88). Singlet oxygen generated from photoactivation of rose bengal inhibits Ca^{2+}-ATPase in cardiac sarcoplasmic reticulum (89).

Hydroxyl radical can damage DNA by altering its component bases or by causing strand breaks (90).

Oxygen radicals are capable of releasing Ca^{2+} from intracellular stores, such as the endoplasmic reticulum and the mitochondria (91). The resultant high concentration of intracellular Ca^{2+} causes activation of enzymes, such as phospholipases.

The integrity of the morphology of cells depends on the organization of membrane myofilaments. Oxygen radicals are capable of damaging the cellular cytoskeleton and causing severe alterations in morphology manifested by bleb formation on the cell surface (91). This can occur as a result of either oxidation of thiols in actin, resulting in aggregation of actin molecules, or enzymatic attack activated by release of Ca^{2+} (91). If the oxidant attack ceases, the damage is reparable and the blebs disappear.

Oxygen radicals can alter collagen (92) and can polymerize hyaluronic acid (93), with consequent alterations in the structure of connective tissue.

Oxygen radicals are chemotactic and promote accumulation of leukocytes (94). It appears that an intermediate chemoattractant may be involved, which is generated by the interaction between superoxide and a tissue component (95). The speed of accumulation of leukocytes attracted by oxidant injury to tissues varies from tissue to tissue. In the cheek pouch of the hamster, it occurs almost immediately (94); in the brain, it is much slower, beginning 4 to 6 h later (14,96) and reaching a peak at about 24 h (14).

VASCULAR EFFECTS OF PRODUCTS OF UNIVALENT REDUCTION OF OXYGEN

Products of univalent reduction of oxygen have pronounced vascular effects (Table 3). These have been most completely studied in the cerebral microcirculation of the cat.

Superoxide, hydrogen peroxide, and hydroxyl radical dilate cerebral arterioles of the cat (40,97). Vasodilation from oxygen radicals has also been reported in the cerebral arterioles of the mouse (98), where the effect seems to depend primarily on hydroxyl radical, in the microcirculation of skeletal muscle of the rat (99), where hydrogen peroxide seems to be the most important mediator, and in the isolated tail artery of the rat or the coronary artery of the dog *in vitro* (100,101). In these

TABLE 3. *Vascular effects of products of univalent reduction of oxygen*

Altered vessel tone
Altered vessel reactivity
Altered endothelium dependent responses
Increased platelet aggregability
Altered endothelial permeability
Destructive lesions of the vessel wall
Reduced oxygen consumption of the vessel wall

tissues, the response has been variably reported to depend on hydroxyl radical or on hydrogen peroxide.

Exogenous hydrogen peroxide dilates cerebral arterioles (97,102), arterioles of skeletal muscle in the rat (99), and isolated thoracic aorta (103), coronary arteries (101), or pulmonary arteries (104). In the cerebral arterioles, the dilation in response to low concentrations of hydrogen peroxide is probably due to generation of hydroxyl radical, since it is inhibited by scavenging the catalytic iron of the Haber-Weiss reaction with deferoxamine (102). Higher concentrations, however, have an additional effect, independent of hydroxyl radical generation (82).

The effect of hydrogen peroxide is mostly due to a direct action on vascular smooth muscle (101), although there may be a contribution from enhanced release of endothelium-derived relaxing factor (EDRF). In pulmonary arteries, hydrogen peroxide activates soluble guanylate cyclase (104); compound I of catalase, a radical intermediate form of the enzyme generated during the peroxidation of hydrogen peroxide, may be a mediator of guanylate cyclase activation (104). In contrast to these findings, hydrogen peroxide inactivates guanylate cyclase in cerebral arterioles, probably by generating a powerful oxidant similar to hydroxyl radical (102). These differences in findings may reflect differences between vascular beds or differences between large vessels and the microcirculation. In some vessels, hydrogen peroxide causes hyperpolarization of vascular smooth muscle, which presumably accounts for the resultant relaxation (105). In cerebral arterioles this effect is probably mediated via opening of an adenosine triphosphate (ATP)-sensitive potassium channel since it is inhibited strongly by pretreatment with inactivators of this channel (unpublished observations).

Some vessels, such as the isolated basilar artery of the dog (106) or the isolated rabbit aorta (107), contract in response to oxygen radicals. In the basilar artery of the dog it was suggested that the secretion of superoxide by the endothelium accounts for the endothelium-dependent vasoconstrictor effects of the calcium ionophore A23187 (106). According to this view, superoxide generated via cyclooxygenase is the endothelium-derived contracting factor generated by the ionophore. The large isolated vessel preparations typically secrete high concentrations of EDRF. Superoxide and other oxygen radicals interact strongly with EDRF with mutual inactivation. Therefore, under these conditions a contracting or vasoconstrictor effect of oxygen radicals may be due to inactivation of a vasodilator rather than due to a direct contracting effect on vascular smooth muscle. In both the basilar artery of the dog and in the rabbit aorta, oxygen radicals cause a large increase in the production of vasoconstrictor prostanoids (106,107). These products of cyclooxygenase are responsible for the observed vasoconstriction in the rabbit aorta (107) but not in the basilar artery (106). Oxygen radicals cause vasoconstriction in isolated perfused lungs, probably because of release of thromboxane A_2 (108).

Oxygen radicals induce severe alterations in the responses of blood vessels to vasoconstrictor and vasodilator agents. In cerebral arterioles, exposure to oxygen radicals diminishes the responsiveness of vascular smooth muscle to the vasoconstrictor effects of hypocapnia (40,97,109) or to the vasodilator effects of hypercapnia and arterial hypotension (110). In isolated rabbit thoracic aorta, the vasoconstrictor effects of catecholamines are diminished because of oxidation of norepinephrine by hydroxyl radical (111). In isolated pulmonary arteries superoxide inactivates guanylate cyclase (55). In cerebral arterioles inactivation of guanylate cyclase by oxygen radicals was mediated by hydroxyl radical or another powerful radical with similar reactivity (56,102).

Of great interest is the effect of oxygen radicals on endothelium-dependent responses (112). These responses are caused by the release of EDRFs, which are short-lived, unstable agents that diffuse to the vascular smooth muscle and cause relaxation. Oxygen radicals eliminate the vasodilation from acetylcholine in cerebral arterioles (54,113,114) and in isolated coronary arteries (101). The mechanism of this effect seems to be multiple. In the cerebral vessels, where oxygen radicals are strongly relaxant, the effect is, in part, due to nonspecific diminished capacity to dilate (113). The major effect, however, is due to either damage to the endothelium, with inability to produce EDRF (114), or destruction of EDRF by direct oxidant attack by the radicals (54,101,115). In the cerebral vessels, this effect seems to be mediated by hydroxyl radical (54). In isolated coronary vessels (101) or in cultured endothelial cells (115), it appears to be more dependent on superoxide. This difference may reflect differences in the EDRF generated by acetylcholine. In cerebral arterioles the EDRF is likely a nitrosothiol (102), while in the coronary arteries and cultured endothelial cells it is free nitric oxide. As noted above, depending on the concentration of EDRF, the effect of oxygen radicals on blood vessels may be modified because of the interaction with EDRF, with resultant mutual inactivation.

Human endothelial cells in culture are injured by exposure to extracellularly generated oxygen radicals and exhibit enhanced platelet adherence (116). Exposure of cerebral vessels to oxygen radicals increases the tendency toward platelet aggregation, although the radicals by themselves may not induce aggregation (117). The enhanced aggregability of platelets under these conditions is demonstrable if one uses a second proaggregatory stimulus, which then induces aggregation more easily. This tendency toward platelet aggregation may be in part the result of elimination of EDRF, which is a strong inhibitor of platelet aggregation (118). It is not known whether prostacyclin, another endothelium-derived powerful inhibitor of platelet aggregation, is also involved. Increased generation of superoxide intracellularly by the administration of menadione inhibited the conversion of PGH_2 to prostacyclin (119). On the other hand, extracellular generation of superoxide and hydrogen peroxide caused a marked increase in prostacyclin secretion by human cultured endothelial cells (116). It is not known whether the location of the increased production of radicals accounts for the difference in results.

Oxygen radicals induce increased endothelial permeability, along with extravasation of plasma proteins and other macromolecules (94,120). In the brain, where the blood-brain barrier normally prevents the leakage of protein from the intravascular compartment, the blood-brain barrier breaks down and protein leaks into the vessel wall as well as into the surrounding brain (120). This, undoubtedly, contributes to edema formation and to increased intracranial pressure.

Exposure of cerebral vessels to oxygen radicals causes discrete destructive lesions of the endothelium and vascular smooth muscle (1,96,97,109,110). The lesions in the endothelium consist of blebs. When the blebs burst into the lumen of the vessel, either spontaneously or in the process of fixation, the lesions are converted to craters. The density of these lesions is about 0.5 to 1/100 μm^2. Their mechanism is not known with confidence; however, they seem very similar to the lesions seen in hepatocytes or white cells in culture, which have been ascribed to destruction of the cytoskeleton of the cell (91). Lesions of the vascular smooth muscle were infrequent and consisted mostly of vacuolization or inclusion bodies.

Following exposure to oxygen radicals *in vivo,* or following incubation with an oxygen radical generating system *in vitro,* cerebral arterioles display reductions in oxygen consumption (110,121), very likely due to the destruction of the mitochondria caused by the radicals.

CEREBRAL VASCULAR EFFECTS OF ACUTE HYPERTENSION

Acute, severe hypertension in cats induces cerebral vascular changes very similar to those caused by oxygen radicals (110). The cerebral arterioles dilate to a very pronounced degree and remain dilated even after the blood pressure returns to the baseline. This sustained dilation clearly indicates that an active mechanism causing relaxation of vascular smooth muscle was initiated. The dilated arterioles have abnormal reactivity. Their vasoconstrictor response to arterial hypocapnia is severely compromised, and the vasodilator response to arterial hypercapnia or arterial hypotension is reduced. They respond with reduced vasodilation to topical nitroprusside, an agent that causes relaxation by directly activating guanylate cyclase in vascular smooth muscle (unpublished observation). Responses to endothelium-dependent vasodilators, such as acetylcholine, bradykinin, and arachidonate, are either severely depressed or, in the case of acetylcholine, converted to a small vasoconstriction (120 and unpublished observations). The depression of the vasodilator responses to endothelium-dependent vasodilators is more pronounced than that due to agents that act directly on the vascular smooth muscle. Using an *in vivo* bioassay technique (122), in which acetylcholine induces the production of EDRF in a cat with a cranial window and in which the effluent is transferred within a few seconds to the brain of a rat subjected to cholinergic blockade, it was shown that EDRF production is eliminated following acute hypertension (unpublished observations). Endothelium-dependent relaxations are also depressed in cerebral and other arteries in animals with chronic hypertension (123,124). This effect is evidently due to the release of an endothelium-derived contracting factor derived from the metabolism of arachidonate via cyclooxygenase (124).

The blood-brain barrier following acute hypertension is compromised, and plasma proteins and other macromolecules leak into the vessel wall and into the extracellular space (125). It has been suggested that the primary site of leakage is small veins (126). However, other experiments using horseradish peroxidase, which is identified by electron microscopy, show extensive leakage into the wall of intracerebral arterioles (125). Leakage of proteins and other macromolecules into the vessel wall has been found in mesenteric vessels of animals subjected to prolonged severe hypertension (127). The administration of SOD, catalase, or their combination or the administration of DMSO inhibited these vascular abnormalities (128), suggesting that oxygen radicals are involved in their mediation.

Following acute hypertension, cerebral and mesenteric arterioles display discrete destructive lesions of the endothelium (110,128). In cerebral vessels lesions of the vascular smooth muscle are much rarer and affect only a small portion of the smooth muscle cells in the vessel wall (110). Endothelial lesions similar to those found in cerebral arterioles in acute hypertension have been described in arteries of rats with chronic genetic hypertension (129). Cerebral arterioles subjected to acute hypertension display a reduction in their oxygen consumption, probably due to damage to mitochondria (110).

SUPEROXIDE GENERATION IN ACUTE HYPERTENSION

Acute severe hypertension induced by intravenous infusion of vasoconstrictor agents in cats induces generation of superoxide in the brain (113). This was demonstrated by the SOD-inhibitable portion of nitroblue tetrazolium, a dye that is reduced by superoxide. Superoxide generation was not the result of the direct effect of the vasoconstrictor agent used to raise blood pressure, because no radical generation was detected if the increase in blood pressure was prevented by controlled bleeding (113). No superoxide generation was seen in the brain under resting conditions (14,113). Interestingly, superoxide generation following acute hypertension continued for at least an hour after the blood pressure had returned to the baseline (113). Superoxide was evidently generated in cells and subsequently escaped into the extracellular space, as shown by the fact that its appearance in the extracellular space was inhibited by irreversible inhibition of the anion channel with phenylglyoxal (113).

One of the sites of generation of superoxide is the vessel wall itself (130). This was shown by a histochemical technique dependent on the oxidation of manganese by superoxide from the divalent to the trivalent state (131). Trivalent manganese then oxidized diaminobenzidine, which precipitated and could be demonstrated by electron microscopy following fixation with osmic acid. Superoxide was shown by this technique in the mitochondria of vascular smooth muscle, in surface lesions of vascular smooth muscle, and in endothelial lesions, as well as extracellularly (130,131). No superoxide could be demonstrated in the brain parenchyma, but this may be due to incomplete penetration of the reagents.

ROLE OF PHAGOCYTIC CELLS IN HYPERTENSION

It has recently been suggested that activated phagocytic cells, particularly monocytes and neutrophils, may contribute to the increase in vascular resistance observed in hypertension and to the organ and tissue injury associated with hypertension (132). So far most of the evidence was obtained in spontaneously hypertensive rats. In this strain, leukocyte counts are elevated and a higher proportion of circulating leukocytes are activated as indicated by secretion of superoxide (132). Activation of leukocytes may be the result of endothelial injury induced by hypertension.

A variety of mechanisms may be involved. Activated

leukocytes have altered rheological properties that may result in increased vascular resistance by mechanical means (133,134). Also, they secrete a variety of products including oxygen radicals, which may have significant vasoactive effects or may inactivate other vasoactive agents and interfere with proper vascular control (135). Also, leukocytes following adhesion to the endothelium may migrate into the tissue and induce tissue injury, in part, by secretion of oxygen radicals.

Relevance to human hypertension is suggested by similar findings by Russian investigators of the increased proportion of activated leukocytes in human hypertensives (136,137) and by the fact that a variety of abnormalities, including reduced concentrations of superoxide dismutase (138), increased sodium cytoplasmic content, perhaps due to inhibition of Na^+,K^+-ATPase (139), and defective Na^+-H^+ antiporter activity resulting in elevated pH (140), have been observed in the leukocytes of hypertensive patients.

ROLE OF OXYGEN RADICALS IN CEREBRAL VASCULAR EFFECTS OF ACUTE HYPERTENSION

There is strong evidence that oxygen radicals are mediators of the cerebral vascular abnormalities resulting from acute hypertension. Pretreatment with topical superoxide dismutase or nitroblue tetrazolium, both of which scavenge superoxide, or with mannitol, a scavenger of hydroxyl radical, inhibits the sustained vasodilation seen after acute hypertension, preserves normal reactivity of cerebral arterioles toward the vasoconstrictor effects of hypocapnia, and reduces the density of the focal endothelial lesions (110). The sustained dilation following acute hypertension is reversed by aftertreatment with topical superoxide dismutase and catalase applied several minutes after termination of the hypertensive episode (113). Similarly, EDRF production is preserved by pretreatment with superoxide dismutase and catalase. Topical application of these enzymes several minutes after the termination of hypertension restores endothelium-dependent relaxation in response to acetylcholine (113).

Pharmacological evidence suggests strongly that oxygen radicals generated by acute hypertension originate from accelerated arachidonate metabolism via PGH synthase. This view is supported by several lines of evidence. First, pretreatment with the cyclooxygenase inhibitors indomethacin or AHR-5850, both of which inhibit superoxide production by PGH synthase in vitro (39), inhibited the sustained vasodilation, abnormal reactivity, and vessel-wall injury secondary to acute hypertension (110). Second, accelerated metabolism of arachidonate induced by topical application of high concentrations of exogenous arachidonate or by topical application of bra-

dykinin reproduced the cerebral vascular abnormalities of acute hypertension (1,40). Both topical arachidonate and bradykinin generate superoxide (14). Superoxide production induced by these agents in the brain is inhibited by indomethacin (14). It appears likely, therefore, that acute hypertension leads to activation of phospholipases, which release arachidonate from endogenous sources, followed by accelerated metabolism of arachidonate, and by generation of superoxide. There is no direct confirmation of this hypothesis.

Polypeptides such as bradykinin are potential candidates as mediators of the activation of phospholipase following acute hypertension. These polypeptides are known to activate phospholipase and to release arachidonate. As noted above, they also generate superoxide (14,41,141).

The possibility that bradykinin itself may be involved in the mediation of the cerebrovascular effects of acute hypertension has not been evaluated. However, its possible participation in the cerebrovascular effects of fluid-percussion brain injury (4), which is also associated with acute hypertension and leads to similar vascular lesions, has been tested. The topical application of a specific antagonist of bradykinin in this condition led to diminished vasodilation and to preservation of the vascular responsiveness of vessels to arterial hypocapnia (142).

The sensory fibers of the trigeminal nerve contain polypeptides that may have effects similar to those of bradykinin (143–146). These nerve fibers are in close proximity to surface vessels of the hemispheres. They contain a variety of polypeptides, including substance P, neurokinin A, calcitonin-gene-related peptide (CGRP), and cholecystokinin-8. There is strong evidence supporting the participation of polypeptides from this source in the vasodilation and increased vascular permeability to proteins in acute hypertension. In cats subjected previously to unilateral trigeminal ganglionectomy, which led to degeneration of the sensory fibers unilaterally, the responses of blood vessels to arterial hypocapnia, arterial hypoxia, and arterial hypercapnia were symmetrical (147). However, the vasodilation in response to severe arterial hypertension was significantly reduced on the denervated side, suggesting that a vasodilator agent present in nerve fibers contributes to this vasodilation (147). Similarly, the extravasation of labeled plasma albumin was less pronounced on the denervated side than on the intact side (147). The hyperemia seen during acute hypertension was also diminished significantly on the denervated side in the hemispheres but not in the brainstem, whose vessels are not innervated by the trigeminal nerve (148).

This effect of trigeminal ganglionectomy could be explained by the interruption of a reflex that involves transmission of sensory input to the brain, with the initiation of efferent impulses through another pathway to the blood vessels. An alternative explanation is that we are dealing with an axon reflex that does not require the participation of the central nervous system. The distinction between these two possibilities was made by testing the response to acute hypertension in animals subjected to trigeminal rhizotomy. In such animals, the response to acute hypertension was symmetrical, indicating that the vasodilation is mediated by an axon reflex (148).

OTHER HYPEREMIC SYNDROMES CAUSED BY OXYGEN RADICALS

There is evidence for the participation of oxygen radicals in abnormal vasodilation associated with other experimental hyperemic syndromes. Fluid-percussion brain injury (4) and prolonged seizures (148) are associated with sustained vasodilation, hyperemia, and vascular changes similar to those seen in acute hypertension. In both of these conditions, it has been shown that oxygen radicals are generated (4,130,149,150) and that they contribute significantly to the abnormal vascular responses. In both conditions, acute hypertension is an important feature. In the case of brain injury, it is known that acute hypertension is essential for the initiation of the cerebrovascular changes (151). A recent preliminary trial of antioxidant therapy with polyethylene glycol conjugated SOD (PEG-SOD) in patients with severe brain injury yielded encouraging results. In these patients the administration of PEG-SOD was associated with a considerably reduced rate of mortality and severe neurological disability (152). In experimental seizures inhibition of the associated hypertension did not affect superoxide production, suggesting that radical production in this condition is independent of the changes in blood pressure (150).

Brain ischemia followed by perfusion is associated with vasodilation, abnormal vascular responses, and breakdown of the blood-brain barrier, all features very similar to those seen in acute hypertension. In this condition there is also evidence for the generation of oxygen radicals (131,153).

It therefore appears that the mechanisms that account for the cerebrovascular abnormalities seen in acute hypertension may be common to a variety of other pathophysiological responses.

IMPLICATIONS FOR HUMAN HYPERTENSION

Considerable interest has been generated recently in the use of antioxidant therapy to inhibit the consequences of cardiovascular disease. Interest has centered mainly on the use of vitamin E, because of its powerful antioxidant activity, its ease of administration, relatively low price, and the apparent absence of side effects.

Two recent prospective epidemiological studies have shown that the ingestion of high doses of vitamin E in men and women was associated with a markedly reduced risk of major coronary artery disease (154,155). The evidence was sufficiently suggestive to initiate a randomized clinical trial to test the effectiveness of vitamin E (156). It should be noted that earlier small clinical trials using vitamin E as an antioxidant yielded negative results.

In view of the evidence of participation of oxidant-mediated vascular injury in hypertension and the fact that hypertension is a major risk factor for coronary disease, and the fact that many hypertension patients die of the consequences of atherosclerotic vascular disease, it is appropriate to consider whether antioxidant therapy has a place in the treatment of hypertensive patients. The epidemiological evidence cited above does not constitute proof of cause and effect association. Also, it is sound therapeutic principle to wait for the results of controlled clinical trials before any form of therapy, even a relatively safe one, can be recommended for general use. Such evidence does not exist at the present time for vitamin E or other antioxidant therapy. It is, therefore, appropriate to wait for the results of controlled trials before such therapy can be recommended.

ACKNOWLEDGMENT

This work was supported by grants HL 21851 and NS 19316 from the National Institutes of Health.

REFERENCES

1. Kontos HA. *Circ Res* 1985;57:508–516.
2. McCord JM, Roy RS. *Can J Physiol* 1982;60:1346–1352.
3. Bulkley GB. *Br J Cancer* 1987;55:66–73.
4. Kontos HA. *CNS Trauma* 1986;3:257–263.
5. Slater TF. *Biochem J* 1984;222:1–15.
6. Taube H. *J Gen Physiol* 1965;49:29–50.
7. Fridovich I. *Science* 1978;201:875–880.
8. Halliwell B, Gutteridge JMC. *Biochem J* 1984;219:1–14.
9. Fridovich I. *Annu Rev Pharmacol Toxicol* 1983;23:239–257.
10. Gebicki JM, Bielski BH. *J Am Chem Soc* 1981;103:7020–7023.
11. Bielski BHJ, Arudi RL, Sutherland MW. *J Biol Chem* 1983;258:4759–4761.
12. Fukuzawa K, Gebicki JM. *Arch Biochem Biophys* 1983;226:242–251.
13. Lynch RE, Fridovich I. *J Biol Chem* 1978;253:4697–4699.
14. Kontos HA, Wei EP, Ellis EF, Jenkins LW, Povlishock JT, Rowe GT, Hess ML. *Circ Res* 1985;57:142–151.
15. Jones DP, Eklow L, Thor H, et al. *Arch Biochem Biophys* 1981;210:505–516.
16. Dorfman LM, Adams GE. *Reactivity of the hydroxyl radical in aqueous solutions.* Washington, DC: US Department of Commerce, National Bureau of Standards, June 1973.
17. Khan AU. *J Phys Chem* 1976;80:2219–2225.
18. Kasha M, Khan AU, Phil D. *Ann NY Acad Sci* 1970;171:5–22.
19. Beckman JS, Beckman TW, Chen J, Marshall PA, Freeman BA. *Proc Natl Acad Sci USA* 1990;87:1620–1624.
20. Chance B, Sies H, Boveris A. *Physiol Rev* 1979;59:527–605.
21. Turrens JF, Boveris A. *Biochem J* 1980;191:421–427.
22. Turrens JF, Freeman BA, Crapo JD. *Arch Biochem Biophys* 1982;217:411–421.

23. Turrens JF, Freeman BA, Levitt JG, et al. *Arch Biochem Biophys* 1982;217:401–410.
24. Forman JJ, Kennedy J. *Arch Biochem Biophys* 1976;173:219–224.
25. Fridovich I. *Adv Neurol* 1979;26:255–259.
26. Massey V, Palmer G, Ballou D. In: Kamin H, ed. *Flavins and flavoproteins*. Baltimore: University Park Press, 1971;349–361.
27. Hamed MY, Silver J, Wilson MT. *Inorg Chim Acta* 1983;80:237–244.
28. Misra H. *J Biol Chem* 1974;249:2151–2155.
29. Cohen G, Heikkila R. *J Biol Chem* 1974;249:2447–2452.
30. Misra HP, Fridovich I. *J Biol Chem* 1972;247:6960–6962.
31. Fridovich I. *J Biol Chem* 1970;245:4053–4057.
32. Betz AL. *J Neurochem* 1985;44:574–579.
33. Batelli MG, Corte ED, Stirpe F. *Biochem J* 1972;126:747–749.
34. Engerson TD, McKelvey TG, Rhyne DB, et al. *J Clin Invest* 1987;79:1564–1570.
35. Yamamoto S. In: Pace-Ascieak C, Granstrom E, eds. *Prostaglandins and related substances*. Amsterdam: Elsevier, 1983;171–202.
36. Lambeir A-M, Markey CM, Dunford HB, et al. *J Biol Chem* 1985;260:14894–14896.
37. Dunford HB. In: Caughy WS, ed. *Biochemical and clinical aspects of oxygen*. New York: Academic Press, 1979;167–176.
38. Land EJ, Swallow AJ. *Biochim Biophys Acta* 1971;234:34–42.
39. Kukreja RC, Kontos HA, Hess ML, Ellis EF. *Circ Res* 1986;59:612–619.
40. Kontos HA, Wei EP, Povlishock JT, Christman CW. *Circ Res* 1984;55:295–303.
41. Holland JA, Pappolla, Wolin MS, Pritchard KA, Rogers NJ, Stemerman MB. *J Cell Physiol* 1990;143:21–25.
42. Kameda K, Ono T, Imai T. *Biochem Biophys Acta* 1979;572:77–82.
43. Kuthan H, Ullrich V. *Eur J Biochem* 1982;126:583–588.
44. Pou S, Pou WS, Bredt DS, Snyder SH, Rosen GM. *J Biol Chem* 1992;267:24173–24176.
45. Heinzel B, John M, Klatt P, Bohme E, Mayer B. *Biochem J* 1992;281:627–630.
46. Rosenblum WI, Nishimura H, Nelson GH. *Am J Physiol* 1992;262:H1343–H1349.
47. Omar HA, Kamal M, Mohazzab H, Mortelliti MP, Wolin MS. *Am J Physiol* 1993;264:L141–L145.
48. Powis G, Svingen BA, Appel P. *Mol Pharmacol* 1981;20:387–394.
49. Bus JS, Aust SD, Gibson JE. *Environ Health Perspect* 1976;16:139–146.
50. Goodman J, Hochstein P. *Biochem Biophys Res Commun* 1977;77:797–803.
51. Thayer WS. *Chem Biol Interact* 1977;19:265–278.
52. Rosen GM, Freeman BA. *Proc Natl Acad Sci USA* 1984;81:7269–7273.
53. Beauchamp C, Fridovich I. *Anal Biochem* 1971;44:276–287.
54. Marshall JJ, Wei EP, Kontos HA. *Am J Physiol* 1988;255:H847–H854.
55. Cherry PD, Omar HA, Farrell KA, Stuart JS, Wolin MS. *Am J Physiol* 1990;259:H1056–H1062.
56. Kontos HA, Wei EP. *Stroke* 1993;24:427–434.
57. Badwey JA, Karnovsky ML. *Annu Rev Biochem* 1980;49:695–726.
58. Bielski BHJ, Chan PC. In: Michelson AM, McCord JM, Fridovich I, eds. *Superoxide and superoxide dismutases*. New York: Academic Press, 1977;409–416.
59. Bielski BHJ, Richter HW. *J Am Chem Soc* 1977;99:3019–3023.
60. Aust SD, Morehouse LA, Thomas CE. *J Free Radicals Biol Med* 1985;1:3–25.
61. McCord JM, Day ED, Jr. *FEBS Lett* 1978;86:139–142.
62. Halliwell B, Gutteridge JMC. *Arch Biochem Biophys* 1986;246:501–514.
63. Minotti G, Aust SD. *J Biol Chem* 1987;262:1098–1104.
64. Harrison PM. *Semin Hematol* 1977;14:55–70.
65. Mazur A, Baez S, Shorr E. *J Biol Chem* 1955;213:147–160.
66. Sirivech S, Frieden E, Osaki S. *Biochem J* 1974;143:311–315.
67. Koppenol WH, Moreno JJ, Pryor WA, Ischiropoulos H, Beckman JS. *Chem Res Toxicol* 1992;5:834–842.
68. Radi R, Beckman JS, Bush KM, Freeman BA. *Arch Biochem Biophys* 1991;288:481–487.
69. Radi R, Beckman JS, Bush KM, Freeman BA. *J Biol Chem* 1991;266:4244–4250.
70. Rosen H, Klebanoff SJ. *J Biol Chem* 1977;252:4803–4810.
71. Fridovich I. *Annu Rev Biochem* 1975;44:147–159.
72. Marklund S. *Proc Natl Acad Sci USA* 1982;79:7634–7638.
73. Karlsson K, Marklund SL. *FEBS Lett* 1985;184:237–239.
74. Frankel EN. *Prog Lipid Res* 1980;19:1–22.
75. Vladimirov YA, Olenev VI, Suslova TB, et al. *Lipid Res* 1980;17:173–249.
76. Hillered L, Ernster L. *J Cereb Blood Flow Metab* 1983;3:207–214.
77. Pryor WA. In: Pryor WA, ed. *Free radicals in biology*, vol 1. New York: Academic Press, 1976;1–49.
78. Trelstad RL, Lawley KR, Holmes LB. *Nature* 1981;289:310–312.
79. Floyd RA, Watson JJ, Wong PK. *J Biochem Biophys Meth* 1984;10:221–225.
80. Grootveld M, Halliwell B. *Biochem J* 1986;237:499–504.
81. Halliwell B, Grootveld M. *FEBS Lett* 1987;213:9–14.
82. Rivett AJ. *Curr Top Cell Regul* 1986;28:291–337.
83. Buchanan JD, Armstrong DA. *Int Rev Radiat Biol* 1978;33:409–414.
84. McCord JM, Russell WJ. In: Cerutti PA, Fridovich I, McCord JM, eds. *Oxy-radicals in molecular biology and pathology*. New York: Alan R. Liss, 1988;27–35.
85. Kono Y, Fridovich I. *J Biol Chem* 1982;257:5751–5754.
86. Blum J, Fridovich I. *Arch Biochem Biophys* 1985;240:500–508.
87. Hodgson EK, Fridovich I. *Biochemistry* 1975;14:5294–5299.
88. Maridonneau I, Braquet P, Garay RP. *J Biol Chem* 1983;258:3107–3113.
89. Kukreja RC, Kearns AA, Zweier JL, Kuppusamy P, Hess ML. *Circ Res* 1991;69:1003–1014.
90. Cochrane CG, Schraufstatter IU, Hyslop PA, et al. In: Cerutti PA, Fridovich I, McCord JM, eds. *Oxy-radicals in molecular biology and pathology*. New York: Alan R. Liss, 1988;125–136.
91. Orrenius S, McConkey DJ, Nicotera P. In: Cerutti PA, Fridovich I, McCord JM, eds. *Oxy-radicals in molecular biology and pathology*. New York: Alan R. Liss, 1988;327–339.
92. Greenwald RW, Moy WW, Lazarus D. *Arthritis Rheum* 1976;19:799.
93. Greenwald RA, Moy WW. *Arthritis Rheum* 1980;23:455–463.
94. Del Maestro RF. *Can J Physiol Pharmacol* 1982;60:1406–1414.
95. Petrone WF, English DK, Wong K, et al. *Proc Natl Acad Sci USA* 1980;77:1159–1163.
96. Christman CW, Wei EP, Kontos HA. *Am J Physiol* 1984;247:H631–H637.
97. Wei EP, Christman CW, Kontos HA, Povlishock JT. *Am J Physiol* 1985;248:H157–H162.
98. Rosenblum WI. *Am J Physiol Heart Circ Physiol* 1983;14:H139–H142.
99. Wolin MS, Rodenburg JM, Messina EJ. *Am J Physiol* 1987;252:H1159–H1163.
100. Lamb FS, Webb RC. *Am J Physiol* 1984;217:H709–H714.
101. Rubanyi GM, Vanhoutte PM. *Am J Physiol* 1986;250:H815–H821.
102. Wei EP, Kontos HA. *Hypertension* 1990;16:162–169.
103. Needleman P, Jakschik B, Johnson EM. *J Pharmacol Exp Ther* 1973;187:324–331.
104. Burke TM, Wolin MS. *Am J Physiol* 1987;21:H721–H732.
105. Beny JL, von der Weid PY. *Biochem Biophys Res Commun* 1991;176:378–384.
106. Katusic ZS, Vanhoutte PM. *Am J Physiol* 1989;257:H33–H37.
107. Tesfamariam B, Cohen RA. *Am J Physiol* 1992;263:H321–H326.
108. Tate RM, Morris HG, Schroeder WR, et al. *J Clin Invest* 1984;74:608–613.
109. Kontos HA, Wei EP, Povlishock JT, Dietrich WD, Magiera CJ, Ellis EF. *Science* 1980;209:1242–1245.
110. Kontos HA, Wei EP, Dietrich WD, et al. *Am J Physiol* 1981;240:H511–H527.
111. Wolin MS, Belloni FL. *Am J Physiol* 1985;249:H1127–H1133.
112. Furchgott RF. *Circ Res* 1983;53:557–573.

113. Wei EP, Kontos HA, Christman CW, DeWitt DS, Povlishock JT. *Circ Res* 1985;57:781–787.
114. Kontos HA, Wei EP, Povlishock JT. *Am J Physiol* 1989;256: H665–H671.
115. Gryglewski RJ, Palmer RMJ, Monada S. *Nature* 1986;320:454–456.
116. Shatos MA, Doherty JM, Hoak JC. *Arteriosclerosis Thrombosis* 1991;11:594–601.
117. Rosenblum WI, Wei EP, Kontos HA. *Texas Heart Inst J* 1982;9: 345–348.
118. Azuma H, Ishikawa M, Sekizaki S. *J Pharmacol* 1986;88:411–415.
119. Barchowsky A, Tabrizi K, Kent RS, Whorton AR. *J Clin Invest* 1989;83:1153–1159.
120. Wei EP, Ellison MD, Kontos HA, Povlishock JT. *Am J Physiol* 1986;251:H693–H699.
121. Levasseur JE, Kontos HA, Ellis EF. *Am J Physiol* 1985;248: H534–H539.
122. Kontos HA, Wei EP, Marshall JJ. *Am J Physiol* 1988;255: H1259–H1262.
123. Mayhan WG, Faraci FM, Heistad DD. *Am J Physiol* 1987;253: H1435–H1440.
124. Luscher TF, Vanhoutte PM. *Hypertension* 1986;8:344–348.
125. Povlishock JT, Kontos HA, Rosenblum WI, et al. *Acta Neuropathol* 1980;51:203–213.
126. Mayhan WG, Heistad DD. *Circ Res* 1986;59:216–220.
127. Giese J. *The pathogenesis of hypertensive vascular disease.* Copenhagen: Munksgaard, 1966.
128. Wilson SK. *Circ Res* 1990;66:722–734.
129. Hazama F, Ozaki T, Amano S. *Stroke* 1979;10:245–252.
130. Povlishock JT, Williams JI, Wei EP, Kontos HA. *FASEB J* 1988;2:A835.
131. Kontos CD, Wei EP, Williams JI, Kontos HA, Povlishock JT. *Am J Physiol* 1992;263:H1234–H1242.
132. Schmid-Schonbein GW, Seiffge D, DeLano FA, Shen K, Zweifach BW. *Hypertension* 1991;17:323–330.
133. Ito BR, Schmid-Schonbein G, Engler RI. *Blood Vessels* 1990;16: 145–166.
134. Lipowsky HH, Usami S, Chen S. *Microvasc Res* 1980;19:297–319.
135. Mugge A, Lopez JAG. *Hypertension* 1991;17:331–333.
136. Ananchenko VG, Vakolyuk RM, Kuznetsov SV, Malashenkova IK, Streitsova TV, Strizhova NV. *Sov Med* 1986;10:3–5.
137. Ananchenko VG, Kuznetsov SV, Vakolyuk RM, Vakolyuk VS, Strizhova NV, Malashenkova IK, Kim IS. *Sov Med* 1988;7:32–35.
138. Rahman I, Nath N. *Indian J Med Res* 1988;88:64–70.
139. Posten L, Sewell RB, Wilkinson SP, et al. *Br Med J* 1981;282: 847–849.
140. Ng LL, Dubley C, Bomford J, Hawley D. *J Hypertens* 1989;7: 471–475.
141. Kontos HA, Wei EP, Kukreja RC, Ellis EF, Hess ML. *Am J Physiol* 1990;258:H1261–H1266.
142. Ellis EF, Holt SA, Wei EP, Kontos HA. *Am J Physiol* 1988;255: H397–H400.
143. Mayberg M, Langer R, Zervas N, et al. *Science* 1982;213:228–230.
144. Liu-Chen LY, Mayberg MR, Moskowitz MA. *Brain Res* 1983;268:162–166.
145. Norregaard TV, Moskowitz MA. *Brain* 1985;108:517–533.
146. McCulloch J, Uddman R, Kingman T, et al. *Proc Natl Acad Sci USA* 1986;83:5731–5735.
147. Moskowitz MA, Wei EP, Saito K, Kontos HA. *Am J Physiol* 1988;255:H1–H6.
148. Sakas DE, Moskowitz MA, Wei EP, et al. *Proc Natl Acad Sci USA* 1989;86:1401–1405.
149. Armstead WM, Mirro R, Leffler CW, Busija DW. *J Cereb Blood Flow Metab* 1988;9:175–179.
150. Bauknight GC Jr, Wei EP, Kontos HA. *Stroke* 1992;23:1512–1514.
151. Wei EP, Dietrich WD, Povlishock JT, Navari RM, Kontos HA. *Circ Res* 1980;46:37–47.
152. Muizelaar JP, Marmarou A, Young HF, Choi SC, Wolf A, Schneider RL, Kontos HA. *J Neurosurg* 1993;78:375–382.
153. Nelson CW, Wei EP, Povlishock JT, Kontos HA, Moskowitz MA. *Am J Physiol* 1992;263:H1356–H1362.
154. Stampfer MJ, Hennekens CH, Manson JE, Colditz GA, Rosner B, Willett WC. *N Engl J Med* 1993;328:1444–1449.
155. Rimm EB, Stampfer MJ, Ascherio A, Giovannucci E, Colditz GA, Willett WC. *N Engl J Med* 1993;328:1450–1456.
156. Women's Health Study Research Group. *J Myocardial Ischemia* 1992;4:27–29.

Hypertension: Pathophysiology, Diagnosis, and Management, Second Edition, edited by J.H. Laragh and B.M. Brenner, Raven Press, Ltd., New York © 1995.

CHAPTER 41

Vascular Smooth Muscle Cell Differentiation and Growth Response in Hypertension

Paolo Pauletto, Riccardo Sarzani, Alessandro Rappelli, Achille C. Pessina, and Saverio Sartore

Arterial hypertension represents a main cardiovascular risk factor not only because of left ventricular hypertrophy and heart failure but also because it accelerates the atherogenic process (1,2) and induces striking structural changes in both large and small arteries (3,4). Hypertension, in fact, may be accompanied by a remodeling of the arterial wall characterized by intimal thickening due to vascular smooth muscle cell (SMC) hyperplasia, and medial hypertrophy due to SMC hypertrophy or hyperplasia (3,5,6). Structural remodeling with spatial rearrangement of SMCs within the media may also occur (4). In all cases, SMCs are thought to play a key role also because they synthesize the extracellular matrix of the arterial wall (7,8), made up of collagen, elastin, proteoglycans, and fibronectin. In hypertension, all vascular components undergo an adaptive process with some potentially beneficial consequences (more strength of the vascular wall to face the increase in pressure) along with some adverse ones (chronic increase in the peripheral resistances, acceleration of atherogenesis, etc.) (9,10). Some data suggest instead that vascular hypertrophy could be an abnormality that precedes or accompanies the development of arterial hypertension (11), thus implying a role for genetic or, perhaps, humoral factors (3).

In large vessels, and sometimes in the resistance vessels, the major contribution to arterial media thickening comes from an increase in the number of SMCs themselves (SMC hyperplasia) or an increase in SMC mass (SMC hypertrophy), or both (6). Hypertrophy of SMC is usually associated with increased DNA content (polyploidy) leading to tetraploid and octaploid SMC formation (3,5,6). In most studies, hypertrophy and polyploidy have been documented in the aorta and other large vessels, even though in some animal models (e.g., rabbit aorta) SMC hyperplasia occurs (12). On the other hand, in small arteries and arterioles of experimental animal models hyperplasia seems to be the most common finding (3,6). Moreover, SMC remodeling without changes in cell number or size has been described at this level (4,13). Hence, SMC can undergo different modifications ranging from remodeling without a real increase in cell mass or cell number, to true cell hyperplasia or cell hypertrophy with polyploidy. The pathophysiological mechanisms underlying these changes are poorly un-

P. Pauletto and A. C. Pessina: Institute of Clinical Medicine, University of Padova, Padova, Italy.

R. Sarzani and A. Rappelli: Institute of Clinical Medicine, University of Ancona, Ancona, Italy.

S. Sartore: Department of Biomedical Sciences, University of Padova; and C.N.R. Unit for Muscle Biology and Physiopathology, Padova, Italy.

derstood. An increase in blood pressure per se certainly plays a role as evidenced by Folkow (14–16) and by others (4,5,7,17), but there is growing evidence that humoral factors also regulate both normal vessel homeostasis and arterial growth in vascular disease (18–22). The same factors are also likely to control SMC differentiation during development and, in postnatal life, normal vessel homeostasis and pathological remodeling (3,15,23). Therefore, it might be that common mechanisms can be responsible for changes occurring in blood vessels during development and in hypertension.

Some basic questions, however, should be addressed: Which mechanisms, apart from blood pressure levels, regulate SMC growth and differentiation in normal vessels? What is the role of SMC differentiation in hypertension? What is the role of peptide growth factors in hypertension? How can vasoactive molecules induce not only changes in blood pressure but also participate in arterial wall remodeling? We will focus on these aspects, trying to summarize the present knowledge in this field.

SMOOTH MUSCLE CELL HOMEOSTASIS IN NORMAL ARTERIES

Growth Control

In analogy with other muscular tissues, SMCs in normal adult arteries show an extremely low replication rate (24). Complex interactions among mechanical, circulating, and tissue factors are likely to regulate the homeostasis of SMC under physiological conditions. The many factors capable of promoting or inhibiting SMC growth, mainly *in vitro,* have been recently reviewed by Schwartz et al. (3) and by Casscells (25). On the whole, there is no conclusive evidence that all these factors could play the same role in SMC regulation *in vivo.* Under culture conditions, growth of quiescent SMCs occurs depending upon the density of cell seeding (26). SMC growth can also be achieved by adding polypeptide growth factors such as platelet-derived growth factor (PDGF), fibroblast growth factor (FGF), or epidermal growth factor (EGF) to the culture medium. On the other hand, other polypeptides, hormones, and vasoactive substances are recognized to act on cultured SMC as growth inhibitors (3,25). The idea that polypeptide factors derived from platelets or leukocytes controlled SMC replication in atherogenesis (27) gave emphasis to the possibility that they also take part in SMC homeostasis. Peptide growth factors regulate cell growth in a lineage- and stage-specific fashion. They are encoded by multigene families (FGF, transforming growth factor [TGF-β]), are developmentally regulated, provoke plasticity of gene expression, and act through autocrine or paracrine mechanisms. As discussed below, in some cases, they act as "competence" factors (PDGF) capable of activating quiescent SMCs or as "progression" factors allowing cell cycle progression (insulinlike growth factor [IGF-I]) after

cell activation. Moreover, they may display a bimodal mechanism of action (TGF-β$_1$), either as growth promoters or as growth inhibitors, depending upon the culture conditions. For many growth factors, multiple receptors and signal transductions have been identified; the gene regulatory regions and the transcription factors involved in these phenomena are partly characterized. Their multiple actions include cell differentiation, production of extracellular matrix, cell attachment, cell migration, thrombosis, and regulation of autocrine synthesis of growth factors and cytokines (3). A comparable variety of actions can be exerted by some hormones, vasoactive substances, and cytokines (3). It is from the interactions of these molecules in the growth factors–hormones–cytokines network that regulation of SMC growth may be achieved. In addition, as discussed below, the expression of many of these factors is induced in vascular disease, and they are thought to play a major role in the remodeling of the arterial wall in hypertension. However, it remains to be established to what extent factors required for SMC growth *in vitro* are also effective *in vivo* conditions.

Taken together, different mechanisms can be hypothesized to explain SMC growth control in normal adult vessels: (a) cell-to-cell contact, in analogy with observations made on cultured SMC, BC3H1 cells, and endothelial cells—the latter cells, however, display some specific molecules controlling cell contact which are lacking in SMC (28); (b) an imbalance between growth promoters and growth inhibitors produced by cells of the arterial wall, such as endothelial cells and SMCs; (c) growth factors derived from blood-borne cells, such as platelets and the monocyte/macrophage cells; (d) the phagocytic activity of scavenger cells (monocytes, macrophages) that degrade debris as well as senescent fibroblasts and SMCs. This, in turn, induces cell proliferation and the laying down of new extracellular matrix. Scavenger cells express specific receptors for advanced glycosylation end products (AGEs). The uptake of AGE-modified proteins induces human monocytes to produce and release tumor necrosis factor (TNF), interleukin-1 (IL-1), and IGF-I (29), which are thought to contribute to the maintenance of normal tissue homeostasis; and (e) at least in the pulmonary bed, differentiation and migration of SMC partly depends on arterial elastolytic activity and an impaired assembly of elastin, respectively (30).

These hypotheses are not mutually exclusive and may represent different parts of a coordinated mechanism of growth control.

The Role of Differentiation

The role played by SMC differentiation in arterial wall homeostasis is less clear. As pointed out by Schwartz and colleagues (3), this topic may represent a major issue in a discussion on SMC growth control. Extensive studies on the phenotypic changes occurring in cultured SMC have been made by the Campbells (31–33). Changes in SMC phenotype observed *in vitro* have been interpreted as due to a "phenotypic modulation." Conversely, SMC *in vivo* under certain pathological conditions involving proliferation/migration of medial SMC into the intima (atherogenesis, balloon injury of endothelium) display a dedifferentiated/"synthetic" SMC phenotype. These cells markedly differ from the differentiated/"contractile" phenotype present in the adult normal vessels. The main characteristics of dedifferentiated/synthetic SMC are the increased size with appearance of large amounts of endoplasmic reticulum; the loss of cytocontractile proteins with expression of new isoforms; changes in the specific activity of some cellular enzyme, (such as increase of cytochrome *c* reductase, acid phosphatase, and β-glucosaminidase, and decrease of acid cholesteryl esterase; increased synthesis of collagen and glycosaminoglycans; increased degradation of very-low-density lipoprotein (VLDL) and β-VLDL; decreased degradation of low-density lipoprotein (LDL); increased esterification and accumulation of cellular cholesterol (34). Moreover, dedifferentiated/synthetic SMCs do not contract and display high susceptibility to proliferate and migrate. It is important to note that synthetic SMC grown *in vitro* can modulate to the contractile phenotype depending on the initial seeding density and factors of the conditioning media (32,35). It is not clear whether the SMC plasticity observed *in vitro* also occurs in intact vessels.

It has been suggested that the achievement of the new morphological and biochemical properties is in some way linked to the ability to respond to mitogens. This would be how SMCs become "activated" and ready for growth. Hedin and Thyberg (36) proposed that fibronectin promotes modulation of SMC from contractile to synthetic phenotype, but replication is not initiated unless SMCs are exposed to mitogens. More recently, type I collagen (37), PDGF (38), and competence growth factors (39) have been reported to induce modulation of cultured SMCs toward the synthetic phenotype. On the other hand, heparin not only inhibits SMC proliferation *in vivo* and *in vitro* (40,41), but also inhibits modulation to a synthetic phenotype (31,42), as judged by the switching in actin isoform expression (42).

The concept that changes in cell phenotype are a prerequisite for SMC growth, although not for migration, is now generally accepted (3,26). Hence, the identification of phenotypic changes of SMCs with development and in normal wall homeostasis is of fundamental importance to the understanding of the changes occurring in vascular disease.

VASCULAR SMOOTH MUSCLE DIFFERENTIATION IN HYPERTENSION

In vivo and *in vitro* studies on SMC differentiation have been performed in normal arteries using a number of specific cytoskeletal, cytocontractile, membrane, and extracellular matrix markers. (For a complete review on this topic, see refs. 26 and 43.) Very little information is available, however, concerning the differentiation of SMCs in hypertensive vessels. In a model of aortic coarctation, Kocher and Gabbiani (44) have found that in the thoracic hypertensive segment above the ligature there was no change in the content of smooth muscle α-actin messenger RNA (mRNA), as compared with controls. By contrast, our data (45) show that in renovascular hypertensive rabbits the majority of aortic SMCs display a partially differentiated profile with respect to myosin isoform expression. In normotensive adult rabbits, SMCs of the partially differentiated type represent a minor cell population accounting for about 4% of the total SMC number in the upper aorta (46). This cell population is characterized by a peculiar myosin isoform content, i.e., coexistence of smooth muscle (SM) and nonmuscle (NM) myosin (45), whereas the large majority of aortic SMCs in adult rabbit aorta (90-day-old animals) express SM-myosin exclusively (47). In the postnatal stage of development (from 3 to 45 days after birth), all aortic SMCs contain both SM and NM myosin (47). Before birth, a different NM myosin isoform content can be observed. Taken together, these findings indicate the existence of three developmental stages in the maturation of the vessel wall as far as myosin isoform expression is concerned: fetal, intermediate (postnatal), and adult (47).

In light of this maturational cell sequence, it appears evident that renovascular hypertension in rabbits is accompanied by a partial recapitulation of an immature SMC phenotype. In Fig. 1 the main changes in SMC phenotypes occurring during an 8-month period of renovascular hypertension are shown. In the earlier stages of hypertension (1–4 months from renal artery stenosis) a striking increase of the intermediate-type SMC population occurs in the aortic media, which is paralleled by the accumulation of medial SMC in the intima (intimal thickening). Intimal cells display the same myosin isoform content peculiar to the intermediate-type SMC found in the underlying media. The later stages of renovascular hypertension (8 months from renal artery stenosis) are characterized by an almost complete disappearance of intermediate-type SMC from both intima and media, and the reappearance of adult-type SMC (Fig. 1).

Despite the moderate increase in blood pressure (140–150 mm Hg), which is generally observed in renovascular hypertensive rabbits, a significant increase in aortic media thickness is consistently found. The increase in mass of the vessel wall is due to SMC hyperplasia, as also reported by others in this animal model (48). It is interesting to note that in other experimental conditions characterized by SMC proliferation and migration, such as atherosclerosis and hyperthyroidism, a marked increase of the SMC population of intermediate type is likewise

Normal aorta (adult rabbit)

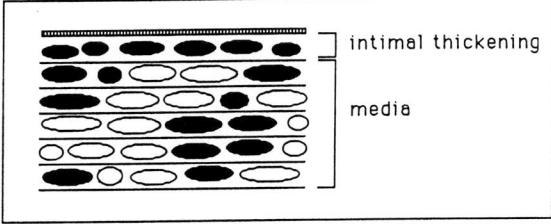

Rabbit aortas after 1–4 months from surgery

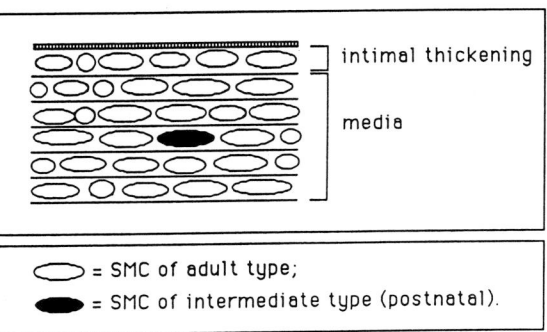

Rabbit aortas after 8 months from surgery

◯ = SMC of adult type;
● = SMC of intermediate type (postnatal).

FIG. 1. Representation of phenotypic changes that rabbit aortic SMCs undergo during development of renovascular hypertension during an 8-month period. Note (1) the marked increase of the intermediate-type SMC population in the media, (2) the appearance of intimal thickening composed of SMC of the same type, and (3) the marked decrease of SMCs of intermediate type at later stages of hypertension.

found (49–51). In hypertensive vessels, changes of SMC at the cytoskeletal level are also accompanied by an increased expression of mRNAs coding for procollagen type I (α-1), procollagen type III (α-1), fibronectin, and PDGF-β receptor compared with normotensive controls (45).

Compared with hypertension, atherosclerosis, and hyperthyroidism, the administration of calcium antagonists (52,53) and sympathetic denervation (43) exert an opposite effect on the size of this SMC population. In fact, intermediate-type SMCs strongly decrease or disappear from the aortic media of adult rabbit in these two experimental conditions.

Although the predominant response of the aortic wall to increased blood pressure involves an increase in intermediate-type SMC, in a few animals the appearance

of fetal-type SMC can be occasionally observed. Experiments performed using angiotensin II (AII) infusion for 2 weeks at either subhypertensive or hypertensive doses have revealed the presence of some fetal SMCs both in the aortic intima and media (in preparation). Therefore, the phenotypic changes that aortic SMCs can undergo might be related to the local level of AII production.

The tendency for increasing the size of the immature SMCs in the vascular wall is also found in another model of hypertension, i.e., the stroke-prone spontaneously hypertensive rats (SHR-SP; 54,55). In comparison with normotensive Wistar-Kyoto (WKY) control rats, SHR-SPs display a marked increase of SMCs showing an immature pattern of myosin isoform expression, both in the aorta and in small coronary arteries (54,55). This phenotypical change can be prevented by diuretic treatment (indapamide or hydrochlorothiazide), despite the scarce effect on lowering of blood pressure and on medial hypertrophy (54,55). This finding indicates that changes in pattern of SMC differentiation can be dissociated from medial thickness and blood pressure levels.

The question of the origin of the immature SMCs found in the aortic wall of hypertensive animals is still open. Some authors have claimed that a process of phenotypic modulation is involved in the formation of such a type of cell, at least in atherosclerosis (26). However, it may be that a dedifferentiation process is responsible for the presence of undifferentiated SMCs in the media (56). Another hypothesis may be put forward relying on the existence of stemlike cells that act as a source of immature SMCs (57). This hypothesis implies the persistence of immature SMCs in the adult arterial wall, i.e., the preexistence of these cells to wall injury. Moreover, Schwartz and colleagues (3) have recently proposed a further variant to the dedifferentiation hypothesis. In their view, two different SMC populations exist in the aortic media: The first cell type can undergo a dedifferentiation process, recapitulating the structural and functional properties peculiar to vascular SMCs of newborn animals (PUP cells); the other one would be relatively unable to change its mature phenotype.

VASCULAR SMOOTH MUSCLE CELL GROWTH IN HYPERTENSION

The Role of Vasoactive Substances

Catecholamines

Catecholamines have trophic activity on blood vessels and stimulate SMC growth *in vitro*. Bevan (12) observed a significant reduction of SMC DNA synthesis in denervated ear arteries of rabbits. Chemical sympathectomy with 6-hydroxydopamine caused a reduction in SMC number in rabbit aortic media (58), and a reduction in SMC cell layers in rat mesenteric arteries (59). Since sympathectomy inhibits the proliferation of SMC, endogenous catecholamines could be implicated in normal cellular turnover of the vessel wall. Many studies indicate that there is a hypernoradrenergic innervation in blood vessels from SHR compared with control WKY rats (60). In SHR, the increased activity of the vascular sympathetic system is found immediately after birth and before the onset of hypertension and could participate in the development and maintenance of both high blood pressure and increased SMC growth (60).

A single injection of phenilephrine, a nonselective agonist of α-adrenergic receptors, does not stimulate DNA synthesis in normal rat aorta (61), whereas administration of the α_1-adrenergic receptor agonist methoxamine induces intimal SMC accumulation in thoracic aorta of chicken (62). It is also interesting to note that α_1-adrenergic receptors appear to mediate in part the increase of aortic DNA synthesis induced by AII infusion in WKY rats (63). Moreover, adrenaline is able to stimulate aortic SMC DNA synthesis in rabbits fed a cholesterol-enriched diet (64).

In vitro, adrenaline (at a minimum concentration of 1 nM), noradrenaline, and isoproterenol (a nonselective agonist for β-adrenergic receptors) stimulate proliferation of rat aortic SMCs (65). Such effect appears to be mediated through β-adrenergic receptors because propranolol, a nonselective β-adrenergic receptor antagonist, inhibits the growth of SMCs induced by epinephrine (65). High concentrations of noradrenaline, similar to those found in proximity of noradrenergic nerve endings, can induce hypertrophy and increase in the number of polyploid SMCs; these effects can be abolished by simultaneous α- and β-adrenergic receptor blockade (66). In subconfluent serum-free cultures, noradrenaline stimulates DNA synthesis (at a minimum concentration of 100 pM), whereas in confluent cultures the effective concentrations are of three orders of magnitude higher (64). Antagonists of α-adrenergic receptors block the growth-promoting effects of catecholamines (64). The results of these studies suggest also that stimulation of β_2-receptors may inhibit SMC growth, in apparent contrast with the results of other authors (64–66). Culture conditions and growth status of SMCs are the most likely explanation for these discrepancies.

It has been suggested that PDGF may be involved in mediating the trophic effects of catecholamines on SMCs. In fact, the in vivo stimulation of α_1-adrenergic receptors induces an increase in the expression of growth-related genes like c-fos, c-myc, and ornithine decarboxylase as well as PDGF-A chain in rat aortic media (61). Furthermore, noradrenaline can up-regulate the number of PDGF-β receptors in cultured SMC. Such an increase can contribute in making SMC more responsive to PDGF-BB (67).

Angiotensin

AII, besides exerting vasoconstriction, has been shown to stimulate hyperthropic or hyperplastic growth of SMCs in vitro and in vivo. Numerous experiments have been performed to study the in vitro effects of AII on SMC growth, but the results are partly conflicting perhaps due to different animal species, type of vessel, and culture conditions.

AII acts by binding to specific receptors present as two main subtypes (AT1 and AT2) on SMC (68). AT1 appears to mediate AII vasoconstriction and is the most represented subtype in adult vessels (about 80% of AII receptors) (69–72). After arterial injury in 15-day-old rats, AT1 increases dramatically, suggesting a specific role for this subtype in SMC proliferation and migration (73). Moreover, the AT1 antagonist DuP 753 blocks AII-induced hypertrophic and hyperplastic growth of cultured SMC derived from WKY and SHR thoracic aorta (74). AT2 is much more abundant in the aorta of fetal or young rats (71), suggesting a role for this AII receptor subtype during vascular development.

AII, at a minimum concentration of 100 nM, was able to induce proliferation of human SMCs from young aorta growing in secondary cultures in the presence of 10% serum (75). In secondary SMC cultures from rat mesenteric artery grown in the presence of 10% fetal bovine serum, an increased cell proliferation was observed in response to lower concentrations of AII (1 nM; 76,77). This effect was blocked using the antagonist saralasin (76,77). In contrast, other authors have reported that various concentrations of AII have only a hypertrophic effect (with polyploidy) on secondary cultures of SMCs prepared from rat thoracic aorta (78,79). It has also been suggested that the hyperplastic response of SMCs to AII depends on the continuous exposure of these cells to factors present in platelet-poor plasma-derived serum (80).

It has been hypothesized that AII, as noradrenaline, has only indirect effects on SMC growth because it would be dependent upon growth factors like PDGF-AA dimers, whose expression is stimulated by vasoconstrictor substances (61,81). AII seems also to be able to induce an increase of SMC PDGF-β receptors, making the cells more responsive to PDGF-BB (67). This in turn stimulates DNA synthesis and cell proliferation (67). In contrast, other studies have shown that AII is able to increase the proliferative response to PDGF-BB only in SMCs from SHR, but not SMCs from normotensive control rats (82). These experiments have also evidenced the role of tumor growth factor-β_1 (TGF-β_1) in AII-induced SMC proliferation (82). On the other hand, studies performed by other groups indicate that the AII-induced secretion of active TGF-β_1 is involved in the inhibition of SMC proliferation (83–85). In these latter studies, SMC proliferation induced by AII seems to be mediated through basic FGF and PDGF-AA (83–85).

Taken together, these studies showed that at least three growth factors are involved in the modulation of SMC growth stimulated by AII. Many other variables, such as the source of SMCs and their growth status in relation to culture conditions, may influence the effects of these factors. The results of recent studies showed that the pathways whereby AII may indirectly stimulate SMC are even more complex. This hormone stimulates confluent and quiescent human SMC from omental vessels to synthesize active endothelin, which reinforces AII stimulation on SMC contractile tone and growth (86). Moreover, AII increases mRNA levels of growth-related proto-oncogenes c-*fos,* c-*myc,* and c-*jun* (87–90) in SMC. This effect, at least in the case of the increase of c-*fos* and phosphoinositide turnover, appears to be mediated through the AT1 receptor (81). In the light of these findings, AII is able to stimulate SMC growth independently from hemodynamic effects.

In vivo studies show that AII has similar growth-promoting effects on SMC (see also Vascular Smooth Muscle Differentiation in Hypertension, above). A continuous subcutaneous infusion of AII in rats is able to induce SMC proliferation in both intact and injured carotid arteries and in aorta as well (91). AII infusion can also induce a moderate increase in aortic gene expression of the PDGF-A chain (61). In addition, vascular and interstitial renal injury present in AII-induced hypertension is associated with increased interstitial expression of PDGF-B chain (92).

Angiotensin converting enzyme (ACE) inhibitors have been used in many studies with various animal models and in man to prevent or reduce increased growth and other pathological changes in arteries (reviewed in 80). Taken together these data add further support for the *in vivo* role of AII in the induction of the vascular changes independently from blood pressure lowering. Other factors, like an increase in kinins or aldosterone, might also be involved in determining the effects of ACE inhibitors.

Vasopressin

Vasopressin, a vasoconstrictor hormone that has been involved in the pathogenesis of hypertension, appears to stimulate rat aortic SMC proliferation *in vitro* (93,94). Species-specific factors present in the serum used for culturing SMCs (20) and the phase of cell cycle can affect vasopressin-induced SMC growth (95). The effect of vasopressin on these cells seems to be mediated by the activation of phospholipase C, through G protein–coupled V_1 receptor (96,97). This in turn leads to an increased synthesis of prostaglandin E_2 (PGE_2) and prostacyclin (PGI_2) (98,99), which act as antiproliferative agents inhibiting the cell cycle progression from late G_1 phase into the S phase (100–102). Some discrepancies about the

effects of vasopressin on SMC growth have been found by Geisterfer and Owens (103). These authors reported a vasopressin-induced hypertrophy but not polyploidy or hyperplasia in quiescent rat aortic SMC (103).

Endothelin

Endothelin is a powerful vasoactive peptide produced by endothelium. Three isoforms of endothelin (ET-1, ET-2, and ET-3), produced from three different genes, have been identified (104). The expression of the three isoforms varies according to endothelial cell type, and the vascular endothelium appears to produce only ET-1 (105). Endothelin acts by binding to the ETA receptor that is highly expressed in SMC (105,106). Recent studies have demonstrated that cultured aortic SMCs obtained by enzymatic digestion of rat and rabbit vascular tissues produce ET (107). Furthermore, other studies have shown that vasoactive hormones (AII, vasopressin) and growth factors (PDGF-AA, TGF-β_1, and EGF) increase the expression of ET mRNA and the secretion of biologically active ET-1 from quiescent SMCs of human omental vessels grown in the absence of serum for 48 hours (108). Endothelial ET-1 or ET-1 secreted from SMC could be involved in the autocrine-paracrine regulation of the muscular tone and of SMC growth, because of their mitogenic effect on SMC (109,110). However, ET appears to require the presence of serum or PDGF to act as a co-mitogen in the stimulation of DNA synthesis (86).

The Role of Polypeptide Growth Factors

The role of growth factors has been mainly defined in vascular restenosis and atherosclerosis, but, as reported above, some growth factors seem to be involved in vascular changes associated with arterial hypertension.

Platelet-Derived Growth Factor

The hypothesis that a PDGF was implicated in the control of SMC growth has been inferred from the observation that a platelet-derived component of serum, but not platelet-poor plasma, is mitogenic for SMC (27). PDGF is a dimeric molecule that is made of two structurally different chains, produced by two similar genes, in different functional combinations: AA, BB, or AB. Endothelial cells and macrophages can produce both PDGF chains, whereas adult SMCs and fibroblasts usually produce only A chains (111). The endothelium releases PDGF-BB in a polarized way from the side adherent to the extracellular matrix, that is the side turned toward the vascular media. It might be hypothesized that the endothelium transduces hormonal and hemodynamic stimuli through the release of PDGF-BB, in order to modulate the trophism and activity of the underlying SMC.

PDGF receptors are made up of two subunits (α and β) that can form homodimeric or heterodimeric receptors in such a way that subunit β binds only PDGF-BB while subunit α binds both PDGF-AA and -AB (112). On SMC and fibroblast cellular membranes, β subunits of PDGF receptor are much more abundant than α subunits, which means that PDGF-BB, one of the most potent mitogens for SMC, is much more effective than PDGF-AA in stimulating SMC (113). The diverse effects of PDGF-AA versus -BB are thus determined by the absolute and relative differences in α and β PDGF receptor subunits present on target cells (113). Despite this fact, PDGF-AA might be an important growth factor for SMC, at least in some circumstances where TGF-β_1 is involved in stimulating SMC growth (114). In fact, TGF-β_1 would be able to influence the effects of PDGF-AA produced by the action of TGF-β_1 itself. Very low amounts of TGF-β_1, i.e., a quantity per cell that induces the maximum proliferative response of human neonatal aortic SMC, can diminish the number of α subunits, the only isoform capable of binding PDGF-A chain (114).

PDGF appears to have a role in mediating the trophic effects of vasoconstrictor substances on SMC. As noted above, *in vivo* stimulation of α_1-adrenergic receptors induces in aortic media the gene expression of PDGF-A chain (61). The induction of PDGF-AA in SMC may mediate the effects of AII *in vivo* and *in vitro* (61,89). Furthermore, interstitial fibrosis in the kidneys of rats given an infusion of AII is associated with increased expression of PDGF-B chain mRNA (92). It is interesting to note that in some conditions, chronic administration of PDGF-BB to subconfluent serum-deprived SMC cultures gives rise to SMC hypertrophy (38). Therefore, in these conditions PDGF-induced cellular hypertrophy in vascular SMC is related to a partial progression of the cell cycle.

Sarzani et al. (115) have observed that an increase in the levels of aortic mRNA for β subunits of PDGF receptor was associated with hypertension induced by the administration of salt and deoxycorticosterone acetate in uninephrectomized rats (DOCA/salt model) (115). In this same animal model the expression of PDGF α receptor, as well as PDGF-A and -B chains, was unchanged (115,116). Increased expression of the β subunit of PDGF receptor seems to be a general feature of hypertensive vessels. In fact, both in SHR (117) and in renovascular hypertensive rabbits (118) an increased expression of this subunit occurs. It is also interesting to note that in both normotensive and hypertensive rats, the expression of the β subunit of PDGF receptor increases in aorta with aging (117), as happens with arterial pressure. These data indicate that during vascular remodeling (development of hypertension and aging) the expression of

genes coding for the ligand/receptor system of PDGF has a different regulation. The increased expression of the β subunit of PDGF receptor also suggests that in the presence of chronic arterial hypertension and in aging, medial SMCs are particularly sensitive to PDGF-BB and/or -AB and, therefore, are more prone to grow.

Noradrenaline and AII seem to be able to induce an increase in PDGF β-receptors of SMC and to potentiate the effect of PDGF-BB on DNA synthesis (67). Other studies have nevertheless demonstrated that AII increases the proliferative response of SMC from SHR *in vitro* to PDGF-BB, whereas this phenomenon would not occur in the SMCs from normotensive rats (82).

Insulinlike Growth Factors

IGF-I and IGF-II are among the best known polypeptide growth factors. They have an insulin-like activity, stimulate cellular growth, and modulate cell differentiation (119). IGF-I, the most important mediator of postnatal growth, exerts its activity through endocrine, autocrine, and paracrine mechanisms (119). The growth hormone (GH) is the main regulator of IGF-I gene expression and synthesis in tissues, whereas IGF-II does not seem to be GH-dependent (119). A paracrine type of regulation of IGF-I expression is suggested by the observations that PDGF and FGF stimulate the production of IGF-I from cultured fibroblasts and SMCs (120,121). IGF-I, which is also synthesized by SMC, acts like a "progression" factor that makes SMCs able to complete their cell cycle after stimulation by PDGF (120–123).

Recently, IGF-I has been implicated in the mechanism(s) underlying the vascular changes associated with arterial hypertension. In a rat model of hypertension produced by infrarenal aortic coarctation, an increase in mRNA level was documented for IGF-I in the aorta above the coarctation, suggesting a specific role for IGF-I in vascular remodeling (124). A down-regulation of mRNA level for IGF-I receptor was also observed but it appears to be secondary to the increased IGF-I expression (125). IGF-I may also have an important role in the accumulation of vascular extracellular matrix because it stimulates the synthesis of various extracellular matrix components, e.g., collagen I and II (126) and elastin (127).

Transforming Growth Factor-β_1

This growth factor generally acts as a growth inhibitor for most cells *in vitro* but, in some conditions, it may behave as a growth factor for SMC by inducing hypertrophy and hyperploidy (128) or hyperplasia (114,129). As already mentioned above, TGF-β_1 at low concentrations induces proliferation of human newborn aortic SMCs

(114). This effect of TGF-β_1 appears to be indirect and mediated by PDGF-AA produced by the SMCs themselves (114). TGF-β_1 by itself would be otherwise able to influence these indirect effects by causing a reduction in number of the α subunits of PDGF receptor, the only one capable of binding PDGF-A chain (114). Therefore, due to down-regulation of α-PDGF receptors, SMCs exposed at relatively high TGF-β_1 concentrations do not proliferate, whereas a proliferative response would occur in the SMCs exposed to relatively low concentrations of TGF-β_1 (114).

It has also been reported that in aortic SMCs from SHRs higher levels of mRNA coding for TGF-β_1 are present than in normotensive controls. These cells can proliferate if they are stimulated by TGF-β_1, whereas cells of normotensive control rats do not (129). These data suggest that aortic SMCs from SHR have a greater sensitivity to the stimulating effects of exogenous TGF-β_1, even if this molecule can potentially be produced in large amounts by SMCs.

Other studies, some of which were carried out on adult human aortic SMC (130), have on the contrary demonstrated that TGF-β_1 inhibits SMC growth, and an autocrine secretion of active TGF-β_1 inhibits SMC proliferation in response to AII (85). The apparently conflicting effects that TGF-β_1 has on SMC seem to depend on TGF-β_1 concentration, culture conditions, animal species, and age. It is likely that part of the discrepancies observed in these studies is related to the type and relative amount of TGF-β_1 receptors in SMC. In fact, while type I receptor mediates the effects of TGF-β_1 on extracellular matrix, type II receptor influences the inhibitory effects of this growth factor on SMC (131,132). Thus, the effects of TGF-β_1 on the metabolism of various components of the vascular extracellular matrix (like different types of collagen, fibronectin, and proteoglycans) might explain its ability to "give shape to the tissues" as well as to induce SMC growth in some circumstances (133–135).

The importance of TGF-β_1 as a mediator of vascular changes is also supported by investigations performed by Sarzani et al. (116,117) on SHR and DOCA/salt rats. These studies have shown an increase in TGF-β_1 expression in the aorta of hypertensive rats, similarly to what happens with aging (116,117). A rapid increase in TGF-β_1 gene expression is also found after intimal-medial injury of rat carotid arteries and in the formation of intimal thickening. This increase is paralleled by an increased expression of fibronectin and collagen I and III (134). Under these experimental conditions, TGF-β_1 infusion caused an increase in DNA synthesis in neointima, suggesting that this factor stimulates SMC growth *in vivo* (134).

As cited above, many studies *in vitro* have shown that the AII-dependent increase in the secretion of active TGF-β_1 has a unique role in mediating AII-induced SMC growth, but there is still controversy whether AII-induced TGF-β_1 stimulates or inhibits SMC growth (82–85).

Nerve Growth Factor

Nerve growth factor (NGF) is a trophic factor that regulates the growth of peripheral sympathetic fibers and sensitive neurons (136). A series of experiments has shown that NGF mRNA levels and NGF of target tissues correlate to the density of sympathetic innervation of the tissue. It appears that a higher expression of NGF not only plays an important role in the noradrenergic innervation of vessels, but can also favor the development of hypertension and vascular changes. The sympathetic innervation, and its trophic effect (partly mediated by PDGF [61]), is more developed in vessels from SHR compared to those from WKY (60). Such an increased sympathetic innervation appears to be secondary to an augmentation of NGF production by the SMCs themselves because aortas and mesenteric arteries from young SHRs contain higher levels of NGF than the corresponding control animals (137). *In vitro,* rat aortic SMCs produce NGF (138). Moreover, the expression and secretion of NGF from SMC can be stimulated by AII and vasopressin, whereas phenylephrine inhibits secretion (138), suggesting a further interaction of these agonists in hypertension-associated SMC growth.

Type-A Natriuretic Peptide

Type-A natriuretic peptide (ANP), also known as atrial natriuretic peptide or atrial natriuretic factor, was isolated for the first time from cardiac atrium (139). Two other peptides with structure and activity similar to that of ANP followed the initial discovery of this factor; these are the type-B natriuretic peptide (BNP), mainly produced by the myocardium and also known as brain natriuretic peptide, and the type-C natriuretic peptide (CNP) (140,141). Three types of atrial natriuretic peptide receptors (NPR) mediate the effects of natriuretic peptides on vascular SMC (142): NPR-A has an intracellular portion with guanilyl cyclase activity and is activated by ANP and BNP; NPR-B is very similar to NPR-A but it is activated by CNP (140,143). The third receptor, NPR-C, also known as the "clearance receptor," does not have an intracellular portion with enzymatic activity similar to NPR-A, and seems to be important for the clearance and buffering of the circulatory levels of NP (140,143), although some biological effects mediated by this receptor can also be demonstrated. ANP has a vasorelaxant activity and also reduces SMC growth *in vivo* and *in vitro* through a high number of NPR (142,143). *In vivo* long-term infusion of nonhypotensive doses of ANP in SHR reduces carotid artery medial thickness and nuclear size, and increases vascular compliance (144). *In vitro,* ANP inhibits rat aortic SMC proliferation in response to serum, and prevents cell hypertrophy in response to AII and TGF-β_1 in quiescent cells (145). Analogues of cyclic guanosine monophosphate (cGMP) and nitric oxide-generating vasodilators, like sodium nitroprussate and dinitrate isosorbide stimulating soluble guanylyl cyclase, can mimic the effects of ANP on SMC growth (145,146), suggesting that ANP activity on these cells is mediated through the NPR-A, via increasing intracellular cGMP concentration. Primary cultures of rat aortic SMCs respond poorly to the antimitogenic effect of ANP and analogues, and this may be related to lower expression of NPR-C, which appears to be involved in the NP-induced SMC growth inhibition (147). The observations that aortic tissue expresses ANP (148) and that subcultured aortic SMC secretes ANP (149) suggest that local production of ANP might have autocrine/paracrine functions.

CNP reduces arterial blood pressure without inducing natriuresis (150). The expression of CNP-specific receptors NPR-B in cultured SMCs (142) and in aortic tissue (151,152) as well as the stimulation of cGMP production by CNP suggest a specific role of this factor on arterial SMC growth. In addition, some endothelial production of CNP has been recently demonstrated (153). It is important to note that TGF-β_1 modulates endothelial and SMC growth and induces a dramatic increase in the expression and secretion of CNP from endothelial cells (153).

Taken together, these data suggest that CNP exerts a local control on SMC tone and growth, regulated by different growth factors. In fact, CNP inhibits SMC proliferation, stimulated by serum or growth factors (PDGF, bFGF, or EGF), more powerfully than ANP (154,155).

CONCLUSIONS

There is a growing evidence that SMC differentiation and proliferation occurring in the maturation of the arterial wall during development and in homeostasis of the adult vessels could be controlled by locally produced or activated autocrine/paracrine molecules, such as growth factors or cytokines. Changes in blood pressure and flow characteristics in the perinatal period are also likely to play an important role in modulating the physiological remodeling of the vessels. The association between hemodynamic stimuli and locally produced vasoactive substances may influence the dynamic interaction of endothelium with SMC and thus the final outcome of the organizing vascular wall. In all circumstances of vascular remodeling changes in the cytoskeleton, proteins of SMC are likely to play a fundamental role in determining smooth muscle plasticity. The fact that the ultrastructural, biochemical, and immunochemical features of SMC in vascular disease (experimental and spontaneous atherosclerosis, balloon injury, hypertension) seem to be comparable to those displayed by SMC grown in *vitro,* or present in developing vascular smooth muscle, has been related to a change in the rate of proliferation. However, the relationship between proliferation and differentiation in the vascular smooth muscle is not clear yet. For some authors, the achievement of a poorly differentiated SMC phenotype is a prerequisite for mitogen responsiveness. For others, modifications of the SMC differentiation pattern seems to be a consequence of vascular injury. Certainly, in some experimental models of SMC proliferation the observed phenotypical changes are only partially related to cell replicative activity.

The study of myosin isoform expression may be particularly helpful in identifying the SMC phenotype involved in vascular diseases. Using this marker of SMC differentiation, we have shown that in the aorta of renovascular hypertensive rabbits and stroke-prone SHR, "immature" SMCs increase markedly and account for the majority of vascular SMCs. At least in hypertensive rabbits, SMC hyperplasia is accompanied by an increased expression of aortic mRNAs coding for fibronectin, procollagen type I (α_1), and PDGF-β receptor, and represents how aortic-wall hypertrophy is achieved. This demonstrates *in vivo* that changes in SMC phenotype and growth run in parallel, possibly through mediators such as growth factors or cytokines in an autocrine/paracrine manner. It is also relevant that similar effects on SMC phenotype and growth have been obtained by infusion of AII in rabbits at hypertensive and at subhypertensive doses. This vasoactive substance has been reported to act as an SMC growth promoter through autocrine production of growth factors and cytokines. In analogy with this observation, it has been reported that in adult rats local sympathetic activity exerts a trophic influence on growth-related gene expression via α_1-adrenergic receptors, acting through stimulation of PDGF-A chain. This event is accompanied by increasing β-actin transcription. Hence, it can be reasonably hypothesized that AII and other vasoactive substances not only play a role in blood pressure regulation but also participate in the remodeling of the arterial wall in hypertension by inducing changes in both SMC phenotype and growth.

ACKNOWLEDGMENTS

This work has also been supported by funds from the Biomedical Association for Vascular Research, Padova, Italy. The authors wish to thank Ms. Lorrie Maas Fusetti for her excellent editing work.

REFERENCES

1. Bondjers G, Glukhova M, Hansson GK, Postnov YV, Reidy MA, Schwartz S. Hypertension and atherosclerosis: cause and effect, or two effects with one unknown cause? *Circulation* 1991;84 (suppl VI):VI-2–VI-16.

2. Pauletto P, Scannapieco G, Pessina C. Sympathetic drive and vascular damage in hypertension and atherosclerosis. *Hypertension* 1991;17(3):75–81.

3. Schwartz SM, Heimark RL, Majesky MW. Developmental mechanism underlying pathology of arteries. *Physiol Rev* 1990;70(4):1177–1209.

4. Mulvany MJ, Aalkjaer C. Structure and function of small arteries. *Physiol Rev* 1990;70:921–961.

5. Owens GK. Influence of blood pressure on development of aortic medial smooth muscle hypertrophy in spontaneously hypertensive rats. *Hypertension* 1987;9:178–187.

6. Owens G, Schwartz S. Alterations in vascular smooth muscle mass in the spontaneously hypertensive rat. Role of cellular hypertrophy, hyperploidy and hyperplasia. *Circ Res* 1982;51:280–289.

7. Leung DYM, Glagov S, Mathews MB. Cyclic stretching stimulates synthesis of matrix components by arterial smooth muscle cells *in vitro*. *Science* 1986;231:405–407.

8. Foldart JM, Rorive GL, Nusgens BV, Lapiere CM. The relationship between blood pressure and aortic collagen metabolism in renal hypertensive rats. *Clin Sci Mol Med Suppl* 1978;55:27s–29s.

9. Unfriend S, Cardinale G, Spector S. Hypertension-induced vascular fibrosis and its reversal by anti-hypertensive drugs. In: Laragh JH, Buhler FR, Seldin OW, eds. *Frontiers in hypertension research*. New York: Springer-Verlag; 1981.

10. Chobanian AV. Corcoran lecture: Adaptative and maladaptative responses of the arterial wall to hypertension. *Hypertension* 1990;15:666–674.

11. Loeb AL, Mandel G, Straw JA, Bean BL. Increased aortic DNA synthesis precedes renal hypertension in rats: an obligatory step? *Hypertension* 1986;8:754–751.

12. Bevan RD. Effect of sympathetic denervation on smooth muscle cell proliferation in the growing rabbit ear artery. *Circ Res* 1975;37:14–19.

13. Mulvany MJ. Abnormalities of resistance vessel structure in essential hypertension: are these important? *Clin Exp Pharmacol Physiol* 1991;18:13–20.

14. Folkow B. The Fourth Volhard Lecture. Cardiovascular structural adaptation: its role in the initiation and maintenance of primary hypertension. *Clin Sci Mol Med Suppl* 1978;55:3S–22S.

15. Folkow B, Grimby G, Thulesius O. Adaptive structural changes of the vascular wall in hypertension and their relation to the control of the peripheral resistance. *Acta Physiol Scand* 1958;44:255–272.

16. Folkow B. Physiological aspects of primary hypertension. *Physiol Rev* 1982;62:347–504.

17. Lowell Langille B. Remodeling of developing and mature arteries: endothelium, smooth muscle, and matrix. *Physiol Rev* 1986;66:710–770.

18. Seifert RA, Schwartz SM, Bowen-Pope DF. Developmentally regulated production of platelet-derived growth factor-like molecules. *Nature* 1984;311:669–671.

19. Naftilan AJ, Pratt RE, Dzau VJ. Angiotensin II induction of c-*fos*, c-*myc* and platelet derived growth factor in vascular smooth muscle cells. *Clin Res* 1988;36:303A.

20. Campbell-Boswell M, Lazzarini Robertson A. Effects of angiotensin II and vasopressin on human smooth muscle cells *in vitro*. *Exp Mol Pathol* 1981;35:265–276.

21. Geisterfer AAT, Owens GK. Hypertrophic response of cultured vascular smooth muscle cells to angiotensin II. *Fed Proc* 1986;45:584.

22. Dzau VJ, Gibbons GH. Cell biology of vascular hypertrophy in systemic hypertension. *Am J Cardiol* 1988;62:30G–35G.

23. Dzau VJ. The role of mechanical and humoral factors in growth regulation of vascular smooth muscle and cardiac myocytes. *Curr Opin Nephrol Hypertens* 1993;2:27–32.

24. Clowes AW, Clowes MM, Reidy MA. Kinetics of cellular proliferation after injury. III. Endothelial and smooth muscle growth in chronically denuded vessels. *Lab Invest* 1986;54:295–303.

25. Casscells W. Smooth muscle cell growth factors. *Prog Growth Factors Res* 1993;3:177–206.

26. Thyberg J, Hedin U, Sjolund M, Palmberg L, Bottger BA. Regulation of differentiated properties and proliferation of arterial smooth muscle cells. *Arteriosclerosis* 1990;10:966–990.

27. Ross R. The pathogenesis of atherosclerosis: a perspective for the 1990s. *Nature* 1993;362:801–809.

28. Pober HS, Contran HS. What can be learned from the expression of endothelial adhesion molecules in tissues? *Lab Invest* 1991;64:301–305.

29. Kirstein M, Aston C, Hintz R, Vlassara H. Receptor-specific induction of insulinlike growth factor I in human monocytes by advanced glycosylation end product-modified proteins. *J Clin Invest* 1992;90(2):439–446.

30. Rabinovitch M. Investigational approaches to pulmonary hypertension. *Toxicol Pathol* 1991;19(4.1):458–469.

31. Campbell-Chamley JH, Campbell GR. What controls smooth muscle phenotype? *Atherosclerosis* 1981;40:347–357.

32. Campbell JH, Kocher O, Skalli O, Gabbiani G, Campbell GR. Cytodifferentiation and expression of α-smooth muscle actin mRNA and protein during primary culture of aortic smooth muscle cells: correlation with cell density and proliferative state. *Arteriosclerosis* 1989;9:633–643.

33. Campbell GR, Campbell JH, Manderson JA, Horrigon S, Rennick RE. A multifunctional mesenchymal cell. *Arch Pathol Lab Med* 1988;112:977–986.

34. Campbell GR, Campbell JH. Smooth muscle phenotypic changes in arterial wall homeostasis: implications for the pathogenesis of atherosclerosis. *Exp Mol Pathol* 1985;42:139–162.

35. Birukov KG, Frid MG, Rogers JD, Shirinsky VP. Synthesis and expression of smooth muscle phenotype markers in primary culture of rabbit aortic smooth muscle cells: influence of seeding density and media and relation to cell contractility. *Exp Cell Res* 1993;204:46–53.

36. Hedin U, Thyberg J. Plasma fibronectin promotes modulation of arterial smooth-muscle cells from contractile to synthetic phenotype. *Differentiation* 1987;33:239–346.

37. Yamamoto M, Yamamoto K, Noumura T. Type I collagen promotes modulation of cultured rabbit arterial smooth muscle cells from a contractile to a synthetic phenotype. *Exp Cell Res* 1993;204:121–129.

38. Blank RS, Owens GK. Platelet-derived growth factor regulates actin isoform expression and growth state in cultures rat aortic smooth muscle cells. *J Cell Physiol* 1990;142:635–642.

39. Kato M, Kyogoku M. Competence growth factors evoke the phenotypic transition of arterial smooth muscle cells. *Ann NY Acad Sci* 1990;598:232–237.

40. Guyton JR, Rosenberg RD, Clowes AW, Karnovsky MJ. Inhibition of rat arterial smooth muscle cell proliferation by heparin: *in vivo* studies with anticoagulant and non-anticoagulant heparin. *Circ Res* 1980;46:625–634.

41. Hoover RL, Rosenberg R, Haering W, Karnovsky MJ. Inhibition of rat arterial smooth muscle cells proliferation by heparin. *Circ Res* 1980;47:578–583.

42. Desmoulière A, Brandt-Rubbia L, Gabbiani G. Modulation of actin isoform expression in cultured arterial smooth muscle cells by heparin and culture conditions. *Arterioscl Thromb* 1991;11:244–253.

43. Sartore S, Scatena M, Chiavegato A, Faggin E, Giuriato L, Pauletto P. Myosin isoform expression in smooth muscle cells during physiological and pathological vascular remodeling. *J Vasc Res* 1994;31:61–81.

44. Kocher O, Gabbiani G. Analysis of α-smooth muscle actin mRNA expression in rat aortic smooth muscle cells using a specific cDNA probe. *Differentiation* 1987;34:201–209.

45. Pauletto P, Giuriato L, Scatena M, Chiavegato A, Sarzani R, Rappelli A, Dessì Fulgeri P, Pessina AC, Sartore S. Hyperplastic growth of aortic smooth muscle cells in renovascular hypertensive rabbits is accompanied by the expansion of an immature cell population. *Circ Res* 1994;74:774–788.

46. Pauletto P, Sartore S, Giuriato L, Scatena M, Guidolin D, Scannapieco G, Pessina AC. Computer-driven assessment of "immature"-type smooth muscle cells in rabbit aorta. *J Hypertens* 1991;9:S180–S181.

47. Giuriato L, Scatena M, Chiavegato A, Tonello M, Scannapieco G, Pauletto P, Sartore S. Non-muscle myosin isoforms and cells heterogeneity in developing rabbit vascular smooth muscle. *J Cell Sci* 1992;101:233–246.

48. Bevan RD. An autoradiographic and pathological study of cellu-

lar proliferation in rabbit arteries correlated with an increase in arterial pressure. *Blood Vessels* 1976;13:100–128.

49. Zanellato AMC, Borrione AC, Tonello M, Scannapieco G, Pauletto P, Sartore S. Myosin isoform expression and smooth muscle cell heterogeneity in normal and atherosclerotic rabbit aorta. *Arteriosclerosis* 1990;10:996–1009.

50. Giuriato L, Scatena M, Chiavegato A, Zanellato AMC, Guidolin D, Pauletto, P, Sartore S. Localization and smooth muscle cell composition of atherosclerotic lesions in Watanabe heritable hyperlipidemic rabbits. *Arterioscl Thromb* 1993;13:347–359.

51. Giuriato L, Borrione AC, Zanellato AMC, Tonello M, Scatena M, Scannapieco G, Pauletto P, Sartore S. Aortic intimal thickening and myosin isoform expression in hyperthyroid rabbits. *Arterioscl Thromb* 1991;11:1376–1389.

52. Pauletto P, Scannapieco G, Borrione AC, Zanellato AMC, Tonello M, Giuriato L, Pessina AC, Dal Palù C, Sartore S. A nifedipine-sensitive smooth muscle cell population is present in the atherosclerotic rabbit aorta. *Arterioscl Thromb* 1991;11:928–939.

53. Pauletto P, Sartore S, Giuriato L, Scatena M, Tonello M, Scannapieco G, Pessina AC, Dal Palù C. Calcium antagonists and vascular smooth muscle cells in atherogenesis. *J Cardiovasc Pharmacol* 1992;19(suppl 2):S8–S16.

54. Contard F, Glukhova M, Sabri A, Marotte F, Sartore S, Narcisse G, Schatz C, Guetz D, Rappaport L, Samuel JL. Comparative effects of indapamide and hydrochlorothiazide on cardiac hypertrophy and vascular smooth-muscle phenotype in the stroke-prone, spontaneously hypertensive rats. *J Cardiovasc Pharmacol* 1993;22:S29–S34.

55. Contard F, Sabri A, Glukhova M, Sartore S, Marotte F, Pomies JP, Guetz D, Samuel J, Rappaport L. Arterial smooth muscle cell phenotypes in stroke-prone spontaneously hypertensive rats. *Hypertension* 1993;22:665–676.

56. Kocher O, Skalli O, Cerruti D, Gabbiani F, Gabbiani G. Cytoskeletal features of rat aortic cells during development. An electronmicroscopic, immunohistochemical, and biochemical study. *Circ Res* 1985;56:829–838.

57. Schwartz SM, Reidy MR, Clowes AW. Kinetics of atherosclerosis: a stem cell model. *Ann NY Acad Sci* 1985;454:292–304.

58. Fronek K, Bloor CM, Amiel D, Chvapil M. Effect of long-term sympathectomy on the arterial wall in rabbits and rats. *Exp Mol Pathol* 1978;28:279–289.

59. Lee RMKW, Triggle CR, Cheung DWT, Coughlin MD. Structural and functional consequence of neonatal sympathectomy on the blood vessels of spontaneously hypertensive rats. *Hypertension* 1987;10:328–338.

60. Head RJ. Hypernoradrenergic innervation: its relationship to functional and hyperplastic changes in the vasculature of the spontaneously hypertensive rat. *Blood Vessels* 1989;26:1–20.

61. Majesky MW, Daemen MJAP, Schwartz SM. α1-Adrenergic stimulation of platelet-derived growth factor A-chain gene expression in aorta. *J Biol Chem* 1990;265:1082–1088.

62. Majesky MW, Reidy MA, Benditt EP, Juchau MR. Focal smooth muscle proliferation in the aortic intima produced by an initiation-promotion sequence. *Proc Natl Acad Sci USA* 1985;82:3450–3454.

63. van Kleef EM, Smits JFM, De Mey JGR, Cleutjens JPM, Lombardi DM, Schwartz SM, Daemen MJAP. α1-Adrenergic blockade reduces the angiotensin II-induced vascular smooth muscle cell DNA synthesis in the rat thoracic aorta and carotid artery. *Circ Res* 1992;70:1122–1127.

64. Nakaki T, Nakayama M, Yamamoto S, Kato R. α1-Adrenergic stimulation and β2-adrenergic inhibition of DNA synthesis in vascular smooth muscle cells. *Mol Pharmacol* 1990;37:30–36.

65. Blaes N, Boissel J-P. Growth stimulating effect of catecholamines on rat aortic smooth muscle cells in culture. *J Cell Physiol* 1983;116:167–172.

66. Printseva OY, Tjurmin AV, Rudchenko SA, Repin VS. Noradrenaline induces the polyploidization of smooth muscle cells: the synergism of second messengers. *Exp Cell Res* 1989;184:342–350.

67. Bobik A, Grinpukel S, Little PJ, Grooms A, Jackman G. Angiotensin II and noradrenaline increase PDGF BB receptors and potentiate PDGF BB stimulated DNA synthesis in vascular smooth muscle. *Biochem Biophys Res Commun* 1990;166:580–588.

68. Bumpus FM, Catt JK, Chiu AT, De Gasparo M, Goodfriend T, Hausain A, Peach MJ, Taylor DG, Timmermans PB. Nomenclature for angiotensin receptors a report of the nomenclature committee of the council for high blood pressure research. *Hypertension* 1991;17:720–721.

69. Wong PC, Hart SD, Zaspel AM, Chiu AT, Ardecky RJ, Smith RD, Timmermans PB. Functional studies of nonpeptide angiotensin II receptor subtype-specific ligands: DuP753 (AII-1) and PD 13177 (AII-2). *J Pharmacol Exp Ther* 1990;255:584–592.

70. Dudley DT, Panek RL, Major TC, Lu GH, Bruns RS, Klinkefus BA, Hodges JC, Weishaar RE. Subclasses of angiotensin II binding sites and their functional significance. *Mol Pharmacol* 1990;38:370–377.

71. Viswanathan M, Tusutsumi K, Correa FMA, Saavedra JM. Changes in the expression of angiotensin receptor subtypes in the rat aorta during development. *Biochem Biophys Res Commun* 1991;179:1361–1367.

72. Chang RS, Lotti VJ. Angiotensin receptor subtype in rat, rabbit and monkey tissues: relative distribution and species dependency. *Life Sci* 1991;49:1485–1490.

73. Viswanathan M, Stromberg C, Seltzer A, Saavedra J. Balloon angioplasty enhanced the expression of angiotensin II AT1 receptors in neointima of rat aorta. *J Clin Invest* 1992;90:1707–1712.

74. Bunkenburg B, Amelsvoort T, Rogg H, Wood JM. Receptor-mediated effects of angiotensin II on growth of vascular smooth muscle cells from spontaneously hypertensive rats. *Hypertension* 1992;20:746–754.

75. Campbell-Boswell M, Robertson AL. Effects of angiotensin II and vasopressin of human smooth muscle cells *in vitro*. *Exp Mol Pathol* 1981;35:265–276.

76. Lyall F, Lever AF, Morton JJ. Vascular hypertrophy and hypertension: a role for growth factors? *Acta Physiol Scand* 1988;133(suppl 571):189–196.

77. Lyall F, Morton JJ, Lever AF, Cragoe EJ. Angiotensin II activates Na-H exchange and stimulates growth in vascular smooth muscle cells. *J Hypertens* 1988;6(suppl 14):S438–S441.

78. Geisterfer AAT, Peach MJ, Owens GK. Angiotensin II induces hypertrophy, not hyperplasia, in cultured rat aortic smooth muscle cells. *Circ Res* 1988;62:749–756.

79. Berck BC, Vekshtein V, Gordon HM, Tsuda T. Angiotensin II stimulated protein synthesis in cultured vascular smooth muscle cells. *Hypertension* 1989;13:305–314.

80. Jackson CL, Schwartz SM. Pharmacology of smooth muscle cells replication. *Hypertension* 1992;20:713–736.

81. Lyall F, Dornan ES, McQueen J, Boswell F, Kelly M. Angiotensin II increases proto-oncogene expression and phosphoinositide turnover in vascular smooth muscle cells via the angiotensin II AT1 receptor. *J Hypertens* 1992;10:1463–1469.

82. Stouffer GA, Owens GK. Angiotensin II induced mitogenesis of spontaneously hypertensive rat-derived cultured smooth muscle cells is dependent on autocrine production of transforming growth factor-β. *Circ Res* 1992;70:820–828.

83. Gibbons GH, Pratt RE, Dzau VJ. Vascular smooth muscle cell hypertrophy vs. hyperplasia. Autocrine transforming growth factor β. Expression determines growth response to angiotensin II. *J Clin Invest* 1992;90:456–461.

84. Itoh H, Mukoyama M, Pratt RE, Gibbons GH, Dzau VJ. Multiple autocrine growth factors modulate vascular smooth muscle cell growth response to angiotensin II. *J Clin Invest* 1993;91:2268–2274.

85. Koibuchi Y, Lee WS, Gibbons GH, Pratt RE. Role of transforming growth factor-β1 in the cellular growth response to angiotensin II. *Hypertension* 1993;21:1046–1050.

86. Weissberg PL, Witchell C, Davenport AP, Hesketh TR, Metcalfe JC. The endothelin peptides ET-1, ET-2, ET-3 and sarafotoxin S6b are co-mitogenic with platelet-derived growth factor for vascular smooth muscle cells. *Atherosclerosis* 1990;85:257–262.

87. Taubman MB, Bradford CB, Izumo S, Tsuda T, Alexander RW, Nadal-Ginard B. Angiotensin II induces c-fos mRNA in aortic smooth muscle. *J Biol Chem* 1989;264:526–530.

88. Naftilan AJ, Pratt RE, Eldridge CS, Lin HL, Dzau VJ. Angiotensin induces c-fos expression in smooth muscle via transcriptional control. *Hypertension* 1989;13:706–711.

89. Naftilan AJ, Pratt RE, Dzau VJ. Induction of platelet-derived growth factor A-chain and c-myc gene expression by angiotensin

II in cultured rat vascular smooth muscle cells. *J Clin Invest* 1989;83:1419–1424.

90. Naftilan AJ, Gilliland GK, Eldridge CS, Kraft AS. Induction of the proto-oncogene c-jun by angiotensin II. *Mol Cell Biol* 1990;10:5536–5540.

91. Daemen MJAP, Lombardi D, Bosman FT, Schwartz SM. Angiotensin II induces smooth muscle cell proliferation in the normal and injured rat arterial wall. *Circ Res* 1991;68:450–456.

92. Johnson RJ, Alpers CE, Yoshimura A, Lombardi D, Pritzl P, Floege J, Schwartz SM. Renal injury from angiotensin II-mediated hypertension. *Hypertension* 1992;19:464–474.

93. Altura BM, Altura BT. Vascular smooth muscle and neurohypophyseal hormones. *Fed Proc* 1977;36:1853–1860.

94. Hamada M, Nishio I, Baba A, Fukuda K, Takeda J, Ura M. Enhanced DNA synthesis of cultured vascular smooth muscle cells from spontaneously hypertensive rats: difference of response to growth factor, intracellular free calcium concentration and DNA synthesizing cell cycle. *Atherosclerosis* 1990;81:191–198.

95. Murase T, Kozawa O, Miwa M, Tokuda H, Kotoyori J, Kondo K, Oiso Y. Regulation of proliferation by vasopressin in aortic smooth muscle cells: function of protein kinase C. *J Hypertens* 1992;10:1505–1511.

96. Nabika T, Valletri PA, Lovenberg W, Beaven MA. Increase in cytosolic calcium and phosphoinositide metabolism induced by angiotensin II and vasopressin in vascular smooth muscle cells. *J Biol Chem* 1985;260:4661–4670.

97. Grillone LR, Clark MA, Godfrey RW, Stassen F, Crooke ST. Vasopressin induces V1 receptors to activate phosphatydilinositol- and phosphatydilcholine-specific phospholipase c and stimulates the release of arachidonic acid by at least two pathways in the smooth muscle cell line. *J Biol Chem* 1988;263:2658–2663.

98. Vallotton MB, Wthrich RP, Lew PD, Capponi AM. Effects of vasopressin and its analogues on rat aortic smooth muscle and renal medullary tubular cells: characterization of receptor subtypes. *J Cardiovasc Pharmacol* 1986;8(suppl 7):S5–S11.

99. Hassid A, Williams C. Vasoconstrictor-evoked prostaglandin synthesis in cultured vascular smooth muscle cells. *Am J Physiol* 1983;245:C278–C282.

100. Huttner JJ, Gwebu ET, Panganamala RV, Milo GE, Cornwell DG. Fatty acids and their prostaglandin derivatives: inhibitors of proliferation in aortic smooth muscle cells. *Science* 1977;197:289–291.

101. Loesberg C, van Wijk R, Zandvergen J, van Aken WG, van Mourik JA, de Groot PHG. Cell cycle-dependent inhibition of human vascular smooth muscle cell proliferation by prostaglandin E1. *Exp Cell Res* 1985;160:117–125.

102. Morisaki N, Kanzaki T, Motoyama N, Saito Y, Yoshida S. Cell cycle-dependent inhibition of DNA synthesis by prostaglandin E2 in cultured rabbit aortic smooth muscle cells. *Atherosclerosis* 1988;71:165–171.

103. Geisterfer AAT, Owens GK. Arginine vasopressin-induced hypertrophy of cultured rat aortic smooth muscle cells. *Hypertension* 1989;14:413–420.

104. Inoue A, Yanagisawa M, Kimura S, Kasuya Y, Miyauchi T, Goto K. The human endothelin family: three structurally and pharmacologically distinct isopeptides predicted by three separate genes. *Proc Natl Acad Sci USA* 1989;86:2863–2867.

105. Lüscher TF, Oemar BS, Boulanger CM, Hahn AWA. Molecular and cellular biology of endothelin and its receptors-Part I. *J Hypertens* 1993;11:7–11.

106. Lüscher TF, Oemar BS, Boulanger CM, Hahn AWA. Molecular and cellular biology of endothelin and its receptors-Part II. *J Hypertens* 1993;11:121–126.

107. Kanse SM, Takahashi K, Warren JB, Perera T, Porta M, Ghatei M, Bloom SR. Production of endothelin by vascular smooth muscle cells. *J Cardiovasc Pharmacol* 1991;17(suppl 7):S113–S116.

108. Resink TJ, Hahn AWA, Scott-Burden T, Powell J, Weber E, Buhler F. Inducible endothelin mRNA expression and peptide secretion in cultured human vascular smooth cells. *Biochem Biophys Res Commun* 1990;168:1303–1310.

109. Komuro I, Kurihara H, Sugiyama T, Takaku F, Yazaki Y. Endothelin stimulates c-fos and c-myc expression and proliferation of vascular smooth muscle cells. *FEBS Lett* 1988;238:249–252.

110. Bobik A, Grooms A, Millar JA, Mitchell A, Grinpukel S. Growth factor activity of endothelin on vascular smooth muscle. *Am J Physiol* 1990;258:C408–C415.

111. Libby P, Warner SJC, Salomon RN, Birinyi LK. Production of platelet-derived growth factor-like mitogen by smooth-muscle cells from human atheroma. *N Engl J Med* 1988;318:1493–1498.

112. Seifert RA, Hart CE, Philiphs PE, Forstrom JW, Ross R, Murray MJ, Bowen-Pope DF. Two different subunits associate to create isoform-specific platelet-derived growth factor receptors. *J Biol Chem* 1989;264:8771–8778.

113. Sachinidis A, Locher R, Vetter W, Tatje D, Hoppes J. Different effects of platelet-derived growth factor isoforms on rat vascular smooth muscle cells. *J Biol Chem* 1990;265:10238–10243.

114. Battegay EJ, Raines EW, Seifert RA, Bowen-Pope DF, Ross R. TGF-β1 induces bimodal proliferation of connective tissue cells via complex control of an autocrine PDGF loop. *Cell* 1990;63:515–524.

115. Sarzani R, Arnaldi G, Chobanian AV. Hypertension-induced changes of platelet-derived growth factor receptor expression in rat aorta and heart. *Hypertension* 1991;17:888–895.

116. Sarzani R, Brecher P, Chobanian AV. Growth factor expression in aorta of normotensive and hypertensive rats. *J Clin Invest* 1989;83:1404–1408.

117. Sarzani R, Arnaldi G, Takasaki I, Brecher P, Chobanian AV. Effects of hypertension and aging on platelet-derived growth factor receptor expression in rat aorta and heart. *Hypertension* 1991;18(suppl III):III-93–III-99.

118. Sarzani R, Paci VM, Pauletto P, Dessi Fulgheri P, Lanari A, Sartore S, Pessina AC, Rappelli A. Platelet-derived growth factor gene expression in renovascular hypertension (abstr). 13th Annual European Conference on Vascular Biology, Venice July 1–4, 1991.

119. Sara VR, Hall K. Insulinlike growth factors and their binding proteins. *Physiol Rev* 1990;70:591–614.

120. Clemmons DR, Shaw DS. Variables controlling somatomedin production by cultured human fibroblasts. *J Cell Physiol* 1983;115:137–142.

121. Delafontaine P, Lou H, Alexander RW. Regulation of insulin-like growth factor-I messenger RNA levels in vascular smooth muscle cells. *Hypertension* 1991;18:742–747.

122. Clemmons DR, Van Wyk JJ. Evidence for a functional role of endogenously produced somatomedinlike peptides in the regulation of DNA synthesis in cultured human fibroblasts and porcine smooth muscle cells. *J Clin Invest* 1985;75:1914–1918.

123. Clemmons DR. Interaction of circulating cell-derived and plasma growth factors in stimulating cultured smooth muscle cell replication. *J Cell Physiol* 1984;121:425–430.

124. Fath KA, Alexander RW, Delafontaine P. Abdominal coarctation increases insulinlike growth factor I mRNA levels in rat aorta. *Circ Res* 1993;72:271–277.

125. Delafontaine P, Bernstein KE, Alexander RW. Insulinlike growth factor I gene expression in vascular cells. *Hypertension* 1991;17:693–699.

126. Goldstein RH, Polliks CF, Pilch PF, Smith BD, Fine A. Stimulation of collagen formation by insulin and insulin-like growth factor I in culture of human lung fibroblasts. *Endocrinology* 1989;124:964–970.

127. Badesch DB, Lee PDK, Parks WC, Stenmark KR. Insulinlike growth factor stimulates elastin synthesis by bovine pulmonary arterial smooth muscle cells. *Biochem Biophys Res Commun* 1989;160:382–387.

128. Owens GK, Geisterfer AAT, Yang Y, Komoriya A. Transforming growth factor β induced growth inhibition and cellular hypertrophy in cultured vascular smooth muscle cells. *J Cell Biol* 1988;107:771–780.

129. Hamet P, Hadrava V, Kruppa V, Tremblay J. Transforming growth factor β1 and effect in aortic smooth muscle cells from spontaneously hypertensive rats. *Hypertension* 1991;17:896–901.

130. Bjorked S. Effects of transforming growth factor β1 on human arterial smooth muscle cells *in vitro*. *Arterioscl Thromb* 1991;11:892–901.

131. Ebner R, Chen RH, Shum L, Lawler S, Zioncheck TF, Lee A, Lopez AR, Derynck R. Cloning of a type I TGF-β1 receptor and

its effect on TGF-β binding to the type II receptor. *Science* 1993;260:1344–1348.

132. Chen R-H, Ebner R, Derynck R. Inactivation of the type II receptor reveals two receptor pathways for the diverse TGFβ activities. *Science* 1993;260:1344–1348.

133. Chen J-K, Hoshi H, McKeehan WL. Transforming growth factor type β specifically stimulates synthesis of proteoglycan in human adult arterial smooth muscle cells. *Proc Natl Acad Sci USA* 1987;84:5287–5291.

134. Majesky MW, Lindner V, Twardzik DR, Schwartz SM, Reidy MA. Production of transforming growth factor β1 during repair of arterial injury. *J Clin Invest* 1991;88:904–910.

135. Schonherr E, Jarvelainen HT, Sandell L, Wight TN. Effects of platelet-derived growth factor and transforming growth factor β1 on the synthesis of a large versicanlike chondroitin sulfate proteoglycan by arterial smooth muscle cells. *J Biol Chem* 1991;266:17640–17647.

136. Levi-Montalcini R. The nerve growth factor 35 years later. *Science* 1987;237:1154–1162.

137. Donohue SJ, Head RJ, Stitzel RE. Elevated nerve growth factor levels in young spontaneously hypertensive rats. *Hypertension* 1989;14:421–426.

138. Creedon D, Tuttle JB. Nerve growth factor synthesis in vascular smooth muscle. *Hypertension* 1991;18:730–741.

139. Bold AJ. Atrial natriuretic factor: a hormone produced by the heart. *Science* 1985;230:767–770.

140. Koller KJ, Goeddel DV. Molecular biology of the natriuretic peptides and their receptors. *Circulation* 1992;86:1081–1088.

141. Nakao K, Ogawa Y, Suga S-I, Imura K. Molecular biology and biochemistry of the natriuretic peptide system. I: Natriuretic peptides. *J Hypertens* 1992;10:907–912.

142. Suga S-I, Nakao K, Kishimoto I, Hosoda K, Mukoyama M, Arai H, Shirakami G, Ogawa Y, Komatsu Y, Nakagawa O, Hama N, Imura H. Phenotype-related alteration in expression of natriuretic peptide receptor in aortic smooth muscle cells. *Circ Res* 1992;71:34–39.

143. Nakao K, Ogawa Y, Suga S-I, Imura H. Molecular biology and biochemistry of the natriuretic peptide system. II: Natriuretic peptide receptors. *J Hypertens* 1992;10:1111–1114.

144. Mourlon-Le Grand MC, Poitevin P, Benessiano J, Duriez M, Michel JB, Levy BI. Effect of a nonhypotensive long-term infusion of ANP on the mechanical and structural properties of the arterial wall in Wistar-Kyoto and spontaneously hypertensive rats. *Arterioscl Thromb* 1993;13:640–650.

145. Itoh H, Pratt RE, Dzau VJ. Atrial natriuretic polypeptide inhibits hypertrophy of vascular smooth muscle cells. *J Clin Invest* 1990;86:1690–1697.

146. Garg UC, Hassid A. Nitric oxide-generating vasodilators and 8-bromo-cyclic guanosine monophosphate inhibit mitogenesis and proliferation of cultured rat vascular smooth muscle cells. *J Clin Invest* 1989;83:1774–1777.

147. Chaill PA, Hassid A. Differential antimitogenic effectiveness of atrial natriuretic peptides in primary versus subcultured rat aortic smooth muscle cells: relationship to expression of ANF-C receptors. *J Cell Physiol* 1993;154:28–38.

148. Gardner DG, Deschepper CF, Baxter JD. The gene for the atrial natriuretic factor is expressed in the aortic arch. *Hypertension* 1987;9:103–106.

149. Westenfelder C, Baranowski EH. Cultured aortic smooth muscle cells (SMC) secrete atrial natriuretic factor (ANF). *Kidney Int* 1990;37:343a.

150. Singo AJ, Clavell AL, Aarhus LL, Burnett JC. Cardiovascular and renoaction of C-type natriuretic peptide. *Am J Physiol* 1992;262:H308–H312.

151. Komatsu Y, Nakao K, Itoh H, Suga S-I, Ogawa Y, Imura H. Vascular natriuretic peptide. *Lancet* 1992;340:622.

152. Furuya M, Takehisa Y, Minamitake Y, Kitajima Y, Hayashi Y, Ohnuma N, Ishihara T, Minamino, Kangawa K, Matsuo H. A novel natriuretic peptide, CNP, potently stimulates cyclic GMP production in rat cultured smooth muscle cells. *Biochem Biophys Res Commun* 1990;170:201–208.

153. Suga S-I, Nakao K, Itoh H, Komatsu Y, Ogawa Y, Hama N, Imura H. Endothelial production of C-type natriuretic peptide and its marked augmentation by transforming growth factor β. *J Clin Invest* 1992;90:12145–12149.

154. Porter JG, Catalano R, McEnroe G, Lewicki JA, Protter AA. C-type natriuretic peptide inhibits growth factor-dependent synthesis in smooth muscle cells. *Am J Physiol* 1992;263:C1001–C1006.

155. Furuya M, Yoshida M, Hayashi Y, Ohnuma N, Minamino N, Kangawa K, Matsuo H. C-type natriuretic peptide is a growth inhibitor of rat vascular smooth muscle cells. *Biochem Biophys Res Commun* 1991;177:927–931.

Blood Pressure Regulation in Normal and Hypertensive States

Part B: Neural and Other Humoral Factors in the Control of Arterial Pressure

Hypertension: Pathophysiology, Diagnosis, and Management, Second Edition, edited by J.H. Laragh and B.M. Brenner, Raven Press, Ltd., New York © 1995.

CHAPTER **42**

The Role of the Central Nervous System in Hypertension

Suzanne Oparil, Yiu-Fai Chen, Kathleen H. Berecek, David A. Calhoun, and J. Michael Wyss

The central nervous system (CNS) plays an important role in the regulation of the cardiovascular system. By controlling both peripheral autonomic nervous system activity and the release of hormones, the CNS acutely

S. Oparil, Y.-F. Chen, and D. A. Calhoun: Vascular Biology and Hypertension Program of the Division of Cardiovascular Disease, Department of Medicine, University of Alabama, Birmingham, Alabama 35294.
 K. H. Berecek: Department of Physiology and Biophysics, and Vascular Biology and Hypertension Program of the Division of Cardiovascular Disease, Department of Medicine, University of Alabama, Birmingham, Alabama 35294.
 J. M. Wyss: Department of Cell Biology, and Vascular Biology and Hypertension Program of the Division of Cardiovascular Disease, Department of Medicine, University of Alabama, Birmingham, Alabama 35294.

modifies blood pressure and heart rate, thus facilitating cardiovascular homeostasis and appropriate responses to the environment. While this moment-to-moment control of the cardiovascular system is well accepted, the role of the CNS in the chronic regulation of the cardiovascular system has been less clear. Early clinical studies suggested that the CNS and peripheral sympathetic nerves were involved intimately in hypertension. However, methods for dissecting the role of non-neural factors, such as the renal pressor system, in the disease tended to precede similar developments in neurobiology, and thus the role of the brain was not pursued as rigorously. During the past 20 years neurobiology has made great progress and has provided important new tools for the investigation of the role of the CNS in hypertension. Using new tract tracing and electron microscopic techniques,

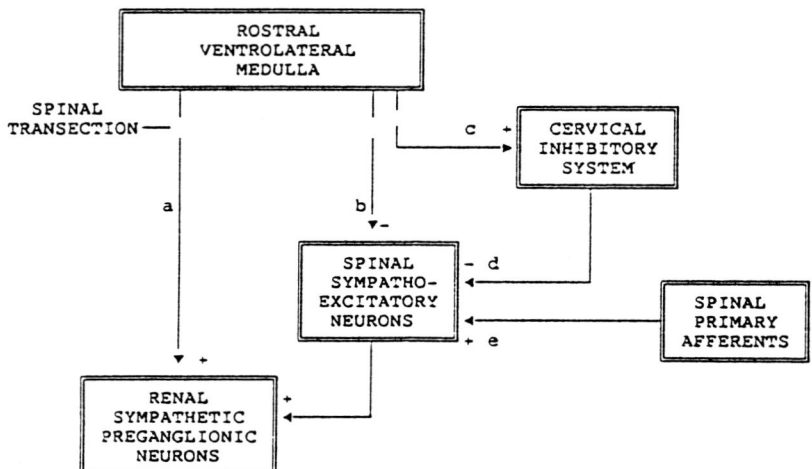

FIG. 1. Poree and Schramm suggest that a combination of inputs from the ventrolateral medulla and cervical spinal cord (spinal sympathoexcitatory neurons) modulates the activity of the renal sympathetic, preganglionic neurons in the thoracic spinal cord and thereby regulates renal function. Activation of the rostral ventrolateral medulla stimulates the preganglionic neurons directly, and indirectly causes inhibition of the sensory feedback (*e*) to these neurons (*b and c, d*). This inhibitory role of the cervical spinal cord is difficult to observe in intact rats, but is obvious after transection of the medullary input to the spinal cord, as shown (*from 3a*). When these pathways are transected, as shown, the inhibitory role of the cervical inhibitory network is revealed. (From ref. 3, with permission.)

researchers have characterized the brain regions that influence the cardiovascular system, and using electrophysiological and pharmacological techniques, they have elucidated the interactions between these nuclei, the peripheral nervous system, and neurohormonal control of the cardiovascular system. Most recently, the use of immunocytochemical techniques and molecular approaches has greatly facilitated these studies. It is now clear that the nervous system contributes directly to some forms of hypertension and plays at least a permissive role in all forms of the disorder. This chapter considers those areas of the CNS that appear to be most important in cardiovascular regulation, then reviews the evidence suggesting that specific neurotransmitter systems in these areas are causally related to the development and/or maintenance of hypertension.

THE SPINAL CORD

The sympathetic nervous system regulates arterial pressure principally by controlling the diameter of resistance vessels. The final common pathway for CNS regulation of the sympathetic nervous system comprises the preganglionic neurons of the thoracic spinal cord, which are condensed into four separate cell groups, the largest of which is the intermediolateral cell column (IML) (1,2). The activity of these neurons is controlled by sensory innervation from the periphery, by descending projections from the brain, and by neurons in the cervical spinal cord which appear to inhibit the access of information to the preganglionic neurons (Fig. 1) (3,4). Abnormalities in the peripheral sensory and spinal cord innervation of the sympathetic preganglionic neurons may play a role in some forms of hypertension, but the CNS innervation of these neurons appears to provide the predominant nervous system contribution to hypertension in most animal models and in humans.

THE MEDULLA

The Nucleus Tractus Solitarius (NTS)

The NTS is the primary site of termination for carotid and aortic baroreceptor afferents (5), and the neurons of the NTS regulate blood pressure by influencing sympathetic nervous system activity and vasopressin release (6). In rats, ablation of the NTS produces fulminating hypertension (7), while in other species NTS lesions cause a less severe form of chronic hypertension (8). In addition to the cardiovascular afferents, the NTS receives several visceral inputs including those from the kidney (9,10). The NTS also receives projections from many cardiovascular regulatory nuclei in diverse brain regions, including telencephalon (11,12), hypothalamus (13,14), cerebellum (15) and brainstem (16) and from the spinal cord (17). Thus, the NTS can influence cardiovascular regulation in response to many sources of information. In the spontaneously hypertensive rat (SHR), the glutaminergic, cholinergic, and atrial natriuretic peptide innervation of the NTS is disturbed, and these abnormalities appear to contribute to the development of hypertension in this model (18,19; also see below).

The NTS projects indirectly to sympathetic preganglionic sympathetic neurons and directly to parasympathetic preganglionic neurons that project to the heart. It also projects both directly and indirectly to the paraventricular nucleus of the hypothalamus and thereby can modify the activity of vasopressin-releasing neurons (20). The NTS projects to the amygdala, where it can influence emotional responses (21).

The Parasympathetic Preganglionic Nuclei

Neurons in the dorsal motor nucleus of the vagus and the nucleus ambiguus project to the heart. While early reports suggested that the cardioinhibitory neurons were located in and around the dorsal motor nucleus of the vagus, more recent reports have localized most of these neurons in the nucleus ambiguus (22). Damage to the nucleus ambiguus results in diminished heart rate control, while stimulation of these neurons elicits bradycardic responses (23–25). Further, 2-deoxy-^{14}C glucose studies in the rat indicate that the nucleus ambiguus is more active than other brain stem nuclei during reflex bradycardia (26). The nucleus ambiguus is involved in blood pressure regulation, probably through connections to pressor areas in the medulla (27). Stimulation of the nucleus ambiguus evokes pressor effects which appear to be independent of the cardioinhibitory response (27), while lesions of the nucleus ambiguus facilitate the development of hypertension in sinoaortic denervated rats (24). Thus, both the dorsal motor nucleus of the vagus and the nucleus ambiguus contain preganglionic neurons that influence the cardiovascular system, but the nucleus ambiguus appears to be the predominant site of origin of the cardiac depressor projections.

The Ventrolateral Medulla

The ventrolateral medulla plays a critical role in the tonic control of vasomotor tone (28–31). Many of the neurons in this region project to the spinal cord, where they innervate the sympathetic autonomic nuclei (28,29). Stimulation of neurons in the rostral ventrolateral medulla elicits increases in heart rate and blood pressure, release of catecholamines from the adrenal medulla and release of arginine vasopressin (AVP) from the neurohypophysis (30). Conversely, reduction in the activity of these neurons, either through permanent lesion or temporary blockade, causes arterial pressure to fall to levels observed following spinal cord transection (31). These studies strongly suggest that neurons in the rostral ventrolateral medulla, including the subretrofacial nucleus, maintain background input to vasomotor centers in the spinal cord, and thereby tonically regulate sympathetic nervous system activity and arterial pressure (Fig. 2) (32). The phenotype of these neurons has not been fully elucidated. Reis and colleagues have focused on adrenergic neurons, while Guyenet and Dampney (33,34) have shown that noncatecholaminergic neurons in this region contribute importantly to vasomotor tone. The latter view is supported by the finding that application of adrenaline to the sympathetic preganglionic neurons reduces, rather than increases, the firing of sympathetic axons (33,35). Further, neurons in the rostral ventrolateral medulla that display pacemaker activity and project to the thoracic spinal cord do not express an adrenergic phenotype (36). At least a portion of the rostral ventro-

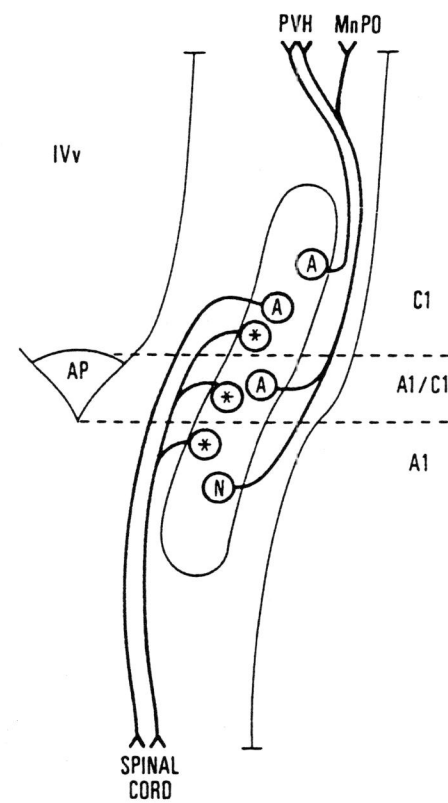

FIG. 2. The ventrolateral medulla sends cholinergic (*A and N*) and noncholinergic (*) projections to the spinal cord and to the hypothalamus, thus directly and indirectly influencing sympathetic nervous system activity. AP, area postrema; IVv, fourth ventricle; MnPO, median preoptic nucleus; PVH, paraventricular hypothalamic nucleus. (From ref. 32, with permission.)

lateral medulla neurons that project to the sympathetic preganglionic neurons use glutamate as a neurotransmitter (37), and these may provide the primary excitatory input from the medulla to the preganglionic neurons.

The neurons in the rostral ventrolateral medulla are innervated by areas of the NTS that receive baroreflex information (38), and lesions in these regions of the NTS produce hypertension. Conversely, unilateral lesions of the rostral ventrolateral medulla do not alter arterial pressure, but do abolish reflex responses to baroreflex stimulation that are mediated via the ipsilateral NTS. The finding that lesions in the C1 area abolish the hypertension elicited by lesions of the NTS lends further support for a role of the rostral ventrolateral medulla in NTS-mediated cardiovascular reflexes (39).

Immediately caudal to the rostral ventrolateral medulla is the A1 area (caudal ventrolateral medulla), which contains noradrenergic neurons (Fig. 2) (32). Stimulation of this region inhibits sympathetic discharge and lowers blood pressure, and lesions in this region elicit hypertension (40,41). Unlike the rostral ventrolateral medulla neurons, the A1 neurons do not have direct access to the spinal cord; instead their inhibitory function is mediated through the rostral ventrolateral neurons (42). The caudal ventrolateral medulla is composed of a rostral segment which plays a major role in the baroreceptor reflex and a caudal segment which inhibits sympathetic activity independent of the baroreflex response (43). Localized, bilateral lesions of the neurons in the rostral ventrolateral medulla completely abolish A1-induced hypotension, suggesting that noradrenaline released by A1 neurons has a powerful inhibitory influence on tonic vasomotor control. The sympathoinhibitory function of the caudal ventrolateral medulla appears to be reduced in the SHR compared with that in normotensive control rats (44). In contrast, the pressor responses to angiotensin injections into the rostral ventrolateral medulla are increased in SHR compared with that in control rats (45).

The Area Postrema

The area postrema lies immediately dorsal to the NTS and receives baroreceptor information. It lacks a blood brain barrier and thus can monitor the circulating concentrations of peptides, including angiotensin II, which stimulate sympathetic nervous system activity. Ablation of the area postrema causes a moderate, sustained decrease in blood pressure in normotensive dogs, while electrical stimulation of this area results in increases in arterial pressure (46). These effects are likely mediated by the projections of the area postrema to cardiovascular regulatory nuclei in the brainstem (47). Lesions of the area postrema prevent deoxycorticosterone-NaCl (DOCA-NaCl) induced hypertension in the rat (48,49) and attenuate spontaneous hypertension in SHR (50), suggesting that this area participates in the pathogenesis of neurogenic hypertension in rats.

THE PONS AND MIDBRAIN

The parabrachial nucleus contributes importantly to arterial pressure regulation. Visceral afferent information projects directly to this nucleus via the NTS (51,52), and individual neurons in the region are influenced by baroreceptor activation (53). The area also receives projections from forebrain regions, including the hypothalamus, ventral forebrain, and cortex (54). These two types of information are integrated by parabrachial neurons which exert visceral control via their efferent connections with the forebrain (particularly limbic and hypothalamic areas), medulla (NTS and reticular formation), and spinal cord (54,55). High-frequency electrical stimulation of some areas within the parabrachial nucleus increases heart rate and arterial pressure in the cat (56). The descending projections of the parabrachial nucleus appears to be important in arterial pressure regulation. Localized stimulation of the parabrachial nucleus results in tachycardia and hypertension that is not eliminated by decerebration above the brainstem. The parabrachial nucleus has a potent modulatory influence on NTS neurons that receive afferent cardiovascular information (57). Further, an intact lateral parabrachial nucleus is necessary for the expression of angiotensin-induced hypertension in the rat (58).

The periaqueductal region of the midbrain also appears to contribute importantly to cardiovascular regulation. Microinjection of excitatory amino acids into this region elicits a cardiovascular defense reaction characterized by skeletal muscle vasodilatation (59). These studies indicate that the periaqueductal gray, which has connections with both the limbic forebrain and the brainstem, may be important in stress-induced hypertension.

THE HYPOTHALAMUS

A number of hypothalamic nuclei containing several different neurotransmitters contribute to cardiovascular regulation (60,61). Many researchers have examined hypothalamic neurotransmitter stores, uptake, release, and receptor mechanisms in various forms of hypertension. Electrophysiological studies have demonstrated that certain hypothalamic nuclei receive cardiovascular sensory input and that stimulation of discrete hypothalamic sites elicits increases or decreases in heart rate, cardiac output, and blood pressure. A critical role of the hypothalamus in hypertension has also been supported by Eilam et al., who demonstrated that transplantation of hypothalamic neurons and glial cells from an SHR to a normotensive rat induces hypertension, while transplantation of similar tissue from a normotensive rat to a normotensive rat has no sustained effect on arterial pressure (Fig. 3) (62).

Pressor Regions

The lateral and posterior hypothalamic areas and the ventrolateral hypothalamic nucleus are generally recognized as sympathoexcitatory regions (63–66). The lateral and posterior hypothalamic areas contain neurons that project directly to the medulla and spinal cord (67,68), and stimulation of the posterior hypothalamic nucleus increases sympathetic nervous system activity and attenuates baroreflex-induced bradycardia (69). In contrast, lesions of this area reduce arterial pressure in renal and DOCA-NaCl hypertensive rats and in SHR (70), and electrical stimulation of the neurons in this region results in greater pressor effects in SHR than in normotensive control rats (71). Neurotransmitter imbalances in the posterior hypothalamus also appear to contribute to hypertension. In the posterior hypothalamic area of SHR compared with that of normotensive control rats, norad-

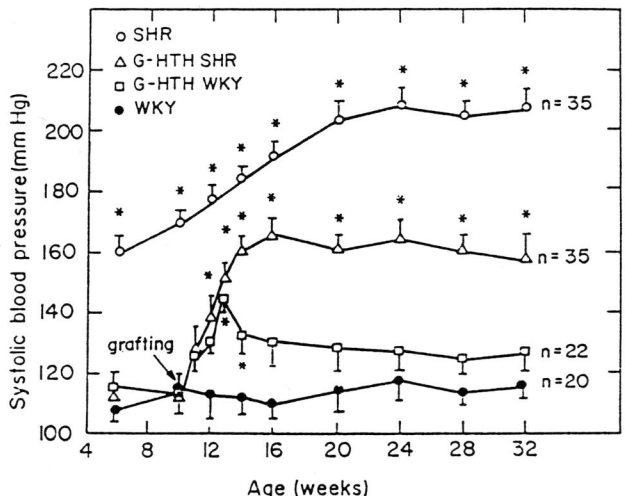

FIG. 3. Changes in systolic arterial pressure in control SHR and control WKY, and in WKY in which neurons from the hypothalamus of embryonic SHR (G-HTH SHR) or WKY (G-HTH WKY) were implanted into the hypothalamus. The WKY transplant caused a transient increase in arterial pressure, but the SHR transplant elicited a much larger and sustained hypertension. (From ref. 62, with permission.)

renergic and cholinergic inputs appear to be activated (72,73), and the ability of gamma-aminobutyric acid (GABA) to inhibit neurons appears to be suppressed (74).

The Paraventricular Nucleus

The paraventricular nucleus of the hypothalamus contributes to the CNS regulation of the cardiovascular system by activation of sympathetic outflow and vasopressin release (75). This nucleus is innervated by medullary neurons that convey baroreflex and cardiovascular information (76–78) and hypothalamic neurons that likely convey both cardiovascular and emotional information (78). The paraventricular nucleus projects reciprocally to the NTS, the vagal parasympathetic nuclei, and the thoracic sympathetic neurons (Fig. 4) (20,79,80).

Several lines of evidence suggest that the paraventricular nucleus contributes to some forms of hypertension. (a) Caverson and Ciriello (81) demonstrated that renal nerve stimulation excites neurons in the paraventricular nucleus, and that the latter neurons modulate the activity of renal sympathetic axons, thus providing a reflex loop for renal control. It is likely that this pathway plays a role in forms of hypertension in which afferent renal nerve activity is altered (82). (b) The activity of these sympathoexcitatory neurons is modulated by blood pressure changes. The metabolic activity of neurons in the paraventricular nucleus is greater in SHR than in normotensive control rats, and when arterial pressure is reduced, the metabolic activity of these neurons is re-

duced in SHR (83). (c) SHR (compared with normotensive control rats) display an increase in basal and K^+ induced release of noradrenaline from terminals in the paraventricular nucleus (84). (d) The paraventricular region appears to be the primary brain target of ouabain-like factors that elicit pressor responses (85). Together, these findings suggest that functional abnormalities in the paraventricular nucleus contribute to hypertension in several rodent models (84).

The Anterior Hypothalamus

Johnson and his colleagues demonstrated that the anteroventral third ventricle (AV3V) region of the hypothalamus is involved in the pathogenesis of hypertension in the rat (86). The single most important component of AV3V is the median preoptic nucleus, which receives afferents from the circumventricular organs, the parabrachial nucleus, the NTS, and catecholaminergic nuclei in the pons and medulla (87,88). Lesions of AV3V cause

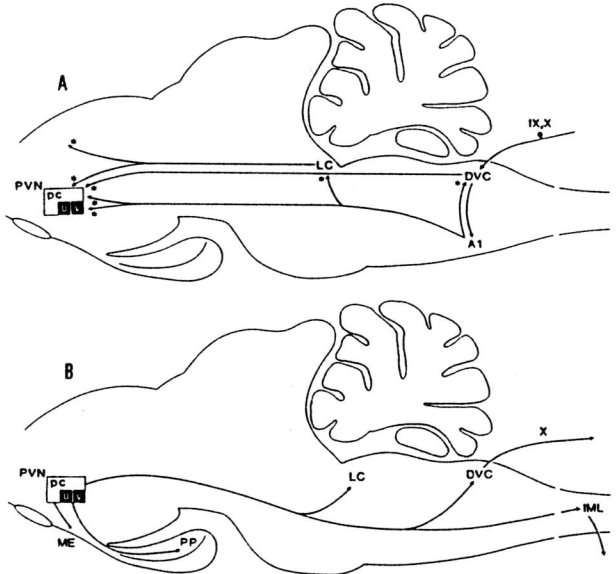

FIG. 4. A: Organization of ascending, predominantly noradrenergic projections (*) to the paraventricular nucleus. **B:** Organization of efferent projections from the paraventricular nucleus which appear to be involved in the central control of cardiovascular function. The parvicellular division of the paraventricular nucleus projects to preganglionic cell groups of both divisions of the autonomic nervous system in the brainstem and spinal cord; to the locus ceruleus; and to the median eminence. Neurons in the magnocellular division of the paraventricular nucleus project directly to the posterior lobe of the pituitary, where they release AVPn into the circulation. A1, A1 catecholaminergic cell group; DVC, dorsal vagal complex; ME, median eminence; IML, intermediolateral cell column of spinal cord; IX, glossopharyngeal nerve; X, vagus nerve; LC, locus ceruleus; PP, posterior pituitary; pc, parvicellular division of the paraventricular nucleus. (From ref. 20, with permission.)

significant decreases in blood pressure and/or prevent the expression of hypertension in most animal models. The major exception to this is the SHR (89). Stimulation of AV3V neurons elicits regionally specific pressor and depressor responses (90). Further, the AV3V region is involved in reflex control of arterial pressure, including the baroreflex (91) and some components of renal reflexes (92). AV3V is also involved in fluid and electrolyte homeostasis (86), likely through atrial natriuretic peptide (ANP) containing neurons within this region (93).

The anterior hypothalamic area, which lies immediately caudal to AV3V, plays an important role in blood pressure control. Electrolytic lesions in this area produce fulminating hypertension in normotensive Sprague-Dawley rats (94), and electrical stimulation of anterior hypothalamic area lowers blood pressure in normotensive animals (95–97). Further, studies in the cat suggest that the anterior hypothalamic area may be a vagal excitatory center (95,96). Both vagal and sympathetic outflow are modified by neurons in this area, since destruction of the anterior hypothalamic area results in an increased pressor response and decreased bradycardia following intravenous injection of phenylephrine (98).

Intracerebroventricular (ICV) NaCl loading reduces the sympathoinhibitory responses elicited by anterior hypothalamic area stimulation (99). Further, the discharge rate of anterior hypothalamic neurons is altered by carotid sinus nerve stimulation (100) or baroreceptor activation in isolated carotid sinus preparations (101). Neurons in this region respond to atrial stretch (102), and noradrenaline release is increased in the anterior hypothalamic area during baroreceptor activation (103). Thus, anterior hypothalamic neurons appear to represent important components of the baroreflex pathway, and reduced baroreceptor-mediated input to these depressor neurons may underlie some forms of spontaneous hypertension (104).

Direct measurement of noradrenaline release from the anterior hypothalamic area in freely moving rabbits demonstrates that chemically induced increases in arterial pressure enhance noradrenaline release from the anterior hypothalamic area, while chemically induced decreases in blood pressure decrease noradrenaline release from this area (105). These changes are opposite in direction to the blood pressure changes observed in the posterior hypothalamic area (a pressor region) of rabbits chal-

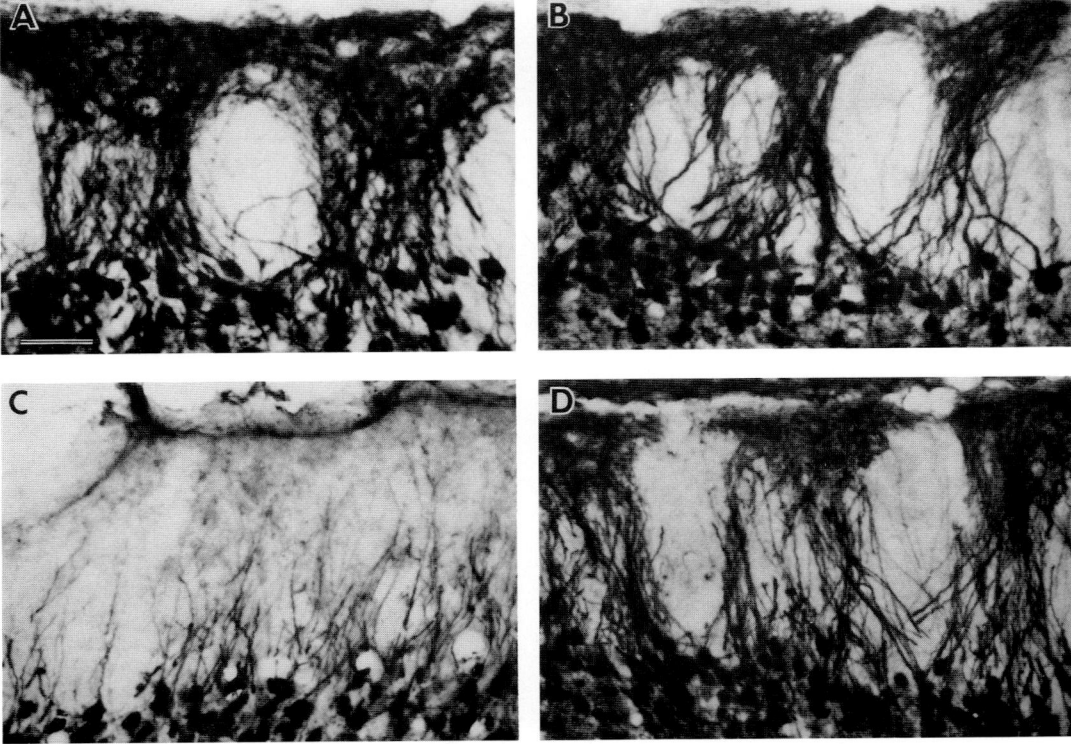

FIG. 5. Photomicrograph depicting the age-related breakdown of apical dendrites in the retrosplenial cortex of the SHR. **A** and **B** display the normal pattern of dendrites in a normotensive Sprague-Dawley (**A**) and a hypertensive SHR (**B**) at 4 months of age. **C** demonstrates the disorganization of the dendrites in a 14-month-old SHR, and **D** demonstrates a normal bundling pattern in a 14-month-old SHR that was normotensive throughout life due to continuous treatment with captopril. In the 12-month-old untreated SHR, the disorganization of these dendrites is associated with a deficit in learning and memory. Lifetime captopril treatment prevents both the breakdown and the cognitive impairment in 12-month-old SHR. Scale bar = 25 μm. (From ref. 117, with permission.)

lenged in the same way. Further, as considered below, microinjection of adrenergic agonists into the anterior hypothalamic area causes depressor responses (an effect that is mediated, in part, by increased local GABA release [106]) that are greater in magnitude in hypertensive than normotensive rats (107). Taken together, these studies strongly suggest that the anterior hypothalamic area plays a role in the sympathoinhibitory control of systemic blood pressure.

THE CEREBRAL CORTEX

Other regions of the forebrain, particularly those cortical and subcortical regions which form the "limbic cortex," also modulate blood pressure (108,109). Four areas, the amygdala (110,111), the septal nuclei (112), the insular cortex (113), and the cingulate cortex (114), have received particular attention as potential cardiovascular regulatory centers. Since these areas are involved in learning, emotional responses (especially the defense reaction), and the integration of information from higher centers, they are likely to be most important in the pathogenesis of hypertension that is related to environmental stress.

Several recent reports have suggested a relationship between hypertension, damage to the cerebral cortex, and cognitive impairment. In mature SHR, the lateral cerebral ventricles display a progressive dilation that appears to compromise the cortical mantle (115). The increase in size of the ventricles is not attenuated by antihypertensive treatment (115). Whatever the relationship between hypertension and ventricular expansion in the SHR, the result is atrophy of the cortical mantle (116). Cortical damage in the SHR is relatively selective for the limbic cortex (117), and structural damage is correlated with an early onset of learning and memory deficits in aging SHR (118). Interestingly, the limbic damage and the cognitive impairment are prevented by lifetime antihypertensive treatment with angiotensin-converting enzyme inhibitors (Fig. 5) (117,118). Pilot studies in normotensive patients with Alzheimer's disease suggest that angiotensin-converting enzyme inhibitors may have similar cognitive effects in humans (119).

NEUROTRANSMITTER-SPECIFIC PATHWAYS

Monoaminergic Mechanisms

Studies of the contribution of the central nervous system to hypertension have focused on the role of central monoaminergic neurons, largely because these neurotransmitters can be easily measured and are known to be involved in peripheral sympathetic nervous system control of cardiovascular function. These studies have demonstrated that (a) alterations in monoaminergic neurons

in the central nervous system accompany hypertension, (b) damage to the monoaminergic system attenuates hypertension in some models, (c) interventions that lower blood pressure often affect central monoaminergic neurons, and (d) dietary NaCl-induced increases in arterial pressure are accompanied by specific alterations in central monoaminergic systems, thus suggesting that central monoaminergic mechanisms play a pathogenetic role in the development of NaCl-sensitive hypertension.

Noradrenaline and Adrenaline

The Spontaneously Hypertensive Rat (SHR) of the Okamoto Strain

The SHR has been used extensively to study genetically determined hypertension and its effects on the cardiovascular system (120,121). Destruction of central noradrenergic neurons with intracerebroventricular 6-hydroxydopamine prevents the subsequent development of hypertension in the SHR (122,123), and monoamine stores and activity in brain regions that are involved in cardiovascular regulation are altered during the developmental phase of hypertension in this model (72,124). In addition, the activity of the catecholamine-synthesizing enzymes dopamine-beta-hydroxylase (DBH) and phenylethanolamine N-methyltransferase (PNMT) are altered in these brain regions in developing SHR, suggesting that altered catecholamine synthesis in critical blood pressure regulating pathways of the brain plays a pathogenic role in the development of hypertension in these rats. Increased arterial plasma noradrenaline levels have also been observed at the onset of blood pressure elevation in the SHR, suggesting that sympathetic outflow from the central nervous system is increased prior to the development of established hypertension, providing a neurogenic basis for the subsequent elevation in blood pressure.

The Role of Central Noradrenaline in NaCl-sensitive Hypertension in SHR

Bilateral renal denervation reduces renal sympathetic tone, prevents Na$^+$ retention, and delays the development of hypertension in young SHR but does not alter these indices in adult SHR with established hypertension (125). Further, in the young SHR, ingestion of a high NaCl diet exacerbates hypertension, increases peripheral sympathetic nervous-system activity, and alters the noradrenaline content of hypothalamic nuclei known to be involved in the blood pressure regulation (126–129). None of these changes is observed in response to oral NaCl loading in normotensive Wistar-Kyoto (WKY) rats or in mature SHR. These findings suggest that in the SHR, sympathetic nervous-system activity is increased during the developmental phase of NaCl-sensitive hypertension and acts as a trigger to set off a series of events that lead to chronic hypertension.

To further delineate the role of the brain in NaCl-sensitive hypertension, our laboratory has characterized two substrains of SHR. One, the NaCl-sensitive SHR (SHR-S), develops marked increases in blood pressure and peripheral sympathetic nervous system activity when fed a high NaCl diet. The other, the NaCl-resistant SHR (SHR-R), is resistant to the pressor effects of dietary NaCl supplementation. SHR-S maintained on a high NaCl diet display increases in arterial pressure and selective decreases in noradrenaline stores in anterior hypothalamus (128,129). These observations led to the hypothesis that dietary NaCl loading increases blood pressure in SHR-S by reducing noradrenaline release from nerve terminals in the anterior hypothalamus, a brain region that exerts an inhibitory influence on sympathetic nervous-system activity and arterial pressure (Fig. 6). To test this hypothesis, we characterized re-

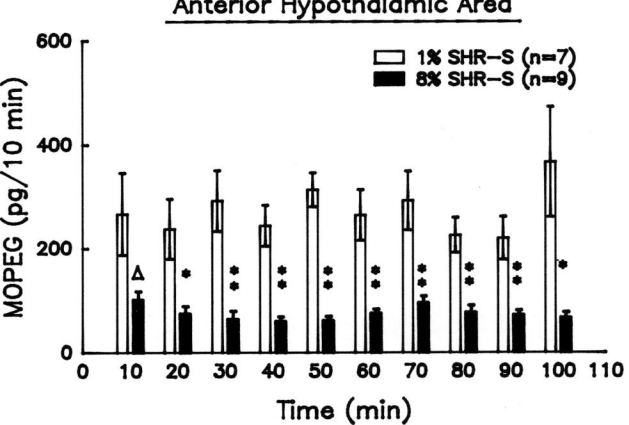

FIG. 7. MOPEG content of each 10-min aliquot of AHA perfusate in 1 percent or 8 percent NaCl-fed SHR-S. Each vertical bar represents the mean ± S.E.M. $\Delta p < 0.1$; *$p < 0.05$; **$p < 0.01$, compared with respective values of the 1 percent NaCl-fed control group. (From ref. 130, with permission.)

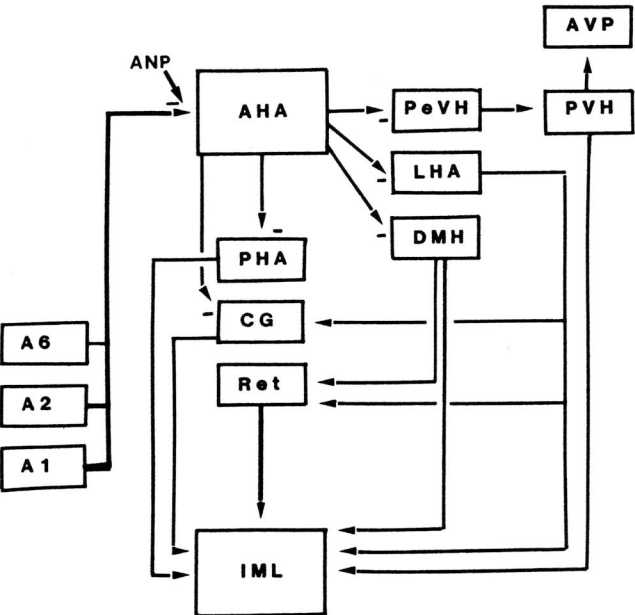

FIG. 6. Schematic representation of the major noradrenergic projections to the anterior hypothalamic area and the major direct and indirect projection from anterior hypothalamic area to "pressor" nuclei. In SHR, increased activity of the inhibitory neuromodulator ANF in anterior hypothalamic area and reduced input from baroreceptor afferents synapsing in brainstem nuclei reduce noradrenaline release in anterior hypothalamic area, resulting in reduced inhibitory control of sympathetic outflow. The (−) indicates synaptic inhibition. A_1, A_2, A_6, brainstem noradrenergic nuclei; AHA, anterior hypothalamic area; AVP, arginine vasopressin release; CG, central gray of the midbrain; DMH, dorsomedial nucleus of the hypothalamus; IML, preganglionic sympathetic nucleus; LHA, lateral hypothalamic area; PeVH, periventricular hypothalamic nucleus; PHA, posterior hypothalamic area; PVH, paraventricular hypothalamic nucleus; Ret, medullary reticular formation. (From ref. 132, with permission.)

gional brain noradrenaline turnover in SHR-S, WKY, and SHR-R fed high and basal NaCl diets. Consumption of an 8 percent NaCl diet increased blood pressure by ~20 mm Hg in SHR-S but had no effect in SHR-R and WKY. The high NaCl diet was associated with a selective decrease in noradrenaline turnover in the anterior hypothalamus of SHR-S on the 8 percent (compared to 1 percent) NaCl diet ($t_{1/2} = 6.3$ hr in 8 percent NaCl fed SHR-S versus 2.3 hr in 1 percent NaCl fed SHR-S; $p < 0.05$). NaCl supplementation had no effect on noradrenaline turnover in any other brain region in SHR-S or in any brain region tested in SHR-R or WKY. A subsequent study tested directly the hypothesis that dietary NaCl supplementation decreases the local release of noradrenaline from nerve terminals in the anterior hypothalamic region of the SHR-S (130). The push-pull microinfusion technique was used to measure basal release of noradrenaline and steady-state levels of 3-methoxy-4-hydroxyphenylglycol (MOPEG, the major metabolite of norepinephrine in brain) in the anterior hypothalamic region of SHR-S and WKY rats. MOPEG levels in the push-pull microperfusate bathing nerve terminals in the anterior hypothalamic region were significantly reduced in SHR-S receiving dietary NaCl supplementation (Fig. 7). MOPEG levels in anterior hypothalamic perfusates of control WKY rats were not affected by dietary NaCl intake. These findings are consistent with the hypothesis that dietary NaCl loading elevates blood pressure in SHR-S by decreasing the release of noradrenaline from noradrenergic nerve terminals in the anterior hypothalamus, thus reducing noradrenergic input to depressor neurons in the anterior hypothalamic area (AHA) and increasing peripheral sympathetic nervous system activity. NaCl-resistant SHR-R and WKY are genetically resistant to these effects of dietary NaCl.

Together with evidence from other laboratories that central α_2 adrenoceptors are altered by changes in dietary NaCl in SHR-S (98,131), these findings led us to hypothesize that the reduction in noradrenaline release in the anterior hypothalamic area of NaCl-loaded SHR-S results in an upregulation of postsynaptic α_2 adrenoceptors in the anterior hypothalamic region. To test this hypothesis, the α_2 adrenoceptor agonist clonidine was microinjected into the anterior hypothalamic area of SHR-S, SHR-R, and WKY fed high or basal NaCl diets, and its effects on blood pressure and heart rate were determined (107,132,133). Clonidine caused dose-dependent, rapid-onset depressor and bradycardic responses that were significantly greater in NaCl-supplemented SHR-S; responses were unaffected by NaCl supplementation in SHR-R and WKY rats. Pretreatment with the selective α_2 adrenoceptor antagonist rauwolscine blocked the depressor and bradycardic effects of clonidine, confirming the α_2 adrenoceptor specificity of the responses. Further, low affinity binding of [³H]-p-aminoclonidine in the anterior hypothalamic region was increased significantly in SHR-S but not in normotensive WKY rats on a high NaCl diet (134). Autoradiographic analysis confirmed that [³H]-p-aminoclonidine binding was increased selectively in the anterior hypothalamic area of NaCl-supplemented SHR-S. In contrast, in the posterior hypothalamic region of SHR-S, α_2-adrenoceptors were significantly reduced during consumption of a high NaCl diet. The high NaCl diet did not alter α_2-adrenoceptors in the medulla, nor did it affect α_1- or β-adrenoceptors in any brain region studied in either strain.

These data suggest that in SHR-S, dietary NaCl supplementation exacerbates hypertension by reducing noradrenaline release from nerve terminals in the anterior hypothalamic area, thereby upregulating α_2-adrenergic receptors and causing withdrawal of sympathoinhibition. We subsequently tested the hypothesis that tonic activation of anterior hypothalamic α_2-adrenergic receptors by chronic local microinfusion of clonidine prevents NaCl-sensitive hypertension in SHR-S by enhancing α_2-adrenergic receptor-mediated sympathoinhibition (135). We observed that chronic microinfusion of clonidine into the anterior hypothalamic area in doses that did not alter blood pressure when administered systemically offset the hypertensive effect of dietary NaCl supplementation and attenuated the enhancing effects of dietary NaCl on left ventricular mass and plasma noradrenaline levels (Fig. 8). These data support the hypothesis that salt-induced hypertension in SHR-S is associated with diminished sympathoinhibitory function of central α_2-adrenergic receptors and that chronic microinfusion of clonidine into the anterior hypothalamic area prevents salt-sensitive hypertension in this model, at least in part, by enhancing α_2-adrenergic receptor-mediated sympathoinhibition.

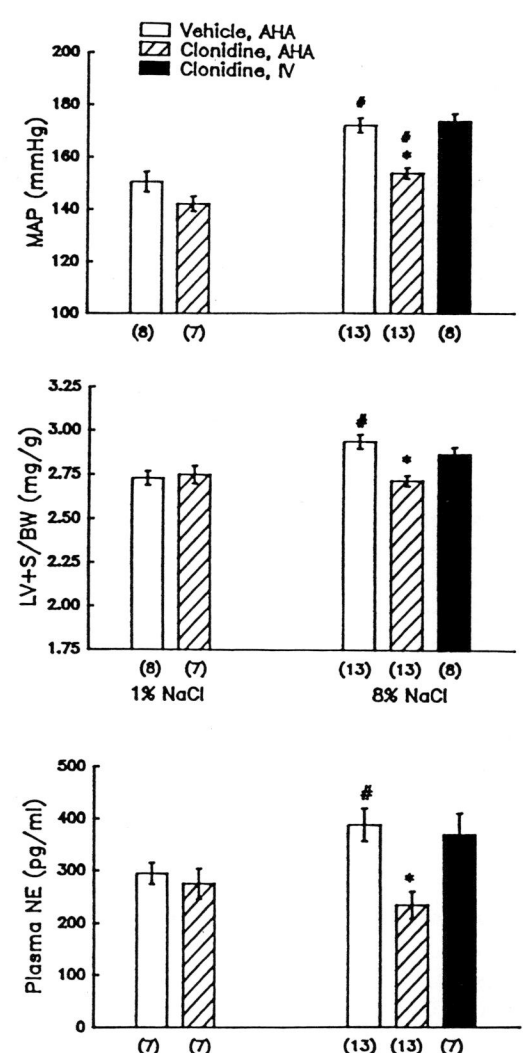

FIG. 8. Effects of chronic microinfusion of clonidine into anterior hypothalamic area (AHA) or femoral vein (IV) on mean arterial pressure (MAP) (*top panel*), weights of left ventricle plus septum/body weight (LV + S/BW) ratio (*middle panel*), and plasma norepinephrine (NE) levels (*bottom panel*). *$p < 0.05$ compared to other groups on same diet; #$p < 0.05$ compared with respective 1 percent NaCl group. (Adapted from ref. 135.)

Mineralocorticoid-induced Hypertension

The Deoxycorticosterone Acetate (DOCA)-NaCl Hypertensive Rat

The DOCA-NaCl hypertensive rat is a model of acquired hypertension in which blood pressure elevations are induced by administration of a high NaCl diet to ordinary laboratory rats treated with the mineralocorticoid DOCA. Central monoaminergic systems are altered in this model: brainstem noradrenaline turnover is decreased, while noradrenaline turnover in the heart and other peripheral tissues and plasma noradrenaline levels are increased, suggesting that peripheral sympathetic nervous system activity is increased (136). This decrease in brainstem noradrenaline turnover rate may reflect a decrease in the activity of central inhibitory noradrenergic pathways, which could result in the activation of the peripheral sympathetic nervous system. The noradrenergic fibers which innervate the NTS and adjacent structures are likely candidates for such a pathway, since chemical or electrical destruction of the NTS of the rat creates a form of hypertension which resembles DOCA-NaCl hypertension. It is important to note that the CNS mechanisms of DOCA-NaCl hypertension are not the same as those of NaCl-sensitive hypertension in the SHR, where reduced noradrenaline release from nerve terminals in the anterior hypothalamic area is the critical factor. There are no differences in endogenous noradrenaline levels or turnover rates in anterior, posterior, or ventral hypothalamic areas, pons, or medulla between DOCA-NaCl hypertensive rats and uninephrectomized Sprague-Dawley controls (137). Further research, including studies performed during the first few days after initiation of DOCA-NaCl treatment, prior to the DOCA-NaCl induced increase in blood pressure, is needed to elucidate the role of CNS in the pathogenesis of DOCA-NaCl hypertension.

Glucocorticoid-induced Hypertension

Glucocorticoid excess is associated with hypertension in humans (Cushing's syndrome) and in animals (138). This type of hypertension is of rapid onset and independent of salt intake and can be inhibited by glucocorticoid antagonists such as RU486 (139). In the periphery, glucocorticoids contribute to the maintenance of hypertension by enhancing the activity of the epinephrine-forming enzyme phenylethanolamine N-methyltransferase (PNMT) (140) and vascular reactivity to norepinephrine and angiotensin II (141). Glucocorticoids also increase the activity of PNMT in hypothalamus, medulla oblongata, and superior cervical ganglion (142). Centrally active PNMT inhibitors lower blood pressure in glucocorticoid-induced hypertension (143). Although it has been reported that elevation of PNMT activity in brain raises blood pressure by increasing sympathetic outflow (144), most studies indicate that sympathetic activity is unchanged or reduced in glucocorticoid-induced hypertension (143,145). Fanelli et al. recently demonstrated that administration of the glucocorticoid betamethasone to Wistar rats induces hypertension associated with alterations in monoamines and metabolites in brain regions known to regulate cardiovascular function, including the rostral ventrolateral medulla, septal and preoptic areas (146).

The Dahl Salt-sensitive (S) Rat

Hypothalamic lesions involving either the periventricular tissue surrounding the anterior third ventricle (AV3V) or the paraventricular-suprachiasmatic region prevent or attenuate the development of hypertension in the Dahl salt-sensitive (S) rat (147). Dahl-S rats display increased hypothalamic noradrenaline and decreased hypothalamic adrenaline content compared with Dahl salt-resistant (R) rats when challenged with a high NaCl diet (148). Noradrenaline turnover in brainstem is higher in Dahl-S rats than in Dahl-R rats on a basal NaCl diet, and is inhibited by high NaCl intake in Dahl-S but not in Dahl-R rats (149). In posterior hypothalamus, noradrenaline turnover is inhibited by high NaCl intake in Dahl-R but not in Dahl-S rats (149). Endogenous noradrenaline levels and turnover rates in anterior, posterior, and ventral hypothalamic areas are not different in Dahl-S rats maintained on basal versus high NaCl diets (137). Dahl-S rats given a high NaCl diet show increases in PNMT activity in the area postrema and nucleus commissuralis compared with Dahl-S rats on normal diets and Dahl-R rats on either diet (150). Further, the density and affinity of the α_2-adrenoreceptors are similar in brain of Dahl-S and Dahl-R strains maintained on either low or high NaCl diets (151). These studies suggest that altered function of brain catecholaminergic neurons during dietary NaCl supplementation contributes to the pathogenesis of hypertension in this model.

The Goldblatt (Renovascular Hypertensive) Rat

Alterations in central noradrenergic pathways are important in the pathogenesis of hypertension induced in the rat by placing a silver clip on one renal artery, whether (the two-kidney, one-clip model 2K, 1C) or not (the one-kidney, one-clip model 1K, 1C) the contralateral kidney is left in place. Hypothalamic tyrosine hydroxylase activity and noradrenaline content are increased after clipping in the 1K1C rat (152), and central 6-hydroxydopamine treatment or lesioning of the posterior hypothalamus prevents or attenuates 1K1C hypertension (70). Peripheral renal denervation in these models attenuates, but does not completely normalize, blood pressure (153–155). This attenuation takes place in the absence of changes in sodium intake or excretion, renin activity, water intake, or renal function (154). The absence of change in indices of efferent renal nerve function following renal denervation has led to the hypothesis that afferent neural feedback from the kidney is important to the establishment and maintenance of hypertension in these models (154). The effects of renal denervation on central noradrenaline stores in the 1K1C hypertensive rat have been examined in order to determine whether interruption of the renal afferent nerves results in a decrease in central sympathetic activity (156,157). Peripheral renal denervation resulted in a selective decrease in hypothalamic noradrenaline content, unaccompanied by changes in noradrenaline or dopamine content in any other brain region studied. Damage of the afferent component of the renal nerves by dorsal rhizotomy of the T_8-L_2 dorsal roots, a method that provides for a permanent loss of renal sensory feedback to the brain and spinal cord but does not damage sympathomotor projections to the kidney, when carried out prior to clipping attenuated the subsequent development of hypertension; when carried out during the maintenance phase of 1K1C hypertension, the intervention produced significant reductions in blood pressure. These data, combined with the finding of a decrease in peripheral sympathetic activity following renal denervation (158), suggest that the renal afferent nerves play a role in the development and maintenance of 1K1C hypertension by modulating monoaminergic activity in brain regions critical for blood pressure control.

Dopamine

Both central and peripheral dopaminergic mechanisms are involved in cardiovascular regulation in normotensive and hypertensive subjects (159,160). In the periphery, activation of dopamine receptors inhibits noradrenaline release from noradrenergic nerve terminals and increases circulating levels of atrial natriuretic peptide (159–161), resulting in vasodilation, bradycardia, and blood pressure reduction. The location of dopaminergic neurons and receptors in the hypothalamus and brainstem suggests that dopamine may be involved in the regulation of nearby cardiovascular control nuclei. The prominence of dopamine projections to the preganglionic sympathetic nuclei of the thoracic spinal cord is consistent with a modulatory effect of dopamine on sympathetic outflow (162). Further, recent studies of Lin and Yang demonstrated that electrical stimulation of the substantia nigra increases striatal dopamine release and induces hypertension and tachycardia in rats, suggesting a possible role of the nigrostriatal dopaminergic system in the integration of cardiovascular information (163).

Quinpirole, a potent and highly selective dopamine D2 agonist that crosses the blood-brain barrier, has been used to define the role of dopaminergic neurons in blood pressure control in normotensive rats (164–168). Intravenous administration of quinpirole decreases arterial pressure and heart rate in pentobarbital-anesthetized Sprague-Dawley rats by inhibiting noradrenaline release from sympathetic nerve endings through peripheral dopamine D2 receptors (165). In contrast, i.v. administration of quinpirole to conscious Sprague-Dawley rats induces a dose-dependent pressor response (166). Pretreatment with i.v. metoclopramide, a dopamine D2 re-

ceptor antagonist that crosses the blood-brain barrier, abolishes the pressor action of quinpirole, whereas pretreatment with i.v. domperidone, a peripherally acting DA D2 antagonist, does not affect this pressor response, suggesting that it is mediated through central D2 dopaminergic system (165). The quinpirole-induced pressor response is dependent on activation of sympathetic outflow and AVP release through the central D2 dopaminergic system.

Alterations in dopaminergic activity in both the brain and the periphery contribute to the development and maintenance of hypertension in humans and in animal models (164,170). Van den Buuse et al. demonstrated that ICV administration of 6-hydroxydopamine to SHR attenuated the subsequent development of hypertension (169). The effect was not diminished by pretreatment with desmethylimipramine, which prevents 6-hydroxydopamine-induced depletion of brain noradrenaline but not dopamine. Thus, central dopaminergic mechanisms play a role in the pathogenesis of hypertension in the SHR. Further, the density of central dopamine D2 receptors is increased in both acquired and genetic models of hypertension in the rat (171,172). The density of [^{3}H]-spiroperidol binding sites is increased in striatum and olfactory tubercle of DOCA/NaCl hypertensive rats and in striatum, olfactory tubercle, frontal cortex, and hypothalamus of SHR (171,172). This may represent upregulation of central D2 receptors as a consequence of reduced central dopaminergic activity in these hypertensive animals. To test this hypothesis, we studied the effect of quinpirole on the release of dopamine and its metabolites from central dopaminergic neurons in normotensive and DOCA/NaCl hypertensive rats using the push-pull microinfusion technique (173). Local administration of quinpirole reduced dopamine metabolites in perfused striatum in both normotensive and DOCA/NaCl hypertensive rats, and i.v. quinpirole caused dopamine stores in the anterior hypothalamus to increase significantly in DOCA/NaCl hypertensive rats but not in controls, presumably due to enhanced quinpirole-induced inhibition of dopamine release through a presynaptic mechanism (173). Quinpirole-induced increments in circulating noradrenaline, adrenaline, and AVP levels were significantly greater in DOCA/NaCl hypertensive rats than in controls. Thus, DOCA/NaCl hypertensive rats exhibited enhanced sympathoadrenal and vasopressinergic responses to a dopamine D2 agonist compared with normotensive controls, providing direct functional evidence for upregulation of central dopamine D2 receptors in DOCA/NaCl hypertensive rats.

Serotonin

Serotonergic neurons in brain have been implicated in the control of blood pressure and the pathogenesis of hypertension. Neuronal cell bodies and nerve terminals containing serotonin are located in areas of brain known to be involved in cardiovascular regulation (174) and descending serotonergic projections which originate in the medulla synapse on preganglionic sympathetic neurons in the spinal cord. Both mRNA and binding corresponding to serotonin receptor subtypes have been found in rat hypothalamic nuclei (anterior, posterior, ventromedial, dorsomedial nuclei) and in regions of brainstem and spinal cord that are important in cardiovascular regulation (175). Further, anatomical and physiological links between serotonergic and noradrenergic neurons in the brain and the spinal cord have been demonstrated (176). The effects of centrally administered serotonin on blood pressure are regionally specific: activation of serotonergic projections from the midbrain to the hypothalamus and from the lateral raphe neurons in the pons (area B3) to the spinal cord cause increases in arterial pressure when activated, while stimulation of more medial B3 neurons causes a depressor response. Chemical depletion of serotonin from these neurons eliminates the cardiovascular responses to stimulation of these regions (177). Microdialysis studies have demonstrated that stimulation of the lateral B3 neurons causes an increase in the release of serotonin in the thoracic spinal cord, suggesting that the pressor response is mediated by a descending serotonergic pathway (178). In contrast, ascending serotonergic projections from the upper brainstem to the hypothalamus appear to mediate depressor responses (177). Serotonin release from neurons in the B3 region rises during increases in arterial pressure but not following decreases in pressure (179), while serotonin release in the NTS rises during acute hypertension and falls during acute hypotension (180). In contrast, noradrenaline release in the NTS decreases in response to both elevation and lowering of blood pressure.

The brain serotonergic system appears to be altered in hypertension. Stores of serotonin and its metabolite 5-hydroxyindoleacetic acid are elevated in the spinal cord, medulla, and pons of the DOCA-NaCl hypertensive rat compared to controls (181). Further, both central and peripheral administration of the serotonin 5-HT$_2$ receptor antagonist ketanserin inhibit NaCl appetite induced by DOCA treatment in the Wistar rat, suggesting that serotoninergic mechanisms may be involved in DOCA-induced salt appetite and hypertension (182). Peripheral and central administration of the 5-HT$_{1\alpha}$ receptor agonist flesinoxan decrease blood pressure and heart rate in both normotensive Wistar rats and SHR, and the sensitivity to flesinoxan is greater in the hypertensive than in the normotensive rats (183). Serotonin synthesis is increased in the pons medulla and spinal cord of 4-week-old SHR compared with WKY controls (184) and ICV administration of the serotonergic neurotoxin, 5,6-dihydroxytryptamine, to 6-week-old SHR retards the subsequent development of hypertension (185), suggest-

ing that alterations in the activity of serotonergic pathways in young SHR contribute to hypertension in the adult. The serotonin contents of the thalamus and medulla, blood pressure, and incidence of stroke are increased in stroke-prone SHR offspring of mothers given high dietary tryptophan (a precursor of serotonin) prior to mating (186), suggesting that dietary tryptophan may affect blood pressure regulation through brain serotonergic pathways. Further, the efficacy of ketanserin, a centrally acting selective antagonist of serotonin 5HT$_2$ receptors, in lowering blood pressure in hypertensive humans gives indirect evidence for the importance of central serotonergic pathways in the maintenance of essential hypertension (187).

Peptide Transmitters

Neuropeptides constitute a highly varied group of proteins consisting of as few as 3 and up to 300 amino acids. They also display a great diversity of function, being involved in such varied processes as reproduction, growth and development, learning and behavior and regulation of autonomic function. In recent years, the role of neuropeptides in central regulation of arterial pressure and in the pathogenesis of hypertension has been the subject of considerable attention (188). Neuropeptides mediate a variety of functions either by an endocrine route or by acting as local modulators of communication between cells. The same peptide may display both paracrine and endocrine activities (189). The availability of sophisticated immunocytochemical and biochemical methods has permitted localization of neuropeptides and their receptors in areas of the brain known to be involved in cardiovascular regulation. Further, several lines of evidence demonstrate that many neuropeptides are co-localized in neurons that express more traditional transmitters (e.g., the catecholamines) and thus may interact with other cardiovascular regulatory pathways. Recent advances in molecular biology have facilitated the understanding of receptor regulation and translational and transcriptional events that underlie the central neural control of the cardiovascular system.

Vasopressin

CNS arginine vasopressin (AVP) plays a role in the control of blood pressure and heart rate in both normotensive and hypertensive animals. ICV administration of AVP produces an increase in arterial pressure and heart rate that can be reversed by a competitive antagonist (190). AVP interacts with neurotransmitters, such as catecholamines, which are involved in arterial blood pressure regulation (191). AVP is also a potent releasing factor for adrenocorticotropic hormone (ACTH) and corticosterone, which in turn act on the cardiovascular system. Agents that inhibit the interaction of AVP with its receptors have cardiovascular effects (192). Further, levels of AVP and its receptor are altered in hypertensive states (193) and increased sensitivity to the pressor effects of AVP has been described in numerous models of hypertension (190). It is unlikely that AVP plays a pathogenic role in hypertension through its peripheral vasoconstrictor and antidiuretic effects, since administration of antagonists to the vascular AVP receptor has failed to cause more than a transient fall in blood pressure in any model of experimental hypertension (194). Instead, AVP in the CNS appears to play a role in hypertension through its ability to increase sympathetic outflow. Most models of hypertension are characterized by sympathetic overactivity (195). In genetic models of hypertension, inborn hyperactivity of the AVP system may lead to central and peripheral sympathetic hyperactivity; in acquired models of hypertension, AVP may serve as the factor linking NaCl and DOCA to the sympathetic nervous system (195). A primary role for AVP in the pathogenesis of DOCA-NaCl hypertension was first suggested by Freidman et al. (196), who found that surgical ablation of the median eminence prevented the development of DOCA-NaCl hypertension, whereas administration of large doses of AVP hastened its onset. Subsequently, elevations in plasma and urinary AVP levels were reported in DOCA-NaCl treated rats in both early and chronic stages of hypertension (197). Immunocytochemical staining of the hypothalamus with an anti-AVP antibody revealed that DOCA-NaCl treated rats had increased numbers of brightly stained cell bodies within the supraoptic and paraventricular nuclei and brightly labeled axons projecting from these nuclei (193). In addition, DOCA-NaCl hypertensive rats display enhanced pressor responsiveness and increased reactivity to AVP in various vascular beds (198,199). Moreover, Brattleboro rats with inherited diabetes insipidus (DI rats) who failed to develop hypertension when treated with DOCA-NaCl did so when AVP was added (200).

AVP appears to contribute to the pathogenesis of DOCA-NaCl hypertension via a CNS mechanism. DOCA-NaCl treated rats show significantly greater increases in blood pressure and heart rate in response to ICV administration of AVP than do control rats (201). The increased sensitivity of DOCA-NaCl treated rats to the CNS effects of AVP has also been demonstrated in microinjection and microiontophoresis studies in the locus ceruleus (201,202). Further, lesions of the paraventricular nucleus, which synthesizes AVP, or the anteroventral region of the third ventricle (AV3V), locus ceruleus, or the area postrema, areas receiving vasopressinergic innervation, prevent or attenuate the development of DOCA-NaCl hypertension (202,203). The finding of increased responsiveness of the DOCA-NaCl hypertensive rats to the CNS effects of AVP suggests that brain AVP receptors may be upregulated in this model.

Swords et al. have recently assessed the effect of *in vivo* and *in vitro* administration of DOCA on AVP binding in the brain (193). The number of AVP binding sites in the hypothalamus of DOCA-NaCl treated rats was increased during the prehypertensive and early hypertensive stages compared to control rats, but not in the established phase of hypertension. The effect of *in vivo* administration of DOCA on AVP binding in rat brain appears to be due to a direct action of DOCA on neuronal AVP receptors, as *in vitro* treatment of primary neuronal-enriched cultures with DOCA also leads to a dose-dependent and time-dependent increase in number of AVP binding sites. Hence, DOCA-induced upregulation of AVP receptors in brain may play a role in the pathogenesis of DOCA-salt hypertension.

Angiotensin II

There is increasing evidence for an intrinsic renin-angiotensin system and local angiotensin II generation in brain (204). Components of the renin-angiotensin system, including mRNA for angiotensinogen, converting enzyme, and renin, have been localized in brain (205). Angiotensin II-immunoreactive cell bodies and fibers, as well as specific angiotensin II receptors, have been identified in areas of the brain that participate in cardiovascular regulation, including the circumventricular organs, paraventricular nucleus of the hypothalamus, locus ceruleus, NTS, area postrema, and medulla (206). The presence of components of the renin-angiotensin system in neuroblastoma cells (207) and primary neuronal-enriched cell cultures (208) and the finding that these cells synthesize immunoprecipitable angiotensin II, which co-migrates with authentic angiotensin II on high-performance liquid chromatography (HPLC), add further support to the concept of local synthesis of angiotensin II in brain.

Brain angiotensin II has been shown to participate in blood pressure and fluid and electrolyte regulation through mechanisms distinct from those in the periphery. These mechanisms involve enhancement of sympathetic outflow, blunting of baroreceptor reflex gain, stimulation of AVP and ACTH release, and increased catecholamine biosynthesis and turnover (209). In addition, brain angiotensin II elicits two behaviors, thirst and NaCl appetite, which are critical in body fluid and electrolyte regulation (210). Increasing evidence suggests that angiotensin II acts as a neurotransmitter in the CNS. Radioreceptor assays have detected specific, high-affinity angiotensin II receptors in nerve terminals (synaptosomes) (211). Iontophoresis of angiotensin II was found to enhance the rate of discharge of 75 percent of the neurons in the subfornical organ. This effect was dose-dependent and antagonized by saralasin. Other studies have shown that angiotensin II activates neurons of the supraoptic and paraventricular nuclei, areas that synthesize and release AVP (212).

Brain angiotensin II appears to play a major role in the pathogenesis of hypertension in the SHR. In comparison to WKY, SHR show increased sympathetic tone and increased AVP and ACTH secretion (213). SHR also show increased levels of angiotensin II-like material in brain and cerebrospinal fluid, increased turnover of angiotensin II in the brain (214), and increased pressor and neuronal responsiveness to central administration of angiotensin II (215). Comparison of primary neuronal-enriched cultures from newborn SHR and WKY has revealed differences in angiotensin II stores, metabolism, and binding between strains (208). The strongest evidence that brain angiotensin II plays a functional role in the pathogenesis of hypertension in SHR comes from the finding that acute or chronic ICV administration of saralasin or angiotensin-converting enzyme (ACE) inhibitors in doses that are ineffective when given systemically significantly attenuates the subsequent development of hypertension (216,217). Early treatment of young SHR with ACE inhibitors prevents the full expression of hypertension later in life even after treatment is stopped (218–220). A possible critical phase sensitive to pharmacological interference with the renin-angiotensin system has been proposed to explain this phenomenon (221). Interference with blood pressure regulation during this phase would alter the long-term course of the disease. Recently, Wu and Berecek have shown that early treatment of SHR with the ACE inhibitor captopril permanently alters the course of hypertension (220). Mating pairs of SHR were treated with captopril and their pups were maintained on captopril until experimentation. Captopril treatment "cured" the hypertension in these rats: Animals treated with captopril throughout fetal and neonatal life had normal blood pressures, whereas animals that had been removed from captopril and the offspring of treated rats had significantly lower blood pressures than sham-treated controls (Fig. 9). The mechanisms underlying the chronic antihypertensive effect of early treatment of SHR with captopril are not known with certainty. The observation that the antihypertensive effect was associated with a decrease in CNS responses to angiotensin I and II suggests that captopril may permanently alter the development of hypertension in SHR through an alteration in the brain renin-angiotensin system. Other possible mechanisms include the remodeling of cardiac and blood vessel structure, an alteration in factors in the pregnant female SHR which may contribute to the full expression of hypertension in their offspring, or a downregulation of angiotensin II receptors in the brain.

Regulation of angiotensin II receptors in SHR is abnormal in a number of tissues, including brain (222,223). ACE inhibitor treatment causes a downregu-

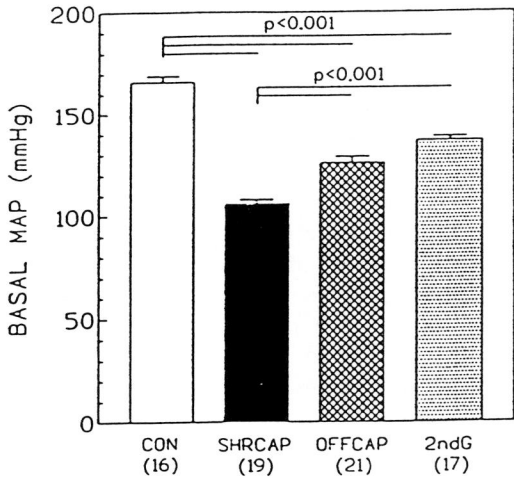

FIG. 9. Basal mean arterial pressure (MAP) of four rat groups at 4 to 6 months of age. Basal MAP was monitored for 4 consecutive days in conscious, freely moving rats. Daily MAP values were averaged for each rat. Data are means ± SEM analyzed by analysis of variance with Bonferroni's posttest procedure. Number of animals is in parentheses. CON, control rats; SHRCAP, spontaneously hypertensive rats that received captopril; OFFCAP, SHRCAP taken off captopril at 2 months; 2nd G, first offspring of OFFCAP rats. (Adapted from ref. 220.)

lation in angiotensin II receptors in brain tissue and primary neuronal cell cultures from SHR, but not from normotensive rat strains (223,224). Recent studies from our own laboratory indicate that endogenous angiotensin II in the anterior hypothalamic area of SHR-S is tonically active in the maintenance of hypertension and suggest that upregulation of type 1 angiotensin II (AT_1) receptors is involved in this process (225,226). Blockade of AT_1 receptors in anterior hypothalamic area by local microinjection of losartan (2-n-butyl-4-chloro-5-(hydroxymethyl)-1-[2′-(1H-tetrazol-5-yl)biphenyl-4-yl)-methyl]imidazole, potassium salt), a highly selective nonpeptide antagonist, caused significant dose-related decreases in mean arterial pressure with unchanged heart rate in SHR-S but not in WKY rats (Fig. 10). The depressor response was enhanced by dietary NaCl supplementation. Further, microinjection of angiotensin II into the anterior hypothalamic area of SHR-S caused a pressor response that was enhanced by dietary NaCl supplementation and blocked by pretreatment with the losartan metabolite EXP 3174. Microinjection of the selective type 2 angiotensin II (AT_2) receptor antagonist PD 123319 into the anterior hypothalamic area did not affect blood pressure or heart rate in SHR-S. These data provide the first demonstration that endogenous angiotensin II in the anterior hypothalamic area participates in the tonic control of blood pressure in SHR and that this effect is mediated by AT_1 receptors. These findings further suggest that endogenous angiotensin II and AT_1

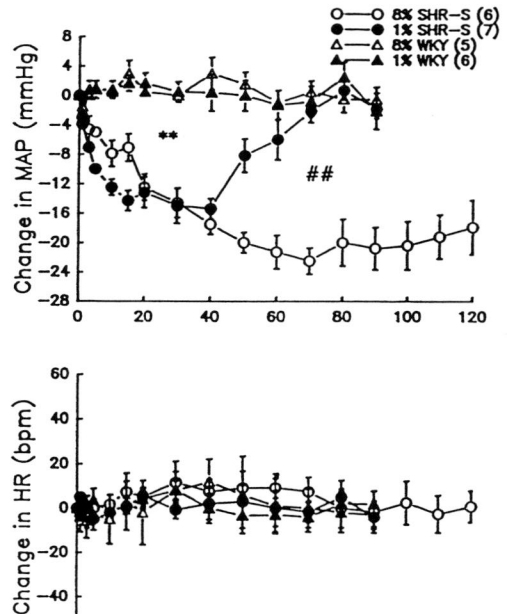

FIG. 10. Effect of microinjection of losartan into the anterior hypothalamic area (AHA) on mean arterial pressure (MAP) and heart rate (HR) in NaCl-sensitive spontaneously hypertensive rats (SHR-S) and Wistar-Kyoto (WKY) rats on 1 percent NaCl and 8 percent NaCl diets. **$p < 0.01$, comparison between WKY and SHR-S on either diet 3–50 minutes after injection; ##$p < 0.01$, comparison between 8 percent NaCl-fed SHR-S and any of other three groups 50–90 minutes after injection. (From ref. 226, with permission.)

receptors in the anterior hypothalamic area are involved in the pathogenesis of NaCl-sensitive hypertension in this model.

Natriuretic Peptides

The Natriuretic Peptide Family

The natriuretic peptide (NP) hormone family consists of three peptides, atrial natriuretic factor (ANF), brain natriuretic peptide (BNP), and type-C natriuretic peptide (CNP), that exhibit a common spectrum of biological activities (227). The biological activity of NP results from binding to cell-surface receptors (NPR-A, NPR-B) with intrinsic ligand-activated guanylate cyclase activities (228). Another class of NP receptors (NPR-C) has a truncated intracellular domain and appears to function in clearing the peptides from the extracellular space (229).

Atrial Natriuretic Factor

ANF was originally isolated from the atrium (230), and initial studies focused on ANF as a hormone of cardiac origin (227). ANF is also found in brain and may function as a neuromodulator that participates in cardiovascular control (231). A complete ANF synthetic, processing, and effector system has been described in rat brain (232,233). ANF-containing cell bodies are found in highest density in the anterior hypothalamic region adjacent to the anteroventral tip of the third ventricle (AV3V) (233), a region involved in the development and maintenance of hypertension and in fluid and electrolyte balance. Regulation of the synthesis, posttranslational processing, and release of ANF in brain appears to be different than in heart (234).

The ANF content of brain regions involved in cardiovascular and volume regulation is altered in several rodent models of hypertension, including the SHR, the Dahl salt-sensitive (Dahl-S) rat, the one-kidney, one-clip (1K1C) and the two-kidney, one-clip (2K1C) renovascular hypertensive rat, and the DOCA-salt hypertensive rat, compared with that in age-matched normotensive controls (235–237). Differences in immunoreactive ANF levels have also been found in neuronal and glial cultures derived from hypothalamus and brainstem of neonatal SHR compared with WKY, suggesting that genetically mediated differences between strains in brain ANF expression appear long before hypertension develops. The ANF content of the hypothalamus, pons, and septum is significantly higher in SHR than in age-matched Wistar-Kyoto (WKY) controls, and application of ANF to brain slices *in vitro* causes markedly greater increases in cyclic guanosine-5'-monophosphate (cGMP) levels in hypothalamus and brainstem of SHR than of WKY. Thus, ANF-sensitive particulate guanylate cyclase activity in the hypothalamus and brainstem is greater in SHR than in WKY rats.

The effects of brain ANF on neuronal excitability and blood pressure are regionally selective—and appear to be diametrically opposite in forebrain versus hindbrain (231). Injection of ANF into the lateral ventricle significantly increases blood pressure in conscious SHR and WKY rats; the pressor responses to ANF are greater in SHR than in WKY (238). In contrast, injection of ANF into the fourth ventricle lowers blood pressure in conscious SHR and WKY rats (239), while injection of ANF into the third ventricle lowers blood pressure and decreases lumbar sympathetic nerve traffic in conscious SHR but not in WKY. In normotensive rats, microinjection of ANF into NTS, cuneate nucleus, or the spinal trigeminal complex decreases blood pressure, while microinjection of ANF into the preoptic suprachiasmatic nucleus increases blood pressure (240,241). Thus, exogenous ANF acts at hindbrain sites, especially NTS, to lower blood pressure, and at anterior hypothalamic sites, to elevate blood pressure. On a cellular level, ANF reduces neuronal excitability in the rat hypothalamus: when applied locally to individual neurons, ANF inhibits the neuronal firing rate (231). ANF may therefore act as an inhibitory neuromodulator in forebrain.

Selective increases in the ANF content of the anterior hypothalamic region have been observed in the salt-sensitive SHR (SHR-S) compared with age matched WKY rats (236). The anterior hypothalamic region contains neurons that have a depressor effect when excited by electrical stimulation or noradrenergic input, and studies from our laboratory have demonstrated a selective reduction in release of endogenous noradrenaline from nerve terminals in the anterior hypothalamic area of SHR-S fed a high NaCl diet (128–130; Fig. 6). We concluded that the resultant reduction in local noradrenergic input to depressor neurons and decreased inhibition of sympathetic outflow from the brain were responsible for NaCl-sensitive hypertension in the SHR-S model.

The regional selectivity of the reduction in anterior hypothalamic noradrenaline release in NaCl-supplemented SHR-S can be explained by either selective diminution in noradrenergic input to the region, as by blunted baroreflex function (104,242,243), or by local overexpression of inhibitory neuromodulator(s) (244). Inhibition of noradrenaline release by a neuromodulator, such as ANF, that is selectively overexpressed in the anterior hypothalamic area of SHR-S could account for the observed localized reduction in noradrenaline release. ANF has been shown to inhibit noradrenaline release in other systems, including peripheral nerve terminals *in vivo* and an adrenal pheochromocytoma (PC-12) cell line *in vitro,* and to reduce the excitability of rat hypothalamic neurons *in vivo* (231,245). Therefore, we hypothesized that the increased ANF that we observed in the anterior hypothalamus of SHR-S produces local tonic inhibition of noradrenaline release, reducing excitation of depressor neurons and thereby elevating blood pressure (231; Fig. 6). According to this hypothesis, blockade of the ANF effect by local microinjection of an anti-ANF antibody would stimulate noradrenaline release, thus exciting depressor neurons in the anterior hypothalamic area, increasing sympathetic nervous system inhibition, and lowering blood pressure. We observed that microinjection of a blocking monoclonal antibody to ANF directly into the anterior hypothalamic area produced significant decreases in blood pressure and heart rate in SHR-S but not in WKY rats (237). This is the first direct demonstration that endogenous brain ANF is involved in the central regulation of blood pressure. Together with previous observations that injection of rat ANF into the lateral ventricle of SHR increases blood pressure and heart rate (238), our finding of a depressor response to blockade of endogenous ANF in the anterior hypothalamic area supports the hypothesis that the increased stores of ANF in the anterior hypothalamus of SHR-S play a functional role in the tonic control of blood pressure. In contrast, anterior hypothalamic ANF

does not appear to participate in blood pressure control in the normotensive WKY rat.

In contrast to its inhibitory effect on forebrain neurons, ANF enhances neuronal excitability in rat hindbrain. Microinjection studies have shown that locally administered ANF produces significant increases in the firing rate of NTS neurons in association with depressor and bradycardic responses in anesthetized Wistar rats (241). Most ANF-responsive sites (86 percent) are located between 0.5 mm rostral and 1.5 mm caudal to the obex, corresponding to the site of termination of baro- and chemoreceptor afferents. Further, neurons that are excited by microinjection of ANF into NTS are also excited by activation of arterial baroreceptors and inhibited by baroreceptor unloading (241). These findings suggest that ANF-induced activation of NTS neurons may mediate the depressor effect associated with arterial baroreceptor reflex activation.

To elucidate the role of endogenous ANF in NTS in the control of blood pressure and baroreflex sensitivity, we have microinjected a blocking monoclonal antibody to ANF into the caudal NTS of conscious, unrestrained SHR and WKY rats and observed the effects on blood pressure and baroreflex-mediated heart rate control. Initial experiments tested the hypothesis that blockade of endogenous ANF in caudal NTS by local microinjection of monoclonal antibody to ANF increases blood pressure in SHR by blocking tonic activation of NTS neurons (246). Microinjection of the antibody into the caudal NTS of conscious, freely moving SHR produced significant increases in blood pressure (Fig. 11); no response was seen in WKY rats. Antibody injections evoked similar pressor responses in both salt-sensitive (SHR-S) and salt-resistant (SHR-R) rats and in SHR-S on both basal (1 percent) NaCl and high (8 percent) NaCl diets (247). The pressor response to the monoclonal antibody decreased progressively in magnitude with increasing distance rostral in the NTS (Fig. 11), consistent with previous observations of co-localization of ANF-responsive sites and sites of termination of baroreceptor and chemoreceptor afferents within the caudal NTS (241). Although ANF and its receptors have been described previously on cell bodies and nerve terminals in the NTS, our finding of a pressor response to blockade of endogenous ANF in the caudal NTS is the first direct evidence for a functional role for endogenous ANF in NTS in blood pressure control (231).

The observation that a pressor response to blockade of ANF in NTS occurred in SHR but not in WKY rats suggests that NTS neurons are tonically activated by ANF in SHR but not in WKY rats. Our data further suggest that this effect is independent of the salt sensitivity of hypertension and of dietary salt intake in the SHR (247). Increased tonic activation of NTS neurons by ANF would tend to lower blood pressure, thus represent-

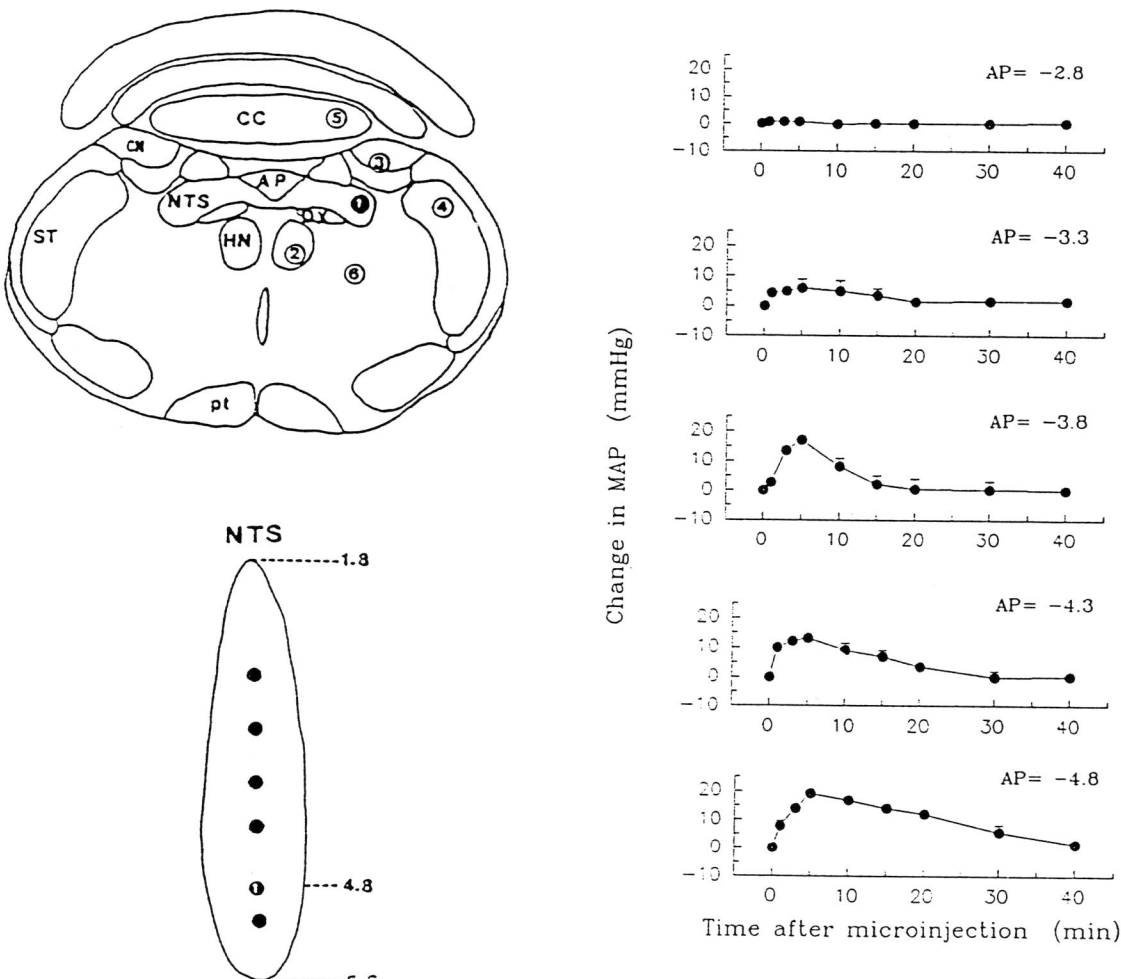

FIG. 11. Top left: Diagrammatic representation of a coronal section through medulla at a level 4.8 mm caudal to interaural line. Increases in mean arterial pressure (MAP) were observed only in response to microinjection of monoclonal antibody to atrial natriuretic peptide into sites in caudal nucleus tractus solitarii (NTS) (*dark area, 1*). No alterations in blood pressure were observed after antibody injections into surrounding areas, including hypoglossal nucleus (*HN, 2*), cuneate nucleus (*CN, 3*), spinal trigeminal nucleus (*ST, 4*), cerebellar cortex (*CC, 5*), or a position 0.6 mm ventral to caudal NTS (*6*). AP, area postrema; DX, dorsal motor nucleus of the vagus; pt, pyramidal tract. **Bottom left:** Longitudinal section of NTS, with solid circles indicating sites of microinjection of antibody. Numbers indicate distance (in mm) caudal to interaural line. **Right:** Effects of microinjection of monoclonal antibody to ANF into caudal NTS (AP = −4.8), mid NTS (AP = −4.3 and −3.8), midrostral NTS (AP = −3.8), and rostral NTS (AP = −2.8) on MAP in SHR. (Adapted from ref. 247.)

ing an inadequate compensation for the elevated blood pressure in SHR (231). Tonic activation of the baroreceptor reflex pathway in SHR under resting conditions could account for the reduced sensitivity of cardiopulmonary and arterial baroreceptor reflexes that has been observed in SHR compared to normotensive control rats. This could represent the central defect in the baroreceptor reflex pathway previously described in SHR (248). As an initial test of this hypothesis, we determined whether ANF receptors in the caudal NTS are involved in baroreceptor reflex control of heart rate in SHR (249).

We studied arterial baroreceptor reflex–mediated changes in heart rate during phenylephrine infusion before and after microinjection of ANF or monoclonal antibody to ANF into caudal NTS of conscious unrestrained SHR-S and WKY rats. The slope of the heart rate/mean arterial pressure relation was significantly less in the SHR-S than in WKY, confirming that baroreceptor reflex control of heart rate is blunted in this hypertensive model. Microinjection of ANF further blunted baroreceptor reflex control of heart rate, while microinjection of the monoclonal antibody enhanced the sensitivity of baroreceptor reflex control of heart rate in SHR-S but not in WKY rats. Further, recent experiments suggest that microinjection of ANF into the NTS also blunts baroreflex control of lumbar sympathetic nerve activity in SHR-S. Thus, endogenous ANF in the caudal NTS appears to modulate baroreceptor reflex control of heart rate and sympathetic outflow in SHR but not in WKY rats (231,249). This is the first direct demonstration that endogenous ANF in the NTS modulates any aspect of baroreceptor reflex function in hypertension.

In summary, in the normotensive WKY, excitation of NTS neurons by baroreflex afferents leads to activation of sympathoinhibitory neurons in NTS and anterior hypothalamic area, strong inhibition of sympathetic nervous system outflow, and a decrease in arterial pressure (231) (Fig. 12). In SHR, brain ANF acts at the levels of the NTS and the anterior hypothalamus to perturb this normal baroreflex regulatory pathway. ANF tonically activates sympathoinhibitory neurons in the caudal NTS of SHR, thereby restraining the rise in arterial pressure, and tonically inhibits baroreflex responsiveness to alterations in blood pressure. Attenuated baroreflex-mediated input to the anterior hypothalamic area, in combination with local inhibition of noradrenaline release from anterior hypothalamic nerve terminals by ANF, reduces activation of sympathoinhibitory neurons in the anterior hypothalamic area. This results in increased sympathetic outflow and higher blood pressure in the SHR. Thus, ANF appears to act at a number of sites in brain to facilitate the development and maintenance of sympathetically mediated hypertension in the SHR model.

Brain Natriuretic Peptide

Brain natriuretic peptide (BNP), a natriuretic peptide that is very similar to ANF in structure and pharmacologic activity, was first isolated from porcine brain (250,251). Subsequent studies revealed that immunoreactive BNP is expressed to a much greater extent in heart of most species than in brain (252). In fact, BNP gene transcripts have not been detected in brain in most spe-

cies examined to date (253). BNP appears to function as a hormone of cardiac origin rather than as a CNS neuropeptide.

Type-C Natriuretic Peptide

Type-C natriuretic peptide (CNP), a natriuretic peptide that is very similar to both ANF and BNP in structure and pharmacologic activity, is expressed predominantly in the CNS (254). CNP is found in brain of most species, including human, at tissue concentrations far greater than those of ANF and BNP, but is found in the blood only in very low concentrations, if at all (255). Further, the ANP-B receptor, which is selectively activated by CNP (256), is expressed at high levels in brain (257). It has been postulated, therefore, that CNP is responsible for most of the CNS effects presently attributed to the NP family and that it functions as a CNS neuropeptide rather than as a circulating hormone. CNP modulates the secretion of luteinizing hormone and stimulates prolactin secretion through actions at the hypothalamic level (258,259). Further, centrally administered CNP evokes a number of responses that differ from those elicited by ANF administered under the same conditions. These include a water drinking response in the rat (260) and a depressor response in the sheep that is accompanied by reductions in circulating cortisol and aldosterone levels and attenuation of the expected baroreflex-mediated heart rate increase (261). These findings are consistent with earlier reports that i.v. administration of CNP results in natriuresis, diuresis, and a decrease in blood pressure (254). The potency of i.v. CNP was approximately 1 percent of the related peptides ANF and BNP (254), suggesting that the hemodynamic effects of peripherally administered CNP may be mediated by the CNS (261). Further investigation is needed to define the mechanism(s) of the depressor response to CNP and its site(s) of action within the CNS.

Endothelin

The endothelins (ET) are a family of 21 amino acid peptides that were first isolated from the media of cul-

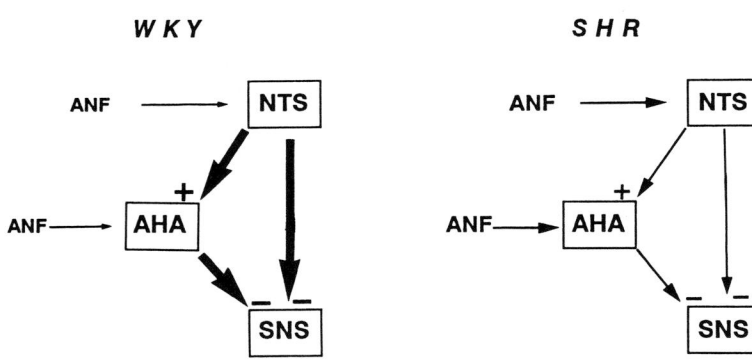

FIG. 12. Schematic representation of mechanisms by which ANF in NTS and anterior hypothalamic area exerts tonic control over sympathetic outflow and blood pressure in SHR but not in WKY. AHA, anterior hypothalamic area; SNS, sympathetic nervous system activity; +, strong activation; +, attenuated activation; −, strong inhibition; −, attenuated inhibition. (From ref. 231, with permission.)

tured endothelial cells (262,263). The three isoforms of ET, designated ET-1, ET-2, and ET-3, are products of separate genes. ET-1 is primarily an endothelial cell product and is the most potent peptide vasoconstrictor known. ET-3 is produced by multiple cell types and has less well-defined functions. ET-3 is thought to be the predominant member of the family produced in brain (264). The ETs express their biological activity by activating two classes of receptors, ET_A, which is found mainly on vascular smooth muscle cells and is relatively selective for ET-1, and ET_B, which is found on a large variety of cell types and is nonselective (264). The ET_A and ET_B receptors are products of different genes.

A complete ET synthetic, processing, and effector system has been identified and characterized in brain (264,265). In human and rat brain, the density of ET gene transcript levels and ET binding sites is highest in hypothalamus, suggesting the possibility of neuroendocrine and cardiovascular regulatory functions. Immunocytochemical and cell fractionation studies have demonstrated ET in neurons and synaptosomes, respectively, suggesting that it may function as a neurotransmitter in brain.

ICV administration of ET-1 in the conscious rat elicits a dose-dependent pressor response accompanied by increases in heart rate, sympathetic outflow, AVP release, and circulating noradrenaline and AVP levels (266). The pressor response to centrally administered ET-1 can be blocked by peripheral administration of a combination of prazosin or a ganglion blocker and an AVP V_1 receptor blocker, confirming its dependence on enhanced AVP and noradrenaline release in the periphery. Further, the ETs have a variety of neuroendocrine effects that are pertinent to cardiovascular function. Injection of ET-3 into the third cerebroventricle of rats exposed to exogenous and endogenous stimuli for drinking inhibits the water drinking response (267); ET-1 stimulates AVP release from the perfused rat hypothalamus (268), and both ET-3 and ET-1 inhibit prolactin release from dispersed anterior pituitary cells *in vitro*. It is likely that endogenous ET has similar neuroendocrine effects *in vivo* since (a) ET-3 is present in high concentrations in the magnocellular neurons of the hypothalamus that project to the median eminence and posterior pituitary (264); (b) the ET content of the hypophyseal system decreases in response to water deprivation in the rat; and (c) passive immunoneutralization of endogenous ET-3 enhances the angiotensin II-induced drinking response (267). The CNS neuronal pathways through which ET acts to elicit a pressor response remain incompletely defined, as are the neurotransmitters involved. Since ET can release monoamines from nerve terminals and activate the renin-angiotensin system, it is possible that monoaminergic and angiotensin-producing neuronal pathways participate in mediating the pressor response to ET in CNS.

Microinjection of exogenous ET into the area postrema of anesthetized rats produces a biphasic (increase followed by decrease) blood pressure response, while application of ET to the ventral surface of the medulla or microinjection into the NTS results in increases in blood pressure, heart rate, and renal nerve activity, indicating the presence of ET receptors in important cardiovascular regulatory pathways (269). ET_A and ET_B receptors have been identified and quantitated in the rat hypothalamus and ventrolateral medulla (269). Decreased densities of ET_A and ET_B receptors, as defined by labeled ET-1 and sarafotoxin 6b binding, have been described in SHR compared with that in WKY rats (269). Other investigators have reported no differences in ET-1 binding to membranes prepared from homogenates of various brain regions of SHR versus WKY (270), and reports of the relative intensity of ET gene transcript levels in SHR versus WKY are inconsistent. Further study is needed to resolve this controversy and to assess the role of endogenous brain ET in the pathogenesis of hypertension.

Steroid Neuromodulators

Estrogens

Reports concerning the role of endogenous estrogen in cardiovascular control and the pathogenesis of hypertension are conflicting. Systemic hypertension is significantly less common in premenopausal women than in men, but the prevalence of essential hypertension in postmenopausal women increases dramatically, reaching levels significantly higher than those in men of comparable age (271). Further, the treatment of stroke-prone SHR with estradiol inhibits the development of hypertension (272), suggesting that estrogen has an important antihypertensive effect. In contrast, in a more recent study, ovariectomy at 4 weeks had no effect on the subsequent development of hypertension in female SHR (273), calling into question the role of estrogen in modulating blood pressure control in the model. Estrogen binding sites have been found in multiple brain regions, including the ventral hypothalamus, para- and periventricular nuclei in the anterior hypothalamus, preoptic area, lateral septum, bed nuclei of the stria terminalis, the amygdala, central gray, raphe nuclei, ventrolateral reticular formation, nucleus ambiguus, dorsal motor nucleus of the vagus, NTS, and nucleus intermediolateralis, which participate in cardiovascular regulation (274,275). Between 50–80 percent of estrogen target cells in the brainstem contain catecholamine fluorescence. These include neurons in the lateral reticular nucleus (group A1), the NTS (group A2), the pons (group A5), locus ceruleus (group A6) and in the vicinity of the lateral lemniscus (group A7). In the hypothalamus, estradiol and dopamine are co-localized in neurons in the arcuate and periventricular nuclei (275). Further, co-localization of estradiol and ANP in neurons of the ventral periventricular nucleus and the preoptic and anterior hypothalamus has been described (276). Recent studies by Petitti et al. (277,278) demonstrated that estradiol administered *in vivo* selectively elevates the number of α_{1B}-adrenoceptors in hypothalamus and preoptic area of ovariectomized female rats and potentiates α_1 adrenoceptor-mediated augmentation of cyclic adenosine monophosphate (cAMP) formation in these brain regions. These data indicate that estrogen regulates the activity of monoaminergic pathways that are involved in the control of blood pressure and electrolyte balance. The role of brain estrogen in the pathogenesis of hypertension needs further investigation.

Androgens

Autoradiographic studies with ^{3}H-dihydrotestosterone have demonstrated nuclear labeling of neurons within brain regions that are involved in cardiovascular regulation, including the ventral hypothalamus, periventricular nucleus, preoptic area, amygdala, dorsolateral septum, bed nuclei of the stria terminalis, central gray, raphe nuclei, catecholamine group A5, nucleus ambiguus, area postrema, dorsal motor nucleus of the vagus, and spinal cord (275,279). Co-localization of dihydrotestosterone and catecholamines has been found in 50–80 percent of catecholaminergic neurons in the pons, the dorsolateral corner of the fourth ventricle, the locus ceruleus, and the arcuate and periventricular nuclei of the hypothalamus (280). The demonstration that androgen and androgen binding sites are present in these critical regions of the brainstem and hypothalamus suggests that androgens may affect the production and release of neurotransmitters and neuropeptides that control cardiovascular function.

A sexually dimorphic pattern of blood pressure in which hypertension develops more rapidly and becomes more severe in the male than in the female has been observed in several forms of hypertension (273,281). The sexually dimorphic pattern of hypertension in the SHR appears to be androgen-dependent, since gonadectomy retards the development of hypertension in young male, but not in female SHR, and administration of testosterone propionate to gonadectomized SHR of both sexes confers a male pattern of blood pressure development (273,282). Stores of noradrenaline in the posterior hypothalamic region are significantly greater in intact male and testosterone-treated SHR of both sexes than in intact or ovariectomized female rats. Whether these androgen-mediated alterations in posterior hypothalamic neurons are a determinant of the androgen-mediated sexual dimorphism of blood pressure is unknown and needs further study.

Adrenocorticoids

Adrenocorticoids contribute to cardiovascular homeostasis and blood pressure regulation via effects on the brain (283,284). Two types of corticoid receptors have been detected and may transduce the cardiovascular effects of these steroids in brain. Mineralocorticoid receptors (Type 1) are located in neurons of the hippocampus, septum, periventricular regions, and a number of discrete neuronal cell groups in the cortex and brain stem, whereas glucocorticoid receptors (Type 2) are located in the paraventricular and supraoptic nuclei, arcuate nucleus, limbic system, cortical and thalamic neurons, and all neurons of the ascending catecholaminergic pathway (275,284–288). Neurons in the paraventricular nucleus and NTS containing a high density of Types 1 and 2 corticoid receptors are involved in the central regulation of blood pressure (275,286).

Intracerebroventricular (ICV) administration of aldosterone or the selective glucocorticoid antagonist RU 38486 increases blood pressure, whereas ICV administration of the glucocorticoid agonist RU 28362 or the mineralocorticoid antagonist RU 28318 decreases blood pressure (289,290). Central administration of RU 28318 also prevents NaCl-induced hypertension in Dahl/JR NaCl-sensitive rats (291). These data suggest that the central mineralocorticoid and glucocorticoid receptor systems mediate opposing actions on the regulation of blood pressure. It was recently shown that in glucocorticoid (betamethasone) treated rats, the increase in blood pressure is associated with an increase in the density of muscarinic receptors in the hypothalamus and anteroventrolateral medulla (292). Choline acetyltransferase activity and choline uptake are decreased in the hypothalamus and anteroventrolateral medulla and increased in the anterior hypothalamic preoptic area in this model. The functional significance of these changes in brain muscarinic cholinergic activity in glucocorticoid-induced hypertension is not fully understood.

Clonidinelike Substance(s)

Clonidine is a clinically useful antihypertensive agent that acts on the CNS to reduce sympathetic outflow (293). Early studies showed that clonidine lowers blood pressures via an agonist action on α_2-adrenergic receptors in the ventrolateral medulla (294,295). Studies utilizing more selective and potent α_2-agonists, such as guanabenz and guanfacine, suggest that a receptor other than the α_2-adrenergic receptor may contribute to the antihypertensive action of clonidine. It has been shown that clonidine binds to imidazoline-specific sites as well as to α_2-adrenergic receptors in the ventrolateral medulla (296). These nonadrenergic clonidine binding sites bind certain imidazoles and imidazolines with high affinity and were thus termed imidazole binding sites (296). Subtypes of these receptors, some of which are recognized by imidazolines but not imidazoles, have been identified (297). I_1-sites are labeled by (^3H) clonidine, whereas I_2-sites are labeled by (^3H idazoxan). The I_2 sites show low affinity for clonidine but high affinity for guanidine compounds. The I_1 imidazoline sites have been localized by receptor autoradiography in cardiovascular regulatory regions of the rat medulla, including the ventrolateral medulla, and in the kidney; these sites are also present in the ventrolateral medulla of the human brain (298). The vasodepressor activity of clonidine appears to be mediated by I_1 imidazoline sites rather than by α_2-adrenergic receptors (299). Much investigative energy has been devoted to identification and characterization of putative endogenous ligands for imidazoline receptors (299). These substances may play a role in the pathogenesis of hypertension and may have therapeutic potential.

HUMAN HYPERTENSION

Increased Sympathetic Nervous System Activity in Primary Hypertension

The nervous system plays a permissive role in all forms of hypertension. Under normal conditions, the baroreflex system maintains arterial pressure at homeostatic levels, but in hypertensive individuals this mechanism resets after chronic exposure to elevated blood pressure. The evidence that the nervous system plays more than a permissive role in primary hypertension is derived from several observations. First, several classes of antihypertensive drugs lower blood pressure by direct action on the CNS. These include α_2-adrenoceptor agonists (e.g., clonidine and guanabenz) which act on hypothalamic and brainstem nuclei, β-adrenoceptor blockers, and angiotensin-converting enzyme inhibitors. Second, the CNS, via the renal nerves, is critically important in adjusting fluid volume and renin release and thereby setting arterial pressure. Environmental and dietary stress can be relayed to the kidney and compromise renal function (300). Further, long-term increases in sympathetic renal nerve activity may damage the intrarenal arterioles and glomeruli. Third, sympathetic nervous system activity is elevated in nearly every form of human and experimental hypertension, and reduction of this activity decreases arterial pressure (301). Chemical or surgical lesions of the sympathetic nervous system lower arterial pressure in most hypertensive individuals. Further, hypertensive patients display exaggerated responses to emotional stimuli. Wallin et al. reported that sympathetic nervous system activity rises in hypertensive subjects who are anticipating a stress (302). No such changes occur in normotensive individuals in the same situation. Together with similar data from hypertensive animals in

which stress causes sustained hypertension (303,304), these data suggest that inappropriate CNS responses to environmental stimuli can contribute to human essential hypertension. Measurement of plasma catecholamine levels and, in particular, regional run-off of norepinephrine indicates that sympathetic nervous system activity is elevated in young hypertensive subjects. Using microneurography to measure muscle sympathetic nervous system activity (MSNA), investigators have demonstrated that sympathetic nervous system activity is elevated in both young subjects in the early stages of hypertension and older subjects with sustained hypertension. Recently, it has been reported that African-Americans with a positive family history of hypertension display greater MSNA responses to stress than whites, which may contribute to the increased incidence of hypertension in blacks. Further, power spectrum analyses of heart rate rhythmicity suggest that sympathetic nervous system activity is increased in hypertensive subjects of all ages.

Norepinephrine Spillover

Prior to the development of microneurography, most researchers measured plasma concentration or urinary excretion of noradrenaline to estimate total sympathetic nervous system activity (305). This approach has several limitations. Of particular concern is the dependence of plasma noradrenaline concentration on both the release and clearance of noradrenaline. The release of noradrenaline reflects sympathetic nervous system activity, but large variations in the clearance of released noradrenaline can introduce fluctuations in plasma concentrations independent of the level of sympathetic activity. Measurement of urinary excretion of noradrenaline introduces additional variability secondary to interindividual differences in the renal clearance of plasma noradrenaline. In spite of these limitations, plasma noradrenaline levels in young hypertensive subjects have consistently been shown to be greater than those levels in age-matched normotensive controls, suggesting that sympathetic nervous system activity is elevated in the developmental stages of hypertension (306,307).

To avoid the confounding influence of variations in noradrenaline clearance, techniques have been developed, based on isotope dilution in plasma, to measure metabolic clearance rates, allowing for estimation of release, or spillover, of noradrenaline into plasma. These techniques can be used to measure whole-body spillover of noradrenaline to provide estimates of overall sympathetic nervous system activation, or to measure organ-specific noradrenaline release for determining regional patterns of sympathetic nervous system activity in humans. Esler et al. have reported that noradrenaline spillover is significantly increased in young (<40 years of age), untreated subjects with primary hypertension, suggesting, like simple plasma noradrenaline measurements, that sympathetic nervous system activity is elevated in the early stages of hypertension (307,308). Measurements of regional noradrenaline release into plasma indicate that this increase in sympathetic nervous system activity in young hypertensives is primarily attributable to increased sympathetic outflow to the kidneys and heart (308). Further, Egan et al. have demonstrated that in NaCl-sensitive hypertensive subjects, a high NaCl diet elevates both arterial pressure and forearm vascular resistance. These alterations are related to increased sympathetic nervous system activity and not to changes in peripheral adrenergic receptors (309).

Microneurography

In the 1960s, Hagbarth and Valbo developed an electrophysiological technique for recording muscle and skin sympathetic nerve activity from peripheral nerves (310). That technique has been used extensively to measure peripheral sympathetic nervous system activity at rest and in response to various interventions. Generally, muscle sympathetic nervous system activity (MSNA) is recorded from the peroneal nerve inferior to the knee. MSNA is thought to originate centrally, since the level of activity is altered by agents that presumably act at receptor sites within the central nervous system (311).

By far, the largest comparison of MSNA in normotensive and hypertensive subjects was by Yamada et al. (312). In this study, 43 normotensive (32 males and 11 females) and 63 hypertensive (48 males and 15 females) Japanese subjects had resting MSNA recorded from the tibial nerve. MSNA was significantly greater in the hypertensive group than the normotensive group, even when the two groups were carefully matched for age. The large number of subjects is the most obvious strength of this study, making its findings particularly compelling. Other investigators have reported MSNA to be increased in the developmental stages of hypertension. Anderson et al. found elevated resting MSNA in 12 young males with borderline or intermittent hypertension compared with that in 15 age-matched normotensive males (313). When MSNA is compared between subjects, it is reported as the number of impulses or "bursts" per minute. In this study, during high dietary NaCl ingestion (400 meq Na^+/day), the subjects with borderline hypertension had 25 ± 1 bursts per minute compared with 16 ± 1 bursts per minute in the normotensive subjects. In a recent study, Floras and Hara found that resting MSNA was significantly greater in young subjects with mild (Stage 1) hypertension (10 males and 2 females) than in age-matched normotensive subjects (11 males) (314). Peripheral vascular resistance in the lower extremities was also greater in the hypertensive subjects. In-

creased MSNA and peripheral vascular resistance were present during two separate recording sessions at least 1 month apart, suggesting that the differences were not due simply to a greater alerting or arousal response by the hypertensive subjects during the initial recording session. The above studies suggest that central sympathetic outflow is increased in both the developmental stages and the established phase of primary hypertension. This increase in sympathetic nerve activity occurs concomitantly with elevations in peripheral vascular resistance in the extremities.

Microneurography has also been used to compare peripheral sympathetic nerve activity in African-Americans and American whites. In a comparison of normotensive subjects, blacks and whites with and without a family history of hypertension (i.e., a first-degree relative with hypertension) had similar resting levels of MSNA (315). Blacks with a positive family history of hypertension, however, had significantly greater increases in mean arterial pressure and MSNA during cold pressor testing than age-matched normotensive whites with or without a family history of hypertension (Fig. 13). Responses in blacks with a negative family history of hypertension tended to be intermediate between blacks with a positive family history and the two white groups. Greater stress-induced increases in MSNA may predispose blacks with a positive family history to develop hypertension. As hypothesized by Folkow, repeated stress-induced vasoconstriction leads to vascular hypertrophy, increased vascular resistance, and a consequent increase in blood pressure (316). Additional studies are necessary to determine if African-Americans manifest greater MSNA responses to other types of stress.

A separate study compared blood pressure and MSNA responses during the cold pressor test in black versus white subjects with established hypertension (317). All subjects were withdrawn from antihypertensive therapy for a minimum of 2 weeks prior to study. Baseline MSNA was similar in the two groups, as were cold-induced changes in blood pressure and MSNA. Unlike young normotensive subjects, blacks with established hypertension did not have greater stress-induced changes in sympathetic nerve activity, suggesting that increased sympathetic responses to stress may contribute to the development of hypertension, but not to the maintenance of established hypertension in African-Americans.

Power Spectrum Analysis

Power spectrum analysis is a computer-based technique that quantifies variability in hemodynamic parameters. Power spectrum analyses of heart rate variability indicate that fluctuations in heart rate are not random, but exhibit periodicities of fairly constant frequency. The first component is synchronous with respi-

Baseline   Cold Stress

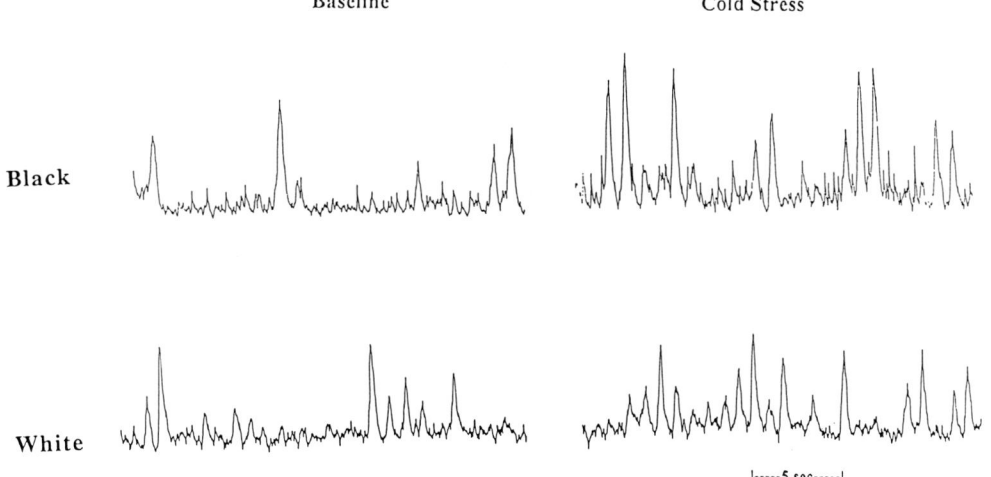

Black

White

|-----5 sec-----|

FIG. 13. Muscle sympathetic nerve activity (MSNA) recorded from the peroneal nerve at rest and during cold pressor testing of a 29-year-old black female and a 26-year-old white male, both with a positive family history of hypertension. Baseline MSNA was similar in the two subjects, but the increase in activity in response to cold stress was greater in the black subject.

ration and occurs at relatively high frequency (0.25 Hz). A second component is identified at a lower frequency (0.1 Hz). The high-frequency variation in the RR interval reflects vagal activity; the low-frequency variation, sympathetic activity (318). Accordingly, by evaluating the relative preponderance of these two frequencies in RR variability, it is possible to estimate the level of vagal and sympathetic activation in humans at rest or during activity. Comparisons of hypertensive subjects with age-matched normotensive controls using power spectrum analysis of heart rate have shown hypertensive subjects to have an increased low frequency/high frequency ratio consistent with greater sympathetic activation (319). Since these reports have included hypertensive subjects of all ages, power spectrum analysis suggests that primary hypertension, regardless of age, is characterized by increased sympathetic nervous system activity.

Medullary Compression

In a subset of patients, there appears to be an association between primary hypertension and localized compression of the ventrolateral medulla (320). In these patients, the posterior inferior cerebellar artery and/or the vertebral artery compresses neurons in cardiovascular regulatory centers, thereby increasing sympathetic nervous system activity. Jannetta et al. reported that successful microvascular decompression of the ventrolateral medulla significantly reduced blood pressure in 33 of 36 hypertensive patients, with 13 requiring no antihypertensive medications postoperatively (320–321). Animal studies and angiographic and autopsy studies in humans have also demonstrated a correlation between vascular compression of the ventrolateral medulla and hyperten-

sion (322–323). Additional studies are needed to clarify this association and its possible role in the development of hypertension.

Tumors such as those described by Cushing (324) and intracerebral ischemia or bleeding can compromise important cardiovascular regulatory centers in the ventral medulla either by exciting tonic vasomotor neurons directly or by limiting their opposing inhibitory innervation. Further, patients undergoing withdrawal from centrally acting agents such as opiates, alcohol, and clonidine (325–327) develop hypertension. These findings indicate a role for the CNS in both the initiation and the maintenance phases of some forms of human hypertension.

Neurological Consequences of Hypertension

Irrespective of etiology, hypertension can alter brain structure and function (304). Hypertension is associated with brain ischemia and/or with local decreases in the density of brain tissue in human subjects (328). Patients in advanced stages of arterial hypertension may display hypertensive encephalopathy, the symptoms of which include severe headache, somnolence, convulsions, vomiting, and visual disturbances (329,330). Recently, Schwartz and colleagues have examined the brains of patients with hypertensive encephalopathy using computed tomography (CT), magnetic resonance imaging (MRI), and single photon emission computed tomography (SPECT) imaging (331). They demonstrated that, irrespective of cause, hypertensive encephalopathy is associated with edema in the occipital cortex and underlying white matter (331) (Fig. 14). Hypertensive encephalopathy develops gradually over days and appears to be

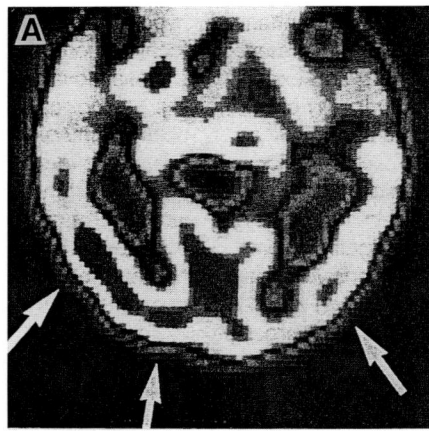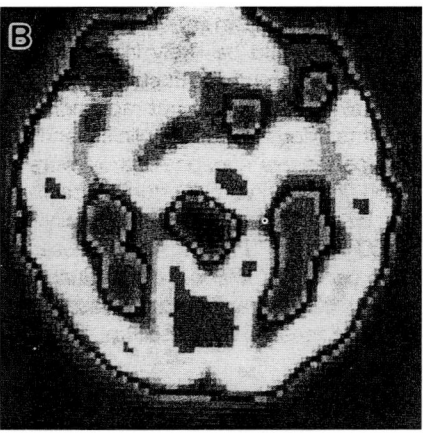

FIG. 14. Two SPECT images from a 23-year-old male with hypertensive encephalopathy due to renal failure (Wegener's granulomatosis). **A** displays increased perfusion in the occipital poles (*dark areas pointed to by the arrows*) and **B** shows the resolution of these abnormalities 10 days after normalization of arterial pressure. (From ref. 331, with permission.)

caused by exaggerated constriction of the brain vasculature in response to systemic hypertension, resulting in ischemia and cytotoxic edema. In contrast, acute, severe hypertensive crisis (e.g., that caused by cocaine abuse) is associated with intracerebral hemorrhages that appear to result from the abrupt pressure increase overwhelming the ability of the brain to autoregulate its vasculature (332,333). These and other studies indicate that cerebral vascular autoregulation normally plays an important protective role in maintaining cerebral blood flow in hypertensive subjects. Finally, a recent population-based study demonstrates that in 85-year-old Swedes, the incidence of vascular dementia is equal to the incidence of Alzheimer's disease, thus demonstrating the importance of chronic antihypertensive treatment for the prevention of CNS damage (334).

ACKNOWLEDGMENTS

The authors thank Leigh Grossman for her secretarial assistance. This work was supported by National Institutes of Health Grants HL 37722, HL 47081, HL 44195, HL 31515, HL 46554, HL 02568, HL 47081, HL 50147 and grants from the American Heart Association, National Center and Alabama Affiliate.

REFERENCES

1. Chung JM, Chung K, Wurster RD. *Brain Res* 1975;91:126–131.
2. Strack AM, Sawyer WB, Marubio LM, Loewy AD. *Brain Res* 1988;455:187–191.
3. Poree LR, Schramm LP. *Brain Res* 1992;599:297–301.
4. Poree LR, Schramm LP. *Brain Res* 1992;599:302–308.
5. Ciriello J, Calaresu FR. *J Autonom Nerv Syst* 1981;3:299–310.
6. Sved AF, Imaizuma T, Talman WT, Reis DJ. *Hypertension* 1985;7:262–267.
7. Ferrario CM, Barnes KL, Bohonek S. *Hypertension* 1981; 3(Suppl 2):112–118.
8. Nathan MA, Reis DJ. *Circ Res* 1977;40:72–80.
9. Wyss JM, Donovan MK. *Brain Res* 1984;298:130–134.
10. Simon OR, Schramm LP. *Brain Res* 1984;290:239–247.
11. Hopkins DA, Holstege G. *Exp Brain Res* 1978;32:529–547.
12. Terreberry RR, Naefsey E. *Brain Res* 1983;278:245–249.
13. Conrad LCA, Pfaff DW. *J Comp Neurol* 1976;169:221–262.
14. Swanson LW. *Brain Res* 1977;128:346–353.
15. Batton RR, Jayaraman A, Ruggiero D, Carpenter MB. *J Comp Neurol* 1977;174:281–306.
16. Chiba T, Doba N. *Brain Res* 1976;102:255–265.
17. Zemlan FP, Leonard CM, Kow LM, Pfaff DW. *Exp Neurol* 1978;62:298–334.
18. Talman WT, Lewis SJ. *Clin Exp Hypertens Part A Theory Pract* 1991;13(5):661–668.
19. Kawata K, Nakan K, Morii N, et al. *Neuroscience* 1985;16:521–546.
20. Sawchenko PE, Swanson LW. *Brain Res Rev* 1982;4:275–325.
21. Ricardo JA, Koh ET. *Brain Res* 1978;153:1–26.
22. Laughton WB, Powley TL. *Am J Physiol* 1987;252:R13–R25.
23. Willette RN, Sarcas PP, Krieger AJ, Sapur HN. *Neuropharm* 1983;22:1071–1079.
24. Machado BH, Brody MJ. *Hypertension* 1988;11:1135–1138.
25. Stuesse SL, Fish SF. *J Comp Neurol* 1984;229:271–278.
26. Gonzalez-Lima F. *Behav Brain Res* 1988;28:325–336.
27. Machado BH, Brody MJ. *Hypertension* 1988;11:602–607.
28. Armstrong DM, Ross CA, Pickel VM, Joh TH, Reis DJ. *J Comp Neurol* 1982;212:173–187.
29. Reis, DJ. *Circulation* 1984;70(Suppl III):31–45.
30. Ross CA, Ruggiero DA, Park DH, et al. *J Neurosci* 1984;4:474–494.
31. Dampney RAL, Goodchild AK, Robertson LG, Montgomery W. *Brain Res* 1982;249:223–235.
32. Tucker DC, Saper CB, Ruggiero DA, Reis DJ. *J Comp Neurol* 1987;259:591–603.
33. Guyenet PG, Stornetta RL. *Brain Res* 1982;235:271–283.
34. Dampney RA, Goodchild AK. *Can J Physiol Pharmacol* 1987;65:1572–1579.
35. Sangdee C, Franz DN. *Neurosci Lett* 1983;37:167–173.
36. Sun MK, Hackett JT, Guyenet PG. *Brain Res* 1988;438:23–40.
37. Morrison SF, Callaway J, Milner TA, Reis DJ. *Brain Res* 1991;562(1):126–135.
38. Dampney RAL, Moon EA. *Am J Physiol* 1980;239:H349–H358.
39. Granata AR, Ruggiero DA, Park DH, Joh TH, Reis DJ. *Am J Physiol* 1985;248:H547–H567.
40. Blessing WW, Reis DJ. *Brain Res* 1982;253:161–171.
41. Imaizumi T, Granata AR, Benarroch EE, Sved AF, Reis DJ. *J Hypertens* 1985;3:491–501.
42. Ross DA, Armstrong DM, Ruggiero DA, Pickel VM, Joh TH, Reis DJ. *Neurosci Lett* 1981;25:257–262.
43. Cravo SL, Morrison SF, Reis DJ. *Am J Physiol* 1991;261(4 Pt 2):R985–R994.
44. Smith JK, Barron KW. *Brain Res* 1990;506(1):153–158.
45. Muratani H, Ferrario CM, Averill DB. *Am J Physiol* 1993;264(2 Pt 2):R388–R395.
46. Ferrario CM, Barnes KL, Szilagyi JE, Brosnihan KB. *Hypertension* 1979;1:235–245.
47. Shapiro RE, Miselis RR. *J Comp Neurol* 1985;234:344–364.

48. Bruner CA, Mangiapane ML, Fink GD, Webb RC. *Hypertension* 1988;11:668–673.
49. Fink GD, Bruner CA, Mangiapane ML. *Hypertension* 1987;9:355–361.
50. Mangiapane ML, Skoog KM, Rittenhouse P, Blair ML, Sladek CD. *Circ Res* 1989;64:129–135.
51. Loewy AD, Burton H. *J Comp Neurol* 1978;181:421–450.
52. Ricardo JA, Koh ET. *Brain Res* 1978;153:1–26.
53. Cechetto DF, Calaresu FR. *Am J Physiol* 1983;245:R811–R819.
54. Fulwiler CE, Saper CB. *Brain Res Rev* 1984;7:229–259.
55. Herbert H, Moga MM, Saper CB. *J Comp Neurol* 1990;293:540–580.
56. Marovitch S, Kamada M, Reis DJ. *Brain Res* 1982;232:57–75.
57. Felder RB, Mifflin SW. *Circ Res* 1988;63:35–49.
58. Fink GD, Pawloski CM, Ohman LE, Haywood JR. *Hypertension* 1991;17:1177–1184.
59. Hilton SM, Redfern WS. *J Physiol (London)* 1986;378:213–228.
60. Calaresu FR, Ciriello J. *Can J Physiol Pharmacol* 1981;59:1274–1277.
61. Cantor EH, Abraham S, Spector S. *Life Sci* 1981;519–526.
62. Eilam R, Malach R, Bergmann F, Segal M. *J Neurosci* 1991;11(2):401–411.
63. Ciriello J, Caverson MM. *Am J Physiol* 1984;247:R872–R879.
64. Buñag RD, Butterfield J, Sasaki S. *Hypertension* 1983;5:460–467.
65. Sasaki S, Buñag RD. *J Cardiovasc Pharmacol* 1982;4:1042–1048.
66. Juskevich JC, Robinson DS, Whitehorn D. *Eur J Pharmacol* 1978;51:429–439.
67. Kuypers HGJM, Maisky VA. *Neurosci Lett* 1973;1:9–14.
68. Schwanzel-Fukuda M, Morrell JI, Pfaff DW. *J Comp Neurol* 1984;226:1–20.
69. Smith JK, Barron KW. *Am J Physiol* 1989;257(*Heart Circ Physiol* 26):H1994–H2000.
70. Buñag RD, Eferakeya AD. *Cardiovasc Res* 1976;10:663–671.
71. Berecek KH, Brody MJ. In: Rascher W, Clugh D, Ganten D, eds. *Proceedings, 4th International Symposium on Rats with Spontaneous Hypertension and Related Studies.* Heidelberg, Stuttgart: Schattauer Verlag, 1981:394.
72. Winternitz SR, Wyss JM, Oparil S. *Brain Res* 1984;324:51–58.
73. Brezenoff HE, Xiao YF. *Life Sci* 1989;45(13):1163–1170.
74. Wible JH, DiMicco JA, Luft FC. *Hypertension* 1989;14:623–628.
75. Ciriello J, Calaresu FR. *Am J Physiol* 1980;239:R137–R142.
76. Patel KP, Schmid PG. *J Auton Nerv Syst* 1988;22:211–219.
77. McKeller S, Loewy AD. *Brain Res* 1981;217:351–357.
78. Ter Horst GJ, Luiten PGM. *Brain Res Bull* 1987;18:191–203.
79. Swanson LW, Kuypers HG. *J Comp Neurol* 1980;194:555–570.
80. Gilbey MP, Coote JH, Fleetwood-Walker S, Peterson DF. *Brain Res* 1982;251:283–290.
81. Caverson MM, Ciriello J. *Am J Physiol* 1988;254:R531–R543.
82. Wyss JM, Aboukarsh N, Oparil S. *Am J Physiol* 1985;250:H82–H86.
83. Krukoff TL, Calaresu FR. *Brain Res* 1984;322:75–82.
84. Qualy JM, Westfall TC. *Am J Physiol* 1988;254:H993–H1003.
85. Jones DL, Lo S. *Pharmacol Biochem Behav* 1990;36(4):979–983.
86. Johnson AK. In: Schrier RW, ed. *Vasopressin.* New York: Raven Press; 1985:319–342.
87. Miselis RR. *Brain Res* 1981;230:1–23.
88. Saper CB, Reis DJ, Jon T. *Neurosci Lett* 1983;42:285–291.
89. Brody MJ, Johnson AK. In: Martini L, Ganong WF, eds. *Frontiers in neuroendocrinology,* vol 6. New York: Raven Press; 1980:249–272.
90. Knuepfer MM, Johnson AK, Brody MJ. *Brain Res* 1984;294:305–314.
91. Mangiapane ML, Brody MJ. *Am J Physiol* 1987;253:R827–R831.
92. Webb RL, Brody MJ. *Clin Exp Hypertens Part A Theory Pract* 1987;9(Suppl 1):47–57.
93. Saper CB, Standaert DG, Currie MG, Schwartz D, Geller DM, Needleman P. *Science* 1985;227:1047–1049.
94. Nathan MA, Reis DJ. *Circ Res* 1975;37:226–235.
95. Folkow B, Johansson B, Oberg B. *Acta Physiol Scand* 1959;47:262–270.
96. Hilton SM, Spyer KM. *J Physiol (Lond)* 1971;218:271–293.
97. Gellman MD, Schneiderman N, Wallach JH, LeBlanc W. *J Auton Nerv Syst* 1981;4:301–317.
98. Meldrum MJ, Xue C-S, Badino L, Westfall TC. *J Cardiovasc Pharmacol* 1985;7:59–65.
99. Miyajima E, Buñag RD. *Am J Physiol* 1985;248:H937–H943.
100. Calaresu FR, Ciriello J. *Am J Physiol* 1980;239:R130–R136.
101. Spyer KM. *J Physiol (Lond)* 1972;224:245–257.
102. Grizzle WE, Johnson RN, Schramm LP, Gann DS. *Am J Physiol* 1975;228:1039–1045.
103. Simon OR, Basuray BN, West WL, Copeland R. *Neuropharm* 1985;24:665–675.
104. Thornton RM, Wyss JM, Oparil S. *Hypertension* 1989;14:518–523.
105. Robinson RL, Dietl H, Bald M, Kraus A, Philippu A. *Naunyn-Schmiedebergs Arch Pharmacol* 1983;322:203–209.
106. Czyzewska-Szafran H, Jastrz:ebski Z, Remiszewska M, Wutkiewicz M. *Eur J Pharmacol* 1991;198(2–3):115–120.
107. Wyss JM, Yang R, Jin H, Oparil S. *J Hypertens* 1988;6:805–813.
108. Folkow B, Hallback-Nordlander M, Martner J, Nordborg C. *Acta Physiol Scand* 1982;116:133–139.
109. Kaada BR. *Acta Physiol Scand* 1951;24(Suppl 83):1–285.
110. Galeno TM, Van Hoesen GW, Brody MJ. *Brain Res* 1984;291:249–259.
111. Iwata J, Chida K, LeDoux JE. *Brain Res* 1987;418:183–188.
112. Calaresu FR, Ciriello J, Mogenson GJ. *J Physiol* 1976;260:515–530.
113. Yasui Y, Breder CD, Saper CB, Cechetto DF. *J Comp Neurol* 1991;303:355–374.
114. Burns SM, Wyss JM. *Brain Res* 1985;340:71–77.
115. Ritter S, Dinh TT, Stone S, Ross N. *Brain Res* 1988;450:354–359.
116. Tajima A, Hans FJ, Livingstone D, et al. *Hypertension* 1993;21:105–111.
117. Wyss JM, Van Groen T. *Cerebral Cortex* 1992;2:468–476.
118. Wyss JM, Fisk G, Van Groen T. *Brain Res* 1992;592:135–140.
119. Sudilovsky A, Cutler NR, Sramek JJ, et al. *Alz Dis Assoc Disorder* 1993;7(2):105–111.
120. Okamoto K, Aoki K. *Jpn Circ J* 1963;27:282–293.
121. Ooshima A, Yamori Y, Okamoto K. *Jpn Circ J* 1972;36:797–812.
122. Haeusler G, Finch L, Thoenen H. *Experientia* 1972;28:1200–1203.
123. Oparil S, Cutilletta AF. *Am J Cardiol* 1979;44:970–978.
124. Saavedra JM, Grobecker H, Axelrod JH. *Circ Res* 1978;42:529–534.
125. Winternitz SR, Katholi RE, Oparil S. *J Clin Invest* 1980;66:971–978.
126. Winternitz SR, Oparil S. *Clin Exp Hypertens* 1982;4:751–760.
127. Winternitz SR, Wyss J, Meadows JR, Oparil S. *Clin Sci Mol Med* 1982;63:339s–342s.
128. Wyss JM, Chen YF, Jin H, Gist R, Oparil S. *Hypertension* 1987;10:313–320.
129. Chen YF, Meng QC, Wyss JM, Jin H, Oparil S. *Hypertension* 1988;11:55–62.
130. Chen CW, Chen YF, Meng QC, Wyss M, Oparil S. *Brain Res* 1991;565:135–141.
131. Koepke JP, Jones S, DiBona GF. *Hypertension* 1988;11:326–333.
132. Oparil S, Meng QC, Chen YF, Yang RH, Jin H, Wyss J. *J Cardiovasc Pharmacol* 1988;12(Suppl 3):S56–S69.
133. Yang R, Jin H, Chen YF, Oparil S, Wyss JM. *J Cardiovasc Pharmacol* 1989;13:162–167.
134. Klangkalya B, Sripairojthikoon W, Oparil S, Wyss JM. *Brain Res* 1988;451:77–84.
135. Jin H, Yang RH, Wyss JM, Chen YF, Oparil S. *Hypertension* 1991;18:224–229.
136. DeChamplain J, Mueller RA, Axelrod J. *Circ Res* 1969;25:285–291.
137. Chen YF, Meng QC, Wyss JM, Jin HK, Rogers CF, Oparil S. *Hypertension* 1990;16:55–62.
138. Krakoff LR. *Cardiol Clin* 1988;6:537–545.
139. Mantero F, Boscaro M. *J Steroid Biochem Mol Biol* 1992;43:409–413.

140. Kennedy B, Elayan H, Ziegler MG. *Hypertension* 1993;21:415–419.
141. Grunfeld JP. *Horm Res* 1990;34:111–113.
142. Moore KE, Phillipson OT. *J Neurochem* 1975;25:289–294.
143. Waeber B, Gavras H, Bresnahan MR, Gavras I, Brunner HR. *Clin Sci* 1983;65:255–261.
144. Black J, Waeber B, Bresnahan MR, Gavras I, Gavras H. *Circ Res* 1981;49:518–524.
145. Brown MR, Fisher LA. *Life Sci* 1986;39:1003–1012.
146. Fanelli M, Nahmod VE, Torres N, et al. *Neurosci Lett* 1992;135:189–192.
147. Brody MJ, Fink GD, Buggy J, et al. In: Meyer P, Schmitt H, eds. *Perspectives in nephrology and hypertension,* vol 6. New York: John Wiley; 1979:76–84.
148. Iwai J, Friedman R, Tassinari L. *Clin Sci Mol Med* 1980;59:263s–265s.
149. Kotchen TA, Blehschmidt NG, Reddy SR. *J Lab Clin Med* 1991;117:383–389.
150. Saavedra JM, Correa FM, Iwai J. *Brain Res* 1980;193:299–303.
151. Periyasamy SM, Rapp JP. *Biochem Pharmacol* 1989;38:3851–3858.
152. Eide I, Myers MR, DeQuattro V, Kolloch R, Eide K, Whigham M. *J Cardiovasc Pharmacol* 1980;2:833–841.
153. Katholi RE, Whitlow PL, Winternitz SR, Oparil S. *Hypertension* 1982;4:II166–174.
154. Katholi RE, Winternitz SR, Oparil S. *Hypertension* 1981;3:404–409.
155. Katholi RE, Whitlow PL, Winternitz SR, Oparil S. *Hypertension* 1982;4:II166–II174.
156. Winternitz SR, Katholi RE, Oparil S. *Hypertension* 1982;4:369–373.
157. Wyss JM, Aboukarsh N, Oparil S. *Am J Physiol* 1986;250:H82–H86.
158. Katholi RE, Winternitz SR, Oparil S. *J Clin Invest* 1982;69:55–62.
159. Cavero I, Massingham R, Lefevre-Borg F. *Life Sci* 1982a;31:939–948.
160. Cavero K, Massingham R, Lefevre-Borg F. *Life Sci* 1982b;31:1059–1069.
161. Haeusler G, Lues I, Minck KO, Schelling P, Seyfried CA. *Eur Heart J* 1992;13(D):129–135.
162. Lindvall O, Bjorklund A, Skagerberg G. *Ann Neurol* 1983;14:255–260.
163. Lin MT, Yang JJ. *Am J Physiol* 1993 (in press).
164. Chen YF, Jin H, Paul R, Nagahama S. *J Pharmacol Exp Ther* 1988;246:485–492.
165. Nagahama S, Chen YF, Lindheimer MD, Oparil S. *J Pharmacol Exp Ther* 1986a;239:426–432.
166. Nagahama S, Chen YF, Lindheimer MD, Oparil S. *J Pharmacol Exp Ther* 1986b;236:735–742.
167. Yang RH, Chen YF, Wyss JM, Oparil S. *Soc Neurosci Abstr* 1988;502.
168. Nagahama S, Chen YF, Oparil S. *Am J Physiol* 1985;249:H64–H70.
169. Van den Buuse M, Versteeg DHG, De Jong W. *Hypertension* 1984;6:899–905.
170. Shigetomi S, Buu NT, Kuchel O. *Hypertension* 1991;17:997–1002.
171. Chiu P, Rajakumar G, Chiu S, Kwan CY, Mishra RK. *Prog Neuropsychopharmacol Biol Psychiatry* 1984;8:665–668.
172. LeFur G, Guilloux F, Kabouche M, Mitrani N, Ferris O, Uzan A. *Dev Brain Res* 1981;1:153–163.
173. Chen YF, Oparil S. *Brain Res* 1987;400:225–231.
174. Dahlstrom A, Fuxe K. *Acta Physiol Scand* 1965;247:1–36.
175. Pompeiano M, Palacios JM, Mengod G. *J Neurosu* 1992;12(2):440–453.
176. Barban JM, Aghajanian GK. *Brain Res* 1981;204:1–11.
177. Chalmers JP, Pilowsky PM, Minson JB, Kapoor V, Mills E, West MJ. *Am J Hypertens* 1988;1:79–83.
178. Ungerstedt U, Herrara-Marschiltz M, Zetterstrom T. *Prog Brain Res* 1982;55:41–49.
179. Aslanian V, Lambas-Senas L, Renaud B. *Life Sci* 1988;43:1031–1038.
180. Bhaskaran D, Freed CR. *J Pharmacol Exp Ther* 1988;245:356–363.
181. Dawson R, Nagahama S, Oparil S. *Neuropharm* 1988;27:417–426.
182. Gentili L, Saija A, Luchetti G, Massi M. *Pharmacol Biochem Behav* 1991;39:171–176.
183. Piianzin AI, Popova NK, Markel AL. *Farmakologiia I Toksikologiia* 1991;54:28–30.
184. Smith ML, Browning RA, Myers JH. *Eur J Pharmacol* 1979;53:301–305.
185. Buckingham RE, Hamilton TC, Robson D. *Eur J Pharmacol* 1976;36:431–437.
186. Ito H, Shiokawa H, Torii M, Suzuki T. *Clin Exp Hypertens Part A Theory Pract* 1991;A13:971–979.
187. Breckenridge A. *Drugs* 1988;36:44–54.
188. Reid JL, Rubin PC. *Physiol Rev* 1987;67:725–749.
189. Morris JF, Chapman DB, Sokol HW. In: Gash DM, Boer GJ, eds. *Vasopressin principles and properties.* New York: Plenum Press; 1987.
190. Berecek KH, Mah SC, Baum P, Hofbauer KG. *J Hypertens* 1984a;2(Suppl 3):29–31.
191. Unger T, Rohmeiss P, Becker H, Ganten D, Lang RE, Petty M. *J Hypertens* 1984;2(Suppl 3):25–27.
192. Hofbauer KG, Mah SC, Baum HP, Hanni H, Wood JM, Kraitz J. *J Cardiovasc Pharmacol* 1984;6:S184–S191.
193. Swords BH, Wyss JM, Berecek KH. In: Jard S, Jamison R, eds. *Vasopressin.* Paris: Colloque Inserm/John Libbey Eurotext Ltd; 1991.
194. Cowley AW, Liard JF. In: Gash DM, Boer GJ, eds. *Vasopressin principles and properties.* New York: Plenum Press; 1987.
195. Gavras H, Gavras I. *J Hypertens* 1989;7:601–606.
196. Friedman SM, Friedman CL, Nakashima M. *Endocrinol* 1960;67:752–759.
197. Mohring J, Mohring B, Petri M, Haack D. *Am J Physiol* 1977;232:F260–F269.
198. Berecek KH, Stocker M, Gross F. *Circulation* 1980;46:619–624.
199. Crofton JT, Share L, Wang BC, Shade RE. *Hypertension* 1980;2:424–431.
200. Berecek KH, Murray RD, Gross F, Brody MJ. *Hypertension* 1982;4:3–12.
201. Berecek KH, Olpe HR, Jones RSG, Hofbauer KG. *Am J Physiol* 1984b;247:H675–H681.
202. Berecek KH. *J Cardiovasc Pharmacol* 1986;8(Suppl 7):S76–S80.
203. Ciriello J, Kline RL, Zhang TX, Caverson MM. *Brain Res* 1984;310:355–359.
204. Harding JW, Wright JW, Speth RC, Barnes CD, eds. *Angiotensin and Blood Pressure Regulation.* San Diego, CA: Academic Press; 1988.
205. Raizada MK, Phillips MI, Sumners C, eds. *Cellular and Molecular Biology of the Renin-Angiotensin System.* Boca Raton, FL: CRC Press; 1993.
206. Lind RW, Swanson LW, Ganten D. *Neuroendocrinol* 1985;40:2–24.
207. Fishman M, Zimmerman E, Slater E. *Science* 1981;214:921–923.
208. Raizada MK, Stenstrom B, Phillips MI, Sumners C. *Am J Physiol* 1984;247:C115–C119.
209. Ganten D, Fuxe K, Phillips MI, Mann JFE, Ganten U. In: *Frontiers in neuroendocrinology,* vol 5. New York: Raven Press; 1978:61–99.
210. Epstein AN, Fitzsimons JT, Rolls BJ. *J Physiol (Lond)* 1970;210:457–474.
211. Bradford HF, *Chemical neurobiology* New York: WH Freeman and Co; 1986:265–310.
212. Sladek CD, Armstrong WE. In: Gash DM, Boer GJ, eds. *Vasopressin: principles and properties.* New York: Plenum Press; 1987:275–333.
213. Dietz R, Schomig A, Haebara H, Mann JF, et al. *Circ Res* 1978;43(Suppl I):98.
214. Hermann K, McDonald W, Unger T, Lang RE, Ganten D. *J Physiol (Paris)* 1984;79:471–480.
215. Casto R, Phillips MI. *Am J Physiol* 1985;249:R341–R347.

216. Unger T, Kaufman-Buhler I, Scholkens BA, Ganten D. *Eur J Pharmacol* 1981;70:467–478.
217. Berecek KH, Okuno T, Nagahama T, Oparil S. *Hypertension* 1983;5:689–700.
218. Giudicelli JF, Freslon JL, Glasson S, Richer C. *Clin Exp Hypertens* 1980;2:1083–1096.
219. Harrap SB, Merwe Van der WM, Griffin SA, Macpherson F, Lever AF. *Hypertension* 1990;16:603–614.
220. Wu JN, Berecek KH. *Hypertension* 1993;22:139–146.
221. Unger T, Retting R. *Hypertension* 1990;16:615–616.
222. Raizada MK, Muther TF, Sumners C. *Am J Physiol* 1984;247:C364–C372.
223. Wilson KM, Magargal W, Berecek KH. *Hypertension* 1988;1(Suppl I):I148–I152.
224. Berecek KH, Swords BH, Lo S, Kirk KA. *J Hypertens* 1992;10:545–552.
225. Yang RH, Jin H, Wyss JM, Oparil S. *Hypertension* 1992;19:475–481.
226. Yang RJ, Jin H, Wyss JM, Oparil S. *Hypertension* 1992;20:755–762.
227. Rosenzweig A, Seidman CE. *Annu Rev Biochem* 1991;60:229–255.
228. Chinkers M, Garbers DL. *Science* 1989;245:1392–1394.
229. Maack TM, Suzuki M, Almeida FA, et al. *Science* 1987;238:675–678.
230. deBold AJ, Borenstein HB, Veress AT, Sonnenberg H. *Life Sci* 1981;28:89–94.
231. Oparil S, Wyss JM. *News in Physiological Sciences* 1993;8:223–228.
232. Gardner DG, Vlasuk GP, Baxter JD, Fiddes JC, Lewicki JA. *Proc Natl Acad Sci* 1987;84:2175–2179.
233. Saper CB, Standaert DG, Currie MG, Schwartz D, Geller DM, Needleman P. *Science* 1985;227:1047–1049.
234. Phillips MI, Kimura B, Wang H, Hoffman WE. *Am J Physiol* 1989;257(Regulatory Integrative Comp Physiol 26):R1393–R1399.
235. Imada T, Takayanagi R, Inagami T. *Biochem Biophys Res Commun* 1985;133:759–765.
236. Jin H, Chen YF, Yang RH, Meng QC, Oparil S. *Hypertension* 1988;11:739–744.
237. Yang RH, Jin H, Chen YF, Wyss JM, Oparil S. *J Clin Invest* 1990;86:1985–1990.
238. Squadrito F, Frisina N, Buemi M, et al. *J Cardiovasc Pharmacol* 1989;13(Suppl 6):527–530.
239. Levin ER, Weber MA, Mills S. *Am J Physiol* 1988;255:H616–H622.
240. McKitrick DJ, Calaresu HR. *Am J Physiol* 1988;255:R182–R187.
241. Ermirio R, Ruggeri P, Cogo CE, Molinari C, Calaresu FR. *Am J Physiol* 1989;256:R577–R582.
242. Calhoun DA, Wyss JM, Oparil S. *Hypertension* 1991;17:363–368.
243. Nakamura Y, Calhoun DA, Chen YF, Wyss JM, Oparil S. *Hypertension* 1993;22:285–291.
244. Jin H, Yang RH, Chen YF, Wyss JM, Oparil S. *Am J Hypertens* 1991;4:449–455.
245. Wong M, Samson WK, Dudley CA, Moss R. *Neuroendocrinol* 1986;44:49–53.
246. Yang RH, Jin H, Wyss JM, Chen YF, Oparil S. *Hypertension* 1992;19:198–205.
247. Yang RH, Jin H, Wyss JM, Chen YF, Oparil S. *Hypertension* 1992;20:242–246.
248. Gonzalez ER, Krieger EJ, Sapru H. *Hypertension* 1983;5:346–352.
249. Jin H, Yang RH, Calhoun D, Wyss JM, Oparil S. *Hypertension* 1992;20:374–379.
250. Sudoh T, Kangawa K, Minamino N, Matsuo H. *Nature* 1988;332:78–81.
251. Minamino N, Aburaya M, Ueda S, Kangawa K, Matsuo H. *Biochem Biophys Res Commun* 1988;155:740–746.
252. Aburaya M, Minamino N, Hino J, Kangawa K, Matsuo H. *Biochem Biophys Res Commun* 1989;165(2):880–887.
253. Steinhelper M. *Circ Res* 1993;72(5):984–991.
254. Sudoh T, Minamino N, Kangawa K, Matsuo H. *Biochem Biophys Res Commun* 1990;68:863–870.
255. Komatsu Y, Nakao K, Suga S, et al. *Endocrinol* 1991;129:1104–1106.
256. Koller KJ, Lowe DJ, Bennett GL, et al. *Science* 1991;252:120–123.
257. Suga S, Nakao K, Itoh H, et al. *J Clin Invest* 1991;90:1145–1149.
258. Huang FLS, Skala KD, Samson WK. *J Neuroendocrinol* 1992;4:325–330.
259. Huang FLS, Skala KD, Samson WK. *J Neuroendocrinol* 1992;4:593–597.
260. Samson WK, Skala KD, Huang FLS. *Brain Res* 1991;568:285–288.
261. Charles CJ, Richards AM, Espiner EA. *Endocrinol* 1992;131:1721–1726.
262. Yanagisawa M, Kurihara H, Kimura S, et al. *Nature* 1988;322:411–415.
263. Rubanyi GM, ed. *Endothelin.* New York: Oxford University Press; 1991.
264. Yoshizawa T, Shinmi O, Giaid A, et al. *Science* 1990;247:462–464.
265. Hoyer D, Waeber C, Palacios JM. *J Cardiovas Pharmacol* 1989;13:S162–S165.
266. Yamamoto T, Kimura T, Ota K, et al. *Am J Physiol* 1992;262:E856–E862.
267. Samson WK, Skala K, Huang FLS, Gluntz S, Alexander B, Gomez-Sanchez CE. *Brain Res* 1991;539:347–351.
268. Shichiri M, Hirata Y, Kanno K, Ohta K, Emori T, Marumo F. *Biochem Biophys Res Commun* 1989;163:1332–1337.
269. Gulati A, Rebello S. *Neuropharm* 1992;31:243–250.
270. Banasik JL, Hosick H, Wright JW, Harding JW. *J Pharmacol Exper Therap* 1991;257:302–306.
271. Hypertension Detection and Follow-up Program Cooperative Group. *Am J Epidemiol* 1977;106:351–361.
272. von Eiff AW, Lutz HM, Gries J, Kretzschmar R. *Brain Res in Cardiology* 1985;80:191–201.
273. Chen YF, Meng QC. *Life Sci* 1991;48:85–96.
274. Stumpf WE, Sar M, Keefer DA. In: Stumpf WE, Grant LD, eds. *Anatomical neuroendocrinology.* Basel: Karger; 1975:104–119.
275. Stumpf WE. *Experientia* 1990;46:13–25.
276. Bidmon HJ, Stumpf WE, Kawamata S, Shirasu K, Gutkowska J, Sar M. *Histochemistry* 1990;94:505–508.
277. Petitti N, Karkanias GB, Etgen AM. *J Neurosci* 1990;10:2841–2849.
278. Petitti N, Etgen AM. *J Neurosci* 1992;12:3869–3876.
279. Sar M, Stumpf WE. In: Stumpf WE, Grant LD, eds. *Anatomical neuroendocrinology.* Basel: Karger; 1975:120–133.
280. Heritage AS, Stumpf WE, Sar M, Grant LD. *Science* 1980;207:1377–1379.
281. Ganten U, Schroder G, Witt M, Zimmermann F, Ganten D, Stock G. *J Hypertens* 1989;7:721–726.
282. Chen YF, Naftilan AJ, Oparil S. *Hypertension* 1992;19:456–463.
283. Myers JH, Bohr DF. In: Mantero F, Biglieri EG, Funder JW, Scoggins BA, eds. *The adrenal gland and hypertension.* New York: Raven Press; Serono Symposia, 1985;27:131–158.
284. Lohmeier TE, Carroll RG. In: Mantero F, Biglieri EG, Funder JW, Scoggins BA, eds. *The adrenal gland and hypertension.* New York: Raven Press; Serono Symposia, 1985;27:159–175.
285. Stumpf WE, Sar M. In: Jones MF, Gillham B, Dallman MF, Chattopadhyay S, eds. *Interaction within the brain-pituitary adrenocortical system.* New York: Academic Press; 1979:137–156.
286. Van Eekelen JA, Kiss JZ, Westphal HM, de Kloet ER. *Brain Res* 1987;436:120–128.
287. Van Eekelen JA, Jiang W, de Kloet ER, Bohn MC. *J Neurosci Res* 1988;21:88–94.
288. Reul JM, de Kloet ER. *Endocrinol* 1985;117:2505–2511.
289. van den Berg DTWM, de Kloet ER, van Dijken HH, de Jong W. *Endocrinol* 1990;126:118–124.
290. Gomez Sanchez EP, Fort C, Thwaites D. *Am J Physiol* 1992;262:E96–E99.
291. Gomez Sanchez EP. *Am J Hypertens* 1991;4:374–381.
292. Torres N, Fanelli M, Alvarez AL, Santajuliana D, Finkielman S, Pirola CJ. *J Endocrinol* 1991;129:269–274.

293. Weber MA, Graettinger WF, Cheung DG. In: Laragh JH, Brenner BM, eds. *Hypertension: pathophysiology, diagnosis, and management.* New York: Raven Press; 1990:2251–2261.
294. Timmermans PB, Schoop AM, Kwa HY, Van Zwieten PA. *Eur J Pharmacol* 1981;70:7–15.
295. Punnen S, Urbanski R, Krieger AJ, Sapru HN. *Brain Res* 1987;422:336–346.
296. Ernsberger P, Meeley MP, Mann JJ, Reis DJ. *Eur J Pharmacol* 1987;134:1–13.
297. Michel MC, Insel PA. *Trends Pharmacol Sci* 1989;10:342–344.
298. Ernsberger P, Meeley MP, Reis DJ. *Brain Res* 1988;441:309–318.
299. Ernsberger P, Meeley MP, Reis DJ. *J Hypertens* 1986;4(Suppl 5):S109–S111.
300. Reis DJ, LeDoux JE. *Circulation* 1987;76:I2–I9.
301. Abboud FM. *Clin Exp Hypertens A* 1984;6:43–60.
302. Wallin BG, Mörlin C, Hjemdahl P. *Acta Physiol Scand* 1987;129:489–497.
303. Reis DJ, Talman WT. Brain lesions and hypertension. In: de Jong W, ed. *Handbook of hypertension: experimental and genetic models of hypertension,* vol 4. Amsterdam: Elsevier; 1984:451–473.
304. Reis DJ. The brain and hypertension. *Arch Neurol* 1988;45:180–182.
305. von Euler US, Hellner S, Purkhold A. *Scand J Clin Lab Invest* 1954;6:54–59.
306. Goldstein DS. *Hypertension* 1983;5:86–99.
307. Esler M, Ferrier C, Lambert G, et al. *Hypertension* 1991;17(Suppl III):III29–III35.
308. Esler M, Jennings G, Korner P, et al. *Hypertension* 1988;11:3–20.
309. Egan BM, Weder AB, Prtrin J, Hoffmann RG. *Am J Hypertens* 1991;4:416–421.
310. Hagbarth K-E, Valbo AB. *Acta Physiol Scand* 1968;74:96–108.
311. Esler MD, Wallin G, Dorward PK, et al. *Am J Physiol* 1991;260:R817–R823.
312. Yamada Y, Miyajima E, Tochikubo O, Matsukawa T, Ishii M. *Hypertension* 1989;13:870–877.
313. Anderson EA, Sinkey CA, Lawton WJ, Mark AL. *Hypertension* 1989;14:177–183.
314. Floras JS, Hara K. *J Hypertens* 1993;11:647–655.
315. Calhoun DA, Mutinga ML, Wyss JM, Oparil S. *Hypertension* 1993;22:412.
316. Folkow BS. *Physiol Rev* 1982;62:347–504.
317. Calhoun DA, Mutinga ML, Wyss JM, Oparil S. *Am J Hypertens* 1993;6:17A.
318. Malliani A, Pagani M, Lombardi F, Furlan R, Guzzetti S, Cerutti S. *Hypertension* 1991;17(Suppl III):III36–III42.
319. Guzetti S, Piccaluga E, Casati R, et al. *J Hypertens* 1988;6:711–717.
320. Jannetta PJ, Segal R, Wolfson SK. *Ann Surg* 1985;201:391–398.
321. Jannetta PJ, Segal R, Wolfson SK Jr, Dujovny M, Semba A, Cook EE. *Ann Surg* 1985;202:253–261.
322. Naraghi R, Gaab MR, Walter GF, Kleineberg B. *J Neurosurg* 1992;77:103–112.
323. Kleinberg B, Becker H, Gaab MR. *Neuroradiology* 1991;33:2–8.
324. Cushing H. *Am J Med Sci* 1902;124:375–400.
325. Gold MS, Kleber HD. In: Lal H, Fielding S, eds. *Psychopharmacology of clonidine.* New York: Alan R Liss, 1981;299–306.
326. Beevers D, Ballan L, Saunders J, Paton A, Walters J. *Contrib Nephrol* 1982;30:92–97.
327. Reid JL, Dargie HK, Davis DS, Wing LMH, Hamilton CA, Dollery CT. *Lancet* 1977;1:1171–1174.
328. Barone FC, Price WJ, White RF, Willette RN, Feuerstein GZ. *Neurosci Biobehav Rev* 1992;16(2):219–233.
329. Chester EM, Agamanolis DP, Banker BQ, Victor M. *Neurology* 1977;28:928–939.
330. Gifford RW. *JAMA* 1991;266:829–835.
331. Schwartz RB, Jones KM, Kalina P, et al. *AJR* 1992;159:379–383.
332. Nag S, Robertson DM, Dinsdale HB. *Lab Invest* 1977;39:150–161.
333. Jacobs IR, Roszler MH, Kelly JK, Klein MA, King GA. *Radiology* 1989;170:223–227.
334. Skoog I, Nilsson L, Palmertz B, Andreasson L, Svanborg A. *New Engl J Med* 1993;328:153–158.

*Hypertension: Pathophysiology, Diagnosis,
and Management, Second Edition,*
edited by J.H. Laragh and B.M. Brenner,
Raven Press, Ltd., New York © 1995.

CHAPTER 43

Cerebral Consequences of Hypertension

J. David Spence

Hypertension is the most important treatable risk factor for cerebral vascular disease: by age 55–60, nearly 40 percent of people in the U.S. have systolic and/or diastolic hypertension (1). In the U.S., stroke[1] ranks third as the underlying cause of death, with approximately 1,000 stroke deaths per 100,000 population by age 70; the economic cost of stroke exceeds a billion dollars annually in the U.S. (2). Most of the neurological consequences of hypertension are vascular, in the form of cerebral hemorrhage or infarction, but the pathogenesis of strokes associated with hypertension is poorly understood, with little understanding of the distinction between small vessel strokes and atherosclerotic strokes. Because these two types of stroke occur and are prevented differently, this chapter will focus on clarifying the distinction between strokes due to small vessel disease and those due to atherosclerosis, and on how antihypertensive drugs differ in

their effects on the pathophysiological processes that affect small and large arterial vessels in different ways.

It has long been known that patients with hypertension are subject to severe consequences resulting from vascular and cardiac changes associated with high blood pressure (3,4). With recent advances in the detection and treatment of high blood pressure, it has become increasingly clear that the arteriolar consequences of hypertension respond very well to the lowering of blood pressure, but that the atherosclerotic consequences are less responsive (5–13). These differential responses to the lowering of blood pressure lead to inferences about the pathogenesis of the vascular consequences that occur in hypertensive patients and lead to new questions about how to further reduce the residual atherosclerotic consequences of hypertension that until now have continued to be resistant to treatment (12).

As recently as the late 1960s, a common indication for hemodialysis was hypertensive renal failure (an arteriolar consequence of hypertension), particularly in blacks (14); half of patients with stroke were victims of hypertensive arteriolar disease (15). Two decades later, in communities where hypertension was extensively detected and treated, the picture had changed dramatically (15). We were able to observe these changes in London, Ontario, because our first computerized axial tomography (CT) scanner was installed at Victoria Hospital in 1976, 2 years before the initiation of a large hypertension detection and treatment program by the University of Western Ontario Department of Family Medicine (16). In the mid 1970s, 500 patients per year were being admitted to our hospital with stroke. By 1977, with the im-

J. D. Spence: Department of Clinical Pharmacology and Neurology, University of Western Ontario, London, N6A 4G5, Canada.

[1] Throughout this chapter use of the term *stroke* will mean cerebral vascular consequences including both infarction and intracerebral hemorrhage; in the clinical setting it is advisable to reserve to the term a deliberately broad meaning such as "sudden onset of a central nervous system deficit" so as to avoid the diagnostic errors that result from the assumption that all such events are vascular. Approximately 15 percent of patients presenting with a "stroke" have nonvascular causes including tumor; postictal paralysis; subdural hematoma; infectious, inflammatory, or even metabolic causes such as hypoglycemia. For this reason the term *cerebral vascular accident,* which assumes a vascular etiology as the patient comes through the door, can lead to serious errors in management.

proved diagnostic accuracy resulting from routine use of CT scanning, it was apparent that half the strokes were a consequence of hypertensive arteriolar disease: of these, approximately three-fourths were due to intracerebral hemorrhage, and approximately one-fourth were due to lacunar infarction.

With the initiation of the Family Medicine project, in which 34 physicians followed 32,124 patients for a period of 5 years, and special hypertension assistants were assigned to half the practices with a view to improving detection and treatment of hypertension, a remarkable "bandwagon effect" was seen in the surrounding area. By 1983, 94 percent of hypertensive patients in the London area were detected, 92 percent were on treatment, and 72 percent were well controlled (17). By 1984, despite an increase in the population by nearly one-third from the late 1970s, and some aging of the population, the number of stroke patients admitted to our hospital was down to 250 per year, and there had been a striking change in the composition of the stroke population: now less than 10 percent of strokes were a consequence of hypertension. In contrast, strokes due to cerebral atherosclerosis (mainly extracranial carotid disease) had not changed. They accounted for 35 percent of 500 strokes per year in 1978 and 70 percent of 250 strokes per year in 1983. Thus, it was apparent that there had been no reduction in atherosclerotic stroke, despite a dramatic decline in strokes due to hypertensive arteriolar disease.

These events had been presaged by Pickering (3) and Russell (18), who pointed out that strokes resulting from high blood pressure were due to hemorrhage and lacunar infarction as manifestations of arteriolar disease, and that treatments to reduce elevated blood pressure should therefore prevent only arteriolar stroke.

These observations highlight the need for a clearer understanding of the way in which hypertension causes vascular damage. Such understanding will improve our se-lection of antihypertensive therapy so that we have a chance of reducing the atherosclerotic complications of hypertension, which until now have been largely unresponsive to treatment.

HYPERTENSIVE ARTERIOLAR DISEASE

Hypertensive Encephalopathy

Since the work of Giese (19), it has been apparent that during severe hypertensive crisis, the apparent vaso-spasm that can be observed experimentally is probably the normal response to markedly increased pressure as part of autoregulation of blood flow to various tissues. As Giese showed, and Skinhoj, Strandgaard, Johansson, and others confirmed (20–22), the apparent areas of va-sodilation are the injured part of the arteriole, while the "spastic" segments are normal. Hypertensive encepha-lopathy appears to be the result of forced vasodilation due to breakthrough of cerebral autoregulation, mark-edly increased cerebral blood flow, engorgement of the brain, and cerebral edema. These changes are associated with areas of cerebral ischemia due to fibrinoid necrosis and occlusion of some small vessels. The occipital cortex appears to be particularly susceptible to edema, perhaps accounting for the cortical blindness and flashing lights that lead to the name of this syndrome when seen in as-sociation with pregnancy (eclampsia). It may be that the cerebral arterioles are particularly susceptible to in-creased pressure because they are thinner than systemic arterioles (Fig. 1), a circumstance which, it is speculated by analogy to giraffes, may be related to the upright pos-ture (23).

One source of confusion in the management of these patients is the mistaken, though widely held, belief that papilledema must be present; this is not the case, since

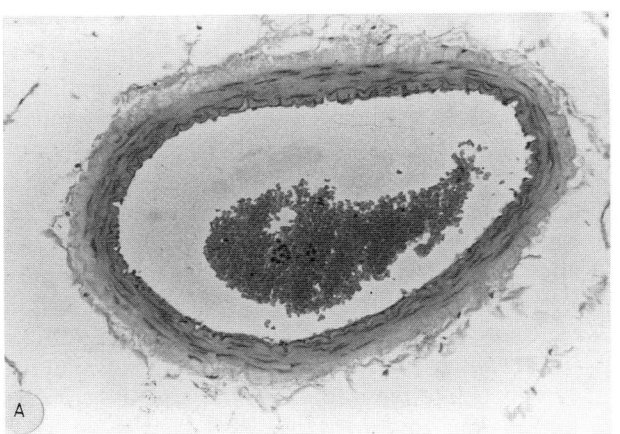 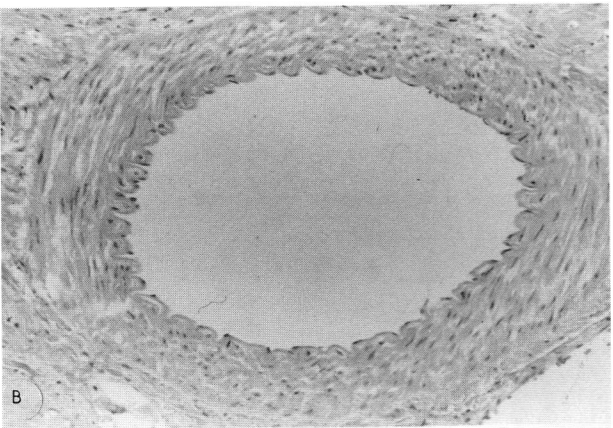

FIG 1. Cerebral arteries are thinner than systemic arteries of similar size. **A:** Cerebral artery. **B:** Mesen-teric artery. (Courtesy of Dr. John C. E. Kaufman, Division of Neuropathology, University of Western Ontario. From ref. 13, with permission.)

papilledema takes time to develop, and not all patients with hypertensive encephalopathy will manifest papilledema at the onset of the problem. Another source of confusion is the notion that hypertensive encephalopathy is seen only in patients with very high blood pressure. On the contrary, during pregnancy this syndrome is seen in young women with only modestly elevated pressure (e.g., 160/100 mm Hg), illustrating an important point that the pressure at which cerebral autoregulation "breaks through" is determined by the level of the previously normal pressures to which the individual's arterioles have been exposed in the recent past. Thus, patients with premorbid pressures at a low normal level will experience breakthrough at modestly elevated pressures, whereas patients with long-standing severe hypertension will tolerate much higher pressures, presumably because of structural adaptation of the arterioles to high pressure (24). Baumbach and Heistad (25) have recently reviewed the evidence for the Mulvaney hypothesis (26) that not only hypertrophy but also arteriolar remodeling occur in hypertension. In our clinic, we have had two patients walk in, with no symptoms or signs of any significant clinical problem, having blood pressures greater than 300/170 mm Hg. This individual tolerance to pressure levels leads to the need for the individualization of target pressures for treatment in the acute management of hypertensive emergencies. For most patients, a target treatment pressure of approximately 120 mm Hg mean arterial pressure (MAP) will be reasonable, but target pressure should be somewhat higher for patients with long-standing severe hypertension, and lower for patients with a recent history of low normal pressures (MAP is calculated from the diastolic plus one-third of the pulse pressure; a MAP of 120 mm Hg therefore represents pressures of about 160/100 or 180/90 mm Hg).

Effects of Antihypertensive Drugs

The selection of which drug to use in the management of this emergency is probably not as important as which not to use. The use of sublingual nifedipine, a popular treatment in many emergency rooms, is to be deplored because, like intramuscular hydralazine (Apresoline), it is uncontrollable once given, and severe hypotension may lead to disastrous results such as cerebral infarction. In addition to reports of stroke resulting from sudden hypotension from intramuscular hydralazine, I am aware of three strokes resulting from the use of "sublingual" nifedipine (in fact, the use of the term *sublingual* is a misnomer for nifedipine as absorption from the buccal mucosa is very slow; the rapid action undoubtedly results from swallowing of nifedipine erroneously administered sublingually on the assumption that its rapid action is related to rapid absorption from the mouth) (27).

Since blood pressure drops more precipitously when it

is very high to begin with, the occurrence of adverse effects should not be surprising. There have also been reports of myocardial ischemia from this practice (28). The management of severe hypertension in the setting of hypertensive encephalopathy or acute stroke should take into account the importance of not suddenly dropping the blood pressure below the threshold for cerebral autoregulation. The use of small repeated intravenous doses (or infusions) of potent intravenous drugs such as hydralazine, diazoxide, sodium nitroprusside; or intravenous beta blockers in combination with vasodilators, under careful observation, is to be preferred in principle (29).

Hypertensive Strokes

Hypertensive arteriolar disease leads to focal dysfunction of the brain of sudden onset (stroke) in at least two ways: hemorrhage due to the rupture of arteriolar microaneurysms that tends to occur in the basal ganglia, thalamus, pons, or cerebellum (Fig. 2); and infarction. The location of these events is perhaps best explained by Hachinski's concept of the vascular centrencephalon (30) (Fig. 3). These events occur in short, straight arteries with few branches, functional end-arteries, supplying the medial and basal portions of the brain and brainstem from the ventral surface, penetrating in the dorsal direction. Since the arteries arise from large basal trunks, the gradation between arterial and capillary pressure occurs over a relatively short distance, requiring the arterioles to withstand high pressures. In contrast, pressures are dissipated in the long, branching, penetrating vessels which perfuse the newer parts of the brain. (In a sense, the cortex is protected by a step-down transformer, while the vascular centrencephalon receives the full brunt of high pressure.)

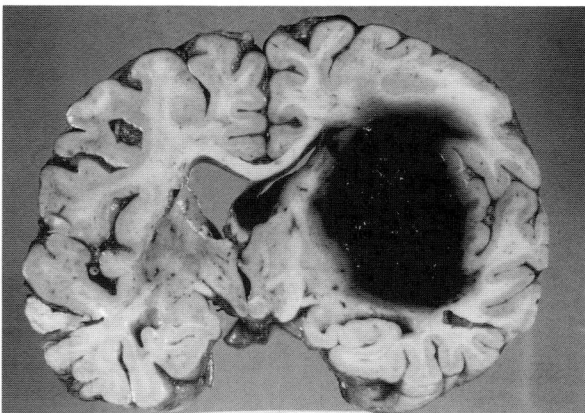

FIG. 2. Coronal section of formalin-fixed brain at the level of the mamillary bodies. Large hemorrhage originating in the putamen. The hematoma has dissected into the adjacent lateral ventricle. Patient is a 57-year-old with long-standing hypertension (A-276-87, SJH). (From ref. 13, with permission.)

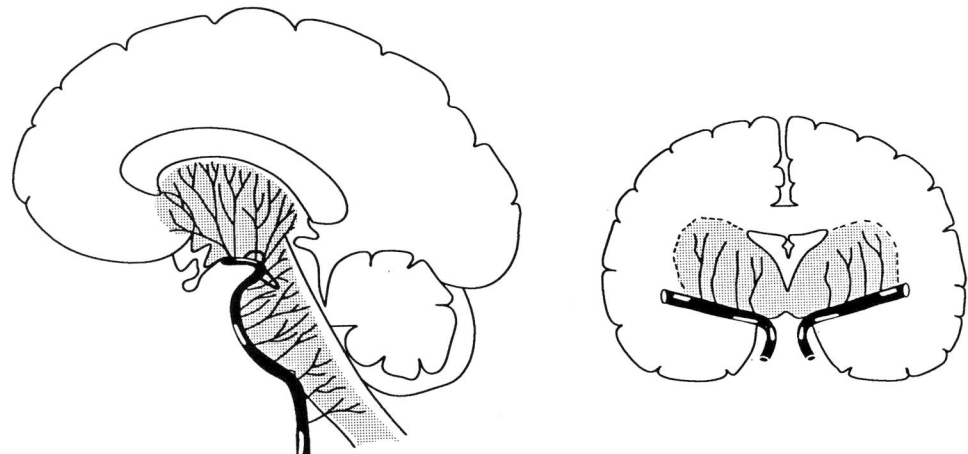

FIG 3. Vascular centrencephalon. (From refs. 13,30, with permission.)

It is very clear that the widespread detection and treatment of hypertension has markedly reduced the occurrence of hypertensive intracerebral hemorrhage. In Victoria Hospital, intracerebral hemorrhage is now less likely to be due to hypertension than to amyloid angiopathy (Fig. 4), a condition of the elderly sometimes associated with Alzheimer's disease (31). Characteristically, the location of these hemorrhages is at the junction of cortex and white matter, often in the posterior parietal lobe (32).

The term *lacunar infarction,* described extensively by Fisher (33), is one that should be reserved for small infarctions due to arteriolar disease (Fig. 5). The lacunes occur as the result of occlusion or stenosis of arterioles and small arteries. Fibrinoid necrosis of the vessel wall results from high blood pressure and is an important feature. Other changes include hyaline degeneration, mi-

croaneurysm formation, and focal hemorrhage. These lesions should not be confused with small infarctions related to embolism of atheromatous debris from proximal larger arteries, particularly the carotid bifurcation. Hypertension is not a necessary condition for the latter events, which are now commonly attributed mistakenly to hypertensive arteriolar disease because of their appearance on CT scans of the brain.

Hachinski et al. (34) have recently described a condition called *leuko-airaiosis,* which may relate in part to hypertensive arteriolar strokes combined with the results of episodes of hypotension in patients with reduced cerebral vascular reserve due to hypertensive thickening of small vessels. This concept is rather similar to one recently enunciated by Floras (35), who discussed nocturnal hypotension below the autoregulatory threshold for myocardial perfusion in connection with the J-shaped

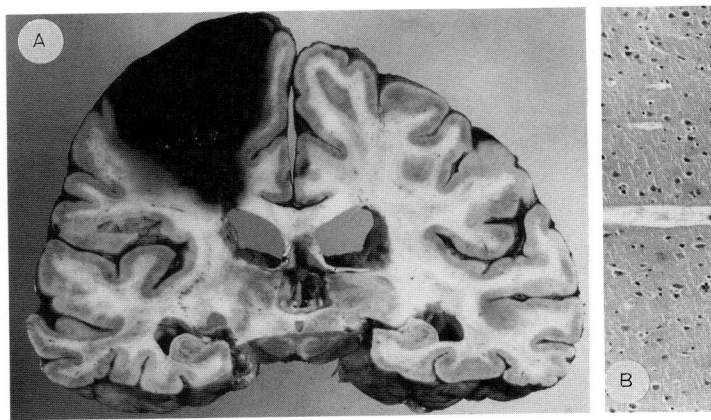
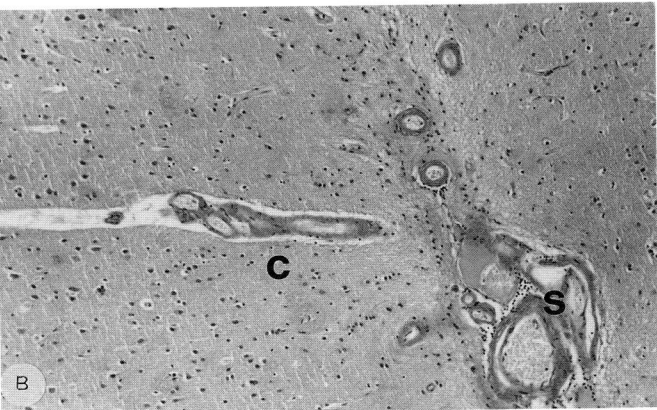

FIG. 4. A: Coronal section of formalin-fixed brain at the level of the pulvinar. Hemorrhage in the left superior parietal lobe which extends to the subarachnoid space. Congophilic angiopathy in a 68-year-old patient. **B:** Photomicrograph of the depth of a sulcus in the occipital cortex; congophilic angiopathy in the vessels of the subarachnoid space (s) and the adjacent cortex (c). Patient was 80 years old, with Alzheimer's disease. (From ref. 13, with permission.)

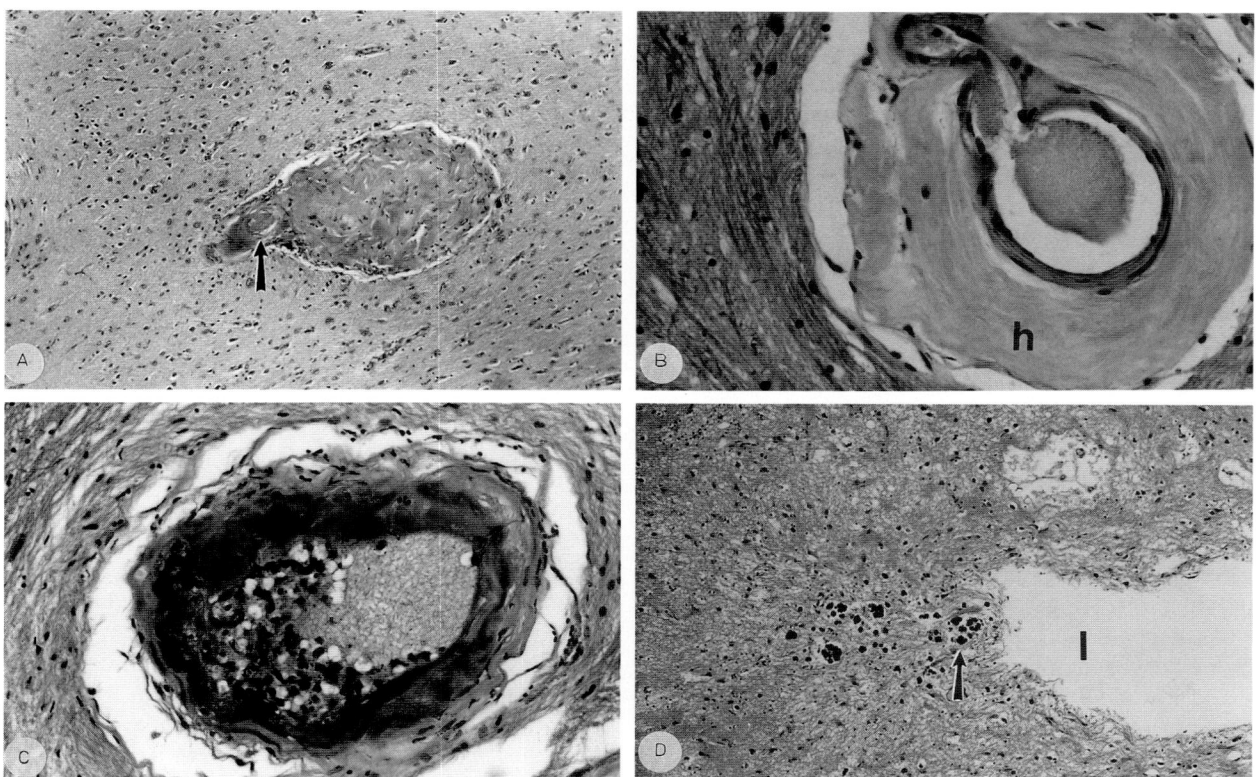

FIG 5. Hypertensive arteriolar disease. **A:** Collagenoid microaneurysm (Charcot-Bouchard) in the thalamus. Vessel of origin (*arrow*). There is surrounding gliosis (100×). **B:** Arteriole in the internal capsule; hyaline degeneration in the wall (h) (300×). **C:** Fibrinoid degeneration in the vessel wall; invasion by macrophages (215×). **D:** Cystic space; edge of a lacune (*left*); there is evidence of previous hemorrhage; hemosiderin-laden macrophage (*arrow*) (90×). (From ref. 13, with permission.)

curve of vascular risk (36). Bulpitt (36) recently reviewed the controversy over the J-shaped curve, which seems unlikely to be caused by effective therapy for hypertension.

Effects of Antihypertensive Drugs

From the evidence reviewed above, it appears to be the lowering of blood pressure itself that prevents hypertensive arteriolar strokes, with little reason for preference among the types of antihypertensive drugs available. However, atherosclerotic stroke is less clearly related to pressure; it seems likely that the prevention of atherosclerotic strokes may require attention to other effects of antihypertensive drugs in addition to the lowering of pressure.

ATHEROSCLEROSIS

Pathogenesis of Atherosclerosis

Since the recent advent of effective therapies for hyperlipidemia (37–39), there has been a resurgence in the popularity of the notion that atherosclerosis is caused by disordered metabolism of lipoproteins and excessive consumption of lipids. While these factors are of indisputable importance, it is well in the setting of the discussion of hypertension and its treatment to keep in mind that hypertension is an important risk factor for atherosclerotic events and that the focal location of atherosclerotic lesions at sites predisposed to perturbations of flow patterns (40) leads to the inescapable conclusion that disturbed flow patterns are important. Thus, in considering how to prevent atherosclerotic complications of hypertension, particularly atherosclerotic events such as embolization of platelet aggregates and atheromatous debris, hemodynamic aspects of hypertension and the effects of antihypertensive drugs on flow disturbances must be considered.

It may be worthwhile to make a distinction between atherosclerosis as a remodeling process by which the artery adapts to changing hemodynamic conditions and to the interaction of vascular geometry with normal flow patterns, and the events associated with disease. Glagov et al. (41) contributed in 1987 the concept that arteries remodel as required to maintain a constant shear rate at the interface between the intima and the bloodstream.

If an area of low shear develops at the near side of a bend or branch, the area will fill in (just as in the case of a river). Similarly, if an area of high shear develops at the far wall, the artery will tend to enlarge away from the high shear rate. The "desired" shear rate has been calculated to be approximately 15 dynes/cm of shear stress (41).

Since hypertension is an important risk factor for atherosclerosis, it is logical to assume that treatment to lower blood pressure will contribute to prevention of atherosclerosis. However, the relationship between hypertension and atherosclerosis is indirect and complicated (12,42).

Hemodynamics and Atherosclerosis

Atherosclerosis can be thought of both as a natural process by which the artery remodels itself to maintain normal shear rates (Fig. 6) and as the result of endothelial injury and repair (43–45). Injury to the endothelium, caused by factors including the occurrence of abnormal high- and low-shear flow patterns, leads to interaction between the arterial wall and platelets, with release of platelet growth factors that results in proliferation of smooth muscle cells in the intima (45). A plaque develops, which further causes flow disturbances. The presence of other aggravating factors such as hyperlipidemia and smoking mitigates against normal repair, leading to the persistence or worsening of lesions. Since the intima is the part of the artery that is exposed to the kinetic energy associated with disturbed flow patterns, it seems logical to pay attention to the effects of antihypertensive drugs on flow patterns in addition to their effects on pressure (12,42).

For some time, the relationship of arterial flow disturbances to the initiation and progression of atherosclerosis has been of interest (46–66). Recently, it has been proposed that arterial flow disturbances may be important not only for the localization of atherosclerosis, but also in the initiation, progression, and complications of atherosclerosis (embolization of platelet thrombus, embolization of atheromatous debris [Fig. 7], and intraplaque hemorrhage or dissection) (67).

Table 1 explores the relationships between hypertension and vascular events in the context of the total fluid energy in the blood. In normal circumstances, blood is thought to flow in a laminar fashion, with the blood moving most quickly in the central (axial) part of the stream and most slowly along the wall. Under these circumstances, most of the total fluid energy in the blood is in the form of pressure energy, and the endothelium is spared from exposure to high velocity gradients along the wall (high shear rates) (52). Thus, under normal circumstances, the endothelium is not exposed to appreciable amounts of kinetic energy, and no endothelial damage results from the flow of blood. In conditions in which flow patterns become disturbed, there is conversion of pressure energy into kinetic energy, and the energy which was present in the blood in the form of pressure now has the potential to injure the vessel lining (52).

Two factors may lead the endothelium to be exposed to kinetic energy. First, the occurrence of bends and branches may bring the fast-moving axial stream into contact with the wall (sites of high shear), and at sites where the fast-moving stream tends to pull away from the wall, abnormal low-shear sites may develop. These are also thought to be potentially important in the pathogenesis of atherosclerosis (48). Thus, the geometry of the vessels may lead to the occurrence of disturbed flow patterns under hemodynamic conditions in which flow would remain laminar in a straight tube. Second, for a tube of a given geometry, what determines whether flow will remain laminar or become nonlaminar (for fluid of a given density and viscosity) is the set of hemodynamic parameters governing the pattern of flow (49–51). For steady flow in straight tubes, factors which tend to increase the occurrence of disturbed flow patterns (e.g., tur-

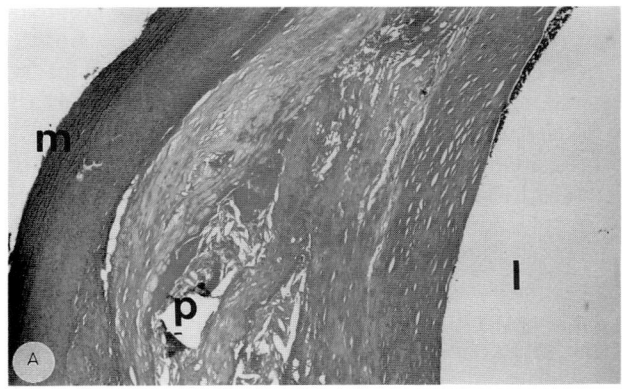
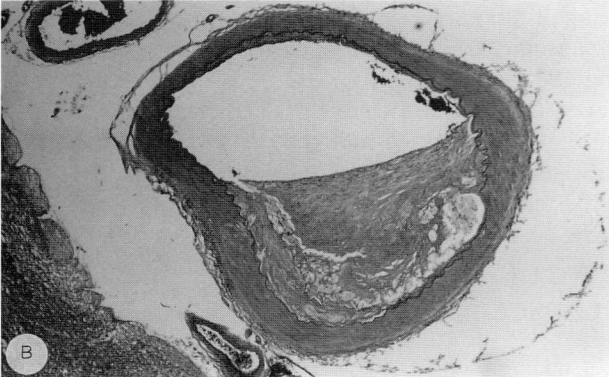

FIG 6. Atherosclerotic vessels. **A:** Endarterectomy specimen; atheromatous plaque in the intima (p); resected portion of the media (m); lumen 1) (30×). **B:** Posterior cerebral artery at the uncus; eccentric atheromatous degeneration (35×). (From ref. 13, with permission.)

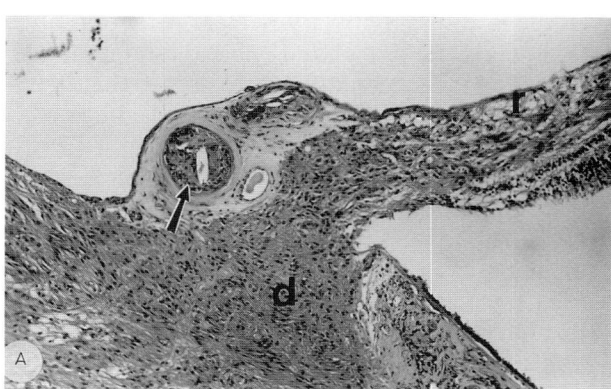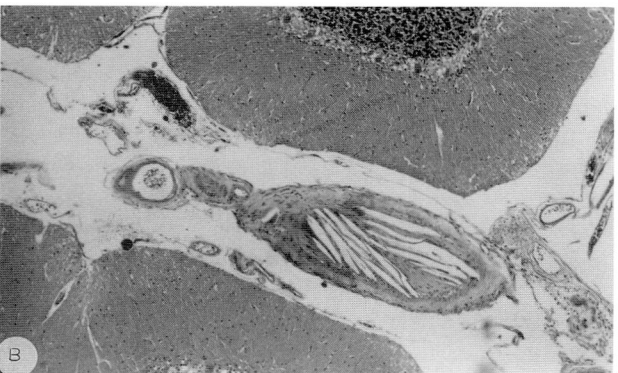

FIG. 7. Atheromatous embolization. **A:** Optic disc; retinal artery plugged with atheromatous debris including cholesterol crystals (*arrow*); gliotic disc (d); retina (r) artifactually torn away from choroid (100×). **B:** Cholesterol crystals in an artery in the subarachnoid space of the cerebellum (55×). (From ref. 13, with permission.)

bulence) include the diameter of the vessel and the velocity and density of the fluid; the main factor tending to diminish the occurrence of turbulence is the viscosity of the fluid (50). Since for a given individual the geometry of the vessels and the density and viscosity of the blood are given, the variable determining the occurrence of nonlaminar flow would be blood velocity, if the prevailing conditions were those of steady flow in straight tubes, as studied by Reynolds (50). In biology, however, the situation is much more complex, since flow is pulsatile and the tubes branch and bend. In these circumstances, the factors that determine the occurrence of disturbed flow pattern are mainly the heart rate and the blood velocity. Roach et al. (53) have shown that for any angle of bifurcation the critical Reynolds number decreases as the angle of bifurcation widens (i.e., the blood has to go more slowly for the flow pattern to remain laminar as the angle widens) and that for pulsatile flow, the fluid has to move even more slowly to remain laminar. Yellin (54) introduced the concept of diastolic damping time and pointed

out that as heart rate increases, the greater is the tendency for transitory flow disturbances at peak systole to become propagated from one cycle to the next and to extend downstream. This concept of diastolic damping time may be particularly important in coronary and cerebral arteries, where most of the flow occurs during diastole (55).

The implication of the above is that slower heart rates contribute to smoother patterns of blood flow, and increased heart rates contribute to disturbed flow patterns. In part, this may arise because increasing the heart rate increases the frequency and speed with which the blood accelerates and decelerates, tending to magnify oscillations in shear along the wall during the transition from forward flow during systole to reverse flow during diastole (48). In this context it is interesting to note that heart rate is an independent predictor of coronary risk in man (68) and also predicts progression of coronary artery disease in a monkey model of stress-induced atherosclerosis (69).

TABLE 1. *Hypertension as a disorder of increased total fluid energy in the circulation: relationship of vascular consequences to kinetic energy versus pressure energy*

Consequences of pressure	Consequences of kinetic energy
Arteriolar consequences	Arterial consequences
Nephrosclerosis	Initiation of atherosclerosis
Brain hemorrhage	Progression of stenosis
Lacunar stroke	Embolization
Hypertensive encephalopathy	Platelet aggregates
Arterial consequences	Atheromatous debris
Aortic cystic medial necrosis	Myocardial infarction
Rupture of aortic aneurysm	Cerebral infarction
Rupture of berry aneurysm	Enlargement of berry aneurysms
Cardiac damage	Dissection of aortic aneurysm
Left ventricular hypertrophy	
Congestive heart failure	

Until recently, the field of hemodynamic theories of atherogenesis has been dominated by the controversy over the question of whether atherosclerosis was caused by high shear or low shear. The proponents of high shear as the important factor suggested that injury to the vascular endothelium by high fluid shear stresses was the focus for the subsequent development of atherosclerosis as a repair process at the site of injury (47). Proponents of the low-shear hypothesis suggested that exposure of the endothelium to low fluid shear stresses may be conducive to the formation of atherosclerosis by adversely affecting the mass transfer of lipids across the arterial wall (48). Most recent evidence supports the localization of large plaques to sites of low shear (58,59), but recently Friedman et al. have proposed a unifying hypothesis, suggesting that both high-shear and low-shear sites may be important, each in different ways (63). They observed that atherosclerosis develops more quickly but to a limited extent at high-shear areas, and more slowly but to a greater extent at low-shear areas. This information, viewed with the work of Glagov et al. (41), leads to the concept of atherosclerosis as a remodeling process, with the shape of the artery changing so as to conform to the flow pattern. Thus, both high- and low-shear areas are subject to development of atherosclerosis, but in different ways, at different rates, and to a different extent.

Fortunately, from the standpoint of prevention, the hemodynamic variables in the upstream parent artery that determine occurrence of both high-shear and low-shear areas downstream in the bifurcation are the same; it is only the location of the flow disturbances that is determined by the geometry of the vessel (62). Since antihypertensive drugs not only lower blood pressure but have other effects that may affect atherosclerosis, these effects should be considered. In addition to adverse effects of antihypertensive drugs on lipoproteins (70,71), there is recent evidence that effects of antihypertensive drugs on arterial flow disturbances may affect atherosclerosis (42,61,64–69,72,73).

Adverse Effects of Antihypertensive Drugs on Lipoproteins

Since about 1980, there has been growing awareness that antihypertensive drugs have adverse effects on lipoprotein patterns. On average, nonselective beta blockers, probably all kaliuretic diuretics, and probably all sympatholytic drugs such as methyldopa tend to increase triglycerides and lower high-density lipoprotein (HDL) cholesterol levels, with the result that the cholesterol/HDL ratio is adversely affected by about 15 percent (12). The magnitude of this adverse effect is placed in perspective by considering that the Lipid Clinics Coronary Prevention Trial (37) achieved a 20 percent reduction in coronary mortality by a 9 percent reduction of cholesterol levels, using diet and cholestyramine. It has been estimated independently by two groups that the magnitude of this adverse effect is enough to completely offset the benefit of treating mild hypertension (70,71). There is some evidence that the relatively cardioselective beta blockers and those with weak intrinsic sympathomimetic activity (ISA) may be neutral with respect to effects on lipids, while alpha blockers, beta blockers with strong ISA, potassium-and-magnesium-sparing diuretics, and possibly angiotensin-converting enzyme (ACE) inhibitors may have beneficial effects on lipoproteins (12). There is as yet no evidence that these effects on lipoproteins are reflected in changes in risk, but it is reasonable to consider the importance of these adverse effects, particularly in patients with hyperlipidemia, diabetes, or with other risk factors.

Effects of Antihypertensive Drugs

The pathogenesis of atherosclerosis and the hemodynamic variables which determine the occurrence of disturbed flow patterns that may lead to not only the initiation and progression of atherosclerosis itself but also to embolic and occlusive complications of atherosclerosis have been reviewed above. The problem is complex. In general, it is likely that increased blood velocity, increased heart rate, and increased acceleration and deceleration of blood would lead to the occurrence of disturbed flow patterns. It is thus of interest to study the effects of cardiovascular drugs on those hemodynamic parameters which may affect patterns of arterial flow.

Since 1973, the author has been involved in the study of the effects of antihypertensive drugs on blood velocity and arterial flow disturbances. Antihypertensive drugs have different effects on blood velocity in the carotid arteries of rhesus monkeys (72) and in the aorta of hypertensive man (61). Using carotid Doppler flow mapping, we showed that hydralazine aggravated, whereas propranolol diminished, the occurrence of abnormal high-velocity patterns thought to be associated with turbulence and vortex formation in patients with carotid stenosis (64). It has since been shown in hypertensive, cholesterol-fed rabbits (66); in broad-breasted turkeys (73); and in socially stressed monkeys (69) that beta blockers significantly reduced the development of atherosclerosis.

All of the foregoing would be of little interest if the treatment of high blood pressure were successful in preventing the atherosclerotic complications related to hypertension. However, this is not the case (5,14,74). The Veterans Administration cooperative study (hydrochlorothiazide-reserpine-hydralazine) (6), the study by Beevers et al. (7) in patients with stroke and hypertension (methyldopa-thiazide), the Australian mild hypertension study (9), and others have shown that by treating hypertension we can prevent progression to malignant hypertension and reduce the risk of death, stroke, renal failure, and congestive heart failure; however, the risk of myocardial infarction is reduced only slightly. McMahon et al. (74) suggested that antihypertensive therapy reduces stroke by 40 percent but reduces myocardial infarction by only 14 percent. Russell (18) pointed out that the strokes that are prevented by the treatment of high blood pressure are not atherosclerotic strokes, but those due to small vessel occlusion (lacunar infarcts) and small vessel rupture (intracerebral hemorrhages). In the Australian study by Morgan et al. (75) of mild hypertension in the elderly, and in the Multiple Risk Factor Intervention Trial (MRFIT) (10), the use of hydrochlorothiazide was associated with increased risk of myocardial infarction. The first two hypertension studies that have shown significant reduction of myocardial infarction were the Hypertension Detection and Follow-Up Program (HDFP) study (8) in which reserpine was widely used along with thiazide, and the Gothenburg study (11), in which first-line therapy was a beta blocker. Thus, if we accept that myocardial infarction is a good marker for atherosclerotic complications of hypertension, it appears that to prevent atherosclerotic strokes, we must begin to pay attention to effects of antihypertensive drugs in addition to the lowering of blood pressure, such as their effects on lipoproteins, blood velocity, and arterial flow disturbances.

The study of complications of human atherosclerosis in relation to selected antihypertensive regimens with different effects on flow patterns will require very large studies. We have begun on studies which look at the simpler question of the progression of atherosclerotic lesions in patients with carotid stenosis. We have developed methods to measure the effects of antihypertensive drugs on arterial flow disturbances (76), and we are developing methods to measure atherosclerosis noninvasively for use as a surrogate outcome in intervention studies (77).

As discussed above, one hemodynamic factor which tends to aggravate flow disturbances is heart rate. In addition to observations from the Framingham Study, showing that increased heart rate is an independent risk factor (56), Kaplan et al. (68) have recently shown in macaques that heart rate is associated with sympathetic activation and lipid levels, and worsening of atherosclerosis in their model of atherosclerosis induced by social stress. Kaplan et al. (69) have recently reviewed the antiatherosclerotic effects of beta-adrenergic blockers, emphasizing protection from the sympathetic arousal due to stress.

In addition, there has been recent interest in the possibility that calcium-channel antagonists (78,79) and ACE inhibitors (80) may also have antiatherosclerotic effects in animal models. There may be additional benefits of ACE inhibitors in myocardial ischemia related to inactivation of free radicals (81,82). There is also some angiographic evidence, though little based on clinical end-points, that calcium-channel antagonists may be antiatheroclerotic in man (83).

In addition to effects on stress responses, lipids, and flow disturbances referred to above, Winther and Trap-Jensen (84) have recently added to the range of possible effects of antihypertensive drugs on atherosclerosis. Their observation is that beta blockers have beneficial effects on platelets, which may be expected to reduce the likelihood of atherosclerosis progression and complications.

Since the great majority of hypertensives (71 percent) have mild hypertension (85), and the complications of hypertension that are due to pressure have already been eliminated to a great extent (15), the prevention of atherosclerosis and its complications remains as the greatest challenge in hypertension. Some recent evidence indicates that beta-adrenergic blockers may reduce atherosclerotic complications in man (86,87), but a great deal of work remains to be done.

VASCULAR ECTASIA IN HYPERTENSION

In some patients, atherosclerosis in combination with hypertension can lead to remarkable enlargement of the arteries. Although this is asymptomatic for the most part, the enlargement of arteries can in some cases cause symptoms. The following case illustrates one such circumstance.

The patient was a 65-year-old woman who was admitted to Victoria Hospital on July 8, 1970, from a local nursing home where she had been living for 2 years in a state of presenile dementia. For several months prior to admission her speech had become more and more dysarthric, she had developed difficulty swallowing, had become incontinent of urine, and her gait had deteriorated progressively. She had diabetes mellitus, treated with a 1,500-calorie diet, and hypertension, for which she was being given methyldopa and hydrochlorothiazide, started in January of 1970, at which time her pressure was 210/110 mm Hg. By the time of admission she was confined to bed because she was unable to walk at all. Her admission was precipitated by a transient ischemic attack with right hemiparesis and weakness of the right ninth and twelfth cranial nerves. Her blood pressure on admission was 160/100 mm Hg, but during the course of the admission it was labile, with pressures as high as 180/130; in part the difficulty in controlling her pressure was related to the difficulty in swallowing her tablets.

Several days after admission, after the right hemiparesis had cleared, her neurological examination revealed dysarthria; confusion; disorientation to time and place; inability to perform rudimentary tests of memory, calculation, or abstraction; pseudobulbar palsy; and bilaterally spastic legs with bilateral extensor plantar responses. With a picture of progressive dementia, incontinence, and gait disturbance, a diagnosis of hydrocephalus was entertained.

An air encephalogram was done which showed considerable dilation of the lateral ventricles, including the temporal horns, and slight enlargement of the fourth ventricle, which was displaced backward along with the aqueduct. The radiologist, Dr. John Allcock, noted a large indentation in the floor of the third ventricle from below and posteriorly, and his initial report raised the question of basilar ectasia. The following day a cerebral angiogram was done after rotating the patient in such a way that the residual air was positioned in the third ventricle; the vertebral injection showed gross elongation and tortuosity of the basilar artery; the report goes on as follows: "There is still some air in the lateral and third ventricles from the previous air study, and in the hanging head view, the indentation previously described in the floor of the third ventricle is again seen, and the basilar artery fits very nicely into this."

The patient was treated with a ventriculoperitoneal shunt and made a remarkable recovery. At her follow-up visit of October 15, 1970, she was walking; was oriented to time, place, and person; was no longer incontinent; and was now able to feed herself and swallow without difficulty. The shunt was functioning normally as judged by palpation of the reservoirs.

This syndrome, sometimes called "Ekbom's other syndrome," had been described by Breig et al. (88) and is one of very few examples of symptoms due to vascular ectasia.

Unfortunately, her blood pressure was not well controlled, and on January 28, 1971, she was readmitted with a blood pressure of 250/150 mm Hg, having suffered a hemorrhage into the right globus pallidus, which ruptured into the lateral ventricle; she did not recover. Thus, both her remarkable syndrome and her terminal event were related to hypertension; her experience makes a good case for control of hypertension in the elderly.

TREATMENT OF HYPERTENSION IN THE ELDERLY

Stamler (89) has recently reemphasized the quantitative nature of the problem of hypertension and the importance of recognizing that systolic hypertension is a more accurate predictor of atherosclerotic risk than is diastolic hypertension:

> The optimal systolic blood pressure (SBP) for adults is a level under 118 mm Hg, and the relationship of systolic blood pressure to risk is continuous, strong, graded and exponential; risk is significantly increased for the 80% of the population who have SBP above optimal . . . and not just for those with frank hypertension.

While it has long been known that systolic hypertension is a significant risk factor for atherosclerotic events, it is only recently that firm evidence has been available to show that treatment of isolated systolic hypertension is clearly beneficial (90).

That study (90) used thiazide diuretic as first-line therapy, and most experts would agree that small doses of thiazide (e.g., 12.5 mg daily of hyrochlorothiazide) would be the treatment of choice for systolic hypertension in the elderly. It is important to keep the dose low to minimize adverse effects such as potassium depletion, gout, glucose intolerance, and aggravation of hyperlipidemia. In a commentary on recent literature, Kaplan (91) suggested that a dose of hydrochlorothiazide of 12.5 mg should be "about right" and speculated that doses as low as 6.25 mg may be suitable. Salt restriction also minimizes potassium depletion, and in patients with significant problems of potassium depletion it is useful to know the stimulated plasma renin status (see below).

Beta-adrenergic blockers, by reducing heart rate, may aggravate systolic hypertension because the increased stroke volume, in combination with a stiff vascular tree, widens pulse pressure. Therefore, addition of a vasodilator such as hydralazine or nifedipine may be preferable to use of a beta blocker without vasodilators in patients with high diastolic pressures who do not respond to diuretic alone. This may be important if Christensen's finding (92) that reduction of pulse pressure is necessary to normalize small artery structure translates from rats to the human condition.

A special problem in the management of hypertension in the elderly is the error in blood pressure measurement related to stiff arteries. Among patients over age 60 who have high diastolic pressures but no signs of end-organ disease, approximately half will have a false elevation of the diastolic pressure by 30 mm Hg or more (93); the magnitude of the cuff artifact is proportional to the stiffness of the arteries (94,95). This may account for a number of cases of elderly patients who do not seem to tolerate reduction of blood pressure toward normal and who suffer symptoms suggesting hypotension at relatively normal pressures (see Chapter 115 for a review of this issue). For the most part, however, even elderly patients with hypertension can be successfully treated; the approach is to use small doses of medication, increase doses cautiously and conservatively, and consider the possibility of secondary hypertension in those patients who are resistant to treatment (96). Since the advent of balloon angioplasty, renovascular hypertension is a common, readily treatable cause of severe resistant hypertension in the elderly. The Systolic Hypertension in the Elderly Program (SHEP) study (90) and other studies have confirmed the benefits of treating even isolated systolic hypertension in the elderly. Neurological adverse effects of antihypertensive drugs can include cerebral dysfunction (fatigue, confusion, hallucinations), neuropathy, and myopathy; they are reviewed elsewhere (13).

ACKNOWLEDGMENTS

I am grateful to my coauthors of previous chapters which are widely quoted here: Dr J. Malcolm Arnold and Dr. Joseph J. Gilbert (60), and Dr. Vladimir C. Hachinski (13), and to the publisher of those chapters, Elsevier, Amsterdam, for permission to quote from and reproduce the figures from those chapters.

REFERENCES

1. Stamler J. High blood pressure in the United States—an overview of the problem and the challenge. In: *Proceedings of the National Conference on High Blood Pressure Education.* National Heart and Lung Institute: 1973;DHEW publication no (NIH)73-486.
2. Kurtzke JF. Epidemiology of cerebrovascular disease. In: McDowell FH, Caplan LR, eds. *Cerebrovascular survey report, National Institute of Neurological and Communicative Disorders and Stroke.* 1985;1-34.
3. Pickering G. Hypertension: causes, consequences and management. London: Churchill Livingstone, 1974;40-62.
4. Kannel WB, Sorlie P. Hypertension in Framingham. In: Paul O ed. *Epidemiology and control of hypertension.* New York: Stratton Intercontinental, 1975;553-570.
5. Samuelsson O, Wilhelmson L, Andersson O, Pennert K, Berglund G. Cardiovascular morbidity in relation to change in blood pressure and serum cholesterol levels in treated hypertension. *JAMA* 1988;258:1768-1776.
6. Veterans Administration Trial on effects of antihypertensive treatment on morbidity in hypertension. Results in patients with diastolic blood pressure averaging 90 through 114 mm Hg. *JAMA* 1970;213:1143-1452.
7. Beevers DG, Fairman MJ, Hamilton M, Harpur JE. Antihypertensive treatment and the course of established cerebral vascular disease. *Lancet* 1973;1:1407-1409.
8. Hypertension Detection and Follow-up Program Cooperative Group. Five-year findings of the Hypertension Detection and Follow-up Program. I. Reduction in mortality in persons with high blood pressure, including mild hypertension. *JAMA* 1979;242:2562-2571.
9. Management Committee of the Australian Therapeutic Trial in Mild Hypertension: the Australian therapeutic trial in mild hypertension. *Lancet* 1980;1:1261-1267.
10. Multiple Risk Factor Intervention Trial Research Group: Multiple Risk Factor Intervention Trial: risk factor changes and mortality results. *JAMA* 1982;248:1465-1477.
11. Berglund G, Sannerstedt R, Andersson O, Wedel H, Wilhelmsen L, Hansson L, Sivertsson R, Wikstrand J. Coronary heart disease after treatment of hypertension. *Lancet* 1978;1:1-5.
12. Spence JD. Antihypertensive therapy and atherosclerosis. In: Rapaport E, ed. *Cardiology update* New York: Elsevier, 1986;137-155.
13. Spence JD, Hachinski VC. Neurological complications of hypertension. In: Goetz C, Tanner CM, Aminoff MJ, eds. *Handbook of clinical neurology,* vol 19 (63): Systemic Diseases, Part I. Amsterdam: Elsevier, 1993;71-91.
14. Rostand SG, Brown G, Kirk KA, Rutsky EA, Dustan HP. Renal insufficiency in treated essential hypertension. *N Engl J Med* 1989;320:684-688.
15. Spence JD. Antihypertensive therapy and prevention of atherosclerotic stroke. *Stroke* 1986;17:808-810.
16. Bass MJ, McWhinney IR, Donner A. Do family physicians need medical assistants to detect and manage hypertension? *Can Med Assoc J* 1986;134:1247-1255.
17. Birkett NJ, Donner A. Prevalence and control of hypertension in an Ontario county. *Can Med Assoc J* 1985;132:1019-1024.
18. Russell RWR. How does high blood pressure cause stroke? *Lancet* 1975;2:1283-1285.
19. Giese J. Acute hypertensive vascular disease. 2. Studies on vascular reaction patterns and permeability changes by means of vital microscopy and colloidal tracer technique. *Acta Path Microbiol Scand* 1964;62:497-517.
20. Skinhoj E, Strandgaard S. Pathogenesis of hypertensive encephalopathy. *Lancet* 1973;1:461-462.
21. Strandgaard S, Olesen J, Skinhoj E, et al. Autoregulation of brain circulation in severe arterial hypertension. *Br Med J* 1973;1:07-510.
22. Johansson B, Strandgaard S, Lassen NA. On the pathogenesis of hypertensive encephalopathy: the hypertensive "breakthrough" of autoregulation of cerebral blood flow with forced vasodilatation, flow increase, and blood-brain barrier damage. *Circ Res* 1974;34(suppl):167-174.
23. Warren JV. The physiology of the giraffe. *Sci Am* 1974;231:96-100,105.
24. Folkow B. Structural factors: the vascular wall. Consequences of treatment. *Hypertension* 1983;5(suppl III):58-62.
25. Baumbach GL, Heistad DD. Adaptive changes in cerebral blood vessels during chronic hypertension. *J Hypertens* 1991;9:87-991.
26. Mulvaney MJ. Structure and function of small arteries in hypertension. *J Hypertens* 1990;8:(suppl 7)s225-232.
27. van Harten J, Burggraaf K, Danhof M, van Brummelen P, Breimer DD. Negligible sublingual absorption of nifedipine. *Lancet* 1987;2:1363-1365.
28. Levitt AD, Zweiffler AJ. Nifedipine, hypotension and myocardial injury. *Ann Int Med* 1988;108:305-306.
29. Spence JD, Del Maestro RF. Hypertension in acute strokes: *Treat Arch Neurol* 1985;42:1000-1002.
30. Hachinski VC, Norris JW. The vascular infrastructure. *The acute stroke.* Philadelphia: FA Davis, 1985;27-40.
31. Gilbert JJ, Vinters HV. Cererbral amyloid angiopathy: incidence and complications in the aging brain. I: Cerebral hemorrhage. *Stroke* 1983;14:915-923.
32. Vinters HV, Gilbert JJ. Cerebral amyloid angiopathy: incidence and complications in the aging brain. II: The distribution of amyloid vascular changes. *Stroke* 1983;14:924-928.
33. Fisher CM. Lacunar infarction. In: Toole JF, Sickert R, Whisnant J, eds. *Cerebral vascular disease* (Sixth Princeton Conference). New York: Grune & Stratton, 1968;232-236.
34. Hachinski VC, Potter P, Merskey H. Leuko-araiosis: an ancient term for a new problem. *Can J Neuro Sci* 1987;13:533-534.
35. Floras JS. Antihypertensive treatment, myocardial infarction, and nocturnal myocardial ischemia. *Lancet* 1988;2:994-996.
36. Bulpitt C. The J-shaped curve in hypertension. *N Engl J Med* 1992.
37. Lipid research clinics program: the lipid research clinics coronary primary prevention trial results. II. The relationship of reduction in incidence of coronary heart disease to cholesterol lowering. *JAMA* 1984;251:365-374.
38. Frick MH, Elo O, Haapa K, et al. Helsinki Heart Study: primary-prevention trial with gemfibrozil in middle-aged men with dyslipidemia: safety of treatment, changes in risk factors, and incidence of coronary heart disease. *N Engl J Med* 1987;317:1237-1245.
39. Brett AS. Treating hypercholesterolemia: how should practicing physicians interpret the published data for patients? *N Engl J Med* 1989;321:676-679.
40. Schwartz CJ, Mitchell JRA. Observations on localization of arterial plaques. *Circ Res* 1962;11:63-73.
41. Glagov S, Zarins CK, Stankunavicius R, Kolettis CJ. Compensatory enlargement of human atherosclerotic coronary arteries. *N Engl J Med* 1987;316:1371-1375.
42. Spence JD. Hemodynamic effects of antihypertensive drugs: possible implications for the prevention of atherosclerosis. *Hypertension* 1984;6(suppl III):163-168.

43. Haust MD. Injury and repair in the pathogenesis of atherosclerotic lesions. In: Jones RJ, ed. *Atherosclerosis*. Berlin, Heidelberg, New York: Springer Publishers, 1970; 12–20.

44. Haust MD, More RH. Development of modern theories on the pathogenesis of atherosclerosis. In: Wissler RW, Geer JC, eds. The pathogenesis of atherosclerosis. Baltimore: Williams and Wilkins, 1972; 1–19.

45. Ross R, Glomset JA. The pathogenesis of atherosclerosis. *N Engl J Med* 1976;295:36–77.

46. Texon M. Hemodynamic basis of atherosclerosis. New York: Hemisphere Publishing Company, 1980.

47. Fry DL. Acute vascular endothelial changes associated with increased blood velocity gradients. *Circ Res* 1968;22:165–167.

48. Caro CG, Fitz-Gerald JM, Schroter RC. Atheroma and arterial wall shear; observation, correlation and proposal of a shear dependent mass transfer mechanism for atherogenesis. *Proc Royal Soc London* (Biology) 1971;107:109–24.

49. Nerem RM, Cornhill JF. The role of fluid mechanics in atherogenesis. *J Biomechan Engin* 1980;102:181–189.

50. Milnor WR. *Hemodynamics*. Baltimore: Williams and Wilkins, 1982.

51. Stein PD, Sabbah HN. Hemorheology of turbulence. *Biorheology* 1980;17:301–309.

52. Burton AC. Kinetic energy in the circulation: streamline flow and turbulence: measurement of arterial pressure. In: *Physiology and Biophysics of the Circulation*. Chicago: Yearbook Medical Publishers, 1972;101–114.

53. Roach MR, Scott S, Ferguson CG. The hemodynamic importance of the geometry of bifurcations in the circle of Willis (glass model studies). *Stroke* 1972;3:255–267.

54. Yellin EL. Laminar-turbulent transition process in pulsatile flow. *Circ Res* 1966;19:791–804.

55. Spence JD. Spectral analysis of carotid vs femoral Doppler velocity patterns: a clue to the genesis of flow disturbances in cerebral arteries? In: Frontiers of engineering in health care: 0000-0355-376. New York: Institute for Electrical Engineering, 1981;355–359.

56. Kannel WB, Kannel CE, Paffenbarger R. Heart rate and cardiovascular mortality in the Framingham study. *Circulation* 1985;72(suppl 3):111–151.

57. Kaplan JR, Manuck SB, Adams MR, Clarkson TB. The effects of beta-adrenergic blocking agents on atherosclerosis and its complications. *Eur Heart J* 1987;8:928–944.

58. Sabbah HN, Khaja F, Hawkins ET, Brymer JF, McFarland TM, van der Bel-Khan J, Doerger PT, Stein PD. Relation of atherosclerosis to arterial wall shear in the left anterior descending coronary artery of man. *Am Heart J* 1986;112:453–458.

59. Zarins CK, Giddens DP, Bharadvaj BK, Sottiurai VS, Mabon RF, Glagov S. Carotid bifurcation atherosclerosis: quantitative correlation of plaque localization with flow velocity profiles and wall shear stress. *Circ Res* 1983;53:502–514.

60. Spence JD, Arnold JMO, Gilbert JJ. Consequences of hypertension and effects of antihypertensive therapy. In: Robertson JIS, ed. *Handbook of Hypertension*, vol. 15. Amsterdam: Elsevier, 1992;621–654.

61. Spence JD. Effects of antihypertensive drugs on blood velocity: implications for atherogenesis. *Can Med Assoc J* 1982;127:721–724.

62. Friedman MH, O'Brien B, Ehrlich LW. Calculations of pulsatile flow through a branch: implications for the hemodynamics of atherosclerosis. *Circ Res* 1975;36:277–85.

63. Friedman MH, Deters OJ, Bargeron CB, Hutchins GM, Mark FF. Shear-dependent thickening of the human arterial intima. *Atherosclerosis* 1986;60:161–171.

64. Spence JD. Effects of hydralazine versus propranolol on blood velocity patterns in patients with carotid stenosis. *Clin Sci* 1983;65:91–93.

65. Spence JD. Effects of antihypertensive drugs on atherogenic factors: possible importance of drug selection in prevention of atherosclerosis. *J Cardiovasc Pharmacol* 1985;7:121–125.

66. Spence JD, Perkins DG, Kline RL, Adams M, Haust MD. Hemodynamic modification of aortic atherosclerosis: Effects of propranolol vs hydralazine in hypertensive hyperlipidemic rabbits. *Atherosclerosis* 1984;50:325–33.

67. Spence JD. Pathogenesis of atherosclerosis: effects of antihypertensive drugs. *J Hum Exp Hypertens* 1989;3(suppl 2):63–68.

68. Kaplan JR, Manuck SB, Clarkson TB. The influence of heart rate on coronary atherosclerosis. *J Cardiovasc Pharmacol* 1987;10(suppl 2):S100–S102.

69. Kaplan JR, Manuck SB, Adams MR, Weingand KW, Clarkson TB. Inhibition of coronary atherosclerosis by propranolol in behaviorally predisposed monkeys fed an atherogenic diet. *Circulation* 1987;76:1363–1372.

70. Woodcock BG, Rietbrock M. Beta-blocker induced changes in the cholesterol: high-density lipoprotein cholesterol ratio and risk of coronary heart disease. *Klinische Wochenschrift* 1984;62:843–849.

71. Ames RP, Hill P. Antihypertensive therapy and the risk of coronary heart disease. *J Cardiovasc Pharmacol* 1982;4(suppl 2):206–212.

72. Spence JD, Pesout AB, Melmon KL. Effects of antihypertensive drugs on blood velocity in rhesus monkeys. *Stroke* 1977;8:589–594.

73. Scannapieco G, Pauletto P, Semplicini A, Dario C, Vescovo G, Mazzucato A, Angelini A, Pessina AC. Evaluation of the efficacy of various hypotensive drugs in broad-breasted white turkeys as an experimental model of arterial hypertension with high catecholamine levels. *Boll Soc Ital Biol Sper* 1983;59:1265–1271.

74. MacMahon SW, Cutler JA, Furberg CD, Payne GH. The effects of drug treatment for hypertension on morbidity and mortality from cardiovascular disease: a review of randomized controlled trials. *Prog Cardiovasc Dis* 1986;29(suppl I):99–118.

75. Morgan T, Adam W, Carney S, Gibbard R, Brown S, Wheeler D. Treatment of mild hypertension in elderly males. *Clin Sci* 1979;57:255s–357s.

76. Spence JD. Quantitative spectral analysis of carotid Doppler: use in measurement of the effects of antihypertensive drugs on arterial flow disturbances. *Clin Invest Med* 1989;12:82–89.

77. Beaudry M, Spence JD. Measurement of atherosclerosis: development of an atherosclerosis severity index, clinical experimental hypertension. *Clin Exp Hypertens Theor Pract* 1989;A11(5,6):943–956.

78. Parmley WW, Blumlein SL, Sievers R. Modification of experimental atherosclerosis by calcium channel blockers. *Am J Cardiol* 1985;55:165B–171B.

79. Weinstein DB, Heider JG. Protective action of calcium channel antagonists in atherogenesis and experimental vascular injury. *Am J Hypertens* 1989;2:205–212.

80. Fleckenstein A, Fleckenstein-Grun G, Frey M, Zorn J. Calcium antagonism and ACE inhibition: two outstandingly effective means of interference with cardiovascular calcium overload, high blood pressure, and arteriosclerosis in spontaneously hypertensive rats. *Am J Hypertens* 1989;2:194–204.

81. Linz KW, Scholkens BA, Han Y-F. Beneficial effects of converting enzyme inhibitor, ramipril, in ischemic rat hearts. *J Cardiovasc Pharmacol* 1986;(suppl 10):S91–S99.

82. Przyklenk K, Kloner RA. Relationships between structure and effects of ACE inhibitors: comparative effects in myocardial ischemic/reperfusion injury. *Br J Clin Pharmacol* 1989;28:167S–175S.

83. Lichten PR, Hugenholtz P, Rafflenbenl W, Jost S, Hecker H, and the INTACT-Study Group. Retardation of the progression of coronary artery disease with nifedipine. Results of INTACT. *Circulation* 1989;(suppl II)80:11–382.

84. Winther K, Trap-Jensen J. Effects of three beta-blockers with different pharmacodynamic properties on platelet aggregation and platelet and plasma cyclic AMP. *Eur J Clin Pharmacol* 1988;35:17–20.

85. Relman AS. Mild hypertension: no more benign neglect. *N Engl J Med* 1980;302:293–294.

86. Olsson G, Rehnqvist N, Sjogren A, et al. Long-term treatment with metoprolol after myocardial infarction: report on three year mortality and morbidity. *JACC* 1985;5:1428–1437.

87. Wikstrand J, Warnold I, Olsson G, Tuomilehto J, Elmfeldt D, Berglund G. Primary prevention with metoprolol in patients with hypertension: Mortality results from the MAPHY study. *JAMA* 1988;259:1976–1982.

88. Breig A, Ekbom K, Greitz, T, Kugelberg E. Hydrocephalus due to elongated basilar artery. A new clinicoradiologic syndrome. *Lancet* 1967;1:874–875.

89. Stamler J. Research opportunities and directions in the blood pres-

sure problem; combining predictors. *Am J Hypertens* 1991;4:646–660.

90. SHEP Cooperative Research Group: prevention of stroke by antihypertensive drug treatment in older persons with isolated systolic hypertension. Final results of the systolic hypertension in the elderly program (SHEP). *JAMA* 1991;265:3255–3264.

91. Kaplan NM. The case for low dose diuretic therapy. *Am J Hypertens* 1991;4:970–971.

92. Christensen KL. Reducing pulse pressure in hypertension may normalize small artery structure. *Hypertension* 1991;18:762–772.

93. Spence JD, Sibbald WJ, Cape RD. Direct, indirect and mean blood pressures in hypertensive patients: the problem of cuff artefact due to arterial wall stiffness and a partial solution. *Clin Invest Med* 1980;2:165–173.

94. Finnegan TP, Spence JD, Wong DG, Wells GA. Blood pressure measurement in the elderly: correlation of arterial stiffness with difference between intraarterial and cuff pressures. *J Hypertens* 1985;3:231–235.

95. Messerli FH, Ventura HO, Amodeo C. Osler's maneuver and pseudohypertension. *N Engl J Med* 1985;312:1548–1551.

96. Spence JD. Stepped care therapy for hypertension is dead, but what will replace it? *Can Med Assoc J* 1989;140:133–1136.

Hypertension: Pathophysiology, Diagnosis,
and Management, Second Edition,
edited by J.H. Laragh and B.M. Brenner,
Raven Press, Ltd., New York © 1995.

CHAPTER 44

The Sympathetic Nervous System and Catecholamine Release and Plasma Clearance in Normal Blood Pressure Control, in Aging, and in Hypertension

Murray Esler

M. Esler: Baker Medical Research Institute, Prahran 3181, Melbourne, Australia.

The historical antecedents of the study of sympathetic nervous system function in human hypertension are the description of the vasomotor nerves (1) and the isolation and synthesis of the adrenal medullary pressor principle, epinephrine (2). Soon after the demonstration by von Euler (3) that the sympathetic nervous transmitter was norepinephrine, and not epinephrine, which had been believed for a time, neurochemical measurements of transmitter release, based on urinary excretion rates, were first applied in patients with essential hypertension in an attempt to quantify the level of sympathetic nervous activity present (4). Subsequent to the development of sensitive radioenzymatic assays for catecholamines (5), an elevated plasma norepinephrine concentration in antecubital venous blood was reported in some patients with essential hypertension (6).

Static measurements of plasma norepinephrine concentration, however, although providing a useful guide to sympathetic nervous system function, have substantial limitations in hypertension research (7). One technical weakness is the dependence of the plasma concentration on the rate at which the transmitter is removed from plasma, after its overflow to the circulation, and not only on sympathetic nerve firing and norepinephrine release. This is well illustrated by kinetic analysis of the basis for the rise in the plasma concentration of norepinephrine with postural stimulation, where decreased norepinephrine plasma clearance and increased norepinephrine release contribute approximately equally (8).

Perhaps the principal limitation of plasma norepinephrine concentration measurements is the fact that all global indices of sympathetic nervous function provide no information on the regional patterning of sympathetic nervous activation in hypertension. This runs contrary to the functional organization of the sympathetic nervous system. With physiological stimuli (7,9,10) and in cardiovascular diseases (7,11) patterning of sympathetic responses is evident, with the sympathetic outflow to some organs being activated, while those to other regions may be unchanged or inhibited. That almost 90 years after Geisbock suggested the nervous system might be involved in the development of essential hypertension (12) the proposition remains somewhat contentious indicates that the available research methodology for testing sympathetic nervous system function in humans has lacked precision.

METHODS OF CLINICAL TESTING OF SYMPATHETIC NERVOUS SYSTEM FUNCTION

To better understand possible neural mechanisms initiating the blood pressure rise in the early phases of essential hypertension, and to study the influence of aging on the sympathetic nervous system, precise knowledge of regional sympathetic nervous function is needed. Individual components of neural control of the circulation have provided a basis for the development of clinical tests of regional sympathetic nervous system function (Table 1). These tests are complementary, not competing methodologies, measuring different aspects of sympathetic nervous function. Clinical microneurography, for recording multiunit sympathetic nerve firing in subcutaneous nerves passing to skin and skeletal muscle, and the measurement of norepinephrine spillover to the circulation using radiotracer methodology are the most analytically powerful techniques. Power spectral analysis of spontaneous, superimposed circulatory rhythms, which in comparison is lacking somewhat in precision, has the virtue of being a noninvasive method.

Clinical Microneurography

This technique provides a method for studying nerve firing rates in subcutaneously distributed sympathetic nerves (13,14). A fine tungsten electrode is inserted through the skin, with positioning of the electrode tip in sympathetic fibers of, most commonly, the common peroneal or median nerves. Multifiber recordings of "bursts" of nerve activity, synchronous with the heart beat, are generated. The method has been widely used to study the sympathetic nervous control of the cardiovascular system (14).

Norepinephrine Spillover Rate Measurements

Neurotransmitter release can be studied clinically using radiotracer-derived measurements of the appearance rate of norepinephrine in plasma, from individual organs or from the body as a whole (15,16). With microneurographic methods for studying sympathetic nerve firing rates, the nerves to skeletal muscle and skin only can be studied. An important limitation in hypertension research is the inaccessibility to testing of the sympathetic nerves to internal organs. Regional norepinephrine spillover measurements help overcome this deficiency.

TABLE 1. *Independent indices of sympathetic nervous system function*

Clinical microneurography (13,14)
Measurement of total and regional norepinephrine spillover (15,16)
Heart rate spectral analysis (17,18)
Cardiovascular response to adrenergic blockade (19,20)

Sympathetic function can be quantified clinically by independent neurophysiological, neurochemical, and pharmacological methodologies, and by analysis of circulatory rhythms. References are shown in parenthesis.

Power Spectral Analysis of Circulatory Rhythms

With this technique, sophisticated mathematical partitioning is used to identify individual superimposed rhythms producing cyclical variation in heart rate and arterial pressure (17,18). Underlying independent high-frequency (approximately 0.3 Hz) and low-frequency (approximately 0.1 Hz) rhythmic influences on heart rate can be recognized. The autonomic nervous system provides the principal effector mechanism for this heart rate variability. The high-frequency component is coupled with the respiratory cycle, determined primarily by vagal function and largely abolished by atropine. Low-frequency variability derives in part from the influence of the cardiac sympathetic nerves and is reduced by β-adrenergic blockade (18). Low-frequency variability in heart rate does not, of course, strictly provide a measure of the rate of firing of the cardiac sympathetic nerves, despite widespread and often uncritical interpretation of the variability measurement in this way. Low-frequency heart rate variability is determined by the combined influences of the intrinsic central nervous oscillation in sympathetic outflow, the gain of the relevant circulatory reflex loops, and the postsynaptic chronotropic responsiveness of the heart.

Pharmacological Autonomic Blockade

Pharmacological blockade of the autonomic nervous system can be used to estimate the prevailing level of neural cardiovascular tone (19,20). The method developed initially was to utilize the fall in arterial pressure after ganglionic blockade to gauge the overall "neurogenic component" in essential hypertension (19). Pharmacological block of the heart with propranolol and atropine (20) has been used to quantify sympathetic nervous and vagal influences on heart rate and cardiac output in early human hypertension. The measured responses, however, are influenced not only by the level of sympathetic nerve firing, but in addition by end-organ responsiveness in the cardiovascular system.

In this chapter results from quantitative neurochemical methodology will primarily be relied upon to describe human sympathetic nervous and adrenal medullary circulatory control in health, with normal aging, and in essential hypertension. Results derived from the complementary neurophysiological, spectral analysis, and pharmacological techniques will provide supplementary information.

SOURCES OF CATECHOLAMINES IN PLASMA

The catecholamines (dopamine, norepinephrine, and epinephrine) are widely distributed in mammalian species. By the turn of the century the origin of circulating epinephrine from the adrenal medulla and its pressor effects were clearly established (2). Its actions as a central nervous system (CNS) neurotransmitter were demonstrated subsequently (21). Norepinephrine, also secreted by the adrenal medulla, only acts as a circulating hormone in limited circumstances (22). Its biological importance is as the major transmitter of the sympathetic nervous system and as a CNS transmitter (23). Dopamine is distributed with norepinephrine and epinephrine in tissues (24), being their precursor, and is an important CNS transmitter (25).

Dopamine is the immediate precursor of norepinephrine (Fig. 1), conversion being by side-chain hydroxylation through the action of dopamine-β-hydroxylase (DβH). Epinephrine is produced from norepinephrine by terminal side-chain methylation, via phenylethanolamine methyltransferase (PNMT) (26). Catecholamines enter plasma principally by overflow of the released neurotransmitter to the circulation or after secretion by the adrenal medulla. The bulk of norepinephrine in plasma originates from sympathetic nerves, and of epinephrine from the adrenal medulla. The source of plasma dopamine remains uncertain.

Norepinephrine

Only a few percent of the norepinephrine entering plasma in humans originates from the adrenal medulla (27). Similarly, only a small component of the norepinephrine plasma pool appears to derive from noradrenergic brain neurons (28). The bulk of norepinephrine in plasma is derived from the sympathetic nervous system, with the sympathetic nerves of the kidneys, skeletal muscle, and the lungs each making a substantial contribution (15 to 30 percent) (7,16). The sympathetic innervation of the liver, gastrointestinal tract, heart, and skin each are responsible for less than 10 percent of the plasma norepinephrine appearance rate (7,16,29).

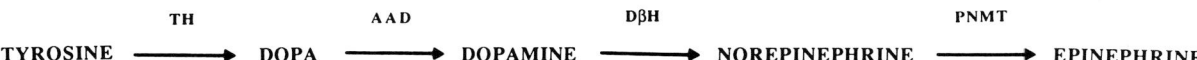

FIG. 1. Pathway for catecholamine biosynthesis, with involved enzymes. TH, tyrosinehydroxylase; AAD, aromatic acid decarboxylase; DβH, dopamine-β-hydroxylase; PNMT, phenylethanolamine methyltransferase; DOPA, 3,4-dihydroxyphenylalanine. (From ref. 7, with permission.)

Epinephrine

Although the majority of plasma epinephrine undoubtedly derives directly from the adrenal medulla, some contribution form extraadrenal chromaffin tissue (30) and from epinephrine coreleased from sympathetic nerves (31–33) is probable. Under certain circumstances, such as in patients with heart failure, regional adrenaline release from organs such as the liver and lungs contributes materially to the epinephrine plasma pool (32). An alternative pathway of epinephrine biosynthesis, utilizing an enzyme other than PNMT, may possibly be involved in extraadrenal epinephrine production (34,35).

Dopamine

The extent to which dopamine in plasma originates from peripherally released transmitter is uncertain. It has proven difficult to demonstrate dopaminergic nerves in which the principal transmitter is dopamine. There has been no demonstration to date that CNS dopamine enters the circulation. The most likely sources of plasma dopamine are precursor dopamine released from sympathetic nerves and the adrenal medulla, and from the synthesis of dopamine by the renal tubules, utilizing dihydroxyphenylalanine (DOPA) extracted from plasma (36).

PLASMA CATECHOLAMINE KINETICS

A special impetus to the development of techniques for studying the rates of overflow of catecholamines to the circulation has been provided by the lack of clinical methods for studying human catecholaminergic neuronal function in inaccessible sites, such as the sympathetic nerves of internal organs and the neurons of the CNS. The inapplicability of electrophysiological neural recording methodologies in contexts such as these has led to a continuing search for alternative techniques, especially biochemical ones.

Whole-Body Norepinephrine Spillover to Plasma

The potential value of norepinephrine release rate measurements as an index of sympathetic nerve firing was seen early. Soon after von Euler (3) categorized the sympathetic transmitter as norepinephrine, Peart (37) described norepinephrine overflow into the venous effluent of an organ (the cat spleen) on electrical stimulation of its nerve supply. This washout of norepinephrine in general is proportional to the rate of sympathetic nerve firing (38–40). The application of isotope dilution methodology to measure total rates of norepinephrine

spillover to plasma was a useful innovation, eliminating the confounding effect of variation in norepinephrine (NE) plasma clearance on plasma norepinephrine concentration. During an intravenous infusion of tritiated NE (15):

$$\text{Total NE Spillover Rate} = {}^3\text{H NE Infusion Rate}/$$
$$\text{Plasma NE Specific Radioactivity.}$$

Rather than the rate of release of norepinephrine from sympathetic nerve varicosities, which is unmeasurable clinically, the norepinephrine spillover rate gives the rate at which released norepinephrine enters plasma; in humans this is approximately 10 percent to 20 percent of the norepinephrine synthesis rate (41). The overall rate of spillover of norepinephrine to plasma (with arterial sampling) in healthy resting humans is 200 to 600 ng/min (Fig. 2). With powerful stimuli to the sympathetic nervous system, such as submaximal aerobic exercise, readings of 1500 to 4000 ng/min are encountered (49,50).

Norepinephrine Plasma Clearance

Norepinephrine is removed from the circulation rapidly, with a plasma clearance of 1.5 to 4.0 L/min (15,43–45) (Fig. 2). Removal of norepinephrine from plasma involves the combined processes of neuronal uptake by sympathetic nerves, extraneuronal uptake by a variety of other tissues, and metabolic conversion by O-methylation, oxidative deamination, and sulfoconjugation (7,26). The rate of plasma clearance is dependent on these cellular mechanisms, in particular neuronal uptake, but also on the cardiac output and regional blood flows (51). The lowering of cardiac output encountered in cardiac failure, and with β-adrenergic adrenoceptor blockade and head-up tilting, for example, is responsible for reduced rates of removal of norepinephrine from the circulation, which contribute to the elevation in plasma norepinephrine concentration (7,8,22,52,53).

Regional Norepinephrine Spillover to Plasma

Global measures of sympathetic function neglect the fact that the sympathetic nervous system shows regional differentiation. With certain reflex responses and in disease states some sympathetic outflows may be activated but others unchanged or inhibited (9–11). Techniques measuring organ-specific norepinephrine release to plasma are available for studying regional sympathetic nervous function in humans. The relationship that in general exists between the sympathetic nerve firing rate of an organ, with electrical stimulation in the physiological range, and the rate of spillover of norepinephrine into its venous effluent provide the experimental justifi-

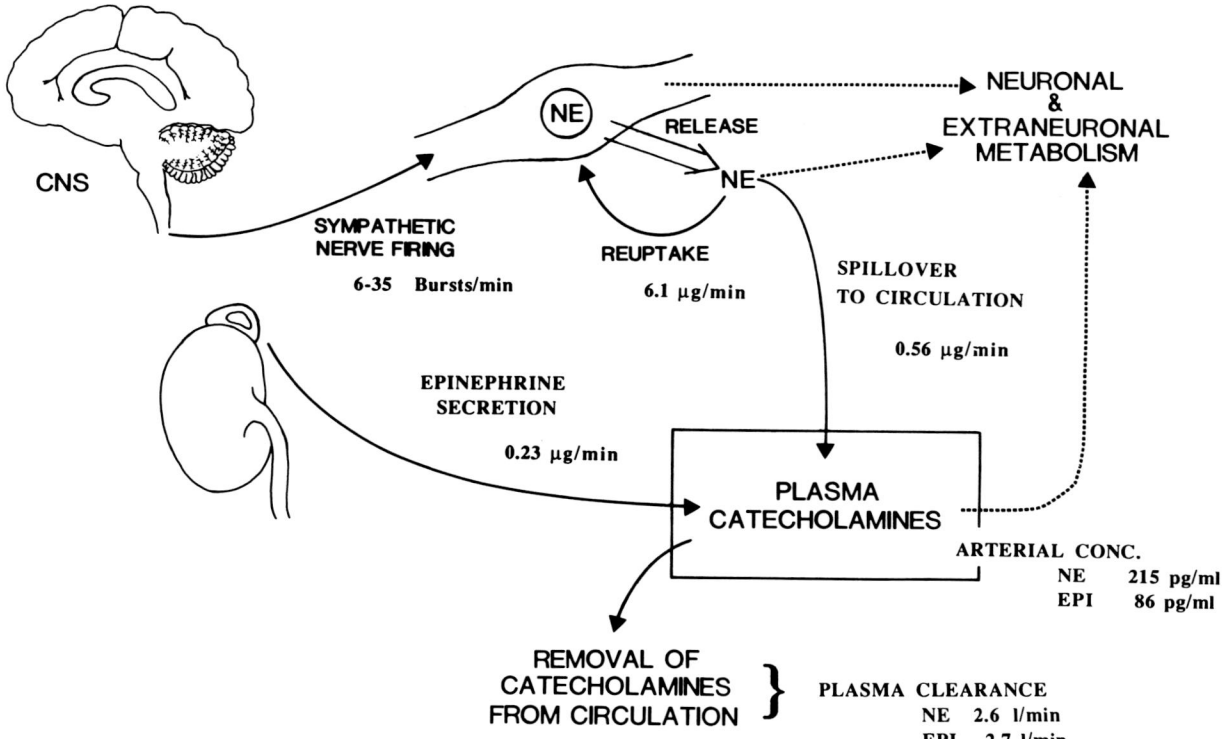

FIG. 2. Scheme of catecholamine kinetics in humans, with typical values at rest for muscle sympathetic nerve firing (13,14,42), rates of norepinephrine neuronal reuptake and spillover to plasma from sympathetic nerves (7,43–47), epinephrine secretion by the adrenal medulla (48), rates of clearance of both catecholamines from plasma (7,43–48), and plasma concentrations (7,43–48), which represent the balance of the dual processes of addition to and removal from plasma.

cation for using measures of regional norepinephrine release as a clinical index of sympathetic nervous tone in individual organs. During constant rate infusion of tritiated norepinephrine, outward flux of endogenous norepinephrine can be measured by isotope dilution (16):

$$\text{Regional NE Spillover} = [(C_V - C_A) + C_A \cdot E] \cdot PF$$

where C_V and C_A are the plasma concentration of norepinephrine in venous and arterial plasma, E is the fractional extraction of tritiated norepinephrine, and PF is the organ plasma flow.

Typical rates of regional spillover of norepinephrine to plasma in healthy human subjects are as follows: for the heart 5 to 25 ng/min, for the kidneys 45 to 140 ng/min, for the gut and liver 10 to 40 ng/min, for the lungs 30 to 120 ng/min, and for skeletal muscle 50 to 130 ng/min (7,16,49,52,54–56). Regional differentiation of human sympathetic nervous responses is evident from organ-specific norepinephrine spillover measurements in a range of clinical contexts, such as the preferential activation of the sympathetic outflows to the heart and kidneys during mental stress (54,57), the preferential activation of the cardiac sympathetic outflow in patients predisposed to ventricular arrhythmias (58), and the selective stimulation of the nerves to the kidneys with dietary so-

dium restriction (55). During submaximal aerobic exercise, noradrenaline spillover from the heart increases by as much as 30-fold (49,50).

Neuronal Reuptake of Norepinephrine

Active removal of norepinephrine from the synaptic cleft after its release, by neuronal reuptake, ensures prompt termination of postsynaptic receptor activation once an appropriate end-organ response has been achieved (59). Thus, most of the norepinephrine released is recaptured by the sympathetic nerve, where it is stored for subsequent release or metabolized to dihydroxyphenylglycol (DHPG) (60). Of the released transmitter escaping reuptake and local metabolism at extraneuronal sites, a fraction (5–20 percent) diffuses unchanged into the circulation (47,61) (Fig. 2). The rate of this spillover of norepinephrine to plasma is dependent on the capacity for neuronal reuptake, increasing substantially if the uptake process is impaired by pharmacological blockade of the norepinephrine transporter with drugs such as the tricyclic antidepressant, desipramine (62,63). Neuronal norepinephrine uptake can be quantified in humans by studying the removal of infused radiolabeled norepinephrine from plasma (since this is in part dependent on uptake into sympathetic nerves), the conversion of the tritiated norepinephrine to the tritiated metabolite, DHPG (occurring intraneuronally after uptake), and the extent to which pharmacological uptake blockade impairs these processes (Fig. 3) (47,61). With sympathetic denervation of the heart, such as is seen with cardiac transplantation and in patients with pure autonomic failure, tritiated norepinephrine uptake by the heart and its processing to tritiated DHPG is at a very low level (64,65). This methodology can be applied in the study of the effects of normal aging on norepinephrine reuptake.

Cotransmitter Release from Human Sympathetic Nerves

With regional venous sampling and application of the Fick principle it is possible to test for organ-specific release of the presumed sympathetic cotransmitters neuropeptide Y (NPY) (66) and epinephrine (31). In contrast to release of the major sympathetic neurotransmitter, cotransmitter release is detected only with some difficulty. Net overflow of NPY to plasma has been reported across the forearm (66) and the human kidney (54) under resting conditions. Overflow of NPY from the heart is not evident at rest in healthy subjects, but becomes readily apparent with high rates of cardiac sympathetic nerve firing, such as in patients with cardiac failure (67).

Epinephrine exists in peripheral tissues, where it appears to have been largely derived from hormone circulating in plasma, not synthesis *in situ* (68,69). Evidence exists that epinephrine within sympathetic nerves, derived from this source, may be released with norepinephrine and act as a cotransmitter facilitating the release of the major neurotransmitter (70). To detect outward flux of epinephrine to plasma, indicative of release of epinephrine from neuronal (and perhaps extraneuronal) stores, in the face of the net extraction of plasma epinephrine, which occurs across all organs except the adre-

nal medulla, radiotracer methodology is needed (32). The principle applied is that the outward flux of epinephrine can be measured from the reduction in the ratio of plasma radiolabeled to unlabeled epinephrine concentration (the isotope dilution) occurring in the passage of blood through an organ. Regional neuronal release of epinephrine in young healthy human subjects is not evident at rest, and can be demonstrated only under special circumstances, such as from the heart with the stimulation of the cardiac sympathetic outflow accompanying aerobic exercise (32), and after loading of the neuronal epinephrine pool by intravenous infusion of epinephrine (71). The functional significance in humans of this neuronally released epinephrine remains uncertain, although its participation in the early pathogenesis of essential hypertension has been suspected (72,73).

Epinephrine Secretion and Plasma Clearance

Epinephrine secretion rates have been estimated in humans utilizing adrenal vein catheterization (27). This value ignores the input to plasma from extraadrenal chromaffin tissue; under resting conditions this appears to constitute a substantial fraction of total epinephrine secretion in humans (30). Also ignored is any input of epinephrine released from sympathetic nerves, although this input to the plasma epinephrine pool must generally be small (31,32).

Epinephrine secretion rate measurements incorporating these possible additional sources can be determined by isotope dilution, similar in principle to the measurement of whole-body norepinephrine spillover rates (48). Epinephrine secretion at rest in humans averages 150 to 350 ng/min. Two- to fourfold increases are seen during aerobic exercise and laboratory mental stress (7,48). Measurements of epinephrine secretion are yet to be made during insulin-induced hypoglycemia in humans, when plasma epinephrine concentrations increase up to 100-fold (22).

INVOLVEMENT OF THE SYMPATHETIC NERVOUS SYSTEM AND CATECHOLAMINES IN NORMAL BLOOD PRESSURE CONTROL

The autonomic nervous system occupies a central position in the normal regulation of the cardiovascular system. This is achieved principally through the effects of the sympathetic nervous system on the function of the heart, large arteries, arterioles, veins, and the kidneys. The parasympathetic nervous system, through vagus nerve regulation of heart rate, plays a subsidiary role. The role played by circulating catecholamines secreted by the adrenal medulla in cardiovascular regulation in general, and blood pressure control in particular, is a contentious issue.

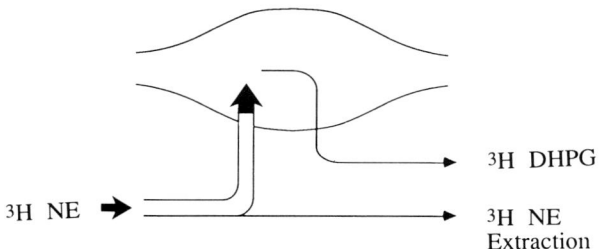

FIG. 3. Principle by which the neuronal uptake of norepinephrine can be quantified in humans, for the whole body (47) or for individual organs (61), by studying the removal of infused radiolabeled norepinephrine from plasma, the subsequent intraneuronal conversion of the tritiated norepinephrine to the tritiated metabolite dihydroxyphenylglycol (DHPG), and the extent to which pharmacological neuronal uptake block reduces these processes.

Threshold Catecholamine Plasma Concentrations for Cardiovascular Actions

To what extent norepinephrine circulating in plasma acts as a hormone is disputed. The most widely held view is that the threshold plasma concentration for norepinephrine's cardiovascular actions is in excess of 1000 pg/ml (22). Such a value is reached only in unusual circumstances, such as at near maximal levels of aerobic exercise, or clinically in patients with pheochromocytoma or myocardial infarction (22). Accordingly norepinephrine is primarily a neurotransmitter, rather than a hormone. An alternative viewpoint, however, would place the norepinephrine threshold plasma concentration appreciably lower, say at 600 pg/ml (74,75), and would suggest a larger role for norepinephrine as a hormone.

In contrast to norepinephrine, epinephrine has important and well-established cardiovascular actions as a hormone. Under resting conditions the prevailing concentration of 20 to 100 pg/ml in arterial plasma is insufficient for direct actions on the heart and blood vessels (22). If the plasma epinephrine concentration doubles or triples, with stimuli such as cigarette smoking or mild mental stress, then the threshold plasma concentration for the cardiovascular actions of epinephrine is exceeded. At higher plasma concentrations (>250 pg/ml), such as with hypoglycemia, epinephrine has powerful hormonal actions on the circulation, producing tachycardia and regional vasoconstriction in most vascular beds (excluding skeletal muscle where β-adrenergic va-

sodilatation predominates). With plasma dopamine, there is general agreement on a lack of physiological effects; the threshold plasma concentration for cardiovascular and natriuretic actions is at least 100 times higher than the plasma concentration at rest (<50 pg/ml) (76).

Sympathetic Nervous Regulation and Dysregulation of Arterial Pressure

The influences of the sympathetic nervous system on normal cardiovascular control are both short- and long-term. Long-term circulatory control involves in particular the regulation of salt and water balance through sympathetic nervous effects on renin secretion and renal tubular reabsorption of sodium (77). Examples of short-term sympathetic nervous circulatory control are the neural modification of venous capacitance, arteriolar resistance, and heart rate with upright posture (78), and the regulation of regional blood flow, in parallel with metabolic and autoregulatory influences on flow, during exercise (79).

Schemes of the organization of circulatory control rightly emphasize the preeminence of reflex blood pressure homeostasis (78). This is achieved, on the afferent side, through arterial and low-pressure receptors, with reflex outputs to the heart, resistance vessels, capacitance vessels, and kidneys. The central nervous system integration of high-pressure baroreceptor influences involves, in

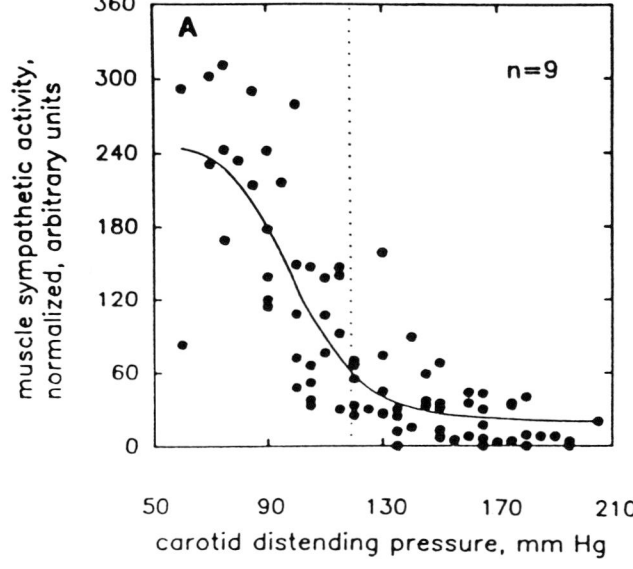

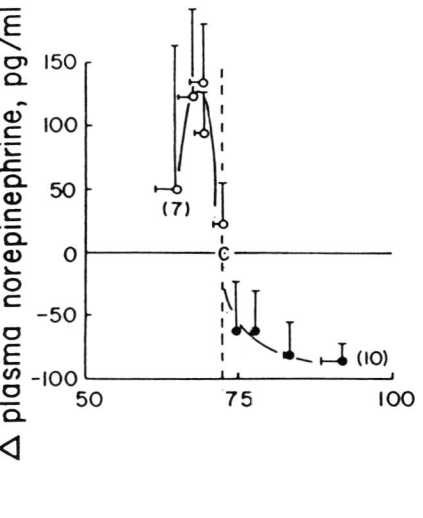

FIG. 4. Influence of the arterial baroreflex on sympathetic nervous system activity in humans, with acute changes in blood pressure produced in the laboratory. **Left panel:** Firing rates in postganglionic sympathetic fibers to skeletal muscle are inversely related to distending pressures in the carotid artery, with changes produced experimentally by neck suction or compression. (From ref. 82, with permission.) **Right panel:** With changes in arterial pressure produced pharmacologically, with both rises and falls around the starting diastolic pressure of 75 mm Hg, change in the plasma concentration of norepinephrine and blood pressure are related inversely. (From ref. 83, with permission.)

particular, the nucleus tractus solitarius of the brainstem (80), while volume receptor projections to the locus coeruleus have been identified (81). Efferent sympathetic activity in human subjects adjusts accurately and appropriately with change in arterial pressure (Fig. 4). With acute changes in blood pressure produced experimentally in the laboratory, a precise relationship can be demonstrated between the magnitude of the pressure change and the sympathetic nervous response, quantified using microneurography or plasma norepinephrine (Fig. 4). To illustrate some of these principles of sympathetic nervous circulatory control, the reflex sympathetic adjustments to upright posture, which achieve BP homeostasis during gravitational challenge, will be described, and then the failure of sympathetic circulatory control that characterizes the simple fainting reaction.

Blood Pressure Regulation During Upright Posture

With sitting and standing, translocation of blood occurs from the intrathoracic area to the distensible veins of the legs and abdomen. It is the reduction in the degree of distension of the cardiopulmonary volume receptors that principally underlies the reflex circulatory response, high pressure arterial baroreceptors apparently making lesser contribution. Reflex sympathetic nervous adjustments occur that lead to increases in total peripheral vascular resistance and venous tone and contribute to the elevation in heart rate (in concert with vagal withdrawal). In human subjects, increased sympathetic outflow to blood vessels of skeletal muscle can be demonstrated by microneurography during head-up tilting (Fig. 5), and the overall rate of spillover of norepinephrine increases. The plasma norepinephrine concentration rises disproportionately, due to concomitant reduction in the rate of removal of norepinephrine from plasma (8,84,85) (Fig. 5). Activation of the renal sympathetic nerves, underlying the renal vasoconstriction and increased secretion of renin, is evident in the increased spillover of norepinephrine into the renal veins (54).

If the reflex increase in sympathetic activity with upright posture is diminished, either blocked pharmacologically or deficient in patients with autonomic insufficiency syndromes, postural hypotension results. The failure of the plasma concentration of norepinephrine to rise with standing or head-up tilting has been used as a diagnostic test to detect autonomic failure in patients with postural hypotension (86). But we find this not to be a reliable indicator, our clinical experience being that an increase in plasma norepinephrine concentration commonly occurs in patients with pure autonomic failure (Table 2). The reason is that there is a large fall in cardiac output and in regional blood flows during orthostasis in patients with autonomic failure, and that this

Muscle Sympathetic Nerve Activity

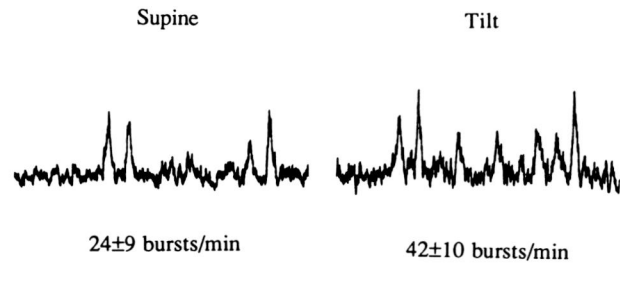

Supine   Tilt

24±9 bursts/min   42±10 bursts/min

Norepinephrine Plasma Kinetics

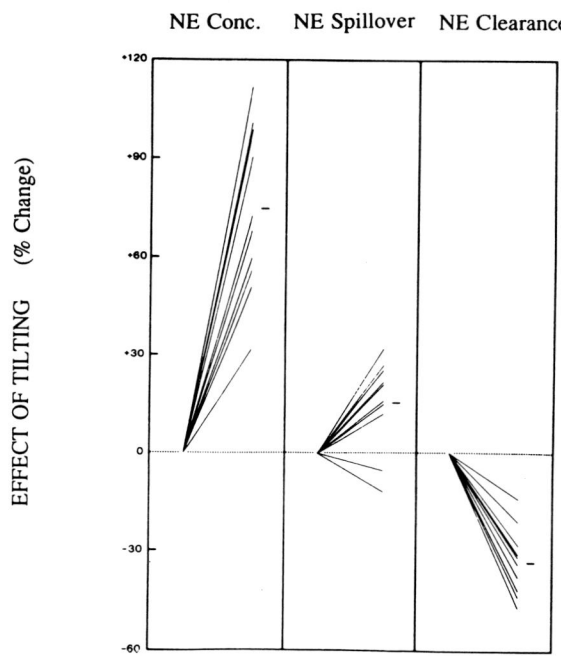

FIG. 5. Activation of the sympathetic nervous system with head-up tilting. **Top panel:** Representative microneurography trace and values from six healthy subjects (mean, SEM) tilted at 40° head-up for 30 minutes. (Unpublished observations from testing performed in collaboration with Dr. J. Thompson.) **Bottom panel:** The rise in plasma norepinephrine concentration with 60 minutes of 40° head-up tilting, in ten patients with untreated essential hypertension, was attributable to both increased spillover of norepinephrine to plasma and lowered norepinephrine plasma clearance. (From ref. 8, with permission.)

TABLE 2. *Effect of head-up tilting on plasma norepinephrine kinetics*

	Healthy subjects	Pure autonomic failure
Change in norepinephrine plasma concentration (pg/ml)	+112 ± 20	+73 ± 29*
Change in norepinephrine plasma clearance (%)	−12 ± 3	−36 ± 4*
Change in total norepinephrine spillover (%)	+24 ± 3	−8 ± 2*

In six patients with pure autonomic failure there was a misleading rise in the plasma concentration of norepinephrine with head-up tilting (30° for 15 min), despite no increase in norepinephrine release, due to a large fall in norepinephrine plasma clearance (means, SED listed). In four of six pure autonomic insufficiency patients the plasma norepinephrine response to tilt was within the range of response found in the eight age-matched healthy subjects. The fall in norepinephrine clearance in these patients is attributable to exaggerated posture-dependent venous pooling and the consequent large fall in cardiac output in the absence of cardiovascular sympathetic innervation. Mean values are shown, with significance of differences between the two groups.
* *p* < .05, Student's *t*-test. (Tabulated from ref. 86, with permission.)

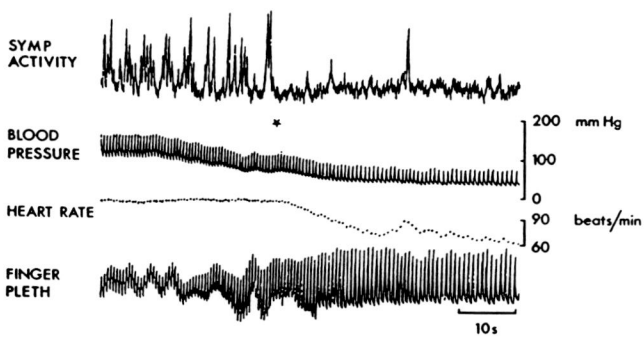

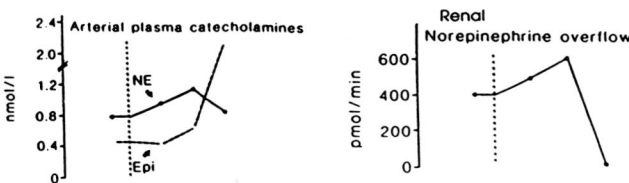

NOREPINEPHRINE MEASUREMENT
% of Baseline

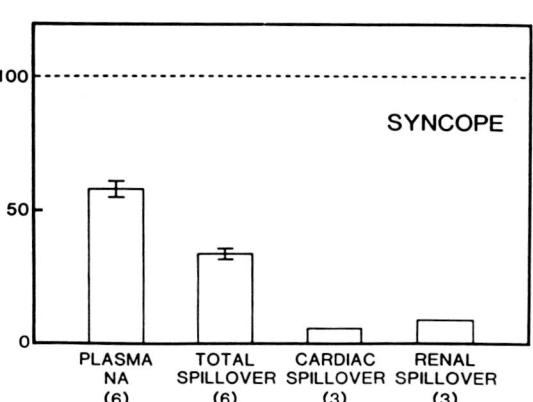

lowers the clearance of norepinephrine from plasma and elevates the plasma concentration in the absence of any increase in norepinephrine release (86) (Table 2).

Simple Fainting Reaction

The fainting reaction is a hypotensive circulatory response that may occur with prolonged standing, or in response to unpleasant experiences, such as venipuncture. Although often appearing to be abrupt in onset when occurring with upright posture as the provocation, there is usually an antecedent phase of borderline circulatory compensation during which sympathetic nervous activation may be subnormal but adrenal medullary release of epinephrine is markedly increased (54).

The sudden blood pressure fall characterizing the faint is a consequence of bradycardia, the source of the term *vasovagal reaction,* since this heart rate slowing was initially thought to be principally vagal in origin, and falling vascular resistance. The fall in vascular resistance almost certainly results from withdrawal of sympathetic nervous vasoconstrictor tone (7,54,87) (Fig. 6). The reduc-

FIG. 6. Inhibition of the sympathetic nervous system during a fainting reaction. **Top panel:** Changes in muscle sympathetic activity, blood pressure, heart rate, and finger pulse plethysmogram with syncope (onset marked by asterisk) occurring during the course of a nitroprusside infusion. (From ref. 87, with permission.) **Middle panel:** A fall in arterial plasma norepinephrine concentration and rise in epinephrine concentration at the onset of syncope occurring during the application of lower body negative pressure, and the associated fall in norepinephrine overflow from the kidney. (From ref. 54, with permission.) **Bottom panel:** In healthy subjects suffering a fainting reaction during percutaneous placement under local anesthesia of a central venous catheter, sympathetic withdrawal to the heart and kidneys was almost complete, based on the marked reduction in regional norepinephrine spillover. Number of subjects given in parenthesis. (From ref. 7, with permission.)

tion in heart rate is also due at least in part to reduced sympathetic activity in the cardiac sympathetic nerves, and not solely to the influence of the vagus. Cardiac sympathetic nerve firing, based on measurements of norepinephrine spillover from the heart, falls to near zero during syncope. Renal sympathetic activity also drops precipitously (Fig. 6) (7,54).

The peripheral receptors subserving the fainting response and the central nervous integration of this afferent input is unclear. The discharge of left ventricular receptors excessively stimulated by a hypercontractile, adrenergically stimulated left ventricular myocardium has been proposed as the trigger for the response, but it is difficult to reconcile this suggestion with the occurrence of vasodepressor syncope in patients having undergone prior cardiac denervation (88).

In recent years, study of orthostatic circulatory responses during diagnostic head-up tilt testing has become part of mainstream, clinical cardiology practice in patients with unexplained syncope (89). The test is commonly applied in those patients in whom Holter monitoring and clinical electrophysiology testing discloses no cardiac arrhythmia. If a pronounced hypotensive response occurs with tilting, the patient's syncopal attacks are then attributed to a pathological fainting response, so-called neurocardiogenic syncope or malignant vasodepressor syndrome. Although neurocardiogenic syncope is held by some to be a common and important condition (89), this is disputed. It has been claimed that diagnostic precision in this area is flawed by a high level of false-positive testing (90), with the use of overly rigorous tilt testing schedules typically involving a relatively prolonged period of tilting, often with a pharmacological challenge.

EFFECTS OF AGING ON THE SYMPATHETIC NERVOUS SYSTEM AND CATECHOLAMINE KINETICS IN HEALTHY HUMAN SUBJECTS

The prevalence of arterial hypertension has been found to increase with age in the majority of countries. Why this occurs is largely a mystery. Researchers have suspected a causal role for the reduction in distensibility of the arterial tree that accompanies aging (91), and for diminishing functional capacity with age in organs, such as the kidney, that are involved in blood pressure regulation (92). Since theories of human hypertension development usually encompass a causal role for the sympathetic nervous system, age-dependent sympathetic nervous dysfunction could possibly be a cause of hypertension in later years. The plasma concentration of the sympathetic neurotransmitter, norepinephrine, does rise with age (93). A review of the influence of aging on sympathetic nervous function in healthy subjects becomes pertinent in this context of possible links between hyper-

tension development and age-dependent changes in sympathetic nervous system function.

Sympathetic Nerve Firing Rates

Efferent sympathetic nerve traffic to skeletal muscle measured by microneurography increases with aging (94,95) (Fig. 7). This occurs in physically active, healthy men and women, and is not attributable to associated obesity or heart disease (96). The cause is unclear, but clinical testing indicates it is unlikely to be defective arterial baroreceptor buffering of sympathetic outflow (96).

This increase in muscle sympathetic nerve firing rate with aging only goes part way toward explaining the age-dependence of plasma norepinephrine concentration values. Sympathetic nerves to skeletal muscle contribute only 20 percent of the total norepinephrine entering plasma (16). Further, sympathetic traffic in internal organs such as the heart and kidney, where nerve recording is not possible, cannot be directly inferred from the finding in muscle since individual regional sympathetic nerve firing rates differ markedly under some conditions (10,97).

Norepinephrine Spillover, Clearance, and Plasma Concentration

The plasma concentration of norepinephrine is higher in older healthy people than in younger ones, increasing by approximately 13 percent per decade (98). This is due to increased spillover of transmitter into the circulation from sympathetic nerves in the elderly (99,100), and to a lesser degree to lowered plasma clearance of norepinephrine (98,99). The increased overflow of norepinephrine to plasma is attributable, at least in part, to elevated rates of sympathetic nerve firing, as evident from the microneurographic recordings from the nerves to skeletal muscle (94,95). Not all sympathetic outflows, the renal sympathetic nerves providing one example (101), participate in this increase in sympathetic nerve firing with age. Spillover of norepinephrine from the heart to the circulation is increased in older subjects (Fig. 7), but in this instance an age-dependent reduction in neuronal norepinephrine reuptake, which facilitates transmitter overflow, may possibly be involved.

Neuronal Reuptake of Norepinephrine

Active removal of released norepinephrine from the synaptic cleft by neuronal reuptake is the principal mechanism by which postsynaptic receptor activation is terminated (26). Most of the norepinephrine released is recaptured by the sympathetic nerve, where it is stored for subsequent release or metabolized to DHPG (60,61).

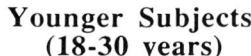

Younger Subjects
(18-30 years)

Older Subjects
(60-75 years)

SPECTRAL ANALYSIS

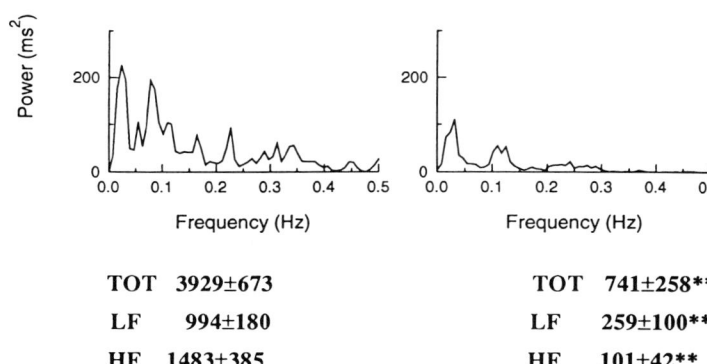

TOT	3929±673		TOT	741±258**
LF	994±180		LF	259±100**
HF	1483±385		HF	101±42**

MICRONEUROGRAPHY

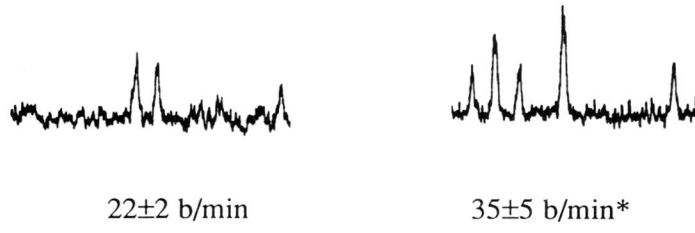

22±2 b/min   35±5 b/min*

FIG. 7. Influence of aging on sympathetic nervous system function at rest. Muscle sympathetic nerve firing rate (**middle panel**) and spillover of the sympathetic transmitter from the heart (**bottom panel**) were higher ($p < .05$) in 12 older than in 21 younger healthy subjects. Despite this evidence of sympathetic nervous activation with aging, spectral analysis of heart rate rhythm disclosed reduced spectral power at all frequencies (**top panel**), including the low-frequency (LF) band associated with sympathetic nervous influence on the heart. This was presumably due in part to reduced adrenoceptor sensitivity and postreceptor signal transduction in the hearts of the older subjects (107). (Unpublished results produced from testing in collaboration with Dr. B. Kingwell and Dr. J. Thompson.)

CARDIAC NORADRENALINE SPILLOVER

11±2 ng/min   21±3 ng/min*

As reduced neuronal reuptake increases the intensity and duration of the noradrenergic response, and facilitates the overflow of the transmitter into plasma (26,62), it is pertinent to ask whether the increased norepinephrine spillover rates and higher plasma norepinephrine concentration values found in older human subjects are due to impaired norepinephrine reuptake.

Neuronal norepinephrine uptake can be quantified in humans by studying the kinetics of norepinephrine and its intraneuronal metabolite, DHPG (Fig. 3) (47). We find the extraction of tritiated norepinephrine across the heart is reduced in healthy human subjects over 50 years of age (Fig. 8). This provides presumptive evidence of reduced neuronal uptake of norepinephrine, since in the heart removal of radiolabeled norepinephrine in transit is largely due to uptake into sympathetic nerves (56). Further evidence of impairment of norepinephrine reuptake with aging is provided by consideration of the relative washout of norepinephrine and DHPG from the sympathetic nerves of the heart into the circulation. Both at rest and during the stimuli of isometric exercise and

difficult mental arithmetic, which activate the sympathetic nervous system, overflow of the intraneuronal metabolite DHPG from the heart is less in older than in younger people, despite higher rates of norepinephrine spillover in those subjects who are older (Fig. 8). These results, strongly suggesting neuronal norepinephrine reuptake is diminished by aging, are in general agreement with earlier studies by Hoeldtke and Cilmi (102), who described in the elderly (a) increased spillover of norepinephrine into the circulation despite normal total body synthesis rates of the transmitter, (b) lower rates of excretion of DHPG in urine, and (c) higher urinary excretion of the extraneuronal norepinephrine metabolite, methoxyhydroxyphenylglycol (MHPG).

Epinephrine Secretion

In elderly human subjects the plasma concentration of epinephrine is either reduced or similar to that in the young (103,104). Our own experience, in a comparison

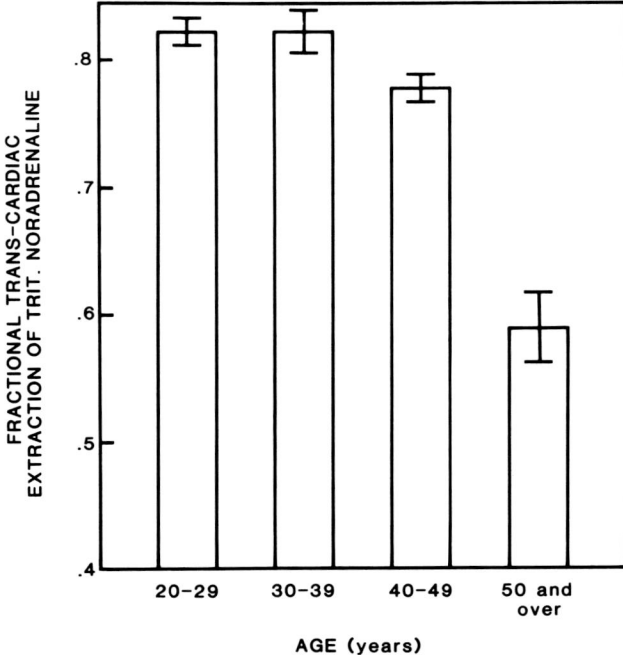

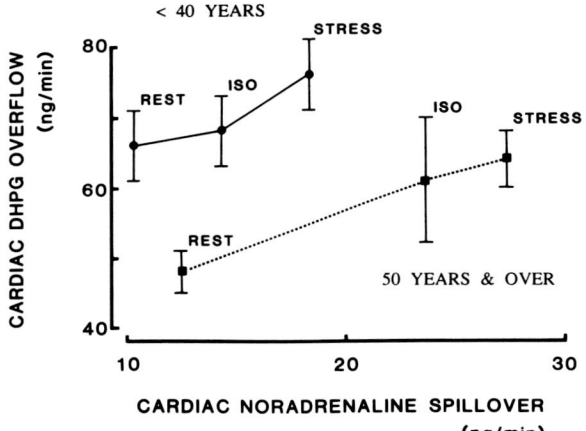

FIG. 8. Evidence of reduced neuronal uptake of noradrenaline in older human subjects. **Top panel:** The fractional extraction of tritiated noradrenaline from plasma in transit through the heart during the course of an intravenous infusion of the tracer, which is largely due to uptake into sympathetic nerves (56), was reduced in 11 men aged 50 years or over ($p < .01$). **Bottom panel:** During sympathetic stimuli that activate the sympathetic nervous system, isometric hand grip (Iso) and difficult mental arithmetic (Stress), overflow of noradrenaline from the heart to plasma was greater in older (>50 years) than in younger men (<40 years), but at each level of cardiac noradrenaline spillover the overflow from the heart of the intraneuronal metabolite DHPG was less in the older men, suggesting that reuptake of the released noradrenaline was reduced. (Unpublished results produced from testing in collaboration with Dr. I. Meredith.)

of healthy men aged 20 to 30 years and 60 to 75 years, is shown in Table 3. The mean epinephrine secretion rate was 78 percent higher in younger subjects. The plasma clearance of epinephrine, much as for norepinephrine, was lower in older subjects (28 percent reduced). The resulting plasma epinephrine concentration was 23 percent higher in younger subjects (Table 3). Clearly, adrenal medullary stimulation does not accompany the sympathetic nervous system activation occurring with aging.

Catecholamine Responses to Stressors

The rise in plasma norepinephrine concentration occurring during reflex stimulation of the sympathetic nervous system, with a range of stressors, has been reported to be greater in older than in younger people (105). Whether this is due to more intense activation of sympathetic nervous outflows, to faulty transmitter reuptake, or to reduced norepinephrine plasma clearance has been unclear. Recent observations with microneurographic recording of muscle sympathetic nerve firing during the application of stressors (106) suggest that reflex increases in nerve traffic may perhaps not be greater in the elderly. Our own unpublished observations with neurochemical measurements during the application of laboratory stressors are in agreement (Fig. 8), and favor reduced neuronal reuptake of the transmitter as the mechanism of higher norepinephrine plasma concentrations during stress.

End-Organ Sensitivity to Catecholamines

Although the available evidence does suggest that aging increases rates of sympathetic nerve firing, at least in some organs, and elevates the synaptic concentration of norepinephrine, this is not necessarily translated into greater adrenergic responses. Factors such as adrenergic receptor subsensitivity or uncoupling can blunt end-organ responsiveness (107). This is illustrated by Fig. 7, which indicates that although the spillover of norepinephrine from the heart is increased in older people at

TABLE 3. *The influence of aging on epinephrine plasma kinetics*

	Age 20–30 years	Age 60–65 years
Secretion (ng/min)	284 ± 30	160 ± 16*
Plasma clearance (L/min)	2.96 ± 0.12	2.15 ± 0.14*
Arterial plasma concentration (pg/mL)	90 ± 9	73 ± 6

Comparison of epinephrine plasma kinetics at rest in 21 younger and 12 older healthy men (means, SEM). Unpublished results produced from testing in collaboration with Dr. D. R. Seals.
*$p < .05$.

rest, heart rate spectral power in the 0.1-Hz band, which is determined in part by efferent sympathetic traffic and represents a functional cardiac neuroeffector response (17,18), is in fact markedly reduced. The heart rate oscillations measured by spectral analysis at 0.1 Hz are dependent not only on efferent sympathetic traffic, but also on the gain of baroreflex arcs, cardiac β-adrenoceptor sensitivity, and postreceptor signal transduction, all of which are reduced in the elderly.

SYMPATHETIC NERVOUS FUNCTION AND CATECHOLAMINE KINETICS IN ESSENTIAL HYPERTENSION

Data drawn from a range of sources, utilizing electrophysiological, neurochemical, circulatory monitoring and pharmacological techniques, now provides compelling evidence that overactivity of the sympathetic nervous system is present in a proportion of patients with essential hypertension, principally younger ones with hypertension in its earlier, developmental phase (8,17, 95,108,109).

Norepinephrine Release, Plasma Clearance, and Plasma Concentration

The plasma concentration of norepinephrine is commonly elevated in essential hypertension. This is due to an increased overall rate of spillover of norepinephrine

to plasma, in younger patients, and not due to a diminution in norepinephrine plasma clearance (110,111). Approximately 50 percent of this increase in total norepinephrine spillover is explicable in terms of increased transmitter overflow from the heart and kidneys (Fig. 9) (8,111). The increased cardiorenal spillover of norepinephrine provides presumptive evidence of increased sympathetic outflow to these organs, since it is not attributable to other factors possibly influencing norepinephrine washout, such as increased blood flows or defective neuronal reuptake of norepinephrine.

Two clinical aspects of human hypertension in its early developmental phase, the hemodynamic pattern and the clinical renin status, are particularly related to neural mechanisms. The changes in the hemodynamics of hypertension as the disease progresses appear to be dictated in part by ongoing changes in the level of cardiac sympathetic stimulation. As demonstrated by the longitudinal studies of Lund-Johansen (112), the high heart rate and cardiac output often present in hypertension in its early phase subsequently give way to normal or reduced values and an arterial pressure elevation based on increased total peripheral vascular resistance. This progressive reduction in cardiac output is partly due to the development of secondary cardiovascular hypertrophy, but it is paralleled by a conspicuous fall in the level of cardiac sympathetic activity with aging in hypertensive patients (Fig. 9). In addition, renal renin release and renin status in essential hypertension appear to be impor-

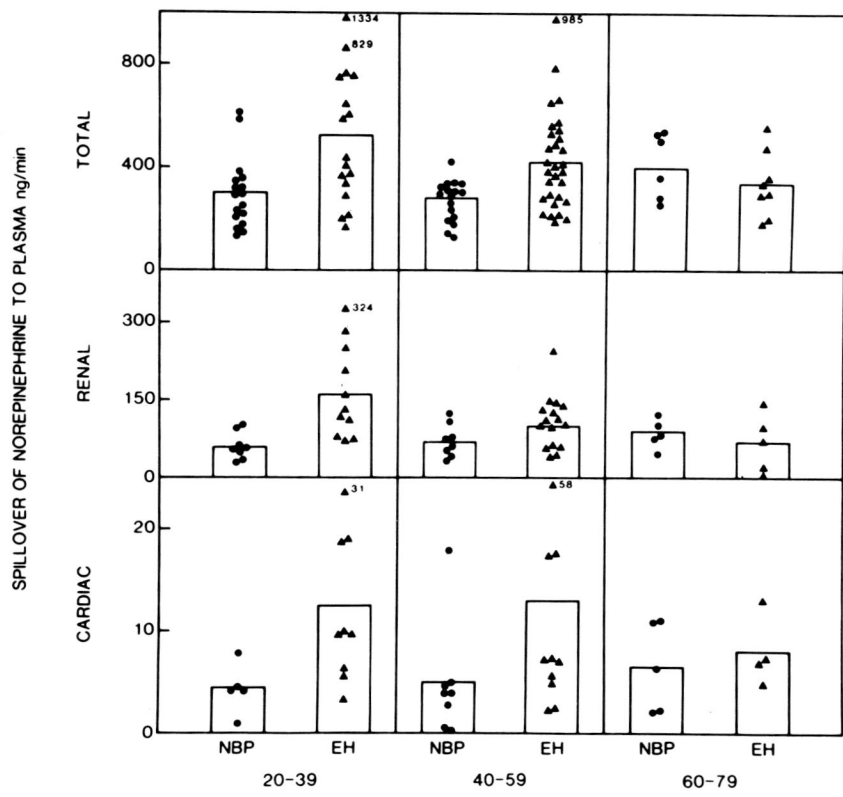

FIG. 9. Total, renal, and cardiac norepinephrine spillover to plasma in patients with essential hypertension (EH) and healthy subjects with normal arterial pressures (NBP), according to age. Increased norepinephrine overflow, for the body as a whole and from the heart and kidneys, was present particularly in younger patients. (From ref. 111, with permission.)

tantly determined by the activity of the renal sympathetic nerves in individual patients. Release of renin from the juxtaglomerular cells of the kidney is under neural control. In young patients with high renin essential hypertension the elevated rates of release of renin from the kidneys and the high plasma renin activity appear to be due to increased renal sympathetic nervous activity. In older patients renal renin release is typically normal or reduced, as are renal norepinephrine spillover values (111).

Sympathetic Nerve Firing and Heart Rate Spectral Analysis

When first measured in patients with essential hypertension, microneurographic recordings suggested that muscle sympathetic nerve firing was normal (14). More recent studies in borderline (108) and established (95) hypertension have provided strong evidence for the presence of increased muscle sympathetic nerve firing. The sympathetic outflow to skin is yet to be studied in human hypertension. With heart rate spectral analysis in essential hypertension, as in healthy subjects, high-frequency (approximately 0.3 Hz) and low-frequency (approximately 0.1 Hz) components of heart rate variability can be delineated. The high-frequency component is linked to respiration, associated in particular with vagal influences and abolished by atropinization. Low-frequency variability derives in part from the cardiac sympathetic nerves, and is reduced by β-adrenergic blockade (17,18). In untreated patients with essential hypertension the low-frequency element has been reported to be enhanced and the high-frequency component to be reduced or absent (17), consistent with the presence of cardiac sympathetic stimulation and parasympathetic withdrawal.

CNS Control of Sympathetic Outflow

The causes of the increased sympathetic nervous activity in essential hypertension remain largely conjectural. Behavioral and life-style factors have been thought possibly to be of importance (9,111). Recent results suggest that the increased sympathetic nerve firing rates present in a proportion of patients with essential hypertension, whatever the initiating mechanism, may possibly derive from increased norepinephrine release in subcortical brain areas. Reports of an elevated norepinephrine concentration in cerebrospinal fluid in essential hypertension (113) constituted the initial clinical observation pointing to possible abnormalities of central monoaminergic neuronal transmission.

Central nervous system noradrenergic mechanisms are of importance in the regulation of sympathetic nervous system responses, including those accompanying stress reactions. Forebrain noradrenergic cell groups are typically sympathoexcitatory and pressor, while the bulbar centers are depressor (80,114–117). The largest group of norepinephrine-containing neurons, estimated to account for not less than 50 percent of the norepinephrine in the brain, is the locus coeruleus and its projections (118). Electrophysiological and anatomical studies carried out in animals provide evidence of connections linking the locus coeruleus, the pressor hypothalamic nuclei, and the amygdala with the sympathetic preganglionic neurons in the thoracolumbar cord, either directly, or more commonly via neuronal groups of the rostral ventrolateral medulla (114–117).

Given the importance of central noradrenergic neurotransmission in influencing sympathetic nervous outflow from the brain, norepinephrine spillover from the brain has been measured in essential hypertension patients, with sampling from high in the internal jugular vein, analogous to the measurement of norepinephrine spillover from peripheral organs. Norepinephrine is released into the cerebrovascular circulation in both hypertensive patients and healthy subjects, apparently from brain neurons rather than cerebrovascular sympathetic nerves (28,119), and despite any obstacle to passage provided by the brain-blood barrier (Fig. 10). Norepinephrine spillover from the brain on average is higher than in healthy subjects, as is the overflow into the internal jugular veins of the lipophilic metabolite DHPG. Cerebral venous scans indicate that the increased overflow of norepinephrine and DHPG is from subcortical brain regions only (119). In patients with an increased spillover of norepinephrine and DHPG from the brain, peripheral sympathetic activity is increased (119). These results suggest that activation of CNS noradrenergic neuronal cell groups, presumably in the forebrain, may mediate the increased sympathetic outflow from the brain in essential hypertension.

Neuronal Reuptake of Norepinephrine

While it is clear that sympathetic nerve firing rates are elevated in a proportion of patients with essential hypertension, studies with radiolabeled norepinephrine indicate that an additional amplification of the neural signal, by faulty neuronal reuptake of the transmitter, occurs in some patients (110,120,121). This has been described in hypertensive patients of all ages, and does not represent an exaggeration of the lesser grade of reduction of norepinephrine reuptake seen with normal aging in healthy people. The mechanism is unclear. While a genetic cause has been suspected, amelioration of the impaired transmitter reuptake has been described with dietary sodium restriction (120).

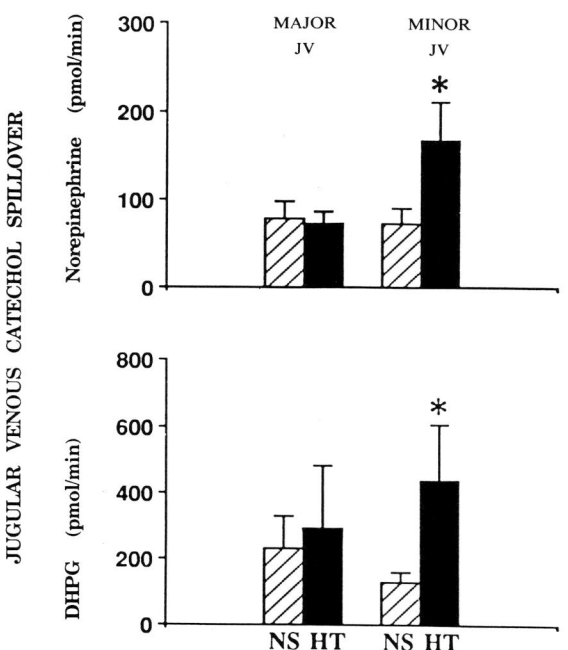

FIG. 10. Bar graph shows catechol spillovers into the cerebrovascular circulation in 18 healthy (NS) and 11 untreated hypertensive (HT) subjects. **Top panel:** Spillover values of noradrenaline obtained by sampling from the "major JV" and "minor JV." The major JV is identified by a cerebral venous sinus scan, and is the internal jugular vein, which receives the superior sagittal sinus and carries the bulk of cortical venous return. The minor JV is the jugular vein derived from the straight sinus, draining predominantly subcortical regions. **Bottom panel:** Spillover values of the lipophilic noradrenaline metabolite DHPG. *$p < .05$ significant difference in noradrenaline and DHPG spillovers into the minor JV between normotensive and hypertensive subjects. (From ref. 119, with permission.)

Release of Epinephrine from Sympathetic Nerves

One theory of the pathogenesis of essential hypertension envisages that stress-induced elevations in the plasma concentration of epinephrine may enlarge the pool of epinephrine present in sympathetic nerves, and, through release of this epinephrine as a cotransmitter, facilitate norepinephrine release and lead to cardiovascular stimulation and the development of arterial hypertension (72,73). The plasma concentration of epinephrine is, however, less commonly elevated in patients with essential hypertension than is the plasma concentration of the sympathetic neurotransmitter norepinephrine (6). Special significance is given within this conceptual framework of hypertension pathogenesis to minimally elevated plasma epinephrine values (72,73).

The first step taken in the testing of the epinephrine hypothesis of essential hypertension was to study the effects of infusion of epinephrine on the release of norepinephrine; typically the plasma concentration of nor-

epinephrine is elevated during an epinephrine infusion (122). However, this does not necessarily represent a presynaptic effect of neuronally released epinephrine on norepinephrine release. Sympathetic nerve firing increases during an epinephrine infusion, possibly due to its vasodilator actions (123). Perhaps more interesting are the sustained aftereffects of epinephrine on norepinephrine release and sympathetic nervous cardiovascular responses. Prolonged increases in heart rate and reflexly induced vasoconstrictor responses have been noted after infusions of epinephrine (124). But again, at this time increased sympathetic nerve firing also occurs, perhaps attributable to an accompanying, long-lasting reduction in central venous pressure (123).

To detect outward flux of epinephrine to plasma, indicative of regional release, in the face of the net extraction of plasma epinephrine that occurs across all organs except the adrenal medulla, radiotracer methodology is needed. The principle applied is that the outward flux of epinephrine can be measured from the reduction in the ratio of plasma radiolabeled to unlabeled epinephrine concentration (the isotope dilution) occurring in the passage of blood through an organ (32). It is now clear that under certain conditions epinephrine can be released by human sympathetic nerves. It has been possible to demonstrate release of epinephrine from the heart in healthy young men, but only with the extreme level of stimulation of the cardiac sympathetic nerves that accompanies aerobic exercise (32), or after loading of the sympathetic nerves by intravenous infusion of epinephrine (125). No release is evident from the resting heart, or during the lesser degrees of activation of the cardiac sympathetic outflow that accompanies isometric exercise and mental challenge. The source of the epinephrine released from the heart is most likely circulating epinephrine secreted by the adrenal medulla and extracted from plasma by the cardiac sympathetic nerves. Findings with the neuronal noradrenaline uptake blocker desipramine demonstrate that the human heart extracts adrenaline from plasma principally by the process of neuronal uptake (69). A report that cardiac tissue contains enzymes capable of synthesizing adrenaline, however, does indicate that some cardiac adrenaline may possibly be synthesized locally (126).

In brief, it is now clear that under certain circumstances epinephrine is released from human sympathetic nerves, and that circulating hormone extracted from plasma is the source of at least some of this neuronally released epinephrine. Preliminary results suggest that the rate of release of epinephrine from sympathetic nerves may, in fact, be normal in patients with essential hypertension (125). The causal chain linking a stress-related elevation of plasma epinephrine concentration to a neurogenic pathogenesis of essential hypertension still remains largely untested, and certainly unproven.

Consequences of Sympathetic Activation: Effects Additional to Hypertension Pathogenesis?

It is possible that the clinical relevance of sympathetic nervous activation in essential hypertension goes beyond the pathogenesis of the hypertension, and extends to hyperlipemia and atherosclerosis development, cardiovascular hypertrophy, ventricular arrhythmias, and to insulin resistance and hyperinsulinemia.

Nonobese patients with essential hypertension characteristically have *insulin resistance and mildly elevated serum insulin values* (127). Whether the peripheral insulin resistance is a cause or a consequence of the hypertension is debated. A viewpoint gaining favor is that the hyperinsulinemia of essential hypertension is a secondary phenomenon, resulting from the underlying hemodynamic abnormalities present. Glucose utilization by skeletal muscle under the influence of insulin, which is the process largely determining measured insulin resistance, is dictated by muscle blood flow (128). Reduced skeletal muscle blood flow in hypertension, resulting either from neural vasoconstriction or from vascular rarefaction, may possibly be the primary cause of the insulin resistance and attendant hyperinsulinemia.

The failure of antihypertensive therapy to reduce the incidence of coronary artery disease in patients with essential hypertension, despite blood pressure reduction, has suggested that *hyperlipidemia* and *atherosclerosis development* might, perhaps, share a common pathogenic mechanism with hypertension. This could possibly be overactivity of the sympathetic nervous system, since in nonhuman primate models of stress-induced atherosclerosis, for example, activation of the sympathetic nervous system has been demonstrated to be a major atherogenic mechanism (129). Sympathetic nervous activation and plasma catecholamine excess have complex effects on blood lipids. A range of possibly atherogenic lipid changes has been demonstrated (130–132). Clearance of chylomicrons in the periphery and of chylomicron remnants by the liver is slowed, leading to prolongation of the postabsorptive phase of chylomicronemia. This change has been attributed to adrenergic vasoconstriction reducing regional blood flows and consequently

chylomicron clearance. Lipolysis in adipose tissue is activated from stimulation of hormone-sensitive lipase. The released free fatty acids serve as a substrate for hepatic lipogenesis. Catecholamine-induced hypercholesterolemia reflects, in part, enhanced cholesterol biosynthesis (130–132).

While *cardiac and arteriolar smooth muscle hypertrophy* in essential hypertension represent in part a reaction to increased work load, the sympathetic nervous system has additional cardiovascular growth-promoting effects. Growth of cardiac myocytes in cell culture is stimulated by catecholamines (133). Given this background, it is perhaps surprising that left ventricular mass and cardiac sympathetic activity appear to be unrelated in hypertensive patients (134). Patients with essential hypertension are prone to *cardiac arrhythmias and sudden death*. The importance of neural mechanisms in a variety of experimental models of arrhythmia development is well established, with stimulation of the cardiac sympathetic outflow predisposing to ventricular tachycardia and ventricular fibrillation (135). Increased cardiac sympathetic nerve firing has also been demonstrated to commonly underlie clinical ventricular arrhythmias (136). The contribution of increased cardiac sympathetic activity to arrhythmogenesis in hypertensive patients, relative to other relevant factors such as underlying coronary atherosclerosis, and left ventricular hypertrophy, which promotes reentrant arrhythmias, is unclear at present.

Effects of Treatment on Sympathetic Function and Plasma Catecholamines

Changes commonly occur in sympathetic nervous system function with drug treatment of hypertension, representing the therapeutic sympathoinhibitory action of the drug, or homeostatic adaptations that oppose the mechanisms of action of the drug, undermining its efficacy as an antihypertensive (Table 4). An example of the former is the reduction in sympathetic nerve firing with clonidine, while the selective activation of the renal sympathetic outflow with diuretics is an example of the latter (Table 4). Elevation of the plasma concentration and urinary excretion of norepinephrine in hypertensive pa-

TABLE 4. *Effects of treatment of hypertension on sympathetic nervous system function and norepinephrine release*

Drug treatment	
Diuretics	Selective activation of renal sympathetic outflow
Hydralazine, minoxidil, nitroprusside, vasodilator calcium antagonists	Reflex sympathetic stimulation
Clonidine, methyl dopa, ganglion blockers	Reduced sympathetic nerve firing
β-Adrenergic blockers	Reduced norepinephrine plasma clearance
ACE inhibitors	Minimal effects
Nonpharmacological treatment	
Reduced dietary energy intake	Sympathetic nervous system inhibition
Low-salt diet	Selective activation of renal sympathetic outflow
Exercise training	Selective renal sympathetic nervous inhibition

From ref. 137, with permission.

tients by drug therapy can cause diagnostic confusion, suggesting a possible diagnosis of pheochromocytoma. Nonpharmacological antihypertensive measures in some instances also modify sympathetic nervous function. Exercise training selectively inhibits renal sympathetic nerve firing (138), while a low-salt diet selectively activates the renal sympathetic outflow (55), much as diuretics do (51) (Table 4).

The Renal Production of Dopamine

The topic of catecholamines and hypertension has a broader context than matters such as epinephrine secretion, neurotransmitter release, and the quantification of sympathetic nervous system function in hypertension, which have been considered so far. This is exemplified by the role of renal tubular dopamine mechanisms in regulating body sodium balance, and the possible disturbance of this process in patients with essential hypertension (139). Dopamine is relatively abundant in the kidney, with existing renal dopamine/norepinephrine tissue concentration ratios exceeding 1:10 (140). While it has been wondered whether this renal dopamine represents dopamine existing as a biosynthetic precursor of norepinephrine in sympathetic nerves, or whether a subset of renal dopaminergic fibers might exist (141), a substantial fraction of the dopamine found in the kidney is extraneuronal, formed in the proximal renal tubules by decarboxylation of DOPA extracted from plasma (36,142).

It seems probable that renal tubular dopamine is involved in the regulation of urinary sodium excretion, representing a natriuretic mechanism (36,142). The possibility that dopamine is causally involved in the pathogenesis of essential hypertension derives from this natriuretic action and evidence that in some patients with essential hypertension renal dopamine production is diminished (139). Reduced urinary dopamine excretion, and dopamine/DOPA urinary excretion ratios have been reported in hypertensive patients on a high-salt diet, and in subjects with normal blood pressure who are genetically predisposed to essential hypertension. There appears to be deficient renal uptake and decarboxylation of DOPA in at least a subset of essential hypertensives, especially those showing undue sensitivity to the pressor effects of dietary sodium (143–145). The evidence is very suggestive, but as yet there is no proof that this is a causal mechanism of their hypertension.

SUMMARY: THE SYNDROME OF NEUROGENIC ESSENTIAL HYPERTENSION

From an extensive series of clinical studies, assessing overlapping aspects of autonomic nervous system and cardiovascular physiology, a picture has emerged of neurogenic initiation of the blood pressure elevation in a substantial proportion of patients with essential hypertension. The patients are young (usually under 40 years) men and women with borderline or mild established hypertension. Typical features of the syndrome are the sympathetic nervous activation, manifest as an increase in muscle sympathetic nerve firing and high rates of spillover of the sympathetic neurotransmitter norepinephrine from the kidneys and heart, coupled with the peripheral expressions of this sympathoexcitation evident in a high plasma renin activity (due to an elevated rate of renal renin release), a high heart rate and in some cases an elevated cardiac output, an accentuated hemodynamic response to pharmacological adrenergic blockade, and heart rate spectral analysis findings suggestive of cardiac sympathetic activation and vagal withdrawal.

The underlying cause remains unclear, although stress and behavioral factors, especially the suppression of hostility, have been suspected. Recent research, based on transmitter washout into the cerebrovascular circulation, suggests that increased release of forebrain norepinephrine, perhaps an expression of behavioral factors, may possibly be the CNS mechanism underlying the sympathetic nervous activation.

It will be important to test for genetic determinants of these observed alterations in sympathetic function in human hypertension. Additional important priorities will be to ascertain what adverse effects additional to the blood pressure elevation, such as myocardial hypertrophy, hyperlipidemia, and atherosclerosis, might derive directly from the sympathetic nervous activation, and to establish whether progression occurs from mild hypertension with neurogenic features in the young, to more severe established hypertension, with apparently normal neural activity, in later years.

REFERENCES

1. Bernard C. *Compte Rendu Soc Biol (Paris)* 1851;3:163–183.
2. Elliot TR. *J Physiol (Lond)* 1905;32:401–467.
3. von Euler US. *Acta Physiol Scand* 1946;12:73–97.
4. von Euler US, Hellner S, Purkhold A. *Scand J Clin Lab Invest* 1954;6:54–59.
5. Engelman K, Portnoy B, Lovenberg W. *Am J Med Sci* 1968;255:259–268.
6. Goldstein DS. *Hypertension* 1983;5:86–99.
7. Esler M, Jennings G, Lambert G, Meredith I, Horne M, Eisenhofer G. *Physiol Rev* 1990;70:963–985.
8. Esler M, Jennings G, Korner P, et al. *Hypertension* 1988;11:3–20.
9. Folkow B. *Physiol Rev* 1982;62:347–504.
10. Janig W, McLachlan EM. *J Auton Nerv Syst* 1992;41:3–14.
11. Esler M, Jennings G, Lambert G. In: Sandler M, Dahlstrom A, Belmaker RH, eds. *Progress in catecholamine research. Part C: Clinical aspects: Proceedings Of The Sixth International Catecholamine Symposium.* Jerusalem, New York: Liss, 1988;95–100.
12. Geisbock F. Cited in Julius S, Esler M, eds. *The nervous system in arterial hypertension.* Springfield, IL: Charles C Thomas, 1976;xii.
13. Hagbarth K-E, Vallbo AB. *Acta Physiol Scand* 1968;74:96–108.
14. Wallin BG, Delius W, Hagbarth K-E. *Circ Res* 1973;33:9–21.
15. Esler M, Jackman G, Bobik A, et al. *Life Sci* 1979;25:1461–1470.

16. Esler M, Jennings G, Korner P, Blombery P, Sacharias N, Leonard P. *Am J Physiol* 1984;247:E21–E28.
17. Guzzetti S, Piccaluga E, Casati R, et al. *J Hypertens* 1988;6:711–717.
18. Axelrod S, Gordon D, Madwed JB, Snidman NC, Shannon DC, Cohen RJ. *Am J Physiol* 1985;249:H867–H875.
19. Doyle AE, Smirk FH. *Circulation* 1955;12:543–552.
20. Julius S, Pascual A, London R. *Circulation* 1971;44:413–418.
21. Hokfelt T, Fuxe K, Goldstein M, Johansson O. *Brain Res* 1974;66:235–251.
22. Cryer PE. *N Engl J Med* 1980;303:436–444.
23. Bloom FE, Hoffer BJ. In: Usdin E, Snyder SL, eds. *Frontiers in catecholamine research.* New York: Pergamon, 1973;637–642.
24. Pierpont GL, De Master EG, Reynolds S, Pederson J, Cohn JN. *J Lab Clin Med* 1985;106:205–210.
25. Carlsson A, Fuxe K, Hamberger B, Lindqvist M. *Acta Physiol Scand* 1966;67:481–497.
26. Kopin IJ. *Pharmacol Rev* 1985;37:333–364.
27. Planz G, Planz R. *Experientia Basel* 1979;35:207–208.
28. Ferrier C, Esler M, Eisenhofer G, et al. *Hypertension* 1992;19:62–69.
29. Eisenhofer G, Smolich JL, Esler MD. *Am J Physiol* 1992;262:L360–L365.
30. Sha S, Tse TF, Clutter WE, Cryer PE. *Am J Physiol* 1984;247:E380–E384.
31. Peronnet F, Nadeau R, Boudreau G, et al. *Am J Physiol* 1988;254:R659–R662.
32. Esler M, Eisenhofer G, Chin J, et al. *Clin Autonom Res* 1991;1:103–108.
33. Eisenhofer G, Smolich JJ, Esler MD. *Naunyn Schmiedebergs Arch Pharmacol* 1992;345:160–171.
34. Elayan HH, Kennedy BP, Ziegler MG. *Cardiovasc Res* 1990;24:53–56.
35. Kennedy B, Elayan H, Ziegler MG. *Am J Physiol* 1990;258:L227–L231.
36. Lee MR. *Clin Sci* 1982;62:439–448.
37. Peart WS. *J Physiol (Lond)* 1949;108:491–501.
38. Blombery PA, Heinzow BGJ. *Circ Res* 1983;53:688–694.
39. Bradley T, Hjemdahl P. *Acta Physiol Scand* 1984;122:369–379.
40. Noshiro T, Saigusa T, Way D, Dorward PK, McGrath BP. *Am J Physiol* 1991;261:F44–F50.
41. Hoeldtke RD, Cilmi KM, Reichard GA Jr, et al. *J Lab Clin Med* 1983;101:772–782.
42. Esler M, Wallin BG, Dorward P, et al. *Am J Physiol* 1991;260:R817–R823.
43. Goldstein DS, Eisenhofer G, Sax FL, Keiser HR, Jopin IJ. *Psychosom Med* 1987;49:591–605.
44. Christensen NJ, Hilsted J, Hegedus L, Madsbad S. *Am J Physiol* 1984;247:E29–E34.
45. Veith RC, Best JD, Halter JB. *J Clin Endocrinol Metab* 1984;59:151–155.
46. McCance AJ, Forfar JC. *Circulation* 1989;80:1642–1651.
47. Eisenhofer G, Esler MD, Meredith IT, Ferrier C, Lambert G, Jennings G. *Clin Sci* 1991;80:257–263.
48. Best JD, Halter JB. *J Clin Endocrinol Metab* 1982;55:263–268.
49. McCance AJ, Forfar JC. *Br Heart J* 1989;61:238–247.
50. Hasking GJ, Esler MD, Jennings GL, Dewar E, Lambert G. *Circulation* 1988;78:516–521.
51. Esler M, Willett I, Leonard P, et al. *J Auton Nerv Syst* 1984;11:125–144.
52. Hasking G, Esler M, Jennings G, Burton D, Johns J, Korner P. *Circulation* 1986;73:615–621.
53. Davis D, Sinoway LI, Robinson J, et al. *Circ Res* 1986;61(suppl 1):I-87–I-90.
54. Tidgren B, Hjemdahl P, Theodorsson E, Nussberger J. *Am J Physiol* 1990;259:F573–F579.
55. Friberg P, Meredith I, Jennings G, Lambert G, Fazio V, Esler M. *Hypertension* 1990;16:121–130.
56. Goldstein DS, Brush JE, Eisenhofer G, Stull R, Esler M. *Circulation* 1988;78:41–48.
57. Esler M, Jennings G, Lambert G. *Psychoneuroendocrinology* 1989;14:477–481.
58. Meredith IT, Friberg P, Jennings GL, et al. *Hypertension* 1991;18:575–582.
59. Hertting G, Axelrod J, Whitby LG. *J Pharmacol Exp Ther* 1962;134:146–153.
60. Eisenhofer G, Goldstein DS, Ropchak TG, Nguyen HQ, Keiser HR, Kopin IJ. *J Auton Nerv Syst* 1988;24:1–14.
61. Eisenhofer G, Smolich J, Esler MD. *Circulation* 1991;84:1354–1363.
62. Chang PG, Krogt JA, van Brummelen P. *Hypertension* 1987;9:647–653.
63. Kahan T, Hjemdahl P, Dahlof C. *Acta Physiol Scand* 1984;122:369–379.
64. Meredith IT, Esler MD, Cox HS, Lambert GW, Jennings GL, Eisenhofer G. *Clin Autonom Res* 1991;1:187–194.
65. Kaye D, Esler M, Kingwell B, Jennings G, McPherson G, Esmore D. *Circulation* 1993;88:1110–1118.
66. Kahan T, Taddei S, Pedrinelli R, Hjemdahl P, Salvetti A. *J Cardiovasc Pharmacol* 1992;19:587–592.
67. Kaye D, Lambert GW, Lefkowits J, Morris M, Jennings G, Esler M. *J Am Coll Cardiol* 1994;in press.
68. Majewski H, Hedler L, Starke K. *Naunyn-Schmiedebergs Arch Pharmacol* 1982;321:20–27.
69. Eisenhofer G, Esler M, Cox H, et al. *J Clin Endocrinol Metab* 1990;70:1710–1720.
70. Adler-Graschinsky E, Langer SZ. *Br J Pharmacol* 1975;53:43–50.
71. Esler M, Thompson J, Jennings G, et al. *Proceedings of the 7th International Catecholamine Symposium.* Amsterdam: Roepers, 1992;87.
72. Majewski H, Tung LH, Rand MJ. *J Cardiovasc Pharmacol* 1981;3:179–185.
73. Brown MJ, Macquin N. *Lancet* 1981;2:1079–1082.
74. Chang PC, Kriek E, van der Krogt JA, Blauw G-J, van Brummelen P. *Clin Sci* 1987;75:469–475.
75. Izzo J. *Hypertension* 1983;5:787–789.
76. Padbury JF, Agata Y, Baylen BG, et al. *J Pediatr* 1987;110:293–298.
77. DiBona G. *Am J Physiol* 1977;233:F73–F81.
78. Korner PI. *Physiol Rev* 1971;51:312–367.
79. Rowell LB. *Human circulation regulation during physical stress.* New York: Oxford University Press, 1986.
80. Chalmers J, Pilowsky P. *J Hypertens* 1991;9:675–694.
81. Svensson TH, Thoren P. *Brain Res* 1979;172:174–178.
82. Rea RF, Eckberg DL. *Am J Physiol* 1987;253:R929–R934.
83. Eckberg DL, Harkins SW, Fritsch JM, Musgrave GE, Gardner DF. *J Clin Invest* 1986;78:366–374.
84. Linares OA, Jacquez JA, Zech LA, et al. *J Clin Invest* 1987;80:1332–1341.
85. Meredith IT, Eisenhofer G, Lambert GW, Jennings GL, Esler MD. *Hypertension* 1992;19:628–633.
86. Ziegler MG, Lake CR, Kopin IJ. *N Engl J Med* 197;296:293–297.
87. Wallin BG, Sundlof G. *J Autonom Nerv Syst* 1982;6:287–291.
88. Scherrer R, Vissing S, Morgan BJ, Hanson P, Victor RG. *N Engl J Med* 1990;322:602–604.
89. Fitzpatrick AP, Theodorakis G, Vardos P, Sutton R. *J Am Coll Cardiol* 1991;17:125–130.
90. Kapoor WN, Brant N. *Ann Intern Med* 1992;116:358–363.
91. Randall O, Esler M, Culp B, Julius S, Zweifler A. *J Lab Clin Med* 1978;91:514–519.
92. Hollenberg NK, Adams DF, Solomon HS, Rashid A, Abrams HL, Merrill JP. *Circ Res* 1974;34:309–316.
93. Ziegler MG, Lake CR, Kopin IJ. *Nature* 1976;261:333–335.
94. Sundlof G, Wallin BG. *J Physiol (Lond)* 1978;274:621–637.
95. Yamada Y, Miyajima E, Tochikubo O, Matsukawa AT, Ishii M. *Hypertension* 1989;13:870–877.
96. Ng AV, Callister R, Johnson DG, Seals DR. *Hypertension* 1993;21:498–503.
97. Wallin BG, Esler M, Dorward P, et al. *J Physiol (Lond)* 1992;453:45–56.
98. Esler M, Skews H, Leonard P, Jackman G, Bobik A, Korner P. *Clin Sci* 1981;60:217–219.

99. Veith RC, Featherstone JA, Linares OA, Halter JB. *J Gerontol* 1986;41:319–324.
100. Rubin PC, Scott PJW, McLean K, Reid JL. *Eur J Clin Invest* 1982;12:121–125.
101. Esler M, Lambert G, Jennings G. In: Amery A, Staessen J, eds. *Handbook of hypertension, vol II. Hypertension in the elderly.* Amsterdam: Elsevier, 1989;85–98.
102. Hoeldtke RD, Cilmi KM. *J Clin Endocrinol Metab* 1985;60:479–484.
103. Weidman P, Beretta-Piccoli C, Ziegler WJ, Keusch G, Gluck Z, Reubi FC. *Kidney Int* 1978;14:619–628.
104. Franco-Morselli R, Elghozi LJ, Joly E, Di Giuilio S, Meyer P. *Br Med J* 1977;2:1251–1254.
105. Young JB, Rowe JW, Pallotta JA, Sparrow D, Landsberg L. *Metabolism* 1980;29:532–539.
106. Ng AV, Callister R, Johnson DG, Seals DR. *Am J Physiol* 1994;in press.
107. Kusiak JW, Pitha J. *Life Sci* 1983;33:1679–1686.
108. Anderson EA, Sinkey CA, Lawton WJ, Mark AL. *Hypertension* 1989;14:177–183.
109. Esler M, Jennings G, Biviano B, Lambert G, Hasking G. *J Cardiovasc Pharmacol* 1986;8(suppl 5):539–544.
110. Esler M, Jackman G, Bobik A, et al. *Hypertension* 1981;3:149–156.
111. Esler M, Lambert G, Jennings G. *Clin Exp Hypertens* 1989;11(suppl 1):75–89.
112. Lund-Johansen P. *J Hypertens* 1989;7(suppl 6):S52–S55.
113. Eide I, Kolloch R, De Quattro V, Miano L, Dugger R, Van der Meulen J. *Hypertension* 1979;1:255–260.
114. Fleetwood-Walker SM, Coote JH. *Brain Res* 1981;205:141–155.
115. van Huysse JW, Bealer SL. *Am J Physiol* 1991;260:R1071–R1076.
116. Huangfu D, Koshiya N, Guyenet P. *Am J Physiol* 1991;261:R393–R402.
117. Koepke JP, Jones S, DiBona GF. *Brain Res* 1987;404:80–88.
118. Foote SL, Bloom FE, Aston-Jones G. *Physiol Rev* 1983;63:844–914.
119. Ferrier C, Jennings GL, Eisenhofer G, et al. *J Hypertens* 1993;11:1217–1227.
120. Kimura S, Miura Y, Adachi M, et al. *Jpn Circ J* 1983;47:1237–1242.
121. Goldstein DS, Horwitz D, Keiser HR, Polinsky RJ, Kopin IJ. *J Clin Invest* 1983;72:1748–1758.
122. Musgrave IF, Bachmann AW, Gordon RD. *J Hypertens* 1984;2(suppl 3):135–137.
123. Persson B, Andersson OK, Hjemdahl P, Wysocki M, Agerwall S, Wallin BG. *J Hypertens* 1989;7:747–756.
124. Floras JS. *Hypertension* 1992;19:1–18.
125. Esler M. *Proceedings of the 7th International Catecholamine Symposium.* Amsterdam: Roepers, 1992;88.
126. Kennedy B, Ziegler MG. *Circulation* 1991;84:891–895.
127. Modan M, Halkin H, Almog S, et al. *J Clin Invest* 1985;75:809–817.
128. Baron AD, Laakso M, Brechtel G, Hoit B, Watt C, Edelman SV. *J Clin Endocrinol Metab* 1990;70:1525–1533.
129. Clarkson TB, Kaplan JR, Adams MR. *Circulation* 1987;76:I-29–I-40.
130. Landsberg L, Young JB. Catecholamines and the adrenal medulla. In: Wilson JD, Foster DW, eds. *Williams textbook of endocrinology.* Philadelphia: WB Saunders, 1992;621–705.
131. Dimsdale JE, Herd JA, Hartley LH. *Psychosom Med* 1983;45:227–232.
132. O'Donnell L, Owens D, McGee C, et al. *Metabolism* 1988;37:910–915.
133. Simpson P, McGrath A. *J Clin Invest* 1983;72:732–738.
134. Esler M, Lambert G, Jennings G. *J Hypertens* 1990;8(suppl 7):S53–S57.
135. Verrier RL, Lown B. *Annu Rev Physiol* 1984;46:155–176.
136. Meredith IT, Broughton A, Jennings GL, Esler MD. *N Engl J Med* 1991;325:618–624.
137. Esler M. In: Bouloux P-M, ed. *Bailliere's clinical endocrinology and metabolism.* Philadelphia: WB Saunders, 1993;415–438.
138. Meredith IT, Friberg P, Jennings GL, et al. *Hypertension* 1991;18:575–582.
139. Kuchel O, Buu NT, Unger T, et al. *J Clin Endocrinol Metab* 1979;48:425–429.
140. Caramona MM, Soares-da-Silva P. *Br J Pharmacol* 1985;86:351–356.
141. Bell C. *Clin Exp Hypertens* 1987;9:955–975.
142. Williams M, Young JB, Rosa RM, et al. *J Clin Invest* 1986;78:1687–1693.
143. Saito I, Takeshita E, Saruta T, et al. *J Hypertens* 1984;2:61–64.
144. Weinberger MH, Luft FC, Henry DP. *Clin Exp Hypertens* 1982;4:719–735.
145. Shikamu R, Yoshimura M, Kabara S, et al. *Life Sci* 1986;38:915–921.

Hypertension: Pathophysiology, Diagnosis, and Management, Second Edition, edited by J.H. Laragh and B.M. Brenner, Raven Press, Ltd., New York © 1995.

CHAPTER 45

Brain Serotonin and Hypertension

Paul M. Pilowsky, Jane B. Minson, Leonard F. Arnolda, and J. P. Chalmers

Serotonin (5-hydroxytryptamine; 5-HT) was first identified in the mammalian brain by Twarog and Page (1) in 1953. In 1956, evidence was provided that serotonin was distributed nonuniformly in the brain, suggesting that it was localized within neurons, and therefore might be a neurotransmitter. The anatomical finding that serotonin neurons and terminals were present in areas of the brain known to be important in the control of blood pressure prompted a number of physiological and pharmacological studies. Among the first, were those by Ito and Schanberg (2) in 1972, who administered parachlorophenylalanine intracerebroventricularly to rats and reported a brief elevation in blood pressure, and studies by Wing and Chalmers (3), who observed reductions in blood pressure in animals with neurogenic hypertension after parachlorophenylalanine administration. Following a prolonged debate as to whether or not central serotonergic neurons exerted a sympathoexcitatory or sym-

pathoinhibitory effect, the advent of more refined physiological and pharmacological techniques has helped to resolve elements of this conflict (4–24). In essence, it has become apparent that there are many distinct groups of serotonin-containing neurons, with different complements of colocalized transmitter chemicals, traversing different pathways in the brain and spinal cord, and having markedly different cardiovascular effects. The recent cloning of serotonin receptors, and their localization in the brainstem and spinal cord, clarifies the situation further, and paves the way for highly specific studies of the role of serotonergic pathways.

MORPHOLOGY OF SEROTONIN-CONTAINING NEURONS IN THE BRAIN

Location of Cell Bodies

In 1964, using a histofluorescence technique, Dahlström and Fuxe (25) were the first to report on the existence and anatomical localization of serotonin-containing neurons in the medulla and spinal cord.

P. M. Pilowsky, J. B. Minson, L. F. Arnolda, J. P. Chalmers: Department of Medicine and Centre for Neuroscience, Flinders University, Adelaide, South Australia 5042.

Serotonin-containing neurons were found in the raphe nuclei, extending rostrally from the medulla oblongata (Figs. 1 and 2). Nine distinct collections of serotonin-containing neurons were found, and are arbitrarily designated B1 to B9. This work has since been confirmed in studies using immunohistochemistry to detect serotonin (26). By the same nomenclature, noradrenaline-containing neuronal cell groups in the brain are designated A1 to A16, and adrenaline-containing groups C1 to C3.

In the brainstem, there are three groups of serotonin-containing neurons: B1, B2, and B3. These groups are located within the nucleus raphe pallidus (B1), the nucleus raphe obscurus (B2), and the nucleus raphe magnus (B3). Two subgroups of the B3 cell group are recognized: a medial group and a lateral group. The medial group is located in the midline of the medulla extending dorsally from the ventral surface. The lateral group is an extension of the medial group. It is found adjacent to the ventral surface of the medulla, immediately lateral to the olivary nuclei and pyramidal tracts. A smaller number of cells, lying on the dorsal surface of the olive, connects the medial and lateral components. Although the two groups appear to be part of the same population of cells, they are considered separately because physiological studies suggest differing functions for neurons at these two sites.

More rostrally are the B4 to B9 cell groups. The B4 cell group is located in the lateral part of the nucleus vestibu-laris lateralis, dorsal to the nucleus prepositus hypoglossi. The B5 cells are in the intermediate part of the nucleus raphe pontis. The B6 and B7 cells are found in the nucleus raphe dorsalis, with the B7 group being by far the larger. The B8 neurons are found in the nucleus centralis superior, and the B9 group is found in and around the medial lemniscus. Additional smaller groups of serotonin-containing neurons have been described in the area postrema and in the subcoeruleus area (26,27).

With the advent of sophisticated tract tracing and immunohistochemical techniques, there has been extensive mapping of serotonin pathways in the brain and spinal cord. Numerous studies have demonstrated the presence of other neurotransmitters within serotonin neurons, and some headway is now being made in monitoring the expression of different genes in serotonin neurons with molecular biological techniques (23,28,29).

Projections of Serotonin-Containing Neurons

The axonal projections of serotonin-containing neurons are extensive (Fig. 1). Axonal varicosities are found throughout the neuraxis, from the cortex to the spinal cord. Sites known to be important in cardiovascular regulation that receive a rich serotonergic input include the sympathetic preganglionic neurons in the spinal cord, the ventral medulla, the nucleus tractus solitarius, the dorsal motor nucleus of the vagus and nucleus am-

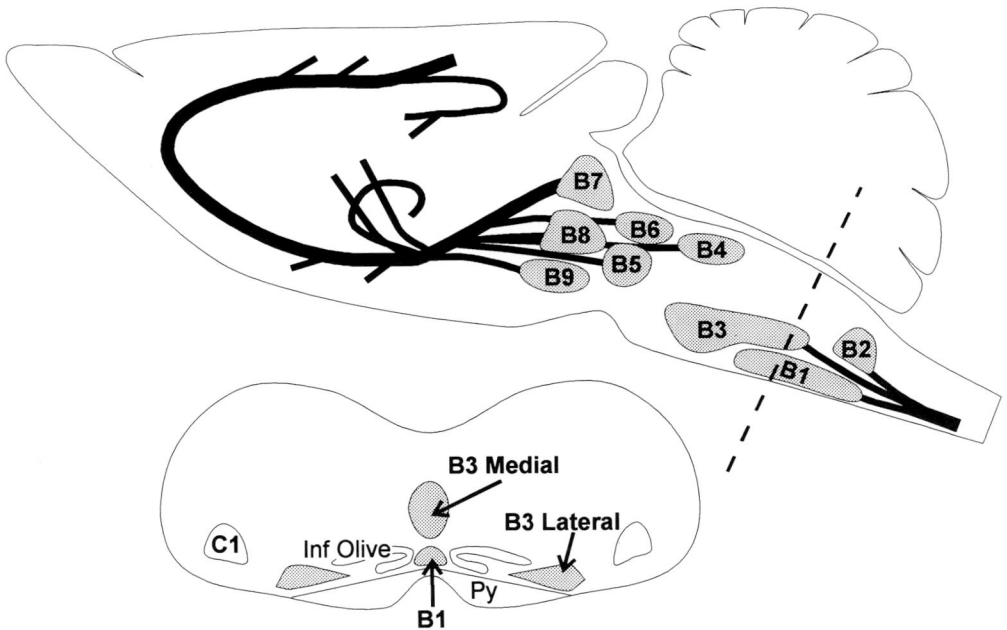

FIG. 1. Two major serotonin pathways are thought to act in the central regulation of blood pressure. From the B7 and B8 serotonin cell groups in the mesencephalon, serotonin projections ascend to the hypothalamus and forebrain. Serotonergic projections arising from the B1, B2, and B3 cell groups project to the spinal cord where they innervate several cell types including sympathetic preganglionic neurons. The B3 cell group has lateral and midline components. The C1 adrenaline cell group is distinct from, and lateral to, the B3 lateral cell group. Inf Olive, inferior olive; Pyr, pyramidal tracts.

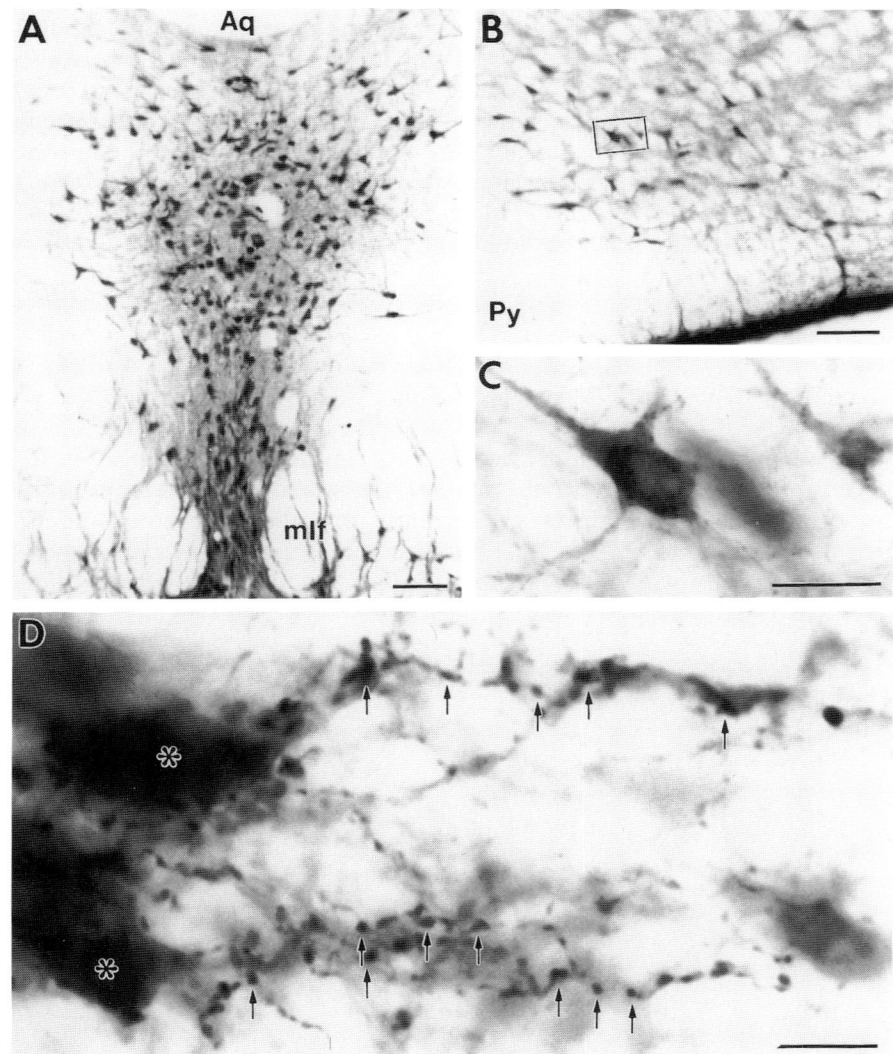

FIG. 2. Light microscopy showing examples of serotonin-immunoreactivity in rat brain and spinal cord. **A:** Serotonin cells in the dorsal raphe (B7) nucleus (see Fig. 1). Most of the cells of this nucleus are located in the midbrain, dorsal to the medial longitudinal fasciculus (mlf). The serotonergic cell population in this nucleus contains about half of all of the serotonin nerve cells in the brain (112). Aq, aqueduct. Bar = 100 μm. **B:** Serotonin cells in the lateral parts of the raphe magnus (B3) nucleus. The serotonin cells in this group lie above the lateral edges of the pyramidal tract (Py; Fig. 1). Many of these cells have spinally projecting axons. These B3 nerve cells are likely to act in the regulation of blood pressure. The effects of changing activity in the area of these nerves is shown in Figs. 3 and 4. Nerve cells in the boxed area are shown enlarged in C. Bar = 100 μm. **C:** Lateral B3 nerve cells enlarged from B. Two cells are in the plane of focus. Bar = 20 μm. **D:** In the T8 thoracic segment of spinal cord the cell bodies of two retrogradely labeled sympathoadrenal nerves in the intermediolateral cell column are marked with an asterisk. Serotonin-immunoreactive fibers with boutons entwine the processes of these sympathoadrenal neurons; many close appositions between the serotonin fibres and the sympathoadrenal nerves are seen (*arrows*). This serotonin input is likely to affect the activity of the sympathoadrenal neurons. Bar = 10 μm.

biguus, the parabrachial nucleus, the locus coeruleus, and many parts of the hypothalamus including the magnocellular, vasopressin-containing neurons of the supraoptic and paraventricular nuclei. Clearly, serotonin-containing neurons are well placed to have a profound influence on the cardiovascular system at numerous afferent, efferent, and integrative sites (4,26).

Ascending Serotonergic Pathways

Most of the ascending projections arise in the dorsal and median raphe nuclei and project to the cortex, hippocampus, amygdala and the hypothalamus, including the suprachiasmatic nucleus, and the supraoptic and paraventricular nuclei (26) (Fig. 1). The suprachiasmatic nucleus receives one of the densest serotonergic inputs in the brain, and neurons in this nucleus that contain vasoactive intestinal polypeptide are prime targets for serotonin inputs (30). Experimental interventions that

affect the activity of neurons in the dorsal and median raphe nuclei produce complex effects on blood pressure that are discussed below. Since these responses can be affected by lesions above *and* below the site of stimulation, it is clear that there must be a suprabulbar relay that in turn causes an alteration in sympathetic outflow.

Descending Serotonergic Pathways

Descending serotonergic projections arise from the midbrain and medullary serotonin cell groups. One prominent pathway arises in the midbrain and projects to the locus coeruleus. Other pathways from the midbrain project to the nucleus tractus solitarius and the medullary raphe nuclei. Bulbospinal serotonin pathways arise from the pontomedullary cell groups B1, B2, and B3 (Figs. 1 and 2). The axons of the bulbospinal serotonergic neurons from synaptic contacts throughout the spinal gray matter. Targets include the dorsal horn, the ventral horn—including phrenic motoneurons in the cervical spinal cord (13)—as well as the intermediolateral cell column in the thoracolumbar spinal cord (31–35). A physiological role for bulbospinal serotonin neurons in blood pressure control has been suggested by ourselves and others. Two components of the bulbospinal serotonin pathways that are likely to be critically important are the B3 lateral cell group, which appears to mediate pressor and sympathoexcitatory responses (15), and the B3 neurons in the midline, which may have a depressor and sympathoinhibitory function (9,20). In addition, there is some evidence that bulbospinal serotonin neurons may play a role in the hypotensive action of α-methyldopa (16,18,20,22,36). These issues are addressed in more detail below.

It is important to note that the B3 lateral cell group is anatomically separate from the C1 adrenaline cell group, which is located more laterally in the rostral ventrolateral medulla (Figs. 1 and 3). It has been suggested that the

lateral area, which incorporates the C1 neurons, should be referred to as the rostral ventrolateral medulla while the more medial aspect of the rostral ventrolateral medulla, which includes the B3 lateral neurons, is referred to as the rostral ventromedial medulla. Some confusion may arise from this terminology because the term *rostral ventromedial medulla* is also used by some authors, especially in the pain literature, to refer to midline neurons (37,38).

Colocalization of Other Neurotransmitters in Serotonergic Neurons

Immunocytochemistry has been used extensively to demonstrate that serotonin-containing neurons also contain a wide range of other neurotransmitters (32,33,39–41). Putative neurotransmitters and/or their synthesizing enzymes that have been localized within

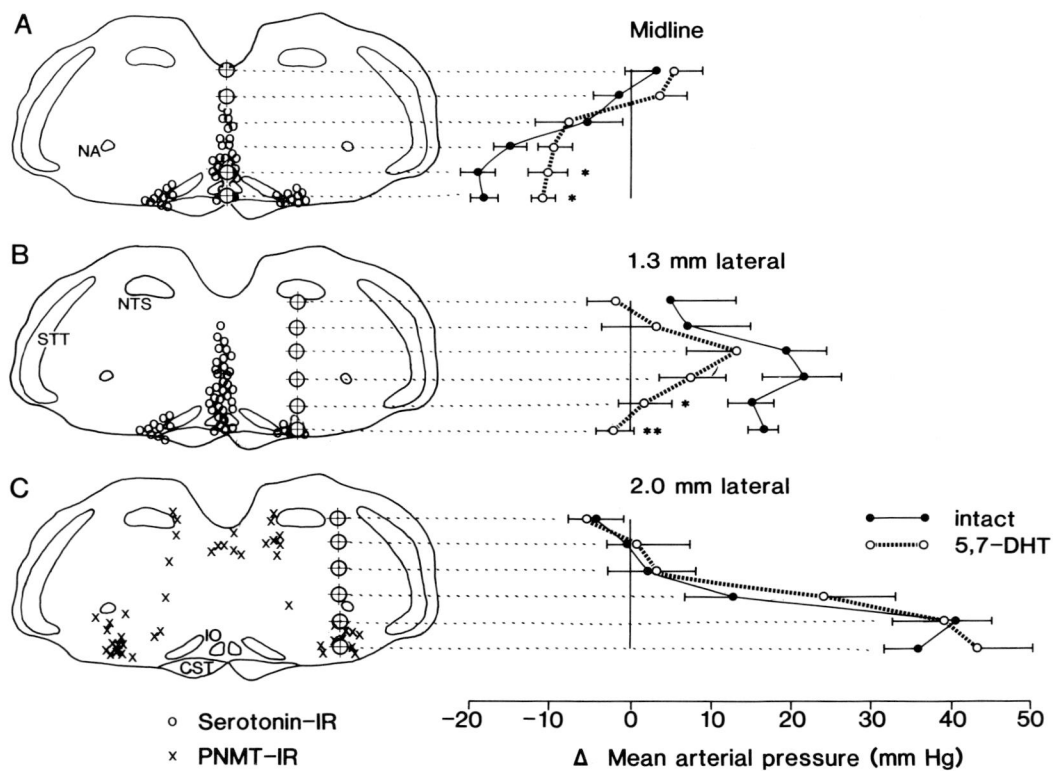

FIG. 3. A comparison of the effects of stimulating the rostral ventrolateral medulla (C1 area) and the rostral ventromedial medulla (B3 lateral area). **Left:** Distribution of serotonin-immunoreactive cell bodies (A,B) and PNMT-immunoreactive cell bodies (C, adrenaline synthesizing) in rat medulla oblongata at the level 1.5 to 2.0 mm rostral to obex. PNMT, phenylethanolamine-N-methyltransferase; CST, corticospinal tract; IO, inferior olive; NA, nucleus ambiguus; NTS, nucleus tractus solitarius; STT, spinal trigeminal tract. **Right:** Changes in mean arterial pressure after l-glu (10 nmol) microinjections in the medulla oblongata at the level 1.5 to 2.0 mm rostral to obex. Serial microinjections were made at 0.5-mm intervals in the midline (A), in a sagittal plane 1.3 mm lateral to the midline (B), and in a sagittal plane 2.0 mm lateral to the midline (C) in intact rats (A, $n = 15$; B, $n = 17$; C, $n = 16$) and in rats treated 14 days earlier with the serotonergic neurotoxin 5,7-DHT i.c.v. (A, $n = 9$; B, $n = 9$; C, $n = 8$). *$p < .05$; **$p < .01$ (ANOVA). (From ref. 15, with permission.)

serotonergic neurons include thyrotropin releasing hormone, substance P, met- and leu-enkephalin, phosphate-activated glutaminase (a glutamate synthesizing enzyme), glutamate, aspartate, and γ-aminobutyric acid (39,42). The recent finding from our laboratory that all serotonergic neurons synthesize glutamate is likely to be highly significant. Previous physiological studies have demonstrated that both transmitters are important in bulbospinal serotonin pathways (10,19,43). It may be that glutamate is the principal neurotransmitter of these neurons, mediating fast synaptic transmission, while serotonin and other co-stored transmitters play a more subtle role in affecting the general level of neuronal excitability (44–46). Physiological studies have demonstrated that these co-stored neurotransmitters subserve a variety of functions, and that they can have different time courses of action. Thus, at a given synapse target, one neurotransmitter may cause opening of an ion channel and generation of a fast postsynaptic potential, while another, co-released neurotransmitter may affect intracellular calcium stores and have a slow, longer-lasting effect on membrane potential (47).

Apart from the physiological role of co-released neurotransmitters, the different combinations of neurotransmitters found within serotonergic neurons may provide additional clues about their function. In the lumbar spinal cord of the rat, neurons that contain serotonin and thyrotropin-releasing hormone and substance P are found in the ventral horn, but not in the intermediolateral cell column. Serotonin-containing axons in the intermediolateral cell column contain thyrotropin-releasing hormone but not substance P, or may contain neither peptide (48). In contrast, in the thoracic spinal cord all combinations of neurotransmitters may be possible (31,33). It remains to be seen if this type of chemical coding reflects an underlying functional code such that, for example, serotonin neurons that contain substance P might be involved in vasoconstrictor pathways but not piloerector pathways.

CLASSIFICATION OF SEROTONIN RECEPTORS

Receptors are classified by their responses to specific agonists and antagonists under conditions of equilibrium in isolated tissue assays. Serotonin receptors are presently classified in three main groups with the recent possibility of a fourth group (49). At the time of writing, several groups, using molecular biological techniques, have reported the existence of at least 13 separate serotonin receptors belonging to seven main groups. The extent to which any of these additional serotonin receptors are expressed and their functional role in central cardiovascular control awaits further investigation.

5-HT1 Receptors

Four subtypes of 5-HT1 receptor have been identified: 5-HT1A, B, C, and D (49,50). All are potently and selectively stimulated by 5-carboxamidotryptamine (5CT). The 5-HT1A receptor can act through a K^+ channel, or by decreasing intracellular adenosine 3′,5′-cyclic monophosphate (cAMP) (49). It is likely to be important at a number of sites. Immunohistochemical studies have shown 5-HT1A receptors to be present as autoreceptors on serotonin neurons in the raphe nucleus (51), while autoradiographic studies have shown receptor binding in the nucleus tractus solitarius. Intracerebroventricular administration of 5-HT1A agonists causes hypertension, tachycardia, and sympathoexcitation (52). Application of drugs in specific brain areas reveals that 5-HT1A receptors are important in the regulation of cardiac parasympathetic preganglionic neurons in the medulla oblongata (53), in the ventrolateral medulla (54,55), in the spinal cord, and in the nucleus tractus solitarius.

The 5-HT1B receptor has recently been identified in humans and shown to be distinct from the 5-HT1D receptor, although their pharmacological properties are virtually indistinguishable. The finding that 5-HT1B and 1D are different receptors is likely to have clinical significance since these are the receptors where the antimigraine drug sumitriptan acts. Human and rodent 5-HT1B receptors display identical binding characteristics for serotonin, but not for a range of other pharmacological agents. This difference in binding characteristics has been shown to be due to a difference of a single amino acid between the two proteins (50).

The 5-HT1C receptor is similar to the 5-HT2 receptor in its pharmacological profile and in the intracellular mechanisms that are used.

5-HT2 Receptors

The 5-HT2 receptors were previously known as D (for dibenzyline) receptors (56). Autoradioradiographic studies have shown 5-HT2 receptors throughout the brain (57,58). α-Methyl-5-HT is an agonist at both 5-HT1C and 5-HT2 receptors. Selective antagonists include ketanserin, ritanserin, pizotifen, LY53857, and, more recently, RP62203. Ketanserin has some affinity for α_1-adrenoceptors and histamine H_1 receptors but only at concentrations 10- to 30-fold higher than those that antagonize 5-HT2 receptors. Intracerebroventricular injection of 5-HT1C/2 receptor agonists causes vasopressin release.

5-HT3 Receptors

The 5-HT3 receptors were previously known as M (for morphine) receptors (56). These receptors are activated by 2-methyl-5-HT and antagonized by cocaine. The 5-HT receptors are found on the carotid body where they mediate the 5-HT-induced increase in carotid sinus nerve discharge (59). The 5-HT3 receptors are also present on the terminals of vagal afferent neurons in the epicardium (60). Stimulation of these receptors mediates the sympathoinhibitory Bezold-Jarisch reflex.

5-HT4 Receptors

5-Methoxytryptamine and renzapride are selective agonists. Activation of 5-HT4 receptors increases intracellular cAMP. No role for 5-HT4 receptors in the central control of blood pressure has been established (49).

CENTRAL SEROTONIN NEURONS AND THE REGULATION OF BLOOD PRESSURE

Pressor and depressor effects on blood pressure have been described in studies investigating serotonin pathways in the brain, but such functional diversity comes as no surprise in the light of the large number of distinct groups of serotonin neurons localized in the brain and their diverse projection patterns (Fig. 1). Investigations relating the function of central serotonergic neurons to blood pressure regulation fall into two broad groups: first, studies where serotonin transmission is altered by manipulations that evoke widespread changes in central serotonin neuron activity, for example, the effects on blood pressure after the administration of serotonergic drugs intracerebroventricularly; and second, studies where a localized manipulation has been used, for example, the microinjection of drug into a discrete brain area, in order to correlate a change in the activity of a particular group of serotonin neurons with a particular cardiovascular event.

Generalized Changes in Central Serotonergic Transmission

Among the early studies of serotonin function in blood pressure regulation were those that sought to remove, either by ablation or depletion, all central serotonin neurons. In these studies, 5,6- and 5,7-dihydroxytryptamine (DHT), neurotoxic analogues of serotonin that cause the selective degeneration of serotonin nerve endings, were injected intracerebroventricularly, and the effects on blood pressure observed. In the rabbit these neurotoxins caused hypertension in the hours immediately after administration (5,61), but in the long-term resulted only in minor hypotension (3) or was without effect on blood pressure (61). These data suggest that the acute hypertensive responses reflect serotonin release from the terminals causing sympathoexcitation, while the long-term effects reflect the destruction of terminals and withdrawal of sympathoexcitation. Other depletion studies, using parachlorophenylalanine, are less clear. In the rat, depletion causes hypertension (2), but hypotension is elicited in the rabbit (62). Unfortunately, the different degrees of ablation or depletion that occur in different projections are hard to control so that the interpretation of these types of studies is difficult.

Serotonin or serotonin agonists have been administered to mimic the activation of groups of serotonin neurons. Generally, centrally administered serotonin acts to elevate blood pressure, but the site of action is difficult to determine. Serotonin administered into the third ventricle elicits larger pressor responses than those after serotonin injection into the lateral or fourth ventricles (63), suggesting an effect of serotonin on hypothalamic structures. Indeed, intracerebroventricularly (i.c.v.) administered serotonin effects can be blocked in part by vasopressin antagonists, so that some of the pressor effects might be due to a release of vasopressin (64). The pressor effects of i.c.v. serotonin are attenuated by cervical transection of the spinal cord, by adrenalectomy, and by adrenergic blocking drugs, so that descending pathways are involved in mediating the responses (65). Further evidence that serotonin facilitates central sympathetic nerve activity comes from studies in which agents that block the central excitatory effects of serotonin are observed to inhibit the sympathetic nerve discharge recorded from peripheral nerves and where these drug effects are abolished after serotonin depletion (66,67). It is likely that the sympathoexcitatory effects of serotonin are mediated through the 5-HT1A receptors described above (52), and selective 5-HT1A receptor agonists, including 8-hydroxy-2-(di-*n*-propylamino) tetralin (8-OH-DPAT), injected at low doses i.c.v. cause sympathoexcitation, tachycardia, and an increase in blood pressure (52,68). High doses i.c.v. and intravenous 8-OH-DPAT inhibit sympathetic activity and lower arterial blood pressure (69,70). Again these studies highlight the difficulties in the interpretation of data in this type of investigation. Do higher drug doses cause different effects through nonselective actions on other receptor types or do the drugs diffuse further in the brain and activate receptors that mediate different functions? Such questions are difficult to answer using these types of studies, and more powerful indications of serotonin function in blood pressure control come from investigations looking at the specific serotonin pathways.

Changes in Specific Serotonin Pathways

Ascending Serotonin Pathways

Serotonin injected directly into the hypothalamus increases blood pressure (71). These observations are consistent with midbrain serotonin neurons (dorsal and median raphe [Figs. 1 and 2]) projecting to the hypothalamus and subserving a pressor function. In support of this hypothesis are electrical stimulation studies, which report an elevation of blood pressure after midbrain raphe stimulation and an attenuation of these effects after the depletion of serotonin or after the direct intrahypothalamic injection of a serotonin antagonist (71–73). These pressor responses are abolished by the transection of the brain rostral to the midbrain, confirming an ascending projection pathway. Transection of the brain caudal to the midbrain also abolishes the responses, demonstrating that a relay descending pathway must be activated for sympathetic activity to be modified.

Descending Serotonin Pathways

More extensive studies of serotonin mechanisms in descending pathways have been undertaken. These stud-

ies have focused on the ventral medulla, which contains many neurons that have axons descending to the spinal cord (4). The B1, B2, and B3 groups of serotonin neurons are among these spinally projecting ventral medullary neurons (Fig. 1). These serotonin neurons innervate the sympathetic preganglionic neurons of the thoracic spinal cord (74,75), so that stimulation of these serotonin neurons directly modifies sympathetic outflow and blood pressure. Stimulation in the area of the lateral B3 serotonin neurons, lying adjacent to the lateral borders of the pyramidal tracts, elicits increases in blood pressure that are largely abolished by pretreatment with 5,7-dihydroxytryptamine to deplete spinal serotonin content (17,76) (Figs. 3 and 4). In contrast to the lateral pressor serotonin neurons, stimulation of the midline raphe cell groups in the medulla causes blood pressure to fall (76,77) (Fig. 3). This heterogeneity in response to stimulation in these two distinct groups of serotonin neurons highlights the problems described above, that is, that different populations of serotonin neurons are likely to

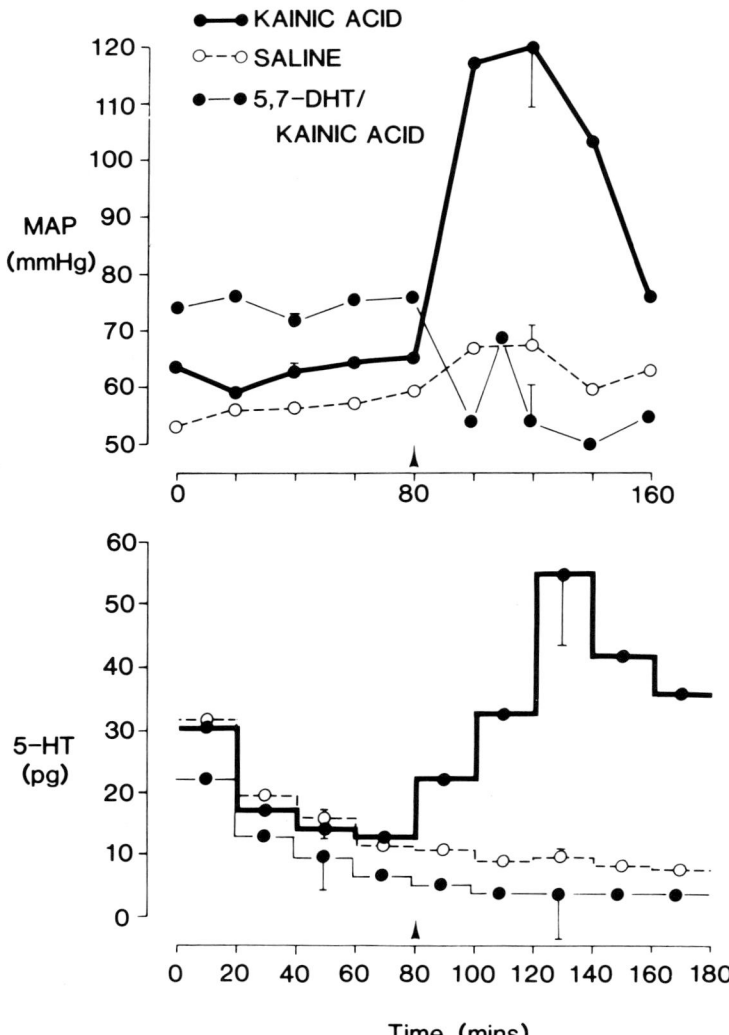

FIG. 4. Microdialysis for serotonin in the rat thoracic spinal cord. **Upper panel:** The effect on mean arterial pressure (mmHg) of bilateral microinjections of kainic acid into the region of the lateral B3 serotonin cells of five normal WKY rats (*black circles* and *thick blacklines*) and of five WKY rats pretreated with the serotonin neurotoxin 5,7-DHT 2 weeks earlier (*black circles* and *thin black lines*). Vehicle-treated rats received microinjections of vehicle alone (*open circles* and *dotted line*). Microinjections were made at 80 minutes (*arrow*). **Lower panel:** The effects on spinal serotonin efflux (pg/20-minute collection period) of bilateral microinjections of kainic acid or vehicle, onto the B3 lateral serotonin cell group. Kainic acid caused a significant increase in blood pressure and spinal serotonin release. Both effects are abolished by prior lesioning of the serotonin neurons with 5,7-DHT. (From ref. 8, with permission.)

subserve different functions. Other investigations suggest the midline medullary serotonin neurons are separate both from the sympathoexcitatory and the sympathoinhibitory neurons and that rather than relaying specific sympathetic information these serotonin nerves act as neuromodulators to set the level of excitability of sympathetic preganglionic neurons (78).

Direct evidence for the involvement of bulbospinal serotonin neurons in cardiovascular control comes from experiments where the release of serotonin from the nerves has been measured. A microdialysis probe, placed in the intermediolateral cell column to detect serotonin in the extracellular fluid, collected more serotonin after stimulation of the rostral ventral medulla in the area of the B3 neurons when there was also an increase in blood pressure (8). Furthermore, prior treatment with 5,7-dihydroxytryptamine depleting spinal cord serotonin abolished both the increase in serotonin release and the increase in blood pressure (8) (Fig. 4). Several studies have addressed the identification of the serotonin receptor likely to mediate the serotonin effects in the spinal cord. In one study the B3 serotonin neurons in the lateral rostral ventral medulla were stimulated before and after the intrathecal administration of different serotonin receptor antagonists (19). Since methysergide (a mixed 5-HT1 and 5-HT2 receptor antagonist) attenuated the response, but ketanserin (a 5-HT2 antagonist) and ICS 205930 and MDL 7222 (both 5-HT3 antagonists) were without effect, the results suggested spinal cord 5-HT1 receptors mediated the sympathoexcitatory effects of B3 serotonin neurons (19). The sympathoexcitatory effects of intrathecally applied serotonin also appear to be 5-HT1 receptor mediated (79), and iontophoresis studies demonstrating that serotonin excites sympathetic preganglionic neurons in the intermediolateral cell column of the spinal cord (80,81) also show that these excitatory responses to serotonin could be blocked by 5-HT1 antagonists (82). It must be noted however, that a serotonin-mediated sympathoinhibition of sympathetic preganglionic neurons is also observed in some studies (82,83). Pharmacological studies suggest 5-HT2 receptors might mediate these sympathoinhibitory effects of serotonin (84).

Other neurotransmitters have been identified within the bulbospinal serotonin neurons, as described above, and it is likely that the cardiovascular effects of the activation of this pathway are the result of postsynaptic events in response to the release of colocalized transmitters, rather than the release of serotonin alone. For example, the spinally projecting sympathoexcitatory B3 serotonin neurons in the ventrolateral medulla all contain phosphate-activated glutaminase (6) and some are likely also to contain substance P (48,85). It is clear that the physiological effects of stimulation of this bulbospinal serotonin pathway is mediated by serotonin and by excitatory amino acid release, since 5-HT1 receptor antago-

nism alone could only attenuate the effects of B3 stimulation, whereas after the administration, in addition, of an excitatory amino acid receptor antagonist, the sympathoexcitatory effects of B3 stimulation were completely abolished (19,86). A functional interaction at these spinal levels between substance P and serotonin in the regulation of sympathetic activity and blood pressure also seems likely (87).

The rostral ventral medulla, as well as being the source of the spinally projecting serotonin neurons, also receives serotonergic inputs from other brain areas. Electrochemical detection has shown that serotonin release increases in the rostral ventral medulla during baroreceptor activation (88), suggesting that the serotonin inputs might have a role in the baroreflex regulation of sympathetic activity. The 5-HT1A receptors have been identified within the rostral ventral medulla, some as somatic autoreceptors on serotonin neurons, as well as postsynaptic receptors on other neurons. Studies suggest that it is these receptors that mediate the sympathoinhibitory effects of 8-OH-DPAT observed in a number of species (54,55), and attention is now focusing on these 5-HT1A receptors in the ventral brainstem as the target of the antihypertensive agent urapidil (see below). Reciprocal inputs between the rostral ventral medullary neurons and the medullary serotonin neurons have been described (89,90), suggestive of a complex interaction between the distinct groups of neurons in the ventral medulla that control sympathetic activity and blood pressure. Clearly, serotonin neurons act within this neural network, but the role for serotonin in this intricate system is still to be elucidated.

SEROTONIN AND EXPERIMENTAL HYPERTENSION

The demonstration of serotonin-containing neurons and nerve terminals in brain regions known to be involved in cardiovascular regulation (see above), has led to considerable interest in a possible role for serotonin-containing neurons in hypertension; however, the role of these neurons is still uncertain.

The Spontaneously Hypertensive Rat

The spontaneously hypertensive rat has been widely studied. There is evidence of increased synthesis of serotonin in this strain but disagreement as to which sites are involved. Thus, the activity of the rate-limiting enzyme in serotonin synthesis, tryptophan hydroxylase, was reported to be increased in the hypothalamus but not in the pons medulla of the spontaneously hypertensive rat (91). However, the rate of serotonin synthesis *in vivo* (estimated by the accumulation of 5-hydroxytryptophane after decarboxylase inhibition) was increased in the pons medulla and spinal cord of spontaneously hypertensive rats but not in the hypothalamus (92). Depletion of serotonin stores with parachlorophenylalanine (93) lowers blood pressure in the spontaneously hypertensive rat while serotonergic neurotoxins have been shown to retard the development of hypertension in this strain (94).

Mills et al. (14) have examined the contribution of bulbospinal serotonergic pathways in the spontaneously hypertensive rat. Intrathecal administration of the nonselective serotonin antagonist, methysergide, attenuated the pressor response elicited by stimulating the B3 region, which contains serotonergic nerves but did not affect resting arterial pressure. In contrast, 2-amino phosphonovaleric acid, an N-methyl-D-aspartate receptor antagonist, did lower arterial pressure in spontaneously hypertensive rats but not in normotensive Wistar-Kyoto (WKY) controls (95). Moreover, 2-amino phosphononvaleric acid attenuated the pressor response elicited by stimulation of either the rostroventromedial medulla including the B3 region or the nearby rostral ventrolateral medulla including the C1 region, which contains bulbospinal adrenaline neurons. These data imply that tonic activation of N-methyl-D-aspartate (NMDA), but not serotonergic receptors in the spinal cord, contributes to hypertension in the spontaneously hypertensive rat. Intraspinal injection of 5,7-DHT to destroy bulbospinal serotonin neurons lowers blood pressure in normotensive rats but not in spontaneously hypertensive rats (96). Thus bulbospinal serotonergic mechanisms do not appear to play a primary role in the pathogenesis of hypertension in the spontaneously hypertensive rat, although other serotonergic pathways may be involved.

Deoxycorticosterone Acetate (DOCA)/Salt Hypertension

Tryptophan hydroxylase was reported to be normal after 8 weeks of deoxycorticosterone/salt hypertension. The time at which measurements are made may be important. Increased levels of serotonin and 5-hydroxyindoleacetic acid were reported in the pons, medulla, and spinal cord of rats within 2 to 4 weeks of commencing treatment (97), but levels were normal in these regions after 5 or more weeks of DOCA/salt (91,97,98). However, intracisternal 5,6-DHT did not affect the development or maintenance of DOCA/salt hypertension (98).

Neurogenic Hypertension

Neurogenic hypertension produced by sinoaortic denervation in the rabbit results in increased levels of serotonin and its breakdown product, 5-hydroxyindoleacetic acid, in the thoracolumbar spinal cord and the pons-medullary region (3). Moreover, intracisternal administration of a serotonin selective neurotoxin, 5,6-DHT, prevented the increase in arterial blood pressure that

follows sinoaortic denervation in the rabbit and lowers blood pressure in established neurogenic hypertension (3).

Renal Hypertension

Serotonin and 5-hydroxyindoleacetic acid levels were unchanged in renal wrap hypertensive rabbits (3) and in two-kidney, two-clip renal hypertension in the rat (99). Serotonergic neurotoxins had no effect on the development of renal wrap hypertension in the rabbit (3) or two-kidney, two-clip hypertension in the rat (99).

While it is clear that central serotonin-containing neurons play a critically important role in the control of blood pressure, their role in experimental models of hypertension is less obvious. This is reflected in the definitive evidence that central serotonergic neurons are important in neurogenic hypertension following sinoaortic denervation in contrast to the lack of data implicating particular serotonin-containing pathways in the spontaneously hypertensive rat, the DOCA/salt rat or the renal wrap hypertensive rabbit.

DRUGS ACTING THROUGH CENTRAL SEROTONIN PATHWAYS

There is evidence that a number of antihypertensive drugs may act through central serotonergic mechanisms.

Methyldopa

Methyldopa has been used in the treatment of hypertension since the early 1960s. It was initially believed that methyldopa lowered blood pressure by acting as a false neurotransmitter (100). It is now believed that methyldopa is first converted to methylnoradrenaline and that this compound lowers blood pressure largely by its agonist activity at central α_2-receptors (101).

There also appear to be important effects of methyldopa on central serotonergic neurons since the serotonin neurotoxin 5,6-DHT attenuates the depressor response to intracisternally administered methyldopa (102). These effects appear to be mediated by medullary neurons. Methyldopa produces a profound and long-lasting fall in blood pressure when injected into the lateral B3 region, which contains bulbospinal serotonin neurons (16,18) (Fig. 5). This hypotensive response is attenuated by pretreatment with another selective serotonin neurotoxin, 5,7-DHT, administered either intracerebroventricularly (16,18) or intraspinally (18). Clearly, other mechanisms are involved since the hypotensive response to methyldopa was attenuated but not abolished by 5,7-DHT (16,18) and because intracerebroventricular administration of the α-antagonist phentolamine also reduced the hypotensive response to methyldopa (16).

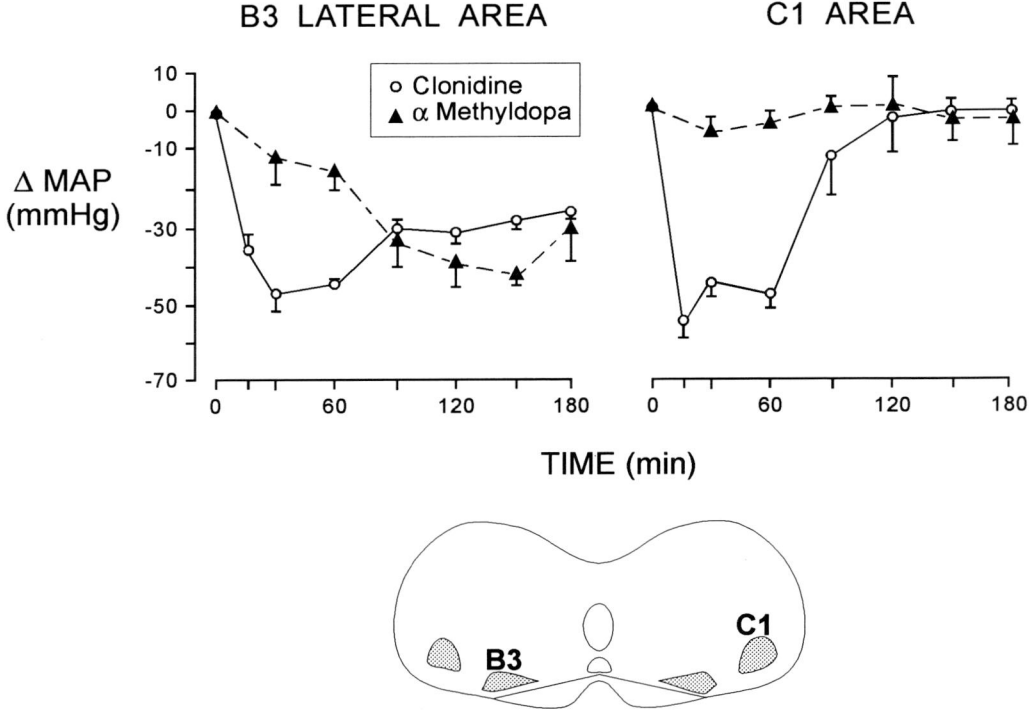

FIG. 5. Changes in mean arterial pressure (MAP) after microinjection of methyldopa or clonidine administered at 0 min into the B3 lateral serotonin area, or into the C1 adrenaline area in anesthetized spontaneously hypertensive rats. Results are mean ± SEM. Methyldopa: B3, $n = 4$; C1, $n = 6$. Clonidine: B3, $n = 7$; C1, $n = 6$. Methyldopa effectively reduces blood pressure when injected into the B3 area, but not the C1. (From ref. 16, with permission.)

Clonidine

Clonidine is another well established centrally acting antihypertensive drug that is believed to act via central α_2-receptors (103) or possibly via imidazoline receptors (104). However, 5,6-DHT attenuates the depressor response to intracisternally administered clonidine (102), suggesting a role for serotonergic neurons. Clonidine elicits hypotensive responses when injected into either the lateral B3 area or the nearby C1 region, which contains adrenaline neurons (16) (Fig. 5). Also, 5,6-DHT attenuates the response to injection of clonidine in the B3 region but does not affect the response to C1 injection (16). Thus it is possible that the hypotensive action of clonidine is mediated in part through serotonergic neurons, possibly because of α_2-receptors or imidazoline receptors located on the cell bodies of the B3 serotonin bulbospinal neurons.

Ketanserin

Ketanserin is an antagonist at both 5-HT2 receptors and at α_1-receptors (103,105). The relative importance of serotonin versus alpha blockade and of central versus peripheral mechanisms of action is controversial (103).

Ritanserin, a 5-HT2 receptor antagonist without alpha-blocking actions, does not lower blood pressure acutely in spontaneously hypertensive rats, suggesting that 5-HT2 blockade alone cannot account for the antihypertensive effect of ketanserin (106). However, chronic ritanserin treatment in spontaneously hypertensive rats does potentiate the depressor response to the α_1-blocker, prazosin (107), suggesting that 5-HT2 receptor blockade might contribute to ketanserin's hypotensive effect. The contribution of central neural mechanisms to the actions of ketanserin is suggested by the lack of tachycardia (106,107) and the decrease in sympathetic nerve activity (107) that accompany the depressor response to ketanserin. Moreover, neither peripheral alpha blockade nor peripheral 5-HT2 receptor blockade can be demonstrated during chronic administration of ketanserin to humans despite the persistent antihypertensive effect (108).

Urapidil

Urapadil is a 5-HT1A agonist with α_1-blocking properties (103). Its hypotensive effects are not due to α_1-blockade alone since urapidil lowers blood pressure further after pretreatment with prazosin to block α_1-

receptors (109). Systemic administration of urapadil lowers sympathetic nerve activity in the cat (110), suggesting that central actions may contribute to its hypertensive effect. Urapidil lowers blood pressure when applied to the intermediate area of the ventral surface of the medulla, suggesting that this might be its central site of action (110). Selective 5-HT1A agonists also lower blood pressure when applied at this site (111), but α-antagonists do not (110). No selective 5-HT1A antagonists exist, but spiperone, which blocks both 5-HT1A and α_1-receptors, abolished the hypotensive response to urapidil in prazosin-pretreated rat (109). Thus urapidil lowers blood pressure by a central effect on 5-HT1A receptors in addition to its peripheral α-antagonist action.

ACKNOWLEDGMENTS

Our laboratory is supported by grants from the National Health and Medical Research Council, the National Heart Foundation, and the National Sudden Infant Death Council of Australia.

REFERENCES

1. Twarog BM, Page IH. Serotonin content of some mammalian tissues and urine and a method for its determination. *Am J Physiol* 1953;175:157–161.
2. Ito A, Schanberg SM. Central nervous system mechanisms responsible for blood pressure elevation induced by p-chlorophenylalanine. *J Pharmacol Exp Ther* 1972;181:65–74.
3. Wing LMH, Chalmers JP. Participation of central serotonergic neurons in the control of the circulation of the unanesthetized rabbit. *Circ Res* 1974;35:504–513.
4. Chalmers JP, Pilowsky PM. Brainstem and bulbospinal neurotransmitter systems in the control of blood pressure. *J Hypertens* 1991;9:675–694.
5. Pilowsky PM, Morris MJ, Kapoor V, West MJ, Chalmers JP. Role of renal nerve activity, plasma catecholamines and plasma vasopressin in cardiovascular responses to intracisternal neurotoxins in the rabbit. *J Auton Nerv Syst* 1986;17:109–120.
6. Minson JB, Pilowsky PM, Llewellyn-Smith IJ, Kaneko T, Kapoor V, Chalmers JP. Glutamate in spinally projecting neurons of the rostral ventral medulla. *Brain Res* 1991;555:326–331.
7. Voss MD, de Castro D, Lipski J, Pilowsky PM, Jiang C. Serotonin immunoreactive boutons form close appositions with respiratory neurons of the dorsal respiratory group in the cat. *J Comp Neurol* 1990;295:208–218.
8. Pilowsky PM, Kapoor V, Minson JB, West MJ, Chalmers JP. Spinal cord serotonin release and raised blood pressure after brainstem kainic acid injection. *Brain Res* 1986;366:354–357.
9. Chalmers JP, Kapoor V, Macrae IM, Minson JB, Pilowsky PM, West MJ. New approaches to the study of bulbospinal (B3) serotonergic neurons in the control of blood pressure. *J Hypertens* 1985;3:S5–S9.
10. Chalmers JP, Pilowsky PM, Minson JB, Kapoor V, Mills EH, West MJ. Central serotonergic mechanisms in hypertension. *Am J Hypertens* 1988;1:79–83.
11. Chalmers JP, Minson JB, Pilowsky PM, et al. Pressor systems from ventrolateral medulla: epinephrine- and serotonin-containing neurons. In: *Progress in catecholamine research*. Part B: central aspects. Sandler M, Dahlstrom A, Belmaker RH, eds. New York: Alan R. Liss, 1988;291–295.
12. Minson JB, Chalmers JP, Drolet G, et al. Central serotonergic mechanisms in cardiovascular regulation. *Cardiovasc Drugs Ther* 1990;4:27–32.
13. Pilowsky PM, de Castro D, Llewellyn-Smith IJ, Lipski J, Voss MD. Serotonin immunoreactive boutons make synapses with feline phrenic motoneurons. *J Neurosci* 1990;10:1091–1098.
14. Mills EH, Minson JB, Chalmers JP. Effects of intrathecal administration of methysergide, phentolamine, and pindolol on pressor responses to electrical stimulation of the rostral ventrolateral medulla. *J Cardiovasc Pharmacol* 1988;11:456–460.
15. Minson JB, Chalmers JP, Caon AC, Renaud B. Separate areas of rat medulla oblongata with populations of serotonin- and adrenaline-containing neurons alter blood pressure after l-glutamate stimulation. *J Auton Nerv Syst* 1987;19:39–50.
16. Drolet G, Aslanian V, Minson JB, Morris M, Chalmers JP. Differences in the central hypotensive actions of alpha-methyldopa and clonidine in the spontaneously hypertensive rat: contribution of neurons arising from the B3 and the C1 areas of the rostral ventrolateral medulla. *J Cardiovasc Pharmacol* 1990;15:118–123.
17. Howe PRC, Kuhn DM, Minson JB, Stead BH, Chalmers JP. Evidence for a bulbospinal serotonergic pressor pathway in the rat brain. *Brain Res* 1983;270:29–36.
18. Minson JB, Choy VJ, Chalmers JP. Bulbospinal serotonin neurons and hypotensive effects of methyldopa in the spontaneously hypertensive rat. *J Cardiovasc Pharmacol* 1984;6:312–317.
19. Mills EH, Minson JB, Chalmers JP. The effect of intrathecal serotonergic antagonists on the pressor response to stimulation of the brainstem in the rat. *Clin Exp Hypertens* 1989;A11:265–276.
20. Macrae IM, Minson JB, Kapoor V, Morris MJ, Chalmers JP. Midline B3 serotonin nerves in rat medulla are involved in hypotensive effect of methyldopa. *J Cardiovasc Pharmacol* 1986;8:381–385.
21. Chalmers JP, Macrae M, Minson JB, Kapoor V. Methyldopa hypotension and ascending projections from midline serotonin (B3) cells in the medulla. *J Hypertens* 1985;3:S111–S112.
22. Chalmers JP, Minson JB, Choy V. Bulbospinal serotonin pressor pathways and hypotensive action of methyldopa in the rat. *Hypertension* 1984;6:II-16–II-21.
23. Riley LA, Jonakait GM, Hart RP. Serotonin modulates the levels of mRNAs coding for thyrotropin-releasing hormone and preprotachykinin by different mechanisms in medullary raphe neurons. *Mol Brain Res* 1993;17:251–257.
24. Brodin E, Linderoth B, Goiny M, et al. In vivo release of serotonin in cat dorsal vagal complex and cervical ventral horn induced by electrical stimulation of the medullary raphe nuclei. *Brain Res* 1990;535:227–236.
25. Dahlström A, Fuxe K. Evidence for the existence of monoamine-containing neurons in the central nervous system. *Acta Physiol Scand* 1964;62:2–55.
26. Steinbusch HWM. Serotonin-immunoreactive neurons and their projections in the CNS. In: Björklund A, Hökfelt T, Kuhar MJ, eds. *Handbook of chemical neuroanatomy*. Amsterdam: Elsevier Science Publishing, 1984;68–125.
27. Steinbusch HWM. Distribution of serotonin-immunoreactivity in the central nervous system of the rat- cell bodies and terminals. *Neuroscience* 1981;6:557–618.
28. Priestley JV, Wotherspoon G, Savery D, Averill S, Rattray M. A combined in situ hybridization and immunofluorescence procedure allowing visualisation of peptide mRNA and serotonin in single sections. *J Neurosci Methods* 1993;48:99–110.
29. Riley LA, Hart RP, Jonakait GM. Both zimelidine and clorgyline decrease preprotachykinin mRNA in adult medullary raphe nuclei. *Mol Cell Neurosci* 1991;2:139–144.
30. Bosler O, Beaudet A. VIP neurons as prime synaptic targets for serotonin afferents in rat suprachiasmatic nucleus: a combined radioautographic and immunocytochemical study. *Neuroscience* 1985;14:749–763.
31. Sasek CA, Wessendorf MW, Helke CJ. Evidence for co-existence of thyrotropin-releasing hormone, substance P and serotonin in ventral medullary neurons that project to the intermediolateral cell column in the rat. *Neuroscience* 1990;35:105–119.
32. Nicholas AP, Pieribone VA, Arvidsson U, Hökfelt T. Serotonin-, substance P- and glutamate/aspartatelike immunoreactivities in medullo-spinal pathways of rat and primate. *Neuroscience* 1992;48:545–559.
33. Wessendorf MW, Elde R. The coexistence of serotonin and substance P-like immunoreactivity in the spinal cord of the rat as

shown by immunofluorescent double labeling. *J Neurosci* 1987;7:2352–2363.

34. Jones SL, Light AR. Termination patterns of serotonergic medullary raphespinal fibers in the rat lumbar spinal cord: an anterograde immunohistochemical study. *J Comp Neurol* 1990;297:267–282.

35. Newton BW, Burkhart AB, Hamill RW. Immunohistochemical distribution of serotonin in spinal autonomic nuclei: II. Early and late postnatal ontogeny in the rat. *J Comp Neurol* 1989;279:82–103.

36. Choy VJ, Chalmers JP. Importance of central serotonin neurons in the hypotensive action of methyldopa in the rat. *Clin Exp Pharmacol Physiol* 1984;11:37–44.

37. Heinricher MM, Kaplan HJ. GABA-mediated inhibition in rostral ventromedial medulla: role in nociceptive modulation in the lightly anesthetized rat. *Pain* 1991;47:105–113.

38. Kaplan H, Fields HL. Hyperalgesia during acute opioid abstinence: evidence for a nociceptive facilitating function of the rostral ventromedial medulla. *J Neurosci* 1991;11:1433–1439.

39. Millhorn DE, Hökfelt T, Seroogy K, Oertel W, Verhofstad AAJ, Wu JY. Immunohistochemical evidence for colocalization of gamma-aminobutyric acid and serotonin in neurons of the ventral medulla oblongata projecting to the spinal cord. *Brain Res* 1987;410:179–185.

40. Miceli MO, Post CA, Van der Kooy D. Catecholamine and serotonin colocalization in projection neurons of the area postrema. *Brain Res* 1987;412:381–385.

41. Leger L, Charnay Y, Dubois PM, Jouvet M. Distribution of enkephalin-immunoreactive cell bodies in relation to serotonin-containing neurons in the raphe nuclei of the cat: immunohistochemical evidence for the coexistence of enkephalins and serotonin in certain cells. *Brain Res* 1986;362:63–73.

42. Bowker RM, Steinbusch HWM, Coulter JD. Serotonergic and peptidergic projections to the spinal cord demonstrated by a combined retrograde HRP histochemical and immunocytochemical staining method. *Brain Res* 1981;211:412–417.

43. Mills EH, Minson JB, Pilowsky PM, Chalmers JP. N-methyl-D-aspartate receptors in the spinal cord mediate pressor responses to stimulation of the rostral ventrolateral medulla in the rat. *Clin Exp Pharmacol Physiol* 1988;15:147–155.

44. Calaresu FR, McKitrick DJ, Weernink EJ. Microinjection of substance P and ACh into rat intermediolateral nucleus elicits cardiovascular responses. *Am J Physiol* 1990;259:R357–R361.

45. Anwyl R. Neurophysiological actions of 5-hydroxytryptamine in the vertebrate nervous system. *Prog Neurobiol* 1990;35:451–468.

46. Elliott P, Wallis DI. Serotonin and L-norepinephrine as mediators of altered excitability in neonatal rat motoneurons studied in vitro. *Neuroscience* 1992;47:533–544.

47. Dun NJ, Wu SY, Shen E, Miyazaki T, Dun SL, Ren C. Synaptic mechanisms in sympathetic preganglionic neurons. *Can J Physiol Pharmacol* 1991;70:S86–S91.

48. Wu WC, Elde R, Wessendorf MW. Organization of the serotonergic innervation of spinal neurons in rats—III. Differential serotonergic innervation of somatic and parasympathetic preganglionic motoneurons as determined by patterns of coexisting peptides. *Neuroscience* 1993;55:223–233.

49. Watson S, Abbott A. Receptor nomenclature supplement. *TIPS* 1992;January:1–36.

50. Oksenberg D, Marsters SA, O'Dowd BF, et al. A single amino-acid difference confers major pharmacological variation between human and rodent 5-HT receptors. *Nature* 1992;360:161–163.

51. Sotelo C, Cholley B, El Mestikawy S, Gozlan H, Hamon M. Direct immunohistochemical evidence of the existence of 5-HT1A autoreceptors on serotoninergic neurons in the midbrain raphe nuclei. *Eur J Pharmacol* 1990;2:1144–1154.

52. Anderson IK, Martin GR, Ramage AG. Central administration of 5-HT activates 5-HT1A receptors to cause sympathoexcitation and 5-HT2/5-HT1c receptors to release vasopressin in anaesthetized rats. *Br J Pharmacol* 1992;107:1020–1028.

53. Ramage AG. Influence of 5-HT$_{1A}$ receptor agonists on sympathetic and parasympathetic nerve activity. *J Cardiovasc Pharmacol* 1990;15:S75–S85.

54. Helke CJ, McDonald CH, Phillips ET. Hypotensive effects of 5-HT receptor activation: ventral medullary sites and mechanisms of action in the rat. *J Auton Nerv Syst* 1993;42:177–188.

55. Laubie M, Drouillat M, Dabiré H, Cherqui C, Schmitt H. Ventrolateral medullary pressor area: site of hypotensive and sympatho-inhibitory effects of 8-OH-DPAT in anaesthetized dogs. *Eur J Pharmacol* 1989;160:385–394.

56. Gaddum JH, Picarelli ZP. Two kinds of tryptamine receptor. *Br J Pharmacol* 1957;12:323–328.

57. Malgouris C, Flamand F, Doble A. Autoradiographic studies of RP 62203, a potent 5-HT2 receptor antagonist. In vitro and ex vivo selectivity profile. *Eur J Pharmacol* 1993;233:29–35.

58. Malgouris C, Flamand F, Doble A. Autoradiographic studies of RP 62203, a potent 5-HT2 receptor antagonist. Pharmacological characterization of [3H]RP 62203 binding in the rat brain. *Eur J Pharmacol* 1993;233:37–45.

59. Yoshioka M. Effect of a novel 5-hydroxytryptamine-antagonist, GR38032F, on the 5-hydroxytryptamine-induced increase in carotid sinus nerve activity in rats. *J Pharmacol Exp Ther* 1989;250:637–641.

60. Veelken R, Sawin IL, DiBona GF. Epicardial serotonin receptors in circulatory control in conscious Sprague-Dawley rats. *Am J Physiol* 1990;258:H466–H472.

61. Head GA, Korner PI. Cardiovascular functions of brain serotonergic neurons in the rabbit as analysed from the acute and chronic effects of 5,6-dihydroxytryptamine. *J Cardiovasc Pharmacol* 1982;4:398–408.

62. Wing LMH, Chalmers JP. Effects of p-chlorophenylalanine on blood pressure and heart rate in normal rabbits and rabbits with neurogenic hypertension. *Clin Exp Pharmacol Physiol* 1974;1:219–229.

63. Lambert G, Friedman G, Buchweitz E, Gerson S. Involvement of 5-hydroxytryptamine in the central control of respiration, blood pressure and heart rate in the anesthetized rat. *Neuropharmacology* 1978;17:807–813.

64. Inoue A, Bunag RD. Sympathetic inhibition and vasopressin mediation during centrally induced responses to serotonin in rats. *J Cardiovasc Pharmacol* 1989;13:902–907.

65. Krstic MK, Djurkovic D. Analysis of cardiovascular responses to central administration 5-hydroxytryptamine in rats. *Neuropharmacology* 1980;19:455–463.

66. Antonaccio MS, Taylor DG. Reduction in blood pressure, sympathetic nerve discharge, and centrally evoked pressor responses by methysergide in anesthetized cats. *Eur J Pharmacol* 1977;42:331–338.

67. McCall RB, Humphrey SJ. Involvement of serotonin in the central regulation of blood pressure: evidence for a facilitating effect on sympathetic nerve activity. *J Pharmacol Exp Ther* 1982;222:94–102.

68. Dedeoglu A, Fisher LA. Central nervous actions of serotonin and a serotonin receptor agonist: cardiovascular excitation at low doses. *J Pharmacol Exp Ther* 1991;257:425–432.

69. McCall RB, Patel BN, Harris LT. Effects of serotonin and serotonin receptor agonists and antagonists on blood pressure, heart rate and sympathetic nerve activity. *J Pharmacol Exp Ther* 1987;242:1152.

70. Fozard JR, Mir AK, Middlemiss DN. Cardiovascular response to 8-hydroxy-2-(di-n-Propylamino) tetralin(8-OH-DPAT) in the rat: site of action and pharmacological analysis. *J Cardiovasc Pharmacol* 1987;9:328–347.

71. Smits JFM, Struyker-Boudier HAJ. Intrahypothalamic serotonin and cardiovascular control in rats. *Brain Res* 1976;127:422–425.

72. Smits JFM, Van Essen H, Struyker-Boudier HAJ. Serotonin-mediated cardiovascular responses to electrical stimulation of the raphe nuclei in the rat. *Life Sci* 1978;23:173–178.

73. Kuhn DM, Wolf WA, Lovenberg W. Pressor effects of electrical stimulation of the dorsal and median raphe nuclei in anesthetized rats. *J Pharmacol Exp Ther* 1980;214:403–409.

74. Bacon SJ, Smith AD. Preganglionic sympathetic neurons innervating the rat adrenal medulla: immunocytochemical evidence of synaptic input from nerve terminals containing substance P, GABA or 5-hydroxytryptamine. *J Auton Nerv Syst* 1988;24:97–122.

75. Llewellyn-Smith IJ, Minson JB, Pilowsky PM, Chalmers JP. There are few catecholamine- or neuropeptide Y-containing synapses in the intermediolateral cell column of rat thoracic spinal cord. *Clin Exp Pharmacol Physiol* 1991;18:111–115.

76. Sawchenko PE, Swanson LW, Steinbusch HWM, Verhofstad

AAJ. The distribution and cells of origin of serotonergic inputs to the paraventicular and supraoptic nuclei of the rat. *Brain Res* 1983;277:355–360.

77. McCall RB, Humphrey SJ. Evidence of GABA mediation of sympathetic inhibition evoked from midline medullary depressor sites. *Brain Res* 1985;339:356–360.

78. McCall RB, Clement ME. Identification of serotonergic and sympathetic neurons in medullary raphe nuclei. *Brain Res* 1989;477: 172–182.

79. Scarisbrick IA, Jones EG, Isackson PJ. Coexpression of mRNAs for NGF, BDNF, and NT-3 in the cardiovascular system of the pre- and postnatal rat. *J Neurosci* 1993;13:875–893.

80. DeGroat WC, Ryall RE. An excitatory action of 5-hydroxytryptamine on sympathetic preganglionic neurons. *Exp Brain Res* 1967;3:299–305.

81. McCall RB. Serotonergic excitation of sympathetic preganglionic neurons: a microiontophoretic study. *Brain Res* 1983;289:121–127.

82. Lewis DI, Coote JH. The influence of 5-hydroxytryptamine agonists and antagonists on identified sympathetic preganglionic neurones in the rat, in vivo. *Br J Pharmacol* 1990;99:667–672.

83. Cabot JB. Raphe inhibition of sympathetic preganglionic neurons. *Science* 1979;203:184–185.

84. Yusof APM, Coote JH. Excitatory and inhibitory actions of intrathecally administered 5-hydroxytryptamine on sympathetic nerve activity in the rat. *J Auton Nerv Syst* 1988;22:229–236.

85. Pilowsky PM, Minson JB, Hodgson AJ, Howe PRC, Chalmers JP. Does substance P coexist with adrenaline in neurones of the rostral ventrolateral medulla in the rat? *Neurosci Lett* 1986;71: 293–298.

86. Mills EH, Minson JB, Drolet G, Chalmers JP. Effect of intrathecal amino acid receptor antagonists on basal blood pressure and pressor responses to brainstem stimulation in normotensive and hypertensive rats. *J Cardiovasc Pharmacol* 1990;15:877–883.

87. Gradin K. Interactions between substance P and serotonergic mechanisms at preganglionic sympathetic nerves in thoracic spinal cord. *Acta Physiol Scand* 1990;138:101–102.

88. Bhaskaran D, Freed CR. Catechol and indole metabolism in rostral ventrolateral medulla change synchronously with changing blood pressure. *J Pharmacol Exp Ther* 1989;249:660.

89. Zagon A. Innervation of serotonergic medullary raphe neurons from cells of the rostral ventrolateral medulla in rats. *Neuroscience* 1993;55:849–867.

90. Chan SHH, Chan YH, Ong BT. Anatomic connections between nucleus reticularis rostroventrolateralis and some medullary cardiovascular sites in the rat. *Neurosci Lett* 1986;71:277–282.

91. Nagaoka A, Lovenberg W. Regional changes in the activities of aminergic enzymes in the brains of hypertensive rats. *Eur J Pharmacol* 1977;43:297–306.

92. Smith ML, Browning RA, Myers JH. In vivo rate of serotonin synthesis in brain and spinal cord of young spontaneously hypertensive rats. *Eur J Pharmacol* 1979;53:301–305.

93. Jarrott B, McQueen A, Graf L, Louis WF. Serotonin levels in vascular tissue and the effects of a serotonin inhibitor on blood pressure in hypertensive rats. *Clin Exp Pharmacol Physiol* 1975;2(suppl):201–205.

94. Buckingham RE, Hamilton TC, Robson D. Effect of intracerebroventricular 5,6-dihydroxytryptamine on blood pressure of spontaneously hypertensive rats. *Eur J Pharmacol* 1976;36:431–437.

95. Mills E, Minson JB, Drolet G, Chalmers JP. Effect of intrathecal amino acid receptor antagonists on basal blood pressure and pressor responses to brainstem stimulation in normotensive and hypertensive rats. *J Cardiovasc Pharmacol* 1990;15:877–883.

96. Howe PRC, Stead BH, Lovenberg W, Chalmers JP. Effects of central serotonin nerve lesions on blood pressure in normotensive and hypotensive rats. *Clin Exp Pharmacol Physiol* 1982;9:335–339.

97. Dawson R Jr, Nagamhama S, Oparil S. Central serotonergic alterations in deoxycorticosterone acetate/NaCl (DOCA/NaCl)-induced hypertension. *Neuropharmacology* 1988;27:417–426.

98. Myers MG, Reid JL, Lewis PJ. The effect of central serotonin depletion on DOCA-saline hypertension in the rat. *Cardiovasc Res* 1974;8:806–810.

99. Trolliet MR, Kurnjek ML, Mikulic L, Basso N, Taquini AC. Development of renovascular hypertension after central serotonin depletion. *Hypertension* 1990;15:I166–I169.

100. Day MD, Rand MJ. A hypothesis for the mode of action of alpha methyldopa in relieving hypertension. *J Pharm Pharmacol* 1963;15:221–224.

101. Reid JL, Elliott HL. Methyldopa. In: Doyle AE, ed. *Handbook of hypertension. vol 5. Clinical pharmacology of antihypertensive drugs.* Amsterdam: Elsevier, 1984;92–112.

102. Head GA, Korner PI, Lewis SL, Badoer E. Contribution of noradrenergic and serotonergic neurons to the circulatory effects of centrally acting clonidine and alpha-methyldopa in rabbits. *J Cardiovasc Pharmacol* 1983;5:945–953.

103. vanZweiten PA, Blauw GJ, vanBrummelen P. Serotonergic receptors and drugs in hypertension. *Pharmacol Toxicol* 1992;70: s17–s22.

104. Ernsberger P, Giuliano R, Willette RN, Reis DJ. Role of imidazole receptors in the vasodepressor response to clonidine analogs in the rostral ventrolateral medulla. *J Pharmacol Exp Ther* 1990;253:408.

105. Hoyer D, Vos P, Closse A, Palacios JM, Engel G, Davies H. [3H]-Ketanserin labels serotonin 5-HT2 and alpha 1-adrenergic receptors in human brain cortex. *J Cardiovasc Pharmacol* 1987;10: S48–S50.

106. Smits J, VanDorsten F, Struyker-Boudier HAJ. Interference of ketanserin with baroreflex control of the circulation in the conscious spontaneously hypertensive rat. *Drugs* 1988;36:55–60.

107. Persson B, Gradin K, Pettersson A, Hedner T. Antihypertensive effects of ketanserin and ritanserin in the spontaneously hypertensive rat. *J Cardiovasc Pharmacol* 1988;11:S22–S24.

108. Blauw GJ, Doorenbos CJ, Bruning TA, van Brummelen P, Van Zwieten PA. Antihypertensive treatment with ketanserin shows no evidence of vascular serotonin₂-receptor and alpha₁-adrenoceptor blockade. *Drugs* 1990;40:42–44.

109. Ramage AG. The mechanism of the sympathoinhibitory action of urapidil: role of 5-HT1A receptors. *Br J Pharmacol* 1991;102: 998–1002.

110. Gillis RA, Dretchen KL, Namath I, et al. Hypotensive effect of urapidil: CNS site and relative contribution. *J Cardiovasc Pharmacol* 1987;9:103–109.

111. Gillis RA, Hill KJ, Kirby JS, et al. Effect of activation of central nervous system serotonin 1A receptors on cardiorespiratory function. *J Pharmacol Exp Ther* 1989;248:851–857.

112. Descarries L, Watkins KC, Garcia S, Beaudet A. The serotonin neurons in nucleus raphe dorsales of adult rat: a light and electron microscope radioantographic study. *J Comp Neurol* 1982;207: 239–254.

Hypertension: Pathophysiology, Diagnosis, and Management, Second Edition, edited by J.H. Laragh and B.M. Brenner, Raven Press, Ltd., New York © 1995.

CHAPTER 46

Role of Vasopressin in Hypertensive Disorders

Irene Gavras and Haralambos Gavras

Much interest has been generated in the last few years over the role of arginine vasopressin (AVP) in cardiovascular regulation. While earlier publications had dealt mostly with the hydroosmotic and direct vasoconstricting actions of this hormone, more recent studies have focused on its effects on the central nervous system (CNS), where it acts as a neurotransmitter and/or modulator of autonomic neurotransmission.

The various effects of AVP are mediated via different vasopressinergic receptors. Two types of AVP receptors have been clearly characterized: the V_1 receptors located on vascular smooth muscle (1) and liver cells (2), and the V_2 receptors located in the renal tubule (3). Stimulation of V_1 receptors produces smooth muscle contraction, i.e., a pressor effect, whereas stimulation of V_2 receptors produces the antidiuretic effect, i.e., reabsorption of free water. The CNS receptors of AVP are not yet well characterized and are probably distinct from the V_1 and V_2 receptor populations (4).

The second messengers activated by these receptors are also different: Stimulation of V_1 receptors involves elevation of intracellular calcium and increased turnover of phosphatidylinositol (5), i.e., intracellular events similar to those following stimulation of α_1-adrenoceptors (6). The effects of the V_2 receptors are mediated via activation of adenylate cyclase and formation of adenine 3',5'-cyclic monophosphate (cyclic AMP) (7).

There is general agreement regarding the mechanism by which AVP contributes to circulatory homeostasis. Stimulation or suppression of AVP release is effected via

two mechanisms: (a) A *volumetric* mechanism: When circulation is compromised either because of diminished blood volume or because of a fall in blood pressure—and thereby a fall of "effective" blood volume—the decreased atrial stretch signals a stimulation of AVP release. Conversely, an expansion in total or "central" blood volume is perceived as a signal for suppression of AVP release. (b) A *hydroosmotic* mechanism, whereby hemoconcentration and increased plasma osmolality signals stimulation of AVP release, whereas hemodilution and hypoosmolality suppress AVP release via osmoreceptors (and, possibly, sodium-sensitive receptors) of the central nervous system. AVP will then exert its pressor action via the V_1-vascular receptors and its free water-retaining action via the V_2-renal tubular receptors, to restore normal blood pressure and osmolality and maintain optimal conditions for circulation.

What is still highly controversial is whether, and how, AVP contributes to acute elevation of blood pressure above normal and/or the development and maintenance of established chronic hypertension. The arguments against a role of AVP in hypertension include the following:

1. The plasma levels of AVP have not been shown to be consistently elevated in any type of chronic hypertension. There is no consistent correlation of plasma AVP concentrations with absolute blood pressure or with changes in blood pressure obtained by various physiological or experimental maneuvers.
2. The highest concentrations of endogenous AVP are encountered in the syndrome of inappropriate antidiuretic hormone secretion, which is not associated with hypertension.
3. Infusion of exogenous AVP in normal intact animals

   I. Gavras, H. Gavras: Hypertension and Atherosclerosis Section, Department of Medicine, Boston University School of Medicine, Boston, Massachusetts 02118.

or humans fails to raise blood pressure. Minimal pressor effect is obtained by excessive rates of infusion that produce blood levels well beyond the physiologic range.

4. Administration of specific antivasopressor AVP antagonists, which can abolish the pressor action of AVP at the vascular receptor level, does not produce change in resting blood pressure in intact animals, normal hydrated human volunteers, or patients with mild to moderate essential hypertension.

This chapter reviews the evidence in support of AVP's contribution to the development and possibly the sustenance of certain forms of hypertension, and addresses the points that question the validity of these arguments.

PLASMA LEVELS OF AVP AND BLOOD PRESSURE

The first argument, i.e., the lack of correlation between AVP concentrations and blood pressure, is strongly reminiscent of similar debates in the mid-1960s regarding the role of the renin-angiotensin system in hypertension. Subsequent classification of essential hypertensives into low-, normal-, and high-renin subgroups, as well as clarification of the reciprocal relationship between plasma renin activity and state of sodium balance by use of specific angiotensin antagonists, finally laid those arguments to rest.

The direct pressor action of AVP on the vasculature depends on a number of variables. Experiments both *in vitro* with vascular strips and *in vivo* with isolated vascular preparations *in situ,* have shown that AVP is the most potent direct vasoconstrictor of the vascular smooth muscle (8,9). Yet, when exogenous AVP is infused into intact animals or humans, extremely high pharmacologic doses are required to produce a minimal rise in blood pressure (10–12).

This apparent insensitivity of the normal subject's vasculature to the vasopressor effect of AVP is mostly attributed to the hormone's action on the baroreflexes; small increases in plasma levels of AVP augment the feedback gain of baroreflexes by increasing their sensitivity, thereby accentuating the decrease in heart rate and cardiac output and offsetting their own pressor effect. This was first demonstrated in conscious dogs with intact baroreflexes, where systemic infusion of exogenous AVP in pharmacologic doses induced progressive decreases in heart rate and cardiac output, with increased peripheral vascular resistance but only modest elevation of arterial pressure at the highest rates. However, after sinoaortic baroreceptor denervation, there was a considerable lowering in the threshold of sensitivity to the pressor action of AVP, accompanied by an increase of as much as 100-fold in its pressor effect. By comparison, there was a four- to fivefold increase in pressor responses to systemically infused norepinephrine or angiotensin II under these conditions (10). These findings were subsequently confirmed and amplified by numerous similar experiments (11,13,14).

In humans, it was shown that plasma concentrations up to 120 pg/ml did not affect blood pressure (12) (normal range is 2.2 ± 1.1 pg/ml). However, when cardiovascular reflexes were impaired due to idiopathic autonomic insufficiency, there was a striking increase in the pressor responsiveness to AVP (15), with only small concurrent increases in the responsiveness to norepinephrine and angiotensin II. Likewise, administration of a hyperosmotic radiopaque material, which increased plasma osmolality, resulted in elevation of AVP with transient pressor response in quadriplegic patients (with severed sympathetic tracts) but not in normal individuals (16). These reports indicated a unique interaction between AVP and the peripheral arterial baroreflex system. They also provided an explanation for the apparent discrepancy between the old observation that the antidiuretic hormone can improve idiopathic orthostatic hypotension (17) and the common knowledge that it does not alter blood pressure when used as substitution therapy in diabetes insipidus.

As with other vasoactive hormones, the sensitivity of various regional vascular beds to the constrictor effect of AVP is widely different: The vasculature of peripheral muscles and skin and of the gastrointestinal tract exhibit the greatest sensitivity to the pressor activity of AVP, whereas the renal, coronary, and cerebral blood vessels are the least sensitive (18–20). Interestingly, this pattern of vascular sensitivity is precisely the opposite from that of angiotensin, which acts most on the vessels of the kidney, brain, and heart and least on the musculocutaneous vasculature (21). However, alterations in autonomic innervation might well alter the vascular-wall sensitivity of a given arterial tree to AVP.

Another important determinant of AVP's pressor activity is its interaction with other vasoactive hormones. At plasma concentrations that are themselves nonpressor, AVP has been reported to raise blood pressure by potentiating the vasoconstricting effect of catecholamines (22). Angiotensin II seems to facilitate the release of AVP, and even small alterations within the physiological range of endogenous angiotensin appear to influence AVP secretion (23,24). Prostaglandins, on the other hand, have been reported to exert either an inhibitory (25) or a facilitatory (26) effect on AVP secretion, with conflicting findings being reported sometimes from the same team of investigators. Based on our studies with intact and nephrectomized animals (27), we proposed the hypothesis that some renal prostaglandins may inhibit, and extrarenal ones may enhance, the release of AVP.

Other neurotransmitters and neuromodulators, including biogenic amines and opioid peptides, may also exert variable effects on neurosecretory neurons or synapses at various levels of the central nervous system, but the exact nature of their effects remains controversial (28–32).

The interaction of AVP with the sympathetic nervous system has been the object of several studies that have shown that the pressor effect of AVP is greatly enhanced by maneuvers that inhibit sympathetic function (33–36). Attempts to further dissect the interaction between vasopressin and various components of the sympathetic nervous system, have shown that the maximal vasopressor potential of AVP can be expressed under conditions of impaired α_1-adrenoceptor function (37). In other words, the one sympathetic component that appears to be mostly responsible for blunting the direct pressor effectiveness of AVP is the α_1-adrenergic activity, and only after its blockade can AVP take over as the primary vasoconstrictor factor. Whether this has anything to do with the fact that both the α_1 and the V_1 receptors on smooth muscle cells share the same intracellular second messenger system remains an interesting speculation.

On the other hand, intact α-adrenoceptor function appears to be a prerequisite for allowing maximal AVP release in response to nonosmotic stimuli, because under conditions of separate or combined α_1 and α_2 inhibition the secretion of AVP is greatly attenuated (35,37). Nevertheless, the role of the central α_1- and α_2-adrenoceptors on the release of AVP remains controversial since there are many conflicting reports (38). The most likely explanation for these discrepancies is that different experimental conditions, such as the use of different anesthetics or lack thereof, can markedly alter or even reverse central nervous system responses to a given stimulus (39). This complex relationship between AVP and various components of the sympathetic system, which affect variably both its release and its pressor effectiveness, is probably one of the main reasons for the well-documented absence of correlation between blood pressure changes and changes in plasma AVP levels induced by various maneuvers, as stated earlier.

The contribution of the hydroosmotic effect (i.e., fluid retention via excessive renal tubular reabsorption) of AVP to blood pressure elevation is another matter of on-going debate. Although the term *volume-expanded hypertension* is still widely used, it is probably a misnomer, since it implies increased intravascular fluid volume with overfilling of the arterial tree. Various theories are proposed from time to time in order to reconcile the concept of volume-expanded hypertension with the fact that blood volume is not expanded in hypertension (40). This term was originally coined to indicate one extreme of a hypothetical bipole, whose other extreme was intense vasoconstriction due to excessive release of renin-angiotensin (41). However, it is now generally accepted that there can be no arterial hypertension without arteriolar constriction and elevation of peripheral vascular resistances. Accordingly, the salt-dependent hypertension, which occupies the opposite end from the renin-dependent type in the above bipole, is also due to vasoconstriction, which in this case is sustained by other (nonrenin) pressor mechanisms (42,43). Excessive retention of fluid does exist in a variety of pathologic conditions; intravascular fluid volume expansion with hemodilution is encountered in a number of metabolic disorders, ranging from water intoxication, to hyponatremic congestive heart failure, to the syndrome of inappropriate antidiuretic hormone secretion, none of which is characterized by hypertension (indeed, the latter syndrome, as mentioned earlier, has been used as one of the arguments against AVP's contribution to hypertension). Expansion of the "third" space, i.e., the extravascular fluid volume, is not related to arterial pressure, as illustrated by the fact that edematous conditions are generally not associated with hypertension.

Therefore, in our view, the only contribution that the renal effect of AVP could have to hypertension is the correction of the hypovolemic state, whenever such state exists, and restoration of normovolemia. This position is not accepted by everyone, as other investigators believe that the antidiuretic activity of AVP is necessary for the development of hypertension. This belief is mainly based on the fact that deamino-8-D-arginine vasopressin (dDAVP) is a synthetic peptide analog of AVP with only agonistic V_2-receptor activity, can restore the capacity of congenitally AVP-deficient rats to develop salt-induced hypertension (see below). However, our thesis is that this hypertensive effect of V_2 agonists is exerted not so much via the renal V_2 receptors, but rather via the central nervous system receptors of AVP, which, although distinct from the classic V_1 and V_2 receptors, can be activated by compounds with both V_1 and V_2 binding characteristics. The data summarized below are consistent with the thesis that the AVP effects most pertinent to hypertension are more likely to be those exerted on the CNS receptors (V_3?).

CONTRIBUTION OF AVP TO VARIOUS TYPES OF HYPERTENSION

A number of studies have investigated the role of AVP in the development and maintenance of various pathogenetically different types of experimental or human hypertension.

Acute Experimental Hypertension

Two types of acute experimental hypertension have been causally linked with excessive stimulation of AVP release.

Acute infusions of hypertonic saline in totally anephric or subtotally nephrectomized animals or deoxycorti-

costerone acetate (DOCA)-salt hypertensive animals induce sharp rises in blood pressure, accompanied by
increases in plasma AVP and catecholamine levels (44–
47). This hypertensive response is characterized by intense vasocontriction with evidence of contracted intravascular fluid volume (42,45). It is reversible in part by
V_1 inhibition and in part by sympathetic blockade, and
is completely abolished when both systems are inhibited,
indicating that it is attributable to vasoconstriction due
partly to the direct pressor effect of AVP and partly to
sympathetic stimulation (44–46).

Acute neurogenic hypertension induced by lesions in
certain areas of the brainstem has also been attributed in
part to AVP stimulation. Lesions of the A_1 area of the
ventrolateral medulla produce an acute severe hypertension leading to pulmonary edema (48). This mostly neurogenic hypertension is attributed to a large extent to
sympathetic overdrive secondary to destruction of sympathoinhibitory neurons (49). However, it was also
found to be partly AVP-dependent as it was accompanied by a surge in AVP release (50,51) and was partly
reversible by systemic administration of an antivasopressor AVP antagonist (50). Likewise, destructive lesions in
the area of the nucleus tractus solitarii (NTS) produced
acute hypertension attributable to both increased sympathoadrenal activity and excessive release of vasopressin (52,53); both catecholamines and AVP were elevated
in the systemic circulation, and either blockade of AVP
or sympathetic inhibition could in part reverse the hypertensive response. In contrast, microinjection of hypertonic saline in the NTS also produced an acute, hypertensive response attributable to disinhibition of
central sympathoinhibitory neurons, but this was not associated with elevation of circulating AVP (54) and
could not be prevented or reversed by systemic AVP
blockade (55). Other CNS manipulations, such as fastigial stimulation (56,57), dorsolateral transection of the
medulla to isolate the NTS (58), or stimulation of certain
hypothalamic regions, such as the AV3V area and paraventricular nuclei, with certain peptides (59) or calcium
ions (60), can also produce acute hypertensive responses
attributable, to a large extent, to central stimulation
of AVP.

Although it is generally accepted that stimulation of
central vasopressinergic neurons must play an important
role in the sequence of events that leads to sympathoexcitatory pressor reactions, it is still unclear whether this
role is limited to a central neuromodulatory action of
AVP on sympathetic neurons or whether AVP's peripheral vasoconstrictor effect also contributes to the blood
pressure rise. Indeed, some of the above-cited studies
have reported that the acute hypertensive response elicited by these maneuvers can be partly reversed or prevented by systemic administration of an antivasopressor
AVP antagonist (50), and others failed to demonstrate
such effect (55).

Furthermore, when exogenous AVP is introduced in
minute amounts directly into certain areas of the CNS, it
also produces an immediate rise in blood pressure (BP).
These amounts would be too small to exert a peripheral
vasopressor effect. Such experiments have used various
techniques such as microinjection or microiontophoresis into well-defined areas of the brainstem (61–63)
or into the cerebral ventricles (64,65), in doses insufficient to induce systemic arterial pressor effects. The resulting rise in BP was invariably characterized by increased sympathetic outflow attributable to activation of
central catecholaminergic neurons (63,65–67).

These data have led us to propose the "ignition key"
theory to describe AVP's role in linking acute salt loading to central sympathetic stimulation (68). According to
this theory, salt loading initially causes a release of AVP,
which acts via descending vasopressinergic pathways
from the periventricular hypothalamic region that are
linked to ascending catecholaminergic neurons of the
dorsal and ventrolateral medulla (69). These complex
neuronal circuits permit the reciprocal influence between peptidergic and aminergic nerve fibers and receptors; moreover, they may be influenced even by systemically circulating substances that might be unable to cross
the blood-brain barrier, because some relevant areas
that are anatomically linked to this circuit (e.g., area
postrema) are considered to lie outside the blood-brain
barrier. Therefore, the major effect on blood pressure of
AVP or its peptide analogs, whether administered (or released) locally into the CNS or systemically in the peripheral circulation, may still be exerted mostly
centrally.

Chronic Experimental Hypertension

The peripheral vasoconstriction and elevated arteriolar resistance of non–renin-dependent hypertension is
maintained by a variety of pressor mechanisms, of which
the most prominent is sympathetic overactivity (42). Experimentally, this hypertension is produced either by inbreeding (strains of rats with genetic predisposition to
hypertension) or by chronic salt loading aided by various
maneuvers such as reduction of renal mass and treatment with DOCA.

The DOCA-salt model is the one in which the role of
AVP has been most extensively investigated (47,70–81).
These studies were spurred by an early experiment demonstrating that small doses of pitressin could accelerate
the development of DOCA-salt hypertension (82). When
measurements of plasma and urine levels of endogenous
AVP became available, they were reported to be elevated
in this model, even though only rarely did plasma AVP
levels correlate with the height of blood pressure (78).
These animals were also found to have increased vascular reactivity to AVP.

Further evidence in support of AVP's pressor contribution to this hypertension was derived from the partial fall of blood pressure in response to systemic administration of an antivasopressor V_1 antagonist (47,71,78). However, other investigators have reported that a V_1 antagonist failed to produce a blood pressure fall in this model (76,77,83–85). This is in accordance with our own experience when we administered the V_1 antagonist in the established phase of hypertension in this model (personal observations, unpublished). As a possible explanation for these discrepancies, it was proposed that AVP may act as a pressor agent only in later stages of DOCA-salt hypertension, when the increased vascular reactivity to it has been well established and when the attenuating influence of baroreflexes has been impaired (75). Although this is possible as a contributory mechanism, our experience with acute salt-induced hypertension suggests that it is more likely that AVP participates to a great extent in the earliest induction phase by acting as the "ignition key," mentioned earlier, that sets in motion the hyperadrenergic response to salt loading.

In an effort to better define the contribution of AVP in the development of DOCA-salt hypertension, several investigators chose also to study this type of hypertension in rats genetically deficient in AVP (71,73,74,76,85–87). They found that it was not possible to induce hypertension in Brattleboro rats with hereditary diabetes insipidus unless the rats were pretreated with exogenous AVP. These rats were also found to have an abnormal baroreflex mechanism, whose sensitivity could be restored to normal by administration of small (nonpressor) doses of AVP (87). Interestingly, the capability of these rats to develop DOCA-salt hypertension could also be restored by treatment with dDAVP, an AVP analog with potent V_2 (renal) agonistic properties but with minimal, if any, V_1 pressor effect (80,87). Moreover, DOCA-salt rats, as mentioned earlier, were also shown to have an exaggerated renal tubular response to AVP (88).

All of these findings led to the conclusion that the antidiuretic property of AVP is necessary to enhance fluid retention and volume expansion in order to produce this type of hypertension, whereas the vasopressor property is not important. And yet, whenever saline intake or blood volume expansion were measured, they were similar in those AVP-deficient animals that did develop some hypertension and those that did not (86). An additional argument in favor of this interpretation was the fact that many studies, as mentioned earlier, failed to demonstrate a blood pressure fall in response to antivasopressor V_1 antagonists in DOCA-salt rats.

However, this interpretation is flawed because it fails to take into account the effects of these peptides on central vasopressinergic receptors. This is best illustrated by attempts to induce DOCA-salt hypertension in Brattleboro rats with or without lesions of the anteroventral region of the third ventricle (AV3V) (73), an area particularly rich in vasopressinergic neurons (89). Whereas

sham-lesioned rats could become hypertensive by DOCA-salt if treated with exogenous AVP, AV3V lesioned ones could not, even though their plasma AVP levels were comparable to those of normal intact rats treated by DOCA-salt. This suggests that AVP exerts its actions through central mechanisms, requiring the integrity of vasopressinergic neurons of the hypothalamus. Lesions in the area postrema, another area linked to AVP's central activity, were also recently reported to prevent the development of DOCA-salt hypertension (90). Taken in conjunction with previously mentioned studies involving manipulation of brain nuclei rich in catecholaminergic neurons and vasopressinergic projections, these findings support the hypothesis that AVP acts on central neural structures to enhance sympathetic outflow, and that DOCA-salt loading and possibly other locally generated neuropeptides stimulate AVP and increase the responsiveness of these neural structures to the central effects of AVP (59,91).

In various models of chronic renal hypertension associated with salt loading, the reports of AVP's contribution can be equally confusing. Such models include the abdominal aortic constriction proximal to the kidneys (92), the two-kidney-one-clip (93), the one-kidney-one-clip (84,94), the subtotally nephrectomized (46,95), and the one-kidney–figure 8–wrapped rats (96), with various degrees of renal insufficiency. In all of these rat models as well as in renal hypertension in dogs (97), AVP has been reported to be elevated at some point in the course of the development of the disease. However, their blood pressure responses to an antivasopressor AVP inhibitor have been inconsistent, with some studies reporting a small drop (95) and others no response at all (46,84). Attempts to clarify the issue by using the genetically AVP deficient Brattleboro rats have in fact added to the controversy: Some investigators could produce one-kidney-one-clip hypertension, albeit of a milder degree, in this strain, without AVP supplementation (86,98,99), suggesting that AVP may not be essential. Others were unable to produce the abdominal aortic constriction type of hypertension (92), unless the rats received exogenous AVP. The fact that AVP analogs with only V_2 (antidiuretic) agonistic properties, such as dDAVP or dVDAVP, could restore the capacity of these rats (92,100), just like the DOCA-salt rats mentioned earlier, to develop severe hypertension has been usually viewed as evidence that the renal tubular activity of AVP is needed for expansion of blood volume in the so-called volume-dependent form of hypertension (98,101); this, despite the lack of consistent data in support of the postulated increase in intravascular fluid volume. The recent information that a V_2 agonist analog can restore the capacity of Brattleboro rats to develop a renin-dependent (as opposed to volume-expanded) type of hypertension, i.e., the type induced by aortic constriction (92), would be even harder to reconcile with this view. In fact, the authors of that article concluded that AVP may act in this setting by sensitizing the arteries to the pressor effect of other vasoconstrictors, such as angiotensin II. Interestingly, neither renal–high salt (102) nor DOCA-salt hypertension (103) could be prevented by chronic antivasopressor AVP inhibition in normal rats.

In contrast, there is a general agreement that the relevance of AVP in experimental malignant phase hypertension is less likely. Plasma AVP levels can be very high in this condition regardless of its pathogenetic origin, i.e., regardless of whether it is the end stage of a DOCA-salt hypertension or of two-kidney-one-clip renovascular hypertension (70,78,93). However, the vasodepressor response to a V_1 antagonist is reported to be minimal (78). It should be kept in mind that both types are characterized by severe vasoconstriction, hemoconcentration, and hypovolemia, with evidence of acute fluid loss (104). Accordingly, the high levels of plasma AVP are probably the result of the cycles of acute diuresis characteristic of the evolution of this syndrome, rather than the cause of the concurrent vasoconstriction. The fact that Brattleboro rats can also develop malignant hypertension is another piece of evidence against a pathogenetic role of AVP in this syndrome (105).

Other salt-dependent models of experimental hypertension in which the role of AVP has been extensively investigated are those with genetic hypertension, such as the various strains of spontaneously hypertensive rats (SHRs) of Okamoto and Aoki (106–111), the Dahl S rats (112), and the Sabra rats (113,114). In some of these the plasma levels of AVP were found to be elevated at various ages (106,107,112). Yet other studies reported depressed levels of AVP in SHRs (115).

Administration of an antivasopressor AVP antagonist has also led to contradictory reports: Some studies reported a fall in blood pressure (106) whereas others failed to confirm such response (109,112). Moreover, as with the salt-loaded models mentioned earlier, continuous infusion of this antagonist in young SHRs from 4 to 13 weeks of age failed to alter the rate or magnitude of increase in blood pressure (116), suggesting that AVP plays no pathogenetic pressor role in SHRs. In this case, however, it could be argued that 4 weeks of age was already too late since by that age SHRs have already higher blood pressures than control Wistar-Kyoto rats, and therefore the possible early neuromodulatory actions of AVP on central sympathetic neurons may have already taken place. In support of this view are reports of abnormal patterns of distribution of central catecholaminergic and vasopressinergic neurons (111) and abnormal central responses (117,118) or content of AVP in brain nuclei of SHRs (108,119) or Sabra rats (113,114).

On the other hand, it has also been suggested that some of these abnormalities could be not the cause but the result of chronically elevated blood pressure in these

models (111). However, it is interesting to note that the genetically AVP deficient Brattleboro rats were also found to have abnormal noradrenergic innervation of hypothalamic nuclei (120), which may indicate that AVP plays a role even in the ontogenesis of normal noradrenergic innervation patterns in the CNS.

Increased pressor responsiveness to AVP has been reported for various genetically hypertensive rats, including SHRs (110) and Dahl S rats (112). This has been suggested as a possible explanation for the fact that even when AVP levels are reported to be elevated, they are not nearly as high as the pharmacologic doses necessary to elicit a pressor response in normal animals, and yet they are incriminated, at least in part, for the maintenance of hypertension in these strains.

In summary, it appears that for all the salt-dependent forms of experimental hypertension, whether acute or chronic, the evidence suggests that AVP may play an important role at least in the early stages of its induction, if not its chronic maintenance. The debate in the literature is mostly as to whether the vasopressor or renotubular properties of the hormone are the sine qua non for the development of hypertension. The prevailing opinion seems to be that the V_2-mediated retention of excessive amounts of water is a prerequisite for the initiation of hypertension because salt-induced hypertension is still widely considered to be volume expanded (despite the lack of convincing evidence for this concept) and because pure V_2 agonists can be substituted for AVP to restore the capacity of AVP-deficient animals to develop hypertension.

Since we have already presented ample evidence that these models of salt-dependent hypertension are in fact characterized by contracted, not expanded, intravascular fluid volume (42,45), we offer an alternative explanation for these findings: Either AVP or dDAVP and dVDAVP (the V_2 agonists) can facilitate the induction of salt-dependent hypertension, not via hydroosmotic action on the renal tubule, but via activation of vasopressinergic CNS receptors. These receptors, which are neither V_1 nor V_2 (4) and are sometimes referred to as V_3, are not yet defined and characterized, but appear to share some of the characteristics from both the V_1 and the V_2 populations, because they respond to selective AVP analogs with either V_1 or V_2 binding properties. It is therefore likely that the substituted dDAVP or dVDAVP in the above experiments acted as a neurotransmitter and/or neuromodulator in Brattleboro rats, rather than as an antidiuretic-volume expander. Accordingly, it is neither the direct vasopressor nor the hydroosmotic action, but rather the CNS effect of AVP—i.e., the modulation of sympathetic neuronal function—that should be considered as the crucial factor in the induction of the various types of salt-dependent hypertension, which are invariably characterized by increased sympathetic outflow.

AVP in Human Hypertension

Most human studies investigating the role of AVP in hypertension are based on measurements of plasma and urine levels in various hypertensive populations. Only a few have also used an antivasopressor V_1 antagonist to evaluate blood pressure responses.

Measurements of plasma AVP levels in essential hypertension have given conflicting results: Generally elevated AVP levels had been reported earlier (121), but a more recent publication from the same team found that only hypertensive men had significantly higher AVP (122). Others found no difference between normals and hypertensives with various degrees of severity in either basal or stimulated AVP (123). Another group reported generally lower AVP levels in essential hypertension and primary hyperaldosteronism, while elevated levels were seen only in malignant hypertension, in which case they were probably the result of salt and fluid loss rather than the cause of hypertension (12). Similar results, i.e., lower AVP levels in low-renin hypertension and primary aldosteronism and higher in malignant hypertension than in normal subjects, were also reported by a group of Japanese authors (124), but these authors interpreted this as evidence that AVP seems to play a role in malignant hypertension only.

In contrast, a Swedish group found that AVP levels are significantly higher in low-renin essential hypertension, as compared to normal-renin hypertensives and to normotensive controls (125,126). Interestingly, the low-renin hypertensives in these studies were also found to have evidence of sympathetic overactivity, which would be consistent with the experimental data cited earlier. Evidence of decreased central dopaminergic activity was also reported by this group in essential hypertensive men (127), a finding particularly interesting in the light of previous animal studies that suggested that AVP release is under constant dopaminergic inhibition (29,30). It is important to note that the findings of increased AVP and decreased dopaminergic activity persisted when these patients were compared with age-matched controls, as some studies have reported normal ranges of AVP to be higher in older subjects (128). In our own studies we found no age-related difference in AVP in normotensive subjects (129), but we detected a significant racial difference between elderly hypertensive patients: Blacks, with presumably low-renin hypertension, had more than twice the average AVP levels of white age-matched hypertensives (130).

In studies exploring the responsiveness of AVP to various manipulations, it was found that hypertensives were no different from normotensives when challenged with phlebotomy, water loading or restriction, or salt restriction, i.e., both volumetric and hydroosmotic challenges (131–134). However, one study suggested that the renal tubular responsiveness to AVP may be diminished, which would require a larger compensatory increase in AVP (135); another pointed out that if AVP response is plotted against the absolute blood pressures it would appear that in hypertensives the relationship is skewed in a manner suggesting increased stimulation in response to blood pressure lowering, which might antagonize the effectiveness of antihypertensive drugs (134).

A consistent feature in all these studies has been the lack of correlation between blood pressure levels and plasma levels of AVP. Indeed, the one pathologic condition with excessively high circulating levels of AVP is the syndrome of inappropriate antidiuretic hormone (SIADH) encountered in various neurologic disturbances, drug reactions, or paraneoplastic syndromes, all of which tend to have normal or low blood pressure, despite evidence of hypervolemia with hemodilution. This has been used as one of the arguments against AVP's pressor contribution to hypertension (136,137). The only known case of SIADH associated with hypertension was recently reported in a young man with neuroblastoma in whom both the metabolic aberrations and the hypertension were reversed after resection of the tumor (138).

The development of one antivasopressor V_1 antagonist for human use helped to further promote our knowledge of the pressor effects of AVP. This highly specific V_1 antagonist is d$(CH_2)_5$Tyr(Me) AVP (139), which in doses of 0.5 mg IV can block the pressor activity of exogenous AVP by over 80% (140). In well-hydrated human volunteers in the resting state, this compound produced no blood pressure change (141,142), suggesting that AVP plays no role in maintaining normotension, as would be expected from previous experimental studies in animals (33). However, in severe salt-induced hypertension of end-stage renal disease (a situation analogous to that of the anephric animal infused with hypertonic saline), where AVP was found to be somewhat higher than normal (143), the V_1 antagonist did produce a modest but consistent fall in supine blood pressure by 9 to 12 mm Hg (140) within 20 to 45 minutes.

In patients with accelerated or malignant hypertension of various causes, the V_1 antagonist produced a small blood pressure fall when given as a first drug; however, if the patients had been pretreated by a sympatholytic agent (clonidine), the AVP antagonist produced a substantial fall of blood pressure up to 18 mm Hg in diastolic (144). The largest falls were observed in patients pretreated with doses of clonidine high enough to suppress plasma norepinephrine levels to the range of 80 pg/ml (normal 250–400 pg/ml). This again is consistent with the animal experiments that have shown AVP to assume an important pressor role only after sympathetic inhibition, thus acting as a backup rather than a primary pressor mechanism in the sustenance of a certain blood pressure level (33). It also confirms the prediction of the above-mentioned study, based on plotting of AVP-pressure relationships in normotensives and hypertensives (134), that the pressor effect of AVP may significantly antagonize the therapeutic effect of antihypertensive drugs.

In mild uncomplicated essential hypertension, the AVP antagonist did not produce cardiovascular effects unless AVP had been stimulated by various maneuvers such as cigarette smoking or sauna (145). In our own experience, patients with mild to moderate hypertension likewise had no blood pressure fall in the supine resting state (141). However, in the standing position the AVP antagonist produced decrements in mean blood pressure averaging 7 to 15 mm Hg, depending on the age and race of the patients: Young and white subjects had the least, whereas elderly and blacks had the most pronounced falls. All elderly patients in this study had subclinical evidence of autonomic insufficiency brought about by specific maneuvers (146). Interestingly, diabetic hypertensive patients with clinical evidence of autonomic neuropathy (who already had mild postural hypotension), after receiving one dose of the AVP antagonist, had no change in supine blood pressure, but exhibited an average postural diastolic blood pressure fall by 44 mm Hg (147). All of these data indicate that AVP plays a major role in sustaining high blood pressure in the upright posture, especially in hypertensives with impaired sympathetic function and/or suppressed renin-angiotensin activity.

A particularly intriguing feature in these studies is the fact that the orthostatic blood pressure fall did not occur immediately upon assuming the erect position, but became apparent at about 1 hour after orthostasis and ambulation (i.e., approximately 2 hours after IV administration of the AVP antagonist), and continued for an additional hour of observation, after which there was a tendency to recovery. This time course cannot be easily explained by a mechanism of direct competitive inhibition of AVP at the vascular wall V_1 receptor level as has been postulated for anephric animals or humans after acute salt-loading. It therefore appears likely that the antagonist may have acted either on the baroreceptors to gradually eliminate the AVP-induced sensitization or through a CNS-mediated mechanism. At this point it is not clear whether peripherally circulating AVP or its peptide analogs can cross the blood-brain barrier; however, some brain regions relevant to the central action of AVP, such as the area postrema and the organum vasculosum of lamina terminalis (OVLT), are believed to lie outside the blood-brain barrier, and would therefore be within reach of circulating AVP and/or its peptide analogs, regardless of these compounds' ability to penetrate other brain regions. It is possible then that the delay in the postural effects of the AVP antagonist may represent the time necessary to interfere with the function of central vasopressinergic neurons.

An additional action of AVP that may or may not play a role in blood pressure regulation, but has received very little attention to date, is the direct vasodilatory effect mediated via extrarenal V_2-like receptors (148–151). The existence of such receptors is still hypothetical, supported by indirect findings with the use of selective AVP agonists and antagonists. There is not enough information at this point to permit speculation as to a possible contribution of this function in blood pressure regulation. The recent development of nonpeptide orally active AVP antagonists effective in humans with selective V_1 (152,153) or V_2 (Dr. T. Sato, Otsuka Pharmaceuticals, personal communication) antagonistic capacity should solve these problems and promote the therapeutic application of the earlier experimental findings.

CONCLUSIONS

It is increasingly being recognized that vasopressin plays an important role in the development and maintenance of several types of hypertension. Much of the controversy regarding the magnitude of this role stems from the assumption that the major pressor function of AVP might be exerted via the V_1 receptors on the vascular wall, and might be expected to correlate with circulating AVP levels. However, the recently accumulated knowledge from both experimental and human studies suggests that this is not the case. In fact, hypertensive conditions where endogenous AVP levels are the highest, such as experimental or human malignant hypertension, are indeed the least AVP-dependent, and in these cases the rise in AVP seems to be simply a reaction to the accompanying hypovolemia and hemoconcentration. The renal tubular (V_2-mediated) action of AVP, which is important in restoring compromised blood volume, is probably also noncontributory to hypertension, since abnormal intravascular volume expansion is not a consistent characteristic of the most AVP-dependent type, i.e., the acute salt-induced hypertension.

The evidence reviewed in this chapter suggests that AVP is part of a highly integrated neurohumoral system, where pressor hormones and autonomic neurons influence each other's actions. Accordingly, the major role of AVP as a hypertensive factor seems to be that of a neuromodulator acting through central nervous system receptors on vasopressinergic and catecholaminergic neurons to alter baroreflex sensitivity and sympathetic outflow. Although the nature of these CNS receptors, occasionally referred to as V_3, has not yet been defined, it appears that they are capable of responding to agents with either V_1 or V_2 binding characteristics, while possessing additional actions (such as learning and memory enhancement [154]) that are apparently unrelated to, and unaffected by, the above characteristics. The recent cloning of genes for AVP and its receptors (155,156) should permit the use of molecular biology techniques for assessment of AVP gene expression in various tissues and models of hypertension and for further characterization of V receptor subtypes.

REFERENCES

1. Schiffrin EL, Genest J. ³H-vasopressin in binding to the rat mesenteric artery. *Endocrinology* 1983;113:409–411.
2. Cantau B, Keppens S, DeWulf H, Jard S. (³H)-vasopressin binding to isolated rat hepatocytes and liver membranes: regulation by GTP and relation to glycogen phosphorylase activation. *J Recept Res* 1980;1:137–168.
3. Guillon G, Butlen D, Cantau B, Barth T, Jard S. Kinetic and pharmacological characterization of vasopressin membrane receptors from human kidney medulla: relation to adenylate cyclase activation. *Eur J Pharmacol* 1982;85:291–304.
4. Knepel W, Homolka L, Vlaskovska M, Nutto D. *In vivo* adrenocorticotropin beta endorphin releasing activity of vasopressin analogues is related neither to pressor nor to antidiuretic activity. *Endocrinology* 1984;114:1797–1804.
5. Mitchell RH, Kirk CJ, Billah MM. Hormonal stimulation of phosphatidylinositol breakdown with particular reference to the hepatic effects of vasopressin. *Biochem Soc Trans* 1979;7:861–865.
6. Litosch I, Sue-Hwa L, Fain JN. Rapid changes in hepatocyte phosphoinositides induced by vasopressin. *J Biol Chem* 1983;258:13727–12732.
7. Jard S. Vasopressin isoreceptors in mammals: relation to cyclic AMP-dependent and cyclic AMP-independent transduction mechanisms. In: Kleinzeller A, Martin BR, eds. *Membrane receptors*. New York: Academic Press, 1983;255–280.
8. Altura BM, Altura TT. Vascular smooth muscle and neurohypophyseal hormones. *Fed Proc* 1977;36:1853–1860.
9. Monos E, Cox RH, Peterson LH. Direct effect of physiological doses of arginine vasopressin on the arterial wall *in vivo*. *Am J Physiol* 1978;234:H167–H172.
10. Cowley AW, Monos E, Guyton AC. Interaction of vasopressin and the baroreceptor reflex system in the regulation of arterial blood pressure in the dog. *Circ Res* 1974;34:505–514.
11. Montani JP, Liard JF, Schoun J, Mohring J. Hemodynamic effects of exogenous and endogenous vasopressin at low plasma concentrations in conscious dogs. *Circ Res* 1980;47:346–355.
12. Morton JJ, Padfield PL. Vasopressin and hypertension. *J Cardiovasc Pharmacol* 1986;8(suppl 7):S101–106.
13. Pullan PT, Johnston CI, Anderson WP, Korner PI. Plasma vasopressin in blood pressure homeostasis and in experimental renal hypertension. *Am J Physiol* 1980;239:H81–H87.
14. Cowley AW Jr, Quillen EW Jr, Skelton MM. Role of vasopressin in cardiovascular regulation. *Fed Proc* 1983;42:3170–3176.
15. Mohring J, Glanzer K, Maciel A, Dusing R, Kramer HJ, Arbogast R, Koch-Weser J. Greatly enhanced pressor response to antidiuretic hormone in patients with impaired cardiovascular reflexes due to idiopathic orthostatic hypotension. *J Clin Pharmacol* 1980;2:367–376.
16. DiPette D, Gavras I, North W, DiPette P, Gavras H. Vasopressin response to hyperosmotic stimulus. Blood pressure effect in normal subjects and in patients with impaired sympathetic system. *Clin Exp Hypertens [Abstract]* 1984;6(4):851–861.
17. Wagner HN Jr, Braunwald E. The pressor effect of the antidiuretic principle of the posterior pituitary in orthostatic hypotension. *J Clin Invest* 1956;35:1412.
18. Heyndrickx BD, Boettcher D, Vatner S. Effects of angiotensin, vasopressin and methoxamine on cardiac function and blood flow distribution in conscious dogs. *Am J Physiol* 1976;231:1579–1587.
19. Schmid PF, Abboud M, Wendling E, Ramberg A, Mark A, Heistad D, Eckstein J. Regional vascular effects of vasopressin: plasma levels and circulatory responses. *Am J Physiol* 1974;227:998–1004.
20. Charocopos F, Hatzinikolaou P, North WG, Gavras H. Systemic

and regional hemodynamic effects of endogenous vasopressin stimulation in rats. *Am J Physiol* 1982;243(*Heart Circ Physiol* 12):H560–H565.
21. Gavras H, Liang C, Brunner HR. Redistribution of regional blood flow after inhibition of the angiotensin-converting enzyme. *Circ Res* 1978;43(suppl I):56–63.
22. Bartelstone HJ, Nasmyth PA. Vasopressin potentiation of catecholamine actions in dog, rat, cat, and rat aortic strip. *Am J Physiol* 1965;208:754.
23. Mitchell LD, Barron K, Brody MJ, Johnson AK. Two possible actions for circulating angiotensin II in the control of vasopressin release. *Peptides* 1982;3:503–507.
24. Brooks VL, Keil LC, Reid IA. Role of the renin-angiotensin system in the control of vasopressin secretion in conscious dogs. *Circ Res* 1986;58:829–838.
25. Hoffman PK, Share L, Crofton JT, Shade RE. The effect of intracerebroventricular indomethacin on osmotically stimulated vasopressin release. *Neuroendocrinology* 1982;34:132–139.
26. Brooks DP, Share L, Crofton JT, Nasjeletti A. Central indomethacin enhances volume-dependent vasopressin release. *Am J Physiol* 1984;247:R1017–R1021.
27. Gavras I, Hatinoglou S, Benetos A, Gavras H. Calcium stimulates vasopressin release. *J Hypertens* 1986;4:451–454.
28. Urano A, Kobayashi H. Effects of noradrenaline and dopamine injected into the supraoptic nucleus on urine flow rate in hydrated rats. *Exp Neurol* 1978;60:140–150.
29. Forsling ML, Ivensen LL, Lightman SL. Dopamine and enkephalin directly inhibit vasopressin release from the neurohypophysis. *J Physiol (Lond)* 1981;319:66.
30. Hatzinikolaou P, Gavras H, North WG, Kohlmann O, Gavras H. Evidence for dopaminergic regulation of vasopressin release in the anephric rat. *J Hypertens* 1984;2:311–315.
31. Ishikawa SE, Schrier RW. Evidence for a role of opioid peptides in the release of arginine vasopressin in the conscious rat. *J Clin Invest* 1981;69:666–672.
32. Share L. Centrally acting humoral factors in the control of vasopressin release. In: Cross BA, Leng G, eds. *The neurohypophysis: structure, function and control. Progress in brain research.* Amsterdam: Elsevier, 1983;425–435.
33. Gavras H, Hatzinikolaou P, North WG, Bresnahan M, Gavras I. Interaction of the sympathetic nervous system with vasopressin and renin in the maintenance of blood pressure. *Hypertension* 1982;4(suppl 3):400–405.
34. Houck PC, Fiksen-Olsen MJ, Britton SL, Romero JC. Role of angiotensin and vasopressin on blood pressure of ganglionic blocked dogs. *Am J Physiol* 1983;244(*Heart Circ Physiol* 13):H115–H120.
35. Paller MS, Linas SL. Role of angiotensin II, alpha-adrenergic system, and arginine vasopressin on arterial pressure in rat. *Am J Physiol* 1984;246(*Heart Circ Physiol* 15):H25–H30.
36. Gardiner SM, Bennett T. The contribution of the autonomic nervous system, the renin-angiotensin system and vasopressin to the maintenance of arterial blood pressure in adrenalectomized Wistar rats. *Clin Sci* 1986;71:357–365.
37. Gavras I, Hatinoglou S, Gavras H. The adrenergic system and the release and pressor action of vasopressin. *Hypertension* 1986;8(suppl II):II-163–II-167.
38. Kimura T, Shoji M, Iitake K, Kozo O, Matsui K, Yoshinaga K. The role of central alpha-1 and alpha-2 adrenoceptors in the regulation of vasopressin release and the cardiovascular system. *Endocrinology* 1984;114:1426.
39. Vlahakos D, Gavras I, Gavras H. Alpha-adrenoceptor agonists applied in the area of the nucleus tractus solitarii in the rat: effect of anesthesia on cardiovascular responses. *Brain Res* 1985;347:372–375.
40. Hamlyn JM, Blaustein MP. Sodium chloride, extracellular fluid volume, and blood pressure regulation. *Am J Physiol* 1986;2(suppl 4):F563–F575.
41. Laragh JH. Vasoconstriction—volume analysis for understanding and treating hypertension: the use of renin and aldosterone profiles. In: Laragh JH, ed. *Hypertension manual.* New York: Yorke Medical Books, 1974;823–849.
42. Gavras H. Possible mechanisms of sodium-dependent hyperten-

sion: volume expansion or vasoconstriction? *Clin Exp Hypertens* [*Abstract*] 1982;4(4&5):737–749.

43. Gavras H. How does salt raise blood pressure? A hypothesis. *Hypertension* 1986;8:83–88.

44. Hatzinikolaou P, Gavras H, Brunner HR, Gavras I. Sodium-induced elevation of blood pressure in the anephric state. *Science* 1980;209:935–936.

45. Hatzinikolaou P, Gavras H, Brunner HR, Gavras I. Role of vasopressin, catecholamines, and plasma volume in hypertonic saline-induced hypertension. *Am J Physiol* 1981;240(*Heart Circ Physiol* 9):H827–H831.

46. DiPette DJ, Gavras I, North WG, Brunner HR, Gavras H. Vasopressin in salt-induced hypertension of experimental renal insufficiency. *Hypertension* 1982;4(suppl II):II-125–II-130.

47. Crofton JT, Share L, Brooks DP. Osmotic stimulation in DOC-salt hypertension: vasopressin and blood pressure. *J Hypertens* 1986;4:307–312.

48. Blessing WW, West MJ, Chalmers J. Hypertension, bradycardia and pulmonary oedema in the conscious rabbit after brainstem lesions coinciding with the A1 group of catecholamine neurones. *Circ Res* 1981;49:959–970.

49. Blessing WW, Reis DJ. Inhibitory cardiovascular function of neurons in the caudal ventrolateral medulla of the rabbit: relationship to the area containing A1 noradrenergic cells. *Brain Res* 1982;253:161–171.

50. Blessing WW, Sved AF, Reis DJ. Destruction of noradrenergic neurones in rabbit brainstem elevates plasma vasopressin, causing hypertension. *Science* 1981;217:661–663.

51. Minson J, Chalmers J, Kapoor V, Cain M, Caon A. Relative importance of sympathetic nerves and of circulating adrenaline and vasopressin in mediating hypertension after lesions of the caudal ventrolateral medulla in the rat. *J Hypertens* 1981;4:273–281.

52. Sved AF. Peripheral pressor systems in hypertension caused by nucleus tractus solitarius lesions. *Hypertension* 1986;8:742–747.

53. Kubo T, Kihara M. Contribution of vasopressin to hypertension caused by baroreceptor denervation and nucleus tractus solitarius lesions in rats. *J Pharmacobiodyn* 1986;9:626–629.

54. Vlahakos D, Gavras H. Central sympathetic stimulation produced by saline application into the nucleus tractus solitarii area of conscious rats. *Neurosci Lett* 1988;92:335–340.

55. Gavras H, Bain GT, Bland L, Vlahakos D, Gavras I. Hypertensive response to saline microinjection in the area of the nucleus tractus solitarii of the rat. *Brain Res* 1985;343:113–119.

56. Delbo A, Sved AF, Reis DJ. Fastigial stimulation releases vasopressin in amounts that elevate arterial pressure. *Am J Physiol* 1983;244:H687–H694.

57. Delbo A, Sved AF, Reis DJ. Inhibitory influences from arterial baroreceptors in vasopressin release elicited by fastigial stimulation in rats. *Circ Res* 1984;54:248–253.

58. Grojec ZZ, Bayorh MA, Zebre RL, Palkovits M, Kopin IJ. Role of catecholamines and vasopressin in cardiovascular responses to bilateral dorsolateral transection of the medulla oblongata in the rat. *Hypertension* 1983;5:908–915.

59. Gruber KA, Eskridge SL, Callahan MF. Activation of the central vasopressin system: a potential factor in the etiology of hypertension. *Klin Wochenschr* 1987;65(suppl 8):82–86.

60. Benetos A, Gavras I, Gavras H. Stimulation of vasopressin by calcium microinjections in the area of the paraventricular nucleus of the hypothalamus. *Brain Res* 1987;412:182–184.

61. Pittman QJ, Lawrence D, McLean L. Central effects of arginine vasopressin on blood pressure in rats. *Endocrinology* 1982;110:1058–1060.

62. Matsuguchi H, Sharabi RM, Gordon FJ, Johnson AK, Schmid PG. Blood pressure and heart rate responses to microinjection of vasopressin into the nucleus tractus solitarius region of the rat. *Neuropharmacology* 1982;2:29–31.

63. Berecek KH, Olpe HR, Hofbauer KG. Responsiveness of locus ceruleus neurons in hypertensive rats to vasopressin. *Hypertension* 1987;9(suppl III):III-110–III-113.

64. Berecek KH, Mah SC, Baum P, Hofbauer KG. Cardiovascular effects of intracerebroventricular injection of vasopressin in unanesthetized normotensive and DOCA-salt hypertensive rats. *Hypertens* 1984;2:29–31.

65. Tan DP, Tsou K. New evidence for neuronal function of vaso-

66. Feuerstein G, Zerbe RL, Faden AI. Central cardiovascular effects of mammalian neurohypophyseal peptides in conscious rats. *Peptides* 1983;4:627–630.

67. Unger T, Rohmeiss P, Becker H, Ganten D, Lang RE, Petty M. Sympathetic activation following central vasopressin receptor stimulation in conscious rats. *J Hypertens* 1984;2:25–27.

68. Gavras I, Mulinari RA, Ribeiro AB, Gavras H. Role of vasopressin in hypertension and heart failure: clinical studies. In: Cowley AW, ed. *Vasopressin; cellular and integrative functions.* New York: Raven Press, 1988;467–479.

69. Sladek CD. Regulation of vasopressin release by neurotransmitters, neuropeptides and osmotic stimuli. *Brain Res* 1983;60:71–90.

70. Mohring J, Mohring B, Petri M, Haack D. Vasopressor role of ADH in the pathogenesis of malignant DOC hypertension. *Am J Physiol* 1977;232:F260–F269.

71. Crofton JT, Share L, Shade RE, Lee-Kwon WJ, Manning M, Sawyer WH. The importance of vasopressin in the development and maintenance of DOC-salt hypertension in the rat. *Hypertension* 1979;1:31–38.

72. Marchetti J, Thibbonier M, Gonzales MF, Corvol P, Menard J. Dynamic study of antidiuretic hormone during benign mineralocorticoid and metacorticoid hypertension. *Acta Endocrinol* 1980;95:444–453.

73. Berecek KH, Barron KW, Webb RL, Brody MJ. Vasopressin-central nervous system interactions in the development of DOCA hypertension. *Hypertension* 1982;4(suppl II):II-131–II-137.

74. Berecek KH, Murray RD, Gross F, Brody MJ. Vasopressin and vascular reactivity in the development of DOCA hypertension in rats with hereditary diabetes insipidus. *Hypertension* 1982;4:3–12.

75. Matsuguchi H, Schmid PG. Pressor response to vasopressin and impaired baroreflex function in DOC-salt hypertension. *Am J Physiol* 1982;242:H44.

76. Burnier M, Biollaz J, Brunner DB, Gavras H, Brunner HR. Alpha and beta adrenoceptor blockade in normotensive and deoxycorticosterone (DOC)-hypertensive rats: plasma vasopressin and vasopressin pressor effect. *J Pharmacol Exp Ther* 1983;224:221–227.

77. Yamamoto J, Yamane Y, Umeda Y, Yoshioka T, Nakai M, Ikeda M. Cardiovascular haemodynamics and vasopressin blockade in DOCA-salt rats. *Hypertension* 1984;6:397–402.

78. Hiwatari M, Abrahams JM, Saito T, Johnston CI. Contribution of vasopressin to the maintenance of blood pressure in deoxycorticosterone-salt induced malignant hypertension in spontaneously hypertensive rats. *Clin Sci* 1986;70:191–198.

79. Chen YF, Lindheimer MD, Oparil S. Increased vasopressinergic activity following DOCA administration in the rat. *Brain Res Bull* 1986;16:93–98.

80. Saito T, Yajima Y, Watanabe T. Involvement of AVP in the development and maintenance of hypertension in rats. In: Yoshida S, Share L, Yagi K, eds. *Antidiuretic hormone.* Baltimore: University Park Press, 1981;215–225.

81. Ouchi Y, Share L, Crofton JT, Iitake K, Brooks DP. Sex difference in the development of deoxycorticosterone-salt hypertension in the rat. *Hypertension* 1987;9:172–177.

82. Friedman SM, Friedman CL, Nakashima M. Accelerated appearance of DCA in rats treated with pitressin. *Endocrinology* 1960;67:752.

83. Okuno T, Winternitz SR, Lindheimer MD, Oparil S. Central catecholamine depletion, vasopressin and blood pressure in the DOCA/NaCl rat. *Am J Physiol* 1983;244:H807–H813.

84. Rabito SF, Carretero OA, Scicli AG. Evidence against a role of vasopressin in the maintenance of high blood pressure in mineralocorticoid and renovascular hypertension. *Hypertension* 1981;3:34–38.

85. Rascher W, Lang RE, Taubitz M, Meffle H, Unger T, Ganten D, Gross F. Vasopressin-induced increase in total peripheral resistance in deoxycorticosterone acetate hypertensive rats is buffered by the baroreceptor reflex. *Clin Sci* 1981;61:153s–156s.

86. Zicha J, Kunes J, Jelinek J. Age-dependent DOCA-salt hyperten-

sion in Brattleboro rats: the role of vasopressin. *Physiol Bohemoslov* 1987;36:33–42.

87. Imai Y, Nolan PL, Johnston CI. Restoration of suppressed baroreflex sensitivity in rats with hereditary diabetes insipidus (Brattleboro rats) by arginine-vasopressin and DDAVP. *Circ Res* 1983;53:140–149.

88. Pettinger WA, Fallet R, Wang Y, Tam LT, Jeffries WB. Enhanced cAMP response to vasopressin in the CCT of DOCA-Na hypertensive rats. *Am J Physiol* 1986;251:F1096–F1100.

89. Sofroniew MV. Vasopressin and oxytocin in the mammalian brain and spinal cord. *Trends Neurosci* 1983;6:467–471.

90. Bruner CA, Mangiapane ML, Fink GD, Webb RC. Area postrema lesion prevents hypertension but not altered vascular reactivity in deoxycorticosterone-salt treated rats [*Abstract*]. *Hypertension* 1987;10:364.

91. Berecek KH. Role of central vasopressin in cardiovascular regulation. *J Cardiovasc Pharmacol* 1986;8(suppl 7):S76–S80.

92. Aperia A, Sahlgren B, Eklof AC, Lundin S, Melin P. Role of arginine-vasopressin for the development of hypertension following aortic constriction. *Acta Physiol Scand* 1986;128:495–499.

93. Mohring J, Mohring B, Petri M, Haack D. Plasma vasopressin concentrations and effects of vasopressin antiserum on blood pressure in rats with malignant two-kidney Goldblatt hypertension. *Circ Res* 1978;42:17–22.

94. Johnston CI, Pullan PT, Walter NMA. Vasoactive peptides in experimental renal hypertension. *Klin Wochenschr* 1978;56(suppl 1):81–85.

95. Lee-Kwon WJ, Share L, Crofton JT, Shade RE. Vasopressin in the rat with partial nephrectomy-salt hypertension. *Clin Exp Hypertens* 1981;3:281–297.

96. Hinojosa C, Shade RE, Haywood JR. Plasma vasopressin concentration in high sodium renal hypertension. *J Hypertens* 1986;4:529–534.

97. Ben LK, Maselli J, Keil LC, Reid IA. Role of renin-angiotensin system in control of vasopressin and ACTH secretions during the development of renal hypertension in dogs. *Hypertension* 1984;6:35–41.

98. Share L, Crofton JT. Contribution of vasopressin to hypertension. *Hypertension* 1982;4(suppl III):III-85–III-92.

99. Woods RL, Johnston CI. The role of vasopressin in hypertension: studies using the Brattleboro rat. *Am J Physiol* 1982;242:F727–F732.

100. Woods RL, Johnston CI. Importance of antidiuretic properties of vasopressin experimental renal hypertension. *Clin Exp Pharmacol Physiol* 1983;80:519–523.

101. Johnston CI. Vasopressin in circulatory control and hypertension. *J Hypertens* 1985;3:557–569.

102. Hinojosa C, Haywood JR. Development of high sodium renal hypertension during chronic blockade of the vascular effects of vasopressin. *J Pharmacol Exp Ther* 1986;238:492–496.

103. Gavras I, Mulinari R, Gavras H. Renin-angiotensin and vasopressin in the development of salt-induced hypertension. *J Hypertens* 1988;6:999–1002.

104. Gavras H, Brunner HR, Laragh JH, Vaughan ED Jr, Koss M, Cote LJ, Gavras I. Malignant hypertension resulting from deoxycorticosterone acetate and salt excess: role of renin and sodium in vascular changes. *Circ Res* 1975;36:300–309.

105. Woods RL, Abrahams JM, Kincaid-Smith P, Johnston CI. Malignant hypertension in Brattleboro (vasopressin-deficient) rats. *J Hypertens* 1983;1:37–43.

106. Crofton JT, Share L, Shade RE, Allen C, Tarnowski D. Vasopressin in the rat with spontaneous hypertension. *Am J Physiol* 1978;135:H361–H365.

107. Mohring J, Kintz J, Schoun J. Studies on the role of vasopressin in blood pressure control of spontaneously hypertensive rats with established hypertension (SHR, stroke-prone strain). *J Cardiovasc Pharmacol* 1979;1:593–608.

108. Mohring J, Schoun J, Kintz J, McNeill R. Decreased vasopressin content in brainstem of rats with spontaneous hypertension. *Naunyn Schmiedebergs Arch Pharmacol* 1980;315:83–84.

109. Filep J, Fejestoth G. Does vasopressin sustain blood pressure in conscious spontaneously hypertensive rats? *Hypertension* 1986;8:514–519.

110. Datar S, Laverty WH, McNeill JR. Clonidine fails to reduce pressor responsiveness of conscious spontaneously hypertensive rats to vasopressin. *Can J Physiol Pharmacol* 1986;64:284–289.

111. Sladek JR Jr, Davis BJ, Sladek CD. Localization of vasopressin-neurophysin and norepinephrine in the supraoptic nucleus of spontaneously hypertensive rats. *Brain Res* 1986;365:293–304.

112. Matsuguchi H, Schmid PG, van Orden D, Mark AL. Does vasopressin contribute to salt-induced hypertension in the Dahl strain? *Hypertension* 1981;3:174–181.

113. Feuerstein G, Zerbe RL, Ben-Ishay D, Kopin IJ, Jacobowitz DM. Catecholamines and vasopressin in forebrain nuclei of hypertension-prone and -resistant rats. *Brain Res Bull* 1981;7:671–676.

114. Feuerstein G, Zerbe RL, Ben-Ishay D, Kopin IJ, Jacobowitz DM. Catecholamines and vasopressin in hindbrain nuclei of hypertension-prone and -resistant rats. *Brain Res* 1982;251:169–173.

115. Rascher W, Weidmann E, Gross F. Vasopressin in the plasma of stroke-prone spontaneously hypertensive rats. *Clin Sci* 1981;61:295–298.

116. Sladek CD, Blair ML, Mangipane M. Evidence against a pressor role for vasopressin in spontaneous hypertension. *Hypertension* 1987;9:332–338.

117. Morris M, Sain LE, Schumacher SL. A reduction of central peptidergic responses in the spontaneously hypertensive rat. *J Hypertens* 1986;4(suppl 1):S177–S178.

118. Nakai M, Yamane Y, Umeda Y, Yamamoto J, Matsui Y. Enhanced vasopressin release upon activation of the central neural mechanism in spontaneously hypertensive rats. *Jpn J Physiol* 1986;36:613–618.

119. Rascher W, Lang RE, Unger T, Ganten D, Gross F. Vasopressin in brain of spontaneously hypertensive rats. *Am J Physiol* 1982;242:H496–H499.

120. Pirozzolo FJ, Hansch EC. Supraoptic nucleus of the Brattleboro rat has an altered afferent noradrenergic input. *Science* 1981;214:347–350.

121. Cowley AW Jr, Cushman WC, Quillen EW Jr, Skelton MM, Langford HG. Vasopressin elevation in essential hypertension and increased responsiveness to sodium intake. *Hypertension* 1981;3(suppl I):I-93–I-100.

122. Cowley AW Jr, Skelton MM, Velasquez MT. Sex differences in the endocrine predictors of essential hypertension. Vasopressin versus renin. *Hypertension* 1985;3(suppl I):I-151–I-160.

123. Davies R, Forsling M, Bulger G, Phillips T. Plasma vasopressin and blood pressure. Studies in normal subjects and in benign essential hypertension at rest and after postural challenge. *Br Heart J* 1983;49:528–531.

124. Ando T, Shimamoto K, Nakahashi Y, Nishitani T, Hosoda S, Ishida H, Yokoyama I, Tanaka S, Iimura O. Plasma antidiuretic hormone levels in patients with normal and low renin essential hypertension, and secondary hypertension. *Endocrinol Jpn* 1983;30:567–570.

125. Skjoto J, Aakesson I, Os I, Kjeldsen SE, Eide I, Leren P. Increased plasma vasopressin and serum uric acid in the low renin type of essential hypertension. *Acta Med Scand* 1984;215:165–172.

126. Os I, Kjeldsen SE, Sdkoto J, Westheim A, Lande K, Aakesson I, Frederichsen P, Leren P, Hjermann I, Eide IK. Increased plasma vasopressin in low renin essential hypertension. *Hypertension* 1986;8:506–513.

127. Os I, Kjeldsen SE, Westheim A, Aakesson I, Norman N, Enger E, Hjermann I, Eide I. Decreased central dopaminergic activity in essential hypertension. *J Hypertens* 1987;5:191–197.

128. Frolkis VV, Golovchenko SF, Medved VI, Frolkis RA. Vasopressin and cardiovascular system in aging. *Gerontology* 1982;28:290–302.

129. Bursztyn MR, Bresnahan M, Gavras I, Gavras H. Effect of aging on vasopressin, catecholamines, and alpha$_2$-adrenergic receptors. *J Am Geriatr Soc* 1990;38:628–632.

130. Bursztyn MR, Bresnahan M, Gavras I, Gavras H. Pressor hormones in elderly hypertensive persons—racial difference. *Hypertension* 1990;15(suppl I):I-88–I-92.

131. Velasquez MT, Menitove JE, Skelton MM, Cowley AW Jr. Hormonal responses and blood pressure maintenance in normal and hypertensive subjects during acute blood pressure loss. *Hypertension* 1987;9:423–428.

132. Velasquez MT, Skelton MM, Cowley AW Jr. Water loading and restriction in essential hypertension. *Hypertension* 1987;9:407–414.

133. Os I, Kjeldsen SE, Westheim A, Jackson MB, Aakesson I, Fredrichsen P, Eide I, Leren P. The effect of sodium depletion and potassium supplementation on vasopressin, renin and catecholamines in hypertensive men. *Acta Med Scand* 1986;220:195–203.

134. Robertson GL, Ganguly A. Osmoregulation and baroregulation of plasma vasopressin in essential hypertension. *J Cardiovasc Pharmacol* 1986;8(suppl 7):S87–S91.

135. Pedersen EB, Danielsen H, Madsen M, Sorensen SS, Thomsen OO. Abnormal vasopressin and aldosterone response to furosemide in essential hypertension. *Acta Med Scand* 1986;219:387–392.

136. Padfield PL, Brown JJ, Lever AF, Morton JJ, Robertson JJ, Robertson JIS. Blood pressure in acute and chronic vasopressin excess. *N Engl J Med* 1981;304:1067–1070.

137. Bartter FC. Vasopressin in blood pressure. *N Engl J Med* 1981;304:1097–1098.

138. Osterman J, Calhoun A, Dunham M, Cullum UX Jr, Clark RM, Stewart DD, Scheithauer BW, Zimmerman EA, Defendini R, Zang X, et al. Chronic syndrome of inappropriate antidiuretic hormone secretion and hypertension in a patient with olfactory neuroblastoma. Evidence of ectopic production of arginine vasopressin by the tumor. *Arch Intern Med* 1986;146:1731–1735.

139. Kruszynski M, Lammek B, Manning N, Seto J, Haldar J, Sawyer WH. [1-(beta-mercapto-beta, beta-cyclopentamethylenepropionic acid 0,2-(0-methyl)tyrosine]arginine-vasopressin and [1-(beta-mercapto-beta,beta-cyclopentamethylene-propionic acid)]arginine-vasopressin, two highly potent antagonists of the vasopressor response to arginine-vasopressin. *J Med Chem* 1980;23:364–368.

140. Gavras H, Ribeiro AB, Kohlman O, Saragoca M, Mulinari RA, Ramos O, Gavras I. Effect of a specific inhibitor of the vascular action of vasopressin in humans. *Hypertension* 1984;6(suppl I):I-156–I-160.

141. Bussien JP, Waeber B, Nussberger J, Schaller MD, Gavras H, Hofbauer K, Brunner HR. Does vasopressin sustain blood pressure of normally hydrated healthy volunteers? *Am J Physiol* 1984;246:H143–H147.

142. Mulinari RA, Saad CI, Kohlmann O Jr, Ribeiro AB, Gavras I, Gavras H. Cardiovascular role of vasopressin in the upright position in normotension and hypertension (Abstract). *Hypertension* 1987;9:557.

143. Papadoliopoulou-Diamandopoulou N, Papagalanis N, Gavras I, Gavras H. Vasopressin in end-stage renal disease: relationship to salt, catecholamines an renin activity. *Clin Exp Theory Pract* 1987;A9:1197–1208.

144. Ribeiro A, Mulinari R, Gavras I, Kohlmann O, Ramos O, Gavras H. Sequential elimination of pressor mechanisms in severe hypertension in humans. *Hypertension* 1986;8(suppl I):I-169–I-173.

145. Waeber B, Nussberger J, Hofbauer KG, Nicod P, Brunner HR. Clinical studies with a vascular vasopressin antagonist. *J Cardiovasc Pharmacol* 1986;8(suppl 7):S111–S116.

146. de Paula RB, Plavnik FL, Rodrigues CIS, de A Rocha F, Kohlmann O Jr, Ribeiro AB, Gavras I, Gavras H. Contribution of vasopressin to orthostatic blood pressure maintenance in essential hypertension. *Am J Hypertens* 1993;6:794–798.

147. Ribeiro AB, Saad CI, Zanella T, Mulinari RA, Kohlmann O Jr, Gavras H. Vasopressin maintains blood pressure in diabetic orthostatic hypotension. *Hypertension* 1988;11(suppl 1):I-217–I-221.

148. Schwartz J, Liard JF, Ott C, Cowley AW Jr. Hemodynamic effects of neurohypophyseal peptides with antidiuretic activity in dogs. *Am J Physiol* 1985;249:H1001–H1008.

149. Williams TDM, Lightman SL, Leadbeater MJ. Hormonal and cardiovascular responses to dDAVP in man. *Clin Endocrinol* 1986;24:89–96.

150. Bichet DG, Razi M, Lonergan M, Arthus M, Papukna V, Kortas C, Barjon J. Hemodynamic and coagulation responses to 1-desamino[8-D-arginine]vasopressin in patients with congenital nephrogenic diabetes insipidus. *N Engl J Med* 1988;318:881–887.

151. Hish AT, Dzau VJ, Majzoub JA, Creager MA. Vasopressin-mediated forearm vasodilation in normal human: evidence for a vascular vasopressin V₂ receptor. *J Clin Invest* 1989;84:418–426.

152. Yamamura Y, Ogawa Hidenori, Chihara T, Kondo K, Onogawa T, Nakamura S, Mori T, Tominaga M, Yabuuchi Y. OPC-21268, an orally effective, nonpeptide vasopressin V1 receptor antagonist. *Science* 1991;252:572–574.

153. Imaizumi T, Harada S, Hirooka Y, Masaki H, Momohara M, Takeshita A. Effects of OPC-21268, an orally effective vasopressin V₁ receptor antagonist in humans. *Hypertension* 1992;20:54–58.

154. DeWied D. Long-term effect of vasopressin on the maintenance of a conditioned avoidance response in rats. *Nature* 1971;233:58–60.

155. Ashen MD, Hartman RD, Barraclough CA, Petersen SL, Hamlyn JM. Vasopressin gene transcripts in mineralocorticoid hypertension: an in situ study. *J Hypertens* 1992;10:1317–1326.

156. Lolait SJ, O'Caroll A-M, McBride OW, Konig M, Morel A, Brownstein MJ. Cloning and characterization of a vasopressin V2 receptor and possible link to nephrogenic diabetes insipidus. *Nature* 1992;357:336–339.

Hypertension: Pathophysiology, Diagnosis,
and Management, Second Edition,
edited by J.H. Laragh and B.M. Brenner,
Raven Press, Ltd., New York © 1995.

CHAPTER **47**

Neuropeptides in Blood Pressure Control

Vera Ralevic and Geoffrey Burnstock

Several lines of evidence implicate the peripheral nervous system in the complex etiology and maintenance of hypertension. A number of studies have focused on the role of sympathetic perivascular nerves with the aim of identifying in hypertension a pathology resulting from a specific malfunction in sympathetic neurotransmission. Despite substantial evidence that sympathetic nerves have a role in hypertension, no one hypothesis sufficiently explains their involvement, suggesting that it may be unreasonable to look for a specific dysfunction occurring in a single class of perivascular nerves. Hence, just as hypertension is recognized to be a multifactorial disease, so should the role of the peripheral nervous system in hypertension be considered in terms of the contribu-

tion of its several constituents. This does not preclude the possibility that the sympathetic nervous system serves as the final common pathway by which neural defects are expressed in hypertension.

Perivascular nerves other than the sympathetic division have received relatively little attention in relation to hypertensive disease. Recent discoveries on the organization of the peripheral nervous system demand that the roles of other nerve types, namely parasympathetic and sensorimotor nerves, and perivascular projections from intrinsic neurons are considered. This in turn highlights the possible importance of neuropeptides in hypertension, since it is now known that, in addition to the classic transmitters noradrenaline (NA) in sympathetic nerves and acetylcholine (ACh) in parasympathetic nerves, perivascular nerves contain a number of cotransmitter substances, including neuropeptides, for which important roles have been identified. Favored packaging of co-

   V. Ralevic and G. Burnstock: Department of Anatomy and Developmental Biology, University College London, London WC1E 6BT, United Kingdom.

transmitters into specific combinations has been identified, with characteristic patterns including neuropeptide Y (NPY) with NA and adenosine 5'-triphosphate (ATP) in sympathetic nerves, vasoactive intestinal polypeptide (VIP) with ACh in parasympathetic nerves, and substance P and calcitonin gene-related peptide (CGRP) in sensorimotor nerves (1).

Cotransmission allows enhanced fine control and complexity of neurotransmission via pre- and postjunctional modulatory mechanisms. Neuromodulation can also take place between transmitters released from adjacent terminals of different populations of nerves and this has been termed "cross-talk." Implicit in this is the recognition of a certain degree of interdependence between different types of perivascular nerves. Some of the controversy in the current literature regarding the role of perivascular nerves in the development and maintenance of hypertension may be explained by the fact that long-term trophic effects are involved. Increases or decreases in perivascular innervation by certain populations of nerves have been shown to produce marked changes in innervation by adjacent populations, a reflection of the remarkable plasticity of the nervous system. In addition, trophic effects of perivascular nerves on development and growth of smooth muscle and the endothelium have been shown. In all of these respects, important roles have been identified for neuropeptides, although little attention has been paid to the implications of this for the pathogenesis of hypertension.

This chapter reviews the roles of neuropeptides as cotransmitters and neuromodulators in the short-term and long-term control of local vascular tone, with the aim of drawing attention to areas where abnormal function might be responsible for causing or maintaining the elevated systemic arterial pressure that is characteristic of hypertension. This discussion will concentrate on peptides as transmitters in the peripheral nervous system, and thus will not include central effects or the renin-angiotensin system. Evidence is presented for a contribution by neuropeptides to the development of hypertensive disease, both directly and through vascular changes associated with diabetes mellitus and the aging process. Emphasis is placed on the fact that the role of perivascular nerves in hypertension must be considered in terms of the balance effected between vasoconstrictor and vasodilator tone, by the short-term modulatory interactions that occur between classes of perivascular nerves, and by their long-term (trophic) effects on nerves, smooth muscle, and endothelial cells.

VASCULAR NEUROEFFECTOR JUNCTION

Perivascular nerves at the adventitial-medial border of most blood vessels form a plexus consisting of an extensive network of branching terminal fibers. These terminal axons are devoid of Schwann cell covering and are rich in varicosities (1–2 μm diameter) separated by intervaricose regions (0.1–0.3 μm diameter) (2). The varicosities are the main sites of storage of neurotransmitters that are released en passant by the depolarizing effect of nerve impulses passing along the axons. Unlike the classic synapse of the skeletal neuromuscular junction and those present in ganglia, a fixed relationship between varicosities and smooth muscle cells is not a feature of the autonomic neuroeffector junction. In addition, there are no features of postjunctional specialization, although prejunctional varicosity membranes sometimes have thickenings. The junctional cleft can vary between 50 and 2000 nm, depending on the size of the vessel, and it has been suggested that the wide cleft predisposes the autonomic neuroeffector junction to both pre- and postjunctional modulatory influences from locally released transmitters from the same or adjacent nerve terminals, or by circulating neurohormones or local agents such as prostanoids, bradykinin, histamine, or angiotensin. The concept of modulatory effects elicited between different classes of perivascular nerves via their transmitters is also referred to as cross-talk (3).

NEUROPEPTIDES IN PERIVASCULAR NERVES

In sympathetic and parasympathetic divisions, neuropeptides are typically co-stored and co-released with the classic transmitters NA and ACh, respectively. In most sensorimotor nerves, classic transmitters do not appear to be present and neuropeptides function as transmitters in their own right. Peptide-containing secretory vesicles can frequently be recognized by electron microscopic techniques on the basis of an electron-dense core, attributable to the fixation of protein within the vesicle. An important difference between peptide transmitters and classic transmitters lies in their synthesis; classic transmitters are synthesized in the nerve terminal. Resupply is therefore rapid, being by local synthesis and reuptake, while resupply of peptides is a longer process involving axonal transport from the cell body (4). Another difference lies in the fact that for neuropeptides there are no mechanisms for reuptake and reuse, imposing constraints on their availability. Characteristic patterns of stimulation, typically of high frequency and long duration, have been associated with the release of peptides from nerves and may be important in relation to the supply, storage, release, and depletion of transmitter in the nerve terminal.

Sympathetic Nerves

The interest directed toward sympathetic nerves as a factor in the pathogenesis of hypertension is unsurprising, given that these make up the most important division of nerves involved in producing vasoconstrictor tone. There is substantial evidence associating an increase in sympathetic nerve activity with the development and maintenance of hypertension, although this is by no means totally resolved. Until recently, this mechanism has been considered almost exclusively in terms of the effects of vasoconstrictor sympathetic catecholamines. However, it is now known that sympathetic nerves release NPY and ATP as cotransmitters together with the classic transmitter NA (Fig. 1). 5-Hydroxytryptamine (5-HT) and opioid peptides have also been identified in sympathetic neurons. In addition, somatostatin has been detected in neurons of sympathetic ganglia (5). Some consideration of the roles of nonpeptide (ATP and 5-HT) as well as peptide transmitters in sympathetic nerves is relevant to the present discussion, since by considering a complete profile of sympathetic neurotransmission peptidergic transmission may be placed in context.

Nonpeptide Sympathetic Cotransmission (NA and ATP)

Early evidence for sympathetic cotransmission was established for NA and ATP in the vas deferens, a tissue with a high density of sympathetic nerves (6,7). Subsequently, numerous studies demonstrated that sympathetic cotransmission of NA and ATP also occurs in many different blood vessels in a variety of species (1,8). Preloading with (^{3}H)-adenosine and measurement of tri-

tium efflux, a measure of ATP release, has shown tetrodotoxin- and guanethidine-sensitive cotransmission of NA and ATP in the rabbit aorta and portal vein (9), the dog basilar artery (10), rabbit pulmonary artery (11), and rabbit mesenteric artery (12). The rabbit saphenous artery provides a classic example of a vessel in which pharmacological manipulations have been used to identify NA and ATP cotransmission (13,14) (Fig. 2). In this vessel, electrical stimulation of sympathetic nerves produces a contractile response, of which less than 30 percent is blocked by the α-adrenoceptor antagonist prazosin. The remainder, the purinergic component, is abolished following desensitization of P_{2x}-purinoceptors with α,β-methylene ATP (13). Furthermore, reserpine treatment, which depletes sympathetic nerves of their catecholamine content, fails to abolish nerve-mediated contractions, whereas destruction of sympathetic nerves with 6-hydroxydopamine (6-OHDA) abolishes nerve-mediated responses (14). Electrophysiological studies have confirmed sympathetic cotransmission of NA and ATP, showing that these act as mediators of the slow depolarization and excitatory junction potential, respectively (15–18).

Considerable variation exists in the relative proportions of NA and ATP acting as cotransmitters in sympathetic nerves. For example, in guinea pig submucosal arterioles, both vasoconstriction and excitatory junction potentials evoked in response to electrical stimulation of sympathetic nerves are mediated exclusively by ATP, with NA assuming the role of a neuromodulator by acting through prejunctional α_2-adrenoceptors to depress transmitter release (19). At the other extreme, in rat mes-

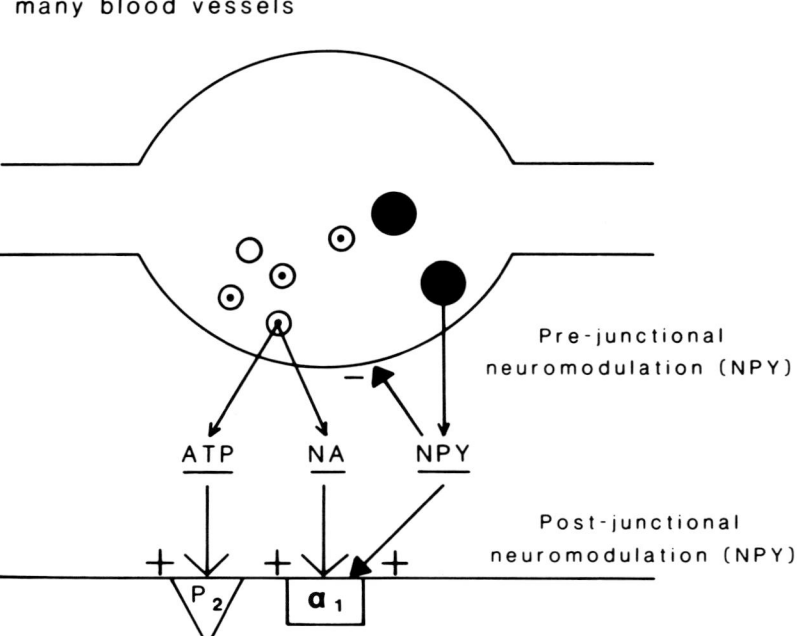

FIG. 1. Schematic representation of sympathetic neurotransmission showing that NA, ATP, and NPY are released as cotransmitters from single nerve varicosities of sympathetic nerves supplying the vas deferens and many blood vessels. NA and ATP, released from small (and large) granular vesicles, act on the smooth muscle to elicit contraction (+) via α_1-adrenoceptors and P_2-purinoceptors, respectively. NPY, preferentially released from large vesicles, generally has little direct action on the muscle cell, but exerts potent neuromodulatory actions: both prejunctional inhibition (−) of the release of NA (and ATP) and postjunctional enhancement of the action of NA. (From ref. 3, with permission.)

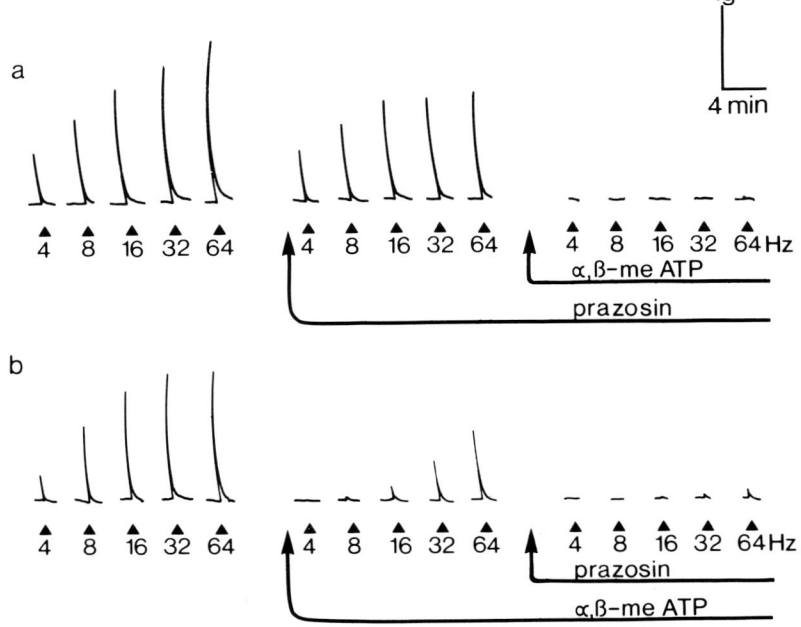

FIG. 2. Contractions produced in the isolated saphenous artery of the rabbit on neurogenic transmural stimulation (0.08–0.1 msec; supramaximal voltage) for 1 sec (a, b) at the frequencies (Hz) indicated (▲). Nerve stimulations were repeated in the presence of 10 μM prazosin added before (a) or after (b) desensitization of the P_2-purinoceptor with α,β-methylene ATP (α,β-Me ATP), as indicated on the figure by the *arrowed lines*. The *horizontal bar* signifies 4 min and the vertical bar 1 g. (From ref. 13, with permission.)

enteric arteries the purinergic component is relatively small (20). In addition, it has been noted that the purinergic component is optimal with short bursts of low-frequency stimulation, whereas longer durations of higher frequency favor adrenergic transmission (13,18, 21,22). The reason for this variation is not entirely clear, but may in part be a reflection of the differential storage of NA and ATP in sympathetic vesicles and the involvement of different classes of vesicle during different stimuli. ATP is co-stored with NA in small and large sympathetic vesicles; the NA/ATP ratio is three to five times higher in small than in large vesicles (23).

Differential prejunctional modulation of the release of NA and ATP by various agents has been shown in the vas deferens and has interesting implications for prejunctional modulation of sympathetic neurotransmission in blood vessels (1,6,23). Both NA and ATP are able to exert prejunctional modulation of sympathetic transmission, NA via prejunctional α_2-adrenoceptors and ATP via P_1-purinoceptors following breakdown to adenosine. Postjunctionally, the effects of NA and ATP released as sympathetic cotransmitters are generally cooperative, since both typically act as vasoconstrictors following release from sympathetic nerves. Postjunctional synergism may occur, having been described in the rat femoral artery, guinea pig and rat portal vein, and the rat mesenteric arterial bed (1,20).

5-HT immunofluorescent nerves have been localized in a number of vessels. However, it seems that in general 5-HT is not synthesized and stored in separate nerves, but is taken up from the blood, probably after release from platelets, and is stored in and released as a "false

transmitter" from sympathetic nerves (24,25). Accordingly, 5-HT immunostaining is lost after surgical and/or chemical sympathectomy (26,27). 5-HT has direct effects on vascular smooth muscle (usually vasoconstriction) and can act as a pre- or postjunctional modulator of sympathetic transmission; it inhibits the release of NA from sympathetic nerve terminals and postjunctionally potentiates the vasoconstrictor effects of NA (28,29).

Neuropeptide Y in Sympathetic Nerves

NPY is a 36-amino-acid peptide, originally isolated from porcine brain (30), that is present in almost all perivascular sympathetic nerves examined so far (31–34). In these nerves the release of both NPY and NA due to electrical stimulation of sympathetic nerve terminals is prevented by guanethidine, while surgical removal of either the stellate ganglion or the superior cervical ganglion, or 6-OHDA treatment, results in attenuated levels of NPY in the cardiovascular system (31,33,35). Electron microscopy and fractionation studies carried out in some nonvascular tissues have demonstrated that NPY is preferentially localized, along with NA and ATP, in large dense-cored vesicles that make up approximately 5 percent of the terminal axon vesicle population (32,36). Most NA is stored separately from NPY in the same nerve endings in small dense-cored vesicles. As with neuronal ATP, the pattern of stimulation appears to be an important determinant of the release of coexisting sympathetic transmitters. For example, in the pig spleen NPY release is optimal at high-frequency intermittent bursts of stimulation (37).

In most vessels NPY released from sympathetic nerves has little direct effect except at high concentrations, and its main role appears to be that of a pre- or postjunctional neuromodulator. In contrast, NPY is a potent constrictor in coronary (38,39), renal (40), cerebral (41–44), and splenic vessels (37,45). A potential role for NPY in hypertension is supported by demonstrations that intra-arterial infusion of synthetic human NPY into the human forearm causes a slowly developing and dose-dependent decrease in forearm blood flow and an increase in venous tone (46). Further, intravenously infused NPY has been shown to produce an increase in mean arterial pressure that was more marked in spontaneously hypertensive rats (SHR) than in controls (47).

Opioid Peptides in Sympathetic Nerves

Opioid peptides are widely distributed in peripheral sympathetic neurons. They are commonly colocalized with NA in cell bodies and fibers and in some cases coexist with NPY. In bovine splenic nerve, NA is found in both small and large dense-cored vesicles, whereas [met]-enkephalin is co-localized only in the large vesicles (48). Similarly, in bovine vas deferens, immunoelectron microscopy and density gradient separations have shown co-localization of peptide and amine exclusively within the large dense-cored vesicles, and both were co-released by transmural stimulation in a guanethidine-sensitive manner (49). The co-storage of enkephalins has been confirmed at an ultrastructural level by direct immuno-gold labeling of large dense-cored vesicles in nerve terminals of pig cerebral arteries and vas deferens (50,51). In the guinea pig heart, the sympatholytic agent 6-OHDA reduced the cardiac enkephalin content (by about 70 percent) (52). In the pig cerebral artery a population of large dense-cored sympathetic vesicles was found to contain dopamine β-hydroxylase, NPY, and enkephalin (51).

Differential innervation by NA, NPY, and dynorphin (DYN) of consecutive segments of the vasculature of the guinea pig skin has been described (53). Three different immunohistochemical classes were identified: neurons supplying the distributing arteries contain NA and NPY; neurons supplying the smaller arteries and some arterioles contain NA, NPY, and pro-DYN–derived peptides; and neurons with NA and pro-DYN–derived peptides, but without NPY, which are distributed almost exclusively to the smallest arterioles and arteriovenous anastomoses (53).

Although opioid receptor agonists have been shown to have direct vasodilator actions in some vessels (54,55), high doses are required and they generally have no direct motor effects. Their main hypotensive and bradycardic responses appear to be mediated via effects on the central nervous system or by prejunctional neuromodulation.

Neuropeptides and Sympathetic Neuromodulation

The major role of NPY released from sympathetic nerves in the vasculature and in the vas deferens appears to be that of a pre- and/or postjunctional modulator of sympathetic transmission, since it has little direct postjunctional action or causes contraction only at high concentrations (32,34,36,41,56,57). At the prejunctional level, NPY has potent inhibitory effects reducing the release of NA and ATP from sympathetic nerves (58–60). The importance of considering perivascular neurotransmission as made up of complex individual elements, and not as a simple mechanistic process, is illustrated in the sympathetic nervous system by a recent study showing differential modulation by NPY of the sympathetic cotransmitters ATP and NA in the guinea pig saphenous artery. Remarkably, NPY was shown to potentiate sympathetic constriction by a selective action on the purinergic component without modifying the noradrenergic component of the response (61).

Postjunctionally, NPY generally acts to enhance the actions of either sympathetic nerve stimulation, or exogenous NA and ATP by actions that are independent of direct effects (36,43,56,57,62–65). The potentiating effect of NPY is not restricted to sympathetic transmitters but can also be observed with responses to histamine (31,66). Contractions to 5-HT and high levels of K^+ ions have also been reported to be potentiated (41,62,63). Postjunctional inhibitory effects of NPY have been demonstrated in canine cerebral arteries, where NPY was shown to suppress the contractile action of exogenously applied NA (44). Binding experiments using a series of C-terminal fragments of NPY led Wahlestedt and co-workers (66,67) to propose the existence of two different receptor subtypes—one postsynaptic (Y_1), the other presynaptic (Y_2) (66,67). However, it appears that some postsynaptic effects of NPY could be mediated by a third class of receptor (see ref. 34).

The involvement of opioid peptides in peripheral neuromodulation is increasingly being recognized. For example, presynaptic inhibitory opioid receptors have been shown to modulate the activity of cardiac sympathetic nerves in many species (see ref. 68) and in several blood vessels, including the rabbit pulmonary artery (69), the rabbit ear artery (70,71), the rabbit mesenteric artery (72,73), the rat mesenteric artery (73), the rabbit portal vein (74), and the rat tail artery (75). Species differences have been shown; for example, agonists selective for subtypes of opioid receptors μ, δ, and κ had no effect on responses to sympathetic nerve stimulation in the perfused rat mesentery (73), while, in contrast, prejunctional inhibitory effects of these agonists have been shown on sympathetic neurotransmission in the rabbit mesenteric artery (72,73). It is interesting to note that in the rabbit mesenteric artery an α_2-adrenoceptor antagonist selectively enhanced the inhibitory effect of a κ-opioid selective agonist on sympathetic transmission, indicative of interactions between prejunctional κ-opioid receptors and α₂-adrenoceptors in this vessel (73).

Parasympathetic Nerves

The distribution of parasympathetic nerves in the cardiovascular system is less extensive than that of sympathetic nerves, with many blood vessels receiving no parasympathetic innervation. ACh is the classic inhibitory transmitter of most parasympathetic nerves, which typically exert opposite actions to the vasoconstrictor effects of sympathetic nerves. Direct vasodilator effects of ACh on vascular smooth muscle cells, however, have been demonstrated in only a few vessels, including the feline posterior auricular artery (76), guinea pig saphenous and coronary arteries (77), and arterioles in the submucous plexus of guinea pig intestine (78). In most other vessels ACh produces relaxations that are entirely dependent on the presence of an intact endothelium (79); in the absence of the endothelium, ACh either has no effect or may cause vasoconstriction. Since it is unlikely that ACh, released from perivascular nerves, would traverse the smooth muscle layer, particularly in large blood ves-

sels, to elicit vasodilatation via endothelial cells, this raises intriguing questions about the functional role of ACh as a vasodilator transmitter in parasympathetic nerves. It is possible that the growing number of putative transmitter substances, including neuropeptides, that have recently been identified in parasympathetic nerves, may have a previously unrecognized importance as mediators of parasympathetic nerve-induced vasodilatation.

Vasoactive Intestinal Polypeptide in Parasympathetic Nerves

In the same way that NPY has been considered to be the main neuropeptide cotransmitter in sympathetic neurons, so has VIP been attributed with a cotransmitter role in cholinergic parasympathetic neurons (80–83) (Fig. 3). The classic evidence for cotransmission of ACh and VIP in certain postganglionic parasympathetic neurons comes from pharmacological studies performed on cat salivary glands (80,84). ACh and VIP are released from the same parasympathetic nerve terminals in response to transmural nerve stimulation. During low-frequency stimulation, ACh is released to cause an increase in salivary secretion from acinar cells and also to

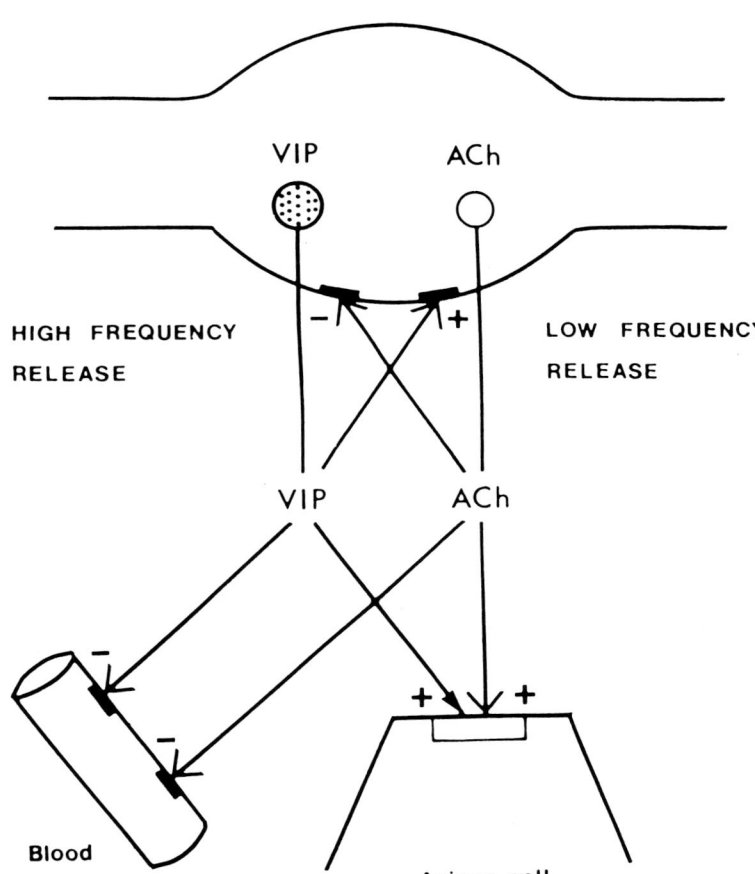

FIG. 3. Parasympathetic neurotransmission. A classic transmitter, acetylcholine (ACh), coexists with vasoactive intestinal polypeptide (VIP) in parasympathetic nerves supplying the cat salivary gland. ACh and VIP are stored in separate vesicles; they can be released differentially at different stimulation frequencies to act on acinar cells and glandular blood vessels. Cooperation is achieved by the selective release of ACh at low impulse frequencies and of VIP at high frequencies. Pre- and postjunctional modulation is indicated. (From ref. 81, with permission.)

elicit some minor dilatation of blood vessels in the gland. VIP is preferentially released at high frequencies to cause marked vasodilatation of blood vessels, and, while it has no direct effect on acinar cells, it acts as a neuromodulator to enhance substantially both the postjunctional effect of ACh on acinar cell secretion and the release of ACh from nerve varicosities via prejunctional receptors. The differential release of ACh and VIP at different frequencies of stimulation may be related to the preferential storage of ACh and VIP in small clear vesicles and in large dense-cored vesicles, respectively, with the latter apparently needing higher frequencies of stimulation to release their transmitter content (80).

Peptide histidine isoleucine (PHI) and VIP are fragments of the same precursor molecule, prepro-VIP, and certain of their amino acid sequences are identical. PHI has been shown to be released, in addition to VIP and ACh from parasympathetic neurons supplying the submandibular salivary gland (82). Double immunostaining has revealed the coexistence of VIP and PHI in cerebrovascular nerve fibers (85). VIP/PHI nerve fibers have also been demonstrated in the rabbit uterine artery, but the physiological significance of this coexistence is not clear since the two peptides are equipotent and their effects are additive.

Other Peptides in Parasympathetic Nerves

Vasodilator nerves to the uterine arteries in the guinea pig contain immunoreactivity to VIP, which coexists with DYN (a peptide contained in the proenkephalin A sequence), NPY, and somatostatin (86). NPY-like immunoreactivity (-LI) has also been reported in some of the choline acetyltransferase (ChAT)/VIP-containing neurons of the parasympathetic ciliary, sphenopalatine, otic (87,88), and pterygopalatine ganglia (89,90), with targets including the iris and cerebral vessels. Double immunostaining has revealed a population of fibers that contains NPY co-localized with VIP in guinea pig (91) and pig (51) cerebral arteries. CGRP-LI has been reported in parasympathetic cholinergic neurons located in the pontine and sacral parasympathetic nuclei and in the ventral horn (see ref. 33). The functional significance of these examples of co-localization remains to be determined.

Nitric Oxide in Parasympathetic Nerves

Autonomic control of penile erection, involving relaxation of the smooth muscle of the corpus cavernosum as well as dilatation of other penile vascular beds, has traditionally been attributed to the vasodilator effects of ACh and VIP released from parasympathetic nerves. Recent evidence suggests that nitric oxide (NO) released from nerves may have an important role in smooth muscle relaxation leading to penile erection. In the rat penis

all of the parasympathetic neurons projecting to the penis are found in the major pelvic ganglion. Positive staining for nitric oxide synthase (NOS) and nicotinamide adenine dinucleotide phosphate-diaphorase (NADPH-d) (now regarded as a marker for NOS) has been shown in many of the neurons of the major pelvic ganglion, axons of the penile cavernous nerve, varicose terminals associated with various tissues of the rat penis, and neuronal plexuses in the adventitial layer of penile arteries (92,93). A functional correlate for this evidence for the presence of NO in nerves has been provided by demonstrations of a role for NO as a vasodilator transmitter of isolated strips of rabbit and human corpus cavernosum and in the bovine penile artery (see ref. 94).

Recently, NOS-containing fibers, shown by lesion studies to arise from parasympathetic cell bodies in the sphenopalatine ganglia, have been localized in the adventitia of cerebral arteries and many of these also contain VIP (see ref. 95). A functional role for perivascular neuronal NO in cerebral arteries has been identified in studies showing that stimulation of adventitial nerve fibers causes vascular relaxation that is attenuated by inhibitors of NOS (96).

Neuropeptides and Parasympathetic Neuromodulation

VIP has no direct effects on acinar cells but acts as a neuromodulator to enhance substantially both the postjunctional effect of ACh on acinar cell secretion and the release of ACh from nerve varicosities via prejunctional receptors (80–82). The functional significance of NPY in some of the ChAT/VIP-containing neurons of the parasympathetic ciliary, sphenopalatine, otic, and pterygopalatine ganglia, or in VIP-containing nerve fibers in cerebral arteries is not known. However, it has been shown that a low dose of NPY may antagonize the vasodilator effects of VIP (97), ACh, and substance P in the guinea pig uterine artery (98). In the rat femoral artery *in vitro* NPY has been shown to attenuate the endothelium-dependent relaxation induced by ACh, but not that evoked by agents thought to act mainly on the smooth muscle (99).

Sensorimotor Nerves

Sensorimotor nerves are widely distributed throughout the cardiovascular system, having been identified extensively in the heart, around large arteries and veins, and in smaller vessels supplying vascular beds (33,100, 101). It is increasingly being recognized that in addition to their afferent (sensory) function, whereby they convey signals from the periphery to the central nervous system, primary sensory afferents have an efferent (motor) function on target tissues that may take place by the well-known "axon reflex" arrangement (102), or by the release of transmitter from the same terminal that is excited by the environmental stimulus (see refs. 103,104). In recognition of their dual afferent and efferent function, the term *sensorimotor* has been used for these nerves (1,105).

Substance P and Calcitonin Gene-Related Peptide in Sensorimotor Nerves

The neuropeptides substance P and CGRP are the principal transmitters of primary sensory afferent nerves and have been shown to coexist in the same perivascular terminals (106–108). Furthermore, with the use of colloidal gold particles of different sizes, they have been shown to coexist in the same large granular vesicles (109,110). Capsaicin sensitivity has been used as a marker for sensory neurons, and the loss of substance P–LI (111–113) and CGRP (106–108,114–116) following capsaicin treatment has been used to map the distribution of peripheral sensory nerve fibers.

The peripheral effects of substance P, namely vasodilatation, plasma extravasation, and release of histamine from mast cells, are consistent with its role as a sensory neurotransmitter and mediator of neurogenic inflammation. Substance P is generally a potent vasodilator both *in vivo* and *in vitro,* and in isolated large arteries relaxation has been shown to be an endothelium-dependent effect (117–121). However, vasoconstriction to substance P (100,122–124), or no effects (100,125), have also been described. CGRP is also a potent vasodilator both *in vivo* and *in vitro* (107,126–130). In most vessels vasodilatation due to CGRP is due to its action on receptors on the vascular smooth muscle; however, in the rat aorta (126,131–133) and in human arteries (134) CGRP has been shown to elicit endothelium-dependent relaxations.

The role of substance P co-localized with CGRP in sensorimotor nerves is problematic. First, there appears to be no correlation between the density of innervation and vascular reactivity; the rat carotid artery, where substance P innervation is very sparse, exhibits a dose-dependent relaxation to substance P, whereas the well-innervated superior mesenteric artery does not (100, 125). Second, in most vessels substance P does not appear to act directly on receptors on the vascular smooth muscle to produce vasodilatation. It does, however, produce potent vasodilatation via receptors on endothelial cells, which lead to the release of NO. While it is possible that substance P released from nerves supplying the microvasculature could produce vasodilatation via endothelial cells, it is most unlikely to reach the endothelium without degradation in larger blood vessels. In this case it may be that the primary role of substance P is either sensory or trophic and not motor.

Direct pharmacological evidence for a motor function of capsaicin-sensitive primary sensory afferents has been shown in the heart and in certain vascular preparations

in vitro. In the guinea pig heart, transmural stimulation of nonadrenergic, noncholinergic (NANC) capsaicin-sensitive neurons causes positive inotrophic and chronotrophic effects that are mediated by CGRP (135–140). In rat mesenteric arteries, overwhelming evidence exists for a role for CGRP as the mediator of vasodilatation following release from sensorimotor nerves. In the presence of guanethidine to block sympathetic transmission, perivascular stimulation of the raised-tone rat mesenteric arterial bed produces a characteristically slow-onset, long-lasting vasodilator response that is capsaicin- and tetrodotoxin-sensitive (125). Vasodilatation is accompanied by the release of CGRP-LI, but not substance P–LI (141–143), and can be inhibited both by the CGRP receptor antagonist (*8–37*) and by desensitization of the CGRP receptor (144), providing compelling evidence that CGRP is the vasodilator sensory neurotransmitter in this vascular bed. Despite the extensive co-localization of substance P–LI with CGRP-LI in sensory nerve fibers in rat mesenteric arteries, substance P is not co-released with CGRP by electrical stimulation at parameters causing release of CGRP and subsequent profound vasodilatation (141), and exogenously applied substance P has little or no direct effect on rat mesenteric arteries. CGRP has also been implicated in neurogenic vasodilatation of the cat cerebral artery (145) and guinea pig main pulmonary artery (146).

Other Peptides in Sensorimotor Nerves

Many other peptides, including neurokinin A (NKA), somatostatin, DYN, galanin, and VIP, have been described in capsaicin-sensitive sensory neurons (see refs. 103,147). Unmyelinated sensory neurons containing cholecystokinin (CCK)/CGRP/DYN/substance P have been shown to project to cutaneous arterioles in guinea pig skin (148). Neurons from the same ganglia that contain CCK/CGRP/substance P innervate arterioles of skeletal muscle; CGRP/DYN/substance P nerve fibers mostly supply the pelvic viscera, and CGRP/substance P fibers run mainly to the heart, large arteries, and veins (148).

Somatostatin has been detected in neurons of sensory ganglia (149) and in capsaicin-sensitive perivascular nerves in the brain (150). It causes vasoconstriction in almost all of the vessels that have been studied, including pial and extracerebral arteries (54,151), mesenteric artery and vein (152), and the portal vein (153). Gastrin-releasing peptide and CCK are present in cerebrovascular nerves (154,155), although there is a lack of evidence for vasomotor effects on the cerebral vasculature. Capsaicin treatment of the guinea pig and trigeminal ganglionectomy of the cat both caused a complete disappearance of CCK-LI in cerebrovascular nerves (156).

Galanin-LI has been detected in CGRP-containing neurons of the dorsal root ganglia (DRG) (157) and in perivascular nerves of the gut (158–160). Its action, if any, on the vasculature is unknown.

There is also evidence for a sensory role for ATP and it has been proposed that ATP may coexist in sensory nerve terminals with substance P and CGRP (1).

Neuropeptides and Sensorimotor Neuromodulation

In addition to their direct effects on blood vessels, pre- and postjunctional neuromodulatory actions have been described for substance P and CGRP. When substance P is injected with CGRP into human skin, it is able to convert the CGRP-mediated long-lasting vasodilatation into a transient response by a mechanism that is dependent on the action of proteases released from mast cells by substance P (161). On the other hand, CGRP potentiates tachykinin-induced plasma protein extravasation in rat and rabbit skin (162). CGRP has been shown to potentiate substance P transmission in the spinal cord by inhibiting a specific substance P–endopeptidase and by increasing the release of substance P from capsaicin-superfused slices of dorsal spinal cord *in vitro* (see ref. 33). By analogy with other systems, it seems likely that modulatory interactions between substance P, CGRP, ATP, and other putative sensory cotransmitters will increasingly be described in the periphery. Galanin has been shown to have an inhibitory action on the positive inotrophic responses due to antidromic activation of peripheral terminals of capsaicin-sensitive neurons in guinea pig atria (163). Somatostatin has been shown to inhibit the release of substance P from sensory nerve endings (164). Somatostatin reduces mesenteric blood flow in the dog and diminishes the vasodilator effect of intraarterial capsaicin (165,166), suggesting that it modulates the activity of sensory-afferent nerve fibers.

Perivascular Nerves Projecting from Intrinsic Neurons

Gut

Projections of fibers from the enteric nervous system have been shown to extend to mesenteric and other local vessels. Perivascular substance P–LI fibers, which are insensitive to capsaicin treatment, have been found supplying arterioles of the distal colon and rectum of rats (167,168) and are likely to have arisen from enteric substance P neurons in the gut. Extensive and detailed studies have allowed a very complete mapping of the complex neuronal markers and projections of enteric neurons (169,170). Several peptidergic substances including NPY, VIP, PHI, substance P, and CGRP have been identified in intrinsic enteric neurons, often coexisting (up to six peptides in the same neuron) with the classic neurotransmitters NA and ACh (170). The pre-

cise roles of the coexisting substances, however, have not for the most part been established, except for the proposed combinations of ACh and substance P in the excitatory nerves and ATP and VIP in the NANC inhibitory neurons involved in peristaltic reflexes. The recent co-localization of NOS and NADPH-d in cultured myenteric neurons of the guinea pig (171), together with evidence for a role for NO in the inhibitory control of some intestinal smooth muscle, and the co-localization of NOS and VIP in neurons of the myenteric plexus (94) raises the possibility of cotransmission of NO/ATP/VIP. Both CGRP and tachykinins stimulate the release of ACh from nerves in the gut (172). The vasodilator effect of VIP in submucosal arterioles of the guinea pig is attributed to the activation of enteric cholinergic vasodilator neurons (173). Other intrinsic interactions are also likely to occur, possibly involving NO.

Heart

Studies of intrinsic cardiac neurons in culture have shown that some of these neurons show immunofluorescence for mixtures of both NPY and 5-HT in different proportions (174). A clue to the physiological significance of this coexistence is that both 5-HT and NPY are potent vasoconstrictors of coronary vessels and may have synergistic actions. ACh and ATP may also be utilized as neurotransmitters by intracardiac neurons (175). In addition, the presence of NOS immunoreactivity and positive staining for NADPH-d have recently been detected in a subpopulation of intrinsic neurons of the guinea pig heart (176), suggesting that complex patterns of coexistence and interactions between a variety of neurotransmitters and NO are likely to occur.

Neurotensin, a tridecapeptide isolated from bovine hypothalamus (177), is present in perivascular nerve fibers in the heart (178,179), brain (180), and kidney (181). The actions of neurotensin are varied; it has been shown to cause vasoconstriction in a number of vessels (182), but has no effect on rat cerebral vessels (151).

Airways

Intrinsic ganglia in the airways are capable of integrating complex local reflex activity (183–185). Intrinsic neurons project from these ganglia to contribute to neuronal regulation of blood vessels in the airways.

Other

Recently, NO together with ATP have been shown to be mediators of NANC vasodilatation of the rabbit portal vein, raising the possibility of NO/ATP cotransmission (186).

Vasopressin-LI nerves have been shown to be present in the vasculature of mammals (187,188). Vasopressin exerts a potent vasoconstriction in all of the vessels in which it has been tested (189,190), probably through a V_1 receptor situated on smooth muscle cells (191).

NEUROPEPTIDES AND INTERACTIONS BETWEEN DIFFERENT TYPES OF PERIVASCULAR NERVES—"CROSS-TALK"

Histochemical studies providing evidence for dense networks of perivascular nerves in many vessels support the concept that reciprocal interactions or "cross-talk" can occur between transmitters released from different nerve types. Cross-talk is not a new concept, having been extensively demonstrated for the classic transmitters NA and ACh (see, for example, ref. 192). However, our knowledge about the extent of this cross-talk appears to be expanding with a rapidity proportional to the increase in number of recently discovered cotransmitter substances contained in perivascular nerves. Exactly how these interactions contribute to various physiological and pathophysiological conditions is not yet fully understood. This section presents evidence for interactions between classes of perivascular nerves with emphasis on the roles of neuropeptides. Clearly, the integrity of any one nerve type will to a greater or lesser extent influence the density and function of other nerve types, with implications for the development of disorders of the control of vascular tone leading to hypertension and other cardiovascular disorders.

Interactions Between Sympathetic and Sensorimotor Nerves

Sympathetic peptide and nonpeptide neurotransmitters have been shown to elicit pre- and postjunctional modulatory effects on sensorimotor neurotransmission (Fig. 4). In the rat mesenteric arterial bed the activity of sensorimotor nerves has been shown to be subject to prejunctional inhibitory neuromodulation by the sympathetic cotransmitters NA (via α_2-adrenoceptors) (193) and NPY (194,195) (Fig. 5), and by adenosine (via A_1-receptors, possibly following breakdown from ATP) (196,197). The inhibitory action of NPY may be quite a general one, since it also inhibits transmission at other NANC terminals (198).

Inhibitory opioid control of primary afferent nerves in the rat hind paw (199) and in capsaicin-sensitive sensory nerves in the guinea pig atria (200,201) have been described. Recently, opioid peptides have been shown to elicit inhibitory effects on sensorimotor nerves in the rat mesenteric arterial bed via opioid receptors of the μ subtype (73,195,202). Furthermore, the opioid receptor an-

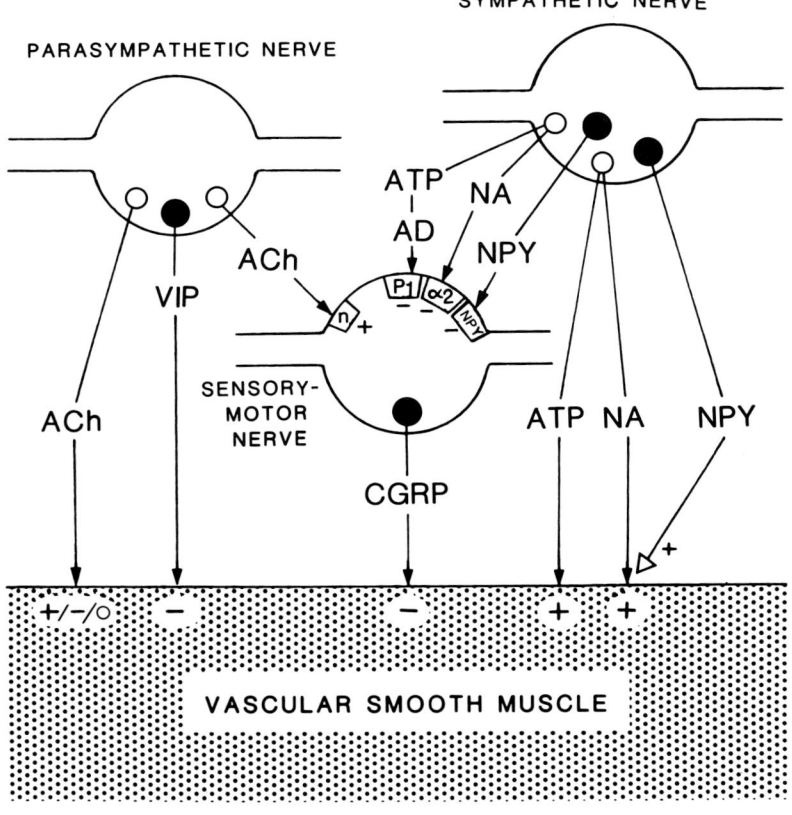

FIG. 4. Schematic representation showing the principal interactions between sympathetic, parasympathetic, and sensorimotor nerves. Sensorimotor neurotransmission is subject to prejunctional inhibitory modulation by adenosine 5'-triphosphate (ATP) (via its breakdown product adenosine [AD]), noradrenaline (NA), and neuropeptide Y (NPY) released from sympathetic varicosities. Acetylcholine (ACh) released from parasympathetic nerves stimulates the release of calcitonin gene-related peptide (CGRP) from sensorimotor nerves. Postjunctional vasoconstrictor (+) and vasodilator (−) responses are indicated. In most vessels ACh has no direct effect (O) on the vascular smooth muscle. Postjunctional potentiation of vasoconstrictor responses to NA by NPY are shown. VIP, vasoactive intestinal peptide; n, nicotinic receptor; P_1, purinoceptor; α_2, adrenoceptor.

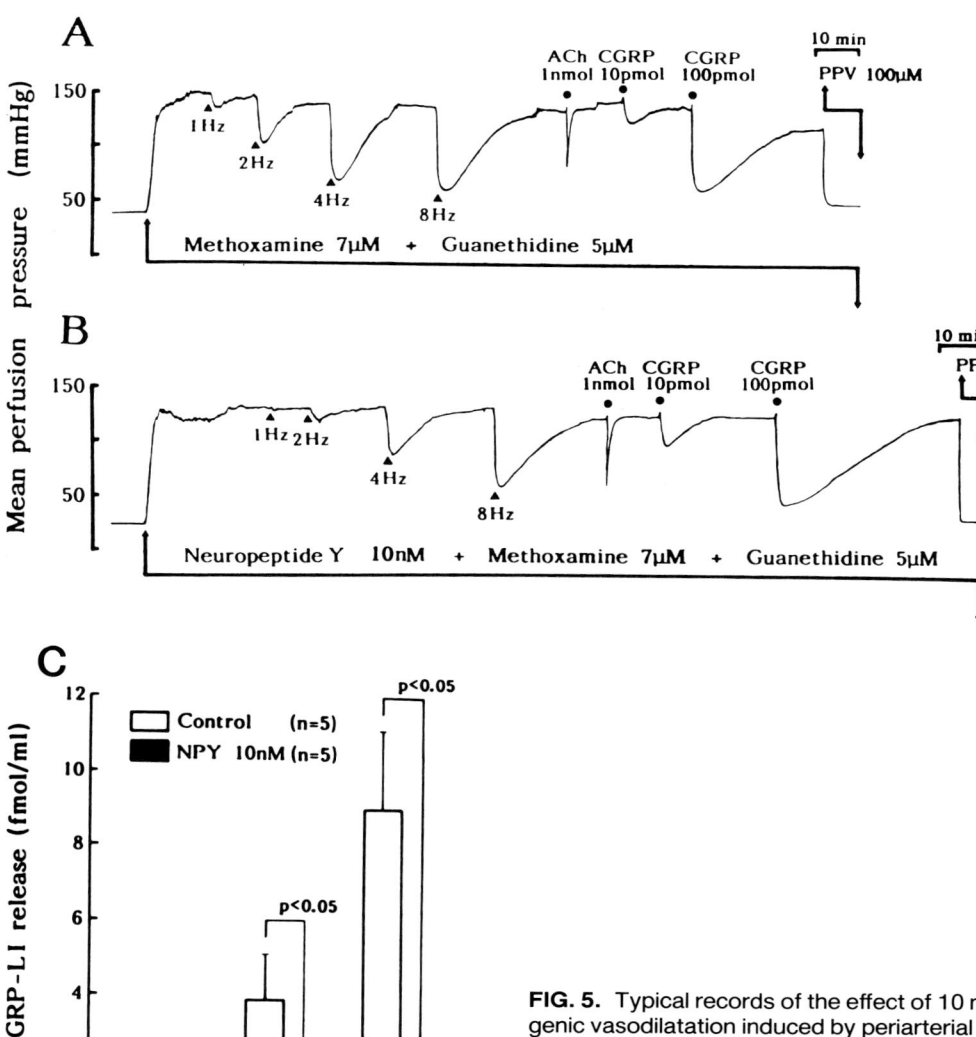

FIG. 5. Typical records of the effect of 10 nM neuropeptide Y (NPY) on neurogenic vasodilatation induced by periarterial nerve stimulation (PNS), and of the effect of bolus infusion of acetylcholine (ACh, 1 nmol) and rat calcitonin gene-related peptide (CGRP, 10 and 100 pmol) in perfused mesenteric vascular beds with active tone produced by 7 μM methoxamine in presence of 5 μM guanethidine. **A:** Responses in absence of NPY. **B:** Responses in presence of 10 nM NPY. PPV, papaverine. **C:** Effect of NPY on neurogenic release of CGRP-like immunoreactivity (CGRP-LI) induced by periarterial nerve stimulation (PNS) in perfused mesenteric vascular beds in the presence of 5 μM guanethidine. (From ref. 194, with permission.)

tagonist, naloxone, potentiated sensorimotor vasodilatation in mesenteric beds from reserpine treated rats (in which sympathetic nerves are depleted of their catecholamine content, but not of other substances such as ATP, NPY and opioids) (202), consistent with an endogenous source of opioid peptides in sympathetic nerves. An alternative source of opioid peptides is represented by enkephalin- and DYN-containing nerves projecting from the gut, as has been shown in guinea pig mesenteric arteries (203).

The modulatory effects of sensorimotor transmitters on sympathetic nerves in the periphery are predominantly postjunctional. The classic sensory neurotrans-

mitters substance P and CGRP have been shown to influence sympathetic transmission in several peripheral systems. For example, substance P can act as a postjunctional neuromodulator in the rat mesenteric bed, where it potentiates vasoconstrictor responses to NA (204). Postjunctional sympathetic neuromodulation has been demonstrated for CGRP in the rat mesenteric arterial bed (142), rat hepatic artery (205), and rabbit ear artery (206), where CGRP attenuated sympathetic vasoconstriction but did not affect the release of NA. Tachykinins have been shown to facilitate transmitter release from sympathetic nerve terminals (207,208), and CGRP seems to have an inhibitory influence, particularly on the release of ATP (209). Facilitatory receptors for NKA and bradykinin on sympathetic nerves have also been described.

Interactions Between Sympathetic and Parasympathetic Nerves

In the uterine cervix, NPY inhibits cholinergic transmission by an action that appears to be presynaptic (210). Prejunctional inhibitory effects of NPY on cholinergic transmission in the guinea pig heart *in vitro* have been shown (211), although it was not determined whether these occurred at the postganglionic terminals or pre- or postsynaptically at the parasympathetic ganglion. Interactions between the vagus and sympathetic nerves on heart rate has also been described in anesthetized dogs, in which prolonged attenuation of the action of the vagus following sympathetic stimulation could be abolished by guanethidine and was demonstrated to be due to the release of NPY from the sympathetic nerves (32,212). Intermittent high-frequency stimulation of cardiac sympathetic nerves was found to be more effective in inhibiting cardiac vagal action than continuous stimulation with the same mean frequency (32). This effect was not mimicked by several other peptides that have been reported to occur in or near the heart, including VIP, somatostatin, neurotensin, vasopressin, and substance P (213).

Recent evidence shows that NO can modulate the activity of sympathetic nerves. An inhibitor of the synthesis of NO reduced NA outflow from sympathetic nerves in the rat mesenteric arterial bed, suggesting that NO can enhance sympathetic neurotransmission (214). In the rabbit coronary artery, maximally relaxing concentrations of NO were found to have no effect on NA release (215). The origin of this NO is not clear; being ubiquitous, its source could be as a transmitter from adjacent parasympathetic or intrinsic NO-containing nerves, or from the vascular endothelium.

Interactions Between Parasympathetic and Sensorimotor Nerves

ACh, via nicotinic receptors, stimulates capsaicin-sensitive sensory neurons in a number of preparations (216–221) (Fig. 4).

PEPTIDES IN ENDOTHELIAL CELLS

Several lines of evidence indicate that endothelial cells are a major site of storage, release, and in some cases synthesis of a number of peptide and nonpeptide substances, including substance P, vasopressin, angiotensin II (AgII), NPY, atrial natriuretic factor, endothelin, 5-HT, ATP, and ACh (see ref. 222). These factors contribute to the control of vascular tone in response to changes in the local environment, for instance in blood flow or oxygenation. It is particularly appropriate that signals generated by the endothelium should be the means by which the caliber of blood vessels is regulated, in view of the central position of endothelial cells as the boundary between the circulation and the rest of the vessel wall. It is well recognized that malfunctions in endothelial cells occur in hypertension; it is possible that these may extend to changes in the content of endothelial vasoactive substances and hence to endothelial-mediated autoregulatory control mechanisms.

Storage and Synthesis of Peptides in Endothelial Cells

Immunocytochemical staining combined with electron microscopy has been used to show the presence of substance P, 5-HT, vasopressin, AgII, endothelin-1, and ChAT in endothelial cells of a variety of blood vessels, including coronary, mesenteric, femoral, renal, pulmonary, and cerebral arteries *in situ* (223–229) and in rabbit aortic endothelial cells in primary culture (230) (Fig. 6). More recently, NPY and atrial natriuretic peptide have been localized in endothelial cells of human umbilical vessels (231). Immunocytochemical staining has proved invaluable for localizing vasoactive substances within endothelial cells, but generally cannot distinguish between their presence as a consequence of intracellular synthesis, or as a result of uptake from the circulation.

Vasopressin

Vasopressin is a potent vasoconstrictor that can elicit endothelium-dependent and -independent relaxation (232,233). It has been demonstrated by immunocytochemistry with electron microscopy that vasopressin immunoreactivity can be localized in the cytoplasm of endothelial cells in rat mesenteric and renal arteries (226). In both of these vessels, about 10 percent of the endothelial cells were immunoreactive for vasopressin. Recently, a higher frequency of staining for vasopressin has been observed in rat pulmonary endothelial cells, with approximately 50 percent of pulmonary endothelial cells revealing vasopressin immunoreactivity (227). In cultured endothelial cells of the rabbit aorta more than 60 percent of cells exhibited co-localization of vasopressin and 5-HT (230). Whether endothelial cells are capable of synthesizing vasopressin from its amino acid precursors or whether the hormone is taken up from the circulation is unknown.

Angiotensin-Converting Enzyme

Angiotensin-converting enzyme (ACE), which is responsible for the conversion of AgI to its vasoactive

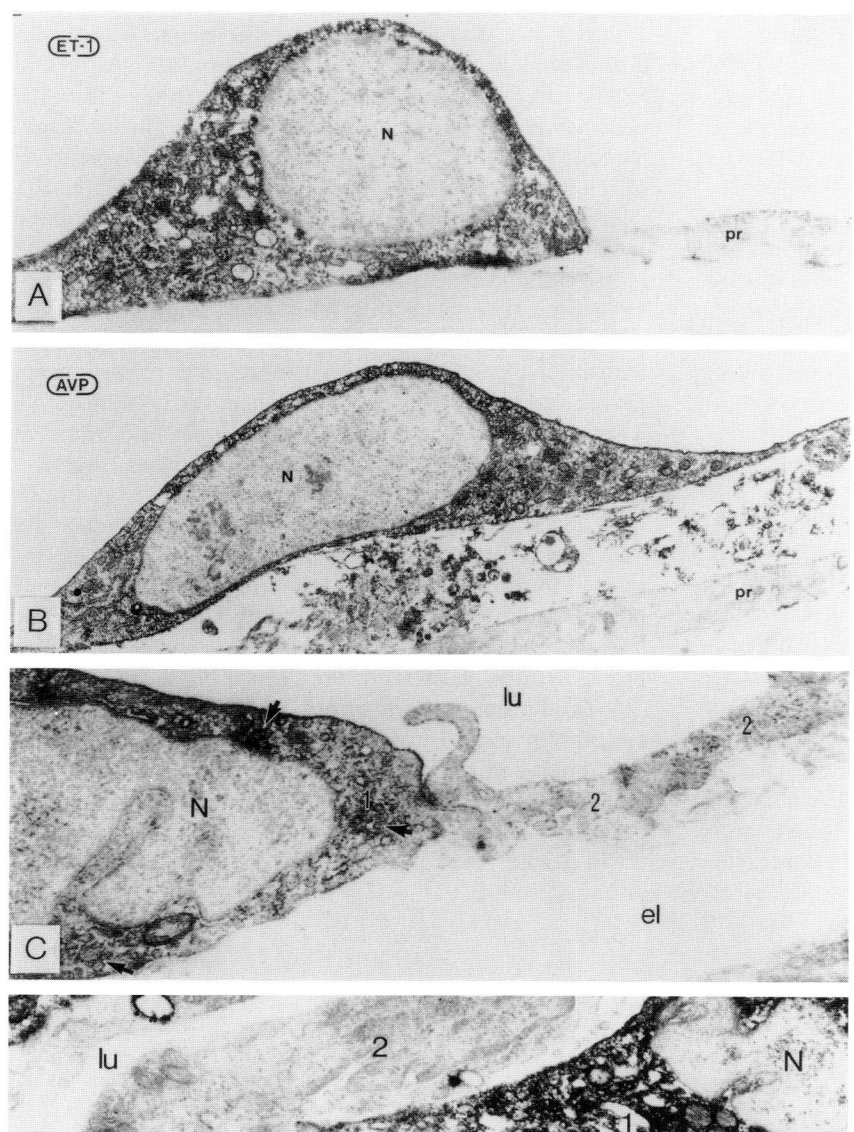

FIG. 6. A, B: Electron micrographs of cultured endothelial cells of rabbit aorta showing cytoplasmic staining of cells positive for endothelin-1 (ET-1) (A) and arginine-vasopressin (AVP) (B). The labeled cells contain numerous organelles. Note the unlabeled nuclei (N) and also the unlabeled neighboring endothelial cell processes (pr). A, ×6000; B, ×6000. **C:** A fragment of rat femoral artery demonstrates a substance P–positive endothelial cell (*1*). Note vesicles (*arrows*) dispersed through the labeled cytoplasm. The nucleus of the cell is unlabeled. Profiles of neighboring endothelial cells are substance P–negative (*2*). **D:** Electron micrograph of rat mesenteric artery. An example of AgII-positive (*1*) and AgII-negative (*2*) endothelial cells; bm, basement membrane. ×11,700. (A, B from ref. 230, with permission; C from ref. 223, with permission; D from ref. 226, with permission.)

product AgII (234), is localized in endothelial cells of capillaries and large arteries and veins throughout the vasculature of the lung, liver, adrenal cortex, pancreas, kidney, and spleen (235). In pulmonary vessels ACE is concentrated on the luminal surface of endothelial cells (234,236); however, evidence also exists for the synthesis of AgII within the vascular wall (237). Intracellular synthesis of AgII and renin expression by bovine aortic endothelial cells have been reported (238,239). Hence, it appears that the AgII immunoreactivity that has been localized in endothelial cells of the rat mesenteric artery (226) is likely to be there as a consequence of synthesis rather than uptake. Interestingly, AgII was not localized in endothelial cells of the rat renal artery (226). This is consistent with an earlier suggestion that endothelial cells of the renal glomerulus may be unique among en-

dothelial cells in that they are not immunoreactive to ACE (237,238).

Substance P

Immunocytochemical studies have shown that substance P and 5-HT are localized, in different proportions, in endothelial cells in coronary, mesenteric, renal, and femoral arteries of the rat (223,224,226). A nonneuronal source of substance P was also demonstrated for intracranial and extracranial feline cephalic arteries in 1985 by Norregaard and Moskowitz (240). These workers found that while sensory denervation of these vessels by trigeminal ganglionectomy caused a complete depletion of substance P–immunoreactive nerve fibers, there was only a 55 percent reduction in the total vessel substance P content. More recently, substance P levels have been measured in isolated endothelium from human cerebral arteries and bovine aorta (241,242). It is not yet clear whether endothelial cells have the capacity to synthesize substance P. Conflicting results have been obtained using passages of endothelial cells in culture but these may reflect inherent problems associated with this technique. Substance P was measured in freshly isolated bovine aortic endothelial cells, but not in primary cultures prepared from the same source (241). On the other hand, substance P was still detectable in a primary culture of bovine cerebral microvessels (at levels of 20 percent of that of freshly isolated cells); thereafter, consecutive passages of these cells revealed similar levels of substance P, suggesting that substance P was being synthesized by the cells (241). Attempts to identify preprotachykinin mRNA, which encodes substance P, within endothelial cells have so far been unsuccessful (241,242).

Endothelin

Endothelial cells are known to produce endothelin, the most potent vasoconstrictor peptide known. This 21-residue peptide has been isolated from porcine aortic endothelial cells, and the complementary DNA of its precursor, preproendothelin, has been cloned and sequenced (243,244). Analysis of the human endothelin gene has revealed three distinct isoforms of endothelin: endothelin-1, endothelin-2, and endothelin-3 (245). Endothelial cells produce exclusively endothelin-1. Co-localization of endothelin-1 with NO within endothelial cells has elegantly been shown by double immunogold labeling (Fig. 7). Endothelin is also expressed in neurons of the human spinal cord and dorsal root ganglia (246). Endothelin is a potent vasoconstrictor, both in isolated vessels and *in vivo*. Characteristic slowly developing and long-lasting vasoconstrictor responses to endothelin have been observed in rabbit skin microvasculature (247), isolated human resistance vessels (248), canine femoral artery and vein (249), porcine coronary artery (244), and rat mesenteric resistance vessels (250,251), while intravenous injection causes a rapid and transient decrease in systemic blood pressure followed by a profound and long-lasting increase in blood pressure in rats (252,253). In the human forearm circulation, endothelin increases peripheral vascular resistance and decreases local blood flow (254). Endothelin may also influence blood pressure indirectly via actions on the autonomic nervous system (255–257) and has been shown to inhibit NA neurotransmission in the guinea pig femoral artery (258) and rat mesenteric artery (256). On the other hand, endothelin may, by potentiating the effects of sympathetic nerve stimulation, NA and 5-HT (256,259–261), contribute to vasospasm. In addition to its vasoconstrictor action, endothelin can elicit vasodilatation in a variety of isolated blood vessels (251,262–267) and in whole animals (268–270).

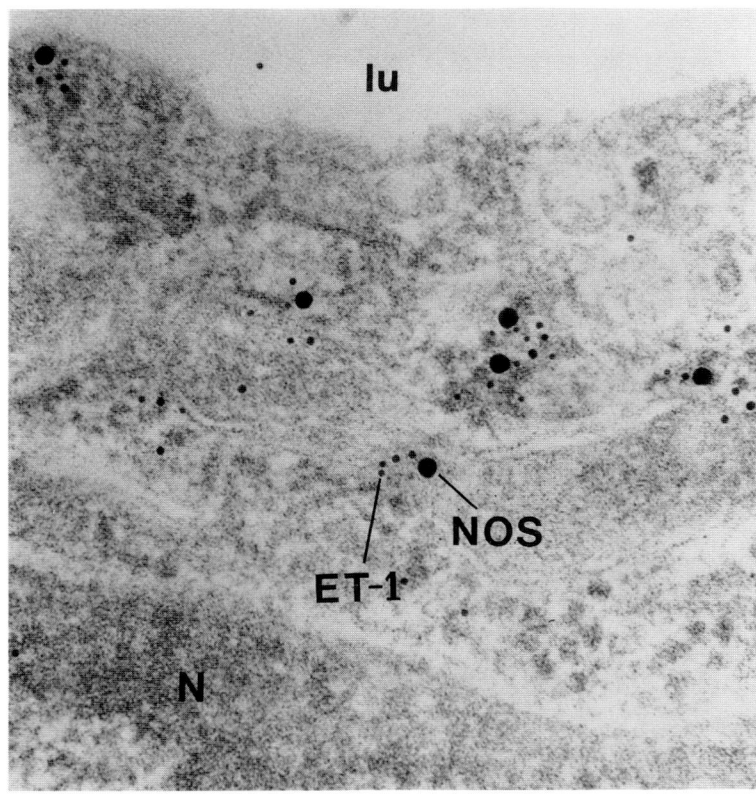

FIG. 7. Electron micrograph of fragment of rabbit aorta. Immunogold labeling shows co-localization of nitric oxide synthase (NOS) (large particles) and endothelin-1 (ET-1) (small particles). N, nucleus; lu, lumen. ×182,000 (Courtesy of A. Loesch.)

Release of Peptides from Endothelial Cells

The physiological relevance of the storage and synthesis of peptide and nonpeptide substances in endothelial cells is that changes in the hemodynamic environment, for instance an increase in blood flow or decrease in oxygenation, triggers their release from endothelial cells. These substances can then act on specific receptors on the same or neighboring endothelial cells to stimulate the release of endothelium-derived relaxing factor (EDRF), which in turn acts on the underlying smooth muscle to produce vasodilatation. Hence, blood vessel tone can be regulated under conditions when an increase in blood flow is desirable to maintain vascular homeostasis.

Substance P, 5-HT, ATP, and ACh, all of which are present in coronary endothelial cells, have been shown to be released during hypoxia from perfused guinea pig and rat hearts (224,225,271). Since substance P, ATP, 5-HT, and ACh elicit coronary vasodilatation via specific receptors on the coronary endothelium (272–275), this provides a mechanism for the hypoxic vasodilator response. The different time course of release of these substances has allowed speculation that 5-HT and ATP, released immediately with the onset of hypoxia, may have a role in initiating the hypoxic vasodilatation, while substance P and adenosine (formed as a breakdown product of ATP) may have a role in maintaining the response (224,273,276).

In the perfused rat hindlimb, an increase in flow has been shown to cause release of substance P into the effluent (277). After removal of the endothelium by perfusion with air bubbles (278), increased flow no longer evoked the release of substance P. Furthermore, denervation of the hindlimb vasculature of substance P–containing nerves by neonatal capsaicin treatment had no effect on flow-induced release of substance P (277), implicating an endothelial and not a neuronal source of this peptide. Substance P is a potent endothelium-

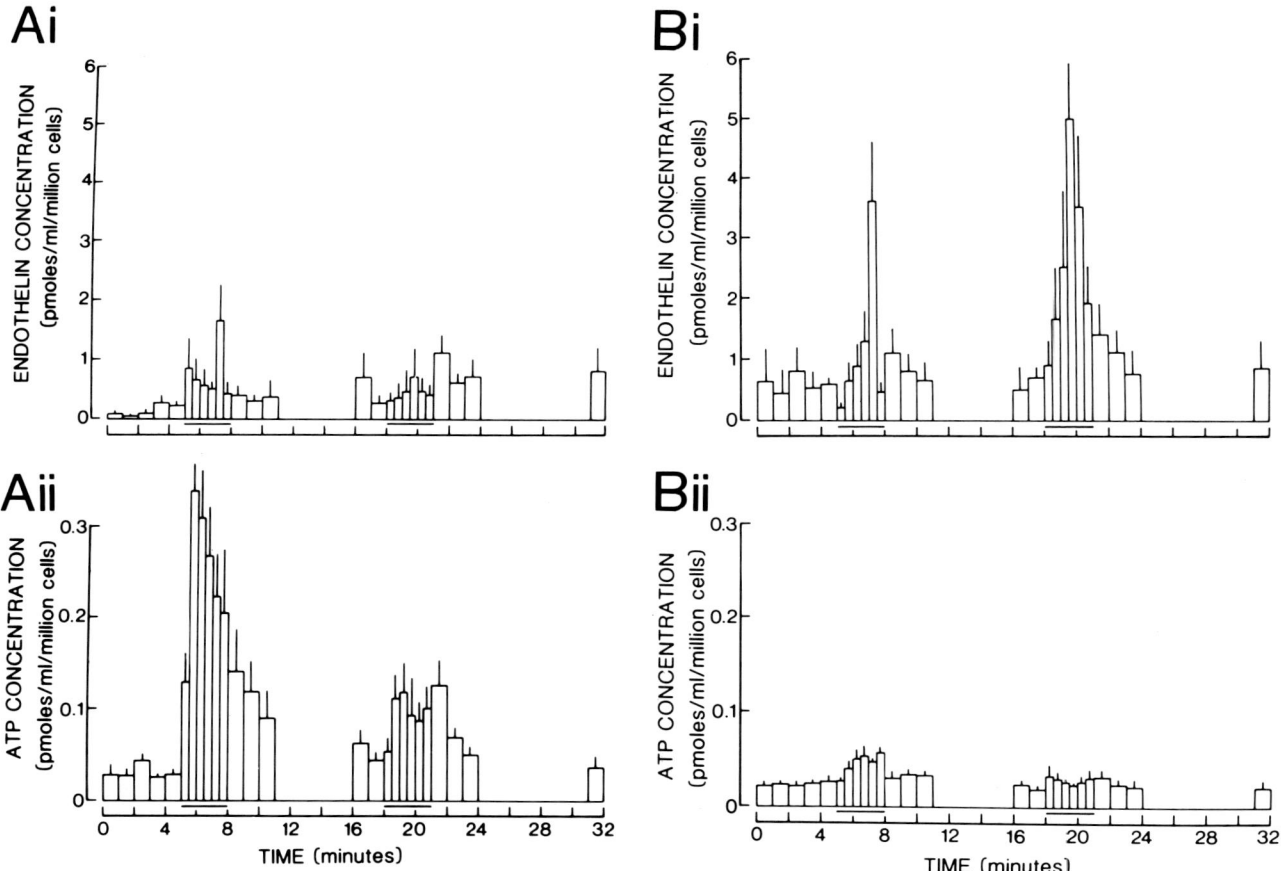

FIG. 8. A: Release of (i) endothelin, and (ii) ATP, by freshly isolated endothelial cells from the thoracic aorta of normoxic rats. Cells were perfused at a low flow rate (0.5 ml min^{-1}) and stimulated twice (with an interval of 10 min) by an increased flow rate (3.0 ml min^{-1}) for 3 min (shown by lines under the x-axis); $n = 4$. **B:** Release of (i) endothelin, and (ii) ATP, by freshly isolated endothelial cells from the thoracic aorta of chronically hypoxic rats. Cells were perfused at a low flow rate (0.5 ml min^{-1}) and stimulated twice (with an interval of 10 min) by an increased flow rate (3.0 ml min^{-1}) for 3 min (shown by lines under the x-axis); $n = 4$. (From ref. 286, with permission.)

dependent vasodilator and has been localized within endothelial cells of the rat femoral artery (223). Hence, it is possible that a physiological role of substance P released from endothelial cells during an increase in flow is to initiate the well-established endothelium-dependent vasodilatation that occurs as a consequence of increased flow. Substance P, ATP, and ACh are released following an increase in the rate of perfusion of columns of human umbilical vein endothelial cells grown on microcarrier beads (279), supporting the view that changes in flow can stimulate the release of these substances from endothelial cells.

In the porcine aorta, endothelin is continuously released in an endothelium-dependent manner, as it is in endothelial cells in culture (280–282). Low levels of circulating endothelin have also been detected in human plasma (283). Despite evidence for the widespread distribution of endothelin receptors (284,285) and its profound and diverse biological activity, the role(s) of endothelin in the cardiovascular system is not well established. Endothelin is unlikely to be responsible for hypoxic vasoconstriction, since the slow time course of the response to endothelin has been proposed to be incompatible with the rapid onset of the hypoxic vasoconstrictor response that occurs in most vessels. Endothelin (together with ATP, but not VIP) has been shown to be released from isolated rabbit aortic endothelial cells in response to an increase in flow (286,287) (Fig. 8). Indeed, changes in flow may modulate the synthesis of endothelin, since increased shear stress was able to induce the synthesis of preproendothelin-1 mRNA in cultured endothelial cells (288).

NEUROPEPTIDES AND LONG-TERM (TROPHIC) CONTROL OF VASCULAR FUNCTION

Changes in innervation involving one class of perivascular nerves have been shown to lead to significant changes in the surviving populations, a reflection of the remarkable plasticity of the peripheral nervous system. In addition, perivascular nerves play a major role in the development of blood vessels via long-term trophic effects on the vascular smooth muscle and endothelium. A number of studies have specifically demonstrated important roles for neuropeptides in these long-term trophic mechanisms. Neuropeptides can induce changes in neuronal excitability at both the pre- and postjunctional level via responses that are less intense but of longer duration than those produced by classic transmitters. Further, many neuropeptides elicit cellular responses via transmembrane signaling systems that are also utilized in cell growth. It has therefore been speculated that certain neuropeptides have trophic effects, being involved

in growth and development of components of the vessel wall, including nerves, smooth muscle, and endothelial cells (103,289–292). This would account for the fact that certain of the neuropeptides that have been identified as cotransmitters in perivascular nerves have been shown to have little direct actions on blood vessels. Hence, long-term interactions that occur between classes of perivascular nerves and the trophic influence of perivascular nerves on the blood vessel wall should be taken into account when considering the contribution of perivascular nerves to physiological or pathophysiological conditions, including hypertension.

Neuropeptides and Plasticity of Perivascular Nerves

Remarkable plasticity of the peripheral nervous system has been shown (see ref. 293). Following elimination of either sensory or sympathetic nerves, the remaining nerve population undergoes changes consistent with marked proliferation of the nerve terminals. The resulting hyperinnervation by the remaining population is ultimately due to the upsetting of a competitive balance between these nerves, supporting the concept that neurotrophic competition plays a major role in establishing innervation levels in target tissues. Clearly, an implication of these reciprocal interactions is that the roles of sympathetic, parasympathetic, and sensorimotor nerves should be equally considered in terms of their contribution to hypertension. In addition, the roles of individual cotransmitters should be considered, since plasticity has been shown to include changes in the proportion of coexisting transmitters within a single population of nerves.

Permanent destruction of capsaicin-sensitive afferent neurons can lead to an increase in the transmitter content and/or innervation density of sympathetic nerve endings (294,295). Conversely, long-term ablation of sympathetic neurons is followed by an increase in the peptidergic afferent innervation (294,296–299). It has also been shown that there is an increase in enteric NPY-containing neurons after long-term loss of sympathetic neurons, possibly representing a long-term compensatory mechanism (300). Fike et al. (301) recently showed that sensory denervation improved sympathetic reinnervation in partially sympathectomized rat superior tarsal smooth muscle. These workers also showed that sustained juvenile sympathectomy was associated with sensory hyperinnervation. Mione et al. (302) have demonstrated that guanethidine treatment reverses the loss of CGRP-LI fibers (but not substance P–LI fibers) caused by neonatal capsaicin treatment, further illustrating the plasticity of expression and interdependence of sympathetic and sensory nerves.

Reciprocal interactions between afferent and sympathetic neurons may be responsible for the decreased mesenteric blood flow seen in adult rats treated neonatally with capsaicin (303), which could reflect hyperactivity of sympathetic vasoconstrictor neurons. Indeed, we have found an increased responsiveness to sympathetic nerve stimulation in mesenteric arterial beds from rats treated neonatally with capsaicin; there was also increased sensitivity to vasoconstrictor responses to NA and potassium chloride (304), suggesting that changes in the vascular smooth muscle had occurred and possibly mimicking the development of hypertension where increased sympathetic activity has trophic influences on smooth muscle development, generally resulting in hypertrophy and hyperplasia.

VIP has been shown to stimulate mitosis, promote neurite outgrowth and enhance the survival of sympathetic neuron precursors or neuroblasts in culture (305). More recently, VIP has been shown to modulate the neurotransmitter phenotype of cultured chick sympathetic neurons (290). An inhibitory sympathetic input to VIP- and neurotensin-containing nerves in the enteric nervous system is suggested by the increases in gut content of these peptides following guanethidine sympathectomy (306). On the other hand, there was an increase in dopamine β-hydroxylase immunoreactivity in nonnoradrenergic (NPY- and VIP-containing) axons supplying the guinea pig uterine artery after chemical sympathectomy with 6-OHDA (307). The number of NPY and VIP axons containing somatostatin also increased after 6-OHDA (307), demonstrating the plasticity of peripheral neurons, which can change their levels of neuropeptides and transmitter-synthesizing enzymes in response to local environmental changes.

Neuropeptides and Long-Term Effects on Vascular Smooth Muscle

There is evidence that a local release of sensory neuropeptides plays a trophic role in postnatal development and maturation of neuromuscular structures, as well as maintenance of tissue integrity and ability of repair in response to injury (see ref. 103). Substance P has been shown to stimulate proliferation of embryonic rat aortic smooth muscle cells (308). Similar findings have been observed with substance P and NKA on cultures of smooth muscle cells from the rat aorta (309). Vasopressin was shown to inhibit or stimulate human arterial smooth muscle cell proliferation, depending on the culture medium (310). Neuropeptides may modulate the expression of certain receptors on the muscle membrane; for instance, CGRP has been shown to increase the synthesis of ACh receptors at vertebrate neuromuscular junction (311,312). Trophic effects of neuropeptides on other cell types have also been described for VIP (313–

315), NPY (316), CGRP (317), NKA (318), substance P and substance K (292,309,318), bombesin (319), bradykinin (320), CCK (321), vasopressin (322), and endothelin (323) (see also 289,291).

Neuropeptides and Long-Term Effects on Endothelial Cells

Recent evidence has suggested that long-term interactions can occur between perivascular nerves and endothelial cells (see ref. 222). Selective manipulation (denervation or chronic stimulation) of specific populations of autonomic or sensory nerves has provided clear evidence for long-term interactions between perivascular nerves and endothelial cells. In a study of the rabbit ear artery, Mangiarua and Bevan (324) showed that surgical denervation to remove sympathetic and sensory nerves resulted in impaired endothelium-dependent vasodilator responses to methacholine. This was not due to an impaired ability of the smooth muscle to relax, since the endothelium-independent vasodilator response to sodium nitroprusside was unaffected. A recent study of the rat mesenteric arterial bed showed that selective destruction of capsaicin-sensitive primary sensory afferents in neonates resulted in adult rats with impaired endothelium-dependent vasodilator responses to ACh (325). In this study, destruction of sympathetic nerves with 6-OHDA had no such detrimental effect on endothelium-dependent vasodilatation, suggesting that sensory neuropeptides may have a trophic influence on endothelial cell development (325). In this respect both CGRP (326) and substance P (292,318) have been shown to have a proliferative effect on endothelial cells in culture.

Chronic stimulation (10 days in vivo) of the rabbit auricular nerve supplying the central ear artery produced marked structural and immunocytochemical changes in the endothelial cells of that vessel; a subpopulation of endothelial cells were found to have developed cytoplasmic protrusions of the apical region, which showed positive immunoreactivity for CGRP and NPY (327) (Fig. 9). Using the same model of chronic stimulation (4–16 days in vivo), a selective impairment of contractile responses to postjunctional stimulation of the P_{2x}-purinoceptor was observed, while constrictor responses to exogenous NA were unaffected (328). A unique study by Taguchi et al. (329) showed that intimal thickening produced by mechanical injury of the dog carotid artery resulted in an increase in substance P–containing nerve fibers as well as in neuron-specific enolase positive nerve fibers, but not in adrenergic or cholinergic fibers. The implication of this is that in addition to trophic effects exerted by perivascular nerves on endothelial cells, a reciprocal trophic effect of endothelial cells on nerves may also take place.

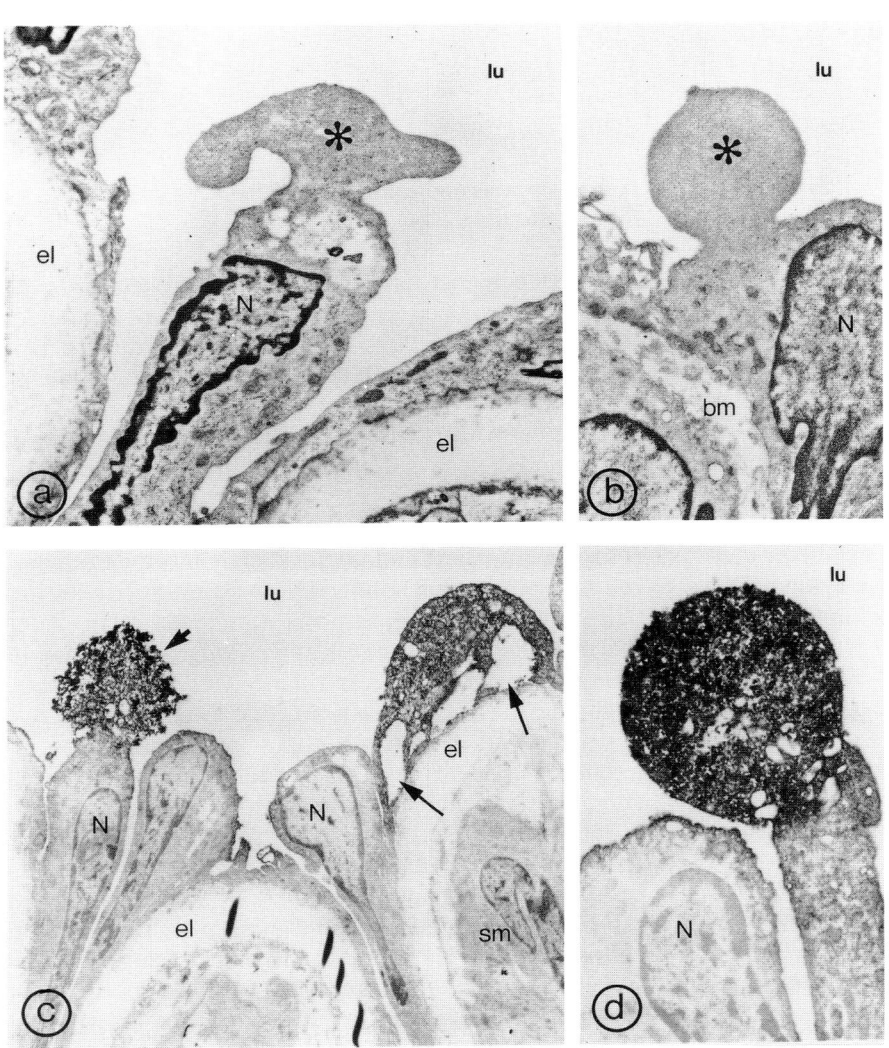

FIG. 9. Conventional electron microscopy (**A, B**) and electron-immunocytochemistry (**C, D**) of rabbit central ear artery following long-term electrical stimulation of perivascular nerves *in vivo*. A, B: Note the differences in shapes of the endothelium-associated protrusions (*asterisks*) and the granular nature of the cytoplasm of the protrusions. N, nucleus; el, elastic lamina; bm, basement membrane; sm, smooth muscle that penetrated into intima; lu, lumen of the artery. C: Note calcitonin gene-related peptide (CGRP)–like immunoreactivity associated with an endothelial cell partially separated from subendothelial cell layer (*longer arrows*). Protrusion at the apical region of another endothelial cell (*short arrow*) also shows CGRP-like immunoreactivity. D: Note neuropeptide Y (NPY)-like immunoreactivity, which is restricted to protrusion at the apical region of endothelial cell. A, B: ×8,000; C: ×6,400; D: ×8,800. (From ref. 327, with permission.)

HYPERTENSION

Hypertension is characterized by an increased peripheral vascular resistance that may be the result of structural and functional changes of the blood vessel wall leading to loss of blood vessel lumen volume. Structural changes in the media have been described, namely hyperplasia and hypertrophy, which would tend to promote the effects of vasoconstrictor substances and attenuate the effects of vasodilator substances. In addition, hypertension is associated with changes in perivascular nerves and endothelial cells. Essential hypertension is a multifactorial disease, with no single factor satisfactorily explaining all aspects of this condition. However, the sympathetic nervous system appears to be involved in essential hypertension in a subgroup of patients, although its specific involvement is unclear (330–332). Evidence in support of a contribution of sympathetic perivascular nerves to hypertension is presented to allow the roles of neuropeptides in hypertension to be put into context. The possible contribution of neuropeptides released as transmitters from sympathetic and other types of perivascular nerves is considered in terms of the development and maintenance of hypertension.

The Sympathetic Nervous System in Hypertension

It is known that there is an increase in sympathetic activity in various experimental models of hypertension, including deoxycorticosterone acetate (DOCA)-salt and SHR (333,334). Electron microscopic examination of sympathetic axon terminals in the sheep renal artery has shown an increase in the number of vesicles and in the size and density of granular cores in chronic renal hypertension (335) (Fig. 10). An increase in NA content and density of NA-containing nerves has been reported in tissues from SHR by many workers (333,336). Enhanced release of NA in SHR has also been seen, for example an increase in ^{3}H-NA from the portal vein and endogenous

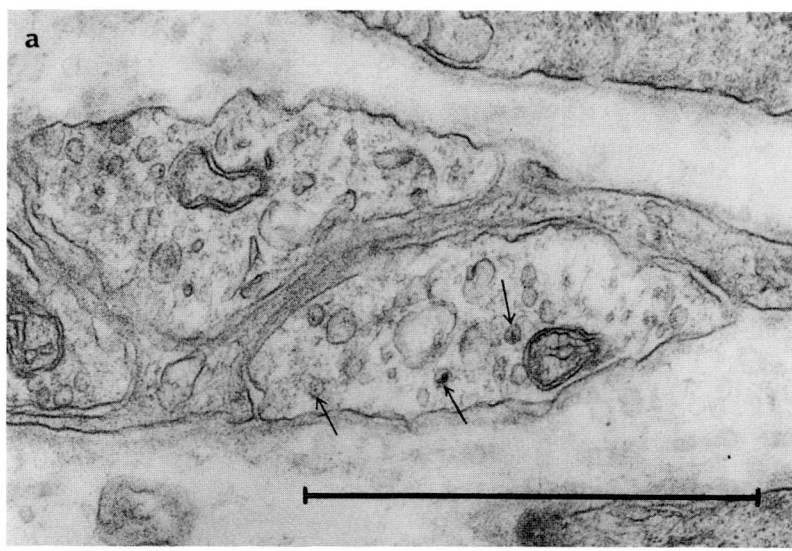

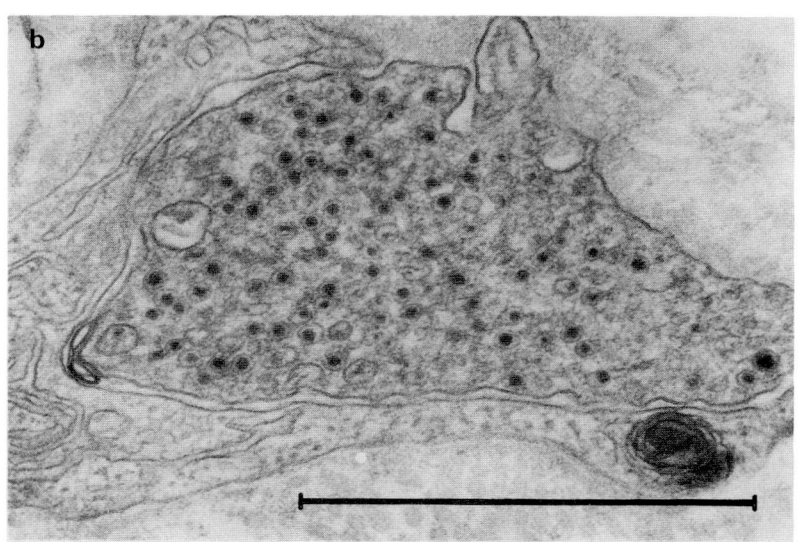

FIG. 10. Electron micrographs of axon profiles in the media of sheep renal artery. A: Axon profiles from a normal animal; note the moderate number of vesicles containing variably sized granular cores (*arrows*). B: Axon profile from sheep with chronic renal hypertension; note the increase in number of vesicles and in size and density of granular cores. Calibration 1 μm. (From ref. 335, with permission.)

NA from the caudal artery and perfused mesenteric arterial bed (337). Enhanced 5-HT release from sympathetic nerves of mesenteric beds from SHR (338) is also consistent with the commonly observed increase in sympathetic activity seen in hypertension. A 5-HT$_2$–receptor blocker, ketanserin, has been reported to reduce blood pressure in patients with essential hypertension (339,340).

Some of the most persuasive evidence for participation of the sympathetic nervous system in hypertension has come from the effects of various sympatholytic procedures where depletion of central and/or peripheral sites of catecholamines prevents or attenuates the development of hypertension in SHR (341), Dahl (salt-sensitive genetic hypertensive) (342,343), and DOCA-salt hypertensive (344) rats. Neonatal sympathectomy

of SHR not only prevented the development of hypertension in young animals, but also reduced the extent to which blood pressure elevation and cardiovascular hypertrophy were seen in adulthood (341,345).

Bevan (346) and Bevan and Tsuru (347) found that sympathetic denervation in young rabbits decreases uptake of ^{3}H-thymidine in the ear artery and inhibits normal proliferation of arterial smooth muscle cells, suggesting that normal development is inhibited by sympathetic denervation. Sympathetic nerves appear to influence the development of normal and hypertrophic vessels by an action that is independent of arterial pressure (348). Consistent with this is the fact that increased sympathetic innervation of SHR occurs immediately after birth and prior to the expression of a hypertensive elevation of blood pressure and medial hypertrophy and hyperplasia

(333,349). Various models of sympathectomy have shown that an incomplete sympathectomy usually results in the development of hypertension in SHR, indicating that the presence of a small portion of sympathetic transmitter appears to be sufficient for the development and maintenance of hypertension in SHR (350). This suggests that it may be the trophic influence of a hyperactive sympathetic nervous system on blood vessels which is crucial to the development of hypertension rather than the increase in pressure per se. A recent study showing that the hypertension produced in rats by administration of an inhibitor of NO (an endogenous vasodilator derived from the endothelium) was not associated with structural changes in mesenteric resistance arteries further suggests that increased pressure per se is not the principal factor responsible for hypertensive alterations in vascular structure (351).

Nerve growth factor (NGF) plays an important role in the development of perivascular nerves and in the continuous dynamic control of transmitter levels and synthesis in mature neurons. Hyperinnervation of the sympathetic nervous system observed in SHR has been discussed in the context of an increase in NGF (333,334,336,352–354). NGF has been shown to be increased in tissues from hypertensive rats at a young age, although the differences disappeared in adulthood (354). Furthermore, elevated levels of NGF in peripheral tissues of SHR (354–356) have been shown which are likely to be responsible for the hyperinnervation and resulting hyperplastic changes, but not exclusively for the elevated blood pressure (356). Studies supporting this hypothesis have shown that chronic NGF treatment leads to changes in vascular innervation and smooth muscle thickness that are similar to those seen in hypertensive rats (356), while antibodies against NGF given to neonatal SHR have been reported to either retard or prevent the development of hypertension in the SHR. In addition, mRNA for NGF has been shown to be markedly elevated in the kidney and mesenteric vasculature (but not in the heart) of SHR (357).

The sympathetic nervous system has also been shown to exert a repressive effect on the nuclear activity of effector cells, since long-term sympathetic denervation results in an increase in the dimensions and proliferative activity of effector cells (358). Osswald and colleagues found that the marked hypertrophy of the saphenous vein of the dog and the rabbit ear artery produced by surgical or chemical sympathectomy was prevented by constant infusion of adenosine or its stable analogue 5'-N-ethylcarboxamidoadenosine (NECA), and was mimicked by the adenosine receptor antagonist dipropylsulfophenylxanthine (DPSPX) (359–361). From these results they advanced the hypothesis that adenosine (resulting from the breakdown of ATP released from sympathetic nerves) is involved in the repressive trophic effects of sympathetic innervation (357,359). However,

how this relates to hypertension and to the recently reported increase in plasma levels of adenosine in conscious SHR (361) is not clear.

The importance of considering nerves in terms of their cotransmitter components and not just as a whole is emphasized by a number of studies showing that hypertension can differentially affect coexisting transmitter substances, changing their relative proportions within the nerve. For example, Rump et al. (362) showed that the pressor response to sympathetic nerve stimulation in the isolated kidney of SHR at 1 Hz is entirely purinergic and is attenuated by prostaglandin E_2 (PGE_2). In addition, evidence has been presented that there is a significantly greater cotransmitter role for ATP with NA in tail arteries of SHRs compared with normotensive rats (17), although other workers have reported that there are no differences (363).

Substantial evidence exists for pre- and postjunctional adrenergic dysfunctions in hypertension, namely impaired prejunctional regulation of sympathetic activity involving α_2-adrenoceptors and enhanced sensitivity of prejunctional β_2-adrenoceptors. A decrease in postjunctional β- and an increase or no change in α_1-receptors have also been shown. This has recently been reviewed (364).

Prejunctional inhibitory adenosine receptors on sympathetic terminals have been implicated in hypertension. For instance, in situ blood-perfused rat mesenteries from SHR were less sensitive than controls to the prejunctional inhibitory effects of adenosine (365). A diminished adenosine-mediated presynaptic inhibition of [^{3}H]NA release from mesenteric arteries of SHR has also been shown (366). Since adenosine is a degradation product of ATP, changes in presynaptic regulation by purines may be a reflection of changes in the amount of ATP released from the sympathetic terminal. A subsensitivity of presynaptic adenosine A_1-receptors has also been shown in caudal arteries of SHR, and one possible explanation advanced for this was down-regulation following overactivity of sympathetic transmission (367). Whatever the cause, it is evident that such a subsensitivity of presynaptic A_1-receptors would contribute to enhanced transmitter release from peripheral terminals and subsequently increase vascular resistance. A reduced sensitivity to the postjunctional vasodilator effects of adenosine has been observed in arterioles of the SHR cremaster muscle (368).

Some evidence exists for changes in parasympathetic neurotransmission in hypertension. For instance, Korner et al. (369) found that the elevated heart rate of hypertensives was the result mainly of parasympathetic inhibition, whereas the results reported by Julius et al. (370) and Julius and Esler (371) suggest a combination of parasympathetic inhibition and sympathetic stimulation. Henquet et al. (372) reported decreased salivary flow in borderline hypertensives, suggesting decreased parasympathetic activity. Evidence for changes in senso-rimotor nerves are discussed in the next subsection.

Neuropeptides in Hypertension

Some of the inconsistencies in the proposal that over-activity of the sympathetic nervous system is responsible for essential hypertension arise from studies showing that in SHR sympathetic overactivity is relatively minor

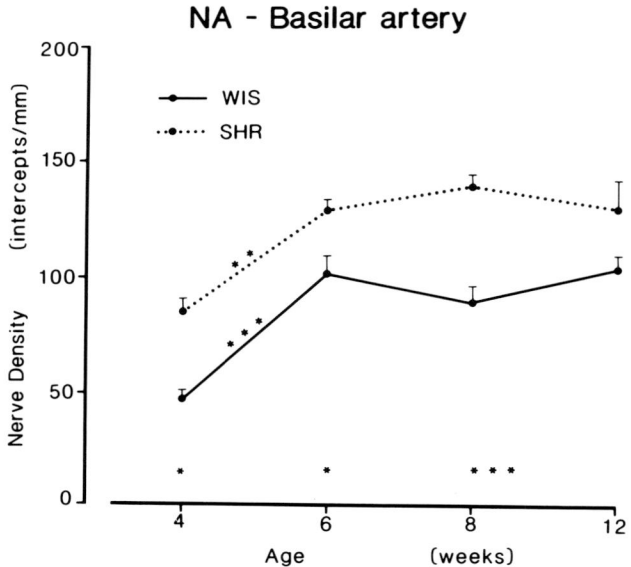

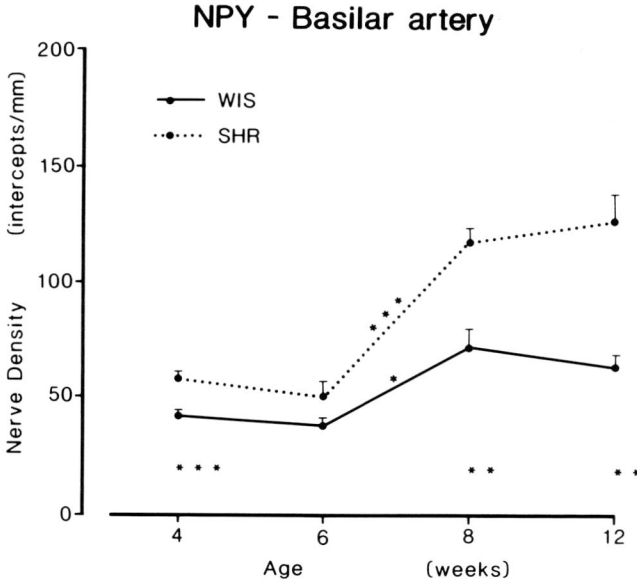

FIG. 11. Graphs showing developmental changes in the density of nerve fibers supplying the basilar artery in normotensive Wistar controls (WIS) and SHR. **A:** NA-containing nerve fibers. **B:** NPY-containing nerve fibers. *$p < .05$, **$p < .01$, ***$p < .001$. (From ref. 373, with permission.)

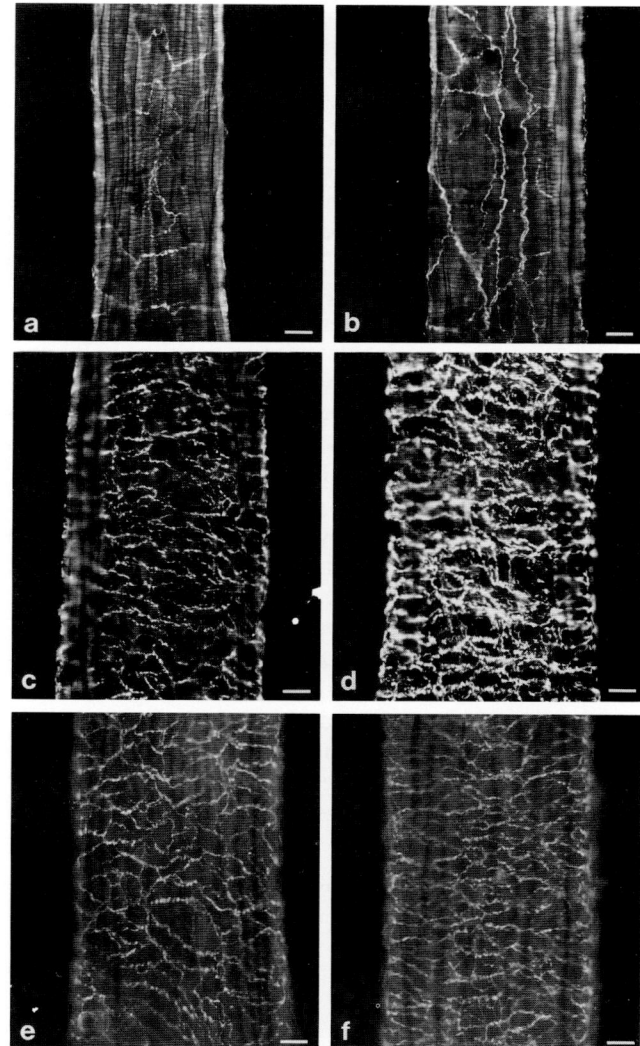

FIG. 12. Photomicrographs showing cerebrovascular nerves containing NA and NPY in normotensive Wistar and spontaneously hypertensive rats (SHR). **A, B:** NA-containing nerve supplying the superior cerebellar artery of 6-week-old Wistar and SHR, respectively. **C, D:** NA-containing nerves supplying the anterior cerebral artery of 4- and 12-week-old SHR, respectively. With the increased density of innervation there are more nerve fibers running close together in perivascular bundles, giving the impression of increased nerve thickness. **E, F:** NPY-containing nerves supplying the anterior cerebral artery of 4-week-old Wistar and SHR, respectively. Bars = 25 μm. (From ref. 373, with permission.)

and seems to diminish as the hypertension progresses. The fact that the stimulus is not maintained may suggest that while it may be important in the initiation, the maintenance depends on longer-term trophic mechanisms. This role may be provided by the neuropeptides present not only in sympathetic nerves but in any one of the other divisions of perivascular nerves.

A number of immunohistochemical studies have shown changes in neuropeptide-containing perivascular nerves in hypertension. An increase in NPY-LI and NA was seen in cerebrovascular nerves of SHR (373) (Figs. 11 and 12); the increase in both NPY and NA was restricted to perivascular nerves, since no change was observed in the sympathetic nerve cell bodies in the superior cervical ganglion from which these nerves arise. An increase in NPY and in VIP nerve density, but no change in substance P nerve density, has been observed in hypertensive rat mesenteric vessels (374,375). Similarly, an increase in catecholamine- and NPY-LI–containing nerve fibers has been shown in cerebral arteries of SHR, but there were no differences in acetylcholinesterase-positive, VIP-, and substance P–containing nerve fibers (376). In a study of peptide-containing nerves around blood vessels of stroke-prone SHR, Lee and co-workers (375) found that the density of substance P–containing nerves was decreased in cerebral arteries of stroke-prone SHR, and this was increased by sympathectomy in contrast to the decrease caused in peripheral vessels. NPY nerve density was higher in peripheral blood vessels of stroke-prone SHR, but not different in cerebral vessels. Sympathectomy abolished peripheral NPY, but had no effect on NPY in cerebral arteries (375). A reduction of NPY levels has been shown in the kidney and renal artery (377). Immunocytochemical quantitation of neuronal NPY levels in superior cervical ganglia of rats showed that there were both fewer

NPY-immunoreactive (IR) ganglia and total numbers of ganglionic cells in SHR (378).

In the tail artery of the SHR, antibodies to NPY depressed the response to sympathetic nerve stimulation but had no effect in controls (379), suggesting that the contribution of NPY to the vascular contractile response to sympathetic stimulation may be enhanced in hypertensive animals. SHRs were shown to be more responsive to the effects of intravenous NPY in increasing mean arterial pressure (47), consistent with the hypothesis that NPY is an important contributor to the development and maintenance of hypertension. In the mesenteric arterial bed of the SHR, prejunctional inhibitory effects of NPY on sympathetic nerve stimulation were attenuated, while postjunctional potentiation was enhanced; these dysfunctions in pre- and postjunctional neuromodulatory mechanisms are cooperative in producing enhanced sympathetic activity and hence increased vascular tone (380) (Fig. 13).

In humans, elevated plasma levels of NPY and NA have been shown in hypertensive subjects (381) and were suggested to be due to an increase in sympathetic nervous activity. Neurogenic hypertension elicited by sinoatrial denervation was associated with an increase in catecholamine levels in plasma in dogs, but there was no increase in NPY (382). This was not due to depletion of

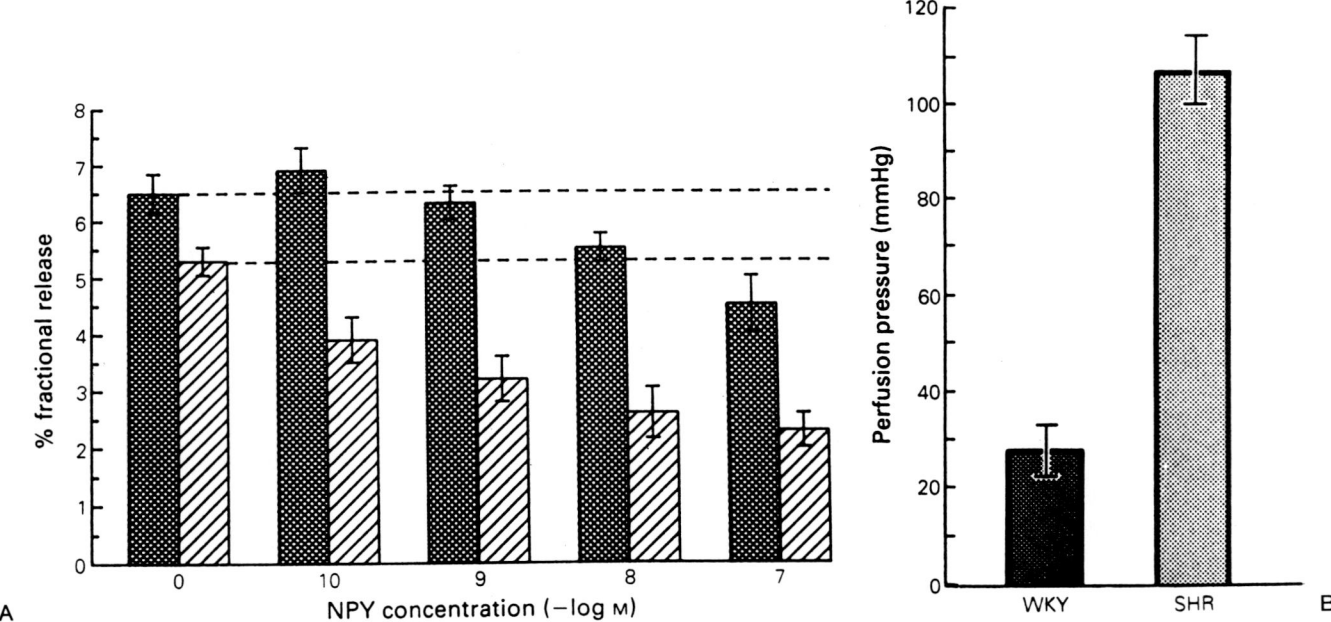

FIG. 13. A: The effect of NPY on the periarterial nerve stimulation (8 Hz)–induced release of endogenous NA from the perfused mesenteric arterial bed of 8- to 10-week-old Wistar-Kyoto (WKY) rats ☐ or spontaneously hypertensive rats (SHR) ▨. Data are plotted as percent fractional release versus NPY concentration. Each bar is the mean ± s.e. mean of five to seven preparations. **B:** The effect of neuropeptide Y (NPY) (10^{-7} M) on the periarterial nerve stimulation (8 Hz)–induced increase in perfusion pressure of the perfused mesenteric arterial bed obtained from 8- to 10-week-old Wistar-Kyoto (WKY) rats or spontaneously hypertensive rats (SHR). Data are plotted as the increase in perfusion pressure in WKY or SHR. Each bar is the mean ± s.e. mean of five to seven preparations. (From ref. 380, with permission.)

NPY pools of sympathetic nerve endings, since activation of sympathetic nerve endings with yohimbine significantly increased plasma NPY-LI levels (382). Kahan et al. (383) have shown a release of NPY from sympathetic nerves in the human forearm in essential hypertension, but did not compare this to controls. On the other hand, it has been shown that the increased plasma levels of NPY-LI and catecholamines in severe hypertension remain after treatment to normotension in man, suggesting that peripheral markers of the sympathetic system in severe hypertension may not be directly related to blood pressure (384).

In the mesenteric arterial bed of the SHR, a substantial decrease in CGRP-containing sensorimotor vasodilator nerves (385,386) has been suggested to contribute to the development of hypertension (Fig. 14); this effect was exacerbated by increasing age and was reversed by chronic treatment with the antihypertensive captopril (387). Moreover, the plasma CGRP concentration is lower in adult SHR than in age-matched normotensive control rats, indicating that release of CGRP from perivascular

nerves may decrease in SHR (388). This deficit in neurogenic vasodilator function may produce an imbalance that could contribute to the development and maintenance of hypertension. In SHR vasodilator responses to exogenous CGRP increased with age, whereas an age-related decrease in vasodilatation was found in control rats; this was suggested to result from increased sensitivity of receptors to CGRP, caused by the decreased release of CGRP from the sensorimotor nerves (386,387). Westfall et al. (380) have also shown a decrease in the duration of sensorimotor vasodilatation in the rat mesenteric bed, but found that responses to exogenous CGRP were also decreased. The endothelium-independent relaxation of isolated basilar arteries to CGRP in stroke-prone SHR has been found to be enhanced (389), possibly as a consequence of primary changes in CGRP-containing sensorimotor nerves.

There is substantial evidence to indicate that defects in endothelial cell function are involved in the pathology of hypertension. It is largely unknown how hypertension affects the content of the many different vasoactive sub-

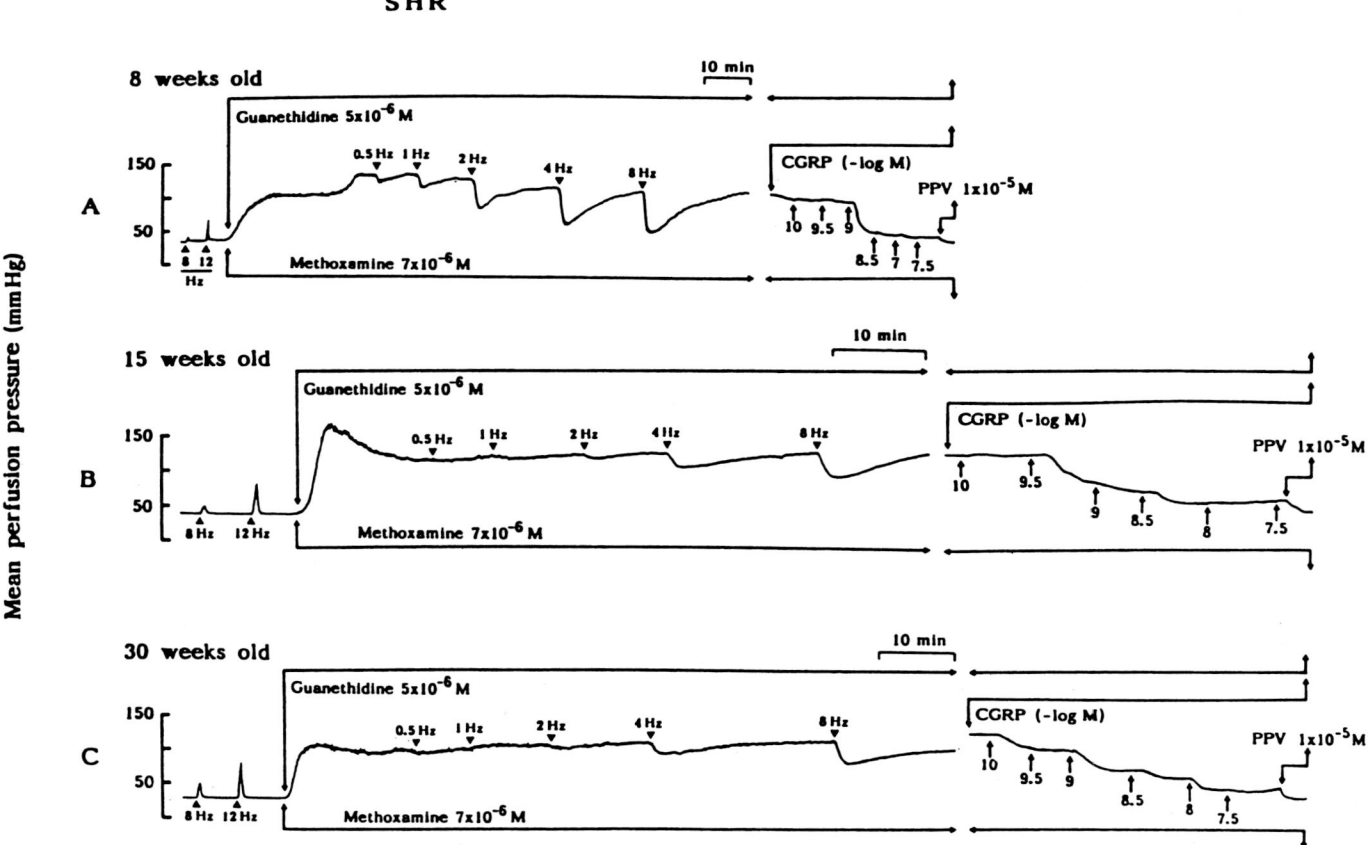

FIG. 14. Typical recordings of age-related changes in pressor response to perivascular nerve stimulation (▲), vasodilator response to perivascular nerve stimulation (▼), and rat calcitonin gene-related peptide (CGRP)–induced vasodilation in the perfused mesenteric vascular beds isolated from 8-week-old (**A**), 15-week-old (**B**), and 30-week-old (**C**) spontaneously hypertensive rats (SHR). PPV, papaverine. (From ref. 385, with permission.)

stances found in endothelial cells. It has been suggested that the vascular wall renin-angiotensin system, of which the endothelium is an integral part, plays an important role in the maintenance of high blood pressure in an animal model of hypertension (390). The potent vasoconstrictor function of endothelin in principle makes it a prime candidate responsible for the development of hypertension. Increased sensitivity to endothelin-1 has been shown in renal arteries of SHR (391). However, in patients with essential hypertension the circulating levels of endothelin do not appear to be increased (392), and a strong link has not yet been established between endothelin and hypertension. In view of the long-term influence of perivascular nerves on endothelial cells, it would be interesting to determine to what extent neural-endothelial interactions are involved in hypertension.

DIABETES

An increased incidence of hypertension and postural hypotension is characteristically present in the diabetic population. Diabetes is known to produce pathological changes in blood vessel structure and function involving nerves (sensory, motor, and autonomic) and endothelial cells. The pathology of diabetic neuropathy has been extensively studied in the streptozotocin-diabetic rat, a model of insulin-dependent diabetes. This model has contributed to evidence that changes in neuropeptides are associated with diabetes, although whether as a cause or consequence of this condition is not yet clear.

In the streptozotocin-diabetic rat, contractile responses of the mesenteric arterial bed (393) and tail artery (394) to sympathetic nerve stimulation were markedly decreased. Perivascular nerves in penile vessels containing VIP and ACh were shown to be seriously damaged or lost in the diabetic impotent man and in streptozotocin-diabetic rats (395–397). In contrast, VIP expression is increased in the diabetic gut (398). A reduction in the expression of VIP and 5-HT, but not NPY and NA, has been demonstrated in perivascular nerves supplying the cerebral blood vessels of streptozotocin-induced diabetic rats (399). In painful diabetic sensory neuropathy there is associated involvement of small myelinated A delta and unmyelinated C fibers. Interestingly, an increase in the relative number of PGP 9.5- (a general neuronal marker), CGRP-, and VIP-immunoreactive fibers has been seen in the skin of rat in early streptozotocin-induced diabetes (400).

In a recent study we have shown that capsaicin-sensitive sensorimotor nerve-induced vasodilator responses were impaired in the rat mesenteric arterial bed from streptozotocin-diabetic rats. Responses to exogenously applied CGRP, the principal vasodilator transmitter in these nerves, were unaffected, indicating that this was not due to changes in postjunctional mechanisms. Vasoconstrictor responses to stimulation of sympathetic nerves were unimpaired. It can be speculated that this dysfunction of sensorimotor nerves, in the presence of unaltered sympathetic activity, could contribute to hypertension in diabetes by shifting the balance of vasodilator to vasoconstrictor neural control in favor of the latter (401).

There is much controversy about the effect of experimental diabetes mellitus on vascular responsiveness to various agents. The reason for this may reside in differences in the species and vessel studied, as well as the mode of inducing diabetes and the time after diabetes induction. Hence, an increased vascular reactivity to α-adrenoceptor agonists, serotonin, K^+, and prostaglandins has been reported in various arteries of rabbit and rat models of diabetes (402–404). An increased vascular reactivity to AgII has also been shown in diabetic rats (405) and humans (406). In contrast, there are several reports indicating no change or diminished contractile responses to these same agonists (393,407–410). These changes may involve receptor up- or down-regulation, or may be due to long-term trophic changes in smooth muscle and endothelial cells.

AGING

The incidence of hypertension increases with age. Hypertension in the elderly is multifactorial, involving changes in perivascular nerves, smooth muscle, and endothelial cells. Neuropeptides may contribute to age-related hypertension directly via changes in perivascular innervation and hence changes in control of vascular tone, or via their trophic effects on components of the blood vessel wall.

An involvement of the sympathetic nervous system may be suggested by the fact that in normotensive subjects levels of plasma NA increase with advancing age (411). Development and aging have been associated with different patterns of change in innervation between different vessels, as well as between different classes of perivascular nerves. Different patterns of change in the development of sympathetic adrenergic nerves have been seen in various vessels from the rabbit, guinea pig, and rat. With few exceptions, after an initial peak there is a decline in adrenergic nerve density with age (373,412,413). Histological evidence shows a loss of nerve terminals in some tissues (413,414), although an increase in nerve density in some rat vessels has also been observed (415). The catecholamine content of the heart (416–419) and some arteries (420–422) is generally reported to decrease with age. Neuronal uptake of NA is generally decreased, as is the function of prejunctional α_2-adrenoceptors. In the rat tail artery, release of NA was reported to increase with age (423). It is possible that the ratio of sympathetic cotransmitters varies with age, as shown in the rat tail artery where the purinergic component was predominant in vessels from young animals (424). In most vessels the postjunctional vasoconstrictor effects of NA are maintained with maturation and aging (see ref. 425). On the other hand, a marked and progressive decrease in β-adrenergic relaxation has been observed with increasing age in animals and in man (426,427). A reduction in the accumulation of 5-HT in perivascular nerves of the rat has been shown to occur in old age (428,429). Aging was associated with a decrease in NPY within individual neurons, as well as with decreased numbers of NPY-LI neurons in rat superior cervical ganglia (378).

The effects of development and age on peptidergic perivascular nerves has been studied in some detail in rat (373,430) and human (431) cerebral vessels, in guinea pig mesenteric, femoral, carotid, and renal arteries (413), and in the rat mesenteric vascular bed (432). A remarkable observation from these studies is that despite the colocalization of transmitters in sensory or sympathetic nerves, there is no apparent correlation between the expression of coexisting transmitters during development.

For instance, CGRP-LI was found earlier than substance P–LI in cerebrovascular nerves, and increased in old age, as did VIP-LI, while the density of substance P–LI nerve fibers did not change (373,430) (Fig. 15). Similarly, NA and NPY underwent different expression in cerebrovascular nerves during development (373,430). In guinea pig mesenteric and carotid arteries, while adrenergic nerve density reached a peak 4 weeks after birth, nerves containing VIP, CGRP, and substance P reached a peak at birth and declined with age, raising the possibility that perivascular neuropeptides may play a trophic role in early development (413). In the developing rat mesenteric vascular bed the appearance of CGRP-LI has been shown to precede the appearance of substance P–LI, NPY-LI, and VIP-LI, leading to the suggestion that CGRP-LI nerves, being the first to innervate the vessels, may act as pioneer fibers to guide the other fibers during development (432).

The impaired sensorimotor vasodilatation seen in the mesenteric bed of the SHR is further reduced with increasing age (385,386,433). This decrease was associated with a decrease in CGRP-LI in mesenteric, femoral, and

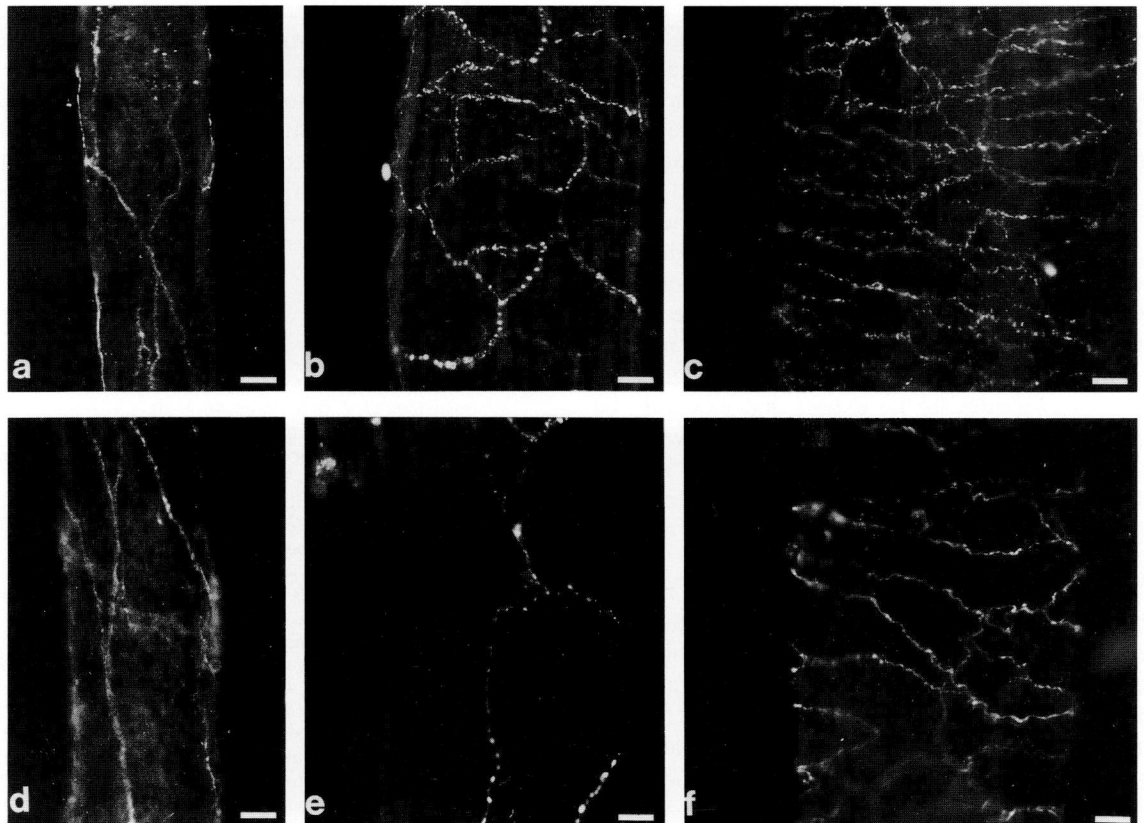

FIG. 15. Photomicrographs of stretch preparations of cerebral arteries showing perivascular nerve fibers at various age stages. VIP-containing nerves in the middle cerebral artery at 1 day (**A**), 8 months (**B**), and 27 months (**C**). CGRP-containing nerve fibers in the posterior cerebral artery at 1 day (**D**), 4 months (**E**), and 27 months (**F**). Nerve density is increased in old age for both VIP and CGRP. Scale bars = 25 μm. (From ref. 430, with permission.)

renal arteries (433). Aging is also known to be associated with a decrease in inflammatory and repair processes (434–436) and an age-related decrease in axon reflexes (434,437), consistent with a reduction in sensory nerves or their function with age.

There is little information about the effect of age on the content or release of peptides from endothelial cells. Evidence for age-related changes in the endothelial content of vasoactive substances is provided by a recent study showing that ATP and endothelin can be released from endothelial cells freshly isolated from old, but not from young rabbit aortas (287). Plasma levels of endothelin increase with age in humans, but the physiological relevance of this has not yet been established (392).

ARE STUDIES IN SMALL ANIMALS RELEVANT TO HUMAN ESSENTIAL HYPERTENSION?

The question has been raised as to how relevant are studies in small experimental animals to human essential hypertension. In answer, there are several things to consider. A basic understanding of mechanisms of blood vessel control is essential to our understanding of the development of cardiovascular disorders, including hypertension. Significantly, virtually all of the landmark discoveries in blood vessel control, including the most recent and widely accepted phenomena of cotransmission and endothelial modulation, were made in isolated animal tissues and were subsequently confirmed in humans. For example, no consideration of sympathetic activity is complete without recognizing the contribution of NPY and ATP as cotransmitters with NA. An obvious advantage of the use of animal models lies in the ability to "dissect out" components of vascular control mechanisms by immunohistochemical, pharmacological, and biochemical techniques, to an extent that can only be approximated in humans. With respect to perivascular nerves, this allows detailed examination of the several different nerve types and their cotransmitter content. This basic understanding of vascular control can then be applied to studies of animal models of disease.

With respect to hypertension, several animal models of hypertension exist, most of which are associated with an increase in sympathetic nervous activity. While it is recognized that human hypertension is a multifactorial disease involving factors other than sympathetic nerves, animal models of hypertension do allow examination of the role of perivascular nerves and endothelial cells to be studied in detail, and significant advances have been made in our understanding of the interplay between perivascular nerves, smooth muscle, and endothelial cells. Current literature on the role of neuropeptides in hypertension and on hypertension associated with aging and diabetes is fragmented and thus does not form a cohesive whole. However, it is clear that selective changes do occur in neuropeptides in these conditions and it is only by mapping out these changes that we will appreciate the part they play in hypertension.

CONCLUSIONS

Several points relevant to the role of neuropeptides in hypertension are raised in this chapter. First, attention is drawn to the fact that neurogenic control of vascular tone is not an exclusive role of the sympathetic nervous system, but also involves parasympathetic and sensorimotor nerves as well as perivascular projections of neurons from intramural ganglia, and by implication a number of different neuropeptides. Second, the roles of cotransmitter substances, including neuropeptides, should be examined in detail in view of their diverse pre- and postjunctional neuromodulatory effects. Third, reciprocal neuromodulatory interactions or cross-talk between classes of perivascular nerves have been identified. Fourth, the interactions that occur between perivascular nerves may be particularly important on a long-term basis in view of the plasticity of the autonomic nervous system. Fifth, peptides that are stored in, and released from, endothelial cells contribute to the control of blood vessel tone. Finally, trophic effects of perivascular nerves on the development of smooth muscle and endothelial cells have been shown. Since all of these are in operation in perivascular neural control, it may be unrealistic to look for a single drug regime to combat hypertension and in this respect research may be better targeted toward cocktails of drugs.

REFERENCES

1. Burnstock G. *Arch Int Pharmacodyn Ther* 1990;304:7–33.
2. Burnstock G. *J Anat* 1986;146:1–30.
3. Burnstock G. *J Cardiovasc Pharmacol* 1987;10:S74–S81.
4. Lundberg JM, Franco-Cereceda A, Lacroix JS, Pernow J. *Blood Vessels* 1991;28:27–34.
5. Luft R, Efendic S, Hökfelt T. *Diabetologia* 1978;14:1–13.
6. Stjärne L. *Rev Physiol Biochem Pharmacol* 1989;112:1–137.
7. Burnstock G. *Neurochem Int* 1990;17:357–368.
8. Burnstock G, Ralevic V. In: Garland CJ, Angus J, eds. *Pharmacology of vascular smooth muscle*. Oxford: Oxford University Press, 1993;in press.
9. Su C. *J Pharmacol Exp Ther* 1975;195:159–166.
10. Muramatsu I, Fujiwara M, Miura A, Sakakibara Y. *J Pharmacol Exp Ther* 1981;216:401–409.
11. Katsuragi T, Su C. *J Pharmacol Exp Ther* 1982;220:152–156.
12. von Kügelgen I, Starke K. *J Physiol (Lond)* 1985;367:435–455.
13. Burnstock G, Warland JJI. *Br J Pharmacol* 1987;90:111–120.
14. Warland JJI, Burnstock G. *Br J Pharmacol* 1987;92:871–880.
15. Sneddon P, Burnstock G. *Eur J Pharmacol* 1984;106:149–152.
16. Suzuki H. *J Physiol (Lond)* 1985;359:401–415.
17. Vidal M, Hicks PE, Langer SZ. *Naunyn Schmiedebergs Arch Pharmacol* 1986;332:384–390.
18. Ramme D, Regenold JT, Starke K, Busse R, Illes P. *Naunyn Schmiedebergs Arch Pharmacol* 1987;336:267–273.
19. Evans RJ, Surprenant A. *Br J Pharmacol* 1992;106:242–249.
20. Ralevic V, Burnstock G. *Circulation* 1991;84:1–14.

21. Kennedy C, Saville V, Burnstock G. *Eur J Pharmacol* 1986;122: 291–300.
22. Evans RJ, Cunnane TC. *Naunyn Schmiedebergs Arch Pharmacol* 1992;345:424–430.
23. von Kügelgen I, Starke K. *Trends Pharmacol Sci* 1991;12:319–324.
24. Kawasaki H, Takasaki K. *J Pharmacol Exp Ther* 1984;229:816–822.
25. Jackowski A, Crockard A, Burnstock G. *Neuroscience* 1989;29: 453–462.
26. Cowen T, Alafaci C, Crockard HA, Burnstock G. *Brain Res* 1986;384:51–59.
27. Gale JD, Cowen T. *Neuroscience* 1988;24:1051–1059.
28. Seabrook JM, Nolan PL. *Eur J Pharmacol* 1983;89:131–135.
29. Medgett IC, Fearn HJ, Rand MJ. *Clin Exp Pharmacol Physiol* 1984;11:343–346.
30. Tatemoto K. *Proc Natl Acad Sci USA* 1982;79:5485–5489.
31. Edvinsson L, Håkanson R, Wahlestedt C, Uddman R. *Trends Pharmacol Sci* 1987;8:231–235.
32. Potter EK. *Pharmacol Ther* 1988;37:251–273.
33. Mione MC, Ralevic V, Burnstock G. *Pharmacol Ther* 1990;46: 429–468.
34. Walker P, Grouzmann E, Burnier M, Waeber B. *Trends Pharmacol Sci* 1991;12:111–115.
35. Lundberg JM. *Arch Int Pharmacodyn* 1990;303:9–19.
36. Stjärne L, Lundberg JM, Åstrand P. *Neuroscience* 1986;18:151–166.
37. Lundberg JM, Rudehill A, Sollen A, Theodorsson-Norheim A, Hamberger B. *Neurosci Lett* 1986;63:96–100.
38. Allen JM, Bircham PMM, Edwards AV, Tatemoto K, Bloom SR. *Regul Pept* 1983;6:247–253.
39. Franco-Cereceda A, Lundberg JM, Dahlof C. *Acta Physiol Scand* 1985;124:361–369.
40. Allen JM, Polak JM, Rodrigo J, Darcy K, Bloom SR. *Cardiovasc Res* 1985;19:570–577.
41. Edvinsson L, Ekblad E, Håkanson R, Wahlestedt C. *Br J Pharmacol* 1984;83:519–525.
42. Edvinsson L, Copeland JR, Emson PC, McCulloch J, Uddman R. *J Cereb Blood Flow Metab* 1987;7:45–57.
43. Hanko JH, Tornebrandt K, Hardebo JE, Kahrstrom J, Nobin A, Owman CH. *J Auton Pharmacol* 1986;6:117–124.
44. Suzuki Y, Shibuya M, Ikegaki I, Satoh S, Takayasu M, Asano T. *Eur J Pharmacol* 1988;146:271–277.
45. Lundberg JM, Rudehill A, Sollevi A, Fried G, Wallin G. *Neuroscience* 1989;28:475–486.
46. Pernow J, Lundberg JM, Kaijser L. *Life Sci* 1987;40:47–54.
47. Miller DW, Tessel RE. *J Cardiovasc Pharmacol* 1991;18:647–656.
48. Fried G, Terenius L, Brodin E, et al. *Cell Tissue Res* 1986;243: 495–508.
49. De Potter WP, Coen EP, De Potter RW. *Neuroscience* 1987;20: 855–866.
50. Thureson-Klein A, Kong JY, Klein RL. *Blood Vessels* 1989;26: 177–184.
51. Kong JY, Thureson-Klein A, Klein RL. *Peptides* 1990;11:565–575.
52. Lang RE, Hermann K, Dietz W, et al. *Life Sci* 1983;32:399–406.
53. Gibbins IL, Morris JL. *J Auton Nerv Syst* 1990;29:137–150.
54. Hanko J, Hardebo JE, Owman C. In: Heistad DD, Marcus ML, eds. *Cerebral blood flow: effects of nerves and neurotransmitters.* Amsterdam: Elsevier, 1982;227–234.
55. El-Sharkawy TY, Al-Shireida MF, Pilcher CWT. *Can J Physiol Pharmacol* 1991;69:846–851.
56. Glover WE. *Clin Exp Pharmacol Physiol* 1985;12:227–230.
57. Pernow J, Saria A, Lundberg JM. *Acta Physiol Scand* 1986;126: 239–249.
58. Dahlöf C, Dahlöf P, Tatemoto K, Lundberg JM. *Naunyn Schmiedebergs Arch Pharmacol* 1985;328:327–330.
59. Lundberg JM, Pernow J, Tatemoto K, Dahlof C. *Acta Physiol Scand* 1985;123:511–513.
60. Ellis JL, Burnstock G. *Br J Pharmacol* 1990;100:457–462.
61. Cheung DW. *Circ Res* 1991;68:1401–1407.
62. Ekblad E, Edvinsson L, Wahlestedt C, Uddman R, Håkanson R, Sundler F. *Regul Pept* 1984;8:225–235.

63. Neild TO. *J Physiol* 1987;386:19–30.
64. Gustafsson H, Nilsson H. *Acta Physiol Scand* 1990;138:503–507.
65. Xia J, Neild TO, Kotecha N. *Br J Pharmacol* 1992;107:771–776.
66. Wahlestedt C, Yanaihara N, Håkanson R. *Regul Pept* 1986;13: 307–318.
67. Wahlestedt C, Grundemar L, Håkanson R, et al. *Ann NY Acad Sci* 1990;611:7–26.
68. Illes P. *Rev Physiol Biochem Pharmacol* 1989;112:139–233.
69. Seelhorst A, Starke K. *Arch Int Pharmacodyn* 1986;281:298–310.
70. Illes P, Pfeiffer N, von Kugelgen I, Starke K. *J Pharmacol Exp Ther* 1985;232:526–533.
71. Bartho L, Amann R, Saria A, Szolcsanyi J, Lembeck F. *Naunyn Schmiedebergs Arch Pharmacol* 1987;336:316–320.
72. Illes P, Ramme D, Starke K. *J Physiol* 1986;379:217–228.
73. Nguyen K, Barrios V, Duckles SP. *Life Sci* 1991;48:931–938.
74. Szabo B, Wichmann T, Starke K. *Eur J Pharmacol* 1987;139: 103–110.
75. Bucher B, Corriu C, Stoclet J-C. *Naunyn Schmiedebergs Arch Pharmacol* 1992;345:37–43.
76. Brayden JE, Bevan JA. *Circ Res* 1985;56:205–211.
77. Keef KD, Bowen SM. *FASEB J* 1988;2:A1814.
78. Neild TO, Shen K-Z, Surprenant A. *J Physiol* 1990;420:247–265.
79. Furchgott RF, Zawadzki JV. *Nature* 1980;88:373–376.
80. Lundberg JM. *Acta Physiol Scand* 1981;suppl 496:1–57.
81. Burnstock G. In: Osborne NN, ed. *Dale's principle and communication between neurones.* Oxford: Pergamon Press, 1983;7–35.
82. Lundberg JM, Fahrenkrug J, Larsson O, Änggård A. *Neurosci Lett* 1984;52:37–45.
83. Campbell G. *Annu Rev Pharmacol Toxicol* 1987;27:51–70.
84. Lundberg JM, Änggård A, Fahrenkrug J, Hökfelt T, Mutt V. *Proc Natl Acad Sci USA* 1980;77:1651–1655.
85. Edvinsson L, McCulloch J. *Regul Pept* 1985;10:345–356.
86. Morris JL, Gibbins IL, Furness JB, Costa M, Murphy R. *Neurosci Lett* 1985;62:31–37.
87. Leblanc GC, Trimmer BA, Landis SC. *Proc Natl Acad Sci USA* 1987;84:3511–3515.
88. Leblanc GC, Landis SC. *J Neurosci* 1988;8:146–155.
89. Kuwayama Y, Emson PC, Stone RA. *Brain Res* 1988;446:219–224.
90. Cavanagh JFR, Mione MC, Burnstock G. *J Cereb Blood Flow Metab* 1989;9(suppl 1):S34.
91. Gibbins IL, Morris JL. *Brain Res* 1988;444:402–406.
92. Burnett AL, Lowenstein CJ, Bredt DS, Chang TSK, Snyder SH. *Science* 1992;257:401–403.
93. Keast JR. *Neurosci Lett* 1992;143:69–73.
94. Rand MJ. *Clin Exp Pharmacol Physiol* 1992;19:147–169.
95. Bredt DS, Snyder SH. *Neuron* 1992;8:3–11.
96. Toda N, Minami Y, Okamura T. *Life Sci* 1990;47:345–351.
97. Morris J. *Peptides* 1990;11:381–386.
98. Fallgren B, Ekblad E, Edvinsson L. *Neurosci Lett* 1989;100:71–76.
99. Grundemar L, Hogestatt ED. *Eur J Pharmacol* 1992;221:71–76.
100. Barja F, Mathison R, Huggel H. *Cell Tissue Res* 1983;229:411–422.
101. Franco-Cereceda A, Henke H, Lundberg JM, Petermann JB, Hökfelt T, Fischer JA. *Peptides* 1987;8:399–410.
102. Lewis T, ed. *The blood vessels of the human skin and their responses.* London: Shaw and Sons, 1927.
103. Maggi CA, Meli A. *Gen Pharmacol* 1988;19:1–43.
104. Szolcsanyi J. *Agents Actions* 1988;23:4–11.
105. Burnstock G. *J Cardiovasc Pharmacol* 1985;7(suppl 3):S137–S146.
106. Gibbins IL, Furness JB, Costa M, MacIntyre I, Hillyard CJ, Girgis S. *Neurosci Lett* 1985;57:125–130.
107. Uddman R, Edvinsson L, Ekblad E, Håkanson R, Sundler F. *Regul Pept* 1986;15:1–23.
108. Lee Y, Takami K, Kawai Y, et al. *Neuroscience* 1985;15:1227–1237.
109. Gulbenkian S, Merighi A, Wharton J, Varndell IM, Polak JM. *J Neurocytol* 1986;15:535–542.
110. Wharton J, Gulbenkian S. *Experientia* 1987;43:821–832.
111. Gamse R, Holzer P, Lembeck F. *Br J Pharmacol* 1980;68:207–213.

112. Furness JB, Papka RE, Della NG, Costa M, Eskay RL. *Neuroscience* 1982;7:447–459.
113. Holzer P, Bucsics A, Lembeck F. *Neurosci Lett* 1982;31:253–257.
114. Gibson SJ, Polak JM, Bloom SR, et al. *J Neurosci* 1984;4:3101–3111.
115. Wanaka A, Matsuyama T, Yoneda S, et al. *Brain Res* 1986;369:185–192.
116. Lundberg JM, Franco-Cereceda A, Hua X, Hökfelt T, Fischer JA. *Eur J Pharmacol* 1985;108:315–319.
117. Pernow B, Rosell S. *Acta Physiol Scand* 1975;93:139–141.
118. Edvinsson L, McCulloch J, Uddman R. *J Physiol (Lond)* 1981;318:251–258.
119. Furchgott RF. *Circ Res* 1983;53:557–573.
120. D'Orleans-Juste P, Dion S, Mizrahi J, Regoli D. *Eur J Pharmacol* 1985;114:9–21.
121. Edvinsson L, Fredholm BB, Hamel E, Jansen I, Verrecchia C. *Neurosci Lett* 1985;58:213–217.
122. Lee TJ-F, Saito A, Berezin I. *Science* 1984;224:898–901.
123. Regoli D, Escher E, Mizrahi J. *Pharmacology* 1984;28:301–320.
124. Regoli D, Escher E, Drapeau G, D'Orleans-Juste P, Mizrahi J. *Eur J Pharmacol* 1984;97:179–189.
125. Kawasaki H, Takasaki K, Saito A, Goto K. *Nature* 1988;335:165–167.
126. Brain SD, Williams TJ, Tippins JR, Morris HR, MacIntyre I. *Nature* 1985;313:54–56.
127. Hanko J, Hardebo JE, Kahrstrom J, Owman C, Sundler F. *Neurosci Lett* 1985;57:91–95.
128. McCulloch J, Uddman R, Kingman TA, Edvinsson L. *Proc Natl Acad Sci USA* 1986;83:5731–5735.
129. McEwan J, Larkin S, Davies G, et al. *Circulation* 1986;74:1234–1247.
130. Abdelrahman A, Pang CY. *Eur J Pharmacol* 1992;217:185–189.
131. Kubota M, Moseley JM, Butera L, Dusting GJ, MacDonald PPS, Martin TJ. *Biochem Biophys Res Commun* 1985;132:88–94.
132. Grace GC, Dusting GJ, Kemp BE, Martin TJ. *Br J Pharmacol* 1987;91:729–733.
133. Fiscus RR, Zhou H-L, Wang X, et al. *Neuropeptides* 1991;20:133–143.
134. Thom S, Hughes AD, Goldberg P, Martin G, Schachter M, Sever PS. *Br J Clin Pharmacol* 1987;24:139–144.
135. Saito A, Kimura S, Goto K. *Am J Physiol* 1986;250:H693–H698.
136. Saito A, Ishikawa T, Kimura S, Goto K. *J Pharmacol Exp Ther* 1987;243:731–736.
137. Miyauchi T, Ishikawa T, Sugishita Y, Saito A, Goto K. *J Cardiovasc Pharmacol* 1987;10:675–682.
138. Ishikawa T, Okamura N, Saito A, Masaki T, Goto K. *Circ Res* 1988;63:726–734.
139. Maggi CA, Chiba T, Giuliani S. *Eur J Pharmacol* 1991;192:85–88.
140. Rubino A. *Gen Pharmacol* 1993;24:539–545.
141. Fujimori A, Saito A, Kimura S, Goto K. *Neurosci Lett* 1990;112:173–178.
142. Kawasaki H, Nuki C, Saito A, Takasaki K. *J Pharmacol Exp Ther* 1990;252:403–409.
143. Manzini S, Perretti F, Tramontana M, et al. *Gen Pharmacol* 1991;22:275–278.
144. Han S-P, Naes L, Westfall TC. *Biochem Biophys Res Commun* 1990;168:786–791.
145. Saito A, Masaki T, Uchiyama Y, Lee TJ-F, Goto K. *J Pharmacol Exp Ther* 1989;248:455–462.
146. Liu SF, Crawley DE, Evans TW, Barnes PJ. *J Pharmacol Exp Ther* 1992;260:541–548.
147. Holzer P. *Rev Physiol Biochem Pharmacol* 1992;121:49–146.
148. Gibbins IL, Furness JB, Costa M. *Cell Tissue Res* 1987;248:417–437.
149. Hökfelt T, Elde R, Johansson O, Luft R, Arimura A. *Neurosci Lett* 1975;1:231–235.
150. Duckles SP, Buck SH. *Brain Res* 1982;245:171–174.
151. Hanko J, Hardebo JE, Owman C. *J Cereb Blood Flow Metab* 1981;1:S346–S347.
152. Tornebrandt K, Nobin P, Owman C. *Peptides* 1987;8:251–256.
153. Jaspan J, Polonski K, Lewis M, Moossa AR. *Diabetes* 1987;28:888–892.
154. Uddman R, Edvinsson L, Owman C, Sundler F. *J Cereb Blood Flow Metab* 1983;3:386–390.
155. McCulloch J, Kelly PAT. *J Cereb Blood Flow Metab* 1984;4:625–628.
156. Liu-Chen LY, Norregaard TV, Moskowitz MA. *Brain Res* 1985;359:166–176.
157. Ju G, Hökfelt T, Brodin E, et al. *Cell Tissue Res* 1987;247:417–431.
158. Ekblad E, Rokaeus A, Håkanson R, Sundler F. *Neuroscience* 1985;16:355–365.
159. Melander T, Hökfelt T, Rokaeus A, Fahrenkrug J, Tatemoto K, Mutt V. *Cell Tissue Res* 1985;239:253–270.
160. Fehér E, Burnstock G. *Neurosci Lett* 1988;92:137–142.
161. Brain SD, Williams TJ. *Nature* 1988;355:73–75.
162. Gamse R, Saria A. *Eur J Pharmacol* 1985;114:61–66.
163. Giuliani S, Amann R, Papini AM, Maggi CA, Meli A. *Eur J Pharmacol* 1989;163:91–96.
164. Gazelius B, Brodin E, Olgart L, Panopoulos P. *Acta Physiol Scand* 1981;113:155–159.
165. Rozsa Z, Jansco G, Varro V. *Naunyn Schmiedebergs Arch Pharmacol* 1984;326:352–356.
166. Rozsa Z, Varro V, Jansco G. *Eur J Pharmacol* 1985;115:59–64.
167. Holzer P, Gamse R, Lembeck F. *Eur J Pharmacol* 1980;61:303–307.
168. Cuello AC, Gamse R, Holzer P, Lembeck F. *Naunyn Schmiedebergs Arch Pharmacol* 1981;315:185–194.
169. Costa M, Furness JB, Gibbins IL. In: Hökfelt T, Fuxe K, Pernow B, eds. *Coexistence of neuronal messengers: a new principle in chemical transmission. Progress in Brain Research.* Amsterdam: Elsevier, 1986;68:217–239.
170. Furness JB, Costa M, eds. *The enteric nervous system.* Edinburgh: Churchill Livingstone, 1987.
171. Saffrey MJ, Hassall CJS, Hoyle CHV, et al. *NeuroReport* 1992;3:333–336.
172. Hedqvist P, Von Euler US. *Acta Physiol Scand* 1975;95:341–343.
173. Galligan JJ, Jiang M-M, Shen K-Z, Surprenant A. *J Physiol (Lond)* 1990;420:267–280.
174. Hassall CJS, Burnstock G. *Brain Res* 1987;422:74–82.
175. Crowe R, Burnstock G. *Circ Res* 1982;16:384–390.
176. Hassall CJS, Saffrey MJ, Belai A, et al. *Neurosci Lett* 1992;143:65–68.
177. Carraway R, Leeman SE. *J Biol Chem* 1973;248:6854–6861.
178. Weihe E, Reinecke M, Forsmann WG. *Cell Tissue Res* 1984;236:527–537.
179. Reinecke M, Weihe E, Carraway RE, Leeman SE, Forssman WJ. *Neuroscience* 1982;7:1785–1795.
180. Chan-Palay V. In: Owman C, Edvinsson L, eds. *Neurogenic control of brain circulation.* Oxford: Pergamon Press, 1977;39–53.
181. Forssman BB, Hock D, Metz J. *Neurosci Lett* 1982;(suppl 10):S183.
182. Quirion R, Rioux F, St-Pierre S, Regoli D. *Life Sci* 1979;25:1969–1973.
183. Coburn RF. *Annu Rev Physiol* 1987;49:573–582.
184. Allen TGJ, Burnstock G. *Br J Pharmacol* 1990;100:261–268.
185. Allen TGJ, Burnstock G. *J Physiol (Lond)* 1990;423:593–614.
186. Brizzolara AL, Crowe R, Burnstock G. *Br J Pharmacol* 1993;109:606–608.
187. Hanley MR, Benton HP, Lightman SL, et al. *Nature* 1984;309:258–261.
188. Jojart I, Joo F, Siklos L, Laszlo FA. *Neurosci Lett* 1984;51:259–264.
189. Nakano J. *Jpn Circ J* 1973;37:363–371.
190. Altura BM, Altura BT. *Fed Proc* 1977;36:1853–1860.
191. Penit J, Faure M, Jard S. *Am J Physiol* 1983;244:E72–E82.
192. Alberts P. *Acta Physiol Scand Suppl* 1982;506:1–39.
193. Kawasaki H, Nuki C, Saito A, Takasaki K. *Brain Res* 1990;506:287–290.
194. Kawasaki H, Chikako N, Saito A, Takasaki K. *Am J Physiol* 1991;261:H683–H690.
195. Li Y, Duckles SP. *Eur J Pharmacol* 1991;195:365–372.
196. Rubino A, Ralevic V, Burnstock G. *Eur J Pharmacol* 1992;220:95–98.
197. Rubino A, Ralevic V, Burnstock G. *J Pharmacol Exp Ther* 1993;267:1100–1104.

198. Vila E, Taberno A, Fernandes F, Salaices M. *Br J Pharmacol* 1992;107:66–72.
199. Lembeck F, Donnerer J. *Eur J Pharmacol* 1985;114:241–246.
200. Giuliani S, Maggi CA, Meli A. *Gen Pharmacol* 1990;21:417–421.
201. Mantelli L, Amerini S, Rubino A, Ledda F. *Eur J Pharmacol* 1990;180:325–330.
202. Ralevic V, Rubino A, Burnstock G. (Unpublished observations).
203. Lindh B, Hokfelt T, Elfvin L-G. *Neuroscience* 1988;26:1037–1071.
204. Gulati N, Huggel H, Gulati OP. *Gen Pharmacol* 1983;14:157–160.
205. Braveit M, Helle KB. *Scand J Clin Lab Invest* 1991;51:395–402.
206. Maynard KI, Saville VL, Burnstock G. *Eur J Pharmacol* 1990;187:171–182.
207. Von Euler US, Hedqvist P. *Acta Physiol Scand* 1974;60:651–653.
208. Lee CM, Iversen LL, Hanley MR, Sandberg BEB. *Naunyn Schmiedebergs Arch Pharmacol* 1982;318:281–287.
209. Ellis JL, Burnstock G. *Br J Pharmacol* 1989;98:707–713.
210. Stjernquist M, Emson P, Owman CH, Sjoberg NO, Sundler F, Tatemoto K. *Neurosci Lett* 1983;39:279–284.
211. Lundberg JM, Hua XY, Franco-Cereceda A. *Acta Physiol Scand* 1984;121:325–332.
212. Franco-Cereceda A, Lundberg JM, Dahlof C. *Acta Physiol Scand* 1985;124:361–369.
213. Kilborn MJ, Potter EK, McCloskey DI. *J Auton Nerv Syst* 1986;17:131–142.
214. Yamamoto R, Wada A, Asada Y, Niina H, Sumiyoshi A. *Naunyn Schmiedebergs Arch Pharmacol* 1993;374:238–240.
215. Cohen RA, Weisbrod RM. *Am J Physiol* 1988;254:H871–H878.
216. Juan H. *Pain* 1982;12:259–264.
217. Chahl LA. *Pharmacol Ther* 1988;37:275–300.
218. Saria A, Martling CR, Yan Z, Theodorsson-Norheim E, Gamse R, Lundberg JM. *Am Rev Respir Dis* 1988;137:1330–1335.
219. Franco-Cereceda A, Saria A, Lundberg JM. *Acta Physiol Scand* 1989;135:173–187.
220. Ralevic V, Khalil Z, Dusting GJ, Helme RD. *Br J Pharmacol* 1992;106:650–655.
221. Li Z, Duckles SP. *J Pharmacol Exp Ther* 1993;264:1305–1310.
222. Ralevic V, Burnstock G. *Neural-endothelial interactions in the control of local vascular tone.* Texas: Landes, 1993.
223. Loesch A, Burnstock G. *Anat Embryol* 1988;178:137–142.
224. Burnstock G, Lincoln J, Feher E, et al. *Experientia* 1988;44:705–707.
225. Milner P, Ralevic V, Hopwood AM, et al. *Experientia* 1989;45:121–125.
226. Lincoln J, Loesch A, Burnstock G. *Cell Tissue Res* 1990;259:341–344.
227. Loesch A, Tomlinson A, Burnstock G. *Anat Embryol* 1991;183:129–134.
228. Tomlinson A, Van Vlijmen H, Loesch A, Burnstock G. *Cell Tissue Res* 1991;263:173–181.
229. Loesch A, Domer FR, Alexander B, Burnstock G. *Brain Res* 1993;611:333–337.
230. Loesch A, Bodin P, Burnstock G. *Peptides* 1991;12:1095–1103.
231. Cai WQ, Bodin P, Sexton A, Loesch A, Burnstock G. *Cell Tissue Res* 1992;272:175–181.
232. Katusic ZS, Shepherd JT, Vanhoutte PM. *Circ Res* 1984;55:575–579.
233. Katusic ZS, Shepherd JT, Vanhoutte PM. *Fed Proc* 1984;43:1084.
234. Ryan JW. In: Jaffe EA, ed. *Biology of endothelial cells.* Boston: Martinus Nijhoff, 1984;317–329.
235. Caldwell PRB, Seegal BC, Hsu KC, Das M, Soffer RL. *Science* 1976;191:1050–1051.
236. Ryan JW, Ryan US, Schultz DR, Whitaker C, Chung A, Dorer EE. *Biochem J* 1975;146:497–499.
237. Dzau VJ. *Am J Med* 1984;77:31–36.
238. Kifor I, Dzau VJ. *Circ Res* 1987;60:422–428.
239. Lilly LS, Pratt RE, Alexander RW, et al. *Circ Res* 1985;57:312–318.
240. Norregaard TV, Moskowitz MA. *Brain* 1985;108:517–533.
241. Linnik MD, Milbury PE, Moskowitz MA. *J Cereb Blood Flow Metab* 1989;9(suppl 1):S683.
242. Linnik MD, Moskowitz MA. *Peptides* 1989;10(5):957–962.
243. Yanagisawa M, Inoue A, Ishikawa T, et al. *Proc Natl Acad Sci USA* 1988;85:6964–6967.
244. Yanagisawa M, Kurihara H, Kimura S, et al. *Nature* 1988;332:411–415.
245. Inoue A, Yanagisawa M, Kimura S, et al. *Proc Natl Acad Sci USA* 1989;86:2863–2867.
246. Giaid A, Gibson SJ, Ibrahim NBN, et al. *Proc Natl Acad Sci USA* 1989;86:7634–7638.
247. Brain SD, Tippins JR, Williams TJ. *Br J Pharmacol* 1988;95:1005–1007.
248. Hughes A, Thom S, Martin G, Sever P. *Clin Sci* 1986;70(suppl 13):88.
249. Miller VM, Komori K, Burnett JCJ, Vanhoutte PM. *Am J Physiol* 1989;257:H1127–H1131.
250. Hiley CR, Douglas SA, Randall MD. *J Cardiovasc Pharmacol* 1989;13(suppl 5):S197–S199.
251. Warner TD, de Nucci G, Vane JR. *Eur J Pharmacol* 1989;159:325–326.
252. De Nucci G, Thomas R, D'Orleans-Juste P, et al. *Proc Natl Acad Sci USA* 1988;85:9797–9800.
253. Miyauchi T, Ishikawa T, Tomobe Y, et al. *Hypertension* 1989;14:427–434.
254. Brain SD, Crossman DC, Buckley TL, Williams TJ. *J Cardiovasc Pharmacol* 1989;13(suppl 5):147–149.
255. Kneupfer MM, Han SP, Trapani AJ, Fok KF, Westfall TC. *Am J Physiol* 1989;257:H918–H926.
256. Tabuchi Y, Ogihara T. *Biochem Biophys Res Commun* 1989;159:1304–1308.
257. Waite RP, Pang CCY. *J Pharmacol Exp Ther* 1992;260:45–50.
258. Wiklundin NP, Oehlen A, Cederqvist B. *Acta Physiol Scand* 1988;134:311–312.
259. Godfraind T, Mennig D, Morel N, Wobo M. *J Cardiovasc Pharmacol* 1989;13(suppl 5):S112–S117.
260. Wong-Dusting HK, La M, Rand MJ. *Clin Exp Pharmacol Physiol* 1990;17:269–273.
261. Yang Z, Richard V, von Segesses L, et al. *Circulation* 1990;82:188–195.
262. Armstead WM, Mirro R, Leffler CV, Busija DW. *Am J Physiol* 1989;257:H707–H710.
263. Baydoun AR, Peers SH, Cirino G, Woodward B. *J Cardiovasc Pharmacol* 1990;15:759–763.
264. Fukuda N, Izumi Y, Soma M, et al. *Biochem Biophys Res Commun* 1990;167:739–745.
265. Hasunuma K, Rodman DM, O'Brien RF, McMurtry IF. *Am J Physiol* 1990;259:H48–H54.
266. Perreault T, De Marte J. *J Cardiovasc Pharmacol* 1991;18:45–50.
267. Namiki A, Hirata Y, Ishikawa M, Moroi M, Aikawa J, Machii K. *Life Sci* 1992;50:677–682.
268. Whittle BJR, Lopez-Belmonte J, Rees DD. *Br J Pharmacol* 1989;98:646–652.
269. Gardiner SM, Compton AM, Bennett T, Palmer RM, Moncada S. *Eur J Pharmacol* 1989;171:237–240.
270. Fozard JR, Part M-L. *Br J Pharmacol* 1992;105:744–750.
271. Paddle BM, Burnstock G. *Blood Vessels* 1974;11:110–119.
272. Cohen RA, Shepherd JT, Vanhoutte PM. *Am J Physiol* 1983;245:H1077–H1080.
273. Hopwood AM, Lincoln J, Kirkpatrick KA, Burnstock G. *Eur J Pharmacol* 1986;165:323–326.
274. Stewart DJ, Holtz J, Pohl U, Bassenge E. *Eur J Pharmacol* 1987;143:131–134.
275. Vials A, Burnstock G. *Br J Pharmacol* 1992;107:604–609.
276. Burnstock G. *Blood Vessels* 1987;24:156–160.
277. Ralevic V, Milner P, Hudlicka O, Kristek F, Burnstock G. *Circ Res* 1990;66:1178–1183.
278. Ralevic V, Kristek F, Hudlicka O, Burnstock G. *Circ Res* 1989;64:1190–1196.
279. Milner P, Kirkpatrick KA, Ralevic V, Toothill V, Pearson J, Burnstock G. *Proc R Soc Lond [Biol]* 1990;241:245–248.
280. Schini V, Hendrickson H, Heublein D, Burnett J Jr, Vanhoutte PM. *Eur J Pharmacol* 1989;165:333–334.
281. Boulanger C, Luscher TF. *J Clin Invest* 1990;85:587–590.
282. D'Orleans-Juste P, Mitchell JA, Wood EG, Hecker M, Vane JR. *Can J Physiol Pharmacol* 1992;70:687–694.

283. Suzuki N, Matsumoto H, Kitada C, et al. *J Cardiovasc Pharmacol* 1989;13(suppl 5):151–152.
284. Koseki C, Imai M, Hirata Y, Yanagisawa M, Masaki T. *Am J Physiol* 1989;256:R858–R866.
285. Masaki T, Yanagisawa M, Goto K, Kimura S, Takuwa Y. In: Rubanyi GM, ed. *Cardiovascular significance of endothelium-derived vasoactive factors.* New York: Futura, 1991;65–81.
286. Bodin P, Milner P, Winter R, Burnstock G. *Proc R Soc Lond [Biol]* 1992;247:131–135.
287. Milner P, Bodin P, Loesch A, Burnstock G. *J Vasc Res* 1992;29:420–425.
288. Yoshizumi M, Kurihara H, Sugiyama T, et al. *Biochem Biophys Res Commun* 1989;161:859–864.
289. Zachary I, Woll PJ, Rozengurt E. *Dev Biol* 1987;124:295–308.
290. Beretta C, Zurn AD. *Dev Biol* 1991;148:87–94.
291. Rozengurt E. *Eur J Clin Invest* 1991;21:123–134.
292. Ziche M, Morbidelli L, Geppetti CA, Dolara P. *Life Sci* 1991;48:PL7–PL11.
293. Burnstock G. In: Timras PS et al., ed. *Plasticity and regeneration of the nervous system.* New York: Plenum Press, 1991;291–301.
294. Terenghi G, Zhang S-Q, Unger WG, Polak JM. *Histochemistry* 1986;86:89–95.
295. Luthman J, Stromberg I, Brodin E, Jonsson G. *Int J Dev Neurosci* 1989;7:613–620.
296. Nielsch U, Keen P. *Eur J Pharmacol* 1987;138:193–197.
297. Aberdeen J, Corr L, Milner P, Lincoln J, Burnstock G. *Neuroscience* 1990;35:175–184.
298. Donnerer J, Amann R, Lembeck F. *Neuroscience* 1991;45:761–765.
299. Mione MC, Cavanagh JFR, Lincoln J, Milner P, Burnstock G. *Neuroscience* 1990;34:369–378.
300. Aberdeen J, Moffitt D, Burnstock G. *Regul Pept* 1991;34:43–54.
301. Fike EA, Simons E, Boswell C, Smith PG. *Exp Neurol* 1992;118:85–94.
302. Mione MC, Cavanagh JFR, Kirkpatrick KA, Burnstock G. *Cell Tissue Res* 1992;268:491–504.
303. Hottenstein OD, Pawlik WW, Remak G, Jacobson ED. *Naunyn Schmiedebergs Arch Pharmacol* 1991;343:179–184.
304. Ralevic V, Karoon P, Burnstock G. (Unpublished observations).
305. Pincus DW, DiCicco-Bloom BE, Black IB. *Nature* 1990;343:564–567.
306. Nelson DK, Service JE, Studelska DR, Brimijoin S, Go VLW. *J Auton Nerv Syst* 1988;22:203–210.
307. Morris JL, Gibbins IL, Furness JB. *J Auton Nerv Syst* 1987;21:15–27.
308. Payan DG. *Biochem Biophys Res Commun* 1985;130:104–109.
309. Nilsson J, von Euler AM, Dalsgaard C-J. *Nature* 1985;315:61–63.
310. Campbell-Boswell M, Robertson AL Jr. *Exp Mol Pathol* 1981;35:265–276.
311. New HV, Mudge AW. *Nature* 1986;323:809–811.
312. Fontaine B, Klarsfeld A, Hökfelt T, Changeux J-P. *Neurosci Lett* 1986;71:59–65.
313. George FW, Ojeda SR. *Proc Natl Acad Sci USA* 1987;84:5803–5807.
314. Haegerstrand A, Jonzon B, Dalsgaard CJ, Nilsson J. *Proc Natl Acad Sci USA* 1989;86:5993–5996.
315. Wollina U, Bonnekoh B, Mahrle G. *Int J Oncol* 1992;1:17–24.
316. Rebuffat P, Malendowica LK, Beloni AS, Mazzochi G, Nussdorfer GG. *Neuropeptides* 1988;11:133–136.
317. Boudard F, Bastide M. *J Neurosci Res* 1991;29:29–41.
318. Ziche M, Morbidelli L, Pacini M, Geppetti P, Alessandri G, Maggi CA. *Microvasc Res* 1990;40:264–278.
319. Rozengurt E, Sinnett-Smith J. *Proc Natl Acad Sci USA* 1983;80:2936–2940.
320. Woll PJ, Rozengurt E. *Growth Factors* 1988;1:75–83.
321. Pfeiffer CJ, Chernenko GA, Kohli Y, Barrowman JA. *Can J Physiol Pharmacol* 1982;60:358–362.
322. Rozengurt E, Legg A, Pettican P. *Proc Natl Acad Sci USA* 1979;76:1284–1287.
323. Takuwa N, Takuwa Y, Yanagisawa M, Yamashita K, Masaki T. *J Biol Chem* 1989;264:7856–7861.
324. Mangiarua EI, Bevan RD. *Eur J Pharmacol* 1986;122:149–152.
325. Miller ME, Scott TM. *Artery* 1990;17:233–247.
326. Haegerstrand A, Dalsgaard C-J, Jonzon B, Larsson O, Nilsson J. *Proc Natl Acad Sci USA* 1990;87:3299–3303.
327. Loesch A, Maynard KI, Burnstock G. *Neuroscience* 1992;48:723–726.
328. Maynard KI, Loesch A, Burnstock G. *Br J Pharmacol* 1992;107:833–836.
329. Taguchi T, Ishii Y, Matsubara F, Tenaka K. *Exp Mol Pathol* 1986;44:138–146.
330. de Champlain J. *Clin Endocrinol Metab* 1977;6:633–655.
331. Abboud FM. *Hypertension* 1982;4(suppl II):II208–II225.
332. Goldstein DS, Kopin IJ. In: Laragh JH, Brenner BM, eds. *Hypertension: pathophysiology, diagnosis, and management.* New York: Raven Press, 1990;711–747.
333. Head RJ. *Blood Vessels* 1989;26:1–20.
334. Head RJ. *Blood Vessels* 1991;28:173–178.
335. Burnstock G, Gannon B, Iwayama T. *Circ Res Suppl* 1970;26–27:II5–II23.
336. Mangiarua EI, Lee RMKW. *Can J Physiol Pharmacol* 1990;68:492–499.
337. Westfall TC, Meldrum MJ, Carpentier S, Naes L, Zhang S-Q. *Blood Vessels* 1987;24:94–99.
338. Kawasaki H, Urabe M, Takasaki K. *Hypertension* 1987;10:321–327.
339. De Cree J, Leempoels J, De Cock W, Verhegen H. *Clin Sci* 1981;61:473S–476S.
340. Anderson A, Morgan T, Dumpys R. *Clin Exp Pharmacol Physiol* 1983;10:331–333.
341. Lee RMKW, Triggle CR, Cheung DNT, Coughlin MD. *Hypertension* 1987;10:328–338.
342. Friedman R, Tassinari LM, Heine M, Iwai J. *Clin Exp Hypertens* 1979;1:779–799.
343. Takeshita A, Mark AL, Brody MJ. *Am J Physiol* 1979;236:H48–H52.
344. Reid JL, Zivin JA, Kopin IL. *Circ Res* 1975;37:569–579.
345. Lee RMKW, Coughlin MD, Cheung DWT. *J Hypertens* 1986;4(suppl 3):S81–S83.
346. Bevan R. *Circ Res* 1975;37:14.
347. Bevan R, Tsuru H. *Circ Res* 1981;49:478–485.
348. Bevan RD. *Am Rev Respir Dis* 1989;140:1478–1482.
349. Scott TM, Pang SC. *J Auton Nerv Syst* 1983;8:25–32.
350. Lee TJ-F. In: Lee RMKW, ed. *Blood vessel changes in hypertension: structure and function.* Boca Raton, FL: CRC Press, 1989;1–18.
351. Dunn WR, Wilson VG. *J Physiol* 1993;467:307P.
352. Folkow B, Hallback M, Lundgren Y, Weiss L. *Acta Physiol Scand* 1972;84:512–523.
353. Lee RMKW, Coughlin M, Tsoporis J, Kwan C-Y, Guan Y-Y, Leenen FHH. *Can J Physiol Pharmacol* 1992;70:1154–1160.
354. Ueyama T, Hamada M, Hano T, Nishio I, Masuyama Y, Furukawa S. *J Hypertens* 1992;10:215–219.
355. Donohue SJ, Head RJ, Stitzel RE. *Hypertension* 1989;14:421–426.
356. Zettler C, Head RJ, Rush RA. *Brain Res* 1991;538:251–262.
357. Falckh PH, Harkin LA, Head RJ. *Clin Exp Pharmacol Physiol* 1992;19:541–545.
358. Azevedo I, Osswald W. *Pharmacol Res* 1992;25:227–236.
359. Albino-Teixeira A, Azevedo I, Branco D, Osswald W. *Eur J Pharmacol* 1990;179:141–149.
360. Osswald W. *J Neural Transm* 1991;34:157–162.
361. Yamada K, Goto A, Ishii M, Yoshioka M, Matsuoka H, Sugimoto T. *Clin Exp Pharmacol Physiol* 1992;19:563–567.
362. Rump LC, Wilde K, Schollmeyer P. *J Hypertens* 1990;8:897–908.
363. Dalziel HH, Machaly M, Sneddon P. *Eur J Pharmacol* 1989;173:19–26.
364. de Chamberlain J. *J Hypertens* 1990;8(suppl 7):S77–S85.
365. Jackson EK. *Am J Physiol* 1987;253:H909–H918.
366. Kubo T, Su C. *Eur J Pharmacol* 1983;87:349–352.
367. Illes P, Rickmann H, Brod I, Bucher I, Stoclet J-C. *Eur J Pharmacol* 1989;174:237–251.
368. Lynch C, Roddick V, Hutchins P. *Microvasc Res* 1989;38:164–174.
369. Korner PI, Shaw J, Uther JB, West MJ, McRitchie RJ, Richards JG. *Circulation* 1973;48:107–117.

370. Julius S, Pascual AV, London R. *Circulation* 1971;44:413–418.
371. Julius S, Esler M. *Am J Cardiol* 1975;36:685–696.
372. Henquet JW, van Baak M, Schols M, Rahn KH. *Eur J Clin Pharmacol* 1982;22:285–288.
373. Dhital KK, Gerli R, Lincoln J, et al. *Brain Res* 1988;444:33–45.
374. Foote J, Robinson J, Scott TM. *J Physiol (Lond)* 1986;377:55P.
375. Lee RMKW, Nagahama M, McKenzie R, Daniel EE. *Hypertension* 1988;11:I117–I120.
376. Kawamura K, Takebayashi S. *Angiology* 1991;42:123–132.
377. Ballesta J, Polak JM, Allen JM, et al. *Regul Pept* 1984;9:323.
378. Gurusinghe CJ, Harris PJ, Abbott DF, Bell C. *Hypertension* 1990;16:63–71.
379. Daly RN, Roberts MI, Ruffolo RR, Hieble JP. *J Hypertens* 1988;6(suppl 4):S535–S538.
380. Westfall TC, Han S-P, Kneupfer M, et al. *Br J Clin Pharmacol* 1990;30:75S–82S.
381. Solt MB, Brown MR, Kennedy B, Kolterman OG, Ziegler MG. *Am J Hypertens* 1990;3:823–828.
382. Tavernier G, Damase-Michel C, Portolan G, Tran M-A, Montastruc J-L. *Naunyn Schmiedebergs Arch Pharmacol* 1992;345:431–436.
383. Kahan T, Taddei S, Pedrinelli R, Hjemdahl P, Salvetti A. *J Cardiovasc Pharmacol* 1992;19:587–592.
384. Edvinsson L, Ekman R, Thulin T. *Regul Pept* 1991;32:279–287.
385. Kawasaki H, Saito A, Takasaki K. *Circ Res* 1990;67:733–743.
386. Kawasaki H, Saito A, Takasaki K. *Brain Res* 1990;518:303–307.
387. Kawasaki H. *Clin Exp Pharmacol Physiol* 1992;19:569–573.
388. Xu D, Wang X, Wang J-P, et al. *Peptides* 1989;10:309–312.
389. Nishimura Y, Usui H, Suzuki A, Kajimoto N, Yamanishi Y. *Jpn J Pharmacol* 1992;59:333–338.
390. Okamura T, Miyazaki M, Inagami T, Toda NN. *Hypertension* 1986;8:560–565.
391. Tomobe Y, Miyauchi T, Saito A, et al. *Eur J Pharmacol* 1988;152:373–374.
392. Miyauchi T, Yanagisawa M, Suzuki N, et al. *Circulation* 1989;80(suppl II):2280.
393. Takiguchi Y, Satoh N, Hashimoto H, Nakashima M. *Blood Vessels* 1988;25:250–260.
394. Hart JL, Freas W, McKenzie JE, Muldoon SM. *J Auton Nerv Syst* 1988;25:49–57.
395. Crowe R, Lincoln J, Blacklay PF, Pryor JP, Lumley JSP, Burnstock G. *Diabetes* 1983;32:1075–1077.
396. Lincoln J, Crowe R, Blacklay PF, Pryor JP, Lumley JSP, Burnstock G. *J Urol* 1987;137:1053–1059.
397. Blanco R, de Tejada IS, Goldstein I, Krane RJ, Wotiz HH, Cohen RA. *J Urol* 1990;144:278–280.
398. Belai A, Lincoln J, Milner P, Crowe R, Loesch A, Burnstock G. *Gastroenterology* 1985;89:967–976.
399. Lagnado MLJ, Crowe R, Lincoln J, Burnstock G. *Blood Vessels* 1987;24:169–180.
400. Karanth SS, Springall DR, Francavilla S, Mirrlees DJ, Polak JM. *Histochemistry* 1990;94:659–666.
401. Ralevic V, Belai A, Burnstock G. *Br J Pharmacol* 1993;110:1091–1097.
402. Scarborough NL, Carrier GO. *J Pharmacol Exp Ther* 1984;231:603–609.
403. MacLeod KM, McNeill JH. *Can J Physiol Pharmacol* 1985;63:52–57.
404. Agrawal DK, McNeill JH. *Can J Physiol Pharmacol* 1987;65:1484–1490.
405. Christlieb AR. *Diabetes* 1974;23:962–970.
406. Christlieb AR, Janka H-U, Kraus BB, et al. *Diabetes* 1976;25:268–274.
407. Sullivan S, Sparks HV. *Am J Physiol* 1979;236:H301–H306.
408. Turlapathy PDMV, Lum G, Altura BM. *Am J Physiol* 1980;239:E412–E421.
409. Pfaffman MA, Ball CR, Darby A, Hilman R. *Am J Physiol* 1982;242:H490–H495.
410. Andersson D, Brunkwall J, Bergqvist D, Edvinsson L. *J Auton Nerv Syst* 1992;37:215–222.
411. Ziegler MG, Lake CR, Kopin IJ. *Nature* 1976;261:333–335.
412. Cowen T, Haven AJ, Wen-Qin C, Gallen D, Franc F, Burnstock G. *J Auton Nerv Syst* 1982;5:317–336.
413. Dhall U, Cowen T, Haven AJ, Burnstock G. *J Auton Nerv Syst* 1986;16:109–126.
414. Amenta F, Mione MC. *J Auton Nerv Syst* 1988;22:247–251.
415. Mione MC, Erdo SL, Kriss B, Ricci A, Amenta F. *J Auton Nerv Syst* 1988;25:27–33.
416. Martinez JL, Vasquez BJ, Messing RB, Jensen RA, Liang KC, McGauch JL. *J Gerontol* 1981;36:280–284.
417. Rappaport EB, Young JB, Landsberg L. *J Gerontol* 1981;36:152–157.
418. Daly RN, Goldberg PB, Roberts J. *J Pharmacol Exp Ther* 1988;245:798–803.
419. Borton M, Docherty JR. *Naunyn Schmiedebergs Arch Pharmacol* 1989;340:139–143.
420. Fouda AK, Atkinson J. *Naunyn Schmiedebergs Arch Pharmacol* 1986;334:37–39.
421. Duckles SP. *Neurobiol Aging* 1983;4:151–156.
422. Handa RK, Duckles SP. *Neurobiol Aging* 1987;8:511–516.
423. Buchholz J, Tsai H, Friedman D, Duckles SP. *J Pharmacol Exp Ther* 1992;260:722–727.
424. Bao JX, Eriksson IE, Stjärne L. *Acta Physiol Scand* 1989;136:287–288.
425. Docherty JR. *Pharmacol Rev* 1990;42:103–125.
426. Pan HY-M, Hoffman BB, Pershe RA, Blaschke TF. *J Pharmacol Exp Ther* 1986;239:802–807.
427. Vanhoutte PM. *J Cardiovasc Pharmacol* 1988;12(suppl 8):S11–S18.
428. Gale JD, Alberts JCJ, Cowen T. *J Auton Nerv Syst* 1989;28:51–60.
429. Cowen T, Thrasivoulou C. *Brain Res* 1990;513:237–243.
430. Mione MC, Dhital KK, Amenta F, Burnstock G. *Brain Res* 1988;460:103–113.
431. Edvinsson L, Edman R, Otteson A, Uddman R. *J Cereb Blood Flow Metab* 1985;5(suppl 1):S545.
432. Scott TM, Woolgar JR. *J Physiol* 1988;399:80P.
433. Li Y, Duckles SP. *Eur J Pharmacol* 1993;236:373–378.
434. Helme RD, McKernan S. *Ann Neurol* 1985;18:505–509.
435. Makinodan T, Kay MMB. *Adv Immunol* 1980;29:287–330.
436. Parkhouse N, LeQuesne PM. *N Engl J Med* 1988;318:1306–1309.
437. Helme RD, McKernan S. In: Chahl LA, Szolcsanyi J, Lembeck F, eds. *Antidromic vasodilatation and neurogenic inflammation.* Budapest: Akademiai Kiado, 1984;303–312.

Hypertension: Pathophysiology, Diagnosis, and Management, Second Edition,
edited by J.H. Laragh and B.M. Brenner,
Raven Press, Ltd., New York © 1995.

CHAPTER 48

Brain Natriuretic Peptide as a Cardiac Hormone in Cardiovascular Disorders

Yoshihiro Ogawa and Kazuwa Nakao

Since the discovery of atrial natriuretic peptide (ANP) in the heart and subsequently in the brain, ANP has been implicated in the control of blood pressure and body fluid homeostasis as a cardiac hormone and as a neuropeptide (1–3). A second natriuretic peptide, originally isolated from the porcine brain in 1988 and thereafter named *brain natriuretic peptide* (BNP) (4), shows a remarkable sequence homology to ANP and has central and peripheral actions similar to those of ANP (5–7). Soon after its discovery in the brain, the role of BNP as a neuropeptide has attracted the interest of many researchers. However, the highest concentration of BNP was found in the heart (8,9), where it works as a cardiac hormone (8–11). In this chapter, we will review the current state of knowledge on BNP as a cardiac hormone with special reference to its implications in cardiovascular disorders.

Y. Ogawa and K. Nakao: Second Division, Department of Medicine, Kyoto University Faculty of Medicine, Kyoto 606, Japan.

STRUCTURE AND BIOSYNTHESIS

Peptide Structure

Porcine BNP is a 26-amino-acid peptide with the 17-residue ring structure formed by an intramolecular disulfide linkage (4), which is the essential part for the biological actions of natriuretic peptides. Using an antiserum against porcine BNP, however, no immunoreactivity was detected in tissue extracts of rats and humans, suggesting the structural divergence of BNP across species. Subsequently, molecular cloning of the gene and isolation of the peptide have revealed that the structure of BNP varies considerably among species (12–21). As shown in Fig. 1, the structure of mammalian ANP is highly conserved except for a single residue substitution in the ring structure (Met^{12} in humans → Ile^{12} in rodents) (1,2). The structure of C-type natriuretic peptide (CNP), a third natriuretic peptide, is identical among species (1,2). By contrast, the major circulating forms of BNP are 26-, 45-, and 32-amino-acid peptides in pigs, rats, and humans, respectively (4,9,10,16,17). Although

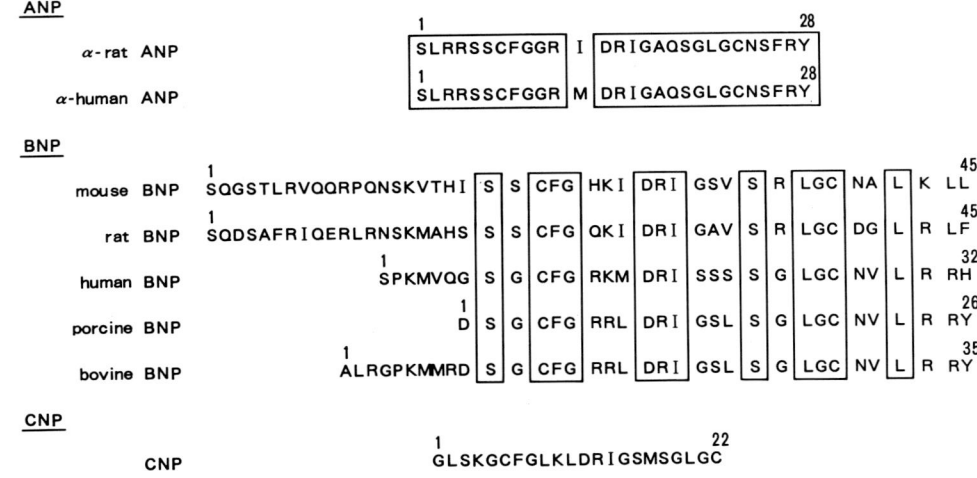

FIG. 1. Amino acid sequences of natriuretic peptides. Amino acid sequences are shown in one-letter code. Identical amino acids are boxed.

mouse BNP is a 45-amino-acid peptide (19,20), there is only a 64 percent sequence homology between rat and mouse peptides. Bovine BNP is a 35-amino-acid peptide, originally isolated from cultured adrenal chromaffin cells as aldosterone secretion inhibitory factor (21). The marked structural divergence of BNP among species is reflected by the species specificity of the biological actions of BNP (22).

Biosynthetic Pathway

The biosynthetic pathway of BNP in the heart has been proposed since the complementary DNAs (cDNAs) and genes for BNP from various species were cloned and sequenced by recombinant DNA techniques (12–15,18–20). As shown in Fig. 2, BNP arises from a single precursor, prepro-BNP molecule translated from the BNP mes-

senger RNA (mRNA). In humans (14,15), for instance, by removal of a hydrophobic 26-amino-acid signal peptide, the 134-amino-acid prepro-BNP is reduced to a 109-amino-acid peptide, pro-BNP. This peptide is further processed to the C-terminal 32-amino-acid human BNP, the principal storage form in the human heart (10,17). The cleaved mature peptide is also the major storage form in the rat and mouse cardiac tissues (the 45-amino-acid peptide) (9,16,20), whereas in the porcine heart, the precursor form (pro-BNP) is predominant (8). Therefore, the processing pattern of BNP in the heart is also divergent among species.

Gene Structure and Chromosomal Localization

The BNP gene is present as a single-copy gene and is organized into three exons separated by two introns in a

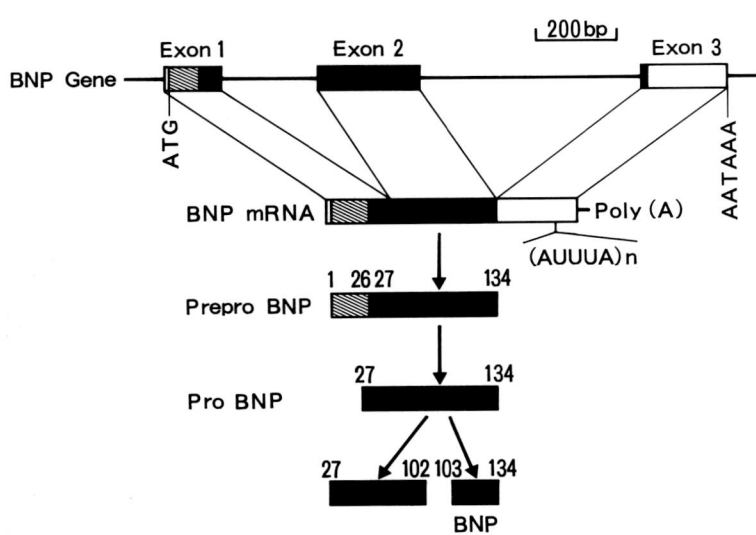

FIG. 2. Schematic representation of the human BNP gene, messenger RNA (mRNA), and precursor. Hatched boxes and closed boxes denote the signal peptide and prohormone sequences, respectively. The AU-rich sequences in the 3'-untranslated region of mRNA are represented by (AUUUA)n. (From ref. 2, with permission.)

similar manner to the ANP gene (15,18–20) (see Fig. 2). In the human BNP gene (15), exon 1 encodes the 5'-untranslated region, the signal peptide, and the first 18 amino acids of prepro-BNP. Exon 2 encodes most of the prohormone sequence, whereas exon 3 encodes the C-terminal 5 amino acids, and further extends to the 3'-untranslated region. The 1.8-kilobase (kb) fragment of the 5'-flanking sequence of the human BNP gene has been cloned and sequenced (23), which demonstrated that it contains an activator protein-1 (AP-1) binding site, a c-myc binding site, and several copies of acute phase regulatory elements. In the 3'-untranslated region of the human BNP mRNA, there are several copies of AUUUA motif which is implicated in mRNA instability (14,15). The AU-rich sequence is also present in BNP mRNA from other species (12–15,18–20), but is not found in ANP mRNA (1,2), suggesting that the BNP gene expression is regulated differently from the ANP gene expression at the posttranscriptional level. The chromosomal localization of the human BNP gene is unclear at present; however, the mouse BNP gene has been assigned to the chromosome 4, which is tightly linked to the ANP gene (19).

SYNTHESIS AND SECRETION IN THE HEART

Normal Heart

Although BNP was first isolated from the porcine brain and was also present in the canine brain (4,24), no significant amount of BNP-like immunoreactivity was detected in brain extracts of rats and humans (9), suggesting that the tissue distribution as well as structure of BNP is divergent among species. Subsequent studies revealed that the highest concentration of BNP is found in the heart rather than in the brain (8,9), and it was demonstrated that BNP is a novel cardiac hormone that is secreted from the porcine heart (8).

The BNP secretion from the heart was closely examined using the isolated perfused rat heart prepared by the Langendorff's method (9,11). As shown in Fig. 3, approximately 60 percent of the BNP secretory rate is maintained even after the atrial removal during the perfusion experiment, while the ANP secretory rate is reduced to less than 5 percent. These observations indicate that BNP is secreted predominantly from the ventricle, whereas ANP is secreted from the atrium. Northern blot analysis and reverse transcription-polymerase chain reaction have also confirmed that BNP occurs mainly in the rat ventricle (11,25). Therefore, BNP is mostly a ventricular hormone in rats, which sharply contrasts to ANP, an atrial hormone.

To determine the major source of BNP in the heart in humans, the plasma BNP concentrations were measured

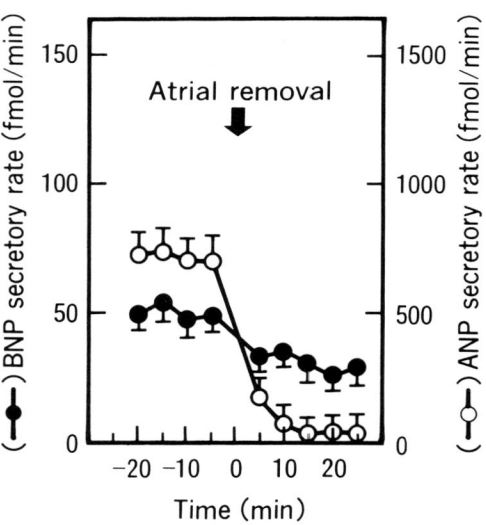

FIG. 3. Time course of BNP (*closed circles*) and ANP (*open circles*) secretory rates from the isolated perfused rat heart before and after atrial removal. (From ref. 11, with permission.)

in blood samples obtained from various sites during cardiac catheterization (10). There is a significant step-up of the plasma BNP concentration in the coronary sinus (CS) compared with that in the aortic root (Ao)

$$(\Delta_{(CS - Ao)}BNP)$$

suggesting that BNP is secreted from the heart through the CS. Furthermore, the step-up of the BNP concentration in the anterior interventricular vein (AIV), which drains the left ventricle but not the atrium

$$(\Delta_{(AIV - Ao)}BNP)$$

is comparable to

$$\Delta_{(CS - Ao)}BNP.$$

Therefore, in humans as well, BNP is a cardiac hormone that is secreted mainly from the ventricle. Northern blot analysis also demonstrated that BNP is synthesized principally in the human ventricles (10,26,27). In healthy controls, the plasma BNP concentration is 0.90 fmol/mL, which is only one-sixth of the plasma ANP concentration (10,28,29) (Figs. 4,5).

The BNP gene seems to be expressed constitutively in the ventricle throughout the course of development. The BNP mRNA levels in ventricles of neonatal rats are comparable with those in adult tissues (25). Similarly, ventricular expression of BNP is unchanged during development in humans (27). The profile of the BNP gene expression during development makes a striking contrast to that of the ANP gene expression; although abundant ANP mRNA and ANP are found in fetal and neonatal ventricles, these levels decline rapidly after the birth (1,2).

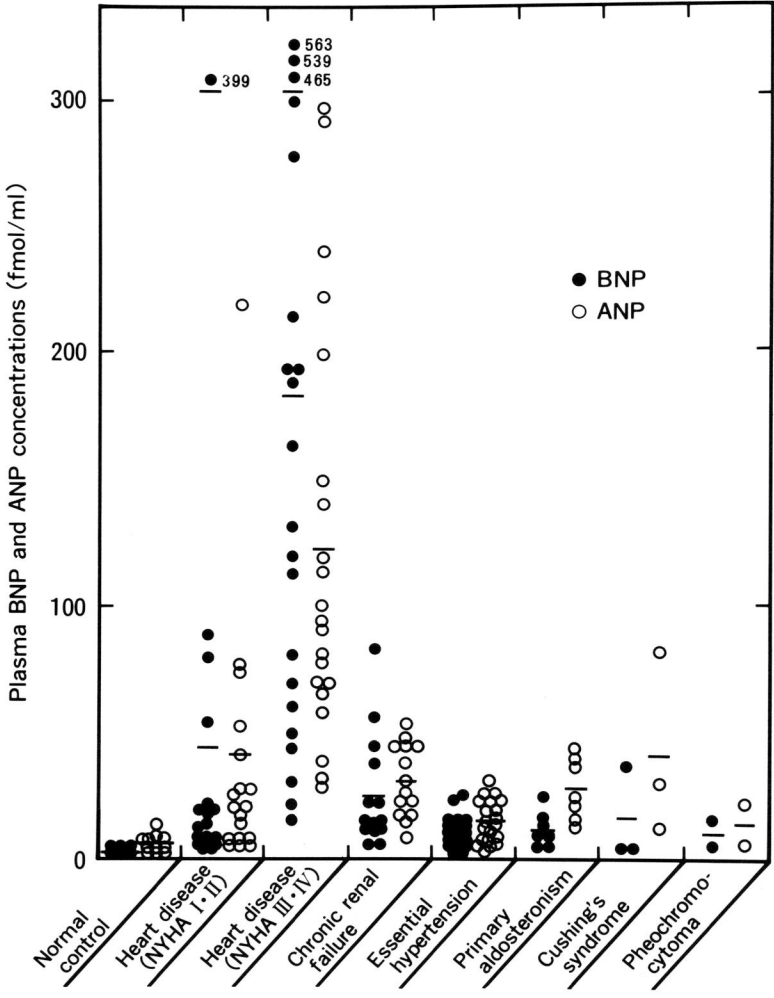

FIG. 4. Plasma BNP (*closed circles*) and ANP (*open circles*) concentrations in healthy controls and in patients with various cardiovascular disorders. (From ref. 29, with permission.)

Diseased Heart

Congestive Heart Failure

The plasma BNP concentrations are remarkably elevated in patients with congestive heart failure (CHF) in proportion to its severity (as much as 300-fold increase as compared with the control), and exceeds the plasma ANP concentration in severe cases [New York Heart Association class (NYHA) III/IV] (10,28,29) (see Figs. 4,5). In those patients, the BNP secretion from the ventricle is markedly augmented, thereby largely contributing to the elevated plasma BNP concentrations (10). Furthermore, the BNP gene expression is upregulated in failing human ventricles (10,26,27). Increased synthesis and secretion of BNP are also observed in hypertrophic (BIO 14.6) and dilated (BIO 53.58) cardiomyopathic hamster strains as compared with the control F1B strain (30). Considering the potent natriuretic, diuretic, and vasorelaxant activities, augmented synthesis and secretion of BNP as well as ANP (1,2) in the ventricle in patients with CHF may represent an important compensatory mechanism of heart failure.

The secretion patterns of BNP vary with underlying cardiac disorders of CHF with different degrees of overload in atria and ventricles (31). In patients with mitral stenosis in whom atria are mainly overloaded, the plasma ANP concentrations are significantly elevated, showing a highly positive correlation with pulmonary capillary wedge pressure (PCWP), whereas the plasma BNP concentrations are slightly elevated. On the other hand, in patients with dilated cardiomyopathy in whom both atria and ventricles are overloaded, the plasma BNP concentrations are remarkably elevated, being highly correlated with left ventricular end-diastolic pressure (LVEDP) as well as PCWP. Therefore, the plasma BNP concentration may reflect the degree of ventricular dysfunction.

However, even in myocytes of hypertrophic cardiomyopathy with normal systolic function, increased expression of BNP in the ventricle was also demonstrated by immunohistochemical analysis of endomyocardial

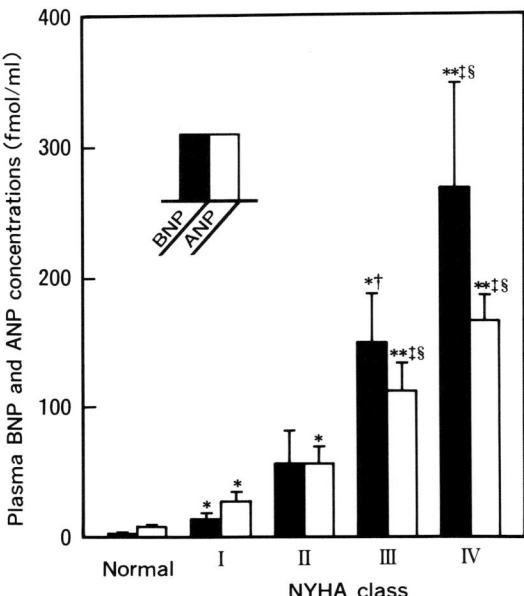

FIG. 5. Plasma BNP (*closed columns*) and ANP (*open columns*) concentrations in healthy controls and in patients with heart disease. NYHA class, the functional classification of the New York Heart Association. *p <.01, **p <.001 compared with values in normal group. †p <.05, ‡p <.01 compared with values in NYHA class I group. §p < .01 compared with values in NYHA class II group. (From ref. 28, with permission.)

biopsy specimen (32). In those patients, the BNP expression levels are highly correlated with myocardial fiber disarray, cardiocyte hypertrophy, and fibrosis. The mechanisms by which augmented synthesis and secretion of BNP are unclear at present, but left ventricular wall stress induced by the histologic changes may be one of the important stimuli to the BNP synthesis and secretion.

Acute Myocardial Infarction

The plasma BNP concentration is also elevated in the early phase of acute myocardial infarction (AMI) (33,34). In patients with AMI, the plasma BNP concentration is remarkably elevated on admission (approximately 20-fold as high as the control), whereas the plasma ANP concentration is slightly elevated (by only threefold) (34) (Fig. 6). Rapid induction of the BNP expression in the ventricle is further observed in rats with AMI produced by coronary artery ligation (35). Accordingly, BNP may be a sensitive marker for cardiac changes associated with AMI. Furthermore, sustained increases in the plasma BNP concentration are often observed in patients with poor prognosis (in patients with anterior infarction, CHF, higher level of maximal creatine kinase-MB isoenzyme, lower left ventricular ejection fraction, etc.) (33,34). In this regard, the plasma BNP concentrations should represent a good indicator of prognosis in patients with AMI.

Hypertensive Disorders

The plasma BNP concentrations are also significantly increased in essential hypertension, primary aldosteronism, and chronic renal failure as compared with the control; it also tends to increase in Cushing's syndrome and pheochromocytoma (29) (see Fig. 4). The increases in the plasma BNP concentration in patients are much more prominent than those in the plasma ANP concentration. This is due mainly to augmented secretion of BNP from the ventricle, but also due in part to the slower clearance of BNP from the circulation than that of ANP (10).

The BNP synthesis and secretion are augmented in ventricles of hypertensive rat models (11,36–38). The

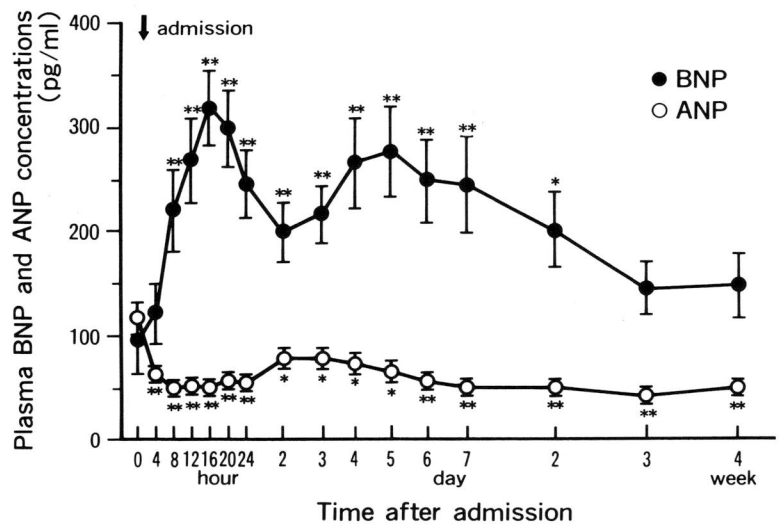

FIG. 6. Time course of plasma BNP (*closed circles*) and ANP (*open circles*) concentrations in patients with AMI. Values are expressed as mean ± SEM. *p <.05, **p <.01 compared with values on admission. (From ref. 34, with permission.)

BNP synthesis is increased in hypertrophied ventricles of spontaneously hypertensive rats (SHR) and of stroke-prone spontaneously hypertensive rats (SHR-SP) (11,36). Furthermore, augmented secretion of BNP is observed in ventricles of SHR-SP or deoxycorticosterone acetate (DOCA)-salt hypertensive rats (11,37,38). In these hypertensive rat models, the BNP expression in the ventricle is increased with the progression of hypertension (36–38), and a positive correlation is observed between plasma BNP concentrations and systolic blood pressure (37). Therefore, BNP should play pathophysiological roles in the establishment of hypertension. Furthermore, the BNP gene expression in the ventricle is already induced at the onset of the hypertensive stage and is preferentially responsive to the development of hypertension as compared with ANP (36). These findings support the concept that BNP represents a sensitive marker of cardiac changes associated with hypertension.

Cellular Mechanisms for Gene Expression

Cellular mechanisms for the BNP gene expression in the ventricle have been studied using primary cultures of neonatal rat cardiocytes. During ventricular cardiocyte hypertrophy evoked by endothelin-1 or phorbol 12-myristate 13-acetate, a protein kinase C (PKC) activator (39,40), induction of the BNP gene is more rapid than that of the ANP gene, being as rapid as that of the proto-oncogene c-fos, one of the immediate early genes (40). The rapid induction of BNP is partially inhibited by staurosporine, an inhibitor of PKC, suggesting that the rapid induction is mediated at least in part by a PKC-dependent pathway. The AP-1 binding site and several copies of acute phase regulatory elements in upstream sequences of the human BNP gene (23) may be involved in the rapid inducibility of BNP in hypertrophied ventricular cardiocytes *in vitro* and possibly in diseased ventricles *in vivo*. Furthermore, the half-life of BNP mRNA is shorter than that of ANP mRNA in cultured ventricular cardiocytes (39,40). This is due at least in part to the protein-synthesis–dependent mechanism probably through the AUUUA motif in the 3′-untranslated region of BNP mRNA. Therefore, the BNP gene expression is regulated differently from the ANP gene expression in the heart, both at transcriptional and posttranscriptional levels.

RECEPTORS AND THERAPEUTIC POTENTIALS

Receptors

The biological responses to acute administration of natriuretic peptides include vasodilation as well as natriuretic and diuretic effects (1,2), and most of the biological actions of natriuretic peptides are thought to be mediated by intracellular cyclic GMP (cGMP) accumulation through the activation of particulate guanylyl cyclase (1,2,41,42). Molecular cloning studies have identified two different natriuretic peptide receptors with guanylyl cyclase activity (GC-A and GC-B) (41,42). These receptors are single transmembrane proteins with guanylyl cyclase catalytic domain in the cytoplasmic regions (41,42). Given the structural divergence of BNP among species (see Fig. 1), BNP from different species has profoundly different effects on guanylyl cyclase activation (42,43), and thus on the biological actions *in vivo* (22). For instance, rat BNP is almost equipotent to rat ANP in natriuresis and vasorelaxation in rats, whereas human BNP has no significant activity (22). Accordingly, it is necessary to perform studies on receptor/ligand specificity within the same species for the elucidation of the biological actions of BNP. The rank order of ligand selectivity for GC-A and GC-B is ANP ≥ BNP ≫ CNP and CNP > ANP ≥ BNP, respectively (41–44). A new subtype of guanylyl cyclase–coupled receptor with the highest affinity to BNP has been suggested to be present (41,42), but has never been cloned.

A third natriuretic peptide receptor, the clearance receptor (C receptor), is also a single transmembrane protein with a very short 37-amino-acid cytoplasmic domain (42,44). This protein is not coupled to the cGMP production, and its primary function is to remove excess natriuretic peptides from the circulation (45). The rank order of ligand selectivity for C receptor is ANP > CNP > BNP (10,42,43,44), which is consistent with the slower clearance of BNP than that of ANP from the circulation (10).

Therapeutic Potentials in Cardiovascular Disorders

Acute administration of BNP (46) as well as ANP (47) can improve left ventricular function in patients with CHF by its prominent natriuretic and vasodilatory activities. As shown in Fig. 7, acute infusion of BNP at a rate of 0.1 μg/kg/min decreases PCWP and systemic vascular resistance (SVR), and increases stroke volume index (SVI), suggesting the beneficial effect of BNP on left ventricular function. Furthermore, the BNP infusion significantly increases urine volume and excretion of sodium and chloride in patients with CHF as compared with the control subjects (46), being in sharp contrast to the previous observation that patients with CHF show blunted natriuretic response to the ANP infusion (47). In addition, BNP exerts a longer duration of actions than ANP, probably due to the longer half-life of BNP in the circulation (10). Therefore, BNP should be a promising agent with different therapeutic applications than ANP.

On the other hand, it has been unclear whether BNP can improve hemodynamics in patients with CHF on a long-term basis. Recent progress in molecular biology

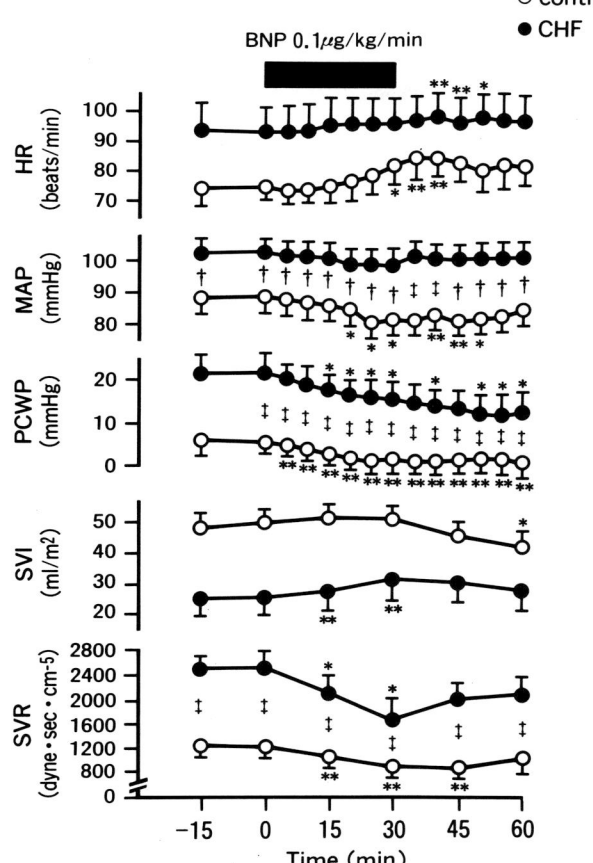

FIG. 7. Serial responses of heart rate (HR), mean systemic arterial pressure (MAP), pulmonary capillary wedge pressure (PCWP), stroke volume index (SVI), and systemic vascular resistance (SVR) during the BNP infusion in patients with congestive heart failure (CHF) and control subjects. *p <.05, **p <.01 compared with values at time 0. †p <.05, ‡p <.01 control versus CHF. (From ref. 46, with permission.)

has permitted the generation of transgenic mice in which the BNP gene is overexpressed in the liver, leading to the chronic elevation of the plasma BNP concentration (20). These transgenic mice show significantly lower blood pressure accompanied by elevated plasma cGMP concentration, despite potential desensitization or down-regulation of peripheral guanylyl cyclase–coupled receptors and/or reduction in intravascular volume. These observations indicate that BNP is involved in the chronic cardiovascular regulation and also suggest the potential usefulness of BNP as a long-term as well as a short-term therapeutic agent in the treatment of cardiovascular disorders.

CONCLUSIONS

Although BNP was originally isolated from the porcine brain, subsequent studies have established that BNP acts mainly as a cardiac hormone, which occurs predom-

inantly in the ventricle. The BNP synthesis and secretion are markedly augmented in ventricles of various cardiovascular disorders such as CHF, AMI, and hypertensive disorders, and the role of BNP as a cardiac hormone has drawn the interest of many basic and clinical investigators. Recent advances in biochemistry, pharmacology, and molecular biology have begun to reveal the molecular mechanisms of BNP, which will facilitate its clinical implications in cardiovascular disorders.

REFERENCES

1. Rosenzweig A, Seidman CE. Atrial natriuretic factor and related peptide hormones. *Annu Rev Biochem* 1991;60:229–255.
2. Nakao K, Ogawa Y, Suga S, Imura H. Molecular biology and biochemistry of the natriuretic peptide system. I: Natriuretic peptides. *J Hypertens* 1992;10:907–912.
3. Nakao K, Morii N, Itoh H, et al. Atrial natriuretic peptide in brain: implication of central cardiovascular control. *J Hypertens* 1986;4: S492–S496.
4. Sudoh T, Kangawa K, Minamino N, Matsuo H. A new natriuretic peptide in porcine brain. *Nature* 1988;332:78–819.
5. Itoh H, Nakao K, Yamada T, et al. Antidipsogenic action of a novel peptide "brain natriuretic peptide" in rats. *Eur J Pharmacol* 1988;150:193–196.
6. Shrakami G, Nakao K, Yamada T, et al. Inhibitory effect of brain natriuretic peptide on central angiotensin II-stimulated pressor response in conscious rats. *Neurosci Lett* 1988;91:77–83.
7. Yamada T, Nakao K, Itoh H, et al. Intracerebroventricular injection of brain natriuretic peptide inhibits vasopressin secretion in conscious rats. *Neurosci Lett* 1988;95:223–228.
8. Saito Y, Nakao K, Itoh H, et al. Brain natriuretic peptide is a novel cardiac hormone. *Biochem Biophys Res Commun* 1989;158:360–368.
9. Ogawa Y, Nakao K, Mukoyama M, et al. Rat brain natriuretic peptide: tissue distribution and molecular form. *Endocrinology* 1990;126:2225–2227.
10. Mukoyama M, Nakao K, Hosoda K, et al. Brain natriuretic peptide as a novel cardiac hormone in humans: evidence for an exquisite dual natriuretic peptide system, atrial natriuretic peptide and brain natriuretic peptide. *J Clin Invest* 1991;87:1402–1412.
11. Ogawa Y, Nakao K, Mukoyama M, et al. Natriuretic peptides as cardiac hormones in normotensive and spontaneously hypertensive rats: the ventricle is a major site of synthesis and secretion of brain natriuretic peptide. *Circ Res* 1991;69:491–500.
12. Porter JG, Arfsten A, Palisi T, Scarborough RM, Lewicki JA, Seilhamer JJ. Cloning of a cDNA encoding porcine brain natriuretic peptide. *J Biol Chem* 1989;264:6689–6692.
13. Kojima K, Minamino N, Kangawa K, Matsuo H. Cloning and sequence analysis of cDNA encoding a precursor for rat brain natriuretic peptide. *Biochem Biophys Res Commun* 1989;159:1420–1426.
14. Sudoh T, Maekawa K, Kojima M, Minamino N, Kangawa K, Matsuo H. Cloning and sequence analysis of cDNA encoding a precursor for human brain natriuretic peptide. *Biochem Biophys Res Commun* 1989;159:1427–1434.
15. Seilhamer JJ, Arfsten A, Miller JA, et al. Human and canine gene homologs of porcine brain natriuretic peptide. *Biochem Biophys Res Commun* 1989;165:650–658.
16. Kambayashi Y, Nakao K, Itoh H, et al. Isolation and sequence determination of rat cardiac natriuretic peptide. *Biochem Biophys Res Commun* 1989;163:233–240.
17. Kambayashi Y, Nakao K, Mukoyama M, et al. Isolation and sequence determination of human brain natriuretic peptide. *FEBS Lett* 1990;259:341–345.
18. Roy RN, Flynn TG. Organization of the gene for iso rANP, a rat B-type natriuretic peptide. *Biochem Biophys Res Commun* 1990;171:416–423.
19. Steinhelper ME. Structure, expression, and genomic mapping of the mouse natriuretic peptide type-B gene. *Circ Res* 1993;72:984–992.

20. Ogawa Y, Itoh H, Tamura N, et al. Molecular cloning of the complementary DNA and gene that encode mouse brain natriuretic peptide and operation of transgenic mice that overexpress the brain natriuretic peptide gene. *J Clin Invest* 1994; in press.

21. Nguyen TT, Lazure C, Babinski K, Chretien M, Ong H, De Lean A. Aldosterone secretion inhibitory factor: a novel neuropeptide in bovine chromaffin cells. *Endocrinology* 1989;124:1591–1593.

22. Kambayashi Y, Nakao K, Kimura H, et al. Biological characterization of human BNP and rat BNP: species-specific actions of BNP. *Biochem Biophys Res Commun* 1990;173:599–605.

23. Ogawa Y, Nakao K, Nakagawa O, et al. Upstream sequences regulating the brain natriuretic peptide gene expression in the heart. *J Hypertens* 1992;20:442 (abst P92).

24. Itoh H, Nakao K, Saito Y, et al. Radioimmunoassay for brain natriuretic peptide (BNP): detection of BNP in canine brain. *Biochem Biophys Res Commun* 1989;158:120–128.

25. Dagnino L, Drouin J, Nemer M. Differential expression of natriuretic peptide genes in cardiac and extracardiac tissues. *Mol Endocrinol* 1991;5:1292–1300.

26. Hosoda K, Nakao K, Mukoyama M, et al. Expression of brain natriuretic peptide gene in human heart: production in the ventricle. *Hypertension* 1991;17:1152–1156.

27. Takahashi T, Allen PD, Izumo S. Expression of A-, B- and C-type natriuretic peptide genes in failing and developing human ventricles: correlation with expression of the Ca^{2+}-ATPase gene. *Circ Res* 1992;71:9–17.

28. Mukoyama M, Nakao K, Saito Y, et al. Increased human brain natriuretic peptide in congestive heart failure. *N Engl J Med* 1990;323:757–758.

29. Mukoyama M, Nakao K, Saito Y, et al. Human brain natriuretic peptide, a novel cardiac hormone. *Lancet* 1990;335:801–802.

30. Tamura N, Ogawa Y, Itoh H, et al. Molecular cloning and characterization of cDNAs for hamster brain and atrial natriuretic peptides: cardiomyopathic hamsters are useful models to investigate the pathophysiological significance of brain and atrial natriuretic peptides. *J Clin Invest* 1994; in press.

31. Yoshimura M, Yasue H, Okumura K, et al. Different secretion patterns of atrial natriuretic peptide and brain natriuretic peptide in patients with congestive heart failure. *Circulation* 1993;87:464–469.

32. Hasegawa K, Fujiwara H, Doyama K, et al. Ventricular expression of brain natriuretic peptide in hypertrophic cardiomyopathy. *Circulation* 1993;88:372–380.

33. Mukoyama M, Nakao K, Obata K, et al. Augmented secretion of brain natriuretic peptide in acute myocardial infarction. *Biochem Biophys Res Commun* 1991;180:431–436.

34. Morita E, Yasue H, Yoshimura M, et al. Increased plasma levels of brain natriuretic peptide in patients with acute myocardial infarction. *Circulation* 1993;88:82–91.

35. Hama N, Itoh H, Shirakami G, et al. Rapid ventricular induction of brain natriuretic peptide gene expression in rats with acute myocardial infarction. *Circulation* 1993;88[Suppl II]:I-442.

36. Dagnino L, Lavigne JP, Nemer M. Increased transcripts for B-type natriuretic peptide in spontaneously hypertensive rats: quantitative polymerase chain reaction for atrial and brain natriuretic peptide transcripts. *Hypertension* 1992;20:690–700.

37. Yokota N, Aburaya M, Yamamoto Y, et al. Increased plasma brain natriuretic peptide levels in doca-salt hypertensive rats: Relation to blood pressure and cardiac concentration. *Biochem Biophys Res Commun* 1990;173:632–638.

38. Kohno M, Horio T, Yoshiyama M, Takeda T. Accelerated secretion of brain natriuretic peptide from the hypertrophied ventricles in experimental malignant hypertension. *Hypertension* 1992;19:206–211.

39. LaPointe MC, Sitkins JR. Phorbol ester stimulates the synthesis and secretion of brain natriuretic peptide from neonatal rat ventricular cardiocytes: a comparison with the regulation of atrial natriuretic factor. *Mol Endocrinol* 1993;7:1284–1296.

40. Nakagawa O, Ogawa Y, Itoh H, et al. Rapid transcriptional activation and early mRNA turnover of brain natriuretic peptide in cardiocyte hypertrophy: evidence for brain natriuretic peptide as an "emergency" cardiac hormone against ventricular overload. *J Clin Invest* 1994; in press.

41. Chinkers M, Garbers DL. Signal transduction by guanylyl cyclases. *Annu Rev Biochem* 1991;60:553–575.

42. Nakao K, Ogawa Y, Suga S, Imura H. Molecular biology and biochemistry of the natiuretic peptide system. II: Natriuretic peptide receptors. *J Hypertens* 1992;10:1111–1114.

43. Koller KJ, Lowe DG, Bennett GL, et al. Aelective activation of the B natriuretic peptide receptor by C-type natriuretic peptide (CNP). *Science* 1991;252:120–123.

44. Suga S, Nakao K, Hosoda K, et al. Receptor seceltivity of natriuretic peptide family, atrial natriuretic peptide, brain natriuretic peptide, and C-type natriuretic peptide. *Endocrinology* 1992;130:229–239.

45. Maack T, Suzuki M, Almeida FA, et al. Physiological role of silent receptors of atrial natriuretic factor. *Science* 1987;238:675–678.

46. Yoshimura M, Yasue H, Morita E, et al. Hemodynamic, renal, and hormonal responses to brain natriuretic peptide infusion in patients with congestive heart failure. *Circulation* 1991;84:1581–1588.

47. Saito Y, Nakao K, Nishimura K, et al. Clinical application of atrial natriuretic polypeptide to patients with congestive heart failure: beneficial effects on left ventricular function. *Circulation* 1987;76:115–124.

Hypertension: Pathophysiology, Diagnosis, and Management, Second Edition,
edited by J.H. Laragh and B.M. Brenner,
Raven Press, Ltd., New York © 1995.

CHAPTER **49**

Molecular Characterization and Regulation of Adrenergic Receptors

Brian Kobilka and Brian B. Hoffman

Cardiovascular function is tightly regulated by the autonomic nervous system. Cardiac muscle, cardiac conducting tissue, and coronary and systemic blood vessels are richly innervated by autonomic nerves. Sensory nerves monitor the volume and pressure status of the heart and blood vessels, as well as the metabolic state of cardiac and systemic tissues. This information is processed by the central nervous system, and impulses sent via the autonomic motor nerves modulate cardiac rate and contractility, as well as coronary and systemic vascular resistance. In addition to these direct controls over the cardiovascular system, the sympathetic nervous system has other effects influencing the cardiovascular system; for example, innervation of the kidney influences fluid and electrolyte balance.

Adrenergic receptors, activated by catecholamines, form the interface between the sympathetic nervous sys-

tem and the cardiovascular system. Sympathetic nerves release the neurotransmitter norepinephrine from nerve terminals; epinephrine is the predominant hormone released from the adrenal medulla. Catecholamines are also important neurotransmitters within the central nervous system. The effect of norepinephrine released from a nerve terminal depends on the type of cell found postsynaptically, the type of receptors on the cell surface, and the type of effector molecules found within the cell.

The importance of adrenergic receptors in the control of cardiovascular function can be appreciated by observing the physiological effects of the administration of agonist or antagonist drugs interacting with these receptors. Pharmacological control over the activity of these receptors has proved useful for a number of acute and chronic cardiovascular disorders such as hypertension, coronary artery disease, acute hypotension, congestive heart failure, and bradyarrhythmias. However, currently available drugs lack the selectivity to permit specific control over highly selected aspects of the cardiovascular system that are regulated by the sympathetic nervous system. Undesirable adverse effects may be due in part to the lack of selectivity of a drug for a particular subtype of receptor, or may be due to the different effects a drug may

B. Kobilka: Departments of Medicine and Molecular and Cellular Physiology, Stanford University School of Medicine, Stanford, California 94304.

B. B. Hoffman: Department of Medicine, Stanford University School of Medicine; and Veterans Affairs Medical Center, Palo Alto, California 94304.

have on different tissues. Also, the effect of many agonist compounds such as clonidine, isoproterenol, and dopamine may be limited by the tendency of cells to adapt to the drug by decreasing the number and/or functional capacity of the receptors for the drug. A better understanding of the complexity of the sympathetic nervous system at the cellular and molecular level may provide new approaches to pharmacologically modulate its activity and that of target cells.

Studying the structure and function of these receptors has been challenging because they are not naturally abundant proteins, and they require a lipid environment to be fully active. The complementary DNA (cDNA) or genomic clones for the major types of adrenergic receptors have recently been obtained. Applying the techniques of molecular biology to the study of G protein–coupled receptors has helped circumvent many of the technical difficulties that had complicated previous efforts at biochemical characterization of these proteins.

ADRENERGIC RECEPTOR SUBTYPES

The adrenergic receptors have been one of the most extensively studied class of G protein–coupled receptors. The diversity of adrenergic receptors was first identified through the physiological responses produced by potency series of a variety of agonists; however, it was the development of radioligand binding assays and multiple selective synthetic agonists and antagonist compounds that provided the critical tools for pharmacological, physiological, and biochemical characterization of these receptors. Based on these studies, it was possible to clearly distinguish four major types of mammalian adrenergic receptors: α_1, α_2, β_1, and β_2. More recent pharmacological studies have demonstrated more subtle distinctions suggesting that there are several subtypes of both α_1- and α_2-receptors (1,2). The first DNA clones for adrenergic receptors were obtained as a result of having amino acid sequence from purified receptor protein for hamster β_2 (3) and α_1 (4), and human α_2 (5) receptors, as well as the turkey erythrocyte β-receptor (6). These DNA clones were then used to design oligonucleotide and cDNA probes to isolate clones coding for other adrenergic receptors by screening DNA libraries under conditions that would permit identification of closely related but potentially different DNA sequences. With this low stringency screening technique it has been possible to obtain a cDNA clone for the human β_1-adrenergic receptor (7), as well as clones for adrenergic receptors that had previously been only partially characterized by pharmacological or physiological studies or not previously recognized. As a result of this cloning work the following receptors have been identified: three subtypes of the α_1-adrenergic receptor (4,8–10), three subtypes of β-adrenergic receptor (β_1, β_2, and β_3) (14), as well as at least three subtypes of α_2-receptor (11–13).

Subtypes of α-adrenergic receptors are a particularly important issue in cardiovascular biology because of the importance of these receptors in blood vessels, where they induce smooth muscle contraction, and in the heart, where α_1-agonists have positive inotropic actions and promote hypertrophy. The nomenclature for α_1-receptor subtypes is confusing because there is no generally agreed upon formal system. There are at least three, and very likely more, subtypes of α_1-receptor. The α_{1A}- and α_{1B}-subtypes were first identified in pharmacological and radioligand binding experiments (15–17). These subtypes were identified as insensitive to irreversible blockade by the alkylating clonidine analogue chlorethylclonidine (α_{1A}) or, on the other hand, susceptible to chlorethylclonidine (α_{1B}-subtype). In addition, the compound WB4101 has a higher affinity for the α_{1A}- than α_{1B}-receptors. In addition, there is evidence suggesting that the chlorethylclonidine-sensitive α_{1A}-receptors are linked to the influx of extracellular Ca^{2+}, whereas α_{1B}-receptors activate phospholipase C, leading to release of intracellular Ca^{2+} via inositol triphosphate (17). There is pharmacological evidence suggesting that smooth muscle contraction induced by catecholamines acts via variable patterns of α_{1A}- versus α_{1B}-receptors in different vascular beds such as aorta, renal artery, and mesenteric artery (18). Subsequently, a number of α_1-receptors have been identified via molecular cloning and expression in transfected cells. The exact correspondence between these different experimental approaches is not yet clear. It appears likely that the pharmacologically identified α_{1B}-receptor corresponds to the cloned α_1-receptor localized to chromosome 5. The α_{1A}-receptor defined pharmacologically may not yet be cloned. In addition, the physiological role of the α_{1C}- and α_{1D}-receptors identified with molecular cloning is uncertain. Future work will help resolve the potential differential expression of these subtypes in various vascular beds and elucidate signal transduction pathways utilized by these receptors. While the overall significance of the heterogeneity of these subtypes for cardiovascular pathophysiology is not yet clear, this area provides considerable promise for the development of highly selective adrenergic drugs with specificities not currently available.

Each of the adrenergic receptors has a preference for a specific G protein or a class of G proteins that can regulate one or more cellular processes. The β_1- and β_2-receptors couple to a G protein (Gs) that stimulates adenylyl cyclase, leading to a rise in intracellular concentrations of adenosine 3',5'-cyclic monophosphate (cAMP). The α_2-receptors couple to a G protein (Gi) that inhibits adenylyl cyclase and also may inhibit Ca^{2+} channels and open K^+ channels. Three types of Gi proteins have been identified: Gi1, Gi2, and Gi3. The interaction between specific Gi's and specific receptor subtypes has not yet been fully characterized. The α_1-adrenergic receptor couples to a G protein (Gq) that activates phospholipase C, leading to enhanced polyphosphoinositide metabolism, releasing diacylglycerol and inositol triphosphate.

There is evidence that some receptors may interact with more than one major type of G protein. For example, stimulation of the α_2-adrenergic receptor overexpressed in cultured cells not only leads to inhibition of adenylyl cyclase but can also lead to activation of phospholipase C, although the physiological significance of these observations is uncertain (19).

COMMON STRUCTURAL FEATURES OF G PROTEIN–COUPLED RECEPTORS

Analysis of the primary amino acid sequence deduced from the cloned DNA sequences provided the first clues to the structure of these membrane proteins. All of the adrenergic receptors cloned thus far share the general features illustrated in Fig. 1, using the β_2-adrenergic receptor as an example. There are seven clusters of 20 or more hydrophobic amino acids that have been proposed to be membrane-spanning domains. The amino terminus lies on the outside of the cell and the carboxyl terminus is in the cytoplasm. The amino terminus has one or more glycosylation sites, and the cytoplasmic domains have amino acid sequences that are potential substrates for a variety of protein kinases, enzymes capable of phosphorylating the receptor. In comparing the sequences of these receptors with each other, the greatest degree of similarity is found in the hydrophobic domains. For ex-

ample, when comparing two closely related receptors such as two subtypes of the α_2-receptor, between 65 and 85 percent of the amino acids in the hydrophobic domains are identical. For less closely related receptors, such as the β-receptors and the α-receptors, only 40 percent to 50 percent of the amino acids in the hydrophobic domains are identical. The most noticeable differences between any two receptors are found in the amino terminus, the third cytoplasmic loop (i-3), and the carboxyl terminus. These regions not only differ in the specific sequence of amino acids, but also in the size of these domains. The function performed by some of these structural domains will be discussed below.

SIGNAL TRANSDUCTION MEDIATED BY G PROTEIN–COUPLED RECEPTORS

In discussing membrane receptors, signal transduction refers to the process of transmitting information across the plasma membrane without the direct transport of molecules across this membrane. In other words, the function of receptors is to detect extracellular hormones or neurotransmitters and to respond by changes in structure. These changes in the receptor structure or conformation can then be detected by intracellular molecules. In the case of the adrenergic receptors the intracellular molecules that detect changes in receptor structure are

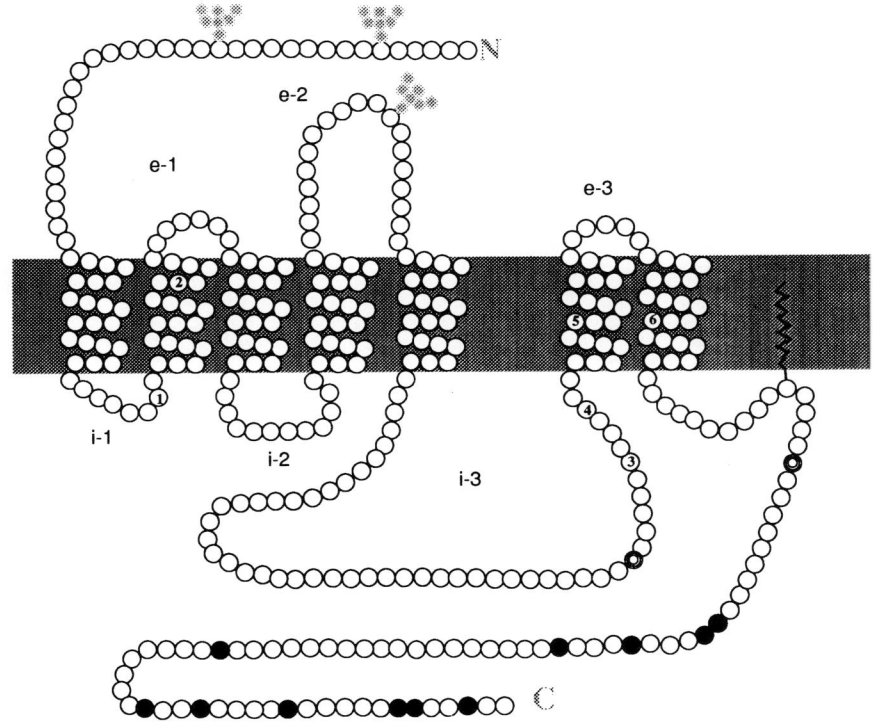

FIG. 1. Structural features of the β_2-adrenergic receptor. The *shaded area* represents the plasma membrane. The extracellular loops between membrane-spanning domains are labeled e-1, e-2, and e-3, and the intracellular loops are labeled i-1, i-2, and i-3. Potential sites for phosphorylation by β-adrenergic receptor kinase (BARK) and protein kinase A (PKA) are defined in the figure.

membrane-associated guanosine triphosphate (GTP)-binding proteins, which are referred to as G proteins (20).

Figure 2 is a diagram of the activation of adenylyl cyclase by a G protein–coupled receptor such as the β_2-receptor, which illustrates some common features of the interactions between receptors and G proteins (21–24). Receptors form complexes with heterotrimeric GTP-binding proteins consisting of α, β, and γ subunits. Formation of this complex alters the properties of both the receptor and the G protein. When the receptor is complexed with a G protein, the receptor often has a higher affinity for agonists. When the G protein forms a com-

plex with an agonist-occupied receptor, the G protein α-subunit exhibits a more rapid rate for the dissociation of GDP and the subsequent binding of GTP. The Gsα-GTP complex dissociates from the receptor and the β- and γ-subunits. The free Gsα-GTP subunit can activate adenylyl cyclase. This stimulation is turned off by the guanosine triphosphatase (GTPase) activity of the α-subunit, leading to the formation of guanosine diphosphate (GDP) by hydrolysis of GTP. The Gsα-GDP reassociates with the $\beta\gamma$-subunits and the cycle can begin again.

The cDNAs for more than 20 G protein α-subunits have been cloned and these α-subunits can be classified

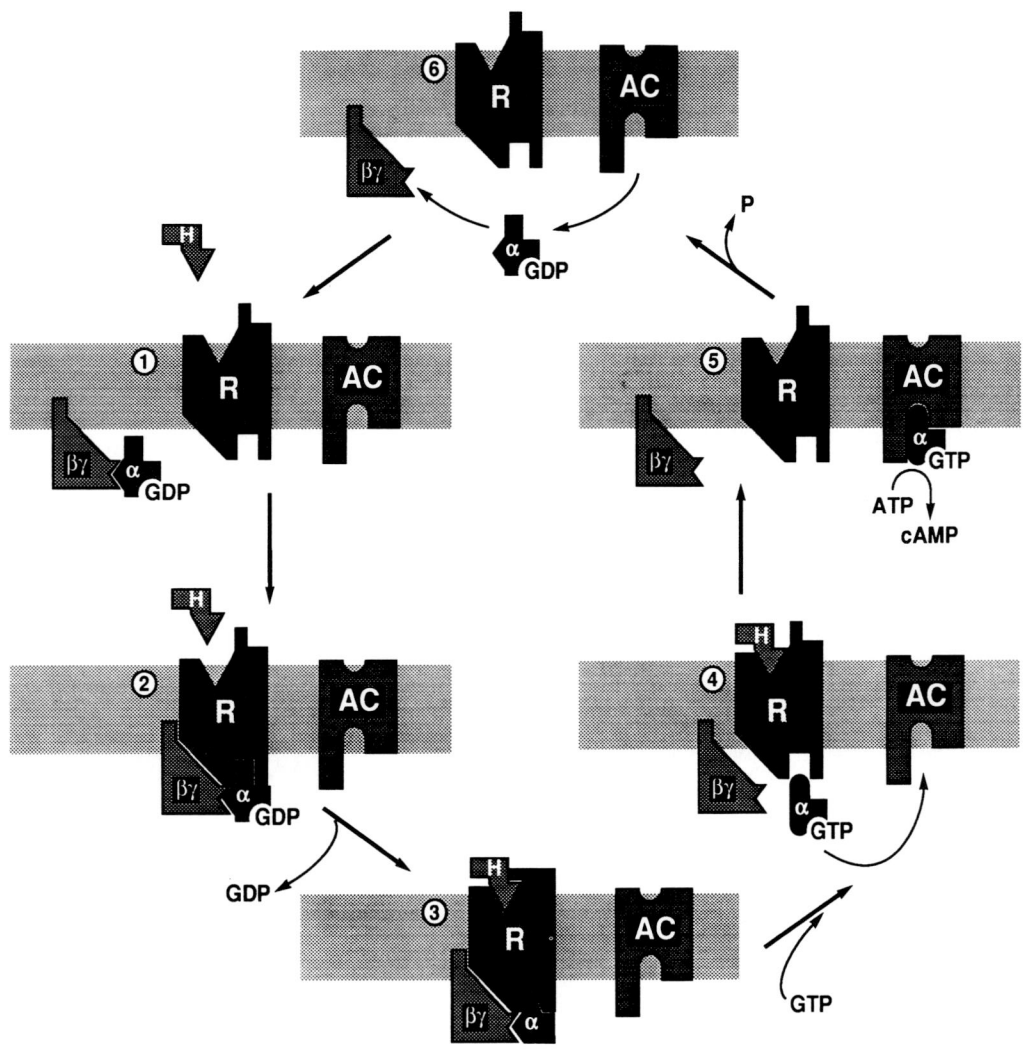

FIG. 2. Activation of Gs by the β-adrenergic receptor. Prior to activation the heterotrimeric form of Gs may not be associated with the receptor (step 1); however, the receptor, which is coupled to Gs, has a higher affinity for the agonist as shown in steps 2 and 3. Agonist induced changes in the receptor are transmitted to Gs and result in the exchange of GDP for GTP on the α-subunit (steps 2–4). Upon binding GTP (step 4), Gs$_\alpha$ assumes an activated conformation, is released from the receptor and from the $\beta\gamma$-subunits, and activates adenylyl cyclase (steps 4,5). Activation of adenylyl cyclase continues until GTP bound to the α-subunit is hydrolyzed to GDP and the α-subunit dissociates from adenylyl cyclase and binds to the $\beta\gamma$-subunits (steps 5,6). R, β-receptor; AC, adenylyl cyclase; H, agonist hormone; α, α-subunit of Gs; $\beta\gamma$, β- and γ-subunits of Gs.

into four large groups on the basis of amino acid homology and functional properties: Gs proteins, Gi proteins, Gq proteins, and G12 proteins (25). Members of the Gs family activate adenylyl cyclase and Ca^{2+} channels. Members of the Gi class of G proteins (Gi1, Gi2, Gi3, and Go) have been observed to inhibit the activity of adenylyl cyclase and to modulate the activity of phospholipase A2, K^+ channels, and Ca^{2+} channels. The Gq proteins stimulate phospholipase C, resulting in the production of the second messengers diacylglycerol and inositol 1,4,5-trisphosphate. The functional role of G12 proteins is not yet known.

The β- and γ-subunits are tightly, but noncovalently, bound to each other. The $\beta\gamma$-dimer is essential for effective activation of the α-subunit by a receptor. However, little is known about the physical interaction between the receptor and the $\beta\gamma$-dimer. There is evidence that mammalian $\beta\gamma$-subunits may play a direct role in activating phospholipase A_2 and some forms of adenylyl cyclase under specific conditions (26,27).

SECOND MESSENGERS

The activation of adenylyl cyclase by Gs leads to the generation of cAMP, which increases the activity of cAMP-dependent protein kinase, also termed protein kinase A (PKA). A common mechanism of conveying messages within the cell is the transfer of phosphates from adenosine triphosphate (ATP) to proteins by kinases such as PKA. Enzymes, channels, and proteins that modify gene expression can be turned on or off by the addition of phosphates by kinases or the removal of phosphates by phosphatases. Protein kinase A modulates a variety of processes involved in cellular metabolism as well as the activity of ion channels. In cardiac tissue, the activity of Ca^{2+} channels is regulated by phosphorylation of the channel protein by PKA. In blood vessels, PKA promotes smooth muscle relaxation, although the molecular mechanism is uncertain.

Activation of phospholipase C following α_1-adrenergic receptor stimulation leads to the cleavage of membrane phospholipids to produce inositol phosphates and diacylglycerol. Inositol phosphates increase the cytoplasmic concentration of intracellular calcium, which activates Ca^{2+}-dependent protein kinases, which in turn regulate the activity of a variety of enzymes and channels. Diacylglycerol activates protein kinase C (PKC), which modulates the activity of cytosolic and nuclear proteins through phosphorylation. For example, both Ca^{2+}-dependent kinases and PKC promote smooth muscle contraction in blood vessels.

STRUCTURAL DOMAINS INVOLVED IN SIGNAL TRANSDUCTION

A great deal has been learned about the relationship between the structural details of adrenergic receptors and their activation with agonists and antagonists as well as the capacity of the receptors to couple to signal transduction pathways. A number of these concepts are reviewed briefly in the following sections.

The Ligand-Binding Domain

Mutagenesis studies indicate that the membrane spanning domains of adrenergic receptors (Fig. 1) are likely to form the ligand-binding site. This differs from other types of plasma membrane receptors such as the low-density lipoprotein (LDL) receptor, the insulin receptor, and the platelet-derived growth factor receptor, where ligand binding takes place on an extracellular domain. Removal of most of the amino terminus by proteolysis (28,29) or by deletion mutations (30) has little effect on the ability of β-adrenergic receptors to bind ligands. Mutagenesis studies have provided extremely valuable information regarding the role of specific amino acids in adrenergic receptors in ligand binding. In experiments utilizing site-directed mutagenesis, specific amino acids in a receptor can be changed as desired using molecular biological techniques. These experiments permit the identification of amino acids involved in key functions of the receptor. Figure 3 illustrates key interactions between specific amino acid residues in the β_2-adrenergic receptor and the β-receptor agonist isoproterenol. The importance of these residues has been demonstrated in a series of experiments combining site-directed mutagenesis with pharmacophore analysis (31–33). The carboxylate group on the aspartate residue in the third hydrophobic domain is believed to act as a counter-ion for the catecholamine nitrogen. When this aspartate residue is changed to a serine, catecholamines are no longer effective agonists (33). However, catecholesters capable of forming hydrogen bonds with the hydroxyl group of the serine are capable of acting as full agonists for this mutant receptor (33). These studies provide support for the hypothesis that the chemical nature of the aspartate residue in the third membrane spanning domain is important in direct interactions with the amine of catechol agonists.

A similar approach has been used to demonstrate the role of serine 204 and 207 in the fifth hydrophobic domain in interacting with the meta- and para-hydroxyls on the catechol ring (31). β_2-Adrenergic receptor mutants were made in which either serine 204 or serine 207 were replaced by alanine. These mutant receptors were expressed in cells and were analyzed for their ability to activate adenylyl cyclase following stimulation by isoproterenol or derivatives of isoproterenol lacking either the para- or the meta-hydroxyl on the catechol ring. Isoproterenol was able to activate both mutant receptors, and the derivatives of isoproterenol lacking the meta- and para-hydroxyls were both effective in activating the wild type β_2-receptor. The β_2-receptor mutant lacking serine 204 could only be activated by isoproterenol and

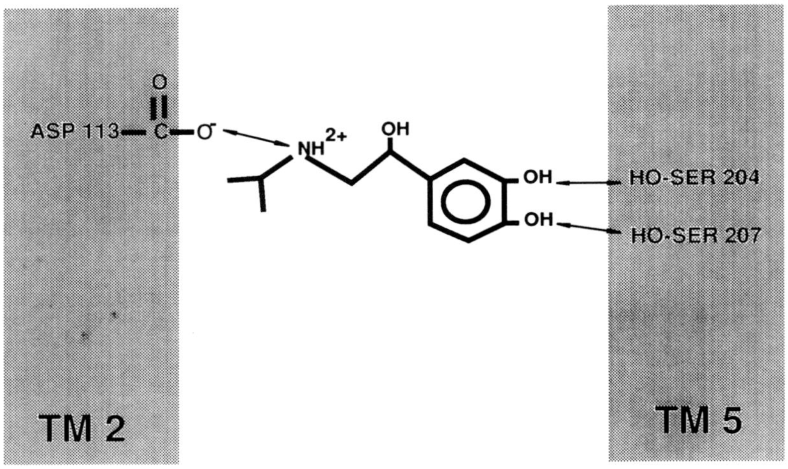

FIG. 3. Sites of interaction between the β_2-adrenergic receptor and the agonist isoproterenol as determined by mutagenesis studies (31). Transmembrane domains 2 and 5 are indicated by the *shaded bars*.

the isoproterenol derivative lacking the para-hydroxyl, but not by the isoproterenol derivative lacking the meta-hydroxyl. Conversely, the β_2-receptor mutant lacking serine 207 could only be activated by isoproterenol and the isoproterenol derivative lacking the meta-hydroxyl, but not by the derivative lacking the para-hydroxyl. These studies provide strong support for the hypothesis that serine 204 forms a hydrogen bond with the meta-hydroxyl of the catechol ring and that serine 207 forms a hydrogen bond with the para-hydroxyl. Mutation of a number of other amino acids in different membrane-spanning domains has also been shown to affect ligand binding (34); however, it is not possible to determine if these mutations affect the binding domain or the overall structure of the protein.

Determinants of Subtype-Specific Ligand Binding

Of enormous therapeutic importance is the specificity with which the various adrenergic receptors recognize drugs with different affinities. A rational understanding of the basis for these different properties of each subtype should be useful in the development of novel drugs with highly selective specificity for the various subtypes. The aspartate and serine residues indicated in Fig. 3 are found in all of the adrenergic receptors. These residues are therefore likely to be important components of the catechol-binding pocket of all of the adrenergic receptors and are not likely to be important for determining differences in binding to subtype specific ligands. Evidence from chimeric receptor studies has suggested that determinants of subtype-specific ligand binding are found on several of the membrane-spanning domains. The seventh hydrophobic domain is important in determining differences in antagonist binding specificity between the β_2- and α_2-adrenergic receptors (35). More recently, it has been observed that changing the phenylalanine at position 412 in the human platelet α_2-adrenergic receptor to asparagine (the amino acid found in the homologous region of the β_2-receptor) results in loss of binding to the β_2-receptor antagonist yohimbine and acquisition of high affinity for the β-receptor antagonists alprenolol, propranolol, and pindolol (36). These studies suggest a direct interaction between subtype-specific ligands and specific amino acids in the seventh membrane-spanning domain of the α_2- and β_2-adrenergic receptor.

Evidence from studies of chimeric receptors formed from pharmacologically closely related β_1- and β_2-receptors suggest that most of the membrane-spanning domains make some contribution to determining ligand-binding specificity (37,38). This contribution may be through allosteric effects or by directly contributing to the binding pocket.

G Protein–Coupling Domains

Mutagenesis studies on adrenergic receptors have revealed that several cytosolic domains are involved in the functional coupling of receptors and G proteins. The study of chimeric receptors constructed from receptors with different G protein–coupling specificities has been valuable in identifying the third cytoplasmic domain as being responsible for determining the specificity of receptor–G protein interactions (35,39,40). The exchange of a 12 amino acid sequence in the amino terminal segment of the third cytoplasmic domain of the muscarinic (M_1) receptor with the sequence from the homologous domain of the turkey β-receptor altered G protein–coupling specificity (39). This chimeric receptor was capable of activating phospholipase C (the property of the muscarinic receptor) as well as adenylyl cyclase (the property of the β-receptor) when bound to the muscarinic agonist acetylcholine, but not to adrenergic receptor agonists. When the second cytoplasmic domain of this chimeric receptor is replaced with the homologous sequence from the turkey β-receptor, the new chimeric receptor fully activates adenylyl cyclase when occupied by acetylcholine, but activation of phospholipase C is reduced. These data indicate that this 12 amino acid peptide of the third intracellular loop along with regions of the second intracellular loop is important for defining G protein–coupling specificity.

Domains within the carboxyl terminus of the third intracellular domain and the amino terminal portion of the carboxyl terminus may also participate in interactions with G proteins (34,40,41). While these domains do not appear to determine specificity of interactions, mutations in these domains modify the efficiency of coupling as determined by the maximal stimulation of adenylyl cyclase and the concentration of agonist required to produce half-maximal stimulation.

Mutations may also lead to receptors that are more efficient in G protein activation (40). When the amino acid sequence REKKAA from the carboxyl end of the third intracellular loop of the α_1-receptor is replaced by KEHKAL from the β_2-receptor, the resulting chimeric receptor exhibited a 100-fold increase in affinity for norepinephrine in ligand binding assays. Furthermore, the median effective concentration (EC_{50}) for activation of phospholipase C is 100-fold lower than the EC_{50} for the wild type α_1-receptor, and the basal level of inositol phosphate turnover in cells expressing this mutant α_1-receptor is twofold higher than the basal level in cells expressing the wild type α_1-receptor (40). These results indicate that natural mutations in G protein–coupled receptors could transform these receptors into potential oncogenes. Chronic stimulation of serotonin 5-HT$_{1c}$ receptors expressed in NIH 3T3 cells leads to the generation of transformed foci in cultured cells (42). Injection of these foci into nude mice leads to the formation of tumors. The *mas* oncogene is an example of a seven-membrane-spanning domain protein that is capable of inducing tumors in nude mice (43).

RECEPTOR REGULATION

Signal transduction by adrenergic receptors is constantly regulated by adjustments in the functional capacity of receptors and in receptor density at the cell surface. For the purposes of this discussion, the term *desensitization* will be used to refer to a variety of processes by which the functional interaction of a receptor and its G protein are impaired, leading to a reduction in the cellular response to a hormone or neurotransmitter. This process usually follows prolonged stimulation of the receptor or related receptors that activate the same G protein.

Desensitization is a clinically important phenomenon that is likely to be part of the normal physiological regulation of adrenergic receptor function. However, in pathological conditions such as chronic lung disease or

congestive heart failure, desensitization may limit the efficacy of hormones, neurotransmitters, or drugs that may otherwise be clinically beneficial. The process of desensitization to a drug is frequently called tachyphylaxis. Better understanding of the mechanism of desensitization may lead to new ways of modifying this process for therapeutic purposes.

The process of desensitization of the β-receptor has been most extensively characterized (44,45). In mechanistic terms, the process of desensitization can be brought about by changes in receptor structure by phosphorylation and by changes in receptor density.

RECEPTOR PHOSPHORYLATION

The functional properties of cellular proteins and enzymes are often regulated by phosphorylation and dephosphorylation. Stimulation of the β-adrenergic receptors leads to changes in the activity of PKA, which is activated by cAMP. PKA recognizes specific amino acid sequences (consensus sequences) on the β_2-receptor and transfers a phosphate from ATP to two serine residues on the protein. A more recently characterized kinase has been identified that phosphorylates receptors only when they are occupied by an agonist. This kinase has been named β-adrenergic receptor kinase (βARK) (46). Mutagenesis studies have characterized the location of functionally important sites for phosphorylation of the β_2-receptor (see Fig. 1) by PKA and βARK (47). Phosphorylation at these sites impairs the ability of the receptor to activate Gs.

Desensitization of the β_2-receptor mediated by βARK and PKA differ in two important ways. First, βARK phosphorylation of the β-receptor is entirely dependent on the presence of agonist. Unoccupied receptor or antagonist-occupied receptor cannot be phosphorylated by βARK. This differs from PKA phosphorylation of the receptor, which does not require agonist occupancy. In fact, PKA phosphorylation of the β_2-receptor may occur following activation of this kinase by other receptors. The second difference in desensitization mediated by these kinases is that phosphorylation of the β_2-receptor by PKA impairs β_2-receptor function directly, whereas the disruption of receptor–G protein interaction following βARK phosphorylation of β_2-receptor requires another protein (48). This protein, which has recently been cloned (49), has been called β-arrestin because of its structural and functional similarity to arrestin, a protein that regulates visual signal transduction. A model comparing PKA- and βARK-mediated desensitization of the β-receptor is illustrated in Fig. 4.

REGULATION OF RECEPTOR DENSITY

Signal transduction by G proteins can be regulated by altering the density of functional receptors at the cell sur-

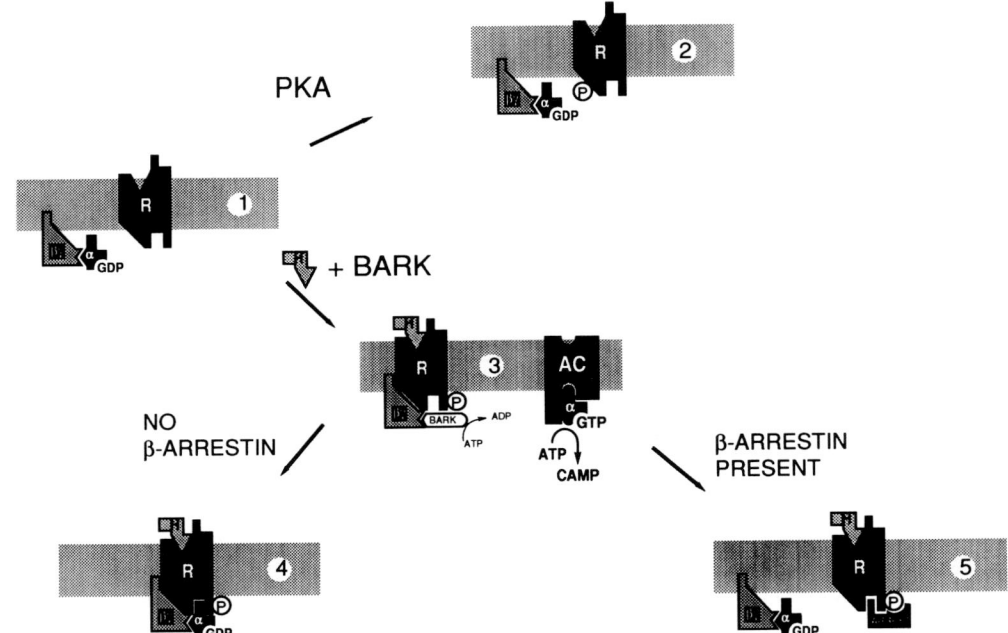

FIG. 4. Different mechanisms of desensitization mediated by β-adrenergic receptor kinase (BARK) and protein kinase A (PKA). **Panel 1:** The nonphosphorylated state. **Panel 2:** Phosphorylation by protein kinase A occurs following activation by PKA through the β-receptor or through stimulation of other receptors coupled to adenylyl cyclase. Phosphorylation of the β-receptor by PKA appears to directly interfere with Gs activation. **Panel 3:** In contrast, phosphorylation of the β-receptor by BARK requires that the receptor be occupied by agonist. BARK phosphorylation is enhanced by βγ-subunits (79,80) and it is possible that the release of the α-subunit following activation by the receptor makes room for BARK to bind to the βγ-subunit. **Panel 4:** Unlike receptor phosphorylated by PKA, receptor phosphorylated by BARK is still capable of activating adenylyl cyclase (4). An additional factor, β-arrestin, binds to the BARK phosphorylated receptor and blocks activation of Gs. R, β-receptor; AC, adenylyl cyclase; H, agonist hormone; α, α-subunit of Gs; βγ, β- and γ-subunits of Gs, BARK, β-adrenergic receptor kinase; ARREST, β-arrestin; P, phosphate.

face. Receptor density can be modified by changes in the rate of synthesis of new receptors. The rate of β_2-receptor mRNA synthesis and destruction are both modulated by intracellular cAMP. The density of β_2-receptors at the cell surface can also be modified by at least two processes that actively remove receptors from the plasma membrane: sequestration, which is a reversible process, and down-regulation, which leads to destruction of receptor protein. The molecular mechanisms involved in these processes have not yet been characterized; however, it is likely that interactions between these receptors and cytoskeletal proteins are involved.

ADRENERGIC MECHANISMS IN AN ANIMAL MODEL OF PHEOCHROMOCYTOMA

An instructive example of adrenergic receptor regulation of particular relevance to hypertension involves experiments conducted in New England Deaconess Hospital (NEDH) rats, which can harbor a transplantable pheochromocytoma. A transplantable pheochromocytoma that secretes predominantly norepinephrine as well

as dopamine and can be passaged in the NEDH strain of rat was developed by Warren and Chute (50). Implantation of pheochromocytoma generally leads to a marked increase in plasma concentrations of catecholamines with norepinephrine increasing from 500–700 pg/ml to 30,000–40,000 pg/ml after about 4 weeks. Systolic blood pressure is generally elevated into the range of 170 to 200 mm Hg. The NEDH rat harboring pheochromocytoma has been used to investigate a number of questions relating to the effects of prolonged exposure to catecholamines including desensitization of responses mediated by catecholamines (51–57), as well as mechanisms of catecholamine-induced cardiomyopathy (58–60), and mechanisms of hypertension in rats harboring pheochromocytomas (60,61).

Relatively little is known about the development of desensitization *in vivo* and the relationship between elegantly demonstrated changes in receptor function and alterations in physiological responses in cells. The rat model of pheochromocytoma has been useful in determining some of these relationships. It has been repeatedly and elegantly demonstrated in cultured cell models that prolonged exposure to catecholamines leads to a blunted ability of cells to subsequently synthesize cAMP in response to subsequent stimulation by agonists. However, the implications of these changes for physiological responses mediated by the desensitized cells has not been extensively characterized. There is enormous redundancy in the cAMP system in many cells. This means that a far less than maximal cAMP response is adequate to activate protein kinase A sufficiently to lead to a full physiological response. For example, prolonged exposure to catecholamines leads to marked down-regulation of β-adrenergic receptors in adipocytes, which is associated with a markedly diminished cAMP response to β-agonists (53,57). However, only a relatively modest increase in cAMP is required to fully activate lipolysis. Even in fat cells whose β-adrenergic receptors are down-regulated by as much as 90 percent, there is still a sufficient cAMP response to catecholamines to activate protein kinase A enough to fully activate lipolysis (57). Consequently, the blunted cAMP response in adipocytes leads to loss in sensitivity of the cells to catecholamines without loss of maximal functioning. In adipocytes, there was no change in the relationship between activation of protein kinase A and lipolysis with desensitization; in other words, the decrease in sensitivity to catecholamines could be fully explained by the blunted cAMP response. For very few desensitized cells has this relationship between β-receptor number, cAMP responses, protein kinase A activation, and physiological response been determined.

Desensitization of α_1-receptor–mediated responses is less well understood than desensitization of responses mediated by β-adrenergic receptors. A number of investigations have examined the effects of catecholamines on the ability of α-receptors to activate inositol phospholipid breakdown in cultured transformed smooth muscle cells (62,63). Activation of protein kinase C in these cells, primarily with phorbol esters, rapidly impairs the ability of α-agonists to activate inositol phospholipid breakdown. These changes are associated with phosphorylation of α_1-receptors. In addition, these investigators found that norepinephrine treatment of these cells rapidly impaired the ability of α-receptors to activate inositol phospholipid breakdown. These changes occurred within minutes. Norepinephrine apparently also induced sequestration of α_1-receptors away from the cell surface as evidenced by decreased [^{3}H]prazosin binding to the treated cells. The changes in receptor binding were paralleled by the rapid phosphorylation of α_1-receptors in the cells. These experiments suggest several analogies with mechanisms of β-adrenergic receptor desensitization.

This animal model of pheochromocytoma has also been useful in the investigation of desensitization of responses mediated by α_1-adrenergic receptors. The ability of the α-receptor agonist phenylephrine to induce con-

traction of aorta isolated from rats harboring pheochromocytoma is markedly impaired (54). Contraction mediated by thromboxane A_2 and angiotensin II receptors is also blunted, indicating that the desensitization induced by pheochromocytoma is heterologous since more than one type of receptor is desensitized (54,60). These results suggests the possibility that there may be alterations in vascular smooth muscle in rats harboring pheochromocytoma other than changes in adrenergic receptors. Indeed, a surprisingly complex and diverse variety of mechanisms are involved in desensitization of α_1-adrenergic responses in blood vessels. For example, the release of endothelium-derived relaxing factor (EDRF) from the endothelium plays an important role in development of desensitization; i.e., prolonged α-adrenergic stimulation of blood vessels leads to enhanced release and action of EDRF in the desensitized arteries (64,65). In addition, prolonged activation of α_1-receptors in vascular smooth muscle leads to down-regulation of protein kinase C, which may serve also to attenuate smooth muscle contraction (66). These results highlight the additional complexity of desensitization of α_1-receptor–mediated responses in blood vessels from rats with pheochromocytoma or in vessels incubated *in vitro* with adrenergic agonists. The potential importance of these regulatory mechanisms in modifying more subtle forms of enhanced sympathetic nervous system activity as may be found in hypertension or congestive heart failure remains to be determined.

Rats harboring pheochromocytoma have been useful in other studies of relevance to hypertension. Catecholamine-induced cardiomyopathies have been found in a variety of settings characterized by catecholamine excess, such as in the use of sympathomimetic drugs or in humans with pheochromocytoma (67,68). These effects have been investigated in a number of experimental models of catecholamine excess (69,70). Indeed, cardiac damage induced by stress has also been observed (71). Catecholamine-induced cardiomyopathy is characterized by multifocal areas of inflammatory infiltrates, enhanced interstitial and replacement fibrosis, and contraction band necrosis. Which adrenergic receptors activated by elevated concentrations of circulating catecholamines produce cardiac damage in rats harboring pheochromocytoma? This problem has been addressed by treating rats implanted with pheochromocytoma with drugs in an effort to prevent the development of cardiomyopathy. Cardiac morphological abnormalities in hearts from rats harboring pheochromocytoma can be quantified with a histological scoring system (58,59). Interestingly, mere normalization of blood pressure with the vasodilator hydralazine does not attenuate the development of cardiomyopathy; consequently, the cardiomyopathy is not due directly to the elevated blood pressure (59). However, the β-receptor antagonist timolol markedly attenuates the development of the cardiomyopathy; indeed, it is more effective than α-adrenergic receptor blockade with phenoxybenzamine (59). These results suggest that excess β-adrenergic stimulation of the heart leads to cardiac damage in pheochromocytoma. The relevance of these finding to humans with pheochromocytoma is uncertain; however, the results raise the question that preoperative preparation with a β-adrenergic antagonist of some patients with pheochromocytoma and also patients with metastatic pheochromocytoma may be useful. The cardiomyopathy found in rats harboring pheochromocytoma is a marked, potentially interesting example of lesions found under more subtle conditions of catecholamine excess.

Studies of adrenergic mechanisms in rats harboring pheochromocytoma have had interesting implications for the role of catecholamine excess in the development of hypertension. There are a number of relatively uncommon causes of secondary hypertension such as Cushing's syndrome, renal artery stenosis, and pheochromocytoma. In terms of mechanism of hypertension, pheochromocytoma would appear to be very straightforward; namely, excess production of catecholamines leads to an increase in peripheral resistance and consequent hypertension. However, there are several clinical observations that suggest that the situation may be more complex. Hypertension in patients with pheochromocytoma may be sustained or intermittent; while it is often assumed that these differences reflect differences in pattern of secretion of catecholamines, this has not been clearly demonstrated. Furthermore, Bravo and colleagues (72) showed that hypertension in patients with pheochromocytoma could be lowered acutely with the α_2-adrenergic agonist clonidine at a dose that had no effect on the circulating concentrations of catecholamines. This result suggested the possibility that the sympathetic nervous system was playing a role in the maintenance of hypertension in pheochromocytoma. NEDH rats harboring pheochromocytomas provide an opportunity to more systematically examine this question than is possible in patients with this rare disease. Indeed, it has been demonstrated that clonidine markedly lowers blood pressure in rats harboring pheochromocytoma, as does a ganglionic blocking drug (61). In addition, the angiotensin-converting enzyme inhibitor captopril also markedly lowers blood pressure in rats harboring pheochromocytoma without decreasing the markedly elevated plasma catecholamine concentrations (60). These studies demonstrate the complex and incompletely understood interplay between adrenergic receptor activation and hypertension.

HETEROLOGOUS REGULATION OF ADRENERGIC RECEPTORS

Not only catecholamines themselves but also a variety of other drugs and hormones may regulate expression of adrenergic receptors in a large number of cells, including cardiomyocytes and vascular smooth muscle cells. These heterologous regulators of adrenergic receptor expression run the gamut from thyroid hormone to antidepressant drugs. The basis for these regulatory mechanisms is beginning to be understood at the molecular level. For example, glucocorticoids have been found to induce transcription of the α_{1B}-receptor gene (73). The mechanism for hypertension in patients with Cushing's syndrome is uncertain and is likely due to several different effects of glucocorticoids such as sodium retention, activation of the renin-angiotensin system, as well as decreased activity of prostaglandin and kallikrein-kinin systems, which ordinarily tend to promote vasodilitation (74). In addition, it has been found, both in experimental models and humans, that glucocorticoids enhance vasoconstriction mediated by catecholamines (75–77). To what extent the recently recognized role of glucocorticoids in regulating expression of α_1-receptors contributes to hypertension remains to be more fully explored.

Activation of protein kinase C by phorbol esters has recently been found to also induce transcription of the α_{1B}-receptor gene in transformed smooth muscle cells (78). These observations raise the possibility that hormonal activation of protein kinase C may also regulate expression of α_1-receptors in vascular smooth muscle cells. This likelihood suggests possible interplay between adrenergic receptors and various signaling systems in the cardiovascular system, such as angiotensin II receptors, which are powerful activators of protein kinase C in smooth muscle.

These are some examples where recent insight into regulation of adrenergic receptor genes may help explain or even predict important regulation of these receptors in cells of the cardiovascular system. As further insights are obtained relating to the genetic control of expression of these receptors, we may expect to discover novel regulatory mechanisms of pathophysiological significance for hypertension.

REFERENCES

1. Bylund DB. *Pharmacol Biochem Behav* 1985;22:835–843.
2. Han C, Abel PW, Minneman KP. *Nature* 1987;329:333–335.
3. Dixon RAF, Kobilka BK, Strader DJ, Benovic JL, Dohlman HG, et al. *Nature* 1986;321:75–79.
4. Cotecchia S, Schwinn DA, Randall RR, Lefkowitz RJ, Caron MG, et al. *Proc Natl Acad Sci USA* 1988;85:7159–7163.
5. Kobilka BK, Matsui H, Kobilka TS, Yang-Feng TL, Francke U, et al. *Science* 1987;238:650–656.
6. Yarden Y, Rodriguez H, Wong SK, Brandt ER, May DC, et al. *Proc Natl Acad Sci USA* 1986;83:6795–6799.
7. Frielle T, Collins S, Daniel KW, Caron MG, Lefkowitz RJ, Kobilka BK. *Proc Natl Acad Sci USA* 1987;84:7920–7924.
8. Schwinn DA, Lomasney JW, Lorenz W, Szklut PM, Fremeau RT Jr, et al. *J Biol Chem* 1990;265:5183–5189.
9. Lomasney JW, Cotecchia S, Lorenz W, Leung WY, Schwinn DA, Yang-Feng TL, Brownstein M, Lefkowitz RJ, Caron MG. *J Biol Chem* 1991;266:6365–6369.

10. Perez Perez DM, Piascik MT, Graham RM. *Mol Pharmacol* 1991;40:876–883.
11. Regan JW, Kobilka TS, Yang-Feng TL, Caron MG, Lefkowitz RJ, Kobilka BK. *Proc Natl Acad Sci USA* 1988;85:6301–6305.
12. Lomasney JW, Lorenz W, Allen LF, King K, Regan JW, et al. *Proc Natl Acad Sci USA* 1990;87:5094–5098.
13. Weinshank RL, Zgombick JM, Macchi M, Adham N, Lichtblau H, Branchek TA, Hartiz PR. *Mol Pharmacol* 1990;38:681–688.
14. Emorine LJ, Marullo S, Briend-Sutren MM, Patey G, Tate K, et al. *Science* 1989;245:1118–1121.
15. Minneman KP. *Pharmacol Rev* 1988;40:87–119.
16. Minneman KP, Han C, Abel PW. *Mol Pharmacol* 1988;33:509–514.
17. Ruffolo RR, Nichols AJ, Stadel JM, Hieble JP. *Pharmacol Rev* 1991;43:475–505.
18. Han C, Li J, Minneman KP. *Eur J Pharmacol* 1990;190:97–104.
19. Cotecchia S, Kobilka BK, Daniel KW, Nolan RD, Lapetina EY, et al. *J Biol Chem* 1990;265:63–69.
20. Iyengar R, Birnbaumer L. *G proteins*. San Diego: Academic Press, 1990.
21. Freismuth M, Casey PJ, Gilman AG. *FASEB J* 1988;3:2125–2131.
22. Ross EM. *Neuron* 1989;3:141–152.
23. Birnbaumer L, Abramowitz J, Brown AM. *Biochem Biophys Acta* 1990;1031:163–224.
24. Bourne H, Sanders DA, McCormick F. *Nature* 1991;349:117–127.
25. Hepler JR, Gilman AG. *Trends Biochem Sci* 1992;17:383–387.
26. Kim D, Lewis DL, Graxialei L, Neer EJ, Gar-Sagi D, Clapham DE. *Nature* 1989;337:557–560.
27. Conklin BR, Chabre O, Wong YH, Federman AD, Bourne HR. *J Biol Chem* 1992;267:31–34.
28. Rubenstein RC, Wong SKF, Ross EM. *J Biol Chem* 1987;262:16655–16662.
29. Wong SKF, Claughter C, Ruoho AE, Ross EM. *J Biol Chem* 1988;263:7925–7928.
30. Dixon RAF, Sigal IS, Candelore MR, Register RB, Scattergood W, et al. *EMBO J* 1987;6:3269–3275.
31. Strader CD, Candelore MR, Hill WS, Sigal IS, Dixon RAF. *J Biol Chem* 1989;264:13572–13578.
32. Strader CD, Candelore MR, Hill WS, Dixon RAF, Sigal IS. *J Biol Chem* 1989;264:16470–16477.
33. Strader CD, Gaffney T, Sugg EE, Candelore MR, Keys R, et al. *J Biol Chem* 1991;266:5–8.
34. Strader CD, Sigal IS, Dixon RAF. *FASEB J* 1989;3:1825–1832.
35. Kobilka BK, Kobilka TS, Daniel K, Regan JW, Caron MG, Lefkowitz RJ. *Science* 1988;240:1310–1316.
36. Suryanarayana S, Daunt DA, Von Zastrow M, Kobilka BK. *J Biol Chem* 1991;266:15488–15492.
37. Frielle T, Daniel KW, Caron MG, Lefkowitz RJ. *Proc Natl Acad Sci USA* 1988;85:9494–9498.
38. Dixon RAF, Hill WS, Candelore MR, Rands E, Diehl R, et al. *Proteins* 1989;6:267–274.
39. Wong SK, Parker EM, Ross EM. *J Biol Chem* 1990;265:6219–6224.
40. Cotecchia S, Exum S, Caron MG, Lefkowitz RJ. *Proc Natl Acad Sci USA* 1990;87:2896–2900.
41. O'Dowd BF, Hnatowich M, Regan JW, Leader WM, Caron MG, Lefkowitz RJ. *J Biol Chem* 1988;263:15985–15992.
42. Julius D, Livelli TJ, Jessell TM, Axel R. *Science* 1989;244:1057–1062.
43. Young D, Waitches G, Birchmeier C, Fasano O, Wigler M. *Cell* 1986;5:711–719.
44. Hausdorff WP, Caron MG, Lefkowitz RJ. *FASEB J* 1990;4:2881–2889.
45. Lefkowitz RJ, Hausdorff WP, Caron MG. *Trends Pharmacol Sci* 1990;11:190–194.
46. Benovic JL, DeBlasi A, Stone WC, Caron MG, Lefkowitz RJ. *Science* 1989;246:235–246.
47. Hausdorff WP, Bouvier M, O'Dowd BF, Irons GP, Caron MG, Lefkowitz RJ. *J Biol Chem* 1989;264:12657–12665.
48. Benovic JL, Kuhn J, Weyland I, Codina J, Caron JG, Lefkowitz RJ. *Proc Natl Acad Sci USA* 1987;84:8879–8882.
49. Lohse MJ, Benovic JL, Codina J, Caron MG, Lefkowitz RJ. *Science* 1990;248:1547–1550.
50. Warren S, Chute RN. *Cancer* 1972;29:327–331.
51. Snavely MD, Motulsky HJ, O'Connor DT, Ziegler MG, Insel PA. *Clin Exp Hypertens* 1982;A4:829–848.
52. Snavely MD, Motlusky HJ, Moustafa E, Mahan LC, Insel PA. *Circ Res* 1982;57:504–513.
53. Tsujimoto G, Manger WM, Hoffman BB. *Endocrinology* 1984;114:1272–1278.
54. Rosenbaum JS, Zera P, Umans VA, Ginsburg R, Hoffman BB. *J Pharmacol Exp Ther* 1986;238:396–400.
55. Tsujimoto G, Honda K, Hoffman BB, Hashimoto K. *Circ Res* 1987;61:86–98.
56. Tsujimoto G, Minegishi A, Ishizaki T, Hoffman BB, Hashimoto K. *J Pharmacol Exp Ther* 1987;242:637–645.
57. Prokocimer PG, Maze M, Vickery R, Hoffman BB. *Endocrinology* 1988;123:528–533.
58. Rosenbaum JS, Billingham ME, Ginsburg R, Tsujimoto G, Lurie K, Hoffman BB. *Am J Cardiovasc Pathol* 1988;1:389–399.
59. Rosenbaum JS, Ginsburg R, Billingham ME, Hoffman BB. *J Pharmacol Exp Ther* 1987;241:354–360.
60. Hu Z-W, Billingham M, Tuck M, Hoffman BB. *Hypertension* 1990;15:210–215.
61. Prokocimer PG, Maze M, Hoffman BB. *J Pharmacol Exp Ther* 1987;241:870–874.
62. Bouvier M, Leeb-Lundberg LM, Benovic JL, Caron MG, Lefkowitz RJ. *J Biol Chem* 1987;262:3106–3113.
63. Leeb-Lundberg LM, Cotecchia S, DeBlasi A, Caron MG, Lefkowitz RJ. *J Biol Chem* 1987;262:3098–3105.
64. Hiremath A, Hu Z, Hoffman BB. *J Cardiovasc Pharmacol* 1991;18:151–157.
65. Hu Z-W, Honda H, Murad F, Hoffman BB. *J Pharmacol Exp Ther* 1992;260:756–761.
66. Hu Z-W, Azhar S, Hoffman BB. *J Cardiovasc Pharmacol* 1992;20:982–989.
67. Kline IK. *Am J Pathol* 1961;38:539–591.
68. Van Vliet PD, Burchell HB, Titus JL. *N Engl J Med* 1966;274:1102–1108.
69. Chappel CI, Rona G, Balazs T, Gàudry R. *Can J Biochem Physiol* 1959;37:35–42.
70. Kahn DS, Rona G, Chappel CI. *Ann NY Acad Sci* 1969;156:285–293.
71. Haggendal J, Johansson G, Jonsson L, Thoren-Tolling K. *Acta Pharmacol Toxicol* 1982;50:58–66.
72. Bravo E, Tarazi RC, Fouad FM, Textor SC, Gifford RW, Vidt DG. *Hypertension* 1982;4(suppl 2):II-193–II-199.
73. Sakaue M, Hoffman BB. *J Clin Invest* 1991;88:385–389.
74. Saruta T, Suzuki H, Handa M, Igarashi Y, Kondo K, Senba S. *J Clin Endocrinol Metab* 1986;62:275–279.
75. Kadowitz PJ, Yard AC. *Eur J Pharmacol* 1971;13:281–286.
76. Yard AC, Kadowitz PJ. *Eur J Pharmacol* 1972;20:1–9.
77. Besse JC, Bass AD. *J Pharmacol Exp Ther* 1966;154:224–238.
78. Hu ZW, Shi XY, Sakaue M, Hoffman BB. *J Biol Chem* 1993;268:3610–3615.
79. Kameyama K, Haga K, Haga T, Kontani K, Katada T, Fukada Y. *J Biol Chem* 1993;268:7753–7758.
80. Pitcher JA, Inglese J, Higgins JB, Arriz JL, Casey PJ, Kim C, Benovic JL, Kwatra MM, Caron MG, Lefkowitz RJ. *Science* 1993;257:1264–1267.

Hypertension: Pathophysiology, Diagnosis, and Management, Second Edition, edited by J.H. Laragh and B.M. Brenner, Raven Press, Ltd., New York © 1995.

CHAPTER 50

Alpha-Adrenergic Receptors in Hypertension

Haralambos Gavras, Diane Handy, and Irene Gavras

Increased activity of the sympathetic nervous system is believed to contribute to hypertension via neurohormonal stimulation of adrenergic receptors (ARs). The ARs are members of the guanidine nucleotide (G) regulatory protein-coupled receptor superfamily (1) and are divided into three major types: α_1, α_2, and β (2). Initially, ARs were characterized according to the functional response to their stimulation or inhibition by various pharmacologic probes (3). Subsequently, they were classified according to their binding affinity to selective radioligands (4). More recently, the use of molecular biology techniques has confirmed the heterogeneity of AR subtypes as products of different genes. This permitted further identification of at least three subtypes for each one, for a total of nine recognized members of the AR family at the time of this writing: α_{1A}, α_{1B}, α_{1C}, α_{2A}, α_{2B}, α_{2C} and β_1, β_2, β_3 (2). All are activated to variable extents by catecholamines or other sympathomimetic amines, which elicit type-specific and tissue-specific responses. This chapter briefly reviews the salient characteristics of the α_1 and α_2 ARs in relation to their contribution to the development and maintenance of hypertension via their tissue-specific effects and/or interaction with other pressor systems.

H. Gavras, D. Handy, and I. Gavras: Hypertension and Atherosclerosis Section, Department of Medicine, Boston University School of Medicine, Boston, Massachusetts 02118.

FUNCTIONAL CHARACTERISTICS OF ALPHA-ADRENERGIC RECEPTORS

Activation of α_1-AR by agonists leads to coupling with a stimulatory G protein, which activates the enzyme phospholipase C, which increases formation of inositol triphosphate and diacylglycerol as the second messengers triggering further biochemical reactions, which regulate calcium-ion flux in the effector cell. Usually, activation of α_2-AR by agonists leads to coupling with an inhibitory G protein (G_i), which inhibits the enzyme adenylyl cyclase and decreases formation of the messenger adenosine 3',5'-cyclic monophosphate (cAMP), thus inhibiting further biochemical reactions (5). However, recent studies of recombinant α_2-AR suggest that certain subtypes may bind to noninhibitory G proteins (see below). Antagonists are substances that bind to the receptor without triggering further intracellular events, while blocking its accessibility to agonists.

Both types of α-AR are widely distributed in various regions of the central nervous system (CNS), as well as in vascular, cardiac, renal, and other tissues, with specific subtypes probably predominating in specific areas. In relation to the sympathetic synapse, the α_2-ARs can be both presynaptic (modulating neurotransmission via a negative feedback mechanism) and postsynaptic (mediating the response of the effector organs), whereas the α_1-ARs are always postsynaptic (6). Their density is believed to be determined by genetic factors, age, and possibly dietary factors (sodium and calcium intake), as well as by the presence of agonists or antagonists, which influence their turnover rates—i.e., agonists accelerate the receptors' metabolism, causing a net loss from cell surfaces (down-regulation), whereas antagonists prolong their half-life, thus increasing their net numbers (up-regulation) (7).

The functional physiologic or pharmacologic response to a given stimulus appears to be qualitatively determined by the effector tissue cell, the receptor subtype, and its anatomic location, including the presynaptic or postsynaptic position in relation to the synaptic cleft of the sympathetic neuron (8,9), and quantitatively determined by the number of available receptors and by their state of affinity, which can be modified by various factors, including cations and guanine nucleotides (10–12). Specifically, the monovalent Na^+ ion decreases the affinity of α_2-AR for agonists, but increases the affinity of α_1-AR; the divalent Ca^{2+} and Mg^{2+} cations increase the affinity of α_2-AR for agonists. These changes may be relevant to the pressor or depressor responses elicited from α-AR by various stimuli. It is generally accepted that the quantitative influence of various factors on a specific receptor type studied in accessible tissues (e.g., peripheral vessels or platelets) can be reasonably extrapolated and applied to the same receptor type elsewhere, e.g., the CNS.

MOLECULAR CHARACTERISTICS AND SIGNALING MECHANISMS OF ALPHA-ADRENERGIC RECEPTORS

The latest and most precise classification of AR subtypes has involved expression of cloned sequences in mammalian cell lines and analysis of receptor/ligand interactions of recombinant proteins, sometimes from different species. Thus, cDNAs and/or genes encoding for the three distinct α_1-AR subtypes and the three distinct α_2-AR subtypes have been cloned, sequenced, and characterized (2,13–27).

Analysis of the predicted protein sequences show that the α-ARs share the common structure of membrane-bound proteins that interact with G proteins; these receptors have seven hydrophobic regions that have been postulated to serve as the transmembrane pocket for ligand binding. An aspartate residue (asp-79) within the second transmembrane domain appears to be the site where Na^+ acts to modulate ligand binding to α_2-AR (28,29). Since this residue is highly conserved among all G protein–linked receptors, it is conceivable that Na^+ may play an even broader role in regulating the functions of several receptors (29). The transmembrane regions are the most highly conserved region of the molecule, with about 70 percent to 77 percent homology within either the α_1 or α_2 class of receptors and about 45 percent ho-

mology between members of the α_1- and α_2-AR class. The homology in amino acid sequences of α-AR subtypes between species can be as high as 89 percent to 90 percent, as shown for the rat and human α_{2A}-AR sequenced by us and others (23,24,26,27).

A common feature of the α_1-AR is the long intracellular C-terminus, which is highly divergent among the subtypes, and contains sites for phosphorylation and palmitoylation. In contrast, the α_2-AR has a short C-terminus and a much larger third cytoplasmic loop, which is highly divergent among the subtypes. It has been suggested that the sites of phosphorylation within this loop of the α_2-AR and in the C-terminus of the α_1-AR may be related to receptor desensitization (30).

Through the various subtypes of G proteins, α_1- and α_2-AR mediate a variety of cellular responses to epinephrine and norepinephrine. The α_{1A}-AR subtype, as mentioned earlier, has been shown to activate phospholipase C via pertussis toxin–insensitive G proteins (31). The activation of phospholipase C causes phosphatidylinositol hydrolysis and the formation of inositol triphosphate, which leads to the release of Ca^{2+} from intracellular stores, and the formation of diacylglycerol, which subsequently activates protein kinase C. Recent work examining the ability of recombinant α_{1B}-AR and α_{1C}-AR to activate phospholipase C indicates that stimulation of the α_{1C}-AR results in a two- to threefold increase in the production of inositol phosphates (32). Other evidence suggests that the α_{1A}-AR can mediate the influx of extracellular Ca^{2+} (33).

In the case of the α_2-AR, several intracellular effects are mediated through the action of pertussis toxin–sensitive G proteins, such as the well-characterized inhibition of adenylyl cyclase (34). In addition, the α_2-ARs have been shown to mediate intracellular Ca^{2+} and K^+ fluxes, activate Na^+/H^+ antiporters, and stimulate phosphatidylinositol hydrolysis (35–37). The existence of multiple receptor/G protein–coupled responses within a given cell line is suggested by several studies that indicate α_2-AR may associate with more than one G protein in a given cell line. Recent studies of recombinant α_2-AR have shown the preferential association of the α_{2C} subtype to G_0 subtypes of G proteins (38), suggesting that the α_{2C} subtype is responsible for Ca^{2+} and K^+ channel regulation, whereas the α_{2A} and α_{2B} subtypes bind to various forms of G_i, G proteins that are responsible for adenylyl cyclase inhibition (39).

ALPHA-ADRENERGIC RECEPTORS IN THE CENTRAL NERVOUS SYSTEM

Mapping of the CNS distribution of α_1- and α_2-AR has been obtained by autoradiography using selective radiolabeled ligands (40–42). Higher densities of α_1-AR were visualized in the lamina V of the cortex, thalamic nuclei, hippocampus, and dentate gyrus, whereas a low and relatively even density was observed throughout the hind brain and spinal cord. The α_2-ARs were found in high concentrations in the periventricular, paraventricular, and arcuate nuclei of the hypothalamus, medial preoptic nucleus and bed nucleus of the stria terminalis, and in brainstem areas such as the nucleus tractus solitarii (NTS), the locus coeruleus (LC), the dorsal parabrachial nucleus, and the cells of the A1 area of the ventrolateral medulla. These brainstem regions are innervated by catecholaminergic neurons involved in continuous cardiovascular regulation and baroreflex control via alterations of sympathetic and parasympathetic outflow. (They are also involved in the integration of cognitive and viscerosensory information and responses to arousal, pain, stress, and anxiety [41]).

A major function of the catecholaminergic neurons in these medullary structures (i.e., the NTS, the LC, the A_1 area, etc.) is the constant tonic inhibition of sympathetic vasoconstrictor tone (43,44). This is shown by the fact that localized destructive maneuvers produce extremely severe and labile "neurogenic" hypertension, whereas systemic administration of drugs that stimulate the central α_2-AR such as clonidine and methyldopa, lowers blood pressure and suppresses the sympathetic drive. Furthermore, direct stimulation of the sympathoinhibitory α_2-AR located in key areas of the hypothalamus or medulla by intracerebral administration of minute amounts of the nonselective agonist norepinephrine (45) or by selective agonists, such as clonidine (46,47) and guanabenz (48), produces a hypotensive effect, whereas inhibition by selective α_2-AR antagonists, such as yohimbine (49), produces a hypertensive reaction, attributable, respectively, to decreased or increased sympathetic outflow.

The capacity of clonidine to suppress the release of norepinephrine by activating the central sympathoinhibitory α_2-AR is the basis of the clonidine suppression test used diagnostically to rule out a pheochromocytoma. In cases of hypertension with elevated circulating norepinephrine levels well beyond the normal range, but less than the typically extreme levels of a pheochromocytoma, it is necessary to separate the excessive sympathetic outflow of, for example, an acute anxiety state or drug withdrawal, from the autonomous oversecretion of catecholamines by an adrenomedullary tumor. Measurement of circulating catecholamines before and 2 or 3 hours after a single oral dose of 0.2 mg clonidine will show a 50 percent or more suppression of norepinephrine of sympathetic neuronal origin, but no change in catecholamines secreted by a tumor.

Of particular interest is the evidence linking salt-induced hypertension with modulation of the central α_2-AR. Ample experimental evidence has implicated increased sympathetic nervous system activity as a major mechanism sustaining salt-dependent hypertension

(50,51). Hypertonic saline introduced intracisternally (52), intracerebroventricularly (53,54), or into the NTS area (55) produces sharp hypertensive reactions attributable to sympathetic activation. Because the sodium ion is known to diminish the affinity of α_2-AR for agonists, both in vitro (10,11) and in vivo (56), we proposed the theory that this effect may be relevant to the mechanism of salt-induced hypertension. Specifically, we proposed that a decrease in the affinity of central α_2-AR for locally occurring natural agonists would result in disinhibition of the tonic sympathoinhibitory action of the catecholaminergic neurons of the brainstem, thus leading to a hyperadrenergic state in the periphery (50). This theory is reinforced by a number of data produced by recent studies. One is the discovery of an endogenous neurotransmitter, a "clonidine displacing substance" (57), a noncatecholamine and nonpeptide that, like clonidine, binds to both α_2-AR and imidazole receptors located in the same areas of the medulla oblongata and produces a hypotensive action via diminished sympathetic drive (58). This naturally occurring α_2-AR agonist binds, like clonidine, to the α_2-AR with a higher affinity than norepinephrine (59). Another is the observation that salt-sensitive animals exposed to high dietary sodium intake develop hypertension associated with diminished agonist neurotransmitter (norepinephrine) in anterior hypothalamic and brainstem regions (60,61) and altered numbers of α_2-AR in these regions (62–66). While there is still debate in the literature as to the exact nature and interpretation of these alterations (i.e., as to whether there is up-regulation in numbers due to diminished availability of agonist or to diminished affinity for agonist, or whether there is down-regulation in numbers, making fewer receptors available for agonists), there is general agreement that the net result of these salt-induced alterations is decreased excitation of inhibitory α_2-AR, leading to withdrawal of sympathoinhibitory CNS neuronal activity and increase in sympathetic output to the periphery (50,67,68).

There is little knowledge regarding the possible role of central α_1-ARs in hypertension, although it is believed that they may somehow affect baroreflex activity, as their density has been reported to be increased in the NTS of animals with genetic hypertension (69). It is also known that spinal cord transection or other lesions leading to noradrenergic denervation cause up-regulation of spinal α_1-AR numbers (70), leading to denervation hypersensitivity. There is even less knowledge at this time as to possible differential roles of various α_2-AR or α_1-AR subtypes that predominate in various brain regions (71–73). We have recently shown multiple α_2-AR–specific mRNA species in brain tissues, suggesting that more than one of the α_2-AR genes may be transcribed in various subregions of the brain (26,74,75). There is also accumulating evidence, as mentioned earlier, that subtypes differ both in their selective ligand recognition properties and the mechanisms of intracellular signal transduction (71,76), but the possible relevance of these findings to hypertensive mechanisms remains to be clarified.

ALPHA-ADRENERGIC RECEPTORS IN THE KIDNEY

Catecholamines of neuronal or adrenomedullary origin contribute to the control of renal vasomotor tone, glomerular filtration, renin secretion, antidiuretic hormone activity, and reabsorption of sodium by the renal tubule.

α_2-ARs are the numerically dominant AR type in the kidney; their density is increased in the kidneys of genetically hypertensive rat models, and it is further augmented by high dietary salt intake (77). In rat, the α_{2B}-AR subtype (initially identified as the α_2-AR in neonatal rat lung, [78]) is the predominant kidney α_2-AR, although all three subtypes are expressed in rat kidney (75).

Of particular interest is the fact that the salt-sensitive inbred models of genetic hypertension (such as spontaneous hypertensive rats [SHRs], Dahl S rats, and Sabra rats, which are generally considered to be the counterpart of salt-sensitive human essential hypertension) not only have increased density of renal α_2-AR (79–82), but tend to further up-regulate their α_2-AR numbers when placed on a high-salt diet (83–85). Yet they are also characterized by various indices of elevated sympathetic nervous system activity, including high levels of circulating plasma catecholamines (85) and increased renal nerve activity (86,87). The inability to down-regulate their renal α_2-AR (88,89) under these conditions may be one of the characteristics of genetically salt-sensitive hypertension, since α_2-ARs tend to increase proximal tubular salt and water retention (90,91), promote renal vasoconstriction (92–94), and influence the glomerular filtration rate. In contrast, in models of acquired salt-induced hypertension there is no increase in the density of renal α_2-AR (84).

The effect of α_2-AR on renin release is controversial, with some studies showing increased renin release after intrarenal α_2-AR blockade (93) and others showing no effect (95). Interestingly, α_2-AR agonists inhibit the antidiuretic effect of vasopressin, whose renotubular V_2 receptors act via stimulation of the same intracellular second messenger, cAMP, that is inhibited by activation of the α_2-AR (96). It is also of particular interest that the antinatriuretic effect of α_2-AR agonists occurs not only via activation of α_2-AR, but also via renal imidazole receptors, which, like those of the CNS, respond to clonidine displacing substances in a way similar to the α_2-AR, in this case by affecting the Na^+-H^+ exchange (97,98).

α_1-ARs have also been reported by some investigators to be elevated in SHRs (84), but others failed to detect differences in α_1-AR density between SHRs and Wistar-Kyoto (WKY) rats (99,100) or increased α_1-AR levels in

other experimental models of genetic hypertension, such as the Dahl S (81) or the Sabra rats (80). There are also conflicting reports as to whether a high salt intake elevates α_1-AR numbers (84) or not (79) in genetically salt-sensitive hypertension.

α_1-ARs are always postjunctional and respond to norepinephrine release after renal sympathetic nerve stimulation to induce vasoconstriction and contribute to sodium and water retention (96). Their selective chronic blockade, however, appears to lead to compensatory proliferation of postjunctional α_2-ARs, which take over the same functions (96).

Taken together, these observations have led some investigators to propose the theory that genetic predisposition to salt-sensitive hypertension may be associated with increased density of renal α-AR and inability to down-regulate α-AR in the face of high sympathetic activity, which would further exaggerate vasoconstriction and renal sodium reabsorption (77,101). It would also appear that renal α_2-AR may be more relevant to hypertension than renal α_1-AR (77,96).

ALPHA-ADRENERGIC RECEPTORS IN HEART AND VASCULATURE

Cardiac function and systemic vascular resistance are under sympathoadrenal control exerted via stimulation of α_1, α_2, and β-AR. Activation of α_1-AR of cardiac myocytes has been implicated in the positive inotropic (102,103) and arrhythmogenic effect (104,105) of catecholamines, as well as the development of myocardial hypertrophy (106,107) and the release of atrial natriuretic peptide (108). Myocardial ischemia or hypoxia leads to increased α_1-AR density in myocytes (108). There are conflicting reports as to whether myocardial α_1-AR numbers are increased or decreased in experimental rat models of genetic or acquired hypertension (101). Regardless, extrapolation from experimental animal studies on the role of α_1-AR in myocardial function, myocardial ischemia, or congestive heart failure may be inappropriate for humans, because density of cardiac α_1-AR seems to differ widely among species, with rats having generally much higher cardiac α_1-AR numbers than man and other mammalians (103,109). It is also likely that the density and distribution of various α_1-AR subtypes in various cardiac structures may differ not only among species, but also within the same species at different ages (110–112). This may explain the wide variability in biochemical and functional responses elicited by various α_1-AR agonists in terms of both magnitude and pattern of response (e.g., dissociation of contractile response from electrophysiological response in rat but not in rabbit [103]).

It is believed that cardiac myocytes do not possess α_2-AR and any α_2-AR properties detected in cardiac tissue would be derived from the coronary vasculature.

Both α_1-AR and α_2-AR mediate vascular smooth muscle contraction (113–115) via a mechanism involving Ca^{2+} channels and intracellular free Ca^{2+} metabolism (116,117), although the contribution of α_1-AR to peripheral vasoconstriction is quantitatively much more important than that of the postsynaptic α_2-AR. The sodium ion alters the affinity of these AR to their agonists in opposite directions: it increases the affinity of α_1-AR but decreases that of α_2-AR, as shown *in vitro* (10–12), and *in vivo* in intact animals with use of selective antagonists and saline infusions (56). The affinity of vascular α_1-AR for agonists differs in different arterial trees (118). Moreover, their density is diminished by agonists, leading to desensitization (76), and their selectivity can be abolished by phenoxybenzamine (119).

It is attractive to attribute the increased vascular reactivity observed in essential hypertension, especially in salt sensitive individuals, to an increase in numbers or affinity of vascular α-AR to catecholamines (120). However, numerous functional studies of α-AR reaction to selective agonists and antagonists have yielded contradictory responses, with no evidence suggesting consistent alterations of numbers or affinity status in hypertensives versus normotensives (101). This issue is further obscured by the fact that the terms *responsiveness* and *sensitivity* are sometimes used by investigators to imply alterations in α-AR numbers or affinity on the basis of an *in vivo* functional response. For example, the greater hypotensive response to a sympatholytic treatment in salt-loaded hypertensive subjects has been interpreted as evidence in support of increased density or affinity of α-AR; however, a functional response is the sum of the blockade of the mechanism predominantly responsible for blood pressure maintenance under those conditions (i.e., sympathetic overdrive) and for a number of compensatory interactions with other vasoactive systems, as well as for the influence of anatomic factors (e.g., vascular smooth muscle hypertrophy). Accordingly, functional responses to specific α-AR agonists and antagonists are useful in the clinical assessment of integrated biological reactions for therapeutic purposes (121), but do not permit conclusions as to α-AR numbers or affinity status.

ALPHA₂-ADRENERGIC RECEPTORS IN PLATELETS

Because platelets are the only readily available human cells for study of the α_2-AR *in vivo*, they have been used extensively for studies of numbers and affinity status under various conditions despite two important limitations, i.e., lack of sympathetic innervation and of cell nucleus, which may alter their capacity to respond to manipulations. Nevertheless, studies with central sympatholytic antihypertensive agents suggest that, as with other tissues, platelet α_2-AR density may also be primarily regulated by sympathetic nerve activity rather than circulating catecholamines (122). The α_2-AR in human platelets belong to the α_{2A}-AR subtype (20,78).

The density of platelet α_2-AR is normally diminished with age (123), probably reflecting down-regulation due to higher circulating norepinephrine levels in the elderly (124), so that any comparisons between normotensives and hypertensives should be made in age-matched subjects. Little is known about possible gender- or race-related differences in α_2-AR characteristics, other than a diminished affinity status of α_2-AR in elderly black normotensives in comparison to their white counterparts or to age- and race-matched hypertensives (125).

Studies on the numbers or affinity of platelet α_2-AR in essential hypertension have yielded conflicting results. Some have reported significant increases in α_2-AR density or functional responsiveness in hypertensives (126,127), in children of hypertensive parents (128,129), or in salt-sensitive normotensives (130); others have found decreased α_2-AR density in hypertensives (131). Some have found that hypertensives do not differ in α_2-AR density from normotensives (132–134), but are unable to down-regulate normally their α_2-AR numbers in the presence of excess agonist (135), whereas others have reported that hypertensives down-regulate normally their platelet α_2-AR in response to elevated catecholamine concentrations (135).

Taken together, these reports suggest that genetically determined hypertension and/or salt-sensitivity may be associated with abnormalities in the numbers or affinity of α_2-AR in platelets, which can be taken to reflect similar alterations in other tissues more relevant to hypertension (CNS, renal, or vascular). However, discrepancies in their results make their interpretation uncertain.

At this stage it appears that little additional progress on the role of α-AR in hypertension can be expected from functional studies *in vivo* or from assessment of α-AR properties by more refined and selective pharmacologic and radioligand binding techniques. Rather, further knowledge is more likely to come from application of molecular biology techniques. The cloning, sequencing, and expression of the gene coding for the human platelet α_2-AR (26,78) was followed by characterization of other α-AR subtypes (2). Early studies have failed so far to detect genetic differences in α_2-AR between normotensives and hypertensives (136,137). However, linkage studies of restriction fragment length polymorphisms (RFLP) are under way, including a recent report of an RFLP in an α_2-AR gene that is associated with hypertension in black subjects (138). Better characterization of α_2-AR subtypes should further enhance these efforts.

REFERENCES

1. Lefkowitz RJ, Caron MG. Adrenergic receptors: models for the study of receptors coupled to guanine nucleotide regulatory proteins. *J Biol Chem* 1988;263:4993–4996.

2. Bylund DB. Subtypes of α_1 and α_2-adrenergic receptors. *FASEB J* 1992;6:832–839.
3. Ahlquist RP. A study of the adrenergic receptors. *Am J Physiol* 1948;153:586–600.
4. Lands AM, Lunduena FP, Buzzo HJ. Differentiation of receptors responsiveness to isoproterenol. *Life Sci* 1967;6:2241–2249.
5. Raymond JR, Hnatowich M, Lefkowitz RJ, Caron MG. Adrenergic receptors. Models for regulation of signal transduction processes. *Hypertension* 1990;15:119–131.
6. Ruffolo RR Jr. Distribution and function of peripheral α-adrenoceptors in the cardiovascular system. *Pharmacol Biochem Behav* 1985;22:827–833.
7. Mahan LC, McKernan RM, Insel PA. Metabolism of alpha- and beta-adrenergic receptors in vitro and in vivo. *Annu Rev Pharmacol Toxicol* 1987;27:215–235.
8. Ruffolo RR, Jr, Sulpizio AC, Nichols AJ, DeMarinis RM, Hieble JP. Pharmacologic differentiation between pre- and postjunctional α_2-adrenoceptors by SK & F 104078. *Naunyn Schmiedebergs Arch Pharmacol* 1987;336:415–418.
9. Van Zwieten PA. Adrenergic and muscarinergic receptors: classification, pathophysiological relevance and drug target. *J Hypertens* 1991;9:(suppl 6):S18–S27.
10. Tsai BS, Lefkowitz RJ. Agonist-specific effects of monovalent and divalent cations on adenylate cyclase-coupled alpha adrenergic receptors in rabbit platelets. *Mol Pharmacol* 1978;14:540–548.
11. Bylund DB, U'Prichard DC. Characterization of α_1- and α_2-adrenergic receptors. *Int Rev Neurobiol* 1983;24:343–431.
12. U'Prichard DC, Mitrius JC, Kahn DJ, Perry BD. The α_2-adrenergic receptor: multiple affinity states and regulation of a receptor inversely coupled to adenylate cyclase. In: Segawa T, et al, eds. *Molecular pharmacology of neurotransmitter receptors.* New York: Raven Press, 1983.
13. Cotecchia S, Schwinn DA, Randall RR, Lefkowitz RJ, Caron MG, Kobilka BK. Molecular cloning and expression of the cDNA for the hamster α_1-adrenergic receptor. *Proc Natl Acad Sci USA* 1988;85:7159–7163.
14. Schwinn DA, Lomasney JW, Lorenz W, Szklut PJ, Fremeau RT Jr, Yang-Feng TL, Caron MG, Lefkowitz RJ, Cotecchia S. Molecular cloning and expression of the cDNA for a novel α_1-adrenergic receptor subtype. *J Biol Chem* 1990;265:8183–8189.
15. Voigt MM, Kispert J, Chin H. Sequence of a rat brain cDNA encoding an alpha-1B adrenergic receptor. *Nucleic Acids Res* 1990;18:1053.
16. Lomasney JW, Cotecchia S, Lorenz W, Leung W-Y, Schwinn DA, Yang-Feng TL, Brownstein M, Lefkowitz RJ, Caron MG. Molecular cloning and expression of the cDNA for the α_{1A}-adrenergic receptor. *J Biol Chem* 1991;266:6365–6369.
17. Perez DM, Piascik MT, Graham RM. Solution phase library screening for the identification of rare clones: isolation of an alpha 1D-adrenergic receptor cDNA. *Mol Pharmacol* 1991;40:876–883.
18. Bruno JF, Wittaker J, Song J, Berelowitz M. Molecular cloning and sequencing of a cDNA encoding a human α_{1A}-adrenergic receptor. *Biochem Biophys Res Commun* 1991;179:1485–1490.
19. Ramarao CS, Denker JMK, Perez DM, Gaivin RJ, Riek RP, Graham RM. Genomic organization and expression of the human α_{1B}-adrenergic receptor. *J Biol Chem* 1992;267:21936–21945.
20. Kobilka BK, Matsui H, Kobilka TS, Yang-Feng TL, Francke U, Caron MG, Lefkowitz RJ, Regan JW. Cloning, sequencing, and expression of the gene coding for the human platelet α_2-adrenergic receptor. *Science* 1987;238:650–656.
21. Regan JW, Kobilka TS, Yang-Feng TL, Caron MG, Lefkowitz RJ, Kobilka BK. Cloning and expression of a human kidney cDNA for an α_2-adrenergic receptor subtype. *Proc Natl Acad Sci USA* 1988;85:6301–6305.
22. Fraser CM, Arakawa S, McCombie WR, Venter JC. Cloning, sequence analysis and permanent expression of a human α_2-adrenergic receptor in chinese hamster ovary cells. *J Biol Chem* 1989;264:11754–11761.
23. Chalberg SC, Duda T, Rhine JA, Sharma RK. Molecular cloning, sequencing and expression of an α_2-adrenergic receptor complementary DNA from rat brain. *Mol Cell Biochem* 1990;97:161–172.
24. Zeng D, Harrison JK, D'Angelo DD, Barber CM, Tucker AL, Lu Z, Lynch KR. Molecular characterization of a rat α_2-B-adrenergic receptor. *Proc Natl Acad Sci USA* 1990;87:3102–3106.
25. Lomasney JW, Lorenz W, Allen LF, King K, Regan JW, Yang-Feng TL, Caron MG, Lefkowitz RJ. Expansion of the α_2-adrenergic receptor family: cloning and characterization of a human α_2-adrenergic receptor subtype, the gene for which is located on chromosome 2. *Proc Natl Acad Sci USA* 1990;87:5094–5098.
26. Flordellis C, Handy DE, Bresnahan MR, Zannis VI, Gavras H. Cloning and expression of a rat brain alpha 2B-adrenergic receptor. *Proc Natl Acad Sci USA* 1991;88:1019–1023.
27. Lanier SM, Downing S, Duzic E, Homcy CJ. Isolation of rat genomic clones encoding subtypes of the α_2-adrenergic receptor. *J Biol Chem* 1991;266:10470–10478.
28. Guyer CA, Horstman DA, Wilson AL, Clark JD, Cragoe EJ Jr, Limbird LE. Cloning, sequencing and expression of the gene encoding of the porcine α_2-adrenergic receptor: Allosteric modulation by Na^+, H^+ and amiloride analogs. *J Biol Chem* 1990;265:17307–17317.
29. Horstman DA, Brandon S, Wilson AL, Guyer CA, Cragoe EJ Jr, Limbird LE. An aspartate conserved among G-protein receptors confers allosteric regulation of α_2-adrenergic receptors by sodium. *J Biol Chem* 1990;265:21590–21595.
30. Lomasney JW, Cotecchia S, Lefkowitz RJ, Caron MG. Molecular biology of α_2-adrenergic receptors: implications for receptor classification and for structure-function relationships. *Biochim Biophys Acta* 1991;1095:127–139.
31. Minneman KP. α_1-Adrenergic receptor subtypes, inositol phosphates and sources of cell Ca^{2+}. *Pharmacol Rev* 1988;40:87–119.
32. Schwinn DA, Page SO, Middleton JP, Lorenz W, Liggett SB, Yamamoto K, Lapetina EG, Caron MG, Lefkowitz RJ, Cotecchia S. The α_{1C}-adrenergic receptor: characterization of signal transduction pathways and mammalian tissue heterogeneity. *Mol Pharmacol* 1991;40:617–626.
33. Tsujimoto G, Tsujimoto A, Suzuki E, Hashimoto K. Glycogen phosphorylase activation by two different α_1-adrenergic receptor subtypes: methoxamine selectively stimulates a putative α_1-adrenergic receptor subtype (α_{1A}) that couples with Ca^{2+} influx. *Molec Pharmacol* 1989;36:166–176.
34. Simon MI, Strathmann MP, Gautman N. Diversity of G-proteins in signal transduction. *Science* 1991;252:802–808.
35. Michel MC, Brass LF, William A, Bokoch GM, LaMorte VJ, Motulsky HJ. α_2-Adrenergic receptor stimulation mobilizes intracellular Ca^{2+} in human erythroleukemia cells. *J Biol Chem* 1989;264:4986–4991.
36. Isom LL, Cragoe EJ, Limbird LE. α_2-Adrenergic receptors accelerate Na^+/H^+ exchange in neuroblastoma X glioma cells. *J Biol Chem* 1986;262:6750–6757.
37. Sweatt JD, Connolly TM, Cragoe EJ, Limbird LE. Evidence that Na^+/H^+ exchange regulates receptor-mediated phospholipase α_2 activation in human platelets. *J Biol Chem* 1986;261:8667–8673.
38. Coupry I, Duzic E, Lanier SM. Factors determining the specificity of signal transduction by guanine nucleotide-binding protein-coupled receptors. II. Preferential coupling of the α_{2C}-adrenergic receptor to the guanine nucleotide binding protein, G_0. *J Biol Chem* 1992;267:9852–9857.
39. Duzic E, Coupry I, Downing S, Lanier SM. Factors determining the specificity of signal transduction by guanine nucleotide-binding protein-coupled receptors. *J Biol Chem* 1992;267:9844–9851.
40. Young WS III, Kuhar MJ. Noradrenergic α_1 and α_2 receptors: light microscopic autoradiographic localization. *Proc Natl Acad Sci USA* 1980;77:1696–1700.
41. Unnerstall JR, Fernandez I, Orensanz LM. The alpha-adrenergic receptor: radiohistochemical analysis of functional characteristics and biochemical differences. *Pharmacol Biochem Behav* 1985;22:895–874.
42. Roudet C, Savasta M, Feuerstein C. Normal distribution of alpha-1-adrenoceptors in the rat spinal cord and its modification after noradrenergic denervation: a quantitative autoradiographic study. *J Neurosci Res* 1993;34:44–53.
43. Reis DJ. Experimental evidence in support of a central neural imbalance hypothesis of hypertension. In: Laragh JH, Buhler FR, Seldin DW, eds. *Frontiers of hypertension research.* New York: Springer-Verlag, 1981;341–343.

44. Hausler G. Central α-adrenoceptors involved in cardiovascular regulation. *J Cardiovasc Pharmacol* 1982;4(suppl 1):572–575.

45. DeJong W. Noradrenaline: central inhibitory control of pressure and heart rate. *Eur J Pharmacol* 1974;29:179–181.

46. Wyss JM, Yang R, Jin H, Oparil S. Hypothalamic microinjection of alpha₂-adrenoceptor agonists causes greater sympathoinhibition in spontaneously hypertensive rats on high NaCl diets. *J Hypertens* 1988;6:805–813.

47. Punnen S, Urbanski R, Krieger AJ, et al. Ventrolateral medullary pressor area: site of hypotensive action of clonidine. *Brain Res* 1987;422:336–346.

48. Koepke JP, Jones S, Dibona GF. Sodium responsiveness of central α₂-adrenergic receptors in spontaneously hypertensive rats. *Hypertension* 1988;11:326–333.

49. Tibirica E, Feldman J, Bousquet P. Differences in the ability of yohimbine to antagonize the hypotensive effect of clonidine in normotensive and spontaneously hypertensive anesthetized rats. *J Pharm Exp Ther* 1988;244:1062–1066.

50. Gavras H. How does salt raise blood pressure? A hypothesis. *Hypertension* 1986;8:83–88.

51. Oparil S. Increased sympathetic nervous system activity in salt-dependent hypertension. In: National Institutes of Health. *USA-Poland Symposium, Cardiovascular Disease.* Washington, DC: U.S. Department of Health and Human Services 1986;41–57.

52. Wei ET, Wu Y. Pressor effects of intracisternal Na⁺ in normotensive and spontaneously hypertensive rats. *Brain Res* 1979;169:605–609.

53. Miyajima E, Bunag RD. Chronic cerebroventricular infusion of hypertonic sodium chloride in rats reduces hypothalamic sympatho-inhibition and elevates blood pressure. *Circ Res* 1984;54:566–575.

54. Benetos A, Bresnahan M, Gavras I, Gavras H. Central catecholamines and alpha-adrenoceptors in acute hypertension induced by intracerebroventricular hypertonic saline. *J Hypertens* 1987;5:699–704.

55. Gavras H, Bain GT, Bland L, Vlahakos D, Gavras I. Hypertensive response to saline microinjection in the area of the nucleus tractus solitarii of the rat. *Brain Res* 1985;343:113–119.

56. Kohlmann O Jr, Gavras I, Biolaz J, Biolaz B, Gavras H. Sodium chloride-induced partial inhibition in vivo of alpha 2-adrenoceptor agonist function. *J Hypertens* 1985;3:269–274.

57. Atlas D, Burstein Y. Isolation and partial purification of a clonidine-displacing endogenous brain substance. *Eur J Pharmacol* 1984;144:287–293.

58. Reis DJ, Morrison S, Ruggiero DA. The C1 area of the brainstem in tonic and reflex control of blood pressure. *Hypertension* 1988;11(suppl I):I-8–I-13.

59. Reis DJ, Regunathan S, Meeley MP. Imidazole receptors and clonidine-displacing substance in relationship to control of blood pressure, neuroprotection, and adrenomedullary secretion. *Am J Hypertens* 1992;5:51S–57S.

60. Wyss JM, Chen Y-F, Jin H, Gist R, Oparil S. NaCl-sensitive SHR exhibit reduced hypothalamic noradrenergic input following NaCl loading. *Hypertension* 1987;10:313–320.

61. Chen Y-F, Meng Q, Wyss JM, Jin H, Oparil S. High NaCl diet reduces hypothalamic norephinephrine turnover in hypertensive rats. *Hypertension* 1988;11:55–62.

62. Morris MJ, Devynck MA, Woodcock EA, Johnston CI, Meyer P. Specific changes in hypothalamic alpha-adrenoceptors in young spontaneously hypertensive rats. *Hypertension* 1981;3:516–520.

63. Cantor EH, Abraham S, Spector S. Central neurotransmitter receptor in hypertensive rats. *Life Sci* 1981;28:519–526.

64. Bresnahan MR, Gavras I, Hatinoglou S, Muller RE, Gavras H. Central alpha-adrenoceptors during the development of hypertension in rats on high and low salt intake. *J Hypertens* 1986;4:719–726.

65. Klangkalya B, Sripairojthikoon W, Oparil S, Wyss JM. High NaCl diet increases hypothalamic α₂-adrenoceptors in SHR. *Brain Res* 1988;457:77–84.

66. Yamada S, Ashizawa N, Nakayama K, Tomita T, Hayashi E. Decreased density of α₂-adrenoceptors in medulla oblongata of spontaneously hypertensive rats. *J Cardiovascular Pharmacol* 1989;13:440–446.

67. Koepke JP, Jones S, DiBona GF. Sodium responsiveness of cen-

68. Oparil S. Central mechanism of hypertension. *Am J Hypertens* 1989;2:474–482.

69. MacLean MR, Phillips MI, Sumners C, Raizada MK. Alpha-1-adrenergic receptors in the nucleus tractus solitarii region of rats with experimental and genetic hypertension. *Brain Res* 1990;519:261–265.

70. Roudet C, Savasta M, Feuerstein C. Normal distribution of alpha-1-adrenoceptors in the rat spinal cord and its modification after noradrenergic denervation: a quantitative autoradiographic study. *J Neurosci Res* 1993;34:44–53.

71. Minneman KP, Atkinson B. Interaction of subtype-selective antagonists with alpha 1-adrenergic receptor-mediated second messenger responses in rat brain. *Mol Pharmacol* 1991;40:523–530.

72. Zilles K, Gross G, Schleicher A, Schildgen S, Bauer A, Bahro M, Schwendemann G, Zech K, Kolassa N. Regional and laminar distributions of alpha 1-adrenoceptors and their subtypes in human and rat hippocampus. *Neuroscience* 1991;40:307–320.

73. Terman BI, Riek RP, Grodski A, Hess HJ, Graham RM. Identification and structural characterization of alpha 1-adrenergic receptor subtypes. *Mol Pharmacol* 1990;37:526–534.

74. Flordellis C, Castellano M, Franco R, Zannis VI, Gavras H. Expression of multiple alpha 2-adrenergic receptor messenger RNA species in rat tissues. *Hypertension* 1990;15:881–887.

75. Handy DE, Flordellis CS, Bogdanova NN, Bresnahan MR, Gavras H. Diverse tissue expression of α₂-adrenergic receptor genes. *Hypertension* 1993;21:861–865.

76. Kiuchi K, Vatner DE, Uemura N, Bigaud M, Hasebe N, Hempel DM, Graham RM, Vatner SF. Mechanisms of alpha 1-adrenergic vascular desensitization in conscious dogs. *Circ Res* 1992;71:1185–1199.

77. Pettinger WA. Renal α₂-adrenergic receptors and hypertension. *Hypertension* 1987;9:3–6.

78. Bylund DB, Ray-Prenger C, Murphy TJ. Alpha 2A and alpha-2B adrenergic receptor subtypes: antagonist binding in tissues and cell lines containing only one subtype. *J Pharmacol Exp Ther* 1988;245:600–607.

79. Pettinger WA, Sanchez A, Saavedra J, Haywood JR, Gandler T, Rodes T. Altered renal alpha₂-adrenergic receptor regulation in genetically hypertensive rats. *Hypertension* 1982;4:II-188–II-192.

80. Parini A, Diop L, Dausse J-P, Ben Ishay D. Sabra rats as a model to differentiate between Na⁺ and GTP regulation of α₂-adrenoceptor densities. *Eur J Pharmacol* 1985;112:97–104.

81. McCaughran JA Jr, Juno CJ, O'Malley E, Rosenthal M. The ontogeny of renal α₁- and α₂-adrenoceptors in the Dahl rat model of experimental hypertension. *J Auton Nerv Syst* 1986;17:1–20.

82. Spripairojthikoon W, Wyss JM. High NaCl diets increase α₂-adrenoceptor mediated increase in renal cortex and medulla of NaCl-sensitive spontaneously hypertensive rats. *Eur J Pharmacol* 1989;167:335–365.

83. Pettinger WA, Gandler T, Sanchez A, Saavedra JM. Dietary sodium and renal alpha₂-adrenergic receptors in Dahl hypertensive rats. *Clin Exp Hypertens* 1982;A4(4&5):819–828.

84. Saiz J, Lara B, Torres A, Sanchez A. Hypertensinogenic factors and renal α-adrenoceptors in young SHR and WKY rats. *Life Sci* 1987;41:2261–2268.

85. Dawson R Jr, Oparil S. Renal catecholamines and α₂-adrenergic receptors in salt-related and genetic hypertension. *Pharmacology* 1987;34:131–142.

86. Norman RA Jr, Dzielak DJ. Role of renal nerves onset and maintenance of spontaneous hypertension. *Am J Physiol* 1982;243:H284–H288.

87. Koepke JP, DiBona GF. High sodium intake enhances renal nerve and antinatriuretic responses to stress in SHR. *Hypertension* 1985;7:357–363.

88. Graham RM, Pettinger WA, Sagalowsky A, Brabson J, Gandler T. Renal alpha-adrenergic receptor abnormality in the spontaneously hypertensive rat. *Hypertension* 1982;4:881–887.

89. Snavely MD, Ziegler MG, Insel PA. Subtype-selective downregulation of rat renal cortical alpha- and beta-adrenergic receptors by catecholamines. *Endocrinology* 1985;117:2182–2189.

90. Young WS, Kuhar MJ. α_2-Adrenergic receptors are associated with renal proximal tubules. *Eur J Pharmacol* 1980;67:493–495.

91. Insel PA, Snavely MD, Healy DP, Munzel PA, Potenza CL, Nord EP. Radioligand binding and functional assay demonstrate postsynaptic alpha$_2$-receptors on proximal tubules of rat and rabbit kidney. *J Cardiovasc Pharmacol* 1985;7(suppl 8):S9–S17.

92. Baines AD. Is there a role for renal α_2-adrenoceptors in the pathogenesis of hypertension? *Can J Physiol Pharmacol* 1987;65:1638–1643.

93. de Leeuw PW, Birkenhager WH. Alpha-adrenoceptors and the kidney. *J Hypertens* 1988;6(suppl 2):S21–S24.

94. Wolff DW, Colindres RE, Strandhoy JW. Unmasking sensitive α_2-adrenoceptor-mediated renal vasoconstriction in conscious rats. *Am J Physiol* 1989;257:F1132–F1139.

95. DiBona GF, Sawin LL. Role of renal α_2-adrenergic receptors in spontaneously hypertensive rats. *Hypertension* 1987;9:41–48.

96. Pettinger WA, Umemura S, Smyth DD, Jeffries WB. Renal alpha 2-adrenoceptors and the adenylate cyclase-cAMP system: biochemical and physiological interactions. *Am J Physiol* 1987;252:F199–F208.

97. Limbird LE. Receptors linked to inhibition of adenylate cyclase: additional signaling mechanisms. *FASEB J* 1988;2:2686–2695.

98. Bidet M, Poujeol P, Parini A. The imidazoline-guanidinium receptor site, a target for some alpha-2 adrenergic agonists, is involved in inhibition of Na$^+$-H$^+$ exchange in renal proximal tubule cells. *J Hypertens* 1991;9(suppl 6):S216–S217.

99. Jeffries WB, Yang E, Pettinger WA. Renal α_1-adrenergic receptor response coupling in spontaneously hypertensive rats. *Hypertension* 1988;12:80–88.

100. Jackson CA, Michel MC, Insel PA. Expression of renal alpha 1-adrenergic receptor subtypes in established hypertension. *J Cardiovasc Pharmacol* 1992;19:857–862.

101. Michel MC, Brodde, O-E, Insel PA. Peripheral adrenergic receptors in hypertension. *Hypertension* 1990;16:107–120.

102. Bruckner R, Mugge A, Scholz H. Existence and functional role of alpha$_1$-adrenoceptors in the mammalian heart. *J Mol Cell Cardiol* 1985;17:639–645.

103. Endoh M, Hiramoto T, Ishihata A, Takanashi M, Inui J. Myocardial alpha 1-adrenoceptors mediate positive inotropic effect and changes in phosphatidylinositol metabolism. Species differences in receptor distribution and the intracellular coupling process in mammalian ventricular myocardium. *Circ Res* 1991;68:1179–1190.

104. Kurz T, Yamada KA, DaTorre SD, Corr PB. Alpha 1-adrenergic system and arrhythmias in ischemic heart disease. *Eur Heart J* 1991;12(suppl F):88–98.

105. Hasumi M, Hiroe M, Fujita N, Hasumi S, Toyosaki T, Nagao H, Hosoda S, Kasajima T, Sekiguchi M. Significant myocardial pathology and increase of alpha 1-adrenergic receptor number affecting the arrhythmogenic condition in cases with ventricular tachycardia. *Heart Vessels Suppl* 1990;5:31–36.

106. Lee HR, Henderson SA, Reynolds R, Dunnmon P, Yuan D, Chien KR. α_1-Adrenergic stimulation of cardiac gene transcription in neonatal rat myocardial cells. Effects on myosin light chain-2 gene expression. *J Biol Chem* 1988;263:7352–7358.

107. Ikeda U, Tsuruya Y, Yaginuma T. Alpha 1-adrenergic stimulation is coupled to myocyte hypertrophy. *Am J Physiol* 1991;260:H953–H956.

108. Benfey BG. Function of myocardial alpha-adrenoceptors. *Life Sci* 1990;46:743–757.

109. Steinfath M, Chen YY, Lavicky J, Magnussen O, Nose M, Rosswag S, Schmitz W, Scholz H. Cardiac alpha 1-adrenoceptor densities in different mammalian species. *Br J Pharmacol* 1992;107:185–188.

110. del Balzo U, Rosen MR, Malfatto G, Kaplan LM, Steinberg SF. Specific alpha 1-adrenergic receptor subtypes modulate catecholamine-induced decreases in ventricular automaticity. *Circ Res* 1990;67:1535–1551.

111. Kimball KA, Cornett LE, Seifen E, Kennedy RH. Aging: changes in cardiac alpha 1-adrenoceptor responsiveness and expression. *Eur J Pharmacol* 1991;208:231–238.

112. Kinami J, Tsuchihashi H, Baba S, Mano F, Maruyama K, Nagatomo T. Alpha 1-adrenoceptor subtypes in the rat ventricular muscle. *J Pharm Pharmacol* 1992;44:97–100.

113. Timmermans PBMWM, Chiu AT, Thoolen MMMC. Calcium handling in vasoconstriction to stimulation of alpha$_1$ and alpha$_2$-adrenoceptors. *Can J Physiol Pharmacol* 1987;65:1649–1657.

114. Young MA, Vatner DE, Knight DR, Graham RM, Homcy CJ, Vatner SF. Alpha-adrenergic vasoconstriction and receptor subtypes in large coronary arteries of calves. *Am J Physiol* 1988;255:H1452–H1459.

115. Holtz J. Alpha-adrenoceptor subtypes in the coronary circulation. *Basic Res Cardiol* 1990;85(suppl 1):81–95.

116. Ruffolo RR Jr, Nichols J, Oriowo MA. Interaction of vascular alpha-1 adrenoceptor with multiple signal transduction pathways. *Blood Vessels* 1991;28:122–128.

117. Lee JY, DeBernardis JF. Alpha 2-adrenergic receptors and calcium: alpha 2-receptor blockade in vascular smooth muscle as an approach to the treatment of hypertension. *Methods Find Exp Clin Pharmacol* 1990;12:213–225.

118. Oriowo MA, Bevan RD, Bevan JA. Variable receptor affinity and tissue sensitivity. *Blood Vessels* 1991;28:115–121.

119. Goncalves J, Nunes JP, Paiva MQ, Guimaraes S. Loss of selectivity of so-called selective α_1-adrenoceptor agonists after phenoxybenzamine. *Naunyn Schmiedebergs Arch Pharmacol* 1988;338:234–238.

120. Jie K, van Brummelen P, Vermeij P, Timmermans PBMWM, van Zwieten PA. α_1- and α_2-Adrenoceptor mediated vasoconstriction in the forearm of normotensive and hypertensive subjects. *J Cardiovasc Pharmacol* 1986;8:190–196.

121. Robertson D, Goldberg MR, Tung C-S, Hollister AS, Robertson RM. Use of alpha$_2$ adrenoceptor agonists and antagonists in the functional assessment of the sympathetic nervous system. *J Clin Invest* 1986;78:576–581.

122. Noshiro T, Miura Y, Kimura S, Meguro Y, Sugawara T, Ohashi H, Takahashi M, Sano N, Watanabe H, Ohzeki T, Shimizu K, Yoshinaga K. Functional relationships between platelet alpha$_2$-adrenoceptors and sympathetic nerve activity in clinical hypertensive states. *J Hypertens* 1990;8:1097–1104.

123. Bursztyn MR, Bresnahan M, Gavras I, Gavras H. Effect of aging on vasopressin catecholamines, and alpha$_2$-adrenergic receptors. *Am Geriatrics Soc* 1990;38:628–632.

124. Hollister AS, Fitzgerald GA, Nadeau JHJ, Robertson D. Acute reduction in human platelet α_2-adrenoceptor affinity for agonist by endogenous and exogenous catecholamines. *J Clin Invest* 1983;72:1498–1505.

125. Bursztyn MR, Bresnahan M, Gavras I, Gavras H. Pressor hormones in elderly hypertensive persons—racial difference. *Hypertension* 1990;15:(suppl I)I-88–I-92.

126. Brodde O-E, Stuka N, Demuth V, Fesel R, Bergerhausen J, Daul A, Bock KD. Alpha- and beta-adrenoceptors in circulating blood cells of essential hypertensive patients: increased receptor density and responsiveness. *Clin Exp Hypertens* 1985;A7:1135–1150.

127. Fritschka E, Kribben A, Haller H, Hoyer J, Thiede H-M, Distler A, et al. Familial aggregation of altered adrenoceptor density and free intracellular calcium in patients with essential hypertension. *J Cardiovasc Pharmacol* 1987;10(suppl 4):S122–S125.

128. Michel MC, Galal O, Stoermer J, Bock KD, Brodde OE. Alpha- and beta-adrenoceptors in hypertension. II. Platelet alpha$_2$- and lymphocyte beta$_2$-adrenoceptors in children of parents with essential hypertension. *J Cardiovasc Pharmacol* 1989;13:432–439.

129. Umemura S, Hirawa N, Hayashi S, Toya Y, Minamisawa K, Iwamoto T, Kihara M, Ishii M. Effect of dietary sodium on platelet alpha$_2$-adrenoceptors in young normotensive men with or without a family history of hypertension. *J Hypertens* 1992;10:1397–1401.

130. Skrabal F, Gruber G, Meister B, Ledochowski M, Doll P, Lang F, Cerny E. Salt sensitivity in normotensives with family history of hypertension: studies of membrane transport, intracellular electrolytes and α_2-adrenergic receptors. *J Hypertens* 1985;3(suppl 3):S25–S28.

131. Jones CR, Elliott HL, Deighton N, Howie CA, Reid JL. Alpha-adrenoceptor number and function in platelets from treated and untreated patients with essential hypertension and age- and sex-matched controls. *J Hypertens* 1985;3(suppl 3):S153–S155.

132. Motulsky H, O'Connor DT, Insel PA. Platelet α_2-adrenergic receptors in treated and untreated essential hypertension. *Clin Sci* 1983;64:265–272.

133. Ashida T, Tanaka T, Yokoughi M, Kuramochi M, Deguchi F, Kimura G, et al. Effect of dietary sodium on platelet α_2-adrenergic receptors in essential hypertension. *Hypertension* 1985;7:972–978.

134. Hollister AS, Onrot J, Lonce S, Nadeau JHJ, Robertson D. Plasma catecholamine modulation of alpha$_2$ adrenoreceptor agonist affinity and sensitivity in normotensive and hypertensive human platelets. *J Clin Invest* 1986;77:1416–1421.

135. Midel MC, Mindermann G, Daul A, Brodde O-E. Effects of antihypertensive therapy on human α- and β-adrenoceptors. *J Hypertens* 1991;9:601–606.

136. Sun L, Schulte N, Pettinger P, Regan JW, Pettinger WA. The frequency of α_2-adrenoceptor restriction fragment length polymorphisms in normotensive and hypertensive humans. *J Hypertens* 1992;10:1011–1015.

137. Zee RYL, Morris BJ, Griffiths LR. Association analyses of RFLPs for the α_2- and β_1-adrenoceptor genes in essential hypertension. *Hypertens Res* 1992;15:57–60.

138. Lockette W, Farrow S. A genetic polymorphism of the alpha-2 adrenergic receptor is associated with essential hypertension and pregnancy induced hypertension in blacks (Abstract). *Hypertension* 1993;21:543.

Hypertension: Pathophysiology, Diagnosis, and Management, Second Edition, edited by J.H. Laragh and B.M. Brenner, Raven Press, Ltd., New York © 1995.

CHAPTER **51**

The Sympathetic Nervous System in Human Hypertension

Ronald G. Victor and Allyn L. Mark

Despite decades of research, there are still large gaps in our understanding of the role of the sympathetic nervous system in human hypertension. This has resulted in large part from the lack of sophisticated methodology for studying the sympathetic nervous system in humans. The application of radiotracer norepinephrine kinetic techniques and of microneurographic methods for direct measurement of sympathetic nerve activity (SNA) in humans has permitted recent insight, but further advances in methodology are needed.

In this chapter, we will review briefly (a) methods for studying the sympathetic nervous system in humans, (b) the mounting evidence for heightened sympathetic activity in human hypertension, (c) potential mechanisms for increased SNA in hypertension, and (d) the potential significance of elevated SNA. Instead of an exhaustive review, we have attempted to highlight recent knowledge from our perspective.

METHODS FOR THE STUDY OF SYMPATHETIC NEURAL ACTIVITY IN HUMAN HYPERTENSION

Plasma Catecholamines

The common method for assessing the activity of the sympathetic nervous system in humans has been measurement of plasma norepinephrine (NE). These measurements have contributed useful information, but they have serious limitations. It is unlikely that these measurements alone will further advance knowledge of the sympathetic neural function. What are these limitations? First, plasma concentrations of NE are influenced by many variables including sympathetic nerve activity, prejunctional modulation of neurotransmitter release, and the clearance, metabolism, and reuptake of NE from the circulation. Measurements of plasma NE do not permit dissection of the components involved in sympathetic neural function. Advocates of the value of plasma NE might argue that measurement of plasma NE provides a measure of "overall" sympathetic activity or tone and is therefore the best single measure of sympathetic function. This prompts mention of the second limitation

R. G. Victor: Department of Internal Medicine, Cardiology Division, University of Texas Southwestern Medical Center, Dallas, Texas 75235.

A. L. Mark: Cardiovascular Center, University of Iowa College of Medicine and the Veterans Administration Medical Center, Iowa City, Iowa 52242.

of these measurements. The use of plasma NE as a measure of overall sympathetic activity assumes that there is such a thing as overall activity of the sympathetic nervous system that can be assessed by one measurement. This assumption treats the sympathetic nervous system as a humoral system. Unfortunately for the study of sympathetic function, the system displays profound regional differences in activity and regulation. Consequently, sympathetic function cannot be assessed by a single measurement such as plasma NE, and further advances in this field will require a combination of techniques, each with its distinctive advantages and disadvantages.

Norepinephrine Spillover

Radioisotope determinations of NE spillover (Fig. 1) have several advantages over measurements of plasma NE concentration as an index of sympathetic neural activity (1–3). The radioisotopic methods avoid the confounding influence of NE clearance from plasma and permit assessment of NE spillover in specific target tissues. Because NE is both extracted and released by all organs, organ NE extraction must be taken into account in the measurement of organ-specific NE spillover rates, which is calculated by the following equation;

$$\text{Organ NE Spillover} = [(C_V - C_A) + C_A(\text{NE}_E)] \times PF$$

where C_V = venous effluent plasma NE concentration,

C_A = arterial plasma NE concentration, NE_E = fractional extraction of [^{3}H]NE, and PF = organ plasma flow (1).

This calculation measures the spillover of NE from an organ into its venous effluent and does not measure the rate of NE release at the neuroeffector junction.

Because the relation between sympathetic nerve discharge and NE spillover from a given target organ can be modulated by several factors (e.g., prejunctional receptors), perhaps the most powerful approach is the combination of regional NE spillover with microneurographic measurement of SNA (4).

Microneurography

The microneurographic method for direct intraneural recording of SNA in humans was developed by Hagbarth and Vallbo about 30 years ago and has been used increasingly as a research tool to study regulation of SNA in cardiovascular states such as hypertension (5–7). Tungsten microelectrodes are inserted percutaneously into peripheral nerves for recording of multiunit and, rarely, single unit sympathetic action potentials. The technique has proved remarkably safe and well tolerated. Evidence that the spontaneous activity is indeed postganglionic efferent SNA and not motor or sensory activity derives from several persuasive observations. First, the activity is eliminated by nerve block proximal but not distal to

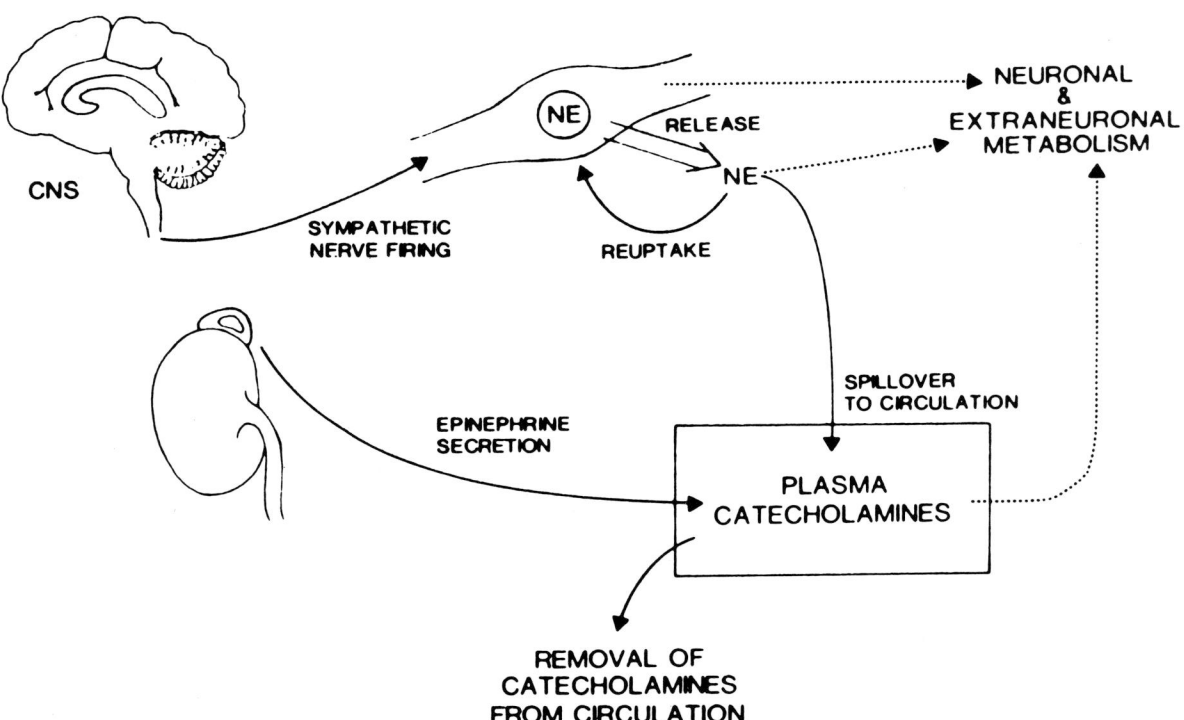

FIG. 1. Schematic depiction of factors influencing plasma levels of catecholamines and the spillover of norepinephrine into the circulation. (From ref. 1, with permission.)

the recording site. Second, the conduction velocity is approximately 1 m/sec, which is similar to that of sympathetic unmyelinated C fibers. Third, the activity is reversibly eliminated by ganglionic blockade.

There are several strengths of the microneurographic method. It readily permits separate recordings of SNA to either skeletal muscle or skin (Fig. 2). This is important because of profound differences in the characteristics and control of muscle versus cutaneous SNA. Parenthetically, separate recording of muscle and skin SNA is difficult to achieve in experimental animals. Thus, microneurography readily permits measurements in conscious humans that are elusive even in anesthetized animals.

Muscle SNA consists of intermittent, pulse synchronous bursts. These bursts tend to occur during spontaneous reductions in arterial pressure and are suppressed during increases in pressure, indicating exquisite baroreceptor modulation of muscle SNA. In addition, there is evidence for potent regulation of muscle SNA by respiratory and chemoreceptor reflexes, muscle and cutaneous afferent input, and neural actions of humoral factors such as angiotensin and insulin. In contrast to the profound baroreflex control of muscle SNA, skin SNA does not appear to be under baroreflex control and is, therefore, not pulse synchronous. Skin SNA is regulated principally by thermal and respiratory reflexes and by central neural influences.

Muscle SNA unquestionably reflects substantially sympathetic noradrenergic vasoconstrictor. There are also hints that muscle SNA may at times transmit sympathetic vasodilator impulses, but this is controversial and it has not been possible to distinguish separate vasoconstrictor and vasodilator activity in recordings of muscle SNA. In contrast, skin SNA consists of several types of impulses: sudomotor, vasoconstrictor, and vasodilator.

The microneurographic method provides dynamic, moment-to-moment recording of SNA. This is a distinctive strength compared to virtually all other methods for measuring sympathetic function in humans. Another strength is the reproducibility of measurements of muscle SNA in a subject (8). There is substantial variability between subjects in resting muscle SNA, but there is surprising reproducibility between recordings from two nerves and sessions in a given subject. The remarkable reproducibility within subjects has permitted use of the method to compare muscle SNA between groups, e.g., normotensive and hypertensive humans. Quantitation of skin SNA is more difficult than muscle SNA. In addition, skin SNA is quite sensitive to arousal and thermal influences and consists of mixed fibers. There has been, to our knowledge, no systematic evaluation of the reproducibility of measurements of skin SNA between sessions.

With a technique as appealing as microneurography, it is incumbent to state its limitations as well as strengths. The method provides no information regarding SNA to critical organs such as the kidney, heart, and brain. Further, although the measurements provide a window on reflex and central neural regulation of muscle and skin SNA, they do not delineate the complex events at the sympathetic neuroeffector junction. Thus, microneurography is a powerful technique that has advanced knowl-

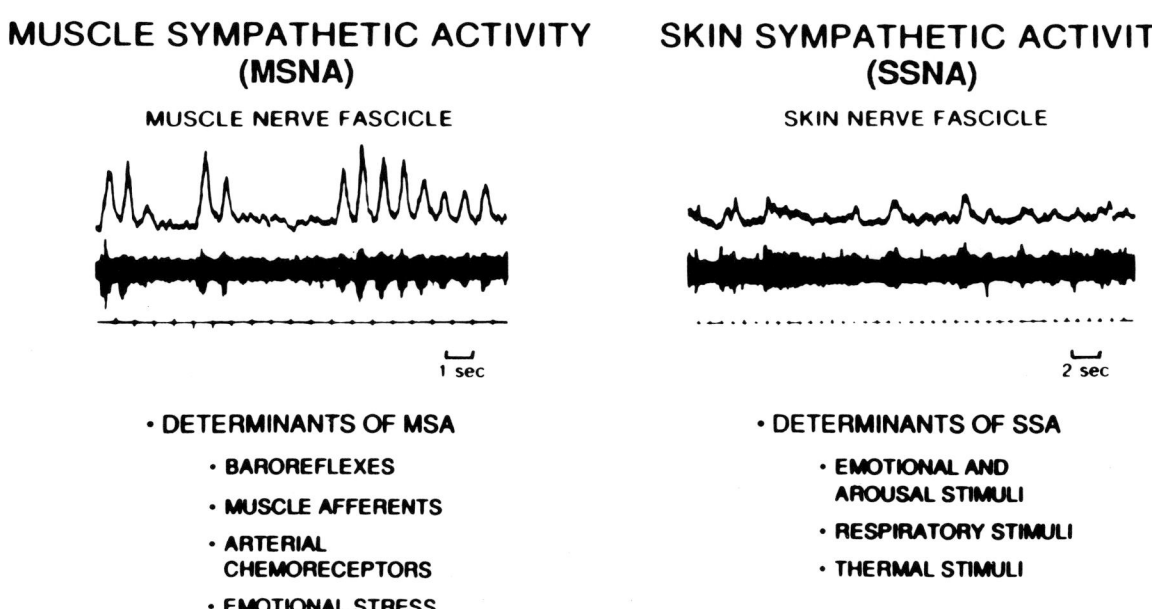

FIG. 2. Recordings showing the differences in characteristics and control mechanisms of sympathetic nerve activity to muscle and skin (see text for description).

edge of sympathetic function in humans, but its value and use rest on recognition of its limitations as well as its strengths.

Positron Emission Tomographic (PET) Imaging

A promising new method for the study of cardiac sympathetic function and innervation is PET imaging using 6-[^{18}F]fluorodopamine. This method has been developed and systematically validated by Goldstein and colleagues in dogs (9) and humans (10). Several radiolabeled sympathomimetic agents have been used to assess cardiac sympathetic innervation with PET. These agents have not been substrates for catecholamine metabolizing enzymes and have not permitted measurement of sympathetic function. The novel feature of Goldstein's method is the use of radiolabeled fluorodopamine. The neuronal uptake and intraneuronal disposition of fluorocatecholamines are qualitatively similar to those of endogenous catecholamines. This feature has permitted use of PET imaging of fluorodopamine for the study of cardiac sympathetic function as well as innervation. In the initial human studies, fluorodopamine produced negligible hemodynamic effects and acceptable radiation exposure. The fluorodopamine was taken up by cardiac sympathetic nerves, translocated from the axoplasm into storage vesicles, metabolized to the fluorinated analogues of NE, and released. This work indicates that thoracic PET scanning after 6-[^{18}F]fluorodopamine injection has the exciting potential to measure cardiac sympathetic function noninvasively in humans. The contribution of this method may be limited by the cost of the equipment and the performance of PET studies. Nevertheless, this development demonstrates again that imaginative use of new technology is increasing the power and sophistication of integrative physiology in humans.

EVIDENCE FOR SYMPATHETIC OVERACTIVITY IN HUMAN HYPERTENSION

Essential Hypertension

After reviewing studies of plasma catecholamines in essential hypertension, Goldstein (11) concluded that most studies revealed elevated plasma NE levels in young hypertensive patients.

Initial microneurographic studies provided no evidence for increased muscle SNA in patients with essential hypertension (12). Several other studies also failed to detect differences in resting muscle SNA in hypertensive and normotensive humans (13,14). In contrast, a number of recent carefully controlled studies from different laboratories have demonstrated heightened resting muscle SNA in humans with essential hypertension (15–20). This has been found in both young mildly hypertensive humans and in older patients with essential hypertension compared with age-matched normotensive humans (Figs. 3 and 4). The reasons for findings of high resting levels of muscle SNA in some but not all studies are not clear, but several factors merit consideration. One factor is sodium intake, which has a profound influence on muscle SNA (15) (Fig. 3). A second factor is body weight. Body weight is a major determinant of resting muscle SNA in healthy humans (21), and decreases in body weight are accompanied by reduction in muscle SNA (22). Thus, differences in body weight may have contributed to differences in muscle SNA in some studies comparing hypertensive and normotensive subjects. However, Floras and Hara (20) found substantial elevations of muscle SNA in mildly hypertensive humans even when compared with weight- and age-matched normotensive subjects.

Thus, there is now evidence from several laboratories for elevated resting muscle SNA in essential hyperten-

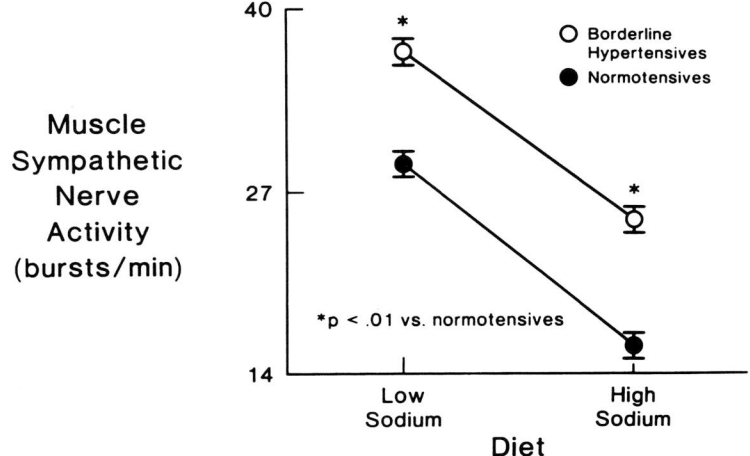

FIG. 3. Muscle sympathetic nerve activity (MSNA) in borderline hypertensive (BHT) and normotensive (NT) humans on low- and high-sodium diets. MSNA declined ($p < .01$) on high-sodium diet, but was higher ($p < .01$) in BHT than in NT subjects on both diets. Entries are mean ± SE. (From ref. 15, with permission.)

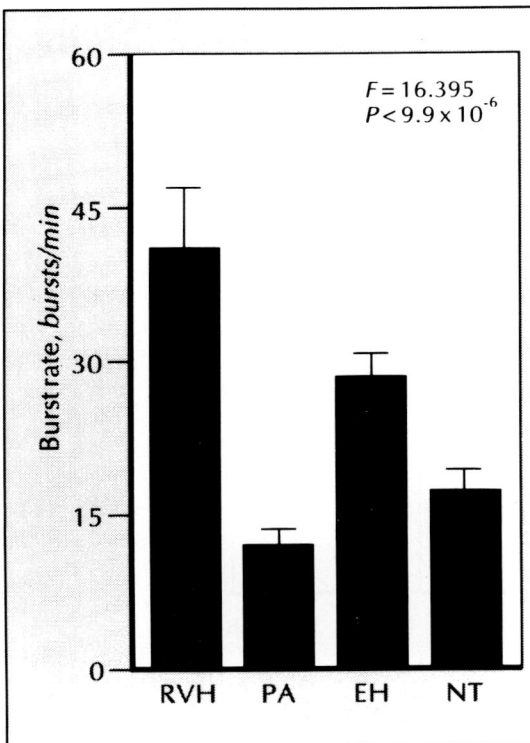

FIG. 4. Muscle sympathetic nerve activity (MSNA) in patients with renovascular hypertension (RVH), primary aldosteronism (PA), and essential hypertension (EH) and in normotensive subjects (NT). MSNA was higher in patients with EH and RVH than in NT subjects, but was reduced in patients with PA. Entries are mean ± SE. (Adapted from ref. 16, with permission.)

sion, particularly in young mildly hypertensive subjects. The elevated muscle SNA is accompanied by elevated limb vascular resistance (20). Moreover, Egan et al. (23) found that mildly hypertensive subjects had elevated plasma NE levels, augmented decreases in limb vascular resistance in response to α-adrenergic blockade, and no increase in α-receptor sensitivity as assessed by responses to NE. Taken together, these studies indicate that mildly hypertensive humans have enhanced sympathetic vasoconstrictor tone in skeletal muscle that results from augmented sympathetic nerve discharge and release of NE and not from exaggerated responses to the neurotransmitter.

Matsukawa et al. (24) demonstrated that patients with accelerated essential hypertension have even greater increases in muscle SNA than do patients with milder hypertension. Interestingly, captopril decreased muscle SNA in the patients with accelerated hypertension, but not in those with mild hypertension. This suggests that the heightened sympathetic activity in accelerated hypertension is linked to activation of the renin-angiotensin system. The findings also suggest that elevated muscle

SNA in mildly hypertensive subjects is not maintained by the renin-angiotensin system and must be related to other mechanisms.

In addition to microneurographic and functional evidence for elevated SNA to skeletal muscle in essential hypertension, Esler and colleagues (1) demonstrated that NE spillover was elevated in essential hypertension, particularly in young hypertensive patients and in normotensive offspring of hypertensive parents. With measurements of regional NE kinetics, the increased spillover emanated mainly from the heart and kidneys (Fig. 5). These observations might help explain the hemodynamic profile of early human hypertension characterized by increased heart rate, cardiac output, and renal vascular resistance.

In discussing the sympathetic nervous system in essential hypertension, mention should be made of a subgroup of patients referred to by Williams and Hollenberg (25) as nonmodulators. These patients are characterized by abnormalities in control of the renin-angiotensin-aldosterone axis in response to changes in salt intake and posture. Interestingly, the nonmodulators have also been found to have abnormalities in control of plasma NE (26). During low salt intake, increases in plasma NE during upright posture were exaggerated in the nonmodulators compared with normotensive controls and to hypertensive patients with normal modulation of the renin-angiotensin-aldosterone system. It is not known if the abnormal regulation of plasma NE reflects alterations in sympathetic neural outflow or in prejunctional modulation of the release of NE from adrenergic nerve endings. It was concluded that the catecholamine abnormalities are a secondary event (26), but the possibility remains that these reflect an independent genetic abnormality and may contribute to altered regulation of the renin-angiotensin-aldosterone system in these patients.

Age, Gender, and Racial Differences in SNA

Resting levels of muscle SNA, like plasma NE, increase with age both in normotensive individuals and in patients with essential hypertension (5,27,28). An important unanswered question is whether the increased sympathetic drive exerts a trophic effect on vascular smooth muscle in large arteries, thereby contributing to the pathogenesis of systolic hypertension in the elderly. Recent studies have implicated gender as another independent determinant of sympathetic nerve activity in normotensive individuals since resting levels of muscle SNA were consistently lower in young women than in young men and in older women compared with older men (27). Whether these gender-related differences in sympathetic activity are related in any way to the pathogenesis of essential hypertension remains to be determined.

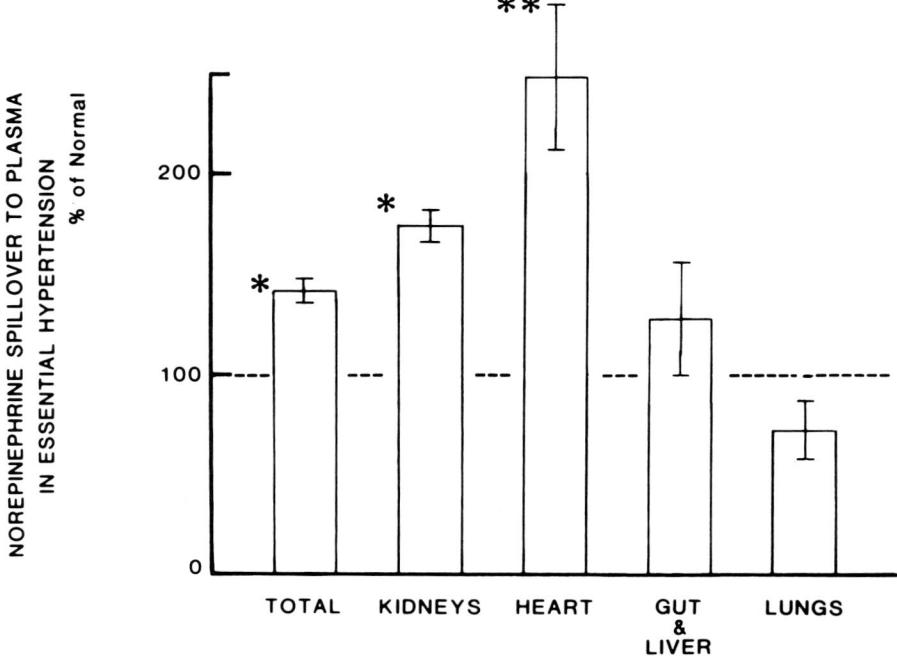

FIG. 5. Norepinephrine spillover data showing evidence for augmented renal and cardiac sympathetic neural outflow in patients with primary hypertension. Entries are mean ± SE. *p < .05 and **p < .01 vs normals. (From ref. 1, with permission.)

Hypertension is more prevalent and is associated with accelerated target organ damage in African-Americans compared with white Americans (29). Laboratory stressors, such as the cold pressor test, produce larger increases in peripheral vascular resistance and blood pressure in normotensive African-American subjects than in white cohorts, suggesting that excessive α-adrenergic vasoconstriction may be involved in the pathogenesis of hypertension in African-Americans (30–34). Calhoun et al. (35,36) recently demonstrated that the heightened blood pressure response to cold pressor stimulation in normotensive African-Americans versus normotensive whites was accompanied by a greater increase in muscle SNA, despite similar increases in heart rate. There were no differences in the baseline levels of muscle SNA between the groups. These observations relate to Folkow's vascular amplifier hypothesis (37) in which repeated activation of the sympathetic nervous system in response to environmental stressors eventually leads to vascular hypertrophy, thereby causing a sustained increase in vascular resistance and chronic hypertension. In this regard, racial differences in hemodynamic responses to cold pressor testing seem to disappear once essential hypertension becomes chronic (38).

Given the importance of this topic as a public health issue, further studies are needed to prove that such differences in sympathetic and blood pressure reactivity are related to race per se rather than to differences in the family history of hypertension or to socioeconomic and/or psychophysiological variables. Another key issue is whether these observations can be generalized to sympathetic stimuli that are encountered frequently in daily life outside of the human physiology laboratory such as exercise, heat stress, and emotional stresses.

Secondary Hypertension

Renovascular Hypertension and Aldosteronism

In patients with renovascular hypertension, increased plasma renin activity and angiotensin II were found to be accompanied by increased muscle SNA (16) (Fig. 4). This sympathetic activation was normalized after percutaneous renal angioplasty. These neurophysiological observations extend previous reports that renovascular hypertension is accompanied by increased plasma levels of NE (39). Taken together, these observations suggest that activation of the renin-angiotensin system increases arterial pressure in part by increasing SNA. The potential mechanisms by which this may occur are described later in this chapter.

In contrast to the elevated SNA in patients with renovascular hypertension, muscle SNA and plasma renin activity were decreased in patients with primary aldosteronism (16) (Fig. 4). In addition, muscle SNA was decreased by administration of the mineralocorticoid fludrocortisone acetate to normotensive subjects (40). This inhibitory influence of mineralocorticoid excess may be explained, in part, by increases in plasma volume and cardiac filling pressure, which result in stimulation of inhibitory cardiopulmonary baroreceptors.

Hypertension in Patients with Chronic Renal Failure

Hypertension occurs in up to 80 percent of patients with chronic renal failure and is a major risk factor for increased cardiovascular morbidity and mortality in this patient population (41). Although this hypertension is thought to be largely volume dependent, it is also accompanied by increased systemic vascular resistance (42), suggesting a potential pathophysiological role for neurohumoral activation. Plasma NE levels in chronic renal failure have varied from low to high. More recently, Converse et al. (43) found that muscle SNA and vascular resistance in the calf were markedly elevated in chronic hemodialysis patients with native kidneys. In contrast, sympathetic activity and vascular resistance were indistinguishable from normal in chronic hemodialysis patients who had undergone bilateral nephrectomy (Fig. 6). These findings suggest that chronic uremia is accompanied by reversible sympathetic activation, which appears to be dependent upon a signal arising in the failing kidney.

The nature of this signal is unknown but it might be related either to uremic toxins acting on renal afferents nerves, which reflexively increase efferent SNA, or to the renal release of humoral substances, such as angiotensin II, which secondarily increase sympathetic outflow. Regardless of the precise mechanism, the findings suggest

that the antihypertensive effect of nephrectomy in some patients with end-stage renal failure may be caused not only by removal of the renal renin-angiotensin system but also by a reduction in sympathetic drive to the peripheral circulation.

Cyclosporine-Induced Hypertension

Cyclosporine A (CsA), the first immunosuppressive agent with relative T-cell specificity, has markedly improved both long-term survival after organ transplantation and the treatment of autoimmune diseases (44,45). However, CsA also has emerged as a new secondary cause of hypertension. Two syndromes have been described: acute hypertension with the initiation of a high dose of CsA, and chronic hypertension with maintenance immunosuppression (46–51). Studies in experimental animals have produced substantial evidence that CsA can cause rapid increases in SNA, thereby producing neurally mediated vasoconstriction and acute hypertension (52–56).

In humans, SNA has not been studied prospectively during the initiation of CsA treatment. However, in several cross-sectional studies muscle SNA has been recorded in patients undergoing chronic immunosuppressive therapy with CsA. Scherrer et al. (57) found that muscle SNA was markedly elevated in heart transplant recipients and in patients with myasthenia gravis receiving CsA (Fig. 7). In contrast, muscle SNA was indistinguishable from normal in both heart transplant recipients and patients with myasthenia who were receiving more traditional immunosuppressive treatment without

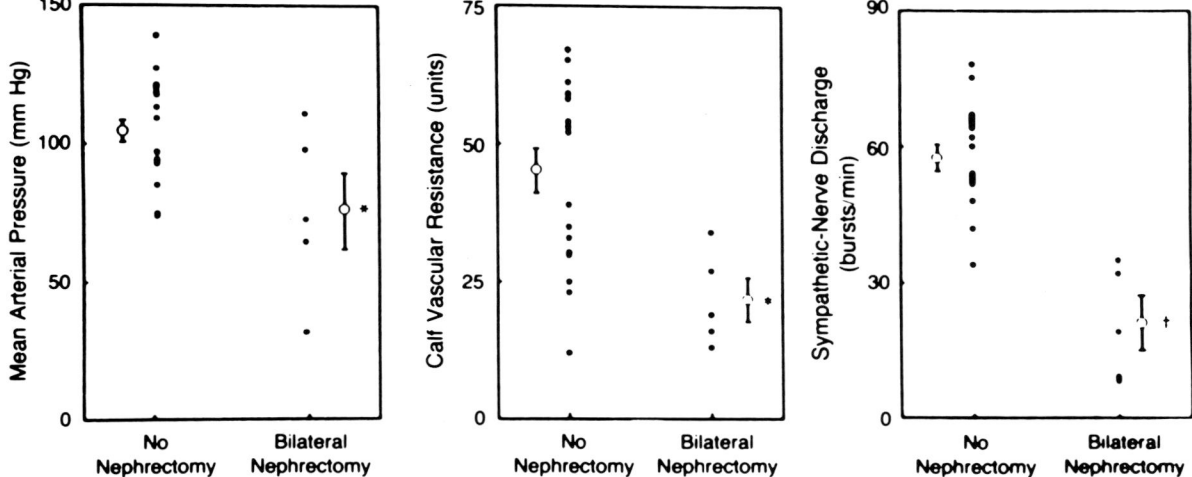

FIG. 6. Mean arterial pressure, calf vascular resistance, and muscle sympathetic nerve discharge (MSNA) in patients with chronic renal failure (CRF) who either had or had not undergone bilateral nephrectomy. Although not shown here, MSNA was much higher in the patients with CRF without nephrectomy than in normal controls (58 ± 3 vs 23 ± 3 bursts/min, respectively; p < .01). In anephric CRF patients, MSNA and calf vascular resistance were indistinguishable from normal controls. (From ref. 43, with permission.)

A.

Heart-Transplant Recipient Taking Cyclosporine

B.

Cyclosporine
(9/16/88)

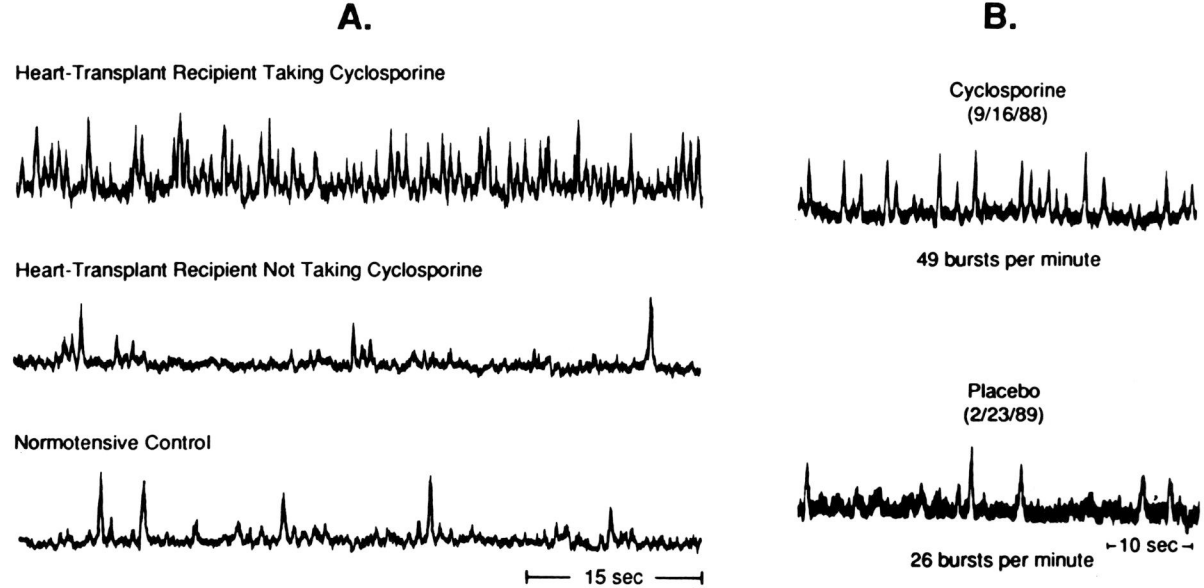

Heart-Transplant Recipient Not Taking Cyclosporine

49 bursts per minute

Normotensive Control

Placebo
(2/23/89)

├── 15 sec ──┤

26 bursts per minute   ├─10 sec─┤

FIG. 7. A: Recordings of MSNA in a heart transplant recipient taking cyclosporine, a heart transplant recipient not taking cyclosporine, and a normotensive control. Summary data (mean ± SE) for MSNA for respective groups of patients were 80 ± 3, 30 ± 4, and 28 ± 4 bursts/min. **B:** Recordings of MSNA in a patient with myasthenia gravis during treatment with cyclosporine and placebo. (Adapted from ref. 57.)

CsA. These observations have been replicated recently (58). In addition, muscle SNA has been found to be elevated in heart-lung transplant recipients receiving CsA (59). These findings are difficult to reconcile with the study of Kaye et al. (60), who found that muscle SNA and renal and total body NE spillover were normal in CsA-treated heart transplant recipients. In another group of CsA-treated heart transplant recipients studied recently by Elam et al. (61), muscle SNA (expressed in bursts/min) was higher than in controls but the magnitude of the elevation was less than in the original cohort studied by Scherrer et al. The variability in the results of these cross-sectional studies may be related in part to antihypertensive medications that may mitigate the sympathoexcitatory effect of CsA. This variability emphasizes the need for controlled, prospective studies of muscle SNA before and during treatment with CsA.

Cocaine-Induced Hypertensive Crisis

Acute hypertensive crisis is one of the cardiovascular complications of cocaine abuse. In addition to the well-known effect of cocaine on peripheral sympathetic nerve terminals to block NE reuptake, a recent study by Jacobsen et al. (62) suggests that intranasal cocaine exerts two directionally opposite effects on muscle SNA in humans: baroreflex-mediated sympathoinhibition (in response to a rapid increase in blood pressure) and central neural sympathoexcitation. In healthy subjects without a his-

tory of cocaine abuse, the sympathoinhibitory effect predominates. However, the sympathoexcitatory action of cocaine was unmasked when the cocaine-induced rise in blood pressure was minimized with a concomitant infusion of nitroprusside. In the setting of recreational cocaine abuse, the sympathoexcitatory action of cocaine might become dominant and amplify the drug's sympathomimetic effects, thereby precipitating a hypertensive emergency, if baroreflex buffering were overcome by an excessively high dose of cocaine or if it were impaired in individuals with conditions such as essential hypertension.

Hypertension in Patients with Baroreflex Failure

Paroxysmal supine hypertension masquerading as pheochromocytoma in patients with baroreflex failure has been described by Aksamit et al. (63) and recently systematically characterized by Robertson et al. (64). A spontaneous surge in blood pressure with an unchanged heart rate suggests the diagnosis, typically in a patient who has a past history of extensive radiation to the neck and thorax, which either destroys the sinoaortic baroreceptors or the elastic elements of the vessel walls in which they are embedded. Microneurographic confirmation of sinoaortic baroreceptor denervation consists of a recording of muscle SNA muscle that is unchanged during increases and decreases in blood pressure produced by infusions of vasoactive drugs (63). In addition, with acute local anesthesia of sinoaortic baroreceptor afferents, the recording of muscle SNA loses its pulse synchronicity (65).

Hypertension in Patients with Obstructive Sleep Apnea

Muscle SNA has recently been measured during sleep in normal humans (66,67). In these studies the normal nocturnal dip in blood pressure was accompanied by decreased muscle SNA during stages 2 to 4 of sleep whereas rapid eye movement (REM) sleep was accompanied by increased muscle SNA, presumably reflecting increased cortical and/or somatomotor arousal.

Arterial hypertension is present in the majority of patients with obstructive sleep apnea (OSA). Studies by Hedner et al. (68) and by Somers et al. (69) suggest that sympathetic neural activation may contribute to daytime as well as nocturnal arterial hypertension in these patients. In patients with OSA, the normal nocturnal decrease in both arterial pressure and muscle SNA is lost and replaced by sudden surges in sympathetic activity and blood pressure in response to repeated episodes of apnea. Furthermore, patients with OSA showed elevated baseline levels of muscle SNA even when awake and breathing. Preliminary data by Crabtree et al. (70) suggest that such long-lasting sympathetic overactivity may be related to resetting and sensitization of the carotid body chemoreflex.

POTENTIAL MECHANISMS LEADING TO SYMPATHETIC OVERACTIVITY

The mechanisms of sympathetic overactivity in human hypertension remain problematic. Nevertheless, there is sufficient evidence to consider several potential mechanisms.

Reflex Mechanisms

Arterial and Cardiopulmonary Baroreflexes

Arterial Baroreflexes

There are abnormalities in arterial baroreceptor control of heart rate in essential hypertension and in normotensive offspring of hypertensive parents. Understandably, this has prompted interest in the concept that elevated levels of muscle SNA in hypertension might result partly from impaired baroreceptor restraint on sympathetic neural outflow. This concept remains problematic. For example, there is evidence from animal studies that abnormalities in baroreceptor control of parasympathetic activity (heart rate) do not necessarily indicate abnormalities in baroreceptor control of sympathetic ac-

tivity and vascular resistance (71,72). It appears that there is greater central nervous system reserve for baroreceptor control of sympathetic compared with parasympathetic mechanisms. In this regard, Rea and Hamdan (14) found that arterial baroreceptor control of muscle SNA was normal in young adults with very mild hypertension. Despite the presence of normal arterial baroreceptor control, the mildly hypertensive subjects exhibited heightened sympathetic neural drive. The finding of heightened sympathetic drive in the presence of normal baroreceptor regulation of muscle SNA suggests that factors other than arterial baroreflexes are responsible for the development of elevated muscle SNA in the earliest stages of essential hypertension (14). In contrast, Matsukawa et al. (17) observed that baroreceptor control of muscle SNA was reduced in humans with either mild or established hypertension. If arterial baroreceptors are involved in elevation of muscle SNA in essential hypertension, they may be more important in the maintenance rather than the development of heightened SNA.

For years it has been held that alterations in baroreceptor reflexes represent adaptive responses to chronic increases in arterial pressure. However, Dahl genetically salt-sensitive rats fed a rigorously low-salt diet display abnormalities in baroreceptor afferent mechanisms in the absence of increases in arterial pressure (73). This finding introduced the concept that alterations in arterial baroreflexes in hypertension might be related in part to genetic abnormalities that precede the increase in arterial pressure. Parmer et al. (74) measured baroreflex control of heart rate in normotensive and hypertensive humans grouped by the presence or absence of a family history of hypertension. In both normotensive and hypertensive groups, baroreflex sensitivity was lower in those subjects with a family history of hypertension (Fig. 8). After controlling for other variables including arterial pressure, a family history of hypertension still had a highly significant influence on baroreflex sensitivity. This suggests that baroreceptor impairment in humans might in part be genetically determined. This could represent a hereditary component in the pathogenesis of essential hypertension.

Cardiopulmonary Baroreflexes

In contrast to arterial baroreflexes, several studies suggest that cardiopulmonary baroreceptor control of sympathetic neural vasoconstrictor activity is enhanced in mildly hypertensive subjects in the supine position. This concept derives from studies of reflex responses to mild lower body negative pressure, which acts mainly to decrease the activity of cardiopulmonary as opposed to arterial baroreceptors. Low levels of lower body negative pressure produce exaggerated increases in muscle SNA

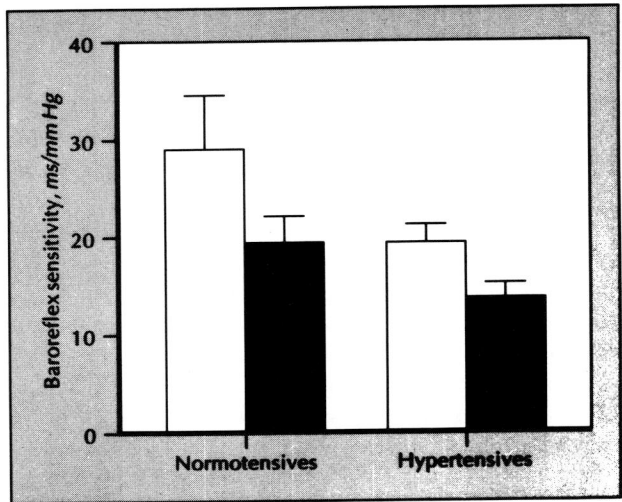

FIG. 8. Baroreflex control of heart interval measured using bolus injections of phenylephrine in normotensive and hypertensive subjects subgrouped by presence (*shaded bars*) or absence (*clear bars*) of a family history of hypertension. A family history of hypertension was associated with a lower baroreflex sensitivity in both groups. (From ref. 38, with permission.)

(14) and forearm vascular resistance (75) in mildly hypertensive humans. These findings suggest that the elevated muscle SNA in mild hypertension is not caused by alterations in cardiopulmonary baroreceptors. Instead, cardiopulmonary baroreceptors may act to buffer a heightened sympathetic neural drive in mild hypertension.

An augmented cardiopulmonary baroreflex in borderline hypertension might help maintain a nocturnal decline in blood pressure during the early phases of essential hypertension (76). Increased cardiopulmonary blood volume during recumbency would be expected to activate this augmented reflex mechanism causing reflex vasodilation and decreased blood pressure. As left ventricular hypertrophy develops, the augmentation of cardiopulmonary baroreflex may be lost. This could contribute to loss of the normal nocturnal decline in arterial pressure during sleep.

Ventricular baroreceptor denervation may be important in the hypertension that accompanies administration of CsA in patients with heart transplantation. These patients have a higher incidence and severity of hypertension than do other groups of patients receiving comparable doses of CsA. This could relate in part to the loss of a buffering influence of ventricular baroreceptors to counter the sympathoexcitatory action of CsA (57).

Arterial Chemoreflexes

Arterial chemoreceptors are potent stimuli to sympathetic activity in response to hypoxia. It has recently been proposed that sensitization of arterial chemoreceptor reflexes may be implicated in heightened sympathetic activation in hypertension. Spontaneously hypertensive rats manifest exaggerated carotid sinus chemoreceptor discharge and reflexes during hypoxia (77,78). Young hypertensive humans have a potentiated ventilatory (79) and muscle SNA (13) response to hypoxia. The potentiated sympathetic neural responses are particularly obvious when the inhibitory influences of thoracic afferents are eliminated during brief apnea. The mechanism(s) of the augmented chemoreceptor function in hypertension is not clear. One possibility involves interaction of baroreceptor and chemoreceptor reflexes. Inhibitory influences from arterial baroreceptors restrain the SNA responses to chemoreceptor stimulation during hypoxia. It has been postulated that impairment in the inhibitory influence of arterial baroreceptors might promote exaggerated SNA responses to hypoxia (80).

It is not known if the chemoreceptor reflex contributes to heightened muscle SNA in hypertension in the absence of hypoxia. Sensitization of chemoreceptor reflexes might, however, contribute importantly to the elevations in muscle SNA and arterial pressure that characterize many patients with obstructive sleep apnea.

Excitatory Reflexes Arising in Renal Afferents

Studies in animals have indicated that the kidney is a sensory organ containing mechanically and chemically sensitive afferent nerves that might be involved in the pathogenesis of hypertension by causing reflex activation of the sympathetic nervous system (81–86). Stimulation of renal afferent nerves with intrarenal administration of uremic toxins (e.g., urea) or ischemic metabolites (e.g., adenosine) in animals reflexively increases efferent SNA and blood pressure (81,82). Furthermore, renal afferent denervation reduces sympathetic overactivity and blood pressure in experimental renovascular hypertension (84,85). Thus, elevated SNA and blood pressure in some patients with end-stage renal disease may be caused in part by uremic toxins acting on excitatory renal afferents in the failing kidney, a mechanism that is eliminated by bilateral nephrectomy (43). In support of this hypothesis, preliminary studies by Campese et al. (*personal communication*) suggest that renal deafferentation (dorsal rhizotomy) may prevent the development of hypertension in rats with experimental renal failure.

Humoral Mechanisms

Insulin Resistance and Obesity

Insulin resistance and hyperinsulinemia have been implicated in the pathogenesis of hypertension secondary to obesity and in essential hypertension. Infusion of insulin while maintaining euglycemia increases plasma NE (87) and muscle SNA (88,89). This sympathoexcitatory effect of insulin can occur with relatively low plasma concentrations (90). This suggests that hyperinsulinemia could contribute to increases in muscle SNA in physiological and pathophysiological states such as obesity and hypertension.

There is striking regional nonuniformity in the sympathoexcitatory actions of insulin. In normotensive rats, insulin increases lumbar but not renal SNA (91), and in normotensive humans insulin increases SNA to muscle (Fig. 9) but not skin (89). Thus, in normotensive states, the sympathoexcitatory actions of insulin are directed to skeletal muscle.

Surprisingly, although insulin increases sympathetic noradrenergic vasoconstrictor activity to skeletal muscle, it produces vasodilation and not vasoconstriction in muscle (88). This reflects a vasodilator action of insulin (possibly endothelial dependent) that normally overrides the sympathetic vasoconstrictor influence. This observation would seem to challenge the concept that a sympathoexcitatory action of insulin contributes to vasoconstriction and hypertension. However, in the presence of insulin resistance and hypertension, the sympathoexcitatory action of insulin is exaggerated and the vasodilator action is attenuated. Under these conditions, the sympathoexcitatory action of insulin might predominate and contribute to increases in vascular resistance and arterial pressure.

Randin et al. (21) recently compared muscle SNA in normotensive obese and lean subjects. The obese subjects, who had higher fasting plasma insulin levels, also had a twofold higher level of muscle SNA. This was observed in the absence of differences in plasma NE levels between groups. Muscle SNA correlated with both body mass index and plasma insulin concentration. These observations and the fact that physiological concentrations of insulin can influence sympathetic activity prompt speculation that hyperinsulinemia may contribute to elevated levels of muscle SNA in obesity and perhaps in essential hypertension even in the absence of obesity.

Angiotensin II

There are several mechanisms by which angiotensin II might increase postganglionic SNA and thereby raise arterial pressure. Angiotensin II acts in the central nervous system and on autonomic ganglia to facilitate sympathetic activity in addition to facilitating sympathetic mechanisms at the neuroeffector junction (92). Matsukawa et al. (93) have demonstrated that angiotensin II attenuates baroreflex control of muscle SNA in humans. As mentioned previously, the renin-angiotensin system appears to contribute importantly to the heightened muscle SNA in accelerated essential hypertension, but not in mild essential hypertension (24). In addition, angiotensin II per se is unlikely to be the primary factor causing elevated muscle SNA in patients with chronic renal failure. The elevated muscle SNA in these patients was dissociated from plasma renin activity and plasma levels of angiotensin II and was not normalized by administration of converting enzyme inhibitors (43).

Epinephrine as an Amplifier and/or Activator SNA

Floras (94) has recently reviewed the mechanisms by which surges of adrenomedullary secretion of epineph-

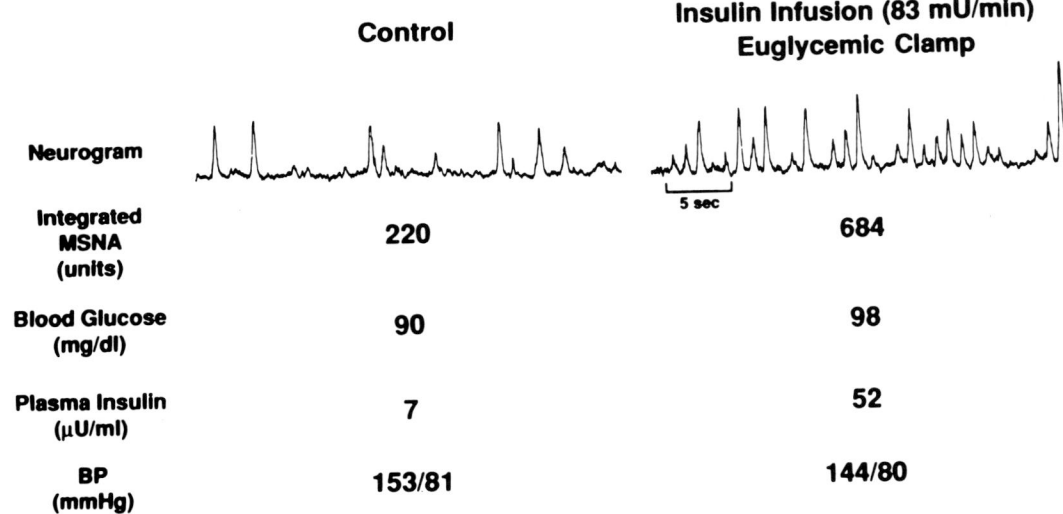

FIG. 9. Segments of record from a normal subject showing that increases in plasma insulin while maintaining euglycemia substantially increase MSNA. Although not shown here, the increase in MSNA was accompanied by vasodilation in the limb, indicating that insulin produces opposing sympathoexcitatory and vasodilator actions. (From ref. 15, with permission.)

rine in response to psychophysiological stressors could contribute to the development of essential hypertension by amplifying sympathetic neurotransmission. These mechanisms include (a) epinephrine-induced stimulation of prejunctional β_2-adrenoceptors, which enhance NE release during sympathetic nerve stimulation; (b) neuronal uptake of circulating epinephrine, which is co-released with NE during sympathetic nerve stimulation; and (c) epinephrine-induced increases in the rate of sympathetic nerve discharge. This last effect, which was studied by Persson et al. (95), may be related to perturbations in arterial and cardiopulmonary baroreflexes in response to the hemodynamic changes induced by increases in plasma epinephrine concentration. These include decreased diastolic blood pressure, which would unload sinoaortic baroreceptors, and decreased central venous pressure, which would unload cardiopulmonary baroreceptors.

Neuronal Signal Transduction Pathways

Nitric Oxide as a Central Sympathetic Neurotransmitter

Recent studies in animal preparations have advanced the concept that neuronal, as well as endothelial, nitric oxide (NO) synthase contributes to the tonic regulation of vasomotor tone and blood pressure (96–105). Several lines of evidence strongly suggest that neuronal NO is a major component of the signal transduction pathways involved in the tonic restraint of central sympathetic neural outflow. The neuronal isoform of NO synthase was identified by staining for nicotinamide adenine dinucleotide phosphate, reduced (NADPH) diaphorase in specific regions of rat brains such as the nucleus tractus solitarius and rostral ventrolateral medulla that are involved in the neural control of blood pressure (96, 97). Neuronal NO synthase is a calcium-calmodulin–dependent enzyme that is activated, for example, when calcium influx through N-methyl-D-aspartate (NMDA) receptor-operated channels is stimulated by L-glutamate, the key inhibitory neurotransmitter in the nucleus tractus solitarius (103). It has been proposed that NO mediates glutaminergic inhibition of central sympathetic outflow. Microinjection of N^G-monomethyl-L-arginine or L-NMMA (which inhibits NO synthase) into the rat nucleus tractus solitarius inhibited the ability of L-glutamate to cause centrally mediated decreases in blood pressure (104).

Further evidence that neuronal NO is involved in the tonic central inhibition of sympathetic outflow in rats, rabbits, and cats is that renal SNA and blood pressure increased with microinjection of L-NMMA into the nucleus tractus solitarius or rostral ventral lateral medulla but not with microinjection into the area postrema or caudal ventrolateral medulla (99–101). In animal

models, the sympathoexcitatory effect of NO inhibition also has been clearly demonstrated during systemic administration of monomethyl arginines (98,102). A key unanswered question is whether these experimental findings can be extrapolated to humans.

Inhibition in tonic NO synthesis has been implicated in the pathogenesis of human essential hypertension (105) as well as in the hypertension of patients with chronic renal failure (106). Asymmetric dimethyl arginine, for example, is a recently identified endogenous circulating inhibitor of NO synthase. This substance is normally excreted by the kidney and accumulates excessively in the plasma of patients with chronic renal failure. Thus, the possibility exists that tonic inhibition of neuronal as well as endothelial NO synthase might contribute to increases in elevated vasomotor tone and blood pressure in patients with chronic renal failure.

Calcineurin as an Inhibitory Signal Transduction Element in the Regulation of Neuronal Excitability

Recent animal studies have suggested that the same cytosolic proteins involved in mediating the immunosuppressive action of drugs such as CsA and FK-506 also mediate immunosuppressive drug-induced renal insufficiency and hypertension (107–110). There is now substantial evidence that in T lymphocytes CsA and FK-506 bind to cytoplasmic receptors termed "immunophilins" and that the drug-immunophilin complexes in turn bind to and inhibit the activity of calcineurin, a calcium-calmodulin–dependent phosphatase (111–115). Inhibition of calcineurin prevents dephosphorylation of transcriptional elements on the interleukin-2 gene, thereby preventing T-cell amplification (and thus preventing organ rejection).

Calcineurin is abundant in brain and other neural tissue (116) where it has been hypothesized to modulate neuronal excitability by regulating the influx of calcium through L-type calcium channels (117,118). In rats, the ability of CsA, FK-506, and their structural analogues to increase renal sympathetic nerve activity and blood pressure and to cause nephrotoxicity is closely correlated with their ability to inhibit the phosphatase activity of brain calcineurin in vitro and to inhibit calcineurin-mediated signaling in isolated T cells (107–110). These correlational studies provide a conceptual framework for the hypothesis that the hypertensive effects of CsA and related immunosuppressant drugs are related in part to sympathetic overactivity. This hypothesis awaits rigorous testing.

Genetic Influences

Although there has been substantial interest in the genetic factors regulating arterial pressure, there has been scant attention to genetic mechanisms influencing the sympathetic nervous system.

Williams et al. (119) examined 109 twin pairs and concluded that genetic influences contributed to more than half of the variability in plasma NE levels. Wallin et al. (120) recently undertook to determine if genetic influences contribute to the large interindividual differences in muscle SNA. Pairs of monozygotic male twins and age-matched unrelated male control subjects underwent microneurographic measurements of muscle SNA. Intrapair differences in muscle SNA were much lower in the twins (1.7 + 0.5 bursts/min; mean + SE) than in the unrelated controls (11.8 + 2 bursts/min) (Fig. 10). This observation strongly suggests that sympathetic neural outflow is controlled genetically. These two studies should prompt the search for the genetic factors influencing sympathetic neural outflow.

POTENTIAL IMPORTANCE OF SYMPATHETIC NEURAL ACTIVATION IN THE PATHOGENESIS OF HUMAN HYPERTENSION

The sympathetic nervous system plays a pivotal role in rapid, short-term alterations in cardiovascular function during physiological states such as exercise and orthostatic stress and during pathophysiological states such as hemorrhagic hypotension. Despite this knowledge and the increasing evidence for sympathetic overactivity in many hypertensive states, the importance of sympathetic activation in the pathogenesis of sustained arterial

hypertension has been challenged on several grounds. This issue has been discussed in an editorial (121) by one of us (A. L. M.) and by Abboud (122). For example, it has been argued that sympathetic overactivity alone is not sufficient to cause hypertension because several disorders with profound sympathetic activation such as heart failure and cirrhosis are not characterized by hypertension. However, the same caveats apply to the renin-angiotensin system. There is heightened activity of the renin-angiotensin system in heart failure and cirrhosis without hypertension. Yet few would challenge the importance of the renin-angiotensin system in the pathogenesis of some forms of sustained hypertension. Hypertension is multifactorial, and increased activity of the sympathetic nervous system interacting with other factors could contribute to hypertension.

It has been suggested that the sympathetic nervous system is important in the moment-to-moment regulation of cardiovascular function but not in the long-term control of arterial pressure. It also has been further suggested that sympathetically mediated vasoconstriction in the peripheral circulation alone cannot cause a persistent elevation in arterial pressure in the absence of alterations in the kidney. It has been argued that the hypertensive effects of neurogenic vasoconstriction would be mitigated by multiple counterregulatory mechanisms including increased natriuresis and diuresis. Given these challenges, it is important to emphasize the neuroeffector mechanisms, other than α-adrenergic vasoconstriction, by which the sympathetic nervous system can influence the long-term regulation of blood pressure.

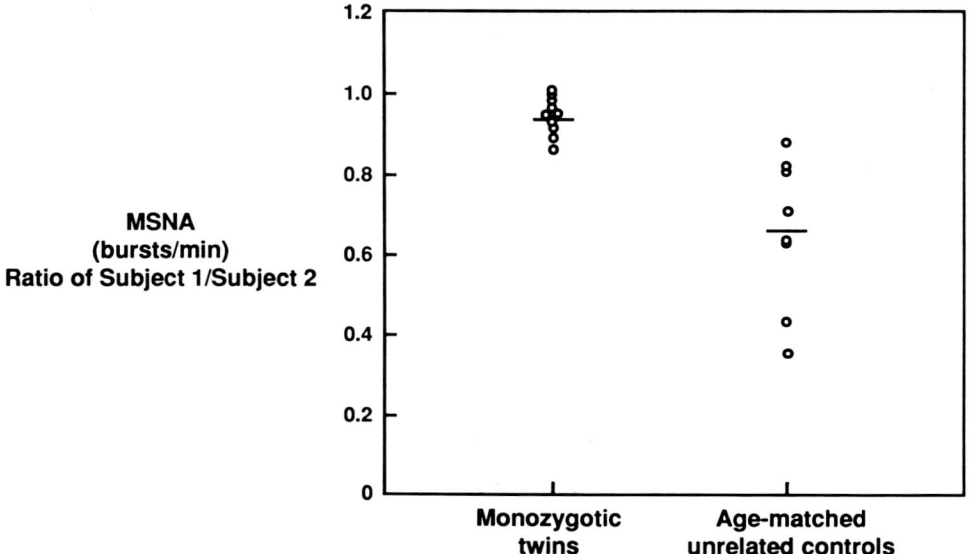

FIG. 10. Comparison of the variability in supine, resting muscle sympathetic nerve activity (MSNA) between pairs of monozygotic twins and pairs of age-matched, unrelated control subjects. The between-subjects variability was much less ($p < .05$) in pairs of twins than in pairs of unrelated controls. (From ref. 120, with permission.)

First, DiBona (123) demonstrated that the renal sympathetic nerves not only cause renal vasoconstriction but also enhance the release of renin and promote reabsorption of sodium and water from the renal tubules. In rats, these effects can occur at low frequencies of renal nerve stimulation that do not affect renal blood flow or glomerular filtration. Thus, low levels of renal SNA can shift the pressure-natriuresis curve and facilitate the maintenance of hypertension by interfering with the ability of the kidney to compensate for an increase in arterial pressure through pressure natriuresis.

Second, the sympathetic nervous system, like the renin-angiotensin system, can exert trophic effects on vascular muscle, which are independent of its hemodynamic effects (124,125). In this regard, recent evidence suggests that patients who chronically abuse the indirect sympathomimetic agent cocaine often develop cardiac and peripheral vascular hypertrophy even in the absence of a sustained elevation in arterial pressure (126–128). This may reflect the trophic effects of sympathetic stimulation. The trophic effects of long-term sympathetic stimulation on blood vessels appear to be greatest during growth and development. Sympathetic overactivity appears to occur during the early stages of hypertension when it is most likely to influence the structure of blood vessels, and thus the long-term regulation of arterial pressure. Structural changes in blood vessels increase vascular resistance and the vasomotor response to vasoconstrictor stimuli so that the effects of the sympathetic nervous system on vasomotor tone and vascular structure interact to increase peripheral vascular resistance and arterial pressure (129).

Third, studies in spontaneously hypertensive rats suggest a role for the sympathetic nervous system in abnormalities of vascular membrane permeability (130). The spontaneously hypertensive rat has an increase in passive permeability of vascular muscle to sodium. This results in augmented vasoconstrictor responses to NE. This abnormality in membrane permeability appears to be related to a genetically determined trophic influence of the sympathetic nervous system. Thus, genetically determined sympathetic influences acting during development can cause long-term alterations in vascular smooth muscle that may contribute to hypertension.

ACKNOWLEDGMENTS

Dr. Victor is supported by funding from the National Heart Lung and Blood Institute (RO-1 HL44010) and from the Extramural Grant Program (Renal Division) of the Baxter Healthcare Corporation. Dr. Victor is an Established Investigator of the American Heart Association. Dr. Mark's research, cited in this review, was supported by grants HL44546, HL24962, and HL14388 from the National Heart, Lung, and Blood Institute; by grant RR59 from the General Clinical Research Centers Program of the National Institutes of Health; and by research funds from the Department of Veterans Affairs. The authors thank Nancy Davin for secretarial assistance.

The authors have drawn on previous reviews of this topic from our laboratories in preparing this chapter and acknowledge the valued contributions of our colleagues to work from our laboratories discussed in this chapter.

REFERENCES

1. Esler M, Jennings G, Lambert G. *Am J Hypertens* 1989;2:140S–146S.
2. Esler M, Ferrier C, Lambert G, Eisenhofer G, Cox H, Jennings G. *Hypertension* 1991;17:III29–III35.
3. Esler M, Lambert G, Jennings G. *J Hypertens* 1990;8:S53–57.
4. Grossmann E, Rea RF, Hoffman A, Goldstein DS. *Am J Physiol* 1991;29:R142–R147.
5. Vallbo AB, Hagbarth K-E, Torebjork HE, Wallin BG. *Physiol Rev* 1979;59:919–957.
6. Wallin BG. In: Stalberg E, Young RR, eds. *Butterworths Int Med Rev, Neurology 1, Clinical Neurophysiology.* London: Butterworths, 1981;145–167.
7. Mark AL. *J Hypertens* 1990;8:S67–S75.
8. Sundlöf G, Wallin BG. *J Physiol (Lond)* 1977;272:383–397.
9. Goldstein DS, Chang PC, Eisenhofer G, Miletech R, Finn R, Bacher J, Kirk KL, Bacharach S, Kopin IJ. *Circulation* 1990;81:1606–1621.
10. Goldstein DS, Eisenhofer G, Dunn BB, Armando I, Lenders J, Grossman E, Holmes C, Kirk KL, Bacharach S, Adams R, Herscovitch P, Kopin IJ. *J Am Coll Cardiol* 1993;22:1961–1971.
11. Goldstein DS. *Hypertension* 1983;5:86–99.
12. Wallin BG, Sundlöf. *Hypertension* 1979;1:67–77.
13. Somers VK, Mark AL, Abboud FM. *Hypertension* 1988;11:608–612.
14. Rea RF, Hamdan. *Circulation* 1990;82:856–862.
15. Anderson EA, Sinkey CA, Lawton WJ, Mark AL. *Hypertension* 1989;14:177–183.
16. Miyajima E, Yamada Y, Yoshida Y, Matsukawa T, Shionoiri H, Tochikubo O, Ishii M. *Hypertension* 1991;17:1057–1062.
17. Matsukawa T, Gotoh E, Hasegawa O, Miyajima E, Shionoiri H, Tochikubo O, Ishii M. *Funct Neurol* 1991;6:113–120.
18. Matsukawa T, Gotoh E, Uneda S, Miyajima E, Shionoiri H, Tochikubo O, Ishii M. *Acta Physiol Scand* 1991;141:157–165.
19. Yamada Y, Miyajima E, Tochikubo O, Matsukawa T, Ishii M. *Hypertension* 1989;13:870–877.
20. Floras JS, Hara K. *J Hypertens* 1993;11:647–655.
21. Randin D, Vollenweider P, Tappy L, Jequier E, Nicod P, Scherrer U. *Diabetes* 1993;42:96A (abstract).
22. Andersson B, Elam M, Wallin BG, Bjorntorp P, Andersson OK. *Hypertension* 1991;18:783–789.
23. Egan B, Panis R, Hinderliter A, Schork N, Julius S. *J Clin Invest* 1987;80:812–817.
24. Matsukawa T, Mano T, Gotoh E, Ishii M. *J Clin Invest* 1993;92:25–28.
25. Williams GH, Hollenberg NK. *Am J Med* 1985;79:3–9.
26. Conlin PR, Braley LM, Menachery AI, Hollenberg NK, Williams GH. *J Clin Endocrinol Metab* 1992;75:1017–1021.
27. Ng AN, Callister R, Johnson DG, Seals DR. *Hypertension* 1993;21:498–503.
28. Yamada Y, Miyajima E, Tochikubo O, Matsukawa T, Ishii M. *Hypertension* 1989;13:870–877.
29. Whelton PK, Klag MJ. *Hypertension* 1989;13:I19–I27.
30. Falkner B, Kushner H, Onesti G, Angelakos ET. *Hypertension* 1981;3:521–527.
31. Murphy JK, Alpert BS, Moes DM, Somes GW. *Hypertension* 1980;2:686–694.
32. Thomas J, Semenya K, Thomas CB, Thomas DJ, Neser WB, Pearson TA, Gillum RF. *J Chronic Dis* 1987;40:721–727.

33. Anderson NB, Myers HF, Pickering T, Jackson JS. *J Hypertens* 1989;7:161–172.
34. Anderson NB, Lane JD, Muranaka M, Williams RB Jr, Houseworth SJ. *Psychosom Med* 1988;50:57–63.
35. Calhoun DA, Mutinga ML, Collins AS, Wyss JM, Oparil S. *Hypertension* 1993;22:801–805.
36. Calhoun DA. *Am J Med Sci* 1992;304:306–311.
37. Folkow BS. *Physiol Rev* 1982;62:347–504.
38. Parmer RJ, Cervenka JH, Stone RA, O'Connor DT. *Circulation* 1990;81:1305–1311.
39. Gordon RD, Backmann AW, Jackson RV, Saar N. *Clin Exp Pharmacol Physiol* 1982;9:277–281.
40. Mion D Jr, Rea RF, Anderson EA, Kahn D, Sinkey C, Mark AL. *Hypertension* 1994:23:123–130.
41. Rostand SG, Brunzell JD, Cannon RO III, Victor RG. *J Am Soc Nephrol* 1991;2:1053–1062.
42. Zucchelli P, Zuccala A. In: Cameron S, Davison AM, Grunfeld J-P, Ritz E, eds. *Textbook of clinical nephrology,* vol 2. Oxford: Oxford University Press, 1992;1458–1467.
43. Converse RL Jr, Jacobsen TN, Toto RD, Jost CMT, Csentino F, Fouad-Tarazi F, Victor RG. *N Engl J Med* 1992;327:1912–1918.
44. Cohen DJ, Loertscher R, Rubin MF, Tilney NL, Carpenter CB, Strom TB. *Ann Intern Med* 1884;101:667–682.
45. Kahan BD, ed. *Cyclosporine: application in autoimmune diseases.* Philadelphia: Grune and Stratton, 1988;3–383.
46. Joss DV, Barrett AJ, Kedra JR, Lucas CF, Desai S. *Lancet* 1982;1:906.
47. Reece DE, Frei-Lahr DA, Sheperd JD, Dorovini-Zis K, Gascoyne RD, Graeb DA, Spinelli JJ, Barnett MJ, Klingemann HG, Herzig GP, et al. *Bone Marrow Transplant* 1991;8:393–401.
48. Thompson ME, Shapiro AP, Johnsen AM, Reeves R, Itzkoff J, Ginchereau E, Hardesty RL, Griffith BP, Bahnson HT, McDonald R Jr. *Transplant Proc* 1983;15(suppl 1):2573–2577.
49. Schachter M. *J Hypertens* 1988;6:511–516.
50. Curtis JJ. *J Am Soc Nephrol* 1992;2(suppl 12):S243–S245.
51. Olivari MT, Antolick A, Ring WS. *J Heart Transplant* 1989;8:34–39.
52. Murray BM, Paller MS, Ferris TF. *Kidney Int* 1985;28:767–774.
53. Moss NG, Powell SL, Falk RJ. *Proc Natl Acad Sci USA* 1985;82:8222–8226.
54. Thomson SC, Tucker BJ, Gabbai F, Blantz RC. *J Clin Invest* 1989;83:960–969.
55. Morgan BJ, Lyson T, Scherrer U, Victor RG. *Hypertension* 1991;18:458–466.
56. Chiu PJ, Vemulapalli S, Sabin C, Rivelli M, Bernardino V, Sybertz EJ. *J Pharmacol Exp Ther* 1992;261:994–999.
57. Scherrer U, Vissing SF, Morgan BJ, Rollins JA, Tindall RSA, Ring S, Hanson P, Mohanty PK, Victor RG. *N Engl J Med* 1990;323:693–699.
58. Lyson T, Morgan BJ, Scherrer U, Victor RG. (Unpublished observation.)
59. Seals DS, Suwarno NO, Joyner MJ, Iber C, Copeland JG, Dempsey JA. *Circ Res* 1993;72:440–454.
60. Kaye D, Thompson J, Jennings G, Esler M. *Circulation* 1993;88:1101–1109.
61. Elam M, Casale R, La Rovere M-T, Mortara A, Tavazzi L. *Eur Heart J* 1993;14:521–525.
62. Jacobsen TN, Snyder RW II, Grayburn PA, Lange RA, Lyson T, Victor RG. *Circulation* 1993;88:1–85.
63. Aksamit TR, Floras JS, Victor RG, Aylward PE. *Hypertension* 1987;9:309–314.
64. Robertson D, Hollister AS, Biaggioni I, Netterville JL, Mosqueda-Garcia R, Robertson RM. *N Engl J Med* 1993;329:1449–1455.
65. Faguis J, Wallin BG, Sundlöf G, Nerhed C, Engelsson S. *Brain* 1985;108:335–350.
66. Hornyak M, Cejuar M, Elam M, Matousek M, Wallin BG. *Brain* 1991;114:1281–1295.
67. Somers VK, Dyken ME, Mark AL, Abboud FM. *N Engl J Med* 1993;328:303–307.
68. Hedner J, Ejnell H, Sellgren J, Hedner T, Wallin G. *J Hypertens* 1988;6:S529–S531.
69. Somers VK, Dyken ME, Abboud FM. *Circulation* 1993;88:1–9.
70. Crabtree D, Morgan B, Skatrud J. *Am Rev Respir Dis* 1993;147:A1015.
71. Guo GB, Thames MD, Abboud FM. *Circ Res* 1983;53:223–234.
72. Mancia G, Ferrari L, Gregorini G, Parati G, Ferrari MC, Pomidossi G, Zanchetti A. *Am J Cardiol* 1979;44:895–902.
73. Mark AL. *Hypertension* 1991;17:186–190.
74. Parmer RJ, Cervenka JH, Stone RA. *Circulation* 1992;85:497–503.
75. Mark AL, Kerber RE. *Hypertension* 1982;4:39–46.
76. Victor RG, Morgan BJ. *Circulation* 1990;82:1057–1059.
77. Przybylski J, Trzebski A, Czyzewski T, Jodkowski J. *Bull Eur Physiopathol Respir* 1982;18:145–154.
78. Fukuda Y, Sato A, Trzebski A. *J Auton Nerv Syst* 1987;19:1–11.
79. Trzebski A, Tafil M, Zoltowski M, Przybylski J. *Cardiovasc Rev* 1982;16:163–172.
80. Somers VK, Mark AL, Abboud FM. *J Clin Invest* 1991;87:1953–1957.
81. Katholi RE, Whitlow PL, Hageman GR, Woods WT. *J Hypertens* 1984;2:349–359.
82. Recordati G, Moss NG, Genovesi S, Rogenes P. *J Auton Nerv Syst* 1981;3:327–351.
83. DiBona GF. *Rev Physiol Biochem Pharmacol* 1982;94:76–181.
84. Faber JE, Brody MJ. *Circ Res* 1985;57:676–688.
85. Katholi RE, Winternitz SR, Oparil S. *J Clin Invest* 1982;69:55–62.
86. Kopp UC. *J Hypertens* 1993;11:765–773.
87. Rowe JW, Young JB, Minaker KL, Stevens AL, Pallotta J, Landsberg L. *Diabetes* 1983;30:219–225.
88. Anderson EA, Balon TW, Hoffman RP, Sinkey CA, Mark AL. *Hypertension* 1992;19:621–627.
89. Berne C, Fagius J, Pollari T, Gjemdahl P. *Diabetologia* 1992;35:873–879.
90. Vollenweider P, Randin D, Tappy L, Jequier E, Nicod P, Scherrer U. *Hypertension* 1993;22:451.
91. Morgan DA, Balon TW, Ginsberg BH, Mark AL. *Am J Physiol* 1993;33:R423–R427.
92. Regolli D, Park WK, Rioux F. *Pharmacol Rev* 1974;26:69–123.
93. Matsukawa T, Gotoh E, Miyajima E, Yamada Y, Shionoiri H, Tochikubo O, Ishi M. *J Hypertens* 1988;6:S501–S504.
94. Floras JS. *Hypertension* 1992;19:1–18.
95. Persson B, Adersson OK, Hjemdahl P, Wysocki M, Agerwall S, Wallin G. *J Hypertens* 1989;7:747–756.
96. Bredt DS, Hwang PM, Synder SH. *Nature* 1990;347:768–770.
97. Iadecola C, Faris PL, Hartman BK, Xu X. *Brain Res* 1993;603:173–179.
98. Sakuma I, Togashi H, Yoshioka M, Saito H, Yanagida M, Tamura M, Kobayashi T, Yasuda H, Gross S, Levi R. *Circ Res* 1992;70:607–611.
99. Togashi H, Sakuma I, Yoshioka M, Kobayashi T, Yasuda H, Kitabatake A, Saito H, Gross SS, Levi R. *J Pharmacol Exp Ther* 1992;262:343–347.
100. Shapoval LN, Sagach VF, Pobegailo LS. *Neurosci Lett* 1991;132:47–50.
101. Harada S, Tokunaga S, Momahara M, Masaki H, Tagawa T, Imaizumi T, Takeshita A. *Circ Res* 1993;72:511–516.
102. Toda N, Kitamurea Y, Okamurura T. *Hypertension* 1993;21:3–8.
103. Garthwaite J, Charles SL, Chess-Williams R. *Nature* 1988;336:385–388.
104. DiPaola ED, Vidal MJ, Nisitico G. *J Cardiovasc Pharm* 1991;17:S269–S272.
105. Panza JA, Casino PR, Kilcoyne CM, Quyyumi AA. *Circulation* 1993;87:1468–1474.
106. Vallance P, Leone A, Calver A, Collier J, Moncada S. *Lancet* 1992;339:572–575.
107. Lyson T, Ermel LD, Belshaw PJ, Alberg DG, Schreiber SL, Victor RG. *Circ Res* 1993;73:596–602.
108. Sigal NH, Dumont FJ, Durette P, Sierkierka JJ, Peterson L, Rich DH, Dunlap BE, Staruch MJ, Melino MR, Koprak S, et al. *J Exp Med* 1991;173:619.
109. Dumont FJ, Staruch MJ, Koprak SL, Siekierka JJ, Lin CS, Harrison R, Sewell T, Kindt VM, Beattie TR, Wyvratt M, Sigal NH. *J Exp Med* 1992;176:751–760.

110. Spencer DM, Wandless TJ, Schreiber SL, Crabtree GR. *Science* 1993;262:1019–1024.
111. Schreiber SL. *Science* 1991;251:283–287.
112. Liu J, Farmer JD Jr, Lane WS, Friedman J, Weissman I, Schreiber SL. *Cell* 1991;66:807–815.
113. Clipstone NA, Crabtree GR. *Nature* 1992;357:695–697.
114. O'Keefe SJ, Tamura J, Kincaid RL, Tocci MJ, O'Neill EA. *Nature* 1991;357:692–694.
115. Klee CB, Crouch TH, Krinks MH. *Proc Natl Acad Sci USA* 1979;76:6270–6273.
116. Steiner JP, Dawson TM, Fotuhi M, Glatt CE, Snowman AM, Cohen N, Snyder SH. *Nature* 1992;358:584–587.
117. Chad JE, Eckert R. *J Physiol (Lond)* 1986;378:31–51.
118. Armstrong DL. *Trends Neurosci* 1989;12:117–122.
119. Williams PD, Puddey IB, Beilin LJ, Vandongen R. *J Clin Endocrinol Metab* 1993;77:794–799.
120. Wallin BG, Kunimoto MM, Sellgren J. *Hypertension* 1993;22:282–284.
121. Mark AL. *N Engl J Med* 1990;323:748–750.
122. Abboud FM. *Hypertension* 1982;4:II208–225.
123. DiBona GF. *Am J Hypertens* 1989;2:119S–124S.
124. Bevan RD. *Hypertension* 1984;6:III-19–III-26.
125. Hart MN, Heistad DD, Brody MJ. *Hypertension* 1980;2:419–423.
126. Brickner ME, Willard JE, Eichorn EJ, Black J, Grayburn PA. *Circulation* 1991;84:1130–1135.
127. Jost CMT, Cigarroa CG, Cooley R, Grayburn PA, Victor RG. *Circulation* 1992;86:I-678.
128. Cigarrora CG, Boehrer JD, Brickner ME, Eichhorn EJ, Grayburn PA. *Circulation* 1992;86:226–231.
129. Korner PI, Bobik A, Angus JA, Adams MA, Friberg P. *J Hypertens* 1989;7:S125–S134.
130. Abel PW, Hermsmeyer K. *Circ Res* 1981;49:1311–1318.

Hypertension: Pathophysiology, Diagnosis, and Management, Second Edition,
edited by J.H. Laragh and B.M. Brenner,
Raven Press, Ltd., New York © 1995.

CHAPTER **52**

Possible Role of the Parasympathetic System in the Pathogenesis and Treatment of Hypertensive Vascular Disease

Peter A. van Zwieten, Maarten G. C. Hendriks, and Tobias A. Bruning

There is little doubt that the pathogenesis of essential hypertension (EHT) is strongly influenced by the autonomic nervous system. In addition, drug treatment of EHT is also based in many cases on the interference of antihypertensive drugs with the sympathetic nervous system. Although still subject to some debate in certain details, evidence for an important role of the sympathetic nervous system in the pathogenesis and maintenance may be summarized as follows. The "excitatory psychoemotional influences" proposed by Folkow (1) to be an important stimulus that may reinforce or sometimes precipitate primary hypertension in persons with a genetic predisposition are now being linked to episodic increases in plasma adrenaline (2). Accordingly, the role of adrenaline released from the adrenal medulla in the genesis of EHT has become an acceptable hypothesis (2). EHT is not associated with a consistent elevation of plasma catecholamines, but there is a clearly increased spillover of noradrenaline from the synapses into the circulating blood of patients with EHT (3). Recently, the hypothesis was put forward (4) that this process is governed by the central nervous system and possibly deranged in hypertensives. More recently, increased sympathetic firing in the neurons of persons with EHT has been established and this finding may be considered as rather direct evidence in favor of a major role of the sympathetic nervous system in EHT (5). Finally, the vascular system of hypertensive humans and animals is known to be hypersensitive to various categories of pressor agents, including α-adrenoceptor stimulants (6).

In an earlier stage it was already clear that several types

P. A. van Zwieten: Departments of Pharmacotherapy and Cardiology, Academic Medical Center, University of Amsterdam, 1105 AZ Amsterdam, The Netherlands.

M. G. C. Hendriks: Department of Pharmacotherapy, Academic Medical Center, University of Amsterdam, 1105 AZ Amsterdam, The Netherlands.

T. A. Bruning: Department of Pharmacotherapy, Academic Medical Center, University of Amsterdam, 1105 AZ Amsterdam, The Netherlands; and Department of Nephrology, University Hospital, 2333 AA Leiden, The Netherlands.

of antihypertensive drugs exert their effects on the cardiovascular system by depressing the activity of the sympathetic nervous system and/or its sequelae. In fact, any element of the sympathetic system can be influenced by drugs: at the central nervous level (central α_2-adrenoceptor stimulants, which depress peripheral sympathetic activity, such as clonidine and α-methyldopa); at the sympathetic ganglia (ganglioplegic agents); at postganglionic sympathetic neurons (peripheral neuron blockers like guanethidine, etc.); by depletion of the intracellular noradrenaline stores (reserpine); and at the level of peripheral adrenoceptors (α- and β-adrenoceptor blocking agents) (7).

Until very recently our research and thinking concerning the role of the autonomic nervous system was merely focused on the sympathetic circuit. However, the autonomic nervous system is composed of both the sympathetic and parasympathetic circuits, which are assumed to maintain equilibrium and homeostasis by means of their mutual, functional antagonism. The emphasis on the sympathetic circuit of the autonomic nervous system is understandable for several reasons. First, sympathetic activation has been known for a long time to be a hypertensive mechanism. Second, the sympathetic system and its various components and elements, including neurotransmitters, adrenoceptors, and even neuronal activity, can be investigated with great sophistication. Finally, as stated above, classical drug therapy of EHT is to a major degree based on compounds that somehow depress sympathetic activation and its sequelae—it is only for a decade now that drugs with other mechanisms such as calcium antagonists or angiotensin-converting enzyme (ACE) inhibitors have played an important role in antihypertensive treatment, and even these newer drugs may interact with certain elements of the sympathetic system in addition to their primary modes of action (8). Another reason why much less attention has been paid to the parasympathetic system is the fact that it is notoriously difficult to obtain quantitative information on parasympathetic neuronal activity *in vivo* (9). Furthermore, drugs interacting with the parasympathetic system have not been developed in such a sophisticated manner as those aiming at the sympathetic neurons and adrenoceptors; no "parasympathetic" drug is known to be a useful antihypertensive.

However, modern developments in the research on the parasympathetic nervous system and drugs interacting with this system have led to a renaissance of interest in its possible role in the pathogenesis, maintenance, and treatment of EHT.

The major innovations in the parasympathetic field, to be discussed below in more detail, may be summarized as follows:

1. the discovery that the vasodilator effect of acetylcholine (ACh) is mediated by endothelium-derived relaxing factor (EDRF) and hence involves the nitric oxide (NO) pathway (10);
2. the much improved knowledge of muscarinic cholinergic receptors and their subtypes, and the development of selective antagonists of certain muscarinic receptor subtypes;
3. improved possibilities for the assessment of parasympathetic neuronal activity *in vivo*.

Before dealing with the role of the parasympathetic nervous system in EHT, we shall briefly summarize the modern insights in these fields of research on the parasympathetic system.

MODERN DEVELOPMENTS IN RESEARCH ON THE PARASYMPATHETIC NERVOUS SYSTEM

Cholinergic Receptors and the NO Pathway

As to be discussed below, acetylcholine (ACh), the neurotransmitter in the parasympathetic nervous system, is a nonselective agonist of the various types of muscarinic (M) receptors. Under *in vivo* conditions ACh will predominantly act as a *vasodilator*. As shown by Furchgott and Zawadski (10), this vasodilator effect requires the presence of endothelial lining. Upon stimulation with ACh the endothelial cells will release EDRF, which was later shown to consist of NO. NO stimulates the enzyme guanylate cyclase and thus enhances the formation of the endogenous vasodilator cyclic guanosine monophosphate (cGMP) (Fig. 1). This indirect vasodilatation caused by ACh has now been recognized as a most important route of signal transduction and it is generally known as the NO pathway (11–13). Functional studies in isolated vessels strongly suggest that the release of EDRF (NO) and hence the vasodilator effect of ACh is mediated by muscarinic receptors of the M_3 type.

In reality the matter is even more complicated. Stimulation of arterial tissue with muscarinic agonists may also result in membrane hyperpolarization of vascular smooth muscle cells, a response that also requires an intact vascular endothelium (14). Several studies have shown that neither endogenous vasodilators nor NO per se provoke membrane hyperpolarization (14). These data suggest that EDRF is not the only endogenous substance released by the vascular endothelium. For this reason the existence of endothelium-derived hyperpolarizing factor (EDHF), a yet-unidentified factor that mediates smooth muscle hyperpolarization and thus vasodilatation, has been proposed.

The direct stimulation of M_1 and possibly also M_3-receptors on vascular smooth muscle cells may also cause vasoconstriction, particularly in vascular preparations of venous origin. ACh may also induce activation of the sympathetic stimuli via the excitation of presynaptic M-receptors.

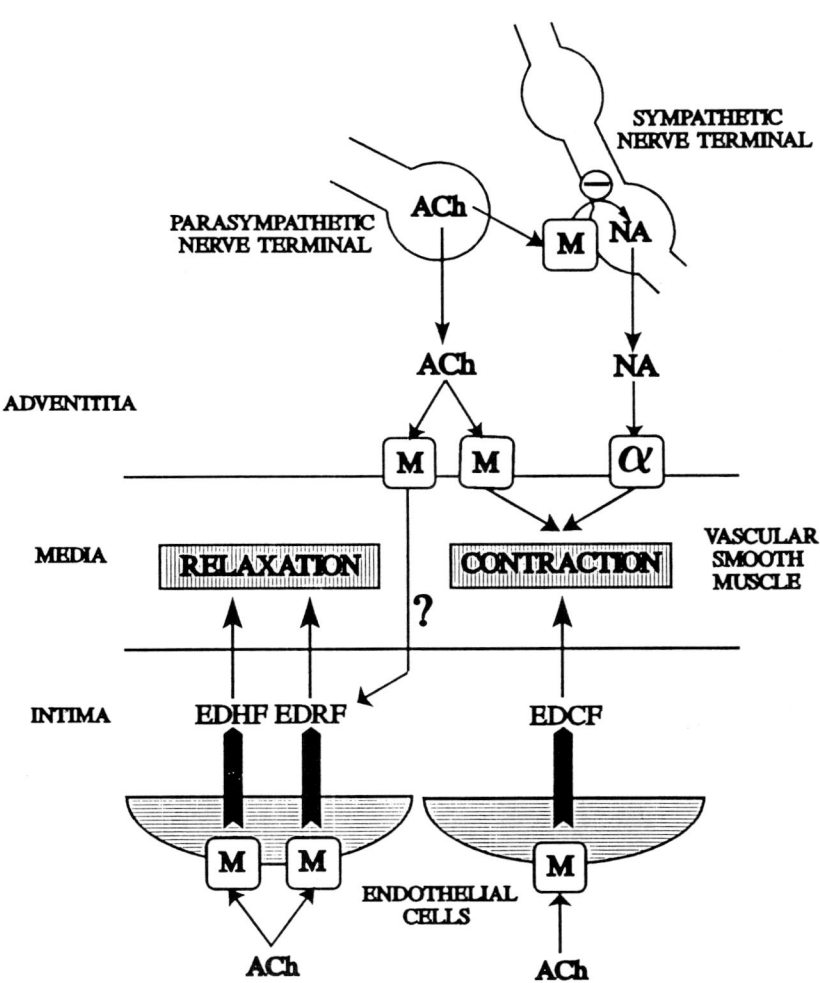

FIG. 1. Schematic representation of the events that take place upon stimulation of the muscarinic receptor in the vascular smooth muscle and the interaction with the sympathetic nervous system. Acetylcholine stimulates muscarinic receptors present in the endothelium, which results in the liberation of EDRF and EDHF, which in turn cause relaxation of the smooth muscle. At the same time another process may take place: acetylcholine may also stimulate another receptor on the endothelium, which may cause smooth muscle contraction via EDCF release. Via stimulation of muscarinic receptors on the sympathetic nervous system, the release of noradrenaline is blocked.

It should be emphasized, however, that the predominant effect of ACh, the result of parasympathetic neuronal activity, is expressed by vasodilatation, mediated by endothelial M_3-receptors and the NO pathway.

Muscarinic Cholinergic Receptors: Agonists and Antagonists

A major innovation in the field of the cholinergic nervous system is the discovery of several subpopulations of muscarinic receptors. Concomitantly, attempts have been made to develop agonists and antagonists that may be selective for particular muscarinic receptor subpopulations, and indeed several compounds that fulfill these conditions are beginning to emerge, especially with respect to the receptor antagonists.

Cholinergic receptors have traditionally been subdivided into muscarinic and nicotinic subtypes owing to the classical work of Sir Henry Dale. The parasympathetic system is intricately associated with muscarinic receptors, which are stimulated by ACh (the neurotransmitter) and by synthetic parasympathomimetic drugs. It is now known that the muscarinic receptors are subdivided into at least three functional subtypes, M_1, M_2, and M_3, and very recently a fourth subtype, M_4, has been submitted to exist (15–18). By means of molecular biological cloning techniques, five molecular subtypes (m_1, m_2, m_3, m_4, m_5) have been identified and analyzed; three of these (m_1, m_2, m_3) correspond to the functional receptors M_1, M_2, M_3, whereas the functional relevance of the m_4 and m_5 structures so far remains unknown (18). The tissues and organs where the various M-receptors have been demonstrated to occur are listed in Table 1. The functional sequelae of stimulation or blockade of these receptor subtypes by appropriate agonists and antagonists are also shown in this table.

A few examples of muscarinic receptor agonists and antagonists of particular M-receptor subtypes are given in Table 2. The overall picture concerning the selectivity of drugs for M-receptor subtypes may be summarized as follows: ACh, the endogenous neurotransmitter and most of the classical parasympathomimetic drugs, such as carbachol, aceclidine, pilocarpine, arecoline, acetyl-β-methacholine and muscarine, are nonselective, which means that they will stimulate several or all M-receptor

TABLE 1. *Various types of muscarinic receptors in different tissues; and the effects of receptor stimulation and blockade by appropriate agonists and antagonists*

Receptor type	Organ/tissue	Stimulation (agonist)	Blockade (antagonist)
M_1	Neurons, ganglia (sympathetic)	Excitation, NA-release ↑	Depression, NA-release ↓
M_2	Heart, coronary arteries	Bradycardia, contractility ↓, contraction	Tachycardia, contractility ↑, relaxation
M_3	Glands, ileum, vessels	Secretion ↑, contraction, relaxation (via EDRF)	Secretion ↓, relaxation

subtypes simultaneously. The experimental compounds McN-A-343, isoarecaidine, and SDZ ENZ 163 display moderate selectivity for M_1-receptors, in particular those in the brain. There is interest in such compounds as a potential treatment of Alzheimer's disease. The compound L-660,863 is assumed to display some selectivity for the M_2-receptor. Selective M_3-receptor agonists are so far not available.

Atropine is the best known nonselective antagonist for the various M-receptor subtypes. Pirenzepine is moderately selective for the M_1-subtype, whereas AF-DX 116, AQ-RA 741, himbacine, and methoctramine are selective for the M_2-subtype. The compounds p-F-HHSiD and to a lesser degree 4-DAMP are selective antagonists for M_3-receptors but they also possess affinity for the M_1 receptor. (For reviews on M-receptors and associated drugs see refs. 15–18.) For chemical structures see Fig. 2.

Biochemical studies have indicated that muscarinic (M_2)-receptors are coupled to adenylate cyclase. In contrast to β-adrenoceptors, which are also coupled to adenylate cyclase, muscarinic receptor stimulation is inhibitory as a result of its involvement of an inhibitory Gi protein, thus causing a decrease in the cellular concentration of cAMP (18).

As in the sympathetic system, the existence of presynaptic muscarinic receptors, besides those at postsynaptic sites, has been demonstrated. Presynaptic M-receptors are assumed to modulate the release of ACh from the parasympathetic nerve endings.

TABLE 2. *Selective antagonists for muscarinic receptor subtypes*

Receptor subtypes	Antagonists
M_1	Pirenzepine
	Telenzepine
M_2	AF-DX 116; AF-DX 237; AQ-RA 741
	Himbacine
	Gallamine
	Pancuronium
	Methoctramine
M_3	4-diphenylacetoxy-N-methylpiperidine (4-DAMP)
	p-F-hexahydro-sila-difenidol (p-FHHSiD)

Potential Therapeutic Use of Selective Muscarinic Receptor Agonists and Antagonists

As mentioned above, there is potential interest in selective M_1-receptor stimulants (such as McN-A-343) for the treatment of Alzheimer's disease. Selective M_2-receptor agonists might be of potential use to reduce heart rate and arteriovenous (A-V) conduction without being accompanied by the well-known side effects of the beta blockers. Selective M_3-receptor stimulants, as yet not available, would be of potential interest as vasodilators and antihypertensives.

Pirenzepine is a selective M_1-receptor antagonist that is used in the treatment of peptic ulcers (17). At least on theoretical grounds such a compound would be preferable to a nonselective antagonist, such as atropine and related drugs. A selective M_2-receptor antagonist might be of use in patients with A-V block; such a drug would act similarly to atropine, without being accompanied by the various noncardiac side effects (ocular, glandular, gastrointestinal, and urogenital). It has been demonstrated that coronary spasm as in Prinzmetal's angina may be governed by parasympathetic activation, probably involving both M_2- and M_3-receptors (19). Again selective antagonists of these two receptor subtypes might be of potential therapeutic value and at least preferable to the nonselective antagonist atropine. With the exception of pirenzepine, none of the more or less selective M-receptor agonists and antagonists has passed the experimental stage.

Assessment of Parasympathetic Activity *in Vivo*

In contrast to the sympathetic neuronal activity, where great progress has been made with respect to its recording *in vivo,* it still remains notoriously difficult to assess and quantify the activity of the parasympathetic nervous system. In the adrenergic system the fate of the neurotransmitters noradrenaline and adrenaline (and their metabolites) can be established by analyzing them in biological fluids. However, this is virtually impossible for acetylcholine (ACh), the neurotransmitter of the cholinergic (parasympathetic) system, which is degraded extremely rapidly *in vivo* as a result of the influence of esterases.

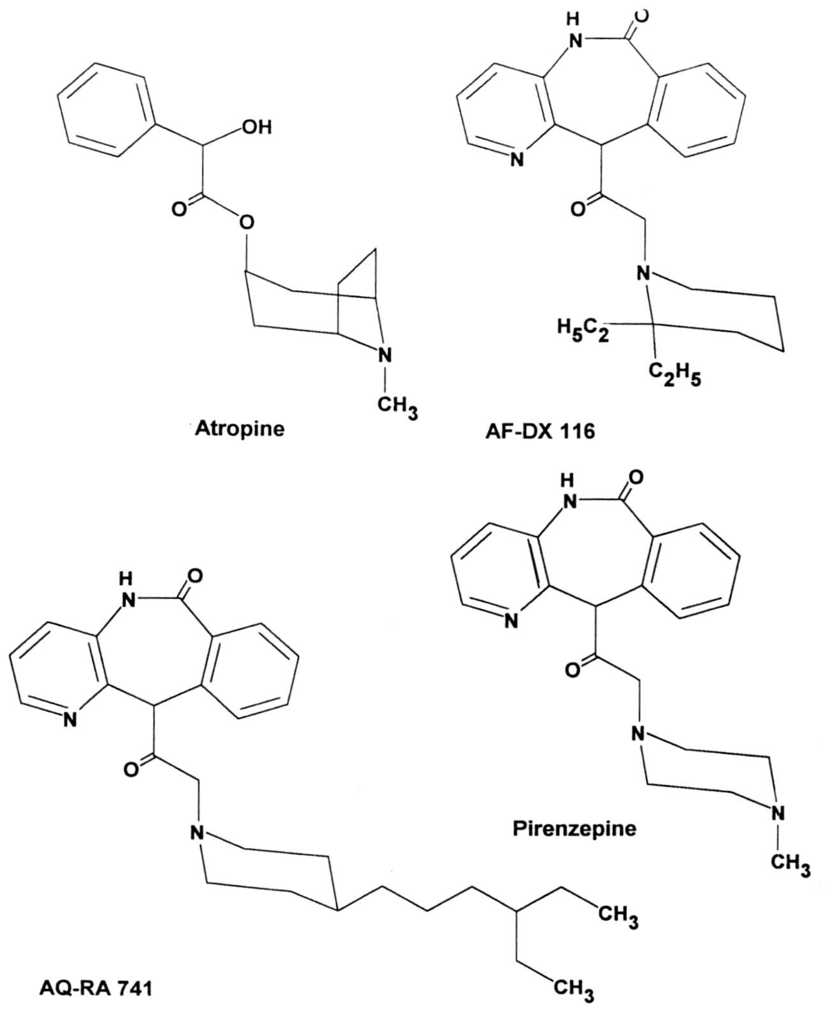

FIG. 2. Chemical structures of some selective and nonselective muscarinic receptor antagonists. Shown are atropine (nonselective), pirenzepine (M_1), AF-DX 116 and AQ-RA 741 (M_2).

Great progress has been made in the direct recording of electric activity of peripheral sympathetic neurons. However, the anatomical location and characteristics of peripheral parasympathetic nerves are such that direct recording, as for sympathetic neurons, hardly appears feasible with the techniques available at present. Indirect information concerning the functional activity of ACh and its possible alterations in disease can be obtained by studying the vasodilator effects of muscarinic receptor agonists, in particular vascular beds (Fig. 1). This vasodilator process may be classified as an indirect one, as discussed above. Indirect relaxation caused by the inhibition of sympathetic outflow has also been demonstrated in animal models and in man. There is no doubt that the vasodilatation caused by muscarinic receptor stimulation should be regarded as a major target of the parasympathetic system. The existence and functional relevance of muscarinic receptors in the human forearm vascular bed was recently confirmed by means of venous occlusion plethysmography (20). Several studies in animal models have already confirmed the presence and functional relevance of muscarinic receptors in various vascular beds, including resistance vessels (14,21–24). Indirect information concerning parasympathetic nervous activity can also be obtained by assessing salivary secretion (25). It should be realized, however, that salivary secretion is governed by the cranial parasympathetic nerves (facial and glossopharyngeal), which have little to do with the cardiovascular system.

More recently the measurement of heart rate variability by means of spectral analysis has become available as a more direct approach to assess parasympathetic activity *in vivo* (26), but the technique is sophisticated and only valid when applied by experienced experts.

POTENTIAL ROLE OF THE PARASYMPATHETIC NERVOUS SYSTEM IN EHT

It seems reasonable to assume that besides the sympathetic system its parasympathetic counterpart also plays

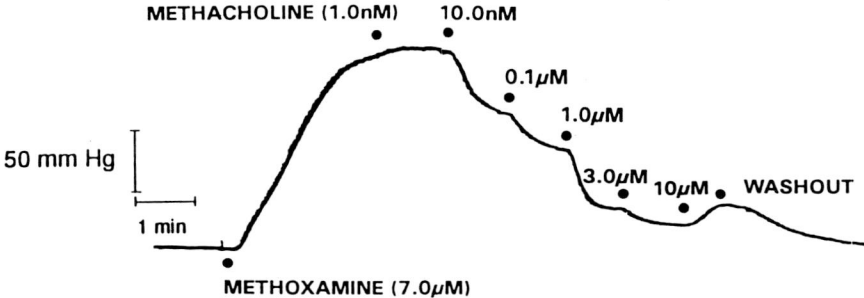

FIG. 3. Endothelium-dependent vaso-dilatation induced by the muscarinic agonist (acetyl-β) methacholine (MCh) in the perfused mesenteric vascular bed preparation taken from a normotensive Wistar-Kyoto rat. Original tracing. The preparations were precontracted with the α_1-adrenoceptor methoxamine and subsequently dilated with MCh. Removal of the endothelium abolishes the endothelium-dependent response.

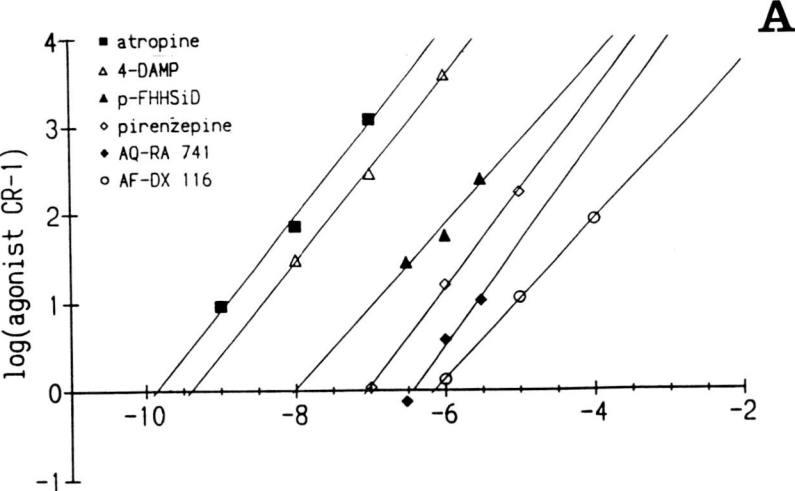

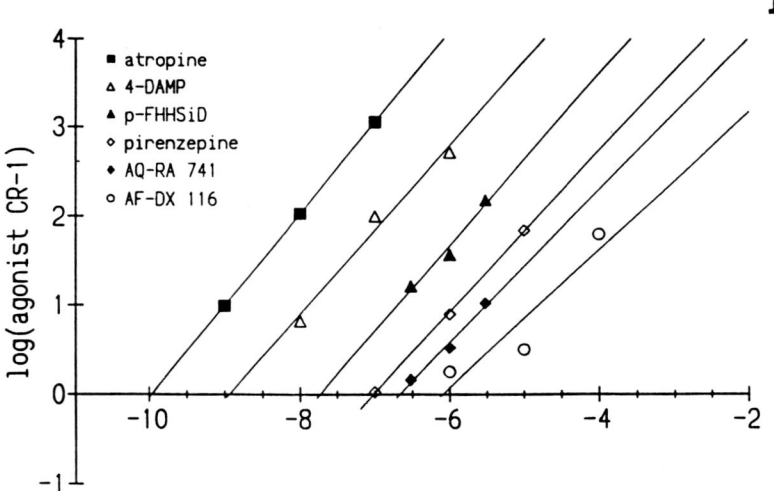

FIG. 4. Effects of various muscarinic receptor antagonists on methacholine-induced, endothelium-dependent vasodilatation in the perfused mesenteric vascular bed preparation (compare Fig. 3), obtained from normotensive Wistar-Kyoto rats (**A**), or from spontaneously hypertensive rats (SHR) (**B**), respectively. The effects of the muscarinic antagonists were quantified by means of Arunlakshana-Schild plots of log (dose-ratio-1) versus log (antagonist concentration). The rank order of pA_2 values, obtained from the X-intercept, for atropine (nonselective), pirenzepine (M_1), AF-DX 116 and AQ-RA 741 (M_2), and 4-DAMP and pFHHSiD (M_3), clearly indicates the presence of the M_3-subtype on the vascular endothelium for both types of preparations (A and B). Data from the authors' department.

a role in EHT. Even if there would be no change per se in the parasympathetic system associated with EHT, the sympathetic/parasympathetic tone ratio is bound to be altered in EHT, since it is now widely accepted that EHT is associated with elevated sympathetic neuronal activity.

Essential Hypertension and the NO Pathway

Soon after the discovery of the NO pathway attempts were made to evaluate its possible role in the pathogenesis and maintenance of EHT. Generalized endothelial damage was submitted as an important and possibly causative mechanism associated with the pathogenesis and maintenance of EHT. Endothelial dysfunction would logically lead to an impairment of the NO pathway and hence to reduced endogenous vasodilator mechanisms. Endothelial dysfunction was indeed demonstrated to occur in large conduit arteries of hypertensive animals. However, no such impairment could be found in resistance vessels of hypertensive rats and other species. Although endothelial dysfunction and an impairment of the NO pathway appear to offer an attractive hypothesis, this issue so far remains subject to controversy and debate (27–29).

Essential Hypertension and Muscarinic Receptors

Owing to the availability of selective muscarinic receptor antagonists for the various subtypes, it has been possible to characterize the M-receptor subtypes in various vascular beds. More recently, a few authors have studied possible changes of vascular M-receptors in the cardiovascular system of hypertensive animals. The results obtained so far may be summarized as follows: In large conduit arteries (aorta, middle cerebral artery, etc.) the M_3-receptor appears to be the predominant receptor subtype as concluded from functional studies with M-receptor subtype antagonists. The characteristics of this receptor are not clearly influenced by the hypertensive state, as concluded from experiments with isolated vessels taken from hypertensive animals (14,21). In isolated resistance arteries, investigated by means of the rat isolated perfused mesenteric arterial bed, the endothelium-mediated vasodilatation induced by ACh and related M-receptor agonists is mediated by the M_3-receptor subtype (Fig. 3). This vasodilatation was counteracted most effectively by M_3-receptor antagonists such as 4-DAMP and p-F-HHSiD, and much less so by pirenzepine (M_1), AF-DX 116, and AQ-RA 741 (both M_2) (14,21) (Fig. 4).

The same pattern was found in the vessels of spontaneously hypertensive rats, indicating that also in hypertensive animals the M_3-receptor subtype is predominant in a functional sense. In the forearm vascular bed of normotensive volunteers we recently demonstrated the

functional relevance of muscarinic receptors by means of venous occlusion plethysmography (20). Accordingly, the vasodilator effect of ACh and that of methacholine (a more stable, nonselective muscarinic receptor agonist) was quantified and then subjected to different types of M-receptor antagonists. A Schild analysis (Fig. 5) was performed, yielding the affinity constants. The affinity constants and rank order of potency of the antagonists, which is atropine (nonselective) > pirenzepine (M_1) > AF-DX 116 (M_2), indicate that cholinergic vasodilatation in this vascular bed is mediated by the M_3-receptor subtype. These experiments will be repeated in hypertensive patients in order to investigate the characteristics of the M-receptor in this vascular bed in the hypertensive state.

Parasympathetic Activity in Essential Hypertension

The few data available point toward a reduced parasympathetic activity in EHT. Accordingly, patients with hyperkinetic borderline hypertension showed a smaller increase in heart rate and cardiac output to atropine than did normotensive controls (30). This finding reflects a diminished basal level of cardiac parasympathetic inhibition. A similar decrease in parasympathetic tone was also found in patients with a normal cardiac output and

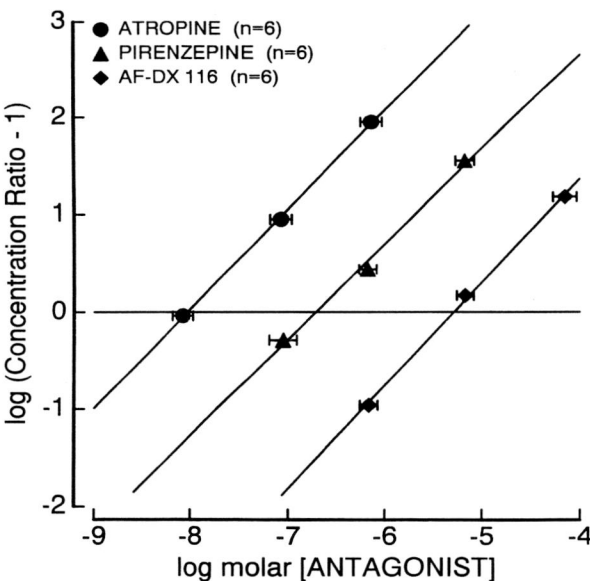

FIG. 5. Schild regressions based on calculated plasma concentrations of the nonselective muscarinic antagonist atropine (pA$_2$ of 8.03 ± 0.03), the M$_1$-selective antagonist pirenzepine (pA$_2$ of 6.71 ± 0.08), and the M$_2$-selective antagonist AF-DX 116 (pA$_2$ of 5.32 ± 0.05), against the methacholine-induced vasodilator response in the human forearm. The affinity constants and rank order of potency—atropine > pirenzepine > AF-DX 116—indicate that cholinergic vasodilatation in this vascular bed is mediated by the M$_3$-receptor subtype (data given in mean ± SEM). Data from the authors' department.

borderline hypertension (31) as well as in patients with established EHT (32).

Spectral analysis of heart rate variability in EHT patients also indicated a reduced parasympathetic activity (26). Bohm et al. (30) found diminished salivary flow rates in patients with borderline hypertension, indicating that the reduction of parasympathetic activity is not limited to the cardiovascular system.

ANTIHYPERTENSIVE DRUGS AND THE PARASYMPATHETIC SYSTEM

Established Antihypertensive Drugs

Several of the older antihypertensive drugs are known to cause adverse reactions that reflect a relative increase in parasympathetic nervous activity, indirectly caused by reduced sympathetic tone. The enhanced parasympathetic activity caused by such drugs includes, for instance, congestion of the nasal mucosa, diarrhea, nausea, and bradycardia. Such adverse reactions are known, for instance, for reserpine, guanethidine, and for the ganglionic blocking agents, all of which reduce sympathetic tone, although via different mechanisms (33).

In addition the ganglionic blocking agents cause direct impairment of peripheral parasympathetic tone as a result of the blockade of parasympathetic ganglia. This effect is counteracted by the simultaneous impairment of sympathetic ganglionic blockade, which is in fact the basis of the therapeutic activity of these old antihypertensive drugs (33).

Regular physical exercise, although not a drug, is known to moderately lower elevated blood pressure and as such is generally recommended as part of the basal, nondrug treatment of EHT. It is a well-known fact that regular physical exercise will shift the parasympathetic/sympathetic tone ratio toward the parasympathetic component. This shift may be the explanation for the blood pressure–lowering effect of this type of intervention.

The currently used antihypertensive drugs, such as beta blockers, diuretics, ACE inhibitors, calcium antagonists, and selective α_1-adrenoceptor antagonists (α_1-blockers) do not directly or indirectly interfere with the parasympathetic nervous system and its receptors.

Drugs Interacting with the Parasympathetic Nervous System as Potential Antihypertensives

If we assume that decreased parasympathetic tone is associated with EHT, this abnormality of autonomic nervous activity may be thought of as a basis for antihypertensive therapy. We already mentioned the beneficial influence of physical exercise in this connection. However, antihypertensive drugs based upon activation of the parasympathetic system still appear to be very remote.

From a theoretical point of view the activation of vascular M_3-receptors with highly selective agonists would be a potential option. Such compounds are unavailable at present, but their design is not necessarily impossible. For such new compounds it will be mandatory to eliminate the various unpleasant gastrointestinal, urogenital, glandular, and ocular side effects caused by the stimulation of M_1- and M_2-receptors. An additional possibility would be the addition of selective M_1- and/or M_2-receptor antagonists to the treatment with an M_3-receptor agonist. Selective M_1- and/or M_2-receptor antagonists, which are indeed available at present, could eliminate the aforementioned undesired effects outside the cardiovascular system.

CONCLUSIONS AND PERSPECTIVES

The evidence for a pathogenetic role of the parasympathetic system in EHT is concluded mostly from indirect experimental approaches. In spite of this the opinion is growing that the parasympathetic system tends to be less active in EHT patients than in normotensives. Even clearer is the shift toward enhanced sympathetic over parasympathetic activity, since evidence for sympathetic hyperactivity in EHT becomes more and more convincing. The sympathetic/parasympathetic activity ratio appears to be changed more clearly than that of the individual components alone. Research in the parasympathetic system, long neglected and subject to stagnation, has now been revived for the reasons discussed above. Muscarinic receptor pharmacology, which has led to the discovery of several interesting new agents, also touches hypertension research. The same holds for the interesting link between vasodilatation caused by ACh (the neurotransmitter in the parasympathetic nervous system) and the recently discovered, highly important NO pathway. Unfortunately, the direct assessment of parasympathetic activity *in vivo* so far remains virtually impossible.

The beneficial effect of physical exercise on EHT as well as the adverse reactions to several older antihypertensive drugs can be readily explained on the basis of alterations in the sympathetic/parasympathetic tone ratio. However, new therapeutic options based on parasympathetic mechanisms are still remote, but not impossible.

In conclusion, it now seems worthwhile to pay more attention in hypertension research to the parasympathetic system, its associated receptors, and drugs acting thereupon (34,35).

REFERENCES

1. Folkow B. Physiological aspects of primary hypertension. *Physiol Rev* 1982;62:347–504.
2. Floras JS. Epinephrine and the genesis of hypertension. *Hypertension* 1992;19:1–18.

3. Julius S, Johnson EH. Stress, autonomic hyperactivity and essential hypertension. An enigma. *J Hypertens* 1985;3(suppl 4):S11–S17.

4. Ferrier L, Esker MD, Eisenhofer G, et al. Increased norepinephrine spillover into the jugular veins in essential hypertension. *Hypertension* 1992;19:62–69.

5. Julius S. Changing role of the autonomic nervous system. *J Hypertens* 1990;8(suppl 7):S59–S65.

6. Van Zwieten PA. Antihypertensive drugs interacting with the sympathetic nervous system and its receptors. In: Antonaccio MJ, ed. *Cardiovascular drug Therapy,* 3rd ed. New York: Raven Press, 1990;37–73.

7. Van Zwieten PA. General introduction: the classification of antihypertensive drugs. In: van Zwieten PA, ed. *Handbook of Hypertension.* Amsterdam: Elsevier 1984;1–5.

8. Van Zwieten PA. Drugs interacting with α-adrenoceptors. *Cardiovasc Drugs Ther* 1989;3:121–133.

9. Mancia G, Ferrari A, Gregorni L, et al. Blood pressure variabilities in normotensive and hypertensive human beings. *Circ Res* 1983;53:96–104.

10. Furchgott RF, Zawadski JV. The obligatory role of endothelial cells in the relaxation of arterial smooth muscle by acetylcholine. *Nature* 1980;288:373–376.

11. Furchgott RF. Role of endothelium in responses of vascular smooth muscle. *Circ Res* 1983;53:557–573.

12. Palmer RMJ, Ferrige AG, Moncada S. Nitric oxide accounts for the biological activity of endothelium-derived relaxing factor. *Nature* 1987;327:524–526.

13. Vallance P, Collier J, Moncada S. Effects of endothelium-derived nitric oxide on peripheral arteriolar tone in man. *Lancet* 1989;2:997–1000.

14. Hendriks MGC. *Endothelium vasodilation in resistance arteries: investigations in various pathological models.* PhD Thesis, University of Amsterdam, 1993.

15. Doods HN, Mathy MJ, Davidesko D, van Charldorp KJ, de Jonge A, van Zwieten PA. Selectivity of muscarinic antagonists in radioligand and in vivo experiments for the putative M_1, M_2 and M_3-receptors. *J Pharmacol Exp Ther* 1987;246:929–934.

16. Eglen RM, Whiting RL. Heterogeneity of vascular muscarinic receptors. *J Auton Pharmacol* 1990;19:233–245.

17. Mutschler E, Moser U, Wess J, Lambrecht L. Muscarinic receptor subtypes: agonists and antagonists. *Prog Pharmacol* 1989;7:13–31.

18. Goyal RK. Muscarinic receptor subtypes. Physiology and clinical implications. *N Engl J Med* 1989;321:1022–1028.

19. Van Zwieten PA, Düren DR, van Charldorp KJ, de Jonge A. Coronary spasm induced by vagal stimulation in rat isolated hearts and during a vasovagal reaction in a patient. *Neth J Cardiol* 1988;1:41–44.

20. Bruning TA, Chang PC, Hendriks MGC, Kuypers EAP, van Zwieten PA. Muscarinic receptor subpopulations in the forearm bed of normotensive humans. European Society of Hypertension, Milan 1993.

21. Hendriks MGC, Pfaffendorf M, van Zwieten PA. Characterization of the muscarinic receptors in the mesenteric vascular bed of spontaneously hypertensive rats. *J Hypertens* 1991;9(suppl 6):S188–S189.

22. Hendriks MGC, Pfaffendorf M, van Zwieten PA. Characterization of the muscarinic receptors in the mesenteric vascular bed of spontaneously hypertensive rats. *J Hypertens* 1993;11:1329–1335.

23. Hendriks MGC, Pfaffendorf M, van Zwieten PA. Characterization of the muscarinic receptor subtype mediating vasodilatation in the rat perfused mesenteric vascular bed preparation. *J Auton Pharmacol* 1992;12:411–420.

24. Hendriks MGC, Pfaffendorf M, van Zwieten PA. The effect of muscarinic receptor alkylation on endothelium-dependent vasodilation in SHR. *Blood Pressure* 1994;in press.

25. Van Hooff M, van Baak MA, Schols M, Rahn KH. Studies of salivary flow in borderline hypertension: effects of drugs acting on structures innervated by the autonomic nervous system. *Clin Sci* 1984;66:599–604.

26. Mancia G, Ferrari A, Gregorni L, Parati G, Pomidossi G, Bertinieri G, Grassi G, DiRienzo M, Pedotti A, Zanchetti A. Blood pressure and heart rate variabilities in normotensive and hypertensive human beings. *Circ Res* 1983;53:96–104.

27. Panza JA, Quyyumi AA, Brush JE, Epstein SE. Abnormal endothelium-dependent vascular relaxation in patients with essential hypertension. *N Engl J Med* 1990;323:22–27.

28. Linder L, Kiowski W, Bühler F, Lüscher TF. Indirect evidence for release of endothelium-derived relaxing factor in human forearm circulation in vivo: blunted response in hypertension. *Circulation* 1990;81:1762–1767.

29. Lüscher TF, Vanhoutte PM. Endothelium-dependent contractions to acetylcholine in the aorta of the spontaneously hypertensive rat. *Hypertension* 1986;8:344–348.

30. Bohm RO, van Baak MA, van Hooff ME, Mooy J, Rahn KH. A long term study of plasma renin activity in borderline hypertension. *J Hypertens* 1987;5:655–661.

31. Julius S, Pascual AV, London R. Role of parasympathetic inhibition in the hyperkinetic type of borderline hypertension. *Circulation* 1971;44:413–418.

32. Korner PI, Shaw J, Uther JB, West MJ, McRuckchie RJ, Richards JG. Autonomic and non-autonomic circulatory components in essential hypertension in man. *Circulation* 1973;48:107–117.

33. Boura ALA, Green AF. Depressants of peripheral sympathetic nerve function. In: van Zwieten PA, ed. *Handbook of Hypertension,* vol 3. Amsterdam, New York, Oxford: Elsevier, 1984;194–238.

34. Van Zwieten PA. The cholinergic nervous system in Hypertension. *Blood Pressure* 1992;1:68–71.

35. Van Zwieten PA, Hendriks MGC. The parasympathetic nervous system and hypertension. *Hypertension Annual* (Current Science, London 1994);in press.

Hypertension: Pathophysiology, Diagnosis, and Management, Second Edition, edited by J.H. Laragh and B.M. Brenner, Raven Press, Ltd., New York © 1995.

CHAPTER 53

Heart Rate Variability and Cardiovascular Risk Assessment

Kenneth M. Stein, Neal Lippman, and Bruce B. Lerman

In 1963, Hon and Lee (1) monitored fetal electrocardiograms during labor and observed that fetal demise was preceded by tachycardia and an "extremely regular" heart rate. Although this observation has profoundly

K. M. Stein, N. Lippman, B. B. Lerman: Division of Cardiology, Department of Medicine, The New York Hospital–Cornell University Medical Center, New York, New York 10021.

affected modern obstetrical practice, the corresponding importance of measures of heart rate variability in adult patients has only recently been recognized. Analysis of heart rate variability, the irregularity of "regular" sinus rhythm, can provide insights into cardiovascular neurohumoral tone and improve our understanding of cardiac pathophysiology (2,3). Following pioneering analyses linking diminished heart rate variability to cardiovascular mortality (4,5), it has become apparent that heart rate variability is inversely related to prognosis in patients with coronary artery disease (6), myocardial infarction (7), and valvular heart disease (8), and that assessment of heart rate variability may improve our ability to stratify risk in these patients.

MEASURES OF HEART RATE VARIABILITY

Definitions of Time and Frequency Domains

A plethora of different measures of heart rate variability has been proposed. (For the most part, use of these techniques has been restricted to the analysis of patients with sinus rhythm; thus, the term *heart rate variability* is usually taken to connote "sinus cycle length variability.") Just as a complex musical chord can be described equally as a sound wave oscillating over time or as a series of individual notes (frequencies), other dynamic signals, including beat to beat variations in heart rate, can be represented in both the time and frequency domains (Fig. 1). Thus, different measures of heart rate variability can be grouped by analytic method as time-domain ("statistical" or "sequence-independent") and frequency-domain ("power spectral") measures. For any given purpose, one or the other of these representations may be more easily interpreted. However, transformation from one domain to the other neither increases nor decreases the information content of the original signal.

Time-Domain Measures

Some of the more common time-domain measures of heart rate variability are (a) the standard deviation (SD) (or variance) of the RR interval (or heart rate); (b) SDANN, the standard deviation of the 5-minute mean RR intervals tabulated over the 288 5-minute periods that comprise the 24-hour day (9); (c) the SD index, the mean of the 5-minute standard deviations of the RR interval tabulated over the 288 5-minute periods that comprise the 24-hour day (10), a measure that is complementary to SDANN; (d) the root-mean-square difference (RMSSD) among successive normal RR intervals; and (e) NN50, the mean hourly number (or pNN50, the proportion) of normal RR intervals whose duration is >50 msec longer than the previous normal RR interval (11). Table 1 lists values for these variables in normal subjects. It should be noted that the range of normal values is particularly wide for RMSSD and pNN50.

Frequency-Domain Measures

Frequency-domain, or "power spectral," analysis of heart rate variability refers to the determination of the specific frequencies at which variations in heart rate occur. The technique yields a curve describing the amplitudes of the individual frequency components of a patient's heart rate variability (Fig. 2). The amplitude of the

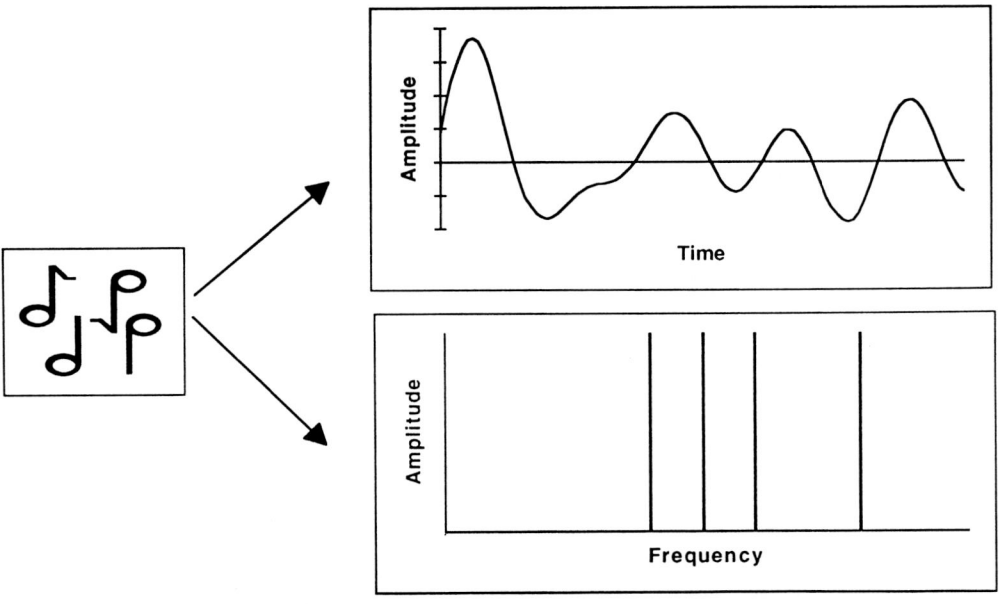

FIG. 1. Time and frequency domains. A musical chord can be described in the time domain as a complex pattern of vibrations over time, or in the frequency domain as the combination of four different notes (frequencies), each of a given amplitude. Although both descriptions are equally valid, and both have the same information content, for any given purpose one of these two representations may be more easily interpreted than its counterpart.

TABLE 1. *Heart rate variability in normal subjects*

		n	Mean	Reference
SD		6	195 ± 31	Myers et al., 1986 (17)
		16	176 ± 40	Cook et al., 1991 (84)
		5	155 ± 54	Dougherty and Burr, 1992 (14)
		17	185 ± 39	Hohnloser et al., 1992 (101)
		20	165 ± 41	Kauffman et al., 1993 (28)
	Total	64	175 ± 40	
			[95% CI: 95–255]	
SDANN		6	170 ± 23	Myers et al., 1986 (17)
		20	154 ± 40	Martin et al., 1987 (56)
		33	149 ± 46	van Hoogenhuyze et al., 1991 (79)
		5	117 ± 58	Dougherty and Burr, 1992 (14)
	Total	64	150 ± 44	
			[95% CI: 61–239]	
SD index		20	76 ± 14	Martin et al., 1987 (56)
		22	68 ± 16	Huikuri et al., 1990 (102)
		33	76 ± 25	van Hoogenhuyze et al., 1991 (79)
		5	79 ± 38	Dougherty and Burr, 1992 (14)
	Total	80	74 ± 21	
			[95% CI: 31–117]	
RMSSD		16	54 ± 22	Cook et al., 1991 (84)
		5	33 ± 20	Dougherty and Burr, 1992 (14)
		17	68 ± 34	Hohnloser et al., 1992 (101)
	Total	38	58 ± 29	
			[95% CI: 0–116]	
pNN50		16	26 ± 12	Cook et al., 1991 (84)
		17	25 ± 13	Hohnloser et al., 1992 (101)
		20	19 ± 9	Kauffman et al., 1993 (28)
	Total	53	23 ± 11	
			[95% CI: 1–45]	

Data are presented as mean ± standard deviation for individual studies, and as mean ± standard deviation with 95% confidence limits of normal values (derived by *t*-test) for aggregate data. SD, standard deviation of RR intervals over 24 hours; SDANN, standard deviation of the 5-minute mean RR intervals over 24 hours; SD index, mean of the 5-minute standard deviations over 24 hours; RMSSD, root-mean successive difference of RR intervals over 24 hours; pNN50, proportion of successive RR intervals differing by >50 msec over 24 hours.

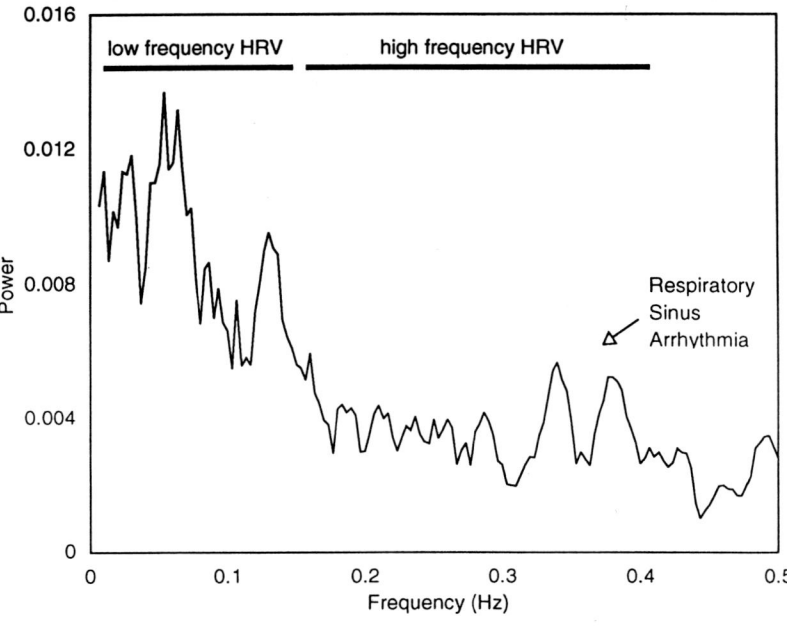

FIG. 2. Heart rate power spectrum. This power spectral representation of heart rate variability, derived during 5 minutes of observation of a patient during supine rest, describes the contribution to overall heart rate variability of oscillations at frequencies ranging up to 0.5 Hz (cycles per second). Using this technique two components of heart rate variability are identified: (a) a high-frequency component (0.15–0.40 Hz), which reflects respiratory sinus arrhythmia, and (b) a low-frequency component (0.04–0.15 Hz).

TABLE 2. *Power spectral analysis of heart rate variability: disparate techniques*

Reference	Analytic method	Duration analyzed	Frequencies analyzed
Pomerantz et al., 1985 (23)	FFT	256 seconds	1) 0.04–0.12 Hz 2) 0.224–0.228 Hz
Myers et al., 1986 (17)	FFT	24 hour	1) 0.0167–0.05 Hz 2) 0.05–0.15 Hz 3) 0.15–0.35 Hz 4) 0.35–0.50 Hz
Pagani et al., 1986 (24)	AR	512 beats	1) ≈0.1 Hz Eq 2) ≈0.25 Hz Eq
Lombardi et al., 1987 (67)	AR	256–512 beats	1) ≈0.09 Hz Eq 2) ≈0.28 Hz Eq
Guzzetti et al., 1988 (44)	AR	512 beats	1) ≈0.1 Hz Eq 2) ≈0.25 Hz Eq
Bigger et al., 1989 (15)	FFT	24 hour	1) 0.15–0.50 Hz 2) <0.50 Hz
Bigger et al., 1989 (16)	FFT	24 hour	1) 0.04–0.15 Hz 2) 0.15–0.40 Hz
Vybiral et al., 1989 (39)	FFT	512 beats	1) ≈0.087 Hz 2) ≈0.25 Hz
Sands et al., 1989 (83)	FFT	256 seconds	0.02–1.0 Hz
Rottman et al., 1990 (41) Bigger et al., 1991 (74) Bigger et al., 1992 (13) Bigger et al., 1993 (75) Kauffman et al., 1993 (28)	FFT	24 hours	1) 0.00001–0.0033 Hz 2) 0.0033–0.04 Hz 3) 0.04–0.15 Hz 4) 0.15–0.40 Hz 5) 0.00001–0.40 Hz
Parati et al., 1990 (45)	FFT	24 hour	1) 0.025–0.07 Hz 2) 0.07–0.14 Hz 3) 0.14–0.35 Hz
Hayano et al., 1990 (65) Hayano et al., 1991 (66)	AR	5 minute	1) 0.04–0.15 Hz 2) 0.25 Hz
Bekheit et al., 1990 (88)	FFT	10 minute	0.04–0.12 Hz
Casolo et al., 1991 (77)	FFT	24 hours	1) 0.04–0.12 Hz 2) 0.22–0.32 Hz
Cook et al., 1991 (84)	FFT	24 hours	1) 0.003–0.40 Hz 2) 0.003–0.04 Hz 3) 0.04–0.15 Hz 4) 0.15–0.40 Hz
Dougherty and Burr, 1992 (14)	AR	24 hour	1) 0.00–0.04 Hz 2) 0.04–0.15 Hz 3) 0.15–0.40 Hz 4) 0.00–0.50 Hz
Kienzle et al., 1992 (27)	FFT	24–48 hours	1) 0.05–0.15 Hz 2) 0.2–0.5 Hz 3) 0–0.5 Hz
Huikuri et al., 1992 (53)	AR	24 hour	1) 0.04–0.15 Hz 2) 0.15–0.40 Hz
Binder et al., 1992 (76) Hohnloser et al., 1992 (101) Stein et al., 1993 (8) Pedretti et al., 1993 (63)	FFT	24 hours	1) 0.01–1.00 Hz 2) 0.04–0.15 Hz 3) 0.15–0.40 Hz
Huikuri et al., 1993 (57)	AR	24 hour	1) <0.0033 Hz 2) 0.0033–0.04 Hz 3) 0.04–0.15 Hz 4) 0.15–0.40 Hz 5) <0.40 Hz
Luria et al., 1993 (71)	AR	24 hours	1) 0–0.05 Hz 2) 0.05–0.20 Hz 3) 0.20–0.35 Hz
Casadei et al., 1993 (89)	AR	512 beats	1) ≈0.1 Hz Eq 2) ≈0.3 Hz Eq

AR, autoregression; FFT, fast Fourier transform.

oscillation (or "power," which is amplitude squared) at any given frequency and the total contribution to heart rate variability contained with a range (or "band") of frequencies can then be analyzed. Following the initial determination of the power spectrum of heart rate fluctuations by Sayers (12), numerous authors have applied power spectral analysis to the measurement of heart rate variability. Although a single fundamental principle underlies this approach, as was the case with time-domain analysis, the specific methodological details used by different authors have varied widely (Table 2); as a result there is no established single technique for determining frequency domain measures of heart rate variability and therefore no clearly established normal values for these measures.

Frequency Categorization of Measures of Heart Rate Variability

Indices of heart rate variability can be organized according to frequency (Fig. 3). Four broad components of

heart rate variability have been defined (13): high frequency (0.15 Hz to 0.40 Hz), low frequency (0.04 Hz to 0.15 Hz), very low frequency (0.0033 Hz to 0.04 Hz), and ultra low frequency (<0.0033 Hz). Although it is natural to organize the frequency-domain indices of heart rate variability according to this scheme, it can also be used to categorize the time-domain variables. Within this conceptual framework, RMSSD and NN50 predominantly measure high-frequency heart rate variability. In fact, these variables are so closely correlated with high-frequency power as measured by power spectral analysis (linear correlation coefficients ranging from 0.87 to 0.99 have been reported [8,14–16]) that they are, for all practical purposes, interchangeable with the power spectral measures. The SD index is sensitive to heart rate fluctuations at frequencies > 0.04 Hz (combined low- and high-frequency variability) (17). The SD index is directly analogous to the total power derived from 5-minute power spectra, and is similar to the total power derived from 2-minute power spectra. SDANN behaves as a low-pass filter with a cutoff frequency of approximately 0.006

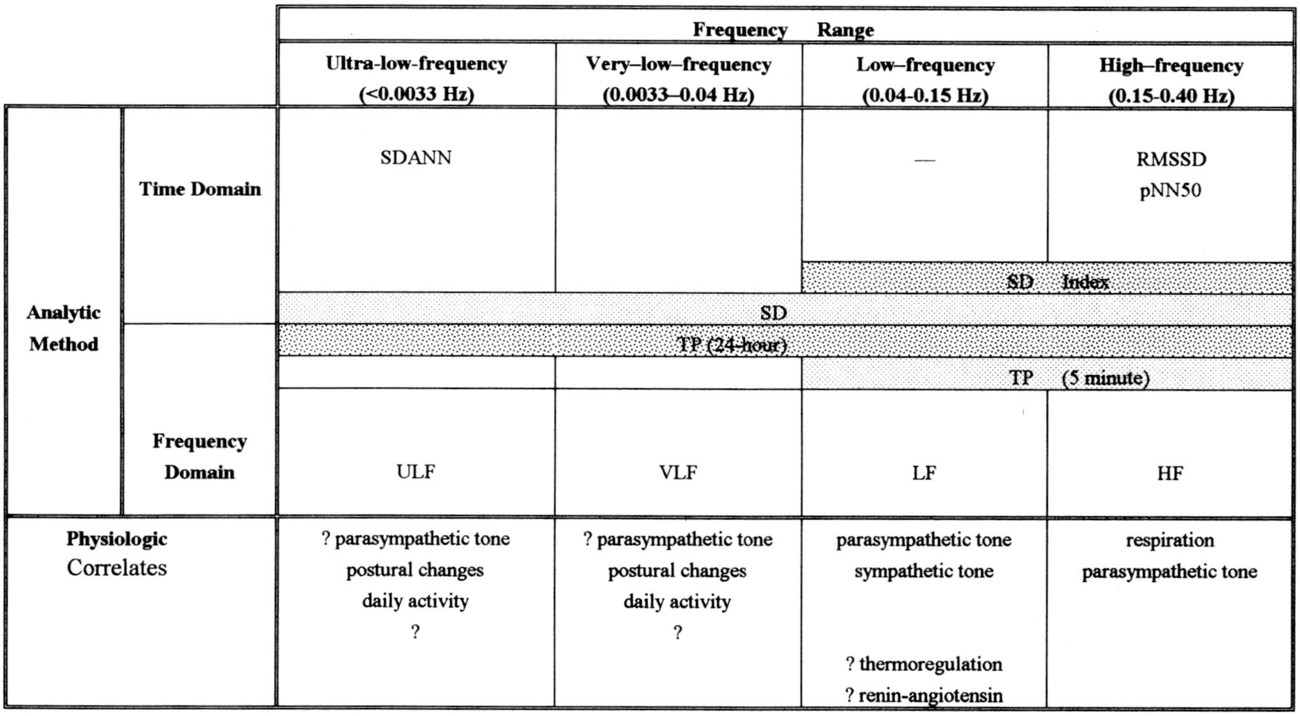

		Frequency Range			
		Ultra–low–frequency (<0.0033 Hz)	Very–low–frequency (0.0033–0.04 Hz)	Low–frequency (0.04-0.15 Hz)	High–frequency (0.15-0.40 Hz)
Analytic Method	Time Domain	SDANN		—	RMSSD pNN50
				SD Index	SD Index
		SD	SD	SD	SD
		TP (24-hour)	TP (24-hour)	TP (24-hour)	TP (24-hour)
				TP (5 minute)	TP (5 minute)
	Frequency Domain	ULF	VLF	LF	HF
Physiologic Correlates		? parasympathetic tone postural changes daily activity ?	? parasympathetic tone postural changes daily activity ?	parasympathetic tone sympathetic tone ? thermoregulation ? renin-angiotensin	respiration parasympathetic tone

FIG. 3. Theoretic relationships among measures of heart rate variability, stratified according to analytic method and frequency content. The high-frequency measures (RMSSD and high-frequency power amplitude) include fluctuations due to respiratory sinus arrhythmia that are mediated by parasympathetic tone. Low-frequency power amplitude reflects lower-frequency fluctuations in heart rate, which result from combined sympathetic and parasympathetic influences. SDANN assesses the dispersion of heart rates among the 288 5-minute intervals that comprise a 24-hour day and reflect ultra-low-frequency heart rate variability. Since most measures of "total" power amplitude are based on averaged 2-minute or 5-minute spectra, these reflect combined low- and high-frequency heart rate variability but do not measure ultra-low-frequency variation. SDANN, standard deviation of the 5-minute mean RR interval; RMSSD, root mean square successive difference of the RR interval; LF, low-frequency power; TP, total-frequency power; HF, high-frequency power; ULF, ultra-low-frequency power; VLF, very-low-frequency power.

Hz (17). The vast majority of power within SDANN is contained in the frequencies below 0.0033 Hz and it may be considered to be a measure of ultra-low-frequency heart rate variability. Twenty-four-hour variance (standard deviation squared) and 24-hour total power are by definition equivalent, and encompass all heart rate variability within the 24-hour day. Ultra-low-frequency fluctuations contribute the vast majority of daily total power and as a result SD and total power are strongly correlated with SDANN and ultra-low-frequency power.

PHYSIOLOGICAL SIGNIFICANCE OF HEART RATE VARIABILITY

Significance of High-Frequency and Low-Frequency Heart Rate Variability

Classification of heart rate variability according to frequency range has proven useful in understanding the physiological determinants of heart rate variability. High-frequency heart rate fluctuations (with a center frequency of 0.224–0.28 Hz, corresponding to ≈ 15 cycles per minute [18]) reflect respiratory sinus arrhythmia (19). These fluctuations, in turn, are predominantly mediated by rhythmic oscillations in vagal tone during the respiratory cycle (20). Their amplitude correlates with parasympathetic tone (21) and they can be abolished by bilateral cooling of the vagi (22) or infusion of atropine (18,23,24) or glycopyrrolate (25).

Low-frequency fluctuations (0.042–0.12 Hz) correspond to Mayer waves in the arterial pulse (blood pressure oscillations at 6–9 cycles per minute) and lower frequency blood pressure fluctuations. These, in turn, result from periodic fluctuations in peripheral vasomotor tone related to thermoregulation (26) and matching of regional perfusion to local metabolic demands. Through the baroreceptor reflex, these oscillations induce compensatory oscillations in heart rate. As a result, low-frequency heart rate variability reflects a complex combined (nonlinear) interaction of the sympathetic and parasympathetic nervous systems: during β-adrenergic blockade, actions that increase parasympathetic tone increase low-frequency power, whereas during parasympathetic blockade, actions that increase sympathetic tone also increase low-frequency power (18,23). However, in intact animals, both selective β- and α-adrenergic blockade increase low-frequency power (25). In the intact preparation it is likely that vagal tone predominates: low-frequency heart rate variability is significantly correlated with high-frequency heart rate variability (8,14), but low-frequency heart rate variability is inversely correlated with measures of plasma catecholamines and muscle sympathetic nerve activity (27). Experimental studies have also suggested that the renin-angiotenisin system may serve to damp low-frequency heart rate fluctua-

tions, which are therefore increased following administration of angiotensin-converting enzyme inhibitors (18,25). However, data in humans are inconclusive (28).

Heart Rate Variability and Sympathetic Tone

Since high-frequency heart rate variability reflects parasympathetic tone and low-frequency heart rate variability reflects combined sympathetic and parasympathetic tone, some authors have proposed that the ratios of low frequency to total power ("normalized" or "fractional" low-frequency power) and the ratio of low-frequency to high-frequency power might be indices of sympathetic tone. However, given the complex nonlinear interactions that lead to low-frequency heart rate variability, until this assumption is assessed by means of direct comparison of heart rate variability with other measures of sympathetic tone (e.g., muscle sympathetic nerve activity), it is more prudent to regard these ratios as indices of sympathovagal balance (24). Although heart rate variability analysis provides relatively pure measures of cardiac parasympathetic tone (measures of high-frequency heart rate variability), it does not provide a correspondingly pure measure of cardiac sympathetic tone.

Very-Low- and Ultra-Low-Frequency Heart Rate Variability

In contrast to low- and high-frequency heart rate variability, the physiology underlying very-low-frequency and ultra-low-frequency heart rate fluctuations is poorly understood. (Despite the fact that over the 24-hour day the bulk of power is contained in these frequency ranges [29,30].) These values are moderately to strongly correlated with measures of low- and high-frequency heart rate variability (8,14–16) and it is thus likely that parasympathetic tone plays a role, but the exact relationship has yet to be defined. Furthermore, these measures are sensitive to alterations in heart rate due to changes in posture and activity.

METHODOLOGICAL ISSUES IN POWER SPECTRAL ANALYSIS

The Heart Rate Tachygram

The first step in power spectral analysis of heart rate variability consists of removing ectopic beats and artifact from the RR interval sequence (see below) and converting the resulting listing of "normal" RR intervals into a function of instantaneous heart rate versus time (Fig. 4A–C). This function is referred to as the heart rate tachygram (or tachogram). To perform this conversion a

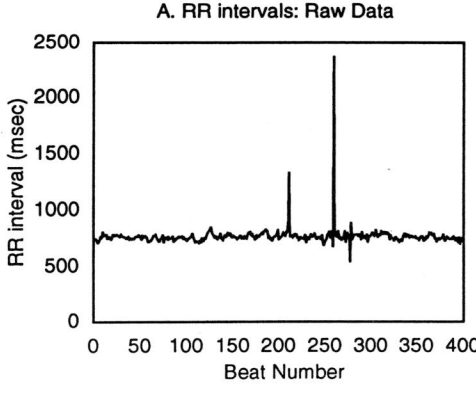

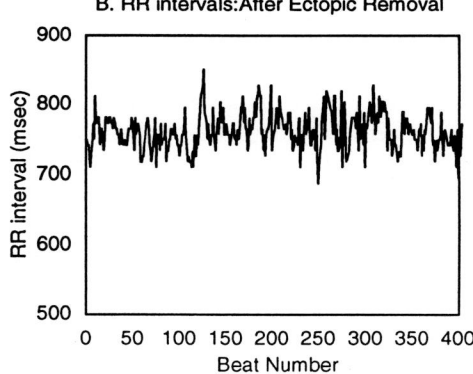

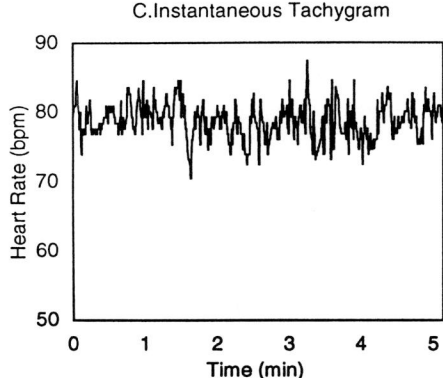

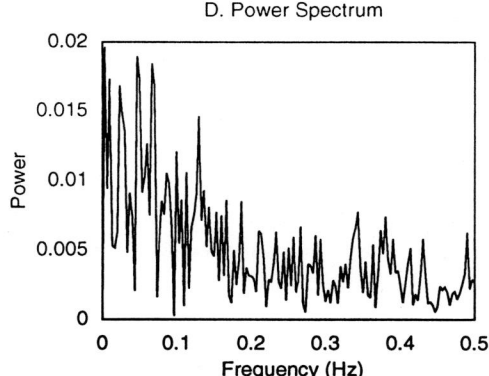

FIG. 4. Derivation of the heart rate power spectrum. **A:** Original RR interval sequence (including a ventricular ectopic beat resulting in a short RR interval followed by a long RR interval. **B:** RR interval sequence following removal of the ectopic beat and interpolation. **C:** The corrected RR interval sequence is resampled at a fixed rate and converted into a tachygram. **D:** Heart rate power spectrum derived from the tachygram.

fixed resampling frequency (typically 2–4 Hz) is chosen. The resampling frequency serves as a "clock"; at each tick of the clock the instantaneous heart rate is computed from the original RR interval sequence. The resulting tachygram will have sharp transitions in heart rate where one RR interval ends and the next one begins. Some authors have advocated the use of smoothing techniques to remove these abrupt transitions that may alter the results of power spectral analysis (31). It is not absolutely necessary to create a heart rate tachygram to do power spectral analysis. An alternative technique views the sequence of RR intervals as a function relating RR interval to the beat number in the sequence. Although the results obtained in this way are not mathematically identical to those obtained when conversion to a tachygram is performed, they appear to be similar for their clinical application (32).

Fourier Analysis

Power spectral analysis relies on a mathematical theorem (Fourier's theorem) that states that any complex periodic signal can be expressed as the sum of a series of appropriately selected functions (e.g., sine and cosine functions). For example, any function $R(t)$ on an interval $[-L, L]$ can be represented as:

$$R(t) = \sum_{n=1}^{\infty} \left[A_n \cos \frac{n\pi t}{L} + B_n \sin \frac{n\pi t}{L} \right] + C$$

Although the mathematics is beyond the scope of this discussion, by extending the interval of this series to become infinite and by using Euler's formula,

$$e^{ix} = \cos (x) + i \sin (x)$$

we can obtain the following expression for $R(t)$:

$$R(t) = \int_{-\infty}^{\infty} r(f) e^{-2\pi i f t} df$$

which is known as the Fourier integral. By solving for the function $r(f)$, we obtain the Fourier transform:

$$r(f) = \int_{-\infty}^{\infty} R(t) e^{2\pi i f t} dt$$

If the units for t are seconds [i.e., if $R(t)$ represents the instantaneous heart rate as a function of time] then the units for f will be cycles per second (or Hertz, abbreviated Hz), and $r(f)$ therefore describes the amplitude of heart rate fluctuations as a function of frequency. Application of the Fourier transform thus allows us to convert an RR interval sequence from the time domain into the frequency domain (Fig. 4D).

Although the above mathematical development has assumed that all the functions involved are continuous, in practice heart rate variability analysis is performed for a discrete function defined by the discrete moments at which the instantaneous heart rate is determined. If the heart rate determination is performed at equally spaced intervals (the sampling interval, Δ) and we have obtained N such samples, then we can convert the Fourier transform into its discrete form:

$$r(f_n) = \Delta \sum_{k=0}^{N-1} R_k e^{2\pi i k n/N}$$

where $r(f_n)$ represents the spectral amplitude at the frequency f_n and R_k represents the kth point in the original data sequence. The contribution to total variability (or "power") within a given frequency range is derived by computing the sum of the squared amplitudes of $r(f)$ within the desired frequency range.

Fast Fourier Transform

In practice, performing the Fourier transform is computationally complex and can require a substantial amount of computer time. For N data points, the number of computations required to compute the Fourier transform is of the order N^2. The fast Fourier transform (FFT) algorithm reduces the number of computations to the order of $N \log_2(N)$, a substantial reduction that makes the performance of spectral analysis possible even using relatively large amounts of data (33). The fundamental frequency (or lowest frequency determined by the FFT algorithm) is determined by the total length T of sampling, and the other frequencies are integer multiples of the fundamental frequency. For example, if a 5-minute (300 second) recording of RR intervals is used, then the fundamental frequency is $1/T = 1/300$ second, or 0.003 Hz, and the amplitudes obtained by the FFT correspond to frequencies of 0.003 Hz, 0.006 Hz, 0.009 Hz, etc. Values for frequencies that are not integral multiples of $1/T$ cannot be determined by the discrete FFT method. The role of the fundamental frequency as the lowest possible frequency that can be determined is particularly relevant when very-low-frequency oscillations in heart rate are being analyzed. In performing measures of ultra-low-frequency heart rate variability, an adequate data collection period must be used to ensure a fundamental frequency below that which is to be measured.

Another important point regarding the FFT algorithm is that it requires the number of input data points, N, to be a power of 2. When the number of data points is not a power of 2, zero padding, in which enough zeroes are appended to the data stream to bring its length up to the next higher power of 2, is used. A problem associated with this technique, however, is that it changes the characteristics of the heart rate function by introducing a period in which the heart rate abruptly falls to 0 beats per minute. A better solution uses the technique of digital resampling to create a heart rate tachygram in which the resampling frequency is chosen to ensure that the number of data points available is always a power of 2.

Nyquist Frequency

If the sequence of data points to be used in heart rate variability analysis is obtained by sampling at a time interval Δ, then the Nyquist critical frequency (f_c) is:

$$f_c = \frac{1}{2\Delta}$$

The *sampling theorem* states that no spectral components at frequencies greater than f_c can be determined by Fourier analysis. Instead, the spectral data that is contained in those frequencies is shifted into the frequencies below the Nyquist frequency, an effect known as "aliasing." Essentially, oscillations that occur at a frequency above the Nyquist frequency are "missed" between successive data samples. Once the data has been collected there is no way to correct for aliasing, although there are some methods for determining the degree to which aliasing affects the results. During long-term electrocardiographic recordings, the electrocardiogram is typically sampled at rates of 128 Hz or more, depending on the equipment used. Although the Nyquist critical frequency of 64 Hz is well above the frequency range at which important variations in heart rate occur, each R wave can be detected with an accuracy of only about 7.8 msec. This inaccuracy in R-wave detection may result in artifactual changes in heart rate variability measures (34), although the optimal frequency for R-wave detection has not been determined.

Data Windowing

When the FFT algorithm is applied to a series of discrete data points, the resultant power spectrum ideally gives power at a series of discrete frequencies. In practice, power may "leak" from one frequency to another, a process termed "spectral leakage." Data windowing, or the application of a window function to the original series of data points, is used to reduce spectral leakage. Many different windowing functions can be used and, as is the case with other aspects of heart rate variability calculations, the optimal windowing function to use (and whether different windowing functions should be used in different circumstances, such as for short versus long collection intervals) has not been rigorously explored, although most authors have employed some form of windowing in their data analysis.

Stationarity

The FFT algorithm assumes that the input data comprises a portion of a periodically repeating, infinitely long, data set whose period is precisely the length of the sampling time. Accordingly, the next data point following the last observed RR interval is assumed to be a repeat of the first RR interval in the sequence. Therefore, to appropriately perform FFT analysis of heart rate variability, the property of stationarity is desirable. In its broadest sense, stationarity implies that there are no changes in any of the statistical properties of the RR interval sequence during the data collection period. If there is a substantial deviation from stationarity, this results in the artifactual introduction of increased high-frequency power in the power spectral calculation. It is thus important to obtain stationary data for heart rate variability analysis. When short time periods are being analyzed, this can be done by ensuring adequate stabilization periods following any acute interventions (e.g., tilt table testing), before collecting the RR interval data. Statistical techniques can be applied to test the stability of the resulting RR interval sequence prior to power spectral analysis. There are no comparably simple solutions to the problem of stationarity when analyzing long (e.g., 24-hour) RR interval sequences.

Autoregression Analysis

As a result of the inherent problems associated with the use of the FFT algorithm, other techniques have been developed for the estimation of power spectra. The most commonly used of these (as applied to heart rate variability analysis) is the autoregression (AR) algorithm. The AR method is a three-step procedure: a time series model of the process to be analyzed is selected, the parameters of the model are estimated from the observed RR interval sequence by a technique known as autocorrelation, and these parameters are then used to compute an "idealized" power spectrum. In practice this technique yields a higher frequency resolution than conventional FFT methods, but the "fit" of this power spectrum to the original data is only as good as the match between the specified model and the actual process. A number of different forms of AR algorithms have been used to determine power spectra in the biomedical sciences; the mathematical development of the techniques is beyond the scope of this discussion (35). Both FFT-based and AR-based techniques have been used to determine frequency-domain measures of heart rate variability. Al-

though there are large theoretic differences between the two techniques (in particular, the AR method may be more applicable for the computation of low-frequency power from short data streams), in practice the two techniques yield highly correlated results (32,36).

Relationship of Frequency-Domain to Time-Domain Measures

The total power (or information) in a signal must be the same whether the signal is analyzed in the time domain (seconds) or the frequency domain (Hz), a result known as *Parseval's theorem*. Mathematically, this is stated as:

$$\text{Total Power} = \int_{-\infty}^{\infty} |R(t)|^2 dt = \int_{-\infty}^{\infty} |r(f)|^2 df$$

where $R(t)$ is the time-domain function (e.g., the RR interval sequence) and $r(f)$ is the frequency-domain representation of the signal (e.g., heart rate power spectrum). We can then interpret the total power of the RR interval spectrum within a given frequency band as a measure of the amount of total RR interval variance contributed by fluctuations within that frequency range. Thus, the amplitudes (square root of power) derived from the heart rate power spectrum are measures (in milliseconds) of the contribution within the specified frequency range to the global standard deviation (the square root of variance) of the RR interval.

Noise and Ectopy

In the ideal set of circumstances, subjects undergoing heart rate variability analysis would remain in sinus rhythm throughout the recording period and the electrocardiograms would be completely free of noise and artifact. In real-world settings, however, this ideal is rarely (if ever) achieved. The patients to whom heart rate variability analysis is most frequently applied, including those with hypertension, ischemic heart disease, congestive heart failure, and valvular heart disease, are likely to have substantial amounts of atrial and ventricular ectopy or even episodes of sustained tachycardia. Prolonged electrocardiographic recording, during which the subject can be expected to engage in the normal activities of daily life, may be subject to large amounts of recording artifact, as can shorter monitoring periods during which the subject undergoes positional changes, such as tilt table testing. Techniques for the correction of ectopic beats and noise must therefore be developed and validated (37,38).

Ectopy, whether ventricular or supraventricular, can affect heart rate variability in two distinct ways. Although heart rate variability analysis is concerned with variations in the sinus cycle length, in practice heart rate variability is measured using the RR intervals because of the greater reliability of QRS detection as compared with P wave detection. Ectopic beats disrupt the RR interval sequence by converting the "sinus" RR intervals into artifactually long or short intervals (see Fig. 4A), thereby changing both time-domain and frequency-domain measures of heart rate variability ("mathematic artifact"). Ectopic beats may also cause "physiological artifact" by, as a result of their effects of hemodynamics, inducing reflex changes in autonomic activity.

Some authors circumvent this problem by removing all periods with ectopy from the analysis (39). However, this method may result in the loss of substantial amounts of data (40) and, when techniques are used to assess the impact of brief interventions, this method may limit the population that can be studied. Furthermore, if ectopic beats vary systematically according to neurohumoral tone, this method may substantially bias the results. More commonly, the approach is to remove ectopic RR intervals (and one or more subsequent intervals to account for reflex changes in autonomic tone) and replace them by "shifting down" all subsequent RR intervals in the sequence, or by linear or cubic-spline interpolation (37,41,42). However, these methods do not result in complete correction of the mathematic artifact created by ectopic beats. Both linear and cubic-spline interpolation result in overestimation of low-frequency power and underestimation of high-frequency power (time-domain measures of heart rate variability may be less sensitive to the effects of ectopy than frequency-domain measures). The ability of any of these techniques to correct for sequential ectopic beats, nonsustained tachycardia, or noise, has not yet been determined. Further, such algorithms have typically treated supraventricular and ventricular ectopic beats as being identical. However, supraventricular premature beats, which are likely to reset the sinus pacemaker and ventricular premature beats, which may not reset the sinus pacemaker, are likely to have different effects on heart rate variability, both from a mathematical and physiological standpoint.

Newer algorithms, such as nonlinear predictive interpolation, a technique based on the mathematics of nonlinear dynamics, which uses ectopy- and noise-free portions of the RR interval sequence to predict what the RR intervals would have been had ectopy or noise not been present in other portions of the data, may improve our ability to correct for ectopy, and may be more effective in correcting for nonsustained tachycardia or noise than simpler methods (43). Future directions include the development of more sophisticated algorithms for ectopy correction, assessment of the differences in artifact created by different types of ectopic beats, and the development of algorithms that differentially process supraventricular and ventricular ectopy, sequential ectopic beats, and signal artifact.

HEART RATE VARIABILITY AND CARDIOVASCULAR PATHOPHYSIOLOGY

Hypertension

There is a paucity of data regarding analysis of heart rate variability as a probe to explore proposed neurohumoral abnormalities in patients with essential hypertension. Patients with mild essential hypertension were found in one study to have increased fractional low-frequency heart rate variability and decreased fractional high-frequency heart rate variability compared with normal subjects. Low-frequency heart rate variability was modestly correlated with diastolic blood pressure, findings compatible with a relative sympathetic predominance in these patients (44). Other studies, however, have failed to confirm these findings (30). On the basis of 24-hour recordings, circadian changes in heart rate variability in patients with mild hypertension are similar to those in control subjects, suggesting that dynamic cardiovascular neurohumoral control is unimpaired in these patients (45,46). Given the heterogeneous nature of essential hypertension, and the likelihood that the mechanism of blood pressure elevation may vary from patient to patient, it is noteworthy that none of these studies separately analyzed subgroups of patients with essential hypertension stratified demographically, metabolically, or according to response to pharmacological therapy.

Vasodepressor Syncope

In recent years, tilt table testing has become an important tool in the evaluation of patients with suspected vasodepressor (neurocardiac) syncope (47). It has been proposed that neurocardiac syncope results when orthostatic stress causes reduced venous return to the heart due to pooling of blood in the capacitance vessels of the lower extremities. The fall in preload is associated with an increase in sympathetic tone (48), resulting in increased cardiac contractility. The forceful contractions of the unloaded left ventricle are hypothesized to activate left ventricular mechanoreceptors that, via unmyelinated vagal afferents, cause a reflex withdrawal of sympathetic tone and increase in parasympathetic tone, leading to sudden vasodilatation (often associated with bradycardia), hypotension, and loss of consciousness (49). In normal volunteer subjects upright tilt produces a shift in spectral power from high- to low-frequency bands (24,39,50). Lipsitz et al. (51) observed an increase in low-frequency and total spectral power with little change in high-frequency power in response to upright tilt in normal subjects. This response was most prominent in younger subjects and was most pronounced in those (clinically normal) subjects who developed syncope during upright tilt. Although the high rate of positive tilt table tests in normal clinical volunteers in this study may limit its clinical applicability, these results are compatible with limited parasympathetic withdrawal and excess of sympathetic tone in response to orthostatic stress in patients with vasodepressor syncope. This is consistent with preliminary results suggesting that the lack of parasympathetic withdrawal, as assessed by the failure of high-frequency heart rate variability to fall during upright tilt, may predict those subjects who will develop syncope in response to tilt table testing (52). Further work is required to determine whether measurement of heart rate variability can be used to further elucidate the mechanisms of vasodepressor syncope or identify patients prone to this disorder.

Ventricular Arrhythmias and Sudden Cardiac Death

Heart rate variability in all frequency bands is reduced in survivors of ventricular fibrillation compared with control subjects (14,17,53). However, whether this abnormality represents a residuum of the cardiac arrest or a risk factor associated with the pathogenesis of the arrhythmia is not yet certain. In an animal model, reduced heart rate variability following myocardial infarction was associated with a higher risk of ventricular fibrillation during combined acute ischemia and exercise (54). Among patients referred for Holter monitoring for any cause, those with reduced heart rate variability have a fourfold increase in risk of sudden cardiac death during 2 years of follow-up (55). Furthermore, patients with ventricular fibrillation during Holter monitoring have markedly lower heart rate variability than normal subjects (56). In one group of patients with a history of life-threatening arrhythmias, heart rate variability was reduced over the hour before clinical episodes of sustained ventricular tachycardia (57). However, other investigators found that time-domain measures of heart rate variability did not change immediately preceding ventricular fibrillation and did not differ from a matched control group with nonsustained ventricular tachycardia (58).

It has been proposed that the observed interaction between abnormal ventricular function, frequent and complex ventricular arrhythmias, and the presence of abnormal heart rate variability supports the hypothesis that abnormalities in neurohumoral tone, manifested by diminished heart rate variability, might be the critical factor linking "substrate" (scarring and fibrosis of the ventricular myocardium) and "trigger" [frequent and complex ventricular premature contractions (VPCs)] in the pathogenesis of sudden cardiac death (59,60). This hypothesis is supported by the observation that the combination of enhanced sympathetic tone and diminished parasympathetic tone lowers the threshold for ventricular fibrillation (61). However, reduced heart rate variabil-

ity is also associated with the presence of late potentials on the signal averaged electrocardiogram (62) as well as inducible sustained monomorphic ventricular tachycardia at electrophysiological study (63) following an acute myocardial infarction. Thus, rather than reflecting a "third factor" in the genesis of sudden cardiac death, reduced heart rate variability might simply be a marker for an abnormal substrate.

HEART RATE VARIABILITY AND PROGNOSIS IN CARDIOVASCULAR DISEASE

Coronary Artery Disease

In 1975, Tibblin et al. (4) found that a simple index of heart rate variability derived from a ten-beat ECG was inversely related to the subsequent risk of death from ischemic heart disease in a large population study, providing the impetus for the study of these measures in patients with ischemic heart disease. It has since become apparent that high-frequency heart rate variability (but not low-frequency heart rate variability) is inversely correlated with the presence of coronary atherosclerosis (64). This relationship is independent of previous myocardial infarction, left ventricular function, and established cardiac risk factors, leading some authors to speculate that diminished vagal tone might play a causative role in atherogenesis (65,66). Although ultra-low-frequency heart rate variability is not correlated with the angiographic severity of coronary artery disease, it is a potent prognostic indicator in patients undergoing coronary angiography, independent of left ventricular ejection fraction or coronary anatomy. Markedly reduced ultra-low-frequency heart rate variability (SDANN < 50 msec) was associated with an 18-fold increase in mortality in this population in the year following cardiac catheterization (6).

Myocardial Infarction

Heart rate variability is markedly reduced within hours following acute myocardial infarction. The extent of reduction correlates with clinical, electrocardiographic, biochemical, and hemodynamic indices of infarct severity, and with prognosis (5,7,13,62,67–72). In these studies, patients with low heart rate variability following myocardial infarction were two to seven times as likely to die than patients with higher heart rate variability. The choice of an "optimal" measure of heart rate variability for risk stratification in this population remains controversial. Bigger and colleagues (13) compared heart rate variability measures in all frequency bands and found that measures of ultra-low- and very-low-frequency heart rate variability had stronger associations with subsequent risk than did measures of high-frequency and low-frequency heart rate variability. Inconsistent effects of infarct location on heart rate variability have been reported (5,16,69–71,73), although the predominant evidence suggests that heart rate variability is higher following inferior than anterior infarction. Heart rate variability increases over the 3 months following the event, but does not return to normal even 1 year following myocardial infarction (74), and heart rate variability 1 year following myocardial infarction remains inversely correlated with outcome (75).

Other Cardiovascular Disease

The prognostic utility of measures of heart rate variability is most clearly defined in populations with ischemic heart disease. However, these techniques have also been applied to patients with congestive heart failure, valvular heart disease, and to patients who have undergone orthotopic cardiac transplantation.

Congestive Heart Failure

The prognostic importance of heart rate variability in patients with congestive heart failure is not well established, although among patients with severe left ventricular dysfunction, patients with diminished ultra-low-frequency heart rate variability (SDANN < 55) have a 20-fold increase in the risk of death while awaiting cardiac transplantation (76). High-frequency, low-frequency, and ultra-low-frequency heart rate variability are markedly reduced in patients with moderate-to-severe congestive heart failure due to both ischemic heart disease and idiopathic cardiomyopathy (77–80). Ultra-low-frequency heart rate variability has also been positively correlated with left ventricular ejection fraction in patients with a history of life-threatening cardiac arrhythmia (14). Likewise, resting left and right ventricular ejection fractions are positively correlated with ultra-low-frequency (but not low-frequency or high-frequency) heart rate variability in patients with nonischemic mitral regurgitation (8). These observations are consistent with chronic parasympathetic withdrawal and sympathetic excitation in patients with functionally significant ventricular dysfunction, independent of the etiology of ventricular dysfunction (81,82).

Valvular Heart Disease

In patients with chronic severe nonischemic mitral regurgitation, ultra-low-frequency heart rate variability (SDANN) was inversely correlated with progression to atrial fibrillation, progression to valve surgery, and mortality. In this population, SDANN was as potent a prognostic indicator as measures of left and right ventricular ejection fraction (8). Reduced heart rate variability (SDANN < 100) was associated with an odds ratio of 6:1 for death or progression to mitral valve surgery in this population.

Cardiac Transplantation

Following orthotopic cardiac transplantation, the functionally denervated transplanted heart shows virtually no heart rate variability, whereas heart rate variability in the recipient atrial remnant tends to return toward normal (80). Although the mechanism is uncertain, the development of transplant rejection is associated with a small but significant increase in heart rate variability (83).

FUTURE DIRECTIONS

Does Heart Rate Variability Have a Role in Directing Therapy?

Although substantial progress has been made in understanding the physiology and prognostic significance of measures of heart rate variability, several critical questions remain unanswered. Foremost is whether interventions designed to increase heart rate variability improve outcome among patients with diminished heart rate variability; along with *identifying* high-risk patients, should measures of heart rate variability be used to *guide* therapy? To answer this question, an improved understanding of the chronic effects of various therapies on heart rate variability as well as proof that measures that modify heart rate variability alter prognosis are required.

Among normal subjects, it has been established that digoxin treatment increases virtually all measures of heart rate variability (without affecting mean heart rate in sinus rhythm) (28), that beta blockers increase low-frequency and high-frequency heart rate variability (11,84), and that transdermal scopolamine increases mean RR interval and standard deviation of the RR interval (85). Enalapril and diltiazem have no effect on heart rate variability in normal subjects (28,84). The effects of drugs among patients with cardiovascular disease remain, for the most part, unexplored. Atenolol increases fractional high-frequency power and decreases fractional low-frequency power in hypertensive subjects (44). Captopril, which improves long-term outcome in patients with coronary artery disease and congestive heart failure, increases high-frequency heart rate variability in this population (86). Following myocardial infarction, metoprolol increases high-frequency heart rate variability and has inconsistent effects on low-frequency heart rate variability (87,88); diltiazem reduces low-frequency heart rate variability, but nifedipine has no effect (88). In contrast, low-dose scopolamine increases low- and high-frequency heart rate variability among patients with recent myocardial infarction (a vagomimetic effect) (63,89). However, although vagal stimulation prevents sudden death in animal models of acute ischemia (90), the clinical utility of this approach is presently unproven. Among patients with frequent and complex ventricular arrhythmias, flecainide (a drug associated with a relatively high risk of proarrhythmia in this population) and propafenone decreased high-frequency heart rate variability, whereas amiodarone had no effect (91).

Does Heart Rate Variability in Atrial Fibrillation Have Any Significance?

Future research is also required to understand the applicability of these techniques to patients with atrial fibrillation. Such patients constitute a significant (and potentially high-risk) minority of patients with hypertension, coronary artery disease, valvular heart disease, and cardiomyopathy. In contrast to the predictive value defined for patients in sinus rhythm, the physiological correlates and prognostic significance of the variability of the ventricular response in atrial fibrillation have not been established. During atrial fibrillation a rapid, irregular atrial input into the atrioventricular (AV) node is "scaled" down to a slower, but still irregular ventricular response. Although the exact mechanism by which the AV node governs the ventricular response to the irregularly irregular impulses of atrial fibrillation is controversial (92,93), this response is modulated by autonomic and neurohumoral factors. Cross et al. (94) demonstrated intact baroreflex control of the heart rate during atrial fibrillation, with the same frequency response as in sinus rhythm. However, if the "scaling" function of the AV node is nonlinear, this would not necessarily lead to the same output frequencies in the heart rate spectrum (95). Thus, although it is plausible that measurements of the variability of this response might have qualitatively similar relationships with neurohumoral tone as do measurements of sinus cycle length variability, this is not at all inevitable. Preliminary data suggest that diminished variability of the ventricular response in chronic atrial fibrillation is associated with an increased clinical event rate among patients with nonischemic mitral regurgitation.

Is Chaos Theory Applicable to Heart Rate Variability Analysis?

Finally, it is worth noting that power spectral measures of heart rate variability based on the Fourier transform use a technique designed for systems with regular oscillations, while statistical and autoregressive power spectral measures use techniques that assume random oscillations. However, heart rate fluctuations are both nonrandom (deterministic) and irregular (aperiodic). Thus, it is likely that newer mathematical techniques de-

signed to analyze deterministic aperiodic ("chaotic") systems will prove useful in the study of heart rate variability (96–98). The feasibility of using such techniques to analyze sinus rhythm has already been demonstrated (99), and preliminary reports suggest that these measures may also prove to be prognostically significant (100).

ACKNOWLEDGMENT

This work was supported in part by NIH Grant HL-44747. Dr. Lerman is an Established Investigator of the American Heart Association.

REFERENCES

1. Hon EH, Lee ST. Electronic evaluation of the fetal heart rate: VIII patterns preceding fetal death, further observations. *Am J Obstet Gynecol* 1963;87:814–826.
2. Malliani A, Pagani M, Lombardi F, Cerutti S. Cardiovascular neural regulation explored in the frequency domain. *Circulation* 1991;84:482–492.
3. Appel ML, Berger RD, Saul JP, Smith JM, Cohen RJ. Beat to beat variability in cardiovascular variables: noise or music? *J Am Coll Cardiol* 1989;14:1139–1148.
4. Tibblin G, Eriksson C-G, Bjuro T, Georgescu D, Svardsudd C. Heart rate and heart rate variability a risk factor for the development of ischaemic heart disease (IHD) in the "Men born in 1913 study"—a ten years follow-up. *ICRS Medical Science* 1975;3:95.
5. Wolf MM, Varigos GA, Hunt D, Sloman JG. Sinus arrhythmia in acute myocardial infarction. *Med J Aust* 1978;2:52–53.
6. Rich MW, Saini JS, Kleiger RE, Carney RM, teVelde A, Freedland KE. Correlation of heart rate variability with clinical and angiographic variables and late mortality after coronary angiography. *Am J Cardiol* 1988;62:714–717.
7. Kleiger RE, Miller JP, Bigger JT Jr, Moss AJ, the Multicenter Post-Infarction Research Group. Decreased heart rate variability and its association with increased mortality after acute myocardial infarction. *Am J Cardiol* 1987;59:256–262.
8. Stein KM, Borer JS, Hochreiter C, Okin PM, Herrold EM, Devereux RB, Kligfield P. Prognostic value and physiologic correlates of heart rate variability in chronic severe mitral regurgitation. *Circulation* 1993;88:127–135.
9. Kleiger RE, Miller JP, Bigger JT Jr, Moss AJ, the Multicenter Postinfarction Research Group. Heart rate variability: a variable predicting mortality following acute myocardial infarction [abstract]. *J Am Coll Cardiol* 1984;3:547.
10. Magid NM, Martin GJ, Kehoe RF, Zheutlin TA, Myers GA, Eckberg DL, Barnett PS, Weiss JS, Lesch M, Singer DH. Diminished heart rate variability in patients with sudden cardiac death [abstract]. *Circulation* 1985;72:241.
11. Ewing DJ, Neilson JMM, Travis P. New method for assessing cardiac parasympathetic activity using 24 hour electrocardiograms. *Br Heart J* 1984;52:396–402.
12. Sayers B McA. Analysis of heart rate variability. *Ergonomics* 1973;16:17–32.
13. Bigger JT Jr, Fleiss JL, Steinman RC, Rolnitzky LM, Kleiger RE, Rottman JN. Frequency domain measures of heart period variability and mortality after myocardial infarction. *Circulation* 1992;85:164–171.
14. Dougherty CM, Burr RL. Comparison of heart rate variability in survivors and nonsurvivors of sudden cardiac arrest. *Am J Cardiol* 1992;70:441–448.
15. Bigger JT Jr, Albrecht P, Steinman RC, Rolnitzky LM, Fleiss JL, Cohen RJ. Comparison of time- and frequency domain-based measures of cardiac parasympathetic activity in Holter recordings after myocardial infarction. *Am J Cardiol* 1989;64:536–538.
16. Bigger JT Jr, LaRovere MT, Steinman RC, Fleiss JL, Rottman JN, Rolnitzky LM, Schwartz PJ. Comparison of baroreflex sensitivity and heart period variability after myocardial infarction. *J Am Coll Cardiol* 1989;14:1511–1518.

17. Myers GA, Martin GJ, Magid NM, Barnett PS, Schaad JW, Weiss JS, Lesch M, Singer DH. Power spectral analysis of heart rate variability in sudden cardiac death: comparison to other methods. *IEEE Trans Biomed Eng* 1986;33:1149–1156.

18. Akselrod S, Gordon D, Ubel FA, Shannon DC, Barger AC, Cohen RJ. Power spectrum analysis of heart rate fluctuation: a quantitative probe of beat-to-beat cardiovascular control. *Science* 1981;213:220–223.

19. Eckberg DL. Human sinus arrhythmia as an index of vagal cardiac outflow. *J Appl Physiol* 1983;54:961–966.

20. Koizumi K, Terui N, Kollai M. Effect of cardiac vagal and sympathetic nerve activity on heart rate in rhythmic fluctuations. *J Auton Nerv Syst* 1985;12:251–259.

21. Fouad FM, Tarazi RC, Ferrario CM, Fighaly S, Alicandri C. Assessment of parasympathetic control of heart rate by a noninvasive method. *Am J Physiol* 1984;246:H838–842.

22. Katonah PG, Jih F. Respiratory sinus arrhythmia: noninvasive measure of parasympathetic cardiac control. *J Appl Physiol* 1975;39:801–805.

23. Pomerantz B, Macaulay RJB, Caudill MA, Kutz I, Adam D, Gordon D, Kilborn KM, Barger AC, Shannon DC, Cohen RJ, Benson H. Assessment of autonomic function in humans by heart rate spectral analysis. *Am J Physiol* 1985;248:H151–153.

24. Pagani M, Lombardi F, Guzzetti S, Rimoldi O, Furlan R, Pizzinelli P, Sandrone G, Malfatto G, Dell'Orto S, Piccaluga E, Turiel M, Baselli G, Cerutti S, Malliani A. Power spectral analysis of heart rate and arterial pressure variabilities as a marker of sympatho-vagal interaction in man and conscious dog. *Circ Res* 1986;59:178–193.

25. Akselrod S, Gordon D, Madwed JB, Snidman NC, Shannon DC, Cohen RJ. Hemodynamic regulation: investigation by spectral analysis. *Am J Physiol* 1985;249:H867–875.

26. Hyndman BW, Kitney RI, Sayers BMcA. Spontaneous rhythms in physiological control systems. *Nature* 1971;233:339–341.

27. Kienzle MG, Ferguson DW, Birkett CL, Myers GA, Berg WJ, Mariano DJ. Clinical, hemodynamic and sympathetic neural correlates of heart rate variability in congestive heart failure. *Am J Cardiol* 1992;69:761–767.

28. Kauffman ES, Bosner MS, Bigger JT Jr., Stein PK, Kleiger RE, Rolnitzky LM, Steinman RC, Fleiss JL. Effects of digoxin and enalapril on heart period variability and response to head-up tilt in normal subjects. *Am J Cardiol* 1993;72:95–99.

29. Kobayoshi M, Musha T. 1/f fluctuation of heartbeat period. *IEEE Trans Biomed Eng* 1982;29:456–457.

30. Mancia G, Ferrari A, Gregorini L, Parati G, Pomidossi G, Bertineri G, Grassi G, diRienzo M, Pedotti A, Zanchetti A. Blood pressure and heart rate variabilities in normotensive and hypertensive human beings. *Circ Res* 1983;53:96–104.

31. Berger RD, Akselrod S, Gordon D, Cohen RJ. An efficient algorithm for spectral analysis of heart rate variability. *IEEE Trans Biomed Eng* 1986;33:900–904.

32. DeBoer RW, Karemaker JM, Strackee J. Comparing spectra for a series of point events particularly for heart rate variability data. *IEEE Trans Biomed Eng* 1984;31:384–387.

33. Press WH, Flannery BP, Teukolsky SA, Vetterling WT. *Numerical recipes in C: the art of scientific computing.* Cambridge: Cambridge University Press, 1988.

34. Merri M, Fadden DC, Mottley JG, Tittlebaum EL. Sampling frequency of the electrocardiogram for spectral analysis of heart rate variability. *IEEE Trans Biomed Eng* 1990;37:99–106.

35. Kay SM, Marple SL Jr. Spectrum analysis—a modern perspective. *Proc IEEE* 1981;69:1380–1411.

36. Cowan MJ, Burr RL, Narayanan SB, Buzaitis A, Strasser M, Busch S. Comparison of autoregression and fast Fourier transform techniques for power spectral analysis of heart period variability of persons with sudden cardiac death before and after therapy to increase heart period variability. *J Electrocardiol* 1992;25:S234–239.

37. Albrecht P, Cohen RJ. Estimation of heart rate power spectrum bands from real-world data: dealing with ectopic beats and noisy data. *Comput Cardiol* 1989:311–314.

38. Malik M, Farrell T, Cripps T, Camm AJ. Heart rate variability in relation to prognosis after myocardial infarction: selection of optimal processing techniques. *Eur Heart J* 1989;10:1060–1074.

39. Vybiral T, Bryg RJ, Maddens ME, Boden WE. Effect of passive tilt on sympathetic and parasympathetic components of heart rate variability in normal subjects. *Am J Cardiol* 1989;63:1117–1120.

40. Myers G, Workman M, Birkett C, Ferguson D, Kienzle M. Problems in measuring heart rate variability of patients with congestive heart failure. *J Electrocardiol* 1992;25S:214–219.

41. Rottman JN, Steinman RC, Albrecht P, Bigger JT Jr, Rolnitzky LM, Fleiss JL. Efficient estimation of the heart period power spectrum suitable for physiologic or pharmacologic studies. *Am J Cardiol* 1990;66:1522–1524.

42. Birkett CL, Kienzle MG, Myers GA. Interpolation over ectopic beats increases low frequency power in heart rate variability spectra. *Comput Cardiol* (IEEE Computer Society Press) 1991:257–259.

43. Lippman N, Stein KM, Lerman BB. Non-linear predictive interpolation: a new method for the correction of ectopic beats for heart rate variability analysis. *J Electrocardiol,* in press.

44. Guzzetti S, Piccaluga E, Casati R, Cerutti S, Lombardi F, Pagani M, Malliani A. Sympathetic predominance in essential hypertension: a study employing spectral analysis of heart rate variability. *J Hypertens* 1988;6:711–717.

45. Parati G, Castiglioni P, Di Rienzo M, Omboni S, Pedotti A, Mancia G. Sequential spectral analysis of 24-hour blood pressure and pulse interval in humans. *Hypertension* 1990;16:414–421.

46. Furlan R, Guzzetti S, Crivellaro W, Dassi S, Tinelli M, Baselli G, Cerutti S, Lombardi F, Pagani M, Malliani A. Continuous 24-hour assessment of the neural regulation of systemic arterial pressure and RR variabilities in ambulant subjects. *Circulation* 1990;81:537–547.

47. Benditt DB, Remole S, Bailin S, Dunnigan A, Asso A, Milstein S. Tilt table testing for evaluation of neurally-mediated (cardioneurogenic) syncope: rationale and proposed protocols. *PACE* 1991;14:1528–1537.

48. Wall BG, Sundlof G. Sympathetic outflow to muscles during vasovagal syncope. *J Auton Nerv Syst* 1982;6:287–291.

49. Abboud FM. Neurocardiogenic syncope. *N Engl J Med* 1993;328:1117–1120.

50. Simpson DM, Wicks R. Spectral analysis of heart rate indicates reduced baroreceptor-related heart rate variability in elderly persons. *J Gerontol* 1988;43:M21–24.

51. Lipsitz LA, Mietus J, Moody GB, Goldberger AL. Spectral characteristics of heart rate variability before and during postural tilt. *Circulation* 1990;81:1803–1810.

52. Lippman N, Stein KM, Lerman BB. Failure to decrease parasympathetic tone during upright tilt predicts a positive tilt table test [abstract]. *Circulation* 1993;88:I-398.

53. Huikuri HV, Linnaluoto MK, Seppanen T, Airaksinen KEJ, Kessler KM, Takkunen JT, Myerburg RJ. Circadian rhythm of heart rate variability in survivors of cardiac arrest. *Am J Cardiol* 1992;70:610–615.

54. Hull SS, Evans AR, Vanoli E, Adamson PB, Stramba-Badiale M, Albert D, Foreman RD, Schwartz PJ. Heart rate variability before and after myocardial infarction in conscious dogs at high and low risk of sudden death. *J Am Coll Cardiol* 1990;16:978–985.

55. Algra A, Tijssen JGP, Roelandt JRTC, Pool J, Lubsen J. Heart rate variability from 24-hour electrocardiography and the 2-year risk for sudden death. *Circulation* 1993;88:180–185.

56. Martin GJ, Magid NM, Myers G, Barnett PS, Schaad JW, Weiss JS, Lesch M, Singer DH. Heart rate variability and sudden death secondary to coronary artery disease during ambulatory electrocardiographic monitoring. *Am J Cardiol* 1987;60:86–89.

57. Huikuri HV, Valkama JO, Airaksinen KEJ, Seppanen T, Kessler KM, Takkunen JT, Myerburg RJ. Frequency domain measures of heart rate variability before the onset of nonsustained and sustained ventricular tachycardia in patients with coronary artery disease. *Circulation* 1993;87:1220–1228.

58. Vybiral T, Glaeser DH, Goldberger AL, Rigney DR, Hess KR, Mietus J, Skinner JE, Francis M, Pratt CM. Conventional heart rate variability analysis of ambulatory electrocardiographic recordings fails to predict imminent ventricular fibrillation. *J Am Coll Cardiol* 1993;22:557–565.

59. Coumel P, Leclerq J-F, Leenhardt A. Arrhythmias as predictors of sudden death. *Am Heart J* 1987;114:929.

60. Kligfield P, Stein KM, Herrold EM. Computer-assisted analysis of Holter recordings. *Ann NY Acad Sci* 1990;601:353.

61. Lown B, Verrier RL. Neural activity and ventricular fibrillation. *N Engl J Med* 1976;294:1165–1170.

62. Farrell TG, Bashir Y, Cripps, Malik M, Poloniecki J, Bennett D, Ward D, Camm AJ. Risk stratification for arrhythmic events in postinfarction patients based on heart rate variability, ambulatory electrocardiographic variables, and the signal-averaged electrocardiogram. *J Am Coll Cardiol* 1991;18:687–697.

63. Pedretti R, Colombo E, Braga SS, Carù B. Influence of transdermal scopolamine on cardiac sympathovagal interaction after acute myocardial infarction. *Am J Cardiol* 1993;72:384–392.

64. Airaksinen KEJ, Ikaheimo MJ, Linnaluoto MK, Niemela M, Takkunen JT. Impaired vagal heart rate control in coronary artery disease. *Br Heart J* 1987;58:592–597.

65. Hayano J, Sakakibara Y, Yamada M, Ohte N, Fujinami T, Yokoyama K, Watanabe Y, Takata K. Decreased magnitude of heart rate spectral components in coronary artery disease: its relation to angiographic severity. *Circulation* 1990;81:1217–1224.

66. Hayano J, Yamada A, Mukai S, Sakakibara Y, Yamada M, Ohte N, Hashimoto T, Fujinami T, Takata K. Severity of coronary atherosclerosis correlates with the respiratory component of heart rate variability. *Am Heart J* 1991;121:1070–1079.

67. Lombardi F, Sandrone G, Pernpruner S, Sala R, Garimoldi M, Cerutti S, Baselli G, Pagani M, Malliani A. Heart rate variability as an index of sympathovagal interaction after acute myocardial infarction. *Am J Cardiol* 1987;60:1239–1245.

68. Cripps TR, Malik M, Farrell TG, Camm AJ. Prognostic value of reduced heart rate variability after myocardial infarction: clinical evaluation of a new analysis method. *Br Heart J* 1991;65:14–19.

69. Casolo GC, Stroder P, Signorini C, Calzolari F, Zucchini M, Balli E, Sulla A, Lazzerini S. Heart rate variability during the acute phase of myocardial infarction. *Circulation* 1992;85:2073–2079.

70. Piplis A, Flather M, Ormerod O, Sleight P. Heart rate variability in acute myocardial infarction and its association with infarct site and clinical course. *Am J Cardiol* 1991;67:1137–1139.

71. Luria MH, Sapoznikov D, Gilon D, Zahger D, Weinstein JM, Weiss AT, Gotsman MS. Early heart rate variability alterations after acute myocardial infarction. *Am Heart J* 1993;125:676–681.

72. Bigger JT Jr, Fleiss J, Rolnitzky LM, Steinman RC. The ability of several short-term measures of RR variability to predict mortality after myocardial infarction. *Circulation* 1993;88:927–934.

73. Flapan AD, Wright RA, Nolan J, Neilson JMM, Ewing DJ. Differing patterns of cardiac parasympathetic activity and their evolution in selected patients with a first myocardial infarction. *J Am Coll Cardiol* 1993;21:926–931.

74. Bigger JT Jr, Fleiss JL, Rolnitzky LM, Steinman RC, Schneider WJ. Time course of recovery of heart period variability after myocardial infarction. *J Am Coll Cardiol* 1991;18:1643–1649.

75. Bigger JT Jr, Fleiss JL, Rolnitzky LM, Steinman RC. Frequency domain measures of heart period variability to assess risk late after myocardial infarction. *J Am Coll Cardiol* 1993;21:729–736.

76. Binder T, Frey B, Porenta G, Heinz G, Wutte M, Kreiner G, Gossinger H, Schmidinger H, Pacher R, Weber H. Prognostic value of heart rate variability in patients awaiting cardiac transplantation. *PACE* 1992;15:2215–2220.

77. Casolo G, Balli E, Fazi A, Gori C, Freni A, Gensini G. Twenty-four-hour spectral analysis of heart rate variability in congestive heart failure secondary to coronary artery disease. *Am J Cardiol* 1991;67:1154–1158.

78. Saul JP, Yutaka A, Berger RD, Lilly LS, Colucci WS, Cohen RJ. Assessment of autonomic regulation in chronic congestive heart failure by heart rate spectral analysis. *Am J Cardiol* 1988;61:1292–1299.

79. van Hoogenhuyze D, Weinstein N, Martin GJ, Weiss JS, Schaad JW, Sahyouni N, Fintel D, Remme WJ, Singer DH. Reproducibility and relation to mean heart rate of heart rate variability in normal subjects and in patients with congestive heart failure secondary to coronary artery disease. *Am J Cardiol* 1991;68:1668–1676.

80. Smith ML, Ellenbogen KA, Eckberg DL, Szentpetery S, Thames M. Subnormal heart period variability in heart failure: effect of cardiac transplantation. *J Am Coll Cardiol* 1989;14:106–111.

81. Eckberg DL, Drabinsky M, Braunwald E. Defective parasympathetic control on patients with heart disease. *N Engl J Med* 1971;285:877–883.

82. Swedberg K, Eneroth P, Kjekshus J, Wilhelmsen L, for the CONSENSUS trial study group. Hormones regulating cardiovascular function in patients with severe congestive heart failure and their relation to mortality. *Circulation* 1990;82:1730–1736.

83. Sands KEF, Appel ML, Lilly LS, Schoen FJ, Mudge GH Jr, Cohen RJ. Power spectrum analysis of heart rate variability in human cardiac transplant recipients. *Circulation* 1989;79:76–82.

84. Cook JR, Bigger JT Jr, Kleiger RE, Fleiss JL, Steinman RC, Rolnitzky L. Effect of atenolol and diltiazem on heart period variability in normal persons. *J Am Coll Cardiol* 1991;17:480–484.

85. Dibner-Dunlap ME, Eckberg DL, Magid NM, Cintron-Trevino NM. The long-term increase of baseline and reflexly augmented levels of human vagal-cardiac nervous activity induced by scopolamine. *Circulation* 1985;71:797–804.

86. Flapan AD, Nolan J, Neilson JMM, Ewing DJ. Effect of captopril on cardiac parasympathetic activity in chronic cardiac failure secondary to coronary artery disease. *Am J Cardiol* 1992;69:532–535.

87. Molgaard H, Mickley H, Pless P, Bjerregaard P, Moller M. Effects of metoprolol on heart rate variability in survivors of acute myocardial infarction. *Am J Cardiol* 1993;71:1357–1359.

88. Bekheit S, Tangella M, el-Sakr A, Rasheed Q, Craelius W, El-Sherif N. Use of heart rate spectral analysis to study the effects of calcium channel blockers on sympathetic activity after myocardial infarction. *Am Heart J* 1990;119:79–85.

89. Casadei B, Piplis A, Sessa F, Conway J, Sleight P. Low doses of scopolamine increase cardiac vagal tone in the acute phase of myocardial infarction. *Circulation* 1993;88:353–357.

90. Vanoli E, DeFerrari GM, Stramba-Badiale M, Hull SS, Foreman RD, Schwartz PJ. Vagal stimulation and prevention of sudden death in conscious dogs with a healed myocardial infarction. *Circ Res* 1991;68:1471–1481.

91. Zuanetti G, Latini R, Neilson JMM, Schwartz PJ, Ewing DJ, the Antiarrhythmic Drug Evaluation Group. Heart rate variability in patients with ventricular arrhythmias: effect of antiarrhythmic drugs. *J Am Coll Cardiol* 1991;17:604–612.

92. Wittkampf FHM, De Jongste MJL, Lie KI, Meijler FL. Effect of right ventricular pacing on ventricular rhythm during atrial fibrillation. *J Am Coll Cardiol* 1988;11:539–545.

93. Meijler FL, Wittkampf FHM. Role of the atrioventricular node in atrial fibrillation. In: Falk RH, Podrid PJ, eds. *Atrial fibrillation: mechanisms and management.* New York: Raven Press, 1992;59–80.

94. Cross S, Lee HS, Jennings K, Rawles J. The integrity and frequency response of the carotid baroreceptor heart-rate reflex. Comparison between sinus rhythm and atrial fibrillation [abstract]. *J Am Coll Cardiol* 1993;21:157A.

95. Thompson JMT, Stewart HB. *Nonlinear dynamics and chaos: geometrical methods for engineers and scientists.* New York: John Wiley, 1986.

96. Denton TA, Diamond GA, Helfant RH, Khan S, Karaguezian H. Fascinating rhythm: a primer on chaos theory and its application to cardiology. *Am Heart J* 1990;120:1419–1440.

97. Stein KM, Lippman N, Kligfield P. Fractal rhythms of the heart. *J Electrocardiol* 1991;24:S72–76.

98. Goldberger A, Rigney D. Sudden death is not chaos. In: Kelso JAS, Mandell AJ, Shlesinger MF, eds. *Dynamic patterns in complex systems.* Singapore: World Scientific Publishers, 1988.

99. Skinner JE, Carpeggiani C, Landisman CE, Fulton KW. Correlation dimension of heartbeat intervals is reduced in conscious pigs by myocardial ischemia. *Circ Res* 1991;68:966.

100. Skinner JE, Pratt CM, Vybiral T. A reduction in the correlation dimension of heartbeat intervals precedes imminent ventricular fibrillation in human subjects. *Am Heart J* 1993;125:731.

101. Hohnloser SH, Klingenheben T, Zabel M, Schroder F, Just H. Intraindividual reproducibility of heart rate variability. *PACE* 1992;15:2211–2214.

102. Huikuri HV, Kessler KM, Terracall E, Castellanos A, Linnaluoto MK, Myerburg RJ. Reproducibility and circadian rhythm of heart rate variability in healthy subjects. *Am J Cardiol* 1990;65:391–393.

Hypertension: Pathophysiology, Diagnosis, and Management, Second Edition,
edited by J.H. Laragh and B.M. Brenner,
Raven Press, Ltd., New York © 1995.

CHAPTER **54**

Psychosocial Stress and Experimental Hypertension

James P. Henry, Joann Liu, and Woerner P. Meehan

PATTERNS OF EMOTIONAL RESPONSE TO PSYCHOSOCIAL STIMULATION

Our emotions mirror our neuroendocrine state, and different patterns of hormonal response are involved in the emotions of anger as opposed to anxiety. The patterns change when anxiety and anger evolve into the depression of defeat. This was elegantly demonstrated by the work of Weiss using two rats yoked together, with identical electrodes on their tails attached to the same shock-delivering device. One rat could escape the shock by responding with a turn of a little wheel in front of it when a warning light came on; for the other rat the shock was inescapable. It had no way of turning the shock off but had to passively accept whatever the other animal experienced. Thus the experiences of the two animals were the same but they differed in the extent of their control (1). This basic work showed that the extent to which a mammal perceives the situation as being under control is of greatest importance in determining the intensity of the emotion experienced. The nature of the emotion is also affected. A mere challenge to control elicits the fight response and anger as the organism makes efforts to ensure that control is retained. But with the eventual perception of loss of effective control, anger progressively evolves into anxiety and fear. When escape by flight is not feasible the panicky and helpless state emerges (2,3).

Using intracranial electrodes to stimulate different parts of the amygdalar nuclear complex of alert unrestrained cats, Stock et al. (4) showed that the fight response with erect ears was elicited by stimulation of the central nucleus. There was a sharp increase of heart rate,

J. P. Henry and J. Liu: Nephrology/Hypertension Division, Drew University of Medicine and Science, Los Angeles, California 90059.
W. P. Meehan: Diabetes/Medicine Division, University of Southern California–Los Angeles Medical Center, Los Angeles, California 90031.

blood pressure, and the peripheral resistance—all typical of the release of norepinephrine. By contrast, stimulation of the basal part of the amygdalar nuclei was associated with the defensive posture of the flight response. The cats flattened instead of raising their ears and they hissed and retracted their heads. These effects are typical of epinephrine and the response changed to one of vasodilation mediated by cholinergic fibers and a more modest increase of heart rate and blood pressure (4).

In work with humans Kadish (5) found that in situations in which there was irritation and resentment, there was an increased ratio of norepinephrine to epinephrine in the urine, and Lovallo et al. (6) have also shown that those experiencing a challenge demanding effort without distress had higher levels of norepinephrine excretion. Similarly, nearly 40 years ago, Elmadjian et al. (7) showed that ice hockey players who were actively competing had a sharp rise in norepinephrine. In contrast, interns at Harvard who were giving lectures to sophisticated critical audiences, a situation in which fear of fail-

ure was likely to be aroused, showed a sharp increase in the release of epinephrine (8).

In situations in which control is lost, the pattern changes and the organism is no longer in the fight-flight mode of anger and anxiety. Instead, the mood is one of depression and helplessness. The sex and maternal drives diminish and there is an arousal of the hypothalamo-pituitary-adrenal (HPA) axis with a loss of effort and an inhibition of the fight-flight program. The behavior is one of submission and acceptance of control from external events; in a social situation this means from those who remain in social control (2,3). In addition to increased levels of adrenocorticotropic hormone (ACTH) and corticosterone, those with loss of control may also have an elevation of prolactin in the plasma. Theorell (9) gives as examples of such a state those who are bereaved by the progressive fatal disease of a close relative or the long distress of subway drivers who have been exposed to a mutilating person-under-train accident.

Thus, important neuroendocrine changes accompany

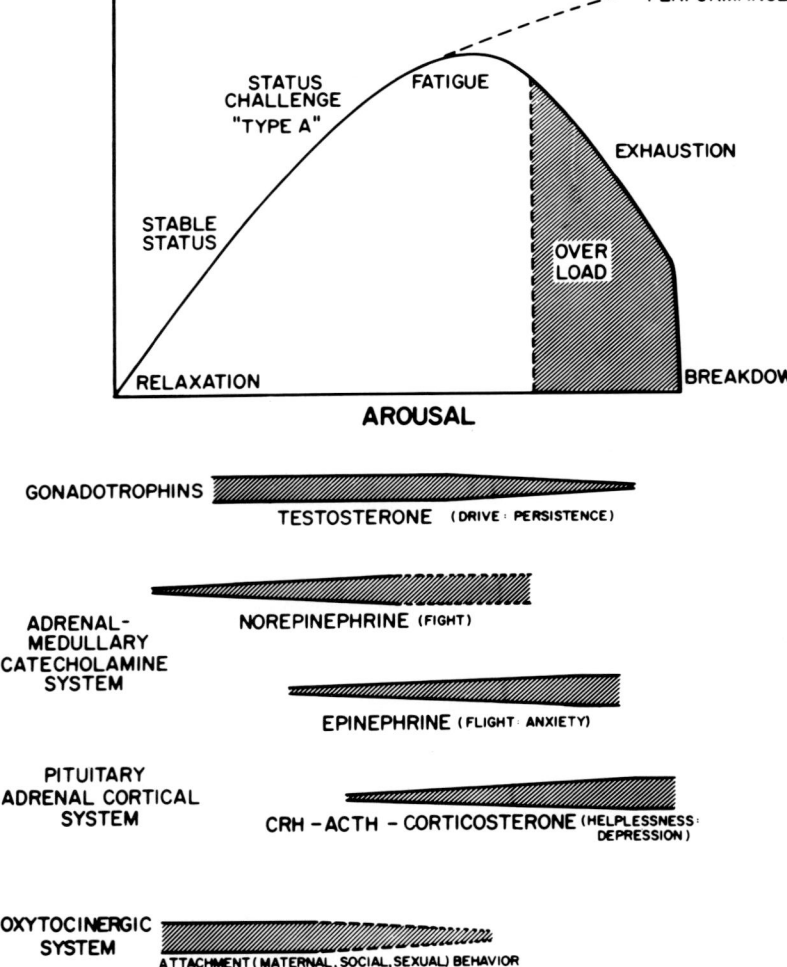

FIG. 1. A theoretical schema based on the curve relating cardiovascular performance to chronic states of arousal. As status and control are increasingly challenged there is a falling off of species preservative activity and an increase of self-preservative effort and the neurotransmitter norepinephrine. As anxiety grows epinephrine and then cortisol rise. Helpless loss of control is associated with arousal of the hypothalamo-pituitary-adrenal (HPA) axis.

the progression from the mere perception of a chronic threat to control to an anxious concern that control may well be lost. In answer to the question of how the mere repetition of neuroendocrine stimulation can bring about disease, it is important to realize that these emotions can be elicited again and again. Further, as a result of prior experience, the responses can leave traces of ever-increasing severity due to sensitization by the repeated confrontations in the social environment. The gradual development of differing pathophysiological conditions such as structural vascular remodeling (10) or adrenal hyperplasia is currently being explained by the differing sustained neuroendocrine patterns that cause the various emotional states.

Figure 1 presents the classic U-shaped relation between arousal, i.e., stress, and performance. It was recently presented in a brief discussion of the biological basis of the stress response (11). It applies to all forms of response to the demand for physical or intellectual effort. Increased arousal in response to increased demand is associated with enhanced performance. But as the performance is progressively upgraded, the organism approaches the point at which the effort is too great; limits are reached and eventually performance drops off. It is critical that the slope of the curve vary according to the individual. It is steeper in those with the resilience of the "born and bred" dominant, and flatter in those who more readily accept defeat. Some are brought close to failure by minor problems; others rarely. In the lower part of the diagram the way in which the various hormones may respond as the curve is traversed is diagrammatically presented. For example, testosterone is reported to increase with successful response to challenge (12). It will fall off eventually as loss of control becomes

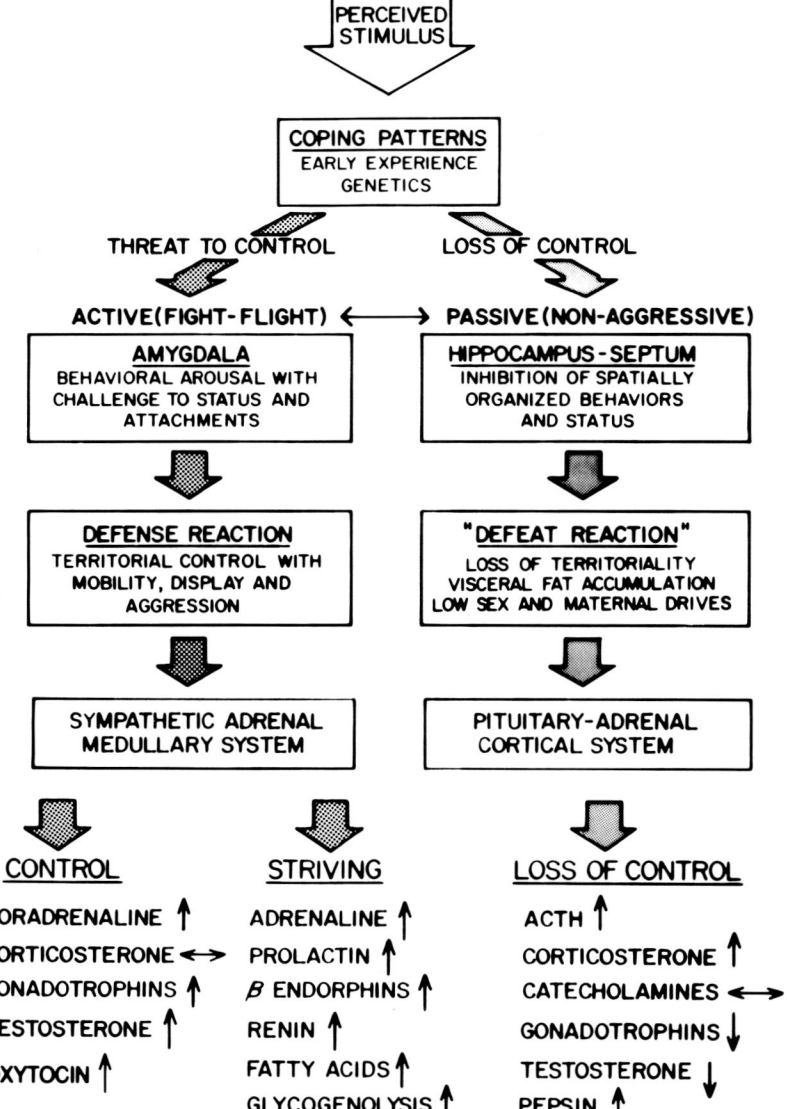

FIG. 2. The defense reaction is activated when the organism is challenged but remains in control. With loss of control there is activation of the HPA axis and the gonadotrophic species preservative system shuts down. Visceral fat accumulates with a cushingoid distribution and there is a shift from active defense to a passive nonaggressive coping style.

imminent. Norepinephrine is the hormone associated with the fighting response to challenge. With the perception that loss of control is increasingly probable, the ratio of the anxiety hormone epinephrine to norepinephrine increases (2,3). As the threat and arousal continue, distress develops and the corticotropin-releasing hormone (CRH)-ACTH-corticosterone, i.e., HPA axis of helplessness and depression, is aroused. These are the hormones classically associated with the Selye general adaptation syndrome (13).

Figure 2 summarizes the same observations in a different form. As the challenge is being met, the organism responds to a threat to its control. The events in the early phases of Fig. 1 are shown in the column on the left in Fig. 2. As the organism runs up the curve, the situation turns to one of striving and the behavior and the neuroendocrine patterns change from those of Cannon's defense reaction to the passive avoidance of Selye's distressed and defeated state. The sympathetic adrenal medullary system gives way to activation of the pituitary adrenal cortical axis (2,11).

EARLY OBSERVATIONS IN CHIMPANZEES, MONKEYS, AND RATS

Prior involvement with animals in rocket flight led to the assignment of the senior author to the supervision of the physiological aspects of the animal phase of Project Mercury. The ensuing 3 years led to the discovery of an unexpected and dramatic hypertension in the flight-trained apes.

The Manned Space Flight program was initiated with the Mercury orbiting capsule project in the early 1960s (14). The objective of this first step to landing a man on the moon was a safe return after orbiting the earth with a man on board. To test the adequacy of the life support system, an animal flight program was established. It was decided to place a chimpanzee in a pressurized couch on the pilot's seat. Because the space was so small, an immature animal weighing 20 to 25 kg had to be used. To establish what effects the weightless state might have on performance, a comprehensive series of operant tasks were imposed on the animal by an expert team of psychologists. Six young males were trained in a series of tasks. Their motivation was controlled by using shock avoidance as well as food pellet and fluid reward. The tasks involved the simultaneous working of two levers. The one on the left imposed a Sidman avoidance task—turning off a light that signaled a shock, while the one on the right had to be activated to postpone a foot shock that would otherwise be delivered every 15 seconds (15). At first the young animals all lived together in a large enclosed space. But as flight time approached they were transferred to small, single cages from which they could be more readily removed and placed in the restraint garment that held them in the training capsule (Fig. 3).

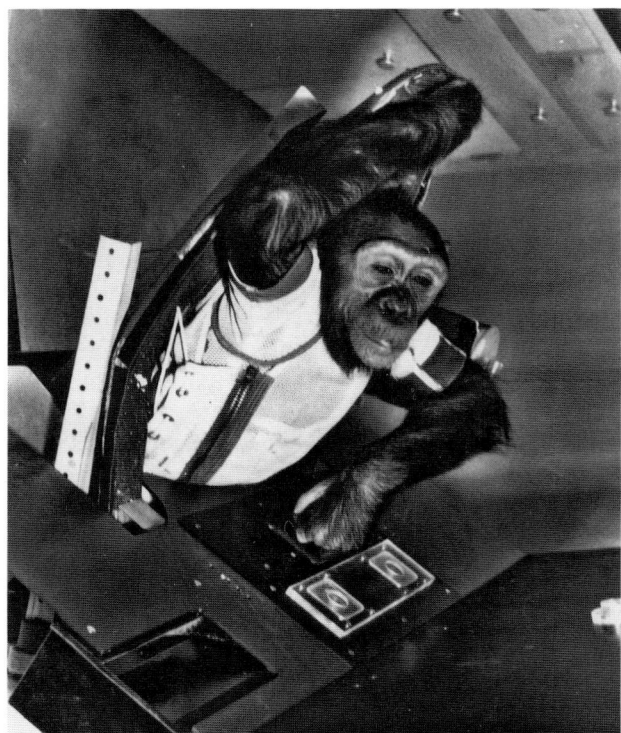

FIG. 3. A young chimpanzee is held in front of his operant task by a nylon restraint suit laced to the couch.

The daily hours of training went on for 15 months starting in the spring of 1960. There was increased rigor in the spring of 1961 as flight time approached. This reached a peak in the summer when two flight animals were selected. At this time, arm cuff measurements of a group of five animals were made at approximately three-month intervals during an 18-month peroid. They rose from a normal 120/90 mm Hg to a plateau of 160/130 mm Hg (Fig. 4). Immediately after the orbital flight, training ceased and the animals were returned to their large home cage. As the figure shows, by the time the last pressures were taken in December 1961 they had returned to near-normal values. These indirect pressures are supported by the flight data. The blood pressure of Enos, the orbital flight chimpanzee, was measured from a tibial arterial catheter for 3 hours before flight and throughout the orbiting experience. It was consistently sustained in excess of 180/140 mm Hg (15).

These pressures were immediately recognized as remarkable for such young animals and a year later a study was initiated at the University of Southern California to determine whether the abnormality had persisted. Two chimpanzees were obtained from the laboratory at Holloman Air Force Base where the training had been conducted. Their pressures were recorded for 2 weeks while undergoing operant training and restraint. One was an experienced trainee and the other was inexperienced. Each was restrained as shown in Fig. 3 for 2 weeks, while

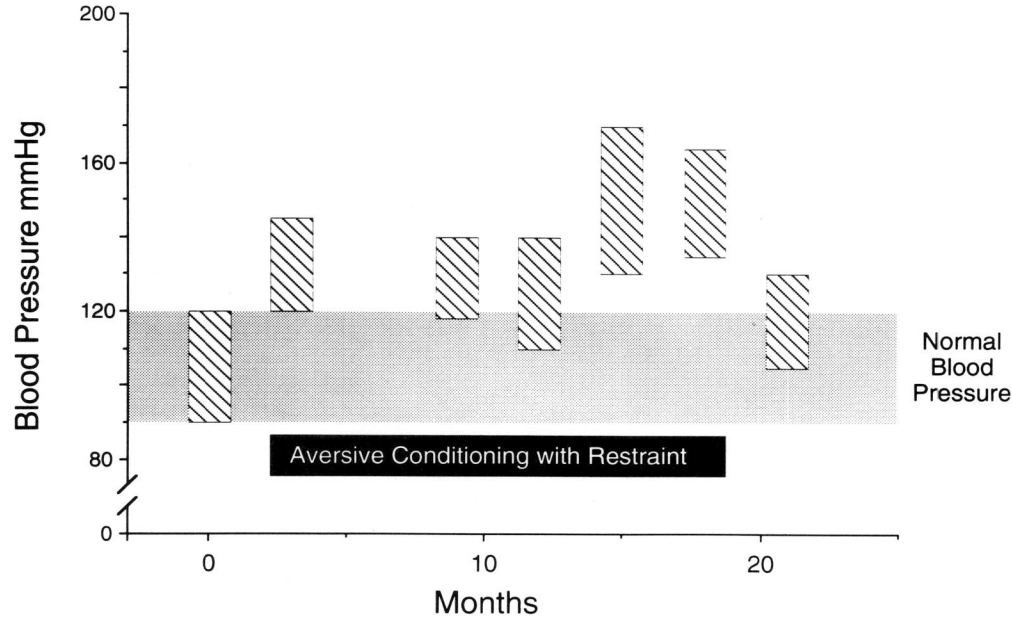

FIG. 4. Mean arm-cuff sphygmomanometric blood pressures of five young chimpanzees were taken at intervals during prolonged training for a Mercury orbiting flight. *Black bar:* Daily aversive conditioning with restraint in a couch. Two months after training was discontinued the pressure returned toward normal.

tibial blood pressures were directly recorded by catheter. The differences were striking. The initial pressure of the experienced animal was 147/76 mm Hg. It increased to 180/142 mm Hg by the seventh day of restraint and subsided to 166/100 mm Hg at the conclusion of the tests on the 14th day (16). Throughout this time the operant conditioning tasks were imposed with foot shock for failure. In all, 20 measures of renal clearance were made on the two animals using para-amino hippuric acid (Fig. 5).

The higher diastolic pressures were accompanied by a reduction of renal blood flow to less than one-half the nonstressed levels ($p = .001$) (17).

Furthermore, the behavior of the trained animal contrasted with the untrained one. Restraint of the untrained animal was accompanied by initial struggles and vocalization. However, the tibial arterial pressure rose from a resting 125/85 mm Hg to only 140/100 mm Hg despite the emotion of forced training. It returned to 125/85 mm Hg when the operant task had been discontinued for 3 days (16). By contrast the trained animal was strikingly "well adapted," calmly eating apples while recording a systolic blood pressure of over 200 mm Hg.

Although the data were limited, these long-term observations of the response of the blood pressure of high-spirited, playful young animals to punishment and restraint is supported by similar data on the blood pressure of children and adults restrained for burn therapy (18). The demanding environment led to a renal vasoconstriction with a sustained high blood pressure. As the months passed, the hypertensive "well-trained" animals ceased

to be agitated, becoming calm and deceptively normal. On the strength of these observations a program was initiated to see if high blood pressure could be induced by psychosocial stress in other mammals, such as mice. The results of this work are summarized below (19).

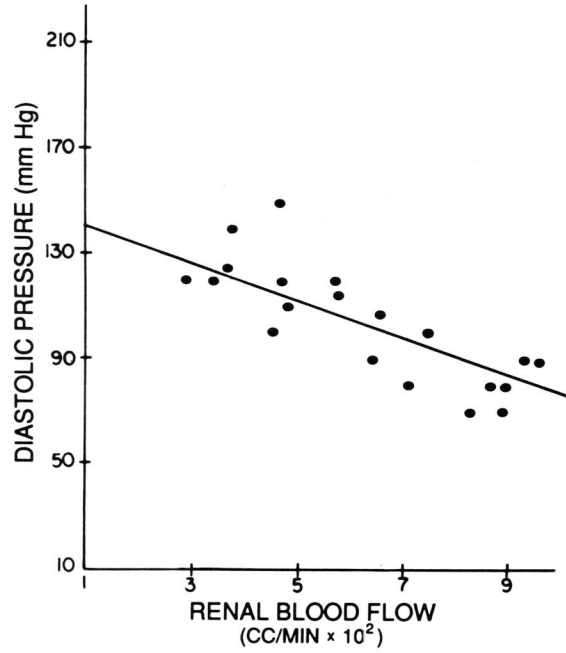

FIG. 5. The relationship of diastolic pressure recorded from a tibial arterial catheter and renal blood flow of chronically restrained chimpanzees. $r = -.84$; $p = .0001$.

The chimpanzee studies were completed in 1964. In 1961 Pickering (20) had already published his theoretical study, *The Nature of Essential Hypertension*. In one chapter he discussed the review by Simonson and Brozek (21) of Russian research on essential hypertension. Furthermore, he visited various Pavlovian dog laboratories and the primate facility at Sukhumi. He notes that there have been several Russian studies with dogs that showed that a stable hypertension will develop in response to the repeated imposition of conflicting stimuli. The work was modeled on the classic Pavlovian paradigm in which a dog was forced to discriminate between a luminous disk and an ellipse. As the ratio of the axes of the ellipse was changed to the point at which the animal could no longer successfully discriminate it from a circle, it would become highly anxious, barking and biting when brought into the experimental room.

Similar emotional breakdown occurred at Sukhumi in a social situation where a dominant male baboon was denied access to a former mate now living with a rival male in the next cage. Over a period of a year the systolic blood pressure of such frustrated animals rose from a normal 120 mm Hg into the 170s. Pickering commented that the Russian work is evidence that "chronic emotional arousal may play an important part in the development of human essential hypertension."

During the same period American investigators attempted to induce chronic hypertension by emotionally arousing monkeys and rats. They arrived at the same conclusions as the Russians. Although it was necessary to use long periods of stimulation, which induced anger and irritation but did not intimidate, it was indeed feasible. For example, Forsyth (22) induced high blood pressure in five out of six chair-restrained rhesus monkeys exposed to shock avoidance. The task forced them to press a lever seconds after a light. Systolic blood pressure rose from the 130s to 150 to 160 mm Hg. Like Pavlov's dogs the monkeys became excited and hyperactive, which suggested to the authors they were "chronically" emotionally aroused, but the pressures did not rise for several months. In parallel work Herd's group used squirrel monkeys. They, too, had to continue for months. Eventually the pressures remained elevated in four out of six animals. They concluded that "reproducible elevations of blood pressure can be associated with behavior" (23).

Six years later Friedman and Dahl (24) exposed Dahl's salt-sensitive rats to daily conflict. They received a shock as an unavoidable consequence of eating. Pellets of food were given in response to pressing a lever at the correct time interval after a light had appeared. The interval was varied unpredictably so that the rat could not achieve a sense of control. After a variable number of lever presses they received a shock deepening the conflict because their responses were being punished in an unpredictable manner. The result of this persistently uncontrollable situation was to induce a 30 to 40 mm Hg elevation of blood pressure.

The above observations were confined to blood pressure. Lawler et al. (25), using borderline hypertensive rats, have extended the work to include pathophysiological observations. Using 3 months of conflict stimuli, which for 2 hours a day imposed the distressing choice of five weak versus one stronger shock, led to a rise in pressure from an already elevated 150 mm Hg to 185 mm Hg. This persisted for 2 further months after cessation of the shocks and was accompanied by severe myocardial fibrosis with myofibrillar degeneration.

Thus, operant conditioning procedures will lead to chronic arousal of the defense-alarm fight-flight response. The long time taken by the subject to become hypertensive under the influence of this reflex suggests, as Lever (26) has recently argued, that some gradual mechanism such as Folkow's (10) slow hypertrophy of the medial layer of the resistance vessels is taking place. The thickening of the vascular wall, i.e., the increase of the ratio of the inner to the outer radius, occurs under the influence of trophic agents whose identity is slowly becoming known. Lever's group (27) has recently proposed a role for angiotensin. Chronic emotional arousal of the solitary animal will, as the preceding work shows, eventually lead to hypertension. But this arousal is being driven by behavioral instrumentation. Will the emotions of chronic psychosocial stimulation in mammals including humans also lead to the hypertensive state?

DOMINANCE AND SUBORDINATION STUDIES IN RATS

The preceding data were obtained from solitary animals that eventually developed high blood pressure when trapped in a situation in which they had to respond to conflicting painful stimuli. The behavioral response could, as Fokkema (28) points out in his study of social behavior and blood pressure, be quite different from the more natural circumstances of social interaction. Using an aortic catheter emerging at the head with a spring to permit the animal to move freely, he obtained significant data on the response to brief dyadic behavioral encounters. In other experiments he intermittently recorded the pressure of catheterized animals that for the rest of the time ran free in a 3 × 2 × 1 meter cage. This was fitted with five nest boxes in which defeated animals could find shelter from further attack. Behavior was categorized as aggressive threat, biting and kicking, and attacking and chasing. Defensive gestures involved the upright posture with forepaws extended, crouched submission, and flight. The major finding was that in such a seminatural situation, territorial and social behavior was highly correlated with the intensity of the blood pressure response; the more aggressive rats had higher blood pressure responses.

Figure 6 shows the blood pressure responses to conflict experiences. With defeat there was a 25 mm Hg rise. Winning an encounter had a less intense effect, i.e., 10 mm Hg. If the animal had previously been defeated, the effect of a victory was also 10 mm Hg. If it had previously been defeated and was then psychosocially stimulated, i.e., threatened by exposure to the now harmless victor penned in a small cage, the mere sight and smell of the victor would raise the former victim's blood pressure by 25 mm Hg.

Fokkema's studies were accompanied by some measurements of plasma norepinephrine, epinephrine, and corticosterone levels. In short dyadic social interactions the height of the blood pressure reaction was related to the height of the catecholamine response. There were higher baseline blood pressures in the rats that showed a higher epinephrine response in a 9-week colony experience. These more aggressive rats had higher baseline norepinephrine and epinephrine levels. Some of them developed a sustained high blood pressure that the author attributed to initiation of Folkow's sequence of structural vascular changes (10). Baseline values of plasma corticosterone were high in both dominant and subdominant animals. Since the higher blood pressures were noted in the subdominant rats, Fokkema thought the corticosterone action might potentiate the response.

The factor of control over the social environment and the continuous effort to gain control and keep it seem important to the regulation of blood pressure. Passive rats that made no effort and outcasts that had been repeatedly defeated often had gastric ulcers, yet they had lower blood pressures than the animals that were still actively competing. The author noted that their situation was analogous to that of rats facing inescapable rather than escapable electric shock (1,29). He concludes that chronic high blood pressure is the result of the attempts of socially active animals to adapt to an environment that is both threatening and demanding.

Certain psychosocial interactions will lead to a fall in blood pressure. Fokkema consistently reported an increase of blood pressure when his rats were challenged but not defeated, remaining able to achieve control (28,30). The typical response was one of aggressive activity with an increase in norepinephrine levels. But in 6 of 11 defeated rats he observed a 5 mm Hg fall in blood pressure (30) and Adams and Blizard (31) report a far more dramatic fall in the course of conflicts staged between a resident-trained Long-Evans "fighter" rat and inbred salt-sensitive S/JR Dahl rats placed in the fighter's cage. In contrast with the S/JR salt-sensitive rat, defeated R/JR salt-resistant rats will not show a fall in pressure (31). This may be because as Eichelman et al. (32) and others have reported, the salt-resistant R/JR strain is more aggressive than the salt-sensitive S/JR strain. Thus, the two Dahl strains differ in their behavior as well as in their response to salt. It was found that after repeated encounters the blood pressure of the salt-sensitive strain would fall by as much as 20 to 40 mm Hg.

The first encounter with the fighter did not lead to such a dramatic fall. It appears that it took time for them to perceive that the Long-Evans rat completely outmatched them. Adams and Blizard (31) note that the submissive gesture of standing erect with the forelimbs limply extended developed in the S/JR rats only in the latter part of the first encounter. However, in subsequent sessions it was assumed immediately on contact. When defeated, the more aggressive R/JR rats also assumed the same submissive posture but their blood pressure did not fall. The genetic factors affecting salt sensitivity apparently affect the control of blood pressure as well.

Pursuing the problem further, Adams and Blizard (31) established that the effects of an electric shock on the S/JR rats was quite different from the effect of confrontation with the fighter. Shocks uniformly caused a rise in the blood pressure. They concluded that there is specificity in the responses to different stressors. Perhaps the

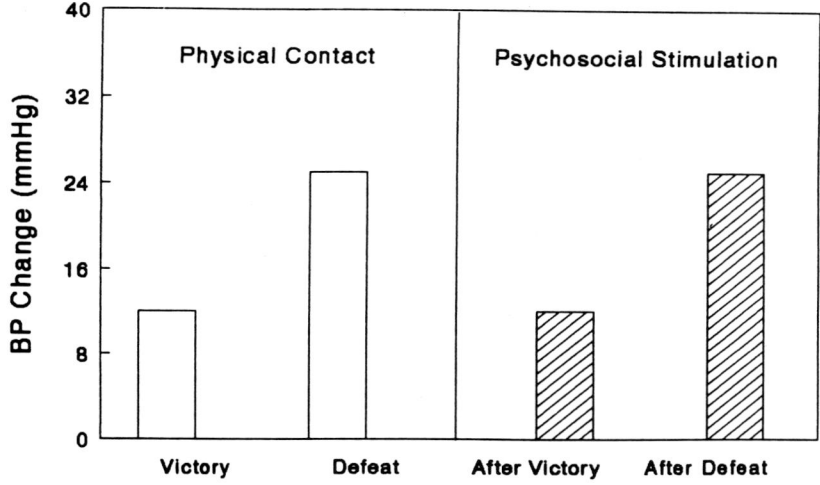

FIG. 6. The blood pressure responses of rats to winning or losing a 10-minute interaction with another rat. The changes after actual physical aggression were no greater than those induced by the psychosocial stimulation of being close to the former rival, now harmless because of confinement to a small cage.

blood pressure decrement seen in the defeated rat is representative of a state of helplessness and depression that is not induced by the type of electric shocks that were used and not as easily induced in the R/JR in spite of defeat.

PSYCHOSOCIAL STRESS AND HYPERTENSION IN RATS

Effects of Conflict Depend on Genetic as well as Environmental Factors

The preceding work with rats shows that sustained elevations of blood pressure do not always follow conflict. Using a complex cage formation that Henry et al. (19) had employed in mice to give high blood pressure, Harrap et al. (33) were surprised to find fighting associated with gastric ulcers, adrenal hypertrophy, and elevated plasma renin and norepinephrine, but not elevation of blood pressure. They concluded that stress due to psychological disturbances will not produce chronic hypertension in the rat. Recently Gelsema et al. (34) have repeated these observations, monitoring the blood pressure by implanted transmitters. This latest methodology led to the same conclusions as those of Harrap et al. Social stress caused adrenal and right and left ventricular hypertrophy but not hypertension. A recent authoritative review of behavioral medicine in hypertension states, "The data in support of the proposition that stress alone could produce hypertension are not compelling" (35), and Lawler's group (25) has suggested that to model human disease it is necessary to use animals that are genetically predisposed to becoming hypertensive.

The complexities of the stress response were discussed above, and evidence was presented that different emotions have different neuroendocrine characteristics (2). Different perceptions of control result in different patterns of neuroendocrine response. The data suggest that the stimulus most effective in raising blood pressure is the continuing conflict that results from a degree of social instability that prevents establishment of a stable dominance heirachy (2). Wexler and Greenberg (36), Ely and Weigand (37), Szilagyi (38), and Mormede et al. (39) have together shown that constantly changing the composition of groups of male rats living in large cages with sexually active females will result in chronic competition, with fighting and an unstable hierachy. The ensuing psychosocial stimulation will lead to various neuroendocrine and cardiovascular changes including a sustained increase in blood pressure. Details of the approach have recently been published and a brief general account of the work and its conclusions follows (40).

Three strains of rats were chosen that differ genetically in their aggressiveness. The first was the WKHA strain developed by Hendley from the spontaneously hyperten-

sive rat (SHR). They are low on the allogrooming that precedes aggression and in active aggression itself (41). Careful observation in our laboratories over a period of months failed to detect any fighting in groups of males and females and no bites were observed at any time either on the tail or rump. The second strain chosen was the Sprague-Dawley albino commonly used in psychosocial studies. They, too, have been closely observed by us. These rats do not bite but the males do show agonistic behavior, such as scratching each other, especially in the mixed groups of males and females. They do not, however, harm each other. We have therefore called them "peaceable." The third strain was the Long-Evans rats. They were used by Adams and Blizard (31) as "fighters" to intimidate the Dahl salt-sensitive S/JR rats because of their "proven level of aggression." In our hands they have lived up to their reputation becoming involved in serious fights. In the course of monitoring the Long-Evans groups a biting score was given to each male: +, if there are a few small scars on the rump or fewer than three bites on the whole body; ++, if one-third of the rump has scars or if there are three to five bites on the whole body; and +++, if more than half of the rump has scars or if there are more than five bites on the whole body. We have called the +++ group "aggressive."

Communal Cages and a Randomization Technique

Four 250 to 300 g experimental males were randomly assigned to each of five stainless steel breeder cages sized $51 \times 61 \times 18$ cm. Four 200 to 250 g females of the same age were added to make up five groups of eight adults each. Since all the females were fertile their reproductive state was one of communal breeding. Control groups were housed in large polyethylene cages. Each held one male and one female. The males remained in the same cage with the same partner while she nursed and was weaned of her young. When the young in the communal cages became pregnant they were removed and housed separately until they had nursed for 3 weeks. The pups were then weaned and the mothers returned at random to one of the breeder groups. When the composition of the breeder groups assigned to the five large communal cages was changed, their ear-punch number was noted. They were then assigned to fresh cages in accordance with a prearranged code so that the groups were constantly changing (42).

The effects of the ensuing unfamiliarity on social interaction and, therefore, in the bite-prone Long-Evans strains, on the extent of scarring on the rump and tail were striking. The percentage of severely scarred animals, i.e., with more than three to four bites on the body, was far greater in those that had been randomized in the communal cages. Five studies of various types, each lasting 4 to 6 months, were completed. Each used five large communal cages. All the experiments had aimed to induce hypertension and pathophysiology. Yet with the exception of the unstable Long-Evans group, the changes were modest and the final, more dramatic changes with this strain were the outcome of a slow trial-and-error process. In other words, only certain genotypes responded with an increase of blood pressure to this social manipulation.

Blood Pressure Response to Psychosocial Stress

Blood pressure was measured indirectly once a month using equipment of the same design as that employed for the studies of mice. These indirect blood pressure measurements using a tail cuff were made only on males. Three measurements were taken to obtain each pressure reading and they were only made several days after any change in social grouping.

Figure 7 summarizes results for the five studies, each of which lasted for upward of half a year. The top line is for the peaceable WKHA strain. Despite the twice weekly changes for $4\frac{1}{2}$ months, which imposed continuous disorder, there was no fighting, and their blood pressure did not differ from the controls. The studies with Long-Evans rats showed that despite their aggressive behavior, when group composition was maintained constant as in the second experiment from the top, there was only a very modest increase of pressure of no more than 5 to 10 mm Hg. In the next two studies cited, which were of the Sprague-Dawley rats, the rats were randomized weekly with ensuing social instability. There was a gradual development of a consistent (10 mm Hg) blood pressure elevation. Repeated and individual analyses of variance (ANOVAs) of the monthly blood pressure showed that, although modest, the pressure changes were highly significant ($p = .0001$). In the final study at the bottom of Fig. 6 the Long-Evans rats were kept in social disorder

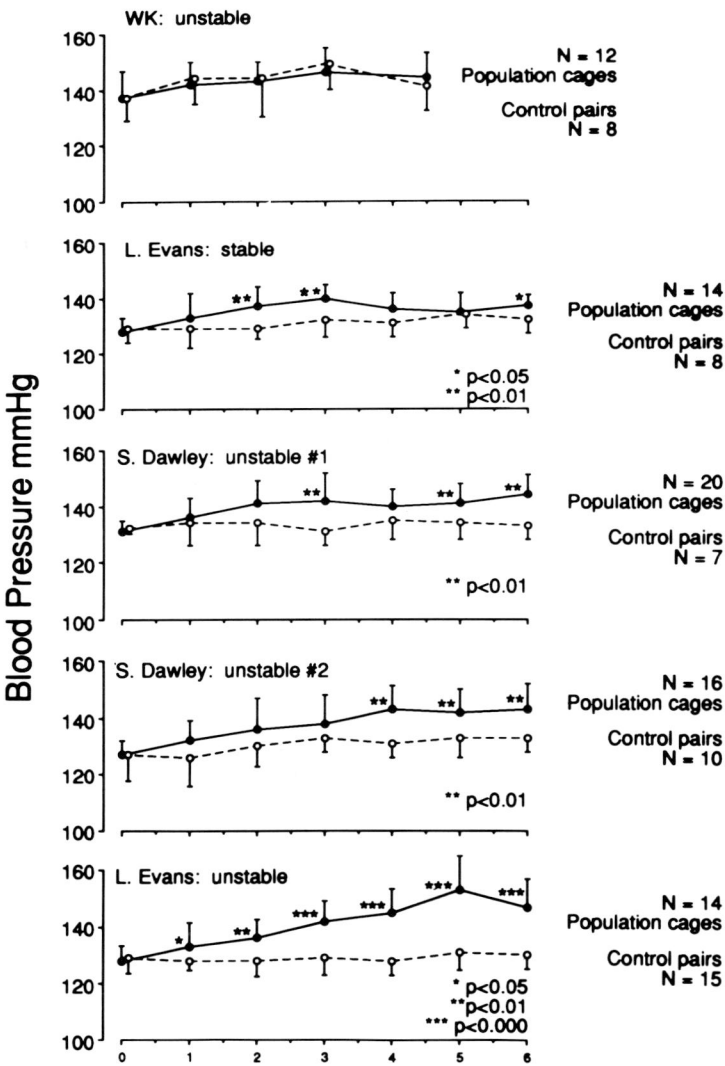

FIG. 7. Line graphs show effects of long-term psychosocial stimulation on blood pressure of male rats in mixed male and female communities (*closed circles*). The Wistar-Kyoto hypertensive rats do not fight; the Sprague-Dawley rats compete and scratch but do not bite; the Long-Evans strain is aggressively competitive, biting freely. These evidences of social stress are more marked in the unstable than in the stable colonies. Controls are male–female dyads in standard cages (*open circles*). *Vertical bars* show standard deviation.

by randomizing the males. They showed a gradual, progressive rise in blood pressure, which attained a highly significant 20 mm Hg differential in the later months.

In addition to the observation of blood pressure by the indirect cuff method, Fig. 8 presents systolic pressure data using the favored carotid artery direct pressure technique (43). Both the second, i.e., the stable, and the fifth, i.e., the unstable, Long-Evans colonies were evaluated. In all cases the animals were left for a day in a shaving-filled box to recover from surgery. All the records displayed on the oscillograph had a dicrotic notch and a pulse pressure ranging from 25 to 35 mm Hg. These pressures taken on conscious animals 24 hours after separation from the colony differed by as much as 25 mm Hg ($p = .001$) from the controls as measured by the same technique.

Heart and Adrenal Weights and Catecholamine Synthetic Enzymes in Socially Stressed Rats

The heart and adrenal weights of both stable and unstable Long-Evans rat colonies increased significantly, reflecting the arousal and social interaction in both sets of colonies. What was not expected was that there was also a significant increase in the heart and adrenal weights of the WKHA rats that had been so peaceable that they bore no tail or rump bites. Also, their blood pressure had remained unchanged from the controls

throughout nearly 5 months of social disorder. These results support the detailed observations of Harrap et al. (33) and Gelsema et al. (34), who reported heart and adrenal hypertrophy despite their failure to induce chronic hypertension in various strains of rats by psychosocial stress.

We have previously used tyrosine hydroxylase (TYOH) and phenylethanolamine-N-methyl transferase (PNMT) in the adrenals as measures of repeated arousal of the sympathetic adrenal medullary system (44). These enzymes are critical for the synthesis of norepinephrine and epinephrine, respectively. In the Sprague-Dawleys there was no significant difference between the levels of TYOH in the communal and paired groups. However, PNMT, which is the enzyme concerned with epinephrine synthesis, was significantly elevated. On the other hand, in the Long-Evans rats the situation was reversed. Here the norepinephrine-related TYOH was significantly elevated but there was no difference between the adrenal PNMT in the communal and the paired groups (40).

Pathophysiological Changes in Socially Stressed Rats

Histological observations were made in the two Sprague-Dawley studies and the incidence of early myocardial fibrosis and mucopolysaccharide deposition in the aortas was determined. The changes were minor but

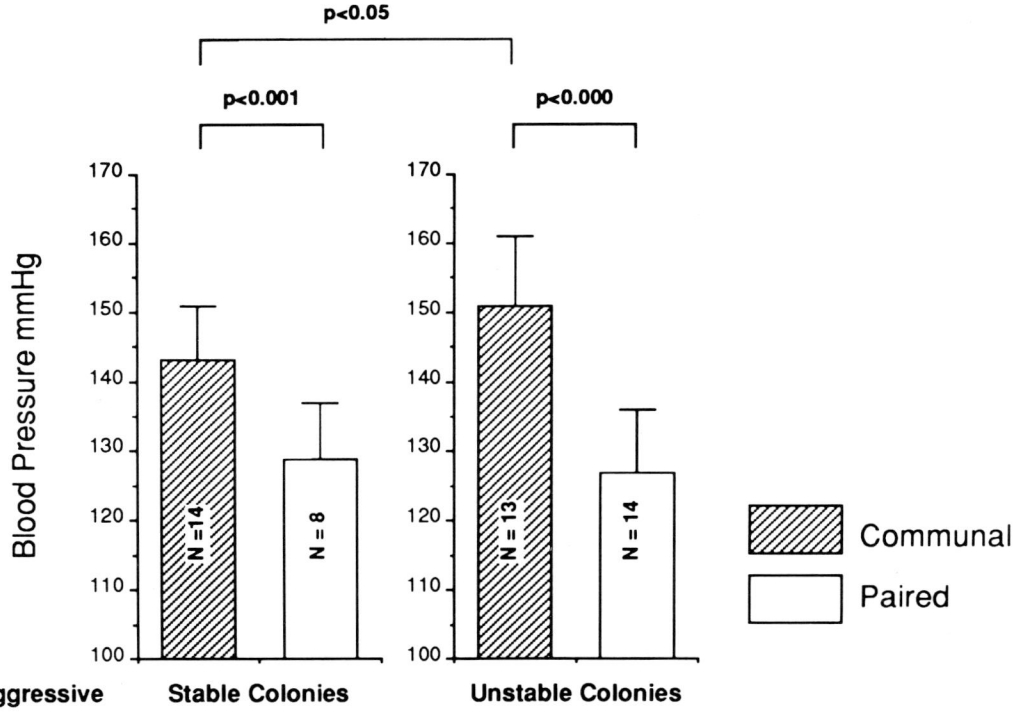

FIG. 8. Bar graph shows confirmation of tail-cuff pressure by direct systolic carotid arterial determinations of stable and unstable Long-Evans rat colonies at termination (6 months). Pressure is higher in the more stressed unstable colonies. *Vertical bars* show standard deviation.

unequivocal. The combined data for the two groups yielded a chi-square test of $p = .03$ for the hearts and $p = .0001$ for the aortas.

In the case of the unstable groups of Long-Evans rats a measure of glomerulosclerosis was added. The myocardial fibrosis and mucopolysaccharide deposition were at the same early stages as was found in the Sprague-Dawley experiments, but the renal damage was quite severe. Approximately a third showed a well-developed atrophy and loss of glomerular capillaries, and in one animal the destruction was severe.

Comments on Psychosocial Stress and Hypertension in Rats

The failure of some studies of psychosocial stress to induce hypertension in rats appears to be due to differences in the genetic and environmental conditions of the experiments. Different strains of rats have different patterns of response to the social environment. Some are more aggressive and these are more likely to develop high blood pressure. The way in which animals relate to each other is critical and if the group is involved in active competition, even if it is a docile strain, an increase in blood pressure will ensue (40).

Rats are highly social and it appears that if a researcher wishes to increase blood pressure, the rats should not be permitted to become familiar with each other and develop a stable hierachy. As long as the group composition is constantly changing, the rats sustain irritable and aggressive relations with each other. If a stable hierachy with a dominant male develops, the subordinates fall into the state of loss of control typical of defeat (3,45). In time they come to accept their position, effort ceases, and their endocrine status becomes normal. This work suggests that it is necessary to use the right strain of animal and the appropriate psychosocial stress in order to induce high blood pressure in normotensive rats.

COMPETITIVE PSYCHOSOCIAL STRESS INDUCES HYPERTENSION IN NORMOTENSIVE MICE

Complex Population Cages and Social Disorder

If the members of a community of male and female mice compete vigorously and persistently for control over access to desiderata such as food, water, a mate, and a safe place to live, a state of chronic high blood pressure develops that closely models human essential hypertension. By controlling the genetic strain, the housing, and the early experience, the intensity of the stress and the resulting hypertension can be modified (40,45).

In our laboratories such a system has been employed for some time. Beginning at the age of 4 months, 16 males and 16 female CBA/USC mice live in complex population cages that consist of seven intercommunicating boxes. Each box is approximately the same size as the standard $27 \times 14 \times 13$ cm opaque polycarbonate vivarium cages in which the male or female controls live. The six similar transparent lucite boxes are connected into a circle by flexible plastic tubes big enough for a mouse to pass through. The boxes are also connected by similarly sized tubes to a central hexagon lucite box with a wire mesh lid (0.5-cm squares), holding sufficient food to last 3 to 4 days and five 250-mL water bottles. The whole system can be mounted on a sliding shelf. Four of the shelves can be assembled into a rack that would fit in a 1.5-m square space.

The narrow tubes provide a continuous challenge to the position of each mouse in the dominance-subordinance hierachy, making it difficult for mice to pass each other and thus forcing one of two entering opposite ends of a tube to back down (46). The central food and water box serves as another area where dominance-subordinance interaction may occur, as in Calhoun's (47) behavioral sinks. The varied escape possibilities provided by the three entrances to each box make the design a modification of the multiple escape pen used by Scott (48) for his studies of fighting mice.

Males derived from separate litters lack the affiliative behavior toward one another that is shown by siblings. Formerly isolated males are even less able to adjust to the presence of others. The addition of females exacerbates male competition. The result is a disordered society in which a would-be dominant puts down opposition by harassing his subordinates, and brief fights and chases disturbing the peace of the colony break out periodically. The result is that normal females fail to raise their young. As males move from one box to another through narrow tubes they are repeatedly forced into tests of dominance or subordinance and all eventually become more or less scarred from nips and bites on the rear. This even applies to dominants because their position is short-lived and all are eventually challenged and exposed to repeated confrontations as they struggle to maintain territory in the multiple entrance box system.

Pathophysiological Changes due to Psychosocial Stress

In mice competing in complex population cages the ensuing hypertension approximates 160 ± 20 mm Hg (SD). The groups have usually been started at 4 months of age with 16 males plus an equal number of females (Fig. 9). At first reversible, the hypertension gradually becomes fixed and progressive arteriosclerosis associated with myocardial fibrosis develops, becoming severe after 6 months (49). Interstitial nephritis also develops, leading to renal failure (50). At least in the initial stages this hypertension results from repeated activation of the sympathetic nervous system and the adrenal content of

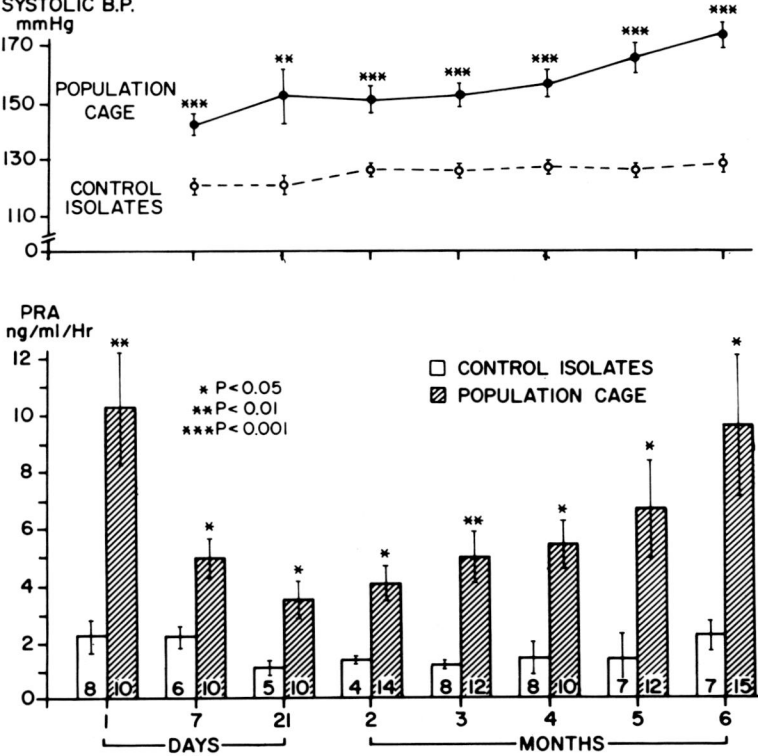

FIG. 9. Longitudinal study of plasma renin activity (PRA) and systolic blood pressure in control isolates and population cage mice. The latter had been previously isolated and then placed in the population cage at 4 months of age. The number of mice in each group is inset in the histograms. *p < .05; **p < .01; ***p < .001.

the catecholamine synthetic enzymes TYOH and PNMT nearly doubles (51). Renin briefly rises to high levels, subsiding after a week to high-normal values (52). Adrenal weight increases by 30%. With time this adrenal cortical hypertrophy may progress to hyperplasia. In addition plasma corticosterone is chronically elevated (2,45).

The picture is one of strong stimulation of the fight-flight response by a challenge that the organism is trying to meet effectively. It involves an arousal of the locus coeruleus as the central amygdalar nuclei respond and norepinephrine levels rise (53).

Arousal of the Sympathoadrenal Medullary System

As threats persist from day to day in an unstable disordered society, further subtle pathological changes gradually develop in the blood pressure control system. One of these shows the striking similarity between psychosocial hypertension in the rodent and in the human (45,52). In the mouse in the early stages of psychosocial stimulation, plasma renin is high (Fig. 9). This parallels the situation in man that Julius (54,55) describes in his discussion of autonomic nervous dysfunction in essential hypertension. In man there is a neurogenic elevation of cardiac activity and increased sympathetic tone to the kidney arterioles and veins that can be abolished by autonomic blockade. The emotionally arousing interactions between male mice in the presence of females in the

complex population cages lead to a doubling of adrenal catecholamine synthetic enzymes within a week (51). This increase is still persisting 6 months later. Plasma catecholamine levels are highest in those with the most social interaction. In mice as in humans and in contrast with the delayed effects of angiotensin-converting enzyme (ACE) inhibitors, β-sympathetic blockade is effective from the beginning of the period of psychosocial stress in the population cage (2,56).

In the human as time goes on the geometrically based vascular reactivity of Folkow (10), critical for the development of primary hypertension, develops gradually. Julius associates this with the changes in responsiveness of heart and blood vessels that are the basis of a transition over the years from a high cardiac output to a high resistance hypertension (54,55). As this progresses renin levels normalize and ACE inhibitors, which have been without influence on the blood pressure despite the high renin and the intense cardiac and vascular adrenergic drive, suddenly become effective. There is evidence that the same mechanisms are at work in mice and that changes in the tissue sensitivity to renin are occurring.

Captopril, Blood Pressure, and Vascular Reactivity in Psychosocially Hypertensive Mice

A collaboration between those working with psychosocial stress in the mouse and renin and vascular research laboratories has revealed the unsuspected

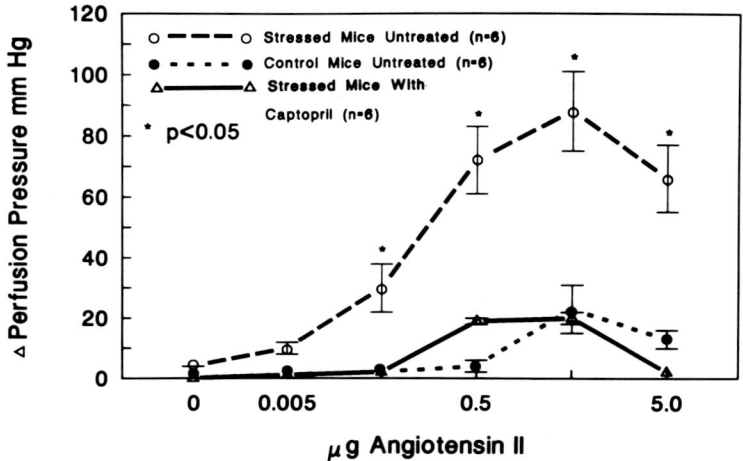

FIG. 10. Study of the vascular reactivity of mice that had become hypertensive as a result of exposure to psychosocial stress for 2 months. At this stage plasma renin is normal and the pressure is responsive to ACE inhibitor. Mean pressor responses of hindquarter vasculature and threshold constrictor responses were elicited at a significantly lower dose of angiotensin II than normal mice. ACE inhibitor abolished this sensitivity. The evidence indicated that hyperresponsiveness to angiotensin II in resistance vessels is critical for maintenance of psychosocial hypertension.

subtleties of the interactions between psychosocial hypertension, the renin-angiotensin system, and ACE inhibitors. Figure 9 presents an early set of observations that were made on socially interacting mice whose renin levels were being studied (52). The diagram shows that during the initial period of excitement plasma renin is at very high levels but that after 3 weeks it has subsided to the high-normal range despite a steadily increasing systolic pressure. The isolated control animals present low-normal renin levels. This pattern is similar to that seen in human essential hypertension and the mice appear to be paralleling the human disease. For example, when an ACE inhibitor was given to mice that had been exposed to psychosocial stress for varying periods, there was no response until the pressure had been elevated for at least a month. It then became highly effective (56). In the accelerated biological time of the short-lived mouse this is equivalent to many months in a human.

The data presented in Fig. 10 suggest that it is not the plasma renin level that is the critical factor in determining a role for angiotensin in the development of hypertension. At 2 months a greatly increased vascular sensitivity to angiotensin II has developed in both the renal and hindquarter vessels. This unexpected increase could explain how hypertension could develop in spite of normal plasma renin levels. The curve with long dashes in Fig. 10 shows the dramatically increased hindquarter vascular reactivity of the untreated chronically stressed mice. The solid curve, which represents those that had been given an ACE inhibitor (started well before they were exposed to the stress), shows that it has abolished this stress-induced hyperresponsiveness to angiotensin II. In the same article, Webb et al. (57) show that this effect of the ACE inhibitor is accompanied by effective control of the psychosocial hypertension.

This work with mice fits with the observations reviewed by Dzau (58) that the ACE inhibitor can be effective despite normal plasma renin levels. It appears that the sympathetic nerve supply to a particular tissue

modulates local renin levels and that the blockade by the ACE inhibitor of local renin-angiotensin systems in the blood vessels, brain, and kidney will mediate the therapeutic effect. As Unger et al. (59) point out, a substantial body of evidence supports the concept that an overactive brain renin system may be a pathogenetic factor in hypertension.

Lever's group (27) has recently shown that the development of Folkow's geometrically based vascular hyperreactivity that lies at the basis of primary hypertension is stimulated by angiotensin. Julius proposes that the sources of the autonomic nervous overactivity that is so critical in the early stages of hypertension are nerve centers such as the amygdalar nuclei (54). The preceding has presented evidence that psychosocial stimulation may be effective in activating the amygdalar and brainstem controls of the sympathetic system and hence in the development of essential hypertension (60).

TELEMETRY AND VIDEOTAPING OF RAT BLOOD PRESSURE AND BEHAVIOR IN COMMUNAL CAGES

The previous sections have presented data on the long-term observations of blood pressure that have been made in rats, mice, and primates during emotionally arousing situations. The instrumentation involved both the direct observation of pressure in the conscious animal by cannulation of an artery and the indirect method using compression of the tail or other extremity and detection of pulsations as the pressure is reduced. In a valuable article giving guidelines on the measurement of blood pressure in rats, Bunag (43) has discussed the pitfalls of both the direct arterial and the tail-cuff techniques. He found it best to combine the repeated use of a thoroughly familiar tail-cuff method with modest preheating and careful restraint. The method should then be validated by comparison with the cannulation of the carotid artery in the conscious animal. In his view all blood pressure differ-

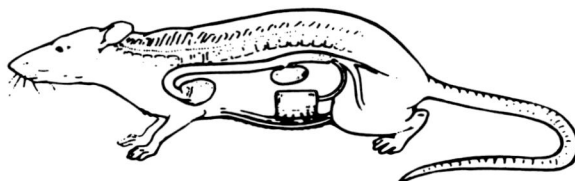

FIG. 11. Implantation of a blood pressure transmitter in a rat is performed by gluing the attached catheter into the descending aorta followed by fixation of the transmitter body to the abdominal musculature.

ences should then be verified by direct measurement of carotid arterial pressure in the same rats.

Especially for the study of psychosocial interactions in a group there are advantages to a method of blood pressure recording that does not disrupt normal behavior. In the tail-cuff method the pressure is measured in circumstances of restraint that resemble the classic human sphygmomanometry in the doctor's office. In the past the main weight of evidence in the study of human hypertension has rested on such indirect blood pressure measurements. The possibility of problems with the ensuing

"white coat" hypertension and the advantages of ambulatory blood pressure recordings are well recognized (61).

Ferrari et al. (62) have recently described the intraarterial pressure alterations that occur during tail-cuff blood pressure measurements in normal as opposed to hypertensive rats (62). They found that even mild heat when combined with restraint together lowered systolic blood pressure in normotensive rats but raised it in hypertensive rats. These differences, which they found when the tail-cuff method is used, cast doubt on this method despite its attractive, easy repetition and noninvasiveness. The disadvantages of direct arterial cannulation with the restraints imposed by it on movement and social interaction have been circumvented to some degree by Fokkema's (28) studies of win-lose dyads. But as Meehan et al. (63) have pointed out, there are clear advantages to a system in which blood pressure sensors are implanted in freely interacting rats living in seminatural colonies made up of males and females.

In 1991, Brockway et al. (64) reported on a new method for continuous chronic measurement and recording of blood pressure, heart rate, and activity in the rat. The approach largely solves the problems discussed

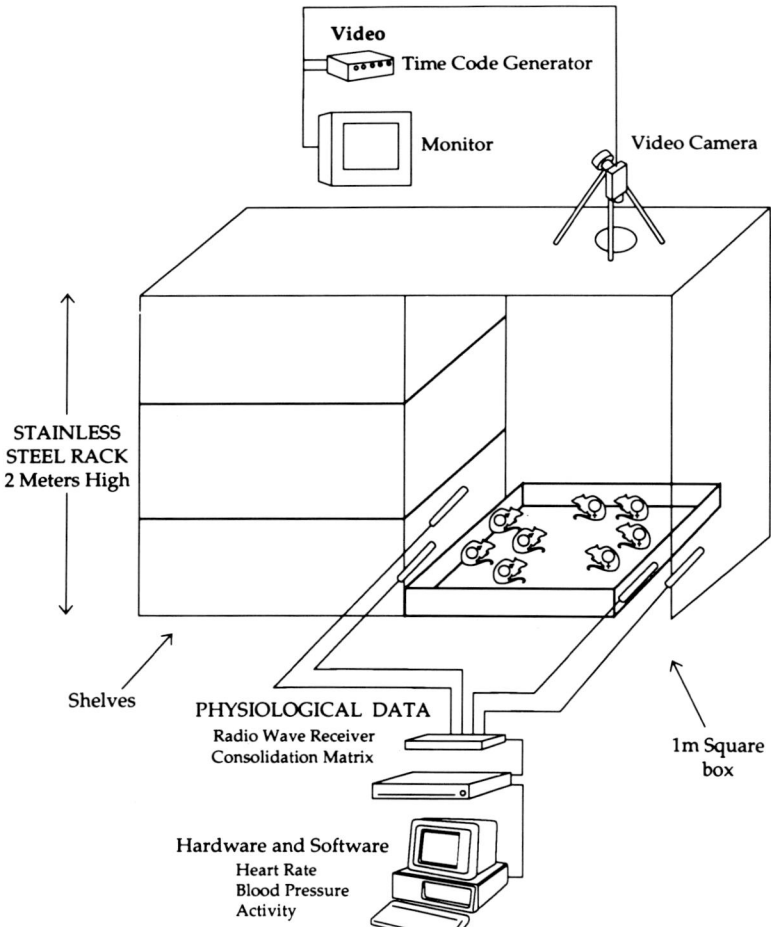

FIG. 12. System for the videotaping of behavior and telemetry of blood pressure of members of a colony of four male and four female rats. The blood pressure signal is received and then processed by a consolidation matrix. It passes by cable to another room where it is stored for processing in a computer. The videotape data are also stored and time coded to correlate behavior with blood pressure.

above. It has undergone extensive trials, and in 1993, Schnell and Wood (65) described the use of this system for measurement of blood pressure and heart rate in conscious, unrestrained marmosets, which are of comparable size to a rat.

The system consists of an implantable radiotelemetry device as sketched in Fig. 11. The body is a cylinder only 1.5 cm long and of the same diameter, weighing 9 g. There is a battery that permits continuous recording for 6 months. A magnetic on/off switch conserves power, extending the working life. The highly stable low-compliance semiconductor strain gauge sensor is actuated by a 0.7-mm diameter 8 to 10 cm fluid-filled catheter. The distal 2 mm of the thin-walled tip is filled with a gel that prevents blood from entering the catheter lumen. An antithrombogenic film applied to the catheter inhibits thrombogenesis. The package is secured to the abdominal wall by a tab and 4–0 braided sutures. The sensing catheter is inserted about 1 cm upstream in the aorta with the aid of a tool made of a split 21-gauge needle bent at an angle. The catheter is secured in place in the aorta by a drop of medical grade (Vetbond) tissue adhesive. A radiofrequency transmitter sends a direct measure of the arterial waveform to antennae located close to the cage. A receiver detects the signal, which is processed by a consolidation matrix and read by a computer. Motor activity is registered by digitalizing the variability of the received signal strength with changes in distance from and orientation of the rat to the receiving antenna.

The implanted rats interact with each other in a 1 m square stainless steel cage that has two lateral compartments, each containing two antennae that are attached to the receiver (Fig. 12). The signals that have been processed by the data acquisition system pass from the consolidation matrix via a cable to another room. There an IBM 80286 compatible computer accepts the data,

which are stored on hard disk for later analysis. Ambient pressure is monitored by a special transducer and subtracted from the reading given by the blood pressure transducer.

Figure 13 is an example of the effects on mean blood pressure when a mature male rat was transferred from an isolation period of 3 weeks to a just-constituted colony of three more males and four females for 3 months. During the 3-week period of isolation the pressure averaged 110 ± 3 mm Hg. The introduction into the colony led to a rise to 119 ± 4 mm Hg ($p < .001$). It then returned to baseline with adjustment to the new social situation that involved weekly randomization of the population. An upward drift to 116 ± 6 mm Hg during the following 2 months paralleled the slow but significant increase noted in the indirect tail-cuff measurements of the other three males in the colony. The increase also paralleled that noted in the two stressed Sprague-Dawley colonies shown in Fig. 6. It would appear that the telemetry animal was experiencing the same increase of blood pressure and presumably the same modest pathophysiological changes as the males in other colonies.

Behavior was followed on videotape. In the communal cage the implanted rat avoided confrontation. Sprague-Dawley rats are peaceable and do not fight but this one was exceptionally quiet. However, it mingled with the others, did not lose weight, and ate and drank normally.

Further work with the telemetry of blood pressure during psychosocial interaction is indicated. Effective demonstration of significant arterial pressure elevation in animals free from the constraint of direct or indirect pressure recording would provide further evidence that chronic psychosocial stress will induce hypertension in normotensive strains of rats.

The relevance of this work to man is discussed by the senior author in chapter 12, *this volume*.

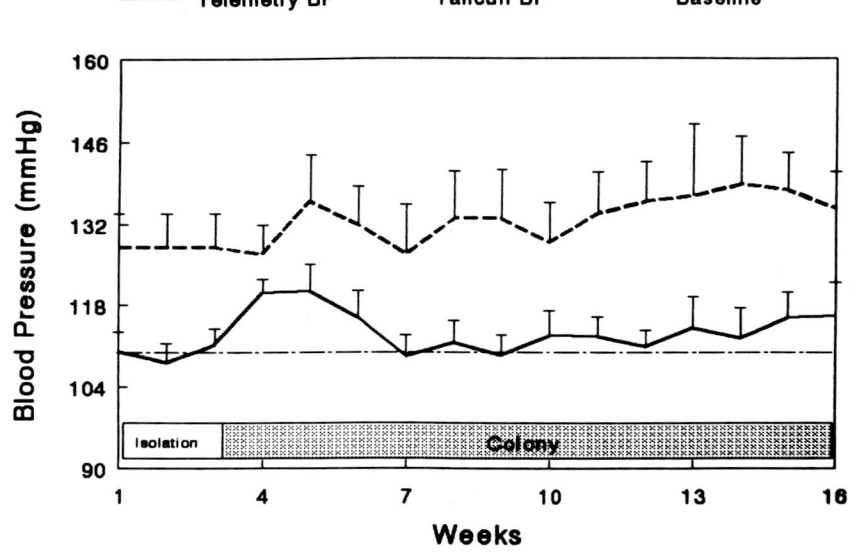

FIG. 13. During isolation the pressure is significantly lower than shortly after placement in a disordered colony but it returns to isolation values. Then there is a gradual rise from the 7th to the 16th week that parallels the indirect tail-cuff measurements of the three other colony males and of the Sprague-Dawley colonies shown in Fig. 6.

REFERENCES

1. Weiss JM. Psychological factors in stress and disease. *Sci Am* 1972;226:104–113.
2. Henry JP. Biological basis of the stress response. *Integr Physiol Behav Sci* 1992;27:66–83.
3. Bohus B, Koolhaas M, de Ruiter AJH, Heijnen CJ. Psycho-social stress: differential alterations in immune system functions and tumor growth. In: Kvetnansky R, McCarty R, Axelrod J, eds. *Stress: neuroendocrine and molecular approaches.* New York: Gordon and Breach, 1992;607–621.
4. Stock G, Schlor KH, Heidt H, Buss J. Psychomotor behavior and cardiovascular patterns during stimulation of the amygdala. *Pfluegers Arch* 1978;376:177–184.
5. Kadish W. Personality traits and the norepinephrine to epinephrine ratio. Master's thesis, Yale University, New Haven, CT, 1983.
6. Lovallo WR, Pincomb GA, Brackett DI, Wilson MF. Heart rate reactivity as a predictor of neuroendocrine responses to aversive and appetitive challenges. *Psychosom Med* 1990;52:17–26.
7. Elmadjian F, Hope JM, Lamson ET. Excretion of epinephrine and norepinephrine under stress. In: Pincus G, ed. *Recent progress in hormone research. Proceedings of the Laurentian Hormone Conference.* New York: Academic Press, 1957;14:513–553.
8. Dimsdale JE, Moss J. Plasma catecholamines in stress and exercise. *JAMA* 1980;243:340–342.
9. Theorell T. Prolactin: A hormone that mirrors passiveness in crisis situations. *Integr Physiol Behav Sci* 1992;27:32–38.
10. Folkow B. Personal and historical perspectives in hypertension, "structural factor" in primary and secondary hypertension. *Hypertension* 1990;16:89–101.
11. deBoer SF, DeBeun R, Slagen JL, Van der Gugten J. Dynamics of plasma catecholamine and corticosterone concentrations during reinforced and extinguished behavior in rats. *Physiol Behav* 1990;47:691–698.
12. Mazur A, Lamb TA. Testosterone, status and mood in human males. *Horm Behav* 1980;14:236–246.
13. Gold PW, Goodwin FK, Chrousos GP. Clinical and biochemical manifestations of depression: relation to the neurobiology of stress. *N Engl J Med* 1988;319:413–420.
14. Meehan JP, Fineg J, Wheelwright CD. Blood pressure instrumentation for the MA-5 flight. In: Henry JP, Mosely JD, eds. *Results of the Project Mercury ballistic and orbital chimpanzee flights.* Washington, DC: NASA SP-39 Office of Scientific and Technical Information National Aeronautics and Space Administration, 1963;55–68.
15. Rohles FH Jr, Grunzke ME, Reynolds HH. Performance aspects of the MA-5 flight. In: Henry JP, Mosely JD, eds. *Results of the Project Mercury ballistic and orbital chimpanzee flights.* Washington, DC: NASA SP-39 Office of Scientific and Technical Information National Aeronautics and Space Administration, 1963;21–24.
16. Meehan JP, Fineg J, Mosely JD. The effect of restraint and training on the arterial pressure of the immature chimpanzee. *Fed Proc* 1964;23:515.
17. Fineg J. Para-aminohippuric acid clearance in the young chimpanzee. Master's thesis, physiology, University of Southern California, 1964.
18. Brizio-Molteni L, Molteni A, Cloutier C, Rainey S. Incidence of post burn hypertension crisis in patients admitted to two burn centers and a community hospital in the United States. *Scand J Plast Reconstr Surg* 1979;13:21–28.
19. Henry JP, Meehan JP, Stephens M. The use of psychosocial stimuli to induce prolonged systolic hypertension in mice. *Psychosom Med* 1967;29:408–432.
20. Pickering G. *The nature of essential hypertension.* London: J. & A. Churchill, 1961.
21. Simonson BE, Brozek J. Russian research on arterial hypertension. *Ann Intern Med* 1959;50:129–184.
22. Forsyth RP. Blood pressure responses to long-term avoidance schedules in the unrestrained rhesus monkey. *Psychosom Med* 1969;31:300–309.
23. Herd JA, Morse WH, Kelleher RT, Jones LG. Arterial hypertension in the squirrel monkey during behavioral experiments. *Am J Physiol* 1969;217:24–29.
24. Friedman R, Dahl LK. The effect of chronic conflict on the blood pressure of rats with a genetic susceptibility to experimental hypertension. *Psychosom Med* 1975;37:402–416.
25. Lawler JE, Barker GF, Hubbard JW, Schaub RG. Effect of stress on the blood pressure and cardiac pathology in rats with borderline hypertension. *Hypertension* 1981;3:496–505.
26. Lever AF. Editorial review. Slow pressor mechanisms in hypertension: a role for hypertrophy of resistance vessels? *J Hypertens* 1986;4:515–524.
27. Lyall F, Morton JJ, Lever AF, Cragoe EJ. Angiotensin II activates Na+H+ exchange and stimulates growth in culture of vascular smooth muscle cells. *J Hypertens* 6(suppl 4):S438–S441.
28. Fokkema DS. Social behavior and blood pressure: a study of rats. Doctorate in natural sciences, Groningen, Netherlands, 1985.
29. Sklar LS, Anisman H. Stress and cancer. *Psychol Bull* 1981;89:369–400.
30. Fokkema DS, Koolhaas JM. Psychosocial stimuli and blood pressure in individual rats. *Physiol Behav* 1985;34:33–38.
31. Adams N, Blizard DA. Defeat and cardiovascular response. *Psychol Rec* 1987;37:349–368.
32. Eichelman B, Dejong W, Williams R. Aggressive behavior in hypertensive and normotensive rat strains. *Physiol Behav* 1973;10:301–307.
33. Harrap SB, Louis WJ, Doyle AE. Failure of psychosocial stress to induce chronic hypertension in the rat. *J Hypertens* 1984;2:653–662.
34. Gelsema AJM, Ruzicka M, Copeland NE. Cardiovascular effects of social stress in a colony of borderline hypertension rats [abstract]. *Hypertension* 1992;20:415.
35. Shepherd JT, Weiss SM, eds. Conference on behavioral medicine and cardiovascular disease. *Circulation* 1987;76(suppl I):I-95–I-100.
36. Wexler BC, Greenberg BP. Pathophysiological differences between paired and communal breeding of male and female Sprague-Dawley rats. *Circ Res* 1987;42:126–132.
37. Ely DL, Weigand J. Stress and high sodium effects on blood pressure and brain catecholamines in spontaneously hypertensive rats. *Clin Exp Hypertens* 1983;5:1559–1587.
38. Szilagyi JE. Psychosocial stress elevates blood pressure via an opioid dependent mechanism in normotensive rats. *Clin Exp Hypertens* 1991;13:1383–1394.
39. Mormede P, Lemaire V, Castanon N, Dulluc J, Laval M, Le Moal M. Multiple neuroendocrine responses to chronic social stress: interaction between individual characteristics and situational factors. *Physiol Behav* 1990;47:1099–1105.
40. Henry JP, Liu J, Nadra WE, Qian CG, Mormede P, Lemaire V, Ely D, Hendley ED. Psychosocial stress can induce chronic hypertension in normotensive strains of rats. *Hypertension* 1993;21:714–723.
41. Hendley ED, Ohlsson WG, Musty RE. Interstrain aggression in hypertensive and/or hyperactive rats: SFR, WKY, WKHA, WHHT. *Physiol Behav* 1992;51:1041–1046.
42. Kelsey JL, Thompson WD, Evans AS. *Methods in observational epidemiology.* New York: Oxford University Press, 1986;257–259.
43. Bunag RD. Measurement of blood pressure in rats. In: de Jong W, ed. *Handbook of hypertension, vol 4: Experimental and genetic models of hypertension.* New York: Elsevier Science Publishers B.V., 1984;1–12.
44. Henry JY, Ely DL, Stephens PM. Changes in catecholamine-controlling enzymes in response to psychosocial activation of the defence and alarm reactions. *Physiol Emotion Psychosom Illness Ciba Found Symp* 1972;225–251.
45. Henry JP, Stephens PM. *Health and the social environment: a sociobiologic approach to medicine.* New York: Springer-Verlag, 1977.
46. Lindzey G, Winston H, Manosevitz M. Social dominance in inbred mouse strains. *Nature* 1961;191:474.
47. Calhoun JB. A "behavioral sink." In: Bliss EL, ed. *Roots of behavior: genetics, instinct and socialization in animal behavior.* New York: Hoeber-Harper, 1962;295–315.
48. Scott JP. Incomplete adjustment caused by frustration of untrained fighting mice. *J Comp Psychol* 1946;39:379.
49. Henry JP, Ely DL, Stephens PM, Ratcliffe HL, Santisteban GA, Shapiro AP. The role of psychosocial factors in the development of

arteriosclerosis in CBA mice: observations on the heart, kidney and aorta. *Atherosclerosis* 1971; 14:203–218.

50. Bennett WM, Walker RG, Henry JP, Kincaid-Smith. Chronic interstitial nephropathy in mice induced by psychosocial stress: potentiation by caffeine. *Nephron* 1983; 34:110–113.

51. Henry JP, Stephens PM, Axelrod J, Mueller RA. Effect of psychosocial stimulation on the enzymes involved in the biosynthesis and metabolism of noradrenaline and adrenaline. *Psychosom Med* 1971; 33:227–237.

52. Vander AJ, Henry JP, Stephens PM, Kay LL, Mouw DR. Plasma renin activity in psychosocial hypertension of CBA mice. *Circ Res* 1978; 42:496–502.

53. Aston JS, Foote SL, Bloom FE. Anatomy and physiology of locus coeruleus neurons: functional implication. In: Ziegler M, Lake CR, eds. *Frontiers of clinical neuroscience: norepinephrine.* Baltimore, MD: William & Wilkins, 1984; 2:92–116.

54. Julius S. Interaction between renin and the autonomic nervous system in hypertension. *Am Heart J* 1988; 116:611–616.

55. Julius S, Johnson EH. Stress autonomic hypertension and essential hypertension: an enigma. *J Hypertens* 1985; 3(suppl):s11–s17.

56. Henry JP, Stephens PM, Vander AJ. Inhibition of angiotensin converting enzyme in CBA mice with psychosocial hypertension. *Clin Exp Hypertens (A)* 1983; 5:87–97.

57. Webb RC, Hamlin NM, Henry JP, Stephens PM, Vander AJ. Captopril, blood pressure and vascular reactivity in psychosocial hypertensive mice. *Hypertension* 1986; 8(suppl I):I-119.

58. Dzau VJ. Autocrine renin-systems in cardiorenal regulation and the pharmacology of ACE inhibitors: In: Sonnenblick EH, Laragh JH, Lesch M, eds. *New frontiers in cardiovascular therapy.* Amsterdam: Excerpta Medica-Elsevier, 1989; 13–28.

59. Unger T, Badoer E, Ganten D, Lang R, Rettig R. Brain angiotensin pathways and pharmacology. *Circulation* 1988; 77(suppl I):40–54.

60. Henry JP, Grim CL. Psychosocial mechanisms of primary hypertension. *J Hypertens* 1990; 8:783–793.

61. Harshfield GA, Pickering TG, Kleinert KD, Blank S, Laragh JH. Situational variations of blood pressure in ambulatory hypertensive patients. *Psychosom Med* 1982; 44(3).

62. Ferrari AU, Daffonchio A, Albergati F, Bertoli P, Mancia G. Intraarterial pressure alterations during tail-cuff blood pressure measurements in normotensive and hypertensive rats. *J Hypertens* 1990; 8:909–911.

63. Meehan WP, Tornatzky W, Miczek K. Blood pressure via telemetry during social stress in freely moving rats. *Soc Neurosci Abstr* 1989; 15.

64. Brockway BP, Mills PA, Azar SH. A new method for continuous chronic measurement and recording of blood pressure. Heart rate and activity in the rat via radio-telemetry. *Clin Exp Hypertens* 1991; 13:885–895.

65. Schnell CR, Wood JM. Measurement of blood pressure and heart rate by telemetry in conscious, unrestrained marmosets. *Am J Physiol* 1993; 33:H1509–1516.

Hypertension: Pathophysiology, Diagnosis, and Management, Second Edition, edited by J.H. Laragh and B.M. Brenner, Raven Press, Ltd., New York © 1995.

CHAPTER 55

The Pathophysiology of the Sympathetic Nervous System in Human Hypertension Studies Using Specific Pharmacological Probes

Peter Bolli, Wolfgang Kiowski, and Fritz R. Bühler

EVIDENCE FOR INCREASED SYMPATHETIC ACTIVITY IN ESSENTIAL HYPERTENSION

Increased sympathetic nervous activity has been implicated in the pathophysiology of essential hypertension (1,2). It has been postulated that the effects of increased sympathetic activity are particularly evident in the early phases, i.e., younger, mild, and borderline hypertensives (3,4), as reflected by an elevated cardiac output and vasoconstriction of the renal and splanchnic, but not of the muscular vascular, beds (5,6), consistent with an increased vasoconstrictor nerve activity in the splanchnic and renal, but normal sympathetic outflow to the muscular vasculature (7). As hypertension progresses, there is a transition to a high vascular resistance–normal cardiac output form of hypertension, partly due to the involvement of adaptive processes (8,9).

P. Bolli: Division of Clinical Pharmacology, Department of Medicine, Health Science Centre, Memorial Medical School, St. John's Newfoundland, Canada A1B 3V6.
F. R. Bühler, W. Kiowski: Department of Research and Division of Cardiology, Department of Internal Medicine, University Hospital, CH-4031 Basel, Switzerland.

Norepinephrine represents the principal neurotransmitter responsible for sympathetic vasoconstriction. Increased plasma norepinephrine concentrations were measured in some, particularly young and mild (10,11) hypertensive patients (4,11–15) and a direct relationship between plasma norepinephrine and blood pressure in some studies was noted (12,16). However, since plasma norepinephrine measurements produced inconsistent results, most likely due to norepinephrine's rapid metabolism, neuronal reuptake, and extraneuronal uptake (17,18), measurement of norepinephrine spillover as a more reliable assessment of sympathetic activity was found to be increased in hypertensives (19). Probably the most convincing evidence for an increased sympathetic nervous system activity being involved in the pathophysiology of essential hypertension is provided by the demonstration of an increased peroneal sympathetic nerve traffic in patients with hypertension (15,20).

Circulating plasma epinephrine, which is less rapidly metabolized, has been used as an indicator for sympathetic nervous system activity, although its importance for the pathophysiology of essential hypertension is uncertain and still debated (21–23). Elevated plasma epinephrine concentrations were observed in all age groups

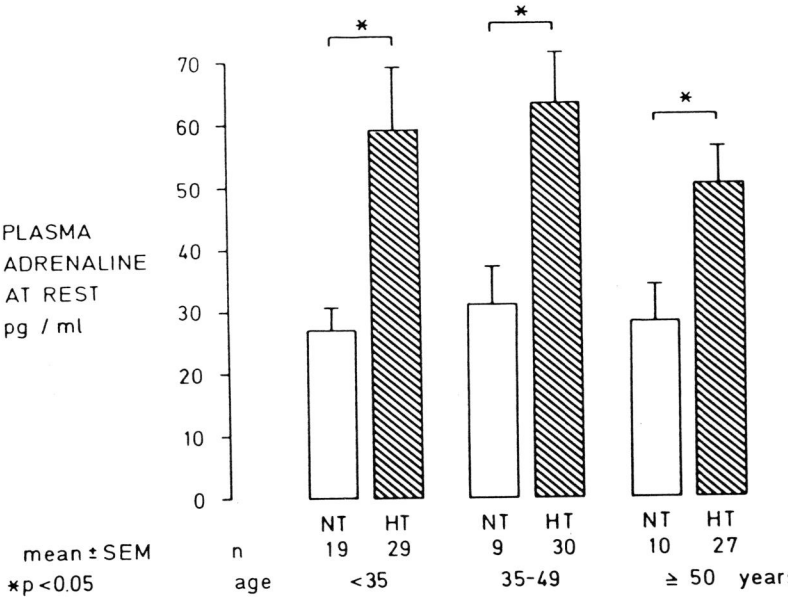

FIG. 1. Plasma adrenaline concentration measured 30 minutes after resting in a supine position between 8 and 10 A.M. in different age groups; 86 hypertensive and 38 normotensive subjects of similar age were studied. (From ref. 70, with permission)

in a fraction of patients with essential hypertension (Fig. 1) (8). Higher plasma epinephrine concentrations were found not only at rest but also during submaximal exercise (Fig. 2) and following cold pressor testing (Fig. 3) (24,25). Plasma epinephrine concentrations were related to diastolic blood pressure (26) and heart rate (8). Therefore, epinephrine concentrations taken as a marker of

sympathetic activity are consistent with the observations made with norepinephrine and supports an increased adrenergic activity in essential hypertension. Recently, the concept of increased adrenergic activity has been expanded to include its potential contribution to the increased coronary risk in hypertensive patients (27).

To prove that increased adrenergic activity is involved

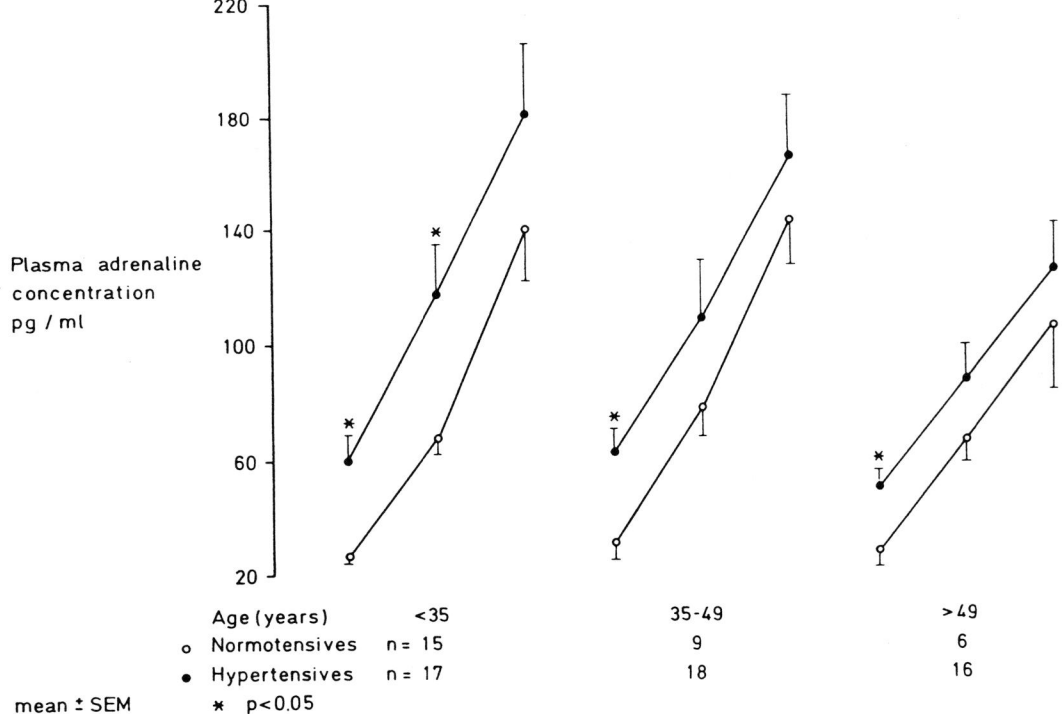

FIG. 2. Plasma adrenaline concentration in normotensive and hypertensive subjects at rest and during graded ergometric exercise. (From ref. 68, with permission)

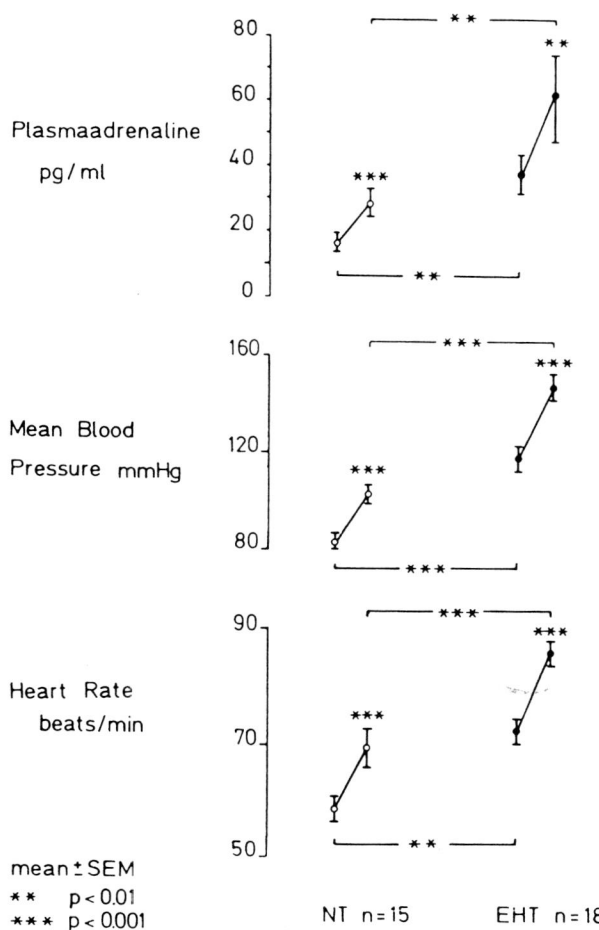

FIG. 3. Effect of cold pressor test on plasma adrenaline, blood pressure, and heart rate in normotensive subjects (NT, *open circles*) and in patients with essential hypertension (EHT, *filled circles*). (From ref. 25, with permission)

in the pathophysiology of essential hypertension thus requires the demonstration of a relationship between (elevated) norepinephrine and epinephrine concentrations and of changes toward restoring a normal hemodynamic pattern following intervention with the sympathetic nervous system. Since α- and β-adrenoceptors are the immediate mediators of norepinephrine- and epinephrine-evoked effects, antagonists and agonists to these receptors represent suitable pharmacological probes. Therefore, the following chapters provide evidence for an increased adrenergic contribution to the pathophysiology of essential hypertension based on studies using pharmacological probes as adrenergic interventions. However, in dealing with results of adrenergic interference, it has to be appreciated that any observations are the end result of often complex hemodynamic interactions and feedback loops of adrenergic transmitter release, and that the evidence derived from the respective experiments has to be weighed against this complex background.

Probably the most indisputable evidence for an adrenergic component to the pathophysiology of essential hypertension is the effectiveness of centrally acting and peripheral α- and β-adrenergic receptor blockers as antihypertensive drugs.

ENHANCED α_1 ADRENOCEPTOR–MEDIATED VASOCONSTRICTION IN ESSENTIAL HYPERTENSION

Elevated peripheral vascular resistance is the main hemodynamic abnormality of essential hypertension (28), particularly in its established form, but also in mild and borderline hypertensives where peripheral vascular resistance is numerically normal but elevated relative to the increased cardiac output (29). The regulation of blood flow through vasoconstrictor and vasodilator mechanisms forms an important part of the overall cardiovascular regulation (30–32). Blood flow depends on vascular tone, which is greatly influenced by the sympathetic nervous system through adrenoceptor stimulation and ultimately by the intracellular free calcium concentration in vascular smooth muscle cells (33). Therefore, factors that determine vascular tone can be directly assessed by measuring alterations in blood flow of regional vascular beds, following pharmacological interventions with stimulation or blockade of adrenoceptor-mediated vascular tone. Since systemic (parenteral or oral) application of adrenergic receptor blockade or stimulation immediately evokes systemic hemodynamic counterregulatory mechanisms, for instance as a response to the blockade-induced fall in blood pressure, the measurement of forearm blood flow using venous occlusion plethysmography (34), combined with intraarterial (brachial artery) infusion of the pharmacological probe, has become a preferred model to study the effects of vasoactive drugs (35) in a relatively "isolated" regional vascular bed (36). A limitation in the interpretation of the results is the fact that the forearm vasculature consists of 90 percent of the arteries that supply the muscle and of only 10 percent of those that supply the skin, which represents the resistance vascular bed proper. Therefore, results obtained in the forearm vascular bed cannot be extrapolated uncritically to other vascular beds. Other vascular beds, although amenable to measurement of blood flow, are hardly accessible for regional infusion of the pharmacological probe.

Early studies by Doyle et al. (37) and Sivertsson and Olander (38) demonstrated a greater vasoconstrictive response to norepinephrine infusions into the forearm and hand circulation, respectively, in hypertensives as compared with normotensives. This increased vasoconstriction to α-adrenoceptor stimulation was repeatedly found in later studies (39,40) and related to some extent to the severity of hypertension (Fig. 4), but whether the en-

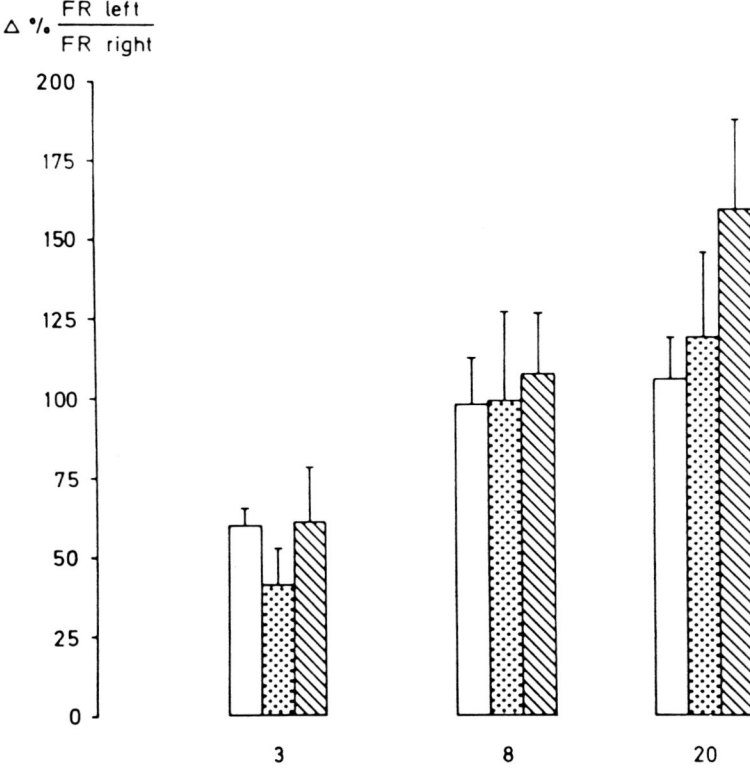

Δ % $\dfrac{FR\ \ left}{FR\ \ right}$

mean ± SEM

Noradrenaline ng / min / 100 ml tissue

FIG. 4. Percentage change in forearm vascular resistance (FR) to intraarterial (brachial artery) infusion of noradrenaline (3,8,20 mm Hg/min/100 ml forearm tissue) in nine normotensive subjects (*open bars*), nine patients with borderline hypertension (*stippled bars*), and nine patients with established hypertension (*hatched bars*). Borderline hypertension = casual BP > 95 mm Hg, intraarterial pressure < 85 mm Hg; established hypertension = casual BP > 95 mm Hg, intraarterial pressure ≥ 85 mm Hg. FR left/FR right = FR infused arm/FR control (noninfused) arm.

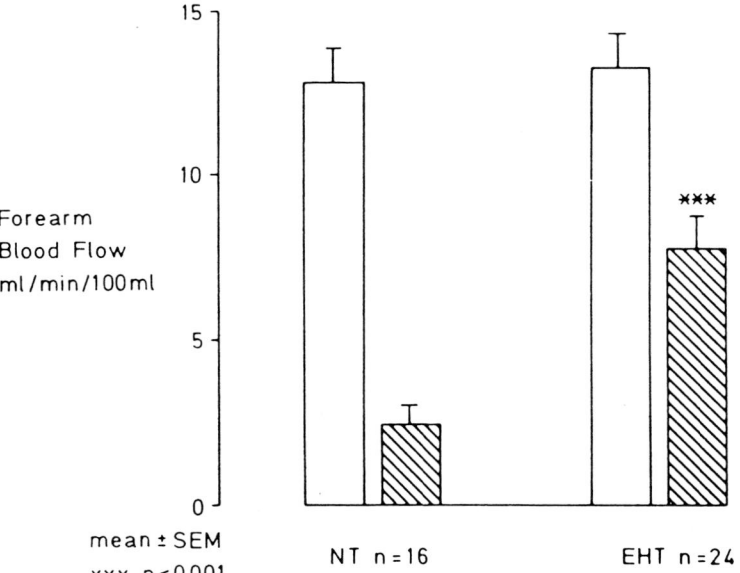

Forearm
Blood Flow
ml / min /100ml

mean ± SEM

*** p < 0.001

NT n = 16   EHT n = 24

FIG. 5. Change in forearm blood flow (FAF) (ml/min/100 ml of forearm tissue) during sodium nitroprusside (0.6 µg/min/100 ml; *open bars*) and prazosin infusion (0.5 µg/min/100 ml; *hatched bars*) in 24 patients with essential hypertension (EHT) and in 16 normotensive subjects (NT). The prazosin-induced increase in FAF was significantly greater in EHT than in NT. (From ref. 41, with permission)

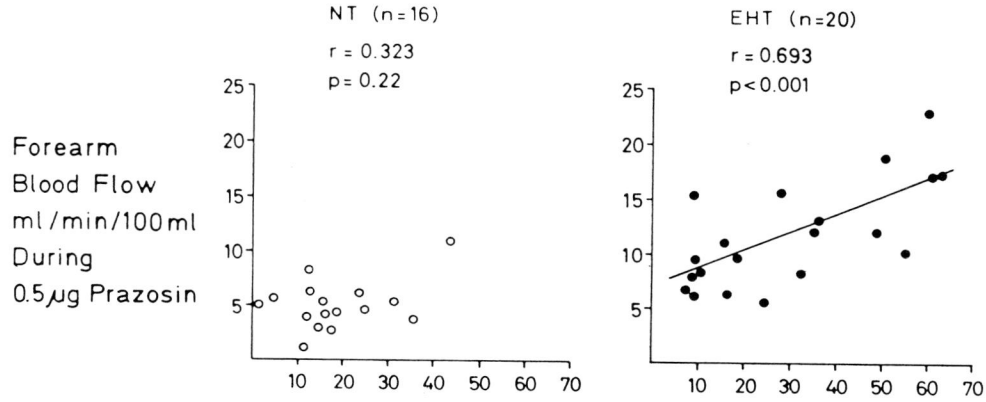

FIG. 6. Relationship between basal plasma epinephrine concentration and forearm blood flow (FAF) during postjunctional alpha-blockade with prazosin (0.5 μg/min/100 ml of forearm tissue) in 20 patients with essential hypertension (EHT; *black circles*) and in 16 normotensive subjects (NT; *open circles*). N EHT, prazosin-induced FAF correlates significantly with plasma epinephrine. (From ref. 4, with permission)

hanced vasoconstrictor response in the hypertensive patients was specific to adrenergic agonism or arose as a general response to any vasoconstrictor stimulation was debated. Therefore, blockade of adrenoceptor-mediated vasoconstriction represents a more specific approach to determine the contribution of increased adrenergic activity to the increased vascular resistance in essential hypertensives. Since vasoconstriction is to a great extent due to postjunctional α_1-adrenoceptor stimulation, α_1-adrenoceptor–mediated vasoconstriction has been investigated by measuring the vasodilator response in the forearm following brachial artery infusion of the α_1-adrenoceptor antagonist prazosin (41). In patients with essential hypertension, the vasodilator response to α_1-adrenoceptor blockade was significantly greater than in age- and gender-matched normotensive subjects as reflected by a greater increase in forearm blood flow in the former (Fig. 5). As the increase in forearm blood flow to non–adrenoceptor-mediated vasodilation with sodium nitroprusside was similar in both groups, the enhanced forearm vasodilator response to prazosin in hypertensive patients can be considered specific for postjunctional α_1-adrenoceptor–mediated vasoconstriction. The direct relationship between resting plasma epinephrine concentration in hypertensives but not in normotensives supports the notion of an increased adrenergically mediated vasoconstriction in patients with essential hypertension (Fig. 6).

Similar results were obtained by Egan et al. (42) using the α-adrenoceptor blocker phentolamine. Intraarterial infusion of phentolamine resulted in a 43 percent greater reduction in forearm vascular resistance in hypertensives as compared with normotensive subjects. Since the hypertensive patients had higher plasma norepinephrine concentrations as compared with their normotensive controls, it can be assumed that their greater adrenergic activity formed part of their increased vascular resis-

tance. In fact, a study by Kiowski et al. (12) showed a relationship between phentolamine-induced forearm vasodilation and plasma noradrenaline concentrations (Fig. 7). Egan et al.'s study also concluded that increased α-adrenergic vasoconstriction in hypertensives does not involve alterations in adrenergic receptors but is due to structural vascular changes (43,44) recently identified as remodeling of the vascular wall (45), which then acts as an amplifier for adrenergic vasoconstrictor stimuli. The presence of structural vascular changes was demonstrated by a greater minimal forearm vascular resistance (after maximal vasodilation following ischemia) in hypertensives in the Egan et al. study and earlier studies (43,44). These vascular changes in hypertensive patients act as an amplifier for any vasoconstrictor substance, as

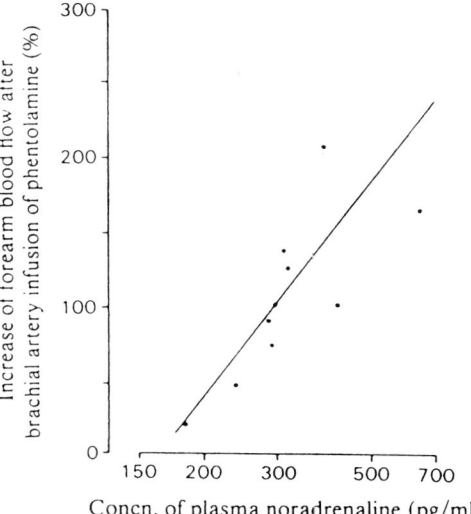

FIG. 7. Relationship of plasma noradrenaline concentration at rest and increase in forearm blood flow after a brachial artery infusion of phentolamine in 11 subjects with essential hypertension ($r = .79$, $p < .01$). (From ref. 12, with permission)

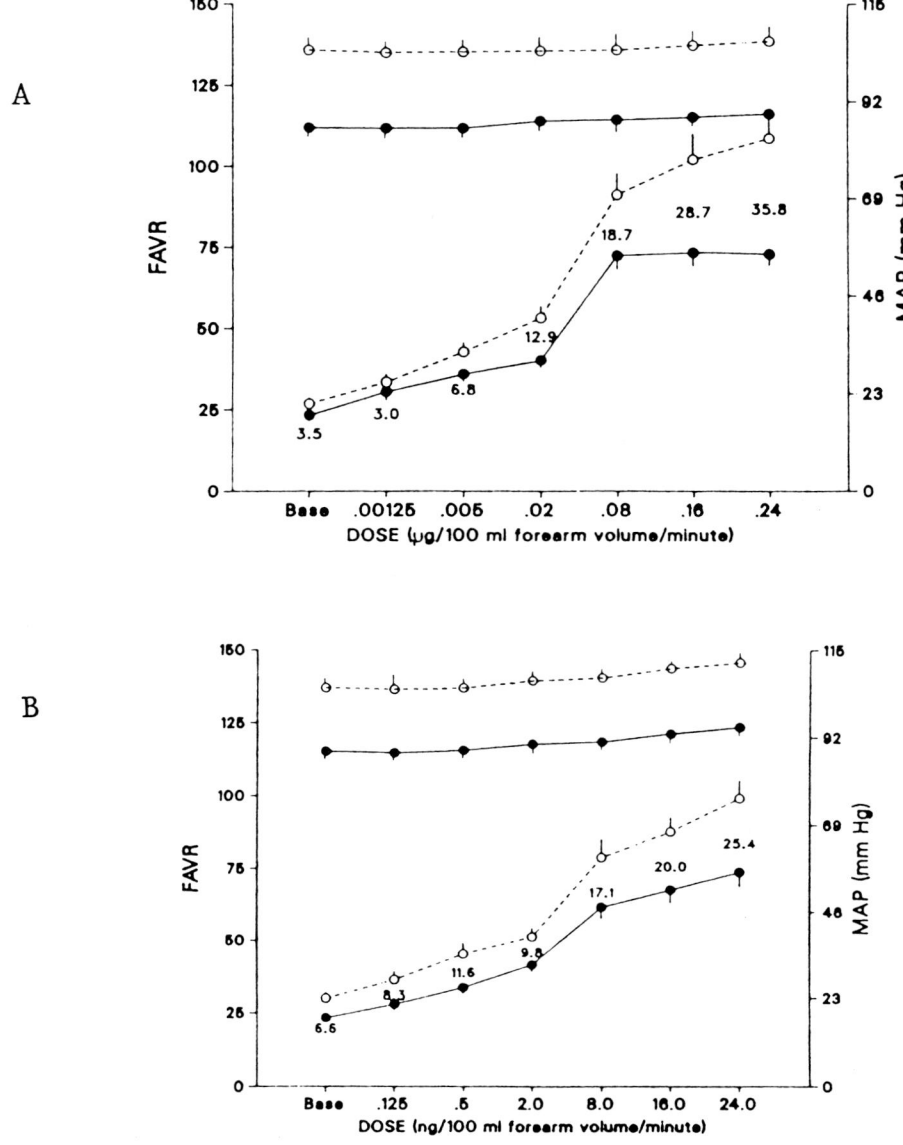

FIG. 8. Forearm vascular resistance (FAVR) and mean arterial pressure (MAP) to increasing concentrations of intraarterially (brachial artery) infused norepinephrine (**A**) and angiotensin II (**B**) in hypertensive patients (*open circles, dotted lines*) and normotensive subjects (*solid circles and lines*). The FAVR response between hypertensives and normotensives was significant ($p < .01$). (From ref. 42, with permission)

shown by equal vasoconstriction responses to norepinephrine and angiotensin II (42) (Fig. 8) and may also explain their greater vasoconstrictor response and blood pressure rise to physical or mental stress.

ROLE OF α-ADRENOCEPTOR–MEDIATED VASOCONSTRICTION FOR ANTIHYPERTENSIVE BETA BLOCKADE

β-Adrenoceptor antagonists interfere with the adrenergic nervous system (46,47). Although the antihyper-

tensive mode of action of beta blockers is complex and not yet fully explained, it involves a reduction of cardiac output. But the antihypertensive response to beta blockade may also involve interference with vasoconstrictor mechanisms (46). In a study comparing hypertensives who responded with those who did not respond to antihypertensive beta blockade with propranolol, the responders were characterized by a greater forearm vasodilator response to alpha blockade with intraarterially infused prazosin, and they also had a significantly (35 percent) higher plasma epinephrine concentration as a marker of increased adrenergic activity (Fig. 9) (48). Following treatment with propranolol, α-adrenoceptor–mediated vasoconstriction was significantly less in the responders as reflected by a smaller increase in forearm blood flow during infusion of prazosin, while there was no change in nonresponders, demonstrating that beta blockade effectively interfered with the enhanced α-adrenoceptor–mediated vasoconstriction. As the fall in heart rate and plasma renin activity was comparable in responders and nonresponders, interference by beta blockade with increased adrenergically induced vasoconstriction appeared to be a decisive factor in lowering of blood pressure in patients with increased adrenergic activity. Since epinephrine activates prejunctional β-adrenoceptors and thus leads to neurotransmitter release

(21) and vasoconstriction (49), blockade of prejunctional β-adrenoceptors, which appears particularly effective in patients with increased adrenergic activity, may represent part of the antihypertensive mechanism of beta blockers.

EPINEPHRINE-INDUCED POSTJUNCTIONAL α_2-ADRENOCEPTOR-MEDIATED VASOCONSTRICTION?

Increased adrenergic activity has been related mainly to the effects of increased norepinephrine, while elevated plasma concentrations of epinephrine have been considered markers of increased adrenergic activity. However, the subdivision of α-adrenoceptors into α_1 and α_2 subtypes (50), and the slightly higher affinity of the latter to epinephrine over norepinephrine, raised the question of whether epinephrine could influence vasoconstriction through stimulation of postjunctional α_2-adrenoceptors (51,52). *In vitro* and animal experiments demonstrated the presence of an autoinhibitory feedback system for neuronal noradrenaline release at the level of the neuroeffector junction, whereby norepinephrine inhibits its own release by stimulating prejunctional α_2-adrenoceptors (53), while postjunctional α_2-adrenoceptors are stimulated by norepinephrine and epinephrine and thereby induce vasoconstriction (54).

The presence of postjunctional α_2-adrenoceptors in man has been shown by the inhibition of the blood pressure response to α-methylnoradrenaline, a relatively selective α_2-adrenoceptor agonist, and by 2-{2-(1,4 benzodioxanyl)}-2-imidazoline (RX 781094), a selective α_2-adrenoceptor antagonist (55). At the vascular level this was demonstrated by a dose-dependent decrease in forearm blood flow to intraarterial infusion of the α_2-adrenoceptor agonist clonidine (Fig. 10) (56) and of the more selective α_2-agonist azepexole (B-HT 933) (57), as well as a dose-dependent decrease in forearm vascular resistance to intraarterial infusion of the α_2-adrenoceptor antagonist yohimbine (Fig. 11) (58) and the inhibition of the azepoxole-induced vasoconstriction with yohimbine but not with the α_1-antagonist doxazosin (Fig. 12) (57).

That epinephrine can induce vasoconstriction through postjunctional α_2-adrenoceptor stimulation is shown by a decrease in forearm blood flow during epinephrine infusion in the presence of postjunctional α_1- and combined β_1- and β_2-adrenoceptor blockade. The specificity of the α_2-adrenoceptor–mediated nature of the vasoconstriction was documented by its inhibition by yohimbine (Fig. 13) (59). Jie et al. (60) found that the postjunctional α_2- as well as the postjunctional α_1-adrenoceptors are stimulated to the same degree by equal concentrations of both epinephrine and norepinephrine,

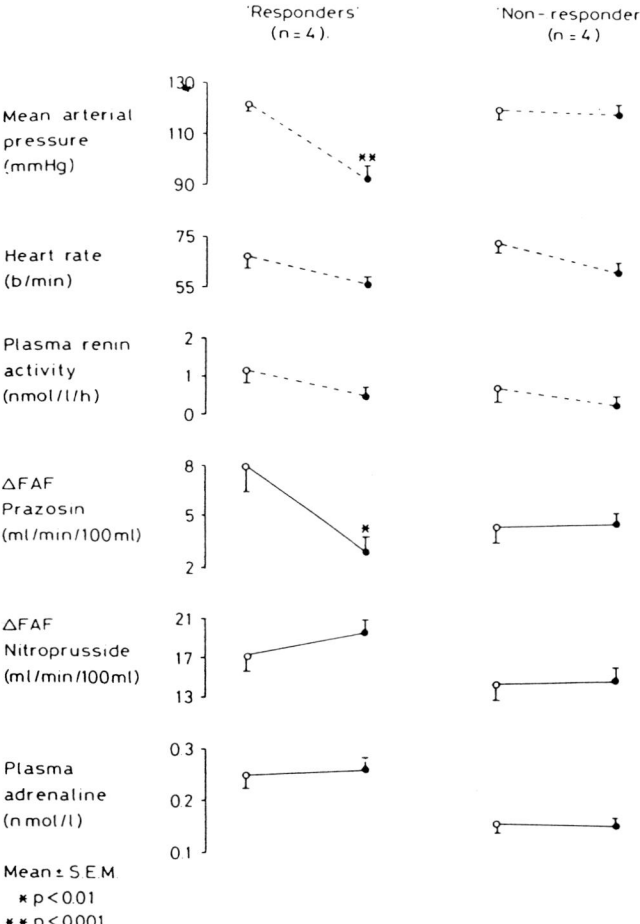

'Responders'
(n = 4)

'Non-responders'
(n = 4)

Mean arterial pressure (mmHg)

Heart rate (b/min)

Plasma renin activity (nmol/l/h)

ΔFAF Prazosin (ml/min/100ml)

ΔFAF Nitroprusside (ml/min/100ml)

Plasma adrenaline (nmol/l)

Mean ± S.E.M.
* p < 0.01
** p < 0.001

FIG. 9. Intraarterial mean blood pressure, heart rate, plasma renin activity, forearm blood flow to postjunctional α-adrenoceptor blockade with prazosin (0.5 μg/min/100 ml tissue) and to nonspecific vasodilation with sodium nitroprusside (0.6 μg/min/100 ml tissue) and plasma adrenaline concentrations before (○) and after (●) 6 weeks of propranolol treatment (320 mg/d) in four "responders" **(left)** and four "nonresponders" **(right)** *p < .05; **p < .01. (From ref. 90, with permission)

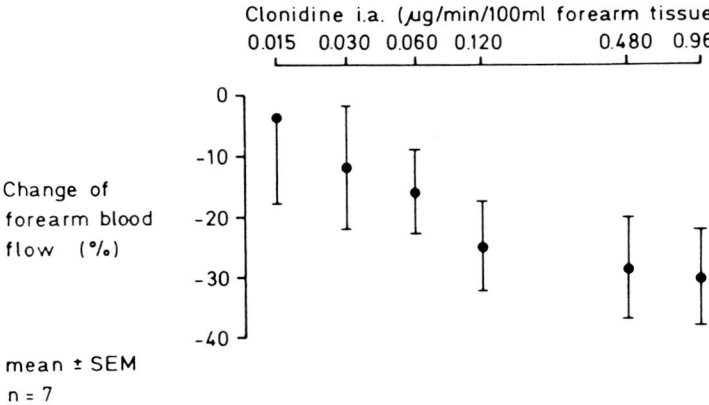

FIG. 10. Decrease in forearm blood flow ($p < .01$; analysis of variance) to increasing doses of intraarterially infused clonidine. The logarithm of the clonidine dose is plotted against the percent changes of forearm blood flow observed during the fifth minute of each clonidine infusion. (From ref. 56, with permission)

as demonstrated by similar decreases in forearm blood flow by both agonists and by a similar partial blocking effect by the α_2-adrenoceptor antagonist yohimbine and the α_1-adrenoceptor antagonist doxazosin, as well as by the complete blocking effect of the combination of both antagonists (Fig. 14). The same authors found that forearm vasoconstriction during low body negative pressure, which by unloading low pressure baroreceptors (61) increases sympathetic efferent activity and raises plasma norepinephrine concentrations (62), was inhibited by α_1-adrenoceptor blockade with doxazosin but not with yohimbine (63). Therefore, the cumulative evidence from all these experiments indicates that both postjunctional α_1- and α_2-adrenoceptors contribute to basal vascu-

lar tone, but that adaptive changes of vascular tone predominantly involve norepinephrine-induced α_1-adrenoceptor–mediated effects.

There is some evidence, although not conclusive, that increased α_2-adrenoceptor–mediated vasoconstriction may contribute to increased vasoconstriction in patients with essential hypertension. A greater vasodilator response to intraarterially infused yohimbine in patients with essential hypertension as compared with normotensive subjects was found to be of similar magnitude as the one observed with α_1-adrenoceptor blockade with prazosin (Fig. 15) (59). The comparable vasodilator response to sodium nitroprusside in hypertensives and normotensives supports the specific nature of the en-

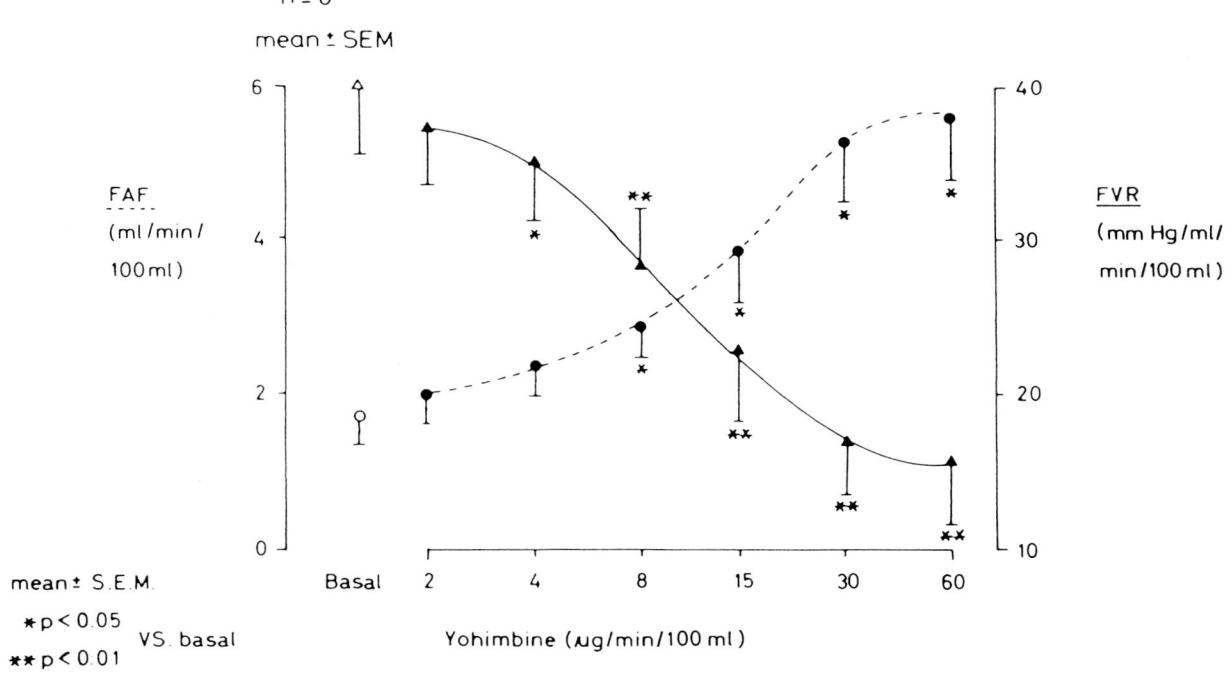

FIG. 11. Forearm vascular resistance (FVR, *solid line*) and forearm blood flow (FAF, *broken line*) to increasing concentrations of intraarterially (brachial artery) infused yohimbine in eight normotensive subjects. (From ref. 91, with permission)

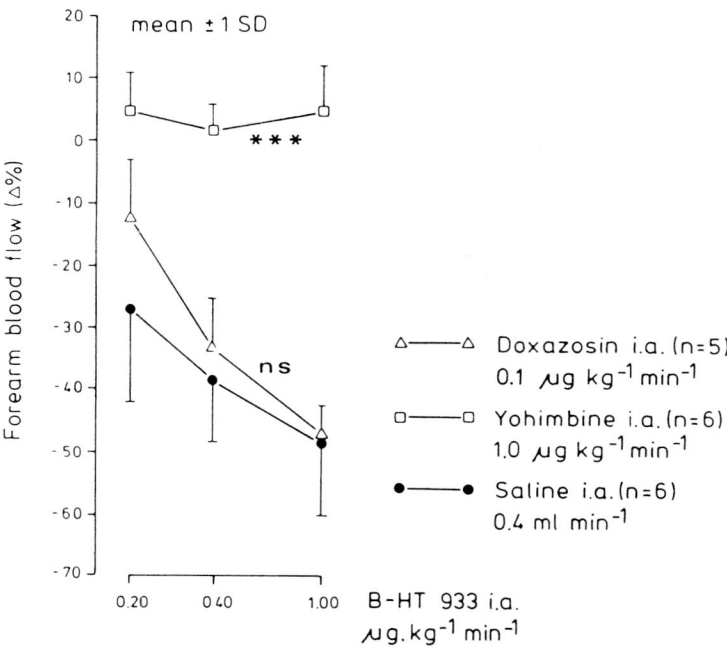

Doxazosin i.a. (n=5)
0.1 μg kg^{-1} min^{-1}

Yohimbine i.a. (n=6)
1.0 μg kg^{-1} min^{-1}

Saline i.a. (n=6)
0.4 ml min^{-1}

B-HT 933 i.a.
μg.kg^{-1} min^{-1}

FIG. 12. Mean percentage changes in forearm blood flow (FBF) during intraarterial (ia) infusion of three cumulative doses of the α_2-agonist B-HT 933 in the presence of saline, yohimbine, and doxazosin. Statistical significance of differences between the infusion with the antagonist compared with the infusion with saline are indicated: ***$p < .001$; ns, not significant. (From ref. 57, with permission)

hanced vasodilator response to α_2-adrenoceptor blockade in hypertensive patients. On the other hand, α_2-adrenoceptor–mediated vasoconstriction has not been found by other investigators (63) to be enhanced in hypertensive patients. One possible reason for this discrepancy could be that plasma epinephrine concentrations in the hypertensive patients of the former study (59) were higher as compared with normotensive subjects (69 ± 31 and 37 ± 13 pg/ml, respectively; mean ± SD; $p < .05$), reflecting an increased sympathetic activity that may

have provided a more favorable condition for demonstrating enhanced α_2-adrenoceptor–mediated vasoconstriction and, hence, a greater vasodilator response to adrenoceptor blockade. Increased adrenergic activity as reflected by higher norepinephrine (12,42) or epinephrine (41) concentrations may be necessary to demonstrate an enhanced α-adrenoceptor–mediated vasoconstrictor contribution to essential hypertension. Similar to other vasoconstrictors, epinephrine-induced forearm vasoconstriction (in the presence of β_1- and β_2- as well as

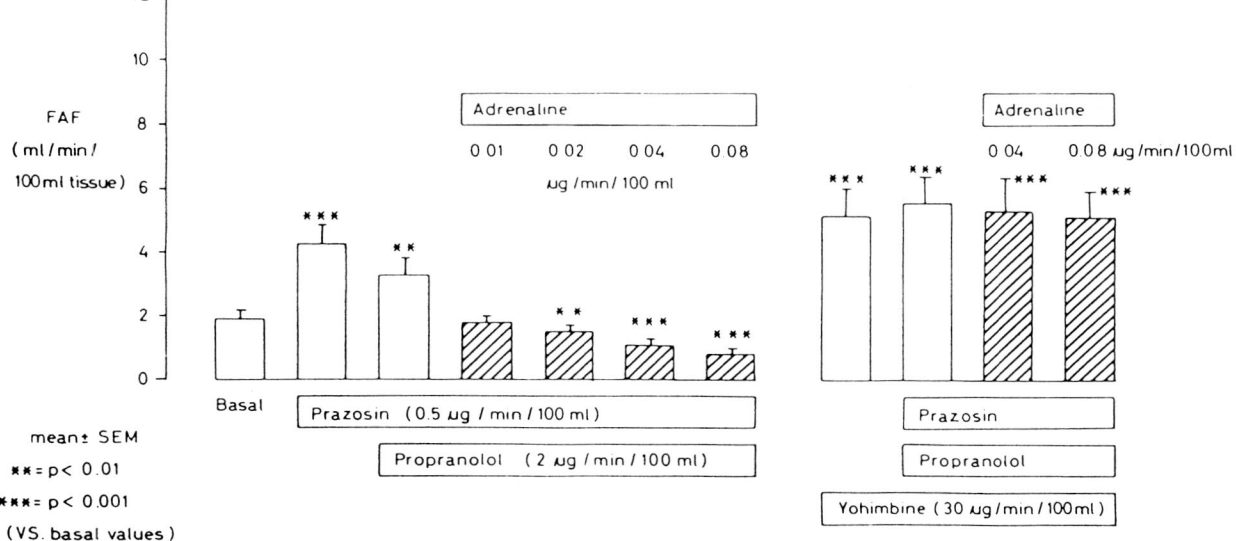

FIG. 13. Forearm blood flow (FAF) responses to increasing doses of intraarterially infused adrenaline (*hatched bars*) during postjunctional α_1-adrenoceptor blockade with prazosin and β-adrenoceptor blockade with propranolol (**left**) and during additional postjunctional α_1-adrenoceptor blockade with yohimbine (**right**) in eight normotensive subjects. (From ref. 91, with permission)

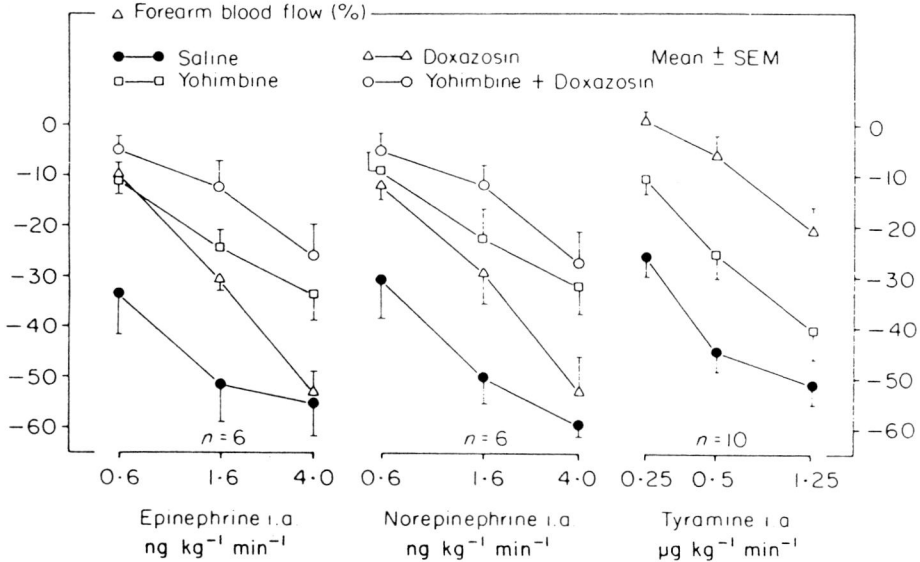

FIG. 14. Mean percentage changes in forearm blood flow in normotensive subjects during intraarterial (i.a.) (brachial artery) infusion of three cumulative doses of epinephrine, norepinephrine, and tyramine in the presence of saline, yohimbine 1.0 μg kg^{-1} min^{-1}, doxazosin 0.1 μg kg^{-1} min^{-1}, and the combination of yohimbine and doxazosin. The epinephrine and norepinephrine infusions were given during a concomitant i.a. infusion of propranolol 1.0 μg kg^{-1} min^{-1}. (From ref. 60, with permission)

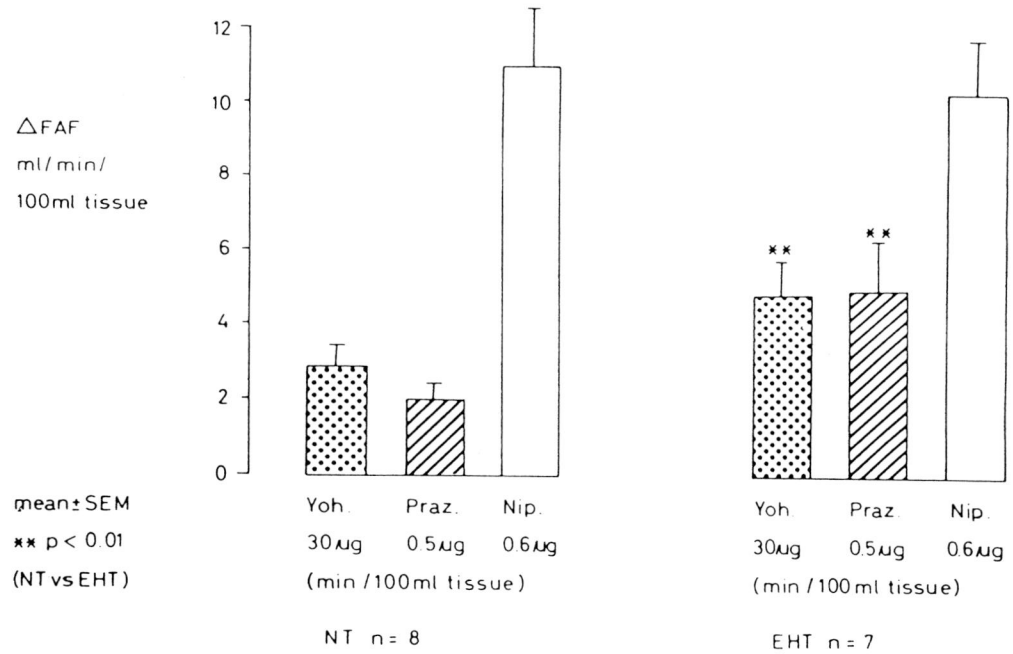

FIG. 15. Increase in forearm blood flow ($\triangle$FAF) following postjunctional α_2-adrenoceptor blockade with intraarterially infused yohimbine (Yoh.; *stippled bars*), α_1-adrenoceptor blockade with prazosin (Praz.; *hatched bars*) and following "nonspecific" (not adrenoceptor-mediated) vasodilation with sodium nitroprusside (Nip.; *blank bars*) in eight normotensive subjects (NT) and seven patients with essential hypertension (EHT). (From ref. 91, with permission)

α_1-adrenoceptor blockade) was greater in patients with essential hypertension as compared with normotensive subjects of comparable age (Fig. 16) (59).

Since norepinephrine regulates its own release through prejunctional α_2-adrenoceptors that, when stimulated, inhibit norepinephrine release (53), it is possible that the contribution of the α_2-adrenoceptor–mediated vasoconstriction may have been underestimated. However, prejunctional α_2-adrenoceptors, if present in the forearm vasculature in man, do not seem to be functionally apparent (64), since there was no change in the venous-arterial norepinephrine difference after infusion of the α_2-adrenoceptor agonist clonidine into the forearm circulation even at concentrations that stimulated postjunctional α_2-adrenoceptors, which, to be stimulated, require higher concentrations of the agonist than the prejunctional α_2-adrenoceptors (Fig. 17) (56). Therefore, this rules out a major influence of prejunctional α_2-adrenoceptors on postjunctional α_2-adrenoceptor-mediated effects. However, other authors have found an increase in plasma norepinephrine concentration following α_2-adrenoceptor blockade with RX 781094 (55); the difference could arise from the fact that in this study the α_2-antagonist was infused intravenously and may have caused reflex sympathetic activation.

Intravenous infusion of epinephrine, reflecting more appropriately increased concentrations of circulating epinephrine, produced differing results. Since the observation that infusion of the α_2-adrenoceptor agonist clonidine reduced facial skin blood flow, which was antagonized by the α_2-adrenoceptor antagonist SK + F86466 but not by the α_1-adrenoceptor antagonist prazosin (65), postjunctional α_2-adrenoceptors are stimulated by sys-temic application of an α_2-agonist and cause vasoconstriction. However, intravenous infusion of epinephrine, in doses that produced plasma concentrations comparable to those observed during mental stress, caused vasodilation in the forearm and an increase in pulse pressure and heart rate (66). Vasodilation in this experimental setting was most likely due to epinephrine-induced stimulation of postsynaptic β_2-receptors on vascular smooth muscle cells (67). Since in the presence of β-adrenoceptor blockade α_2-adrenoceptor–mediated vasoconstriction becomes apparent (Figs. 13 and 16) (59), reduction of β-adrenoceptor–mediated function, as occurs with older age (Fig. 18) and in patients with essential hypertension (68–73), thus conceivably could shift the vascular effects of epinephrine to an α_2-adrenoceptor–mediated vasoconstriction (74). Since epinephrine and norepinephrine stimulate both subtypes of α-adrenoceptors to the same degree when infused at the same concentrations (Fig. 14) (60), but physiological epinephrine concentrations are five to eight times lower than those of norepinephrine, the latter probably will predominate and cause postjunctional α_1-adrenoceptor–mediated vasoconstriction under regular, everyday conditions. However, it is conceivable that conditions that are associated with very high concentrations of epinephrine could override β-adrenoceptor–mediated vasodilation and cause postjunctional α_2-adrenoceptor–mediated vasoconstriction (75). High concentrations of circulating epinephrine could occur during prolonged mental and physical stress (68,76), exposure to cold (77), pain or anxiety (78), or in patients with pheochromocytoma; the pale faces of these patients could reflect epinephrine-induced α_2-adrenoceptor–mediated vasoconstriction (65).

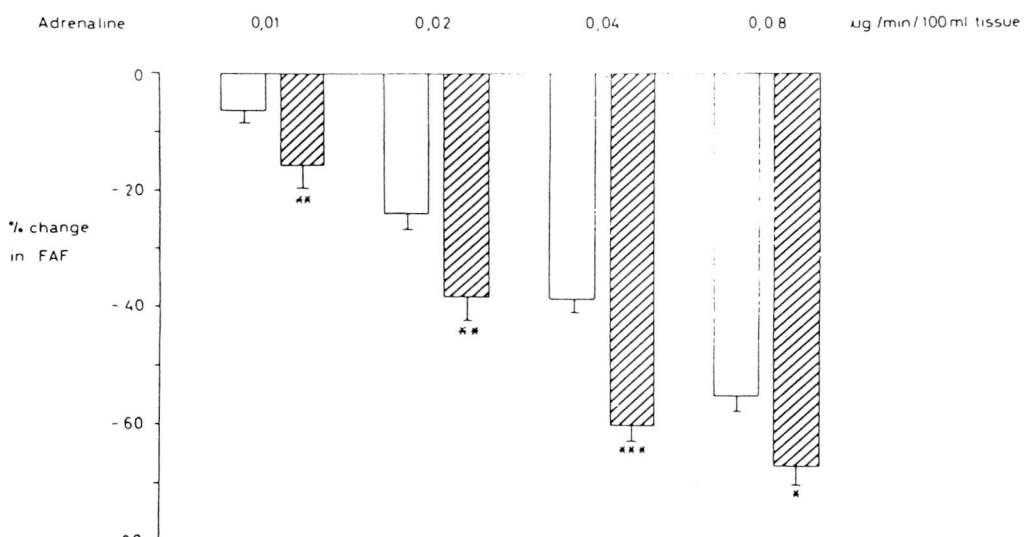

FIG. 16. Decrease in forearm blood flow (FAF) (% of basal flow) to increasing doses of intraarterial adrenaline (0.01, 0.02, 0.04, and 0.08 µg/min/100 ml tissue) in eight normotensive subjects (*open bars*) and seven patients with essential hypertension (*hatched bars*). Mean ± SEM, *p < .05; **p < .001 (normotensive vs essential hypertensive subjects). (From ref. 90, with permission)

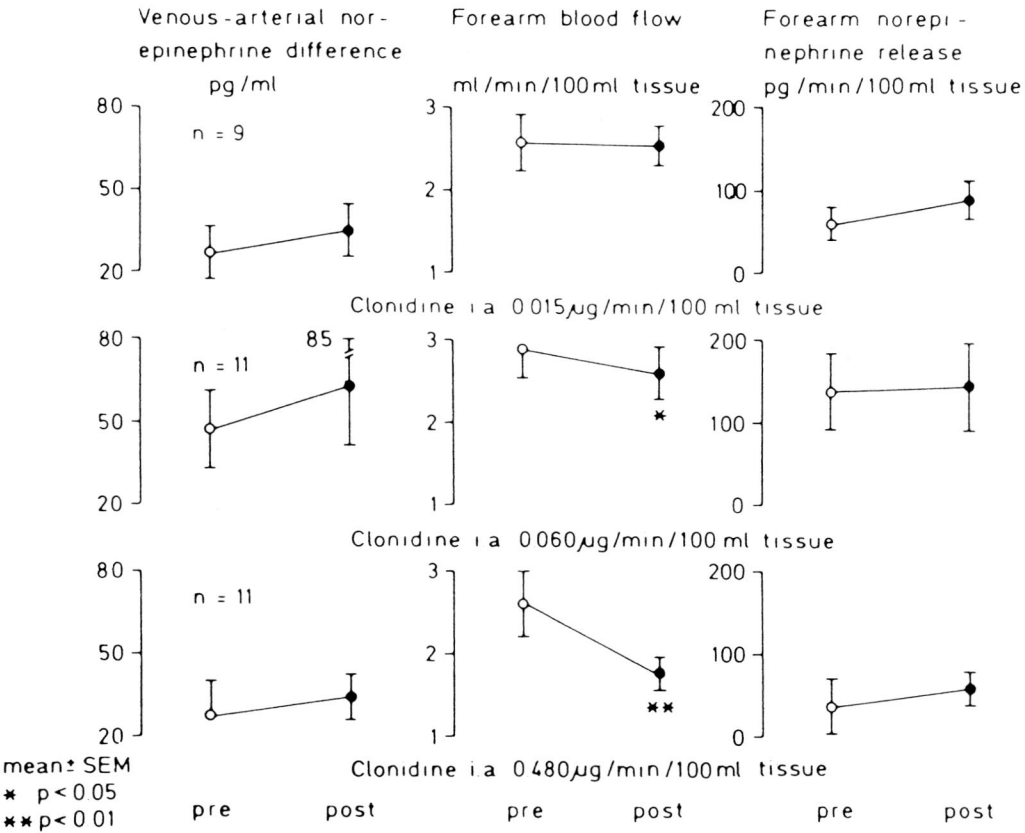

FIG. 17. Venous-arterial norepinephrine difference (**left**), forearm blood flow (**middle**), and forearm norepinephrine release (**right**) in 11 normotensive subjects, before and after brachial artery infusion of the α_2-adrenoceptor agonist clonidine. (From ref. 92, with permission)

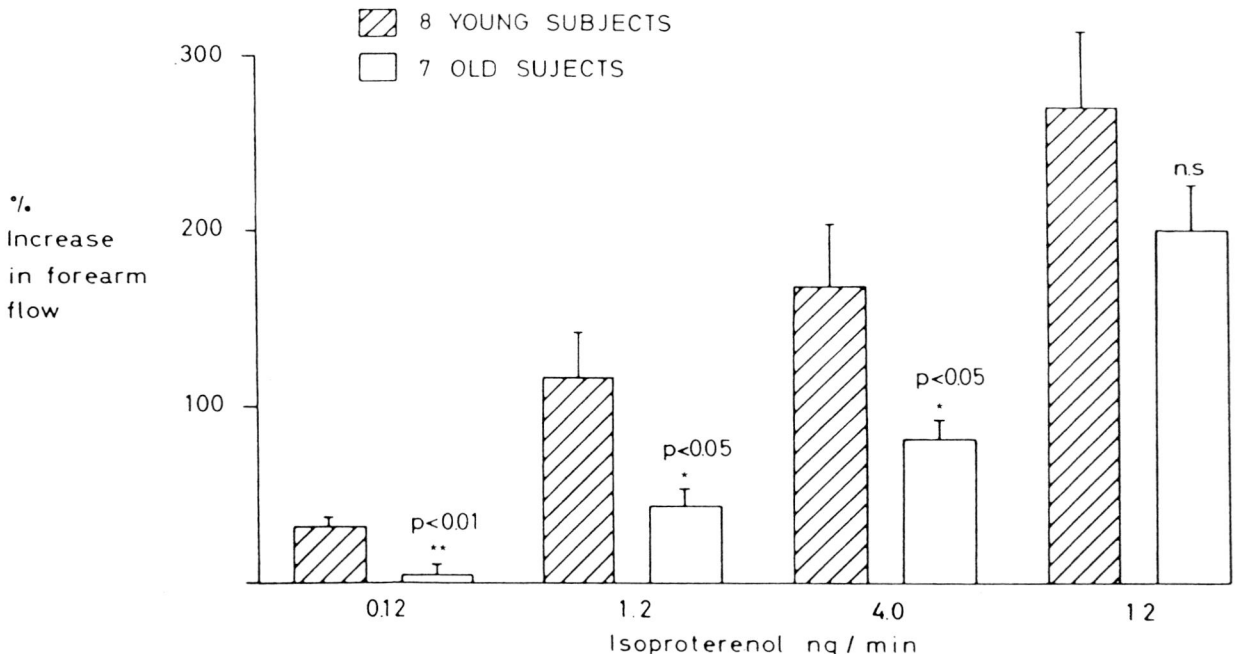

FIG. 18. Percent increase (±SEM) in forearm blood flow during intraarterial infusion of isoproterenol in eight young (*blank bars*) and seven old (*hatched bars*) normal subjects. Statistical significance of differences between young and old subjects: *$p < .05$; **$p < .01$; ns, not significant. (From ref. 70, with permission)

THE FUNCTIONAL CONNECTION OF ADRENOCEPTOR-MEDIATED AND CALCIUM INFLUX–DEPENDENT VASOCONSTRICTION

Vascular tone and hence vascular resistance are ultimately determined by intracellular free-calcium concentration, which transforms phosphate-bound energy into mechanical contraction of the vascular smooth muscles (33). Therefore, blockade of calcium influx to the vascular smooth muscle cells by infusion of calcium antagonists results in a greater forearm vasodilator response than does blockade of α-adrenoceptors. Calcium influx–dependent, like adrenoceptor-mediated vasoconstriction, is enhanced in patients with essential hypertension, as demonstrated by the greater increase in forearm blood flow following intraarterial infusion of calcium antagonists (Fig. 19). The sympathetic nervous system via adrenoceptor-mediated mechanisms plays an important role in cellular calcium handling. Depolarization by norepinephrine, as well as more selective α_1- and α_2-adrenoceptor agonists, acts through receptor-operated calcium channels or receptor-mediated mechanisms, respectively, participating in subcellular calcium mobilization (79–81). Stimulation of α_1-adrenoceptors mediates calcium release, possibly from the sarcoplasmatic reticulum, and thereby initiates further calcium-induced calcium release (82). α_2-Adrenoceptor stimulation may modulate calcium uptake by acting on a receptor-operated calcium channel that can be blocked by calcium antagonists (83). In patients with essential hypertension, chronic calcium antagonist treatment reduced the α_2-adrenoceptor–mediated increase in forearm vascular resistance caused by the α_2-agonist azepexole (Fig. 20) (84). The interaction of sympathetic activity and calcium handling appears to be reflected by the enhanced α-adrenoceptor–mediated as well as calcium influx–dependent vasoconstriction in essential hypertension, which both relate to the degree of adrenergic activity (41,85).

Elevated intracellular free-calcium concentrations were found in platelets of patients with essential hypertension, and there is a direct relationship between intracellular free calcium concentration and blood pressure (86). This relationship may point to a derangement in the cellular handling of calcium in patients with essential hypertension (87). The handling of calcium by platelets may simulate that of vascular smooth muscle cells, since both share a number of common features (88) related to vasoconstriction. This is shown by parallel changes in platelet free-calcium concentration and calcium influx–dependent vasoconstriction during antihypertensive treatment with acebutolol or calcium entry blockade with nitrendipine (89) as shown in Fig. 21. The treatment-induced fall in blood pressure was associated

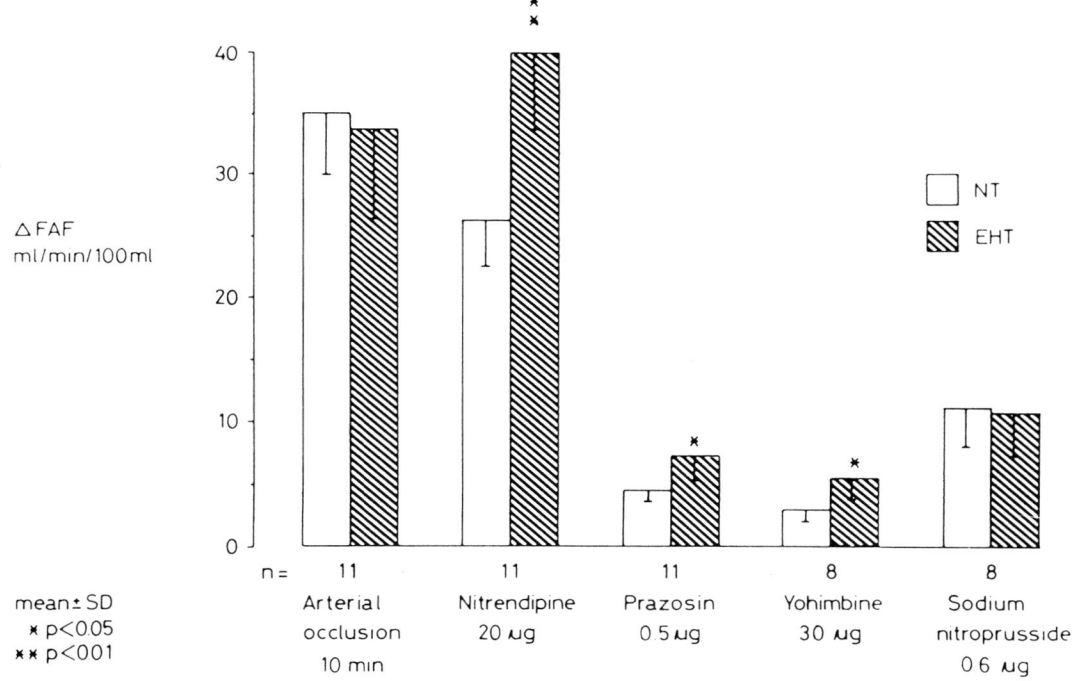

FIG. 19. Mean (±SD) increase in forearm blood flow (Δ FAF) to calcium entry blockade with nitrendipine, to α_1- and α_2-blockade with prazosin and yohimbine, respectively, as well as to "nonspecific" vasodilation after 10-min forearm ischemia (arterial occlusion) and to sodium nitroprusside. Drugs were infused into the left brachial artery and doses are indicated in μg/min/100 ml forearm tissue. Patients with essential hypertension are shown in hatched bars, and age- and sex-matched normotensive control subjects in open bars. *$p < .05$; **$p < .01$. (From ref. 93, with permission)

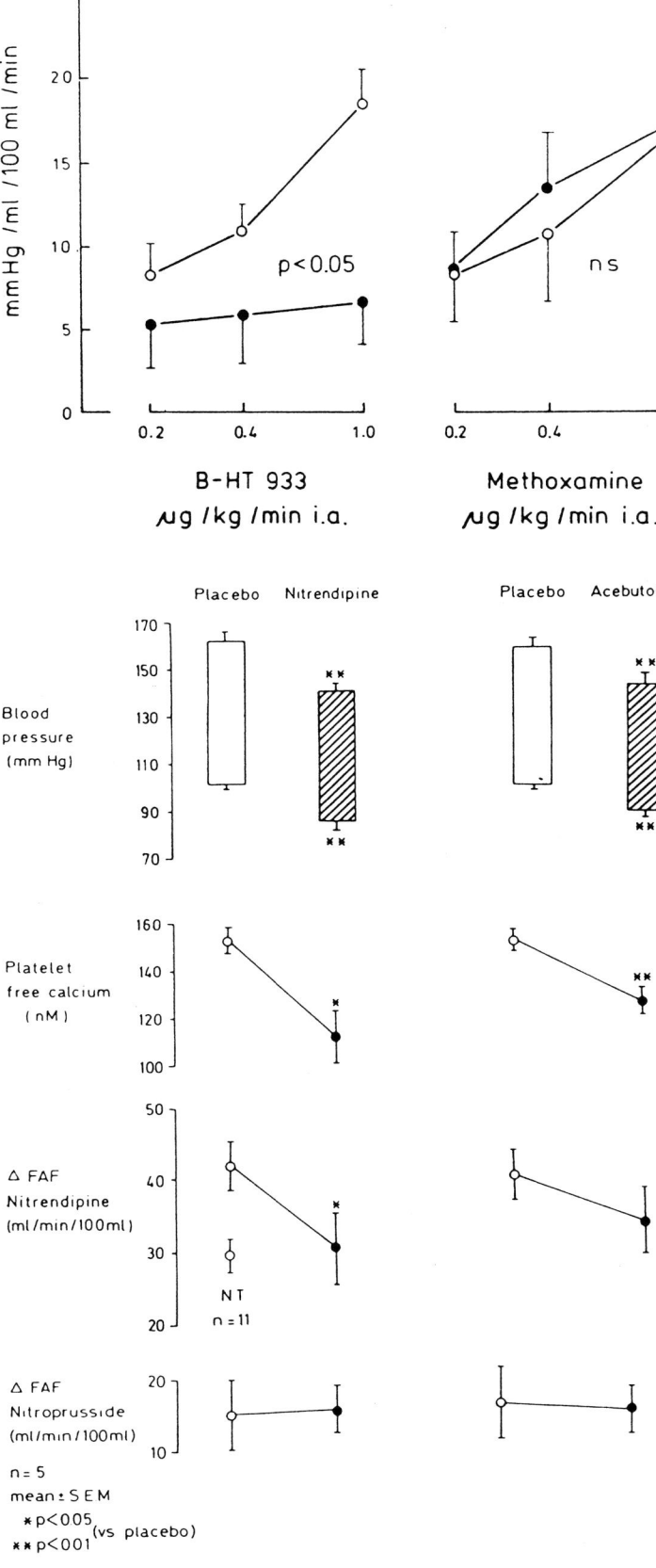

FIG. 20. Mean changes in forearm vascular resistance during intraarterial (i.a.) infusion of three cumulative doses of the α_2-adrenoceptor agonist B-HT 933 (azepexole) and the α_1-adrenoceptor agonist methoxamine during placebo (*open circles*) and during chronic treatment with the calcium antagonist PY 108-068 (*filled circles*) in five hypertensive patients. Calcium entry blockade inhibited α_2- but not α_1-adrenoceptor–mediated vasoconstriction. (From ref. 84, with permission.)

FIG. 21. Blood pressure, platelet free calcium concentration, and increase in forearm blood flow (ΔFAF) in response to intraarterial nitrendipine (20 μg/100 ml forearm volume) and to intraarterial sodium nitroprusside (1.2 μg/100 ml forearm tissue). Measurements were done during placebo (*open symbols*) and after 6 weeks of antihypertensive therapy with nitrendipine or acebutolol (*filled symbols*). NT indicates the increase in forearm blood flow to intraarterial infusion of nitrendipine obtained in 11 normotensive subjects. (From ref. 89, with permission)

with a decrease in the elevated platelet-free calcium concentration and with a normalization of the previously enhanced calcium influx–dependent vasoconstriction, demonstrating the close relationship between platelet-free calcium concentration and vascular resistance. Since nonspecific vasodilation with sodium nitroprusside was not influenced by antihypertensive treatment, this underlines the specificity of treatment-induced changes in calcium influx–dependent vasoconstriction by adrenergic as well as calcium entry blockade. This could indicate that at the level of the vascular smooth muscle cells normalization of the intracellular free calcium concentration and of the enhanced calcium influx–dependent vasoconstriction are important features associated with antihypertensive response. Whether this is a primary phenomenon or occurs as a consequence of the fall in blood pressure remains to be investigated further.

SUMMARY AND CONCLUSIONS

Increased adrenergic activity as reflected by higher norepinephrine and epinephrine plasma concentrations as well as by increased sympathetic nerve traffic in patients with essential hypertension has been documented. That increased adrenergic activity could be involved in the pathophysiology of essential hypertension requires the demonstration of a relationship between increased adrenergic activity and hemodynamic variables, in particular increased vascular resistance, which leads to an elevation in blood pressure. Intervention with the sympathetic nervous system leads to changes toward restoring normal blood pressure and/or a normal hemodynamic pattern.

Since systemic interference with the sympathetic nervous system leads to activation of hemodynamic counterregulatory mechanisms induced by a fall in blood pressure, investigations determining the mechanisms that relate increased sympathetic activity to increased vascular resistance have been done mostly in the regional vascular bed of the forearm. By infusing the interventional drug into the brachial artery, systemic effects caused by the interventional drug can largely be avoided. Using venous occlusion plethysmography, forearm blood flow can be measured and forearm vascular resistance can be calculated. Although observations made in the forearm vascular bed cannot be readily extrapolated to other vascular beds, they facilitate determining mechanisms through which an increased sympathetic activity can lead to increased vascular resistance and the respective effects of interventional pharmacological probes.

α_1-Adrenoceptor blockade by infusion of prazosin or doxazosin into the forearm circulation revealed an enhanced α_1-adrenoceptor–mediated vasoconstrictor component in hypertensive patients, which relates to indices of increased adrenergic activity. Increased α_1-

adrenoceptor–mediated vasoconstriction is considered to be mediated by structural vascular changes such as remodeling of the vascular wall, which amplifies the response to the increased adrenergic vasoconstrictor stimulus.

Postjunctional α_2-adrenoceptor–mediated vasoconstriction has been identified with the use of α_2-adrenoceptor agonists such as clonidine or azepexole and by the vasodilator effect with the α_2-adrenoceptor antagonist yohimbine. α_2-Adrenoceptor–mediated vasoconstriction has been found to be enhanced in patients with essential hypertension and with evidence for increased adrenergic activity as demonstrated by their greater forearm vasodilator response to yohimbine.

Norepinephrine and epinephrine infused at equal concentrations induce a comparable α_1- and α_2-adrenoceptor–mediated vasoconstriction. However, since physiological concentrations of norepinephrine are higher, vascular tone and increased vascular resistance in hypertension are principally determined by norepinephrine. Epinephrine's α_1 and α_2-adrenoceptor-mediated vasoconstrictor effect is countered by its mainly β_2-adrenoceptor–mediated vasodilation. Therefore, the contribution of increased epinephrine concentration to hypertension remains debatable, although it is conceivable that increased concentrations of epinephrine, such as in patients with pheochromocytoma or during mental stress, could lead to epinephrine-induced vasoconstriction mediated by postjunctional α_1- as well as α_2-adrenoceptors, particularly if β-receptor–mediated function is reduced, such as in hypertension or in older age.

Vascular tone and hence vascular resistance are ultimately determined by the intracellular free calcium concentration in vascular smooth muscle cells. Therefore, calcium influx–dependent vasoconstriction is greater than α-adrenoceptor–mediated vasoconstriction, but, similarly to the α-adrenoceptor–mediated vasoconstriction, is also enhanced in patients with essential hypertension. There is a functional relationship between calcium influx–dependent and adrenergically induced vasoconstriction, since stimulation of α_1- as well as α_2-adrenoceptors increases intracellular free calcium concentration. Calcium entry blockade reduces α_2- but not α_1-adrenoceptor–mediated vasoconstriction, demonstrating receptor-operated calcium entry into the cells by the former. This connection between enhanced α-adrenoceptor–mediated and calcium influx–dependent vasoconstriction in essential hypertension is underlined by their direct relationship with indices of increased adrenergic activity.

ACKNOWLEDGMENTS

The authors greatly acknowledge the important contributions made by Drs. Wolfgang Amann, Boa Hua Ji,

Lennart Hulthen, Lily Linder, Franco B. Muller, and Peter Van Brummelen, as well as the technical and secretarial assistance of Ms. B. Libsig, Ms. A. De S. Pinto, and Ms. Beverly Bungay.

REFERENCES

1. De Quattro V, Miura Y. Neurogenic factors in human hypertension: mechanism or myth. *Am J Med* 1973;55:362–378.
2. DeChamplain J. The contribution of the sympathetic nervous system to arterial hypertension. *Can J Physiol Pharmacol* 1978;56:341–353.
3. Julius S, Pascual AV, London R. Role of parasympathetic inhibition in the hyperkinetic type of borderline hypertension. *Circulation* 1971;44:413–418.
4. Esler M, Julius S, Zweifler A, Randall O, Harburg E, Gardiner H, DeQuattro V. Mild high-renin essential hypertension: neurogenic human hypertension? *N Engl J Med* 1977;296:405–411.
5. Folkow B. Physiological aspects of primary hypertension. *Physiol Rev* 1982;62:347–504.
6. Conway J. Hemodynamic aspects of essential hypertension in humans. *Physiol Rev* 1984;64:617–660.
7. Folkow B, Di Bona GF, Hjemdahl P, Thoren PH, Wallin BG. Measurements of plasma norepinephrine concentrations in human primary hypertension—a word of caution on their applicability for assessing neurogenic contributions. *Hypertension* 1983;5:399–403.
8. Buhler FR, Kiowski W, Landmann R, van Brummelen P, Amann FW, Bolli P, Bertel O. Changing role of beta and alpha adrenoreceptor-mediated cardiovascular responses in the transition from a high cardiac output into a high peripheral resistance phase in essential hypertension. In: Laragh JH, Buhler FR, Seldin DW, eds. *Frontiers in hypertension research.* New York: Springer, 1981;316–426.
9. Lund-Johansen P. Central haemodynamics in essential hypertension at rest and during exercise: a 20 year follow-up study. *J Hypertens* 1989;7(suppl 6):S52–S55.
10. Goldstein DS. Plasma norepinephrine in essential hypertension: a study of the studies. *Hypertension* 1981;3:48–52.
11. Goldstein DS. Plasma catecholamines and essential hypertension: an analytical review. *Hypertension* 1983;3:86–99.
12. Kiowski W, van Brummelen P, Buhler FR. Plasma noradrenaline correlates with α-adrenoreceptor-mediated vasoconstriction and blood pressure in patients with essential hypertension. *Clin Sci* 1979;57:177s–180s.
13. Goldstein DS, McCarty R, Polinsky RJ, Kopin IJ. Relationship between venous plasma norepinephrine and sympathetic neural activity. *Hypertension* 1983;5:552–559.
14. Esler M, Zweifler, Randall O, Julius S, DeQuattro V. Agreements among three different indices of sympathetic nervous system activity in essential hypertension. *Mayo Clin Proc* 1977;52:379–382.
15. Wallin GB, Sundlof G, Ericksson GM, Dominiak P, Girbecker H, Lindblad LE. Plasma noradrenaline correlates to sympathetic nerve activity in normotensive man. *Acta Physiol Scand* 1981;3:69–73.
16. Louis WJ, Doyle AE, Anavekar SN. Plasma norepinephrine levels in essential hypertension. *N Engl J Med* 1973;288:599–601.
17. Esler M. Testing neural control of the circulation in patients: plasma catecholamines. In: Zanchetti A, Tarazi RC, eds. *Handbook of hypertension, vol 8: Pathophysiology of hypertension.* Regulatory Mechanisms. Elsevier, Amsterdam: 1986;216–236.
18. Hjemdahl P. Physiological aspects on catecholamine sampling. *Life Sci* 1987;41:841–844.
19. Esler M, Jennings G, Biviano B, Lambert G, Hasking G. Mechanism of elevated plasma noradrenaline in the course of essential hypertension. *J Cardiovasc Pharmacol* 1986;8(suppl 5):S39–S43.
20. Anderson EA, Sinkey CA, Lawton WJ, Mark AL. Elevated sympathetic nerve activity in borderline hypertensive humans: evidence from direct intraneural recordings. *Hypertension* 1989;14:177–183.
21. Adler-Graschinsky E, Langer SZ. Possible role of a beta-adrenoreceptor in the regulation of noradrenaline release by nerve stimulation through a positive feed back mechanism. *Br J Pharmacol* 1975;53:43–50.
22. Brown MJ, Macquin I. Is adrenaline the cause of essential hypertension? *Lancet* 1981;2:1079–1082.
23. Brown MJ, Causon RC, Barnes VF, Brennan P, Barnes G, Greenberg G. Urinary catecholamines in essential hypertension: results of 24-hour urine catecholamine analyses from patients in the Medical Research Council trial for mild hypertension and from matched controls. *Q J Med* 1985;55:637–651.
24. Bolli P, Amann FW, Hulthen L, Kiowski W, Buhler FR. Elevated plasma adrenaline reflects sympathetic overactivity and enhanced alpha adrenoreceptor-mediated vasoconstriction in essential hypertension. *Clin Sci* 1981;61(suppl 7):161s–164s.
25. Buhler FR, Bolli P, Hulthen UL, Amann FW, Kiowski W. Alpha-adrenoceptors, adrenaline, and exaggerated vasoconstriction response to stress in essential hypertension. *Chest* 1983;83(suppl):304–306.
26. Cousineau D, Lapointe L, De Champlain J. Circulating catecholamines and systolic time intervals in normotensive and hypertensive patients with and without left ventricular hypertrophy. *Am Heart J* 1978;96:229–234.
27. Julius S. Sympathetic hyperactivity and coronary risk in hypertension. *Hypertension* 1993;21:886–893.
28. Freis ED. Hemodynamics of hypertension. *Physiol Rev* 1960;40:27–54.
29. Lund-Johansen P. Hemodynamics in hypertension at rest and during exercise. *J Cardiovasc Pharmacol* 1987;10(suppl 11):S1–S5.
30. Alam M, Smirk FH. Blood pressure raising reflexes in health, essential hypertension and renal hypertension. *Clin Sci* 1938;3:259–266.
31. Goldenberg M, Pines KL, Baldwin E, Greene DG, Roh CE. The haemodynamic response of man to norepinephrine and epinephrine and its relation to the problem of hypertension. *Am J Med* 1948;5:792–806.
32. Pickering GW, Kissin M. The effects of adrenaline and of cold on the blood pressure in human hypertension. *Clin Sci* 1936;2:201–207.
33. Kuriyama H, Yto Y, Suzuki H, Kitamura K, Itoh T. Factors modifying contraction relaxation cycle in vascular smooth muscles. *Am J Physiol* 1982;243:H641–H642.
34. Greenfield ADM, Whitney RJ, Mowbray JF. Methods for the investigation of peripheral blood flow. *Br Med Bull* 1963;19:101.
35. Roddie IC, Wallace WFM. Methods for the assessment of the effects of drugs on the arterial system in man. *Br J Clin Pharmacol* 1979;7:317–323.
36. Bolli P, Kiowski W, Buhler FR. The contribution of alpha-1 and alpha-2 adrenoreceptor mediated vasoconstriction in essential hypertension: assessed by forearm venous occlusion plethysmography. In: Safar M, ed. *The cardiovascular system in essential hypertension.* Dordrecht, Boston, Lancaster: Martinus Nijhoff, 1988;233–252.
37. Doyle AE, Fraser JRE, Marshall RJ. Reactivity of forearm vessels to vasoconstrictor substances in hypertensive and normotensive subjects. *Clin Sci* 1959;18:441–453.
38. Sivertsson R, Olander R. Aspects of the nature of the increased vascular resistance and increased "reactivity" to noradrenaline in hypertensive subjects. *Life Sci* 1968;7(part I):1291–1297.
39. Phillipp TH, Distler A, Cordes U. Sympathetic nervous system and blood pressure control in essential hypertension. *Lancet* 1978;2:959–963.
40. Meier A, Weidmann M, Grimm G, Keusch G, Gluck Z, Minder I, Ziegler WH. Pressor factors and cardiovascular pressure responsiveness in borderline hypertension. *Hypertension* 1981;3:367–372.
41. Amann FW, Bolli P, Kiwski W, Buhler F. Enhanced alpha-adrenoreceptor-mediated vasoconstriction in essential hypertension. *Hypertension* 1981 3(suppl I):I-119–I-123.
42. Egan B, Panis R, Hinderliter A, Schork N, Julius S. Mechanism of increased alpha adrenergic vasoconstriction in human essential hypertension. *J Clin Invest* 1987;80:812–817.
43. Folkow B. Cardiovascular structural adaptation; its role in the ini-

tiation and maintenance of primary hypertension. *Clin Sci Mol Med* 1978;55:3s–22s.

44. Sivertsson R. The hemodynamic importance of structural vascular changes in essential hypertension. *Acta Physiol Scand Suppl* 1970;343:1–56.

45. Baumbach GL, Heistad DD. Remodelling of cerebral arterioles in chronic hypertension. *Hypertension* 1989;13:968–972.

46. Tarazi RZ, Dustan HP. Beta adrenoreceptor blockade in hypertension. *Am J Cardiol* 1972;29:633.

47. Langer SZ, Cavero I, Massinghan R. Recent development in noradrenergic neurotransmission and its relevance to the mechanism of action of certain antihypertensive agents. *Hypertension* 1980;2:372–383.

48. Bolli P, Amann FW, Burkart F, Buhler FR. Role of alpha-adrenoceptor-mediated vasoconstriction for anti-hypertensive beta blockade. *J Cardiovasc Pharmacol* 1982;4:S162–S167.

49. Majewski H, McCulloch MW, Rand MJ, Story DF. Adrenaline activation of prejunctional beta-adrenoceptors in guinea-pig atria. *Br J Pharmacol* 1980;71:435.

50. Starke K. Alpha adrenoceptor subclassification. *Rev Physiol Biochem Pharmacol* 1981;88:199–236.

51. Yamaguchi I, Kopin IJ. Differential inhibition of alpha-1 and alpha-2 adrenoceptor-mediated pressure responses in pithed rats. *J Pharmacol Exp Ther* 1980;214:275–281.

52. Lee JY, Walsh GM, Heilman RD, Radzialowski FM. Differential blocking effects of prazosin and yohimbine or vasopressor responses to sympathetic nerve stimulation and intravenous noradrenaline in the pithed rat. *Res Commun Chem Pathol Pharmacol* 1984;43:97–112.

53. Langer SZ. Presynaptic regulation of the release of catecholamines. *Pharmacol Rev* 1980;32:337–362.

54. Timmermans PBMWM, van Zwieten PA. The postsynaptic alpha-2 adrenoceptor *J Auton Pharmacol* 1981;1:171–183.

55. Elliot HL, Reid JL. Evidence for post junctional vascular alpha adrenoceptors in peripheral vascular regulation in man. *Clin Sci* 1983;65:237–241.

56. Kiowski W, Hulthen VL, Ritz R, Buhler FR. Prejunctional alpha-2 adrenoceptors and norepinephrine release in the forearm of normal humans. *J Cardiovasc Pharmacol* 1985;7(suppl 6):144–148.

57. Jie K, van Brummelen P, Vermey P, Timmermans PBMWM, van Zwieten PA. Identification of vascular postsynaptic alpha-1 and alpha-2 adrenoceptors in man. *Circ Res* 1984;54:447–452.

58. Bolli P, Erne P, Kiowski W, Ji BH, Amann FW, Buhler FR. Important contribution of post junctional alpha-2 adrenoceptor-mediated vasoconstriction to arteriolar tone in man. *J Hypertens* 1983;1(suppl 2):257–259.

59. Bolli P, Erne P, Ji BH, Block LH, Kiowski WE, Buhler FR. Adrenaline induces vasoconstriction through post-junctional alpha-2 adrenoceptors and this response is enhanced in patients with essential hypertension. *J Hypertens* 1984;2(suppl 3):115–118.

60. Jie K, van Brummelen P, Vermey P, Timmermans PBMWM, van Zwieten PA. Post-synaptic alpha-1 and alpha-2 adrenoceptors in human blood vessels: interactions with exogenous and endogenous catecholamines. *Eur J Clin Invest* 1987;17:174–181.

61. Zoller RP, Mark AL, Abboud FM, Schmid PG, Heistad DD. The role of low pressure baroreceptors in reflex vasoconstrictor responses in man. *J Clin Invest.* 1972;51:2967–2972.

62. Grassi G, Gavazzi C, Capozi A, Galva MD, Picotti GB, Mancia G. Alterations in plasma adrenaline in response to reflex vasodilation of sympathetic vasoconstrictor tone to skeletal muscle. *J Hypertens* 1984;2(suppl 3):131–133.

63. Jie K, van Brummelen P, Vermey P, Timmermans PBMWM, van Zwieten PA. Alpha-1 and alpha-2 adrenoceptor mediated vasoconstriction in the forearm of normotensive and hypertensive subjects. *J Cardiovasc Pharmacol* 1986;8:190–196.

64. Fitzgerald GA, Watkins J, Dollery CT. Regulation of norepinephrine release by peripheral alpha-2 receptor stimulation. *Clin Pharmacol Ther* 1981;29:160–167.

65. Brown MJ. Adrenaline and adrenoceptors in hypertension. *Pharmacol Toxicol* 1988;63(suppl 1):16–20.

66. Kjeldsen SE, Petrin J, Weder AB, Julius S. Contrasting effects of epinephrine on forearm hemodynamics and aterial plasma norepinephrine. *Am J Hypertens* 1993;6:369–375.

67. Freyschuss U, Hjemdahl P, Juhlin-Dannfelt, Linde B. Cardiovascular and metabolic responses to low dose adrenaline infusion: an invasive study in humans. *Clin Sci* 1986;70:199–206.

68. Bertel O, Buhler FR, Kiowski W, Luetold BE. Decreased beta-adrenoceptor responsiveness as related to age, blood pressure and plasma catecholamines in patients with essential hypertension. *Hypertension* 1980;2:130–138.

69. Fleisch JH. Age-related changes in the sensitivity of blood vessels to drugs. *Pharmacol Ther* 1980;8:477–487.

70. Buhler FR. Elevated plasma adrenaline, age-related decrease in beta-adrenoceptor-mediated cardiovascular functions and increase in alpha-receptor-mediated vasoconstriction in essential hypertension. In: Fuxe K, ed. *Wenner-Gren Center International Symposium Series, vol 33, Central Adrenaline Neurons.* Oxford and New York: Pergamon Press, 1976;305–316.

71. London GM, Safar ME, Weiss YA, Milliez PL. Isoproterenol sensitivity and total body clearance of propranolol in hypertensive patients. *J Clin Pharmacol* 1976;16:174.

72. Vestal RE, Wood AJJ, Shand DG. Reduced beta-adrenoceptor sensitivity in the elderly. *Clin Pharmacol Ther* 1979;25:181.

73. Conway J. Effect of age on the response to propranolol. *Int J Clin Pharmacol* 1970;4:148.

74. Goldberg MR, Robertson D. Evidence for the existence of vascular alpha-2 adrenergic receptors in humans. *Hypertension* 1984;6:551–556.

75. Robertson D, Garland AJ, Robertson RM, Nies AS, Shand DG, Oates JA. Comparative assessment of stimuli that release neuronal and adrenomedullary catecholamines in man. *Circulation* 1979;59:637–643.

76. Buhler FR, Bertel O, Kiowski W. Plasma noradrenaline and adrenaline and beta-adrenoceptor responsiveness in renin subgroups of essential hypertension. *Clin Sci Mol Med* 1978;55:57–60.

77. Bolli P, Amann FW, Hulthen L, Kiowski W, Buhler FR. Elevated plasma adrenaline reflects sympathetic overactivity and enhanced alpha adrenoceptor-mediated vasoconstriction in essential hypertension. *Clin Sci* 1981;61(suppl 7):161–164.

78. Bertel O, Buhler FR, Baitsch G, Ritz R. Plasma adrenaline and noradrenaline in patients with acute myocardial infarction. *Chest* 1982;82:64–68.

79. Haeusler G. Contraction of vascular muscle as related to membrane potential and calcium fluxes. *J Cardiovasc Pharmacol* 1985;7(suppl 6):S3–S8.

80. Holck M, Gerold M. Calcium entry blockers inhibit vasoconstrictor responses to sympathetic nerve stimulation mediated by alpha-1 adrenoceptors. *Naunyn Schmiedebergs Arch Pharmacol* 1985;330:22–32.

81. Van Breeman C. Blockade of membrane calcium fluxes by lanthanum in relation to vascular smooth muscle contractility. *Int Arch Physiol Biochem.* 1969;77:710–717.

82. Leijten P, Saida K, van Breemen C. Norepinephrine induced intracellular Ca^{2+} release from vascular smooth muscle. *J Cardiovasc Pharmacol* 1985;7(suppl 6):S38–S42.

83. Van Zwieten PA, van Meel JCA, Timmermans PBMWM. Functional interaction between calcium antagonists and the vasoconstriction induced by the stimulation of postsynaptic alpha-2 adrenoceptors. *Circ Res* 1983;52:177–180.

84. Jie K, Van Brummelen P, Vermey P, Timmermans PBMWM, van Zwieten PA. Influence of calcium entry blockade on alpha-1 and alpha-2 adrenoceptor-mediated vasoconstriction in the forearm of hypertensive patients. *Eur J Clin Pharmacol* 1987;32:115–120.

85. Hulthen UL, Bolli P, Amann FW, Kiowski W, Buhler FR. Enhanced vasodilation in essential hypertension by calcium channel blockade with verapamil. *Hypertension* 1982;4(suppl II):26–31.

86. Erne P, Bolli P, Buergisser E, Buhler FR. Correlation of platelet calcium with blood pressure. Effect of antihypertensive therapy. *N Engl J Med* 1984;310:1084–1088.

87. Robinson BF. Altered calcium handling as a cause of primary hypertension. *J Hypertension* 1984;2:453–460.

88. Niederman R, Pollard TD. Human platelet myosin. II. In vitro assembly and structure of myosin filaments. *J Cell Biol* 1975;67:72–92.

89. Bolli P, Erne P, Hulthen VL, Ritz R, Kiowski W, Ji BH, Buhler FR. Parallel reduction of calcium-influx-dependent vasoconstric-

tion and platelet-free calcium concentration with calcium entry and beta-adrenoceptor blockade. *J Cardiovasc Pharmacol* 1984;6(suppl 7):996–1001.

90. Bolli P, Kiowski W, Amann FW, Buhler FR. Adrenaline and enhanced vasoconstriction in patients with essential hypertension. *Pharmacol Toxicol* 1988;suppl 1:41–44.

91. Bolli P, Kiowski W, Erne P, Amann FW, Hulthen VL, Muller FB, Buhler FR. The role of catecholamines and calcium in the regulation of blood flow in normotensive subjects and in patients with essential hypertension. *J Cardiovasc Pharmacol* 1987;10(suppl 5): 34–44.

92. Kiowski W, Hulthen L, Bolli P, Ritz R, Buhler FR. Failure of prejunctional alpha-2 adrenoceptor stimulation to reduce norepinephrine release in normal man. *Gen Pharmacol* 1983;14:173.

93. Buhler FR, Bolli P, Erne P, Kiowski W, Muller FB, Hulthen UL, Ji BH. Adrenoceptors, calcium, and vasoconstriction in normal and hypertensive humans. *J Cardiovasc Pharmacol* 1985;7(suppl 6):130–136.

Hypertension: Pathophysiology, Diagnosis, and Management, Second Edition, edited by J.H. Laragh and B.M. Brenner, Raven Press, Ltd., New York © 1995.

CHAPTER **56**

Disorders of Autonomic Cardiovascular Regulation: Baroreflex Failure, Autonomic Failure, and Orthostatic Intolerance Syndromes

David Robertson

Abnormalities in the function of the autonomic nervous system can give rise to an astonishing array of cardiovascular abnormalities. Some of these disorders have pathognomonic features, but many more may subtly mimic other diseases and present major diagnostic challenges. It is important to recognize that autonomic disorders can present as hypertensive emergencies, chronic hypertension, bradycardia, tachycardia, arrhythmias, orthostatic intolerance, chronic hypotension, headache, syncope, and anemia (Table 1). For this reason, they must enter into the differential diagnoses of a large portion of the diseases encountered by the hypertension specialist. A young physician may be tempted to smile indulgently at the extensive listing of presentations in Table 1, but in 20 years of practice he will see himself miss an underlying autonomic diagnosis behind most, if not all, of these presentations.

The disorders of autonomic cardiovascular regulation may be classified as shown in Table 2. In this chapter, only some of the most dramatic and commonly encountered diseases are discussed. More extensive reviews of the diagnosis and treatment of autonomic disorders have recently appeared, and the interested reader is referred to them (1–5).

BAROREFLEX FAILURE

The syndrome of baroreflex failure in human subjects has remained poorly defined in spite of many decades of animal and clinical studies of baroreceptor and autonomic function (6–9). The principal reason for this is that studies have been confined to characterization of single cases (10–14). The recent development of centers for referral of patients with autonomic disorders is allowing investigative groups to develop experience in the recognition of the clinical spectrum of such problems.

In health, the arterial baroreflexes buffer changes in blood pressure so that excessive excursions of pressure above or below the normal range are avoided (15–17). Baroreceptors in the carotid sinus send information about stretch of the vessel wall through the glossopharyngeal (ninth cranial) nerve to the brainstem (18). Similar baroreceptors in the aortic arch and other great vessels of the thorax transmit analogous information through the vagus (tenth cranial) nerve to the same

D. Robertson: Clinical Research Center, Departments of Medicine, Pharmacology, and Neurology, Vanderbilt University, Nashville, Tennessee 37232-2195.

TABLE 1. *Cardiovascular manifestations of autonomic disorders*

	AF	BF	OI	PAS
Malignant hypertension	+	+	−	−
Accelerated hypertension	+	++	−	−
Chronic hypertension	−	++	−	−
Supine hypertension	++	+	−	−
Labile hypertension	−	+++	−	−
Orthostatic hypotension	+++	+/−	+	−
Supine hypotension	+/−	+/−	+/−	+/−
Episodic hypotension	+	+++	++	+++
Postprandial hypotension	+++	−	−	−
Bradycardia	+	+/−	−	−
Episodic bradycardia	−	+/−	+/−	+++
Tachycardia	−	+/−	++	−
Episodic tachycardia	−	+++	++	−
Orthostatic tachycardia	−	+	+++	−
Supraventricular tachyarrhythmia	+/−	+/−	+	−
Ventricular tachyarrhythmia	−	+/−	+	−
Syncope	+++	+	++	+++
Angina pectoris	+	+	−	−

AF, autonomic failure; BF, baroreflex failure; OI, orthostatic intolerance; PAS, paroxysmal autonomic syncopes.

brainstem nuclei (19). In addition, information concerning blood volume in the thorax is sensed by low-pressure receptors and much of this cardiopulmonary receptor input also traverses the vagus nerve on the way to the medulla (7). The brain structures receiving virtually all this input are the commissural, dorsolateral, and medial portions of nucleus of the solitary tract (20,21).

Thus, abnormalities in the relevant vascular baroreceptors, in the glossopharyngeal and/or vagal nerves, or in the brainstem could all lead to baroreflex failure. Among approximately 500 patients referred to Vanderbilt University's Autonomic Dysfunction Center for severe autonomic problems, we identified 11 patients with arterial baroreflex failure (Table 3). The evidence for baroreflex failure was the documentation of an inability of pressor and depressor drug infusions to cause reflex bradycardia and tachycardia, respectively, in an individual in whom wide and parallel excursions of heart rate and blood pressure occurred in response to endogenous factors such as sedation and stress (Table 4). This was confirmed in most cases by historical, physical, and physiological information.

The patients were aged 24 to 62 years. Five were men and six were women. Reasons for referral included evaluation for essential hypertension, suspicion of pheochromocytoma, inability to successfully achieve control of hypertension, and recognition that the integrity of glossopharyngeal or vagal nerves had been compromised. The clinical characteristics of the patients are shown in Tables 3, 4, and 5.

There were several etiologies for the baroreflex abnormalities in the study subjects (Table 3). One patient had surgical section of a glossopharyngeal nerve for intracta-

ble glossopharyngeal neuralgia in the setting of an old contralateral neck injury that apparently involved damage to the glossopharyngeal and vagal nerves on that side. Three patients had undergone surgery and irradiation for throat carcinoma without immediate complication, but in the months following radiotherapy, symptoms of volatile temperament and especially raised blood pressure developed. Four patients had the familial paraganglioma syndrome, a genetic disorder in which affected individuals develop multiple benign non–catecholamine-producing tumors of the carotid body, glomus jugulare, and glomus vagale (22). These tumors are deleterious by virtue of their physical damage to the glossopharyngeal and nearby nerves. One patient had marked cell loss in both nuclei of the solitary tract, due to a degenerative neurological disorder involving medullary and higher central nervous system structures; the etiology in this patient is known from autopsy results following death from pneumonia approximately 1 year after his evaluation on our

TABLE 2. *Differential diagnosis of orthostatic hypotension*

Autonomic disorders
  Bradbury-Eggleston syndrome (primary autonomic failure)
  Shy-Drager syndrome (multiple system atrophy)
  Riley-Day syndrome (familial dysautonomia)
  Dopamine-β-hydroxylase deficiency
  Baroreflex failure
  Acute pandysautonomia
  Secondary autonomic neuropathies
Hypovolemic disorders
  Hemorrhage or plasma loss
  Overdiuresis
  Overdialysis
  Idiopathic hypovolemia
Endocrinologic disorders
  Addison's disease
  Hypoaldosteronism
  Pheochromocytoma
  Renovascular hypertension
Vascular insufficiency
  Varicose veins
  Absent venous valves
  Arteriovenous malformations
Vasodilator excess
  Mastocytosis (histamine, prostaglandin D_2)
  Hyperbradykininism (bradykinin)
  Carcinoid (bradykinin)
  Hypermagnesemia
Paroxysmal autonomic syncopes
  Glossopharyngeal syncope
  Micturition syncope
  Carotid sinus syndrome
  Swallow syncope
  Cough syncope
  Bezold-Jarisch reflex activation
Miscellaneous
  Drugs and toxins
  Stokes-Adams attacks
  Mitral valve prolapse syndrome
  Gastrectomy
  Hypokinesia, weightlessness, bed rest

TABLE 3. *Baroreflex failure: patient characteristics*

Patient	Age/sex	Presentating diagnosis	Observation	Etiology
1	47/F	Blood pressure lability	8 yr	Glossopharyngeal section
2	58/M	Hypertension	5 yr	Neck irradiation
3	51/F	Possible pheochromocytoma	6 yr	Neck irradiation
4	62/M	Hypertension	6 yr	Neck irradiation
5	56/M	Episodic hypertension	4 yr	Bilateral carotid tumor
6	28/F	Tachycardia + hypertension	3 yr	Bilateral carotid tumor
7	24/F	Blood pressure lability	3 yr	Bilateral carotid tumor
8	43/M	Hypertensive crisis	1 yr	Bilateral carotid tumor
9	33/M	Severe hypertension	0.5 yr	Bilateral NTS destruction
10	60/F	Emotional lability	8 yr	Unknown
11	59/F	Volatile hypertension	5 yr	Unknown

NTS, nucleus of the solitary tract.

unit (23). Finally, in two patients, no obvious explanation for the baroreflex failure could be identified and they are thus classified as idiopathic.

After diagnosis, each patient was monitored for excursions of blood pressure, heart rate, and plasma catecholamine levels (24). Twelve normal subjects were also monitored at the General Clinical Research Center. In the course of this evaluation, supine and upright blood pressure was measured at 4-hour intervals and during symptomatic episodes. The baroreflex failure patients were further contrasted in terms of some variables with a group of essential hypertensives and another group with severe autonomic failure due to the Bradbury-Eggleston syndrome. Plasma catecholamines were measured during supine and upright postures, and, in the patients, during symptomatic attacks. A battery of physiological and pharmacological tests was also carried out (25).

Clonidine at an oral dosage of 0.1 mg was administered to determine to what degree α_2-adrenoceptor stimulation could reduce sympathetic activity as reflected in plasma norepinephrine and sphygmomanometric blood pressure (14). In seven patients the relative efficacy of phenoxybenzamine (10–80 mg/d), clonidine (0.3–2.4 mg/d), and placebo were assessed. In the other four patients, systematic trials of phenoxybenzamine and clonidine were not carried out.

The defining feature of baroreflex failure was an ability to modify heart rate by stress (increase in heart rate) or sedation (decrease in heart rate), with no tachycardic response to an exogenous vasodilator and no bradycardic response to the pressor effect of phenylephrine (26). In terms of these variables there was no overlap between the baroreflex failure patients and our normal subjects (Table 6). There was even less overlap between the baroreflex failure patients and patients with severe autonomic failure due to the Bradbury-Eggleston syndrome (Table 5).

All patients had hypertension, either constantly or episodically. The three patients demonstrating sustained hypertension were all individuals who had had acute re-

TABLE 4. *Baroreflex failure: cardiovascular characteristics*

Patient	Blood pressure		Heart rate		Norepinephrine		Phe ΔHR	Nitro ΔHR
	Max	Min	Max	Min	Max	Min		
1 (47/F)	170/139	78/69	120	76	2400	170	−1	+1
2 (58/M)	230/168	80/50	109	65	1309	242	0	0[a]
3 (51/F)	171/128	77/60	121	69	2110	152	0	+1
4 (62/M)	164/131	73/57	120	75	2440	117	0	0
5 (56/M)	248/128	95/70	147	74	1690	224	−1	0
6 (28/F)	201/144	58/47	158	91	2660	162	−2	0
7 (24/F)	176/134	70/50	130	94	2340	111	−1	+2
8 (43/M)	280/145	80/55	153	70	2030	155	0[a]	0
9 (33/M)	215/135	90/70	118	75	514	261	−2[a]	+4
10 (60/F)	230/130	96/75	123	61	1572	274	0	+1
11 (59/F)	171/138	72/61	148	59	1280	112	−2[a]	+4
12 (52/F)[b]	250/160	78/60	144	68	1510	168	—	—
13 (41/M)[c]	230/130	55/44	120	—	1160	360	0	0
Normals	136/80	104/62	96 ± 8	60 ± 8	524 ± 32	242 ± 22	−13 (−7 to −21)	+16 (+9 to +28)

Phe, phenylephrine; Nitro, nitroprusside.
[a] Estimated from Valsalva maneuver.
[b] From ref. 13, with permission.
[c] From ref. 10, with permission.
Reprinted from *N Engl Med*, with permission (ref. 9).

TABLE 5. *Baroreflex failure: clinical characteristics*

Patient	Labile HBP	Headache	Diaphoresis	Flushing	Emotional Volatility
1	+	−	+	+	+
2	+	+	+	+	++
3	+	−	+	+	+
4	+	−	+	+	+
5	+	+	+	+	+
6	+	+	+	+	++
7	+	+	+	+	++
8	+	+	+	+	++
9	+	−	+	+	−
10	+	+	+	+	+
11	+	+	+	+	+
12[a]	+	−	+	+	++
13[b]	+	+	+	+	−

[a] From ref. 13, with permission.
[b] From ref. 10, with permission.

section of their second carotid body tumor (chemodectoma). These patients had had their initial carotid tumor resection several years previously without experiencing any hypertension or symptoms suggestive of baroreflex failure. Yet with resection of the second tumor, and consequent loss of what appeared to be minimal residual glossopharyngeal and vagal nerve function, the full power of neurogenic hypertension was manifest. For 24 to 72 hours, severe (220–280 mm Hg systolic) and unremitting hypertension was present. During this initial period, episodes of normal or low blood pressure were not seen. Only in subsequent days did the severity of hypertension moderate and an episodic hypertensive pattern appear.

In individuals whose baroreflex failure developed more gradually (for example, those in whom it appeared

months to years after neck irradiation), no initial phase of sustained hypertension was observed, at least so far as could be determined by history and review of medical records. Nevertheless, episodic hypertension was prominent and did not completely resolve in any patient during the period of follow-up observations (6 months to 8 years). Most patients had no fall in blood pressure on standing (unless they were receiving phenoxybenzamine or were volume depleted) and, in at least four cases, systolic blood pressure rose 10 to 30 mm Hg with assumption of upright posture.

A typical episode of hypertension is shown in Fig. 1. This episode was preceded by 2 hours of essentially normal blood pressure and was precipitated by a cold pressor test. Blood pressure continued to climb for about 10 minutes after the test stimulus was removed, resulting

TABLE 6. *Comparison of blood pressure, heart rate, and catecholamine values in patients with baroreflex failure, autonomic failure, and essential hypertension*

	Normal (n = 12)	Baroreflex failure (n = 11)	Autonomic failure[a] (n = 12)	Essential hypertension (n = 8)
Mean arterial pressure (mm Hg)	85 ± 10	141 ± 32*	69 ± 10*†	128 ± 16*
Plasma norepinephrine (pg/ml)	524 ± 32	1840 ± 320*†	28 ± 3*†	570 ± 41
Plasma epinephrine (pg/ml)	32 ± 5	110 ± 21*†	10 ± 3*†	38 ± 6
Plasma dopamine (pg/ml)	28 ± 6	64 ± 12*	11 ± 4†	32 ± 7
Urinary norepinephrine (μg/day)	32 ± 5	79 ± 9*†	4 ± 2*†	39 ± 7
Urinary epinephrine (μg/day)	9 ± 3	39 ± 9*†	4 ± 2*†	10 ± 7
Urinary dopamine (μg/day)	239 ± 29	299 ± 33	154 ± 13*†	277 ± 29
Cold pressor test (Δ in systolic, mm Hg)	+24 ± 7	+56 ± 14*	−2 ± 6*†	+33 ± 8
Clonidine Δ BP (systolic mm Hg)	−12 ± 5	−54 ± 14*†	+12 ± 4*†	−26 ± 7
Clonidine Δ plasma norepinephrine	−70 ± 28	−242 ± 48†	−2 ± 6*†	−106 ± 24
Phenylephrine Δ HR (mean ± SEM)	−13 ± 4	−1 ± 1*†	−1 ± 1*†	−9 ± 4

[a] Patients with autonomic failure caused by the Bradbury-Eggleston syndrome (2).

*$p < .05$ (vs normal subjects); † $p < .05$ (vs patients with essential hypertension); autonomic failure patients differed significantly from baroreflex failure patients in all variables reported except phenylephrine-induced bradycardia.

Mean arterial pressure, estimated as 2× diastolic pressure plus systolic pressure, divided by 3.

Reprinted from *N Engl J Med,* with permission (ref. 9).

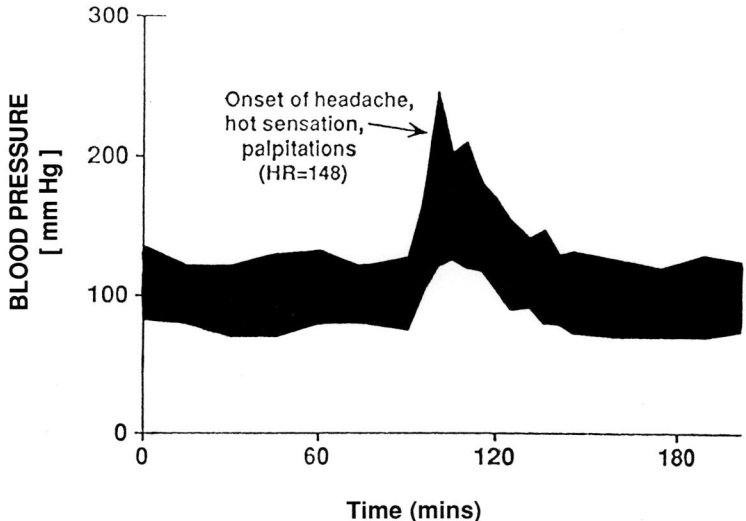

FIG. 1. Blood pressure monitoring over a 200-minute period in a 43-year-old man approximately 2 weeks following surgical removal of a second carotid body tumor, 5 years after removal of the initial (contralateral) carotid body tumor. While blood pressure was being monitored at normal baseline levels, a cold pressor test with immersion of the hand in ice water for 60 seconds was performed. The blood pressure immediately rose and continued to rise for several minutes following discontinuation of the cold stimulus. The symptoms appeared during this time and resolved as blood pressure and heart rate returned to normal over the succeeding half-hour. On some occasions, paroxysms of similar magnitude occurred without obvious exogenous causative stimuli. Reprinted from *N Engl J Med*, with permission (ref. 9).

in a doubling of baseline supine pressure, but ultimately returned to baseline. Similar episodes could be precipitated by even minor mental arousal, such as mental arithmetic calculations.

It is noteworthy that nine patients specifically complained of increased nervousness or emotional lability since the onset of their illness, and ten patients gave such a history in response to specific questioning about it. This symptom was particularly prominent in the subjects who had the greatest blood pressure elevations, and nervousness was worse during blood pressure elevations than in intervening periods. During blood pressure elevations, patients also experienced a sensation of warmth or flushing, palpitations, and, in the severest episodes, also headache and diaphoresis. The full clinical presentation of these symptoms closely resembled those observed in patients with pheochromocytoma (27). The di-

agnosis of pheochromocytoma was seriously considered at some point in virtually all these patients, but was ruled out in some cases by computed tomography (CT) scanning, meta-iodo-benzylguanidine (MIBG) scanning, venous norepinephrine sampling, or arteriography, and in all patients by follow-up demonstrating stability or improvement in hypertensive episodes over time.

Mean extremes of blood pressure during inpatient monitoring are shown in Fig. 2. It is noteworthy that peak blood pressures were much higher in the patients than in normal subjects, while at the same time, some patients had minimal blood pressures (usually at night) that were lower than those observed in the normal subjects.

Heart rate generally paralleled blood pressure, with the same wide excursions (Table 2 and Fig. 3). It is noteworthy, however, that two patients had minimal heart rates

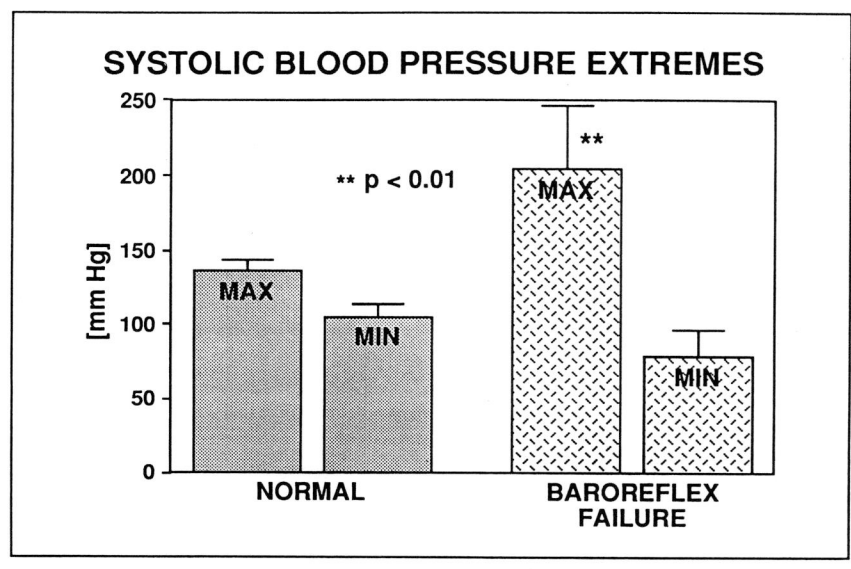

FIG. 2. Extremes of blood pressure recorded during monitoring in a metabolic ward. Patients and normal subjects were at rest and ambulatory, but no vigorous exercise was permitted. MAX, maximum; MIN, minimum. *Asterisks* indicate significant differences from normal subjects.

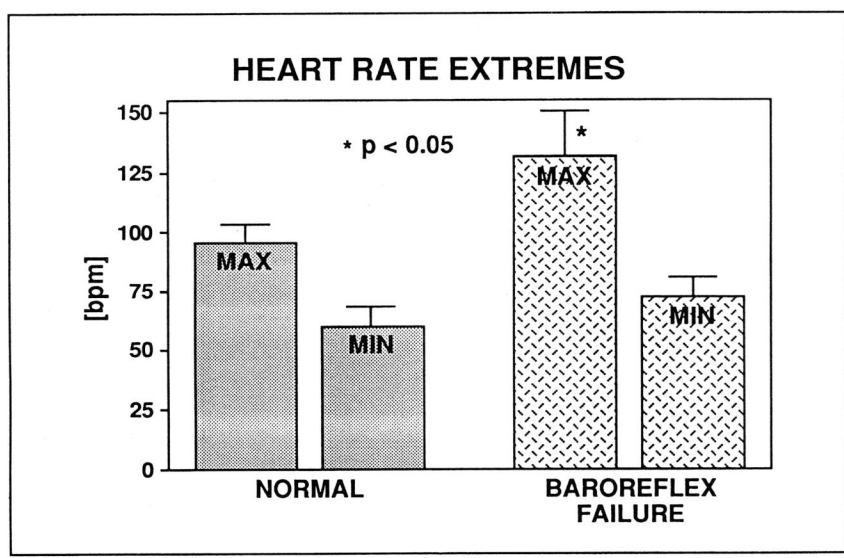

FIG. 3. Extremes of heart rate recorded during monitoring on a metabolic ward. Conditions were as described in Fig. 2. MAX, maximum; MIN, minimum.

above 90 beats per minute (bpm). This could have reflected partial loss of efferent parasympathetic control of heart rate due to damage to the right vagus nerve.

Dramatic excursions of plasma norepinephrine levels paralleled the blood pressure changes and, to a slightly lesser extent, the heart rate changes (Table 4 and Fig. 4). The peak norepinephrine levels in these patients were significantly higher than those of normal subjects. Many normal subjects would not be able to achieve such high plasma norepinephrine levels, even with treadmill exercise, a potent sympathetic nervous system stimulus (24).

Plasma epinephrine levels were also elevated during most attacks, in three patients to greater than 200 pg/ml. Urinary catecholamines averaged 118 μg per 24 hours, more than twice normal. With fractionation of urine,

both norepinephrine and epinephrine components were above average.

The cold pressor test elicited a much greater response in the baroreflex failure patients than in the normal subjects (Fig. 5). In some cases, the cold pressor test set in motion a hypertensive paroxysm that continued for many minutes after the removal of the stimulus.

The effect of clonidine (0.1 mg po) was equally dramatic (Fig. 6). The depressor response was twice that seen in normal subjects. Considerable variation in the response to clonidine was seen, depending on the initial blood pressure level. During periods of hypertension, the clonidine-induced fall in blood pressure was much greater than during quiescent periods.

Clonidine consistently reduced plasma norepineph-

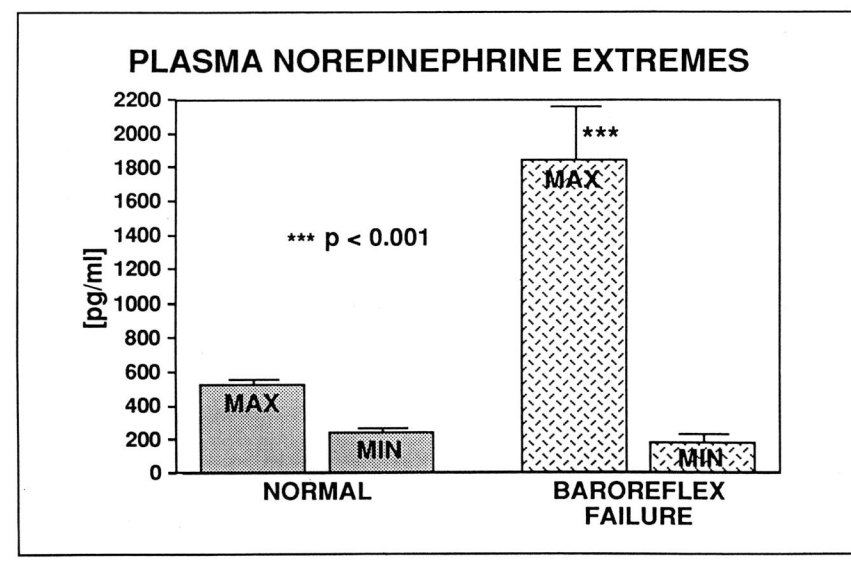

FIG. 4. Extremes of plasma norepinephrine recorded during monitoring on a metabolic ward. Conditions were as described in Fig. 2. MAX, maximum; MIN, minimum.

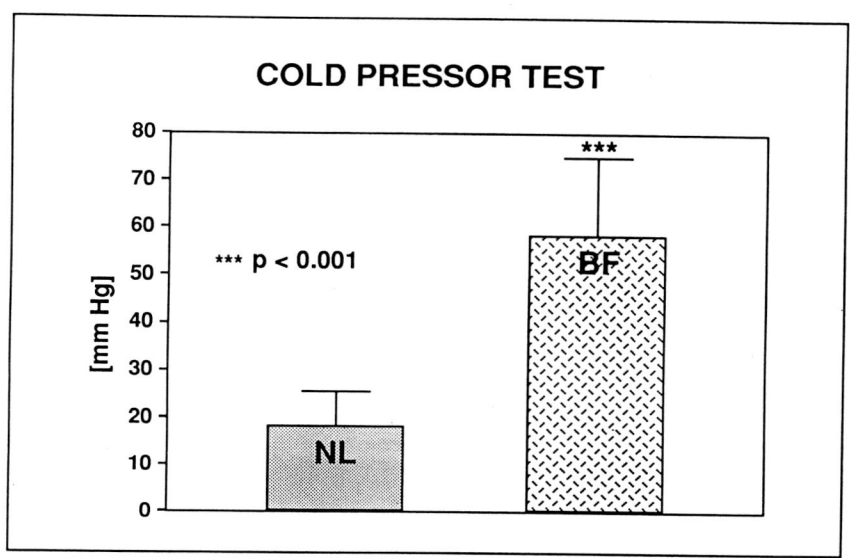

FIG. 5. Rise of the systolic blood pressure in response to the cold pressor test in baroreflex failure (BF) patients and normal subjects (NL).

rine levels in each of the ten subjects in whom the latter was monitored. The mean plasma norepinephrine level before clonidine was 422 ± 141 pg/mL and 2 hours after clonidine had fallen to 180 ± 47 pg/mL.

Responses to other pharmacological interventions were largely predictable. The heart rate response to propranolol (10 mg iv) was dependent on the prevailing level of sympathetic activation; there was little response during periods when blood pressure and heart rate were low, but during episodes of tachycardia, significant heart rate reduction was seen. The mean fall in rate after propranolol was 12 bpm in the baroreflex failure patients with a range of 8 to 38 bpm. Atropine (0.04 mg/kg) did not greatly increase heart rate except when patients had normal or low blood pressures and heart rate immediately prior to its administration. The mean rise in heart rate in

response to atropine was 10 bpm, with a range of 7 to 15 bpm. Tyramine (at doses of 1000 to 3000 μg iv) in three patients had little pressor or tachycardic effect, perhaps because of the high circulating levels of norepinephrine. However, at boluses of 4500 to 6000 μg, heart rate increases of 15, 22, and 30 bpm were observed.

The severity of the hypertension in some subjects required constant antihypertensive therapy, so that systematic assessment of the efficacy of drugs versus placebo could not be determined. In seven patients, however, it was possible to make systematic comparisons of the efficacy of clonidine, phenoxybenzamine, and placebo. The results of these trials are shown in Table 7. Clonidine, albeit over a very wide dosage range, was effective in reducing both the frequency and severity of attacks, whereas phenoxybenzamine attenuated pressor severity

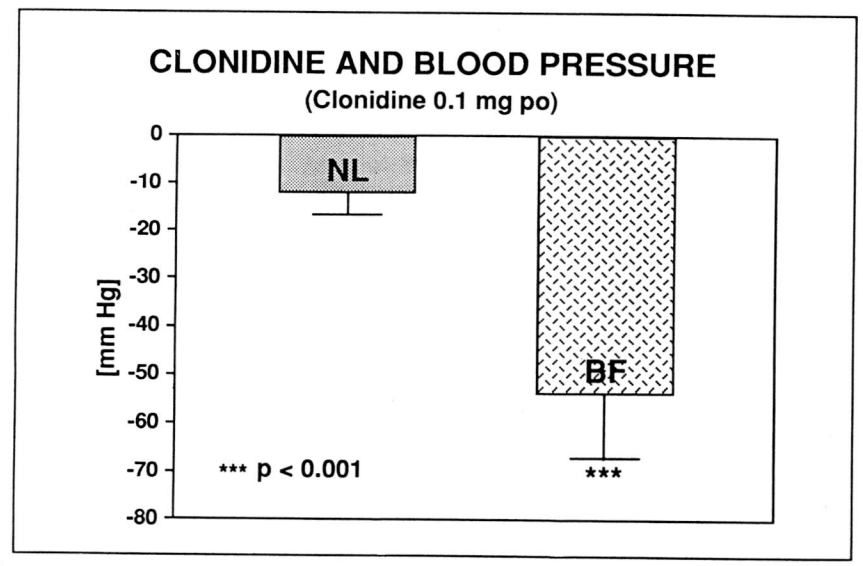

FIG. 6. Fall of the systolic blood pressure in response to clonidine 0.1 mg orally in baroreflex failure (BF) patients and normal subjects (NL). (From ref. 9, with permission.)

TABLE 7. Baroreflex failure: therapy

	Attacks (number/day)	Systolic BP rise (mm Hg)	HR rise (mm Hg)
No therapy	4.7 ± 1.1	92 ± 23	58 ± 9
Phenoxybenzamine (10–80 mg/d)	4.4 ± 1.2	37 ± 21*	62 ± 14
Clonidine (0.3–2.4 mg/d)	0.9 ± 0.3**	32 ± 16*	33 ± 6**

* $p < .05$; ** $p < .01$. Reprinted from N Engl J Med, with permission (ref. 9).

without limiting the unwanted tachycardia or reducing the frequency of attacks. Three patients had orthostatic hypotension while receiving phenoxybenzamine, whereas this side effect occurred in only one patient receiving clonidine. It is noteworthy that supine blood pressure was lower between attacks as well as during attacks in patients receiving either drug. Eight patients were ultimately able to be placed on clonidine patches prior to discharge from the hospital. One patient was treated with methyldopa, but an unusually large dose (3,750 mg po daily) was required for blood pressure control.

Over time, many patients were able to be tapered to lower doses of clonidine, and after a period of 2 to 4 years, two patients discontinued clonidine and found that attacks and symptoms could be controlled most of the time with diazepam 5 mg t.i.d. Breakthrough episodes of hypertension still occur intermittently in these patients during stress.

The powerful role of baroreflexes in blood pressure control in human subjects was shown by Kezdi and co-workers (28,29), who transiently blocked carotid baroreflex function by infiltrating the carotid sinus region with procaine. In normal subjects, as well as patients with essential hypertension, there was only a modest (≈ 10–20 mm Hg) pressor effect when the first side was blocked. However, as soon as the local anesthetic had been infiltrated into the second side, a powerful increase in blood pressure (≈ 75 mm Hg) and heart rate (≈ 50 bpm) occurred. Over the next hour this effect gradually went away as the procaine was absorbed and metabolized. In the course of this investigation, several patients developed systolic blood pressures greater than 300 mm Hg. Thus, the studies of Kezdi and co-workers provided early evidence that when patients with baroreflex nerve lesions were ultimately identified, they would manifest severe hypertension.

Guz and co-workers (30) made similar observations in two normal subjects and one patient. In 1985, Fagius and colleagues (31) injected local anesthetic at the base of the skull in two volunteers, thereby interrupting afferent baroreceptor activity and afferent and efferent vagal activity. An altered pattern of muscle sympathetic nerve traffic and an enhanced sympathetic nerve traffic were

observed. In another study Holton and Wood (32) found that following carotid body removal and consequent sinus denervation, hypoxia due to breathing 10% oxygen caused immediate and marked hypertension and tachycardia. Blood pressure lability continued during the follow-up period (43 and 61 weeks), indicating the chronicity of the hemodynamic abnormality.

Our results indicate that defective baroreceptor function, which may occur in a variety of clinical circumstances, causes severe volatile hypertension (Table 8). The correlation of elevations in plasma norepinephrine with pressor episodes suggests that these episodes are caused by sympathetic nervous system activation that is unrestrained by normal inhibitory influences. The possibility that vasopressin or other humoral pressor agents might also be released was not addressed in our study. A spectrum of clinical symptoms may accompany the hypertension, including headache, palpitations, a hot sensation (pale "flushing"), diaphoresis, and emotional lability (Table 5). At the other extreme, the hypertension may be only moderate and ancillary symptoms minimal or absent. Our patients closely resembled the case reported by Kuchel et al. (13) and that reported by Aksamit et al. (10), whose characteristics are reported as patients 12 and 13 in Table 4 and 5.

There are several potential reasons for the heterogeneity in the clinical expression of baroreflex failure. First, the severest symptoms occur when the baroreflex interruption is sudden, for example, after surgery or injury. Indeed, in the first 24 to 72 hours after such nerve injury, the hypertension can be constant and may require the continuous infusion of nitroprusside or phentolamine. One of our patients (#8) experienced several apneic spells during the first 24 hours. Subsequently, the lability of the blood pressure may be more prominent, and after weeks the episodes of hypertension may become less frequent and the symptoms associated with them less dramatic.

An additional explanation for the heterogeneity of presentation may be the degree of baroreflex impairment in the individual patient. We did not encounter hyper-

TABLE 8. Clinical features of baroreflex failure

Acute baroreflex failure (days)
  Severe continuous hypertension
  Incapacitating headache
  Flushing
  Tachycardia
  Marked anxiety
  Emotional volatility
  Very elevated plasma and urinary catecholamines
Chronic baroreflex failure
  Blood pressure volatility with hypertension and hypotension
  Concomitant blood pressure and heart rate excursions
  Headache and flushing during hypertensive spells
  Elevated catecholamines during hypertensive episodes
  Emotional volatility

tension in any patient in this series after unilateral damage only, although in the two patients with idiopathic baroreflex failure, the bilaterality was able to be inferred only by functional measures. Even with bilateral nerve damage, there may be differing degrees of involvement of glossopharyngeal and vagal nerves, which are in close approximation throughout much of their passage through the neck. In one previously reported case of baroreflex failure, there was evidence for bilateral functional impairment of the aortic baroreflex fibers carried in the vagus nerves, while cardiopulmonary reflex fibers, presumably traveling in the same nerve bundles, appeared to be spared (10).

It is noteworthy that lesser degrees of baroreflex dysfunction have been detected with hemodynamic monitoring during or soon after carotid endarterectomy or carotid body surgery (33–35). The true incidence of long-term elevations of blood pressure or chronic lability of blood pressure after such operative procedures is not known, but it seems unlikely that large increases in blood pressure occur commonly.

On the other hand, the observation that 3 of the 11 patients in our study had had prior neck irradiation may indicate that undergoing this therapeutic procedure should be carefully followed for development of abnormal blood pressure control. We (14) and Aksamit et al. (10) have reported previous baroreflex failure patients who had had irradiation. To our knowledge, no systematic assessment of blood pressure volability or hypertension in this patient population has ever been undertaken.

The two patients in this report that we have classified as idiopathic warrant special consideration. It is possible that the etiology of their dysfunction may lie in the medulla (36), although no abnormality was detected in this structure by CT scanning or magnetic resonance imaging in one of these subjects (these tests were not carried out in the second patient), but a medullary abnormality could easily be missed by such testing. It is possible that these patients could have a disorder similar to those previously described by Page (37), Kuchel and co-workers (13), and other investigators (38–41). Vascular compression of medullary structure has also been proposed as an etiology of some cases of hypertension (42).

It is interesting to speculate about how, in the face of major damage to arterial baroreflex nerves, severe orthostatic hypotension is avoided. Many textbooks suggest that these reflexes are the principal means by which blood pressure in the upright posture is maintained. The simplest explanation is that some cardiopulmonary reflex information is still being integrated, but our studies do not ascertain this. Alternatively, we have to assume that some compensatory mechanism comes into play during assumption of upright posture. In this regard, one could imagine that cardiovascular control nuclei in the medulla might receive input concerning posture from a number of nonbaroreflex sensory sources. For example,

visual cues from the occipital cortex or other sites in the visual pathways leading from the retina might provide positional information; the cerebellum might provide input about position and so might the neurovestibular system. These inputs collectively might compensate for the absence of baroreflexes in our subjects. Their role might be more prominent in severe baroreflex failure than in milder baroreflex failure, and patients with the latter might, in fact, be more susceptible to orthostatic intolerance.

The clinical presentation of baroreflex failure bears an immediate and striking resemblance to the presentation of pheochromocytoma (27), and, therefore, differentiation from this disorder is very important. In the 1980s, Bravo et al. (43) proposed that hypertensive patients with high norepinephrine levels could be differentiated from pheochromocytoma by the ability of clonidine to suppress plasma norepinephrine levels in the former but not the latter. Bravo et al. used 0.3 mg clonidine rather than 0.1 mg for this purpose and measured the norepinephrine at 3 hours rather than 2 hours as we did here. Nevertheless, our patients demonstrated a similar level of norepinephrine suppression (57 percent) even with the smaller dose of clonidine. Therefore, a fortiori, clonidine testing should be an effective diagnostic test in baroreflex failure. This also raises the possibility that some individuals with high norepinephrine levels of uncertain etiology now being followed with pheochromocytoma ruled out might have baroreflex failure as the cause of their volatile hypertension (43).

In conclusion, baroreflex failure in human subjects has a range of presentations, varying from acute onset of a hypertensive crisis, requiring intensive care unit admission and treatment with nitroprusside, to a chronic volatility of blood pressure and heart rate with hypertensive surges in response to stress, punctuated by periods of normal or even low blood pressure during rest (Table 8). Emotional volatility, of unknown cause, frequently accompanies this syndrome. Differentiating this syndrome from other causes of labile hypertension is essential in devising effective treatment. It is likely that baroreflex failure is significantly underdiagnosed.

PHEOCHROMOCYTOMA

Pheochromocytoma is treated exhaustively elsewhere in this volume. It is briefly dealt with here because of its resemblance to severe baroreflex failure. At our institution, pheochromocytoma and baroreflex failure seem to occur with prevalences of the same order of magnitude, but much further study will be required to develop more precise and reliable information about incidence.

Like baroreflex failure, pheochromocytoma can present with severe chronic or episodic hypertension, accompanied by headache, sweating, and palpitations. In occasional patients, pheochromocytoma can also present as orthostatic hypotension, which can be mild to severe. The latter can actually be confused clinically with autonomic failure of the Bradbury-Eggleston type, but urinary catecholamines definitively distinguish these two disorders.

BRADBURY-EGGLESTON SYNDROME

In 1925, Bradbury and Eggleston, in a landmark paper, described the clinical presentation of autonomic failure. Their first patient appeared to have a selective neuropathy involving both the sympathetic and parasympathetic nervous systems. Their study led to recognition of almost all the clinical features we currently associate with autonomic failure. This syndrome is often referred to as idiopathic orthostatic hypotension or pure autonomic failure.

This degenerative disorder of the autonomic nervous system presents in middle to late life. The adrenal medulla is relatively spared until quite late in the disease. The initial clinical abnormality in men is usually impotence, but more commonly it is orthostatic hypotension that brings the patient to the attention of his/her physician. Other features commonly present are reduced sweating (hypohidrosis), nasal stuffiness, bladder and bowel dysfunction, and mild anemia, the latter presumably due to reduced erythropoietin production because of inadequate β_2-adrenoceptor stimulation of release of this hormone (23). Rarely, patients may have such severe orthostatic hypotension that angina pectoris may occur, often in the absence of significant coronary atherosclerosis. In perhaps 3 percent of patients, hypotension may result in such severe underperfusion of the head that seizures may supervene.

The orthostatic hypotension in the Bradbury-Eggleston syndrome is often extraordinarily severe. It is greatest early in the day and after a large meal. In questionable cases where the diagnosis of orthostatic hypotension is being considered, it is especially important that supine and upright blood pressure be assessed in the hour following a large meal. In mildly affected individuals, orthostatic hypotension may be present only during this period. In other patients it may be present in the morning but not later in the day, after climbing a flight of stairs or walking up a hill, but not before. Pressure tends to be lower when individuals are at high altitude or when they hyperventilate. Intercurrent urinary tract infection or pneumonia, even if accompanied only by small temperature elevations, greatly reduce blood pressure. Increased environmental temperature also lowers blood pressure. Most patients learn to avoid the hot summer weather.

In the most severely affected patients, the upright blood pressure may be 60/30 mm Hg or lower. It is obvious that the sphygmomanometer is inadequate to estimate true intraarterial blood pressure in such cases. For this reason, in severely affected patients, it is useful to monitor disease severity with the *standing time,* which is defined as the length of time a patient can stand motionless before the onset of symptoms of orthostatic hypotension. In patients with the Bradbury-Eggleston syndrome, standing motionless is considerably more stressful on the cardiovascular system than walking, since in the latter situation the pumping action of calf muscles helps venous return during this activity. The most common symptoms of orthostatic hypotension in these patients are dizziness or lightheadedness, dimming or tunneling of vision, and pain or discomfort in the back of the neck or head. In a small number of patients, slurred speech may be the presenting symptom. As soon as the patient's herald symptom of orthostatic hypotension appears, he or she is allowed to sit down and the number of elapsed seconds is recorded. If the patient is able to stand for 3 minutes without the onset of symptoms, it is assumed that a reliable blood pressure determination can be made and a sphygmomanometric blood pressure measurement at that point is obtained.

The standing time is primarily of value in monitoring individuals who are unable to stand motionless for as long as 3 minutes. The importance of the standing time is that many individuals who have an increase in standing time from 30 to 120 seconds may have a substantial increase in functional capacity, even though they may have no change in their level of upright blood pressure as assessed by the sphygmomanometer. A patient with a standing time under 30 seconds usually cannot live alone, while a patient with a standing time greater than 60 seconds generally can. Thus, the standing time determination greatly facilitates the management of the most severely affected patients with the Bradbury-Eggleston syndrome.

The orthostatic hypotension in the Bradbury-Eggleston syndrome is frequently accompanied by supine hypertension, even when the patient is not taking pressor medications. However, even when the supine hypertension is quite severe, cardiac function is well maintained, and contractility may even be raised in some circumstances. Nocturia is an invariable accompaniment of the Bradbury-Eggleston syndrome in its severe form and may cause the patient to get up as many as eight times per night to pass substantial volumes of urine. Conversely, there may be little urine production during the day time, while the patient is seated or walking around. The cause of the nocturia is not known with certainty, but increased levels of atrial natriuretic factor and improved perfusion of the kidneys during the nocturnal sleeping period have been most frequently suggested. Clearly, head-up tilt, which reduces the nocturnal blood pressure, can lessen the volume of urine excreted during the night. The extent to which delayed gastric emptying and reduced gastrointestinal motility might contribute to nocturnal diuresis has never been fully evaluated.

It is noteworthy that patients with the Bradbury-Eggleston syndrome do not usually have fevers as high as healthy subjects; nevertheless, any fever will significantly reduce blood pressure and consequently decrease the functional capacity of the patient. A sudden decline in functional mobility in a patient with Bradbury-Eggleston syndrome is strongly suggestive of intercurrent infection, usually of the urinary tract. The basal metabolic rate is typically reduced in these patients. There is marked hypersensitivity to all pressor and depressor stimuli, especially sympathomimetic amines and vasopressin.

Because the diagnosis of the Bradbury-Eggleston syndrome is one of exclusion, it is quite difficult to make. While it is relatively easy with plasma and urinary catecholamine determinations, sweat testing, and nerve conduction studies to assess the generality and specificity of the autonomic deficits, a greater difficulty is differentiating the Bradbury-Eggleston syndrome from the Shy-Drager syndrome (see below). In some cases, the autonomic abnormalities may appear before the other neurological deficits, so characteristic of the Shy-Drager syndrome, appear. Mild extrapyramidal symptoms have developed in one of our patients who had carried the diagnosis of Bradbury-Eggleston syndrome for over 5 years. Whether this heralds full-blown Shy-Drager syndrome or the fortuitous association of his original diagnosis with Parkinson's disease remains unknown. Because of patients such as this, it is unwise to make the diagnosis of Bradbury-Eggleston syndrome unless one has followed the patient for several years without seeing the development of cerebellar, extrapyramidal, or other evidence of central nervous system degeneration.

The pathology of the Bradbury-Eggleston syndrome has not been elucidated, but there is known to be a loss of postganglionic sympathetic and parasympathetic neurons. Extremely low levels of plasma norepinephrine (sometimes less than 10 percent of normal) may be seen.

Patients with the Bradbury-Eggleston syndrome have a generally good prognosis; many live for 20 years or longer after the onset of their disease. Since the disease has its onset relatively late in life, it is not uncommon for patients with the Bradbury-Eggleston syndrome to live into their 80s or 90s. The most common cause of death in these patients is pulmonary embolus.

SECONDARY DYSAUTONOMIAS

A large number of pathological processes capable of producing peripheral neuropathy can also potentially produce autonomic neuropathy (44,45). Many such disorders have been identified and studied. Usually the au-

tonomic impairment is mild to moderate and it seldom dominates the presentation of the primary illness.

Perhaps the most common cause of secondary autonomic dysfunction is diabetes mellitus (46–53). Although sensory fibers are usually affected first, subtle autonomic abnormalities may be discovered quite early in some diabetics. Orthostatic hypotension usually is a relatively late development. In some long-term diabetics, the autonomic involvement can be widespread and quite severe. All signs and symptoms of autonomic failure may be present, but gastrointestinal ones, especially diarrhea and gastroparesis, appear to be relatively more common in diabetic autonomic dysfunction than other forms of autonomic dysfunction. Autonomic neuropathy develops more slowly in diabetics whose glucose is well controlled. Gastroparesis in diabetic patients may improve with erythromycin (54).

A practical difficulty in patients with diabetic autonomic neuropathy and orthostatic hypotension is the powerful vasodepressor effect of insulin itself in these subjects (55–58). It is noteworthy that food is also vasodepressor, and the combined effects of insulin and food may make blood pressure almost impossible to keep under control. Unfortunately, neither of these effects is widely recognized by practicing physicians.

Pathological study reveals that affected diabetic patients have segmental loss of myelin, axon degeneration, and vacuolization and degeneration in the intermediolateral column of the spinal cord and the sympathetic ganglia. There is also a loss of myelinated fibers. Mononuclear cells and mast cells are sometimes in the vicinity of local neural involvement. There is hope that pancreatic transplants will have a beneficial impact on the course of autonomic neuropathy in diabetes (59,60).

Other disorders may present with secondary autonomic neuropathy, including tabes dorsalis, porphyria, pernicious anemia, the Wernicke-Korsakoff syndrome, and amyloidosis (61). Amyloidosis as a cause of autonomic failure is by no means rare, and any patient in whom no primary or secondary diagnosis has been made should be evaluated for amyloidosis.

Malignancies, especially bronchogenic carcinoma (62), may present with autonomic neuropathy and adrenoceptor hypersensitivity (63). The abnormality may respond to radiation and chemotherapeutic regimens in proportion to the change in tumor size. Finally, patients with a variety of spinal cord lesions, whether induced by disease or injury, may have marked autonomic impairment.

SHY-DRAGER SYNDROME

The Shy-Drager syndrome is a form of multiple system atrophy attended by autonomic failure (64). The multiple system atrophies include a number of poorly differentiated degenerative neurological disorders (Table 9), not all of which are attended by clinically recognized autonomic dysfunction. Patients with the Shy-Drager syndrome typically have extensive autonomic failure with concomitant impairment in the cerebellar, extrapyramidal, pontine, and medullary neurological systems. The autonomic failure of the Shy-Drager syndrome can be viewed predominantly as a central defect with an inability to engage peripheral sympathetic and parasympathetic postganglionic neurons. Although the cause remains unknown, antibodies have recently been discovered in the spinal fluid of patients with the Shy-Drager syndrome that bind specifically to rat locus coeruleus (65).

Patients with the Shy-Drager syndrome have a much worse prognosis than those with the Bradbury-Eggleston syndrome, usually surviving only about 10 years after onset; on the other hand, Bradbury-Eggleston patients commonly survive beyond 20 years, and have attained a greater age at death than the general population.

In addition to extrapyramidal features (bradykinesia, tremor, rigidity) and cerebellar abnormalities, Shy-Drager patients may have laryngeal stridor and sleep apnea, which occasionally dominate the clinical presentation. Loud snoring is common.

Antiparkinsonian medications are occasionally of benefit, but are rarely as efficacious as in true Parkinson's disease. Management of orthostatic hypotension is similar to that in the Bradbury-Eggleston syndrome.

Autonomic abnormalities sometimes occur in Parkinson's disease, but most authorities do not consider this to be the Shy-Drager syndrome if the neuropathology shows clear evidence of the Lewy body eosinophilic inclusions typical of Parkinson's disease. This distinction is not always easy to make on clinical grounds, as is illustrated by the substantial number (more than 10 percent) of Parkinson's disease patients coming to autopsy in the United Kingdom who are discovered to lack Lewy bodies and hence seem to fall into one of the multiple system atrophies. Nevertheless, it seems clear that even typical Lewy body Parkinson's disease may be accompanied by a range of autonomic problems (66).

TABLE 9. *The multiple system atrophies*

Shy-Drager syndrome
  Autonomic failure and striatonigral degeneration
  Olivopontocerebellar atrophy
    Congenital ataxia
    Early-onset progressive ataxia
    Autosomal dominant progressive ataxia
    Periodic ataxia
    Adult-onset progressive ataxia
  Steele-Richardson-Olszewski syndrome
  Huntington's disease
  Adrenomyeloneuropathy

DOPAMINE-β-HYDROXYLASE DEFICIENCY

Dopamine-β-hydroxylase (DBH) (EC 1.17.14.1) is required for conversion of dopamine to norepinephrine. However, tyrosine hydroxylase rather than DBH is the rate-limiting step in norepinephrine synthesis under almost all circumstances in man. Even in situations of high sympathetic activation, such as prolonged treadmill exercise, norepinephrine and epinephrine remain the predominant circulating catecholamines, with minimal step-up in plasma dopamine levels (67). Thus, in healthy subjects under ordinary circumstances, DBH activity is sufficient for the needs of autonomic cardiovascular regulation.

There are occasional patients, however, in whom neuronal DBH activity is inadequate (68,69). These individuals have the syndrome of severe DBH deficiency (68). The survival of individuals with essentially complete absence of norepinephrine into adulthood strongly suggests that individuals with partial enzyme deficiency will also be found. Unlike earlier recognized forms of autonomic failure, this disorder was localized to a discrete enzymatic defect, which enabled investigators to approach its treatment more rationally than had heretofore been possible.

DBH is unique among the catecholamine synthesizing enzymes in being located almost exclusively in the chromaffin granules of the adrenal medulla and the large dense-core synaptic vesicles of noradrenergic neurons (70–72). It is found in both peripheral and central noradrenergic and adrenergic neurons. DBH exists both in the dimeric and tetrameric forms, with two copper atoms per monomeric subunit (73,74). The four subunits are linked by disulfide bridges into two dimers, which are joined to each other by noncovalent bonds. The copper is essential for enzyme activity. DBH also requires molecular oxygen and ascorbic acid for enzyme activity. DBH is not substrate-specific, since it oxidizes almost any phenylethylamine to its corresponding phenylethanolamine (including the hydroxylation of tyramine into octopamine) and converts the α-methyldopa metabolite, α-methyldopamine, to α-methylnorepinephrine. The K_m of this enzyme for dopamine is approximately 5 ± 10^{-3} M (75).

DBH occurs in both a soluble and a membrane-bound form (76). These are present in approximately equal amounts in the vesicle. The soluble enzyme is released into the synaptic cleft at the time of vesicular exocytosis and is presumably the source of the enzyme present in blood. Much study has gone into the identification of the differences between these two forms (77). Current evidence suggests that both forms of DBH originate from a single gene and that the soluble form is derived from the membrane bound form (78). The sequence of DBH complementary DNA (cDNA) was reported by Lamouroux et al. (79). The polypeptide chain contained 603 amino acids corresponding to an unmodified protein of 64,862 daltons, preceded by a cleaved signal peptide of 25 residues. Kobayashi and co-workers (80) subsequently showed that there is a single DBH gene of approximately 23 kb and that it is composed of 12 exons, with exon 12 providing two alternative polyadenylation sites.

A syndrome characterized by severe orthostatic hypotension, noradrenergic failure and ptosis of the eyelids was simultaneously recognized in the United States (68) and in the Netherlands (69). Based on a battery of biochemical and physiological tests, it was determined that this disorder was due to a deficiency of DBH. The characteristics of patients with DBH deficiency are distinct from previously recognized forms of autonomic dysfunction (Table 10) and in some cases the anamnesis is so characteristic as to provide the diagnosis. DBH deficiency differs from familial dysautonomia (81) and various other autonomic disorders seen in adults (2) in that the peripheral defect can be localized to the noradrenergic and adrenergic tissues. There is virtual absence of norepinephrine and epinephrine, coupled with greatly increased dopamine in plasma, cerebrospinal fluid, and urine (68,69). Furthermore, there is no evidence of other neurological defects, either central or peripheral (82). The full clinical spectrum of DBH deficiency is still not known, because of the limited number of patients who have been reported. The description here is based primarily on the data in the first six published cases (68,69,83–86) (Table 3). It is likely that many features not currently recognized will ultimately be found to be associated with the disorder as the number of reported cases increases. Conversely, some abnormalities found in individual patients may ultimately prove to be fortuitous associations.

Parents of DBH deficient patients have appeared normal (68,86), but a history of spontaneous abortions and stillbirths has been noted among siblings of affected patients (69). The perinatal period in DBH-deficient subjects has sometimes been particularly difficult (68,69,85). Delay in opening of the eyes (2 weeks in one case) may occur (85) and ptosis of eyelids has occurred in most infants (68,69,85,87). The infants have occasionally been so sickly at birth that parents were advised their

TABLE 10. *Dopamine-β-hydroxylase deficiency*

Severe orthostatic hypotension
Nasal stuffiness
Ptosis of the eyelids
Retrograde ejaculation in males
Complicated perinatal course
    Hypothermia
    Hypoglycemia
    Hypotension
Plasma dopamine/norepinephrine ratio much greater than 10
Absent or undetectable urinary norepinephrine and
    epinephrine

survival was unlikely (68). Although records are incomplete in some cases, it appears that hypotension, hypoglycemia, and hypothermia have occurred primarily in the first year of life (69). The causes of hypoglycemia and hypothermia are not fully understood at present, but epinephrine has a well-characterized caloric effect in animals, and excessive dopamine may reduce temperature in animals. Vomiting occurred four times in the first year of life in one patient (69). Sometimes seizures have occurred, probably because of hypoglycemia or hypotension (85,87). DBH-deficient patients have had markedly reduced ability to exercise because of postural hypotension occurring with exertion (68,86). The syncope associated with this postural hypotension has led to trials of anticonvulsive medications (68), even though the electroencephalogram did not suggest a seizure disorder and efficacy was not observed.

Symptoms have generally worsened considerably in late adolescence and early adulthood (85,86,88). Patients complain of profound orthostatic hypotension, especially early in the day and during hot weather or after alcohol ingestion. There is greatly reduced exercise tolerance, ptosis of the eyelids, nasal stuffiness (68,85), and prolonged or retrograde ejaculation (85,86); the retrograde ejaculation is recognized by the presence of semen in the postejaculation urine void. Presyncopal symptoms include dizziness, blurred vision, dyspnea, nuchal discomfort, and, occasionally, chest pain. Some patients have adopted novel strategies for maintaining upright posture. One patient crossed his legs at a 30° angle and leaned his torso 30° forward, placing his right hand on his right anterior thigh for support (85). Sexual maturation has been normal, with menarche occurring at ages 12 to 14 (68,86,87).

On physical examination, patients have a low normal supine blood pressure and a normal heart rate but an upright blood pressure less than 80 mm Hg systolic. Heart rate rises on standing, but certainly inadequately when one considers the magnitude of the hypotension in the upright posture. Patients are usually unable to stand motionless more than 30 seconds. Pupils are somewhat small but respond to light and accommodation. Parasympatholytics usually dilate the eye appropriately, but in two patients homatropine has failed to do so (69,87). There is usually ptosis of the eyelids. Joints may be hyperflexible (87) or hyperextensible (85). In particular, sweating, a sympathetic nonnoradrenergic function, is normal.

These patients are easily differentiated from those with familial dysautonomia (Riley-Day syndrome). Cholinergic sensitivity as assessed by the ophthalmic response to conjunctival administration of 2.5% methacholine was normal in that there was no response. Intradermal histamine evoked a typical flare reaction, whereas this does not occur in familial dysautonomia. These patients are further distinguished from familial dysautonomia in that the DBH-deficient patients have (a) normal tearing, (b) intact corneal and deep tendon reflexes, (c) normal sensory function, and (d) normal senses of taste and smell. Also, subjects thus far recognized have not been of Ashkenazi Jewish extraction.

There have been other clinical abnormalities in these patients that bear a still uncertain relationship to the pathology as we understand it. Two of six subjects have evidence of mild renal failure (85,86) and at least two patients have experienced recurrent hypomagnesemia (82,85). One patient developed atrial fibrillation at age 40 (85) which proved remarkably resistant to therapy.

Patients with DBH deficiency have had such striking abnormalities in catecholamine metabolism that they are readily distinguishable from patients with all other known disorders. The combination of minimal or undetectable plasma norepinephrine with a five-to tenfold elevation of plasma dopamine is probably pathognomonic of the disorder (Table 4). Indeed, perhaps the only other disorder in which plasma dopamine exceeds plasma norepinephrine is Menkes kinky hair disease, a dramatic illness associated with profound mental retardation (89). Menkes syndrome is an X-linked recessive disorder characterized by early growth retardation, stubby and white hair, hypopigmentation, arterial rupture and thrombosis, urinary tract diverticulae, and focal cerebral and cerebellar degeneration. Survival beyond 10 years is rare, and brain damage is usually severe.

DBH deficiency would probably have been recognized earlier were it not for the fact that most medical centers tend to measure norepinephrine and epinephrine but not dopamine in the evaluation of patients with autonomic dysfunction. Without comparative details about the levels of norepinephrine and dopamine and the patterns of their respective metabolites, the special nature of the enzymatic defect in this disorder can be entirely missed. Such patients were probably considered to have an atypical form of the Bradbury-Eggleston syndrome or idiopathic orthostatic hypotension (90). In addition, commonly used radioenzymatic methods for catecholamine determinations have the disadvantage of a small, but significant, crossover of dopamine into epinephrine. Because of normally low levels of dopamine, this is usually of minor practical importance. However, in a setting of elevated dopamine levels, as present in DBH deficiency, a proportion of dopamine may be erroneously measured as epinephrine (68).

Plasma dopamine levels in DBH-deficient subjects approximate plasma norepinephrine levels in normal subjects, but with greater variability. This is believed to occur because dopamine, rather than norepinephrine, is being stored and released by noradrenergic neurons in DBH-deficient subjects. For this reason, plasma dopamine levels respond to various stimuli that would elicit an increase in plasma norepinephrine levels in normal subjects. For example, a change from supine to upright posture will double or triple the plasma dopamine level. Likewise, the administration of a central suppressant of sympathetic activity such as clonidine (91) will greatly reduce the plasma dopamine level. Plasma dopamine levels have thus been shown to be greatly elevated by insulin hypoglycemia (69), edrophonium (69), tyramine (68), tilt (69,86), and upright posture (68). Perhaps because of high levels of dopamine, plasma prolactin is low in this disorder (82). It is noteworthy that plasma dopa levels are also raised two- to threefold while the enzyme dopa decarboxylase is also normal in plasma (69).

Norepinephrine metabolites have been low or absent in plasma, urine, and cerebrospinal fluid (CSF). Conversely, dopamine metabolites such as homovanillic acid and 3-methoxytyramine are raised. Determination of whether or not norepinephrine exists at all in patients with DBH deficiency must await further investigations and improvements in assay methodology. A low, but apparently detectable, level of vanillylmandelic acid (VMA) was found in the urine of three patients (68,86), and a low, but detectable, level of methoxyhydroxyphenylglycol (MHPG) was found in the CSF of another patient (69). In other patients, these metabolites have been beneath the limits of detection of the assay. Whether these reflect genuine differences in pathology or the limitations of the respective assays remains to be seen. Skin biopsies in three subjects have not shown staining for DBH but tyrosine hydroxylase was present in all (68,86). In the two subjects in whom data have been reported, neuropeptide Y, calcitonin gene-related peptide, substance P, and vasoactive intestinal peptide have all been present (86).

Tests of autonomic function also provide diagnostic information of great specificity. In DBH deficiency, autonomic tests that measure sympathetic noradrenergic and adrenergic function are uniformly abnormal. Cold pressor testing (immersion of a hand in ice water for 1 min) causes either a fall or no change in blood pressure. Isometric handgrip exercise (sustained handgrip for 3 min) fails to increase blood pressure significantly. The Valsalva maneuver results in a profound fall in blood pressure together with an increase in heart rate reflecting parasympathetic withdrawal. The phase IV overshoot of the Valsalva maneuver does not occur. Hyperventilation causes a fall in blood pressure, as is also the case in patients with the Bradbury-Eggleston syndrome. In contrast to the absence of sympathetic activation, the presence of sweating underscores the integrity of sympathetic cholinergic fibers. Moreover, parasympathetic function is preserved since these patients have normal sinus arrhythmia. This selective sympathetic noradrenergic impairment is quite characteristic of DBH deficiency. Other forms of autonomic failure have both sympathetic and parasympathetic involvement (90,92,93).

DBH deficiency shares many pharmacological features of other forms of autonomic failure. There is a severalfold hypersensitivity to α_1-adrenoceptor agonists and β-adrenoceptor agonists. This is also found in other forms of autonomic failure and represents a compensatory receptor up-regulation as a result of the chronic relative depletion of catecholamines (94). This phenomenon is analogous to other forms of "denervation hypersensitivity." Tyramine is an indirectly acting pressor amine that will induce norepinephrine release from adrenergic nerve terminals. Tyramine, in intravenous doses of 2 to 3 mg, will raise plasma norepinephrine and blood pressure in normal subjects and in patients with other types of autonomic failure (94), but no blood pressure elevation occurred even with 6 to 8 mg of tyramine in DBH-deficient subjects. Plasma dopamine, instead of norepinephrine, is increased following the administration of tyramine in these patients.

Propranolol, a β-adrenoceptor antagonist, does not lower the basal heart rate in these patients, but pindolol, a β-antagonist with sympathomimetic properties, raises heart rate significantly. Intravenous atropine raises heart rate by 40 to 60 bpm. The respiratory arrhythmia that occurs in the baseline state in DBH deficiency disappears with the administration of atropine. Taken together, these observations imply normal parasympathetic, but defective sympathetic, control of heart rate. It is also of interest that atropine elicits a much more pronounced pressor effect in DBH-deficient subjects than in normal subjects (68,69).

Clonidine acts on α_2-adrenoceptors or imidazoline receptors in the brainstem to reduce sympathetic outflow and lower blood pressure (91). It can also exert peripheral pressor effects by stimulation of vascular α_2-adrenoceptors (95). DBH-deficient patients have no fall in seated mean arterial pressure following the administration of clonidine, probably reflecting the fact that in these patients, blood pressure is not maintained by sympathetic tone. On the contrary, dramatic increases in blood pressure are seen with higher doses of this agent. It is noteworthy that heart rate decreases in DBH-deficient patients following the administration of clonidine, even though blood pressure does not fall, consistent with the postulated central parasympathetic component in clonidine-induced bradycardia.

Finally, direct measurements of sympathetic nerve traffic to the vasculature of the skeletal muscle have been carried out using microneurography in a patient with DBH deficiency (96). They confirm that sympathetic neural traffic is present and regulated in a qualitatively normal fashion.

DBH-deficient patients have been difficult to treat using standard therapeutic approaches for autonomic failure. Most have failed empirical therapy with anticonvulsant agents prior to diagnosis. Fludrocortisone, at dosages of 0.1 to 0.8 mg daily, has been used to raise blood pressure with some benefit (68), but marked orthostatic hypotension still occurs. Likewise, indomethacin (50 mg four times daily) has been of limited benefit in raising blood pressure in these subjects; furthermore, one patient had aggressive ideation on this drug (85). Monoamine oxidase inhibition (tranylcypromine) has produced paranoid ideation (85). There is some pressor response to phenylpropanolamine (25 and 50 mg), presumably owing to the denervation hypersensitivity of the patients' vascular α-adrenoceptors (85).

Because both plasma dopa and dopamine levels were elevated in DBH-deficient patients, the vasodepressor effects of dopamine, either through direct vasodilatation or by means of a diuretic effect at the level of the kidney, were proposed as possible explanations for the striking severity of low blood pressure in these patients (97,98). It was hypothesized that if dopa and dopamine were reducing blood pressure in DBH-deficient subjects, the administration of metyrosine (α-methyl-para-tyrosine), might prove therapeutic (85). Metyrosine blocks tyrosine hydroxylase, the enzyme leading to the synthesis of dopa. This results in reduced levels of dopamine and norepinephrine, and therefore blood pressure falls in normal subjects, particularly when the subject is in the upright posture. We hypothesized that our patients might have such high dopamine levels that paradoxical pressor effects might occur. Since metyrosine is depressor in healthy individuals, a failure of metyrosine to affect blood pressure, or a reduction in blood pressure with metyrosine, would not support a contribution of dopamine to the low blood pressure in our patients. On the other hand, a rise in blood pressure with metyrosine would suggest that dopa and dopamine were indeed exerting depressor effects and that these effects could be attenuated by an agent that reduced manufacture and release of dopamine. In the event, metyrosine given in doses used to treat pheochromocytoma exerted a dramatic pressor effect which appeared to correlate with the metyrosine-associated reduction in urinary dopamine excretion (83).

In spite of this initially favorable response to metyrosine, much more experience with it will be required before it can be recommended for treatment. Patients receiving metyrosine experienced significant sedation; one patient experienced a dystonic reaction (83) but fortunately responded promptly to a 10 mg intravenous dose of diphenhydramine.

The most effective therapy in these patients so far has been dihydroxyphenylserine (DOPS) (83). We administered DOPS in the hope that it would result in an endogenous conversion (by dopa decarboxylase) of the drug to norepinephrine. This might occur because DBH is not needed for the conversion of DOPS to norepinephrine and, thus, this enzyme could be bypassed in the patients in whom it is defective. There would be an increase in plasma norepinephrine following the administration of DOPS.

The administration of DOPS to patients with DBH deficiency has resulted in dramatic increases in blood pressure and concomitant restoration of plasma and urinary levels of norepinephrine toward normal (83,84). There has been an associated modest decline in dopamine levels, as though the novel provision of norepinephrine to intraneuronal sites might be reducing the activity of tyrosine hydroxylase through feedback inhibition. The increase in plasma norepinephrine was highly correlated with the increase in mean arterial blood pressure. Standing time was greatly increased following DOPS.

We could not be certain whether *de novo* synthesis of norepinephrine from DOPS occurred in neuronal tissues or in extraneuronal tissues, since dopa decarboxylase activity is present in many extraneuronal tissues. However, long-term treatment with DOPS in this disorder is associated with intraneuronal restoration of norepinephrine, which is released upon assuming the upright posture. Thus, DOPS in DBH deficiency appears to be far more effective than any other therapy for any form of autonomic dysfunction (83,84,86,87).

DBH deficiency is clearly a rare disease in adults, but it could be more common in the perinatal period. Medical histories of DBH deficient patients include near-fatal illness during the neonatal period due to hypotension, hypoglycemia, and hypothermia. We suspect that many DBH deficient infants succumb undiagnosed at this point, never reaching childhood and adulthood.

Prior to recognition of DBH deficiency, it was assumed that humans could not live without norepinephrine. Yet, stretching current assay methodology to the limit, it is not certain that any norepinephrine at all is present in the severely affected individuals we have studied; if it is present in plasma, it is less than 1% of normal (99). Since norepinephrine and its receptor sites have long been postulated to play a role in a number of psychiatric disorders, the generally normal (85,87) or near-normal (86) mood and mental status of DBH-deficiency subjects so far encountered has elicited great interest among investigators in the area of depression and schizophrenia.

Shortly after DBH was recognized as an important step in catecholamine synthesis, attempts were made to treat hypertension with DBH inhibitors. Disulfiram (Antabuse), a copper chelator, was early recognized to inhibit DBH. Early clinical studies also demonstrated that fusaric acid and its precursor bupicomide could lower blood pressure in hypertensive subjects and decrease serum DBH activity (75). However, tachycardia and increased excretion of urinary catecholamines were observed. This apparent contradiction can be explained by the fact that fusaric acid apparently stimulates the release of catecholamines from the adrenal gland. More specific and potent DBH inhibitors are currently being tested as antihypertensive agents. As in our patients, inhibition of DBH following the administration of SKF 102698 to rats results in a decrease in plasma and tissue norepinephrine associated with an increase in dopamine levels (100). Also, as our results with metyrosine suggest, the hypotensive effects of specific DBH inhibitors may be related to both a decrease in norepinephrine and an increase in dopamine with its attendant vasodilatory and natriuretic effects. Such agents might be uniquely efficacious antihypertensive and antiarrhythmic agents.

DBH deficiency and its successful treatment by DOPS encourages us to hope that other autonomic disorders may one day also yield to genuinely effective therapeutic interventions.

ORTHOSTATIC INTOLERANCE SYNDROMES

The Bradbury-Eggleston syndrome and the Shy-Drager syndrome tend to occur in middle to older age groups. However, it is not uncommon to encounter mild orthostatic intolerance in younger individuals, especially girls and women from the ages of 15 to 40. The orthostatic intolerance is sometimes characterized by mild orthostatic hypotension, but, more commonly, orthostatic tachycardia is a more constant feature. It is likely that a very large number of pathological processes have this presentation as their final common denominator. Perhaps for this reason, an extraordinary multiplicity of names have been used to characterize one or more subgroups of these patients. Some of these names are shown in Table 11. Some of the terms in Table 11 have been used broadly to categorize all patients described in this section, whereas others relate more specifically to a more or less well-defined subgroup. An attempt to list possible etiologic subgroups is made in Table 12. It is likely that many other etiologies for orthostatic intolerance also exist.

Orthostatic hypotension is present in approximately 10 percent of patients with mitral valve prolapse as de-

TABLE 11. *Orthostatic intolerance syndromes*

Vasoregulatory asthenia
Neurocirculatory asthenia
Mitral valve prolapse syndrome
Postural orthostatic tachycardia syndrome
Orthostatic tachycardia plus
Idiopathic hypovolemia
Hyperadrenergic orthostatic hypotension
Sympathotonic orthostatic hypotension
Sympathicotonic orthostatic hypotension
Distal dysautonomia
Orthostatic intolerance
Soldier's heart
DaCosta syndrome
Postural tachycardia

TABLE 12. *Proposed etiologies of orthostatic intolerance syndromes*

Mitral valve prolapse
Hypovolemia
Hypercoupled β-adrenoceptors
Postinfectious autonomic neuropathy
Partial dysautonomia
Venous valvular incompetence
Inferior vena cava syndrome
Dumping syndrome
Mastocytosis

termined by a click and/or murmur on physical examination or echocardiographic examination (101). Usually the orthostatic hypotension is of milder degree than that encountered in true autonomic failure syndromes such as those discussed above. However, occasional patients have very severe orthostatic hypotension requiring treatment.

As many as 30 percent of patients with the mitral valve prolapse syndrome have dramatic orthostatic tachycardia even though orthostatic hypotension itself may not be present or may be present only after meals. Careful studies have shown that many patients with the mitral valve prolapse syndrome have a 5 percent to 8 percent reduction in blood volume (102,103). This reduction in blood volume may explain the hypotension and tachycardia sometimes seen. It may also explain the high normal or slightly raised plasma norepinephrine levels commonly found in these subjects. However, the cause of the reduced blood volume in the mitral prolapse syndrome is by no means certain. There has been speculation that excessive atrial natriuretic factor might somehow be involved in the pathogenesis of the disorder, but not all patients with mitral valve prolapse have the "raise" atrial natriuretic factor levels. This issue needs further study, however, since even those who do not have raised atrial natriuretic factor levels may have hormone levels that are inappropriately high considering their level of blood volume reduction. It is noteworthy that many patients with similar clinical symptoms do not necessarily have concomitant mitral prolapse (104–107).

There has long been speculation that the mitral valve prolapse syndrome constitutes a dysautonomia (108). Indeed, some evidence for β-adrenoceptor abnormalities has been found in a small number of these patients (109). That there might be a genetic defect leading to supercoupled β-adrenoceptors in the heart and vasculature in some patients with this disorder is intriguing, especially in view of recent evidence that such mechanisms may give rise to thyroid and fertility problems (110–112). However, it appears that the vast majority of patients with the mitral valve prolapse syndrome do not have any failure in the autonomic nervous system (113) but rather have excessive sympathetic activity that is attempting to compensate for the reduced blood volume. So long as the cause of the mitral valve prolapse is unknown, treatment is likely to remain difficult. One school of thought suggests that distal sympathetic failure may be primary in this disorder and that blood volume reduction is secondary to that altered sympathetic activity. For this reason, very low doses of clonidine (0.05 mg po b.i.d.) have been employed with apparent symptomatic benefit in occasional patients. More commonly, however, these patients have been treated successfully with fludrocortisone (0.1–1.0 mg po q.d.) and, in individuals in whom the tachycardia is the predominant symptoms, pindolol (5 mg po t.i.d.). Very low doses of phenobarbital (15–30 mg) have been helpful in some patients (H. Cecil Coghlan, *personal communication*). Through judicious use of these various agents, it is usually possible to manage the mitral valve prolapse syndrome successfully.

MAST CELL ACTIVATION DISORDER

Disorders of abnormal mast cell activation or proliferation are probably much more common than is generally appreciated (114). They often present similarly to the orthostatic intolerance syndromes discussed above. These syndromes are commonly grouped and referred to as mastocytosis. Experience at Vanderbilt University Medical Center suggests that severe mastocytosis is at least as common as severe autonomic failure, but it is much less frequently diagnosed. A major reason for this is that many patients with mastocytosis do not manifest the chronic urticaria described in textbooks and some may also lack the erythematous acneiform papular lesions, even though they may have flushing. Typical symptoms of mastocytosis are (a) flushing, pruritus, and paresthesias; (b) palpitations with or without chest pain; (c) dyspnea and dizziness; (d) syncope (in one-third of cases), usually disproportionate to the hypotension measured; (e) headaches; and (f) intermittent nausea, vomiting, or diarrhea. Blood pressure may be high or low but chronic abnormalities in blood pressure are not seen. With large mast cell degranulations there may be sufficient heparin released to affect clotting time and the partial thromboplastin time (PTT).

These symptoms are often provoked by exercise, by emotional stimuli, by narcotics, and by heat. The diagnosis is made by measuring urinary methylhistamine and urinary prostaglandin D_2; one or both of these should be dramatically raised in a 4-hour urine collection made immediately following an attack. About 75 percent of mastocytosis cases are sporadic while the rest are usually familial in an autosomal dominant pattern. Chronically, H_1- and H_2-antagonists are used initially. If these are insufficient, aspirin is begun at a cautiously low level and advanced stepwise until plasma salicylate levels of 20 to 30 mg/percent are obtained. Occasionally, severe attacks of mastocytosis may result in a profound fall in blood pressure and can be life-threatening. These attacks respond best to intravenous infusion of epinephrine at 2 to 8 μg/min intravenously, which acts at least in part by inhibiting mast cell degranulation.

ACKNOWLEDGMENTS

This work was supported in part by grants from the National Aeronautics and Space Administration (NCC 2-696 and NAG 5-563) and the National Institutes of Health (RR00095, HL44589, HL37961).

REFERENCES

1. Robertson D. In: Melmon KL, Morelli H, eds. *Clinical pharmacology.* New York: McGraw-Hill 1992;84–93.
2. Robertson D, Biaggioni I, eds. *Disorders of the autonomic nervous system.* London: Harwood, 1994; in press.
3. Streeten DHP. *Orthostatic disorders of the circulation.* New York: Plenum, 1987.
4. Low PA. *Clinical autonomic disorders: evaluation and management.* Boston: Little, Brown, 1993.
5. Bannister R. *Autonomic failure.* Oxford: Oxford University Press, 1993.
6. Eckberg DL, Sleight P. *Human baroreflexes in health and disease.* Oxford: Clarendon Press, 1992.
7. Mark AL, Mancia G. In: Shepherd JT, Abboud FM, eds. *Handbook of physiology,* 2nd ed. Bethesda: American Physiological Society 1983;795–818.
8. Persson PB, Kirchheim HR, eds. *Baroreceptor reflexes.* Berlin: Springer-Verlag, 1991.
9. Robertson D, Hollister AS, Biaggioni I, Netterville JL, Mosqueda-Garcia R, Robertson D. The diagnosis and treatment of baroreflex failure. *N Engl J Med* 1993;329.
10. Aksamit TR, Floras JS, Victor RG, Aylward PE. *Hypertension* 1987;9:309–314.
11. Ford FR. *Johns Hopkins Med J* 1957;100:14–16.
12. Hsu CY, Olanoff L. *Am J Med* 1984;76:A49.
13. Kuchel O, Cusson JR, Larochelle P, Buu NT, Genest J. *J Hypertens* 1987;5:277–283.
14. Robertson D, Goldberg MR, Hollister AS, Wade D, Robertson RM. *Am J Med* 1983;74:193–199.
15. Cowley AW, Liard JF, Guyton AC. *Circ Res* 1973;32:564–576.
16. Abbound FM, Eckberg DL, Johannsen UJ, Mark AL. *J Physiol* 1979;286:173–184.
17. Ferguson DW, Abboud FM, Mark AL. *J Clin Invest* 1985;76:2265–2274.
18. Brodal A. *Hjernenervene.* Copenhagen: Munksgaard, 1957;1–31.
19. Magnus O, Koster M, Van der Drift JHA. In: De Jong W, ed. *Hypertension and brain mechanisms, progress in brain disease.* Amsterdam: Elsevier/North-Holland Biomedical Press, 1977; 199–218.
20. Page I. *Hypertension mechanisms.* Orlando: Grune and Stratton, 1987;707–719.
21. Reis DJ, Doba N. *N Engl J Med* 1972;287:1354–1355.
22. van Barrs FM, Cremers CWRJ, van den Broek P, Veldman JE. *Acta Otolaryngol* 1981;91:589–593.
23. Biaggioni, 1994; in press.
24. Robertson D. In: Baughman KL, Greene BM, eds. *Clinical diagnostic manual for the house officer.* Baltimore: Williams and Wilkins, 1981;86–101.
25. Robertson D, Johnson GA, Robertson RM, Nies AS, Shand DG, Oates JA. *Circulation* 1979;59:637–643.
26. Robertson D, Goldberg MR, Hollister AS, Wade D, Robertson RM. *Am J Med* 1984;76:A49–A58.
27. Manger WM, Gifford RW Jr. *Pheochromocytoma.* New York: Springer-Verlag, 1977.
28. Kezdi P. *Arch Intern Med* 1954;91:26–34.
29. Lampen H, Kezdi P, Kopperman E. *Z Kreislaufforsch* 1949;38: 726–737.
30. Guz A, Noble MIM, Widdicombe JG, Trenchard D, Mushin WW, Makey AR. *Clin Sci* 1966;30:161–170.
31. Fagius J, Wallin BG, Sundlof G, Nerhed C, Engelsson S. *Brain* 1985;108:423–483.
32. Holton P, Wood JB. *J Physiol* 1965;181:365–378.
33. Bove EL, Fry WJ, Gross WS, Stanley JC. *Surgery* 1979;85:633–637.
34. Wade JG, Larson CP Jr, Hickey RF, Ehrenfeld WK, Severinghaus JW. *N Engl J Med* 1970;282:823–829.
35. Towne JB, Bernhard VM. *Surgery* 1980;88:575–580.
36. Doba H, Reis DJ. *Circ Res* 1974;34:293.
37. Page I. *Am J Med Sci* 1935;190:9–14.
38. Atuk NO, Evans CH. *N Engl J Med* 1972;287:1356.
39. Chamontin B, Senard JM, Amar J, Doazan JP, Guittard J, Montastruc JL, et al. *Arch Mal Coeur* 1989;82:1143–1146.
40. Funck-Brentano C, Pagny J-Y, Menard J. *Br Heart J* 1987;57: 487–489.
41. Langford HG, Sanford R, Smith R, Currier R, Johnson W, Klein R, Baggett J. *J Hypertens* 1987;5(suppl 5):S467–S469.
42. Jannetta PJ, Segal R, Wolfson SK Jr. *Ann Surg* 1985;201:391–398.
43. Bravo EL, Tarazi RC, Fouad FM, Vidt DG, Gifford RW Jr. *N Engl J Med* 1981;305:623–626.
44. Finley JP, Tibbles JAR. *J Pediatr* 1982;100:409–412.
45. Ingall TJ, McLeod JG, Tamura N. *Muscle Nerve* 1990;13:70–76.
46. Cryer PE, Weiss S. *Arch Neurol* 1976;33:275–277.
47. Cryer PE, Silverberg AB, Santiago JV, Shah SD. *Am J Med* 1978;64:407–416.
48. Cryer PE. *Metabolism* 1980;29:1186–1189.
49. Ewing DJ. *Clin Sci Mol Med* 1978;55:321–327.
50. Ewing DJ, Campbell IW, Clarke BF. *Q J Med* 1980;49:95–108.
51. Ewing DJ, Clarke BF. *Diabetes Care* 1986;9:648–665.
52. Schumer M, Burton G, Burton C, Crum D, Pfeifer MA. *Am J Med* 1988;85:137–146.
53. Watkins PJ. *N Engl J Med* 1990;322:1078–1079.
54. Janssens J, Peeters TL, Vantrappen G, Tack J, Urbain JL, De Roo M, Muls E, Bouillon R. *N Engl J Med* 1990;322:1028–1031.
55. Luft F, von Euler US. *J Clin Invest* 1953;32:1065–1069.
56. Miles DW, Hayter CJ. *Clin Sci* 1968;34:419–430.
57. Christensen NJ. *Diabetologia* 1983;25:377–381.
58. Brown RT, Polinsky RJ, Baucom CE. *Clin Neuropharmacol* 1989;12:227–231.
59. Solders G, Wilczek H, Gunnarson R, Tyden G, Persson A, Groth CG. *Lancet* 1987;2:1232–1235.
60. Kennedy WR, Navarro X, Goetz FC, Sutherland DER, Najarian JS. *N Engl J Med* 1990;322:1031–1037.
61. Alvarez WC, Roth G. *Mayo Clin Proc* 1935;10:483–489.
62. Park DM, Johnson RH, Crean GP, Robinson JF. *Br Med J* 1972;3:510–511.
63. Hui KKP, Conolly ME. *N Engl J Med* 1981;304:1473–1476.
64. Polinsky RJ. In: Jankovic J, Tolosa E, eds. *Parkinson's disease and movement disorders.* Baltimore: Williams & Wilkins 1993;191–204.
65. Polinsky RJ, McRae A, Baser SM, Dahlström A. *J Neurol Sci* 1991;106:96–104.
66. Tanner CM, Goetz CG, Klawans HL. In: Koller WC, ed. *Handbook of parkinson's disease.* New York: Dekker, 1992;185–215.
67. Robertson D, Johnson GA, Robertson RM, Nies AS, Shand DG, Oates JA. *Circulation* 1979;59:637–643.
68. Robertson D, Goldberg MR, Onrot J, Hollister AS, Thompson JC, Wiley R, Robertson RM. *N Engl J Med* 1986;314:1494–1497.
69. Man in't Veld AJ, Boomsma F, Moleman P, Schalekamp MADH. *Lancet* 1987;1:183–187.
70. Goldstein M. *Pharmacol Rev* 1976;18:77–91.
71. Kaufman S, Friedman S. *Pharmacol Rev* 1965;17:71–100.
72. Axelrod J. *Pharmacol Rev* 1972;24:233–243.
73. Sabban EL, Goldstein M. *J Neurochem* 1984;43:1663–1668.
74. Sabban EL, Kuhn LJ, Levin BE. *J Neurosci* 1987;7:192–200.
75. Nagatsu T. In: Boulton RR, Baker GB, eds. *Neuromethods I.* Clifton, NJ: Humana, 1986;79–116.

76. Sokoloff RL, Frigon RP, O'Connor DT. *J Neurochem* 1985;44: 411–420.
77. O'Connor DT, Frigon RP, Stone RA. *Mol Pharmacol* 1979;16: 529–538.
78. Dhawan S, Duong LE, Ornberg RL, Fleming PJ. *J Biol Chem* 1987;262:1869–1875.
79. Lamouroux A, Vigny A, Faucon Biguet N, Darmon MC, Franck R, Henry JP, Mallet J. *EMBO J* 1987;6:3931–3937.
80. Kobayashi K, Kurosawa Y, Fujita K, Nagatsu T. *Nucleic Acids Res* 1989;17:1089–1102.
81. Axelrod FB, Pearson J. *Am J Dis Child* 1984;138:947–954.
82. Laragh J, Brenner BM, eds. *Hypertension: pathophysiology, management, and diagnosis.* New York: Raven Press, 1990.
83. Biaggioni I, Robertson D. *Lancet* 1987;2:1170–1172.
84. Man in't Veld AJ, Boomsma F, van den Meiracker AH, Schalekamp MADH. *Lancet* 1987;2:1172–1175.
85. Biaggioni I, Goldstein DS, Atkinson T, Robertson D. *Neurology* 1990;40:370–373.
86. Mathias CJ, Bannister RB, Cortelli P, Heslop K, Polak JM, Raimbach S, Springall DR, Watson L. *Q J Med* 1990;75:617–633.
87. Man in't Veld AJ, Boomsma F, van den Meiracker AH, Julien C, Lenders J, Schalekamp MA. *J Hypertens* 1988;6(suppl 4):547–549.
88. Robertson D, Perry SE, Hollister AS, Robertson RM, Biaggioni I. *Hypertension* 1991;18:1–8.
89. Hoeldtke RD, Cavanaugh ST, Hughes JD, Mattis-Graves K, Hobnell E, Grover WD. *Pediatr Neurol* 1988;4:23–26.
90. Bradbury S, Eggleston C. *Am Heart J* 1925;1:73–75.
91. Robertson D, Goldberg MR, Tung CS, Hollister AS, Robertson D. *J Clin Invest* 1986;78:576–571.
92. Shy GM, Drager GA. *Arch Neurol* 1960;2:511–527.
93. Schatz IJ. *Orthostatic hypotension.* Philadelphia: FA Davis, 1986;1–128.
94. Robertson D, Hollister AS, Carey EL, Tung CS, Goldberg MR, Robertson RM. *J Am Coll Cardiol* 1984;3:850–856.
95. Robertson D, Goldberg MR, Hollister AS, Wade D, Robertson RM. *Am J Med* 1983;74:193–199.
96. Rea RF, Biaggioni I, Robertson RM, Haile V, Robertson D. *Hypertension* 1990;15:107–112.
97. Kuchel O, Debinski W, Larochelle P. *N Engl J Med* 1986;315: 1357–1358.
98. DiBona GF. *Fed Proc* 1986;45:2871–2877.
99. Goldstein DS, Polinsky RJ, Garty M, Robertson D, Brown RT, Biaggioni I, Stull R, Kopin IJ. *Ann Neurol* 1989;26:558–563.
100. Ohlstein EH, Kruse LI, Ezekiel M, et al. *Clin Pharmacol Ther* 1975;18:145–153.
101. Santos AD, Mathew PK, Hilal A, et al. *Am J Med* 1981;71:746–750.
102. Gaffney FA, Bastian BC, Lane LB, et al. *Am J Cardiol* 1983;52: 316–320.
103. Blomqvist CG. *Hypertension* 1987;8:772–730.
104. Barach JH. *Arch Intern Med* 1925;35:151–165.
105. Bjure A, Laurell H. *Lakareforen Forhandl* 1927;33:1–23.
106. Fouad FM, Tadena-Thome L, Bravo EL, Tarazi RC. *Ann Intern Med* 1986;104:298–303.
107. Hoeldtke RD, Dworkin GE, Gaspar SR, Israel BC. *Neurology* 1989;39:34–40.
108. Mares A, Davies AO, Taylor AA. *Clin Pharmacol Ther* 1990;47: 371–381.
109. Davies AO, Mares A, Pool JL, et al. *Am J Med* 1987;82:193–201.
110. Lefkowitz RJ. *Nature* 1993;365:603–604.
111. Parma J, Duprez L, Van Sande J, Cochaux P, Gervy C, Mockel J, Dumont J, Vassart G. *Nature* 1993;365:649–651.
112. Shenker A, Laue L, Kosugi S, Meredino JJ Jr, Minegishi T, Cutler GB Jr. *Nature* 1993;365:652–654.
113. Schatz IJ. *Arch Intern Med* 1990;144:1037–1041.
114. Roberts LJ, Oates JA. In: Wilson JD, Foster DW, eds. *Williams textbook of endocrinology.* Philadelphia: Saunders, 1985;1363–1379.

SECTION V

Blood Pressure Regulation in Normal and Hypertensive States

Part B: Neural and Other Humoral Factors in the Control of Arterial Pressure

Hypertension: Pathophysiology, Diagnosis, and Management, Second Edition, edited by J.H. Laragh and B.M. Brenner, Raven Press, Ltd., New York © 1995.

CHAPTER 57

Eicosanoids and Hypertension

John Quilley, Caroline P. Bell-Quilley, and John C. McGiff

This chapter is entitled "*Eicosanoids and Hypertension*" because the term *prostaglandin* denotes only products of the cyclooxygenase pathway and is, therefore, restrictive. But the term *eicosanoid* is comprehensive because it refers to all of the C-20 metabolites generated by the three pathways and originating from either arachidonic acid, eicosapentaenoic acid, or dihomo-γ-linolenic acid.

PATHWAYS OF ARACHIDONIC ACID METABOLISM

Three pathways for the enzymatic conversion of arachidonic acid (AA) have been identified: cyclooxygenases, lipoxygenases, and cytochrome P-450–dependent monooxygenases(1). These oxygenases produce an array of AA metabolites with a wide diversity of biological activity. AA (20:4) is not the only substrate; eicosapentaenoic acid (EPA) (20:5) and dihomo-γ-linolenic acid (20:3) can be metabolized by cyclooxygenase to form prostaglandins (PG) of the 3 and 1 series (e.g., PGE_3 and PGE_1), respectively (2). AA is the usual substrate, and the

production of the 3 and 1 series prostanoids is minimal unless dietary manipulation of fatty acid intake is undertaken, the exception being populations such as the Eskimo whose diet provides large quantities of EPA from marine sources (3).

The first step, considered to be rate limiting for eicosanoid biosynthesis, is deacylation, the release of esterified AA from phospholipids, by the actions of phospholipases A_2, C, and D (4–6) (Fig. 1). Release of AA from phospholipids by lipases may be inhibited by lipocortin (calpactin), which binds to the phospholipid substrate (7) and prevents its being acted upon by phospholipase. Cholesterol esters and triglycerides can also serve as sources of AA. Further, AA can be donated by cells to contiguous cells, as may be the case for renal collecting tubules that are able to generate large quantities of PGE_2 in response to antidiuretic hormone (ADH), neighboring cells serving as donors of AA to collecting tubules (6). A general concept regarding prostaglandin production is that storage in the cell of origin does not occur. Synthesis of prostaglandins is associated with their immediate release into the extracellular compartment. However, AA products generated by cytochrome P-450 monooxygenases may be incorporated into tissue lipids (8), from which storage sites they are released to act as either intracellular messengers or in an autocrine or paracrine man-

J. Quilley, C. P. Bell-Quilley, J. C. McGiff: Department of Pharmacology, New York Medical College, Valhalla, New York 10595.

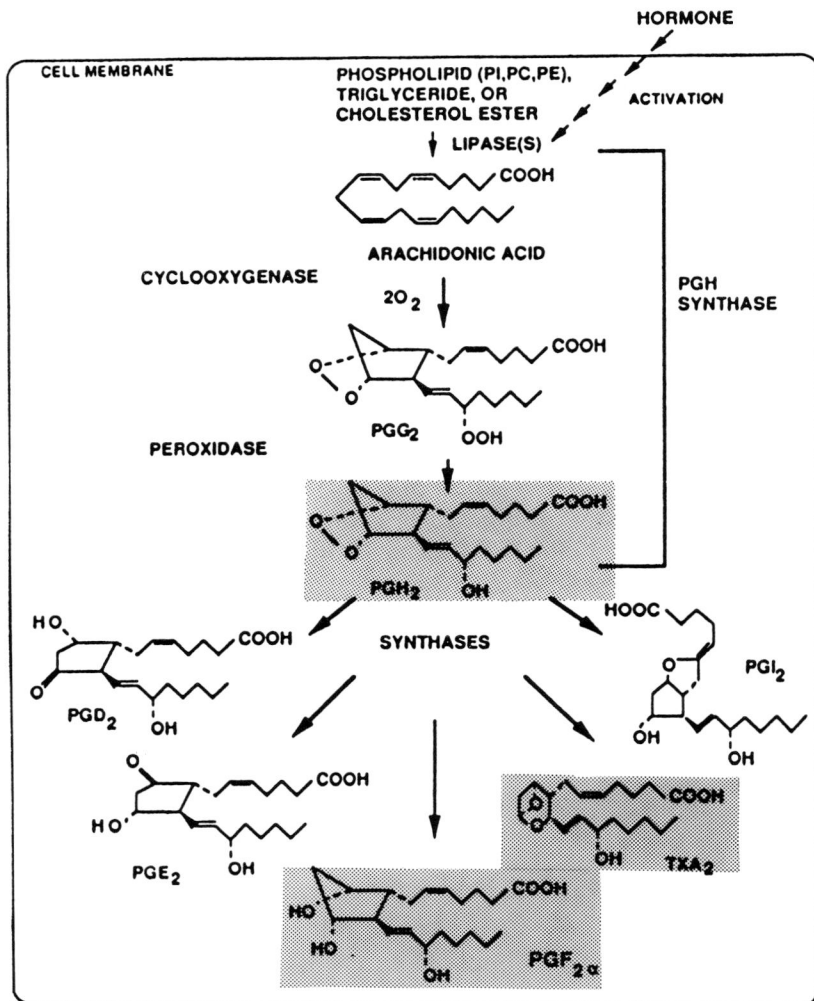

FIG. 1. Hormone-activated prostanoid biosynthesis in a model cell. Although all products of the "cyclooxygenase pathway" are shown, usually only one prostanoid is formed as a major product by a given cell type. PGH, prostaglandin endoperoxide; PI, PC, and PE, phosphatidylinositol, -choline, and -ethanolamine, respectively; PGG₂, PGD₂, PGE₂, and PGF₂α, prostaglandins G₂, D₂, E₂ and F₂α, respectively; PGI₂, prostacyclin; TxA₂, thromboxane A₂. *Stippling* identifies the prohypertensive prostanoids in contrast to PGI₂ and PGE₂, the antihypertensive prostanoids. (From ref. 6, with permission.)

ner. Further, while in storage in membrane-associated phospholipids, they affect, presumably, membrane properties such as fluidity (9).

Phospholipase can be activated by a variety of stimuli, including circulating and local hormones, neurotransmitters, membrane perturbations, and mechanical disruption. Hormonal stimulation can result in the activation of more than one type of lipase (6). For example, angiotensin II receptors are coupled to both phospholipase A_2 and phospholipase C (10). In most tissues the effects of angiotensin II are mediated by the phospholipase C cascade that is preceded by activation of specific angiotensin receptors (AT_1), resulting in a transmembrane signal that is transduced by guanosine triphosphate (GTP)-binding proteins, the G proteins. These G proteins, then, stimulate effector systems; the most prominent, relative to the actions of angiotensin II, is phospholipase C (10). G proteins also regulate binding affinity of angiotensin II to its receptor as well as coupling of the receptor to its effector. Activation of phospholipase C results in the formation of inositol-

1,4,5-trisphosphate (IP_3) and diacylglycerol from phosphatidyl inositol-4,5-bisphosphate (PIP_2) (11). IP_3 causes mobilization of intracellular Ca^{2+} from the endoplasmic reticulum and initiates the influx of extracellular Ca^{2+}. The resultant increase in intracellular Ca^{2+} activates phospholipase A_2 to release AA. Phospholipase A_2 can also be stimulated to release AA independently of prior activation of phospholipase C (6). In addition, AA is released in the phospholipase C cascade as the result of sequential activities of diacylglycerol lipase and monoglyceride lipase, acting on diglycerides and monoglycerides, respectively (6).

The major signaling system for angiotensin II, as indicated, is phospholipase C, notable exceptions being those in the glomerular mesangium and proximal tubules of the kidney (10). In the proximal tubules, adenylyl cyclase is integral to a mechanism subserving the antinatriuretic action of angiotensin II and considered "unique to the kidney." In this setting, decreased levels of adenosine 3',5'-cyclic monophosphate (cAMP) induced by angiotensin II are associated with decreased activity of protein kinase A, which, in turn, reduces phosphorylation of the Na^+/H^+ exchanger (antiporter), thereby diminishing an inhibitory influence on the exchanger and promoting increased proximal tubular sodium reabsorption (10). An eicosanoid-dependent step, thus far not identified, may participate in this sequence by reducing cAMP levels in the proximal tubules and/or by modifying directly the activity of the Na^+/H^+ exchange mechanism. In contrast to the exchanger, which is stimulated by picomolar concentrations of angiotensin II, nanomolar concentrations produce natriuresis through a mechanism acting independently of adenylyl cyclase and mediated by a nonprostaglandin eicosanoid generated by a cytochrome P-450 oxygenase (P-450-AA) (12). In this sequence, phospholipase A_2 is responsible for releasing AA from phospholipids. The prevalent renal phospholipase A_2 is a large (110 kDa) cytosolic protein, activated by a rise in cytosolic Ca^{2+}, showing specificity for phospholipids having arachidonate acylated at the Sn-2 position and responsive to stimulation by hormones (13). Within the kidney, zonal stratification of phospholipase A_2 has been reported and resembles that of cyclooxygenase, the highest activity being present in the papilla and the lowest in the cortex (14). Bradykinin, as well as angiotensin II, has the capacity to stimulate renal phospholipase A_2 (14). In the rat made diabetic and hypertensive with streptozo-

tocin, the renal vasodilator response to bradykinin was attenuated, associated with greatly reduced phospholipase A_2 activity and diminished release of PGE_2 into the renal venous effluent (14). Phospholipase activity has also been reported to be altered in experimental and genetic models of hypertension, although the relationship of these findings to hypertension is uncertain (15).

The release of AA in response to high concentrations of angiotensin II in the proximal tubular fluid, as noted, results in transformation of AA to a cytochrome P-450 product, reported to be 5,6-epoxyeicosatrienoic acid (5,6-EET), a labile and potent eicosanoid that has been shown to increase cytosolic Ca^{2+} (12) (Fig. 2). This epoxide can assume vasoactive properties after an additional transformation step by cyclooxygenase to one or more prostaglandin analogues such as 5,6-epoxy PGE_1 (16). The effect of angiotensin II on proximal tubular epoxygenase activity is specific. Thus, parathyroid hormone and epidermal growth factor also increase formation of P-450-AA metabolites that affect proximal tubular transport, but do not elevate 5,6-EET levels in this nephron segment (17). Rather, they increase formation of 20-hydroxyeicosatetraenoic acid (20-HETE) (Fig. 2), the ω-hydroxylase product of the cytochrome P-450 system (17) and the principal eicosanoid produced by the medullary thick ascending limb of Henle's loop (mTALH) of

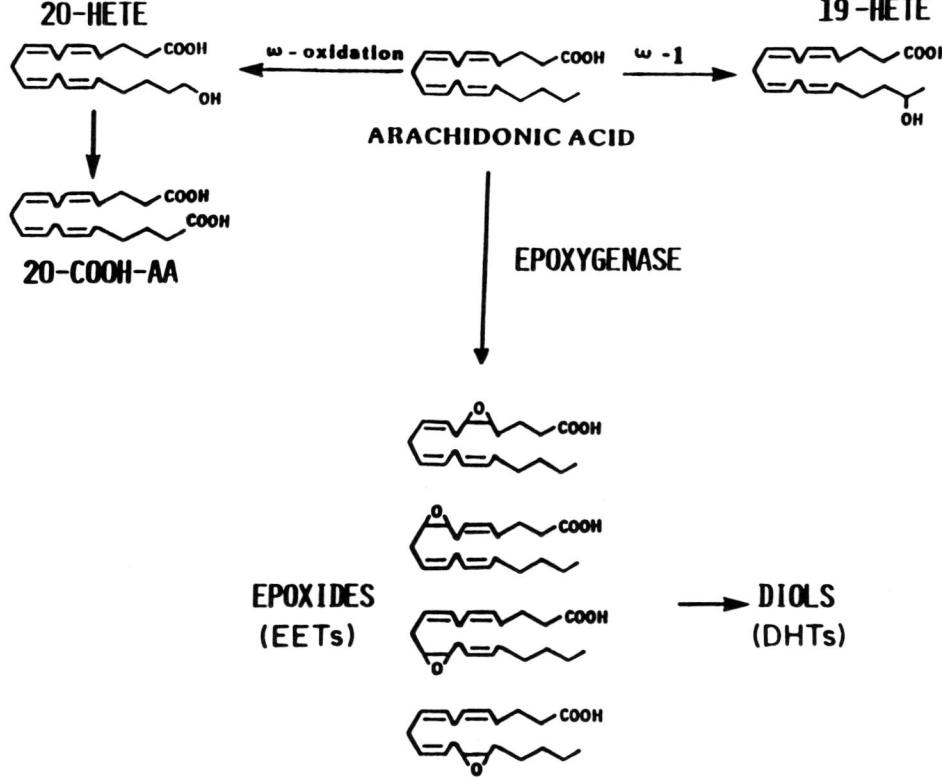

FIG. 2. Cytochrome P-450 metabolites of arachidonic acid. The epoxides from *top* to *bottom* are 5,6; 8,9; 11,12; and 14,15. These give rise to the vicinal diols or dihydroxy compounds, DHTs.

the rabbit (9). ADH also stimulates cytochrome P-450–dependent oxygenation of AA and interacts with the resultant P-450-AA metabolites in both the collecting ducts and the mTALH (18–20).

Cyclooxygenase and lipoxygenases, in the presence of oxygen, catalyze hydrogen removal, rearrangement of double bonds, and insertion of oxygen to produce unstable intermediates of AA, the hydroperoxyeicosatetraenoic acids (HPETEs), which give rise to their corresponding hydroxy acids, the HETEs (21). Cyclooxygenase activity results in the formation of 11-HPETE, the cyclization of which yields PGG_2, which, in turn, undergoes peroxidation to yield PGH_2, the precursor of prostaglandins and thromboxane. The cyclooxygenase and hydroperoxidase activities have not been separated and are attributed to a single enzyme complex (6). Therefore, the more accurate designation of this enzyme is PGH synthase, not cyclooxygenase, as the end product of the sequential operation of a single enzyme complex, embracing both cyclooxygenase and peroxidase activities, is PGH_2. However, cyclooxygenase will be used throughout this chapter because of familiarity and general usage. The principal prostaglandins—D_2, E_2, $F_{2\alpha}$, and I_2—and thromboxane A_2 (TxA_2) are generated by enzymic transformation of PGH_2 (Fig. 1). The proportions of these products will depend upon the relative abundance of the specific transforming enzymes and cofactors in a given tissue. Tissue injury and disease, particularly in association with invasion by the cells of inflammation, will change the profile of eicosanoids generated by that tissue.

One of the more interesting recent developments, having multiple ramifications in the areas of the physiology and pathophysiology of blood pressure regulation, as well as drug development, is the identification of an inducible form of cyclooxygenase (COX), designated COX-2 (PGH synthase-2), the constitutive form of the enzyme being COX-1 (PGH synthase-1) (22). These cyclooxygenase isozymes demonstrate approximately 75% homology. COX-1 is the principal enzyme in most organs and cell lines and is the dominant, if not the only, form present in the adult kidney under physiological conditions (6). COX-2 can be induced by cytokines released during inflammation, cell injury, and repair. The levels of messenger RNA (mRNA) of COX-1 and COX-2 genes are expressed differently with respect to magnitude and time (6,23). COX-2 mRNA increases precipitously from undetectable levels, peaks within 1 to 3 hours, and rapidly returns to low levels, whereas COX-1 mRNA shows a much slower onset and levels persist for much longer periods than those of COX-2.

Glucocorticoids have been shown to suppress expression of COX-2 on exposure of mice to lipopolysaccharide (endotoxin) (22). Indeed, the degree of hypotension and circulatory embarrassment that is produced after administration of endotoxin can be greatly potentiated by

adrenalectomy and, contrarily, can be reduced by treatment with drugs that suppress prostaglandin synthesis, either glucocorticoids or aspirin-like compounds. The failure of some aspirin-like drugs to affect prostaglandin synthesis, as, for example, in the gravid uterus (24) and in certain disease states, may reflect elevation of COX-2 levels in these conditions. Differences in susceptibility of COX-1 and COX-2 to inhibition by aspirin-like drugs may "underlie the unique pharmacological profiles of different" antiinflammatory drugs and may determine the capacity of aspirin-like drugs to elevate blood pressure more readily in some species than in others, as well as determine age- and sex-related differences in the blood pressure-elevating capabilities of aspirin-like drugs (6). For example, for the more frequently used drugs of this class, several have a lower potency relative to COX-2 as compared to COX-1. Cytokines, particularly interleukin-1 (IL-1) and tumor necrosis factor, have been identified as major factors contributing to the expression of COX-2. Further, they may exert this effect through a prior action on the inducible form of nitric oxide synthase (25). IL-1 has been reported to reduce blood pressure, an effect presumably having some dependency on a prostaglandin component, as the natriuretic action of IL-1 and the tumor necrosis factor are dependent on production of PGE_2 (26).

The hydroperoxy fatty acids formed by the various lipoxygenase enzymes include 5-, 8-, 12-, and 15-HPETEs and the corresponding HETEs (27). A dehydrase transforms 5-HPETE to an unstable 5,6-epoxide or leukotriene A_4 (LTA_4), which is the precursor of leukotrienes. Hydrolase activity converts LTA_4 to LTB_4. Glutathione-transferase is the first step in the formation of the peptido leukotrienes. LTC_4 is converted to LTD_4 by γ-glutamyl-transpeptidase; LTD_4, in turn, can be transformed in some tissues to LTE_4. In addition to the leukotrienes, 12-HPETE generated by several tissues can be transformed into hydroxy epoxide metabolites, the hepoxilins (28). Hepoxilins have been shown to promote insulin secretion, calcium mobilization, and to act as second messengers.

The third pathway of AA oxygenation is via cytochrome P-450–dependent monooxygenases, which require molecular oxygen and nicotinamide adenine dinucleotide phosphate, reduced (NADPH) (29). This system metabolizes AA to generate epoxides 5,6-, 8,9-, 11,12-, and 14,15-epoxyeicosatrienoic acids (EETs) and their corresponding vicinal diols, the dihydroxyeicosatrienoic acids (DHTs), as well as mono-HETEs (Fig. 2). The initial studies on the biological effects of the P-450-AA products demonstrated potent vasoactivity and the capacity to influence transport processes (18,30), properties strongly suggesting that they participate in blood pressure control. The mono-HETE, 12(R)-HETE, possesses an interesting biological profile: inhibition of renin release (31) and Na^+,K^+–adenosine triphosphatase

(ATPase) (9) and involvement in the vascular response to injury (32).

AA metabolites, formed in response to hormonal stimulation, act as local modulators by either moderating or amplifying effects of the hormone and, in some instances, mediating the action of the hormone (33). Once released from tissue storage in phospholipids, triglycerides, or cholesterol esters (Fig. 1), AA is rapidly metabolized to a variety of products depending upon the tissue, the species, and the stimulus as well as the presence of injury, stress, or disease (34). For example, within the vasculature, eicosanoid production varies (a) longitudinally, the larger vessels producing predominantly PGI_2 and the microvasculature synthesizing mainly PGE_2, and (b) transversely, the endothelium generating PGI_2, P-450-AA products, and lipoxygenase-derived HETEs, a different profile from that of vascular smooth muscle (9,35,36). Similarly, there are zonal variations within the kidney with respect to cyclooxgenase activity, which is much higher in the medulla and papilla than in the cortex (37), corresponding to regional variations in phospholipase activity (14).

Cytochrome P-450–dependent monooxygenases, capable of metabolizing AA, are found in the renal tubules and in blood vessels, including the endothelium and smooth muscle (9). In the nephron, not only is there segmentation of transport function and hormonal responsiveness, but also segmentation of AA metabolism with respect to pathways (cyclooxygenase versus P-450 monooxygenases) and eicosanoid productive capacity (9). For example, the cortical collecting tubules have a large capacity to generate prostaglandins, whereas proximal tubules and the mTALH normally have a negligible capacity to form prostaglandins but metabolize AA via P-450 monooxygenases to EETs and HETEs (6,12,38). The mTALH, which plays a critical role in salt and water metabolism, has been shown to generate three principal P-450-AA products (38): 1,20-eicosatetraenedioic acid (20-COOH-AA) and 19- and 20-hydroxyeicosatetraenoic acids (19- and 20-HETEs), all of which possess the capability to affect transport function of renal tubules, either by inhibiting the Na^+,K^+-$2Cl^-$ cotransporter, the target of "loop diuretics" such as furosemide, or by affecting the activity of Na^+,K^+-ATPase (20,38). It should be recalled that Na^+,K^+-ATPase (the Na^+ pump) is ultimately responsible for all active sodium transport intrarenally. Consequently, eicosanoids, which are capable of affecting the activity of the Na^+ pump, have particular significance for the development and maintenance of certain forms of hypertension (18).

Tissue variations in AA metabolism also become apparent when comparing platelets, neutrophils, and endothelial cells. Platelets produce almost exclusively TxA_2 via cyclooxygenase and 12-(S)HETE via 12-lipoxygenase (39), whereas neutrophils synthesize predominantly AA metabolites via 5-lipoxygenase (40). In contrast, most endothelial cells synthesize PGI_2 and PGE_2, the lipoxygenase products 12- and 15-HETEs, as well as P-450-AA metabolites (41,42).

GENERATION OF PROSTAGLANDINS BY BLOOD VESSELS

The capacity of blood vessels to generate prostacyclin (PGI_2) is essential to the integrity of the endothelium and contributes to the regulation of vasomotion (36). Production of vascular prostacyclin can be reduced by other AA metabolites arising from lipoxygenases and, possibly, cytochrome P-450 monooxygenases. The earliest *in vitro* studies on prostacyclin production recognized the potential inhibitory properties of 12- and 15-HETEs on prostacyclin synthase (36,43). A recent study by Lin et al. (44) of rats made hypertensive by constriction of the aorta between the origin of the renal arteries demonstrated the importance of interactions of cyclooxygenase and lipoxygenase pathways to blood pressure homeostasis. Vascular prostacyclin production was greatly reduced by 12-HETE. Coincident with the development of hypertension and increased vascular reactivity, the levels of 12-HETE increased in the aorta, associated with enhanced vascular production of PGH_2, the vasoconstrictor prostaglandin endoperoxide. On the other hand, PGE_2, the prototypical eicosanoid modulator, can suppress the activity of lipoxygenases, as first shown by Kuehl et al. (45) for 5-lipoxygenase activity in neutrophils. Further, the vascular actions of angiotensin II that are expressed through 12- and 15-HETEs (46) acting as second messengers are, presumably, subject to modulation by PGE_2 by virtue of an inhibitory action of PGE_2 on lipoxygenase activity (45).

Under conditions of stress, such as anesthesia and surgery, volume depletion, and systemic disease, prostaglandin production, chiefly by the vasculature, will be directed toward maintaining organ function in the face of potentially detrimental stimuli. This is exemplified by the effects of inhibition of prostaglandin synthesis on the renal circulation in anesthetized dogs (47), subject to laparotomy or to any potentially noxious influence that stimulates the renin-angiotensin system. A precipitous increase in renovascular resistance occurs in response to nonsteroidal antiinflammatory drugs (NSAIDs), such as indomethacin, only in surgically stressed animals. In contrast, in resting normal dogs, indomethacin does not affect renal blood flow even at doses that are toxic. In the hypertensive state, particularly with the progression of vascular disease, the renal circulation becomes increasingly dependent on prostaglandin-related mechanisms and, therefore, susceptible to the negative vascular effects of aspirin-like drugs (48). Under conditions of tissue damage such as the multiple forms of glomerulonephritis, hydronephrosis, endothelial injury, and vasculitis associated with severe hypertension, an abnormal profile of eicosanoids is produced by blood vessels because of endothelial dysfunction, the presence of invading white cells, and deposition of platelets at the site of endothelial injury. Endothelial damage with concomitant reduction of PGI_2 synthesis, the latter, perhaps, mediated by 12-HETE, can lead to platelet clumping and adhesion to the vascular wall and increased PGH_2 and TxA_2 synthesis, thereby shifting the balance (PGI_2 vs TxA_2 and PGH_2) toward proaggregatory, vasoconstrictor products (36). This is considered to be a major determinant of the development of toxemia of pregnancy (49). The interactions of these products of AA metabolism hold the key to understanding the balance of forces, both pro- and antihypertensive, the shift of which contributes to elevation of blood pressure (Fig. 3).

Eicosanoids are major contributors to the outcome of the dynamic interactions that determine whether blood pressure is maintained at normotensive levels. Further, there are species of eicosanoids that are clearly prohypertensive, acting either directly, such as TxA_2, by constricting blood vessels (50), or indirectly, such as 12-HETE, by inhibiting production of vasodilator eicosanoids (44). The extent of the eicosanoid network is evident from the effects of the principal modulator eicosanoid, PGE_2, that not only dampens pressor system activity, including the renin-angiotensin, ADH, and adrenergic nervous systems, but also amplifies the vasodilator-diuretic activity of the kallikrein-kinin system (51,52). The pressor systems, such as the interdependent sympathetic nervous and ADH–renin-angiotensin systems, when stimulated, act in concert to retain salt and water and increase vascular resistance (53). Expansion of body fluid volume and increased vascular tone will go unchecked in the face of defects in specific pathways of AA metabolism normally engaged to counteract the influence of prohypertensive stimuli. The contribution of eicosanoids to the regulation of blood pressure will now be considered, as they modulate the renin-angiotensin and autonomic nervous systems, amplify the depressor kallikrein-kinin system, and affect salt and water balance.

PROSTAGLANDINS AS MODULATORS

Prostaglandins Modulate Pressor Hormones

The ability of prostaglandins to moderate the vasoconstrictor-antidiuretic action of pressor hormones was demonstrated more than two decades ago (54). Infusion of angiotensin II into the canine renal artery released prostaglandins from the kidney associated with blunting of the vasoconstrictor and salt and water retaining effects of the peptide (55). The original studies were conducted before the discovery by Vane (56) that aspirin-like drugs inhibited prostaglandin synthesis. Therefore, the relationship between infusion of angiotensin II and release of prostaglandins had to be regarded as an interesting correlation. A cause-and-effect relationship in terms of antagonism of the renal actions of angiotensin II by prostaglandins was established only after the demonstration that inhibition of cyclooxygenase by aspirin-like drugs enhanced the renal vasoconstrictor and sodium-retaining actions of angiotensin II (57). Moreover, after inhibition of prostaglandin synthesis, the heightened renal response to angiotensin II could be dampened by coadministration of PGE_2 (58). In this study, the modulatory action of PGE_2 on the renal vasoconstrictor response to angiotensin II was compared in spontaneously hypertensive rats (SHRs) and Wistar-Kyoto (WKY) rats and was shown to be deficient in the SHR. The infusion of either PGE_2 or PGI_2 blunted the renal vasoconstrictor effect of angiotensin II in the WKY but not in the SHR. As no differences were observed in either number or affinity of glomerular PGE_2 and PGI_2 receptors, a defective signaling system, perhaps involving adenylyl cyclase, was proposed to underlie the impaired buffering capacity of prostaglandins in the SHR. The antagonistic effect of PGE_2 on the actions of angiotensin II, presumably, is related to the capacity of PGE_2 to inhibit formation of lipoxygenase products, principally 12- and 15-HETEs (45). Thus, inhibition of lipoxygenase activity prevented several effects of angiotensin II such as stimulation of aldosterone secretion (59) and inhibition of renin release (60). Lipoxygenase inhibitors also attenuated angiotensin II–induced elevations in blood pressure in normotensive rats and lowered blood pressure in renovascular hypertensive rats, a renin-dependent form of hypertension (61). In support of these studies on the importance of one or more lipoxygenase products to the vascular actions of angiotensin II, Bell-Quilley et al. (46) have shown that the negative renal hemodynamic effects of angiotensin II can be prevented by inhibition of renal lipoxygenases.

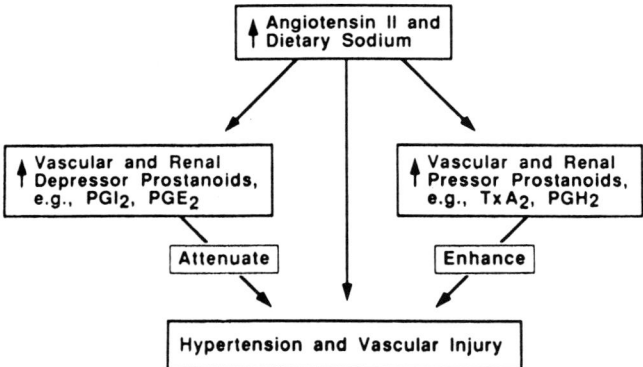

FIG. 3. Prostanoid-mediated prohypertensive and antihypertensive mechanisms in rats with severe angiotensin II–salt hypertension.

Close examination of the interactions of pressor hormones and prostaglandins will reveal some aspects of the mechanisms involved. In response to either angiotensin II or norepinephrine, prostaglandin concentrations in renal venous blood increased rapidly—within 90 seconds—by 50- to 100-fold (62). Inasmuch as prostaglandins are not stored, this represents *de novo* synthesis. The initial studies were conducted in the kidney because of the central role of renal mechanisms in blood pressure control. The modulatory role of prostaglandins in opposing pressor hormones has been subsequently extended to the general circulation, as it was demonstrated that all blood vessels are capable of generating eicosanoids (36,63).

The role of prostaglandins as local hormones that modulate pressor systems is exemplified in the participation of prostaglandin-dependent mechanisms in the acute circulatory response to renal artery stenosis (64). Within 2 to 4 minutes after constricting a canine renal artery, prostaglandins are released into the venous blood of the ischemic kidney and within 7 minutes prostaglandins appear in the venous blood of the uninvolved or contralateral kidney (Fig. 4). As the primary renal prostaglandins do not survive passage across the lungs (65,66), their appearance in the venous effluent of the contralateral kidney cannot be explained by their production in the ischemic kidney. Rather, activation of prostaglandin synthesis by the nonischemic kidney depended on stimulation of the renin-angiotensin system.

Plasma renin activity and angiotensin II levels in the circulating blood had increased by severalfold at the time of elevated prostaglandin levels in the nonischemic kidney. As angiotensin II can stimulate renal prostaglandin production, it was concluded that angiotensin II released prostaglandins from the contralateral kidney as well as from the ischemic kidney. Further, a prostaglandin mechanism is involved in renin release from the ischemic kidney. That is to say, prostaglandins can function as prohypertensive agents by promoting renin release while simultaneously acting to counteract the local renal effects of blood pressure elevating systems. This apparent paradox can be resolved by recognizing that (a) elevation of arterial blood pressure mediated by stimulation of the renin-angiotensin system is directed toward restoration of blood flow to the ischemic kidney, which initially "sees" low perfusion pressures; and (b) in the face of elevated angiotensin II levels, renal blood flow and salt excretion would be further reduced in the ischemic kidney but for the counteracting action of vasodilator prostaglandins, as well as other eicosanoids such as 5,6-EET acting on the proximal tubules (12). The interplay of blood pressure regulating systems set in motion by constriction of a renal artery finally results in restoration of blood flow to the ischemic kidney associated with a renal perfusion pressure that has returned to preconstriction levels distal to the renal artery stenosis and elevated prox-

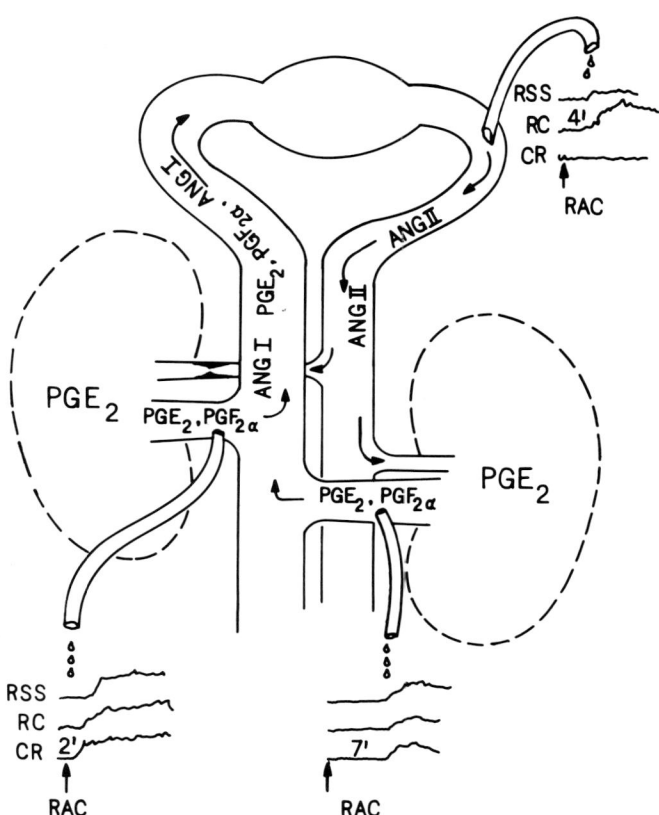

FIG. 4. The effect of right renal arterial constriction on prostaglandin release by the ischemic and contralateral kidneys. Three banks of organs continuously sampled venous blood of each kidney and aortic blood for changes in concentrations of prostaglandins. Within 2 minutes (2') after constriction of the right renal artery, prostaglandins (PGE$_2$ and PGF$_{2\alpha}$) appeared in venous blood of the ischemic kidney as indicated by contraction of the three assay organs (*lower left*). Within 7 minutes (7') after induction of renal ischemia, the contralateral kidney released prostaglandin-like substances probably mediated by angiotensin II (*lower right,* see text). The assay organs monitoring aortic blood (*upper right*) contracted in a manner consistent with increased generation of angiotensin(s) (contraction of RC, primarily). Thoracic caval and renal venous blood, obtained at the time of peak activity of the assay organs, were extracted and purified; PGE$_2$ and PGF$_{2\alpha}$ were recovered from samples of renal venous blood. Caval plasma showed greater than tenfold increase in renin activity. RSS, rat stomach strip; RC, rat colon; CR, chick rectum.

imally, the latter reflecting systemic hypertension. The hypertension, therefore, represents a compensatory mechanism to restore blood flow to an ischemic kidney. Local release of eicosanoids aid in this effort by limiting the effects of angiotensin II on renal function, possibly by inhibiting production of 12-HETE, the putative second messenger that mediates the renovascular actions of angiotensin II (46). In addition, eicosanoid-related mechanisms operating within renal tubular segments modulate the effects of angiotensin II on tubular transport (10,12).

Prostaglandins Interact with the Kallikrein-Kinin System

Prostaglandins subserve antihypertensive mechanisms not only by opposing the blood pressure–elevating effects of pressor systems, but also by augmenting and mediating the vasodilator-diuretic actions of the kallikrein-kinin system (52). Peptide-induced formation of prostaglandins by blood vessels results in changes in the intensity and range of the vascular effects of peptides (33). Further, prostaglandins are involved in the activation of the kallikrein-kinin, neurohypophyseal, and renin-angiotensin systems. Thus, in addition to the extensively studied prostaglandin component in renin release (67–69), there is evidence that a prostaglandin-dependent mechanism participates in the regulation of kallikrein (70) and ADH release (71).

Kinins dilate arteries and arterioles by stimulating production of several vasodilator mediators of endothelial origin, chiefly nitric oxide (NO) and AA metabolites arising from cyclooxygenase and cytochrome P-450 monooxygenases (72–74). Interactions involving kinins and prostaglandins were first observed in the canine kidney (75) and resulted in a spate of studies with variable conclusions regarding the importance of a putative prostaglandin component in the vascular action of kinins. The degree of participation of prostaglandins in the vascular responses to kinins has been attributed to (a) the dose and manner of administration (bolus versus infusion) of kinins, (b) the species studied, and (c) the state of salt and water balance of the animal (76,77).

The contribution of prostaglandin-related mechanisms to the renal effects of bradykinin was studied in the canine blood-perfused isolated kidney (72). This preparation eliminates extrarenal factors, thereby facilitating analysis of renal kinin-prostaglandin interactions. The prostaglandin component of the renal vasodilator action of bradykinin, estimated by comparing the vasodilator effects of the peptide before and after inhibition of prostaglandin synthesis, was 30%. The diuretic action of bradykinin was entirely dependent on a prostaglandin component, in contrast to kinin-induced natriuresis, which was expressed only after inhibition of prostaglandin synthesis. Mullane and Moncada (78) have followed the time course of the prostaglandin component of the renal vasodilator action of bradykinin. They demonstrated that kinin-induced vasodilation became increasingly prostaglandin-dependent after 2 minutes of infusion.

Recent studies have addressed several components that are responsible for the vasodilator responses to kinins. In particular, the NO component has been examined and found to be either negligible in the rat heart (79) or to represent a significant component, albeit one of several, in the rat kidney (74). Cachofeiro et al. (80) found that the renal vasodilator response of the SHR to brady-kinin was only 50% dependent on a NO component, as determined by the capacity of nitroarginine to reduce the kinin-induced vasodilation. Inhibition of NO synthase by nitroarginine was complete, as the attendant increase in guanosine 3',5'-cyclic monophosphate (cGMP) produced by bradykinin was abolished. The several components of the renal vasodilatation produced by bradykinin in the normotensive rat have been analyzed and can be resolved in terms of a minor prostaglandin component and two major components, one NO, and the other, cytochrome P-450-AA metabolites (74). An important issue to be resolved is whether these several vascular components change in a predictable fashion in the face of hypertension, either experimental or genetic.

Renal kinins and AA products act in concert to regulate renal blood flow and its zonal distribution. That intrarenal blood flow distribution is dependent upon kinin and prostaglandin interactions was demonstrated by (a) inhibition of kallikrein with aprotinin and (b) prostaglandin synthesis with indomethacin. Either intervention prevented the zonal redistribution of increased renal blood flow from cortex to medulla produced by an angiotensin-converting enzyme inhibitor (81). Renal papillary blood flow appears to be regulated independently of cortical blood flow through both the kallikrein-kinin and renin-angiotensin systems acting in a reciprocal manner to increase and decrease, respectively, blood flow to the papilla (82). These observations on regulation of renal medullary and papillary blood flow are important to the urinary concentrating mechanism and the excretion of a dilute urine. There is evidence that the interactions of these hormonal pressor and depressor systems within the renal tubular system affect the excretion of urine in a manner analogous to their interactions within the vasculature to regulate renal hemodynamics (83). The evidence for their participation in the regulation of extracellular fluid volume will now be reviewed.

Eicosanoids Affect Salt and Water Balance

Kinin-prostaglandin interactions are favored by conditions existing in the distal nephron and collecting tubules (83). In response to ADH, kallikrein, synthesized in connecting tubule cells (84) of the distal nephron, has been reported to enter the tubular fluid and the renal interstitial space where it liberates kinins from kininogen (85). Kinins stimulate release of PGE_2 from the cells lining the collecting tubules into tubular and vascular compartments (86). PGE_2 then inhibits the hydroosmotic effect of ADH and augments medullary blood flow, actions that favor the excretion of dilute urine (87).

In addition to regulating water excretion, prostaglandins can affect sodium chloride excretion by a direct action on tubular function, as well as indirectly by influencing changes in renal hemodynamics. A direct effect of prostaglandins on tubular transport was demonstrated by increased urinary recovery of microinjected ^{22}Na in response to PGE$_2$, also given by microinjection into the renal tubules (88). PGE$_2$ and PGI$_2$ have been shown to inhibit sodium transport at several sites in the nephron (89,90).

The natriuretic action of high concentrations of angiotensin II in the proximal tubules may depend, as noted, on the formation of 5,6-EET, which has also been shown to inhibit arginine vasopressin (AVP)–induced water flow in the rabbit cortical collecting ducts (19). As this inhibitory effect of 5,6-EET on the action of AVP is cyclooxygenase-dependent, it may be expressed through induction of PGE$_2$ formation by the epoxide (91). Alternatively, 5,6-EET may be transformed via cyclooxygenase to a PGE$_1$ analogue that acts in concert with PGE$_2$ to inhibit the hydroosmotic effect of ADH (91).

Untransformed AA and PGE$_2$ have been reported to modulate K$^+$ efflux in the cortical collecting tubules (92). Further, as reviewed previously, AA metabolites, 20-HETE and 20-COOH-AA, generated by cytochrome P-450 monooxygenase in mTALH (38), can inhibit the Na$^+$,K$^+$-2Cl$^-$ cotransporter in a furosemide-like manner (20). Studies performed under physiological conditions also point to participation of eicosanoid-dependent mechanisms in the control of extracellular fluid volume (93). This finding is in accord with the view that renal eicosanoids "affect several aspects of the countercurrent system in concert to effect regulation of water excretion" (87). Finally, it is important to recognize that AA metabolites generated by the cytochrome P-450 system also act as modulators of sodium, potassium, and chloride transport at several sites in the nephron, including the mTALH, proximal tubules, and collecting duct (12,19,20). The cytochrome P-450 system, via metabolism of AA and steroids, may prove to be of the greatest importance in regulating the ionic composition of body fluids. Indeed, evidence to be reviewed indicates that inhibition of formation of AA metabolites arising from this system can prevent blood pressure elevation in the young SHR, an effect associated with natriuresis (94).

Prostaglandins Modulate the Autonomic Nervous System

The modulatory role of prostaglandins is also evident upon considering their interactions with the activity of the autonomic nervous system, particularly in terms of neurotransmitter release. While this function has been most intensively studied for adrenergic-mediated responses, other systems, such as dopaminergic and cholinergic, are also subject to prostaglandin regulation, both peripherally and centrally (95,96). An effect of prostaglandins of the E series on adrenergic neurotransmission at both pre- and postjunctional sites was recognized

early in studies of the possible biological roles of prostaglandins (97). PGE$_2$ was found to exert an inhibitory effect on norepinephrine release from postganglionic nerve terminals in response to nerve stimulation at a number of neuroeffector sites (98), including the heart, kidney, and blood vessels (99).

Renal adrenergic innervation is dense and has a wide range of functional implications, including regulation of GFR, renal blood flow and its distribution, tubular transport, and renin secretion among others (100). Local mechanisms, including those having a prostaglandin component, have been shown to modulate the response to enhanced activity of the sympathetic nervous system, prejunctionally, by affecting release of norepinephrine, and, postjunctionally, by affecting the response to norepinephrine (97–99).

PGE$_2$, under physiological conditions, acts principally prejunctionally to inhibit norepinephrine release from adrenergic nerve endings. The evidence for this has been obtained primarily from studies of the vascular response of the kidney to nerve stimulation and is as follows: Infusion of PGE$_2$ attenuated the renal vasoconstrictor response to nerve stimulation to a greater extent than to injected norepinephrine (101). Moreover, dampening of renal vasoconstriction induced by exogenous PGE$_2$ was correlated with diminished output of norepinephrine (99). Contrariwise, inhibition of prostaglandin synthesis potentiated the renal vasoconstrictor effect of nerve stimulation associated with enhanced norepinephrine release, which effects could be reversed by administered PGE$_2$. Further, AA mimicked the inhibitory action of PGE$_2$ on constriction of the renal vasculature induced by nerve stimulation (99,102). The release of prostaglandins by nerve stimulation was independent of mechanical events (98) and, in keeping with a neuromodulatory role, prostaglandins were synthesized in amounts considerably above basal levels in response to sympathetic nerve stimulation (103), supporting the hypothesis that the local release of PGE$_2$ served in a negative feedback mechanism modulating norepinephrine outflow (104). Inhibition of norepinephrine release by PGE$_2$ is closely related to restricting Ca^{2+} entry into the nerve terminal, as release of norepinephrine from adrenergic terminals in response to depolarization induced by the action potential is "absolutely dependent upon extracellular Ca^{2+}" (99). Although much of the released prostaglandin appeared to be of extraneuronal origin (release from postjunctional effector cells being evoked as part of the effector response), there was also indirect evidence for release from nerves (98,99).

A prejunctional inhibitory action of PGE$_2$ on adrenergic neurotransmission can be demonstrated even when PGE$_2$ constricts the vasculature under nonphysiological experimental conditions such as the rat isolated kidney perfused with an artificial solution (105). On the other hand, PGF$_{2\alpha}$ and prostacyclin did not affect neurotransmitter release under these experimental conditions. Neither did U-46619, the thromboxane-prostaglandin endoperoxide mimetic. PGE_2 also exhibited inhibitory prejunctional effects on norepinephrine release in the isolated kidney of the rabbit, a species that does not demonstrate the paradoxical vasoconstrictor response of the rat isolated kidney to PGE_2 (102). Moreover, prostaglandin-dependent mechanisms act prejunctionally under conditions approaching the physiological, as evidenced by the enhanced release of norepinephrine produced by stimulating the renal nerves when prostaglandin synthesis was inhibited in the blood-perfused kidney of the anesthetized rat (106).

Norepinephrine releases PGE_2 from the kidney by activating renal α_1-adrenoceptors linked to phospholipase A_2, by a GTP-binding, pertussis toxin–sensitive G protein (98), an effect that can be separated from the resulting vasoconstriction. In other neuroeffector sites, such as the heart, prostaglandin production in response to norepinephrine is likely mediated by phospholipase C linked to β_1-adrenergic receptors (98). These prostaglandin-dependent mechanisms are thought to act in concert with other modulators such as prejunctional α_2-adrenoceptors that regulate norepinephrine release independently of prostaglandins (98,99).

The positive effect of β_1-adrenergic receptor stimulation on prostaglandin synthesis is, itself, subject to modulation by cAMP (107). Thus, inhibition of prostaglandin synthesis has been reported to be produced by cAMP (108), which levels are increased by stimulation of cardiac β_1-adrenergic receptors (107). The inhibitory effect of cAMP on prostaglandin synthesis has been related to suppression of cytosolic Ca^{2+}, which, in turn, reduces availability of AA, secondarily to decreasing the activity of Ca^{2+}-dependent phospholipases (109).

In contrast to the inhibitory effects of PGE_2 and PGI_2 on sympathetic neuroeffector responses, $PGF_{2\alpha}$ was found to be facilitatory (110), suggesting that this effect might contribute to its pressor action. However, the small quantities of $PGF_{2\alpha}$ released from nerve endings make it unlikely that its presynaptic facilitatory effect has significance for blood pressure regulation. Potentiation of the responses to sympathetic nerve stimulation via primarily a presynaptic effect also has been suggested for TxA_2, based on the observation that the thromboxane mimic, endoperoxide analogue U46619, facilitates the responses to nerve stimulation (111). An additional mechanism for stimulation of thromboxane-induced vasoconstriction may operate through the parasympathetic nervous system, as cholinergic stimulation of the lung has been reported to evoke a thromboxane-dependent pulmonary vasoconstriction (112).

In terms of blood pressure regulation, the balance between the inhibitory and stimulatory effects of eicosanoids at pre- and postjunctional sites needs to be evaluated. A deficiency of prostaglandin mechanisms that

brake adrenergic vasoconstriction may exist in hypertensive humans. *In vivo* studies indicate that the overall effect of inhibition of prostaglandin synthesis with aspirin-like drugs is stimulation of sympathetic nervous activity based on increased urinary excretion (113) and enhanced turnover of norepinephrine in the absence of an effect on its metabolism or uptake (114).

Baroreceptor and Chemoreceptor Reflexes

It has been known for some time that PGI_2 affects sensory nerve activity. PGI_2 has been shown to activate cardiac afferent C fibers and to cause vagally mediated bradycardia and hypotension via the Bezold-Jarisch reflex (115,116). However, the concentrations of PGI_2 required to elicit this response are relatively high. Because PGI_2 is unlikely to act as a circulating hormone, in view of the very low blood levels reported under basal conditions (117), the physiological significance of this reflex has been questioned. Indeed, inhibitors of prostaglandin synthesis do not cause a resetting of the reflex. Nonetheless, the response to other agents that stimulate this cardiac reflex can be modulated by PGI_2 (118). Furthermore, locally generated prostacyclin within the vasculature, rather than circulating prostacyclin, may act on cardiovascular reflexes. Captopril also potentiates the reflex, an effect abolished by indomethacin (118). Although prostaglandin levels were not measured in this study, increased local PGI_2 release from the vascular wall provides an explanation for the resetting of cardiac reflexes after inhibiting angiotensin-converting enzyme with captopril.

In addition to an effect on cardiac chemoreceptors, prostaglandins, together with kinins, participate in the activation of renal chemoreceptors (119). This reflex is activated by renal artery stenosis and results in increased blood pressure and an associated increase in sympathetically mediated vasoconstriction in the mesenteric and hindquarter vascular beds. This overall pressor effect occurs despite the concomitant inhibition by prostaglandins of transmitter release from sympathetic terminals. Thus, prostaglandins participate in renal-cardiovascular integration by modulating the activity of chemoreceptor afferent nerves.

The resetting of arterial baroreceptors by a prostaglandin-dependent mechanism has been reported recently and has important implications for cardiovascular control and the development of hypertension (120). The resetting of arterial baroreceptors is accomplished by decreasing their sensitivity that results in elevated blood pressure through removal of a baroreceptor-mediated suppressive influence on efferent sympathetic nerve activity centrally. A deficiency of prostaglandin production, specifically PGI_2, has been implicated in the resetting of arterial baroreceptors and, thereby, the maintenance of hypertension, i.e., a prostaglandin-dependent mechanism increases baroreceptor sensitivity (121) and its removal permits resetting of the barorecep-tor at a higher level of arterial pressure. Thus, barorecep-tors located in the aortic arch and carotid sinus respond to increased arterial pressure with enhanced afferent nerve activity that results in reflex bradycardia and vaso-dilatation as a consequence of increased parasympa-thetic nervous activity and decreased sympathetic ner-vous activity. Increased endothelial production of PGI_2, resulting from mechanical deformation of the vascular wall, has been hypothesized to sensitize baroreceptors and to initiate the events that counter elevations in blood pressure. Thus, application of either PGI_2 or AA to the isolated carotid sinus dose-dependently increased baro-receptor activity, an effect that was abolished after either inhibition of cyclooxygenase or removal of the endothe-lium (122,123). Moreover, baroreceptor function was shown to be impaired in chronic hypertension and in other conditions of endothelial dysfunction associated with diminished conversion of AA to PGI_2 by the iso-lated carotid sinus (124). A defect in PGI_2 synthesizing capacity associated with resetting of baroreceptors ex-plains the failure of cyclooxygenase inhibition to influ-ence baroreceptor activity in hypertensive rabbits, whereas application of PGI_2 enhanced this activity (124).

THE ROLE OF EICOSANOIDS IN THE DEVELOPMENT AND MAINTENANCE OF HYPERTENSION

Definition of the variable, and sometimes opposing, roles of eicosanoids in the development and mainte-nance of hypertension is difficult because of the multi-plicity of eicosanoid products, the diversity of their bio-logical effects, and the interactions of products derived from different pathways of AA metabolism. These difficulties are apparent when attempting to interpret the effects of aspirin-like drugs on blood pressure regulation. Inhibition of prostaglandin synthesis with NSAIDs not only diminishes antihypertensive prostanoids, result-ing in fluid retention and increased vascular resis-tance, but also decreases formation of prohypertensive mediators such as TxA_2 and $PGF_{2\alpha}$ (125). In addition, prostaglandin-dependent mechanisms subserve renin re-lease, the putative secretagogue being either PGI_2 or its active metabolite, 6-keto-PGE_1 (69). Thus, the particular effect of inhibition of prostaglandin synthesis with a NSAID on blood pressure depends on the predominance of either prohypertensive or antihypertensive prosta-noids in the hypertensive subject or in the model of hy-pertension under study (126) (Fig. 3). Further complicat-ing the interpretation of the effects of NSAIDs on blood pressure are the following considerations: (a) the other pathways of AA metabolism, namely, lipoxygenases and cytochrome P-450–dependent monooxygenases, may be enhanced when the activity of the cyclooxygenase path-way is reduced (45); (b) inhibition of cyclooxygenase may not only reduce prostanoid formation but may also prevent the further metabolism of some cytochrome P-450-AA products by cyclooxygenase to compounds that have a different biological profile from the parent com-pound (9); and (c) NSAIDs have many effects unrelated to inhibition of cyclooxygenase, since they can affect calcium movement, cyclic nucleotide metabolism, prostaglandin-catabolizing enzymes, and activity of phospholipases (127).

Similarly, the use of thromboxane synthase inhibitors as tools for addressing the role of TxA_2 in hypertension is complicated, as blockade of TxA_2 synthesis may result in redirection of endoperoxide metabolism to vasodila-tor prostanoids and, secondly, will not prevent the ac-tions of the intermediate endoperoxides, which, like TxA_2, are potent vasoconstrictors. However, compari-son of the effects of thromboxane synthase inhibitors and TxA_2/PGH_2 receptor antagonists permits partial resolu-tion of these problems (128). It is now apparent that in some forms of experimental hypertension, TxA_2/PGH_2 receptors play a pivotal role in the elevation of blood pressure (126). The bulk of the evidence, however, sug-gests that AA metabolites may play a protective role in limiting the elevation of blood pressure by (a) maintain-ing the renal and other regional circulations in the face of progressively severe systemic disease involving the cardiovascular system (47), (b) contributing to a reduc-tion in extracellular fluid volume as a result of natriuretic and diuretic properties, and (c) attenuating the cardio-vascular and renal responses to pressor stimuli and am-plifying those responses to kinins and other blood pressure–lowering hormones. Thus, when prohyperten-sive systems are activated, prostaglandin biosynthesis is stimulated and acts as a brake. Consequently, in the event of a defect in synthesis of antihypertensive prosta-glandins, elevation of blood pressure may ensue (129). Nonetheless, there is evidence for increased prohyper-tensive AA product formation in several forms of hyper-tension, e.g., TxA_2, 19- and 20-HETEs in the SHR (94); PGH_2 in salt/angiotensin II–induced hypertension (126); and the lipoxygenase product, 12-HETE, associ-ated with diminished PGI_2, in aortic coarctation (44) in which increased formation of prohypertensive P-450-AA metabolites has also been reported (130).

Are Aspirin-Like Drugs Prohypertensive?

As noted, prostaglandins contribute to the mainte-nance of the renal circulation under stressful conditions when the renin-angiotensin system and the sympathetic nervous system are activated (47), whereupon the ad-ministration of NSAIDs may precipitate acute renal failure (48). In rabbits with renal hypertension, inhibition of prostaglandin synthesis resulted in the development of malignant hypertension (48). However, the obvious thought that arises is: if prostaglandins are important to the maintenance of normotension, then inhibition of synthesis by chronic administration of NSAIDs should result in elevation of blood pressure. This has been shown only in rabbits receiving 15 mg/kg/day of indomethacin for more than a week, a dose not tolerated by other species, including the rat (129). In this study, blood pressure elevation did not occur unless inhibition of prostaglandin synthesis exceeded 80%, as measured by reduced conversion of AA to prostaglandins in renal slices of treated animals. Consequently, the degree of inhibition of prostaglandin synthesis required to elevate blood pressure by NSAIDs is rarely, if ever, achieved because of the large reserve in prostaglandin synthesizing capacity. Moreover, the true contribution of prostaglandins may only become apparent under the stress of disease or during depletion of extracellular fluids, when an increase in prostaglandin synthesis is required. Thus, Abe et al. (131) have shown that in essential hypertensive patients on a low-sodium diet, which reduces blood pressure, the administration of indomethacin elevated blood pressure to levels observed on a normal-sodium diet. In most studies in humans, changes in blood pressure in response to NSAIDs were either small or absent. However, systemic vascular resistance increased after treatment with NSAIDs. The elevated total peripheral vascular resistance, however, was offset by compensatory mechanisms resulting in reduced cardiac output such that blood pressure changes were minimal (132).

NSAIDs will produce greater increases in regional vascular resistances if tissue and circulating levels of pressor hormones are elevated (47). Under these circumstances the vasoconstrictor and salt- and water-retaining effects of blood pressure elevating hormonal and neural systems will be unopposed by vasodilator-natriuretic prostaglandins. The operation of these countervailing systems can be seen in the response of normotensive subjects to infusion of angiotensin II or vasopressin (133,134). After indomethacin treatment, administration of either pressor hormone produced a greater increase in vascular resistance than in the absence of NSAID treatment. There are hypertensive models, however, such as those characterized by increased formation of vasoconstrictor prostanoids, particularly TxA_2, and the prostaglandins endoperoxides (PGG_2 and PGH_2), that will respond to NSAIDs by a reduction in blood pressure (126). Nasjletti and co-workers have described in detail these circumstances in several experimental models in rats, chiefly those associated with renal ischemia as an initiating factor (126,135).

The recent discovery of an inducible form of cyclooxygenase (COX-2), having a different spectrum of responsiveness to inhibition by NSAIDs, provides an explana-

tion for the lesser sensitivity to NSAIDs in conditions such as pregnancy (6). Thus, some of the most frequently used NSAIDs in experimental studies can be expected to be less effective as an inhibitor of COX-2 as compared with COX-1 (6). Finally, the fact that a NSAID can cause a reduction in blood pressure or modify one or more features of the hypertensive state/model does not permit the conclusion that it does so by eliminating a vasodilator-natriuretic prostaglandin. This statement is based on the recent observation that AA metabolites generated by cytochrome P-450 monooxygenases can assume vasoactive properties or acquire a different profile of vasoactivity after an additional step involving transformation by cyclooxygenase (136). These observations mandate the qualification that misleading conclusions may result from the use of NSAIDs to identify the participation of prostaglandins in experimental and human forms of hypertension. For example, the initiating lesion may be increased AA metabolism by cytochrome P-450 monooxygenases. These P-450-AA metabolites show varying abilities to be metabolized further by cyclooxygenase, a step that can substantially modify their capacity to affect blood pressure. If a NSAID is then given and an effect on blood pressure is produced, the conclusion that a prostaglandin is the responsible agent would be incorrect, as the primary lesion resides in enhanced production of cytochrome P-450-derived AA products with cyclooxygenase acting in a permissive capacity (94,136).

Toxemia of Pregnancy

A role for eicosanoids in the development of hypertension as a result of decreased production of antihypertensive prostanoids in the face of increased activity of blood pressure elevating systems is exemplified in preeclampsia, the hypertension of pregnancy (137). During normal pregnancy, activity of the renin-angiotensin system is elevated and appears to be offset by enhanced prostaglandin synthesis. Thus, plasma levels and urinary excretion of prostaglandins and their metabolites are increased substantially and associated with a reduction in the vascular response to angiotensin II (49), which may be reversed by the administration of cyclooxygenase inhibitors (138). However, the administration of low-dose aspirin has been reported to reduce pregnancy-induced hypertension and further reduce the vascular effects of angiotensin II (139). Because low-dose aspirin affects thromboxane production by platelets while having a relative sparing action on vascular prostacyclin synthesis, this effect of aspirin has been attributed to favoring PGI_2 synthesis versus TxA_2 production. The promotion of thromboxane synthase inhibitors for the treatment of preeclampsia is based on a similar rationale, i.e., reduced formation of TxA_2 associated with redirection of endoperoxides to PGI_2 and PGE_2 production. Thus, Fitzgerald et al. (140) have reported that a relative deficiency in prostacyclin biosynthesis precedes the onset of hypertension in pregnancy.

In normal pregnant women in whom prostaglandin and thromboxane production are increased, the ratio of vasodilator (PGE$_2$ and PGI$_2$) to vasoconstrictor (TxA$_2$) prostanoids remains higher than the ratio found in women with pregnancy-induced hypertension (141), to whom the administration of low-dose aspirin should promote restoration of the balance. Indeed, in women who remain sensitive to the pressor effects of angiotensin II during pregnancy and exhibit relatively decreased plasma levels of 6-keto-PGF$_{1\alpha}$ and PGE$_2$, low-dose aspirin may reduce the sensitivity to angiotensin II (142). Contrariwise, where low-dose aspirin failed to attenuate the pressor effect of angiotensin II, the occurrence of pregnancy-induced hypertension was 100 percent (143). These findings, therefore, suggest that measurements of prostaglandin and/or their metabolites, e.g., 2,3-dinor-6-keto-PGF$_{1\alpha}$, may be used to identify women at risk of developing preeclampsia (140). Additional evidence for a protective role of prostaglandins in pregnancy is provided by studies in the pregnant SHR, in which urinary excretion and blood levels of PGE$_2$ increase to maximum just before parturition. At this time, the rats become normotensive for several days, after which hypertension returns in the early postpartum period (144). However, despite the abundance of evidence supporting the concept that prostaglandins participate in the reduced sensitivity to vasoconstrictor substances in pregnancy, some studies of vascular responsiveness in pregnant animals fail to support this view. Thus, indomethacin did not increase vasoconstrictor responses to angiotensin II in the *in situ* blood perfused mesentery of the pregnant rat (145).

In addition to changes in prostanoid production, a recent study has shown that excretion of P-450-AA metabolites is altered during pregnancy (146). Normal pregnancy was associated with increased urinary excretion of 8,9- and 11,12-DHT; excretion of 11,12-DHT was increased further in women with pregnancy-induced hypertension. However, the significance of these findings is unknown. Their evaluation will require pharmacological probes that possess greater selectivity and lower toxicity than are now available to alter the activity of the cytochrome P-450 system.

Prostaglandins and Thromboxane in Human and Experimental Hypertension

To evaluate the role of renal and systemic eicosanoids in hypertension, urinary excretion of primary prostaglandins, presumed to reflect intrarenal synthesis, has been measured while urinary excretion of stable metabolites has been used as an index of systemic production.

There is evidence that a state of prostaglandin deficiency (another subset of essential hypertension?) may characterize some hypertensive subjects. Tan et al. (147) first reported a reduction in the urinary excretion of PGE$_2$ in essential hypertension. Abe et al. (148) showed that the ability to increase prostaglandin synthesis in response to stimulation (in this case, furosemide) was impaired in hypertensive subjects. Reduced excretion of 6-keto-PGF$_{1\alpha}$, the stable hydrolysis product of prostacyclin, has also been reported in human hypertension (149). On the other hand, as discussed, increased formation of prohypertensive eicosanoids, TxA$_2$ and PGH$_2$, may contribute to elevation of blood pressure (150), particularly when the renin-angiotensin system is stimulated. For example, the capacity of angiotensin II to release TxA$_2$ and other prostanoids from the isolated rabbit kidney was greatly increased by suprarenal aortic coarctation associated with enhancement of the renal vasoconstrictor action of angiotensin II (151).

Nasjletti and Mistry have advanced the concept that, in renin-dependent forms of hypertension, elevation of blood pressure is mediated, in part, by prohypertensive prostanoids, of which PGH$_2$ is the most prominent (126). The availability of TxA$_2$/PGH$_2$ receptor antagonists allows identification of the contribution of prohypertensive prostanoids to the hypertension (135). In rats made hypertensive by constricting the aorta between the origin of the renal arteries, the participation of prohypertensive prostanoids is evident in the first several weeks, coincident with activation of the renin-angiotensin system (135). During this initial period, blockade of TxA$_2$/PGH$_2$ receptors produced a marked drop in blood pressure, which was not the case later when renin levels had returned to normal. Moreover, according to Nasjletti, the administration of TxA$_2$/PGH$_2$ antagonists to rats with mineralocorticoid-salt hypertension, a low-renin state, should be without effect at any stage because production of TxA$_2$ and PGH$_2$ is not increased. In contrast, indomethacin should elevate blood pressure in mineralocorticoid-salt hypertension, as antihypertensive prostanoids should predominate under these conditions (135). These predictions were fulfilled and forced the conclusion that the antihypertensive prostaglandin-dependent mechanism subserved by PGE$_2$ and PGI$_2$ in mineralocorticoid-salt hypertension is a secondary response to elevation of blood pressure.

The relative combination of pro- and antihypertensive prostanoids to the development of hypertension varies with the model and the species. In human hypertension, variations in the ratio of antihypertensive/prohypertensive eicosanoids occur, depending on (a) the severity of the disease, (b) the etiology as, for example, renovascular, and (c) the state of salt and water balance. A question raised by these considerations is whether changes in prostaglandin production are primary or secondary to the development of hypertension. Increased AA metabolism may be the result of hypertension, as reduction of blood pressure in hypertensive patients normalized excretion of urinary PGE$_2$ (152). However, the studies of Tan et al. (147) and Abe et al. (148) cited above, suggest subsets of hypertensive subjects in whom a deficiency of prostaglandin-dependent antihypertensive mechanisms precedes and determines the onset of hypertension. Therefore, the issue concerning a primary versus secondary role for eicosanoids in the development of hypertension remains unresolved and awaits the availability of pharmacological probes such as PGE$_2$ and PGI$_2$, specific receptor antagonists analogous to TxA$_2$/PGH$_2$ receptor antagonists.

Studies of animal models of hypertension suggest a role for eicosanoids in the development and maintenance of hypertension. Tobian et al. (153) have provided evidence of an imbalance of prohypertensive versus antihypertensive prostanoids in the vasculature and kidneys of Dahl S (salt-sensitive) rats, i.e., synthesis of TxA$_2$ was increased while that of PGE$_2$, PGD$_2$, and PGI$_2$ was reduced (153). Moreover, when this strain of rat was switched from a normal-salt to a high-salt diet, the increment in PGE$_2$ was approximately half that observed in the Dahl R (salt-resistant) rat, a strain in which blood pressure is unaffected by salt intake (154). In support of this observation, Rapp and his colleagues have reported a reduction in the urinary excretion of PGE$_2$ in the Dahl S rat before any overt increase in blood pressure (155).

A thromboxane-related mechanism may contribute to the onset of hypertension in the SHR, as Shibouta et al. (156) demonstrated enhanced renal TxA$_2$ synthesis in response to angiotensin II during the developmental phase, but not the established phase, of hypertension. A TxA$_2$ receptor antagonist reversed the increased renal vascular resistance and the decreased glomerular filtration rate (GFR) in SHRs that were 6 weeks old, an age when increased excretion of urinary TxB$_2$ was observed. Further, TxA$_2$ synthase inhibitors have been found to delay or prevent the development of hypertension in the young SHR (157). It is important to recognize that the use of TxA$_2$ synthase inhibitors may not provide a reliable estimate of the role of TxA$_2$ in the development of hypertension as (a) inhibition of TxA$_2$ formation may result in diversion of the precursor endoperoxide, PGH$_2$, to PGI$_2$ and PGE$_2$, which may exert an antihypertensive effect; and (b) inhibition of TxA$_2$ formation may facilitate expression of the vasoconstrictor action of prostaglandin endoperoxides (128). Therefore, the use of TxA$_2$ receptor antagonists to evaluate the participation of TxA$_2$ in hypertension would be more appropriate than TxA$_2$ synthase inhibitors to avoid the above factors complicating the interpretation of the results. This information can be gained by comparing the effects of TxA$_2$ synthase inhibitors to those of TxA$_2$/PGH$_2$ receptor antagonists, as described previously (128).

Sessa et al. (158) have used a direct approach to answer the question of whether TxA$_2$ is involved in the onset of hypertension in the SHR, one based on changes in the activity of TxA$_2$ synthase from 5 to 20 weeks of age. The young SHR showed enhanced capacity to generate TxA$_2$, compared with age-matched WKY rats or the adult SHR. As TxA$_2$ synthase is a cytochrome P-450 hemoprotein, the level of the enzyme can be regulated by manipulating the availability of heme, specifically by depleting heme through induction of heme oxygenase, which catabolizes heme (159). Increased heme oxygenase activity produced by treatment with stannous chloride decreased heme and P-450 content associated with diminished TxA$_2$ synthase activity and reduced blood pressure in the 7-week-old SHR. Increased synthesis of P-450–derived AA metabolites in the young SHR may also contribute to the renal hemodynamic and excretory abnormalities (160). In keeping with these other studies (160,161), which indicated a burst of P-450–dependent oxygenase activity and enhanced formation of P-450-AA metabolites during the developmental phase of hypertension, Sessa et al. (158) also demonstrated the greatest TxA$_2$ synthase activity in the young SHR. The time course of elevated TxA$_2$ synthase activity and P-450-AA production coincided with the functional findings noted above by Shibouta et al. (162) and is in agreement with other reports showing depression of GFR and increased renal vascular resistance, as well as a tendency to retain salt and water during this period in the young SHR (163,164).

Dietary Unsaturated Fatty Acids and Hypertension

Additional evidence for an eicosanoid component in the development of experimental and human hypertension arises from consideration of studies based on manipulating dietary fatty acids. These studies have used several approaches: (a) essential fatty acid (EFA)-deficient diets to reduce formation of AA metabolites; (b) increasing dietary linoleic acid, the precursor of AA, in order to increase AA metabolites, particularly PGE$_2$ and PGI$_2$; and (c) increasing dietary EPA to reduce formation of the 2-series prostanoids and TxA$_2$ and to increase the 3-series prostanoids, particularly TxA$_3$. The replacement of TxA$_2$ by TxA$_3$, a less potent thromboxane, and PGI$_2$ by PGI$_3$, an equipotent prostacyclin, is the rationale for the use of EPA (165). Thus, it was recognized that populations ingesting EPA from marine sources experienced lowered rates of cardiovascular disease (including hypertension), which was attributed primarily to reduced platelet activity. However, the mechanisms underlying the hypotensive effects of manipulating dietary fatty acids is by no means clear and may be the consequence of multiple changes. Moreover, there is evidence that those ingesting diets high in EPA are at risk for bleeding diathesis (166).

Normotensive rats fed a diet deficient in EFAs demonstrated impaired ability to excrete a salt load associated with reduced excretion of PGE$_2$ (167). When dietary salt was increased, elevation of blood pressure occurred. Salt-induced hypertension in EFA-deficient rats was corrected when the major source of endogenous AA, linoleic acid, was added to the diet. Dietary linoleic acid also has been shown to protect against salt-induced hypertension in Dahl S rats (168), although olive oil produced a similar decrease in blood pressure, an effect presumably independent of changes in prostanoid formation (169). Nonetheless, a relative deficiency in antihypertensive prostanoids has been described in Dahl S rats (155). Increased dietary linoleic acid resulted in an initial fall in blood pressure in Dahl S rats given salt; it also delayed the development, and reduced the severity, of hypertension associated with an increase in renal papillary PGE_2 levels (168).

Increasing intake of EPA has variable effects on blood pressure, although, in most studies, dietary intake of EPA was increased by feeding crude fish oil or a mixture of polyunsaturated fatty acids. Lam et al. (170) have fed pure EPA to SHRs, thereby preventing the development of hypertension in the young SHR, an effect that could be reversed when EPA was withdrawn. Further, oral administration of EPA to the adult SHR (i.e., during the established phase of hypertension) resulted in a rapid and large fall in blood pressure. Administration of EPA and docosahexenoic acid in the form of mackerel to patients with mild essential hypertension reduced serum TxB_2 levels and lowered blood pressure (171). Elevation of blood pressure to the pretreatment levels occurred when a normal diet was reinstituted. However, diminished TxA_2 synthesis did not appear to account for the hypotensive effect of this fish diet, since continued intake of diet containing lower levels of EPA and docosahexenoic acid resulted in a sustained reduction in blood pressure, despite the return of serum TxB_2 to normal levels. Similarly, the fall in blood pressure could not be attributed to an increase in PGI_2 production, which was only transiently increased, returning to control levels while blood pressure continued to fall for the duration of fish oil supplementation (172).

In conclusion, the benefit of diets containing EPA is probably the result of multiple effects on the AA cascade, including (a) new product formation, such as TxA_3 replacing TxA_2; (b) altered enzyme function (e.g., decreased generation of leukotrienes); (c) modification of eicosanoid receptor activity; and (d) increased membrane fluidity and decreased blood viscosity.

Cytochrome P-450–Related AA Metabolism in the SHR

The discovery that mTALH forms AA metabolites via a cytochrome P-450–dependent pathway (30) and that these P-450-AA metabolites affect salt and water metabolism and act on blood vessels (18) raises the possibility that alterations in circulating levels or local production of P-450-AA metabolites may be involved in regulation of blood pressure. In hypertension induced by suprarenal aortic coarctation, production of cytochrome P-450-AA metabolites by the mTALH was increased more than twofold (130). When hypertension did not occur in response to coarctation, cytochrome P-450–dependent metabolism of AA was not increased. Increased formation of P-450-AA metabolites in the mTALH, a segment of the nephron that is particularly vulnerable to hypoxia, has been proposed to serve a defensive role by limiting energy expenditure in this renal segment. This proposal was compelling, as P-450-AA metabolites were shown to be capable of inhibiting Na^+,K^+-ATPase, a major determinant of energy expenditure in transporting epithelia. Moreover, an AA product of the cytochrome P-450 system that reduces the activity of Na^+,K^+-ATPase in mTALH has been postulated to account for the exaggerated natriuresis observed in response to volume expansion in hypertension.

Abnormalities of Na^+,K^+-ATPase activity have been described in both essential (173) and experimental (174) hypertension. However, when the principal P-450–derived AA metabolites of the mTALH, 20-HETE, and 20-COOH-AA were studied in terms of their effects on ion channels in this nephron segment, they were shown to mimic the action of furosemide, not the digitalis glycoside ouabain, and, therefore, interacted with the Na^+,K^+-$2Cl^-$ cotransporter rather than the Na^+ pump (20). Any effect of either 20-HETE or 20-COOH-AA on Na^+,K^+-ATPase activity would be secondary to its action on the furosemide-sensitive cotransporter on the luminal surface. However, in other segments of the nephron, P-450-AA metabolites may inhibit Na^+,K^+-ATPase. In any event, the production of 20-HETE and 20-COOH-AA in response to an insult would reduce the energy requirements of the mTALH. Deficient formation of the ω-hydroxylase products, 20-HETE and 20-COOH-AA, might result in enhanced Na^+ and Cl^- reabsorption because of their ability to inhibit the Na^+,K^+-$2Cl^-$ cotransporter. Indeed, just such a lesion has been proposed to account for increased Cl^- reabsorption in the salt-sensitive Dahl hypertensive rat (175). The deficiency in formation of 20-HETE was corrected by induction of ω-hydroxylase activity. Moreover, the elevated blood pressure returned to normal. If confirmed, this finding should inaugurate the era of the rational treatment of hypertension (heretofore empirical): identify primary derangement in terms of an enzyme, normalize enzyme activity, and restore normal levels of blood pressure.

A "renal lesion," resulting in inappropriate retention of NaCl, is thought to be the underlying defect in essential hypertension (176). Blood pressure elevation is compensatory in order to increase renal perfusion pressure, thereby promoting excretion of sodium chloride and correcting the underlying abnormality, salt retention. In hypertension, the pressure-natriuresis curve has shifted to the right; that is, for a given increment of renal perfusion pressure, less sodium chloride is excreted. Several products of the third pathway of AA metabolism have been incriminated in just such an initiating event in the animal model, the SHR, considered to resemble most closely human essential hypertension (94). These AA products of cytochrome P-450 monooxygenase metabolism, which are produced in excess by the SHR, are prohypertensive in the rat; 20-HETE constricts renal blood vessels (177) and 19-HETE stimulates Na^+,K^+-ATPase (178). The manner in which P-450-AA metabolites participate in the elevation of blood pressure may depend specifically on the renal hemodynamic effects of the cyclooxygenase-derived metabolites of 20-HETE, which are vasoconstrictors in the rat. The study of Roman and Kaldunski (179) provides the rationale for this proposal, as they have reported that the rightward shift of the pressure-natriuresis relationship in the SHR could be accounted for by reduced blood flow to the papilla, secondary to elevation of renal medullary vascular resistance (179). Decreased papillary blood flow, secondary to increased production of 20-HETE, would reduce medullary and papillary interstitial pressure and, thereby, promote sodium chloride reabsorption by altering the balance of forces across the nephron segments actively involved in Na^+ and Cl^- reabsorption, such as the mTALH.

In the SHR during the development of hypertension (between 5 and 13 weeks of age), renal metabolism of AA by cytochrome P-450–dependent monooxygenases is increased, as indicated by the capacity of renal cortical and medullary microsomes to generate P-450-AA products when compared with those obtained from the WKY rat (94). Further, the distribution of cytochrome P-450-AA metabolic activity along the nephron is altered in the SHR and varies during the development of hypertension, at which time (first 12 weeks) there is a greater capacity to synthesize 20-HETE (180). These differences are not apparent once hypertension is established. Nonetheless, renal cytochrome P-450 content is elevated during the developmental phase and remains high in the established phase of hypertension (161).

Blood pressure can be normalized in the SHR if production of P-450-AA products is reduced by attacking the cytochrome P-450 enzyme complex through stimulating the enzyme, heme-oxygenase, that degrades heme-containing enzymes, including cytochromes. Selective depletion of renal cytochrome P-450, accomplished by inducing heme oxygenase with tin, given as $SnCl_2$, spares extrarenal cytochrome P-450 and is therefore less toxic than other inducers of heme oxygenase such as $CoCl_2$ (159). $SnCl_2$ produces activation of the heme oxygenase gene, resulting in increased renal heme oxygenase mRNA levels of more than 20-fold in the rat kidney within 8 hours of $SnCl_2$ administration (181). As heme oxygenase regulates the availability of heme for cyto-

chrome P-450, depletion of cytochrome P-450 produces diminished AA metabolism via this pathway. In 7-week-old SHRs, a 4-day treatment with $SnCl_2$ significantly reduced blood pressure associated with increased heme oxygenase activity and reduced cytochrome P-450 content, which was reflected in decreased production of renal AA metabolites (94). However, $SnCl_2$ treatment was without effect on blood pressure in WKY rats or in 20-week-old SHRs, an age when renal cytochrome P-450–dependent metabolism of AA was no different from that seen in WKY rats.

The effect of tin appears to be mediated via actions on renal heme oxygenase activity, since concomitant treatment with tin-protoporphyrin (an inhibitor of heme oxygenase) markedly reduced the blood pressure–lowering effect of $SnCl_2$ in the SHR. These results indicate that one or more cytochrome P-450–dependent AA metabolites participate in the elevation of blood pressure in the SHR.

ACKNOWLEDGMENTS

The authors wish to thank Melody Steinberg for preparation of this manuscript and editorial assistance. This work was supported by NIH grants RO1-HL 25394 and Program Project grant PO1-HL 34300.

REFERENCES

1. Schwartzman M, Carroll MA, Ibraham NG, Ferreri NR, Songu-Mize E, McGiff, JC. Renal arachidonic acid metabolism: the third pathway. *Hypertension* 1985;7(suppl I):I-136–I-144.
2. Codde JP, Beilin LJ. Prostaglandins and experimental hypertension: a review with special emphasis on the effect of dietary lipids. *J Hypertension* 1986;4:675–686.
3. Dyerberg J, Bang HO, Stofferson E, Moncada S, Vane JR. Eicosapentaenoic acid and prevention of thrombosis and atherosclerosis. *Lancet* 1978;2:117–119.
4. Damas J, Bourdon V, Neuray J, Deby A. Bradykinie et biosynthese des prostaglandins *in vitro*. *CR Soc Biol* 1973;167:187.
5. Billah MM, Lapetina EG, Cuatrecasas P. Phospholipase A_2 and phospholipase C activities of platelets. *J Biol Chem* 1980;255:10227–10231.
6. Smith WL. Prostanoid biosynthesis and mechanisms of action. *Am J Physiol* 1992;263:F181–F191.
7. Davidson FF, Dennis EA, Powell M, Glenney JR Jr. Inhibition of phospholipase A_2 by "lipocortins" and calpactins. *J Biol Chem* 1987;262:1968–1705.
8. Capdevila JH, Kishore V, Dishman E, Blair IA. A novel pool of rat liver inositol and ethanolamine phospholipids contains epoxyeicosatrienoic acids (EETs). *Biochem Biophys Res Commun* 1987;146:638–644.
9. McGiff, JC. Cytochrome P-450 metabolism of arachidonic acid. *Annu Rev Pharmacol Toxicol* 1991;31:339–369.
10. Douglas JG, Hopfer U. Novel aspect of angiotensin receptors and signal transduction in the kidney. *Annu Rev Physiol* 1994;in press.
11. Abdel-Latif AA. Calcium-mobilizing receptors, polyphosphoinositides, and the generation of second messengers. *Pharmacol Rev* 1986;38:227–272.
12. Madhun ZT, Goldthwait DA, McKay D, Hopfer U, Douglas JG. An epoxygenase metabolite of arachidonic acid mediates angiotensin II-induced rises in cytosolic calcium in rabbit proximal tubule epithelial cells. *J Clin Invest* 1991;88:456–461.

13. Gronich JH, Bonventre JV, Nemenoff RA. Purification of a high-molecular-mass form of phospholipase A_2 from rat kidney activated at physiological calcium concentrations. *Biochem J* 1990;271:37–43.

14. Quilley J, Sarubbi D, McGiff JC. Influence of diabetes mellitus on renal vascular responses to bradykinin. *Agents Actions* 1992;38:31–35.

15. Limas C, Limas CJ. Enhanced renomedullary prostaglandin synthesis in spontaneously hypertensive rats: role of a phospholipase A_2. *Am J Physiol* 1979;236:H65–H72.

16. Carroll MA, Garcia MP, Falck JR, McGiff, JC. 5,6-epoxyeicosatrienoic acid, a novel arachidonate metabolite. *Circ Res* 1990;67:1082–1088.

17. Omata K, Abraham NG, Schwartzman ML. Renal cytochrome P-450-arachidonic acid metabolism: localization and hormonal regulation in SHR. *Am J Physiol* 1992;262:F591–F599.

18. Schwartzman M, Ferreri NR, Carroll MA, Songu-Mize E, McGiff JC. Renal cytochrome P450-related arachidonate metabolite inhibits (Na^+-K^+)ATPase. *Nature* 1985;314:620–622.

19. Hirt DL, Capdevila J, Falck JR, Breyer MD, Jacobson HR. Cytochrome P450 metabolites of arachidonic acid are potent inhibitors of vasopressin action on rabbit cortical collecting duct. *J Clin Invest* 1989;84:1805–1812.

20. Escalante B, Erlij D, Falck JR, McGiff JC. Effect of cytochrome P450 arachidonate metabolites on ion transport in rabbit kidney loop of Henle. *Science* 1991;251:799–802.

21. Lands WEM. The biosynthesis and metabolism of prostaglandins. *Annu Rev Physiol* 1979;41:633–642.

22. Masferrer JL, Seibert K, Zweifel B, Needleman P. Endogenous glucocorticoids regulate an inducible cyclooxygenase enzyme. *Proc Natl Acad Sci USA* 1992;89:3917–3921.

23. Simmons DL, Xie W, Chipman JG, Evett GE. Multiple cyclooxygenases: cloning of a mitogen-inducible form. In: *Prostaglandins, leukotrienes, lipoxins, and PAF*. Bailey JM, ed. New York: Plenum, 1991;67–78.

24. Terragno NA, Terragno A, Pacholczyk D, McGiff JC. Prostaglandins and the regulation of uterine blood flow in pregnancy. *Nature* 1974;249:57–58.

25. Salvemini D, Misko TP, Masferrer JL, Seibert K, Currie MG, Needleman P. Nitric oxide activates cyclooxygenase enzymes. *Proc Natl Acad Sci USA* 1993;90:7240–7244.

26. Beasley D, Dinarello CA, Cannon JG. Interleukin-1 induces natriuresis in conscious rats: role of renal prostaglandins. *Kidney Int* 1988;33:1059–1065.

27. Samuelsson B. Leukotrienes: mediators of immediate hypersensitivity reactions and inflammation. *Science* 1983;220:568–575.

28. Pace-Asciak CR. Hepoxilins. *Gen Pharmacol* 1993;24:805–810.

29. Morrison AR, Pascoe N. Metabolism of arachidonate through NADPH-dependent oxygenase of renal cortex. *Proc Natl Acad Sci USA* 1981;78:7375–7378.

30. Ferreri NR, Schwartzman M, Ibraham NG, Chander PN, McGiff JC. Arachidonic acid metabolism in a cell suspension isolated from rabbit renal outer medulla. *J Pharmacol Exp Ther* 1984;231:441–448.

31. Quilley CP, McGiff JC. Isomers of 12-hydroxy-5,8,10,14-eicosatetraenoic acid reduce renin activity and increase water and electrolyte excretion. *J Pharmacol Exp Ther* 1990;254:774–780.

32. Proctor KG, Shatkin S Jr, Kaminski PM, Falck JR, Capdevila JH. Modulation of arteriolar blood flow by inhibitors of arachidonic acid oxidation after thermal injury: possible role for a novel class of vasodilator metabolites. *Circulation* 1988;77:1185–1196.

33. McGiff JC. Interactions of prostaglandins with the kallikrein-kinin and renin-angiotensin systems. *Clin Sci* 1980;59:105s–116s.

34. McGiff JC. Prostaglandins, prostacyclin and thromboxanes. *Annu Rev Pharmacol Toxicol* 1981;21:479–509.

35. Gerritsen ME, Cheli CD. Arachidonic acid and prostaglandin endoperoxide metabolism in isolated rabbit and coronary microvessels and isolated and cultivated coronary microvessel endothelial cells. *J Clin Invest* 1983;72:1658–1671.

36. Moncada S, Vane JR. Pharmacology and endogenous roles of prostaglandin endoperoxides, thromboxane A_2 and prostacyclin. *Pharmacol Rev* 1979;30:293–320.

37. Larsson C, Anggard E. Regional differences in the formation and metabolism of prostaglandins in the rabbit kidney. *Eur J Pharmacol* 1973;21:30–36.

38. Carroll MA, Sala A, Dunn CE, McGiff JC, Murphy RC. Structural identification of cytochrome P450-dependent arachidonate metabolites formed by rabbit medullary thick ascending limb cells. *J Biol Chem* 1991;266:12306–12312.

39. Woolard PM. Sterochemical difference between 12-hydroxy-5,8,10,14-eicosatetraenoic acid in platelet and psoriatic lesions. *Biochem Biophys Res Commun* 1986;136:169–176.

40. Borgeat P, Samuelsson B. Metabolism of arachidonic acid in polymorphonuclear leukocytes. *J Biol Chem* 1979;254:7865–7869.

41. Revtyak G, Johnson AR, Campbell WB. Cultured bovine coronary arterial endothelial cells synthesize HETEs and prostacyclin. *Am J Physiol* 1988;254:C8–C19.

42. Oyekan AO, McGiff JC, Quilley J. Cytochrome P-450-dependent vasodilator responses to arachidonic acid in the isolated, perfused kidney of the rat. *Circ Res* 1991;68:958–965.

43. Greenwald JE, Bianchine JR, Wong L. The production of the arachidonate metabolite HETE in vascular tissue. *Nature* 1979;281:588–589.

44. Lin L, Balazy M, Pagano PJ, Nasjletti A. Hyperexpression of PGH_2-mediated mechanism of vascular contraction in hypertensive rats: relation to lipoxygenase and prostacyclin synthase activities. *Circ Res* 1994;74:197–205.

45. Kuehl FA Jr, Dougherty HW, Ham EA. Interactions between prostaglandins and leukotrienes. *Biochem Pharmacol* 1984;33:1–5.

46. Bell-Quilley CP, Lin Y-S R, Hilchey SD, Drugge ED, McGiff JC. Renovascular actions of angiotensin II in the isolated kidney of the rat: relationship to lipoxygenases. *J Pharmacol Exp Ther* 1993;267:676–682.

47. Terragno NA, Terragno DA, McGiff JC. Contribution of prostaglandins to the renal circulation in conscious, anesthetized, and laparotomized dogs. *Circ Res* 1977;40:590–595.

48. Romero JC, Strong CG. The effect of indomethacin blockade of prostaglandin synthesis on blood pressure of normal rabbits and rabbits with renovascular hypotension. *Circ Res* 1977;40:35–41.

49. Goodman RP, Killam AP, Brash AR, Branch RA. Prostacyclin production during pregnancy: comparison of production during normal pregnancy and pregnancy complicated by hypertension. *Am J Obstet Gynecol* 1982;142:817–822.

50. McGiff JC, Quilley CP. Thromboxane A_2 and prostaglandin mediators in hypertension. In: Neri Serneri GG, et al., eds. *Thromboxane A_2 and other vasoconstrictors in clinical conditions*. Florence: Scientific Press, 1993;91–105.

51. McGiff JC, Nasjletti A. Kinins, renal function and blood pressure regulation. *Fed Proc* 1976;35:172–174.

52. McGiff JC, Crowshaw K, Itskovitz HD. Prostaglandins and renal function. *Fed Proc* 1974;33:39–47.

53. McGiff JC, Nasjletti A. Renal prostaglandins and the regulation of blood pressure. In: Kahn RH, Lands WEM, eds. *Prostaglandins and cyclic AMP*. New York: Academic Press, 1973;119–151.

54. McGiff JC, Crowshaw K, Terragno NA, Lonigro AJ. Renal prostaglandins: possible regulators of the renal actions of pressor hormones. *Nature* 1970;227:1255–1257.

55. McGiff JC, Crowshaw K, Terragno NA, Lonigro AJ. Release of a prostaglandinlike substance into renal venous blood in response to angiotensin II. *Circ Res* 1970;26,27(suppl I):I-121–I-130.

56. Vane JR. Inhibition of prostaglandin synthesis as a mechanism of action for aspirinlike drugs. *Nature (New Biol)* 1971;231:232–235.

57. Aiken JW, Vane JR. Intrarenal prostaglandin release attenuates the renal vasoconstrictor activity of angiotensin. *J Pharmacol Exp Ther* 1973;184:678–687.

58. Chatziantoniou C, Arendshorst WJ. Impaired ability of prostaglandins to buffer renal vasoconstriction in genetically hypertensive rats. *Am J Physiol* 1992;263:F573–F580.

59. Nadler JL, Natarajan R, Stern N. Specific action of the lipoxygenase pathway in mediating angiotensin II-induced aldosterone synthesis in isolated adrenal glomerulosa cells. *J Clin Invest* 1987;80:1763–1769.

60. Antonipillai L, Nadler J, Horton R. Angiotensin feedback inhibi-

tion on renin is expressed via the lipoxygenase pathway. *Endocrinology* 1988;122:1277–1281.

61. Nozawa K, Tuck ML, Golub M, Eggena P, Nadler JL, Stern N. Inhibition of lipoxygenase pathway reduces blood pressure in renovascular hypertensive rats. *Am J Physiol* 1990;259:H1774–H1780.

62. Chiba S, Quilley CP, McGiff JC. Decreased vascular responsiveness produced by angiotensin-converting enzyme inhibitors in the rat isolated kidney. *Hypertension* 1982;4:II-80–II-85.

63. Terragno DA, Crowshaw K, Terragno NA, McGiff JC. Prostaglandin synthesis by bovine mesenteric arteries and veins. *Circ Res* 1975;36,37(suppl I):I-76–I-80.

64. McGiff JC, Crowshaw K, Terragno NA, et al. Prostaglandinlike substances appearing in canine renal venous blood during renal ischemia: their partial characterization by pharmacologic and chromatographic procedures. *Circ Res* 1970;27:765–782.

65. Vane JR. Release and fate of vasoactive hormones in the circulation. *Br J Pharmacol* 1969;35:209–242.

66. McGiff JC, Terragno NA, Strand JC, Lee JB, Lonigro AJ, Ng KKF. Selective passage of prostaglandins across the lung. *Nature* 1969;223:742–745.

67. Weber PC, Larsson C, Anggard E, et al. Stimulation of renin release from rabbit renal cortex by arachidonic acid and prostaglandin endoperoxides. *Circ Res* 1976;39:868–874.

68. Larsson C, Weber P, Anggard E. Arachidonic acid increases and indomethacin decreases plasma renin activity in the rabbit. *Eur J Pharmacol* 1974;28:391–394.

69. McGiff JC, Spokas EG, Wong PY-K. Stimulation of renin release by 6-oxo-prostaglandin E_1 and prostacyclin. *Br J Pharmacol* 1982;75:137–144.

70. Vio CP, Churchill L, Terragno A, McGiff JC, Terragno NA. Arachidonic acid stimulates renal kallikrein release in isolated rat kidney. *Clin Sci* 1982;63:235s–237s.

71. Yamamoto M, Share L, Shade RE. Vasopressin release during ventriculocisternal perfusion with prostaglandin E_2 in the dog. *J Endocrinol* 1976;71:325–331.

72. McGiff JC, Itskovitz HD, Terragno NA. The actions of bradykinin and eledoisin in the canine isolated kidney: relationships to prostaglandins. *Clin Sci Mol Med* 1975;49:125–131.

73. Messina EJ, Weiner R, Kaley G. Inhibition of bradykinin vasodilation and potentiation of norepinephrine and angiotensin vasoconstriction by inhibitors of prostaglandin synthesis in skeletal muscle of the rat. *Circ Res* 1975;37:430–437.

74. Fulton D, McGiff JC, Quilley J. Contribution of NO and cytochrome P450 to the vasodilator effect of bradykinin in the rat kidney. *Br J Pharmacol* 1992;107:722–725.

75. McGiff JC, Terragno NA, Malik KU, Lonigro AJ. Release of prostaglandin E-like substance from canine kidney of bradykinin: comparison with eledoisin. *Circ Res* 1972;31:36–43.

76. Lonigro AJ, Hagemann MH, Stephenson AH, Fry CL. Inhibition of prostaglandin synthesis by indomethacin augments the renal vasodilator response to bradykinin in the anesthetized dog. *Circ Res* 1978;43:447–455.

77. Blasingham MC, Nasjletti A. Contribution of renal prostaglandins to the natriuretic action of bradykinin in the dog. *Am J Physiol* 1979;237:F182–F187.

78. Mullane KM, Moncada S. Prostacyclin mediates the potentiated hypotensive effect of bradykinin following captopril treatment. *Eur J Pharmacol* 1980;66:355–365.

79. Quilley J, McGiff JC, Fulton D, Balazy M, Mahboubi K. Nitric oxide-independent coronary vasodilator effect of bradykinin. Abstract, Council for High Blood Pressure Research, 47th Annual Fall Conference and Scientific Sessions, 1993.

80. Cachofeiro V, Sakakibara T, Nasjletti A. Kinins, nitric oxide and the hypotensive effect of captopril and ramiprilat in hypertension. *Hypertension* 1992;19:138–145.

81. Abe Y, Miura K, Imanishi M, et al. Effects of an orally active converting enzyme inhibitor (YS-980) on renal function in dogs. *J Pharmacol Exp Ther* 1980;214:166–170.

82. Roman RJ, Kaldunski ML, Scicli AG, Carretero OA. Influence of kinins and angiotensin II on the regulation of papillary blood flow. *Am J Physiol* 1988;255:F690–F698.

83. McGiff JC, Itskovitz HD, Terragno A, Wong PY-K. Modulation

84. Vio CP, Figueroa CD. Subcellular localization of renal kallikrein by ultrastructural immunocytochemistry. *Kidney Int* 1985;28:36–42.

85. Kauker ML, Crofton JT, Share L, Nasjletti A. Role of vasopressin in regulation of renal kinin excretion in Long-Evans and diabetes insipidus rats. *J Clin Invest* 1984;73:824–831.

86. Garcia Perez A, Smith WL. Apical-basolateral membrane asymmetry in canine cortical collecting tubule cells. Bradykinin, arginine vasopressin, prostaglandin E_2 interrelationships. *J Clin Invest* 1984;74:63–74.

87. Stokes JB. Integrated actions of renal medullary prostaglandins in the control of water excretion. *Am J Physiol* 1981;240:F471–F480.

88. Kauker ML. Prostaglandin E_2 effect from the luminal side on renal tubular ^{22}Na efflux: tracer microinjection studies. *Proc Soc Exp Biol Med* 1977;154:274–277.

89. Stokes JB. Effect of prostaglandin E_2 on chloride transport across the rabbit thick ascending limb of Henle. *J Clin Invest* 1979;61:495–502.

90. Iino Y, Brenner BM. Inhibition of Na transport by prostacyclin (PGI_2) in rabbit cortical collecting tubule. *Prostaglandins* 1981;22:715–721.

91. Carroll MA, Balazy M, Margiotta P, Falck JR, McGiff JC. Renal vasodilator activity of 5,6-epoxyeicosatrienoic acid depends upon conversion by cyclooxygenase and release of prostaglandins. *J Biol Chem* 1993;268:12260–12266.

92. Wang W, Cassola A, Giebisch G. Arachidonic acid inhibits the secretory K^+ channel of cortical collecting duct of rat kidney. *Am J Physiol* 1992;262:F554–F559.

93. Neri-Serneri GG, Masotti G, Castellani S, Scarti L, Sciagra R. Factors affecting excretion of renal prostaglandins. A study with hypertonic sodium and glucose infusions in normal female subjects. In: Dunn MJ, Patrono C, Cinotti GA, eds. *Prostaglandins and the kidney.* New York: Plenum Press, 1983;189–195.

94. Sacerdoti D, Escalante B, Abraham NG, McGiff JC, Levere RD, Schwartzman ML. Treatment with tin prevents the development of hypertension in spontaneously hypertensive rats. *Science* 1989;243:388–390.

95. Dun NJ. Inhibition of acetylcholine release by prostaglandin E_1 in the rabbit superior cervical ganglion. *Neuropharmacology* 1980;19:1137–1140.

96. Westfall TC, Kitay D. The effects of prostaglandins on the release of [^3H] dopamine from superfused slices of rat striatum following electrical stimulation. *Proc Soc Exp Biol Med* 1977;155:305–307.

97. Hedqvist P, Brundin J. Inhibition by prostaglandin E_1 of noradrenaline release and of effector response to nerve stimulation in the cat spleen. *Life Sci* 1969;8:389–395.

98. Malik KU. Interaction of arachidonic acid metabolites and adrenergic nervous system. *Am J Med Sci* 1988;295:280–286.

99. Malik KU, Sehic E. Prostaglandins and the release of the adrenergic transmitter. In: Kalsner S, Westfall TC, eds. *Presynaptic receptors and the question of autoregulation of neurotransmitter release.* New York: Ann NY Acad Sci 1990;604:222–236.

100. DiBona GF. The functions of the renal nerves. *Rev Physiol Biochem Pharmacol* 1982;94:75–181.

101. Lonigro AJ, Terragno NA, Malik KU, McGiff JC. Differential inhibition by prostaglandins of the renal actions of pressor stimuli. *Prostaglandins* 1973;3:595–606.

102. Malik KU, McGiff JC. Modulation by prostaglandin of adrenergic transmission in the isolated perfused rabbit and rat kidney. *Circ Res* 1975;36:599–609.

103. Khan MT, Malik KU. Modulation by prostaglandins of the release of [^3H]noradrenaline evoked by potassium and nerve stimulation in the isolated rat heart. *Eur J Pharmacol* 1982;78:213–218.

104. McGiff JC, Crowshaw K, Terragno NA, Malik KU, Lonigro AJ. Differential effect of noradrenaline and renal nerve stimulation on vascular resistance in the dog kidney and the release of a prostaglandin E-like substance. *Clin Sci* 1972;42:223–233.

105. Rump LC, Schollmeyer P. Effects of endogenous and synthetic prostanoids, the thromboxane A_2 receptor agonist U-46619 and

arachidonic acid on [³H]-noradrenaline release and vascular tone in rat isolated kidney. *Br J Pharmacol* 1989;97:819–828.

106. Inokuchi K, Malik KU. Attenuation by prostaglandins of adrenergically-induced renal vasoconstriction in anesthetized rats. *Am J Physiol* 246:R228–R235.

107. Williams JL Jr, Malik KU. Inhibitory modulation by cAMP of isoproterenol-induced prostacyclin synthesis in rabbit heart. *Am J Physiol* 1989;257:R771–R780.

108. Malmsten C, Granstrom E, Samuelsson B. Cyclic AMP inhibits synthesis of prostaglandin endoperoxide (PGG₂) in human platelets. *Biochem Biophys Res Commun* 1976;68:569–576.

109. Minkes M, Stanford N, Chi M M-Y, et al. Cyclic adenosine 3′,5′-monophosphate inhibits the availability of arachidonate to prostaglandin synthetase in human platelet suspensions. *J Clin Invest* 1977;59:449–454.

110. Kadowitz PJ, Sweet CS, Brody MJ. Potentiation of adrenergic venomotor responses by angiotensin, prostaglandin $F_{2\alpha}$ and cocaine. *J Pharmacol Exp Ther* 1971;176:167–173.

111. Trachte GJ. Thromboxane agonist (U46619) potentiates norepinephrine efflux from adrenergic nerves. *J Pharmacol Exp Ther* 1986;237:473–477.

112. Altiere RJ, Kiritsy-Roy J, Catravas JD. Acetylcholine-induced contractions in isolated rabbit pulmonary arteries: role of thromboxane A₂. *J Pharmacol Exp Ther* 1986;236:535–541.

113. Junstad M, Wennmalm A. Increased renal excretion of noradrenaline in rats after treatment with prostaglandin synthesis inhibitor indomethacin. *Acta Physiol Scand* 1972;85:573–576.

114. Fredholm BB, Hedqvist P. Indomethacin-induced increase in noradrenaline turnover in some rat organs. *Br J Pharmacol* 1975;54:295–300.

115. Chapple DJ, Dusting GJ, Hughes R, Vane JR. Some direct and reflex cardiovascular actions of prostacyclin (PGI₂) and prostaglandin E₂ in anaesthetized dogs. *Br J Pharmacol* 1980;68:437–447.

116. Hintze TH, Kaley G, Panzenbeck MJ. Mechanisms of reflex bradycardia and hypotension by metabolites of arachidonic acid in the cat. *Br J Pharmacol* 1984;82:117–125.

117. Blair IA, Barrow SE, Waddell KA, Lewis PJ, Dollery CT. Prostacyclin is not a circulating hormone in man. *Prostaglandins* 1982;23:579–589.

118. Panzenbeck MJ, Tan W, Hajdu MA, Zucker IH. Prostaglandins mediate the increased sensitivity of left ventricular reflexes after captopril treatment in conscious dogs. *J Pharmacol Exp Ther* 1988;244:384–390.

119. Faber JE. Role of prostaglandins and kinins in the renal pressor reflex. *Hypertension* 1987;10:522–532.

120. Chapleau MW, Hajduczok G, Abboud FM. Mechanisms of resetting arterial baroreceptors: an overview. *Am J Med Sci* 1988;295:327–334.

121. Chapleau MW, Hajduczok G, Abboud FM. Paracrine role of prostanoids in activation of arterial baroreceptors: an overview. *Clin Exp Hypertens [A]* 1991;A13(5):817–824.

122. McDowell TS, Axtelle TS, Chapleau MW, Abboud FM. Prostaglandins in carotid sinus enhance baroreflex in rabbits. *Am J Physiol* 1989;257:R445–R450.

123. Chen HI, Chapleau MW, McDowell TS, Abboud FM. Prostaglandins contribute to activation of baroreceptors in rabbits. *Circ Res* 1990;67:1394–1404.

124. Xie P, Chapleau MW, McDowell TS, Hajduczok G, Abboud FM. Mechanism of decreased baroreceptor activity in chronic hypertensive rabbits. *J Clin Invest* 1990;86:625–630.

125. Miller MJS, Quilley J, McGiff JC. Eicosanoid-dependent mechanisms and the regulation of blood pressure. In: Zanchetti A, Tarazi RC, eds. *Handbook of hypertension*, vol 8. New York: Elsevier, 1986;578–602.

126. Mistry M, Nasjletti A. Prostanoids as mediators of prohypertensive and antihypertensive mechanisms. *Am J Med Sci* 1988;295:263–267.

127. Flower RJ. Drugs which inhibit prostaglandin biosynthesis. *Pharmacol Rev* 1974;26:33–67.

128. Quilley J, McGiff JC, Nasjletti A. Role of endoperoxides in arachidonic acid-induced vasoconstriction in the isolated perfused kidney of the rat. *Br J Pharmacol* 1989;96:111–116.

129. Colina-Chourio J, McGiff JC, Nasjletti A. Effect of indomethacin on blood pressure in the normotensive unanaesthetized rabbit: possible relation to prostaglandin synthesis inhibition. *Clin Sci* 1979;57:359–365.

130. Carroll MA, Schwartzman M, Baba M, Miller MJS, McGiff JC. Renal cytochrome P-450-related arachidonate metabolism in rabbit aortic coarctation. *Am J Physiol* 1988;255:F151–F157.

131. Abe K, Tsunoda K, Yasujima M, et al. Implication of renal prostaglandins in pathogenesis of essential hypertension. *Adv Prostaglandin Thromboxane Leukotriene Res* 1985;15:461–468.

132. Wennmalm A. Influence of indomethacin on the systemic and pulmonary vascular resistance in man. *Clin Sci Mol Med* 1978;54:141–145.

133. Negus P, Tannen RL, Dunn MJ. Indomethacin potentiates the vasoconstrictor actions of angiotensin II in normal man. *Prostaglandins* 1976;12:175–180.

134. Glanzer K, Prussing B, Dusing R, Kramer HJ. Hemodynamic and hormonal responses to 8-arginine vasopressin in healthy man: effects of indomethacin. *Klin Wochenschr* 1982;60:1234–1239.

135. Lin L, Mistry M, Stier CT Jr, Nasjletti A. Role of prostanoids in renin-dependent and renin-independent hypertension. *Hypertension* 1991;17:517–525.

136. Carroll MA, Garcia MP, Falck JR, McGiff JC. Cyclooxygenase dependency of the renovascular actions of cytochrome P450-derived arachidonate metabolites. *J Pharmacol Exp Ther* 1992;260:104–109.

137. Pedersen EB, Christensen NJ, Christensen P, et al. Preeclampsia—a state of prostaglandin deficiency? *Hypertension* 1983;5:105–111.

138. Everett RB, Worley RJ, MacDonald PC, Gant N. Effect of prostaglandin synthetase inhibitors on pressor response to angiotensin II in human pregnancy. *J Clin Endocrinol Metab* 1978;46:1007–1010.

139. Sanchez-Ramos L, O'Sullivan MJ, Garrido-Calderon J. Effect of low-dose aspirin on angiotensin II pressor response in human pregnancy. *Am J Obstet Gynecol* 1987;156:193–194.

140. Fitzgerald DJ, Entman SS, Mulloy K, FitzGerald GA. Decreased prostacyclin biosynthesis preceding the clinical manifestation of pregnancy-induced hypertension. *Circulation* 1987;75:956–963.

141. Minuz P, Covi G, Paluani F, et al. Altered excretion of prostaglandin and thromboxane metabolites in pregnancy-induced hypertension. *Hypertension* 1988;11:550–556.

142. Spitz B, Magness RR, Cox SM, Brown CEL, Rosenfeld CR, Gant NF. Low-dose aspirin. I. Effect on angiotensin II pressor responses and blood prostaglandin concentrations in pregnant women sensitive to angiotensin II. *Am J Obstet Gynecol* 1988;159:1035–1043.

143. Brown CEL, Gant NF, Cox K, Spitz B, Rosenfeld CR, Magness RR. Low-dose aspirin. II. Relationship of angiotensin II pressor responses, circulating eicosanoids, and pregnancy outcome. *Am J Obstet Gynecol* 1990;163:1853–1861.

144. Terragno A, Zamarano B, McGiff JC, Vio CP, Terragno NA. Correlation between arterial wall synthesis of prostaglandin and blood pressure in spontaneously hypertensive rats and Wistar-Kyoto rats. In: Lewis PJ, Moncada S, O'Grady J, eds. *Prostacyclin in pregnancy*. New York: Raven Press, 1983;109–113.

145. Chu ZM, Beilin LJ. Mechanisms of vasodilatation in pregnancy: studies of the role of prostaglandins and nitric-oxide in changes of vascular reactivity in the *in situ* blood perfused mesentery of pregnant rats. *Br J Pharmacol* 1993;109:322–329.

146. Catella F, Lawson JA, Fitzgerald DJ, FitzGerald GA. Endogenous biosynthesis of arachidonic acid epoxides in humans: increased formation in pregnancy-induced hypertension. *Proc Natl Acad Sci USA* 1990;87:5893–5897.

147. Tan SY, Sweet P, Mulrow PJ. Impaired renal production of prostaglandin E₂: a newly identified lesion in human essential hypertension. *Prostaglandins* 1978;15:139–149.

148. Abe K, Yasujima M, Chiba S, Irokawa N, Ito T, Yoshinaga K. Effect of furosemide on urinary excretion of prostaglandin E in normal volunteers and patients with essential hypertension. *Prostaglandins* 1977;14:513–521.

149. Weber PC, Scherer B, Held E, Siess W, Stoffel H. Urinary prosta-

glandins and kallikrein in essential hypertension. *Clin Sci* 1979;57:259s–261s.

150. Hornych A, Safar M, Bariety J, Simon A, London G, Levenson J. Thromboxane B₂ in borderline and essential hypertensive patients. *Prostaglandins Leukotrienes Med* 1983;10:145–155.

151. Miller MJS, McNeill H, Westlin WF, Carroll MA, McGiff JC. Exaggerated renal thromboxane and prostaglandin release by angiotensin II in suprarenal aortic coarctation hypertension. *Pharmacol Res* 1989;21:201–210.

152. Masotti G, Castellani S, Passavanti G, Scarti L, Neri Serneri GG. Blood pressure normalization restores normal renal prostaglandin production in essential hypertension. *Contrib Nephrol* 1985;49:179–184.

153. Tobian L, Uehara Y, Iwai J. Prostaglandin alterations in barely hypertensive Dahl S rats. *Trans Assoc Am Physicians* 1985;98:378–383.

154. Tobian L, Johnson MA, Ganguli M, Goto A, Iwai J. Prostaglandin E₂ (PGE₂) in renal papilla in NaCl hypertension. *Prog Lipid Res* 1981;20:501–503.

155. Sustarsic DL, McPartland RP, Rapp JP. Developmental patterns of blood pressure and urinary protein, kallikrein, and prostaglandin E₂ in Dahl salt-hypertensive-susceptible rats. *J Lab Clin Med* 1981;98:599–606.

156. Shibouta Y, Terashita Z-I, Inada Y, Nishikawa K, Kikuchi S. Enhanced thromboxane A₂ biosynthesis in the kidney of spontaneously hypertensive rats during development of hypertension. *Eur J Pharmacol* 1981;70:247–256.

157. Stier CT, Itskovitz HD. Thromboxane A₂ and the development of hypertension in spontaneously hypertensive rats. *Eur J Pharmacol* 1988;146:129–135.

158. Sessa WC, Abraham NG, Escalante B, Schwartzman ML. Manipulation of cytochrome P-450 dependent renal thromboxane synthase activity in spontaneously hypertensive rats. *J Hypertens* 1989;7:37–42.

159. Kappas A, Maines MD. Tin: a potent inducer of heme oxygenase in kidney. *Science* 1976;192:60–62.

160. Schwartzman ML, Abraham NG, Sacerdoti D, Escalante B, McGiff JC. Effect of acute and chronic treatment of tin on blood pressure in spontaneously hypertensive rats. *Tohoku J Exp Med* 1992;166:85–91.

161. Sacerdoti D, Abraham NG, McGiff JC, Schwartzman ML. Renal cytochrome P-450-dependent metabolism of arachidonic acid in spontaneously hypertensive rats. *Biochem Pharmacol* 1988;37:521–527.

162. Shibouta Y, Inada Y, Terashita Z, Nishikawa K, Kikuchi S, Shimamoto K. Angiotensin-II-stimulated release of thromboxane A₂ and prostacyclin (PGI₂) in isolated, perfused kidneys of spontaneously hypertensive rats. *Biochem Pharmacol* 1979;28:3601–3609.

163. Bierwaltes WH, Arendshorst WJ, Klemmer PJ. Electrolyte and water balance in young spontaneously hypertensive rats. *Hypertension* 1982;4:908–915.

164. Dilley JR, Stier CT Jr, Arendshorst WJ. Abnormalities in glomerular function in rats developing spontaneous hypertension. *Am J Physiol* 1984;246:F12–F20.

165. Needleman P, Raz A, Minkes MS, Ferrendelli JA, Sprecher H. Triene prostaglandins: prostacyclin and thromboxane biosynthesis and unique biological properties. *Proc Natl Acad Sci USA* 1979;76:944–948.

166. Jorgensen KA, Nielsen AH, Dyerberg J. Hemostatic factors and renin in Greenland eskimos on a high eicosapentaenoic acid intake. *Acta Med Scand* 1986;219:473–479.

167. Cox JW, Rutecki GW, Francisco LL, Ferris TF. Studies of the effects of essential fatty acid deficiency in the rat. *Circ Res* 1982;51:694–702.

168. Tobian L, Ganguli M, Johnson MA, Iwai J. Influence of renal prostaglandins and dietary linoleate on hypertension in Dahl S rats. *Hypertension* 1982;4(suppl II):149–153.

169. Ganguli MC, Tobian L, Iwai J. Reduction of blood pressure in salt-fed Dahl salt-sensitive rats with diets rich in olive oil, safflower oil or calcium biophosphate but not with calcium carbonate. *J Hypertens* 1986;4:S168–S169.

170. Lam BK, Marcinkiewicz E, Quilley J, et al. Hypotensive effects of eicosapentaenoic acid (EPA) and its influence on eicosanoid metabolism in spontaneously hypertensive rats. *J Hypertens* 1986;4(suppl 3):S453–S455.

171. Singer P, Berger I, Luck K, Taube C, Naumann E, Godicke W. Long-term effect of mackerel diet on blood pressure, serum lipids and thromboxane formation in patients with mild essential hypertension. *Atherosclerosis* 1986;62:259–265.

172. Knapp HR, FitzGerald GA. The antihypertensive effects of fish oil. A controlled study of polyunsaturated fatty acid supplements in essential hypertension. *N Engl J Med* 1989;320:1037–1043.

173. de Wardener HE, Clarkson EM. Concept of natriuretic hormone. *Physiol Rev* 1985;65:658–759.

174. Postnov YU, Reznikova M, Boriskina G. Na-K-adenosine triphosphatase in the kidney of rats with renal hypertension and spontaneously hypertensive rats. *Pflugers Arch* 1976;362:95–99.

175. Roman RJ, Ma Y-H, Frohlich B, Markham B. Clofibrate prevents the development of hypertension in Dahl salt-sensitive rats. *Hypertension* 1993;21:985–988.

176. Guyton AC. The surprising kidney-fluid mechanism for pressure control—its infinite gain! *Hypertension* 1990;16:725–730.

177. Ma Y-H, Gebremedhin D, Schwartzman ML, et al. 20-Hydroxyeicosatetraenoic acid is an endogenous vasoconstrictor of canine renal arcuate arteries. *Circ Res* 1993;72:126–136.

178. Escalante B, Falck JR, Yadagiri P, Sun L, Laniado-Schwartzman M. 19(s)-Hydroxyeicosatetraenoic acid is a potent stimulator of renal Na⁺-K⁺-ATPase. *Biochem Biophys Res Commun* 1988;152:1269–1274.

179. Roman RJ, Kaldunski ML. Renal cortical and papillary blood flow in spontaneously hypertensive rats. *Hypertension* 1988;11:657–663.

180. Omata K, Abraham NG, Escalante B, Laniado Schwartzman M. Age-related changes in renal cytochrome P-450 arachidonic acid metabolism in spontaneously hypertensive rats. *Am J Physiol* 1992;262:F8–F16.

181. Da-Silva J-L, Tiefenthaler M, Park E, Escalante B, Schwartzman ML, Abraham NG. Tin mediated heme oxygenase gene activation and cytochrome P450 arachidonate hydroxylase inhibition in spontaneously hypertensive rats. *Am J Med Sci* 1993;in press.

Hypertension: Pathophysiology, Diagnosis,
and Management, Second Edition,
edited by J.H. Laragh and B.M. Brenner,
Raven Press, Ltd., New York © 1995.

CHAPTER 58

The Kallikrein-Kinin System as a Regulator of Cardiovascular and Renal Function

Oscar A. Carretero and A. Guillermo Scicli

Both genetic and environmental factors participate in the regulation of blood pressure and in the etiology of hypertension. They act via intermediary phenotypes that control cardiac output and total peripheral resistance, and hence blood pressure (Fig. 1). Vasoactive systems are an important component of these intermediary phenotypes. They can act as local hormones (intracrine, autocrine, and paracrine) or as endocrine and neuroendocrine systems. We use the term *intracrine* to indicate hormones that act within the cells that synthesize them, such as products of proto-oncogenes. The term *autocrine* is used to indicate hormones that act on the cell membrane receptors where they are produced, such as growth factors. The term *paracrine* denotes hormones that act near the site where they are produced but have no systemic effects, such as kinins, eicosanoids, nitric oxide (NO), and endothelium-derived hyperpolarizing factor (EDHF). *Endocrine* refers to hormones such as aldosterone that are released into the extracellular fluid

and act on distant target tissues. Finally, *neuroendocrine* hormones such as catecholamines are released by neurons and act near to or distant from the site of release (Fig. 2).

Blood pressure is the result of a balance between vasopressor and vasodepressor systems. Alteration of this equilibrium may result in (a) hypertension, (b) effective antihypertensive treatment, or (c) hypotension and shock. Changes in this balance could be due to (a) genetic factors such as mutations in one of the genes of the vasoactive system, or genes that regulate the expression of these systems, and/or (b) environmental factors that alter synthesis and release of vasoactive hormones. Endocrine and neuroendocrine vasopressor systems, such as the renin-angiotensin system, aldosterone, and catecholamines, play a well-established and important role in the regulation of blood pressure and in the pathogenesis of some forms of secondary hypertension.

The role of vasodepressor systems is less well established; however, recent evidence suggests that they play an important role in the regulation of blood pressure, the pathogenesis of hypertension and the antihypertensive effects of inhibitors of angiotensin I–converting enzyme (ACE), neutral endopeptidase 24.11 (NEP-24.11), and perhaps metalloendopeptidase 24.15 (MEP-24.15) (1–

O. A. Carretero and A. G. Scicli: Hypertension and Vascular Research Division, Department of Medicine and Heart and Vascular Institute, Henry Ford Hospital, Detroit, Michigan 48202.

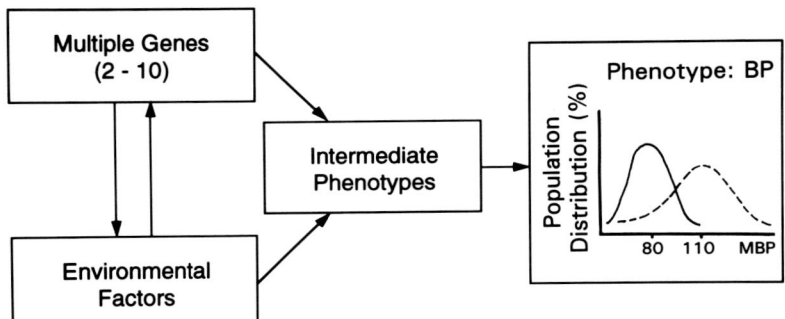

FIG. 1. Schematic representation of the interactions among genetic and environmental factors. Intermediary phenotypes such as low, normal, or high renin or urinary kallikrein are the result of this interaction. These intermediary phenotypes in turn affect blood pressure by increasing vascular resistance and/or cardiac output. As a consequence of the increase in blood pressure, the curve showing the blood pressure distribution in a population is flattened and shifted to the left. (From ref. 165, with permission.)

4). Vasodepressor hormones such as kinins, eicosanoids, endothelium-derived relaxing factor (EDRF), and EDHF act as local hormonal systems, opposing the effects of vasopressor systems. Some vasodepressor systems such as atrial natriuretic factor (ANF) and brain (BNP) and C-type (CNP) natriuretic peptides may act as both endocrine and local hormones. Here we will review the kinin-generating system and the role of kinins in (a) regulation of local blood flow, (b) water and sodium excretion, (c) regulation of blood pressure, (d) hypertension, (e) the antihypertensive effect of ACE inhibitors, (f) the vascular effect of ACE inhibitors, (g) the cardioprotective effect of ACE inhibitors, and (h) the effect of neutral endopeptidase 24.11.

THE KININ-GENERATING SYSTEM

Kininogenases such as glandular and plasma kallikreins are enzymes that generate kinins by hydrolyzing substrates known as kininogens, which circulate at high concentrations in plasma. Kinins are rapidly destroyed by a group of peptidases known as kininases (Fig. 3). Plasma and glandular (tissue) kallikrein are the two most potent kininogenases known; however, they are completely different enzymes. Plasma kallikrein, also known as Fletcher factor, is found in the zymogen form (prekallikrein) and differs from glandular kallikrein in its biochemical, immunological, and functional characteristics (Table 1). It preferentially releases bradykinin from high-

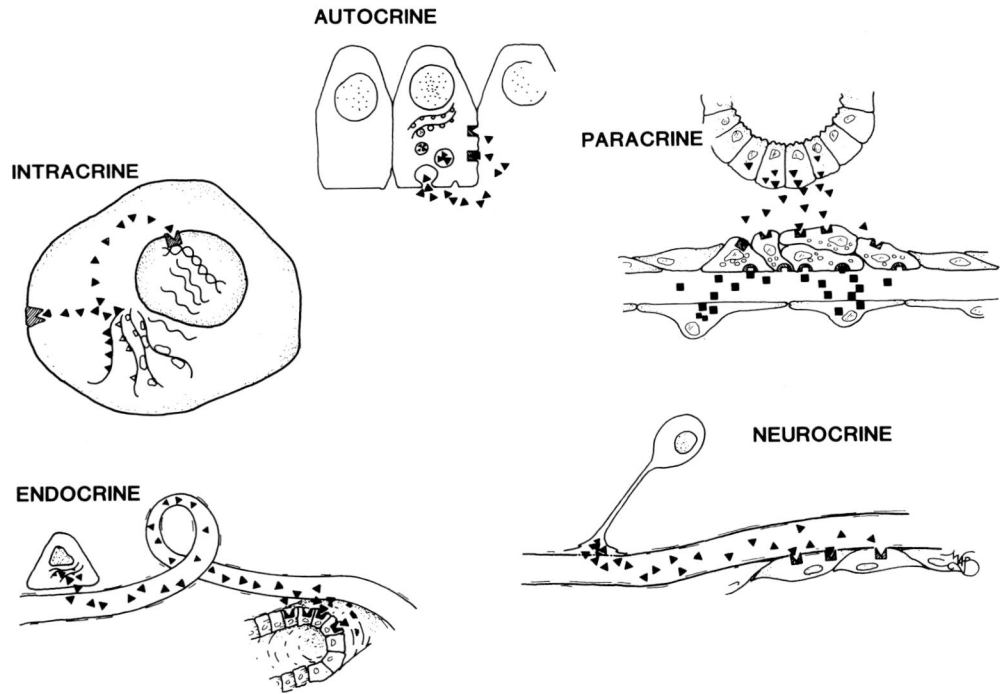

FIG. 2. Mechanisms of hormone action. Autocrine hormones act on the same cell that releases them; intracrine hormones are released and act within the cell; paracrine hormones are released by one cell and act on contiguous or neighboring cells; endocrine hormones are transported by the blood to distant cells; neurocrine hormones are released by a neuron terminal and act on a neighboring or distant cell. (From ref. 166, with permission.)

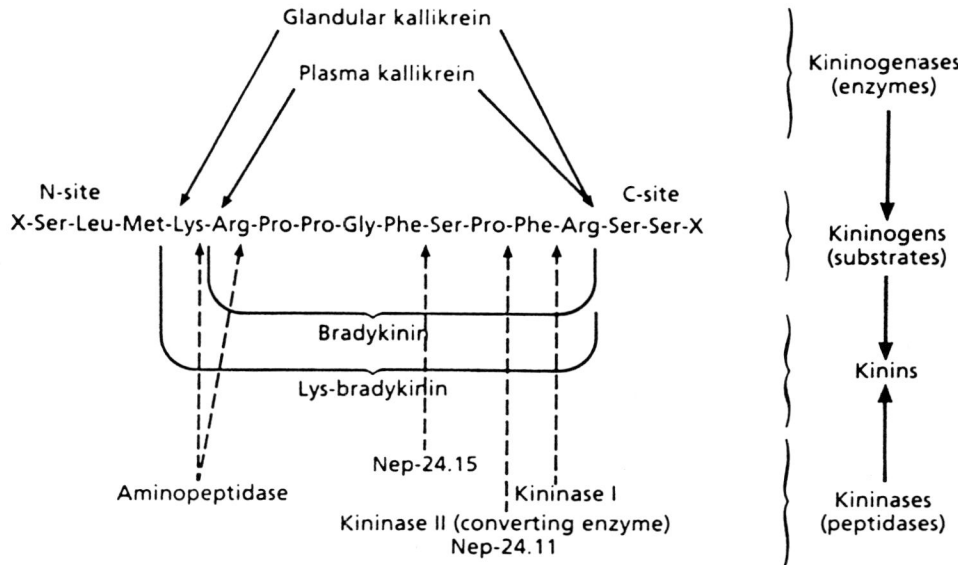

FIG. 3. Site of kininogen cleavage (*solid arrows*) by the main kininogenases (glandular and plasma kallikrein). The *broken arrows* indicate sites of kinin cleavage by kininases (kininase I, kininase II, neutral endopeptidases 24.11 and 24.15, and aminopeptidases). (Modified from ref. 1.)

molecular-weight kininogen (HMWK), also known as Fitzgerald factor; together with HMWK and Hageman factor, it is involved in coagulation, fibrinolysis, and possibly activation of the complement system. The plasma kallikrein-HMWK system, through the release of bradykinin, could be involved in the local regulation of blood flow and in some of the effects of ACE inhibitors. (For a review of the plasma kallikrein-HMWK system, see refs. 5–7).

Glandular or tissue kallikrein (hereafter referred to as glandular kallikrein, or simply kallikrein) belongs to a family of serine proteases with very high homology; the genes encoding for these enzymes are tightly clustered, arranged in tandem on the same chromosome (Fig. 4). The number of family members varies widely among mammals; it is estimated that the kallikrein family con-

tains at least 3 genes in humans, 20 in the rat, and 23 to 30 in the mouse, many of them pseudogenes (8). Despite the high homology of the amino acid composition of the serine proteases encoded by the glandular kallikrein gene family, some are not kininogenases and act on entirely different substrates. For example, tonin, a rat enzyme of the kallikrein family, hydrolyzes angiotensinogen and generates angiotensin II; prostate-specific antigen, a human enzyme of the kallikrein family, hydrolyzes semenogelin, a high-molecular-weight seminal vesicle protein (9,10). We have recently isolated a new member of the kallikrein family from the submandibular gland (11,12). This protease produces contraction of isolated aortic rings and (like tonin) also generates angiotensin II, suggesting that localized regions of variability are important in determining substrate specificity and possibly func-

TABLE 1. *Characteristics of plasma and glandular kallikrein*

	Plasma kallikrein	Glandular kallikrein
Molecular weight (daltons)	100,000	24,000–44,000
Substrate(s)	HMWK	LMWK and HMWK
Kinin released	Bradykinin	Lys-bradykinin[a]
Inhibited by SBTI	Yes	No
Function	Coagulation	Regulation of organ blood flow?
	Fibrinolysis	Water and electrolyte excretion?
	Inflammation?	Blood pressure homeostasis?
	Complement activation?	
	Blood pressure homeostasis?	

HMWK, high-molecular-weight kininogen; LMWK, low-molecular-weight kininogen; SBTI, soybean trypsin inhibitor.
[a] Rat glandular kallikrein releases bradykinin.

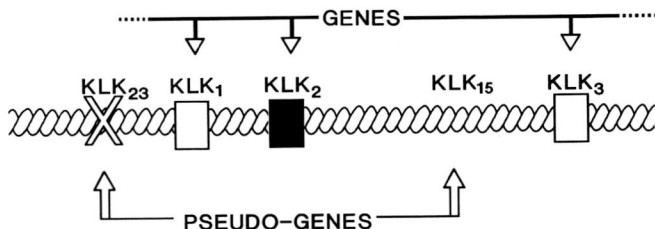

FIG. 4. The genes encoding members of the kallikrein family are situated together on the same chromosome [chromosome 7 in the mouse and the long arm of chromosome 19 (19q13.2-q13.4) in humans]. The kallikrein genes are located in tandem separated by 5,000 to 12,000 bases. They may be derived from a common ancestor. Duplication and recombination of this hypothetical primordial gene would have permitted separate copies to evolve into their complex current structures. Some genes are nonfunctional (pseudogenes). (From ref. 13, with permission.)

tion of all enzymes of the kallikrein family. (For a review of the molecular biology of the glandular kallikrein-kininogen system, see refs. 13–15.)

True glandular kallikrein is encoded by a single gene having five exons and four introns. Other members of the kallikrein gene family have a similar exonic and intronic structure, with the splice junctions completely

conserved. The 5' and 3' flanking regions have a high homology among the various genes; however, gene regulation and site of expression are different, suggesting that small variations in the nucleotide sequence of the 5' region are important in the regulation of expression. The true kallikrein gene is expressed mainly in the submandibular gland, pancreas, and kidney; however, using the polymerase chain reaction we have shown the presence of mRNA in vascular tissue, heart, and adrenal glands, although in smaller amounts (16,17). Kallikrein and kallikreinlike enzymes have also been found in the arteries and veins (18), heart (19), brain (20), pituitary gland (21,22), pancreas (23), intestine (24,25), salivary and sweat glands (26), spleen (27), adrenal glands (28), blood cells (17), and the exocrine secretions of these structures (Fig. 5). Some of them are probably true glandular kallikrein, while others may be separate members of the kallikrein family.

There is immunoreactive glandular kallikrein in plasma, primarily the inactive form; however, a small portion is in the active form (29–33). In humans (34) and rabbits (35), 50 percent or more of urinary kallikrein is the inactive or zymogen form, while in rats most is in the active form (36). Glandular kallikrein can release kinins from both low-molecular-weight kininogen (LMWK) and HMWK. Patients with congenital deficiency of

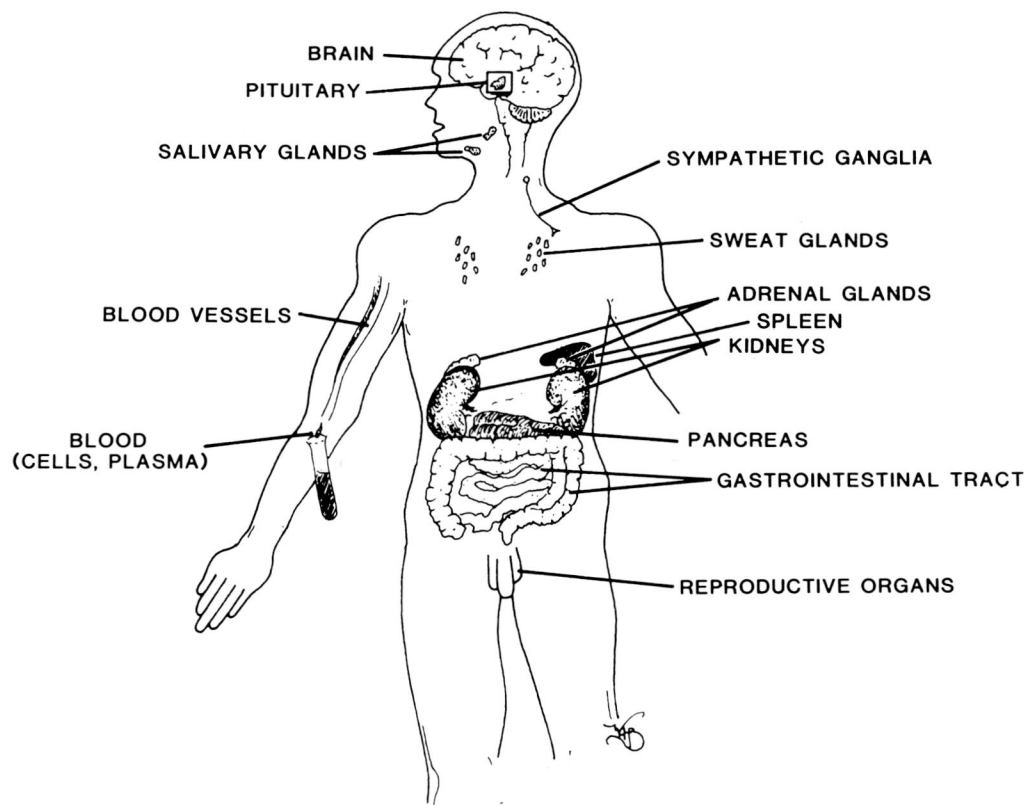

FIG. 5. Locations of mRNA and/or glandular kallikrein. (From ref. 1, with permission.)

plasma HMWK (Fitzgerald trait) have normal amounts of kinins in their blood (37). Glandular kallikrein releases Lys-bradykinin, although rat urinary kallikrein is an exception since it releases bradykinin (38,39).

Kininogens (kallikrein substrates) are the precursors of kinins. In plasma there are two main forms, characterized as LMWK and HMWK (40,41). In addition to releasing kinins, kininogens are potent inhibitors of cysteine proteinases such as calpain and cathepsins H, L, and B (42–44). In the rat there is a third kininogen known as t-kininogen because it releases kinins when incubated with trypsin but not with tissue or plasma kallikrein. It is one of the main acute reactants of inflammation in the rat. All kininogens are also inhibitors of thiol proteases, such as cathepsin M and H and calpains (45–48). In addition, HMWK is involved in the early stages of surface-activated coagulation (intrinsic coagulation pathway) (5,7,49).

Kininases are peptidases that are found in blood and other tissues. They hydrolyze kinins and other peptidic hormones (50). The best known is angiotensin-converting enzyme or kininase II (ACE), which converts angiotensin I to II and inactivates kinin substance P and other peptides (50,51). Another important kininase is neutral endopeptidase 24.11 (NEP-24.11), also known as enkephalinase, which not only hydrolyzes kinins and enkephalins but also destroys ANF, BNP, and endothelin (52,53). Research performed in our laboratory suggests that it may be the most important renal kininase, at least in the rat (54). Other kininases include MEP-24.15, aminopeptidases, and carboxypeptidases; however, it is not known whether they play an important role in the degradation of kinins *in vivo*. After inhibition of most of these enzymes *in vivo*, plasma concentrations of endogenous kinins do not increase significantly and their half-life remains less than 20 seconds, suggesting that other peptidases are also important in kinin metabolism (55).

Kinins are oligopeptides containing the sequence of bradykinin in their structure and act mainly as local hormones, since they circulate at very low concentrations (1 to 50 fmol/ml) and are rapidly hydrolyzed by kininases. In tissues such as the kidney, heart, and aorta, kinin concentrations are higher (100 to 350 fmol/g) (56). However, it is difficult to be certain that kinins are not generated by plasma kallikrein, which has been activated during the process of extracting the peptide from the tissue. Eicosanoids, endothelium-derived nitric oxide (EDNO), EDHF, tissue plasminogen activator (tPA), and cytokines mediate at least some of the effects of exogenously administered kinins (Fig. 6) (57–61). Whether or not endogenous kinins are present in various tissues at concentrations that can cause the release of most of these mediators needs to be studied further. At least two subtypes of kinin receptors have been well characterized using analogues of bradykinin, B_1 and B_2 (62,63). B_1 receptors are not present in normal tissues but are synthesized *de novo* during tissue injury, inflammation, and administration of lipopolysaccharides (such as endotoxin). In some species, such as rabbits, they mediate contraction of the isolated aorta and relaxation of mesenteric arteries. The main agonist for this receptor is des-Arg^9-bradykinin. B_2 receptors mediate most of the effects of bradykinin and are the main receptors for the agonists bradykinin and Lys-bradykinin. This receptor has recently been cloned and appears to belong to the family of seven transmembrane receptors linked to G-proteins (64). Studies using kinin analogues with agonistic and

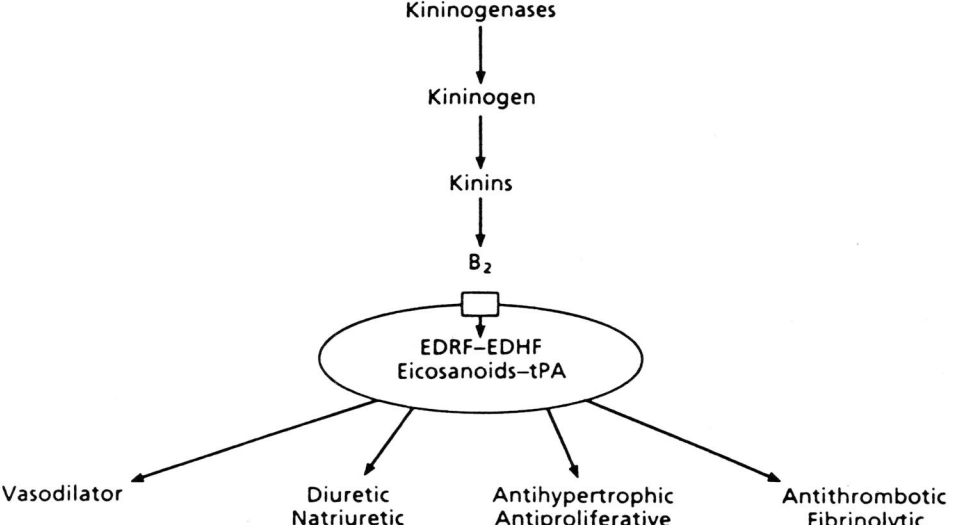

FIG. 6. Mechanism of kinin generation and effects of kinins, either directly or via various intermediaries (EDRF, EDHF, eicosanoids and tPA). (From ref. 165, with permission.)

antagonistic properties in various tissues suggest the existence of other subtypes of receptors (65–68). Stewart and Vavrek (69) discovered that substitution of D-phenylalanine for proline at position 7 of bradykinin converts it into a specific antagonist for B_1 and B_2 receptors. Further modifications have resulted in a very potent B_2 receptor antagonist with effects of extended duration *in vivo*, DArg^0-Hyp^3-Thi^5-DThi^7-Oic^8-bradykinin or Hoe 140 (70), which has become an important tool for studies of the role of kinins in various experimental situations.

KININS IN THE REGULATION OF LOCAL BLOOD FLOW

The development of antibodies to kinins and kallikrein, as well as kinin antagonists and kininase inhibitors, has allowed researchers to study the role of kinins in various physiological and pathological conditions. Kinins play a role in the local regulation of blood flow in the submandibular gland (which is rich in glandular kallikrein), uteroplacental complex, and kidney (71–74). In rats nephrectomized 48 hours earlier to exclude the renal renin-angiotensin system, use of an angiotensin I–converting enzyme (kininase II) inhibitor significantly increased blood flow in the submandibular gland but did not affect blood pressure. In contrast, 10 minutes after sympathetic stimulation of the gland to increase kallikrein secretion in the vascular compartment, the ACE inhibitor markedly decreased blood pressure and increased kinin concentrations in arterial blood (33,75). Changes in both blood flow and blood pressure were blocked by antibodies to kinins and glandular kallikrein. The effect of the ACE inhibitor on basal glandular blood flow was also blocked by a kinin antagonist, DArg^0-Hyp^3-Thi^{5,8}-DPhe^7-bradykinin (20 μg) (71). At this dose the antagonist caused no significant change in blood flow when the ACE inhibitor was not administered, whereas at a higher dose (100 μg/min) basal blood flow decreased significantly. These data suggest that in organs rich in glandular kallikrein, kinins play a role in the regulation of basal blood flow. Studies using kinin antibodies and antagonists clearly indicate that kinins act as paracrine hormones, regulating blood flow within the gland. They also indicate that the effect of ACE inhibitors on blood flow is mediated by kinins (71). In nephrectomized pregnant rabbits infused with an angiotensin antagonist to block the uterine renin-angiotensin system, ACE inhibitors increased both uterine and placental blood flow and immunoreactive prostaglandin E_2 (PGE$_2$), whereas these effects were blocked by a kinin antibody (72). This suggests that endogenously generated kinins may play a role in the regulation of uterine blood flow, either directly or through release of prostaglandins.

Blocking endogenous kinins by administration of low doses of a kinin antagonist, DArg^0-Hyp^3-Thi^{5,8}-DPhe^7-bradykinin, into the renal artery of sodium-depleted dogs did not affect blood pressure but did decrease renal blood flow and autoregulation of the glomerular filtration rate (GFR) (76). The changes in renal blood flow were blocked by prior inhibition of angiotensin I–converting enzyme, suggesting that either they were mediated by renin release due to an agonistic effect of the antagonist, or renal kinins may have increased when ACE (kininase II) was inhibited, thereby competing more effectively with the antagonist. The changes in GFR autoregulation were not altered by the ACE inhibitor and may have been due to a change in either the relationship between afferent and efferent glomerular arteriolar resistance or else the coefficient of filtration (76).

Using the same kinin antagonist, we examined the role of kinins in the regulation of outer cortical and papillary blood flow using a laser-Doppler flowmeter (73). The antagonist lowered papillary blood flow without altering outer cortical blood flow, suggesting that intrarenally formed kinins are important in regulating papillary blood flow. This study also showed that renin plays an important role in the regulation of papillary blood flow, since after kinins were blocked, enalaprilat increased flow significantly. We also found that when enalaprilat (a kininase II inhibitor) and phosphoramidon (an NEP-24.11 inhibitor) were administered simultaneously, papillary blood flow increased by 50 percent, compared with 25 percent for either one separately. These increases were blocked by the kinin antagonist, indicating that the augmented papillary blood flow induced by both ACE and NEP-24.11 inhibitors is mediated by increased kinin concentrations in the interstitial space. In this study no consistent effect on water or sodium excretion was observed; however, water excretion tends to decrease in animals treated with the antagonist.

Seino et al. (74) reported that a kinin antagonist lowered renal blood flow in anesthetized rats. Zimmerman et al. (77) reported that when kallikrein excretion was stimulated by sodium deprivation in dogs, the kinin antagonist (given intrarenally) blocked part of the effect of enalaprilat on renal blood flow. They concluded that although blockade of the renin-angiotensin system accounted for a significant portion of the increase in renal blood flow caused by the ACE inhibitor, a substantial component was contributed by endogenous kinins. Nakagawa and Nasjletti (78) reported similar results in rats, except that the kallikrein-kinin system was stimulated by administration of deoxycorticosterone.

In conclusion, although data regarding the role of kinins in the regulation of renal blood flow are inconsistent, in general they suggest that under basal conditions the role of kinins may be minor; however, when the kallikrein-kinin system is stimulated by low sodium intake or mineralocorticoids, or when endogenous kinin degradation is inhibited, kinins appear to participate in the regulation of renal blood flow. In addition, the data suggest that kinins play an important role in the regulation of papillary blood flow, and that during reduction of renal perfusion pressure, kinins may aid in regulation of the GFR. In the submandibular gland and uteroplacental complex, kinins appear to play an important role in the regulation of blood flow, especially when ACE is inhibited.

KININS IN THE REGULATION OF WATER AND ELECTROLYTE EXCRETION

Renal kallikrein is located in the connecting cells of the connecting tubule; it is released in significant amounts in this segment of the nephron and excreted in the urine (Fig. 7) (35,79,80). Kallikrein releases kinins into the lumen of the distal nephron, either from filtered kininogen or kininogen produced in the principal cells of the distal nephron (81,82). Kinin receptors are also present in the collecting duct (83). In addition, kallikrein is released on the basolateral side of the nephron, where it may liberate kinins from plasma kininogens (84). The interstitial renal fluid contains a high concentration of kinins (85). The role of kinins in the regulation of water and sodium excretion has been studied by either increasing intrarenal kinins or blocking kinins. Kauker showed that infusion of kinins into the late proximal nephron doubled excretion of simultaneously administered ^{22}Na (86), and that part of this effect was mediated by prostaglandins (87). The same investigator has shown that infusion of a kinin antagonist into the late proximal nephron reduced ^{22}Na recovery significantly (88). After systemic administration of phosphoramidon, an inhibitor of NEP-24.11 (which is a major kininase in the nephron), urinary excretion of kinins doubled; diuresis increased by 15 percent and natriuresis by 37 percent (54). Although these data support the hypothesis that increased kinins in the nephron participate in intrarenal control of water and electrolyte excretion, it is also possible that the effect of this peptidase inhibitor is mediated by blocking hydrolysis of other peptides such as ANF (89).

Pollock et al. (90) found that while infusion of aprotinin inhibited the enzymatic activity of urinary kallikrein, it did not affect acute water or electrolyte excretion in euvolemic and sodium- or water-expanded rats. A transient decrease in sodium excretion has been observed during aprotinin administration in mineralocorticoid-treated rats (91). Infusion of kinin antibodies into saline-expanded rats resulted in decreased sodium excretion (92); however, caution should be used in interpreting this finding, since antibodies may stimulate release of histamine, cause an anaphylactoid reaction, or form a high-molecular-weight complex with kininogen, which is then deposited in the nephron, any of which might alter water and sodium excretion. To avoid these problems, we use Fab fragments of kinin antibodies, which are rapidly distributed in the extracellular fluid and excreted by the kidney; moreover, they do not form high-molecular-weight complexes or activate complement and other proteolytic systems in plasma, thus reducing the risk of anaphylactoid reactions. In unanesthetized rats, the Fab fragments blocked 70 percent of the effect of an injection of 100 ng bradykinin on blood pressure and appeared rapidly in the urine, suggesting that they block the effect of kinins not only in the vascular and interstitial spaces but also in the lumen of the distal nephron. Using these Fab fragments and a kinin antagonist, we studied a model in which the renal kallikrein-kinin system is stimulated, namely, deoxycorticosterone acetate (DOCA)-salt–treated rats (93). Both the Fab fragments and kinin antagonist significantly decreased urine volume and increased urinary osmolarity; however, only the Fab fragments significantly lessened urinary sodium excretion. Neither altered blood pressure, renal blood flow, or GFR. The antidiuretic effect of the Fab fragments and kinin antagonist may be due to blockade of kinins in the vascular-interstitial space of the kidney, since the antagonist is likely hydrolyzed in the proximal tubule and does not reach the lumen of the distal nephron. On the other hand, the antinatriuretic effect of Fab fragments of kinin antibodies on sodium excretion may be due to blockade of kinins in both the vascular-interstitial and urinary compartments, or only due to

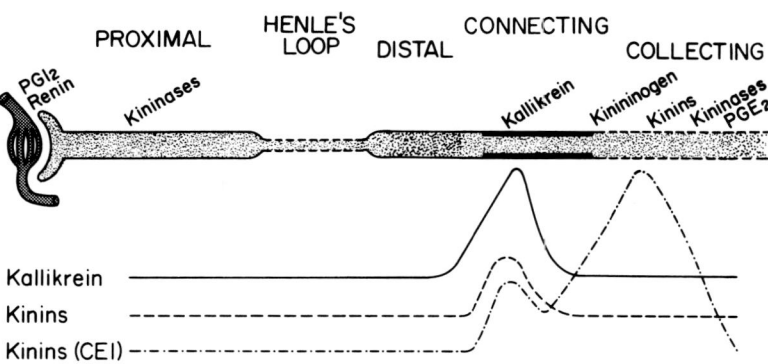

FIG. 7. Location of the renal kallikrein-kinin system in the nephron. Lines at the bottom of the figure represent the site of secretion of kallikrein (*continuous line*) and the site of kinin release (*dashed line*) in the urinary compartment. Kinins (CEI) followed by a *dashed line* with intercalated points indicate the site of kinin formation during treatment with ACE inhibitors. (Modified from ref. 167.)

blockade in the latter, since the antibody appeared in the urine and the antidiuretic effect was not observed with the antagonist. Thus kinins may aid in the regulation of water and sodium excretion when the kallikrein-kinin system is stimulated.

In normal nonanesthetized rats, inhibition of kinin release in the lumen of the nephron by Fab fragments of monoclonal antibodies to kallikrein causes urinary PGE_2, urinary volume (UV), and urinary sodium excretion ($U_{Na}V$) to decrease. The changes in UV and $U_{Na}V$ correlate with those of PGE_2, suggesting that the natriuretic and diuretic effects of kinins are mediated in part by PGE_2 (94).

In vitro, stimulation of the release of EDRF from endothelial cells by bradykinin or acetylcholine increases guanosine 3',5'-cyclic monophosphate (cGMP) content and inhibits Na^+ transport by cortical collecting duct cells (95). *In vivo,* stimulation of EDRF release by bradykinin results in natriuresis and diuresis without affecting the GFR (96). In conclusion, kinins acting as local hormones play a role in the regulation of renal hemodynamic and excretory function, either directly or via the release of PGE_2 and EDRF.

KININS AS REGULATORS OF BLOOD PRESSURE

Kinins circulate in concentrations of approximately 5 to 50 pg/ml of blood (37). These concentrations need to be increased to at least 100 pg in humans (97) and 1,000 pg in rats (98) to cause acute decreases in blood pressure. Although blood kinin concentrations may increase in some physiological and pathological situations, they seldom reach levels that could explain changes in blood pressure, save for exceptional experimental conditions such as stimulation of the sympathetic nerve of the submandibular gland in animals treated with ACE inhibitors (see section on blood flow regulation). Thus kinins would have to be acting as paracrine hormones, regulating local vascular resistance and organ function.

We have shown that arteries and veins contain a kallikreinlike enzyme, and that both vascular tissue and smooth muscle in culture contain mRNA for glandular kallikrein (16,18). Recently Oza et al. (99) reported that vascular smooth muscle in culture releases both glandular kallikrein and kininogen. Thus the components of the kallikrein-kinin system are present in vascular tissue, where they could play an important role in the regulation of blood pressure.

Benetos et al. (100) reported that in rats, high doses of the kinin antagonist Hyp^3-$Thi^{5,8}$-$DPhe^7$-bradykinin (1 mg/rat) increased blood pressure by 13 mm Hg in most animals tested, while a vasodepressor effect was observed in some. At smaller doses (though still sufficient to block exogenous bradykinin), the same antagonist did not alter normal blood pressure. We used a similar antagonist but with DArg residue added to the N-terminal, which Beierwaltes et al. (101) have shown has roughly three times the antagonist activity in the dog hindlimb compared with the peptide Benetos et al. used. When injected into the ascending aorta at high doses (4 mg/kg), it produced a transient biphasic response: first a small pressor effect, followed by a depressor effect (102). While kinins also induce biphasic effects in blood pressure in rats, they first cause a decrease, followed by an increase. The pressor effect of kinins is primarily due to the release of catecholamines by the adrenal glands (103). Kinins can also stimulate release of renin, vasopressin, prostaglandins, and histamine (104–106). To determine whether the pressor effect of the antagonist is due to agonist activity, we tested whether it could be abolished by adrenalectomy, nephrectomy, ganglionic and α and β blockers, a V_1 vasopressin receptor antagonist, H_1 and H_2 histamine receptor blockers, or indomethacin, a prostaglandin synthesis inhibitor; however, we found that it was not affected by any of them, and, conversely, that the depressor effect was blocked by indomethacin and nephrectomy, suggesting that it is caused by release of prostanoids from the kidney (102).

The above studies are compatible with the hypothesis that kinins play a role in the regulation of blood pressure. However, in order to demonstrate the pressor effect, the kinin antagonist has to be used at much higher doses than those needed to block the vasodepressor effect of exogenous bradykinin. High doses may be needed to displace kinins bound to tissue receptors. We must be cautious in interpreting these data, since we cannot rule out the possibility that these kinin antagonists have a vasopressor effect that is unrelated to kinin-blocking activity. Studies by our group using kinin antibodies or their Fab fragments showed that although they partially block the vasodepressor effect of kinins, they cause no acute changes in blood pressure.

Chronically blocking the effect of kinins by infusing a kinin antagonist in normal rats does not increase blood pressure (107,108), suggesting that in normal situations kinins are not a major contributor to the regulation of blood pressure. While rats with a deficiency of kininogen (the kinin precursor) or chronic blockade of the kallikrein-kinin system do not have hypertension, they are more sensitive to the hypertensinogenic effect of salt, deoxycorticosterone plus salt (DOCA-salt), and nonpressor doses of angiotensin II (109–112). However, these studies need to be confirmed before we can be sure kinins oppose potent hypertensive stimuli such as salt, mineralocorticoids, or angiotensin II. At present, using a protocol similar to that reported by Katori and Majima (110), we have not been able to confirm that blockade of kinins with high doses of Hoe 140 makes subpressor doses of angiotensin II hypertensive (Nanba M, Scicli AG, and Carretero OA, unpublished results).

THE KALLIKREIN-KININ SYSTEM IN HUMAN AND EXPERIMENTAL HYPERTENSION

The hypothesis that hypertension results from either an excess of vasopressor substances or a deficiency of vasodepressor substances has stimulated research on the role of the kallikrein-kinin system in the pathogenesis of various types of human and experimental hypertension. The kidney, considered one of the most important determinants in the long-range control of blood pressure, has both vasopressor (renin-angiotensin system) and vasodepressor components (kallikrein-kinin-prostaglandin system). These vasoactive substances could participate in the kidney's capacity to regulate excretion of sodium and water.

Several reports indicate that urinary kallikrein excretion is decreased in essential hypertension in man and in various experimental models of hypertension. However, these results are not universal, as some reports indicate that urinary kallikrein excretion is not altered in essential hypertension unless the kidney has been damaged (for a review, see ref. 1). The reasons for this discrepancy are not known; however, it is interesting to note that many hypertensive patients exhibit normal kallikrein excretion, whereas others have conspicuously low amounts of kallikrein (113). On the other hand, in children with a positive family history of hypertension, there is a negative relationship between blood pressure and kallikrein excretion (114). Berry et al. (115) reported that urinary kallikrein excretion is one of the major genetic markers associated with a family history of essential hypertension. These studies support the hypothesis that the kallikrein-kinin system could also be altered and thus participate in the pathogenesis of essential hypertension.

In an epidemiological study involving a large population of normal children and their mothers, there was a significant familial clustering of urinary kallikrein concentration (esterase activity) (116,117). It was significantly lower in black children than in whites and was found to vary with the season (lower in summer) and time of day (highest in the morning). Families with the lowest mean kallikrein concentrations tended to have higher blood pressure, suggesting a concomitant genetic influence on both blood pressure and kallikrein excretion. In this regard, it is interesting to note that urinary kallikrein excretion is decreased in three different models of genetically hypertensive rats developed by selective inbreeding on the basis of blood pressure (118-120). Perhaps one of the genetic loci that control blood pressure is linked to another that controls renal kallikrein. At present, it is not clear whether these are concomitant but functionally unrelated phenomena, or whether the decrease in kallikrein excretion is a pathogenetic factor in the development of hypertension. Another possibility is that kallikrein excretion is decreased secondary to the increase in blood pressure; however, decreased urinary kallikrein is seen in normotensive children of patients with essential hypertension and also in rats of the New Zealand genetically hypertensive strain as well as in rats bred to be susceptible to the hypertensive effect of salt (Dahl salt-sensitive rats) prior to the development of hypertension (113,118–121). Furthermore, restriction fragment length polymorphisms (RFLP) in the glandular kallikrein gene family have been found in spontaneously hypertensive rats (SHR) compared to Wistar-Kyoto rats (WKY); however, in this study it was not determined whether or not RFLPs were linked to hypertension (122). We have recently found that SHR also exhibit RFLPs compared to brown Norway rats. We studied 32 recombinant inbred substrains of rats derived from these two strains and found that in those that inherited the kallikrein RFLP from SHR, systolic, diastolic, and mean blood pressure were significantly greater than in those that inherited it from the brown Norway progenitor strain (123). These findings suggest that structural alterations in the kallikrein gene family or closely linked genes may have the capacity to affect blood pressure.

Urinary kallikrein excretion is decreased in Dahl salt-sensitive rats (118). It may be that a decrease in kallikrein-kinin system activity alters sodium and water excretion in susceptible rats and thereby promotes hypertension during high sodium intake. It is even possible that similar defects occur in some patients with essential hypertension and very low urinary kallikrein excretion. Kallikrein excretion and renal tissue kallikrein are also decreased in renovascular hypertension (121,124,125), whereas they are increased in hypertension resulting from excess mineralocorticoids, such as primary aldosteronism and DOCA-salt hypertension (121,126–128).

In conclusion, urinary kallikrein excretion is frequently decreased in humans and experimental animals with primary or secondary hypertension, with the exception of mineralocorticoid-induced hypertension in which kallikrein excretion is normal or increased. It has not yet been proven that the decrease in kallikrein excretion indicates lessened intrarenal formation of kinins, or that it contributes to the pathogenesis of hypertension.

ROLE OF KININS IN THE ANTIHYPERTENSIVE EFFECT OF ANGIOTENSIN-CONVERTING ENZYME INHIBITORS

Inhibition of kinin degradation may contribute to the antihypertensive effect of ACE inhibitors (Fig. 8). While blockade of angiotensin II formation appears to be important in this regard, the role of kinins is less well established. Orally active ACE inhibitors are effective antihypertensive agents, not only in high-renin hypertension but also in clinical and experimental models in which the

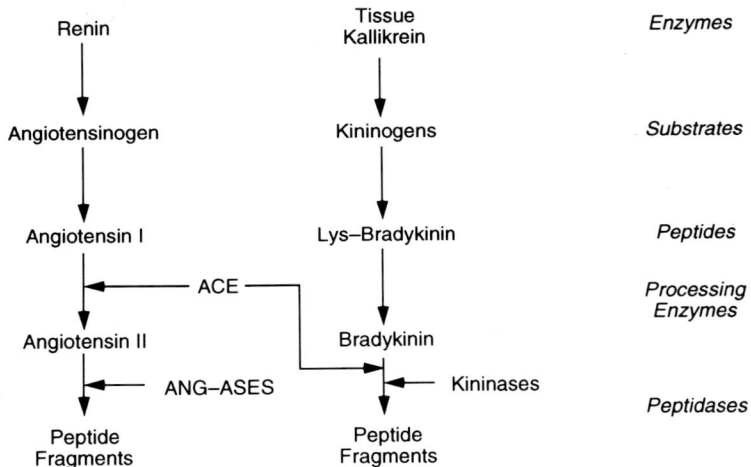

FIG. 8. Schematic representation of the renin-angiotensin and kallikrein-kinin systems. In both systems, a substrate is cleaved by an enzyme of restricted specificity, releasing a peptide that is either already active (Lys-bradykinin, bradykinin) or inactive (angiotensin I). Upon further processing by a specific peptidase, angiotensin I is converted to a vasoactive peptide (angiotensin II). Vasoactive peptides are in turn inactivated by peptidases. Angiotensin-converting enzyme is common to both systems but has different roles: it processes angiotensin I to angiotensin II and is the main kinin-inactivating peptidase. (From ref. 165, with permission.)

renin-angiotensin system has not been pathogenetically implicated (129,130). Thus some effects of ACE inhibitors may be mediated by local renin-angiotensin systems, kinins, or some other as-yet-undetermined mechanism, since ACE can hydrolyze other peptides.

Plasma kinins are unchanged or moderately increased after administration of ACE inhibitors (1). Kinins in the urine have been reported to increase more consistently after ACE inhibitors, indicating that their concentration in renal tissue likewise increases (54,131–134). This in turn may contribute to the antihypertensive effect of ACE inhibitors by altering renovascular resistance and increasing sodium and water excretion.

Many studies have been performed to determine the role of kinins in the antihypertensive effect of ACE inhibitors. Aprotinin, an inhibitor of kallikrein and other proteases, blocks the acute antihypertensive effect of captopril in patients with low- and normal-renin essential hypertension (135). The influence of aprotinin could be due to inhibition of kinin formation or other effects. In SHR and rats with two-kidney, one-clip (2K1C) renovascular hypertension, the acute antihypertensive effects of ACE inhibitors are partially blocked by high-titer antibodies against kinins (136–138), which, however, do not alter their vasodepressor effect in sodium-depleted normotensive rats. Benetos et al. (139) reported that the acute antihypertensive effect of ACE inhibitors in 2K1C rats could be reversed by about 30 percent with a kinin antagonist.

We assessed the influence of kinins on the acute antihypertensive effect of enalaprilat in rats with severe hypertension induced by aortic ligation between the renal arteries (140). In this model, renin plays an important role in the pathogenesis of hypertension (129); however, acute and severe hypertension can produce endothelial damage that may lead to activation of plasma kallikrein and increased kinin formation. We found that enalaprilat lowered mean blood pressure by 48 ± 6 mm Hg in the control group (Fig. 9). In rats treated with the kinin

antagonist, enalaprilat decreased mean blood pressure by only 21 ± 4 mm Hg, which is a significant difference ($p < .01$); however, kinin concentrations in arterial plasma were not significantly altered by the ACE inhibitor (41 ± 10 vs. 68 ± 20 pg/ml). As indicated earlier, if mean blood pressure in the unanesthetized rat is to be decreased, kinins in arterial blood must reach at least 1,000 pg/ml (98). Thus the effect of the ACE inhibitor may be due to an increase in tissue kinins, which could act as a paracrine hormonal system regulating vascular resistance. There is also evidence that in the anesthetized dog, kinins may play a role in the acute hypotensive effect of ACE inhibitors through the release of prostaglandins (141). In conclusion, these studies suggest that some acute effects of ACE inhibitors on blood flow and blood pressure are mediated by kinins, which affect local and peripheral vascular resistance either directly or through release of prostaglandins and EDRF(s). Moreover, kinin antagonists have recently been shown to block some of the chronic antihypertensive effects of ACE inhibitors in renovascular and DOCA-salt hypertension but not in SHR (108,142).

ROLE OF KININS IN THE VASCULAR PROTECTIVE EFFECT OF ANGIOTENSIN-CONVERTING ENZYME INHIBITORS

After removing the endothelium from the carotid artery by passing a catheter with an inflated balloon, the smooth muscle cells are activated and begin to proliferate in the media; they then migrate across the internal elastic lamina into the intima, where they proliferate further to produce neointimal hyperplasia. ACE inhibitors have been shown to inhibit this neointima formation (143,144). Blocking kinins or inhibiting NO synthesis suppresses the protective effect of the ACE inhibitor, suggesting that it may be mediated by a local increase in kinins that may stimulate the release of EDRF, perhaps

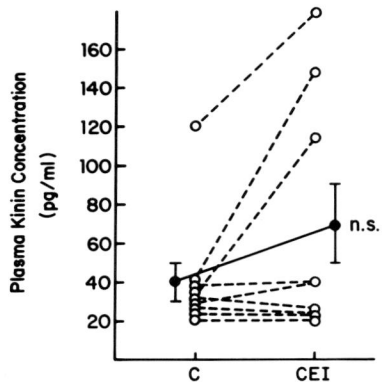

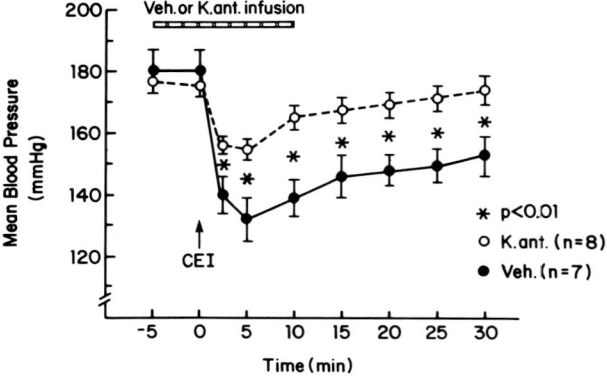

FIG. 9. Plasma kinin concentrations before (C) and 10 minutes after administration of an ACE inhibitor (enalaprilat, 60 μg/kg) in rats with severe hypertension. *Open circles* represent individual rats; *closed circles* are mean values (±SEM) of the entire group (**top**). Effect of ACE inhibitors (enalaprilat, 60 μg/kg) on mean blood pressure of rats with severe hypertension given either kinin antagonist (K ant; 40 μg/kg/min) or vehicle (VEH; 0.9 percent NaCl). Values are mean ± SEM (**bottom**). (From ref. 140, with permission.)

from the vascular smooth muscle cells (107,145). Blocking the effect of angiotensin II with a receptor antagonist has also been shown to inhibit neointima formation (146). These studies suggest that there is a balance among factors that stimulate and inhibit neointima formation, and that alteration of this balance in favor of neointima inhibition, either by blocking kinin degradation and formation of angiotensin II or by suppressing angiotensin II at the level of the receptor, will inhibit neointima formation.

ROLE OF KININS IN THE CARDIOPROTECTIVE EFFECT OF ANGIOTENSIN-CONVERTING ENZYME INHIBITORS

ACE inhibitors have been shown to reverse left ventricular hypertrophy in essential hypertension and in various experimental models. This decrease is partly due to reduced afterload; however, it has been postulated that this antihypertrophic effect may be independent of the decrease in blood pressure. A decrease in angiotensin II formation, which stimulates various proto-oncogenes and growth factors, may participate in the antihypertrophic effect of ACE inhibitors independent of its effect on blood pressure. The cardiac kallikrein-kinin system may also participate in the effect of ACE inhibitors on the heart. Recently it was shown that doses of ACE inhibitors that do not decrease blood pressure reverse left ventricular hypertrophy in rats with hypertension due to aortic coarctation (147). However, to be certain that the doses used do not decrease blood pressure, direct 24-hour blood pressure measurements are needed. The effects of ACE inhibitors on cardiac hypertrophy were reversed by a kinin antagonist, suggesting that kinins mediate this effect either directly or by the release of EDRF or PGI₂ (148). However, using a very similar protocol, we have not been able to confirm that blocking kinins reverses the antihypertrophic effect of ACE inhibitors (149). Capillary length and density increase in hearts of SHR treated with an ACE inhibitor at both antihypertensive and non-antihypertensive doses; since there is evidence that angiotensin II has angiogenic effects (150), this effect of the ACE inhibitor may be due to kinins (151). However, these investigators did not determine whether the effect of ACE inhibitors was blocked by a kinin antagonist. In conclusion, further studies are needed to determine whether doses of ACE inhibitors that do not decrease blood pressure reverse cardiac hypertrophy, and whether kinins participate in this effect.

During myocardial ischemia followed by sympathetic nerve stimulation, kinins in coronary sinus blood increase significantly (152). An ACE inhibitor was shown to reduce myocardial infarct size after ischemia-reperfusion in dogs and rabbits whereas an angiotensin II antagonist (losartan) did not (153). In nephrectomized dogs in which infarction was induced by occlusion of the coronary artery for 90 minutes, blockade of local angiotensin II formation with protease inhibitors had no significant effect on myocardial infarct size despite decreased angiotensin II release. Captopril did not alter local angiotensin II formation but did increase bradykinin and reduce infarct size, suggesting that kinins were responsible for the effect of the ACE inhibitor on infarct size (154). Similarly, when low doses of the ACE inhibitor ramiprilat (which had no systemic effect) were infused into the left coronary artery in dogs, they reduced the size of the infarct caused by ligation of the descending branch of the left coronary artery (155). This cardioprotective effect of ramiprilat was mimicked by bradykinin and abolished by coadministration of a kinin antagonist. Similarly, there is evidence that local inhibition of angiotensin II formation and kinin degradation with an ACE inhibitor ameliorates the cardiac arrhythmias induced by digoxin or reperfusion (156).

In conclusion, in patients with heart failure, ACE inhibitors have been shown not only to improve cardiac function and increase survival but also to decrease the rate of myocardial reinfarction (157). The mechanism of this decrease is not known; however, since ACE inhibitors may block kinin degradation in the coronary circulation, one hypothesis is that kinins stimulate the release of EDRF and PGI_2, which in turn are important inhibitors of platelet aggregation. Since kinins are potent stimulators of the release of tPA (61,158), it is also possible that this potentiation of tPA release may in turn activate plasmin and fibrinolysis. Although the exact mechanism of action of ACE inhibitors in reinfarction is not known, these hypotheses open up a new and exciting area of cardiovascular research.

ROLE OF KININS IN THE ANTIHYPERTENSIVE EFFECT OF NEUTRAL METALLOENDOPEPTIDASE EC3.4.24.11 (NEP-24.11) INHIBITORS

The effects of NEP-24.11 inhibitors, like those of ACE inhibitors, are probably due to blockade of the hydrolysis of a variety of peptides; some lower blood pressure, such as ANF, kinins, enkephalins, and endorphins, while others may increase blood pressure, among them angiotensin, endothelin, neurotensin, and perhaps vasopressin (for a review, see ref. 159), but in any event the final result is a decrease in blood pressure (160). The prevailing hypothesis is that these substances lower blood pressure by inhibiting the hydrolysis of ANF. However, NEP-24.11 is an important kininase in both the kidney and brain (54,159). In our laboratory, Ura et al. (54) have shown that NEP-24.11 is the main renal kininase in the rat and that acute inhibition of this enzyme by phosphoramidon resulted in an increase in urinary kinins and sodium and water excretion; however, it did not alter plasma kinins (55). We propose that the saluretic effect of phosphoramidon may be mediated by an increase in renal kinins and ANF. Smits et al. (161) reported that thiorphan, which is also an NEP-24.11 inhibitor, potentiated the acute effects of ANF on water and sodium excretion, and that these effects were blocked completely by a kinin antagonist. At the dose infused, ANF had no effect on blood pressure. However, it has also been reported that the acute natriuretic effect of NEP-24.11 inhibitors is blocked by ANF antisera (162). In normotensive humans, UK 79300, also an NEP-24.11 inhibitor, increased urinary sodium, water, ANF, and cGMP excretion when administered twice at 12-hour intervals (163). At the dose used, the inhibitor caused no changes in blood pressure; however, plasma renin activity and aldosterone were significantly decreased while a small increase in plasma ANF was observed. (Kinins were not measured in this study.) These studies support the hypothesis that the natriuretic and diuretic effects of NEP-24.11 inhibitors are mediated by an increase in both ANF and renal kinins, which may act synergistically. It is not clear whether an increase in plasma and/or renal ANF is needed for these effects.

Sybertz et al. (2,89) and Seymour et al. (3) have reported that inhibition of NEP-24.11 in DOCA-salt hypertension has an acute antihypertensive effect. In this model, plasma ANF is increased; however, the NEP-24.11 inhibitor did not cause a further increase in ANF and yet polyclonal antiserum to ANF blocked most of the antihypertensive effect of NEP-24.11 while the kinin antagonist had no effect (2). In SHR, NEP-24.11 inhibitors also had an antihypertensive effect, though it was less than in DOCA-salt rats (3) and in some cases the inhibitor took 3 days to lower blood pressure. In humans it has been reported that NEP inhibitors have an antihypertensive effect, which was more pronounced in black patients (164).

In conclusion, NEP inhibitors may be useful in the treatment of hypertension and perhaps heart failure. Their hypertensive effect is probably due to a direct vasodilator action of ANF and the combined natriuretic effect of both ANF and kinins. However, the role of other vasoactive peptides that may be cleaved by NEP-24.11 cannot be completely excluded.

SUMMARY

Local (intracrine, autocrine, and paracrine), endocrine, and neuroendocrine hormonal systems are important components of the many factors that regulate cardiovascular and renal function. Hypertension may result from alteration of the balance among these various systems. Changes in this balance could be due to genetic factors such as (a) mutations in one of the genes of the vasoactive system, or genes that regulate the expression of these systems, and/or (b) environmental factors. These changes may alter synthesis, release, inactivation, and/or sensitivity of one or more vasoactive hormones.

Endocrine and neuroendocrine vasopressor hormonal systems, such as the renin-angiotensin system, aldosterone, and catecholamines, play a well-established and important role in the regulation of blood pressure and the pathogenesis of some secondary forms of hypertension, and perhaps essential hypertension as well. The role of vasodepressor hormones, such as kinins, eicosanoids, and endothelium-derived relaxing factor (EDRF), is less well established. Part of the difficulty involved in determining their function is the fact that they act mainly as autocrine/paracrine hormones. However, there is increasing evidence that vasodepressor hormones not only play an important role in the regulation of blood pressure and renal function but may also participate in opposing remodeling of the cardiovascular system.

This chapter primarily reviewed the role of kinins, which are oligopeptides containing the sequence of bradykinin. They are generated from precursors known as kininogens by enzymes such as glandular (tissue) and plasma kallikrein. Some of the effects of kinins are mediated via autocoids such as eicosanoids, EDRF, endothelium-derived hyperpolarizing factor (EDHF), and/or tissue plasminogen activator (tPA). Acting via these mediators, kinins play an important role in the regulation of cardiovascular and renal function as well as of some of the cardiovascular and renal effects of angiotensin-converting enzyme (ACE) and neutral endopeptidase 24.11 (NEP-24.11) inhibitors.

A study of Utah families revealed that a dominant allele kallikrein gene expressed as high urinary kallikrein excretion was associated with a decreased risk of essential hypertension. Also, a restriction fragment length polymorphism (RFLP) that distinguishes the kallikrein gene family of one strain of spontaneously hypertensive rats (SHR) from normotensive brown Norway rats has been identified; in recombinant inbred substrains derived from these SHR and brown Norway strains, the RFLP marking the kallikrein gene family of the SHR cosegregated with an increase in blood pressure. While rats with a deficiency of kininogen (the kinin precursor) or chronic blockade of the kallikrein-kinin system do not have hypertension, they are more sensitive to the hypertensinogenic effect of salt, deoxycorticosterone plus salt (DOCA-salt), and angiotensin II, suggesting that kinins oppose these hypertensive stimuli; however, these studies need to be confirmed.

In the kidney, kinins have a natriuretic and diuretic effect. There is evidence that renal kinins participate in the regulation of papillary blood flow and that they exert both natriuretic and diuretic effects. Kinins interacting with atrial natriuretic factor (ANF) mediate some of the natriuretic and diuretic effects of NEP-24.11 inhibitors, since these effects are blocked by either kinin receptor antagonists or ANF antibodies. Also, kinin antagonists block the increases in papillary blood sodium and water excretion caused by ACE inhibitors, suggesting that suppressing renal kinin degradation mediates part of their effect. In some experimental models of hypertension, blocking kinins with antibodies or receptor antagonists decreases the acute antihypertensive effect of ACE inhibitors by up to one-third; moreover, kinin antagonists have recently been shown to block some of the chronic antihypertensive effects of ACE inhibitors in renovascular and DOCA-salt hypertension but not in SHR.

ACE inhibitors inhibit neointima formation; this effect is partially blocked by a kinin antagonist or by agents that suppress nitric oxide synthesis. The cardiac antihypertrophic effects of ACE inhibitors have also been reported to be due to kinins; however, these results have not been confirmed. The decrease in infarct size produced by treatment with ACE inhibitors is also reversed by kinin antagonists. In addition, it is reasonable to speculate that in heart failure secondary to infarction, prevention of re-infarction by treatment with ACE inhibitors is at least partially mediated by kinins. Since kinins are known to stimulate the endothelial release of PGI_2 and EDRF—both of which inhibit platelet aggregation—and since kinins also stimulate the release of tPA, which may activate plasminogen, all of these effects will lead to decreased thrombus formation. Thus, although the ultimate function of kinins has not been completely demonstrated, they could play an important role in the regulation of cardiovascular and renal function as well as many of the beneficial effects of inhibitors of zinc metalloendopeptidases such as ACE and NEP-24.11.

ACKNOWLEDGMENT

This research was supported in part by NIH grant HL 28982.

REFERENCES

1. Carretero OA, Scicli AG. Kinins paracrine hormone. *Kidney Int* 1988;34(suppl 26):S-52–S-59.
2. Sybertz EJ Jr, Chiu PJS, Watkins RW, Vemulapalli S. Neutral metalloendopeptidase inhibition: a novel means of circulatory modulation. *J Hypertens* 1990;8(suppl 7):S161–S167.
3. Seymour AA, Norman JA, Asaad MM, Fennell SA, Swerdel JN, Little DK, Dorso CR. Renal and depressor effects of SQ 29,072, a neutral endopeptidase inhibitor, in conscious hypertensive rats. *J Cardiovasc Pharmacol* 1990;16:163–172.
4. Genden EM, Molineaux CJ. Inhibition of endopeptidase-24.15 decreases blood pressure in normotensive rats. *Hypertension* 1991;18:360–365.
5. Colman RW. Patho-physiology of kallikrein system. *Ann Clin Lab Sci* 1980;10:220–226.
6. Kaplan AP, Silverberg M. The coagulation-kinin pathway of human plasma. *Blood* 1987;70:1–15.
7. Sundsmo JS, Fair DS. Relationships among the complement, kinin, coagulation and fibrinolytic systems in the inflammatory reaction. *Clin Physiol Biochem* 1983;1:225–284.
8. Clements JA. The glandular kallikrein family of enzymes: tissue-specific expression and hormonal regulation. *Endocr Rev* 1989;10:393–419.
9. Boucher R, Demassieux S, Garcia R, Genest J. Tonin, angiotensin II system. *Circ Res* 1977;41:26–29.
10. Lilja H. A kallikreinlike serine protease in prostatic fluid cleaves the predominant seminal vesicle protein. *J Clin Invest* 1985;76:1899–1903.
11. Yamaguchi T, Carretero OA, Scicli AG. A novel serine protease with vasoconstrictor activity coded by the kallikrein gene S3. *J Biol Chem* 1991;266:5011–5017.
12. Yamaguchi T, Carretero OA, Scicli AG. A potent vasoconstrictor in the rat submandibular gland. *Hypertension* 1991;17:101–106.
13. Carretero OA, Carbini LA, Scicli AG. The molecular biology of the kallikrein-kinin system: I. General description, nomenclature and the mouse gene family. *J Hypertens* 1993;11:693–697.
14. Scicli AG, Carbini LA, Carretero OA. The molecular biology of the kallikrein-kinin system: II. The rat gene family. *J Hypertens* 1993;11:775–780.
15. Carbini LA, Scicli AG, Carretero OA. The molecular biology of the kallikrein-kinin system: III. The human kallikrein gene family and kallikrein substrate. *J Hypertens* 1993;11:893–898.
16. Saed GM, Carretero OA, MacDonald RJ, Scicli AG. Kallikrein messenger RNA in rat arteries and veins. *Circ Res* 1990;67:510–516.

17. Nolly H, Saed G, Carretero OA, Scicli G, Scicli AG. Adrenal kallikrein. *Hypertension* 1993;21:911–915.
18. Nolly H, Scicli AG, Scicli G, Carretero OA. Characterization of a kininogenase from rat vascular tissue resembling tissue kallikrein. *Circ Res* 1985;56:816–821.
19. Nolly H, Carbini LA, Scicli G, Carretero OA, Scicli AG. A local kallikrein-kinin system is present in rat hearts. *Hypertension* (in press).
20. Chao J, Chao L, Swain CC, Tsai J, Margolius HS. Tissue kallikrein in rat brain and pituitary: regional distribution and estrogen induction in the anterior pituitary. *Endocrinology* 1987;120:475–482.
21. Clements JA, Matheson BA, MacDonald RJ, Funder JW. The expression of the kallikrein gene family in the rat pituitary: oestrogen effects and the expression of an additional family member in the neurointermediate lobe. *J Neuroendocrinol* 1989;1:199–203.
22. Powers CA, Nasjletti A. A major sex difference in kallikreinlike activity in the rat anterior pituitary. *Endocrinology* 1984;114:1841–1844.
23. Frey EK, Kraut H, Werle E. *Kallikrein Padutin* (English transl. 1977 ed. by R Vogel), Stuttgart: Ferdinand Enke Verlag, 1950.
24. Zimmermann A, Geiger R, Kortmann H. Similarity between a kininogenase (kallikrein) from human large intestine and human urinary kallikrein. *Hoppe Seylers Z Physiol Chem* 1979;360:1767–1773.
25. Schachter M, Longridge DJ, Wheeler GD, Mehta JG, Uchida Y. Immunocytochemical and enzyme histochemical localization of kallikrein-like enzymes in colon, intestine, and stomach of rat and cat. *J Histochem Cytochem* 1986;34:927–934.
26. Hilton SM. The physiological role of glandular kallikreins. In: Erdös EG, ed. *Handbook of experimental pharmacology, Vol. 25; Bradykinin, kallidin and kallikrein.* New York: Springer-Verlag, 1970;389–399.
27. Chao J, Chao L, Margolius HS. Isolation of tissue kallikrein in rat spleen by monoclonal antibody-affinity chromatography. *Biochim Biophys Acta* 1984;801:244–249.
28. Scicli G, Nolly H, Carretero OA, Scicli AG. Glandular kallikrein-like enzyme in adrenal glands. *Adv Exp Med Biol* 1989;247B:217–222.
29. Rabito SF, Scicli AG, Carretero OA. Immunoreactive glandular kallikrein in plasma. In: Gross F, Vogel G, eds. *Enzymatic release of vasoactive peptides.* New York: Raven Press, 1980;247–256.
30. Rabito SF, Scicli AG, Kher V, Carretero OA. Immunoreactive glandular kallikrein in rat plasma: a radioimmunoassay for its determination. *Am J Physiol* 1982;242:H602–H610.
31. Geiger R, Clausnitzer B, Fink E, Fritz H. Isolation of an enzymatically active glandular kallikrein from human plasma by immunoaffinity chromatography. *Hoppe Seylers Z Physiol Chem* 1980;361:1795–1803.
32. Lawton WJ, Proud D, Frech ME, Pierce JV, Keiser HR, Pisano JJ. Characterization and origin of immunoreactive glandular kallikrein in rat plasma. *Biochem Pharmacol* 1981;30:1731–1737.
33. Scicli AG, Ørstavik TB, Rabito SF, Murray RD, Carretero OA. Blood kinins after sympathetic nerve stimulation of the rat submandibular gland. *Hypertension* 1983;5(suppl I):I-101–I-106.
34. Pisano JJ, Corthorn J, Yates K, Pierce JV. The kallikrein-kinin system in the kidney. *Contrib Nephrol* 1978;12:116–125.
35. Omata K, Carretero OA, Itoh S, Scicli AG. Active and inactive kallikrein in rabbit connecting tubules and urine during low and normal sodium intake. *Kidney Int* 1983;24:714–718.
36. Noda Y, Yamada K, Igic R, Erdös EG. Regulation of rat urinary and renal kallikrein and prekallikrein by corticosteroids. *Proc Natl Acad Sci USA* 1983;80:3059–3063.
37. Scicli AG, Mindroiu T, Scicli G, Carretero OA. Blood kinins, their concentration in normal subjects and in patients with congenital deficiency in plasma prekallikrein and kininogen. *J Lab Clin Med* 1982;100:81–93.
38. Alhenc-Gelas F, Marchetti J, Allegrini J, Corvol P, Menard J. Measurement of urinary kallikrein activity. Species differences in kinin production. *Biochim Biophys Acta* 1981;677:477–488.
39. Mindroiu T, Scicli G, Perini F, Carretero OA, Scicli AG. Identi-

fication of a new kinin in human urine. *J Biol Chem* 1986;261:7407–7411.
40. Jacobsen S. Substrates for plasma kinin-forming enzymes in human, dog and rabbit plasmas. *Br J Pharmacol* 1966;26:403–411.
41. Jacobsen S. Separation of two different substrates for plasma kinin-forming enzymes. *Nature* 1966;210:98–99.
42. Müller-Esterl W, Fritz H, Machleidt W, Ritonja A, Brzin J, Kotnik M, Turk V, Kellermann J, Lottspeich F. Human plasma kininogens are identical with α-cysteine proteinase inhibitors. Evidence from immunological, enzymological and sequence data. *FEBS Lett* 1985;182:310–314.
43. Ohkubo I, Kurachi K, Takasawa T, Shiokawa H, Sasaki M. Isolation of a human cDNA for α2-thiol proteinase inhibitor and its identity with low molecular weight kininogen. *Biochemistry* 1984;23:5691–5697.
44. Sueyoshi T, Enjyoji K, Shimada T, Kato H, Iwanaga S, Bando Y, Kominami E, Katunuma N. A new function of kininogens as thiol-proteinase inhibitors: inhibition of papain and cathepsins B, H and L by bovine, rat and human plasma kininogens. *FEBS Lett* 1985;182:193–195.
45. Barlas A, Okamoto H, Greenbaum LM. T-kininogen—the major plasma kininogen in rat adjuvant arthritis. *Biochem Biophys Res Commun* 1985;129:280–286.
46. Furuto-Kato S, Matsumoto A, Kitamura N, Nakanishi S. Primary structures of the mRNAs encoding the rat precursors for bradykinin and T-kinin. Structural relationship of kininogens with major acute phase protein and α1-cysteine proteinase inhibitor. *J Biol Chem* 1985;260:12054–12059.
47. Okamoto H, Greenbaum LM. Kininogen substrates for trypsin and cathepsin D in human, rabbit and rat plasmas. *Life Sci* 1983;32:2007–2013.
48. Okamoto H, Greenbaum LM. Pharmacological properties of T-kinin (isoleucyl-seryl-bradykinin) from rat plasma. *Biochem Pharmacol* 1983;32:2637–2638.
49. Kaplan AP, Silverberg M, Ghebrehiwet B, Atkins P, Zweiman B. The kallikrein-kinin system in inflammation. *Adv Exp Med Biol* 1989;247:125–136.
50. Erdös EG. Kininases. In: Erdös EG, ed. *Handbook of experimental pharmacology, Vol. XXV Suppl: Bradykinin, kallidin and kallikrein.* Berlin: Springer-Verlag, 1979;427–487.
51. Erdös EG. Angiotensin I converting enzyme. *Circ Res* 1975;36:247–255.
52. Skidgel RA, Schulz WW, Tam L-T, Erdös EG. Human renal angiotensin I converting enzyme and neutral endopeptidase. *Kidney Int* 1987;31(suppl 20):S-45–S-48.
53. Vijayaraghavan J, Scicli AG, Carretero OA, Slaughter C, Moomaw C, Hersh LB. The hydrolysis of endothelins by neutral endopeptidase 24.11 (enkephalinase). *J Biol Chem* 1990;265:14150–14155.
54. Ura N, Carretero OA, Erdös EG. Role of renal endopeptidase 24.11 in kinin metabolism in vitro and in vivo. *Kidney Int* 1987;32:507–513.
55. Ishida H, Scicli AG, Carretero OA. Role of angiotensin converting enzyme and other peptidases in in vivo metabolism of kinins. *Hypertension* 1989;14:322–327.
56. Campbell DJ, Kladis A, Duncan A-M. Bradykinin peptides in kidney, blood, and other tissues of the rat. *Hypertension* 1993;21:155–165.
57. Cherry PD, Furchgott RF, Zawadzki JV, Jothianandan D. Role of endothelial cells in relaxation of isolated arteries by bradykinin. *Proc Natl Acad Sci USA* 1982;79:2106–2110.
58. Vane JR, Änggård EE, Botting RM. Regulatory functions of the vascular endothelium. *N Engl J Med* 1990;323:27–36.
59. Vanhoutte PM. Endothelium and control of vascular function. State of the art lecture. *Hypertension* 1989;13:658–667.
60. Tiffany CW, Burch RM. Bradykinin stimulates tumor necrosis factor and interleukin-1 release from macrophages. *FEBS Lett* 1989;247:189–192.
61. Smith D, Gilbert M, Owen WG. Tissue plasminogen activator release in vivo in response to vasoactive agents. *Blood* 1985;66:835–839.
62. Regoli D. Pharmacology of bradykinin and related kinins. *Adv Exp Med Biol* 1983;156:569–584.

63. Regoli D, Rhaleb NE, Drapeau G, Dion S, Tousignant C, D'Orléans-Juste P, Devillier P. Basic pharmacology of kinins: pharmacologic receptors and other mechanisms. *Adv Exp Med Biol* 1989;247:399–407.

64. McEachern AE, Shelton ER, Bhakta S, Obernolte R, Bach C, Zuppan P, Fujisaki J, Aldrich RW, Jarnagin K. Expression cloning of a rat B2 bradykinin receptor. *Proc Natl Acad Sci USA* 1991;88:7724–7728.

65. Regoli D, Rhaleb N-E, Dion S, Drapeau G. New selective bradykinin receptor antagonists and bradykinin B2 receptor characterization. *Trends Pharmacol Sci* 1990;11:156–161.

66. Burch RM, Farmer SG, Steranka LR. Bradykinin receptor antagonists. *Med Res Rev* 1990;10:237–269.

67. Regoli D, Rhaleb N-E, Drapeau G, Dion S. Kinin receptor subtypes. *J Cardiovasc Pharmacol* 1990;15(suppl 6):S30–S38.

68. Saha JK, Sengupta JN, Goyal RK. Effect of bradykinin on opossum esophageal longitudinal smooth muscle: evidence for novel bradykinin receptors. *J Pharmacol Exp Ther* 1990;252:1012–1020.

69. Stewart JM, Vavrek RJ. Bradykinin competitive antagonists for classical kinin systems. *Adv Exp Med Biol* 1986;198A:537–542.

70. Wirth K, Hock FJ, Albus U, Linz W, Alpermann HG, Anagnostopoulos H, Henke S, Breipohl G, König W, Knolle J, Schölkens BA. Hoe 140 a new potent and long acting bradykinin-antagonist: in vivo studies. *Br J Pharmacol* 1991;102:774–777.

71. Berg T, Carretero OA, Scicli AG, Tilley B, Stewart JM. Role of kinin in regulation of rat submandibular gland blood flow. *Hypertension* 1989;14:73–80.

72. Seino M, Carretero OA, Albertini R, Scicli AG. Kinins in regulation of uteroplacental blood flow in the pregnant rabbit. *Am J Physiol* 1982;242:H142–H147.

73. Roman RJ, Kaldunski ML, Scicli AG, Carretero OA. Influence of kinins and angiotensin II on the regulation of papillary blood flow. *Am J Physiol* 1988;255:F690–F698.

74. Seino M, Abe K, Nushiro N, Omata K, Kasai Y, Yoshinaga K. Effects of a competitive antagonist of bradykinin on blood pressure and renal blood flow in anesthetized rats. *J Hypertens* 1988;6:867–871.

75. Ørstavik TB, Carretero OA, Johansen L, Scicli AG. Role of kallikrein in the hypotensive effect of captopril after sympathetic stimulation of the rat submandibular gland. *Circ Res* 1982;51:385–390.

76. Beierwaltes WH, Carretero OA, Scicli AG. Renal hemodynamics in response to a kinin analogue antagonist. *Am J Physiol* 1988;255:F408–F414.

77. Zimmerman BG, Raich PC, Vavrek RJ, Stewart JM. Bradykinin contribution to renal blood flow effect of angiotensin converting enzyme inhibitor in the conscious sodium-restricted dog. *Circ Res* 1990;66:234–240.

78. Nakagawa M, Nasjletti A. Renal function as affected by inhibitors of kininase II and of neutral endopeptidase 24.11 in rats with and without desoxycorticosterone pretreatment. *Adv Exp Med Biol* 1989;247:495–499.

79. Omata K, Carretero OA, Scicli AG, Jackson BA. Localization of active and inactive kallikrein (kininogenase activity) in the microdissected rabbit nephron. *Kidney Int* 1982;22:602–607.

80. Scicli AG, Carretero OA, Hampton A, Cortes P, Oza NB. Site of kininogenase secretion in the dog nephron. *Am J Physiol* 1976;230:533–536.

81. Scicli AG, Gandolfi R, Carretero OA. Site of formation of kinins in the dog nephron. *Am J Physiol* 1978;234:F36–F40.

82. Figueroa CD, MacIver AG, Mackenzie JC, Bhoola KD. Localisation of immunoreactive kininogen and tissue kallikrein in the human nephron. *Histochemistry* 1988;89:437–442.

83. Tomita K, Pisano JJ. Binding of [3H]bradykinin in isolated nephron segments of the rabbit. *Am J Physiol* 1984;246:F732–F737.

84. Vio CP, Churchill L, Rabito SF, Terragno A, Carretero OA, Terragno NA. Renal kallikrein in venous effluent of filtering and non-filtering isolated kidneys. *Adv Exp Med Biol* 1983;156B:897–905.

85. Siragy HM, Jaffa AA, Margolius HS. Stimulation of renal interstitial bradykinin by sodium depletion. *Am J Hypertens* 1993;6:863–866.

86. Kauker ML. Bradykinin action on the efflux of luminal 22Na in the rat nephron. *J Pharmacol Exp Ther* 1980;214:119–123.

87. Kauker ML. Kallidin effect on renal tubular function in meclofenamate- and vehicle-pretreated rats. *Proc Soc Exp Biol Med* 1990;193:60–64.

88. Kauker ML, Gisi PJ, Zawada ET. Renal kinins and sodium transport: influence of a bradykinin receptor antagonist (BKRA) (abstract). *FASEB J* 1990;4:A990.

89. Sybertz EJ, Chiu PJS, Vemulapalli S, Watkins R, Haslanger MF. Atrial natriuretic factor-potentiating and antihypertensive activity of SCH 34826. An orally active neutral metalloendopeptidase inhibitor. *Hypertension* 1990;15:152–161.

90. Pollock DM, Butterfield MI, Ader JL, Arendshorst WJ. Dissociation of urinary kallikrein activity and salt and water excretion in the rat. *Am J Physiol* 1986;250:F1082–F1089.

91. Nasjletti A, McGiff JC, Colina-Chourio J. Interrelations of the renal kallikrein-kinin system and renal prostaglandins in the conscious rat. Influence of mineralocorticoids. *Circ Res* 1978;43:799–807.

92. Marin Grez M. The influence of antibodies against bradykinin on isotonic saline diuresis in the rat. Evidence for kinin involvement in renal function. *Pflugers Arch* 1974;350:231–239.

93. Düsing R, Struck A, Göbel BO, Weisser B, Vetter H. Effects of n-3 fatty acids on renal function and renal prostaglandin E metabolism. *Kidney Int* 1990;38:315–319.

94. Saitoh S, Scicli AG, Carretero OA. Effect of inhibiting renal kallikrein on PGE2, water and sodium excretion. *Kidney Int* (submitted).

95. Stoos BA, Carretero OA, Farhy RD, Scicli G, Garvin JL. Endothelium-derived relaxing factor inhibits transport and increases cGMP content in cultured mouse cortical collecting duct cells. *J Clin Invest* 1992;89:761–765.

96. Lahera V, Salom MG, Fiksen-Olsen MJ, Romero JC. Mediatory role of endothelium-derived nitric oxide in renal vasodilatory and excretory effects of bradykinin. *Am J Hypertens* 1991;4:260–262.

97. Bönner G, Preis S, Schunk U, Toussaint C, Kaufmann W. Hemodynamic effects of bradykinin on systemic and pulmonary circulation in healthy and hypertensive humans. *J Cardiovasc Pharmacol* 1990;15(suppl 6):S46–S56.

98. Salgado MCO, Rabito SF, Carretero OA. Blood kinin in one-kidney, one clip hypertensive rats. *Hypertension* 1986;8(suppl I):I-110–I-113.

99. Oza NB, Schwartz JH, Goud HD, Levinsky NG. Rat aortic smooth muscle cells in culture express kallikrein, kininogen, and bradykininase activity. *J Clin Invest* 1990;85:597–600.

100. Benetos A, Gavras I, Gavras H. Hypertensive effect of a bradykinin antagonist in normotensive rats. *Hypertension* 1986;8:1089–1092.

101. Beierwaltes WH, Carretero OA, Scicli AG, Vavrek RJ, Stewart JM. Competitive analog antagonists of bradykinin in the canine hindlimb. *Proc Soc Exp Biol Med* 1987;186:79–83.

102. Carbonell LF, Carretero OA, Madeddu P, Scicli AG. Effects of a kinin antagonist on mean blood pressure. *Hypertension* 1988;11(suppl I):I-84–I-88.

103. Staszewska-Barczak J, Vane JR. The release of catecholamines from the adrenal medulla by peptides. *Br J Pharmacol Chemother* 1967;30:655–667.

104. Beierwaltes WH, Carretero OA. Kallikrein and kinins independently stimulate renin release from isolated rat glomeruli. *Adv Exp Med Biol* 1986;198:265–272.

105. Johnson AR, Erdös EG. Release of histamine from mast cells by vasoactive peptides. *Proc Soc Exp Biol Med* 1973;142:1252–1256.

106. Terragno NA, Lonigro AJ, Malik KU, McGiff JC. The relationship of the renal vasodilator action of bradykinin to the release of a prostaglandin E-like substance. *Experientia* 1972;28:437–439.

107. Farhy RD, Carretero OA, Ho K-L, Scicli AG. Role of kinins and nitric oxide in the effects of angiotensin converting enzyme inhibitors on neointima formation. *Circ Res* 1993;72:1202–1210.

108. Bao G, Gohlke P, Qadri F, Unger T. Chronic kinin receptor

blockade attenuates the antihypertensive effect of ramipril. *Hypertension* 1992;20:74–79.

109. Majima M, Yoshida O, Mihara H, Muto T, Mizogami S, Kuribayashi Y, Katori M, Oh-Ishi S. High sensitivity to salt in kininogen-deficient Brown Norway Katholiek rats. *Hypertension* 1993;22:705–714.

110. Katori M, Majima M. Induction of hypertension by a low dose of angiotensin II in kininogen-deficient Brown-Norway Katholiek rats (abstract). *Hypertension* 1993;22:430.

111. Madeddu P, Glorioso N, Anania V. Chronic blockade of bradykinin receptors in angiotensin-treated rats (abstract). *Hypertension* 1993;22:430.

112. Majima M, Katori M, Hanazuka M, Mizogami S, Nakano T, Nakao Y, Mikami R, Uryu H, Okamura R, Mohsin SSJ, Oh-Ishi S. Suppression of rat deoxycorticosterone-salt hypertension by kallikrein-kinin system. *Hypertension* 1991;17:806–813.

113. Carretero OA, Scicli AG. The renal kallikrein-kinin system in human and in experimental hypertension. *Klin Wochenschr* 1978;56(suppl I):113–125.

114. Williams RR, Hunt SC, Hasstedt SJ, Berry TD, Wu LL, Barlow GK, Stults BM, Kuida H. Definition of genetic factors in hypertension: a search for major genes, polygenes, and homogeneous subtypes. *J Cardiovasc Pharmacol* 1988;12:S7–S20.

115. Berry TD, Hasstedt SJ, Hunt SC, Wu LL, Smith JB, Ash KO, Kuida H, Williams RR. A gene for high urinary kallikrein may protect against hypertension in Utah kindreds. *Hypertension* 1989;13:3–8.

116. Zinner SH, Margolius HS, Rosner B, Keiser HR, Kass EH. Familial aggregation of urinary kallikrein concentration in childhood: relation to blood pressure, race and urinary electrolytes. *Am J Epidemiol* 1976;104:124–132.

117. Zinner SH, Margolius HS, Rosner B, Kass EH. Stability of blood pressure rank and urinary kallikrein concentration in childhood: an eight-year follow-up. *Circulation* 1978;58:908–915.

118. Carretero OA, Amin VM, Ocholik T, Scicli AG, Koch J. Urinary kallikrein in rats bred for their susceptibility and resistance to the hypertensive effect of salt. A new radioimmunoassay for its direct determination. *Circ Res* 1978;42:727–731.

119. Carretero OA, Polomski C, Hampton A, Scicli AG. Urinary kallikrein, plasma renin and aldosterone in New Zealand genetically hypertensive (GH) rats. *Clin Exp Pharmacol Physiol* 1976; 3(suppl):55–59.

120. Carretero OA, Scicli AG, Piwonska A, Koch J. Urinary kallikrein in rats bred for susceptibility and resistance to the hypertensive effect of salt and in New Zealand genetically hypertensive rats. *Mayo Clin Proc* 1977;52:465–467.

121. Keiser HR, Geller RG, Margolius HS, Pisano JJ. Urinary kallikrein in hypertensive animal models. *Fed Proc* 1976;35:199–202.

122. Woodley-Miller C, Chao J, Chao L. Restriction fragment length polymorphisms mapped in spontaneously hypertensive rats using kallikrein probes. *J Hypertens* 1989;7:865–871.

123. Pravenec M, Kren V, Kunes J, Scicli AG, Carretero OA, Simonet L, Kurtz TW. Cosegregation of blood pressure with a kallikrein gene family polymorphism. *Hypertension* 1991;17:242–246.

124. Carretero OA, Oza NB, Scicli AG, Schork A. Renal tissue kallikrein, plasma renin and plasma aldosterone in renal hypertension. *Acta Physiol Latinoam* 1974;24:448–452.

125. Shkhvatsabaya IK, Nekrasova AA, Chernova NA, Khukharev VV. Kinin system of the kidneys in pathogenesis of hypertensive disease [Russ]. *Ter Arkh* 1973;45:71–77.

126. Holland OB, Chud JM, Braunstein H. Urinary kallikrein excretion in essential and mineralocorticoid hypertension. *J Clin Invest* 1980;65:347–356.

127. Margolius HS, Horwitz D, Geller RG, Alexander RW, Gill JR Jr, Pisano JJ, Keiser HR. Urinary kallikrein excretion in normal man. Relationships to sodium intake and sodium-retaining steroids. *Circ Res* 1974;35:812–818.

128. Seino M, Abe K, Otsuka Y, Saito T, Irokawa N, Yasujima M, Ciba S, Yoshinaga K. Urinary kallikrein excretion and sodium metabolism in hypertensive patients. *Tohoku J Exp Med* 1975;116:359–367.

129. Carretero OA, Kuk P, Piwonska S, Houle JA, Marin-Grez M. Role of the renin angiotensin system in the pathogenesis of severe hypertension in rats. *Circ Res* 1971;29:654–663.

130. Marks ES, Bing RF, Thurston H, Swales JD. Vasodepressor property of the converting enzyme inhibitor captopril (SQ 14 225): the role of factors other than renin-angiotensin blockade in the rat. *Clin Sci* 1980;58:1–6.

131. Clappison BH, Anderson WP, Johnston CI. Role of the kallikrein-kinin system in the renal effects of angiotensin-converting enzyme inhibition in anaesthetized dogs. *Clin Exp Pharmacol Physiol* 1981;8:509–513.

132. McCaa RE. Studies in vivo with angiotensin I converting enzyme (kininase II) inhibitors. *Fed Proc* 1979;38:2783–2787.

133. Nasjletti A, Colina-Chourio J, McGiff JC. Disappearance of bradykinin in the renal circulation of dogs. Effects of kininase inhibition. *Circ Res* 1975;37:59–65.

134. Vinci JM, Horwitz D, Zusman RM, Pisano JJ, Catt KJ, Keiser HR. The effect of converting enzyme inhibition with SQ20,881 on plasma and urinary kinins, prostaglandin E and angiotensin II in hypertensive man. *Hypertension* 1979;1:416–426.

135. Overlack A, Stumpe KO, Heck I, Ressel C, Kühnert M, Krück F. Identification of angiotensin II- and kinin-dependent mechanisms in essential hypertension. In: Philipp T, Distler A, eds. *Hypertension: mechanisms and management.* Berlin: Springer-Verlag, 1980;183–191.

136. Carretero OA, Miyazaki S, Scicli AG. Role of kinins in the acute antihypertensive effect of the converting enzyme inhibitor, captopril. *Hypertension* 1981;3:18–22.

137. Carretero OA, Ørstavik TB, Rabito SF, Scicli AG. Interference of converting enzyme inhibitors with the kallikrein-kinin system. *Clin Exp Hypertens [A]* 1983;5:1277–1285.

138. Carretero OA, Scicli AG, Maitra SR. Role of kinins in the pharmacological effects of converting enzyme inhibitors. In: Horovitz ZP, ed. *Angiotensin converting enzyme inhibitors. Mechanisms of action and clinical implications.* Baltimore: Urban & Schwarzenberg, 1981;105–121.

139. Benetos A, Gavras H, Stewart JM, Vavrek RJ, Hatinoglou S, Gavras I. Vasodepressor role of endogenous bradykinin assessed by a bradykinin antagonist. *Hypertension* 1986;8:971–974.

140. Carbonell LF, Carretero OA, Stewart JM, Scicli AG. Effect of a kinin antagonist on the acute antihypertensive activity of enalaprilat in severe hypertension. *Hypertension* 1988;11:239–243.

141. Pontieri V, Lopes OU, Ferreira SH. Hypotensive effect of captopril. Role of bradykinin and prostaglandinlike substances. *Hypertension* 1990;15(suppl I):I-55–I-58.

142. Carretero OA. High-mineralocorticoid conditions: kinins (paracrine hormones) in the regulation of renal function and blood pressure (chap. 123). In: Mornex R, Jaffiol C, Leclèrc J, eds. *Progress in endocrinology. The Proceedings of the Ninth International Congress of Endocrinology, Nice 1992.* London: Parthenon, 1993; 536–540.

143. Powell JS, Müller RKM, Rouge M, Kuhn H, Hefti F, Baumgartner HR. The proliferative response to vascular injury is suppressed by angiotensin-converting enzyme inhibition. *J Cardiovasc Pharmacol* 1990;16(suppl 4):S42–S49.

144. Osterrieder W, Müller RKM, Powell JS, Clozel J-P, Hefti F, Baumgartner HR. Role of angiotensin II in injury-induced neointima formation in rats. *Hypertension* 1991;18(suppl II):II-60–II-64.

145. Farhy R, Ho K-L, Carretero OA, Scicli AG. Kinins mediate the antiproliferative effect of ramipril in rat carotid artery. *Biochem Biophys Res Commun* 1992;182:283–288.

146. Kauffman RF, Bean JS, Zimmerman KM, Brown RF, Steinberg MI. Losartan, a nonpeptide angiotensin II (Ang II) receptor antagonist, inhibits neointima formation following balloon injury to rat carotid arteries. *Life Sci* 1991;49:PL-223–PL-228.

147. Schölkens BA, Linz W, Martorana PA. Experimental cardiovascular benefits of angiotensin-converting enzyme inhibitors: beyond blood pressure reduction. *J Cardiovasc Pharmacol* 1991;18(suppl 2):S26–S30.

148. Linz W, Schölkens BA. A specific B2-bradykinin receptor antagonist HOE 140 abolishes the antihypertrophic effect of ramipril. *Br J Pharmacol* 1992;105:771–772.

149. Rhaleb N-E, Yang X-P, Scicli AG, Carretero OA. Role of kinins and nitric oxide in the antihypertrophic effect of ramipril. *Hypertension* 1994 (in press).

150. Fernandez LA, Twickler J, Mead A. Neovascularization produced by angiotensin II. *J Lab Clin Med* 1985;105:141–145.

151. Unger T, Mattfeldt T, Lamberty V, Bock P, Mall G, Linz W, Schölkens BA, Gohlke P. Effect of early onset angiotensin converting enzyme inhibition on myocardial capillaries. *Hypertension* 1992;20:478–482.

152. Shimamoto K, Miura T, Miki T, Iimura O. Activation of kinins on myocardial ischemia. *Agents Actions* 1992;38:90–97.

153. Hartman JC, Wall TM, Hullinger TG, Shebuski RJ. Reduction of myocardial infarct size in rabbits by ramiprilat: reversal by the bradykinin antagonist HOE 140. *J Cardiovasc Pharmacol* 1993;21:996–1003.

154. Noda K, Sasaguri M, Ideishi M, Ikeda M, Arakawa K. Role of locally formed angiotensin II and bradykinin in the reduction of myocardial infarct size in dogs. *Cardiovasc Res* 1993;27:334–340.

155. Martorana PA, Kettenbach B, Breipohl G, Linz W, Schölkens BA. Reduction of infarct size by local angiotensin-converting enzyme inhibition is abolished by a bradykinin antagonist. *Eur J Pharmacol* 1990;182:395–396.

156. Linz W, Martorana PA, Grotsch H, Qi BY, Schölkens BA. Antagonizing bradykinin (BK) obliterates the cardioprotective effects of bradykinin and angiotensin-converting enzyme (ACE) inhibitors in ischemic hearts. *Drug Dev Res* 1990;19:393–408.

157. Pfeffer MA, Braunwald E, Moyé LA, Basta L, Brown EJ Jr, Cuddy TE, Davis BR, Geltman EM, Goldman S, Flaker GC, Klein M, Lamas GA, Packer M, Rouleau J, Rouleau JL, Rutherford J, Wertheimer JH, Hawkins CM, on behalf of the SAVE Investigators. Effect of captopril on mortality and morbidity in patients with left ventricular dysfunction after myocardial infarction. Results of the survival and ventricular enlargement trial. *N Engl J Med* 1992;327:669–677.

158. Gertz SD, Kurgan A. Tissue plasminogen activator and selective coronary vasodilation (letter). *Am J Cardiol* 1988;62:173.

159. Kosoglou T, Herron JM, Chen R, Given BD, Sybertz EJ, Affrime MB. Antihypertensive effect of the atriopeptidase inhibitor SCH 34826 in essential hypertension [abst 2201]. *Circulation* 1990;82(suppl III):III-554.

160. Itoh H, Nakao K, Mukoyama M, Saito Y, Yamada T, Shirakami G, Arai H, Hosoda K, Suga S-I, Yoshida I, Imura H. Preparation of monoclonal antibodies against brain natriuretic peptide and their application to radioimmunoassay and passive immunization. *Endocrinology* 1990;127:1292–1300.

161. Smits GJ, McGraw DE, Trapani AJ. Interaction of ANP and bradykinin during endopeptidase 24.11 inhibition: renal effects. *Am J Physiol* 1990;258:F1417–F1424.

162. Stunkard AJ, Harris JR, Pederson NL, McClearn GE. The bodymass index of twins who have been reared apart. *N Engl J Med* 1990;322:1483–1487.

163. Samuels GMR, Barclay PL, Peters CJ, Ellis P. Atriopeptidase inhibitors, a novel class of drug that raises levels of endogenous atrial natriuretic factor—the preclinical pharmacology of UK-69,578 [abstract]. *J Am Coll Cardiol* 1989;13:75A.

164. Brownie AC, Alfano J, Gallant S. Rat models of experimental hypertension: their adrenocortical components. In: Biglieri EG, Melby JC, eds. *Endocrine hypertension.* New York: Raven Press, 1990;29–69.

165. Carretero OA. Kinins: local hormones in regulation of blood pressure and renal function. *Choices Cardiol* 1993;7(suppl 1):10–14.

166. Carretero OA, Scicli AG. Local hormonal factors (intracrine, autocrine and paracrine) in hypertension. *Hypertension* 1991;18(suppl I):I-58–I-69.

167. Carretero OA, Scicli AG. Kallikrein. In: Massry SG, Glassock RJ, eds. *Textbook of nephrology,* vol 1. Baltimore: Williams and Wilkins, 1983;2.34–2.39.

Hypertension: Pathophysiology, Diagnosis, and Management, Second Edition,
edited by J.H. Laragh and B.M. Brenner,
Raven Press, Ltd., New York © 1995.

CHAPTER 59

Receptors of Natriuretic Peptides: Structure, Function, and Regulation

Thomas Maack

Atrial natriuretic factor (ANF), or atrial natriuretic peptide (ANP), is a polypeptide hormone secreted mainly by the heart atria in response to increases in atrial stretch or atrial pressure. ANP is a member of the natriuretic peptide family, which includes brain natriuretic peptide (BNP) and C-type natriuretic peptide (CNP). ANP has multiple and rather well-defined actions on the mammalian organism. In the kidney, ANP exerts renal hemodynamic and tubular actions that lead to increases in urinary excretion of fluid and electrolytes. In the cardiovascular system, ANP acts as a strong antagonist of vasoconstriction with a weak agonist (vasoconstrictive) action of its own. Moreover, ANP reduces cardiac output by decreasing plasma volume, an effect that is due mainly to an increase in capillary hydraulic permeability. This increase leads to a shift of fluid from the intra-

vascular to the interstitial compartment. ANP also affects other endocrine functions, acting essentially as a counterregulatory hormone, particularly of the renin-angiotensin-aldosterone system. These combined systemic actions of ANP contribute to the regulation of plasma volume and blood pressure. A review on the functions of natriuretic peptides is provided elsewhere in this volume. For a recent inclusive review on ANP and its receptors with extensive bibliography the reader is directed to ref. 1.

There are two major biochemically and functionally distinct classes of receptors for natriuretic peptides—guanylate cyclase (GC) and clearance (C) receptors (1,2). Figure 1 depicts schematically the structures, ligand binding, and major cellular roles of the receptors that will be considered in this chapter. GC receptors of atrial peptides (also denominated type I, B-ANF, NPRA, or NPRB receptors) are part of a family of membrane-bound guanylate cyclases (3). Two distinct subtypes of

---

T. Maack: Department of Physiology, Cornell University Medical College, New York, New York 10021.

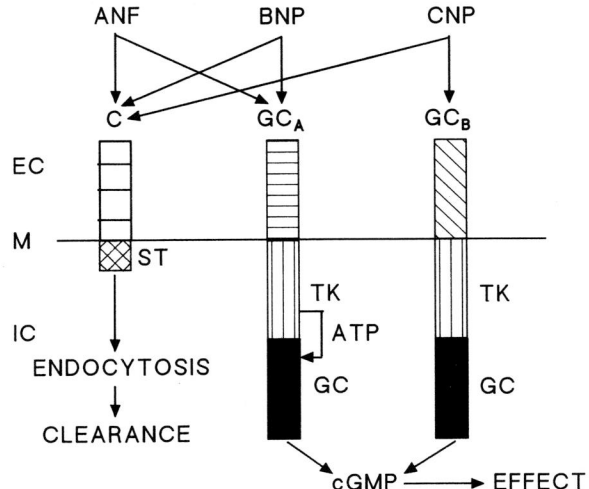

FIG. 1. Schematic representation of the structure of receptors for natriuretic peptides. Guanylyl cyclase (GC_A and GC_B) receptors have an extracellular binding domain (EC), a single transmembrane (M) span, and an intracellular portion (IC) that contains a C-terminal guanylyl cyclase (GC) sequence and a protein kinaselike (TK) sequence. The IC domains of GC_A and GC_B receptors are practically identical, but the amino acid sequences of the EC domains are substantially different. This confers some specificity for ligand binding, GC_A receptors binding with high affinity ANP (ANF) and BNP, whereas GC_B receptors bind only CNP with high affinity. The TK domain of the GC_A, and probably of the GC_B, receptor is a negative modulator of the GC domain. Ligand binding promotes an allosteric interaction of ATP with this domain, leading to derepression and activation of guanylyl cyclase. This activation leads to the generation of cGMP, the main, if not sole, second messenger of the effects of natriuretic peptides. Clearance (C) receptors are also single-span transmembrane receptors, whose main characteristic is a very short intracellular tail (ST). This structural property is shared by all known clearance and/ or transport receptors. C receptors, which have an important role in removing natriuretic peptides from the circulation, bind all of the members of this family with high affinity. The ligand (ANF, BNP, or CNP) is internalized by C receptor–mediated endocytosis, and delivered to lysosomes where it is completely hydrolyzed to constituent amino acids. (See text for more detailed description and references.)

GC receptors—A (GC_A) and B (GC_B)—are involved in mediating the effects of natriuretic peptides. The GC_A receptor is the physiological receptor for ANP, and possibly also for BNP, whereas GC_B receptors are in all likelihood involved in mediating the effects of CNP (3). C receptors (also denominated type II receptors), the other major class of atrial peptide receptors, bind with high affinity all members of the natriuretic peptide family. They are biochemically unrelated to GC receptors and do not mediate the major known end-organ effects of natriuretic peptides. On the other hand, C receptors have an important role in the metabolic clearance and regulation of plasma levels of natriuretic peptides, hence their name of clearance receptors (1,2).

In this noninclusive review, I first briefly address the structure and molecular biology of natriuretic peptides receptors, and then focus on the function, second messengers, dynamics, and regulation of these receptors.

STRUCTURE AND BIOCHEMISTRY OF RECEPTORS OF NATRIURETIC PEPTIDES

Guanylyl Cyclase Receptors

The biochemistry and structure of GC receptors is unique among polypeptide hormone receptors. GC receptors are integral membrane proteins of 120 to 180 kDa with GC activity that is activated by ligand (ANP, BNP, or CNP) binding in the presence of adenosine triphosphate (ATP). This leads to the generation of guanosine 3',5'-cyclic monophosphate (cGMP), the main second messenger of the effects of natriuretic peptides (3–8). The GC_A receptor has an extracellular binding domain of approximately 440 amino acids containing six cysteine residues and six potential N-glycosylation sites. The receptor has a single putative membrane spanning domain and a cytoplasmic portion that contains approximately 565 amino acids. The sequence of approximately 250 amino acids comprising the carboxyl portion of the cytoplasmic domain has very strong homology with soluble GCs and a weaker but still significant homology with brain adenylyl cyclase (7).

The high degree of homology with GC is consistent with the early findings showing that ANP-specific binding and particulate (membrane-bound) GC activity cannot be separated by biochemical purification procedures (4). Moreover, studies with recombinant GC_A receptors have shown that deletion of the GC-like sequence abolishes ligand-induced generation of cGMP (9), and expression of C-terminal sequences of GC_A receptors showed GC activity (10). The meaning, if any, of the limited homology of the carboxyl terminus of GC_A receptors with adenylyl cyclase is unknown.

Interposed between the putative transmembrane domain and the GC sequence, there is an approximately 250 amino acids span with significant homology (31 percent) to the protein kinase domain of the platelet-derived growth factor (PDGF) receptor, with an extremely high (approximately 90 percent) conservation of protein kinase consensus sequences (3,7,9,11). In spite of this homology, GC_A receptors do not show detectable kinase activity (12). Nevertheless, as will be described below, the protein kinaselike sequence has an important negative modulatory role on the GC activity of the receptor (7,11).

The amino acids sequence of GC_A receptors is very well conserved among different tissues and animal species with more than 95 percent amino acid identity among mouse, rat, and human GC_A receptors (3). The gene for rat GC_A receptors expands for 17.5 kilobases with 22 exons interposed by 21 introns. The four domains of the receptor, namely, extracellular, transmembrane, protein kinaselike, and catalytic GC domains, are encoded by exons 1–6, 7, 8–15, and 16–22, respectively (13).

GC_B receptors are structurally very similar to GC_A receptors, and the amino acid sequence of the cytoplasmic domains of these two receptors are practically identical (5,14). The major differences reside in the extracellular binding domain in which there is only 40 percent identity of amino acids between GC_A and GC_B receptors (3). This divergence may explain the different specificity for ligand binding between these two receptor subtypes (see below).

GC_A (and probably GC_B) receptors exist as oligomers (dimers or, most likely, tetramers) in the cell membrane (15), and it is believed that contrary to other receptors with a single span transmembrane region, this is a constitutive property that is not altered by ligand binding (16). The biochemical nature of GC receptors described above implies that, contrary to many other polypeptide hormone receptors, these receptors do not need the intervention of other proteins (e.g., G proteins) for receptor-effector (enzyme) coupling upon ligand binding. However, activation of GC receptors depends on the presence of ATP, a phenomenon that in all likelihood is determined by an allosteric interaction of this nucleotide with the protein kinaselike domain of the receptor (9,17).

Clearance Receptors

Clearance (C) receptors, which make up the other major class of ANP receptors, are by far the most abundant, amounting in some instances (e.g., cultured vascular smooth muscle cells, fibroblasts, lung, kidney cortex) to more than 95 percent of the total population of ANF receptors (1,2,18). C receptors do not generate cGMP upon ligand binding and do not modulate or interfere with cGMP generation by GC receptors (19,20). C receptors were the first of the ANF receptor classes to be fully characterized biochemically (21). They are homodimers of approximately 120 kDa (60 kDa under reducing conditions), containing 496 amino acids per subunit. Similarly to GC receptors, C receptors have a putative single transmembrane domain, and a large extracellular binding domain. The extracellular domain of bovine vascular smooth muscle C receptors has considerable homology (33 percent) with that of GC_A receptors, but no significant amino acid sequence homology with other known proteins. C receptors, similarly to GC receptors, have conserved five cysteine residues and potential glycosylation sites in the extracellular domain. The outstanding structural characteristic of C receptors is their very short

cytoplasmic domain of only 37 amino acids. Short cytoplasmic domains are a rule for all known clearance and/or transport receptors whose molecular structure has been elucidated (e.g., low-density lipoprotein [LDL], asialoglycoprotein, mannose 6 phosphate, and transferrin receptors). The amino acid sequence of C receptors is extremely well conserved in nature. Thus, the amino acid sequences of bovine aortic smooth muscle cells and human kidney C receptors are practically identical (21,22). The structure of the bovine C receptor gene comprises eight exons distributed over a large span of 85 kilobases. Exons 1–6, 7, and 8 code for the extracellular, transmembrane, and cytoplasmic domains, respectively (23).

TISSUE DISTRIBUTION OF ANP RECEPTORS

Atrial natriuretic peptide receptors are found in all tissues and cells studied to date, and are most prevalent in kidney, vasculature, adrenal, lung, intestine, and brain (see ref. 1 for bibliography). We are far from understanding the meaning of this widespread localization of GC and C receptors. Moreover, reports in the literature present contradictory evidence regarding the relative expression of atrial peptide receptors in different tissues. It is likely that the apparent disparities in this regard are due, at least in part, to differences in species (e.g., rat, monkey, or human), experimental preparation (e.g., cultured cells versus freshly isolated cells or tissues), and detection procedures (e.g., autoradiography, ligand binding, cGMP generation, mRNA determination by Northern blotting or *in situ* hybridization).

Cardiovascular Tissues

In vascular tissues, ANP receptors are present in endothelial and smooth muscle cells, and in fibroblasts. In culture conditions, C receptors are the predominant class, constituting greater than 90 percent of the total population of atrial peptide receptors (20,24). Moreover, the density of C receptors in cultured vascular smooth muscle cells may be as high as 500,000 to 600,000 receptors/cell, the highest density for a polypeptide-hormone receptor described to date (2). Vascular smooth muscle and endothelial cells in culture also contain a significant amount of GC receptors, but the subtypes differ. Thus, culture vascular smooth muscle cells express a predominance of functional GC_B over GC_A receptors, whereas the only detectable functional CC receptor in cultured endothelial cells is the GC_A receptor (25,26). Interestingly, in membranes obtained from vascular smooth muscle cells from fresh aortic tissue, the proportion of GC receptor subtypes is reverted, i.e., there are more GC_A than GC_B receptors. Moreover, the density of C receptors in these membranes is substantially lower than that in membranes of cultured vascular smooth muscle cells from the aorta (26).

The predominance of GC_B over GC_A receptors in cultured vascular smooth muscle cells may be due to the rapid proliferative state in which these cells were studied. This finding may be of pathophysiological interest, because in conditions such as atherosclerosis and hypertension there is a marked proliferation of vascular smooth muscle cells. cGMP and natriuretic peptides have been demonstrated to exert a growth-inhibitory action in vascular smooth muscle, as well as in other cultured cells (27,28). Furthermore, CNP, the specific ligand for GC_B receptors, has been shown to be produced by endothelial cells (29). On the basis of these findings it has been postulated that there is local modulation of vascular cell growth by natriuretic peptides, particularly by CNP (27,30). The overexpression of GC_B receptors in rapidly proliferating vascular smooth muscle cells may reflect such a modulatory event. Direct evidence that this is the case is, however, not yet available. In any event, the differential expression of GC receptor subtypes in cultured and fresh vascular smooth muscle cells points out that great care should be exercised in extrapolating distribution of receptor subtypes found in cell cultures to the corresponding tissue *in vivo*.

GC_A and C receptors were also detected in heart myocardial and endocardial cells. It has been reported that the amount of mRNA for C receptors in heart tissue is greater than in any other of the analyzed tissues, including vasculature and kidney (31). This led the authors to speculate that a great proportion of ANP secreted by the heart atria is removed by C receptors before it reaches the circulation. This finding obtained by *in situ* hybridization studies on postmortem tissue in a monkey is not consistent, however, with autoradiographic studies in the rat, which found a relatively sparse population of ANP receptors in the heart, compared with that in the vasculature, kidneys, and lung (32). The presence of GC receptors in myocardial cells is also not easy to assess functionally because most data show a lack of a direct effect of ANP on heart contractility.

Kidneys

As shown in Fig. 2, glomeruli have the highest density of ANP binding sites in the kidney, but ANP receptors are also present in renal arterioles, in the outer medulla, and in the papilla (32–35). In rat kidney cortex and glomeruli more than 95 percent and 70 percent of the total population of ANP receptors, respectively, are C receptors (36,37). Both classes of ANP receptors in glomeruli are mostly localized to podocytes, a somewhat surprising finding because the role of these cells in the modulation of the known glomerular effects of ANP is unknown. Nevertheless, GC_A and C receptors are also present in

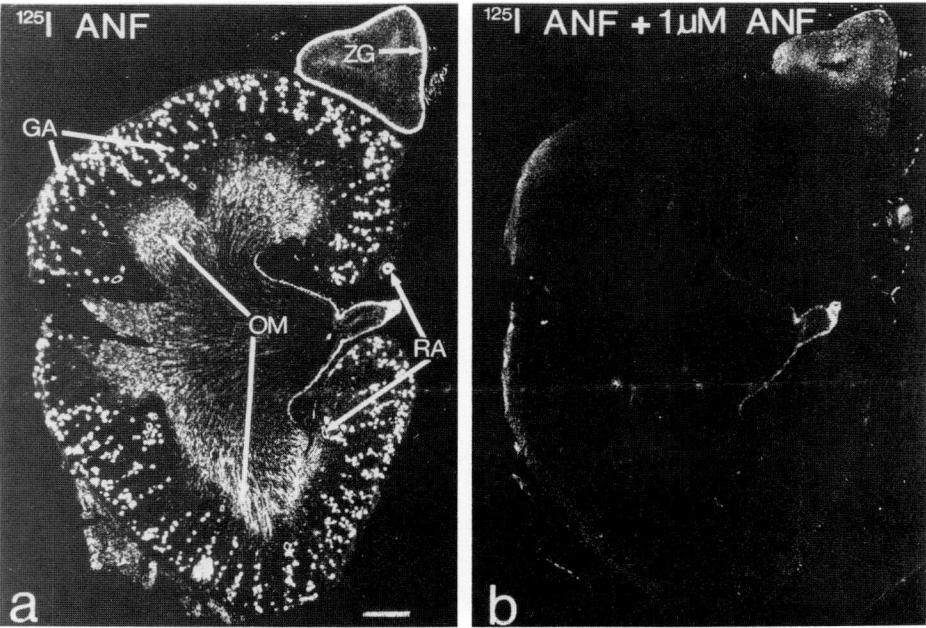

FIG. 2. Autoradiographic localization of specific binding of ANP in kidney and adrenal. Dark field photomicrograph of autoradiograms of guinea pig kidney, and adrenal sections incubated with 150 pM ^{125}I-ANF$_{1-28}$ (**A**), and its serial pair (**B**) incubated with the same concentration of ^{125}I-ANF$_{1-28}$ in presence of excess (1 μM) unlabeled ANF$_{1-28}$ (nonspecific binding). Radioligand binding appears as white silver grains. In the kidney section, the high density of specific binding is present in glomeruli (GA), renal arteries (RA), and outer medulla (OM). In the adrenal cortex, the zona glomerulosa (ZG) is clearly outlined by a dense array of silver grains (From ref. 35, with permission).

mesangial cells, and possibly in glomerular endothelial cells (38–42).

In the renal medulla, ANP receptors are distributed in bundles of descending vasa recta, inner medullary collecting duct (IMCD), and renomedullary interstitial cells (43–45). ANP-induced generation of cGMP in the kidney is quantitatively most prominent in glomeruli and renomedullary interstitial cells, and to a smaller extent in IMCD cells (41,45). Some degree of ANP-induced cGMP generation or presence of mRNA for GC_A receptors has been detected in practically every renal tubular structure, including proximal tubules (44). The physiological significance of these very low levels of GC_A receptor mRNA or of ANP-induced cGMP generation remains to be determined. Nevertheless, the presence of GC_A receptors in glomeruli, renal vasculature, proximal tubules, and IMCDs is consistent with the physiological effects of ANP on these kidney structures (1). The function of the large density of GC_A receptors and of ANP-induced generation of cGMP in renomedullary interstitial cells is unknown.

CNP binding and cGMP generation studies in the rat indicate that, in normal conditions, GC_B receptors are not expressed in mature kidney tissues. However, Northern blot analysis of tissue obtained from humans has revealed the presence of small but significant amounts of mRNA of GC_B receptors in the kidney. The significance of this finding remains to be elucidated (46).

Ligand binding studies in the intact rat kidney have demonstrated that C receptors are present in all regions of the kidney (cortex, medulla, and papilla), with the highest density in the cortex and in glomeruli (34,36). Consistent with this finding, studies with human kidney tissue revealed the presence of mRNA for C receptors in all of these regions (22,46). However, C receptors are apparently absent from epithelial structures of the inner medulla (37). The large density of C receptors in glomerular and renal vascular structures is consistent with the important role of these receptors in removing natriuretic peptides from the circulation, as these structures receive a large proportion (approximately 25 percent) of the cardiac output.

Adrenals

There is an abundant expression of ANP receptors in adrenal zona glomerulosa (Fig. 2) and in isolated zona glomerulosa cells, a finding that is consistent with the major inhibitory effect of ANP on aldosterone secretion by these cells (35,47). There is some controversy as to whether or not C receptors are expressed in these cells, but if present, their density is far smaller than that of GC_A receptors (47). GC_B and C receptors have also been detected in the adrenal medulla and adrenal chromaffin cells (31,48). The physiological role of these receptors in the adrenal medullary cells, if any, is not known.

STRUCTURE-BINDING RELATIONSHIPS

GC_A receptors are the true, and possibly only, biological receptors proper of ANP (2,3,25). Thus, GC_A receptors have a very high affinity (K_d in the subnanomolar range) for ANP (and also for BNP) but a very low affinity for CNP (25,42). On the other hand, GC_B receptors have an extremely low affinity (K_d in the micromolar range) for ANP, a slightly higher but still low affinity for BNP, and a moderately high affinity for CNP (25,49). Thus, GC_B receptors are likely to be the physiologically relevant receptors of CNP but not for ANP or BNP. Unfortunately, the lack of knowledge of the physiological roles of BNP and CNP precludes a functional interpretation of the different affinities of GC receptor subtypes for members of the natriuretic peptide family.

GC_A receptors have rather stringent structural requirements for ligand binding. Disruption of the disulfide bridge, deletion of C-terminal Phe-Arg-(Tyr), or amino acid deletions or substitutions within the ring structure of ANP impair binding to GC_A receptors and, consequently, generation of cGMP and end-organ effects of the hormone (20,36,50–52). On the other hand, C receptors bind all members of the natriuretic peptide family with very high affinity, such that there is receptor occupancy even at physiological plasma concentrations of these peptides (34,36,53). Nevertheless, the affinity for BNP is lower than that for ANP, a finding that may explain the lower metabolic clearance rate of the former (25).

Synthetic deleted analogues of ANP may serve both as specific markers and as blockers of C receptors under experimental conditions. Among the synthetic truncated analogues of ANP developed to date, des [Gln^{18},Ser^{19},Gly^{20},Leu^{21},Gly^{22}]$rANP_{4-23}$-NH_2, simply referred to as C-ANF_{4-23}, became the prototype of a specific ligand for C receptors (36,53). Apparently the minimal amino acid sequence necessary for binding to C receptors comprises the 11–15 sequence of the native ANP molecule, namely, Arg^{11},Ile^{12},Asp^{13},Arg^{14},Ile^{15} (54,55). This is an unusual property, since receptors generally have been thought to have much more stringent structural requirements for their ligands. Nevertheless, C receptors are unable to bind peptides not related to the family of atrial peptides and are, therefore, specific for ANP, BNP, and CNP.

SECOND MESSENGERS AND ANP EFFECTS

cGMP as a Second Messenger

Atrial natriuretic peptide markedly increases cGMP in target cells, tissues, and in plasma (1–14). Moreover, analogues of cGMP mimic ANP vasorelaxant and sodium transport inhibitory effects (4,56–60). These data, and the finding that GC receptors contain guanylyl cyclase in their molecules, provide rather unequivocal evidence that cGMP is the major, if not sole, second messenger of the effects of natriuretic peptides.

Nevertheless, some investigators still question whether cGMP is the only important second messenger of ANP actions. In many instances this contention is based on experimental evidence that is difficult to interpret. For example, it has been shown that there is a poor correlation between the ability of peptide analogues to increase cGMP in cultured rat aortic smooth muscle cells and the vasorelaxant effect of these analogues in preconstricted strips of the rat aorta (61). As pointed out above, however, the major subtype of GC receptor expressed in cultured vascular smooth muscle cells from the rat aorta is the GC_B receptor, which is insensitive to ANP, whereas in the intact aorta the major subtype is the GC_A receptor, the only known receptor that mediates ANP effects (26). Consequently, comparisons between the potency of peptide analogues to increase cGMP in cultured vascular smooth muscle cells and their potency to induce vasorelaxation may not be meaningful. Another example is the large differences between the K_d of binding and the median effective dose (ED_{50}) of the cGMP-generating effect of ANP in many preparations, the latter being one to two orders of magnitude greater than the former. Different experimental conditions in which these parameters are measured are likely to explain this discrepancy. The K_d of binding is usually determined at subphysiological temperatures in either intact cells or membranes, whereas the ED_{50} of the cGMP-generating effect is determined at 37 degrees C in intact cells. In a recent study we have demonstrated that the K_{off} of ANP from GC_A receptors in intact cells at near physiological temperatures is much greater than would be predicted from binding experiments in nonphysiological conditions (42). If this is taken into account, binding isotherms and dose-response curves of the cGMP-generating effect of ANP are likely to be entirely consistent with this nucleotide being the major second messenger of ANP actions. Finally, it is somewhat difficult to reconcile the efferent arteriolar vasoconstrictive and the aldosterone-lowering effect of ANP with the generation of cGMP. This nucleotide is not known to produce vasoconstriction or to counteract angiotensin-induced increase in aldosterone production by adrenal zona glomerulosa cells. Nevertheless, it has been recently shown that HS-142-1, a specific GC receptor antagonist, blocks both of these effects of ANP (62,63).

Other Possible Second Messengers

Some investigators have suggested that inhibition of cAMP or activation of phospholipase C and phosphoinositide turnover may be primary events of the cellular actions of ANP in some tissues (64–67). Some studies indicate that ANP inhibits adenylyl cyclase activity via activation of a pertussis toxin–sensitive G_i protein in practically all membrane preparations tested, including those derived from vascular tissues, glomeruli, and nephron segments (except proximal tubules) (68). This effect was reported to occur at ANP concentrations lower than those necessary to activate guanylyl cyclase or increase cGMP. Other investigators, however, failed to detect inhibition of cAMP by ANP in glomeruli, mesangial cells, and several nephron segments, including IMCD (41,57,69). ANP may also increase phosphoinositide turnover (66,67). In cultured IMDC, ANP increases IP_3 via activation of phospholipase C at concentrations lower ($<10^{-9}$ M) than those needed to stimulate cGMP. This effect is blunted by an inhibitor of protein kinase C, and also at higher concentrations of ANP, or by addition of exogenous cGMP (67). At present, it is not possible to clearly interpret the diverse cellular events referred to above. However, these findings suggest that cellular mediation of ANP effects may be significantly more complex than initially envisioned. It is possible that inhibition of cAMP and/or increase in phosphoinositide turnover may be secondary effects involved in the termination rather than initiation of ANP effects. Indeed, inhibition of cAMP and increase in IP_3 formation usually elicits actions (e.g., vasoconstriction, proximal tubule increase in sodium reabsorption) that are opposite to the primary effects of ANP (vasorelaxation, natriuresis).

It has been speculated that the effects of ANP on second messengers other than cGMP are mediated by C receptors (64,65). However, data in this regard are contradictory (see Other Possible Functions of C Receptors, below). The issue of ANP induction of second messengers other than cGMP and receptor subtypes that may be involved in this process remain to be fully elucidated.

Cellular Mechanisms of ANP Effects

Figure 3 schematically depicts the cellular mechanisms by which cGMP may mediate some of the known actions of ANP. In several cell types, ANP and cGMP reduce agonist or depolarization-induced increases in cytosolic Ca^{2+}, but the exact mechanism(s) of this process is unknown (70–72). This effect is independent of extracellular calcium and sodium and, therefore, is not mediated via membrane calcium channels or the Na-Ca exchange antiporter (73). cGMP has been shown to activate sarcolemmal Ca^{2+}–adenosine triphosphatase (ATPase), an action that may explain in part the ANP-induced decrease in cytosolic Ca^{2+} in vascular smooth muscle cells (74,75). In adrenal glomerulosa cells, ANP decreases a delayed calcium current through the L-channels, but this effect is apparently not related to the inhibition of aldosterone secretion (76). In IMCD, and in cultured vascular smooth muscle and endothelial cells,

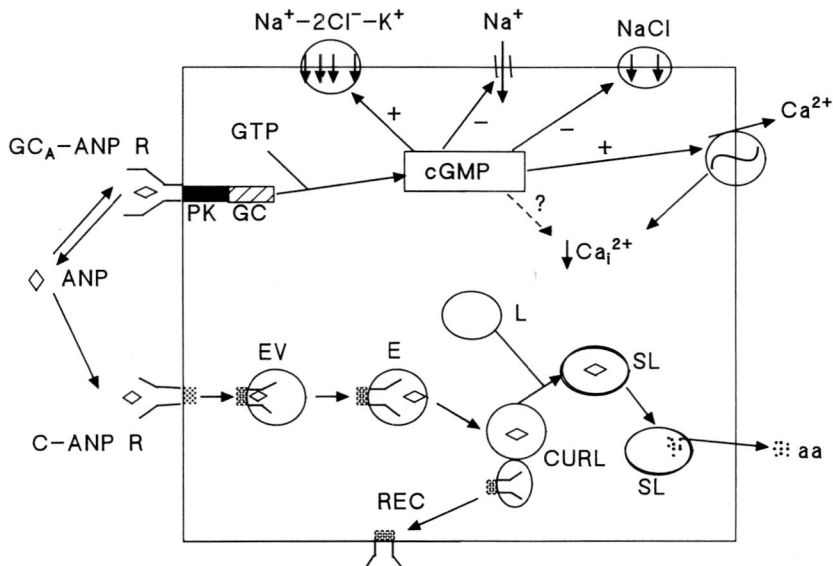

FIG. 3. Schematic representation of the cell physiology of GC$_A$ and C receptors. C receptors (C-ANF R) have as a main systemic function the removal of ANP from the circulation, a function that is performed by receptor-mediated endocytosis (EV, endocytic vesicles; E, endosomes; CURL, compartment for uncoupling receptor-ligand complexes), delivery of ANP to lysosomes (L, primary lysosomes; SL, secondary lysosomes), where it undergoes hydrolysis to amino acids (aa), which are then released to the medium. Internalized receptors recycle (REC) to the cell membrane. GC$_A$ receptors (GC$_A$-ANF R) mediate the systemic effects of ANP, and cGMP is the main second messenger of these actions. Some of the indicated cellular mechanisms for cGMP-mediated events are stimulation of Ca^{2+}ATPase, leading to decreases in cytosolic Ca^{2+}; inhibition of amiloride-sensitive Na$^+$ transport, and of thiazide-sensitive NaCl cotransport; stimulation of furosemide-sensitive Na$^+$-2Cl$^-$-K$^+$ cotransport; and less well defined (*dashed arrow*) intracellular events that lead to a decrease in cytosolic calcium. (From ref. 18, with permission.)

ANP and cGMP stimulate a furosemide-sensitive Na-2Cl-K cotransporter (58,77,78). This action may explain in part the increase in sodium secretion observed in isolated perfused IMCD (58). ANP and cGMP also inhibit amiloride-sensitive uptake of Na$^+$ in LLC-PK$_1$ and IMCD cells (57,59). This event, as well as the vascular smooth muscle effects of cGMP, may be due to stimulation of cGMP-activated protein kinase(s) (75). There is also evidence in cortical collecting ducts of the kidney removed from mineralocorticoid-treated rats, that ANP (and cGMP) inhibits a thiazide-sensitive neutral NaCl cotransport (56).

In intact animals ANP effects are not inhibited and may even be potentiated by amiloride and thiazides, suggesting that inhibition of amiloride-sensitive Na$^+$ uptake or of thiazide-sensitive NaCl reabsorption is either not a main mechanism of the natriuretic effect of ANP, or that this action may be mild and easily overcome by other effects of ANP (79–81). An explanation for the additive natriuretic effects of ANP and these diuretics may reside on renal hemodynamic or proximal tubular effects of ANP that lead to an increase in sodium load to distal nephron segments. Under normal conditions, this increase is partly compensated by an augmented distal reabsorption via amiloride-sensitive sodium channels and/

or via thiazide-sensitive NaCl transport. In the presence of amiloride or thiazides this compensation is removed, resulting in a potentiation of ANP natriuretic effect. Moreover, in some preparations such as in glomeruli, adrenal glomerulosa, and rabbit aorta segments, amiloride potentiates the cGMP-generating effect of ANP and enhances its vasorelaxant and aldosterone-lowering effects, possibly by decreasing the off-rate of the ligand from GC$_A$ receptors (42,82–84).

The experimental maneuvers that are necessary to elicit detectable actions of ANP *in vitro* have contributed to the difficulties of directly assessing the cellular mechanisms of action of ANP. Thus, although ANP leads to changes in enzymatic activities and second messengers in cells and tissues not previously stimulated by other agents, end-cellular, tissue, or organ effects of ANP (e.g., decrease in sodium reabsorption by renal epithelial cells, vasorelaxation in smooth muscle cells, inhibition of aldosterone secretion by adrenal glomerulosa cells) are usually undetectable under these conditions in *in vitro* preparations. These end-effects become apparent only under stimulated conditions, such as when sodium reabsorption is initially increased by mineralocorticoid pretreatment or angiotensin II infusion, isolated vascular strips are initially constricted by vasopressor agents, or aldosterone synthesis is increased by angiotensin II, potassium, or other agents (reviewed in ref. 1). Under these conditions it becomes rather difficult to separate primary from secondary events, and to assess unequivocally the primary cellular mechanisms by which ANP and cGMP (or other putative second messengers) exert their cellular actions. Many of the present apparent contradictions in the literature on cellular mechanisms of action of ANP, and on the involvement of different receptor subtypes and second messengers, result from this experimental problem. On the other hand, the lack of detectable endcellular effects of ANP under basal conditions is not simply due to the insensitivity of the experimental procedures, but it likely reflects the true nature of ANP as a counterregulatory hormone. Thus, early studies in intact animals have shown that in normotensive intact animals, ANP has little or no effect on peripheral vascular resistance while it markedly decreased this parameter in renin-dependent models of hypertension (1).

FUNCTIONS OF C RECEPTORS

Clearance Function

The discovery of the clearance function of C receptors originated from structure-function–binding studies in an isolated perfused rat kidney preparation (36). Figure 4 illustrates some of the results of this study. The top panel shows that a specific ligand of C receptors, $C\text{-}ANF_{4-23}$, displaced more than 95 percent of bound radiolabeled ANF_{1-28} in whole kidney tissue and in the kidney cortex. The bottom panel shows that $C\text{-}ANF_{4-23}$, at concentrations that led to the occupancy of more than 95 percent of renal receptors of ANP, did not have intrinsic biological effects of its own and did not antagonize the effects of ANP in the isolated kidney preparation (36). This finding was interpreted to indicate that the bulk of the renal receptors of ANP is biologically silent, i.e., they do not mediate any of the known renal or vascular effects of ANP. However, as shown in Fig. 5, when administered to intact rats, $C\text{-}ANF_{4-23}$ increases plasma levels of endogenous ANF and, consequently, elicits natriuretic and blood pressure-lowering effects that accompany, *pari passu*, the rise and fall in plasma levels of endogenous hormone (36,53). Several subsequent studies by independent groups of investigators confirmed the finding that *in vivo* blockade of C receptors by specific ligands increases plasma levels of endogenous ANP, an increase that elicits natriuretic and blood pressure-lowering effects in rats (1,54,85,86), ovine fetuses (87), and dogs (88). These results are consistent with the postulate that C receptors mediate the removal of ANF from the circulation. From these studies it was postulated that C receptors act as a hormonal buffer system to impede large inappropriate fluctuations in plasma levels of ANP (36).

Definitive evidence that C receptors have a main role in the metabolic clearance of ANP was obtained in pharmacokinetic experiments in the rat, showing that *in vivo* blockade of these receptors by $C\text{-}ANF_{4-23}$ results in a major decrease in the metabolic clearance of ANP (89). In these experiments $C\text{-}ANF_{4-23}$ reduced the volume of distribution at steady state (V_{ss}) and metabolic clearance rate (MCR) of administered $^{125}I\text{-}ANP_{1-28}$ in a dose-related manner with maximal doses (10 $\mu g \cdot min^{-1}$/kg BW) reducing V_{ss} to one-third and MCR to one-fourth of their control values. From these data it was possible to estimate the relative proportion of unoccupied C receptors in rats. With normal plasma levels of endogenous ANP, occupied C receptors amounted to less than 1 percent of the total amount of C receptors, suggesting that in physiological conditions there is a very large reserve of unoccupied C receptors in the rat. The large reserve of unoccupied C receptors, their very high affinity for ANP, and their strategic localization in tissues and cells that receive a large proportion of the cardiac output (see above), contribute to the efficient clearance function of these receptors.

In vivo blockade of C receptors by $C\text{-}ANF_{4-23}$ also markedly reduced the appearance of $^{125}I\text{-}ANF_{1-28}$ hydrolytic products (^{125}I-monoiodotyrosine, and free ^{125}I) in plasma, demonstrating that C receptors mediate the hydrolysis of ANP (89). The delayed nature of the appearance of labeled hydrolytic products in plasma and the blockade of this phenomenon by $C\text{-}ANF_{4-23}$ are consistent with the postulate that C receptors mediate the metabolism of ANP by a mechanism of receptor-mediated endocytosis followed by lysosomal hydrolysis of ligand. Subsequent studies in cell cultures demonstrated that this is indeed the case (see below).

Interactions of C Receptor and Neutral Endopeptidase (NEP)–Mediated Metabolism of ANP

In addition to its elimination by C receptors, ANP is also subject to inactivation by neutral metalloendopeptidase (NEP, E.C. 3.4.24.11), a protease that hydrolyses mainly the $Cys^7\text{-}Phe^8$ peptide bond resulting in an inactive ring open metabolite of ANP (90). Membrane-bound NEP is found in very high concentrations at the brush border of proximal renal tubules, but is also widely distributed at smaller concentrations in several other tissues (90,91). When administered to intact animals, NEP inhibitors potentiate the effects of ANP, and are able to exert mild natriuretic and, in some instances, blood pressure lowering effects (86,92–96). Whether or not the effects of NEP inhibitors are entirely due to an inhibition of ANP metabolism is still not certain. In normal conditions, most investigators find that these inhibitors have little if any effect on plasma levels of endogenous ANP (93). Moreover, NEP is known to hydrolyze several other

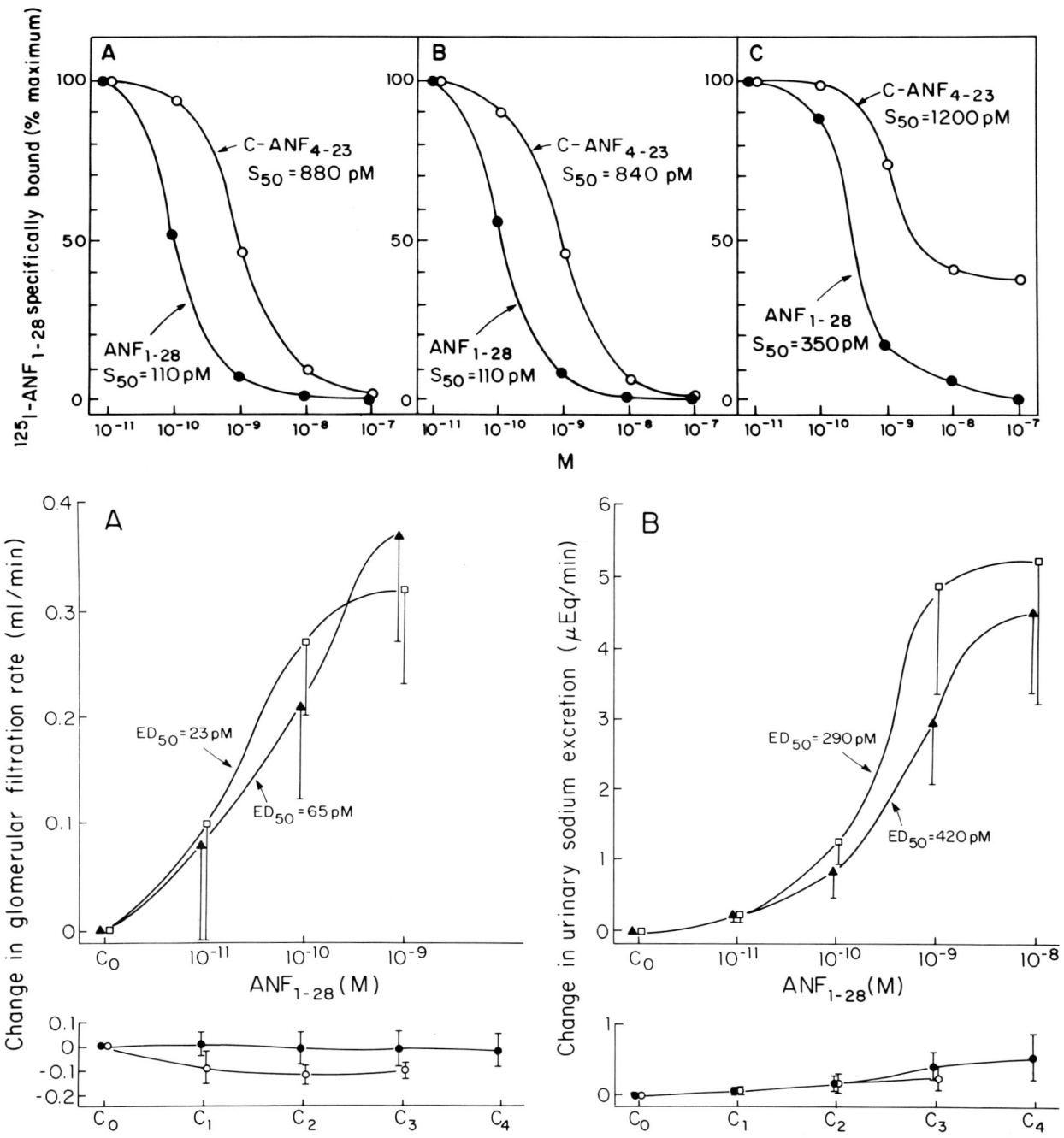

FIG. 4. C receptors constitute the overwhelming majority of total ANP receptors, and do not mediate renal effects of ANP in the isolated perfused rat kidney. **Top:** Competition for binding between ^{125}I-ANF$_{1-28}$ and unlabeled ANF$_{1-28}$ or C-ANF$_{4-23}$, a specific ligand of C receptors, in whole kidney (A), kidney cortex (B), and papilla (C). C-ANF$_{4-23}$, displaces >98 percent of specific binding of ^{125}I-ANF$_{1-28}$ in whole kidney and kidney cortex, and approximately 60 percent in the papilla. This indicates that the overwhelming majority of ANP receptors in the rat kidney are C receptors. **Bottom:** Effects of time control (*closed circles*), ANF$_{1-28}$ (*closed triangles*), C-ANF$_{4-23}$ (*open circles*), and ANF$_{1-28}$ + C-ANF$_{4-23}$ (*open squares*) on glomerular filtration rate (A) and sodium excretion (B) in the isolated perfused rat kidney. Results show that C-ANF$_{4-23}$ at a dose (0.1 μM) that led to the occupancy of >98 percent of ANP receptors in whole kidney tissue and kidney cortex kidney (top) did not have effects on its own and did not alter the dose-response curve of ANF$_{1-28}$ on glomerular filtration rate and sodium excretion or on any other measured renal function parameter (36). These data indicated that C receptors are biologically silent, in the sense that they do not mediate the known renal and vascular effects of ANP. A major function of C-ANF receptors is to remove ANP from the circulation. (See also text and Fig. 5 and 6.) (From ref. 36, with permission.)

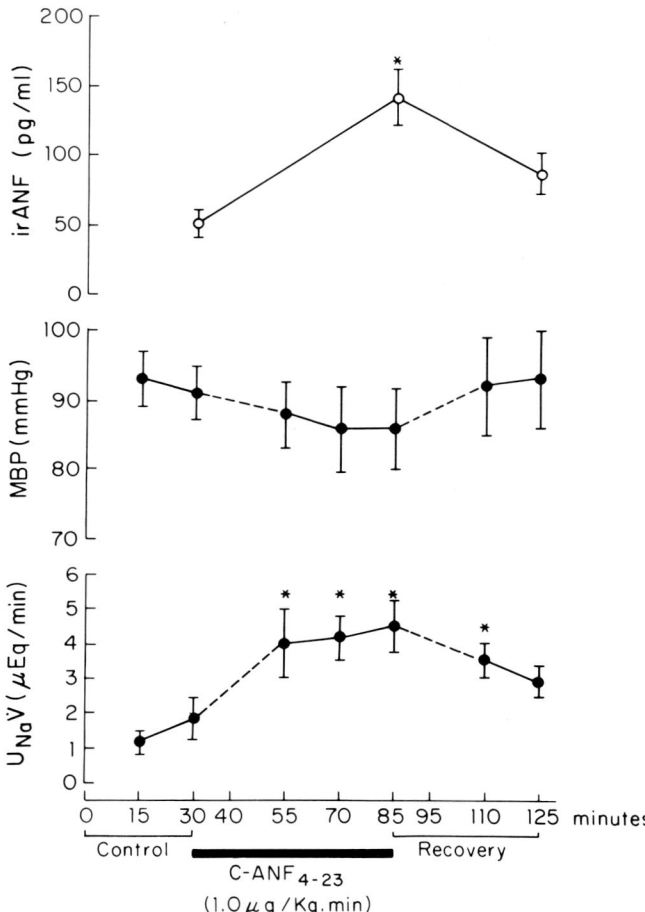

FIG. 5. Effects of blockade of C receptor on plasma levels of ANP, blood pressure, and natriuresis in the rat. C-ANF$_{4-23}$, a specific ligand of C receptors, increases plasma levels of immunoreactive (ir) ANF, which, in turn, leads to an increase in sodium excretion (U$_{Na}$V) and a decrease in mean arterial blood pressure (MBP). Together with the results shown in Fig. 4, these data indicate that C receptors have a main clearance function, and suggest a novel experimental and possibly therapeutic approach to increase plasma levels of endogenous ANP. (From ref. 36, with permission.)

peptides that may have vasorelaxant and natriuretic effects. Among these peptides, bradykinin may be of particular interest because bradykinin receptor antagonists and bradykinin antibodies were shown to almost completely block the potentiating effects of NEP inhibitors on ANP-induced natriuresis in the rat (92,96).

The predominance of C receptors in mediating the metabolic clearance of ANP in normal conditions does not exclude that in certain conditions, particularly when C receptors are nearly saturated, NEP plays an important role in the metabolism of ANP. Thus, NEP inhibitors were shown to further increase plasma levels of ANP when these levels are initially elevated by infusion of the peptide or in pathological conditions, such as in conges-

tive heart failure in experimental animals and humans (85,86,95,97). Recently it was shown that a combination of blockade of C receptors by specific ligands (C-ANF$_{4-23}$ or C-ANF$_{11-15}$), and administration of NEP inhibitors (phosphoramidon or thiorphan-like compounds) has an exquisitively synergistic effect in decreasing the metabolic clearance of ANP in rats (55,98). Figure 6 gives an example of results that demonstrate the synergistic action between C receptor blockade and NEP inhibition. C-ANF$_{11-15}$ alone, similarly to C-ANF$_{4-23}$, decreases the MCR of ^{125}I-ANF$_{1-28}$ by almost threefold and slightly increases the half-time of elimination ($t_{\frac{1}{2}}$) of ANP from the circulation. Phosphoramidon alone has no effect on MCR or $t_{\frac{1}{2}}$ of ^{125}I-ANF$_{1-28}$. However, in combination with C-ANP$_{11-15}$, phosphoramidon further reduces the MCR of ^{125}I-ANF$_{1-28}$ to approximately 15 percent of its normal value and increases its $t_{\frac{1}{2}}$ more than threefold. The combination of C receptor blockade and NEP inhibition practically abolishes the metabolic clearance of ANP, except for the obligatory removal of this polypeptide by glomerular filtration (55).

The above findings may have important potential therapeutic implications in the treatment of cardiovascular and renal diseases. Thus, NEP inhibitors have shown beneficial, albeit mild, effects in hypertension and congestive heart failure (99–102). C receptor ligands were not yet tested in humans, mainly because of the lack of oral bioavailability of these peptidic compounds. The experimental data in experimental animals suggest that the potentially most useful approach would be to therapeutically combine the administration of NEP inhibitors with C receptor ligands. The discovery that very small linear peptides are effective ligands of C receptors raises the hope that they may serve as models for the development of orally active substances.

Other Possible Functions of C Receptors

The finding that C receptors have an important clearance function does not preclude per se that they may also mediate other functions of ANP. As pointed out above, some investigators postulate that C receptors mediate effects of ANP via inhibition of adenosine 3′,5′-cyclic monophosphate (cAMP) or increase in IP$_3$ generation. Results described above demonstrate that C receptors do not mediate any of the known end-organ renal and vascular effects of ANP (vasorelaxation, renal hemodynamic, and excretory effects), or its aldosterone-lowering effect. Based mostly on experiments using C-ANF$_{4-23}$ or other C receptor ligands, some authors have claimed that C receptors mediate the growth inhibitory action of ANP, but results in this regard are conflicting (27,64). GC receptors continue to be the most likely candidate for this effect because cGMP is known to inhibit cellular

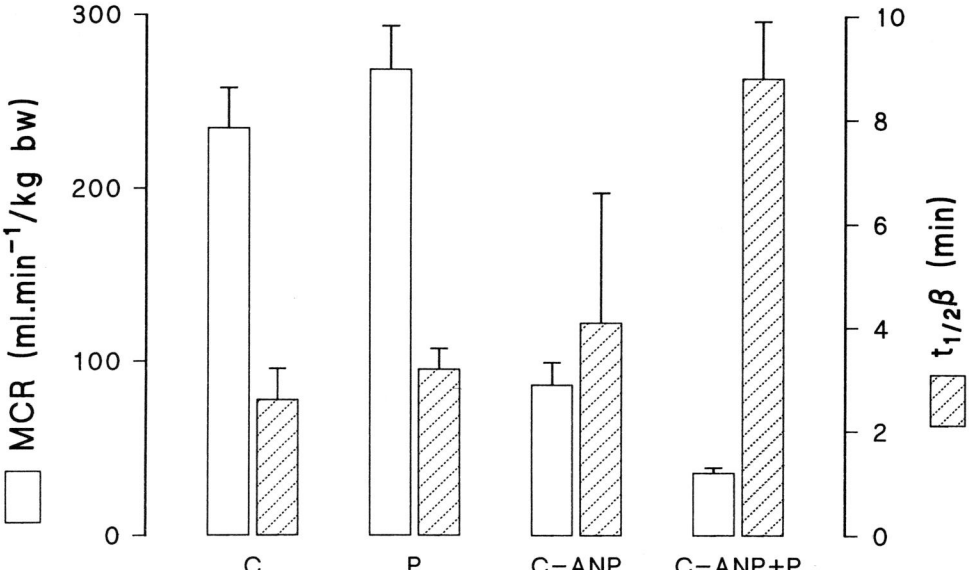

FIG. 6. The synergistic role of C receptors and neutral endopeptidase in the metabolic clearance of ANP. The metabolic clearance rate (MCR) and plasma elimination half time ($t_\frac{1}{2}\beta$) of ^{125}I-ANP$_{1-28}$ was determined in anesthetized rats under control (C) conditions, with inhibition of neutral endopeptidase (NEP) by phosphoramidon (P), with blockade of C receptors by C-ANP$_{11-15}$ (C-ANP), or by a combination of these procedures (C-ANP + P). In control conditions, MCR of ^{125}I-ANP$_{1-28}$ is very high and $t_\frac{1}{2}$ is very fast. Inhibition of NEP alone (P) has no effects on these parameters. Blockade of C receptors (C-ANP) leads to a major decrease in MCR and a slight increase in $t_\frac{1}{2}$ of ^{125}I-ANP$_{1-28}$. Addition of NEP inhibition to C receptor blockade (C-ANP + P) produce a major synergistic effect, further decreasing MCR and increasing $t_\frac{1}{2}$ by threefold. These data confirmed that under normal conditions, C receptors have the major role in removing ANP from the circulation. While NEP has little effect on this process in normal conditions, it markedly potentiates the effects of C receptors when they are nearly saturated. The data also suggest that combination of C receptor blockade and NEP inhibition is the most effective manner of prolonging the effects of ANP. (Based on data from ref. 55.)

growth. Some investigators also postulate that ANP inhibits endothelin, thyroglobulin, progesterone, testosterone, or catecholamine release via C receptors from different types of cultured cells (64). Inhibition of secretion of hormones and other effects of natriuretic peptides could be elicited by decreases in cAMP instead of an increase in cGMP because in both circumstances there may be a decrease in cystosolic calcium concentration. However, in many instances, ANP-induced decrease in cAMP has been shown to be secondary to cGMP, as a result of cGMP-stimulated activation of phosphodiesterases (103,104). Nevertheless it is possible, albeit not proven, that an unidentified novel receptor class or a subtype of the C receptor class is responsible for some of the above observations. Thus, although it cannot be ruled out that C receptors, or a subtype of C receptors, may mediate some effects of ANP, at present the only unequivocally established function of these receptors is to mediate the removal of ANP from the circulation. Further work is needed to clarify the involvement of receptor subtypes in the mediation of some of the less well defined effects of ANP, particularly its generic *in vitro* action of inhibiting secretory processes.

Cellular Mechanisms of the Clearance Function of C Receptors

The cellular mechanisms of the clearance function and dynamics of C receptors were elucidated by experiments in cultured vascular smooth muscle cells (105). Figure 7 shows results of steady-state experiments on the cellular dynamics of surface C receptor–radioligand complexes in cultured vascular smooth muscle cells. Panel A shows that surface C receptors are internalized at a rate of 5 percent of occupied receptors/min when cells are warmed from 4 to 37 degrees C under continuous exposure to saturating concentrations of radioligand (^{125}I-ANF$_{1-28}$). This results in an initial (first 15 min) decrease by half of the density of surface C receptors (panel A). Panels B and C show that the initial decrease in membrane-bound radioligand corresponds initially to the appearance of radioactivity in the intracellular compartment and then, after a short lag time, to the appearance of labeled hydrolytic products in the medium. Internalized C receptors are rapidly replenished in the time course of the experiment as shown by the finding that

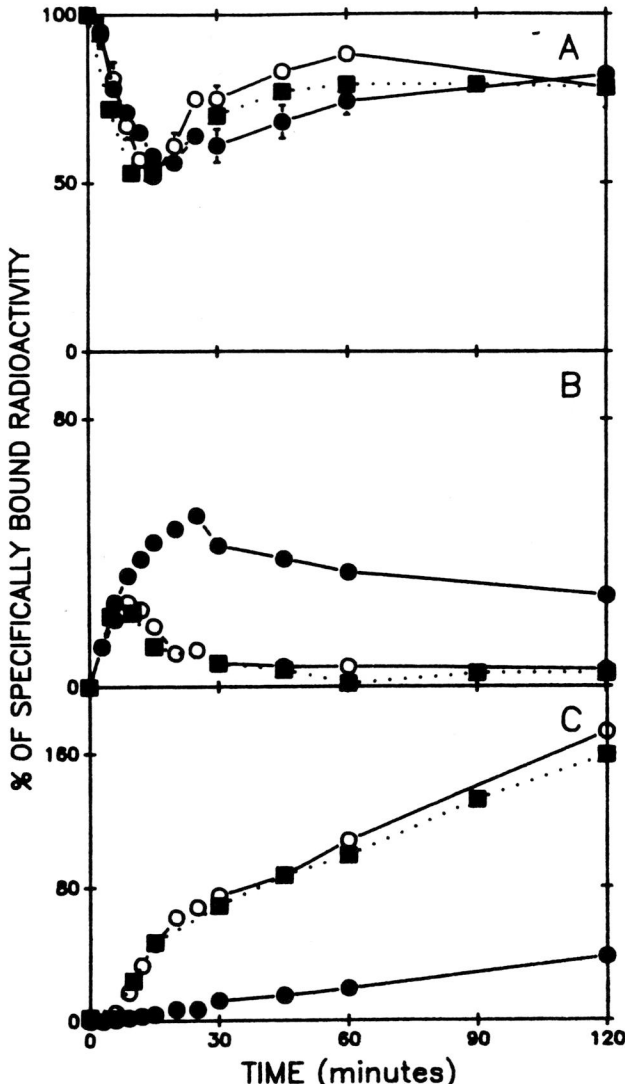

FIG. 7. C receptor–mediated endocytosis and lysosomal hydrolysis of ANP; C receptor recycling. Confluent monolayers of cultured bovine aortic smooth muscle cells were initially equilibrated with saturating concentrations of ^{125}I-ANP$_{1-28}$ at 4 degrees C. Then, cells were warmed to 37 degrees C to initiate the endocytic process in the continuous presence of saturating concentrations of radioligand. Radioactivity bound to the cell membrane (**A**) is a measure of the density of surface C receptors at each time of incubation (density at time zero, approximately 250,000 receptor sites/cell). Radioactivity in the cell interior, and degradation products (^{125}I and ^{125}I-monoiodotyrosine) are shown in **B** and **C**, respectively. Experiments were performed in control conditions (*open circles*), or in the presence of 10 mM NH$_4$Cl, a lysosomotropic weak base that inhibits lysosomal hydrolysis of peptides (*closed circles*), or in the presence of 0.1 mM cycloheximide, a protein synthesis inhibitor (*squares*). The results show that C receptors are endocytosed together with bound ANP, and that internalized ANP undergo lysosomal hydrolysis. Moreover, internalized C receptors are recycled to the cell surface, so as to mediate more than one cycle of ANP internalization and lysosomal hydrolysis. (See text for a more detailed description.) (From ref. 105, with permission.)

the density of surface C receptors returns to near control levels by 30 min (panel A). This replenishment process is not affected by cycloheximide, a protein synthesis inhibitor, indicating that it is not dependent on synthesis *de novo* of receptors, but on recycling of internalized receptors. Results in panel C show that by 120 min, 160 percent of the radioactivity initially bound to surface C receptors appears as hydrolytic products in the medium, further demonstrating that each surface C receptor mediates more than one cycle of ligand internalization and hydrolysis. ^{125}I-ANF$_{1-28}$ internalized together with C receptors is delivered to lysosomes where it is hydrolyzed to completion, and the hydrolytic products (amino acids) are then released to the medium. This is demonstrated by the finding that NH$_4$Cl, a lysosomotropic weak base that impedes the action of lysosomal acid hydrolases, almost completely blocks the appearance of radiolabeled hydrolytic products (^{125}I, and ^{125}I-monoiodotyrosine) in medium (panel C), resulting in the accumulation of radioligand in the cell interior (panel B).

Rapid and almost complete receptor recycling explains why, contrary to other polypeptide hormone receptors, C receptors do not undergo rapid homologous (ligand-induced) down-regulation (2,37,39,105). It is of interest that C receptors are, however, down-regulated by exposure of cells to angiotensin II and by ANP-induced increase in cGMP, but the physiological meaning of this phenomenon remains to be elucidated (106,107). A noteworthy characteristic of the processes of internalization and recycling of C receptors is that they are constitutive in nature, i.e., they do not depend on ligand binding (105). In this sense, C receptors behave as a "turning wheel," continuously moving bound ANP to the cell interior, where it is hydrolyzed within lysosomes.

DYNAMICS OF GC$_A$ RECEPTORS AND RECEPTOR-LIGAND COMPLEXES

GC$_A$ Receptors Are Bona Fide Membrane-Resident Proteins that Do Not Internalize or Mediate Lysosomal Hydrolysis of ANP

Recent studies from my laboratory in cultured glomerular mesangial and renomedullary interstitial cells from the rat have shown that, contrary to C receptors and most other polypeptide hormone receptors, the GC$_A$ receptor is a bona fide membrane-resident protein that does not internalize and does not mediate lysosomal hydrolysis of ANP at substantive rates (42). Figure 8 shows results of experiments in which the lack of changes in intracellular concentration of GC$_A$ receptors in glomerular mesangial cells is contrasted with the increase (internalization), and then the subsequent decrease (recycling), in the intracellular concentration of C receptors.

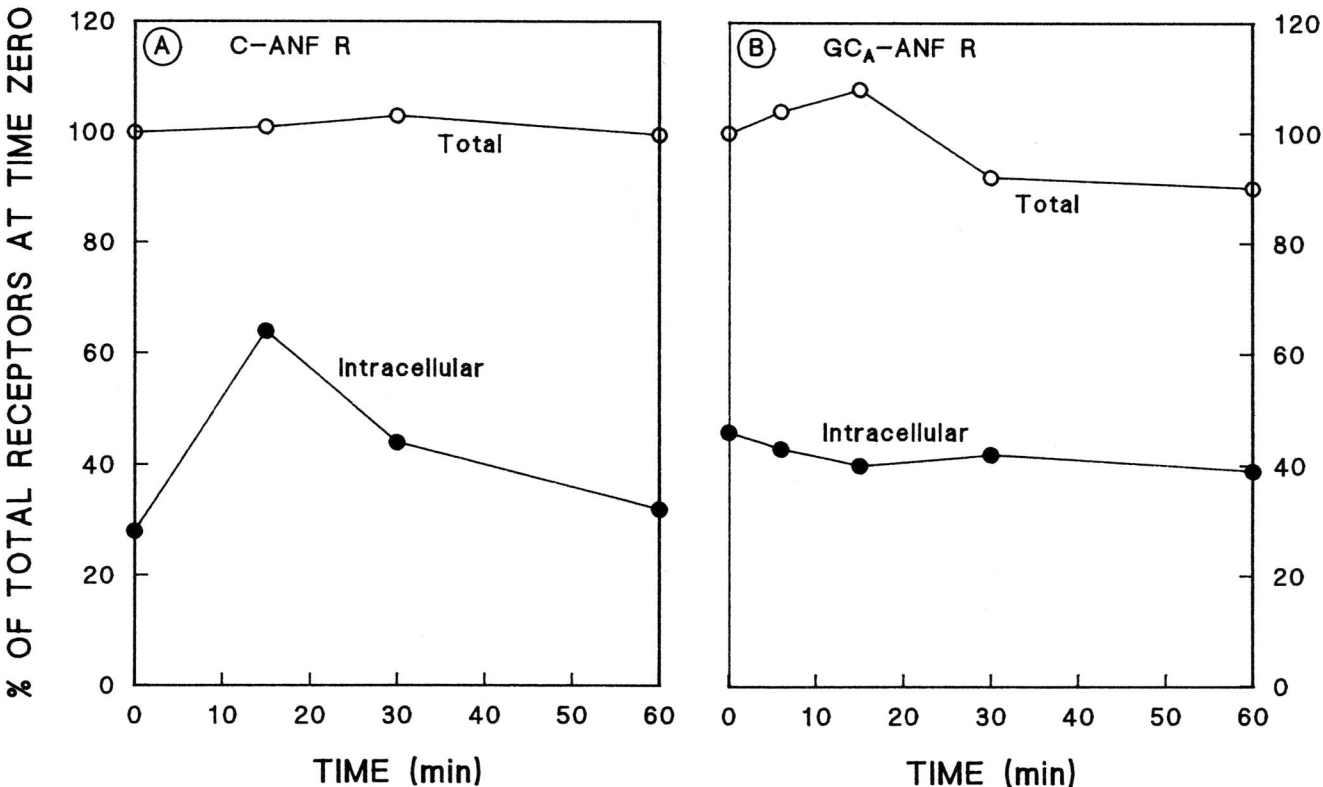

FIG. 8. Cellular dynamics of C and GC_A receptors. Experiments were performed in cell monolayers of cultured bovine aortic smooth muscle cells (C receptors) and rat glomerular mesangial cells (GC_A receptors) exposed to saturating concentrations of ANP. Receptors were solubilized from cells in control conditions (total cell receptors) or after removal of surface receptor by trypsin (intracellular receptors) after each time period of exposure to ANP. The total cell (membrane + intracellular) concentration of C and GC_A receptors remains constant, showing that these receptors are not down-regulated by continuous exposure of the cells to saturating concentrations of ANP. The concentration of intracellular C receptors first rises (internalization) and then returns to basal levels (recycling), in a mirror image of the initial fall and then replenishment of surface C receptors (see Fig. 7A). In contrast, under the same conditions, the intracellular concentration of GC_A receptors remains nearly constant, showing that they are not internalized at substantive rates. (From ref. 18; data from ref. 42 and 105.)

In addition, GC_A receptors in glomerular mesangial, renomedullary interstitial, and neuroblastoma cells fail to mediate significant lysosomal hydrolysis of ANP, even when exposed to the ligand for prolonged periods of time (42,108). Finally, recombinant GC_A receptors transfected into 293 cells also fail to internalize or mediate lysosomal hydrolysis of ANP, confirming that lack of substantive endocytosis is a generic property of these receptors (Maack, T., Silva, M., and Porter, G., *unpublished results*).

The lack of endocytosis of GC_A receptors is consistent with the unique molecular characteristics of these receptors. Thus, as described earlier in this chapter, GC_A receptors, contrary to other polypeptide hormone receptors, contain binding sites (extracellular domain) and the enzyme effector (guanylate cyclase) in the same molecule (Fig. 1). This implies that ligand effects do not necessarily depend on receptor mobility in the plane of the membrane (2,42), which may lead to the entrapment of these receptors in coated pits or other endocytic sites. Moreover, the cytoplasmic domain of GC_A receptors does not contain signals that are usually associated with rapid receptor internalization, such as the NPXY sequence (where X is any amino acid) or aromatic amino acids (Y or P) near the transmembrane domain (2,5,7).

Endocytosis plays an important role in regulating the density of most membrane receptors because, in many instances, a significant proportion of internalized receptors is destroyed together with their ligands within lysosomes. In this case, exposure to high concentration of ligand leads to a prolonged decrease in the cell surface density of these receptors (down-regulation). In view of the efficient recycling of internalized receptors this is not the case for C receptors, as discussed above. For a different reason, namely lack of substantial rates of internalization, homologous down-regulation of GC_A receptors is also not expected to occur. This is indeed the case, as demonstrated by the *in vivo* and *in vitro* experiments showing that high levels of ANP fail to down-regulate GC_A receptors and/or the cGMP response in glomeruli or papillae from the rat (37,41).

Termination of the Interaction of ANP with GC_A Receptors

Endocytosis of receptor-ligand complexes is believed to contribute to the termination of the biological effects of ligands. In the absence of internalization, other process(es) must account for the termination of the interaction of ANP with GC_A receptors. Recently, we found that one of these processes is a rapid dissociation of receptor-ligand complexes when ANP binds to GC_A receptors at physiological, but not at subphysiological, temperatures (42). Figure 9 compares the temperature dependence of the off-rate (K_{off}) of ANP from GC_A receptors in glomerular mesangial cells and from C receptors from the same cell type, or from cultured vascular smooth muscle cells. As can be seen, the dissociation of radiolabeled ANP from both receptors at 4 degrees C is very slow, less than 1.5 percent/min. At 37 degrees C, the dissociation of ANP from C receptors increases modestly to 5 percent/min, an increase that is expected on thermodynamic grounds by the rise in temperature alone. In contrast, there is a disproportionate increase in the offset of ANP from GC_A receptors between 30 and 37 degrees C, resulting in a K_{off} at 37 degrees C that is greater than 85 percent/min. The Q_{10} of the dissociation of ANP from GC_A receptors between 30 and 37 degrees C is >6.8, whereas between 4 and 30 degrees C it is only 2 to 3 (42). These results demonstrate the existence of a physiological process that markedly increases the dissociation of ANP from GC_A receptors. This process depends on active metabolism because it is detectable only in intact cells at physiological temperatures. As will be described below it is possible, even likely, that ATP mediates this sudden increase in receptor-ligand dissociation.

Amiloride, at high concentrations (0.5 mM), mark-

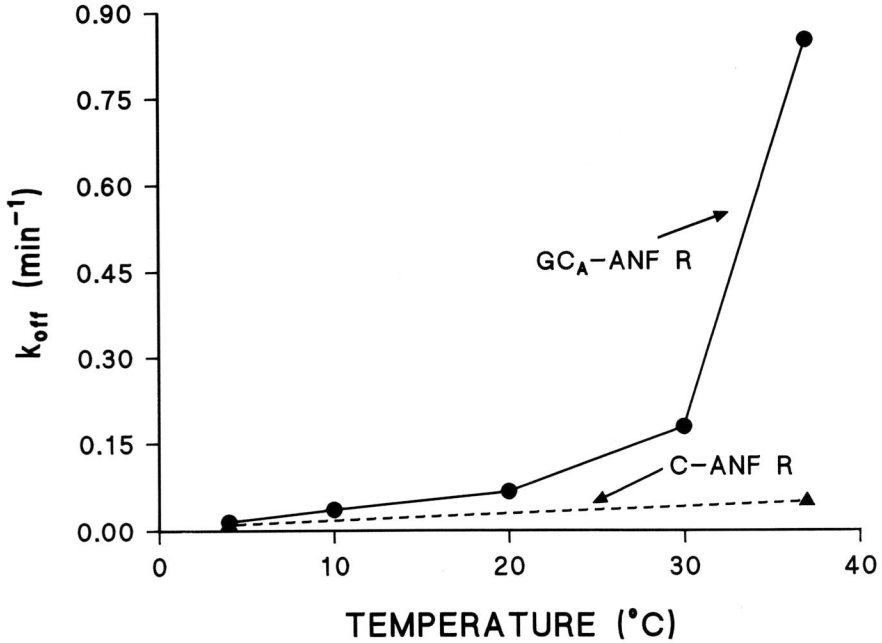

FIG. 9. Temperature dependence of the off-rate (K_{off}) of ANP from surface GC_A and C receptors in intact cells. Dissociation of ^{125}I-ANP_{1-28} from GC_A and C receptors in cultured glomerular mesangial or bovine aortic smooth muscle cells was measured at several temperatures. The dissociation rates of radioligand from GC_A and C receptors at 4 degrees C are similar and very slow, consistent with the almost nearly identical affinities of these two receptors for ANP at low temperatures. As the temperature rises there is only a relatively small increase in K_{off} of ANP from C receptors. The same is true for GC_A receptors at up to 20 degrees C, but then the K_{off} of ANP from these receptors increases dramatically, particularly between 30 and 37 degrees C. At the physiological temperature of 37 degrees C, the K_{off} from GC_A receptors is >85 percent/min, whereas it is <5 percent/min from C receptors. The slow off-rate of ligand from C receptors allows for a sufficient resident time of ANP on these receptors to undergo the process of endocytosis. The rapid off-rate of ANP from GC_A receptors contributes to a prompt termination of ANP biological responses. (From ref. 18, with permission; data from ref. 42.)

edly decreases the K_{off} of ANP from GC_A receptors in glomerular mesangial cells by more than tenfold (42). Earlier studies have shown that amiloride competes with an interaction of ATP with GC_A receptors in membranes of bovine adrenal zona glomerulosa cells (109,110). In these studies it was also shown that ATP increases the K_{off} of ANP more than it increases K_{on}, resulting in an increase in the apparent equilibrium dissociation constant (K_d). Moreover, ATP magnifies the ANP-induced increase in guanylate cyclase activity and in cGMP (9,17,110). It has been postulated that there is an (allosteric) interaction of ATP with the protein kinaselike domain of GC_A receptors (17,110). The results taken as a whole are consistent with the hypothesis that the rapid dissociation of ANP from GC_A receptor in intact cells at physiological temperatures is mediated by ATP (42). Further studies are needed, however, to understand the basic biochemical and physiological mechanisms of this process. In addition, dephosphorylation of GC_A receptors upon ligand binding may also participate importantly in the desensitization and termination of ANP effects (111).

SUMMARY AND CONCLUSIONS

Figure 10 depicts schematically the functional properties of receptor-ligand interactions for ANP and their role in stimulus-response homeostasis and control of plasma levels of ANP. ANP is secreted by the heart atria in response to stimuli that increase atrial stretch or pressure (central venous and arterial blood pressures). These end effects of ANP (e.g., increase in salt excretion, vasorelaxation, decrease in plasma volume) result from its interaction with GC_A receptors to generate cGMP. The effects, by a classical feedback mechanism, will prevent further secretion and increase in plasma levels of ANP. At this point it is important for the organism to rapidly remove excess ANP from the circulation, a function that is primarily accomplished by the interaction of ANP with C receptors, which are specialized to remove the hormone from the circulation by receptor-mediated endocytosis and lysosomal metabolism. Neutral endopeptidase plays a secondary role in the removal of ANP from the circulation under normal conditions, but markedly potentiates C receptor–mediated metabolism of ANP

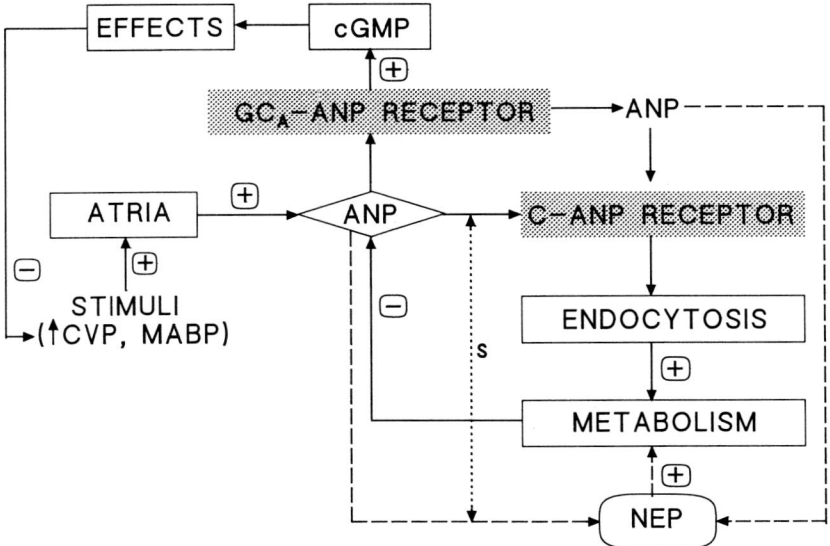

FIG. 10. Schematics of the role of ligand-receptor interactions on ANP homeostasis. (See text for description.) ANF in the *diamond* in the center of the figure represents plasma levels of ANP, which are increased by stimuli that promote atrial secretion of the hormone (CVP, central venous pressure; MABP, mean arterial blood pressure). Plasma levels of ANP are decreased by C receptor–mediated endocytosis and lysosomal metabolism. Thus C receptors behave as a hormonal buffer system to impede large inappropriate fluctuations in plasma levels of ANP, and to promptly remove ANP from the circulation once the stimuli for secretion are terminated. In normal conditions, neutral endopeptidase (NEP) has a small role in the metabolism of circulating ANP, but it potentiates the primary effect of C receptors. The interaction of ANP with GC_A receptors leads to generation of cGMP, organ effects, and a classical systemic negative feedback control of ANP secretion. The termination of ANP effects at the cellular level is due to a rapid decrease in receptor affinity upon ligand binding at physiological temperatures, resulting in a rapid off-rate of ANP from GC_A receptors. ANP released by GC_A receptors can then be removed by C receptor–mediated metabolism, and to a smaller extent by NEP hydrolysis. The combination of these events is likely to result in an efficient effect when plasma concentrations of ANP rise, and a prompt termination of effects when plasma concentrations of the hormone fall.

when plasma levels of endogenous ANP are elevated (e.g., congestive heart failure) or when C receptors are nearly saturated. Blockade of C receptors by specific ligands together with inhibition of neutral endopeptidase represents a novel approach to increase plasma levels of endogenous ANP. This approach may be of potential therapeutic value in the treatment of cardiovascular and renal diseases. In the overall homeostasis of the system it is also important to rapidly terminate hormonal responses, a process that is accomplished, at least in part, by a rapid dissociation of ANP from GC_A receptors.

The major differences between the dynamics of GC_A and C receptors described in this chapter are consistent with the specialized role of these receptors in the mammalian organism. The efficiency of the clearance role of C receptors is favored by a slow dissociation of ANP from these receptors. This increases the resident time of the ligand on surface receptors, permitting the relatively slow endocytic process to internalize ANP, and eventually deliver it to lysosomes, where it is hydrolyzed. The slow dissociation has the disadvantage of decreasing the number of unoccupied C receptors at the cell surface. However, because of the great excess of C receptors relative to normal plasma concentrations of ANP, and the efficiency of the receptor recycling process, this decrease is not normally rate limiting for the clearance of the hormone. On the other hand, GC_A receptors are bona fide membrane-resident proteins that do not internalize or mediate lysosomal hydrolysis of ligand. These receptors mediate the major biological effects of ANP, a process that does not depend per se on receptor internalization. A fast dissociation of ANP from GC_A receptors may be an important component of the stimulus-response homeostasis for this hormone. Thus, when the free concentration of ANP falls, a fast dissociation favors a rapid termination of the response. The dissociated hormone can then be rapidly removed by the abundant C receptors. A fast dissociation rate also increases the availability of unoccupied GC_A receptors, whose density, contrary to that of C receptors, is limited. Thus, the fast dissociation of surface receptor–ligand complexes favors a heightened response to ANP when plasma levels increase. ATP is likely to play a major modulatory role in this process because it increases ligand offset (and to a smaller degree onset), and at the same time magnifies the ANP-induced increase in guanylate cyclase activity. The combination of these events is likely to result in an efficient effect when plasma concentrations of ANP rise, and a prompt termination of effects when plasma concentrations of the hormone fall.

The great strides made in the past years in the understanding of natriuretic peptides and their receptors, in all likelihood, unveiled just the tip of the iceberg of this important regulatory system. The full physiological and pathophysiological implications of the homeostatic cycle of receptor-ligand interactions, as well as the physiological role of BNP and CNP, are far from being fully understood. Future research on molecular structure, as well as on cell, organ, and systemic functions of natriuretic peptide receptors, is expected to further elucidate complex mechanisms involved in pressure-volume homeostasis. This may open new therapeutic avenues for the treatment of cardiovascular and renal diseases, including hypertension.

ACKNOWLEDGMENT

This work is supported by National Institutes of Health grant HL 50996.

REFERENCES

1. Atlas SA, Maack T. Atrial natriuretic factor. In: Windhager EE, ed. *Handbook of Physiology: Renal Physiology.* New York: Oxford University Press, 1992;1577–1673.
2. Maack T. Receptors of atrial natriuretic factor. *Annu Rev Physiol* 1992;54:11–27.
3. Garbers DL, Wong SK-F. Receptor guanylyl cyclases. *J Clin Invest* 1992;90:299–305.
4. Murad F. Cyclic guanosine monophosphate as a mediator of vasodilation. *J Clin Invest* 1986;78:1–5.
5. Schulz S, Singh S, Bellet RA, Singh G, Tubb DJ, Chin H, Garbers DL. The primary structure of a plasma membrane guanylate cyclase demonstrates diversity within this new receptor family. *Cell* 1989;58:1155–1162.
6. Lowe DG, Chang MS, Hellmiss R, Chen E, Singh S, Garbers DL, Goeddel DV. Human atrial natriuretic peptide receptor defines a new paradigm for second messenger signal transduction. *EMBO J* 1989;8:1377–1384.
7. Chinkers M, Garbers DL, Chang MS, Lowe DG, Chin HM, Goeddel DV, Schulz S. A membrane form of guanylate cyclase is an atrial natriuretic peptide receptor. *Nature* 1989;338:78–83.
8. Lucarini AR, Arrighi P, Favilla S, Simonini N, Salvetti A. The influence of dopamine-1 receptor blockade on the humoral and renal effects of low-dose atrial natriuretic factor in human hypertensives. *J Hypertens* 1989;7(suppl 6):S230–S231.
9. Chinkers M, Garbers DL. The protein kinase domain of the ANP receptor is required for signaling. *Science* 1989;245:1392–1394.
10. Thorpe D, Morkin E. The carboxyl region contains the catalytic domain of the membrane form of guanylyl cyclase. *J Biol Chem* 1992;265:14717–14720.
11. Koller KJ, deSauvage FJ, Lowe DG, Goeddell DV. Conservation of kinaselike domain is essential for activation of the natriuretic peptide receptor family. *Mol Cell Biol* 1992;12:2581–2590.
12. Larose L, Rondeau J-J, Ong H, De Lean A. Phosphorilation of atrial natriuretic factor R1 receptor by serine/threonine protein kinases: evidence for receptor regulation. *Mol Cell Biol* 1992;115:203–211.
13. Yamaguchi M, Rutledge LJ, Garbers DL. The primary structure of the rat guanylyl cyclase A/atrial natriuretic peptide receptor gene. *J Biol Chem* 1990;265:20414–20420.
14. Chang MS, Lowe DG, Lewis M, Hellmiss R, Chen E, Goeddel DV. Differential activation by atrial and brain natriuretic peptides of two different receptor guanylate cyclases. *Nature* 1989;341:68–72.
15. Meloche S, Ong H, De Lean A. Functional heterogeneity of atrial natriuretic factor receptor in bovine adrenal zona glomerulosa is explained by an amiloride-sensitive high affinity molecular complex. *J Biol Chem* 1987;262:10252–10258.
16. Chinkers M, Wilson EM. Ligand-independent oligomerization of natriuretic peptide receptors. *J Biol Chem* 1992;267:18589–18597.
17. Chinkers M, Singh S, Garbers DL. Adenine nucleotides are required for activation of rat atrial natriuretic peptide receptor/gu-

anylyl cyclase expressed in a baculovirus system. *J Biol Chem* 1991;266:4088–4093.

18. Maack T, Okolicany J, Koh GY, Price DA. Functional properties of atrial natriuretic factor receptors. *Semin Nephrol* 1993;13:50–60.

19. Leitman DC, Murad F. Comparison of binding and cyclic GMP accumulation by atrial natriuretic peptides in endothelial cells. *Biochim Biophys Acta* 1986;885:74–79.

20. Schenk DB, Johnson LK, Schwartz K, Sista H, Scarborough RM, Lewicki JA. Distinct atrial natriuretic factor receptor sites on cultured bovine aortic smooth muscle and endothelial cells. *Biochem Biophys Res Commun* 1985;127:433–442.

21. Fuller F, Porter JG, Arfsten AE, Miller J, Schilling JW, Scarborough RM, Lewicki JA, Schenk DB. Atrial natriuretic peptide clearance receptor. Complete sequence and functional expression of cDNA clones. *J Biol Chem* 1988;263:9395–9401.

22. Porter JG, Arfsten A, Fuller F, Miller JA, Gregory LC, Lewicki JA. Isolation and functional expression of the human atrial natriuretic peptide clearance receptor cDNA. *Biochem Biophys Res Commun* 1990;171:796–803.

23. Saheki T, Mizuno T, Iwata T, Saito Y, Nagasawa T, Mizuno KU, Ito F, Ito T, Hagiwara H, Hirose S. Structure of the bovine atrial natriuretic peptide receptor (type C) gene. *J Biol Chem* 1991;266:11122–11125.

24. Muller FB, Erne P, Raine AE, Bolli P, Linder L, Resink TJ, Cottier C, Buhler FR. Atrial antipressor natriuretic peptide: release mechanisms and vascular action in man. *J Hypertens Suppl* 1986;4:109–114.

25. Suga S, Nakao K, Hosoda K, Mukoyama M, Ogawa Y, Shirakami G, Arai H, Saito Y, Kambayashi Y, Inouye K. Receptor selectivity of natriuretic peptide family, atrial natriuretic peptide, brain natriuretic peptide, and C-type natriuretic peptide. *Endocrinology* 1992;130:229–239.

26. Suga S, Nakao K, Kishimoto I, Kiminori H, Mukoyama M, Arai H, Shirakami G, Ogawa Y, Komatsu Y, Nakagawa O, Hama N, Imura H. Phenoty-related alteration in expression of natriuretic peptide receptors in aortic smooth muscle cells. *Circ Res* 1992;71:34–39.

27. Porter JG, Catalano R, McEnroe G, Lewicki JA, Protter AA. C-type natriuretic peptide inhibits growth factor-dependent DNA synthesis in smooth muscle cells. *Am J Physiol Cell Physiol* 1992;263:C1001–C1006.

28. Appel RG. Mechanism of atrial natriuretic factor-induced inhibition of rat mesangial cell mitogenesis. *Am J Physiol Endocrinol Metab* 1990;259:E312–E318.

29. Stingo AJ, Clavell AL, Heublein DM, Wei CM, Pittelkow MR, Burnett JC Jr. Presence of C-type natriuretic peptide in cultured human endothelial cells and plasma. *Am J Physiol Heart Circ Physiol* 1992;263:H1318–H1321.

30. Itoh H, Pratt RE, Dzau VJ. Atrial natriuretic polypeptide inhibits hypertrophy of vascular smooth muscle cells. *J Clin Invest* 1990;86:1690–1697.

31. Wilcox JN, Augustine A, Goeddel DV, Lowe DG. Differential regional expression of three natriuretic peptide receptor genes within primate tissues. *Mol Cell Biol* 1991;11:3454–3462.

32. Bianchi C, Gutkowska J, Thibault G, Garcia R, Genest J, Cantin M. Radioautographic localization of 125I-atrial natriuretic factor (ANF) in rat tissues. *Histochemistry* 1985;82:441–452.

33. Koseki C, Hayashi Y, Torikai S, Furuya M, Ohnuma N, Imai M. Localization of binding sites for alpha-rat atrial natriuretic polypeptide in rat kidney. *Am J Physiol Renal Fluid Electrolyte Physiol* 1986;250:F210–F216.

34. Suzuki M, Almeida FA, Nussenzveig DR, Sawyer D, Maack T. Binding and functional effects of atrial natriuretic factor in isolated rat kidney. *Am J Physiol Renal Fluid Electrolyte Physiol* 1987;253:F917–F922.

35. Mantyh CR, Kruger L, Brecha NC, Mantyh PW. Localization of specific binding sites for atrial natriuretic factor in peripheral tissues of the guinea pig, rat, and human. *Hypertension* 1986;8:712–721.

36. Maack T, Suzuki M, Almeida FA, Nussenzveig D, Scarborough RM, McEnroe GA, Lewicki JA. Physiological role of silent receptors of atrial natriuretic factor. *Science* 1987;238:675–678.

37. Martin ER, Lewicki J, Scarborough RM, Ballerman BJ. Expres-sion and regulation of ANP receptors subtypes in rat renal glomeruli and papillae. *Am J Physiol Renal Fluid Electrolyte Physiol* 1989;257:F649–F657.

38. Bianchi C, Gutkowska J, Thibault G, Garcia R, Genest J, Cantin M. Distinct localization of atrial natriuretic factor and angiotensin II binding sites in the glomerulus. *Am J Physiol Renal Fluid Electrolyte Physiol* 1986;251:F594–F596.

39. Chansel D, Pham P, Nivez MP, Ardaillou R. Characterization of atrial natriuretic factor receptors in human glomerular epithelial and mesangial cells. *Am J Physiol Renal Fluid Electrolyte Physiol* 1990;259:F619–F627.

40. Norling LL, Vaughan CA, Chevalier RL. Maturation of cGMP response to ANP by isolated glomeruli. *Am J Physiol Renal Fluid Electrolyte Physiol* 1992;262:F138–F143.

41. Ballermann BJ, Hoover RL, Karnovsky MJ, Brenner BM. Physiologic regulation of atrial natriuretic peptide receptors in rat renal glomeruli. *J Clin Invest* 1985;76:2049–2056.

42. Koh GY, Nussenzweig DR, Okolicany J, Price DA, Maack T. Dynamics of atrial natriuretic factor-guanylate cyclase receptors and receptor-ligand complexes in cultured glomerular mesangial and renomedullary interstitial cells. *J Biol Chem* 1992;267:11987–11994.

43. Bianchi C, Gutkowska J, Garcia R, Thibault G, Genest J, Cantin M. Localization of 125I-atrial natriuretic factor (ANF)-binding sites in rat renal medulla. A light and electron microscope autoradiographic study. *J Histochem Cytochem* 1987;35:149–153.

44. Terada Y, Moriyama T, Martin BM, Knepper MA, Garcia-Perez A. RT-PCR microlocalization of mRNA for guanylyl cyclase-coupled ANF receptor in rat kidney. *Am J Physiol Renal Fluid Electrolyte Physiol* 1991;261:F1080–F1087.

45. Fontoura BMA, Nussenzveig DR, Pelton KM, Maack T. Atrial natriuretic factor receptors in cultured renomedullary interstitial cells. *Am J Physiol Cell Physiol* 1990;258:C692–C699.

46. Jamison RL, Canaan-Kühl S, Pratt R. The natriuretic peptides and their receptors. *Am J Kidney Dis* 1992;20:519–530.

47. Meloche S, Ong H, Cantin M, De Lean A. Affinity cross-linking of atrial natriuretic factor to its receptor in bovine adrenal zona glomerulosa. *J Biol Chem* 1986;261:1525–1528.

48. Heisler S, Morrier E. Bovine adrenal medullary cells contain functional atrial natriuretic peptide receptors. *Biochem Biophys Res Commun* 1988;150:781–787.

49. Koller KJ, Lowe DG, Bennett GL, Minamino N, Kangawa K, Matsuo H, Goeddel DV. Selective activation of the B natriuretic peptide receptor by C-type natriuretic peptide (CNP). *Science* 1991;252:120–123.

50. Leitman DC, Andresen JW, Catalano RM, Waldman SA, Tuan JJ, Murad F. Atrial natriuretic peptide binding, cross-linking, and stimulation of cyclic GMP accumulation and particulate guanylate cyclase activity in cultured cells. *J Biol Chem* 1988;263:3720–3728.

51. Scarborough RM, Schenk DB, McEnroe GA, Arfsten A, Kang LL, Schwartz K, Lewicki JA. Truncated atrial natriuretic peptide analogs. Comparison between receptor binding and stimulation of cyclic GMP accumulation in cultured vascular smooth muscle cells. *J Biol Chem* 1986;261:12960–12964.

52. Scarborough RM, McEnroe GA, Arfsten A, Kang LL, Schwartz K, Lewicki JA. D-amino acid-substituted atrial natriuretic peptide analogs reveal novel receptor recognition requirements. *J Biol Chem* 1988;263:16818–16822.

53. Maack T, Suzuki M, Nussenzveig DR, Owada A, Scarborough RM, Lewicki JA, Almeida FA. Clearance receptors of atrial natriuretic factor. In: Needleman P, ed. *Biological and molecular aspects of atrial factors.* New York: Alan R. Liss, 1988;57–76.

54. Okolicany J, McEnroe GA, Gregory LC, Lewicki JA, Maack T. Effects of small C-ANF receptor ligands on plasma levels of atrial natriuretic factor, blood pressure and renal function in the rat. *Can J Physiol Pharmacol* 1991;69:1561–1566.

55. Okolicany J, McEnroe GA, Koh GY, Lewicki JA, Maack T. Clearance receptor and neutral endopeptidase-mediated metabolism of atrial natriuretic factor. *Am J Physiol Renal Fluid Electrolyte Physiol* 1992;263:F546–F553.

56. Nonoguchi H, Sands JM, Knepper MA. ANF inhibits NaCl and fluid absorption in cortical collecting duct of rat kidney. *Am J Physiol Renal Fluid Electrolyte Physiol* 1989;256:F179–F188.

57. Zeidel ML, Silva P, Brenner BM, Seifter JL. cGMP mediates effects of atrial peptides on medullary collecting duct cells. *Am J Physiol Renal Fluid Electrolyte Physiol* 1987;252:F551–F559.
58. Rocha AS, Kudo LH. Atrial peptide and cGMP effects on NaCl transport in inner medullary collecting duct. *Am J Physiol Renal Fluid Electrolyte Physiol* 1990;259:F258–F268.
59. Cantiello HF, Ausiello DA. Atrial natriuretic factor and cGMP inhibit amiloride-sensitive Na+ transport in the cultured renal epithelial cell line, LLC-PK1. *Biochem Biophys Res Commun* 1986;134:852–860.
60. Winquist RJ. Possible mechanisms underlying the vasorelaxant response to atrial natriuretic factor. *Fed Proc* 1986;45:2371–2375.
61. Budzik GP, Firestone SL, Bush EN, Connolly PJ, Rockway TW, Sarin VK, Holleman WH. Divergence of ANF analogs in smooth muscle cell cGMP response and aorta vasorelaxation: evidence for receptor subtypes. *Biochem Biophys Res Commun* 1987;144:422–431.
62. Oda S, Sano T, Morishita Y, Matsuda Y. Pharmacological profile of HS-142-1, a novel nonpeptide atrial natriuretic peptide (ANP) antagonist of microbial origin. II. Restoration by HS-142-1 of ANP-induced inhibition of aldosterone production in adrenal glomerulosa cells. *J Pharmacol Exp Ther* 1992;263:241–245.
63. Okolicany J, Price DA, Matsuda Y, Maack T. HS-142-1 is a powerful antagonist of the renal effects of ANF (Abstr). *J Am Soc Nephrol* 1992;3:443.
64. Levin ER. Natriuretic peptide C-receptor: more than a clearance receptor. *Am J Physiol Endocrinol Metab* 1993;264:E483–E489.
65. Anand-Srivastava MB, Sairam MR, Cantin M. Ring-deleted analogs of atrial natriuretic factor inhibit adenylate cyclase/cAMP system. Possible coupling of clearance atrial natriuretic factor receptors to adenylate cyclase/cAMP signal transduction system. *J Biol Chem* 1990;265:8566–8572.
66. Hirata M, Chang CH, Murad F. Stimulatory effects of atrial natriuretic factor on phosphoinositide hydrolysis in cultured bovine aortic smooth muscle cells. *Biochim Biophys Acta* 1989;1010:346–351.
67. Berl T, Mansour J, Teiltebaum I. ANP stimulates phospholipase C in cultured RMICT cells: roles of protein kinases and G protein. *Am J Physiol Renal Fluid Electrolyte Physiol* 1991;260:F590–F595.
68. Anand Srivastava MB, Vinay P, Genest J, Cantin M. Effect of atrial natriuretic factor on adenylate cyclase in various nephron segments. *Am J Physiol Renal Fluid Electrolyte Physiol* 1986;251:F417–F422.
69. Nonoguchi H, Knepper MA, Manganiello VC. Effects of atrial natriuretic factor on cyclic guanosine monophosphate and cyclic adenosine monophosphate accumulation in microdissected nephron segments from rats. *J Clin Invest* 1987;79:500–507.
70. Chartier L, Schiffrin EL. Role of calcium in effects of atrial natriuretic peptide on aldosterone production in adrenal glomerulosa cells. *Am J Physiol Endocrinol Metab* 1987;252:F485–F489.
71. Hassid A. Atriopeptins decrease resting and hormone-elevated cytosolic Ca in cultured mesangial cells. *Am J Physiol Renal Fluid Electrolyte Physiol* 1987;253:F1077.
72. Meyer Lehnert H, Tsai P, Caramelo C, Schrier RW. ANF inhibits vasopressin-induced Ca^{2+} mobilization and contraction in glomerular mesangial cells. *Am J Physiol Renal Fluid Electrolyte Physiol* 1988;255:F771–F778.
73. Winquist RJ, Faison EP, Waldman SA, Schwartz K, Murad F, Rapoport RM. Atrial natriuretic factor elicits an endothelium-independent relaxation and activates particulate guanylate cyclase in vascular smooth muscle. *Proc Natl Acad Sci USA* 1984;81:7661–7664.
74. Popescu LM, Panoiu C, Hinescu M, Nutu O. The mechanism of cGMP-induced relaxation in vascular smooth muscle. *Eur J Pharmacol* 1985;107:393–394.
75. Rashatwar SS, Cornell TL, Lincoln TM. Effects of 8-bromo-cGMP on calcium levels in vascular smooth muscle cells: possible regulation of calcium ATPase by cGMP-dependent protein kinase. *Proc Natl Acad Sci USA* 1987;83:5685–5691.
76. Isales CM, Lewicki JA, Nee JJ, Barrett PQ. ANP-(7,23) stimulates a DHP-sensitive Ca^{2+} conductance and reduces cellular cAMP via a cGMP-independent mechanism. *Am J Physiol Cell Physiol* 1992;263:C334–C342.

77. ODonnell ME. Regulation of Na-K-Cl cotransport in endothelial cells by atrial natriuretic factor. *Am J Physiol Cell Physiol* 1989;257:C36–C44.
78. Owen NE, Bush EN, Holleman W, ODonnell ME. Effect of atrial natriuretic factor on Na+-K+-Cl−cotransport of vascular smooth muscle cells. *Hypertension* 1987;10(2):PI128–133.
79. Blaine EH, Seymour AA, Marsh EA, Napier MA. Effects of atrial natriuretic factor on renal function and cyclic GMP production. *Fed Proc* 1986;45:2122–2127.
80. Levy M. Comparative effects of diuretics and atrial peptide in chronic caval dogs. *Am J Physiol Renal Fluid Electrolyte Physiol* 1990;258:F768–F774.
81. Nushiro N, Abe K, Seino M, Yoshinaga K. Interaction between ANP and amiloride in renal tubular sodium handling in anesthetized rabbits. *Am J Physiol Renal Fluid Electrolyte Physiol* 1988;254:F521–F526.
82. Linz W, Albus U, Wiemer G, Breipohl G, Knolle J, Scholkens BA. Amiloride potentiates the vascular effects of atrial natriuretic factor. *J Hypertens Suppl* 1988;6:300–302.
83. Iwata T, Hardee E, Frohlich ED, Cole FE. Amiloride enhances atrial natriuretic factor stimulation of cGMP accumulation in rat glomeruli. *Peptides* 1989;10:575–579.
84. De Lean A. Amiloride potentiates atrial natriuretic factor inhibitory action by increasing receptor binding in bovine adrenal zona glomerulosa. *Life Sci* 1986;39:1109–1116.
85. Kukkonen P, Vuolteenaho O, Ruskoaho H. Basal and volume expansion-stimulated plasma atrial natriuretic peptide concentrations and hemodynamics in conscious rats: effects of SCH 39.370, an endopeptidase inhibitor, and C-ANF-(4-23), a clearance receptor ligand. *Endocrinology* 1992;130:755–765.
86. Wilkins MR, Needleman P. Effect of pharmacological manipulation of endogenous atriopeptin activity on renal function. *Am J Physiol Renal Fluid Electrolyte Physiol* 1992;262:F161–F167.
87. Castro R, Ervin MG, Leake RD, Ross MG, Fisher DA. Effect of a ring-deleted atrial natriuretic factor analogue on ovine fetal renal and cardiovascular function. *Pediatr Res* 1991;29:342–346.
88. Perrella MA, Aarhus LL, Heublein DM, Lewicki JA, Burnett JC Jr. Biologic role of atrial natriuretic factor clearance receptor in congestive heart failure. *Am J Physiol Heart Circ Physiol* 1993;265:H401–H408.
89. Almeida FA, Suzuki M, Scarborough RM, Lewicki JA, Maack T. Clearance function of type C receptors of atrial natriuretic factor in rats. *Am J Physiol Regul Integr Comp Physiol* 1989;256:R469–R477.
90. Stephenson SL, Kenny AJ. The hydrolysis of alpha-human atrial natriuretic peptide by pig kidney microvillar membranes is initiated by endopeptidase-24.11. *Biochem J* 1987;243:183–187.
91. Ronco P, Pollard H, Galceran M, Delauche M, Schwartz JC, Verroust P. Distribution of enkephalinase (membrane metalloendopeptidase, E.C. 3.4.24.11) in rat organs. Detection using a monoclonal antibody. *Lab Invest* 1988;58:210–217.
92. Bralet J, Mossiat C, Gros C, Schwartz JC. Thiorphan-induced natriuresis in volume-expanded rats: roles of endogenous atrial natriuretic factor and kinins. *J Pharmacol Exp Ther* 1991;258:807–811.
93. Koepke JP, Tyler LD, Trapani AJ, Bovy PR, Spear KL, Olins GM, Blaine EH. Interaction of non-guanylate cyclase-linked atriopeptin receptor ligand and endopeptidase inhibitor in conscious rats. *J Pharmacol Exp Ther* 1989;249:172–176.
94. Blake DW, McGrath BP, Donnan GB, Smart S, Way D, Myers KA, Fullerton M. Influence of cardiac failure on atrial natriuretic peptide responses in patients undergoing vascular surgery. *Eur J Anaesthesiol* 1991;8:365–371.
95. Northridge DB, Jardine AG, Alabaster CT, Barclay PL, Connell JM, Dargie HJ, Dilly SG, Findlay IN, Lever AF, Samuels GM. Effects of UK 69 578: a novel atriopeptidase inhibitor. *Lancet* 1989;2:591–593.
96. Smits GJ, McGraw DE, Trapani AJ. Interaction of ANP and bradykinin during endopeptidase 24.11 inhibition: renal effects. *Am J Physiol Renal Fluid Electrolyte Physiol* 1990;258:F1417–F1424.
97. Richards AM, Crozier IG, Kosoglou T, Rallings M, Espiner EA, Nicholls MG, Yandle TG, Ikram H, Frampton C. Endopeptidase 24.11 inhibition by SCH 42495 in essential hypertension. *Hypertension* 1993;22:119–126.

98. Chiu PJS, Tetzloff G, Romano MT, Foster CJ, Sybertz EJ. Influence of C-ANF receptor and neutral endopeptidase on pharmacokinetics of ANF in rats. *Am J Physiol Regul Integr Comp Physiol* 1991;260:R208–R216.

99. Singer DR, Markandu ND, Buckley MG, Miller MA, Sagnella GA, MacGregor GA. Dietary sodium and inhibition of neutral endopeptidase 24.11 in essential hypertension. *Hypertension* 1991;18:798–804.

100. Helin K, Tikkanen I, Tikkanen T, Saijonmaa O, Sybertz EJ, Vemulapalli S, Sariola H, Fyhrquist F. Prolonged neutral endopeptidase inhibition in heart failure. *Eur J Pharmacol* 1991;198:23–30.

101. Bevan EG, Connell JMC, Doyle J, Carmichael HA, Davies DL, Lorimer AR, McInnes GT. Candoxatril, a neutral endopeptidase inhibitor: efficacy and tolerability in essential hypertension. *J Hypertens* 1992;10:607–613.

102. Northridge DB, Jardine A, Henderson E, Dilly SG, Dargie HJ. Increased circulating atrial natriuretic factor concentrations in patients with chronic heart failure after inhibition of neutral endopeptidase: effects on diastolic function. *Br Heart J* 1992;68:387–391.

103. MacFarland RT, Zelus BD, Beavo JA. High concentrations of a cGMP-stimulated phosphodiesterase mediate ANP-induced decreases in cAMP and steroidogenesis in adrenal glomerulosa cells. *J Biol Chem* 1991;266:136–142.

104. Sandberg K, Bor M, Ji H, Carvallo PM, Catt KJ. Atrial natriuretic factor activates cyclic adenosine 3',5'-monophosphate phospho-diesterase in *Xenopus laevis* oocytes and potentiates progesterone-induced maturation via cyclic guanosine 5'-monophosphate accumulation. *Biol Reprod* 1993;49:1074–1082.

105. Nussenzveig DR, Lewicki JA, Maack T. Cellular mechanisms of the clearance function of type C receptors of atrial natriuretic factor. *J Biol Chem* 1990;265:20952–20958.

106. Kato J, Lanier-Smith KL, Currie MG. Cyclic GMP down-regulates atrial natriuretic peptide receptors on cultured vascular endothelial cells. *J Biol Chem* 1991;266:14681–14685.

107. Chabrier PE, Roubert P, Lonchampt MO, Plas P, Braquet P. Regulation of atrial natriuretic factor receptors by angiotensin II in rat vascular smooth muscle cells. *J Biol Chem* 1988;263:13199–13202.

108. Delporte C, Poloczek P, Tastenoy M, Winand J, Christophe J. Atrial natriuretic peptide binds to ANP-R$_1$ receptors in neuro-blastoma cells or is degraded extracellularly at the Ser-Phe bond. *Eur J Pharmacol Mol Pharmacol* 1992;227:247–256.

109. Meloche S, McNicoll N, Liu B, Ong H, De Lean A. Atrial natriuretic factor R1 receptor from bovine adrenal zona glomerulosa: purification, characterization, and modulation by amiloride. *Biochemistry* 1988;27:8151–8158.

110. Larose L, McNicoll N, Ong H, De L. Allosteric modulation by ATP of the bovine adrenal natriuretic factor R1 receptor functions. *Biochemistry* 1991;30:8990–8995.

111. Potter RL, Garbers DL. Dephosphorylation of the guanylyl cyclase-A receptor causes desensitization. *J Biol Chem* 1992;267:14531–14534.

Hypertension: Pathophysiology, Diagnosis,
and Management, Second Edition,
edited by J.H. Laragh and B.M. Brenner,
Raven Press, Ltd., New York © 1995.

CHAPTER **60**

Urodilatin

Mark Gunning and Barry M. Brenner

As a prominent regulatory arm of volume homeostasis in man, the natriuretic peptides are intimately involved in the field of hypertension. Since the description in 1980 by De Bold et al. (40) of natriuretic activity of an atrial extract when given to bioassay rats, we have learned much about the physiologic regulation of salt and water balance by these peptides. Initially the peptides were identified in the atria and hence the name atrial natriuretic peptide (ANP). However, it soon became apparent that other organ systems were capable of synthesizing ANP and that this synthesis could be induced in various pathophysiological states of intravascular volume excess. Furthermore, new members of the natriuretic peptide family (brain natriuretic peptide [BNP] and C-type natriuretic peptide [CNP]) were identified and their roles complementing the better described role of ANP are currently being defined. A full description of the natriuretic peptide system, including ANP, BNP and CNP is to be found in the chapters 48, 59, and 61.

LOCALIZATION

Observations in the mid-1980s demonstrated that ANP or an ANP-like substance was found in the kidney;

this was originally presumed to reflect peptide taken up by the kidney from the circulation. However, in 1988 the identification of a natriuretic peptide in human urine that was identical to ANP except for the addition of a 4 amino acid amino terminal tail led to the hypothesis that a natriuretic peptide was in fact synthesized by the kidney. This peptide was termed urodilatin, is identical to $ANP_{(95-126)}$, and is the topic of this chapter.

Sakamoto et al. (1) demonstrated in the kidney the presence of ANP-like immunoreactivity, which was predominantly found in the cortex. This ANP-like immunoreactivity eluted chromatographically at a position coincident with low molecular weight ($\sim$3 kDa) ANP, and not the higher molecular weight (13 kDa) pro-ANP. The ANP-like immunoreactivity was decreased by prior water deprivation of the animals and could be washed out of the kidney by saline perfusion, both of which features suggested that the peptide may have had its origins in the heart. In 1986 Marumo et al. (2) were able to show the existence of two forms of ANP circulating in human plasma (high and low molecular weight) but the presence of only one such peak of activity in the urine. The single peak in the urine was of a molecular weight similar to the low molecular weight peak seen in plasma, and coeluted from Sephadex 75 columns with synthetic ANP. The observations of McKenzie et al. (3), who localized ANP-like immunoreactivity to the distal tubules and collecting tubules of the kidney, provided the strongest evidence that the kidney generated an ANP-like substance (Fig. 1). Using a specific antibody to $rANP_{(102-126)}$ they examined tissues from the kidney, the atria, the adrenal medulla, and the pituitary. The antibody used was 100 percent cross-reactive with $rANP_{(102-126)}$ and with

M. Gunning: Department of Medicine, Harvard Medical School; Renal Division, Department of Medicine, New England Deaconess Hospital and Joslin Diabetes Center, Boston, Massachusetts 02215.

B. M. Brenner: Renal Division, Department of Medicine, Brigham and Women's Hospital, and The Harvard Center for the Study of Kidney Disease, Harvard Medical School, Boston, Massachusetts 02115.

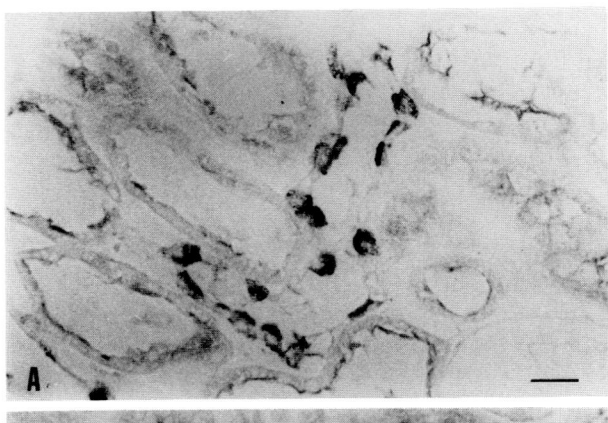

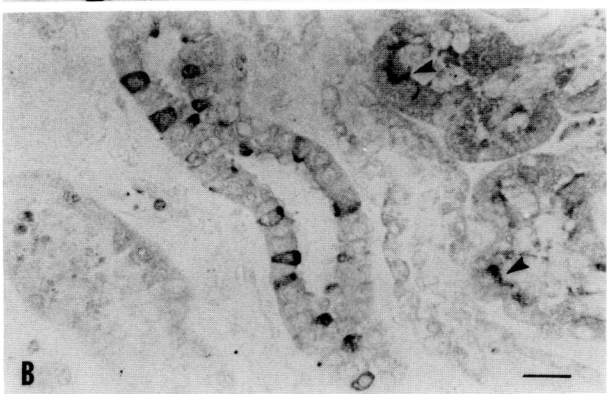

FIG. 1. ANP-like immunoreactivity staining in mammalian renal tissues demonstrating the localization of the ANP antibody to the intercalated cells of the collecting ducts and in particular to the apical region of these cells. **A:** Porcine kidney. Intense ANP-like immunoreactivity is observed in intercalated cells of a cortical collecting tubule. **B:** Human kidney. ANP-like immunoreactivity staining is seen in intercalated cells of a juxtamedullary collecting duct and in the brush border of proximal convoluted tubules (arrowheads). (From ref. 38, with permission.)

rANP$_{(96-126)}$, but less reactive (28 percent with ANP$_{(103-123)}$). They reported the presence of ANP in each of these tissues and in particular noted intense and homogeneous staining in the collecting ducts. Within the collecting ducts of the rat kidney the intercalated cells were stained to the exclusion of the principal cells. In contrast, considerably less intense and more diffuse staining was seen in the region of the proximal tubules, suggesting that this reflected uptake of the peptide from the glomerular filtrate rather than specific localization of the peptide to the proximal tubular cells.

Others have examined the kidney systematically for evidence of ANP synthesis. The production and secretion of the complete 126 amino acid pro-ANP from both adult and neonatal rat kidney cells in culture have been demonstrated (4). In these studies the cortical connecting tubule cells were thought to be the most likely sites of synthesis of this pro-ANP (5). Greenwald et al. (6) localized the production of the ANP prohormone (defined by

both C and N terminal immunoreactivity, and a molecular weight of ~12 kDa) to the distal cortical tubule and failed to demonstrate the peptide in glomeruli, proximal tubules, or inner medullary collecting ducts. The identity of this peptide as true ANP prohormone and not BNP or CNP precursor was established by the finding of messenger RNA (mRNA) specific for ANP in both rat kidney and in kidney cell cultures (7). Furthermore, a smaller peptide, immunoreactive with antibody directed against ANP$_{(103-126)}$, was found that was said to have a molecular weight of ~3 kDa. The full identity of this peptide was not established by sequencing but it is reasonable to believe that it may represent urodilatin, derived from a different processing of the ANP prohormone in the distal cortical tubule. Ritter et al. (5) have shown that the peptide, secreted by the cortical connecting tubule cells in culture, is also a potent stimulator of guanosine 3',5'-cyclic monophosphate (cGMP) accumulation in cultured inner medullary collecting duct (IMCD) cells. Finally, Dean and Greenwald (8) have recently presented their preliminary findings that CNP is also synthesized in the kidney, and that CNP-like immunoreactivity is found in the same regions of the kidney as the CNP-specific mRNA. These regions include but are not limited to those regions in which ANP-like immunoreactivity is also found.

STRUCTURE OF URODILATIN

Schulz-Knappe et al., who had earlier identified ANP$_{(99-126)}$ as the chief circulating form of ANP (which they termed cardiodilatin) (9), identified urodilatin for the first time in human urine (10). In their studies they analyzed the dominant form of biologically active (as defined by an *in vitro* vascular smooth muscle relaxation assay) natriuretic peptide found in the urine. Examining the product of lyophilizing 1000 L of human urine they identified a peptide that by both bioassay and specific radioimmunoassay (RIA) resembled ANP. On further purification and on amino acid sequence analysis of this peptide they demonstrated that the peptide was in fact identical to ANP except for the presence of a four amino acid (Thr-Ala-Pro-Arg) extension at the amino terminal end (Fig. 2). Since this four amino acid extension was not likely to be the result of renal processing of circulating ANP$_{(99-126)}$, they concluded that the peptide was of renal origin and named it urodilatin. Thus, as shown in Fig. 2, urodilatin is an amino terminally extended form of ANP$_{(99-126)}$ and therefore its basic 17-member ring structure and the carboxyterminal tail are identical to those of ANP. The cleavage of the 126 amino acid pro-ANP molecule at a (Leu-Thr) site four amino acids upstream from the usual Arg-Ser cleavage site results in the generation of this peptide. It is suggested that the kidney therefore produces pro-ANP and processes it differ-

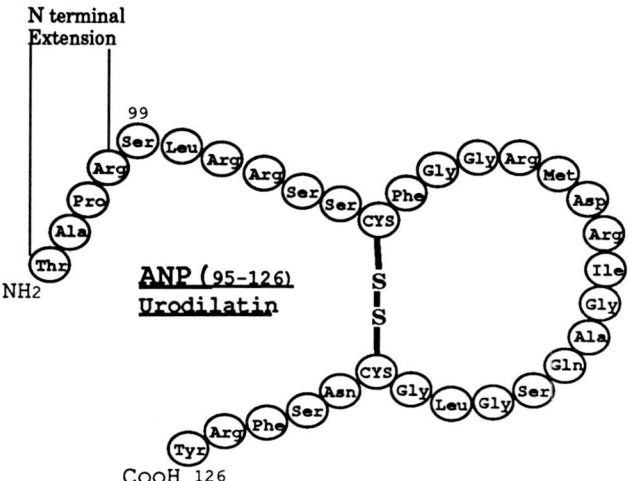

FIG. 2. Schematic representation of the structure of urodilatin. The structure is identical to hANP$_{(99-126)}$ except for the addition of the four amino acids (95–98) at the aminoterminus. (Modified from ref. 39.)

ently from the manner in which it is processed by the atria. Urodilatin may therefore also be referred to as ANP$_{(95-126)}$.

Others have been able to confirm the presence of more than one peak of ANP-like immunoreactivity, only one of which coeluted with ANP$_{(99-126)}$, another eluting in the same position on high-performance liquid chromatography (HPLC) as urodilatin (11,12). A specific antibody recognizing urodilatin to the exclusion of ANP$_{(99-126)}$ is now available and studies using it suggest that urodilatin is indeed found in the urine (13).

Many investigators examining ANP-like immunoreactivity in the urine have established the presence of at least two peaks of activity. Marumo et al. (2) found evidence of the presence of the high molecular weight form of the hormone, pro-ANP. Others have identified ANP$_{(99-126)}$ as well as what have been thought to be degradative fragments. Some investigators have failed to identify ANP$_{(99-126)}$ in the urine. Thus, it remains unclear whether or not significant amounts of the circulating ANP$_{(99-126)}$ are filtered at the glomerulus and found in the urine. However, it appears unlikely that any biologically active filtered ANP$_{(99-126)}$ would be found in the urine as the activity of the endopeptidase (E.C.3.4.24.11), among other degradative enzymes, is very high in the brush border of the renal tubules. This enzyme cleaves the ring structure of ANP$_{(99-126)}$, thereby ensuring loss of bioactivity.

REGULATION OF URODILATIN SECRETION

The foregoing suggests that the synthesis of urodilatin occurs in the kidney. The fact that urodilatin is identical

to the final 32 amino acids of pro-ANP suggests that the synthesis of urodilatin is carried out in a manner similar to that of ANP except that the cleavage site is moved to a site four amino acids upstream. Thus, urodilatin is a posttranslationally modified product of the same gene that encodes pro-ANP. Little is as yet known about the regulation of this secretion of urodilatin. However, the demonstration that urodilatin secretion by the kidney is regulated lends further credence to the idea that urodilatin is an independent and important regulator of renal function, and in particular of sodium and volume homeostasis.

In Vivo

Urodilatin is excreted with a circadian rhythm that parallels the daily rhythm of urinary sodium excretion (14). This basal regulation of urodilatin excretion was identified in studies of normal men using antibodies specific for urodilatin (Fig. 3). Furthermore, when challenged with an acute isotonic saline load, an increase in urodilatin excretion accompanied the resultant natriuresis. The authors found a significant correlation between urodilatin and sodium excretion in these subjects. In these studies no significant alterations in plasma ANP were apparently recorded. Thus the authors inferred that the major modulator of post–saline infusion natriuresis was the secretion of urodilatin.

In separate studies using dogs, results have suggested that urinary urodilatin excretion correlates better with urinary sodium excretion than does plasma ANP concentration under basal conditions and after volume expansion by saline infusion. Generally this correlation held true when the volume-expanding effects of saline infusion were mimicked by left atrial distension by a balloon, inferring, therefore, that urodilatin is the more likely regulator of the natriuresis of saline expansion (13). Finally, in these studies the effect of cardiac denervation was examined in an effort to determine whether a cardiac signal for urodilatin secretion was necessary for the response to volume expansion. In cardiac denervated dogs the correlations between urodilatin and sodium excretion were, if anything, enhanced, suggesting that a stimulus of noncardiac origin may be responsible for the regulation of urodilatin secretion. The data presented in this paper, while statistically significant, should be taken with some caution as they represent simply observations of correlations. Therefore, while consistent with the hypothesis that urodilatin may be important in regulating sodium excretion, they do not necessarily demonstrate this.

The role of cerebral control of sodium excretion and urodilatin secretion has been addressed in a paper by Emmeluth et al. (15), who recently attempted to separate the effects of cerebral sodium concentration and periph-

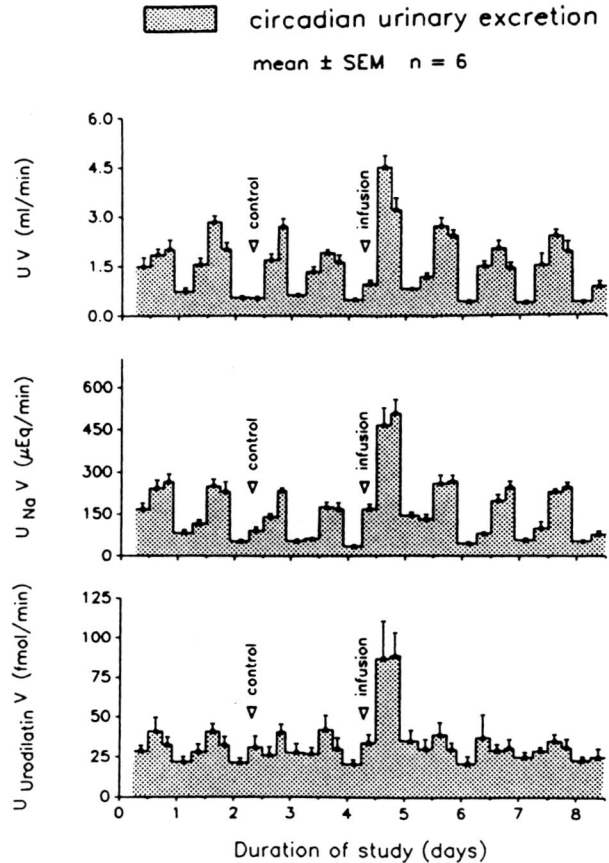

circadian urinary excretion

mean ± SEM   n = 6

FIG. 3. Circadian rhythm of urodilatin excretion and modulation of its excretion rate by volume expansion in human volunteers. Six healthy human volunteers were studied for nine days. Midnight each day is denoted by the X-axis labels. Urine volume (**top panel**), urine sodium excretion (**middle panel**), and urodilatin excretion (**lowest panel**) are shown. Infusion of 2 L isotonic saline over 25 min was given on day 5. (From ref. 14, with permission.)

eral volume expansion. They showed that by increasing the circulating plasma sodium concentration in the brain (hypertonic saline infusion in the carotids) but not systemically, the urodilatin concentration in the urine increased fourfold (and urinary sodium excretion 34-fold) compared with no change in urodilatin concentration and only a modest natriuresis (urinary sodium excretion increased 12-fold) when isotonic saline was infused. Therefore, the brain appeared capable of responding to the local stimulus of hypertonicity/hypervolemia by increasing the secretion of urodilation secretion by the kidney. The intervening signal transduction steps remain to be elucidated and could clearly be of either neural or humoral origin.

In Vitro

The localization of the presence of ANP-like peptide to the cortical collecting duct region of the kidney has

stimulated work with cultured cells from this region of the kidney in an effort to understand the intracellular regulation of synthesis and secretion of this peptide from these cells. Forskolin, a potent stimulator of adenylate cyclase activity, adenosine 3′,5′-cyclic monophosphate (cAMP), and phosphodiesterase inhibition by iso-butyl-methyl-xanthine all inhibit the secretion of the peptide, presumably by increasing intracellular cAMP levels. Phorbol esters (which stimulate secretion of ANP from atrial myocytes) and cGMP have no effect on peptide secretion from these cells (5). Greenwald et al. (6) have examined kidneys from nephrotic rats and found them to be deficient in their processing of $ANP_{(1-126)}$ resulting in the secretion from these cells in culture of the intact pro-ANP rather than the shorter ∼3 kDa peptide.

RENAL ACTION OF URODILATIN

The suggested synthesis and secretion of urodilatin in the kidney, its detection in urine, and the failure to detect its presence in the plasma prompt the hypothesis that this system is entirely confined to the kidney and operates in a paracrine or autocrine manner. Localization of its synthesis to the distal nephron, in particular the cortical collecting ducts, indicates that its effects should be manifest either in that segment of the nephron or further downstream from it, i.e., in the medullary collecting ducts. While the outer medullary collecting ducts are insensitive to natriuretic peptides and are not involved in sodium homeostasis, the IMCD has been clearly shown to be sensitive and responsive to natriuretic peptides. ANP infusion or volume expansion causes an inhibition of sodium reabsorption in the IMCD (16,17). The presence of highly specific guanylate cyclase–linked receptors for ANP in IMCD has also been established (18,19). Gunning et al. (20) have further shown that urodilatin is equipotent with $ANP_{(99-126)}$ in terms of its ability to inhibit Na^+ transport–dependent oxygen consumption in cells of the IMCD and that it is a potent stimulator in these cells of cGMP accumulation. Others have confirmed the stimulation of cGMP accumulation in the IMCD and have further shown that whereas the IMCD is equally sensitive to ANP and urodilatin, the glomerulus is less sensitive to urodilatin than to ANP (21). Valentin et al. (28) have shown that urodilatin and ANP exhibit virtually equal affinity for the natriuretic peptide receptors in the IMCD, and that they are equally effective in stimulating cGMP accumulation.

The glomerulus expresses an abundance of natriuretic peptide (NP) receptors on each of its three cell types but is anatomically upstream from the proposed site of synthesis of urodilatin. Other segments of the nephron (the proximal tubule, the loop of Henle) have been shown to express low levels of guanylate cyclase–linked natriuretic peptide receptors. The functional significance of these receptors remains to be shown. It seems most likely that the glomerular receptors' prime function is to respond to circulating natriuretic peptides and they are most likely involved in regulating the vascular effects of natriuretic peptides on the kidney. By contrast the IMCD is the most likely prime renal target for urodilatin produced and secreted by the kidney.

ANP inhibits sodium transport through the IMCD cell by closing the amiloride-sensitive epithelial sodium channel, which is expressed on the luminal surface (22). Amiloride inhibits sodium transport through this channel by a direct effect on the channel protein. Sonnenberg et al. (23) infused ANP or amiloride into the microcatheterized IMCD (i.e., luminal application only) in order to determine whether an effect of these agents could be found when applied luminally. Observing the effect on sodium reabsorption along the IMCD they noted that 10 nM ANP or 200 μM amiloride each inhibited IMCD sodium reabsorption by 50 percent (23). These data suggested that the NP receptors may be located on the luminal surface of the cell. It is of note in this respect that Gunning et al. (18) were unable to determine the polarity of the receptor localization in their studies characterizing the ANP receptors in the IMCD as they used cell suspensions in which the polarity of the cell population was not maintained (18). In patch clamp studies that addressed the question of whether ANP would inhibit the cation channel in cultured IMCD cells, the ANP was applied to the accessible luminal or apical surface of the cells (24). Notwithstanding this apical application of the peptide the cells were immediately sensitive to ANP, as shown by their response of cation channel closure, the cellular mechanism responsible for the inhibition of sodium reabsorption in this segment.

For urodilatin to act in the IMCD, the sodium reabsorbing epithelia of that segment must come in contact with the peptide via an interaction with cell surface receptors. If the peptide is carried in the conventional manner in the plasma (as ANP and BNP are), then the receptors should be on the basolateral surface of the cell. However, if the peptide is secreted into the tubule lumen then one might expect the receptor to be located on the luminal surface of the responsive downstream cells. Since the latter mode of delivery appears likely for urodilatin, this predicts that natriuretic peptide receptors may be expressed on the luminal surface of IMCD cells. The data of Sonnenberg et al. (23) and Light et al. (24) discussed above appear to confirm the likelihood that receptors are present on the luminal surface of the IMCD cells. Since circulating endogenous and infused natriuretic peptides also have an effect on the IMCD sodium reabsorptive capacity, receptors must also be expressed on the basolateral surface of the cell. The proposed luminal membrane localization in the nephron of a receptor for a bioactive peptide has precedent among other peptide hormones. Receptors for vasopressin and dopamine have been identified on the luminal cell surface (25). Whether the natriuretic peptide receptor mechanism is a single molecular entity in the apical membrane or part of a regulatory subunit of the sodium channel or some other transport protein remains to be elucidated.

While urodilatin may have as its prime target the IMCD, it should be noted that the IMCD is responsive to circulating natriuretic peptides also. Through the observation of many different functional parameters it has been established that the IMCD is responsive in equal measure both in vivo and in vitro to ANP, BNP, and urodilatin (26). This is presumably because the single class of receptor in the IMCD has similar affinity for, and is equally responsive to, all three of these natriuretic peptides (20,21,27,28). It remains to be established, however, which of the natriuretic peptides actually come into intimate contact with the IMCD. That the IMCD is sensitive to ANP and BNP is supported by the following observations: (a) systemically infused ANP (or BNP), in spite of being filtered and degraded as it traverses the proximal tubule, has a marked effect in generating a natriuresis in vivo, suggesting that it is active on the IMCD via a basolateral receptor mechanism; and (b) phosphoramidon, which inhibits the breakdown of ANP and BNP by endopeptidase E.C. 3.4.24.11., but has no effect on the survival of the "protected" urodilatin, does result in the generation of a natriuresis correlated with only a subtle increase in plasma ANP level, when given by infusion into animals (29). This latter observation suggests that rises in plasma ANP well within the range that occurs in normal physiology do have an effect on the IMCD that is separate and distinct from that which can be attributed to urodilatin. These data coupled with the observations that CNP is only a poor natriuretic agent, and that CNP does not stimulate particulate guanylate cyclase, suggest that the guanylate cyclase–linked receptor in the IMCD is the GC-A type of receptor originally cloned and sequenced by Chinkers et al. (30).

Thus, the IMCD appears to be responsive to urodilatin via a guanylate cyclase–linked receptor that recognizes ANP, BNP, and urodilatin (but not CNP). The location of this receptor remains unknown; there is good reason to speculate that it may be expressed on both membranes of the IMCD, since this cell type is responsive both to circulating peptide and urinary peptide. This may be a dynamic process with the expression of the receptor on either membrane varying in response to local or other conditions. The expression of the receptor on the luminal surface may suggest an intimate relationship between this protein and either the sodium channel or some other regulatory or transport protein.

EFFECTS OF URODILATIN

The effects of urodilatin on renal and nonrenal physiology have been inferred from studies in which the peptide has been infused into experimental animal or human subjects. Since this form of natriuretic peptide has not been identified in plasma, and is thought to be localized to the kidney, the relevance of these studies to normal physiology is not clear. Nevertheless, since urodilatin may be produced locally in organs other than the kidney (though no evidence of this has yet been shown), and since its effects on some aspects of physiology have been shown to be different from those of ANP, they are reviewed here.

In general the effects of urodilatin are qualitatively similar to those of ANP, causing vasodilation and natriuresis. In humans Saxenhofer et al. (31) demonstrated a greater sensitivity of the vascular and renal responses to urodilatin than to ANP. The diminished renal response to ANP, however, may in part be explained by the reduction in blood pressure that occurred in the ANP group and not in the urodilatin group. Hildebrandt et al. (32) confirmed this impression of increased renal sensitivity to urodilatin. They showed in dogs that the natriuresis and diuresis resulting from intrarenal arterial infusion of urodilatin was greater than that resulting from equimolar ANP infusion, even when renal perfusion pressure was maintained constant. In healthy volunteers urodilatin infusion caused a markedly more pronounced and prolonged reduction in pulmonary vascular pressures than ANP. This effect, coupled with an enhancement in cardiac index, may be beneficial in the treatment of heart failure (33). ANP is only poorly effective in heart failure and thus this observation may prove therapeutically useful. Riegger et al. (34) also demonstrated in dogs that while urodilatin levels in urine were not elevated in experimental heart failure, the response of natriuresis, diuresis, and reduction in pulmonary vascular pressures were marked after urodilatin infusion. Abassi et al. (35) have similarly shown a greater response to urodilatin than to ANP in rats with congestive heart failure secondary to aorta-caval fistula formation, a model of high output heart failure. Finally, in a model of renal failure that has been used previously to study the effects of ANP in rescuing the postischemic kidney, urodilatin combined with dopamine treatment was shown to be superior to other modalities of treatment used (36). It should be noted that dopamine was needed to maintain mean arterial pressure, which fell during urodilatin infusion.

The foregoing early experimental results point to the possibility that urodilatin may be a safer and more effective treatment for restoring renal function in congestive heart failure (in which the kidney has consistently been found to be hyporesponsive to ANP) and in acute renal failure. Of note one group has already reported on the therapeutic/prophylactic use of urodilatin infusion in heart transplant recipients in an effort to minimize postoperative renal dysfunction. Patients receiving urodilatin in this trial needed less hemodialysis and less furosemide to maintain fluid balance, and had lower serum creatinines and blood urea nitrogen concentrations, as well as having lower central venous pressures, than did control subjects (37).

SUMMARY

The natriuretic peptide system, which at one time represented an appealingly simple model of volume homeostasis, has over the last decade proved itself to be a most elaborate and complex system. The identification to date of three different gene products (ANP, BNP, and CNP) related to this family, and the further definition of different processing of at least one of these products (urodilatin), underlines this new complexity. The emerging data with respect to urodilatin show much promise toward defining a paracrine or autocrine mode of operation of the natriuretic peptide system in an organ that is intimately involved in the regulation of salt and water loss. Much work needs yet to be done in defining the regulation and action of this system more closely and in particular in defining its relationship with both the renin-angiotensin-aldosterone system and the other natriuretic peptide systems. The identification of the inner medullary collecting duct as the probable major site of action of this peptide has suggested that these cells may be unique in that they are likely to express natriuretic peptide receptors on both luminal and basolateral membranes. Finally, the regulation of the secretion of urodilatin provides some intriguing views of the potential for cerebral (and not cardiovascular) control of this natriuretic system.

REFERENCES

1. Sakamoto M, Nakao K, Kihara M, Morii N, Sugawara A, Suda M, Shimokura M, Kiso Y, Yamori Y, Imura H. Existence of atrial natriuretic polypeptide in kidney. *Biochem Biophys Res Commun* 1985;128:1281–1287.
2. Marumo F, Sakamoto H, Ando K, Ishigami T, Kawakami M. A highly sensitive radioimmunoassay of atrial natriuretic peptide (ANP) in human plasma and urine. *Biochem Biophys Res Commun* 1986;137(1):231–236.
3. McKenzie JC, Tanaka I, Misono KS, Inagami T. Immunocytochemical localization of atrial natriuretic factor in the kidney, adrenal medulla, pituitary, and atrium of rat. *J Histochem Cytochem* 1985;33(8):828–833.
4. Ritter D, Needleman P, Greenwald J. Synthesis and secretion of an atriopeptinlike protein in rat kidney cell culture. *J Clin Invest* 1991;87(1):208–212.
5. Ritter D, Chao J, Needleman P, Tetens E, Greenwald JE. Localization, synthetic regulation, and biology of renal atriopeptinlike prohormone. *Am J Physiol* 1992;263 (*Renal Fluid Electrolyte Physiol, 32*):F503–509.
6. Greenwald JE, Needleman P, Wilkins MR, Schreiner GF. Renal synthesis of atriopeptinlike protein in physiology and pathophysiology. *Am J Physiol* 1991;260(*Renal Fluid Electrolyte Physiol, 29*):F602–F607.
7. Greenwald JE, Ritter D, Tetens E, Rotwein PS. Renal expression of the gene for atrial natriuretic factor. *Am J Physiol* 1992;263 (*Renal Fluid Electrolyte Physiol, 32*):F974–978.
8. Dean AD, Greenwald JE. Localization and regulation of c-type natriuretic peptide (CNP) in the kidney. *J Am Soc Nephrol* 1993;4(3):436.
9. Forssmann K, Hock D, Herbst F, Schulz-Knappe P, Talartschik J, Scheler F, Forssman WG. Isolation and structural analysis of the circulating human cardiodilatin (alpha ANP). *Klin Wochenschr* 1986;64(24):1276–1280.
10. Schulz-Knappe P, Forssmann K, Herbst F, Hock D, Pipkorn R, Forssmann WG. Isolation and structural analysis of "urodilatin,"

a new peptide of the cardiodilatin-(ANP)-family, extracted from human urine. *Klin Wochenschr* 1988;66:752–759.

11. Solc J, Bauer K, Timnik A, Solcova A, Dohlemann C, Strom TM, Weil J. Combination of high-performance liquid chromatography and radioimmunoassay for the measurement of urodilatin and alpha-hANP in the urine of healthy males. *Life Sci* 1991; 48(25):2451–2456.

12. Bauer K, Solc J, Timnik A, Solcova A, Weil J. Urodilatin and atrial natriuretic peptide are present in the urine of healthy neonates and young infants. *Biol Neonate* 1992;62(2–3):96–99.

13. Goetz K, Drummer C, Zhu JL, Leadley R, Fiedler F, Gerzer R. Evidence that urodilatin, rather than ANP, regulates renal sodium excretion. *J Am Soc Nephrol* 1990;1:867–874.

14. Drummer C, Fiedler F, Konig A, Gerzer R. Urodilatin, a kidney-derived natriuretic factor, is excreted with a circadian rhythm and is stimulated by saline infusion in man. *J Am Soc Nephrol* 1991;1: 1109–1113.

15. Emmeluth C, Drummer C, Gerzer R, Bie P. Roles of cephalic Na+ concentration and urodilatin in control of renal Na+ excretion. *Am J Physiol* 1992;262(*Renal Fluid Electrolyte Physiol, 31*):F513–516.

16. Jamison RL, Sonnenberg H, Stein JH. Questions and replies: role of the collecting tubule in fluid, sodium, and potassium balance. *Am J Physiol* 1979;237:F247–F261.

17. Sonnenberg H, Honrath U, Chong CK, Wilson DR. Atrial natriuretic factor inhibits sodium transport in medullary collecting duct. *Am J Physiol* 1986;250(*Renal Fluid Electrolyte Physiol, 19*): F963–F966.

18. Gunning ME, Ballermann BJ, Silva P, Brenner BM, Zeidel ML. Characterization of ANP receptors in rabbit inner medullary collecting duct cells. *Am J Physiol* 1988;255(*Renal Fluid Electrolyte Physiol, 24*):F324–F330.

19. Gunning M, Silva P, Brenner BM, Zeidel ML. Characteristics of ANP-sensitive guanylate cyclase in inner medullary collecting duct cells. *Am J Physiol* 1989;256(*Renal Fluid Electrolyte Physiol, 25*): F766–F775.

20. Gunning ME, Otuechere G, Zeidel ML. Mechanism of urodilatin (ANP$_{95-126}$; Uro) inhibition of Na+ transport in rabbit inner medullary collecting duct (IMCD) cells. *J Am Soc Nephrol* 1991;2(3): 402(A).

21. Koike J, Nonoguchi H, Terada Y, Tomita K, Marumo F. Effect of urodilatin on cGMP accumulation in the kidney. *J Am Soc Nephrol* 1993;3(10):1705–1709.

22. Zeidel ML, Kikeri D, Silva P, Burrowes M, Brenner BM. Atrial natriuretic peptide inhibits conductive sodium uptake by rabbit inner medullary collecting duct cells. *J Clin Invest* 1988;82:1067–1074.

23. Sonnenberg H, Honrath U, Wilson DR. In vivo microperfusion of inner medullary collecting duct in rats: effect of amiloride and ANF. *Am J Physiol* 1990;259(*Renal Fluid Electrolyte Physiol, 28*): F222–226.

24. Light DB, Schweibert EM, Harlson KH, Stanton BA. Atrial natriuretic peptide inhibits a cation channel in renal inner medullary collecting duct cells. *Science* 1989;243:383–385.

25. Ando Y, Tabei K, Asano Y. Luminal vasopressin modulates transport in the rabbit cortical collecting duct. *J Clin Invest* 1991;88(3):952–959.

26. Schulz-Knappe P, Honrath U, Forssmann WG, Sonnenberg H. Endogenous natriuretic peptides: effect on collecting duct function in rat kidney. *Am J Physiol* 1990;259(*Renal Fluid Electrolyte Physiol, 28*):F415–418.

27. Gunning M, Ballermann BJ, Silva P, Brenner BM, Zeidel ML. Brain natriuretic peptide: interaction with renal ANP system. *Am J Physiol* 1990;258(*Renal Fluid Electrolyte Physiol, 27*):F467–F472.

28. Valentin JP, Sechi LA, Qui C, Schambelan M, Humphreys MH. Urodilatin binds to and activates renal receptors for atrial natriuretic peptide. *Hypertension* 1993;21(4):432–438.

29. Lafferty HM, Gunning M, Silva P, Zimmerman MB, Brenner MB, Anderson S. Enkephalinase inhibition increases plasma atrial natriuretic peptide levels, glomerular filtration rate, and urinary sodium excretion in rats with reduced renal mass. *Circ Res* 1989;65: 640–646.

30. Chinkers M, Garbers DL, Chang M-S, Lowe DG, Chin H, Goeddel DV, Schulz S. A membrane form of guanylate cyclase is an atrial natriuretic peptide receptor. *Nature* 1989;338:78–83.

31. Saxenhofer H, Raselli A, Weidmann P, Forssmann WG, Bub A, Ferrari P, Shaw SG. Urodilatin, a natriuretic factor from kidneys, can modify renal and cardiovascular function in men. *Am J Physiol* 1990;259(*Renal Fluid Electrolyte Physiol, 28*):F832–F838.

32. Hildebrandt DA, Mizelle HL, Brands MW, Hall JE. Comparison of renal actions of urodilatin and atrial natriuretic peptide. *Am J Physiol* 1992;262(*Regulatory Integrative Comp Physiol, 31*): R395–399.

33. Kentsch M, Ludwig D, Drummer C, Gerzer R, Muller EG. Haemodynamic and renal effects of urodilatin in healthy volunteers. *Eur J Clin Invest* 1992;22(5):319–325.

34. Riegger GA, Elsner D, Forssmann WG, Kromer EP. Effects of ANP-(95-126) in dogs before and after induction of heart failure. *Am J Physiol* 1990;259(*Heart Circ Physiol, 28*):H1643–1648.

35. Abassi ZA, Powell JR, Golomb E, Keiser HR. Renal and systemic effects of urodilatin in rats with high-output heart failure. *Am J Physiol* 1992;262(*Renal Fluid Electrolyte Physiol, 31*):F615–621.

36. Shaw S, Weidmann P, Zimmermann A. Urodilatin, not nitroprusside, combined with dopamine reverses ischemic acute renal failure. *Kidney Int* 1992;42(5):1153–1159.

37. Hummel M, Kuhn M, Bub A, Bittner H, Kleefeld D, Marxen P, Schneider B, Hetzer R, Forssmann WG. Urodilatin: a new peptide with beneficial effects in the postoperative therapy of cardiac transplant recipients. *Clin Invest* 1992;70(8):674–682.

38. McKenzie JC, Scott JN, Inagami T. Immunohistochemical localization of atrial natriuretic peptide in the developing and adult mammalian kidney. *Am J Anat* 1991;190:182–191.

39. Gunning ME, Brenner BM. Natriuretic peptides and the kidney: current concepts. *Kidney Int* 1992;42(suppl 38):S127–S131.

40. De Bold AJ, Borrenstein HB, Veress AT, Sonnenberg H. A rapid and potent natriuretic response to intravenous injection of atrial myocardial extract in rats. *Life Sci* 1981;28:89–94.

Hypertension: Pathophysiology, Diagnosis, and Management, Second Edition,
edited by J.H. Laragh and B.M. Brenner,
Raven Press, Ltd., New York © 1995.

CHAPTER **61**

Physiological Studies of the Natriuretic Peptide Family

John A. Lewicki and Andrew A. Protter

The observation that the myocardial atrium contains a natriuretic, diuretic and vasorelaxant substance was first reported by deBold in 1981 (1). Following the discovery of this natriuretic factor, several groups isolated atrial natriuretic peptide (ANP) in pure form and determined its amino acid sequence. This discovery helped to explain prior observations that the cardiac atria contain secretory granules whose granularity changes as a function of central fluid volume (2,3). This finding focused particular attention on the role of the heart in regulating cardiovascular homeostasis. In the decade following the isolation of ANP, a number of laboratories have devoted attention toward defining the fundamental properties of this peptide. These efforts have fueled our current understanding of the regulation of ANP gene expression, biosynthesis, and secretion; the identity of specific ANP receptors; the definition of the renal, cardiovascular, and endocrine actions of the peptide, including its potential

therapeutic applications; and the role of ANP in both normal and pathophysiological states.

In recent years, two peptides structurally related to ANP have been purified and characterized (see Fig. 1). Brain natriuretic peptide (BNP) was initially isolated from porcine brain, however, this peptide has been determined to be most prevalent in the cardiac ventricle. The finding that the biosynthesis and circulating levels of this peptide are markedly enhanced under conditions of cardiac stress suggests that BNP acts in concert with ANP to modulate cardiovascular homeostasis. Investigation is active toward further defining the actions of BNP. C-type natriuretic peptide (CNP) was also isolated from brain. CNP appears to be localized throughout the central nervous system (CNS) and its recent identification in peripheral tissues has led to emerging interest in defining the fundamental biologic roles of this newly described peptide.

The structures of these three members of this "natriuretic peptide family" are shown in Fig. 1. ANP, BNP, and CNP share common structural features including a 17 amino acid ring structure formed by disulfide bonds

J. A. Lewicki and A. A. Protter: Scios Nova, Inc., Mountain View, California 94043.

ANP   SLRRSSCFGGRMDRIGAQSGLGCNSFRY

BNP   SPKMVQGSGCFGRKMDRISSSSGLGCKVLRRH

CNP   GLSKGCFGLKLDRIGSMSGLGC

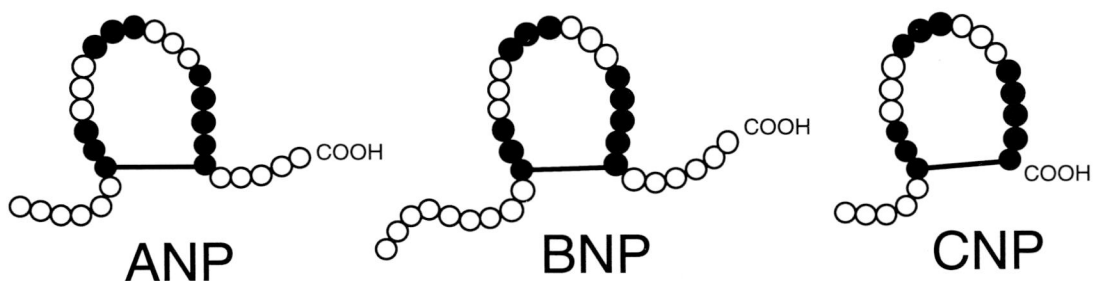

ANP   BNP   CNP

FIG. 1. The amino acid sequences of the human natriuretic peptides. Amino acid residues conserved between the peptides are shaded. The position of the disulfide bond forming the 17 amino acid ring structure in each of the natriuretic peptides is indicated in the schematic on the bottom. ANP: 28 amino acid form—ANP_{99-126}; BNP: 32 amino acid form—$hBNP_{32}$; CNP: 22 amino acid form—CNP_{22}.

with 11 of the 17 amino acids within the ring conserved. This chapter summarizes our current knowledge of the regulation and function of these members of the natriuretic peptide family, ANP, BNP, and CNP, including their role in physiology and disease. Also included is a review of compounds that modulate natriuretic peptide metabolism and clearance. These "clearance inhibitors" have been used as tools to probe the function of the natriuretic peptides and have been tested for their therapeutic potential. Finally, this chapter aims to convey the fact that ongoing, intensive investigation into the role of the natriuretic peptides promises to further advance our understanding of how this novel peptide family acts in concert with other hormones and neurotransmitters to regulate the cardiovascular system.

ATRIAL NATRIURETIC PEPTIDE

Cardiac Synthesis and Secretion of ANP

The heart is the principal source of circulating ANP. Greater than 95 percent of the circulating ANP pool is derived from the cardiac atria, although the cardiac ventricles synthesize significant amounts of ANP as well, particularly under conditions associated with ventricular hypertrophy. Two hallmarks of ANP production by atrial tissue include regulated secretion from secretory granules and proteolytic processing to yield the mature active peptide hormone.

As with many other peptide hormones, the processing of ANP involves proteolysis to remove a secretion signal sequence as well as a pro-peptide portion (see Fig. 2). Amino acid sequences inferred from ANP DNA clones (4–8) resulted in the elucidation of the complete primary *in vitro* translation product of ANP. These studies revealed that the mature 28 amino acid ANP peptide is derived from the carboxyl-terminal end of a high molecular weight precursor protein, preproANP. In human atria, following translation of the 151 amino acid preproANP molecule, the 25 amino acid signal sequence is removed and the 126 amino acid ANP protein, termed proANP or ANP_{1-126}, is stored in post-Golgi secretory granules (9,10). Upon stimulation for ANP release, the atrial secretory granules fuse to the cell surface and release their contents. ProANP is the major form of ANP that can be characterized from rat (11) and human (12) tissue or cellular extracts (13) or from rat cardiac perfusate (14) with only trace amounts of the mature ANP_{99-126} detectable. However, the major form of ANP within the circulation and human coronary sinus is ANP_{99-126}, indicating that additional proteolytic processing of ANP_{1-126} must occur (15–18). It remains unclear whether this proteolytic event occurs immediately prior to, during, or after secretion.

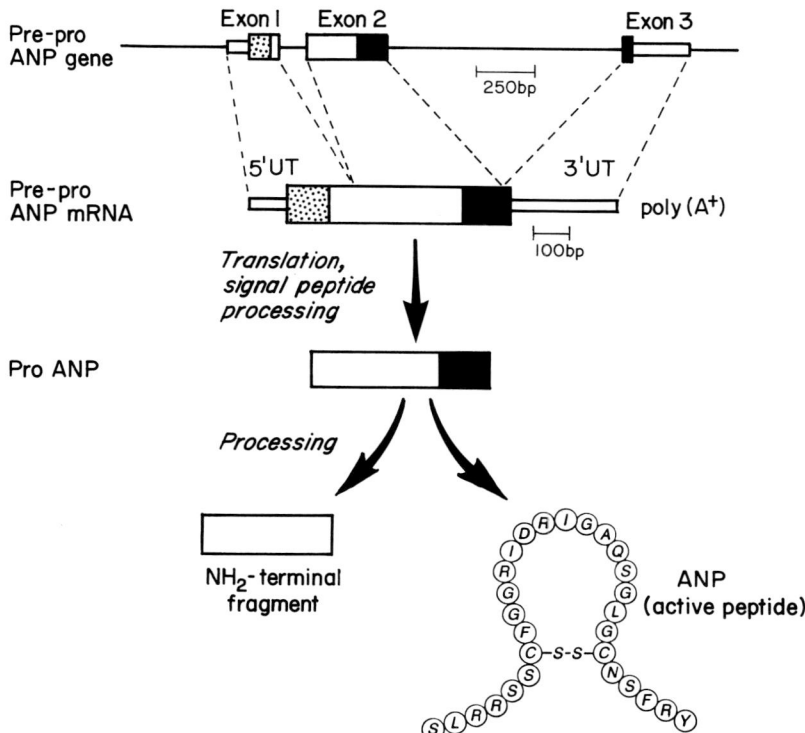

FIG. 2. ANP gene structure and expression, processing of pro-ANP, and release of ANP.

In contrast to the regulated release of ANP from atrial secretory granules, a constitutive secretory pathway appears to mediate the release of ANP from normal cardiac ventricles. Whereas both neonatal atrial and ventricular cardiocytes synthesize and secrete ANP, only the atrial cells store significant amounts of secretory granule-bound peptide (13). The absence of secretory granules from the process of ventricular production of ANP is reflected in decreased storage of ANP in ventricular tissue compared with atria when normalized for total production rates (19). As will be discussed later, BNP is also secreted from the ventricles in a constitutive manner and the process of constitutive ventricular secretion of ANP and BNP contributes profoundly to the circulating pool of these two peptides in the setting of ventricular hypertrophy.

As noted previously, ANP_{99-126} is the primary circulating form of ANP in all species. An alternative form of $hANP_{99-126}$ with an unusual antiparallel dimeric structure, termed β-hANP, has been characterized from atrial extracts and human plasma (20,21). Several studies have shown that the appearance of β-hANP is greatly induced in states of volume overload, for example congestive heart failure, where the expression of ANP is known to be quite high (22–27). It has been suggested that β-hANP formation results from alternative posttranslational processing in the setting of high levels of ANP biosynthesis. β-hANP has been shown to possess ANP agonist activity in a variety of *in vitro* and *in vivo* assays (20,28–30).

However, it remains unclear whether β-hANP represents an active ANP peptide within the circulation as it appears to be rapidly converted in the blood to monomeric ANP_{99-126} (31). The physiological significance of β-hANP is not known at this time; however, it is a major, and in some cases predominant, circulating form of ANP in patients with congestive heart failure (26,27).

An alternative carboxyl-terminal peptide derived from ANP_{1-126} has been purified from human urine and characterized as ANP_{95-126}, a 4 amino acid amino-terminal extended form of ANP_{99-126} (32). It is unlikely that this extended form of ANP, known as urodilatin, is derived from the plasma pool. Studies by several groups (33–35) highlight the kidney as a source for production of proANP-like material, which presumably could be proteolytically processed in a tissue-specific manner to ANP_{95-126} by local kidney proteases. Cell studies indicate that ANP_{95-126} is essentially equipotent to ANP_{99-126} with regard to receptor activation (29,36), and *in vivo* studies (37,38) demonstrating potent renal actions suggest that ANP_{95-126} may act as a paracrine hormone to modulate renal function.

The amino-terminal fragments of proANP, ANP_{1-98}, ANP_{1-30}, and ANP_{31-67} also circulate in the blood at significant concentrations (39–41). *In vitro* and *in vivo* studies in animals and humans (42–44) suggest ANP_{1-30} and ANP_{31-67} may possess some natriuretic and diuretic activity. However, the significance of these findings is uncertain at present.

Regulation of ANP Gene Expression

Tissue-Specific Gene Expression

Isolation of the ANP gene from human (45–47), mouse (47), and rat (48) species has permitted analysis of regions involved in the regulation of tissue-specific gene expression. The 5′ region of DNA flanking the ANP gene is highly conserved between rat, mouse, and human, consistent with an important regulatory function for this region. Field (49) demonstrated atrial-specific gene expression of SV40 T antigen when the ANP gene promoter, encompassed within a 500 base pair fragment flanking the 5′ end of the ANP gene, was fused to DNA encoding the protein and expressed in transgenic mice. Cell transcription studies (50,51) characterizing expression of a chloramphenicol acetyltransferase marker gene as controlled by fragments of the 5′ flanking region of the ANP gene suggest that tissue-specific expression results from a combination of positive regulatory elements acting in cardiac cells and negative regulatory elements acting in noncardiac cells. A small 68 base pair sequence from the 5′ flanking region (-400 to -333) has been shown to promote cardiac cell-specific expression. These reports indicate that genetic information conferring cardiac-specific gene expression is probably contained within the DNA 5′ to the ANP gene.

Physiological Regulation of Gene Expression

While cardiac volume overload and the resulting atrial stretch are directly associated with the release of ANP (52–54), little is known about how these physiological stimuli affect ANP gene expression at the cellular and molecular level. An association has been noted between water-electrolyte balance and ANP gene expression as water deprivation in rats results in a decrease in atrial ANP mRNA levels (7,55,56). Conversely, increased salt intake results in higher ANP mRNA levels (57,58). Similarly, acute stimulation of plasma volume overload results in a significant increase in atrial and ventricular ANP mRNA levels (59). While it is not known how cardiac volume affects ANP gene expression, the application of tension directly onto rat atriocytes results in a significant stimulation of ANP release as well as ANP mRNA synthesis, suggesting that ANP gene expression is directly regulated by atrial stretch (60).

Cardiac Hypertrophy and Atrial Natriuretic Peptide Gene Expression

The elevation of plasma ANP in states associated with chronic cardiac distension and ventricular hypertrophy results from increased atrial as well as ventricular expression of ANP mRNA. Ventricular expression of ANP mRNA is greatly induced in rats with experimental cardiac hypertrophy produced by abdominal aortic constriction (61). As a percentage of atrial ANP mRNA, ventricular ANP mRNA increases from 1.1 percent in control rats to about 30 percent in rats with experimental cardiac hypertrophy. Similarly, it has been shown that ventricular ANP mRNA levels increase significantly in a variety of different rat models of chronic volume overload-induced cardiac stretch, including deoxycorticosterone acetate-salt treatment and aortocaval fistula (59,62). Cardiac disease associated with hypertrophy in humans is also associated with markedly increased expression of ANP mRNA (12,63–65). Myocardial hypertrophy is associated with the expression of various protooncogenes including c-fos (62) and c-jun (for review [66]) which form a complex, termed AP-1, and activate transcription of specific genes through interactions with a defined DNA recognition sequence, termed TRE (67–69). The ANP gene contains three potential AP-1 recognition sites (between -357 and -222 relative to the site of transcription initiation) and cell transcription studies suggest that this DNA region mediates c-fos and c-jun activation of the ANP gene (70). Volume overload-induced cardiac hypertrophy is associated with ventricular expression of several fetal-specific genes including beta myosin heavy chain, alpha actin, and the MB isozyme of creatine kinase. The observation that a high level of ventricular ANP expression also occurs in the fetus but not in adults without cardiac disease, suggests a common regulatory mechanism for these genes (71–73).

Regulation of ANP Release

Atrial release of ANP is regulated primarily by atrial pressure. Perfusion of isolated heart (14,74–77) preparations have demonstrated that discrete increases in atrial pressure stimulate a proportional increase in ANP release from both right and left atria. Experimental manipulations to increase venous return (preload) or arterial resistance (afterload) in an isolated heart lung preparation increase atrial pressure and stimulate ANP release (76). Studies in whole animals demonstrate that a rapid stimulation of ANP release can be achieved by increased atrial pressures brought about by acute plasma volume expansion (78–85), balloon catheter mitral obstruction (86), or arterial occluding cuffs (87). Transmural rather than intramural atrial pressure is required to stimulate ANP release as experimental cardiac tamponade inhibits volume expansion–induced release of ANP (53,88). Application of tension directly to rat atriocytes stimulates ANP release suggesting that a stretch-dependent regulatory process is intrinsic to atrial cells (60). Similar control release mechanisms appear to be operational in humans as increasing atrial pressure by plasma volume expansion (89–91) or water immersion (92,93) has been shown to elevate plasma ANP.

The pressure-induced release of ANP exhibited by isolated cardiac tissue indicates that innervation is not required for secretion; however, denervation has been shown to significantly impair release of ANP in response to volume (94) or osmotic (95,96) stimulation. In addition, hypophysectomy significantly blunts plasma volume expansion–induced ANP release (84,94). Paradoxically, heart transplant recipients exhibit an enhanced released of ANP compared with normal volunteers in response to acute volume expansion (97) and head out water immersion (93). Thus neuronal regulation of atrial ANP release is complex and poorly understood, and may involve both stimulatory and inhibitory influences working in concert with the changes in atrial pressure.

ANP release can be stimulated by a variety of vasoactive hormones including vasopressin (98), neuropeptide Y (NPY) (99), angiotensin II (100), and endothelin (101); effects mediated in part by their pressor actions. However, angiotensin II can stimulate ANP release independent of atrial pressure changes (102). Similarly, endothelin has been shown to stimulate ANP mRNA synthesis and secretion in cultured atrial cells, isolated heart, and isolated atrial preparations (103–107), suggesting that endothelin has a direct stimulatory effect on atrial ANP release.

ANP Receptors

Two functional classes of high-affinity cell surface receptors for the natriuretic peptides have been described: "biological" receptors which, upon ligand activation, mediate the primary physiological actions of the natriuretic peptides, and "clearance" receptors which mediate cellular internalization and degradation of bound ligand thereby regulating natriuretic peptide metabolism (see Fig. 3).

Biological Receptors

Two natriuretic peptide biological receptors have been described: a guanylyl cyclase-A (GC-A) receptor and a guanylyl cyclase-B (GC-B) receptor (108). Cellular, receptor binding, and molecular studies of receptor structure and function have revealed much about the actions of these receptors (see chapter by Maack entitled "ANP Receptors-Functional and Structural Characteristics," *this volume*). Ligand binding to an extracellular binding domain results in the activation of an intracellular guanylyl cyclase domain which catalyzes the formation of guanosine 3'5'-cyclic monophosphate (cGMP) from guanosine 5'-triphosphate (GTP). A second intracellular region, termed the *kinase homology domain* because of its structural homology with known tyrosine kinase proteins (109), is believed to contain an ATP binding site, and studies suggest that in the absence of ligand binding, this region inhibits the activity of the guanylyl cyclase domain. While there is considerable homology between the extracellular regions of GC-A and GC-B receptor, there is exquisite specificity as ANP and BNP both stimulate the GC-A receptor whereas CNP specifically activates only the GC-B receptor. The GC-A and GC-B receptors differ in both their ligand specificity and tissue distribution, underscoring the possibility for fundamental differences in the biological actions of ANP or BNP compared with CNP.

Clearance Receptors

The clearance receptor (110) shows some structural homology to the biological receptors in the extracellular domain but is distinct from the biological receptors in that the clearance receptor has a relatively short intracellular region with no guanylyl cyclase domain. Unlike the biological receptors which can discriminate ANP and

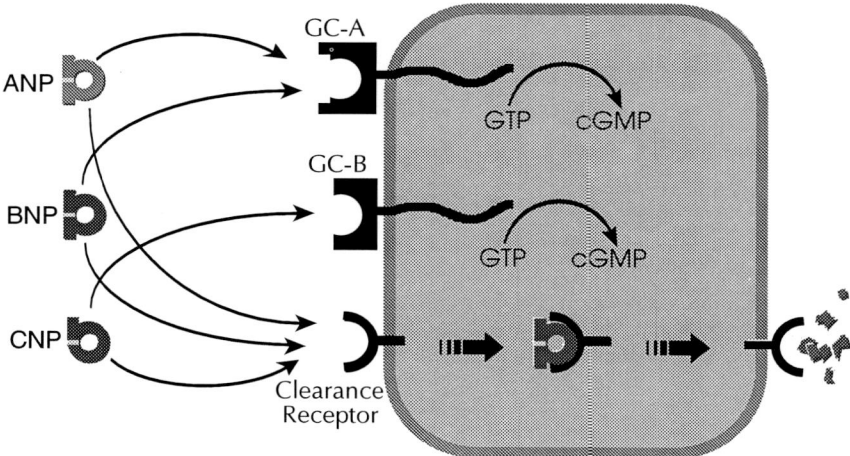

FIG. 3. Binding of the natriuretic peptides to the biological (guanylyl cyclase) and clearance (C-ANP) receptors. The binding specificity of the natriuretic peptides, ANP and BNP, bound to the GC-A receptor and CNP bound to the GC-B receptor, combined with the unique tissue distribution between the GC-A and GC-B receptors is consistent with the possibility of the fundamentally distinct biological activity of ANP and BNP compared to that of CNP. All three of the natriuretic peptides bind to the clearance receptor with high affinity; however, the 14-fold lower affinity of BNP compared with that of ANP for the clearance receptor may contribute to the longer circulating half-life of BNP.

BNP from CNP, the clearance receptor is more promiscuous with regard to ligand recognition and binds all three natriuretic peptides with high affinity. As originally demonstrated by Maack et al. (111) and reviewed later in this chapter, the clearance receptor mediates much of the metabolic degradation of the endogenous natriuretic peptides.

Biologic Actions of ANP

Since the initial discovery of ANP, a plethora of studies have been directed at defining the biologic effects of the hormone on target tissues. These studies have provided a basis for understanding the role of ANP in normal physiology and under pathophysiological conditions. Although our understanding of the physiological role of ANP and other natriuretic peptides is still in its infancy, a pattern has emerged from these studies which suggests that ANP acts in close concert with other hormonal systems, particularly the renin-angiotensin-aldosterone (RAA) system, to regulate fluid volume and blood pressure homeostasis (see Fig. 4). Indeed, ANP opposes many of the direct biological actions of angiotensin II and decreases circulating levels of renin, angiotensin II, and aldosterone. Thus, ANP can be viewed as a physiologic antagonist of the RAA system. Although the current understanding is not as advanced, ANP also antagonizes actions of many other hormones, such as endothelin, vasopressin, and mineralocorticoids and neurotransmitters.

The integrated response of an organism to administration of ANP is the product of a complex interplay between distinct renal, vascular, and endocrine actions of the hormone (see Fig. 4). Administration of ANP to animals or humans elicits a natriuresis and diuresis, a decrease in mean arterial blood pressure, and often a suppression of plasma renin and aldosterone (112–115). These responses occur as a consequence of both direct and indirect actions of ANP and vary in magnitude as a function of the physiological or pathophysiological state of the organism, the dose of ANP administered, the mode and/or length of its administration, and the activity of the hormonal and neurotransmitter systems that counter its activity. As a result, it has often been difficult to ascertain the fundamental mechanisms underlying many of the biological effects of ANP. The following section describes our current state of knowledge concerning the primary biological actions of ANP.

Renal Effects

ANP increases both the absolute and fractional excretion of sodium and water in virtually all experimental animal models and in humans (see Fig. 5) (116–118).

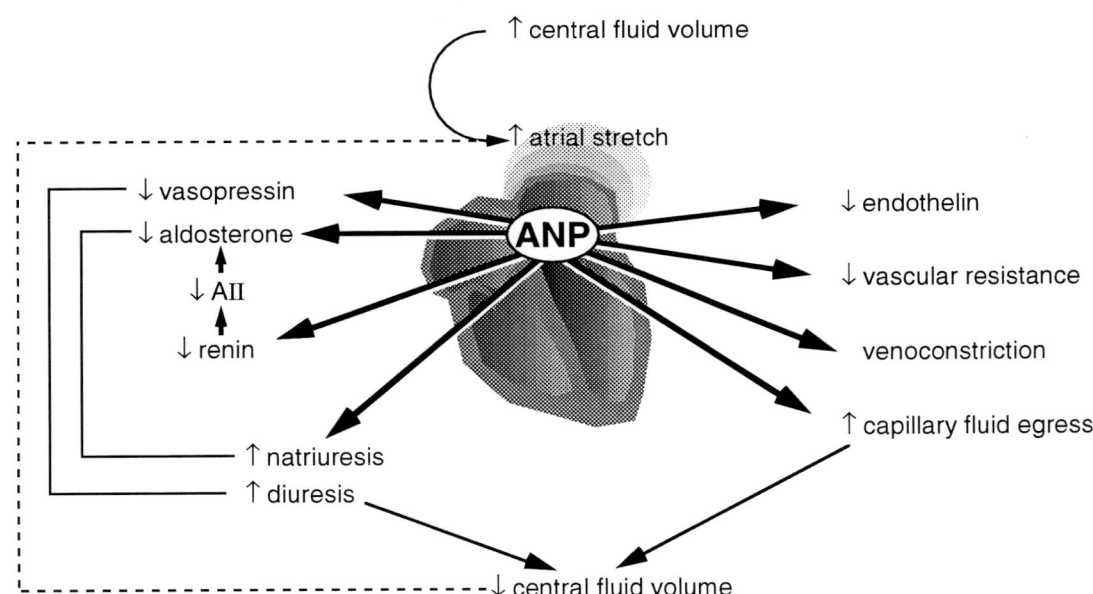

FIG. 4. A schematic representation of the fundamental biological actions of ANP. Increases in central blood volume lead to atrial stretch, which is believed to promote the release of ANP from atrial stores into the circulation. Following its release into the circulation, ANP elicits a spectrum of vascular, renal, and endocrine actions, all of which serve to reduce the elevated central fluid volume. As noted by the dashed line, the reduction in central fluid volume serves as a negative feedback to relieve the atrial stretch and reduce ANP secretion. A number of lines of evidence, reviewed in the section on the "Role of the Natriuretic Peptides in Physiology and Disease," implicate ANP in the physiological regulation of central fluid volume through the mechanisms depicted in this figure.

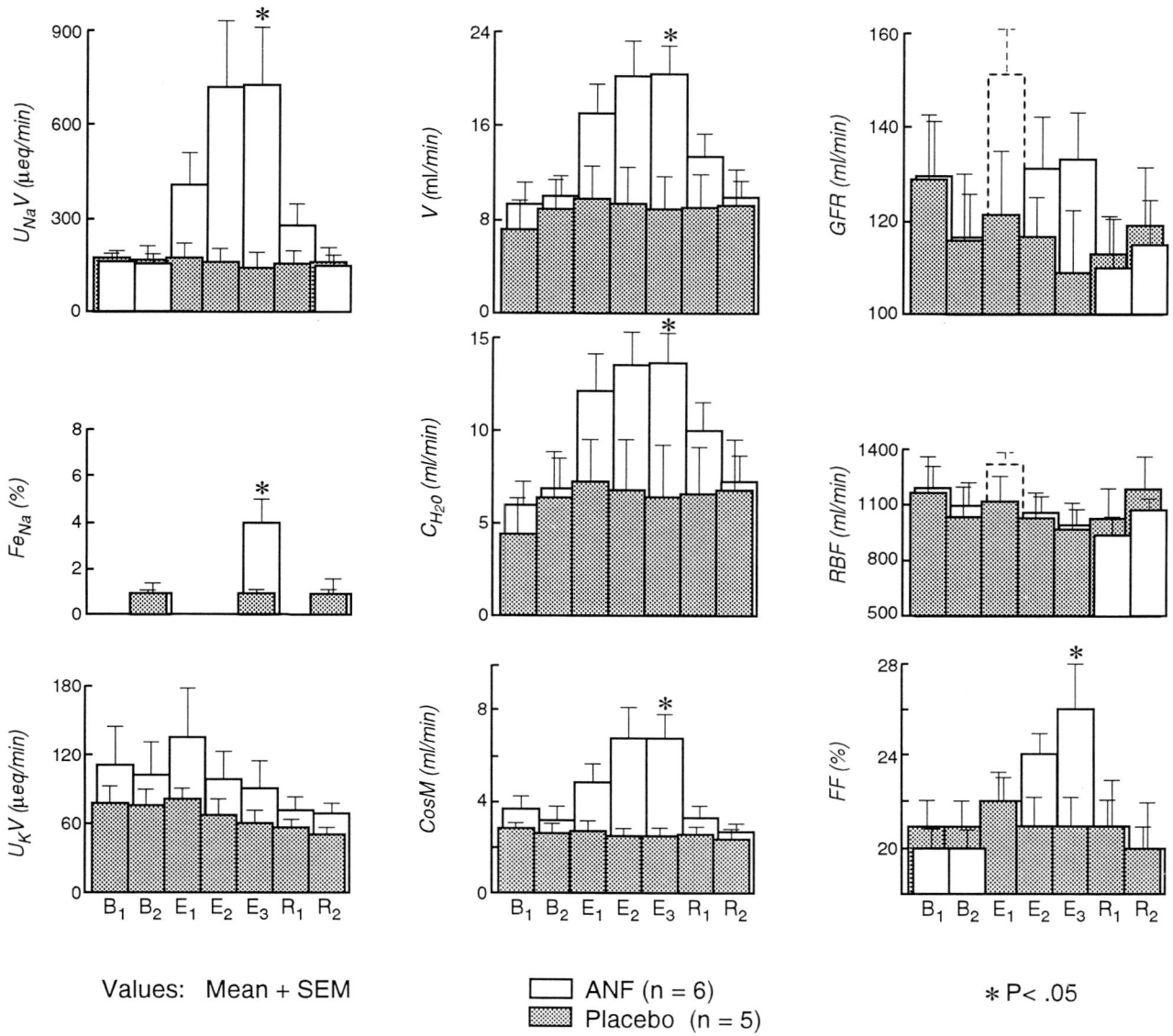

Values: Mean + SEM

☐ ANF (n = 6)
▨ Placebo (n = 5)

* P< .05

FIG. 5. Renal effects of ANP in normal human subjects. Open bars indicate subjects (*n* = 6) who received constant infusion of synthetic rat ANP at a rate of 100 ng/kg/minute during the 60-minute experimental period (E_1 to E_3); shaded bars indicate control subjects (*n* = 5) receiving vehicle alone. All parameters that increased during ANP infusion (*p < 0.05) returned to baseline (B) values during the recovery (R) period. (From ref. 117, with permission.)

There is general agreement that the mode of action of ANP differs from that of any other known natriuretic substance and that both renal hemodynamics effects and direct inhibitory actions on tubular reabsorption of sodium contribute to this activity.

One of ANP's most notable actions is to increase the glomerular filtration rate (GFR) and filtration fraction, even when there is a modest decrease in renal blood flow or blood pressure (Fig. 4) (118–122). ANP increases GFR by enhancing glomerular hydrostatic pressure which results from the differential effect of ANP on the tonus of the resistance vessels of the glomerulus

(118,119,121,123–125). ANP dilates the afferent arteriole, particularly when it is under the influence of vasoconstriction substances, but, somewhat paradoxically, constricts the efferent arteriole. The ANP-mediated constriction of the efferent arteriole is dependent on the presence of extracellular calcium, while afferent arteriolar relaxation occurs independent of extracellular calcium (119,126,127). It has also been reported that ANP increases the glomerular ultrafiltration coefficient (K_f), a factor that could contribute to the increase in GFR (124).

In addition to increasing the filtered load of sodium, other hemodynamic and tubular mechanisms contribute to ANP's natriuretic and diuretic actions. In particular, evidence has pointed to actions of ANP on deep nephrons that disrupt normal glomerulo-tubular balance. For example, ANP has been shown to decrease inner-medullary hypertonicity (128). This effect has been documented by measuring the cortico-medullary concentration of solutes from animals infused with ANP (129). The mechanisms underlying the decrease in inner-medullary hypertonicity remain to be fully elucidated (130–132). But whatever the mechanism, the renal medullary washout appears to contribute prominently to the maintenance of the natriuretic actions of ANP.

ANP possesses direct actions on renal tubules to inhibit sodium reabsorption. In particular, ANP has been shown to inhibit sodium uptake in the inner-medullary collecting duct (133,134). The mechanism of this action is probably an inhibition of amiloride-sensitive sodium channels (135–138). Specific ANP receptors that lead to cyclic GMP accumulation are associated with this structure. ANP not only inhibits sodium and chloride reabsorption in the inner-medullary collecting duct, but may also stimulate a furosemide-sensitive secretion of sodium and chloride into the tubular lumen (139). This may explain the high concentration of sodium in the urine following administration of ANP (120).

ANP inhibits sodium and water reabsorption in other tubular segments generally under conditions of heightened stimulus for sodium reabsorption. ANP has been reported to counteract the sodium-retaining effects of angiotensin II and norepinephrine in the proximal tubule of the rat (140,141) and to decrease sodium reabsorption in cortical collecting ducts isolated from mineralocorticoid-treated rats (142). These observations suggest that ANP effectively antagonizes the actions of stimulatory agonists in the proximal tubule and cortical collecting duct. Furthermore, ANP is likely to blunt distal tubular and cortical collecting duct sodium reabsorption indirectly by inhibiting aldosterone secretion.

It has been established that a number of factors can override the natriuretic effect of ANP. For instance, the ability of ANP to induce a natriuresis is contingent on an adequate renal perfusion pressure and is blunted when the perfusion pressure is abnormally low (120,143–146). Increased activity of the RAA system or increased renal sympathetic nerve activity may also attenuate the renal actions of ANP (147,148). These factors likely contribute to the blunted renal response to ANP that is observed in pathophysiological states like heart failure (see below).

Vascular Effects

Administration of ANP to animals and humans elicits a decrease in blood pressure (1,117,149,150). ANP decreases blood pressure acutely generally when high doses (0.1–1.0 µg/kg/min) of the peptide are administered by infusion or bolus injection. This acute, hypotensive re-

sponse to ANP is apparent in both normotensive and hypertensive states, and is particularly prominent during heightened RAA activity (151).

Several distinct mechanisms contribute to the acute hypotensive actions of ANP. ANP relaxes isolated blood vessels that have been preconstricted by agonists such as norepinephrine, vasopressin, angiotensin II, and endothelin, but does not affect, or may even slightly constrict, isolated vessels under normal resting tone (119,152–154). The likely molecular mechanism underlying the vasorelaxant effect of ANP is its high-affinity binding to ANP receptors on vascular smooth muscle which leads to a stimulation of the receptor-coupled guanylate cyclase with an associated increase in intracellular cyclic GMP accumulation. Cyclic GMP is known to initiate a cascade of events that causes the relaxation of vascular smooth muscle (155). Since ANP is able to directly stimulate cyclic GMP formation in vascular smooth muscle, its vasorelaxant activity does not require an intact endothelial lining (152).

Despite its vasorelaxant properties, ANP does not diminish peripheral vascular resistance in intact animals in a reproducible manner. Rather, most studies have shown the vascular effect of ANP to be more complex than originally anticipated, and the peptide may even exert some regional vasoconstriction *in vivo* (119,156,157). While the overall contribution of ANP's direct vascular actions to its hypotensive properties is unlikely to be important under normal conditions, ANP's vasorelaxant action probably contributes importantly in states when the sympathetic nervous or RAA systems are activated, as in heart failure.

A more consistent association has been established between acute ANP-mediated reductions in cardiac output and blood pressure, which likely results from several factors. It is well documented that ANP increases hematocrit by shifting fluid from the intravascular compartment to the interstitium (158,159). ANP achieves this unidirectional flow of fluid by increasing capillary hydraulic permeability (160,161). The resultant decrease in circulating blood volume likely contributes to the reduction in cardiac output observed upon both acute and chronic infusion of the peptide. An ANP-mediated reduction in venous return may also contribute to the reduced cardiac output. The decrease in venous return may result from an ANP-mediated venoconstriction which provides a resistance barrier to venous return and increases hydrostatic pressure in capillaries leading to a fluid efflux (see Fig. 4) (162–165). ANP has also been reported to have a vagomimetic action and/or interactions with baroreflex mechanisms which could contribute to the observed changes in cardiac output and to the apparent lack of reflex tachycardia.

It should be emphasized that the hemodynamic responses to acute ANP administration differ from those observed during chronic infusion. It has been reported that chronic infusions of ANP, at doses that do not detectably increase plasma ANP levels, cause a decrease in blood pressure that is often sustained throughout the infusion period (166,167). In these studies, peripheral vascular resistance is at control values after several days of infusion, although the hypotension persists. It has been suggested that reductions in effective blood volume contribute most significantly to the chronically maintained hypotensive state. Since low-dose infusion of ANP may, in part, reproduce normal, physiological fluctuations in plasma ANP levels, these studies support a physiological role for ANP in the maintenance of plasma volume (see below).

Endocrine Effects

ANP blocks the secretion and opposes the action of several classes of hormones, including components of the renin-angiotensin-aldosterone system, endothelin, and vasopressin (116,122,168,169). In addition, ANP inhibits the activity of the sympathetic nervous system under many conditions (145).

The pattern of effects on hormone secretion appears to be one of blunting basal and/or stimulated release, suggesting an overall modulatory role for ANP. These effects occur even when low doses of the peptide are administered to animals or humans.

Renin Release

Intravenous infusion of ANP elicits a decrease in plasma renin activity (PRA) associated with a decrease in renin secretion rate, although this effect is not observed under all conditions in a reproducible manner. The influence of ANP on plasma renin activity involves mostly a complex interplay between indirect actions of ANP on the vasculature, kidney, and baroreflex pathways, and also, perhaps, direct effects on renin-secreting juxtaglomerular (JG) cells of the kidney.

Several primary actions of ANP indirectly influence renin secretion. For example, ANP-induced increases in GFR, along with a disruption of glomerulo-tubular balance, leads to an increase in sodium delivery to the macula densa, an event known to decrease renin secretion. The key contribution of hemodynamic events to this response has been documented in experiments showing that ANP does not inhibit renin release when renal blood flow is impeded by clamping the renal artery or in the nonfiltering kidney (143,170). Other indirect mechanisms that could affect renin secretion include afferent arteriolar dilation, which may increase hydraulic pressure on the stretch-sensitive JG cells, and effects on efferent renal sympathetic nerve activity, which would change the baroreflex-mediated renin response to changes in blood pressure (171–173).

A number of investigations have attempted to discern the direct effects of ANP on renin release. These studies have yielded conflicting results as ANP inhibits renin release in certain preparations but does not change, or even stimulate, renin release in others. These data suggest that while ANP may modulate renin release directly, the influence of ANP on renin release in intact animals is dominated by hemodynamic and renal variables (174).

Aldosterone Secretion

ANP inhibits aldosterone secretion evoked by a number of secretagogues. Inhibition of aldosterone secretion by ANP complements its renal natriuretic action, although the physiological relevance of this effect has not been established. ANP blocks agonist-induced release of aldosterone in cultured adrenal glomerulosa cells, and administration of ANP to animals and humans lowers plasma aldosterone levels (116,168,169,175). ANP inhibits the early pathway of aldosterone biosynthesis (cholesterol to pregnenolone) and, while results are conflicting, ANP may also inhibit the late pathway conversion of corticosterone to aldosterone (175–177).

The cellular basis for the ANP inhibition of aldosterone biosynthesis has not been resolved. ANP receptors have been identified on adrenal glomerulosa cells and the peptide has been reported to inhibit adenylate cyclase, stimulate guanylate cyclase, and block calcium channels in these cells (178,179). It is conceivable that any, or all, of these pathways may be coupled to the inhibition of aldosterone secretion. Furthermore, the specific inhibitory pathway utilized by ANP may differ as a function of the aldosterone secretagogue. Indeed, it has been suggested that the ANP-mediated decreases in cyclic adenosine monophosphate (cAMP) blunt ACTH-stimulated aldosterone secretion, while ANP interference with intracellular calcium fluxes underlies its inhibition of angiotensin II and K+-stimulated aldosterone secretion. Although it has been reported that ANP's aldosterone inhibitory action is not mimicked by cyclic GMP analogs, the recent finding that a specific antagonist of the guanylate cyclase-coupled ANP-A receptor (see below) blocks aldosterone secretion suggests that intracellular cyclic GMP may play a permissive role in modulating this response.

Endothelin Release

ANP has been shown to inhibit agonist-induced endothelin release from cultured cells and intact aorta (180,181). The effect appears to be dose-dependent and is also exhibited by other members of the natriuretic peptide family (182). ANP inhibits endothelin release from cultured endothelial cells derived from the thoracic aorta or umbilical vein following stimulation with angiotensin or thrombin. The same effect is observed using preparations of isolated aorta. The molecular mechanism of ANP inhibition of endothelin release has not been determined, but may involve cyclic GMP metabolism.

Central Nervous System Effects

ANP and its familial counterparts have been identified and localized in the central nervous system (CNS), along with specific ANP receptors (for review see Imura et al. [183]). ANP infusion studies into the brain have afforded insights into the central effects of the peptide. As in the periphery, a pattern has emerged in which ANP opposes many of the central actions of angiotensin II. Intracerebroventricular infusion of ANP inhibits angiotensin II and deprivation-induced salt and water intake in rats. Furthermore, ANP inhibits angiotensin II-induced pressor effects in the CNS and blunts the secretion of arginine vasopressin (184,185). Thus, ANP's primary actions in the CNS oppose the conservation of salt and water and are consistent with ANP's peripheral actions to regulate fluid volume and cardiovascular homeostasis.

BRAIN NATRIURETIC PEPTIDE (BNP)

Brain natriuretic peptide (BNP), initially purified and characterized from porcine brain extracts, exhibits natriuretic, diuretic, and smooth muscle relaxant activities similar to those of ANP (186). BNP is 32 amino acids in length and shows significant structural similarity to ANP including the characteristic 17 amino acid ring structure formed by an intramolecular disulfide bridge (see Fig. 1). BNP appears to be equipotent, or perhaps slightly less potent, than ANP in activating the guanylyl cyclase-A receptor; however, the possibility that BNP may interact with its own distinct receptor cannot yet be excluded (187,188). Human BNP has an approximately 14-fold lower affinity for the clearance receptor than does hANP (12,187). While many of the general biological actions of BNP are similar to that of ANP, differences concerning sites of synthesis, regulation of biosynthesis, and metabolism suggest a unique function for BNP.

BNP Structure

Following the isolation of porcine BNP, the structure of human BNP was determined through the characterization of cDNA and genomic clones encoding the peptide (189,190). Analysis of the amino acid sequence inferred from DNA clones to human BNP revealed that a peptide of 32 amino acids, corresponding to porcine BNP, is located in the carboxyl-terminal part of a 134 amino acid primary translation product, termed human preproBNP. Subsequent removal of a 26 amino acid signal sequence from preproBNP yields a 108 amino acid precursor protein termed $proBNP_{1-108}$. Analogous to the processing of ANP, the mature 32 amino acid BNP peptide, termed BNP_{32}, is released proteolytically from this larger propeptide.

Amino acid sequences of BNP from numerous species including dog, sheep, and rat (190,191) reveal that, unlike ANP and CNP, the structure of BNP is poorly conserved through evolution. Consistent with this are the observations of significant species-specific differences in the activity of rat, human, and porcine BNPs (192). For example, human BNP is relatively inactive in rats but exhibits significant renal and vascular effects in conscious cynomolgus monkeys and humans. Conversely, rat BNP shows significant activity in the rat but is relatively inactive in monkeys (193). This species specificity has made pharmacological studies of human BNP problematic.

Biosynthesis of BNP

Although BNP was originally isolated from the brain, its principal site of synthesis appears to be the heart. Unlike ANP, which is produced primarily in the cardiac atria, stored in secretory granules, and released in a regulated manner into the blood in response to pressure-induced atrial stretch, BNP is made primarily by the cardiac ventricle and is released into the blood in a constitutive fashion (12,194).

The ventricle appears to be the primary site of BNP biosynthesis in all species. Analysis of ANP and BNP mRNA levels from normal human heart tissue indicates that the ventricle contains approximately 70–77 percent of the total cardiac BNP mRNA yet only 3–3.5 percent of the total cardiac ANP mRNA (12,194). The expression of the BNP gene is increased markedly upon conditions of ventricular hypertrophy, and ventricular BNP probably accounts for over 90 percent of the total cardiac BNP mRNA in patients with severe heart failure (63). Consistent with the increase in the expression of BNP mRNA, the circulating level of BNP peptide has been shown to be dramatically elevated in the setting of congestive heart failure (CHF) (12). Thus ventricular hypertrophy results in increased ventricular expression of both ANP and BNP as well as increased circulating levels of these two peptide hormones. There are actually two distinct circulating forms of BNP in both normal individuals and heart failure patients, a high molecular weight form corresponding to proBNP (BNP_{1-108} or γ-BNP) and a low molecular weight mature form, BNP_{32} (12,195). In some instances the amount of circulating proBNP is greater than that of BNP_{32} (195). The significance of the high circulating amounts of the proBNP form is not clear, however the "pro" portion of the molecule may confer upon the BNP peptide hormone an extended plasma half-life thereby potentiating its biological actions. It is not known whether the high molecular weight form of plasma BNP constitutes a circulating pool of BNP destined to be proteolytically processed to the $hBNP_{32}$ form.

Biological Actions of BNP

Studies using experimental animals have shown the pharmacological actions of BNP to be qualitatively similar to those of ANP. Thus the spectrum of actions ascribed to ANP, including effects on the kidney (natriuresis and diuresis), the vasculature (hypotension and decreased intravascular fluid volume), and hormone balance (decreased plasma renin and aldosterone) have also been demonstrated upon BNP administration to experimental animals and humans (196).

BNP may elicit quantitatively different effects than ANP, particularly in pathophysiological settings. For instance, in a cohort of patients with severe congestive heart failure, BNP treatment decreased pulmonary capillary wedge pressure and systemic vascular resistance and increased cardiac index (197). These patients showed a robust increase in urine and sodium excretion rates, comparable to the renal response observed in normal volunteers. While congestive heart failure patients treated with ANP give a similar cardiovascular response profile, their renal response is blunted significantly. While more evidence is needed to substantiate this finding, the more prominent renal effects of BNP could potentially be related to the peptide's decreased avidity for the two principal metabolic clearance pathways for the natriuretic peptides within the kidney and other peripheral organs, the protease neutral endopeptidase 24.11, and the clearance receptor. Consistent with this latter possibility, the circulating half-life for human BNP has been determined to be 8–22 minutes, whereas ANP has a circulating half-life of 1–4 minutes.

The spectrum of beneficial cardiac and renal effects associated with BNP coupled with the observation that cardiac expression and circulating levels of BNP are elevated in the setting of congestive heart failure suggest that ventricular release of BNP may represent a natural corrective response to the cardiovascular imbalance associated with this condition.

C-TYPE NATRIURETIC PEPTIDE (CNP)

C-type natriuretic peptide is the most recently described member of the natriuretic peptide family. Although very little is known of the basic biological actions of CNP, knowledge of its structure and unique specificity for the GC-B receptor (see Fig. 3) supports the hypothesis that its actions are fundamentally different from those of ANP and BNP.

CNP was initially isolated from porcine brain and determined to be 22 amino acids in length (198). CNP is structurally related to ANP and BNP as 11 of the 17 amino acids within its disulfide bridged core are identical to ANP and BNP (see Fig. 1). In contrast to ANP and BNP, the structure of CNP terminates at the second cysteine residue of the disulfide ring and the peptide lacks a carboxyl-terminal extension. A second form of CNP, termed CNP_{53}, has been isolated from porcine brain extract, and amino acid sequence characterization has revealed the peptide to be 53 amino acids in length with CNP_{22} at its carboxyl-terminus.

DNA clones encoding CNP have been isolated from human (199), porcine (200), and rat (201) species. Analysis of the primary amino acid sequence inferred from these studies indicates that the initial translation product, preproCNP, is 126 amino acids in length, and processing to mature forms involves at least two proteolytic cleavage steps: initial removal of a 23 amino acid signal sequence yielding a 103 amino acid prohormone ($proCNP_{103}$) and subsequent proteolytic processing to yield one of two mature peptide forms, CNP_{53} or CNP_{22}. As with ANP and BNP, mature CNP peptide is derived by proteolytic processing from the carboxyl end of a precursor protein. Comparison of primary amino acid sequences of CNP from a variety of species has shown that the molecule is extraordinarily well conserved throughout evolution.

Biologic Actions of CNP

CNS Effects of CNP

As already mentioned, CNP was originally isolated from the brain and studies have shown that it is more abundant in the brain than either ANP or BNP and has a distribution within the brain distinct from ANP and BNP; the greatest amount is present in the cerebellum, hypothalamus, and thalamus regions (183,202). Similarly, CNP is more abundant in cerebrospinal fluid than ANP and BNP (203). While low levels of CNP have been detected in the blood (204), the majority of CNP appears to be restricted to the brain (183,202,205). Primary rat neuronal cultures have been shown to be more responsive to CNP than ANP as judged by cyclic GMP accumulation, suggesting that these cell types express more of the CNP-specific guanylyl cyclase receptor (termed GC-B) than the receptor for ANP (GC-A) (206). Intracerebroventricular infusion of CNP into sheep induces a rapid fall in mean arterial blood pressure (207), an effect consistent with the intravenous CNP infusion studies described below (204,208).

Peripheral Effects

Little is known about the peripheral action of CNP. Administration of CNP has been reported to elicit a hypotensive response (more potent than ANP) associated with decreased arterial pressure and decreased cardiac output (204,208). No significant renal effects (diuresis and natriuresis) have been documented. Based upon these studies it has been speculated that CNP decreases arterial pressure and cardiac output by decreasing venous return, an effect consistent with the observation that CNP relaxes preconstricted canine veins (209). However, other studies in dogs and rats have failed to demonstrate potent hypotensive actions of CNP (198,210). While the *in vivo* actions of CNP remain unclear, the lack of a natriuretic and diuretic response by the kidney supports the notion that the effects of CNP are fundamentally distinct from those of ANP and BNP.

Antimitogenic Activity of CNP

Agents that induce (e.g., ANP or sodium nitroprusside) or mimic (e.g., 8-bromo-cyclicGMP) guanosine 3′5′-cyclic monophosphate (cGMP) have been shown to inhibit DNA synthesis and/or cell proliferation in endothelial cells (211), vascular smooth muscle cells (212–215), and mesangial cells (216,217). Several studies have demonstrated that CNP is a more effective stimulant of cGMP production than either ANP or BNP in a variety of vascular smooth muscle cell types, consistent with the finding that these cells contain much more GC-B than GC-A (187,218,219). As a result, CNP is more potent than ANP in inhibiting DNA synthesis when cells are stimulated by a variety of growth factors associated with vascular hyperplasia. As shown in Fig. 6, CNP inhibits DNA synthesis induced by a number of vascular smooth muscle cell mitogens such as basic fibroblast growth factor (FGF), platelet-derived growth factor (PDGF-BB), epidermal growth factor (EGF), and heparin-binding EGF-like growth factor (HBEGF) by 60–80 percent. CNP is approximately 20-fold more potent than ANP as an antimitogen. Thus, CNP appears to inhibit mitogen-induced DNA synthesis in a manner which is independent of the growth factor stimulant, suggesting that CNP could play an important pathophysiological role in regulating vascular tissue organization. In a recent study, CNP has been shown to inhibit the growth of vascular smooth muscle cells *in vivo* in an air-induced vascular injury model of neointimal smooth muscle cell hyperplasia (220). CNP appears to be produced within certain endothelial cell beds, suggesting a possible paracrine

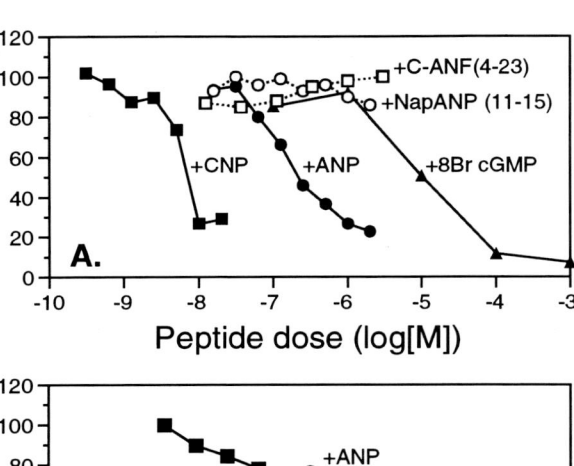

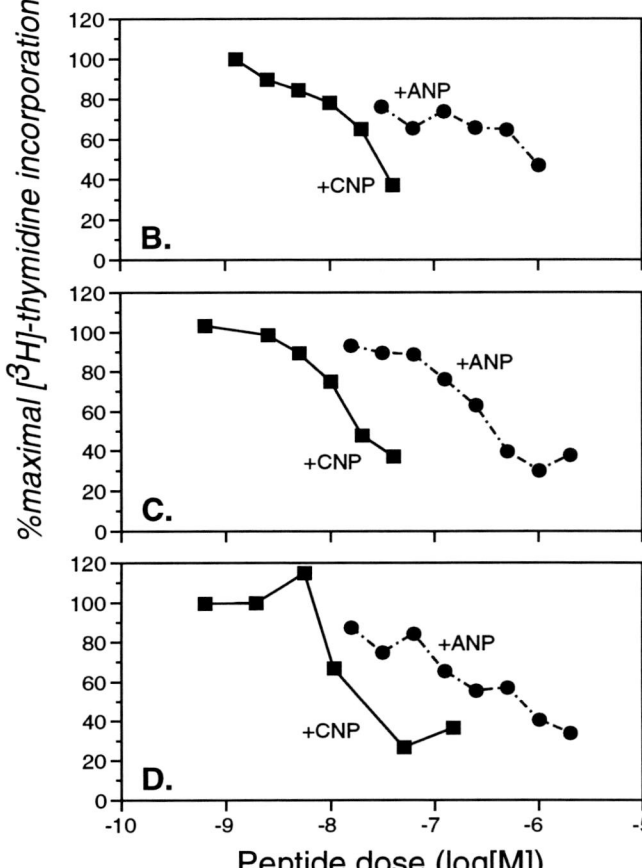

FIG. 6. ANP and CNP inhibit DNA synthesis, as measured by [3H]-thymidine incorporation, in bovine aortic smooth muscle cells stimulated with bFGF (panel **A**), PDGF (panel **B**), EGF (panel **C**), or HB-EGF (panel **D**). In these cells, CNP is approximately 20-fold more potent than ANP as an antimitogenic agent, consistent with the greater cGMP response elicited by CNP as compared with ANP. Furthermore, the antimitogenic effects of 8-bromo-cGMP and the lack of effects of two C-ANP receptor-specific ligands, C-ANP(4-23) and N-[2-naphthoxyacetyl isonipecotyl]-rANP$_{109-113NH2}$ (see panel A) suggest that the antimitogenic effects are mediated through cGMP derived from natriuretic peptides' guanylyl cyclase receptor. (From ref. 219, with permission.)

function of the peptide in regulating vascular tissue organization and possibly vascular tone.

MODULATORS OF NATRIURETIC PEPTIDE CLEARANCE

Two distinct clearance pathways are responsible for the removal of circulating natriuretic peptides in all species (see Fig. 7). While the role of these pathways has been most extensively characterized with respect to the metabolism of ANP, circulating levels of both BNP and CNP are also presumably modulated by these pathways. The majority of ANP clearance occurs via the C-ANP receptor, which rapidly binds and internalizes the peptide to lysosomal compartments where it is then degraded (111,221,222). The C-ANP receptor pool has sufficient capacity to bind most circulating ANP and is responsible for a rather large volume of distribution of the peptide (221,223). Proteolysis by neutral endopeptidase 24.11 (NEP) also contributes to the removal of ANP from the circulation (224,225). NEP is responsible also for degrading filtered ANP within the tubules of the kidney. This enzymatic pathway may contribute most significantly to ANP clearance under pathophysiological conditions in which plasma ANP is already elevated (226).

Compounds that block either the receptor-mediated clearance of ANP or inhibit NEP have been developed and used as probes to examine the physiological significance of these two degradative pathways. These same compounds have been evaluated as therapeutic agents because of their unique ability to increase plasma and/or urine levels of ANP. Clearance receptor inhibitors and NEP inhibitors are inactive when exposed to isolated tissues, thus confirming that they do not bind directly to the biological receptors of ANP. Although several recent reports have noted that clearance receptor ligands affect intracellular events within several cultured cell lines (227,228), it has not been established whether or not this represents a direct or indirect activity of these compounds.

Effects of Clearance Receptor Blockers

The C-ANP receptor plays a primary physiological role in regulating circulating concentrations of the natriuretic peptides. A series of studies has revealed that physiologic stimuli affect the density of clearance receptors. For example, rats deprived of water have been reported to exhibit an increase in the density of clearance receptors in renal glomeruli, and rats maintained on a low sodium diet exhibit a decrease in receptor density (229,230). The administration of a high-salt diet has also been shown to modulate ^{125}I-ANP binding and the volume of distribution of ANP, presumably by altering clearance receptor density. The guanylate cyclase-coupled receptors of ANP may also modulate C-ANP receptor density as increases in intracellular cyclic GMP have been reported to downregulate C-ANP receptor density (231–233).

The structural requirements for ligand binding to C-ANP receptors have been defined and are less stringent than those required for binding to the biological receptors of ANP. A number of specific ligands of C-ANP re-

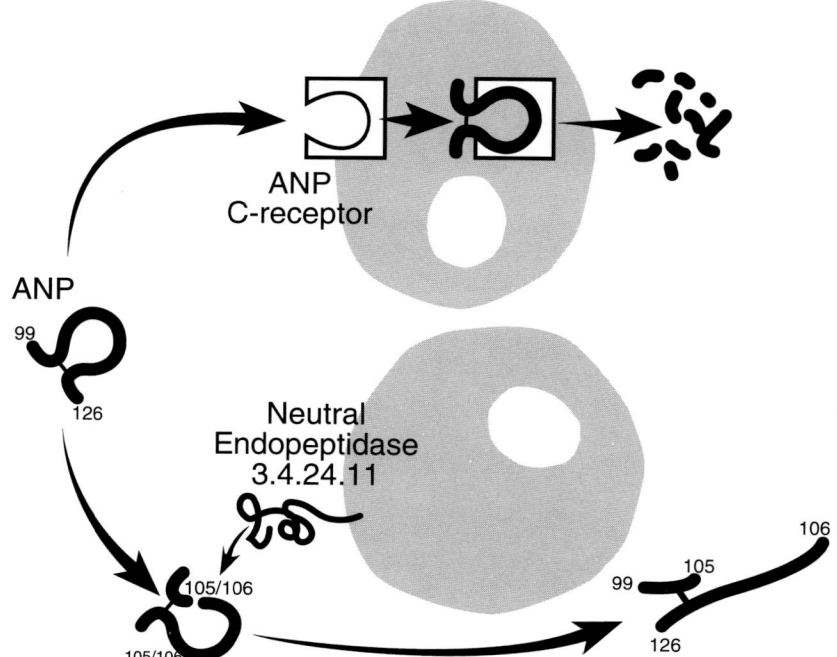

FIG. 7. Schematic of the principal cell surface pathways of ANP metabolism and clearance: the ANP clearance receptor and neutral endopeptidase 3.4.24.11. The clearance receptor binds to the natriuretic peptides and mediates their cellular internalization and subsequent lysosomal degradation. Neutral endopeptidase cleaves the natriuretic peptides resulting in their inactivation. Agents that block the clearance receptor or the neutral endopeptidase enzyme have been shown to increase circulating ANP and promote endogenous ANP activity.

ceptors, which represent fragments of native ANP, have been designed and employed to examine the role of this receptor *in vitro* and *in vivo*. The three most commonly used C-ANP receptor inhibitors are des[Gln^{116},Ser^{117},Gly^{118}, Leu^{119},Gly^{120}]rANP$_{102-126}$NH$_2$, referred to as C-ANP(4-23), des[Phe^{106}Gly^{107}Leu^{121}Gly^{122}]ANP$_{103-126}$(SC46,542), and 2-naphthoxyacetyl-isonipecotyl ANP$_{109-114-NH2}$.

Administration of clearance receptor ligands by infusion results in a decrease in the volume of distribution and metabolic clearance rate of ANP in normal animals (221,223,234,235). Plasma ANP has generally been noted to increase coincident with the decreased metabolic clearance of ANP (111,235–241). While few studies have examined the contribution of the clearance receptor to the metabolic clearance of ANP under pathophysiological conditions, the observation that C-ANP(4-23) infusion elevates ANP levels in dogs with ventricular

pacing-induced heart failure suggests that the clearance receptor contributes to ANP metabolism even when plasma ANP levels are elevated chronically (242).

The increase in plasma ANP that occurs when C-ANP receptor inhibitors are administered (0–300 percent) is generally accompanied by renal, hemodynamic and endocrine effects. These studies demonstrate that small changes in plasma ANP levels have significant biological consequences, consistent with a physiologic role of ANP. Infusion of C-ANP(4-23), or smaller clearance receptor blockers, usually elicits an increase in GFR and urine and sodium output, a decrease in blood pressure, and suppression of the RAA system (see Fig. 8) (111, 236,243,244). Infusion of C-ANP receptor ligands also increases the renal and hemodynamic response to low-dose infusion of ANP in rats and fetal sheep (245,246). Several laboratories have failed to note renal or hemody-

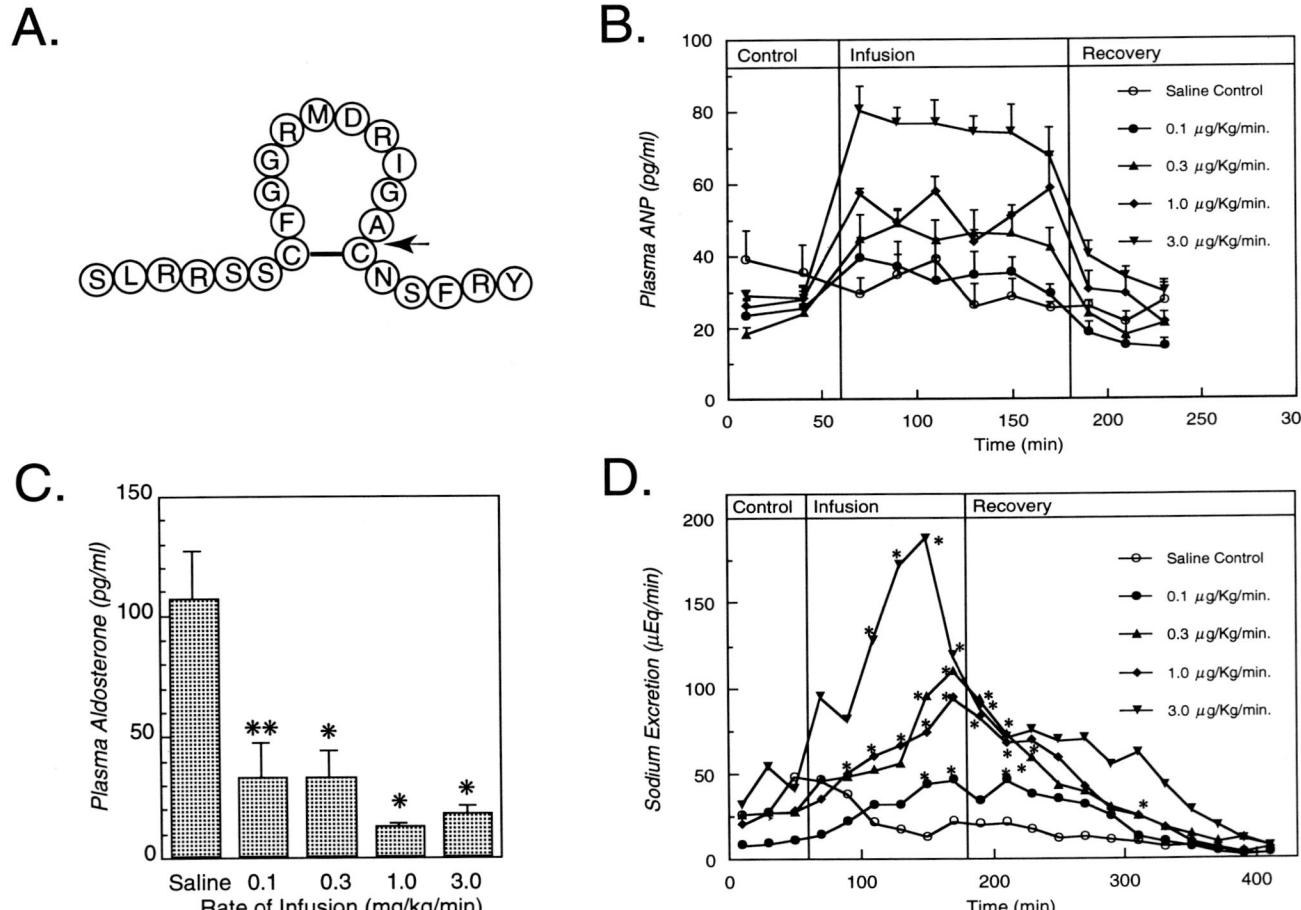

FIG. 8. Effects of clearance receptor–specific ligand infusion on plasma ANP, urinary sodium, and aldosterone. The clearance receptor–specific ligand, des[Gln^{116},Ser^{117},Gly^{118},Leu^{119},Gly^{120}]rANP$_{102-126}$NH$_2$, termed C-ANP(4-23) (panel **A**), was infused at 0.1, 0.3, 1.0, and 3.0 μg/kg/minute into conscious dogs and the response compared to that from saline as a control. Each point represents the mean observation in four dogs. C-ANP(4-23) infusion increases plasma ANP (panel **B**; *$p < 0.05$ compared with control), decreases plasma aldosterone (panel **C**, *$p < 0.05$ and **$p < 0.01$ compared with control), and increases urinary sodium excretion (panel **D**, *$p < 0.01$ compared with control). See Gregory et al. (235). The arrow in panel A indicates where amino acid residues Gln^{116},Ser^{117},Gly^{118},Leu^{119},Gly^{120} were deleted from rANP$_{102-126}$ to form C-ANP(4-23).

namic effects induced by acute or chronic administration of C-ANP receptor ligands, however, suggesting that the biological actions of these compounds may depend on the physiological state of the organism (238,239,242). At present, there is no published data of the effects of clearance receptor ligands in humans.

Effects of Neutral Endopeptidase Inhibitors

Neutral endopeptidase 24.11 (NEP) is a cell surface peptidase that has been implicated in the metabolism of a variety of peptide hormones with diverse biological actions including ANP, BNP, CNP, substance P, bradykinin, angiotensin I, angiotensin II, and others (for a review, see [247]). NEP cleaves ANP between Cys^{105} and Phe^{106} and inactivates the peptide. NEP also cleaves other peptide bonds of ANP coincident with the enzyme's specificity for the A-amino bond of hydrophobic amino acids. *In vitro* studies (248) with purified rabbit NEP enzyme suggests that BNP is less susceptible to degradation by NEP, while CNP appears to be the most sensitive of the natriuretic peptides to NEP cleavage. NEP activity is prevalent in the brush border of the proximal tubule of the kidney. Incubation of ANP with isolated renal brush border membranes results in a rapid cleavage of the peptide at the Cys^{105}, Phe^{106} bond, suggesting that NEP is responsible for the renal catabolism of ANP. NEP is also associated with membranes of brain, lung, seminal vesicles, intestine, and endothelium and a soluble form has been detected in the plasma (247). NEP probably contributes to the vascular and pulmonary clearance of ANP.

Inhibitors of NEP were initially designed to block the degradation of the enkephalins and were assessed for their analgesic properties. The finding that ANP is a substrate for NEP stimulated the development of newer, orally active NEP inhibitors which block NEP activity at low nanomolar concentrations *in vitro*. These inhibitors have been used to investigate the overall contribution of NEP to the metabolic inactivation of ANP and have been evaluated for their possible utility in treating cardiovascular disease (249–254).

Administration of NEP inhibitors, even at high doses, does not increase plasma ANP levels in a reproducible manner. Rather, most NEP inhibitors have been reported to increase plasma ANP in models with high ambient plasma ANP levels. NEP inhibitors increase plasma ANP levels in rat, dog, and hamster models of congestive heart failure (255–258), in deoxycorticosterone acetate (DOCA)/salt hypertensive rats (239,259, 260), and in rats with reduced renal mass (261). NEP inhibitors also elevate plasma ANP levels in normal volunteers and in patients with established congestive heart failure. These observations are consistent with the hypothesis that NEP plays a secondary role in the metabolic clearance of ANP under most normal conditions, but may contribute significantly to the clearance of ANP under pathophysiological conditions when existing clearance receptors may be partially saturated by high endogenous circulating concentrations of ANP and BNP.

Administration of NEP inhibitors elicits a natriuresis, diuresis, and increases in urinary concentrations of ANP and cyclic GMP in most experimental animal models and in humans (226,252,256,262,263). By inhibiting the proteolytic degradation of ANP within the proximal tubules, NEP inhibitors may allow the peptide to reach distal sites of action in the kidney, thus contributing to the observed natriuresis and diuresis. As mentioned above, NEP has been implicated in the metabolism of a diverse group of peptides suggesting that some of the effects of NEP inhibitors may be mediated by molecules other than ANP and BNP. For example, several reports have established that NEP inhibitors block the degradation of kinins within the kidney, which may contribute substantially to the natriuretic and diuretic effects of NEP inhibitors. In several experimental models the renal effects of NEP inhibitors are abolished upon administering specific bradykinin antagonists (264,265), or, alternatively, are mimicked by administering bradykinin itself (266).

NEP inhibitors variably affect blood pressure. These compounds lower blood pressure in the DOCA/salt hypertensive rat, a model of elevated plasma ANP, and suppress RAA activity. The decrease in blood pressure in this model is accompanied by a decrease in cardiac output. NEP inhibitors also decrease blood pressure in the spontaneously hypertensive rat and sodium-replete sheep, but are typically devoid of antihypertensive effects in normotensive animals. NEP inhibitors have been reported to be ineffective in reducing blood pressure when administered chronically.

Recently, significant attention has been devoted to examining the possible therapeutic utility of NEP inhibitors in congestive heart failure and hypertension. In contrast to C-ANP receptor inhibitors, specific NEP inhibitors exhibit good oral bioavailability and thus are attractive candidates for this purpose. Although results have been somewhat inconsistent, studies using NEP inhibitors in CHF have revealed some beneficial hemodynamic, renal, and endocrine effects (254,267). Coincident with these biologic actions, NEP inhibitors generally increase urinary and plasma ANP and cyclic GMP. Whether these actions will be sufficient to warrant widespread use of NEP inhibitors in heart failure is unclear. To date, no data has been published to validate the use of NEP inhibitors in hypertension. Nevertheless, the possibility that NEP inhibitors, used alone or in combination with other agents, will be useful in treating these cardiovascular disorders is still being actively investigated.

ROLE OF THE NATRIURETIC PEPTIDES IN PHYSIOLOGY AND DISEASE

The overall contribution of the natriuretic peptides to cardiovascular and fluid volume homeostasis under normal and pathophysiological conditions has been a topic of intense investigation. Although the functions of BNP and CNP are just now being defined, a number of lines of evidence, reviewed below, imply that ANP plays a physiological role in affecting the acute, and perhaps chronic, regulation of intravascular fluid volume. A complete understanding of the role of ANP is compromised, however, by the fact that, in addition to the natriuretic peptides, a number of other hormones and neurotransmitters contribute to the complex regulation of cardiovascular and fluid volume homeostasis. By interacting with, and often opposing the actions of ANP, these factors have made it difficult to ascertain the precise contribution of ANP.

The first line of evidence that supports a physiological role of ANP has been gained via our insights into the factors regulating the biosynthesis and release of ANP. As outlined already in this chapter, the release of ANP from storage granules within the atrium is strictly regulated. Increases in central fluid volume distend the atrial walls, leading to the controlled release of ANP into the circulation. This regulated mechanism of secretion of ANP fulfills a paradigm that is common to other hormones and factors that control normal physiologic processes. The evidence that ANP release is modulated by hormones like angiotensin and endothelin, as well as the sympathetic nervous system (SNS), provides yet further support for the hypothesis that ANP acts in concert with these agents to control cardiovascular and fluid volume balance. Nevertheless, these observations, by themselves, cannot be used to substantiate a physiologic role for the peptide.

Further support for a physiological role of ANP is garnered from observations that blood volume expansion causes an acute increase in circulating levels of ANP which correlates temporally with the natriuretic, diuretic, and hormonal effects of this intervention in humans and others species (268–271). In general, the magnitude of the increase in plasma ANP correlates with the magnitude of the renal and hormonal responses, and notably with increases in plasma and urinary concentrations of cyclic GMP, the intracellular mediator of ANP action (272–276). Resection of the atrial appendages blunts the natriuretic response to acute volume expansion in anesthetized rats. Active or passive immunization to ANP also abolishes the renal, hormonal, and cyclic GMP responses to acute volume expansion (277–280) and causes an antinatriuresis and increase in blood pressure under basal conditions in experimental animals (281,282). Finally, administration of a newly identified antagonist of ANP biological receptors, HS-142-1, abro-

gates the renal responses to acute volume expansion (283,284).

A number of studies have shown that the administration of low doses of ANP, which change circulating levels of ANP to the same degree as observed during acute volume-induced atrial distention (50–200 percent), causes cardiovascular, renal, and endocrine effects that would serve to reduce central fluid volume. The magnitude of the effects of low-dose ANP even may be underestimated, as reductions in central venous pressure caused by the administration of exogenous ANP could activate the sympathetic nervous system by unloading cardiopulmonary baroreflex receptors, thus counteracting the effects of the peptide. These data serve as yet further evidence that ANP contributes to the acute regulation of central fluid volume and blood pressure.

The potential role of the natriuretic peptides in the chronic control of fluid volume and blood pressure is not well understood. In general, plasma ANP levels are elevated in patients on a high salt diet and likely contribute to chronic fluid volume regulation. Nevertheless, the overall importance of the natriuretic peptides relative to other physical, neural, and hormonal systems in the chronic control of fluid volume is still unclear.

Hypertension

The natriuretic, diuretic, and hypotensive actions of ANP and BNP suggest a role for these peptides in blood pressure homeostasis. By opposing the vasoconstrictive actions of angiotensin, endothelin, and norepinephrine and the sodium-retaining actions of the RAA system, the natriuretic peptides may play a physiologic role in blood pressure regulation, particularly under circumstances when the RAA and sympathetic nervous systems are activated. In addition, ANP's role in regulating central fluid volume contributes prominently to its ability to regulate blood pressure.

Consistent with a role for ANP in blood pressure regulation is the finding that ANP levels in atrial tissue are elevated in hypertensive Dahl salt-sensitive and spontaneously hypertensive rate (SHR) (285–291). In addition, hypertension appears to augment circulating levels of ANP. For instance, in both the one-kidney, one-clip and DOCA salt-sensitive rat models in which hypertension is induced by volume overload, plasma levels of ANP are elevated (292). In DOCA salt-sensitive rats, the increase in ANP levels suggests that ANP plays a major role in the natriuresis which represents an "escape" from the sodium-retaining effects of mineralocorticoid excess (293).

Numerous laboratories have observed that ANP is elevated from 50–100 percent in hypertensive patients compared with normotensive individuals (294–299), although some studies have failed to support this (300–

303). In hypertensive patient populations, plasma ANP levels have been correlated with systolic or mean blood pressure (i.e., severity of hypertension) (298, 299,304,305). Accordingly, the failure of some studies to detect increased plasma ANP levels in hypertensives may be indicative of cohorts with relatively mild hypertension.

Further support for a role of ANP in hypertension is garnered from observations that acute and chronic infusion of ANP, at low doses which produce only small or undetectable increases in plasma ANP, significantly reduces blood pressure in hypertensive animal models (306,307). In general, the acute antihypertensive effects are more evident in animal models in which the RAA and/or sympathetic nervous systems are activated (i.e., two-kidney, one-clip rat) as compared to models of volume-overload (i.e., one kidney, one-clip). The short-term effect in the two-kidney, one-clip rat is accounted for by a reduction in peripheral vascular resistance, again reflecting the potency of ANP as an antagonist of vaso-constrictive substances. Acute (308–310) as well as chronic (5-day) (311) administration of low-dose ANP into patients with essential hypertension also reduces blood pressure toward normotensive values. In spite of these early promising studies, the development of synthetic ANP as a potential antihypertensive agent has been inhibited by its lack of oral bioavailability.

Congestive Heart Failure

As noted previously, congestive heart failure is associated with a marked increase in the level of expression of the genes encoding ANP and BNP. ANP and BNP expression is increased in the myocardial atria, and, most notably, within the ventricle. Coincident with the increased tissue expression of the two peptides, plasma levels of ANP and BNP increase markedly. Whereas the circulating concentration of BNP is about 20 percent that of ANP in normals, BNP levels may exceed those of ANP in patients with Stage IV CHF (see Fig. 9). Presumably the ventricle contributes a large percentage of the BNP to the circulation of CHF patients as plasma BNP has been shown to correlate tightly with increases in left ventricular end-diastolic volume and ventricular mass. The overall contribution of atrial and ventricular stores of ANP to the plasma pool in CHF is somewhat more controversial, although the plasma ANP levels track increases in atrial filling pressures (312,313). In CHF patients, most of the circulating ANP is the ANP$_{1-28}$ species, although modest amounts of pro-ANP$_{1-126}$ are detectable. In contrast, significant amounts of both BNP$_{1-32}$ and pro-BNP are observed in the plasma of CHF patients. The possibility that other tissues, like the lung, may contribute to the plasma pool of ANP and BNP in CHF can not be excluded.

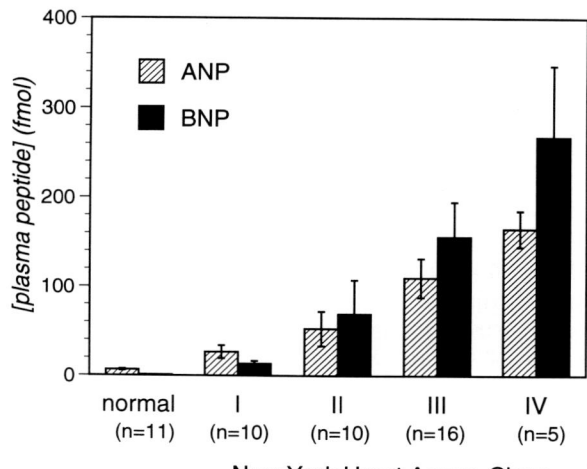

FIG. 9. Elevated levels of plasma ANP and BNP in patients with congestive heart failure compared with normal subjects. Patients are grouped by severity of disease according to the New York Heart Association guidelines. (Drawn from data in ref. 318.)

Paradoxically, in spite of elevated circulating levels of ANP in the CHF setting, evidence suggests a relative deficiency of myocardial ANP in CHF. For example, elevation of atrial pressure by acute volume expansion in dogs with experimental CHF (314) and by exercise in CHF patients (313) results in a blunted induction of ANP release compared with normal animals. Nevertheless, the observations that increases in central blood volume cause further secretion of ANP, and findings that measures which unload the heart acutely reduce plasma ANP levels, imply that the secretory dynamics of ANP are preserved, at least qualitatively, in CHF.

The role of endogenous ANP and BNP in the pathophysiology of CHF is still unclear. It has been proposed that secretion of ANP and BNP by the failing heart provides a compensatory response of the failing heart to combat the fluid overload. This may be true despite the fact that the kidney is generally refractory to ANP in the setting of CHF, although the possibility that BNP may be more active in CHF cannot be excluded. Indeed, the level of sodium and fluid retention could be greater in the absence of these two peptides. Consistent with this latter possibility is the finding that infusion of a neutralizing monoclonal antibody to ANP in a rat model of CHF causes an antinatriuresis, a decrease in cardiac output, and an increase in peripheral systemic resistance (315). Similarly, administration of the ANP antagonist HS-142-1 promotes marked antinatriuresis in a canine model of CHF. The observations that clearance receptor blockers and NEP inhibitors provide at least some hemodynamic and/or renal benefit in the setting of CHF, presumably by modulating circulating or local renal levels of the natriuretic peptides, provide yet further support for a protective role for the natriuretic peptides in CHF.

ANP and BNP as Markers of Ventricular Dysfunction

Numerous studies demonstrate elevated ANP levels in congestive heart failure patients that correlate with cardiac filling pressure (312) and pulmonary capillary wedge pressure (313). Studies have also shown that ANP peptides derived from the amino-terminus of proANP$_{1-126}$, including proANP$_{1-98}$ (316,317) and proANP$_{31-67}$ (40), are also elevated in the blood of patients with heart disease and the levels correlate with the severity of disease as defined by the New York Heart Association classification and left ventricular function. The finding that proANP$_{1-98}$ is significantly elevated above control levels in patients with proven ventricular dysfunction by radionuclide angiography yet without symptoms of heart failure (NYHA class I) suggests that it might be a useful and specific marker for early stage disease (316).

Several studies (12,318–320) have demonstrated circulating BNP levels elevated significantly in patients with congestive heart failure when compared with disease-free individuals. Several-hundred-fold increases in plasma BNP levels have been reported in heart disease patients (see Fig. 9 from reference [318]). Increases in circulating BNP levels have been shown to correlate significantly with the severity of disease when classified by the NYHA guidelines (12,318,319).

Recently, plasma BNP levels have been shown to correlate significantly with the degree of left ventricular dysfunction as measured by echocardiography (320). A subset of patients treated with the angiotensin-converting enzyme (ACE) inhibitor captopril had lower BNP levels and an increase in left ventricular ejection fraction after 6 months compared to a placebo-treated control group. These studies suggest that circulating BNP levels may also be a valuable diagnostic for ventricular dysfunction. In light of the Survival and Ventricular Enlargement (SAVE) study demonstrating that patients with low ejection fractions benefitted from long-term treatment with ACE inhibitors in terms of improved survival, reduced reinfarction incidence, and slower rate of progression to chronic heart disease, a rapid, simple, and inexpensive diagnostic to identify appropriate individuals for treatment should be most useful. The relative value of using ANP peptides versus BNP as a diagnostic marker for ventricular function must await more detailed studies although the fact that BNP is released from the ventricles suggests it may be a more specific marker of ventricular dysfunction.

Therapeutic Applications

Cardiac insufficiency in the setting of CHF triggers a compensatory neurohormonal response (activation of the RAA axis and SNS) to preserve perfusion of vital vascular beds, but which also increases pulmonary and systemic pressures, fluid retention, and leads, ultimately, to further reductions in cardiac output. The novel biological actions of ANP which oppose fluid retention and elevate blood pressure prompted researchers to investigate the peptide in this clinical setting. These studies have revealed that ANP when administered as a bolus (321) or continuous infusion (117,159,322) decreases both pulmonary capillary wedge pressure and systemic vascular resistance and increases cardiac output. These changes occur without a concomitant increase in heart rate and little or no decrease in blood pressure. The cardiac and hemodynamic effects are rapid and can be detected within 5 minutes after administration of the peptide. Although at present the precise way in which ANP acts in heart failure is not completely defined, the data suggest that the peptide affects both preload and afterload by promoting both arterial and venous dilation without directly affecting the myocardium. This is consistent with the observations that the vasodilatory actions of the peptide are most profound when the RAA and SNS systems are activated.

Despite the favorable hemodynamic effects of ANP, enthusiasm has waned toward using this peptide to treat CHF and other edematous states. This lack of enthusiasm arises, in large part, from observations that the renal actions of ANP are blunted substantially in these clinical settings (117,159,323). In contrast to its effects in normal volunteers, ANP has been shown to exert little or no natriuretic and diuretic activities in patients with CHF. Several mechanisms have been proposed to explain this blunted renal effect, including: reduced renal blood flow; activation of neurohumoral pathways (e.g., renin-angiotensin, endothelin, and norepinephrine) that blunt ANP's cellular actions; downregulation or prior occupancy of biological receptors of ANP in the face of elevated circulatory levels of the peptide; and upregulation of metabolic clearance pathways (see below).

The possible use of other natriuretic peptides, or modulators of ANP clearance, to treat CHF has been raised by recent reports in the literature. For instance, a recent study in a small cohort of CHF patients demonstrated that a short intravenous infusion of BNP improves left ventricular function (increased stroke volume index), hemodynamic status (decreased pulmonary capillary wedge pressure and systemic vascular resistance), and, in sharp contrast to findings with ANP, markedly enhances the urinary output of sodium and water (197). Nevertheless, further studies will be required to substantiate this finding. Recent reports have also identified urodilatin (ANP$_{95-126}$) as an agent which may provide hemodynamic, renal, and endocrine benefit in the setting of heart failure (324). Finally, the potential use of inhibitors of ANP clearance in this clinical setting, such as neutral endopeptidase inhibitors, is being explored actively.

Supraventricular Tachyarrhythmias

Plasma ANP levels rise during supraventricular tachycardia and then fall when sinus rhythm is restored (325–332). While increased ANP has been correlated with increased atrial pressure resulting from cardiac arrhythmias (332–334), several animal and human studies have observed tachycardia-associated ANP induction in the absence of elevated atrial pressure, suggesting that the stimulus to release ANP may result from direct effects on atrial tissue tension (335–338). The natriuresis and diuresis associated with cardiac tachyarrhythmias have been attributed at least in part to the direct renal effects of the ANP induced by these cardiac events; this is consistent with the observation that other known actions of ANP including increased glomerular filtration rate, increased hematocrit, and decreased aldosterone and vasopressin are also associated with cardiac tachycardia (331,339).

Acute Renal Dysfunction

A reduction in nephron number associated with chronic renal failure with a constant dietary sodium load results in an increase in plasma fluid volume and an increase in atrial pressure which stimulates ANP release. Elevated levels of circulating ANP have been documented in patients with edematous chronic renal failure (340–344), and, predictably, decreasing fluid load by ultrafiltration and dialysis results in a rapid decrease in circulating ANP (342,345–350). Evidence suggests that ANP released in this setting increases natriuresis per functioning nephron as a compensatory response to restore plasma fluid volume homeostasis (351). In rats with experimental chronic renal failure induced by partial (5/6) nephrectomy, ANP was shown to increase GFR, a striking observation as the reduced renal mass associated with this experimental model results in an elevated single nephron glomerular filtration rate as a compensatory response (352). Thus ANP can further promote renal function thereby supplementing endogenous compensatory mechanisms in the setting of renal dysfunction.

Therapeutic Applications

Intrinsic acute renal failure (ARF) is a complex clinical syndrome associated with a rapid decline in kidney function often resulting from ischemic stress associated with trauma, sepsis, postoperative complications, and adverse effects from certain therapeutic treatments. Kidney ischemia resulting from inadequate blood supply develops from excessive renal vasoconstriction induced by production of and/or increased sensitivity to vasocon-

strictive agents (e.g., endothelin, angiotensin II, thromboxane A2, norepinephrine, and adenosine), decreased production of vasodilators (e.g., endothelial-derived relaxing factor [EDRF] and prostacyclin), and activation of the inhibitory potential of tubular glomerular feedback (353). In addition, the accumulation of cellular debris (protein casts) in renal tubules raises tubular pressure, thereby inhibiting glomerular filtration.

The potential therapeutic use of ANP in the setting of ischemic acute renal failure has received much attention given its renal actions in opposing vasoconstrictors and stimulating GFR. ANP treatment of rats with kidney ischemia induced by renal artery clamping (354,355) or norepinephrine-induced renal artery vasoconstriction (356,357) has been shown to decrease tissue damage and promote renal function. To improve the clinical relevance of the animal model, one study delayed ANP treatment for 48 hours following norepinephrine-induced ischemia, and showed increased renal function and decreased tissue damage in the ANP-treated group (357). The ability of ANP to restore glomerular filtration in these animal models may reflect (a) direct vascular effects of ANP (vasodilation of the afferent renal artery and vasoconstriction of the efferent renal artery) resulting in increased glomerular hydraulic pressure, (b) inhibition of the negative influence of tubular glomerular feedback, and (c) ANP-induced increases in urine flow, which serves to remove tubular debris. Various strategies have been successfully used to oppose the hypotensive effects of ANP seen in some experimental models of ARF in animals. In one animal study, dopamine effectively inhibited ANP-induced hypotension yet did not affect the renal protective effects demonstrated by ANP treatment (357). A second approach was shown in a rat renal artery clamp model of ARF in which it was demonstrated that mannitol synergizes with ANP to promote GFR, thereby allowing lower nonhypotensive doses of ANP to be used which remained renal-protective (358).

Recent clinical reports appear to confirm the beneficial renal effects seen in these initial experimental animal studies. In a recent placebo-controlled study in patients with established acute renal failure, ANP treatment, administered either intravenously or by infusion directly into the renal artery, was shown in a statistically significant manner to increase GFR as measured by creatinine clearance and to decrease the need for dialysis (359). In a second study in heart transplant patients, a clinical setting with a high incidence of renal failure, prophylactic ANP$_{95-126}$ treatment over a 4-day period was associated with significantly improved renal function compared with untreated historical control patients as measured by decreased plasma creatinine and serum urea and a lower incidence of dialysis (360). Thus the ability of ANP to promote kidney function in the setting of acute renal dysfunction suggests a therapeutic value of ANP as a novel renal protective agent.

Renal transplant studies in dogs have shown that ANP in the kidney storage bath (361) or intravenous infusion into organ recipients (362) resulted in beneficial renal effects. In addition, ANP promoted transplanted kidney function in the setting of acute renal allograft rejection in a canine model (363). In spite of these as well as other (364) positive studies of experimental renal transplant in animals, various treatment protocols exploring therapeutic benefits in human renal transplant patients have thus far been equivocal (365–367).

CONCLUSIONS

The natriuretic peptides likely play a fundamental role in the regulation of vascular hemodynamics, including vascular fluid volume and pressure. Our understanding of the biological properties of this hormonal system is most advanced with respect to the biological actions of ANP. Responding to atrial stretch from fluid overload, the cardiac atria release ANP, which exerts a wide variety of renal, hormonal, and vascular actions to decrease vascular fluid volume. In its role in maintaining vascular fluid homeostasis, ANP acts to counterbalance the renin-angiotensin-aldosterone system, endothelin, vasopressin, and various actions of the sympathetic nervous system. Disease states resulting in chronic cardiac overload (chronic renal failure, congestive heart failure, hypertension) induce a state of increased ANP release, and in advanced disease states resulting in cardiac hypertrophy and decreased cardiac output, the heart recruits the ventricle to produce BNP to act in concert with ANP in an effort to reduce fluid stress on the heart and increase cardiac performance. The dramatic elevation of circulating ANP and BNP in response to increased cardiac stress in the setting of congestive heart failure, together with the peptide's actions to promote fluid loss and promote cardiac function, is consistent with an important protective function of these natriuretic peptides in this disease.

The unique receptor specificity of CNP suggests that the biological actions of this peptide will be fundamentally different from ANP and BNP. The antimitogenic effects of CNP (as well as the other natriuretic peptides) may reveal a new physiological function of the natriuretic peptides related to regulation of vascular tissue remodeling. Studies to define the actions of CNP as well as how these actions are integrated with ANP and BNP promise to be an exciting avenue of research.

Our current knowledge of the natriuretic peptide family suggests a widespread role in both normal physiology and disease. Thus, the therapeutic potential of compounds that mimic the actions of the natriuretic peptide hormones or that promote endogenous natriuretic peptide activity for the treatment of heart failure, hypertension, renal failure, and other diseases not discussed in this chapter such as asthma (356–358), remains great and the focus of much attention. In the 12 years since the discovery of ANP, research into the natriuretic peptides has offered a deeper understanding of how the body regulates vascular fluid volume and pressure. Nevertheless, this field is still in its infancy and further research of the natriuretic peptide family promises to add new insights into fundamental mechanisms of cardiovascular homeostasis.

REFERENCES

1. deBold AJ, Borenstein HB, Veress AT, Sonnenberg HA. *Life Sci* 1981;28:89–94.
2. Kisch B. *Exp Med Surg* 1956;114:99–112.
3. Jamieson JD, Palade GE. *J Cell Biol* 1964;23:151–172.
4. Yamanaka M, Greenberg B, Johnson L, et al. *Nature* 1984;309(5970):719–722.
5. Maki M, Takayanagi R, Misono KS, Pandey KN, Tibbetts C, Inagami T. *Nature* 1984;309(5970):722–724.
6. Kangawa K, Tawaragi Y, Oikawa S, et al. *Nature* 1984;312(5990):152–155.
7. Nakayama K, Ohkubo H, Hirose T, Inayama S, Nakanishi S. *Nature* 1984;310(5979):699–701.
8. Seidman CE, Duby AD, Choi E, et al. *Science* 1984;225(4659):324–326.
9. Bloch KD, Scott JA, Zisfein JB, et al. *Science* 1985;230(4730):1168–1171.
10. Shields PP, Glembotski CC. *J Biol Chem* 1988;263(17):8091–8098.
11. Glembotski CC, Oronzi ME, Li XB, et al. *Endocrinol* 1987;121(3):843–852.
12. Mukoyama M, Nakao K, Hosoda K, et al. *J Clin Invest* 1991;87(4):1402–1412.
13. Bloch KD, Seidman JG, Naftilan JD, Fallon JT, Seidman CE. *Cell* 1986;47(5):695–702.
14. Lang RE, Tholken H, Ganten D, Luft FC, Ruskoaho H, Unger T. *Nature* 1985;314(6008):264–266.
15. Schwartz D, Geller DM, Manning PT, et al. *Science* 1985;229(4711):397–400.
16. Thibault G, Lazure C, Schiffrin EL, et al. *Biochem Biophys Res Commun* 1985;130(3):981–986.
17. Theiss G, John A, Morich F, et al. *FEBS Lett* 1987;218(1):159–162.
18. Yandle T, Crozier I, Nicholls G, Espiner E, Carne A, Brennan S. *Biochem Biophys Res Commun* 1987;146(2):832–839.
19. Ogawa Y, Nakao K, Mukoyama M, et al. *Circ Res* 1991;69(2):491–500.
20. Kangawa K, Fukuda A, Kubota I, Hayashi Y, Minamitake Y, Matsuo H. *J Hypertens Suppl* 1984;2(3):S321–S323.
21. Akimoto K, Miyata A, Kangawa K, Koga Y, Hayakawa K, Matsuo H. *J Clin Endocrinol Metab* 1988;67(1):93–97.
22. Miyata A, Toshimori T, Hashiguchi T, Kangawa K, Matsuo H. *Biochem Biophys Res Commun* 1987;142(2):461–467.
23. Marumo F, Kurosawa T, Takeda S, Katoh Y, Hasegawa N, Ando K. *Klin Wochenschr* 1988;66(15):675–681.
24. Ando K, Hirata Y, Emori T, et al. *J Clin Endocrinol Metab* 1990;70(6):1603–1607.
25. Sugawara A, Nakao K, Morii N, et al. *Biochem Biophys Res Commun* 1988;150(1):60–67.
26. Sugawara A, Nakao K, Morii N, et al. *J Clin Invest* 1988;81(6):1962–1970.
27. Naruse M, Hiroe M, Naruse K, et al. *Am J Hypertens* 1990;3(2):105–110.
28. Chino N, Yoshizawa-Kumagaye K, Noda Y, Watanabe TX, Kimura T, Sakakibara S. *Biochem Biophys Res Commun* 1986;141(2):665–672.

29. Heim JM, Kiefersauer S, Fulle HJ, Gerzer R. *Biochem Biophys Res Commun* 1989;163(1):37–41.

30. Kambayashi Y, Kawabata T, Hara S, et al. *FEBS Lett* 1986;206(2):313–318.

31. Itoh H, Nakao K, Shiono S, et al. *Biochem Biophys Res Commun* 1987;143(2):560–569.

32. Schulz-Knappe P, Forssmann K, Herbst F, Hock D, Pipkorn R, Forssmann WG. *Klin Wochenschr* 1988;66(17):752–759.

33. Ritter D, Needleman P, Greenwald JE. *J Clin Invest* 1991;87(1):208–212.

34. Ramirez G, Saba SR, Dietz JR, Vesely DL. *Kidney Int* 1992;41(2):334–341.

35. Greenwald JE, Ritter D, Tetens E, Rotwein PS. *Am J Physiol* 1992;263(5 Pt 2):F974–F978.

36. Valentin JP, Sechi LA, Qui C, Schambelan M, Humphreys MH. *Hypertension* 1993;21(4):432–438.

37. Saxenhofer H, Raselli A, Weidmann P, et al. *Am J Physiol* 1990;259(5 Pt 2):F832–F838.

38. Bestle MH, Bie P. *Acta Physiol Scand* 1993;149(1):77–83.

39. Winters CJ, Sallman AL, Meadows J, Rico DM, Vesely DL. *Biochem Biophys Res Commun* 1988;150(1):231–236.

40. Winters CJ, Sallman AL, Baker BJ, Meadows J, Rico DM, Vesely DL. *Circulation* 1989;80(3):438–449.

41. Ngo L, Wyeth RP, Bissett JK, et al. *Am Heart J* 1989;117(2):385–390.

42. Martin DR, Pevahouse JB, Trigg DJ, Vesely DL, Buerkert JE. *Am J Physiol* 1990;258(5 Pt 2):F1401–F1408.

43. Denker PS, Vesely DL, Gomez-Sanchez CE. *J Steroid Biochem Mol Biol* 1990;37(4):617–619.

44. Vesely DL, Douglass MA, Dietz JR, et al. *Clin Res* 1993;41(2):117A.

45. Greenberg BD, Bencen GH, Seilhamer JJ, Lewicki JA, Fiddes JC. *Nature* 1984;312(5995):656–658.

46. Nemer M, Chamberland M, Sirois D, et al. *Nature* 1984;312(5995):654–656.

47. Seidman CE, Bloch KD, Klein KA, Smith JA, Seidman JG. *Science* 1984;226(4679):1206–1209.

48. Argentin S, Nemer M, Drouin J, Scott GK, Kennedy BP, Davies PL. *J Biol Chem* 1985;260(8):4568–4571.

49. Field LJ. *Science* 1988;239(4843):1029–1033.

50. Wu J, LaPointe MC, West BL, Gardner DG. *J Biol Chem* 1989;264(11):6472–6479.

51. Wu JP, Kovacic-Milivojevic B, Lapointe MC, Nakamura K, Gardner DG. *Mol Endocrinol* 1991;5(9):1311–1322.

52. Schiebinger RJ, Linden J. *Circ Res* 1986;59(1):105–109.

53. Edwards BS, Zimmerman RS, Schwab TR, Heublein DM, Burnett J, Jr. *Circ Res* 1988;62(2):191–195.

54. Ruskoaho H, Tholken H, Lang RE. *Pflueg Arch* 1986;407(2):170–174.

55. Takayanagi R, Tanaka I, Maki M, Inagami T. *Life Sci* 1985;36(19):1843–1848.

56. Zisfein JB, Matsueda GR, Fallon JT, et al. *J Mol Cell Cardiol* 1986;18(9):917–929.

57. Lattion AL, Aubert JF, Fluckiger JP, Nussberger J, Waeber B, Brunner HR. *Am J Physiol* 1988;255(2 Pt 2):H245–H249.

58. Iwao H, Fukui K, Kim S, et al. *Am J Physiol* 1988;255(2 Pt 1):E129–E136.

59. Lattion AL, Michel JB, Arnauld E, Corvol P, Soubrier F. *Am J Physiol* 1986;251(5 Pt 2):H890–H896.

60. Gardner DG, Wirtz H, Dobbs LG. *Am J Physiol* 1992;263(2 Pt 1):E239–E244.

61. Day ML, Schwartz D, Wiegand RC, et al. *Hypertension* 1987;9(5):485–491.

62. Izumo S, Nadal-Ginard B, Mahdavi V. *Proc Natl Acad Sci USA* 1988;85(2):339–343.

63. Takahashi T, Allen PD, Izumo S. *Circ Res* 1992;71(1):9–17.

64. Fischer TA, Haass M, Dietz R, et al. *Clin Sci* 1991;80(4):285–291.

65. Saito Y, Nakao K, Arai H, et al. *Biochem Biophys Res Commun* 1987;148(1):211–217.

66. Komuro I, Yazaki Y. *Annu Rev Physiol* 1993;55(75):55–75.

67. Bohmann D, Bos TJ, Admon A, Nishimura T, Vogt PK, Tjian R. *Science* 1987;238(4832):1386–1392.

68. Chiu R, Boyle WJ, Meek J, Smeal T, Hunter T, Karin M. *Cell* 1988;54(4):541–552.

69. Sassone-Corsi P, Lamph WW, Kamps M, Verma IM. *Cell* 1988;54(4):553–560.

70. Kovacic-Milivojevic B, Gardner DG. *Mol Cell Biol* 1992;12(1):292–301.

71. Wei YF, Rodi CP, Day ML, et al. *J Clin Invest* 1987;79(5):1325–1329.

72. Wu JP, Deschepper CF, Gardner DG. *Am J Physiol* 1988;255(3 Pt 1):E388–E396.

73. Tsuchimochi H, Kurimoto F, Ieki K, et al. *Circulation* 1988;78(4):920–927.

74. Dietz JR. *Am J Physiol* 1987;252(3 Pt 2):R498–R502.

75. Bilder GE, Schofield TL, Blaine EH. *Am J Physiol* 1986;251(5 Pt 2):F817–F821.

76. Onwochei MO, Snajdar RM, Rapp JP. *Am J Physiol* 1987;253(5 Pt 2):H1044–H1052.

77. Ruskoaho H, Vuolteenaho O, Leppaluoto J. *Endocrinol* 1990;127(5):2445–2455.

78. Schwab TR, Edwards BS, Heublein DM, Burnett J Jr. *Am J Physiol* 1986;251(2 Pt 2):R310–R313.

79. Anderson JV, Christofides ND, Bloom SR. *J Endocrinol* 1986;109(1):9–13.

80. Verburg KM, Freeman RH, Davis JO, Villarreal D, Vari RC. *Am J Physiol* 1986;251(5 Pt 2):R947–R956.

81. Kohno M, Clegg KB, Sambhi MP. *Hypertension* 1987;10(2):171–175.

82. John A, Stasch JP, Neuser D, Hirth C, Morich FJ. *Life Sci* 1986;38(22):1991–1997.

83. Eskay R, Zukowska-Grojec Z, Haass M, Dave JR, Zamir N. *Science* 1986;232(4750):636–639.

84. Dietz JR, Nazian SJ. *Am J Physiol* 1988;255(4 Pt 2):R534–R538.

85. Pettersson A, Ricksten SE, Towle AC, Hedner J, Hedner T. *Acta Physiol Scand* 1988;133(4):513–518.

86. Ledsome JR, Wilson N, Courneya CA, Rankin AJ. *Can J Physiol Pharmacol* 1985;63(6):739–742.

87. Metzler CH, Lee ME, Thrasher TN, Ramsay DJ. *Endocrinol* 1986;119(5):2396–2398.

88. Mancini GB, McGillem MJ, Bates ER, Weder AB, DeBoe SF, Grekin RJ. *Circulation* 1987;76(4):884–890.

89. Yamaji T, Ishibashi M, Takaku F. *J Clin Invest* 1985;76(4):1705–1709.

90. Sagnella GA, Markandu ND, Shore AC, MacGregor GA. *Lancet* 1985;2(8466):1208–1211.

91. Kimura T, Abe K, Ota K, et al. *J Clin Endocrinol Metab* 1986;62(5):1003–1010.

92. Anderson JV, Millar ND, O'Hare JP, Mackenzie JC, Corrall RJ, Bloom SR. *Clin Sci* 1986;71(3):319–322.

93. Myers BD, Peterson C, Molina C, et al. *Am J Physiol* 1988;254(4 Pt 2):F562–F573.

94. Zamir N, Haass M, Dave JR, Zukowska-Grojec Z. *Proc Natl Acad Sci USA* 1987;84(2):541–545.

95. Morris M, Alexander N. *Endocrinol* 1988;122(1):373–375.

96. Jiao JH, Baertschi AJ. *Proc Natl Acad Sci USA* 1993;90(16):7799–7803.

97. Geny B, Piquard F, Follenius M, et al. *Am J Physiol* 1993;265:F112–F118.

98. Itoh H, Nakao K, Yamada T, et al. *Endocrinol* 1987;120(5):2186–2188.

99. Baranowska B, Gutkowska J, Lemire A, Cantin M, Genest J. *Biochem Biophys Res Commun* 1987;145(2):680–685.

100. Dietz JR. *Proc Soc Exp Biol Med* 1988;187(3):366–369.

101. Garcia R, Lachance D, Thibault G. *J Hypertens* 1990;8(8):725–731.

102. Volpe M, Atlas SA, Sosa RE, et al. *Circ Res* 1990;67(3):774–779.

103. Suzuki E, Hirata Y, Kohmoto O, et al. *Circ Res* 1992;71(5):1039–1048.

104. Fukuda Y, Hirata Y, Taketani S, et al. *Biochem Biophys Res Commun* 1989;164(3):1431–1436.

105. Horio T, Kohno M, Takeda T. *Metabolism* 1993;42(1):94–96.

106. Mantymaa P, Leppaluoto J, Ruskoaho H. *Endocrinol* 1990;126(1):587–595.

107. Winquist RJ, Scott AL, Vlasuk GP. *Hypertension* 1989;14(1):111–114.

108. Garbers DL. *Pharmacol Ther* 1991;50(3):337–345.
109. Koller KJ, de Sauvage FJ, Lowe DG, Goeddel DV. *Mol Cell Biol* 1992;12(6):2581–2590.
110. Schenk DB, Phelps MN, Porter JG, Fuller F, Cordell B, Lewicki JA. *Proc Natl Acad Sci USA* 1987;84(6):1521–1525.
111. Maack T, Suzuki M, Almeida FA, et al. *Science* 1987;238(4827):675–678.
112. Maack T, Camargo MJ, Kleinert HD, Laragh JH, Atlas SA. *Kidney Int* 1985;27(4):607–615.
113. Atlas SA. *Recent Prog Horm Res* 1986;42(49):207–249.
114. Cantin M, Genest J. *Endocr Rev* 1985;6(2):107–127.
115. Needleman P, Greenwald JE. *N Engl J Med* 1986;314(13):828–834.
116. Maack T, Marion DN, Camargo MJ, et al. *Am J Med* 1984;77(6):1069–1075.
117. Cody RJ, Atlas SA, Laragh JH, et al. *J Clin Invest* 1986;78(5):1362–1374.
118. Huang CL, Lewicki J, Johnson LK, Cogan MG. *J Clin Invest* 1985;75(2):769–773.
119. Camargo MJ, Kleinert HD, Atlas SA, Sealey JE, Laragh JH, Maack T. *Am J Physiol* 1984;246(4 Pt 2):F447–F456.
120. Camargo MJ, Atlas SA, Maack T. *Life Sci* 1986;38(26):2397–2404.
121. Dunn BR, Ichikawa I, Pfeffer JM, Troy JL, Brenner BM. *Circ Res* 1986;59(3):237–246.
122. Burnett J Jr, Granger JP, Opgenorth TJ. *Am J Physiol* 1984;247(5 Pt 2):F863–F866.
123. Atlas SA, Kleinert HD, Camargo MJ, et al. *Nature* 1984;309(5970):717–719.
124. Fried TA, McCoy RN, Osgood RW, Stein JH. *Am J Physiol* 1986;250(6 Pt 2):F1119–F1122.
125. Loutzenhiser R, Hayashi K, Epstein M. *J Pharmacol Exp Ther* 1988;246(2):522–528.
126. Maack T, Kleinert HD. *Biochem Pharmacol* 1986;35(13):2057–2064.
127. Marin-Grez M, Fleming JT, Steinhausen M. *Nature* 1986;324(6096):473–476.
128. Maack T. In: Puschett JB, Greenberg A, eds. *Diuretics II*. New York: Alan R. Liss; 1986:242–249.
129. Davis CL, Briggs JP. *Am J Physiol* 1987;253(4 Pt 2):F679–F684.
130. Maack T. *Biologically active atrial peptides.* New York: Raven Press; 1987:109–118.
131. Kiberd BA, Larson TS, Robertson CR, Jamison RL. *Am J Physiol* 1987;252(6 Pt 2):F1112–F1117.
132. Mendez RE, Dunn BR, Troy JL, Brenner BM. *Kidney Int* 1988;34(1):36–42.
133. Sonnenberg H, Honrath U, Chong CK, Wilson DR. *Am J Physiol* 1986;250(6 Pt 2):F963–F966.
134. Sonnenberg H. *Fed Proc* 1986;45(7):2106–2110.
135. Cantiello HF, Ausiello DA. *Biochem Biophys Res Commun* 1986;134(2):852–860.
136. Light DB, Schwiebert EM, Karlson KH, Stanton BA. *Science* 1989;243(4889):383–385.
137. Zeidel ML. *Annu Rev Physiol* 1990;52(59):747–759.
138. Zeidel ML, Kikeri D, Silva P, Burrowes M, Brenner BM. *J Clin Invest* 1988;82(3):1067–1074.
139. Rocha AS, Kudo LH. *Am J Physiol* 1990;259(2 Pt 2):F258–F268.
140. Harris PJ, Thomas D, Morgan TO. *Nature* 1987;326(6114):697–698.
141. Garvin JL. *Am J Physiol* 1992;263(4 Pt 2):F581–F585.
142. Nonoguchi H, Sands JM, Knepper MA. *Am J Physiol* 1989;256(1 Pt 2):F179–F186.
143. Sosa RE, Volpe M, Marion DN, et al. *Am J Physiol* 1986;250(3 Pt 2):F520–F524.
144. Cogan MG. *Am J Physiol* 1986;250(4 Pt 2):F710–F714.
145. Freeman RH, Davis JO, Vari RC. *Am J Physiol* 1985;248(4 Pt 2):R495–R500.
146. Seymour AA, Smith S, Mazack EK. *Am J Physiol* 1987;253(2 Pt 2):F234–F238.
147. Bie P, Wang BC, Leadley R Jr, Goetz KL. *Am J Physiol* 1990;258(5 Pt 2):R1101–R1107.
148. Koepke JP, Jones S, DiBona GF. *Am J Physiol* 1987;252(5 Pt 2):R1019–R1023.
149. Kleinert HD, Volpe M, Odell G, et al. *Hypertension* 1986;8(4):312–316.
150. Crozier IG, Nicholls MG, Ikram H, Espiner EA, Gomez HJ, Warner NJ. *Lancet* 1986;2(8518):1242–1245.
151. Garcia R, Gutkowska J, Cantin M, Thibault G. *Hypertension* 1987;9(1):88–95.
152. Winquist RJ, Faison EP, Waldman SA, Schwartz K, Murad F, Rapoport RM. *Proc Natl Acad Sci USA* 1984;81(23):7661–7664.
153. Garcia R, Thibault G, Cantin M, Genest J. *Am J Physiol* 1984;247(1 Pt 2):R34–R39.
154. Kleinert HD, Maack T, Atlas SA, Januszewicz A, Sealey JE, Laragh JH. *Hypertension* 1984;6(2 Pt 2):I143–I147.
155. Murad F. *J Clin Invest* 1986;78(1):1–5.
156. Shen YT, Young MA, Ohanian J, Graham RM, Vatner SF. *Circ Res* 1990;66(3):647–661.
157. Woods RL, Anderson WP. *Am J Physiol* 1990;259(4 Pt 2):R813–R822.
158. Almeida FA, Suzuki M, Maack T. *Life Sci* 1986;39(13):1193–1199.
159. Saito Y, Nakao K, Nishimura K, et al. *Circulation* 1987;76(1):115–124.
160. Huxley VH, Tucker VL, Verburg KM, Freeman RH. *Circ Res* 1987;60(2):304–307.
161. Huxley VH, Meyer D Jr. *Am J Physiol* 1990;259(5 Pt 2):H1351–H1356.
162. Trippodo NC, Cole FE, Frohlich ED, MacPhee AA. *Circ Res* 1986;59(3):291–296.
163. Chien YW, Frohlich ED, Trippodo NC. *Am J Physiol* 1987;252(5 Pt 2):H894–H899.
164. Lee RW, Goldman S. *Am J Physiol* 1989;256(3 Pt 2):H760–H765.
165. Mizelle HL, Gaillard CA, Manning RD, Hall JE. *Am J Physiol* 1992;262(1 Pt 2):R120–R125.
166. Parkes DG, Coghlan JP, McDougall JG, Scoggins BA. *Am J Physiol* 1988;254(4 Pt 2):H811–H815.
167. Gaillard CA, Mizelle HL, Montani JP, Brands MW, Hildebrandt DA, Hall JE. *Am J Physiol* 1990;259(5 Pt 2):R973–R980.
168. Kudo T, Baird A. *Nature* 1985;312(5996):756–757.
169. Chartier L, Schiffrin E, Thibault G, Garcia R. *Endocrinol* 1984;115(5):2026–2028.
170. Opgenorth TJ, Burnett J Jr, Granger JP, Scriven TA. *Am J Physiol* 1986;250(5 Pt 2):F798–F801.
171. Thoren P, Mark AL, Morgan DA, O'Neill TP, Needleman P, Brody MJ. *Am J Physiol* 1986;251(6 Pt 2):H1252–H1259.
172. Imaizumi T, Takeshita A, Higashi H, Nakamura M. *Am J Physiol* 1987;253(5 Pt 2):H1136–H1140.
173. Ehmke H, Persson P, Fischer S, Hackenthal E, Kirchheim H. *Pflueg Arch* 1989;413(3):261–266.
174. Ehmke H, Persson PB, Just A, et al. *Am J Physiol* 1992;263(3 Pt 2):R529–R536.
175. Goodfriend TL, Elliott ME, Atlas SA. *Life Sci* 1984;35(16):1675–1682.
176. Campbell WB, Currie MG, Needleman P. *Circ Res* 1985;57(1):113–118.
177. Schiebinger RJ, Kem DC, Brown RD. *Life Sci* 1988;42(8):919–926.
178. Barrett PQ, Isales CM. *Endocrinol* 1988;122(3):799–808.
179. McCarthy RT, Isales CM, Bollag WB, Rasmussen H, Barrett PQ. *Am J Physiol* 1990;258(3 Pt 2):F473–F478.
180. Opgenorth TJ, Novosad EI. *Eur J Pharmacol* 1990;191(3):351–357.
181. Kohno M, Horio T, Ikeda M, et al. *Kidney Int* 1992;42(4):860–866.
182. Kohno M, Horio T, Yokokawa K, Kurihara N, Takeda T. *Hypertension* 1992;19(4):320–325.
183. Imura H, Nakao K, Itoh H. *Front Neuroendocrinol* 1992;13(3):217–249.
184. Samson WK. *Neuroendocr* 1985;40(3):277–279.
185. Samson WK, Aguila MC, Martinovic J, Antunes-Rodrigues J, Norris M. *Peptides* 1987;8(3):449–454.
186. Sudoh T, Kangawa K, Minamino N, Matsuo H. *Nature* 1988;332(6159):78–81.

187. Suga S, Nakao K, Hosoda K, et al. *Endocrinol* 1992;130(1):229–239.
188. Lowe DG, Fendly BM. *J Biol Chem* 1992;267(30):21691–21697.
189. Sudoh T, Maekawa K, Kojima M, Minamino N, Kangawa K, Matsuo H. *Biochem Biophys Res Commun* 1989;159(3):1427–1434.
190. Seilhamer JJ, Arfsten A, Miller JA, et al. *Biochem Biophys Res Commun* 1989;165(2):650–658.
191. Kojima M, Minamino N, Kangawa K, Matsuo H. *Biochem Biophys Res Commun* 1989;159(3):1420–1426.
192. Kambayashi Y, Nakao K, Kimura H, et al. *Biochem Biophys Res Commun* 1990;173(2):599–605.
193. Seymour AA, Asaad MM, Abboa-Offei BE, Rovnyak PL, Fennell S, Rogers WL. *J Pharmacol Exp Ther* 1992;262(1):60–70.
194. Hosoda K, Nakao K, Mukoyama M, et al. *Hypertension* 1991;17(6 Pt 2):1152–1155.
195. Tateyama H, Hino J, Minamino N, et al. *Biochem Biophys Res Commun* 1992;185(2):760–767.
196. Holmes SJ, Espiner EA, Richards AM, Yandle TG, Frampton C. *J Clin Endocrinol Metab* 1993;76(1):91–96.
197. Yoshimura M, Yasue H, Morita E, et al. *Circulation* 1991;84(4):1581–1588.
198. Sudoh T, Minamino N, Kangawa K, Matsuo H. *Biochem Biophys Res Commun* 1990;168(2):863–870.
199. Tawaragi Y, Fuchimura K, Tanaka S, Minamino N, Kangawa K, Matsuo H. *Biochem Biophys Res Commun* 1991;175(2):645–651.
200. Tawaragi Y, Fuchimura K, Nakazato H, et al. *Biochem Biophys Res Commun* 1990;172(2):627–632.
201. Ohyama Y, Miyamoto K, Saito Y, Minamino N, Kangawa K, Matsuo H. *Biochem Biophys Res Commun* 1992;183(2):743–749.
202. Ueda S, Minamino N, Aburaya M, Kangawa K, Matsukura S, Matsuo H. *Biochem Biophys Res Commun* 1991;175(3):759–767.
203. Kaneko T, Shirakami G, Nakao K, et al. *Brain Res* 1993;612(1–2):104–109.
204. Stingo AJ, Clavell AL, Heublein DM, Wei CM, Pittelkow MR, Burnett J Jr. *Am J Physiol* 1992;263(4 Pt 2):H1318–H1321.
205. Minamino N, Makino Y, Tateyama H, Kangawa K, Matsuo H. *Biochem Biophys Res Commun* 1991;179(1):535–542.
206. Sumners C, Tang W. *Am J Physiol* 1992;262(5 Pt 1):C1134–C1143.
207. Charles CJ, Richards AM, Espiner EA. *Endocrinol* 1992;131(4):1721–1726.
208. Clavell AL, Stingo AJ, Wei CM, Heublein DM, Burnett J Jr. *Am J Physiol* 1993;264(2 Pt 2):R290–R295.
209. Wei CM, Aarhus LL, Miller VM, Burnett J Jr. *Am J Physiol* 1993;264(1 Pt 2):H71–H73.
210. Morita H, Hagiike M, Horiba T, et al. *Jpn J Physiol* 1992;42(2):349–353.
211. Itoh H, Pratt RE, Ohno M, Dzau VJ. *Hypertension* 1992;19(6 Pt 2):758–761.
212. Garg UC, Hassid A. *J Clin Invest* 1989;83(5):1774–1777.
213. Itoh H, Pratt RE, Dzau VJ. *J Clin Invest* 1990;86(5):1690–1697.
214. Kariya K, Kawahara Y, Araki S, Fukuzaki H, Takai Y. *Atheroscler* 1989;80(2):143–147.
215. Abell TJ, Richards AM, Ikram H, Espiner EA, Yandle T. *Biochem Biophys Res Commun* 1989;160(3):1392–1396.
216. Garg UC, Hassid A. *Am J Physiol* 1989;257(1 Pt 2):F60–F66.
217. Appel RG. *Am J Physiol* 1990;259(3 Pt 1):E312–E318.
218. Furuya M, Takehisa M, Minamitake Y, et al. *Biochem Biophys Res Commun* 1990;170(1):201–208.
219. Porter JG, Catalano R, McEnroe G, Lewicki JA, Protter AA. *Am J Physiol* 1992;263(5 Pt 1):C1001–C1006.
220. Furuya M, Aisaka K, Miyazaki T, et al. *Biochem Biophys Res Commun* 1993;193(1):248–253.
221. Almeida FA, Suzuki M, Scarborough RM, Lewicki JA, Maack T. *Am J Physiol* 1989;256(2 Pt 2):R469–R475.
222. Nussenzveig DR, Lewicki JA, Maack T. *J Biol Chem* 1990;265(34):20952–20958.
223. Okolicany J, McEnroe GA, Koh GY, Lewicki JA, Maack T. *Am J Physiol* 1992;263(3 Pt 2):F546–F553.
224. Olins GM, Spear KL, Siegel NR, Zurcher-Neely HA. *Biochim Biophys Acta* 1987;901(1):97–100.
225. Koehn JA, Norman JA, Jones BN, LeSueur L, Sakane Y, Ghai RD. *J Biol Chem* 1987;262(24):11623–11627.
226. Trippodo NC, Gabel RA, Harvey CM, Asaad MM, Rogers WL. *J Cardiovasc Pharmacol* 1991;18(3):308–316.
227. Levin ER, Frank HJ. *Am J Physiol* 1991;261(2 Pt 2):R453–R457.
228. Levin ER. *Am J Physiol* 1993;264(4 Pt 1):E483–E489.
229. Kollenda MC, Vollmar AM, McEnroe GA, Gerbes AL. *Am J Physiol* 1990;258(4 Pt 2):R1084–R1088.
230. Michel H, Meyer-Lehnert H, Backer A, Stelkens H, Kramer HJ. *Kidney Int* 1990;38(1):73–79.
231. Rathinavelu A, Isom GE. *Biochem J* 1991;276(Pt 2):493–497.
232. Kato J, Lanier-Smith KL, Currie MG. *J Biol Chem* 1991;266(22):14681–14685.
233. Kato J, Currie MG. *Eur J Pharmacol* 1992;225(2):113–117.
234. Chiu PJ, Tetzloff G, Romano MT, Foster CJ, Sybertz EJ. *Am J Physiol* 1991;260(1 Pt 2):R208–R216.
235. Gregory LC, Scarborough RM, Metzler CH, McEnroe GA, Maack T, Lewicki JA. *J Cell Biochem Suppl* 1988;12A:23.
236. Maack T, Almeida FA, Suzuki M, Nussenzveig DR. *Contrib Nephrol* 1988;68(65):58–65.
237. Jin H, Chen YF, Yang RH, Jackson RM, Oparil S. *J Appl Physiol* 1990;68(6):2413–2418.
238. Kukkonen P, Vuolteenaho O, Ruskoaho H. *Endocrinol* 1992;130(2):755–765.
239. Seymour AA, Norman JA, Asaad MM, et al. *J Pharmacol Exp Ther* 1991;256(3):1002–1009.
240. Koepke JP, Tyler LD, Blehm DJ, Schuh JR, Blaine EH. *Hypertension* 1990;16(6):642–647.
241. Koepke JP, Tyler LD, Mehta PP, et al. *Am J Hypertens* 1990;3(8 Pt 1):622–627.
242. Perrella MA, Aarhus LL, Heublein DM, Lewicki JA, Burnett JC. *Am J Physiol* 1993;265:H401–H408.
243. Vemulapalli S, Chiu PJ, Brown A, Griscti K, Sybertz EJ. *Life Sci* 1991;49(5):383–391.
244. Okolicany J, McEnroe GA, Gregory LC, Lewicki JA, Maack T. *Can J Physiol Pharmacol* 1991;69(10):1561–1566.
245. Castro R, Ervin MG, Leake RD, Ross MG, Fisher DA. *Pediatr Res* 1991;29(4 Pt 1):342–346.
246. Koepke JP, Tyler LD, Trapani AJ, et al. *J Pharmacol Exp Ther* 1989;249(1):172–176.
247. Erdos EG, Skidgel RA. *FASEB J* 1989;3(2):145–151.
248. Kenny AJ, Bourne A, Ingram J. *Biochem J* 1993;291(Pt 1):83–88.
249. Gerbes AL, Vollmar AM. *Life Sci* 1990;47(14):1173–1180.
250. Schwartz JC, Gros C, Lecomte JM, Bralet J. *Life Sci* 1990;47(15):1279–1297.
251. Sybertz EJ. *Clin Nephrol* 1991;36(4):187–191.
252. Pham I, el Amrani AI, Fournie-Zaluski MC, Corvol P, Roques B, Michel JB. *J Cardiovasc Pharmacol* 1992;20(6):847–857.
253. Murohara Y, Johnston CI. *Clin Exp Pharmacol Physiol* 1992;19(5):380–383.
254. Elsner D, Muntze A, Kromer EP, Riegger GA. *Am J Cardiol* 1992;70(4):494–498.
255. Tikkanen I, Helin K, Tikkanen T, et al. *J Pharmacol Exp Ther* 1990;254(2):641–645.
256. Helin K, Tikkanen I, Tikkanen T, et al. *Eur J Pharmacol* 1991;198(1):23–30.
257. Cavero PG, Margulies KB, Winaver J, Seymour AA, Delaney NG, Burnett J Jr. *Circulation* 1990;82(1):196–201.
258. Smits GJ, McGraw DE, Trapani AJ, Blaine EB. *J Pharmacol Exp Ther* 1990;254(1):176–179.
259. Seymour AA, Fennell SA, Swerdel JN. *Hypertension* 1989;14(1):87–97.
260. Sybertz EJ, Chiu PJ, Vemulapalli S, Watkins R, Haslanger MF. *Hypertension* 1990;15(2):152–161.
261. Lafferty HM, Gunning M, Silva P, Zimmerman MB, Brenner BM, Anderson S. *Circ Res* 1989;65(3):640–646.
262. Jin H, Mathews C, Chen YF, et al. *Am J Hypertens* 1992;5(4 Pt 1):210–218.
263. Wilkins MR, Settle SL, Stockmann PT, Needleman P. *Proc Natl Acad Sci USA* 1990;87(16):6465–6469.

264. Smits GJ, McGraw DE, Trapani AJ. *Am J Physiol* 1990;258(5 Pt 2):F1417–F1424.
265. Bralet J, Mossiat C, Gros C, Schwartz JC. *J Pharmacol Exp Ther* 1991;258(3):807–811.
266. Legault L, Cernacek P, Levy M, Maher E, Farber D. *J Clin Invest* 1992;90(4):1425–1435.
267. Northridge DB, Jardine AG, Findlay IN, Archibald M, Dilly SG, Dargie HJ. *Am J Hypertens* 1990;3(9):682–687.
268. Epstein M, Loutzenhiser RD, Friedland E, Aceto RM, Camargo MJ, Atlas SA. *J Hypertens Suppl* 1986;4(2):S93–S99.
269. Epstein M, Loutzenhiser R, Friedland E, Aceto RM, Camargo MJ, Atlas SA. *J Clin Invest* 1987;79(3):738–745.
270. Ogihara T, Shima J, Hara H, et al. *Life Sci* 1986;38(26):2413–2418.
271. Anderson JV, Donckier J, McKenna WJ, Bloom SR. *Clin Sci* 1986;71(2):151–155.
272. Weil J, Lang RE, Suttmann H, Rampf U, Bidlingmaier F, Gerzer R. *Klin Wochenschr* 1985;63(24):1265–1268.
273. Hamet P, Tremblay J, Pang SC, et al. *J Hypertens Suppl* 1986;4(2):S49–S56.
274. Ruskoaho H, Lang RE, Toth M, Ganten D, Unger T. *Eur Heart J* 1987;8(109):99–109.
275. Gerbes AL, Arendt RM, Gerzer R, et al. *Eur J Clin Invest* 1988;18(4):425–429.
276. Bell GM, Atlas SA, Pecker M, Sealey JE, James G, Laragh JH. *Clin Sci* 1990;79(4):371–376.
277. Hirth C, Stasch JP, John A, et al. *J Cardiovasc Pharmacol* 1986;8(2):268–275.
278. Stasch JP, Hirth C, Kazda S, Wohlfeil S. *Eur J Pharmacol* 1986;129(1–2):165–168.
279. Stasch JP, Hirth C, Kazda S, Neuser D. *Life Sci* 1988;42(5):511–516.
280. Greenwald JE, Sakata M, Michener ML, Sides SD, Needleman P. *J Clin Invest* 1988;81(4):1036–1041.
281. Naruse M, Obana K, Naruse K, et al. *Biochem Biophys Res Commun* 1985;132(3):954–960.
282. Sasaki A, Kida O, Kato J, et al. *Hypertension* 1987;10(3):308–312.
283. Morishita Y, Sano T, Ando K, et al. *Biochem Biophys Res Commun* 1991;176(3):949–957.
284. Sano T, Morishita Y, Yamada K, Matsuda Y. *Biochem Biophys Res Commun* 1992;182(2):824–829.
285. Hirata Y, Ganguli M, Tobian L, Iwai J. *Hypertension* 1984;6(2 Pt 2):I148–I155.
286. Snajdar RM, Rapp JP. *Hypertension* 1985;7(5):775–782.
287. Tanaka I, Inagami T. *J Hypertens* 1986;4(1):109–112.
288. Gutkowska J, Kuchel O, Racz K, Buu NT, Cantin M, Genest J. *Biochem Biophys Res Commun* 1986;136(1):411–416.
289. Takayanagi R, Imada T, Grammer RT, Misono KS, Naruse M, Inagami T. *J Hypertens Suppl* 1986;4(3):S303–S307.
290. Higa T, Kitamura K, Miyata A, Kangawa K, Matsuo H, Tanaka K. *Jpn Circ J* 1985;49(9):973–979.
291. Imada T, Takayanagi R, Inagami T. *Biochem Biophys Res Commun* 1985;133(2):759–765.
292. Genest J, Larochelle P, Cusson JR, Gutkowska J, Cantin M. *Hypertension* 1988;11(2 Pt 2):I3–I7.
293. Ballermann BJ, Bloch KD, Seidman JG, Brenner BM. *J Clin Invest* 1986;78(3):840–843.
294. Sugawara A, Nakao K, Sakamoto M, et al. *Lancet* 1985;2(8469–70):1426–1427.
295. Sagnella GA, Markandu ND, Shore AC, MacGregor GA. *Lancet* 1986;1(8474):179–181.
296. Wambach G, Gotz S, Suckau G, Kaufmann W. *Klin Wochenschr* 1986;64(6):53–57.
297. Kohno M, Yasunari K, Matsuura T, Murakawa K, Takeda T. *Am Heart J* 1987;113(5):1160–1163.
298. Montorsi P, Tonolo G, Polonia J, Hepburn D, Richards AM. *Hypertension* 1987;10(6):570–576.
299. Ganau A, Devereux RB, Atlas SA, et al. *J Am Coll Cardiol* 1989;14(3):715–724.
300. Yamaji T, Ishibashi M, Sekihara H, Takaku F, Nakaoka H, Fujii J. *J Clin Endocrinol Metab* 1986;63(4):815–818.
301. Larochelle P, Cusson JR, Gutkowska J, et al. *Br Med J* 1987;294(6582):1249–1252.
302. Nilsson P, Lindholm L, Schersten B, Horn R, Melander A, Hesch RD. *Lancet* 1987;2(8564):883–885.
303. Zachariah PK, Burnett J Jr, Ritter SG, Strong CG. *Mayo Clin Proc* 1987;62(9):782–786.
304. Sagnella GA, Markandu ND, Buckley MG, et al. *Am J Hypertens* 1988;1(2):112–118.
305. Sugawara A, Nakao K, Kono T, et al. *Hypertension* 1988;11(2 Pt 2):I212–I216.
306. Garcia R, Gutkowska J, Genest J, Cantin M, Thibault G. *Proc Soc Exp Biol Med* 1985;179(4):539–545.
307. Garcia R, Thibault G, Gutkowska J, et al. *Proc Soc Exp Biol Med* 1985;179(3):396–401.
308. Richards AM, Nicholls MG, Ikram H, Webster MW, Yandle TG, Espiner EA. *Lancet* 1985;1(8428):545–549.
309. Weidmann P, Gnadinger MP, Ziswiler HR, et al. *J Hypertens Suppl* 1986;4(2):S71–S83.
310. Janssen WM, de Jong PE, van der Hem GK, de Zeeuw D. *Br Med J* 1986;293(6543):351–353.
311. Janssen WM, de Zeeuw D, van der Hem GK, de Jong PE. *Hypertension* 1989;13(6 Pt 1):640–646.
312. Burnett J Jr, Kao PC, Hu DC, et al. *Science* 1986;231(4742):1145–1147.
313. Raine AE, Erne P, Burgisser E, et al. *N Engl J Med* 1986;315(9):533–537.
314. Redfield MM, Edwards BS, McGoon MD, Heublein DM, Aarhus LL, Burnett J Jr. *Circulation* 1989;80(3):651–657.
315. Drexler H, Hirth-Dietrich C, Stasch JP, et al. *Cardiovasc Res* 1991;25(7):558–564.
316. Lerman A, Gibbons RJ, Rodeheffer RJ, et al. *Lancet* 1993;341(8853):1105–1109.
317. Mathisen P, Hall C, Simonsen S. *Scand J Clin Lab Invest* 1993;53(1):41–49.
318. Mukoyama M, Nakao K, Saito Y, et al. *N Engl J Med* 1990;323(11):757–758.
319. Mukoyama M, Nakao K, Saito Y, et al. *Lancet* 1990;335(8692):801–802.
320. Motwani JG, McAlpine H, Kennedy N, Struthers AD. *Lancet* 1993;341(8853):1109–1113.
321. Giles TD, Quiroz AC, Roffidal LE, Marder H, Sander GE. *Clin Pharmacol Ther* 1991;50(5 Pt 1):557–563.
322. Riegger AJ, Kromer EP, Kochsiek K. *Dtsch Med Wochenschr* 1985;110(42):1607–1610.
323. Eiskjaer H, Bagger JP, Danielsen H, et al. *Int J Cardiol* 1991;33(1):61–74.
324. Kentsch M, Ludwig D, Drummer C, Gerzer R, Muller-Esch G. *Eur J Clin Invest* 1992;22(10):662–669.
325. Obata K, Yasue H, Horio Y, et al. *Am Heart J* 1987;113(5):845–847.
326. Anderson JV, Gibbs JS, Woodruff PW, Greco C, Rowland E, Bloom SR. *J Hypertens Suppl* 1986;4(2):S137–S141.
327. Crozier IG, Ikram H, Nicholls MG. *Clin Exp Pharmacol Physiol* 1987;14(7):597–604.
328. Nicklas JM, DiCarlo LA, Koller PT, et al. *Am Heart J* 1986;112(5):923–928.
329. Oliver JR, Twidale N, Lakin C, Cain M, Tonkin AM. *Br Heart J* 1988;59(4):458–462.
330. Christensen G, Bugge JF, Ilebekk A, Kiil F. *Am J Physiol* 1989;256(6 Pt 2):R1245–R1249.
331. Kojima S, Fujii T, Ohe T, et al. *Am J Cardiol* 1988;62(9):576–579.
332. Ellenbogen KA, Rogers R, Walsh M, Mohanty PK. *Am Heart J* 1988;116(5 Pt 1):1233–1238.
333. Roy D, Paillard F, Cassidy D, et al. *J Am Coll Cardiol* 1987;9(3):509–514.
334. Burnett J Jr, Osborn MJ, Hammill SC, Heublein DM. *J Clin Endocrinol Metab* 1989;69(4):881–884.
335. Schiebinger RJ, Linden J. *Am J Physiol* 1986;251(5 Pt 2):H1095–H1099.
336. Tan SY, Nolan J, Craig K, Swainson CP. *J Intern Med* 1993;233(5):415–417.
337. Christensen G, Ilebekk A, Aakeson I, Kiil F. *Acta Physiol Scand* 1988;134(2):263–270.
338. King KA, Ledsome JR. *Am J Physiol* 1991;261(1 Pt 2):H22–H28.

339. Tsai RC, Yamaji T, Ishibashi M, et al. *Am J Cardiol* 1988;61(15): 1260–1264.

340. Rascher W, Tulassay T, Lang RE. *Lancet* 1985;2(8450):303–305.

341. Hasegawa K, Matsushita Y, Inoue T, Morii H, Ishibashi M, Yamaji T. *J Clin Endocrinol Metab* 1986;63(4):819–822.

342. Wilkins MR, Wood JA, Adu D, Lote CJ, Kendall MJ, Michael J. *Clin Sci* 1986;71(2):157–160.

343. Saxenhofer H, Gnadinger MP, Weidmann P, et al. *Kidney Int* 1987;32(4):554–561.

344. Walker RG, Swainson CP, Yandle TG, Nicholls MG, Espiner EA. *Clin Sci* 1987;72(1):19–24.

345. Anderson JV, Raine AE, Proudler A, Bloom SR. *J Endocrinol* 1986;110(2):193–196.

346. Ando R, Matsuda O, Miyake S, Yoshiyama N. *Nephron* 1988;50(3):225–228.

347. Tonolo G, McMillan M, Richards AM, et al. *Nephron* 1990;55(1):58–62.

348. de Chatel R, Mako J, Toth M, Barna I, Lang RE. *Int Urol Nephrol* 1991;23(2):177–183.

349. Larochelle P, Beroniade V, Gutkowska J, et al. *Clin Invest Med* 1987;10(4):350–354.

350. Shenker Y, Port FK, Swartz RD, Gross MD, Grekin RJ. *Life Sci* 1987;41(13):1635–1644.

351. Smith S, Anderson S, Ballermann BJ, Brenner BM. *J Clin Invest* 1986;77(4):1395–1398.

352. Cole BR, Kuhnline MA, Needleman P. *J Clin Invest* 1985;76(6): 2413–2415.

353. Brezis M, Epstein FH. *Annu Rev Med* 1993;44:27–37.

354. Shaw SG, Weidmann P, Hodler J, Zimmermann A, Paternostro A. *J Clin Invest* 1987;80(5):1232–1237.

355. Nakamoto M, Shapiro JI, Shanley PF, Chan L, Schrier RW. *J Clin Invest* 1987;80(3):698–705.

356. Schafferhans K, Heidbreder E, Grimm D, Heidland A. *Nephron* 1986;44(3):240–244.

357. Conger JD, Falk SA, Hammond WS. *Kidney Int* 1991;40(1):21–28.

358. Lieberthal W, Sheridan AM, Valeri CR. *Am J Physiol* 1990;258(5 Pt 2):F1266–F1272.

359. Rahman N, Kim G, Mathews A, et al. *J Ann Soc Nephrol* 1993;4: 323A.

360. Hummel M, Kuhn M, Bub A, et al. *Clin Invest* 1992;70(8):674–682.

361. Marumo F, Masaki Y, Ida T, Sato K, Ando K. *Transplant* 1991;51(5):982–986.

362. Lewis R, Janney R, Osgood R, McAndrew J, Verani R, Fried T. *Kidney Int* 1989;36(4):562–569.

363. Lewis R, Sprayberry S, Ghobrial R, Peirce C, Verani R, Corriere JN. *J Urol* 1993;150(3):1010–1013.

364. Gianello P, Ramboux A, Poelart D, et al. *Transplant* 1989;47(3): 512–515.

365. Bozkurt F, Kirste G, Leipziger J, Schollmeyer P, Drexler H, Keller E. *Transplant Proc* 1987;19(5):4192–4195.

366. Ratcliffe PJ, Richardson AJ, Kirby JE, Moyses C, Shelton JR, Morris PJ. *Kidney Int* 1991;39(1):164–168.

367. Sands JM, Neylan JF, Olson RA, O'Brien DP, Whelchel JD, Mitch WE. *J Am Soc Nephrol* 1991;1(9):1081–1086.

Hypertension: Pathophysiology, Diagnosis, and Management, Second Edition,
edited by J.H. Laragh and B.M. Brenner,
Raven Press, Ltd., New York © 1995.

CHAPTER 62

Endogenous Digitalis-Like Factors in Hypertension

Francis J. Haddy and Vardaman M. Buckalew, Jr.

It is generally agreed that the pathophysiology of essential hypertension involves some abnormality of renal function, probably a defect in renal sodium excretion. Although it is apparent that such a defect would lead to plasma volume expansion, it is far from clear how this abnormality would lead to chronic elevation of blood pressure. One widely discussed theory holds that chronic plasma volume expansion could cause hypertension by altering the plasma concentration of a humoral factor (or factors) involved in the regulation of renal sodium excretion. This hypothesis suggests that natriuretic hormone is a digitalislike factor that could cause hypertension by its inotropic effects on the heart and blood vessels. The hypothesis has recently received support from studies that suggest the source and chemical nature of the digitalislike substance. This chapter briefly presents the historical background and then reviews studies that suggest the digitalislike substance is a steroid, ouabain, or a substance closely related to ouabain, and that it comes from the adrenal cortex. The chapter then concludes with a discussion of its role in hypertension and other conditions.

F. J. Haddy: Department of Physiology, Uniformed Services University of the Health Sciences, Bethesda, Maryland 20814.

V. M. Buckalew, Jr.: Department of Internal Medicine, Section on Nephrology, Bowman Gray School of Medicine of Wake Forest University, Winston-Salem, North Carolina 27157.

BRIEF HISTORICAL SURVEY

In 1961, de Wardener et al. (1) suggested that a third factor, a circulating natriuretic hormone, participates in the regulation of sodium excretion by the kidney following intravenous administration of saline. In 1969, Kramer et al. (2) suggested that this third factor is a Na,K–adenosine triphosphatase (ATPase) inhibitor. Buckalew et al. (3) then showed that saline loaded dogs have a substance in their plasma that inhibits sodium transport across epithelial membranes. Haddy and Overbeck (4) then suggested that this Na,K-ATPase–inhibiting natriuretic hormone participates in the genesis of volume-expanded hypertension. They suggested this because, as might be predicted from the action of an inhibitor, blood vessels from dogs with one-kidney, one-wrapped hypertension had reduced Na,K pump activity (5) and hearts from rats with one-kidney, one-clip hypertension has reduced Na,K-ATPase activity (6,7) (both models are volume expanded). The production of such changes with low potassium or the cardiac glycosides produces vasoconstriction, increased cardiac contractility, and increased blood pressure (8–13). Pamnani et al. (14–16) later showed that the reduced Na,K pump activity in blood vessels could be mimicked in normal blood vessel by applying plasma from dogs with acute volume expansion (14), one-kidney, one-wrapped hypertension (15,16), and other types of volume-expanded hypertension (16). Since the action of the plasma on blood vessels was similar to the action of ouabain, the term *ouabain-like* appeared in the literature (17). The term *digitalis-like* appeared when Gruber et al. (18) showed that the plasma Na,K-ATPase inhibitor seen during acute volume expansion cross-reacts with digoxin antibodies.

Several laboratories then found an inhibitor in the plasma of patients with essential hypertension, particularly of the low renin variety. Data were presented indicating that the plasma of some patients with essential hypertension contains an inhibitor of the Na,K pump (19) and of Na,K-ATPase (20), the latter correlating with blood pressure. The plasma level of the inhibitor increases with the sodium intake, particularly in hypertensive subjects, and the level correlates with blood pressure (21,22). A positive bioassay for an inhibitor of the vascular Na,K pump was obtained in black male patients with low renin hypertension but not in black male patients unselected with respect to renin status (23–25).

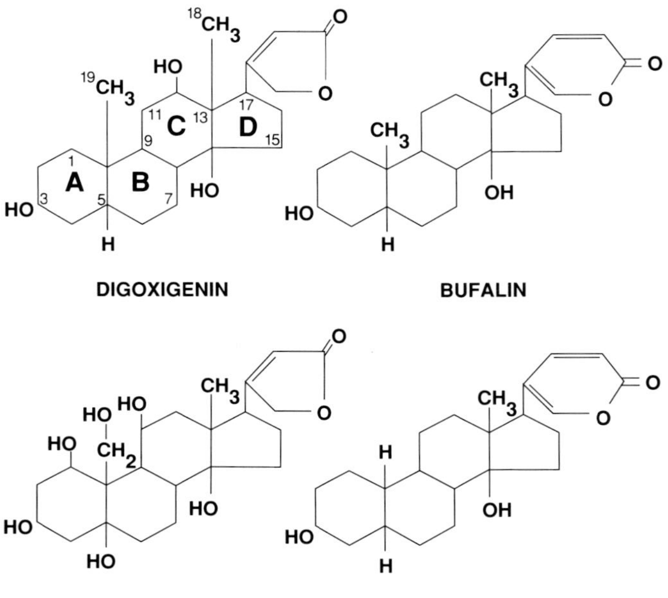

THE RECENT PROPOSAL THAT THE ENDOGENOUS CIRCULATING NA,K-ATPase INHIBITOR IS OUABAIN

Over the years, many laboratories have attempted to establish the chemical structure of the circulating endogenous Na,K-ATPase inhibitor. A surprising turn of events was the announcement in 1991 that the agent in plasma from volume-expanded humans is ouabain (26,27) (Fig. 1). The report was surprising because no mammalian tissue has been shown to have the enzyme 14β-hydroxylase, which is required to attach a hydroxyl group to the 14 position on the steroid ring, and a hydroxyl group in this position is essential for the biological activity of ouabain. Furthermore, no mammalian tissue has been shown to be capable of synthesizing rhamnose, the carbohydrate portion of the plant ouabain (although rhamnose is not essential for ouabain activity, it may be imperative in determining its solubility and therefore its tissue distribution, its ability to penetrate cells, and its influence on intracellular events).

On the other hand, the evidence summarized by Hamlyn and Manunta (28) is persuasive. According to them, the processing of 2 tons of human plasma from volume-expanded subjects, using intact cells in assay systems and/or performing several different types of assays in tandem to reduce the number of false positive results, ultimately led to the identification of ouabain as the "ouabainlike" substance. Several lines of evidence supported their claim. First, the primary mass of the protonated ion by high-resolution mass spectroscopy is identical to the calculated value for ouabain. Thus, the elemental composition of the endogenous compound is $C_{29}H_{45}O_{12}$. Furthermore, the fragmentation patterns of the native and acetylated derivatives of the human compound and ouabain are identical. Second, the number

FIG. 1. The aglycones (genins) of four steroids are shown. The classic cardiac glycosides ouabain and digoxin have rhamnose and three digitoxose, respectively, attached at position 3. Both of these glycosides (or some closely related analogue) have recently been isolated from body fluids and tissues of normal mammalian species. Bufalin closely resembles resibufogenin, a compound isolated from skin and body fluids of toads. A similar compound, 19-norbufalin, has been isolated from human cataractous lens.

and reactivity of the hydroxyl groups to acetylation in the human compound correspond to those for ouabain. Third, the human plasma compound has been shown to bind reversibly with high affinity to purified Na,K-ATPase at the cardiac glycoside binding site. Moreover, binding affinities for the human compound and ouabain are modulated in a similar manner by ionic ligands, and the occupation of the binding site by the human compound leads to the inhibition of Na,K-ATPase by stabilization of the E_2P intermediate, a property that is unique to the cardiac glycosides. Fourth, the cardiotonic and vasopressor actions of ouabain and the human compound in the guinea pig are indistinguishable (29). Fifth, the human compound and commercial ouabain co-elute in a variety of chromatographic systems known to be capable of resolving stereoisomers of ouabain, including those that contain isomers of rhamnose. Sixth, the human compound was 100 percent cross-reactive with polyclonal antibodies raised against a series of ouabain conjugates in the rabbit. Further, the antibodies were ouabain specific in that they demonstrated minimal cross-reactivity with known adrenocortical, ovarian, and testicular steroids as well as other cardiac glycosides (30). Hamlyn and Manunta admit that ouabain is remarkably distinct from other compounds previously described in mammals with respect to fusion of the A-D rings in the steroid nucleus in a *cis-trans-cis* configuration, to the presence of rhamnose, and to a singly unsaturated five-member lactone ring at C17.

Hamyln and Manunta (28) have addressed the possibility that ouabain in mammals might be derived from the food chain. They found very little change in the circulating ouabain level in subjects on total parenteral nutrition. This may not be a critical experiment, however, since exogenous ouabain has been shown to be preferentially taken up by the adrenal, and may be released in response to volume expansion (31,32).

Hamlyn and Manunta (28) also summarize measurements of plasma ouabain in various states associated with altered blood pressure/volume regulation using either a radioimmunoassay (RIA) or ouabain antibodies in an enzyme-linked immunosorbent assay (ELISA). Their antibodies show minimal cross-reactivity with known adrenocortical, testicular, and ovarian steroids but cross-react to various degrees (0.5–5 percent) with other cardenolides and bufodienolides. Measured values in man are elevated in hypothyroidism, congestive heart failure, essential hypertension, Conn's syndrome, chronic renal failure, and salt loading (33). Measured values in animals are elevated in obesity with hypertension and deoxycorticosterone acetate (DOCA)-saline hypertension. Surprisingly, they are not elevated by acute saline loading in dogs (34) or in reduced renal mass saline hypertension, the classical model of low renin, volume-expanded hypertension in which it is most easy to demonstrate the inhibitor using a whole cell assay method (16). It should be noted that these measurements of plasma ouabain were by RIA or ELISA using an antibody that is not 100 percent specific for ouabain, not by the rigorous assay method used in originally identifying the plasma inhibitor as ouabain. Therefore, one cannot be entirely certain that the measurement is in fact the level of ouabain.

Recent physiological data support the notion that the inhibitor could be ouabain. It has been known for some time that ouabain and other cardiac glycosides will raise blood pressure in man, dog, and guinea pig (8,11,35–40) following acute administration. Ouabain does not raise blood pressure in the rat on short-term intravenous administration (40) but it does during chronic administration (intraperitoneal injection for a number of days) (41).

The proposal that the circulating endogenous Na,K-ATPase inhibitor is ouabain has not been confirmed and evidence has appeared that makes the proposal suspect. For example, Naomi et al. (42) measured the affinities of seven different antisera directed against digoxin for a human plasma digitalislike compound and developed an immunological profile ("fingerprint") for this compound. Since they obtained an identical profile from the serum of pregnant women, neonatal cord blood, and in subjects with renal or hepatic failure, they concluded that the same digitalislike compound was present in these sera. Neither ouabain nor lysophosphatidyl choline showed profiles resembling this digitalislike compound. The bufalin profile was similar but not identical.

P. A. Doris (*personal communication*) failed to confirm the consistent presence of authentic ouabain in plasma from normal human subjects. Ouabain immunoreactivity, however, could most often be detected in simple extracts of plasma. However, when the immunoreactivity was characterized, only a small portion of it coincided with ouabain. Perhaps the inhibitor is structurally similar to but not identical to ouabain and digoxin and therefore cross-reacts with certain antibodies to both ouabain and digoxin.

OTHER EVIDENCE THAT THE INHIBITOR IS A STEROID

The case for a steroidal structure of the endogenous circulating Na,K-ATPase inhibitor receives support from other sources. Lichtstein and colleagues (43) suggest that the agent might be a steroidal dienolide derivative, closely related to the cardiac glycosides. They showed that the ouabainlike compound in toad skin is 3-hydroxy-14,15-epoxy-20,22-dienolide glycoside (resibufogenin). They also present evidence that a ouabain-like compound in bovine plasma also may be a steroid, with a structure similar to that of the toad skin compound (44). More recently, Lichtstein and colleagues (45) have purified a compound from human cataractous lens of the eye they have tentatively identified as 19-norbufalin (Fig. 1). Bufalin, a bufodienolide closely related to resibufogenin (Fig. 1), does in fact have the physiological actions expected of a Na,K pump inhibitor; it blocks potassium vasodilation, potentiates norepinephrine vasoconstriction, increases vascular resistance, increases left ventricular dp/dt, raises arterial pressure, and produces natriuresis and diuresis (46,47). The finding of a bufalinlike compound in human tissue is surprising since steroids of this type had been found previously only in amphibians.

LaBella and co-workers (48) have described a series of hydroxy progesterone derivatives that bind to the digitalis receptor. Chloramadinone acetate, a clinically used progestin, has the greatest binding potency, and it also inhibits Na,K-ATPase from several sources and the Na,K pump in skeletal muscle, heart muscle, and red blood cells. However, it does not cross-react with digoxin antiserum or increase cardiac contractility. Wieland et al. (49) do not consider the latter to be negative evidence; they point out that simple glycosidation transforms chlormadinol acetate into a cardioactive steroid, i.e., one that increases cardiac contractility, perhaps by interfering with cellular uptake. More recently, a derivative, 14β-hydroxyprogesterone, has been shown not only to inhibit Na,K-ATPase but also to increase contraction of isolated heart muscle and cause vasoconstriction in isolated conduit vessels (50).

Goto et al. (51) processed 2 tons of human urine and isolated two urinary digitalislike factors, one indistinguishable from digoxin (Fig. 1), and a second similar to ouabain (52). The origin of this urinary digoxin is unknown, but Hamlyn and Manunta (28) suggest a dietary source. Similarly, Shaikh et al. (53) purified a factor from bovine adrenal that was indistinguishable from digoxin by mass sectroscopy, and Weinberg et al. (54) isolated two factors from peritoneal dialysate that resembled ouabain and digoxin. Cloix et al. (55,56) identified a factor in the urine of hypertensive subjects and their relatives that they feel is a unique glycosteroid. The factor is natriuretic, inhibits Na,K-ATPase in a dose-response paralleled to ouabain, and binds preferentially to the E_2 configuration of the enzyme. Weiler et al. (57) characterized a low molecular weight Na,K-ATPase inhibitor in human urine and found that it shares some but not all properties with ouabain. Tamura et al. (58) described a compound in pig urine that is similar to but distinct from ouabain, digoxin, and an adrenal factor.

Haupert and collaborators (59) have recently proposed that their factor isolated from bovine hypothalamus is a stereoisomer of ouabain. Previous physiological characterization of this hypothalamic factor showed some similarities to the digitalis glycosides (it inhibits ^{86}Rb uptake of human red blood cells [RBCs], the hydrolysis of para-nitrophenolphosphate by Na,K-ATPase, a reaction that requires only the E_2 conformation of the enzyme, and ouabain binding to its receptor on toad bladder Na,K-ATPase) (60,61). It is for the most part, however, unlike ouabain in its other studied characteristics. It does not support phosphorylation of Na,K-ATPase and even antagonizes it. It has different ligand requirements for binding and has a higher binding affinity than ouabain. It inhibits Ca-ATPase of sarcoplasmic reticulum and demonstrates no cross-reactivity with digoxin antibodies. Its binding to Na,K-ATPase demonstrates positive cooperatively when the enzyme is inserted into liposomes (ouabain demonstrates negative cooperatively in this same preparation) (62). As a result, its dose response in several assays is steeper than that for ouabain. It is not known whether this factor circulates in plasma. It should be noted that the physiological characteristics of this hypothalamic factor were determined using crude (i.e., impure) preparations of the factor. It remains to be proved that the stereoisomer does, in fact, have distinct physiological effects.

Finally, indirect evidence that the inhibitor is steroidal in nature comes from studies of canrenone, a metabolic product of spironolactone used as an antihypertensive agent in France. It can compete with ouabain for binding to Na,K-ATPase and it lowers the blood pressure and reverses vascular Na,K pump inhibition in a model of hypertension clearly shown to have elevated circulating levels of a digitalislike factor (reduced renal mass saline hypertension in the rat), but has no effect on blood pressure in the spontaneously hypertensive rat (SHR) model, where levels appear to be normal (63,64). Renal excretion of water and sodium does not change. Canrenone also lowers blood pressure and raises red cell Na,K-ATPase activity in some patients with essential hypertension (65).

Thus, the case for a steroidal structure continues to increase in strength.

SOURCE OF THE INHIBITOR

The tissue studies of Haupert and Sancho (66), de Wardener and Clarkson (67), Morgan et al. (68), and others suggested that a circulating Na,K pump inhibitor comes from the hypothalamus. Lesions of the hypothalamus in experimental animals in fact reduce the blood level of the Na,K pump inhibitor (16,69–71), pituitary tumors in human increase it (72), and central administration of hypertonic saline (73,74), a dopamine receptor agonist (75) or angiotensin II (76), triggers its release into the blood. Digitalislike activity had been identified in human cerebrospinal fluid (77–80).

Pamnani et al. (16) and Bealer et al. (71) showed that anteroventral third ventricular (AV3V) lesions abolish the Na,K pump responses to acute volume expansion in the rat; i.e., the usual decrease in Na,K pump activity is no longer seen after an AV3V lesion and neither is the usual increase in the plasma concentration of the inhibitor (16,71). AV3V lesions produce similar changes in rats with reduced renal mass-saline and DOCA-salt hypertension, while at the same time ameliorating the hypertension (69,70).

While these and other observations, particularly those of Takahashi et al. (74,81), Ihara et al. (82), and Yamada et al. (83,84) are compatible with the hypothalamus as the source of the inhibitor, they are also compatible with the possibility that the hypothalamus simply accumulates or influences the agent secreted from another source, such as the adrenal glands. An adrenal origin would support the notion that the inhibitor is a steroid, similar in structure to the cardiac glycosides, which are known to bind to and inhibit Na,K-ATPase.

A number of studies in addition to those cited above suggest that the adrenal is the source of the inhibitor (28,85–97). In 1988, Tamura et al. (86) reported the finding of a putative steroid in bovine adrenal gland that appears to have biological and immunological activities almost identical to digoxin in several assay systems. This inhibitory activity was also found in the plasma of normal and Dahl salt-sensitive (S) rats, in aqueous extracts of their kidneys and liver (but not in extracts of other tissues) (87), and in the urine of rats with reduced renal mass and one-kidney, one-clip hypertension (but not in the urine of SHRs and Dahl S rats and their controls [88]).

Shaikh et al. (53) isolated digoxin immunoreactive factors from bovine adrenal cortex, and Vinge et al. (89) showed that dexamethasone suppressed and adrenocorticotropic hormone (ACTH) increased circulating levels of a digoxin immunoreactive factor. Ludens et al. (90) found the highest ouabain immunoreactivity in the adrenal cortex of the rat; removal of the adrenals caused a 50 percent decrease in the circulating level.

Doris (91–93) developed a digoxin radioimmunoassay and showed that this assay was able to detect in rat plasma a material that was digoxin immunoreactive; the animals had never been treated with cardiac glycoside drugs. He showed that in rats consuming increased sodium chloride, plasma levels of this material were markedly increased (91,92). The cross-reactivity of his antiserum indicated that this immunoreactivity was unlikely to be other endogenous steroids (91–93). He identified the adrenal as the tissue containing the greatest concentration of the digoxinlike material and showed that adrenalectomy produced a significant reduction in the levels of the material in plasma (91). Quartered rat adrenal explants were shown also to release material that was recognized by his anti-digoxin antiserum. The same medium was found to possess the ability to inhibit the binding of tritiated ouabain to erythrocytes, indicating that receptor as well as antiserum recognition was present (94). Digoxin immunoreactivity and ouabain binding competing activity were also present in medium conditioned by the steroidogenic murine adrenal cell line, Y1. High-performance liquid chromatography (HPLC) fractionation of this medium showed that a single peak contained the largest amount of these two activities and also had the largest capacity for inhibiting the ion translocation action of the sodium pump.

Hamlyn and Manunta (28) summarize their studies indicating that ouabain is present in rat, human, and canine adrenal tissue and is secreted from bovine adrenocortical cells in tissue culture. When the adrenal glands are removed from the normal rats, the plasma levels of ouabain are lower than in matched pair-fed control animals. There appears to be a continuous arteriovenous gradient of ouabain across the adrenal gland of conscious chronically cannulated dogs (95). In these experiments the ouabain content of the adrenal venous effluent is three- to fivefold greater than that of the arterial blood entering the gland, suggesting active secretion of ouabain against a concentration gradient. Finally, elevated plasma levels of ouabain have been found in hypertensive patients with adrenocortical tumors (primary aldosteronism) (28,96,97). Removal of the tumors was associated with the normalization of plasma ouabain level and the remission of the hypertension.

Collectively, these findings support the notion that the adrenal cortex is a major source of the inhibitor and that it has the structure of a steroid. However, in many cases, ouabain was measured as ouabain immunoreactivity present in simple solid-phase cartridge extracts of samples. Such an approach may be useful in assuring that certain characterized materials are excluded from the extract (e.g., digoxin), but it cannot guarantee that uncharacterized materials with similar polarity are removed. The uncharacterized materials may be present in sufficient quantity and possess sufficient cross-reactivity in the ouabain immunoassay to result in false ouabain levels. Such uncharacterized cardiac glycosidelike materials have been described by both Hamlyn and Manunta (28) and Doris (98) in plasma and adrenal cortex, respectively. They may well cross-react with antibodies to both ouabain and digoxin and be of physiological significance with respect to fluid balance and hypertension. Doris has in fact described a non-ouabain, non-digoxin material that he finds to be the major peak of the cardiac glycoside material from the adrenal cortex (Doris PA, *personal communication*). Simple extracts of adrenal cortical cell conditioned media have both digoxin and ouabain immunoreactivity (Doris's ouabain antiserum is highly specific and is unable to recognize physiological levels of known steroids unrelated to the cardiac glycosides. Cross-reactivity with pregnenolone, corticosterone, and aldosterone are all less than 0.01 percent and with progesterone less than 0.025 percent. Cross-reactivity with digoxin is 4.5 percent and with ouabagenin is 56.2 percent).

WHAT IS ITS ROLE IN HYPERTENSION?

About 60 percent of hypertensive subjects are salt sensitive, i.e., their blood pressure rises with dietary sodium chloride supplementation and falls with dietary sodium chloride restriction (99). About half of these subjects have low renin hypertension (essential hypertension, renal parenchymal disease, type 1 diabetes mellitus, primary aldosteronism, acromegaly) and about half have normal or high renin hypertension (nonmodulating essential hypertension, characterized by a failure of renal blood flow to increase with salt loading and a reduced ability to excrete a salt load) (99). Common to all is retention of sodium and water on a high-salt diet. It is hypothesized that the water retention translates into hypertension via the digitalislike factor(s) (DLF). In this hypothesis (4,100) (Fig. 2), increased intravascular volume due to impaired excretion of sodium and water by the kidney is sensed by the central circulation, leading to the release of an endogenous digitalislike substance(s). Like the cardiac glycosides, this substance increases cardiac contractility, constricts blood vessels, and reduces tubular reabsorption of sodium. The increased blood pressure and reduced sodium reabsorption result in excretion of the excess volume. An agent with this

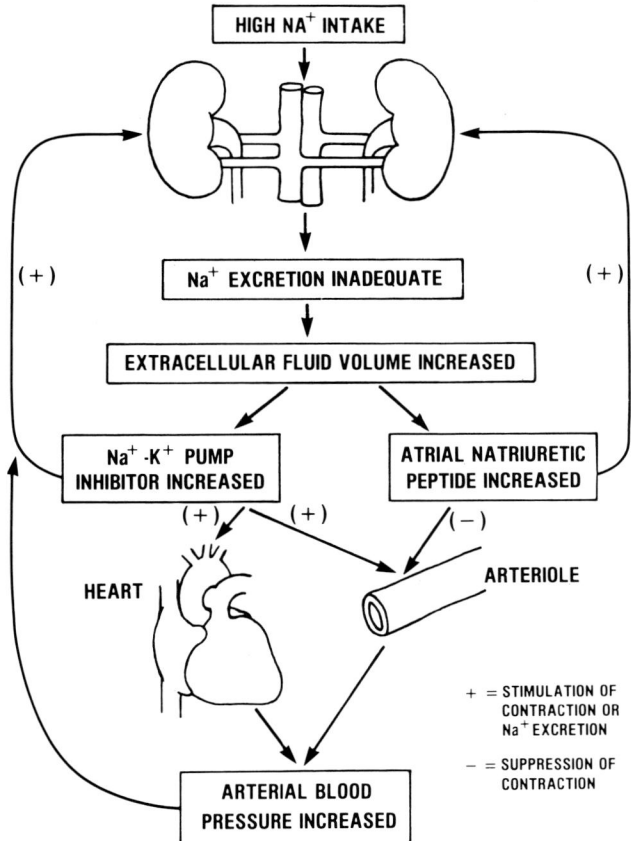

FIG. 2. One explanation for the increase in arterial blood pressure seen when sodium excretion does not keep pace with sodium intake. An increase in pressure in the central circulation stimulates the release of a Na-K pump inhibitor, which through actions on cardiovascular muscle, leads to increased contractile activity and hence arterial pressure. This, along with its action on the renal tubule, tends to normalize volume via diuresis. The rise in pressure in the central circulation also increases the release of the atrial natriuretic peptide, which also tends to reverse this sequence by increasing the ability of the kidney to excrete sodium and water. Thus, according to this view, the elevated pressure is in part generated by a Na-K pump inhibitor acting on heart and blood vessels and is in part compensated by pressure, a sodium pump inhibitor, and atrial natriuretic peptide acting on the kidney. +, stimulation of contraction or Na excretion; −, suppression of contraction. (From ref. 118, with permission.)

combination of properties represents an effective way to rid the body of the extra salt and water; the increase in blood pressure delivers more salt and water to the renal tubules from which they are rejected for reabsorption and excreted. The actions of such an agent would help explain why populations prone to low-renin hypertension (black and elderly persons), who excrete a sodium load more slowly than normal when normotensive, excrete the load faster than normal when hypertensive. The existence of an endogenous digitalislike substance would also help explain why, in volume-expanded hyperten-

sion, extracellular fluid volume returns almost to normal levels in the steady state. Multiple systems control intravascular volume (renin-angiotensin-aldosterone, vasopressin, atrial natriuretic factor, digitalislike substance) and provide a backup in the event of damage to, or deletion of, any one system. However, the penalty of activating the digitalislike natriuretic system is hypertension.

The cellular mechanism by which an endogenous DLF might cause hypertension is gradually being clarified. The high concentration of potassium and the low concentration of sodium in the intracellular fluid relative to extracellular fluid results from the active transport of sodium and potassium ions across the cell membrane (Fig. 3) (101). Na,K-ATPase is the enzymatic transport system—the Na,K pump—that moves three sodium ions outward for each two potassium ions moved inward. The Na,K-ATPase pump is inhibited by lowering the extracellular potassium concentration or the intracellular sodium concentration. It is also inhibited by digitalis glycosides and, according to the hypothesis, by an endogenous digitalislike factor that binds to a receptor site on the enzyme. Since the transport rates of the two ions are not equal, reduction of the pump rate results in a reduction of the negative charge inside the cell and hence depolarization. In vascular smooth muscle, depolarization increases calcium permeability of the membrane and calcium influx increases, resulting in vasoconstriction. It also increases the sensitivity of the muscle to vasoconstrictor agents such as norepinephrine (NE).

Since intraventricular administration of ouabain acutely raises blood pressure (102,103), hypertension might also occur from increased central DLF. Hypothalamic levels of DLF (Na,K-ATPase inhibitory activity) are increased in Milan hypertensive rats (104), SHRs (105), and rats with reduced renal mass drinking saline (106). High dietary sodium increases hypothalamic DLF concentrations (107) and blunts the increase of blood pressure from centrally administered ouabain in SHR (108). The mechanism by which central DLF might raise blood pressure chronically is not known. Based on ouabain's effect, activation of the sympathetic nervous system could be involved. Although a rationale for implicating a cholinelike hypothalamic Na,K-ATPase inhibitor in hypertension has recently been proposed (109), a model of chronic hypertension involving central inhibition of Na,K-ATPase has not been reported.

Since neuronal NE reuptake involves an Na-driven cotransport system dependent on intracellular Na concentration, Na,K-ATPase inhibition could increase the steady-state concentration of neurotransmitter in the synaptic cleft (110), leading to an increased sympathetic tone. Na,K-ATPase inhibition may also increase NE release by adrenergic nerves (111). These effects could be important both centrally and peripherally.

The effects of ouabain on the circulation give some clues as to the role of endogenous DLF in causing hyper-

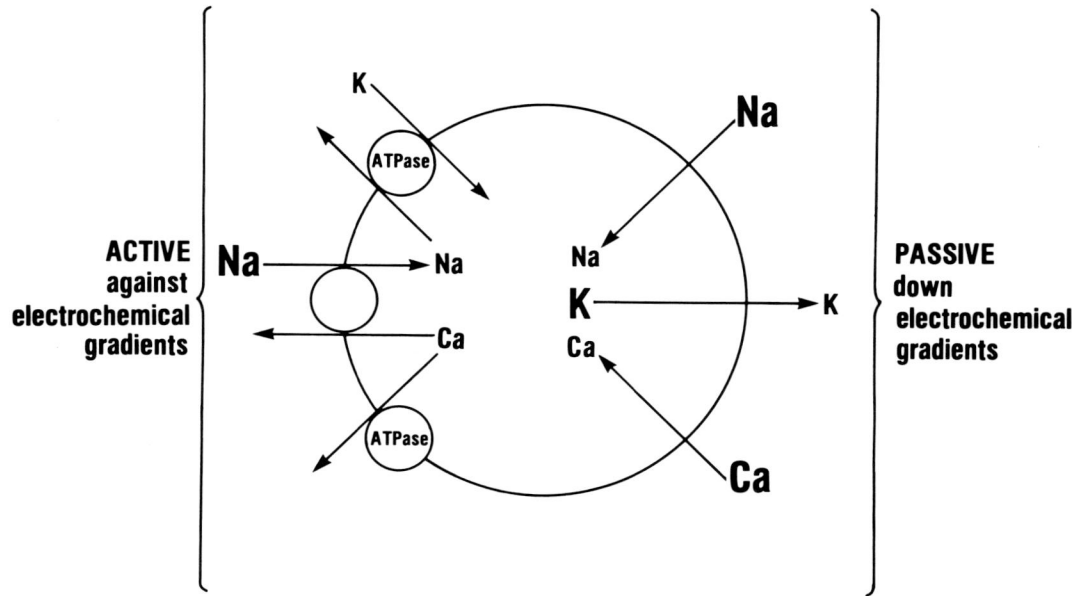

FIG. 3. Schematic of vascular smooth muscle cell depicting passive and active fluxes of Na$^+$, K$^+$, and Ca^{2+}. (From ref. 101, with permission.)

tension and to the nature of a hypertension-causing DLF. Both ouabain and digoxin administration increase pressor responsiveness to exogenous NE both in normotensive and hypertensive subjects (112–114), more so in the former (113). Perhaps this is because the responsiveness of the hypertensive to NE is greater in the first place (114). The digoxin-induced increase in pressor responsiveness to NE in normotensive subjects is greater in those without a family history of hypertension (115).

Chronic digoxin administration to humans does not cause hypertension (112), whereas chronic intraperitoneal ouabain causes chronic hypertension in rats (41). Acute administration of bufalin in rats causes a larger rise in blood pressure than acute equimolar doses of ouabain (47). These observations raise the possibility of marked species variations perhaps in part related to rapidity and completeness of binding, and suggest that all pump inhibitors are not alike with regard to their ability to raise blood pressure. Further clarification of these issues may provide additional insights into how an endogenous DLF might cause hypertension.

If it is assumed that ouabain antibodies cross-react with the most important circulating DLF, be it ouabain or some analogue of ouabain, then the circulating levels of this factor are in the subnanomolar to low nanomolar range (28,116). Some consideration, therefore, has been given to the mechanism by which subnanomolar concentrations of a pump inhibitor could cause blood pressure elevations (110). Since the binding affinity of Na,K-ATPase for ouabain is around 10^{-9} M, low nanomolar concentrations of ouabain would be expected to cause some low-level inhibition of the enzyme. Calculations

recently presented by Blaustein (110) indicate that an 8 percent increase in intracellular sodium concentration secondary to Na,K-ATPase inhibition can lead to a 26 percent increase in intracellular calcium concentration. The increased intracellular calcium concentration will lead to increased sequestering of calcium in the endoplasmic/sarcoplasmic reticulum with about a 2,500-fold amplification. Increased sequestering provides more calcium when calcium-dependent processes are activated causing augmentation of processes such as vascular smooth muscle contraction, inhibition of nitric oxide synthesis, and release of endothelin (110). Thus, low nanomolar concentrations of ouabain or an equally potent analogue could account for the increased pressor reactivity observed in normotensive and hypertensive subjects given digitalis glycosides as discussed above.

In some hypertensive models (e.g., SHR, DOCA-salt) and in some patients with heritable essential hypertension, the primary transport defect in blood vessels may be increased permeability of the vascular smooth muscle cell membrane to sodium. Superimposition of the digitalislike factor on this defect, subsequent to increased sodium intake and decreased sodium excretion, would amplify the effect of the primary defect on internal sodium concentration; it would rise to higher levels because the Na,K pump could not now compensate as well for the increased inward leak of sodium (117,118) (Fig. 4).

This hypothesis (Fig. 2), generated as outlined in the brief historical survey above, has been strengthened and expanded by recent studies in both animals and man. As noted above, chronic Na,K-ATPase inhibition with

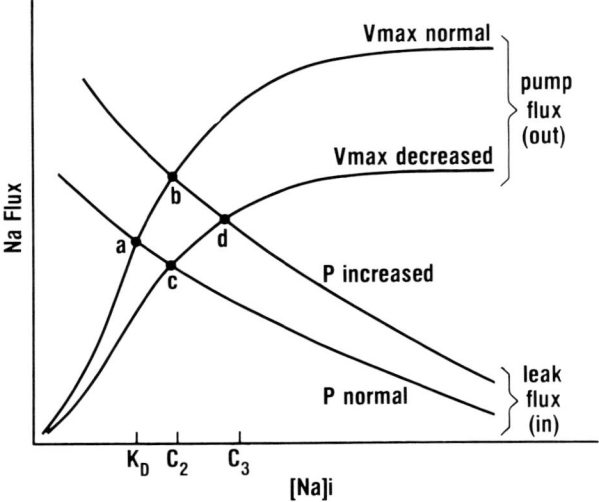

FIG. 4. The hypothetical effects of increased sodium permeability, decreased sodium pump activity, or both on the relationship of sodium flux to intracellular sodium concentration ([Na$_i$]) in vascular smooth muscle. Pump flux (active sodium efflux) is defined as the ouabain-sensitive sodium flux, and leak flux (passive sodium flux) is here defined as ouabain-insensitive sodium flux. The pump is assumed to be operating maximally at each level of [Na$_i$]. The normal steady state (point a) occurs where pump efflux equals leak flux. A new steady state (point b) would be reached at a higher [Na$_i$](C$_2$) if sodium permeability (P) increased without a sufficiently large increase in the pump flux. A new steady state (point c) with increased [Na$_i$](C$_2$) would also occur if the pump flux decreased without change in P (point c, C$_2$). If P increased and the pump flux decreased simultaneously, a new steady state would occur (point d) at an even higher [Na$_i$] (point C$_3$). (From ref. 119, with permission.)

ouabain or bufalin has been shown to cause hypertension in animals, either alone (39,120,121), or in combination with mineralocorticoids (122). Elevated levels of the inhibitor have been found in two additional models of low renin hypertension (123–125), including a model of insulin-dependent diabetes mellitus (124,125). Reduced renal mass saline hypertensive rats were found to have increased plasma ouabain immunoreactivity (126) (contrasting with the findings of Hamlyn and Manunta [28]), increased plasma ouabain displacing activity (127), and increased urinary excretion of digitalislike substance (120,128), and immunizing the rats against ouabain reduced the hypertension and aortic hypertrophy (126). On the other hand, DOCA-salt hypertension in the rat, a model known to have elevated levels of an inhibitor (70,129), did not respond to immunization against digoxin (129). SHR was shown to have increased ouabain displacing activity (127) and the Munster strain of spontaneously hypertensive rat greater than 6 months of age was shown to have increased Na,K-ATPase inhibiting activity (130); the latter was suggested to be secondary to organ damage requiring increased natriuresis to

maintain sodium homeostasis since it occurred after the development of hypertension.

Recent studies in the human continue to implicate a sodium pump inhibitor in hypertension. Similar to the findings reported by Hamlyn and Manunta (28), Naruse et al. (131) found increased plasma level of immunoreactive ouabain in essential hypertension, primary aldosteronism, Cushing's syndrome, pheochromocytoma, acromegaly, and chronic renal failure, and treatment reduced the level. However, bilateral adrenalectomy failed to reduce the level and there was no arteriovenous difference across the adrenal, suggesting to the authors that the adrenal is not likely the major source of the agent.

Recent studies of patients with essential hypertension, like older ones (19,20,22–25,132–135), reveal elevated levels of inhibitors in plasma, particularly in subjects with low plasma renin activity and presumably positive sodium and water balance (136–140). The latter might result from enhanced proximal tubular sodium reabsorption (138), particularly in the presence of a high salt intake. Plasma inhibitory activity correlates with platelet calcium (141). Black subjects may be at a disadvantage; their red blood cells normally have decreased Na,K pump activity and increased sodium content (142,143) and, when hypertensive, this improves with a low-sodium diet (142) or diuretics (144). Acute volume expansion with intravenous saline causes an increase in plasma Na,K-ATPase inhibitory activity, which correlates with a decrease in plasma renin activity, an increase in blood pressure, and forearm arterial and venous constriction (145).

Takahashi et al. (146) measured plasma and urine endogenous digitalislike substance in an adult population in Japan and implicated it in the hypertension associated with excess sodium intake, aging, and obesity. Increased dietary salt intake decreased RBC Na,K pump activity and increased RBC sodium in salt-sensitive but not salt-insensitive subjects (147). However, Spieker et al. (148) were unable to discriminate between essential and secondary hypertension with Na,K-ATPase inhibitory activity of plasma; the activity was elevated in some of both types of patients.

Takahashi et al. (149) suggest that digoxinlike substances are involved in the hypertensive mechanism in patients with insulin resistance. They studied digoxinlike immunoreactivity in male patients with impaired glucose tolerance. Plasma immunoreactivity correlated with serum insulin levels and diastolic blood pressure, suggesting to them that the digitalislike immunoreactivity is the determinant of the hypertension associated with hyperinsulinemia, i.e., insulin resistance.

It is useful to determine which patients are sensitive to salt since this guides therapy in the direction of a salt-restricted diet, diuretics, or both. Salt sensitivity is now determined by observing the change in blood pressure on switching from a low- to a high-salt diet or vice versa. Espinel (150) goes further and determines a salt hypertension threshold, i.e., the salt intake that raises pressure. This is accomplished with a salt step test in which blood pressure is successively observed on unrestricted salt, restricted salt, and then during stepwise increases in salt intake. It would be helpful to have a faster method to determine salt sensitivity. Iwaoka et al. (138) suggest that lithium clearance, a measure of proximal tubular sodium reabsorption, can predict salt sensitivity without salt loading. The same may be the case for the plasma level of the sodium pump inhibitor. Both suggestions need evaluation.

OTHER CONDITIONS

Graves et al. (151) studied patients with renal failure and found that serum and dialysate digitalislike factors increase with sustained volume expansion and correlate with weight and blood pressure. The factor was not ouabain or digoxin but was like that previously found in amniotic fluid. Schoner et al. (152) found an ouabainlike substance in hemofiltrate from patients with uremia, which was not identical with ouabain. Their studies in pig adrenal revealed ouabain and more hydrophilic inhibitors cross-reacting with ouabain antibody, consistent with the adrenal as a source of several ouabainlike substances.

Gusdon et al. (153) demonstrated an elevated digoxinlike factor in preeclampsia. Subsequently, Graves and Williams (154) associated an endogenous ouabainlike factor with pregnancy-induced hypertension. The question was quickly considered by others (155–157). Poston et al. (156) found that plasma digoxin immunoreactivity increases in normal pregnancy but is elevated beyond this in pregnancy-induced hypertension only at 28 to 30 weeks of gestation. Although the level is persistently elevated in some women with pregnancy-induced hypertension, it cannot be used as a predictor of pregnancy-induced hypertension (158). More recent studies reveal increased red blood cell sodium content and decreased ouabain-binding sites in pregnancy-induced hypertension (159) and increased plasma Na,K-ATPase inhibitor in preeclampsia, especially when the preeclampsia is severe and with preexisting renal disease (a digoxin radioimmunoassay did not reveal the inhibitor) (160).

Increased levels of digoxin immunoreactivity (161–163) and leukocyte sodium transport inhibitory activity (164) have been reported in serum of neonates. An endogenous digitalislike substance was recently partially purified from cord blood; it cross-reacts with digoxin antibodies and appears to be the same agent found in adult plasma (165–167).

Increased levels of plasma digitalislike factor have been found under a variety of other conditions. For example, it has been reported to increase during insulin-induced hypoglycemia, and the magnitude of the increase is augmented by salt or fluid loading (168). It has also been reported to increase during percutaneous transluminal angioplasty in patients with coronary stenosis (169), during cardiac catheterization (170), and during high-altitude exposure (171). In the former two cases, the levels correlated with hemodynamic factors such as cardiac output, left atrial pressure, and pulmonary congestion, as if release was an attempt to compensate.

Koga et al. (172) showed that mild exercise decreases plasma endogenous digitalislike substance in hypertensive individuals, perhaps by decreasing plasma volume (173). Thus, digitalislike substance may participate in the mechanism by which exercise lowers blood pressure.

SUMMARY

The evidence that certain types of hypertension, particularly of the low renin variety, result in part from a circulating Na,K-ATPase inhibitor continues to mount. So does the evidence that the inhibitor is a steroid produced either in the adrenal, the hypothalamus, or both. Effort should now be directed at evaluating the proposal that the inhibitor is ouabain or a closely related compound. Effort should also be directed at determining its precise role in primary and secondary hypertension and at devising methods to combat its deleterious effects. Evidence suggests that, since its release is tied to volume expansion, salt-restricted diets and diuretics would reduce the blood level of the inhibitor and thus the blood pressure. When reduction of blood volume is not complete, other methods might be needed. Antibodies to the inhibitor, potassium, and pharmacological agents such as canrenone, which compete with binding of the inhibitor to Na,K-ATPase, should receive additional attention.

REFERENCES

1. de Wardener HE, Mills IH, Clapham WF, Hayter CJ. Studies on the efferent mechanism of the sodium diuresis which follows the administration of intravenous saline in the dog. *Clin Sci* 1961;21: 249–258.
2. Kramer H, Gonick H, Paul W. Third factor: Inhibitor of Na$^+$,K$^+$-ATPase? In: *Proceedings of the Fourth International Congress on Nephrology.* New York: Karger, 1969;373.
3. Buckalew VM, Martinez FJ, Green WE. The effect of dialysates and ultra-filtrates of plasma of saline-loaded dogs on toad bladder sodium transport. *J Clin Invest* 1970;49:926–935.
4. Haddy FJ, Overbeck HW. The role of humoral agents in volume expanded hypertension. *Life Sci* 1976;19:935–947.
5. Overbeck HW, Pamnani MB, Akera T, Brody TM, Haddy FJ. Depressed function of a ouabain-sensitive sodium-potassium pump in blood vessels from renal hypertensive dogs. *Circ Res* 1976;38(suppl 2):II48–II52.
6. Clough DL, Pamnani MB, Overbeck HW, Haddy FJ. Decreased

myocardial Na,K-ATPase in rats with one-kidney, Goldblatt hypertension. *Fed Proc* 1977;36:491.

7. Clough DL, Pamnani MB, Haddy FJ. Decreased myocardial Na$^+$,K$^+$-ATPase activity in one-kidney, one clip hypertensive rats. *Am J Physiol* 1983;245:H244–H251.

8. Vatner SF, Higgins CB, Franklin D, Braunwald E. Effects of a digitalis glycoside on coronary and systemic dynamics in conscious dogs. *Circ Res* 1971;28:470–479.

9. Brender D, Vanhoutte PM, Shepherd JT. Potentiation of adrenergic venomotor responses in dog by cardiac glycosides. *Circ Res* 1969;25:597–606.

10. Brace RA, Anderson DK, Chen WT, Scott JB, Haddy FJ. Local effects of hypokalemia on coronary resistance and myocardial contractile force. *Am J Physiol* 1974;227:590–597.

11. Haddy FJ, Scott JB. Mechanism of the acute pressor action of hypokalemia, hypomagnesemia, and hypo-osmolality. *Am Heart J* 1973;85:655–661.

12. Anderson DK, Roth SA, Brace RA, Radawski D, Haddy FJ, Scott JB. Effect of hypokalemia and hypomagnesemia produced by hemodialysis on vascular resistance in canine skeletal muscle: role of potassium in active hyperemia. *Circ Res* 1972;31:165–173.

13. Chen WT, Brace RA, Scott JB, Anderson DK, Haddy FJ. The mechanism of the vasodilator action of potassium. *Proc Soc Exp Biol Med* 1972;140:820–824.

14. Pamnani MB, Clough DL, Huot SJ, Haddy FJ. Sodium potassium pump activity in experimental hypertension. In: Vanhoutte PM, Leusen I, eds. *Vasodilatation.* New York: Raven Press 1981;391–403.

15. Pamnani M, Huot S, Steffen R, Haddy FJ. Evidence for a humoral Na$^+$ transport inhibiting factor(s) in one-kidney, on wrapped hypertensive dog. *Physiologist* 1980;23(4):91.

16. Pamnani M, Huot S, Buggy J, Clough D, Haddy F. Demonstration of a humoral inhibitor of the Na$^+$-K$^+$ pump in some models of experimental hypertension. *Hypertension* 1981;3(suppl II):II96–II101.

17. Haddy F, Pamnani M, Clough D. The sodium-potassium pump in volume expanded hypertension. *Clin Exp Hypertens* 1978–79;1(3):295–336.

18. Gruber KA, Whitaker JM, Buckalew VM Jr. Endogenous digitalislike substance in plasma of volume-expanded dogs. *Nature* 1980;287:743–745.

19. Poston L, Sewell RB, Wilkinson SP, Richardson PJ, Williams R, Clarkson EM, MacGregor GA, de Wardener HE. Evidence for a circulating sodium transport inhibitor in essential hypertension. *Br Med J* 1981;282:847–849.

20. Hamlyn JM, Ringel R, Schaeffer J, Levinson PD, Hamilton BP, Kowarski AA, Blaustein MP. A circulating inhibitor of (Na$^+$+K$^+$) ATPase associated with essential hypertension. *Nature* 1982;300:650–652.

21. deWardener HE, MacGregor GA, Clarkson EM, Alaghband-Zakdeh J, Bitensky L, Chayen J. Effect of sodium intake on ability of human plasma to inhibit renal Na$^+$-K$^+$-adenosine triphosphatase in vitro. *Lancet* 1981;1:411–412.

22. Hasegawa T, Masugi F, Ogihara T, Kumahara Y. Increase in plasma ouabainlike inhibitor of Na$^+$,K$^+$-ATPase with high sodium intake in patients with essential hypertension. *J Clin Hypertens* 1987;3:419–429.

23. Burris JF, Pamnani MB, Huot SH, Jemionek FJ, Fries ED, Haddy FJ. Sodium-potassium (Na$^+$-K$^+$) pump activity in low renin essential hypertension. *Clin Res* 1982;30:733a.

24. Pamnani MB, Haddy FJ. Characteristics of hypertensive patients with increased plasma Na$^+$+K$^+$ pump inhibitory activity. *Clin Exp Hypertens* [A] 1985;A7:755–768.

25. Pamnani MB, Burris JF, Jemionek JF, Huot SJ, Price M, Fries ED, Haddy FJ. Humoral Na$^+$-K$^+$ inhibitory activity in essential hypertension and in normotensive subjects after volume expansion. *Am J Hypertens* 1989;2:524–531.

26. Hamlyn JM, Blaustein MB, Bova S, DuCharme DW, Harris DW, Mandel F, Matthews WR, Ludens JH. Identification and characterization of ouabainlike compound from human plasma. *Proc Natl Acad Sci USA* 1991;88:6259–6263.

27. Mathews WR, DuCharme DW, Hamlyn JM, Harris DW, Mandel F, Clark MA, Ludens JH. Mass spectral characterization of an endogenous digitalislike factor from human plasma. *Hypertension* 1991;17:930–935.

28. Hamlyn J, Manunta P. Ouabain, digitalislike factors and hypertension. *J Hypertens* 1992;10(suppl 7):S99–S111.

29. Bova S, Blaustein MP, Ludens JH, Harris DW, DuCharme DW, Hamlyn JM. Effects of an endogenous ouabainlike compound on heart and aorta. *Hypertension* 1991;17:944–950.

30. Harris DW, Clark MA, Fisher JF, Hamlyn JM, Kolbasa KP, Ludens JH, Ducharme DW. Development of an immunoassay for endogenous digitalislike factor. *Hypertension* 1991;17:936–943.

31. Huang X, Huang BS, Harmsen E, Leenen FHH. Effects of chronic ouabain on BP and plasma and tissue ouabainlike activity (OLA) in rats. *Hypertension* 1993;22:432.

32. Kitano S, Morimoto S, Koh E, Ogihara T. The adrenals release accumulated exogenous oubain at volume expansion in reduced renal mass hypertensive rats. *Hypertension* 1993;22:432.

33. Manunta P, Hamilton BP, Price E, Hamlyn JM. High dietary intake of sodium increases plasma ouabain levels in normal man. *J Hypertens* 1992;10(suppl 4):S96.

34. Ludens JH, Clark MA, Kolbasa KP, Hamlyn JM. Digitalislike factor and ouabainlike compound in plasma of volume-expanded dogs. *J Cardiovasc Pharmacol* 1993;22(suppl 2):S38–S41.

35. Williams MH Jr, Zohman LR, Ratner AC. Hemodynamic effects of cardiac glycosides on normal human subjects during rest and exercise. *J Appl Physiol* 1958;13:417–421.

36. DeMots H, Rahimtoola SH, McAnulty JH, Porter GA. Effects of ouabain on coronary and systemic vascular resistance and myocardial oxygen consumption in patients without heart failure. *Am J Cardiol* 1978;41:88–93.

37. Songu-Mize E, Nash CB, Elam JT, Caldwell RW. Metabolism and cardiac action of a polar aminocardenolide and digoxin in the conscious dog. *J Pharmacol Exp Ther* 1983;226:65–70.

38. Dogan A, Eliades D, Swindall BT, Pamnani MB, Haddy F. A comparison of the hemodynamic effects of bufalin and ouabain in dog, rat, and guinea pig. *FASEB J* 1992;6:A1253.

39. Haddy F, Pamnani M, Eliades D, Swindall B, Chen S, Dogan A, Yuan C. A comparison of the effects of two putative endogenous Na$^+$,K$^+$-ATPase inhibitors on cardiorenal function in the dog, rat, and guinea pig. In: Puschett JB, Greenberg A, eds. *Diuretics IV: chemistry, pharmacology and clinical applications.* Amsterdam: Elsevier Science Publishers BV, 1993;685–688.

40. Pamnani M, Haddy F, Eliades D, Swindall B. A comparison of the acute effects of two putative endogenous Na$^+$,K$^+$-ATPase inhibitors on cardiorenal function in the dog and rat. *Hypertension* 1991;17:438–439.

41. Yuan CM, Manunta P, Hamlyn JM, Chen S, Bohen E, Yeun J, Haddy FJ, Pamnani MB. Long-term ouabain administration produces hypertension in rats. *Hypertension* 1993;22:178–187.

42. Naomi S, Graves S, Lazarus M, Williams GH, Hollenberg NK. Variation in apparent serum digitalislike factor levels with different digoxin antibodies: the "immunochemical fingerprint." *Am J Hypertens* 1991;4:795–801.

43. Lichtstein D, Kachalsky S, Deutsch J. Identification of a ouabainlike compound in toad skin and plasma as a bufodienolide derivative. *Life Sci* 1986;38:1261–1270.

44. Tal DM, Katchalsky S, Lichtstein D, Karlish SJD. Endogenous "ouabainlike" activity in bovine plasma. *Biochem Biophys Res Commun* 1986;135:1–8.

45. Lichtstein D, Gati I, Samuelov S, Berson D, Rozenman Y, Landau L. Identification of digitalislike compounds in human cataractous lenses. *Eur J Biochem* 1993;216:261–268.

46. Eliades D, Swindall B, Johnston J, Pamnani M, Haddy F. Hemodynamic effects of bufalin in the anesthetized dog. *Hypertension* 1989;13:690–695.

47. Pamnani MB, Chen S, Bryant HJ, Schooley JF Jr, Eliades DC, Yuan CM, Haddy FJ. Effects of three sodium-potassium adenosine triphosphatase inhibitors. *Hypertension* 1991;18:316–324.

48. LaBella FS, Bihler I, Templeton J, Ryung-Soon K, Hnatowich M, Rohrer D. Progesterone derivatives that bind to the digitalis receptor: effects of Na$^+$,K$^+$-ATPase and isolated tissues. *Fed Proc* 1985;44:2806–2811.

49. Weiland J, Schwabe K, Hübler D, Schonfeld D, Repke KR. Glycosidation of chlormadinol acetate alters its actions on Na$^+$/K$^+$-

transporting ATPase and cardiac contractility: a contribution to the endogenous digitalis problem. *J Enzym Inhib* 1987;2:31–36.

50. Bose D, Elliot D, Kobayashi T, Templeton JF, Kumar VPS, La-Bella FS. 14 beta-hydroxyprogesterone binds to the digitalis receptor, inhibits the sodium pump and enhances cardiac contractility. *Br J Pharmacol* 1988;93:453–461.

51. Goto A, Ishiguro T, Yamada K, Ishii M, Yoshioka M, Eguchi C, Shimora M, Sugimoto T. Isolation of a urinary digitalislike factor indistinguishable from digoxin. *Biochem Biophys Res Commun* 1990;173:1093–1101.

52. Goto A, Yamada K, Yagi N, Hui C, Nagoshi H, Sasabe M, Yoshioka M. Digitalislike factors from human urine. *J Cardiovasc Pharmacol* 1993;22(suppl 2):S58–S59.

53. Shaikh IM, Lau BWC, Siegfried BA, Valdes R Jr. Isolation of digoxin-like immunoreactive factors from mammalian adrenal cortex. *J Biol Chem* 1991;266:13672–13678.

54. Weinberg U, Dolev S, Werber MM, Shapiro MS, Shilo L, Shenkman L. Identification and preliminary characterization of two human digitalislike substances that are structurally related to digoxin and ouabain. *Biochem Biophys Res Commun* 1992;188:1024–1029.

55. Cloix JF, Crabos M, Wainer IW, Ruegg U, Seiler M, Meyer P. High yield purification of a urinary Na$^+$ pump inhibitor. *Biochem Biophys Res Commun* 1985;131:1234–1240.

56. Cloix J-F, Crabos MC, Grichois ML, Meyer P. An endogenous digitalislike compound extracted from human urine: biochemical and chemical studies. *Can J Physiol Pharmacol* 1987;65:1522–1527.

57. Weiler E, Gonick H, Prins B, Purdy R, Weber M. Characterization of a low molecular weight Na-K-ATPase inhibitor of urinary origin. *Clin Res* 1991;39:23a.

58. Tamura M, Konishi F, Inagami T. A novel endogenous sodium-pump inhibitor in pig urine: purification and comparison with the inhibitor purified from bovine adrenal glands. *J Cardiovasc Pharmacol* 1993;22(suppl 2):S47–S50.

59. Tymiak AA, Norman JA, Bolgar M, DiDonato GC, Lee H, Parker WL, Lo L-C, Berova N, Nakanishi K, Haber E, Haupert GT Jr. Physicochemical characterization of a ouabain isomer isolated from bovine hypothalamus. *Proc Natl Acad Sci USA* 1993;90:8189–8193.

60. Haupert GT Jr, Carilli CT, Cantley LC. Hypothalamic sodium-transport inhibitor is a high-affinity reversible inhibitor of Na$^+$-K$^+$-ATPase. *Am J Physiol* 1984;247:F919–F924.

61. Haupert GT Jr. Characteristic of the Na$^+$-K$^+$-ATPase inhibitor from hypothalamus. *Prog Biochem Pharmacol* 1988;23:10–21.

62. Anner BM, Rey HG, Moosmayer M, Meszoely I, Haupert GT Jr. Hypothalamic Na$^+$-K$^+$-ATPase inhibitor characterized in two-sided liposomes containing pure renal Na$^+$-K$^+$-ATPase. *Am J Physiol* 1990;258:F144–F153.

63. Pamnani MB, Whitehorn WV, Clough DL, Haddy FJ. Effects of canrenone on blood pressure in rats with reduced renal mass. *Am J Hypertens* 1990;3:188–195.

64. Haddy FJ, Pamnani MB. Pharmacologic agents for the *in vivo* detection of vascular sodium transport defects in hypertension. *Life Sci* 1987;41:2685–2696.

65. Semplicini A, Buzzaccarini F, Ceolotto G, Marzola M, Mozzato MG, Giusto M, Campagnolo M, Simonella C, Pessina AC. Effects of canrenoate on red cell sodium transport and calf flow in essential hypertension. *Am J Hypertens* 1993;6:295–301.

66. Haupert GT Jr, Sancho JM. Sodium transport inhibitor from bovine hypothalamus. *Proc Natl Acad Sci USA* 1979;76:4658–4660.

67. de Wardener HE, Clarkson EM. Concept of natriuretic hormone. *Physiol Rev* 1985;65:658–759.

68. Morgan K, Lewis MD, Spurlock G, Collins PA, Foord SM, Southgate K, Scanlon MF, Mir MA. Characterization and partial purification of the sodium-potassium ATPase inhibitor released from cultured rat hypothalamic cells. *J Biol Chem* 1985;260:13595–13600.

69. Huot SJ, Pamnani MB, Clough DL, Buggy J, Bryant HJ, Harder DR, Haddy FJ. Sodium-potassium pump activity in reduced renal-mass hypertension. *Hypertension* 1983;5(suppl 1):94–100.

70. Songu-Mize E, Bealer SL, Caldwell RW. Effect of AV3V lesions

on development of DOCA-salt hypertension and vascular Na$^+$-pump activity. *Hypertension* 1982;4:575–580.

71. Bealer SL, Haywood JR, Gruber KA, Buckalew VM Jr, Fink GD, Brody MJ, Johnson AK. Preoptic-hypothalamic periventricular lesions reduce natriuresis to volume expansion. *Am J Physiol* 1983;244:R51–R57.

72. Deray G, Rieu M, Devynck MA, Pernollet MG, Chanson P, Luton JP, Meyer P. Evidence of an endogenous digitalislike factor in the plasma of patients with acromegaly. *N Engl J Med* 1987;316:575–580.

73. Jandhyala BS, Ansari AF. Elevation of sodium levels in the cerebral ventricles of anaesthetized dogs triggers the release of an inhibitor of ouabain-sensitive sodium, potassium ATPase into the circulation. *Clin Sci* 1986;70:103–110.

74. Takahashi H, Matsusawa M, Suga K, Ikegaki I, Nishimura M, Yoshimura M, Ihara N, Yamada H, Sano Y. Hypothalamic digitalislike substance is released with sodium-loading in rats. *Am J Hypertens* 1988;1:146–151.

75. Jandhyala BS, Lokhandwala MF, Kivlighn SD, Ansari AF, De Feo ML. Intracisternal administration of pergolide, a dopamine receptor agonist, triggers the release of an inhibitor of ouabain-sensitive sodium, potassium-dependent adenosine triphosphatase and enhances vascular reactivity in anaesthetized dogs. *Clin Sci* 1987;73:183–188.

76. Buckley JP, Doursout M-F, Liang Y-Y, Chelly JE. Central angiotensin II mechanisms and the sodium pump. *J Hypertens* 1986;4(suppl 6):S465–S467.

77. Halperin J, Schaeffer R, Valdez L, Malave S. Ouabainlike activity in human cerebrospinal fluid. *Proc Natl Acad Sci USA* 1983;80:6101–6104.

78. Halperin JA, Martin AM, Malave S. Increased digitalislike activity in human cerebrospinal fluid after expansion of the extracellular fluid volume. *Life Sci* 1985;37:561–566.

79. Halperin JA, Riordan JF, Tosteson DC. Characteristics of an inhibitor of the Na$^+$/K$^+$ pump in human cerebrospinal fluid. *J Biol Chem* 1988;263:646–651.

80. Lichtstein D, Minc D, Bourrit A, Deutsch J, Karlish SJD, Belmaker H, Rimon R, Palo J. Evidence for the presence of "ouabain-like" compound in human cerebrospinal fluid. *Brain Res* 1985;325:13–19.

81. Takahashi H, Matsusawa M, Ikegaki I, Suga K, Nishimura M, Yoshimura M, Yamada H, Sano Y. Digitalislike substance is produced in the hypothalamus but not in the adrenal gland in rats. *J Hypertens* 1988;6(suppl 4):S345–S347.

82. Ihara N, Yuri K, Yamada H, Sano Y. Immunohistochemical studies in the distribution of endogenous digitalislike substance (EDLS)-containing neurons in the rat hypothalamus, with special consideration on the possibility of their coexistence with posterior lobe hormones. *Arch Histol Cytol* 1988;51:35–42.

83. Yamada H, Ihara N, Takahashi H, Yoshimura M, Sano Y. Distribution of the endogenous digitalislike substance (EDLS)-containing neurons labeled by digoxin antibody in hypothalamus and three circumventricular organs of dog and macaque. *Brain Res* 1992;584:237–243.

84. Yamada H, Naruse M, Naruse K, Demura H, Takahashi H, Yoshimura M, Ochi J. Histological study on ouabain immunoreactivities in the mammalian hypothalamus. *Neurosci Lett* 1992;141:143–146.

85. Pernollet MG, Ali RM, Meyer P, Devynck M-A. Are the circulating digitalislike compounds of adrenal origin? *J Hypertens* 1986;4(suppl 6):S382–S384.

86. Tamura M, Lam T-T, Inagami T. Isolation and characterization of a specific endogenous Na$^+$,K$^+$-ATPase inhibitor from bovine adrenal. *Biochemistry* 1988;27:4244–4253.

87. Lam SK, Tamura M, Inagami T. Distribution of a specific inhibitor of the Na$^+$-pump in the tissues of rat. *FASEB J* 1993;7:A533.

88. Tamura M, Lam SK, Inagami T. Detection of a specific Na-pump inhibitor in urine from experimental hypertensive rats. *FASEB J* 1993;7:A533.

89. Vinge E, Erfurth EMT, Lundin S. Effects of adrenal function tests on the levels of endogenous digitalislike substances and some pituitary hormones. *Acta Endocrinol* 1993;128:29–34.

90. Ludens JH, Clark MA, Robinson FG, DuCharme DW. Rat adre-

nal cortex is a source of a circulating ouabainlike compound. *Hypertension* 1992;19:721–724.

91. Doris PA. Immunological evidence that the adrenal gland is the source of an endogenous digitalislike factor. *Endocrinology* 1988;123:2440–2444.

92. Doris PA. Digoxinlike immunoreactive factor in rat plasma: effect of sodium and calcium intake. *Life Sci* 1988;42:783–790.

93. Doris PA, Kilgore MW, Durham D, Alberts D, Stocco DM. An endogenous digitalis factor derived from the adrenal gland: studies of adrenocortical tumor cells. *Endocrinology* 1989;125:2580–2586.

94. Doris PA, Stocco DM. An endogenous digitalislike factor derived from the adrenal gland: studies of adrenal tissue from various sources. *Endocrinology* 1989;125:2573–2579.

95. Boulanger BR, Lilly MP, Hamlyn JM, Laredo J, Shurtleff D, Gann DS. Ouabain is secreted by the adrenal gland in awake dogs. *Am J Physiol* 1993;264:E413–E419.

96. Masugi P, Ogihara T, Hasegawa T, Tomii A, Nagano M, Higashimori K, Kumahara K, Terano Y. Circulating factor with ouabainlike immunoreactivity in patients with primary aldosteronism. *Biochem Biophys Res Commun* 1986;135:41–45.

97. Masugi F, Ogihara T, Hasegawa T, Sakaguchi K, Kumahara Y. Normalization of high plasma level of ouabainlike immunoreactivity in primary aldosteronism after removal of adenoma. *J Hum Hypertens* 1988;2:17–20.

98. Doris PA. Characterization and scattered binding analysis of adrenal of digitalislike material. *Life Sci* 1992;50:1935–1941.

99. Williams GH, Hollenberg NK. Sodium-sensitive essential hypertension: emerging insights into an old entity. *J Am Coll Nutr* 1989;8:490–494.

100. Blaustein MP. Sodium ions, calcium ions, blood pressure regulation, and hypertension: a reassessment and a hypothesis. *Am J Physiol* 1977;232:C165–C173.

101. Haddy FJ. Abnormalities of membrane transport in hypertension. *Hypertension* 1983;5(suppl V):66–72.

102. Caldwell RW, Songu-Mize E, Bealer SL. The vasopressor response to centrally administered ouabain. *Circ Res* 1984;55:773–779.

103. Jacomini LCL, Elghozi JL, Dagher G, Devynck MA, Meyer P. Central hypertensive effect of ouabain in rats. *Arch Int Pharmacodyn* 1984;267:310–318.

104. Ferrandi M, Minotti E, Salardi S, Florio M, Bianchi G, Ferrari P. Characteristics of ouabainlike factor from Milan hypertensive rats. *J Cardiovasc Pharmacol* 1993;22(suppl 2):S75–S78.

105. Millett JA, Holland SM, Alaghband-Zadeh J, de Wardener HE. Na-K-ATPase-inhibiting and glucose 6-phosphate dehydrogenase-stimulating activity of plasma and hypothalamus of the Okamoto spontaneously hypertensive rat. *J Endocrinol* 1986;108:69–73.

106. Holland S, Millett J, Alaghband-Zadeh J, de Wardener H, Pamnani M, Haddy F. Cytochemically detectable glucose-6-phosphate dehydrogenase-stimulating/Na-K-ATPase-inhibiting activity of plasma and hypothalamus in reduced renal mass hypertension. *Am J Hypertens* 1991;4:315–320.

107. Leenen FHH, Harmsen E, Yu H, Ou C. Effects of dietary sodium on central and peripheral ouabainlike activity in spontaneously hypertensive rats. *Am J Physiol* 1993;264:H2051–H2055.

108. Leenen FHH, Huang BS, Harmsen E. Role of brain ouabain-like activity in the central effects of sodium in rats. *J Cardiovasc Pharmacol* 1993;22(suppl 2):S72–S74.

109. de Wardener HE, Holland S, Alaghband-Zadeh J, Morris HR, Panico M, Etienne A. A possible connection between an increased concentration of a cyto-chemically detectable substance in the hypothalamus of the spontaneously hypertensive rat and certain cerebral cholinergic disturbances. *J Cardiovasc Pharmacol* 1993;22(suppl 2):S109–S111.

110. Blaustein MP. Physiological effects of endogenous ouabain: control of intracellular Ca^{2+} stores and cell responsiveness. *Am J Physiol* 1993;264:C1367–C1387.

111. Cress LW, Freas W, Haddy F, Muldoon SM. Effects of bufalin on norepinephrine turnover in canine saphenous vein. *Hypertension* 1991;18:516–522.

112. Guthrie GP Jr. Effects of digoxin on responsiveness to the pressor

actions of angiotensin and norepinephrine in man. *J Clin Endocrinol Metab* 1984;58:76–80.

113. Yamagi I, Kibuchi K, Nishimura M, Nozawa A, Hasegawa T, Kobayakawa H, Komura H, Iimura O. The role of Na,K-ATPase inhibitor on pressor responsiveness in patients with benign essential hypertension. *Am J Hypertens* 1990;3:176–181.

114. Saito T, Takizawa T, Nakatuska T, et al. Role of sodium transport system of cell membrane on pressor response to infused noradrenaline in essential hypertension. *Abstracts of the International Society of Hypertension* 1992;312.

115. Wada A, Kibuchi K, Shimazaki M, et al. Attenuated digoxin induced enhancement of pressor response to infused norepinephrine in young normotensive subject with a family history of essential hypertension. *Abstracts of the International Society of Hypertension* 1992;353.

116. Gottlieb SS, Rogowski AC, Weinberg M, Krichten CM, Hamilton BP, Hamlyn JM. Elevated concentrations of endogenous ouabain in patients with congestive heart failure. *Circulation* 1992;86:420–425.

117. Haddy FJ, Pamnani MB, Clough DL. Pathophysiological role of cation transport and natriuretic factors in hypertension. *Hypertension* 1987;10(suppl I):I-101–I-107.

118. Haddy FJ. Ionic control of vascular smooth muscle cells. *Kidney Int* 1988;34(suppl 25):S-2–S-8.

119. Clough DL, Pamnani MB, Huot SH, Haddy FJ. Myocardial Na^+,K^+-ATPase activity in Dahl salt sensitive and resistant rats. *Clin Exp Hypertens* 1985;A7:573–584.

120. Oshimoto Y, Shimamoto K, Nakagawa M, Masuda A, Satoh S, Imura O. The pressor mechanism in reduced renal mass hypertensive rat, a model of volume dependent hypertension. *Abstracts of the International Society of Hypertension* 1992;S128.

121. Pamnani MB, Chen S, Yuan C, Haddy FJ. Chronic effects of bufalin, a sodium, potassium-ATPase inhibitor, in rats. *Hypertension* 1993;21:557.

122. Sekihara H, Yazaki Y, Kojima T. Ouabain as an amplifier of mineralocorticoid-induced hypertension. *Endocrinology* 1992;131:3077–3082.

123. Tepel M, Theilmeier G, Bachmann J, Ganten D, Rahn KH, Zidek W. Increased cytosolic $[Na^+]_i$ and reduced Na-K-ATPase activity in transgenic rats TGR (m REN2) 27. *Hypertension* 1993;21:542.

124. Chen S, Yuan C, Schooley JF Jr, Haddy FJ, Pamnani MB. A consistent model of insulin-dependent diabetes mellitus hypertension. *Am J Hypertens* 1992;5:671–680.

125. Chen S, Yuan C, Clough D, Schooley J, Haddy FJ, Pamnani MB. Role of digitalislike substance in the hypertension of streptozotocin-induced diabetes in reduced renal mass rats. *Am J Hypertens* 1993;6:397–406.

126. Yamada K, Goto A, Nagoshi H, Omata M. Evidence for the participation of ouabainlike compound (OLC) in reduced renal mass (RRM)-saline hypertension; studies in rats immunized against ouabain. *Hypertension* 1993;21:577.

127. Goto A, Yamada K, Yagi N, Nagoshi H, Chen H, Sugimoto T. Novel concepts on the role of ouabainlike compounds in hypertension. *Abstracts of International Society of Hypertension* 1992;S50.

128. Kimira K, Shima H, Tsuda K, Tanigawa L, Nishio I. Purification of EDLS and of its contribution to hypertension. *Abstracts of the International Society of Hypertension* 1992;S128.

129. Wagener OE, Zeiss CR, del Greco F, Quintanilla AP. Antidigoxin-antibody raised in rats with DOCA-salt hypertension does not alter blood pressure or renal Na,K-ATPase. *FASEB J* 1990;4:A702.

130. Spieker C, Rahn K-H, Zidek W. Age-dependent secretion of a Na^+,K^+-ATPase inhibitor in spontaneously hypertensive rats. *Abstracts of the International Society of Hypertension* 1992;S156.

131. Naruse K, Naruse M, Tanabe A, Yoshimoto T, Watanabe Y, Kurimoto F, Demura H. Does plasma immunoreactive ouabain originate in adrenal gland? *Hypertension* 1993;21:551.

132. Umeda T, Naomi S, Inoue J, Ohno M, Miura F, Hamasaki S, Iwaoka T, Sato T. Assay of a circulating sodium pump inhibitor in patients with essential hypertension and normotensive subjects. *Clin Exp Hypertens [A]* 1987;A9:1209–1219.

133. Iwaoka T, Nugent CA, Umeda T, Sato T. (Na⁺+K⁺)ATPase inhibitors and intracellular electrolytes in essential hypertension. *Jpn Heart J* 1987;28:695–705.

134. Devynck MA, Pernollet MG, Rosenfeld JB, Meyer P. Measurement of digitalislike compound in plasma: application in studies of essential hypertension. *Br Med J* 1983;287:631–634.

135. Moreth K, Renner D, Schoner W. A quantitative receptor assay for "digitalislike" compounds in serum. Demonstration of raised concentrations in essential hypertension and correlation with arterial blood pressure. *Klin Wochenschr* 1987;65:179–184.

136. Musca A, Cammarella I, Ferri C, Bellini C, Ruggeri R, Santucci A, Balsano F. Natriuretic hormones in young hypertensives and in young normotensives with or without a family history of hypertension. *Am J Hypertens* 1992;5:592–599.

137. Goto A, Yamada K, Ishii M, Sugimoto T. Digitalislike activity in human plasma; relation to blood pressure and sodium balance. *Am J Med* 1990;89:420–426.

138. Iwaoka T, Umeda T, Miura F, Inoue J, Sasaki M, Naomi S, Sato T. Renal sodium handling and sodium transport inhibitor in salt-sensitive essential hypertension. *J Hypertens* 1991;9:49–54.

139. Keane P, Burgess E, Watanabe M, Wong T. Plasma sodium-potassium ATPase inhibition activity in low- and normal-renin hypertension. *Am J Hypertens* 1991;4:9–13.

140. Gonick HC, Weiler EWJ, Khalil-Manesh F, Weber MA. Predominance of high molecular weight plasma Na⁺-K⁺-ATPase inhibitor in essential hypertension. *Am J Hypertens* 1993;6:680–687.

141. Sang K, Pernollet M-G, Meyer P, Devynck M-A. Plasma digitalis-like activity and cytosolic Ca²⁺ in essential hypertension. *Am J Hypertens* 1990;3:171–175.

142. Lijnen P, Buyamba-Kabangu J-R M, Fagard R, Staessen J, Amery A. Erythrocyte concentrations and transmembrane fluxes of sodium and potassium in essential hypertension: role of intrinsic and environmental factors. *Cardiovasc Drugs Ther* 1990; 4(suppl 2):321–333.

143. Aviv A, Aladjem M. Essential hypertension in blacks: epidemiology, characteristics, and possible roles of racial differences in sodium, potassium, and calcium regulation. *Cardiovasc Drugs Ther* 1990;4(suppl 2):335–342.

144. Quintanilla AP, Wagener OE. Diuretics and cations transport in hypertensive blacks. *Cardiovasc Drugs Ther* 1990;4(suppl 2): 383–387.

145. Borghi C, Boschi S, Munarini A, Mussi A, Costa FV, Ambrosioni E. Short-term plasma renin activity suppression by saline and release of a plasma endogenous Na/K ATPase inhibitor in essential hypertension. *Am J Hypertens* 1990;3:98–104.

146. Takahashi H, Matsusawa M, Okaboyashi H, Suga K, Ikegaki I, Nishimura M, Yoshimura M. Endogenous digitalislike substance in adult population in Japan. *Am J Hypertens* 1988;1:168s–172s.

147. Saito T, Onuma N, Yamamoto M, et al. Salt sensitivity and cellular sodium influx in essential hypertension. *Abstracts of the International Society of Hypertension* 1992;312.

148. Spieker C, Rahn EH, Zidek W. Na⁺,K⁺-ATPase inhibition in plasma from essential and secondary hypertensives. *Abstracts of the International Society of Hypertension* 1992;329.

149. Takahashi H, Matsusawa M, Nishimura M, Nakanishi T, Yoshimura M. Digoxinlike immunoreactivity may contribute to hyperinsulinemia-associated hypertension in patients with glucose intolerance. *J Cardiovasc Pharmacol* 1993;22(suppl 2):S22–S24.

150. Espinel CH. The salt step test: its usage in the diagnosis of salt-sensitive hypertension and in the detection of the salt hypertension threshold. *J Am Coll Nutr* 1992;11:526–531.

151. Graves SW, Glatter KA, Lazarus JM, Williams GH, Hollenberg NK. Volume expansion in renal failure patients: a paradigm for a clinically relevant [Na,K]ATPase inhibitor. *J Cardiovasc Pharmacol* 1993;22(suppl 2):S54–S57.

152. Schoner W, Heidrich-Lorsbach E, Kirch U, Ahlemeyer B, Sich B. Purification and properties of endogenous ouabainlike substances from hemofiltrate and adrenal glands. *J Cardiovasc Pharmacol* 1993;22(suppl 2):S29–S31.

153. Gusdon JP, Buckalew VM, Hennessy JF. A digoxin-like immunoreactive substance in preeclampsia. *Am J Obstet Gynecol* 1984;150:83–85.

154. Graves SW, Williams GH. An endogenous ouabainlike factor associated with hypertensive pregnant women. *J Clin Endocrinol Metab* 1984;59:1070–1074.

155. Valdes R. Endogenous digoxin-immunoactive factor in human subjects. *Fed Proc* 1985;44:2800–2805.

156. Poston L, Morris JF, Wolfe CD, Hilton PJ. Serum digoxin-like substances in pregnancy-induced hypertension. *Clin Sci* 1989;77: 189–194.

157. Tranquilli AL, Mazzanti L, Bertoli E, Romanini C. Sodium/potassium-adenosine triphosphatase on erythrocyte ghosts from pregnant women and its relationship to pregnancy-induced hypertension. *Obstet Gynecol* 1988;71:627–630.

158. Poston L. Sodium transport inhibitors in pregnancy-induced hypertension. *Cardiovasc Drugs Ther* 1990;4(suppl 2):351–356.

159. Miyamoto S, Makino N, Shimokawa H, Akazawa K, Wake N, Nakano H. The characteristics of erythrocyte Na⁺ transport systems in normal pregnancy and pregnancy-induced hypertension. *J Hypertens* 1992;10:367–372.

160. Spieker C, Kisters K, Niedner W, Rahn KH, Zidek W. A circulating Na⁺,K⁺-ATPase inhibitor in preeclampsia. *Abstracts of the International Society of Hypertension* 1992;329.

161. Ebara H, Suzuki S, Nagashima K, Koizumi T, Nishida A, Kanbe Y, Kuroume T. Digoxin- and digitoxinlike immunoreactive substances in amniotic fluid, cord blood, and serum of neonates. *Pediatr Res* 1986;20:28–31.

162. Koren G, Farine D, Maresky D, Taylor J, Heyes J, Soldin S, MacLeod S. Significance of the endogenous digoxinlike substance in infants and mothers. *Clin Pharmacol Ther* 1984;36:759–764.

163. Lupoglazoff JM, Jacqz-Aigrain E, Guyot B, Chappey O, Blot Ph. Endogenous digoxinlike immunoreactivity during pregnancy and at birth. *Br J Clin Pharmacol* 1993;35:251–254.

164. Morris JF, McEachern MD, Poston L, Smith SE, Mulvany MJ, Hilton PJ. Evidence for an inhibitor of leucocyte sodium transport in the serum of neonates. *Clin Sci* 1987;73:291–297.

165. Balzan S, Ghione S, Biver P, Goazzetti P, Montali U. Partial purification of endogenous digitalislike compound(s) in cord blood. *Clin Chem* 1991;37:277–281.

166. Montali U, Balzan S, Ghione S. Purification of endogenous digitalislike factor(s) from cord blood of neonate by immunoaffinity chromatography. *Biochem Int* 1991;25:853–859.

167. Montali U, Balzan S, Ghione S. Purification of endogenous digitalislike factors (EDLF) from neonate and adult plasma by immunoafine chromatography. *Abstracts of the International Society Hypertension* 1992;278.

168. Graves SW, Adler G, Stuenkel C, Sharma K, Brena A, Majzoub J. Increases in plasma digitalislike factor activity during insulin-induced hypoglycemia. *Neuroendocrinology* 1989;49:586–591.

169. Delva P, Barbieri E, Devynck MA, Capra C, Pernollet MA, Meyer P, Destro G, Zardini P, Lechi A. Increase in plasma digitalislike activity during percutaneous transluminal coronary angioplasty in patients with coronary stenosis. *Life Sci* 1990;47: 385–389.

170. Delva P, Devynck M-A, Degan M, Pernollet M-G, Capra C, Meyer P, Lechi A. Correlations between plasma levels of an endogenous digitalislike substance and haemodynamic parameters measured during cardiac catheterization. *J Hypertens* 1988; 6(suppl 4):S348–S350.

171. De Angelis C, Farrace S, Urbani L, Procu S, Ferri C, D'Amelio R, Santucci A, Balsano F. Effect of high altitude exposure on plasma and urinary digoxinlike immunoreactive substance. *Am J Hypertens* 1992;5:600–607.

172. Koga M, Ideishe M, Matsusaki M, Tashiro E, Kinoshita A, Ikeda M, Tanaka H, Shindo M, Arakawa K. Mild exercise decreases plasma endogenous digitalislike substance in hypertensive individuals. *Hypertension* 1992;19(suppl II):II231–II236.

173. Arakawa K. Antihypertensive mechanism of exercise. *J Hypertens* 1993;11:223–229.

Hypertension: Pathophysiology, Diagnosis, and Management, Second Edition, edited by J.H. Laragh and B.M. Brenner, Raven Press, Ltd., New York © 1995.

CHAPTER 63

Endogenous Ouabain in the Pathogenesis of Hypertensive and Cardiovascular Disorders

John M. Hamlyn, Paolo Manunta, and Bruce P. Hamilton

It is indicative of the diverse personality of biology that ouabain, a cardiac glycoside discovered over a century ago in Africa and used widely by clinicians and scientists, would be found in the circulation of normal man in physiologically significant amounts. Even more strange is the notion that this unusual steroid is likely to be endogenous to mammals and may have a significant role in long-term blood pressure regulation in man and in the rat. This chapter presents the background for this topic and reviews recent data. Other reviews are also available (1–9).

It is well known that certain plants synthesize *Digitalis* glycosides and bufodieneolides. Of greater significance, although less well recognized, is the fact that endogenous bufodieneolides are present in the tissues and plasma of some amphibians (10,11). Therefore, the synthesis of cardiotonic steroids that have stereochemical and other structural features quite distinct from common adrenocortical, testicular, and ovarian steroids is not simply the domain of the plant kingdom.

Preparations from plants and amphibians that contain the prototypical steroids shown in Fig. 1 have been used

for thousands of years by various societies including the ancient Egyptians, Romans, Chinese, and more recently by Western civilizations for pest control, as well as for homicidal, suicidal, and therapeutic purposes (12). Although there are over 400 naturally occurring cardiotonic steroids now recognized, ouabain was discovered and named by Arnaud in 1888 as the active principle in the water soluble extract of the bark of the African tree *Acokanthera schimperi* (13). Such extracts, as well as those from *Strophanthus gratus* (14), were used by Maasai and other African and Polynesian tribesmen as arrow poisons. Clinically, preparations enriched in ouabain as well as the pure compound itself have been used for the treatment of shock (15), congestive heart failure, and certain arrthymias. Due to the poor oral bioavailability of ouabain (16), the knowledge of its actions in man arises primarily from acute intravenous usage. The improved oral bioavailability, slower clearance, and the development of immunoassay methods to quantitate plasma levels of *Digitalis* glycosides such as digoxin were key factors that have contributed to diminished clinical use of ouabain.

J. M. Hamlyn and P. Manunta: Department of Physiology, School of Medicine, University of Maryland, Baltimore, Maryland 21201.

B. P. Hamilton: Department of Medicine, School of Medicine, University of Maryland and VA Medical Center, Baltimore, Maryland 21201.

CARDIAC GLYCOSIDES AS VASOPRESSOR AGENTS

The hemodynamic effects of the acute intravenous administration of cardiac glycosides to normal man have

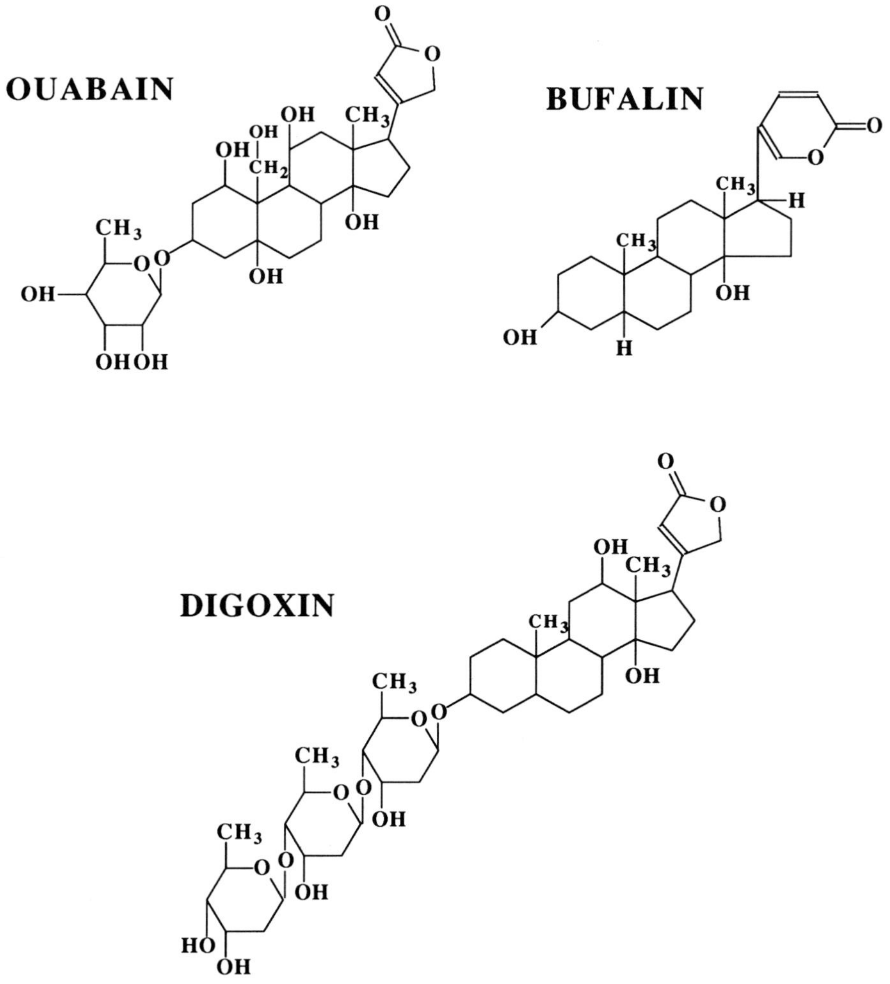

OUABAIN

BUFALIN

DIGOXIN

FIG. 1. Prototypical structures of commonly used cardiotonic steroids. Shown are ouabain, bufalin, and digoxin. Each compound is composed of the basic steroid nucleus with either a five- or six-member lactone ring linked at C17. Ouabain and digoxin are glycosides due to the presence of one or more sugars linked via C3.

been fairly well studied. Most studies have shown a modest increase of total peripheral arterial resistance associated with small increases of blood pressure (17–20). In individuals with compromised cardiac reflexes, frank hypertension may be observed (21). Recognition of the acute vasopressor action of ouabain led to early use in the treatment of shock where it raises blood pressure (15). In patients with congestive heart failure, the administration of cardiac glycosides may in some instances lead to a decrease of total peripheral resistance (20). The vasodilation is mediated via reflex withdrawal of peripheral sympathetic nerve activity that follows increased cardiac output and dominates the underlying vasopressor activity that results from the direct actions of these glycosides on the cellular elements of the vascular wall. Thus, the acute actions of these agents on peripheral vascular resistance and blood pressure are dependent upon the nature of the preexisting conditions within the cardiovascular system.

Although the effects of acute administration of cardiac glycosides on blood pressure seem clear, prolonged therapy with orally active cardenolides such as digoxin has

not been observed to induce sustained hypertension in man (18,22). Moreover, the administration of various cardiac glycosides does not, according to most published studies, induce hypertension in animals (23–26). Thus, not only is the chronic pressor activity of these agents in the normal state questionable, but there is evidence that certain digitalis preparations when used chronically may be antihypertensive in man. For example, the treatment of severe essential hypertension with digitoxin was found to either normalize blood pressure or lower blood pressure substantially and reduce the requirement for other antihypertensive medications (27). The basis of the therapeutic effect has not been determined.

Cardiac glycosides such as digoxin potentiate the pressor response to a variety of peptidic and nonpeptidic vasoconstrictors *in vivo* and *in vitro* (18,28,29). However, the persistence of normotension in patients receiving chronic digoxin therapy suggests that either increased vascular reactivity alone is not sufficient to cause hypertension in man or that it is not present during prolonged administration. There is some evidence that the coadministration of cardiac glycosides with subpressor amounts of either aldosterone or deoxycorticosterone acetate amplifies the hypertensinogenic activity of the latter steroids in animals (26,30). The converse argument, that other agents present in subpressor amounts unmask the pressor effects of cardiac glycosides, has not been considered. There is also evidence that the kidney influences the chronic pressor effects of cardiac glycosides. While prolonged administration of digoxin does not raise the blood pressure of normal rats, it induces hypertension in animals with reduced renal mass (31). Thus, the hypertensinogenic property of some cardiac glycosides is linked with some as yet unrecognized intrinsic renal abnormality as well as with acquired deficits secondary to mild mineralocorticoid excess. Therefore, there is considerable interest, given the prominent role of the kidney in long-term blood pressure regulation, that humoral sodium pump inhibitors, and cardiac glycosides in particular, may activate a novel mechanism relevant to the pathogenesis of essential hypertension.

HUMORAL SODIUM TRANSPORT INHIBITORS IN HYPERTENSION

Increased circulating levels of sodium pump inhibitors have been implicated in the pathogenesis of hypertension (32,33). Some of the best evidence for the presence of a humoral inhibitor of sodium pumps in essential hypertension comes from ion transport measurements. There is fairly consistent evidence that the incubation of lymphocytes and vascular tissue in the plasma of patients with essential hypertension tends to diminish sodium pump–mediated ion fluxes (34–40). Usually, the inhibitory effect is greatest when the plasma originates from patients who exhibit either low plasma renin activity or who are salt-sensitive, although the majority of patients with essential hypertension may be affected (36,41–44). However, measurable differences in cellular sodium transport in patients or in normotensives with a family history of essential hypertension may not be universal (45). As noted elsewhere, the nature of ion transport experiments, and the fact that most are not performed at equilibrium, can lead to predictable systematic underestimates of the effects of humoral inhibitors (7). Other studies have shown that washed red cells and lymphocytes from patients with essential hypertension may show reduced active sodium transport compared with cells from normotensive individuals when incubated in artificial media (40,42–44). There are several possible interpretations of this result including the likelihood that the binding and/or effect of any in vivo humoral inhibitor may linger in vitro for several hours because the inhibitor (like ouabain) may tend to dissociate slowly, especially from highly cardenolide-sensitive sodium pumps. Nevertheless, the use of living cells, as opposed to broken membranes containing Na,K–adenosine triphosphatase (ATPase), has provided most of the consistent evidence

thus far for the association of humoral sodium pump inhibitors with essential hypertension.

Ion transport studies also form the backbone of hard evidence for humoral sodium pump inhibitors in experimental hypertension. Elevated circulating levels of a sodium pump inhibitor have been reported in several low-renin rat models, including 1K1W and 1K1C, and in reduced renal mass hypertension (46,47). Moreover, as with the human studies, cross-incubation experiments indicate that the depressed sodium pump activity characteristic of some arteries harvested from hypertensive animals can be transferred to normal vessels by incubation in the plasma extracts from hypertensive animals.

Increased plasma levels of a sodium transport inhibitor have also been reported in the deoxycorticosterone acetate (DOCA)-salt rat and pig (48–50). The rise in plasma inhibitor levels precedes DOCA-salt hypertension, indicating that the inhibitor is not secondary to hypertension (49). In addition to ion flux measurements, assay techniques including ouabain binding, Na,K-ATPase activity, and cardiac glycoside specific antibodies have been used to probe for endogenous sodium pump inhibitors. The results of such studies, while more subject to false positives than the ion flux procedures, are generally supportive of the concept of elevated humoral inhibitor levels in hypertension or in salt-loaded patients (51–59).

The notion that chronically increased plasma levels of a sodium pump inhibitor account for a portion of the elevated peripheral vascular resistance in hypertension and the evidence that some digoxin antibodies may partially cross-react with an endogenous sodium pump inhibitor have prompted studies in which these agents were administered to hypertensive rats and patients with eclampsia. In most cases, powerful depressor actions have been observed (53,60–64). Although the mechanism of the depressor effect remains to be proven, it may be relevant that commercial preparations of digoxin-specific Fab fragments such as Digibind are able to bind ouabain with fairly high affinity. Thus, sequestration of endogenous ouabain may be one mechanism that accounts for their antihypertensive actions (64). Moreover, it may also explain part of their therapeutic effect in some digitalis-toxic patients with congestive heart failure, individuals likely to have high endogenous levels of ouabain (65). More importantly, the implication that the elevated blood pressures in some patients may depend acutely upon the presence of circulating ouabain or digitalislike entity requires further investigation but appears to be a particularly encouraging result.

PURIFICATION AND IDENTIFICATION OF HUMAN OUABAIN

All attempts to purify endogenous inhibitors of sodium pumps have depended upon a screening assay that

TABLE 1. *Characterized sodium pump inhibitors in mammals*

Source	Assay type[a]	Identity	Comments	Reference
Human plasma	A, B, C, D, F	Ouabain	Probable adrenal origin; found in all mammalian tissues tested	28,69–75
Bovine hypothalamus	A, B, C, D	Not determined MW < 1000 Da Zwitterion	Not shown to circulate CNS specific factor?	76
Human urine	A, B, C, E	Digoxin	Source unknown	77
	A, B, C, G	Steroidal?	Source unknown	78
Bovine adrenal	A, B, C	Unknown	Ouabain-like	79

[a] Where indicated, the material isolated shows significant activity in one or more of the following assays: A, Na,K-ATPase; B, receptor-mediated binding of ^{3}H-ouabain; C, ouabain-sensitive ion transport; D, cardiotonic, increased df/dt; E, cross-reacts with digoxin antibodies; F; cross-reacts 100% with ouabain antibodies; G, natriuresis. Where assays are not indicated, a specific test has not been reported. In some instances the requirement for endogenous material may be too great to be feasible. This is a relevant issue for natriuresis, an assay system that is not considered to be specific for sodium pump inhibitors (assay G). The cross-reactivity of ouabain or ouabain-like materials in digoxin immunoassays may be too low to be determined with the material available (assay E).

employs some exploitable property of the sodium pump (66). Although speculation for the existence of endogenous inhibitors of the sodium pump can be traced back over several decades (67,68), in practical terms the critical significance of the initial screening method is still not widely understood as the key to meaningful progress. Assays such as natriuresis and force production by cardiac tissue, while arguably more physiological than a receptor denuded of its *in vivo* environment with detergents, are not specific, require large amounts of material, and are time-consuming. If ion transport measurements provide the backbone of reasonable evidence for physiologically relevant humoral inhibitors of the sodium pump, it would seem that the use of these techniques would be more likely to lead to important molecules. Indeed, the results from cell-based ion transport and receptor assays have been the most successful; they have led to semi-pure and pure materials being obtained from plasma, urine, and brain (Table 1), and have resulted in the identification of plasma ouabain and a probable urinary digoxin (69,75,77). While it seems likely that an acute dietary source does not explain the presence of ouabain in the human circulation, the origin of the urinary digoxin has not been determined. However, the wide variety of plants that may produce digitalis glycosides and their known oral bioavailability in man (80) and cattle (81) implicate this possibility.

Numerous independent lines of evidence indicate that the human plasma compound is ouabain: (a) The primary mass of the protonated ion, obtained by high-resolution mass spectroscopy (585.295), is identical within experimental error to the calculated value for ouabain (585.291). Thus, the elemental composition of the endogenous compound is $C_{29}H_{45}O_{12}$. (b) The fragmentation patterns of the native and acetylated derivatives of the human compound and ouabain are identical (69,75). (c) The number of acetylatable hydroxyl groups and their reactivity in the human compound correspond with those in commercial ouabain. (d) The human plasma compound binds reversibly with high affinity to purified Na,K-ATPase at the cardiac glycoside-binding site. Moreover, the binding affinities for the human compound and ouabain are modulated in a similar manner by ionic ligands (70). (e) The occupation of the binding site by the human compound leads to inhibition of the Na,K-ATPase by stabilization of the E_2P intermediate, a mechanism of inhibition that is unique to the cardiac glycosides (70). (f) The dissociation rate constant from the dog kidney Na,K-ATPase, a sensitive index of structural and stereochemical differences between cardiac glycosides, is identical for ouabain and the endogenous human material (70). (g) The cardiotonic and vasopressor actions of ouabain and the human compound in the isolated guinea pig atrium are indistinguishable (28). (h) The human compound and commercial ouabain coelute in variety of chromatographic systems known to resolve stereoisomers of ouabain including those containing rhamnose-isomers (75). (i) The human compound cross-reacts 100 percent with ouabain-specific polyclonal antibodies raised against a series of ouabain conjugates in the rabbit (82). Therefore, the aforementioned criteria establish the identity of the human plasma compound as ouabain beyond reasonable doubt (83).

BIOSYNTHESIS

The implications of the structural data raise several issues. Ouabain is distinct from other common steroids previously described in mammals because the C-D rings of the steroid nucleus are fused in a *cis* configuration due to 14β-hydroxylation. Second, the sugar at C3 is a deoxy sugar that is probably rhamnose for the following reasons: First, as noted above, the human ouabain dissociates from dog kidney Na,K-ATPase at a rate identical to that of commercial ouabain under the same reaction conditions while it is known that the presence, nature, and configuration of the sugar markedly influences this rate (84). Similarly, the time constants for the wash in and wash out of the cardiotonic effect in guinea pig heart are the same for commercial and endogenous ouabain (28). Second, the mobility or human and commercial ouabain in various chromatographic systems known to resolve rhamnose isomers is identical (75). Collectively, these and other data suggest that the sugar in the endogenous human compound is rhamnose itself. Why this particular sugar is used preferentially is not yet understood. Another reason for ouabain's distinction from other common steroids is that there is a singly unsaturated five-membered lactone ring at C17. Thus, the presence of all three structural features in a molecule of putative mammalian origin is unanticipated and remarkable.

Several lines of evidence indicate that ouabain is endogenous to mammals. (a) The oral bioavailability of ouabain in man is <5 percent (16). Therefore, high levels of ouabain would have to be present in the normal diet to account for the observed circulating levels. The minimal oral bioavailability is also shared by the rat and probably many other animals (16) that encompass the spectrum from carnivore to herbivore. (b) Patients maintained on semisynthetic diets for periods of 7 days had plasma levels indistinguishable from those on their normal diets (69). According to published reports, the half-time for the urinary clearance of intravenously administered ouabain in man is 19 to 24 h (85). Therefore, in the parenteral experiments, the plasma concentration should have declined by at least seven half-lives if dietary intake were the source. (c) The human adrenal is enriched in ouabain. In the rat, the adrenal content is independent of different dietary and therapeutic conditions including the elevated plasma levels secondary to chronic infusions of ouabain (71,86–88). (d) The plasma levels of ouabain in the rat are lower following bilateral adrenalectomy than their matched pair-fed controls (69). In addition, in rats that undergo selective removal of the adrenal medulla, the plasma levels of ouabain are normal, suggesting that the adrenal cortex is an important source of circulating ouabain (72). (e) The adrenal gland of conscious chronically cannulated afebrile dogs generates an arteriovenous gradient of ouabain; the concentration of ouabain in the adrenal venous effluent is three- to fivefold greater than that of the arterial blood entering the gland. Thus, the canine adrenal actively secretes ouabain that is probably derived from ongoing biosynthesis (89). (f) Elevated plasma levels of ouabain have been found in two hypertensive patients with adrenocortical tumors. In one patient, the venous/arterial gradient was 15 across the normal adrenal and approximately 100 across the tumor-bearing gland (87). In both patients a unilateral adrenalectomy was associated with the normalization of plasma ouabain and the remission of hypertension, re-

sults compatible with those observed previously (90,91). (g) We have obtained evidence that cultured human and bovine adrenocortical cells secrete ouabain (69,92). The secretion appears, in some cell lines, to be increased by vasopressin as well as α_1-adrenoceptor agonists (92). Further, as these cells secrete ouabain in amounts that exceed their cell content by up to tenfold, it is apparent that the cellular ouabain is replaced by *de novo* synthesis as it is secreted. Therefore, these data strongly imply the existence of the enzymatic machinery required for 14β-hydroxylation within the adrenal cortex.

Collectively, the aforementioned data make a compelling case that the adrenal cortex is a source of ouabain in man and the rat and support the claim that ouabain is an important endogenous mammalian counterpart to the exogenous *Digitalis* glycosides. Whether there are other sites of ouabain biosynthesis is not known. Recently, Leenen and colleagues (93) have suggested that the rat brain may be a source of circulating "ouabainlike" activity. This hypothesis is based upon indirect measurements of plasma ouabain that appeared to be modestly lower following 2 weeks of adrenalectomy in spontaneously hypertensive rats (SHRs) replaced with glucocorticoids and mineralocorticoids. However, ouabain is present in all mammalian tissues tested, including the CNS and pituitary, and the total body burden may be a significant reservoir that may minimize the decline in plasma levels in short-term studies following adrenalectomy (69,71,72,87). Further, there is as yet no compelling evidence that the presence of ouabain in nonadrenal tissue is due to anything other than secondary accumulation. Marked tissue sequestration follows the bolus intravenous administration of large doses of ouabain and digoxin in the rat (94). There is also some evidence that the adrenal may contain immunoreactive factors that cross-react weakly with digoxin antibodies (95–97). These adrenal factors are less polar than ouabain in C18 reverse-phase chromatography and it is possible that they are partially hydoxylated intermediates in the synthesis of ouabain.

Hope that the elucidation of the pathway for the synthesis of cardiac glycosides in mammals would benefit from the elucidation of the pathway in plants has been frustrated by the fact that the details of many key steps in plants have not been delineated. However, there is evidence in plants that cholesterol and related steroids are precursors for the steroid nucleus, whereas the lactone ring may be formed from the condensation of two molecules of acetate (98).

OUABAIN AS A LINK BETWEEN RENAL FUNCTION AND HYPERTENSION?

Measurements of plasma ouabain are now available in normal man and for a variety of different disorders including several forms of human hypertension. Results from our laboratory suggest that in normal man the mean plasma ouabain concentration determined by radioimmunoassay lies between 0.29 and 0.44 nM. Measurements made by enzyme-linked immunosorbent techniques tend to indicate higher values in the range of 0.6 to 1.0 nM (65,89,99–103). It is noteworthy that these two results bracket the calculated concentration of ouabain (0.6 nM) based upon the mass of recovered pure material obtained from donor plasma used for the isolation and identification of ouabain (69). Therefore, there is probably no meaningful significance to the difference between the assay formats, such differences being common in immunoassay systems that purport to measure the same compound (cf. atrial peptides, etc.). However, the control data do indicate that absolute values from different techniques may not be strictly comparable, whereas differences within an assay system, e.g., controls versus patients, reflect quantifiable changes. It is also of interest that the ambient concentration of ouabain in man is only modestly below the therapeutic concentration (1–3 nM) of digoxin (104). As the affinity of the human cardiac Na,K-ATPase for ouabain appears to be twofold higher than that for digoxin (105), it appears that circulating ouabain levels may have some tonic actions on the heart, vasculature, and other tissues in normal man. This action may be especially pronounced in patients with congestive heart failure because the plasma levels of ouabain are similar to or, in many cases, exceed those for digoxin (67,106,107).

Preliminary measurements of ouabain in several forms of chronic hypertension suggest that the circulating concentration is raised. The magnitude of most of the increases ranges from approximately 30 percent to 200 percent (69,90,91,100,102,103). Preliminary data from one recent study suggest that the raised plasma levels in essential hypertension decline with antihypertensive therapy (108). Altered plasma levels are also found in several states associated with fluid and electrolyte disturbances (69,87,90,100,102). These include hyper- and hypothyroidism, renal failure, and Conn's syndrome. However, studies in normal individuals given fluorinef, the relationship with cardiac filling pressures in patients with congestive heart failure, and the changes with interdialytic weight changes in patients with chronic renal failure suggest that ouabain responds to volume alteration in a manner distinct from both the atrial peptides and the renin angiotensin-aldosterone system (65,101,102). Thus, many of the key physiological and cellular mechanisms that influence circulating levels of ouabain remain to be elucidated.

Plasma levels of ouabain are modestly raised in patients with chronic renal failure (102). This suggests that the urinary clearance of ouabain may be less influential than anticipated by previous studies in normal man (85). Indeed, recent studies in man suggest that a maximum of 33 percent of an intravenous ouabain load is excreted

via the kidney (16). Clearly, there are important nonrenally mediated pathways for the clearance of plasma ouabain in these patients.

Is it conceivable that ouabain is a link between renal function, sodium intake, and the incidence of hypertension in Western acculturated societies? It is well recognized that the incidence of essential hypertension increases with age. Also well known is the process, beginning around the second decade of life in man, that results in the progressive loss of nephrons. Recent studies by Yuan et al. (109) indicate the presence of two interesting phenomena that suggest that some of these events may be connected. First, the prolonged administration of low doses of ouabain to normal rats results in the induction of maintained hypertension characterized by normal plasma renin activity and aldosterone (86,109). Moreover, the hypertension develops slowly after a latent or prehypertensive period of 7 to 10 days and reaches a plateau around the fourth or fifth week (86,109,110). Treatment with ouabain antibodies or the discontinuation of the administered ouabain reverses the elevated blood pressure (86). The normal plasma renin and aldosterone suggest that this model of hypertension is neither overtly volume expanded nor contracted. Second, although ouabain-induced hypertension occurs in normal rats without preexisting renal impairment, a feature that distinguishes this experimental model from many others, the surgical removal of nephrons exacerbates the hypertension. Loss of 25 percent of the nephrons potentiated the normal blood pressure response to ouabain by approximately 72 percent (109).

The extent to which modest loss of nephrons may amplify the hypertensinogenic actions of ouabain in man is unknown and would depend in part upon the demonstration that prolonged elevation of plasma ouabain either induces or is associated with hypertension. The former experiments, to our knowledge, have not been described. There is, however, accumulating evidence for the latter suggestion. For example, excessive secretion of ouabain appears to be a feature of some hypertensive patients with adrenocortical adenomas (87,90,91,111). In two patients, removal of the offending tumors was associated with normalization of plasma ouabain and significant decreases in blood pressure (87). In both patients the finding of severe hypertension preoperatively with modestly elevated plasma ouabain suggests that this steroid may have powerful chronic pressor actions in man. Similar results have been described in cases where there is defined primary aldosteronism (90,91). In addition to the evidence that plasma ouabain may be elevated in rare hypertensive disorders, there is some indication that patients with essential hypertension may exhibit circulating levels that are raised on average two- to threefold (108,112,113). Therefore, there is a reasonable indication that ouabain is associated with essential hypertension and an expectation that the loss of nephrons in man may augment the pressor action of ouabain, although the experimental confirmation of this latter point is likely to be a challenge.

Preliminary studies with different age groups suggest that higher mean plasma ouabain values tend to be present in older groups (65,99). The genesis of the increase in circulating levels is unclear but may be related to nephron loss, given that the kidney appears to be a significant clearance route for ouabain in normal man. In addition, there is evidence that the intake of sodium chloride influences plasma levels of ouabain. Addition of 10 g of NaCl to the diet of 13 normal men was associated with a 13.5-fold average increase in plasma ouabain by the third day of the diet (99). Therefore, the specter is raised that the age-associated rise in plasma ouabain may be in part secondary to impaired renal clearance of this steroid and co-associated with increased sodium sensitivity. Moreover, both phenomena may be secondary to progressive nephron loss. The elevated plasma ouabain levels as well as increasing sensitivity to the pressor effect of this steroid may therefore represent a link in the relationship between age and the incidence of hypertension in societies where the dietary intake of sodium chloride exceeds ordinary physiological requirements.

MECHANISMS OF OUABAIN-INDUCED HYPERTENSION: A ROLE FOR SODIUM PUMPS?

A simple scheme outlining some of the possible mechanisms for ouabain-induced hypertension is illustrated in Fig. 2. The scheme revolves around the integrated participation of vascular, renal, and possibly CNS mechanisms.

The pressor action of ouabain may involve direct interaction with cellular elements of the vascular wall, especially in "cardiac glycoside-sensitive" species (13, 106,107,114). A direct local action has appeared less plausible in the rat because some previous studies indicate that pharmacological concentrations of ouabain are required to influence tone significantly (115). Moreover, the insensitivity of the rat vasculature to cardiac glycosides seems to parallel recent observations that the predominant sodium pump isoform in cultured aortic vascular smooth muscle cells appears to be an α_1-like isoform that would be expected to bind ouabain with low affinity (116). Therefore, the interpretation of these and several other studies suggests that circulating levels of ouabain would not be expected to interact with vascular smooth muscle cell sodium pumps in this species. Three recent observations challenge this impression. First, one study has suggested that the species specificity of the endogenous ouabain in the rat may be slightly different from human ouabain (117). Because the extracts used in these experiments were highly impure, and the Na,K-ATPase assay used is known to be subject to false positives, the possibility that some other co-present component may account for the difference has not been excluded. Second, studies of the contractility of isolated vascular preparations from the rat show that concentration of ouabain in the low nanomolar range markedly potentiate stimulated tone (118). Third, the growth of rat vascular smooth muscle cells in culture is increased by the presence of nanomolar concentrations of ouabain in the culture fluid (119). Collectively, these data indicate

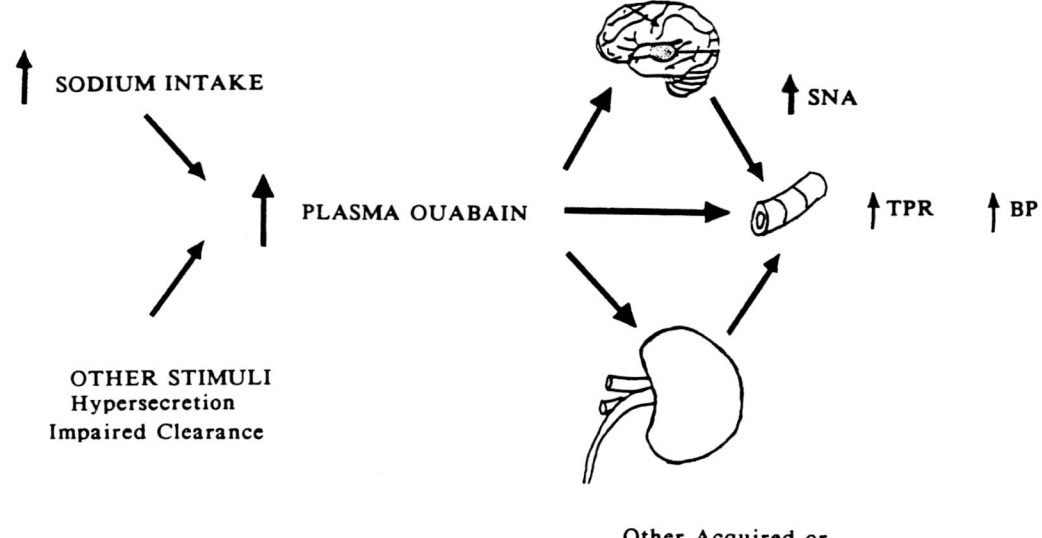

FIG. 2. Probable tissue mechanisms involved in ouabain-induced hypertension. See text for details. SNA, sympathetic nerve activity; TPR, total peripheral vascular resistance. (From ref. 7, with permission.)

that there are functional mechanisms in the vascular wall of the rat that interact with ouabain at concentrations appropriate to ambient circulating levels. The mechanisms involved and their relevance to ouabain-induced hypertension appear to be important issues for future research.

The brain may have a role in ouabain-induced hypertension. Electrolytic lesions of the anteroventral third ventricle (AV3V) in the rat block DOCA-salt or reduced renal mass–saline hypertension. The lesioned animals of both models appear to have plasma sodium pump inhibitor levels similar to those of normal animals (47,50). These and other data emphasize the presence of an important functional link between sodium transport inhibitors and hypertension and reveal the involvement of hypothalamic neurons known to be critical to the onset and maintenance of several forms of experimental hypertension (120).

The acute intracerebroventricular administration of digoxin or ouabain causes peripheral vasoconstriction in skeletal coronary vascular beds and raises blood pressure and heart rate in dogs and rats (54,121). However, the significance of the CNS effects may be tempered by the relative difficulty with which many polar drugs cross the blood-brain barrier. The presence of ouabain in many areas of the rat brain (Manunta and Hamlyn, unpublished data 1992) indicates either the existence of a central ouabain system independent of that in the periphery or the presence of a specific transport mechanism for polar cardiac glycosides in the blood-brain barrier (122). Huang et al. (123) have suggested that the ouabainlike activity present in the rat brain is functional. Based upon experiments that include the effects of acute CNS administration of ouabain as well as digoxin Fab fragments, they claim that brain ouabain is involved in the sympathoexcitatory and pressor effects of intracerebroventricular hypertonic saline (123). Thus, there are clear cardiovascular effects following the instillation of ouabain into the CNS and there is accumulating evidence for the functional mobilization of endogenous ouabain in the brain and the consequences of its blockade. Further, there may be some access of circulating ouabain to hypothalamic or brainstem pathways where the blood-brain barrier may be less prominent. However, there is as yet no conclusive evidence that the CNS plays either a permissive or primary role in this model of hypertension.

The kidney has been repeatedly implicated in the pathogenesis of many forms of hypertension. Acute administration of high doses of ouabain into the kidney induces natriuresis and is associated with inhibition of Na,K-ATPase (124–127). No studies have investigated the hemodynamic consequences of the prolonged renal infusion of ouabain at doses that do not change systemic levels. Therefore, the significance of the kidney in ouabain-induced hypertension can only be considered at present in terms of its role in the sequestration and clearance of ouabain and the indication that reduced nephron number augments the hypertension induced by ouabain.

The plasma levels of ouabain in hypertensive rats receiving prolonged administration of this steroid via daily intraperitoneal injections are no different from vehicle-injected animals when sampling is performed 23 to 24 h after the last injection (109). Therefore, the markedly elevated plasma levels observed in the first hour following injection are cleared rapidly, a portion of which appears in the urine. While the plasma levels of ouabain measured under those experimental conditions do not exhibit any relationship with blood pressure, kidney levels are significantly correlated with that parameter. Whether the increased renal ouabain has some impact on the function of the kidney that is relevant to the generation of hypertension has not been investigated, and the intrarenal site that accumulates ouabain in the rat is not known. However, studies that investigate the reversibility of the hypertension in this model have shown that the kidney level declines to normal associated with the return to normotension (86).

The surgical removal of nephrons in an otherwise normal kidney potentiates ouabain-induced hypertension. However, measurements of plasma ouabain, made 24 h following the last injection of ouabain, indicate no differences between normal animals and the groups with reduced nephron number. Therefore, the basis for the amplification of ouabain-induced hypertension by reduced nephron number does not appear to be secondary to the overt impairment of renal ouabain clearance (109). Rather, it indicates the probable loss of an unidentified renal component that in some way opposes the pressor action of ouabain (and perhaps other hypertensinogenic factors). Nevertheless, it should be recalled that plasma ouabain levels are significantly elevated in patients with chronic renal failure (102). Therefore, there is a relationship between renal clearance and plasma levels that can be observed under those albeit severe conditions. Thus, there are data that indicate that the kidney is important to this model and it seems likely that acquired or inherited defects in renal function may have significant impact on the circulating and pressor effects of ouabain.

Some antihypertensive agents may interfere with the pressor action of ouabain and provide clues to its mechanism and treatment. Despite the fact that spironolactone and canrenone are effective antialdosterone agents, and are antihypertensive where there is mineralocorticoid excess, there is no evidence that their antihypertensive efficacy in essential hypertension is related to this property. Both spironolactone and its primary metabolite canrenone appear to be effective in many patients with essential hypertension as well as in the ouabain-induced hypertensive rat (86,128–132). Moreover, canrenone therapy has been shown to decrease the vasopressor action of ouabain in the human leg (131). The efficacy with which canrenone reverses ouabain-induced hypertension in the rat strongly implies that the antihypertensive action of these antialdosterones involves altered metabolism of ouabain. The mechanism has been suggested to involve a reduction in the binding of ouabain to the sodium pump and, consistent with that notion, spironolactone would be expected to and apparently does antagonize digitalis toxicity in man (133–135). This suggests that certain antialdosterones may in some manner block the binding of endogenous ouabain to the cardiac glycoside receptor (136). Whether such a mechanism would account for the antihypertensive action of spironolactone has not been determined. However, the data suggest the interaction of certain antialdosterone with the endogenous ouabain system is a new and significant phenomenon and represents an exciting area for the development of new, more specific, therapeutic agents that may have widespread utility.

Given the nature and pharmacology of ouabain, it seems almost heretical to wonder whether sodium pumps are the first link in the chain to ouabain-induced hypertension. The sodium pump in most animal species can bind a variety of cardiac glycosides. The phenomenon occurs in primitive animals such as *Hydra vulgaris*, brine shrimp (*Artemia salinas*), and mammals such as man (137,138), species that diverged over 600 million years ago. In man and rat, there are three chromosomally dispersed genes that express distinct isoforms termed α_1, α_2, and α_3 (139–143). Two other genes have also been detected in man (140,142). It is readily apparent that the cardiac glycoside-binding site has been conserved, suggesting that this function has been and continues to be a valuable trait. Both the rat and mouse α_1-isoform are ouabain "resistant," that is, they bind ouabain with very low affinity (144). However, the α_2- and α_3-isoforms in the rat bind ouabain with high affinity and confer sensitivity to those tissues that express these receptor isoforms. Moreover, the sensitivity of the rat α_3-isoform is quantitatively similar to that in man (105,139,145). Therefore, the distribution of these isoforms in CNS, skeletal muscle, and adipose tissue, their differential expression during development, and their high affinity for cardiac glycosides suggests that these receptors are the logical if unproven determinants of the physiological role of endogenous ouabain in the rat (146–150).

A series of experiments that seems to cast doubt about sodium pumps as being the sole class of physiologically significant receptors for ouabain is the finding that equivalent doses of digoxin do not induce hypertension in normal rats (110). Therefore, it is clear that the response to digoxin and ouabain are different in the rat, and a class of receptors specific for ouabain has not been excluded as the basis for this phenomenon. It is also possible that ouabain and digoxin interact with the same receptor, but that the binding of digoxin does not activate the pressor mechanism under normal conditions. There are no direct data that discriminate between these possibilities at present, although the antihypertensive actions of digitoxin in man alluded to earlier seem to favor the latter possibility.

HYPERTENSIVE PHENOTYPES INVOLVING OUABAIN

Essential hypertension is often considered to be the result of the aberrant function of several distinct mechanisms involved in blood pressure control. Several mechanisms may be active in the same patient, each contributing variably to the final phenotype. Some of the evidence for multiple phenotypes arises from the observations that different antihypertensive agents are often effective as monotherapy in different individuals (151). Expecting that ouabain-induced hypertension (i.e., a single hypertensive phenotype) would respond to spironolactone and not to other antihypertensive agents with quite different mechanisms of action, we arranged to test this notion (152). In the study, a variety of commonly used agents were administered individually for 12 days to ouabain-hypertensive rats using doses corresponding to those used maximally in man and normalized for body weight. At the end of the 12-day period, the animals treated with either canrenone, captopril, or metoprolol were all normotensive, whereas blood pressure remained elevated in the animals treated with most other agents. While the efficacy of canrenone was anticipated, the response to the angiotensin-converting enzyme (ACE) inhibitor and the beta blocker is surprising given that there is no evidence either for renin excess or increased cardiac output in this form of hypertension (109). Therefore, a straightforward interpretation of the data is that ouabain heightens the dependence of blood pressure on renin in this model. Arguably of more significance to the identification of multiple phenotypes with therapeutic agents is the observation that mechanistically distinct agents may be effective in the same hypertensive phenotype where the kidney is believed to have no inherited or acquired defects. The implications of this result led us to consider the possible existence of four simple hypertensive phenotypes based on either augmented sensitivity to ouabain or excessive circulating levels. This analysis is presented below.

The general scheme presented in Fig. 2 envisages that diets high in salt raise circulating ouabain. If the rise is sufficiently high and sustained, hypertension results. The role of sodium in this scheme explains the first paradox, that is that ouabain-induced hypertension is not itself sodium-sensitive. The second paradox is that elevated sodium transport inhibitors historically have been detected most often in low-renin hypertension. To explain the second paradox it is necessary to add only an inherited or acquired renal defect predisposing to sodium retention, such defects being common in those experimental models. The environment/genotype/phenotype relationships for the situation discussed above are shown in Table 2. The first phenotype is a low-renin (ACE-insensitive) form of salt-sensitive hypertension that responds to salt restriction and/or diuretics, as well as agents that antagonize ouabain (i.e., spironolactone).

A second phenotype results from a primary excess of ouabain secondary to an adrenocortical tumor or investigator-initiated infusion. Here, plasma renin activity (PRA) and the degree of salt-sensitivity are expected to be entirely normal. This form of hypertension should respond paradoxically to spironolactone as well as ACE inhibitors or sympatholytics. Diuretics are likely to be less effective in this phenotype because there is no co-present renal or other abnormality predisposing to sodium retention (152). The third phenotype results from an inherited defect that causes abnormally low renal clearance of ouabain. This leads to a tendency to raised levels of plasma ouabain and the development of a normal renin form of hypertension that is not salt-sensitive because the remaining renal handling of sodium is entirely normal. Spironolactone, ACE inhibitors, or sympatholytics are likely to be effective agents in the treatment of this phenotype. The fourth phenotype has hypertension associated with either normal or modestly

raised levels of plasma ouabain. The basis for hypertension in this model is an increased sensitivity to the pressor actions of ouabain that is secondary to the loss of nephrons that occurs with aging. Therefore, we suggest that this phenotype is likely to be found more frequently in older individuals co-associated with some degree of sodium sensitivity. This form of hypertension would be partly salt and diuretic-sensitive but would exhibit some response to sympatholytics or inhibition of ACE. Other phenotypes that involve ouabain and inappropriate activity of renin or the sympathetic nervous system as well as intermediate or overlapping forms of those presented in Table 2 are also likely but are not discussed here. The point of this type of analysis is to emphasize the potential for ouabain to induce hypertension that is phenotypically and therapeutically heterogeneous. It should be apparent that the presentation of the actual phenotype is determined less by ouabain itself and more by the presence and magnitude of genetic or acquired abnormalities in renal function. In addition, this analysis, as well as the accumulating experimental and clinical data, predict that the development of highly specific therapeutic agents against the ouabain system, or even the induction of active immunity against ouabain itself, will be an effective means to reduce the incidence and severity of hypertension.

TABLE 2. *Four hypertensive phenotypes predicted to involve ouabain*

Type	Environment	+	Genotype (renal)	=	Phenotype	Therapy[a]	Reference
1	↑ Na intake		Defective Na excretion		↓ PRA ↑ Salt sensitivity ↑ Ouabain Hypertension	Diuretics Salt restriction Spironolactone CCB Sympatholytics ACE-I	30,69,99,152
2	↔ Na intake; ouabain secreting tumor		Normal		↔ PRA ↔ Salt sensitivity ↑ Ouabain Hypertension	Spironolactone ACE-I Sympatholytics CCB Diuretics	87,111
3	↔ Na intake		↓ Ouabain clearance		↔ PRA ↔ Salt sensitivity ↑ Ouabain Hypertension	Spironolactone ACE-I Sympatholytics CCB Diuretics	
4	↔ Na intake; age-induced nephron loss; reduced renal mass		? Normal		↔↓ PRA ↔↑ Salt sensitivity ↔↑ Ouabain ↑ Ouabain sensitivity Hypertension	Spironolactone ACE-I Sympatholytics CCB	109,129

ACE-I, angiotensin-converting enzyme inhibitors; CCB, calcium channel blockers; ↑, increased or high; ↔, unchanged or normal; ↓, decreased or low.
[a] Therapeutic agents are shown in descending order of expected efficacy when used as monotherapy for each phenotype. Spironolactone is considered as an ouabain antagonist. Canrenone is expected to have similar effects to spironolactone. Prolonged use of spironolactone may be undesirable in some individuals; therefore, ACE inhibitors or sympatholytics would be effective for control in phenotypes 2 to 4. Phenotypes 1, 3, and 4 are believed to be indistinguishable from many patients with essential hypertension.

SUMMARY

Links between circulating sodium pump inhibitors and hypertension were proposed approximately 17 years ago (32,33). Subsequent work has led to the isolation and identification of ouabain that is endogenous to the human circulation. The hemodynamic actions of ouabain, the renal modulation of its clearance and pressor actions, and the impact of salt intake on circulating levels all suggest that this unusual steroid has the hallmarks of a new endocrine system of relevance to long-term blood pressure regulation.

ACKNOWLEDGMENTS

We thank Cardiovascular Diseases Research and Analytical Services from the Upjohn Company for the collaboration that led to the discovery of ouabain. We also thank Dr. Mordecai P. Blaustein for fostering this research. Supported in part by a fellowship award from the American Italian Nephrology Society (PM), an American Heart Association Established Investigator award (JMH), the Veterans Administration (BPH), and the UMAB Bressler Research Foundation.

REFERENCES

1. Hilton P. N Engl J Med 1986;314:222–229.
2. Graves SW. CRC Crit Rev Clin Lab Sci 1986;23:177–200.
3. Poston L. Clin Sci 1987;72:647–655.
4. Kramer HJ, Meyer-Lehnert H, Michel H, Predel HG. Am J Hypertens 1991;4:81–89.
5. Schoner W. Clin Exp Hypertens 1992;A14(5):767–814.
6. Goto A, Yamada K, Yagi N, Yoahika M, Sugimoto T. Pharmacol Rev 1992;44:377–399.
7. Hamlyn JM, Manunta P. J Hypertension 1992;10(suppl 7):S99–S111.
8. Ruegg UT. Experentia 1992;48:1102–1106.
9. Blaustein MP. Am J Physiol 1993;264:C1367–C1387.
10. Siperstein MD, Murray AW, Titus E. Arch Biochem Biophys 1957;67:154–160.
11. Lichtstein D, Kachalsky S, Deutsch J. Life Sci 1986;38:1261–1270.
12. Greeff K, Schadewaldt H. In: Greeff K, ed. Cardiac glycosides, part I: experimental pharmacology. New York: Springer-Verlag, 1981;1–12.
13. Arnaud A. Compte Rend Acad Sci Paris 1888;106:1011–1014.
14. Arnaud A. Compte Rend Acad Sci Paris 1888;107:179–182.
15. Horton JAG, Davison MHA. Br J Anaesth 1955;27:139–144.
16. Strobach H, Wirth KE, Rojsathaporn K. Naunyn Schmiedebergs Arch Pharmacol 1968;334:496–500.
17. Cappuccio FP, Markandu ND, Sagnella GA, MacGregor GA. Postgrad Med J 1986;62:265–268.
18. Guthrie GP Jr. J Clin Endocrinol Metab 1984;58:76–80.
19. Kramer HJ, Glanzer K, Freitag T, Schonfeld J, Sorger M, Schlebusch H, Dusing R, Kruck F. Klin Wochenschr 1984;63:32–36.
20. Mason DT, Braunwald E. J Clin Invest 1964;43:532–543.
21. Kumar R, Yankopoulos NA, Abelman WH. Chest 1973;63:105–107.
22. Smith TW, Haber E. N Engl J Med 1973;289:1010–1015.
23. Overbeck HW. Proc Soc Exp Biol Med 1981;167:506–513.
24. Overbeck HW, Pamnani MB, Ku DD. Proc Soc Exp Biol Med 1980;164:401–404.
25. Nirasawa Y, Temma K, Fink GD, Akera T. Life Sci 1985;37:767–774.
26. Spence CD, Coghlan JP, Whitworth JA, Scoggins BA. Clin Exp Pharmacol Physiol 1989;16:211–222.
27. Abarquez RF. Acta Medica Philippina 1967;series 2, 3:161–170.
28. Bova S, Blaustein MP, Ludens JH, Harris DW, DuCharme DW, Hamlyn JM. Hypertension 1991;17:944–950.
29. Brender D, Vanhoutte PM, Shepherd JT. Circ Res 1969;25:597–606.
30. Sekihara H, Yazaki Y, Kojima T. Endocrinology 1992;131:3077–3082.
31. Fujimura A, Ebara A, Yaoka O. Jpn J Hypertension 1984;7:49(abstract).
32. Haddy FJ, Overbeck H. Life Sci 1976;19:935–948.
33. Blaustein MP. Am J Physiol 1977;232:C165–C173.
34. Poston L, Sewell RB, Wilkinson SP, et al. Br Med J 1981;282:847–849.
35. MacGregor GA, Fenton S, Alaghband-Zadeh J, Markandu ND, Roulston JE, deWardener HE. Br Med J 1981;283:1355–1357.
36. Edmonson RPS, MacGregor GA. Br Med J 1981;282:1267–1269.
37. Moreth K, Renner D, Schoner W. Klin Wochenschr 1987;65:179–184.
38. Kuske R, Moreth K, Renner D, Wizemann V, Schoner W. Klin Wochenschr 1987;65:(suppl 8):53–59.
39. Kresinski JM, Godon JP, Rorive GL. Clin Exp Hypertens 1985;A7:721–733.
40. Pamnani MB, Burris JF, Jemionek JF, Huot SJ, Price M, Freis ED, Haddy FJ. Am J Hypertens 1989;2:524–531.
41. Forrester TE, Alleyne GAO. Br Med J 1981;283:5–7.
42. Stokes GS, Monaghan JC, Middleton A, Gunn J, Marwood JF. Klin Wochenschr 1985;63:42–44.
43. Morgan T, Meyers J, Fitzgibbon W. Clin Exp Hypertens 1981;3:641–653.
44. Edmonson RPS, Thomas RD, Hilton PJ, et al. Lancet 1975;1:1003–1005.
45. Gudmundsson T, Andersson O, Herlitz H, Jonsson O, Naucler J, Wikstrand J, Berglund G. J Cardiovasc Pharmacol 1984;6:S35–S41.
46. Pamnani MB, Haddy FJ. Prog Biochem Pharmacol 1988;23:35–45.
47. Huot SJ, Pamnani MB, Clough DL, Buggy J, Bryant HJ, Harder DR, Haddy FJ. Hypertension 1983;5(suppl I):94–100.
48. Hamlyn JM, Ashen MD, Forrest B, Rogowski AC, White RJ. Prog Biochem Pharmacol 1988;23:22–34.
49. Hamlyn JM. J Endocrinol 1989;122:409–420.
50. Songu-Mize E, Bealer SL, Caldwell RW. Hypertension 1982;4:575–580.
51. Hamlyn JM, Ringel R, Schaeffer JS, et al. Nature 1982;300:650–652.
52. deWardener HE, Fenton S, Alaghband-Zadeh J, MacGregor GA. Contrib Nephrol 1982;30:185–191.
53. Kojima I, Yoshihara S, Ogata E. Life Sci 1982;30:1775–1781.
54. Devynck MA, Pernollet MG, Cloix JF, et al. Clin Exp Hypertens 1984;A6:441–453.
55. Yamaji I, Kikuchi K, Nishimura M, et al. Am J Hypertens 1990;3:176–181.
56. Umeda T, Naomi S, Inoue J, et al. Clin Exp Hypertens 1987;A9:1209–1219.
57. Nishio I, Shima H, Tsuda K, Hano T, Masuyama Y. J Hypertens 1988;6(suppl 4):S216–S218.
58. Shima H, Nishio I, Tsuda K, et al. Jpn J Med 1989;28:165–169.
59. Takahashi H, Matsusawa M, Okabayashi H, et al. Am J Hypertens 1988;1:168S–172S.
60. Goodlin RC. N Engl J Med 1988;318:518–519.
61. Kunes J, Stolba P, Pohlova I, Jelinek J, Zicha J. Clin Exp Hypertens 1985;7:707–720.
62. Huang CT, Smith RM. Life Sci 1984;35:115–118.
63. Mann JFE, Miemitz R, Ganten U, Ritz E. J Hypertens 1987;5:543–549.
64. Balzan S, Montali U, Biver P, Ghione S. J Hypertens 1991;9(suppl 6):S304–S305.

65. Gottlieb SS, Rogowski AC, Weinberg M, Krichten CM, Hamilton BP, Hamlyn JM. *Circulation* 1992;86:420–425.
66. Hamlyn JM. *ISI Atlas of Pharmacology* 1988;2:339–344.
67. Szent-Gyorgyi A. *Chemical physiology of contraction in body and heart muscle.* New York: Academic Press, 1953;135.
68. Labella FS, Templeton J, Bose D. *Proc West Pharmacol Soc* 1987;30:365–371.
69. Hamlyn JM, Blaustein MP, Bova S, et al. *Proc Natl Acad Sci USA* 1991;88:6259–6263.
70. Hamlyn JM, Harris DW, Ludens JH. *J Biol Chem* 1989;64:7395–7404.
71. Hamlyn JM, Harris DW, Resau J, Ludens JH. *FASEB J* 1990;4(4):A295, abstr 171.
72. Ludens JH, Clark MA, Robinson FG, DuCharme DW. *Hypertension* 1992;19:721–724.
73. Ludens JH, Clark MS, DuCharme DW, et al. Purification of an endogenous digitalis-like factor for structural analysis. *Hypertension* 1991;17:923–929.
74. Hamlyn JM, Harris DW, Clark MA, Rogowski AC, White RJ, Ludens JH. *Hypertension* 1989;13:681–689.
75. Mathews WR, DuCharme DW, Hamlyn JM, et al. *Hypertension* 1991;17:930–935.
76. Haupert GT. *Prog Biochem Pharmacol* 1988;23:10–21.
77. Goto A, Ishiguro T, Yamada K, et al. *Biochem Biophys Res Comm* 1990;173:1093–1101.
78. Cloix J-F, Crabos M, Grichois MI, Meyer P. *Can J Physiol Pharmacol* 1987;65:1522–1527.
79. Tamura M, Lam T-T, Inagami T. *Biochemistry* 1988;27:4244–4253.
80. Smith TW, Haber E. *N Engl J Med* 1973;289:1063–1072.
81. Thomas DL, Quick MP, Morgan RP. *Vet Record* 1987;120:300–301.
82. Harris DW, Clark MA, Fisher JF, et al. *Hypertension* 1991;17:936–943.
83. Sandor T, Idler DR. In: Idler DR ed. *Steroids in nonmammalian vertebrates.* New York: Academic Press, 1972;6–36.
84. Yoda A. *Ann NY Acad Sci* 1974;242:598–616.
85. Selden R, Smith TW. *Circulation* 1972;45:1176–1182.
86. Manunta P, Hamilton BP, Rogowski AC, Pruce E, Hamlyn JM. *J Hypertens* 1992;10(4):S79, abstr P67.
87. Manunta P, Evans G, Hamilton BP, Gann D, Resau J, Hamlyn JM. *J Hypertens* 1992;10(4):S27, abstr P36.
88. Manunta P, Ashen MD, Rogowski AC, Pinnaparpaglia P, Hamilton BP, Hamlyn JM. *J Hypertens* 1992;10(4):S128, abstr P99.
89. Boulanger BR, Lilly MP, Hamlyn JM, Shurtleff D, Gann DS. *FASEB J* 1992;6(4):A1186, abstr 1446.
90. Masugi F, Ogihara T, Hasegawa T, et al. *Biochem Biophys Res Comm* 1986;135:41–45.
91. Masugi F, Ogihara T, Hasegawa T, Sakaguchi K, Kumahara Y. *J Hum Hypertens* 1988;2:409–420.
92. Laredo J, Hamlyn JM. *Endocrine Soc Abstracts, 74th Annual Meeting,* San Antonio, Texas 1992;71, abstr 79.
93. Leenen FHH, Harmsen E, Yu H, Yuan B. *Am J Physiol* 1993;265:H421–H424.
94. Dutta S, Marks BH. *Life Sci* 1966;5:915–920.
95. Pernollet MG, Ali RM, Meyer P, Devynck M-A. *J Hypertens* 1986;4(suppl 6):S382–S384.
96. Doris PA, Stocco DM. *Endocrinology* 1989;125:2573–2579.
97. Shaikh IM, Lau BWC, Siegfried BA, Valdes R. *J Biol Chem* 1991;266:13672–13678.
98. Reichstein T. *Die Naturwissenschaften* 1967;3:53–76.
99. Manunta P, Hamilton BP, Pruce E, Hamlyn JM. *J Hypertens* 1992;10(4):S96, abstr P81.
100. Donner TW, Hamilton BP, Manunta P, Valente WA, Hamlyn JM. *74th Annual Endocrine Soc Meeting,* San Antonio, Texas 1992;129, abstr 312.
101. Hohl AS, Hamilton BP, Hamlyn JM. *Endocrine Soc Abstr* 1990;233:abstr 835.
102. Schaeffer JS, Talartschik J, Koch KM, Rogowski AC, Manunta P, Hamlyn JM. *J Am Soc Nephrol* 1991;2(3):348, abstr 34P.
103. Argento NB, Hamilton BP, Valente WA, Hamlyn JM. *Hypertension* 1991;18:425, abstr P110.

104. Chamberlain DA. *Postgrad Med* 1974;50:29–35.
105. Brown L, Erdmann E. *Arch Int Pharmacodyn Ther* 1984;27:229–240.
106. Woolfson RG, Hilton PJ, Poston L. *Hypertension* 1990;15:583–590.
107. Woolfson RG, Poston L. *Hypertension* 1991;17:619–625.
108. Naruse K, Naruse M, Tanabe A, et al. *Hypertension* 1993;21:551, abstr 93.
109. Yuan C, Manunta P, Hamlyn JM, et al. *Hypertension* 1993;22:178–187.
110. Manunta P, Rogowski AC, Hamilton BP, Hamlyn JM. *Hypertension* 1992;20(3):404, abstr P32.
111. Evans JG, Manumta P, Hamlyn JM, Hamilton BP, Gann DS. *Abstracts of the 75th Endocrine Society Meeting,* Las Vegas, Nevada 1993;291, abstr 961.
112. Masugi F, Ogihara T, Hasegawa T, Kumahara Y. *Clin Exp Hypertens* 1987;A9:1233–1242.
113. Goto A, Yamada K, Yagi N, Nagoshi H, Hui C, Sugimoto T. *J Hypertens* 1992;10(suppl 4):S50, abstr P52.
114. Lang S, Blaustein MP. *Circ Res* 1980;46:463–470.
115. Aalkjaer C, Mulvany MJ. *J Physiol* 1985;362:215–231.
116. Medford RM, Hyman R, Ahmad M, et al. *J Biol Chem* 1991;266:18308–18312.
117. Ferrandi M, Minotti E, Salardi S, Floriio M, Bianchi G, Ferrari P. *Am J Physiol* 1992;263:F739–F748.
118. Weiss DN, Podberesky D, Heidrich J, Blaustein MP. *Biophys J* 1993;64:abstr A261.
119. Goulomb E, Hill MR, Brown RG, Keiser HR. *Am J Hypertension* 1993;6:79A, abstr 1022.
120. Brody MJ, Fink GD, Buggy J, Haywood JR, Gordon FJ, Johnson AK. *Circ Res* 1978;43:I-2–I-13.
121. Garan H, Smith TW, Powell WJ Jr. *Fed Proc* 1973;32:718.
122. Kurihara A, Suzuki H, Sawada Y, Sugiyama Y, Iga T, Hanano M. *J Pharmaceut Sci* 1988;77:347–352.
123. Huang BS, Harmsen E, Yu H, Lennen F. *Circ Res* 1992;71:1059–1066.
124. Yates NA, McDougall JG. *Br J Pharmacol* 1993;108:627–630.
125. Pamnani MB, Chen S, Bryant HJ, et al. *Hypertension* 1991;18:316–324.
126. Hook JB. *Proc Soc Exp Biol Med* 1969;131:731–734.
127. Toretti J, Hendler E, Weinstein E, Longnecker RE, Epstein FH. *Am J Physiol* 1972;222:1398–1405.
128. Henry M, Wehrien M, Pelletier B, Capron M-H. *Am J Cardiol* 1990;65:36K–38K.
129. Pamnani MB, Whitehorn WV, Clough DL, Haddy FJ. *Am J Hypertens* 1990;3:188–195.
130. Vargas F, Haro JM, Jodar E, Soler A, Garcia del Rio C. *J Pharm Pharmacol* 1988;41:335–338.
131. Semplicini A, Buzzaccarini F, Ceolotto G, et al. *Am J Hypertens* 1993;6:295–301.
132. Manunta P, Tyzack J, Hamilton BP, Hamlyn JM. *Hypertension* 1993;22:432, abstr 55.
133. Selye H, Krajny M, Savoie L. *Science* 1969;164:842–843.
134. Finotti P, Palatini P. *J Pharmacol Exp Ther* 1981;217:784–790.
135. Yeh BK, Chaing BN, Sung PK. *Am Heart J* 1976;92:308–314.
136. Garay RP, Diez J, Nazarate C, et al. *Naunyn Schmeidebergs Arch Pharmacol* 1985;329:311–315.
137. Canfield VA, Xu K-Y, D'Aquila T, Shyjan AW, Levenson R. In: *The sodium pump: recent developments. Soc Gen Physiol* 1991;46(Pt2):231–236.
138. Baxter-Lowe LA, Guo JZ, Bergstrom EE, Hokin LE. *FEBS Lett* 1989;257:181–187.
139. Sweadner KJ. *Biochim Biophys Acta* 1989;988:185–220.
140. Sverdlov ED, Monastyrskaya GS, Broude NE, et al. *FEBS Lett* 1987;217:275–278.
141. Shull GE, Greeb J, Lingrel JB. *Biochemistry* 1986;25:8125–8132.
142. Shull MM, Lingrel JB. *Proc Natl Acad Sci USA* 1987;84:4039–4043.
143. Takeyasu K, Lemas V, Fambrough DM. *Am J Physiol* 1990;28:C619–C630.
144. Repke KRH, Est M, Portius HJ. *Biochem Pharmacol* 1965;14:1785–1802.

145. Blanco G, Berberian G, Beauge L. *Biochim Biophys Acta* 1990;1027:1–7.
146. Adam-Vizi V, Ligeti E. *J Physiol (Lond)* 1984;353:505–521.
147. Vizi ES, Oberfrank F, Bernath S, Lichtstein D. *Neuropharmacology* 1987;26:1541–1544.
148. Powis DA. *J Auton Pharmacol* 1983;3:127–154.
149. Tsuda K, Tsuda S, Shima H, Masuyama Y. *Am J Hypertens* 1989;2:465–467.

150. Taddei S, Salvetti A, Pedrinelli R. *J Hypertens* 1988;6(suppl 4):S357–S359.
151. Nuitta E, Cusi D, Colombo R, et al. *Am J Hypertens* 1988;1:364–371.
152. Tyzack J, Manunta P, Hamilton BP, Hamlyn JM. *Abstracts of the 75th Endocrine Society Meeting,* Las Vegas, Nevada 1993;377, abstr 1305.

Hypertension: Pathophysiology, Diagnosis, and Management, Second Edition, edited by J.H. Laragh and B.M. Brenner, Raven Press, Ltd., New York © 1995.

CHAPTER **64**

The Nitric Oxide System in Circulatory Homeostasis and its Possible Role in Hypertensive Disorders

Jason G. Umans and Roberto Levi

The discovery of a physiological role for nitric oxide (NO) as a modulator of vascular relaxation is a recent and exciting chapter in our quest to understand the control of blood pressure and the aberrations caused by hypertension. It is now known, for instance, that basal and stimulated synthesis of this potent, locally acting vasodilator contributes to both the short and long-term regulation of arterial pressure. NO, the active moiety of endothelium-derived relaxing factor (EDRF), serves as an important intercellular mediator in the vasculature, kidney, endocrine system, and central nervous system. Accordingly, NO may modulate vascular resistance, sodium balance, and arterial pressure by multiple mechanisms, whereas impairment of NO synthesis may contribute to the genesis or perpetuation of hypertension. Although appreciation of the cardiovascular role of NO is quite recent, a vast and often confusing literature has appeared describing its effects in humans and animals. This chapter will focus on the pharmacology of NO, as well as on selected recent investigations that bear on its role in several aspects of blood pressure regulation.

HISTORICAL PERSPECTIVE

The recognition of NO as an endogenous vasoactive mediator has been extensively reviewed (1,2). In 1980, Furchgott and Zawadski reported their seminal observation that relaxation of isolated rabbit aorta by acetylcholine was strictly dependent on the vascular endothelium (3). Subsequently, they demonstrated that endothelial cells elaborate an extremely labile nonprostanoid vasodilator, which they termed EDRF. The factor was released in the basal state by unstimulated endothelium and its release could be stimulated further by a wide variety of pharmacological vasodilators including muscarinic agonists, histamine, bradykinin, substance P, thrombin, α_2-adrenergic agonists, and calcium ionophores, as well as by the physiological stimulus of flow-

   J. G. Umans: Assistant Professor of Medicine and Clinical Pharmacology, Section of Nephrology, University of Chicago, Chicago, Illinois 60637.
   R. Levi: Professor of Pharmacology, Department of Pharmacology, Cornell University Medical College, New York, New York 10021.

induced shear stress. Furchgott and his colleagues used the EDRF inhibitors hemoglobin and methylene blue to demonstrate further a role for basal EDRF synthesis in modulating the vascular response to vasoconstrictor stimuli (4).

The above studies were quickly associated with other observations made in the 1970s and early 1980s; mainly that vascular relaxation by a number of agents, including organic nitrates, nitroprusside, acidified nitrite, and nitric oxide was mediated by accumulation of cyclic guanosine 3':5' monophosphate (cGMP) (5). The effect of all these nitrovasodilators could be inhibited by methylene blue, methemoglobin, or hemoglobin (6). It was then noted that EDRF acted in a manner similar to the above nitrovasodilators in stimulating cGMP accumulation which, together with its vasodilator effect, could be inhibited by these same agents (7).

In an unrelated series of investigations, Stuehr and Marletta demonstrated the arginine-dependent synthesis of a reactive species later shown to be NO, by detecting its stable degradation products, nitrate and nitrite, after macrophage stimulation (8,9). Further, Hibbs and associates noted that the synthesis of this reactive species could be inhibited by guanidino-substituted derivatives of L-arginine (10,11). Following the suggestion by Furchgott and the demonstration by Ignarro (12) that EDRF might, in fact, be nitric oxide, Palmer and co-workers reported a series of cascade bioassay experiments demonstrating that an NO-like compound was released from cultured endothelial cells; and suggested that NO could best account for the observed bioactivity of EDRF (13). Ignarro and co-workers, studying native endothelium from pulmonary artery and vein, arrived at the same conclusion (14). Palmer (15), Sakuma (16), and their respective colleagues next demonstrated that NO synthesis by endothelial cells is arginine-dependent. Since that time, multiple NO synthases have been characterized, their genes identified, and rapid progress has been made to identify alterations in NO synthesis and effect in many conditions including hypertensive disorders.

NO BIOSYNTHESIS AND ITS REGULATION

The NO synthases are complex, multicomponent oxidases that form NO from the terminal guanidino nitrogens of their substrate, arginine, in a five electron oxidation using molecular oxygen, along with nicotinamide adenine dinucleotide phosphate (reduced form) (NADPH) as cosubstrate, and flavin adenine dinucleotide (FAD), flavin mononucleotide (FMN), heme, calmodulin, and tetrahydrobiopterin as co-factors. The genes for three distinct enzymes have been cloned, sequenced, and localized to different human chromosomes; the endothelial NO synthase (eNOS) to chromosome 7, a neuronal form (nNOS) to chromosome 12, and an inducible form (iNOS) to chromosome 17 (17,18).

The endothelial enzyme (19) is calcium-calmodulin regulated, exhibiting low basal activity when endothelial cell cytosolic free calcium concentrations are at resting levels, and maximal activity at the cytosolic free calcium levels, which are achieved following stimulation by vasodilator agonists (20). The endothelial enzyme possesses consensus sequences suggesting a site that might be phosphorylated by protein kinase A, as well as a myristoylation site that contributes to enzyme association with cell membranes. The neuronal enzyme (21) is widely distributed outside of the central nervous system, with marked structural diversity between different tissues. It is likewise activated by the effect of calcium-mobilizing neurotransmitters (22). In contrast, the inducible form of the enzyme (23) binds calmodulin in a calcium-independent manner and therefore exhibits a high level of activity even at trace basal cytosolic calcium concentrations. This enzyme is expressed in macrophages and in a wide variety of tissue and cell types, including vascular smooth muscle (24,25), following exposure to bacterial endotoxin or a number of inflammatory mediators.

VASCULAR PHARMACOLOGY OF NO

The vascular pharmacology of endogenously synthesized NO is largely predicted by the known effects of nitrovasodilators such as glyceryl trinitrate, sodium nitroprusside, molsidomine (through its active metabolite SIN-1), and a number of S-nitrosothiols. These agents all act as NO donors, activating the cytosolic form of vascular smooth muscle guanylyl cyclase leading to cGMP accumulation. This results in relaxation of preconstricted vascular preparations, with or without endothelium, and rightward shifts in the dose–effect curves for a variety of vasoconstrictor agonists. Indeed, vascular relaxation by these agents relates directly to the quantity of NO liberated and is both proportional and temporally related to cGMP accumulation (26). The vasodilation appears to be mediated both by impairment of vasoconstrictor-induced calcium mobilization (or by enhanced calcium resequestration) in vascular smooth muscle as well as by diminished calcium sensitivity of the contractile apparatus (27,28).

As noted, NO is released by vascular endothelium at a low basal rate, buffering the effects of endogenous or exogenous vasoconstrictors. Indeed, endothelial denudation or pharmacological maneuvers that interfere with the generation, transit, or effect of endothelium-derived NO all augment the potency and efficacy of vasoconstrictor agonists. Thus, assessing the magnitude of the enhanced vasoconstriction following NO inhibition serves as the basis for design of most experiments to determine contributions of basal NO release. The pharmacological probes most often reported in such studies may be classified as agents that compete with arginine as substrate for the enzyme, compounds that interact with the enzyme or deplete its obligate co-factors (29), substances that scavenge NO during its brief extracellular transit, or agents that inactivate smooth muscle guanylyl cyclase to interfere with NO's ultimate vasodilator effect. In contrast, those compounds that stabilize NO by depleting superoxide anion, stabilize cGMP by inhibiting its phosphodiesterases, or in some cases, supplemental L-arginine to augment substrate for NO synthesis all may enhance the effects of basal or stimulated NO synthesis.

The guanidino-substituted analogs of L-arginine are the best studied of the NO synthesis inhibitors, including N$^\omega$-methyl-arginine (NMA), N$^\omega$-nitro-arginine [and its more soluble ester precursor N$^\omega$-nitro-arginine methyl ester (L-NAME)], and others. These analogs (but not their D-isomers) all compete with arginine as substrate for NOS, thus appearing more efficacious in the setting of relative arginine lack. The initial interactions of these inhibitors with NO synthases appear to follow competitive kinetics and all are initially reversible on addition of excess L-arginine. However, prolonged treatment with NMA alkylates the enzyme; the NOS inhibition due to sustained nitroarginine exposure is only poorly reversed by subsequent addition of arginine (30).

Hemoglobin, other heme-containing compounds, and the bacterial pigment pyocyanin all form poorly dissociable adducts with free NO, thus scavenging it during its brief extracellular transit from endothelial cell to vascular smooth muscle. The predicted nitrosyl-heme products have been detected by electron paramagnetic resonance spectroscopy, further supporting the proposed mechanism of action for these agents. All of these compounds may antagonize the effect of both basal and vasodilator-stimulated NO release.

Methylene blue and a number of other oxidizing agents not only antagonize the effects of endothelium-dependent vasodilators, but, to a somewhat lesser extent, the effects of synthetic nitrovasodilators as well. The action of methylene blue is mediated by local generation of superoxide anion (31), which both inactivates NO in transit and oxidatively inactivates smooth muscle guanylyl cyclase, thus blocking vascular relaxation.

VASODEPRESSOR EFFECTS OF NO *IN VIVO*

The nitrovasodilators exert direct hypotensive effects, *in vivo*, principally because of decrements in systemic vascular resistance that are associated with increases in circulating levels of cGMP; observations that are consistent with predictions based on their actions *in vitro*. In this respect, phosphodiesterase inhibitors potentiate this hypotensive effect, presumably by inhibiting intracellu-

lar cGMP hydrolysis (32). Similarly, the vasodilating and hypotensive effects of muscarinic cholinergic agonists are associated with dose-dependent increases in circulating cGMP (33), which are in large part NO-mediated.

The above observation, as well as the hypotensive effects of other agents shown to be endothelium-dependent vasodilators *in vitro*, suggest that not only basal, but also pharmacologically stimulated endothelial NO synthesis may lower arterial blood pressure. Regional variations in the response to NO-mediated vasodilators can be attributed to differences in the distribution of receptor populations among various vascular beds (34). Finally, inhibition of NO synthesis interferes with the hypotensive effect of acetylcholine (ACh), principally by shortening the duration of ACh-induced hypotension, with little effect on the maximal fall in blood pressure (35). Since dietary or enzymatic arginine depletion may augment the apparent efficacy of the inhibitory arginine analogs, there appears to be some role for circulating arginine in maintaining the acute hypotensive effect of EDRF-releasing vasodilators.

PRESSOR EFFECT OF ACUTE NO-SYNTHESIS INHIBITION

Several groups reported, and many have since confirmed, that acute administration of NO-synthase inhibitors to anesthetized or awake animals results in significant, dose-dependent, and long-lasting pressor effects in guinea pig (36), rabbit (37) and rat (38) (Fig. 1). Administration of lower, subpressor doses of inhibitors potentiates the pressor responses to infused angiotensin II (AII), norepinephrine, or arginine vasopressin in conscious rats (39). The direct pressor effects of NOS inhibition were selectively blunted or reversed by excess L-arginine and were associated with a reflex bradycardia. Many workers found it surprising that inhibition of a single, widely distributed but locally acting vasodilator system could result in profound elevations of arterial pressure and were puzzled as to why the pressure increments were not rapidly corrected by homeostatic mechanisms. Thus, whereas the acute hypertensive effect of NO inhibition surely depended upon a vascular effect involving withdrawal of a generalized basal vasodilator mechanism, additional actions at sites other than the resistance vasculature were postulated. Indeed, NO appears to inhibit postganglionic sympathetic nerve activity as well as preganglionic activity to the adrenal, to modulate carotid baroreceptor sensitivity, to alter vascular capacitance so as to decrease mean circulatory filling pressure (40), and to alter renin release. All of these effects are blocked by NO synthase inhibitors (see below).

Inhibition of NO synthesis or effect does not appear to contract most vascular tissues from normotensive animals *in vitro* in the absence of other vasoconstrictor stim-

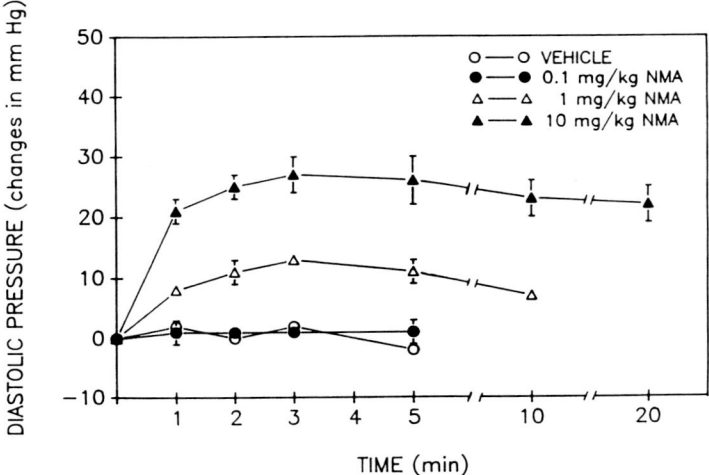

FIG. 1. Pressor effects of NMA (iv bolus, at the doses indicated) in anesthetized guinea pigs. Baseline systolic and diastolic blood pressure were 75 ± 3 and 51 ± 3 mm Hg. (From ref. 36, with permission.)

uli. The extent to which NO inhibitors augment vascular contraction varies among different vasoconstrictor agents and appears greatest at submaximal levels of vasoconstrictor tone. In accord with this background is a report suggesting the "compensatory release" of NO by the perfused mesentery exposed to increasing vasoconstrictor tone, as evidenced by increased production of nitrite together with augmented vasoconstriction following NOS inhibition (41). This notion of compensatory NO release, due likely to increased shear stress in constricted vessels under constant flow conditions, provides an appealing mechanism of vascular adaptation to increments in blood pressure. Indeed, in one report, the pressor effect of NOS inhibition was shown to depend on the basal level of vascular tone, the effect being diminished in rats made hypotensive by ganglionic blockade or pithing and restored or augmented by increasing infusions of phenylephrine (42). Others have failed to confirm these observations, the pressor effect following beta-adrenergic blockade, ganglionic blockade, or pithing being preserved (43). More recently, however, the role of enhanced NO synthesis as a compensatory mechanism has been demonstrated convincingly in several hypertensive animal models (see below).

CHRONIC INHIBITION OF NO *IN VIVO*

The profound cardiovascular effects of acute NO synthase inhibition led investigators to study chronic inhibition of the enzyme, and this has resulted in development of an important and unique model of persistent hypertension. Oral administration of L-NAME to Munich-Wistar rats for 4 to 6 weeks resulted in progressive severe hypertension, renal vasoconstriction, and impaired renal function. After 1 week of inhibition, the hypertension was partially reversible by intravenous L-arginine. Like-

wise, following 2 months' treatment, a 2-week drug-free period only partially reversed the hypertension. Plasma renin activity was elevated at the end of the study, but the hypertension was only partly attenuated by the angiotensin II antagonist losartan, and renal histology was notable both for segmental glomerular sclerosis and for microvascular changes consistent with malignant hypertension (44). Administration of L-NAME for 2 months produced persistent hypertension, associated with increased glomerular pressure, decreased glomerular capillary ultrafiltration coefficient, and single nephron glomerular filtration rate (GFR), as well as glomerular sclerosis and proteinuria (45). Other investigators have confirmed the persistence of hypertension with chronic administration of NO synthase inhibitors to rats, though some suggest a greater role for endogenous AII in the genesis of hypertension (46,47) and others suggest more prompt and complete reversal of the hypertension with either L-arginine administration (48) or discontinuation of the inhibitor (49). More recently, Manning and co-workers administered L-NAME continuously to dogs, resulting in hypertension that persisted over 11 days (50). Initially, there was augmentation of the pressor response to phenylephrine, which did not persist; retention of salt and water was only transient. Clearly, the duration of treatment, presence of renal microvascular lesions, alterations in pressor responsiveness, salt and water balance, and degree of reversibility are all important variables in these studies and will be key to comparing results from differing experimental protocols in the future. Most importantly, genetically normal animals may be rendered chronically, and even malignantly, hypertensive without surgical or dietary interventions by mechanistically well-defined agents that chronically interfere with NO synthesis. Further study of these models and their interactions with other forms of experimental hypertension may provide important insights into hypertensive disorders in humans.

CENTRALLY MEDIATED HEMODYNAMIC EFFECTS OF NO AND NO INHIBITION

The identification of NO as a messenger within the central nervous system and the stimulation of NO synthesis by activation of N-methyl-D-aspartic acid (NMDA) receptors (22) suggested that central alterations in NO effect may contribute to the integrated responses that follow systemic NO synthase inhibition. Activation of baroreflex mechanisms by cardiopulmonary afferent projections to the nucleus tractus solitarius (NTS) in rats depends upon activation of soluble guanylyl cyclase, suggesting a role of endogenous NO (51). Further, unilateral injection of an NO donor into this nucleus results in systemic hypotension and bradycardia (52). Similar micro-injection of NMA into NTS of rabbits increased arterial pressure, sympathetic outflow and, in sinoaortic de-afferented and vagotomized animals, increased heart rate as well (53). Shapoval and colleagues (54) found effects of NO in the ventrolateral medulla of cats to be complex: Increased NO in the rostral ventrolateral medulla decreased blood pressure and renal sympathetic outflow, whereas increased NO in the caudal ventrolateral medulla blocked these effects. These actions were blocked by methylene blue and opposing effects were obtained following local injection of NMA. Collectively, these results suggest that NO serves as an important central mediator of baroreflex function, especially when stimulated by cardiopulmonary afferents.

Intravenous administration of NMA to anesthetized

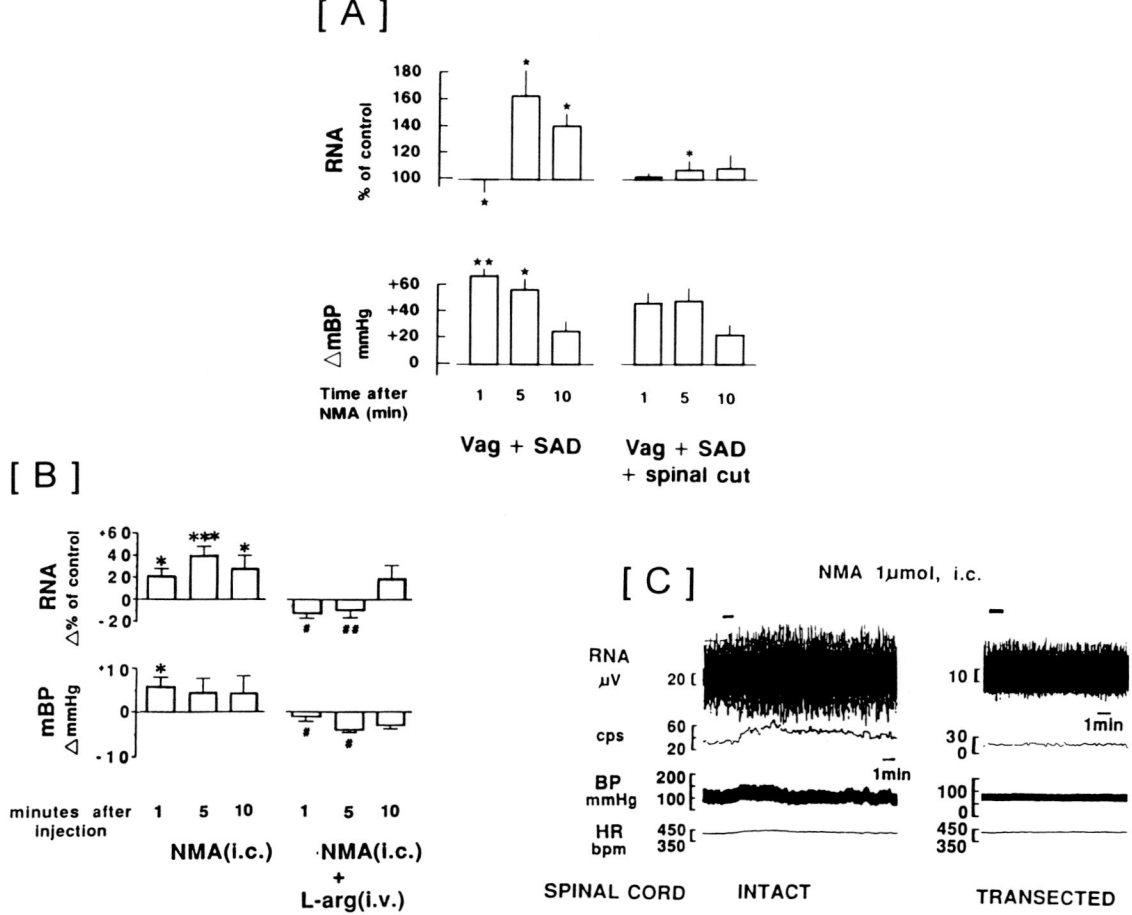

FIG. 2. **A:** Time courses of changes in renal sympathetic nerve activity and mean arterial pressure elicited by NMA (50 μmol/kg, iv bolus) in anesthetized rats with baroreceptor deafferentation, both before and after high cervical spinal cord transection. **B:** Time courses of changes in renal sympathetic nerve activity and mean arterial pressure elicited by NMA (1 μmol/kg, intracisternally), either alone or in combination with L-arginine (500 μmol/kg iv) in anesthetized rats with baroreceptor deafferentation. **C:** Tracings showing the effects of NMA (1 μmol, intracisternal injection) in the anesthetized rat with baroreceptor deafferentation, both before and after high cervical spinal cord transection. Recordings from top to bottom are actual renal sympathetic nerve activity (RNA), discharge rate of RNA, blood pressure, and heart rate. (A from ref 55; B and C from ref. 56, with permission.)

and baroreceptor denervated rats increased renal sympathetic nerve activity in spite of markedly increased blood pressure (55). High cervical cord transection blunted the pressor effect of NMA and blocked the increase in renal nerve activity, pointing to central contributions of NO synthase inhibition to the pressor response and augmented sympathetic outflow following systemic NMA (Fig. 2). Further, low doses of intracisternal NMA markedly augmented renal nerve activity and increased arterial pressure, albeit minimally; both of these actions could be blocked by cervical transection or by arginine administration (56). Collectively, these results underscore important contributions of central nervous system, as well as vascular, NO to the control of blood pressure and modulation of sympathetic tone. They further suggest that the hemodynamic effects of acute systemic NO synthesis inhibition involve both central and peripheral actions.

ROLE OF NO IN RENAL MECHANISMS OF ARTERIAL PRESSURE REGULATION

As reviewed elsewhere (57), long-term adaptation to hypertensive stimuli is mediated primarily through renal homeostatic mechanisms. The ability of chronic NO-synthesis inhibition to produce sustained hypertension associated with structural renal lesions suggests altered renal responses to increased perfusion pressure and to volume excess. Although it is not surprising that eNOS is expressed in renal vasculature, recent studies have also identified the neuronal isoform within the kidney, including the macula densa (58,59); moreover, renal tubular cells exhibit constitutive NOS activity as well as an inducible NOS following cytokine exposure (60,61). These localizations of various NO synthases within the kidney suggest possible roles for NO in modulating renin release, regulating glomerular perfusion, and altering tubular function.

NO and Glomerular Hemodynamics

Following acute inhibition of NO synthesis with NMA, micropuncture studies demonstrated graduated effects on glomerular hemodynamics as a function of dose (62). A very low intrarenal dose of NMA resulted in a small increment in afferent arteriolar resistance with only a minor fall in single nephron GFR and no change in efferent resistance, glomerular capillary hydraulic pressure, or ultrafiltration coefficient (K_f). Increasing the dose produced similar effects on pressure and resistance, but also decreased K_f, whereas systemic administration of pressor doses of NMA led to glomerular hypertension and efferent arteriolar vasoconstriction. The effect on K_f is consistent with work demonstrating mesangial cell responses to exogenous NO (63). There is also evidence for

a selective effect of NO in the afferent arteriole. In this respect, Ito and colleagues (64) performed elegant microperfusion studies that demonstrated selective afferent arteriolar NO synthesis during AII-induced vasoconstriction, thus accounting for the well-known increased sensitivity of the efferent arteriole to this vasoconstrictor.

Contributions of NO to Pressure Natriuresis

The acute hypertensive response to systemic NOS inhibition also results in a prompt but transient increase in urinary sodium excretion. This is consistent with the "pressure–natriuresis" evoked by a variety of vasopressors. However, when renal perfusion pressure is not permitted to increase, NOS inhibition is prolonged, or when subpressor doses of NOS inhibitors are infused either systemically or intrarenally, a profound antidiuretic and antinatriuretic effect is revealed (65,66). Such data imply a key role for intrarenal NO synthesis in mediating the natriuretic response to acute elevations in renal perfusion pressure. Indeed, Suzuki and colleagues (67) noted that acute increases in renal perfusion pressure by a subrenal aortic clamp in renal-denervated rats not only augmented sodium excretion, but also increased the urinary excretion of nitrate and nitrite, the stable degradation products of NO. In accord with these results, unilateral intrarenal infusion of very low doses of L-NAME blunted the acute natriuresis and diuresis that otherwise followed increased renal perfusion pressure in dogs (68) (Fig. 3). More recently, Majid and co-workers (69) extended these results by demonstrating that intrarenal L-NAME decreased the slope of the pressure–natriuresis curve in dogs, an effect that was not altered by coadministration of the AII antagonist losartan. NO may facilitate normal pressure natriuresis by an effect on the medullary circulation; i.e., dilation of these vessels may permit more efficient transmission of increased perfusion pressure to the renal interstitium. In this respect, doses of L-NAME that impair sodium excretion and urine flow decrease renal interstitial hydrostatic pressure (70). Similarly, infusion of nitroarginine directly into the renal medullary interstitium also decreased urine flow and sodium excretion, without any changes in GFR (71). Thus, intrarenal synthesis of NO appears to be crucial in mediating the hemodynamic changes resulting in natriuresis and diuresis due to increased perfusion pressure. Impaired NO synthesis, possibly in the renal medullary circulation, may therefore underlie the defective pressure natriuresis that often attends persistent hypertension. That this is so is suggested by two recent studies in hypertensive animal models. It was found that supplemental L-arginine restores blunted pressure–natriuresis in hypertensive Dahl salt-sensitive rats ingesting a high-salt diet (72). Moreover, it was found that L-arginine normal-

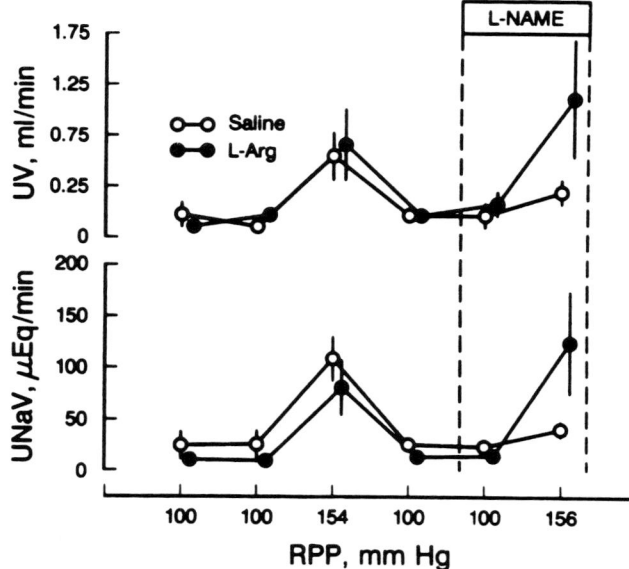

FIG. 3. Effects of two consecutive elevations of renal perfusion pressure (RPP) on urinary flow (UV) and sodium excretion (UNaV) before and during intrarenal infusion of L-NAME in dogs receiving intrarenal saline or L-arginine. L-NAME abolishes the natriuresis and diuresis that accompany increased RPP, its effect being reversed by concurrent infusion of L-arginine. (From ref. 68, with permission.)

izes the blunted pressure–natriuresis that is observed in renally denervated and hormonally clamped spontaneously hypertensive rats (SHRs) (73). Interestingly, L-arginine was without effect in the Wistar-Kyoto (WKY) rat, whereas pressure natriuresis in this normotensive control, but not in the SHR, was blunted by NMA. These latter results may be interpreted to suggest that pressure natriuresis normally depends on NO synthesis, which is not limited by substrate availability. In the hypertensive SHR, however, limited NO synthesis, due in part to lim-

ited substrate availability, results in the observed defect in sodium excretion. In summary, defects in renal NO synthesis contribute to impaired salt excretion and thus to the maintenance of hypertension in two genetic animal models of this disorder.

Contributions of NO to Salt Balance

Just as NO facilitates natriuresis in response to increased renal perfusion pressure, it also appears important in mediating salt excretion following extracellular volume expansion. In dogs, intrarenal infusion of very low doses of L-NAME attenuated the natriuresis, diuresis, and decreased proximal tubular resorption that normally accompany acute isotonic expansion of extracellular fluid volume (74). Also, rats placed on a high-salt diet for 2 weeks increase the urinary excretion of the NO degradation products nitrate and nitrite, their excretion increasing in proportion to that of sodium (75) (Fig. 4). Furthermore, the renal response to NMA infusion was augmented in these salt-loaded rats, again supporting the notion that volume expansion had increased NO synthesis to facilitate natriuresis and maintain normal blood pressure. Of further interest, increasing dietary sodium intake from 80 to 300 mEq/day in dogs unmasks a hypertensive effect of previously nonhypertensive doses of L-NAME (76). Conversely, these latter data could be interpreted to demonstrate that NOS inhibition unmasks the hypertensive effect of moderate increments in dietary salt intake. Finally, in spite of the hypertension, L-NAME increased net positive salt balance in these dogs on a high-salt diet. Collectively, these results reveal an intimate linkage between dietary sodium, volume expansion, and renal NO synthesis, which may bear importantly on the pathogenesis of salt-sensitive forms of hypertension.

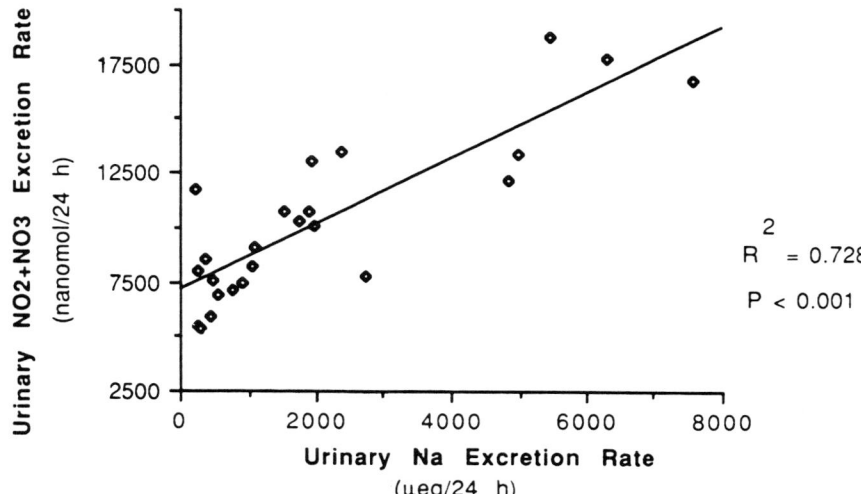

$R^2 = 0.728$

$P < 0.001$

FIG. 4. Correlation of urinary nitrate plus nitrite excretion with urinary sodium excretion in rats receiving normal or high salt (1 percent NaCl as drinking water) diets. (From ref. 75, with permission.)

Contributions of NO to the Regulation of Renin Secretion

Renin secretion, the rate-limiting step in systemic AII production, is principally controlled by three mechanisms: tubular salt delivery to the macula densa, renal sympathetic nerve activity, and a local baroreceptor mechanism sensitive to afferent arteriolar stretch. It now appears that NO may play an important role, in concert with a number of other paracrine factors, in mediating cell-cell communication within the juxtaglomerular apparatus (JGA) and in transducing the tubular signal to the granular (secretory) cell. NO can be synthesized in the macula densa as well as in JGA arteriolar endothelial cells and may act either on granular cells or on the extraglomerular mesangial cells, which are physically interposed between the macula densa and the granular cells. The multiple sites of possible NO synthesis or action within the JGA lead to contrasting hypotheses regarding the effects of this factor on renin release.

L-NAME increases plasma renin activity in the anesthetized rat with fixed renal perfusion pressure and beta-adrenergic blockade, suggesting tonic inhibition of renin release by NO (77). Such an action is supported by studies in renal cortical slices in which NMA increased the basal rate of renin release whereas L-arginine inhibited isoproterenol-stimulated renin release. In the same studies, mellitin-stimulated renin release was found to be inhibited by exogenous nitrovasodilators (78). Likewise, the NO donor nitroprusside has been reported to inhibit renin secretion by isolated juxtaglomerular granular cells (79). In contrast, L-NAME inhibited renin release in the isolated perfused rat kidney, suggesting a stimulatory role of endogenous NO (80). A better perspective on these apparently conflicting results is provided by data from recent studies of mouse juxtaglomerular cells in primary culture. These studies reveal two distinct effects of NO on renin secretion: a potent, transient cGMP-mediated inhibitory effect and a long-lasting stimulatory effect mediated by an uncharacterized calcium-dependent pathway (81). Similarly, Xe and colleagues (82) reported both stimulatory and inhibitory effects of NO on renin secretion in the isolated perfused JGA depending on which cells in the preparation were directly exposed to exogenous L-arginine or nitroarginine. In summary, although there is evidence that NO participates in the regulation of renal renin secretion, its role *in vivo* is still unclear.

ENDOTHELIAL DYSFUNCTION IN HYPERTENSION

Many have reasoned that endothelial dysfunction may act in a manner similar to NO synthase inhibition to augment pressor responses and cause hypertension by impairing the vasodilator effector limb of an important homeostatic pathway. Also, high pressures, per se, might impair endothelial NO synthesis, contributing to the perpetuation of established hypertension, whatever its initial cause. To this end, there have been many studies assessing the effect of hypertension, and its subsequent pharmacological control, on vasodilator agonist-induced endothelium-dependent relaxation, *in vivo, in situ,* or *in vitro.* Observations in a number of rat models of hypertension, including the New Zealand and Dahl strains and animals made hypertensive by the one-kidney–one-clip method, by aortic coarctation, or by administration of DOCA with high salt, all demonstrate marked impairment of endothelium-dependent aortic relaxation, some decreased sensitivity to nitrovasodilators, and restoration of relaxation following normalization of blood pressure (83–85).

Diederich and colleagues (86) noted impaired ACh-induced endothelium-dependent relaxation of norepinephrine-preconstricted, isolated, mesenteric resistance arteries from stroke-prone SHRs, despite well-preserved responses to nitrovasodilators. ACh-induced relaxation normalized following cyclooxygenase inhibition. They concluded that stimulated release of an endothelium-derived prostanoid vasoconstrictor served to mask normal endothelium-dependent relaxation in this preparation. This observation was explored further by Li and Bukoski (87), who noted that synthesis of this cyclooxygenase-dependent endothelium-derived vasoconstrictor could only be demonstrated when norepinephrine was used as the preconstrictor agent for these *in vitro* protocols. Not only was ACh-induced relaxation impaired in some SHR microvascular preparations, but L-NAME's ability to augment norepinephrine-induced vasoconstriction was diminished as well, suggesting an additional defect in basal NO synthesis (88). By contrast, Angus and colleagues (89) failed to observe any decrement in ACh-induced relaxation in small mesenteric arteries from SHRs, or to identify a similar defect in subcutaneous resistance vessels from humans with essential hypertension. Collectively, these and other studies suggest alterations in endothelial function in vessels from some hypertensive animals; nevertheless, some caution is required in the mechanistic interpretation of differing results from *in vitro* studies of tissue from SHR models of hypertension.

Many studies purport to assess "the activity of the NO system" by measuring ACh or vasodilator-stimulated endothelium-dependent relaxation. The interpretation of such studies may be problematic (90); moreover, it is unclear whether impaired vasodilator-stimulated NO synthesis actually predicts any changes in the basal elaboration of NO. Basal NO synthesis may, indeed, be much more relevant to modulation of blood pressure *in vivo.*

A fundamentally different aspect of NO modulation

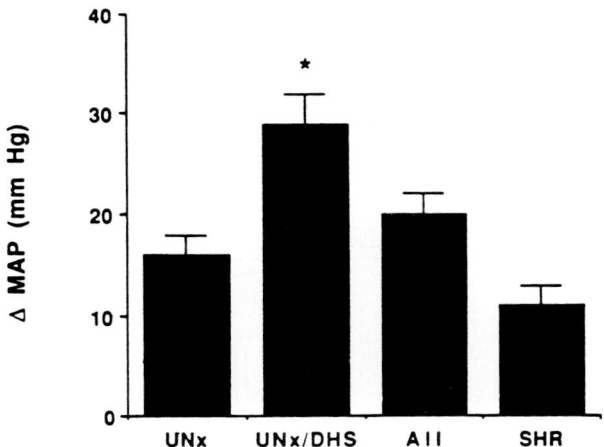

FIG. 5. Pressor effects of NMA (0.11 mg/kg/min, iv) in normotensive uninephrectomized rats (UNx, baseline MAP 112 ± 4 mm Hg), in uninephrectomized rats made hypertensive by DOCA and a high-salt diet (UNx/DHS, baseline MAP 139 ± 2 mm Hg), in rats made hypertensive by infusion of angiotensin II (AII, baseline MAP 134 ± 3 mm Hg), and in spontaneously hypertensive rats (SHR, baseline MAP 164 ± 4 mm Hg). *$p < 0.05$ vs. UNx. (From ref. 93, with permission.)

of vascular function in experimental hypertension was assessed by Pucci and colleagues (91), who noted that aortic rings from above a coarctation in hypertensive rats exhibited slowly developing contractile responses to L-NAME whereas (abdominal aortic) rings from below the coarctation, or rings from DOCA-salt hypertensive rats, did not. They further noted enhanced pressor responses to L-NAME but not to phenylephrine in aorta-coarcted rats compared with controls, even though blood pressure had been made comparable using losartan. These results suggested a compensatory activation of NO-mediated vasodilation in this model of hypertension.

Mesenteric arterial rings, obtained from a DOCA-salt rat model of volume-dependent hypertension and studied *ex vivo,* exhibit normal KCl or norepinephrine-induced vasoconstriction and normal ACh, isoproterenol, or nitroprusside-induced vasodilation when compared with rings from normotensive controls (92). Yet, endothelial denudation or NO synthesis inhibition selectively unmasks enhanced vasoconstrictor responses in rings from such hypertensive animals, suggesting that basal endothelial NO synthesis is augmented in this model. The increased NO synthesis is apparently compensatory for a while, preventing increases in vascular contractility and peripheral resistance during the development of DOCA-salt hypertension.

Similarly, *in vivo* protocols that assess basal NO synthesis by measuring the magnitude of the acute pressor response to infused NMA suggest that NO synthesis is augmented in hypertensive uninephrectomized DOCA-salt loaded rats. By contrast, no such increase was found in rats made equally hypertensive with infused angiotensin II, in hypertensive SHRs, or in normotensive uninephrectomized controls (93) (Fig. 5). This latter study suggests a selective augmentation of NO synthesis to blunt vascular resistance in volume-dependent as compared with vasoconstrictor-induced hypertension. This important observation has been extended by studies in the Dahl-Rapp salt-sensitive rat on a high salt diet, which manifests an augmented pressor response to NMA and normalization of blood pressure (or prevention of hypertension) following dietary supplementation with L-arginine or L-citrulline, despite continued ingestion of a high-salt diet (94) (Fig. 6). No similar hypotensive effect of L-arginine supplementation was observed in the SHR. Importantly, urinary cGMP was augmented in normotensive Dahl salt-resistant rats ingesting a high-salt diet and similar excretion rates were only observed in the salt-sensitive rats when they received supplemental arginine. Such data support a role of augmented NO synthesis in the normal adaptation to volume loading as well as suggest pathophysiological substrate limitation to interfere with this homeostatic augmentation of NO synthesis in this hypertensive animal model. More recently, these

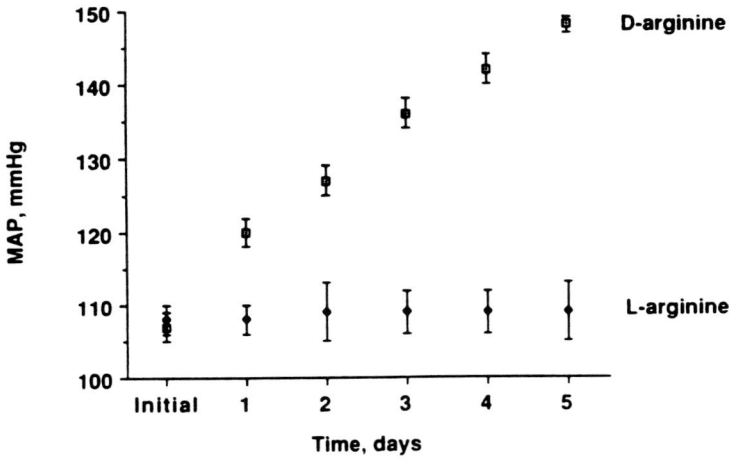

FIG. 6. Effect of oral arginine (1.25 g/L drinking water) on MAP of unrestrained SS/Jr rats switched from a 0.3 percent to 8.0 percent NaCl diet. L-arginine completely blocked the hypertension due to the high-salt diet, whereas D-arginine did not. Urinary excretion of cGMP was higher in the rats receiving L-arginine as was the pressor effect of subsequently administered NMA. (From ref. 94, with permission.)

same workers reported that dexamethasone, administered in doses sufficient to inhibit the induction of NO synthase activity by endotoxin, not only augmented the development of salt-sensitive hypertension in SS/Jr rats but also blocked the protective effect of L-arginine supplementation in these animals (95). This latter finding supports a role for inducible NOS in the vascular adaptation to salt loading in the Dahl rat.

STUDIES IN HUMANS

The first direct evidence that EDRF modulates basal vascular tone in humans was obtained by Collier and Vallance, who demonstrated that large veins on the dorsum of the hand were constricted following endothelial damage due to local infusion of distilled water (96). Subsequently, studies utilizing plethysmographic measurement of forearm blood flow and vascular resistance have demonstrated the vasoconstrictor effect of NMA infused into the brachial artery, as well as its ability to inhibit endothelium-dependent vasodilation of this forearm circulation (97). This latter experimental approach has led to assessment of endothelial function in hypertensive patients. Panza and co-workers (98) noted similar forearm basal blood flow in patients with essential hypertension and in normotensive control subjects. However, the vasodilator response to intrabrachial ACh was blunted in the hypertensive patients, whereas NMA inhibited ACh-induced vasodilation only in the normotensive subjects. They further reported that infusion of L-arginine augmented ACh-induced vasodilation in normotensive, but not in essential, hypertensive subjects, suggesting that NO synthesis is substrate-limited only in normotensive persons (99). Pharmacological normalization of blood pressure failed to rapidly restore the endothelial defect in previously hypertensive patients (100), whereas indomethacin improved ACh forearm vasodilation in both normotensive and essential hypertensive subjects, suggesting the simultaneous elaboration of a prostanoid vasoconstrictor substance in this model (101). These observations are consistent with those made in several animal models.

Intravenous L-arginine has long been used as a provocative agent in endocrine assessment. However, its hemodynamic effects have only been assessed quite recently. Infusion of 30 g L-arginine to normotensive subjects lowered mean arterial pressure and total peripheral resistance, increased heart rate and cardiac output, and resulted in concomitant elevations of plasma citrulline and cGMP as well as of urinary nitrate plus nitrite (102) (Fig. 7). The latter three markers suggest that arginine infusion augments NO synthesis. The same authors (103) noted similar hypotensive and vasodilator responses following L-arginine infusion in patients with essential and secondary hypertension. These systemic he-

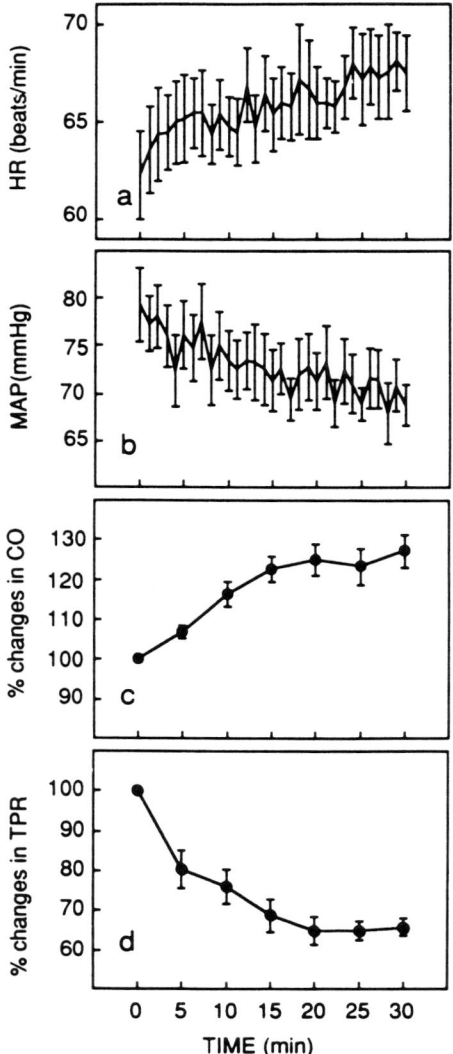

FIG. 7. Effect of L-arginine administration to ten normotensive volunteers on heart rate (HR), mean arterial pressure (MAP), cardiac output (CO), and total peripheral resistance (TPR). (From ref. 102, with permission.)

modynamic responses following arginine infusion to hypertensive subjects stand in apparent contrast with those obtained by Panza and co-workers (99) in studies of the local forearm circulation. Although it is still unclear whether intravenous arginine may exert hemodynamic effects indirectly, rather than by providing additional substrate for NO synthase, these early results appear to support substrate limitation of basal and stimulated NO synthesis in at least some human vascular beds. This might suggest an important species difference since, as already noted, NO synthesis in normotensive rats does not appear to be limited by substrate availability. An alternative interpretation would call attention to the relative abundance of dietary sodium in most human diets, possibly resulting in augmented renal NOS activity and substrate-dependent activity even in the absence of clinical hypertension. Attention to these kinds of experimental details will be key to reconciling future mechanistic studies in animals with results of clinical investigation.

ALTERED NO SYNTHESIS IN DISEASE

Hypertension is common in patients with endstage renal failure. Blood pressure normalization with routine dialysis and ultrafiltration suggest a major contribution of volume expansion to hypertension in this functionally anephric population. Another potential contribution to hypertension in these patients was suggested by Vallance and co-workers (104), who made the important discovery that asymmetric dimethylarginine, an inhibitor of NOS with potency similar to NMA (105), is synthesized endogenously and accumulates in patients with renal failure. However, a causal link of this endogenous NOS inhibitor with hypertension in these patients or in other human disorders remains to be demonstrated.

Renal allograft recipients often manifest treatment-refractory hypertension, most commonly linked to the chronic administration of cyclosporin A. Cyclosporine contributes not only to hypertension, but to renal vasoconstriction so severe as to decrease GFR. Since cyclosporine is toxic to endothelial cells in culture, it has been suggested that endothelial dysfunction may contribute to the vasoconstriction and hypertension that often attend its use. Indeed, Diederich and colleagues (106), as well as others, noted that chronic cyclosporine administration impaired endothelium-dependent relaxation of rat renal arteries. Such an impairment is manifested *in vivo* as inhibition of ACh-induced vasodilation, natriuresis, diuresis, and cGMP excretion in rats treated with cyclosporine (107). However, it remains unclear whether cyclosporine impairs basal NO synthesis in humans. For instance, Gaston et al. have demonstrated that the hypotensive effect of infused L-arginine is preserved in renal allograft recipients receiving cyclosporine, whereas the arginine-induced renal vasodilation is not (108).

As discussed elsewhere in this text, the profound physiological vasodilation that accompanies normal pregnancy is associated with augmented synthesis of NO and evidence of cGMP-mediated vasodilation (109,110). Preeclampsia, a hypertensive disorder unique to human pregnancy, is accompanied by pathognomonic lesions of glomerular endothelial cells (111) and may be principally an endothelial cell disorder (112). NO production is impaired in umbilical vessels from preeclamptic pregnancies (113). McCarthy and co-workers (114) demonstrated impaired endothelium-dependent relaxation of subcutaneous resistance arteries from women with preeclampsia that, however, was not due to altered NO synthesis. Pascoal and colleagues have made similar observations in small omental arteries obtained from preeclamptic women undergoing cesarean deliveries (115). Most recently, Baylis and Engels (116) reported that chronic NOS inhibition in pregnant rats leads to a syndrome of hypertension, proteinuria, and poor fetal outcome reminiscent of human preeclampsia. More detailed animal studies, with careful pathological investigation, will be necessary to delineate further a pathological role of impaired NO synthesis in hypertensive pregnancy.

CONCLUSIONS

Nitric oxide is an important vasodilator whose synthesis in the vasculature serves to buffer the effects of various vasoconstrictor stimuli. It serves also in the central nervous system to mediate some baroreflex functions, and in the kidney to regulate glomerular hemodynamics and renin secretion, as well as to facilitate natriuresis in response to increased pressure or volume expansion. By these varied mechanisms, it is now clear that NO contributes importantly to both the short- and long-term regulation of blood pressure. Nitric oxide synthesis is abnormal in a variety of animal models of hypertension, and possibly in some human hypertensive disorders. Whereas, in some cases impaired NO synthesis or endothelial dysfunction may be a result of hypertension, in other cases it may contribute to the initiation or perpetuation of hypertension. Finally, pharmacological inhibition of NO synthesis provides a new experimental model of hypertension that is associated with structural renal lesions and renal dysfunction. Blood pressure is elevated in this model by a direct effect on the resistance vessels, by diminished venous capacitance, by altered sympathetic outflow, by enhanced salt-sensitivity, and by defective pressure–natriuresis. In little more than a decade since Furchgott first suggested its existence, there is now compelling evidence, still accruing at an explosive rate, that NO is a key mediator in both the normal and pathophysiological control of blood pressure.

REFERENCES

1. Ignarro LJ. *Biochem Pharmacol* 1991;41:485–490.
2. Moncada S. *Pharmacol Rev* 1991;43:109–142.
3. Furchgott RF, Zawadski. *Nature* 1980;288:373–376.
4. Martin W, Furchgott RF, Villani GM, Jothianandan D. *J Pharmacol Exp Ther* 1986;237:529–538.
5. Waldman SA, Murad F. *Pharmacol Rev* 1987;39:163–196.
6. Gruetter CA, Gruetter DY, Lyon JE, Kadowitz PJ, Ignarro LJ. *J Pharmacol Exp Ther* 1981;219:181–186.
7. Rapoport RM, Murad F. *Circ Res* 1983;52:352–357.
8. Stuehr DJ, Marletta MA. *Proc Natl Acad Sci USA* 1985;82:7738–7742.
9. Miwa M, Stuehr DJ, Marletta MA, Wishnok JS, Tannenbaum SR. *Carcinogenesis* 1987;8:955–958.
10. Hibbs JB Jr, Taintor RR, Vavrin Z. *Science* 1987;235:473–476.

11. Hibbs JB Jr, Vavrin Z, Taintor RR. *J Immunol* 1987;138:550–565.
12. Ignarro LJ, Byrns RE, Woods KS. *Circulation* 1986;74:II-287.
13. Palmer RMJ, Ferrige AG, Moncada S. *Nature* 1987;327:524–526.
14. Ignarro LJ, Buga GM, Wood KS, Byrns RE, Chaudhuri G. *Proc Natl Acad Sci USA* 1987;84:9265–9269.
15. Palmer RMJ, Ashton DS, Moncada S. *Nature* 1988;333:664–666.
16. Sakuma I, Stuehr D, Gross SS, Nathan C, Levi R. *Proc Natl Acad Sci USA* 1988;85:8664–8667.
17. Nathan C. *FASEB J* 1992;6:3051–3064.
18. Nathan C, Xie Q-W. *J Biol Chem* 1994. (In press).
19. Lamas S, Marsden PA, Li GK, Tempst P, Michel T. *Proc Natl Acad Sci USA* 1992;89:6348–6352.
20. Loeb AL, Izzo NJ, Johnson RM, et al. *Am J Cardiol* 1988;62:36G–40G.
21. Bredt DS, Hwang PM, Glatt CE, Lowenstein C, Reed RR, Snyder SH. *Nature* 1991;351:714–718.
22. Garthwaite J, Charles SL, Chess-Williams R. *Nature* 1988;336:385–388.
23. Xie Q-W, Cho HJ, Calaycay J, et al. *Science* 1992;256:225–228.
24. Busse R, Muslch A. *FEBS Lett* 1990;275:87–90.
25. Beasley D. *Am J Physiol* 1990;259:R38–R44.
26. Feelisch M, Noack EA. *Eur J Pharmacol* 1987;139:19–30.
27. Twort CHC, van Breemen C. *Circ Res* 1988;62:961–964.
28. Nishimura J, van Breemen C. *Biochem Biophys Res Commun* 1989;163:929–935.
29. Stuehr DJ, Fasehun OA, Kwon NS, et al. *FASEB J* 1991;5:98–103.
30. Olken NM, Marletta MA. *Biochemistry* 1993;32:9677–9685.
31. Moncada S, Palmer RMJ, Gryglewski RJ. *Proc Natl Acad Sci USA* 1986;83:9164–9168.
32. Pearl RG, Rosenthal MH, Murad F, Ashton JPA. *Anesthesiology* 1984;61:712–715.
33. Honma M, Ui M. *Eur J Pharmacol* 1978;47:1–10.
34. Thomas GR, Thiemermann C, Walder C, Vane JR. *Br J Pharmacol* 1988;95:986–992.
35. Aisaka K, Gross SS, Griffith OW, Levi R. *Biochem Biophys Res Commun* 1989;163:710–717.
36. Aisaka K, Gross SS, Griffith OW, Levi R. *Biochem Biophys Res Commun* 1989;160:881–886.
37. Rees DD, Palmer RMJ, Moncada S. *Proc Natl Acad Sci USA* 1989;86:3375–3378.
38. Umans JG, Lindheimer MD, Barron WM. *Am J Physiol* 1990;259:F293–F296.
39. Conrad KP, Whittmore SL. *Am J Physiol* 1992;262:R1137–R1144.
40. Glick MR, Gehman JD, Gascho JA. *Am J Physiol* 1993;265:H47–H51.
41. Gross SS, Aisaka K, Levi R. *Br J Pharmacol* 1992;107:282P.
42. Vargas HM, Ignarro LJ, Chaudhuri G. *Eur J Pharmacol* 1990;190:393–397.
43. Pegoraro AA, Carretero OA, Sigmon DH, Beierwaltes WH. *Hypertension* 1992;19:643–647.
44. Ribeiro MO, Antunes E, de Nucci G, Lovisolo SM, Zatz R. *Hypertension* 1992;20:298–303.
45. Baylis C, Mitruka B, Deng A. *J Clin Invest* 1992;90:278–281.
46. Jover B, Herizi A, Ventre F, Dupont M, Mimran A. *Hypertension* 1993;21:944–948.
47. Pollock DM, Polakowski JS, Divish BJ, Opgenorth TJ. *Hypertension* 1993;21:660–666.
48. Ikeda K, Gutierrez OG Jr, Yamori Y. *Clin Exp Pharmacol Physiol* 1992;19:583–586.
49. Gardiner SM, Kemp PA, Bennett T, Palmer RM, Moncada S. *Eur J Pharmacol* 1992;213:449–451.
50. Manning RD Jr, Hu L, Mizelle HL, Montani J-P, Norton MW. *Hypertension* 1993;22:40–48.
51. Lewis SJ, Machado BH, Ohta H, Talman WT. *Eur J Pharmacol* 1991;203:327–328.
52. Machado BH, Bonagamba LG. *Eur J Pharmacol* 1992;221:179–182.
53. Harada S, Tokunaga S, Momohara M, et al. *Circ Res* 1993;72:511–516.
54. Shapoval LN, Sagach VF, Pobegailo LS. *Neurosci Lett* 1991;132:47–50.
55. Sakuma I, Togashi H, Yoshioka M, et al. *Circ Res* 1992;70:607–611.
56. Togashi H, Sakuma I, Yoshioka M, et al. *J Pharmacol Exp Ther* 1992;262:343–347.
57. Guyton AC. *Science* 1991;252:1813–1816.
58. Wilcox CS, Welch WJ, Murad F, et al. *Proc Natl Acad Sci USA* 1992;89:11993–11997.
59. Mundel P, Bachmann S, Bader M, et al. *Kidney Int* 1992;42:1017–1019.
60. Ishii K, Chang B, Kerwin JF Jr, Wagenaar FL, Huang Z-J, Murad F. *J Pharmacol Exp Ther* 1991;256:38–43.
61. Markewitz BA, Michael JR, Kohan DE. *J Clin Invest* 1993;91:2138–2143.
62. Deng A, Baylis C. *Am J Physiol* 1993;264:F212–F215.
63. Schultz PJ, Tayeh MA, Marletta MA, Raij L. *Am J Physiol* 1991;261:F600–F606.
64. Ito S, Arima S, Ren YL, Juncos LA, Carretero OA. *J Clin Invest* 1993;91:2012–2019.
65. Johnson RA, Freeman RH. *Hypertension* 1992;19:333–338.
66. Lahera V, Salom MG, Miranda-Guardiola F, Moncada S, Rovero JC. *Am J Physiol* 1991;261:F1033–F1037.
67. Suzuki H, Ikenaga H, Hishakawa K, Nakaki T, Kato R, Saruta T. *Clin Sci* 1992;82:631–634.
68. Salom MG, Lahera V, Miranda-Guardiola F, Romero JC. *Am J Physiol* 1992;262:F718–F722.
69. Majid DS, Williams A, Navar LG. *Am J Physiol* 1993;264:F79–F87.
70. Nakamura T, Alberola AM, Granger JP. *Hypertension* 1993;21:956–960.
71. Mattson DL, Roman RJ, Cowley AW Jr. *Hypertension* 1992;19:766–769.
72. Patel A, Layne S, Watts D, Kirchner KA. *Hypertension* 1993;22:863–869.
73. Ikenaga H, Suzuki H, Ishii N, Itoh H, Saruta T. *Kidney Int* 1993;43:205–211.
74. Alberola A, Pinilla JM, Quesada T, Romero JC, Salom MG, Salazar FJ. *Hypertension* 1992;19:780–784.
75. Schultz PJ, Tolins JP. *J Clin Invest* 1993;91:642–650.
76. Salazar FJ, Alberola A, Pinilla JM, Romero JC, Quesada T. *Hypertension* 1993;22:49–55.
77. Sigmon DH, Carretero OA, Beierwaltes. *Am J Physiol* 1992;263:F256–F261.
78. Beierwaltes WH, Carretero OA. *Hypertension* 1992;19:(II)68–73.
79. Greenberg SG, Xe XR, Briggs JP, Schnermann JB. *J Am Soc Nephrol* 1992;3:544.
80. Gardes J, Poux JM, Gonzalez MF, Alhenc-Gelas F, Menard J. *Life Sci* 1992;50:987–993.
81. Schricker K, Kurtz A. *Am J Physiol* 1993;265:F180–F186.
82. Xe XR, Greenberg SG, Schnermann JB, Briggs JP. *FASEB J* 1993;7:A221.
83. Winquist RJ, Bunting PB, Baskin EP, Wallace AA. *J Hypertens* 1984;2:541–546.
84. Lockette W, Otsuka Y, Carretero OA. *Hypertension* 1986;8:II61–II66.
85. Lüscher TF, Vanhoutte PM, Raij L. *Hypertension* 1987;9:III193–III197.
86. Diederich D, Yang Z, Bühler FR, Lüscher TF. *Am J Physiol* 1990;258:H445–H451.
87. Li J, Bukoski RD. *Circ Res* 1993;72:290–296.
88. Li F, Joshua IG. *Clin Exp Hypertens B* 1993;15:511–526.
89. Angus JA, Dyke AC, Jennings GL, et al. *Kidney Int* 1992;41:S73–S78.
90. Angus JA, Lew MJ. *J Hypertens* 1992;10:S179–S186.
91. Pucci ML, Miller KB, Dick LB, Guan H, Lin L, Nasjletti A. *FASEB J* 1993;7:A548.
92. Bockman CS, Jeffries WB, Pettinger WA, Abel PW. *Hypertension* 1992;20:304–313.
93. King AJ, Mercer P, Troy JL, Brenner BM. *J Am Soc Nephrol* 1991;2:1072–1077.
94. Chen PY, Sanders PW. *J Clin Invest* 1991;88:1559–1567.
95. Chen PY, Sanders PW. *Hypertension* 1993;22:812–818.
96. Collier J, Vallance P. *Br J Pharmacol* 1989;97:639–641.

97. Calver A, Collier J, Moncada S, Vallance P. *J Hypertens* 1992;10: 1025–1031.
98. Panza JA, Casino PR, Kilcoyne CM, Quyyumi AA. *Circulation* 1993;87:1468–1474.
99. Panza JA, Casino PR, Badar DM, Quyyumi AA. *Circulation* 1993;87:1475–1481.
100. Panza JA, Quyyumi AA, Callahan TS, Epstein SE. *J Am Coll Cardiol* 1993;21:1145–1151.
101. Taddei S, Virdis A, Mattei P, Salvetti A. *Hypertension* 1993;21: 929–933.
102. Hishikawa K, Nakaki T, Tsuda M, et al. *Jpn Heart J* 1992;33:41–48.
103. Hishikawa K, Nakaki T, Suzuki H, Kato R, Saruta T. *J Hypertens* 1993;11:639–645.
104. Vallance P, Leone A, Calver A, Collier J, Moncada S. *Lancet* 1992;339:572–575.
105. Stuehr DJ, Gross SS, Sakuma I, Levi R, Nathan CF. *J Exp Med* 1989;169:1011–1020.
106. Diederich D, Yang Z, Luscher TF. *J Am Soc Nephrol* 1992;2: 1291–1297.
107. Gallego MJ, Lopez Farre A, Riesco A, et al. *Am J Physiol* 1993;264:H708–H714.
108. Gaston RS, Schlessinger SD, Sanders PW, Barker CV, Curtis JJ, Warnock DG. *J Am Soc Nephrol* 1993;4:550.
109. Conrad K, Joffe G, Kruszyna H, et al. *FASEB J* 1993;7:566–571.
110. Molnar M, Hertelendy F. *Am J Obstet Gynecol* 1992;166:1560–1567.
111. Gaber LW, Spargo BH, Lindheimer MD. *Clin Obstet Gynaecol* 1994. (In press).
112. Roberts JM, Taylor RN, Musci TJ, Rodgers GM, Hubel CA, McLaughlin MK. *Am J Obstet Gynecol* 1989;161:1200–1204.
113. Pinto A, Sorrentino R, Sorrentino P, et al. *Am J Obstet Gynecol* 1991;164:507–513.
114. McCarthy AL, Woolfson RG, Raju SK, Poston L. *Am J Obstet Gynecol* 1993;168:1323–1330.
115. Pascoal I, Lindheimer MD, Nalbantian-Brandt C, Moawad A, Umans JG. *Hypertens Pregnancy* 1994. (In press).
116. Baylis C, Engels K. *Clin Exp Hypertens B* 1992;11:117–129.

Hypertension: Pathophysiology, Diagnosis, and Management, Second Edition,
edited by J.H. Laragh and B.M. Brenner,
Raven Press, Ltd., New York © 1995.

CHAPTER 65

L-Arginine and Nitric Oxide in the Regulation of Blood Pressure

Paul W. Sanders, Pei Yen Chen, Robert S. Gaston, and David G. Warnock

Arterial tone is dependent upon the net effect of competing vasoconstricting and vasodilating influences. One of these vasodilators, nitric oxide (NO), plays a major role in blood pressure regulation. NO is produced endogenously by a family of NO synthases that utilize L-arginine as substrate. Exogenous administration of organic nitrates, such as nitroglycerin and isosorbide dinitrate, and sodium nitroprusside directly enhances NO activity. NO, whether of endogenous or exogenous origin, achieves vasodilation via activation of soluble guanylate cyclase, which initiates a cascade of events resulting in smooth muscle cell relaxation. Not surprisingly, derangement of endogenous nitrovasodilator pathways can produce both hypertension and hypotension. Diminished NO production is involved in the pathogenesis of salt-sensitive hypertension in the Dahl/Rapp rat, in cyclosporine-related posttransplant hypertension, and in hypertension experienced by patients on chronic dialysis. Conversely, excess NO, stimulated by bacterial endotoxin and cytokines, may account for hypotension during septic shock or cytokine-based therapy of malignancy. While NO is involved in memory (1–3), nonadrenergic noncholinergic nerve fiber transmission (4), macrophage-induced cytotoxicity (5,6), platelet aggregation (6) and bleeding time (7), insulin release (8), smooth muscle growth and proliferation (9), and renal hemodynamics (10–12), this chapter describes the biochemistry and metabolism of NO in pathophysiological conditions—sodium-dependent states, atherosclerotic models, sepsis, and other diseases—in which this important vasodilator appears to play a predominant role. Improved understanding of L-arginine:NO pathways offers the hope of new therapeutic modalities for use in human disease.

ENDOTHELIUM-DERIVED RELAXING FACTOR

Classic hypotheses regarding the pathogenesis of hypertension typically suggested derangement of one or more vasoconstrictor pathways. However, the discovery of endothelium-derived relaxing factor (EDRF) by Furchgott and Zawadski (13) in 1980 allowed formula-

    P. W. Sanders, P. Y. Chen, R. S. Gaston, and D. S. Warnock: Nephrology Research and Training Center and Division of Nephrology, Departments of Medicine and Physiology, University of Alabama at Birmingham, and Veterans Affairs Medical Center, Birmingham, Alabama 35294.

tion of a novel concept: systemic blood pressure might reflect the net contribution of both vasodilator and vasoconstrictor influences. In these classic experiments, preconstricted arterial ring preparations with intact endothelium relaxed when stimulated with acetylcholine *ex vivo*. However, if the endothelium was absent or damaged, acetylcholine exerted no vasodilatory effect on the preconstricted arterial ring preparations. These experiments documented the existence of an important vasodilatory substance secreted by acetylcholine-stimulated endothelial cells. Subsequently, EDRF was shown to be NO or an endogenously produced NO-generating compound (both referred to as endogenous NO in this chapter).

NO is recognized as a potent vascular smooth muscle relaxant (14). EDRF was initially thought to be NO because certain vasodilators, including sodium nitroprusside, nitroglycerin, and isosorbide dinitrate, relaxed smooth muscle by either donating NO spontaneously or interacting with cysteine to yield s-nitrosocysteine, which then donates NO (14,15). In addition, EDRF demonstrated several properties very similar to NO, including a very short half-life in solution (14), inactivation by superoxide anions and prolongation of activity with addition of superoxide dismutase (16,17), and inhibition of activity by heme-containing proteins (hemoglobin, myoglobin) and methylene blue (14). Moreover, both sodium nitroprusside and EDRF induced vascular relaxation via the same mechanism of guanosine 3':5'-cyclic monophosphate (cGMP)-mediated dephosphorylation of myosin light chains (18). Discovery that mammalian cells can produce nitrate strengthened the contention that EDRF was, indeed, NO (5,19,20). Finally, using a chemiluminescence technique to detect and quantify NO production, and arterial strips as a bioassay for EDRF production, Palmer and associates demonstrated that NO was released by endothelium and accounted for the biologic properties of EDRF (21). Ignarro and colleagues (22) independently reached the same conclusions. Thus, EDRF and NO are now accepted as synonymously designating the same endogenous nitrovasodilator.

PHYSIOLOGY OF NO

Biochemistry and Biologic Effects

To understand how NO regulates blood pressure, and what factors modify its activity, a review of the chemistry and metabolism of NO is required. Possessing an odd number of electrons in a molecular orbital shared by both the nitrogen and oxygen atoms, NO is by definition a highly reactive free radical (14). As one would predict, given the exquisite reactivity and rapid metabolism of this substance, the predominant biologic effects of NO

are exerted locally, and its specific effects are dependent on the amount of NO present as well as its site of production. For example, NO produced by macrophages has a predominant role in cytotoxicity. NO can interact with superoxide anion to form peroxynitrite ($ONOO^-$), a potent oxidant that under certain conditions, such as reperfusion after anoxia, may be produced in sufficient quantities to induce tissue damage (23). Another cytotoxic effect of NO is nitrosation and inactivation of iron-containing enzymes of the mitochondrial electron-transport chain (14,24). Alternatively, NO produced in the arterial wall results primarily in vasorelaxation; because of its rapid oxidation in the arterial lumen, the vasodilatory actions of NO are exerted primarily in an autocrine or paracrine fashion.

In vascular smooth muscle, NO acts as a novel second messenger to induce vasodilation. By binding to the heme moiety of the soluble form of guanylate cyclase, NO activates the enzyme (Fig. 1) (14,15,25,26). Guanylate cyclase catalyzes the conversion of guanosine triphosphate (GTP) to cGMP, which in turn activates cGMP-dependent protein kinase (14,27). This kinase phosphorylates phospholamban, a regulatory protein for the Ca^{2+}-adenosine triphosphatase (ATPase) in the sarcoplasmic reticulum (28,29). The Ca^{2+}-ATPase decreases intracellular calcium concentration, which ultimately leads to dephosphorylation of myosin light chains and consequent smooth muscle relaxation (30). Spontaneous oxidation to form nitrite and nitrate is the major mode of inactivation of NO (3). NO production in biologic systems may be quantified by measurement of these oxidative products in plasma and urine (31–33), and by measurement of urinary cGMP excretion (12).

L-Arginine is the metabolic precursor of nitrite and nitrate in mammalian cells (5,34); importantly, NO is the intermediate in this reaction (35) and D-arginine does not serve as a precursor. Nitrogen in the guanidinium group of L-arginine serves as a source of nitrate biosynthesis in humans. Using L-[*guanidino*-$^{15}N_2$]-arginine, ^{15}NO has been shown to be derived from either of these two labeled nitrogen atoms of L-arginine (31,32). Studies of NO synthesis have shown that an intermediate, N^{ω}-hydroxy-L-arginine, is produced, followed by the generation of NO and L-citrulline (36).

Nitric Oxide Synthases

Characterization

A novel family of enzymes, termed NO synthases, catalyzes NO production from L-arginine *in vivo*. There are two basic categories of these enzymes (Fig. 2). A *constitutive* form of NO synthase requires calcium and calmodulin to produce NO. The activity of this enzyme is therefore increased by hormones, such as acetylcholine

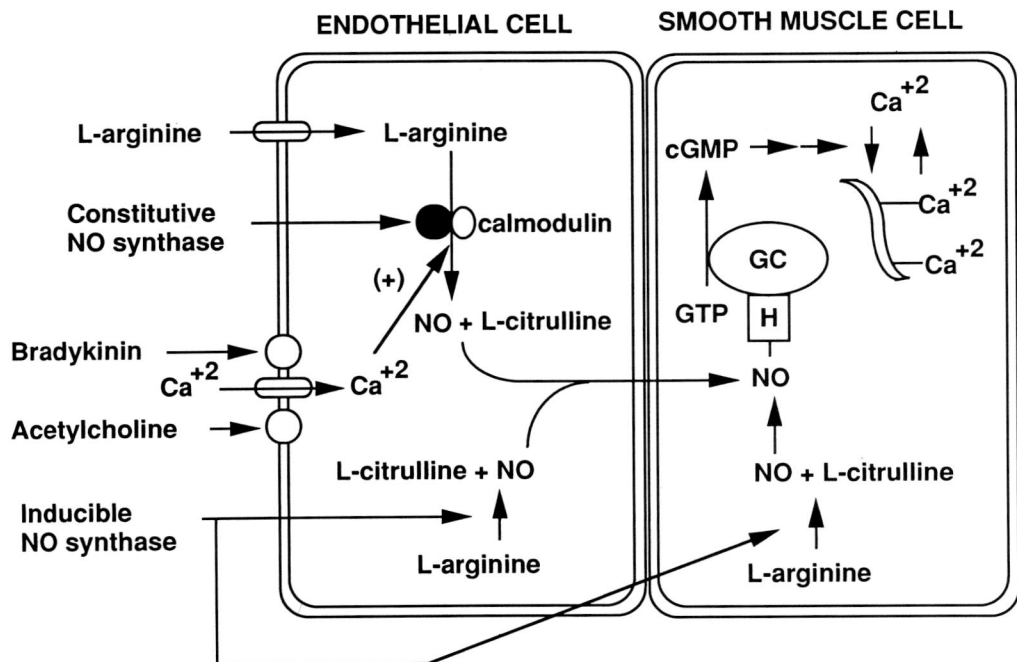

FIG. 1. Model of NO production in the arterial wall. In response to an increase in cytosolic calcium from hormones such as bradykinin or acetylcholine, calmodulin is activated and in turn stimulates the constitutive NO synthase to synthesize NO. NO diffuses into adjacent smooth muscle, where it binds to and activates guanylate cyclase (GC), which produces cGMP. Production of cGMP initiates a series of enzymes that decrease cytosolic calcium concentration and relax the contractile elements of the cell. Smooth muscle relaxation results. Also present in these cells, but under different regulatory control, is the inducible NO synthase. This system, when fully activated, produces NO in excess of 1,000-fold the amount produced by the constitutive NO synthase. The illustration also depicts transport of L-arginine. As expected, this amino acid transport system is stimulated in macrophages generating NO. Availability of L-arginine may become rate-limiting when NO production is maximally stimulated (60). (From ref. 52, with permission.)

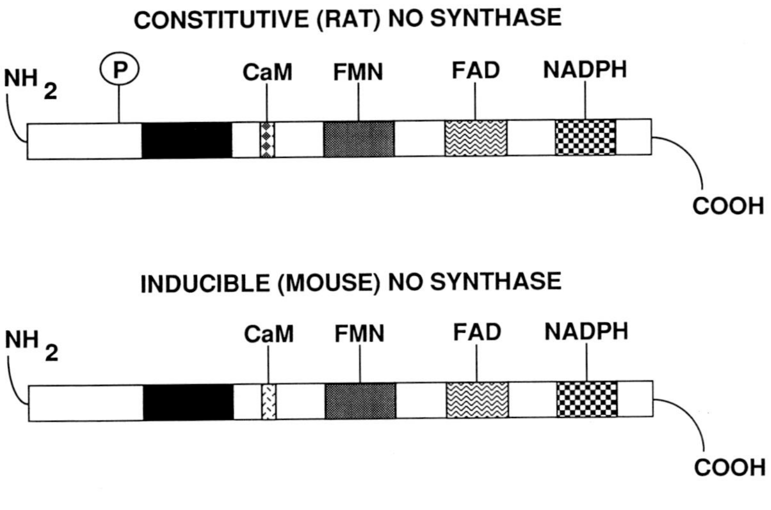

FIG. 2. Constitutive (rat brain) and inducible (mouse macrophage) NO synthases (41,44,47). Sequences of these NO synthases are 51 percent homologous. Portions of the C-terminus, which contains binding sites for nicotinamide adenine dinucleotide phosphate (reduced form) (NADPH), flavin adenine dinucleotide (FAD), and flavin mononucleotide (FMN), are conserved and share homology with rat cytochrome P-450 reductase, an enzyme that also uses NADPH and flavins to effect electron transfer. Thus, an important role for electron transfer in the function of the NO synthases is suggested. A calmodulin-binding site (*CaM*) and at least one phosphorylation (*P*) site are found on the constitutive NO synthase. The blackened area on the NO synthases represents the purported binding site for L-arginine.

and bradykinin, that bind to receptors and increase intracellular calcium concentration (13,14,20,26,27,37, 38). The second type of NO synthase is *inducible* and may either be calcium-independent or calcium-dependent (26,27,37,39,40). Hecker and associates (39) demonstrated that NO can be produced using substrates other than L-arginine. However, it appears that all NO synthases except the inducible, calcium-dependent form generate NO from L-homoarginine and L-arginine–containing small peptides.

Three cloned enzymes currently comprise the family of NO synthases (41–47). The first NO synthase was cloned from rat cerebellum (bNOS), and is a cytosolic, soluble constitutive enzyme that requires calcium and calmodulin; its activity is modulated by a variety of hormones including acetylcholine and bradykinin (41). The bNOS isoform is also present in the macula densa and serves an important role in tubuloglomerular feedback (48). This isoform also possesses at least one phosphorylation site that regulates enzyme activity (37,41,49). Bredt and coworkers (37) showed that cyclic adenosine monophosphate (cAMP)-dependent protein kinase, protein kinase C, and calcium/calmodulin–dependent protein kinases phosphorylate different serine moieties on the constitutive enzyme. Activation of protein kinase C decreased activity of this NO synthase, presumably by serine phosphorylation. Thus, intracellular second messengers that activate protein kinase C, such as the phosphoinositide signaling system (48), can modulate the constitutive NO synthase. Another constitutive NOS is found predominantly in endothelial cells, hence the term *endothelial NO synthase* (eNOS) (42,45,46). This enzyme resembles bNOS, but possesses a myristylated amino terminal glycine, a posttranslational modification that allows the enzyme to remain attached to the cytosolic face of the cell membrane (46,50). The third NO synthase is inducible (iNOS); its expression is promoted by a variety of factors including cytokines (40,43,44,47). NO synthases are present in at least a dozen cell types throughout the body (51,52). Both inducible and constitutive NO synthases are found in vascular endothelium, whereas only the inducible form is found in vascular smooth muscle cells (53). Thus, under certain conditions, NO production by smooth muscle cells may contribute to relaxation in an autocoid fashion.

Co-Factors

Sequence homology exists between the various isoforms of NO synthase and cytochrome P-450 reductase, an enzyme that also uses reduced nicotinamide adenine dinucleotide phosphate (NADPH) and flavins and is involved in electron transfer (41,52). All of the NO synthases effect the five-electron oxidation of L-arginine to form NO and L-citrulline. The co-factor requirement

for these enzymes is therefore significant. Interestingly, bNOS and eNOS have been considered to be calmodulin-dependent, whereas iNOS is calmodulin-independent. However, the iNOS sequence has a putative calmodulin-binding site, implying that it too is calmodulin-dependent. If the affinity for calmodulin is exceptionally high so that it is not released once it binds to the enzyme, then this isoform would appear to be functionally independent of calmodulin (43,44,47). Several other co-factors, especially tetrahydrobiopterin (BH4), are also required. Enzymes involved in synthesis of BH4 are shown in Fig. 3.

Gross and Levi (54–56) demonstrated that synthesis of NO from iNOS can be inhibited by use of 2,4-diamino-6-hydroxypyrimidine (DAHP), a selective inhibitor of GTP cyclohydrolase I, which is the rate-limiting enzyme in BH4 synthesis. These investigators concluded that co-induction of BH4 synthesis with iNOS was required to induce synthesis of NO in vascular smooth muscle. Cytokines have also been shown to stimulate BH4 synthesis in human endothelial cells by inducing GTP cyclohydrolase I; since the constitutive NOS also require BH4, the activity of these enzymes may be increased by this mechanism (56). These data also suggest that a defect in synthesis of BH4 could alter NO generation.

All of the NO synthases are stereoselective, utilizing L-arginine but not D-arginine as the substrate to produce NO (5,34,35,52,55–57). This amino acid substrate is vital in NO production *in vivo*. Depletion of L-arginine attenuates endothelium-dependent relaxation in bovine intrapulmonary arterial rings (58). Addition of L-arginine to aortic ring preparations stimulates endothelium-

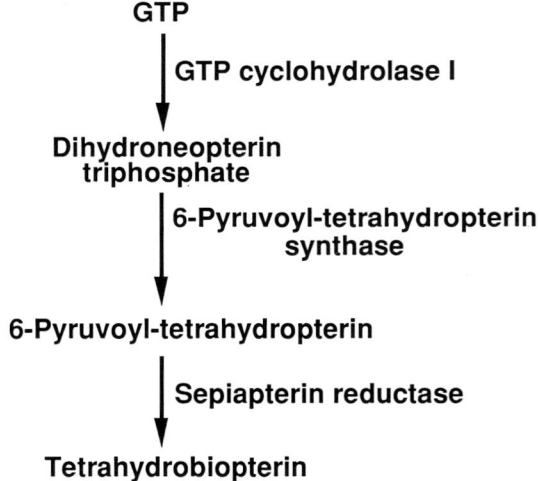

FIG. 3. Synthesis of tetrahydrobiopterin. GTP cyclohydrolase I, which has been cloned in the rat (139), is the first enzyme of this pathway and is induced by cytokines (140). Sepiapterin reductase, which has also been cloned in the rat (141), appears to be constitutively expressed (140). 6-Pyruvoyl-tetrahydro-biopterin synthase has not yet been cloned in the rat.

TABLE 1. *Inhibitors of nitric oxide synthases*

Class of inhibitor	Examples	NO synthase affected	
		Constitutive	Inducible
L-arginine analogs	L-NMMA, L-NA, L-NAME	+	+
Nucleotide-requiring flavoprotein inhibitors	Diphenyleneiodonium	+	+
Trascription inhibitors	Dexamethasone, TGF-β	−	+
Calmodulin inhibitors	Trifluoperazine	+	−

NO, nitric oxide; L-NMMA, N$^\omega$-methyl-L-arginine; L-NA, N$^\omega$-nitro-L-arginine; L-NAME, N$^\omega$-nitro-L-arginine; TGF-β, transforming growth factor-beta.

dependent and endothelium-independent vascular relaxation (59). In macrophages induced to synthesize NO, L-arginine transport is simultaneously stimulated (60) and can potentially become a rate-limiting step in NO generation (52,61). Thus, adequacy of substrate provision may play an important role in specific models of vascular disease.

Inhibitors

Several classes of compounds can inhibit NO synthases (Table 1). Perhaps the best known inhibitors are L-arginine analogs that have asymmetrical substitutions on the guanidinium nitrogen atoms (5,14,20,26,38,57, 62). N$^\omega$-methyl-L-arginine (L-NMMA) is one of the most widely used compounds in this class of competitive inhibitors (14,20,26,57,62–64). Interestingly, the inhibitory activity of this asymmetrical methyl-substituted arginine is not seen with N$^\omega$, N$^{\omega\prime}$, dimethyl-L-arginine, which has methyl groups on both guanidinium nitrogen atoms. Presumably, the inhibitory compound must contain a free NH$_2$- group to provide optimal steric specificity for binding to the enzyme (64). Gross and colleagues (65) have shown that both constitutive and inducible forms of NO synthase can be inhibited by the asymmetrically substituted arginine analogs. N$^\omega$-nitro-L-arginine (L-NA) is 100-fold more potent than L-NMMA as an inhibitor of the constitutive NO synthase. However, equimolar amounts of L-NMMA inhibit the inducible NO synthase to a greater extent than L-NA. Diphenyleneiodonium and similar compounds that inhibit nucleotide-requiring flavo-proteins inhibit both inducible and constitutive NO synthases (66). Dexamethasone prevents the expression of the inducible, but does not alter the constitutive, NO synthase (26,51). Transforming growth factor-beta (TGF-β) (67) and interleukin-10 (IL-10) (68) also prevent expression of the inducible NO synthase. On the other hand, inhibitors of calmodulin, such as trifluoperazine, block the constitutive (calmodulin-dependent) NO synthase, but do not affect the inducible calcium-independent enzyme (69,70). These selective inhibitors of NO synthase may be used to determine the contributions of specific isoforms to altered NO production in given situations.

EXOGENOUS NITROVASODILATORS

Nitric oxide-generating compounds have been used to treat patients for decades, so the concept of NO as a vasodilator is familiar to most clinicians. These compounds include organic nitrates, such as nitroglycerin and isosorbide dinitrate, and sodium nitroprusside (14,15,26,27). Whereas sodium nitroprusside releases NO spontaneously, organic nitrates produce NO only after biotransformation of cellular cysteine to form the labile product, s-nitrosocysteine (14,15,27,71,72). *In vivo,* tolerance develops to organic nitrates, but not nitroprusside, via a process related primarily to a decrease in availability of cellular cysteine (71,72). Interestingly, removal of endogenous NO by denuding the endothelium or inhibition of NO synthase results in supersensitivity of adjacent vascular smooth muscle to exogenous nitrovasodilators. This heightened response is apparently related to enhanced availability of soluble guanylate cyclase following removal of its tonic stimulation by endogenous NO (6). These observations demonstrate that both exogenous and endogenous nitrovasodilators interact with the same intracellular receptor (soluble guanylate cyclase) to alter the final common pathway of phosphorylation and dephosphorylation of myosin light chains.

ENDOGENOUS NO IN HYPERTENSION AND VASCULAR DISEASE

L-Arginine Analogs and Hypertension

L-Arginine analogs, by inhibiting NO synthases, can serve as chemical probes of NO production (5,14,20,26, 38,57,62–65). Addition of L-NMMA to arterial rings *ex vivo* prevents EDRF-induced vasodilation in a concentration-dependent fashion (73). Intravenous infusion of L-NMMA produces rapid and concentration-dependent increases in blood pressure in humans (74) and other mammals (11,12,14,26,63); this increase can be reversed with intravenous L-arginine. L-NMMA decreases blood flow to a variety of arterial beds including the renal, mesenteric, and internal carotid arteries (11). Chronic oral ingestion of arginine analogs, including L-NMMA and

N$^\omega$-nitro-L-arginine (L-NAME), produces sustained increases in blood pressure in rats (26,75–78). Histologic changes compatible with malignant nephrosclerosis occurred in rats with prolonged exposure to high concentrations of these analogs (78). Chronic L-NAME infusion has also been shown to reduce cGMP content of resistance vessels, reduce NO generation, and enhance the vasoconstrictor response to norepinephrine (77). Alternatively, infusion of acetylcholine, by stimulating endothelial cell release of NO, produces a concentration-dependent decrease in blood pressure that correlated with increased urinary cGMP excretion, an index of NO production (12). These studies show that NO is an important determinant of resting arteriolar tone and modulates systemic blood pressure *in vivo*.

Salt-Sensitive Hypertension, L-Arginine, and NO

In human and animal studies, there appears to be a genetic predisposition in some, but not all, subjects to develop hypertension in response to an increase in dietary sodium chloride (NaCl) intake (79–82). However, dissection of the etiologic factors conferring salt-sensitivity has proved difficult. A compelling and relevant model of low-renin hypertension has been developed by the pioneering work of Lewis K. Dahl, who produced from the Sprague-Dawley line two strains of rats that are either susceptible or resistant to the hypertensive effects of a high-salt (8.0 percent NaCl) diet (83). These Dahl salt-susceptible and salt-resistant strains have been completely inbred by John P. Rapp to yield

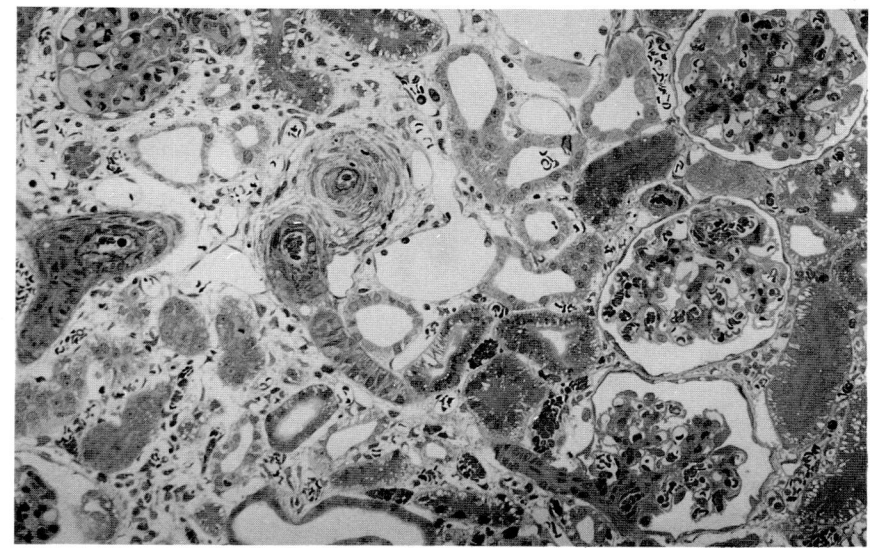

A

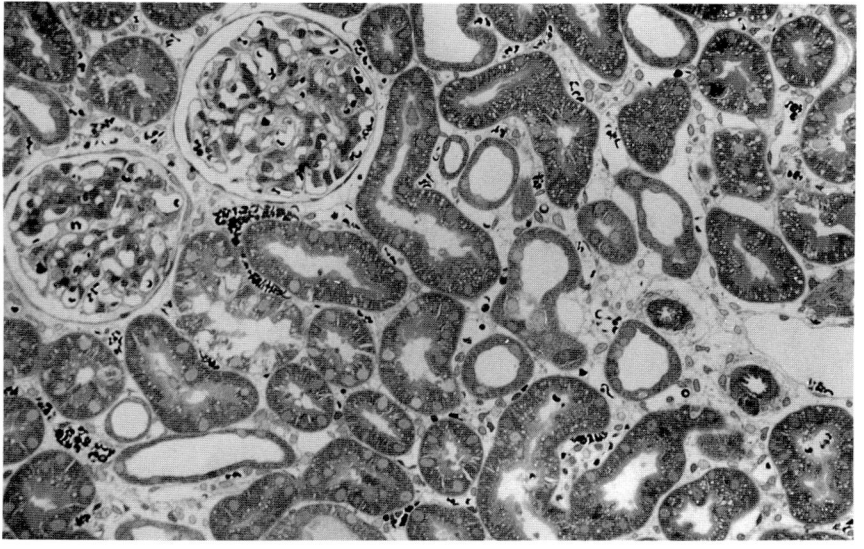

B

FIG. 4. Light micrograph showing renal cortex from untreated SS/jr (*top panel*) and SS/jr rats treated with L-arginine (*bottom panel*). Both rats had been maintained on 8 percent sodium chloride chow for 3 weeks. Without L-arginine supplementation, interlobular arteries and preglomerular arterioles (*arrows*) were thickened, and expansion of the glomerular mesangial spaces was apparent (*arrowheads*). In striking contrast, renal morphology of the L-arginine–treated rats was normal. (Hematoxylin-eosin stain, ×300) (From ref. 84, with permission.)

two strains that are each homozygous at all genetic loci, thus fixing the characteristics of the strains (83). Dahl/Rapp rat strains may thus be characterized as either salt-sensitive (SS/jr) or salt-resistant (SR/jr). On an 8.0 percent NaCl diet, young SS/jr rats rapidly and uniformly develop low-renin hypertension and die within weeks (84). The major cause of death in these SS/jr animals appears to be renal failure from arteriolosclerosis, glomerulosclerosis, and arteriosclerosis, a histologic appearance identical to hypertensive nephrosclerosis in humans (Fig. 4) (84). In contrast, SR/jr rats remain normotensive despite a high salt intake, with well-preserved renal function.

The etiology of salt-sensitive hypertension in SS/jr rats is unknown, but is probably polygenic in origin. One potential cause is sodium retention. Chen and Sanders (*unpublished observations*) and others (85–87) have shown a relative inability of SS/jr rats to increase sodium excretion in the face of a salt load. Interstrain renal transplantation using SS/jr and SR/jr rats has suggested that kidneys from SS/jr rats promote the development of hypertension (83). Using restriction fragment length polymorphism (RFLP) analysis of the renin gene, Rapp and coworkers (88) have shown that a genetic polymorphism in the renin gene co-segregates with the hypertensive condition in the F_2 offspring of S and R rats. These authors have suggested that an abnormality of the renin gene or alleles genetically linked to the renin locus account for 25 percent of the blood pressure differences between S and R rats. While recognizing that other animal models of hypertension can be employed to study the pathogenesis of hypertension, the Dahl/Rapp strains provide a unique means to investigate the pathogenesis of hereditary salt-sensitive hypertension and salt resistance, and may ultimately be very useful in understanding human low-renin essential hypertension in defined, relatively homogeneous populations such as is seen in black patients (80). In this instance, this model of salt-sensitive hypertension is one example in which the L-arginine:NO pathways appear to be deranged in hypertensive vascular disease (Table 2).

An increase in NO production is an important compensatory mechanism that occurs when dietary salt intake is increased. Chen and Sanders have demonstrated that SR/jr rats (along with other Sprague-Dawley rats) augment NO production in response to increased dietary salt, whereas SS/jr rats do not (89). However, dietary L-arginine supplementation in SS/jr rats on a high-salt diet increases NO production (as demonstrated by increased urinary excretion of nitrite/nitrate and cGMP) and completely prevents hypertension and renal failure (52,76,84,89). Renal morphology in L-arginine–treated SS/jr rats is normal and identical to that observed in SR/jr rats on the same high-salt diet (84,89). Concomitant administration of dexamethasone (76), an inhibitor of iNOS (26,51,90), abolished the antihypertensive effect of L-arginine in SS/jr rats on a high-salt diet (Fig. 5), as well as the increase in urinary excretion of cGMP and nitrate. These findings suggest that salt-sensitive hypertension in the SS/jr strain may be due to a genetic defect in the endogenous nitrovasodilator pathway. Addition of L-arginine corrects the deficient NO production that accompanied the high-salt diet; the underlying defects in NO production and/or effectiveness in SS/jr rats are being actively studied.

Patel et al. (91) have shown that a blunted pressure-natriuresis response characterizes salt-sensitive hypertension in SS/jr rats. Dietary supplementation with L-arginine did not affect the normotensive SR/jr rats, but normalized the pressure-natriuretic response in SS/jr rats on an 8-percent NaCl diet. This effect could also be demonstrated in short-term studies performed before there was any hypertension-induced renal damage, and

TABLE 2. *Vascular disorders potentially related to L-arginine:NO pathways*

Hypertension and arteriolosclerosis
Dahl/Rapp salt-sensitive rat
Human essential and low-renin hypertension
End-stage renal failure
Cyclosporine
Hypercholesterolemic atherosclerosis
Hypotension
Septic shock
Cytokine-associated

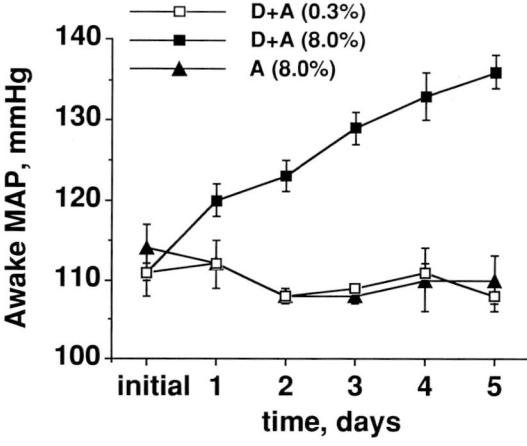

FIG. 5. Graph of daily mean arterial pressures (MAP) obtained from conscious, unrestrained rats. On a high-salt diet, L-arginine supplementation [group A (8.0 percent)] prevented development of hypertension. Administration of dexamethasone, 5 μg/day, to SS/jr rats on a low-salt diet [group D + A (0.3 percent)] did not increase blood pressure. Blood pressure did, however, increase rapidly despite administration of L-arginine in SS/jr rats on the high-salt chow given dexamethasone, 5 μg/day [group D + A (8.0 percent)]. (From ref. 76, with permission.)

was associated with improved autoregulation of glomerular filtration rate (91). In conscious dogs, infusion of L-NAME also attenuated the natriuretic response to salt loading, indicating that systemic hypertension during chronic L-NAME treatment is in part secondary to extracellular fluid volume expansion associated with renal salt retention (92).

In another genetic model of hypertension, the spontaneously hypertensive rat (SHR), L-arginine treatment neither prevents nor corrects hypertension (89). Instead of defective NO production, Nakazono and associates (93) have suggested excessive consumption of NO due to overproduction of superoxide radicals by xanthine oxidase; infusion of oxypurinol lowers blood pressure in these rats. Lee and Webb found that there was greater inhibition of NO production by L-NAME in stroke-prone SHR rats than in Wistar-Kyoto (WKY) control rats, consistent with an overproduction and consumption of NO in the SHR model of hypertension (94). Certainly, alteration of the L-arginine:NO pathways is not responsible for all forms of hypertension. For example, L-arginine does not reduce blood pressure in the deoxy-corticosterone acetate (DOCA)-salt model of hypertension (95).

Interestingly, intravenous infusion of L-arginine in humans lowers systemic blood pressure in patients with essential hypertension and in normal volunteers (96–98). Blood pressure decreases to a greater extent in hypertensive subjects compared to normotensive controls (96–98). L-Arginine concomitantly increases plasma concentration of cGMP and urinary nitrate, supporting the precursor role of this amino acid in NO production in humans (96,97). Of note, plasma catecholamines and renin did not change during L-arginine infusion in humans, and plasma aldosterone levels fell during the infusions (96). The systemic and renal vasodilatory responses to L-arginine have also been shown to be independent of prostaglandin synthesis (99). Patients with essential hypertension possess a defect in endothelium-dependent vasorelaxation, but have preserved endothelium-independent vasodilation (100,101). Because hypertension itself decreases endothelium-dependent vasodilation (74), and L-NMMA infusion has a blunted effect on forearm blood flow in hypertensive subjects (102), determining a cause-and-effect relationship in humans is difficult. However, the studies of Chen and Sanders with prehypertensive Dahl/Rapp rats suggest that a defect in NO production is responsible for salt-sensitive hypertension (89).

Hypertension in End-Stage Renal Failure

Other forms of acquired hypertension may be due to interruption of NO-dependent vasodilation. Vallance and associates (103) have suggested that accumulation of N$^\omega$-dimethyl-L-arginine, an L-arginine analog with an asymmetric dimethyl substitution of a guanidinium nitrogen atom, promotes hypertension in patients on dialysis. This compound inhibits both inducible and constitutive NO synthases in a dose-dependent fashion, and its intravenous infusion into guinea pigs increases blood pressure in a concentration-dependent fashion (103). The clinical significance of these observations is uncertain because the plasma concentration of this inhibitor in patients with renal failure (4.0 ± 0.05 μM) is much lower than the amount required to inhibit significantly both types of NO synthases. Nevertheless, the idea proposed is worthy of further exploration. Several guanidino compounds besides creatinine accumulate in renal failure (104); potentially, these compounds could either inhibit the synthesis of NO, as does N$^\omega$-dimethyl-L-arginine, or serve as a substrate for NO generation.

Nitric Oxide and Renal Hemodynamics

A definite but transient increase in renal blood flow and glomerular filtration rate in response to amino acid infusions is a well-described phenomenon in both animals and humans (105–108). More recently, it has become evident that renal hyperfiltration may not represent a universal response to protein loading, but rather a more specific effect of certain amino acids. While alanine and branched-chain amino acids do not elicit such changes (109,110), administration of the single amino acids L-glycine and L-arginine may result in renal hemodynamic alterations identical to those previously described with mixed amino acid infusions (109,110). In the study by Gaston and coworkers (111) L-arginine, but not branched-chain amino acids, reduced blood pressure and renal vascular resistance, and increased renal blood flow.

Mechanisms underlying the altered renal hemodynamics with different amino acid infusions remain poorly defined. Several investigators have reported the involvement of glucoregulatory hormones (insulin, glucagon, growth hormone, and somatostatin) as mediators of the phenomenon associated with both mixed amino acid and L-arginine infusions (112–114). Krishna and coworkers found that indomethacin, but not enalapril, prevented the response to an oral protein load, supporting a role for vasodilatory prostaglandins (115). Intrarenal kinin production also appears to be involved in the vasodilatory response to amino acids (116). Recently, several lines of evidence have linked NO generation to amino acid–induced renal hyperfiltration. King and coworkers (117) found that L-NMMA abolished the renal response to L-glycine and mixed amino acids in the Munich-Wistar rat, while Tolins and Raij documented a similar effect of L-NMMA in rats using a 10 percent solution of mixed amino acids (118). Cernadas et al. reported data confirming abrogation of the renal response to both L-arginine and L-glycine in the rat by pretreatment with N$^\omega$-nitro-L-arginine, an inhibitor of NO synthase (119). These data imply that NO is essential for the renal hyperemic and hyperfiltration responses to amino acid infusion, reflecting either the role of L-arginine as substrate for NO synthesis, or activation of NO synthase by another amino acid (glycine) or group of amino acids.

Cyclosporine and Hypertension

Another form of acquired, low-renin, salt-sensitive hypertension occurs in patients receiving cyclosporine (120). Cyclosporine damages vascular endothelium and produces intense vasoconstriction, especially of the renal vasculature (96,121). Dinh-Xuan et al. (122) demonstrated that cyclosporine inhibits endothelium-dependent vasorelaxation but does not affect relaxation to exogenous nitrovasodilators; loss of endogenous nitrovasodilator activity from endothelial damage potentially contributes not only to hypertension but also to cyclosporine-induced renal insufficiency. Gaston and colleagues (111) demonstrated a specific loss of the renal vasodilatory response to L-arginine infusion in stable hypertensive renal transplant recipients treated with cyclosporine, as compared to normotensive controls and transplant recipients treated with azathioprine.

In addition to inducing hypertension, cyclosporine attenuates the renal response to amino acid infusion in rats and man. De Nicola and coworkers (123) found that chronic cyclosporine administration to rats decreased renal NO synthase activity, and that this defect was associated with preglomerular vasoconstriction. Cairns et al. (124) studied renal hemodynamics in nine cyclosporine-treated renal allograft recipients and nine similar patients not receiving cyclosporine during a 2-hour infusion of mixed amino acids. Glomerular filtration rate and renal plasma flow increased by approximately 20 percent in the noncyclosporine group, and did not change in the cyclosporine group. These findings were corroborated by Rondeau and coworkers (125) using a similar protocol, and by Nunley and colleagues with oral protein loading (126). Neither study, however, evaluated blood pressure or renal vascular resistance. In the study of Gaston et al. (111), an increase in renal blood flow and glomerular filtration rate in response to L-arginine was observed in the azathioprine-treated patients; the renal plasma flow response was similar to that noted in normal humans, with an exaggerated glomerular filtration response in transplant recipients. Branched-chain amino acids did not affect any parameter, suggesting a specific effect of L-arginine. Consistent with previous studies, subjects receiving cyclosporine-based immunosuppression did not demonstrate altered renal hemodynamics in response to infusion of either amino acid, but still manifested a fall in systemic blood pressure during the L-arginine infusions (111). These results are consistent with a specific inhibitory effect of cyclosporine on vasodilation that is more pronounced in the renal than the systemic circulation.

Nitric Oxide and Hypercholesterolemia

In hypercholesterolemia, chronic impairment of effective NO generation appears to play an important role in abnormal vasodilatory responses in both the coronary and peripheral circulations (127–129). L-Arginine supplementation not only restores EDRF activity (128,129), but has also been proposed to have an anti-atherogenic effect in hypercholesterolemic rabbits (128). While these studies might be faulted because systemic blood pressure and dietary salt intake were not carefully evaluated, it does appear that the hypercholesterolemic rabbit, like the SS/jr rat on a high-salt diet, shows marked improvement in vascular vasodilatory tone with dietary L-arginine supplementation.

It is somewhat surprising that provision of pharmacologic amounts of substrate (e.g., L-arginine) would overcome a deficiency in NO production in the SS/jr rat and hypercholesterolemic rabbit. In this setting of apparent L-arginine "deficiency", Harrison and coworkers have reported that the release of NO from the aorta is actually increased in the hypercholesterolemic rabbit (17,129). This discrepancy is even more marked when the circulating levels of L-arginine (100–200 μM) (52,76) are compared to the substrate affinities of the NO synthases (1–3 μM) (27,37,41,43,44,47). One answer to this dilemma is provided by the observation that hypercholesterolemia enhances endothelial production of superoxide anion (17,129). In this setting, NO is rapidly consumed and other oxygen radicals are generated that may cause tissue damage and contribute to atherosclerotic changes as well as hypertensive arteriosclerosis. As noted previously, similar overproduction of superoxide radicals occurs in the SHR model of hypertension (93), but not in the SS/jr model of salt-sensitive hypertension (Chen and Sanders, *unpublished observations*). Another possibility is that the uptake of L-arginine into endothelial cells is somehow deranged in the hypertensive SS/jr rat, cyclosporine toxicity, and hypercholesterolemia. This thesis would account for the improvement of vasodilatory responses in these models with pharmacologic supplementation of L-arginine, but would not account for the apparent overproduction of NO and therefore substrate consumption in the rabbit model of hypercholesterolemia. It is also conceivable that specific NO synthase isoforms or even the enzymes involved in co-factor synthesis could be genetically abnormal and contribute to the pathogenesis of salt-sensitive hypertension and hypercholesterolemia-induced atherosclerosis in specific experimental models.

ENDOGENOUS NO IN HYPOTENSION

Some hypotensive conditions are associated with stimulation of the inducible L-arginine:NO pathway. NO has been implicated in hypotension from endotoxic shock, as lipopolysaccharide induces the calcium-independent NO synthase in the arterial wall (20,51,64,130). L-NMMA, 20 mg/kg, reverses endotoxin-induced hypotension in dogs, whereas L-arginine, 400 mg/kg, returns blood pressure to its original low levels (131). In a rat model of endotoxic shock, an intravenous bolus of L-NMMA, 3 mg/kg, did not reverse hypotension; an intermediate dose, 30 mg/kg, restored normotension; and a high dose, 300 mg/kg, aggravated the hypotension resulting in death of all rats tested. The authors of this latter study hypothesized that high doses of L-NMMA, by inhibiting both inducible and constitutive NO synthases, effectively block NO production in all vascular beds, producing tissue hypoperfusion and death (132). Whether NO synthase inhibitors are useful clinically is uncertain. Anecdotal experience in two patients with septic shock demonstrated improvement in blood pressure and hemodynamic profile after acute administration of L-NMMA (133). Platelet count fell in both patients. The authors were unable to determine whether L-NMMA produced this side effect, but certainly NO plays an important role in platelet function (7,26). Infusion studies of L-arginine in a larger group of 15 patients with septic shock demonstrated pulmonary and peripheral vasodilation (134). There appeared to be a beneficial effect on oxygen delivery and uptake, and an improvement in the perfusion/ventilation imbalance that characterizes severe septic shock. Further studies are required to define the beneficial effects of diminishing NO synthesis in septic shock with L-arginine antagonists or even dexamethasone, versus enhancing NO synthesis by the provision of additional substrate and co-factors for NO synthase activity.

A variety of cytokines affect NO production. Interferon-γ (IFNγ), tumor necrosis factor-alpha (TNF-α), interleukin-1 (IL-1), and interleukin-2 (IL-2) stimulate production of NO from L-arginine in humans and other mammals (31,67,68,130,135,136). It is interesting to note that NO appears to regulate the expression of vasoconstrictors and growth factors during normoxia and hypoxia (137), and that L-arginine supplementation reduces the intimal hyperplastic response to balloon catheter injury of the rabbit aorta (138). As expected, NO plays a central role in hypotension associated with cytokine infusion. Kilbourn and associates (135) injected TNF-α into dogs and produced hypotension that corrected with a single bolus of L-NMMA, 4.4 mg/kg. Other cytokines, such as IL-10 (68) and TGF-β (67), inhibit NO production. Therefore, the potential roles of cytokines and the interactions with NO and other vasoactive factors in the pathogenesis of vascular disease will continue to be a fertile area of research.

CONCLUSIONS

Ample evidence has accumulated over the past decade documenting that NO is a novel second messenger, important in the control of resting blood pressure. While conventional wisdom has attributed hypertension to defects in vasoconstrictor pathways, derangement in the L-arginine:NO pathways may cause certain types of hypertension, primarily of the salt-sensitive, low-renin variety. Alteration of endogenous nitrovasodilator production may be responsible for hypertension and renal failure in a genetic model of salt-sensitive hypertension in rats, hypertension in patients with end-stage renal disease, cyclosporin-related hypertension, as well as hypotension associated with sepsis and cytokine production and therapy. The use of organic nitrates and nitroprusside produces vasorelaxation through the same guanylate cyclase system used by endogenous NO. Additional knowledge regarding the physiology and pathophysiology of the L-arginine:NO pathways in blood pressure regulation should provide new tools that may prove to be of clinical benefit.

ACKNOWLEDGMENTS

This work was supported by a George M. O'Brien Kidney and Urological Research Centers Program (National Institutes of Health P50DK-39258), National Institutes of Health DK-46199, and the Research Service of the Department of Veterans Affairs.

REFERENCES

1. Bredt DS, Hwang PM, Snyder SH. *Nature* 1990;347:768–770.
2. Schuman EM, Madison DV. *Science (Wash DC)* 1991;254: 1503–1506.
3. Snyder SH, Bredt DS. *Sci Am* 1992;266:68–71.
4. Bult H, Boeckxstaens GE, Pelckmans PA, Jordaens FH, van Maercke YM, Herman AG. *Nature* 1990;345:346–347.
5. Hibbs JB, Taintor RR, Vavrin Z. *Science (Wash DC)* 1987;235: 473–476.
6. Moncada S, Rees DD, Schulz R, Palmer RMJ. *Proc Natl Acad Sci USA* 1991;88:2166–2170.
7. Remuzzi G, Perico N, Zoja C, Corna D, Macconi D, Viganò G. *J Clin Invest* 1990;86:1768–1771.
8. Schmidt HHHW, Warner TD, Ishii K, Sheng H, Murad F. *Science (Wash DC)* 1992;255:721–723.
9. Garg UC, Hassid A. *J Clin Invest* 1989;83:1774–1777.
10. Baylis C, Harton P, Engels K. *J Am Soc Nephrol* 1990;1:875–881.
11. Gardiner SM, Compton AM, Bennett T, Palmer RMJ, Moncada S. *Hypertension* 1990;15:486–492.
12. Tolins JP, Palmer RMJ, Moncada S, Raij L. *Am J Physiol* 1990;258:H655–H662.

13. Furchgott RF, Zawadzki JV. *Nature* 1980;288:373–376.
14. Ignarro LJ. *Annu Rev Pharmacol Toxicol* 1990;30:535–560.
15. Murad F. *J Clin Invest* 1986;78:1–5.
16. Gryglewski RJ, Palmer RMJ, Moncada S. *Nature* 1986;320:454–456.
17. Mügge A, Elwell JH, Peterson TE, Harrison DG. *Am J Physiol Cell Physiol* 1991;260:C219–C225.
18. Rapoport RM, Draznin MB, Murad F. *Nature* 1983;306:174–176.
19. Green LC, Ruiz de Luzuriaga K, Wagner DA, et al. *Proc Natl Acad Sci USA* 1981;78:7764–7768.
20. Marletta MA. *Trends Biochem Sci* 1989;14:488–492.
21. Palmer RMJ, Ferrige AG, Moncada S. *Nature* 1987;327:524–526.
22. Ignarro LJ, Buga GM, Wood KS, Byrns RE, Chaudhuri G. *Proc Natl Acad Sci USA* 1987;84:9265–9269.
23. Beckman JS, Beckman TW, Chen J, Marshall PA, Freeman BA. *Proc Natl Acad Sci USA* 1990;87:1620–1624.
24. Lancaster JR. *Am Sci* 1992;80:248–259.
25. Arnold WP, Mittal CK, Katsuki S, Murad F. *Proc Natl Acad Sci USA* 1977;74:3203–3207.
26. Moncada S, Palmer RMJ, Higgs EA. *Pharmacol Rev* 1991;43:109–142.
27. Murad F, Ishii K, Förstermann U, et al. *Adv Second Messenger Phosphoprotein Res* 1990;24:441–448.
28. Cornwell TL, Lincoln TM. *J Biol Chem* 1989;264:1146–1155.
29. Cornwell TL, Pryzwansky KB, Wyatt TA, Lincoln TM. *Mol Pharmacol* 1991;40:923–931.
30. Darnell J, Lodish H, Baltimore D. Actin, myosin, and intermediate filaments: Cell movements and cell shape. In: *Molecular cell biology.* 2nd ed. New York: Scientific American Books; 1990:859–902.
31. Hibbs JB, Westenfelder C, Taintor R, et al. *J Clin Invest* 1992;89:867–877.
32. Leaf CD, Wishnok JS, Tannenbaum SR. *Biochem Biophys Res Commun* 1989;163:1032–1037.
33. Suzuki H, Ikenaga H, Hishikawa K, Nakaki T, Kato R, Saruta T. *Clin Sci* 1992;82:631–634.
34. Iyengar R, Stuehr DJ, Marletta MA. *Proc Natl Acad Sci USA* 1987;84:6369–6373.
35. Marletta MA, Yoon PS, Iyengar R, Leaf CD, Wishnok JS. *Biochemistry* 1988;27:8706–8711.
36. Stuehr DJ, Kwon NS, Nathan CF, Griffith OW, Feldman PL, Wiseman J. *J Biol Chem* 1991;266:6259–6263.
37. Bredt DS, Ferris CD, Snyder SH. *J Biol Chem* 1992;267:10976–10981.
38. Brenner BM, Troy JL, Ballermann BJ. *J Clin Invest* 1989;84:1373–1378.
39. Hecker M, Walsh DT, Vane JR. *FEBS Lett* 1991;294:221–224.
40. Pollock JS, Förstermann U, Mitchell JA, et al. *Proc Natl Acad Sci USA* 1991;88:10480–10484.
41. Bredt DS, Hwang PM, Glatt CE, Lowenstein C, Reed RR, Snyder SH. *Nature* 1991;351:714–718.
42. Janssens SP, Shimouchi A, Quertermous T, Bloch DB, Bloch KD. *J Biol Chem* 1992;267:14519–14522.
43. Lowenstein CJ, Glatt CS, Bredt DS, Snyder SH. *Proc Natl Acad Sci USA* 1992;89:6711–6715.
44. Lyons CR, Orloff GJ, Cunningham JM. *J Biol Chem* 1992;267:6370–6374.
45. Nishida K, Harrison DG, Navas JP, et al. *J Clin Invest* 1992;90:2092–2096.
46. Sessa WC, Harrison JK, Barber CM, et al. *J Biol Chem* 1992;267:15274–15276.
47. Xie Q-W, Cho HJ, Calaycay J, et al. *Science (Wash DC)* 1992;256:225–228.
48. Wilcox CS, Welch WJ, Murad F, et al. *Proc Natl Acad Sci USA* 1992;89:11993–11997.
49. Nakane M, Mitchell J, Förstermann U, Murad F. *Biochem Biophys Res Commun* 1991;180:1396–1402.
50. Pollock JS, Klinghofer V, Förstermann U, Murad F. *FEBS Lett* 1992;309:402–404.
51. Salter M, Knowles RG, Moncada S. *FEBS Lett* 1991;291:145–149.
52. Sanders PW. *J Nephrol* 1992;5:23–30.
53. Knowles RG, Salter M, Brooks SL, Moncada S. *Biochem Biophys Res Commun* 1990;172:1042–1048.
54. Gross SS, Levi R. *J Biol Chem* 1992;267:25722–25729.
55. Hattori Y, Gross SS. *Biochem Biophys Res Commun* 1993;195:435–441.
56. Werner-Felmayer G, Werner ER, Fuchs D, et al. *J Biol Chem* 1993;268:1842–1846.
57. Sakuma I, Stuehr DJ, Gross SS, Nathan C, Levi R. *Proc Natl Acad Sci USA* 1988;85:8664–8667.
58. Gold ME, Bush PA, Ignarro LJ. *Biochem Biophys Res Commun* 1989;164:714–721.
59. Schini VB, Vanhoutte PM. *Circ Res* 1991;68:209–216.
60. Bogle RG, Baydoun AR, Pearson JD, Moncada S, Mann GE. *Biochem J* 1992;284:15–18.
61. Sato H, Fujiwara M, Bannai S. *J Leukocyte Biol* 1992;52:161–164.
62. Gold ME, Wood KS, Byrns RE, Fukuto J, Ignarro LJ. *Proc Natl Acad Sci USA* 1990;87:4430–4434.
63. Rees DD, Palmer RMJ, Moncada S. *Proc Natl Acad Sci USA* 1989;86:3375–3378.
64. Stuehr DJ, Marletta MA. *Proc Natl Acad Sci USA* 1985;82:7738–7742.
65. Gross SS, Stuehr DJ, Aisaka K, Jaffe EA, Levi R, Griffith OW. *Biochem Biophys Res Commun* 1990;170:96–103.
66. Stuehr DJ, Fasehun OA, Kwon NS, et al. *FASEB J* 1991;5:98–103.
67. Ding A, Nathan CF, Graycar J, Derynck R, Stuehr DJ, Srimal S. *J Immunol* 1990;145:940–944.
68. Cunha FQ, Moncada S, Liew FY. *Biochem Biophys Res Commun* 1992;182:1155–1159.
69. Bredt DS, Snyder SH. *Proc Natl Acad Sci USA* 1990;87:682–685.
70. Förstermann U, Pollock JS, Schmidt HHHW, Heller M, Murad F. *Proc Natl Acad Sci USA* 1991;88:1788–1792.
71. Kukovetz WR, Holzmann S. *Eur J Pharmacol* 1990;38:S9–S14.
72. Mülsch A, Busse R, Bassenge E. *Eur J Pharmacol* 1988;158:191–198.
73. Rees DD, Palmer RMJ, Hodson HF, Moncada S. *Br J Pharmacol* 1989;96:418–424.
74. Dohi Y, Thiel MA, Bühler FR, Lüscher TF. *Hypertension* 1990;16:170–179.
75. Baylis C, Mitruka B, Deng A. *J Clin Invest* 1992;90:278–281.
76. Chen PY, Sanders PW. *Hypertension* 1993;22:812–818.
77. Deng LY, Thibault G, Schiffrin EL. *Clin Exp Hypertens* 1993;15:527–537.
78. Ribeiro MO, Antures E, de Nucci G, Zatz R. *Hypertension* 1991;20:298–308.
79. Dustan HP, Curtis JJ, Luke RG, Rostand SG. *Am J Cardiol* 1987;60:731–771.
80. Grim CE, Wilson TW, Nicholson GD, Hassell TA, Fraser HS, Grim CM. *Hypertension* 1990;15:803–809.
81. Tobian L. *Am J Nephrol* 1983;3:80–87.
82. Ward R. Familial aggregation and genetic epidemiology of blood pressure. In: Laragh JH, Brenner BM, eds. *Hypertension: pathophysiology, diagnosis and management.* New York: Raven Press; 1990:81–100.
83. Rapp JP, Dene H. *Hypertension* 1985;7:340–349.
84. Chen PY, St. John PL, Abrahamson DR, Sanders PW. *Lab Invest* 1993;68:174–184.
85. Greene AS, Yu ZY, Roman RJ, Cowley AW. *Am J Physiol* 1990;258:H508–H514.
86. Kirchner KA. *J Am Soc Nephrol* 1990;1:180–186.
87. Roman RJ, Kaldunski ML. *Hypertension* 1991;17:1018–1024.
88. Rapp JP, Wang S, Dene H. *Science (Wash DC)* 1989;243:542–544.
89. Chen PY, Sanders PW. *J Clin Invest* 1991;88:1559–1567.
90. Auguet M, Lonchampt M-O, Delaflotte S, Goulin-Schulz J, Chabrier PE, Braquet P. *FEBS Lett* 1992;297:183–185.
91. Patel A, Layne S, Watts D, Kirshner K. *Hypertension* 1993;22:863–869.
92. Salazar FJ, Alberola A, Pinilla JM, Romero JC, Quesada T. *Hypertension* 1993;22:49–55.
93. Nakazono K, Watanabe N, Matsuno K, Sasaki J, Sato T, Inoue M. *Proc Natl Acad Sci USA* 1991;88:10045–10048.
94. Lee L, Webb RC. *Hypertension* 1992;19:435–441.

95. Scanlon PH Jr, Dzielak DJ, Hester RL, Kirchner KA. *Clin Res* 1991;39:807A.
96. Hishikawa K, Nakaki T, Suzuki H, Kato R, Saruta T. *J Hypertens* 1993;11:639–645.
97. Hishikawa K, Nakaki T, Tsuda M, et al. *Jap Heart J* 1992;33:41–48.
98. Nakaki T, Hishikawa K, Suzuki H, Saruta T, Kato R. *Lancet* 1990;336:696.
99. Napathorn S, Chaiyabutr N, Buranakari C, et al. *Nephron* 1992;60:220–225.
100. Linder L, Kiowski W, Bühler FR, Lüscher TF. *Circulation* 1990;81:1762–1767.
101. Panza JA, Quyyumi AA, Brush JE, Epstein SE. *N Engl J Med* 1990;323:22–27.
102. Calver A, Collier J, Moncada S, Vallance P. *J Hypertens* 1992;10:1025–1031.
103. Vallance P, Leone A, Calver A, Collier J, Moncada S. *Lancet* 1992;339:572–575.
104. May RC, Kelly RA, Mitch WE. Pathophysiology of uremia. In: Brenner BM, Rector FC Jr, eds. *The kidney.* vol II. 4th ed. Philadelphia: WB Saunders; 1991:1997–2018.
105. Bosch JR, Saccaggi A, Lauer A, Ronco C, Belledonne M, Glabman S. *Am J Med* 1983;75:943–950.
106. Castellino P, Coda B, DeFronzo RA. *Am J Physiol Renal Fluid Electrolyte Physiol* 1986;251:F132–F140.
107. Meyer TW, Ichikawa I, Zatz R, Brenner BM. *Trans Assoc Am Phys* 1993;96:76–83.
108. Pitts RF. *Am J Physiol* 1944;142:355–365.
109. Castellino P, Levin R, Shohat J, DeFranzo RA. *Am J Physiol Renal Fluid Electrolyte Physiol* 1990;258:F992–F997.
110. Claris-Appiani A, Assaei BM, Tirelli AS, Cavanna G. *Kidney Int* 1988;33:91–94.
111. Gaston RS, Schlessinger SD, Sanders PW, Barker C, Curtis JJ, Warnock DG. (Submitted for publication) 1993.
112. Castellino P, Giordano C, Pema A, DeFronzo RA. *Am J Physiol Renal Fluid Electrolyte Physiol* 1988;255:F444–F449.
113. Hirschberg R, Kopple JD. *Kidney Int* 1987;32:382–387.
114. Wada L, Don BR, Schambelan M. *Am J Physiol Renal Fluid Electrolyte Physiol* 1991;260:F787–F792.
115. Krishna GG, Newell G, Miller E, et al. *Kidney Int* 1988;33:578–583.
116. Jaffa AA, Vio CP, Silva RH, et al. *J Clin Invest* 1992;89:1460–1468.
117. King AJ, Troy JL, Anderson S, Neuringer J, Gunning M, Brenner BM. *J Am Soc Nephrol* 1991;1:1271–1277.
118. Tolins JP, Raij L. *Hypertension* 1991;1991:17.
119. Cernadas MR, Lopes-Farre A, Riesco A, et al. *J Pharm Exp Ther* 1992;263:1023–1029.
120. Curtis JJ, Luke RG, Jones P. *Am J Med* 1988;85:134–138.
121. Abraham JS, Bentley FR, Garrison RN, Cryer HM. *Transplant Proc* 1991;23:356–359.
122. Xuan ATD, Fan TPD, Higenbottam TW, Wallwork J. *Transplant Proc* 1990;22:1723–1725.
123. De Nicola L, Thomson SC, Wead LM, Brown MR, Gabbai FB. *J Clin Invest* 1993;92:1859–1865.
124. Cairns HS, Raval U, Neild GH. *Transplantation* 1988;46:79–82.
125. Rondeau E, Paillard F, Peraldi MN, et al. *Kidney Int* 1993;44:165–172.
126. Nunley R, Comstock T, Posner M, Marshall C, Sica DA. *Transplantation* 1991;51:190–193.
127. Chowienczyk PJ, Watts GF, Cockcroft JR, Rotter JM. *Lancet* 1992;340:1430–1432.
128. Cooke JP, Singer AH, Tsao P, Zera P, Rowan RA, Billingham M. *J Clin Invest* 1992;90:1168–1172.
129. Ohara Y, Peterson T, Harrison DG. *J Clin Invest* 1993;91:2546–2551.
130. Busse R, Mülsch A. *FEBS Lett* 1990;275:87–90.
131. Kilbourn RG, Jubran A, Gross SS, et al. *Biochem Biophys Res Commun* 1990;172:1132–1138.
132. Nava E, Palmer RMJ, Moncada S. *Lancet* 1991;338:1555–1557.
133. Petros A, Bennett D, Vallance P. *Lancet* 1991;338:1557–1558.
134. Lorente JA, Landin L, De Pablo R, Renes E, Liste D. *Crit Care Med* 1993;21:1287–1295.
135. Kilbourn RG, Gross SS, Jubran A, et al. *Proc Natl Acad Sci USA* 1990;87:3629–3632.
136. Stuehr D, Marletta MA. *J Immunol* 1987;139:518–525.
137. Kourembanas S, McQuillan LP, Leung GK, Faller DV. *J Clin Invest* 1993;92:99–104.
138. McNamara DB, Aurora H, et al. *Biochem Biophys Res Commun* 1993;193:291–296.
139. Hatakeyama K, Inoue Y, Harada T, Kagamiyama H. *J Biol Chem* 1991;266:765–769.
140. Werner ER, Werner-Felmayer G, Fuchs D, et al. *J Biol Chem* 1990;265:3189–3192.
141. Citron BA, Milstien S, Gutierrez JC, Levine RA, Yanak BL, Kaufman S. *Proc Natl Acad Sci USA* 1990;87:6436–6440.

Hypertension: Pathophysiology, Diagnosis, and Management, Second Edition,
edited by J.H. Laragh and B.M. Brenner,
Raven Press, Ltd., New York © 1995.

CHAPTER 66

Endothelin in Cardiovascular Homeostasis

Gabor M. Rubanyi

Endothelin is the most potent endogenous vasoconstrictor substance known. Therefore, it was postulated early on that the peptide is involved in the regulation of the cardiovascular system in health and disease. Indeed, injection of endothelin into animals resulted in a sustained elevation of arterial blood pressure. Originally it was thought that endothelins modulate arterial blood pressure due solely to their direct effect on vascular smooth muscle. However, studies in the past five years revealed that endothelins can interfere with several homeostatic mechanisms (heart and renal function, central and peripheral nervous system, endocrine systems, water and ion balance) involved in the complex control of the cardiovascular system. The data briefly reviewed in this chapter predominantly originate from studies where synthetic endothelins were applied exogenously to isolated cells and tissues or into intact animals. However, detection of changes in endogenous endothelin expression and production and recent availability of selective tools (i.e., receptor antagonists, antiendothelin antibodies, and endothelin biosynthesis inhibitors) opened the possibility to analyze the potential physiological and pathological role of endogenously produced endothelin peptides. This review attempts to summarize the data suggesting the involvement of endothelins in cardiovascular homeostasis, either by their direct effect on blood vessels (local regulation of vascular tone) or indirectly via interactions with cardiac and renal function, and central and peripheral neural and endocrine control mechanisms.

   G. M. Rubanyi: Berlex Biosciences, Cardiovascular Research, Richmond, California 94804.

THE DISCOVERY OF ENDOTHELINS

Key discoveries in the past 15 years revealed that endothelial cells synthesize and release vasorelaxant (e.g., prostacyclin and endothelium-derived relaxing factor [EDRF]) (1,2) and vasoconstrictor (endothelium-derived contracting factors [EDCF]) (3,4) substances. In 1982, an improperly designed bioassay study led to the discovery of a peptidergic EDCF (5). The idea was to test the biological activity of the culture medium of bovine aortic endothelial cells on isolated pig coronary arteries. It was expected that cultured endothelial cells release EDRF into the culture medium, which will then relax the smooth muscle preparation. Because of the extreme lability of EDRF, no relaxing activity was observed when the culture medium was added to the smooth muscle preparation; the donor (endothelial cells) and acceptor (smooth muscle) were in two different laboratories. In-

stead, the culture medium triggered slowly developing and long-lasting contraction of vascular smooth muscle, which could not be attributed to any known vasoconstrictor mediators and was shown to be of peptidergic nature (Fig. 1) (5). This pioneering observation was confirmed in subsequent studies (6,7). In 1987, Masaki and his colleagues (8) isolated, purified, sequenced, and synthesized this peptidergic EDCF, which they named *endothelin*.

The 21-amino-acid peptide endothelin has no similarity in its sequence to the known peptides of mammalian origin. However, half a year later, the sequence of a rare snake venom, sarafotoxin, was reported to be very similar to that of endothelin (9). One of the most remarkable steps in the progress of endothelin research, following its discovery, was the identification of isotypes of endothelin. Analysis of human genomic sequence revealed the existence of three distinct genes of endothelin,

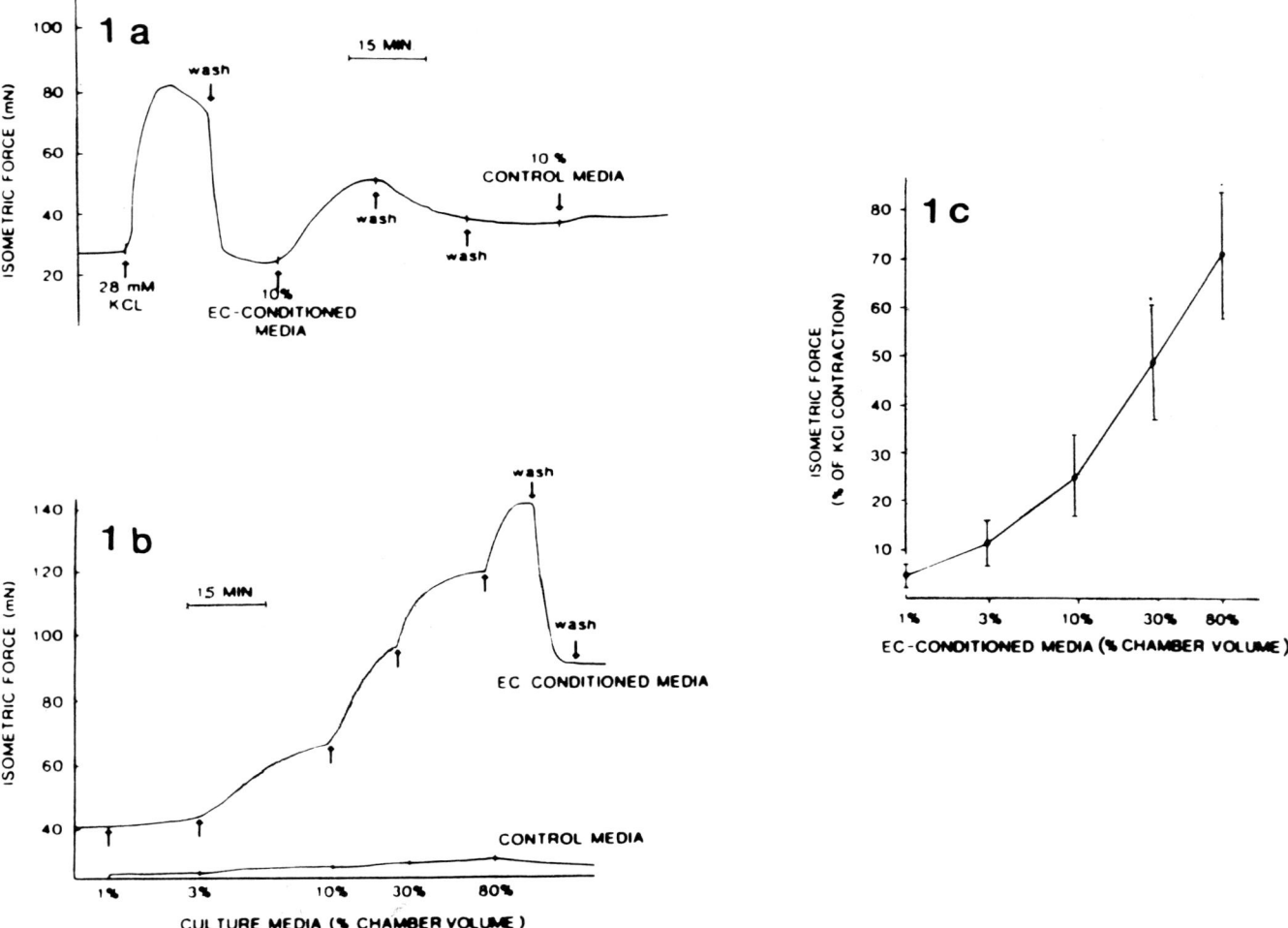

FIG. 1. Discovery of the peptidergic endothelium-derived contracting factor by bioassay, later identified as the 21-amino-acid peptide endothelin. Conditioned media from cultured endothelial cells (EC) evoke concentration-dependent long-lasting contractions of isolated strips of porcine coronary arteries without endothelium. (From ref 5, with permission.)

which encode three distinct endothelin peptides (10) named *endothelin-1* (ET-1), *endothelin-2* (ET-2), and *endothelin-3* (ET-3).

EXPRESSION, PRODUCTION AND ELIMINATION OF ENDOTHELINS IN THE CIRCULATION

Before reviewing the biological actions of endothelins relevant to cardiovascular homeostasis, evidence of their production *in vitro* and *in vivo* will be briefly summarized. Cellular synthesis of the endothelin isoforms has been analyzed in cultured cells, tissue samples, and whole animals by several different techniques. The techniques cover both gene transcription as assessed by messenger ribonucleic acid (mRNA) content, as well as mRNA translation into a protein product.

Cell Culture

The expression of the various genes for endothelin were examined in cultured cells using northern blot analysis. The gene for endothelin-1 has been found to be con-stitutively expressed in cultured endothelial and epithelial cells and in various human cells of carcinoma origin (8,11–15). Exposure of cultured endothelial cells to various inducing agents, some of which increase intracellular calcium and/or activate protein kinase C (PKC), have been found to result in a several-fold increase in preproendothelin-1 mRNA levels (10,14–17) (Fig. 2).

Cellular synthesis of preproendothelin isoforms was also analyzed by quantitation of accumulated protein products of mRNA translation. This is normally accomplished by immunological detection techniques such as radioimmunoassay (RIA) or enzyme-linked immunoabsorption assay (ELISA) of cell culture media. Currently, the ET-1 isoform, and in some cases its protein precursor, pro (big) endothelin-1, have been detected in the culture media of endothelial, epithelial, and carcinoma cells derived from different tissues and organs from several species (16,18,19,21–25). Inducing agents that increase the ET-1 mRNA levels several-fold results in smaller but significant increases in the corresponding protein products (11,17–21). The only cells to date that have been found to produce the immunologically reactive ET-2 peptide are monkey Cos-7 kidney cells (23).

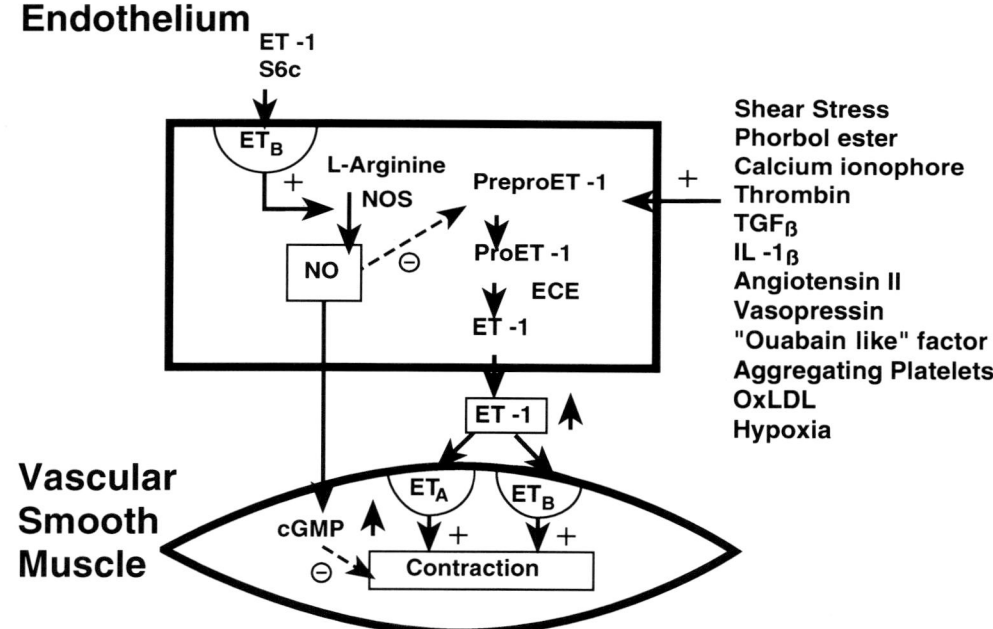

FIG. 2. Biosynthesis and action of endothelin-1 (ET-1) in the blood vessel wall. A variety of factors (*right*) stimulate the expression of ET-1 gene (prepro-ET-1), biosynthesis (conversion of inactive 38-amino-acid pro ET-1 to the 21-amino-acid bioactive ET-1 via the metallo endopeptidase endothelin-converting enzyme [ECE]) and release of ET-1 from endothelial cells. ET-1 acts on underlying vascular smooth muscle eliciting contraction via ET_A and ET_B receptor subtypes. ET-1 and the selective ET_B receptor agonist sarafotoxin-6c (S6c) also act on endothelial cell ET_B receptors, stimulating the synthesis of nitric oxide (NO) from L-arginine by the enzyme nitric oxide synthase (NOS). NO inhibits biosynthesis of ET-1 in endothelial cells, antagonizes smooth-muscle contraction via elevation of cyclic guanosine monophosphate (cGMP), and inhibits platelet aggregation. ET-1 can also induce growth/proliferation (mitogenesis) of endothelial and smooth muscle cells (*not shown*) and interfere with adrenergic neurotransmission in the blood vessel wall by inhibiting norepinephrine (NE) release from nerve endings but potentiating the postjunctional effect of NE on α-adrenoceptor in the smooth muscle cell (*not shown*).

Immunologically reactive ET-3 has been found in culture media from canine tracheal epithelial cells (25).

Tissues *In Situ*

Preproendothelin mRNA was identified by northern analysis and *in situ* hybridization in many tissues from various species (14,15,26–28). For example, mouse and rat intestine express a 2.5-kb transcript thought to be that of ET-1, whereas the kidney, brain, and eye display a 3.7-kb transcript (presumably ET-3), and the lung appears to possess both (14). In addition, ET-1 mRNA has been localized in neuronal cell bodies of the human spinal cord and dorsal root ganglia (27) and in porcine paraventricular nuclear neurons (29), suggesting a neuromodulatory role for endothelin. To date, northern blot analysis has revealed ET-2 gene expression only in the mouse intestine (26).

The protein products of endothelin gene expression have also been detected in many tissue homogenates (30–35). Using RIA or ELISA techniques, the predominant form detected has been reported to be ET-1 and the levels vary from 0.02 pmol/g tissue in rat pituitary to 2.45 pmol/g tissue in porcine renal inner medulla. In almost all tissues tested, ET-3 was detected at significantly lower levels than ET-1 or ET-2. However, in some tissues, relatively high ET-3 levels were detected. These tissues included rat pituitary, in which ET-3 levels were four times higher than were ET-1 levels; in rat inner medulla, in which equal amounts of ET-1 and ET-3 were detected; and in rat intestine, in which ET-3 levels were approximately one-half of the ET-1 levels.

The question of cellular production within tissues has also been addressed with immunohistochemistry (27,31,34,36–39). Using this technique to probe tissue slices derived from the vascular system with immuno-

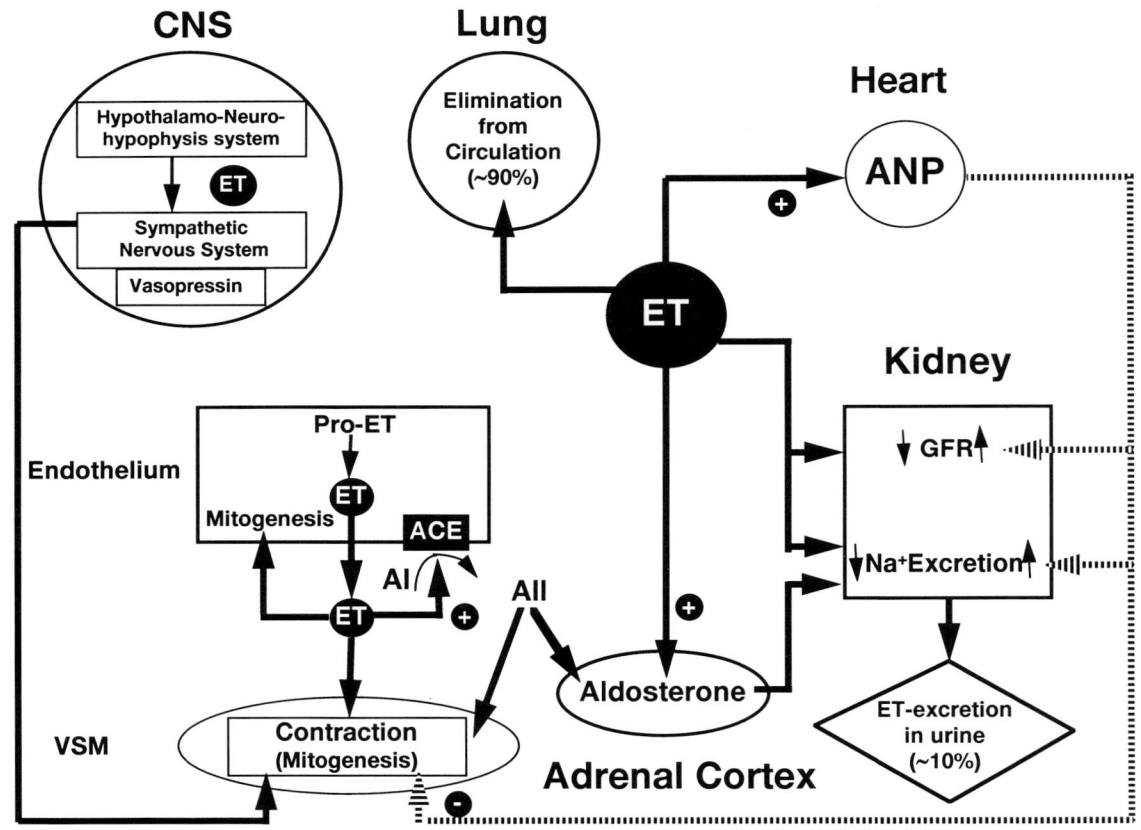

FIG. 3. Local (direct) and neuroendocrine (indirect) control of vascular smooth muscle (VSM) tone and kidney function by ET-1. ET-1 produced locally by vascular endothelium contracts and induces mitogenesis of underlying smooth muscle and acts synergistically on vascular tone and VSM mitogenesis with angiotensin II (AII). ET-1 produced in the kidney reduces glomerular filtration rate (GFR) and sodium (Na⁺) excretion directly and also indirectly via aldosterone secretion from the adrenal cortex (stimulated by ET-1, AII, and sympathetic nerve activation). Atrial natriuretic peptide (ANP) is released by ET-1 from the heart and antagonizes the effects of ET-1 on vascular tone and kidney function. Although ET-1 acts predominantly in a local paracrine/autocrine fashion, elevated circulating plasma ET-1 (potentially derived via slow release from endothelial cells and via rapid release from the neurohypophysis) may act in an endocrine fashion as well. ET-1 is cleared from the circulation, predominantly via the lung (~90 percent) and also by the kidney (~10 percent). ACE, angiotensin-converting enzyme.

fluorescent antibodies, it was determined that endothelin production is localized to human endothelial cells, with no production by vascular smooth muscle cells.

Endothelin in the Plasma, Urine, and Cerebrospinal Fluid

Endothelin-1 synthesis has been shown to occur in vascular endothelial cells that line the blood vessels. Significant quantities of ET-1 are detected in circulating plasma in several species, including human (40–45). The circulating concentrations of ET-1 are in the low picomolar range.

In addition to the circulating peptide, immunoreactive endothelin has been detected in human urine (46). It was found that concentrations of endothelin were on average sixfold higher in urine samples than in plasma. Similarly, endothelin is present in normal human cerebrospinal fluid at levels that are significantly greater (about sevenfold) than in plasma (47,48). Endothelin has also been quantitated in bronchial lavage fluid, where the levels were elevated during the bronchospastic phase of an asthma attack and returned to basal levels after recovery (49).

Elimination of Endothelins from the Circulation

The plasma half-life of the endothelins is short. In the anesthetized rat ~60 percent of intravenously injected ET-1 or ET-3 is removed from the circulation within the first minute (50). The role of the lungs in the removal of circulating endothelin was demonstrated by De Nucci et al. (51), who found that more than 50 percent of infused ET-1 was removed by the lungs after one passage. Although the lung removes ~90 percent of circulating endothelins, excretion via the kidney, and to a smaller extent via the liver, also contributes to the elimination of the peptides from the circulation (Fig. 3). The characteristically long-lasting pressor responses evoked by endothelin in whole animals is thus not due to their persistence in the plasma, but rather to the slow dissociation from the receptors.

The neutral endopeptidase 24.1.1. cleaves ET-1 and ET-3. This enzyme has been identified in rat kidneys (52). Initial cleavage of ET-1 occurs between Ser^5 and Leu^6 within one of the intramolecular loops, while the action against ET-2 and ET-3 is initiated between Asp^{18} and Ile^{19} in the C-terminus.

BIOLOGICAL ACTIONS OF ENDOTHELINS IN THE CARDIOVASCULAR SYSTEM

Hemodynamic Actions

Intravenous infusion of ET-1 causes rapid and transient vasodilation followed by profound and long-lasting increase in blood pressure (8,53–57). The vasodilator effect of endothelin is due to activation of the vascular endothelium, which leads to the formation of prostacyclin (58) and endothelium-derived nitric oxide (58,59); the vasoconstriction is predominantly mediated by the ET_A receptor subtype on vascular smooth muscle. However, in some vascular beds activation of ET_B receptors also causes vasoconstriction both *in vitro* and *in situ* (discussed below in further detail).

Endothelin not only exerts direct vasoconstrictor effects but also is able to potentiate at threshold and subthreshold concentrations contractile responses to other vasoconstrictor substances such as norepinephrine and serotonin (60–62). In addition, the presence of small amounts of other vasoconstrictor substances (e.g., norepinephrine, serotonin, ouabainlike factor) amplified the vasoconstrictor response to ET-1 (8,63–65). Thus, even small (subthreshold) amounts of locally produced endothelin may act as a regulator of vascular tone and reactivity in the circulation.

Effects on the Heart

Soon after the discovery that endothelins evoke sustained vasoconstriction, evidence that endothelins have direct effect on cardiac tissue has been demonstrated (66,67). Endothelin-specific high-affinity binding sites were identified in cardiac myocytes (68), cardiac membranes (69–71), and at the atrioventricular node (72). The direct cardiac actions of endothelins include positive inotropic and chronotropic effects as well as prolongation of action potential duration. Endothelins also affect heart function indirectly via profound coronary vasoconstriction.

Positive Inotropic Effect

The positive inotropic effect of ET-1 has been described for isolated human, guinea pig, and rat atria (73); and ferret (74), and rabbit (75) papillary muscles. This inotropic effect of ET-1 is detectable in electrically driven isolated atrial and papillary muscle preparations, but it is usually masked in intact animal studies because of the secondary negative inotropic effects associated with coronary vasoconstriction (76).

Positive Chronotropic Effect

Intravenous injection of ET-1 causes bradycardia that is secondary to the accompanying reduction on coronary flow (77). In isolated, spontaneously beating atrial preparations, however, ET-1 causes a dose-dependent increase in heart rate (78).

Action Potential Duration

The positive inotropic response is accompanied by a prolongation of the cardiac action potential (75). In rabbit papillary muscle, for example, 10 nM ET-1 lengthens the action potential duration by 16 percent (75).

Endothelin-1 and the Coronary Circulation

Endothelins are potent coronary vasoconstrictors. In anesthetized dogs, for example, bolus intracoronary injection of 30 pmol/kg ET-1 reduces coronary blood flow by ~90 percent and may even cause total coronary artery occlusion (79). This effect has been observed in several animal species (76,80–82). Coronary veins are more sensitive than are coronary arteries, and the effect is endothelium-independent (83). Large subepicardial coronary arteries appear to be more sensitive than endocardial vessels (76).

The coronary vasoconstrictor effect of ET-1 can have serious consequences on heart function. These include a decrease in segmental shortening, an increase in end-diastolic pressure, electrocardiographic signs of myocardial ischemia, a net release of lactate and at higher doses, ventricular fibrillation and death (76,77,84,85). Several

pharmacological interventions, including the administration of nitroglycerine and calcium antagonists, attenuate the constrictor response in large as well as in small vessels.

Isolated Large Arteries and Veins

Since the pioneering observations with the peptidergic endothelium-derived vasoconstrictor on porcine and bovine coronary arteries (5) and the bioassay of the isolated peptide on porcine coronary arteries (8), numerous studies in the past 5 years confirmed that ET-1 is the most potent endogenous substance known to induce contraction of isolated blood vessels. The majority of studies also confirmed the original observation that ET-1 induced slowly developing and long-lasting contraction, which is very difficult to wash out. After the cloning (86,87) and classification (88) of endothelin receptor subtypes, it has been established that these contractions are initiated by binding of endothelins to the ET_A receptor subtype as evidenced by the presence of ET_A receptors on vascular smooth muscle (86), and the order of potency of the various ET isoforms (ET-1 = ET-2 > ET-3) (88) (see Fig. 2). In contrast, ET-1 and ET-3 are equipotent in evoking endothelium-dependent relaxation in isolated blood ves-

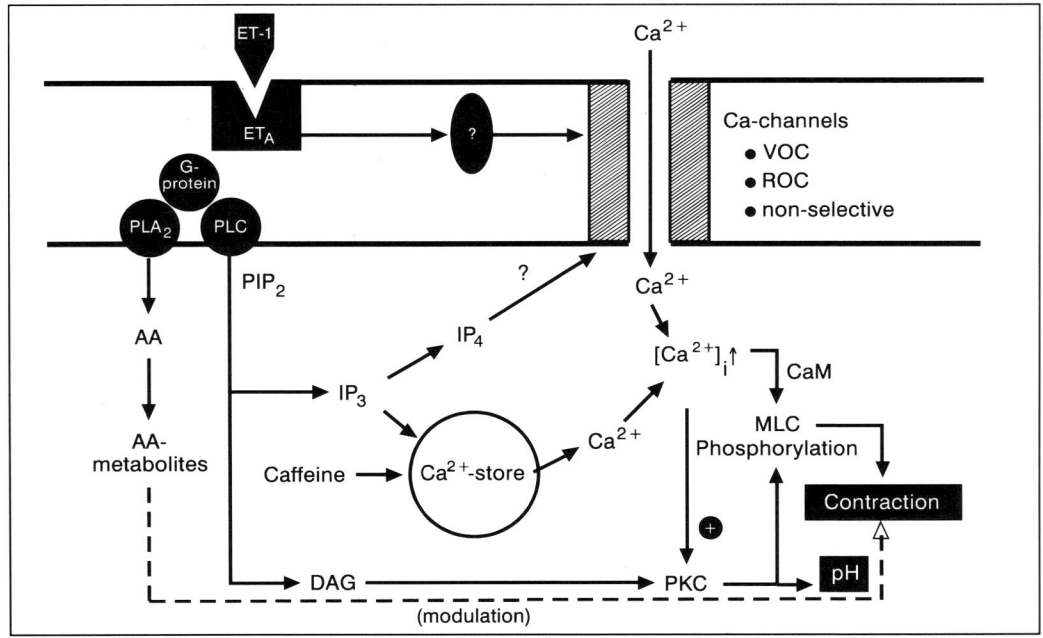

FIG. 4. Signal transduction mechanisms involved in ET-1-induced contraction of vascular smooth muscle (VSM). Binding to a specific membrane receptor (ET_A) ET-1 activates (1) influx of extracellular calcium (Ca^{2+}) into VSM cells (the link between receptor binding and Ca^{2+} channel opening is still unknown); and (2) phosphatidylinositol (PI) hydrolysis via a G-protein and phospholipase C (PLC). PLA_2, phospholipase A_2; AA, arachidonic acid; IP_3, 1,4,5-inositol trisphosphate; DAG, sn1,2diacylglycerol; IP_4, 1,3,4,5inositol tetrakisphosphate; PKC, protein kinase C; Cam, calmodulin; MLC, myosin light chain; VOC, voltage-operated calcium channel; ROC, receptor-operated calcium channel.

sels (89) and depressor response (vasodilation) in intact animals (10), suggesting that these actions are mediated by the ET_B receptor subtype (see Fig. 2). Discovery of selective ligands and antagonists for the ET_A and ET_B receptor subtypes (90–105) provided the necessary tools to characterize vascular actions of endothelins. Using these tools, recent studies demonstrated that the ET_B receptor subtype can also mediate vasoconstriction (90–92).

Although the majority of studies were performed on isolated large arteries, several studies compared the effect of endothelin on large arteries and veins. In general, these studies found that ET-1 is 3 to 10 times more potent in veins than in arteries (106–108).

Signal Transduction Mechanisms in Vascular Smooth Muscle

The activation of vascular smooth muscle via the ET_A receptor subtype is associated with (a) G-protein-linked activation of phospholipase C and subsequent increase of phosphatidylinositol turnover; (b) increased influx of extracellular Ca^{2+} and release of Ca^{2+} from intracellular stores (c) activation of protein kinase C; and (d) stimulation of Na^+/H^+ exchange and alteration of intracellular pH (109,110) (Fig. 4). In some tissues ET-1 can stimulate phospholipase A2 as well, and the consequent generation of arachidonic acid and its metabolites, modulate the biological action of endothelins (see Fig. 4). In addition to the immediate biological response (i.e., contraction), these signal transduction pathways (particularly elevation of Ca^{2+}, change in pH, and activation of PKC) can induce changes in gene expression (e.g., c-fos, c-jun, etc.) involved in cell growth and proliferation (111). Indeed, several studies demonstrated that endothelin can induce growth/proliferation of vascular smooth muscle cells (112), fibroblasts (113), and mesangial cells (114) which may have cardiovascular consequences.

Isolated Microvessels and Microcirculation

Elevation of systemic arterial blood pressure after intravenous injection of ET-1 (see section on hemodynamic actions, above) suggested that in addition to large arteries and veins, endothelin is also a potent vasoconstrictor in resistance arterioles. Direct proof for this hypothesis was provided by studies on isolated arterioles (115). In studies on microcirculation *in situ,* the vasoconstrictor effect of topical application of endothelins was demonstrated by measuring changes in regional blood flow or the diameter of microvessels (116–119). Some studies with cells isolated from microvessels (endothelial cells or pericytes) provided indirect evidence for the effect of endothelins in the microcirculation (120–123).

KIDNEY

Of particular interest in the context of blood pressure regulation is the fact that endothelin has significant effects on the kidney (i.e., decrease in renal plasma flow and glomerular filtration rate) in a concentration range at which no hemodynamic changes occur (124). As the kidney plays a crucial role in the regulation of ion and water balance, plasma volume and osmolarity, these effects may be important for the "indirect" control of cardiovascular homeostasis (see Fig. 3).

ENDOTHELIN AND THE NEURAL CONTROL OF THE CARDIOVASCULAR SYSTEM

Central Nervous System

Endothelins may be involved in the central (nervous) regulation of the cardiovascular system. The following experimental evidence supports this hypothesis: (a) endothelin gene expression and mature endothelin production can be detected in the brain; (b) specific endothelin-binding sites are identified in various regions of the brain; and (c) intracerebroventricular (ICV) injection of endothelins cause significant cardiovascular changes.

Endothelin Expression and Production in the Brain

Ribonucleic acid (RNA) blot hybridization provided evidence of endothelin gene expression in a variety of regions of the human brain (125), but the hypothalamus having the highest density of cells containing preproendothelin mRNA. The presence of immunoreactive (ir) ET-1 and ET-3 was detected in porcine brain (126). Endothelin-3 is produced in the magnocellular neurons of the hypothalamo-neurohypophyseal system (127).

Using highly specific and sensitive radioimmunoassays irET-1 and irET-3 were found in human cerebrospinal fluid (128). The concentration of irET-3 was 150 percent higher than that of irET-1.

Circulating plasma ET-1 level increases rapidly with upright posture and decreases with volume expansion in humans. The site of release was postulated to be the neurohypophysis or anteroventral hypothalamus. This sudden change in circulating irET level is in sharp contrast to the slow and delayed production of ET-1 in the circulation by the endothelium, suggesting a different mechanism of peptide release from the central nervous system.

Endothelin Binding Sites in the Brain

Autoradiograms of $[^{125}I]$ET-1 binding in the rat brain demonstrated that endothelin receptors are predominantly localized in the brain stem, basal ganglia, and cerebellum (129). In addition, specific ET-1 binding sites were identified in nuclei which are involved in the central nervous regulation of the cardiovascular system: nuclei of the anteroventral hypothalamus, the supraoptic nucleus, and the subfornical organ. Endothelin-1 binding sites were also detected on rat pituitary cell membranes (130).

Biological Actions of Endothelin in the Brain

Siren and Feuerstein (131) demonstrated that ICV injection of ET-1 (30 pmol/kg) produced profound pressor and vasoconstrictor response. Similar observations were made after microinjection of ET-1 into the area postrema (AP) of anesthetized rats (132) and into cerebral ventricles of conscious rats (133,134) and conscious rabbits (135).

In parallel with increased mean arterial blood pressure, ICV infusion of ET-1 increased plasma catecholamine and arginine vasopressin levels (AVP), and enhanced renal sympathetic nerve activity (133–135). V1-vasopressinergic receptor antagonists (e.g., TMe-AVP), α-adrenergic receptor antagonists (e.g., prazosin), and ganglionic blockade (e.g., pentolinium, hexamethonium) attenuated or completely abolished the pressor response (133–135), suggesting that centrally administered ET-1 activates the sympathoadrenal and AVP systems, which mediate the central pressor response.

Systemic administration of ET-1 increased the activity of subfornical organ (SFO) neurons which have projections to the paraventricular nucleus (PVN) of the hypothalamus. Systemic ET-1 (50–100 pmol/kg) injection activates vasopressin and oxytocin-secreting neurons in the PVN and supraoptic nucleus (SON) (136). Since ET-1 does not cross blood-brain barrier (i.e., cannot act directly in PVN and SON), it should act on SFO, which lacks this barrier. Indeed, in animals where SFO has been lesioned, systemic ET-1 had little or no effect on vasopressin- and oxytocin-releasing neurons (136).

When administered into the third cerebral ventricle, ET-3 dose-dependently inhibited water intake in conscious rats exposed to exogenous and endogenous stimuli for drinking (160). Selective ET-3 antibody (injected into the third ventricle) potentiates angiotensin-II-induced water drinking, suggesting that endogenous ET-3 plays a role in the central control of fluid and electrolyte homeostasis.

Peripheral Reflex Control of the Cardiovascular System

In addition to their direct action on blood vessels (local control) and indirect action on circulation via stimulation of central sympathoadrenal and vasopressinergic mechanisms (central control), endothelins were reported to also effect peripheral cardiovascular reflex mechanisms.

Adrenergic Neurotransmission in the Blood Vessel Wall

In isolated perfused rat mesenteric arteries subthreshold (for direct vascular contraction) doses of ET-1 (10^{-11}–10^{-10} M) significantly enhanced exogenous norepinephrine-induced vasoconstriction but inhibited periarterial (transmural) nerve-stimulation-induced vasoconstriction (137). These studies suggested that in subpressor doses, ET-1 modulates adrenergic neuroeffector mechanisms: facilitates it at the postjunctional site and inhibits it prejunctionally. Indeed, ET-1 inhibited transmural electrical stimulation-induced [^{3}H]NE release in the same preparation (137).

Similarly, perivascular nerve-stimulation-induced [^{3}H]NE release was suppressed but exogenous norepinephrine-induced vasoconstriction was potentiated by ET-1 in isolated guinea pig pulmonary artery (138).

However, studies in human healthy volunteers showed that intraarterial infusion of low concentrations of ET-1 (1 pmol/min) had no effect on sympathetic nerve activation (evoked by lower body negative pressure) or exogenous norepinephrine-induced vasoconstriction in the forearm (139,140).

Baroreflex

Local exposure of the vascularly isolated and endothelium-denuded carotid sinus of anesthetized dogs to ET-1 (10^{-7} M) produced vasoconstriction and suppression of baroreceptor activity (141). At lower concentration (10^{-8} M), ET-1 caused only vasoconstriction, suggesting that at higher doses ET-1 acts directly on baroreceptor nerve fibers. Such an action could limit the buffering capacity of the baroreflex and promote hypertension.

Baroreflex sensitivity was attenuated by intravenous infusion of 40 fmol/kg/min ET-1 in conscious dogs, but it was not affected by 400 fmol/kg/min ET-1 (142). Intravenous bolus injection of ET-1 (0.3–3.0 nmol/kg) had no significant effect on baroreceptor activity in anesthetized rats (143). In conscious rats, intravenous ET-1 (0.67 nmol/kg) did not alter baroreceptor reflex control of sympathetic efferent nerve activity or heart rate (144).

In contrast to topical (desensitization) and systemic intravenous application (desensitization or no effect), injection of ET-1, ET-2, or ET-3 (25 pmol/kg) into the cisterna magna in conscious normotensive rats caused significant increase of baroreceptor sensitivity by affecting the vagal but not the sympathetic component of the baroreflex (i.e., methylatropine, but not atenolol, prevented the facilitation) (145).

Activation of the baroreflex stimulates endothelin release into the plasma (146). The results of studies in normal subjects and in patients with primary autonomic failure (no baroreflex), showed that activation of baroreflex stimulates the release of endothelin into plasma (probably from the neurohypophysis), and they suggest that impaired endothelin release may contribute to orthostatic hypotension of patients with primary autonomic failure (146).

ENDOTHELIN AND ENDOCRINE CONTROL OF THE CARDIOVASCULAR SYSTEM

Renin-Angiotensin-Aldosterone System

Renin

Both *in vitro* and *in vivo* studies suggest that endothelin can modulate the secretion of renin from the juxtaglomerular cells (JGC) of the renal cortex. However, these studies lead to apparently opposite results: *in vitro* ET-1 invariably suppresses renin secretion, while injection of ET-1 into animals either does not affect or increases plasma renin activity (PRA).

Endothelin-1 suppresses renin secretion from isolated perfused rat kidney (147), rat kidney cortical slices (148,149), isolated rat glomeruli (150), and dispersed rat JGC (149,151,152). In isolated perfused rat kidney, ET-3 also suppressed renin release (163). Endothelin-1 suppressed not only basal but also isoproterenol-induced release of renin from isolated JGC (149,151).

In contrast to findings *in vitro*, systemic injection of pressor doses (>0.2 nM/kg) of ET-1 to anesthetized (154,155) or conscious dogs (156,157) caused significant elevation of PRA. Subpressor doses of ET-1 caused no changes in PRA in conscious rats (158) or even significantly reduced it in anesthetized dogs (155) and conscious normal and cirrhotic rats (159). Similar observations were made in healthy human volunteers, where infusion of 0.4 pmol/kg/min ET-1, which elevated plasma irET-1 to levels similar to that found in several pathological conditions, increased diastolic blood pressure, reduced heart rate and renal plasma flow, and increased renal vascular resistance but had no effect on PRA (160,161). Similar to the *in vitro* findings, infusion of ET-1 (1–4 ng/kg/min) directly into the renal artery decreased renin release significantly in anesthetized dogs (162) and in anesthetized rats (148). In conscious rats, ET-1 antiserum decreased PRA and increased urinary sodium excretion (163). Subcutaneous infusion of ET-1 for a week (0.2 mg/kg/hr) lowered PRA in rats (164).

Angiotensin-Converting Enzyme

Although angiotensin-converting enzyme (ACE) inhibitors do not affect the conversion of pro ET-1 to ET-

1 (165), several studies suggest interaction between the two systems. Infusion of ET-1 (5 pmol/kg/min) for 7 days into rats caused sustained increase in mean arterial blood pressure without changes in plasma angiotensin II level. Co-infusion of captopril (1 mg/kg/hr) prevented ET-1-induced hypertension, suggesting that elevation of blood pressure is caused either by ET-1-induced stimulation of the renin-angiotensin system (166) or that existing levels of angiotensin-II "permit" or facilitate ET-1-induced vasoconstriction (167,168).

Another potentially important interaction between endothelin and the renin-angiotensin system was identified by Kawaguchi et al. (169,170). In cultured pulmonary arterial endothelial cells, ET-1 dose-dependently increased conversion of angiotensin I to angiotensin II by an enalapril-sensitive mechanism. Endothelin-1 (10^{-8} M) stimulates ACE activity 2.5-fold in these cells (170).

Angiotensin II

Angiotensin II is one of the most potent stimulators of ET-1 synthesis/release (171). Angiotensin II and ET-1 act synergistically to induce vasoconstriction, vascular smooth muscle cell proliferation, and aldosterone secretion from the adrenal cortex (172).

Aldosterone

Tissue autoradiography studies revealed significant [^{125}I]ET-1 binding in the medulla and zona glomerulosa (but not in zona fasciculata or reticularis) of the rat adrenal gland (173,174). Similar specific ET-1 binding was demonstrated in cultured bovine adrenal glomerulosa cells (172,175,176) and in porcine, human, and rat adrenal gland (189).

In bovine adrenal glomerulosa cells, ET-1 stimulates aldosterone (but not cortisol) secretion with an EC50 of 300 pM (172). Angiotensin II is a more potent agonist (EC50, 40 pM). Endothelin-1 potentiates Ang II-induced aldosterone secretion (172). Endothelin-1 was more potent than ET-3, suggesting that ET_A receptor subtype mediates the effect in this tissue (175,176).

In good agreement with these *in vitro* observations, systemic injection of ET-1 *in vivo* elevated plasma aldosterone levels in anesthetized dogs (178,179) and in conscious rats (180).

Arginine Vasopressin (AVP)

AVP Stimulates ET-1 Synthesis/Release

Infusion of AVP to conscious dogs increased plasma irET-1 levels significantly (181). Arginine vasopressin stimulates endothelin production in human mesangial cells (182), in rat mesangial cells (183), in cultured bovine aortic endothelial cells (184), and in primary cultures of rabbit endometrial cells (197). In freshly harvested rabbit aortic endothelial cells, endothelin and AVP are colocalized (185,186). In human mesangial cells AVP-induced mitogenic action is apparently mediated by ET-1, since ET-1-antibody suppressed the mitogenic action of AVP (182). In cultured bovine endothelial cells AVP-induced ET-1 production is mediated by V1-vasopressinergic receptors (184). Arginine vasopressin induces ET-1 gene expression in cultured bovine carotid endothelial cells (187).

Endothelins Stimulate AVP Secretion in the Neurohypophysis and Elevate Plasma Levels of AVP

Infusion of ET-1 (30 ng/kg/min) to conscious dogs increased circulating plasma levels of AVP (179). Infusion of ET-1 (20 ng/kg/min) for 1 hour decreased renal blood flow and blocked the antidiuretic effect of AVP in conscious dogs (154,188). Intravenous infusion of 40 fmol/kg/min ET-1 for 40 minutes caused decrease in mean arterial blood pressure, baroreceptor sensitivity, pressor response to NE and Ang II, and decreased circulating plasma levels of AVP (189). Infusion of higher doses of ET-1 (400 fmol/kg/min) increased blood pressure and circulating levels of AVP, suggesting that changes in blood pressure modulate AVP secretion (189).

However, studies with centrally injected (i.e., into the third ventricle) endothelins lead to different conclusions. Intracerebroventricular injection of ET-3 (11 and 23 pmol) caused two- and five- to sevenfold elevation of plasma AVP, respectively, and inhibited stimulated water drinking (160). Intracerebroventricular application of ET-1 caused increase in mean arterial blood pressure which is mediated at least in part by vasopressin (i.e., vasopressinergic receptor blockade decreased the pressor response) (134,190,191). These findings suggested that ET-1-induced AVP secretion from the CNS and consequent elevation in circulating plasma levels of AVP contribute to the pressor response to ET-1. Indeed, systemic injection of ET-1 (50–100 pmol) enhanced the activity of neurons in the subfornical organ (SFO) (which lack the blood-brain barrier), and stimulated the secretion/release of AVP (and oxytocin) (136). Microinjection of ET-1 (5 pmol) into SFO increased the activity of vasopressinergic neurons in the neurohypophysis (192). Thus, both systemically or centrally injected ET-1 can increase AVP secretion in the hypothalamo-neurohypophysial system.

Endothelin-1 and ET-3 potentiate membrane depolarization-induced AVP release from isolated nerve endings of the posterior pituitary via ET_A receptor activation (193). The same nerve endings contain irET, the level of which is regulated by homeostatic mechanisms involved in water balance (192). Endothelin-1 (10^{-9}–10^{-8} M) stimulates AVP release from perfused rat hypothalamus,

which can be blocked by the Ca^{2+}-antagonist nicardipine (194). Immunoreactive ET-3 is present in the median eminence and in the anterior and neurointermediate lobes of the hypothalamus at concentrations much higher than in the aorta (127). ET-1 and ET-3 stimulates release of AVP from rat supraoptic nucleus in vitro (in brain slices) with equal potency, suggesting that ET_B receptor subtype may mediate the response (191).

Interaction Between the Biological Actions of Endothelins and AVP

Several reports indicate potential interactions between the biological actions of endothelins and AVP. In general, endothelin and AVP act synergistically as vasoconstrictors, but endothelin appears to inhibit the effect of AVP on renal collecting tubules.

In isolated mouse kidney cortical collecting tubules (CCT), outer medullary collecting tubules (OMCT), and inner medullary collecting tubules (IMCT), ET-1 (10^{-10}–10^{-8} M) inhibited AVP-induced cyclic adenosine monophosphate (cAMP) accumulation (208). Endothelin-1 had no effect on AVP-induced cAMP accumulation in cortical and medullary ascending limbs of the Henle loop, or parathormone-, calcitonin-, glucagon- and isoproterenol-induced changes in cAMP in OMCT (195). These authors postulated that the observed effects of ET-1 may have the physiological function of maintaining urine volume via antagonism of AVP-induced reduction of urine volume, to counteract the decrease in renal plasma flow (RPF) and glomerular filtration rate (GFR) by ET-1. Similarly, in freshly prepared rat renal papillary tubules, endothelins inhibit AVP-induced cAMP accumulation. Endothelin-1 and ET-3 were equieffective, suggesting that the ET_B receptor subtype mediates the effects (196). Infusion of ET-1 to rats causes diuresis, despite decrease in RPF and GFR (197). In isolated perfused rat IMCT segments, ET-1 (10^{-10}–10^{-8} M) reversibly inhibited AVP-induced osmotic water permeability without affecting AVP-stimulated urea permeability or db-cAMP-induced osmotic water permeability. These studies suggest that endothelin acts at these cells at sites prior to cAMP production in the AVP-induced signal transduction pathway (197).

In contrast to the renal collecting ducts, ET-1 potentiates the vasoconstrictor action of AVP in perfused rabbit ear artery (198), and the pressor effect of AVP in pregnant rats (199).

Atrial and Brain Natriuretic Peptide (ANP and BNP)

Effect of Endothelins on ANP/BNP Secretion

Endothelin-1 stimulates the release of atrial natriuretic peptide (ANP) from isolated rat atrial myocytes (200), neonatal rat cardiomyocytes, and fetal rat hypothalamic cell cultures (201), rat atria (202), cultured fetal rat diencephalic neurons (203), perfused rat heart (204,205), superfused rat atria (206), isolated rat atria (207), cultured rat neonatal cardiac myocytes on beads (208), and cultured rat atrial myocytes (209). Endothelin-1 also stimulates the release of brain natriuretic peptide (BNP) from rat atrial and ventricular cardiomyocytes (210).

Endothelin-1-induced ANP release from rat atrial myocytes was significantly higher in cells isolated from spontaneously hypertensive rats (SHR) than from normotensive Wistar-Kyoto (WKY) rats (200). Similarly, ET-1 stimulates basal and stretch-induced ANP release from perfused hearts, which was more pronounced in hearts from SHR than from WKY rats (204).

The ANP secretion stimulation by ET-1 in cardiac myocytes involves elevation of cytosolic Ca^{2+} (206,208) and activation of PKC (204,205,208).

In good agreement with the *in vitro* studies, intravenous injection of ET-1 elevates circulating plasma ANP levels in conscious newborn calves (211), in conscious normal and cirrhotic rats (212), in conscious dogs (213,214), in anesthetized rats (143), in conscious rats (207), and in anesthetized, bilaterally nephrectomized rats (215). In anesthetized rats, ET-1 injection elevates plasma irBNP (215).

In several of these studies only pressor doses of ET-1 elevated plasma ANP or BNP levels, which correlated well with increases in mean arterial pressure (210,211). Indeed, subpressor doses of ET-1 had no effect on plasma ANP level on conscious dogs (40 pmol/kg) and in conscious newborn calves (214), suggesting that in contrast to *in vitro* studies (where ET-1 acted directly on cardiac myocytes), *in vivo* the stimulus for ANP secretion is right atrial stretch due to elevated blood pressure and right atrial pressure. However, in conscious rats ET-1 (0.3–3.0 nmol/kg) caused increase in plasma ANP with and without elevation of right atrial pressure, suggesting that ET-1 can act directly on atrial myocytes *in vivo* as well (143). In conscious dogs a subpressor dose of ET-1 (40 fmol/kg/min) reduced blood pressure and increased plasma ANP (213).

Effect of ANP on ET-1 Production

The majority of studies showed that ANP effectively reduced ET-1 production in cultured cells. ANP was found to inhibit angiotensin II or thrombin induced ET-1 secretion from cultured bovine aortic endothelial cells (229), cultured rat mesangial cells (230,231), cultured HUVECs (233) isolated porcine aorta (232) and cultured human endothelial cells (234).

Interaction Between the Biological Actions of ET-1 and ANP/BNP

Atrial natriuretic peptide is a potent vasodilator and via stimulation of natriuresis reduces plasma volume and osmolarity. Theoretically, these actions of the peptide can counteract the vasoconstrictor and renal effects (reduction of RPF, GFR, and consequently of natriuresis and diuresis) of ET-1. Indeed, several studies showed that ANP (and BNP) effectively antagonizes the biological actions of ET-1 both *in vitro* and *in vivo*.

In cultured vascular smooth muscle cells, ANP antagonized the mitogenic activity of ET-1 and ET-3 (222). Blood pressure increases after ICV injection of ET-1 was effectively attenuated by coinjection of BNP (223). Similarly, coinjection of BNP reduces centrally applied ET-1-induced elevation of plasma AVP level (224). Intravenous infusion of ET-1 caused pressor response in conscious rats which was reduced by coinjection of ANP (143). Atrial natriuretic peptide also inhibited ET-1-induced renal vasoconstriction (225). In anesthetized and nephrectomized rats ANP-antibody prevented ET-1(25 ng/kg/min)-infusion-induced increase in hematocrit (hemoconcentration and reduction of plasma volume via protein extravasation) but facilitated the increase in mean arterial blood pressure (215). These findings suggested that ET-1-induced ANP secretion attenuates the pressor response and mediates the capillary permeability increase of the peptide. Indeed, earlier studies suggested that ANP release may mediate the initial transient depressor response to bolus injection of ET-1 in rats (226). However, Fozard and Part (200) demonstrated that ANP plays no role in the vasodilator response to ET-1 in SHR.

There are a few studies showing that ET-1 can also effectively antagonize the biological actions of ANP. In cultured rat diencephalic glia cells, ET-1 and ET-3 stimulate mitogenesis and inhibit ANP-induced cyclic guanosine monophosphate (cGMP) elevation (227). Since ET-1 and ET-3 were equipotent, the ET_B receptor subtype was postulated to mediate these effects.

Endothelin-1 also effectively antagonized the cardiovascular (depressor response), renal (natriuresis and diuresis), and endocrine (AVP, renin, aldosterone) effects of ANP *in vivo* (228).

POTENTIAL INTEGRATED PHYSIOLOGICAL SIGNIFICANCE OF ENDOTHELINS IN THE CARDIOVASCULAR SYSTEM

Based on the data reviewed above, several potential physiological mechanisms can be proposed where endothelins may contribute to cardiovascular homeostasis.

Maintenance of Basal Vascular Tone

Endothelin is produced by cultured endothelial cells at a slow basal rate, and, although its expression can be stimulated by various agonists, facilitation of endothelin release is detectable only several hours after stimulation. There is no evidence that endothelin is stored in endothelial cells, so its release may be directly connected to its *de novo* synthesis. Because of its high vasoconstrictor potency and long-lasting action, the continuous release of small amounts of endothelin could contribute to the maintenance of vascular tone. An important feature of endothelin-induced vascular contraction is that it can be inhibited by most known vasodilator agents and by the potent endogenous vasodilator EDRF (NO) (see Fig. 2). If basal tone is maintained by endothelin, it may be balanced by the tonic release of EDRF under physiological conditions, and it should be effectively antagonized by local vasodilator mechanisms in case of increased metabolic requirements. An imbalance between the production of endothelin and EDRF could lead to pathologically elevated vascular tone.

Hemostasis

Thrombin is a potent stimulator of endothelin biosynthesis and release. One may speculate that, in the event of blood coagulation, thrombin-induced release by endothelin and the consequent long-lasting vasoconstriction triggered by the peptide contributes to hemostasis, a role thus far attributed primarily to serotonin released from activated platelets. This mechanism may be especially effective in the case of endothelial dysfunction (i.e., loss of EDRF production), since thrombin is also a potent stimulant of EDRF release.

Vascular Remodeling

In addition to regulation of local vascular tone, endothelin may also modulate vascular smooth muscle growth/proliferation. Endothelin is a smooth muscle mitogen and may therefore mediate growth and remodeling of the blood vessel wall. Endothelin may stimulate smooth muscle proliferation indirectly by facilitating the (local) production of another potent mitogen, angiotensin II (Ang II). It is possible that, in addition to the pathological consequences of its excessive production (i.e., vasospasm, hypertension), the maintenance of basal vascular tone and structure, as well as contribution to hemostasis, represents important physiological roles of the peptide.

Indirect Control of Vascular Tone and Plasma Volume via Interaction with Neuroendocrine and Paracrine Mechanisms

Endothelins may play a role in the control of vascular tone by a variety of indirect mechanisms as well (see Fig. 3), including (a) modulation of central control mechanisms (via enhancing sympathetic nerve activity or vasopressin release and baroreceptor sensitivity) by endo-

thelin produced in the CNS or acting on areas of CNS lacking the blood-brain barrier (e.g., SFO); (b) endothelin released in the vicinity of baroreceptors (carotid sinus, aortic arch, etc.) may suppress their activity; (c) modulation of adrenergic neurotransmission in chromaffin cells (adrenal medulla) and in the blood vessel wall can lead to an increased/decreased liberation of norepinephrine, respectively, and augmentation of postsynaptic effect of the neurotransmitter; and (d) local modulation of the synthesis/release of other endothelium-derived vasoactive substances (EDRF, PGI_2) and Ang II.

The known effects of endothelin on renal function suggest a synergistic action with aldosterone (i.e., antinatriuresis) but via a different mechanism. Exogenous administration of endothelin causes a dose-dependent decrease in GFR. Corresponding reductions in urine flow and sodium excretion occur, leading to Na^+ retention, increased plasma osmolality and volume (see Fig. 3). These latter changes can influence cardiovascular function (e.g., blood pressure), independent of changes in vascular tone.

Functional Antagonism with ANP

Endothelin is a potent secretagogue for ANP release. This observation may be physiologically relevant because some of the known biological actions of ANP oppose those of endothelin (see Fig. 3).

In the kidney, endothelin has a potent antinatriuretic effect, while ANP evokes natriuresis. Similarly, endothelin and ANP have opposing effects on renal blood flow and on peripheral vascular resistance and blood pressure. Atrial natriuretic peptide effectively antagonizes endothelin-induced vasoconstriction and its actions in the CNS. Based on these findings, one may speculate that ANP represents a negative feedback mechanism against endothelin-induced renal and vascular effects.

Regulation of Water Balance

Water loss simulates compensatory mechanisms, which include increased sympathetic activity (via baroreceptor inhibition) and secretion of vasopressin or antidiuretic hormone (ADH) via stimulation of osmoreceptors in the central nervous system (Fig. 5). Inhibition of baroreceptors can also stimulate the release of ADH. Both mechanisms will reduce water excretion in the kidney with resultant normalization of plasma volume. Local production of endothelin (either in peripheral tissues or the central nervous system) may contribute to these regulatory (homeostatic) pathways in several ways (see Fig. 5): (a) inhibition of baroreceptor function; (b) constriction of glomerular afferent arterioles; (c) decreasing

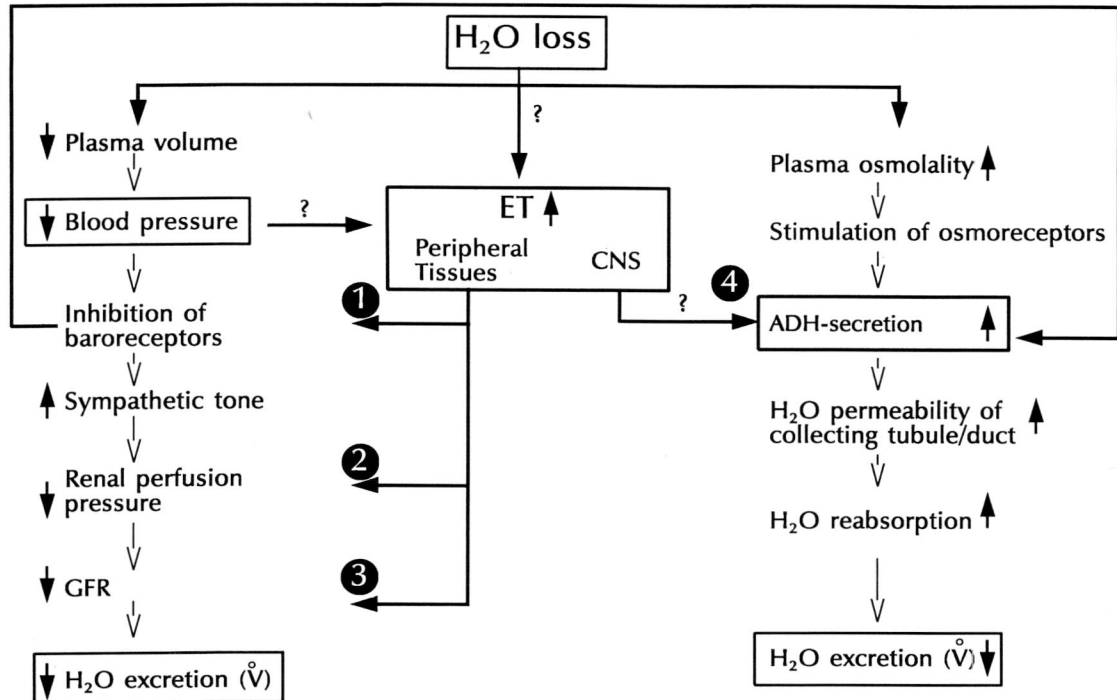

FIG. 5. Potential role of endothelins (ET) in the regulation of water balance. CNS, central nervous system; ADH, antidiuretic hormone (vasopressin); V, diuresis. (From Rubanyi GM (ed.). *Endothelin.* New York: Oxford University Press, 1991, with permission.)

GFR in the kidney; and (d) effects on vasopressin (ADH) secretion (via a central mechanism or through baroreceptor resetting). An increase in circulating endothelin was reported in severe hypotension (e.g., cardiogenic, endotoxin, and hemorrhagic shock) and release of endothelin from the neurohypophysis during water deprivation. These data suggest that endothelin may be involved in compensatory homeostatic mechanism controlling water balance. The demonstration that centrally applied (or produced) ET-3 and ET-1 can inhibit water intake further supports this hypothesis.

CONCLUSIONS

The discovery of a peptidergic EDCF produced by cultured endothelial cells and the determination of its structure and molecular biology generated worldwide interest and exponential growth in research activity.

These studies demonstrated that endothelin(s) can be formed in many cells of the body, as well as the endothelium, and thus have the potential for many of the effects suggested by *in vitro* and *in vivo* studies. Endothelin appears to function predominantly as a local rather than a circulating hormone. These autocrine and paracrine actions suggest that endothelin has the potential to regulate vascular tone; to modulate cardiovascular reflexes and renal function; and to affect renin, aldosterone, vasopressin, and atrial natriuretic peptide release.

Despite the speculations on their potential role in cardiovascular homeostasis, the true significance of endothelins in health and disease remains to be established. Recent developments, however, raise the possibility that these important questions will be answered in the near future. Cloning of the endothelin receptors; characterization of endothelin-converting enzyme; and the availability of specific receptor antagonists, monoclonal antibodies, and converting enzyme inhibitors provided the long-awaited necessary tools to study further the physiological and pathological significance of this unique peptide family.

REFERENCES

1. Moncada S, Gryglewski R, Bunting S, Vane JR. *Nature* 1976;263:663–665.
2. Furchgott RF, Zawadzki JV. *Nature* 1980;288:373–376.
3. DeMey JG, Vanhoutte PM. *Circ Res* 1982;51:439–447.
4. Rubanyi GM, Lorenz RR, Vanhoutte PM. *J Physiol (Lond)* 1986;364:45–56.
5. Hickey KA, Rubanyi GM, Paul R, Highsmith RF. *Am J Physiol* 1985;248(Cell Physiol 17):C550–C555.
6. Gillespie MN, Owasoyo JO, McMurtry IF, O'Brien RF. *J Pharmacol Exp Ther* 1986;236:339–343.
7. O'Brien RF, Robbins RJ, McMurtry IF. *J Cell Physiol* 1987;132:263–270.
8. Yanagisawa M, Kurihara H, Kimura S, Tomobe Y, Kobayashi M, Mitsui Y, Yazaki Y, Goyo K, Masaki T. *Nature* 1988;332:411–415.
9. Kloog Y, Sokolovsky M. *Trends Pharmacol Sci* 1989;10:212–214.

10. Inou A, Yanagisawa M, Kimura S, Kasuya Y, Miyauchi T, Goto K, Masaki T. *Proc Natl Acad Sci U S A* 1989;86:2863–2867.
11. Emori T, Hirata Y, Ohta K, Shichiri M, Marumo F. *Biochem Biophys Res Commun* 1989;160:93–100.
12. Inoue A, Yanagisawa M, Takuwa Y, Mitsui Y, Kobayashi M, Masaki T. *J Biol Chem* 1989;264:14954–14959.
13. Itoh Y, Yanagisawa M, Ohkubo S, et al. *FEBS Lett* 1988;231:440–444.
14. MacCumber M, Ross C, Glaser B, Snyder S. *Proc Natl Acad Sci U S A* 1989;86:7285–7289.
15. Sunnergren K, Word R, Sambrook J, MacDonald P, Casey M. *Mol Cell Endocrinol* 1990;68:R7–R14.
16. Kurihara H, Yoshizumi M, Sugiyama T, et al. *Biochem Biophys Res Commun* 1989;159:1435–1440.
17. Yoshizumi M, Kurihara H, Sugiyama T, et al. *Biochem Biophys Res Commun* 1989;161:859–864.
18. Hexum T, Hoeger C, Rivier J, Baird A, Brown M. *Biochem Biophys Res Commun* 1990;167:294–300.
19. Orlando C, Brandi ML, Peri A, et al. *Endocrinology* 1990;126:1780–1782.
20. Schini VB, Hendrickson H, Heublein DM, Burnett JC Jr, Vanhoutte PM. *Eur J Pharmacol* 1989;165:333–334.
21. Suzuki N, Matsumoto H, Kitada C, Kimura S, Fujino M. *J Biochem* 1989;106:736–741.
22. Takahashi K, Brooks R, Kanse S, Ghatei M, Kohner E, Bloom S. *Diabetes* 1989;38:1200–1202.
23. Kosaka T, Suzuki N, Matsumoto H, et al. *FEBS Lett* 1989;249:42–46.
24. Shichiri M, Hirata Y, Emori T, et al. *FEBS Lett* 1989;253:203–206.
25. Black PN, Ghatei MA, Takahashi K, et al. *FEBS Lett* 1989;255:129–132.
26. Saida K, Mitsui Y, Ishida N. *J Biol Chem* 1989;264:14613–14616.
27. Giaid A, Gibson S, Ibrahim N, et al. *Proc Natl Acad Sci U S A* 1989;86:7634–7638.
28. Bloch K, Eddy R, Shows T, Quertermous T. *J Biol Chem* 1989;264:18156–18161.
29. Yoshizawa T, Shinmi O, Giaid A, et al. *Science* 1990;247:462–464.
30. Kitamura K, Tanaka T, Kato J, Eto T, Tanaka K. *Biochem Biophys Res Commun* 1989;161:348–352.
31. Shinmi O, Kimura S, Sawamura H, et al. *Biochem Biophys Res Commun* 1989;164:587–593.
32. Matsumoto H, Suzuki N, Onda H, Fujino M. *Biochem Biophys Res Commun* 1989;164:74–80.
33. Yanagisawa M, Inoue A, Ishikawa T, et al. *Proc Natl Acad Sci U S A* 1988;85:6964–6968.
34. Haegerstrand A, Hemsen A, Gillis C, Larsson O, Lundberg J. *Acta Physiol Scand* 1989;137:541–542.
35. Kitamura K, Tanaka T, Kato J, Ogawa T, Eto T, Tanaka K. *Biochem Biophys Res Commun* 1989;162:38–44.
36. Hiroe M, Hirata Y, Marumo F, et al. *Peptides* 1989;10:1281–1282.
37. Cintra A, Fuxe K, Anggard E, Tinner B, Staines W, Agnati L. *Acta Physiol Scand* 1989;137:557–558.
38. Yoshizawa T, Kimura S, Kanazawa I, Uchiyama Y, Yanagisawa M, Masaki T. *Neurosci Lett* 1989;102:179–184.
39. Rozengurt N, Springall D, Polak J. *J Pathol* 1990;160:5–8.
40. Botelho-Parker LH. Tissue specific production and action of endothelins. *Presented at the FASEB Endothelin Symposium.* Washington, DC, April 1990.
41. Morel DR, LaCroix JS, Hemsen A, Steinig DA, Pittet J, Lundberg JM. *Eur J Pharmacol* 1989;167:427–428.
42. Pernow J, Lundberg J. *Acta Physiol Scand* 1989;137:553–554.
43. Saito Y, Nakao K, Shirakami G, et al. *Biochem Biophys Res Commun* 1989;163:1512–1516.
44. Suzuki N, Miyauchi T, Tomobe Y, Matsumoto H, Goto K, Masaki T, Fujino M. *Biochem Biophys Res Commun* 1990;167:94–947.
45. Yoshimi H, Hirata Y, Fukuda Y, et al. *Peptides* 1989;10:805–808.
46. Berbinschi A, Ketelslegers JM. *Lancet* 1989;2:46.
47. Hirata Y, Matsunaga T, Ando K, Furukawa T, Tsukagoshi H,

48. Hoffman A, Keiser HR, Grossman E, Goldstein DS, Gold PW, Kling M. *Lancet* 1989;2:1519.
49. Nomura A, Uchida Y, Kambyama M, et al. *Lancet* 1989;2:747–748.
50. Anggard E, Galton S, Rae G. *J Cardiovasc Pharmacol* 1989;13:S46–S49.
51. De Nucci G, Thomas GR, Dorleans-Juste P. *Proc Natl Acad Sci* 1988;85:9797–9800.
52. Vijayaraghana J, Scicli AG, Carretero O. *J Biol Chem* 1990;265:14150–14155.
53. Liu JJ, Gu XH, Casley DJ, Nayler WG. *J Cardiovasc Pharmacol* 1990;5:436–443.
54. Miyauchi T, Yanagisawa M, Tomizawa T, et al. *Lancet* 1989;1:53.
55. Moravec CS, Reynolds EE, Stewart RW, Bond M. *Biochem Biophys Res Commun* 1989;159:14–18.
56. Nayler WG. *J Appl Cardiol* 1989;4:495–504.
57. Hom G, Schutt W, Rubanyi GM. In: Rubanyi GM, Vanhoutte PM, eds. Endothelium-derived contracting factors. Basel: Karger; 1990:98–103.
58. Nayler WG. *Trends Pharmacol Sci* 1990;11:96–99.
59. Nayler WG, Gu XH, Casley DJ, Panagiotopoulos S, Liu J, Mottram PL. *Biochem Biophys Res Commun* 1989;163:1270–1274.
60. Tabuchi Y, Nakamaru M, Rakugi H, Nagano M, Ogihara T. *Biochem Biophys Res Commun* 1989;159:1304–1308.
61. Yang Z, Richard V, von Segesser L, et al. *Circulation* 1990;82:188–195.
62. Dohi Y, Hahn AWA, Boulanger Ch, Buhler FR, Luscher TF. *Hypertension* 1992;19:131–137.
63. Simonson MJ, Wann S, Mene P, et al. *J Clin Invest* 1989;83:708–712.
64. Watanabe T, Suzuki N, Shimatmoto N, Jujino M, Imada A. *Nature* 1990;344:114.
65. Yamasaki H, Niwa M, Yamashita K, et al. *Eur J Pharmacol* 1989;168:247–250.
66. Hu JR, Von Harsdof R, Lang RE. *Eur J Pharmacol* 1988 (1988);158:275–278.
67. Ishikawa TM, Yanagisawa M, Kimura S, Goto K, Masaki T. *Am J Physiol* 1988;255(Heart Circ Physiol 24):H970–H973.
68. Hirata Y, Yoshima H, Emori T. *Biochem Biophys Res Commun* 1989;160:228–234.
69. Gu XH, Casley DJ, Nayler WG. *J Cardiovasc Pharmacol* 1989;13(suppl 5):S171–173.
70. Gu XH, Casley DJ, Nayler WG. *Eur J Pharmacol* 1989;162:509–510.
71. Gu XH, Casley DJ, Cincotta M, Nayler WG. *Eur J Pharmacol* 1990;177:205–209.
72. Yamasaki H, Niwa M, Yamashita K. *Eur J Pharmacol* 1989;168:247–250.
73. Davenport AP, Kaumann PA, Hall JA, Nunez DJ, Brown MJ. *Br J Pharmacol* 1989;96:102.
74. Shah AM, Lewis MJ, Henderson AH. *Eur J Pharmacol* 1989;163:365–367.
75. Watanabe T, Kusomoto K, Kitayoshi T, Shimamoto N. *J Cardiovasc Pharmacol* 1989;13(suppl 5):108–111.
76. Clozel JP, Clozel M. *Circ Res* 1989;65:1193–1200.
77. Karazatowska-Prolopczuk E, Wennmalm A. *Circ Res* 1990;66:46–54.
78. Ishikawa T, Yanagisawa M, Kimura S, Goto K, Masaki T. *Pflugers Arch* 1989;413:108–110.
79. Kurihara H, Yamaoki K, Nagai R. *Life Sci* 1989;44:1937–1943.
80. Chester AH, Dashwood MR, Clarke JG. *Am J Cardiol* 1989;63:1395–1398.
81. Kasuya Y, Ishirawa T, Yanagisawa M. *Am J Physiol* 1989;257(Heart Circ Physiol 26):H1828–1835.
82. Kasuya Y, Takuwaa Y, Yanagisawa M. *Biochem Biophys Res Commun* 1989;161:1049–1055.
83. Cocks TM, Faulkner NL, Sudhir K, Angus J. *Eur J Pharmacol* 1989;171:17–24.
84. Ezra D, Goldstein RE, Czaja JF, Feuerstein GZ. *Am J Physiol* 1989;257(Heart Circ Physiol 26):H339–H343.
85. Hom G, Touhey B, Rubanyi GM. *J Cardiovasc Pharmacol* 1992;19:194–200.

Marumo F. *Biochem Biophys Res Commun* 1990;166:1274–1278.

86. Arai H, Hori S, Aramori I, Ohkubo H, Nakainshi S. *Nature* 1990;348:730–732.
87. Sakurai T, Yangisawa M, Takuwa Y, et al. *Nature* 1990;348:732–735.
88. Masaki T, Angus J, Rubanyi GM, et al. *Pharmacol Rev* [in press].
89. Warner TD, Mitchell JA, DeNucci G, Vane JR. *Cardiovasc Pharmacol* 1989;167:41–47.
90. Clozel M, Gray GA, Breu V, Loffler BM, Osterwalder R. *Biochem Biophys Res Commun* 1992;186:867–873.
91. Harrison VJ, Randriantsoa A, Schoeffter P. *Br J Pharmacol* 1992;105:511–513.
92. Moreland S, McMullen DM, Delaney CL, Lee VG, Hunt JT. *Biochem Biophys Res Commun* 1992;184:100–106.
93. Williams DL Jr, Jones KL, Pettibone DJ, Lis EV, Clineschmidt BV. *Bioclin Biophys Res Commun* 1991;175:556–561.
94. Ihara M, Noguchi K, Saeki T, et al. *Life Sci* 1992;50:247–255.
95. Ihara M, Saeki T, Funabashi K, et al. *J Cardiovasc Pharmacol* 1991;19(suppl 7):S119–S121.
96. Nakamichi K, Ihara M, Kobayashi M, Saeki T, Ishikawa K, Yano M. *Biochem Biophys Res Commun* 1992;182:144–150.
97. Hiley CR, Cowley DJ, Pelton JT, Hargreaves AC. *Biochem Biophys Res Commun* 1992;184:953–959.
98. Webb ML, Dickinson KE, Delaney CL, et al. *Biochem Biophys Res Commun* 1992;185:887–892.
99. Ohlstein EH, Arleth A, Bryan H, Elliott JD, Sung CP. *Eur J Pharmacol* 1992;225:347–350.
100. Atkinson RA, Pelton JT. *FEBS Lett* 1992;296:1–6.
101. Krystek SJ, Bassolino DA, Bruccoleri RE, et al. *FEBS Lett* 1992;299:255–261.
102. Miyata S, Fukami N, Neya M, Takase S, Kiyoto S. *J Antibiot (Tokyo)* 1992;45:788–791.
103. Miyoto S, Hasimoto M, Fujie K, et al. *J Antibiot (Tokyo)* 1992;45:1041–1046.
104. Bazil MK, Lappe RW, Webb RL. *J Cardiovasc Pharmacol* 1992;20:940–948.
105. Meyer P, Flammer J, Luscher TF. *Invest Ophthalmol Vis Sci* (in press).
106. Cocks TM, Faulkner NL, Sudhir K, Angus J. *Eur J Pharmacol* 1989;171(1):17–24.
107. Costello KB, Stewart DJ, Baffour R. *Eur J Pharmacol* 1990;186(2–3):311–314.
108. Yang Z, Bauer E, Von Segesser L, et al. *J Cardiovasc Pharmacol* 1990;16(4):654–660.
109. Rubanyi GM, Parker-Bothelo LH. *FASEB J* 1991;5:2713–2720.
110. Brock T, Danthuluri R. In: Rubanyi GM, ed. *Endothelin.* New York, NY: Oxford University Press; 1992:103–125.
111. Simonson M, Dunn M. *FASEB J* 1990;4:2989–3000.
112. Komuro I, Kurihara H, Sugiyama I, Yoshizumi M, Takaku F, Yazaki Y. *FEBS Lett* 1988;238:249–252.
113. Takuwa N, Takuwa Y, Yanagisawa M, Yamashita K, Masaki T. *J Biol Chem* 1989;264:7856–7861.
114. Simonson MS, Wann S, Mene P, et al. *J Clin Invest* 1989;83:708–712.
115. Deng LY, Schiffrin EL. *Can J Physiol Pharmacol* 1991;69:798–804.
116. Fortes ZB, Costa SG, Nucci G, Nigro D, Scivoletto R, Carvalho MH. *Clin Exp Hypertens* [A] 1990;12:47–61.
117. De Carvalho MH, Nigro D, Scivoletto R, et al. *Hypertension* 1990;15(2 suppl):168–171.
118. Boric MP, Donoso V, Fournier A, et al. *Eur J Pharamcol* 1990;190:123–133.
119. Randall MD, Edwards DH, Griffith TM. *Br J Pharmacol* 1990;101:781–788.
120. Vigne P, Marsault R, Breittmayer JP, Frelin C. *Biochem J* 1990;266:415–420.
121. Vigne P, Ladoux A, Frelin C. *J Biol Chem* 1991;266:5925–5928.
122. Frelin C, Ladoux A, Marsault R, Bigne P. *J Cardiovasc Pharmacol* 1991;17(suppl 7):S131–133.
123. Ishibashi M, Haizuka H, Tsukamura T, Furue H, Yamaji T. *Am J Hypertens* 1992;5:772–774.
124. Miller WL, Redfield MM, Burnett JC Jr. *J Clin Invest* 1989;83:317–320.
125. Lee ME, De La Monte SM, Ng SC, Bloch KD. *J Clin Invest* 1990;86:141–147.
126. Shinmi O, Kimura S, Sawamura T, et al. *Biochem Biophys Res Commun* 1989;164:587–593.
127. Samson WK, Skala K, Huang. *Brain Res* 1991;539(2):347–351.
128. Ando K, Hirata Y, Togashi K, Kawakami M, Marumo F. *J Cardiovasc Pharmacol* 1991;17(suppl 7):S434–436.
129. Koseki C, Imai M, Hirata Y, Yanagisawa M, Masaki T. *Neurosci Res* 1989;6:581–585.
130. Calvo J, Gonzalez R, De Carvalho LF, et al. *Endocrinology* 1990;126:2288–2295.
131. Siren AL, Feuerstein G. *Neuropeptides* 1989;14:231–236.
132. Ferguson AV, Smith P. *Regul Pept* 1990;27:75–85.
133. Kawano Y, Yoshida K, Yoshimi H, Kuramochi M, Omae T. *J Hypertens Suppl* 1989;7:S22–23.
134. Yamamoto T, Kimura T, Ota K, et al. *J Cardiovasc Pharmacol* 1991;17(suppl 7):S316–318.
135. Matsumura K, Abe I, Tsuchihashi T. *Hypertension* 1991;17(6 Pt 2):1192–1196.
136. Wall KM, Ferguson AV. *Brain Res* 1992;586:111–116.
137. Nakamaru M, Tabuchi Y, Rakugi H, Nagano M, Ogihara T. *J Hypertens Suppl* 1989;7:S132–133.
138. Wiklund NP, Ohlen A, Wiklund CU, et al. *Acta Physiol Scand* 1989;137:399–407.
139. Harrison VJ, Randriantsoa A, Schoeffter P. *Br J Pharmacol* 1992;105:511–513.
140. Cockcroft JR, Clarke JG, Webb DJ. *Br J Clin Pharmacol* 1991;31:521–524.
141. Chapleau MW, Hajduczok G, Abboud FM. *Am J Physiol* 1992;263:R103–108.
142. Nakamoto H, Suzuki H, Murakami M, et al. *J Hypertens* 1991;9:337–344.
143. Ohman KP, Hoffman A, Keiser HR. *Acta Physiol Scand* 1990;138:549–556.
144. Kneupfer MM, Han SP, Trapani AJ, Fok KF, Westfall TC. *Am J Physiol* 1989;257:H918–H926.
145. Itoh S, Van Den Buuse M. *Am J Physiol* 1991;260:H1106–H1112.
146. Kaufmann H, Oribe E, Oliver JA. *Lancet* 1991;338(8782–8783):1542–1545.
147. Munter K, Hackenthal E. *J Hypertens Suppl* 1989;7:S276–S277.
148. Matsumura Y, Hisaki K, Ohyama T, et al. *Eur J Pharmacol* 1989;166:577–580.
149. Moe O, Tejedor A, Campbell WB, Alpern RJ, Henrich WL. *Am J Physiol* 1991;260:E521–E525.
150. Rakugi H, Nakamaru M, Saito H, Higaki J, Ogihara T. *Biochem Biophys Res Commun* 1988;155:1244–1247.
151. Takagi H, Hisa H, Satoh S. *Biochem Biophys Res Commun* 1988;157:1164–1168.
152. Takagi M, Tsukada H, Matsuoka H, Yagi S. *Am J Physiol* 1989;257:E833–838.
153. Stier CT Jr, Quilley CP, McGiff JC. *J Pharmacol Exp Ther* 1992;262:252–256.
154. Miller WL, Redfield MM, Burnett JC Jr. *J Clin Invest* 1989;83:317–320.
155. Otsuka A, Mikami H, Katahira K, et al. *Acta Endocrinol (Copenh)* 1989;121:361–364.
156. Goetz KL, Wang BC, Madwed JB, et al. *Am J Physiol* 1988;255:R1064–1068.
157. Nakamoto H, Suzuki H, Murakami M, et al. *Clin Sci* 1989;77:567–572.
158. Madeddu P, Troffa C, Glorioso N, et al. *J Cardiovasc Pharmacol* 1989;14:818–825.
159. Claria J, Jimenez W, La Villa G, et al. *Acta Physiol Scand* 1991;141:305–308.
160. Gasic S, Wagner OF, Vierhapper H, Nowotny P, Waldhausl W. *J Cardiovasc Pharmacol* 1992;19:176–180.
161. Vierhapper H, Wagner O, Nowotny P, Waldhausl W. *Circulation* 1990;81:1415–1418.
162. Chou SY, Dahhan A, Porush JG. *Am J Physiol* 1990;259:F645–F652.
163. Yamada K, Yoshida S. *J Cardiovasc Pharmacol* 1991;17(suppl 7):S290–S292.
164. Mazzocchi G, Malendowicz LK, Nussdorfer GG. *Peptides* 1990;11:763–765.
165. Komuro IH, Kurihara T, Sugiyama M, et al. *FEBS Lett* 1988;238:249–252.

166. Mortensen LH, Fink GD. *Hypertension* 1992;19:676–680.
167. Yasujima M, Abe K, Kanazawa M, et al. *Tohoku J Exp Med* 1991;163:219–227.
168. Takeshita H, Nishikibe M, Yano M, Ikemoto F. *Clin Exp Pharmacol Physiol* 1991;18:661–669.
169. Kawaguchi H, Sawa H, Yasuda H. *J Mol Cell Cardiol* 1990;22:830–842.
170. Kawaguchi H, Sawa H, Yasuda H. *J Hypertens* 1991;9:171–174.
171. Scott-Burden T, Resink TJ, Hahn AWA, Vanhoutte PM. *J Cardiovasc Pharmacol* 1991;17(suppl 7):S96–S100.
172. Cozza EN, Chiou S, Gomez CE. *Am J Physiol* 1992;262:R85–R89.
173. Kohzuki M, Johnston CI, Chai SY, et al. *Clin Exp Pharmacol Physiol* 1989;16:239–242.
174. Koseki C, Amai M, Hirata Y, et al. *J Cardiovasc Pharmacol* 1989;13:S153–S154.
175. Cozza EN, Gomez Shanchez CE, Foecking MF, Chiou S. *J Clin Invest* 1989;84:1032–1035.
176. Gomez Sanchez CE, Cozza EN, Foecking MF, Chiou S, Ferris MW. *Hypertension* 1990;15:744–747.
177. Davenport AP, Nunez DJ, Brown MJ. *Clin Sci* 1989;77:129–131.
178. Miller WL, Redfield MM, Burnett JC Jr. *J Clin Invest* 1989;83:317–320.
179. Goetz K, Wang BC, Leadley R Jr, et al. *Am J Physiol* 1988;255:R1064–1068.
180. Mazzocchi G, Malendowicz LK, Nussdorfer GG. *Peptides* 1990;11;763–765.
181. Emmeluth C, Bie P. *Acta Physiol Scand* 1992;146:197–204.
182. Bakris GL, Fairbanks R, Traish AM. *J Clin Invest* 1991;87:1158–1164.
183. Sakamoto H, Sasaki S, Nakamura Y, Fushimi K, Marumo F. *Kidney Int* 1992;41:350–355.
184. Emori T, Hirata Y, Ohta K. *Hypertension* 1991;18(2):165–170.
185. Milner P, Bodin P, Loesch A, Burnstock G. *Biochem Biophys Res Commun* 1990;170:649–656.
186. Loesch A, Bodin P, Burnstock G. *Peptides* 1991;12(5):1095–1103.
187. Imai T, Hirata Y, Emori T, et al. *Hypertension* 1992;19:753–757.
188. Goetz K, Wang BC, Leadley R Jr, et al. *Proc Soc Exp Biol Med* 1989;191:425–427.
189. Nakamoto H, Suzuki H, Murakami M, et al. *J Hypertens* 1991;9:337–344.
190. Kawao Y, Yoshida K, Yoshimi H, Kuramochi M, Omae T. *J Hypertens Suppl* 1989;7:S22–S23.
191. Yamamoto T, Kimura T, Ota K. *Am J Physiol* 1992;262:E856–E862.
192. Wall KM, Nasr M, Ferguson AV. *Brain Res* 1992;570:180–187.
193. Ritz MF, Stuenkel EL, Dayanithi G, Jones R, Nordmann JJ. *Proc Natl Acad Sci U S A* 1992;89:8371–8375.
194. Schichiri M, Hirata Y, Kanno K, Ohta K, Emori T, Marupoma F. *Biochem Biophys Res Commun* 1989;163(3):1332–1337.
195. Tomita K, Nonoguchi H, Marumo F. *J Clin Invest* 1990;85:2014–2018.
196. Woodcock EA, Land S. *Clin Exp Pharmacol Physiol* 1992;19(5):384–387.
197. Oishi R, Nonoguchi H, Tomita K, Marumo F. *Am J Physiol* 1991;261:F951–F956.
198. Wong Dusting HK, La M, Rand MJ. *J Cardiovasc Pharmacol* 1991;17:S236–S238.
199. Molnar M, Hertelendy F. *Life Sci* 1990;47:1463–1468.
200. Fozard JR, Part ML. *Eur J Pharmacol* 1990;180:153–159.
201. Gardner DG, Newman ED, Nakamura KK, Nguyen KP. *Am J Physiol* 1991;261:E177–E182.
202. Hu JR, Berninger UG, Lang RE. *Eur J Pharmacol* 1988;158:177–178.
203. Levin ER, Isackson PJ, Hu RM. *Endocrinology* 1991;128:2925–2930.
204. Mantymaa P, Leppaluoto J, Ruskoaho H. *Endocrinology* 1990;126:587–595.
205. Pitkanen M, Mantymaa P, Ruskoaho H. *Eur J Pharmacol* 1991;195:307–315.
206. Schiebinger RJ, Gomez Sanchez CE. *Endocrinology* 1990;127:119–125.
207. Stasch JP, Hirth Dietrich C, Kazda S, Neuser D. *Life Sci* 1989;45:869–875.
208. Uusimaa PA, Hassinen IE, Vuolteenaho O, Ruskoaho H. *Endocrinology* 1991;130:864–869.
209. Fukuda Y, Hirata Y, Yoshimi H, et al. *Biochem Biophys Res Commun* 1988;155:167–172.
210. Horio T, Kohno M, Takeda T. *Clin Exp Pharmacol Physiol* 1992;19:575–582.
211. Amadieu Farmakis M, Davicco MJ, Giry J, Barlet JP. *J Dev Physiol* 1991;16:51–56.
212. Claria J, Jimenez W, Arroyo V, et al. *Kidney Int* 1991;40:182–187.
213. Nakamoto H, Suzuki H, Murakami M, et al. *J Hypertens* 1991;9:337–344.
214. Tsuchiya K, Naruse M, Sanaka T, et al. *Life Sci* 1990;46:59–65.
215. Valentin JP, Gardner DG, Wiedemann E, Humphreys MH. *Hypertension* 1991;17:864–869.
216. Hu RM, Levin ER, Pedram A, Frank HJ. *J Biol Chem* 1992;267:17384–17389.
217. Kohno M, Horio T, Yokokawa K, Kurihara N, Takeda T. *Hypertension* 1992;19:320–325.
218. Kohno M, Yokokawa K, Horio T, et al. *Circ Res* 1992;70:241–247.
219. Kohno M, Horio T, Yokokawa K, Kurihara N, Takeda T. *Hypertension* 1992;19:320–325.
220. Kohno M, Yasunari K, Yokokawa K, et al. *J Clin Invest* 1991;87:1999–2004.
221. Saijonmaa O, Ristimaki A, Fyhrquist F. *Biochem Biophys Res Commun* 1990;173:514–520.
222. Neuser D, Zaiss S, Stasch JP. *Eur J Pharmacol* 1990;176:241–243.
223. Makino S, Hashimoto K, Hirasawa R, et al. *Brain Res* 1990;534:117–121.
224. Makino S, Hashimoto K, Hirasawa R, Hattori T, Ota Z. *J Hypertens* 1992;10:25–28.
225. Suzuki E, Hirata Y, Matsuoka H, et al. *J Hypertens* 1991;9:927–934.
226. Winquist RJ, Scott AL, Vlasuk GP. *Hypertension* 1989;14:111–114.
227. Levin ER, Frank HJ, Pedram A. *J Neurochem* 1992;58:659–666.
228. Ota K, Kimura T, Shoji M, et al. *Am J Physiol* 1992;262:E135–E141.

Hypertension: Pathophysiology, Diagnosis, and Management, Second Edition,
edited by J.H. Laragh and B.M. Brenner,
Raven Press, Ltd., New York © 1995.

CHAPTER 67

Adenosine in Cardiovascular Homeostasis and the Pharmacologic Control of its Activity

Italo Biaggioni and Rogelio Mosqueda-Garcia

Adenosine is an intermediate product of the metabolism of adenosine triphosphate (ATP). As such, it is produced in virtually every cell when metabolic demands exceed oxygen supply (Fig. 1). Once released into the interstitium, adenosine is quickly transported back into cells by an energy-dependent uptake mechanism (1) as part of a purine salvage pathway, designed to maintain intracellular levels of ATP. Extracellular levels of adenosine have been shown to increase during hypoxia in several tissues (2), suggesting that release of adenosine during ischemia may overwhelm adenosine uptake and metabolism. Because most of its actions are mediated through cell surface receptors, the importance of endogenous adenosine as a physiologic modulator depends on its interstitial concentrations and, therefore, may be enhanced during situations of increased cell work and ischemia. Extracellular adenosine, however, is short-lived. It is quickly deaminated to inactive inosine by adenosine deaminase and is transported back into cells by this active uptake

mechanism. The effectiveness of this adenosine transport system is species-dependent and is particularly active in humans. Accordingly, the half-life of adenosine in human blood is probably less than 1 second (3).

Adenosine receptors were initially identified and classified according to their effect on adenylate cyclase (4). A_1 receptors, initially shown to inhibit adenylate cyclase, are now known to interact with a variety of second-messenger systems, including potassium channels and phospholipase C, through coupling with G_i and perhaps other guanine nucleotide binding proteins. Two subtypes of adenosine A_2 receptors have been identified, A_{2a} and A_{2b}. Both subtypes activate adenylate cyclase via coupling to G_S proteins (5). A_1, A_{2a}, and A_{2b} receptors have been cloned (6–8). A third type of adenosine receptor, A_3, has also been cloned. It is similar to A_1 receptors in that it also inhibits adenylate cyclase, but it differs from A_1 receptors in its rank order of potencies for agonists and its lower affinity for some methylxanthines (9). This receptor type facilitates mast cell activation (10) but its function in other organ systems remains unclear. Adenosine receptors share significant sequence homology and have the classic 7 transmembrane domains structure of Gprotein-coupled receptors.

I. Biaggioni and R. Mosqueda-Garcia: Clinical Research Center and Division of Clinical Pharmacology, Departments of Medicine and Pharmacology, Vanderbilt University, Nashville, Tennessee 37232.

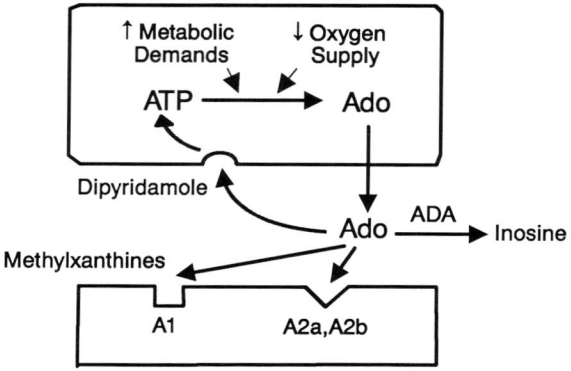

FIG. 1. Outline of the metabolic pathways of adenosine. Adenosine (*Ado*) is formed from breakdown of ATP when metabolic demands in the cell outweigh oxygen supply and is released to the interstitium. The final step in the formation of adenosine from AMP depends on the enzyme 5'-nucleotidase (Not shown is the formation of adenosine from *S*-adenosyl-homocysteine). Interstitial adenosine is quickly transported inside cells through an energy-dependent system to restore intracellular levels of ATP. Interstitial and intracellular adenosine can be deaminated to inosine by adenosine deaminase (*ADA*). Uptake and deamination limit the half-life of adenosine and its effectiveness. Interstitial adenosine acts on at least two adenosine receptors, originally characterized by their ability to inhibit (A_1) or activate (A_2) adenylate cyclase. Two subtypes of adenosine A_2 receptors, A_{2a} and A_{2b}, have been cloned.

Differences in adenosine metabolism and adenosine receptors have been found in hypertensive states. We first review these differences and their significance to hypertension. We then examine the several cardiovascular and autonomic actions of adenosine that are relevant to blood pressure regulation (Table 1). We also discuss the effect of altering adenosine mechanisms, either with adenosine receptor antagonists or uptake inhibitors, on cardiovascular regulation. We end by exploring the potential use of adenosine agonists in the treatment of hypertension. On specific subjects, the reader is directed to more comprehensive reviews than we can offer here.

DIFFERENCES IN ADENOSINE RECEPTORS AND ADENOSINE METABOLISM IN HYPERTENSIVE STATES

A decreased responsiveness of adenylate cyclase to adenosine has been found in myocardial sarcolemma and aorta of spontaneously hypertensive rats (SHR) compared with Wistar-Kyoto (WKY) rats (11). This phenomenon, however, was not specific for adenosine receptors, because it was also found with other G-protein-coupled receptors that activate adenylate cyclase and by non-receptor activators of cyclase such as NaF and forskolin (11). A diminished affinity of central adenosine A_1 receptors for antagonists and for the low affinity state of agonists has also been found in stroke-prone SHR compared with WKY rats (12). The differences in agonist and antagonists binding were abolished by the addition of guanosine triphosphate (GTP) analogues, suggesting that this alteration is due to a defective G protein or by an altered coupling between G protein and adenosine A_1 receptors (12). No differences in coding sequences or levels of expression of A_1 receptor mRNA were found between SHR and normotensive rats (13), confirming that differences in agonist and antagonist affinity are not mediated by structural changes at the receptor level. It has been proposed that these differences in A_1 receptor coupling explain the decreased inhibition of noradrenergic neurotransmission by adenosine in efferent nerves and the decreased hypotensive actions of adenosine in the nucleus tractus solitarii (NTS) in SHR compared with WKY rats (12) (see below). This, however, would imply that adenosine-induced inhibition of noradrenergic neurotransmission is mediated by the low-affinity state of the receptor, because this was the main difference found between SHR and WKY rats (12). Likewise, the hypotensive actions of adenosine in the nucleus tractus solitarii are thought to be mediated by A_2, rather than A_1, receptors (14). Therefore, the physiological relevance of the differences in receptor-effector coupling found in SHR is not defined.

TABLE 1. *Cardiovascular effects of adenosine*

Organ	Action	Receptor type	Effect on blood pressure	Reference
Vascular smooth muscle endothelium?	Vasodilation[a]	A_{2a}/A_{2b}	↓	24
Sinoatrial and Atrioventricular Node	Sinus slowing, AV prolongation	A_1	↓	19
Kidney	↓ Renin release	A_1	↓	52
Vasculature	↑ Renin release	A_2?	↑	66
Sympathetic efferent nerves	↓ Norepinephrine release	A_1	↓	70
Brainstem (Nucleus tractus solitarii)	↓ Sympathetic activity	A_{2a}	↓	94,96
Renal afferents	↑ Sympathetic activity	?	↑	124,125
Arterial chemoreceptors	↑ Sympathetic activity	A_2	↑	123,132,133
Myocardial afferents	↑ Sympathetic activity	A_1	↑	139,141,142
Skeletal muscle afferents	↑ Sympathetic activity	?	↑	150,151

[a] Adenosine can produce vasoconstriction in certain vascular beds; see text.

In contrast to the changes found in A_1 receptor binding, no differences in the uptake of adenosine by the lung have been found in SHR compared with WKY rats (15). Similarly, no consistent differences in adenosine uptake binding were found in the kidney, heart, or platelets of SHR compared with WKY rats (16) or in adenosine deaminase activity in the brain of SHR compared with WKY rats (17). Therefore, whereas there are significant differences in adenosine metabolism between animal species (3,18), no consistent dissimilarities have been found between hypertensive and normotensive animals.

CARDIOVASCULAR EFFECTS OF ADENOSINE

Adenosine acts at A_1 receptors in the sinus node and the atrioventricular (AV) node, producing sinus slowing and AV node prolongation, respectively. Both actions are mediated through opening of potassium channels, but one may predominate over the other depending on the species studied (19). AV prolongation after intravenous adenosine is prominent in humans and accounts for its efficacy in the treatment of supraventricular tachycardias involving the AV node (20). Adenosine has negative inotropic actions in atrial muscle, probably through A_1 receptors. In ventricular muscle, adenosine does not have negative inotropic actions under resting conditions, but it opposes the positive chronotropic, inotropic, and arrhythmogenic actions of adrenergic agonists in vitro (21). The importance of this action in vivo remains controversial (22), but under certain clinical conditions, endogenous adenosine may oppose catecholamine-mediated ventricular tachycardia (23).

Adenosine is also a potent vasodilator by acting on A_{2a} or A_{2b} receptors, depending on the vascular bed and species studied (24). Adenosine receptors activate adenylate cyclase and decrease intracellular free calcium in vascular smooth muscle (25). The increase in cyclic adenosine monophosphate (AMP) activates cyclic AMP-dependent kinase, which phosphorylates myosin light chain kinase, making it less effective to phosphorylate myosin light chain, hindering the actin–myosin interaction required for muscle contraction. It is not clear if this mechanism alone explains adenosine-induced vasodilation. For example, the vasodilator actions of adenosine are attenuated by glibenclamide in the isolated heart (26) and in the whole animal in vivo (27), suggesting that ATP-sensitive potassium channels may also be involved in this action. It is not known, however, if adenosine activates ATP-sensitive potassium channels directly, and very high doses of glibenclamide, reaching toxic levels, are sometimes required to attenuate the vasodilator actions of adenosine in vivo (28).

It is also unclear if endothelial cells contribute to adenosine-induced vasodilation. Endothelial cells possess A_2 receptors that activate adenylate cyclase (29).

Studies using intracoronary infusion of radiolabeled adenosine have shown that most of the radioactivity remains in the endothelial cells (30), implying that the endothelium acts as a barrier between the intravascular space and the underlying vascular smooth muscle cells. Likewise, infusion of adenosine linked to macromolecules, thereby less likely to cross the endothelial barrier, still produces coronary vasodilation (31). In vitro and animal studies, however, have produced conflicting results as to whether adenosine-induced vasodilation is endothelium-dependent (32–34). Even in studies showing endothelium dependency, it is unclear if adenosine-induced vasodilation is mediated by the endothelium-dependent relaxing factor nitric oxide or other endothelium-dependent factors not yet characterized (35).

Considering its vasodilatory actions and that interstitial adenosine may accumulate during hypoxia, adenosine has long been proposed as a mediator of reactive hyperemia. This hypothesis has been tested in animals using adenosine receptor antagonists or adenosine deaminase to block endogenous adenosine and adenosine uptake blockers to potentiate endogenous adenosine. Current evidence does not support a role of adenosine in the regulation of local blood flow under resting conditions or during nonischemic exercise (36). During conditions of ischemia, however, adenosine does seem to contribute to reactive hyperemia in the heart (37) and skeletal muscle in animals (38,39). Endogenous adenosine may also contribute to postischemic reactive hyperemia in the human forearm (40).

Whereas adenosine is a vasodilator in most vascular beds, it produces transient vasoconstriction in the kidney (41). Even if adenosine is administered intrarenally as a continuous infusion, renal blood flow decreases initially but then returns toward baseline, or even above baseline, values (42). This decrease in renal blood flow is primarily due to constriction of afferent arterioles in cortical glomeruli, is mediated through A_1 receptors, and involves a complex interaction with angiotensin II. Angiotensin II antagonists prevent the renal vasoconstriction produced by adenosine, and, conversely, adenosine receptor antagonists prevent the renal vasoconstriction effects of angiotensin II (43). More recently, adenosine has been shown to produce vasoconstriction in other vascular beds (44). Adenosine produces transient pulmonary vasoconstriction in sheep (45) and cats (46) in vivo, but this effect has not been observed in humans (47) and may, therefore, be species-dependent. Vasoconstriction by adenosine has also been observed in vitro in the rat hepatic circulation (48) and, inconsistently, in primate coronary artery strips (49). Vasoconstriction in these vascular beds is characterized by rapid tachyphylaxis and is mediated by adenosine-induced release of thromboxanes or endoperoxides (45,48). This phenomenon resembles the endothelium-derived vasoconstriction observed with acetylcholine in other preparations (50), but it is not known if adenosine-induced vasoconstriction is endothelium-dependent or if it is mediated through other cell types. Likewise, neither the adenosine receptor type involved nor the physiological importance of these actions has been defined.

EFFECTS OF ADENOSINE ON THE KIDNEY AND ON THE RENIN-ANGIOTENSIN SYSTEM

Intrarenal infusion of adenosine produces dilation of efferent arterioles and afferent vasoconstriction, leading to a decrease in glomerular filtration rate. In contrast to the transient renal artery vasoconstriction observed during continuous intrarenal infusion of adenosine, the decrease in glomerular filtration rate is sustained for the duration of the infusion and will lead to a decrease in urine output (51). Glomerular filtration rate and urine output returns promptly toward baseline values after discontinuation of the infusion, and renal blood flow markedly increases (51).

Adenosine is a potent inhibitor of renin release via A_1 receptors (42,52,53). There is pharmacologic evidence that A_2 receptors are present in kidney slices and stimulate rather than inhibit renin release in vitro (54). Studies using non-selective A_1/A_2 antagonists, however, have shown that the A_1-mediated inhibition of renin predominates in vivo; adenosine antagonists potentiate the increase in renin release produced by sodium restriction (55), furosemide (56), hydralazine (57), and suprarenal aortic constriction (58). Furthermore, the specific adenosine receptor antagonist 1,3-dipropryl-8-sulfophenylxanthine (DPSPX) increased plasma renin activity in conscious unrestrained rats (57), suggesting that even under basal physiologic conditions, endogenous adenosine tonically inhibits renin release. In humans caffeine potentiates the increase in plasma renin activity produced by hydralazine, presumably by blocking endogenous adenosine (59). Selective antagonism of A_1 receptors also increases basal plasma renin activity in humans (60).

Inhibition of renin release by endogenous adenosine may be relevant to renin-dependent hypertension inasmuch as caffeine has been shown to worsen hypertension in two-kidney, one-clip rats (61). Studies with adenosine receptor antagonists suggest that adenosine not only inhibits renin release but also antagonizes the slow pressor effect of angiotensin II (62). Furthermore, plasma levels of adenosine are significantly increased in rats with renin-dependent hypertension (61,63). The source of this increased circulating adenosine is not known, but angiotensin II has been found to release adenosine from rat lung (64). In this animal model of hypertension, therefore, endogenous adenosine seems to act as a physiologic negative feedback mechanism of the renin-angiotensin system, whereby adenosine is released under conditions of increased renin, acts as a break to renin release, and opposes angiotensin actions.

However, it has recently been reported that intrabrachial adenosine releases angiotensin II from the human coronary bed (65) and the forearm (66). This effect is blocked by theophylline and is not reproduced by nitroprusside, suggesting that it is mediated by adenosine receptors and it is unrelated to a vasodilation (66). Forearm ischemia also induced the release of renin and angiotensin II, an effect that was blocked by intraarterial theophylline, suggesting that endogenous adenosine, released during ischemia, mediated this effect (65). This effect is probably mediated by A_2 receptors, analogous to the increase in renin release produced by A_2 receptors in renal slices (54). In the kidney the higher affinity of adenosine for A_1 receptors probably overwhelms any effect of A_2 receptors, so that the net effect is inhibition of renin release by adenosine. It is possible that the lack of A_1 receptors in the vasculature unmasks an A_2-mediated renin release in the human forearm. This paradoxic response contradicts the postulated inhibition role of adenosine on renin release. The importance of this phenomenon, however, remains unclear. Intraarterial captopril blocked adenosine-induced angiotensin II release from the forearm without enhancing adenosine-induced forearm vasodilation (66), suggesting that the release of angiotensin II was not sufficient to impair adenosine vasodilation. On the other hand, blockade of angiotensin AT_1 receptors with losartan potentiated the vasodilation produced by the adenosine A_2 agonist DPMA (N6-[2-(3,5-dimethoxyphenyl)-2-(2-methyl phenyl) ethyl] adenosine) in rats (67).

EFFECTS OF ADENOSINE ON AUTONOMIC CARDIOVASCULAR CONTROL

Presynaptic Effects of Adenosine on Efferent Nerves

Adenosine has been shown to inhibit neurotransmitter release through putative presynaptic receptors in both the brain and the periphery (68,69). This is true of practically all neurotransmitters studied, including norepinephrine (70). Several studies have found that the inhibition of norepinephrine release by exogenous adenosine is impaired in SHR compared with WKY rats (71–74). Endogenous adenosine, however, did not affect electrically-stimulated norepinephrine release from mesenteric arteries of normotensive rats (75) or SHR (73) in vivo, probably due to the lack of significant adenosine release in this model (73). It is possible, however, that endogenous adenosine may participate in the regulation of adrenergic neurotransmission in vivo in other tissues with greater metabolic demands (e.g., the heart) (76), especially under conditions of ischemia. Of interest, Taddei et al. (77) recently reported that intrabrachial administration of theophylline significantly potentiated sympathetically mediated forearm vasoconstriction, suggesting that endogenous adenosine inhibits adrenergic neurotransmission *in vivo* in humans. It remains to be determined if the decreased sensitivity to the presynaptic inhibitory actions of adenosine found in SHR contributes to the development or maintenance of hypertension.

Whereas the inhibitory effects of adenosine on neurotransmitter release have been documented in most efferent nerves, adenosine was found to enhance the vasoconstrictive effects of transmural nerve stimulation in guinea pig pulmonary arteries (78). It was suggested that this effect was partially due to presynaptic stimulation of norepinephrine release. However, in this and in a handful of other experimental models, adenosine was found to produce postsynaptic potentiation of norepinephrine-induced vasoconstriction (79,80). Therefore, even though adenosine may increase the vasoconstriction induced by nerve stimulation, in most tissues this action can be attributed to postsynaptic effects rather than to presynaptic enhancement of neurotransmitter release.

Ganglionic Transmission

A few studies have investigated the effect of adenosine on ganglionic neurotransmission, and most of them show an inhibitory effect. Adenosine inhibits the release of acetylcholine presynaptically and blocks calcium currents postsynaptically in the rat superior cervical ganglion (81). Adenosine may also inhibit neurotransmission in the cat parasympathetic vesical ganglia (82). Indirect evidence suggests that intravenous adenosine inhibits ganglionic transmission *in vivo* in anesthetized rats (83). However, adenosine has been found to increase the pressor effects of nicotine in rats, presumably by enhancing the effects of nicotine in sympathetic ganglia (84). The mechanisms that would explain this apparent effect have not been elucidated.

Effects of Adenosine on the Central Nervous System

A growing number of studies suggest that adenosine acts as neuromodulator of central cardiovascular regulation. Adenosine is released from nerve terminals by depolarization (85) and acts on A_1 and A_2 adenosine receptors. The existence and distribution of these receptors in relevant central nervous system (CNS) cardiovascular nuclei have been documented by autoradiographic and radioligand binding techniques (86). Key elements in the metabolism of adenosine have also been documented within the CNS, including adenosine deaminase (87,88) and an energy-dependent high affinity uptake mecha-

nism (89). These may be involved in the removal of synaptically released adenosine.

Direct administration of adenosine within the CNS has provided further evidence of the potential cardiovascular regulatory role of this substance. Earlier studies documented that intracerebroventricular (ICV) administration of adenosine evoked dose-related reductions in blood pressure and heart rate that were antagonized by caffeine (90,91). These effects were likely the result of a decrease in sympathetic tone (92). More recent studies have attempted to elucidate the specific brain nuclei that mediate these cardiovascular changes. Because the highest density of adenosine uptake sites in the CNS has been observed in the NTS (87,93) and this nucleus is of primary importance in reflex cardiovascular function, it is not surprising that many studies have focused on the characterization of the effects of adenosine in the NTS. Microinjection of adenosine into the caudal part of the pars medialis of the NTS evokes a dose-related decrease in blood pressure, heart rate (94–96), and renal sympathetic nerve activity (97) (Fig. 2). These responses are blocked by the adenosine antagonists caffeine and DPSPX (94,96).

The cardiovascular effects of adenosine in the NTS seem to involve A_2 receptors. On an equimolar basis, 5'-N-ethylcarboxamido-adenosine (NECA) was more potent than $(-)-N^6$-(R-phenyl-isopropyl)-adenosine (PIA), which in turn was more potent than adenosine in producing cardiovascular changes in the NTS (94). Microinjection of the selective A_{2a} adenosine receptor agonist CGS-21680 into the caudal NTS evoked similar actions (14), and administration of agents that increase cyclic

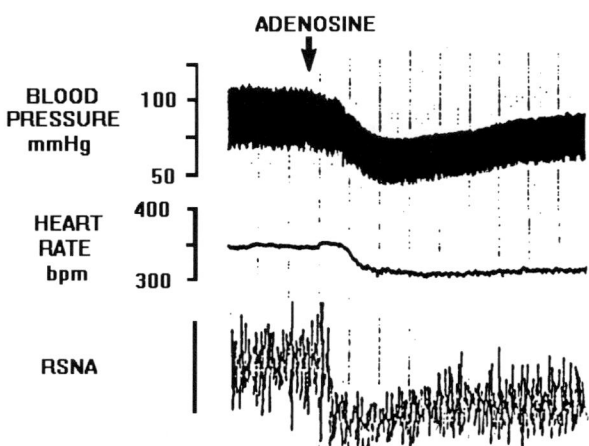

FIG. 2. Cardiovascular effects of adenosine in the nucleus tractus solitarii. Effect of microinjection of adenosine (2.3 nmol/60 nl) into the nucleus tractus solitarii of rat brainstem. Adenosine lowers blood pressure, heart rate, and renal sympathetic nerve activity (*RNSA*) in this model. These effects are similar to those obtained with excitatory amino acid glutamate.

AMP, such as isoproterenol or cyclic AMP itself, also decreased blood pressure and heart rate (98).

At least two other sites within the CNS may also contribute to the cardiovascular effects of ICV adenosine. The area postrema (AP) is a circumventricular organ that lacks a complete blood–brain barrier and is, therefore, susceptible to systemic circulating agents. Microinjection of adenosine into the AP evokes potent hypotensive and bradycardic effects (94), with concomitant reductions in renal sympathetic nerve activity (97). Neuronal cell groups located in the spinal cord also participate in cardiovascular regulation (99), and intrathecal administration of adenosine or NECA at the T8–T10 vertebral level results in hypotensive and bradycardic effects (100). The cardiovascular actions of adenosine in the brain, however, are site-specific. No significant cardiovascular effects are observed if adenosine is microinjected into rostral regions of the NTS (101), into sites lateral or ventrolateral to the caudal NTS (91), into regions of the ventrolateral medulla (94), into the lateral hypothalamus and raphe magnus (91), or into lower segments of the spinal cord (i.e., lumbar) (102).

A detailed analysis of the hemodynamic effects of adenosine in the brainstem have raised fundamental questions about the mechanism of action by which this purine affects neuronal cardiovascular function. In general, adenosine has been considered an inhibitory neuromodulator; local iontophoretic application of adenosine inhibits spontaneous neuronal firing in cerebral cortex, hippocampus, thalamus, cerebellum and superior colliculus (103), depresses excitatory synaptic transmission in the olfactory cortex and the hippocampus (104), and inhibits the release of both excitatory and inhibitory neurotransmitters in the brain, including acetylcholine (105), serotonin (106), norepinephrine (70,107), dopamine (108), γ-amminobutyric acid (GABA) (109), and glutamate (110,111).

Given the neuroinhibitory actions of adenosine, its effects in the NTS pose an apparent paradox. In this nucleus, excitatory neurotransmitters, such as glutamate, decrease blood pressure, heart rate, and sympathetic nerve activity (112). These effects are strikingly similar to those of adenosine and opposite to those of GABA, a putative inhibitory neuromodulator (113). These observations suggest that adenosine exerts excitatory actions in the NTS and raise the possibility of an interaction between adenosine and glutamate. Accordingly, it was found that while the intra-NTS administration of the adenosine antagonist DPSPX inhibited the cardiovascular effects of intra-NTS adenosine, it had no effect on glutamate actions. In contrast, kynurenic acid, a glutamate-receptor antagonist, inhibited the effects of both adenosine and glutamate (96). These results suggest that the hemodynamic effects of adenosine may be mediated, at least partially, by an interaction with glutamate in the NTS. It could be proposed, for example, that aden-

osine produces direct activation of glutamate receptors. However, the adenosine analogue PIA did not displace radiolabeled glutamate from its receptors in studies using radioligand binding techniques in rat brainstem membranes that included the NTS. Similarly, glutamate did not displace radiolabeled PIA (100). These results suggest that the interaction observed between adenosine and glutamate cannot be explained at the level of the receptor.

However, the possibility that the cardiovascular actions of adenosine in the NTS is explained by modulation of glutamate levels is supported by recent studies using in vivo microdialysis techniques (96). Perfusion of adenosine through a stereotaxically implanted microdialysis cannula increased the concentrations of interstitial glutamate in the NTS in a dose-dependent manner (Fig. 3). This effect correlated with decreases in arterial blood pressure. The exact mechanism by which adenosine increases the release of glutamate remains to be established. Adenosine could release glutamate directly from the synaptic terminal, could suppress an inhibitory circuit that tonically restrains glutamate release, or could inhibit glutamate uptake or metabolism.

The increase in glutamate levels evoked by adenosine in the NTS is at variance with the reported reduction of glutamate levels produced by adenosine in slices of rat dentate gyrus (111), in hippocampal pyramidal cells, and in hippocampal slices (110). Also, it seems to contradict the widely held view of adenosine acting as an inhibitory neuromodulator. Increasing numbers of studies, however, are finding that adenosine enhances the release of some neurotransmitters and exerts neuroexcitatory actions. For example, adenosine enhanced postsynaptic field potentials evoked by electrical stimulation in recordings from the granular cell layer of guinea pig hippocampal slices at concentrations ranging from 10 nM to 1 μM (114). Higher concentrations produced the classical inhibitory effects of adenosine. These excitatory effects of adenosine in the hippocampus have also been observed by others (115). They could be attributed to activation of A_2 receptors (116) and may involve glutamate release (117). Activation of A_{2a} receptors in rat striatum also increases the release of dopamine (118) and acetylcholine (119). Taken together, these experiments seem to indicate that activation of A_2 adenosine receptors, in areas such as the hippocampus and the NTS, increases the release of neurotransmitters and enhances neuronal excitability. It remains to be established whether this is a widespread phenomenon in the CNS or if it is restricted to the nuclei studied to date.

The physiologic relevance of the cardiovascular effects of adenosine in the CNS has recently been explored. Considering that afferent fibers that relay baroreceptor information make their first synapse in the NTS and that excitatory amino acids such as glutamate may play a role in NTS neurotransmission, it could be postulated that

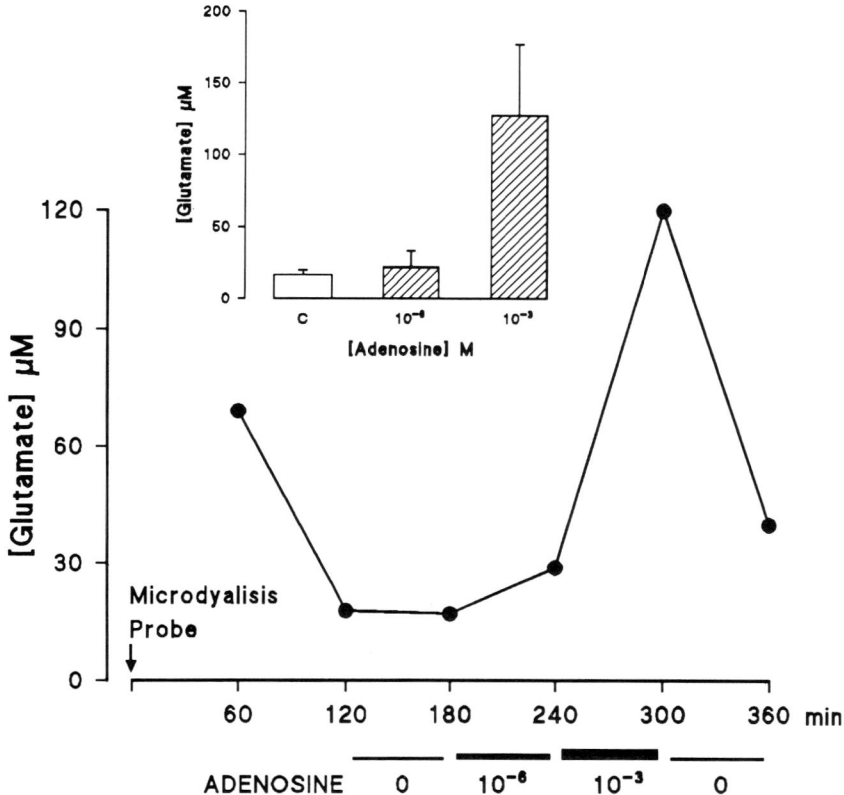

FIG. 3. Effect of adenosine on glutamate release the nucleus tractus solitarii *in vivo*. Increase in glutamate release by adenosine in nucleus tractus solitarii (*NTS*) of rabbits. *Arrow* indicates stereotaxic implantation of microdialysis probe in right NTS. Either artificial cerebrospinal fluid or increasing concentrations of adenosine (10^{-6} and 10^{-3} M) were perfused through the microdialysis probe for 60-minute periods while collecting perfusate for glutamate measurements. **Insert** shows average data.

adenosine is involved in the regulation of baroreflex function. Consistent with this hypothesis, both the intra-NTS microinjection of DPSPX and the intracisternal or intravenous administration of caffeine inhibited the baroreflex-mediated bradycardia elicited by phenylephrine (120). A similar inhibition by caffeine of baroreflex-mediated bradycardia has also been documented in humans (see below) (121). Overall, these results strongly suggest that endogenous adenosine has a facilitatory role on baroreflex activation, presumably by facilitating glutamate release.

The role of CNS adenosine on hypertension is, however, less well understood. Tseng et al. (122) found reduced hypotensive effects after intra-NTS microinjection of adenosine in SHRs compared to WKY rats. It could be postulated that a decrease in the hypotensive effects of endogenous adenosine in the SHR (i.e., by differences in receptor coupling) may lead to increased levels of arterial blood pressure. Although these are intriguing possibilities, it is not clear what role, if any, the central modulatory actions of adenosine play in the development or maintenance of genetic hypertension.

Effects of Adenosine on Afferent Nerves

In contrast to the significant inhibitory actions of adenosine on efferent nerves, there is growing evidence that adenosine produces a widespread excitation of afferent fibers. Indeed, we are not aware of any instance in which adenosine inhibits afferent nerves. The first evidence that adenosine may excite afferent nerves was provided more than a decade ago by McQueen and Ribeiro (123) and Katholi et al. (124). Katholi et al. found that intrarenal infusion of adenosine increased plasma norepinephrine and blood pressure in dogs, in association with an increase in renal afferent nerve activity (Fig. 4). Furthermore, the pressor response to intrarenal adenosine was abolished by renal nerve section, indicating that these effects were due to adenosine-induced activation of renal afferent fibers (124). Infusion of adenosine into the renal pelvis produced identical but earlier hemodynamic and neural responses, suggesting that adenosine chemosensitive fibers are located within or near the renal pelvis (124). Intrarenal infusion of adenosine deaminase, used to lower endogenous adenosine concentration, decreased blood pressure in one-kidney, one-clip rats but not in normotensive rats, suggesting that activation of renal afferent nerves by endogenous adenosine may be relevant to the development of hypertension in this model (125). However, chronic intrarenal infusion of adenosine has no sustained effect on blood pressure in awake normotensive rats, SHR (126), or dogs (127). Therefore, it is unclear if the activation of renal afferents by adenosine is of importance in other forms of hypertension.

McQueen and Ribeiro showed that adenosine also excites the arterial chemoreceptors located in the carotid bodies and aortic arch that are involved in the modulation of respiration. Intracarotid injections of adenosine in cats (128) and rats (129) increase carotid sinus nerve activity, implying carotid body chemoreceptor activation. This effect is independent of the vascular effects of adenosine and is also observed in the isolated superfused cat carotid (130) and aortic (131) bodies. This effect is blocked by 8-phenyltheophylline and is thought to be mediated through A_2 receptors (128). Arterial chemoreceptor activation appears particularly prominent in humans and may explain most of the cardiovascular effects of intravenous adenosine in this species. Intravenous adenosine produces a dramatic increase in minute ventilation in humans. This effect is probably explained by activation of arterial chemoreceptors because adenosine increases blood pressure and stimulates respiration if injected into the aortic arch at a site proximal to the origin of the carotid arteries but decreases blood pressure and has no effect on ventilation when infused into the descending aorta (132,133) (Fig. 5A). These effects are antagonized by theophylline (134,135) and caffeine (136,137) and are potentiated by dipyridamole (138), implying that they are mediated by extracellular adenosine receptors. Furthermore, the pressor effect of adenosine is not observed in patients with autonomic failure, implying that it is due to sympathetic activation (133) (Fig. 5B).

Similarly, intracoronary administration of adenosine increases systemic blood pressure in patients with intact autonomic innervation but not in patients with transplanted, and therefore denervated, hearts (139). This suggests that adenosine stimulates myocardial afferent nerves resulting in sympathetic activation. Less dramatic increases in blood pressure have been reported in other studies involving intracoronary infusion of adenosine in humans (140), but recent animals studies have provided direct evidence of this effect; Montano et al. (141) found that epicardial application of adenosine increases afferent impulse activity from cardiac nerves in cats. A study in sinoaortic denervated and vagotomized dogs, using intracoronary administration of selective adenosine analogues, suggests that the sympathoexcitation produced

by intracoronary adenosine is mediated by A_1 receptors (142). It has been proposed, therefore, that adenosine activates cardiac chemosensitive fibers that form the afferent limb of a sympathetic reflex. It is unclear, however, how much of this effect can be explained by adenosine activation of cardiac sensory afferents evoking pain (143). For example, intraarterial administration of adenosine into the forearm evokes ischemiclike pain, an effect not produced by nitroprusside and, therefore, unrelated to vasodilation (144). Intravenous administration of adenosine in humans can produce chest discomfort, which has been described by volunteers as resembling that of myocardial angina (145) or peptic ulcer (146). Selective intracoronary infusions have confirmed that adenosine can activate sensory afferents located in the heart (140,147). It has been proposed, therefore, that endogenous adenosine, released locally during ischemia, plays an important role in the production of anginal pain. In agreement with this hypothesis, theophylline decreases the severity of exercise-induced chest pain in patients with stable angina (140).

Afferent fibers are also located in skeletal muscle and are activated by isometric exercise, forming the afferent limb of a reflex that results in sympathetic activation and increased blood pressure (148). This exercise pressor reflex has been extensively studied in the human forearm using direct recordings of efferent muscle sympathetic nerve activity (MSNA). It has been shown that voluntary isometric handgrip increases MSNA and blood pressure in humans, in part due to activation of these afferents (149). Intraarterial injection of adenosine into the forearm also increases MSNA and blood pressure, mimicking the exercise pressor reflex (150,151). The sympathoexcitation produced by intrabrachial adenosine in humans is not seen with intrabrachial nitroprusside and, therefore, is unrelated to vasodilation (150). Equivalent painful stimuli produced significantly less increases in MSNA than intrabrachial adenosine (151), suggesting that the change in MSNA produced by intrabrachial adenosine cannot be totally explained by activation of sensory afferents. Chemosensitive afferent fibers involved in the exercise pressor reflex are slow-conducting group IV C-fibers (152) that share the same morphologic and electrophysiologic characteristics of sensory afferent fibers. It is likely, therefore, that adenosine activates both sensory and muscle metaboreceptors in the human forearm. A previous animal study found that adenosine activated only a small proportion of muscle afferents (153), suggesting that this phenomenon predominates in humans.

It is possible, therefore, that adenosine accumulates in skeletal muscle during exercise and activates muscle metaboreceptors, contributing to the initiation of the exercise pressor reflex in humans. In support of this hypothesis, intrabrachial administration of theophylline attenuates the increase in sympathetic activity and in blood pressure produced by sustained handgrip (151). In

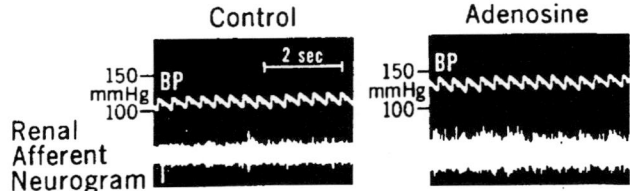

FIG. 4. Activation of Renal Afferents by Adenosine. Effect of infusion of adenosine into the renal artery of an α-chloralose-anesthetized dog on systemic arterial blood pressure (BP) and renal afferent neurogram. (From ref. 124, with permission.)

these studies the exercise pressor reflex was evoked by sustained handgrip at 30 percent of maximal voluntary contraction. This level of muscle contraction produces local ischemia due to compression of arteries by the exercising muscle. It cannot be concluded, therefore, that endogenous adenosine mediates the cardiovascular and neural responses during nonischemic exercise as it apparently does during ischemic exercise.

PHARMACOLOGIC MODULATION OF ADENOSINE MECHANISMS

Drugs that interact with adenosine mechanisms are among the most commonly used in clinical practice. Caffeine and theophylline act as adenosine receptor antagonists in humans (135), and dipyridamole potentiates the actions of adenosine (138) by blocking its uptake. These drugs can be used in humans as pharmacologic probes to gain insight into the role of endogenous adenosine in physiologic and pathophysiologic situations. Doubts about their specificity limit the conclusions than can be derived from their use. More potent and specific adenosine antagonists and uptake inhibitors have been developed and may soon be available for human use. An additional confounding factor is introduced when these drugs are given by systemic administration. In this case, they will interact with adenosine mechanisms throughout the body. As we have seen, adenosine has multiple, and sometimes conflicting, actions. The net effect of systemic blockade of adenosine receptors, or of inhibition of adenosine uptake, therefore, will be the result of a complex interaction between these multiple actions. These limitations need to be considered when reviewing the studies presented below.

Potentiation of Endogenous Adenosine

Dipyridamole is among the 50 most commonly prescribed drugs in the United States. Dipyridamole is an inhibitor of the active nucleoside transport system and, therefore, blocks cellular uptake of adenosine. Dipyridamole is a potent adenosine uptake inhibitor, with a K_i in the 10- to 300-nM range for most animal species, including humans (154). Rats, however, are relatively insensitive to dipyridamole, with a K_i of 3 to 12 μM, making this drug a less useful tool in this species. In agreement with its inhibitory actions on adenosine uptake, dipyridamole potentiates the cardiovascular actions of intravenous adenosine by approximately fourfold in humans (138). Because dipyridamole is a bidirectional blocker of the transport system, it may also prevent adenosine release and may not increase endogenous interstitial adenosine (154). However, studies have estimated an increase in interstitial adenosine by dipyridamole during ischemia (155). The most prominent actions of dipyridamole, coronary vasodilation and inhibition of platelet aggregation, can therefore be ascribed to potentiation of endogenous adenosine. Dipyridamole, however, can have other mechanisms of actions. It is a phosphodiesterase inhibitor, with an IC_{50} of 1 μM (156). These concentrations are higher than those required to inhibit adenosine uptake but are within the plasma levels found in humans of 0.1 to 10 μM (154,157). Finally, some studies suggest that dipyridamole induces the release of prostacyclin, but the importance of this putative action is questionable in humans (157). The best evidence that dipyridamole acts by increasing the actions of endogenous adenosine in humans is that its effects may be blocked by adenosine antagonists (158,159).

The hemodynamic effects of intravenous dipyridamole in humans are those of a vasodilator, reducing systemic vascular resistance and producing a near maximal coronary vasodilation (160). Systolic blood pressure either decreases (160), remains unchanged (158), or increases (159), while diastolic blood pressure decreases (158,160). Blood pressure is maintained despite systemic and regional vasodilation because of an increase in heart rate and cardiac output (160). The simplest interpretation of these hemodynamic changes is that heart rate increases due to baroreflex-mediated sympathetic activation. It has recently been described, however, that intravenous dipyridamole increases minute ventilation and sympathetic activity (161,162), suggesting that dipyridamole activates arterial chemoreceptors. This mechanism, however, may not completely explain the sympathetic activation produced by intravenous dipyridamole because suppression of peripheral chemoreceptor drive by inhalation of 100 percent oxygen abolished the increase in ventilation produced by dipyridamole, but not the increase in sympathetic activity. Excitation of other afferent fibers and vasodilation-mediated baroreflex activation probably also contributes to dipyridamole-induced sympathetic activation.

Dipyridamole can potentially be used to enhance endogenous adenosine in situations in which the accumulation of this nucleoside may be beneficial, such as during myocardial ischemia (163). The systemic effects of dipyridamole, however, may be counterproductive. A pharmacologic agent that would selectively increase adenosine in the ischemic tissue would be advantageous. That was the rationale in developing AICA riboside (Acadesine) as a therapeutic agent in myocardial ischemia (164,165). Acadesine increases the levels of endogenous adenosine in ischemic tissues but is pharmacologically silent in nonischemic tissues. The reason for this selectivity is that it requires active ATP catabolism to function. The precise mechanism of action has not been established fully. Acadesine is a weak inhibitor of adenosine deaminase and adenosine kinase, actions that would raise extracellular adenosine levels by decreasing its metabolism. Acadesine is converted to its 5'-monophosphate metabolite ZMP, which is also a weak inhibitor of AMP deaminase. This will prevent the conversion of AMP to IMP, and the excess AMP then contributes to adenosine formation, whereas IMP would have been converted to inactive inosine. The K_i of Acadesine and it metabolites for blockade of these enzymes is in the low millimolar range. Early human studies have shown promising results in decreasing adverse cardiac events in patients undergoing elective coronary artery bypass graft surgery (166).

Antagonism of Endogenous Adenosine

Caffeine and related methylxanthines exert several pharmacological actions that affect, among others, the cardiovascular, renal, respiratory, and central nervous system. Initially, it was thought that effects on calcium mobilization (167) or inhibition of phosphodiesterases (168) could be responsible for the pharmacologic effects of caffeine. However, subsequent studies have indicated that the major effects of caffeine in humans are exerted via antagonism of adenosine receptors (169), even though other mechanisms cannot be totally excluded (170). Caffeine is a nonselective and relatively weak antagonist of adenosine receptors in vitro ($K_i \approx 40$ to 50 μM). Plasma concentrations of caffeine in vivo can reach 40 μM after oral administration (135). Of interest, the concentrations of caffeine reached in the CNS are equivalent to those found in plasma (171). Also, its main metabolite paraxanthine (1,7-dimethylxanthine) is as potent as caffeine (1,3,7-trimethylxanine) as an adenosine receptor antagonist (135). In contrast, the in vitro concentrations of caffeine needed to produce inhibition of phosphodiesterases range between 0.2 and 1 mM, and the threshold for calcium mobilization is 250 μM (170). These data suggest that methylxanthines act as adenosine receptor antagonists. In agreement with this, caffeine and theophylline block the actions of intravenous adenosine in humans (134–137), and, more importantly, chronic caffeine consumption produces apparent up-regulation of platelet adenosine receptors in humans (135), as would be expected for an antagonist.

Tolerance may develop rapidly for many of caffeine actions. Decreased cardiovascular and locomotor effects of caffeine are seen within 1 to 3 days (170,172). Similar tolerance has been also observed with other methylxanthines. As with many agents that produce tolerance, a withdrawal syndrome has been described for caffeine. In humans, caffeine withdrawal is characterized by headache, irritability, nervousness, and decreased energy and may be due to up-regulation of adenosine receptors.

The cardiovascular effects of caffeine have been studied in some detail. In caffeine-naive normotensive subjects, the acute administration of 250 mg of caffeine (equivalent to 2 cups of coffee) increases blood pressure by approximately 10 to 14 mm Hg and plasma norepi-

nephrine, epinephrine, and renin by 75, 207, and 57 percent, respectively (173). A biphasic effect on heart rate, bradycardia followed by tachycardia, is also present. As mentioned before, after 3 to 4 days of chronic caffeine administration (250 mg three times a day), there are not appreciable effects on cardiovascular function (172). Changes in baroreflex function and in central sympathetic tone are likely involved in the acute pressor effect of caffeine. The acute oral administration of caffeine reduced baroreflex sensitivity in caffeine-free normotensive subjects from a basal of 31 ± 7 msec/mm Hg to 11 ± 2 msec/mm Hg 30 minutes after caffeine (121). The administration of caffeine has also been shown to increase muscle sympathetic nerve activity by approximately 138 percent (174). Overall, these results indicate that several prohypertensive factors are set in motion by the presence of caffeine, including an increase in renin levels, inhibition of cardiovascular reflex adaptative mechanisms (decreased baroreflex function), and activation of pressor sympathetic mechanisms (increase in plasma catecholamines and neural sympathetic function).

Because of these observations, it has been considered important to assess the effects of caffeine in hypertension (175). Overall, the hemodynamic response to acute caffeine in hypertensive subjects seems to be less than in normotensive controls. In borderline hypertensive subjects, the response to caffeine (250 mg) was characterized by a modest increase in systolic blood pressure (9 ± 3 mm Hg) without a change in diastolic pressure (175). Although there was a slight rise in plasma norepinephrine, there were no changes in plasma epinephrine or in plasma renin levels. Although there are no studies addressing the effects of caffeine on baroreflex function and in central sympathetic function in human hypertension, experiments in hypertensive animals also indicate an important relationship between adenosine, renin, and caffeine in cardiovascular control. As mentioned before, adenosine levels are elevated in the two-kidney, one-clip renovascular hypertensive rat and may provide a partial compensation for the elevated renin activity (61). When caffeine is administered in these animals, not only does tolerance to its cardiovascular effects not develop, but blood pressure importantly increases above the already basal hypertensive levels. A high proportion of these animals develop malignant hypertension and die (63). Although there are no extensive clinical data evaluating caffeine effects in humans with renovascular hypertension, one recent study indicated that acute intravenous administration of caffeine failed to increase renal vein renin in the stenotic side of subjects with renovascular hypertension (176).

From these and other reports, it appears that the increase in blood pressure after caffeine administration results from antagonism of adenosine at different levels, including the kidney and the CNS. It is particularly intriguing that a continuous intraperitoneal infusion for 1 week of the specific adenosine antagonist DPSPX produced significant hypertension in normotensive Wistar rats whereas a controlled infusion had no effect (177). Tolerance to the cardiovascular effects of DPSPX was not apparent in this study. However, it is not clear what, if any, would be the clinical significance of these actions. Caffeine is one of the most extensively used pharmacologic agents in the world. It has been estimated that more than 1 billion kilograms of coffee are consumed annually in the United States (178). Epidemiologic studies, however, suggest that the medical risks associated with coffee consumption are relatively low. A study in about 10,000 hypertensive subjects found no increased risk in mortality, cerebrovascular accidents, or cardiovascular diseases in relation to the consumption of coffee (179). Similarly, moderate consumption of coffee does not increase the risk of myocardial infarction (180). The data in heavy caffeine drinkers are conflicting and often confounded by smoking and ethanol consumption. Finally, some reports have suggested the presence in coffee of an agent that induces hypercholesterolemia, and that may explain the elevation of blood cholesterol in coffee drinkers in Nordic European countries (181).

A more recent consideration has been the potential implications caffeine ingestion in nonregular drinkers during periods of stress. An increase in coffee consumption is observed during heightened occupational demand or during conflicting emotional settings. Because stress per se is a factor known to increase blood pressure, its combination with coffee (particularly in nonregular coffee drinkers) may have a significant clinical effect. There are, however, very few studies addressing the cardiovascular effects of coffee consumption and stress. The few available reports indicate that an additive pressor effect results from the combination of caffeine and mental stress (182,183). Importantly, the combination of these two factors may increase blood pressure to hypertensive levels (184). At the present time, we have no information about the long-term effects of consumption of coffee during periods of stress, nor do we know whether tolerance to coffee can be overcome by increasing ingestion of coffee during stressful situations. Clearly, additional research is necessary to address the potential deleterious medical effects of the combination of coffee and stress.

ADENOSINE AND ADENOSINE ANALOGUES AS POTENTIAL THERAPEUTIC AGENTS IN HYPERTENSION

Because adenosine dilates most vascular beds, depresses sinus node automaticity, and inhibits norepinephrine and renin release, adenosine could be considered

an ideal antihypertensive agent. Indeed, intravenous adenosine lowers blood pressure in most animal species without the reflex activation of sympathetic or renin mechanisms characteristic of other vasodilators (47). Furthermore, intravenous adenosine produces significant hypotension in SHR, which is diminished after ganglionic blockade (126), implying that in vivo inhibition of sympathetic tone contributes to the hypotensive action of adenosine in the SHR. Intravenous adenosine is also a potent hypotensive agent in anesthetized humans (185). In this setting, adenosine-induced hypotension is characterized by reduced systemic vascular resistance in parallel with increased cardiac output and only a moderate increase in heart rate. This is probably due to the lack of the compensatory activation of the sympathetic and renin systems (47), thus providing remarkably stable hypotension without tachyphylaxis or rebound hypertension. Its usefulness, however, has been hampered by the renal and myocardial effects of adenosine. Intravenous adenosine, given to anesthetized patients after coronary artery bypass surgery, decreased renal blood flow, glomerular filtration rate and urine output (51). These effects are most likely caused by preglomerular vasoconstriction and probably reflect transient hemodynamic changes rather than structural renal damage because they are completely reversed to a transient hyperemia upon discontinuation of the infusion. Perhaps of greater importance are the cardiac effects of intravenous adenosine. Adenosine produces significant coronary vasodilation whereas equivalent hypotensive doses of nitroprusside do not (186). Coronary vasodilation can be seen even at small intravenous doses that produced little if any effect on blood pressure (187). Although this effect may be beneficial in some patients, recent studies in patients undergoing coronary artery bypass surgery demonstrated that, when used to control hypertension in the immediate postoperative period, adenosine produced ST segment depression whereas nitroprusside did not (188). Adenosine-induced myocardial ischemia in this setting is probably related to its coronary vasodilating effect, eliciting a "coronary steal" phenomenon, similar to that seen with intravenous dipyridamole.

Given the significant hypotension produced by intravenous adenosine, there has been great interest in developing adenosine analogues for the treatment of hypertension. In reviewing results from adenosine analogues, it must be noted that anesthesia may significantly alter the cardiovascular effects of adenosine. For example, the hypotensive effects of intravenous adenosine are enhanced in anesthetized rats, and bradycardia is observed only in anesthetized but not in conscious rats (189). These differences are probably explained by the impairment of autonomic reflexes produced by anesthesia. Even greater differences are found between anesthetized and conscious humans (see below). Also, virtually all studies of adenosine analogs have been performed in rats

(190–198), an issue that may be important when we discuss potential species differences in the cardiovascular effects of adenosine.

A_1-selective agonists are potent antihypertensive agents in normotensive and spontaneously hypertensive rats (190,191,199). The mechanism of this hypotensive action is unclear. Indirect evidence suggests that A_1 agonists do not produce significant vasodilation in rats (190). However, A_1 agonists significantly decrease plasma renin activity (190,199) and heart rate (190,191,199) in rats. The bradycardia is thought to contribute to the hypotensive effects of these agents in rats by lowering cardiac output (190).

Perhaps because of the profound bradycardia produced by A_1 agonists in rats, the development of adenosine agonists as antihypertensives has focused on A_2-selective agonists (191,195,196,198). A_2 agonists produce a decrease in blood pressure due to systemic vasodilation with no apparent negative effects on myocardial contractility (192). On the contrary, cardiac output increases mostly due to a significant tachycardia (190–192,199). There is also a marked increase in plasma renin activity (190,199). The increases in heart rate and plasma renin activity can be explained almost completely by reflex activation of the sympathetic nervous system because they are abolished by β-adrenergic blockade (190,192). The hemodynamic and humoral effects of A_2-selective agonists in rats, therefore, are those of a pure vasodilator.

A potential problem in relying solely on rat studies to determine the hypotensive actions of adenosine is the significant species differences found in the cardiovascular effects of this nucleoside. The depressant effect of adenosine on AV nodal conduction, for example, is greater in guinea pig hearts than in rat and rabbit hearts, whereas the reverse applies to the sinoatrial slowing. These differences are probably explained by a lower number of binding sites for A_1 receptors in guinea pig compared with rat or rabbit atrial membranes (19,200). The overall hemodynamic responses to adenosine analogues may also differ between species. In contrast to the profound bradycardia and lack of vasodilation produced by A_1-selective agonists in anesthetized rats (191), Gerencer et al. (199) found that the A_1-selective agonist CHA (N^6-cyclohexyladenosine) produced significant systemic vasodilation and hypotension in dogs. No significant effect on myocardial contractility was observed. On the contrary, cardiac index and heart rate increased significantly. Both these effects were abolished by cardiac autonomic blockade with combined β-adrenergic and cholinergic antagonists, implying that CHA was acting as a pure vasodilator eliciting reflex sympathetic activation. PR interval, measured during atrial pacing, shortened significantly in contrast to the AV block expected for an A_1 agonist. This effect was also abolished by autonomic blockade. The A_2-selective agonist PAA had an identical hemodynamic profile. The hemodynamic profile of A_1-selective agonists in the dog is that of an arteriolar vasodilator and is totally different from that observed in rats. In particular, the profound bradycardia observed in rats is not found in dogs.

Perhaps of greater significance to the development of clinically effective antihypertensive adenosine analogues are the differences in the hemodynamic effects of adeno-

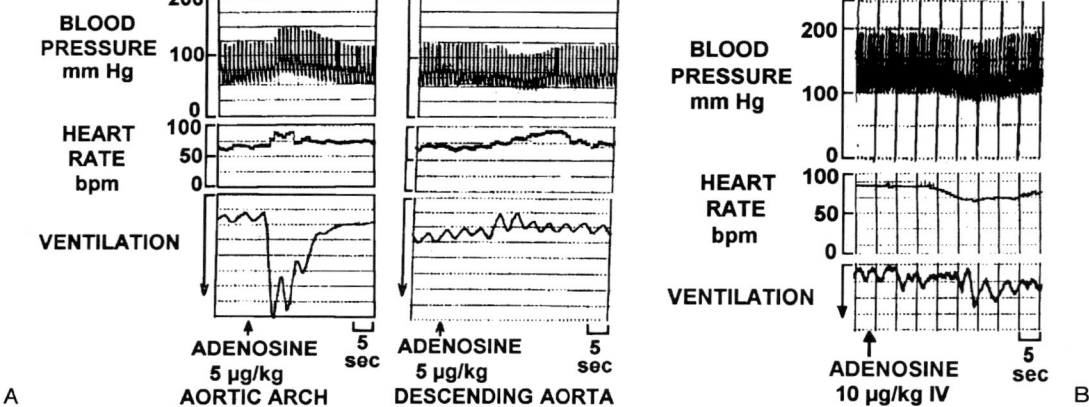

FIG. 5. Cardiovascular and respiratory effects of adenosine in humans. A. Differential effects of bolus injections of adenosine in humans, depending on the site of administration. Adenosine increases blood pressure and stimulates ventilation when infused into the aortic arc proximal to the origin of the carotid arteries (left panel), but lowers blood pressure and has no effect on ventilation when infused into the descending aortic (right panel). These different effects are likely due to activation of aortic chemoreceptors as shown in animal models. B. Effects of adenosine in the absence of functional autonomic reflexes. Adenosine lowers blood pressure and produces bradycardia in patients with primary autonomic failure, implying that the pressor effect found in normal subjects is due to a sympathetic reflex. (Data from ref. 133, with permission.)

sine in humans compared with most other animal species. Intravenous adenosine lowers blood pressure in virtually all animal models. In contrast, intravenous adenosine increases heart rate, systolic blood pressure, sympathetic efferent nerve activity (201), and plasma catecholamines (138) in conscious humans (Fig. 6). The cardiovascular effects of adenosine in conscious humans are completely caused by sympathetic activation because adenosine produces hypotension and bradycardia in patients with degeneration of the autonomic nervous system (133) (Fig. 5). This notable sympathetic activation is not explained by compensatory baroreflex mechanisms triggered by vasodilation, because it is significantly greater than that produced by intravenous nitroprusside at equivalent vasodilator doses (201). The effects of intravenous adenosine in conscious humans can be explained to a large extent by arterial chemoreceptor activation; adenosine increases blood pressure and stimulates respiration if infused into the aortic arch at a site proximal to the origin of the carotid arteries but decreases blood pressure and has no effect on ventilation when infused into the descending aorta (132,133). The extremely short half-life of adenosine in humans may contribute to the magnitude of arterial chemoreceptor activation during intravenous administration; plasma concentrations of adenosine, and its effectiveness, will be greatest near the site of injection (e.g., coronary arteries, carotid bodies) and will decrease exponentially at more distant sites (e.g., peripheral vasculature). However, given the magnitude of adenosine-induced sympathetic activation in humans, it is unlikely that longer-acting adenosine analogues will be devoid of sympathoexcitatory effects. Prolonging the half-life of adenosine with dipyridamole, for example, did not alter the hemodynamic profile of intravenous adenosine; tachycardia, increased blood pressure, and respiratory stimulation still predominated whereas hypotension was not observed (138).

Because the receptor type that mediates the sympathoexcitatory effects of adenosine is not known, it is difficult to predict whether A_1- or A_2-selective agonists will be more useful in lowering blood pressure in humans. Perhaps because of its predominance in humans, only a handful of studies have examined these excitatory effects in animals. This paucity of animal studies has limited our understanding on the molecular mechanisms of the excitatory actions of adenosine. A_2 receptors appear to mediate the activation of arterial chemoreceptors (128), and A_{2a} receptors may be involved in the neuroexcitatory actions of adenosine in the NTS (14) and in other CNS nuclei. However, the sympathoexcitatory effects of intracoronary adenosine are reportedly mediated through A_1 receptors (142). Clearly more studies are needed in this area before adenosine analogues are developed in a rational manner. Significant knowledge will be gained by the development of selective agonists and antagonists that can be used experimentally in humans.

ACKNOWLEDGMENT

This chapter was supported in part by grants HL14192 (Specialized Center of Research in Hypertension) and RR00095 (Clinical Research Center) from the National Institutes of Health.

REFERENCES

1. Jarvis SM. *Mol Pharmacol* 1986;30:659–665.
2. Bockman EL, McKenzie JE. *Am J Physiol* 1983;244:H552–H559.
3. Moser GH, Schrader J, Deussen A. *Am J Physiol* 1989;256:C799–C806.
4. Londos C, Cooper DMF, Wolff J. *Proc Natl Acad Sci* 1980;77:2551–2554.
5. Feoktistov I, Biaggioni I. *Mol Pharmacol* 1993;43:909–914.
6. Libert F, Schiffmann SN, Lefort A, et al. *EMBO J* 1991;10:1677–1682.
7. Maenhaut C, Van Sande J, Libert F, et al. *Biochem Biophys Res Commun* 1990;173:1169–1178.
8. Rivkees SA, Reppert SM. *Mol Endocrinol* 1992;6:1598–1604.
9. Zhou Q-Y, Li C, Olah ME, Johnson RA, Stiles GL, Civelli O. *Proc Natl Acad Sci USA* 1992;89:7432–7436.
10. Ramkumar V, Stiles GL, Beaven MA, Ali H. *J Biol Chem* 1993;268:16887–16890.
11. Anand-Srivastava MB. *Biochem Pharmacol* 1988;37:3017–3022.
12. Matias A, Zimmer FJ, Lorenzen A, Keil R, Schwabe U. *Eur J Pharmacol* 1993;244:223–230.
13. Ungerer M, Obermaier-Skrobranek B, Lohse MJ. *Eur J Pharmacol* 1992;226:381–382.
14. Barraco RA, El-Ridi MR, Ergene E, Phillis JW. *Brain Res Bull* 1991;26:59–84.
15. Bottiglieri DF, Robertson D, Jackson EK. *Hypertension* 1988;12:102–107.
16. Williams EF, Udofia UP, Brooks GR, Hawk NN. *Life Sci* 1990;46:1007–1012.
17. Davies LP, Hambley JW, Johnston GAR. *Neurochem Int* 1987;10:533–536.
18. Jarvis SM, Hammond JR, Paterson ARP, Clanachan AS. *Biochem J* 1982;208:83–88.
19. Froldi G, Belardinelli L. *Circ Res* 1990;67:960–978.

HEART RATE	65 ± 4	97 ± 6	bpm
BLOOD PRESSURE	128 ± 4 / 69 ± 4	138 ± 4 / 63 ± 5	mmHg
C.V.P.	4 ± 1	4 ± 1	mmHg
VENTILATION	7.8 ± 0.7	14.8 ± 1.2	L/min
M.S.N.A	198 ± 52	452 ± 92	Units

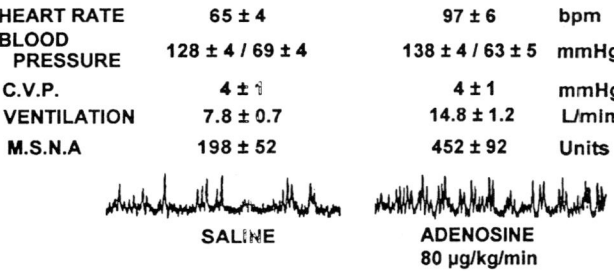

SALINE   ADENOSINE
                80 µg/kg/min

FIG. 6. Increase in sympathetic nerve activity produced by adenosine in humans. Figure shows effect of saline or adenosine on heart rate, blood pressure, central venous pressure (*C.V.P.*), minute ventilation, and muscle sympathetic nerve activity (*M.S.N.A.*) in normal volunteers. Adenosine was infused intravenously as a constant infusion. Sympathetic nerve activity was measured through an electrode placed in a peroneal nerve. (Data from ref. 201, with permission.)

20. Bellardinelli L, Linden J, Berne RM. *Prog Cardiovasc Dis* 1989;32:73–97.
21. Dobson JG Jr, Ordway RW, Fenton RA. *Am J Physiol* 1986;251: H455–H462.
22. Seitelberger R, Schutz W, Schlappack O, Raberger G. *Naunyn Schmiedebergs Arch Pharmacol* 1984;325:234–239.
23. Lerman B. *Circulation* 1993;87:382–390.
24. Webb RL, Sills MA, Chovan JP, Balwierczak JL, Francis JE. *Cardiovasc Drug Rev* 1992;10:26–53.
25. Bradley AB, Morgan KG. *Am J Physiol* 1985;248:H109–H117.
26. Daut J, Maier-Rudolph W, von Beckerath N, Mehrke G, Gunther K, Goedel-Meinen L. *Science* 1990;247:1341–1344.
27. Belloni FL, Hintze TH. *Am J Physiol* 1991;261:H720–H727.
28. Yoneyama F, Yamada H, Satoh K, Taira N. *Eur J Pharmacol* 1992;213:199–204.
29. Des Rosiers C, Nees S. *Naunyn Schmiedebergs Arch Pharmacol* 1987;336:94–98.
30. Nees S, Herzog V, Becker BF, Bock M, Des Rosiers C, Gerlach E. *Basic Res Cardiol* 1985;80:515–529.
31. Olsson RA, Davis CC, Khouri EM. *Life Sci* 1977;21:1343–1350.
32. Rubanyi G, Vanhoutte PM. *J Cardiovasc Pharmacol* 1985;7: 139–144.
33. Konishi M, Su C. *Hypertension* 1983;5:881–886.
34. Yen M-H, Wu C-C, C W-F. *Hypertension* 1988;11:514–518.
35. Headrick JP, Berne RM. *Am J Physiol* 1990;259:H62–H67.
36. Klabunde RE, Laughlin MH, Armstrong RB. *J Appl Physiol* 1988;64:108–114.
37. Berne RM. *Circ Res* 1980;47:807–813.
38. Dobson JG Jr, Rubio R, Berne RM. *Circ Res* 1971;29:375–384.
39. Schwartz LM, McKenzie JE. *Am J Physiol* 1990;259:H1295–H1304.
40. Costa F, Angel M, Cavalcante J, Haile V, Biaggioni I. *Circulation* 1992;86:
41. Osswald H. *Naunyn Schmiedebergs Arch Pharmacol* 1975;288: 79–86.
42. Osswald H. *Trends Pharmacol Sci* 1984;5:94–97.
43. Hall JE, Granger JP, Hester RL. *Am J Physiol* 1986;250:F917–F923.
44. Biaggioni I. *Hypertension* 1992;20:457–465.
45. Biaggioni I, King LS, Enayat N, Robertson D, Newman JH. *Circ Res* 1989;65:1516–1525.
46. Neely CF, Pellack D, Kadowitz P. *FASEB J* 1989;3:A280 (abst).
47. Edlund A, Sollevi A, Linde B. *Clin Sci* 1990;79:131–138.
48. vom Dahl S, Wettsetin M, Gerok W, Haussinger D. *Biochem J* 1990;270:39–44.
49. Nakane T, Chiba S. *Heart Vessels* 1990;5:71–75.
50. Auch-Schwelk W, Katusic ZS, Vanhoutte PM. *Hypertension* 1990;15:699–703.
51. Zall S, Milocco I, Ricksten SE. *Anesth Analg* 1993;76:493–497.
52. Tagawa H, Vander AJ. *Circ Res* 1970;26:327–338.
53. Jackson EK. *Annu Rev Pharmacol Toxicol* 1991;31:1–35.
54. Churchill PC, Churchill MC. *J Pharmacol Exp Ther* 1985;232: 589–594.
55. Kuan C-J, Wells JN, Jackson EK. *J Pharmacol Exp Ther* 1989;249:110–116.
56. Paul S, Jackson EK, Robertson D, Branch R, Biaggioni I. *J Pharm Exp Ther* 1989;251:183–187.
57. Kuan C-J, Wells JN, Jackson EK. *Circ Res* 1990;66:637–646.
58. Deary G, Branch RA, Jackson EK. *Naunyn Schmiedebergs Arch Pharmacol* 1989;339:690–696.
59. Brown NJ, Porter J, Ryder D, Branch RA. *J Pharmacol Exp Ther* 1991;256:56–61.
60. van Buren M, Bijlsma JA, Boer P, van Rijn HJM, Koomans HA. *Hypertension* 1993;22:728–734.
61. Ohnishi A, Li P, Branch RA, Biaggioni I, Jackson EK. *Hypertension* 1988;12:152–161.
62. Ohnishi A, Li P, Branch RA, Holycross B, Jackson EK. *J Clin Invest* 1986;80:13–16.
63. Ohnishi A, Branch RA, Jackson K, Biaggioni I, Deray G, Jackson EK. *J Clin Invest* 1986;78:1045–1050.
64. Bottiglieri DF, Kost CK Jr, Jackson EK. *J Cardiovasc Pharmacol* 1990;16:101–106.
65. Taddei S, Salvetti A. *J Hypertens* 1992;10(suppl 7):S165–S172.
66. Taddei S, Virdis A, Favilla S, Salvetti A. *Hypertension* 1992;19: 672–675.
67. Smits GJ, Kitzen JM, Perrone MH, Cox BF. *Hypertension* 1993;22:221–230.
68. Dunwiddie TV. *Int Rev Neurobiol* 1985;27:63–139.
69. White TD. *Pharmacol Ther* 1988;38:129–168.
70. Wakade AR, Wakade TD. *J Physiol* 1978;282:35–49.
71. Kamikawa Y, Cline WH, Su C. *Eur J Pharmacol* 1980;66:347–353.
72. Kubo T, Su C. *Eur J Pharmacol* 1983;879:349–352.
73. Jackson EK. *Am J Physiol* 1987;253:H909–H918.
74. Illes P, Rickmann H, Brod I, Bucher B, Stoclet JC. *Eur J Pharmacol* 1989;174:237–251.
75. Kuan C-J, Jackson EK. *Am J Physiol* 1988;255:H386–H393.
76. Richardt G, Waas W, Kranzhofer R, Mayer E, Schomig A. *Circ Res* 1987;61:117–123.
77. Taddei S, Pedrinelli R, Salvetti A. *Circulation* 1990;82:2061–2067.
78. Wiklund NP, Cederqvist B, Gustafsson LE. *Br J Pharmacol* 1989;96:425–433.
79. Hedqvist P, Fredholm BB. *Naunyn Schmiedebergs Arch Pharmacol* 1976;293:217–223.
80. Gustafsson LE. *Acta Physiol Scand* 1981;111:263–268.
81. Henon BK, McAfee DA. *J Physiol* 1983;336:601.
82. Akasu T, Shinnick-Gallagher P, Gallagher JP. *Nature* 1984;311: 62.
83. Delle M, Ricksten SE, Delbro D. *Anesth Analg* 1988;67:307–312.
84. von Borstel RW, Evoniuk GE, Wurtman RJ. *J Pharmacol Exp Ther* 1986;236:344–349.
85. Bender AS, Wu PH, Phillis JW. *J Neurochem* 1980;35:629–640.
86. Goodman RR, Snyder SH. *J Neurosci* 1982;2:1230–1241.
87. Marangos PF, Patel J, Clark-Rosenberg R, Martino AM. *J Neurochem* 1982;39:184–191.
88. Nagy J, Labella LA, Buss M, Daddona PE. *Science* 1984;224: 166–168.
89. Bender AS, Wu PH, Phillis JW. *J Neurochem* 1981;36:651–660.
90. Hedner T, Hedner J, Wessberg P, Jonasson T. *Neurosci Lett* 1982;33:147–151.
91. Barraco R, Phillis JW, Campbell WR, Marcantonio DR, Salah RS. *Neuropharmacology* 1986;25:675–680.
92. Laborit H, Manzo-Fay G, Baron C, Hasni H. *Res Commun Chem Pathol Pharmacol* 1990;68:307.
93. Deckert J, Bisserbe JC, Klein E, Marangos PJ. *J Neurosci* 1957;8: 2338–2347.
94. Tseng CJ, Biaggioni I, Appalsamy M, Robertson D. *Hypertension* 1988;11:191–197.
95. Barraco RA, Janusz CJ, Polasek PM, Parizon M, Roberts PA. *Brain Res Bull* 1988;20:129–132.
96. Mosqueda-Garcia R, Tseng CJ, Appalsamy M, Beck C, Robertson D. *Hypertension* 1991;18:494–502.
97. Mosqueda-Garcia R, Appalsamy M, Robertson D. *Neuroscience* 1989;15:1178.
98. Barraco RA, Janusz CJ. *Med Sci Res* 1988;16:977–979.
99. Galosy RA, Clarke LK, Vasko MR, Crawford IL. *Neurosci Behav Rev* 1981;5:137–175.
100. Mosqueda-Garcia R, Tseng CJ, Beck C, McCormick M, Robertson D. In: Kunos G, Ciriello J, eds. New York: Springer-Verlag; 1991:165–180.
101. Barraco RA, Polasek PM, Janusz CJ, Campbell WR, Schoener EP. *Gen Pharmacol* 1987;18:405–416.
102. Sosnowski M, Stevens CW, Yaksh TL. *J Pharmacol Exp* 1989;250:915–922.
103. Phillis JW, Kostopoulou GW, Limacher JJ. *Can J Physiol Pharmacol* 1974;52:1226–1229.
104. Dunwiddie TV, Proctor WR. In: Gerlach E, Becker BF, eds. Berlin: Springer-Verlag, 1987;499–508.
105. Fredholm BB, Duner-Engstrom M, Fastbom J, et al. In: Gerlach E, Becker BF, eds. Berlin: Springer-Verlag, 1987;499–508.
106. Feuerstein TJ, Bar KL, Lucking CH. *Naunyn Schmiedebergs Arch Pharmacol* 1988;338:664–670.
107. Phillis JW, Barraco RA. *Adv Cyclic Nucleotide Protein Phosphorylation Res* 1985;19:243–257.
108. Michaelis ML, Michaelis EK, Myers SI. *Life Sci* 1979;27:2083–2092.

109. Hollins C, Stone TW. *Br J Pharmacol* 1980;69:107–112.
110. Corradetti R, LoConte G, Moroni F, Passani MB, Pepeu G. *Eur J Pharmacol* 1984;104:19–26.
111. Dolphin AC, Archer ER. *Neurosci Lett* 1983;43:49–54.
112. Talman WT. *Neurosci Lett* 1989;102:247–252.
113. Kubo T, Kihara M. *Neurosci Lett* 1988;89:156–160.
114. Nishimura S, Mohri M, Okada Y, Mori M. *Brain Res* 1990;525: 165–169.
115. Ameri A, Jurna I. *Brain Res* 1991;546:69–78.
116. Sebastiao AM, Ribeiro JA. *Neurosci Lett* 1992;138:41–44.
117. Sakurai T, Okada Y. *J Physiol* 1992;446:380P.
118. Zeiterstrom T, Fillen M. *Eur J Pharmacol* 1990;180:137–143.
119. Brown SJ, James S, Reddington M, Richardson PJ. *J Neurochem* 1990;55:31–38.
120. Mosqueda-Garcia R, Tseng CJ, Appalsamy M, Robertson D. *Eur J Pharmacol* 1989;174:119–122.
121. Mosqueda-Garcia R, Tseng CJ, Biaggioni I, Robertson RM, Robertson D. *Clin Pharmacol Ther* 1990;48:568–574.
122. Tseng CJ, Mosqueda-Garcia R, Appalsamy M, Robertson D. *Clin Res* 1988;36:264A (abst).
123. McQueen DS, Ribeiro JA. *Br J Pharmacol* 1981;74:129–136.
124. Katholi RE, Hageman GR, Whitlow PL, Woods WT. *Hypertension* 1983;5(Suppl I):I-149–I-154.
125. Katholi RE, McCann WP, Woods WT. *Hypertension* 1985;7: I88–I93.
126. Ohnishi A, Biaggioni I, Deray G, Branch RA, Jackson EK. *Hypertension* 1986;8:391–398.
127. Hall JE, Granger JP. *Am J Physiol* 1986;250:F32–F39.
128. McQueen DS, Ribeiro JA. *Br J Pharmacol* 1986;88:615–620.
129. Monteiro EC, Ribeiro JA. *Naunyn Schmiedebergs Arch Pharmacol* 1987;335:143–148.
130. Runold M, Cherniack NS, Prabhakar NR. *Resp Physiol* 1990;80: 299–306.
131. Runold M, Cherniack NS, Prabhakar NR. *Neurosci Lett* 1990;113:111–114.
132. Watt AH, Reid PG, Stephens MR, Routledge PA. *Br J Clin Pharmacol* 1987;23:486–490.
133. Biaggioni I, Olafsson B, Robertson RM, Hollister AS, Robertson D. *Circ Res* 1987;61:779–786.
134. Maxwell DL, Fuller RW, Conradson T-B, et al. *Acta Physiol Scand* 1987;131:459–465.
135. Biaggioni I, Paul S, Puckett A, Arzubiaga C. *J Pharmacol Exp Ther* 1991;258:588–593.
136. Smits P, Boekema P, De Abbreu R, Thien T, van't Laar A. *J Cardiovasc Pharmacol* 1987;10:136–143.
137. Smits P, Lenders JWM, Thien T. *Clin Pharmacol Ther* 1990;48: 410–418.
138. Biaggioni I, Onrot J, Kincaid D, Hollister AS, Robertson D. *Life Sci* 1986;39:2229–2236.
139. Cox DA, Vita JA, Treasure CB, Fish RD, Selwyn AP, Ganz P. *J Clin Invest* 1989;84:592–596.
140. Crea F, Pupita G, Galassi AR, et al. *Circulation* 1990;81:164–172.
141. Montano N, Lombardi F, Ruscone TG, Contini M, Guazzi M, Malliani A. *Cardiologia* 1991;36:953–959.
142. Dibner-Dunlap ME, Kinugawa T, Thames MD. *Am J Physiol* 1993;265:H395–H400.
143. Bleehan T, Keele CA. *Pain* 1977;3:367–377.
144. Sylven C, Jonzon B, Fredholm B, Kaijser L. *Cardiovasc Res* 1988;22:674–678.
145. Sylven C, Jonzon B, Edlund A. *Eur Heart J* 1989;10:48–54.
146. Watt AH, Lewis DJM, Horne JJ, Smith PM. *Br Med J* 1987;294: 10–12.
147. Langerqvist B, Sylven C, Beermann B, Helmius G, Waldenstrom A. *Cardiovasc Res* 1990;24:609–613.
148. Mitchell JH, Kaufman MP, Iwamoto GA. *Annu Rev Physiol* 1983;45:229–242.
149. Mark AL, Victor RG, Nerhed C, Wallin BG. *Circ Res* 1985;57: 461–469.
150. Costa F, Biaggioni I. *J Pharmacol Exp Ther* 1993;267:1369–1374.
151. Costa F, Biaggioni I. *J Clin Invest* 1994;93: in press.
152. Kaufman MP, Rybicki KJ, Waldrop TG, Mitchell JH. *J Appl Physiol* 1984;56:1265–1271.
153. Rotto DM, Kaufman MP. *J Appl Physiol* 1988;64:2306–2313.
154. Newby AC. *Biochem J* 1986;237:845–851.
155. Knabb RM, Gidday JM, Ely SW, Rubio R, Berne RM. *Am J Physiol* 1984;247:H804–H810.
156. Weishaar RE, Burrows SD, Kobylarz DC, Quade MM, Evans DB. *Biochem Pharmacol* 1986;35:787–800.
157. FitzGerald GA. *N Engl J Med* 1987;316:1247–1257.
158. Sollevi A, Ostergren J, Fagrell B, Hjemdahl P. *Acta Physiol Scand* 1984;121:165–171.
159. Smits P, Straatman C, Pijpers E, Thien T. *Clin Pharmacol Ther* 1991;50:529–537.
160. Brown BG, Josephson MA, Petersen RB, et al. *Am J Cardiol* 1981;48:1077–1085.
161. Engelstein E, Somers V, Clary MP, Lerman B, Rea RF. *Circulation* 1992;86:I-368.
162. Lucarini AR, Picano E, Marini C, Favilla S, Salvetti A, Distante A. *Chest* 1992;102:444–447.
163. Van Belle H. *Cardiovasc Res* 1993;27:68–76.
164. Mauser M, Hoffmeister HM, Nienaber C, Schaper W. *Circ Res* 1985;56:220–230.
165. Gruber HE, Hoffer ME, McAllister DR, et al. *Circulation* 1989;80:1400–1411.
166. Leung J, Stanley T, Matthew J, et al. *J Am Coll Cardiol* 1992;19: 112A.
167. Katz AM, Repke DI, Hasselbach W. *J Biol Chem* 1977;252: 1938–1949.
168. Butcher RW, Sutherland EW. *J Biol Chem* 1962;237:1244–1250.
169. Rall TW. *Pharmacologist* 1982;24:277–287.
170. Daly JW. In: In: Garatini S, ed. New York: Raven Press; 1991: 97–150.
171. Biaggioni I, Paul S, Robertson D. *Clin Chem* 1988;34:2345–2348.
172. Robertson D, Wade D, Workman R, Woosley RL, Oates JA. *J Clin Invest* 1981;67:1111–1117.
173. Robertson D, Frolich JC, Carr RK, et al. *N Engl J Med* 1978;298: 181–186.
174. Mosqueda-Garcia R, Robertson D, Robertson RM. In: In: Garatini S, ed. New York: Raven Press, 1991:157–176.
175. Robertson D, Hollister AS, Kincaid D, et al. *Am J Med* 1984;77: 54–60.
176. Postma CT, Smits P, Rosenbusch G, Thien T. *Am J Hypertens* 1991;4:951–954.
177. Matias A, Albino-Teixeira A, Pol:onia J, Azevedo I. *Eur J Pharmacol* 1991;193:101–104.
178. Somani SM, Gupta P. *Int J Clin Pharmacol Ther Toxicol* 1988;26:521–533.
179. Hypertension Detection and Follow-up Program Cooperative Group. *JAMA* 1979;242:2562–2571.
180. Heyden S, Tyroler HA, Heiss G, Hames CG, Bartel A. *Arch Intern Med* 1978;138:1472–1475.
181. Tverdal A, Stensvold I, Solvoll K, Foss OP, Lung-Larsen P, Bjartveit K. *Br Med J* 1990;300:566–569.
182. Lane JD, Williams RB. *Psychophysiology* 1985;22:648–655.
183. France C, Ditto B. *J Behav Med* 1988;11:473–482.
184. Pincomb GA, Lovallo WR, Passey RB, Wilson MF. *Am J Cardiol* 1988;61:798–802.
185. Sollevi A, Lagerkranser M, Irestedt L, Gordon E, Lindquist C. *Anesthesiology* 1984;61:400–405.
186. Owall A, Sollevi A. *Acta Anaesthesiol Scand* 1991;35:216–220.
187. Owall A, Ehrenberg J, Brodin LA, Juhlin-Dannfelt A, Sollevi A. *Acta Anaesthesiol Scand* 1993;37:140–148.
188. Zall S, Kirno K, Milocco I, Richsten S-E. *Anesth Analg* 1993;76: 498–503.
189. Biaggioni I, Bennett B, Patel B, Jackson EK, Robertson D. *Clin Res* 1987;35:373A.
190. Webb RL, McNeal RB Jr, Barclay BW, Yasay GD. *J Pharmacol Exp Ther* 1990;254:1090–1099.
191. Francis JE, Webb RL, Ghai GR, et al. *J Med Chem* 1991;34: 2570–2579.
192. Webb RL, Barclay BW, Graybill SC. *J Pharmacol Exp Ther* 1991;259:1203–1212.
193. Milavec-Krizman M, Wagner H̄, Kralj A, Evenou JP, Gadient F. *Nucleosides Nucleotides* 1991;10:1127–1129.

194. Trivedi BK, Blankley CJ, Bristol JA, et al. *J Med Chem* 1991;34:1043–1049.
195. Matsuda A, Shinozaki M, Yamaguchi T, et al. *J Med Chem* 1992;35:241–252.
196. Abiru T, Miyashita T, Watanabe Y, Yamaguchi T, Machida H, Matsuda A. *J Med Chem* 1992;35:2253–2260.
197. Kogi K, Uchibori T, Aihara K, Yamaguchi T, Abiru T. *Jpn J Pharmacol* 1991;57:153–165.
198. Abiru T, Yamaguchi T, Watanabe Y, Kogi K, Aihara K, Matsuda A. *Eur J Pharmacol* 1991;196:69–76.
199. Gerencer RZ, Finegan BA, Clanachan AS. *Br J Pharmacol* 1992;107:1048–1056.
200. Musser B, Morgan ME, Leid M, Murray TF, Linden J, Vestal RE. *Eur J Pharmacol* 1993;246:105–111.
201. Biaggioni I, Killian TJ, Mosqueda-Garcia R, Robertson RM, Robertson D. *Circulation* 1991;83:1668–1675.

Blood Pressure Regulation in Normal and Hypertensive States

Part D: Calcium and Magnesium in Blood Pressure Regulation

Hypertension: Pathophysiology, Diagnosis,
and Management, Second Edition,
edited by J.H. Laragh and B.M. Brenner,
Raven Press, Ltd., New York © 1995.

CHAPTER **68**

Blood Pressure and Calcium and Magnesium Intake

William R. Harlan and Linda C. Harlan

Calcium and magnesium intake have been linked to blood pressure regulation for many years. These linkages have been made at the cellular level and, more recently, through numerous observational and intervention studies. In subjects over 50 years of age, associations were reported between decreased heart disease or hypertension and water hardness, a characteristic of water dependent on its calcium and magnesium content. The first reports described an association between soft-water areas and an increase in heart disease relative to disease in hard-water areas. The ecological associations were supplemented in the 1980s by more structured observational studies that confirmed a small, though fairly consistent, relationship between dietary calcium and blood pressure. These associations were developed generally from studies with dietary questionnaires that were not primarily designed to investigate this relationship, although the relationship was found in a number of different populations and age groups when studied cross-sectionally. Similar associations were reported for magnesium and blood pressure. These populational findings have been buttressed by animal studies that have also disclosed an inverse association between blood

pressure and calcium or magnesium. Based on these observations, interventional trials have been conducted to study the clinical efficacy of increasing calcium or magnesium intake. This chapter presents a review of the clinical and epidemiological studies relating calcium and magnesium to blood pressure. Supplementation studies conducted during pregnancy and those conducted in patients also receiving antihypertensive medications are not included.

CALCIUM AND MAGNESIUM INTAKE FROM WATER

Interest in calcium and magnesium was initially provided by epidemiological studies suggesting a protective effect of water hardness on the development of cardiovascular disease (1–3). The geographic distribution of mineral-rich water corresponded to lower rates of all cardiovascular disease, including stroke and hypertension, and it was inferred that this protective effect came from the water hardness. Hard water contains magnesium and calcium. Soft water contains few minerals, but has greater capacity for leaching minerals such as lead from the reservoirs and pipelines. In localities with mineral-rich water, water supplies can add substantial amounts of calcium and magnesium to the diet. Important amounts of lead may be ingested in soft-water areas that have pipe and/or soldered connections with high lead content, and lead levels have been linked, in turn, with

W. R. Harlan: Division of Disease Prevention, National Institutes of Health, Bethesda, Maryland 20892.

L. C. Harlan: Division of Cancer Prevention and Control, National Cancer Institute, National Institutes of Health, Bethesda, Maryland 20892.

elevated blood pressure (4). Regulations in the United States now prohibit the use of lead-containing pipes or solder in new buildings.

These ecological relationships were stronger in the United Kingdom than elsewhere, but were also found in the United States and Canada (1–3). However, there were exceptions to these patterns. It was apparent the assessment of calcium and magnesium intake were variable and incomplete and were relatively remote from the individual physiological response. Individual intake of water varies, as does the proportion of an individual's total mineral intake that is derived from water. Foods and supplements account for considerable daily mineral intake. Moreover, the specificity of the relationship was questioned, because other ecological and geographic variations might explain the observed patterns of cardiovascular morbidity and mortality. Animal experiments produced inconsistent results, although they generally supported the geographic relationship (5). Population-based studies of dietary intake have provided a more complete and proximate measure of the intake of these cations and their relationships to blood pressure.

DIETARY CALCIUM INTAKE

Approximately 99 percent of the calcium in the body is found in the bones, with the remaining 1 percent in extracellular fluids (6). The Recommended Dietary Allowance (10th edition) (RDA) for calcium was increased to 1,200 mg per day for individuals age 11 to 24 years. For adults age 25 and older the RDA remained at the same level, 800 mg per day. The primary reason given for the increase in the calcium RDA for the 11- to 24-year-olds was concern related to calcium intake and the need to insure bone mineral density during growth. Absorption of calcium is highly variable. Both nutritional and physiological influences affect the absorption. Most notably, vitamin D enhances the absorption of calcium, and estrogens maintain calcium in bone.

An analysis of the National Health and Nutrition Examination Survey II, 1976–1980, found the majority of calcium in the diet (>55 percent) comes from dairy products (7). Other good sources of calcium are broccoli and green leafy vegetables, such as kale and collard greens. The 1989 and 1990 Continuous Survey of Food Intake for Individuals (CSFII) estimates of mean intake of calcium for adults, age 19 and over, are 827 and 622 mg per day for men and women, respectively (8). Calcium intake varies by race and socioeconomic status (9). The United States Department of Agriculture has estimated the intake of calcium to be 640 mg for white women and 452 mg for African-American women (9). A study of African-American adults by Gerber et al. (9) reported that after adjusting for age and energy intake, calcium

intake is greater with higher socioeconomic status in both men and women.

A large number of observational studies have been reported in which dietary calcium intake was related inversely to blood pressure. The design has generally been cross-sectional with relationships being sought from assessments done concurrently, but there are some longitudinal studies. Study populations included both men and women as well as a number of different racial/ethnic groups: Japanese-Americans, Puerto Ricans, African-Americans, and nonminority white persons. The age range included individuals from 20 through 80 years. Direct comparisons across studies are difficult. Each study adjusted for different covariates, and different methods were used to collect the dietary and nondietary data. Lengthy food frequency questionnaires, brief food frequency questions, diet records, and 24-hour dietary recalls have all been used to assess dietary calcium. Although many of these studies used data not primarily collected to study this relationship, the intake estimates are probably not influenced greatly by varying precision of the instruments used. Calcium, unlike many other nutrients, is found in large amounts in a relatively small number of foods consumed regularly in the United States (10). Food frequency questionnaires with as few as ten food items have been found to adequately quantify calcium intake (11). However, confounding effects from other nutrients contained in these foods is a greater problem. It is often not possible to separate the effects of calcium from those of other nutrients found in the same foods. Also, dietary patterns associated with low calcium intake may include increased intake of other foods, such as alcohol, that have the reverse effect on blood pressure. Of equal concern are the relationships between age or socioeconomic status and blood pressure and the parallel associations with calcium intake. The difficulty in disentangling specific causal effects of a single nutrient from these confounding factors is difficult in all observational studies but especially so in cross-sectional analyses.

There have been more than 30 reports on observational studies of calcium and blood pressure. The earliest report by Langford and Watson found, in African-American schoolgirls, an association between low calcium intake and low urinary ratio of sodium to calcium (12). The next report of an association between calcium and blood pressure came in 1982 when McCarron and co-workers (25) reported a lower calcium intake in hypertensives than normotensives. Since that time there have been numerous reports. Most report an inverse relationship, although some find a positive association while others find no association. Analyses of the National Health and Nutrition Examination Survey I (NHANES I) highlight the difficulty of comparing reported observational studies. Using the same data set, different authors report different findings. Exclusion criteria, covariates included, and methods used by the authors varied. McCarron et al. included men and women 18 to 74 years old with no history of hypertension and the analysis did not use the sample design and weighting factors (13). These authors found higher intakes of calcium were associated with lower systolic blood pressures and lower absolute risk of hypertension. Another analysis of the NHANES I data included men and women 18 to 74, excluding only individuals who were on treatment for hypertension or were on a special diet. The sample design and weight factors were accounted for in the analysis. The sample was stratified by gender and adjusted for a large number of covariates. Included in the covariates was serum calcium. At least one author has suggested this was overadjusting (14). Calcium was positively related to systolic blood pressure in men and inversely related to diastolic blood pressure in women (15). In an analysis of older Americans an inverse association between calcium and systolic blood pressure was found in women only (16). Gruchow et al. (17), in an unstratified analysis of the NHANES I data, found no association, after adjusting for age, race, and body mass index. Sempos et al. (18) excluded those under 40 years of age and respondents who regularly or occasionally used antihypertensive agents. Mean blood pressures were examined by quintile of calcium intake; the only significant association was for African-American men.

Overall, the observational studies more often reported an inverse relationship between calcium and either systolic or diastolic blood pressure. Some authors have suggested an nonlinear relationship between calcium and blood pressure, which might help to explain the conflicting results seen in the observational studies. Others have suggested possible effect modifiers, such as dietary sodium, potassium, or vitamin D.

Two interesting prospective studies have been reported. In one prospective study of dietary nutrients and blood pressure, the Nurses' Health Study, the risk of developing hypertension over a 4-year period was investigated (19). More than 58,000 women completed a food frequency questionnaire and were followed for incidence of self-reported hypertension. During those 4 years 3,275 incident cases of hypertension were reported. After controlling for age, body mass index, and alcohol consumption, both calcium and magnesium intake were inversely associated with the risk of hypertension. In another prospective study, an inverse relationship was reported between the blood pressure in infants at 1, 6, and 12 months and prenatal maternal calcium intakes (20).

DIETARY MAGNESIUM INTAKE

The most recent RDA for magnesium for adults, age 19 and over, is 280 mg for women and 350 mg for men

(6). Magnesium intake has reportedly declined substantially since the turn of the century, when it was estimated to be 475 to 500 mg per day (21). Estimates from 1978 to 1985 place average intake at 225 to 318 mg per day. The 1989 and 1990 CSFII mean intake for adults, age 19 and over, is 283 mg per day for men and 215 mg per day for women (8). Green leafy vegetables are good sources of magnesium, as are nuts, legumes, and grains that have not had the germ and/or outer layers removed. Magnesium is found in many unprocessed foods, but can be lost in processing (6). Meat, fish, and milk are low in magnesium and, except for bananas, fruits are relatively poor sources as well. Only about 50 percent of ingested magnesium is absorbed, although absorption varies (6).

Magnesium has been used for many years to prevent convulsions in preeclamptic women, and the blood pressure-lowering effect of magnesium on pregnancy-induced hypertension was a clinical standby before the advent of hypotensive agents. These observations led investigators to examine the association between dietary magnesium and blood pressure. Several careful studies have produced provocative findings (19,22,23). The 46 hypertensives in McCarron's (22) study had lower dietary intakes of both calcium and magnesium. Hypertensives reported a dietary intake of 206 mg per day compared with 261 mg per day for normotensives. In a careful study of actual intake, scientists in Newfoundland asked subjects to prepare twice the usual servings of food (24). The second serving was placed in a container and analyzed for five electrolytes. When dietary magnesium was compared, hypertensives ($n = 48$) consumed 155 mg per day compared with 173 mg per day for normotensives ($n = 125$).

The prospective Nurses' Health Study reported magnesium was related to the development of hypertension. Over 3,000 of the 58,000 nurses developed hypertension over a 4-year period (19). After adjusting for age, Quetelet's index, alcohol, magnesium, and calcium, no other mineral was found to be a significant predictor of hypertension.

SUMMARY OF OBSERVATIONAL STUDIES

The majority of the observational studies have found an inverse relationship between blood pressure and calcium or magnesium or both. Although fewer studies have been published relating dietary magnesium to blood pressure, an inverse relationship is generally reported. However, there may be publication bias. Studies that show no association between calcium or magnesium and blood pressure may be less likely to be published. The relationship in these studies is not especially strong and lessens with adjustment for covariables or changes in study group composition as illustrated by the varying results with different analyses of the NHANES data.

A major concern with the associations between food intake and blood pressure is the lack of specificity for a nutrient effect. Foods are consumed rather than nutrients and it is seldom possible to separate the effects of the various nutrients contained in the food or to account for the effects of nutrients *not* consumed when a particular dietary pattern is followed. Adjustments for total caloric intake, salt use, and alcohol consumption only partially account for these nutrient effects and there may be other unknown confounding factors that could explain the relationship. Interventional studies using specific nutrient supplements and assessing food and nutrient intake can address some of these issues. The use of a randomized controlled design provides for a balance of confounding factors across the interventional and control groups, and further strengthens the inferences.

CALCIUM INTERVENTION STUDIES

Mechanisms

Many explanations have been offered for the inverse relationship between dietary calcium intake and blood pressure. Other chapters in this book discuss these potential physiological mechanisms. However, it is useful to sketch potential mechanisms and their relevance in the context of interventional studies, because these mechanisms may help to explain the findings.

Only a subgroup of persons given increased calcium responded with a drop in blood pressure, and these individuals have been classified as calcium-responsive. Presumably, those whose blood pressure is calcium-responsive require a somewhat higher calcium intake in order to maintain normal blood pressure. There is no means of determining those who are calcium responders except by testing the blood pressure response to increased intake. Therefore, these responsive individuals are usually identified in subgroup analysis after the trial is concluded. Several explanations for responsiveness have been offered. Perhaps the simplest explanation is a direct calcium effect on sodium balance. Increased calcium intake acts to increase sodium excretion in the urine, and thereby decrease pressure. It would be useful to know whether calcium sensitivity and sodium sensitivity of blood pressure to dietary intake are characteristics of the same individual. Equally important is whether these sensitivities vary or remain constant on repeated challenges of the same individual. Such determinations would clarify whether these sensitivities are inherent within individuals and whether linkages exist between sodium and calcium handling and blood pressure.

Considerable attention has been directed toward increased calcium or magnesium intake and the resultant changes in hormonal levels of calcium-regulating hormones, in renin-angiotensin, and in the interaction between the two hormonal systems. These alterations have been explored by Resnick and co-workers and are elaborated elsewhere in this volume. It has been proposed that urinary calcium wasting is an underlying defect in calcium-sensitive hypertension. A normal or increased calcium intake offsets this hypercalciuria and moderates the hormonal imbalance. This mechanism implies that the blood pressure changes result from the hormonal alterations rather than from a direct calcium effect. The hormonal changes could also change blood pressure through an effect on sodium metabolism. Some findings support this mechanism. Persons whose blood pressure responds to increased calcium intake are reported to have higher levels of parathyroid hormone, which may directly or indirectly influence blood pressure.

The cellular effects of calcium on vascular tone have been responsible for much of the interest in calcium intake and blood pressure and seem to provide a physiological explanation and biological plausibility for the epidemiological observations. Although this explanation may have validity, several concerns should be noted. The cellular mechanism is physiologically remote from dietary intake. The levels of total and ionized calcium are closely regulated by hormones, so that wide variations in calcium intake are not matched by major changes in the concentration of calcium surrounding the cells. Intuitively, it is difficult to directly link calcium intake and cellular events except through hormonal changes. This does not imply that cellular calcium flux and levels of cytosolic calcium ion are not important in determining vascular tone or in regulating blood pressure. Rather, considerably more evidence is needed to support a proximate physiological mechanism.

Summary of Clinical Trials

At least 29 clinical trials of calcium supplementation and blood pressure have been published (25–53). These are summarized in Table 1. Both normotensive and hypertensive individuals have been included in studies, with ages ranging from 16 through 86, and different racial/ethnic groups have been participants. The vast majority of these trials used calcium supplementation rather than dietary modification. The dose of calcium administered has varied from 1.0 to 1.5 g with the usual dose being 1 g. The lengths of the interventions have been from 5 days to 4 years. In addition, several clinical trials investigated blood pressure response to calcium supplementation during pregnancy. We will briefly review 29 published calcium and blood pressure intervention trials. Calcium trials during pregnancy and those conducted only on patients receiving thiazides will not be included. Studies are presented by year of publication, with the dietary modification and sodium-loading studies presented last (Table 1).

An early report of the blood pressure effect of calcium supplementation was derived from a study primarily intended to study osteoporosis (25). Postmenopausal women were enrolled in the study and randomized to receive 1.0 to 1.2 g of calcium in addition to placebo, synthetic salmon calcitonin, or stanozolol. The women were followed for 2 years. Women receiving calcium and stanozolol had an increase in their mean arterial pressure. Women receiving calcium and salmon calcitonin had a decrease in their pressure, while those receiving calcium and placebo experienced no change.

A study conducted in Guatemala by Belizan et al. (26) investigated calcium supplementation in a population of 28 men and 29 women who were given 1 g calcium supplementation or a placebo by random allocation. One observer made all blood pressure measurements during the 22-week trial. Women receiving calcium supplements had a 5.6 percent decrease in diastolic blood pressure, stabilizing after 9 weeks, and men a 9 percent decrease stabilizing after 6 weeks.

McCarron and Morris (27) recruited 48 hypertensives and 32 normotensive subjects to participate in a double-blind, calcium supplement–placebo crossover trial. Subjects were given 1000 mg of calcium or placebo for 8 weeks, followed by a 4-week washout period, and then crossed over to either placebo or supplementation. Hypertensive subjects experienced a decrease in blood pressure, but no decrease was observed in normotensive subjects. These authors, using a decline of 10 mm Hg in standing systolic blood pressure as the definition of calcium-sensitive individuals, identified 21 hypertensives and 6 normotensive subjects as calcium-sensitive. However, retrospective subgroup analyses in a clinical trial is hazardous when the subgroup response differs from the overall response.

Data from a 4-year calcium supplementation study of osteoporosis were used to examine the effect of supplemental calcium on blood pressure (28). Women were assigned randomly to calcium supplementation (1.5 g) or placebo. In the 34 hypertensives, a 13 mm Hg decrease in systolic blood pressure was reported in the calcium-supplemented group and a 7 mm Hg increase in the unsupplemented group. No significant changes were seen in the normotensive group. Each woman completed multiple food records (19 to 20 per year) during the final 3 years of the study. When dietary calcium intake was compared, hypertensives, whether supplemented or unsupplemented, tended to have lower dietary calcium intakes than normotensive, but this difference was not statistically significant. This study has the longest duration of calcium supplementation trials and, additionally, food records were recorded frequently. Thus, the finding of blood pressure decrease in hypertensive women is especially noteworthy.

Thirty-two subjects were randomly assigned to 1.5 g calcium or placebo in a 4-week, double-blind trial (29).

Diastolic blood pressures were between 88 and 95 mm Hg, and antihypertensive medications known to affect calcium were discontinued 2 weeks prior to the trial. More than 80 percent of the subjects were black. Based on a "diet history" that used both a food frequency questionnaire and a 24-hour recall, subjects had an average dietary intake of calcium of less than 750 mg per day. Although the 4-week blood pressure did not differ from the baseline values, supine systolic blood pressure in the calcium-supplemented group was actually higher at the second week. There was no change in the blood pressures of the placebo group. When responses within the calcium group were compared, those with increased blood pressure had higher urinary calcium concentrations and higher reported sodium intakes at baseline than those with a decrease or no change in their blood pressure. This study and several other studies have been characterized as being too brief and with inadequate sample size to detect an effect on blood pressure (30,31).

Ninety mildly hypertensive subjects, defined as having three annual systolic readings of 140 mm Hg or higher and/or diastolic readings of 90 mm Hg or higher during the 7 to 9 years prior to the study, were recruited for a double-blind calcium supplementation–placebo study (32). The 77 men and 13 women were randomly assigned to receive 1 g of calcium or a placebo. Blood pressure measurements at 6 and 12 weeks of the study showed a significant decrease in diastolic blood pressure and a small, nonsignificant decrease in systolic pressure. Further analysis showed the decrease to be confined to those individuals with a higher initial parathyroid hormone (PTH) level. It has been suggested that calcium responders may be identified by having higher PTH levels and hypercalciuria, and this study offers support for this view.

Other relative short-term studies reported no reduction in mean blood pressure with calcium supplementation when sodium or potassium intake was controlled (33,34). This finding could be attributable to the blunting of calcium supplementation when sodium or potassium intake is decreased.

Many studies listed in Table 1 have small samples and report variable responses to calcium supplementation, and the conflicting findings from these reports have been attributed to inadequate sample size to detect modest blood pressure effects. Cutler and Brittain (14) performed a metanalysis of trials to overcome the problem of numerous underpowered studies. They reported a small decrease in systolic pressure of 1.8 mm Hg when studies were combined. Another characteristic of many smaller studies is the lack of blood pressure decrease in normotensive persons but a decrease in hypertensive persons. When the effect size is small, it is more difficult to find statistically significant effects with lower pressures.

Morris and McCarron (35) reported on a study of

TABLE 1. *Clinical trials of calcium supplementation and blood pressure*

Location of population	Sample size/age	Patient conditions and study design	Ca^{2+} dose/duration	Results
Oregon (25) 1981	$n = 81$ postmenopausal	Osteoporosis	1–1.2 g 2 years	↓ BP with Ca/salmon calcitonin ↓ in DBP
Guatemala (26) 1983	$n = 57$ Age 18–35	S/P	1 g 22 weeks	
Oregon (27) 1985	$n = 48$ HTN $n = 32$ normal Age 21–70	NTN HTN CR	1 g 8 weeks	↓ in HTN; no change in NTN
Wisconsin (28) 1985	$n = 81$ normal $n = 34$ Rx HTN Age 35–65	NTN Rx HTN S/P	1.5 g 4 years	↓ in HTN; no change in NTN
North Carolina (29) 1986	$n = 32$ Age 18–75	High NTN Mild HTN S/P;D-B	1.5 g 6 weeks	↑ in SBP
England (30) 1986	$n = 8$ Age 20–43	NTN CR	1.8 g Controlled diet 1 week	No change
Netherlands (31) 1986	$n = 58$ women Age 20–23	NTN S/P;D-B	1.5 g Controlled diet 6 weeks	No change
Netherlands (32) 1986	$n = 90$ mild HTN Age 16–29	D-B	1 g 12 weeks	↓ in DBP
Australia (33) 1986	$n = 47$ HTN $n = 48$ NTN Mean age: placebo 60 ± 3 10 mmol 53 ± 5 20 mmol 59 ± 3	NTN; HTN S/P	10 mmol 20 mmol 2 months	No change
Italy (48) 1986	$n = 18$ Mean age 43 ± 9	Mild HTN S/P;D-B;CR	1 g 15 weeks	↓ in standing SBP
Italy (34) 1986	$n = 23$ Mean age 42.6 ± 8.6	M/M HTN S/P;D-B;CR	1 g 8 weeks	No change
Japan (49) 1986	$n = 14$ Mean age: 71 (Ca^{2+}), 73 (Ca^{2+}, D$_3$)	HTN	2 g Ca^{2+} 2 g Ca^{2+} plus D$_3$ 8 weeks	↓ in SBP Ca^{2+} No change Ca^{2+} plus D$_3$
Indiana (50) 1987	$n = 75$ men Age 19–52	NTN S/P	1.5 g 12 weeks	↓ in SBP ↓ in DBP
South Dakota (44) 1987	$n = 24$ women Mean age 57 ± 9.5	Mild HTN	1 g 12 weeks	↓ in SBP
Greece (46) 1987	$n = 18$ Age 25–60	M/M HTN S/P;CR	1 g 5 days	↓ in SBP
England (43) 1987	$n = 18$ Age 28–65	M/M HTN S/P;D-B;CR	1.6 g 1 month	No change
Italy (51) 1987	$n = 8$ Mean age 40 ± 3	Mild HTN S/P;D-B;CR	1 g 3 weeks	No change
Italy (52) (51) 1988, 1987	$n = 15$ Mean age 41 ± 2	Mild HTN S/P;D-B	1 g; low Ca^{2+} diet 4 weeks	No change
California (47) 1991	$n = 19$ Age 30–65	Mild HTN D-B;CR	1.2 g 3 months	No change
Japan (45) 1991	$n = 9$ Age 65–86	HTN CR	1 g 8 weeks	↓ in mean pressures
Oregon (35) 1992	$n = 103$ Age 50–80	HTN D-B	1 g 12/48 weeks	no mean different @ 12 wks
Indiana (36) 1992	$n = 42$ Mean age; placebo 35.9 ± 15.7 Rx 32.3 ± 10.7	HTN D-B	1.5 g 8 weeks	↓ in mean pressures

TABLE 1. *Continued.*

Location of population	Sample size/age	Patient conditions and study design	Ca^{2+} dose/duration	Results
US multicenter (37) 1992	$n = 237$ Ca^{2+} $n = 234$ placebo Age 30–54	S/P;D-B	1 g 6 months	No change
Denmark (53) 1993	$n = 30$ Age 42–75	UnRx HTN S/P;D-B;CR	2 g 12 weeks	Placebo ↓ larger
New Jersey (38) 1988	$n = 50$ Age 21–65	NTN High Ca^{2+} diet CR	1150 mg dietary Ca^{2+} 8 weeks	↓ in SBP
Netherlands (39) 1990	$n = 60$ Age 19–23	NTN D-B	1180 mg vs 95 mg Ca^{2+} mild K$^+$/Mg^{2+} varied 6 weeks	Small ↓ in SBP
Washington (40) 1992	$n = 13$ men Age 46–75	HTN CR	0.4 vs 1.5 g dietary calcium 4 weeks	No change
New York (41) 1986	$n = 8$ Mean age 53 ± 4	HTN Hi vs low salt diet	2 g 1 month	Smaller ↑ in salt sensitive; larger in salt insensitive
Japan (42) 1989	$n = 27$ Age 39–67	Borderline HTN D-B Salt loaded	300 mEq Na$^+$ 2.16 g 1 week	Smaller ↑ in BP

M/M HTN, mild/moderate hypertension; NTN, normotensive; S/P, supplement/placebo; D-B double-blind;
CR, crossover.

calcium supplementation in individuals aged 50 to 80 years with mildly elevated blood pressure. At 12 weeks there was no difference in the mean blood pressures between those on placebo and those on 1 g of calcium carbonate (600 mg elemental calcium). However, 42 of the 103 study subjects had a decrease in blood pressure of at least 5 mm Hg and were continued on calcium supplementation. Their pressures remained lower through the 48 week study. After completion of 48 weeks of calcium supplementation, 12 of these subjects were given placebos for 12 weeks. Systolic blood pressures increased significantly. The authors suggest that although general use of calcium in older individuals may not be warranted, there are individuals who respond to calcium supplementation and whose lowered blood pressure can be maintained for at least a year.

In a 1.5-g calcium double-blind supplementation study Lyle (36) followed 42 adults with diastolic blood pressures of 85 to 104 mm Hg. The calcium supplementation group had a lower mean pressure at 8 weeks than did the placebo regardless of baseline total serum calcium levels.

The Trials of Hypertension Prevention study (TOHP) measured the efficacy of nonpharmacological intervention for individuals with high-normal diastolic blood pressure (80 to 89 mm Hg) (37). The study investigated the effect of weight reduction, sodium reduction, stress management, usual care, calcium supplementation, magnesium supplementation, potassium, fish oil, or placebo on blood pressure. Some 237 subjects were given 1 g calcium per day. Compared with those on placebo, the calcium-supplemented group had no significant change in either systolic or diastolic blood pressure. This carefully performed study measured blood pressure using blinded observers and followed the participants for 6 months. The absence of a significant effect on blood pressure provides evidence that calcium supplementation has little or no efficacy in lowering blood pressure of individuals with high normal pressures, a group for whom nonpharmacological intervention is desirable.

Using dairy products, Bierenbaum and co-workers (38) supplemented the diets of 50 free-living volunteers in a crossover trial. A decline in systolic blood pressure of 5 mm Hg was found during the dairy product supplementation. No change in diastolic pressure was noted.

A 6-week study used modified milk as a means of investigating the relationship between calcium intake and blood pressure (39). Participants were instructed to consume a low-calcium diet (<500 mg/day) while receiving one of the milks. The authors reported a small but significant difference in the systolic blood pressures of normotensive young women drinking "normal" milk with 1180 mg of calcium compared with those drinking milk with 95 mg of calcium at 3 weeks of the study. At 6 weeks a small difference remained, but was not statistically significant. The "mineral poor" milk also had only 580 mg of potassium and 10 mg of magnesium compared with 1650 mg of potassium and 110 mg of magnesium in the "mineral rich" milk.

A crossover study by Kynast-Gales and Massey (40), which varied consumption of dairy products, showed no blood pressure differences for hypertensive men consuming 1500 mg versus 400 mg of dairy products. In this study blood pressures were measured both in the laboratory and through the use of ambulatory monitoring devices.

Resnick et al. (41) investigated the effect of calcium supplementation in hypertensives on high- and low-sodium diets. Eight hypertensives were placed on high (200 mmol) and low (50 mmol) sodium chloride diets for 2 months each. Subjects received 2 g calcium or placebo for 1 month on each diet. On the low-sodium diet, calcium had no effect on blood pressure in either salt-sensitive or salt-insensitive subjects. Salt-sensitive subjects on the high-sodium diet had a smaller increase in blood pressure compared with placebo. The salt-insensitive subjects on a high-sodium diet had a larger increase in blood pressure on calcium than on placebo.

Saito et al. (42) studied the effect of calcium on borderline hypertensives given a high-salt diet. Diets of the participants in this study were controlled. All electrolytes remained constant. Dietary calcium was maintained at 250 mg per day and only the sodium varied: low (50 mEq), usual (150 mEq), and high (300 mEq). Subjects were assigned to calcium supplementation or placebo group and consumed the high- and low-sodium diets for 7 days each with a 7-day usual diet between. Neither the calcium nor placebo group had a significant change in blood pressure at the end of the low-sodium diet. However, at the end of the 7 days on the high-sodium diet the placebo group had a significant increase in their blood pressure, while the calcium group had no change. These studies included small numbers of subjects and were directed toward elucidating mechanisms, but they indicate the potential importance of sodium balance and sodium sensitivity in demonstrating a calcium effect.

When the trials listed in Table 1 are taken together, there is not a consistent blood pressure response to calcium supplementation. A metanalysis of some of these studies suggests a decrease with calcium supplementation but the confidence interval was large and included unity. The large and well-conducted TOHP study found no significant effect. Certain individuals may be calcium sensitive, while others are not. However, there is no independent assessment for calcium responsiveness that would identify, prospectively, candidates for this management. McCarron (54) has suggested that the differing results of supplementation studies are due, in part, to differences in individual threshold "set points." These threshold set points vary by age and gender, and are affected by other factors, such as alcohol. The influence of calcium on blood pressure is not strictly linear in all groups.

MAGNESIUM INTERVENTION STUDIES

Mechanisms

Magnesium is the primary intracellular divalent cation. Studies of animals provided diets deficient in mag-

nesium have found an increased systemic vascular resistance and hypertension (55). Magnesium in large doses (15 mmol Mg^{2+} and above) may have a pharmacological effect to lower blood pressure. Magnesium supplementation may act by restoring diuretic action and lowering blood pressure when individuals are magnesium or potassium depleted. The pharmacological action of magnesium has been attributed to intracellular inhibition of calcium activity, effectively acting as an intracellular calcium blocker. Plasma levels of magnesium are not as closely regulated as are levels of calcium, and dietary and other influences may alter plasma levels. This provides a more proximate effect by which intake might affect cellular metabolism. Measurement of serum magnesium levels also affords an estimate of compliance and absorption.

Summary of Clinical Trials

At least ten clinical trials have studied the effect of magnesium supplementation on blood pressure (37,56–62). These studies are presented in Table 2. Studies are included only if diuretics were not part of the intervention so as to avoid the confounding effects of magnesium or potassium depletion on blood pressure response. The studies are presented in Table 2 by year of publication and include information on country where the study was conducted, sample size, subjects' ages, study design, dose, length of supplementation, and effect on blood, pressure.

Cappuccio et al. (56) found no effect on blood pressure with a 15 mmol per day magnesium supplement. Seventeen subjects with supine diastolic blood pressures between 90 and 114 mm Hg and receiving no antihypertensive medications were randomized to a double-blind, supplementation-placebo, crossover study. During the 1 month of active treatment there was a significant increase in serum magnesium concentration. However, there were differences in blood pressure between magnesium-supplemented subjects and placebo controls.

Twenty-one men with a mean blood pressure of 111 mm Hg were enrolled in a nonrandomized magnesium supplementation study (57). After 4 weeks of observation, supplementation with 15 mmol of magnesium was begun for 4 weeks. The men received placebos for 4 weeks following the magnesium supplementation. A significant decrease in mean blood pressure was reported during the magnesium supplementation with a significant increase during the placebo phase. In another nonrandomized supplementation study, Zemel et al. (58) reported no significant differences in pressure after 3 months of supplementation with 40 mmol of magnesium.

In a potassium-magnesium study conducted in India, Patki et al. (59) randomized 37 adults with a mean age of

TABLE 2. *Clinical trials of magnesium supplementation on blood pressure*

Population	Sample size	Design	Magnesium dose	Results
England (56) 1985	$n = 17$ Age 33–66	M/M HTN S/P;D-B;CR	15 mmol 1 month	No change
Japan (57) 1986	$n = 21$ men Mean age 44 ± 7	M/M HTN	600 mg 4 weeks	↓ in mean BP
Michigan (58) 1990	$n = 13$ Age 20–69	Mild HTN S/P;D-B	40 mmol 3 months	No change
India (59) 1990	$n = 37$ Mean age 49.9 ± 7.6	Mild HTN Mild HTN Hi NTN	K^+ 30 mmol K^+ 30 mmol & Mg^{2+} 10 mmol 8 weeks	K ↓ in BP K^+ & Mg^{2+} no added change
Sweden (60) 1991	$n = 71$ Mean age; 60 ± 9.4 Rx, 62 ± 7.8 placebo	S/P;D-B 6 months	15 mmol 6 months	No change overall; ↓ BP in low urinary Mg^{2+} pt
US multicenter (37) 1992	$n = 227$ Mg^{2+} $n = 234$ placebo Age 30–54	S/P;D-B	15 mmol 6 months	No change
Italy (62) 1992	$n = 14$ Age 35–60	M/M HTN S/P;D-B	15 mmol 6 months	No change
Sweden (61) 1993	$n = 17$ Mean age 50 ± 6	HTN S/P;D-B;CR	15 mmol/30 mmol/40 mmol 3 wks each 21 weeks	↓ in BP

M/M HTN mild/moderate hypertension; NTN, normotensive; S/P, supplement/placebo; D-B double-blind; CR, crossover.

49.9 years in a double-blind, supplement-placebo trial. The subjects had diastolic blood pressure between 90 and 110 mm Hg and were on no antihypertensive medications for the 4 weeks prior to the supplementation study. The trial was conducted over 32 weeks with an initial washout period of 4 weeks. Subjects were given each of three preparations (one at a time): placebo, potassium 30 mmol per day, or potassium 30 mmol per day plus magnesium 10 mmol per day, for an 8-week period, with a 2-week washout period between preparations. The authors concluded that the 30 mmol per day of potassium lowered blood pressure, but there was no additional lowering with magnesium, although the lack of a full factorial design left the effect of magnesium alone unanswered.

Lind et al. (60) selected 77 subjects with mild hypertension or high normal blood pressure for a 6-month placebo controlled trial. These authors report that when all subjects were analyzed together there was no hypotensive effect of magnesium. Only subjects whose pretreatment urinary excretion of magnesium was low or individuals with high pretreatment potassium experienced a decrease in their systolic and diastolic blood pressure.

Seventeen subjects with diastolic blood pressure of 90 mm Hg or greater were recruited into a study of magnesium double-blind, supplementation-placebo crossover (61). Subjects were randomly assigned to either placebo or supplement. The supplementation consisted of 15 mmol per day of magnesium for 3 weeks, followed by 30 mmol per day for 3 weeks, and 40 mmol per day for 3 weeks, for a total of 9 weeks of supplementation. The

mean of both systolic and diastolic blood pressures began to decline as soon as the 30 mmol magnesium supplementation began. When subjects on 40 mmol per day of magnesium were compared with subjects in the placebo group, the magnesium group had significantly lower mean systolic and diastolic pressures. However, the therapeutic potential at higher levels of magnesium intake is problematic because diarrhea is frequent and hypovolemia may occur.

The largest study of magnesium supplementation is the Trial of Hypertension Prevention (TOHP) (37). In TOHP, a 15-mmol magnesium supplement was given to 227 individuals with diastolic blood pressures between 80 and 89. This treated group was compared with 234 individuals randomized to receive placebos. After 6 months of supplementation, no change was found in the blood pressures of subjects on magnesium supplementation compared with those on placebo.

Excluding studies of patients on diuretics and receiving magnesium, the data from clinical trials are not very promising for the use of oral magnesium as a hypotensive agent. The increases in serum magnesium measured in some studies provide an intermediate assessment that magnesium was absorbed. Of the eight studies in Table 2, six found no change in blood pressure while two found a decrease in pressure (37,56–62). However, it should be noted that the sample sizes were small in all studies except TOHP, in which no effect was noted. A dose of 15 mmol was used most often because of the adverse effects of higher doses. The only dose-ranging study found a hypotensive effect at 40 mmol, a dose associated with frequent side effects and unlikely to be generally useful for long-term management of blood pressure. Despite the overall lack of response of blood pressure to magnesium supplementation, it has been suggested that selected individuals or subgroups may be responsive. Individuals deficient in magnesium because of low dietary intake or diuretic therapy may experience blood pressure lowering, and supplementation may be useful in these circumstances.

THERAPEUTIC IMPLICATIONS

Nonpharmacological therapy through dietary modification or nutrient supplementation would be an important and useful approach to prevention of hypertension, to management of modest elevations of blood pressure, and to enhancement of pharmacological treatment. The observational studies of oral calcium and magnesium have suggested that these minerals might have useful potential to decrease blood pressure. However, the clinical trial data are conflicting when calcium or magnesium supplements have been tested in a randomized, controlled design, the evidential standard for attributing specific causal effect. For magnesium supplementation at levels of 15 mmol of Mg^{2+} daily, the majority of trials find no significant effect. Inadequate sample size and poor standardization of blood pressure assessment may have impaired the power to find small but statistically significant blood pressure responses in most of these studies. But the largest study, TOHP, did not find a significant change in blood pressure and was performed over 6 months by investigators experienced in blood pressure standardization and assessment of adherence (37). Moreover, there are troublesome "laxative" effects of magnesium that may limit practical use with supplementation at 15 mmol (600 mg) or higher of magnesium. Therefore, oral magnesium supplementation alone cannot be recommended as an effective means to lower blood pressure. Short-term use in magnesium-depleted persons, especially during diuretic therapy, may augment blood pressure lowering of these agents.

Calcium intake of 1.0 to 1.5 g per day through dietary modification or supplementation with calcium tablets also appears promising from observational studies. Calcium intake is also related to prevention and management of other conditions. Osteoporosis and bone mineral density can be improved by intakes of 1 g per day or more, which should be maintained from adolescence through late adult life. There is also putative but unproven benefit in preventing colorectal cancer and perhaps breast cancer. These considerations speak to the need for increasing calcium intake that is currently below these levels.

With respect to blood pressure, the clinical trial findings when calcium intake is increased are conflicting, but there is a trend toward a positive effect with calcium supplements of 1.0 to 1.5 g per day. The findings have been highly variable across studies and within studies, but the largest study (TOHP) found no significant blood pressure lowering at 600 mg per day. Investigators have analyzed their data retrospectively and found a subgroup of "calcium responders." These responders had a persistently lower blood pressure on calcium supplementation in contrast to others who experienced no change or had an increase in pressure. An analogy to salt sensitivity has been made, but similar practical problems arise. There is no independent and prospective means of identifying those whose blood pressure will respond to calcium, just as there is no means of determining salt sensitivity before actually implementing therapy or experimental study. Hypertension has a complex etiology with multiple factors responsible for its development and maintenance. Thus, it would be expected that certain subgroups of individuals might be responsive to an intervention while others would not. However, there are practical limitations with respect to research and practice related to post hoc designation of responsive individuals. Design of studies of efficacy need a means of identifying possible responsiveness before initiating a trial of therapy. Similarly, if only selected individuals benefit, there should be a selection of patients to receive the therapy before initiating treatment unless the therapy has been shown to have an important benefit on all potential recipients. Diuretics and other pharmacological agents have a generally beneficial effect on all treatment candidates.

Based on the data and experience available, calcium supplementation or increased dietary intake of calcium-rich foods would not be recommended for treatment of hypertension nor specifically for prevention of hypertension. Reliance on this approach would not be appropriate given the uncertain response in unselected individuals and the lack of means of determining a priori who might respond. However, increasing calcium intake for the general population has other benefits with few risks. Therefore, a recommendation that calcium intake be maintained at 1.0 to 1.5 g per day through dietary intake or supplements or both can be made for adolescents and adults. This level should be sufficient to achieve a blood pressure lowering response in those who are responsive.

REFERENCES

1. Neri LC, Johansen HL. Water hardness and cardiovascular mortality. *Ann NY Acad Sci* 1978;304:203–219.
2. Stitt FW, Crawford MD, Clayton DC, Morres JN. Clinical and biochemical indicators of cardiovascular disease among men living in hard and soft water areas. *Lancet* 1973;1:122–126.
3. Schroeder HA. Relation between mortality from cardiovascular disease and treated water supplies: variations in states and 163 largest municipalities of the United States. *JAMA* 1960;172:1902–1908.
4. Masironi R, Kortyohann SR, Pierce JO, Schamschula RC. Calcium content of river water, trace element concentrations in

toenails and blood pressure in village population in New Guinea. *Sci Total Environ* 1976;6:41–53.

5. Schwartz J. The relationship between blood lead levels and blood pressure. Presentation to the Royal Society of Canada Commission on Lead in the Environment, US Environmental Protection Agency, Washington, DC, 1985.

6. National Research Council (U.S.). *Recommended dietary allowances*, 10th ed. Washington, DC: National Academy Press, 1989.

7. Block G, Dresser CM, Hartman AM, Carroll MD. Nutrient sources in the American diet: quantitative data from the NHANES II survey. I. Vitamins and minerals. *Am J Epidemiol* 1985;122:13–26.

8. Continuing Survey of Food Intake by Individuals 1989 and 1990. USDA Public Use Data Tape.

9. Gerber AM, Sherman JA, Ammerman AS, Keenan NL, Garrett JM, Strogatz DS, Haines PS. Socioeconomic Status and electrolyte intake in black adults: the Pitt county study. *Am J Public Health* 1991;81:1608–1612.

10. *Dietary intake source data, United States, 1971–1974.* DHEW publication no. 79-1221, Washington, DC: US Government Printing Office, 1979.

11. Cummings SR, Block G, McHenry K, Baron RB. Evaluation of two fold frequency methods of measuring dietary calcium intake. *Am J Epidemiol* 1987;127:796–802.

12. Langford HG, Watson RL. Electrolytes, environment and blood pressure. *Cli Sci Mol Med* 1973;45:111S–113S.

13. McCarron DA, Morris CD, Henry HJ, Stanton JL. Blood pressure and nutrient intake in the United States. *Science* 1984;224:1392–1398.

14. Cutler JA, Brittain E. Calcium and blood pressure: an epidemiologic perspective. *Am J Hypertens* 1990;3:137S–146S.

15. Harlan WR, Hull AL, Schmouder RL, Landis JR, Thompson FE, Larkin FA. Blood pressure and nutrition in adults: the National Health and Nutrition Examination Survey. *Am J Epidemiol* 1984;120:17–28.

16. Harlan WR, Hull AL, Schmouder RL, et al. High blood pressure in older Americans: the First National Health and Nutrition Examination Survey. *Hypertension* 1984;6:802–809.

17. Gruchow HW, Sobocinski KA, Barboriak JJ. Alcohol, nutrient intake and hypertension in US adults. *JAMA* 1985;253:1567–1570.

18. Sempos C, Cooper R, Dovar MG, Johnson C, Drizd T, Yetley E. Dietary calcium and blood pressure in National Health and Nutrition Examination Surveys I and II. *Hypertension* 1986;8:1067–1074.

19. Witteman JCM, Willett WC, Stampfer MJ, Colditz GA, Sacks FM, Speizer FE, Rosner B, Hennekens CH. A prospective study of nutritional factors and hypertension among US women. *Circulation* 1989;80:1320–1327.

20. McGarvey S, Zinner SH, Willett WC, Rosner B. Maternal prenatal dietary potassium, calcium, magnesium and infant blood pressure. *Hypertension* 1991;17:218–224.

21. Altura BM, Altura BT. Cardiovascular risk factors and magnesium: relationships to atherosclerosis, ischemic heart disease and hypertension. *Magnes Trace Elem* 1991–92;10:182–192.

22. McCarron DA. Calcium and magnesium nutrition in human hypertension. *Ann Intern Med* 1983;98:800–805.

23. Karppanen H, Tanskanen A, Tuomelehto J, et al. Safety and effects of potassium and magnesium containing low sodium salt mixtures. *J Cardiovasc Pharmacol* 1984;6:S236–S243.

24. Fowdor JG, Rusted IE. Electrolyte profiles in a hypertensive population: the Newfoundland study. *Clin Invest Med* 1987;10:586–591.

25. McCarron DA, Chestnut CH, Cole C, Baylink DJ. Blood pressure response to the pharmacologic management of osteoporosis. *Clin Res* 1981;29:274A.

26. Belizan JM, Villar J, Pineda O, Gonzalez AE, Sainz E, Garrera G, Sibrian R. Reduction of blood pressure with calcium supplementation in young adults. *JAMA* 1983;249:1161–1165.

27. McCarron DA, Morris CD. Blood pressure response to oral calcium in persons with mild to moderate hypertension. *Ann Intern Med* 1985;103:825–831.

28. Johnson NE, Smith EL, Freudenheim JL. Effects on blood pressure of calcium supplementation of women. *Am J Clin Nutr* 1985;42:12–17.

29. Bloomfield RL, Young LD, Zurek G, Felts JH, Straw MK. Effects of oral calcium carbonate on blood pressure in subjects with mildly elevated arterial pressure. *J Hypertens* 1986;4(suppl 5):S351–S354.

30. Cappuccio FP, Markandu ND, Beynon GW, Shore AC, MacGregor GA. Effect of increasing calcium intake on urinary sodium excretion in normotensive subjects. *Clin Sci* 1986;71:453–456.

31. van Beresteyn ECH, Schaafsma G, deWaard H. Oral calcium and blood pressure: a controlled intervention trial. *Am J Clin Nutr* 1986;44:883–888.

32. Grobbee DE, Hoffman A. Effect of calcium supplementation on diastolic blood pressure in young people with mild hypertension. *Lancet* 1986;2:703–707.

33. Nowson C, Morgan T. Effect of calcium carbonate on blood pressure. *J Hypertens* 1986;4:S673–S675.

34. Zoccali C, Mallamaci F, Delfion D, Ciccarelli M, Parlongo S, Iellamo D, Moscato D, Maggiore Q. Long-term calcium supplementation in essential hypertension: a double-blind, randomized, crossover study. *J Hypertens* 1986;4:S676–678.

35. Morris CD, McCarron DA. Effect of calcium supplementation in an older population with mildly increased blood pressure. *Am J Hypertens* 1992;5:230–237.

36. Lyle RM. Does baseline serum total calcium level influence the blood pressure response to calcium supplementation? A double-blind study. *Neth J Med* 1992;41:48–55.

37. The Trials of Hypertension Prevention Collaborative Research Group. The effects of nonpharmacologic interventions on blood pressure of persons with high normal levels. Results of the Trials of Hypertension Prevention. Phase I. *JAMA* 1992;267:1213–1220.

38. Bierenbaum ML, Wolf E, Besgeier G, Maginnis WP. Dietary calcium: a method of lowering blood pressure. *Am J Hypertens* 1988;1:149s–152s.

39. van Bersteijn ECH, van Schaik M, Schaafsma G. Milk: does it affect blood pressure? A controlled intervention study. *J Intern Med* 1990;228:477–482.

40. Kyrast-Gales SA, Massey LK. Effects of dietary calcium from dairy products on ambulatory blood pressure in hypertensive men. *J Am Diet Assoc* 1992;92:1497–1501.

41. Resnick LM, DiFabio B, Marion R, James GD, Laragh JH. Dietary calcium modifies the pressor effects of dietary salt intake in essential hypertension. *J Hypertens* 1986;4:S679–S681.

42. Saito K, Sano H, Furuta Y, Fukuzaki H. Effect of oral calcium on blood pressure response in salt-loaded borderline hypertensive patients. *Hypertension* 1989;13:219–226.

43. Cappuccio FP, Markandu ND, Singer DRJ, Smith SJ, Shore AC, MacGregor GA. Does oral calcium supplementation lower high blood pressure? A double-blind study. *J Hypertens* 1987;5:67–71.

44. Gilliland M, Zawada ET, McClung D, TerWee J. Preliminary report: natriuretic effect of calcium supplementation in hypertensive women over forty. *J Am Coll Nutr* 1987;6:139–143.

45. Takagi Y, Fukase M, Takata S, Fujimi T, Fujita T. Calcium treatment of essential hypertension in elderly patients evaluated by 24 H monitoring. *Am J Hypertens* 1991;4:836–839.

46. Lasaridis AN, Kaisis CN, Zananiri KI, Syganis CD, Tourkantonis AA. Oral calcium supplementation promotes renal sodium excretion in essential hypertension. *J Hypertens* 1987;5:S307–S309.

47. Tanji JL, Lew EY, Wong GY, Treguboff C, Ward JA, Amsterdam EA. Dietary calcium supplementation as a treatment for mild hypertension. *J Am Board Fam Pract* 1991;4:145–150.

48. Strazzullo P, Siani A, Guglielmi S, DiCarlo A, Galletti F, Cirillo M, Mancini M. Controlled trial of long-term calcium supplementation in essential hypertension. *Hypertension* 1986;8:1084–1088.

49. Ogihara T, Saito H, Tabuchi Y, Hashizume K, Kumahara Y. The hypotensive effect of long-term oral calcium loading in elderly hypertensive patients: the importance of endogenous vitamin D_3 suppression. *J Hypertens* 1986;4:S685–S687.

50. Lyle RM, Melby CL, Hyner GC, Edmondson JW, Miller JZ, Weinberger MH. Blood pressure and metabolic effects of calcium supplementation in normotensive white and black men. *JAMA* 1987;257:1772–1776.

51. Siani A, Strazzullo P, Guglielmi S, Mancini M. Clinical studies of the effects of different oral calcium intakes in essential hypertension. *J Hypertens* 1987;5:S311–S313.

52. Siani A, Pasquale G, Guglielmi S, Parcioni D, Giacco A, Iacone A, Mancini M. Controlled trial of low calcium versus high calcium intake in mild hypertension. *J Hypertens* 1988;6:253–256.

53. Galloe AM, Graudal N, Moller J, Bro H, Jorgensen M, Christensen HR. Effect of oral calcium supplementation on blood pressure in patients with previously untreated hypertension: a randomized, double-blind, placebo-controlled, crossover study. *J Hum Hypertens* 1993;7:43–45.

54. McCarron DA. Epidemiological evidence and clinical trials of dietary calcium's effect on blood pressure. *Contrib Nephrol* 1991;90:2–10.

55. Chrysant SG, Ganousis L, Chrysant C. Hemodynamic and metabolic effects of hypomagnesemia in spontaneously hypertensive rats. *Cardiology* 1988;75:81–89.

56. Cappuccio FP, Markandu ND, Beynon GW, Shore AC, Sampson B, MacGregor GA. Lack of effect of oral magnesium on high blood pressure: a double-blind study. *Br Med J* 1985;291:235–238.

57. Motoyama T, Sano H, Suzuki H, Kawaguch K, Saito K, Furuta Y, Fukuzaki H. Oral magnesium treatment and the erythrocyte sodium pump in patients with essential hypertension. *J Hypertens* 1986;4:S682–S684.

58. Zemel PC, Zemel MB, Urberg M, Douglas FL, Geiser R, Sowers JR. Metabolic and hemodynamic effects of magnesium supplementation in patients with essential hypertension. *Am J Clin Nutr* 1990;51:665–669.

59. Patki PS, Singh J, Gokhale SV, Bulakh PM, Shrotri DS, Patwardhan B. Efficacy of potassium and magnesium in essential hypertension: a double-blind, placebo controlled, crossover study. *BJM* 1990;301:521–523.

60. Lind L, Lithell H, Pollare T, Ljunghall S. Blood pressure response during long-term treatment with magnesium is dependent on magnesium status. *Am J Hypertens* 1991;4:674–679.

61. Widman L, Wester PO, Stegmayr BK, Wirell M. The dose-dependent reduction in blood pressure through administration of magnesium. *Am J Hypertens* 1993;6:41–45.

62. Ferrara LA, Iannuzzi R, Castaldo A, Iannuzzi A, Dello Russo A, Mancini M. Long-term magnesium supplementation in essential hypertension. *Cardiology* 1992;81:25–33.

Hypertension: Pathophysiology, Diagnosis,
and Management, Second Edition,
edited by J.H. Laragh and B.M. Brenner,
Raven Press, Ltd., New York © 1995.

CHAPTER 69

Calcium and Calcium-Regulatory Hormones in Hypertension

James R. Sowers, Paul R. Standley, Michael L. Tuck, and Jeffrey L. Ram

A considerable body of evidence suggests a relationship between abnormalities of calcium (Ca^{2+}) metabolism and hypertension (1–31). Indeed, investigation of factors regulating cellular Ca^{2+} ($[Ca^{2+}]_i$) function may be of seminal importance in understanding the mechanisms underlying hypertension. Regulation of $[Ca^{2+}]_i$ is especially important in vascular smooth muscle (VSM) tissue, as $[Ca^{2+}]_i$ is essential in the generation and maintenance of active tension (31–37). As reviewed in this chapter, there is evidence that $[Ca^{2+}]_i$ is abnormally high in some cell types in human hypertension. Most measurements in people have been made in accessible cells such as platelets, erythrocytes, and lymphocytes, and these data have

been extrapolated to what may be occurring in vascular tissue. Evidence that this extrapolation is legitimate is garnered from studies in animal models of hypertension, also reviewed in this chapter, indicating that Ca^{2+} function is abnormal in VSM tissue. In this chapter, normal VSM Ca^{2+} metabolism is reviewed initially, and then $[Ca^{2+}]_i$ function is discussed in the context of animal and human hypertension.

NORMAL VASCULAR SMOOTH MUSCLE $[Ca^{2+}]_i$ METABOLISM

The concentration of Ca^{2+} in the extracellular fluid is regulated in the range of 1.2 mM (31). In contrast, in the vascular smooth muscle cell (VSMC) (31–37), as in many other cell types (2–20), $[Ca^{2+}]_i$ is in the range of 50 to 200 nM. The largest pool of total intracellular Ca^{2+} is in the millimolar range and is largely bound by sarcoplasmic reticulum, mitochondria, and Ca^{2+} binding proteins, principally calmodulin, which serve not only to

J. R. Sowers, P. R. Standley, J. L. Ram: Division of Endocrinology, Metabolism, and Hypertension, Wayne State University, Detroit, Michigan 48201.
M. L. Tuck: Department of Medicine, UCLA School of Medicine, and Endocrinology Division, VA Medical Center, Sepulveda, California 91343.

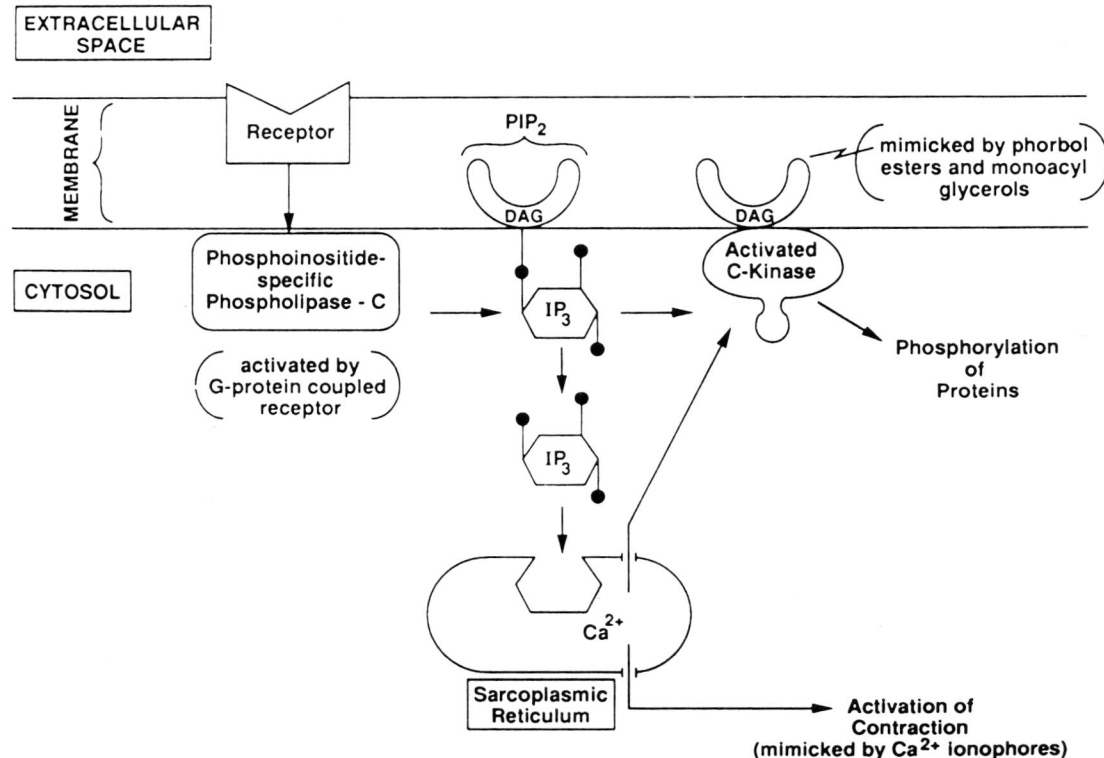

FIG. 1. Schematic diagram of the roles of phospholipase C and its substrates in VSMC. DAG, diacyl-glycerol; IP₃, inositol triphosphate; PIP₂, phosphatidylinositol, 4,5-bisphosphate. (From ref. 1, with permission.)

buffer $[Ca^{2+}]_i$, but also to modulate many of the cellular events mediated by $[Ca^{2+}]_i$ changes (Fig. 1). In VSMC as in other eukaryotic cells, the principal Ca^{2+} transport systems are in the plasma membrane, the sarcoplasmic reticulum, and the mitochondria.

PLASMA MEMBRANE Ca^{2+} TRANSPORT

VSMC plasma membranes possess both voltage-sensitive and receptor-operated Ca^{2+} channels (31–37). Voltage-sensitive Ca^{2+} channels become functional as the plasma membrane is depolarized; inward Ca^{2+} currents become at about −40 mV and reach a maximum around 0 mV. Voltage-sensitive Ca^{2+} channels can be divided into at least two subtypes: one type is activated by small depolarizations and is inactivated quickly (T-type); the other type opens for a more sustained period but requires a larger depolarization to become active (L-type). L-type channels are much more sensitive to dihydropyridine Ca^{2+} channel blockers than are T-type channels. Voltage-sensitive Ca^{2+} channels also provide a mechanism by which $[Ca^{2+}]_i$ can be regulated by other cations. For example, opening of potassium channels can produce membrane hyperpolarization and reduce conductance of voltage-gated Ca^{2+} channels (38,39). Accordingly, Ca^{2+}-activated K channels may serve as a

feedback mechanism to cellular Ca^{2+} entry (37). Additionally, there is evidence from patch clamp studies that both α-adrenergic and β-adrenergic agonists may attenuate current through these channels (40).

RECEPTOR-OPERATED Ca^{2+} CHANNELS

In addition to voltage-operated Ca^{2+} channels, receptor-operated Ca^{2+} channels are present in the VSMC plasma membrane (31,41), although these channels may be limited primarily to large arteries and may be sparse or absent in arterioles (37,41). Substantial data supporting the presence of receptor-operated Ca^{2+} channels comes from investigations where pharmacological blockers of L-type (voltage-gated) Ca^{2+} channels had very little effect on agonist stimulated Ca^{2+} influx (37,42). These data collectively suggest the presence of plasmalemmal Ca^{2+} channels sensitive to norepinephrine, vasopressin, angiotensin II, endothelin and other hormones (42,43). There is some evidence that the inositol-phosphate pathway is an important second messenger system in mediating receptor-operated Ca^{2+} channel opening in response to hormones (32,43). In contrast, protein kinase C activation can either depress (44) or accentuate (45) influx of Ca^{2+} through voltage-operated channels.

The mechanisms by which neurotransmitters and hormones increase Ca^{2+} influx into VSMC are often complex. For example, in patch-clamp recordings of the activity of individual Ca^{2+} channels in VSMC, the effect of norepinephrine on Ca^{2+} influx may involve steady depolarization with an increase in opening probability of the Ca^{2+} channels (46). In contrast, in another study involving VSMC from rat portal vein, norepinephrine reduced L-type current but increased T-type current (47), both actions presumably mediated by an α-adrenergic mechanism (40).

Endothelin-induced Ca^{2+} influx in VSM appears to be mediated by voltage-dependent channels (48,49) as well as nonvoltage-mediated channels (50,51). In a cultured rat aortic cell line, vasopressin activates a nonspecific cation current (52), as well as inhibits an L-type Ca^{2+} channel, a response similar to that produced by endothelin in some cells (50). Angiotensin II enhances voltage-dependent Ca^{2+} current in portal vein VSMC (53), and serotonin activates voltage-dependent Ca^{2+} current in basilar artery VSMC (39). Thus, hormonal effects on Ca^{2+} influx involve complex mechanisms that appear to be tissue specific.

INTRACELLULAR ORGANELLE RELEASE OF Ca^{2+}

Organelles, particularly the sarcoplasmic reticulum (SR), function as Ca^{2+} pumps or storage sites, and smooth muscle contractile agonists can trigger a rise in $[Ca^{2+}]_i$ by causing release of Ca^{2+} from the SR and other organelles. The second messenger for release of Ca^{2+} from the SR is generally inositol triphosphate (IP_3) (54) (Fig. 1). As detailed in a prior review, agonist binding to a VSMC receptor activates phospholipase C via a guanosine triphosphate (GTP)-regulated protein. Phospholipase C catalyzes the hydrolysis of phosphatidylinositol 4,5-biphosphate (PIP_2) to form IP_3 and diacylglycerol (DAG). IP_3 diffuses to the SR where it triggers Ca^{2+} release and subsequent Ca^{2+}-activated physiological events (i.e., VSMC contraction). The existence of "Ca^{2+} release" channels in the SR is supported by the observation that IP_3 induces Ca^{2+} release from skinned porcine coronary artery cells (55,56), presumably by opening a receptor-operated Ca^{2+} channel. This IP_3 effect is a GTP-dependent process and is inhibited by pertussis toxin (58). In contrast, caffeine, adenosine triphosphate (ATP), and ryanodine release Ca^{2+} from the SR by a mechanism that does not require GTP and is insensitive to pertussis toxin (59–61).

Another VSM intracellular Ca^{2+}-storing organelle is the mitochondria. Mitochondria normally store much less Ca^{2+} than SR; however, in states of VSMC injury the mitochondria may act as an important pump for Ca^{2+} regulation.

MECHANISMS INVOLVED IN REDUCING VASCULAR SMOOTH MUSCLE $[Ca^{2+}]_i$

Maintenance of $[Ca^{2+}]_i$ at a level 10^4-fold lower than extracellular Ca^{2+} is important in allowing VSM to maintain resting tone (1). Maintenance of a physiologically low $[Ca^{2+}]_i$ is a dynamic process that is achieved by the concerted effects of a variety of mechanisms operating at various subcellular levels. The three major mechanisms by which VSM $[Ca^{2+}]_i$ is maintained at a physiologically low level include (a) uptake into SR and to a lesser extent mitochondria by specific Ca^{2+}–adenosine triphosphatases (ATPases), (b) ATP-dependent Ca^{2+} transport (Ca^{2+}-ATPase) across the cell membrane, and (c) Na^+-Ca^{2+} exchange across the cell membrane (1).

The Ca^{2+}-ATPase in SR is the primary mechanism whereby the SR takes up Ca^{2+} (63–67). Sarcoplasmic reticulum isolated by density gradient centrifugation from bovine pulmonary artery contains a Ca^{2+}-transport ATPase of molecular weight 100,000 that is antigenically related to the Ca^{2+}-pump of cardiac SR (64). SR Ca^{2+}-ATPase is regulated, in part, by adenosine 3',5'-cyclic monophosphate (cAMP), calmodulin and guanosine 3',5'-cyclic monophosphate (cGMP) (37,64). VSMC SR Ca^{2+}-ATPase also appears to be pH sensitive, as alkaline pH results in a conversion of the Ca^{2+} binding site to a higher affinity state (32,68). In cardiac SR at a saturating external Ca^{2+} level, the activity of the Ca^{2+}-ATPase pump demonstrates a sigmoidal pH dependence with maximal values in the pH range of 6.0 to 6.5 range, half-maximal value at pH 7.2, and minimal activity at pH 8.0 (69). It has also been demonstrated that ATP-dependent Ca^{2+} accumulation into reconstituted SR proteoliposomes is increased when a proton ionophore is added (37,65). Further, Ca^{2+} uptake into these proteoliposomes is accompanied by internal alkalinization (65). This collective evidence suggests that SR Ca^{2+}-ATPase is a counterpart to protons and is most active when the SR internal hydrogen ion concentration is high (37). Although not as much is known about mitochondrial Ca^{2+} transport, this process appears to involve a high-capacity, low-affinity process (62).

In contrast to the SR Ca^{2+}-ATPase, the plasma membrane Ca^{2+}-ATPase is a 130,000-dalton protein (64). Furthermore, the plasma membrane Ca^{2+}-ATPase activity level is much more dependent upon binding to calmodulin than is the SR Ca^{2+}-ATPase (67). Plasma membrane Ca^{2+}-ATPase may also be stimulated by protein kinase C (66), and is inhibited by vanadate (67). Because the plasmalemmal Ca^{2+}-ATPase has high affinity for Ca^{2+}, this pump is very instrumental in maintaining $[Ca^{2+}]_i$ at a low physiological level (1,70). This high-affinity, lower-capacity system pumps Ca^{2+} out of the cell in exchange for protons (i.e., Ca^{2+} out, $2 H^+$ in) (1,37). Following an increase in $[Ca^{2+}]_i$, the binding of Ca^{2+} to calmodulin induces a conformational change, and the Ca_4-calmodulin complex then stimulates Ca^{2+}-ATPase activity, thus providing the compensatory increase in the rate of calcium efflux (1). The plasmalemmal Ca^{2+}-ATPase pump is also phosphorylated and concomitantly stimulated by cGMP-dependent mechanisms (71,72). Additional control mechanisms include inhibition by IP_3 (73) and stimulation by insulin (possibly genomic) (1,74,75) and genomically by 1,25-dihydroxy vitamin D_3 (75,76).

Another potentially important mechanism for the maintenance of physiological levels of VSM $[Ca^{2+}]_i$ is the Na^+-Ca^{2+} exchange. The Na^+-Ca^{2+} exchanger appears to be important in handling quantitatively large Ca^{2+} movements associated with depolarization and repolarization (71,77). In a quantitative study of the Na^+ dependence of Ca^{2+} efflux, one group found that while Na^+-independent efflux (i.e., Ca^{2+}-ATPase dependent) reached its maximum when $[Ca^{2+}]_i$ was 0.6-1 μM, Na^+-dependent efflux increased monotonically even above 1 μM $[Ca^{2+}]_i$ (71). At approximately 500 nM $[Ca^{2+}]_i$ (levels achieved with agonists), Na^+-dependent efflux is the predominant mechanism for removal of $[Ca^{2+}]_i$ to the exterior of the VSMC. However, at 50 to 100 nM $[Ca^{2+}]_i$ (basal levels), and at submaximal responses to agonists, Na^+-independent efflux is predominant. Thus, maximal agonist-induced (e.g., angiotensin and vasopressin) increases in $[Ca^{2+}]_i$ lead to an efflux of Ca^{2+} via the Na^+-Ca^{2+} exchange (78–80). The level of Na^+-Ca^{2+} exchange activity is also regulated by $[Na^+]_i$ as evidenced by the observation that when $[Na^+]_i$ is increased by ouabain, Ca^{2+} entry upon removal of external Na^+ is increased (79,80). The apparent K_m for Ca^{2+} with respect to Na^+-Ca^{2+} exchange is 1.5 to 15 μM (81), and the maximal transport velocity is threefold to sixfold greater for the sarcolemmal Na^+-Ca^{2+} exchange than for the sarcolemmal Ca^{2+}-ATPase (82). Thus, Na^+-Ca^{2+} exchange is a high-capacity Ca^{2+} transport system that becomes predominant when $[Ca^{2+}]_i$ rises above 500 nM, whereas the Ca^{2+}-ATPase transport system has a lower capacity and is the predominant mechanism of Ca^{2+} efflux mechanism associated with basal physiological levels of $[Ca^{2+}]_i$ (1,83).

EFFECTS OF VSMC pH ON $[Ca^{2+}]_i$

A role of VSMC pH in regulating $[Ca^{2+}]_i$ is supported by observations that cellular alkalinization with NH_4Cl caused a rise in $[Ca^{2+}]_i$ in a VSMC line (37,84). This increase in Ca^{2+} was not dependent upon an external source, but rather appeared to come from a vasopressin-sensitive intracellular source (37,84). It has been suggested (37) that cell alkalinization increases IP_3 levels with consequent activation of IP_3-sensitive Ca^{2+} channels (84). However, it has also been shown that alkalinization-induced Ca^{2+} release in bovine endothelial cells is not accompanied by changes in either basal or ATP-stimulated IP_3 formation (85). There is also evidence that cell alkalinization enhances the sensitivity of the SR to IP_3, as documented in platelets (86), and that increased cell alkalinization can alter the affinity of the Ca^{2+} release channel for Ca^{2+} with a resultant increase in the release of Ca^{2+} (87). Acute decreases in cellular pH—whether by use of high CO_2 media or by NH_3Cl washout—results in a VSMC $[Ca^{2+}]_i$ transient, apparently by release from an intracellular storage site other than SR (37).

Changes in VSMC pH may also modulate the rate at which $[Ca^{2+}]_i$ transients induced by other mechanisms return to basal levels. Indeed, increased cell pH may stimulate the plasmalemmal as well as the SR Ca^{2+}-ATPase pump (1,37,75), Na^+-Ca^{2+} exchange (37), and reuptake of Ca^{2+} by the SR via a Ca^{2+}-H^+ exchanging ATPase (37,75,87). In contrast, during cell acidification, VSMC $[Ca^{2+}]_i$ extrusion and reuptake mechanisms are decreased and Ca^{2+} transients following acidification are much more prolonged than those observed following alkalinization (37).

G-PROTEIN REGULATION OF $[Ca^{2+}]_i$

A family of cell membrane-associated proteins, the G proteins, mediate many of the cellular activities of guanosine triphosphate (GTP) (1,88) (Fig. 2). The G protein family consists of α, β, and γ subunits. In the inactive state, guanosine diphosphate (GDP) is bound to the α-subunit. Upon activation (i.e., with agonist binding to a receptor complex), GDP is released and replaced by GTP and the α-subunit dissociates from the G-protein complex (1,88,89). GTP-α then diffuses into the cell cytoplasm where it can modulate various cellular mechanisms. Subsequently, intrinsic guanasine triphosphatase (GTPase) activity of the α-subunit hydrolyses GTP to GDP, allowing α to bind to the G-protein $\beta\gamma$ complex, to start the process over again. Many G proteins exist; perhaps the most studied are the G_s, known to stimulate the activity of adenylate cyclase; G_i, an inhibitor of adenylate cyclase; and G_k, an activator of cardiac potassium channels (88,89). In VSMC the G proteins mediate the coupling mechanisms of receptors to the activation of second messengers, including cAMP and inositol phosphate (88–90), and to VSMC biological functions such as Ca^{2+}-related contraction (91,92). G proteins exert their effects on VSMC $[Ca^{2+}]_i$ and related functions by increasing Ca^{2+} release from SR and intracellular storage sites (91,93,94) and possibly by modification of Ca^{2+} channels themselves (1,92). Thus, G proteins may affect many of the Ca^{2+}-related functions in VSMC, including the sensitivity of contractile proteins to Ca^{2+}, the release

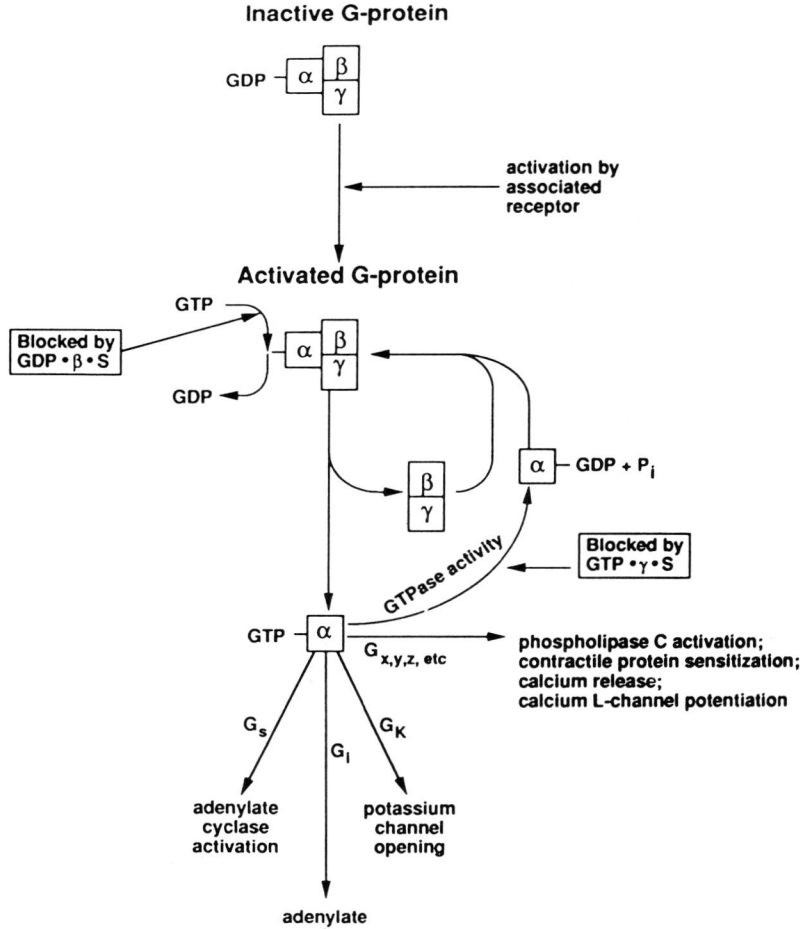

FIG. 2. Schematic diagram of the mechanism of activation of G proteins and several of their possible roles in VSMC. (From ref. 1, with permission.)

of Ca^{2+} from SR, and the activity of voltage-dependent Ca^{2+} channels.

PROTEIN KINASE C REGULATION OF $[Ca^{2+}]_i$

As previously reviewed (1), diacylglycerols (DAG) produced by hydrolysis of PIP_2 (Fig. 2) have two putative signaling roles: (a) it can be further cleaved to release arachidonic acid, which serves as a precursor for synthesis of prostaglandins and related lipid-signaling molecules; and (b) it can activate protein kinase C (PKC), which can then phosphorylate a number of cellular proteins (93). The subsequent effects of PKC-stimulated protein phosphorylation includes the activation of plasma membrane Na^+-H^+ exchange, thereby affecting cellular pH as well as $[Ca^{2+}]_i$ (93). In VSMC, PKC also activates plasma membrane Ca^{2+}-ATPase (94) and myosin light chain (95). Thus, the PKC pathway, which Ca^{2+} plays an important role in activating, many accordingly provide an additional mechanism to regulate VSM tension (1).

ROLE OF CALCITROPHIC HORMONES IN MAINTENANCE OF CALCIUM HOMEOSTASIS

Of the calcitrophic hormones, parathyroid hormone (PTH) and the biologically active vitamin D metabolites appear to be the most important in regulation of blood pressure. PTH is an 84 amino acid linear polypeptide with a molecular weight of 9500. All of the structural information necessary for its biological activity exists in the 34 amino acids at the amino terminus (92). In target tissues, PTH binds to a membrane receptor and exerts many of its metabolic actions by activation of adenylate cyclase (92), catalyzing formation of cAMP from ATP. The cAMP binds to a specific cAMP-binding protein coupled to protein kinase A (PKA). The subsequent phosphorylation of cellular proteins, in turn, triggers tissue-specific physiological responses.

Vitamin D and its metabolites are steroid hormones that are biochemically related to cholesterol (92,95,96). Human vitamin D is derived from two sources: (a) photoconversion of 7-dehydrocholesterol to vitamin D_3 (cholecalciferol) in the epidermis under the influence of ultraviolet radiation, and (b) dietary sources containing vitamin D_2 (ergocalciferol) (95,96). Vitamin D_2 and D_3 lack biological activity and must undergo metabolic transformation for activation (95,96). The first step in activation involves 25-hydroxylation by microsomal enzymes in the liver. The product of this reaction, 25(DH)-D_3, is a weakly active metabolite that undergoes a second hydroxylation step in renal tubules to form 1,25-$(OH)_2$-D_3, the most active form of vitamin D. PTH, prolactin, estrogen, and growth hormone all may increase this mitochondrial 1-hydroxylase activity and yield greater production of 1,25$(OH)_2$-D_3. This active D metabolite binds to a receptor in the target cells and causes transcription of the specific genes that code for proteins including a Ca^{2+}-binding protein called calbindin-D involved in the intracellular transport of Ca^{2+} (95,96). 1,25$(OH)_2D_3$ influences the proliferation and differentiation of normal and tumor cells, and like the glucocorticoids and estrogens, it also has immunoregulatory activities (96,97).

PARATHYROID HYPERTENSIVE FACTOR (PHF)

This putative hypertensive factor, produced by the parathyroid glands but not related structurally or biochemically to PTH, may contribute to the development of high blood pressure in some segments of the hypertensive population (98–100). PHF has been reported to be increased in low renin essential hypertension with salt sensitivity (9,98,99). This characteristic presumably is related to the fact that PHF can decrease urinary sodium excretion. Furthermore, PHF has been reported to increase cell $[Ca^{2+}]_i$ and is correlated in experimental deoxycorticosterone acetate (DOCA)-salt hypertension and in essential hypertension with increased cell $[Ca^{2+}]_i$ (100). PHF, like PTH, has been shown to be stimulated by low plasma Ca^{2+} and to be suppressed by Ca^{2+} supplementation (99). These properties make PHF a candidate hypertensinogenic factor in conditions of salt-sensitive, low-renin hypertension. However, considerable work remains to characterize this factor as a true hypertensinogen factor in human essential hypertension.

CALCITONIN GENE–RELATED PEPTIDE (CGRP)

CGRP is a 37 amino acid peptide found extensively throughout the peripheral and central nervous system (101–105). The importance of CGRP actions in regulating the cardiovascular system is indicated by the fact that peripheral administration of CGRP causes vasodilation and positive chronotropic and inotropic effects (101–105). Additionally, CGRP binding in the intima and me-

dia of coronary arteries and heart valves has been demonstrated autoradiographically (105,106). Thus, the release of CGRP from vascular and cardiac nerve fibers may play a functional role in the neurogenic regulation of VSM tone and cardiac contractility.

HYPERTENSION ASSOCIATED WITH HYPERPARATHYROIDISM

Hypertension is often present in disorders in which hyperparathyroidism (hPTH) (with or without hypercalcemia) is present (107–114). In a number of reports since 1980, the prevalence of systolic and diastolic hypertension in these cases has varied from approximately 25 to 75 percent (107–110). In those reports in which information from normocalcemic control subjects was included, the occurrence of hypertension in hPTH was approximately twice that expected for sex-, age-, and race-matched populations (112–114).

Although a number of mechanisms have been suggested to explain the increased prevalence of hypertension associated with hPTH, the current consensus is that the pathogenesis of hypertension associated with hPTH is multifactored and remains poorly understood (112–114). It appears that many of these patients have essential hypertension with associated family histories of hypertension. Factors reported to impact on the higher prevalence of hypertension in hPTH include the degree of elevation of PTH, degree and chronicity of hypercalcemia, levels of phosphate and magnesium, older age, and renal impairment.

There is an accumulating body of evidence that PTH or its related analogue parathyroid hormone-related protein (PTHrp) has significant effect on blood pressure regulation. In one large study (111), serum phosphate levels in hypertensive patients were significantly less than in the normotensive group, suggesting that the hypertensive group had greater PTH-mediated tissue effects than the normotensive group of hPTH patients. Consistent with this concept is the observation that blood pressure returned to normal in a significant proportion of hypertensive patients following surgical correction of the hyperparathyroid state (111–114).

A role of PTH in causing hypertension is suggested by several lines of evidence. PTH levels have been reported to be elevated in untreated hypertensives as well as in animal models of hypertension (3,4,10–12,14,17,20–22,94,115–117). Chronic infusion of PTH (human amino terminal peptide 1-34 PTH) in normal individuals resulted in a reversible rise in blood pressure to hypertensive levels (118). In contrast, acute infusion of PTH—or PTHrp—consistently resulted in vasodilation and a reduction in blood pressure (119,120).

In vitro studies exploring the actions of PTH and PTHrp on VSMC suggest a possible explanation for the disparate clinical study results. PTH and PTHrp appear to share the same membrane receptors on VSMC (121). PTHrp is also present in significant amounts in VSMC (121), and vasoactive peptides such as angiotensin II, endothelin, and norepinephrine can modulate its synthesis. These results suggest that PTHrp may act in a pericranial fashion to mediate vasoconstrictor activity. Conversely, PTH can decrease angiotensin II and vasopressin-induced intracellular Ca^{2+} transients (116,117). It has been suggested that conditions in which there is a chronic elevation of PTH and PTHrp may be associated with desensitization to their vasodilatory responses and relatively unopposed vasoconstriction responses (116).

It appears that the relationship between hypertension and hPTH is related to a relatively high incidence of essential hypertension. The mean age at the time of diagnosis of hPTH is between 50 and 55 years, an age at which the prevalence of hypertension is at least 20 percent (122,123). Accordingly, at least 50 percent of individuals with hPTH and hypertension may have essential hypertension, that is causally unrelated to the hPTH (122). Consistent with this notion is the observation that over 50 percent of hPTH patients successfully treated surgically remain hypertensive (110,111,124,125). Indeed, some studies have even documented the development of hypertension following successful parathyroid surgery (125). Also, studies of medical management of hPTH with agents that lower serum Ca^{2+} have not resulted in improvement of hypertension.

PSEUDOHYPOPARATHYROIDISM

Individuals with various PTH-resistance syndromes have an increased prevalence of hypertension (4,126, 127). Patients with these disorders develop secondary hyperparathyroidism usually in the presence of hypocalcemia. In a limited number of patients, Brickman et al. (4) have observed that correction of hypocalcemia does not reverse hypertension. The mechanism of the hypertension is poorly defined although studies do suggest altered sympathetic nervous system activity (especially abnormal dopaminergic regulatory mechanisms) (126) and altered circadian rhythms of blood pressure (127).

RENAL INSUFFICIENCY AND SECONDARY HYPERPARATHYROIDISM

A close relationship between serum Ca^{2+} concentration and blood pressure has been observed in both individual patients as well as groups of individuals with end-stage renal disease treated with hemodialysis (122). In this regard, dialysis with a high Ca^{2+} concentration in the dialysate can reduce or block the occurrence or severity of postdialysis hypotension. Furthermore, patients with end-stage renal disease have an augmented pressor re-

sponse to acute Ca^{2+} infusion (128,129). A linear relationship has been observed between levels of intact PTH and mean arterial pressure (130). PTH levels were also highly correlated with levels of platelet $[Ca^{2+}]_i$ (130). Treatment with alfacalcidol lowered plasma PTH, platelet $[Ca^{2+}]_i$, and blood pressure. Calcitriol or alfacalcidol had previously been shown to decrease PTH secretion and blood pressure in patients with chronic renal disease (131).

VITAMIN D METABOLISM AND HYPERTENSION

$1,25-(OH)_2-D (D_3)$ has been suggested to have a hypertensive effect (11,12,20,21). In this regard, DNA binding receptors for D_3 have recently been demonstrated in VSMC (132,133). Minghetti and Norman (97) presented an extensive review of the various genomic actions of the DNA-binding receptor for the hormone D_3 and summarized its regulate gene expression for VSMC differentiation and proliferation. Additionally, Walters et al. (134) have observed that nanomolar quantities of D_3 cause a threefold increase in cardiomyocyte Ca^{2+} uptake. Indeed, this effect on $[Ca^{2+}]_i$ may account for the effect D_3 to increase vascular tone (135).

ABNORMALITIES IN CELLULAR Ca^{2+} METABOLISM IN HYPERTENSION

In essential hypertension there is evidence for an array of alterations of the Ca^{2+} regulatory system including increased cell $[Ca^{2+}]_i$, increased Ca^{2+} uptake and decreased removal of $[Ca^{2+}]_i$ (1). Increased $[Ca^{2+}]_i$ is directly related via increases in myosin light chain phosphorylation to an increase in active tension and therefore could directly contribute to the development of hypertension (1,136–147). In this regard a number of laboratories have reported elevated platelet $[Ca^{2+}]_i$ and a positive relationship with elevated blood pressure in hypertensives (see ref. 1 for review). Indeed, a positive correlation between blood pressure and platelet $[Ca^{2+}]_i$ has also been reported in normotensive individuals (116). Also, antihypertensive therapy has been reported to reduce platelet $[Ca^{2+}]_i$, and we have recently observed that platelet $[Ca^{2+}]_i$ is actually lower in diabetic hypertensive patients treated with calcium antagonists and angiotensin-converting enzyme (ACE) inhibitors than in normotensive diabetics and controls (Fig. 3). These observations suggest that basal platelet $[Ca^{2+}]_i$ levels are generally higher in hypertensives but may be affected dramatically by antihypertensive therapy.

A number of possibilities exist to explain the higher $[Ca^{2+}]_i$ observed in essential hypertension. For example, individuals with hypertension have been reported to display reduced binding of Ca^{2+} to erythrocyte membranes

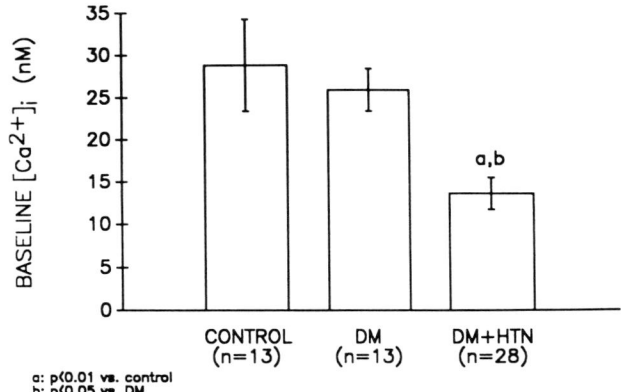

a: p<0.01 vs. control
b: p<0.05 vs. DM

FIG. 3. Baseline [Ca^{2+}]$_i$ in fura-2 loaded platelets derived from subjects in three study groups, including normal controls, nonhypertensive type II diabetics, and treated hypertensive type II diabetics.

as compared to normotensives (148,149). A reduction in Ca^{2+} binding to inner cell membranes could indirectly cause an increase in [Ca^{2+}]$_i$, as it results in reduced potassium conductance, membrane depolarization, and activation of voltage-operated Ca^{2+} channels (150).

There is also evidence that cell membrane Ca^{2+}-ATPase may function in a reduced state in hypertension, either due to an intrinsic defect in the pump itself or inadequate activation (151–156). The V_{max} for Ca^{2+}-ATPase in the platelet membranes is lower in essential hypertensives (156). Since the level and distribution of calmodulin is normal in hypertensive individuals (155), the observed reduction in the V_{max} may reflect (a) impaired calmodulin binding kinetics or (b) an intrinsic abnormality in the expression of the pump, leading to reduced calmodulin activation of Ca^{2+}-ATPase. Such an abnormality of platelet membrane Ca^{2+}-ATPase with reduction in calmodulin activation of Ca^{2+}-ATPase has been observed in hypertensive individuals (154). Others have observed a reduced affinity of the pump for cytosolic Ca^{2+} in a subgroup of patients with essential hypertension (157). Others have suggested that there may be a circulating inhibitor of the membrane Ca^{2+}-ATPase pump in essential hypertension (6).

Increased cell [Ca^{2+}]$_i$ could theoretically relate to increased intracellular Na$^+$ [Na$^+$]$_i$ altered Na$^+$/Ca^{2+} exchange (81,145,158–161). The Na$^+$/Ca^{2+} exchanger moves one Ca^{2+} ion across the plasma in exchange for three or four Na$^+$ ions moving in the opposite direction. The Na$^+$/Ca^{2+} exchanger normally functions to transport Ca^{2+} from the intracellular to extracellular space (145). Theoretically, significant increases in [Na$^+$]$_i$ would result in inhibition of Na$^+$/Ca^{2+} exchange increasing [Ca^{2+}]$_i$. The [Na$^+$]$_i$, in turn, is predominantly regulated by the activity of plasma membrane Na$^+$,K$^+$-ATPase (159). Endogenous regulators of the Na$^+$,K$^+$-ATPase include ouabain (162,163) and perhaps other

circulating factors (6,164). In this regard, elevations in endogenous Na$^+$,K$^+$-ATPase inhibitors have been reported in essential hypertension (165), and abnormalities of the Na$^+$-Ca^{2+} exchanger per se have been inferred in experimental hypertension (145,166).

Another transport abnormality in hypertensives that has been extensively studied by Aviv and Livne (8) is that of altered Na$^+$-H$^+$ exchange. Activity of the Na$^+$-H$^+$ exchanger has been reported to be elevated in hypertensive states (8,35,37,168,175). Increases in activity of the Na$^+$-H$^+$ exchanger may be secondary to increases in [Na$^+$]$_i$ and [Ca^{2+}]$_i$ or may reflect a primary abnormality in membrane transport mechanisms in hypertension. Another disturbance in cellular metabolism that has been observed in hypertension is that of increased platelet cAMP—an abnormality that predisposes to exaggerated agonist-evoked [Ca^{2+}]$_i$ responses (176). Thus, there are a number of cellular metabolic and transport abnormalities that may characterize the disease known as essential hypertension.

CALCIUM, INSULIN, AND BLOOD PRESSURE

The recently recognized relationship between insulin resistance, hyperinsulinemia, and high blood pressure may be mediated through alterations in calcium metabolism (177–180). Many conditions such as obesity, diabetes mellitus, and essential hypertension have common abnormalities in insulin function and calcium metabolism. Insulin is now recognized as a risk factor for hypertension, glucose intolerance, dyslipidemia, and atherosclerosis (181). As insulin resistance is found in lean hypertensive subjects, hypertension per se can be associated with insulin resistance independent of body weight or other confounding variables. The fact that insulin resistance and insulin levels correlate with blood pressure suggest a causal role for insulin in the onset or maintenance of hypertension (182). Under experimental conditions insulin has been shown to alter sodium transport (183), sympathetic nervous system activity (184,185), and vascular tone. Insulin increases sodium reabsorption by direct effects on the renal tubules (183), but it is questionable if this effect leads to chronic sodium retention, volume expansion, and hypertension. Acute insulin infusion in normals increases catecholamine levels (184) and regional sympathetic activity as determined by microneurography (185). However, despite this sympathetic stimulation, the acute vascular effect of insulin is vasodilation with decreased forearm vascular resistance. The contrasting effects of insulin to raise sympathetic activity yet reduce vascular resistance suggest that insulin can have properties of both a vasoconstrictor and a vasorelaxant.

Recent research has linked both hypertension and diabetes to common defects in calcium metabolism. Hypercalcuria is found in insulin-deficient streptozotocin diabetic rats (186) due to specific defects in renal tubular calcium reabsorption. Increased cell levels of calcium and reduced Ca-ATPase activity are found in skeletal muscle cells, in bone cells, and in erythrocytes from rats with insulin resistance (187). In humans, induced hyperinsulinemia leads to exaggerated urinary calcium excretion and diabetic subjects have hypercalcuria, decreased duodenal calcium transport, and low serum ionized calcium (20,186). Studies have found elevated cytosolic calcium in platelets from subjects with Type 2 diabetes mellitus (8,20). Interestingly, several of the defects in renal and gastrointestinal calcium metabolism and cytosolic calcium reported in diabetics are also found in patients with essential hypertension (1–8). Several mechanisms may explain the link between abnormal calcium homeostasis and hypertension in diabetes. Higher levels of free 1,25-dihydroxyvitamin D reported in diabetics could increase calcium uptake in both cardiac tissue and vascular smooth muscle. Insulin may also directly alter the vascular smooth muscle calcium signal leading to changes in vascular tone.

Although the role of insulin as a regulator of calcium metabolism remains controversial, several effects of insulin have been reported on calcium mobilization and transport. Insulin has direct effects on calcium metabolism in skeletal tissue (188,189), cardiac muscle cells (190), adipocytes (191) and kidney tissue (192). Direct effects of insulin on calcium channels have been demonstrated in cultured skeletal muscle cells. In primary cultured rat embryo hindlimb muscle cells, incubation with insulin inhibits depolarization-induced calcium inward current (189). In cultured human muscle cells, more prolonged (2 weeks) treatment with insulin potentiates 40 mMK^+ induced ^{45}Ca uptake (188). These studies suggest that insulin alters calcium transport in several tissues including vascular smooth muscle. Whether insulin alone modulates levels of cytosolic calcium is less certain. In the studies of Draznin et al. (193), insulin incubated for 24 hours with isolated adipocytes in a glucose medium caused an elevation in cytosolic calcium that was blocked by verapamil, suggesting effects on calcium influx.

When insulin is administered *in vivo* or added to an *in vitro* preparation, most studies find acute vasodilation. Hypotension sometimes occurs with insulin treatment in diabetic patients with the complications of diabetic neuropathy (194). Infusion of increasing doses of insulin by the hyperinsulinemic euglycemic clamp method in controls produced a significant increase in leg blood flow (195) and, interestingly, this response is attenuated in obese subjects, suggesting resistance to insulin's action on blood vessels.

Insulin added to *in vitro* vascular preparations attenuates vasoconstriction induced by norepinephrine in resistance beds such as the isolated perfused rat tail (196).

Yagi et al. (197) performed extensive studies with rabbit femoral arteries and veins showing that 30 minute incubations with insulin dose-dependently inhibited norepinephrine and angiotensin II-induced contractions.

Other reports have described potential hypertensive effects of insulin. Yanagisawa-Miwa et al. (198) observed an enhancing effect of insulin on contraction to a thromboxane A_2 analogue in porcine coronary artery. In alloxan- and streptozotocin-induced diabetic animals, insulin reverses diabetes-induced vascular contractility (199) and long-term insulin therapy (8–12 weeks) has been shown to increase vascular contractility to high potassium (200). Numerous studies have shown that both Type 1 and Type 2 diabetic patients whether normotensive or hypertensive with or without complications have enhanced blood pressure responses to administration of angiotensin II and norepinephrine (201). The cause of this enhanced vascular reactivity in diabetes mellitus is unknown, but could relate to abnormal vascular calcium metabolism.

Several studies investigating the mechanism for insulin-induced vasodilation have shown that it attenuates the effects of angiotensin II, arginine vasopressin and serotonin on the calcium signal for contractility in vascular smooth muscle cells. Standley et al. (36) demonstrated in a cultured vascular smooth muscle cell line (a7r5), that insulin decreased arginine vasopressin-induced inward current in receptor-operated and in voltage dependent calcium channels resulting in a 55 percent reduced peak cytosolic calcium response. Similar results from this laboratory were found in vessels from Zucker Obese rats. Thus, insulin decreases agonist-mediated intracellular calcium transients through reducing calcium fluxes. This potential vasorelaxant mechanism of insulin has been further studied with angiotensin II. Saito et al. (202) reported that insulin added alone to vascular smooth muscle cells has no effect on cytosolic calcium, but that it inhibited dose-dependently angiotensin II-induced peak cytosolic calcium responses by up to 50 percent. In this study, an additional mechanism for insulin's effect on calcium was noted to be through inhibition of inositol triphosphate-releasable intracellular calcium stores. Kahn et al. (203) examined the effect of insulin in individual vascular smooth muscle cells using photomicroscopy to measure contraction. Preincubation with insulin attenuated angiotensin II- and serotonin-induced contractions in a dose-dependent manner. Serotonin-induced intracellular calcium transients were inhibited by insulin and this effect was blocked by verapamil and ouabain, indicating an effect of insulin on calcium channels and the Na-K pump. As insulin has been shown to increase the activity of the Na^+-K^+-pump (204,205), it was proposed that insulin stimulation of the Na^+-K^+-pump leads to hyperpolarization of the cell and reduced calcium influx through the voltage-operated calcium channels.

Insulin also regulates cell calcium levels by altering the activity of the Ca-ATPase membrane pump. Levy et al. (187) found that insulin increased Ca-ATPase activity in a variety of tissues. However, in both human and experimental diabetes, there is a generalized reduction in Ca-ATPase activity (31,187) that might indicate a resistance to insulin's normal effect on this pump. Reduced calcium efflux through this pathway would lead to calcium accumulation in vascular smooth muscle cells and provide an explanation for the high tissue levels of calcium, increased vascular reactivity and high incidence of hypertension in diabetes mellitus. Insulin also stimulates the Na^+/H^+ antiporter transport system (206) and this transport pathway has been shown to be elevated in diabetes and hypertension and linked to abnormal calcium metabolism (8).

Thus, the abnormal insulin function that has been broadly described in hypertension and diabetes could provide the missing link between the well-known observations of defective calcium metabolism and increased vascular resistance seen in these conditions. One possibility is that insulin is normally operative as a vasodilator acting as an antagonist to vasoconstrictor substances by reducing calcium transients. With chronic exposure to levels of insulin above physiologic as seen in diabetes and hypertension, there might be a desensitization of its acute relaxant effect resulting in a shift in vascular tone towards vasoconstriction with increased vascular resistance and hypertension.

REFERENCES

1. Ram JL, Standley PR, Sowers JR. Calcium function in vascular smooth muscle and its relationship to hypertension. In: Epstein M, ed. *Calcium antagonists and the kidney.* St. Louis: Hanley & Belfus, 1993:29–48.
2. Sowers JR, Standley PR, Zemel PC. Calcium and hypertension. *J Lab Clin Med* 1989;114:228–248.
3. Brickman AS, Nyby MD, von Hungen K, Eggena P, Tuck ML. Calcitropic hormones, platelet calcium, and blood pressure in essential hypertension. *Hypertension* 1990;16:515–522.
4. Brickman AS, Stern N, Sowers JR. Hypertension in pseudohypoparathyroidism. *Am J Med* 1988;85:785–792.
5. Lind L, Hvarfner A, Palmer M, Grimeluin L, Aberstrom G, Ljunghall S. Hypertension in primary hyperparathyroidism in relation to histopathology. *Eur J Surg* 1991;157:457–459.
6. Linder A, Kenny M, Miacham AJ. Effects of a circulating factor in patients with essential hypertension on intracellular free calcium in normal platelets. *N Engl J Med* 1987;316:509–513.
7. Postnov Y. An approach to the explanation of cell membrane attraction in primary hypertension. *Hypertension* 1990;15:332–337.
8. Aviv A, Livne A. The Na^+/H^+ antiport, cytosolic free Ca^{2+}, and essential hypertension: a hypothesis. *Am J Hypertens* 1988;1:410–413.
9. Pang PKT, Lewanczuk RZ. Parathyroid origin of a new circulating hypertensive factor in spontaneously hypertensive rats. *Am J Hypertens* 1989;2:898–902.
10. Resnick LM. Uniformity and diversity of calcium metabolism in hypertension a conceptional framework. *Am J Med* 1987;82(suppl 1B):16–25.
11. Resnick LM, Muller FB, Laragh JH. Calcium-regulating hormones in essential hypertension: relations to plasma renin activity and sodium metabolism. *Ann Intern Med* 1986;105:649–654.
12. Resnick LM, Laragh JH, Sealey JE. Divalent cations in essential hypertension. Relations between serum ionized calcium, magnesium and plasma renin activity. *N Engl J Med* 1983;309:808–819.
13. Erne P, Hermsmeyer K. Intracellular vascular muscle Ca^{2+} modulation in genetic hypertension. *Hypertension* 1989;14:145–151.
14. Zidek W, Vetter H. Cellular calcium metabolism in primary hypertension. *Klin Wochenschr* 1987;65:155–160.
15. Cooper RS, Shamsi N, Katz S. Intracellular calcium and sodium in hypertensive patients. *Hypertension* 1987;9:224–229.
16. Vincenzi FF, Morris CD, Kinsel LB, Kenny M, McCarron DA. Decreased calcium pump adenosine triphosphate in red blood cells of hypertensive subjects. *Hypertension* 1986;8:1058–1066.
17. Sowers JR, Zemel MB, Bronstein RA. Erythrocyte cation metabolism in preeclampsia. *Am J Obstet Gynecol* 1989;161:441–445.
18. Levy J, Zemel MB, Sowers JR. Role of cellular calcium metabolism in abnormal glucose metabolism and diabetic hypertension. *Am J Med* 1989;87(suppl 6A):7–15.
19. Draznin B. Cytosolic calcium and insulin resistance. *Am J Kidney Dis* 1993;21(6):32–38.
20. Resnick LM. Calcium metabolism in hypertension and altered metabolic disorders. *Diabetes Care* 1991;14:505–520.
21. Sowers JR. Dietary calcium effects in salt-sensitive hypertension. *Clin Nutr* 1989;8:158–163.
22. Feinleib M, Lenfantoc, Miller SA. Hypertension and calcium. *Science* 1984;226:384–386.
23. Draznin B. Cytosolic calcium. A new factor in insulin resistance. *Diabetes Res Clin Pract* 1991;11:141–146.
24. Draznin B. Cytosolic calcium and insulin resistance. *Am J Kidney Dis* 1993;21(6):32–38.
25. Resink TJ, Tbachuk VA, Erne P, Buhler FR. Platelet membrane calmodulin-stimulated calcium-adenosine triphosphatase: altered activity in essential hypertension. *Hypertension* 1986;8:159–166.
26. Hvarfner A, Larsson R, Morlin C, Rastad J, Wide L, Akeratrom G, Ljunghall S. Cytosolic free calcium in platelets: relationship to blood pressure and indices of systemic calcium metabolism. *J Hypertens* 1988;6:71–77.
27. Shore AC, Booker J, Sagnella G, Markandu ND, MacGregor GA. Serum ionized calcium and pH: effects of blood storage, some physiological influences and a comparison between normotensive and hypertensive subjects. *J Hypertens* 1987;5:499–505.
28. McCarron DA. Calcium metabolism and hypertension. *Kidney Int* 1989;35:717–736.
29. Oshima T, Matsuura H, Matsumoto K, Kido K, Kajerjama G. Role of cellular calcium in salt sensitivity of patients with essential hypertension. *Hypertension* 1988;11:703–707.
30. Shingu T, Matamira H, Kusaka M, Inone I, Yuasa A, Shingu TT, Ishida T, Kajirjama G. Significance of intracellular free calcium and magnesium and calcium-regulating hormones with sodium chloride loading in patients with essential hypertension. *J Hypertens* 1991;9:1021–1028.
31. Ram JL, Standley PR, Sowers JR. Hypertension, insulin function and calcium. In: Draznin B, ed. Diabetes and atherosclerosis-molecular basis and clinical aspects. New York: Elsevier, 1993:291–305.
32. Cappone AM, Lew PD, Valloton MB. Cytosolic free calcium levels in monolayers of cultured rat aortic smooth muscle cells: effects of angiotensin II and vasopressin. *J Biol Chem* 1985;260:7836–7842.
33. Van Breemen C, Cauvin C, Johns A, Leijten P, Hiromichi Y. Ca^{2+} regulation of vascular smooth muscle. *Fed Proc* 1986;45:2746–2751.
34. Carafoli E. Intracellular calcium homeostasis. *Annu Rev Biochem* 1987;56:395–433.
35. Batlle DC, Godinich MJ, Lapointe MS, Munoz E, Carone F, Mehring N. Extracellular Na^+ dependency of free cytosolic Ca^{2+} regulation in aortic vascular smooth muscle cells. *Am J Physiol* 1991;261:6845–6856.
36. Standley PR, Zhang F, Ram JL, Sowers JR. Insulin attenuates vasopressin-induced calcium transients and a voltage-dependent calcium response in rat vascular smooth muscle cells. *J Clin Invest* 1991;88:1230–1236.
37. Daugirdas JT, Batlle DC. Interactions of pH_i and Ca^{2+} in vascular smooth muscle tissue. *J Lab Clin Med* 1992;119(6):667–675.

38. Cox RH. K(+)-channel activators in vascular smooth muscle. *Prog Clin Biol Res* 1990;334:171–185.

39. Nelson MT, Pallak JB, Worley JF, Standen NB. Calcium channels, potassium channels, and voltage dependence of arterial smooth muscle tone. *Am J Physiol* 1990;259:C3–18.

40. Droogans G, Declerck I, Custiels R. Effect of adrenergic agonists on Ca²⁺ channel currents in single vascular smooth muscle cells. *Pfluegers Arch* 1987;409:7–12.

41. Cauvin C, Weir SW, Buhler FR. Differences in Ca²⁺ handling along the arterial tree: an update including studies in human mesenteric resistance vessels. *J Cardiovasc Pharmacol* 1988;12(suppl 6):S10–S15.

42. Cauvin C, Lakeman S, Cameron J, Hwang O, Van Breeman C. Differences in norepinephrine activation and diltiazem inhibition of calcium channels in isolated rabbit aorta and mesenteric resistance vessels. *Circ Res* 1985;56:822–828.

43. Ruegg UT, Wallsnofer A, Weir S, Cauvin C. Receptor-operated calcium-permeable channels in vascular smooth muscle. *J Cardiovasc Pharmacol* 1989;14(suppl 6):S49–S58.

44. Galizzi J-P, Qar J, Fosset M, Van Rengerghem C, Ladunski M. Regulation of calcium channels in aortic muscle cells by protein kinase C activators (diacylglycerol and phorbol esters) and by peptides (vasopressin and bombesin) that stimulate phosphoinositol breakdown. *J Biol Chem* 1987;262:6947–6950.

45. Litten RX, Suba EX, Roth BL. Effects of a phorbolester on rat aortic contraction and calcium influx in the presence and absence of BAYk8644. *Eur J Pharmacol* 1987;149:185–191.

46. Nelson MT, Standen NB, Brayden JE, Worley JF III. Noradrenalin contracts arteries by activating voltage-dependent calcium channels. *Nature* 1988;336:382–385.

47. Pacaad P, Loirand G, Mironneau C, Mironneau J. Opposing effects of noradrenaline on the two classes of voltage-dependent calcium channels of single vascular smooth muscle cells in short term primary culture. *Pflugers Arch* 1987;410:557–559.

48. Goto K, Kasurja Y, Matsuki N, Takuwa Y, Kurihara H, Ishikawa T, Kimura S, Yonagisawa M, Masaki T. Endothelin activates the dihydripyridine-sensitive, voltage-dependent Ca²⁺ channel in vascular smooth muscle. *Proc Natl Acad Sci USA* 1989;86:3915–3918.

49. Inene Y, Oike M, Nakao K, Kitamura K, Kuriyama H. Endothelin augments unitary-calcium channel currents on the smooth muscle cell membrane of guinea pig portal vein. *J Physiol* 1990;423:171–191.

50. Van Renterghem C, Vigne P, Barhanin J, Schmid-Alliana A, Frelin C, Lazduneki M. Molecular mechanism of action of the vasoconstrictor peptide endothelin. *Biochem Biophys Res Commun* 1988;157:977–985.

51. Wagner-Mann C, Sturek M. Endothelin mediates Ca influx and release in porcine coronary smooth muscle cells. *Am J Physiol* 1991;260:C771–C777.

52. Van Renterghem C, Romey G, Lazdunski M. Vasopressin modulates the spontaneous electrical activity in aortic cells (line A7r5) by acting on three different types of ionic channels. *Proc Natl Acad Sci USA* 1988;85:9365–9369.

53. Ohya Y, Speralakis N. Involvement of a GTP-binding protein in stimulating action of angiotensin II on calcium channels in vascular smooth muscle cells. *Circ Res* 1991;68:763–771.

54. Kitazawa T, Kabarjashi S, Horiuti K, Somlyo AV, Somlyo AP. Receptor-coupled, permeabilized smooth muscle: role of the phosphatidylinositol cascade, G-proteins, and modulation of the contractile response to Ca²⁺. *J Biol Chem* 1989;264:5339–5342.

55. Suematsu E, Hirata M, Hashimoto T, Kuriyama H. Inositol 1,4,5-triphosphate releases Ca²⁺ from intracellular store sites in skinned single cells of porcine coronary artery. *Biochem Biophys Res Commun* 1984;120:481–485.

56. Yamamoto H, Van Breeman C. Inositol 1,4,5-triphosphate releases calcium from skinned cultured smooth muscle cells. *Biochem Biophys Res Commun* 1985;130:270–274.

57. Walker JW, Somlyo AV, Goldman YE, Somlyo AP, Trentham DR. Kinetics of smooth and skeletal muscle activation by laser pulse photolysis of caged inositol 1,4,5-triphosphate. *Nature* 1987;327:249–252.

58. Saida K, Van Breeman C. GTP requirement for inositol-1,4,5-triphosphate-induced Ca²⁺ release from sarcoplasmic reticulum in smooth muscle. *Biochem Biophys Res Commun* 1987;144:1313–1316.

59. Van Breeman C, Saida K, Yamamoto H, Hwang K, Twart C. Vascular smooth muscle sarcoplasmic reticulum. Function and mechanisms of Ca²⁺ release. *Ann NY Acad Sci* 1988;522:60–73.

60. Smith JS, Cornoado R, Meissner G. Sarcoplasmic reticulum continues adenine nucleotide-activated calcium channels. *Nature* 1985;316:446–449.

61. Ito K, Ikemoto T, Takakura S. Involvement of Ca²⁺ influx-induced Ca²⁺ release in contraction of intact vascular smooth muscles. *Am J Physiol* 1991;261:H1464–1470.

62. Gunter TE, Pfeiffer DR. Mechanisms by which mitochondria transport calcium. *Am J Physiol* 1990;259:C134–143.

63. Grover AK. Ca-pumps in smooth muscle: one in plasma membrane and another in endoplasmic reticulum. *Cell Calcium* 1985;6:227–236.

64. Eggermont JA, Vrolix M, Raeymaekers L, Wuytack F, Casteils R. Ca²⁺-transport ATPases of vascular smooth muscle. *Circ Res* 1988;62:266–278.

65. Levy D, Seigneuret M, Bluzat A, Rigaad JL. Evidence for proton countertransport in reconstituted proteoliposomes with low ionic permeability. *J Biol Chem* 1990;265:19524–19534.

66. Fukudu T, Orgurusu T, Furulsawa K, Shigekawa M. Protein kinase C-dependent phosphorylation of sarcolemmal Ca²⁺-ATPase isolated from bovine aortic smooth muscle. *J Biochem* 1990;108:629–634.

67. Sun H-T, Yoshida Y, Imai S. A Ca²⁺-activated Mg²⁺-dependent ATPase with high affities for both Ca²⁺ and Mg²⁺ in vascular smooth muscle macrosomes: comparison with plasma membrane Ca²⁺-ATPase isolated from bovine aortic smooth muscle. *J Biochem* 1990;108:629–634.

68. Nakamura J. pH and temperature resolve the kinetics of two pools of calcium bound to the sarcoplasmic reticulum Ca²⁺-ATPase. *J Biol Chem* 1989;264:17029–17031.

69. Dixon DA, Haynes DH. The pH dependence of the cardiac sarcolemmal Ca²⁺-transporting ATPase: evidence that the Ca²⁺ translocator bears a doubly negative charge. *Biochim Biophys Acta* 1990;1029:274–284.

70. Furakawa KI, Tawada Y, Shigekawa M. Regulation of the plasma membrane Ca²⁺ pump by cyclic nucleotides in cultured vascular smooth muscle cells. *J Biol Chem* 1988;263:8058–8065.

71. Furukawa KI, Nakamura H. Cyclic GMP regulator of the plasma membrane (Ca²⁺-Mg²⁺) ATPase in vascular smooth muscle. *J Biochem* 1987;101:290.

72. Baltensperger CM, Carafoli E, Chiesi M. The Ca²⁺-pumping ATPase and the major substrates of the cGMP-dependent protein kinase in smooth muscle sarcolemma are distinct entities. *Eur J Biochem* 1988;172:7–16.

73. Popescu LM, Hinescu ME, Musat S, Ionescu M, Pistritzu F. Inosital triphosphate and the contraction of vascular smooth muscle cells. *Eur J Pharmacol* 1986;123:167–169.

74. Sowers JR. At the cutting edge. Insulin resistance and hypertension. *Mol Cell Endocrinol* 1990;74:87–89.

75. Carafoli E. The calcium pumping ATPase of the plasma membrane. *Annu Rev Physiol* 1991;53:531–547.

76. Kawashima H. Receptor for 1,25 dihydroxy vitamin D in a vascular smooth muscle cell line derived from rat aorta. *Biochem Biophys Res Commun* 1987;146:1–6.

77. Blaustein MP, Ahida T, Goldman MF, Wier WG, Hamlyn JM. Sodium/calcium exchange in vascular smooth muscle: a link between sodium metabolism and hypertension. *Ann NY Acad Sci* 1986;448:199–216.

78. Smith JB. Angiotensin-receptor signalling in cultured vascular smooth muscle cells. *Am J Physiol* 1986;250:F759–769.

79. Smith JB, Smith L. Extracellular Na⁺ dependence of changes in free Ca²⁺, 45 Ca²⁺ efflux, and total cell Ca²⁺ produced by angiotensin II in cultured aortic muscle cells. *J Biol Chem* 1987;262:17455–17460.

80. Nabel EG, Berk BC, Brock TA, Smith TW. Na⁺-Ca²⁺-exchange in cultured vascular smooth muscle cells. *Circ Res* 1988;62:486–493.

81. Matlib MA. Na⁺-Ca²⁺ exchange in sarcolemmal membrane vesicles of dog mesenteric artery. *Am J Physiol* 1988;255:C223–C330.

82. Slaughter RS, Shevell JL, Felix JP, Garcia ML, Kaczarowski GJ.

High levels of sodium-calcium exchange in vascular smooth muscle sarcolemmal membrane vesicles. *Biochemistry* 1989;28:3995–4002.

83. Bova S, Goldman WF, Yauan X-J, Blaustein MP. Influence of Na⁺ gradient on Ca²⁺ transients and contraction in vascular smooth muscle. *Am J Physiol* 1990;259:H409–H423.

84. Siskind MS, McCoy CE, Chobanean A, Schwartz JH. Regulation of intracellular calcium by cell pH in vascular smooth muscle cells. *Am J Physiol* 1989;256:C234–240.

85. Danthuluri NR, Kim D, Brock TA. Intracellular alkalinization leads to Ca²⁺ mobilization from agonist-sensitive pools in bovine aortic endothelial cells. *J Biol Chem* 1990;265:19071–19076.

86. Brass LF, Joseph SK. A role for inositol triphosphate in intracellular Ca²⁺ mobilization and granule secretion in platelets. *J Biol Chem* 1985;260:15172–15179.

87. Schultz I, Thevenod F, Dehlinger-Kremer M. Modulation of intracellular free Ca²⁺ concentration by IP₃-sensitive and IP₃-insensitive nonmitochondrial Ca²⁺ pools. *Cell Calcium* 1989;283:658–660.

88. Breitweiser GE. G-protein-mediated ion channel activation. *Hypertension* 1991;17:684–692.

89. Birnbaumer L. G-proteins in signal transduction. *Annu Rev Pharmacol Toxicol* 1991;30:675–705.

90. Kondo K, Kozawa O, Takusulai K, Oiso Y. Ca²⁺ influx stimulated by vasopressin is mediated by phosphoinositide hydrolysis in rat smooth muscle cells. *Biochem Biophys Res Commun* 1989;161:677–682.

91. Nishimura J, Kolber M, Van Breeman C. Norepinephrine and GTP-gamma-S increase myofilament Ca²⁺ sensitivity in alpha toxin permeabilized arterial smooth muscle. *Biochem Biophy Res Commun* 1988;157:677–683.

92. Sowers JR, Zemel PC, Standley PR. Calcium metabolism and dietary calcium in salt sensitive hypertension. *Am J Hypertens* 1991;4:557–563.

93. Nishizuka Y. Studies and perspectives of protein kinase C. *Science* 1986;97:305–312.

94. Fujiwara T, Itoh T, Kubotu Y, Kuriyama H. Effects of guanosine nucleotides on skinned smooth muscle tissue of the rabbit mesenteric artery. *J Physiol* 1989;408:535–547.

95. Bell NH. Vitamin D-endocrine system. *J Clin Invest* 1985;76:1–6.

96. DeLuca HF. The vitamin D story: a collaborative effort of basic science and clinical medicine. *FASEB J* 1987;2:224–236.

97. Minghetti PP, Norman AW. 1,25 (OH)₂-vitamin D₃ receptors: gene regulation and genetic circuitry. *FASEB J* 1988;2:3043–3053.

98. Lewanczuk RZ, Resnick LM, Blumenfield J. A new circulating hypertensive factor in human essential hypertension. *J Hypertens* 1990;8:105–108.

99. Pang PKT. Satellite symposium of the International Society of Hypertension on the parathyroid hypertensive factor. Madrid, June 13, 1992. *J Cardiovasc Pharmacol* 1992; special issue.

100. Lewanczuk RZ, Benishin CG, Pang PKT. Parathyroid hypertensive factor decreases urinary sodium excretion in normotensive rats (abstr). 14th Scientific Meeting of the International Society of Hypertension, Madrid, June 13, 1992. *J Hypertens* 1992;12(suppl 4):90.

101. Braun SC, Williams TJ, Tippins JR, Morris HR, MacIntyre I. Calcitonin gene-related peptide is a potent vasodilator. *Nature* 1965;313:54–56.

102. Fisher LA, Kikkawa DO, Rivier JE, Amara SG, Evans RM, Rosenfield MG, Vale WW, Brown MR. Stimulation of noradrenergic sympathetic outflow by calcitonin gene-related peptide. *Nature* 1983;305:534–537.

103. Lundbert JM, Franco-Cereceda A, Hua X, Hokfelt T, Fischer JA. Co-existence of substance P and calcitonin gene-related peptide immunoreactivities in sensory nerves in relation to cardiovascular and bronchoconstrictor effects of capsaicin. *Eur J Pharmacol* 1985;108:315–321.

104. Tippins JR, Morris HR, Panico M, Etienne T, Bevis P, Girgis S, MacIntyre I, Azria M, Attinger M. The myotropic and plasma-calcium modulating effects of calcitonin gene-related peptide. *Neuropeptides* 1984;4:425–430.

105. Signal S, Franco-Cereceda A, Henke H, Lundberg JM, Fischer JA. Specific receptor and cardiovascular effects of calcitonin, a gene-related peptide. *Endocrinology* 1986;119:381–389.

106. Mulderry PB, Ghatei MA, Rodrigo J, Allen JM, Rosenfeld MG, Polak JM, Bloom SR. Calcitonin gene-related peptide in cardiovascular tissues of the rat. *Neuroscience* 1985;14:947–954.

107. Heath H, Hodgson SF, Kennedy MA. Primary hyperparathyroidism. Incidence, morbidity and potential economic impact in a community. *N Engl J Med* 1980;302:189–193.

108. Nainby-Luxmoore JC, Langford HG, Nelson NC, Watson RL, Barnes TY. A case-comparison study of hypertension and hyperparathyroidism. *J Clin Endocrinol Metab* 1982;55:303–306.

109. Zawada ET, Brickman AS, Maxwell MH, Tuck M. Hypertension associated with hyperparathyroidism is not responsive to angiotensin blockade. *J Clin Endocrinol Metab* 1980;50:912–915.

110. Ringe J-D. Reversible hypertension in primary hyperparathyroidism. Pre- and postoperative blood pressure in 75 cases. *Klin Wochenschr* 1984;62:465–469.

111. Daniels J, Goodman AD. Hypertension and hyperparathyroidism. *Am J Med* 1983;75:17–23.

112. Nikkila MT, Jaaristo JJ, Kovivula TA. Clinical and biochemical features in primary hyperparathyroidism. *Surgery* 1989;105:148–153.

113. Lind L, Hvarfner A, Palmer M, Grimelius L, Akerstrom G, Ljunghall S. Hypertension in primary hyperparathyroidism in relation to histopathology. *Eur J Surg* 1991;157:457–459.

114. Uden P, Chan A, Duh Q-Y, Siperstein A, Clark OH. Primary hyperparathyroidism in younger and older patients: symptoms and outcome of surgery. *World J Surg* 1992;19:791–798.

115. Stern N, Lee DBN, Silis V, et al. Effects of high calcium intake on blood pressure and calcium metabolism in young SHR. *Hypertension* 1984;6:639–646.

116. Brickman AS, Nyby M, von Hunger K, Eggena P, Tuck ML. Parathyroid hormone, platelet calcium and blood pressure in normal subjects. *Hypertension* 1991;18:176–182.

117. Sowers JR, Zemel P, Standley P, Kraniak J, Zemel MB. Role of calcium in modulating salt sensitivity. In: Rettig R, Ganten D, Luft FC, eds. *Salt and hypertension.* Berlin: Springer-Verlag, 1989;169–175.

118. Hulter HN, Melby JC, Peterson JC, Cooke CR. Chronic continuous PTH infusion results in hypertension in normal subjects. *J Clin Hypertens* 1986;4:360–370.

119. Wang HH, Drugge ED, Yen YC, Blumenthal MR, Pang PKT. Effects of synthetic parathyroid hormone on hemodynamic and regional blood flows. *Eur J Pharmacol* 1984;97:209–215.

120. Roca-Cusachs A, Dipette DJ, Nickols GA. Regional and systemic hemodynamic effects of parathyroid hormone-related protein: preservation of cardiac function and coronary renal flow with reduced blood pressure. *J Pharmacol Exp Ther* 1991;256:110–118.

121. Hongo T, Kupfer J, Enomoto H, Sharifi B, Giannella-Neto D, Forrester JS, Singer FR, Glotzman D, Hendy GN, Pirola C, Fagin JA, Clemens TL. Abundant expression of parathyroid hormone-related protein in primary rat aortic smooth muscle cells accompanies serum-induced proliferation. *J Clin Invest* 1991;88:1841–1847.

122. Sowers JR, Tuck ML. Hypertension associated with diabetes mellitus, hypercalcemic disorders, acromegaly and thyroid disease. *Clin Endocrinol Metab* 1981;10(3):631–650.

123. Sowers JR. Hypertension in the elderly. *Am J Med* 1987;82(suppl 1B):1–8.

124. Diamond TW, Botha JR, Wing J, Meyers AM, Kalk WJ. Parathyroid hypertension. A reversible disorder. *Arch Intern Med* 1986;146:1709–1712.

125. Sanco JJ, Rouco J, Riera-Vidal R, Sitges-Serra A. Long-term effects of parathyroidectomy for primary hyperparathyroidism on arterial hypertension. *World J Surg* 1992;16:732–736.

126. Sowers JR, Brickman A, Asp ND, Jasberg K, Magnone S. Altered dopaminergic modulation of prolactin and aldosterone secretion in pseudohypoparathyroidism. *J Clin Endocrinol Metab* 1981;52:914–918.

127. Sowers JR, Brickman AS. Arcadian blood pressure, renin, aldosterone, cortisol and prolactin levels in hypertensive pseudohypoparathyroid patients. *J Clin Endocrinol Metab* 1982;55:1202–1208.

128. Moore WT, Smith LH. Experience with calcium infusion test in parathyroid disease. *Metabolism* 1963;12:447–452.

129. Weidman NP, Massry SG, Coburn JW, et al. Blood pressure effects of acute hypercalcemia: studies in patients with chronic renal failure. *Ann Intern Med* 1972;76:741–747.

130. Raine AEG, Bedford L, Simpson AWM, Ashley CC, Brown R, Woodhead JS, Ledingham JGG. Hyperparathyroidism, platelet intracellular calcium and hypertension in chronic renal failure. *Kidney Int* 1993;43:700–705.

131. Lind L, Wengle B, Wide L, Sorensen O, Ljunghall S. Hypertension in primary hyperparathyroidism. Reduction of blood pressure by long-term treatment with vitamin D (alphcalcidol). *Am J Hypertens* 1988;1:397–402.

132. Koh E, Marimoto S, Fukus K, Itoh K, Hironaku T, et al. 1,25-dihydroxyvitamin D_3 binds specifically to rat vascular smooth muscle cells and stimulates their proliferation in vitro. *Life Sci* 1988;42:215–223.

133. Merke J, Hofmann W, Goldsmidt D, Tirz E. Demonstration of 1,25(OH)$_2$ vitamin D_3 receptors and actions in vascular smooth muscle cells in vitro. *Calcif Tissue Int* 1987;41:112–114.

134. Walters MR, Ilenchuls TT, Claycomb WC. 1,25-dihydroxyvitamin D_3 stimulates [$^{45}Ca^{2+}$] uptake by cultured adult rat ventricular cardiac muscle cells. *J Biol Chem* 1987;262:2536–2541.

135. Bukoski RD, DeWan P, McCarron DA. 1,25(OH)$_2$ vitamin D_3 modifies growth and contractile function of vascular smooth muscle of spontaneously hypertensive rats. *Am J Hypertens* 1989;2:553–556.

136. Sommerville LE, Harlshorne DJ. Intracellular calcium and smooth muscle contraction. *Cell Calcium* 1986;7:353–364.

137. Nishimura J, vanBreemen C. Direct regulation of smooth muscle contractile elements by second messengers. *Biochem Biophys Res Commun* 1989;163:929–935.

138. Hai C-M, Murphy RA. Ca^{2+}, crossbridge phosphorylation and contraction. *Annu Rev Physiol* 1989;51:285–298.

139. Sugirjama T, Yoshizumi M, Takaku F, Yazalai Y. Abnormal calcium handling in vascular smooth muscle cells of spontaneously hypertensive rats. *J Hypertens* 1990;8:369–375.

140. Perry PA, Webb RC. Agonist-sensitive calcium stores in arteries from steroid hypertensive rats. *Hypertension* 1991;17:603–611.

141. Soloviev AI, Bershtein SA. The contractile apparatus in vascular smooth muscle cells of spontaneously hypertensive rats possess increased calcium sensitivity: the possible role of protein kinase C. *J Hypertens* 1992;10:131–136.

142. Reuter H. Sodium-calcium exchange: ins and outs of Ca^{2+} transport. *Nature* 1991;349:567–568.

143. Ashida T, Blaustein MP. Regulation of cell calcium and contractility in mammalian smooth muscle: the role of sodium-calcium exchange. *J Physiol (Lond)* 1990;392:617–635.

144. Rusch NJ, DeLucena RG, Wooldridge TA, England SK, Cowley AW. A Ca^{2+}-dependent K^+ current is enhanced in arterial membranes of hypertensive rats. *Hypertension* 1992;19:301–307.

145. Rimbold CM, Richard H, Chen XL. Na^+-Ca^{2+} exchange, myoplasmic Ca^{2+} concentration, and contraction of arterial smooth muscle. *Hypertension* 1992;19:308–313.

146. Livne AA, Akaronovitz O, Paran E. Higher Na^+-H^+ exchange rate and more alkaline intracellular pH set-point in essential hypertension: effects of protein kinase modulation in platelets. *J Hypertens* 1991;9:1013–1019.

147. Erne P, Bolli P, Burgisser E. Correlation of platelet calcium with blood pressure: effect of antihypertensive therapy. *N Engl J Med* 1984;310:1084–1088.

148. Postnov YV, Orlov SN, Shevchenko A, Adler AM. Altered sodium permeability, calcium binding and Na-K-ATPase activity in the red blood cell membrane in essential hypertension. *Pflugers Arch* 1977;381:263–269.

149. Orlov SN, Postnov YV. Ca^{2+} binding and membrane fluidity in essential and renal hypertension. *Clin Sci* 1982;63:281–284.

150. Robinson BF. Altered calcium handling as a cause of primary hypertension. *J Hypertens* 1984;2:453–460.

151. Moore L, Hurwitz L, Davenport GR, Landon EJ. Energy dependent calcium uptake activity of microsomes from the aorta of normal and hypertensive rats. *Biochem Biophys Acta* 1975;413:432–443.

152. Kwan CY, Belbeck L, Daniel EE. Abnormal biochemistry of vas-

153. Postnov YV, Orlov SN, Reznikova MB, Rjazhsky GG, Pokudin NI. Calmodulin distribution and Ca^{2+} transport in the erythrocytes of patients with essential hypertension. *Clin Sci* 1984;66:459–465.

154. Resink TJ, Tkachuk VA, Erne P, Buhler FR. Platelet membrane calmodulin-stimulated calcium-adenosine triphosphatase. Altered activity in essential hypertension. *Hypertension* 1986;8:159–166.

155. Vincenzi FF, Morris CD, Kinsel LB, Kenny M, McCarron DA. Decreased calcium pump adenosine triphosphatase in red blood cells of hypertensive subjects. *Hypertension* 1986;8:1058–1066.

156. Takaya J, Lasker N, Bamforth R, Gutkin M, Byrd LH, Aviv A. Kinetics of Ca^{2+}-ATPase activation in platelet membranes of essential hypertensives and normotensives. *Am J Physiol* 1990;258:C988–C994.

157. De la Sierra A, Hannaert P, Ollivier J-P, Senn N, Garay R. Kinetic study of the Ca^{2+} pump in erythrocytes from essential hypertensive patients. *J Hypertens* 1990;8:285–293.

158. Bova S, Goldman WF, Yuan X-J, Blaustein MP. Influence of Na^+ gradient on Ca^{2+} transients and contraction in vascular smooth muscle. *Am J Physiol* 1990;259(Heart Circ Physiol):H409–H423.

159. Ashida T, Blaustein MP. Regulation of cell calcium and contractility in mammalian smooth muscle: the role of sodium-calcium exchange. *J Physiol (Lond)* 1990;392:617–635.

160. Aaronson PI, Benham CD. Alterations in [Ca^{2+}]$_i$ mediated by sodium-calcium exchange in smooth muscle cells isolated from the guinea-pig ureter. *J Physiol (Lond)* 1989;416:1–18.

161. Reuter H. Sodium-calcium exchange: ins and outs of Ca^{2+} transport. *Nature* 1991;349:567–568.

162. Woolfson RG, Hilton PJ, Poston L. Effects of ouabain and low sodium on contractility of human resistance arteries. *Hypertension* 1990;15:583–590.

163. Ludens JH, Clark MA, DuCharme DW, Harris DW, Lutzke BS, Mandel F, Mathews WR, Sutter DM, Hamlyn JM. Purification of an endogenous digitalis-like factor from human plasma for structural analysis. *Hypertension* 1991;17:923–929.

164. Navran SS, Allain G, Garcia HF, Allen JC, Seidel CL. Serotonin-induced Na^+/K^+ pump stimulation in vascular smooth muscle cells. Evidence for coupling to multiple receptor mechanisms. *J Pharmacol Exp Ther* 1991;256:297–303.

165. Hamlyn JM, Ringle R, Schaeffer J, Levinson PD, Hamilton BP, Kowarski AA, Blaustein MP. A circulating inhibitor of (Na+K)-ATPase associated with essential hypertension. *Nature* 1982;300:650–652.

166. Thompson LE, Rinaldi GJ, Bohr DF. Decreased activity of the sodium-calcium exchanger in tail artery of stroke-prone spontaneously hypertensive rats. *Blood Vessels* 1990;27:197–201.

167. Livne A, Veitch R, Grinstein S, Balfe JW, Marquez-Julio A, Rothstein A. Increased platelet Na^+-H^+ exchange rates in essential hypertension: application of a novel test. *Lancet* 1987;1:533–536.

168. Oshima T, Matsuura H, Kido K, et al. Intralymphocytic sodium and free calcium and plasma renin in essential hypertension. *Hypertension* 1988;12:26–31.

169. Schmouder RL, Weder AB. Platelet sodium-proton exchange is increased in essential hypertension. *J Hypertens* 1989;7:325–330.

170. Wheling M, Kasmayr J, Theisen K. The Na^+-H^+ exchanger is stimulated and cell volume increased in lymphocytes from patients with essential hypertension. *J Hypertens* 1991;9:519–524.

171. Rosskopf D, Morgenstern E, Schloz W, Osswald U, Siffert W. Rapid determination of the elevated Na^+-H^+ exchange in platelets of patients with essential hypertension using an optical swelling assay. *J Hypertens* 1991;9:231–238.

172. Tokudome G, Tomonari H, Gardner JP, et al. Variations in the apparent pH set point for activation of platelet Na-H antiport. *Hypertension* 1990;16:180–189.

173. Livne AA, Aharonozitz O, Paran E. Higher Na^+-H^+ exchange rate and more alkaline intracellular pH set-point in essential hypertension: effect of protein kinase C modulation in platelets. *J Hypertens* 1989;7:325–330.

174. Ng LL, Fennell DA, Dudley C. Kinetics of the human leucocyte

Na$^+$-H$^+$ antiport in essential hypertension. *J Hypertens* 1990;8:533–537.

175. Goldsmith DJA, Tribe RM, Poston L, et al. Leucocyte intracellular pH and Na$^+$-H$^+$ exchange activity in essential hypertension: an *in vitro* study under physiological conditions. *J Hypertens* 1991;9:645–653.

176. Mazeaud MM, LeQuan Sang K-H, DeVynck M-A. Platelet cyclic AMP in essential hypertension. *J Hypertens* 1989;7:501–506.

177. Defronzo RA, Ferrannini E. Insulin resistance: A multifaceted syndrome responsible for NIDDM, obesity, hypertension, dyslipidemia and atherosclerosic heart disease. *Diabetes Care* 1991;14:173–194.

178. Ferrannini E, Buzzigoli G, Bonadona R, et al. Insulin resistance in essential hypertension. *N Engl J Med* 1987;317:350–357.

179. Corry DB, Tuck ML. Hypertension and diabetes. Seminars in Nephrology 1991;11:561–570.

180. Haffner SM. Editorial: Insulin and blood pressure: fact or fantasy? *J Clin Endocrinol Metab* 1993;76(3):541–543.

181. Reaven GM. Treatment of hypertension. Focus on prevention of coronary heart disease. *J Clin Endocrinol Metab* 1993;76(3):537–540.

182. Lind L, Lithell H, Pollare T. Is it hyperinsulinemia or insulin resistance that is related to hypertension and other metabolic cardiovascular risk factors? *J Hypertens* 1993;11(suppl 4):S11–S16.

183. DeFronzo RA, Cooke CR, Andres R, et al. The effects of insulin on renal handling of sodium, calcium and phosphate in man. *J Clin Invest* 1975;55:845–855.

184. Rowe JW, Young JB, Minaker KL, Stevens AL, Pallotta J, Landsberg L. Effect of insulin and glucose infusions on sympathetic nervous activity in normal man. *Diabetes* 1981;30:219–225.

185. Anderson EA, Hoffman RP, Balon TW, Sinkey CA, Mark AL. Hyperinsulinemia produces both sympathetic neural activation and vasodilation in normal humans. *J Clin Invest* 1991;87:2246–2252.

186. Resnick LM. Hypertension and abnormal glucose homeostasis. Possible role of divalent ion metabolism. *Am J Med* 1989;87(6A):17S–22S.

187. Levy J, Zemel MB, Sowers JR. Role of cellular calcium metabolism in abnormalities in glucose metabolism and diabetic hypertension. *Am J Med* 1989;87(suppl 6A):7–16.

188. Desnuelle C, Askanas V, Engel WK. Insulin enhances development of voltage-dependent calcium channels in aneurally cultured human muscle. *J Neurochem* 1987;49:1133–1138.

189. Wu F, Zieler K. Calcium currents in rat myoballs and their inhibition by insulin. *Endocrinology* 1989;125:2563–2572.

190. Gupta MP, Makino N, Khatter K, Dhalla NS. Stimulation of Na/Ca exchange in heart sarcolemma by insulin. *Life Sci* 1986;39:1077–1083.

191. Pershadsingh HA, McDonald JM. Direct addition of insulin inhibits a high affinity Ca^{2+}-ATPase in isolated adipocyte plasma membranes. *Nature* 1979;281:495–497.

192. Levy J, Gavin JR III, Morimoto S, Hammerman MR, Avioli LV. Hormonal regulation of (Ca^{2+} + Mg^{2+})ATPase activity in canine renal basolateral membrane. *Endoclinology* 1986;119:2405–2411.

193. Draznin B, Kao M, Sussman KE. Insulin and glyburide increase cytosolic free Ca^{2+} concentrations in isolated rat adipocytes. *Diabetes* 1987;36:174–178.

194. Page M, Watkins PJ. Provocation of postural hypotension by insulin in diabetic autonomic neuropathy. *Diabetes* 1976;25:90–95.

195. Laakso M, Edelman SV, Brechtel G, et al. Decreased effect of insulin to stimulate skeletal muscle blood flow in obese man. *J Clin Invest* 1990;85:1844–1852.

196. Alaxander WD, Oake RJ. The effect of insulin on vascular reactivity to norepinephrine. *Diabetes* 1977;26:611–614.

197. Yagi, Takata S, Kiyokawa H. Effects of insulin on vasoconstrictive responses to norepinephrine and angiotensin II in rabbit femoral artery and vien. *Diabetes* 37:1064–1067.

198. Yanagisawa-Misa A, Ito H, Sugimoto T. Effects of insulin on vasoconstriction induced by thromboxane A2 in porcine coronary artery. *Circulation* 1990;81:1654–1659.

199. Head RJ, Longhurst PA, Panek RL, Stizel RE. A contrasting effect of the diabetic state upon the contractile responese of aortic preparations from the rat and rabbit. *Br J Pharmacol* 1987;91:275–286.

200. Pfaffman MA, Ball CR, Darby A, Hilman R. Insulin reversal of diabetes-induced inhibition of vascular contractility in the rat. *Am J Physiol* 1982;242:H490–H495.

201. Tuck ML, Corry DB, Trujillo A. Salt sensitive blood pressure and exaggerated vascular reactivity in the hypertension of diabetes mellitus. *Am J Med* 1990;88:210–216.

202. Saito F, Hori M, Fittingoff M, Tuck ML. Insulin attenuates agonist-mediated calcium mobilization in cultured rat vascular smooth muscle cells. *J Clin Invest* 1993;92:1161–1167.

203. Kahn AM, Seidel CL, Allen JC, O'Neil RG, Shelat H, Song T. Insulin reduces contraction and intracellular calcium concentration in vascular smooth muscle. *Hypertension* 1993;22:735–742.

204. Omatsu-Kanbe M, Kitasato H. Insulin stimulates the translocation of Na$^+$/K$^+$-dependent ATPase molecules from intracellular stores to the plasma membrane in frog skeletal muscle. *Biochem J* 1990;272:727–733.

205. Rosic NK, Standeart ML, Pollet RJ. The mechanism of insulin stimulation of (Na$^+$,K$^+$)-ATPase transport activity in muscle. *J Biol Chem* 1985;260:6206–6212.

206. Moore RD. Stimulation of Na:H exchange by insulin. *Biophys J* 1981;33:203–210.

Hypertension: Pathophysiology, Diagnosis, and Management, Second Edition, edited by J.H. Laragh and B.M. Brenner, Raven Press, Ltd., New York © 1995.

CHAPTER 70

Ionic Disturbances of Calcium and Magnesium Metabolism in Essential Hypertension

Lawrence M. Resnick

At present, the clinical expression and consequences of cardiovascular syndromes such as hypertension cannot be traced to an easily identifiable primary defect, properly termed the "cause" of the disease. This is so for a number of reasons. One reason is that the expression of the disease is not the disease itself, but merely a sign of the disease—hypertension being an abnormal physical sign of an underlying pathophysiological process, whose nature and extent are still undefined. Second, the elevated blood pressure readings that currently define hypertension clinically may derive from different "causes" in different populations or even in different individuals; hence, the heterogeneity of hypertension. This dual problem, hypertension as only one sign of an as yet undefined underlying process, and the number of different pathophysiological processes that may result in the indistinguishable, chronically elevated blood pressures we collectively call hypertension, is also apparent in current trends in hypertension research. One approach no longer seeks underlying "causes," and focuses on identifying epidemiologically defined "risk factors." Another approach utilizes the modern techniques of molecular biology to search for an ultimate genetic lesion as the basis for hypertension. We sought to develop a conceptual framework of hypertensive cardiovascular disease in which the influence of varying environmental and genetically determined factors are integrated into a common pathophysiological setpoint of altered cell and organ system function, resulting in the clinical expression of hypertension and/or any other of the allied clinical conditions deriving from this same underlying functional "lesion."

Our approach focuses on the role of steady-state cellular ion activity as a final common pathway mediating cellular responsiveness to a wide variety of external stimuli. Methodologically, the development of nuclear magnetic resonance (NMR) spectroscopic techniques, in addition to previously available fluorescent spectroscopy, has allowed for the precise, consistent measurement of a variety of intracellular mineral ion species, including pH, sodium, potassium, intracellular free magnesium, and cytosolic free calcium (1–4) (Figs. 1 and 2). Utilizing these NMR techniques, we have described altered extracellular and intracellular distributions of divalent cations

L. M. Resnick: Division of Endocrinology and Hypertension, Wayne State University Medical Center, Detroit, Michigan 48201.

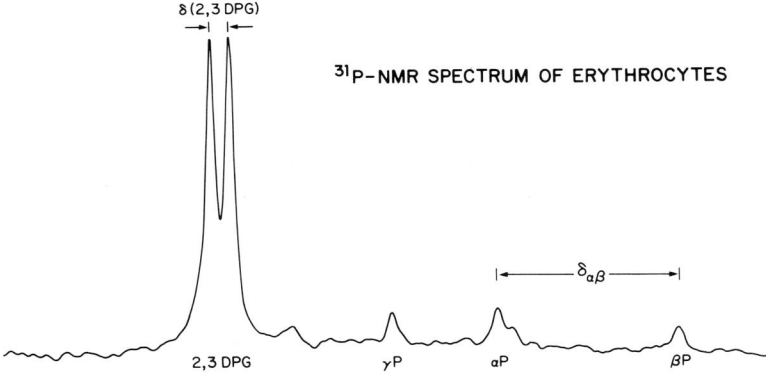

³¹P–NMR SPECTRUM OF ERYTHROCYTES

FIG. 1. ^{31}P-nuclear magnetic resonance spectrum of red blood cells. 2,3 DPG, 2,3 diphosphoglycerate; δ(2,3 DPG), chemical shift difference of 2,3 DPG; αP, βP, γP = α, β, and γ phosphoryl resonances of ATP; $\delta_{\alpha\beta}$, chemical shift difference of α- and β-phosphoryl resonances of ATP.

such as calcium and magnesium in different forms of hypertensive disease. We have been impressed by the relation of these different ion defects to differing activities of well-recognized pressor hormone systems such as the renin-angiotensin-aldosterone system, thereby reflecting the heterogeneity of underlying hypertensive mechanisms. We have also been impressed by the presence of these mineral ion defects not only in hypertension per se, but to a greater or lesser extent in other cardiovascular and metabolic aspects of what has been termed "Syndrome X," including obesity, insulin resistance, hyperinsulinemia, type II, noninsulin-dependent diabetes mellitus (NIDDM), and left ventricular hypertrophy (5,6). These observations have led us to formulate an ionic hypothesis of cardiovascular and metabolic disease, in which the predisposition to, and/or the actual presence of hypertension, together with any or all of its allied syndromes referred to above (more descriptively termed "generalized cardiovascular and metabolic disease," or GCMD) all derive from an underlying defect in steady-state cell mineral ion activity, characterized at least in part by excess cytosolic free calcium (Cai) and reciprocally suppressed intracellular free magnesium (Mgi) levels.

According to the ionic hypothesis, this abnormal intracellular ion environment, although common to all forms of hypertensive disease, reflects different hormonal and environmentally induced mechanisms in different individuals. Thus, in salt-sensitive, low renin forms of hypertension, excess Cai derives from calcium-hormone–mediated, cellular calcium uptake from the extracellular space. Conversely, in salt-insensitive, renin-dependent hypertension, the same excess Cai derives instead from angiotensin II–mediated release of calcium into the cytosol from IP$_3$-sensitive intracellular stores. All hypertension is then a combination, to varying degrees, of these two general calcium-related mechanisms.

Last, other environmental-dietary factors besides dietary salt, such as calcium or magnesium intake, or even sugar, can also affect blood pressure homeostasis, as well as the onset of associated cardiovascular and metabolic syndromes. This results to the extent that they can influence cellular ion activity, either directly or indirectly, by stimulating or suppressing those hormone systems normally controlling the disposition of these ions into or out of various cell systems. Altogether then, hypertension becomes merely one clinical expression of a common cellular ionic defect, which may also be manifested in different tissues independently of the blood pressure, as insulin resistance and hyperinsulinemia, as left ventricular hypertrophy, as increased platelet aggregation, and as accelerated atherosclerotic disease. Pathophysiologically, it is the metabolic setpoint of ion-active hormone systems, genetically defined, but environmentally modified on a day-to-day basis, that determines the contribution of, e.g., dietary calcium or magnesium to blood pressure. Thus, the same maneuver, such as salt loading or calcium or magnesium supplementation, may in different people cause pressure to rise, to fall, or to remain unchanged according to the ambient hormonal environment.

This chapter reviews the evidence for ionic, hormonal, and environmental disturbances of calcium and magnesium metabolism in hypertension. An attempt will be made to integrate these discrete defects into an overall pathophysiological scheme in accordance with the hypotheses mentioned above. Figure 3 illustrates this overall approach, in which various hormone systems

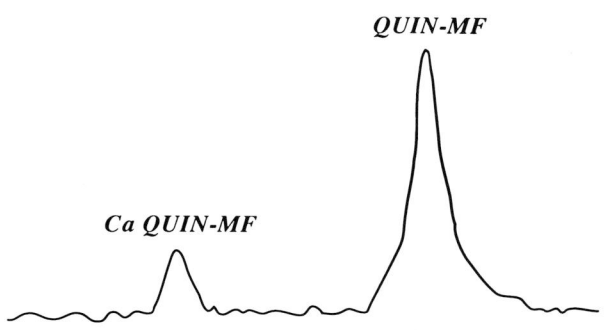

FIG. 2. ^{19}F-nuclear magnetic resonance spectrum of the intracellular probe, QUIN-MF, both free (peak labeled QUIN-MF) and calcium-bound (peak labeled Ca-QUIN-MF).

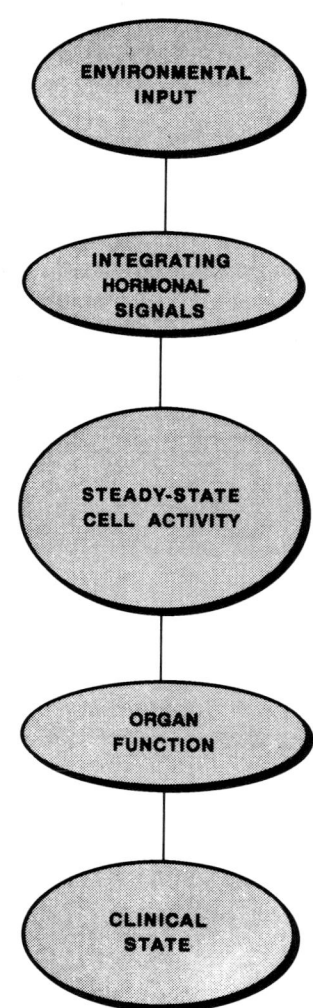

FIG. 3. Diagram depicting the hierarchy of physiological regulation, in which steady-state cellular ion activity plays a central role, mediating the effects of environmental signals and the hormonal factors interpreting those signals at the cellular level, and resulting in altered organ system function and clinical status.

transduce environmental signals at the cellular level, thereby altering ambient steady-state cell ion content. These ion activities, in turn, determine the functional characteristics of each organ system, resulting in the clinical states we recognize as normal or pathological.

INTRACELLULAR CALCIUM AND MAGNESIUM METABOLISM IN HYPERTENSION

Cellular Ions as Determinants of Blood Pressure and Metabolic Disturbances

That extracellular calcium is required for cardiac muscle contraction has been known for over a century (7).

However, the involvement of intracellular calcium in regulating the contractile properties of muscle, and thus peripheral vascular tone and blood pressure, has been appreciated only within the past few decades (8). In smooth muscle, initiation of contraction is associated with depolarization of the plasma membrane triggering a characteristic slow, calcium-mediated current, elevating cytosolic free calcium levels (9). Increased calcium binding to calmodulin results, which in turn activates myosin light-chain kinase (10), beginning a cascade of molecular rearrangements leading to myofilament shortening and what physiologically we observe as contraction, or in vascular smooth muscle, as vasoconstriction. Furthermore, muscle relaxation is also a calcium-dependent process, associated with calcium sequestration into intracellular storage sites such as the sarcoplasmic reticulum (11). Hence, alterations in the ability of cells to adequately accumulate and/or reversibly sequester cytosolic free calcium will necessarily affect the force of contraction (and peripheral vascular tone) generated as well as the ability of muscles to relax. It follows, therefore, that peripheral vascular tone, cardiac systolic function and diastolic relaxation, and blood pressure should be quantitatively determined, at least in part, by steady-state cytosolic free calcium concentrations. For blood pressure, this was clinically demonstrated in 1984, when levels of both systolic and diastolic blood pressure were shown to be closely and directly related to cytosolic free calcium levels measured in human platelets from normotensive and hypertensive subjects (12).

It is also now appreciated that the role of calcium in stimulus-contraction coupling and relaxation is itself modified and dependent on the steady-state activities intracellularly of other mineral ion species, including magnesium, potassium, and hydrogen ion activities (13–15). When measured concomitantly, higher cytosolic free calcium levels are inversely proportional to intracellular free magnesium and intracellular potassium levels, and maneuvers that alter the amount of one ionic species tend to proportionately affect the others as well (16,17). Indeed, cellular magnesium depletion is associated with increases in vascular tone and/or blood pressure similar to the effects of an induced cellular calcium excess (18). In addition, experimentally induced extracellular potassium depletion is associated with increased vascular tone, and the presence of intracellular potassium deficiency has been documented in cells from hypertensive subjects (19,20). Similarly, dietary potassium supplementation can ameliorate the incidence of strokes in experimental animals (21), and spontaneous intake of higher potassium-containing diets was also associated with fewer strokes in elderly individuals (22). Magnesium competes for binding with calcium on calmodulin, stimulates plasma membrane sodium-potassium ATPase, allosterically enhances calcium-activated potassium channel activity, and participates in sarcoplasmic reticular calcium sequestration from the cytosol, all of these actions tending to inhibit or offset the depolarizing and cell-stimulating effects of excess cytosolic free calcium. Hence, cellular magnesium deficiency would tend to promote and exaggerate calcium-induced cell stimulation in general, and vasoconstriction in particular. These effects of primary magnesium depletion have indeed been observed (23). Similarly, cellular acidosis and alkalosis routinely lead to altered cytosolic free calcium levels, as well as to a modification of calcium's ability to stimulate contraction (24,25). These interrelationships among the various mineral ions intracellularly are mediated at the cellular level by those multiple membrane pump mechanisms responsible for maintaining the gradients of these ions across cell membranes. These include Na^+-K^+ ATPase, Na-Ca exchange, $Na^+/K^+/Cl$ cotransport, Na^+/H^+ exchange, Na^+/Mg^+ exchange, Ca^{2+} ATPases, and others, each of which have been the focus of much attention in trying to identify markers or primary defects responsible for different forms of hypertensive disease. Although each of the above ion species and ion pumps may contribute to the pathophysiology of hypertension, this review will focus on the divalent cations, calcium and magnesium. Additionally, we will focus on cellular levels of these divalent cations, since changes in steady-state ion activities, rather than often compensatory changes in flux rates or ion pump activities per se, are more likely to result in altered cell function, and thus in an altered resulting physiological and clinical state.

Intracellular free calcium and magnesium content are not only involved in regulating cardiac and smooth muscle contractile function, but are critical to cellular responses to a wide variety of external stimuli, including stimulus-secretion coupling in endocrine cells, neurotransmitter release from nerve terminals both centrally and peripherally, and renal excretory function (26). As such, endocrine, neural, and renal aspects of blood pressure homeostasis are all determined, at least in part, by the steady-state divalent cation content of body tissues. Additionally, on this basis, the now well-known metabolic and cardiac conditions associated with, but often independent of the presence of hypertension itself, such as hyperinsulinemia, insulin resistance, obesity, NIDDM, left ventricular hypertrophy, and accelerated atherosclerotic disease, would also be predicted to depend on these same intracellular ion activities—the higher the cytosolic free calcium or the lower the free magnesium, the more severe should be the lesion. Accumulating evidence supports these predictions, and leads to the concept of intracellular ion defects as a common cellular lesion underlying the epidemiological link between hypertension and these more general cardiovascular risk factors.

Abnormalities of Cai and Mgi in Hypertension and Related Disorders—The Mechanism of Syndrome X

The first definitive demonstration of consistently altered cytosolic calcium ion activity was reported a decade ago by Swiss workers, using the then newly described fluorescent dye technology to measure intracellular free ion content in platelets of normotensive and hypertensive subjects (12). That this was not just an epiphenomenon was suggested by the close, direct relation between the height of the blood pressure and the intracellular free calcium concentration. Furthermore, antihypertensive drug therapy reduced blood pressure and cytosolic free calcium levels in parallel. These results have led to an extensive investigation of cellular calcium abnormalities in hypertension, and increased cytosolic free calcium content has now been reported as characteristic of hypertension in a wide variety of cell types, including white blood cells (27), erythrocytes (28), and vascular smooth muscle (29) (Fig. 4).

The mechanism(s) responsible for this cellular calcium abnormality remains unknown. Indeed, the presence of elevated cytosolic free calcium in hypertension may result from and reflect different underlying defects in different patient populations suffering from different forms of hypertension. Intrinsic cellular defects, such as an abnormal Na^+/H^+ exchange protein demonstrating altered allosteric cooperative properties (30,31), an abnormally suppressed Ca^{2+} ATPase activity (32,33), and generalized biophysical abnormalities of membrane function (34–36), have all been reported. Alternatively, a role for extrinsic, circulating factors has been suggested by investigations of digitalis-like factors, recently confirmed as oubain in humans (37–39), of calcium-related hormones such as 1,25 dihydroxyvitamin D (40–43) and

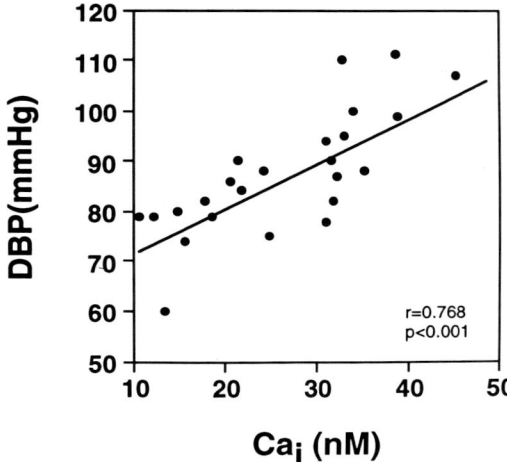

FIG. 4. Relation of diastolic blood pressure (DBP) to basal fasting cytosolic free calcium concentrations (Cai) in peripheral red blood cells of normal and hypertensive subjects.

the newly described parathyroid hypertensive factor (PHF) (44,45), and of already recognized pressor hormone systems such as the renin-angiotensin-aldosterone system (46). Faced with this plethora of proposed factors and mechanisms, we have proposed a scheme (see below) in which the apparently uniform elevations of cytosolic free calcium in hypertension derive from variable contributions of two basic mechanisms, either involving accumulation of cellular calcium from the extracellular space, or calcium release from intracellular stores (47). This cellular calcium-based classification of hypertension has clinical consequences, and parallels the physiological classification scheme of Laragh based on considerations of volume vis-à-vis constrictor mechanisms operative in blood pressure homeostasis (48) (see below).

At the same time as the role of intracellular free calcium in hypertension was being defined, our group reported parallel, reciprocal findings when measuring intracellular free magnesium (49). Utilizing NMR spectroscopic techniques developed by Gupta (1) to noninvasively measure cellular ion content, we observed a close, consistent, inverse relation between both systolic and diastolic blood pressures, and the intracellular free magnesium content of erythrocytes in normotensive and essential hypertensive subjects (Fig. 5). In parallel with and reciprocally opposite to the results with free calcium, successful antihypertensive therapy was associated with an increase in free magnesium levels back toward normotensive values. Dynamically, this inverse relation between the height of the blood pressure and intracellular free magnesium was also observed in experimental animals, both normotensive and with different induced forms of hypertension, in whom different diets decreasing or increasing free magnesium resulted in opposite

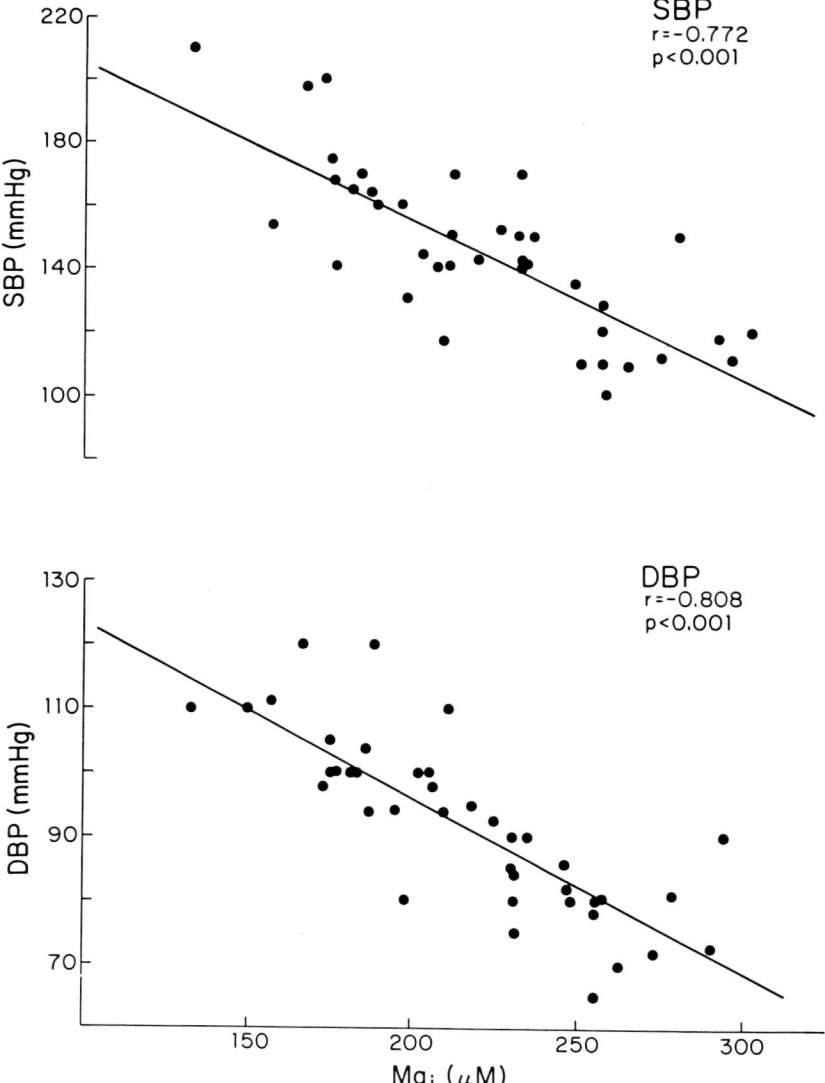

FIG. 5. Relation of systolic (SBP) and diastolic (DBP) blood pressures to basal fasting intracellular free magnesium concentrations (Mgi) in peripheral red blood cells of normal and hypertensive subjects.

parallel increased or decreased blood pressure. Similar, confirmatory results have been found by Japanese workers in both erythrocytes and vascular smooth muscle of experimental hypertensive rat models (50). Although the mechanism(s) of this cellular magnesium deficiency in hypertension is unknown, it is clearly linked to the parallel excess cellular calcium that has received more attention in the literature. Thus, magnesium depletion increases tissue calcium content (51). Indeed, we have observed an inverse relation between intracellular free magnesium levels and free calcium levels when these two ions were measured concomitantly in cells from the same subject (52). Altogether, regardless of the primacy of either ionic lesion, or of their underlying mechanisms, it is now clear that the elevated blood pressures defining the presence of clinical hypertension are consistently and quantitatively characterized by increased steady-state cytosolic free calcium levels, and reciprocally suppressed free magnesium levels.

The potential significance of these reciprocal deviations in cellular free calcium and magnesium levels in hypertension became more apparent when intracellular ion levels were also evaluated in comparison with other aspects of hypertensive disease. Thus, echocardiographically determined left ventricular (LV) mass was also closely and directly related to basal erythrocyte free calcium levels while being inversely related to free magnesium levels (53). Indeed, these relations, derived from red blood cell measurements, were statistically stronger than the relation of LV mass to the blood pressure itself, further supporting the relevance of this altered ion "profile." Additionally, the metabolic defects of hyperinsulinemia and insulin resistance associated with essential hypertension, and which, like left ventricular hypertrophy, may occur independently of elevated blood pressure values, were also investigated and analyzed concomitantly with intracellular ions. The presence of insulin resistance in hypertension was first suggested by consistently hyperinsulinemic responses of hypertensive, compared with normotensive, subjects to a standard oral glucose tolerance test (Fig. 6). Although the cellular mechanism(s) underlying the insulin resistance of hypertension remain unclear, it became apparent that, similar to the other ion-linked abnormalities in hypertension, the insulinemic response to glucose loading was also closely related to fasting, basal ion levels intracellularly. Specifically, the lower the free magnesium and the higher the free calcium, the greater was the hyperinsulinemic response to glucose (54) (Fig. 7). So over and over again, the levels of cytosolic free calcium and of free magnesium were closely and oppositely related to whichever aspects of hypertensive disease were evaluated, the height of the blood pressure itself, the extent of cardiac hypertrophy, or the degree of hyperinsulinemia reflecting peripheral insulin resistance.

These observations led to a hypothesis linking insulin

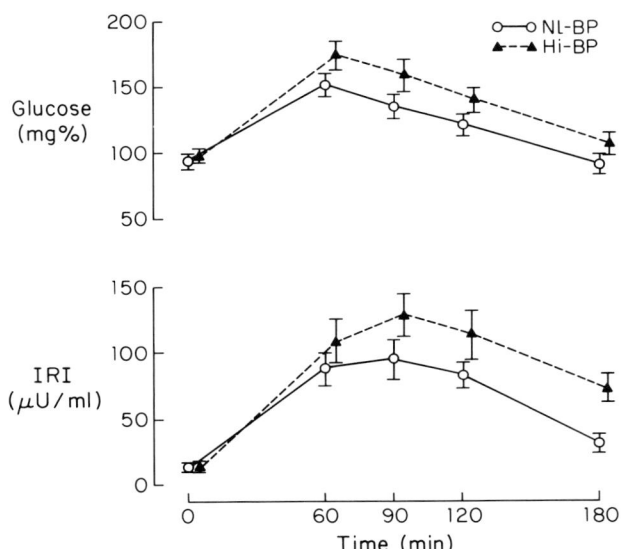

FIG. 6. Oral glucose tolerance tests in normal and essential hypertensive subjects, showing the time course of both glucose and insulin (IRI) responses.

resistance and hypertension on a cellular ionic basis (55). Rather than trying to explain how hypertension predisposes to or itself causes insulin resistance, as some authors have suggested (56,57), or, conversely, how insulin resistance and hyperinsulinemia as a primary lesion predisposes to hypertension, as others think (58), we believe it more likely that the link between each abnormality derives from a common abnormal intracellular ionic environment, of which they are each different organ system expressions (Fig. 8).

The Ionic Hypothesis of Cardiovascular and Metabolic Disease

The prevalence of this altered intracellular divalent cation "profile" has now been extended to include other clinical conditions predisposing to and/or associated with hypertension, such as obesity and NIDDM. When analyzed in these conditions, similar deviations of intracellular ions were observed. Thus, obesity, even in the absence of overt hypertensive disease, is associated with increased levels of cytosolic free calcium, although free magnesium values were only modestly reduced (28). In red cells from subjects with NIDDM, abnormalities of divalent cation levels were similar to those found in essential hypertension, consisting of an excess of cytosolic free calcium and of a reciprocal suppression of free magnesium (28). These alterations were also observed when the degree of cardiac hypertrophy was compared to cellular ion content. In NIDDM as well, the higher the cytosolic free calcium, the greater was the left ventricular mass index (59). These data led to an extension of the earlier hypothesis that insulin resistance and hyperten-

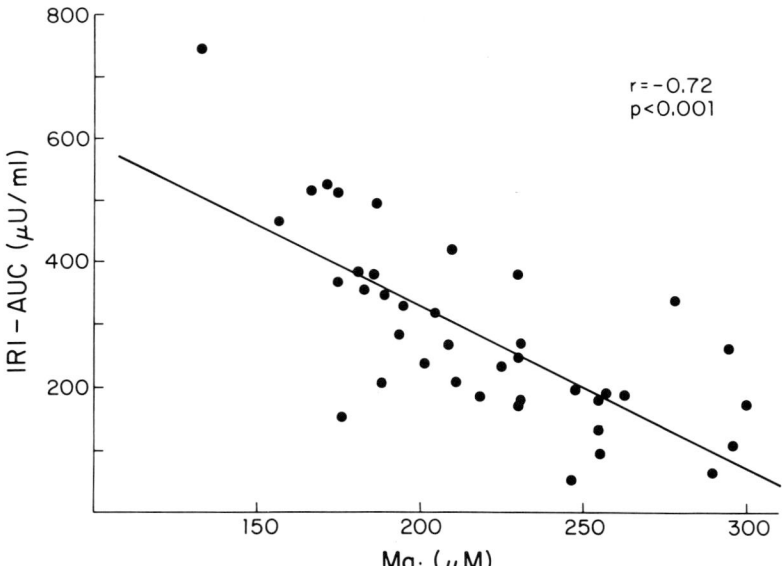

FIG. 7. Relation of the integrated insulinemic response to oral glucose loading (IRI-AUC) to basal fasting intracellular free magnesium concentrations in normal and hypertensive subjects.

sion each reflected a similar abnormal intracellular ionic environment. In its present form, the ionic hypothesis of cardiovascular and metabolic disease attempts to explain the clinical and epidemiological linkage of different syndromes, usually considered distinct, as a consequence of their common derivation from and/or reflection of altered steady-state cell ion activity (Fig. 9).

Why did measurements of ions in red cells so closely predict the physiological measurements of blood pressure, left ventricular mass, and hyperinsulinemia, which represent diverse tissue functions and cell types, and to which red cells do not directly contribute? It seemed reasonable to suggest that the ambient ion activities measured in the red cell somehow reflected altered cellular ionic activity in other tissues as well. This led to the further question: What would be the expected consequences if all cells of the body were affected similarly? The answer points to altered cellular ion content as at least one possible basis underlying the pathophysiology not only of hypertension, but of those other cardiovascular, neural, and metabolic abnormalities associated with hypertension and characteristic of aging populations in Western civilization. We have collectively termed these abnormalities *generalized cardiovascular and metabolic disease* (GCMD).

According to what is already known in the literature,

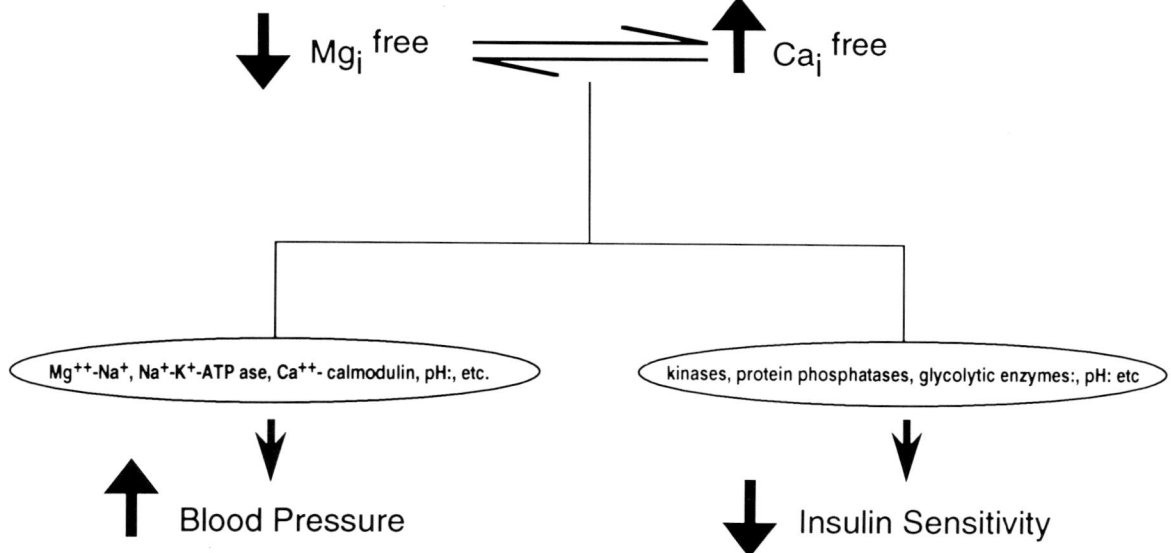

FIG. 8. Hypothetical scheme in which both hypertension and insulin resistance are related by virtue of their common origin, reflecting primary disturbances in cellular divalent cation regulation.

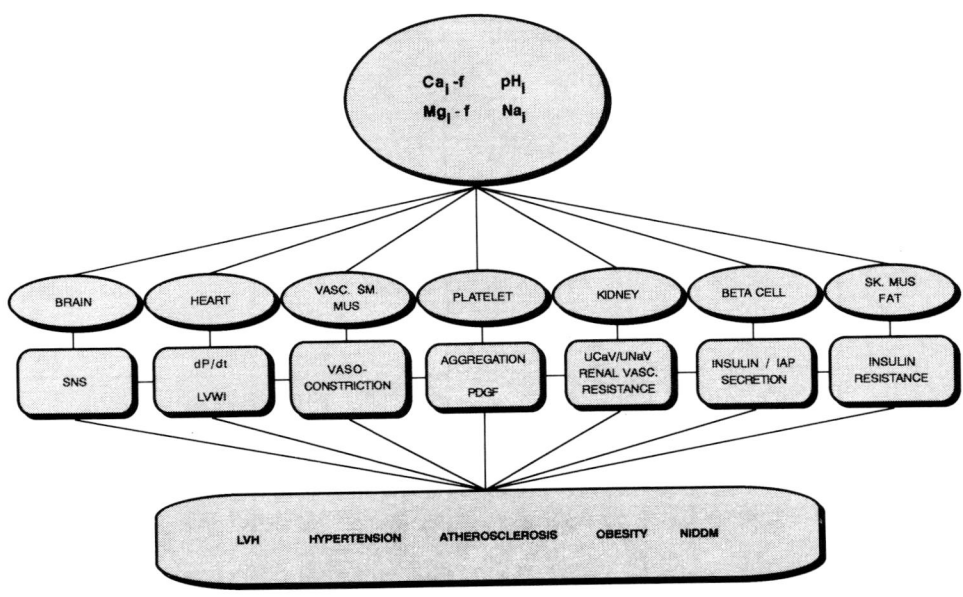

FIG. 9. Ionic hypothesis of cardiovascular and metabolic disease, in which multiple clinical components (*bottom*) represent different clinical manifestations of shared cellular ion abnormalities (*top*) expressed differently in different organ systems (*middle*) (see text).

increased cytosolic free calcium can cause cellular insulin resistance (60–63). In pancreatic beta cells, as in almost all endocrine secretory cells [parathyroid hormone (PTH) and renal renin secretion being notable exceptions], increasing free calcium content stimulates hormone secretion and sensitizes cells to other stimuli as well (26). Hence insulin resistance, as well as hyperinsulinemia, are expected consequences of a primary excess of cytosolic free calcium (64). Similar to stimulus-secretion coupling in endocrine tissue, neurotransmitter release is also potentiated in the presence of increased cytosolic free calcium and/or lower free magnesium concentrations (26), consistent with and perhaps helping to explain the numerous studies demonstrating increased central and peripheral sympathetic activity in hypertension (57,65). Cardiac and smooth muscle contraction are directly enhanced by increased intracellular free calcium, leading to and consistent with the increased peripheral vasoconstriction characteristic of all hypertension, and the increased wall stress, enhanced contractility, and decreased diastolic relaxation characteristic of early hypertensive heart disease (66,67). Platelet aggregation is also potentiated by excess cellular calcium or cellular magnesium deficiency, with the consequent release of vascular growth factors, accelerating thrombosis, and atherosclerosis (68,69). Magnesium deficiency can di-

rectly potentiate the formation of cholesterol-laden atherosclerotic plaques (70), and calcium excess can directly result in the vascular calcification also characteristic of the atherosclerotic process.

Altogether, based on the twofold findings (a) that cellular calcium excess and/or magnesium deficiency can directly result in the pathophysiological vascular, cardiac, and metabolic properties of essential hypertension, and (b) that these cellular ionic lesions are indeed present, not only in hypertension itself, but also, to a greater or lesser extent, in those states associated with and predisposing to hypertension, such as obesity and NIDDM, we formulated the ionic hypothesis of cardiovascular and metabolic disease. According to this hypothesis, all cells exhibit a common intracellular lesion, which while perhaps differing in the ultimate genetic substrate and environmental precipitants among different population groups, is expressed phenotypically as excess cytosolic free calcium and suppressed free magnesium [as well as decreased intracellular potassium (19) and pH (71)] levels. As a consequence of this altered cellular ion activity, steady-state cell function, and hence the specific functions associated with different organ systems, are also altered. Clinically, this appears, again as modified by other environmental and genetic factors, as clinical hypertension, along with cardiac hypertrophy, insulin resistance, hyperinsulinemia, and accelerated atherosclerosis. Certain consequences of this model include: (a) each organ system manifestation of the same ionic lesion may be at least partially independent of the expression of the same ionic defect by another tissue. Thus, (b) the ionic hypothesis helps to explain the persistence of cardiac hypertrophy, and of accelerated coronary atherosclerotic disease despite apparently good control of elevated blood pressures. It also helps to resolve the now needless controversies arising from the assignment of primacy of one clinical expression vis-à-vis another. In this formulation, for example, (c) altered insulin action and hypertension do not so much "cause" one another as merely represent different tissue manifestations of similar "primary" cellular ionic lesions. This model also predicts (d) that maneuvers that succeed in ameliorating the intracellular ionic lesion will necessarily benefit many, if not all, of its different clinical expressions. Thus, lowering intracellular cytosolic free calcium and/or elevating free magnesium levels ought to coordinately lower elevated blood pressure, improve peripheral insulin resistance, decrease left ventricular hypertrophy, decrease platelet aggregation, and retard the atherosclerotic process. Published and ongoing studies with calcium channel antagonists suggest that this may indeed be the case.

EXTRACELLULAR REGULATION OF INTRACELLULAR IONS

The above-described ionic hypothesis may serve to unify previous approaches by emphasizing the role of steady-state cellular ion activity as a common basis for better understanding the variety of other cardiovascular and metabolic syndromes associated with hypertension. It remains to be understood, however, what in turn is responsible for these abnormalities of cellular ion content in hypertension and its allied conditions. Most efforts in this area have focused on intracellular factors, including genetic mechanisms, membrane pumps, phosphorylating and dephosphorylating enzyme cascades,

and other intracellular regulating factors such as G-proteins, phospholipases, and arachidonic acid derivatives. Less emphasis has been placed on the influence on intracellular ions of extracellular ions, small molecules, and of the circulating hormonal species that serve to regulate their distribution between extracellular and intracellular spaces. As opposed to the uniformly altered intracellular environment common to the many clinically linked conditions above, we have hypothesized that reciprocating activities of different extracellular dietary-linked hormonal factors cause this common intracellular ionic "profile," and help us to understand and to classify at the cellular level the heterogeneity of hypertensive mechanisms characterizing clinical hypertensive disease (Fig. 10). Furthermore, this approach corresponds to and parallels the volume-vasoconstriction analysis of hypertension introduced over two decades ago by Laragh (72). The above considerations were based on the investigation (a) of basal fasting serum ionized calcium and magnesium levels in essential hypertensive subjects in relation to the activity of the renin-angiotensin system and calcium regulating hormones; (b) of intracellular and extracellular mineral ion content in subjects on low and high dietary salt intakes, in relation to calcium regulating hormones; and (c) of intracellular free calcium and magnesium content in response to an oral glucose tolerance test, in relation to circulating glycosylated hemoglobin levels, and after *in vitro* incubation with differing concentrations of glucose and insulin.

Extracellular Distribution of Divalent Cations and Their Regulating Hormones

Early evidence suggesting a link between divalent cation metabolism and the heterogeneity of hypertension came from studies in which extracellular circulating ionized calcium and magnesium levels were measured in essential hypertensive subjects who had been classified a priori on the basis of renin-sodium profiling (73). This clinically validated method provides information on an individual basis of the relative contribution to the blood

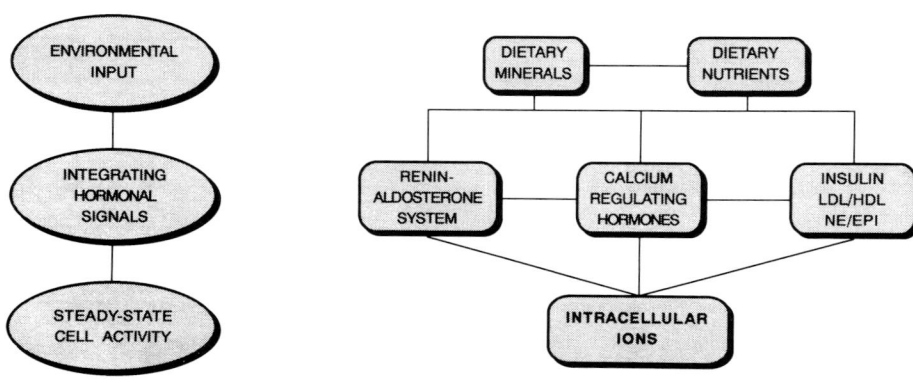

FIG. 10. The extracellular regulation of intracellular ion homeostasis by dietary minerals and nutrients, mediated by their respective hormone systems.

pressure of angiotensin-dependent vis-à-vis sodium-volume–dependent factors (72). Serum-ionized calcium levels were directly related to renin status. Although all values were within the normal range of the test, low renin subjects exhibited significantly lower ionized calcium levels compared to normotensive or other hypertensive subjects. Conversely, inappropriately high renin activity levels were associated with circulating ionized calcium levels that were higher than average levels among normotensive or hypertensive groups. Serum magnesium levels were also deviated within the normal range among different renin subgroups of hypertensive subjects, but in an opposite, reciprocal manner—the higher renin group having the lowest magnesium values (Fig. 11). To determine the biological significance of these small deviations in circulating ion levels within the normal range, parathyroid hormone (PTH), calcitonin, and 1,25 dihydroxyvitamin D (1,25 D) levels were also measured in relation to the renin system activity among essential hypertensive subjects (41). Consistent with the lower measured ionized calcium levels in low renin hypertensives, these subjects displayed higher circulating PTH and 1,25 D values, and reciprocally lower calcitonin levels, compared to normotensive or other hypertensive individuals. Opposite results characterized the high renin subjects—lower PTH and 1,25 D levels, and higher calcitonin values. Even independently of the assignment of renin status, a continuous, inverse relation was observed between the absolute value of plasma renin activity and

circulating 1,25 D levels (Fig. 12). Hence, in the basal state, the activity of the renin-angiotensin system was linked to that of various calcium-regulating hormone species. Furthermore, different renin-defined pathophysiological types of essential hypertension were characterized by parallel deviations in extracellular calcium and magnesium ionic and hormonal metabolism in both directions away from normotensive values. Low renin subjects display a calcium "profile" suggestive of an extracellular calcium deficiency, whereas an extracellular calcium surfeit is suggested among high renin subjects.

To reconcile the uniform deviations of intracellular ion content present in all hypertension-excess cytosolic free calcium and suppressed free magnesium values with the heterogeneous deviations of extracellular calcium and magnesium metabolism among different forms of hypertensive disease, a model was proposed in which the intracellular ion abnormalities of hypertension derive to a variable extent in different subjects, and/or in different circumstances in the same subject, from two basic pathophysiological mechanisms (47,74) (Fig. 13). One mechanism is dependent on cellular calcium accumulation from the extracellular space, the other on calcium release into the cytoplasm from intracellular stores. In both cases, the result is the excess cytosolic free calcium characteristic of hypertension. However, the first mechanism, operative in the low renin hypertensive state (referred to as a type I defect) would result in an inverse

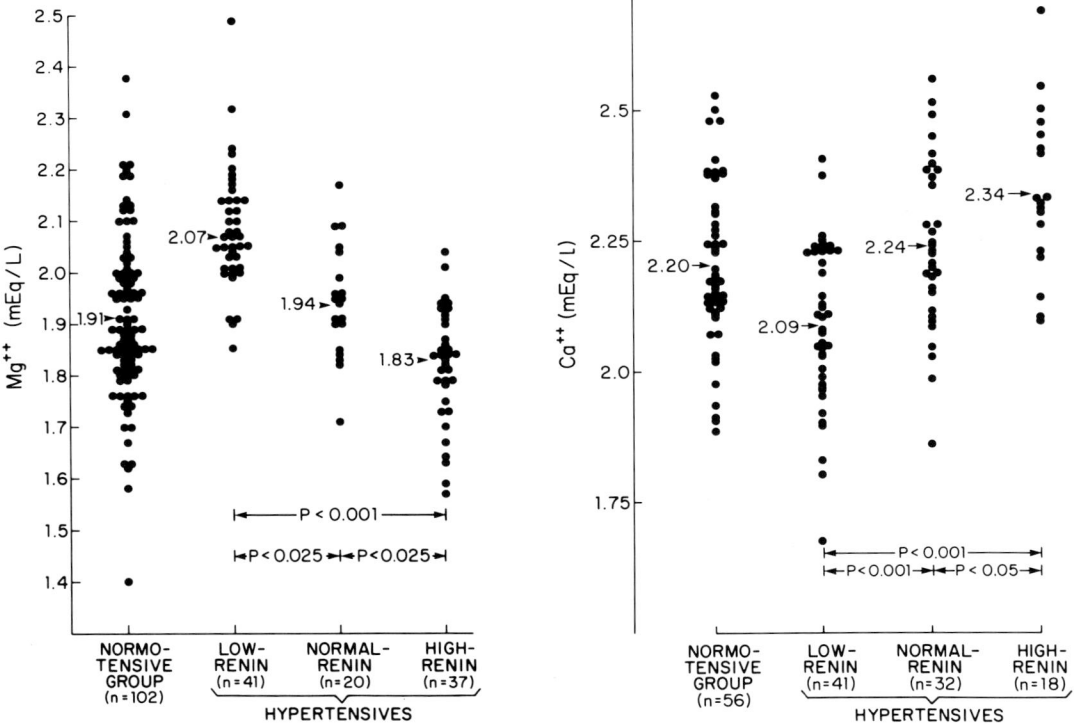

FIG. 11. The distribution of serum magnesium (Mg²⁺, *left*), and of serum ionized calcium (Ca²⁺, *right*) in normotensive subjects and in different renin subgroups of essential hypertensive subjects.

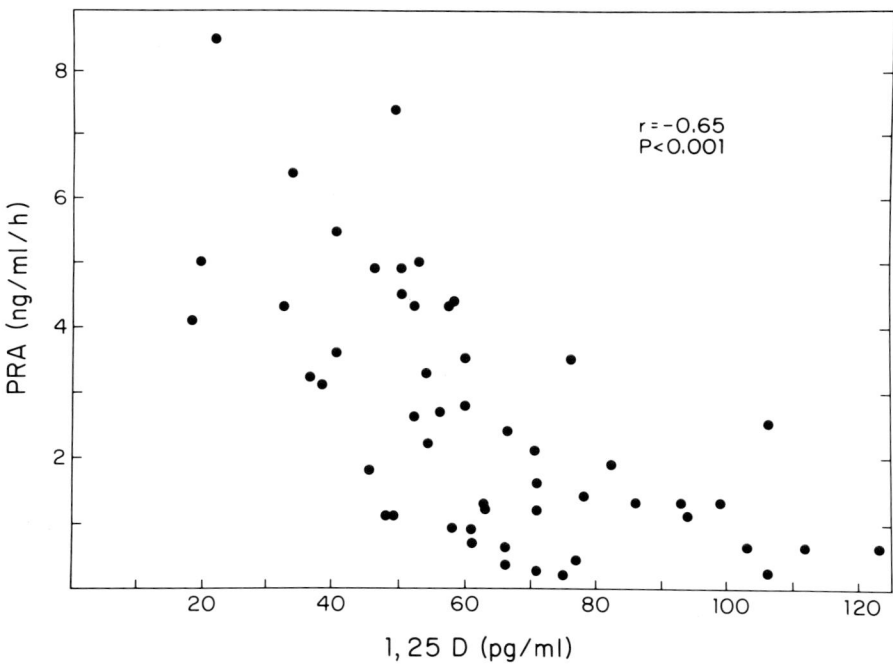

FIG. 12. The relation of plasma renin activity values (PRA) to circulating 1,25 dihydroxyvitamin D levels (1,25 D).

relation between extracellular and intracellular calcium, lower extracellular calcium being the mirror image of higher intracellular levels. This mechanism would predict an inverse relation between blood pressure [proportional to intracellular free calcium (12)] and serum ionized calcium. This has been demonstrated (75). It also would predict the enhanced antihypertensive efficacy of calcium channel blockade in low renin individuals, since their pressure, according to this model, is more dependent on extracellular calcium transport intracellularly.

This has also been verified (76). The second mechanism, operative in high renin hypertension (referred to as a type II defect), would result in a direct relation of extracellular and intracellular free calcium because the cell plasma membrane under circumstances of intracellular cytosolic calcium excess would serve to increase its export extracellularly. Here, blood pressure and serum-ionized calcium should be directly related, as has been demonstrated in high renin subjects (75).

Although angiotensin II directly releases calcium from

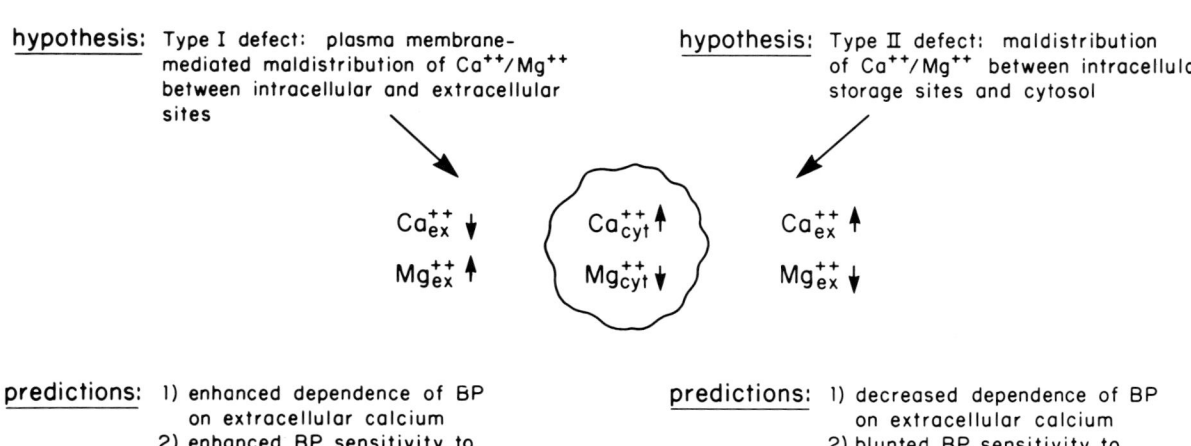

FIG. 13. Cellular hypothesis in which the classification of hypertension on the basis of plasma renin activity is associated with different calcium/magnesium lesions, the case of low renin hypertension representing an exaggerated cellular calcium accumulation from the extracellular space (type 1 defect), and high renin hypertension representing angiotensin II-dependent exaggerated calcium release from intracellular stores.

intracellular sarcoplasmic reticulum (77) into the cytoplasm, and presumably mediates renin-dependent, high renin hypertension, what factor(s) mediates the excess cellular accumulation of calcium from the extracellular space in the low renin state? Consistent with the predominance of dietary salt sensitivity of blood pressure in low renin subjects (72) as well as the preferential hypotensive action of oral calcium supplementation in this form of hypertensive disease (78), the blood pressure, hormonal, and cellular ionic effects of dietary salt and calcium were investigated.

Extracellular Calcium-Dependent Hypertension: Dietary Salt, Dietary Calcium, and the Role of Calcium-Regulating Hormones

The pressor response to dietary and intravenously administered salt loading is dependent on hormone-mediated cellular calcium uptake from the extracellular space. This conclusion is based on clinical data as well as data from experimental animal models. When essential hypertensive subjects were studied under metabolic balance conditions and placed on low (10 mEq/day) and high (210 mEq/day) dietary salt intakes for 1 week each, a relation was observed between the ability of salt to elevate pressure and the concomitant salt-induced changes in circulating serum-ionized calcium: the more the ionized calcium fell in the extracellular space, the greater was the pressor response (40) (Fig. 14). Identical results were also obtained by other groups and in longer-term salt-loading studies among outpatient essential hypertensives (16,79). As initially hypothesized (40), it is now clear that the lowering of extracellular calcium levels

with salt loading is a mirror image reflection of reciprocal salt-induced elevations in cytosolic free calcium levels, now reported by different groups in peripheral blood cells, as well as platelets (16,17). Furthermore, consistent with this model, calcium-channel–blocking drugs are especially effective in low renin, salt-sensitive states (80–82), in which they reverse the cellular ionic effects of dietary salt (Fig. 15).

These results are also supported by animal studies. For example, the genetic Dahl S rat, a salt-sensitive model of hypertension, exhibits a suppression of plasma renin activity and of extracellular ionized calcium, findings paralleling those in man after salt loading, especially in the low renin, salt-sensitive essential hypertensive subject. Additionally, in the normal dog, although no consistent or significant blood pressure changes result from either acute intravenous saline infusions alone or from calcium infusions maintaining calcium levels within the normal range, when both calcium and saline are co-administered in the same amounts, significant elevations in pressure routinely result. Furthermore, this pressor response to combined saline-calcium infusions can be blocked by the prior administration of a calcium-channel–blocking agent (83). Chronically, the hypotensive action of calcium-channel–blocking drugs are potentiated in salt-dependent forms of hypertensive disease (84). Altogether, these data strongly suggest the critical role of cellular calcium uptake from the extracellular space as the mechanism of salt-related forms of hypertensive disease.

Interestingly, and consistent with the multiple ionic defects observed in hypertension, the cellular ionic effects of dietary salt loading are not limited to changes in the distribution of calcium ions, but apply in a coordi-

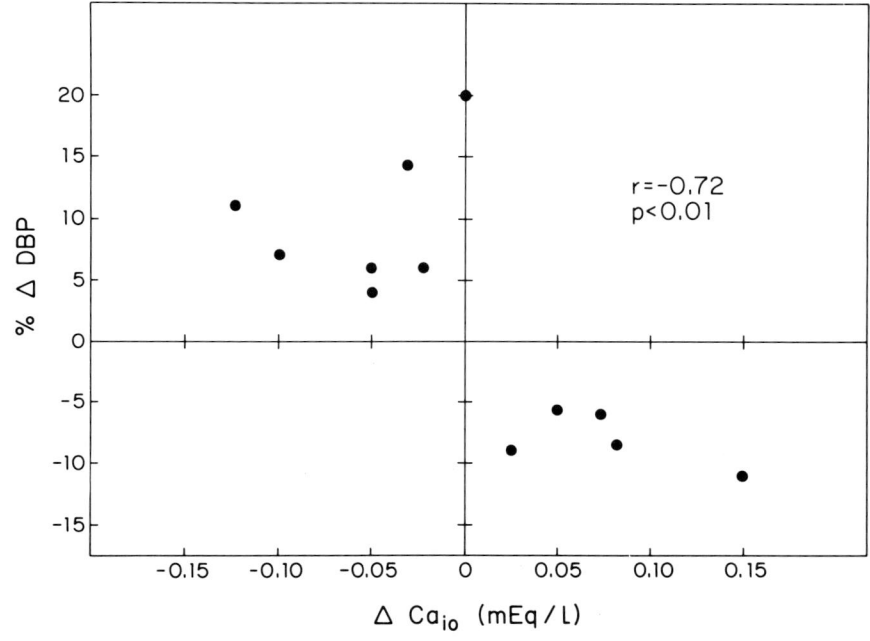

FIG. 14. The relation of the pressor response to dietary salt loading (percent ΔDBP) in essential hypertensive subjects to salt-induced changes in serum-ionized calcium levels (ΔCa-io).

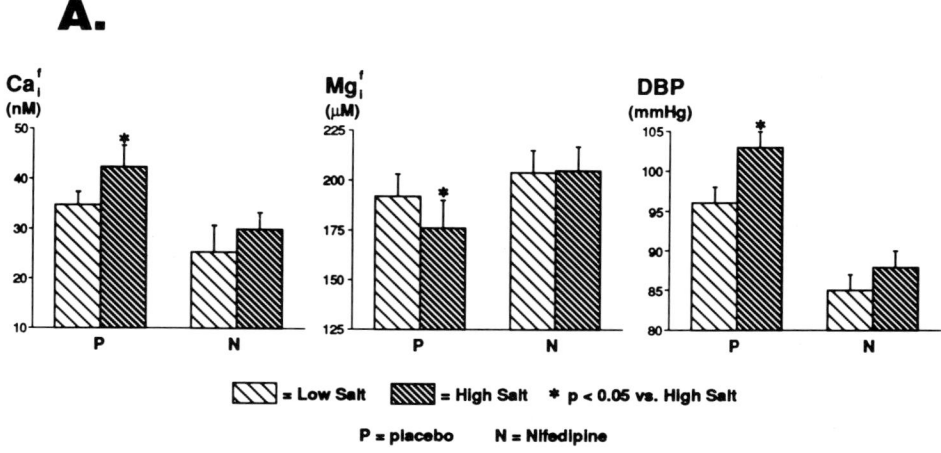

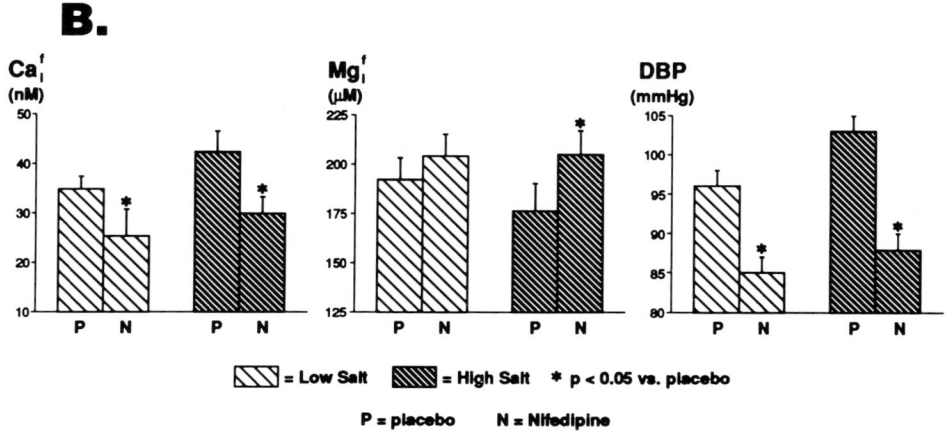

FIG. 15. Ionic responses to low- and high-salt diets in essential hypertensive subjects on placebo (*P*) vs. nifedipine (*N*) therapy (*top,* **A**). **B** shows same data reorganized to show the greater effects of nifedipine on high vs. low salt intakes in the same hypertensive subjects. Cai, cytosolic free calcium; Mgi, intracellular free magnesium; DBP, diastolic blood pressure.

nate manner to other mineral ion species as well. Thus, the ability of salt to alter blood pressure was also related to its ability to suppress intracellular free magnesium, to lower intracellular pH, and to cause an exaggerated rise in intracellular sodium content. Similarly, calcium channel blockade reverses not only the excess cytosolic free calcium induced by salt, but also restores intracellular magnesium and pH to average normotensive levels (85). Although it cannot be determined which of these ions is of overriding or primary importance, it seems that cellular sodium content per se is less important in mediating the pressure response because calcium channel blockade may not restore intracellular sodium levels toward normal, and may even exacerbate salt-induced cellular sodium elevations.

On the basis of the above data, the question, why does dietary salt exert a pressor effect in only some, approximately 40 to 70 percent, of hypertensive individuals, but not in others?, can be restated as the question, what factors, present in some, but not all, hypertensive subjects

mediate the cellular ionic and pressor effects of dietary salt? These factors, once identified, if causally related to salt-dependent hypertension, ought to be expressed differentially in response to salt exposure and to be quantitatively proportional to the resultant pressor response. At present, it seems that those circulating hormonal substances normally participating in the physiological regulation of extracellular calcium metabolism also serve to concomitantly regulate cellular access to calcium. Although the involvement of a variety of calcium-regulating hormones in blood pressure homeostasis has been recently reviewed (42), it is important here to highlight the role of at least two such factors, 1,25 D and the recently described PHF.

In parallel with the ability of salt to induce changes in circulating ionized calcium, especially among salt-sensitive subjects, was a similar effect of salt to stimulate circulating 1,25 D levels. Indeed, the more salt elevated 1,25 D levels, the more the pressure went up (40). This has been confirmed in normotensive and borderline hypertensive subjects as well (86). If, rather than being merely an epiphenomenon, this salt-induced differential stimulation of 1,25 D contributes to the variable pressor effects of salt, then maneuvers that suppress 1,25 D levels ought to offset the ability of salt to raise pressure. This was the rationale of early attempts to lower blood pressure by increasing intake of calcium (87).

Using an oral calcium supplementation regimen of 500 mg four times daily, the pressor effect of salt was indeed blunted (88). This "antisalt" possibility was raised in the first report of the hypotensive effect of oral calcium supplementation seven decades ago (89). This effect of calcium to offset salt-induced hypertension was associated with a parallel suppression of salt-induced stimulation of 1,25 D levels (Fig. 16). The response to calcium was heterogeneous, and although salt-sensitive patients exhibited a significant depressor response, no effects or even pressor responses were observed in non–salt-sensitive patients (88). When extended over a 6-month period in free living essential hypertensives, a similar linkage of salt and calcium was noted. The greater the average 24-hour urine sodium excretion, reflective of average salt intake, the greater was the hypotensive response to calcium (90) (Fig. 17). This has been demonstrated by other workers in human hypertension

as well (91,92), and is supported by both epidemiological (93) and animal studies (94). Thus, in a Canadian study, blood pressures were measured in people who were classified according to their dietary sodium as well as calcium intakes. Among subjects with higher dietary calcium intakes, there was no relation between salt intake and blood pressure. However, subjects with deficient calcium intakes exhibited a significant, positive relation between dietary salt and blood pressure (93). This supports a role for calcium hormones such as 1,25 D in the hypertensive process because elevations of 1,25 D, with attendant potentiated cellular calcium uptake (see below), are an expected and appropriate response to lower calcium intakes. Similarly, when blood pressures were recorded in spontaneously hypertensive rats (SHR) on diets containing low and high sodium and calcium content, it was found that pressures were lowest on the higher calcium diets, regardless of sodium content (94). Salt loading in the salt-sensitive Dahl S rat, in parallel with human low renin hypertension, is also associated with elevated circulating 1,25 D levels (95). Furthermore, increased dietary calcium intakes preferentially lower blood pressure in salt-dependent, DOCA-NaCl rats, but not in renin-dependent, two kidney, one clip (2K, 1C) Goldblatt hypertensive rats (96) (Fig. 18). The

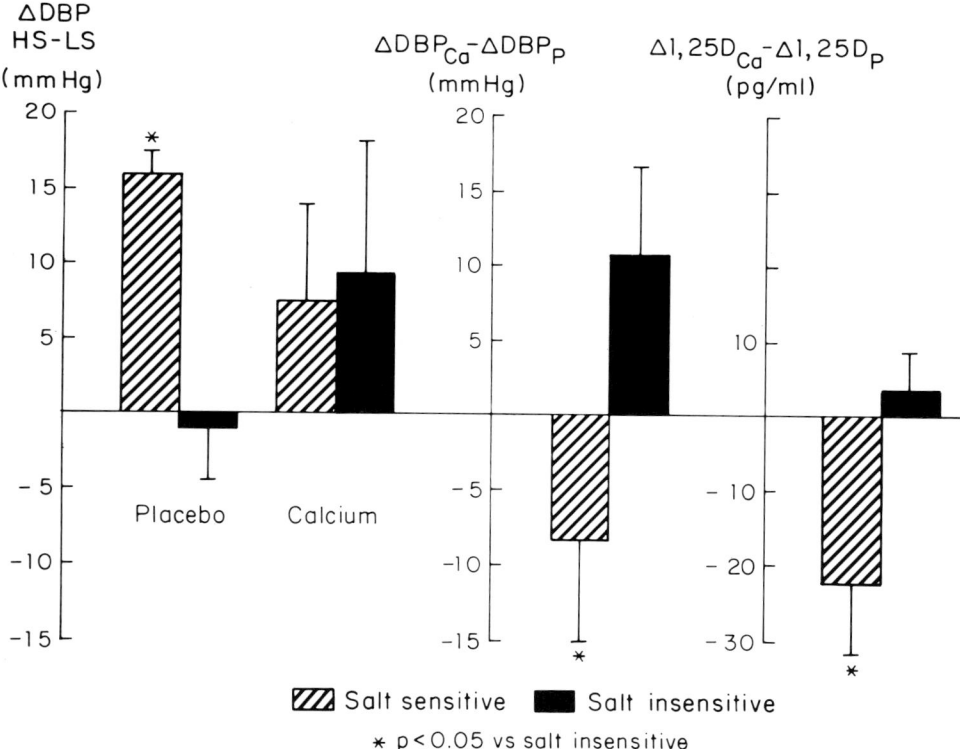

FIG. 16. The effects of oral calcium supplementation on the diastolic blood pressure (ΔDBP) and 1,25 dihydroxyvitamin D effects of dietary salt loading (HS-LS). $\Delta DBP_{Ca} - \Delta DBP_P$ = difference in the effect of high- vs. low-salt diets on blood pressure in subjects taking calcium vs. placebo treatments. $\Delta 1,25D_{Ca} - \Delta 1,25D_P$ = difference in the effect of high- vs. low-salt diets on 1,25 dihydroxyvitamin D levels in subjects taking calcium vs. placebo treatments.

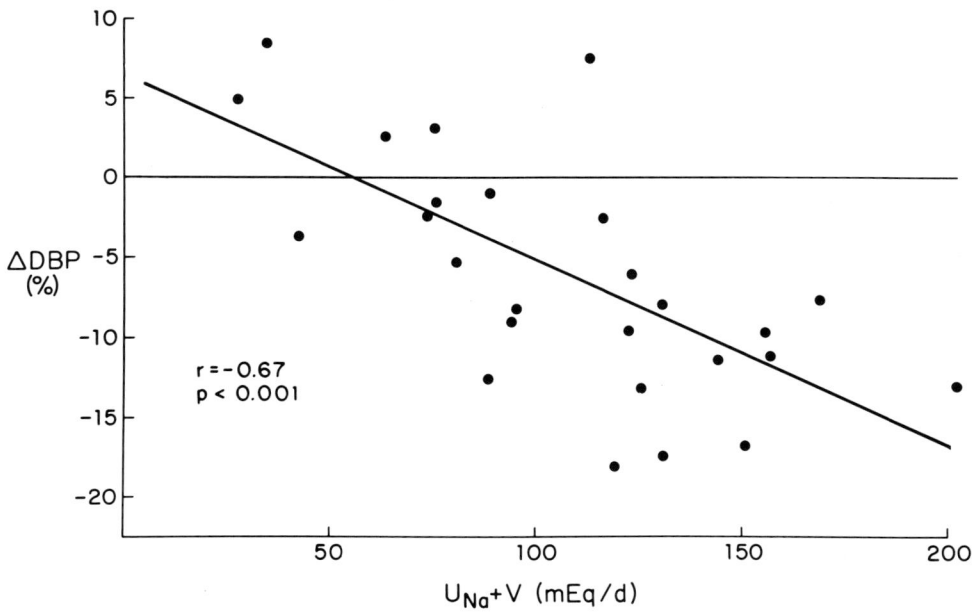

FIG. 17. Relation of the blood pressure effects of long-term therapy with oral calcium supplementation (ΔDBP) to the average level of urinary sodium excretion (UNa + V) over that time.

ability of calcium to lower pressure in elderly human hypertensives, in whom low renin, salt-sensitive mechanisms predominate, has also been linked to circulating 1,25 D levels (97).

Altogether, these studies thus support the reciprocal, opposing effects of dietary salt and calcium on blood pressure. It appears that the ability of salt to elevate blood pressure, as well as of calcium to lower it, both derive from their reciprocal actions on circulating levels of calcium hormones such as 1,25 D; salt elevating pressures by stimulating 1,25 D, and calcium offsetting the salt effect by suppressing 1,25 D. Thus 1,25 D, appropriately elevated in the face of a dietary calcium deficiency and exacerbated by excess dietary salt, may be a critical mediator of hypertension under these circumstances, and may reciprocally explain the hypotensive action of calcium supplementation—each dietary mineral acting to raise or lower blood pressure, respectively, by raising or lower circulating 1,25 D levels in the circulation. Failure to appreciate the predominant effect of oral calcium

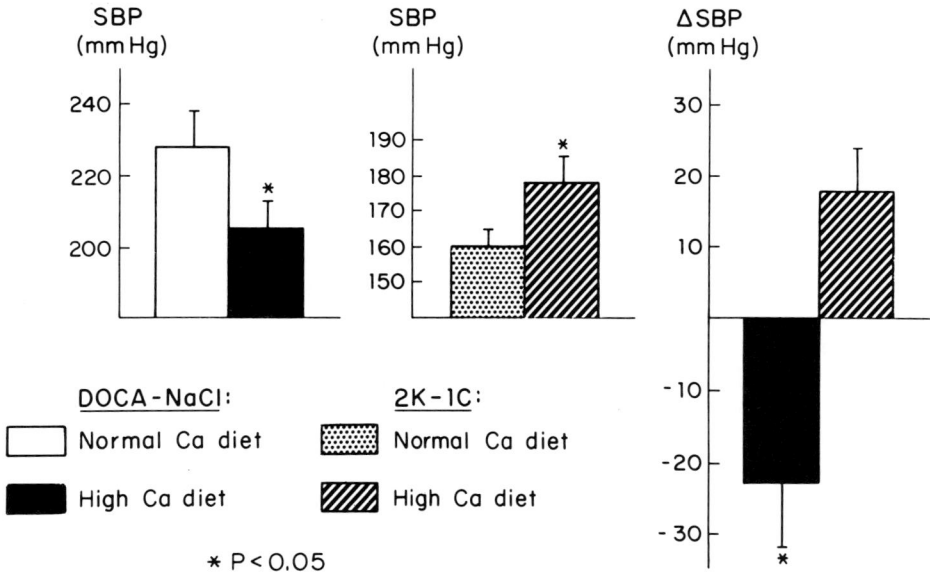

FIG. 18. Differential blood pressure (SBP) effects of increased dietary calcium intake on salt-sensitive (DOCA-NaCl) vs. renin-dependent (2K-1C) forms of experimental hypertension.

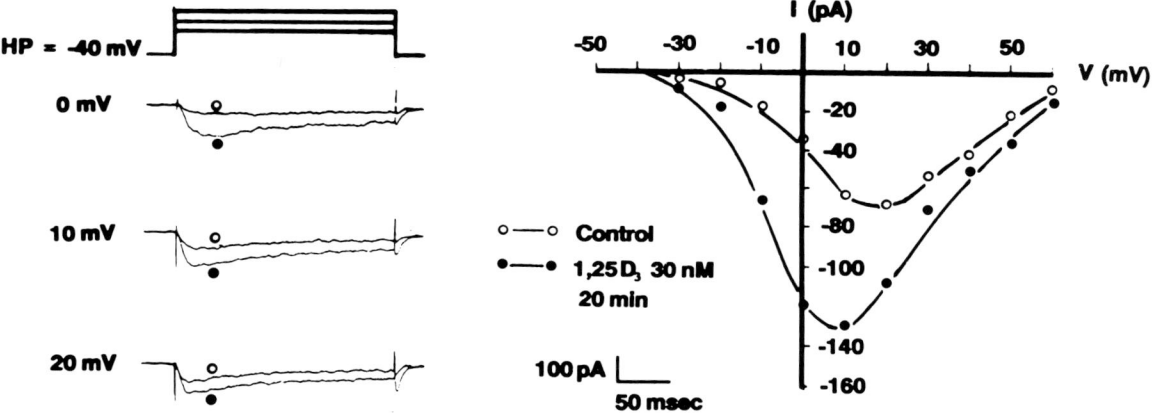

FIG. 19. Electrophysiological effects of 1,25 dihydroxyvitamin D (1,25 D) on L-type calcium channel current in isolated vascular smooth muscle cells.

supplementation in salt-sensitive hypertension, rather than uniformly in all forms of hypertensive disease, may perpetuate needless controversies and continue to obscure those clinical situations and subjects for whom dietary calcium represents a reasonable nonpharmacological antihypertensive therapy, especially in circumstances where dietary salt restriction is unsuccessful or contraindicated.

These clinically derived data can now be better understood as a result of more basic physiological studies in which the presence of vitamin D hormone receptors have been documented in vascular smooth muscle cells (98–100) and in heart (101), where 1,25 D serves to directly increase cellular calcium uptake (102). Indeed, vitamin D–induced vascular calcification, although perhaps operating by a steroid receptor–independent mechanism (103), was a model system used by Fleckenstein to study the vascular protective effects of calcium-channel–blocking agents (104). 1,25 D can also potentiate the vasoconstrictive effects of acute pressor hormone administration, and chronically can itself raise blood pressure at circulating levels considered within the normal range (105). At the cellular level, it has now been shown in patch clamp experiments that 1,25 D stimulates L-channel calcium current, and concomitantly elevates FURA-2 measured levels of cytosolic free calcium in these cells (43) (Fig. 19). Altogether, then, since (a) higher basal circulating 1,25 D levels are observed among low renin, black, and/or salt-sensitive individuals, which (b) are further elevated by dietary salt loading in salt-sensitive subjects, and which (c) are suppressed by oral calcium supplementation predominantly among these same individuals, it therefore seems reasonable to identify 1,25 D tentatively as at least one potential mediator of salt-sensitive hypertension in man.

More recently, similar findings were observed with PHF. This substance was originally identified in SHR, but not in Wistar-Kyoto (WKY) rats as a delayed pressor activity of dialyzed plasma extracts. It is currently defined as a bioassayable pressor activity, as well as by its action to increase ^{45}Ca uptake in vascular smooth muscle (106). On the basis of transplant and *in vitro* incubation studies, it appears that PHF originates in the parathyroid gland, from cells distinguishable from PTH-secreting chief cells by unique staining characteristics (107–109). PHF levels are elevated in DOCA-NaCl, but not 2K, 1C hypertensive rats, suggesting that hypertension per se cannot explain these findings (110). Recently, PHF activity has been reported in human hypertension (44), and may account for the differential ability of hypertensive versus normotensive serum to elevate cytosolic free calcium *in vitro* (111). Clinically, PHF appears to predominate among low renin and salt-sensitive essential hypertensive patients (45) (Fig. 20). It has also been identified in patients exhibiting the hypertension associated with primary hyperparathyroidism, in whom preoperative PHF levels predicted the blood pressure response to parathyroidectomy (112,113). It is interesting to note that even within the normotensive population, PHF levels were significantly higher among black compared to white subjects, and were also inversely related to plasma renin activity values. When studied prospectively, dietary salt loading was associated with a reciprocal suppression of plasma renin activity and stimulation of PHF-like activity. The basal level of PHF predicting the pressor response to salt—the higher the PHF, the greater the salt—induced a rise in blood pressure (45). Last, semipurified PHF extracts directly suppress plasma renin activity and reciprocally stimulate 1,25 D levels (114).

Altogether, therefore, these data support, according to our hypothesis, a reciprocating coordinate regulation of cellular calcium homeostasis by the renin-angiotensin system and calcium-regulating hormones (Fig. 21). Renin system activity, via angiotensin II, elevates cytosolic free calcium by promoting calcium release from intracel-

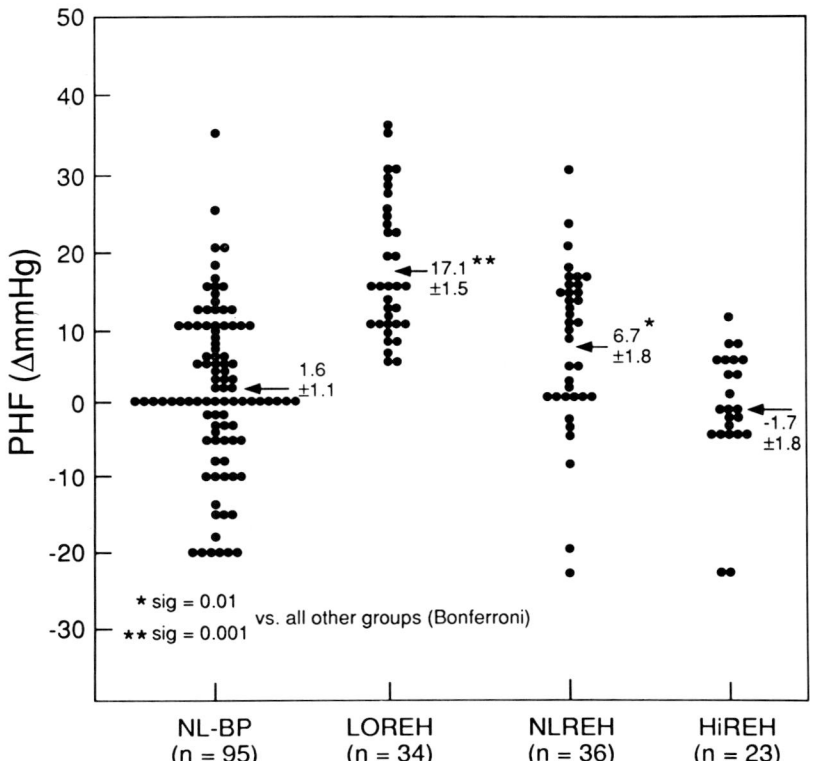

FIG. 20. Parathyroid hypertensive factor (PHF) levels in normotensive subjects and in different renin subgroups of essential hypertensive subjects.

lular stores; this action reciprocating with the action of circulating calcium-related substances such as 1,25 D and PHF, which elevate cytosolic free calcium by promoting cellular calcium uptake from the extracellular space. The above calcium-regulating hormones appear to mediate at least one mechanism of hypertension altering the steady-state relationship between intracellular and extracellular calcium by promoting cellular calcium accumulation from the extracellular space. This mechanism predominates in salt-sensitive forms of hyperten-

sive disease and is associated with suppression of plasma renin activity. This extracellular calcium–dependent form of hypertension may also be offset pharmacologically by calcium-channel–blocking drugs and physiologically by increasing dietary calcium intake. These mechanistic observations have practical implications as well. They suggest that calcium-channel antagonists as well as calcium supplementation itself should be particularly effective in salt-sensitive hypertensive patients groups, which is in accord with clinical experience (see above).

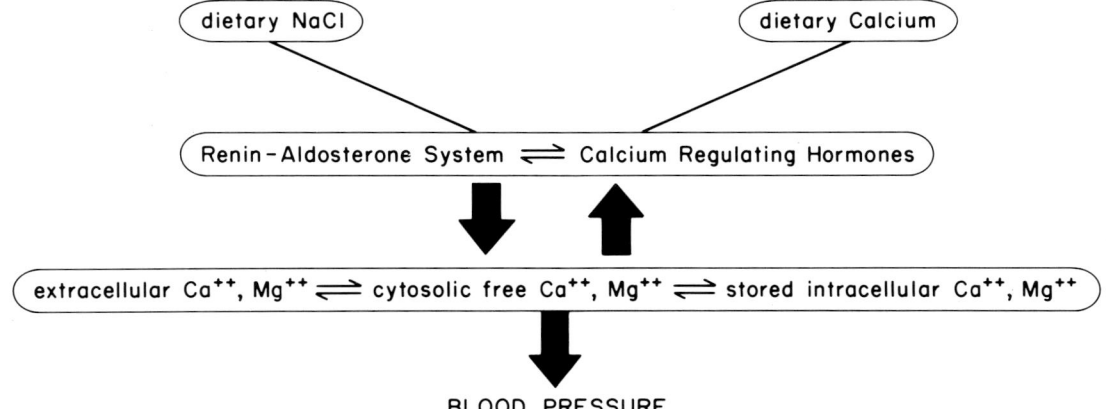

FIG. 21. Reciprocal linked influences of dietary salt and calcium intake on blood pressure, both mediated by their effects on the renin-angiotensin system and on calcium-regulating hormones, to alter the steady-state relation of free intracellular calcium and magnesium levels.

Indeed, recent data suggest an additive antihypertensive effect of calcium supplementation combined with calcium-channel blockade in these subjects (115).

Role of Glucose and Insulin Metabolism in Regulating Intracellular Ions

The intracellular ionic environment may also be influenced by alteration of environmentally derived nutrients and their regulating hormones. Experiments over four decades ago studying insulin effects on free water clearance demonstrated an insulin-induced renal sodium retention, and the link between renal ion handling (116), cellular ion content (117), and insulin action has recently received increasing attention. Although many accumulated data have focused on the effects of insulin itself, less emphasis has been placed on what appears to be an independent contribution of glucose to cellular ion content.

Following the oral ingestion of a glucose load, extracellular calcium levels have been reported to decline (118). Similar changes have been observed in circulating magnesium and potassium as well. Utilizing NMR spectroscopic techniques, our group measured intracellular levels of free magnesium, pH, sodium, and free calcium levels in erythrocytes of normal human subjects, as well as in cells of individuals with essential hypertension and type II NIDDM, before and after oral glucose loads. We found consistent responses in normal individuals, but not in those with hypertension. Specifically, intracellular free magnesium levels initially fell whereas intracellular free calcium levels reciprocally rose over the 180 minutes following oral glucose ingestion. Additionally, intracellular pH and intracellular sodium levels rose transiently (119). In obese normotensive subjects, a delayed exaggerated rise in intracellular calcium and fall in magnesium were observed. In hypertensive and diabetic subjects, oral glucose loading produced no significant changes in either free magnesium or calcium values. These data raised the questions: (a) To what extent are oral glucose–induced changes in cellular ion content a reflection of the direct actions of glucose per se, or rather the effects of insulin or other humoral or neural-mediated responses to glucose ingestion?, and (b) What is the relation, if any, between the cellular ionic responses to oral glucose and the insulin resistance and hyperinsulinemia of hypertension?

To investigate further the role of glucose and/or insulin in altering cellular ion metabolism, we directly assessed their individual effects on cellular ion content *in vitro* in normal human red blood cells. Glucose itself, in a specific, dose- and time-dependent manner, elevated cytosolic free calcium and reciprocally suppressed intracellular free magnesium and pH levels, thus reproducing the altered intracellular ionic "profile" of hypertension

(120) (Fig. 22, left). Interestingly, preliminary experiments in red cells obtained from essential hypertensive subjects reveal a blunting of these glucose-induced ionic effects. Since glucose transport in red cells is independent of insulin action, these data suggest a primary cellular ionic defect, rather than altered insulin action, as the cause of the abnormal cellular responses to oral glucose loads noted above. The physiological relevance of this effect was suggested by the threshold concentration of glucose exerting these effects, 10 mM or 180 mg percent, which approximates the renal threshold, or T_m, for glucose excretion. Furthermore, among a mixed sample of normotensive and hypertensive patients, the basal fasting cytosolic free calcium level was directly related to ambient glycated hemoglobin levels (unpublished data)—the greater the HbA1C value, the higher the fasting Cai level. Since none of these subjects was diabetic, and since their HbA1C values, reflective of long-term average blood glucose levels, were within a range considered normal, these observations strongly suggest that circulating extracellular glucose values, even within the normal range, may be one physiological determinant of basal fasting steady-state cytosolic free calcium levels, and thus of calcium-dependent basal vascular tone, blood pressure, and neural and cardiac tissue responsiveness. As such, these data may also help to explain the biological basis underlying the epidemiological observation that glucose values, even within normal limits, correlate with and predispose to the incidence of peripheral vascular and coronary artery disease.

Insulin itself also has primary ionic effects in a variety of cells, including red cells, in which glucose transport, as noted above, is insulin-independent (the red cell possessing a GLUT-1 glucose transporter). In the red cell insulin, opposite to glucose, elevates intracellular free magnesium, but also increases cytosolic free calcium and sodium levels (121,122) (Fig. 22, right). This not only supports a primary role of insulin in cellular ion homeostasis, but also suggests that the presence of insulin receptors in these cells should not, therefore, be considered vestigial. Similar experiments in red cells taken from essential hypertensive subjects demonstrate a blunting of the magnesium-elevating action of insulin, despite a persistence of its calcium-stimulating effects (123). This dissociation between insulin effects on magnesium vis à vis calcium may help to explain the physiological action of insulin in normal subjects as a vasodilator substance, whereas at the same time, vasoconstrictive responses to insulin have been observed in hypertensive subjects (124–126). These data also suggest that the definition of insulin resistance itself may need to be modified. Rather than merely a reflection of altered peripheral glucose uptake and disposition, it appears that insulin resistance is also an ionic phenomenon, even in tissues such as the red cell that do not demonstrate any insulin effects on glucose uptake or disposition. Indeed, it may be prefera-

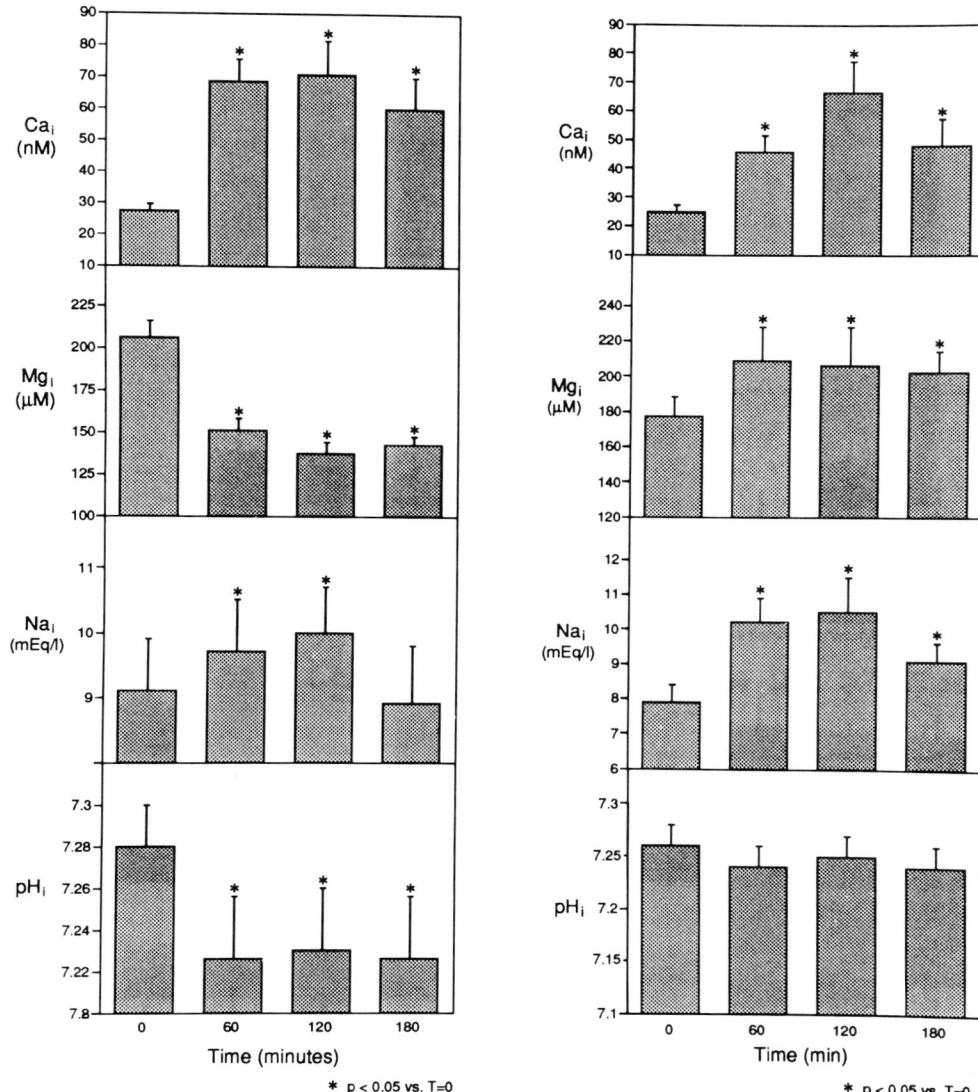

FIG. 22. *In vitro* ionic effects of hyperglycemia (*left*) and of insulin (*right*) on normal peripheral red blood cells. Cai, cytosolic free calcium; Mgi, intracellular free magnesium; Nai, intracellular sodium; pHi, intracellular pH.

ble to define insulin resistance in ionic terms, which can better explain the cellular linkage between this phenomenon and the vascular consequences associated with it, such as hypertension and atherosclerotic vascular disease.

SUMMARY: CELLULAR IONIC INTERPRETATION OF THE VASOCONSTRICTION–VOLUME ANALYSIS OF HYPERTENSION

More than two decades ago (72), Laragh proposed a physiological analysis of hypertension based on two different qualitative mechanisms. This scheme suggested that all diastolic hypertension may be considered as

made up of differing quantitative contributions of two general underlying mechanisms, one dependent on the vasoconstrictive activity of the renin-angiotensin system, and the other dependent on volume factors that are sensitive to dietary salt intake. Measurement of plasma renin activity together with 24-hour urine sodium excretion (grossly reflective of average dietary salt intake) in an individual patient provides an estimate of the relative importance of renin vis-à-vis sodium–volume factors in maintaining the elevated pressure. By utilizing the renin–sodium "profile," it has been possible to provide an individualized approach to therapy, in which the dietary or drug choices offered can be matched to the predominant underlying pathophysiological factors, i.e., to make the "punishment fit the crime," so to speak.

Based on the data now available, it appears that this physiological scheme can be understood and restated in equivalent cellular ionic terms. We have emphasized the following concepts: (a) the critical role of steady-state ion activity in determining the setpoint of cellular function generally, thus affecting concomitantly the state of vasoconstriction, cardiac contractility, renal excretory function, platelet aggregation, endothelial cell function, insulin secretion, and peripheral insulin sensitivity; (b) the role of hormonal integrating signals in transducing environmental dietary mineral and nutrient signals at the cellular level by altering the steady-state relation of extracellular to intracellular ions, and of intracellular cytosolic free ions to compartmentalized ion stores; and (c) hypertension as one of many clinical expressions of altered cellular ion activity, other components of GCMD or "Syndrome X" being other tissue-specific manifestations of the same process.

The apparently uniform intracellular ionic lesion characterizing hypertension as well as its allied clinical conditions must be reconciled with the more obvious extracellular diversity of ion distributions in different forms of hypertensive disease. This led to the formulation of an overall hypothesis in which all hypertension derives from quantitatively variable contributions in different subjects, of two general ionic mechanisms. These mechanisms are defined by the extent to which the ionic lesion is dependent on excess cellular calcium accumulation from the extracellular space vis-à-vis excess calcium release from intracellular sites. Extracellular calcium-dependent hypertension is determined by circulating calcium and nutrient-related hormones, as well as by circulating levels of nutrients themselves, such as glucose. As such, this mechanism underlies the phenomenon of dietary salt sensitivity and of the ability of calcium-channel antagonists as well as of oral calcium supplementation to preferentially offset salt-related forms of clinical and experimental hypertension. This form of hypertension is thus analogous to and helps to explain the sodium–volume component of Laragh's volume–vasoconstriction model. Intracellular calcium-dependent hypertension is analogous to the renin-dependent, angiotensin II–mediated vasoconstrictive component of the volume–vasoconstriction analysis. The cellular ionic mechanism is determined by the ability of angiotensin II to cause an IP_3-dependent release of calcium into the cytosol from intracellular stores. As such, this mechanism not only explains the preferential hypotensive efficacy of antirenin therapy with, for example, converting enzyme inhibitors, direct renin inhibitors, and beta blockers, but also explains the lesser salt sensitivity of high-renin compared to low-renin subjects, since the high-renin state is not associated with an excess of those other hormonal mediators of the salt-sensitive state, such as 1,25 D, which are present to a greater extent in the low-renin subject.

Also explained in the cellular ionic model, paralleling the volume–vasoconstriction model, is the normally reciprocating relationship of the two cellular ionic mechanisms. For example, an increased intake of dietary salt might normally result in a salt-dependent 1,25 D–mediated entry of calcium from outside the cell. This would then be compensated for by a suppression of renin activity [juxtaglomerular renin release being suppressed by increased cell calcium entry, (127)], lower angiotensin II levels, and thus a compensatory shift in the intracellular steady-state calcium equilibrium to decrease endoplasmic reticulum calcium release and thereby modulate the initial increased extracellular calcium entry. In normal subjects and in salt-insensitive hypertensive subjects, no net change in cytosolic free calcium occurs, and the blood pressure does not change. This is the picture of the normal subject on a high-salt diet. Similarly, an increase in renal renin secretion would, by increasing circulating angiotensin II levels, increase intracellular calcium release. The resultant transiently increased cytosolic free calcium level would be offset by an appropriate stimulation of plasma membrane calcium ATPase and other pump and channel mechanisms to bring cytosolic free calcium back to normal steady-state values. At the same time, the resultant increased net extrusion of cell calcium would produce a transient rise in steady-state extracellular calcium, thereby suppressing those hormones, such as 1,25 D and PHF, that contribute to extracellular calcium transport intracellularly. The net result, once again, would be normal cytosolic free calcium levels and normal blood pressure in the setting of high plasma renin activity. This is the picture of a normal subject on a low-salt diet.

When either of the above mechanisms operates at an abnormally high level, inappropriate for the physiological state, or when both mechanisms operate in the same direction simultaneously, the homeostatic balance between them may break down. Thus, in salt-sensitive subjects, either an excessive calcium hormone response (of 1,25 D, PHF, or other factors), or a deficient suppression of renin [the nephron heterogeneity hypothesis (48)] results in an imperfectly buffered accumulation of calcium from the extracellular space, a net rise in cytosolic free calcium, and a rise in blood pressure. Conversely, the use of angiotensin II in salt-loaded experimental hypertension and, clinically, bilateral renal artery stenosis (in which both mechanisms are present), may each result in more severe, or even malignant, hypertension, pulmonary edema, etc., because under these conditions the cell would have no way to buffer the rise in cellular calcium, calcium accumulating in the cytosol from both extracellular and intracellular storage sites. This may also be the cause of the vascular cell death and calcification, as shown by Fleckenstein (104), in the presence of excess vitamin D (extracellular calcium entry) together with nicotine (intracellular calcium release). It is therefore tempting to assign a more general role to the renin-angiotensin system and to calcium-regulating hormones in the regulation of intracellular as well as extracellular mineral ion homeostasis.

REFERENCES

1. Gupta R, Benovic J, Rose J. The determination of the free magnesium level in the human red blood cell by ^{31}P-NMR. *J Biol Chem* 1978;253:6172–6176.
2. Gupta R, Gupta P. Direct observation of resolved resonances from intra- and extracellular sodium 23 ions in NMR studies of intact cells and tissue using dysprosium (III) tripolyphosphate as paramagnetic shift reagent. *J Magn Reson* 1982;47:344–350.
3. Moon RB, Richards JH. Determination of intracellular pH by ^{31}P magnetic resonance. *J Biol Chem* 1973;248:7276–7278.
4. Veniero J, Gupta RK. NMR measurement of intracellular potassium in the perfused normotensive and spontaneously hypertensive rat aorta by a multinuclear subtraction procedure. *Am J Hypertens* 1992;5:733–739.
5. Resnick LM. Ionic basis of hypertension, insulin resistance, vascular disease, and related disorders: mechanism of Syndrome X. *Am J Hypertens* 1993;6:123s–134s.
6. Reaven G, Hofman B. A role for insulin in the aetiology and course of hypertension. *Lancet* 1987;2:435–436.
7. Ringer S. A third contribution regarding the infusion of the inorganic constituents of the blood on the ventricular contraction. *J Physiol (Lond)* 1883;4:222–225.
8. Kuriyama H, Uyshi I, Sueuk H, Kitamura A, Itoh T. Factors modifying contraction-relaxation cycle in vascular smooth muscles. *Am J Physiol* 1982;243:H641–H662.
9. Bean BP, Sturek M, Pugg A, Hermsmeyer K. Calcium channels in muscle cells isolated from rat mesenteric arteries: modulation by dihydropyridine drugs. *Circ Res* 1986;59:229–235.
10. Adelstein RS, Eisenberg E. Regulation and kinetics of the actin-myosin ATP interaction. *Annu Rev Biochem* 1980;49:921–956.
11. Inesi G. Mechanism of calcium transport. *Annu Rev Physiol* 1985;47:573–601.
12. Erne P, Bolli P, Burgissen E, Buhler F. Correlation of platelet calcium with blood pressure: effect of antihypertensive therapy. *N Engl J Med* 1984;319:1084–1088.
13. Altura BM, Altura BT, Carella A. Mg^{2+}-Ca^{2+} interaction in contractility of vascular smooth muscle: Mg^{2+} versus organic calcium channel blockers on myogenic tone and agonist-induced responsiveness of blood vessels. *Can J Physiol Pharmacol* 1987;65:729–745.
14. Langer GA. The effect of pH on cellular and membrane calcium binding and contraction of myocardium. *Circ Res* 1985;57:374–382.
15. Schwarz W, Passow H. Ca^{2+}-activated K$^+$ channels in erythrocytes and excitable cells. *Annu Rev Physiol* 1983;45:359–374.
16. Shingu T, Matsuura H, Kusaka M, et al. Significance of intracellular free calcium and magnesium and calcium-regulating hormones with sodium chloride loading in patients with essential hypertension. *J Hypertens* 1991;9:1021–1028.
17. Resnick L, Gupta R, Lewanczuk R, Pang P, Laragh J. Intracellular ions in salt-sensitive essential hypertension: possible role of calcium regulating hormones. In: Morii, ed. *Calcium regulating hormones I. Role in diseases and aging,* vol. 90. Tokyo: Springer-Verlag; 1991:88–93.
18. Altura BM, Altura BT, Gebrewold A. Magnesium deficiency and hypertension: correlation between magnesium-deficient diets and microcirculatory changes in situ. *Science* 1984;223:1315–1317.
19. Resnick LM, Veniero JC, Gupta RK, Laragh JH. Assessment of intracellular potassium and sodium in hypertension and diabetes by nuclear magnetic resonance spectroscopy. *J Hypertens* 1993;11(Suppl 5):S473.
20. Rinaldi G, Bohr DF. Potassium-induced relaxation of arteries in hypertension: modulation by extracellular calcium. *Am J Physiol* 1989;25:H707–712.
21. Tobian L, Lange J, Ulm K, Wold L, Iwai J. Potassium reduces cerebral hemorrhage and death in hypertensive rats even when BP is not lowered. *Hypertension* 1985;7(Suppl 2):I110–I114.
22. Khaw KT, Barrett-Connor E. Dietary potassium and stroke-associated mortality: a 12-year prospective population study. *N Engl J Med* 1987;316:235–240.
23. Altura BM. Magnesium and the regulation of contractility of vascular smooth muscle. *Adv Microcirc* 1982;11:77–113.
24. Allen DG, Orchard CH. The effects of changes of pH on intracellular calcium transients in mammalian cardiac muscle. *J Physiol (Lond)* 1983;335:555–567.
25. Davies TA, Weil G, Simons ER. Simultaneous flow cytometric measurements of thrombin-induced cytosolic pH and Ca^{2+} fluxes in human platelets. *J Biol Chem* 1990;265:11522–11526.
26. Rubin RP. The role of calcium in the release of neurotransmitter substances and hormones. *Pharmacol Rev* 1970;22:389–427.
27. Bing RG, Heagerty AM, Jackson JA, Thurston H, Swales JD. Leucocyte ionized calcium and sodium content and blood pressure in humans. *Hypertension* 1986;8:483–488.
28. Resnick L, Gupta R, Bhargava K, Gruenspan H, Alderman M, Laragh J. Cellular ions in hypertension, diabetes, and obesity: a nuclear magnetic resonance spectroscopic study. *Hypertension* 1991;17:951–957.
29. Papageorgiou P, Morgan KP. Intracellular free Ca^{2+} is elevated in hypertrophic aortic muscle from hypertensive rats. *Am J Physiol* 1991;29:H507–H515.
30. Livne AA, Aharonovitz O, Paran E. Higher Na$^+$-H$^+$ exchange rate and more alkaline intracellular pH setpoint in essential hypertension: effects of protein kinase modulation in platelets. *J Hypertens* 1991;9:1013–1019.
31. Canessa M, Morgan K, Semplicini A. Genetic differences in lithium-sodium exchange and the regulation of the sodium-hydrogen exchanger in essential hypertension. *J Cardiovasc Pharmacol* 1988;12(Suppl 3):S92–S98.
32. Vincenzi F, Morris C, Kissal LB, Kenny M, McCarron DA. Decreased calcium pump adenosine triphosphatase in red blood cells of hypertensive subjects. *Hypertension* 1986;8:1058–1066.
33. Postnov YV, Orlov SN, Reznikova MB, Rjazhsky GG, Pokudin NI. Calmodulin distribution and Ca^{2+} transport in the erythrocytes of patients with essential hypertension. *Clin Sci* 1984;66:459–463.
34. Tsuda K, Tsuda S, Minatogawa Y, Iwahashi H, Kido R, Yiu M. Decreased membrane fluidity of erythrocytes and its relevance to renin profile in essential hypertension. *Jpn Circ J* 1988;52:1301–1308.
35. Dominiczak AF, Lazar DF, Das SK, Bohr DF. Lipid bilayer in genetic hypertension. *Hypertension* 1991;18:748–757.
36. Adeoya AS, Bing RF, RIN. Erythrocyte calcium-stimulated, magnesium-activated adenosine 5'-triphosphatase activity in essential hypertension. *J Hypertens* 1992;10:651–656.
37. Matthews WR, DuCharme DW, Hamlyn JM, et al. Mass spectral characterization of an endogenous digitalislike factor from human plasma. *Hypertension* 1991;17:930–935.
38. Hamlyn JM, Ringel R, Schaeffer J, et al. A circulating inhibitor of (Na$^+$ + K$^+$) ATPase associated with essential hypertension. *Nature (Lond)* 1982;300:650–652.
39. Hamlyn JM. Increased levels of a humoral digitalis-like factor in deoxycorticosterone acetate-induced hypertension in the pig. *J Endocrinol* 1989;122:409–420.
40. Resnick L, Nicholson J, Laragh J. Alterations in calcium metabolism mediate dietary salt sensitivity in essential hypertension. *Trans Assoc Am Physicians* 1985;98:313–321.
41. Resnick L, Muller F, Laragh J. Calcium regulating hormones in essential hypertension: relation to plasma renin activity and sodium metabolism. *Ann Intern Med* 1986;105:649–654.
42. Resnick L. Calciotropic hormones in human and experimental hypertension. In: Laragh J, Brenner B, Kaplan N, eds. *Endocrine mechanisms in hypertension.* New York: Raven Press; 1989:265–297. (*Perspectives in hypertension;* vol 2).
43. Shan J, Resnick LM, Lewanczuk RZ, Karpinski E, Li B, Pang PKT. 1,25 Dihdroxyvitamin D as a cardiovascular hormone: effects on calcium current and cytosolic free calcium in vascular smooth muscle cells. *Am J Hypertens* 1993;6(In press).
44. Lewanczuk R, Resnick L, Blumenfeld J, Laragh J, Pang P. A new circulating hypertensive factor in the plasma of essential hypertensive subjects. *J Hypertens* 1990;8:105–108.

45. Resnick LM, Lewanczuk RZ, Laragh JH, Pang PKT. Parathyroid hypertensive factor-like activity in human essential hypertension: relationship to plasma renin activity and dietary salt sensitivity. *J Hypertens* 1993;11:1235–1241.

46. Laragh J, Resnick L. Recognizing and treating two types of long-term vasoconstriction in hypertension. *Kidney Int* 1988;34(Suppl 25):S162–S174.

47. Resnick LM, Laragh JH. Calcium metabolism and hypertension: clinical evidence and cellular hypothesis. In: Aoki K, ed. *Essential hypertension* 2. Tokyo: Springer-Verlag; 1989:353–372.

48. Sealey J, Blumenfeld J, Bell M, Pecker M, Sommers S, Laragh J. Presidential address. On the renal basis for essential hypertension: nephron heterogeneity with discordant renin secretion and sodium excretion causing a hypertensive vasoconstriction-volume relationship. *J Hypertens* 1988;6:763–777.

49. Resnick L. Intracellular free magnesium in erythrocytes of essential hypertension: relation to blood pressure and serum divalent cations. *Proc Natl Acad Sci (USA)* 1984;81:6511–6515.

50. Matsuura T, Kohno M, Kanayama Y, et al. Decreased intracellular free magnesium in erythrocytes of spontaneously hypertensive rats. *Biochem Biophys Res Commun* 1987;143:1012–1017.

51. Stephenson E, Podolsky R. Regulation by magnesium of intracellular calcium movement in skinned muscle fibers. *J Gen Physiol* 1977;69:17–35.

52. Resnick L, Gupta R, Laragh J. RBC cytosolic free calcium levels in hypertension: relation to blood pressure and other cations. *Am J Hypertens* 1990;3:59A.

53. Resnick L, Roman M, Gupta R, Devereux R, Laragh J. Intracellular cation determinants of left ventricular mass. *Am J Hypertens* 1990;3:15A.

54. Resnick L, Gupta R, Gruenspan H, Alderman M, Laragh J. Hypertension and peripheral insulin resistance: mediating role of intracellular free magnesium. *Am J Hypertens* 1990;3:373–379.

55. Resnick L. Hypertension and abnormal glucose homeostasis: possible role of divalent ion metabolism. *Am J Med* 1989;87(Suppl 6A):17S–22S.

56. Julius S, Gudbrandsson T, Jamerson K, Shahab ST, Andersson O. The hemodynamic link between insulin resistance and hypertension. *J Hypertens* 1991;9:983–986.

57. Julius S, Gudbrandsson T, Jamerson K, Andersson O. The interconnection between sympathetics, microcirculation and insulin resistance in hypertension. *Blood Pressure* 1992;1:9–19.

58. Reaven G. Insulin resistance, hyperinsulinemia, hypertriglyceridemia, and hypertension: parallels between human disease and rodent models. *Diabetes Care* 1991;14(3):195–202.

59. Barbagallo M, Resnick LM, Gruenspan H, Devereux RB, Laragh JH. Glucose vs. insulin as determinants of left ventricular mass in non-insulin dependent diabetes mellitus (NIDDM). *J Hypertens* 1992;10(Suppl 4):S101.

60. Draznin B, Sussman K, Kao M, Lewis D, Sherman N. The existence of an optimal range of cytosolic free calcium for insulin-stimulated glucose transport in rat adipocytes. *J Biol Chem* 1987;262:14385–14388.

61. Draznin B, Sussman K, Eckel R, Kao M, Yost T, Sherman N. Possible role of cytosolic free calcium in mediating insulin resistance of obesity and hyperinsulinemia. *J Clin Invest* 1988;82:1848–1852.

62. Draznin B. Cytosolic calcium: a new factor in insulin resistance? *Diabetes Res Clin Pract* 1991;11:141–146.

63. Levy J, Zemel MB, Sowers JR. Role of cellular calcium metabolism in abnormal glucose metabolism and diabetic hypertension. *Am J Med* 1989;87(Suppl):7S–15S.

64. Hellman B, Sehlin J, Taljedal JB. Calcium and secretion: distinction between two pools of glucose-sensitive calcium in pancreatic islets. *Science* 1976;194:1421–1423.

65. Rocchini A, Key J, Bondie D. The effect of weight loss on the sensitivity of blood pressure to sodium in obese adolescents. *N Engl J Med* 1989;321:580–585.

66. Altura BM, Altura BT. Magnesium ions and contraction of vascular smooth muscles: relationship to some vascular diseases. *Fed Proc* 1981;40:2672–2679.

67. Jelicks LA, Gupta RK. NMR measurement of cytosolic free calcium, free magnesium, and intracellular sodium in the aorta of the normal and spontaneously hypertensive rat. *J Biol Chem* 1990;265:1394–1400.

68. Ahn YS, Jy W, Harrington W, Shanbaky N, Fernandez LF, Haynes DH. Increased platelet calcium in thrombosis and related disorders and its correction by nifedipine. *Thromb Res* 1987;45:135–143.

69. Shanbaky NM, Ahn Y, Jy W, Harrington W, Fernandez L, Haynes DH. Abnormal aggregation accompanies abnormal platelet Ca^{2+} handling in arterial thrombosis. *Thromb Haemostasis* 1987;57:1–10.

70. Altura BM, Brust M, Bloom S, Barbour R, Stempack J, Altura B. Magnesium dietary intake modulates blood lipid levels and atherogenesis. *Proc Natl Acad Sci (USA)* 1990;87:1840–1844.

71. Resnick L, Gupta R, Sosa R, Corbett M, Laragh J. Intracellular pH in human and experimental hypertension. *Proc Natl Acad Sci (USA)* 1987;84:7663–7667.

72. Laragh JH. Vasoconstriction-volume analysis for understanding and treating hypertension: the use of renin and aldosterone profiles. *Am J Med* 1973;55:261–274.

73. Resnick L, Laragh J, Sealey J, Alderman M. Divalent cations in essential hypertension. Relations between serum ionized calcium, magnesium, and plasma renin activity. *N Engl J Med* 1983;309:888–891.

74. Resnick L. Uniformity and diversity of calcium metabolism in hypertension: a conceptual framework. *Am J Med* 1987;82(Suppl 1B):16–26.

75. Hunt SC, Williams RR, Kuida H. Different plasma ionized calcium correlations with blood pressure in high and low renin normotensive adults in Utah. *Am J Hypertens* 1991;4:1–8.

76. Resnick L, Nicholson J, Laragh J. Calcium, the renin-angiotensin system, and the hypotensive response to nifedipine. *Hypertension* 1987;10:254–258.

77. Smith J, Smith L. Extracellular Na^+ dependence of changes in free Ca^{2+}, Ca^{2+} efflux, and total cell Ca^{2+} produced by angiotensin II in cultured arterial muscle cells. *J Biol Chem* 1987;262:17455–17460.

78. Resnick L. Role of calcium and magnesium in the therapy of human hypertension. In: Laragh J, Brenner B, ed. *Hypertension: pathophysiology, diagnosis, and management,* vol 2. New York: Raven Press; 1989:2037–2059.

79. Oshima T, Matsuura H, Matsumoto K, Kido K, Kajiyama G. Role of cellular calcium in salt sensitivity of patients with essential hypertension. *Hypertension* 1988;11:703–707.

80. Hall C, Hungerford S. Prevention of DOCA-salt hypertension with the calcium blocker nitrendipine. *Clin Exp Hypertens A* 1983;5:721–728.

81. Resnick L, Laragh J. Renin, calcium metabolism, and the pathophysiologic basis of antihypertensive therapy. *Am J Cardiol* 1985;56:68H–74H.

82. Resnick L, Nicholson J, Laragh J. The antihypertensive effects of calcium channel blockade: role of sodium and calcium metabolism. *J Cardiovasc Pharm* 1988;12(Suppl 6):S114–S116.

83. Nicholson J, Resnick L, Cigarroa J, Marion D, Vaughan EJ, Laragh J. The pressor effect of sodium-volume expansion is calcium mediated. *Am J Hypertens* 1991;4:904–908.

84. Iriuchijima J. Effect of calcium antagonist nifedipine on blood pressure of various hypertensive rats. *Hiroshima J Med Sci* 1980;29:15–19.

85. Resnick L, Gupta R, Laragh J. Calcium channel blockade reverses salt sensitivity: role of intracellular ions. *Clin Res* 1990;38:259A.

86. Hughes G, Oexmann M, Margolius H, Epstein S, Bell N. Normal vitamin D and mineral metabolism in essential hypertension. *Am J Med Sci* 1988;296:252–259.

87. Resnick L, Sealey J, Laragh J. Short and long-term oral calcium alters blood pressure (BP) in essential hypertension. *Fed Proc* 1983;42:300(abst).

88. Resnick L, DiFabio B, Marion R, James G, Laragh J. Dietary calcium modifies the pressor effects of dietary salt intake in essential hypertension. *J Hypertens* 1986;4(Suppl 6):S679–S681.

89. Addison W. The use of calcium chloride in arterial hypertension. *Can Med Assoc J* 1924;14:1059–1061.

90. Resnick L, Nicholson J, Laragh J. Calcium metabolism and es-

sential hypertension—relation to altered renin system activity. *Fed Proc* 1986;45:2739–2745.

91. Zemel M, Gualdoni S, Walsh M, et al. Effects of sodium and calcium on calcium metabolism and blood pressure regulation in hypertensive black adults. *J Hypertens* 1986;4(Suppl 5):S364–S366.

92. Saito K, Sano H, Furuta Y, Fukuzaki H. Effect of oral calcium on blood pressure response in salt-loaded borderline hypertensive patients. *Hypertension* 1989;13:219–226.

93. Hamet P, Daignault-Gelinas M, Lambert J, et al. Epidemiological evidence of an interaction between calcium and sodium intake impacting on blood pressure: a Montreal study. *Am J Hypertens* 1992;5:378–385.

94. McCarron D, Lucas P, Schneidman R, Druecke T. Blood pressure development of the spontaneously hypertensive rat following concurrent manipulation of dietary Ca and Na: relation to intestinal Ca fluxes. *J Clin Invest* 1985;76:1147–1154.

95. Kotchen T, Oh C, Whitescarver S, Resnick L, Gertner J, Blehschmidt N. Calcium and calcium regulating hormones in the "prehypertensive" Dahl salt sensitive rat. *Am J Hypertens* 1989;2:749–753.

96. Resnick LM, Sosa RE, Corbett ML, Gestner JM, Sealey JE, Laragh JH. Effects of dietary calcium on sodium-volume vs. renindependent forms of experimental hypertension *Trans Assoc Amer Physicians* 1986;99:172–179.

97. Ogihara T, Saito H, Tabuchi Y, Hashizume K, Kumahara Y. The hypotensive effect of long-term oral calcium loading in elderly hypertensive patients: the importance of endogenous vitamin D suppression. *J Hypertens* 1986;4(Suppl 6):S685–S687.

98. Merke J, Hofmann W, Goldenschmidt D, Ritz E. Demonstration of 1,25 (OH0)2 vitamin D receptors and actions in vascular smooth muscle cells in vitro. *Calcif Tissue Int* 1987;41:112–114.

99. Kawashima O. Receptor for 1,25 dihydroxyvitamin D in a vascular smooth muscle cell line derived from rat aorta. *Biochem Biophys Res Commun* 1987;146:1–6.

100. Berger U, Wilson P, McClelland RA, et al. Immunocytochemical detection of 1,25-dihydroxyvitamin D receptors in normal human tissues. *J Clin Endocrinol Metab* 1988;67:607–613.

101. Walters M, Wicki D, Riggle P. 1,25 Dihydroxy-vitamin D3 receptors identified in the rat heart. *J Mol Cell Cardiol* 1986;18:67–72.

102. Bukoski R, Xue H, McCarron D. Effect of 1,25(OH)₂ vitamin D3 and ionized calcium on ⁴⁵Ca uptake by primary cultures of aortic myocytes of spontaneously hypertensive and Wistar-Kyoto normotensive rats. *Biochem Biophys Res Commun* 1987;146:1330–1335.

103. Baran DT, Kelly M. Lysophosphatidylinositol: a potent mediator of 1,25 dihydroxyvitamin D-induced increments in hepatocyte cytosolic calcium. *Endocrinology* 1988;122:930–934.

104. Fleckenstein A, Frey M, Zorn J, Fleckenstein-Grun G. Experimental basis of long-term therapy of arterial hypertension with calcium antagonists. *Am J Cardiol* 1985;56:3H–14H.

105. Bukoski RD, Xue H. On the vascular inotropic action of 1,25-(OH)₂ vitamin D₃. *Am J Hypertens* 1993;6:389–396.

106. Lewanczuk R, Wang J, Zheng Z, Pang P. Effect of spontaneously hypertensive rat plasma on blood pressure and tail artery calcium uptake in normotensive rats. *Am J Hypertens* 1989;2:26–31.

107. Kaneko T, Ohtani R, Lewnaczuk R, PKT P. A novel cell type in the parathyroid gland of spontaneously hypertensive rats. *Am J Hypertens* 1989;2:549–552.

108. Pang PKT, Lewanczuk RZ. Parathyroid origin of a new circulating hypertensive factor in spontaneously hypertensive rats. *Am J Hypertens* 1989;2:898–904.

109. Neuser D, Schulte-Brinkmann R, Kazda S. Development of hypertension in WKY rats after transplantation of parathyroid glands from SHR/SP. *J Cardiovasc Pharmacol* 1990;16:971–974.

110. Lewanczuk RZ, Pang PKT. Parathyroid hypertensive factor is present in DOCA-salt but not two-kidney-one-clip hypertensive rats. *Am J Hypertens* 1991;4:802–805.

111. Barbagallo M, Gupta RK, Lewanczuk RZ, Pang PKT, Resnick LM. Serum mediated intracellular calcium changes in normotensive and hypertensive red cells: role of parathyroid hypertensive factor (PHF). *J Cardiovasc Pharmacol* 1994;23(Suppl 2):S14–S17.

112. Lewanczuk RZ, Pang PKT. Expression of parathyroid hypertensive factor in hypertensive primary hyperparathyroid patients. *Blood Pressure* 1993;2:22–27.

113. Lind L, Ljunghall S. Hypertension, primary hyperparathyroidism and the parathyroid hypertensive factor. *Blood Pressure* 1993;2:4–5.

114. Lewanczuk RZ, Benishin CG, Pang PKT. Parathyroid hypertensive factor (PHF) decreases urinary sodium excretion (UNaV) in normotensive rats. *J Hypertens* 1992;10(Suppl 4):S115.

115. Resnick LM, Nicholson JP, Gupta RK, Laragh JH. Interactive effects between oral calcium supplementation and calcium antagonist therapy in essential hypertension. *J Hypertens* 1993;11(Suppl 5):S472.

116. DeFronzo R, Cooke C, Andres R. The effect of insulin on the renal handling of sodium, potassium, calcium, and phosphate in man. *J Clin Invest* 1975;55:845–855.

117. Zierler K, Wu F. Insulin acts on Na, K, and Ca currents. *Trans Assoc Am Physicians* 1988;101:320–325.

118. Rosenbloom A. Serum calcium and magnesium decline during oral glucose tolerance testing in children and adolescents with preclinical diabetes less than in normals. *Metabolism* 1977;26:1033.

119. Resnick L, Gupta R, Gruenspan H, Laragh J. Intracellular ion response to glucose tolerance: Relation of hypertension, obesity, and insulin resistance. *Circulation* 1988;78(Suppl II):II–570.

120. Resnick L, Barbagallo M, Gupta R, Laragh J. Ionic basis of hypertension in diabetes: role of hyperglycemia. *Hypertension* 1991;18:395.

121. Barbagallo M, Gupta RK, Resnick LM. Cellular ionic effects of insulin in normal human erythrocytes: a nuclear magnetic resonance study. *Diabetologia* 1993;36:146–149.

122. Barbagallo M, Gupta RK, Resnick LM. Independent effects of hyperinsulinemia and hyperglycemia on intracellular sodium in normal human red cells. *Am J Hypertens* 1993;6:264–267.

123. Barbagallo M, Gupta RK, Laragh JH, Resnick LM. Ionic effects of insulin in normal and hypertensive erythrocytes: towards an ionic definition of insulin resistance. *J Hypertens* 1993;11(Suppl 5):S399.

124. Anderson EA, Hoffman RP, Balon TW, Sinkey CA, Mark AL. Hyperinsulinemia produces both sympathetic neural activation and vasodilatation in normal humans. *J Clin Invest* 1991;87:2246–2252.

125. Anderson EA, Gudbjornsdottir S, Elam M, Sellgren J, Mark AL. Insulin causes vasoconstriction and increases arterial pressure in obese, insulin resistant hypertensive humans. *Hypertension* 1992;20:409(abst).

126. Anderson EA, Mark AL. The vasodilator action of insulin. Implications for the insulin hypothesis of hypertension. *Hypertension* 1993;21:136–141.

127. Churchill PC. Second messengers in renin secretion. *Am J Physiol* 1985;249:F175–F184.

Hypertension: Pathophysiology, Diagnosis, and Management, Second Edition, edited by J.H. Laragh and B.M. Brenner, Raven Press, Ltd., New York © 1995.

CHAPTER 71

Calcium Metabolism in Experimental Genetic Hypertension

Daniel C. Hatton, Eric W. Young, Richard D. Bukoski, and David A. McCarron

Calcium (Ca^{2+}) plays a central role in the regulation of vascular smooth muscle contraction. Since elevated peripheral resistance is the hallmark of hypertension, it follows that aberrations of Ca^{2+} metabolism at either the cellular or systemic level may be involved in the pathogenesis of hypertension. This possibility is evident in the many studies that have found reductions of blood pressure with dietary Ca^{2+} supplementation in experimental models of hypertension (1). Further evidence of the connection between Ca^{2+} and hypertension can be found in the pertinent chapters on epidemiology, Ca^{2+}-regulating hormones in human hypertension, and the various human and experimental forms of secondary hypertension in this book.

While a variety of alterations in cellular and systemic

Ca^{2+} handling have been described in experimental hypertension, the causal link remains speculative at this time. This chapter will describe the alterations in Ca^{2+} handling that have been identified in vascular smooth muscle and other cell types isolated from experimental models of genetic hypertension. Systemic Ca^{2+} metabolism will then be reviewed and the possible connections between altered systemic Ca^{2+} metabolism and elevated blood pressure will be explored. Finally, likely mechanisms through which Ca^{2+} metabolism alters blood pressure will be examined.

EXPERIMENTAL MODELS OF GENETIC HYPERTENSION

The most commonly studied model of experimental genetic hypertension is the Aiko-Okamoto spontaneously hypertensive rat (SHR). Although the SHR is an imperfect model of human essential hypertension, it does appear that alterations of Ca^{2+} metabolism found in human hypertension are closely approximated in the SHR. In considering the SHR, care must be taken when comparing results to its normotensive control strain, the

D. C. Hatton and D. A. McCarron: Department of Medicine, Division of Nephrology and Hypertension, Oregon Health Sciences University, Portland, Oregon 97201.

E. W. Young: Nephrology Section, VA Medical Center, Ann Arbor, Michigan 48105.

R. D. Bukoski: Department of Internal Medicine, University of Texas Medical Branch at Galveston, Galveston, Texas 77555.

Wistar-Kyoto (WKY) rat. Kurtz and Morris (2) have provided evidence that suggests that considerable phenotypic variation exists within both the SHR and the normotensive WKY strains that may be dependent on the breeder supplying the animals. This problem appears to relate to improper pure-breeding of the WKY strain when a normotensive control was needed at the outset of the SHR strain in the 1960s (3). For this and other reasons, the value of the SHR as a research tool remains questionable. Nonetheless, it remains the most important experimental model of genetic hypertension and forms the basis for most of the discussion in this chapter. Considerable emphasis is placed on the age and sex of the animals used in the studies as systemic Ca^{2+} handling may change over the life of the animal. As always, it is imperative to take into account the breeding history of the animals when evaluating any study utilizing SHR and WKY.

Several other experimental models of genetic hypertension have been studied to a limited extent in the area of Ca^{2+} metabolism. The Lyon hypertensive rat (LH), derived from the Sprague-Dawley rat, has been studied with regard to the sensitivity of its blood pressure to oral Ca^{2+}. It has been demonstrated that parathyroidectomy prevents the rise in blood pressure in the LH (4) as it does in the SHR (5,6). While the results make the LH a promising model for study of alterations in Ca^{2+} regulation and blood pressure, the SHR has been studied more frequently, apparently because of its widespread availability. Another genetic model of hypertension, the Milan hypertensive and normotensive strains of rat, have produced some interesting results that largely complement the SHR, although this model has been studied only infrequently outside the laboratory where it was developed. The Dahl salt-sensitive and resistant strains are genetic models of hypertension and normotension respectively; but enhanced salt intake is required for the expression of hypertension. Some information exists about Ca^{2+} metabolism in this strain. Finally, nongenetic experimental models of hypertension have several notable alterations in Ca^{2+} metabolism that may be pertinent to the pathogenesis of these particular forms of secondary hypertension.

In general, genetic models of hypertension are characterized by elevated total peripheral resistance in the presence of normal cardiac output (7). Arterial pressor responses both to infusions of contractile agonists (8) and to psychological stress (9) have been found to be significantly greater in the SHR than in the WKY. These findings have been interpreted to indicate that the elevated total peripheral resistance may be a reflection of altered reactivity due to either structural changes in the vasculature or functional changes of vascular smooth muscle. Because Ca^{2+} is a primary regulator of vascular smooth muscle function, it has been proposed that cellular defects in the metabolism of this cation may result in functional abnormalities (10–13). In the discussion that follows, Ca^{2+} metabolism at the systemic and cellular level will be evaluated for its role in hypertension.

VASCULAR SMOOTH MUSCLE Ca^{2+} METABOLISM

While regulation of Ca^{2+} metabolism at the whole animal level is centered around maintaining serum levels of ionized Ca^{2+} in the millimolar range, parallel systems of the cell are set to maintain intracellular Ca^{2+} at a level of approximately 100 nM. Thus a 10,000-fold gradient of ionized Ca^{2+} across the cell membrane is present and functionally utilized by the cell as a mechanism of signal transduction. Ca^{2+} is believed to be directly involved in the contraction of vascular smooth muscle through a myosin light chain–linked mechanism (14,15). A transient rise in free intracellular Ca^{2+} allows binding of Ca^{2+} to the Ca^{2+} regulatory protein calmodulin, forming a complex that activates myosin light chain kinase. This enzyme subsequently catalyses the phosphorylation of myosin light chains, which stimulates actomyosin adenosine triphosphatase (ATPase) activity. In addition to this primary role as a regulator of contractile activity, Ca^{2+} is also required as a co-factor in the generation of other second messengers. For example, Ca^{2+} is required for full activation of phospholipase C, which hydrolyzes inositol bis-phosphate, initiating the production of the inositol polyphosphates (IP$_3$ and IP$_4$) and diacylglycerol (16). These second messengers act to induce the release of Ca^{2+} from the sarcoplasmic reticulum (17,18) and presumably to activate Na^+-H^+ exchange (19,20). In addition, Ca^{2+} is required for activation of the enzyme protein kinase C that has been proposed to modulate a number of cell functions. Included are the phosphorylation of key actin binding proteins that may play a role in vascular smooth muscle contractile regulation (14) and translation of growth factor signals to the proliferative response (21).

It is believed that elevations in intracellular Ca^{2+} are brought about through at least two pathways. It is known that activator Ca^{2+} can be released from internal stores, such as the sarcoplasmic reticulum (17,18) and that Ca^{2+} can enter the cell from the extracellular space either by passive leak (22,23) or through distinct Ca^{2+} channels that are activated by changes in membrane potential produced either pharmacologically or electrically (24,25). Recent work with the intracellular Ca^{2+} indicators, aequorin (26,27) and the bapta-derivative fluorescent compounds fura-2 (28,29) and Indo-1 (30), indicates that the rise in Ca^{2+} induced in vascular smooth muscle by agonists is transient in nature. Specifically, it has been observed that a peak concentration is reached within a minute of activation and that this falls off over time to reach a lower, yet elevated steady-state level.

Obviously if Ca^{2+} enters the cell to trigger intracellular events, its gradient across the cell membrane must be re-established for the cell to return to a resting, inactivated state. It is currently believed that removal of this cation from the myoplasm occurs by both active and facilitated processes. The presence of membrane bound, calmodulin-dependent, Ca^{2+}-ATPase activity in vascular smooth muscle has now been described by several investigators (31–34). These results, coupled with reports that subcellular membrane fractions of vascular smooth muscle are capable of ATP-supported Ca^{2+} uptake (11,35–39), strongly suggest that a Ca^{2+} pump is functional in both the sarcolemma and the sarcoplasmic reticulum. In addition to the Ca^{2+} pump, facilitated transport of Ca^{2+} out of the cell by a Na^+-Ca^{2+} exchange mechanism has also been proposed to play a major role in regulating cellular Ca^{2+} in vascular tissue (38). Although there is both physiological and biochemical evidence in support of the presence of a Na^+-Ca^{2+} exchange system (39–42), the magnitude of its contribution to Ca^{2+} regulation is not currently well understood.

In summary, the vascular smooth muscle cell has available a large transcellular gradient of Ca^{2+} that can be used for translating extracellular signals into functional activity. It is imperative that the smooth muscle cell maintain this gradient for normal function. It is not surprising, therefore, that redundant systems exist for achieving this end (i.e., Ca^{2+} uptake by intracellular organelles, and Ca^{2+} extrusion across the cell membrane via both the Ca^{2+} pump and the Na^+-Ca^{2+} exchange process). When considering a disorder such as hypertension, which is characterized in part by altered vascular reactivity, it is logical to propose that dysfunction of one or some of these Ca^{2+} regulatory mechanisms may result in altered cell activation. For example, there could be enhanced contractile activity as a result of sustained activation of a Ca^{2+} channel. Or, vascular tone may be sustained because of an impairment in vasorelaxation caused by a depressed rate of Ca^{2+} extrusion. This could occur secondary to defective Ca^{2+}/calmodulin stimulation of Ca_{2+}-ATPase, for example. Furthermore, Ca^{2+}-dependent regulation of second messenger generation may be altered such that there could be altered growth patterns in the cell secondary to altered growth factor signal processing. Thus investigators have sought to determine whether Ca^{2+} metabolism is altered in vascular smooth muscle of hypertensive animals, and whether these alterations are translated into dysfunctional contractile or proliferative responses.

ENDOTHELIAL CELL Ca^{2+} METABOLISM

Over the past several years it has become increasingly apparent that the endothelial lining of blood vessels plays an important role in regulating vascular tone. Rather than acting as a passive barrier between the blood and the surrounding tissue as previously thought, the endothelium is a sophisticated structure that synthesizes and releases a variety of substances that, among other things, have vasoactive effects on the underlying smooth muscle cells. The vasoactive effects include vasodilatory influences mediated by endothelium-derived relaxing factor (EDRF), believed to be nitric oxide (NO), prostaglandins, and a putative endothelium-derived hyperpolarizing factor (EDHF), as well as vasoconstrictor substances mediated predominantly by endothelins. Depending upon the balance between vasoconstrictive and vasodilatory forces, the endothelium has the potential to have substantial impact on vascular tone and, hence, the hypertensive process.

As with vascular smooth muscle, Ca^{2+} homeostasis is critical for orchestrating endothelial cell function (for a review, see 43). Activation of endothelial cells by an agonist is commonly mediated through guanosine 5'-triphosphate (GTP)-binding regulatory proteins (44) with subsequent activation of second messengers such as inositol 1,4,5-triphosphate, diacylglycerol, and adenosine 3':5'-cyclic phosphate (cyclic AMP) (45). This results in an initial spike of intracellular Ca^{2+} due to liberation of intracellular Ca^{2+} from the endoplasmic reticulum (46,47). The initial sharp increase in Ca^{2+} is followed by an extended plateau phase that is critically dependent upon influx of Ca^{2+} from extracellular sources (48). Reductions of Ca^{2+} below normal dose-dependently compromise the magnitude of the plateau phase, resulting in a reduction in the synthesis and release of EDRF (49,50).

The extracellular Ca^{2+} appears to enter the endothelial cell through a Ca^{2+}-permeable, nonselective cation channel activated by a receptor, a second messenger such as IP_4 (43), or depletion of Ca^{2+} stores in the endoplasmic reticulum (51). Although there do not appear to be any voltage-dependent Ca^{2+} channels on endothelial cells, Ca^{2+} influx is modulated by membrane potential (52,53). Ca^{2+} influx is facilitated by a potassium current that serves to hyperpolarize the cell, thus increasing the electrochemical gradient for Ca^{2+} which, ultimately, facilitates extracellular Ca^{2+} entry into the cell (54).

Perturbations of extracellular Ca^{2+} have significant ramifications for the synthesis and release of EDRF precisely because extracellular Ca^{2+} levels determine free cytosolic Ca^{2+} levels (49). Synthesis of EDRF from L-arginine by NO synthase varies with free cytosolic Ca^{2+} levels because it is a Ca^{2+}/calmodulin-dependent process (49,55). Likewise, release of EDRF depends upon free cytosolic Ca^{2+} levels. The importance of extracellular Ca^{2+} is particularly apparent in the context of flow-dependent vasodilation where there is continuous modulation of Ca^{2+} influx by mechanical stimulation of the blood vessel (56). Using mesenteric resistance vessels mounted in a myograph, Bevan and Joyce (50) showed that decreasing extracellular Ca^{2+} caused a dose-dependent reduction in flow-induced vasodilation. They found similar results for reductions in the extracellular sodium chloride concentration. However, simultaneous reduction of both sodium chloride and Ca^{2+} did not compromise flow-dependent vasodilation, suggesting that there was a unique interaction of sodium chloride and Ca^{2+} on flow-dependent vasodilation.

Removal of the endothelium alters intracellular free Ca^{2+} levels in the underlying vascular smooth muscle (VSM), suggesting the endothelial function modulates Ca^{2+} homeostasis in VSM (57). Thus, Ca^{2+} metabolism of endothelial cells can have significant implications for Ca^{2+} homeostasis in the vasculature and resultant vascular tone. Since endothelial cells handle Ca^{2+} in much the same way as vascular smooth muscle cells (VSMCs), many of the same subcellular mechanisms that are suspected to be defective in VSMCs from hypertensive models need to be evaluated in endothelial cells as well.

VASCULAR SMOOTH MUSCLE Ca^{2+} METABOLISM IN HYPERTENSION

There is considerable evidence of disordered Ca^{2+} metabolism in tissues and cells from SHR as well as humans with essential hypertension. These results have indicated that cells from hypertensive subjects are unable to effectively defend cellular Ca^{2+} homeostasis, leading to the suggestion that defective cellular Ca^{2+} metabolism is a pathogenic factor in hypertension (58). Much of that evidence comes from work on cells isolated from blood. Platelets, erythrocytes, lymphocytes, and thymocytes have all been shown to have elevated intracellular Ca^{2+} levels and/or larger Ca^{2+} transients to agonists (59–62). Much of this work is predicated on the assumption that these cells may act as surrogates for vascular smooth muscle cells and may be indicative of Ca^{2+} metabolism in vessels. However, there is no conclusive evidence that this is the case.

Some of the earliest work that examined Ca^{2+} metabolism of vascular smooth muscle of the SHR involved the measurement of Ca^{2+} uptake capacity of isolated subcellular membrane fractions (11,12,35–38). While the results have not been entirely consistent, the general consensus has been that there is depressed ATP-dependent Ca^{2+} uptake capacity in both crude microsomal fractions of aorta and in more purified sarcolemmal fractions of the mesenteric artery bed. On the basis of these results, it has been suggested that the vascular myocyte may not be able to maintain normal levels of intracellular Ca^{2+} or to properly remove Ca^{2+} after activation in the hypertensive animal. However, the interpretation of these data is not necessarily as straightforward as it may seem. For example, problems of purity of the membrane fractions with respect to organelle content and the disruptive changes that they may undergo during the isolation process have been recognized (63). Furthermore, values of Ca^{2+} uptake are generally

normalized to protein content of the vesicular preparation. However, there is clear evidence that vascular smooth muscle of conduit arteries of the SHR is hypertrophied (64). Therefore, consistently depressed values of Ca^{2+} uptake may simply reflect increased protein content per unit area of membrane. In addition, these experiments have measured Ca^{2+} uptake capacity of subcellular fractions prepared from conduit vessels despite the fact that this diameter artery is not thought to contribute significantly to resistance to blood flow (65). Thus the applicability of findings of depressed Ca^{2+} uptake capacity by subcellular fractions of conduit arteries to mechanisms underlying the altered reactivity of resistance arteries is not clear.

Influx of ^{45}Ca into both intact tissue and in cultured vascular smooth muscle cells has been examined in the SHR. There are reports that both basal and agonist-stimulated influx of ^{45}Ca are elevated in resistance vessels of the SHR (23). In larger conduit arteries, ^{45}Ca uptake has been found to be elevated or not different between the SHR and WKY depending on the age of the animal (11,36). Furthermore, when primary cultures of aortic myocytes were examined, it was observed that ^{45}Ca uptake was elevated in cells of the hypertensive rat (66). When taken at face value these results suggest that the cell membrane of the SHR smooth muscle cell is hyperpermeable to Ca^{2+}. However, this interpretation may be oversimplified. At times longer than 1 minute, it is likely that backflux of the isotope complicates interpretation of the influx measurement and prevents kinetic assessment of unidirectional flux across the cell membrane (67). More likely, influx measured over a longer period of time reflects the sum of passive flux into the cell, rapid filling of readily accessible storage pools, and active extrusion out of the cell across the cell membrane. Furthermore, complications also arise when accounting for the noncellular trapping of label within the extracellular space and nonspecific binding to the extracellular matrix (67). Thus experiments using ^{45}Ca may be most efficiently applied toward the assessment of exchangeable pools of intracellular Ca^{2+} in intact muscle or cultured cells.

In order to circumvent problems associated with tracer experiments, several groups have employed Ca^{2+}-sensitive intracellular probes, such as fura-2 and Indo-1, to assess both basal levels of intracellular Ca^{2+} and the magnitude and time course of transient agonist-induced changes. Most of the work studying vascular smooth muscle of the SHR and WKY has been carried out using cultured aortic myocytes and variable results have been reported. Sugiyama et al. (28) have found that basal Ca^{2+} is elevated in both primary and multiply passaged cells of the SHR. Nabika et al. (30) have reported that Ca^{2+} concentration is not elevated in the cells of the SHR under basal conditions although agonist-induced transients are significantly increased.

In contrast to these results, Bukoski et al. (29) have found that free Ca^{2+} in primary cultures of mesenteric artery myocytes of the SHR and WKY are not different and neither are agonist-induced alterations. They have also measured Ca^{2+} in intact mesenteric resistance arteries using fura-2 and have been unable to detect any difference in intracellular Ca^{2+} levels between the SHR and WKY. The latter results raise the possibility that vascular smooth muscle cells in culture undergo changes in Ca^{2+} metabolism that prevent them from accurately reflecting the *in vivo* situation. To test this possibility, Bukoski (68) measured intracellular Ca^{2+} in intact mesenteric resistance arteries, in primary cultures of vascular myocytes, and in passaged myocytes. The results indicate very little difference in intracellular Ca^{2+} in intact resistance arteries or primary cultures of myocytes between SHR and WKY. However, passaged myocytes exhibited elevated intracellular Ca^{2+} and hyperresponsiveness to angiotensin II, suggesting that a change in the phenotype of the VSM may be responsible for alterations in Ca^{2+} handling. These results are commensurate with the observations of Storm et al. (69), who examined intracellular Ca^{2+} in pancreatic arterioles. They found no evidence of elevated basal intracellular in arterioles from stroke-prone spontaneously hypertensive rats (SHRSP) nor was there evidence of altered responsiveness of potential-operated Ca^{2+} channels as has been hypothesized for the SHR (70–72). Changes in Ca^{2+} homeostasis that have been observed in larger vessels may be related to phenotypic changes in VSM induced by elevated blood pressure. Papageorgiou and Morgan (73) found that elevated intracellular Ca^{2+} in hypertrophied aortic vascular smooth muscle cells was associated with phenotypic signs of active growth.

In summary, ^{45}Ca uptake by isolated subcellular membrane fractions, ^{45}Ca flux into intact tissue and cultured cells, and more direct assessment of intracellular Ca^{2+} using intracellular fluorescent probes have been used to address the question of whether cellular Ca^{2+} metabolism of vascular smooth muscle is abnormal in the SHR. Although this research has been ongoing for nearly two decades, our understanding of whether differences in levels of free intracellular Ca^{2+} are present in the SHR and whether dysfunction of cellular transport processes might underlie these potential differences is not complete. An equally pertinent question is whether the defects that have been described to date, i.e., attenuated ATP-supported ^{45}Ca uptake by subcellular fractions, increased basal and agonist-induced influx, and perhaps modestly elevated levels of free intracellular Ca^{2+}, are manifest in altered contractile function.

IS ALTERED Ca^{2+} METABOLISM REFLECTED BY ALTERED FUNCTIONAL PROPERTIES?

Much of the experimental evidence examining vascular function in the SHR has been gathered using the aorta, superior mesenteric and caudal arteries, and the portal vein. However, it is known that significant resistance to blood flow is not generated by vessels with luminal diameters greater than approximately 300 and that up to 70 percent of peripheral resistance can be accounted for by vessels with diameters between 100 and 200 (74–76). Thus consideration of whether changes in vascular smooth muscle functional activity contribute to hypertension should be theoretically restricted to contractile properties measured in true resistance arteries.

It has been consistently observed that active tension generation (force per unit length of vessel) is elevated in resistance arteries of the SHR. However, this difference is not present if active wall stress (tension normalized to cross-sectional area of the vessel wall) is calculated instead (77). The apparent difference in tension development by the vessel from the hypertensive animal is therefore the result of the presence of structural changes and does not reflect a difference in the intrinsic ability of the muscle cell to contract. This finding alone indicates that the contractile proteins are likely to be intact and that excitation-contraction coupling mechanisms, including changes in free intracellular Ca^{2+}, function normally in the SHR.

Aside from contractile force–generating ability, another functional difference that may alter vascular tone in the hypertensive animal is an increase in sensitivity of the vessels to contractile agonists or a decrease in sensitivity to vasodilatory agents. Both nerve activity and endothelial activity influence the sensitivity to agonists. If sensitivity to norepinephrine is determined in the presence of the neuronal amine pump inhibitor, cocaine, or in chemically sympathectomized vessels, the SHR exhibits slightly increased sensitivity to the catecholamine (78,79). Interestingly, this has also been reported in the tail artery by Webb and Vanhoutte (80). While these latter reports indicate that there may be a difference in the intrinsic sensitivity of the vascular smooth muscle to norepinephrine, in the presence of an intact sympathetic nerve terminal no functional differences would be present. Thus the suggested relevance of this finding to enhanced reactivity observed *in vivo* is questionable. On the other hand, the apparent intrinsic difference may be related to impaired endothelial function. Falloon et al. (81) reported that isolated mesenteric resistance vessels from SHR mounted in a pressurized system show increased sensitivity to norepinephrine compared to WKY and that the difference is eliminated by destruction of the endothelium. The data suggest that either the response to norepinephrine is antagonized by release of vasodilators from the endothelium and the release of vasodilators is compromised in the SHR or norepinephrine causes the release of a constricting agent from the endothelium in the SHR that is not present in the WKY.

Considerable evidence for the release of a constrictive agent from SHR endothelium has emerged from studies showing that acetylcholine-induced vasorelaxation is impaired in the SHR (82,83). Relaxation can be improved by indomethacin, suggesting that the vasoconstrictive substance is a prostaglandin (84). However, it is unlikely that acetylcholine is causing the release of the vasoconstrictor. More likely, vasoconstrictor release is caused by the agonist that is used to precontract the vessels. For example, when vasopressin is used instead of norepinephrine to precontract the vessel, there is no evidence of a vasoconstrictive substance being released from the endothelium when acetylcholine is used to relax the vessel (85).

In addition to the above-mentioned parameters, it has been observed that after removal of Ca^{2+} from the cell with the Ca^{2+} chelating agent EGTA, resistance arteries of the SHR exhibit increased sensitivity to Ca^{2+} when it is added back in the presence of norepinephrine (86,87). These results indicate that there may indeed be increased sensitivity of vascular smooth muscle of the SHR to Ca^{2+}. This may play a role in the hypertensive state. However, when Ca^{2+} sensitivity was measured using the same experimental paradigm in resistance arteries of the human essential hypertensive, the opposite result was found (88). Vessels from the hypertensive subjects actually exhibited a depressed sensitivity to Ca^{2+}, suggesting that this property does not reflect a basic defect central to dysfunction of vascular smooth muscle in hypertension. Furthermore, it can be argued that experiments that employ EGTA may actually be uncovering a differential sensitivity of the hypertensive muscle cell to the effect of stripping away Ca^{2+}, rather than an intrinsic defect in cell function.

Finally, an increase in spontaneous rhythmic activity has been reported in the mesenteric resistance artery of the SHR (89), as well as in the tail artery of the stroke-prone variation of the SHR (90,91). This finding has been interpreted to indicate that there may be a pacemaker locus within the cell membrane that is present in the SHR and is either not present or is suppressed in the WKY. Furthermore, it has been proposed that the cellular mechanism responsible for this effect may contribute to the increased reactivity of vascular smooth muscle that has been described *in vivo*. Although these findings are promising, until the cellular events that underlie this phenomenon are defined, its relationship to intrinsic cellular defects in Ca^{2+} metabolism remains speculative.

In summary, there appear to be only minor differences in the intrinsic contractile properties of resistance arteries of the SHR and WKY. There may be more pronounced differences in vasodilation either as a consequence of endothelial influences or aberrations in Ca^{2+} extrusion, making it more difficult for the vessel to relax. Additional data need to be gathered to assess the extent and nature of the differences in vasorelaxation between experimental models and their controls.

Another possibility to be considered is that whereas only minor differences in intrinsic contractile ability of vessels of the SHR and WKY are detectable *in vitro*, the vessel may demonstrate altered reactivity *in vivo* secondary to neural and/or humoral influences. Nerve activity could be catecholaminergic or peptidergic whereas humoral factors could be either platelet-associated growth factors or hormones responsible for Na^+ or Ca^{2+} metabolism of the whole animal.

In contrast to the findings that reactivity of isolated resistance arteries does not reflect the apparent alterations in Ca^{2+} metabolism that have been described, a consistent observation has been that resistance vessels of the SHR demonstrate increased medial thickness. In the smaller artery this appears to result from a hyperplastic event (92). The stimulus for the increased proliferation in the resistance vessel is unknown. One hypothesis is that there is an increase in micropermeability of the endothelial barrier to serum-borne mitogens or platelet-derived growth factors as a result of elevated transmural pressure (93). Furthermore, there are reports that indicate that vascular smooth muscle of the SHR and SHRsp demonstrates increased growth rates in culture (94), suggesting that they respond to growth factors in an intrinsically different manner. It is therefore intriguing to speculate that the subtle alterations in cellular Ca^{2+} metabolism that have been discussed may manifest themselves in enhanced rates of cell growth and not altered reactivity. Alternatively, the differences in Ca^{2+} metabolism may reflect properties of growing vessels. In either case, the result would be an effectively narrowed lumen that would produce greater resistance to blood flow in the SHR than in the WKY in the face of any given stimulus, as proposed by Folkow (7). Obviously, additional investigation will be required before definitive statements can be made.

SYSTEMIC Ca^{2+} METABOLISM IN EXPERIMENTAL HYPERTENSION

Many reports document abnormalities of Ca^{2+} metabolism at the systemic level in the SHR as well as in human hypertension and other forms of experimental hypertension. However, there is disagreement as to the interpretation of these abnormalities. One view holds that the hypertensive animal has difficulty conserving whole body Ca^{2+} and is relatively "Ca^{2+} deficient" compared to the appropriate normotensive control animal. However, others interpret the same data to indicate an inappropriate surfeit of whole body Ca^{2+} in the hypertensive animal. While there is little doubt that Ca^{2+} handling is altered in experimental models of genetic hypertension, the meaning of the defects requires careful analysis.

The specific manifestations of abnormal Ca^{2+} metabolism that have been reported in experimental hypertension include low concentration of serum ionized Ca^{2+}, elevated concentration of serum parathyroid hormone, hypercalciuria, alterations of intestinal Ca^{2+} absorption and vitamin D production, and elevated serum calcitonin concentration. Ultimately, these findings are reflected in total body and bone Ca^{2+} balance. As before, the majority of published evidence comes from the SHR. Because blood pressure and Ca^{2+} handling are dependent on the age and sex of the animal studied, it is important to keep track of these variables in evaluating the experimental evidence in this area.

Serum Ca^{2+}

In the male SHR, a small but significant decrease in serum-ionized Ca^{2+} has been reported in animals between 8 and 45 weeks of age by several investigators (95–100). In the female SHR, depressed serum-ionized Ca^{2+} has also been reported in 5- and 13-week-old rats (100), and decreased ultrafilterable Ca^{2+} (which is 80 percent ionized serum Ca^{2+}) was found in 23-week-old animals (101). Although the fasting or fed status of the animals at the time of blood drawing was not specified in all of these reports, it appears that decreased serum-ionized Ca^{2+} is more likely to be found if the animals are in a fasted state. Parathyroidectomized, 25- to 26-week-old female SHR had no difference in fasting serum-ionized Ca^{2+} (101), indicating that absent parathyroid function obliterates the difference in fasting serum-ionized Ca^{2+}. Similarly, no difference in serum-ionized Ca^{2+} was detected between very young (25 days old) male and female SHR and WKY (102). The SHR used in the latter study were considered to be prehypertensive as there was no detectable elevation in blood pressure. Thus it appears that serum-ionized Ca^{2+} is initially normal in the SHR but falls as the animal ages. Possible reasons for low serum-ionized Ca^{2+} in SHR include decreased intestinal Ca^{2+} absorption, increased renal Ca^{2+} excretion, depressed kidney or bone response to parathyroid hormone (PTH), and elevated calcitonin levels. Evidence for each of these possibilities is presented in subsequent sections.

Decreased serum-ionized Ca^{2+} has also been found in the uninephrectomized deoxycorticosterone acetate (DOCA)-salt hypertensive rat relative to its sham-operated control (100). Similarly, low serum-ionized Ca^{2+} has been reported in human essential hypertension (103–105) and in some patients with primary aldosteronism (106).

Parathyroid Function

Serum PTH has been found either to be elevated in the SHR or not different from the WKY, apparently as a function of the specific assay used. When elevated, it has been proposed to be a secondary response to the low serum-ionized Ca^{2+}. For example, Stern et al. (96) found

that carboxy-terminal PTH was measurable in 43 percent of 6-week-old male SHR and in 55 percent of 10-week-old male SHR, whereas all WKY of the same ages had undetectable C-terminal PTH. In this study, serum-ionized Ca^{2+} was significantly lower in 10-week-old SHR than in WKY. Bindels et al. also found elevated immunoreactive PTH and decreased serum-ionized Ca^{2+} in 8-week-old SHR although another assay for intact PTH showed no difference between SHR and WKY (95). Similarly, a midmolecule PTH assay did not detect a difference between 13- to 15-week-old SHR and WKY (107), and an intact-whole molecule assay did not detect a difference in SHR and WKY from 6 to 20 weeks (108). Interestingly, the latter study also found no differences in PTH levels of SHR and WKY using immunoassays with antibodies directed toward both carboxy and amino terminal fragments.

In contrast, McCarron et al. (97) reported that amino-terminal PTH was significantly elevated in male SHR at 18, 24, and 29 weeks of age and that a C-terminal assay also revealed a higher serum PTH concentration in the SHR at 29 weeks of age. Likewise, DiPette et al. (99) found a significant elevation of amino-terminal PTH in 14- to 16-week-old SHR. Since glomerular filtration rate is consistently normal in SHR at these ages, it is unlikely that reduced clearance of immunoreactive but biologically inert PTH fragments accounts for the elevated PTH levels. Furthermore, morphologic investigations have demonstrated that SHR exhibit parathyroid gland hyperplasia, suggesting that chronic stimulation of the parathyroid cells may exist (109). Elevated serum PTH levels have also been reported in humans with essential hypertension (110–116), or gestational hypertension (117) in those at genetic risk for hypertension (118), and individuals with primary aldosteronism (106). Furthermore, PTH has been found to be significantly correlated with both blood pressure in hypertensive individuals (113,116) and renal failure patients (119) and with left ventricular weight in untreated hypertensive subjects (120).

Although serum PTH may be elevated in the SHR in response to a decreased serum-ionized Ca^{2+}, end-organ responsiveness to the hormone may be abnormal. Reduced renal responsiveness to PTH is suggested by findings of hypercalciuria (see below), decreased basal and stimulated $1,25(OH)_2$ vitamin D_3 production (see below), and low to normal urinary and nephrogenous cyclic AMP (101,121–123), all in the face of apparently elevated immunoreactive PTH. Moreover, infusion of PTH caused a smaller increment in serum-ionized Ca^{2+} in 13-week-old male SHR than in WKY (124). The diminished response in the SHR may be due to downregulation of renal PTH receptors as a consequence of chronically elevated circulating PTH. DiPette et al. (99) found that PTH receptor levels in the SHR were only 60 percent of that observed in WKY tissue. Thus, it would appear that failure of the SHR to increase serum-ionized Ca^{2+} adequately results in chronic elevation of circulating PTH and a subsequent downregulation of renal PTH receptors.

Another line of evidence that suggests that parathyroid gland function and PTH play a role in hypertension are observations that parathyroidectomy in weanling rats attenuates the rate of rise of blood pressure in the SHR (5,6,57,125), the stroke-prone SHR (126,127), and the LH strain of genetically hypertensive rat (4). Furthermore, transplantation of parathyroid glands between SHR and WKY results in an elevation of blood pressure in the WKY (125–130). The reduction in blood pressure with parathyroidectomy is accompanied by enhanced contractile responses to norepinephrine in isolated vessels from the SHR (57,130,131) that are attenuated by removal of the endothelium (57,130).

The study of Gairard et al. (6) found that blood pressure was lowered even though serum Ca^{2+} levels were maintained within normal limits by feeding the parathyroidectomized rats a diet containing an elevated Ca^{2+} content. It should be noted that the parathyroidectomized rats grew more slowly than the control animals in this study, introducing the confounding variable of body mass into the analysis. Unfortunately, no allowance for this factor was made, making clear interpretation of the results difficult. Although this work has been interpreted to indicate that PTH may play a direct role in the development of hypertension, it is unlikely that this hormone has direct vascular effects because PTH appears to be without cardiovascular effects at physiological concentrations and acts as a vasodilator at supraphysiological concentrations (132–134).

Vitamin D

Vitamin D regulation appears to be abnormal in the SHR and may partially explain disordered Ca^{2+} homeostasis in the strain. Serum measurements of $1,25(OH)_2$ vitamin D_3 in young male SHR are variously reported to be normal (91,135–138) or elevated (95,101,139) compared to the WKY. However, at 11 to 13 weeks of age, normal (98,140,141) or decreased serum levels of $1,25(OH)_2$ vitamin D_3 begin to appear in the SHR (109,142–145) as they are developing hypertension. Low or even normal serum $1,25(OH)_2$ vitamin D_3 concentrations may be inappropriate because SHR have been reported to have low serum-ionized Ca^{2+} (95–97), low serum phosphorus (95,146), and, perhaps elevated PTH (95–97,109), all of which would be expected to stimulate $1,25(OH)_2$ vitamin D_3 production. Serum 25-(OH) vitamin D_3 tends to be normal or elevated in the SHR indicating that substrate depletion cannot account for the low $1,25(OH)_2$ vitamin D_3 (135,142,147). Additional evidence for altered vitamin D metabolism in the SHR is

indicated by subnormal increments in serum $1,25(OH)_2$ vitamin D_3 in response to PTH (137,144), cyclic AMP (144), phosphate depletion (144,145), and Ca^{2+} depletion (143). Furthermore, on a vitamin D–deficient diet, the SHR but not the WKY develops hypocalcemia and a low serum concentration of $1,25(OH)_2$ vitamin D_3 (147). The decreased serum concentration of $1,25(OH)_2$ vitamin D_3 in the SHR may be explained entirely by decreased production because metabolic clearance of the hormone is the same in the SHR and WKY (107).

Although some studies have suggested that the SHR displays intestinal resistance to the effects of $1,25(OH)_2$ vitamin D_3 (126,141,148), others have found a normal (143) or enhanced (149) intestinal response to the hormone. Lucas et al. (143) found that Ca^{2+} flux across isolated duodenal segments increased to normal in the SHR when they were given supplemental $1,25(OH)_2$ vitamin D_3. Similarly, the calcemic response to systemic PTH infusion is restored to normal in the SHR with the administration of $1,25(OH)_2$ vitamin D_3 (124).

Calcitonin

Although the relationship between calcitonin and blood pressure has not been extensively studied as yet, several investigators have reported that serum calcitonin concentration is elevated in the SHR. Bindels et al. (95) found elevated serum calcitonin in the 8-week-old SHR, whereas Patel and Hsu (150) have reported elevated calcitonin in 16-week-old SHR but not in younger animals. Primary hypersecretion of calcitonin is a potential explanation for the low ionized Ca^{2+} and hypercalciuria (see below) seen in the SHR. Alternatively, calcitonin may be elevated secondary to other pathological events. Certainly more work needs to be done in this area.

Calcitonin Gene-Related Peptide

Although it is not considered a Ca^{2+} regulating hormone, calcitonin gene-related peptide (CGRP) appears to be responsive to Ca^{2+} status (151) and it is a potent vasodilator. This 37 amino-acid neuropeptide results from alternative processing of the calcitonin gene. It is widely distributed in the central and peripheral nervous systems (152). Intravenous infusion of CGRP produces marked hypotension through a reduction in total peripheral resistance (153,154). Central nervous system administration of CGRP produces variable effects depending upon the dose and site of administration. For example, injection of 0.2 pmol CGRP into the nucleus tractus solitarius produces a depressor response, whereas 2 pmol results in a pressor response (155). Likewise, injections into the central nucleus of the amygdala resulted in a pressor response but intrathecal injections caused a reduction in blood pressure (156,157). Given the vasoactive properties of CGRP and its presence in central and peripheral nervous system sites involved in cardiovascular regulation, CGRP may be involved in the alterations in blood pressure that characterize hypertension, particularly since circulating levels are lower in the SHR than the WKY (158).

Ca^{2+} Excretion

Urinary Ca^{2+} excretion is increased in the mature SHR although there is controversy as to whether the hypercalciuria reflects primary intestinal hyperabsorption or a primary renal leak. In the growing animal, 24-hour urinary Ca^{2+} excretion has been reported as decreased (95,102), not different (97,101,124,129), and increased (101,146,159) relative to the WKY. However, longitudinal studies indicate that hypercalciuria develops by 17 weeks of age in the male SHR (97) and by 25 to 26 weeks of age in the female SHR (96). McCarron et al. (97) found elevated urinary Ca^{2+} excretion in male SHR at 17, 22, 28, and 43 weeks of age with concurrently low serum-ionized Ca^{2+} and high serum PTH. The hypercalciuria of these animals was interpreted to reflect a primary renal leak in that urinary Ca^{2+} excretion was increased in the face of a diminished filtered load of Ca^{2+} and an increased level of PTH, which should stimulate tubular Ca^{2+} reabsorption. Hypercalciuria persisted when 18- to 20-week old male SHR were placed on a low Ca^{2+} diet, providing additional evidence for a renal leak or abnormal humoral regulation of renal Ca^{2+} excretion (160).

In contrast to the above evidence, which supports the idea of a primary renal Ca^{2+} leak, Lau et al. (101) propose that the hypercalciuria occurs because of primary intestinal hyperabsorption of Ca^{2+}. In part, this hypothesis is based on the finding of diminished Ca^{2+} excretion after fasting in 8- to 14-week-old male and 23-week-old female SHR in the presence of normal urinary cyclic AMP. The latter parameter was used to estimate PTH activity because it was not measured directly. However, it must be recalled that hypercalciuria in 24-hour urine collections occurs in animals older than those studied and that urinary cyclic AMP may not be appropriately elevated in the SHR because of target organ resistance to PTH (161). Lau et al. (101) also reported that the older female SHR has greater intestinal Ca^{2+} absorption and total body Ca^{2+} balance than the WKY, which supports a primary intestinal problem. However, as discussed below, much evidence runs counter to these balance studies, leaving the question unresolved.

The distinction between renal and absorptive hypercalciuria in the mature SHR is important because of what it implies about the overall Ca^{2+} status of the hypertensive animal, i.e., a relative deficit or surfeit of Ca^{2+} compared to the normotensive control animal. In the idealized situation, a primary renal Ca^{2+} leak implies hypercalciuria and depressed serum-ionized Ca^{2+} in the fasting state, elevated serum PTH and urinary cyclic AMP, parathyroid hyperplasia, and negative or corrected Ca^{2+} balance in the SHR relative to the WKY (162). Primary intestinal hyperabsorption of Ca^{2+} implies normal urinary Ca^{2+} excretion and serum-ionized Ca^{2+} in the fasting state, suppressed parathyroid function and gland size, and positive or corrected Ca^{2+} balance in the SHR relative to the WKY (162). In short, renal hypercalciuria is consistent with whole animal Ca^{2+} deficiency and absorptive hypercalciuria is consistent with Ca^{2+} excess in the SHR. Notably, intestinal Ca^{2+} absorption should theoretically be increased in both states. Given the heterogeneity of the WKY and, to a lesser extent the SHR strains, it must be acknowledged that both Ca^{2+} deficit and surfeit states may exist for the SHR depending on the source of the animals (2). Another possibility is that Ca^{2+} balance of the SHR changes relative to the WKY as the animal ages.

Hypercalciuria has also been reported in the Milan hypertensive rat (MHS) as compared with its normotensive control (163). Hypercalciuria in the MHS appears to be due to a renal leak, indirectly suggesting that the same pathophysiology applies to the SHR. Impaired tubular reabsorption in the MHS may be secondary to reduced renal Ca^{2+}-ATPase activity (164). The Dahl salt-sensitive hypertensive rat also demonstrates hypercalciuria, which appears to be on a renal basis (165). Similarly, renal hypercalciuria has long been recognized with mineralocorticoid-induced hypertension (166). Finally, several studies have found evidence for renal hypercalciuria in human essential hypertension, which is independent of urinary sodium excretion or filtered load of Ca^{2+} (110,167–171).

Intestinal Ca^{2+} Transport and Absorption

Perhaps no aspect of systemic Ca^{2+} metabolism in the SHR has produced such contradictory information as the measurement of intestinal Ca^{2+} transport and absorption. Unfortunately, knowledge of Ca^{2+} absorption alone does not reveal the overall Ca^{2+} status of the organism because intestinal hyperabsorption would be predicted for both renal and absorptive calciurias in their pure forms. Therefore, measurements of net intestinal Ca^{2+} absorption must be related to concurrent determinations of Ca^{2+} excretion and balance. On the other hand, measurement of Ca^{2+} transfer across isolated intestinal segments or cells provides information about the actual transport mechanisms, but may not be strictly related to overall net absorption.

At the cellular level, Ca^{2+} metabolism is altered in freshly isolated proximal enterocytes from the SHR as compared with the WKY. Ca^{2+} influx and cellular Ca^{2+} pools are reduced in SHR enterocytes (138). Furthermore, the Ca^{2+} efflux constant is reduced in the SHR

(172). Addition of ouabain or removal of sodium from the enterocyte incubation media obliterates the difference in efflux rate constant between SHR and WKY primarily by reducing the efflux rate in the WKY. The results suggest that baseline Na^+/Ca^{2+} exchange is reduced in the SHR. Moreover, the finding of reduced Ca^{2+} influx and cellular pool size indicates a primary Ca^{2+} uptake problem in the SHR. These cellular phenomena may underlie abnormal Ca^{2+} absorption in the SHR.

A number of studies have been performed using the everted duodenal gut sac technique, which measures net active and passive transfer of radiolabeled Ca^{2+} from the mucosal to the serosal surface. Different investigators have found either no difference (96,148), decreased (135,136), or increased (148) duodenal Ca^{2+} transport in the SHR. The reason for the marked discrepancies is unclear, but Schedl et al. (173) have consistently found decreased transport in SHR obtained from three different breeders, arguing that the source of the animals is not a sufficient explanation for the conflicting results. Similarly, *in vivo* techniques for measuring duodenal radioactive Ca^{2+} transfer have indicated both increased (148) and decreased (136) absorption in the SHR.

Slightly more consistent results have been obtained from measurements of duodenal Ca^{2+} transport by the modified Using apparatus, which provides a direct measurement of active Ca^{2+} flux. With this technique, electrochemical Ca^{2+} gradients are eliminated by voltage clamping the preparation and exposing the mucosal and serosal surfaces to the same physiological concentration of nonradioactive Ca^{2+}. Using chamber measurements of mucosal-to-serosal and net fluxes across the isolated duodenum were significantly decreased in the 12- to 14-week-old SHR and in the 24-week-old SHR maintained on a low Ca^{2+} diet (142,143). On normal Ca^{2+} diets, there was no difference between SHR and WKY in unidirectional and net Ca^{2+} fluxes in older 24- (143) and 35- (174) week-old animals. However, the SHR develops renal hypercalciuria by this age, suggesting that the duodenal Ca^{2+} transport in the older SHR may be inadequate to compensate for increased urinary losses.

The basis for impaired Ca^{2+} transport in the SHR may be attributable to reduced levels of Ca^{2+} binding proteins important in the transport process. Roullet et al. (141) found that both calbindin-D9K and calmodulin are reduced in young SHR. Likewise, Cloney et al. (140) found reduced calbindin-D9K as well as reduced intestinal alkaline phosphatase, another $1,25(OH)_2$ vitamin D_3–dependent protein important in Ca^{2+} absorption. In both studies, calbindin-D9K decreased with age in the WKY, and, in the Roullet et al. (141) study, calcitriol was significantly correlated with calbindin-D9K levels. However, in the SHR, calbindin-D9K was reduced despite elevated calcitriol in one study (140) and normal calcitriol levels in the other (141). This outcome suggests

resistance of the duodenal enterocyte to $1,25(OH)_2$ vitamin D_3 in the SHR.

Several investigators have performed metabolic balance studies on the SHR and WKY in order to determine whole animal net Ca^{2+} absorption and retention. Stern et al. (96) found no difference in cumulative Ca^{2+} retention between SHR and WKY rats 6 to 10 weeks of age. Rather, their data suggest a trend for reduced cumulative Ca^{2+} absorption in the SHR. Similarly, Lau et al. (101) found reduced fractional Ca^{2+} absorption and a trend for reduced absolute Ca^{2+} absorption and retention in 10-week-old male SHR rats studied over 6 days. Bindels et al. (95) reported no difference in Ca^{2+} absorption in 6- and 8-week-old male SHR. By contrast, hyperabsorption of Ca^{2+} was found in 3-week-old prehypertensive male and female SHR (102), and in mature 25- and 50-week-old female SHR (101). Hsu et al. (122) estimated net Ca^{2+} absorption by measuring urinary Ca^{2+} excretion following an oral load of radiolabeled Ca^{2+} and found increased Ca^{2+} absorption in 13- to 16-week-old male SHR. Assuming that all of these studies purporting to measure whole animal Ca^{2+} absorption are valid, a very confusing and inconsistent picture results. Given the inherent difficulty in performing accurate balance studies in rats, it is tempting to look at other measures of cumulative Ca^{2+} balance.

Bone

Since bone is the largest store of Ca^{2+} in the body, measurement of bone Ca^{2+} content and mineralization may provide an accurate index of whole animal Ca^{2+} balance. Bone Ca^{2+} content was not different between SHR and WKY at 6 and 18 weeks of age (95,123), but was found to be significantly reduced in the SHR at 23 and 54 weeks of age (143,175). Similarly, ash weights of the femur were normal in the 6-week-old male SHR (90), but reduced in the 26-week-old male SHR (176). One study of hydralazine-treated female SHR reported increased fractional bone mass and Ca^{2+} density at 1 year of age (101).

More thorough analyses of the histomorphometric characteristics of SHR bone indicate a pattern of deficits consistent with chronic bone resorption along with a reduced structural load (177). Examination of proximal tibial metaphysis and epiphyseal growth plate and midtibial shaft of 26-week-old SHR indicated a number of deficits in the SHR including growth plate thickness, longitudinal growth rate, trabecular bone volume, trabecular thickness and number, perostal and endocortical apposition rate, and bond formation rate as well as disordered osteoclast activity (177). A similar reduction in bone volume and trabecular thickness was found in an earlier study (178). Overall, the results are consistent with chronic exposure to elevated levels of circulating PTH along with reduced structural load on the bone, perhaps because of the lower cumulative weight gain in the SHR (177).

Thus in the male SHR bone Ca^{2+} is normal in early life, but falls below WKY as the animals reach late adolescence and early adulthood. Reduced bone Ca^{2+} and mineralization in the male SHR suggests reduced Ca^{2+} retention over time mediated by decreased Ca^{2+} absorption or increased excretion.

Integrated View of Systemic Ca^{2+} Metabolism in the SHR

From the above information about systemic Ca^{2+} metabolism in experimental hypertension, it is possible to make some general statements and tentative conclusions about overall Ca^{2+} status. If nothing else, it is clear that indices of Ca^{2+} and mineral metabolism change over the life of the SHR relative to the WKY control. It appears that low ionized serum Ca^{2+} and perhaps hyperparathyroidism consistently appear early in the life of the SHR. Intestinal Ca^{2+} absorption or transport has been found to be decreased in most studies, perhaps secondary to reduced levels of Ca^{2+} binding proteins, whereas urinary Ca^{2+} excretion is not commensurately decreased. Serum $1,25(OH)_2$ vitamin D_3 is either normal or elevated in the young SHR, but falls below WKY values at approximately 12 weeks of age. Older animals (greater than 17 weeks of age) develop overt hypercalciuria, intestinal absorption fails to increase in step, and a detectable fall in bone calcification appears shortly thereafter (approximately 24 weeks of age). Given that multiple systems involved in whole animal Ca^{2+} homeostasis are altered throughout the life of the SHR, it is relevant to consider whether these are isolated phenomena or whether they play a role in the abnormally elevated blood pressure that characterizes this animal.

RELATIONSHIP BETWEEN Ca^{2+} METABOLISM AND HYPERTENSION

It has been argued that a systemic Ca^{2+} deficiency resulting from biochemical alterations in transmembrane Ca^{2+} transport in multiple systems may play a causal role in hypertension. Experimental support for this hypothesis comes from more than 70 studies that have found that oral Ca^{2+} supplementation lowers blood pressure in the SHR and other experimental models of hypertension (for a review, see 1). In humans, approximately two-thirds of Ca^{2+} supplementation studies have found a reduction in blood pressure (179–216).

To date, the most convincing evidence suggests that Ca^{2+} supplementation may lower blood pressure through a modulatory action on sympathetic nervous system activity. There are consistent reports of altered sympathetic nervous system activity associated with variations in dietary Ca^{2+}. Increased dietary Ca^{2+} reverses the increased blood pressure induced by sodium chloride while reducing circulating catecholamines. Lower circulating catecholamines are likely due to increased hypothalamic norepinephrine (NE) levels and a pursuant reduction of sympathetic nervous system outflow (217–219). Restricting dietary Ca^{2+} has the opposite effect in both normotensive and hypertensive rats (220–226).

In addition to altered sympathetic nervous system outflow, blood pressure responses to NE are modified by dietary Ca^{2+}. Pressor responses are reported to be potentiated by restricted Ca^{2+} diets and dampened by high Ca^{2+} diets. Hatton et al. (227,228) reported diminished pressor responses to exogenous NE in SHR on high Ca^{2+} diets. The reduced pressor response did not occur to angiotensin II, suggesting that it was not due to a generalized change in vascular responsiveness. Doris (229), Kageyama et al. (230–232), Baksi (221), and Peuler (233) have reported similar results with regard to NE.

The reduced responsiveness to NE may be related to altered adrenergic receptor activity. Hatton et al. (228) demonstrated that dietary Ca^{2+} specifically modulates the α-1 adrenergic receptor. Blockade of α-1 adrenergic receptors with phentolamine or prazosin eliminated the difference in blood pressure that prevailed in animals on high and low Ca^{2+} diets. Blockade of α-2, β-1, or β-2 adrenergic receptors had no such effect. Likewise, pharmacologic reduction of blood pressure with CGRP, sodium nitroprusside, or the converting enzyme inhibitor captopril had no differential effect on blood pressure. The results of this study strongly suggest that dietary Ca^{2+} modifies the α-1 adrenergic receptor. The nature of the effect remains to be determined, but there may be a difference in receptor expression or affinity. Divalent cations such as Ca^{2+} have been reported to increase the affinity of adrenergic receptors for their ligands (234).

The response of vasoactive humoral factors to Ca^{2+} supplementation is just beginning to be investigated and the early focus has been on the calciotropic hormones $1,25(OH)_2$ vitamin D_3 and PTH. In this regard it should be restated that PTH is a vasodilator at high concentrations and appears to be without effect on vascular smooth muscle at physiological concentrations (132–134). Nevertheless, the outcome of parathyroidectomies and transplantation of parathyroid glands between SHR and WKY suggests that the parathyroid gland is important in the development of hypertension in the SHR. One possible explanation for the paradoxical relation between the known actions of PTH and the apparent importance of the parathyroid gland in hypertension is a proposed parathyroid hypertensive factor described by Pang and Lewanczuk (125). This hypertensinogenic substance is responsive to dietary Ca^{2+} (235) and is reported to be elevated in human and experimental models of hypertension (236). When injected into normotensive animals, the substance causes an elevation in blood pressure with a time lag of about 60 min. Although preliminary descriptions of the molecular structure of this compound have been reported (237), the full structure of the substance has not yet been identified.

On the other hand, PTH may exert an effect on blood pressure by stimulating the synthesis and release of $1,25(OH)_2$ vitamin D_3. Receptors for $1,25(OH)_2$ vitamin D_3 are present in vascular tissue (238,239) and calcitriol has been shown to stimulate Ca^{2+}-ATPase in VSM, suggesting that $1,25(OH)_2$ vitamin D_3 may play a role in regulating cellular Ca^{2+} metabolism (240,241). Exposure to $1,25(OH)_2$ vitamin D_3 potentiates the norepinephrine-stimulated Ca^{2+} transient in intact mesenteric resistance arteries as well as isolated VSM cells (242,243). Furthermore, maximal force generation is enhanced in vessels from both hypertensive and normotensive animals injected with $1,25(OH)_2$ vitamin D_3 (244–246).

Despite evidence of direct effects on VSM, observations of elevated blood pressure as a consequence of administration of $1,25(OH)_2$ vitamin D_3 have been inconsistent. Neither Bukoski et al. (242) or Hatton et al. (246) found elevated blood pressure as a consequence of exposure to calcitriol although in both cases enhanced vascular contractility was evident in isolated vessels from animals given $1,25(OH)_2$ vitamin D_3 injections. On the other hand, Shimosawa et al. (247) did observe a potentiation of pressor responses to both NE and angiotensin II in animals treated with calcitriol or the noncalcemic analogue 22-oxacalcitriol for 14 days. With daily injections over a 28-day period, Bukoski and Xue found evidence of sustained elevations in blood pressure in normotensive Wistar rats (248). However, chronic administration of $1,25(OH)_2$ vitamin D_3 in SHR produced only a transient elevation in blood pressure after 5 weeks of treatment, suggesting a modest effect of the hormone on blood pressure (249).

Another possible explanation for the inverse relationship between Ca^{2+} regulating hormones and blood pressure is that the regulating hormones are simply a marker of reduced serum-ionized Ca^{2+} and it is the reduction in serum-ionized Ca^{2+} that is responsible for elevated blood pressure. According to this scheme, ionized Ca^{2+} could act directly on either endothelial cells or vascular smooth muscle cells to alter vascular tone. Bohr and his colleagues have most clearly delineated the potential role of extracellular Ca^{2+} on vascular smooth muscle function. Several years ago, Bohr (250) showed that increasing extracellular Ca^{2+} diminished vascular reactivity in isolated vessels through a reduction of ionic flux across the cell membrane. Since then, Bohr and coworkers (251–257) have shown that the membrane stabilizing effect of extracellular Ca^{2+} is much more pronounced in hypertension. This has led to the suggestion (256) that there is

a generalized defect or deficit in the Ca^{2+} binding protein of the plasma membrane in hypertension, and that this defect is responsible for a lack of membrane stability.

The stabilizing effect of extracellular Ca^{2+} on the vascular smooth muscle cell may be reinforced by release of EDRF (256). As outlined above, the synthesis and release of EDRF is directly dependent upon extracellular Ca^{2+} levels. Consequently, optimal release of EDRF will depend, to some extent, on maintaining adequate levels of extracellular Ca^{2+}. Assuming that serum-ionized Ca^{2+} levels are depressed in SHR, as would be indicated by elevated PTH levels, it would be predicted that EDRF release would be reduced in SHR.

Although the ultimate lesions responsible for altered Ca^{2+} metabolism in the SHR are not known, it has been proposed that there is a defect in some aspect of cellular Ca^{2+} handling that is common to all cell types including vascular smooth muscle, renal tubular cells, and intestinal epithelial cells. According to this hypothesis, both the relative Ca^{2+} deficient state and the hypertensive condition would arise from this same pancellular defect in Ca^{2+} handling. The candidates include defective Ca^{2+} binding proteins such as calmodulin, altered Ca^{2+} pump activity, and/or sodium pump activity. There is evidence of Ca^{2+}-sensitive deficits in each of these cellular components in the SHR. Porsti et al. found that potassium-induced relaxation of mesenteric arterial rings was augmented by Ca^{2+} supplementation in SHR (258). Since ouabain was able to prevent the relaxation, the difference between diet groups was attributed to increased Na-K-ATPase activity. This outcome is consistent with the notion of a reciprocal relationship between intracellular Ca^{2+} and Na-K-ATPase activity; as intracellular Ca^{2+} declines, Na-K-ATPase activity increases (259).

Porsti et al. (260) as well as Wuorela et al. (261) have observed an increase in the maximal velocity of Ca^{2+} transport by "inside-out" red blood cell vesicles from SHR on Ca^{2+} supplemented diets. The greater velocity of Ca^{2+} transport is indicative of increased Ca^{2+}-ATPase activity. Wuorela et al. (261) also reported that nitroprusside-induced relaxation of NE-contracted mesenteric arterial rings was enhanced in Ca^{2+}-supplemented animals, perhaps as a consequence of an increased ability to extrude Ca^{2+} from the cell.

The increased ability of vessels to relax following Ca^{2+} supplementation is an important finding. Previous studies of isolated vessels from Ca^{2+}-supplemented animals concentrated on maximal contractility as the measure of vascular function. Either no change or even enhanced contraction following Ca^{2+} supplementation was typically found (262–265). However, in examining relaxation, an entirely different picture emerges. Here it can more clearly be seen that Ca^{2+} supplementation has an impact on the vasculature commensurate with an *in vivo* finding of lowered blood pressure.

An impact of dietary Ca^{2+} on calmodulin may explain

these outcomes. Using duodenal enterocytes, Roullet et al. (266) have observed that calmodulin levels are lower in the SHR than in the WKY, and that increasing dietary Ca^{2+} eliminates that difference. Subsequent work indicates that dietary Ca^{2+} can actually upregulate calmodulin levels (C. Roullet, *personal communication*, 11/93). Correction of a defect in calmodulin activity by Ca^{2+} could provide a mechanism whereby a multitude of molecular and cellular processes might be modified. Calmodulin plays a pivotal role in intracellular Ca^{2+} regulation and could be responsible for diet-induced variations in Ca^{2+}-ATPase (267,268), an enzyme of critical importance to extrusion of Ca^{2+} from the cell and therefore of vasorelaxation.

While the final analysis of the contribution of distributed Ca^{2+} metabolism to the overall pathophysiology of human essential hypertension may show that it is only one of multiple factors that give rise to elevated blood pressure in the human, continued research should be conducted in this area to critically test the hypothesis.

REFERENCES

1. Hatton DC, McCarron. Dietary calcium and blood pressure in experimental models of hypertension: a review. *Hypertension* (In press).
2. Kurtz TW, Morris RC. Biological variability in Wistar-Kyoto rats: implications for research with the spontaneously hypertensive rat. *Hypertension* 1987;10:127–131.
3. St Lezin E, Simonet L, Pravenec M, Kurtz TW. Hypertensive strains and normotensive 'control' strains. How closely are they related? *Hypertension* 1992;19:419–424.
4. Pernot F, Schleiffer R, Berthelot A, Vincent M, Sassard J, Gairard A. Parathyroidectomy and development of genetic hypertension in the Lyon rat strain. *Clin Exp Hypertens* 1986;A8:133–134.
5. Schleiffer R, Pernot F, Gairard A. Parathyroidectomy, cardiovascular reactivity and calcium distribution in aorta and heart of spontaneously hypertensive rats. *Clin Sci* 1986;71:505–511.
6. Gairard A, Berthelot A, Schleiffer R, Pernot F. Parathyroidectomy significantly decreases hypertension in spontaneously hypertensive and deoxycorticosteroid-saline treated rats. *Can J Physiol Pharmacol* 1981;60:208–212.
7. Folkow B. Physiological aspects of primary hypertension. *Physiol Rev* 1982;62:347–504.
8. Folkow B, Hallback M, Jones JV, Sutter M. Dependence on external calcium for the noradrenaline contractility of the resistance vessels in spontaneously hypertensive and renal hypertensive rats as compared to normotensive controls. *Acta Physiol Scand* 1977;101:84–97.
9. Hatton DC, Buchholz RA, Fitzgerald RD. Autonomic control of heart rate and blood pressure in SHR during aversive classical conditioning. *Comp Physiol Psych* 1981;95:978–990.
10. Bohr DF, Webb RC. Vascular smooth muscle membrane in hypertension. *Annu Rev Pharmacol Toxicol* 1988;28:389–409.
11. Bhalla RC, Webb RC, Ashley T, Brock T. Calcium fluxes, calcium binding and adenosine 3′,5′-monophosphate dependent protein kinase activity in aorta of spontaneously hypertensive and Wistar normotensive rats. *Mol Pharmacol* 1978;14:468–477.
12. Kwan CY, Belbeck L, Daniel EE. Abnormal biochemistry of vascular smooth muscle plasma membranes isolated from hypertensive rats. *Mol Pharmacol* 1980;77:137–140.
13. Bukoski RD, McCarron DA. Calcium and hypertension. In: Baker PF, ed. *Handbook of experimental pharmacology.* Berlin: Springer-Verlag; 1988.
14. Rasmussen H, Takuwa Y, Park S. Protein kinase C in the regula-

tion of vascular smooth muscle contraction. *FASEB J* 1987;1: 177–185.
15. Rembold CM, Murphy RA. Myoplasmic calcium, myosin phosphorylation, and regulation of the crossbridge cycle in swine arterial smooth muscle. *Circ Res* 1986;58:803–815.
16. Berridge MJ. Inositol triphosphate and calcium mobilization. *J Cardiovasc Pharmacol* 1986;8(Suppl 8):S85–S90.
17. Somlyo AV, Bond M, Somlyo AP, Scarpa A. Inositol trisphosphate–induced calcium release and contraction in vascular smooth muscle. *Proc Natl Acad Sci USA* 1985;82:5231–5235.
18. Yamamoto H, van Breemen C. Inositol-1,4,5-trisphosphate releases calcium from skinned cultured smooth muscle cells. *Biochem Biophys Res Commun* 1985;130:270–274.
19. Kahn AM, Shelat H, Allen JC. Na^+-H^+ exchange is present in sarcolemmal vesicles from dog superior mesenteric artery. *Am J Physiol* 1986;250:H313–H319.
20. Williamson JR. Inositol lipid metabolism and intracellular signalling mechanisms. *News Physiol Sci* 1986;1:72–76.
21. Rozengurt E, Mendoza SA. Early stimulation of Na^+-H^+ antiport, Na^+-K^+ pump activity and Ca^{2+} fluxes in fibroblast mitogenesis. *Curr Topics Membr Trans* 1986;27:163–191.
22. Kageyama Y, Suzuki H, Hayashi K, Saruta T. Effects of calcium loading on blood pressure in spontaneously hypertensive rats: attenuation of vascular reactivity. *Clin Exp Hypertens* 1986;A8: 355–370.
23. Cauvin C, Hwang BS, Yamamoto M, van Breemen C. Effects of dihydropyridines on tension and calcium-45 influx in isolated mesenteric resistance vessels from spontaneously hypertensive and normotensive rats. *Am J Cardiol* 1987;59:116B–122B.
24. Bean BP, Sturek M, Puga A, Hermsmeyer K. Calcium channels in muscle cells isolated from rat mesenteric arteries. Modulation by dihydropyridine drugs. *Circ Res* 1986;59:229–235.
25. Sturek M, Hermsmeyer K. Calcium and sodium channels in spontaneously contracting vascular muscle cells. *Science* 1986;233:475–478.
26. Morgan JP, Morgan KG. Alterations of cytoplasmic calcium levels in smooth muscle by vasodilators in the ferret. *J Physiol (Lond)* 1980;57:539–551.
27. Defeo TT, Morgan KG. Calcium-force relationships as detected with aequorin in two different vascular smooth muscles of the ferret. *J Physiol (Lond)* 1985;369:269–282.
28. Sugiyama T, Yoshizumi M, Takaku F, et al. The elevation of the cytosolic ions in vascular smooth muscle cells in SHR: measurement of the free calcium ions in single living cells by laser microfluorospectrometry. *Biochem Biophys Res Commun* 1986; 141:340–345.
29. Bukoski RD, DeWan P, McCarron DA. Intracellular Ca^{2+} in cultured aortic myocytes and mesenteric resistance vessels of spontaneously hypertensive and Wistar-Kyoto rats. *FASEB J* 1988;2: A503.
30. Nabika T, Velletri PA, Beaven MA, Endo J, Lovenberg W. Vasopressin-induced calcium increased in smooth muscle cells from spontaneously hypertensive rats. *Life Sci* 1985;37:579–584.
31. Chiesi M, Gasser J, Carafoli E. Properties of the Ca-pumping ATPase of sarcoplasmic reticulum from vascular smooth muscle. *Biochem Biophys Res Commun* 1984;124:797–805.
32. Eggermont JA, Vrolix M, Raeymaekers L, Wuytaek F, Casteels R. Ca^{2+} transport ATPase of vascular smooth muscle. *Circ Res* 1988;62:266–278.
33. Furukawa K, Nakamura H. Characterization of the [Ca^{2+}, Mg^{2+}]-ATPase purified by calmodulin-affinity chromatography from bovine aortic smooth muscle. *J Biochem* 1984;96:1343–1350.
34. Sumida M, Okuda H, Hamada M. Ca^{2+}, Mg^{2+}-ATPase of microsomal membranes from bovine aortic smooth muscle. Identification and characterization of an acid-stable phosphorylated intermediate of the Ca^{2+}, Mg^{2+}-ATPase. *J Biochem* 1984;96:1365–1374.
35. Aoki K, Yamashita Y, Tomita N, Tazumi K, Hotta K. ATPase activity and Ca binding ability of subcellular membranes of arterial smooth muscle in spontaneously hypertensive rat. *Jap Heart J* 1974;15:180–181.
36. Shibata S, Kochii M, Taniguchi T. Calcium fluxes and binding in the aortic smooth muscle from the spontaneously hypertensive rat. *Blood Vessels* 1975;12:279–289.

37. Webb RC, Bhalla RC. Altered calcium sequestration by subcellular fractions of vascular smooth muscle from spontaneously hypertensive rats. *J Mol Cell Cardiol* 1976;8:651–661.

38. Blaustein MP. Sodium ions, calcium ions, blood pressure regulation and hypertension: a reassessment and hypothesis. *Am J Physiol* 1977;232:C165–C173.

39. Smith JB, Smith L. Extracellular Na$^+$ dependence of changes in free Ca^{2+}, ^{45}Ca^{2+} efflux, and total cell Ca^{2+} produced by angiotensin II in cultured arterial muscle cells. *J Biol Chem* 1987;262:17455–17460.

40. Ashida T, Blaustein MP. Regulation of cell calcium and contractility in mammalian arterial smooth muscle: the role of sodium-calcium exchange. *J Physiol* 1987;392:617–635.

41. Matlib MA, Schwartz A, Yamori Y. A Na$^+$-Ca^{2+} exchange process in isolated sarcolemmal membranes of mesenteric arteries from WKY and SHR rats. *Am J Physiol* 1985;249:C166–C172.

42. Nabel EG, Berk BC, Brock TA, Smith TW. Na$^+$-Ca^{2+} exchange in cultured vascular smooth muscle cells. *Circ Res* 1988;62:486–493.

43. Himmel HM, Whorton AR, Strauss HC. Intracellular calcium, currents, and stimulus-response coupling in endothelial cells. *Hypertension* 1993;21:112–127.

44. Flavahan NA, Vanhoutte PM. G-proteins and endothelial responses. *Blood Vessels* 1990;27:218–229.

45. Fain JN, Wallace MA, Wojcikiewicz RJH. Evidence for involvement of guanine nucleotide-binding regulatory proteins in the activation of phospholipases by hormones. *FASEB J* 1988;2:2569–2574.

46. Buchan KW, Martin W. Bradykinin induces elevations of cytosolic calcium through mobilization of intracellular and extracellular pools in bovine aortic endothelial cells. *Br J Pharmacol* 1991;102:35–40.

47. Jaffe EA, Grulich J, Weksler BB, Hampel G, Watanabe K. Correlation between thrombin-induced prostacyclin production and inositol trisphosphate and cytosolic free calcium levels in cultured human endothelial cells. *J Biol Chem* 1987;262:8557–8565.

48. Dolor RJ, Hurwitz LM, Mirza Z, Strauss HC, Whorton AR. Regulation of extracellular calcium entry in endothelial cells: role of the intracellular calcium pool. *Am J Physiol* 1992;262:C171–C181.

49. Lopez-Jaramillo P, Gonzalez MC, Palmer RMJ, Moncada S. The crucial role of physiological Ca^{2+} concentrations in the production of endothelial nitric oxide and the control of vascular tone. *Br J Pharmacol* 1990;101:489–493.

50. Bevan JA, Joyce EH. Calcium dependence of flow-induced dilation. Cooperative interaction with sodium. *Hypertension* 1993;21:16–21.

51. Schilling WP, Cabello OA, Rajan L. Depletion of the inositol 1,4,5-triphosphate-sensitive intracellular Ca^{2+} store in vascular endothelial cells activates the agonist-sensitive Ca^{2+}-influx pathway. *Biochem J* 1992;284:521–530.

52. Schilling WP. Effect of membrane potential on cytosolic calcium of bovine aortic endothelial cells. *Am J Physiol* 1989;257:H778–H784.

53. Lückhoff A, Busse R. Calcium influx into endothelial cells and formation of endothelium-derived relaxing factor is controlled by the membrane potential. *Pfluegers Arch* 1990;416:305–311.

54. Busse R, Fichtner H, Lückhoff A, Kohlhardt M. Hyperpolarization and increased free calcium in acetylcholine-stimulated endothelial cells. *Am J Physiol* 1988;255:H965–H969.

55. Busse R, Mulsch A. Calcium-dependent nitric oxide synthesis in endothelial cytosol is mediated by calmodulin. *FEBS Lett* 1990;265:133–136.

56. Shen J, Luscinskas FW, Connolly A, Dewey CF, Gimbrone MA. Fluid shear stress modulates cytosolic free calcium in vascular endothelial cells. *Am J Physiol* 1992;262:C384–C390.

57. Schleiffer R, Xue H, McCarron D, Bukoski R. Effect of chronic subacute parathyroidectomy on blood pressure and resistance artery contractility in the spontaneously hypertensive rat. *J Hypertens* 1993;11:709–716.

58. McCarron DA. Calcium metabolism and hypertension. *Kidney Int* 1989;35:717–736.

59. Orlov SN, Pokudin NI, Postnov YV. Calcium transport in erythrocytes of rats with spontaneous hypertension. *J Hypertens* 1986;6:829–837.

60. Oshima T, Young EW, Hermsmeyer K, McCarron DA. Modification of platelet and lymphocyte calcium handling and blood pressure by dietary sodium and calcium in genetically hypertensive rats. *J Lab Clin Med* 1992;119:151–158.

61. Oshima T, Young EW, McCarron DA. Abnormal platelet and lymphocyte calcium handling in prehypertensive rats. *Hypertension* 1991;18:111–115.

62. Bruschi G, Bruschi ME, Caroppo M, Orlando G, Pavarani C, Cavatorta A. Intracellular free [Ca^{2+}] in circulating lymphocytes of spontaneously hypertensive rats. *Life Sci* 1984;35:535–542.

63. Allen JC, Bukoski RD. Current status of vascular smooth muscle subcellular calcium regulation. In: Crass ML, Barnes PT, eds. *Vascular smooth muscle: metabolic, ionic and contractile mechanisms.* New York: Academic Press; 1982:99–134.

64. Owens GK, Schwartz SM. Alterations in vascular smooth muscle mass in the spontaneously hypertensive rat. Role of cellular hypertrophy, hyperplasty and hyperplasia. *Circ Res* 1982;51:280–289.

65. Mulvany MJ. Do resistance vessel abnormalities contribute to the elevated blood pressure of spontaneously hypertensive rats? *Blood Vessels* 1983;20:1–22.

66. Bukoski RD, Xue H, McCarron DA. Effect of 1,25(OH)$_2$ vitamin D$_3$ and ionized Ca^{2+} on ^{45}Ca uptake by primary cultures of aortic myocytes of spontaneously hypertensive and Wistar Kyoto normotensive rats. *Biochem Biophys Res Commun* 1987;146:1330–1335.

67. Jones AW. Content and fluxes of electrolytes. In: Bohr D, Somlyo AP, Sparks HV, eds. *Handbook of physiology: the cardiovascular system. vol II. vascular smooth muscle.* Bethesda: American Physiological Society; 1980:253–299.

68. Bukoski RD. Intracellular Ca^{2+} metabolism of isolated resistance arteries and cultured vascular myocytes of spontaneously hypertensive and Wistar-Kyoto normotensive rats. *J Hypertens* 1990;8:37–43.

69. Storm DS, Stuenkel EL, Webb RC. Calcium channel activation in arterioles from genetically hypertensive rats. *Hypertension* 1992;20:380–388.

70. Bruner CA, Webb RC. Increased vascular reactivity to Bay K 8644 in genetic hypertension. *Pharmacology* 1990;41:24–35.

71. Asano M, Aoki K, Matsuda T. Contractile effects of Bay K 8644, a dihydropyridine calcium agonist, on isolated femoral arteries from spontaneously hypertensive rats. *J Pharmacol Exp Ther* 1986;239:198–205.

72. Sada T, Koike H, Ikeda M, Sato K, Ozaki H, Karaki H. Cytosolic free calcium of aorta in hypertensive rats: chronic inhibition of angiotensin converting inhibitor. *Hypertension* 1990;16:245–251.

73. Papageorgiou P, Morgan KG. Intracellular free Ca^{2+} is elevated in hypertrophic aortic muscle from hypertensive rats. *Am J Physiol* 1991;260:H507–H515.

74. Chilian WM. Distribution of vascular resistance in the coronary microcirculation. In: Halpern W, et al., eds. *Second international symposium on resistance arteries.* Ithaca, NY: Perinatology Press; 1988:34–40.

75. Fronek K, Zweifach BW. Microvascular pressure distribution in skeletal muscle and the effect of vasodilation. *Am J Physiol* 1975;228:791–796.

76. Shapiro HM, Stromberg DD, Lee DR, Wiederhielm CA. Dynamic pressures in the pial artery microcirculation. *Am J Physiol* 1971;221:279–283.

77. Mulvany MJ, Halpern W. Contractile properties of small arterial resistance vessels in spontaneously hypertensive and normotensive rats. *Circ Res* 1977;41:19–26.

78. Mulvany MJ, Aalkjaer C, Christensen J. Changes in noradrenaline sensitivity and morphology of arterial resistance vessels during development of high blood pressure in spontaneously hypertensive rats. *Hypertension* 1980;2:664–671.

79. Whall CW, Myers MM, Halpern W. Norepinephrine sensitivity, tension development and neuronal uptake in resistance arteries from spontaneously hypertensive and normotensive rats. *Blood Vessels* 1980;17:1–15.

80. Webb RC, Vanhoutte P. Sensitivity to noradrenaline in isolated tail arteries from spontaneously hypertensive rats. *Clin Sci* 1979;57:315–335.

81. Falloon BJ, Bund SJ, Tulip JR, Heagerty AM. In vitro perfusion studies of resistance artery function in genetic hypertension. *Hypertension* 1993;22:486–495.

82. Lüscher TF, Vanhoutte PM. Endothelium-dependent contractions to acetylcholine in the aorta of the spontaneously hypertensive rat. *Hypertension* 1986;8:344–348.

83. Tesfamaraiam B, Halpern W. Endothelium-dependent and endothelium-independent vasodilation in resistance arteries from hypertensive rats. *Hypertension* 1988;11:440–444.

84. Lüscher TF, Aarhus LL, Vanhoutte PM. Indomethacin improves the impaired endothelium-dependent relaxations in small mesenteric arteries of the spontaneously hypertensive rat. *Am J Hypertens* 1990;3:55–58.

85. Li J, Bukoski RD. Endothelium-dependent relaxation of hypertensive resistance arteries is not impaired under all conditions. *Circ Res* 1993;72:290–296.

86. Mulvany MJ, Korsgaard N, Nyborg N. Evidence that the increased calcium sensitivity of resistance vessels in spontaneously hypertensive rats is an intrinsic defect of their vascular smooth muscle. *Clin Exp Hypertens* 1981;3:749–761.

87. Mulvany MJ, Nyborg N. An increased calcium sensitivity of mesenteric resistance vessels in young and adult spontaneously hypertensive rats. *Br J Pharmacol* 1980;71:585–596.

88. Aalkjaer C, Heagerty AM, Petersen KK, Swales JD, Mulvany MJ. Evidence for increased media thickness, increased neuronal uptake, and depressed excitation-contraction coupling in isolated resistance vessels from essential hypertensives. *Circ Res* 1987;61:181–186.

89. De Mey JG, Boonen HCM, Struyker-Boudier HAJ. Rhythmic contractile activity in resistance-sized arteries of spontaneously hypertensive rats. In: Halpern W, et al., eds. *Second international symposium on resistance arteries.* Ithaca, NY: Perinatology Press; 1988:336–341.

90. Meyers JH, Lamb FS, Webb RC. Norepinephrine-induced phasic activity in tail arteries from genetically hypertensive rats. *Am J Physiol* 1985;248:H419–H423.

91. Bruner CA, Meyers JH, Sing CF, Jokelainen PT, Webb RC. Genetic association of hypertension and vascular changes in stroke-prone spontaneously hypertensive rats. *Hypertension* 1986;8:904–910.

92. Owens GK, Schwartz SM, McCanna M. Evaluation of medial hypertrophy in resistance vessels of spontaneously hypertensive rats. *Hypertension* 1988;11:198–207.

93. Owens GK, Reidy MA. Hyperplastic growth response of vascular smooth muscle cells following induction of acute hypertension in rats by aortic coarctation. *Circ Res* 1985;57:695–705.

94. Kanbe T, Nara Y, Tagami M, Yamuri Y. Studies of hypertension-induced vascular hypertrophy in cultured smooth muscle cells from spontaneously hypertensive rats. *Hypertension* 1983;5:887–892.

95. Bindels RJM, van den Broek LAM, Jongen MJM, Hackeng WHL, Lowik CWGM, van Os CH. Increased plasma calcitonin levels in young spontaneously hypertensive rats: role in disturbed phosphate homeostasis. *Pfluegers Arch* 1987;408:395–400.

96. Stern N, Lee DBN, Silis V, et al. Effects of high calcium intake on blood pressure and calcium metabolism in young SHR. *Hypertension* 1984;6:639–646.

97. McCarron D, Yung NN, Ugoretz BA, Krutzik S. Disturbances of calcium metabolism in the spontaneously hypertensive rat: attenuation of hypertension by calcium supplementation. *Hypertension* 1981;43:I162–I167.

98. Wright GL, Torasson MA, Barbe JS, Crouse W. The concentrations of ionic and total calcium in plasma of the spontaneously hypertensive rat. *Can J Physiol Pharmacol* 1980;58:1494–1499.

99. DiPette DJ, Christenson W, Nickols MA, Nickols GA. Cardiovascular responsiveness to parathyroid hormone (PTH) and PTH-related protein in genetic hypertension. *Endocrinology* 1992;130:2045–2051.

100. Wright GL, Rankin GO. Concentrations of ionic and total calcium in plasma of four models of hypertension. *Am J Physiol* 1982;243:H365–H370.

101. Lau K, Chen S, Eby B. Evidence for an intestinal mechanism in hypercalciuria of the spontaneously hypertensive rat. *Am J Physiol* 1984;247:E625–E633.

102. Lau K, Langman CB, Gafter U, Dudeja PK, Brasitus TA. Increased calcium absorption in prehypertensive spontaneously hypertensive rat. *J Clin Invest* 1986;78:1803–1090.

103. Folsom AR, Smith CL, Prineas RJ, Grim RH. Serum calcium fractions in essential hypertension and matched normotensive controls. *Hypertension* 1986;8:11–15.

104. McCarron DA. Low serum concentrations of ionized calcium in patients with hypertension. *N Engl J Med* 1982;307:226–228.

105. Resnick LM, Laragh JH, Sealey JE, Alderman MH. Divalent cations in essential hypertension: relation between serum ionized calcium, magnesium, and plasma renin activity. *N Engl J Med* 1983;309:888–891.

106. Resnick LM, Laragh JH. Calcium metabolism and parathyroid function in primary aldosteronism. *Am J Med* 1986;78:385–390.

107. Young EW, Hsu CH, Patel S, Simpson RU, Konanicky P. Metabolic degradation and synthesis of calcitriol in the spontaneously hypertensive rat. *Am J Physiol* 1987;252:E778–E782.

108. Pang PKT, Harvey S, Doris PA. Plasma parathyroid hormone during the development of spontaneous hypertension in rats. *Can J Physiol Pharmacol* 1987;65:2386–2414.

109. Merke J, Slotkowski A, Mann H, Lucas PH, Drüeke T, Ritz E. Abnormal 1,25(OH)$_2$D$_3$ receptor status in genetically hypertensive rats. *Kidney Int* 1987;31:303.

110. McCarron D, Pingree PA, Rubin RJ. Enhanced parathyroid function in essential hypertension: a homeostatic response to a urinary calcium leak. *Hypertension* 1980;2:162–168.

111. Strazzullo P, Nunziata V, Cirillo M. Abnormalities of calcium metabolism in essential hypertension. *Clin Sci* 1983;65:137.

112. Grobbee DE, Hofman A. Effect of calcium supplementation on diastolic blood pressure in young people with mild hypertension. *Lancet* 1986;2:703–707.

113. Brickman AS, Nyby MD, von Hungen K, Eggena P, Tuck ML. Calcitropic hormones, platelet calcium, and blood pressure in essential hypertension. *Hypertension* 1990;16:515–522.

114. Reichel H, Liebethal R, Hense HW, Schmidt-Gayk H, Ritze E. Disturbed calcium metabolism in subjects with elevated diastolic blood pressure. *Clin Invest* 1992;70:748–751.

115. Papagalanis N, Kourti A, Tolis A, et al. Effect of intravenous calcium infusion on indices of activity of the parathyroid glands and on urinary calcium and sodium excretion in normotensive and hypertensive subjects. *Am J Hypertens* 1993;6:59–65.

116. Grobbee DE, Hackeng WHL, Birkenhäger, Hofman A. Raised plasma intact parathyroid hormone concentrations in young people with mildly raised blood pressure. *Br Med J* 1988;296:814–816.

117. Van Overloop B, Treisser A, Coumaros G, Schleiffer R, Gairard A. Decreased ionized calcium and increased parathyroid hormone in the serum of mild gestational hypertensive patients at the third trimester: a link between calcium metabolism and hypertension in pregnancy. *Clin Exp Hypertens Preg* 1992;B11(2 & 3):233–247.

118. Van Hooft IMS, Grobbee DE, Frölich M, Pols HAP, Hofman A. Alterations in calcium metabolism in young people at risk for primary hypertension. The Dutch Hypertension and Offspring Study. *Hypertension* 1993;21:267–272.

119. Raine AEG, Bedford L, Simpson AWM, et al. Hyperparathyroidism, platelet intracellular free calcium and hypertension in chronic renal failure. *Kidney Int* 1993;43:700–705.

120. Duprez D, Bauwens F, de Buyzere M, et al. Relationship between parathyroid hormone and left ventricular mass in moderate essential hypertension. *J Hypertens* 1991;9(Suppl 6):S116–S117.

121. McCarron DA. Impaired nephrogenous cAMP response in the spontaneously hypertensive rat. *Kidney Int* 1983;23:106.

122. Hsu CH, Chen PS, Smith DE, Yang CS. Pathogenesis of hypercalciuria in spontaneously hypertensive rats. *Miner Electrolyte Metab* 1986;12:130–141.

123. McCarron DA, Shneidman RJ, Lee DM. Ca^{2+} defects in experimental hypertension: SHR's renal response to chronic infusion of human PTH (1-34). *Kidney Int* 1987;32:S249–S253.

124. Hsu CH, Patel S, Young EW. Calcemic response to parathyroid

hormone in spontaneously hypertensive rats: role of calcitriol. *J Lab Clin Med* 1987;110:682–689.

125. Pang PKT, Lewanczuk RZ. Parathyroid origin of a new circulating hypertensive factor in spontaneously hypertensive rats. *Am J Hypertens* 1989;2:898–902.

126. Mann JFE, Wiecek A, Bommer J, Ganten U, Ritz E. Effects of parathyroidectomy on blood pressure in spontaneously hypertensive rats. *Nephron* 1987;45:46–52.

127. Kazda S, Garthoff B, Hirth C, Preis W, Stasch J. Parathyroidectomy mimics the protective effect of calcium antagonist nimodipine in salt loaded stroke-prone hypertensive rats. *J Hypertens* 1986;4(Suppl 3):S483–S485.

128. Neuser D, Schulte-Brinkman R, Kazda S. Development of hypertension in WKY rats after transplantation of parathyroid glands from SHR/SP. *J Cardiovasc Pharmacol* 1990;6:971–974.

129. Neuser D, Schulte-Brinkman R, Kazda S. Influence of transplantation of parathyroid glands on blood pressure development in stroke prone spontaneously hypertensive rats and in normotensive Wistar Kyoto rats. *Clin Exp Hypertens Theory Prac* 1991;A13(3):325–338.

130. Pernot F, Schleiffer R, Vincent M, Sassard J, Gairard A. Parathyroidectomy in the Lyon hypertensive rat: cardiovascular reactivity and aortic responsiveness. *J Hypertens* 1990;8:1111–1117.

131. Schleiffer R, Gairard A. Influence of parathyroidectomy on aortic responsiveness to noradrenaline in spontaneously hypertensive rats. *Arch Int Pharmacodyn Ther* 1988;292:189–202.

132. Pang PKT, Tenner TE, Yee JA, Yang M, Janssen HF. Hypotensive action of parathyroid hormones preparations on rats and dogs. *Proc Natl Acad Sci (USA)* 1980;77:675–678.

133. Nickols GA. Increased cAMP in cultured vascular smooth muscle cells and relaxation of aortic strips by parathyroid hormone. *Eur J Pharmacol* 1985;116:137–144.

134. Schleiffer R, Helwig JJ, Pernot F, Gairard A. Vascular effects of calcitonin and parathyroid hormone. In: Doepfner W, ed. *Calcitonin—1984.* Amsterdam: Excerpta Medica; 1985:15–24.

135. Schedl HP, Miller DL, Pape JM, Horst RL, Wilson HD. Calcium and sodium transport and vitamin D metabolism in the spontaneously hypertensive rat. *J Clin Invest* 1984;73:980–986.

136. McCarron DA, Lucas PA, Schneidman RJ, Drüeke T. Blood pressure development of the spontaneously hypertensive rat after concurrent manipulations of Ca^{2+} and Na^{+}: relation to intestinal fluxes. *J Clin Invest* 1985;76:1147–1154.

137. Kawashima H. Altered vitamin D metabolism in the kidney of the spontaneously hypertensive rat. *Biochem J* 1986;237:893–897.

138. Roullet C, Drüeke T, Lacour B, McCarron D. Ca^{2+} influx of isolated enterocytes in adult SHRs and WKYs. *Circulation* 1986;74:331.

139. Drüeke T, Lucas PA, Bourgouin P, et al. Changes in calcitriol status and related parameters in the young hypertensive rat. *Kidney Int* 1988;33:294.

140. Cloney DL, Gray RW, Bruns ME, et al. Intestinal vitamin D-dependent calbindin-D_{9k} and alkaline phosphatase in spontaneously hypertensive rats. *Am J Physiol* 1991;260:G691–G697.

141. Roullet CM, Roullet JB, Duchambon P, et al. Abnormal intestinal regulation of calbindin-D9K and calmodulin by dietary calcium in genetic hypertension. *Am J Physiol* 1991;261:F474–F480.

142. Schedl HP, Miller DL, Horst RL, Wilson HD, Natarajan K, Conway T. Intestinal calcium transport in the spontaneously hypertensive rat: response to calcium depletion. *Am J Physiol* 1986;250:G412–G419.

143. Lucas PA, Brown RC, Drüeke T, Lacour B, Metz JA, McCarron DA. Abnormal vitamin D metabolism, intestinal calcium transport, and bone calcium status in the spontaneously hypertensive rat compared with its genetic control. *J Clin Invest* 1986;78:221–227.

144. Young EW, Patel SR, Hsu CH. Plasma 1,25-$(OH)_2$ vitamin D_3 response to parathyroid hormone, cyclic AMP, and phosphorus depletion in the spontaneously hypertensive rat. *J Lab Clin Med* 1986;6:562–566.

145. Kurtz TW, Portale AA, Morris RC. Evidence for a difference in vitamin D metabolism between spontaneously hypertensive and Wistar-Kyoto rats. *Hypertension* 1986;8:1015–1020.

146. Hsu CH, Chen PS, Caldwell RM. Renal phosphate excretion in spontaneously hypertensive and Wistar Kyoto rats. *Kidney Int* 1984;25:789–795.

147. Hsu CH, Yang CS, Patel SR, Stevens MG. Calcium and vitamin D metabolism in spontaneously hypertensive rats. *Am J Physiol* 1987;253:F712–F718.

148. Toraason MA, Wright GL. Transport of calcium by duodenum of spontaneously hypertensive rat. *Am J Physiol* 1981;241:G344–G347.

149. Gafter U, Eby B, Martin C, Lau K. Response of spontaneously hypertensive rats to 1,25$(OH)_2D_3$ in vivo. *Kidney Int* 1986;30:497–502.

150. Patel S, Hsu C. Calcitriol synthesis is decreased in spontaneously hypertensive rats. *Kidney Int* 1988;33:304.

151. DiPette DJ, Westlund KN, Holland OB. Dietary calcium modulates spinal cord content of calcitonin gene-related peptide in the rat. *Neurosci Lett* 1988;95:335–340.

152. Okimura Y, Chihara K, Abe H, et al. Calcitonin gene-related peptide-like immunoreactivity in the central nervous system and peripheral organs of rats. *Regul Pept* 1987;17:327–337.

153. Gardiner SM, Compton AM, Bennett T. Regional hemodynamic effects of calcitonin gene-related peptide. *Am J Physiol* 1989;256:R332–R338.

154. DiPette DJ, Schwarzenberger K, Kerr N, Holland OB. Systemic and regional hemodynamic effects of calcitonin gene-related peptide. *Hypertension* 1987;9(Suppl III):III142–III146.

155. Vallejo M, Lightman S, Marshall I. Central cardiovascular effects of calcitonin gene-related peptide: interaction with noradrenaline in the nucleus tractus solitarius of rats. *Exp Brain Res* 1988;70:221–224.

156. Brown MR, Gray TS. Peptide injections into the amygdala of conscious rats: effects on blood pressure, heart rate and plasma catecholamines. *Regul Pept* 1988;21:95–106.

157. Rochford J, Yashpal K, Henry JL. Intrathecal administration of calcitonin gene-related peptide (CGRP) increases heart rate and decreases arterial pressure in the urethane anesthetized rat. *Brain Res Bull* 1990;25:809–816.

158. Xu D, Wang X, Wang J-P, et al. Calcitonin gene-related peptide (CGRP) in normotensive and spontaneously hypertensive rats. *Peptides* 1989;10:309–312.

159. Ayachi S. Increased dietary calcium lowers blood pressure in the spontaneously hypertensive rat. *Metabolism* 1979;28:1234–1238.

160. Grady JR, Dorow J, McCarron DA. Urinary calcium excretion and cAMP response of the spontaneously hypertensive rat to Ca^{2+} deprivation. *Clin Res* 1983;31:330A.

161. Scoggins BA. Hypertension: role of the hypothalamic-pituitary-adrenal axis. *News Physiol Sci* 1987;2:132–135.

162. Coe FL, Favus MJ. Disorders of stone formation. In: Brenner BM, Rector FC, eds. *The kidney.* 3rd ed. Philadelphia, W. B. Saunders; 1986:1403–1422.

163. Cirillo M, Galletti F, Corrado MF, Strazzullo P. Disturbances of renal and erythrocyte calcium handling in the Milan hypertensive strain. *J Hypertens* 1986;4:443–449.

164. Bianchi G, Ferrari P, Salvati P, et al. A renal abnormality in the Milan hypertensive strain of rats and in humans predisposed to essential hypertension. *J Hypertens* 1986;4:533–536.

165. Umenura S, Smyth DD, Nicar M, Rapp JP, Pettinger WA. Altered calcium homeostasis in Dahl hypertensive rats: physiological and biochemical studies. *J Hypertens* 1986;4:19–26.

166. Kurtz TW, Morris RC. Dietary chloride as a determinant of disordered calcium metabolism in salt-dependent hypertension. *Life Sci* 1985;36:921–929.

167. McCarron DA, Morris CD. Blood pressure response to oral calcium in persons with mild to moderate hypertension. *Ann Intern Med* 1985;103:825–831.

168. Young EW, Morris CD, McCarron DA. Urinary calcium excretion in essential hypertension. *J Lab Clin Med* 1992;120:624–632.

169. Zoccali C, Mallamaci F, Postorino M, et al. Hyperfiltration and calcium metabolism in essential hypertension. *Am J Hypertens* 1991;4:944–950.

170. Luft FC, Zemel MB, Sowers JA, Fineberg NS, Weinberger MH. Sodium bicarbonate and sodium chloride: effects on blood pres-

sure and electrolyte homeostasis in normal and hypertensive man. *J Hypertens* 1990;8:663–670.

171. Pan WH, Tseng WP, You FJ, Tai Y, Chou J. Positive relationship between urinary sodium chloride and blood pressure in Chinese health examinees and its association with calcium excretion. *J Hypertens* 1990;8:873–878.

172. McCarron DA, Lucas P, Lacour B, Drüeke T. Ca^{2+} efflux rate constant in isolated SHR enterocytes. *Kidney Int* 1986;29:252.

173. Schedl HP, Wilson HD, Reeves CP. Duodenal Ca transport is lower in the spontaneously hypertensive (SH) than the Wistar-Kyoto (WKY) control rat independently of breeder. *Clin Res* 1987;35:893A.

174. Gafter U, Kathpalia S, Zikos D, Lau K. Ca fluxes across duodenum and colon of spontaneously hypertensive rats: effect of 1,25(OH)$_2$D$_3$. *Am J Physiol* 1986;251:F278–F282.

175. Metz JA, Karanja N, McCarron DA. Bone mineral density in spontaneous hypertension: differential effects of dietary calcium and sodium. *Am J Med Sci* 1990;300:225–230.

176. Izawa Y, Sagara K, Kadota T, Makita T. Bone disorders in spontaneously hypertensive rat. *Calcif Tissue Int* 1985;37:605–607.

177. Wang T, Hsu J, Jee WS, Matthews JL. Evidence for reduced cancellous bone mass in the spontaneously hypertensive rat. *Bone Miner* 1993;20:251–264.

178. Yamori Y, Fukuda S, Tsuchikura S, Ikeda K, Nara Y, Horie R. Stroke-prone SHR (SHRSP) as a model for osteoporosis. *Clin Exper Hypertens Theory Prac* 1991;A13(5):755–762.

179. Belizan JM, Villar J, Pineda O, et al. Reduction of blood pressure with calcium supplementation in young adults. *JAMA* 1983;249:1161–1166.

180. Luft FC, Aronoff GR, Sloan RS, Fineberg NS, Weinberger MH. Short-term augmented calcium intake has no effect on sodium homeostasis. *Clin Pharmacol Ther* 1986;39:414–419.

181. Tabuchi Y, Ogihara T, Hashizume K, Saito H, Kumahara Y. Hypotensive effect of long-term oral calcium supplementation in elderly patients with essential hypertension. *J Clin Hypertens* 1986;3:254–262.

182. Lyle RM, Melby CL, Hyner GC, Edmondson JW, Miller JZ, Weinberger MH. Blood pressure and metabolic effects of calcium supplementation in normotensive white and black men. *JAMA* 1987;257:1772–1776.

183. Lasaridis AN, Kaisis CN, Zananiri KI, Syrganis CD, Tourkantonis AA. Oral calcium supplementation promotes renal sodium excretion in essential hypertension. *J Hypertens* 1987;5:S307–S309.

184. Bierenbaum ML, Wolf E, Bisgeier G, Maginnis WP. Dietary calcium: a method of lowering blood pressure. *Am J Hypertens* 1988;1:149s–152s.

185. Gilliland M, Zawada ET, McClung D, TerWee J. Preliminary report: natriuretic effect of calcium supplementation in hypertensive women over forty. *J Am Coll Nutr* 1987;6:139–143.

186. Vinson JA, Mazur T, Bose P. Comparison of different forms of calcium on blood pressure of normotensive young males. *Nutr Rep Int* 1987;36:497–505.

187. Tabuchi Y, Ogihara T, Hashizume K, Saito H, Kumahara Y. Hypotensive effect of long-term oral calcium supplementation in elderly patients with essential hypertension. *J Clin Hypertens* 1986;3:254–262.

188. Takagi Y, Fukasa M, Takata B, Fujimi T, Fujita T. Calcium treatment of essential hypertension in elderly patients evaluated by 24 H monitoring. *Am J Hypertens* 1991;4:836–839.

189. Van Beresteijn ELH, Van Schaulk M, Schaafsma G. Milk: does it affect blood pressure? A controlled intervention study. *J Intern Med* 1990;228:477–480.

190. Buonopane GJ, Kilara A, Smith JS, McCarthy RD. Effect of skim milk supplementation on blood cholesterol concentration, blood pressure, and triglycerides in a free-living human population. *J Am Coll Nutr* 1992;11:56–67.

191. Belizan JM, Villar J, Zalzar A, Rojas L, Chan D, Bryce GF. Preliminary evidence of the effect of calcium supplementation on blood pressure in normal pregnant women. *Am J Obstet Gynecol* 1983;146:175–180.

192. Villar J, Repke J, Belizan JM, Pareja G. Calcium supplementation reduces blood pressure during pregnancy: results of a randomized clinical trial. *Obstet Gynecol* 1987;70:317–322.

193. López-Jaramillo P, Narváez M, Weigel RM, Yepez R. Calcium supplementation reduces the risk of pregnancy-induced hypertension in an Andes population. *Br J Obstet Gynaecol* 1989;96:648–655.

194. López-Jaramillo P, Narváez M, Yépez R. Effect of calcium supplementation on the vascular sensitivity to angiotensin II in pregnant women (letter). *Am J Obstet Gynecol* 1987;156:261–262.

195. Marya RK, Rathee S, Manrow M. Effect of calcium and vitamin supplementation on toxemia of pregnancy. *Gynecol Obstet Invest* 1987;24:38–42.

196. Belizan JM, Villan J, Gonzalez L, Campodonica L, Berjel E. Calcium supplementation to prevent hypertensive disorders of pregnancy. *N Engl J Med* 1991;325:1389–1405.

197. Knight KB, Keith RE. Calcium supplementation on normotensive and hypertensive pregnant women. *Am J Clin Nutr* 1992;55:891–895.

198. Saito K, Sano H, Furata Y, Fukuzaki H. Effect of oral calcium on blood pressure response in salt-loaded borderline hypertensive patients. *Hypertension* 1989;13:219–226.

199. Saito K, Sano H, Furuta Y, et al. Calcium supplementation in salt-depleted hypertension. *Contrib Nephrol* 1991;90:25–35.

200. Weinberger MH, Wagner UL, Fineberg NS. The blood pressure effects of calcium supplementation in humans of known sodium responsiveness. *Am J Hypertens* 1993;6:799–805.

201. Lyle RM. Does baseline serum total calcium level influence the blood pressure response to calcium supplementation? A double-blind study. *Netherlands J Med* 1992;41:48–55.

202. Meese RB, Gonzalez DG, Casparian JM, Ram CVS, Pak CYC, Kaplan NM. Failure of calcium supplements to relieve hypertension. *Am J Med Sci* 1987;294:219–224.

203. Grobbee DE, Hofman A. Calcium supplementation lowers blood pressure in young mildly hypertensive subjects: a randomized, controlled trial. *Lancet* 1986;ii:703–707.

204. Bloomfield RL, Young LD, Zurek G, Felts JH, Straw MK. Effects of oral calcium carbonate on blood pressure in subjects with mildly elevated arterial pressure. *J Hypertens* 1986;4(Suppl 5):s351–s354.

205. Strazzullo P, Siani A, Guglielmi S, et al. Controlled trial of long-term oral calcium supplementation in essential hypertension. *Hypertension* 1986;8:1084–1088.

206. Thomsen K, Nilas L, Christiansen C. Dietary calcium intake and blood pressure in normotensive subjects. *Acta Med Scand* 1987;222:51–56.

207. Siani A, Strazzullo P, Guglielmi S, et al. Controlled trial of low calcium versus high calcium intake in mild hypertension. *J Hypertens* 1988;6:253–256.

208. Cappuccio FP, Markandu ND, Singer DRJ, Smith SJ, Shore AC, MacGregor GA. Does oral calcium supplementation lower high blood pressure? A double blind study. *J Hypertens* 1987;5:67–71.

209. Van Beresteyn ECH, Schaafsma G, De Waard H. Oral calcium and blood pressure: a controlled intervention trial. *Am J Clin Nutr* 1986;44:883–888.

210. Nowson C, Morgan T. Effect of calcium carbonate on blood pressure in normotensive and hypertensive people. *Hypertension* 1989;13:630–639.

211. The effects of non-pharmacologic interventions on blood pressure of persons with high normal levels. *JAMA* 1992;267:1213–1220.

212. Kawasaki N, Matsui K, Ito M, et al. Effect of calcium supplementation on the vascular sensitivity to angiotensin II in pregnant women. *Am J Obstet Gynecol* 1985;153:576–582.

213. Morris CD, McCarron DA. Effect of calcium supplementation in an older population with mildly increased blood pressure. *Am J Hypertens* 1992;5:230–237.

214. Singer DRJ, Markandu ND, Cappuccio FP, et al. Does oral calcium lower blood pressure: a double-blind study. *J Hypertens* 1985;3:661–671.

215. Zoccali C, Mallamaci F, Delfino D, et al. Long-term oral calcium supplementation in essential hypertension: a double-blind, randomized, crossover study. *J Hypertens* 1990;4(Suppl 6):S676–S678.

216. Zoccali C, Mallamaci F, Delfino D, et al. Double-blind randomized, crossover trial of calcium supplementation in essential hypertension. *J Hypertens* 1988;6:451–455.

217. Oparil S, Chen YF, Jin HK, Yang RH, Wyss JM. Dietary Ca^{2+} prevents NaCl-sensitive hypertension in spontaneously hypertensive rats via sympatholytic and renal effects. *Am J Clin Nutr* 1991;54:227S–236S.

218. Wyss JM, Chen Y-F, Meng QC, Jin HK, Jirakulsomchok S, Oparil S. Dietary Ca^{2+} prevents NaCl-induced exacerbation of hypertension and increases hypothalamic norepinephrine turnover in spontaneously hypertensive rats. *J Hypertens* 1989;7:711–719.

219. Yang R-H, Jin H, Chen Y-F, Oparil S, Wyss JM. Dietary Ca^{2+} supplementation prevents the exaggerated responsiveness of anterior hypothalamic α_2-adrenoceptors in NaCl-loaded spontaneously hypertensive rats. *J Cardiovasc Pharmacol* 1989;13:162–167.

220. Metz JA, Karanja N, Torok J, McCarron DA. Modification of total body fat in spontaneously hypertensive rats and Wistar-Kyoto rats by dietary calcium and sodium. *Am J Hypertens* 1988;1:58–60.

221. Baksi SN. Blood pressure and hypothalamic norepinephrine and dopamine in calcium-deficient rats. *Am J Hypertens* 1989;2:462–464.

222. Baksi SN, Hughes MJ. Alteration of adrenal catecholamine levels in the rat after dietary calcium and vitamin D deficiencies. *J Auton Nerv Sys* 1984;11:393–396.

223. Hagihara M, Togari A, Matsumoto S, Nagatsu T. Dietary calcium deprivation increased the levels of plasma catecholamines and catecholamine-synthesizing enzymes of adrenal glands in rats. *Biochem Pharmacol* 1990;39:1229–1231.

224. Luft FC, Ganten U, Meyer D, et al. Effect of high calcium diet on magnesium, catecholamines, and blood pressure of stroke-prone spontaneously hypertensive rats. *Proc Soc Exp Biol Med* 1988;187:474–481.

225. Scrogin KE, Hatton DC, McCarron DA. The interactive effects of dietary sodium chloride and calcium on cardiovascular stress responses. *Am J Physiol* 1991;261:R945–R949.

226. Felicetta JV, Beck FWJ, Metz JA, McCarron DA, Sowers JR. Diet and catecholamines in the spontaneously hypertensive rat. *J Hypertens* 1986;4(Suppl 5):S55–S57.

227. Hatton DC, Scrogin KE, Metz JA, McCarron DA. Dietary calcium alters blood pressure reactivity in spontaneously hypertensive rats. *Hypertension* 1989;13:622–629.

228. Hatton DC, Scrogin KE, Levine D, Feller D, McCarron DA. Dietary calcium modulates blood pressure through an α-1 adrenergic mechanism. *Am J Physiol* 1993;264:F234–F238.

229. Doris PA. Interactions between sodium and calcium intake and blood pressure responses to norepinephrine and parathyroid hormone. *Horm Metab Res* 1988;20:163–167.

230. Kageyama Y, Suzuki H, Arima K, Saruta T. Oral calcium treatment lowers blood pressure in renovascular hypertensive rats by suppressing the renin-angiotensin system. *Hypertension* 1987;10:375–382.

231. Kageyama Y, Suzuki H, Hayashi K, Saurta T. Effects of calcium loading on blood pressure in spontaneously hypertensive rats: attenuation of the vascular reactivity. *Clin Exp Hypertens* 1986;A8:355–370.

232. Kageyama Y, Suzuki H, Arima K, Kondo K, Saruta T. Effects of calcium loading in DOCA-salt hypertensive rats. *Jpn Circ J* 1987;51:1315–1324.

233. Peuler JD. Contrasting hemodynamic effects of high oral calcium in genetic models of salt-sensitive hypertension. *Clin Exp Hypertens* 1991;A13:709–717.

234. Rouot BM, U'Prichard DC, Snyder SH. Multiple α_2-noradrenergic receptor sites in rat brain: selective regulation of high-affinity [^{3}H]clonidine binding by guanine nucleotides and divalent cations. *J Neurochem* 1980;34:374–384.

235. Lewanczuk RZ, Chen A, Pang PTK. The effect of dietary calcium on blood pressure in spontaneously hypertensive rats may be mediated by parathyroid hypertensive factor. *Am J Hypertens* 1990;3:349–353.

236. Resnick LM, Gupta RK, Lewanczuk RZ, Pang PKT, Laragh JH. Intracellular ions in salt-sensitive essential hypertension: possible role of calcium-regulating hormones. *Contrib Nephrol* 1991;90:88–93.

237. Benishin CG, Lewanczuk RZ, Pang PKT. Isolation and characterization of parathyroid hypertensive factor (PHF). *J Hypertens* 1990;8(Suppl 3):S98 (abst).

238. Koh E, Morimoto S, Fukuo K, et al. 1,25-Dihydroxyvitamin D_3 binds specifically to rat vascular smooth muscle cells and stimulates their proliferation in vitro. *Life Sci* 1988;42:215–223.

239. Mitsuhashi T, Morris RC, Ives HE. 1,25-Dihydroxyvitamin D_3 modulates growth of vascular smooth muscle cells. *J Clin Invest* 1991;87:1889–1895.

240. Kawashima H. 1,25-Dihydroxyvitamin D_3 stimulates Ca-ATPase in a vascular smooth muscle cell line. *Biochem Biophys Res Commun* 1988;150:1138–1143.

241. Inoue T, Kawashima H. 1,25-Dihydroxyvitamin D_3 stimulates $^{45}Ca^{2+}$ uptake by cultured vascular smooth muscle cells derived from rat aorta. *Biochem Biophys Res Commun* 1988;152:1388–1394.

242. Bukoski RD, Xue H, McCarron DA. Effect of 1,25(OH)$_2$ vitamin D_3 and ionized Ca^{2+} on ^{45}Ca uptake by primary cultures of aortic myocytes of spontaneously hypertensive and Wistar Kyoto normotensive rats. *Biochem Biophys Res Commun* 1987;146:1330–1335.

243. Xue H, McCarron DA, Bukoski RD. 1,25(OH)$_2$ vitamin D_3-induced ^{45}Ca uptake in vascular myocytes cultured from spontaneously hypertensive and normotensive rats. *Life Sci* 1991;49:651–659.

244. Bukoski RD, DeWan P, McCarron DA. 1,25(OH)$_2$ vitamin D_3 modifies growth and contractile function of vascular smooth muscle of spontaneously hypertensive rats. *Am J Hypertens* 1989;2:553–556.

245. Bukoski RD, Wang D, Wagman DW. Injection of 1,25-(OH)$_2$ vitamin D_3 enhances resistance artery contractile properties. *Hypertension* 1990;16:523–531.

246. Hatton DC, Xue H, DeMerritt JA, McCarron DA. 1,25(OH)$_2$ vitamin D_3-induced alterations in vascular reactivity in the SHR. *Am J Med Sci* (In press).

247. Shimosawa T, Ando K, Fujita T. Enhancement of vasoconstrictor response by a noncalcemic analogue of vitamin D_3. *Hypertension* 1993;21:253–258.

248. Bukoski RD, Xue H. On the vascular inotropic action of calcitriol. *Am J Hypertens* 1993;6:388–396.

249. Bukoski RD, Li J, Bo J. Effect of long-term administration of 1,25(OH)$_2$ vitamin D_3 on blood pressure and resistance artery contractility in the spontaneously hypertensive rat. *Am J Hypertens* 1993;6:944–950.

250. Bohr DF. Vascular smooth muscle: dual effect of calcium. *Science* 1963;139:597–599.

251. Dominiczak AF, Lazar DF, Das AK, Bohr DF. Lipid bilayer in genetic hypertension. *Hypertension* 1991;18:748–757.

252. Bohr DF. What makes the pressure go up? A hypothesis. *Hypertension* 1981;3(Suppl II):II160.

253. Rinaldi G, Bohr DF. Potassium-induced relaxation of the arteries in hypertension: modulation by extracellular calcium. *Am J Physiol* 1989;256:H707–H712.

254. Furspan PB, Rinaldi GJ, Hoffman K, Bohr DF. Dietary calcium and cell membrane abnormality in genetic hypertension. *Hypertension* 1989;13:727–730.

255. Bohr DF, Wu CC. Mechanisms of calcium relaxation of vascular smooth muscle. *Am J Physiol* 1991;261:H1411–H1416.

256. Dominiczak AF, Bohr DF. Cell membrane abnormalities and the regulation of intracellular calcium concentration in hypertension. *Clin Sci* 1990;79:415–423.

257. Furspan PB, Bohr DF. Calcium-related abnormalities in lymphocytes from genetically hypertensive rats. *Hypertension* 1986;8(Suppl II):II123–II126.

258. Porsti I, Arvola P, Wuorela H, Vapaatalo H. High calcium diet augments vascular potassium relaxation in hypertensive rats. *Hypertension* 1992;19:85–92.

259. Shiffman FH, Bose R. A role of calcium in altered sodium ion transport of hypertensives? *Life Sci* 1988;42:1573–1581.

260. Porsti I, Arvola P, Wuorela H, et al. Effects of a high calcium diet and deoxycorticosterone on vascular smooth muscle responses in spontaneously hypertensive rats. *J Hypertens* 1990;8:835–841.

261. Wuorela H, Arvola P, Porsti I, Siltaloppi E, Saynavalammi P, Vapaatalo H. The effect of high calcium intake on Ca^{2+} ATPase

and the tissue Na:K ratio in spontaneously hypertensive rats. *Naunyn Schmied Arch Pharmacol* 1992;345:117–122.

262. Hatton DC, Muntzel M, McCarron DA, Pressley M, Bukoski RD. Early effects of dietary calcium on blood pressure, plasma volume, and vascular reactivity. *Kidney Int* 1988;34:16–18.

263. Porsti I. Arterial smooth muscle contractions in spontaneously hypertensive rats on a high-calcium diet. *J Hypertens* 1992;10:255–263.

264. Pernot F, Schleiffer R, Bergmann C, Vincent M, Sassard J, Gairard A. Dietary calcium, vascular reactivity, and genetic hypertension in the Lyon rat strain. *Am J Hypertens* 1990;3:846–853.

265. Ambrozy SL, Shehin SE, Chiou C-Y, Sowers JR, Zemel MB. Effects of dietary calcium on blood pressure, vascular reactivity and vascular smooth muscle calcium efflux rate in Zucker rats. *Am J Hypertens* 1991;4:592–596.

266. Roullet CM, Roullet J-B, Duchambon P, et al. Abnormal intestinal regulation of calbindin-D9K and calmodulin by dietary calcium in genetic hypertension. *Am J Physiol* 1991;261:F474–F480.

267. Cox JA, Comte M, Stein EA. Activation of human erythrocyte Ca^{2+}-dependent Mg^{2+}-activated ATPase by calmodulin and calcium: quantitative analysis. *Proc Natl Acad Sci* 1982;79:4265–4269.

268. Drüeke TB. Mechanisms of action of calcium absorption: factors that influence bioavailability. In: Langford H, Levine B, Ellenbogen L, eds. *Nutritional factors in hypertension.* New York: Alan R Liss; 1990:155–173.

Hypertension: Pathophysiology, Diagnosis,
and Management, Second Edition,
edited by J.H. Laragh and B.M. Brenner,
Raven Press, Ltd., New York © 1995.

CHAPTER **72**

Role of Magnesium in the Pathogenesis of Hypertension Updated: Relationship to its Actions on Cardiac, Vascular Smooth Muscle, and Endothelial Cells

Burton M. Altura and Bella T. Altura

B. M. Altura: Departments of Physiology and Medicine,
SUNY Health Science Center at Brooklyn, Brooklyn, New
York 11203.
  B. T. Altura: Department of Physiology, SUNY Health Science Center at Brooklyn, Brooklyn, New York 11203.

Over the past 10 years, numerous experimental, epidemiological, and clinical studies have appeared in the literature that point to an important role for magnesium ions (Mg^{2+}) in the etiology of cardiovascular pathology (1–13). Dietary deficiency in Mg as well as abnormalities in Mg metabolism appear to play important roles in ischemic heart disease (IHD), congestive heart failure, sudden cardiac death, a number of cardiac arrhythmias, vascular complications in diabetes mellitus (DM) and preeclampsia-eclampsia, and hypertension. The major risk factors for IHD and acute myocardial infarction, namely hypertensive vascular disease, diabetic vascular disease, insulin resistance, atherosclerosis, and vasospasm, may be reflections of abnormal dietary deficiency, and improper metabolism, of Mg. Since much of the problem in hypertension and DM vascular complications is related to alterations in cardiac hemodynamics and bioenergetics, vascular tone, vascular reactivity, and atherosclerosis, the effects Mg^{2+} exert on cardiac function and bioenergetics, blood vessels, and the atherosclerotic process are reviewed. However, as this chapter is an update of the one we wrote 5 years ago (14), we have chosen to focus on the literature of the past 7 to 8 years and will refer the reader to our earlier review of this area where appropriate. Inasmuch as Mg^{2+} is known to impact upon divalent cation metabolism and transport in vascular smooth muscle (VSM) and endothelial cells (1–

3,5,6,15–17), we have also chosen to review some of this information and to examine some recent data on subcellular compartmentation of Ca^{2+} and Mg^{2+}.

DISTRIBUTION, ABSORPTION, AND EXCRETION OF MAGNESIUM

Approximately 21–28 g of magnesium, 60 percent of which is a relatively nonexchangeable component of bone, is found in the adult body of man. An additional 20 percent resides in the skeletal muscles. As a soft tissue cation, Mg ranks second to potassium (K) in quantity; it also resembles K in distribution. Cells contain about 38 percent of the total Mg in the body; 1 to 2 percent resides in the extracellular component. Approximately 35 percent of the Mg in plasma is thought to be bound nonspecifically to proteins. The exact proportions of these fractions have been difficult to determine precisely and until recently there was no way to make rapid blood, serum, or plasma ionized Mg determinations.

The advent of a new ion-selective electrode (ISE) for extracellular Mg^{2+} measurements (see below) has allowed for the determination of ionized whole blood, serum, and plasma Mg^{2+} in normal healthy human volunteers and diseased subjects. These data indicate that ionized serum or plasma Mg^{2+} normally is about 71 percent of the total Mg.

With the normal diet, 30 to 40 percent of the ingested Mg^{2+} is absorbed via the jejunum and ileum. Under normal circumstances, the kidney is the prime regulator of Mg balance in the body. Three to 6 percent of the filtered load is excreted by the kidneys. About 25 percent of the filtered Mg is reabsorbed in the proximal tubule and 50 to 60 percent in the thick ascending loop of Henle. The mechanisms controlling Mg absorption in the kidney, however, remain unknown. A number of physiological and pharmacological factors can influence renal handling of magnesium, as summarized in Table 1.

ROLES OF Mg IN CELL METABOLISM

Two major roles for Mg exist in biological systems: (a) it can form chelates with various intracellular anionic ligands, e.g., adenosine 5′-triphosphate (ATP), and (b) it

TABLE 1. *Physiological and pharmacological factors influencing renal handling of magnesium*

Factors stimulating Mg^{2+} reabsorption	Factors inhibiting Mg^{2+} reabsorption
Low plasma Mg	High plasma Mg
Low plasma Ca	High plasma Ca
High TF_{Mg}	Unfavorable transepithelial voltage
Favorable transepithelial voltage	Volume expansion
Volume depletion	Salt, osmotic diuresis
PTH	Alcohol
Calcitonin	Loop diuretics
ADH	Thiazides
K-sparing diuretics	Cisplatin
	Gentamycin
	Cyclosporine

TF_{Mg}, threshhold for filtration; PTH, parathyroid hormone; ADH, antidiuretic hormone.

TABLE 2. *Physiological functions of magnesium*

Enzyme functions	Structural functions	Membrane functions	Calcium antagonist
7 Glycolytic enzymes	Proteins	Hormone-receptor binding	Muscle contraction/relaxation
4 TCA cycle enzymes	Polyribosomes	Gating of Ca^{2+} channels	Neurotransmitter release
Membrane-bound ATPases	Nucleic acids	Transmembrane flux of ions	Action potential conduction
Kinases—creatine kinase	Mitochondria	Adenylate cyclase system	In nodal tissue
Alkaline phosphatase	Multienzyme complexes, e.g.	Ca^{2+}-Ca^{2+} Release	
12 Photosynthetic enzymes	G-Proteins, NMDA		

TCA, tricarboxylic acid; ATPases, adenosine triphosphatases; NMDA, *N*-Methyl-D-aspartic acid.

can compete with Ca^{2+} for binding sites on membranes (external and internal) and proteins (6,50,51).

Mg^{2+} catalyzes or activates more than 325 enzymes in the body and is pivotal in the transfer, storage, and utilization of energy (50,51). It activates phosphate groups and reactions that involve ATP. The intracellular level of free Mg^{2+} ($[Mg^{2+}]_i$) serves to regulate intermediary metabolism through activation of such rate-limiting enzymes as hexokinase, pyruvate dehydrogenase, enolase, and creatinine phosphokinase. Mg^{2+} can cause a conformational change during catalytic processes (e.g., Na^+-K^+-ATPase) by promoting aggregation of multienzyme complexes (e.g., aldehyde dehydrogenase) or by a mixture of mechanisms [e.g., F_1-ATPase (246)].

Within the cell nucleus, Mg^{2+} regulates DNA synthesis. Large numbers of Mg^{2+} ions are bound to the pentose-phosphate backbone of DNA. By regulating DNA and RNA (i.e., RNA synthetase, mRNA attachment to ribosomes, etc.) synthesis and structure, Mg^{2+} plays a vital role in regulating cell growth, reproduction, and membrane structure (51,247,248). The role of magnesium in regulating cell membrane permeability, transmembrane electrolyte flux, and cell adhesion is becoming widely accepted and this is generating considerable interest (50,249,250). Magnesium's role in regulating mitochondrial membrane permeability has long been recognized (251).

PHYSIOLOGICAL ROLES OF MAGNESIUM

As a consequence of its numerous biochemical cellular activities, Mg plays a pivotal role in control of neuronal activity, cardiac excitability, neuromuscular transmission, muscular contraction, vasomotor tone, blood pressure, and peripheral blood flow (Table 2). By competing with Ca^{2+} for membrane-binding sites and by modulating calcium binding and release from the sarcoplasmic reticulum (SR) membranes, Mg^{2+} can act to maintain low resting levels of $[Ca^{2+}]_i$ and trigger muscle contraction or relaxation.

Besides controlling membrane permeability, Mg^{2+} can affect the electrical properties of cellular membranes. At cell membranes, internal Mg^{2+} can regulate ion flux through voltage-gated, acetyl-choline–activated, Ca^{2+}-activated and ATP-activated K^+ channels. Alterations in $[Mg^{2+}]_i$ and extracellular Mg^{2+} ($[Mg^{2+}]_o$) can result in alterations in action and resting potentials in certain cell types. Cardiac and vascular smooth muscle cell membranes are particularly vulnerable to deficits in $[Mg^{2+}]_o$ (see below). Deficits in $[Mg^{2+}]_o$ can also result in elevation in $[Ca^{2+}]_i$ in these excitable cells.

IMPORTANCE OF CARDIAC EVENTS IN HYPERTENSIVE VASCULAR DISEASE

Hypertension is clearly a hemodynamic abnormality. Any factors that result directly or indirectly in a sustained increase in either blood flow or vascular resistance will result in an increased intravascular pressure. The many diverse factors (e.g., neural, humoral, ionic, etc.) that interact to disturb pressure–flow–resistance relationships will serve to define the type and etiology of hypertension (Table 3). Irrespective of the etiology or vari-

TABLE 3. *Major factors determining level of arterial blood pressure*

1. Total peripheral vascular resistance
   General vasomotor control
   Local vasomotor control mechanisms
   Neurohumors
   Hormones
   Local tissue hormones
   Ions
2. Cardiac output
   Heart rate
   Pacemaker frequency
   Cardiac sympathetic and cholinergic discharge
   Neurohumors
   Stroke volume
   Systolic volume
   Ventricular ejection
   Diastolic volume
   Coronary blood flow
   Ventricular distensibility
   Cardiac sympathetic discharge
   Ventricular filling pressure
   Venous capacity
   Blood volume
   Neurohumors
   Speed of ejection
3. Aortic compliance
4. Diastolic arterial blood volume

TABLE 4. *Cytosolic free Mg²⁺ concentration in nucleated mammalian tissues and cells*

Tissue/cell (method)	$[Mg^{2+}]_i$ (mM/L)	Authors
Rat skeletal muscle (electrode, enzymatic)	1.0–2.8	Gunther and Dorn (18)
Rat brain (binding, aconitate hydratase)	1.0–1.5	Velaso et al. (19)
Rat brain (³¹P-NMR)	0.8–1.2	Vink et al. (20,21)
	0.5–0.85	Altura and Gupta (22)
		Altura et al. (23)
Human brain (³¹P-NMR)	0.3–0.5	Taylor et al. (24)
Rat liver (binding, aconitate hydratase)	1.0–1.5	Velaso et al. (19)
Rat liver (enzymatic, null point)	0.3–1.6	Gunther and Dorn (18)
		Corkey et al. (25)
Rat liver (Mag-fura-2)	0.59	Raju et al. (26)
Pancreatic acinar cells	1.36	Lennard and Singh (27)
Rat aorta (Mag-fura 2)	0.4–0.8	Zhang et al. (28)
Human aortic endothelial cells (Mag-fura-2)	0.3–0.6	Zhang et al. (29)
Canine cerebral vascular muscle (Mag-fura-2)	0.4–0.7	Altura et al. (30)
Rat astrocytes, Type 2 (Mag-fura-2)	0.08–0.27	Babu et al. (31)

able (e.g., electrolyte alterations, defects in ion transport, neurogenic mechanisms, overproduction of neurohumors, increased vascular reactivity to constrictors, decreased vascular reactivity to dilators, genetics, obesity, diet, lipids, renal alterations, atherogenesis, diabetes, etc.), the result will be a raised systemic arterial blood pressure and hypertensive vascular disease. Of these variables, two, namely, the cardiac output (CO) and the ratio of mean arterial blood pressure (MAP) to output (or resistance), are quite important and have attracted a great deal of attention. Since measured arterial blood pressure (BP) in the formula BP = CO × TPR (total peripheral resistance) can be due to either an increased resistance or elevated flow, it has become clear that the level of CO in etiology, maintenance, and treatment of high blood pressure is very important (149).

Recent experimental and clinical findings reveal that the intracellular and extracellular concentration of Mg^{2+} can affect, in diverse ways, directly and indirectly, the major factors that determine the level of arterial blood pressure (Table 3).

It is also becoming clear that one can not consider the importance of Mg^{2+} to the hypertensive disease process without also considering its interaction with other cations, particularly K^+, Ca^{2+}, Na^+, and H^+.

INTRACELLULAR Mg²⁺ LEVELS IN VARIOUS CELL AND TISSUE TYPES

Although total cellular Mg can be easily and accurately determined by atomic absorption spectroscopy, including that present in cardiac and vascular smooth muscle, it has been difficult to determine precisely the total intracellular free-Mg, probably because of its binding to ionic constituents and intracellular organelles and the lack of techniques to assess it. Recently, however, a number of new techniques, including specific-sensitive

TABLE 5. *Intracellular free Mg²⁺ levels in mammalian cardiac cells*

Cardiac tissue	$[Mg^{2+}]_i$	Method	Authors
Perfused guinea pig heart	0.8	³¹P-NMR	Gupta and Moore (32)
	2.5	³¹P-NMR	Wu et al. (33)
Sheep Purkinje fibers	3.5	ISEs	Hess et al. (34)
Sheep ventricular muscle	3.1	ISEs	Hess et al. (34)
Ferret ventricular muscle	3.0	ISEs	Hess et al. (34)
	0.4–0.9	ISEs	Blatter and McGuigan (35)
Perfused rat heart	0.6–0.7	³¹P-NMR	Reiner et al. (36)
			Barbour et al. (37,38)
			Altura et al. (39,40)
	0.6–0.7	³¹P-NMR	Kirkels et al. (44)
	0.6–0.9	³¹P-NMR	Headrick and Willis (41)
Rat cardiac myocytes	0.5–0.6	³¹P-NMR	Wittenberg et al. (42)
			Gupta and Wittenberg (43)
Perfused ferret heart	1.2	³¹F-NMR	Kirschenlohr et al. (45)
Rat heart	0.86	Mag-fura-2	Murphy et al. (46)

³¹P-NMR, ³¹P-nuclear magnetic resonance; ISE, ion-selective electrode.

Mg^{2+} microelectrodes, ^{31}P-nuclear magnetic resonance (NMR) spectroscopy, ^{19}F-NMR spectroscopy, and molecular fluorescent probes have been utilized with some success to assess intracellular free Mg^{2+} concentration in a number of cell and tissue types (see Table 4). These studies reveal that intracellular free Mg^{2+} concentrations in many nucleated mammalian cells, so far examined, appear to range from 0.4 to 2.8 mM/L; adult myocardial muscle cells appear to have the widest range of measured intracellular free Mg^{2+} levels, 0.50–3.5 mM/L (see Table 5). The more recent (e.g., 1987–1993) values obtained by ^{31}P-NMR, ^{19}F-NMR, and Mag-fura-2 are of particular interest (0.5–1.2 mM/L) (e.g., Table 5) because, until the appearance of these studies, it was believed that free intracellular Mg^{2+} concentration in cardiac muscle was about 2.5–3.5 mM/L, which could lead to serious errors with respect to cardiac Mg^{2+} levels in pathophysiological states and to the mechanism(s) responsible for controlling free cytosolic Mg^{2+} in cardiac myocytes. With respect to rat and canine vascular smooth muscle and human vascular endothelial cells, the studies using the fluorescent probe, Mag-fura-2, indicate that the intracellular free Mg^{2+} concentration is between 0.4 and 0.8 mM/L (6,12,13,28–30,47,48), or approximately the same as that in cardiac muscle. One recent study employing ^{31}P-NMR spectroscopy on intact rat aorta indicates that with this probe the $[Mg^{2+}]_i$ is somewhat lower than that found with the fluorescent probe (49). Data utilizing ^{19}F-NMR or Mg^{2+} selective microelectrodes are not yet available for vascular muscle or endothelial cells.

ASSOCIATION OF INTRACELLULAR Mg^{2+} AND K^+

Regulation of K^+ Transport by Mg^{2+}

It is clear that the cellular distribution of Mg resembles that of K (for review, see ref. 50). Mg is essential for stabilizing the intracellular K and its transport across cell membranes (for reviews see refs. 50,51). Most of the studies indicate a close correlation between the intracellular K^+ concentration and the intracellular Mg^{2+} concentration under a wide range of pathophysiological situations of Mg depletion. The data suggest, albeit mostly indirectly, that Mg^{2+} can, to a large extent, regulate the cellular and subcellular distribution and the intracellular concentration of K^+.

A review of the literature of the past two decades clearly reveals that experimental dietary Mg deficiency (in different mammals) usually results in a loss of intracellular K^+ from various organs and cells so far studied, e.g., the myocardium, skeletal muscle, liver, kidney, red blood cells, and lymphocytes. The more severe losses in cellular Mg^{2+} and K^+ appear to take place in muscle cells, e.g., cardiac and skeletal muscle (see data in Table II in ref. 50).

Evidence from both *in vivo* and *in vitro* experiments indicates that ventricular slices obtained from Mg^{2+}-deficient rats and human atrial cells in culture, containing different concentrations of Mg^{2+}, suggest that most of the K^+ loss and Na^+ gain is a consequence of Mg's action on the Na^+-K^+ membrane pumps (52–55). Interestingly, the concomitant elevations observed in tissue Ca^{2+} and Na^+, together with the reductions in Mg^{2+} and K^+ in these Mg^{2+}-deficient tissues and cells, resemble rather closely the electrolyte changes noted recently in experimentally injured myocardial cells and in tissues from sudden death ischemic heart disease, acute myocardial infarction (AMI), and essential hypertension in patients (2,6,11,12,50,51,56).

Interaction of K^+ and Mg^{2+} in Heart Muscle

It would appear from some clinical observations that IHD following a long history of angina, in particular, results in the greatest reductions in myocardial Mg^{2+} and K^+ concentrations (see Tables III and IV in ref. 50), leading us to believe that ischemia (e.g., hypoxia, anoxia) in and around the coronary arteries and arterioles is somehow involved in the electrolyte shifts. The latter events may aid in explaining why coronary arteries excised from victims of sudden death ischemic heart disease exhibit greater reductions in Mg concentrations than does the myocardium itself (57–59). Is there experimental and/or clinical evidence that could be utilized to support the notion that ischemic events will result in loss of myocardial and coronary vascular muscle K and Mg?

As early as 1967 (60), it had been demonstrated that asphyxia can result in rapid (within 30 seconds) and progressive loss of myocardial total Mg. Over the intervening 25 years, it has been clearly demonstrated that asphyxia, anoxia, coronary ligation, or cardiac surgery can result in rapid loss of myocardial Mg and K followed by elevations in myocardial Na^+ and Ca^{2+} (2,44,54–56,61–63).

Although it is not clear as to which of these elements is the first to change (i.e., this could be intracellular, compartmental, and/or at the membrane), Lehr and coworkers have presented a great deal of experimental evidence in animals to suggest that Mg may be the first cation to change in the myocardium in hypoxic-induced injury to the heart (64,65). Moreover, these experiments suggest that after appropriate myocardial insults, provoked by diverse means, total Mg loss can occur within 30 to 60 min after the insult. However, since recent experiments on perfused working rat hearts suggest that Mg^{2+} can cross the cardiac membranes in less than 3 min (36–40), some Mg^{2+} loss probably occurs very quickly after an insult. Does the loss in Mg^{2+}, therefore, set in motion the observed concomitant cellular alterations in K^+, Na^+, and Ca^{2+}? And how do such myocardial cation

TABLE 6. *Actions of cytosolic Mg²⁺ in cardiac and vascular smooth muscle*

Action	References
1. Cellular bioenergetics and membrane pumps	3,6,14,36–40,43, 44,50,53,55,56
2. Block inward Ca²⁺ currents (slow channels)	2,6,13,28,39,50,53, 55,56,66–69,71, 75,96–99
3. Reduce; slow Na⁺ current	70
4. Modify action potential duration via action on K⁺ channels	71,82–87,100
5. Modification of ion channel behavior	72,73,101
6. Modulate tension development, force of contractility, and cardiac output	2,5,6,13,14,28, 36–40,55,56,59, 61,63,67,75,76, 78,89,99

changes affect cardiac excitability, coronary vascular tone, and blood flow?

Recent work from several laboratories is beginning to suggest that Mg²⁺ can affect cardiac excitability and contractility by a number of cellular pathways (Table 6), e.g., cellular bioenergetics and membrane pumps (3,6,14,36–40,42–44,50,53,55,56), Ca²⁺ channels (slow channels) (6,14,45,56,66–74), Ca²⁺ release and uptake from the sarcoplasmic reticulum (SR) (75–81), rectification of K⁺ channels (71,82–87), conduction, voltage and tension oscillation (2,11,54–56,61,63,78,90–95), and the contractile apparatus, e.g., myosin adenosine triphosphatase (ATPase), light chain myosin kinase, calmodulin, cross-bridging, etc. (56,76–78). Although a number of these aspects are beyond the scope of this chapter, certain aspects are discussed below.

A number of drugs, which are discussed subsequently in this review as well as elsewhere (1,4,6,7,9,11–14,22,23,30,51,54,56,88,92,102), often cause Mg and K wasting and losses of these two cations. For example, even though digitalis toxicity results in reduction in cardiac Mg and K, the cardiotoxicity can be rapidly reversed by Mg²⁺ replacement therapy (4,9,51,54,88,92,102), not K⁺. It should also be pointed out here that the diuretics that promote Mg²⁺ loss, discussed in Table 1 and elsewhere (see ref. 14, for review), also pro-

mote renal loss of K⁺. Hypertension, both clinically and experimentally produced, has long been associated with alterations in cellular K movements (14,50,103). We now know that hypertension in both animals and humans is often also associated with hypomagnesemia in plasma and tissues.

An early, rapid loss of myocardial and, probably also coronary vascular muscle Mg²⁺ as a primary event in the subsequent loss of K⁺, and tissue gain of Ca²⁺ and Na⁺, after hypertensive-related myocardial ischemic events may then be followed by cellular depletion of phosphagen levels (see data in Table VI, ref. 50). Not only has this been observed for the myocardium in asphyxia and anoxic events, but also after coronary ligation, and transplantation or cardiac surgery performed for hypertensive-related vascular disorders (41,44,50,60, 62,104–108). In some studies, there is a close parallel between the temporal changes in total Mg content and phosphagen levels (see data in Tables V and VI in ref. 50). Since 65 to 93 percent of the intracellular Mg²⁺ is normally thought to be bound to ATP (in the form of MgATP), depending upon cell type, a rapid depletion of phosphagen content could result in a loss of cellular Mg. On the other hand, a rapid loss of cellular Mg could result in a simultaneous breakdown of phosphagens and their cellular loss. Using ³¹P-NMR and perfused working rat hearts, we have demonstrated that reduction in cardiac [Mg²⁺]ᵢ can result in loss of phosphocreatine (PCr) and ATP (40) as well as acidification of the cytosol (e.g., Table 7). We have recently noted very similar effects on intracellular free Mg, PCr, and intracellular pH (pHi) in brains of rats administered either alcohol (23) or cocaine (22). Both alcohol and cocaine induced brain ischemia. Since ischemia results in local tissue metabolism leading to an elevation in H⁺ concentration, and a reduction in pHi is known to result in cellular losses of both Mg²⁺ and ATP, there would be further reductions in both constituents. The latter has, indeed, been recently demonstrated by our group using rat perfused, working hearts and ³¹P-NMR (ref. 40, *unpublished data*) (Table 7). However, several investigators have demonstrated a rise in free cytosolic Mg²⁺ in response to loss in ATP levels as a consequence of ischemia (41,44,46,104,106). Since the increase in [Mg²⁺]ᵢ was less

TABLE 7. *Effects of low extracellular Mg²⁺ (0.3 mM) on cytoplasmic phosphates, phosphorylation potential, intracellular free Mg²⁺, and intracellular pH in working rat perfused hearts*

[Mg²⁺]ₒ (mM)	Pᵢ (mM)	ATP (mM)	PCr (mM)	CPP (mM⁻¹)	[Mg²⁺]ᵢ (μM)	pHi
1.2	4.7 ± 1.2	6.8 ± 0.1	9.2 ± 0.5	38.4 ± 10.2	651 ± 55	7.14 ± 0.044
0.3	13.9 ± 3.5*	4.7 ± 0.1*	6.3 ± 0.7*	7.6 ± 2.0*	426 ± 54*	7.00 ± 0.050†

Adapted from ref. 40. Values are means ± SEM.
* $p < 0.01$; † $p < 0.05$.
[Mg²⁺]ₒ, extracellular Mg²⁺; Pᵢ, intracellular phosphorus; ATP, adenosine 5′-triphosphate; PCr, phosphocreatine; CPP, cytoplasmic phosphorylation potential; [Mg²⁺]ᵢ, intracellular free Mg²⁺; pHi, intracellular pH.

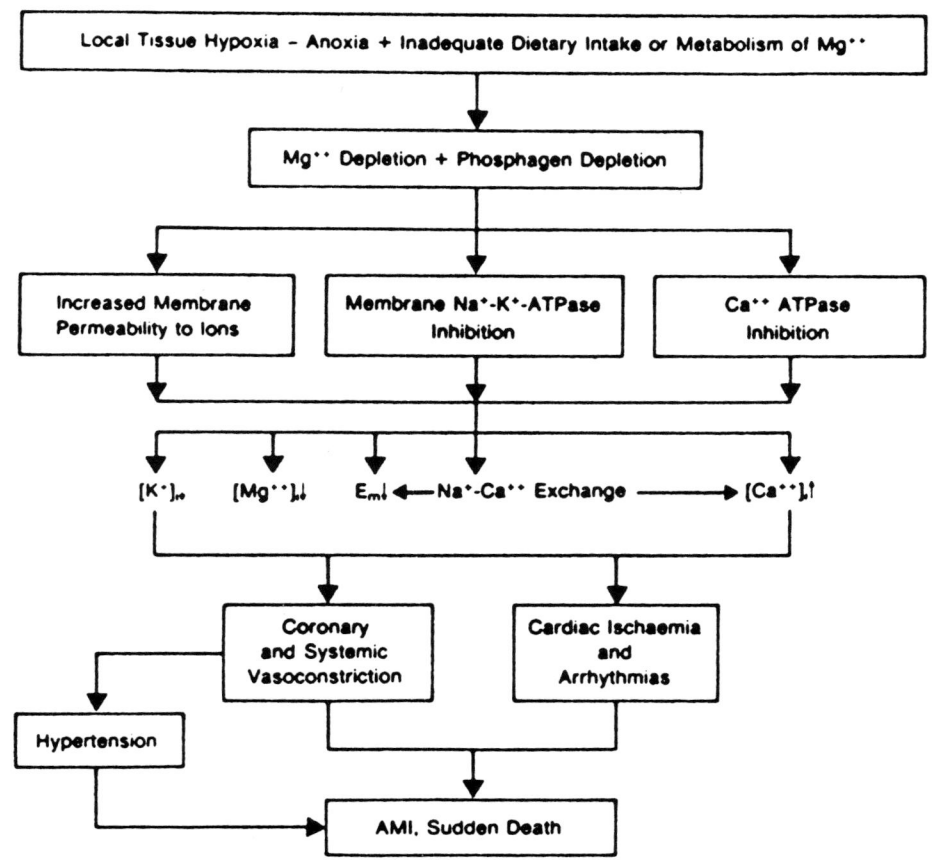

FIG. 1. Hypothetical scheme for the dysfunction of normal cardiovascular tone and cardiac rhythm by deficits in dietary Mg^{2+} intake and inadequate metabolism of Mg^{2+}. (From ref. 50, with permission.)

than that calculated for ATP loss, this might suggest either a net loss of $[Mg^{2+}]_i$ or a binding to cell organelles.

Interaction of K^+ and Mg^{2+} in Blood Vessels

The additional question to be resolved is what role such electrolyte changes, particularly Mg^{2+}–K^+ interactions, and phosphagen alterations play in alterations of coronary, cerebral, and peripheral vascular tone, which may in themselves lead to hypertensive vascular disease, unstable angina pectoris, coronary vasospasm, and stroke (e.g., Fig. 1). Could the latter be the primary rather than the secondary event, either leading to or contributing to the observed cardiac arrhythmias, strokelike events, etc., often observed in hypertensive subjects?

Mg and K do, indeed, appear to interact in important ways to control vascular tone and reactivity (108–111). Acute withdrawal of, or reduction in, $[K^+]_o$ produces relaxation of basal tone in isolated coronary arteries, whereas acute withdrawal of $[Mg^{2+}]$ produces contraction of these blood vessels (110). The magnitude of coronary contraction obtained on withdrawal of $[Mg^{2+}]_o$ is dependent upon the $[K^+]_o$; the higher the $[K^+]_o$, the greater the contraction. The precise ratio of $[K^+]_o/$

$[Mg^{2+}]_o$ appears to be important in dictating the degree of contraction (maximal response) and sensitivity [median effective concentration, (EC_{50})] of canine coronary vascular smooth muscle cells to serotonin (5-HT) (110).

Withdrawal or lowering the $[Mg^{2+}]_o$ or $[K^+]_o$ can also produce spasms of cerebral arteries and arterioles. The lower the extracellular concentration of either Mg^{2+} or K^+, the greater the magnitude of cerebral arterial contraction. These cerebrovascular contractions induced by lowering either the $[Mg^{2+}]_o$ or $[K^+]_o$ cannot be antagonized or attenuated by the known pharmacological antagonists. These ionic alterations all result in an increased Ca uptake that seems to be associated with the degree of vasospasm. Using ion-selective electrodes (ISEs) to assess extracellular ionized Mg (IMg^{2+}) and ionized K^+, we have recently found that the $[K^+]_o/[Mg^{2+}]_o$ ratio is important in preeclampsia in pregnant women (113). It is of interest to note that a combination of a K and Mg salt mixture seems to be of considerable therapeutic potential in SHR (114).

MYOCARDIAL ACTIONS OF Mg^{2+}

During the past decade, a number of reviews on different aspects of this important and still unresolved subject have appeared (2,5,6,9,11,14,39,43,54,61,63,67, 74,78,92). Therefore, our remarks will be directed to pertinent reports that have appeared since 1985, except in some instances.

Some Electrophysiological Actions

Since much of the electrophysiological actions of Mg^{2+} have also been reviewed recently (2,11,14,54,61,78,92), we will restrict our remarks to only a few relevant, recent findings. It has now been amply demonstrated that hypoxic-induced depolarization (117), digitalis-induced oscillatory afterpotentials (88), reperfusion arrhythmias (5,8,9,11,54,55,92,93,102,120), the calcium paradox (78), K^+-induced depolarization (11,82–87,92,119), as well as fibrillation (11,56,121) can all be prevented or ameliorated by elevation in $[Mg^{2+}]_o$. It is now known that the distortions produced in the cardiac action potentials in these pathophysiological situations are dependent upon the inward current attributed to Ca^{2+} (55,56,66,69,71,81,84). As reviewed above, it has been demonstrated that the $[Mg^{2+}]_i$ can block inward Ca^{2+} currents (66–68,88). Whether or not a prominent effect of Mg^{2+} on K^+ currents is playing a role in these pathophysiological events remains to be studied.

With respect to nodal tissue, the earlier idea that Mg^{2+} can modulate chronotropicity of the sinoatrial node (122–124) was confirmed and extended by Opthof and coworkers (125–127), using the isolated sinoatrial node preparations of the guinea pig and rabbit. In addition to demonstrating a negative chronotropic effect for Mg^{2+}, these investigators found that the major effects of Mg^{2+} on this tissue appear to be a decrease in the rate of diastolic depolarization and production of pacemaker shifts. The negative chronotropicity of elevated Mg^{2+} has been confirmed recently in intact dogs, baboons, and rats, as well as perfused rat hearts (38,39,89,128,129).

It now appears from data generated in the past few years that cytosolic free Mg^{2+} modifies the cardiac action potential by exerting effects on at least three different K^+ channels (71,82,87). Overall, these findings on resting membrane potentials, action potentials, and pacemaker cells would seem to suggest that physiological concentrations of Mg^{2+} (a) are important in regulating membrane-dependent electrical changes, (b) can act as modulators of conduction, and (c) stabilize membranes of cardiac muscle cells and pacemaker cells.

Cardiac Contractility and Bioenergetics

Mg^{2+} ions are important for regulation of Na^+ and K^+ transport across cell membranes, including those found in cardiac and vascular smooth muscle cells (2,14–16,50–53,56,70,78,130,131). Mg^{2+} activates a Na^+, K^+ ATPase pump that in turn plays a major role in regulat-

ing Na^+, K^+-transport (131). Loss of cardiac cellular Mg^{2+} has been demonstrated to decrease the activity of the pump (but not affect the number of Na^+, K^+-pump sites) (132) and to result in loss of critically important phosphagens: MgATP and PCr (6,14,40,50,60,74,133, 134). We have reported that 4 to 8 weeks of Mg deficiency in rats (serum Mg fell from 1.85 to 0.72 mg percent) resulted in significant falls in adenosine 5'-diphosphate (ADP), mitochondrial oxygen consumption, creatine phosphokinase (mitochondrial and myofibrillar), and several acid extractable phospholipid precursors from left ventricular cardiac muscle (123). Using isolated perfused rat hearts, reflectance spectroscopy, and ^{31}P-NMR, we have found that rapid, acute reductions in $[Mg^{2+}]_o$ can induce concomitant rapid decreases in contractile force, coronary flow, as well as reductions in PCr, pHi, and free intracellular Mg^{2+} (Table 7), and decreases in the steady-state levels of oxymyoglobin and the extent of oxidized cytochrome aa_3 (40,135,136); elevations in $[Mg^{2+}]_o$, i.e., above 1.2 mM Mg^{2+}, resulted in increases in inotropic activity for a short time, elevations in coronary flow and PCr, rises in pHi, and rises in the steady-state levels of oxymyoglobin and the extent of oxidized cytochrome aa_3 (36–39,135).

Thus, under conditions where cellular Mg^{2+} is depleted, Na^+-K^+ pump activity, phosphagen stores, pHi, and cardiac cellular bioenergetics will be compromised, leading to alterations in resting membrane potentials (e.g., membrane depolarization); ion transport dysfunctions (e.g., loss of K^+, gain of Na^+ and Ca^{2+}); and loss of contractile force and cardiac output (e.g., Fig. 1).

Hypoxia-Ischemia

During the past decade, a considerable amount of interest has been generated with respect to salutary effects of Mg^{2+} on mechanical and electrophysiological recovery after myocardial ischemia or anoxia in animals and humans (1–14,39,40,44,54,57,62–65,78,89,92–95,102, 104–106,117,118,120,121,136), as well as in drug-induced arrhythmias, myocardial infarction, and congestive heart failure (see references in 2,9,10,11,54,56, 63,137). However, it is not clear as to how these beneficial actions of Mg arise. For example, does loss of extracellular ionized Mg^2 and/or cytosolic free cardiac muscle Mg^{2+} promote arrhythmogenesis? If so, is this a consequence of ionic changes in cardiac muscle and/or coronary vascular muscle (50)? Does hypoxia per se promote arrhythmogenesis without alterations in $[Mg^{2+}]_i$ or $[Mg^{2+}]_o$? Recent observations support the reverse (54, 55,78,92,98). It has been shown with ion-selective microelectrodes that graded degrees of hypoxia will produce reversible decreases in intracellular, free $[Mg^{2+}]_i$ (34). Interestingly, this same group as well as others have found that elevating $[Mg^{2+}]_o$ from 0.5–10.0 mM/L results in a reversible increase of $[Mg^{2+}]_i$ in cardiac cells (34,36–40,100). Others have reported, in a preliminary communication, that a similar elevation in $[Mg^{2+}]_o$ also increases efflux of $^{28}Mg^{2+}$ from isolated rat hearts (138). However, during ischemia the rate of $^{28}Mg^{2+}$ efflux was retarded markedly, but was not seen on reperfusion after ischemia (138). Above, we indicated that ischemia per se could provoke either a loss or a rise in cytosolic $[Mg^{2+}]_i$ with falling ATP levels. At present, it is not completely clear how Mg^{2+} exerts its beneficial cardiac actions. At the very least, the beneficial actions of Mg^{2+} are clearly multifactorial in nature (Table 6). In conclusion, it is apparent that Mg^{2+} exerts direct actions on cardiac muscle cells and on cardiac bioenergetics and modulates stability and excitability of these cell membranes, attributes that would be important tools in the therapy of hypertension.

MAGNESIUM METABOLISM AND HYPERTENSIVE DISEASE

Although it was first demonstrated in 1925 by Blackfan and Hamilton (139) that infusion of a Mg salt could reverse hypertension in some patients, this concept was not taken seriously until relatively recently. Experimentally, it is now known that dietary Mg deficiency can produce hypertension (140–143; Berthelot et al., *personal communication*) and aggravate preexisting hypertension (141–146). A number of reports, reviewed below, have appeared that indicate that intravenous infusion or systemic or oral administration of Mg salts can lower the arterial blood pressure of renal hypertensives, essential hypertensives, pregnancy-induced hypertensives, diuretic-induced hypertensives, drug-induced hypertensives, and alcohol-induced hypertensives. Arterial blood pressure was significantly lowered in at least two of these studies after only 3 to 5 weeks of Mg supplementation (147,148). But what is the evidence for a role for Mg in hypertensive vascular disease? And, do hypertensive animals and patients present with significant hypomagnesemia?

Evidence for Role of Mg in Hypertensive Vascular Disease

Experimental

With respect to a link between Mg and experimental hypertension, several reports are available utilizing various animal models. For example, experiments have been carried out using dietary deficiency of Mg in rats, spontaneously hypertensive rats (SHRs), audiogenic stress in rats, deoxycorticosterone acetate (DOCA)-salt induced hypertension in rats, and pulmonary hypertension in rats induced with monocrotaline or hypoxia. In 1984, it was reported that 12 weeks of mild dietary deficiency of Mg could induce elevation of blood pressure and constriction of arterioles, venules, and precapillary sphincters in the microcirculation (140); the milder the dietary depletion of Mg, the less the elevation in arterial blood pressure and the less the peripheral vasoconstriction. Using SHRs, it has been demonstrated that they have lower red blood cell and plasma Mg levels than either Wistar controls or Wistar-Kyoto (WKY) rats (150–154, Table 8). From a number of these studies, it is also clear that SHRs exhibit elevated serum Ca/Mg ratios (e.g., 14,150,151). The latter would tend to elevate arteriolar tone, increase peripheral vascular reactivity, and increase peripheral vascular resistance. More recently, Ng and coworkers, using the fluorescent probe mag-fura-2 to measure intracellular free Mg ($[Mg^{2+}]_i$), reported that aortic smooth muscle cells as well as striated muscle cells in these SHRs exhibited lowered levels of $[Mg^{2+}]_i$ (47).

In 1981, it was first suggested by Altura and Altura (155) that vascular smooth muscle cells from SHR may have decreased membrane permeability to $[Mg^{2+}]_o$, lowered $[Mg^{2+}]_i$, and altered Ca^{2+}-Mg^{2+} exchange and membrane-binding sites (155). At that time, we also noted that elevation of extracellular Mg^{2+} ($[Mg^{2+}]_o$) exerted very little in the way of a relaxant action on SHR blood vessels, indicating an underlying defect in vascular Mg^{2+} metabolism and calcium handling at the plasma and intracellular membranes (155). Furthermore, we suggested that these defects are probably inherited (140). More recently, this hypothesis has received support from three

TABLE 8. *Serum magnesium levels in spontaneously hypertensive rats (SHR)*

Normotensive		SHR			
Serum Mg (mM/L)	No. of animals	Serum Mg (mM/L)	No. of animals	Age (wk)	Reference No.
1.24 ± 0.057	34	0.92 ± 0.24	29*	14–16	150
0.88 ± 0.04	12	0.78 ± 0.03	12†	11	151
0.86 ± 0.02	8	0.79 ± 0.01	8†	8	152
2.02 ± 0.07		1.08 ± 0.05	30*	19–21	154

Values are means ± SEM.
* $p < 0.001$.
† $p < 0.05$.

different types of studies in human subjects, one study done in intact humans with mild hypertension (156) and two done on plasma membranes of red blood cells obtained from patients with high blood pressure (157,158). Fujita and coworkers (156) clearly found an attenuated vasodilator response to administration of Mg in subjects with borderline hypertension compared to controls, whereas Mattingly and colleagues (157) noted that red blood cell (RBC) plasma membranes from hypertensives did not handle Mg^{2+} as did similar RBC membranes from controls. Paolisso and his colleagues reported that erythrocyte membranes of essential hypertensive patients exhibit decreased permeability to $[Mg^{2+}]_o$ (158).

If hypertension is, in part, due to imbalance in transport of Mg^{2+} across plasma membranes, one should see alterations in either its transport per se and/or alterations in cellular content and subcellular distribution of this divalent cation in blood vessels and the myocardium. In 1986, Wallach and Verch (159) reported that several tissues from SHRs demonstrated significantly lowered levels of Mg (e.g., heart, lungs, kidney, bone). In 1991, using SHRs Jelicks and Gupta reported that intracellular free Mg^{2+} concentration is decreased in these hypertensive rat hearts concomitant with an elevation in P_i and a decrease in the cytosolic phosphorylation potential (161). More recently, others using rats stressed with noise, to induce high blood pressure, found that both the heart and blood vessels exhibited significantly lowered levels of Mg concomitant with elevations in Ca content (141,142,160). The work of others on isolated RBC membranes, obtained from hypertensive subjects, suggests rather strongly that Mg^{2+} is not bound (or probably transported) in the same manner as in normal RBC membranes (157). However, to our knowledge good experimental data on Mg^{2+} transport across either vascular smooth muscle or cardiac myocyte plasma membranes from hypertensive subjects or animals are not available. No data are available on subcellular transport of $[Mg^{2+}]_i$ in tissues of hypertensive animals or humans.

If Mg is important in the etiology and pathophysiology of hypertensive vascular disease, one might expect less than normal Mg intake to exacerbate a preexisting hypertensive state and excess Mg intake to lower arterial blood pressure. As expected, SHRs as well as DOCA-salt maintained rats and audiogenic-stressed rats fed diets low in Mg intake clearly exhibit an exacerbation of arterial blood pressure (141,142,144,145,160). Oral and parenteral administration of Mg^{2+} can lower blood pressure in SHRs, audiogenic-stressed animals, and DOCA-salt maintained hypertensive animals (6,10,14,41,142,144, 145,160,162,163). In addition, it has also been demonstrated that Mg can attenuate elevations in arterial blood pressure induced by nonspecific stressors (164).

Is there evidence to indicate that there is a genetic predisposition to hypertension that is Mg- and sex-linked? In the past 5 years, a group in Japan published several

reports that suggest that male children of parents with a genetic history of familial hypertension exhibit significant deficits in red blood cell Mg content (202,203). In these studies of junior high school students there was an inverse relationship between arterial blood pressure and red blood cell intracellular Mg content. These are the first studies to support the suggestion we made in 1984 (140) that there probably is a close relationship between genetic control of tissue $[Mg^{2+}]_i$ and a predisposition for high blood pressure.

Rats made pulmonary hypertensive either by feeding a plant extract, monocrotaline, or by subjection to experimental hypoxia, exhibit significant attenuation of pulmonary hypertension and right ventricular hypertrophy when fed Mg salts (165–170). In addition, in a series of experiments, we have demonstrated that pulmonary vascular muscle and endothelial cell hyperplasia, characteristic of pulmonary hypertension, can be almost completely prevented by feeding rats higher than normal Mg intake in their diets (166–168). Such findings, which remain to be demonstrated in humans with pulmonary hypertension, suggest that Mg^{2+} may exert effects on collagen and elastin deposition as well as the enzymes and growth factors involved in the hyperplastic process observed in pulmonary hypertension.

Very recently, Laurant and coworkers (163) using rats with DOCA-salt hypertension found that Mg-enriched diets not only reduced mean arterial blood pressure but increased the generation of PGI_2 (prostacycline) in their aortas. This was not seen in control animals. An increased synthesis of PGI_2 in peripheral blood vessels and tissues would, in itself, tend to lower arterial blood pressure, as it is a powerful vasodilator substance and acts to prevent platelet aggregation. Such an observation lends support to the hypothesis suggested a few years ago by Nadler et al. (171), from studies in hypertensive human subjects, that prostanoids may be the target site for Mg^{2+}. They reported that administration of the cyclooxygenase inhibitor, indomethacin, to these patients prevented the beneficial blood pressure–lowering action of Mg. It is of interest to point out here that the potency of the vasodilator action of PGI_2 and eicosanoids on peripheral blood vessels is controlled by the concentration of Mg^{2+} (172,173).

Whether or not the primary effects of Mg deficiency are on Ca^{2+} release and on membrane binding in vascular smooth muscle and cardiac myocytes (2,6,10,14,28, 39,50,75,96), and the secondary actions are on modulation of synthesis of vasodilator (and/or vasoconstrictor) substances, is not clear. However, it is clear that in those cases in which electrolyte contents and fluxes have been examined, Ca is always also altered. However, data on other electrolytes are beginning to point toward the importance of other ions like phosphate in Mg deficiency–induced hypertension (134,174). We have demonstrated that rats that develop severe hypertension, as a consequence of implanting large doses of DOCA (and feeding NaCl), exhibit serum hypomagnesemia and hypophosphatemia concomitant with elevation in serum Ca (10,14). Such animals fed Mg (in the form of Mg aspartate HCl) show marked attenuation of the high blood pressure and a restoration of both the serum and Mg and phosphate levels to normal. Since hypophosphatemia, in itself, has been shown to cause hypertension (134,174), one must raise the possibility that alterations in phosphate metabolism may play an important role in certain forms of Mg deficiency–induced hypertension. In any event, the experimental findings, gathered from numerous laboratories over the past 10 years, support the hypothesis offered more than 15 years ago that defects in Mg metabolism and deficits in dietary intake of Mg are probably important contributing factors to several forms of experimental hypertension (150,175).

Clinical

There have been at least 28 independent studies demonstrating that patients with hypertension of diverse etiologies can exhibit hypomagnesemia either in serum and/or tissues (14). On average, patients with long-term essential hypertension appear to exhibit at least a 15 percent deficit in total serum Mg (14). Reports by Petersen et al. (176), Resnick et al. (177), Dyckner and Wester (178), Touyz et al. (179,181), Paolisso et al. (182), and Shingu et al. (183) clearly demonstrate inverse correlations between total serum (or tissue) Mg concentration and arterial blood pressures. Other studies provide evidence for the idea that certain hypertensive patients exhibit reduced urinary excretion of Mg that is inversely correlated to diastolic blood pressure (14).

The average 15 percent deficit in total Mg mentioned above, which we calculated from 24 different studies in the literature (14), would represent a loss of 125 μM from the serum. If this represented a deficit of free, ionized $[Mg^{2+}]_i$, it would be enough to produce constriction of arterioles in the splanchnic and skeletal muscle vasculatures (14,140–142); 125 μM $[Mg^{2+}]_o$ is known to induce vasodilation of arterioles in these microvasculatures, at least in the rat (184–186).

A number of epidemiologic studies support a rather strong inverse relationship between dietary intake of Mg (or vegetables high in Mg) and systolic arterial blood pressures (1,2,4,14,150,187–192). However, at least one epidemiologic study carried out in Belgium did not find an inverse relationship between dietary Mg intake and systemic arterial blood pressure (193). Although several studies found that Mg treatment of hypertensives lowered arterial blood pressure significantly (e.g., 148,156, 171,178,182,194–196), several studies could not confirm a beneficial effect of Mg supplementation, even in mild, untreated hypertensives (197–200). A number of

confounding factors could, however, account for these differences in efficacy. In some beneficial studies, Mg oxide was used with great effect (148); in others where no significant effects were observed, Mg aspartate was usually the salt used. In addition, in a number of the studies, in which no significant effects on arterial blood pressure were observed, the Mg supplementation either failed to alter the serum level of Mg or failed to increase significantly the urinary output of Mg; this might signify differences in basal Mg balance and/or metabolism among the groups of subjects. Moreover, there was often no change in either red blood cell Mg or plasma renin activity (199), suggesting possibly that the dose of Mg given either was too small (e.g., only 10 mmol/day) or was not given long enough (e.g., only 8 weeks). An attenuated vasodilator response, first noticed in SHR rats (155) and seen clinically recently in some subjects with borderline hypertension (156), supports the latter hypothesis. It must also be entertained that since all of the previous studies assessed only total Mg (TMg), but not ionized Mg (IMg^{2+}), the former parameter to guide therapeutic efficacy may not be reliable. Recently, we have found that even borderline hypertensives usually exhibit significantly depressed serum ionized, but not total, Mg levels (*unpublished data*). Moreover, pregnant women with transient hypertension during labor clearly exhibit deficits in IMg^{2+}, but not TMg, which is related to the incidence of hypertension (201). In addition, it is clear from the positive results obtained so far that oral Mg supplementation seems to be of particular benefit in hypertensive subjects who are receiving traditional nonpotassium-sparing diuretics (178,195,196) and that irrespective of the therapy used to treat hypertensive subjects, an alleviation of the high blood pressure is always associated with elevation in the levels of RBC intracellular free Mg (177).

Ionized Intracellular Free Magnesium Ions are Lowered in Vascular Smooth Muscle and Blood Cells in Hypertensive Animals and Humans

If a deficit in intracellular free Mg is important in the etiology of hypertensive vascular disease, then vascular smooth muscle cells, blood cells (i.e., RBCs and platelets), as well as whole blood, plasma, and serum from both hypertensive animals and human subjects with hypertensive vascular disease would be expected to demonstrate such intracellular as well as extracellular losses of Mg^{2+}. A number of studies employing ^{31}P-NMR spectroscopy, the fluorescent probe mag-fura-2, and unique Mg^{2+} ion-selective electrodes support this supposition (13,47,49,56,145,153,177,181,205,230,231,252,255, 256). At least two of these studies demonstrate a close correspondence between RBC $[Mg^{2+}]_i$ and serum $[Mg^{2+}]_o$ but not total Mg in essential hypertensive and noninsulin-dependent diabetes mellitus (NIDDM) subjects (230,231). Figure 2 illustrates such a relationship in NIDDM hypertensive patients. Although this new data is only for a limited number of patients, it certainly strengthens the idea that hypertensive vascular disease is most probably associated with a "true" defect in intracellular free Mg.

Evidence for Role of Mg in Diabetic Vascular Disease

Experimental

Several studies have been published during the past decade on experimental diabetes mellitus, its vascular effects, and Mg (2,6,9,10,14,56,150,155). Streptozotocin-induced DM in rats is clearly associated with an intense magnesuria, glycosuria, and polyuria (136). The increase in urinary Mg concentration parallels the degree of glycosuria. This supports and extends numerous previous findings that DM can result in hypomagnesemia (2,4,6,9,14,155,205–209). Basal tension of aortas and portal veins excised from rats administered alloxan steadily increased from the first through the eighth week as the degree of diabetes (assessed by serum glucose, triglycerides, cholesterol, and creatinine) became progressively worse (150,210). These studies also demonstrated alterations in vascular reactivity associated with elevated serum Na/Ca and Ca/Mg ratios. Twenty to 25 percent of the latter alloxan-diabetic rats exhibited significant elevations in arterial blood pressure by the eighth week after treatment (150). This is particularly interesting since long-term DM in humans results in hypertension in 40 to 80 percent of patients (14,207). Elevation of $[Mg^{2+}]_o$ failed to relax the diabetic rat aortas; diabetic venous smooth muscle also demonstrated little response to high concentrations of Mg^{2+} (14,155,210). Most importantly, the diabetic vessels of these rats showed marked eleva-

tions in total exchangeable and membrane-bound calcium (211). Such data overall lend support to the concept that the vascular membranes in diabetic subjects probably have undergone alterations in their Mg-Ca exchange sites and permeability to $[Mg^{2+}]_o$ (155). But are these divalent cation, permeability, and membrane alterations a result of the diabetic state or are they linked to the etiology of the syndrome? Boquist and coworkers (212,213) have found that alloxan and streptozotocin can produce direct alterations in membrane permeability to mouse liver mitochondria *in vitro*. High concentrations of alloxan reduced efflux of endogenous Mg^{2+}, K^+, and adenine nucleotides, efflux of accumulated Ca^+, K^+-uptake inhibition, loss of membrane potential, and swelling. We were particularly interested to learn from these studies that the loss of Mg^{2+} preceded the release of accumulated Ca^{2+}, which parallels the efflux of K^+ and swelling. This thus resembles very closely what has been observed for Mg-K-Ca interactions and control of vascular homeostasis (2,6,50,108). In addition, animal studies have indicated that there is increased glucagon stimulation (214), decreased insulin secretion (215), and reduced insulin uptake in low $[Mg^{2+}]_o$ (216). It will be important to extend such studies with alloxan and streptozotocin to isolated blood vessels and electrolyte transport across the vascular walls.

Clinical

With respect to clinical observations in diabetes mellitus, there appears to be a strong growing association between it, hypertension, and abnormal glucose tolerance (182,205,217). Control of diabetes mellitus is inversely related to Mg deficiency (204,206,207,218–220). Diabetic retinopathy is clearly associated with a state of Mg deficiency (14,218,221,222). Interestingly, insulin-dependent diabetes mellitus as well as NIDDM are associated with reduced total serum and intracellular levels

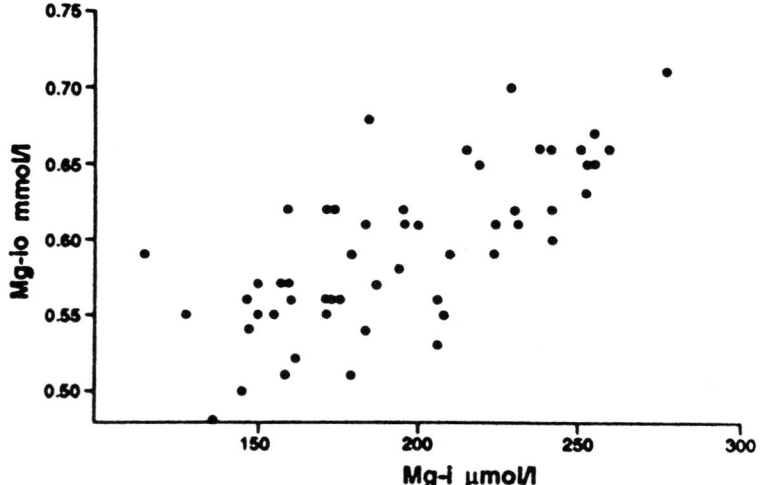

FIG. 2. Relation of serum ionized magnesium values (Mg-io) to intracellular levels of free magnesium. Mg$_i$, intracellular free magnesium levels. Mg-io and Mg$_i$ were significantly related. $r = 0.728$ ($p < 0.001$). (From ref. 231, with permission.)

of Mg (14,207,223–228,231) and increased urinary loss of Mg (24,207,229). Even though all of the subjects investigated did not always exhibit simultaneous reduction in serum total Mg and intracellular free Mg, oral Mg treatment improved control of both insulin-dependent DM (226) and NIDDM (182,227).

We have utilized a new ISE for ionized magnesium to measure serum IMg^{2+} in fasting subjects with and without NIDDM, and compared these values to levels of serum TMg and intracellular free Mg^{2+} analyzed in RBCs by ^{31}P-NMR spectroscopy (230,231). Both IMg^{2+} and intracellular free Mg^{2+}, but not TMg, were significantly reduced in NIDDM compared with nondiabetic controls. A close relationship was noted between serum IMg^{2+} and intracellular free Mg^{2+} ($r = 0.73$, $p < 0.001$) (Fig. 2). We therefore hypothesize that Mg deficiency, both extracellular and intracellular, is a characteristic of chronic stable mild NIDDM, and may predispose subjects to the excess cardiovascular morbidity of the diabetic state. Moreover, by adequately reflecting cellular Mg metabolism rather than total serum Mg levels, IMg^{2+} measurements may provide a more readily available tool than has heretofore been available to analyze Mg metabolism in a variety of vascular related diseases.

Mg AND ATHEROGENESIS—IMPORTANT LINK BETWEEN VASCULAR DISEASE, HYPERTENSION, AND ISCHEMIC HEART DISEASE

Hypercholesterolemia has been widely accepted as a high-risk factor for development of atherosclerosis, hypertension, and ischemic heart disease (3,10,232), particularly since cholesterol-rich diets lead to deposition of lipids in blood vessel walls and an atherosclerotic-like state in experimental animals (233). Increased blood levels of lipoproteins are thought to lead eventually to endothelial cell injury or denudation with concomitant uptake of the former molecules (234,235). However, it is not clear how the lipoproteins and Ca^{2+} gain access to the normally and relatively impermeable arterial walls. Approximately 35 years ago, it was suggested that use of intramuscular $MgSO_4$ in patients with coronary insufficiency might lower serum B-lipoproteins and result in improvement of the clinical condition (236). It has been known for some time that Mg deficiency is associated with a number of dyslipidemias (3,10,28,237–242). We have recently found that dietary deficiency of Mg in rabbits (compatible with the reduced dietary intake of Mg seen in the adult population of the Western world) exacerbates atherogenesis and lipid deposition in arterial muscle, and stimulates (or activates) macrophages of the reticuloendothelial system (RES) (243,244). In addition, we demonstrated that pretreatment of animals with orally administered Mg aspartate HCl: (a) attenuated the atherosclerotic process markedly, (b) lowered serum cholesterol and triglycerides in normal as well as atherosclerotic animals, and (c) attenuated elevated Ca in the arterial wall. In addition, in these studies, we noted that the extent of the atherogenic lesions was, in fact, poorly correlated with the level of serum cholesterol and highly dependent on the level of dietary Mg. It would appear from these new, quantitative data that dietary Mg intake plays an important modulatory role in controlling lipid metabolism in the arterial wall. Many of these results have been confirmed recently by others (245). In recent studies, we have noted that oral Mg administration to rabbits with developing atherosclerosis, in the arterial walls, can reverse a large part of the atherogenesis (246a). Such new experiments lend support to the hypothesis that early intervention with higher than normal dietary intake of Mg could attenuate the incidence of atherogenesis.

HARDNESS OF DRINKING WATER, SOIL MAGNESIUM CONTENT, AND HYPERTENSIVE VASCULAR DISEASE

Ever since the work of Kobayashi in Japan in 1957, it has been suggested that the hardness of drinking water may be associated with the prevention of cardiovascular ailments (1,8,10,57,59,257–260). Controversy has, however, arisen regarding such an association (261). It has often been taken for granted that "hardness of water" implies a high content of Mg^{2+}. If one ingests about 2.4 liters of water per day in total fluid intake (e.g., soft drinks, fruit juices, beverages, water, etc.), then depending upon the area of residence, the Mg^{2+} intake may vary from as little as 2 mg/day (e.g., in South Africa, Newfoundland) to as much as 175 mg/day [e.g., in a very-hard-water area of California (258,260,262)].

Water hardness is primarily dependent on the calcium and magnesium concentrations (260); if hard-water geographic areas around the world are considered, one can find very-hard-water areas (>400 mg/L Mg^{2+}) but the Mg^{2+} level can be very low in certain regions (e.g., <6 mg/L) (258,260,262). So, one can indeed have hard water (e.g., large amounts of Ca^{2+}) without much Mg^{2+}. This has been the problem in attempting to correlate many of the epidemiologic studies in hard- versus soft-water areas. A hardness of 100 is considered average. Thus, water having a 600 hardness is very hard; indeed, this occurs in France and Italy, and despite this the water may contain a very low concentration of Mg^{2+} (e.g., only 16 mg/L in Lille, France) (258). It is clear from several studies done to date (14,257,258), in which either water hardness or Mg^{2+} levels were carefully ascertained, that there is an inverse relationship between water hardness or Mg^{2+} and arterial blood pressure (and hypertensive vascular disease) (263–266). The lower the hardness of

Mg in these studies, the higher the arterial blood pressure. Although several additional epidemiologic studies also exist (e.g., ref. 266), these in the main either did not accurately assess water hardness (or Mg content) or utilized boys and girls rather than middle-aged men and women. So, there does appear to be an inverse correlation between hardness of water or Mg content and incidence (development?) of hypertension.

If one arbitrarily divides the United States into Eastern and Western halves, the measured soil Mg content, on average, in the Eastern U.S. is about one-third that of the Western U.S. (e.g., 2,300 vs. 7,800 μg/g [Mg], $p < 0.001$) (261). The calculated water hardness of the Eastern U.S., on average, is one-half that of the Western U.S. (e.g., 81 ± 56 vs. 154 ± 71 μg/g, means $\pm$ SD, $p < 0.001$) (261). Although the death rate for cardiovascular diseases in the Eastern U.S. is significantly higher than that of the Western U.S. (429 ± 39 vs. 366 ± 32, $p < 0.001$, 1979 figures), noncardiovascular death rates are equivalent (261). Similar phenomena have been observed in Canada, Finland, and South Africa (1,258,260,262,267,268). Leary and Reyes (262) published findings from 12 magisterial districts in South Africa demonstrating that as the concentration of Mg in the drinking water in various geographical regions was found to be less and less, the death rate from ischemic heart disease was seen to rise more and more. Studies such as these (1,258,260,267,268) suggest that there may be an important relationship between dietary Mg intake and the incidence of hypertensive vascular disease.

DIETARY Mg INTAKE, Mg DAILY REQUIREMENTS, FOOD SUPPLY, AND CARDIOVASCULAR-HYPERTENSIVE DISEASE

At the turn of the century in the United States, ingestion of magnesium was about 450–485 mg/day

TABLE 9. Effects of food preparation on magnesium loss

Food	Mg (mg/kg)	% Mg loss
Potatoes		
Baked in skin	290	0
Boiled	240	17
Peas		
Fresh	330	0
Boiled	210	36
Carrots		
Raw	120	0
Cooked	70	36
Cabbage		
Raw	170	0
Boiled	70	59
Brussels sprouts		
Raw	280	0
Boiled	110	61

TABLE 10. Refining and processing foods results in severe loss of magnesium contents

Food	Mg (mg/kg dry wt)	% Mg loss
Molasses	170–250	0
White sugar	2	98.8–99.2
Wheat	1500–1670	0
Flour	210–299	80.1–87.4
Corn	644	0
Starch	22	96.6
Unpolished rice	1477	0
Polished rice	251	83.0

(269,270). The most recent figures indicate that these values are now much lower (e.g., men $\sim$ 185 to 260 mg/day; women $\sim$ 172 to 235 mg/day, $n = 25,264$) (259). If we accept that the recommended daily allowance (RDA) = 350 mg/day, these values represent dietary deficits of 90–178 mg/day. Surveys in Europe and North America reveal just as alarming deficits in dietary intake of Mg (e.g., men $\sim$ 189–262 mg/day; women $\sim$ 143–283 mg/day, $n = 3,400$); these values represent deficits of 67–161 mg/day (259). If we accept the idea of some investigators that the current RDA (i.e., 350 mg/day for men, 300 mg/day for women) recommended by the U.S. National Academy of Sciences is too low (4,259,269) and that it should be 450–500 mg/day (4,269,271), the deficits become very pronounced, thereby placing the American population at risk for development of disease processes, particularly when numerous physiological functions (Table 2) could be curtailed or compromised.

In addition to a probable dietary deficiency of Mg in the average human subject's daily food supply in North America and Europe, it should be stressed that we tend to forget that when foods (containing Mg) are cooked and processed (or refined), most food staples lose more than 65 percent of the Mg content (Tables 9 and 10). Such a situation results in further reductions in dietary intake of Mg.

According to epidemiologic studies in which dietary variables were assessed in 615 human subjects by the 24-hr recall method, Mg had the strongest association with blood pressure (272). During the past decade, a reduction in the consumption of fruits, vegetables, and unprocessed cereals has been observed globally (259,273). Together with this, there has been an increased consumption of processed food and a marked fall in Mg intake (4,259,271). Is the known amelioration and decreased incidence of hypertension in human subjects placed on vegetarian diets (192,259,273,274) a consequence of the increased dietary intake of Mg? Legumes, nuts, beans, green leafy vegetables, and unprocessed cereals, which form the basis of vegetarian diets, are rich in Mg (Tables 9 and 10). Considerable data have now accumulated to demonstrate that a variety of coronary heart diseases and myocardial ischemic syndromes, such

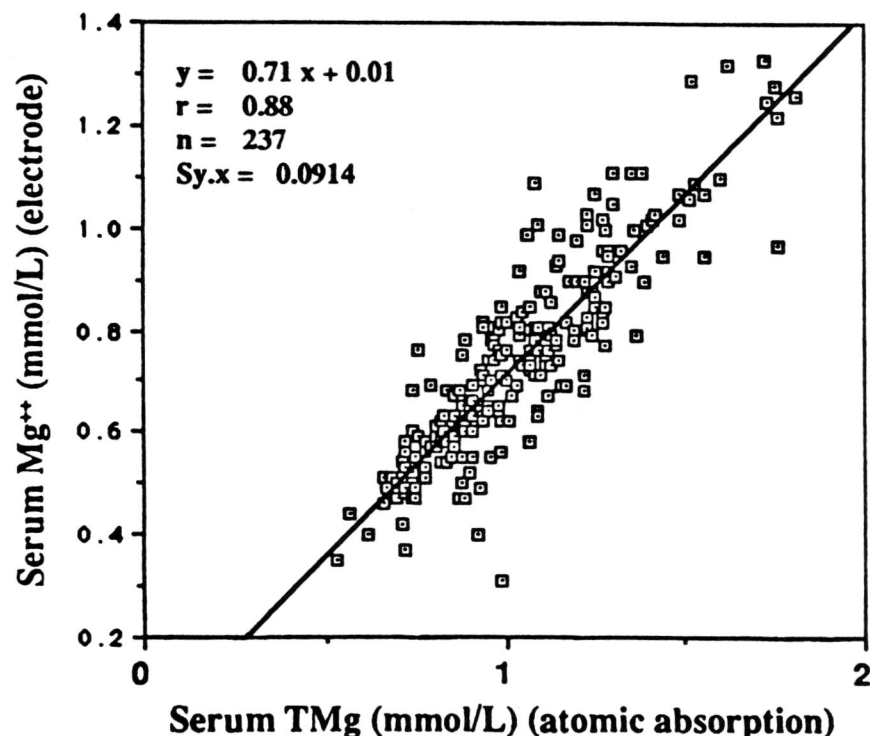

$$y = 0.71 x + 0.01$$
$$r = 0.88$$
$$n = 237$$
$$Sy.x = 0.0914$$

FIG. 3. Serum IMg^{2+} versus serum total magnesium (TMg). Correlation of Mg^{2+} [ion-selective electrode (ISE)] with TMg (atomic absorption) on serums taken from normal faculty and staff, students, and patients undergoing cardiac surgery.

as unstable angina pectoris, sudden-death ischemic heart disease, acute myocardial infarction, torsades des pointes, and cardiomyopathies, are often associated with profound losses in myocardial Mg, ionized Mg as well as total body Mg (1,3–13,50,51,63,64,95,112,137,155,257, 258,269,271,275–280).

SERUM IONIZED MAGNESIUM IN CARDIOVASCULAR-HYPERTENSIVE DISEASE AND HOSPITALIZED PATIENTS

Although chronic serum hypomagnesemia has often been associated with multiple clinical cardiovascular disorders, serum total Mg (TMg) has not always been reduced, leaving clinicians and experimentalists to conclude that Mg may not be important in cardiovascular disease. Previous studies have been hindered by the use of TMg as a reflection of Mg homeostasis. TMg is a measurement of all Mg in the serum, including Mg that is bound to proteins and anions as well as "free" biologically active, ionized Mg (IMg^{2+}).

Using the new ISEs (281), it has now been demonstrated by three different laboratories that IMg^{2+}, but not TMg, is usually significantly depressed (12–50 percent) in ischemic heart disease, cardiac arrhythmias, acute myocardial infarction, NIDDM, renal-hypertensive disease, and essential hypertension; the magnitude of the deficit in IMg^{2+} often being dependent upon the cardiovascular disease and its severity (56,201,230,231,253–255,281–285).

IMg^{2+}, in contrast to TMg, data recently obtained from cardiopulmonary bypass patients (who in the main had a history of hypertensive vascular disease) indicates a wide scatter about the regression line (Fig. 3) that in our opinion most likely reflects differences in Mg^{2+} binding to anions from serum sample to serum sample (283,284). This type of data suggests that TMg determinations cannot be used to predict the biologically active IMg^{2+} values. This probably represents a clear indication that the IMg^{2+} level should prove to be a valuable diagnostic and prognostic parameter in critical care and acute medical-cardiovascular settings.

ASSOCIATION BETWEEN Mg LEVELS, CERTAIN DRUG TOXICITIES, CHRONIC ALCOHOLISM, AND HYPERTENSION

A number of disease states that result in elevation of arterial blood pressure are often associated with decreased levels of serum IMg^{2+}/TMg and/or tissue $[Mg^{2+}]_i$/TMg (1,4,6,7,9–11,50,54,56,63,143,208, 257,258,269,271,281). Chronic alcoholism, often leading to hypertensive vascular disease, appears to be associated with serum, myocardial, and vascular tissue loss of both bound and free Mg (14,23,30,134,143,281,286–290). In addition, 60 to 80 percent of chronic alcoholics develop high blood pressure, which remains to be explained (143,291–293). Recent experimental findings suggest that a continued and progressive loss of cellular ionized Mg may set into motion the alcohol-induced hypertension (143,289).

Hypomagnesemia Associated With Cyclosporine, Organ Transplantation, Cisplatin, and Calcium-Induced Hypertension

Toxicities of certain drugs, for example cyclosporine, which is widely used to suppress immune function prior to organ transplantation, and cisplatin, widely used to treat testicular cancer, appear to be associated with a high frequency of hypomagnesemia and concomitant hypertension and/or intense peripheral vasoconstriction, namely, a Raynaud-type syndrome (1,6,7,11,14,50, 54,56,253,255,257,280,294,295–297). Renal transplant recipients exhibit marked deficits in serum IMg^{2+} compared to control, healthy subjects, with very little change in either TMg or serum ionized calcium (ICa^{2+}) (253,255). The serum IMg^{2+} level correlates inversely with the cyclosporine trough level. The ratio of ICa^{2+}/ IMg^{2+}, a sign of potential peripheral vasoconstriction, is elevated in these renal patients (253,255) and correlates positively with the cyclosporine trough level. These ionic alterations could contribute significantly to cyclosporine-induced hypertension and nephrotoxicity. Accelerated atherosclerosis observed after renal transplantation may relate to alterations in IMg^{2+}, which are associated with atherogenesis in other models (243,244).

Hypercalcemic hypertension also appears to be associated with a hypomagnesemic state (298). Whether or not the latter is associated with a deficit in IMg^{2+} is not known. It will be important, in the near future, to try to correlate the degree of peripheral vasoconstriction in these syndromes with the degree of cellular Mg^{2+} depletion.

END-STAGE RENAL DISEASE, DIALYSIS, UREMIA, Mg METABOLISM, AND HYPERTENSION

In the United States, atherosclerotic disease is the leading cause of death in patients with end-stage renal disease, whether treated by hemodialysis or continuous ambulatory peritoneal dialysis (CAPD) (299).

In healthy individuals, more than 75 percent of plasma Mg is filtered by the kidney; however, 65 percent of filtered Mg is reabsorbed in the loop of Henle (300). Dialysate Mg in standard solutions is absent or in the range of 0.25–0.4 mM/L because of the fear of producing hypermagnesemia in a population that lacks the ability to excrete Mg via glomerular filtration (301). Studies of tissue total Mg content in uremia patients are contradictory. For example, skeletal muscle TMg has been reported to decrease in some reports (302,303), whereas bone TMg has been reported to increase (304,305).

Recent studies employing ^{31}P-NMR spectroscopy (306) and ion-selective electrodes (254) in uremia subjects indicate that both tissue and serum demonstrate deficits in free Mg^{2+}. The percent of TMg that was ionized (percent IMg^{2+}) in serum of both hemodialysis and CAPD patients was low compared with that of controls (254). The mean ICa^{2+}/IMg^{2+} ratios were significantly elevated in both types of uremic patients. We conclude that both hemodialysis and CAPD patients have deficits in mean IMg^{2+} (and probably cellular $[Mg^{2+}]_i$) at the present levels of Mg in dialysates, and that the percent IMg^{2+} is low, resulting in masking of hypomagnesemia by normal or high TMg levels. Whether the observed increases in ICa^{2+}/IMg^{2+} ratios, associated with atherogenesis in animal models (243,244), contribute to cardiovascular-hypertensive disease in uremic-dialysis patients remains to be investigated.

VASOSPASM, Mg DEFICIENCY, AND HYPERTENSION

Several clinical entities, including hypertension of unknown origin, preeclampsia-eclampsia of pregnancy, alcohol-induced hypertension, diabetes-mellitus–induced hypertensive vascular disease, congestive heart failure, drug-induced hypertensive vascular diseases, and several types of ischemic heart disease (IHD) are associated with hypomagnesemia, as indicated above. A number of these hypertensive vascular diseases (e.g., primary hypertension, preeclampsia, DM, IHD), as reviewed above, often have the highest incidence in geographic regions that contain Mg^{2+}-poor water and/or Mg^{2+}-poor soil.

Mg Ions, Vascular Contractility, and Basal Vascular Tone

Magnesium ions have been shown to directly alter baseline tension or tone of blood vessels (2,5,6,14,50, 75,115,129,140,144,155). Decrements in extracellular Mg^{2+} result, in a concentration-dependent manner, in rapid elevations in contractile tension development in a variety of mammalian arteries and arterioles. Elevation in $[Mg^{2+}]_o$ concentration, on the other hand, above the physiological level inhibits spontaneous mechanical activity and lowers baseline tension; none of these findings can be attributed to changes in osmolarity or the release or synthesis of any known vasoactive substance.

We have shown previously that these elevations in mechanical activity are lowered markedly when external Ca^{2+} ions are lowered or chelated (28,155,175,208, 320,326). Such findings suggest that some influx of extracellular Ca^{2+} ions is necessary for these contractile responses. In addition, a variety of neurohumoral agents that induce contraction in vascular smooth muscle exhibit heightened contractile responses as external Mg^{2+} is lowered, and depressed or attenuated contractile activity is observed as $[Mg^{2+}]_o$ is elevated (2,5, 6,50,57,59,155,172,175,185,208,257,307,321). How are these actions of $[Mg^{2+}]_o$ brought about?

Mg^{2+} and Ca Channels

Evidence indicates that Mg^{2+} can regulate Ca^{2+} flux across the vascular smooth muscle cell membranes as well as its release from intracellular storage sites (2,5,6, 13,14,17,28,50,75,96,108–110,141,143,155,175,208, 252,307–309,315–321,326–382). Since a change in cytosolic free Ca^{2+} concentration is a very important second messenger in facilitation of contraction or relaxation, it may be physiologically relevant that Mg^{2+} regulate the activity of vascular smooth muscle cells by competing with Ca^{2+} and modulating the level of cytosolic free intracellular Ca^{2+}.

Acute administration of Mg in animals and humans induces hypotension and peripheral vasodilation (1,2,5,6). This vasodilator effect has been attributed, at least in part, to its Ca^{2+} channel-blocking property as well as modulation of intracellular free Ca^{2+} in vascular smooth muscle cells (2,3,28,96,155).

Influence of $[Mg^{2+}]_o$ on $[Ca^{2+}]_i$ and $[Mg^{2+}]_i$ in VSM and Endothelial Cells

Intracellular free Mg^{2+} is a cofactor for numerous enzymes and signal-transduction proteins and regulates bioenergetics and ion transport (Table 2). Thus, it seems desirable to know whether or not changes in external Mg concentration can alter intracellular free Mg^{2+} in vascular smooth muscle cells. It also seems desirable to know whether or not changes in external Mg^{2+} concentration can also alter the subcellular distribution of both intracellular compartmentalized Ca^{2+} and Mg^{2+}.

During the past ten years, it has become quite apparent that the endothelial cell layer plays an active and important role in modulating vascular tone by synthesizing and releasing a variety of endothelial-derived relaxant factors (EDRFs). Several different groups have now shown that these EDRFs are modulated by the extracellular concentration of Mg^{2+} (15,16,329–331). A rise of intracellular free Ca^{2+} concentration is known to be closely coupled to the synthesis and release of prostacyclin, EDRFs, and cell contraction in response to a number of agonists or physical stimuli. It is now well established that intracellular Ca^{2+} release in endothelial cells can be mediated by activation of plasma membrane receptors coupled to phospholipase C and generation of 1,4,5 inositol-trisphosphate or IP_3. However, the contribution of Ca^{2+} release via non–IP_3-dependent or Ca^{2+} release mechanisms in endothelial cells remains controversial. It would thus be of importance to define the role,

if any, of Mg^{2+} in Ca^{2+}-induced Ca^{2+} release in endothelial cells.

With these points in mind, we have undertaken a series of studies using cultured rat aortic and canine cerebral vascular smooth muscle cells as well as human aortic cells to define the role of external Mg in modulation of intracellular Ca^{2+} and intracellular Mg^{2+}, and their compartmentation, if any, in vascular muscle and endothelial cells. For these ongoing studies, we are directly measuring intracellular $[Ca^{2+}]_i$, and intracellular $[Mg^{2+}]_i$, and mapping the intracellular free calcium and Mg distribution via Ca^{2+} and Mg^{2+} imaging in single cells, similar to imaging techniques recently described (28,39,332). Aortic smooth muscle cells from rats as well as canine cerebral vascular smooth muscle cells were isolated and cultured in Dulbecco's modified Eagle's medium at 37 degrees centigrade in a humidified atmosphere composed of 95 percent air–5 percent CO_2. The intima of the blood vessels were rubbed gently with wire to rub off the endothelial cells (EC). Experiments were done to compare primary cultured cells to cells passed several times to determine whether this made a difference. In addition, a human aortic endothelial cell line obtained from the National Institutes of Health was utilized (17).

Immunohistochemical staining with a monoclonal antibody recognizing exclusively α-smooth muscle actinin indicates that over 96 percent of our cultures are pure vascular smooth muscle cells.

Changes in intracellular free Ca^{2+} were measured with the Ca^{2+} fluorescence indicator fura-2. This molecular probe has a high affinity for Ca^{2+} over Mg^{2+} and other divalent cations. A ratiometric technique was used to estimate intracellular free Ca^{2+} (332). All cells were loaded with 2 μM fura-2 acetoxymethyl ester, the cell-permeant form of fura-2 in the culture media for 60 min. After loading of the molecular fluorescent probe, the cells were perfused with media containing different concentrations of free Mg^{2+} and Ca^{2+}. Both ionic extracellular Mg^{2+} and Ca^{2+} concentrations were measured with ion-selective electrodes (283,284).

Background fluorescence for both excitation wavelengths was acquired from blanks for each experiment and subtracted from each pair of images separately before ratioing. Fluorescence ratios were obtained by dividing the 340-nm image by the 380-nm image. Intracellular free Ca^{2+} was calculated according to Grynkiewicz et al. (333). Particular care was taken to minimize photobleaching of the probe. Experiments were undertaken in total darkness and exposure to excitation light was less than 2 min in all experiments.

Aortic Smooth Muscle

Most of the vascular smooth muscle cells in primary cultures appeared spindle-shaped in 1.2 mM normal external Mg²⁺ concentration. The resting distribution of intracellular free Ca²⁺ appeared heterogeneous within the cells by ratio-image analysis. The perinuclear region, arbitrarily chosen as the central ellipsoid area in the widest part of the cell, revealed the most brightness, reflecting a relatively higher Ca²⁺ than the peripheral cytoplasmic area. This observation of a $[Ca^{2+}]_i$ gradient in the vascular muscle cell suggests that the plasma membrane and discrete localized processes, within the perinuclear area, may regulate intracellular free Ca²⁺ activity subcellularly (Fig. 4).

In order to probe the effects of $[Mg^{2+}]_o$ on intracellular free Ca²⁺, the extracellular Mg²⁺ concentrations in the media were altered. Somewhat to our surprise, removal of extracellular Mg after only 5 min of washing had dramatic effects on cell fluorescence and geometry (332). Removal of extracellular Mg²⁺ resulted in an increase in free intracellular Ca²⁺ concomitant with a rounding or contraction of the cells. Reduction in $[Mg^{2+}]_o$ to zero mM resulted in approximately a 6-fold increment in $[Ca^{2+}]_i$ (332). To examine the changes produced under physiological conditions, $[Mg^{2+}]_o$ was lowered to 0.3 mM, the lowest ionized physiological level seen clinically (281,283,284). This maneuver raised $[Ca^{2+}]_i$ about 3.5-fold. However, a heterogeneous distribution of $[Ca^{2+}]_i$ was still evident when $[Mg^{2+}]_o$ was lowered to 0.3 mM,

even though $[Ca^{2+}]_i$ in the peripheral cytoplasmic region was increased. Although the changes of cell geometry induced by contraction could influence the accuracy of $[Ca^{2+}]_i$ measurements, the ratioed image reflects an absolute increase in $[Ca^{2+}]_i$.

In contrast to lowering $[Mg^{2+}]_o$, elevation of Mg²⁺ to 4.8 mM (i.e., four times normal) was found to decrease $[Ca^{2+}]_i$ from about 95 nM to about 72 nM showing relatively less of an influence on $[Ca^{2+}]_i$ compared to $[Mg^{2+}]_o$ removal (332).

These observations support our previous findings in intact and isolated blood vessels that indicate that reduction in $[Mg^{2+}]_o$ results in spasm of blood vessels, elevation of basal tone, and increments in spontaneous mechanical activity. The intracellular free Ca²⁺ changes brought about by varying $[Mg^{2+}]_o$ clearly indicate the dependence of $[Ca^{2+}]_i$ and basal $[Ca^{2+}]_i$ upon $[Mg^{2+}]_o$.

To obtain further insights into the existence and nature of these regulatory processes, aortic cells were exposed to media in which both $[Ca^{2+}]_o$ and $[Mg^{2+}]_o$ were omitted (332). It was anticipated that such a maneuver would reveal the steady-state distribution of intracellular free Ca²⁺ across the sarcolemma and intracellular organelle membranes. A strong dependence of the $[Mg^{2+}]_o$-induced increment of $[Ca^{2+}]_i$ upon $[Ca^{2+}]_o$ was observed as exemplified by the marked lowering of $[Ca^{2+}]_i$ from

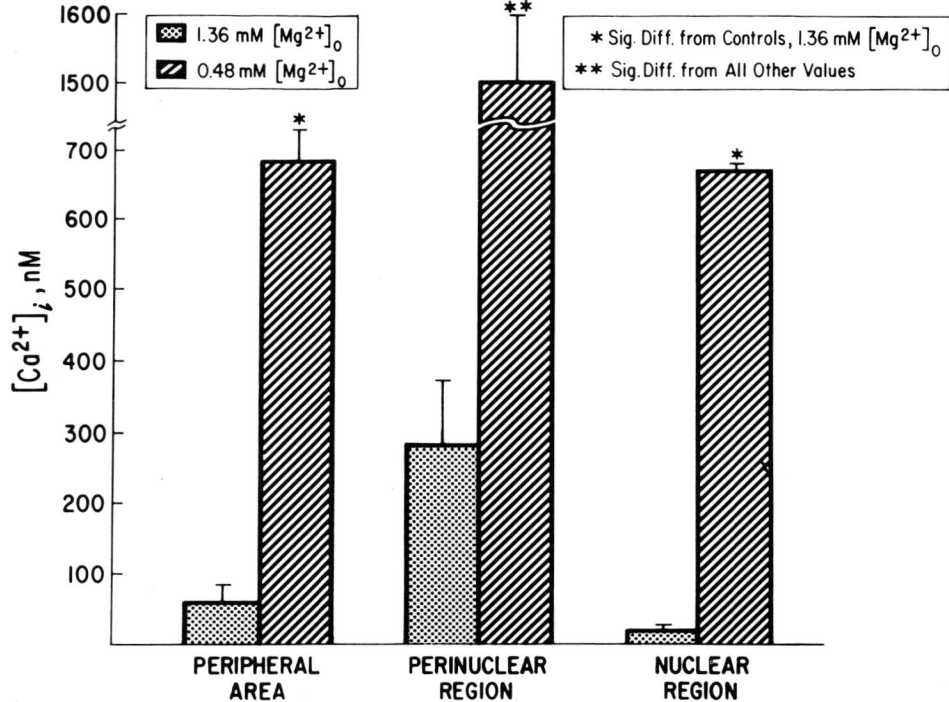

FIG. 4. Effects of reduction in $[Mg^{2+}]_o$ on subcellular pools of $[Ca^{2+}]_i$ in perinuclear, peripheral, and nuclear subcellular region of canine cultured cerebral vascular smooth muscle (VSM) cells. Cells were imaged using fura-2. □ = Normal 1.36 mM $[Mg^{2+}]_o$; ▨ = 0.48 mM $[Mg^{2+}]_o$, *p < 0.001 versus controls, 1.36 mM $[Mg^{2+}]_o$, **p < 0.01 versus other values. Extracellular free $[Mg^{2+}]$ was measured using ISE. (From ref. 13, with permission.)

approximately 92 nM to about 3 nM. This represents about a 200-fold decrement compared with cells treated by $[Mg^{2+}]_o$ withdrawal alone. The $[Ca^{2+}]_i$ gradient thus completely disappears in the absence of $[Ca^{2+}]_o$. Although removal of both $[Ca^{2+}]_o$ and $[Mg^{2+}]_o$ could be interpreted as resulting in dye leakage from the cells, these data also suggest that both divalent cations are needed for maintaining membrane permeability and integrity of these cells.

Cerebral Vascular Smooth Muscle

Turning to cultured canine cerebral vascular smooth muscle cells, the mean basal $[Ca^{2+}]_i$ is about 90 nM, similar to that obtained in rat aortic smooth muscle cells. But we found the range of $[Ca^{2+}]_i$ in the cells to be from 10 to 270 nM (334, *unpublished data*). Since these cells are primary cells, not from a cell line, different smooth muscle cell phenotypes of different stages of the cell cycle and/or chronological age could account for such variations in $[Ca^{2+}]_i$.

Since we have demonstrated that basal tone of cerebral vascular smooth muscle cells are very sensitive to external $[Mg^{2+}]_o$ (109,111,115), it was of great interest to determine if small physiological decrements in $[Mg^{2+}]_o$ would alter $[Ca^{2+}]_i$ incrementally.

Our data indicate that as external Mg^{2+} is lowered from the brain physiological level of 1.3 mM, stepwise, to 0.48 mM Mg^{2+}, the intensity of the fluorescence increases dramatically, suggesting, that the $[Ca^{2+}]_i$ levels are rising incrementally. It is also apparent that the intensity of the fluorescence varies from one part of the cell to another with the perinuclear area showing the greatest intensity (e.g., Fig. 4).

Our data show that stepwise decrements of $[Mg^{2+}]_o$, via perfusion of the cultured cells with different $[Mg^{2+}]_o$-deficient solutions, resulted in stepwise elevations in $[Ca^{2+}]_i$ in a concentration-dependent manner. These findings suggest that regulation of $[Ca^{2+}]_i$ by $[Mg^{2+}]_o$ may be a general cellular property of vascular smooth muscle cells. A relatively small change of $[Mg^{2+}]_o$ from 1.36 mM to 1.07 mM, which can be seen in normal human cerebrospinal fluid (CSF), elevated $[Ca^{2+}]_i$ significantly to about 215 nM, an approximately 2.5-fold increase over basal levels. Further decreases in $[Mg^{2+}]_o$ resulted in larger increments in $[Ca^{2+}]_i$ in as little as 2 min of exposure. Compared to rat aortic smooth muscle cells, canine cerebral VSM cells are clearly more sensitive to alteration of $[Mg^{2+}]_o$.

In other experiments (334, *unpublished data*), we found that a decrease in $[Mg^{2+}]_o$ from 1.3 to 0.48 mM doubled the basal value of $[Ca^{2+}]_i$ within 2 min, and elevation of $[Ca^{2+}]_i$ occurred much more quickly compared to that observed with smaller, stepwise lowering of $[Mg^{2+}]_o$. However, similar to the previous results noted

above, $[Ca^{2+}]_i$ did not seem to remain in a steady state, and an elevated $[Ca^{2+}]_i$ was maintained for at least 22 min of observation.

Such findings suggest two important things: (a) a dependence of the time course of $[Ca^{2+}]_i$ rise upon $[Mg^{2+}]_o$; and (b) a role for Mg^{2+} as a regulatory ligand that could regulate cellular processes much more rapidly than thought heretofore.

Intracellular Free Mg^{2+} Measurements

For measurements of intracellular free Mg^{2+}, we used the fluorescent probe, mag-fura-2, after the work of Raju and colleagues published in 1989 (26). As with fura-2, background fluorescence for both excitation wavelengths was acquired from blanks for each experiment and subtracted from each pair of images separately before ratioing. Fluorescence ratios were obtained by dividing the 335-nM image by the 370-nM image. Intracellular free Mg^{2+} was then calculated according to Raju et al. (26). Particular care was taken here to minimize photobleaching of the probe.

The fluorescent intensity in a single VSM cell could be recorded with high resolution (28). Like that seen for fura-2, there was a clear heterogeneous distribution of the probe, again with the perinuclear area showing the greatest fluorescent intensity (e.g., Fig. 5). When the cells were exposed to elevated $[Mg^{2+}]_o$ for only 2 to 5 min, the mag-fura-2 fluorescence intensity increased considerably, and once again displayed a clear heterogeneous distribution with the perinuclear areas exhibiting the greatest brightness (e.g., Fig. 5).

The calculated intracellular free Mg^{2+}, i.e., 0.63 ± 0.09 mM, indicates that the basal level of ionized Mg in these cells is about 600 μM. However, when the external Mg^{2+} is elevated 4-fold, the basal level of $[Mg^{2+}]_i$ rises about 2.5-fold to about 1.63 ± 0.08 mM. The $[Mg^{2+}]_i$ to $[Mg^{2+}]_o$ ratio falls significantly from 0.5 to 0.3. These rises of $[Mg^{2+}]_i$ are maintained for at least 60 min.

Since we have shown clearly (*vide supra*) that elevation of $[Mg^{2+}]_o$ to 4.8 mM decreased intracellular free Ca^{2+} to about 70 nM, overestimation of $[Mg^{2+}]_i$ caused by interference with excess Ca^{2+} seems very unlikely. The dissociation of the Mg-fura-2 complex is about 65 μM, which is clearly much higher than the nanomolar levels of $[Ca^{2+}]_i$ we have observed.

Thus, the increases in $[Mg^{2+}]_i$, recently reported, may be of significant physiological relevance, because $[Mg^{2+}]_i$ in the millimolar range is known to fit Michaelis-Menten K_m values for many cellular enzyme systems, and clearly exerts potent inhibition on Ca channel activity. We propose that increased $[Mg^{2+}]_i$ maintains low $[Ca^{2+}]_i$, thus preventing peripheral vasoconstriction (or vasospasm) and hypertension.

Since Mg^{2+} affects binding of Ca^{2+} to other probes like

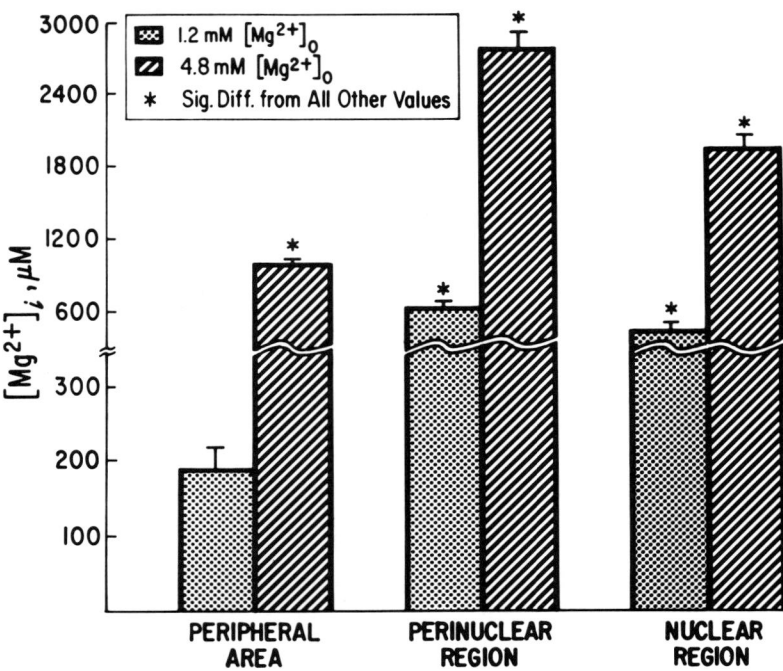

FIG. 5. Effects of elevation in $[Mg^{2+}]_o$ on subcellular compartmentation of $[Mg^{2+}]_i$ in cultured rat aortic smooth muscle cells. Cells were imaged using mag-fura-2. □ = normal 1.2 mM $[Mg^{2+}]_o$; ▨ = 4.8 mM $[Mg^{2+}]_o$. *$p < 0.01$ versus all other values. (From ref. 13, with permission.)

aequorine, a widely used bioluminescent indicator, an exact knowledge of $[Mg^{2+}]_i$ would be required for aequorine experiments measuring $[Ca^{2+}]_i$ (see ref. 13 for further discussion).

Exactly how elevation in $[Mg^{2+}]_o$ produces rapid rises in cellular $[Mg^{2+}]_i$ is not clear. However, irrespective of the exact underlying molecular mechanisms, our findings of a fine regulation of $[Ca^{2+}]_i$ as well as $[Mg^{2+}]_i$ by $[Mg^{2+}]_o$ suggest that Mg^{2+}'s role as a cellular regulator in VSM cells may be physiologically relevant.

The fine responses in $[Ca^{2+}]_i$ and its subcellular distribution suggest that changes in $[Mg^{2+}]_o$ could induce substantial potentiation or inhibition of vascular contraction, and thus regulate regional blood flow and its distribution much more finely than believed until now.

$[Mg^{2+}]_o$ AND INTRACELLULAR FREE CALCIUM IN ENDOTHELIAL CELLS

Magnesium ions play a well-known inhibitory role in caffeine-mediated Ca^{2+} release from the SR in muscle cells, in general, but little is known regarding the effects of Mg^{2+} in endothelial cells (EC). Recent studies, including our own, indicate that Mg^{2+} may be involved in regulation of Ca^{2+} homeostasis in endothelium since changes of extracellular $[Mg^{2+}]_o$ affect release of endothelial-derived relaxant factors, and nitric oxide, from endothelium (15–17,329–331). It would thus be important to define the interaction of Mg^{2+} and caffeine in the regulation of $[Ca^{2+}]_i$ in endothelium and thus elucidate the mechanisms of intracellular Ca^{2+} release in endothelial cells. For such experiments, we utilized a hu-

man aortic endothelial cell line obtained from the National Institutes of Health (17). The cells were loaded with Fura-2 for 60 min as for the VSM cells. The cells were superfused with media containing 1.2 or 0.3 mM $[Mg^{2+}]_o$ in the presence and absence of 10 mM caffeine.

It seems clear from these studies that, unlike VSM cells, EC do not exhibit enhanced Ca^{2+} influx as $[Mg^{2+}]_o$ is lowered. Moreover, high concentrations of caffeine, an ER-SR releaser of Ca^{2+}, exert no effects (17). However, if Mg was lowered simultaneously with the addition of 10 mM caffeine, there was a considerable increase in fluorescence.

Our results indicate that the basal level of intracellular free Ca^{2+} in human ECs is similar to that seen in VSMs, i.e., about 75 nM. Lowering $[Mg^{2+}]_o$ or adding 10 mM caffeine caused insignificant changes in basal $[Ca^{2+}]_i$ (17).

However, treatment with 10 mM caffeine in 0.3 mM $[Mg^{2+}]_o$ resulted in significant elevation of Ca^{2+}, or about a 7-fold increment. Such a large magnitude in elevation of $[Ca^{2+}]_i$ suggests that the caffeine-sensitive pool is large compared to the intracellular Ca^{2+} content in endothelial cells.

Pretreatment of the EC with 1 mM Ni^{2+} partially inhibited the caffeine-induced Ca^{2+} release in EC exposed to 0.3 mM Mg^{2+}, suggesting that filling or emptying of caffeine-sensitive intracellular pools may be associated with Ca^{2+} entry (17). Such Ca^{2+} movements across the plasma membrane of EC may thus be regulated by Mg^{2+}. It is thus possible that changes in extracellular ionized Mg^{2+} concentration (281,283,284) could induce substantial potentiation or inhibition of endothelial functions, and play important roles in hypertensive-vascular disease.

Mg²⁺ DEFICIENCY INDUCES FORMATION OF FREE RADICALS IN CARDIAC MUSCLE, VASCULAR MUSCLE, AND ENDOTHELIAL CELLS

Exactly how Mg deficiency promotes cardiovascular damage is uncertain. Over the past decade, information has been gathered to implicate the generation of oxygen-free radicals in ischemic/reperfusion injury of several vascular regions, including the myocardium, skeletal muscle, and the splanchnic tract (338,339). These highly reactive free radical molecules (e.g., superoxide anions and hydroxyl radicals) are generated in the body by reduction of oxygen. Normally, in a healthy subject, different scavenger systems, present in the blood and tissues, remove these free radicals before they can induce cell damage.

During the past five years, several investigators have performed experiments, both *in vivo* and *in vitro*, that suggest that Mg-deficient states can result in formation

of lipid peroxidation products (340–347). These lipid peroxidation products apparently appear within 7 to 21 days after initiating a Mg deficiency state in rats and hamsters. Cardiomyopathic lesions appear to become prominent after 14 days for the hamster model and approximately 21 days for the rat model (348). However, using a perfused rat heart model, exposed to low $[Mg^{2+}]_o$, hearts start to fail after 5 to 10 min (40). Cultured endothelial cells produce oxygen radicals extracellularly after exposure to a Mg-deficient environment (e.g., 0.4 mM/L) for 5 days (345), but the cellular viability appears to become compromised after only 15 min of exposure to low $[Mg^{2+}]_o$ (345), as has been found in the perfused rat heart (40). Despite what appears to be discrepant, temporal relationships, several different antioxidants afford complete protection against myocardial necrosis in these animal models (341–343,345), strengthening the idea that free radicals are important in Mg deprivation-induced vascular injury.

In addition, oxidative modification of lipoproteins is a well-recognized step in atherogenesis (349), and Mg deficiency results in alterations in plasma lipoproteins and triglycerides (63,238,239–245). Moreover, a new study has clearly demonstrated that Mg levels affect the suscep-

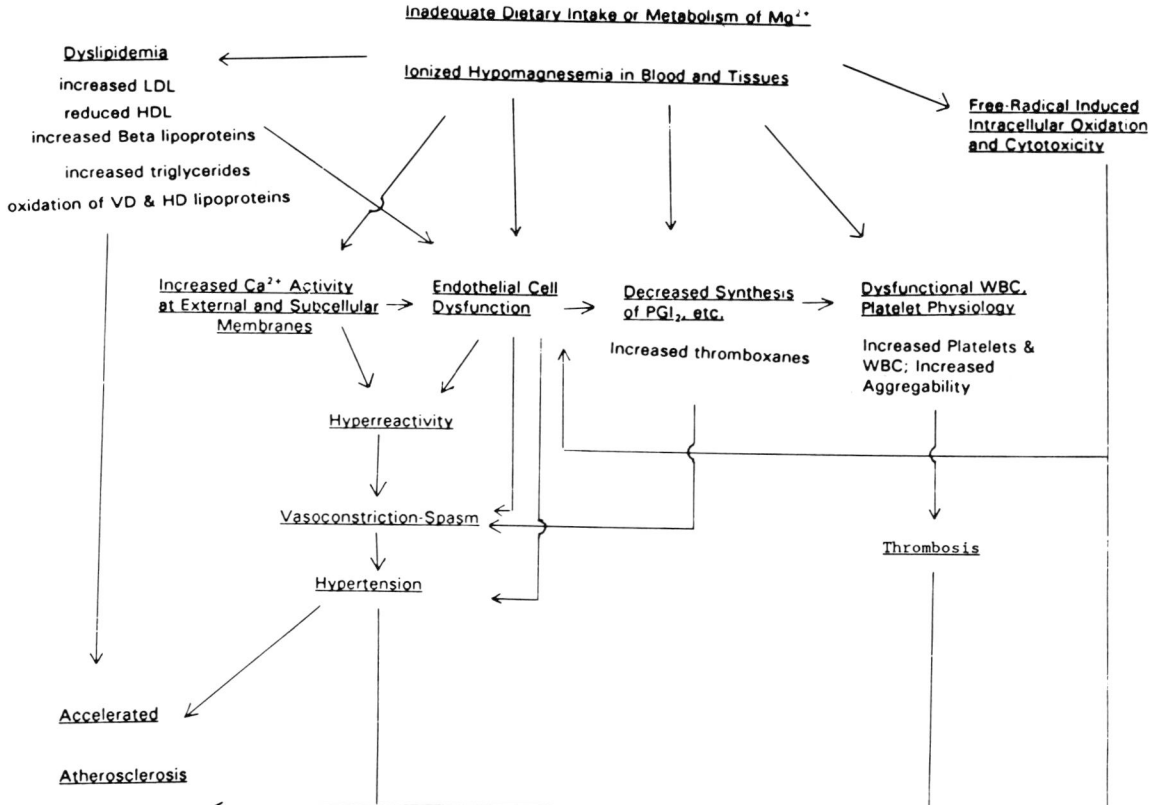

FIG. 6. Hypothetical scheme whereby inadequate dietary intake or metabolism of Mg²⁺ (along with that presented in Fig. 1) could lead to vasospasm, hypertension, atherosclerosis, and intravascular thrombosis.

tibility of lipoproteins to peroxidation (346). Oxidized lipoproteins [e.g., oxidized very-low-density lipoproteins (VLDL) and low-density lipoproteins (LDL)] are clearly cytotoxic to cells in culture (348,349). Moreover, it has recently been demonstrated *in vivo* that Mg deficiency elevates circulating levels of the inflammatory cytokines [interleukin-1 (IL-1), IL-6, and tumor necrosis factor-alpha (TNF-α)] and endothelin concomitant with appearance of lipid peroxidation products and myocardial damage (350). Collectively, such data suggest that the vascular injury seen in atherogenesis and hypertensive disease that often leads to IHD could indeed all be brought about by Mg-deficient states preceding these syndromes; at the very least, hypertension-induced Mg deficiency would exacerbate the vascular injury and pose a risk factor for IHD and stroke.

Whether or not the above animal experiments prove to hold for the human subject will have to await further study. Nevertheless, such data provide an important, missing link needed to explain vascular injury in Mg-deficient states.

Having the above new data on free-radical–induced intracellular oxidation and cytotoxicity, in conjunction with the scheme in Fig. 1, allows us to propose the hypothetical scheme illustrated in Fig. 6 to demonstrate how inadequate dietary intake or metabolism of Mg^{2+} could result in vasospasm, hypertension, atherosclerosis, and vascular thrombosis.

Mg^{2+}—THE NATURALLY OCCURRING OR MIMIC Ca^{2+} ANTAGONIST

Much emphasis has often been placed on the use and design of drugs that can antagonize or prevent the access of activator, free calcium ions (Ca^{2+}) to the contractile apparatus in muscles, including cardiac myocytes and vascular smooth muscle cells. These so-called Ca^{2+} antagonists (i.e., Ca^{2+} entry blockers, slow channel-blocking agents) have been suggested as therapeutic agents for the treatment of a variety of cardiac and vascular disorders, including angina, cardiac arrhythmias, hypertension, strokes, transient ischemic attacks, cerebrovasospasm, migraine, and Raynaud's phenomenon. This suggestion is based primarily on the assumption that these Ca^{2+} antagonists will produce peripheral, coronary, and cerebral vascular dilation and restore normal cardiac rhythm. Most of these drugs are not without risk and may not result in vasodilation.

In the 1970s, we demonstrated that Mg^{2+} clearly affected uptake, distribution, and content of Ca^{2+} in vascular smooth muscle cells (2,6,75,96,155,208,257,319–321). We also suggested that Mg^{2+} might be the naturally occurring Ca^{2+} antagonist (2,6,75,96,155,208,257,319–321,351). During the past ten years, this idea seems to have caught the attention of numerous investigators and clinicians (4,5,7–9,11,53,63,67,103,146,153,159,

179,196,202,275,279,287,298,300,312,323,352,353). Is Mg^{2+} a naturally occurring or mimic Ca^{2+} antagonist? By definition, if a drug prevents only uptake of Ca^{2+} into cells, it can be labeled a Ca^{2+} antagonist (133). Although this simple definition is being contested at the present time, Mg^{2+}, by current standards, can be labeled a weak Ca^{2+} antagonist bcause it is several orders of magnitude less potent than verapamil, nifedipine, and other dihydropyridine Ca^{2+} antagonists (5,321). However, in the cardiovascular system, Mg^{2+}, unlike most other Ca^{2+} antagonists, can act on voltage-regulated channels, receptor-operated channels, and leak-operated channels (320,321), possibly making it an ideal cardiac and vascular muscle Ca^{2+} antagonist.

At vascular membranes, Mg^{2+} can (a) block Ca^{2+} entry and lower peripheral and cerebral vascular resistance, (b) regulate release of Ca^{2+} from SR, (c) improve peripheral and cerebral blood flows, (d) relieve cerebral, coronary, and peripheral vasospasm, and (e) lower arterial blood pressure (provided that enough Mg^{2+} is administered). At cardiac membranes it can (a) slow heart rate, (b) decrease oxygen demand, (c) act as an antiarrhythmic agent, (d) increase cellular bioenergetics, (e) preserve high-energy phosphates, (f) protect mitochondrial function against Ca^{2+} overload, (g) reduce infarct size, and (h) protect against free-radical formation.

CONCLUSIONS

The data reviewed herein are consistent with the hypothesis that the extracellular Mg^{2+} concentration, membrane Mg, and intracellular level of Mg^{2+} exert regulatory roles in cardiac hemodynamics, vascular tone, and vascular reactivity (or peripheral vascular resistance); these factors probably have an important functional role in control of Ca^{2+} uptake, subcellular content, and distribution in smooth, endothelial, and cardiac muscle cells. Certain vascular disease states (hypertensive-related), e.g., hypertension, sudden death ischemic heart disease, IHD, preeclampsia-eclampsia, stroke, congestive heart failure, and diabetes mellitus, are associated with a deficiency of plasma and tissue ionized free Mg^{2+}—the vascular and blood pressure changes here being, at least in part, reflections of the direct cardiac and vascular actions of the lack, or reduction, of element 12.

The prime factors for setting the dysfunctional cardiac and vascular events into motion are inadequate dietary intake, inadequate metabolism of Mg, hypoxia–ischemia, cell injury, or drug-induced alterations in cellular Mg^{2+} metabolism and renal loss in Mg^{2+}.

ACKNOWLEDGMENTS

We are grateful to our longtime collaborators, Asefa Gebrewold, Aimin Zhang, Toni P.-O. Cheng, Lawrence

M. Resnick, and Raj K. Gupta who aided us immensely throughout the past 7 to 10 years, as well as to the National Institutes of Health. This work was supported in part by United States Public Health Service Research Grant AA-08674.

REFERENCES

1. Altura BM, Altura BT. New perspectives on the role of magnesium in the pathophysiology of the cardiovascular system. 1. Clinical aspects. *Magnesium* 1985;4:226–244.
2. Altura BM, Altura BT. New perspectives on the role of magnesium in the pathophysiology of the cardiovascular system. II. Experimental aspects. *Magnesium* 1985;4:245–271.
3. Altura BM. Ischemic heart disease and magnesium. *Magnesium* 1988;7:57–67.
4. Seelig M. Cardiovascular consequences of magnesium deficiency and loss: pathogenesis, prevalence and manifestations—magnesium and chloride loss in refractory potassium repletion. *Am J Cardiol* 1989;63:4G–21G.
5. Sjogren A, Edvinsson L, Fallgren B. Magnesium deficiency in coronary artery disease and cardiac arrhythmias. *J Int Med* 1989;226:213–222.
6. Altura BM, Altura BT. Magnesium and the cardiovascular system: experimental and clinical aspects updated. In: Sigel A, ed. *Metal ions in biological systems. vol 26: compendium on magnesium and its role in biology, nutrition, and physiology.* New York: Marcel Dekker; 1990:359–416.
7. Salem M, Munoz R, Chernow B. Hypomagnesemia in critical illness. A common and clinically important problem. *Crit Care Clin* 1991;7:225–252.
8. Eisenberg MJ. Magnesium deficiency and sudden death. *Am Heart J* 1991;10:269–280.
9. Purvis JR, Movahed A. Magnesium disorders and cardiovascular diseases. *Clin Cardiol* 1992;15:556–568.
10. Altura BM, Altura BT. Cardiovascular risk factors and magnesium: relationship to atherosclerosis, ischemic heart disease and hypertension. *Magnesium Trace Elem* 1992;10:182–192.
11. Arsenian MA. Magnesium and cardiovascular disease. *Prog Cardiovasc Dis* 1993;35:271–310.
12. Altura BM, Altura BT. Magnesium and cardiovascular diseases. In: Berthon G, ed. *Handbook on metal-ligand interactions in biological fluids.* Vol 2; Part 5, Chapter 3, Section B, New York: Marcel Dekker; 1994 (in press).
13. Altura BM, Zhang A, Altura BT. Magnesium, hypertensive vascular diseases, atherogenesis, subcellular compartmentation of Ca^{2+} and Mg^{2+} and vascular contractility. *Miner Electrolyte Metab* 1993;19:323–336.
14. Altura BM, Altura BT. Role of magnesium in the pathogenesis of hypertension: relationship to its actions on cardiac and vascular smooth muscle. In: Laragh JH, Brenner BM, eds. *Hypertension: pathophysiology, diagnosis, and management.* vol I. New York: Raven Press; 1990:1003–1025.
15. Zhang A, Altura BT, Altura BM. Endothelial-dependent differences in responsiveness of rat aortic smooth muscle to reduction in extracellular magnesium and sodium ions. *Magnesium Trace Elem* 1990;9:186–190.
16. Zhang A, Altura BT, Altura BM. Endothelial-dependent sexual dimorphism in vascular smooth muscle: role of Mg^{2+} and Na^+. *Brit J Pharmacol* 1992;105:305–310.
17. Zhang A, Cheng TP-O, Altura BT, Altura BM. Mg^{2+} and caffeine-induced intracellular Ca^{2+} release in human vascular endothelial cells. *Br J Pharmacol* 1993;109:291–292.
18. Gunther T, Dorn F. Die intrazellulaire Mg-Ioenaktivitat in verscheiden Saugertierzellen. *Z Natur* 1971;26b:176–177.
19. Velaso D, Guynn RW, Oskarsson M, Veech RL. The concentration of the free and bound magnesium in rat tissues. *J Biol Chem* 1973;248:4811–4819.
20. Vink R, McIntosh TK, Demediuk P, Faden AI. Decrease in total and free magnesium concentration following traumatic brain injury in rats. *Biochem Biophys Res Commun* 1987;149:594–599.
21. Vink R. Magnesium and brain trauma. *Magnesium Trace Elem* 1992;10:1–10.
22. Altura BM, Gupta RK. Cocaine induces intracellular free Mg deficits, ischemia and stroke as observed by in vivo ^{31}P-NMR of the brain. *Biochim Biophys Acta* 1992;1111:271–274.
23. Altura BM, Altura BT, Gupta RK. Alcohol intoxication results in rapid loss in free magnesium in brain and disturbances in brain bioenergetics: relation to cerebrovasospasm, alcohol-induced strokes, and barbiturate anesthesia-induced deaths. *Magnesium Trace Elem* 1992;10:122–135.
24. Taylor JS, Vieneron DB, Murphy-Boesch J, et al. Free magnesium levels in normal human, brain and brain tumors: ^{31}P chemical-shift imaging measurements at 1.5T. *Proc Natl Acad Sci USA* 1991;88:6810–6814.
25. Corkey B, Duszynski J, Rich T, Matschinsky B, Williamson JR. Regulation of free and bound magnesium in rat hepatocytes and isolated mitochondria. *J Biol Chem* 1986;261:2567–2574.
26. Raju R, Murphy E, Levy LA, Hall RD, London RE. A fluorescent indicator for measuring cytosolic free magnesium. *Am J Physiol* 1989;256:C540–C548.
27. Lennard R, Singh J. Effects of secretagogues on intracellular free calcium and magnesium concentrations in rat pancreatic acinar cells. *Gen Pharmacol* 1992;23:903–908.
28. Zhang A, Cheng TP-O, Altura, Altura BT, Altura BM. Extracellular magnesium regulates intracellular free Mg^{2+} in vascular smooth muscle cells. *Pfluegers Arch Eur J Physiol* 1992;421:391–393.
29. Zhang A, Cheng TP-O, Altura BT, Altura BM. Regulatory effects of extracellular Mg^{2+} on intracellular-free Mg^{2+} in human endothelial cells. (Submitted for publication).
30. Altura BM, Zhang A, Cheng TP-O, Altura BT. Ethanol promotes rapid depletion of intracellular free Mg in cerebral vascular smooth muscle cells: possible relation to alcohol-induced behavioral and stroke-like effects. *Alcohol* 1993;10:563–566.
31. Babu AN, Change TP-O, Zhang A, Altura BT, Altura BM. Low concentrations of ethanol deplete astrocytes of intracellular free magnesium. *Brain Res Bull* 1994 (in press).
32. Gupta RK, Moore RD. ^{31}P-NMR studies of intracellular free Mg^{2+} in intact frog skeletal muscle. *J Biol Chem* 1980;255:3987–3993.
33. Wu ST, Pieper GM, Sakany JM, Eliot RS. Measurement of free magnesium in perfused and ischaemic arrested heart muscle. A quantitative phosphorus-^{31} nuclear magnetic resonance and multi-equilibria analysis. *Biochem* 1981;20:7399–7403.
34. Hess P, Metzeger P, Weingart R. Free magnesium in sheep, ferret, and frog striated muscle as measured with ion selective microelectrodes. *J Physiol* 1982;333:173–188.
35. Blatter LA, McGuigan JAS. Free intracellular magnesium concentration in ferret ventricular muscle measured with ion selective micro-electrodes. *Q J Exp Physiol* 1986;71:467–473.
36. Reiner SD, Barbour RL, Dowd TL, Gupta RK, Altura BM. Effects of magnesium sulfate on hemodynamics and intracellular Mg and cardiac bioenergetics as assessed by ^{31}P-NMR. *FASEB J* 1988;2:A774.
37. Barbour RL, Reiner SD, Dowd TL, Gupta RK, Altura BM. ^{31}P-NMR and reflectance spectroscopy studies characterizing the positive inotropic effects of elevated extracellular magnesium. *FASEB J* 1989;3:250.
38. Barbour RL, Altura BM, Reiner SD, et al. Influence of Mg^{2+} on cardiac performance, intracellular free Mg^{2+} and pH in perfused hearts as assessed by ^{31}P nuclear magnetic resonance spectroscopy. *Magnesium Trace Elem* 1992;10:99–116.
39. Altura BM, Barbour RL, Reiner SD, et al. Influence of Mg^{2+} on distribution of ionized Ca^{2+} in vascular smooth muscle and on cellular bioenergetics and intracellular free Mg^{2+} and pH in perfused hearts probed by digital imaging microscopy, ^{31}P-NMR and reflectance spectroscopy. In: Zakhari S, Witt E, eds. *Imaging techniques in alcohol research.* National Institute on Alcohol Abuse and Alcoholism; Monograph 21. Washington, DC: 1992:235–272.
40. Altura BM, Barbour RL, Dowd TL, Wu F, Altura BT, Gupta RK. Low extracellular magnesium induces intracellular free Mg deficits, ischemia, depletion of high-energy phosphates and cardiac failure in intact working rat hearts: a ^{31}P-NMR study. *Biochim Biophys Acta Molec Dis* 1993;1182:329–332.
41. Headrick JP, Willis RJ. Cytosolic free magnesium in stimulated, hypoxic, and underperfused rat heart. *J Molec Cell Cardiol* 1991;23:991–999.

42. Wittenberg BA, Doeller JE, Gupta RK, White RL. Measurement of sarcolemmal permeability and intracellular pH, free magnesium, and high energy phosphates of isolated heart cells. In: Clark WA, Decker RS, Borg TK, eds. *Biology of isolated adult cardiac myocytes*. Amsterdam: Elsevier; 1988:118–130.

43. Gupta RK, Wittenberg BA. ^{31}P-NMR studies of isolated heart cells: effects of myoglobin activation. *Am J Physiol* 1991;261: H1155–H1163.

44. Kirkels JH, Van Echteld CJA, Ruigrok TJC. Intracellular magnesium during myocardial ischemia and reperfusion: possible consequences for postischemic recovery. *J Molec Cell Cardiol* 1989;21:1209–1218.

45. Kirschenlohr HL, MetCalfe JC, Morris PG, Rodrigo GC, Smith GA. Ca^{2+} transient, Mg^{2+}, and pH measurement in the cardiac cycle by ^{19}F-NMR. *Proc Natl Acad Sci USA* 1988;85:9017–9021.

46. Murphy E, Steenbergen C, Levy LA, Raju B, London RE. Cytosolic free magnesium levels in ischemic rat heart. *J Biol Chem* 1989;264:5622–5627.

47. Ng LL, Davies JE, Ameen M. Intracellular free-magnesium levels in vascular smooth muscle and striated muscle cells of the spontaneously hypertensive rat. *Metabolism* 1992;41:722–777.

48. Quamme GA, Dai L-J, Rabkin SW. Dynamics of intracellular free Mg^{2+} changes in a vascular smooth muscle cell line. *Am J Physiol* 1993;265:H281–H288.

49. Jellicks LA, Gupta RK. Measurement of cytosolic free calcium, free magnesium and intracellular sodium in the aorta of the normal and spontaneously hypertensive rat. *J Biol Chem* 1990;265: 1394–1400.

50. Altura BM, Altura BT. Magnesium, electrolyte transport and coronary vascular tone. *Drugs* 1984;28(Suppl 1):120–142.

51. Aikawa JK. *Magnesium: its biologic significance*. Boca Raton, FL: CRC Press; 1981.

52. Borchgrevink PC, Ryan MP. Effects of magnesium, ouabain and bumetanide on ^{86}rubidium uptake in a human atrial cell line. *Br J Pharmacol* 1988;95:614–618.

53. Ahmad A, Bloom S. Sodium pump and calcium channel modulation of Mg-deficiency cardiomyopathy. *Am J Cardiovasc Pathol* 1989;2:277–283.

54. Keller PK, Aronson RS. The role of magnesium in cardiac arrhythmias. *Prog Cardiovasc Dis* 1990;32:433–448.

55. Tosaki A, Szerdahelyi P, Engelman RM, Das DK. Effects of extracellular magnesium manipulation on reperfusion-induced arrhythmias and myocardial ion shifts in isolated ischemic reperfused hearts. *J Pharmacol Exp Ther* 1993;267:1045–1053.

56. Altura BM, ed. Workshop and Symposium on Magnesium in Clinical Medicine and Therapeutics, La Jolla, CA, 1991. *Magnesium Trace Elem* 1992;10:59–304.

57. Altura BM. Sudden-death ischemic heart disease and dietary magnesium intake: is the target site coronary vascular smooth muscle? *Med Hypotheses* 1979;5:843–849.

58. Crawford J, Crawford MD. Prevalence and pathological changes in ischemic heart disease in a hard-water and soft-water area. *Lancet* 1967;i:229–232.

59. Turlapaty PDMV, Altura BM. Magnesium deficiency produces spasms of coronary arteries: relationship to etiology of sudden-death ischemic heart disease. *Science* 1980;208:198–200.

60. Hochrein H, Kuschke HJ, Zagga Q, Fahl F. Das Verhalten der intracellularen Magnesium-Konzentration in Myokard bei Insuffizienz, Hypoxie and Kammerflimmern. *Klin Wochenschr* 1967;45:1093–1096.

61. Shine KI. Myocardial effects of magnesium. *Am J Physiol* 1979;237:H413–H423.

62. Ferrari F, Albertini A, Curello S, et al. Myocardial recovery during post-ischaemic reperfusion: effects of nifedipine, calcium and magnesium. *J Molec Cell Cardiol* 1986;18:487–498.

63. Rasmussen HS. Justification for magnesium therapy in acute ischaemic heart disease. Clinical and experimental studies. *Danish Med Bull* 1993;40:84–99.

64. Lehr D. Magnesium and cardiac necrosis. *Magnesium Bull* 1981;3:178–191.

65. Guideri A, Lehr D, Horowitz S. Enhanced incidence of isoproterenol-induced ventricular fibrillation in the magnesium-deficient rat. *J Am Coll Nutr* 1985;4:139–156.

66. Agus Z, Kelepouris E, Dukes T, Morad M. Cytosolic magnesium modulates calcium channel activity in mammalian ventricular cells. *Am J Physiol* 1989;256:H452–H455.

67. White RE, Hartzell HC. Magnesium ions in cardiac function. Regulator of ion channels and second messengers. *Biochem Pharmacol* 1989;38:859–867.

68. Wu J, Lipsius SI. Effects of intracellular Mg^{2+} on T- and L-type Ca^{2+} currents in single atrial myocytes. *Am J Physiol* 1990;259: H1842–H1850.

69. Dichtl A, Vierling W. Inhibition by magnesium of calcium inward current in heart ventricular muscle. *Eur J Pharmacol* 1991;204:243–248.

70. Albitz R, Magyar J, Nilius B. Block of single cardiac sodium cells by intracellular magnesium. *Eur Biophys J* 1990;19:19–23.

71. Agus Z, Morad M. Modulation of cardiac ion channels by magnesium. *Annu Rev Physiol* 1991;53:299–307.

72. O'Rourke B, Backx PH, Marban E. Phosphorylation-independent modulation of L-type calcium channels by magnesium-nucleotide complexes. *Science* 1992;257:243–248.

73. O'Rourke B. Ion channels as sensors of cellular energy. Mechanisms of modulation by magnesium and nucleotides. *Biochem Pharmacol* 1993;46:1103–1112.

74. Gupta RK, Wittenberg BA. ^{19}F Nuclear magnetic resonance studies of free calcium in heart cells. *Biophys J* 1993;65:2547–2558.

75. Altura BM, Altura BT. Role of magnesium ions in contractility of blood vessels and skeletal muscle. *Magnesium Bull* 1981;3(Suppl 1A):102–114.

76. Altura BM, ed. American Physiological Society Symposium: role of magnesium in regulation of muscle contraction, April 4, 1980, Anaheim, CA. *Fed Proc* 1981;40:2654–2679.

77. Guillain F, Champel P, LaCapere J-J, Gingold M-P. Role of Mg^{2+} ions in several steps at the sarcoplasmic reticulum ATPase cycle. *Curr Top Cell Regul* 1984;24:397–407.

78. Chapman RA, Tunstall J. The calcium paradox of the heart. *Progr Biophys Molec Biol* 1987;50:67–96.

79. Vierling W, Seibel K, Reiter M. Voltage-dependent calcium release in guinea pig cardiac ventricular muscle as antagonized by magnesium and calcium. *Basic Res Cardiol* 1987;82:415–427.

80. Chiese M, Inesi G. Mg^{2+} and Mn^{2+} modulation of Ca^{2+} transport and ATPase activity in sarcoplasmic reticulum vesicles. *Arch Biochem Biophys* 1981;208:586–592.

81. White RE, Hartzell HC. Effects of intracellular free magnesium on calcium current in isolated cardiac myocytes. *Science* 1988;239:778–780.

82. Horie M, Irisawa H, Noma A. Voltage-dependent magnesium block of adenosine-triphosphate sensitive potassium channel in guinea-pig ventricular cells. *J Physiol (Lond)* 1987;387:251–272.

83. Matsuda H, Saigusa A, Irisawa H. Ohmic conductance through the inwardly rectifying K channel and blocking by internal Mg^{2+}. *Nature* 1987;325:156–159.

84. Vandenberg CA. Inward rectification of potassium channel in cardiac ventricular cells depends on internal magnesium ions. *Proc Natl Acad Sci USA* 1987;84:2560–2564.

85. Horie M, Irisawa H. Rectification of muscarinic K^+ current by magnesium ions in guinea pig atrial cells. *Am J Physiol* 1987;253: H210–H214.

86. Matsuda H. Open-state substructure of inwardly rectifying potassium channels revealed by magnesium block in guinea-pig heart cells. *J Physiol (Lond)* 1988;397:237–258.

87. Ishijara K, Mitsuye T, Noma A, Takano M. The Mg^{2+} block and intrinsic gating inward rectification of K^+ current in guinea pig myocytes. *J Physiol (Lond)* 1989;419:297–320.

88. Moe BM. On the therapeutic mechanism of Mg^{2+} in digitoxic arrhythmias and the role of cardiac glycosides in Mg depletion. *Magnesium* 1984;3:8–20.

89. Friedman HS, Nguyen TN, Mokroaui AM, Barbour RL, Murakawa T, Altura BM. Effects of magnesium chloride on cardiovascular dynamics in the neurally intact dog. *J Pharmacol Exp Ther* 1987;243:126–130.

90. Harris MNE, Crowther A, Jupp RA, Aps C. Magnesium and coronary revascularization. *Br J Anesth* 1988;60:779–783.

91. Chen H, Bando S, Nakaya Y. Alterations of cardiac conduction refractoriness in humans following intravenous administration of magnesium sulfate. *Tokushima J Exp Med* 1988;35:13–20.

92. Dubey A, Solomon R. Magnesium, myocardial ischaemia and arrhythmias. The role of magnesium in myocardial infarction. *Drugs* 1989;37:1–7.

93. Bril A, Rochette L. Prevention of reperfusion-induced ventricular arrhythmias in isolated rat heart with magnesium. *Can J Physiol Pharmacol* 1990;68:694–699.

94. Nattel S, Turmel N, Macleod R, Solymoss BC. Actions of intravenous magnesium on ventricular arrhythmias caused by acute myocardial infarction. *J Pharmacol Exp Ther* 1991;259:939–946.

95. England MR, Gordon G, Salem M, Chernow B. Magnesium administration and dysrhythmias after cardiac surgery. A placebo-controlled, double-blind, randomized trial. *JAMA* 1992;268:2395–2402.

96. Turlapaty PDMV, Altura BM. Extracellular magnesium ions control calcium exchange and content of vascular smooth muscle. *Eur J Pharmacol* 1978;52:421–423.

97. Manzini S, Parlani M, Astolfi M, Maggi CA, Meli A. Positive-inotropic effect of Mg^{2+} in a K^+-depolarized iosprenaline-reactivated guinea-pig ventricular strip. *Gen Pharmacol* 1986;17:159–165.

98. Miyame S. Influence of magnesium and extracellular calcium reduction on ouabain-treated sinoatrial node cells in rabbit heart. *Pharmacol Toxicol* 1989;65:192–197.

99. Hall SK, Fry CH. Magnesium affects excitation, conduction and contraction of isolated mammalian cardiac muscle. *Am J Physiol* 1992;263:H622–H633.

100. Quamme G, Rabkin S. Cytosolic free magnesium in cardiac myocytes: identification of a Mg^{2+}-influx pathway. *Biochem Biophys Res Commun* 1990;167:1406–1412.

101. Gelband CH, Ishikawa T, Post JM, Keef KD, Hume JR. Intracellular divalent cations block smooth muscle K^+ channels. *Circ Res* 1993;73:24–34.

102. Wester PO. Electrolyte balance in heart failure and the role for magnesium ions. *Am J Cardiol* 1992;70:44C–49C.

103. Singh RB, Rastogi SS, Mehta PJ, Cameron EA. Magnesium metabolism in essential hypertension. *Acta Cardiol* 1989;44:313–322.

104. Hara A, Matsumura H, Abdiko Y. Beneficial effect of magnesium on the isolated perfused rat heart during reperfusion after ischaemia: comparison between pre-ischaemic and post-ischaemic administration of magnesium. *Naunyn-Schmied Arch Pharmacol* 1990;342:100–106.

105. Sommers KE, Ohkado A, Simplaceanu E, Koretsky AP, Ho C, del Nido PJ. The role of magnesium in postischemic cardiac dysfunction. *Surgery* 1992;112:159–165.

106. Borchgrevink PC, Bergan AS, Bakoy OE, Jynge P. Magnesium and reperfusion of ischemic rat heart as assessed by ^{31}P-NMR. *Am J Physiol* 1989;256:H195–H204.

107. Greve G, Bakoy OE, Holten T, Jynge P, Saetersdal T. Reversibility of mild to moderate ischemic injuries in the isolated rat heart. A characterization by ^{31}P-NMR and by physiological and ultrastructural indices. *Am J Pathol* 1993;142:1279–1289.

108. Altura BM, Altura BT. Interactions of Mg and K on blood vessels. Aspects in view of hypertension: review of present status and new findings. *Magnesium* 1984;3:175–194.

109. Altura BT, Altura BM. Interactions of Mg and K on cerebral vessels. Aspects in view of stroke: review of present status and new findings. *Magnesium* 1984;3:195–211.

110. Murakawa T, Altura BT, Altura BM. Importance of magnesium and potassium concentration on basal tone and 5-HT induced on interactions in canine coronary artery. *Br J Pharmacol* 1988;94:325–334.

111. Murakawa T, Altura BT, Altura BM. Extracellular magnesium and potassium concentrations interact to modulate tone and reactivity of isolated canine cerebral vascular muscle. *Magnesium* 1990;9:79–93.

112. Singh BN, Hollenberg NK, Poole-Wilson PA, Robertson JIS. Diuretic-induced potassium and magnesium deficiency: relation to drug-induced QT prolongation, cardiac arrhythmias and sudden death. *J Hypertens* 1992;10:301–316.

113. Handerwerker SM, Altura BT, Altura BM. Ionized serum magnesium and potassium levels in pregnant women with preeclampsia and eclampsia. *J Reprod Med* 1994 (in press).

114. Mervaala EMA, Himberg J-J, Laakso J, Tuoimainen P, Karppanen H. Beneficial effects of a potassium- and magnesium-enriched salt alternative. *Hypertension* 1992;19:535–540.

115. Altura BT, Altura BM. Withdrawal of magnesium causes vasospasm while elevated magnesium produces relaxation of tone in cerebral arteries. *Neurosci Lett* 1980;20:323–327.

116. Seelig JM, Wei EP, Kontos HA, Choi SC, Becker DP. Effect of changes in magnesium ion concentration on cat cerebral arteries. *Am J Physiol* 1983;245:H22–H26.

117. Woods WT, Champman GD. Preservation of resting potential by magnesium in hypoxic canine cardiac cells. *Magnesium* 1985;4:96–101.

118. Keren A, Dorian P, Davy JM, Opie LH. Effects of magnesium on ischemic and reperfusion arrhythmias in the rat heart and electrophysiologic effects of hypermagnesemia in the anesthetized dog. *Cardiovasc Drugs Ther* 1988;2:637–645.

119. Ito J, Ehara T. Mg inhibits voltage and tension oscillations but potentiates twitch in depolarized myocardium. *Am J Physiol* 1987;253:H248–H253.

120. Shattock MJ, Hearse DJ, Fry CH. The ionic basis of the anti-ischemic and anti-arrhythmic properties of magnesium in the heart. *J Am Coll Nutr* 1987;6:27–33.

121. Billman GE, Hoskins RS. Prevention of ventricular fibrillation with magnesium sulfate. *Eur J Pharmacol* 1988;158:167–171.

122. Reiter M, Noe J. Die Bedutung von Calcium, Magnesium, Kalium and Natrium fur die rhythmische Erregungschildung im Sinusknoten des Warmbluterherzens. *Pfluegers Arch Ges Physiol* 1959;269:366–374.

123. Toda N, West TC. Interaction between Na, Ca and Mg and vagal stimulation in the SA node of the rabbit. *Am J Physiol* 1967;212:424–430.

124. Turlapaty PDMV, Carrier OJR. Influence of magnesium on calcium-induced responses of atrial and vascular muscle. *J Pharmacol Exp Ther* 1973;187:86–98.

125. Opthof T, Mackaay AJC, Bleeker WK, Houtkooper JM, Abels R, Bouman LN. Dependence on the chronotropic effects of calcium, magnesium and sodium on temperature and cycle length in isolated rabbit atria. *J Pharmacol Exp Ther* 1980;212:183–189.

126. Opthof T, Mackaay AJC, Bleeker WK, Jongsma HJ, Bouman LN. Magnesium and sinus node function. *Magnesium Bull* 1981;3:54–59.

127. Opthof T, Mackaay AJC, Bleeker WK, Jongsma HJ. Differences between rabbit sinoatrial pacemakers in the response to Mg, Ca and temperature. *Cardiovasc Res* 1983;17:526–532.

128. James MFM, Cork RC, Dennett JE. Cardiovascular effects of magnesium sulphate in the baboon. *Magnesium* 1987;6:314–324.

129. Nagai I, Gebrewold A, Altura BT, Altura BM. Magnesium salts exert direct vasodilator effects on rat cremaster muscle microcirculation. *Arch Int Pharmacodyn Ther* 1988;294:194–214.

130. Flatman PW. Mechanism of magnesium transport. *Ann Rev Physiol* 1991;53:259–271.

131. Skou JC. Enzymatic basis for active transport of Na^+ and K^+ across cell membranes. *Physiol Rev* 1965;45:596–617.

132. Fisher PWF, Giroux A. Effects of dietary magnesium on sodium-potassium pump action in the heart of rats. *J Nutr* 1987;117:2091–2095.

133. Fleckenstein A. *Calcium antagonism in heart and smooth muscle.* New York: Wiley-Interscience; 1983.

134. Brautbar N, Altura BM. Hypophosphatemia and hypomagnesemia result in cardiovascular dysfunction: theoretical basis for alcohol-induced cellular injury. *Alcohol Clin Exp Res* 1987;11:118–126.

135. Wu F, Barbour RL, Altura BT, Altura BM. Influence of elevated versus low extracellular magnesium on hemodynamics and bioenergetics in perfused rat hearts. *FASEB J* 1988;2:A702.

136. Wu F, Zou LY, Altura BT, Barbour RL, Altura BM. Low extracellular magnesium results in cardiac failure in isolated perfused rat hearts. *Magnesium* 1992;10:364–373.

137. Altura BM, Altura BT. Biochemistry and pathophysiology of congestive heart failure: is there a role for magnesium? *Magnesium* 1986;5:134–143.

138. Maguire ME, Crome R, Hearse DJ, Manning AS. Efflux of ^{28}Mg

from isolated rat heart: effect of ischemia, temperature and Mg concentration. *Magnesium* 1985;4:206 (Abst).

139. Blackfan KD, Hamilton B. Treatment of hypertensive disease. *Boston Med Surg J* 1925;193:617–628.

140. Altura BM, Altura BT, Gebrewold A, Ising H, Gunther T. Magnesium-deficiency and hypertension: correlation between magnesium-deficient diets and microcirculatory changes in situ. *Science* 1984;223:1315–1317.

141. Altura BM, Altura BT, Gebrewold A, Ising H, Gunther T. Noise-induced hypertension and magnesium in rats: relationship to microcirculation and calcium. *J Appl Physiol* 1992;72:194–202.

142. Altura BM, Altura BT, Gebrewold A, Ising H, Gunther T. Extraaurale Wirkungen chronischer Larmbelastung auf Blutdruck, Mikrozirkulation und Elektrolyte bei Ratten: Beeinflussung durch Mg²⁺. In: Ising H, Kruppa B, eds. *Larm und Krankheit—noise and disease.* Stuttgart: Gustav Fischer Verlag; 1993:65–90.

143. Altura BM, Altura BT. Role of magnesium and calcium in alcohol-induced hypertension and strokes as probed by in-vivo television microscopy, digital image microscopy, optical spectroscopy, ³¹P-NMR spectroscopy and a unique Mg²⁺ ion selective electrode. *Alcohol Clin Exp Res* 1994 (In press).

144. Berthelot A, Exposito J. Effects of dietary magnesium on the development of hypertension in the spontaneously hypertensive rat. *J Am Coll Nutr* 1983;4:345–353.

145. Chrysant SG, Ganousis L, Chrysant C. Hemodynamic and metabolic effect of hypomagnesemia in spontaneously hypertensive rats. *Cardiology* 1988;75:81–89.

146. Weaver K. Pregnancy-induced hypertension and low birth weight in magnesium-deficient ewes. *Magnesium* 1986;5:191–200.

147. Karppanen H, Janskanen A, Tuomilehto J, et al. Safety and effects of potassium- and magnesium-containing low sodium salt mixtures. *J Cardiovasc Pharmacol* 1984;6:S236–S243.

148. Motoyama T, Sano H, Fukuzaki H. Oral magnesium supplementation in patients with essential hypertension. *Hypertension* 1989;13:227–232.

149. Genest J, Kuchel O, Hamet P, Cantin M. *Hypertension.* 2nd ed. New York: McGraw-Hill; 1983.

150. Altura BM, Altura BT. Influence of magnesium on vascular smooth muscle and serum biochemical parameters from diabetic and hypertensive rats. *Magnesium* 1983;2:253–266.

151. Henrotte J-G, Santarromana M, Bourdon R. Concentrations en magnesium calcium et zinc du plasma et des erythrocytes de rats spontanement hypertendus. *CR Seances Acad Sci* 1985;300:431–436.

152. Berthelot A, Meyers E, Luthringer C, Exinger F. Etude de quelques parametres du metabolisme du magnesium chez le rat spontanement hypertendu. *Magnesium* 1985;4:280–282.

153. Matsura J, Kona M, Kanayama Y, et al. Decreased intracellular magnesium in erythrocytes of spontaneously hypertensive rats. *Biochem Biophys Res Commun* 1987;143:1012–1017.

154. Boeckh-Haebisch EMA. Nifedipine, its action on the cationic concentrations in heart vessels, skeletal muscle and blood in tissues of normotensive and spontaneously hypertensive rats (SHR). *Gen Pharmacol* 1988;19:407–416.

155. Altura BM, Altura BT. Magnesium ions and contraction of vascular smooth muscles: relationship to some vascular diseases. *Fed Proc* 1981;40:2672–2679.

156. Fujita T, Ito Y, Ando K, Noda H, Ogota E. Attenuated vasodilator response to Mg²⁺ in young patients with borderline hypertension. *Circulation* 1990;82:384–393.

157. Mattingly MT, Bizezinski WA, Wells IC. Decreased cell membrane magnesium in some essential hypertension patients. *Clin Exp Hypertens Part A Theory Pract* 1991;A13:65–82.

158. Paolisso G, Passariello N, Agambato S, et al. Impaired insulin-mediated erythrocyte magnesium accumulation in essential hypertension. *Clin Sci* 1987;73:535–539.

159. Wallach S, Verch RL. Tissue magnesium in spontaneously hypertensive rats. *Magnesium* 1986;5:33–38.

160. Altura BM, Altura BT, Gebrewold A, Ising H, Gunther T. Extraaurale Larmwirkungen auf Blutdruck, Mikrozirkulation und Electrolyte bei Ratten. *Bundesgesundheitsblatt* 1992;35:135–139.

161. Jelicks LA, Gupta RK. Intracellular free magnesium and high energy phosphates in the perfused normotensive and spontane-ously hypertensive rat heart. A ³¹P-NMR study. *Am J Hypertens* 1991;4:131–136.

162. Dipette D, Simpson, Guntipali J. Systemic and regional hemodynamic effects of acute magnesium administration in the normotensive and hypertensive state. *Magnesium* 1987;6:136–149.

163. Laurant P, Moussard C, Alber D, Henry JC, Berthelot A. In vivo and in vitro magnesium effects on aortic prostacylin generation in DOCA-salt hypertensive rats. *Prostag Leukotr Essent Fatty Acids* 1992;47:183–186.

164. Ising H, Bertschat F, Ibe K, Stooby V, Goosen MC, Hengst G. Stress-induced Ca/Mg shifts and vascular responses in animals and man: comparison to electrolyte alterations in myocardial infarction patients. *Magnes Bull* 1986;8:95–103.

165. Mathew R, Gloster ES, Altura BT, Altura BM. Magnesium aspartate HCL attenuates monocrotaline induced pulmonary artery hypertension. *Clin Science* (Lond) 1988;75:661–667.

166. Mathew R, Altura BT, Altura BM. Strain differences in pulmonary hypertensive response to monocrotaline alkaloid and the beneficial effect of oral magnesium treatment. *Magnesium* 1989;8:110–116.

167. Mathew R, Altura BM. Magnesium and the lungs. *Magnesium* 1988;7:173–187.

168. Mathew R, Gloster ES, Altura BT, Altura BM. Pulmonary vasculature in monocrotaline-induced hypertensive rats on magnesium therapy. *Microcirc Endothelium Lymphatics* 1990;6:267–283.

169. Lu C-Y, Wang D-Y. Effects of dietary magnesium on pulmonary vascular reactivity and chronic hypoxic pulmonary hypertension in rats. *J Tongji Med Univ* 1991;11:1–5.

170. Mathew R, Altura BM. Role of magnesium in lung diseases, asthma, allergy and pulmonary hypertension. *Magnesium Trace Elem* 1992;10:220–228.

171. Nadler JL, Goodson S, Rude R. Evidence that prostacyclin mediates the vascular action of magnesium in humans. *Hypertension* 1987;9:379–383.

172. Altura BM, Altura BT. Vascular smooth muscle and prostaglandins. *Fed Proc* 1976;35:2360–2366.

173. Altura BM, Altura BT, Waldemar Y. Prostaglandin-induced relaxations and contractions of arterial smooth muscle: effects of magnesium ions. *Artery* 1976;2:326–336.

174. Lau K, Oasa C. Interactions between Mg and blood pressure. In: Massry SG, Maschio G, Ritz E, eds. *Phosphate and mineral metabolism.* New York: Plenum Press; 1984:275–290.

175. Altura BM, Altura BT. Magnesium and vascular tone and reactivity. *Blood Vessels* 1978;15:5–16.

176. Petersen B, Schrell M, Christiansen C, Transbol IB. Serum and erythrocyte magnesium in normal elderly Danish people. *Acta Med Scand* 1977;201:31–34.

177. Resnick LM, Gupta RK, Laragh JH. Intracellular free magnesium in erythrocytes of essential hypertension: relation to blood pressure and serum divalent cations. *Proc Nat Acad Sci USA* 1984;81:6511–6515.

178. Dyckner T, Wester PO. Effect of magnesium on blood pressure. *Br Med J* 1983;286:1847–1849.

179. Touyz RM, Milne FJ, Seiffel HC, Reinach SG. Magnesium, calcium, sodium and potassium status in normotensive and hypertensive-Johannesburg patients. *S Afr Med J* 1987;72:377–381.

180. Touyz RM, Milne FJ, Reinach SG. Platelet and erythrocyte Mg²⁺, Ca²⁺, Na⁺, K⁺ and cell membrane adenosine triphosphatase activity in essential hypertension in blacks. *J Hypertens* 1992;10:571–578.

181. Touyz RM, Milne FJ, Reinach SG. Intracellular Mg²⁺, Ca²⁺, Na⁺, K⁺ in platelets and erythrocytes of essential hypertension patients: relation to blood pressure. *Clin Exp Hypertens Part A Theory Pract* 1992;A14:1189–1209.

182. Paolisso G, DiMaro G, Cozzolino T, et al. Chronic magnesium administration enhances oxidative glucose metabolism in thiazide treated hypertensive patients. *Am J Hypertens* 1992;5:681–686.

183. Shingu T, Matsuura H, Kusaka M, et al. Significance of intracellular free calcium and magnesium and calcium-regulating hormones with sodium chloride loading in patients with essential hypertension. *J Hypertens* 1991;9:1021–1028.

184. Nagai I, Gebrewold A, Altura BT, Altura BM. Magnesium salts

exert direct vasodilator effects on rat cremaster muscle microcirculation. *Arch Intern Pharmacodyn Ther* 1988;294:194–214.

185. Nishio A, Gebrewold A, Altura BT, Altura BM. Comparative effects of magnesium salts on reactivity of arterioles and venules to constrictor agents: an *in situ* study. *J Pharmacol Exp Ther* 1988;246:859–865.

186. Nishio A, Gebrewold A, Altura BT, Altura BM. Comparative vasodilator effects of magnesium salts on rat mesenteric arterioles and venules. *Arch Intern Pharmacodyn Ther* 1989;298:139–163.

187. McCarron DA. Calcium and magnesium nutrition in human hypertension. *Ann Intern Med* 1983;98:800–805.

188. Kesteloot H. Urinary cations and blood pressure-population studies. *Ann Clin Res* 1984;16(Suppl):72–80.

189. M'buyamaba-Kabangu JR, Lijnen P, Staessen J, et al. Relationship between blood pressure and urinary sodium, potassium, calcium and magnesium in Nantu of Zaire. *J Hypertens* 1986;4:27–30.

190. Joffres MR, Reed DM, Yano K. Relationship of magnesium intake and other dietary factors to blood pressure: the Honolulu Heart Study. *Am J Clin Nutr* 1987;45:469–475.

191. McGarvey ST, Zinner SH, Willet WC, Rosner B. Maternal prenatal dietary potassium, calcium, magnesium and infant blood pressure. *Hypertension* 1992;17:218–224.

192. Miller WL, Crabtree BF, Evans DK. Exploratory study of the relationship between hypertension and diet diversity among Saba islanders. *Public Health Rep* 1992;107:426–432.

193. Staesen J, Bulpitt C, Fagard R, Joosens JV, Lijnen P, Amery A. Four urinary cations and blood pressure: a population study in two Belgian towns. *Am J Epidemiol* 1988;117:676–687.

194. Wester PO, Dyckner T. Magnesium and hypertension. *J Am Coll Nutr* 1987;6:321–328.

195. Reyes AJ, Leary WP, Acosta-Barrios TN, Davis WH. Magnesium supplementation in hypertension treatment with hydrochlorothiazide. *Curr Ther Res* 1984;36:322–340.

196a. Hattori S, Saito K, Sano H, Fukuzaki H. Intracellular magnesium deficiency and effect of oral magnesium on blood pressure and red cell sodium transport in diuretic-treated hypertensive patients. *Jap Circ J* 1988;52:1249–1256.

196b. Lind L, Lithell H, Pollare T, Ljunghall. Blood pressure response during long-term treatment with magnesium is dependent on a magnesium-status. A double-blind, placebo-controlled study in essential hypertension and in subjects with high-normal blood pressure. *Am J Hypertens* 1991;4:674–679.

197. Cappuccio FP, Markandu ND, Benynon GW, Shore AC, Sampson B, MacGregor GA. Lack of effect of oral magnesium on high blood pressure; a double blind study. *Br Med J* 1985;291:235–238.

198. Henderson DG, Schierue J, Schudt J. Effect of magnesium supplementation on blood pressure and electrolyte concentrations in hypertensive patients receiving long-term diuretic treatment. *Br Med J* 1986;293:664–665.

199. Nowson CA, Morgan TO. Magnesium supplementation in mild hypertensive patients on a moderately low sodium diet. *Clin Exp Pharmacol Toxicol* 1989;16:299–302.

200. Ferrara LA, Ianuzzi R, Castaldo A, Ianuzzi A, Dell Russo A, Mangini M. Long-term magnesium supplementation in essential hypertension. *Cardiol* 1992;81:25–33.

201. Handwerker SM, Altura BT, Royo B, Altura BM. Ionized magnesium and calcium levels in umbilical cord serum of pregnant women with transient hypertension during labor. *Am J Hypertens* 1993;6:542–545.

202. Shibutani Y, Sakamoto K, Katsuno S, Yoshimoto S, Matsuura T. Serum and erythrocyte magnesium levels in junior high school students: relation to blood pressure and a family history of hypertension. *Magnesium* 1988;7:188–194.

203. Shibutani Y, Sakamoto K, Satsuno S, Yoshmimoto S, Matsurra T. Relation of serum and erythrocyte magnesium levels to blood pressure and a family history of hypertension. *Acta Paediatr Scand* 1990;79:316–321.

204. Paolisso G, Passariello N, Agambato S, et al. Impaired insulin-mediated erythrocyte magnesium accumulation in essential hypertension. *Clin Science* 1987;73:535–539.

205. Resnick LM, Gupta RK, Gruenspan H, Alderman MH, Laragh JH. Hypertension and peripheral insulin resistance: possible mediating role of intracellular free magnesium. *Am J Hypertens* 1990;3:373–379.

206. Levin GE, Mather HM, Pilkington TRE. Tissue magnesium status in diabetes mellitus. *Diabetologia* 1981;21:131–134.

207. Altura BM, Halevy S, Turlapaty PDMV. Vascular smooth muscle in diabetes and its influence on the reactivity of blood vessels. *Adv Microcirc* 1979;8:118–150.

208. Altura BM. Magnesium and regulation of contractility of vascular smooth muscle. *Adv Microcirc* 1982;11:77–113.

209. Resnick LM. Hypertension and abnormal glucose homeostasis: possible role of divalent ion metabolism. *Am J Med* 1989;87:6A–17S.

210. Turlapaty PDMV, Altura BM. Magnesium ions and contraction of alloxan-diabetic vascular muscle. *Artery* 1980;6:375–384.

211. Turlapaty PDMV, Altura BT, Altura BM. Ca^{2+} uptake and distribution in alloxan-diabetic rat arterial and venous smooth muscle. *Experientia* 1980;36:1298–1299.

212. Nelson L, Boquist L. Effects of alloxan and streptozotocin on calcium transport in isolated mouse liver mitochondria. *Cell Calcium* 1982;3:191–198.

213. Boquist L. Alloxan effects on mitochondria: study of oxygen consumption, fluxes of Mg^{2+}, Ca^{2+}, and K^+ and adenine nucleotides, membrane potential and volume changes in vitro. *Diabetologia* 1984;27:379–386.

214. Leclercq-Meyer V, Marchand J, Malaiise WJ. The effect of calcium and magnesium on glucagon secretion. *Endocrinology* 1973;93:1360–1370.

215. Gueux E, Rassiguier Y. The effect of magnesium deficiency on glucose stimulated insulin secretion in rats. *Horm Metab Res* 1983;15:594–597.

216. Gould MK, Chaudry IH. The action of insulin on glucose uptake by isolated rat soleus muscle. *Biochim Biophys Acta* 1970;215:249–257.

217. Jarrett RH, Keen H, McCartney M, et al. Glucose tolerance and blood pressure in two population samples: the relation to diabetes mellitus and hypertension. *Int J Epidemiol* 1978;7:15–24.

218. NcNair P, Christiansen C, Madsbad S, et al. Hypomagnesemia, a risk factor in diabetic retinopathy. *Diabetes* 1978;27:1075–1078.

219. Fujii S, Takemura T, Wada M, Akai T, Okuda K. Magnesium levels in plasma, erythrocyte and urine in patients with diabetes mellitus. *Horm Metab Res* 1982;14:161–162.

220. Sjögren A, Floren CH, Nilsson A. Magnesium deficiency in IDDM related to level of glycosylated hemoglobin. *Diabetes* 1986;35:459–463.

221. Wada M, Jujii S, Takemura T, Seki J, Akai T. Magnesium levels and diabetic retinopathy. *Magnes Bull* 1983;1:12–14.

222. Hatwal A, Gujral AS, Bhatia RPS, Agrawal JK, Bajpai HS. Association of hypomagnesemia with diabetic retinopathy. *Acta Ophthalmol* 1989;67:714–716.

223. Bachem V, Strobel B, Jastram U, Jannsen EG, Paschen K. Magnesium and diabetes. *Magnes Bull* 1980;1:35–39.

224. Johansson G, Danielson BG, Ljunghall S, Wibell L. Evidence for a disturbed magnesium metabolism in diabetes mellitus. *Magnes Bull* 1981;2:178–180.

225. Jenkins LL, Rohn R. Distribution of copper, magnesium and zinc in plasma and cellular components of blood from type 1 diabetic children. *Clin Chem* 1986;32:1089.

226. Sjögren A, Floren E, Nilsson A. Magnesium, potassium and zinc deficiency in subjects with Type II diabetes mellitus. *Acta Med Scand* 1988;224:461–465.

227. Paolisso G, Sgambato S, Pizza G, Passariello N, Varicchio M, D'Onofrio F. Improved insulin response and action by chronic magnesium administration in aged NIDDM subjects. *Diab Care* 1989;12:265–269.

228. Sheehan JP. Magnesium deficiency and diabetes mellitus. *Magnesium Trace Elem* 1992;10:215–219.

229. Tuvemo T, Gebre-Medhin M. The role of trace elements in juvenile diabetes mellitus. *Pediatrics* 1983;12:213–219.

230. Resnick LM, Altura BT, Gupta RK, Laragh JH, Altura BM. Serum ionized magnesium in essential hypertension and non-insulin diabetes mellitus: relation to intracellular free magnesium. *Clin Res* 1992;40:285A.

231. Resnick LM, Altura BT, Gupta RK, Laragh JH, Alderman MH, Altura BM. Intracellular and extracellular magnesium depletion

in type 2 (non-insulin-dependent) diabetes mellitus. *Diabetologia* 1993;36:767–770.

232. Dawber T. *The Framingham Study. The epidemiology of atherosclerosis.* Cambridge: Harvard University Press; 1980.

233. Ross R, Harker L. Hyperlipidemia and atherosclerosis. *Science* 1976;193:1084–1100.

234. Ross R. The pathogenesis of atherosclerosis. *N Engl J Med* 1986;314:488–500.

235. Lee KT, Onodera K, Janaka K, eds. Atherosclerosis: II. Recent progress in atherosclerosis research. *Ann NY Acad Sci* 1990;598:1–598.

236. Malkiel-Shapiro B. Further observations on parenteral magnesium sulphate therapy in coronary heart disease. A clinical appraisal. *S Afr Med J* 1958;32:1211–1215.

237. Bersohn I, Witwisrand MB, Oeloese PJ, Potehefstroom BS. Correlations of serum magnesium and serum cholesterol levels in South African Bantu and European subjects. *Lancet* 1957;i:1020–1021.

238. Rayssiguier Y. Magnesium, lipids and vascular diseases. *Magnesium* 1986;5:182–190.

239. Rayssiguier Y. Magnesium and lipids in cardiovascular disease. *J Am Coll Nutr* 1986;5:507–519.

240. Jaya P, Kurup PA. Magnesium deficiency and metabolism of lipids in rats fed cholesterol-free and cholesterol containing diet. *Indian J Biochem Biophys* 1987;24:92–95.

241. Davis WH, Leary WP, Reyes AJ, Olhaberry JV. Monotherapy with magnesium increases abnormally low high density lipoprotein cholesterol: a clinical assay. *Curr Ther Res* 1984;36:341–346.

242. Rasmussen HS, Autrup P, Golstein K, et al. Influence of magnesium substitution therapy on blood lipid composition in patients with ischemic heart diseases. *Arch Intern Med* 1989;149:1050–1053.

243. Altura BT, Brust M, Gebrewold A, Barbour RL, Bloom S, Altura BM. Oral administration of magnesium lowers serum cholesterol and triglycerides and ameliorates atherogenesis rabbits. *Fed Proc* 1987;46:977.

244. Altura BT, Brust M, Bloom S, Barbour RL, Stempak JK, Altura BM. Magnesium dietary intake modulates blood lipid levels. *Proc Natl Acad Sci USA* 1990;87:1840–1844.

245. Orimo H, Ouchi Y. The role of calcium and magnesium in the development of atherosclerosis. Experimental and clinical evidence. *Ann NY Acad Sci* 1990;598:444–457.

246. Garfinkel D, Garfinkel L. Magnesium and regulation of carbohydrate metabolism at the molecular level. *Magnesium* 1988;7:249–261.

246a.Yeh Q, Altura BT, Barbour RL, Altura BM. Dietary magnesium intake modulates atherosclerosis in rabbits. *FASEB J* 1990;4:A1155.

247. Vernon WB. The role of magnesium in nucleic acid and protein metabolism. *Magnesium* 1988;7:234–248.

248. Cameron IL, Smith NKR. Cellular concentration of magnesium and other ions in relation to protein synthesis, cell proliferation and cancer. *Magnesium* 1989;8:31–44.

249. Gunther T. Biochemistry of magnesium and calcium at membranes. In: Itokawa Y, Durlach J, eds. *Magnesium in health and disease.* London: Lubbey; 1989:3–10.

250. Gunther T. Biochemical bases of the therapeutic actions of magnesium. *Magnes Bull* 1991;13:46–52.

251. Altura BM, Durlach J, Seelig MS, eds. *Magnesium in cellular processes and medicine.* Basel: Karger; 1987.

252. Resnick LM, Gupta RK, Bhargava KK, Gruenspan H, Alderman MH, Laragh JR. Cellular ions in hypertension, diabetes and obesity: a nuclear magnetic resonance study. *Hypertension* 1991;17:951–957.

253. Markell MS, Altura BT, Barbour RL, Altura BM. Ionized and total magnesium levels in cyclosporin-treated renal transplant recipients: relationship with cholesterol and cyclosporin levels. *Clin Sci* 1993;85:315–318.

254. Markell MS, Altura BT, Sarn Y, et al. Deficiency of serum ionized magnesium in patients on hemodialysis or peritoneal dialysis. *ASAIO J* 1993;39:M801–M804.

255. Markell MS, Altura BT, Sarn Y, Barbour RL, Friedman EA, Altura BM. Relationship of ionized magnesium and cyclosporine level in renal transplant recipients. *Ann NY Acad Sci* 1994 (In press).

256. Touyz RM, Schiffrin EL. The effect of angiotensin II on platelet intracellular free magnesium and calcium ion concentrations in essential hypertension. *J Hypertens* 1993;11:551–558.

257. Altura BM, Altura BT. Mg, Na and K interactions and coronary heart diseases. *Magnesium* 1982;1:241–265.

258. Altura BM, Altura BT. Magnesium-calcium interactions and contraction of arterial smooth muscle in ischemic heart diseases, hypertension and vasospastic disorders. In: Wester P, ed. *Electrolytes and the heart.* New York: Trans Medica; 1983.

259. Marier JR. Magnesium content of the food supply in the modern day world. *Magnesium* 1986;5:1–8.

260. Marier JR, Neri LC, Anderson TW. Water hardness, human health, and the importance of magnesium. Ottawa: National Research Council of Canada; 1979:119. Report no 17581.

261. Masironi R. Geochemistry and cardiovascular diseases. *Philos Trans R Soc London* 1979;288:193–203.

262. Leary WP, Reyes AJ. Magnesium and sudden death. *S Afr Med J* 1983;64:697–698.

263. Stitt FW, Crawford MD, Clayton DG, et al. Clinical and biochemical indicators of cardiovascular disease among men living in hard and soft water areas. *Lancet* 1973;i:122–126.

264. Masironi R, Koritoyohann SR, Pierce JO, Schamshula RG. Calcium content of river water, trace element concentrations in toenails and blood pressure in village populations in New Guinea. *Sci Total Environ* 1976;6:41–53.

265. Puddu V, Menotti A, Signoretti P. Drinking water and cardiovascular disease. *Am Heart J* 1980;99:534–540.

266. Levine AI, Novikov YV, Plitiman SI, Noarov YA, Lastochlima KO. Effects of water in varying degrees of hardness on cardiovascular system. *Grig Sanit* 1981;10:16–19.

267. Altura BM. Magnesium and regulation of contractility. *Adv Microcirc* 1982;8:77–113.

268. Marier JR, Neri LC. Quantifying the role of magnesium in the interrelationship between human mortality/morbidity and water hardness. *Magnesium* 1985;4:53–59.

269. Seelig MS. *Magnesium deficiency in the pathogenesis of disease.* New York: Plenum Press; 1980.

270. Marier JR. Quantitative factors regarding magnesium status in the modern-day world. *Magnesium* 1982;1:3–15.

271. Altura BM, Brodsky MA, Elin RJ, Gyms JA, Resnick LM, Seelig MS. Magnesium: growing in clinical importance. *Patient Care* 1994;28:130–150.

272. Joffres MR, Reed DM, Yano K. Relationship of magnesium intake and other dietary factors to blood pressure: the Honolulu Heart Study. *Am J Clin Nutr* 1987;45:469–475.

273. Rouse IL, Beillin LJ, Armstrong BK, Vandongen R. Blood pressure-lowering effect of a vegetarian diet. *Lancet* 1983;1:5–10.

274. Melby CL, Goldflies DG, Toohey ML. Blood pressure differences in older black and white long-term vegetarians and nonvegetarians. *J Am Coll Nutr* 1993;12:262–269.

275. Kugiyama K, Yasue H, Okumura K, et al. Suppression of exercise-induced angina by magnesium sulfate in patients with variant angina. *J Am Coll Cardiol* 1988;12:1177–1183.

276. Durak I, Sahin A, Yurtarslanj Z, Sonel A. Analysis of calcium, zinc, magnesium, iron and copper content in myocardium and stenotic mitral valves. *Am J Cardiol* 1989;64:1392–1394.

277. Miyagi H, Yasue H, Okumura K, Ogawa H, Goto K, Oshima S. Effect of magnesium on anginal attack induced by hyperventilation in patients with variant angina. *Circulation* 1989;79:597–602.

278. Gottlieb SS, Baruch L, Kukin ML, Bernstein JL, Fisher ML, Packer M. Prognostic importance of the serum magnesium concentration in patients with congestive heart failure. *J Am Coll Cardiol* 1990;16:827–831.

279. Singh RB, Mori H, Kummerow FA. *Nutrition in coronary heart disease.* Moradabad, India: ICN Publications; 1991.

280. Millane TA, Jennison SH, Mann JM, Holt DW, McKenna WJ, Camm AJ. Myocardial magnesium depletion associated with prolonged hypomagnesemia: a longtitudinal study in heart transplant recipients. *J Am Coll Cardiol* 1992;20:806–812.

281. Altura BM, Lewenstam A, eds. Unique magnesium-sensitive ion selective electrodes. *Scand J Clin Lab Invest* 1994;54(Suppl 217).

282. Altura BT, Altura BM, Tranbaugh RF, et al. Plasma ionized magnesium measurements in human subjects during cardiopulmonary bypass: possible relationship to hypotension after cardio-

plegia and coronary spasm postperfusion. *Magnesium Trace Elem* 1990;9:325.

283. Altura BT, Shirey T, Young CC, et al. A new method for the rapid determination of ionized Mg²⁺ in whole blood, serum and plasma. *Methods Find Exp Clin Pharmacol* 1992;14:297–304.

284. Altura BT, Altura BM. Measurement of ionized magnesium in whole blood, plasma and serum with a new ion-selective electrode in healthy and diseased human subjects. *Magnesium Trace Elem* 1992;10:90–98.

285. Brookes CIO, Fry CH. Ionised magnesium and calcium in plasma from healthy volunteers and patients undergoing pulmonary bypass. *Br Heart J* 1993;69:404–408.

286. Wacker WEC. *Magnesium and man.* Cambridge: Harvard University Press; 1980.

287. Berkelhammer C, Bear RA. A clinical approach to common electrolyte problems. 4. Hypomagnesemia. *Can Med Assoc J* 1985;132:360–368.

288. Cronin RE, Knochel JP. Magnesium deficiency. *Adv Intern Med* 1983;38:509–533.

289. Altura BM, Altura BT. Peripheral and cerebrovascular actions of ethanol, acetaldehyde and acetate: relationship to divalent cations. *Alcohol Clin Exp Res* 1987;11:99–111.

290. Shane SR, Flink EB. Magnesium deficiency in alcohol addiction and withdrawal. *Magnesium Trace Elem* 1992;10:263–268.

291. Altura BM. Cardiovascular effects of alcohol and alcoholism. American Society of Pharmacology and Experimental Therapeutics Symposium, April 1981, Atlanta. *Fed Proc* 1982;41:2437–2464.

292. Beilin LJ, Puddey IB. Alcohol and essential hypertension. *Alcohol* 1984;19:191–195.

293. Potter JF, Bannen LT, Beevers DG. Alcohol and hypertension. *Br J Addict* 1984;79:365–372.

294. June CH, Thompson CB, Kennedy MS, Loughran JP Jr, Degg HJ. Correlation of hypomagnesemia with the onset of cyclosporine-associated hypertension in marrow transplant patients. *Transplantation* 1986;41:47–51.

295. Doll DC, Ringenberg QS, Yarbro JW. Vascular toxicity associated with antineoplastic agents. *J Clin Oncol* 1986;4:1405–1417.

296. Buckley JE, Clark VL, Meyer TJ, Pearlmen NW. Hypomagnesemia after cisplatin combination chemotherapy. *Arch Intern Med* 1987;144:2347–2348.

297. Sartori S, Nielsen I, Tassinari D, Rigolin F, Arcudi D, Abbasciano V. Changes in intracellular magnesium concentrations during cisplatin chemotherapy. *Oncol* 1993;50:230–234.

298. Zawada ET, Brautbar N. The possible role of magnesium in hypercalcemia hypertension. *Magnesium* 1984;3:132–137.

299. US Renal Data Systems. USRDS 1992 annual data report. Bethesda, MD: National Institutes of Health, National Institute of Diabetes and Digestive and Kidney Diseases; August 1992.

300. Elin RJ. Magnesium metabolism in health and disease. *Dis Month* 1988;34:161–218.

301. Valporean ML, Van Stone JC. Dialysate magnesium. *Semin Dialysis* 1993;6:46–51.

302. Lim P, Chir B, Dong S, Khoo OT. Intracellular magnesium depletion in CRF. *N Engl J Med* 1969;280:981–984.

303. Bergstrom J, Alverstrand A, Furst P, Hultman E, Widstam-Atorps U. Muscle intracellular electrolytes in patients with chronic uremia. *Kidney Int* 1983;24(Suppl 16):S153–S160.

304. Berlyne GM, Ben-Ari J, Szwarcberg J, Kaneti J, Danovitch GM, Kaye M. Increase in bone Mg content in renal failure in man. *Nephron* 1973;9:90–93.

305. Alfrey AC, Miller NL. Bone magnesium pools in uremia. *J Clin Invest* 1973;3019–3027.

306. Nishida A, Shapiro JI, Chan L. Effects of uremia on cytosolic free magnesium [Mg²⁺]ᵢ and energy metabolism in skeletal muscle. *Kidney Int*, Abstracts of the American Society of Nephrology 25th Annual Meeting, Baltimore, November 1992.

307. Goldstein S, Zsoter TJ. The effect of magnesium on the response of smooth muscle to 5-hydroxytryptamine. *Br J Pharmacol* 1978;62:507–514.

308. Fujiwara M, Kitagewa H, Kurahashi K. Effects of magnesium on contractile responses induced by electrical transmural stimulation in rabbit thoracic aorta. *Br J Pharmacol* 1978;63:51–56.

309. Greenberg S. Effect of prostacyclin and 9α, 11-α-epoxymethanoprostaglandin H₂ on calcium and magnesium fluxes and tension development in canine intralobular pulmonary arteries and veins. *J Pharmacol Exp Ther* 1981;219:326–337.

310. Foley DH. Magnesium withdrawal diminishes responses of rabbit coronary and femoral arterial smooth muscle to adenosine and sodium nitroprusside. *Magnesium* 1983;2:125–131.

311. Satoh Y, Okayama H, Keitoku M, Maruyama Y, Takishima T. The effect of Mg²⁺ on isolated human coronary arterial contraction. *J Appl Cardiol* 1988;3:111–120.

312. Kimura T, Yasue H, Sakaino N, Rokutanda M, Jougasaki M, Araki H. Effects of magnesium on the tone of isolated human coronary arteries. Comparison with diltiazem and nitroglycerin. *Circul* 1989;79:1118–1124.

313. Szabo C, Dora E, Frago M, Horvath I, Kovah AGB. Noradrenaline induces rhythmic contractions of feline middle cerebral artery at low extracellular magnesium concentration. *Blood Vessels* 1990;27:373–377.

314. Corr L, Burnstock G, Poole-Wilson P. Magnesium inhibits the responses to neuropeptide Y in the rabbit coronary artery. *J Mol Cell Cardiol* 1991;23:231–235.

315. Noguera MA, D'Ocon MP. Different and common intracellular-calcium stores mobilized by noradrenaline and caffeine in vascular smooth muscle. *Naunyn-Schmied Arch Pharmacol* 1992;345:333–341.

316. Noguera MA, D'Ocon MP. Modulatory role of magnesium on the contractile response of rat aorta to several agonists in normal and calcium-free medium. *J Pharm Pharmacol* 1993;45:697–700.

317. Gonzalez C, Cruz MA, Gallardo V, Varela J. Magnesium and potassium ions on tone and reactivity of human placental chorionic veins. *Gen Pharmacol* 1991;22:1121–1125.

318. Noguero MA, D'Ocon MP. Amplifying effect of serotonin on contractile responses in rat aorta and depletion of intracellular Ca-stores. *Gen Pharmacol* 1993;24:619–626.

319. Altura BM, Altura BT. Magnesium modulates calcium entry and contractility in vascular smooth muscle. In: Ohnishi T, Endo M, eds. *The mechanism of gated calcium transport across biological membranes.* New York: Academic Press; 1981:137–145.

320. Altura BM, Altura BT, Carella A, Turlapaty PDMV. Ca²⁺ coupling in vascular smooth muscle: Mg²⁺ and buffer effects on contractility and membrane Ca²⁺ movements. *Can J Physiol Pharmacol* 1982;60:459–482.

321. Altura BM, Altura BT, Carella A, Gebrewold A, Murakawa T, Nishio A. Mg²⁺-Ca²⁺ interaction in contractility of vascular smooth muscle: Mg²⁺ versus organic calcium channel blockers on myogenic tone and agonist-induced responsiveness of blood vessels. *Can J Physiol Pharmacol* 1987;65:729–745.

322. Chadda KD, Schultz NA. Magnesium deficiency and coronary vasospasm: role in sudden cardiac death. *Magnesium* 1982;1:84–94.

323. Bloom S. Coronary arterial lesions in Mg-deficient hamsters. *Magnesium* 1985;4:82–95.

324. Chang C, Varhghese J, Downey J, Bloom S. Mg-deficiency and myocardial infarct size in dogs. *J Am Coll Cardiol* 1985;5:280–289.

325. Buja LM, Burton KP, Hagler HK, Willerson JT. Quantitative x-ray microanalysis of the elemental composition of individual myocytes in hypoxic rabbit myocardium. *Circulation* 1983;68:872–882.

326. Altura BM, Altura BT. Magnesium and contraction of arterial smooth muscle. *Microvasc Res* 1974;7:145–155.

327. Altura BM, Altura BT. Magnesium withdrawal and contraction of arterial smooth muscle: effects of EDTA, EGTA and divalent cations. *Proc Soc Exp Biol Med* 1976;152:752–755.

328. Zhang A, Carella A, Altura BT, Altura BM. Interactions of magnesium and chloride ions on tone and contractility of vascular muscle. *Eur J Pharmacol* 1991;203:223–235.

329. Altura BT, Altura BM. Endothelial-dependent relaxation in coronary arteries requires magnesium ions. *Br J Pharmacol* 1987;91:449–451.

330. Ku DD, Ann HS. Magnesium deficiency produces endothelium-dependent vasorelaxation to canine coronary arteries. *J Pharmacol Exp Ther* 1987;241:961–966.

331. Gold ME, Buga GM, Wood KS, Byrns RE, Chaudhuri G, Ignarro LI. Antagonistic modulatory roles of magnesium and calcium on

release of endothelium-derived relaxing factors and smooth muscle tone. *Circ Res* 1990;66:355–366.

332. Zhang A, Cheng TP-O, Altura BM. Magnesium regulates intracellular free ionized calcium concentration and cell geometry in vascular smooth muscle cells. *Biochim Biophys Acta Molec Cell Res* 1992;1134:25–29.

333. Grynkiewicz G, Penie M, Jsien RY. A new generation of Ca^{2+} indicators with greatly improved fluorescence properties. *J Biol Chem* 1985;260:3440–3450.

334. Zhang A, Cheng TP-O, Altura BT, Altura BM. Reduction in extracellular ionic activity of magnesium induces elevation and oscillation of intracellular free calcium ($[Ca^{2+}]_i$) in canine cerebral vascular smooth muscle cells. *FASEB J* 1992;6:A1950.

335. Popescu LM, de Bruijn WC, Zelck U, Ionescu N. Intracellular distribution of calcium in smooth muscle. Facts and artifacts: a correlation of cytochemical, biochemical and x-ray microanalysis. *Findings Morphol Embryol* 1980;26:251–258.

336. Gunther T. Functional compartmentation of intracellular magnesium. *Magnesium* 1986;5:53–59.

337. Altura BM, Zhang A, Cheng TP-O. Effects of extracellular magnesium ($[Mg^{2+}]_o$) on intracellular free ionized magnesium concentration ($[Mg^{2+}]_i$) and its regulation in vascular smooth muscle cells. *FASEB J* 1992;6:1790.

338. Cochrane CG, Gimbrone MA Jr, eds. *Biological oxidants: generation of injurious consequences.* New York: Academic Press; 1992.

339. Yellon DM, Jennings RB, eds. *Myocardial protection. The pathophysiology of reperfusion and reperfusion injury.* New York: Raven Press; 1992.

340. Manfouz M, Kummerow FA. Effect of magnesium deficiency on delta-6-desaturase activity and fatty acid composition of rat liver microsomes. *Lipids* 1989;24:727–732.

341. Freedman AM, Altrakchi AH, Cassidy MM, Weglicki WB. Magnesium deficiency-induced cardiomyopathy: protection by vitamin E. *Biochem Biophys Res Commun* 1990;170:1102–1106.

342. Freedman AM, Cassidy MM, Weglicki WB. Captopril protects against myocardial injury induced by magnesium deficiency. *Hypertension* 1991;18:142–147.

343. Atrakchi AH, Bloom S, Dickens BF, Mak IT, Weglicki WB. Hypomagnesemia and isoproterenol cardiomyopathies: protection by probucol. *Cardiovasc Pathol* 1992;1:155–160.

344. Kummerow FA. Hypothesis: possible role of magnesium and calcium in the development of structure and function of the plasma membrane in mammalian cells and in human diseases. *J Am Coll Nutr* 1992;11:410–425.

345. Dickens BF, Weglicki WB, Li &-S, Mak IT. Magnesium deficiency in vitro enhances free radical-induced intracellular oxidation and cytotoxicity in endothelial cells. *FEBS Lett* 1992;311:187–191.

346. Rayssiguier Y, Gueux E, Bussiere L, Durlach J, Mazur A. Dietary magnesium affects susceptibility of lipoproteins and tissues to peroxidation in rats. *J Am Coll Nutr* 1993;12:133–127.

347. Guex E, Cubizolles C, Bussiere L, Mazur A, Rassiguier Y. Oxidative modification of triglyceride-rich lipoproteins in hypertriglyceridemic rats following magnesium deficiency. *Lipids* 1993;28:573–575.

348. Ross R. Atherosclerosis: a defense mechanism gone awry. *Am J Pathol* 1993;143:987–1002.

349. Morel DW, Chisolm GM. Antioxidant treatment of diabetic rats inhibits lipoprotein oxidation and toxicity. *J Lipids Res* 1989;30:1827–1834.

350. Weglicki WB, Phillips TM, Fredman AM, Cassidy MM, Dickens BF. Magnesium-deficiency elevates circulating levels of inflammatory cytokines and endothelin. *Molec Cell Biochem* 1992;118:105–111.

351. Altura BM, Altura BT. General anesthetics and magnesium ions as calcium antagonists on vascular smooth muscle. In: Weiss GB, ed. *New perspectives on calcium antagonists.* Washington, DC: American Physiological Society; 1981:131–145.

352. Iseri LT, French JH. Magnesium: nature's physiologic calcium blocker. *Am Heart J* 1984;108:188–193.

353. Levine BS, Coburn JW: Magnesium, the mimic antagonist of calcium. *N Engl J Med* 1984;310:1253–1255.

Blood Pressure Regulation in Normal and Hypertensive States

Part E: Molecular-Genetic Factors in Hypertension

Hypertension: Pathophysiology, Diagnosis, and Management, Second Edition, edited by J.H. Laragh and B.M. Brenner, Raven Press, Ltd., New York © 1995.

CHAPTER 73

Membrane Carriers Related to Intracellular Calcium Regulation

Ernesto Carafoli, Michele Chiesi, and Paolo Gazzotti

The signaling function of Ca^{2+} demands its modulation at submicromolar concentration levels. This is accomplished through the reversible complexation by specific binding proteins, which are present in the cytosol, organized in nonmembranous structures, or intrinsic to membranes. The most intensively studied class of Ca^{2+}-binding proteins has calmodulin and troponin C as its best-known members; proteins of this class repeat a structural model first established on the crystal structure of parvalbumin—that is, a 12-amino-acid Ca^{2+}-binding loop flanked by two α-helices perpendicular to each other. The calmodulin-type proteins undergo conformational changes upon binding of Ca^{2+}; that is, they become more hydrophobic on the surface and thus become able to transmit to target the Ca^{2+} information. Thus, the Ca^{2+}-binding proteins of the calmodulin-troponin-C type play the very important role of processing the Ca^{2+} signal. That they contribute to the overall Ca^{2+}-buffering power of cells is obvious. However, their Ca^{2+}-buffering role is evidently limited quantitatively by their total amount in cells: It can be calculated that calmodulin can buffer a maximum of 8 μM Ca^{2+}, whereas troponin C could buffer up to 6 μM and 80 μM Ca^{2+} in heart and skeletal muscles, respectively (1). These values are significant but may fall short of the requirements, particularly in cells where large amplitude movements of Ca^{2-} can be physiologically expected (e.g., muscles). Other Ca^{2+}-binding proteins, different from the parvalbumin-calmodulin-troponin-C group, are thus present in cells and, in fact, play the most important role in the buffering of Ca^{2+}. These proteins are intrinsic to membranes and move Ca^{2+} back and forth between cells and the extracellular ambient, as well as between cellular compartments. It is self-evident that the quantitative limitations of the soluble Ca^{2+}-binding proteins do not apply to the membrane-intrinsic Ca^{2+} (carrier) proteins. Even if present in very minute amounts, these proteins could buffer very large amounts of Ca^{2+}, provided that they complex it at one side of a membrane, transport it across, and "return" uncomplexed for the next binding and transport cycle. Normal eukaryotic cells contain several Ca^{2+}-carrying, membrane-intrinsic proteins (Fig. 1). They are found in the plasma membrane, in endo(sarco)plasmic reticulum, and in the inner membrane of the mitochondria. Since the functional cycle of cells demands both

E. Carafoli and P. Gazzotti: Laboratory of Biochemistry, Swiss Federal Institute of Technology (ETH), 8092 Zurich, Switzerland.
M. Chiesi: Department of Research, Pharmaceutical Division, Ciba-Geigy, Ltd., 4002 Basel, Switzerland.

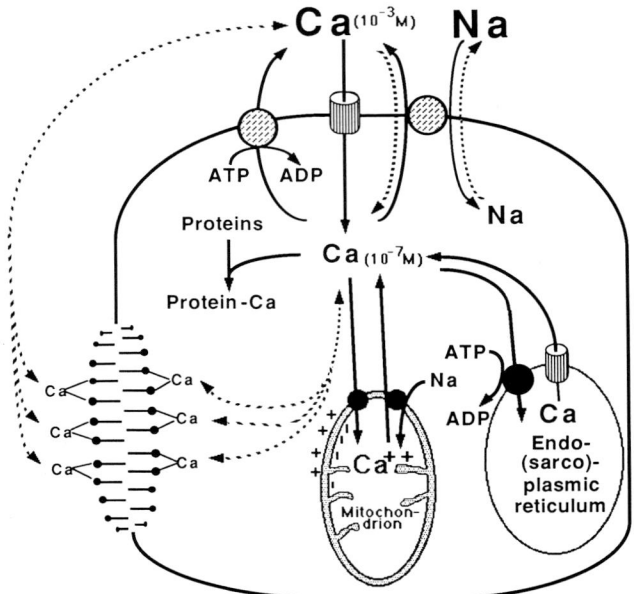

FIG. 1. Systems for the control of Ca²⁺ in eukaryotic cells. The scheme shows the soluble Ca²⁺-binding proteins and the membrane-intrinsic Ca²⁺-binding and transport proteins. The Ca²⁺-transporting systems in the lysosomes and in the Golgi membranes are only poorly known and are thus not shown.

high- and low-affinity regulation of Ca²⁺, some of those carrier proteins interact with Ca²⁺ with high affinity, whereas some react with low affinity. The high-affinity control is performed by adenosine triphosphatases (ATPases), whereas the low-affinity control chooses from among a number of other transporting modes (Table 1).

In this chapter, a succinct description will be offered of the systems that transport Ca²⁺ across the plasma and the organellar membranes. Although the general principles of membrane transport of Ca²⁺ are valid for all cells, differences exist in the relative importance of the various systems and perhaps even in their mechanisms. Given the special importance of (smooth) muscle to hypertension, particular attention will be paid to the aspects that are typical of, or of particular importance to, muscles.

CALCIUM TRANSPORT IN THE PLASMA MEMBRANE

Three Ca²⁺-transporting systems are located in the plasma membrane: a channel, an ATPase, and a Na⁺–

Ca²⁺ exchanger. The channel is the system responsible for the controlled influx of Ca²⁺ into cells; the other two systems are responsible for Ca²⁺ export. Under some circumstances, however, the Na⁺–Ca²⁺ exchanger can also operate in the direction of Ca²⁺ influx.

The Calcium Channel

The Ca²⁺ channel has been known for decades, but the most significant contributions to its understanding have only come recently, following the introduction of the patch-clamp technique, which has permitted the study of single channels. A direct outcome of the work on single channels has been the discovery that several Ca²⁺-channel types exist, differing in electrophysiological properties (2). At present, four channel types have been identified: the L, the N, the T, and the P. The most common is the L type, which is the classic channel on which most pharmacological studies have been performed. It is "gated" by the electrical potential across the plasma membrane, with Ca²⁺ currents becoming evident as the transmembrane potential increases from the resting level of about −70 mV to about −40 mV: the current peaks at about 0 mV. The openings of the L-type Ca²⁺ channels produce currents of relatively long duration and allow the passage of about 3×10^6 Ca²⁺ ions per second (the duration of the opening event, however, is much shorter).

A number of compounds of pharmacological importance to the field of hypertension have been found to block the L-type channels. They are collectively referred to as *Ca²⁺ antagonists* (3). The best known among them are the *dihydropyridines,* of which a large number of derivatives have been prepared, with different lipophilicity, tissue specificity and affinity, and metabolic properties. The finding that lipophilicity increases the effectiveness of dihydropyridines is normally taken as an indication that they act on the channel from the lipid phase of the membrane. Also important as L-channel blockers are tertiary amines such as verapamil, as well as some benzothiazepines (diltiazem).

The N- and T-type channels are less well characterized and their pharmacological reactivity is virtually unknown (a toxin, omega-conotoxin, has been found to block the N channels). The T channels, which open at more negative transmembrane potentials than do the L channels, are responsible for short-duration currents.

TABLE 1. *Ca²⁺-transporting systems in cell membranes*

Transporting mode	Membrane system	Ca²⁺ affinity
ATPases	Plasma membrane and endo(sarco)plasmic reticulum (Golgi? lysosomes?)	High
Exchangers (Na⁺–Ca²⁺)	Plasma membrane and mitochondria	Low
Channels	Plasma membrane and endo(sarco)plasmic reticulum	Low
Electrophoretic uniporters	Mitochondrial inner membrane	Low

The N channel is only found in nervous tissues: It is opened by very large depolarizations from negative transmembrane potentials. One important aspect of the L channels is the positive regulation by a cAMP-dependent phosphorylation process. The phenomenon offers obvious therapeutic possibilities in heart pharmacology (4) and in fact mediates, in part, the positive inotropic effect of β-agonists. (However, see the discussion below on the Ca^{2+}-ATPase of the plasma membrane.) The effect of the phosphorylation is the increase in the probability of channel opening: Under optimal stimulation conditions, up to 70 percent of the total channels may be found in the open state as opposed to only about 10 percent under nonstimulated (i.e., nonphosphorylated) conditions.

When considering the plasma membrane of cells like heart or skeletal muscle as a whole, the density of the Ca^{2+} channels is much lower than that of the Na^+ channel. However, in specialized plasma membrane domains (e.g., the T system in skeletal muscle cells), the channel is very abundant. This finding has been instrumental in the success of the isolation attempts, which have used labeled dihydropyridines to tag the channel (5,6). The isolated channel appears to be a complex structure, consisting of two α subunits of about 170 kDa, one β subunit of 55 kDa, and one γ subunit of about 30 kDa (a δ subunit has also been suggested). The isolated complex has recently been incorporated into planar phospholipid bilayers, forming a 20-pS channel that retains the functional characteristics of the L channels in the native membranes (7). An important development of the isolation work has been the determination of the primary structure of the dihydropyridine receptor in the Ca^{2+} channel from skeletal muscles (8). The largest subunit of the channel (170 kDa), which contains the dihydropyridine receptor, has been sequenced using DNA cloning techniques. The subunit is homologous with the voltage-dependent sodium channel both in amino acid sequence and in the putative transmembrane topology, containing four units of homology spanning the membrane. Each of the four units, which are assumed to surround the ionic channel, contain six presumably α-helical transmembrane stretches. The fourth of the six putative α helices in every repeat contains five or six Arg or Lys residues, which may represent the voltage sensor. The total number of amino acids in the receptor is 1,873, corresponding to a M_r of 212,018. The discrepancy with the previously accepted Mr of about 170,000 may be due to proteolytic effects or to inaccuracies in the electrophoretic method of Mr determination. The homology with the sodium channel, whose channel function can be expressed by cDNA corresponding to the large polypeptide of 260 kDa (9), suggests that the dihydropyridine receptor itself is a Ca^{2+} channel. However, Ca^{2+} entry through the channel is not essential for contraction in skeletal muscle, suggesting that the receptor may have another function; that is, it may be a voltage sensor involved in excitation-contraction coupling to release Ca^{2+} from the sarcoplasmic reticulum (see below).

The Na^+–Ca^{2+} Exchanger

The Na^+–Ca^{2+} exchanger is a large-capacity Ca^{2+}-transporting system, which is particularly active in excitable tissues (e.g., heart). Although its main function is accepted to be the export of Ca^{2+}, there is general agreement that under certain conditions the system can also mediate Ca^{2+} influx, at least in heart cells. Most of the knowledge currently available on the exchanger derives from work on heart and the giant axon of the squid (10,11). Early experiments have indicated that the carrier operates electrogenically, exchanging three Na^+ for one Ca^{2+}: Therefore, it responds not only to the Na^+ and Ca^{2+} gradients across the plasma membrane but also to the transmembrane electrical potential. An important development, which has permitted the precise determination of the biochemical parameters of the process, has been the successful measurement of the exchange reaction in isolated heart sarcolemmal vesicles (12). Sarcolemmal vesicles have now become the method of choice for the biochemical study of the reaction: They have allowed researchers to establish conclusively that the cation stoichiometry of the carrier is one Ca^{2+} for three Na^+ and that the K_m (Ca^{2+}) of the system is disappointingly high (5 μM or more). This point is of particular importance for the functioning of the system *in vivo* because it is difficult to see how the carrier could ever become significantly activated under the conditions presumably prevailing *in vivo* (i.e., 100–200 nM free Ca^{2+}). Although the concentration of free Ca^{2+} in the cytoplasm (e.g., in heart) undoubtedly fluctuates during the functional cycle of cells, values in excess of 1 μM seem unrealistic. The possibility, of course, exists that the properties of the exchanger may have become altered during the separation of the sarcolemmal vesicles, but it seems more likely that endogenous factors, some of which are possibly still unknown, activate the system (i.e., increase its Ca^{2+} affinity) *in vivo*. The putative endogenous activating factors include acidic phospholipids and limited proteolysis (10), but it must also be mentioned that Mg, at the concentrations presumably present *in vivo*, depresses the Ca^{2+} affinity of the system (13). Of particular interest in this connection is the finding (14) that the Ca^{2+} affinity of the exchanger in heart sarcolemmal vesicles is increased by a kinase-linked phosphorylation process. Recent work (15) has extended the latter findings to the giant axon of the squid, showing a large activation of the exchange reaction under conditions that would favor its kinase-linked phosphorylation. After a long succession of conventional identification and purification attempts (16,17), the cardiac exchanger has recently been cloned

(17b). The protein has 11 putative transmembrane domains and a very large unit (more than 400 residues) protruding into the cytosol between transmembrane domains 5 and 6. This unit contains a calmodulin binding domain (however, the exchanger is not known to be calmodulin-sensitive) (17c) and a Ca^{2+} binding site (17d). Surprisingly, the deletion of this large intracellular unit only depresses the activity of the exchanger by about 50 percent (17e).

A number of inhibitors, most of which are amiloride derivatives, have been described (18), but none shows the necessary inhibitory specificity for the exchanger. In principle, the exchanger would be an ideal candidate for pharmacological attempts to influence the cellular homeostasis of Ca^{2+}. An additional problem is the fact that the exchanger is enzymatically silent: tests of its function must therefore use reconstituted phospholipid vesicles (19)—obviously a much more difficult task than the measurement of enzymatic activities in membrane-free systems.

One last point worth mentioning in this discussion of the Na^+–Ca^{2+} exchanger, in view of the particular importance of (vascular) smooth muscle to hypertension, is the existence and the role of the exchanger in the latter tissue. The existence of the exchanger in the plasma membrane of smooth muscle has traditionally been viewed as a controversial issue, although there is general agreement that the system, if present, is of low activity (20). Recent work on isolated plasma membrane vesicles has conclusively documented the exchanger in vascular smooth muscle (21,22), myometrium (23), ileal smooth muscle (24), and tracheal smooth muscle (25). These recent contributions have confirmed that the activity of the system is much lower than the activity in heart sarcolemma.

The Ca^{2+}-ATPase of the Plasma Membrane

The third Ca^{2+}-transport system present in the plasma membrane is an ATPase that pumps Ca^{2+} out of the cell (26). It is now generally assumed that the enzyme is present in all eucaryotic plasma membranes. Although the general mechanistic prototype of the ATPase appears to be that extensively studied on the erythrocyte, some plasma membranes (e.g., those of liver) (27) may contain an enzyme with slightly different properties. It may also be mentioned in this context that recent work on the primary structure of the enzyme using DNA cloning techniques has revealed several isoforms of the ATPase (see below).

The pump is a high-affinity enzyme, which interacts with Ca^{2+} with a K_m well below 1 μM. Thus, the pump is ideally qualified to export Ca^{2+} continuously from the cell, although, at variance with the Na^+–Ca^{2+} exchanger, it does so with a low total transport capacity, of the order of 0.5 nmoles per milligram of membrane protein per second. This value may be adequate to satisfy the Ca^{2+} export requirements of nonexcitable cells (e.g., erythrocytes) but is likely to be insufficient in other cell types (e.g., heart); this explains the presence of an active Na^+–Ca^{2+} exchanger in these cells.

The pump belongs to the ATPases of the P class; that is, it forms an aspartyl-phosphate during the reaction cycle (28). Its reaction mechanism is thus analogous to that of the Ca^{2+}-ATPase of sarcoplasmic reticulum. Since the latter will be described in some detail below, no detailed mechanistic discussion will be offered here. It is worth mentioning, however, that the Ca^{2+}/ATP stoichiometry of the plasma membrane pump is 1, whereas that of the sarcoplasmic reticulum pump is 2. The plasma membrane pump is a target of calmodulin stimulation (29,30); however, at variance with other enzyme targets where calmodulin acts by promoting phosphorylation, the activation in this case is due to the direct interaction of calmodulin with the pump. The stimulation by calmodulin is predominantly on the Ca^{2+} affinity of the enzyme: The K_m shifts from 10–20 μM in the absence of the activator to about 0.4–0.5 μM in its presence. A number of treatment alternatives to calmodulin, studied in detail on the purified enzyme, activate the ATPase in a way similar to calmodulin. Among them is the exposure to acidic phospholipids (including the phosphorylated derivatives of phosphatidylinositol), or polyunsaturated fatty acids and a controlled treatment with a number of proteases, particularly trypsin (31–33).

The interaction with calmodulin has permitted the isolation of the ATPase, first from erythrocytes (34) and then from a number of other plasma membranes, including those of heart (35) and smooth muscle (36), using calmodulin affinity chromatography. The purified enzyme (37) is a single polypeptide of about 140 kDa that reproduces the functional properties of the enzyme *in situ*, including the transport of Ca^{2+} with optimal efficiency in reconstituted liposomes. The reconstituted system has permitted researchers to conclude that the Ca^{2+}/ATP stoichiometry of the enzyme is 1, as opposed to the analogous enzyme of sarcoplasmic reticulum, whose stoichiometry is 2 (see below). It has also shown that the pump operates as an obligatory proton exchanger (38), although the stoichiometry of the exchange (i.e., electroneutral or electrogenic) is still open.

One very interesting aspect of the ATPase, both in the membrane environment and in the purified state, is the phosphorylation by the cyclic adenosine monophosphate (cAMP)-dependent kinase (39,40). The phosphorylation activates the enzyme, thus potentiating the efflux of Ca^{2+} from cells: Taken together with the activation of the Ca^{2+} channels described above, this shows that the effect of cAMP is not the undirectional activation of any given Ca^{2+}-transporting system of the plasma membrane (i.e., the Ca^{2+} channel) but is, instead, the overall increase of the flux of Ca^{2+} across it. Phosphorylation of the pump by protein kinase C has also been repeatedly reported, but its functional effect (an activation) is not as evident as that of the cAMP-dependent kinase. Protein kinase C phosphorylates the pump at least two sites, one of them located within the calmodulin-binding domain (40b).

Work using a combination of labeling and proteolysis techniques (41) has identified the calmodulin-binding domain next to the C-terminus of the ATPase molecule. The domain resembles the calmodulin-binding domains of other calmodulin-modulated enzymes (e.g., myosin light-chain kinase) in its propensity to form an amphiphilic helix and in its strong basic character. The complete primary structure of the enzyme was first deduced from the DNA of a teratoma cell library (42): its molecular architecture in the plasma membrane is shown schematically in Fig. 2. This isoform of the pump contains 1,220 amino acids, corresponding to a M_r of 134,683. Asp 475 forms the acyl phosphate during the reaction cycle, and Lys 601 binds the ATP antagonist fluorescein isothiocyanate (FITC). Acidic sequences have been recognized at the two sides of the calmodulin-binding domain. These sequences have been found to contain Ca^{2+} binding sites (40c), and could indeed play a role in the binding of Ca^{2+} and in regulating the interaction of calmodulin with the pump. The calmodulin binding domain has been shown to interact with the main body of the pump during the resting state at two sites close to the active site (40c,40d). This maintains the pump in the inhibited state: calmodulin presumably swings its binding domain away, relieving the inhibition. Of the ten hydrophobic domains, four are located in the N-terminal portion of the pump, and six are located in the C-terminal portion. The midportion of the pump (about 500 residues) contains no hydrophobic domains. The residue phosphorylated by the cAMP-dependent kinase is Ser 1178, located on the C-terminal side of the calmodulin-binding domain. As mentioned above,

screening of cDNA libraries made with RNA from different tissues (e.g., muscle, brain, intestinal mucosa) has shown that numerous isoforms of the pump exist. In humans, four genes have been identified and located on chromosomes 1, 12, χ, and 3. Additional isoform diversity is produced by alternative splicing of primary transcripts. Although at the protein level only a limited number of isoforms have so far been detected, mRNA analysis has identified well over 20 isoforms (40f). At the present time, two of the gene products termed 1 and 4 appear to be expressed in equivalent amounts in all human tissues examined (housekeeping genes). The other two gene products are instead transcribed in a tissue-specific way, brain being the favored tissue for their expression. As for the alternative splicing, it occurs at two preferred locations in the molecule: site A is in the N-terminal region, site C within the calmodulin-binding domain (40g,40h).

CALCIUM TRANSPORT SYSTEMS OF MITOCHONDRIA AND THEIR FUNCTIONAL ROLE

Two intracellular compartments—the sarcoplasmic reticulum and the mitochondria—have the ability of sequestering Ca^{2+} by means of energy-dependent processes. This was first reported in 1961 (43,44). The role of sarcoplasmic (endoplasmic) reticulum as the main regulator of the cytosolic free Ca^{2+} level has been clearly demonstrated (45,46) (see below). On the other hand, the exact function of the mitochondrial Ca^{2+} transport systems is still a matter for debate. The modes of Ca^{2+} transport in mitochondria, as well as their functional role, will be briefly discussed here.

The Mitochondrial Ca^{2+} Uniporter

Mitochondria isolated from almost all sources can actively transport Ca^{2+} across the inner membrane into their matrix (47–49). The driving force for this active transport is the electrical potential generated across the inner membrane during oxidation of metabolic substrates by the respiratory chain or during hydrolysis of ATP by the coupling ATPase. The electrophoretic nature of the Ca^{2+}-transport process has been clearly shown using mitochondria in which the respiratory chain and the ATPase are both inhibited. These mitochondria can still accumulate Ca^{2+} in response to a diffusion potential generated across the inner membrane by a gradient of K^+ in the presence of the neutral ionophore valinomycin (50). The observed stoichiometry of two K^+ released per Ca^{2+} accumulated indicates that the Ca^{2+} carrier is working as a uniporter (51). The net transfer of two charges per Ca^{2+} transported is also consistent with the results obtained using other experimental approaches.

The uptake of Ca^{2+} via the uniporter can be reversed

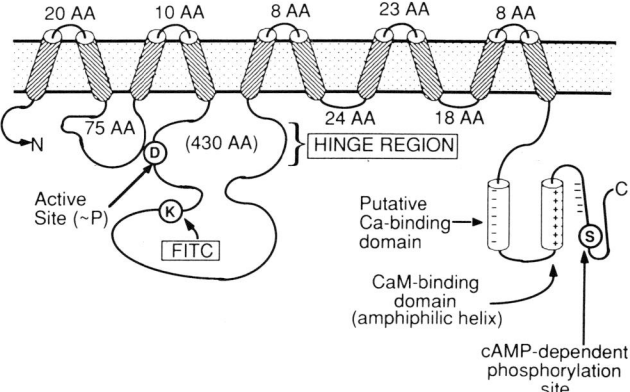

FIG. 2. A schematic representation of the membrane architecture of the plasma membrane Ca^{2+}-ATPase.

by lowering the membrane potential. The efflux of Ca^{2+} that occurs under deenergized conditions is prevented by inhibitors of Ca^{2+} transport through the uniporter, indicating that the efflux occurs via reversal of the uniporter.

In respiring mitochondria, in the absence of electroneutrally permeant anions, net Ca^{2+} transport is accompanied by the extrusion of protons by the respiratory chain, with a stoichiometry of $2H^+/Ca^{2+}$ (52). Under these conditions the uptake of Ca^{2+} is relatively limited (about 90 nmoles per milligram of protein), since the extrusion of H^+ by the respiratory chain causes alkalinization of the matrix and a decrease in membrane potential. In the presence of phosphate, which enters mitochondria electroneutrally via a H^+-phosphate symport, the high pH gradient formed during the uptake of Ca^{2+} is dissipated and more Ca^{2+} (up to 2 micromoles per milligram of protein) can enter the matrix, where it forms an insoluble complex with phosphate (53). The Ca^{2+}-phosphate complex can be seen as electron-opaque granules in the electron microscope (54).

The kinetic parameters of the mitochondrial Ca^{2+}-uniporter depend strongly on the experimental conditions, particularly on the ionic strength and Mg^{2+} concentration (55–57). Relatively low K_m values for external Ca^{2+} (between 1 and 5 μM) are obtained in media of low ionic strength in the absence of Mg^{2+}, whereas higher values (15–40 μM) are found under more physiological conditions in the presence of Mg^{2+} and high ionic strength. The apparent maximum velocity (V_{max}) reported for heart mitochondria is between 100 and 1,000 nmoles Ca^{2+}/min per milligram of protein. The Ca^{2+} uniporter is inhibited by the hexavalent ruthenium complex ruthenium red (58).

The chemical nature of the mitochondrial Ca^{2+} uniporter is still a matter for debate. A soluble Ca^{2+}-binding glycoprotein has been isolated, and it has been shown that antibodies against this 42-kDa protein inhibit the uptake of Ca^{2+} in liver mitochondria (59,60). Since the glycoprotein is not an integral protein, it has been postulated that it could work as a superficial Ca^{2+} receptor in the transport system. A 6-kDa Ca^{2+}-binding protein (calciphorin) that can move Ca^{2+} into an organic phase in a ruthenium red sensitive fashion has also been isolated (61).

The Na^+-Ca^{2+} Exchanger

Na^+-induced release of Ca^{2+} from preloaded mitochondria was first shown in 1974 (62). It was later found that the efflux is mediated by a presumably electroneutral Na^+–Ca^{2+} exchanger that is present in the inner membrane of mitochondria of most mammalian tissues (63,64). The Na^+-induced Ca^{2+} release is an active process because Ca^{2+} ions must exit against the electrochemical gradient of Ca^{2+} present in energized mitochondria.

The energy for the release of Ca^{2+} is provided by the electrochemical gradient of Na^+, and the release occurs without collapsing the membrane potential. The carrier is specifically inhibited by some Ca^{2+} antagonists (e.g., diltiazem, $K_i 7$ μM) and by lanthanides (65,66), but the sensitivity to lanthanides is about 30 times lower than that of the uniporter. The Na^+–Ca^{2+} exchanger, whose activity is much lower than that of the uniporter, is optimally measured after inhibition of the influx pathway with ruthenium red; it is particularly active in mitochondria isolated from excitable tissues such as heart (V_{max}: about 20 nmoles Ca^{2+}/min per milligram of protein, at Na^+ concentration 10 mM) but has low activity (about 5–10 nmoles/min per milligram of protein) in nonexcitable tissues. The affinity of the exchanger for internal Ca^{2+}, obtained by measuring the intramitochondrial free Ca^{2+} concentration with the so-called null-point Ca^{2+} titration technique, is about 6 μM (67). Half-maximal activation of the Ca^{2+} efflux rate catalyzed by the exchanger is observed at 4–5 mM Na^+. Although the relationship linking the Ca^{2+} efflux rate to the Na^+ concentration is strongly sigmoidal, significant changes of cytosolic Na^+ are presumably necessary to induce an evident activation of the exchanger in vivo.

Functional Role of the Ca^{2+}-Transport Systems in Mitochondria

The magnitude of the membrane potential generated by respiring mitochondria in vivo is assumed to be around 160 mV (68). Hence, Ca^{2+} should attain electrochemical equilibrium across the inner membrane at a free concentration ratio of about 10^5. Since the cytosolic Ca^{2+} concentration is between 10^{-7} and 10^{-6} M, the intramitochondrial free Ca^{2+} in vivo should be about 10^{-2} M. However, experiments using electron-probe x-ray microanalysis (EPMA) in quickly frozen tissues (45,46) have shown that in smooth muscle cells (and also in other cell types) the intramitochondrial Ca^{2+} is much lower, approximately 2 nmoles per milligram of mitochondrial protein (i.e., about 2 mM). Assuming a ratio of mitochondrial free Ca^{2+} to total Ca^{2+} of about 10^{-3} (67), the EPMA measurements indicate that the intramitochondrial free Ca^{2+} is about 2 μM. This value is about four orders of magnitude lower than that predicted from the electrochemical equilibrium of Ca^{2+} in energized mitochondria but is consistent with the low uniporter affinity for Ca^{2+} found in isolated mitochondria. It clearly indicates that mitochondria are unlikely to play a significant role in the physiological regulation of cytoplasmic Ca^{2+}. This conclusion is also supported by experiments that show no significant increase in mitochondrial Ca^{2+} during maximal contraction in smooth muscle (69).

However, the mitochondrial Ca^{2+}-transport systems can be activated in vivo under pathological conditions that allow cytosolic Ca^{2+} to increase much above the physiological level. Mitochondria can then accumulate and store large amounts of Ca^{2+} in the form of an insoluble Ca^{2+} phosphate complex without significant alterations to the ionic concentration of Ca^{2+} in the matrix (70,71). If the injured cells recover before mitochondria are irreversibly damaged, the excess Ca^{2+} accumulated by mitochondria will be gradually released back to the cytoplasm. Since Ca^{2+} will have to be dissolved from the precipitated phosphate salt deposits, it is likely that the release will occur slowly (i.e., at a rate compatible with the exporting capacity of the plasma membrane systems). In other words, the ability of mitochondria to accumulate large quantities of Ca^{2+} and phosphate is an essential safety device that prevents deleterious increases of Ca^{2+} in the cytoplasm of injured cells (71).

Recently, it has become gradually accepted that the most important role of the mitochondrial Ca^{2+} transport systems in healthy cells is the regulation of the intramitochondrial Ca^{2+}-dependent dehydrogenases (72). It is now known that in higher animals at least three intramitochondrial dehydrogenases—pyruvate dehydrogenase phosphate phosphatase, NAD^+-dependent isocitrate dehydrogenase, and 2-oxoglutarate dehydrogenase—can be activated severalfold by increasing the concentration of free Ca^{2+} from 0.1 to 1.0 and above, with half-maximal activation at about 1 μM free Ca^{2+} (Fig. 3). Therefore, a relatively small increase of cytoplasmic Ca^{2+}, sufficient to slightly activate the uniporter, may change the intramitochondrial free Ca^{2+} and regulate the rate of oxidative phosphorylation by regulating the activity of the Ca^{2+}-dependent dehydrogenases. Whether matrix Ca^{2+} can be increased sufficiently in this way by

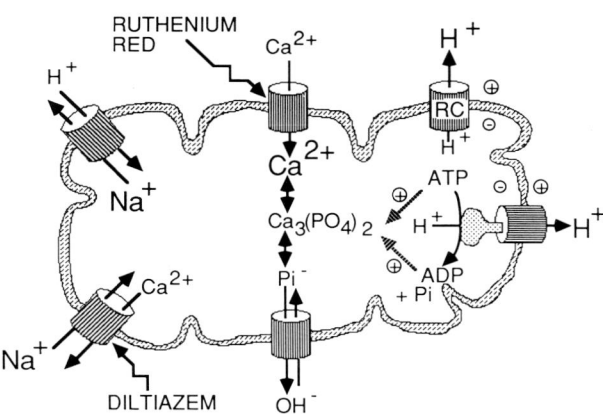

FIG. 4. The membrane carriers involved in the transport of Ca^{2+} in and out of the mitochondria. RC, respiratory chain.

physiological effectors is an open question. A general summary of the Ca^{2+}-transporting systems of mitochondria and of the carriers and reactions related to them is presented in Fig. 4.

CALCIUM TRANSPORT ACROSS THE MEMBRANE OF SARCOPLASMIC (ENDOPLASMIC) RETICULUM

In mammalian striated muscles, including the heart, most of the excitatory Ca^{2+} derives from the sarcoplasmic reticulum (SR); this justifies a detailed description of the functional and molecular characteristics of the Ca^{2+}-transporting systems in the organelle. The SR consists basically of two continuous elements: (a) a system of longitudinal tubules that surrounds the myofibrils, and (b) the terminal cisternae [i.e., the enlarged saclike structures that are in contact with the plasma membrane and, in particular, with its tubular invaginations (the transverse tubular system, also called the *T system*)]. Terminal cisternae and the T system form a junctional gap with a width of 10–20 nm (73,74). The cleft is crossed by periodic densities (called *feet*) that join the two membranes and that are thought to play a crucial role in excitation-contraction coupling (75). The cisternal elements of the SR contain a filamentous interior matrix, whereas the longitudinal system is virtually empty (76). The filaments are made up of a very acidic Ca^{2+}-binding protein of M_r about 63,000. The protein is named *calsequestrin* (77) and binds nearly 1 μmol of Ca^{2+} per milligram (30–40 mole of Ca^{2+}/mole of calsequestrin) with low affinity (the dissociation constant is about 800 μM). The rapid release and subsequent reaccumulation of Ca^{2+} by the SR are responsible for the contraction and relaxation of the myofilaments. This performance is made possible by two Ca^{2+}-transporting systems: a Ca^{2+}-pump and Ca^{2+}-release channels. The Ca^{2+} pump (ATPase) translocates Ca^{2+} from the cytosol

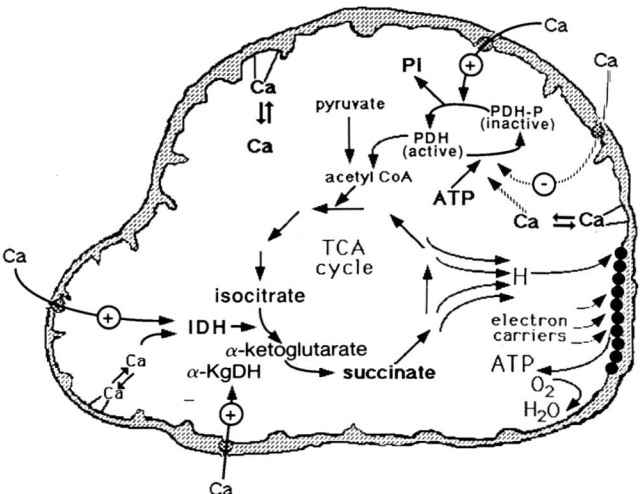

FIG. 3. Calcium control of some of the dehydrogenases of the mitochondrial matrix. PDH, pyruvate dehydrogenase; IDH, isocitrate dehydrogenase (NAD-dependent); α-KgDH, ketoglutarate dehydrogenase.

into the lumen of the SR at a rate that is compatible with the physiological requirements of relaxation. The ATPase is distributed all along the SR, with the exception of the portion adjacent to the gap junctions (78). Most of the Ca^{2+} in the luminal space is stored in the cisternal compartments, where it is buffered by calsequestrin. Excitation of muscle cells—induced, for instance, by the depolarization of the plasma membrane during the action potential (79)—causes the opening of Ca^{2+}-release channels localized on the cisternal compartments (80), massive Ca^{2+} efflux, and contraction of the myofilaments. Ca^{2+} stores that are similar to those of the SR and that can release physiologically relevant amounts of Ca^{2+} in response to chemical transmitters have been described also in various smooth muscles and in nonmuscle cells. In fact, it has been observed that an organelle (named *calciosome*), possibly separated from the (endoplasmic) reticulum, is present in a variety of cell types (81). Such an organelle contains a Ca^{2+} pump, a calsequestrinlike protein, and Ca^{2+}-release channels, and it could thus act as a rapid regulator of the intracellular Ca^{2+} homeostasis.

The Ca^{2+}-Pumping ATPase of Sarcoplasmic Reticulum

The Ca^{2+}-ATPase is the principal protein component of the SR. The protein consists of a polypeptide chain of about 105,000 Da (82) with a pronounced amphiphilic character. A hydrophilic portion protrudes from the cytoplasmic surface of the membrane, and a hydrophobic core is inserted into the membrane bilayer. The membrane architecture is thus analogous to that of the Ca^{2+}-ATPase of the plasma membrane (see Fig. 2). Proteolytic fragmentation and subsequent isolation of five cytoplasmic segments have permitted the determination of the amino acid sequence of most of the hydrophilic portion of the enzyme, on which the active sites (such as the adenine-nucleotide-binding and fluorescein isothiocyanate-binding sites and the phosphorylation site) are localized (83–85). The full sequence of the Ca^{2+} pump has been deduced from its complementary DNA sequence (86). The predicted secondary structure and the membrane topography thus obtained indicate three distinct domains: (a) a hydrophobic portion made up of 10 putative transmembrane helices (M1–M10); (b) a stalk made up of a pentahelical amphipathic piece; and (c) three globular cytoplasmic regions, which contain the adenine-nucleotide-binding domains, the phosphorylation domains, and the transduction domains. Several isoforms of the Ca^{2+} pump have been identified in muscular tissue by immunologic techniques (87,88), and two separate genes have been identified, encoding the isoforms present in fast-twitch and slow-twitch muscle and named SERCA1 and SERCA2 (89). The SERCA1 gene encodes two alternatively spliced transcripts that differ in their

C-termini and are developmentally regulated (SERCA1a and SERCA1b are found in adult skeletal and neonatal skeletal muscle, respectively). The SERCA2 gene also encodes two alternatively spliced isoforms; one is present in slow twitch and cardiac muscle (SERCA2a) whereas the other is expressed in smooth muscle and in nonmuscle cells (SERCA2b) (89a). In spite of their differences, the predicted secondary structures of the two isoforms lead to a similar topographical mapping of the pump, indicating similar mechanisms of action.

The principal characteristics of the catalytic and transport cycle of the ATPase of fast skeletal muscle SR have been clarified. As already mentioned, SR membranes accumulate 2 moles of Ca^{2+} per mole of ATP hydrolyzed (90). Each ATPase molecule contains one reactive catalytic site (91,92) and a class of high-affinity Ca^{2+}-binding sites (K_d of about 10^{-6} M) exposed to the cytosolic face. They are stoichiometrically correlated to the catalytic site in a 2:1 ratio (93) and display a cooperative behavior along with a major conformational change of the protein. Direct measurements of Ca^{2+}-binding with rapid filtration techniques (94) have shown that the binding to a first set of sites induces a conformational change that renders a second set of sites available for Ca^{2+}-binding (93,94). During ATP utilization a phosphorylated intermediate form of the enzyme appears transiently; that is, the terminal phosphate of ATP is transferred to the aspartic acid residue typical of the catalytic site (95,96). The phosphoenzyme is formed very rapidly, but only if the high-affinity Ca^{2+}-binding sites presumed to be located near the center of transmembrane sequences M4, M5, M6, and M8 (96a,96b) are saturated (97). Ca^{2+} ions bound to negatively charged groups become rapidly internalized (occluded) after enzyme phosphorylation by bound ATP (98). In fact, lanthanum or ethylene glycol bis(aminoethyl ether)tetraacetic acid (EGTA) displace Ca^{2+} from these sites before, but not after, phosphoenzyme formation. Ca^{2+} is then released into the lumen of the SR before hydrolytic cleavage of the phosphoenzyme takes place. The inwardly oriented Ca^{2+} binding sites (which are exposed to the lumen but are inaccessible from the cytoplasm) have much lower Ca^{2+} affinity, so that high Ca^{2+} concentrations can be attained in the lumen. The vectorial translocation process can be visualized as the passage through a turnstile where access to the Ca^{2+} translocation site alternates between cytoplasmic and luminal sides (96a). The activation of the turnstile leading to the disruption of the high-affinity sites could be coupled to the conformational changes that are known to occur during the transition between the high-energy and the low-energy forms of the phosphorylated intermediate (the E_1–P and E_2–P states, respectively). To complete the transport cycle, the phosphoenzyme then undergoes hydrolytic cleavage and the enzyme returns to the original conformation. Whether the Ca^{2+} pump is intrinsically electrogenic or whether the transport reaction includes the co- or counter transport of specific compensating ions is still open to question. Experiments carried out on reconstituted ATPase preparations have shown that the process of Ca^{2+}-pumping produces separation of charges across the membrane (99,100). Native SR membranes, however, are very permeable to a variety of cations and anions that cross the membrane via independent channels, which would rapidly compensate for any electrogenic property of the pump.

All the steps involved in the transport cycle are fully reversible, and it is indeed possible to utilize the dissipation of the transmembrane Ca^{2+} gradient *in vitro* to induce ATP synthesis (101). The reversal of the Ca^{2+} pump involves the binding of Pi and the formation of phosphorylated intermediates that are chemically equivalent to those formed by utilization of ATP. In principle, reversal of the Ca^{2+} pump could account for a rapid Ca^{2+} release from the SR, but it is doubtful that the reversal could occur under physiological conditions.

A schematic summary of the organization of SR in the muscle fiber and of the molecular architecture of SR's Ca^{2+} uptake and release systems is presented in Fig. 5.

Physiological Regulation of the Ca^{2+} Pump

In cardiac muscle, the activation of a cAMP-dependent protein kinase leads to the massive stimulation of the Ca^{2+}-pumping activity of the SR (102–104).

The stimulation provides an explanation for the mediation by cAMP of some of the most important heart effects of catecholamines:

1. *Abbreviation of the systole.* The SR removes more efficiently and rapidly the Ca^{2+} ions from the cytosol (i.e., from the myofilaments), thus improving the relaxation kinetics.
2. *Positive inotropism.* The Ca^{2+} gradient across the SR membrane (i.e., the amount of rapidly releasable Ca^{2+}) is increased by the stimulation of the pump.

However, additional phosphorylation processes catalyzed by the cAMP-dependent kinase [such as the phosphorylation of the voltage-dependent Ca^{2+} channels and of the Ca^{2+} pump of the plasma membrane (see above), as well as the phosphorylation of troponin-I and of the myosin light chains] could also contribute to the regulation of contractility. In the heart SR membrane, the intrinsic protein phospholamban is selectively phosphorylated by the cAMP-dependent kinase. Phospholamban is functional also in the regulation of muscles other than the heart (105): Cross-reactivity studies with phospholamban-specific monoclonal antibodies have shown it to be present in slow-contracting skeletal muscles and in some smooth muscles (106) but absent from fast-twitch skeletal muscles. In addition to the cAMP-dependent protein kinase, phospholamban is also a substrate for two other kinases, namely, the calmodulin-dependent kinase (107,108) and protein kinase C (109,110): the

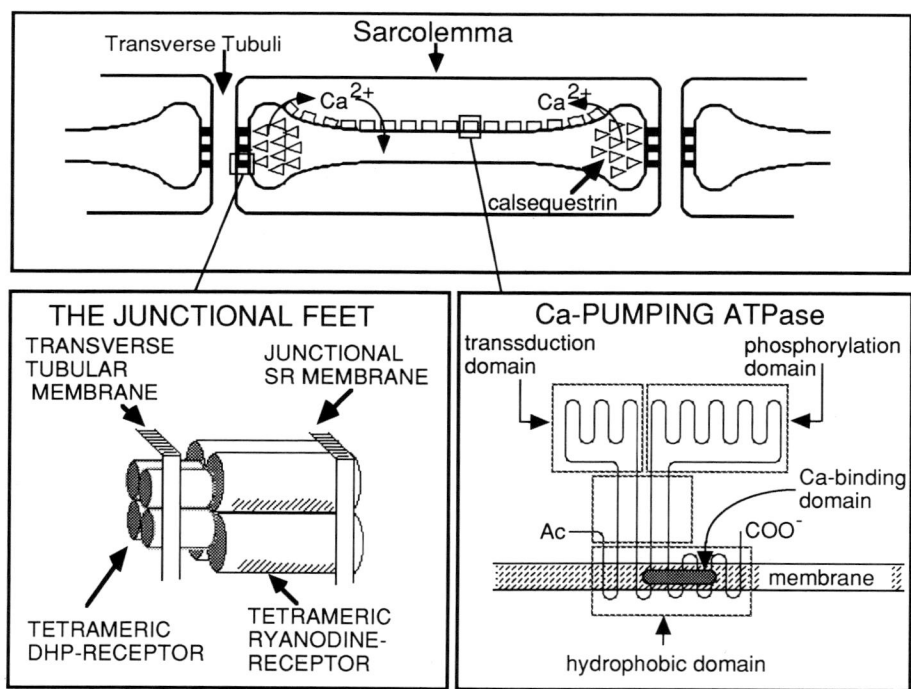

FIG. 5. The functional organization of SR in the muscle fiber, and the molecular architecture of the Ca^{2+}-transporting systems of SR.

physiological effect of the calmodulin-dependent phosphorylation is apparent in conditions of high frequency of contraction, whereby Ca^{2+} sequestration by the SR needs to be increased without change in cAMP levels. Under these conditions, the activation of the calmodulin-dependent kinase is probably related to the time average increase of intracellular Ca^{2+}. The phosphorylation of phospholamban by protein kinase C is unlikely to have physiological implications. Phospholamban phosphorylation is combined with the stimulation of Ca^{2+}-pumping activity, the effects of the cAMP-dependent kinases and of the calmodulin-dependent kinases being additive. Phospholamban is an amphiphilic molecule composed of 53 amino acids with a M_r of 6080 (112). It has a very high content of α-helix probably interrupted into two portions in the central region. The C-terminus is highly hydrophobic and most likely anchors the protein to the membrane. A hydrophilic N-terminus region of about 30 amino acids is assumed to protrude from the membrane into the cytosolic space. The hydrophilic portion contains several positively charged amino acids that confer to the unphosphorylated protein a rather alkaline character (pI value of about 10) (113) and two adjacent phosphorylation sites (a Ser and a Thr) that are selectively phosphorylated by the cAMP-dependent and the calmodulin-dependent kinases, respectively (111,112, 114). The protein has a strong tendency to form pentameric complexes not only in the membrane but also in solution (114a). Dissociation into monomers occurs only under extreme conditions, such as boiling in sodium dodecyl sulfate (SDS). Site-directed mutagenesis has shown that cysteine residues in the hydrophobic transmembrane domain are important in the stabilization of the pentameric structure even though no disulfide bonds are involved (114b).

Phospholamban can be viewed as an endogenous inhibitor of the Ca^{2+} ATPase activity. Its controlled proteolytic digestion causes stimulation of the pump, supporting the inhibitory role (114c). A monoclonal antibody directed to the hydrophilic portion of cardiac phospholamban mimics the effect of phospholamban phosphorylation and stimulates directly the Ca^{2+} pump (115). Reconstitution studies with isolated ATPase and either native (115a,115b) or synthetic (115c) phospholamban have shown that (a) phospholamban, in its unphosphorylated form, inhibits the ATPase, and that (b) its phosphorylation relieves the inhibition. Kinetically, phosphorylation of phospholamban exerts a dual effect on the Ca^{2+} pump: it increases the V_{max} of the Ca^{2+}-translocation reaction by affecting the rate of decomposition of the phosphorylated intermediate of the Ca^{2+}-ATPase (116), and it induces an increase in the apparent affinity of the enzyme for Ca^{2+}. The latter effect is very important at the physiological submicromolar free Ca^{2+} concentrations. The coupling efficiency of the Ca^{2+}-

transport system is not affected by phospholamban. The mechanism of inhibition probably involves changes in the positive and negative charges in the vicinity of the Ca^{2+} binding sites (116a,116b). Upon phosphorylation the pI value of phospholamban shifts from about 10 down to less than 6 (104). This shift induces an appreciable change in the electrostatic membrane potential. This could influence the concentration of Ca^{2+} in the vicinity of the membrane and thus affect the apparent affinity of the ATPase for Ca^{2+} (116a). In addition to these charge effects, a specific interaction between phospholamban and the ATPase is also likely to occur, as long ago proposed (117,118). The existence of a specific phospholamban-binding domain on the ATPase has been recently demonstrated with a heterobifunctional radioactive cross-linking agent attached to the hydrophilic portion of isolated phospholamban (118a). After photoactivation in the presence of the solubilized ATPase, the label was found to be associated to a domain just C-terminal to the catalytic aspartyl residue. The phospholamban-binding domain is present also in the fast-twitch muscle isoform of the SR ATPase (118a). Thus, the regulation of the SR ATPase in fast- and slow-twitch muscles depends on the differential expression of the regulatory protein phospholamban rather than on intrinsic differences between the ATPase isoforms.

The Ca^{2+}-Release Channels of Sarcoplasmic Reticulum

In striated muscles, the rate of Ca^{2+} release is about three orders of magnitude higher than that of Ca^{2+} uptake (119), indicating that a channel rather than a carrier-linked enzymatic process is involved. A considerable amount of information on the molecular components involved has recently become available. Crucial to the developments have been (a) the availability of radioactive ryanodine, a neutral plant alkaloid that interferes with the channel function in the submicromolar range (120), and (b) rapid kinetic methods to resolve the Ca^{2+}-release process in the millisecond range. Ryanodine receptors (the common name given to these intracellular Ca^{2+}-release channels) were originally described in the sarcoplasmic reticulum of skeletal (type 1) and cardiac (type 2) muscle. Two genes encoding the skeletal and cardiac muscle ryanodine receptor have been cloned (120a). The proteins encoded are 66 percent identical and display a M_r of about 560,000. The ryanodine receptors have been reconstituted into black lipid membranes and shown to form Ca^{2+}-release channels with characteristics similar to those of the native form. Opening of the channel requires low concentrations of Ca^{2+} ions in the cytosolic space (micromolar to submicromolar range), thus explaining the well-known phenomenon of Ca^{2+}-induced Ca^{2+} release, in which physiological concentrations of Ca^{2+} induce rapid Ca^{2+} release from the cisternal elements of the sarcoplasmic reticulum. The channel is activated by micromolar concentrations of nucleotides such as ATP and is inhibited by high concentrations of Mg and/or Ca^{2+}. Caffeine induces rapid Ca^{2+} release also in the absence of the stimulatory low concentrations of Ca^{2+} ions, and its action is enhanced by nucleotides. Thus, caffeine behaves as a Ca^{2+} "analog": Ryanodine binds to the channel slowly and with very high affinity (K_d of about 5–10 nM) in the open state (123). Ryanodine-modified channels are then locked in an open state of reduced conductance insensitive to Mg (123). Under such conditions, the sarcoplasmic reticulum loses the ability to accumulate (and thus to release) excitatory Ca^{2+} ions. In fact, ryanodine is known to cause a gradual decline of the contractile force in cardiac muscle. The cardiac ryanodine receptor is apparently sensitive to lower concentrations of Ca^{2+}, and less sensitive to inhibition by Mg and ruthenium red, than the skeletal muscle counterpart (123,124).

Electron micrographs of the isolated channel of skeletal muscle SR show a fourfold symmetry, which suggests that the functional unit could be composed of a complex of four identical subunits with an M_r of about 2,000,000 (121). This structure resembles that described for the feet projections connecting the cisternal compartments with the T system. In fact, ryanodine receptors, Ca^{2+}-release channels, and feet projections have now been found to be identical (121,122). Thus, the release site is restricted to the specialized junctional region that lacks Ca^{2+}-ATPase molecules and is in direct contact with the T system. The molecular components of the T system interacting with the Ca^{2+}-release channel are not known, but a very likely candidate could be the dihydropyridine (DHP) receptor (see above). The highest concentration of DHP receptors has been found in the T system of fast skeletal muscle (125), a tissue where Ca^{2+} fluxes across the plasma membrane play no role in excitation-contraction coupling. In fact, in skeletal muscle, only a minor portion of the DHP receptors represents functional Ca^{2+} channels (126). They may serve another purpose in the T-tubular system—for instance, as the voltage sensor that couples depolarization of the plasma membrane with the opening of the intracellular Ca^{2+}-release SR channels (8,127). Strong support for this interesting hypothesis comes from the observation that DHPs inhibit intramembrane charge movements at the level of the plasma membrane during depolarization and, concomitantly, also inhibit the process of Ca^{2+} release from the cisternae (127,128). This agrees with the fact that excitation-contraction coupling in fast skeletal muscle does not require Ca^{2+} entry via voltage-sensitive Ca^{2+} channels. On the other hand, contraction of cardiac muscle (where most DHP receptors are functional Ca^{2+} channels) requires extracellular Ca^{2+} and Ca^{2+} entry. In heart, the opening of the Ca^{2+}-release channels localized on the sarcoplasmic reticulum is apparently dependent on the occupancy of high-affinity Ca^{2+}-binding sites (Ca^{2+}-induced Ca^{2+} release) (129).

In addition to Ca^{2+} ions, other intracellular messengers could play a role in the activation of Ca^{2+} release from intracellular Ca^{2+} stores in tissues different from heart and skeletal muscle. Inositol trisphosphate (IP_3) has been proposed as the link between receptor-mediated activation of phospholipase C and Ca^{2+} mobilization from the endoplasmic reticulum (or calciosome; see above) in a variety of cell types (130), including vascular smooth muscles (131). The IP_3-gated Ca^{2+}-channels (or IP_3 receptors) constitute a second distinct class of intracellular Ca^{2+}-release channels. The IP_3 receptors appear to be ubiquitous whereas the ryanodine receptors are considered to be more restricted in their expression (i.e., muscles and brain). The involvement of IP_3 in the activation of Ca^{2+} release in striated muscles seems unlikely (132). Experiments on the kinetic properties of IP_3-induced Ca^{2+} release using caged IP_3 indicate that the phenomenon is too slow to play a significant role in the rapid regulation of intracellular Ca^{2+} in striated muscles, whereas it is consistent with the contraction kinetics of smooth muscles (133). In addition to the IP_3-sensitive channels, some smooth muscles also contain channels with characteristics similar to those described above for the skeletal muscle. In most smooth muscles, maximal contractions can be supported by Ca^{2+} deriving from the sarcoplasmic reticulum on agonist activation. Such contractions, however, are transient in nature if extracellular Ca^{2+} is removed. In fact, stress maintenance in smooth muscles is critically dependent on the slow influx of Ca^{2+} via voltage-dependent or receptor-operated Ca^{2+} channels (134).

REFERENCES

1. Carafoli E. Intracellular calcium homeostasis. *Annu Rev Biochem* 1987;56:395–433.
2. Nilius B, Hess P, Lansmann JB, Tsien RW. A novel type of cardiac calcium channel in ventricular cells. *Nature* 1985;316:433–446.
3. Fleckenstein A. *Calcium antagonism in heart and smooth muscle.* New York: John Wiley; 1973.
4. Reuter H, Stevens DF, Tsien RW, Yellen G. Properties of single calcium channels in cardiac cell culture. *Nature* 1982;297:501–504.
5. Borsotto M, Barhanin J, Norman RI, Lazdunski M. Purification of the dihydropyridine receptor of the voltage-dependent Ca channel from skeletal muscle transverse tubules using ^{3}H-PN200-100. *Biochem Biophys Res Commun* 1984;122:1354–1366.
6. Curtis BM, Catterall WA. Purification of the calcium antagonist receptor of the voltage-sensitive calcium channel from skeletal muscle transverse tubules. *Biochemistry* 1984;23:2113–2118.
7. Flockerzi V, Oeken H-J, Hofmann F, Pelzer D, Cavalie A, Trautwein W. Purified dihydropyridine-binding site from skeletal muscle t-tubules is a functional calcium channel. *Nature* 1986;323:66–68.

8. Tanabe T, Takeshima H, Mikani A, et al. Primary structure of the receptor for calcium channel blockers from skeletal muscle. *Nature* 1987;328:313–318.

9. Noda M, Ikeda T, Suzuki H, et al. Expression of functional sodium channels from cloned cDNA. *Nature* 1986;322:826–828.

10. Philipson KW. Sodium-calcium exchange in plasma membrane vesicles. *Annu Rev Physiol* 1985;47:561–571.

11. Shenn SS, Blaustein MP. Sodium/calcium exchange and regulation of cell calcium and contractility in cardiac muscle, with a note about vascular smooth muscle. In: Fozzard HA, et al, eds. *The heart and cardiovascular system.* New York: Raven Press; 1986:509–535.

12. Reeves JP, Sutko JL. Sodium-calcium exchange in cardiac membrane vesicles. *Proc Natl Acad Sci (USA)* 1979;76:590–594.

13. Trosper TL, Philipson KD. Effects of divalent and trivalent cations on Na$^+$–Ca^{2+} exchange in cardiac sarcolemmal vesicles. *Biochim Biophys Acta* 1983;731:63–68.

14. Caroni P, Carafoli E. The regulation of the Na$^+$/Ca^{2+} exchanger of heart sarcolemma. *Eur J Biochem* 1983;132:451–460.

15. Di Polo R, Beauge L. In squid axons, ATP modulated Na$^+$–Ca^{2+} exchange by a Ca^{2+}-Cai-dependent phosphorylation. *Biochim Biophys Acta* 1987;897:347–354.

16. Soldati L, Longoni S, Carafoli E. Solubilization and reconstitution of the Na$^+$/Ca^{2+} exchanger of cardiac sarcolemma. Properties of the reconstituted system and tentative identification of the protein(s) responsible for the exchange activity. *J Biol Chem* 1985;260:13321–13327.

17a. Barzilai A, Spanier R, Rahamimoff H. Isolation, purification and reconstitution of the Na$^+$-gradient-dependent Ca^{2+} transporter (Na$^+$/Ca^{2+} exchanger) from brain synaptic plasma membranes. *Proc Natl Acad Sci USA* 1984;81:6521–6525.

17b. Nicoll DA, Longoni S, Philipson KD. Molecular cloning and functional expression of the cardiac sarcolemmal Na$^+$–Ca^{2+} exchanger. *Science* 1992;250:562–565.

17c. Li Z, Nicoll DA, Collins A, et al. Identification of a peptide inhibitor of the cardiac sarcolemmal Na$^+$–Ca^{2+} exchanger. *J Biol Chem* 1991;266:1014–1020.

17d. Matsuoka S, Nicoll DA, Reilly RF, Hilgemann DW, Philipson KD. Initial localization of regulator. *Biochemistry* 1993;90:3870–3874.

17e. Nicoll DA, Philipson KD. Molecular studies of the cardiac sarcolemmal sodium-calcium exchanger. *Ann NY Acad Sci* 1991;639:181–189.

18. Siegl PKS, Cragoe EJ, Trumble MJ, Kaczorowski J. Inhibition of sodium-calcium exchange in membrane vesicles and papillary preparations from guinea-pig heart by analogs of amiloride. *Proc Natl Acad Sci USA* 1984;81:3238–3242.

19. Miyamoto H, Racker E. Solubilization and partial purification of the Ca^{2+}/Na$^+$ antiporter from the plasma membrane of bovine heart. *J Biol Chem* 1980;255:2656–2658.

20. Brading AF, Lategau TW. Na-Ca exchange in vascular smooth muscle. *J Hypertension* 1985;3:109–116.

21. Matlib MA, Reeves JP. Solubilization and reconstitution of the sarcolemmal Na$^+$/Ca^{2+} exchange system of vascular smooth muscle. *Biochim Biophys Acta* 1987;904:145–148.

22. Bingham-Smith J, Cragoe EJ, Smith L. Na$^+$/Ca^{2+} antiport in cultured arterial smooth muscle cells. *J Biol Chem* 1987;262:11988–11994.

23. Grover AK, Kwan CY, Rangachari PK, Daniel EE. Na-Ca exchange in smooth muscle plasma membrane-enriched fractions. *Am J Physiol* 1979;244:C158–C165.

24. Morel N, Godfraind T. Sodium-calcium exchange in smooth muscle microsomal fractions. *Biochem J* 1984;218:421–427.

25. Slaughter RS, Welton AF, Morgan DW. Sodium-calcium exchange in sarcolemmal vesicles from tracheal smooth muscle. *Biochim Biophys Acta* 1987;904:92–104.

26. Schatzmann HJ. The calcium pump of erythrocytes and other animal cells. In: Carafoli E, ed. *Membrane transport of calcium.* London: Academic Press; 1982:41.

27. Lotersztajn S, Hanoune J, Pecker F. A high affinity calcium stimulated magnesium-dependent ATPase. Dependence on an endogenous protein activator distinct from calmodulin. *J Biol Chem* 1981;256:11209–11215.

28. Pedersen PL, Carafoli E. Ion motive ATPases. *TIBS* 1987;12:146–150, 186–189.

29. Gopinath RM, Vincenzi FF. Phosphodiesterase protein activator mimics red blood cell cytoplasmic activator of (Ca^{2+} − Mg^{2+}) ATPase. *Biochem Biophys Res Commun* 1977;77:1203–1209.

30. Jarrett HW, Penniston JT. Partial purification of the Ca^{2+} − Mg^{2+} ATPase activator from human erythrocytes: its similarity to the activator of 3′:5′-cyclic nucleotide phosphodiesterase. *Biochem Biophys Res Commun* 1977;77:1210–1216.

31. Niggli V, Adunyah ES, Penniston JT, Carafoli E. Purified (Ca^{2+} − Mg^{2+})-ATPase of the erythrocyte membrane. Reconstitution and effect of calmodulin and phospholipids. *J Biol Chem* 1981;256:345.

32. Niggli V, Adunyah ES, Carafoli E. Acidic phospholipids, unsaturated fatty acids and proteolysis mimic the effect of calmodulin on the purified erythrocyte Ca^{2+}-ATPase. *J Biol Chem* 1981;256:8588–8592.

33. Stieger J, Schatzmann HJ. Metal requirement of the isolated red cell Ca-pump ATPase after elimination of calmodulin dependence by trypsin attack. *Cell Calcium* 1981;2:601–616.

34. Niggli V, Penniston JT, Carafoli E. Purification of the (Ca^{2+} + Mg^{2+}) ATPase from human erythrocyte membranes using a calmodulin affinity column. *J Biol Chem* 1979;254:9955–9958.

35. Caroni P, Carafoli E. The Ca^{2+}-pumping ATPase of heart sarcolemma. Characterization, calmodulin dependence, and partial purification. *J Biol Chem* 1981;256:3263–3270.

36. Wuytack F, DeSchutter G, Casteels R. Purification of (Ca^{2+} + Mg^{2+})-ATPase from smooth muscle by calmodulin affinity chromatography. *FEBS Lett* 1981;129:297–300.

37. Carafoli E, Zurini M. The Ca^{2+}-pumping ATPase of plasma membranes. Purification, reconstitution and properties. *Biochim Biophys Acta Rev Bioenerg* 1982;683:279–301.

38. Niggli V, Sigel E, Carafoli E. The purified Ca^{2+} pump of human erythrocyte membranes catalyzes an electroneutral Ca^{2+}:H$^+$ exchange in reconstituted liposomal systems. *J Biol Chem* 1982;257:2350–2356.

39. Caroni P, Carafoli E. Regulation of Ca^{2+}-ATPase of heart sarcolemma by a phosphorylation/dephosphorylation process. *J Biol Chem* 1981;256:9371–9373.

40a. Neyses L, Reinlib LP, Carafoli E. Phosphorylation of the Ca^{2+} pumping ATPase of heart sarcolemma and erythrocyte plasma-membrane by the cAMP-dependent protein kinase. *J Biol Chem* 1985;60:10283–10287.

40b. Wang KKW, Wright LC, Machan CL, Allen BG, Conigrave AD, Roufogalis BD. Protein kinase C phosphorylates the carboxyl terminus of the plasma membrane Ca^{2+}-ATPase from human erythrocytes. *J Biol Chem* 1991;266:9078–9085.

40c. Hoffmann F, James P, Vorherr T, Carafoli E. The C-terminal domain of the plasma membrane Ca^{2+} pump contains three high affinity Ca^{2+} binding sites. *J Biol Chem* 1993;268:10252–10259.

40d. Falchetto R, Vorherr T, Brunner J, Carafoli E. The plasma membrane Ca^{2+} pump contains a site that interacts with its calmodulin binding domain. *J Biol Chem* 1991;266:2930–2936.

40e. Falchetto R, Vorherr T, Carafoli E. The calmodulin binding site of the plasma membrane Ca^{2+} pump interacts with the transduction domain of the enzyme. *Protein Science* 1992;1:1613–1621.

40f. Stauffer T, Hilfiker H, Carafoli E, Strehler EE. Quantative analysis of alternative splicing options of human plasma membrane calcium pump genes. *J Biol Chem* 1993;268:25993–26003.

40g. Carafoli E. The Ca^{2+} pump of the plasma membrane. *J Biol Chem* 1992;267:2115–2118.

40h. Carafoli E. Calcium pump of the plasma membrane. *Physiol Rev* 1991;71:129–153.

41. James P, Maeda M, Fischer R, et al. Identification and primary structure of a calmodulin binding domain of the Ca^{2+} pump of human erythrocytes. *J Biol Chem* 1988;263:2905–2910.

42. Verma AK, Filoteo AG, Stanford DR, et al. Complete primary structure of human plasma membrane Ca^{2+} pump. *J Biol Chem* 1988;263:14152–14159.

43. Hasselbach W, Makinose M. Die Calciumpumpe der "Erschlaffungsgrana" des Muskels und ihre Abhängigkeit von der ATPspaltung. *Biochem Z* 1961;333:518–528.

44. Vasington FD, Murphy JV. Active binding of calcium by mitochondria. *Fed Proc* 1961;20:146.

45. Somlyo AP, Somlyo AV, Shuman H, Endo M. Calcium and monovalent ions in smooth muscle. *Fed Proc* 1982;41:2883–2890.

46. Somlyo AP, Bond M, Somlyo AV. Calcium content of mitochondria and endoplasmic reticulum in liver frozen rapidly *in vivo*. *Nature* 1985;314:622–625.

47. Carafoli E, Crompton M. Calcium ions and mitochondria. In: Duncan CJ, ed. *Calcium in biological systems*. Cambridge: Cambridge University Press; 1976:89–115.

48. Crompton M. The regulation of mitochondrial calcium transport in heart. In: Shamoo AE, ed. *Current topics in membrane and transport*. New York: Academic Press; 1985;25:231–276.

49. Nicholls DG, Akerman K. Mitochondrial calcium transport. *Biochim Biophys Acta* 1982;683:57–88.

50. Scarpa A, Azzone GF. The mechanism of ion translocation in mitochondria. Coupling of K^+ efflux with Ca^{2+} uptake. *Eur J Biochem* 1970;12:328–355.

51. Akerman KEO. Charge transfer during valinomycin-induced Ca^{2+} uptake in rat liver mitochondria. *FEBS Lett* 1978;93:293–296.

52. Brand MD, Chen C-H, Lehninger AL. Stoichiometry of H^+ ejection during respiration-dependent accumulation of Ca^{2+} by rat liver mitochondria. *J Biol Chem* 1976;251:968–974.

53. Rossi CS, Lehninger A. Stoichiometric relationship between accumulation of ions by mitochondria and the energy-coupling sites in the respiratory chain. *Biochem Z* 1964;228:698–713.

54. Greenawalt JW, Rossi CS, Lehninger AL. Effect of active accumulation of calcium and phosphate ions on the structure of rat liver mitochondria. *J Cell Biol* 1964;23:21–38.

55. Vinogradov A, Scarpa A. The initial velocities of calcium uptake by rat liver mitochondria. *J Biol Chem* 1973;248:5527–5531.

56. Crompton M, Sigel E, Salzman M, Carafoli E. A kinetic study of the energy-linked influx of Ca^{2+} into heart mitochondria. *Eur J Biochem* 1976;69:429–434.

57. McMillin-Wood J, Wolkowicz PE, Chu A, Tate CA, Goldstone MA, Entman ML. Calcium uptake by two preparations of mitochondria from heart. *Biochim Biophys Acta* 1980;591:251–265.

58. Moore CI. Specific inhibition of mitochondrial Ca^{2+} transport by ruthenium red. *Biochem Biophys Res Commun* 1971;42:298–305.

59. Carafoli E, Sottocasa G. The Ca^{2+} transport system of the mitochondrial membrane and the problem of the Ca-carrier. In: Ernster L, Estabrook, Slater, eds. *Dynamics of energy-transducing membranes*. Amsterdam: Elsevier; 1974:455–469.

60. Panfili E, Sandri G, Sottocasa GL, Lunazzi G, Liut G. Specific inhibition of mitochondrial Ca^{2+} transport by antibodies directed to the Ca-binding glycoprotein. *Nature* 1976;264:185–186.

61. Ambudkhar IS, Kima PE, Shamoo AE. Characterization of calciphorin, the low molecular weight calcium inophore, from rat liver mitochondria. *Biochim Biophys Acta* 1984;771:165–170.

62. Carafoli E, Tiozzo R, Lugli G, Crovetti F, Kratzing C. The release of calcium from heart mitochondria by sodium. *J Mol Cell Cardiol* 1974;6:361–371.

63. Crompton M, Capano M, Carafoli E. The sodium-induced efflux of calcium from heart mitochondria. A possible mechanism for the regulation of mitochondrial calcium. *Eur J Biochem* 1976;69:429–434.

64. Crompton M, Moser R, Ludi H, Carafoli E. The interrelations between the transport of sodium and calcium in mitochondria of various mammalian tissues. *Eur J Biochem* 1978;82:25–31.

65. Vaghy PL, Johnson DJ, Matlib M, Wang T, Schwartz A. Selective inhibition of Na^+-induced Ca^{2+} release from heart mitochondria by diltiazem and Ca antagonist drugs. *J Biol Chem* 1982;257:6000–6002.

66. Crompton M, Heidi I, Baschera C, Carafoli E. The resolution of calcium fluxes in heart and liver mitochondria using the lanthanides series. *FEBS Lett* 1979;104:352–354.

67. Coll KE, Joseph SK, Corkey BE, Williamson JR. Determination of the matrix free Ca^{2+} concentration and kinetics of Ca^{2+} efflux in liver and heart mitochondria. *J Biol Chem* 1982;257:8696–8704.

68. Hoek JB, Nicholls DG, Williamson JR. Determination of mitochondrial motive force in isolated hepatocytes. *J Biol Chem* 1980;255:1458–1564.

69. Bond M, Shuman H, Somlyo AP, Somylo AV. Total cytoplasmic calcium in relaxed and maximal contracted rabbit portal vein smooth muscle. *J Physiol (Lond)* 1984;357:185–201.

70. Somlyo AP, Somlyo AV, Shuman H. Electron probe analysis of vascular muscle: composition of mitochondria, nuclei and cytoplasm. *J Cell Biol* 1979;81:316–335.

71. Carafoli E. Membrane transport and the regulation of the cell calcium levels. In: Cowley RA, Trump BF, eds. *Pathophysiology of shock, anoxia, and ischemia*. Baltimore: Williams & Wilkins; 1985:95–111.

72. Denton RM, McCormack JG. The calcium sensitive dehydrogenases of vertebrate mitochondria. *Cell Calcium* 1986;7:377–386.

73. Franzini-Armstrong C. Membrane systems in muscle fibers. In: GH Bourne, ed. *The structure and function of muscle; vol 1*. New York: Academic Press; 1972:532.

74. Franzini-Armstrong C. Structure of sarcoplasmic reticulum. *Fed Proc* 1980;39:2403–2409.

75. Eisenberg BR, Eisenberg RS. The T-SR junction in contracting single skeletal muscle fibers. *J Gen Physiol* 1982;79:1–9.

76. Meissner G. Isolation and characterization of two types of sarcoplasmic reticulum vesicles. *Biochim Biophys Acta* 1975;389:5168.

77. MacLennan DH, Wong PTS. Isolation of a calcium sequestering protein from sarcoplasmic reticulum. *Proc Natl Acad Sci USA* 1971;68:1231–1235.

78. Jorgensen AO, Shen AC-Y, MacLennan DH, Tokuyasu KT. Ultrastructural localization of the $Ca^{2+} + Mg^{2+}$-dependent ATPase of sarcoplasmic reticulum in rat skeletal muscle by ferritin labeling of ultrathin frozen sections. *J Cell Biol* 1982;92:409–416.

79. Huxley AF. The activation of striated muscle and its mechanical response. *Proc Roy Soc Lond* [Biol] 1971;178:1–11.

80. Winegrad S. The intracellular site of calcium activation of contraction in frog skeletal muscle. *J Gen Physiol* 1970;55:77–88.

81. Volpe P, Krause KH, Hashimoto S, et al. Calciosome, a cytoplasmic organelle: the IP3-sensitive Ca store of non-muscle cells? *Proc Natl Acad Sci USA* 1988;85:1091–1095.

82. MacLennan DH. Purification and properties of an adenosine triphosphatase from sarcoplasmic reticulum. *J Biol Chem* 1970;245:4508–4518.

83. Allen G. Primary structure of the calcium ion-transporting adenosine triphosphatase of rabbit skeletal sarcoplasmic reticulum. *Biochem J* 1980;187:545–616.

84. Allen G, Green NM. Primary structures of cystein-containing peptides from the calcium ion-transporting adenosine triphosphatase of rabbit sarcoplasmic reticulum. *Biochem J* 1978;173:393–402.

85. Klip A, Reithmeier RAF, MacLennan DH. Alignment of the major tryptic fragments of the adenosine triphosphatase from sarcoplasmic reticulum. *J Biol Chem* 1980;255:6562–6567.

86. MacLennan DH, Brandl CJ, Korczak B, Green NM. Amino-acid sequence of a Ca-Mg-dependent ATPase from rabbit muscle SR, deduced from its complementary DNA sequence. *Nature* 1985;316:696–700.

87. DeFloor PH, Levitsky D, Biryvkowa T, Fleischer S. Immunological dissimilarity of the Ca-pump protein of skeletal and cardiac muscle SR. *Arch Biochem Biophys* 1980;200:196–205.

88. Zubrzycka-Gaarn E, MacDonald G, Phillips L, Jorgensen AD, MacLennan DH. Inositol trisphosphate, a novel second messenger in cellular signal transduction. *J Bioenerg Biomembr* 1984;16:441–464.

89. Brandl CJ, Green NM, Korczak B, MacLennan DH. Two Ca ATPase genes: homologies and mechanistic implications of a deduced amino acid sequence. *Cell* 1986;44:597–607.

89a. Lytton J, MacLennan DH. Molecular cloning of cDNA from human kidney coding for two alternatively spliced products of the cardiac Ca-ATPase gene. *J Biol Chem* 1988;263:15024–15029.

90. Hasselbach W. Relaxing factor and the relaxation of muscle. *Prog Biophys Biophys Chem* 1964;14:167–222.

91. Barrabin H, Scofano H, Inesi G. Adenosine triphosphatase site stoichiometry in sarcoplasmic reticulum vesicles and purified enzyme. *Biochemistry* 1984;22:1542–1548.

92. Mitchinson C, Wilderspin A, Trinnaman B, Green NM. Identification of a labelled peptide after stoichiometric reaction of fluorescein isothiocyanate with the Ca^{++}-dependent adenosine triphosphatase of sarcoplasmic reticulum. *FEBS Lett* 1982;146:87–92.

93. Inesi G, Kurzmack M, Coan C, Lewis D. Cooperative calcium binding and ATPase activation in sarcoplasmic reticulum vesicles. *J Biol Chem* 1980;255:3025–3031.

94. Dupont Y. Low-temperature studies of the sarcoplasmic reticulum calcium pump mechanism of calcium binding. *Biochim Biophys Acta* 1982;688:75–87.

95. Bastide F, Meissner G, Fleischer S, Post RL. Similarity of the active site of phosphorylation of the ATPase for transport of sodium and potassium ions in kidney to that for transport of calcium ions in sarcoplasmic reticulum of muscle. *J Biol Chem* 1973;248: 8385–8391.

96. Degani C, Boyer P. A borohydride reduction method for characterization of the acyl phosphate linkage in proteins and its application to sarcoplasmic reticulum adenosine triphosphatase. *J Biol Chem* 1973;248:8222–8226.

96a.Clarke DM, Loo TW, Inesi G, MacLennan DH. Location of high affinity Ca-binding sites within the predicted transmembrane domain of the sarcoplasmic reticulum Ca-ATPase. *Nature* 1989;339:476–478.

97. Froehlich J, Taylor E. Transient-state kinetic studies of sarcoplasmic reticulum adenosine triphosphatase. *J Biol Chem* 1975;250: 2013–2021.

98. Verjovski-Almeida S, Kurzmack M, Inesi G. Partial reactions in the catalytic and transport cycle of sarcoplasmic reticulum ATPase. *Biochemistry* 1978;17:5006–5013.

99. Zimmniak P, Racker E. Electrogenicity of Ca^{2+}-transport catalyzed by the Ca^{2+}-ATPase from sarcoplasmic reticulum. *J Biol Chem* 1978;253:4631–4646.

100. Chiesi M, Inesi G. ATP dependent fluxes of manganese and hydrogen ions in SR vesicles. *Biochemistry* 1980;19:2912–2918.

101. Makinose M, Hasselbach W. ATP synthesis by the reverse of the sarcoplasmic calcium pump. *FEBS Lett* 1971;12:271–272.

102. Kirchberger MA, Tada M, Katz AM. Adenosine 3':5'-monophosphate-dependent protein kinase-catalyzed phosphorylation reaction and its relationship to calcium transport in cardiac sarcoplasmic reticulum. *J Biol Chem* 1974;249:6166–6173.

103. Tada M, Kirchberger MA, Katz AM. Phosphorylation of a 22,000-dalton component of the cardiac sarcoplasmic reticulum by adenosine 3':5'-monophosphate-dependent protein kinase. *J Biol Chem* 1975;250:2640–2647.

104. Gasser J, Chiesi M, Carafoli E. Concerted phosphorylation of the 26 kDa phospholamban oligomer and of the low molecular weight phospholamban subunits. *Biochemistry* 1986;25:7615–7623.

105. Suzuki T, Lui P, Wang JH. The use of monoclonal antibodies for the species and tissues distribution of phospholamban. *Cell Calcium* 1986;7:41–47.

106. Jorgensen AP, Jones LR. Immunoelectron microscopical localization of phospholamban in adult canine ventricular muscle. *J Cell Biol* 1986;104:1343–1352.

107. LePeuch CJ, Haiech J, Demaille JG. Concerted regulation of cardiac SR Ca-transport by cAMP-dependent and Ca-calmodulin-dependent phosphorylations. *Biochemistry* 1979;18:5150–5157.

108. Bilegikjian LM, Kranias EG, Potter JD, Schwartz A. Studies on phosphorylation of canine cardiac SR by calmodulin-dependent protein kinase. *Circ Res* 1981;49:1356–1363.

109. Limas CJ. Phosphorylation of cardiac SR by a Ca-activated phospholipid-dependent protein kinase. *Biochem Biophys Res Commun* 1980;96:1378–1383.

110. Movsesian MA, Nishikawa M, Adelstein RS. Phosphorylation of phospholamban by Ca-activated phospholipid-dependent protein kinase. *J Biol Chem* 1984;259:8029–8032.

111. Wegener AD, Jones LR. Phosphorylation-induced mobility shift in phospholamban in SDS-polyacrylamide gels. *J Biol Chem* 1984;259:1834–1841.

112. Fuji J, Ueno A, Kitano K, Tanaka S, Tada M, Kadama M. Complete complementary DNA-derived amino acid sequence of canine cardiac phospholamban. *J Clin Invest* 1987;79:301–304.

113. Jones LR, Zimmerman HK, Wilson WW, Gurd FR, Wegener AD. Purification and characterisation of phospholamban from canine cardiac SR. *J Biol Chem* 1985;260:7721–7730.

114. Wegener AD, Zimmerman HK, Liepnieks J, Jones L. Proteolytic cleavage of phospholamban purified from canine cardiac SR vesicles. *J Biol Chem* 1986;261:5154–5159.

114a.Simmerman HK, Lovelace DE, Jones LR. Secondary structure of detergent-solubilized phospholamban, a phosphorylatable, oligomeric protein of cardiac sarcoplasmic reticulum. *Biochim Biophys Acta* 1989;997:322–329.

114b.Fujii J, Maruyama K, Tada M, MacLennan DH. Expression and site-specific mutagenesis of phospholamban. *J Biol Chem* 1989;264:12950–12955.

114c.Kirchberger MA, Borchman D, Kasinathan C. Proteolytic activation of the canine cardiac sarcoplasmic reticulum calcium pump. *Biochemistry* 1986;25:5484–5492.

115. Suzuki T, Wang SH. Stimulation of bovine cardiac SR Ca-pump and blocking of phospholamban phosphorylation and dephosphorylation by a phospholamban monoclonal antibody. *J Biol Chem* 1986;261:7018–7023.

115a.Inui M, Chamberlain BK, Saito A, Fleischer S. The nature of the modulation of Ca-transport as studied by reconstitution of cardiac sarcoplasmic reticulum. *J Biol Chem* 1986;261:1794–1800.

115b.Kim HW, Steenaart NA, Ferguson DG, Kranias EG. Functional reconstitution of the cardiac sarcoplasmic reticulum Ca-ATPase with phospholamban in phospholipid vesicles. *J Biol Chem* 1990;265:1702–1709.

115c.Vorherr T, Wrzosek A, Chiesi M, Carafoli E. Total synthesis and functional properties of the membrane-intrinsic protein phospholamban. *Protein Science* 1993;2:339–347.

116. Tada M, Yamada M, Ohmori F, Kuzuya T, Inui M, Abe H. Transient state kinetic studies of Ca^{2+} dependent ATPase and calcium transport by cardiac sarcoplasmic reticulum. Effect of cyclic AMP-dependent protein kinase catalyzed phosphorylation of phospholamban. *J Biol Chem* 1980;255:1982–1985.

116a.Chiesi M, Schwaller R. Involvement of electrostatic phenomena in phospholamban-induced stimulation of Ca-uptake into cardiac sarcoplasmic reticulum. *FEBS Lett* 1989;244:241–244.

116b.Xu Z-C, Kirchberger MA. Modulation of polyelectrolytes of canine cardiac microsomal calcium uptake and the possible relationship to phospholamban. *J Biol Chem* 1989;264:16644–16651.

117. Tada M, Ohmori F, Yamada M, Abe H. Mechanism of the stimulation of Ca^{2+} dependent ATPase of cardiac sarcoplasmic reticulum by adenosine 3':5'-monophosphate dependent protein kinase. *J Biol Chem* 1979;254:319–326.

118. Hicks MJ, Shigekawa M, Katz AM. Mechanism by which cyclic adenosine 3':5'-monophosphate dependent protein kinase stimulates calcium transport in cardiac sarcoplasmic reticulum. *Circ Res* 1979;44:384–391.

118a.James P, Inui M, Tada M, Chiesi M, Carafoli E. Nature and site of phospholamban regulation of the Ca-pump of sarcoplasmic reticulum. *Nature (London)* 1989;342:90–92.

119. Martonosi A. Biochemical and clinical aspects of SR function. *Curr Top Membr Transp* 1972;3:83–197.

120. Pessah IN, Francini AE, Scales DJ, Waterhouse AL, Casida SE. Calcium-ryanodine receptor complex. *J Biol Chem* 1986;261: 8643–8648.

120a.Otsu K, Willard HF, Khanna VK, Zorzato F, Green NM, MacLennan DH. Molecular cloning of cDNA encoding the Ca-release channel of rabbit cardiac SR. *J Biol Chem* 1990;265:13472–13483.

121. Lai FA, Erickson HP, Rousseau E, Lim Q, Meissner G. Purification and reconstitution of the Ca-release channel from skeletal muscle. *Nature* 1988;331:315–319.

122. Inui M, Saito A, Fleischer S. Purification of the ryanodine-receptor and identity with feet structures of junctional terminal cisterne of SR from fast skeletal muscle. *J Biol Chem* 1987;262: 1740–1747.

123. Imagawa T, Smith JS, Coronado R, Campbell KP. Purified ryanodine receptor from skeletal muscle SR is the Ca-permeable pore of the Ca-release channel. *J Biol Chem* 1987;262:16636–16643.

124. Somlyo AV, Gonzalez-Serratos H, Shuman H, McClellan G, Somlyo AP. Calcium release and ionic changes in the sarcoplasmic reticulum of tetanized muscle: an electron-probe study. *J Cell Biol* 1981;90:577–594.

125. Fosset M, Saimrich E, Delpont E, Lazdunski MI. Nitrendipine receptors in skeletal muscle. *J Biol Chem* 1983;258:6086–6092.

126. Schwartz LM, McCleskey EW, Almers W. DHP-receptors in

muscle are voltage-dependent but most are not functional calcium channels. *Nature* 1985;314:747–751.

127. Rios E, Brum G. Involvement of DHP-receptors in EC-coupling in skeletal muscle. *Nature* 1987;325:717–720.

128. Melzer W, Schneider MF, Simon BJ, Szucs G. Intermembrane charge movement and Ca-release in frog skeletal muscle. *J Physiol (Lond)* 1986;373:481–511.

129. Fabiato A, Fabiato F. Use of chlortetracycline fluorescence to demonstrate Ca-induced Ca release from SR of skinned cardiac cells. *Nature* 1979;281:146–148.

130. Berridge MJ, Irvine RF. Monoclonal antibodies to the Ca^{2+} + Mg^{2+}-dependent ATPase of sarcoplasmic reticulum, identify polymorphic forms of the enzyme and indicate the presence in

the enzyme of a classical high-affinity Ca^{2+} binding site. *Nature (Lond)* 1984;312:315–321.

131. Somlyo AV, Bond M, Somlyo AP, Scarpa A. IP3-induced Ca-release and contraction in vascular smooth muscle. *Proc Natl Acad Sci USA* 1985;82:5231–5235.

132. Volpe P, Di Virgilio F, Pozzan T, Salviati G. Role of IP3 in E-C coupling in skeletal muscle. *FEBS Lett* 1986;197:1–4.

133. Walker SW, Somlyo AV, Goldman YE, Somlyo AP, Trentham DR. Kinetics of smooth and skeletal muscle activation by laser pulse photolysis of caged IP3. *Nature* 1987;327:249–252.

134. Ratz PH, Murphy RA. Contributions of intracellular and extracellular Ca pools to activation of myosin phosphorylation and stress in swine carotid media. *Circ Res* 1987;60:410–421.

Hypertension: Pathophysiology, Diagnosis, and Management, Second Edition,
edited by J.H. Laragh and B.M. Brenner,
Raven Press, Ltd., New York © 1995.

CHAPTER **74**

Lessons from Experimental Genetic Hypertension

Patrizia Ferrari and Giuseppe Bianchi

The main objective of studying animal models of arterial hypertension is to furnish an experimental and theoretical foundation for understanding its different aspects in humans. The major obstacle in attempting to accomplish this objective is our ignorance regarding the pathogenic mechanisms of hypertension. In fact, although at the clinical level the picture appears rather uniform, the causes of human essential hypertension (EH) are very likely heterogeneous and multifactorial and involve many possible genetic, biochemical, and physiological mechanisms. Therefore, the lack of precise criteria for separating different subgroups of patients makes comparisons with the various animal models very difficult.

How can one assess the relevance of a given animal model if so little is known about the corresponding hu-

man disease? One possible way of circumventing this problem is to measure as many biochemical and physiological factors as possible in humans and then compare the same spectrum of characteristics in a given animal model and its appropriate control. If we examine different types of secondary hypertension such as those that can be induced in animals by different types of renal or adrenal manipulations, by administration of corticoids, and by psychological stress, we have to admit that these known factors or mechanisms of hypertension produce similar blood pressure changes both in rat and in man. Hence, it is possible to assume that as far as the "genetic" type of hypertension is concerned, similarities could also be found, provided that the primary mechanism triggering the whole series of events can be identified.

With the development of the molecular biology approach to primary hypertension, the possible relationship between DNA polymorphism and blood pressure abnormalities in rats together with the sequence of events going from particular DNA polymorphism to the

P. Ferrari: PRASSIS, Sigma Tau Research Institute, 20019 Milan, Italy.
G. Bianchi: University of Milan, Division of Nephrology and Hypertension, S. Raffaele Hospital, 20132 Milan, Italy.

development of hypertension in the different rat models may be studied. In this way we may have precise molecular abnormalities with their biochemical activities to use as markers in humans to detect if a subset of patients might have similar genetic molecular mechanisms as the cause of its hypertension.

Other chapters of this book deal with molecular biology and genetics of rat and human primary hypertension. This chapter briefly summarizes the most relevant abnormalities so far detected in different rat models at the level of cell membranes, kidney function, hormonal, cardiovascular, and nervous systems. We shall try to establish parallelism with analogous findings in human primary hypertension.

At present there are at least eight strains of rat considered to be models of different forms of genetic hypertension. A full description of each can be found in ref. 1. Our discussion is limited to the following: Okamoto's spontaneously hypertensive rats (SHRs); the Milan hypertensive strain (MHS); the Lyon hypertensive strain (LH); the New Zealand genetically hypertensive strain (GH); the Dahl's rats selected for sensitivity (DS) and resistance (DR) to dietary salt-induced hypertension; and the inbred strains (SS/Jr and SR/Jr), subsequently derived from the latter, by Rapp and Dene (2).

CELL MEMBRANE ALTERATIONS AND MOLECULAR MECHANISMS

Over the last 20 years extensive studies were carried out to discover one or more genetic markers to be used either for diagnosis or as intermediate phenotypes to clarify the primary molecular mechanisms leading to EH. As alterations in cell transport of ions especially at the renal and vascular levels may be one of the genetic mechanism causing hypertension, the study of ion transport systems across the cell membranes may furnish useful results both for the comprehension of the organ abnormalities responsible for "essential" forms of hypertension and for the detection of genetic markers.

Research in this area has been mainly carried out on red or white blood cells (RBC, WBC), on the assumption that these cells carry the genetic message responsible for the abnormalities of those cells (renal, vasal, nervous) more directly involved in BP regulation. Moreover, many of these studies have been carried out in genetic animal models of hypertension to overcome the problem of genetic heterogeneity of human population. In fact, in animal models it is possible to distinguish whether these alterations are (a) just secondary adjustments of the cell machinery to a primary, presently undiscovered, alteration; (b) genetically linked to a primary alteration but without any direct role in the development of hypertension; (c) determined by a pleiotropic effect of a single gene affecting, in parallel, both blood cells and organ cells (renal, nervous, vascular) involved in BP regulation.

Spontaneously Hypertensive Rats

In SHRs both increased (3) and normal (4) intracellular Na (Na_i) have been reported in RBC and WBC, when compared with normotensive Wistar-Kysto (WKY) rats. Two reasons can be found to explain this discrepancy. First, the development of high blood pressure in SHRs is very rapid after weaning (5) and this makes it difficult to detect some cell alterations that are primary and not due to secondary readjustment to the BP increase. Second, the diffusion among different laboratories of the SHR strain occurred before the achievement of homozygosis at all loci; therefore, it has been demonstrated that these substrains of SHRs differ in their genetic background (6). The variety of the results obtained by different groups can be therefore explained on the basis of this heterogeneity.

De Mendoca et al. (7) observed that Na_i increased in SHR RBCs (but not in those of WKY) only after an acute or chronic Na load, suggesting either a reduced ability of the cell to extrude Na_i or an increased Na influx. In line with these results, net Na extrusion has been reported to be decreased (7), and Na passive permeability increased in SHR RBCs (8–11). A possible explanation for the relationship between Na_i and Na transports has been furnished by Rosati et al. (12), who found a reduced affinity of Na-K cotransport for the internal Na in young and adult SHRs RBC, as previously described in humans (13), and a 50 percent decrease of the maximal Na-K pump rate in adult SHRs (12). From these results it has been speculated that an increase in cell Na content does not adequately stimulate the Na-K cotransport; therefore, a transient cell Na retention may occur in adult SHRs.

The presence of a circulating Na-K pump inhibitor that might be secondarily increased in adult SHRs could be responsible for cell pump inhibition, as reported by Jones et al. (14). However, no conclusive evidence of altered Na-K pump activity has been provided in SHRs. In fact, the pump was also reported to be either increased in heart, vasculature (15,16), and renal preparations from young SHRs (17), or equal (18), or even reduced in renal tissue of adult SHRs as compared with WKY rats (19,20). The circulating inhibitor may be washed out during cell or enzyme preparation, or there may be compensatory increase of the number of pump sites (21); both possibilities may explain these discrepancies.

More recently, a widespread abnormality of the Na-H exchange system has been reported in different tissues of SHR rats. Na-H exchange activity has been found to be increased in thymocytes (22), lymphocytes (23), neutrophils (24), platelets (25), vascular smooth muscle cells (26,27), and brush-border membrane vesicles from kidney cortex (28). The alteration of Na-H exchange has also been demonstrated to be present in intact segments of mesenteric arteries of SHRs, even before the development of hypertension (29). An increase of Na-H exchange in the vascular smooth muscle cells can contribute to the abnormal cell growth (30) and the enhanced vasoreactivity to angiotensin II (27,31) observed in SHRs. At the renal level, the increased rate of Na-H exchange found in vesicles prepared from young SHRs may account for the renal defect in Na excretion documented in this strain (32).

SHRs and humans also both show alterations of intracellular Ca and Ca transport. Ca binding to the inner cell membrane was found to be decreased (33,34) and intracellular Ca concentration was found to be increased in SHRs when measured in lymphocytes (35), platelets (36), and whole perfused kidney by the nuclear magnetic resonance (NMR) technique (37). Moreover, SHR RBC membranes showed a consistent reduction of the Ca-pump transport activity (38,39), a finding also confirmed in synaptosomes (40), which indicates that an extensive membrane alteration of the interaction between calmodulin and Ca pump is present in this rat model, as it is in humans. Given the role played by Ca in the mechanisms of contraction and reactivity of smooth muscle cells and nerve terminals, this cell Ca transport abnormality may be related to the development of hypertension (41).

Clearly a wide spectrum of cellular dysfunctions can be detected in different tissues of SHRs both before and after the development of hypertension, all being possibly involved in causing and/or sustaining the rise of blood pressure. However, at present we lack a clear cause-effect relationship between all these cell alterations and the possible molecular mechanisms causing them. Some findings have been considered to be relevant to this questions. (a) An increase in plasma membrane microviscosity found in RBCs, liver, nerves, and heart has been claimed to be involved in causing ion transport alterations in SHR. However, recently a study on the cosegregation of membrane microviscosity and blood pressure in F_2 hybrids, obtained by crossing stroke-prone SHRs (SHRs-SP) with WKY rats, failed to find any correlation between these two traits (42). (b) An enhanced phosphatidylinositide (PI) turnover in SHR cell membranes (43,44) has been regarded as a defect related to the abnormal Ca binding and transport and involved in the modulation of the transmembrane signal transduction via diacylglycerol (DAG) and Protein Kinase C (PkC) activation (45). Postnov (46) developed this topic both in SHRs and human essential hypertensives, demonstrating that most of the cellular alterations typical of hypertension can be reproduced by inducing kinase activation (12-O-Tetradecanoylphorbol-13-acetate-[TPA]-

dependent) by DAG. PkC activity has been found increased either in erythrocytes (47), platelets (48), or brain tissue (49) of SHRs as compared with WKY, suggesting a widespread presence of this biochemical alteration in SHRs. A primary genetic link between PkC activity alteration and cell membrane ion abnormalities has been suggested by a study on restriction fragment length polymorphism (RFLP) of DNA on the proto-oncogene loci for c-src and c-fos genes in SHR and WKY. Kotelevtsen et al. (50) found a polymorphism in the loci of the c-src and c-fos genes of SHR and WKY rats and demonstrated the existence of a cosegregation in (SHR × WKY) F_2 hybrids of c-src alleles with both the rate of the Na-K cotransport and the RBC Ca content (50). This suggests that the c-src locus itself, or some other locus close to it, may determine the increased Na-K cotransport and Ca content in SHR RBC. The link between these traits and hypertension remains to be determined, since in the F_2 population c-src gene polymorphism has not been measured together with blood pressure.

Dahl Sensitivity Rats

The ion transports have been studied both in DS/Jr and DS rats as function of the Na diet. McCormick et al. (51) found an increased RBC Na_i, a similar ouabain-sensitive Rb uptake, and a faster ouabain-insensitive Rb uptake in fresh RBC from prehypertensive DS rats on a low-Na diet. In parallel, the ability of DS plasma to displace the ^{3}H-ouabain binding, taken as an index of the presence of a circulating ouabainlike factor (OLF), was found increased as compared with DR rats (51). Na-loaded RBC of DS rats maintained on a high-Na diet showed an increased rate of the Na-K cotransport than those of DR rats (52). A detailed study on the kinetic characteristics of RBC ion transports was performed by Zicha and Duhm (53) on DS/Jr and DR/Jr rats, before and after the development of hypertension, on both a high- and low-Na diet. The kinetic parameters of the Na-K pump were similar in DS and DR rats at low Na diet, but the pump V_{max} increased in adult DS rats fed a high-Na diet (53). Similarly, only on a high-Na diet did DS rats show a significant increase of the cotransport V_{max} when compared with DR rats (53). Since adult DS rats maintained on a high-Na diet showed an increased intracellular Na concentration and an increased Na leak, the faster rate of cotransport might be secondary to this increase of the intracellular Na (53).

As previously reported for SHRs, DS rats shows an increased RBC Na-H exchange when made hypertensive by a high Na diet (54). Similarly, Ca uptake measured in isolated thoracic aorta was found to be increased in DS rats after 4 weeks on a high-Na diet (55), suggesting that also in DS rats cell Ca handling may be altered.

Na-K pump activity and the abundance of its mRNA,

measured in isolated proximal tubuli, were found similar in young prehypertensive DS and DR rats, but increased twofold in DS rats after high-Na diet (56). Since DS rats were found to lack the capacity to down-regulate the Na,K-adenosine triphosphatase (ATPase) activity in response to dopamine (56), it has been suggested that the increased Na,K-ATPase response to Na in DS rats may be due to an impaired renal response to dopamine.

Lyon Hypertensive and New Zealand Genetically Hypertensive Strains

Data concerning membrane abnormalities in the LH and GH are very scanty. No significant alterations of the net Na extrusion and Na,K-ATPase activity were observed in RBCs and renal tissue of LH (52,57). Similarly, the Na influx did not differ in RBCs of hypertensive (GH) and normotensive (GN) New Zealand rats (58).

Milan Hypertensive Strain

To identify the primary molecular defect that produces in MHS rats the peculiar increase in tubular Na reabsorption (59), we have, first, identified those alterations that can be considered primitive to the hypertension (i.e., present before its development), second, demonstrated that such alterations are primarily determined and genetically associated with the hypertension, and third, demonstrated that they are present not only in RBC but also in renal tubular cells, where their pathophysiological role would be more relevant.

Regarding the first point, RBCs of MHS and Milan normotensive strain (MNS) rats have been studied at different ages. The MHS rats have a reduced cell volume and intracellular Na content at all ages, a faster Na-K cotransport up to 60 days of age, and a decreased Na-K pump activity after the development of hypertension (60). The faster Na-K cotransport of MHS RBC is likely due to a higher affinity for intracellular Na (61). Moreover, the smaller cell volume and the faster Na-K cotransport were demonstrated to be (a) primarily determined in the stem cells of MHS rats by bone marrow transplantation experiments (62) and (b) genetically associated to MHS hypertension by genetic cross-breeding (62). Also in a few recombinant inbred (RI) strains we showed that the RBC cotransport rates correlated with blood pressure levels (63). These RBC abnormalities of MHS rats may also be relevant to the development of hypertension, since similar alterations are present in renal (64–66) and vascular cells (67), confirming the validity of the RBC for studying the molecular alterations present in other cell types.

By manipulating the RBC membrane, we have found a link between altered cotransport and the membrane skeleton, since the smaller volume and the higher affinity

for Na of MHS cotransport are maintained in emptied and resealed ghosts (68), while the difference in cotransport kinetics disappears in inside-out vesicles (IOV) deprived of the membrane skeleton (68). Moreover, cross-immunization with ghosts and membrane skeletons between MHS and MNS rats revealed an immunogenic difference in a 105-kDa membrane skeleton protein (69). This protein was identified to be *adducin* (70), an α-β heterodimer with subunits of MW 103,000 (α) and 97,000 (β) (71). Using MHS antisera to screen a mouse cDNA expression library, a positive clone coding for a portion of β-adducin cDNA was identified (72). The rat full-length β-adducin and α-adducin cDNA was successively isolated and characterized (72,73). Comparison of MNS and MHS nucleotide sequences, revealed, for the α-adducin subunit, a thymine-adenine transversion in the codon for amino acid 316, resulting in a phenylalanine-tyrosine (F-Y) substitution (73). A similar comparison for the β-adducin subunit revealed an adenine-guanine transition in the codon for amino acid 529, resulting in a glutamine-arginine (Q-R) substitution (73).

Some degree of adducin polymorphism in MNS had already been noted when studying the antibody response of the two strains to membrane skeleton injections (69). The characterization of the genotypes confirmed this phenomenon in the β sequence. Namely, all the MHS rats studied were YY for α and RR for β adducins, while the MNS strain was homozygotic for α-adducin (FF) but polymorphic for the β-adducin (QQ, QR, and RR) (73), suggesting that, in spite of the high inbreeding of more than 60 generations, something had prevented the achievement of homozygosis at the β-adducin locus in the normotensive strain. The reasons for this continued heterozygosity in the MNS may include either a recent point mutation, optimization of biological fitness, and/or selection for low blood pressure. The first two possibilities were discarded because evidence of the polymorphism in MNS was first obtained 5 years earlier. Moreover, when RR and QQ genotypes were selected into separate MNS substrains, no significant differences were found in their reproduction, litter size, body growth, sex ratios, or blood pressure. Conversely, when the systolic blood pressure of QQ, QR, and RR MNS rats were measured, the QR genotype displayed a significant lower blood pressure than the other two (74). Therefore, we are left with the possibility that the persistence of heterozygosis in MNS may be due to the selection for the lowest blood pressure.

As previously stated, adducin is a membrane skeletal protein involved in many cell functions, since it is able to bind calmodulin and phosphatidylserine in a Ca-dependent way (71), favors the assembling of the actin-spectrin complex (71), and, as recently proposed, can be included in the family of the MARKS proteins that are involved in cellular signal transduction triggered by the protein kinase A–dependent cell phosphorylation (75). Considering that a molecular alteration of the adducin heterodimers might affect the stability and function of the cell membrane skeleton and that MHS renal and red blood cells are characterized by specific ion transport abnormalities, it is very likely that adducin polymorphism could represent a primary genetic molecular mechanism of the cell dysfunctions responsible for hypertension in MHS.

MHS rats also show other cell differences compared with MNS rats that are also present in SHRs and in humans. Ca-ATPase has been found to be reduced both in ghosts (76) and in basolateral renal vesicles of MHS rats (77), and, as in SHRs, the Ca binding and the Ca transport in IOV is decreased (78) and intralymphocytic Ca is increased in MHS rats (79). Moreover, in MHS rats, the activity of a Ca-dependent protease, calpain, is tenfold greater in RBCs and twofold greater in renal tissue that in MNS rats, because of a reduced amount of its endogenous inhibitor calpastatin (80). This enzymatic alteration, however, should not be involved in the development of hypertension, since in (MHS × MNS) F_2 hybrids it has been possible to dissociate the blood pressure levels from the cell calpain activity (81).

Humans and Rats

After the first demonstration by Losse et al. (82) of an increased RBC Na_i in primary forms of hypertension, many other groups found similar results both in EH (83,84) and in normotensive offspring of hypertensive parents (85,86). However, an inverse correlation between RBC Na_i and BP levels in offspring of hypertensive parents (87) or even reduced Na_i both in EH and adolescent with positive familiarity for hypertension (88,89) has been recently described. Differences in methodology, genetics, or a different reactivity of cells obtained by hypertensive patients can be involved in causing these discrepancies. However, since Na_i is ultimatively determined by the overall equilibrium among the different Na transports, it cannot be considered as a genetic marker for EH but only as a possible mirror of more relevant disturbances of the ion transport systems.

Na passive permeability was found to be increased in the RBC of EH studied by Garay et al. (90) and the author estimated a frequency between 10 percent and 30 percent in the Caucasian population of this cell alteration. However this Na "leak" cannot be defined as a specific Na pathway or a Na channel in RBC and no alterations of selective Na channels have been demonstrated at kidney or smooth muscle levels in EH. Therefore, an alteration of this pathway could not be easily associated with a determined genetic abnormality.

Na-K-Cl cotransport was found reduced (91), normal (92), or increased (93) in EH as compared with matched controls. Studying the kinetic parameters of RBC in EH

and normotensive controls, it was found that (a) the V_{max} is family-aggregate (93), and it is under genetic control (94); (b) the V_{max} in EH as compared with normotensives is highly variable, being higher, lower, or equal (95); (c) the regulatory ability to handle Na_i was found decreased (lower affinity for Na_i) in 20 percent to 40 percent of EH (96).

To try to understand the apparent discrepancy of the results on V_{max}, our group has studied the distribution of the RBC Na-K-Cl cotransport in 348 never-treated EH and 123 normotensive controls without familiarity for hypertension (97). Normotensives showed an unimodal distribution, while a bimodal distribution was detected in EH with the lower mode comparable with that of normotensives, and the higher accounting for 28 percent of total EH population (97), suggesting the existence of a heterogeneity for cotransport only in EH. In a second study we have also considered the interfamilial correlation of different RBC transport systems and Na_i (98). Na_i and the Na-K pump were found highly and significantly correlated between spouses, suggesting a strong influence of environment on these parameters. Conversely, Na-K cotransport was found to correlate between midparents and offspring, and not between spouses, only in the hypertensive families, indicating that in this subset of population only this phenotypic trait has greater genetic polymorphism (98). Moreover, a direct correlation between erythrocyte Na-K cotransport and renal sodium excretion after furosemide administration has been demonstrated (99). This finding clearly suggests that the Na-K cotransport activity in erythrocytes and the luminal renal membrane (where the furosemide receptor is located) are somehow linked, and a genetic mechanism may be responsible for this parallelism as shown in MHS rats.

Na-Li countertransport shows familial aggregation and high heritability (98,100); therefore, it is one of the most important candidates for the genetic marker of EH. Na-Li exchange has been found usually increased in at least one portion of EH (100) also identified as "nonmodulators" with respect to the ability to modify the Na-dependent vascular and adrenal responsiveness to angiotensin II (101). The same familial study, previously reported on Na-K cotransport (98), showed that there is a highly significant correlation between midparent and offspring values of RBC Na-Li countertransport both in normotensive and hypertensive families, confirming the high degree of genetic components controlling this pathway. A characterization of the Na-H exchange in EH has been done on platelets and leukocytes. Ng et al. (102) found an increased Na-H exchange in leukocytes of hypertensive patients, without any difference in the affinity for H, as compared with the controls. Livne et al. (103) demonstrated that hypertensive patients with their BP controlled by the treatment have a lower Na-H exchange measured in platelets than untreated patients, confirming an association between altered Na-H exchange and hypertension, but raising the possibility that such an alteration might be only secondary to the pathology. Lifton et al. (104) did not find any genetic linkage between RLFP of the gene of Na-H exchange (APNH) and the Na-Li countertransport locus, and APNH and hypertension in 93 hypertensive sibling pairs, where pedigree analysis revealed the existence of a major gene responsible for elevated countertransport. Therefore, it is unlikely that a mutation at the APNH locus can contribute both to the variability of Na-Li countertransport and to the pathogenesis of hypertension in this population.

Activity of the Na-K pump has been found to be reduced in RBC and white blood cells of hypertensive patients (84,105). Its dependence on humoral factors, such as the circulating pump inhibitor (106,107), and environmental factors, such as diet (108), makes it difficult to assess whether an alteration of the Na-K pump reflects a genetic disturbance of the cell membrane in hypertension.

Other cell abnormalities observed in essential hypertension include reduced Ca binding to the cell membrane (109), increased intracellular Ca content (110,111), and reduced activity of the calmodulin-dependent Ca pump (112), among many others. However, no clear evidence has been provided in humans for a particular genetically determined alteration correlated with hypertension, probably because of multigenic and multifactorial dependence of this pathologic trait.

In conclusion, it can be speculated that there are a number of patients with—or prone to develop—hypertension characterized, as in MHS rats, by a reduced Na_i and a faster RBC Na-K cotransport. In these subjects the faster Na transport across cell membranes could cause an increased renal tubular Na reabsorption that might be the key event in the hypertensive process. In keeping with this hypothesis, Weder (113) and our group (97) have demonstrated a correlation between fractional excretion of lithium and urate and RBC Na-Li countertransport and Na-K cotransport in essential hypertensives, suggesting that those subjects with greater Na transport across RBC membrane have also faster Na reabsorption. Accordingly, a direct correlation between erythrocyte cotransport and renal Na excretion after furosemide has been recently demonstrated by our group (99).

On the other hand, similarities between SHRs and human subjects can be recognized when considering subgroups of hypertensives in which alterations of the ion transport systems are in keeping with cellular Na retention, as in the so-called cotransport minus (114) and pump minus (105) subjects. In these subjects the hypertensive role played by a given cell alteration could be expressed in those organs or tissues, such as nerves and vasculature, where an increased Na_i causes hyperactivity and contraction.

Other biochemical and functional cell alterations, such as those concerning Ca handling (109) and PI turnover (115), also seem to be common to certain rat strains and humans.

RENAL MECHANISMS

The role of the kidney in the development of genetic hypertension has been extensively studied in three different rat models and, at least for one strain, the MHS, it is possible to analyze the methodological and theoretical problems involved in the detection of the primary molecular mechanism responsible for the renal alteration involved in the regulation of blood pressure.

The following points will be discussed in detail:

1. The effect of renal transplantation on blood pressure.
2. The different types of renal pressor mechanisms at work in the different strains of rats evaluated by (a) studies on isolated kidneys, with special regard to the pressure-natriuresis curve, and (b) studies on the whole animal.
3. The biochemical-cellular mechanisms underlying renal mechanisms in at least one of these strains.

Spontaneously Hypertensive Rats

The renal contribution to the development and maintenance of hypertension in the SHR was supported by the demonstration that kidneys transplanted from SHRs, but not from WKY rats, raised blood pressure in F_1 hybrid rats obtained by crossing SHRs and WKY rats (116). Furthermore, Rettig et al. (116–118) demonstrated that a very significant portion of the blood pressure difference between a substrain of SHR (the stroke-prone SHR developed in Heidelberg) and its control WKY strain was due to a primary kidney alteration, even though other extrarenal mechanisms could contribute to the blood pressure difference between the two strains.

Isolated SHR kidney, perfused with an artificial medium containing albumin and compared with those of WKY rats, showed, at any pressure, lower values of plasma flow, glomerular filtration rate (GFR), urinary sodium, fractional excretion of sodium (FENa), and fractional excretion of lithium (FELi) as an estimation of proximal tubular resorption, while the fractional handling of Na and H_2O at the distal sites of the nephron was similar in the two kidney strains at all pressures (119). When albumin was omitted from the perfusion, there was a marked increase in urinary Na in the kidneys of the two strains (more than 20 times the values in presence of albumin) and the values of the SHR kidney were higher than those of WKY (119). GFR was also higher in SHR kidney while the FENa was similar and FELi tended to be lower than that seen in presence of albumin; however, the difference was small (119). In young rats (4 weeks old), the SHR kidney showed an increased vascular resistance, a higher FENa at any pressure, and a leftward shift of the pressure-natriuresis curve, as compared with WKY (120).

When isolated SHR and WKY kidneys were perfused *in situ* with blood (121), using a procedure that minimizes nervous and hormonal differences between the two strains (122,123), young rats (3–5 weeks old) showed, at any pressure, a similar GFR and renal plasma flow (RPF), while the excretion of Na and H_2O was shifted toward the right in SHR as pressure increased (121). In adult rats (10–20 weeks old) a greater shift and a lower slope of the pressure-natriuresis curve was observed in SHR (124), while no difference in GFR, renal blood flow (RBF), or peritubular and glomerular capillary pressure was detected. In spite of the similar changes in whole renal and cortical blood flow, the increase of papillary blood flow with increasing perfusion pressure was not as high in SHR as in WKY (125). This phenomenon was present both in young rats (3–5 weeks old) and in adult rats, where it was more marked. A lower papillary blood flow would explain the decrease of the medullary interstitial hydrostatic pressure. This reduction in medullary pressure, in presence of the renal capsule, would be transmitted to the whole kidney. Moreover, since interstitial hydrostatic pressure and tubular reabsorption are strictly related, it was proposed that the rightward shift of the pressure-natriuresis curve in SHR can be due to the decreased interstitial hydrostatic pressure (126,127). As the medullary blood flow derives exclusively from the perfusion of the juxtamedullary nephrons, it was logical to study the pressure-diameter relationship of the preglomerular vasculature of the adult SHR and the WKY juxtamedullary nephrons, under controlled conditions and after blockade of the vascular tone with a low-calcium solution. The tone in SHR preglomerular vessels was greater than that in WKY (128,129). Low-calcium solution abolished this difference while indomethacin had no effect. This study was carried out on the isolated kidney perfused with a physiological salt solution (128). According to these results it has been recently demonstrated that an inverse correlation between the diameter of renal afferent arterioles and an F_2 hybrid population obtained by crossing SHR with WKY (130). Arendshorst et al. (32,131–133) studied the role of the kidney in the pathogenesis of hypertension in SHR. Their major findings were the following:

1. In the whole animal, as compared with WKY, 6-week-old SHRs were moderately hypertensive and had a reduced GFR and RBF and an increased renal vascular resistance (32). At 12 to 14 weeks of age, when hypertension is fully developed in SHR, GFR and RBF were similar in the two strains (132,134).

The reduction of GFR at a young age seemed to be due to enhanced tubuloglomerular feedback, reduced ultrafiltration coefficient, and glomerular plasma flow (132).

2. The renal vascular tone in young SHRs was more dependent on angiotensin-converting enzyme activity than in WKY (133). The vascular reactivity to angiotensin II was enhanced in SHR, and indomethacin abolished the strain difference in the renal response to angiotensin (135).

3. Exaggerated salt and water renal retention occurred during the development of hypertension in young SHR in relation to age-matched WKY (136).

The major discrepancy between the results obtained by Arendshorst et al. (32,131–133) in the whole animal and those obtained by Roman (121,124) with isolated kidney *in situ* concerns the lack of differences in RBF and GFR between young SHR and WKY, as reported by the latter group. However, according to Roman and Kaldunski (125), the greater tubular reabsorption in SHR was secondary to a lower renal interstitial pressure, which, in turn, was due to a lower papillary blood flow. Therefore, the increase in the preglomerular vascular tone of the juxtamedullary nephrons could be the primary cause of the shift of the pressure-natriuresis curve.

In conclusion, all these findings suggest that the pressor effect of the SHR kidney after transplantation might be due to an increased tone of the preglomerular vessels even though a primary difference in tubular handling of Na and H_2O between SHR and WKY may not be entirely excluded. The enhanced renal vascular tone in SHR may certainly be influenced by the sympathetic drive to the kidney and could partly explain the discrepancy between the data obtained from the whole animals and those obtained from the isolated kidney.

Kallikrein, renin, different arachidonic acid metabolites, mineralocorticoid hormones, and catecholamine may all have an influence on both the vascular tone and the tubular reabsorption of Na and H_2O (137). As synthesis and activity of these substances in SHR and WKY kidneys have been shown to be different (138–140), it is not possible to rule out that the shift of the pressure-natriuresis curve in SHR can be due to some primary alteration of one of these hormonal pathways. Whatever the primary mechanism is, the experiments of kidney transplantation clearly indicate that it must be an intrarenal mechanism.

Dahl Sensitivity Rats

There are two strains of Dahl rats—one (DS/Jr) that is fully inbred and the other (DS) that seems not yet fully inbred (141). Unfortunately, kidney cross-transplantation experiments have been carried out only in the second strain (142–145). Because of the peculiarity of these rats, which develop hypertension only when fed with a high-sodium diet (146), the pressor secondary kidney changes could be excluded. So far, the results of two research groups demonstrated that the predisposition to develop hypertension, or at least a portion of it, could be transplanted with the kidney from DS to DR rats on either low- or high-sodium diet. However, on a high-sodium diet, DS rats developed hypertension independently of the type of transplanted kidney (DS or DR), even though DS rats receiving a DS kidney showed slightly higher BP levels than when receiving a DR kidney (142–145). Therefore, besides the primary renal mechanism, some other extrarenal mechanisms must be at work in DS rats receiving a high-sodium diet.

In artificial perfusion medium the function (GFR, RBF, Na, and H_2O excretion) of DS and DR kidneys did not seem to differ, with the exception of vascular resistance, which was higher in the DS kidney (147). When perfused with whole blood both *in vitro* (148) and *in situ* (122), GFR and Na excretion were lower while renal vascular resistance was higher in DS when perfused at the same hydrostatic pressure of DR. The kidneys from animals on high-sodium diet showed greater differences in function than the kidneys from animals on low-sodium diet (122). Kidney function differences were also seen in the whole animal when measured in Dahl rats purchased from Brookhaven (DS) as compared to Dahl rats inbred by John Rapp (DS/Jr) (123). In fact, the GFR of the latter was definitely lower (−39 percent), compared with its control (DR/Jr), while this difference was less (−25 percent) when GFR of DS was compared with GFR of DR. This small difference was due to the high variability of the DS values that may reflect the genetic heterogeneity of the DS rats produced in Brookhaven (141). The marked decrease of total GFR in DS/Jr rats, together with a much greater heterogeneity of single-nephron GFR, may be due to the progressive glomerular disease described by Sterzel et al. (149), which also causes proteinuria in this strain.

A careful study of the pressure-natriuresis relationship was carried out on the kidney perfused *in situ* with blood and under well-controlled hormonal and nervous influences (123). This study showed that on low-salt diet both DS and DS/Jr kidneys required higher renal perfusion pressure to excrete the same amount of sodium. On a high-salt diet, a shift toward the right of the pressure-natriuresis curve of DS/Jr rather than a change in the slope was observed. The same changes were observed for GFR, while RBF was not statistically different in the four strains at all the perfusion pressures and was well autoregulated on the low-salt diet, while on the high-salt diet RBF tended to be lower in DS/Jr than in DR/Jr. The same authors studied the excretion of NaCl and H_2O handling in the different portions of the nephron (150). Proximal tubular and collecting duct reabsorption was

found to be lower, while loop of Henle reabsorption was higher in DS/Jr as compared to DR/Jr. When DS were compared with DR the same changes were observed but they reached the statistical significance only for the Henle's loop data.

Cortical and papillary blood flow and renal interstitial pressure were similar in DR/Jr and DS/Jr on low-salt diet at all the perfusion pressures (123), became lower in DS/Jr than in DR/Jr on high-salt diet at increasing perfusion pressures. In view of these findings, which demonstrate an impairment of the DS kidney's ability to excrete Na^+ (rightward shift of the pressure-natriuresis curve, increased tubular Na^+ reabsorption), it has been suggested that this intrinsic renal defect may trigger the release of a saluretic substance able, on one hand, to normalize the Na handling but, on the other, responsible for the systemic increase of vascular resistance (151). The first experiment, using parabiotic techniques, supported this hypothesis (152), demonstrating that when DR and DS rats, on a high-Na diet, were joined by parabiosis, DR developed a marked hypertension while DS showed BP levels lower than those of single DS or DS + DS rats (152). This first observation was further confirmed by other experiments that suggested the renal origin of this hypertensive factor (153), whose chemical nature has not yet been identified. The biological activity of this factor seems to be related to the Na-K pump inhibition (154) that leads to an increase of reactivity and contractility in nerve terminals and smooth muscle cells (see sections Cell Membrane Alterations and Molecular Mechanisms, above, and Hormones and Humoral Factors, below).

Milan Hypertensive Strain

Kidney cross-transplantations performed in both young and adult Milan rats demonstrated that MHS kidneys carry a message capable of initiating hypertension (155,156). The following studies on renal function and body fluid metabolism showed that this pressor role is probably due to an intrinsic defect in the transtubular Na reabsorption. GFR and urinary flow were greater while plasma and renal renin were lower in young MHS than in MNS of the same age, and these differences tended to disappear as hypertension was fully developed in MHS (157,158). Balance studies showed a renal Na retention in MHS during the development of hypertension (157). Micropuncture studies in young MHS and MNS showed that the single nephron GFR was greater in MHS, which also showed a greater whole kidney GFR, a blunted tubuloglomerular feedback mechanism, and an increased renal interstitial hydrostatic pressure (159). After a few days, when a 20–mm Hg blood pressure difference between MHS and MNS was present, the renal interstitial pressure difference became similar in the two strains, glomerular tubular feedback became more activated in MHS, and the difference in the whole and single-nephron GFR tended to disappear. The maintenance of a normal Na balance, despite a faster GFR, could be due to an increased tubular reabsorption as demonstrated by experiments on isolated perfused kidneys.

When the function of isolated kidneys from young (4 weeks old) MHS and MNS was studied *in vitro* by using an artificial medium plus albumin and 1 mM Ca^{2+}, the following results were obtained (160,161): GFR, urinary flow, overall tubular sodium reabsorption, and kidney O_2 consumption were greater, while vascular resistance was lower in the MHS kidney.

The pressure-natriuresis curves expressed as the relation between perfused pressure and fractional excretion of Na (162) were similar in young MHS and MNS; however, it must be noted that, because of the much higher level of GFR in MHS, the tubular Na load was much higher in MHS than in MNS (102 vs 52 mmol/min/g kidney weight) in order to achieve the same urinary Na excretion (2 mmol/min/g kidney weight). Kidneys removed from adult animals showed almost the same functional differences, except for vascular resistances, which were similar in the two strains, and the pressure-natriuresis curve (expressed as the relation between perfusion pressure and fractional excretion of Na), which was shifted toward the right in MHS (162). Taken together, these results support the notion that a primary increase of tubular reabsorption in MHS may cause both the renal functional changes observed *in vitro* and the greater pressure effect after kidney transplantation. To gain further information about the mechanisms underlying tubular reabsorption in MHS, the effects of three diuretics—amiloride, hydrochlorothiazide, and bumetanide—were tested on the same isolated kidney preparation, using kidneys removed from young MHS and MNS (163). The tubular effect of bumetanide in MHS kidneys was much greater and it appeared at a lower concentration as compared with the effect of bumetanide in the MNS kidney or to the effect of the other two diuretics in the MHS kidney. Also, the natriuretic effect of ouabain (10^{-3} M) was much greater in MHS than in the MNS isolated kidney (164); however, this difference appeared only when ouabain was given to kidneys after 75 minutes of *in vitro* perfusion, but it was not present when ouabain was given after only 15 minutes of perfusion. It must be noted here that the natriuretic response to hydrochlorothiazide was similar in MHS and MNS at the two time-intervals of perfusion. Therefore, it was likely that perfusion *in vitro* of isolated MHS kidneys removed some factors that prevent the full tubular action of ouabain (164). Consistent with these findings, there is other evidence supporting the presence of higher levels of a circulating ouabainlike factor (OLF) in MHS than in MNS (165) such as the reduction of Na-K pump ac-

tivity in adult RBC of adult hypertensive MHS. Recently, we purified by high performance liquid chromatography (HPLC) OLF from hypothalamus and adrenals of adult MHS and MNS and we found a five- to tenfold increase of the OLF yield from MHS than MNS tissues (166).

Looking at the cell mechanisms that can underlie such renal dysfunction, peculiar alterations of tubular cell ion transports can be detected; it was shown that the Na/H countertransport in brush-border vesicles (167), the Na-K cotransport in luminal membrane of the tick ascending limb (168), and the activity of the Na,K-ATPase detected either in purified enzyme (169) or in proximal and ascending limb isolated tubuli (170) were all working at a faster rate in MHS than in MNS preparations. Therefore, it is possible to find ion transport abnormalities at the cell level that are in keeping with the overall organ dysfunction.

Humans and Rats

The studies carried out so far on the role of the kidney in human essential hypertension can be summarized as follows:

1. Kidney transplantation can normalize blood pressure in patients with renal failure caused by malignant hypertension (171).
2. Patients receiving kidneys removed from donors with normotensive parents required less antihypertensive therapy to control posttransplant hypertension than those receiving kidneys removed from donors with hypertensive patients. These statistical differences were still present after taking into account possible confounding factors such as kidney function, rejection crisis, or immunosuppressive therapy (172). These findings suggest that the kidney may possess an intrinsic pressor-depressor mechanism that is possibly under genetic control.

In offspring of hypertensive patients, renal blood flow, GFR, and the excretion of a sodium load may be increased (173,174), whereas urinary kallikrein (175) and plasma renin (173) may be decreased when compared with offspring of normotensive parents. These differences were seen in some subgroups of patients but not in all patients; some may show opposite changes when compared with controls (176). The relationship between changes in Na balance and renal blood flow may be different in subgroups of hypertensive patients as compared with another subgroup (nonmodulators versus modulators) (101), thus suggesting some heterogeneity of the renal mechanisms regulating blood flow and Na excretion in EH. However, the results obtained in animal models can help in understanding the variety of renal functional changes described in human essential hypertension.

In all animal models in which renal transplantation experiments have been performed, the kidney carries the pressor message, even when removed from animals in the prehypertensive phase (118). Since similar observations have been made in transplanted patients, there is strong support for the hypothesis that in humans some primary intrinsic renal abnormalities affect cell and, in turn, organ function, influencing the overall body BP regulation. Considering the different aspects of renal functions in the three rat models cited, it is clear that, besides the common pressor role of the kidney, different renal functional alterations trigger the development of hypertension. In Dahl rats an apparently normal kidney became hypertensive when challenged with a Na load through a humoral mechanism. A similar mechanism may also be at work in subjects prone to develop hypertension because of an abnormal sensitivity to Na.

Spontaneously hypertensive rats show a more complex picture of the possible renal primary alterations, since either renal vascular tone and renal volume regulation or hormonal factors (angiotensin II) seem impaired. In particular, if a genetic relationship between angiotensin II response and blood pressure development could be demonstrated, this intrarenal defect might be also similar to that of a subset of human hypertensive patients, since 30 percent of EH have been estimated to be non-modulators like SHRs (101). On the other hand, SHRs may represent the animal model closer to those subgroups of patients in whom a decrease of GFR and RPF seems to occur at the earlier stages of hypertension or in the prehypertensive phase (176).

In the Milan strain a primary tubular alteration of Na reabsorption seems to be the cause of the hypertensive process. A subset of normotensive subjects is prone to develop hypertension because of a positive familiarity for this disease (173,174), and MHS rats show many similar functional characteristics. In particular, from the overall kidney function (increased GFR and tubular reabsorption) to the cell alterations (faster Na-K cotransport in RBC), the picture is strictly superimposable in the two species, supporting the concept that both in MHS and in at least one subgroup of patients a common pathophysiological mechanism is operating.

HORMONES AND HUMORAL FACTORS

Spontaneously Hypertensive Rats

Signs of hyperplasia and hypertrophy of the adenohypophysis adrenocorticotropic hormone (ACTH)-producing cells (177) and of the adrenal glomerulosa and fasciculata zones (178) have been observed in SHRs, suggesting a hyperfunctional status of these areas. In agreement with these findings, basal, ACTH, and KCl-stimulated plasma levels of aldosterone and corticosterone were higher, while plasma renin activity was lower in SHR as compared with WKY (179). This suggests that a moderate elevation of aldosterone and corticosterone, and the concomitant hypertropy, could be ascribed to hyperresponsiveness to ACTH and KCl of adrenals in adult SHRs.

More recently, a biochemical abnormality in the enzymatic pathway leading to an enhanced production of adrenal corticosteroids has been documented in SHRs. In fact, the activity of 6β-hydroxylase, an enzyme involved in steroidogenesis, has been found to be increased sixfold in the kidney and twofold in the liver of adult SHRs as compared with WKY rats (180). Since 6β-OH-corticosterone seems to increase Na transport across epithelia, it has been suggested that this alteration of the steroid metabolism may contribute to BP elevation in SHR by affecting renal Na retention.

The reduced plasma renin activity (PRA) in SHR (179,181–183) could be a consequence of the increased steroidogenesis in SHRs at the hypertensive age. Vascular renin has been claimed to have a hypertensive role in SHR, since the interconversion of the inactive to active renin in the arterial wall (184) is increased in this strain, and might be responsible for the increased vasospasm and vascular resistance in these rats.

An increased plasma vasopressin concentration was described in adult SHRs (185,186), supporting a role for it in the maintenance of hypertension. As reported for other strains of hypertensive rats, urinary kallikrein (total and active) was found to be suppressed in 4- to 15-week-old SHRs (187,188), and it has been suggested that an early defect in the kallikrein activity in SHRs could contribute to the development of hypertension. In line with this early observation, the study of RFLP on SHR genomic DNA using kallikrein probes revealed polymorphism in five different regions, indicating possible differences in tissue kallikrein genes or in their regulatory regions in SHR (189).

The possible pathophysiological role of a circulating Na-K pump inhibitor in this strain is still under investigation. Some findings support the notion that this substance may be increased. As already cited in our discussion on cell membrane alterations, the inhibition of the cell Na-K pump and the increase of Na$_i$ are indirect evidence for the presence of this substance. Moreover, using a cytochemical technique, Millet et al. (190) revealed an enhanced inhibitory activity of SHR plasma on the Na,K-ATPase activity.

Besides the presence of a circulating pump inhibitor, in recent years some attention has been addressed to the existence of another substance with possible hypertensive activity, produced by parathyroid glands (191). In fact, parathyroidectomy performed in young SHRs prevents the development of hypertension (192,193) and parathyroid cross-transplantation from SHR-SP to WKY produces hypertension in the latter strain (194). Partial purification from plasma and characterization of this factor suggest that it is different from parathormone (PTH), is peptidic in nature, is directly produced by specialized parathyroid cells (195), increases Ca uptake in vascular smooth muscle cells (VSMC), and potentiates the actions of various vasopressor substances (196).

The atrial content of atrial natriuretic peptide (ANP) was found to be reduced (197), although as hypertension progressed, its plasma levels increased (198). Renal responsiveness to ANP (199), as well as the secretion of ANP in response to a chronic Na load, is in fact increased (200). It seems, therefore, that an increased turnover of ANP in SHRs could be compensating for an otherwise reduced Na and water elimination.

Interest has increased in recent years in the association between obesity, impaired glucose tolerance or type 2 diabetes, and hypertension (201). In particular, much evidence supports the existence of a reduced sensitivity to insulin both in human and animal hypertension. In this respect, it has been found that SHRs have an impaired oral glucose tolerance (202,203), hyperinsulinemia, and elevated plasma insulin in response to oral glucose (203) as compared with WKY rats. Therefore, it has been proposed that hyperinsulinemia in SHR may contribute to the genesis of hypertension. However, all the in vivo studies cited above have been conducted in anesthetized or restrained rats in which stressful conditions may have influenced the glucose metabolism. Recently, Buchanan et al. (204) showed that the insulin effect on hepatic glucose output and peripheral glucose clearance measured in conscious, unrestrained rats is similar in WKY and SHR rats at 10 weeks of age, when hypertension is already developed in SHR. These data therefore tend to exclude a primary participation of insulin resistance in SHR development of hypertension.

Dahl Sensitivity Rats

In DS rats an altered steroidogenesis with an increased production of 18-OH-deoxycorticosterone (DOC) has been demonstrated and found to be genetically associated with hypertension (205). Recently, a polymorphism for the allele of the 11β-hydroxylase has been demonstrated between DS and DR rats (206). This polymorphism co-segregates with an increased adrenal capacity to synthesize 18-OH-DOC and blood pressure. DR rats carry the 11β-hydroxylase allele that is associated with a reduced capacity to produce 18-OH-DOC and encodes five amino acid substitutions in the 11β-hydroxylase protein (206). Therefore, it has been suggested that the salt resistance of DR rats may be due to the reduced ability to produce 18-OH-DOC.

The plasma and renal renin activities measured both in vivo and in isolated perfused kidney (148) were clearly lower in DS than in DR rats, independent of the Na diet (207) and rat age (208). Plasma vasopressin (AVP) levels were found to be similar in DS and DR rats on low-Na diet and only slightly increased in DS rats after 6 to 8 weeks on an 8 percent Na diet (209). Urinary kallikrein excretion was found to be lower in DS rats than in DR rats (210).

As far as it concerns the presence in DS rats of a hypertensive circulating substance responsible for the elevation of BP when transferred through parabiosis to DR rats (152), no direct evidence has been provided so far for the presence of an Na,K-ATPase inhibitor in Dahl's rat plasma. However, the original finding of a pressor effect of DS serum was further confirmed by Hirata et al. (211). Also, it has been shown that DS rats have an increased atrial content of ANP to which they are markedly hyporesponsive at the renal level (212,213). These two defects, which are also present before a clear blood pressure rise is observed (213), are thought to be genetically determined (214) and, in any case, consistent with the renal natriuretic defect of DS rats.

Lyon Hypertensive Strain

Plasma renin activity is higher in LH than Lyon low pressure strain LL before the development of hypertension (215); then, the differences tend to disappear with increasing age. Also, urinary DOC is increased in young LH rats (216). However, it is difficult to establish whether these enhanced PRA and DOC levels are primary or secondary to other pressor mechanisms, since an enhanced sympathetic drive (see section Neural Mechanisms, below) is present in this strain and may account for the hormonal alterations of LH rats. In particular, an increased renal synthesis of thromboxane A_2 (TxA_2), due to increased activity of the Tx synthetase, has been observed in young LH rats (217). This alteration is magnified by adrenergic stimulation. In fact, renal prostanoid secretion from isolated kidneys of LH rats has been found increased by 10- to 20-fold by norepinephrine, as compared with LN and LL kidneys. Since the in vivo turnover of norpinephrine is increased in kidney cortex of young LH rats (218), the combination of an enhanced TxA_2 renal production and adrenergic drive can be involved in the enhanced renal resistance and lower GFR observed in LH hypertension (219).

Vasopressin does not seem to be particularly involved in hypertension in this strain, since both LH and LL rats showed increased AVP as compared with LN (220). The thyroid and its hormones may be involved in this form of hypertension, since surgical thyroidectomy has a more marked hypotensive effect in LH than in LN strain (221). A hyperresponsiveness to thyroid hormones or the effect of partial parathyroidectomy during thyroid ablation could explain the role of the thyroid in LH hypertension.

New Zealand Genetically Hypertensive Strain

A slight suppression of the renin-angiotensin-aldosterone system is present in the young-adult GH compared with New Zealand normotensive (NR) rats (222), and only in older GH animals (27 weeks) do plasma renin and aldosterone increase, probably as a consequence of renal damage (223). Vasopressin could have some involvement in sustaining GH hypertension, since an increased pressor responsiveness to exogenous vasopressin has been documented in GH rats (224). However, the significance of this finding is unclear, since GH rats also exhibit a hyperresponsiveness to angiotensin II (224). An altered renal prostaglandin metabolism has been described as a contributing factor to GH hypertension (225). However, Baer et al. (226) demonstrated that this altered metabolism is not associated with GH hypertension, since it is present only in male rats.

Milan Hypertensive Strain

Plasma renin activity is suppressed in young prehypertensive MHS, and the differences with MNS rats tend to disappear as hypertension develops (157). In adult hypertensive MHS rats, signs of adrenal hypertrophy appear (227) accompanied by an increase of plasma corticosterone and, in 3-month-old MHS rats, of plasma aldosterone (227). The reasons for this increased steroidogenesis in MHS are not clear. Recently, reduced activity of the hepatic 11β-hydroxysteroid dehydrogenase (11β-HSD) with a reduced gene expression has been found in young prehypertensive MHS (228). However, at a renal level where an alteration of 11β-HSD activity and gene expression might play a pathophysiological role, no differences between MHS and MNS were detected (228). Therefore, it is difficult to find a clear relationship between the impaired epatic 11β-HSD activity in MHS and the pathogenesis of this form of hypertension.

Urinary kallikrein (229) and plasma ADH (230) are suppressed in young MHS rats compared with MNS rats.

The following observations suggest the presence of a higher level of circulating OLF in MHS than in MNS: a low PRA either before or after the development of hypertension in MHS (157), a lower Na-K pump activity in erythrocytes as hypertension develops in MHS (60), an increased renal interstitial pressure in MHS before the development of hypertension that becomes similar to that of MNS 1 week after the development of hypertension (159), the enhanced natriuretic activity of ouabain in MHS isolated perfused kidney (164), and the increased Na,K-ATPase inhibitory activity of MHS

plasma (165). These indirect data have now been confirmed by the direct measurement of the amount of OLF extracted and purified by HPLC from the hypothalama and adrenals of MHS, which was found to be five- to tenfold higher than in MNS (166).

Humans and Rats

A comparative overview of the hormonal patterns of the different hypertensive rat strains yields the following findings:

1. The rate of steroidogenesis, which in hypertensive men can be normal or sometimes increased (231), usually appears to be increased in rat models after the development of hypertension, when signs of adrenal hypertrophy or hyperplasia also appear. The pressor role of these hormones may thus be concerned with maintenance of hypertension.
2. Except for GH and Lyon strains, PRA is usually suppressed in hypertensive rats. A decreased PRA in prehypertensive stages could be due, as in MHS and Dahl rats, to an intrarenal abnormality of the Na and water excretion. Human subjects prone to develop hypertension show many analogies with these rat models regarding renal function, Na and water excretion, and hormonal patterns (232,233). The reduced PRA seen in adult SHRs is most likely a consequence of the hypertensive status. Since low PRA is also reported for subgroups of hypertensive patients, a similar negative feedback mechanism may be at work also in humans.
3. Concerning natriuretic factors, two different considerations must be made for ANP and the Na-K pump inhibitor: ANP is now well accepted to be a hormone having regulatory activities on the body fluid balance, and it seems to be more involved in the acute phases of volume alterations (234) as a consequence of primary organ dysfunction in kidney, heart, and the nervous system.

NEURAL MECHANISMS

The presence of a circulating Na-K pump inhibitor has been indirectly demonstrated also in hypertensive subjects. This plasma factor seems to possess the same characteristics as those described for the factor detected in MHS, SHR, and Dahl strains. It is therefore likely that such a plasma factor may have some role in sustaining high blood pressure in those forms of essential hypertension where a primary renal defect is present.

The notion that altered neurogenic mechanisms can be involved in the development and/or maintenance of human EH is popular, but the complexity of the sympathetic nervous regulation and its dependence on both the central neural control and the peripheral cardiovascular responses make it difficult to understand whether neural functional alterations are localized at central or peripheral levels or whether they are due to an abnormal vascular reactivity to normal stimuli.

In genetic animal models in which the functional alterations of both the central and peripheral nervous system can be measured before and after the development of hypertension, it is possible to better understand the basis for these neural defects.

Spontaneously Hypertensive Rats

Much evidence indicates that one of the major factors accounting for the development of SHR hypertension is increased sympathetic nerve traffic (235). Alterations of the central nervous system (CNS) neuroanatomical organization in SHRs have been described (236), and recently the involvement of the area postrema region in determining the increase of blood pressure has been suggested since its ablation in 4-week-old SHRs attenuates the development of hypertension (237).

Altered central catecholaminergic mechanisms seem also to contribute to the development of SHR hypertension. The activities of tyrosine-hydroxylase, dopamine-beta-hydroxylase (DBH), and phentolamine-N-methyl-transferase (PNMT) have been found to be increased in the brain of young SHRs (4–5 weeks old) (238,239). Central norepinephrine (NE) turnover increases with age in SHR (239), while at the periphery in the kidney and skeletal muscle it is increased in the prehypertensive phases and reduced after hypertension is established (240). The effect of mental stress on pressor responses (241) and the dependence of these responses on Na intake (242) were also claimed as further evidence of an increased central hyperactivity in response to the environmental stimuli in these animals. An increased responsiveness of central α_2-adrenergic receptors in SHR to high-sodium intake has been observed and demonstrated to affect the neural control of renal function (243).

An exaggerated vasoconstrictor response to sympathetic nervous stimulation (SNS) has also been described in SHRs (244–246). Because neural mechanisms, central regulation, and receptor organization are involved in vascular hyperresponsiveness, all these aspects have been investigated, showing a wide spectrum of alterations: increased sensitivity to central stimuli (247); greater release of catecholamines at the periphery (244,248–250); structural vascular wall abnormalities (251); and altered adrenoceptor mechanisms at the effector organs (252,253), which have been observed mainly in young borderline hypertensive rats.

Further evidence for a primary involvement of SNS was found by Campbell et al. (254) in an experiment of cross-transplantation between 2-week-old SHRs and WKY rats of a section of caudal artery into the anterior eye chamber. They demonstrated that the SHR-altered membrane potential of the vascular smooth muscle cells was present only when a trophic sympathetic influence of the same strain was maintained.

A contributing factor to the maintenance of hypertension should be the reduced sensitivity of the SHR baroreflex as age increases and blood pressure rises (255,256). As demonstrated by Andresen et al. (257), this is probably due to a primary defect present in the baroreceptors themselves and not to structural wall changes.

Dahl Sensitivity Rats

Many parallels can be demonstrated between SHRs and Dahl rats concerning the possible contribution of neural mechanisms to the promotion of hypertension. Stressful conditions also promote the development of hypertension in DS rats when maintained on low-Na diet (258). Moreover, lesions of the anteroventral third ventricle attenuate the BP rise of DS rats maintained on a high-Na diet (259), suggesting that NaCl-induced hypertension in this strain requires the integrity of this region and is partially related to a reduced vasopressin excretion.

Similarly to SHRs, DS rats show increased PNMT activity in brainstem epinephrine neurons after a high-Na diet (260), indicating an involvement of this central area in BP regulation as a function of Na metabolism.

In plasma, basal levels of catecholamines did not differ between DS and DR rats, but DS responded to stress stimuli with a higher secretion of both NE and epinephrine (261). Other studies directed at evaluating the role of SNS at the peripheral level showed that the peripheral chemical sympathectomy prevents the BP rise in DS rats, whatever the Na diet (262). The increased vascular resistance due to Na diet is reduced in isolated hindquarters of DS rats' sympathetic denervation (263), and the contribution of neurogenic mechanisms to the determination of pressure-flow curves accounts for 50 percent of the increased vascular resistance produced by high-Na intake. However, renal denervation performed before switching from low- to high-Na diet did not prevent or attenuate the development of hypertension in DS rats (264), suggesting that the mechanisms involved in the Na sensitivity and hypertension in DS rats are independent of the renal neurogenic control. Moreover, peripheral, but not central, α-adrenoceptor alterations could participate in the DS hypertension, since the number of renal α_2-receptors is enhanced in DS rats as compared with DR rats both at low- and high-Na diet, while in the brain the receptor density and affinity are the same in the two strains (265).

Lyon Hypertensive Strain

Many findings support the notion that hypertension in this strain is, at least in part, due to an early increase of sympathoadrenal activity; PNMT activities both at the central level and in the adrenal glands (266), DBH activity in the superior cervical ganglia (267), and urinary excretion of adrenaline (268) are increased in young (5-week-old) LH rats. These differences tend to disappear during growth, and all parameters are normalized by 21 weeks of age (268). Moreover, similar alterations of sympathoadrenal activity have recently been described in neonatal LH rats (269), which exhibited a decreased activity in central dopaminergic neurons and an enhanced maturation of adrenals. At the periphery the involvement of SNS activity in LH hypertension was studied by measuring norepinephrine turnover in different organs both in 5- and 2-week-old LH, LN, and LL rats (218). NE turnover at the cardiac level is reduced in LH rats, but it is increased in the kidney and in the adrenals, supporting other results of an enhanced neurogenic activity that modulates renal function in this strain (219).

The cardiovascular reactivity of LH rats to neuromediators (NE, epinephrine, angiotensin II) also seems to be enhanced, especially in adult rats with well-established hypertension (270).

Others (271) have shown that the baroreflex sensitivity, measured after phenylephrine injections, increased with age more markedly in normotensive control strains than in LH rats, thereby confirming the presence of a general impairment of baroreceptor resetting, as described for other generically hypertensive rats.

New Zealand Genetically Hypertensive and Milan Hypertensive Strains

These two strains do not exhibit any clear evidence of a neurogenic participation in the development of hypertension. The few reports on GH rats concerning this aspect fail to demonstrate hyperresponsiveness to stress in terms of NE and epinephrine plasma levels (272,273).

In MHS rats, no signs of pressor hyperresponsiveness to stress have been detected (274). Moreover, the low frequency of heart rate and the increased cardiac vagal tone suggest an enhanced cardiac depressor sympathetic drive (274). Plasma levels of catecholamines determined under very controlled conditions did not differ in young and adult MHS and MNS rats (275). No alterations of central α-receptors were found in MHS rats, whereas in the kidney the number of α_2-receptor binding sites decreased with the development of hypertension (276), supporting the hypothesis of a secondary down-regulation due to the primary increase in renal Na reabsorption.

HUMANS AND RATS

The participation of the central or sympathetic nervous system in the development of hypertension is a quite common feature in some strains, even though in at least two rat models (MHS and GH) this evidence is not present. This is in agreement with other studies that failed to find clear differences in catecholamine metabolism, plasma catecholamine levels (277), and baroreflex activity (278) in hypertensive patients.

To try to link the alterations in CNS and SNS activities described in some rat strains and subgroups of hypertensive patients with a primary cell abnormality that may influence organ function in different districts, the following observation can be relevant: a primary alteration of Na or Ca transport in neurons or nerve terminals (Na-K pump or Ca pump inhibition, Na-H exchange, or Na passive permeability increases) can lead to transient or chronic enhancement of intracellular Na and, in turn, of Ca. These are mechanisms that can lead to (a) an increased catecholamine release, (b) reuptake, and (c) turnover (279). These are indications that an excessive Na intake may facilitate neurogenic vasoconstriction in those animal models and humans that are genetically susceptible to salt hypertension (280,281). Moreover, a greater depolarization of vascular muscle cells due to, for instance, Na-K pump inhibition may account for hyperresponsiveness to neurotransmitters (282). There may also be a similar membrane defect responsible for adrenoceptor changes, since down- and up-regulation of α-adrenoceptors have been demonstrated to be Na-dependent (283). In the CNS the increased receptor sensitivity to neuropeptides may also be due to changes mediated by ion transport systems, for instance, an enhanced Na-H exchange activation due to angiotensin II (284,285).

Therefore, at present it is impossible to establish whether the SNS or CNS abnormalities so far described both in man or in rats are the result of a generalized primary defect(s) in cell membrane regulation of ion transports, which also produces changes in the nervous cells, or are the result of a primary defect in a more specific function of these cells, including their complex intercellular connections. In this regard it is relevant to recall here the kidney transplantation experiments in SHR or Dahl rats described above. How we can reconcile a primary role of the nervous system with the fact that, at least in SHR, the most significant portion of hypertension can be transplanted with the kidney?

HEART

Modification of the structure or function of the heart in human hypertension has been regarded as either (a) a secondary response to an increased cardiac load or (b) a primary modification that by itself can cause hypertension (286). Moreover, it is unclear whether the regression of left ventricular hypertrophy induced by antihypertensive drugs actually abolishes the risk associated with increased cardiac size (287). Regarding the first point, in some hypertensive strains of rat, heart size is already increased at this age, whereas in others the increase is secondary to the development of hypertension (288). However, in strains whose heart size is increased at birth it is not possible to say whether these modifications are actually primary since their blood pressure is already above normal at birth (289). In humans it has been shown that the cardiac mass measured by echocardiography may be larger in offspring of hypertensive patients as compared to those of normotensive patients (290).

However, due to the well-known greater pressor responsiveness to different environmental stimuli in the offspring of hypertensive parents, as compared to those of normotensive parents (291), it is not possible to exclude an influence of afterload on such a difference in left ventricular mass. Studies on animal models (particularly SHR) suggest that the following factors may result in left ventricular hypertrophy during the stages preceding or accompanying the development of genetic forms of hypertension:

1. An increase in afterload that may be present even in the uterus or soon after birth (289). During this period the heart may be particularly sensitive to afterload differences for various reasons. One of them may be the presence of mitotic myocyte divisions, which cease sometime after birth (292,293).

2. A greater sensitivity of myocytes to physical, humoral, or neural factors. For instance, the adenylate cyclase response to isoproterenol is significantly higher in the heart of newborn SHRs than in that of newborn WKY rats (294), and the phosphoinositide turnover has been recently demonstrated to be enhanced after NE stimulation in SHR, suggesting a role in the SHR hypertrophy possibly mediated by an altered cell Ca handling (295).

3. A greater sympathetic drive to the heart, which may be a part of the increased sympathetic activity causing the hypertensive state in SHRs, as suggested by some authors (see Neural Mechanisms, above).

4. Higher levels of circulating growth factors, which may be particularly effective in the cardiovascular system (296,297).

At present we do not know whether all these causes work together or separately in the different animal strains or in humans. Certainly they must be regarded as possible explanations of the enlargement of left ventricular mass detected before and during the development of hypertension.

There are, however, strains of rat (MHS and LH) in which no difference in heart weight is present before the development of hypertension and in which the increase of left ventricular mass seems to parallel the increase of blood pressure (288,298). In this respect, the possibility that cardiac hypertrophy is a phenomenon not genetically linked to the mechanism leading to hypertension has been raised by recent experiments performed both in SHR (299) and MHS rats (Casari et al., unpublished results), demonstrating that the left ventricular weight to body weight ratio is not correlated with the blood pressure levels measured in an F_2 hybrid population obtained by crossing the parental hypertensive (SHR or MHS) and normotensive (WKY or MNS) strains. It is, therefore, possible that genetic factors different from those involved in causing hypertension have a permissive role in the development of cardiac hypertrophy. In both adult rats and humans an increase of ventricular mass is due to increased myocyte size and proliferation of connective tissue elements (300). Compensatory neovascularization occurs during the early phases of cardiac hypertrophy in the SHR (301); however, this process is insufficient to maintain normal vascularization levels, and a significant decrease in capillary density occurs in older rats (302,303). These processes, together with a structural narrowing of the coronary vascular bed (304), are probably the causes of the increased risk associated with the enlarged heart.

Many studies have been performed, mainly in SHRs, regarding the effect of antihypertensive therapy on heart structure and performance (305–308). In general these studies show that the normalization of blood pressure does not fully normalize the heart weight, thus confirming that other factors, besides afterload, are involved in cardiac hypertrophy. Moreover, the reduction of heart weight is mainly due to increased reduction of tissue in the ventricular wall (300). This may furnish some experimental basis for the clinical observation that the normalization of blood pressure through antihypertensive therapy does not normalize cardiac morbidity or mortality (309).

CONCLUSIONS

Whatever physiological and biochemical variables we consider, we may find some similarities between rats and humans with genetic or essential hypertension, provided that appropriate subgroups of patients are selected. According to this approach, the following subgroups of EH can be recognized: subjects with low plasma renin, with low or high RBC cotransport, subjects with normal or high Na-Li countertransport, and "modulators or "nonmodulators." However, it is not clear whether such subgroups represent the tails of a normal distribution or whether they are nosologic entities with peculiar genetic and biochemical mechanisms. To prove the existence of this new clinical entity we need to demonstrate that these biochemical, cellular, or organic dysfunctions are accompanied by precise genetic-molecular abnormalities that may explain such dysfunctions. Indeed, the complexity of the interactions existing in the human population between genetic and environmental factors that influence the levels of blood pressure hampers the attempt to study the mode of genetic transmission of these variables in the individual member of a family tree. We may approach this problem by taking advantage of the existence of animal models in which an appropriate genetic characterization is possible, and where the sequence of events going from a given genetic abnormality to arterial hypertension may be clarified. In this way it is possible to have a theoretical background to be applied to human studies.

Our research group, following this approach, has verified that mutations in the membrane skeleton protein adducin are associated with the blood pressure variations of the Milan hypertensive rat strain (74). Furthermore, we previously demonstrated that cell membrane skeleton influences the functional characteristics of MHS cells in terms of volume and Na-K cotransport activity (61,68) and that these characteristics are genetically associated with MHS hypertension (62). We are now currently involved in studying the relationship between the molecular alterations of adducin and its cell functional role in determining its pressor effect in MHS. Studies on the polymorphism of the adducin gene in those patients selected according to the criteria of biochemical and functional similarities with Milan rats (97–99) are in progress. The same approach can be proposed for the identification and characterization of the genetic mechanisms underlying hypertension in the other rat models and those patients who share with them the same cellular and organ dysfunctions.

REFERENCES

1. Lovenberg W, Horan M, eds. Genetic rat models hypertension. *Guidelines for breeding, care and use. Hypertension* 1987;9 (suppl I).
2. Rapp JP, Dene H. *Hypertension* 1985;7:340–349.
3. Berglund G, Singstrom L, Lundin S, Karlberg BE, Herlitz H. *Clin Sci* 1981;61:313–316.
4. Duhm J, Gobel BO, Beck FX. *Hypertension* 1983;5:642–652.
5. Okamoto K, Yamori Y, Oshima A, et al. In: Okamoto K. ed. *Spontaneous hypertension its pathogenesis and complications.* Tokyo: Igaru Shoin, 1972;1–8.
6. Louis WJ, Howes LG. *J Cardiovasc Pharmacol* 1990;6(suppl 7): S1–S5.
7. De Mendoca M, Knorr A, Grichois ML, Ben-Ishay D, Garay R, Meyer P. *Kidney Int* 1982;21(suppl II):S69–S75.
8. Feig PU, Mitchell PP, Boylan IW. *Hypertension* 1985;7:423–429.
9. Wiley JS, Hutchinson JS, Mendelsohn FAO, Doyle AE. *Clin Exp Pharmacol Physiol* 1980;7:527–530.
10. Friedman SM, Friedman CL. *Circ Res* 1976;39:433–441.
11. Harris AL, Guthe CC, Van't Veer F, Bohr DF. *Hypertension* 1984;6:42–48.
12. Rosati C, Meyer P, Garay RP. *Hypertension* 1986;8:379–385.
13. Cusi D, Fossali E, Piazza A, et al. *Am J Hypertens* 1991;4:725–734.
14. Jones RB, Patrick J, Hilton PJ. *Clin Sci* 1981;61:313–316.
15. Dufilho DM, Devynck MA, Beugras JP, Meyer P. *J Cardiovasc Pharmacol* 1984;6:273–278.
16. Friedman SM. *Hypertension* 1979;1:572–582.
17. Cangiano JL, Rodriguez-Sargent C, Opava-Stitzer S, Martinez-Maldonado M. *Proc Soc Exp Biol Med* 1984;177:240–246.
18. Garg LC, Narang N. *J Lab Clin Med* 1985;106:43–46.
19. Postnov YU, Reznikova M, Boriskina G. *Pflugers Arch* 1976;362:95–99.
20. Chen CC, Lin-Shiau SY. *Eur J Pharmacol* 1986;122:311–319.
21. Blaustein MP. *Hypertension* 1984;6:445–453.
22. Feig PU, D'Occhio MA, Boylan JW. *Hypertension* 1987;9:282–288.
23. Saleh AM, Batlle DC. *J Clin Invest* 1990;85:1734–1739.
24. Feig PU, D'Occhio MA, Boylan JW. *J Hypertens* 1986;5:S224–S226.
25. Feig PU. *Am J Hypertens* 1990;3:927–932.
26. Kobayashi A, Nara Y, Nishio T, Mori C, Yamori Y. *J Hypertens* 1990;8:153–157.
27. Berck BG, Vallega G, Musslin AJ, Gordon HM, Canessa M, Wayne AR. *J Clin Invest* 1989;83:822–829.
28. Morduchowicz GA, Sheikh-Amad D, Jo OD, Nord EP, Lee DBN, Yanagawa N. *Kidney Int* 1989;36:576–581.
29. Foster CD, Honeyman TW, Scheid CR. *Am J Physiol* 1992;262: H1657–H1662.
30. Mahnensmith RL, Aronson PS. *Circ Res* 1985;56:773–788.
31. Resink TJ, Scott-Burder T, Baur U, Bürgin M, Bühler FR. *Hypertension* 1989;14:293–303.
32. Dilley JR, Stier CT, Arendshorts WJ. *Am J Physiol* 1984;246: F12–F20.
33. Postnov YU, Orlov SN, Gulak PV. *Pflugers Arch* 1976;365:257–263.
34. Devynck MA, Pernollet MG. *Hypertension* 1981;3:397–403.
35. Bruschi G, Bruschi ME, Caroppo M, Orlandini G, Pavarani C, Cavatorta A. *Life Sci* 1984;35:535–542.
36. Tepel M, Husseini S, Wischniowski H, Zidek W. *Am J Hypertens* 1992;5:740–743.
37. Dowd TL, Gupta RK. *J Biol Chem* 1992;267:3637–3643.
38. Orlov SN, Pokudin NI, Postnov YD. *Pflugers Arch* 1983;63:43–45.
39. Adeyoa AS, Norman RI, Bing RF. *Clin Sci* 1989;77:395–400.
40. Kravtsov GM, Orlov SN, Pokudin NI, Postnov YV. *Clin Sci* 1983;65:126–135.
41. Rasmussen H, Barrett PQ. *Physiol Rev* 1984;64:938–984.
42. McLaren Y, Kreutz R, Lindpaintner K, et al. *J Hypertens* 1993;11:25–30.
43. Koutouzov S, Marche P, Cloix JF, Meyer P. *Am J Physiol* 1882;243:H590–H587.
44. Heagerty AM, Qllerenshaw JD, Swales JD. *Br J Pharmacol* 1986;89:803–807.
45. Berridge MJ. *Hypertension* 1984;220:33–45.
46. Postnov YV. *Hypertension* 1990;15:332–337.
47. Kravtsov GM, Dulin NO, Postnov YV. *J Hypertens* 1988;6:853–857.
48. Takaori K, Itoh S, Kanayama Y, Takeda T. *Biochem Biophys Res Commun* 1986;141:769–773.
49. Kravtsov GM, Dulin NO, Postnov YV. *Bull Exp Biol Med* 1989;68:42–43.
50. Kotelevtsen YV, Spitkovski DD, Orlov SN, Postnov YV. *J Hypertens* 1989;7(suppl 6):S112–S113.
51. McCormick CP, Hennessy JF, Rauch AL, Vardaman MB. *Am J Hypertens* 1989;2:604–609.
52. De Mendoca M, Knorr A, Grichois ML, et al. *Klin Wochenschr* 1985;63(suppl III):66–69.
53. Zicha J, Duhm J. *Hypertension* 1990;15:612–627.
54. Pontremoli R, Spalvins A, Menachery A, Torielli L, Canessa M. *Kidney Int* 1992;42:1355–1362.
55. Vasdev S, Prabhakaran V, Sampson CA. *Hypertension* 1990;15: 183–189.
56. Nishi A, Celsi G, Aperia A. *Am J Physiol* 1993;264:F448–F452.
57. Biol MC, Vincent M, Sassard J. *Arch Int Physiol Biochim* 1979;87:291–296.
58. Wiley JS, Hutchinson JS, Mendelsohn FAO, Doyle AE. *Clin Exp Pharmacol Physiol* 1980;7:527–530.
59. Ferrari P, Barber BR, Torielli L, Ferrandi M, Salardi S, Bianchi G. *Hypertension* 1987;10(suppl I):I-32–I-36.
60. Ferrari P, Ferrandi M, Torielli L, Canessa M, Bianchi G. *J Hypertens* 1987;5:199–206.
61. Ferrari P, Torielli L, Cirillo M, Salardi S, Bianchi G. *J Hypertens* 1991;9(8):703–711.

62. Bianchi G, Ferrari P, Trizio D, et al. *Hypertension* 1985;7:319–325.

63. Ferrari P, Torielli L, Barber BR, Soldati L, Duzzi L, Bianchi G. *Proceedings of 14th Scientific Meeting of the International Society of Hypertension* (abstract) P29 Madrid, 14–18 June, 1992.

64. Beck F, Bianchi G, Dorge A, Rick R, Schramm M, Thurau K. *J Hypertens* 1983;1(suppl 2):38–39.

65. Parenti P, Hanozet G, Bianchi G. *Hypertension* 1986;8:932–939.

66. Ferrari P, Nussdorfer G, Torielli L, Salvati P, Tripodi MG, Niutta E, Bianchi G. In: Hofman A, Grobbee DE, Schalekamp MADH, eds. *Renal function and cell characteristics during the development of essential and genetic hypertension.* Amsterdam: Elsevier, 1987;63–67.

67. Vallega G, Atkinson W, Tsai E, Torielli, Canessa M. *FASEB J* 1989;J3:A1187.

68. Ferrari P, Torielli L, Salardi S, Rizzo A, Bianchi G. *Biochim Biophys Acta* 1992;1111:111–119.

69. Salardi S, Saccardo B, Borsani G, et al. *Am J Hypertens* 1989;2:229–237.

70. Gardner K, Bennett V. *J Biol Chem* 1986;261:1339–1348.

71. Gardner K, Bennett V. *Nature* 1987;328:359–362.

72. Tripodi G, Piscone A, Borsani G, et al. *Biochem Biophys Res Commun* 1991;177:3:939–947.

73. Tripodi G, Casari G, Baralle FE, Bianchi G. *Proceedings of Sixth European Meeting on Hypertension* (Abstract) 769 Milan, 4–7 June, 1993.

74. Bianchi G, Tripodi G, Casari G, et al. *Proceedings of Sixth European Meeting on Hypertension* (Abstract) 65 Milan, 4–7 June, 1993.

75. Aderem A. *Cell* 1992;71:713–716.

76. Vezzoli G, Elli A, Tripodi G, Bianchi G, Carafoli E. *J Hypertens* 1985;3:645–648.

77. Gmaj P, Bianchi G, Murer H. *Biochem Biophys. Acta* 1988;941:187–197.

78. Cirillo M, Galletti F, Corrado MF, Strazzullo C. *J Hypertens* 1986;4:443–449.

79. Bruschi G, Bruschi ME, Orlandini G, Cavatorta A, Broghetti A, Ferrandi M, Bianchi G. *J Hypertens* 1985;3(suppl 3):S45–S47.

80. Pontremoli S, Melloni E, Salamino F. *Biochem Biophys Res Commun* 1986;138:1370–1375.

81. Soldati L, Molinari I, Salardi S, Barber BR, Ruggiero M, Serra F, Bianchi G. *Biochem Biophys Res Commun* 1991;175(2):468–491.

82. Losse H, Wehmeyer H, Wessel F. *Klin Wochenschr* 1960;38:393–402.

83. Aderounmu AF, Salako LA. *Eur J Clin Invest* 1979;9:369–375.

84. Edmonson RP, Thomas RD, Hilton PJ, Patrick J, Jones NF. *Lancet* 1975;1:1003–1005.

85. Ambrosioni E, Costa FV, Montebugnoli L, Tartagni F, Mangnani B. *Clin Sci* 1981;61:181–186.

86. Pedersen KE, Nielson JR, Kjaer K, Kiltgaard NA, Johansen T. *J Hypertens* 1983;1(suppl 2):132–134.

87. Wessel F. In: Zumkley H, Losse H, eds. *Intracellular electrolytes and arterial hypertension.* New York: Goerg Thieme Verlag, 1980;85–90.

88. Simon G, Conklin DJ. *J Hypertens* 1986;4:71–75.

89. Cusi D, Tripodi G, Alberghini E, et al. In: Bianchi G, Carafoli E, Scarpa A, eds. *Membrane pathology.* New York: Academy of Science, 1986;576–578.

90. Garay RP, Nazaret C. *Clin Sci* 1985;69:613–624.

91. Garay RP, Dagher G, Pernolett MG, Dewynck MA, Meyer P. *Nature* 1980;284:281–283.

92. Canessa M, Brugnara C, Cusi D, Tosteson DC. *J Gen Physiol* 1986;87:113–142.

93. Cusi D, Barlassina C, Ferrandi M, Lupi P, Ferrari P, Bianchi G. *Clin Exp Hypertens* 1981;3:871–994.

94. Lewitter FI, Canessa M. *Am J Hum Genet* 1985;36:5–172.

95. Canessa M, Bize J, Spalvins A, Falkner B, Katz E. *J Clin Hypertens* 1986;2:101–108.

96. Price M, Hannaert P, Dagher G, Garay RP. *Hypertension* 1984;6:352–359.

97. Cusi D, Fossali E, Piazza A, et al. *Am J Hypertens* 1991;4:725–734.

98. Cusi D, Barlassina C, Tripodi G, et al. *J Hypertens* 1987;5:S255–S256.

99. Cusi D, Niutta E, Barlassina C, et al. *J Hypertens* 1993;in press.

100. Canessa M, Solomon H, Falkner B, Adragna N, Ellison RC. In: Villareal H, Sambhi MP, eds. *Topics in pathophysiology of hypertension.* Boston: Martinus Nijoff, 1984;78–87.

101. Williams GH, Tuck ML, Sullivan JM, Dluhy RG, Hollenberg NK. *Am J Med* 1982;72:907–914.

102. Ng LL, Fennel DA, Dudley C. *J Hypertens* 1990;8:667–673.

103. Livne A, Balfe JW, Veitch R, Marquez-Julio A, Grinstein S, Rohstein A. *Lancet* 1987;1:533–536.

104. Lifton RP, Hunt SC, Williams RR, et al. *Hypertension* 1991;17:8–14.

105. Diez J, Hannaert P, Garay R. *Am J Physiol* 1987;252:H1–H6.

106. Poston L, Sewell RB, Wilkinson SP, et al. *Clin Res* 1981;282:847–849.

107. de Wardener HE, Clarkson EM. *Physiol Rev* 1985;65:658–759.

108. Wald H, Epstein FH, Popovtzer MM. *Proc Soc Exp Biol Med* 1983;172:291–296.

109. Postnov YU, Orlov SN, Pokudin NI. *Pflugers Arch* 1979;379:191–195.

110. Erne P, Bolli P, Burgisser E, Buhler FR. *N Engl J Med* 1984;310:1084–1088.

111. Bruschi G, Bruschi ME, Caroppo M, Orlandini G, Spaggiari M, Cavatorta A. *Clin Sci* 1985;68:179–184.

112. Resink TJ, Tkachuk VA, Erna P, Buhler FR. *Hypertension* 1986;8:159–166.

113. Weder A. *N Engl J Med* 1986;314:198–201.

114. Garay RP, Nazaret C, Hannaert P, Price M. *Eur J Clin Invest* 1983;13:311–320.

115. Marche P, Koutouzov S, Girard A, Elgozi JL, Meyer P, Ben-Ishay D. *Hypertension* 1986;8:983–989.

116. Rettig R, Folberth C, Stauss H, et al. *Hypertension* 1990;15:429–435.

117. Rettig R, Folberth C, Stauss H, et al. *Am J Physiol* 1990;258:F606–F611.

118. Rettig R, Folberth C, Graf C, Kopf D, Stauss H, Unger T. *Clin Invest Med* 1991;14:6:492–498.

119. Firth JD, Raine AEG, Ledingham JGG. *Clin Sci* 1989;76:335–341.

120. Salvati P, Ferrario RG, Bianchi G. *J Hypertens* 1987;5(suppl 5):S253–S237.

121. Roman RJ. *Hypertension* 1987;9(suppl III):130–136.

122. Roman RJ. *Am J Physiol* 1986;251:F57–F65.

123. Roman RJ, Kaldunski ML. *Am J Physiol* 1991;261:R595–R602.

124. Roman RJ, Cowley Jr. AW. *Am J Physiol* 1985;248:F119–F205.

125. Roman RJ, Kaldunski ML. *Hypertension* 1988;11:6:657–663.

126. Roman RJ. *Am J Hypertens* 1990;3:893–900.

127. Cowley AW Jr. *Physiol Rev* 1992;72:1:231–300.

128. Gebremedhim D, Fenoy FJ, Harder DR, Roman RJ. *Hypertension* 1990;16:648–654.

129. Skov K, Mulvany J, Korsgaard N. *Hypertension* 1992;20:821–827.

130. Mulvany J. *Proceedings of Sixth European Meeting on Hypertension* (Abstract) 537 Milan, 4–7 June, 1993.

131. Arendshorst WJ. *Circ Res* 1979;44:344–349.

132. Dilley JR, Arendshorst WJ. *Am J Physiol* 1984;247:F672–F679.

133. Arendshorst WJ, Chatziantoniou C, Daniels F. *Kidney Int* 1990;38(suppl 30):S92–S96.

134. Arendshorst WJ, Beierwaltes WH. *Am J Physiol* 236;5:F246–F251.

135. Chatziantoniou C, Daniels FH, Arendshorst WJ. *Am J Physiol* 1990;259:F372–F382.

136. Beierwaltes WH, Arendshorst WJ, Klemmer PJ. *Hypertension* 1982;4:908–917.

137. Cowley Jr AW, Roman JR, Kreiger JE. *Clin Exp Pharmacol Physiol* 1991;18:21–27.

138. Shibouta YZ, Terashita Z, Inada Y, Nishikawa K, Kikuchi S. *Eur J Pharmacol* 1981;70:247–256.

139. Sinaiko A, Mirkin B. *Circ Res* 1974;34:693–696.

140. Berecek KH, Schwertschlag U, Gross F. *Am J Physiol* 1980;238(7):H287–H293.

141. O'Dowd BF, Rapp JP. *Hypertension* 1991;18:9–11.

142. Dahl LH, Heine M, Thompson K. *Proc Soc Exp Biol Med* 1972;140:852–856.

143. Dahl LK, Heine M, Thompson K. *Circ Res* 1974;34:94–101.

144. Dahl LK, Heine M. *Circ Res* 1975;36:692–696.

145. Morgan DA, DiBona GF, Mark AL. *Hypertension* 1990;15:436–442.
146. Dahl LK, Knudsen KD, Heine M. *Circ Res* 1968;22:11–18.
147. Steele TH, Challoner-Hue L. *Am J Physiol* 1988;254:F533–F539.
148. Tobian L, Lange J, Azar S, et al. *Circ Res* 1978;43(suppl I):192–197.
149. Sterzel RB, Luft FC, Gao Y, et al. *Kidney Int* 1988;33:1119–1129.
150. Roman RJ, Kaldunski M. *Hypertension* 1991;17:1018–1024.
151. de Wardener HE, MacGregor GA. *Kidney Int* 1980;18:1–9.
152. Dahl LH, Knudsen KD, Heine M, Leitl G. *J Exp Med* 1967;126:687–699.
153. Knudsen KD, Dahl LH, Heine M, Leitl G. *J Exp Med* 1969;129:507–522.
154. de Wardener HE, Clarkson EM. *Physiol Rev* 1985;65:658–759.
155. Bianchi G, Fox U, Di Francesco DF, Bardi U, Radice M. *Clin Sci Mol Med* 1973;45(suppl I):135s–139s.
156. Bianchi G, Fox U, Di Francesco DF, Giovannetti AM, Pagetti D. *Clin Sci Mol Med* 1974;47:435–448.
157. Bianchi G, Baer PG, Fox U, Duzzi L, Pagetti D. *Circ Res* 1975;36/37(suppl I):153–161.
158. Ferrari P, Cusi D, Barber BR. *Clin Sci* 1982;63:61s–64s.
159. Boberg U, Persson EG. *Am J Physiol* 1986;16:F967–F974.
160. Salvati P, Pinciroli GP, Bianchi G. *J Hypertens* 1984;2(suppl 3):351–353.
161. Salvati P, Ferrario RG, Parenti P, Bianchi G. *J Hypertens* 1987;5:31–38.
162. Salvati P, Ferrario RG, Bianchi G. *J Hypertens* 1987;5(suppl 57):S253–S237.
163. Salvati P, Ferrario RG, Bianchi G. *Kidney Int* 1990;37:1084–1089.
164. Foulkes R, Ferrario RG, Salvati P, Bianchi G. *Clin Sci* 1992;82:185–190.
165. Holland SM, Millett J, Alaghband-Zadeh J, de Wardener HE, Ferrari P, Bianchi G. *Hypertension* 1987;9:498–503.
166. Ferrandi M, Minotti E, Salardi S, Florio M, Bianchi G, Ferrari P. *Am J Physiol* 1992;263:F739–F748.
167. Hanozet GM, Parenti P, Salvati P. *Biochim Biophys Acta* 1985;819:179–186.
168. Ferrandi M, Salardi S, Parenti P, et al. *Biochim Biophys Acta* 1990;1021:13–20.
169. Parenti P, Villa G, Hanozet GM, Ferrandi M, Ferrari P. *FEBS Lett* 1991;290(1,2):200–204.
170. Melzi ML, Bertorello A, Fukuda Y, Muldin I, Sereni F, Aperia A. *Am J Hypertens* 1989;2:563–566.
171. Curtis JJ, Luke RG, Dustan HP. *N Engl J Med* 1983;309:1009–1053.
172. Guidi E, Bianchi G, Rivolta E, et al. *Nephron* 1985;41:14–21.
173. Bianchi G, Cusi D, Gatti M, et al. *Lancet* 1979;1:173–177.
174. Bianchi G, Cusi D, Barlassina C, et al. *Kidney Int* 1983;23:870–875.
175. Louis WJ, Tabei R, Spector S. *Lancet* 1971;2:1283–1286.
176. Muldoon MF, Terrell DF, Bunker CH, Manuck SB. *Am J Hypertens* 1993;6:76–88.
177. Tabei R, Maruyama T, Kumada M, Okamoto K. In: Okamoto K, ed. *Spontaneous Hypertension*. Tokyo: Igaku Shoin, Ltd., 1972;185–193.
178. Tsuchivama H, Suigihara H, Kawai K. In: Okamoto K, Ed. *Spontaneous Hypertension*. Tokyo: Igaku Shoin, Ltd., 1972;177–184.
179. Sowers J, Tuck M, Asp ND, Sollars E. *Endocrinology* 1981;108:1216–1221.
180. Watlington CO, Kramer LB, Schuetz EG, et al. *Am J Physiol* 1992;262:F927–F931.
181. Freeman RH, Davis JO, Versano-Aharon N, Weinberger MH. *Circ Res* 1975;37:66–71.
182. Herlitz H, Lundin S, Hennig M, Aurell M, Karlberg BE, Berglund G. *Clin Exp Hypertens* 1982;A4(6):15–35.
183. Shiono K, Sokabe H. *Am J Physiol* 1976;231:1295–1299.
184. Mizuno K, Watari H, Tani M, Fukuchi S. *Clin Exp Theory Pract* 1985;A7(12):1707–1717.
185. Mohring J, Kintz J, Schoun J. *J Cardiovasc Pharmacol* 1979;1:593–608.
186. Saito T, Yajima Y, Sato K, Watanabe T. *Jpn Heart* 1979;20(suppl 1):322–324.

187. Ader JL, Pollock DM, Butterfield MI, Arendshorst. *Am J Physiol* 1985;248:F369–F403.
188. Ader JL, Tran-Van T, Alaghband-Zadeh J, de Wardener HE. *Am J Physiol* 1987;252:F964–F969.
189. Woodley-Miller C, Chao J, Chao L. *J Hypertens* 1989;7:865–871.
190. Millet JA, Holland SM, Alaghband-Zadeh J, de Wardener HE. *J Endocrinol* 1985;201:358–361.
191. Pang PKT, Benishin CG, Lewanczuk RZ. *Am J Hypertens* 1991;4:472–477.
192. Schleiffer R, Berthlot A, Pernot F, et al. *Jpn Circ J* 1981;45:1272–1279.
193. Mann JFE, Wiecek A, Bommer J, et al. *Nephron* 1987;45:47–52.
194. Neuser D, Schulte-Brinkmann R, Kazda S. *J Cardiovasc Pharmacol* 1990;16:971–974.
195. Kaneko T, Ohtani R, Lewanczuk RZ, Pang PKT. *Am J Hypertens* 1989;2:549–552.
196. Lewanczuk RZ, Wang J, Zhang SR, Pang PKT. *Am J Hypertens* 1989;2:26–31.
197. Sonnenberg H, Milojevic S, Chong CK, Veres AT. *Hypertension* 1983;5:672–675.
198. Takayanagi R, Imada T, Grammer RT, Misono KS, Naruse M, Inagami T. *J Hypertens* 1986;4(suppl 4):S303–S307.
199. Pang SC, Huang M-C, Tremblay J, et al. *Clin Sci* 1985;69:721–726.
200. Morii N, Nakao K, Kihara M, et al. *J Hypertens* 1986;4(suppl 3):S317–S319.
201. Ferrari P, Weidmann P. *J Hypertens* 1990;8:491–500.
202. Yamori Y, Ohtaka M, Ueshima H, et al. *Jpn Circ J* 1978;42:841–847.
203. Mondon CE, Reaven GM. *Metab Clin Exp* 1988;37:303–305.
204. Buchanan TA, Sipos GF, Marilejo N, Liu C, Campese VM. *Am J Physiol* 1992;262:E14–E19.
205. Rapp JP, Dahl LK. *Endocrinology* 1972;90:1435–1446.
206. Cicila GT, Rapp JP, Wang J-M, Lezin ES, Ng SC, Kurtz TW. *Nature Gen* 1993;3:346–353.
207. Iwai J, Dahl LK, Knudsen KD. *Circ Res* 1973;32:678–683.
208. Rapp JP, McPartland RP, Sustarsic DL. *Biochem Genet* 1980;18:1087–1092.
209. Matsuguchi H, Schmid PG, Van Orden D, Mark AL. *Hypertension* 1981;3:174–181.
210. Rapp JP, Tan SY, Margolius HS. *Endocr Res Commun* 1978;5:1:35–41.
211. Hirata Y, Tobian L, Simon G, Iwai J. *Hypertension* 1984;6:709–716.
212. Hirata Y, Ganguli N, Tobian L, Iwai J, Dahl S. *Hypertension* 1984;6(suppl I):I-148–I-155.
213. Snajdar RM, Rapp JP. *Hypertension* 1985;7:775–782.
214. Snajdar RM, Dene H, Rapp JP. *Endocrinology* 1987;120:2512–2520.
215. Vincent M, Dupont J, Sassard J. *Clin Sci Mol Med* 1976;50:103–107.
216. Gomez-Sanchez CE, Bataillard A, Vincent M, Sassard J. *J HTA* 1987;5(suppl 5).
217. Geoffroy J, Benzoni D, Vincent M, Sassard J. *Hypertension* 1990;16:655–661.
218. Sautel M, Sacquet J, Vincent M, Sassard J. *Am J Physiol* 1988;255:H736–H741.
219. Liu LK, Aissa AH, Laréal MC, Benzoni D, Vincent M, Sassard J. *Hypertension* 1991;17:296–302.
220. Gauqueilin G, Gharib C, Vincent M, et al. *J Cardiovasc Pharmacol* 1984;6:94–98.
221. Vincent M, Bornet H, Berthezene F, Dupont J, Sassard J. *Clin Sci Mol Med* 1978;54:391–395.
222. Gresson CR, Bird DL, Simpson FO. *Life Sci* 1973;12:393–399.
223. Carretero OA, Polomski C, Hampton A, Scicli AG. *Clin Exp Pharmacol Physiol* 1976;3:55–59.
224. Crofton JT, Share L, Baer PG, Allen CM, Wang BC. *Clin Exp Hypertens* 1981;3:975–989.
225. Armstrong JM, Blackwell GJ, Flower RJ, McGiff JC, Mullane KM, Vane JR. *Nature* 1976;260:582–584.
226. Baer PG, Cagen LM. *Hypertension* 1981;3:257–261.
227. Mantero F, Nussdorfer GG, Robba C, Opocher G, Ferrari P, Bianchi G. *J Hypertens* 1983;1(suppl 2):150–152.
228. Stewart PM, Whorwood CB, Valentino R, et al. *J Hypertens* 1993;11:349–354.

229. Porcelli G, Bianchi G, Croxatto HR. *Proc Soc Exp Biol Med* 1975;149:983–986.
230. Bianchi G, Cusi D, Barlassina C, et al. *Ric Clin Lab* 1980;10:163–170.
231. Fraser R, Brown JJ, Lever AF, Robertson JIS. In: Genest J, Kuchel O, Hamet P, Cantin M, eds. *Hypertension,* 2nd ed. New York: McGraw-Hill, 1983;338–348.
232. Bianchi G, Cusi D, Gatti M, et al. *Lancet* 1979;1:173–177.
233. Bianchi G, Cusi D, Barlassina C, et al. *Kidney Int* 1983;23:870–875.
234. Maack T, Camargo MJF, Kleinert HD, Laragh J, Atlas SA. *Kidney Int* 1985;27:607–615.
235. Judy WV, Watanabe MD, Henry DP, Besch HR Jr, Murphy WR, Hockl GM. *Circ Res* 1976;38(suppl II):II-21–II-29.
236. Nelson DO, Boulant JA. *Brain Res* 1981;226:119–130.
237. Mangiapane ML, Skoog KM, Rittenhause P, Blair ML, Sladek CD. *Circ Res* 1989;64:129–135.
238. Nagaoka A, Lovenberg W. *Eur J Pharmacol* 1977;43:297–306.
239. Saavedra JM, Grobecker H, Axeirod J. *Circ Res* 1978;42:529–534.
240. Patel KP, Kleine RL, Mercer PF. *Hypertension* 1981;3:682–690.
241. Hallback M, Folkow B. *Acta Physiol Scand* 1974;90:684–698.
242. Ely DL, Friberg P, Nilsson H, Folkow B. *Acta Physiol Scand* 1985;123:159–169.
243. Koepke JP, Jones S, DiBona JF. *Hypertension* 1988;11:326–333.
244. Lokhandwala MF, Eikenburg DC. *Life Sci* 1983;33:1527–1542.
245. Finch L, Haeusler G. *Blood Vessels* 1978;11:145–158.
246. Lais LT, Brody MJ. *Eur J Pharmacol* 1978;47:177–189.
247. Juskevich JC, Robinson DS, Whitehorn D. *Eur J Pharmacol* 1978;51:429–439.
248. Ekas RD, Lokhandwala MF. *Am J Physiol* 1981;241:R379–R384.
249. Masuyama Y, Tsuda K, Kuchi M, Nishio I. *J Hypertens* 1986;4(suppl 3):S189–S192.
250. Tsudi K, Kuchi M, Nishio I, Masuyama Y. *J Hypertens* 1986;4(suppl 3):S193–S195.
251. Folkow B. *J Hypertens* 1986;4(suppl 3):S51–S56.
252. Pettinger WA, Sanchez A, Saavedra J, Haywood JR, Gandler T, Roders T. *Hypertension* 1982;4(suppl II):II-188–II-192.
253. Knorr A, Muller B, Kazda S. *Biochem Pharmacol* 1983;32:2639–2642.
254. Campbell GR, Campbell JC, Short N, Robinson RB, Hermsmeyer K. *Hypertension* 1981;3:534–543.
255. Struyker-Boudler HAJ, Evenwel RT, Smits JFM, Van ESSEN H. *Clin Sci* 1982;62:589–594.
256. Gonzales ER, Krieger AJ, Sapru HN. *Hypertension* 1983;5:346–352.
257. Andresen MC, Khhraus JM, Brown AM. *Circ Res* 1978;43:728–738.
258. Friedman R, Iwai J. *Science* 1976;193:161–162.
259. Goto A, Ganguli M, Tobian L, Johnson MA, Iwai J. *Am J Physiol* 1982;243:H614–H618.
260. Saavedra JM, Correa FM, Iwai J. *Brain Res* 1980;193:229–303.
261. Saavedra JM, McCarty R, Fernandez-Pardal J, Giucheney P, Weise V, Iwai J. *Proceedings of Fourth International Symposium on rats with spontaneous hypertension* (Abstract) 28 Heidelberg, 1–4 September, 1981.
262. Takeshita A, Mark AL, Brody MJ. *Am J Physiol* 1979;236:H48–H52.
263. Takeshita A, Mark AL, Iwai J, Prochaska J. *Circ Res* 1978;43(suppl 1):I86–I91.
264. Osborn JL, Roman RJ, Ewens JD. *Hypertension* 1988;11:523–528.
265. Periyasamy SM, Rapp JP. *Biochem Pharmacol* 1989;38:21:3851–3858.
266. Renaud B, Fourniere S, Denoroy L, Vincent M, Pujol JF, Sassard J. *Brain Res* 1978;159:149–159.
267. Denoroy L, Fourniere S, Vincent M, Renaud B, Pujol JF, Sassard J. *Brain Res* 1979;163:60–64.
268. Peyrin L, Cottet-Emard JM, Renaud B, Vincent M, Sassard J. *Clin Exp Hypertens* 1980;2:2:297–307.
269. Denoroy L, Sautel M, Sacquet J, Vincent M, Sassard J. *Neurosci Lett* 1985;58:165–170.
270. Yoccoz D, Vincent M, Hyvert P, Sassard J. *Eur Heart J* 1982;3(suppl C):9–13.
271. Feng Su D, Cerrutti C, Barres C, Vincent M, Sassard J. *Am J Physiol* 1986;251:H1111–H1117.
272. McCarty R. *Proceedings of Fourth International Symposium on rats with spontaneous hypertension* (Abstract) 116 Heidelberg, 1–4 September, 1981.
273. McGregor DD, Montgomery JC, Jones DR, Phelan EL. *Clin Exp Pharmacol Physiol* 1976;3:121–125.
274. Hallback M, Jones JV, Bianchi G, Folkow B. *Acta Physiol Scand* 1977;99:208–216.
275. Ferrari P, Picotti GB, Bondiolotti GP, Caravaggi AM, Bianchi G. *Clin Sci* 1981;61:199s–202s.
276. Parini C, Diop L, Ferrari P, Bondiolotti GP, Dausse JP, Bianchi G. *Hypertension* 1987;10:505–511.
277. Goldstein DS. *Fed Proc* 1984;43:57–61.
278. Bevegsard S, Castenfors J, Danielson M. *Scand J Clin Lab Invest* 1977;37:495–501.
279. Langer SZ. *Pharmacol Rev* 1981;32:337–362.
280. Winternitz SR, Oparil S. *Clin Exp Hypertens* 1982;A4(4/5):751–760.
281. Kirkendall WM, Connor WE, Abboud FM, Ratogi SP, Anderson TA, Fry M. *J Lab Clin Med* 1976;87:418–423.
282. Mulvany MJ. *J Hypertens* 1985;3:429–436.
283. Snavely MD, Insel PA. *Mol Pharmacol* 1982;22:532–546.
284. Owen NE. *J Cell Biol* 1986;103:2053–2060.
285. Grinstein S, Rothstein A. *J Membr Biol* 1986;90:1–12.
286. Freis ED. *Physiol Rev* 1960;40:27–54.
287. Frohlich ED. *N Engl J Med* 1987;317:831–833.
288. Pang SC, Long C, Poirer M, et al. *J Hypertens* 1986;4(suppl 3):S119–S122.
289. Gray SD. *Clin Exp Hypertens Theory Pract* 1984;A6:4:755–781.
290. Radice M, Alli C, Avanzini F, et al. *Am Heart J* 1986;111:115–120.
291. Folkow B. *Physiol Rev* 1982;62:347–504.
292. Walter SV, Hamet P. *Hypertension* 1986;8:520–525.
293. Van der Laarse A, Bloys van Treslong CHF, Vliegen HW, Ricciardi L. *Cardiovasc Res* 1987;21:223–229.
294. Blumenthal SJ, McConnaughey MM, Iams SG. *Clin Exp Hypertens* 1982;4:883–901.
295. Kawaguchi H, Shoki M, Sano H, et al. *J Mol Cell Cardiol* 1992;24:1003–1010.
296. Greenberg S, Gaines K, Sweat D. *Am J Physiol* 1981;241:H421–H430.
297. Hamet P, Tremblay J, Pang SC, Walter SV, Wen Y-I. *Can J Physiol Pharmacol* 1985;63:380–386.
298. Bianchi G, Barber BR, Ferrari P. In: de Jong W, ed. *Experimental and genetic models of hypertension.* Amsterdam: Elsevier, 1984;4:328–349.
299. Michel MC, Casto R, Printz M, Insel PA. *Proceedings of 14th Scientific Meeting of the International Society of Hypertension* (Abstract) P44 Madrid, June 14–19, 1992.
300. Frohlich ED. In: Genest J, Kuchel O, Hamet P, Cantin M, eds. *Hypertension: physiopathology and treatment,* 2nd ed. New York: McGraw-Hill, 1983;791–810.
301. Anversa P, Melissari M, Beghi C, Olivetti G. *Am J Physiol* 1984;246:H739–H746.
302. Engelmann GL, Vitullo JC, Gerrity RG. *Circ Res* 1987;60:487–494.
303. Odek-Ogunde M. *Lab Invest* 1982;46:54–60.
304. Friberg P, Nordlander M, Lundin S, Folkow B. *Acta Physiol Scand* 1985;125:1–11.
305. Sen S, Tarazi RC, Bumpus FM. *Cardiovasc Res* 1977;11:427–433.
306. Pegram BL, Ishise S, Frohlich ED. *Cardiovasc Res* 1982;16:40–46.
307. Sen S, Tarazi RC, Bumpus FM. *Hypertension* 1980;2:169–176.
308. Horinaka S, Frohlich ED. *Cardiovasc Res* 1992;26:396–400.
309. Staessen J, Cattaert A, Fagard R, Lijnen P, Vanhees L, Amery A. In: Genest J, Kuchel O, Hamet P, Cantin M, eds. *Hypertension: physiopathology and treatment,* 2nd ed. New York: McGraw-Hill, 1983;1069–1093.

*Hypertension: Pathophysiology, Diagnosis,
and Management, Second Edition,*
edited by J.H. Laragh and B.M. Brenner,
Raven Press, Ltd., New York © 1995.

CHAPTER **75**

Possible Genetic Lesions in Experimental and Clinical Forms of Essential Hypertension

Theodore W. Kurtz

The results of studies in twins, natural and adopted siblings, and in other family structures have shown that 20 to 60 percent of the population variability in blood pressure is genetically determined (1,2). Studies in animal models of spontaneous hypertension have also demonstrated that genetic factors can contribute to increased blood pressure (2). Based on these observations, investigators have begun to search for genetic determinants of increased blood pressure and have recently implicated a number of molecular variants in the pathogenesis of human and experimental forms of spontaneous hypertension. In this chapter, we review evidence suggesting the involvement of specific genes in the pathogenesis of essential hypertension, and provide perspectives for interpreting the results of molecular genetic studies of high blood pressure.

EXPERIMENTAL HYPERTENSION

In the spontaneously hypertensive rat (SHR) and in the Dahl salt-sensitive rat, a limited number of genes may be largely responsible for the increased blood pres-

T. W. Kurtz: Department of Laboratory Medicine, University of California–San Francisco, 505 Parnassus Avenue, Room L-518, San Francisco, California 94143.

sure (2–7). Accordingly, the prospects for identifying primary genetic determinants of hypertension in the SHR and Dahl models appear promising. It may also prove feasible to search for genetic determinants of increased blood pressure in other rat models such as the Milan and Lyon hypertensive strains (8–10). In contrast, in animal models in which a large number of minor genes interact to cause increased blood pressure, it will be much more difficult to dissect out the primary genetic causes of hypertension. For example, in some mouse models of hypertension, multiple minor genes appear to be responsible for the increased blood pressure (11).

In F2 and backcross populations derived from matings of normotensive rats and hypertensive rats, linkage approaches can be used to search for chromosome regions that contain genes contributing to spontaneous hypertension (12). In these studies, one determines whether the blood pressure of F2 or backcross progeny that inherit a given genetic marker from the hypertensive progenitor strain is different from the blood pressure of progeny that inherit the corresponding genetic marker from the normotensive progenitor strain. With this kind of approach, one can investigate the relationship between blood pressure and the inheritance of DNA markers for anonymous genes scattered throughout the genome, or for candidate genes suspected to be involved in hypertension.

In recent genetic studies in segregating populations derived from SHR or Dahl rats, it has been reported that blood pressure regulatory genes may be located in or near a variety of loci including renin (10,13–16), angiotensin-converting enzyme (ACE) (17–20), atrial natriuretic peptide receptor (20), 11β-hydroxylase (21), and neuropeptide Y (22). Positive results have also been reported in blood pressure linkage studies of the Y chromosome (23,24), the Sa gene (25–28) a kallikrein-related gene (29), and genes of the major histocompatibility complex (30). It should be recognized, however, that linkage studies of segregating populations cannot definitively implicate a specific locus in the pathogenesis of a multifactorial disorder like hypertension. Positive linkage results could be reflecting blood pressure effects of genes that are very distant from the candidate locus being tested. Even a gene that accounts for 25 percent of the hypertension may not be reliably mapped to a well-defined chromosome region because the 95 percent confidence intervals for the estimated map locations can encompass large sections of chromosome (12,31). Therefore, it is important to interpret blood pressure linkage studies with considerable caution.

THE EXAMPLE OF RENIN

Renin is one of the most widely studied candidate genes for hypertension. The possibility that inherited variation in renin gene function might contribute to genetic hypertension was originally suggested by linkage studies of blood pressure in F2 and backcross populations derived from inbred Dahl salt-sensitive and Dahl salt-resistant rats (13,14). Rapp and colleagues (13,14) found the blood pressures of F2 and backcross progeny that inherited the renin allele from the Dahl salt-sensitive rat to be greater than the blood pressures of progeny that inherited the renin allele of the Dahl salt-resistant rat. Although these findings might suggest that sequence differences in or near the renin gene contribute to the greater blood pressure in salt-sensitive rats versus salt-resistant rats, such findings could actually reflect the blood pressure effect of a gene that is millions of base-pairs of DNA away from the renin locus. In fact, several lines of evidence suggest that the renin allele of the salt-sensitive strain may actually promote lower blood pressure than the renin allele of the salt-resistant strain.

Dahl's original strain of Brookhaven salt-sensitive (S) rats was derived and continues to be maintained by selective breeding of animals that exhibit severe hypertension on a high NaCl diet (32,33). In this strain, the recurrent selective breeding of rats that exhibit severe hypertension on a high NaCl diet should have promoted fixation of the major alleles that determine salt-sensitive hypertension. However, despite the intense selection pressure to fix alleles for salt-sensitive hypertension, it is interesting to note that with respect to the renin gene, Brookhaven Dahl salt-sensitive rats carry more than one allele and the population is in Hardy-Weinberg equilibrium (34). Some Dahl salt-sensitive rats carry the renin allele characteristic of the Dahl salt-resistant (R) rat (34). This suggests that the renin locus is unlikely to be of primary importance in the pathogenesis of salt-sensitive hypertension, at least in the Dahl model.

The linkage studies implicating the renin gene in the hypertension of Dahl salt-sensitive rats are also difficult to reconcile with the fact that plasma renin activity is lower in Dahl salt-sensitive rats than in Dahl salt-resistant rats (35,36). In segregating populations derived from Dahl rats, no physiological mechanism has been identified that could logically explain the linkage reported between the renin allele of the salt-sensitive rat and increased blood pressure. Furthermore, in genetic studies of SHR and of Lyon hypertensive rats, it is interesting to note that the renin allele that co-segregates with increased blood pressure more closely resembles the renin allele of the Dahl salt-resistant rat than of the Dahl salt-sensitive rat (10,15,37). DNA sequence analysis has revealed differences in the renin genes of Dahl salt-sensitive and salt-resistant strains but the differences are largely confined to noncoding regions of unknown functional significance (38). It remains to be determined whether the sequence differences in the noncoding regions contribute to differential regulation of renin gene activity in Dahl salt-sensitive and salt-resistant rats.

Congenic strains have recently been used to directly investigate the role of renin gene polymorphisms in the difference in blood pressure between Dahl salt-sensitive and salt-resistant rats. To determine whether transfer of the S renin gene into the R strain confers an increase in blood pressure in the R strain, St. Lezin et al. (39) used backcross breeding and genomic selection techniques to derive a congenic R strain that carries the renin gene of the S strain. Analysis of multiple DNA fingerprint and microsatellite polymorphisms confirmed that this congenic R strain is genetically identical to the progenitor R strain except for the S renin gene and a short length of associated chromosome. In a preliminary study, the blood pressure of the congenic R strain with the S renin allele appeared to be slightly lower than that of the progenitor R strain (39). This suggests that transfer of the S renin allele into the R strain is not sufficient to cause an increase in BP in the R strain and raises the possibility that the S renin allele may actually promote lower BP than the R renin allele. Although these findings do not suggest a pathogenetic role for renin polymorphisms in the Dahl model of hypertension, they do provide support for the concept that sequence variation in or near the renin gene can contribute to inherited variations in blood pressure. The contrasting results of the renin gene studies in the Dahl congenic strains versus those in the segregating F2 and backcross populations underscore the need to interpret linkage studies of hypertension with caution.

THE EXAMPLE OF 11β-HYDROXYLASE

In most rat studies in which DNA polymorphisms have been linked to inherited variations in blood pressure, the polymorphisms have not been linked to inherited variations in defined biochemical processes known to be capable of affecting blood pressure. Most of the polymorphisms that have been linked to the regulation of blood pressure have involved DNA sequences without any known function. To date, 11β-hydroxylase is the only gene identified in an experimental animal model in which coding sequence mutations have been logically related to inherited variation in blood pressure *and* to Mendelian variation in a specifically defined biochemical process that has the capacity to affect blood pressure, in this case the synthesis of the mineralocorticoid 18-hydroxydeoxycorticosterone (18-OH-DOC) by 11β-hydroxylase (21).

In a classic series of studies in the Dahl S and R strains, Rapp and Dahl (40–42) found that strain differences in the adrenal capacity to synthesize 18-OH-DOC co-segregated with strain differences in blood pressure. The adrenal gland of the Dahl R rat was found to produce less 18-OH-DOC than that of the Dahl S rat and circulating levels of 18-OH-DOC were found to be lower in Dahl R rats than in Dahl S rats. Accordingly, it was suggested that genetically determined alterations in the synthesis of this mineralocorticoid contributed to the differences in blood pressure between the Dahl S and R strains. Given that administration of physiological amounts of 18-OH-DOC to NaCl-fed rats can increase blood pressure (43), it is reasonable to suspect that differences in the production of 18-OH-DOC between Dahl S and R rats might contribute to their differences in blood pressure.

Recently, Cicila et al. (21) have found that in genetic studies in Dahl S and R rats fed a high-NaCl diet, 11β-hydroxylase polymorphisms co-segregate with blood pressure and with strain differences in the adrenal capacity to synthesize 18-OH-DOC. The Dahl R rat carries an 11β-hydroxylase allele that (a) differs from those of 12 other rat strains, (b) is associated with a uniquely reduced capacity to synthesize 18-OH-DOC, and (c) encodes 5 amino acid substitutions in the 11β-hydroxylase protein (21). Matsukawa et al. (44) have found that transfection of COS cells with 11β-hydroxylase complementary DNA (cDNA) from the Dahl R strain is associated with significantly lower conversion of DOC to 18-OH-DOC than transfection with 11β-hydroxylase cDNA from the Dahl S strain (44). Thus, the differences in 11β-hydroxylase sequence between Dahl salt-sensitive and salt-resistant rats appear to be of functional significance.

The Dahl R rat was derived by recurrent selective breeding of Sprague-Dawley rats that displayed normal blood pressure despite being fed a high-NaCl diet (45). Given that most of the Sprague-Dawley rats in Dahl's original colony displayed increased blood pressure when exposed to large amounts of NaCl, and given that large amounts of NaCl can increase blood pressure in many other strains of rats, the robust salt-resistance of the Dahl R strain constitutes an unusual cardiovascular phenotype (46–48). The findings of Cicila et al. (21) suggest that in the Dahl R rat, the resistance to NaCl-induced increases in blood pressure may be due in part to reduced 18-OH-DOC synthesis stemming from mutations in 11β-hydroxylase. Although Dahl originally suggested that intrinsic renal factors were largely responsible for the difference in blood pressure between the salt-sensitive and salt-resistant strains, recent kidney transplant studies by Morgan et al. (49) have clearly shown that humoral factors may contribute to the strain differences in blood pressure. While the studies of Cicila and co-workers indicate that genetically induced alterations in 11β-hydroxylase activity may contribute to the relative salt-resistance of the R rat, they do not provide an explanation for the dramatic salt-sensitivity of the S rat.

MISCELLANEOUS CANDIDATE GENES IN EXPERIMENTAL HYPERTENSION

Based on linkage studies in segregating populations derived from SHR, Dahl, and Lyon hypertensive rats, investigators have proposed a variety of candidate genes for hypertension. However, none of the candidate polymorphisms has been linked to a biochemical perturbation that could logically explain the genetic linkage to increased blood pressure. For example, it has been reported that blood pressure is greater in F2 rats that inherit the ACE allele of the stroke-prone SHR than in F2 rats that inherit the ACE allele of the normotensive Wistar-Kyoto (WKY) rat (17,18). However, plasma ACE is lower in rats that inherit the ACE allele of the stroke-prone SHR than in rats that inherit the ACE allele of the WKY strain (50). Unless the lower plasma ACE in stroke-prone SHR is associated with greater tissue ACE, it will be difficult to logically connect the ACE polymorphism to hypertension. In humans, it appears that circulating levels of ACE are directly related to tissues levels of ACE, at least in white blood cells (51).

In SHR, the S_A gene has emerged as a particularly intriguing candidate gene for hypertension. The S_A gene, which is located on rat chromosome 1, was discovered by Iwai and Inagami by differential hybridization analysis of kidney cDNA libraries from SHR and WKY rats (26,52,53). The expression of the S_A gene is much greater in kidneys of SHR than in WKY (52). In segregating populations derived from crosses of SHR and a variety of normotensive strains, linkage studies have indicated that the S_A allele of the SHR co-segregates with an increase in blood pressure (25–27). In addition, Samani et al. (27) have shown that the S_A polymorphism that co-segregates with increased blood pressure also co-segregates with increased renal expression of the messenger RNA for the S_A gene (27). The S_A gene has also been reported to co-segregate with blood pressure in an F2 population derived from Dahl salt-sensitive rats and normotensive Lewis rats (28). Although the function of the S_A gene is unknown, the observations that S_A gene polymorphisms co-segregate with blood pressure and with the level of S_A gene expression in the kidney make it an attractive candidate gene for hypertension.

SEX CHROMOSOME GENES AND EXPERIMENTAL HYPERTENSION

Recent studies in F2 populations have raised the possibility that genes on the sex chromosomes may contribute to inherited variations in blood pressure (17,24). However, apart from the influence of male sex and female sex on blood pressure, the influence of X and Y chromosomal genes on blood pressure has not been uniformly clear (18,54,55). The studies of Turner et al. (23) in congenic strains provide the strongest evidence for a role of sex linked genes in the pathogenesis of experimental hypertension. These investigators have found that transfer of the Y chromosome from a WKY strain into an SHR strain can decrease blood pressure in the SHR strain. They have also found that transfer of the Y chromosome from an SHR strain into a WKY strain can increase blood pressure in the WKY strain. Although genetic studies of F2 populations derived from the SHR have not uniformly revealed an effect of the Y chromosome on blood pressure, such variable results may stem from the use of different rat strains with different genetic backgrounds (23,24,54–56). Regardless of the results of studies in F2 populations, the experiments with the congenic strains of SHR and WKY provide a compelling basis for further investigation of the role of Y chromosome genes in hypertension.

HUMAN ESSENTIAL HYPERTENSION

Essential hypertension is believed to be a multifactorial disorder caused by the interaction of a variety of genetic and environmental factors (57). Segregation analyses have provided little evidence to suggest that single gene defects account for even a modest fraction of cases of essential hypertension. Nevertheless, it is conceivable that in some families, single gene defects may be largely responsible for inherited forms of essential hypertension. That is, in some families with essential hypertension, increased blood pressure might be transmitted in a simple

Mendelian fashion. In such families, traditional linkage studies could be used to identify a gene responsible for a subtype of essential hypertension just as they have been used to identify the molecular defect in glucocorticoid remediable aldosteronism (58). However, despite numerous attempts to subgroup patients with essential hypertension according to various biochemical and physiological characteristics, simple Mendelian forms of increased blood pressure have not been readily identified. Thus, the prospects of detecting specific subgroups in which apparent essential hypertension is transmitted in a simple Mendelian fashion would seem quite limited. Accordingly, in subjects with essential hypertension, the search for genetic determinants of increased blood pressure will primarily involve a search for susceptibility genes rather than genes that are necessary or sufficient for essential hypertension.

GENETIC ANALYSIS OF THE RENIN-ANGIOTENSIN SYSTEM IN ESSENTIAL HYPERTENSION

Sib-pair linkage studies and case-control studies have recently implicated the angiotensinogen gene on chromosome 1 in the pathogenesis of essential hypertension (59). In one of the most comprehensive molecular genetic studies conducted to date, Jeunemaitre et al. (59) found a 33 percent excess of shared angiotensinogen alleles among Caucasian male sibling pairs with essential hypertension as defined by diastolic blood pressures greater than 100 mm Hg or by the need for treatment with two or more antihypertensive drugs. No excess of shared angiotensinogen alleles was observed among female sibling pairs with essential hypertension. Jeunemaitre et al. also found that a specific molecular variant in the angiotensinogen gene (designated T235) was associated with increased blood pressure and increased plasma levels of angiotensinogen. Taken together, these findings strongly suggest that a blood pressure regulatory locus exists in or near the angiotensinogen locus on chromosome 1. Based on these data and a number of important assumptions, Jeunemaitre et al. estimated that mutations in the angiotensinogen gene might be predisposing factors for increased blood pressure in at least 3 to 6 percent of hypertensives in Salt Lake City with onset of hypertension before age 60 (59).

Although the data implicating a role for angiotensinogen in essential hypertension are compelling, it should be recognized that sib-pair linkage studies and association studies cannot by themselves definitively establish that a specific genetic variant is responsible for a modestly increased risk for high blood pressure. Even if the results of the linkage and association studies of the angiotensinogen gene in essential hypertension are confirmed, they could still be reflecting blood pressure effects of another gene linked to the angiotensinogen locus rather than angiotensinogen itself. That is, an unknown allele that promotes increased blood pressure might be in linkage disequilibrium with the angiotensinogen variant associated with essential hypertension. In such a case, genetic approaches would not be capable of pinpointing the true culprit responsible for the increased susceptibility to hypertension. Here the biochemical and physiological studies take on considerable importance as they can provide functional data to support the pathogenetic role of one genetic variant over another. In the case of the angiotensinogen gene and hypertension, it has been emphasized that the T235 variant is also associated with increased plasma concentration of angiotensinogen and this may offer a biochemical connection to the increased blood pressure (59).

Sib-pair studies and association studies have also been used to investigate whether the renin gene and the gene for ACE might contribute to increased risk for essential hypertension (60–67). Studies in Caucasian subjects have failed to reveal any consistent relationship between these genes and the pathogenesis of increased blood pressure. It should be emphasized, however, that genetic studies of complex disorders like hypertension may be particularly prone to generating false-negative results (68). It is difficult to exclude a pathogenetic role for a given candidate gene in all subgroups of patients with essential hypertension. For example, a specific molecular variant might not influence blood pressure in subjects consuming a normal or high-potassium diet while it could confer increased risk for hypertension in subjects consuming a low potassium diet. In addition, the results of genetic studies in Caucasians may differ from those in other groups. In a recent population study in black subjects of Afro-Caribbean origin, Barley et al. (63) found evidence of a modest association between increased blood pressure and a 5.0 kb BglI restriction fragment length polymorphism (RFLP) in the renin gene. While this finding remains to be confirmed and is subject to alternative interpretations, it raises the possibility that molecular variation in the renin-angiotensin system might confer increased risk for essential hypertension in some ethnic groups but not in others.

MISCELLANEOUS CANDIDATE GENES IN ESSENTIAL HYPERTENSION

In addition to genes of the renin-angiotensin system, a variety of other molecular markers have been tested in genetic studies of essential hypertension. Some of the genes that have been examined include those coding for haptoglobin (69,70), insulin (71), the insulin receptor (71), a sodium-proton antiporter (72), MNS blood group antigens (73), the estrogen receptor (74), and antigens of the major histocompatibility complex (MHC) (75). While several of these loci represent interesting targets

for genetic studies of high blood pressure, evidence for their involvement in essential hypertension is nonexistent or weak relative to the evidence implicating the angiotensinogen gene. Genetic studies of these loci have been subject to various limitations such as (a) sole dependence on case-control methods that are susceptible to generating spuriously positive genetic associations unrelated to disease pathogenesis (76), (b) dependence on sib-pair linkage analyses that have limited power for detecting susceptibility loci for multifactorial disorders (77,78), (c) use of patient populations that have not been well-characterized with respect to blood pressure or environmental factors known to affect blood pressure, (d) dependence on data from a single population or ethnic group, or (e) lack of evidence that the variant allele or gene marker of interest is related to alterations in an intermediate phenotype (e.g., a hormone level) that could logically affect blood pressure. In Brazilian populations, both sib-pair linkage and case-control studies have implicated genes of the MHC in hypertension (75). In these studies, however, no intermediate phenotypes have been identified that might account for a connection between genes of the MHC and hypertension and the findings remain to be confirmed in separate studies in independent populations.

In addition to using molecular markers in genetic studies of hypertension, some investigators have studied the genetics of certain quantitative traits that may be related to increased blood pressure (candidate intermediate phenotypes) (79). For example, cross-sectional studies have shown an association between low urinary excretion of kallikrein and increased blood pressure, and statistical genetic studies have suggested that urinary excretion of kallikrein is partially determined by a major gene (80,81). Thus, it is conceivable that identification of a major gene controlling kallikrein excretion may result in the identification of a gene involved in hypertension. Red cell sodium-lithium countertransport (SLC) is another putative intermediate phenotype for hypertension that has been extensively studied (82–84). However, the functional relevance of SLC to blood pressure control is unclear and the notion that this system is involved in the pathogenesis of hypertension remains highly speculative. To effectively explore the role of these kinds of candidate intermediate phenotypes in genetic susceptibility to hypertension, it will be important to identify molecular markers related to these phenotypes.

SUMMARY

Because hypertension is an arbitrarily defined multifactorial disorder and blood pressure is a highly variable and complex phenotype, molecular genetic studies of essential hypertension should be interpreted with caution. Results may vary depending on the manner in which hypertension is defined, the methods used to measure blood pressure, criteria used to define statistical significance, the genetic backgrounds of the study subjects, and a wide range of environmental factors. These concerns are similar to those encountered in biochemical and physiological studies of hypertension. However, in contrast to traditional biochemical and physiological measurements, DNA sequence information cannot be secondarily altered by the effects of high blood pressure.

In the genetic studies that have been conducted to date, it has not been possible to conclusively establish a role for specific molecular variants in the pathogenesis of primary hypertension. Although multiple chromosome regions have been identified that may contain genes contributing to high blood pressure, and a potential role for angiotensinogen variants in essential hypertension appears promising, much more work will be required to pinpoint molecular sequences that promote hypertension. Gene targeting studies may ultimately provide the most direct opportunity for testing the role of specific nucleotide changes in the pathogenesis of hypertension (85).

ACKNOWLEDGMENTS

This work was supported by grants from the National Institutes of Health (Hypertension Program Project PO1 HL35018), Bethesda, Maryland; the American Heart Association, National Center, Dallas, Texas; the American Heart Association, California Affiliate, Inc., Burlingame, California; and the Max and Victoria Dreyfus Foundation, New York, New York.

REFERENCES

1. Ward R. In: Laragh JH, Brenner BM, eds. *Hypertension: pathophysiology, diagnosis, and management.* New York: Raven Press, 1990;81–100.
2. Rapp JP. In: Genest J, Kuchel O, Hamet P, Cantin M, eds. *Hypertension, pathophysiology and treatment.* New York: McGraw-Hill, 1983;582–598.
3. Tanase H. *Exp Anim* 1979;28:519–530.
4. Knudsen KD, Dahl LK, Thompson K, Iwai J, Heine M, Leitl G. *J Exp Med* 1970;132:976–1000.
5. Yen TT, Yu P, Roeder H, Willard PW. *Heredity* 1974;33:309–316.
6. Ikeda K, Nara Y, Nabica T, et al. *Clin Exp Pharmacol Physiol* 1991;18:593–597.
7. Kurtz TW, Casto R, Simonet L, Printz M. *Hypertension* 1990;16:718–724.
8. Bianchi G, Barber BR, Ferrari P, Duzzi L. *Hypertension* 1987;9(suppl I):I-30–I-33.
9. Vincent M, Sassard J. *Hypertension* 1987;9(Suppl I):I-27–I-29.
10. Dubay C, Vincent M, Samani NJ, et al. *Nature Genet* 1993;3:354–357.
11. Schlager G. In: De Jong W, eds. *Handbook of hypertension: experimental and genetic models of hypertension.* North-Holland: Elsevier, 1984;192–199.
12. Lander ES, Botstein D. *Genetics* 1989;121:185–199.
13. Rapp JP, Wang S-M, Dene H. *Science* 1989;243:542–544.
14. Rapp JP, Wang SM, Dene H. *Am J Hypertens* 1990;3:391–396.
15. Kurtz TW, Simonet L, Kabra PM, Wolfe S, Chan L, Hjelle BL. *J Clin Invest* 1990;85:1328–1332.
16. Pravenec M, Simonet L, Kren V, et al. *Genomics* 1991;9:466–472.
17. Hilbert P, Lindpainter K, Beckmann JS, et al. *Nature* 1991;353:521–529.
18. Jacob HJ, Lindpaintner K, Lincoln SE, et al. *Cell* 1991;67:213–224.
19. Nara Y, Nabika T, Ikeda K, Sawamura M, Endo J, Yamori Y. *Biochem Biophys Res Commun* 1991;181:941–946.
20. Deng Y, Rapp JP. *Nature Genet* 1992;1:267–272.
21. Cicila GT, Rapp JP, Wang J-M, St. Lezin E, Ng SC, Kurtz TW. *Nature Genet* 1993;3:346–353.
22. Katsuya T, Higaki J, Zhao Y, et al. *Biochem Biophys Res Commun* 1993;192:261–267.
23. Turner ME, Johnson ML, Ely DL. *Hypertension* 1991;17:1097–1103.
24. Ely DL, Turner ME. *Hypertension* 1990;16:277–281.
25. Iwai N, Kurtz TW, Inagami T. *Biochem Biophys Res Commun* 1992;188:64–69.
26. Lindpaintner K, Hilbert P, Ganten D, Nadal-Ginard B, Inagami T, Iwai N. *J Hypertens* 1993;11:19–23.
27. Samani NJ, Lodwick D, Vincent M, et al. *J Clin Invest* 1993;92:1099–1103.
28. Harris EL, Dene H, Rapp JP. *Am J Hypertens* 1993;6:330–334.
29. Pravenec M, Kren V, Kunes J, et al. *Hypertension* 1991;17:242–246.
30. Pravenec M, Klir P, Kren V, Zicha J, Kunes J. *J Hypertens* 1989;7:217–222.
31. Darvasi A, Weinreb A, Minke V, Weller JI, Soller M. *Genetics* 1993;134:943–951.
32. Rapp JP. *Hypertension* 1982;4:753–763.
33. Rapp JP. *Hypertension* 1987;9(suppl I):I–21.
34. O'Dowd BF, Rapp JP. *Hypertension* 1991;18:9–11.
35. Rapp JP, Tan SY, Margolius HS. *Endocrine Res Commun* 1978;5:35–41.
36. Rapp JP, McPartland RP, Sustarsic DL. *Biochem Genet* 1980;18:1087–1096.
37. Rapp JP, Dene H, Deng AY. *J Hypertens* 1994;12:119–125.
38. Alam KY, Wang Y, Dene H, Rapp JP. *Clin Exp Hypertens* [A] 1993;15:599–614.
39. St. Lezin E, Wong A, Wang JM, et al. *Hypertension* 1993;22:421(Abstract).
40. Rapp JP, Dahl LK. *Endocrinology* 1972;90:1435–1446.
41. Rapp JP, Dahl LK. *Endocrinology* 1971;88:52–65.
42. Rapp JP, Dahl LK. *Biochemistry* 1976;15:1235–1242.
43. Carroll J, Komanicky P, Melby JC. *J Steroid Biochem* 1981;14:989–995.
44. Matsukawa N, Nonaka Y, Higaki J, et al. *J Biol Chem* 1993;266:9117–9121.
45. Dahl LK, Heine M, Tassinari L. *J Exp Med* 1962;115:1173–1190.
46. Meneely GR, Tucker RG, Darby WJ, Auerbach SH. *J Exp Med* 1953;98:71–79.
47. Preuss MB, Preuss HG. *Lab Invest* 1980;43:101–107.
48. Smith-Barbaro PA, Quinn MR, Fisher H, Hegsted DM. *Proc Soc Exp Biol Med* 1980;165:283–290.
49. Morgan DA, DiBona GF, Mark AL. *Hypertension* 1990;15:436–442.
50. Kreutz R, Hubner N, Fernandez-Alfonso MS, Ganten D, Nadal-Ginard B, Lindpaintner K. *Hypertension* 1993;22:442 (Abstract).
51. Costerousse O, Allegrini J, Lopez M, Alhenc-Gelas F. *Biochem J* 1993;290:33–40.
52. Iwai N, Inagami T. *Hypertension* 1991;17:161–169.
53. Szpirer C, Riviere M, Szpirer J, et al. *J Hypertens* 1993;11:919–925.
54. Vincent M, Kaiser MA, Orea V, Lodwick D, Samani NJ. *Hypertension* 1994;23:161–166.
55. St. Lezin EM, Pravenec M, Mark AL, Kurtz TW. *Hypertension* 1993;submitted.
56. Tanase H, Suzuki Y, Ooshima A, Yamori Y, Okamoto K. *Jpn Circ J* 1970;34:1197–1212.
57. Kurtz TW, Spence MA. *Am J Med* 1993;94:77–84.
58. Lifton RP, Dluhy RG, Powers M, et al. *Nature* 1992;355:262–265.

59. Jeunemaitre X, Soubrier F, Kotelevtsev YV, et al. *Cell* 1992;71: 169–180.
60. Naftilan AJ, Williams R, Burt D, et al. *Hypertension* 1989;14:614–618.
61. Soubrier F, Jeunemaitre X, Rigat B, Houot A-M, Cambien F, Corvol P. *Hypertension* 1990;16:712–717.
62. Zee RYL, Ying LH, Morris BJ, Griffiths LR. *J Hypertens* 1991;9: 825–830.
63. Barley J, Carter ND, Cruickshank JK, et al. *J Hypertens* 1991;9: 993–996.
64. Jeunemaitre X, Rigat B, Charru A, Houot AM, Soubrier F, Corvol P. *Hum Genet* 1992;88:301–306.
65. Jeunemaitre X, Lifton RP, Hunt SC, Williams RR, Lalouel JM. *Nature Genet* 1992;1:72–75.
66. Harrap SB, Davidson HR, Connor JM, et al. *Hypertension* 1993;21:455–460.
67. Schmidt S, van Hooft IMS, Grobbee DE, Ganten D, Ritz E. *J Hypertens* 1993;11:345–348.
68. Risch N. *Genet Epidemiol* 1990;7:41–45.
69. Luft FC, Weinberger MH, Miller JZ, Fineberg NS, Christian JC, Grim CE. *Clin Exp Hypertens* [*A*] 1987;A9:174.
70. Weinberger MH, Miller JZ, Fineberg NS, Luft FC, Grim CE, Christian JC. *Hypertension* 1987;10:443–446.
71. Ying LH, Zee RY, Griffiths LR, Morris BJ. *Biochem Biophys Res Commun* 1991;181:486–492.
72. Lifton RP, Hunt SC, Williams RR, Pouyssegur J, Lalouel JM. *Hypertension* 1991;17:8–14.
73. Miller JZ, Grim CE, Conneally PM, Weinberger MH. *Hypertension* 1979;1:493–497.
74. Lehrer S, Rabin J, Kalir T, Schachter BS. *Hypertension* 1993;21: 439–441.
75. Gerbase-DeLima M, DeLima JJ, Persoli LB, Silva HB, Marcondes M, Bellotti G. *Hypertension* 1989;14:604–609.
76. Cooper DN, Clayton JF. *Hum Genet* 1988;78:299–312.
77. Risch N. *Am J Hum Genet* 1990;46:229–241.
78. Greenberg DA. *Am J Hum Genet* 1993;52:135–143.
79. Williams RR, Hunt SC, Hasstedt SJ, et al. *J Cardiovasc Pharmacol* 1988;12(suppl 3):S7–S20.
80. Scicli AG, Carretero OA. *Kidney Intl* 1986;29:120–130.
81. Berry TD, Hasstedt SJ, Hunt SC, et al. *Hypertension* 1989;13:3–8.
82. Canessa M, Adragna N, Solomon HS, Connolly TM, Tosteson DC. *N Engl J Med* 1980;302:772–776.
83. Turner ST, Michels VV. *Hypertension* 1991;18:183–190.
84. Hasstedt SJ, Wu LL, Ash KO, Kuida H, Williams RR. *Am J Hum Genet* 1988;43:14–22.
85. Smithies O. *Trends Genet* 1993;9:112–116.

Hypertension: Pathophysiology, Diagnosis, and Management, Second Edition, edited by J.H. Laragh and B.M. Brenner, Raven Press, Ltd., New York © 1995.

CHAPTER **76**

The Search for the Genetic Basis of Blood Pressure Variation in Rats

John P. Rapp

Blood pressure is known to have a significant genetic component in several species of animals and in humans (1). Rodent models for genetic hypertension are especially well developed (1,2). In all species, blood pressure behaves as a quantitative (polygenic) trait. That is, blood pressure per se shows continuous variation, and discrete phenotypes are not generally discernible by studying the frequency distributions for blood pressure. Continuous variation is the consequence of the additive effects of genes (alleles) at multiple genetic loci that influence blood pressure. Polygenic inheritance for blood pressure makes sense, since blood pressure is influenced by multiple biochemical and physiologic systems, each of which may have its own genetic inputs. The challenge is to characterize exactly what these multiple genetic inputs are. A paradigm for doing this will be given.

BASIC GENETIC CONCEPTS

Selection for a Quantitative Trait

Figure 1 shows diagrammatically how a quantitative trait, such as blood pressure, responds to selective breed-

J. P. Rapp: Department of Medicine, Medical College of Ohio, Toledo, Ohio 43699.

ing in animal experimentation. All the high- and low-blood-pressure strains of rodents were developed basically in this way. The blood pressures of a large, outbred (heterogeneous), base population of animals (e.g., rats) is obtained. Several pairs of animals with the highest blood pressure are bred to each other, and the blood pressures of the offspring are determined, and again the selection and breeding for high blood pressure is practiced. Repeating this procedure for several generations concentrates the genes for high blood pressure into a high selected line. Similarly, a line is selected for low blood pressure, to provide a contrasting line.

Usually, at some point in the selective breeding it is desirable to practice inbreeding in order to fix the characteristics of the line. An allele is said to be "fixed" if it is homozygous in all animals of a line or strain. For example, the albino allele has been fixed in many stocks of laboratory rats. Once 20 brother–sister matings are performed, the line is considered to be fully inbred and is designated as an *inbred strain*. Inbreeding forces homozygosity to occur to the point where essentially all loci are homozygous. Once an allele is fixed in the homozygous state in a strain, there is no possibility of genetic variation at this locus unless either (a) a mutation occurs (very rare) or (b) outside breeding stock carrying a different allele at the locus in question is introduced.

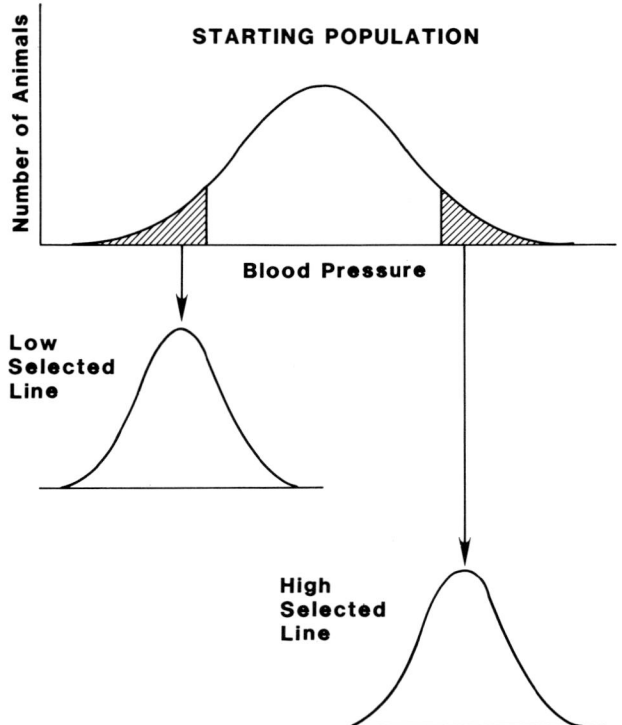

FIG. 1. Diagrammatic representation of the effects of selective breeding for a quantitative trait—in this case, blood pressure. Genes for blood pressure are assumed to be segregating in the starting population. Animals in the upper and lower tails of the frequency distribution of the starting population carry high numbers of plus and minus alleles, respectively. Plus alleles increase blood pressure, whereas minus alleles decrease blood pressure. Repeated selective breeding concentrates the plus and minus alleles in their respective high- and low-blood-pressure selected lines. Since selective breeding tends to fix the genes involved in the homozygous state, the variance of the selected lines is lower than that of the starting population. (From ref. 1, with permission.)

Thus, all individuals from an inbred strain are genetically identical to one another, and their genetic characteristics are constant over time. Experimentally, these properties are highly advantageous.

Strain Comparisons

Given a high-blood-pressure strain and a contrasting low-blood-pressure strain, the obvious first thing to do to find the mechanisms responsible for the blood pressure differences is to compare strains for biochemical, physiological, and morphological traits that may be causing the blood pressure differences. How to interpret any such differences found immediately poses an important problem of interpretation. There are basically three ways by which such strain differences can arise: (a) the result of the selective breeding process; (b) the result of genetic drift; (c) the secondary consequence of blood pressure differences.

There are several ways to minimize the possibility that one is looking at a consequence of hypertension. A developmental study is sometimes useful; that is, one expects that a genetic trait that causes high blood pressure should be present in young animals before they develop significant hypertension. Most often it is found that the trait of interest and blood pressure diverge concomitantly with age between the high- and low-blood-pressure strains, and the developmental study does not really clearly define a cause-and-effect relationship. If a strain characteristic is the result of hypertension, then it should be present in outbred normotensive animals that are made hypertensive by other means (e.g., deoxycorticosterone acetate [DOCA]-salt hypertension, renal hypertension, etc.). Conversely, drug therapy that prevents hypertension in the high-blood-pressure strain would be expected to minimize strain difference in traits that are the consequences of hypertension. By far, the best way to be sure that one is not dealing with the consequences of hypertension is to search for discrete traits that follow Mendelian inheritance. That way, one can infer a specific genotype for each rat from the phenotype. Since genotypes are determined at fertilization, they cannot be secondary consequences of blood pressure differences. The problem of how to find such favorable discrete Mendelian traits will be addressed below.

Genetic drift refers to the chance selection and fixation of contrasting alleles in contrasting high- and low-blood-pressure strains. The base population from which the high and low strains were selected is said to be polymorphic at a given locus if two or more alleles at the given locus are present with reasonable frequencies in the population. If a locus is polymorphic in the base population, then one, or the other, of the alleles *must* be fixed in the high- and low-blood-pressure strains as the strains are inbred. If, by chance, each strain fixes a different allele, then the strains will show a genetic difference that is completely unrelated to blood pressure.

Genetic differences between strains selectively bred to have high and low blood pressure also arise as a consequence of the selection. The selection and inbreeding process concentrates the alleles for high blood pressure in the high line and the alleles for low blood pressure in the low line. Obviously, this creates differences in the biochemical–physiological systems controlled by these genes, and such genetic differences will be causally related to blood pressure differences.

The problem is how to (a) find genetic traits that are causally related to blood pressure differences and (b) differentiate these from effects of genetic drift and consequences of blood pressure differences. The solution is to show that a strain-specific trait co-segregates in genetic experiments with blood pressure. A general paradigm for doing this has been developed (3), and the most useful aspects of this paradigm involving Mendelian traits will be reiterated here. To understand the application of co-segregation analysis with regard to identifying the genes controlling blood pressure, some fundamental properties of Mendelian and polygenic traits must be reviewed.

Mendelian Inheritance

A *segregating population* is one in which different alleles have combined at random to yield all possible genotypes. For our purposes, the most useful segregating population is an F_2 population derived from two inbred strains. Let the locus A have two alleles, A_1 and A_2; let parental strain P_1 have the homozygous genotype A_1A_1; and let parental strain P_2 have the homozygous genotype A_2A_2. If a $P_1 \times P_2$ cross is made to produce F_1 hybrids (genotype A_1A_2) and then F_1 hybrids are crossed ($F_1 \times F_1$), the resulting F_2 population will have genotypes A_1A_1, A_1A_2, and A_2A_2 in the Mendelian ratio of 1:2:1 as shown below:

Parental strain P_1 ——— Parental strain P_2
Genotype: A_1A_1 ——— Genotype: A_2A_2

F_1 hybrid
Genotype: A_1A_2

F_1 animals can produce gametes carrying either allele A_1 or A_2, and these combine in all possible ways to form zygotes in the ratio $1A_1A_1:2A_1A_2:1A_2A_2$ as follows:

		Gametes from male	
		A_1	A_2
Gametes from	A_1	A_1A_1	A_1A_2
female	A_2	A_1A_2	A_2A_2

Polygenic (Quantitative) Traits

A *quantitative trait* is one that shows continuous variation; that is, discrete nonoverlapping phenotypes are

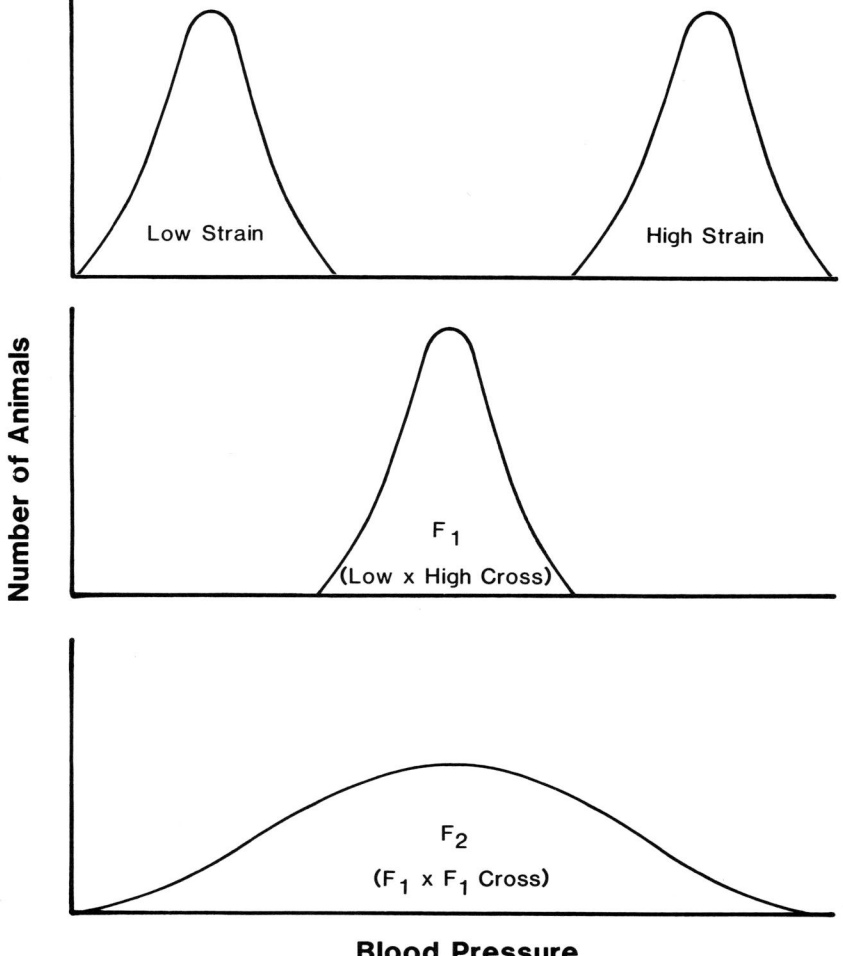

FIG. 2. Diagrammatic representation of the frequency distributions of blood pressure for low- and high-blood-pressure parental strains (**upper panel**), their F_1 hybrid population (i.e., a low × high strain cross) (**center panel**), and an F_2 population (i.e., $F_1 \times F_1$ cross) (**lower panel**). It is assumed that there is no dominance or epistatic effects on blood pressure.

not discernible. Blood pressure is such a trait; people and animals show a continuous spectrum of blood pressures from low to high. This continuous variation is the net result of alleles at many genetic loci impinging on blood pressure, each gene exerting positive or negative incremental effects.

Figure 2 shows diagrammatically how blood pressure is likely to behave in genetic crosses of high- and low-blood-pressure inbred strains. In Fig. 2 it is assumed that genes have only additive effects on blood pressure. This is a reasonable first approximation, but, in reality, effects of dominance (interaction of alleles) and epistasis (interaction of nonalleles) are possible. Because the parental strains are inbred, all animals within a parental strain are homozygous at essentially all genetic loci, and so within the strain the animals are genetically identical to one another. Thus, the variance in blood pressure within each

parental strain is due only to environmental (nongenetic) factors. Also note that in Fig. 2 the variance of the F_1 population is equal to that of the parental strains. The variance of blood pressure among F_1 animals is due only to environmental (nongenetic) variation, since all F_1 animals are genetically identical to one another. Within the F_1 population, all animals are genetically identical because (a) at all loci for which the inbred (homozygous) parental strains carry different alleles, all F_1 animals will be heterozygous, and (b) at loci for which the parental strains carry the same allele, all F_1 animals will be homozygous and identical to the parents. The mean of the F_1 population falls halfway between the two parental means because F_1 hybrids get one allele from each parent at the loci influencing blood pressure, and, on the average, the net effects of such plus alleles (from the high parental strain) and minus alleles (from the low-blood-pressure strain) will be the midparental value.

Note, in Fig. 2, that although the F_2 population has a mean at the midparental value (like the F_1 population), it has a variance larger than the parental or F_1 populations. This is because alleles at the multiple loci influencing blood pressure are segregating at random with regard to one another. This generates a wide range of new genotypes that are associated with a wide range of phenotypes (blood pressures). The principle of how this comes about can be illustrated as follows by considering two loci (locus A and locus B) influencing blood pressure, each with two alleles (A_1 for low blood pressure, A_2 for high blood pressure, B_1 for low blood pressure, and B_2 for high blood pressure). Consider what happens to these alleles in forming F_1 and F_2 populations:

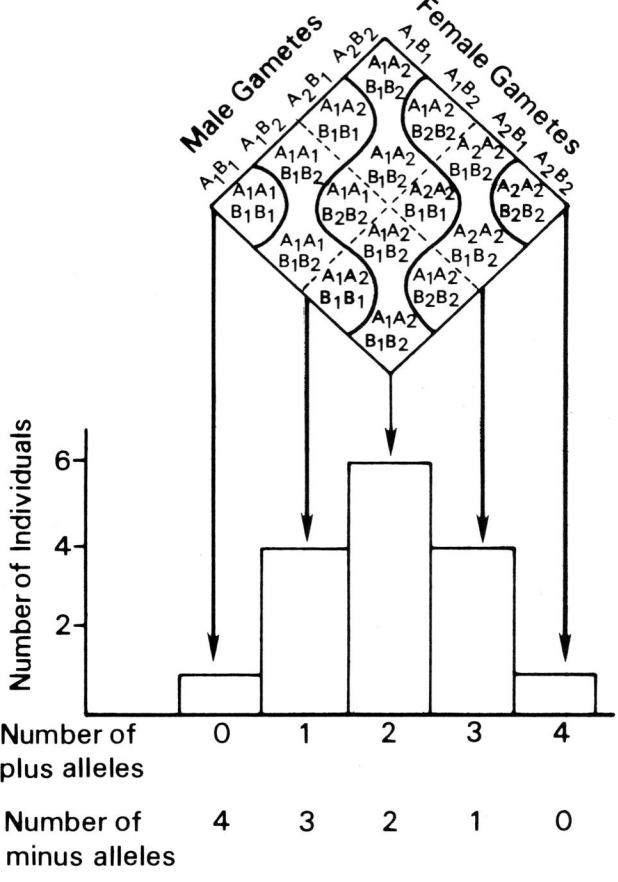

FIG. 3. Diagram showing the possible genotypes for two genetic loci (A and B), each having two alleles (A_1 or A_2 and B_1 or B_2) in an F_2 population derived from crossing inbred parental strains with the genotypes $A_1A_1B_1B_1$ and $A_2A_2B_2B_2$; alleles A_1 and B_1 are minus alleles (lower blood pressure) and A_2 and B_2 are plus alleles (increase blood pressure). See text for explanation. (From ref. 1, with permission; redrawn from ref. 4.)

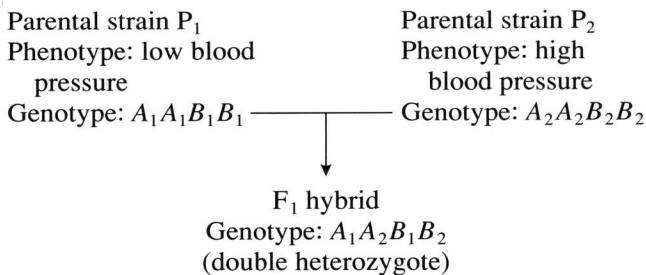

Parental strain P_1
Phenotype: low blood pressure
Genotype: $A_1A_1B_1B_1$ ———————

Parental strain P_2
Phenotype: high blood pressure
Genotype: $A_2A_2B_2B_2$

F_1 hybrid
Genotype: $A_1A_2B_1B_2$
(double heterozygote)

F_1 animals can form gametes of the following types: A_1B_1, A_1B_2, A_2B_1, A_2B_2, and these combine in all possible ways in an F_2 population to form zygotes as shown in Fig. 3. Examination of Fig. 3 shows that only one of 16 animals has the parental genotype for the lowest blood pressure (i.e., all four minus alleles $A_1A_1B_1B_1$), four of 16 animals have genotypes carrying three minus and one plus alleles, six of 16 animals have two minus and two plus alleles, four of 16 animals have one minus and three plus alleles, and only one of 16 animals has the parental genotype for the highest blood pressure (i.e., all four plus alleles $A_2A_2B_2B_2$). Thus, if the blood pressure of an individual is the net effect of all plus and minus alleles over loci A and B, blood pressure phenotypes will form a histogram as shown at the bottom of Fig. 3. If there were more than two loci, the number and complexity of genotypes in the F_2 population would increase dramatically and the phenotypic classes would become impossible to differentiate, leading to an essentially continuous distribution as depicted for the F_2 population in Fig. 2.

IDENTIFYING THE GENES FOR CONTROLLING BLOOD PRESSURE

Co-segregation Analysis

It can be seen from the above discussion that the continuous blood pressure distributions are the result of multiple discrete effects of many genetic loci. These loci are, of course, following the laws of discrete Mendelian inheritance, but their individual unique effects are not discernible by measuring blood pressure. The fundamental way to identify individual genes causing blood pressure differences is to find Mendelian traits that co-segregate with blood pressure (3). For example, suppose it is possible to determine the genotype of rats at the A locus in an F_2 population where two alleles A_1 and A_2 are segregating. There will be three genotypes A_1A_1, A_1A_2, A_2A_2 in the ratio of 1:2:1. If locus A codes for a gene that

influences blood pressure or is located on a chromosome near (i.e., genetically linked to) a gene that influences blood pressure, then the blood pressure of rats with genotypes A_1A_1, A_1A_2, A_2A_2 will differ significantly among themselves. If on the other hand alleles at locus A and the genes that influence blood pressure are segregating independently of each other, then the blood pressure of the rats with genotypes A_1A_1, A_1A_2, A_2A_2 will not be statistically different.

Candidate Phenotypes

Before the invention of molecular biology, the only way to genotype rats for co-segregation analysis was to look for biochemical or physiological traits (intermediate phenotypes) that might be inherited in Mendelian fashion and then to perform a co-segregation analysis using such traits. With few exceptions these phenotypes were not clearly inherited as discrete Mendelian traits and thus their usefulness in genetic analysis was compromised on theoretical grounds (3) as well as in practice. The intermediate phenotypes utilized in genetic analysis of the rat models that gave evidence for co-segregation with blood pressure have been reviewed (5), but with the exception of steroid profiles in Dahl rats (see below), none of the intermediate phenotypes led to the discovery of a genetic locus of known function influencing blood

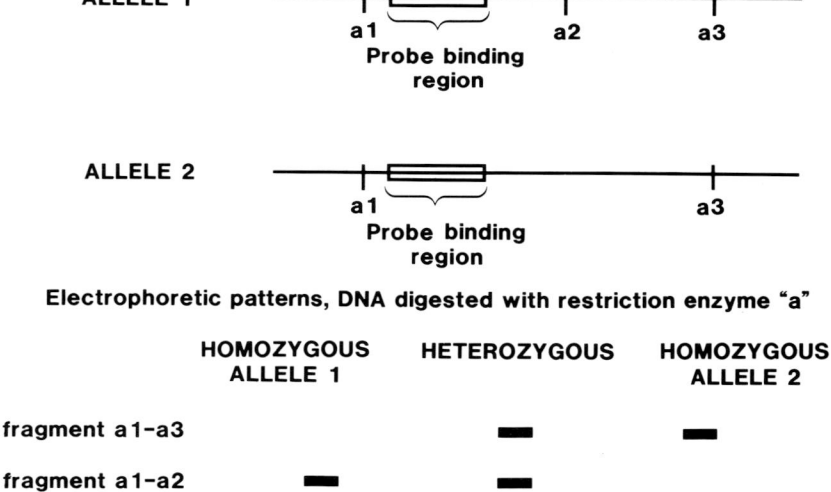

FIG. 4. Mechanism for the generation of restriction fragment length polymorphism (RFLP). The specific sites in the DNA of two different alleles (1 or 2), which are cut by the restriction enzyme a, are labeled a_1, a_2, and a_3. Different-sized fragments of DNA are generated depending on the presence or absence of restriction enzyme sites. Since site a_2 is lacking in allele 2, alleles 1 and 2 yield different-sized pieces of DNA that contain the "probe binding region." The lower half of the figure shows the electrophoretic patterns from the three possible genotypes involving alleles 1 and 2. The patterns are obtained by autoradiography after digestion of genomic DNA with restriction enzyme a, agarose gel electrophoresis to separate DNA fragments, blotting the DNA from the gel onto a filter (so-called Southern blot), and hybridization of the filter to a radioactive cloned DNA (probe) with high base sequence identify to the genomic DNA at the position designated as the probe binding region. The probe binds to the target genomic DNA by complementary base pairing.

pressure. This is because most of the traits studied were really not Mendelian or because the traits did not easily lead to obvious single candidate genes.

Molecular Genetic Analysis

The key to genetic analysis is accurate genotyping, i.e., determining which alleles at a genetic locus are carried by an individual. Molecular biological methods are available to do this by studying DNA directly. Two important techniques are analysis of restriction fragment length polymorphisms (RFLPs) or analysis of simple sequence repeats (SSRs), also called microsatellites.

Restriction Fragment Length Polymorphisms

Restriction endonucleases are enzymes that cut double-stranded DNA at specific sites determined by the base sequence of the DNA. The principle of RFLP analysis is given in Fig. 4. Allele 1 in Fig. 4 has three sites, a_1, a_2, and a_3, at which restriction enzyme a will cut the DNA. A cloned piece of DNA that can be radioactively labeled (i.e., a probe) can be used to detect by Southern blot analysis (6) a specific base sequence of DNA that is complementary to the probe; this DNA is designated the probe binding region in Fig. 4. The genomic DNA extracted from any tissue (usually liver) is digested with a restriction enzyme and the DNA fragments generated are separated by agarose gel electrophoresis. The digested and electrophoresed DNA is transferred to a nitrocellulose membrane that is then hybridized to the radioactive probe. The probe can be made to anneal to the DNA to which it is complementary, and an autoradiograph of the filter will show the position of the DNA to which the probe binds, i.e., the fragment between a_1 and a_2 for allele 1. Allele 2 has sites a_1 and a_3, but lacks a_2. The piece of DNA binding to the probe (fragment between a_1 and a_3) is longer for allele 2 than the corresponding fragment from allele 1 (fragment between a_1 and a_2). The longer fragment migrates more slowly on gel electrophoresis and shows up as a separate band on the autoradiograph. The lower half of Fig. 4 shows the autoradiographic binding pattern expected for DNA from animals homozygous for allele 1, homozygous for allele 2, and the heterozygote that shows bands characteristic for both alleles 1 and 2 because it carries a copy of each allele. Besides mutations that cause alteration in the DNA base sequence in a specific restriction site (and therefore loss of the site), band patterns on Southern blots can be changed by insertions or deletions, variable sizes of tandem repeats, or by inversions of the DNA segment. Such mutations also change the length of DNA fragments generated by restriction enzymes. An example of a restriction fragment, length polymorphism is shown in Fig. 5 for the rat renin

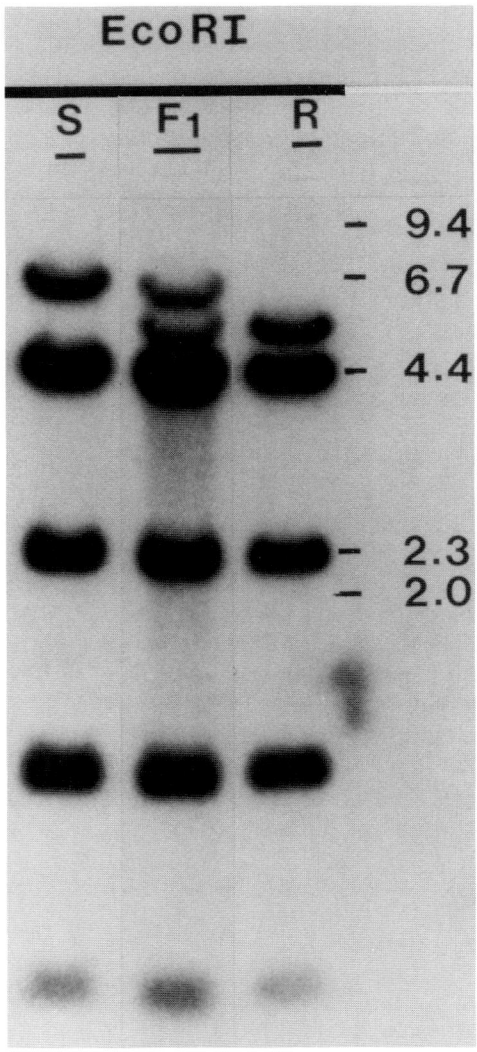

FIG. 5. Autoradiograph of Southern blot of genomic DNA from R, F₁ (R × S cross) and S rats digested with restriction enzyme *Eco* RI. The probe was a full-length complementary DNA (cDNA) for the rat renin gene. Four pieces are identical in size for the three different genotypes but the largest piece has a different mobility in S and R rats. F₁ rats show both the unique S and the unique R bands since they have copies of both the S and R renin alleles. The scale is in kilobases (kb). (From ref. 7, with permission.)

alleles in Dahl salt hypertension-sensitive (S), Dahl salt hypertension-resistant (R) rats and their F₁ hybrid.

Simple Sequence Repeats

DNA of eukaryotes is riddled with simple sequence repeated elements (8–11). A common type is the dinucleotide repeat $(CA)_n$. Such repeated elements occur in introns and in the nontranslated DNA flanking many genes; they are quite variable in length among individu-

ALLELE

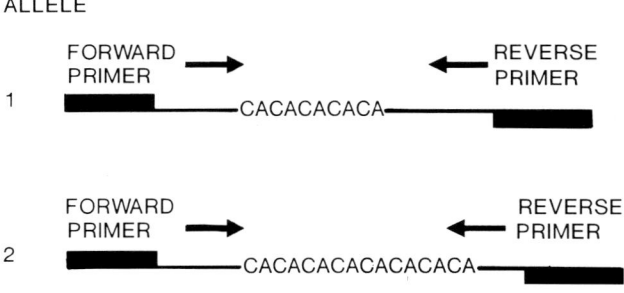

LENGTH OF PCR PRODUCTS: ALLELE 1 < ALLELE 2

FIG. 6. Amplification of DNA around a dinucleotide repeated element $(CA)_n$ by the polymerase chain reaction (PCR). The length of the PCR product depends on the length of the DNA between the primers. Thus allele 1 (*top*) yields a shorter product then allele 2 (*bottom*).

als in a species and thus they serve as superb genetic markers. An efficient way to utilize the SSR is shown in Fig. 6. If the DNA sequence around the repeated element is known, the DNA region containing the repeated element can be amplified by the polymerase chain reaction. This involves melting the double-stranded DNA to produce single strands, annealing specific oligonucleotide primers to the single-stranded DNA, replication of the DNA by DNA polymerase, and repeating the process through 25 or more cycles. This results in a logarithmic amplification of the target DNA to the point where the product(s) can be separated by electrophoresis and visualized by either radioactive labeling or straining techniques. As indicated in Fig. 6, if the length of the repeated elements varies the size of the products vary, giving rise to allele-specific bands of different mobility on gel electrophoresis as shown in Fig. 7.

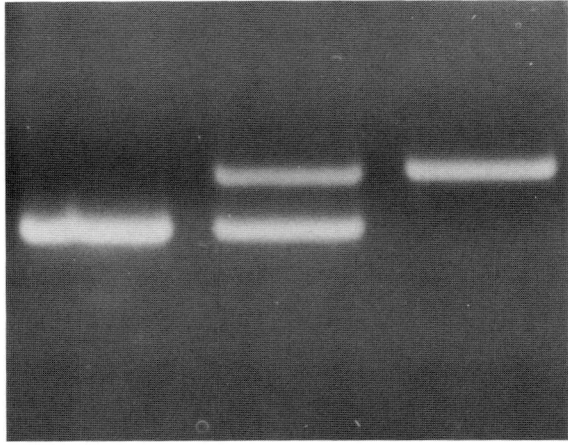

FIG. 7. Agarose gel electrophoresis of PCR products containing a simple sequence repeated element of variable length. *Left lane,* homozygote for shorter allele; *center lane,* heterozygote; *right lane,* homozygote for larger allele. (Photograph courtesy of Dr. Alan Deng.)

CANDIDATE GENES

One strategy for identifying the genes for hypertension is the candidate gene approach. Based on what is known about the biochemical and physiological regulation of blood pressure there are numerous obvious candidate genetic loci, genetic variations in which blood pressure can theoretically be altered. To test the candidate, one merely has to identify DNA variants in or near the alleles at the locus of interest between hypertensive and normotensive strains of rats and determine if these alleles co-segregate with blood pressure. A positive co-segregation result is necessary, but not sufficient, to establish the candidate as a cause of blood pressure differences (see below).

Renin

Renin is an obvious candidate gene. The renin alleles in Dahl salt-sensitive (S) and Dahl salt-resistant (R) rats are easily typed on the basis of an RFLP (Fig. 5). Figure 8 shows the blood pressure distributions of S and R rats and F_2 rats derived from an S × R cross and fed a high-salt diet. Table 1 gives the blood pressure of F_2 rats categorized by renin genotype. There were highly significant

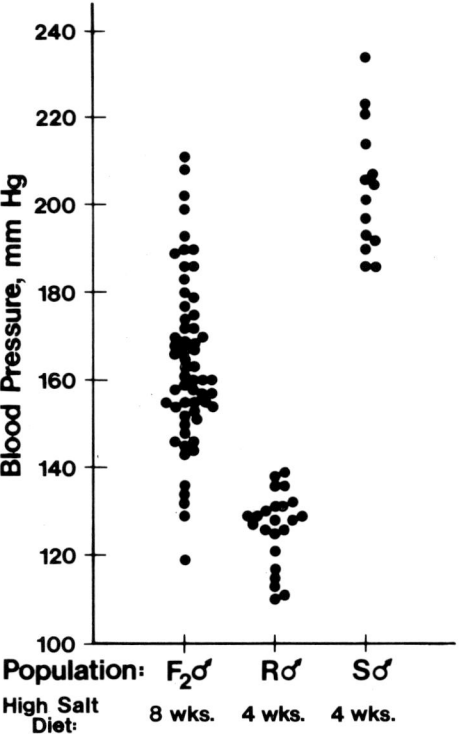

FIG. 8. Scatter diagram of blood pressure for S and R rats and an F_2 population derived from S and R. Data are for males fed high-salt diet; similar data were obtained for females. (From ref. 12, with permission.)

TABLE 1. *Data for blood pressure, heart weight, body weight, and number of rats classified by renin genotype for F_2 rats obtained from crossing S and R rats*[a]

Renin genotype, by sex	Blood pressure (mm Hg)	Heart weight (mg)	Body weight (g)	Heart weight/body weight (mg/g)
Males				
Ren^r/Ren^r 12	148.7 ± 4.3	1314 ± 29	335 ± 5.0	3.93 ± 0.094
Ren^r/Ren^s 28	165.6 ± 3.5	1364 ± 20	336 ± 3.0	4.06 ± 0.063
Ren^s/Ren^s 19	171.0 ± 4.3	1438 ± 24	334 ± 7.2	4.45 ± 0.175
Females				
Ren^r/Ren^r 12	154.4 ± 6.4	980 ± 28	235 ± 2.1	4.17 ± 0.13
Ren^r/Ren^s 27	163.9 ± 3.6	995 ± 17	230 ± 2.1	4.33 ± 0.08
Ren^s/Ren^s 14	174.8 ± 6.2	1026 ± 25	225 ± 5.0	4.59 ± 0.17
Probabilities				
Sex	NS	<.001	<.001	.033
Genotypes	<.001	.005	NS	.001
Interaction	NS	NS	NS	NS

[a] Males were fed a high-salt (8% NaCl) diet for 8 weeks from weaning; females, for 11 weeks. In F_2 rats the blood pressure response of females to salt is slower than that of males, and thus it was necessary to feed a high-salt diet longer to females than to males in order to achieve the same blood pressure levels for the two sexes. Values are means ± SEM. The symbol *Ren* is used to denote the renin locus. The R-rat allele is designated *Ren^r*, and the S-rat allele is designated *Ren^s*. Data were analyzed for differences among genotypes by a 2 × 3 factorial analysis of variance. NS, not significant (i.e., $p > .1$) (From ref. 12, with permission.)

differences among renin genotypes, i.e., S and R renin alleles co-segregate with blood pressure (12,13). The conclusion is that structural differences in the renin gene, or structural differences at a locus linked to the renin gene, cause blood pressure differences in S and R rats. The renin locus is on rat chromosome 13 (14).

Is it really the renin gene that is at fault? Surprisingly, recent evidence suggests that the renin gene is only acting as a marker for an unknown linked gene. The DNA base sequence in the coding and 5′-regulatory regions of S and R renin alleles are identical (15). Regulatory elements can be far outside the immediate 5′-flanking region, so the sequence data do not rule out mutations in remote renin regulatory sites. Thus, although a region around renin on rat chromosome 13 certainly influences blood pressure in Dahl rats, a definite assignment of this effect to renin is not possible based on available data.

Another problem with renin as a candidate gene in Dahl rats is that there is no obvious logical intermediate phenotype to explain the genetic association with blood pressure. S rats have low plasma and renal renin (16–18), whereas genetically regulated high renin would be expected to cause hypertension. The lower renin is presumably the result of volume expansion in S rats (19). There is evidence, however, that S rats do not suppress the renin-angiotensin system on high-salt diet whereas R rats do (18).

Steroid 11β-Hydroxylase

In contrast to renin, the data relating genetic variants in steroid 11β-hydroxylase to blood pressure is more complete. Originally it was observed that Dahl S and R

rats had markedly different steroid biosynthetic activities at the following branch point in steroidogenesis (20,21):

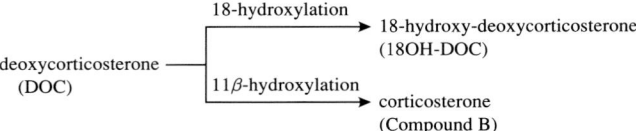

S rats had an increased rate of 18-hydroxylation and a decreased rate of 11β-hydroxylation compared with R rats, but the total of the products 18OH-DOC + B were equal between strains. The ratio of 18OH-DOC/[18OH-DOC + B] produced from DOC *in vitro* by adrenal tissue easily differentiated S and R rats, and F_1 (S × R) rats had an intermediate steroid ratio. The 18OH-DOC/[18OH-DOC + B] ratio was inherited as a Mendelian codominant trait (Fig. 9), and this co-segregated with blood pressure with an effect of about 15 mm Hg between alternate homozygous genotypes in salt-fed F_2 rats (20). Moreover, S rats had a twofold increase in plasma levels of 18OH-DOC (17,22,23), and exogenously administered 18OH-DOC is a moderately hypertensinogenic steroid (24,25).

It is known that the enzyme called 11β-hydroxylase in fact catalyzes both 11β- and 18-hydroxylation of DOC (21,26). The gene for 11β-hydroxylase has, therefore, been analyzed by using the techniques of molecular biology. It has been found that an RFLP for 11β-hydroxylase co-segregates with both the 18OH-DOC/[18OH-DOC + B] ratio and blood pressure using Dahl rats (27). Also, five separate base changes in the coding sequence of 11β-hydroxylase between S and R rats were found that result in amino acid substitutions (27,28). By making chimeric

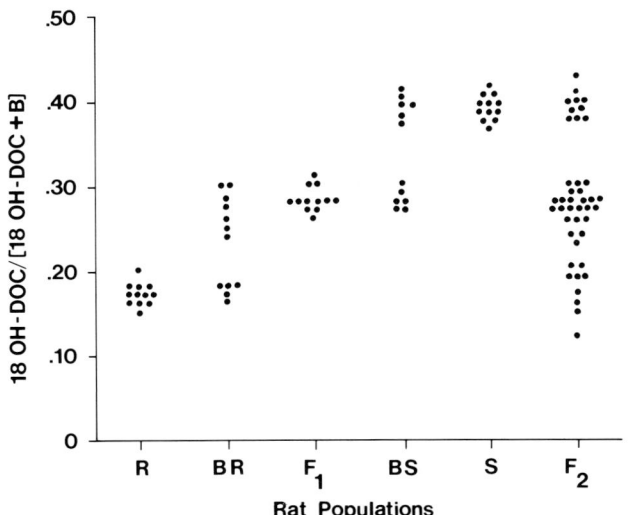

FIG. 9. Scatter diagram of steroid ratio 18OH-DOC/[18OH-DOC + B] obtained by *in vitro* incubation of rat adrenals with DOC precursor. R, Dahl salt resistant; BR, backcross to R obtained by crossing $F_1 \times R$; F_1, hybrid obtained by crossing $S \times R$; BS, backcross to S obtained by crossing $F_1 \times S$; S, Dahl salt sensitive; F_2, obtained by crossing $F_1 \times F_1$. Note that the steroid ratio segregates 1:1 in BR and BS populations and 1:2:1 in the F_2 rats. (Representative data redrawn from ref. 20, with permission.)

genes between S and R 11β-hydroxylase alleles and expressing the genes in COS cells, it was shown that the substitutions at amino acids 381 and/or 384 accounted for the strain-specific steroid profiles. The other amino acid substitutions had no effect on steroid profile (28).

Other Candidate Genes

An anonymous gene (called the SA gene) that is expressed more in the kidneys of spontaneously hypertensive rats (SHRs) than in Wistar-Kyoto (WKY) control rats, was cloned by Iwai and Inagami (29). RFLP analysis has subsequently shown co-segregation of the SA gene with systolic blood pressure in crosses involving SHR (30–32) and Dahl S rats (33). The SA gene co-segregated with about 10 mm Hg of blood pressure in crosses involving SHR and more than 20 mm Hg in a cross with Dahl S rats. The SA gene is on chromosome 1 (32). Its function is unknown. Thus whether the SA gene is acting as merely a marker for a chromosomal region, or is a true candidate, is ambiguous.

Using a panel of recombinant inbred strains derived from SHRs and brown Norway rats it was found that the gene for tissue kallikrein co-segregated with systolic blood pressure and accounted for about 10 mm Hg (34). The tissue kallikrein locus is on chromosome 1 (35) as is the SA gene noted above. SA is closely linked to skeletal myosin light chain 2 (MYL2) (32), which is over 50 centimorgans from kallikrein (35). Thus, the two loci are far

enough apart on chromosome 1 to behave independently. (If two loci are far apart on the same chromosome, they behave as though they were on separate chromosomes [i.e., they segregate independently] because of frequent chromosomal crossing-over between loci [see below].)

SHRs are thermosensitive compared to WKY rats, which led to the examination of heat shock proteins. Using recombinant inbred strains derived from SHRs and brown Norway rats it was found that heart shock protein 70 (hsp 70) co-segregated with blood pressure, accounting for about 11 mm Hg of blood pressure (36). The hsp 70 is located on rat chromosome 20 near the rat major histocompatibility complex (RT1). A congenic strain of SHR carrying the brown Norway region of chromosome 20 with RT1 was developed and showed a 26 mm Hg lower blood pressure than the original SHR (36), confirming the recombinant inbred strain data.

Recently guanylyl cyclase A (GCA) (i.e., atrial natriuretic peptide receptor) was found to co-segregate with systolic blood pressure accounting for from 13 to 18 mm Hg in various crosses involving Dahl rats (37). GCA is on rat chromosome 2 (38).

The neuropeptide Y locus on rat chromosome 4 has recently been implicated to influence blood pressure by co-segregation analysis in an F_2 population derived from SHR and WKY (39). The blood pressure effect was about 10 mm Hg.

There is evidence in the SHR model for a blood pressure effect of the Y chromosome, increased systolic blood pressure of about 20 mm Hg being associated with the SHR Y chromosome. In this case the data are based on co-segregation analysis as well as congenic strains carrying contrasting Y chromosomes (40,41).

GENOME SCANNING

The genetic loci controlling a quantitative trait such as blood pressure are referred to as quantitative trait loci (QTL). The QTL have specific chromosomal locations and specific, but unknown, identities and functions. Besides guessing at what the QTL might be (the candidate gene approach given above), it is possible to genotype a segregating rat population for many anonymous genetic markers distributed throughout the whole genome (in the rat there are 20 autosomes, and X and Y sex chromosomes), in order to determine which markers co-segregate with blood pressure. The markers that do co-segregate with blood pressure indicate a chromosomal region containing a QTL. For genome scanning to work, a reasonably large number of polymorphic genetic markers are required. The simple sequence repeats generated by polymerase chain reaction (PCR) are ideal for this purpose.

Figure 10 shows the relationship during meiosis between a marker locus (locus M with alleles M_1 and M_2)

DUPLICATED
MEIOTIC CHROMOSOMES
AT SYNAPSE

MEIOTIC PRODUCTS
(Gametes)

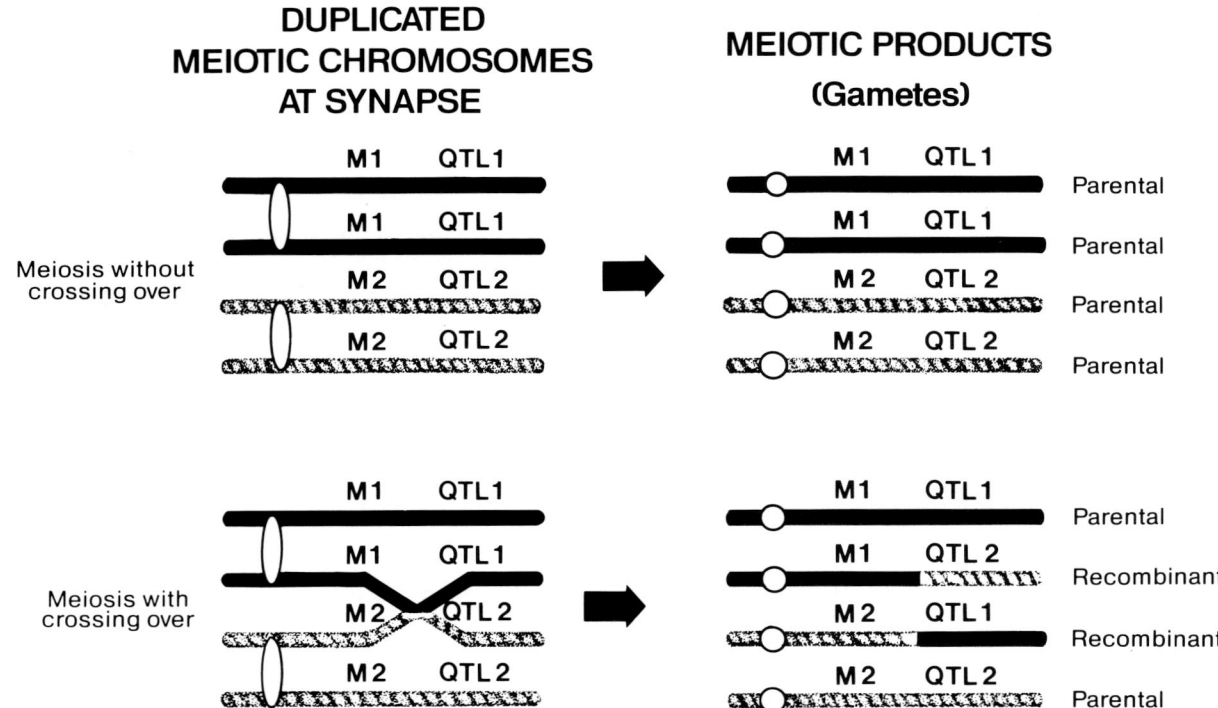

FIG. 10. Relationships during meiosis between a marker locus (locus M) with alleles M_1 and M_2, and a quantitative trait locus (QTL) for blood pressure (locus QTL) with alleles QTL_1 and QTL_2. The meiosis depicted is in an F_1 heterozygote obtained by crossing two inbred strains, one strain with genotype M_1QTL_1 and the other M_2QTL_2 (parental genotypes).

and a QTL (locus QTL with alleles QTL_1 for low blood pressure, and allele QTL_2 for high blood pressure). Note in the upper part of Fig. 10 without chromosomal crossing-over, that in all gametes M_1 remains associated with QTL_1 and M_2 remains associated with QTL_2, that is, they retain the coupling associations present in the parental genotype. In this case, the M_1 allele will co-segregate with lower blood pressure (because it marks the QTL_1 allele) and the M_2 allele will co-segregate with higher blood pressure (because it marks the QTL_2 allele).

In the lower part of Fig. 10 half of the gametes retain the parental relationships between marker and QTL alleles, but in the other half of the gametes the relationships are reversed due to chromosomal crossing-over. M_1 and QTL_2 are inherited together and M_2 and QTL_1 are inherited together. This will obviously degrade the relationship of M_1 with low blood pressure and M_2 with high blood pressure in a co-segregation analysis.

The frequency of crossing-over between loci is a function of the chromosomal distance between them, the greater the distance the more frequently crossing-over will occur. If the marker is very close to the QTL, it will serve as an accurate marker. As the chromosomal distance between the QTL and the marker increase, the signal (blood pressure effect co-segregating with the marker) will decrease because of crossing-over. Figure 11 shows

the relationship between the effect of a QTL observed to be associated with a linked marker locus as a function of frequency of crossing-over (genetic distance) between the QTL and the marker.

Genome scanning was performed on an F_2 population derived from stroke prone SHRs and WKY rats. A marker on chromosome 10 did co-segregate with blood pressure (38,43). Since the marker was close to the locus for angiotensin converting enzyme (ACE), interest was immediately focused on ACE as the candidate in this region. The ACE locus was subsequently shown to co-segregate with blood pressure in another F_2 population derived from stroke prone SHR and WKY (44) as well as in an F_2 population derived from Dahl S rats (37). The effect associated with the ACE locus was about 10 to 20 mm Hg depending on the conditions of the experiments.

A genome scan of an F_2 population derived from Lyon hypertensive (LH) and Lyon normotensive (LN) rats yielded significant blood pressure associations for the renin locus and carboxypeptidase B. The latter contains an informative SSR and serves as marker locus for an unknown QTL (45). Carboxypeptidase B is on chromosome 2 (35), but it is too far from the candidate gene GCA (noted above) to be detecting blood pressure effects of that part of chromosome 2 (Deng and Rapp, unpublished observations).

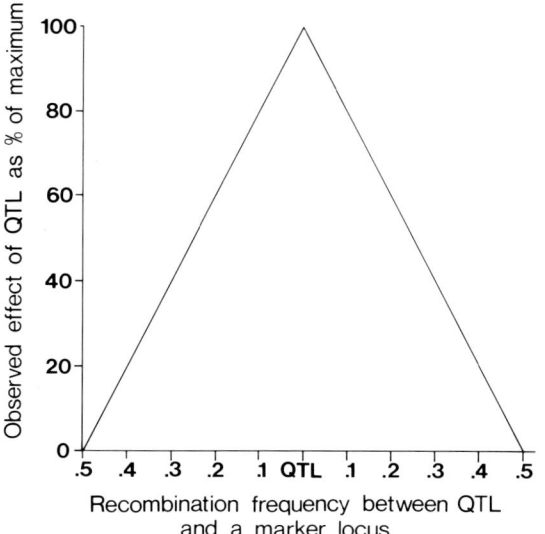

FIG. 11. Relationship between the phenotypic effect of a quantitative trait locus (QTL) observed to co-segregate with a marker locus as a function of the recombination frequency between the marker locus and the QTL. The recombination frequency is the proportion of recombinant gametes produced by chromosomal crossing-over to the total number of gametes produced. The observed effect of the QTL decreases as a function of $(1-2r)$, where r = recombination frequency (42). The horizontal axis represents genetic distance between the QTL and the marker as measured by the recombination frequency. Marker loci can be on either side of the QTL.

CONVERGENCE OF GENOME SCANNING AND CANDIDATE GENE APPROACHES

Because blood pressure is influenced by so many physiological systems (cardiovascular, nervous, renal, and endocrine), there are many candidate genes. As numerous candidate genes are tested for co-segregation with blood pressure the data take on the characteristics of a genome scan, that is, there are many markers on different chromosomes and so eventually one will be found to co-segregate with blood pressure by virtue of linkage to an unknown QTL. Conversely, if numerous anonymous chromosomal markers are studied, and one is found to co-segregate with blood pressure, it is quite likely that some gene of the cardiovascular, nervous, renal, or endocrine systems that can be construed as a candidate will be linked to the marker.

The premise of the two approaches is different. For candidate genes it is assumed that the candidate may actually be the QTL; for the genome scan it is assumed that the marker locus is not the QTL. Either approach eventually leads to candidate loci. This does not mean that the candidate is the QTL, only that it passes the co-segregation test and may be the QTL.

DEFINITIVE IDENTIFICATION OF A QUANTITATIVE TRAIT LOCUS (QTL)

Proof that a candidate gene is in fact a QTL for blood pressure ultimately has to rest on more than a co-segregation analysis. First, DNA variation in the coding or regulatory regions of the alleles in question has to exist and be shown to result in phenotypes that make biological sense with regard to influencing blood pressure. Second, it has to be shown in the whole animal that such DNA variants and their resulting phenotypes actually do cause blood pressure effects. The latter is approximated by constructing congenic strains that differ in only small chromosomal regions of interest carrying the contrasting candidate alleles. Congenic strains are produced by standard genetic techniques (46) involving crossing two contrasting strains, and then repeated backcrossing to one strain always selecting as breeder animals heterozygous for the gene of interest. This is followed by two generations of selective breeding to fix the alternate allele in the homozygous state. Ultimately this procedure yields two strains genetically identical except for the chromosomal region on which selection was made. If, for example, these strains differ in blood pressure then this confirms the chromosomal region manipulated as one carrying a QTL.

Construction of congenic strains for chromosomal regions of interest will no doubt often be necessary in narrowing down and identifying regions of chromosomes carrying a QTL. Once this is done "candidate DNA variants" within this region have to be found. Then the ultimate test will be to duplicate these very specific mutations in an inbred strain by homologous recombination in transgenic rats and to show that blood pressure of the transgenic rats differs from the parental strain. This will avoid the ambiguity associated with the many genetic loci contained in the chromosomal regions that are manipulated in congenic strains. At present such experiments with homologous recombination involve the use of embryo stem cells, which are available only for mice.

It is well to appreciate that no QTL for blood pressure has been definitely identified in rats. With the exception of 11β-hydroxylase, the existing data only achieve the first step of identifying chromosomal regions that co-segregate with blood pressure in an initial screening procedure. For 11β-hydroxylase, specific DNA variants and a biologically meaningful intermediate phenotype are known. Still lacking is the demonstration that creating such specific DNA variants experimentally in whole animals by homologous recombination alters blood pressure.

REFERENCES

1. Rapp JP. Genetics of experimental and human hypertension. In: Genest J, Kuchel O, Hamet P, Cantin M, eds. *Hypertension, patho-*

physiology and treatment, 2nd ed. New York: McGraw-Hill, 1983;582–598.

2. Lovenberg W, Horan M. *Hypertension* 1987;9(suppl I):I1–I42.
3. Rapp JP. *Hypertension* 1983;5(suppl I):I198–I203.
4. Mather K, Jinks JL. *Biomedical genetics,* 2nd ed. Ithaca, NY: Cornell University Press, 1971;4.
5. Rapp JP. *Hypertension* 1991;18(suppl I):I18–I28.
6. Southern EM. *J Mol Biol* 1975;98:503–517.
7. Wang S-M, Rapp JP. *Mol Endocrinol* 1989;3:288–294.
8. Weber JL, May PE. *Am J Hum Genet* 1989;44:388–396.
9. Weber JL. *Genomics* 1990;7:525–530.
10. Hillebrand CE, Moyzis PK. *Genomics* 1991;10:807–815.
11. Beckman JS, Weber JL. *Genomics* 1992;12:627–631.
12. Rapp JP, Wang S-M, Dene H. *Science* 1989;243:542–544.
13. Rapp JP, Wang S-M, Dene H. *Am J Hypertens* 1990;3:391–396.
14. Pravenec M, Simonet L, Kren V, et al. *Genomics* 1991;9:466–472.
15. Alam KY, Wang Y, Dene H, Rapp JP. *Clin Exp Hypertens* 1993;15:599–614.
16. Dene H, McIlwain C, Rapp JP. *Clin Exp Hypertens* 1989;A11:1585–1594.
17. Rapp JP, Tan SY, Margolias HS. *Endocr Res Commun* 1987;5:35–41.
18. Bouhnik J, Richoux JP, Huang H, Savoie F, Baussant T, Alhenc-Gelas F, Corvol P. *Clin Sci* 1992;83:13–22.
19. Overbeck HW, Ku DD, Rapp JP. *Hypertension* 1981;3:306–312.
20. Rapp JP, Dahl LK. *Endocrinology* 1972;90:1435–1446.
21. Rapp JP, Dahl LK. *Biochemistry* 1976;15:1235–1242.
22. Rapp JP, Dahl LK. *Nature* 1972;237:338–339.
23. Nicholis MG, Brown WCB, May GD, Mason PA, Fraser R. *J Steroid Biochem* 1979;10:67–70.
24. Rapp JP, Knudsen KD, Iwai J, Dahl LK. *Circ Res* 1973;32,33(suppl I):I139–I149.
25. Oliver JT, Birmingham MK, Bartova A, Lim P, Chan TH. *Science* 1973;182:1249–1251.
26. Nonaka Y, Okamoto M. *Eur J Biochem* 1991;202:897–902.
27. Cicila GT, Rapp JP, Wang JM, St. Lezin E, Ng SC, Kurtz TW. *Nature Genetics* 1993;3:346–353.
28. Matsukawa N, Nonaka Y, Higaki J, Nagano M, Mikami M, Ogihara T, Okamoto M. *J Biol Chem* 1993;268:9117–9121.
29. Iwai N, Inagami T. *Hypertension* 1991;17:161–169.
30. Iwai N, Kurtz TW, Inagami T. *Biochem Biophys Res Commun* 1992;188:64–69.
31. Iwai N, Inagami T. *J Hypertens* 1992;10:1155–1157.
32. Lindpaintner K, Hilbert P, Ganten D, Nodal-Ginard B, Inagami T, Iwai N. *J Hypertens* 1993;11:19–23.
33. Harris EL, Dene H, Rapp JP. *Am J Hypertens* 1993;6:330–334.
34. Pravenec M, Kren V, Kunes J, Scicli AG, Carretero OA, Simonet L, Kurtz TW. *Hypertension* 1991;17:242–246.
35. Serikawa T, Kuramoto T, Hilbert P, et al. *Genetics* 1992;131:701–721.
36. Hamet P, Kong D, Pravenec M, et al. *Hypertension* 1992;19:611–614.
37. Deng Y, Rapp JP. *Nature Genetics* 1992;1:267–272.
38. Jacob HJ, Lindpaintner K, Lincoln SE, et al. *Cell* 1991;67:213–224.
39. Katsuya T, Higaki J, Zhao Y, Miki T, Mikami H, Serikawa T, Ogihara T. *Biochem Biophys Res Commun* 1993;192:261–267.
40. Ely DL, Turner ME. *Hypertension* 1990;16:277–281.
41. Ely DL, Daneshvar H, Turner ME, Johnson ML, Salisbury RL. *Hypertension* 1993;21:1071–1075.
42. Soller M, Brody T. *Theor Appl Genet* 1976;47:35–39.
43. Hilbert P, Lindpaintner K, Beckmann JS, et al. *Nature* 1991;353:521–529.
44. Nara Y, Nabika T, Ikeda K, Sawamura M, Endo J, Yamori Y. *Biochem Biophys Res Commun* 1991;181:941–946.
45. Dubay C, Vincent M, Samani N, et al. *Nature Genetics* 1993;3:354–357.
46. Green EL. *Genetics and probability in animal breeding experiments.* New York: Oxford University Press, 1981.

Hypertension: Pathophysiology, Diagnosis,
and Management, Second Edition,
edited by J.H. Laragh and B.M. Brenner,
Raven Press, Ltd., New York © 1995.

CHAPTER 77

Transgenic Rats and Experimental Hypertension

Sigrid Hoffmann, Martin Paul, Hidenori Urata,
Jürgen Wagner, and Detlev Ganten

The application of molecular genetic methods in hypertension research provides qualitatively new insights into the pathophysiology of primary hypertension. Several candidate genes for hypertension, such as the genes for components of the renin-angiotensin system, have been cloned and well studied in cell culture systems and especially in rat models with genetic spontaneous hypertension. The causes of primary hypertension, however, remain unknown. The reasons are that the genetics of hypertension are very complex and the long-term influence of environmental factors confounds the genotype–phenotype relationship individually. The inherent limitation of previous methods used for studies on the cause of primary hypertension becomes more and more apparent. To dissect the complex interactions among different genetic and environmental factors contributing to the development of hypertension, well-defined experimental animal models are mandatory.

A qualitatively new, powerful tool to address such questions is the use of transgenic animal models. In these animals, overexpression or suppression of individual candidate genes involved in hypertension permits a systematic testing of gene function, regulation, and its relationship to a specific phenotype in the context of a whole organism and during development. Using tissue-specific and cell type–specific promotors it has become possible to study the physiological consequences of gene expression in particular areas of the cardiovascular system.

With the availability of transgenic technology, it is for the first time possible to study the *in vivo* regulation and function of human genes in a rat model. Preclinical studies of drugs such as renin inhibitors that specifically interact with the human renin-angiotensin system could be conducted in these specific rat models for human hypertension. This would considerably facilitate drug development and reduce ethical and financial problems involved in primate experimentation.

This chapter will discuss the strategies for generation of transgenic animals and give an overview of the transgenic models for experimental hypertension that exist to date.

S. Hoffmann, H. Urata, J. Wagner, and D. Ganten: Max-Delbrück Center for Molecular Medicine, 13125 Berlin-Buch, Germany.
M. Paul: German Institute for Blood Pressure Research.

STRATEGIES FOR GENERATION OF TRANSGENIC ANIMALS

Transgenic animals have integrated in their genome a foreign, experimentally introduced DNA, which is, in most cases, spatially and temporally correctly expressed and is stably transmitted through subsequent progeny in a Mendelian fashion. The transgenic technique was established in mice as early as 1980 (1). The mouse is the most extensively used species for transgenic experiments. Reasons include that the mouse genome is one of the best characterized and the establishment of transgenic mice is cheaper and easier to perform than in other species. In hypertension research, however, rats may be more appropriate models because they offer several advantages over mice. Methodological approaches of whole animal physiology and pharmacology for characterization of the animals is much easier to perform in rats than in mice. In addition there are several genetically hypertensive rat lines already available which provide a body of reference data. But methodological difficulties in producing transgenic rats limited, for a long time, the application of transgenic experiments in this species. The first transgenic experiments in cardiovascular research were, therefore, performed in mice (2–5). Since Mullins et al., however, established in 1990 the first transgenic rat harboring the mouse renin gene (TGRRen-2) new avenues for hypertension research were opened (5).

Today several techniques for introduction of the transgene into the germ line are established in mice, including the direct microinjection of the cloned DNA into the pronucleus of fertilized eggs (6–8), the use of retroviral vectors for transfection of preimplantative embryos (9,10), and the transfection of embryonic stem cells that colonize the germ line of foreign embryos (11,12). The direct microinjection of DNA into fertilized eggs is the most commonly used technique and the only one that has been successfully applied to generate transgenic animals in different species like rats, sheeps, cows, rabbits, and pigs (13). The use of embryonic stem cells has gained growing importance because it is the only technique available to produce transgenic "knock out" models (see below). To date, this technique is restricted to mice because embryonic stem cell cultures are not available in other species.

Several detailed methodological descriptions for the construction of transgenic mice by microinjection are available (7,8,14). Principally the steps of transgenic procedure in mice and in rats are very similar (Fig. 1). Superovulation is induced by hormonal treatment of premature females. The fertilized eggs are collected from females 10–12 hours after mating. At this stage the male and the female pronuclei are still individualized. Microinjection of 1–2 pl (2 ng/µl) DNA into the male pronucleus is performed under a microscope using micromanipulators. The eggs are kept in position by a glass pi-

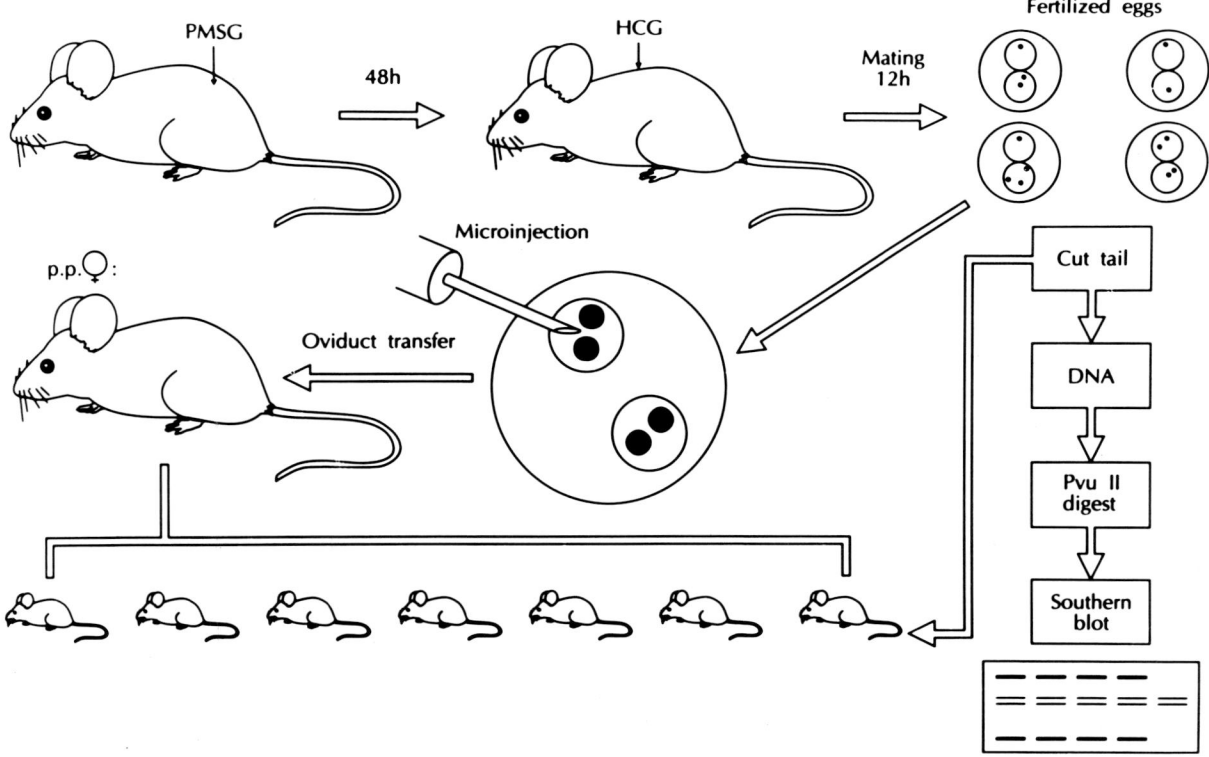

FIG. 1. Flowsheet for the generation of transgenic rats.

pette, filled with oil under light vacuum. The DNA is injected through a thin glass pipette (diameter, 1 μm). The eggs are then transferred into oviducts of pseudopregnant females, obtained by mating with males previously sterilized by vasectomy. One of the critical problems in establishing transgenic rats was the lack of knowledge on superovulation in this species. For the induction of superovulation in mice, pregnant mare serum gonadotropin (PMSG) that possesses activity of folliclestimulating hormone (FSH) and of luteotropic hormone (LH) is used. For effective induction of superovulation in rats, however, a specific ratio between FSH and LH activity is necessary that cannot be provided by PMSG (15–18). According to Armstrong (19), the application of 2 U highly purified FSH from porcine pituitary in combination with 0.4 International Units (IU) human chorionic gonadotropin (2 IU HCG) over a period of 48 hours succeeded in obtaining a superovulatory response of 60–100 eggs per female. This hormone is applied using minipumps that are implanted subcutaneously because of the short half-life of FSH (20).

By variation in the design of the DNA construct, several applications of the transgenic approach are possible. A large number of transgenic studies have been carried out to examine the tissue-specific expression of foreign genes (3,21,22) and the identification of cis-acting DNA sequences necessary for an appropriate spatial and temporal gene expression. For this approach, regulatory sequences are attached to genes of an easily scorable enzymatic marker as the luciferase or *lacZ* gene, which can be used to monitor the promotor activity (23–25).

The functions of genes can be studied by overexpressing or suppressing these genes in the whole body or in single tissues only. In overexpression experiments the genomic DNA is injected or the transgene is designed by linking the cDNA to a tissue-specific, inducable or developmental regulated promotor (26,27). This approach is especially valuable for testing the function of human genes and for the creation of disease models in rats caused by the overexpression of human genes.

Several approaches for suppression of specific host genes in transgenic models have been developed more recently. The most powerful technique is the "knock out" of genes by homologous recombination between a specific host gene in embryonic stem cells (ES) and an adequately inactivated or mutated gene that is introduced into ES cells by electroporation or microinjection. Successfully modified ES cells are transferred into the inner cell mass of blastocysts, which results in the development of chimeric animals (11,28,29). In these models, specific genes are inactivated in each cell throughout the development and provide indirect information about the normal function of these genes. Moreover, transgenic models for human diseases caused by single gene defects can be created. Another approach includes the inhibition of the translation of a specific gene in a particular tissue

by microinjection of antisense DNA or ribozymes linked to a tissue-specific promotor (30,31). Finally, conditionally or inducible genetic systems for killing specific cell lineages in transgenic animals (e.g., those specialized for the production of a specific gene) have been generated. For this purpose, cytotoxic genes (32,33) or the thymidinkinase (*tk*) gene from the herpes simplex virus (34,35), attached to cell type-specific promoters, have been used. Expression of the cytotoxic gene directly causes cell death. The expression of the *tk* gene, however, is only toxic in the presence of certain nucleoside analogues such as gancyclovir; therefore, cell death may be induced by application of gangcyclovir to the animals.

Another application of transgenic technique is targeted oncogenesis. By attaching tissue-specific or cell type–specific promotors to a potent oncogene like the SV40 T antigene gene, the creation of specific tumor models is possible (32,33). In such a way, several disease models relevant for cardiovascular research have been established (36–40). In this way, rare and difficult-to-culture cell types such as juxtaglomerular cells can be immortalized. A set of renin-expressing cells that could be useful for *in vitro* studies on the renin promotor region could be obtained (37).

TRANSGENIC ANIMALS DEVELOPING HYPERTENSION

One of the best analyzed systems contributing to the development of the hypertensive phenotype is the renin-angiotensin system (RAS). The genes expressing all the components of this system (angiotensinogen, renin, angiotensin-converting enzyme [ACE], and angiotensin II receptors) have been cloned in several species including human and intensively analyzed. Many successfully used drugs in human hypertension act on the basis of inhibition of components of this system, for example, ACE inhibitors. Genetic linkage studies have recently demonstrated that the components of the renin-angiotensin system are associated with hypertension (41–44). For this reason components of the RAS were the first to be analyzed in transgenic mice and rats.

Transgenic Mice Harboring the Rat Renin and Angiotensinogen Gene

Okhubo established in 1990 two transgenic mice lines expressing the rat renin or the rat angiotensinogen gene driven by the mouse metallothionein-1 (MT-1) promoter (45). MT-1 is a strong promoter, induced by ZnSO4 application; it directs the expression of the gene mainly in the liver. Both transgenic lines were normotensive. Mating these two transgenic lines created a new transgenic line expressing both the rat renin and the rat angiotensinogen 3 in the liver. These mice developed hypertension with a mean blood pressure of 125.8 mm Hg in males and 131.8 mm Hg in females compared with 95.2 mm Hg or 105.2 mm Hg in mice carrying only one of these transgenes. It has been reported that mouse angiotensinogen is not cleaved by rat renin (46). This explains the normotensive phenotype of rat renin mice. Normotension in rat angiotensinogen mice is in contrast to the results of Kimura et al. (47), who reported on a hypertensive transgenic mouse line expressing the rat angiotensinogen gene under the control of the native promoter in considerable amounts in the liver and brain (Fig. 2).

Nevertheless, the hypertensive transgenic line carrying the MT-1 rat renin and MT-1 rat angiotensinogen gene provided the first model for generation of hypertension in mice that is caused by the combined action of two exogeneous genes of a foreign species.

The Hypertensive Transgenic Rat TGR(mREN2)27

In 1990, Mullins et al. created the first transgenic rat in hypertension research (5). These rats carried the entire DBA/2J Ren 2d gene including the 5.3 and 9.5 kb of the 5′ and 3′ flanking sequences, respectively. This construct was chosen because its tissue-specific expression was previously demonstrated in transgenic mice (3) and, therefore, high expression in appropriate tissues could be expected. Several lines expressing the transgene and with fulminant hypertension were established and have now been characterized (transgenic rat lines TGR[mREN2]) (48). In heterozygous male TGR(mREN2)27, blood pressure increased shortly after weaning at 5 weeks of

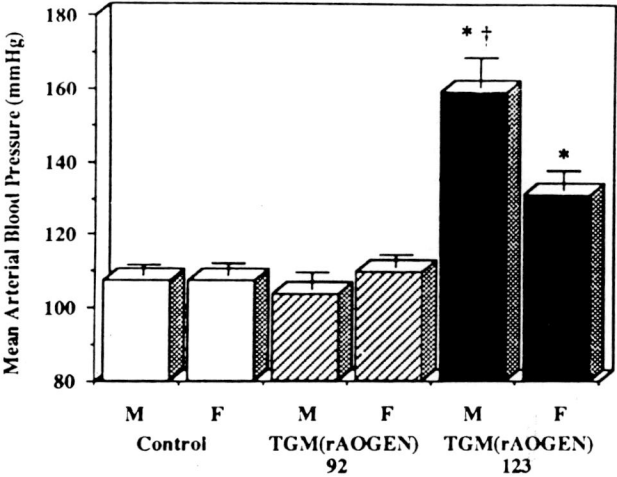

FIG. 2. Transgenic mice (TGM[rAOGEN]) harboring the entire rat angiotensinogen including 1.6 kb of 5′ flanking sequence. TGM(rAOGEN)123 expressing a substantial amount of the transgene in liver and brain developed hypertension. TGM(rAOGEN)93 expressing considerable amounts of the transgene only in the brain don't develop a hypertension phenotype.

age, and a maximal value of approximately 240 mm Hg was reached at 10 weeks of age (49). Homozygous TGR(mREN2)27 develop even higher blood pressure and show a high mortality rate without treatment with ACE inhibitors (49). The highest expression of the Ren-2 gene was found in the adrenal gland, whereas the kidney (which expresses highest renin levels in rats and human) showed only low renin levels, which could have been influenced by feedback inhibition (50). Tissue renin protein concentrations paralleled the mRNA measurements, i.e., tissue renin was demonstrated to be low in the kidney and high in the adrenal gland. The plasma RAS was not stimulated and the concentrations of active renin, angiotensin I (ANG I), ANG II, and angiotensinogen were unchanged or even suppressed when compared with that of control animals (4,5,49), characterizing these rats as a low-renin-hypertension model. In contrast, the concentration of plasma inactive renin (prorenin) is much higher in TGR(mREN2)27 than in control rats. The main source of plasma inactive renin in TGR(mREN2)27 was probably the adrenal glands, because its concentration was reduced by 80 percent after bilateral adrenalectomy (50). Moreover, isolated adrenal cells of these transgenic rats secrete considerable amounts of inactive, but also active, renin (51). The physiological significance of the high plasma inactive renin is currently under investigation. The fact that the elevated blood pressure decreased to nearly normotensive values after adrenalectomy supports an important role for this organ in the development of hypertension. The potential role of the adrenal gland in hypertension in these animals was further investigated by measuring the concentrations of adrenal steroids. Results indicated that the urinary excretion of deoxycorticosterone, corticosterone, and aldosterone was significantly elevated in young TGR(mREN2)27 during the developmental phase of hypertension, but not in adult animals (52). These data support the hypothesis that adrenal expression of the transgene stimulates corticosteroid production and increases its sensitivity to ACTH.

Although the role of the adrenal gland has generated the most interest in the investigation of hypertensive mechanisms in this transgenic model, increased production of renin or ANG II in other organs may equally contribute to the phenotypic alterations. Recently, studies investigating the cardiovascular system in these animals have been carried out. Hilgers et al. (48) used an isolated hindlimb preparation to demonstrate that the vasculature of the transgenic animals produced increased amounts of ANG II, which is most likely due to overexpression of the transgene in the vascular wall. Sensitive ribonuclease (RNase) protection assays indeed have shown that Ren-2 expression was markedly increased in blood vessels (34). The hearts of the transgenic animals show marked pathological changes including hypertrophy and fibrosis (53). This can be partially explained by the dramatically elevated blood pressure levels, but there are clearly additional effects. Current studies focus on the investigation of the cardiac function in these animals and its cellular basis.

Transgenic Animals Expressing the Human Renin Gene

Tissue-specific regulation of human renin was initially studied in transgenic mice (57BL/6) using a genomic construct of the gene with 3.0 kb of 5'-flanking regions and 1.2 kb of downstream sequences (54). The transgene in these animals was correctly spliced and showed a tissue-specific expression pattern in the kidney and was also expressed in other cardiovascular organs. Human renin protein was detected in the juxtaglomerular apparatus of the kidney by the use of a monoclonal antibody specific to human renin, demonstrating not only correct tissue-specific but also cell-specific expression (21).

A construct containing the entire human renin gene has been microinjected into pronuclei of fertilized rat oocytes from outbred Sprague-Dawley/WKY hybrids. The construct comprised a total length of 17.6 kb after stripping it from vector-encoded sequences (22). Two rat lines could be obtained which transmitted the transgene to their progeny. These transgenic rats produced and secreted active human renin into their plasma, as has been determined by an immunoradiometric assay using monoclonal antibodies specific for human renin. The plasma level of active human renin in one line was slightly less than in humans, whereas in the other line, active human renin exceeded about 12 times the levels found in humans. Transgene expression was found to be highest in the kidney, but was also present in extrarenal tissues such as the lung or the gastrointestinal tract (22). On the cellular level, *in situ* hybridization showed that human renin expression under basal conditions is confined to the juxtaglomerular apparatus.

To examine the question whether the presence of the transgene interferes with production of endogenous renin, plasma rat renin concentration was also determined, but no significant differences existed between transgenic rats and negative controls. Also, no alterations in other components of the RAS such as angiotensin II or angiotensinogen could be detected. In addition, both rats strains were normotensive. These negative findings can be explained by the fact that human renin does not interact with rat angiotensinogen except at very high doses. To investigate how the human renin transgene responds to physiological stimuli of renin secretion, animals were sodium-depleted by placement on a low-sodium diet for 3 days. In plasma, active human renin levels increased by about 11-fold, similar to the increase in rat renin. This indicates that the transgene

is regulated by sodium depletion and does not interfere with rat renin production even under stimulated conditions.

Transgenic Animals Expressing the Human Angiotensinogen Gene

A genomic human angiotensinogen gene construct, comprising 5 exons, 4 introns, 1.3 kb of 5'-flanking region, and 2.4 kb of 3'-flanking region, was used to generate transgenic mice as well as rats carrying the human angiotensinogen transgene (4,22,55). In transgenic mice, expression of the transgene could be detected predominantly in the liver, and to a lesser extent in the brain, kidney, heart, and other organs (4,55). Four lines of transgenic rats were obtained. Human angiotensinogen was secreted into the plasma in all rats but the levels markedly varied between the lines ranging from 120 μg/ml up to 5 mg/ml. All four lines exceeded plasma angiotensinogen levels in humans, which is approximately 60 μg/ml. Despite the high plasmatic levels, these animals were normotensive, indicating that human angiotensinogen did not interact with rat renin at the concentration found in these animals (22). Compared to transgene negative controls, rat angiotensinogen levels as well as angiotensin II levels were not significantly different from levels measured in the transgenics. Transgene expression was highest at the appropriate sites in the liver, where it was expressed in the parenchyma as demonstrated by *in situ* hybridization (22). Transgene expression detected in the kidney and the gastrointestinal tract was approximately tenfold lower. These findings are in contrast to a previously described transgenic mouse strain carrying the human angiotensinogen gene. Here, human angiotensinogen was expressed as high in the kidney as in the liver in contrast to humans, where kidney angiotensinogen is low (54,56). Human renin and angiotensinogen in transgenic rats have been shown to be expressed highest in the kidney and the liver, respectively. In addition, expression can also be demonstrated in extrarenal and extrahepatic tissues. The coexpression of human transgenes in crossbred transgenic animals carrying both genes in these organs supports the possibility of local angiotensin I production due to the interaction of human proteins. The functional role of such human-dependent tissue-specific RAS remains to be established.

Species-specificity of the Human Renin Substrate Reaction in Transgenic Rats

Despite the high expression of the human transgenes, rats carrying either the human renin or human angiotensinogen gene remained normotensive as an indication of the species-specificity of the human renin substrate reaction. As demonstrated by the unaltered levels of angiotensin II in both human renin and angiotensinogen transgenic rats, rat renin did not react with human angiotensinogen nor did human renin with rat angiotensinogen. Blood pressure remained unaltered when the human specific renin inhibitor Ro 42-5892 was given as a bolus injection to sodium-depleted TGR(hREN)1936 rats, whereas the angiotensin II receptor antagonist lowered blood pressure by about 20 mm Hg. The species-specificity of the human renin substrate reaction in the transgenic rats could further be demonstrated by injection of recombinant human renin into rats carrying the human angiotensinogen gene. Here, at a dosage of 5 μg renin I/ml/h, blood pressure rapidly increased from 142 ± 4 mm Hg to 192 ± 8 mm Hg. Addition of the human renin inhibitor Ro 42-5892 rapidly normalized the blood pressure to pretreatment values. Human renin at this dosage did not elicit a hypertensive response in transgene negative controls, indicating that the blood pressure increase was due to the interaction of human renin with human angiotensinogen. Infusion of rat renin in equipressor doses raised blood pressure as well. However, in this case, Ro 42-5892 remained without any effect, whereas DuP 753 (10 mg/kg) normalized blood pressure rapidly. This supports the finding that angiotensin II formation in this case originated from the reaction of rat renin with rat angiotensinogen (Fig. 3).

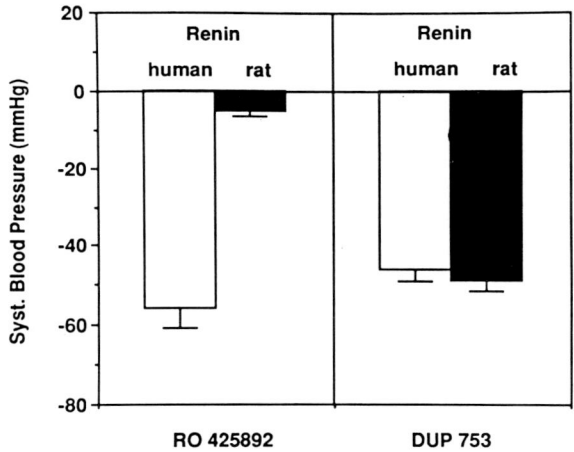

FIG. 3. Species-specificity of the human renin-angiotensin interaction in transgenic rats is demonstrated by the effects of the human renin inhibitor RO 425892. Recombinant human renin or partially purified rat renin was infused in equipressor doses to raise blood pressure from normotensive values to approximately 190–200 mm Hg in rats transgenic for human angiotensinogen. A subsequent infusion of RO 425892 (1 mg/kg body weight, i.v.) normalized blood pressure only in transgenic rats that had been given human renin, but had no effect after i.v. rat renin. Infusion of the angiotensin II receptor antagonist DuP 753 (10 mg/kg body weight, i.v.) lowered blood pressure rapidly in both instances. Human renin did not raise blood pressure in nontransgenic controls, nor was blood pressure reduced below normal by RO 425892 or DuP 753 when applied in controls. Syst, systolic.

TRANSGENIC MICE DEVELOPING HYPOTENSION

Transgenic Mice Harboring the Transthyretin/ANF Gene

Steinhelper et al. developed in 1990 a transgenic mouse line carrying the atrial natriuretic factor (ANF) gene (57). ANF is a peptide hormone synthesized predominantly by atrial cardiomyocytes and is known to be involved in the control of cardiovascular functions by rapid natriuretic and diuretic effects as well as reduction in arterial blood pressure after acute administration. The liver-specific mouse transthyretin (TTR) promoter was used to drive the expression of the ANF gene in transgenic mice. The mouse ANF promoter enables continuous expression of ANF in the liver and, therefore, was chosen in order to study the effects of chronically elevated ANF. Plasma immunoreactive ANF concentration was elevated eightfold in transgenics as compared with nontransgenic litter mates and this elevation resulted in a significantly lower mean atrial pressure (78.9 mm Hg). This hypotensive phenotype did not exhibit difference in heart rate nor significant changes in fluid or electrolyte balance as compared with nontransgenic controls. Therefore, the origin of hypotension in the TTR/ANF transgenic mice may partly be due to nonrenal actions of ANF such as a direct influence on the heart and vasculature.

Transgenic Mice Expressing an Antisense Angiotensinogen Fusion Gene

The first successful approach of transgenic antisense technology in hypertension research was reported by Pedrazzini in 1993 (58). To block the RAS by inhibiting the angiotensinogen synthesis in the liver, he introduced an antisense angiotensinogen gene driven by the liver-specific phospoenolpyruvate carboxykinase gene promoter into the germ line of mice. The resulting transgenic mice had significantly lower plasma angiotensinogen concentration and a significant reduction in blood pressure as compared with nontransgenic controls.

FUTURE RESEARCH TARGETS

The establishment of transgenic rats carrying candidate genes for cardiovascular diseases has without doubt opened new avenues in hypertension research. One focus of future experiments will be the testing of new candidate genes. Other genes of the renin-angiotensin system, ACE, angiotensin II receptor, and human heart chymase have been cloned (59) and are available for transgenic experiments. Human heart chymase is the most potent and specific AII-forming enzyme described so far. Since it is found only in hearts of human but not in hearts of other species, the development of transgenic rats expressing human heart chymase is of great interest and is ongoing in our laboratory.

Another important target for transgenic hypertension research will be the endothelin peptide family. The members of this family (endothelin I, II, and III) are thought to play an important role in cardiovascular regulation. Despite extensive biochemical, pharmacological, and molecular biological studies, their ultimate role *in vivo* remains elusive. Recently the establishment of transgenic rats expressing human endothelin-2 genes has been reported (60). These animals will provide important tools for the study of endothelin function and regulation.

Particular emphasis is now being applied to direct transgene expression in specific organs, such as the heart or the vascular wall, in order to study the role of tissue-renin-angiotensin system specifically. For this purpose, research has focused on the identification of tissue-specific promotor sequences that direct the expression into the heart and into the vascular wall, for instance (23,61–63). In addition to these overexpression models, research efforts are now being directed to the development of transgenic rats in which the gene under investigation is suppressed by antisense, ribozyme, or cell-ablating approaches.

The development of embryonic stem cell culture of rats as a precondition for the creation of "gene knock out" models in rats is, therefore, one of the main research foci.

The combination of different transgenic lines by mating or successive microinjections would allow the establishment of specific models for cardiovascular research with known multigenetic defects that could imitate the complexity of hypertension more realistically.

These experiments provide exciting new model systems to study clinical issues that heretofore had been difficult if not impossible to address. Better information about the genetic causes of hypertension will permit a causal therapy and prevention instead of palliative treatment as is applied today.

REFERENCES

1. Gordon JW, Scangos GA, Plotkin DJ, et al. *Proc Natl Acad Sci USA* 1980;77:7380–7384.
2. Tronik D, Dreyfus M, Babinet Ch, Rougeon F. *EMBO J* 1987;6: 983–987.
3. Mullins JJ, Sigmund CD, Kane-Haas C, McGowan RA, Gross KW. *EMBO J* 1989;8:4065–4072.
4. Fukamiza A, Seo MS, Hatae T, et al. *Biochem Biophys Res Commun* 1989;165:826–832.
5. Mullins JJ, Peters J, Ganten D. *Nature* 1990;344:541–544.
6. Babinet C, Morello D, Renard JP. *Genome* 1989;31:938–949.
7. Gordon JW, Ruddle FH. *Methods Enzymol* 1983;101:411–433.
8. Hogan B, Costantini F, Lacy E. *Manipulating the mouse embryo: a laboratory manual.* Cold Spring Harbor Laboratory, Cold Spring Harbor, New York; 1986.
9. Jaenisch R, Jahner D, Nobis P, et al. *Cell* 1981;24:519.
10. Soriano P, Cone RD, Mulligan RC, Jaenisch R. *Science* 1986;234: 1409.
11. Robertson EJ. *Biol Reprod* 1991;44:238–245.
12. Williams DA. *Bone Marrow Transplantation* 1990;5:141–144.
13. Brem G, Brenig B, Godman M. *Zuchthygiene* 1985;20:251.
14. Brinster RL, Chen HY, Trumbauer ME, Yagle MK, Palmiter RD. *Proc Natl Acad Sci USA* 1985;82:4438–4442.
15. Young WY, Yuen BH, Moon YS. *Gamete Res* 1987;16:109–120.
16. Leveille MC, Armstrong DT. *Gamete Res* 1989;23:127–138.
17. Jong-Ho L, Kang DJ, Park CS. *Korean J Anim Sci* 1988;30:714–719.
18. Yun YW, Yuen BH, Moon YS. *Biol Reprod* 1988;39:279–286.
19. Armstrong DT, Siuda A, Opavsky MA, Chandrasekhar Y. *Biology of Reproduction* 1989;40:54–62.
20. Bogdanove EM, Gay VL. *Endocrinol* 1969;84:1118–1138.
21. Fukamizu A, Hatae T, Kon Y, et al. *Biochem J* 1991;278:601–603.
22. Ganten D, Wagner J, Zeh K, et al. *Proc Natl Acad Sci USA* 1992;89:7806–7810.
23. Rindt H, Gulick J, Knottst S, Neumann J, Robbins J. *J Biol Chem* 1993;268:5332–5338.
24. Parsons WJ, Richardson JA, Graves KH, Williams RS, Moreadith RW. *Proc Natl Acad Sci USA* 1993;90:1726–1730.
25. Parmacek MS, Vora AJ, Shen T, Barr E, Jung F, Leiden JM. *Mol Cell Biol* 1992;12:1967–1976.
26. Cuthbertson RA, Klintworth GK. *Lab Invest* 1988;58:484–502.
27. Jami J. *Nouv Rev Fr Hematol* 1988;30:7–11.
28. Evans MJ. *Mol Biol Med* 1989;6:557–565.
29. Mansour SL. *Genetic Analysis Techniques and Applications* 1990;7:219–227.
30. Katsuki M, Sato M, Kimura M, Yokoama M, Kobayashi K, et al. *Science* 1988;241:593–595.
31. Moxham CM, Hod Y, Malbon CC. *Science* 1993;260:991–995.
32. Behringer RR, Mathews LS, Palmiter RD, Brister RL. *Genes Dev* 1988;2:453–461.
33. Palmiter RL, Behringer RR, Quaife CJ, Maxwell F, Maxwell IH, Brinster RL. *Cell* 1987;50:435–443.
34. Borrelli E, Heyman RA, Sawchenko PE, Evans RM. *Nature* 1989;339:538–541.
35. Heyman RA, Borelli E, Lesley J, et al. *Proc Natl Acad Sci USA* 1989;86:698–2702.
36. Field LJ. *Science* 1988;239:1029–1033.
37. Behringer RR, Peschon JJ, Messing A, et al. *Proc Natl Acad Sci USA* 1988;85:2648–2652.
38. Jacob HJ, Sigmund CD, Shockley TR, Gross KW, Dzau VJ. *Hypertension* 1991;17:1167–1172.
39. Yee SP, Mock D, Maltby V, et al. *Proc Natl Acad Sci USA* 1989;86: 5873–5877.
40. Edwards JG, Smith CK, Santerre RF, Bales K, et al. *Abstracts of the scientific conference on the molecular biology of the normal, hypertrophied and failing heart.* Pacific Grove, California, August 4–8, 1993.
41. Cambien F, Poirier O, Lecerf L, Evans A, et al. *Nature* 1992;359: 641–645.
42. Hilbert P, Lindpainter K, Beckmann JS, Serikawa T, Soubrier F, Duhay C, et al. *Nature* 1991;353:521–529.
43. Jacob HJ, Lindpaintner K, Lincoln SE, et al. *Cell* 1991;67:213–224.
44. Jeunemaitre X, Soubrier F, Kotelevtsev YV, Lifton RP, Williams CS, et al. *Cell* 1992;71:169–180.
45. Ohkubo H, Kawakami H, Takumi T, Arai H, et al. *Proc Natl Acad Sci* 1990;87:5153–5157.
46. Oliver W, Gross F. *Proc Soc Exp Biol* 1966;122:923–926.
47. Kimura S, Mullins J, Bunnemann B, et al. *EMBO J* 1992;11:821–827.
48. Hilgers KF, Peters J, Sommer M, et al. *Hypertension* 1992;19:687–691.
49. Bader M, Zhao Y, Sander M, et al. *Hypertension* 1992;19:681–686.
50. Peters J, Münter K, Bader M, Hackenthal E, Mullins JJ, Ganten D. *J Clin Invest* 1992;91:251–257.

51. Sander M, Bader M, Djavidani B, et al. *Endocrinol* 1992;131:807–814.
52. Ganten D, Takahashi S, Lindpaintner K, Mullins JJ. *Hypertension* 1991;18:III-108–III-114.
53. Bachmann S, Peters J, Engler E, Ganten D, Mullins J. *Kidney Int* 1992;41:24–36.
54. Takahashi S, Fukamizu A, Hasegawa T, et al. *Biochem Biophys Res Commun* 1991;180:1103–1109.
55. Sigmund CD, Jones CA, Kane CM, Wu C, Lang JA, Gross KW. *Circ Res* 1992;70:1070–1079.
56. Takahashi S, Fukamizu A, Hatae T, et al. *J Vet Med Sci* 1992;54:1191–1193.
57. Steinhelper ME, Cochrane KL, Field LJ. *Hypertension* 1990;16:301–307.
58. Pedrazzini T, Pascal C, Aubert JF, Brunner H-R. *Scientific conference on molecular biology of the normal, hypertrophied and failing heart*. Pacific Grove, California; August 4–8, 1993 (abst 65).
59. Urata H, Kinoshita A, Misono KS, Bumpus FM, Husain A. *J Biol Chem* 1990;265:22348–22357.
60. Paul M, Zimmermann F, Ruf P, Zintz M, Meier D, Yanagisawa M. *Arch Pharmacol* 1993;347(suppl):R93(abst).
61. Shani M. *Nature* 1985;314:283–285.
62. Subramaniam A, Jones WK, Gulick J, Wert S, Neumann J, Robbibs J. *J Biol Chem* 1991;266:24613–24620.
63. Lee KJ, Ross RS, Rockman HA, et al. *J Biol Chem* 1992;267:15875–15885.

The Kidneys and the Renin-Angiotensin Aldosterone Axis: Role in Sodium-Volume Homeostasis and Arterial Tone in Pathogenesis of Hypertension

Hypertension: Pathophysiology, Diagnosis,
and Management, Second Edition,
edited by J.H. Laragh and B.M. Brenner,
Raven Press, Ltd., New York © 1995.

CHAPTER 78

The Dominant Role of the Kidneys in Long-Term Arterial Pressure Regulation in Normal and Hypertensive States

Arthur C. Guyton, John E. Hall, Thomas G. Coleman,
R. Davis Manning, Jr., and Roger A. Norman, Jr.

   A. C. Guyton, J. E. Hall, T. G. Coleman, and R. D. Manning, Jr.: Department of Physiology, University of Mississippi Medical Center, Jackson, Mississippi 39216.
   R. A. Norman, Jr.: Director of Clinical Research, North Mississippi Medical Center, Tupelo, Mississippi 38801.

This chapter discusses the tremendous importance of the kidneys in controlling the long-term level of arterial pressure. It is our specific goal to demonstrate that a renal-fluid volume mechanism for pressure control (in contradistinction to the kidneys' renin-angiotensin system) is so powerful that it allows the kidneys to override virtually all other mechanisms for long-term pressure control (1–4).

THE RENAL-FLUID VOLUME MECHANISM FOR PRESSURE CONTROL

Pressure Diuresis and Pressure Natriuresis Provide a Powerful Mechanism for Pressure Control

When the arterial pressure rises above normal, the increased pressure has a direct effect on the kidneys to cause increased urinary output of both fluid volume and salt. These effects are called, respectively, *pressure diuresis* and *pressure natriuresis.* Any continued excess loss of body fluid volume will eventually return the pressure to normal because adequate fluid volume is a necessary requirement for the circulatory system to function.

Though most researchers in the fields of renal and hypertension physiology have recognized that pressure diuresis and pressure natriuresis can play a role in pressure control, many have suggested that these effects are of only minor importance rather than a dominating factor. One reason for their believing this has been the type of experiment illustrated in Fig. 1A, an experiment run hundreds of times in many laboratories.

Figure 1A shows the effects on the circulation and on urinary output caused by rapidly increasing the blood volume in dogs (5). Blood was transfused equal to approximately 40 percent of the dog's own blood volume (an increase in blood volume equal to four units of blood in human beings); the blood was given over a time interval of only 4 minutes. Yet, as illustrated by the lowermost curve, the arterial pressure rose very little, only 12 percent to 15 percent despite this massive and very rapid increase in blood volume. However, it should be remembered that for short-term control of the arterial pressure, the nervous system has extremely powerful pressure control reflexes such as the baroreceptor reflexes, reacting within seconds to readjust the arterial pressure back toward its initial level. Therefore, observe in Fig. 1B exactly the same experiment as in Fig. 1A but performed this time in dogs whose nervous systems had been totally blocked (5). Note, that without the interference of the rapidly acting nervous pressure reflexes, the increase in volume caused an extreme and instantaneous 125 percent increase in pressure, not the mild increase observed when the nervous pressure control reflexes were functional.

Also important in Fig. 1B is the subsequent time course of arterial pressure and urinary output following the transfusion. As long as the arterial pressure stayed above the original control value, the urinary output remained above normal. One can understand that this excess renal loss of water and salt can accumulate over hours or weeks until eventually the accumulated loss will of necessity return the arterial pressure back to normal.

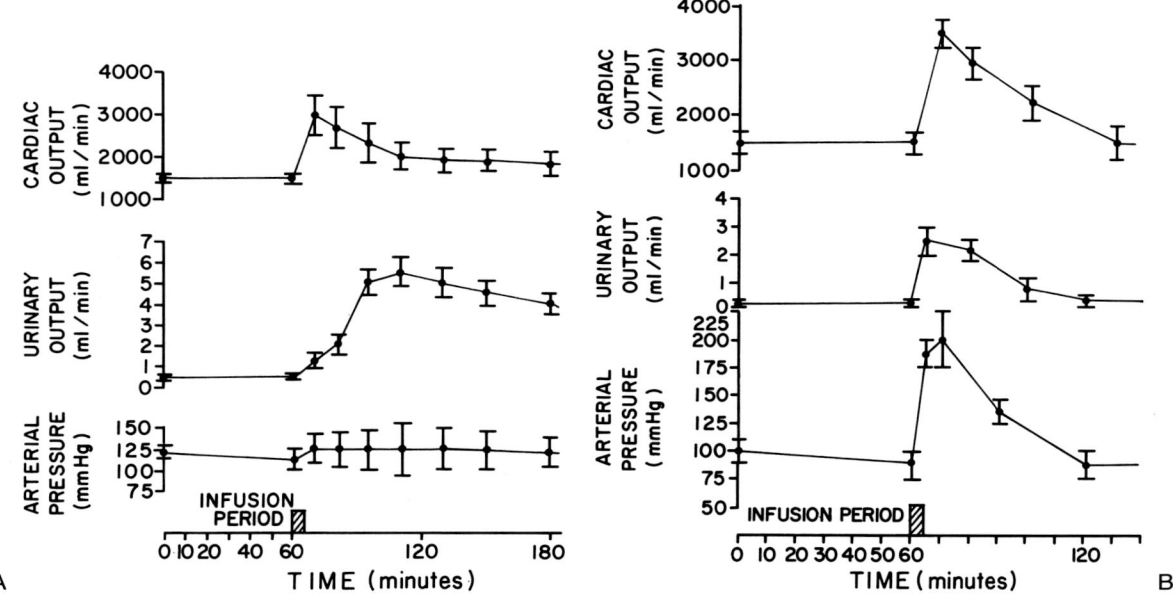

FIG. 1. Effect of transfusing a volume of blood into dogs equal to approximately 40% of the dog's own blood volume in a period of 4 minutes under two different conditions: **(A)** with intact cardiovascular nervous reflexes; **(B)** after destruction of the nervous system to block all cardiovascular nervous reflexes. (From ref. 5, with permission.)

The "Renal Function Curve" Demonstrates the Quantitative Effect of Changes in Arterial Pressure on Urinary Output

The quantitative characteristics of pressure diuresis and natriuresis are expressed by the so-called renal function curve illustrated in Fig. 2 (6,7). Normally, excess arterial pressure has approximately the same proportional effect on both fluid volume loss and sodium loss. Therefore, the curve, although shown in Fig. 2 for fluid volume output, is approximately correct for sodium output as well.

Figure 2 shows that fluid output falls to zero at a mean arterial pressure of about 50 to 60 mm Hg. At the other extreme, fluid output is about seven times normal when the mean arterial pressure rises to 200 mm Hg. A similar renal function curve can be drawn for sodium excretion.

Arterial Pressure is Controlled to That Level at which Fluid Output Equilibrates with Fluid Intake

Note also in Fig. 2 the dashed line, which represents the normal net intake of fluid volume. The "net intake" is that amount of fluid volume that must be excreted by the kidneys to maintain body fluid balance; that is, it is the total intake minus fluid lost from the body by nonrenal routes.

Especially important is the point in the figure, labeled "equilibrium pressure," where the net intake line crosses the renal function curve. It is only at this unique pressure level that the renal fluid output is exactly equal to the net intake. At any other pressure, the fluid volume of the body will be either increasing or decreasing. For instance, at a pressure of 150 mm Hg, fluid output is three times the intake, representing a rapid decrease of body fluid volume. The diagram also demonstrates that the volume will continue to decrease until the pressure falls all the way back to the equilibrium pressure level. Therefore, if ever the pressure rises above the equilibrium pressure level, there will be continual diminishment of body fluid volume until such time that the blood volume falls low enough literally to force the arterial pressure down to the equilibrium pressure level—not part way to the equilibrium pressure, but all the way.

Conversely, when the arterial pressure falls below the equilibrium pressure, the net intake is greater than the output, and the body continues to accumulate fluid, eventually driving the arterial pressure up to the equilibrium pressure.

Experiments have shown that this fluid volume mechanism will usually bring the pressure to a steady-state level within a week or so, with most of the effect occurring within the first 3 to 5 days (8–11). The reason for the slowness of the effect is that a large amount of body fluid volume cannot be accumulated instantaneously or lost instantaneously. Furthermore, multiple readjustments in the other arterial pressure control mechanisms—the nervous controls, for instance—must also take place before the full effect can be established.

Thus, it is mathematically impossible for the arterial pressure to remain indefinitely at any other pressure level besides the equilibrium level defined by the point where the renal function curve crosses the net fluid intake level.

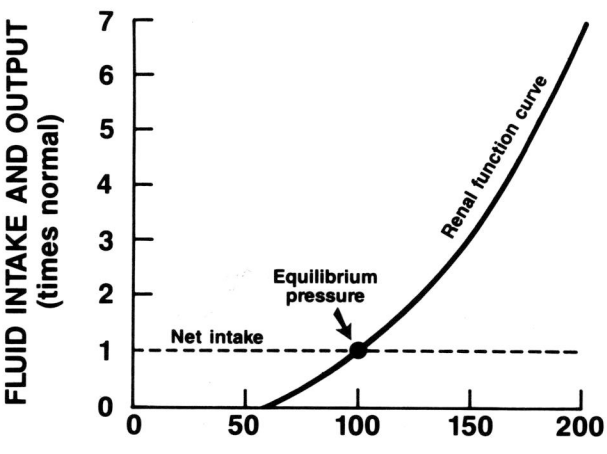

FIG. 2. A graphic method for equating the renal function curve with the net fluid intake level, showing the equilibration of fluid intake and output at the equilibrium-pressure level. The renal-fluid volume mechanism for pressure control will always return the long-term level of arterial pressure to the equilibrium pressure level. (Modified from ref. 13.)

The Relationship of Body Salt Balance to the Equilibration Process

Thus far, we have discussed the effect of fluid volume instead of body salt for controlling arterial pressure. However, it is common knowledge that salt intake in the diet and salt retention by the kidneys is almost always more important in determining the arterial pressure level than is fluid volume intake. How does one reconcile this importance of salt with the fluid volume equilibration process illustrated in Fig. 2? The answer is that an increase in extracellular fluid volume almost always occurs when there is an increase in extracellular salt (12). For instance, when excess salt is eaten or excess salt is reabsorbed by the renal tubules, the thirst mechanism causes a parallel amount of water usually to be ingested to go along with the salt. Also, if ever the salt concentration in the extracellular fluid becomes excessive, antidiuretic hormone is secreted within minutes, and the kidneys then retain still additional quantities of water to match the excessive salt in the extracellular fluid. Thus, the determining factor for buildup of the extracellular fluid volume is almost always initial accumulation of salt.

Because of this parallel relationship between salt and fluid volume retention one can construct an equilibration diagram for salt intake and output to control arterial pressure that is almost identical to the fluid intake and output diagram of Fig. 2.

The Renal-Fluid Volume Mechanism for Pressure Control Has an Infinite Gain Characteristic

Note especially in Figs. 1A and 2 that the arterial pressure eventually returns *all the way* back to the equilibrium pressure level, not merely part of the way. The effectiveness of a feedback control system is expressed in terms of its feedback gain. When the renal-fluid volume mechanism corrects an abnormal pressure all the way back to the equilibrium pressure level, this amounts to infinite correction of the pressure abnormality. Therefore, the renal-fluid volume mechanism is said to have an "infinite gain" characteristic for controlling arterial pressure.

Comparative Pressure Controlling Characteristics of the Renal-Fluid Volume Mechanism and Other Pressure Controllers

Figure 3 illustrates the approximate feedback gains for eight separate arterial pressure control mechanisms at different time intervals after a sudden abnormal change in arterial pressure occurs (13). Note that the times are expressed on a semi-log scale in seconds, minutes, hours, and days. It is clear from this diagram that the three nervous control mechanisms—the *baroreceptor, chemoreceptor,* and *central nervous system ischemic mechanisms*—are all activated within the first few seconds after any sudden appearance of abnormal pressure. Therefore, it is mainly the nervous control mechanisms that play the immediate role in returning the arterial pressure back toward the normal level. Next are several hemodynamic and endocrine mechanisms, including (a) the renin-angiotensin-vasoconstriction mechanism, (b) stress relaxation of the vascular walls, and (c) fluid shift through the capillary membranes between the interstitium and the blood. After several hours, the renal-fluid volume mechanism (also called the renal-blood volume-pressure control mechanism) begins to become effective; along with this, aldosterone secretion by the adrenal glands plays a helping role to make the renal-fluid volume mechanism more effective. Within a few days to a week or so, the fluid volume mechanism reaches almost full effectiveness, that is, it has almost attained its infinite gain characteristic.

When two or more competing control systems attempt to adjust the arterial pressure to different levels, the degree of effectiveness of each respective control system is

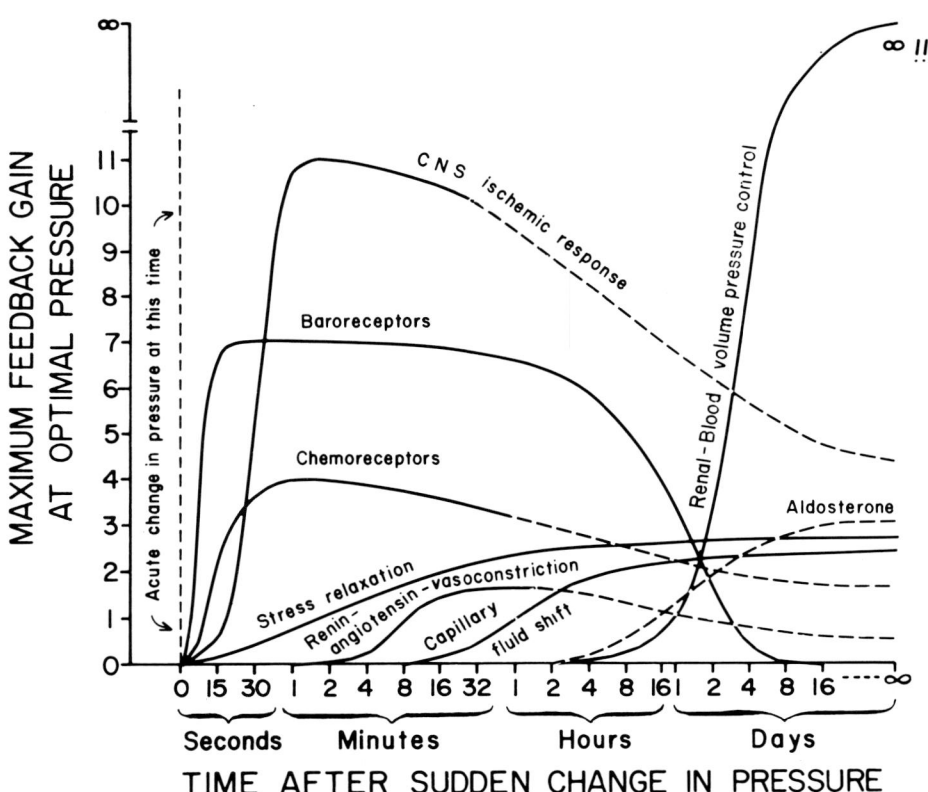

FIG. 3. Approximate degree of activity, expressed as feedback gain, of several arterial pressure control systems at various times after a sudden change in arterial pressure. Note the infinite gain of the renal-volume mechanism for pressure control. (From ref. 13, with permission.)

directly proportional to the gain of that system. Note in Fig. 3 that only the renal fluid-volume mechanism ever has infinite gain, but this infinite gain is reached only after an interval of time. Therefore, one can see that in the first seconds, minutes, hours, and even several days after abnormal pressure occurs, the other pressure control mechanisms besides the renal fluid-volume mechanism often play the more important roles in pressure control, such as to prevent the loss of life after acute hemorrhage or to prevent a stroke when some temporary factor attempts to elevate the pressure too high. On the other hand, the fluid volume mechanism, because of its infinite gain, eventually becomes the control system that determines either entirely or almost entirely the long-term arterial pressure level.

Two Basic Determinants in the Renal-Fluid Volume Pressure Control Mechanism

A full understanding of Fig. 2 will make it clear that the long-term arterial pressure level can be changed *only* by changing one or both of the two determining factors in that figure (13):

1. the level of net intake,
2. the rightward or leftward degree of shift of the different segments of the renal function curve along the arterial pressure axis.

Figure 4 illustrates how changing one or both of these determinants can change the level at which the arterial

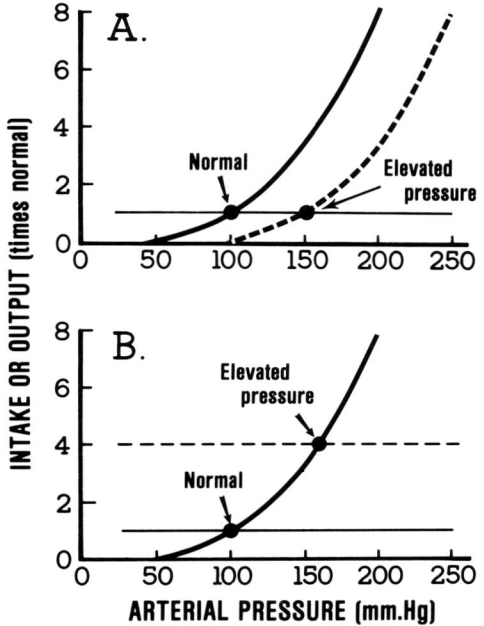

FIG. 4. Illustration of the two ways by which the long-term arterial pressure level can be altered: (**A**) by shifting the renal function curve to a different pressure range; (**B**) by changing the level of intake. (From ref. 14, with permission.)

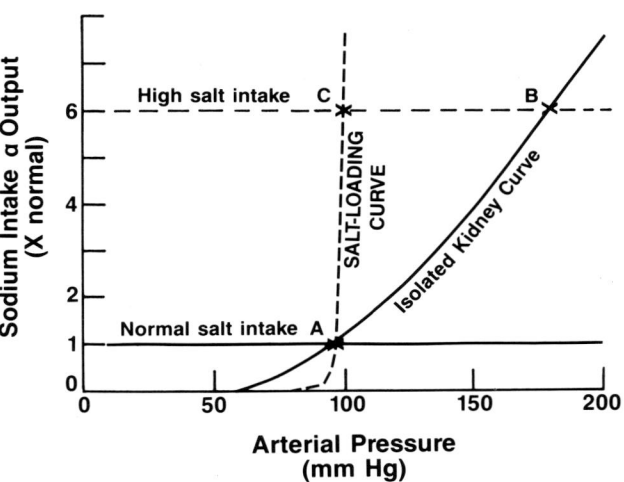

FIG. 5. Equating the isolated kidney renal function curve and the salt-loading renal function curve with two levels of salt intake. At normal salt intake both curves equilibrate with the intake at exactly the same arterial pressure level, but this is not true at high salt intake. (Modified from ref. 13.)

pressure will stabilize (14). Figure 4A shows the normal net intake level and the normal renal function curve (the solid curve). Then, to the right is a function curve for abnormal kidney function (the dashed curve), illustrating that in this case only at a very high arterial pressure will these kidneys excrete enough water and salt to match the intake. Thus, if for pathological reasons the kidneys change their characteristics so that the renal function curve becomes shifted to the right, the arterial pressure will thereafter stabilize at the shifted point shown in the figure labeled "elevated pressure," not at the normal pressure level.

Figure 4B shows a change in the second determinant, in this case an increase in the net intake to four times normal (the dashed line). The point at which the new intake level crosses the renal function curve is at a different equilibrium pressure from the normal, and there will be a new level of pressure stabilization.

The Salt-Loading Type of Renal Function Curve—Role of the Renin-Angiotensin System

The renal function curves shown in Figs. 2 and 4 are typical of those recorded in the isolated perfused kidney in which the arterial pressure is raised or lowered acutely and no other factor besides pressure changes are affecting kidney output. However, it is not practical to record renal function curves of this type in the intact living animal. Therefore, another type of renal function curve has been employed even more effectively to study the events of arterial pressure control. This is the salt-loading renal function curve, also called in some publications the chronic renal function curve (13,15).

The typical salt-loading renal function curve is illustrated by the dashed curve in Fig. 5. This type of curve is constructed using the following procedure (16): Each level on the curve represents the steady-state relationship between mean arterial pressure and urinary sodium output. To achieve the different levels of sodium output, the animal is given successively new levels of sodium intake, each lasting for several days until the animal reaches sodium balance (that is, until sodium output equals intake); then the stabilized mean arterial pressure is measured and plotted against the sodium intake and output. Then, the animal is started on another level of sodium intake for several days, repeating the same process for multiple points on the curve. Plotting all these points for normal kidneys gives the very steep curve called the sodium-loading renal function curve illustrated by the dashed curve in Fig. 5. But why is this curve so steep in comparison with the curve recorded in the isolated kidney? When an intact animal is loaded with different levels of sodium, not only does the animal's mean arterial pressure change but multiple hormonal and electrolyte changes occur as well. Thus, pressure changes are not the only factor affecting renal sodium output when one records the salt-loading type of renal function curve. Instead the changes in sodium output are caused by multiple factors acting on the kidneys, including pressure changes, hormonal changes, changes in extracellular electrolyte concentrations, and possibly other factors as well.

The Salt-Loading Renal Function Curve is the Appropriate Curve to Use When Analyzing Long-Term Regulation of Arterial Pressure

The salt-loading renal function curve can be used for analyzing chronic pressure regulation in the same way that the isolated kidney renal function curve is used for analyzing acute pressure regulation. This is illustrated in Fig. 5, which shows two renal function curves: (a) the isolated kidney renal function curve and (b) the salt-loading renal function curve (dashed curve). The figure

also shows a lower horizontal solid line representing the normal salt intake and an upper dashed line for high intake. The normal intake line and the isolated kidney renal function curve (the solid curve) equilibrate at point A, predicting that the arterial pressure normally should stabilize at the pressure level of point A. Note that the salt-loading renal function curve also passes through point A. Therefore, using the salt-loading renal function curve to predict the long-term level of normal arterial pressure will give exactly the same value.

Now let us change the salt intake to the high level illustrated by the upper dashed line. This equates with the isolated kidney renal function curve at point B and with the salt-loading renal function curve at point C. Which of these two points predicts the long-term chronic arterial pressure level, point B or point C? The answer is point C. The reason is that the effects of hormonal and electrolyte changes on kidney salt output must be considered along with the effects of pressure when analyzing long-term pressure regulation, not merely the acute pressure effect alone. Since all of these combined factors go into the makeup of the salt-loading renal function curve, it is clear that it is the salt-loading renal function curve that is important in analyzing long-term chronic pressure regulation.

The Renin-Angiotensin-Aldosterone System is the Principal Cause of the Difference Between the Isolated Acute Kidney Renal Function Curve and the Chronic Salt-Loading Renal Function Curve

Why is the chronic salt-loading renal function curve almost vertical in the normal animal, having a slope about 20 times as great as the acute renal function curve recorded from the isolated kidney? The experiment illustrated in Fig. 6 helps to answer this. The "normal" curve in this figure is approximately the same as the salt-loading renal function curve for normal dogs shown in Fig. 5. The numbers in parentheses adjacent to the re-

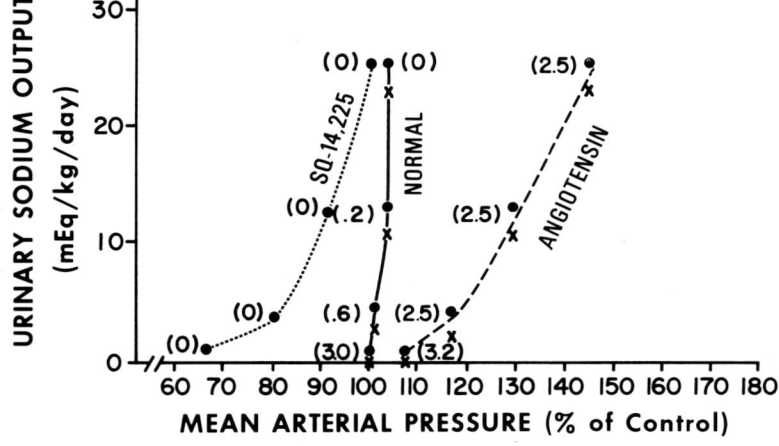

FIG. 6. Salt-loading renal function curves recorded in three separate series of dogs under three respective conditions: normal dogs, dogs receiving the converting enzyme inhibitor captopril (SQ-14,225), and dogs receiving continuous infusion of angiotensin. The numbers in parentheses represent the calculated levels of circulating angiotensin, considering the normal level to be 1.0. (From ref. 13, with permission.)

corded points are plasma concentrations of circulating angiotensin II at the different levels of sodium output, as calculated from plasma renin activity levels (13). Note that at the lowermost point for the "normal" curve the concentration of angiotensin was calculated to be three times normal. However, at the uppermost point, the angiotensin was calculated to be 0, showing a decreasing angiotensin as one proceeds from the bottom to the top of the curve.

Now, study the other two curves. The curve to the right was measured in the same way as the normal salt-loading renal function curve but in animals that received continuous infusion of angiotensin II; this kept the circulating level of angiotensin II nearly constant and at a high level during the many days of the experiment. Note that the upper portion of this curve is shifted far to the right along the pressure axis, but at the lowest level of sodium output the lower tip of this curve is almost coincident with the lower tip of the normal curve.

The curve to the left in Fig. 6 was recorded in the same manner as the other two curves, except that now the converting enzyme inhibitor captopril (SQ-14,225) was infused continually throughout the experiment to block the formation of angiotensin II; the result was an angiotensin II concentration always maintained at zero. Note that the lowermost portion of this curve is shifted far to the left whereas the upper tip of the curve (at high sodium level) is almost coincident with the upper tip of the normal curve.

Thus, the left-hand curve in the figure is the salt-loading renal function curve for an animal with no circulating angiotensin II, and the right-hand curve is for an animal with a constantly elevated level of angiotensin II. For the normal curve, the angiotensin II changes progressively at different levels of sodium intake, beginning at the bottom with a high level of circulating angiotensin (a value of 3.0) and proceeding to zero angiotensin at the top. One can see that when an animal is on a very low level of salt intake, with a concomitant high level of naturally formed angiotensin II, the normal kidney is actually operating on the bottom of the high angiotensin curve. Then, when the animal is on very high salt intake, with concomitant decrease in angiotensin to zero, the kidney then operates on the zero angiotensin curve. Thus the "normal" curve is very steep because of the feedback effects of the renin-angiotensin control system to alter sodium retention by the kidneys.

The Renin-Angiotensin System Allows the Normal Person to Eat Very Small or Very Large Amounts of Salt with Very Little Change in Arterial Pressure

We can now return to the role of the renin-angiotensin system and its relationship to the renal-fluid volume mechanism for pressure control, and ask the simple

question: What is the importance of the renin-angiotensin system in the regulation of arterial pressure in the normal animal or normal person? To help answer this, Fig. 7 replots the data of Fig. 6 after transposing the axes—now showing sodium intake on the abscissa and mean arterial pressure on the ordinate. The lowermost curve shows the effects caused by administering captopril (SQ-14,225) to cause zero circulating angiotensin, and the uppermost curve shows the effects of high circulating angiotensin caused by continuous infusion of angiotensin. The center curve is for the normal animal. Note the extreme range of sodium intake and yet almost no change in arterial pressure in the normal animal. But in both the other conditions, when the renin-angiotensin system was unable to change its level of activity, the pressure changed ten times as much.

Almost identical studies to those illustrated for dogs by the middle curve of Fig. 7 have been run by Murray et al. (17) in normal human beings, with virtually the same results. The salt intake was varied over several days from 10 to 1,500 mEq sodium per day, and the pressure changed only a few millimeters of mercury despite the 150-fold change in salt intake.

Therefore, in normal arterial pressure regulation, the interaction of the renin-angiotensin system with the renal-fluid volume mechanism for pressure control provides an excellent example of how a pressure-regulating subsystem (the renin-angiotensin system) can modify a primary system (the fluid volume system) to achieve ad-

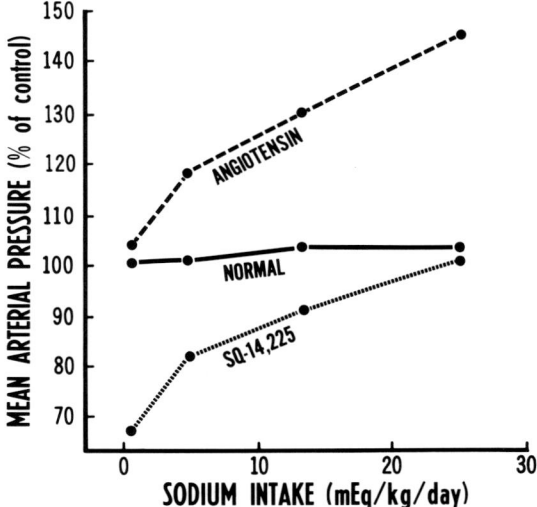

FIG. 7. Replot of the data in Fig. 6 but with sodium intake represented on the abscissa and mean arterial pressure on the ordinate. The *solid curve* demonstrates that when the renin-angiotensin system is functioning normally, a person or an animal can increase or decrease sodium intake as much as 50-fold without significant alteration of the arterial pressure. The other two curves demonstrate that this is not true when the renin-angiotensin system is blocked by captopril infusion or angiotensin infusion. (Modified from ref. 13.)

ditional optimization—in this case to allow the aborigines of central Australia and Brazil to have normal arterial pressures despite sodium intakes of only a few milliequivalents per day, and yet also to allow persons who eat several hundred milliequivalents of salt per day such as residents of northern Japan also to have normal arterial pressures for many of their early years (before secondary effects of the excess sodium might cause hypertension).

Use of Salt-Loading Renal Function Curves for Predicting Long-Term Arterial Pressures in Multiple Different Kidney Conditions

Figure 8 illustrates the approximate salt-loading chronic renal function curves for different kidney conditions. Several of these curves have been measured in detail at multiple levels of salt loading. Others have been measured and/or estimated at only a few isolated points and the curves constructed from these points.

Note also in Fig. 8 two horizontal lines depicting, respectively, a low level of sodium intake and a high level. Some of the salt-loading curves are very steep, such as for the normal person. When this is true, the level of salt intake makes very little difference in the predicted pressure level because the function curve crosses the low and high salt intake lines at approximately the same pressure.

On the other hand, in several abnormal kidney conditions, such as renal medullary lesions, reduced renal mass, infusion of aldosterone, infusion of angiotensin, and reduced glomerular filtration coefficient, one can see that the arterial pressure is quite "salt-sensitive"; that is,

the pressure changes greatly when the level of salt intake changes.

Salt-loading renal function curves can be quite useful in predicting the effects of many therapeutic agents for treating hypertension. This is currently being explored in a series of studies by Kimura and his colleagues (18,19) at the National Cardiovascular Institute in Japan. In patients who have salt-sensitive types of hypertension, the natriuretic drugs (diuretics) are almost always effective in reducing the arterial pressure. In those patients who have salt-insensitive hypertension (steep slope of the salt-loading renal function curve), the natriuretic drugs are not very effective; for these types of hypertension, the therapy must shift the curve to the left in Fig. 8. The types of drugs that have this effect, based on preliminary information, are those that directly vasodilate the renal arteries or function indirectly by blocking the renin-angiotensin system—especially the converting enzyme inhibitors (20).

HOW DOES INCREASED FLUID VOLUME INCREASE THE ARTERIAL PRESSURE AND CAUSE HYPERTENSION?

Many hypertension research workers have had difficulty in understanding the long-term increase in arterial pressure in response to increased extracellular fluid volume because even in severe essential hypertension the extracellular fluid volume, blood volume, and cardiac output are usually very near to normal. Instead, it is total peripheral resistance that is increased instead of extracellular fluid volume, blood volume, and cardiac output. If this is true, then how can the renal-fluid volume mechanism possibly be implicated as the major cause of the high pressure? To provide a starting point for answering this question, let us summarize data collected in multiple experiments caused by volume loading in animals with reduced kidney excretion capability.

During Development of Volume-Loading Hypertension, the Extracellular Fluid Volume and Blood Volume Increase First, Followed by Increased Arterial Pressure and Even Later by Increased Total Peripheral Resistance

Figure 9 summarizes the approximate average results of multiple volume-loading experiments performed over a period of weeks in dogs (8,10,11,13). Kidney mass had already been reduced to about 30 percent of normal by removing the poles of one kidney and the entire second kidney. Then on day 0 isotonic saline infusion was started to increase the salt intake to approximately five to six times normal. The figure shows that many factors

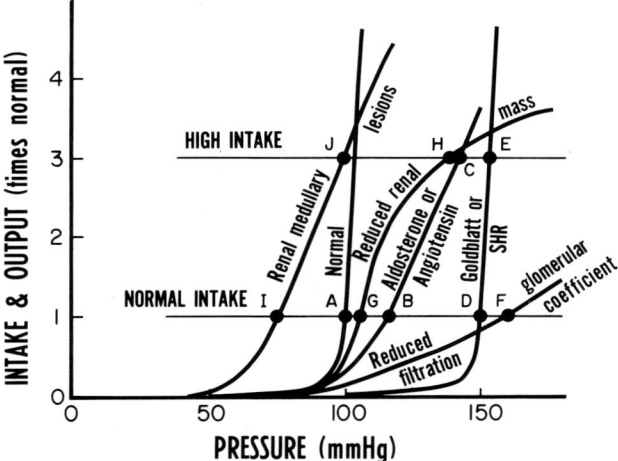

FIG. 8. Equilibration of multiple salt-loading renal function curves for different kidney conditions with normal salt intake and high salt intake. Note that for some renal conditions the equilibration pressure changes greatly with the level of salt intake, whereas for other conditions the equilibrium pressure changes hardly at all. (From ref. 13, with permission.)

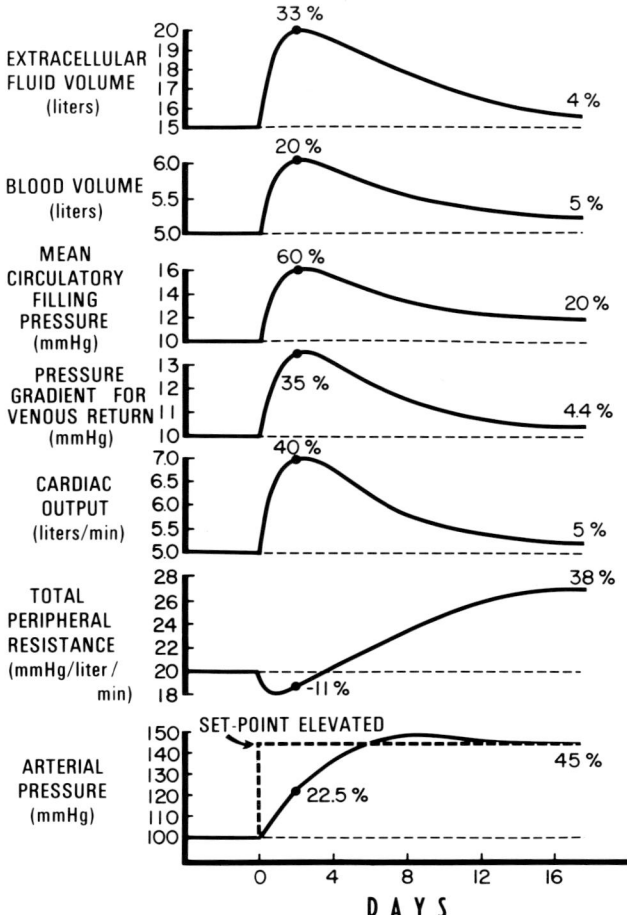

FIG. 9. Approximate transient hemodynamic changes that occurred in dogs during the development of volume-loading hypertension. Approximately 70% of the renal mass had been removed several weeks in advance. Then, after day 0, isotonic saline solution was continuously infused intravenously at a rate about five times the normal salt intake of the animals. (From ref. 13, with permission.)

changed as hypertension developed, as described in the following subsections.

The Fluid Volumes, Cardiac Output, and Mean Circulatory Filling Pressure Increase Initially

At the onset of hypertension, five factors increased greatly almost exactly in parallel with each other, shown by the five uppermost curves of the figure for (a) extracellular fluid volume, (b) blood volume, (c) mean circulatory filling pressure, (d) pressure gradient for venous return, and (e) cardiac output. However, by the end of 10 days to 2 weeks, which was also when the hypertensive pressure had reached a steady-state level, four of these five factors had returned to within about 5 percent of normal, the exception being the mean circulatory filling

pressure, which stabilized at a value about 20 percent above normal.

Significance of the Continued Elevation of the Mean Circulatory Filling Pressure

The mean circulatory filling pressure is the pressure that exists in all parts of the circulation when the heart has been stopped and the blood volume has become redistributed in the system until all pressures are at equilibrium. It is the elevated mean circulatory filling pressure during volume loading that keeps extra blood flowing from the periphery to the heart and therefore keeps driving the heart to maintain, in the steady state, a slightly elevated cardiac output (21).

The importance of the mean circulatory filling pressure in multiple types of hypertension has been demonstrated. It has been found to be elevated in spontaneously hypertensive rats; renal wrap hypertensive dogs; one-kidney, one-clip hypertensive dogs; angiotensin infusion hypertensive dogs; aldosterone infusion hypertensive dogs; volume-loading hypertensive dogs; and in several different types of acute hypertension such as norepinephrine infusion hypertension, hypertension caused by compression of the brain, and hypertension caused by occluding the two common carotid arteries to elicit the carotid sinus reflex (13). Yet in the chronic stages of virtually all of these different types of hypertension the blood volume has only rarely been measured to be increased more than 5 percent to 10 percent above normal, and in some hypertension the volume is even below normal. This suggests that it is not increased blood volume alone that causes, or attempts to cause, increased return of blood to the heart in hypertension. Instead, it is the ratio of the blood volume to the physical capacity of the circulation, as expressed by the mean circulatory filling pressure, that does this (22). The fact that the mean circulatory filling pressure is high in all types of hypertension even though most often the blood volume is only slightly increased, or perhaps normal or even low, suggests that the actual physical capacity and/or capacitance of the circulatory system has been reduced in most hypertensive states, either as a result of continuous vascular muscle contraction or as a result of structural reduction of the vascular dimensions. Under such conditions, even a normal blood volume is sufficient to overfill the system, giving an elevated mean circulatory filling pressure and ultimate hypertension.

Total Peripheral Resistance Increases Secondarily During Development of Volume-Loading Hypertension

Especially interesting are the changes in total peripheral resistance that occur during development of volume-loading hypertension. During the first several days, as shown in Fig. 9, the total peripheral resistance decreases, but after 3 to 4 days it has returned to normal; subsequently it rises far above normal, increasing almost as much percentage-wise as the arterial pressure had already risen. Thus, two separate phases in the changes in total peripheral resistance are significant. Most of the initial decrease in total peripheral resistance was explained by Cowley and Guyton (23), who performed this same volume-loading type of hypertension in dogs whose baroreceptor nerves had been sectioned. In these dogs the initial decrease in total peripheral resistance did not occur. Therefore, the initial decrease in total peripheral resistance was mainly caused by peripheral arteriolar dilatation resulting from baroreceptor reflex activation when the arterial pressure began to rise.

Total Peripheral Resistance Increases After the Hypertension Has Already Developed in Volume-Loading Hypertension

The lowermost panel of Fig. 9 illustrates the arterial pressure rise at the onset of volume-loading hypertension. Because the total peripheral resistance decreased initially, the early rise in arterial pressure was caused entirely by the initial increase in cardiac output, not even to the slightest extent by increased total peripheral resistance; the total peripheral resistance at this time was actually reduced.

Yet, during the ensuing week and a half after the hypertension had already reached or almost reached full height, the fluid volumes and the cardiac output all fell almost all the way back toward normal while the total peripheral resistance increased. Thus, the hypertension converted from a high cardiac output hypertension to a high total peripheral resistance hypertension.

Conversion of the Initial High Cardiac Output Hypertension to a Permanent High Total Peripheral Resistance Hypertension Is Caused Mainly by Autoregulation

"Autoregulation" means automatic readjustment of local tissue blood flow back to or near to normal whenever it becomes too high or too low. In most tissues, autoregulation is believed to result from the following mechanism: When the blood flow to a tissue becomes greater than normal, the excess flow delivers increased amounts of oxygen and/or other nutrients to the tissues and also removes greater quantities of carbon dioxide and other metabolic products from the tissues (24). For reasons that are not completely established, the delivery of extra oxygen and other nutrients and/or excess removal of the metabolic end products causes the blood vessels to constrict.

Therefore, one can readily understand that when the arterial pressure rises and increases tissue blood flow above normal, this local autoregulatory process occurs in almost all parts of the body, leading to constriction of the local blood vessels. This constriction, in turn, decreases the venous return of blood to the heart, thus decreasing cardiac output back near to normal, but at the same time increases the total peripheral resistance instead.

One immediately sees the applicability of the autoregulatory principle to the events illustrated in Fig. 9. At the onset of the volume-loading hypertension, the blood flow to the tissues (the cardiac output) was very great. But then, during the 2 weeks of the experiment, the blood flow decreased progressively back toward normal while the total peripheral resistance increased and maintained the arterial pressure in the hypertensive state.

Without going into details, a large number of physiological experiments and histologic studies have shown that the increase in total peripheral resistance during the first hours of the autoregulation process is caused by contraction of the smooth muscle in the arteriolar walls mainly in response to increased tissue oxygen or decreased metabolic end products (24–27). But, then, over a period of days and weeks, the data show progressive anatomical hypertrophy of the arteriolar walls that convert the initial vasoconstrictive increase in resistance into a structural increase in resistance (28–32).

High-Volume States are Not Always Associated with Hypertension

Several research workers have pointed out specific high-volume states that are not associated with hypertension. Sometimes, they have incorrectly used these to support the concept that increased body-fluid volume has little to do with the development of hypertension. However, in all or virtually all such instances, the reason why the high extracellular fluid volume or blood volume occasionally does not cause hypertension is quite well known (33–35). To give a single example, let us understand the high blood volume that occurs in heart failure and other heart debilities (33). In acute cardiac debility, the arterial pressure initially falls, which in turn causes the kidney output of water and salt to become acutely reduced. This, in turn, causes a buildup of body fluid, increasing both the extracellular fluid volume and blood volume. If the heart debility is not too great, the increase in blood volume will eventually return the cardiac output and arterial pressure back to normal despite the weakened heart, at which time the kidneys begin again to function normally. Obviously, the increased volume in this instance simply brings the circulation from a hypodynamic state up to a normal state, rather than promoting the hyperdynamic state of hypertension.

Excess Body Sodium Causes Hypertension Only When It Increases the Extracellular Fluid Volume

The causal relationship between excess sodium retention and hypertension is well known. Yet what is the mechanism by which excess sodium causes the hypertension? Theoretically it would be possible for excess sodium to cause hypertension in several different ways. One would be to cause secondary fluid retention in the body and thus cause volume-loading hypertension, as we have already discussed in this chapter. Other possible mechanisms would be (a) a direct effect of sodium to constrict the arterioles throughout the body, (b) indirect effects of sodium to alter the secretion of hormones that affect the circulation, and (c) altering neural control of the circulation.

To test the relative importance of sodium acting through the volume mechanism versus its other possible effects, Norman et al. (36) increased the total exchangeable sodium in animals about 20 percent. In half the animals, plasma sodium concentration was increased an average of 23 mEq/L by hemodialysis using a high-sodium dialysate, while extracellular fluid volume was maintained at normal levels by ultrafiltration. In the second group, plasma sodium concentration was kept at normal levels during dialysis, while extracellular fluid volume was expanded 20 percent by infusion. Figure 10 illustrates the results from these two separate procedures. The solid points on the graph show the effect on arterial pressure of increasing the exchangeable sodium but without an increase in extracellular fluid volume. The arterial pressure rose from a mean level of 93 mm Hg to a mean level of 98 mm Hg, a rise that was not statistically significant. On the other hand, when the volume was allowed to increase along with the exchangeable sodium, the pressure rose from a mean value of 96 mm Hg to a mean value of 142 mm Hg, an increase of 46 mm Hg. Thus, this experiment suggested very strongly that virtually all, if not all, of the effect of sodium to cause hypertension results from the secondarily increased extracellular fluid volume caused by the high body sodium.

In another series of experiments, Manning et al. (37) employed in dogs a combination of hypotonic saline infusion along with administration of small amounts of antidiuretic hormone to increase the blood volume to approximately 25 percent above normal even though the plasma sodium concentration fell from 144 mEq/L all the way down to 123 mEq/L. The arterial pressure rose an average of 47 percent; thus, a severe volume-loading hypertension occurred despite the fall in sodium concentration far below normal. If sodium concentration per se rather than volume were the important factor, the pressure should have declined rather than have risen. Therefore, again the results suggest that sodium concentration per se is of little or no importance. Instead, it is the vol-

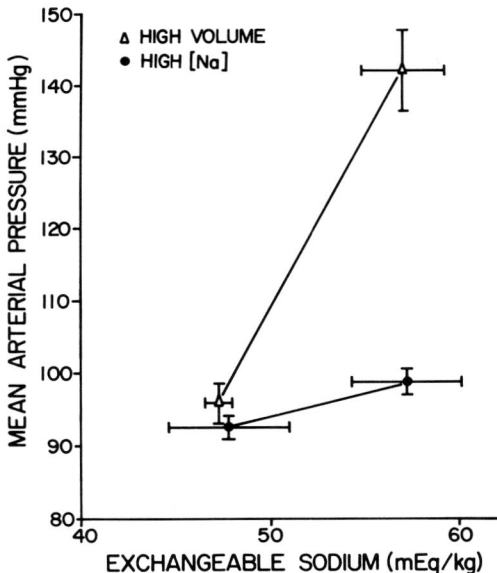

FIG. 10. Effect of different levels of exchangeable sodium in two series of sheep: (●) when the sheep were dehydrated so that they could not increase their extracellular fluid volume along with the increasing exchangeable sodium; (△) when the extracellular fluid volume of the sheep was allowed to increase along with the increase in exchangeable sodium. (From ref. 36, with permission.)

ume increase that accompanies salt retention that is important.

THE RESISTANCE AXIS FOR CAUSING HYPERTENSION—CHRONIC HYPERTENSION OCCURS FOLLOWING AN INCREASE IN RESISTANCE ONLY WHEN THIS OCCURS BETWEEN THE HEART AND THE KIDNEY TUBULES

This section answers the question, Under what conditions can an increase in peripheral resistance cause persistent, chronic hypertension? Let us begin by listing those types of increases in resistance that are known to be followed by the development of persistent hypertension: (a) coarctation of the aorta above the kidneys (29,30), (b) increased renal arterial resistance (38), (c) increased renal afferent arteriolar resistance (39), and (d) increased glomerular membrane resistance (decreased filtration coefficient) (40).

A primary increase in the resistance in other arteries of the body besides those listed above ordinarily will not cause chronic hypertension. In fact, specific studies by multiple researchers on constriction of the aorta below the kidneys, constriction of the arteries to the limbs, or chronic constriction of the arteries to the head have

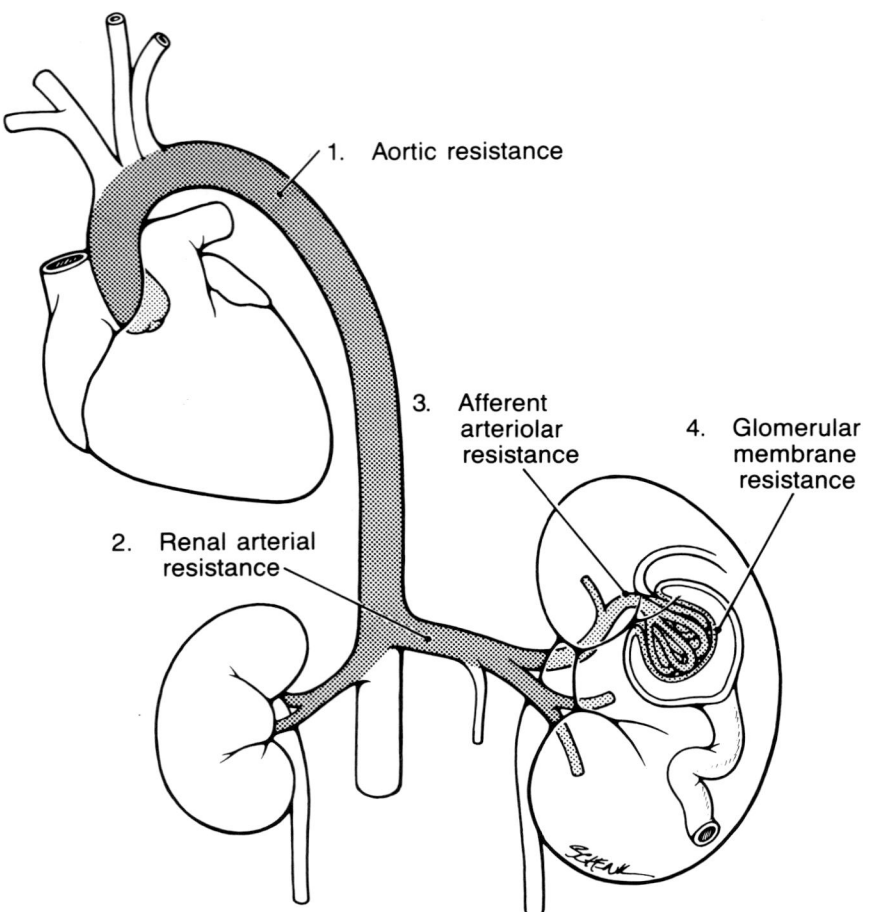

FIG. 11. The resistance axis of hypertension. An increase in resistance at any point in the *shaded area* of this figure will invariably cause chronic hypertension. An increase in resistance at any other point in the circulation has not been proved to cause chronic hypertension. (From A. C. Guyton, Collected Illustrations, Department of Physiology and Biophysics, University of Mississippi Medical Center.)

failed to elicit long-term hypertension. Therefore, Fig. 11 illustrates what we have named the "resistance axis of hypertension." This figure shows a shaded area from the root of the aorta all the way to the glomerular membrane, including the glomerular membrane itself. At any point along this course, increased resistance seems invariably to cause persistent hypertension, which seems not to be true for increases in arterial resistance anywhere else within the circulatory system.

To develop this thesis still further, Fig. 12 illustrates the approximate effects on arterial pressure and cardiac output of different levels of total peripheral resistance in multiple clinical conditions (13). Note specifically that it is not arterial pressure that is altered by the different abnormal total peripheral resistances, but instead the cardiac output. In fact, the cardiac output in each instance is almost the exact reciprocal of the total peripheral resistance in each instance while the arterial pressure is normal. However, note very carefully the following point: *None of the clinical conditions represented in Fig. 12 is known to affect the resistance significantly anywhere along the resistance axis of hypertension illustrated in Fig. 11.*

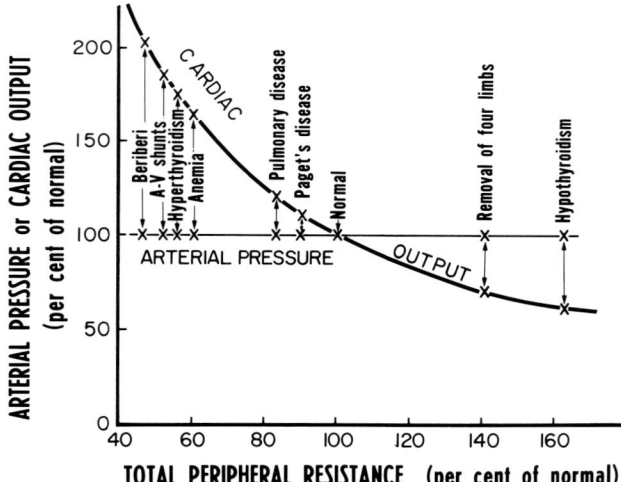

FIG. 12. Relationship of total peripheral resistance to both arterial pressure and cardiac output in different clinical conditions, but when the increase in resistance does not include increased resistance anywhere along the "resistance axis of hypertension." This figure illustrates an inverse relationship between total peripheral resistance and cardiac output but no definitive effect of total peripheral resistance change on arterial pressure. (From ref. 13, with permission.)

THE BODY CANNOT CONTROL ARTERIAL PRESSURE LONG-TERM IN THE ABSENCE OF THE RENAL-FLUID VOLUME MECHANISM FOR PRESSURE CONTROL

In Fig. 3, which compares the feedback gains of most of the important arterial pressure-regulating mechanisms, only the renal-fluid volume mechanism was shown to have infinite gain. It is this infinite gain feature that allows this mechanism to override all the other pressure regulators of the body. Yet, another question must still be asked: Are all the other pressure control mechanisms capable of controlling the arterial pressure long-term without a functioning renal-fluid volume pressure control mechanism?

We initially studied this question in the 1960s and 1970s using mathematical computer models of the circulatory pressure control systems. In these models it was possible to eliminate the renal-fluid volume pressure controller by simply writing the appropriate equations (41). When this was done, the systemic arterial pressure drifted steadily in one direction or another. And when the slightest abnormality of the circulation was instituted—such as a slight increase in rate of salt intake—the rate of arterial pressure drift became very rapid, reaching a pressure so high in the case of excess salt intake that it culminated in congestive heart failure and fulminating edema within a few weeks. But this was only a mathematical model.

In 1984, Hall and his coworkers (42) succeeded in developing an animal experimental model in which the renal-fluid volume mechanism for pressure control was prevented from functioning. This was achieved by using an electronically controlled servocontrol mechanism to activate automatically a hydraulic constrictor around the aorta above the renal arteries whenever the renal arterial pressure attempted to rise above the original control value. Thus, this procedure maintained the renal arterial pressure always at its original control level. Therefore, when the central arterial pressure became elevated, the kidneys did not experience this pressure rise and could not respond with increased fluid loss. Figure

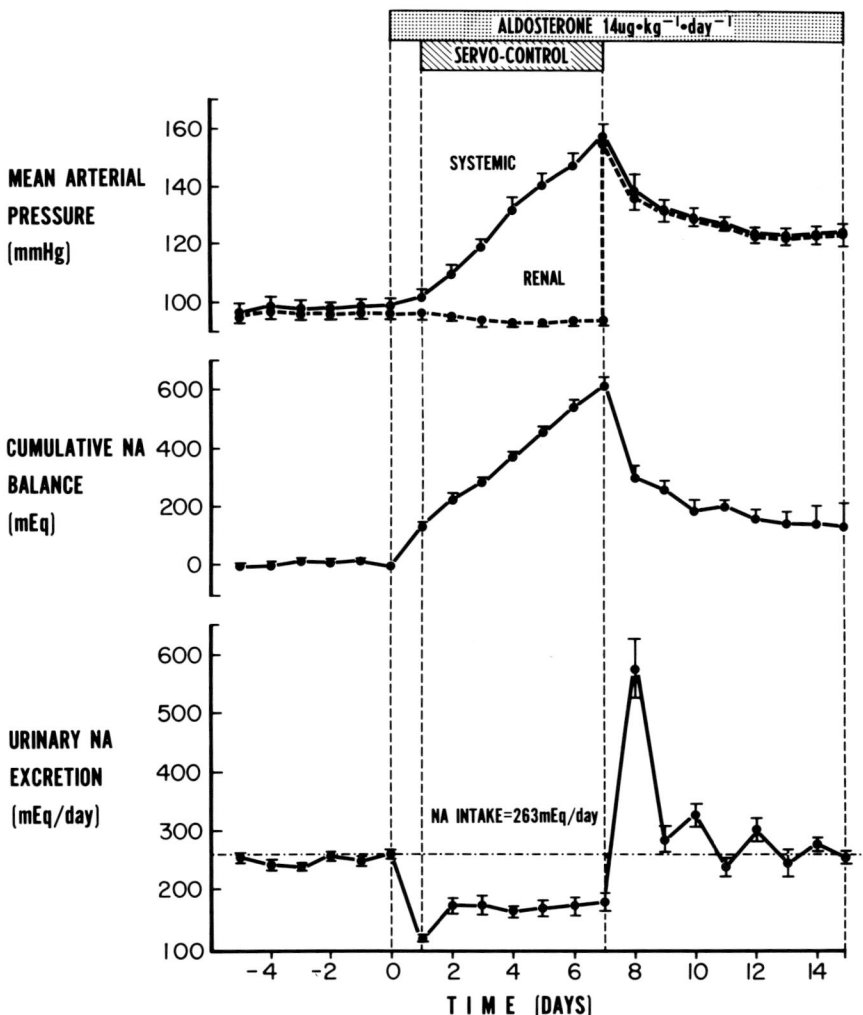

FIG. 13. Effect of aldosterone on mean arterial pressure, cumulative sodium balance, and urinary sodium excretion under two sequential conditions: for 7 days during which time the renal arterial pressure was prevented from rising by an electronic servocontrol device; for another 8 days after removing the servocontrol so that the renal arterial pressure then rose to equal the systemic arterial pressure. Note the inability of the circulatory system to achieve a steady-state pressure level when the renal-fluid volume feedback mechanism was blocked. (From ref. 42, with permission.)

13 illustrates the results of a study using this technique, as follows: To cause salt retention, dogs were given a continuous infusion of aldosterone for slightly over 2 weeks. During the first part of the aldosterone infusion, the renal servocontrol mechanism was used to keep the renal arterial pressure exactly at its control level, as illustrated by the dashed curve in the top panel of the figure, even though the animal's systemic arterial pressure increased steadily. In the absence of any increase in renal pressure the kidneys could not excrete the excess amounts of salt reabsorbed by the renal tubules in response to the aldosterone. Consequently, the sodium balance (middle panel) showed continued accumulation of sodium without any relief. At the end of 7 days, the dogs were already developing signs of congestive heart failure. At this time, the servocontrol mechanism was turned off, and the renal arterial pressure was allowed to rise to equal the systemic arterial pressure. Instantaneously, the kidneys began to excrete the excess salt (shown by the lowest panel). During the next week the arterial pressure returned to the lower level that was appropriate to maintain fluid balance for the rate of aldosterone infusion. Thus, it was clear from this experiment that the renal-fluid volume mechanism allowed the circulatory system to escape from the sodium accumulation effects of aldosterone, because the rising pressure acted on the kidneys to cause pressure natriuresis, thus balancing out the sodium-retaining effects of the aldosterone.

Hall and his colleagues (43,44) also performed this same experiment using other stresses on the circulation. The results were the same, namely uncontrolled increase in arterial pressure culminating in congestive heart failure when the renal-fluid volume mechanism for pressure control was blocked from functioning.

Therefore, animal experiments as well as computer model theory all demonstrate that it is impossible for the other pressure control mechanisms of the circulation, when acting independently of the renal-fluid volume mechanism, to control the arterial pressure in a stable manner over a long period of time.

ESSENTIAL HYPERTENSION ALMOST CERTAINLY IS A VOLUME-LOADING TYPE OF HYPERTENSION

Figure 14 illustrates two typical salt-loading renal function curves drawn from clinical data in essential hypertensive patients, showing definitive shift of the curves in the hypertensive direction (45). One of the essential hypertension curves is almost exactly parallel to the normal curve but shifted to a higher pressure range. This type of curve is typical of the non–salt-sensitive type of essential hypertension, because changing the salt intake changes the arterial pressure hardly at all, illustrated by the very slight pressure change from point A to point B. The other curve shows a much less steep slope, a shift

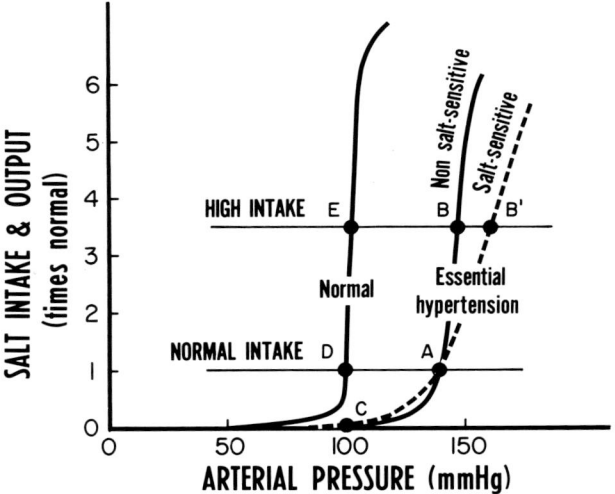

FIG. 14. Salt-loading renal function curves for the normal person, the non–salt-sensitive essential hypertensive person, and the salt-sensitive essential hypertensive person, showing also equilibration of these curves with either normal or high salt intake. (From ref. 13, with permission.)

from point A to point B'; this is characteristic of salt-sensitive hypertension, because changing the level of salt intake in this instance does have a pronounced effect on the arterial pressure.

Observe in Fig. 14 that both of the essential hypertensive salt-loading renal function curves are shifted into a far higher than normal arterial pressure range. Therefore, in each type of patient the renal-fluid volume mechanism for pressure control is set to a higher than normal pressure range. This explains why essential hypertensive patients undergoing anesthesia often exhibit anuria when the arterial pressure falls to normal, a widely observed principle in the practice of anesthesiology; a normal pressure is simply too low to maintain normal urinary output of water and salt.

Therefore, essential hypertension almost certainly is a volume-loading type of hypertension caused by failure of the kidneys to eliminate enough salt and water at normal pressure levels. However, because of the usual slowness in the development of essential hypertension, developing over a period of many years, and with the pressure rising only a few millimeters per year, one usually finds no evidence that the person has gone through the volume-loading phase that precedes by only a few days to weeks the secondary conversion to the increased total peripheral resistance phase that then lasts for the remainder of the person's lifetime (46,47).

A Possible Smooth Muscle–Genetic Theory for Volume-Loading Essential Hypertension

In recent years, many investigators have suggested that hypertension begins as a genetic abnormality of vascular smooth muscle throughout the body (48). The thesis is that a genetic abnormality of ion transport through the smooth muscle cell membrane causes arteriolar constriction everywhere in the body, thus increasing the total peripheral resistance. It is almost universally suggested that the increase in total peripheral resistance is the primary cause of the hypertension. Yet we have seen from the analyses in this chapter that any increase in total peripheral resistance that does not cause retention of salt and water by the kidneys cannot cause hypertension. On the other hand, if the genetic smooth muscle abnormality increases the degree of constriction of the afferent arterioles of the kidneys at the same time that it also causes increased constriction everywhere else in the body, this would indeed cause hypertension. However, note especially that it is increased arteriolar resistance in the kidneys that is the essential step in causing the persistent hypertension, not the increase in total peripheral resistance throughout the body, for the hypertension would have developed in response to renal fluid retention even if there had been no increase in vascular resistance anywhere else in the body besides in the renal arterioles.

Unfortunately, there is almost no absolute evidence that such a genetic–smooth muscle–renal-volume-loading mechanism actually occurs in human essential hypertension. Yet Gothberg (39) has demonstrated in the spontaneously hypertensive rat that the basic renal afferent arteriolar resistance is indeed greatly increased in at least this one type of genetically hypertensive animal. Furthermore, since this spontaneous rat hypertension is genetically inherited, it is possible that the increased afferent arteriolar resistance results from a genetic factor. The question that is unanswered is whether this results from a generalized smooth muscle genetic abnormality in the entire body or from some specific genetically determined local change in the kidney afferent arterioles themselves.

Even though it has not been possible to test in animal experiments the genetic concepts discussed above, the same genetic concepts have been tested in a mathematical computer model of the circulation (49). Intriguingly, when all arteriolar resistances of the entire body are increased in the model, including increases in both afferent and efferent resistances in the kidneys, the computer results are very similar to those of essential hypertension. But, *if the increase in renal afferent resistance is left out while the resistance is increased in all the other arterioles of the body, no hypertension will occur!*

SUMMARY

The thesis of this chapter has been that the renal-fluid volume mechanism for arterial pressure regulation is so powerful that it literally dominates all long-term pressure regulation. This is true because, under almost all condi-tions, this mechanism has infinite feedback gain for controlling arterial pressure, whereas none of the other arterial pressure–regulating mechanisms has this characteristic. In fact, both animal experiments and computer analyses suggest that all the other pressure-regulating mechanisms operating together do not, in the absence of the renal-fluid volume pressure-regulating mechanism, have the capability to maintain the arterial pressure in the normal range for longer than a few days at most.

An important feature of the renal-fluid volume mechanism is that in the long-term chronic state almost unmeasurable increases in extracellular fluid volume, blood volume, and cardiac output seem to be sufficient to cause marked elevation of the arterial pressure. A physiological mechanism that allows these very small increases in volumes and cardiac output to increase the arterial pressure markedly is the phenomenon of peripheral blood flow autoregulation. The autoregulation process does not change the level to which the arterial pressure will rise, for that is determined by the renal-fluid volume mechanism; what it does do is to reduce very, very greatly the amounts of increased extracellular fluid volume, blood volume, and cardiac output required to achieve the elevated pressure level. It does this by converting the initial high cardiac output hypertension caused by excess volume loading into a high peripheral resistance hypertension while returning the cardiac output and fluid volume so near to normal that abnormal values are difficult to detect.

The renin-angiotensin system interacts with the renal-fluid volume mechanism for pressure control in an especially unique and valuable manner: it allows the normal animal or normal human being to eat tremendously varying amounts of salt from day to day or week to week without causing major variations in arterial pressure. The reason for this is that when one eats excessive amounts of salt the level of circulating angiotensin decreases markedly, which in turn causes the kidneys to shift the renal function curve to a lower pressure range. Therefore, even though the increased salt intake does have a direct effect to increase the blood pressure, the shift of the function curve in the opposite direction provides about 90 percent compensation in the degree of pressure rise that actually occurs. Thus, the renin-angiotensin system functions as a very valuable *subsystem* of the renal-fluid volume mechanism for pressure control to stabilize the pressure level in the face of tremendous changes in the salt in the diet from as little as one-tenth normal to as high as ten times normal.

REFERENCES

1. Guyton AC. *Hypertension* 1992;19:I2–I8.
2. Guyton AC. *Science* 1991;252:1813–1816.
3. Guyton AC. *Am J Physiol* 1990;259:R865–877.
4. Guyton AC. *Hypertension* 1990;16:725–730.

5. Dobbs WA, Prather JW, Guyton AC. *Am J Cardiol* 1971;27:507–512.
6. Selkurt EE, Hall PW, Spencer MP. *Am J Physiol* 1949;159:369–378.
7. Thompson DD, Pitts RF. *Am J Physiol* 1952;168:490–499.
8. Langston JB, Guyton AC, Douglas BH, Dorsett PE. *Circ Res* 1963;12:508–513.
9. Douglas BH, Guyton AC, Langston JB, Bishop VS. *Am J Physiol* 1964;207:669–671.
10. Coleman TG, Guyton AC. *Circ Res* 1969;25:152–160.
11. Manning RD Jr, Coleman TG, Guyton AC, Norman RA Jr, McCaa RE. *Am J Physiol* 1979;236:R40–R47.
12. Young DB, Pan YJ, Guyton AC. *Am J Physiol* 1977;232:R145–R149.
13. Guyton AC. *Arterial pressure and hypertension.* Philadelphia: WB Saunders, 1980.
14. Guyton AC. *Textbook of medical physiology.* Philadelphia: WB Saunders, 1991.
15. Guyton AC, Coleman TG, Cowley AW, Scheel KW, Manning RD, Norman RA. *Am J Med* 1972;52:584–594.
16. DeClue JW, Guyton AC, Cowley AW, Coleman TG, Norman RA, McCaa RE. *Circ Res* 1978;43:503–512.
17. Murray RH, Luft FC, Bloch R, Weyman AE. *Proc Soc Exp Biol Med* 1978;159:432–436.
18. Kimura G, Saito F, Deguchi F, et al. *J Hypertens* 1986;4:S192–S194.
19. Kimura G, Saito F, Kojima S, et al. *Hypertension* 1987;10:11–15.
20. Hall JE, Guyton AC, Smith MJ, Coleman TG. *Am J Physiol* 1980;239:F271–F280.
21. Guyton AC. *Physiol Rev* 1955;35:123–129.
22. Richardson TQ, Stallings JO, Guyton AC. *Am J Physiol* 1961;201:471–474.
23. Cowley AW Jr, Guyton AC. *Circ Res* 1975;36:536–546.
24. Johnson PC, Ed. *Autoregulation of blood flow.* New York: American Heart Association, 1964.
25. Jones RD, Berne RM. *Circ Res* 1964;15(suppl I):I30–I38.
26. Guyton AC, Ross JM, Carier RO Jr, Walker JR. *Circ Res* 1964;14:60–69.
27. Granger HJ, Guyton AC. *Circ Res* 1969;25:379–388.
28. Lassen N. *Physiol Rev* 1959;39:183–238.
29. Wakim KG, Slaughter O, Clagett OT. *Proc Mayo Clin* 1948;23:347–351.
30. Patterson GC, Shepherd JT, Whelan RF. *Clin Sci* 1957;16:627–632.
31. Stanek KA, Coleman TG, Murphy WR. *Hypertension* 1987;9:611–618.
32. Folkow B, Hallback M, Lundgren Y, Sivertsson R, Weiss L. *Circ Res* 1973;32/33:I2–I38.
33. Friedberg CK. *Diseases of the heart,* 3rd ed. Philadelphia: WB Saunders, 1966;254.
34. Manning RD, Guyton AC. Conditions which can prevent the development of volume-loading hypertension. In: Seki K, Casley-Smith JR, Andreoli TE, eds. *Edema: recent advances.* Tokyo: 1984;271–279.
35. Manning RD. *Am J Physiol* 1987;252:F91–F98.
36. Norman RA, Coleman TG, Wiley TL, Manning RD, Guyton AC. *Am J Physiol* 1975;229:1068–1072.
37. Manning RD Jr, Guyton AC, Coleman TG, McCaa RE. *Am J Physiol* 1979;236:H314–H322.
38. Goldblatt H. *Physiol Rev* 1947;27:120–165.
39. Gothberg G. *Structural adaptation of the renal vascular bed in rats.* Goteberg: Department of Physiology, University of Goteborg, 1982.
40. Friedberg CK. *Diseases of the heart,* 3rd ed. Philadelphia: WB Saunders, 1966;1513–1515.
41. Guyton AC, Hall JE, Manning RD Jr, Norman RA Jr, DeClue JW. A systems analysis of volume regulation. In: *Alfred Benzon Symposium XI.* Copenhagen: Munksgaard, 1978;283.
42. Hall JE, Granger JP, Smith MJ, Premen AJ. *Hypertension* 1984;6:I183–I192.
43. Hall JE, Granger JP, Hester RL, Coleman TG, Smith MJ, Cross RB. *Am J Physiol* 1984;246:F627–F634.
44. Hall JE, Montani JP, Woods LL, Mizelle HL. *Am J Physiol* 1986;250:F907–F916.
45. Guyton AC, Coleman TG, Young DB, Lohmeier TE, DeClue JW. *Annu Rev Med* 1979;31:15–27.
46. Tarazi RC, Dustan HP, Frohlich ED. *Circulation* 1969;40:357–363.
47. Frohlich ED. Hemodynamics of hypertension. In: Genest J, Koiw E, Kuchel O, eds. *Hypertension.* New York: McGraw-Hill, 1977;15.
48. Postnov YV, Orlov SN. Alteration of cell membranes in primary hypertension. In: Genest J, Kuckel O, Hamet P, Cantin M, eds. *Hypertension,* 2nd ed. New York: McGraw-Hill, 1983;95–107.
49. Guyton AC, Hall JE, Montani J-P. *Acta Physiol Scand* 1988;133(suppl 571):163–174.

Hypertension: Pathophysiology, Diagnosis, and Management, Second Edition, edited by J.H. Laragh and B.M. Brenner, Raven Press, Ltd., New York © 1995.

CHAPTER 79

Salt Intake and Cardiac Hypertrophy

Roland E. Schmieder and Alfred H. Beil

Sodium homeostasis profoundly influences the cardiovascular system in normotensive and hypertensive subjects (1–3). After considerable progress has been made in defining the relationship between dietary salt intake and blood pressure, more recent attention has been focused on the relationship between dietary salt intake and another predictor of cardiovascular morbidity: left ventricular hypertrophy (LVH).

CLINICAL SIGNIFICANCE OF LEFT VENTRICULAR HYPERTROPHY

Left ventricular hypertrophy is related to cardiovascular morbidity and mortality independently of other risk factors, including hypertension. Data from the Framingham cohort showed that LVH as established by electrocardiographic evidence cannot be considered a compensatory process only, but should be viewed as a powerful independent risk factor for congestive heart failure, coronary artery disease, and sudden death (4–6).

The introduction of echocardiography in clinical praxis has made possible the noninvasive estimation of left ventricular mass. Autopsy studies have confirmed the validity of *in vivo* estimates of left ventricular mass by echocardiography (7–9).

R. E. Schmieder and A. H. Beil: Department of Internal Medicine IV, University of Erlangen-Nürnberg, Nürnberg, Germany.

Upper limits when measurements are made according to the recommendations of the American Society of Echocardiography for left ventricular mass, left ventricular mass/body surface area, and left ventricular mass/height are, respectively, 294 g, 150 g/m^2, and 163 g/m in men; and 194 g, 120 g/m^2, and 121 g/m in women (10).

Echocardiography has been shown to be far more sensitive than electrocardiography for detecting increases in left ventricular mass (11,12). As a consequence, in epidemiologic studies the prevalence of LVH is higher if analyzed by echocardiography than by electrocardiography. In 3.2 percent of Framingham Study participants ages 30 to 62 (13) and 5 percent of hypertensive subjects of the Hypertension Detection and Follow-up Program (14), evidence of LVH was found using electrocardiography. Estimates obtained by echocardiography are much higher. Prevalence ranged from 3 to 10 percent in normotensive subjects to 25 to 30 percent in hypertensives (10,15–17).

The clinical significance of LVH detected by echocardiography is well established: In a follow-up study performed on 140 hypertensive men, cardiovascular risk increased fourfold, independently of hypertension, cigarette smoking, and serum cholesterol, when LVH was shown to be present by echocardiography (18). A multiple regression analysis of data from a prospective study revealed that for any particular blood pressure, echocardiographic evidence of LVH raised the cardiovascular risk by 2.1 (19). Similar to other cardiac prog-

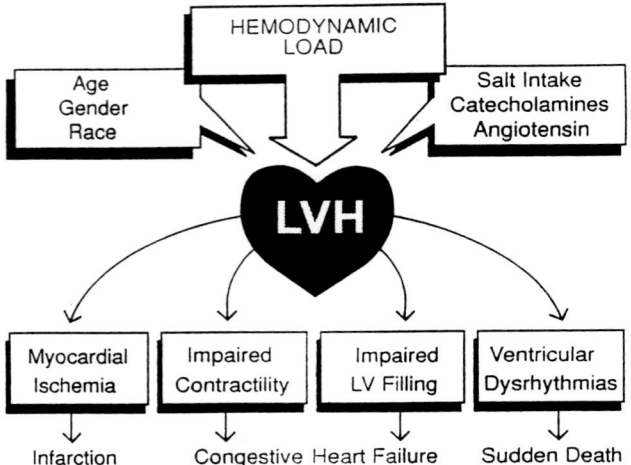

FIG. 1. Relation between relative wall thickness and sodium excretion. (From ref. 46, with permission.)

nostic factors (such as severity of coronary artery disease, left ventricular ejection fraction, sex, and age), echocardiographic evidence of LVH was shown to be an independent predictor of prognosis in more than 600 subjects whose coronary vessels and ejection fraction had been examined by angiography (20).

The observation that LVH is a risk factor per se can be explained by a variety of negative effects on myocardial structure and function caused by LVH (Fig. 1): As the ventricle becomes hypertrophic, available coronary flow is often exceeded by the demands for cellular oxygen supply. The capillary vessel density does not progress at the same rates as left ventricular mass does, and structural changes in coronary vessels impair coronary dilatation capacity (21–23). Thus, a reduction in coronary flow because of coronary artery disease may lead to a mismatch between supply and demand and contributes to myocardial ischemia and infarction (24,25). As a consequence, prognosis after myocardial infarction is worse in patients with LVH than in those without (26).

Blake and coworkers (27), by applying rest and exercise radionuclide angiography and echocardiography, demonstrated that high left ventricular mass is independently associated with exercise left ventricular dysfunction. The reduced left ventricular ejection fraction at peak exercise was the result of an exercise-induced increase in end-systolic chamber volume, associated with a diminished augmentation of cardiac output. Furthermore, left ventricular diastolic function, too, has been found to be impaired in patients with LVH (28). Diastolic dysfunction can even appear before LVH is present and before the appearance of systolic impairment. Reduced filling performance in the state of LVH is due to increasingly poor distensibility and protracted relaxation of the myocardium (28–31). Hypertensive patients with

LVH and normal coronary arteries show more frequent and more severe ventricular arrhythmias than those without LVH and normotensive healthy controls (32–34). These findings may explain the 2.5-fold increase in the incidence of cardiac sudden death in patients with electrocardiographic detected LVH (35).

SALT INTAKE AS A DETERMINANT OF LEFT VENTRICULAR HYPERTROPHY

In hypertensives, elevation of blood pressure imposes a pressure load on the left ventricle, thereby eliciting myocardial hypertrophy in the left ventricle and, according to recent results, also the right ventricle (36,37). However, in patients with mild hypertension, who represent more than 10 percent of the population, a given increase in afterload does not necessarily result in a linear increase in left ventricular mass proportionate to the pressure load. This suggests other possible contributing determinants, such as age, sex, race, obesity, blood viscosity, and neuroendocrinic stimulation, all of which have been reported to participate in the process of left ventricular adaptation (37–44).

In 1988 Schmieder et al. (45) evaluated several clinical, hemodynamic, and endocrine factors that were prone to modifying the adaptation of left ventricular structure in 42 patients with mild essential hypertension. Dietary salt intake assessed by sodium excretion over 24 hours was shown to be a powerful determinant of posterior wall thickness, relative wall thickness, and left ventricular mass. In contrast, diastolic pressure, body mass index, hematocrit, and epinephrine were found to be weaker determinants of left ventricular structure. In this study, it was therefore first reported that salt intake estimated by sodium excretion is one of the strongest predictors of posterior wall thickness and relative wall thickness independent of other variables (Figs. 2 and 3).

A similar study was performed in 66 middle-aged white male patients, all with never-treated mild essential hypertension (WHO stage I or II) (46). Analysis of this more homogeneous study population revealed significant correlations between sodium excretion and diastolic diameter of the left ventricle and with left ventricular mass. Again, dietary sodium intake was identified as the strongest determinant of cardiac structural adaptation to a persistent increase in arterial pressure. According to these results, dietary sodium intake must be regarded as a blood pressure–independent determinant of LVH in patients with essential hypertension. Since these two studies comprised previously treated and untreated, male and female, and black and white patients, one must presume that dietary salt intake participates in the hypertrophic process independently of sex, race, or duration of hypertension.

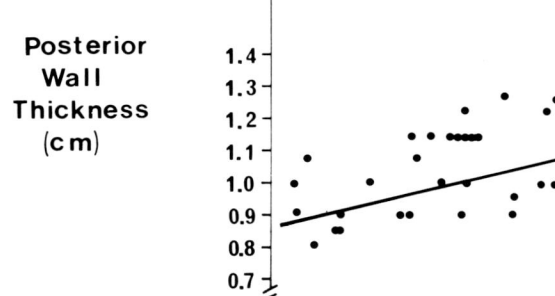

FIG. 2. Relation between posterior wall thickness and sodium excretion. (From ref. 46, with permission.)

Recently, we confirmed blood pressure–independent effects of dietary salt intake on myocardial hypertrophy in a hypertensive study population (untreated mild to moderate essential hypertension) for the first time by using ambulatory blood pressure monitoring (and not casual blood pressure) as a diagnostic tool for evaluation of the hemodynamic afterload. Sodium excretion over 24 hours correlated with relative wall thickness ($r = .41$, $p = .0125$) but not with ambulatory blood pressure values. Multiple regression analysis identified sodium excretion ($\beta = .40$, $p < .02$) in this homogeneous hypertensive group as an independent determinant for relative wall thickness, which is the classic pattern of LVH in hypertensive heart disease (unpublished data).

Data supporting these implications were presented by du Cailar et al. (47), who studied the influence of salt intake (estimated by urinary sodium excretion) on left ventricular mass in 91 never-treated patients with essential hypertension and 50 normotensive subjects. In both study groups left ventricular mass was positively correlated with urinary sodium excretion; however, the intercept with the ordinate axis was higher in the hypertensive than in the normotensive group. In other words, for a given level of salt intake, hypertensive patients have

a higher left ventricular mass index than normotensive subjects. This emphasizes the pathogenetic role of both sodium and arterial pressure in cardiac structural adaptation. In this study patients with higher concentric LVH were characterized by surprisingly lower mean arterial pressure and similar known duration of hypertension, but higher urinary sodium excretion than subjects with a lower degree of LVH.

Another great body of evidence that dietary sodium intake is an independent direct correlate of left ventricular mass was given by Daniels and colleagues (48), who studied 104 adolescents with essential hypertension. This study is noteworthy in two ways: first, because it was the first to determine the impact of dietary salt intake on LVH in a population of children and adolescents with essential hypertension—38.5 percent of the young patients were found to have LVH; and second, because dietary sodium intake was not only assessed by measurement of 24-hour sodium excretion, but also estimated via observation by a trained dietician of foods consumed and calculation of sodium intake from the known sodium composition of each food. With both methods salt intake was found to be a powerful and blood pressure–independent determinant of LVH, thus confirming pre-

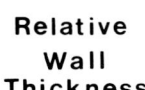

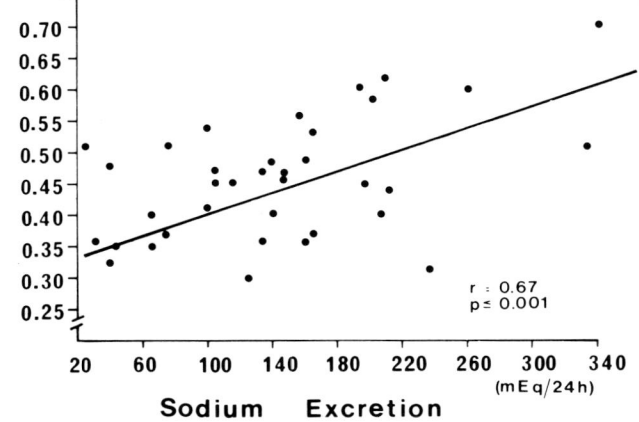

FIG. 3. Cardiac hypertrophy. Possible determinants and its influence on cardiovascular morbidity. (From ref. 46, with permission.)

vious studies using only 24-hour sodium excretion for assessment of dietary salt intake.

These data are mirrored by similar findings using animal models. Kihara et al. (49), in an attempt to elucidate the effect of chronic salt loading on heart size and biochemical composition, examined left ventricular weight and blood pressure in male Wistar-Kyoto rats who were given drinking water of a different salt content (1 percent NaCl vs tap water) over a period of 7 months. Left ventricular weight was significantly greater in the salt group than in the control groups, although there was no difference in blood pressure between the groups. Biochemical analysis of the myocardium revealed an increase in noncollagenous protein/DNA ratio and total collagen content as well as decreased DNA concentration in the left ventricle of the salt group compared with the control. Thus, hypertrophy rather than hyperplasia of myocardial cells with concomitant activation of collagen synthesis took place in this model of salt-induced cardiac hypertrophy.

De Simone et al. (50) studied the effect of different salt intakes on left ventricular mass in rats with two kidney–one clip hypertension by using echocardiography. Again, in multivariate analysis left ventricular mass was related directly to salt intake (31 percent), independently of blood pressure.

To assess the role of dietary sodium (Na^+) with or without chloride (Cl^-) on the development of LVH, Sprague-Dawley rats with two kidney–one clip hypertension were given different forms of diets for 4 weeks after clipping (51): normal sodium chloride (Na^+ 77 mmol/L and Cl^- 77 mmol/L drinking water), sodium citrate (Na^+ 77 mmol/L and Cl^- 0 mmol/L) and low sodium chloride (Na^+ 0 mmol/L and Cl^- 0 mmol/L). Blood pressure was similar in all hypertensive rats regardless of the diet. Hypertensive rats on normal sodium chloride and sodium citrate diet showed identical LVH (left ventricular weight per body weight), whereas no LVH occurred in animals on a low-salt diet, and this despite a similar blood pressure level. Thus, in this model, too, sodium per se emerges as a modulator of the left ventricular response to hypertension. The anion linked to Na^+ does not influence the effect of sodium on hypertension and LVH.

HOW SALT INTAKE COULD MODIFY LEFT VENTRICULAR MASS

What, then, are the precise pathogenetic mechanisms linking dietary salt intake to LVH? Numerous neural, hormonal, and hemodynamic stimuli have been implicated in cardiac muscle growth, including α- and β-adrenergic agonists, the renin-angiotensin-aldosterone system, thyroxine, glucagon, and insulin.

At present, interest focuses on three different mech-

anisms: the sympathetic nervous system, the renin-angiotensin-aldosterone system, and fluid-volume homeostasis.

Sympathetic Nervous System

Increased cardiac sympathetic nerve activity and elevated levels of circulating catecholamines could be a primary effector initiating LVH. In cardiac myocytes, α-adrenergic receptors are present and stimulation of these leads to positive inotropic and chronotropic effects (52,53). Significant myocardial hypertrophy developed after norepinephrine infusion into dogs, independent of changes in arterial blood pressure, intracardiac pressures, and cardiac work (54,55). In an attempt to provide evidence that cardiac hypertrophy in response to norepinephrine is directly mediated by stimulation of myocardial adrenoceptors, Zierhut and Zimmer (56) treated rats with norepinephrine or norfenephrine (α-agonists), simultaneously reversing changes in functional parameters with verapamil. The addition of verapamil did not prevent the development of cardiac hypertrophy, thus indicating that cardiac hypertrophy was directly mediated by stimulation of α- and β-adrenoceptors.

High salt intake enhances the activity of the sympathetic nervous system to various stress stimuli (57), and consequently, the structural effects of sympathetic activation may be augmented after an increase in sodium intake.

However, animal studies have failed to confirm such a close relationship. In male Wistar rats increased saline intake produced concentric LVH without any increase in blood pressure (58). Cardiac neuronal sympathetic activity as assessed through measurement of catecholamine turnover rates and tyrosine hydroxylase activity did not increase during the development of saline-induced cardiac hypertrophy (58). In this study, the absence of increases in filling pressures, cardiac sympathetic neuronal activity, or pressure load during the development of sodium-induced cardiac hypertrophy argues against the hypothesis that salt intake exerts its trophic action on myocardial cells via the sympathetic nervous system. These results indicate that in this type of hypertrophy sodium may directly influence cellular mechanisms involved in the regulation of left ventricular mass (LVM).

Renin-Angiotensin-Aldosterone System

Angiotensin II acts via a variety of mechanisms on cardiac tissue. The indirect cardiovascular effects of angiotensin II include central nervous system actions, increased sympathetic activity achieved by inhibition of norepinephrine uptake in the presynaptic space, stimulation of aldosterone synthesis and release, decreased renal excretion of Na^+, and increase of vascular tone (59). The direct cardiac actions of angiotensin II are mediated by membrane receptors and are coupled to effector responses by nucleotide-binding proteins, thereby stimulating cardiac contractility, and the augmentation of protein synthesis, resulting in cardiac hypertrophy (for review see ref. 59).

A linear relationship between angiotensin II level and LVH in patients with essential hypertension was observed (60) but needs to be reconfirmed in a larger population. Indirect support for a direct growth-stimulating action of angiotensin II on myocardial cells comes from a study that found a close relationship between glomerular filtration rate and left ventricular structure: hypertensive patients with glomerular hyperfiltration had significantly increased left ventricular mass (61). Since glomerular hyperfiltration in these patients suggests vasoconstriction at the efferent site of the glomerulum that is mediated by angiotensin II, the common denominator for the association of glomerular hyperfiltration with LVH might be increased renin–angiotensin II stimulation.

Physiologically, high salt intake leads to a suppression of the renin–angiotensin II–aldosterone system. However, the suppressor effect of salt loading on the renin-angiotensin II-aldosterone system is diminished in nearly one-half of the population with essential hypertension (62). Thus, inappropriately elevated angiotensin II levels (in relation to sodium homeostasis), which prevail in this subpopulation, may account for the increase in left ventricular mass.

Fluid-Volume Homeostasis

Analysis of the interaction of sodium intake and blood volume reveals that a high dietary salt intake could accelerate LVH by chronically expanding intravascular volume, thereby increasing preload to the left ventricle. Indeed, total blood volume has been documented to be a determinant of LVH (39). Since intracellular and extracellular fluid volume state appeared to be dependent, at least to some extent, on sodium balance, an interaction with left ventricular dimensions should be expected (63). Data presented so far on salt-induced cardiac hypertrophy indicate that dietary sodium intake modulates the diastolic diameter in normotensive subjects (47) and in patients with never-treated mild essential hypertension (46), whereas in patients at a later stage of hypertensive disease sodium intake determines the degree of wall thickness (45) and of relative wall thickness, i.e., concentric LVH (45,47).

Other Mechanisms

Recently, tremendous effort has been made to elucidate the role of intracellular pH in cellular structural ad-

aptation. Meanwhile, there is evidence that an increase in pH is a necessary signal for the initiation of growth and development in many cell types (59). Intracellular pH is in large part controlled by the Na^+-H^+ exchange system (64).

Strazzullo and coworkers (65) studied the relationship between lymphocyte Na^+-H^+ exchange activity and left ventricular mass in hypertensive patients. Na^+-H^+ exchange activity was significantly and directly associated with left ventricular mass. Our own data (unpublished) in patients with essential hypertension do not favor such a straightforward relationship between Na^+-H^+ exchange and LVH, since no significant correlation was observed between both parameters. Düsing et al. (66) found a positive correlation between sodium-chloride intake and the Na^+-H^+–exchange activity, possibly leading to a rise in intracellular pH and growth stimulation. These preliminary but promising data warrant further investigation in this area.

THERAPEUTIC CONSEQUENCES

Experimental Data

Left ventricular hypertrophy has been shown to be associated with a decline in the maximum velocity of cardiac muscle shortening that usually correlates with the decreased Ca^{2+}–adenosine triphosphatase (ATPase) activity of myosin. During development of myocardial hypertrophy the myosin isozymic pattern changes: cardiac myosin isozymes shift from a faster migrating type V_1 to a form that migrates more slowly, V_3 (67–72).

Sen and Young (67), in an attempt to throw light on the role of dietary sodium in modulation of myosin isozymic pattern, treated renal hypertensive rats (two kidney–one clip) with a sodium-deficient diet. Renal hypertension was associated with an increase in the V_3 component. There was a dramatic change in the myosin isozyme distribution pattern after treatment with low sodium. Six weeks of low-sodium therapy in renal hypertensive rats resulted in a significant increase in V_1 and a decrease in V_3, thus demonstrating that the altered myosin isozymic pattern can be normalized by a low-sodium diet.

Clinical Data

What are the clinical implications arising from all these findings? Is general salt restriction warranted? So far only a few preliminary studies have addressed the question of whether salt restriction leads to a reduction in left ventricular mass in patients.

Ferrara et al. (73) evaluated the effect of short-term (12-week) salt depletion on left ventricular mass in hypertensive patients. They compared the effects of chlorthalidone therapy with those of severe restriction of salt intake. Ten men with mild to moderate hypertension underwent severe restriction of salt intake (less than 2 g daily) followed by diuretic therapy (chlorthalidone, 25 mg/day), or vice versa. Echocardiographic measurements have shown that either low-sodium intake or diuretic treatment produced a significant reduction in left ventricular mass in a period as brief as 6 weeks. The correlation found between left ventricular mass and an observed fall in blood pressure and cardiac workload may have accounted for changes in left ventricular mass. However, such a close correlation was not found in other studies (74). Therefore, Ferrara and colleagues concluded that a factor other than hypertension, namely salt intake, has been involved in the regression of left ventricular mass.

More recently, data presented by the Treatment of Mild Hypertension Study (TOMHS) Research Group (75) showed a significant correlation between reduced salt intake and left ventricular mass in the whole study group; salt restriction was the only factor (for instance not blood pressure fall) that was significantly correlated with reduction in left ventricular mass ($\beta = .123$). In patients on antihypertensive therapy a change in left ventricular mass was produced by a decrease in salt intake, blood pressure fall, and weight loss, whereas in the placebo group only the decrease of diastolic blood pressure was determinant. As long as comprehensive clinical data are lacking, any specific "antitrophic" action of salt restriction beyond that associated with the blood pressure–lowering effect remains to be proven before general guidelines can be given.

SUMMARY

Left ventricular hypertrophy has been found to be significantly related to morbidity and mortality independently of other risk factors, thus representing an important determinant for target-organ damage in cardiovascular disease. There is a close relationship between the development and persistence of LVH and sodium homeostasis. The higher sodium intake, the greater was left ventricular mass in normotensive and, most relevant, in hypertensive subjects. The pathophysiology of this blood pressure–induced link between salt intake and myocardial hypertrophy is currently under investigation, with special interest in the sympathetic nervous system, the renin-angiotensin-aldosterone system, and fluid-volume homeostasis.

At present, salt restriction cannot in general be recommended as effective strategy to reverse LVH in hypertensive patients. Nevertheless, high salt intake should be considered a possible reason for persisting LVH in the presence of good blood pressure control.

REFERENCES

1. Ambard L, Beaujard E. *Arch Gen Med* 1904;1:520–525.
2. Fries ED. *Circulation* 1976;53:589–594.
3. Messerli FH, ed. *The heart and hypertension,* 1st ed. New York: Yorke Medical Books, 1986.
4. Kannel WB. *Am J Med* 1983;75(suppl 3A):4–11.
5. Kannel WB, Gordon T, Offut D. *Ann Intern Med* 1969;71:89–105.
6. Gordon T, Kannel WB. *JAMA* 1971;215:1617–1625.
7. Devereux RB, Lutas EM, Casale PN, et al. *J Am Coll Cardiol* 1984;4:1222–1230.
8. Devereux RB, Reichek N. *Circulation* 1977;55:613–618.
9. Devereux RB, Alonso DR, Lutas EM, et al. *Am J Cardiol* 1986;57:450–458.
10. Levy D, Anderson KM, Savage DD, Kannel WB, Christiansen JC, Castelli WP. *Ann Intern Med* 1988;108:7–13.
11. Reichek N, Devereux RB. *Circulation* 1981;63:1391–1398.
12. Woythaler JN, Singer SL, Kwan OL, et al. *J Am Coll Cardiol* 1983;2:305–311.
13. Kannel WB, Gordon T, Offut D. *Ann Intern Med* 1969;71:89–105.
14. Hypertension Detection And Follow-Up Program Cooperative Group. *JAMA* 1979;242:2562–2571.
15. Hammond IW, Devereux RB, Alderman MH, et al. *J Am Coll Cardiol* 1986;7:639–650.
16. Savage DD, Drayer JIM, Henry WL, et al. *Circulation* 1979;59:623–632.
17. Devereux RB, Alonso DR, Lutas EM, Pickering TG, Harshfield GA, Laragh JH. In: Ter Keurs HEDJ, Schipperheyn JJ, eds. *Cardiac left ventricular hypertrophy.* The Hague: Martinus Nijhoff, 1983;16–37.
18. Casale PN, Devereux RB, Milner M, et al. *Ann Intern Med* 1986;105:173–178.
19. Koren MJ, Uhn RJ, Laragh JH, Devereux RB. *Ann Intern Med* 1991;114:345–352.
20. Cooper RS, Simmons BE, Castaner A, Santhanam V, Ghali J, Mar M. *Am J Cardiol* 1990;65:441–445.
21. Strauer BE. *Am J Cardiol* 1979;44:999–1006.
22. Marcus ML, Harrison DG, Chilian WM, et al. *Circulation* 1987;75(suppl I):19–25.
23. Tomanek RJ, Palmer PJ, Pieffer GH, et al. *Circ Res* 1986;58:38–46.
24. Weinberger MH. *Hypertension* 1990;16:201–211.
25. Neill WA, Fluir-Lundeed JH. *Am J Cardiol* 1979;44:746–753.
26. Ghali JK, Liao Y, Simmons B, Castaner A, Cao G, Cooper RS. *Ann Intern Med* 1992;117:831–836.
27. Blake J, Devereux RB, Borer JS, Szulc M, Pappas TW, Laragh JH. *Am J Med* 1990;88:477–485.
28. Gibson DG, Trail TA, Hall RJC, Brown DJ. *Br Heart J* 1979;41:54–59.
29. Smith VE, Schulman P, Karimeddini MK, White WB, Meeran MK, Katz AM. *J Am Coll Cardiol* 1985;5:869–874.
30. Inouye I, Massie BM, Loge D, Simpson P, Tubau JF. *Am J Cardiol* 1984;53:1583–1587.
31. Phillips RA, Goldman ME, Ardeljan M, Arora R, Eison HB, Buyan Y, Krakoff LR. *J Am Coll Cardiol* 1989;14:979–985.
32. Messerli FH, Ventura HO, Elizardi DJ, Dunn FG, Frohlich ED. *Am J Med* 1984;77:18–22.
33. Schmieder RE, Messerli FH. *Am Heart J* 1992;123:89–95.
34. McLenachan JM, Henderson E, Morris KI, Dargie HJ. *N Engl J Med* 1987;317:787–792.
35. Kannel WD. *Am J Med* 1983;75(suppl 3A):4–11.
36. Nunez BD, Messerli FH, Amodeo C, Garavaglia GE, Schmieder RE, Frohlich ED. *Am Heart J* 1987;14:813–818.
37. Devereux RB, Savage DD, Sachs I, Laragh JH. *Am J Cardiol* 1983;51:171–176.
38. Messerli FH, Schlant RC. *Am J Med* 1983;75(suppl 3A):1–3.
39. Messerli FH, Sundgaard-Riise K, Ventura HO, Dunn FG, Oigman W, Frohlich ED. *Arch Intern Med* 1984;144:477–481.
40. Yamori Y, Mori C, Nishio T, et al. *Am J Cardiol* 1979;44:964–969.
41. Messerli FH, Sundgaard-Riise K, Reisin ED, et al. *Ann Intern Med* 1983;99:757–761.

42. Devereux RB, Pickering TG, Cody RJ, Laragh JH. *J Clin Hypertens* 1987;3:87–103.
43. Frohlich ED, Tarazi RC. *Am J Cardiol* 1979;44:959–963.
44. Devereux RB, Savage DD, Drayer JI, Laragh JH. *Hypertension* 1982;4:524–531.
45. Schmieder RE, Messerli FH, Garavaglia GE, Nunez BD. *Circulation* 1988;78(4):951–956.
46. Schmieder RE, Grube E, Impelmann V, Rüddel H, Schulte W. *Z Kardiol* 1990;79:557–564.
47. Du Cailar G, Ribstein J, Daures JP, Mimran A. *Am J Physiol* 1992;263:H177–181.
48. Daniels SD, Meyer RA, Loggie MH. *Circulation* 1990;82:1243–1248.
49. Kihara M, Utagawa N, Mano M, Nara Y, Horie R, Yamori Y. *Heart Vessels* 1985;1:212–215.
50. De Simone G, Devereux RB, Camargo JF, Wallerson DC, Laragh JH. *Circulation* 1990;92(suppl III):13.
51. Pasquie JL, Jover B, Du Cailar G, Mimran A. *J Am Coll Cardiol* 1993;21:469A.
52. Buxton ILO, Brunton LL. *Am J Physiol* 1986;251:H307–H313.
53. Brown JH, Buxton IL, Brunton LL. *Circ Res* 1985;57:532–537.
54. Laks MM, Morardy F, Swan HJC. *Chest* 1973;64:75–78.
55. King BD, Sack D, Kichuk MR, Hintze TH. *Hypertension* 1987;9:582–590.
56. Zierhut W, Zimmer HG. *Circ Res* 1989;65:1417–1425.
57. Skrabal F, Anbock J, Hartnagl H. *Lancet* 1981;2:895–900.
58. Fields NG, Yuan B, Leenen FH. *Circ Res* 1991;68:745–755.
59. Morgan HE, Baker KM. *Circulation* 1991;83:13–25.
60. Schmieder RE, Messerli FH, Garavaglia GE, Nunez BD, MacPhee AA, Re NR. *Am J Med* 1988;84(suppl 3A):136–139.
61. Schmieder RE, Messerli FH, Garavaglia G, Nunez B. *JAMA* 1990;264:2775–2780.
62. Hollenberg NK. *Contrib Nephrol* 1984;43:102–113.
63. Sullivan JM, Ratts TE, Schoeneberger AA, Samaha JK, Palmer ET. *Am J Clin Nutr* 1979;32:2410–2415.
64. Moolenaar WH. *Annu Rev Physiol* 1986;48:363–376.
65. Strazzullo P, De Simone G, Celentano A, Iao R, Ragone E, Pagano E, Tammaro P, Cane M. *J Hypertens* 1991;9(suppl 6):S306–S307.
66. Düsing R, Göbel BO, Hoffmann G, Siffert W, Vetter H. *J Am Soc Nephrol* 1992;3:518(abstract).
67. Sen S, Young DR. *Hypertension* 1986;8:918–924.
68. Lompre AM, Mercadier JJ, Wisnewsky C, et al. *Dev Biol* 1981;84:286–290.
69. Mercadier JJ, Lompre AM, Wisnewsky C, et al. *Circ Res* 1981;49:525–532.
70. Gorza L, Pauletto P, Pessin AC, Sartore S, Schiaffino S. *Circ Res* 1981;49:1003–1009.
71. Litten RZ, Martin BJ, Low RP, Alpert NR. *Circ Res* 1982;50:856–864.
72. Rupp H, Jacob R. *Can J Physiol Pharmacol* 1982;60:1098–1103.
73. Ferrara LA, De Simone G, Pasanisi F, Mancini M, Mancini M. *Hypertension* 1984;6:755–759.
74. Drayer JIM, Gardin JM, Weber MA. *Chest* 1983;84:217–221.
75. Liebson P, Prineas R, Grandits G, Dianzumba S, Grimm R. *Circulation* 1992;86(suppl I):599(abstract).

Hypertension: Pathophysiology, Diagnosis, and Management, Second Edition, edited by J.H. Laragh and B.M. Brenner, Raven Press, Ltd., New York © 1995.

CHAPTER 80

The Juxtaglomerular Apparatus: A Morphologic Perspective

Luciano Barajas, Eduardo C. Salido, Li Liu, and Kenneth V. Powers

At the hilus of the renal glomerulus the thick ascending limb of the Henle loop (TALH) of the same nephron contacts the glomerular vascular pole. At the site of contact the TALH is anatomically different from the rest of the TALH. The most obvious difference is the close proximity of the nuclei of the tubular cells at the site of contact. This condensation of nuclei was recognized by light microscopists (1) and accounts for the name *macula densa* (MD) given by Zimmermann (2) to this region of the nephron (Figs. 1–3). Cells with morphologic features of MD cells are found situated peripheral to the region of the MD in contact with the vascular component (3–6) (Fig. 3). The functional significance of these cells is unknown, but the observation that nitric oxide synthase immunoreactivity is displayed not only by the MD cells in contact with the vascular component but also by these nonjuxtaglomerular "macular" cells located in the free wall of the TALH (see section on Macula Densa) indicates functional similarities.

The vascular structures at the hilus of the glomerulus consist of the afferent and efferent arterioles and the region between the arterioles containing a group of cells known as the Goormaghtigh cells. This component of the vascular pole, containing the Goormaghtigh cells, is continuous with the glomerular mesangium; thus the term *extraglomerular mesangium* (EM) was proposed to

designate this region and extraglomerular mesangial cells to refer to the Goormaghtigh cells (7). The EM was described with the light microscope by Zimmermann (2), who called it the "Polkissen." Oberling and Hatt (8) made the first ultrastructural description of this region and referred to it as the "lacis" because of the lace-like appearance that the extraglomerular mesangial cell processes and the interlacing intercellular spaces give this region. These various names (extraglomerular mesangium, lacis, Polkissen, Goormaghtigh cell field) are currently used to designate this region.

A unique and morphologically distinct cell type with both smooth muscle and endocrine characteristics is found in the glomerular arterioles and extraglomerular mesangial region. These cells are the site of synthesis and storage of renin (9). They are more abundant in the afferent arteriole as it approaches the glomerulus and they may also be found in the afferent arteriole away from the glomerulus, as far as its junction with the interlobular artery. These renin-containing cells can also be seen in the EM and in the efferent arteriole.

It has been proposed that the MD (tubular component) and the adjacent structures of the vascular pole, the afferent and efferent arterioles, and EM (vascular component) constitute an anatomical and functional unit that is known as the juxtaglomerular apparatus (JGA). The renin-containing cells are referred to as the juxtaglomerular (JG) cells. The unique anatomical relationships of the JGA are central to considerations of the tubular control of renin secretion (10,11) and tubuloglomerular feedback mechanisms (12–14).

L. Barajas, E. C. Salido, L. Liu, and K. V. Powers: Department of Pathology, Harbor-UCLA Medical Center, Torrance, California 90509.

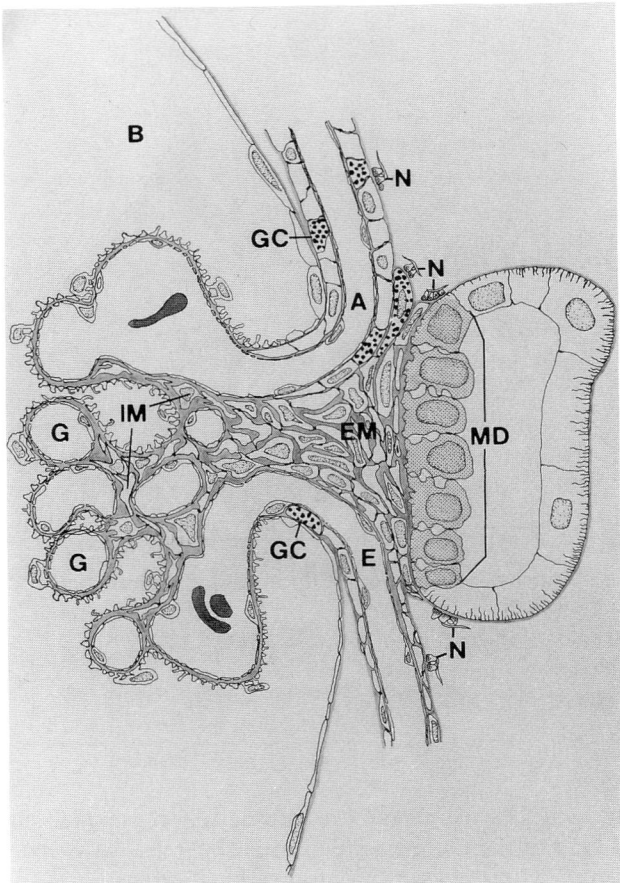

FIG. 1. Diagram of the juxtaglomerular apparatus of the rat illustrating the tubular and vascular components. The tubular component consists of a specialized region of the thick ascending limb of Henle, the macula densa (MD). The vascular component consists of the afferent (A) and efferent (E) arterioles and the extraglomerular mesangium (EM) (also known as the lacis, "group of cells of Goormaghtigh," and "Polkissen"). The MD is in contact with the EM. The EM is continuous with the intraglomerular mesangium (IM). Granular cells (GC) are seen in the walls of the glomerular arterioles and are most abundant in the afferent arteriole. The vascular and tubular components are innervated by sympathetic nerves (N). B, Bowman's space; G, glomerular capillary.

MACULA DENSA (TUBULAR COMPONENT)

The MD is located within the terminal portion of the TALH (15) and adjacent to the vascular pole of the glomerulus. The height of the cells of the MD varies with the species. They are taller than the unmodified cells in the rest of the TALH in the rabbit (16). In the mouse (Fig. 2) and in the rat (Fig. 3) the MD cells differ less in their height from the rest of the TALH. In all species their height is related to the development of the extracellular spaces. The mitochondria of the MD cells are also smaller and differently shaped and their basolateral membranes are simpler than those of the unmodified

TALH. The mitochondria also appear to be dispersed in the cytoplasm instead of concentrated at the base of the cells near the basolateral membranes, as is the case with the TALH.

The contact of the MD with the vascular component is extensive and mandatory with the EM, although it also exists, to a variable extent, with the afferent and efferent arterioles (3). The surface of the MD facing the EM also differs from the comparable surface of the rest of the TALH. At the site of contact the basilar profile of the MD cells appears irregular and borders a space that varies in width and separates the MD from the EM. Basement membrane material, also of variable width and density, is seen in this space extending between the irregularities of the MD basilar surface and into the EM. It appears that the basement membrane at the MD-EM interface is continuous with the intercellular basement membrane or basement membrane–like material seen in the intercellular spaces of the EM. The basement membrane of the unmodified TALH, in contrast, appears to have a more consistent thickness. Examination of the MD-EM basement membrane with the scanning electron microscope shows the distinct appearance of the EM-MD interface (17). Although in the rest of the tubules the basement membrane appears as a smooth wall, at the site of contact between the MD and the EM it is replaced by a complex array of tunnels, pleats, and brid-

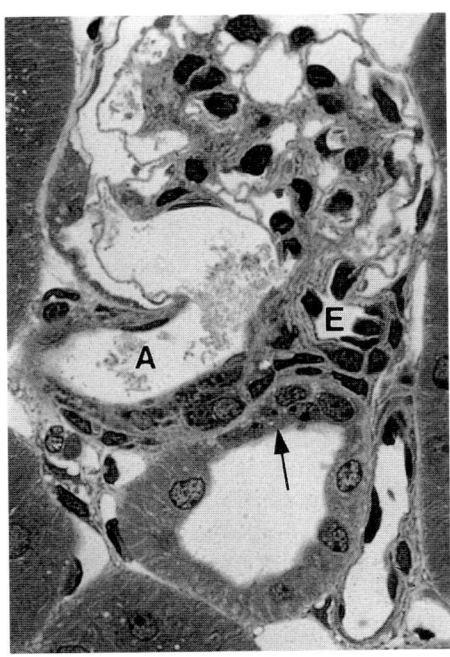

FIG. 2. Light micrograph of the juxtaglomerular apparatus of the mouse. The vascular and tubular components are illustrated. The extraglomerular mesangial cells can be seen between the afferent (A) and efferent (E) arterioles and in contact with the macula densa (*arrow*). ×850. (From ref. 6, with permission.)

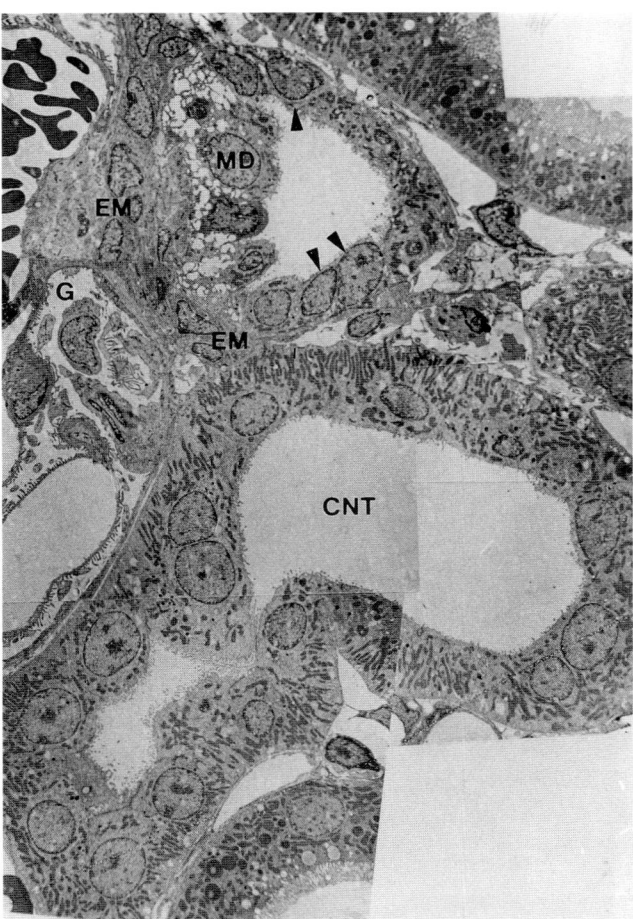

FIG. 3. The connecting tubule (CNT) is seen establishing contact with the extraglomerular mesangium (EM). The macula densa (MD) shows prominent lateral intercellular spaces. Note the macula densa–like cells, the perimacular cells, not in contact with the vascular component (*arrowheads*). G, Glomerulus. ×880. (From ref. 6, with permission.)

ges that gradually blend with the smooth basement membrane of the contiguous TALH (Fig. 4). Although interpretation of these observations is difficult at this time, given the drastic nature of the techniques used to visualize the MD-EM basement membrane, they clearly illustrate the special relationship of the distal nephron with the glomerulus at the JGA. The replacement of the smooth and continuous basement membrane of the TALH with a network-like structure at the site of contact of the MD with the EM, albeit under special experimental conditions, suggests that the structure of this interface favors not only the anchoring of the MD to the EM but also the exchange of information (chemical, physical, or of some other type) between the tubular and vascular components.

Another anatomical feature distinguishing the MD from the rest of the TALH is the existence of wide lateral intercellular spaces (LISs) separating the MD cells at the

site of contact with the EM (Fig. 3). The significance of the capillary-deprived EM in the generation of the LIS is underscored by the absence of LIS between the MD-like cells (perimacular cells) not in contact with the EM (Fig. 3). In the rest of the TALH the LISs are closed. Experimental evidence points toward a functional significance of the LIS. Whereas under normal fixation conditions the LISs are usually open wide, in mannitol or furosemide-induced diuresis the LISs narrow (16,18).

These changes in LIS width during diuresis are consistent with observations made by direct visualization of perfused nephron segments that include the MD. Using differential-interference-contrast microscopy, it was observed that reduction of the osmolality of the perfusion fluid widened the LIS and increased the height of the MD cells (19). With furosemide or mannitol-induced diuresis the MD is expected to have an increased osmolality that would result in the narrowing of the LIS. Therefore, the closure of the LIS observed under diuresis, in fixed tissues, is compatible with the interference microscopy results obtained in *in vitro* microperfused MD preparations. The significance of the LISs is still unclear; changes in their width might be related to the assumed water-permeability of the MD as compared with the relative water impermeability of the unmodified TALH. There are also marked histochemical differences between the MD and the rest of the TALH (20). Among the important ones are the low levels of Na, K-ATPase in the MD compared with the rest of the TALH (21–23). There are also differences between the MD and the unmodified TALH regarding the presence of Tamm-Horsfall (TH) glycoprotein. TH is absent from the MD in contrast to its presence along the luminal and basolateral aspects of the plasma membrane of the TALH (24,25). It has been suggested, based on the *in vitro* properties of TH (26), that the viscosity and gel formation of TH along the plasma membrane might restrict water movement across the TALH and be responsible for the relative water impermeability of the TALH. Uromodulin, a glycoprotein with immunosuppressive properties, has been shown to be identical to TH (27). Thus, TH may play an immunoregulatory role by binding to and affecting the activity of a variety of cytokines, such as interleukin-1 and tumor necrosis factor (28).

Epidermal growth factor (EGF) has been immunolocalized by light and electron microscopy in the TALH and distal convoluted tubule (DCT) of the mouse kidney; it is absent from the MD (29,30) (Fig. 5). Immunoelectron microscopy disclosed EGF immunoreactivity along the luminal plasma membrane and apical vesicles of the cells of the TALH and DCT (29). Relatively large amounts of prepro-EGF mRNA in the mouse kidney have been demonstrated not only by dot and Northern blot analysis but also by *in situ* hybridization (31). *In situ* hybridization with a prepro-EGF cDNA probe revealed the presence of EGF mRNA in the same segments of the

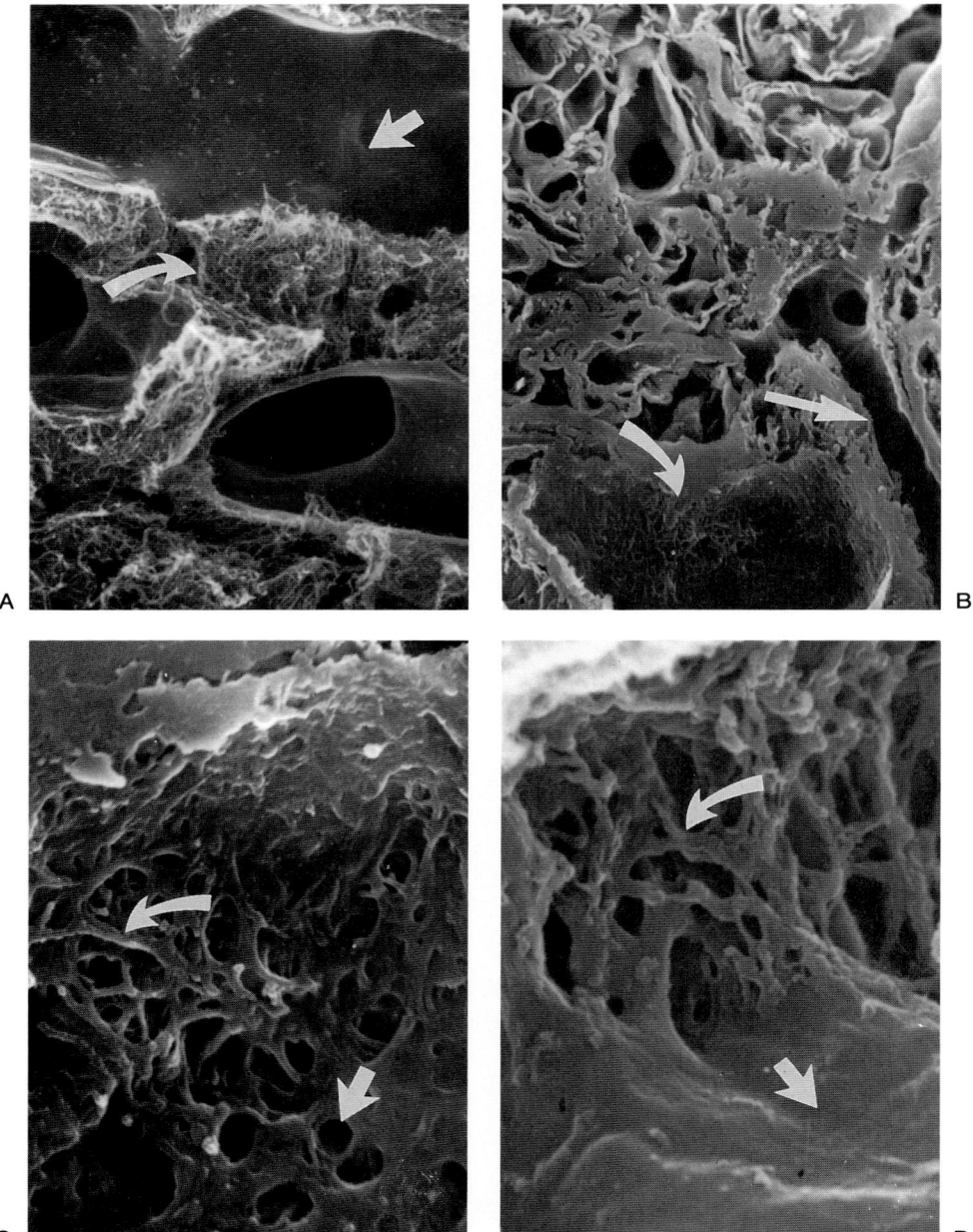

FIG. 4. A: Normal tubular (probably proximal) basement membranes (*short arrow*) have a smooth inner (luminal) surface and are separated by fibrillar interstitial connective tissue (*curved arrow*). ×1,000. **B:** A normal acellular, freeze cracked glomerulus with macula densa basement membrane (*curved arrow*) and arteriole (*arrow*) exposed, respectively, in cross and longitudinal sections. ×1,000. **C:** Higher magnification of the macula densa basement membrane in Fig. 4B. Notice the frequent shallow variably sized tunnels (*arrow*) with occasional pleats and bridges (*curved arrow*). ×5,000. **D:** A macula densa that shows prominent bridge formation (*curved arrow*). This complexity gradually blends into the smooth surface of the TALH basement membrane (*arrow*) opposite the macula densa. ×8,000. (From ref. 16, with permission.)

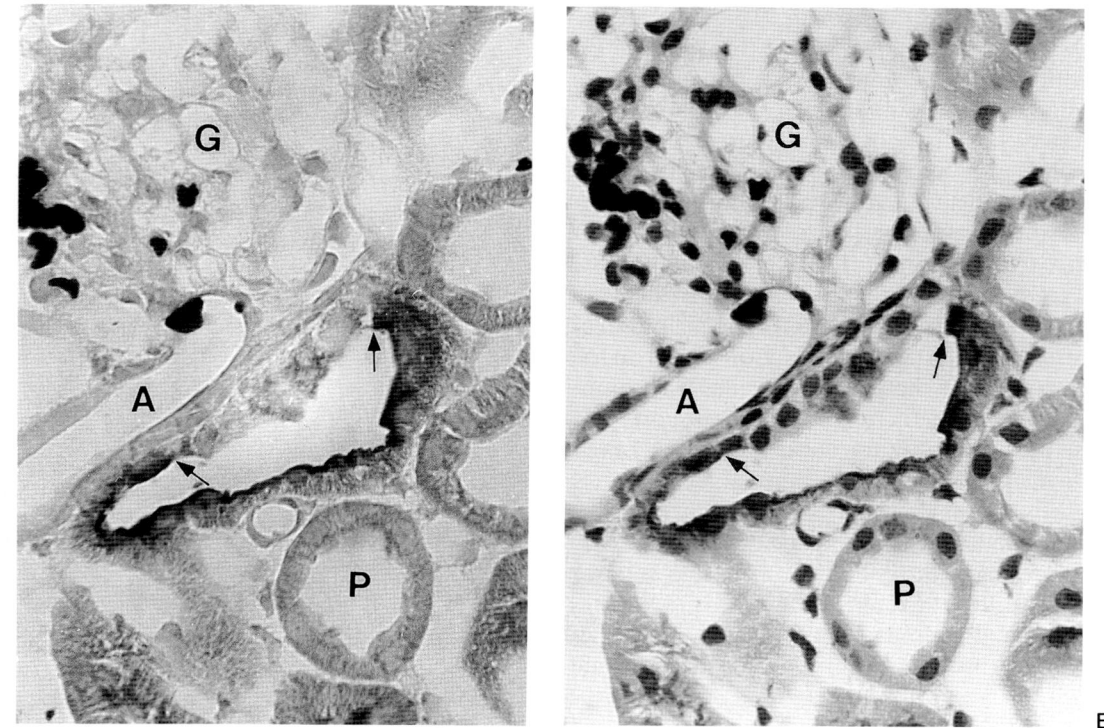

FIG. 5. A: Epidermal growth factor immunoreactivity is absent in the macula densa (between *arrows*) but can be seen in the luminal aspect of the rest of the TALH. **B:** The same area counterstained with hematoxylin shows the condensation of nuclei characteristic of the macula densa. A, afferent arteriole; G, glomerulus; P, proximal tubule. ×750. (From ref. 6, with permission.)

nephron showing EGF immunoreactivity, namely the TALH and the DCT (6,32). Epidermal growth factor mRNA was absent from the MD (Fig. 6). The immunocytochemical and *in situ* hybridization data mentioned above are consistent with the concept that EGF is synthesized in the kidney as a transmembrane prepro-EGF molecule as suggested by analysis of the EGF cDNA (33,34). There is relatively little known about the function of EGF and its precursor in the kidney. Epidermal growth factor has a mitogenic effect on renal tubular cells and in a variety of cultured cell preparations (35,36). Thus, it could be proposed that EGF plays a developmental and regenerative role in the urinary tract. Epidermal growth factor has been shown also to induce an increase in transmembrane ion fluxes in cultured fibroblasts (37). Changes in urine flow and ionic composition have been reported after the infusion of EGF into sheep renal arteries (38). These observations suggest a possible role for EGF in membrane transport in the distal nephron. It has also been suggested that the EGF precursor could function as a receptor (39). If, indeed, EGF functions as a receptor, the nature of the ligand is unknown.

The recent localization of nitric oxide synthase (NOS) in the MD suggests a possible role of nitric oxide (NO) in juxtaglomerular function. The MD displays strong im-

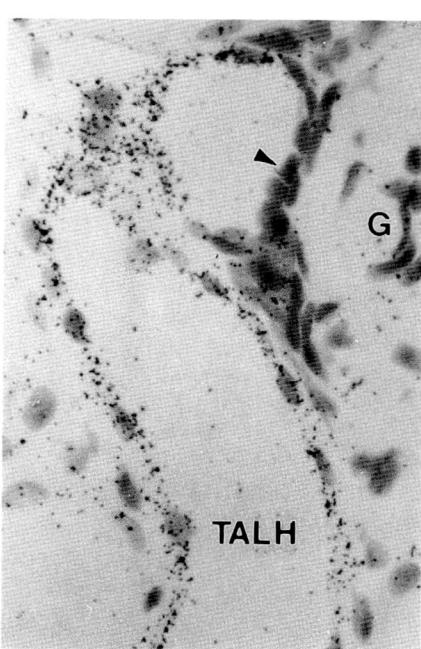

FIG. 6. *In situ* hybridization of prepro-EGF mRNA in the mouse kidney. Note the presence of labeled cells (dark grains) in the thick ascending limb of Henle (TALH), whereas the macula densa cells (*arrowhead*) lack specific hybridization. G, glomerulus. Prepro-EGF cDNA probe labeled with ^{3}H by nick translation. ×700. (From ref. 6, with permission.)

munoreactivity for NOS (Fig. 7) and the enzymatic activity of NOS has been demonstrated in that location using the nicotinamide adenine dinucleotide phosphate (NADPH) diaphorase technique (Fig. 8) (40,41). Both reactions may be seen in cells contiguous to the juxtaglomerular MD (42) as well as in other cells of the TALH. This is consistent with ultrastructural observations of cells morphologically similar to those of the MD located in the free portion of TALH peripheral to the MD. NOS mRNA expression has also been demonstrated in the MD (40). These morphologic observations are consistent with the possible action of NO on the vascular component of the juxtaglomerular apparatus. The results of micropuncture studies support this view because they strongly suggest that arginine-derived NO is implicated in the juxtaglomerular feedback response (41).

The unique characteristics and location of the MD prompted Goormaghtigh (43,44) to propose a role for the MD in the control of renin release. This notion received experimental support with the work of Vander and Miller (45), in which the composition of the distal

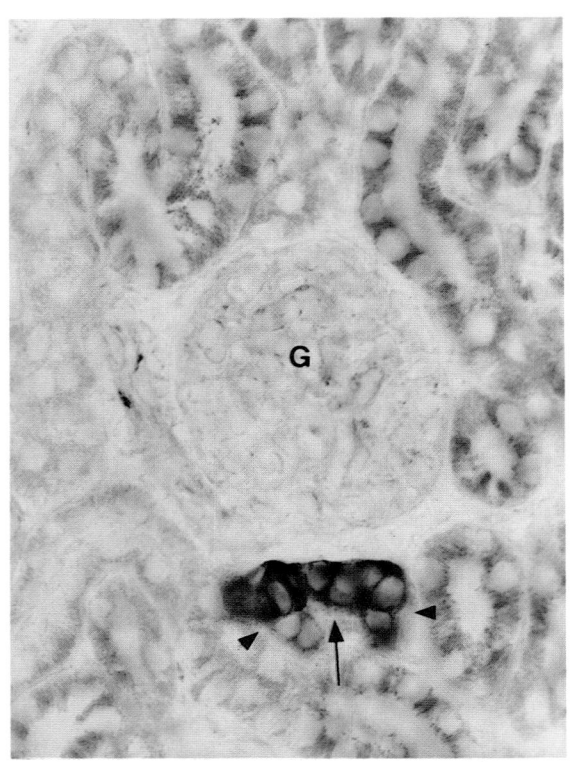

FIG. 8. NADPH diaphorase enzyme activity in the macula densa (*arrow*) of the juxtaglomerular apparatus of the rat kidney. Also note the enzymatic activity of the macular cells, in the free wall of the tubule and contiguous to the macula densa in contact with the vascular component (*arrowheads*). G, glomerulus. ×540.

tubular fluid was changed by means of diuretics. More recently, an *in vitro* preparation has been used in which microdissected single juxtaglomerular apparatuses, including the tubular segment containing the MD, were perfused with solutions that varied in their sodium chloride content (46). A decrease in the sodium chloride concentration at the MD resulted in a stimulation of the rate of renin release. These results are in agreement with Vander and Miller's conclusion that a low sodium chloride load sensed at the MD increases renin release.

VASCULAR COMPONENT

The vascular component consists of the afferent and efferent arterioles and the extraglomerular mesangial region (Goormaghtigh cell field, lacis, Polkissen). Included in the vascular component are the smooth muscle cells of the glomerular arterioles, the extraglomerular mesangial (Goormaghtigh) cells, which are functionally and structurally integrated with the glomerular mesangial cells, and the renin-containing granular cells known as the juxtaglomerular cells (JGCs). The JGCs are located in the wall of the glomerular arterioles and are interspersed

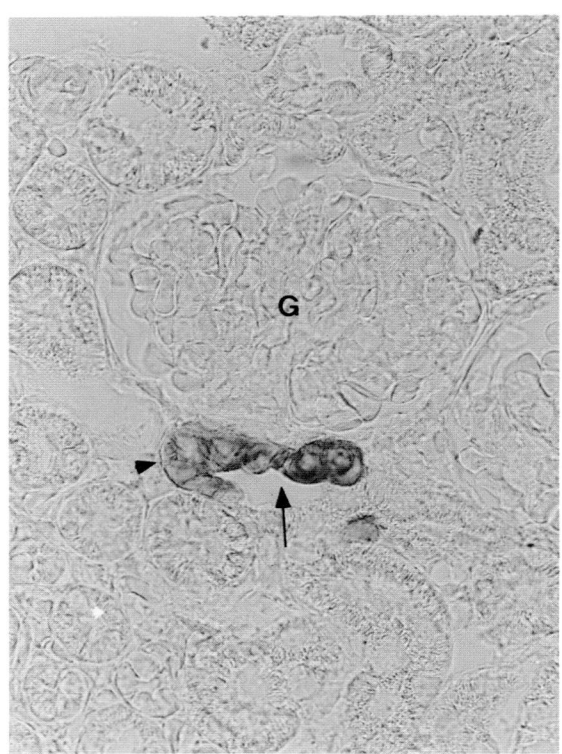

FIG. 7. Immunocytochemical localization of nitric oxide synthase (NOS) in the macula densa cells (*arrow*) of the JGA of rat kidney with polycolonal antiserum against type I NOS (1:1000). Note the positive reaction for NOS in macular cells in the free wall of the TALH (*arrowheads*). G, glomerulus. Avidin biotinylated immunoperoxidase complex (ABC) method (vector), ×540. (Antibodies to NOS provided by Drs. J. S. Pollock and H. H. H. W. Schmidt.)

among the smooth muscle cells and occasionally found within the extraglomerular mesangium. Identified as modified smooth muscle cells since their discovery with the light microscope more than half a century ago (47), their smooth muscle characteristics have been clearly shown with the electron microscope. They show myofibrils and attachment bodies in amounts that appear to be in reverse proportion to their degree of granularity. In addition, electrophysiological studies have shown that the JGC do not differ significantly in their active and passive membrane properties from the vascular smooth muscle cells of the afferent arteriole. Furthermore, they show spontaneous transient depolarizations similar to those described for vascular smooth muscle (48).

The endocrine nature of these cells was also noticed by light microscopists. Goormaghtigh (43,44) pointed to the endocrine features of the JGC and suggested that they were the source of renin. Secretory activity was suggested by later electron microscopic studies that showed a well-developed endoplasmic reticulum containing electron-dense material and membrane-bound cytoplasmic granules originating in the Golgi apparatus (49,50). Granules of different sizes and shapes were observed in the JGC with the electron microscope (Fig. 9). Based on morphologic observations in several species, it was proposed that the large "mature" granules were derived from small granules present in the Golgi cisternae. These small granules have a characteristic shape and a crystalline substructure. They have been called protogranules and are thought to be precursors of the mature granules because intermediate granular forms are observed, which may include accumulations of protogranules. In some species such as man and monkey, the protogranules show sharp angles that make them so morphologically distinct that their presence is of value in the diagnosis of diseases involving the JGC such as JG tumors.

The demonstration of a good correlation between the degree of granularity of the JGA and the renin content of the kidney in normal and experimental conditions provided indirect evidence that the JGCs contained renin (51,52). Antisera against partially purified renin was distinctly localized in the JG granules by Edelman and Hartroft (53) in 1961. Cook (54) was able to extract renin from the JGCs by means of a micropipette, providing evidence that renin was located in the JGC.

With the purification of the various components of the renin-angiotensin system, specific antibodies have been produced. These antibodies have been extensively used in conjunction with improved immunocytochemical methods, which permitted their immunolocalization at the ultrastructural level. The results of these immunocytochemical studies have confirmed and expanded previous knowledge about the distribution of renin and added new information on the localization of the other components of the renin-angiotensin system. Renin can be im-

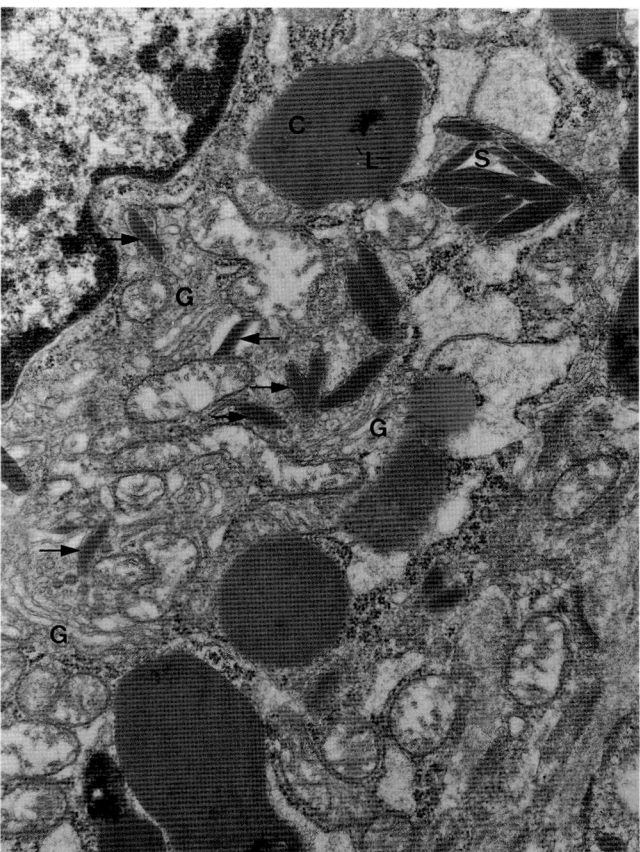

FIG. 9. Portion of the cytoplasm of a granular cell from the juxtaglomerular apparatus of a patient with renovascular hypertension. Rhomboid-shaped protogranules (*arrows*) are seen within the cisternae of the Golgi apparatus (G). A sac (S) containing multiple protogranules and vesicles is seen at the *upper left.* Near it is a conglomerate (C). Lines of fusion (L) of the protogranules are present in the conglomerate and in the *upper right* sac. ×30,000. (From ref. 49, with permission.)

munolocalized readily in the glomerular arterioles at a site, the JGC (Fig. 10A), where *in situ* hybridization studies found renin mRNA (Fig. 10B) and thus confirmed the JGC as a site of renin production (55).

As already mentioned, the proportion of smooth muscle fibrils and secretory granules vary greatly among the JGCs, resulting in considerable JGC heterogeneity. In general, there is a reverse proportion in the amount of granularity and fibrils, which correlates with the amount of renin and myosin immunoreactivity (56). The variation in renin and myosin immunoreactivity in the JGCs ranges from JGCs without myosin immunoreactivity but strong renin immunoreactivity, seen closest to the glomerulus, to those cells displaying myosin but not renin immunoreactivity, which are indistinguishable from smooth muscle cells (57). However, the majority of the JGCs show both types of immunoreactivity.

Renin has been immunolocalized ultrastructurally in granules of the JGCs (Fig. 11) and interestingly the JGC

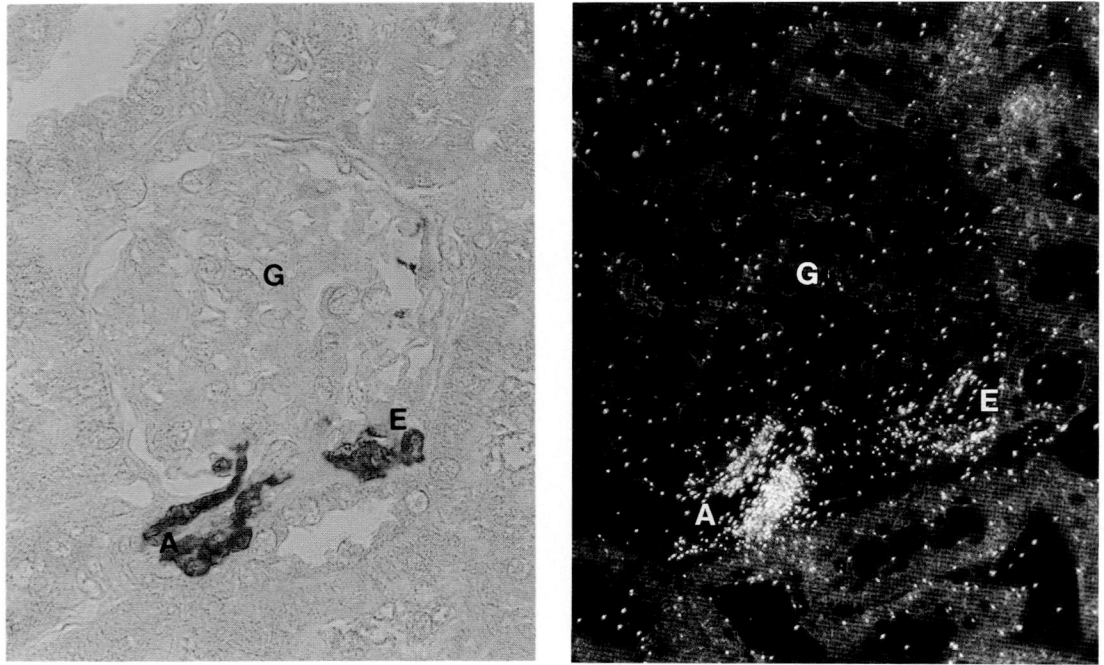

FIG. 10 A: Immunocytochemical localization of renin in the JGC of the rat afferent and efferent arteriole. Avidin biotinylated horseradish peroxidase complex (ABC) method (vector), ×540. (Renin antibody provided by T. Inagami.) **B:** *In situ* hybridization with renin mRNA in rat kidney. The label is concentrated in the juxtaglomerular cells. Dark field microscopy. ×450. A, afferent arteriole; E, efferent arteriole; G, glomerulus. Renin antisense RNA probe labeled with ^{35}S and obtained from cDNA (provided by K. R. Lynch).

exhibits immunoreactivity not only to renin but also to angiotensin II (58,59). By immunoelectron microscopy, using double labeling with colloidal gold particles of different sizes, renin and angiotensin II were found not only in the same cell but also in the same granule (60). In the control situation, there were fewer particles corresponding to angiotensin II than there were corresponding to renin. In renal ischemia there were more angiotensin II particles and fewer renin particles immunolocalized in the JG granules. The presence of renin and angiotensin II in the JG granule implies their possible cosecretion into the periarteriolar interstitium and a local paracrine action of angiotensin II. The local action of the peptide could lead to vasoconstriction of the glomerular arterioles. In this manner, angiotensin II could mediate the effector response in tubuloglomerular feedback mechanism as proposed by Thurau (13).

There is, however, no agreement as to the role of angiotensin II in tubuloglomerular feedback. Review of physiological data obtained with different methodologies supports the view that angiotensin II does not mediate tubuloglomerular feedback because stimuli that augment the tubuloglomerular feedback response also reduced renin secretion and, presumably, angiotensin II formation and/or secretion (20). The lack of a role for angiotensin II in the tubuloglomerular feedback re-

sponse is also suggested by the low density of angiotensin II receptors in the afferent arteriole (assuming that the afferent arteriole is the effector site of tubuloglomerular feedback). Angiotensin II receptors are concentrated in the glomerulus, with a decrease in density as the location of the glomeruli approach the medulla, and in the medulla, predominantly in the region of the vasa recta in the outer medulla (61). The presence of high receptor densities in the vasa recta is in agreement with a role of angiotensin II in medullary hemodynamics (62).

At least two subtypes of angiotensin II receptors have been recently demonstrated. Studies in the human have shown the presence of type 2 angiotensin II receptor exclusively on the large preglomerular vessels, whereas the type 1 angiotensin II receptor is present in the glomeruli, the outer medulla, and presumably the small vessels and the tubulointerstitium (63). Other recent investigations emphasize that type 1 angiotensin II receptor subtype is the predominant receptor subtype in rat and human kidney. *In situ* hybridization studies on type 1 angiotensin II receptor (AT1) gene expression in the rat kidney have shown AT1 mRNA in glomeruli, vasa recta, and arteries of the adult rat (64). Investigations using reverse transcription and polymerase chain reaction (RT-PCR) on microdissected rat renal tubular segments, glomeruli, vasa recta vascular bundles, and arcuate arteries indicate

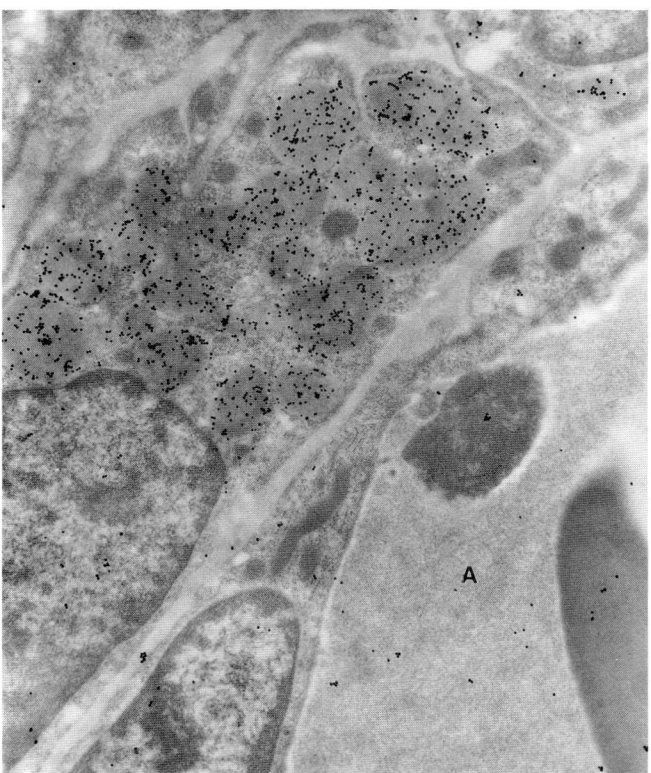

FIG. 11. Juxtaglomerular granular cells in wall of afferent arteriole (A). Section treated with immunogold technique using renin antiserum. Numerous gold particles are observed in the juxtaglomerular cell granules. (Renin antiserum provided by Dr. T. Inagami.) ×15,650.

relatively high amounts of AT1 receptor mRNA in the glomerulus, proximal tubules, cortical collecting ducts, and vasculature (65). Applying also RT-PCR to the localization of AT1 mRNA in the rat kidney, other investigators have found the glomerulus to present the highest expression of AT1 mRNA followed by the renal papilla, the renal cortex, and the renal medulla (66). In this same study, *in situ* hybridization disclosed a high concentration of AT1 mRNA in the extraglomerular mesangium but little in the afferent arteriole. This interesting finding may be a reflection of the continuity of the intraglomerular with the extraglomerular mesangium and of the similarities of the mesangial cells present in both locations. It is also of interest that treatment with angiotensin I–converting enzyme (ACE) inhibitors results in expression of AT1 in the afferent arteriole at the level of the JGCs (66).

Although the localization of angiotensin II receptors in the small preglomerular vessels remains unclear, the afferent arteriole contracts when exposed to angiotensin II *in vivo* in the rat split hydronephrotic kidney (67), and on blood perfused juxtamedullary nephrons, exogenous or locally generated angiotensin II–induced vasoconstriction of the afferent arteriole (68). It appears, there-

fore, that the afferent arteriole is responsive to the vasoconstrictive effects of angiotensin II, and thus locally generated angiotensin II, produced by whatever mechanism, could participate in glomerular hemodynamics.

There is controversy about the origin of the angiotensin II observed in the JGC. Some authors favor internalization following receptor binding or nonspecific pinocytosis rather than its endogenous formation (60,69), since angiotensin I has not been localized in the JG cell in normal or ischemic kidneys. Angiotensin I immunoreactivity, however, has been shown in animals treated with ACE inhibitors (70). The observation that cultured JGCs (71) from neonatal cats contain renin, ACE, and angiotensin I and II supports the view that the JGC may contain most of the components of the renin-angiotensin system. The presence of angiotensinogen in the JGC, however, remains uncertain. Angiotensinogen has been reported in the particulate fractions of homogenates of kidney cortex (72). Although angiotensinogen mRNA has been identified in rat kidneys (73–75), there is no total agreement as to its distribution. Whereas Campbell and Habener (74) found the highest levels of angiotensinogen mRNA in the renal cortex and progressively lower levels in the outer medulla and the inner medulla, Fried and Simpson (75) found angiotensinogen mRNA predominantly in the medulla. *In situ* hybridization studies have shown angiotensinogen mRNA to be localized primarily in the proximal tubule with some localization also occurring in the distal tubule and glomeruli (76). More recent investigations, which have been already mentioned, using RT-PCR on microdissected renal structures, confirm the predominant localization of angiotensinogen mRNA in the proximal tubules with a small amount present in glomeruli and vasa recta (65). These results are consistent with the predominant cortical localization of angiotensinogen. In any event it seems likely that there is a local angiotensin-generating mechanism in the kidney that uses both plasma-derived and tissue-derived components (77,78).

The distribution of renin and renin gene expression changes during the development. Gomez et al. (79) have shown that kidney renin mRNA levels are 7.9-fold higher in the newborn than in the adult animal. This difference corresponded with the difference in the concentration of renin in the kidney and a change in the distribution of renin-containing cells. In the newborn kidney, renin-containing cells were observed throughout the entire length of the afferent arterioles and interlobular arteries, whereas in the adult they were confined to the proximity of the glomerulus. The significance of this change of the distribution of renin in the kidney and of the renin-angiotensin system in general on renal development is currently under investigation.

For more than two decades, the JG granules have been known to have lysosomal properties such as the incorporation of exogenous tracers (80) and the presence of acid phosphatase activity (81,82). Using ultrastructural immunocytochemistry, Taugner and associates (83) have confirmed the presence of acid phosphatase. They also demonstrated the presence of another lysosomal enzyme, cathepsin B (84), which is able to activate renin *in vitro* (85). It is possible that this enzyme activates renin prior to secretion. Renin has been localized by immunoelectron microscopy in the mature granules and protogranules. Taugner and associates (86,87) investigated the intracellular processing of renin in relation to the assumed stages of granule maturation. Using antisera against different portions of the prosegment of human renin, they showed that the prosegment of renin is mainly localized to the protogranules, whereas renin itself is localized largely in the mature granules. This observation suggests that the activation of renin in the JGC occurs mainly prior to the "maturation" of the granule, namely in the protogranules. The morphologic basis of renin release by the JGC remains uncertain. In situations associated with high renin release such as after adrenalectomy (88), sodium depletion (89), and in acute renal failure (90), invaginations of the plasma membrane associated with extracellular condensations of electron-dense material has been interpreted as indicating exocytosis. The loss of membrane particles in freeze fracture surfaces after renal nerve stimulation also has been viewed as indicating exocytosis (91). Physiological evidence has been presented supporting the concept that renin may be also secreted by a mechanism other than exocytosis (92). Regardless of the mechanism, renin is most likely released to the interstitium and enters the circulation through the capillaries (93).

Extraglomerular Mesangium (Cells of Goormaghtigh, Lacis, Polkissen)

The EM is located between the afferent and efferent arterioles and has a roughly conical shape, with the base facing the MD and the tip being continuous with the glomerular mesangium. The Goormaghtigh cells extend laterally, forming a rim around the MD and can be seen interposed between the glomerular arterioles and the MD. No capillaries or nerve fibers penetrate this region. Goormaghtigh cells (EM cells) are small with a scanty cytoplasm. They appear as flattened cylinders three-dimensionally, with abundant processes at both ends (94). An interstitium containing basement membrane–like material separates the EM cells. They are, however, extensively coupled by gap junctions between themselves, with the cells of the glomerular mesangium and the glomerular arterioles. The abundance of gap junctions within this region has been documented by several authors (95–98). There are no gap junctions between the MD and extraglomerular mesangium in spite of their extensive interface. The location of the EM makes it crucial for the transmission of the "signal" from the MD to the

vascular component of the JGA. Gap junctions are regions of the plasma membrane containing transmembrane channels that permit the passage of ions and low molecular weight substances (99). They are the site of electrical coupling of cells.

It is unknown to what extent junctional communication participates in JGA function but the distribution of gap junctions is of interest in the tubuloglomerular feedback mechanism. The presence of gap junctions between the EM cells and the cells of the afferent and efferent arterioles and the glomerular mesangium suggests that they could be involved in the spread of the "signal" throughout the vascular component of the JGA and thereby reach the effector site(s) of tubuloglomerular feedback. Gap junctions are seen not only between granular JG cells, Goormaghtigh cells, arteriolar smooth muscle cells, and glomerular mesangial cells, but also between the endothelial and smooth muscle cells and the JG granular cells (100). This suggests the possibility of a bidirectional signal transfer from the arteriolar wall to the lumen.

The functional coupling between the MD and the extraglomerular mesangium is supported by the morphometric studies of Schnabel and Kriz (101), who observed that changes in the body fluid volume induced parallel variations in the size of the EM interstitium and the LIS of the MD. In the volume-expanded animals the EM interstitium and LIS were wider, whereas in the volume-depleted animals they were narrower than in the controls. These changes in LIS and in EM width correlate inversely with tubuloglomerular feedback sensitivity.

Kriz and Sakai (102) have proposed that the extraglomerular mesangium with the terminal portion of the afferent arteriole and the initial portion of the efferent arteriole functions as an integrating stretch receptor of signals from the contiguous urinary space, muscle, and granular cells of the afferent and efferent arterioles and the MD. Supporting this concept are the potential contractile properties of the EM cells, as implied by the presence of microfilaments, and their connection to the other cells of the vascular component by gap junctions. Their hypothesis also rests heavily upon the ultrastructural evidence that, in addition to the anchoring of the MD to the extraglomerular mesangium and adjacent portions of the glomerular arterioles, there is also a tight connection of the arterioles and extraglomerular mesangium to the reflexion of the glomerular basement membrane into the periglomerular basement membrane. In this manner, taking into consideration its contractile nature, the EM would not only serve as a closure device for the vascular pole but also might be able to transduce changes in tension from regions contiguous with it to the afferent and efferent arterioles. Kriz and Sakai proposed that a mechanical component might also be part of the MD signal. With the base of the MD firmly anchored in the extraglomerular mesangium and the cell height restricted by membrane cytokeratins, an increase in the lateral space volume between MD cells would also increase the tension in the extraglomerular mesangium. A decrease in LIS volume would, accordingly, diminish tensions transmitted to the extraglomerular mesangium from the MD.

It has been suggested that the fluid balance of the EM depends not only on the MD flow, but also on the transport of fluid from the glomerular afferent arteriole. Supporting this view is the presence of endothelial fenestrations in the wall of the afferent arteriole facing the extraglomerular mesangium and JGCs (103). It could also be speculated that renin might reach the glomerular circulation via the fenestrated endothelium of the glomerular afferent arteriole. Rosivall and Taugner (104) have used ferritin particles as a tracer of fluid movement in the JGA. Twenty-five seconds after the injection of ferritin, the density pattern of particles in the extraglomerular mesangium showed a gradient from the afferent arteriole to the region close to the MD. No ferritin was seen in

the region of the efferent arteriole. These observations together with the calculated pressure gradients were interpreted as indicating the presence of a variable bulk fluid flow into the extraglomerular mesangium from the afferent arteriole, glomerular capillaries, and urinary spaces. These flows could affect interstitial fluid composition in the EM and thereby influence juxtaglomerular function.

THE INNERVATION OF THE JUXTAGLOMERULAR APPARATUS

Nerves were described in the JGA by early investigators using light microscopic methods (105). Their distribution was uncertain but their assumed significance was underscored by the term *neuromyoarterial juxtaglomerular apparatus* coined by Goormaghtigh (106) to refer to the JGA. Using a variety of methods it has been shown

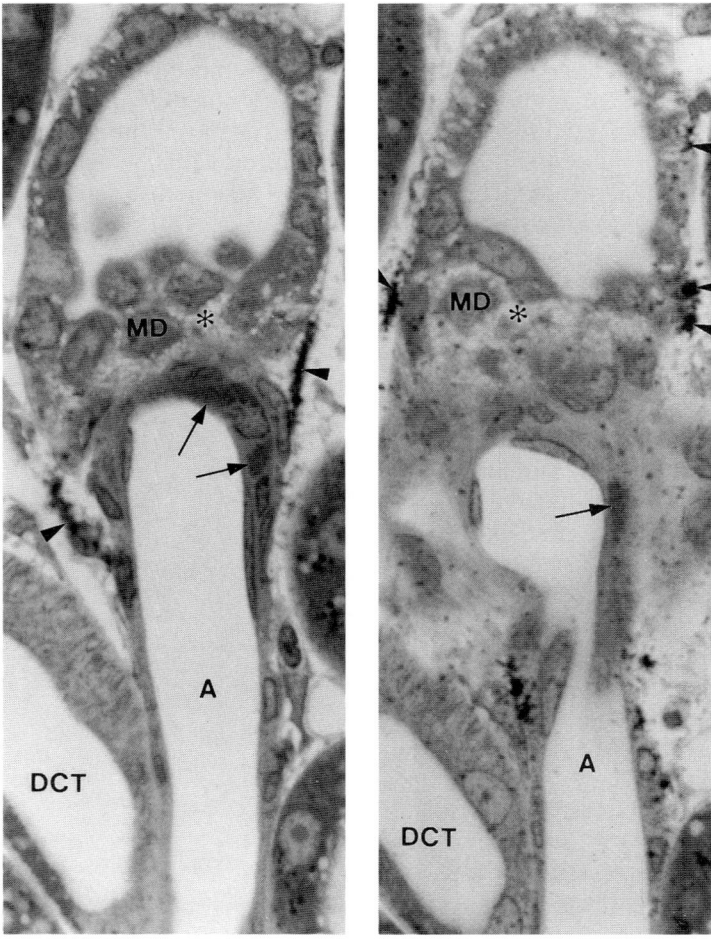

FIG. 12. Autoradiograms of sequential sections of a rat juxtaglomerular region. Monoaminergic nerves (*arrowheads*) are labeled with tritiated norepinephrine. **A:** The nerves can be followed from the afferent arteriole (A) to the periphery of the macula densa (MD). **B:** The nerves can be seen overlapping the afferent arteriole (A) and the periphery of the macula densa (MD), indicating likely sites of neuroeffector contact. Note the contact of the late distal convoluted tubule (DCT) with the afferent arteriole. *Arrows,* renin granules; *asterisk,* lateral intercellular spaces. Toluidine blue. ×1,300. (From ref. 6, with permission.)

that both the tubular and vascular components are innervated (4,5,107,108). Although the MD cells are not innervated, the contact of nerves with perimacular ("intermediary") cells has been described ultrastructurally (4,5) and by light microscopic autoradiography (108) (Fig. 12). With the electron microscope, neuroeffector contacts have been seen on the afferent and efferent arterioles and much less frequently with the extraglomerular mesangium. Serial section electron microscopy disclosed that many cells of the vascular component are not individually innervated (109). However, neural stimuli could reach the noninnervated cells via gap junctions present between the cells of the vascular component. Neural stimuli could also reach the glomerular mesangium through the gap junctions linking the extraglomerular with the glomerular mesangium. Neuroeffector contacts can be easily found on the juxtaglomerular granular cells. This observation is in agreement with the established role of the sympathetic nervous system on the control of renin secretion (10). It has become apparent that the renal sympathetic nerves might also have a direct effect on the renal tubules (110).

Quantitative studies using autoradiography indicate that all major segments of the nephron receive a certain amount of innervation (111). Although the overall greatest amount of innervation occurs on the proximal tubule, the TALH shows the highest density of nerves. Additional investigations have disclosed that the premacular region of the TALH has the highest concentration of innervation, followed by the TALH at the level of the JGA and the post-MD region (112). The relative abundance of TALH innervation and its distribution provides anatomical support for the physiological evidence that renal nerve activity might modulate renin secretion by a nonneural mechanism, most likely involving the MD (113). This view is supported by micropuncture studies showing that renal nerve stimulation directly affects sodium, water, and potassium transport (114,115). Consequently, nerve-mediated changes in the composition of the fluid reaching the MD would affect renin secretion. The level of renal nerve stimulation appears to determine whether the renal nerves act on the JGC directly or through a nonneural pathway (116). It is of interest to note that in spite of the abundant innervation of the TALH, including the perimacular cells bordering the MD, previous investigations failed to demonstrate a role for the renal nerves in tubuloglomerular feedback (117). Only recently, studies in the acutely denervated rat have disclosed reduced TGF sensitivity after denervation (118).

Dopamine-containing nerves have been found on the glomerular arterioles of the dog (119,120) and the existence of a dopaminergic vasodilatory innervation has been proposed. Vasoactive intestinal peptide (VIP)-immunoreactive fibers have been demonstrated in the kidney in association with the renal artery and its branches (121,122). Less frequently they can be seen in

association with the afferent arterioles in the dog and rat. In the rat, VIP-immunoreactive fibers have been observed close to the vascular pole (122). VIP-immunoreactive nerves also may have a vasodilatory effect. Nerves containing neuropeptide Y, which has a vasoconstrictive effect, have been found in the juxtaglomerular apparatus of a variety of species (123).

OTHER TUBULOVASCULAR RELATIONSHIPS

In addition to the special relationship of the MD with the vascular component of the JGA, other parts of the distal nephron are seen very frequently, although not always, in "contact" with the glomerular vessels. The significance of these tubulovascular relationships remains to be proven. A frequent and often extensive contact of the pre-JGA TALH with the efferent arteriole in the rat has been reported (124,125). Faarup (125) stated almost 30 years ago that the distal nephron, in its intercalated portion, contacted the afferent arteriole, which in some instances belonged to the same nephron. Using semithin plastic-embedded serial sections we have observed the very frequent contact of the connecting portion of the distal nephron with the afferent arteriole (Fig. 13) and on occasion with the extraglomerular mesangium (Fig. 3) (6). There was variation with the level of the nephron.

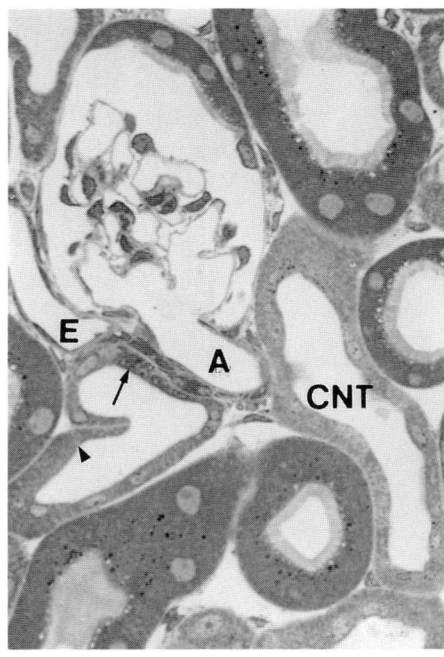

FIG. 13. Juxtaglomerular apparatus of mouse. Afferent arteriole (A), efferent arteriole (E), extraglomerular mesangium between the arterioles. *Arrow,* macula densa; connecting tubule (CNT) in contact with the afferent arteriole. The thick ascending limb of Henle extends beyond the macula densa followed by the transition (*arrowhead*) to the convoluted portion. ×470. (From ref. 6, with permission.)

In all superficial and midcortical nephrons the afferent arteriole was contacted by a connecting tubule (CNT). In all the midcortical nephrons ($n = 15$) and most of the superficial nephrons (13 of the 15), the CNT belonged to the same nephron whereas in the remaining two superficial nephrons the afferent arteriole was in contact with the CNT of another nephron. In 11 of the 15 juxtamedullary nephrons surveyed, the CNT was seen to be in contact with an afferent arteriole and only eight of these were found to belong to the same nephron (6). These contacts between connecting tubule and afferent arteriole of the same nephron have recently been confirmed using computer assisted three-dimensional reconstructions (126). The functional validity of such contacts has received support from the recent observations by Morsing et al. (127), using micropuncture, that blocking distal fluid flow decreases the sensitivity of the tubuloglomerular feedback system while enhancing the final constrictor effect on the afferent arteriole (127).

The CNT has been shown by microdissection (128–130) and histochemical studies (131,132) to contain kallikrein. This protease activates renin *in vitro* (133). Kallikreins and kinins have been shown to stimulate renin secretion from preparations of isolated rat glomeruli with the afferent arteriole attached (134,135). Localization of renin and kallikrein in the same section, using the immunoperoxidase technique and two different chromogens, has shown a frequent and close proximity of the renin-containing cells of the afferent arteriole and the kallikrein-containing cells of the CNT (136). It can be speculated that if kallikrein reaches the interstitium, it might activate renin. It also might lead to the formation of kinins, which could affect the vascular tone of the afferent arteriole. Contact between the kallikrein-containing tubule and afferent arteriole have been also reported in the human kidney (137).

Immunoreactivity to kallikrein has been found in cells located at the Bowman's capsule near the vascular pole in the sheep (138) and *in situ* hybridization studies have shown kallikrein mRNA in the same location (139). These cells, named *peripolar cells,* are frequently seen in sheep and have been described in a variety of other species (140–143), although they appear to be rare. The peripolar cells may be seen in close anatomical proximity to the renin-containing cells of the juxtaglomerular apparatus. The possibility of a functional relationship between the peripolar cells and the JGA has been suggested. Whether a renin-kallikrein interaction occurs is a matter of speculation, although the rarity of the peripolar cells in some species detracts from their possible significance, at least in those species.

ACKNOWLEDGMENTS

The skillful assistance of Shirley Slye and Joanne Ong in the preparation of the chapter is gratefully acknowledged. This work is supported by grant RO1 HL 18340 from the National Heart, Lung, and Blood Institute.

REFERENCES

1. Peter K. *Anat Anz* 1907;30(suppl):114.
2. Zimmermann KW. *A Mikrosk Anat Forsch* 1933;32:176–278.
3. Christensen JA, Bohle A. *Virchows Arch [A]* 1978;379:143–150.
4. Gorgas K. In: Coupland RE, Forssmann WG, eds. *Peripheral neuroendocrine interaction.* New York: Springer-Verlag, 1978;144–152.
5. Gorgas K. *Adv Anat Embryol Cell Biol* 1978;54:14–84.
6. Barajas L, Salido EC, Powers KV. In: Persson AEG, Boberg U, eds. *The juxtaglomerular apparatus.* Amsterdam: Elsevier, 1988;7–26.
7. Barajas L. *J Ultrastruct Res* 1970;33:116–147.
8. Oberling C, Hatt PY. *Ann Pathol Anat* 1960;5:441–474.
9. Barajas L. *Am J Physiol* 1979;237:F333–F343.
10. Davis JO, Freeman RH. *Physiol Rev* 1976;56:1–56.
11. Briggs JP, Schnermann J. *Renal Physiol* 1986;9:193–203.
12. Guyton AC, Langston JB, Navar G. *Circ Res* 1964;15(suppl I):I-187–I-194.
13. Thurau K. *Am J Med* 1964;36:698–719.
14. Wright FS, Briggs JP. *Physiol Rev* 1979;59:958–1006.
15. Kaissling B, Peter S, Kriz W. *Cell Tissue Res* 1977;182:111–118.
16. Kaissling B, Kriz W. *Kidney Int* 1982;22:S9–S17.
17. Bonsib SM. *J Ultrastruct Molec Struct Res* 1986;97:103–108.
18. Alcorn D, Anderson WP, Ryan GB. *Renal Physiol* 1986;9:335–347.
19. Kirk KL, Bell PD, Barfuss DW, Ribadeneira M. *Am J Physiol* 1985;248:F890–F894.
20. Briggs JP, Schnermann J. *Annu Rev Physiol* 1987;49:251–273.
21. Beeuwkes R, Rosen S. *J Histochem Cytochem* 1975;11:828–839.
22. Beeuwkes R, Rosen S. *Curr Top Membr Transp* 1980;13:343–354.
23. Kashgarian M, Biemesderfer D, Caplan M, Fobush B. *Kidney Int* 1985;28:899–913.
24. Hoyer JR, Sisson SP, Vernier RL. *Lab Invest* 1979;41:168–173.
25. Sikri KL, Foster CL, Bloomfield FJ, Marshall RD. *Biochem J* 1979;181:525–532.
26. Stevenson FK, Cleave AD, Kent PW. *Biochem Biophys Acta* 1971;236:59–66.
27. Pennica D, Kohr WJ, Kuang WJ, et al. *Science* 1987;236:83–88.
28. Hession C, Decker JM, Sherblom AP, et al. *Science* 1987;237:1479–1484.
29. Salido EC, Fisher DA, Barajas L. *J Ultrastruct Molec Struct Res* 1986;91:105–113.
30. Salido EC, Barajas L, Lechago J, Laborde NP, Fisher DA. *J Histochem Cytochem* 1986;34:1155–1160.
31. Rall LB, Scott J, Bell GI, et al. *Nature* 1985;313:228–231.
32. Salido EC, Yen PH, Shapiro LJ, Fisher DA, Barajas L. *Am J Physiol* 1989;256:F632–F638.
33. Gray A, Dull TJ, Ullrich A. *Nature* 1983;303:722–725.
34. Scott J, Urdea M, Quiroga M, et al. *Science* 1983;221:236–240.
35. Norman J, Badie-Dezfooly B, Nord EP, et al. *Am J Physiol* 1987;253:F299–F309.
36. Wilson PD, Horster MF. *Am J Physiol* 1983;13:C166–C174.
37. Rozengurt E, Heppel LA. *Proc Natl Acad Sci USA* 1975;72:4492–4495.
38. Scoggins BD, Butkus A, Coghlan JP, et al. In: Labrie F, Proulx L, eds. *Endocrinology.* New York: Elsevier, 1984;573–576.
39. Pfeffer S, Ullrich A. *Nature* 1985;313:184.
40. Mundel P, Bachmann S, Bader M, et al. *Kidney Int* 1992;42:1017–1019.
41. Wilcox CS, Welch WJ, Murad F, et al. *Proc Natl Acad Sci USA* 1992;89:11993–11997.
42. Bachman S, Mundel P, Kriz W. *J Am Soc Nephrol* 1992;3:540(Abstract).
43. Goormaghtigh N. *J Pathol Bacteriol* 1945;57:392–393.
44. Goormaghtigh N. *Rev Belge Sci Med* 1945;16:65–155.
45. Vander AJ, Miller R. *Am J Physiol* 1964;207:537–546.
46. Skott O, Briggs JP. *Science* 1987;237:1618–1620.
47. Ruyter JHC. *Z Mikrosk Anat Forsch* 1925;2:242–248.

48. Buhrle CP, Nobiling R, Taugner R. *Am J Physiol* 1985;249: F272–F281.
49. Barajas L, Latta H. *Anat Rec* 1965;151:321.
50. Barajas L. *J Ultrastruct Res* 1966;15:400–413.
51. Hartroft PM, Hartroft WS. *J Exp Med* 1953;97:415–429.
52. Hartroft WS, Hartroft PM. *Fed Proc* 1961;20:845–854.
53. Edelman R, Hartroft PM. *Circ Res* 1961;9:1069–1077.
54. Cook WF. In: Fisher JW, ed. *Hormones and the kidney.* London: Academic Press, 1971;117–128.
55. Deschepper CF, Mellon SH, Cumin F, Baxter JD, Ganong WF. *Proc Natl Acad Sci USA* 1986;83:7552–7556.
56. Taugner R, Rosivall L, Buehrle CP, Groeschel-Stewart U. *Cell Tissue Res* 1987;248:579–588.
57. Taugner R, Nobiling R, Mertz R, Taugner F, Bührle CP, Hackenthal E. *Cell Tissue Res* 1988;252:687–690.
58. Celio MR, Inagami T. *Proc Natl Acad Sci USA* 1981;78:3897–3900.
59. Taugner R, Hackenthal E. *Histochemistry* 1981;72:499–509.
60. Cantin M, Gutkowska J, Lacasse J, et al. *Am J Pathol* 1984;115: 212–224.
61. Mendelsohn FAO, Dunbar M, Allen A, Chou ST, Millan MA, Aguilera G, Catt J. *Fed Proc* 1986;45:1420–1425.
62. Chou S-Y, Faubert PF, Porush JG. *Fed Proc* 1986;45:1438–1443.
63. Groene HJ, Simon M, Fuchs E. *Am J Physiol* 1992;262:F326–F331.
64. Tufro-McReddie A, Harrison JK, Everett AD, Gomez RA. *J Clin Invest* 1993;91:530–537.
65. Terada Y, Tomita K, Nonoguchi, Marumo F. *Kidney Int* 1993;43:1251–1259.
66. Kakinuma Y, Fogo A, Inagami T, Ishikawa I. *Kidney Int* 1993;43:1229–1235.
67. Steinhausen M, Sterzel RB, Fleming JT, Kuhn R, Weis S. *Kidney Int* 1987;31(suppl 20):S64–S73.
68. Casellas D, Jover B, Dupont M. *J Am Soc Nephrol* 1990;1: 662(abstract).
69. Taugner R, Mannek E, Nobiling R, et al. *Histochemistry* 1984;81:39–45.
70. Naruse K, Inagami T, Celio MR, Workman RJ, Takii Y. *Hypertension* 1982;4(suppl II):II70–II74.
71. Rightsel WA, Okamura T, Inagami T, et al. *Circ Res* 1982;50: 822–829.
72. Morris BJ, Johnston CI. *Biochem J* 1976;154:625–637.
73. Campbell DJ, Habener JF. *J Clin Invest* 1986;78:31–39.
74. Campbell DJ, Habener JF. *J Hypertension* 1986;4(suppl 6): S385–S387.
75. Fried TA, Simpson EA. *Am J Physiol* 1986;250:F374–F377.
76. Ingelfinger JR, Zuo WM, Fon EA, Ellison KE, Dzau VJ. *J Clin Invest* 1990;85:417–423.
77. Campbell DJ. *J Hypertens* 1985;3:199–207.
78. Navar LG, Rosivall L, Carmines PK, Oparil S. *Fed Proc* 1986;45: 1448–1453.
79. Gomez RA, Lynch KR, Chevalier RL, et al. *Am J Physiol* 1988;254:F582–F587.
80. Latta H, Manusbach AB. *J Ultrastruct Res* 1962;6:562–572.
81. Fisher ER. *Science* 1966;152:1752–1753.
82. Lee JC, Hurley S, Hopper J. *Lab Invest* 1966;15:1459–1476.
83. Taugner R, Whalley A, Angermuller S, Buhrle CP, Hackenthal E. *Cell Tissue Res* 1985;239:575–587.
84. Taugner R, Buhrle CP, Nobiling R, Kirschke H. *Histochemistry* 1985;83:103–108.
85. Takahashi S, Murakami K, Miyake Y. *J Biochem* 1982;91:419–422.
86. Taugner R, Murakami K, Kim S-J. *Histochemistry* 1986;85: 107–109.
87. Taugner R, Kim S-J, Murakami K, Waldherr R. *Histochemistry* 1987;86:249–253.
88. Peter S. *Cell Tissue Res* 1976;168:45–53.
89. Hill PA, Coghlan JP, Scoggins BA, Ryan GB. *Pathology* 1983;15: 463–473.
90. Ryan GB, Alcorn D, Coghlan JP, Hill PA, Jabobs R. *Kidney Int* 1982;22:S3–S8.
91. Taugner R, Forssmann WG, Billich H, Boll U, Ganten D, Seller H. In: Coupland RE, Forssmann WG, eds. *Peripheral neuroendocrine interaction.* Berlin: Springer-Verlag, 1978;153–163.
92. Fray JCS, Lush DJ, Valentine AND. *Fed Proc* 1983;42:3150–3154.
93. Morgan T, Davis J, Gillies A. *Kidney Int* 1982;22:S63–S66.
94. Spanidis A, Wunsch H, Kaissling B, Kriz W. *Anat Embryol* 1982;165:239–252.
95. Biava CG, West M. *Am J Pathol* 1966;49:679–721.
96. Pricam C, Humbert F, Perrelet A, Orci L. *J Cell Biol* 1974;63: 349–354.
97. Boll HU, Forssmann WG, Taugner R. *Cell Tissue Res* 1975;161: 459–469.
98. Taugner R, Schiller A, Kaissling B, Kriz W. *Cell Tissue Res* 1978;186:279–285.
99. Beyer EC. *Int Rev Cytol* 1993;137C:1–37.
100. Taugner R, Kirchheim H, Forssmann WG. *Cell Tissue Res* 1984;235:319–325.
101. Schnabel E, Kriz W. *Anat Embryol* 1984;170:217–222.
102. Kriz W, Sakai T. In: Persson AEG, Boberg U, eds. *The juxtaglomerular apparatus.* Amsterdam: Elsevier, 1988;27–37.
103. Rosivall L, Taugner R. *Cell Tissue Res* 1986;243:525–533.
104. Rosivall L, Taugner R. In: Persson AEG, Boberg U, eds. *The juxtaglomerular apparatus.* Amsterdam: Elsevier, 1988;7–26.
105. DeMuylder CG. *The "neurility" of the kidney. A monograph on nerve supply to the kidney.* Springfield, IL: Thomas, 1952.
106. Goormaghtigh N. *C R Soc Biol* 1937;124:293–296.
107. Barajas L. *Fed Proc* 1978;37:1192–1201.
108. Barajas L, Powers K. *J Hypertens* 1984;2(suppl 1):3–12.
109. Barajas L, Muller J. *J Ultrastruct Res* 1973;43:107–132.
110. DiBona GF. *Rev Physiol Biochem Pharmacol* 1982;94:76–181.
111. Barajas L, Powers K, Wang P. *Am J Physiol* 1984;247:F50–F60.
112. Barajas L, Powers K. *Am J Physiol* 1988;24:F340–348.
113. Thames MD, DiBona GF. *Circ Res* 1979;44:645–652.
114. DiBona GF, Sawin LL. *Am J Physiol* 1982;243:F576–F580.
115. Bencsath P, Szenasi G, Takacs L. *Am J Physiol* 1985;249:F308–F314.
116. Thames MD. *J Hypertens* 1984;2(suppl 1):57–66.
117. Takabatake T, Yasuyuki U, Katsuroh O, Huttori N. *Am J Physiol* 1990;258:F980–F985.
118. Kurkus J, Thorup C, Morsing P, Person AEG. *Acta Physiol Scand* 1993;149:119–120.
119. Bell C. *Neuroscience* 1982;7:1–8.
120. Dinerstein RJ, Vannice J, Henderson RC, Roth LJ, Goldberg LI, Hoffmann PC. *Science* 1979;205:497–499.
121. Barajas L, Sokolski KN, Lechago J. *Neurosci Lett* 1983;43:263–269.
122. Knight DS, Beal JA, Yuan ZP, Fournet TS. *Anat Rec* 1987;219: 193–203.
123. Ballesta J, Polak JM, Allen JM, Bloom SR. *Histochemistry* 1984;80:483–485.
124. Barajas L, Latta H. *Lab Invest* 1963;12:257–269.
125. Faarup P. *Acta Anat* 1965;60:20–38.
126. Dorup J, Morsing P, Rasch R. *Lab Invest* 1992;67:761–769.
127. Morsing P, Velazquez H, Ellison, Wright FS. *Acta Physiol Scand* 1993;148:63–68.
128. Tomita K, Endou H, Sakai F. *Pflugers Arch* 1981;389:91–95.
129. Omata K, Carretero OA, Scicli AG, Jackson BA. *Kidney Int* 1982;22:602–617.
130. Proud D, Knepper MA, Pisano JJ. *Am J Physiol* 1983;244:F510–F515.
131. Figueroa CD, Caorsi I, Subiabre J, Vio CP. *J Histochem Cytochem* 1984;32:117–121.
132. Figueroa CD, Caorsi I, Vio CP. *J Histochem Cytochem* 1984;32: 1238–1240.
133. Sealey JE, Atlas SA, Laragh JH. *Am J Med* 1978;65:994–1000.
134. Beirwaltes WH, Prada J, Carretero OA. *Hypertension* 1985;7:27–31.
135. Beirwaltes WH, Prada J, Carretero OA. *Am J Physiol* 1985;248: F757–F761.
136. Barajas L, Powers KV, Carretero O, Scicili AG, Inagami T. *Kidney Int* 1986;29:965–970.
137. Vio CP, Figueroa CD, Caorsi I. *Am J Hypertens* 1988;1:269–271.
138. Gall JAM, Alcorn D, Coghlan JP, Johnston CI, Ryan GB. *Proceedings of the IXth Int Cong of Nephrol* 1984;451(abstract).
139. Xiong W, Chao L, Chao J. *Kidney Int* 1989;35:1324–1329.
140. Gardiner DS, Lindop GBM. *Histopathology* 1985;9:675–685.
141. Hanner RH, Ryan GB. *J Anat* 1980;130:445–455.
142. Ryan GB, Coghlan JP, Scoggins BA. *Nature* 1979;277:655–656.
143. Ryan GB, Alcorn D, Coghlan JP, Hill PA, Jacobs R. *Kidney Int* 1982;22(suppl 12):S3–S8.

Hypertension: Pathophysiology, Diagnosis, and Management, Second Edition, edited by J.H. Laragh and B.M. Brenner, Raven Press, Ltd., New York © 1995.

CHAPTER 81

Neural Control of Renal Function: Role in Human Hypertension

Gerald F. DiBona and Ulla C. Kopp

Efferent renal sympathetic nerve activity (ERSNA) is elevated in human essential hypertension as well as in several forms of experimental hypertension in animals. It is known that ERSNA has significant effects on all major aspects of renal function. This chapter presents the evidence in support of a role for the renal nerves in the control of kidney function in hypertension.

NEURAL CONTROL OF RENAL FUNCTION—NORMAL PHYSIOLOGY

Renal Neuroanatomy

Interest in the functional significance of the renal nerves has increased steadily since the application of ultrastructural, histofluorescent, and histochemical techniques provided a more definitive description of the intrinsic innervation of the kidney (1). It is now known that there is extensive and exclusive adrenergic innervation of the afferent and efferent glomerular arterioles, proximal and distal renal tubules, ascending limb of Henle's loop,

G. F. DiBona and U. C. Kopp: Department of Internal Medicine, University of Iowa College of Medicine, Iowa City, Iowa 52242.

and juxtaglomerular apparatus. Within the nephron, the greatest relative density of innervation is in the thick ascending limb of Henle's loop, followed by the distal convoluted tubule and the proximal tubule. Although there appears to be renal nerves that contain dopamine, the evidence supporting the presence of renal nerves that utilize dopamine as a true neurotransmitter remains controversial (2–7).

Physiological Effects

With this more complete understanding of the ultrastructure of the intrinsic renal innervation, there has been a growing interest in the effects produced by alterations in ERSNA on various aspects of overall renal function. From an extensive body of experimental evidence, derived largely from studies in animals (2–7), it is known that renal sympathetic nerve activity significantly influences many important aspects of renal function (Table 1). Using direct electrical renal nerve stimulation, application of graded frequencies produces frequency-dependent changes in renal blood flow and glomerular filtration rate, renal tubular sodium and water reabsorption, and renin secretion. In general, the frequency-response relationship for increases in renin secretion rate

TABLE 1. *Renal responses to graded renal nerve stimulation*

RNS (Hz)	RSR	$U_{Na}V$	GFR	RBF
0.25	0	0	0	0
0.50	↑	0	0	0
1.00	↑	↓	0	0
2.50	↑	↓	↓	↓

RNS, renal nerve stimulation; RSR, renin secretion rate; $U_{Na}V$, urinary sodium excretion; GFR, glomerular filtration rate; RBF, renal blood flow.

is to the left of that for increases in renal tubular sodium and water reabsorption, which in turn is to the left of that for decreases in renal blood flow and glomerular filtration rates (Fig. 1).

In most mammalian species, the frequency-dependent decreases in renal blood flow and increases in renal vascular resistance caused by increases in ERSNA are predominantly mediated by renal vascular α_1-adrenoceptors (8). However, there is evidence for a small but definite contribution of renal vascular α_2-adrenoceptors in the rabbit (9).

The renal sympathetic nerves can regulate urinary sodium and water excretion by (a) changing renal hemodynamics (e.g., renal blood flow, glomerular filtration rate) through changes in renal vascular resistance, (b) changing renin release from the juxtaglomerular granular cells with increased formation of angiotensin II, or (c) through a direct effect on the innervated renal tubules (10). With respect to the influence of renal nerve stimulation on glomerular filtration rate, there is an additional contribution from the concomitant stimulation of angiotensin II production, which acts on glomerular mesangial cells to affect glomerular filtration rate via alterations in glomerular capillary ultrafiltration coefficient (11), the product of glomerular capillary surface area (regulated by mesangial cell contractility), and glomerular capillary hydraulic permeability.

Increases or decreases in ERSNA, at frequencies that do not alter renal perfusion pressure, total renal blood flow or its distribution, or glomerular filtration rate, cause parallel changes in net renal tubular sodium and water reabsorption with reciprocal changes in urinary water and sodium excretion. That is, increases in ERSNA increase net renal tubular sodium and water reabsorption and decrease urinary water and sodium excretion, whereas decreases in ERSNA decrease net renal tubular sodium and water reabsorption and increase urinary water and sodium excretion. The changes in renal tubular sodium and water reabsorption occur throughout the nephron in rough proportion to the density of tubular innervation and are mediated via α_1-adrenoceptors located on the peritubular membranes in the dog (12), rat (13,14), and rabbit (15) kidneys. In microdissec-

tion studies of the rat nephron, α_1-adrenoceptors have been localized to the proximal convoluted and proximal straight tubules in addition to the medullary and cortical thick ascending limb of Henle's loop and the distal convoluted tubule; they were not found in the cortical and outer medullary collecting ducts (16). A current formulation of the cellular mechanism of action of the neurotransmitter of the renal nerves, norepinephrine, on tubular sodium reabsorption is as follows: α_1-adrenoceptor activation increases intracellular calcium concentration with subsequent activation of the calcium/calmodulin–dependent protein phosphatase 2B, calcineurin, which is capable of dephosphorylating Na^+,K^+–adenosine triphosphatase (ATPase) from its inactive phospho-Na^+,K^+-ATPase to its active dephospho-Na^+,K^+-ATPase form (17). The increased activity of Na^+,K^+-ATPase increases the movement of intracellular sodium across the basolateral cell membrane to the extracellular space. This creates a more favorable gradient for the entry of extracellular sodium across the apical cell membrane to the intracellular space. The net effect is an increase in transepithelial sodium transport.

ERSNA can influence renin secretion rate from the kidney by a variety of mechanisms (2–7), either directly or by interacting with the renal tubular macula densa and vascular baroreceptor mechanisms for renin secretion (Tables 1 and 2). At frequencies of renal sympathetic nerve stimulation (≤0.25 Hz) that do not affect renal hemodynamics, urinary sodium excretion, or basal renin secretion rate, the renin secretion rate response to nonneural stimuli (i.e., baroreceptor and macula densa mechanisms) is augmented. This important interaction

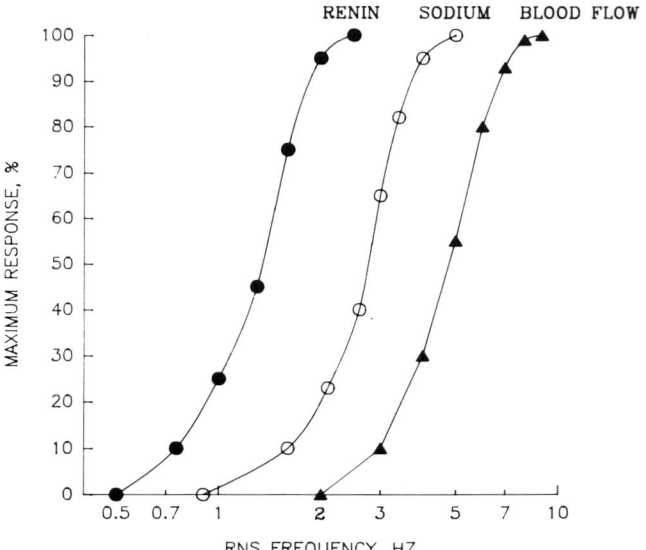

FIG. 1. Relationship of effects of renal sympathetic nerve stimulation on responses of renin secretion (increase), urinary sodium excretion (decrease), and renal blood flow (decrease).

TABLE 2. *Neural control of renin secretion rate[a]*

Renal nerve stimulation frequency (Hz)	Mechanism of increase in renin secretion rate
0.25	Modulation of nonneural mechanisms
0.50	Direct neural release from juxtaglomerular granular cells without alterations in stimuli to macula densa receptor or baroreceptor
1.00	Alteration in stimulus to macula densa receptor
2.50	Alteration in stimulus to baroreceptor

[a] Effects become additive as frequency of renal nerve stimulation increases.

(18) functions such that when there is strong stimulation to the renal vascular baroreceptor (markedly reduced renal arterial pressure), augmentation of the renin secretion rate response is achieved with very low frequencies of renal sympathetic nerve stimulation. Conversely, at lesser degrees of renal vascular baroreceptor stimulation (lesser decreases in renal arterial pressure), higher frequencies of renal sympathetic nerve stimulation are required for augmentation of the renin secretion rate. At slightly higher frequencies of renal sympathetic nerve stimulation (0.5 Hz), the renin secretion rate is increased without alterations in renal hemodynamics or urinary sodium excretion, and, thus, there is no change in input stimuli to the baroreceptor or macula densa receptor mechanisms for renin secretion. This increase in the renin secretion rate is due to direct stimulation of β_1-adrenoceptors located on juxtaglomerular granular cells (2–7). At a frequency of renal sympathetic nerve stimulation (1.0 Hz) that increases renal tubular sodium reabsorption (lowers urinary sodium excretion) without changing renal hemodynamics, the renin secretion rate is further increased, possibly reflecting an interactive contribution from the tubular macula densa receptor mechanism. At frequencies of renal sympathetic nerve stimulation (>2.0 Hz) that produce renal vasoconstriction with decreases in renal blood flow, glomerular filtration rate, and urinary sodium excretion, the increase in the renin secretion rate derives from a complex interaction between all three mechanisms involved in the regulation of renin secretion and involves both β_1- and α_1-adrenoceptors, with renal prostaglandins being coupled in series to the α_1-adrenoceptor–mediated renal vasoconstriction (2–7).

As is evident, the renal sympathetic nerves participate in the regulation of several renal functions felt to be importantly involved in hypertension; among them are the control of renal hemodynamics (renal blood flow and vascular resistance, glomerular filtration rate), renal tubular reabsorption of sodium and water, and the renin secretion rate.

ROLE OF RENAL NERVES IN HYPERTENSION

Increased ERSNA in Human and Experimental Hypertension

Increased renal vascular resistance with a reduction in renal blood flow is commonly observed in patients with essential hypertension. There is clear evidence that ERSNA is increased in human subjects with essential hypertension and that it contributes to the observed abnormal renal hemodynamic pattern. Hollenberg (19) demonstrated that the increase in renal blood flow (and decrease in renal vascular resistance) in response to the renal arterial administration of the α-adrenoceptor antagonist phentolamine was significantly greater in human subjects with essential hypertension than in normotensive control subjects. This finding indicates that, in human essential hypertension, there is increased sympathetic vasoconstrictor influence on the renal vasculature. In agreement with these findings, Lorelius et al. (20) showed that splanchnic blockade increased renal blood flow (and decreased renal vascular resistance) in patients with essential hypertension but not in normotensive control subjects. Esler et al. (21) have demonstrated that norepinephrine spillover to plasma, an index of total sympathetic nervous system activity, is increased in human essential hypertensive subjects and that this increase derives in large part from a significant increase in renal norepinephrine spillover, an accurate index of ERSNA. Therefore, there is compelling evidence for an important contribution of the increase in ERSNA to the abnormal renal hemodynamics observed in human essential hypertension. In this regard it is important to note that renal vascular reactivity to norepinephrine administration is normal in patients with essential hypertension (22).

In addition, sympathetic nerve activity to skeletal muscle resistance vessels [muscle sympathetic nerve activity (MSNA)] is increased in essential hypertension (23,24). Furthermore, arterial baroreflex control of MSNA in essential hypertensive patients is normal, suggesting that the increased MSNA in essential hypertension is a result of central neural mechanisms and not of impaired arterial baroreceptor input (25).

Both ERSNA and MSNA are influenced by dietary NaCl intake, being higher during low than high dietary NaCl intake (26).

In addition to evidence for increased ERSNA in human essential hypertension there is direct evidence for increased ERSNA in experimental hypertension. In the spontaneously hypertensive rat (SHR), arguably the most relevant animal model for human essential hypertension, single fiber measurements of ERSNA have demonstrated that ERSNA is significantly higher in SHR than the normotensive control Wistar-Kyoto (WKY) rats (27).

Effect of Renal Denervation in Experimental Hypertension

Strong evidence for the participation of the renal nerves in hypertension derives from the studies of complete renal denervation in several experimental forms of hypertension in animals. For the most part, the technique employed produced a combined surgical-pharmacological disruption of the entire renal nerve population, both afferent and efferent; this is referred to as complete renal denervation. Table 3 shows the various experimental forms of hypertension in animals in which complete renal denervation delayed the development and/or attenuated the magnitude of hypertension (28,29). The uniform effect of complete renal denervation on the hypertension in such a diverse group of experimental forms of hypertension in several different species would seem to indicate a universally important role for the renal nerves in hypertension.

In several of the models the effect of the complete renal denervation on the hypertensive process was associated with changes in renal function characteristic of decreases in ERSNA. For example, the effect of complete renal denervation to delay the development of the hypertension in SHR (30) was associated with an increase in the fraction of the ingested sodium excreted in the urine (denervation natriuresis), and the subsequent development of hypertension was paralleled by a return of renal tissue norepinephrine content toward normal (evidence of renal reinnervation) and a decrease in the fraction of the ingested sodium excreted in the urine. Additional studies have shown that the development of efferent renal sympathetic innervation is accelerated in SHR and that inhibition of sympathetic function ameliorates renal vascular and parenchymal damage independent of systemic hypertension (31).

The issue of whether the effect of complete renal de-

nervation, with sections of both afferent and efferent renal neural pathways, is mediated by interruption of afferent or efferent renal nerve activity has been studied by more direct techniques involving selective interruption of the afferent renal neural pathways. Thoracolumbar dorsal rhizotomy to produce selective afferent renal denervation attenuated the severity of hypertension in rats with one-kidney, one-clip (1K,1C) and two-kidneys, one-clip (2K,1C) Goldblatt hypertension and in dogs with chronic aortic coarctation hypertension (32). However, no such effect was seen SHR (32), indicating that the antihypertensive effect of complete renal denervation in SHR was mediated by interruption of efferent renal neural pathways.

The effect of selective afferent renal denervation in Goldblatt hypertensive rats is mediated by a central feedback mechanism involving a reduction in hypothalamic norepinephrine stores, which results in a decrease in peripheral sympathetic nervous system activity, thereby reducing arterial pressure. These results indicate that afferent renal nerves, conveying information from renal sensory receptors to the neuraxis, are important modulators of central integrative centers involved in the regulation of peripheral sympathetic nervous system activity in this model of hypertension.

Renorenal reflexes (33,34), mediated by both renal mechanoreceptors and chemoreceptors and important in the coordination of renal excretory activity between the two kidneys, are impaired in SHR (35). This impairment is related to the effect of arterial pressure on the kidney as the abnormality is not present in young prehypertensive SHRs or in treated SHRs who are normotensive (36). Renorenal reflexes are also impaired in (2K,1C) Goldblatt hypertensive rats (37).

The development of hypertension produced by intrarenal norepinephrine infusion in rats is not affected by bilateral renal denervation, suggesting that nonneural, possibly hormonal, pathways mediate the hypertension in this model (38).

It is of interest that bilateral renal denervation has divergent effects in two genetic models of NaCl-sensitive hypertension: it prevents the development of hypertension in borderline hypertensive rat (BHR) (39) but has no effect in Dahl NaCl-sensitive (S) rats (40). This suggests that either the kidney of the BHR and the Dahl S respond differently to changes in ERSNA or that the characteristics of ERSNA are different in BHR and Dahl S.

TABLE 3. *Animal models of experimental hypertension in which complete renal denervation delays or prevents the development of hypertension*

Spontaneously hypertensive rat (SHR)
Stroke-prone SHR
NaCl-sensitive SHR
New Zealand SHR
Borderline hypertensive rat (BHR)
Goldblatt 1 kidney, 1 clip (rat)
Goldblatt 2 kidney, 1 clip (rat)
Aortic coarctation (dog, rat)
Aortic nerve transection (rat)
Sinoaortic denervation–NaCl (rabbit)
DOCA-NaCl rat
DOCA (miniature swine)
Grollman renal wrap (rat)
Low sodium, 1 kidney (rat)
Angiotensin II (rat)

Causes of Increased ERSNA in Hypertension

Although altered arterial baroreceptor function has been viewed as a potential mechanism for the increases in ERSNA and MSNA in hypertension, the finding that MSNA is increased in essential hypertensive patients at a time when arterial baroreceptor regulation of MSNA is normal strongly supports the view that the heightened sympathetic neural drive in hypertension in humans is of central neural origin.

In terms of central neural mechanisms for increased sympathetic neural activity in hypertension, Folkow (41) has identified three major interdependent causative elements in the physiology of primary hypertension: hereditary predisposition (genetic factor), environmental influences, and structural cardiovascular adaptations to the increase in arterial pressure. Of the environmental influences, two major factors have been identified: excitatory environmental (psychoemotional) stress and dietary NaCl intake. Environmental stress may be translated into increased sympathetic nervous system activity via the limbic-hypothalamic-bulbar autonomic centers. Environmental stress can induce chronic hypertension in normotensive Sprague-Dawley rats (42). Increased dietary NaCl intake can augment sympathetic nervous system activity responses to environmental stress (43). The development of hypertension in rats with a genetic predisposition to hypertension is accelerated by high dietary NaCl intake alone (44) or by environmental stress alone (45); however, the combination of genetic predisposition, high dietary NaCl intake, and environmental stress results in more severe hypertension than any factor alone (46). Complete renal denervation delays the onset of chronic stress hypertension (39), further emphasizing the important role of the renal nerves in the pathophysiology of hypertension.

In the SHR (47) as well as two NaCl-sensitive genetic forms of hypertension, the Dahl (48) and BHR (49), there is an increased response to environmental stress characterized by enhanced pressor, tachycardic, and renal sympathoexcitatory responses in association with a significant antidiuresis and antinatriuresis. In addition, increased dietary NaCl intake leads to even greater responses to environmental stress (47–49). The renal excretory responses are mediated by the increase in ERSNA as they are abolished by prior bilateral renal denervation (47–49). Thus, these studies indicate an important interaction between genetic predisposition to hypertension and the environmental influences of stress and increased dietary NaCl intake. This interaction results in increases in ERSNA of central neural origin (50,51), which contribute to the maintenance of hypertension via the changes produced in renal function.

The mechanisms by which peripheral (including renal) sympathetic outflow is increased in NaCl-sensitive hypertension are related to an NaCl-induced alteration in central nervous system mechanisms that govern peripheral sympathetic nerve activity (Fig. 2). The increased arterial pressure and ERSNA in SHR (47) and BHR (49) in response to increased dietary NaCl intake is associated with a decrease in norepinephrine concentration (52) and turnover (53) in the anterior hypothalamic

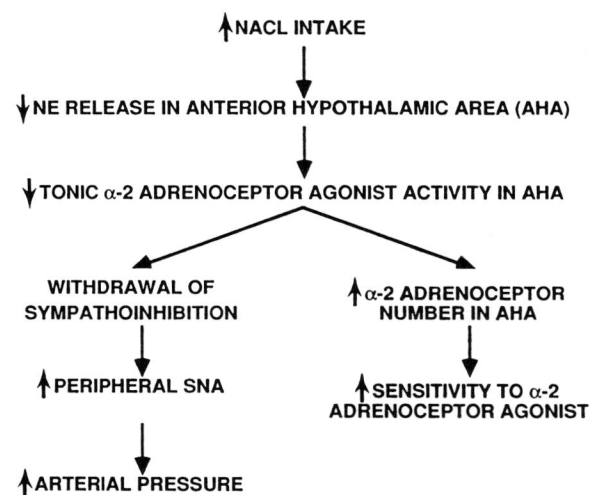

FIG. 2. Diagram outlining the central nervous system mechanisms involved in NaCl-sensitive hypertension. NE, norepinephrine; SNA, sympathetic nerve activity.

area. In addition, the release of norepinephrine in the anterior hypothalamic area is decreased (54). This suggests that increased dietary NaCl intake produces a specific decrease in norepinephrine synthesis in the anterior hypothalamic area. As norepinephrine serves as an agonist for anterior hypothalamic area α_2-adrenoceptors, which serve to tonically suppress peripheral sympathetic outflow, the decrease in local concentration of the natural agonist would result in an increase in peripheral (including renal) sympathetic outflow, thus contributing to NaCl-sensitive hypertension. The decrease in the local concentration of norepinephrine, the natural agonist of anterior hypothalamic area α_2-adrenoceptors, was found to lead to the following events: increased number (upregulation) of anterior hypothalamic area α_2-adrenoceptors (55) and increased responsiveness to central administration of α_2-adrenoceptor agonists (56,57). Central administration of α_2-adrenoceptor agonists produces greater decreases in arterial pressure, heart rate, and ERSNA in both SHR (58) and BHR (59) when they are consuming a high compared with a normal or low dietary NaCl intake. Thus, increased dietary NaCl intake, via an alteration in the central nervous system mechanisms that regulated peripheral sympathetic outflow, results in a withdrawal of tonic sympathoinhibition leading to increases in peripheral sympathetic outflow.

The BHR has been studied extensively as a model of interaction between genetic predisposition to hypertension and increased dietary NaCl intake leading to increased arterial pressure via activation of (renal) sympathetic neural pathways. The BHR is a genetic model of environmentally induced hypertension. The BHR is the first filial offspring of an SHR × WKY mating and possesses genetic information from both the normotensive WKY and the hypertensive SHR parent. As described by

Lawler and colleagues (60), the BHR become permanently hypertensive when subjected to a time-limited period of exposure to environmental stress (45) or to increased dietary sodium intake (44). Renal denervation, performed early but not late, can prevent the development of environmental stress-induced hypertension in BHR (39).

Exaggerated natriuresis is a phenomenon observed in hypertensive animals and humans whereby the natriuretic response to intravenous isotonic saline loading is enhanced over that seen in normotensive controls. The exaggerated natriuresis is accompanied by an exaggerated withdrawal of ERSNA in SHR (61–63); this exaggerated withdrawal of ERSNA contributes to the exaggerated natriuresis because it is attenuated by prior renal denervation. Since increased dietary sodium intake causes the BHR to exhibit one characteristic of the phenotype of the hypertensive SHR parent, i.e., a sustained increase in arterial pressure, it was of interest to determine whether other features of the hypertensive SHR parent phenotype were also expressed by the increased dietary sodium intake. BHR, when maintained on a 1 percent NaCl diet, did not exhibit an increase in arterial pressure, an exaggerated natriuretic response to isotonic saline loading, or an augmented response to acute environmental stress. In contrast, BHR given an 8 percent NaCl diet demonstrated an increase in arterial pressure in association with an exaggerated natriuretic response to isotonic saline loading. The exaggerated natriuresis was associated with an exaggerated withdrawal of ERSNA, and prior renal denervation diminished the exaggerated natriuretic response, indicating its dependence, in part, on the withdrawal of ERSNA. In addition, they demonstrated an augmented response to acute environmental stress with greater increases in heart rate, mean arterial pressure, and ERSNA, and a greater decrease in urinary sodium excretion, which was dependent on intact renal innervation (48). The responsiveness of central nervous system α_2-adrenoceptors is enhanced as reflected by greater responses of arterial pressure, heart rate, and ERSNA to the intracerebroventricular administration of guanabenz, an α_2-adrenoceptor agonist (59). The expression of these responses in BHR made hypertensive by 8 percent NaCl dietary intake, similar to those observed in the hypertensive SHR parent, but not in normotensive BHR on a 1 percent NaCl dietary intake or the normotensive WKY parent (47,49), suggests that these dietary NaCl–inducible responses are genetically conveyed to the BHR by the SHR in latent forms.

Similar effects of environmental stress on renal function have been observed in human subjects. In response to environmental stress, both normotensive and hypertensive human subjects exhibit increased arterial pressure, heart rate, and renal vascular resistance, and decreased renal blood flow, glomerular filtration rate, urinary flow rate, and sodium excretion (64–70). There is also increased spillover of norepinephrine into the renal vein as a reflection of increased ERSNA, with an increased renin secretion rate and increased muscle sympathetic nerve activity (64,68). It is important to note that the decreases in urinary flow rate and sodium excretion as well as the increase in renin secretion rate are occurring in the face of a combination of an increase in arterial pressure and an increase in ERSNA. Since the increase in arterial pressure would by itself increase urinary flow rate and sodium excretion and decrease renin secretion, it is evident that the increase in ERSNA is dominant over the rise in arterial pressure and accounts for the observed findings.

The clinical relevance of an important interaction between dietary NaCl intake and stimuli that cause reflex activation of the sympathetic nervous system in hypertension is illustrated by a study by Lawton and colleagues (71). The arterial pressure, renal blood flow, and renal vascular resistance responses of borderline hypertensive and normotensive subjects to changing from supine to upright posture were measured during consumption of both low and high dietary NaCl intakes. This orthostatic stress is known to produce reflex sympathetic activation. In normotensive subjects, the decreases in diastolic arterial pressure and the increases in renal vascular resistance with assumption of upright posture were similar on both low and high dietary NaCl intakes. However, in borderline hypertensive subjects, the results were different. On low dietary NaCl intake, diastolic arterial pressure did not decrease and the increase in renal vascular resistance with assumption of upright posture was not significantly greater than that observed in normotensive subjects on low dietary NaCl intake. However, on high dietary NaCl intake, diastolic arterial pressure increased and the increase in renal vascular resistance with assumption of upright posture was significantly greater than that observed in normotensive subjects on high dietary NaCl intake. The rise in renal vascular resistance was in excess of that required for a normal renal blood flow autoregulatory response to the increase in arterial pressure, as it resulted in a significant decrease in renal blood flow. Therefore, a high dietary NaCl intake produced an augmented renal vasoconstrictor response to orthostatic stress in borderline hypertensive subjects. Since orthostatic stress is known to produce reflex activation of the sympathetic nervous system, and borderline hypertensive subjects may be conjectured to have a genetic predisposition to hypertension, the congruence of these findings in human subjects with those of NaCl-sensitive genetic hypertensive rats given a high dietary NaCl intake and subjected to acute environmental stress is noteworthy.

The majority of patients with chronic renal failure being maintained with hemodialysis therapy are hypertensive. Measurements of MSNA demonstrate that nonnephrectomized hemodialysis patients had increased

MSNA, arterial pressure, and calf vascular resistance compared with nephrectomized hemodialysis patients whose values were similar to those of normal subjects (72). These observations suggest that chronic renal failure may be accompanied by reversible (i.e., by bilateral nephrectomy) sympathetic activation, which may be contributing to the hypertension and appears to be mediated by an afferent signal arising in the failing kidneys. Thus, as with certain experimental animal forms of hypertension, afferent renal nerve activity may tonically increase peripheral sympathetic outflow in patients with chronic renal failure.

Renal Effects of Increased ERSNA Contributing to Hypertension

A major hypothesis for the development of hypertension is that abnormal renal function is critical for the initiation, development, or maintenance of primary hypertension (73). The maintenance of sodium and water balance by the kidneys is believed to be primary in long-term control of arterial pressure. An increase in arterial pressure leads to an increased urinary sodium and water excretion with consequent reduction of blood volume until arterial pressure is returned to normal. In hypertension, it is hypothesized that factors disrupt the maintenance of sodium and water balance by the kidneys such that an elevated arterial pressure is required to reestablish and maintain normal sodium and water balance. Several types of renal dysfunction could contribute to the hypertensive state, including increased renal vascular resistance, increased renal retention of sodium and water, and increased release of renin, catecholamines, or other vasoactive substances. As presented above, ERSNA is known to be important in the physiological regulation of these renal functions. Thus, excessive ERSNA could contribute to these postulated renal dysfunctions, which in turn produce renal sodium and water retention and result in the requirement for an increased arterial pressure in order to reestablish and maintain normal sodium and water balance.

By virtue of their potential for producing renal sodium and water retention, all of the effects of ERSNA are capable of contributing to the initiation, development, and maintenance of hypertension. In this regard, Roman and Cowley (74), in anesthetized surgically prepared normotensive rats, demonstrated that the prevailing level of ERSNA in the intact renal nerves is sufficient to significantly attenuate the diuretic and natriuretic response to increases in renal perfusion pressure (pressure diuresis and natriuresis); at every level of renal perfusion pressure, fractional excretion of water and sodium was higher following complete renal denervation than when renal innervation was intact. This attenuation of the pressure diuresis and natriuresis relationship by ERSNA has also

been shown in normotensive dogs (75,76) and is dependent on activation of intrarenal α_1-adrenoceptors located on renal tubules (75). More importantly, in SHR wherein ERSNA is known to be elevated, renal denervation leads to normalization of pressure diuresis and natriuresis (77,78). In addition, acute renal denervation in SHR results in a decrease in renal vascular resistance, an increase in renal blood flow and glomerular filtration rate, a diuresis and natriuresis, and an attenuation in the sensitivity of the tubuloglomerular feedback system (77–79). Thus, in SHR, ERSNA exerts a tonic influence on the kidney with the likelihood that enhanced responsiveness of the tubuloglomerular feedback system is a mediator of the excess renal sodium and water retention and the abnormal pressure diuresis and natriuresis, thus contributing to the maintenance of the hypertension.

As the kidneys receive approximately 20 percent of cardiac output, changes in renal blood flow and renal vascular resistance can make substantial contributions to changes in total peripheral resistance. In established human essential hypertension, total peripheral resistance is increased; in the kidneys, renal blood flow is decreased, renal vascular resistance is increased, and there is evidence of increased neural renal vasoconstrictor tone. It is likely that early in the course of hypertension, the renal vasculature undergoes mainly autoregulatory adjustments that involve only modest increases in mainly preglomerular and overall renal vascular resistance, with preservation of the glomerular filtration rate. As hypertension progresses, there is progressive structural adaptation of the renal vascular bed so that, in order to maintain the glomerular filtration rate, postglomerular vascular resistance is increased, resulting in substantial increases in overall renal vascular resistance. The structural adaptation (vascular narrowing) is related to medial thickening with an increased wall/lumen ratio and is seen functionally as enhanced contractile strength and renovascular reactivity to renal nerve stimulation or norepinephrine (80).

Based on initial observations that the renal α_2-adrenoceptor number was increased in certain forms of experimental hypertension (81,82), it was proposed that renal α_2-adrenoceptors were important mediators of the renal functional responses to the increased ERSNA that contributes to the development of the hypertension (83). It was further proposed that a genetically determined alteration of renal α-adrenoceptors may be an important pathophysiological component in genetic forms of experimental hypertension (83). However, physiological studies demonstrated that the renal vasoconstrictor and antinatriuretic responses to renal nerve stimulation as well as adrenergic agonists in SHR were mediated by renal α_1-adrenoceptors and not by α_2-adrenoceptors (14). Similar studies by others confirmed this (84) and demonstrated that the same situation prevailed in other genetic as well as nongenetic forms of experimental hypertension [stroke-prone SHR (SHR-SP), deoxycorticosterone acetate (DOCA)-NaCl, 2K,1C Goldblatt] (85). Subsequent studies have demonstrated that neither renal α_1- nor α_2-adrenoceptor number co-segregated with arterial pressure in the F_2 generation of WKY × SHR hybrids (86) and that the renal α_{1A}-α_{1B}-adrenoceptor ratio was similar in WKY, SHR, and F_1 rats transplanted with a kidney from either strain (87). Thus, these studies refute the original hypothesis and indicate that genetically determined alterations of renal α-adrenoceptor numbers do not play an important role in the development of hypertension in the SHR or other forms of experimental hypertension. Additional studies in the NaCl-sensitive strain of SHR (SHR-S) demonstrated that increased dietary NaCl intake increased arterial pressure in SHR-S but not in the NaCl-resistant strain of SHR (SHR-R), whereas the renal α_2-adrenoceptor number increased similarly in both SHR-S and SHR-R (88). Therefore, NaCl-induced increases in arterial pressure are independent of up-regulation of the renal α_2-adrenoceptor number in SHR-S. Moreover, development of hypertension is not associated with increases in the renal α_1- nor α_2-adrenoceptor number in 2K,1C or 1K,1C Goldblatt hypertension or DOCA-NaCl hypertension (89). Thus, there is little evidence in support of the hypothesis that renal α_2-adrenoceptors are important mediators of the renal functional responses to the increased ERSNA that contributes to the development of the hypertension.

Renal Dopaminergic Defect in Hypertension

Although there are nerves within the kidney that contain dopamine, the evidence that dopamine serves as a true neurotransmitter within the kidney remains controversial (90). The main source of renal dopamine derives from conversion of circulating L-dihydroxyphenylalanine (L-DOPA) to dopamine by aromatic L-amino acid decarboxylase (L-AAAD) located predominantly in the proximal renal tubular epithelial cells (91,92). Inhibition of L-AAAD decreases urinary dopamine excretion (93). High NaCl intake increases and low NaCl intake decreases urinary L-DOPA and dopamine excretion in parallel, supporting the view that high NaCl intake increases delivery of L-DOPA to proximal tubular epithelial cell uptake sites, resulting in increased renal cortical dopamine production (94). Dopamine possesses diuretic, natriuretic, and renal vasodilator actions (90,95) and is capable of inhibiting the Na^+-H^+ exchange in the proximal tubule (96,97) and Na^+,K^+–adenosine triphosphatase (ATPase) in the proximal tubule (98), medullary thick ascending limb (99), and cortical collecting duct (100). These responses are mediated by a synergistic action on dopamine (DA) DA_1- and DA_2-receptors in proximal tu-

bule segments (101) and DA_1 receptors in medullary thick ascending limb (99) and cortical collecting duct (100). The DA_1 receptors are coupled to adenyl cyclase with generation of adenosine 3′,5′-cyclic monophosphate (cAMP), which, *in vitro*, can decrease both Na^+-H^+ exchange (102) and Na^+,K^+-ATPase activity (103).

Since inhibitors of L-AAAD attenuate the natriuretic response to NaCl loading (104), it has been proposed that the renal dopamine system serves as a paracrine or autocrine system to regulate renal tubular sodium reabsorption, thereby contributing to the renal regulation of sodium balance (90,95,105). The diuretic and natriuretic responses to dopamine administration are attenuated in two genetic forms of experimental hypertension, SHR (106) and Dahl (107), wherein excessive renal sodium retention contributes to the hypertension. Each of these models has been characterized by a defect in coupling of renal tubular DA_1-receptors to the adenyl cyclase–cAMP system, which results in a decreased production of cAMP and less inhibition of both Na^+-H^+ exchange and Na^+,K^+-ATPase activity (108–110). Increased dietary NaCl intake in young Dahl-S leads to a transient exaggerated increase in proximal tubular Na^+,K^+-ATPase activity, whereas in adult Dahl-S it results in a failure of proximal tubular Na^+,K^+-ATPase activity to normally suppress. Thus, these defects in the coupling between dietary NaCl intake, renal cortical dopamine metabolism, and the regulation of proximal tubular Na^+,K^+-ATPase activity favor renal sodium retention in both young and adult Dahl-S rats.

As a result of these various studies, the concept of a defect in renal dopamine production has been advanced as a potential mechanism for the development of hypertension, especially NaCl-sensitive hypertension. Studies in human subjects demonstrate that, during NaCl loading, NaCl-resistant hypertensive subjects showed no increase in blood pressure and a substantial increase in urinary dopamine excretion, whereas NaCl-sensitive subjects showed an 11–mm Hg increase in blood pressure and no increase in urinary dopamine excretion (111). These findings were present in the first-degree normotensive relatives of the hypertensive patients, suggesting that the abnormality of renal dopamine production in the hypertensive patients is inherited and not acquired as a consequence of the hypertensive process (112,113). The urinary excretion pattern of high L-DOPA, low dopamine, and low dopamine/L-DOPA ratio suggests that delivery of L-DOPA to the renal tubules is normal or increased but that uptake and/or conversion to dopamine is defective in NaCl-sensitive hypertensives (114).

The enlarging body of evidence suggests that a renal dopaminergic defect may contribute to hypertension, especially NaCl-sensitive forms of hypertension, by impairing the ability of the kidney to excrete sodium in response to increases in dietary sodium intake.

SUMMARY

There is a substantial and enlarging body of evidence supporting the view that increased ERSNA plays an important role in the initiation, development, and maintenance of human essential hypertension. An abnormality in renal function is a central issue in the initiation, development, and maintenance of hypertension. Increased ERSNA produces substantial alterations in renal function: decreases in renal blood flow, glomerular filtration rate, urinary flow rate, and sodium excretion, and increases in renal vascular resistance and renin secretion. In experimental animal forms of hypertension, ERSNA is increased and renal denervation delays or prevents the development of hypertension. An alteration in central nervous system mechanisms that govern peripheral sympathetic outflow, including ERSNA, contributes to NaCl-sensitive forms of genetic hypertension. ERSNA is increased in human essential hypertension and contributes to the observed decrease in renal blood flow and increase in renal vascular resistance. Other renal functional abnormalities observed in human essential hypertension, such as reductions in glomerular filtration rate and renal sodium retention, are well-recognized responses to increased ERSNA.

ACKNOWLEDGMENTS

This work was supported by National Institutes of Health grants DK 15843, HL 44546, HL 14388, American Heart Association grant-in-aid 890693, and by grants from the Veterans Administration.

REFERENCES

1. Barajas L, Liu L, Powers K. *Can J Physiol Pharmacol* 1992;70: 735–749.
2. DiBona GF. *Rev Physiol Biochem Pharmacol* 1982;94:76–181.
3. Kopp UC, DiBona GF. In: Fisher JW, ed. *Kidney hormones*, vol 3. London: Academic Press, 1986;621–660.
4. DiBona GF. *Miner Electrolyte Metab* 1989;15:4–96.
5. Kopp UC, DiBona GF. In: Zucker IH, Gilmore JP, eds. *Reflex control of the circulation.* Boca Raton: CRC, 1991;493–528.
6. Kopp UC, DiBona GF. In: Seldin DW, Giebisch G, eds. *The kidney—physiology and pathophysiology.* New York: Raven, 1992;1157–1204.
7. Kopp UC, DiBona GF. In: Maggi CA, ed. *Nervous control of the urogenital system,* vol 3. London: Harwood, 1993;143–196.
8. DiBona GF. *J Cardiovasc Pharmacol* 1985;7(suppl 8):S18–S23.
9. Hesse IFA, Johns EJ. *J Auton Pharmacol* 1984;4:145–152.
10. Schuster VL. *Fed Proc* 1986;45:1444–1447.
11. Blantz RC, Konnen KS, Tucker BJ. *J Clin Invest* 1976;57:419–434.
12. Osborn JL, Holdaas H, Thames MD, et al. *Circ Res* 1983;53: 298–305.
13. Johns EF, Manitius J. *Br J Pharmacol* 1986;89:91–97.
14. DiBona GF, Sawin LL. *Hypertension* 1987;9:41–48.
15. Hesse IFA, Johns EJ. *J Physiol* 1984;352:527–538.
16. Cohen HT, Takemoto F, Satoh T, et al. *Can J Physiol Pharmacol* 1992;70:1016–1020.
17. Aperia A, Ibarra F, Svensson L-B, et al. *Proc Natl Acad Sci USA* 1992;89:7394–7397.
18. Kopp UC, DiBona GF. *Am J Physiol* 1984;246:F620–F626.
19. Hollenberg NK. *Medicine* 1975;54:29–44.
20. Lorelius LE, Lofroth PO, Morlin C, et al. *Scand J Clin Lab Invest* 1978;38:233–240.
21. Esler M, Jennings G, Lambert G, et al. *Physiol Rev* 1990;70:963–985.
22. Gombos EA, Hulet WH, Bopp D, et al. *J Clin Invest* 1962;41: 203–210.
23. Anderson EA, Sinkey CA, Lawton WJ, et al. *Hypertension* 1989;14:177–183.
24. Yamada Y, Miyajima E, Tochikubo O, et al. *Hypertension* 1989;13:870–877.
25. Rea RF, Hamdan M. *Circulation* 1990;82:856–862.
26. Friberg P, Meredith I, Jennings G, et al. *Hypertension* 1990;16: 121–130.
27. Thorén P, Ricksten S-E. *Clin Sci* 1979;57:197s–199s.
28. Janssen BJA, Smits JFM. *Miner Electrolyte Metab* 1989;15:74–82.
29. Wyss JM, Oparil S, Sripairojthikoon W. *Can J Physiol Pharmacol* 1992;70:759–770.
30. Winternitz SR, Katholi RE, Oparil S. *J Clin Invest* 1980;66:971–978.
31. Gattone VH, Evan AP, Overhage JM, et al. *J Hypertens* 1990;8: 423–428.
32. Oparil S, Sripairojthikoon W, Wyss JM. *Can J Physiol Pharmacol* 1987;65:1548–1558.
33. Kopp UC. *Can J Physiol Pharmacol* 1992;70:750–758.
34. Kopp UC. *J Hypertens* 1993;11:765–773.
35. Kopp UC, Smith LA, DiBona GF. *Hypertension* 1987;9:69–75.
36. Kopp UC, Smith LA. *Hypertension* 1989;13:430–439.
37. Kopp UC, Buckley-Bleiler RL. *Hypertension* 1989;14:445–452.
38. Janssen BJA, Van Essen H, Vervoort-Peters LHTM, et al. *J Hypertens* 1989;7:447–455.
39. Lawler JE, Sanders BJ, Cox RH, et al. *Clin Exp Hypertens* 1989;A11:1549–1563.
40. Wyss JM, Sripairojthikoon W, Oparil S. *Can J Physiol Pharmacol* 1987;65:2428–2432.
41. Folkow B. *Physiol Rev* 1982;62:347–504.
42. Henry JP, Liu Y-L, Nadra WE, et al. *Hypertension* 1993;21:714–723.
43. Winternitz SR, Oparil S. *Clin Exp Hypertens* 1982;A4:751–760.
44. Lawler JE, Sanders BJ, Chen Y-F, et al. *Clin Exp Hypertens* 1987;A9:1713–1731.
45. Lawler JE, Barker GF, Hubbard JW, et al. *Hypertension* 1981;3: 496–505.
46. Ely DL, Wiegand J. *Clin Exp Hypertens* 1982;A5:1559–1587.
47. Koepke JP, DiBona GF. *Hypertension* 1985;7:357–363.
48. DiBona GF, Jones SY. *Hypertension* 1991;17:44–53.
49. Koepke JP, Jones S, DiBona GF. *Hypertension* 1988;11:334–338.
50. Koepke JP, Jones S, DiBona GF. *Circ Res* 1986;58:241–248.
51. Koepke JP, Jones S, DiBona GF. *Brain Res* 1987;404:80–88.
52. Wyss JM, Chen YF, Jin H, et al. *Hypertension* 1987;10:313–320.
53. Chen Y-F, Meng Q, Wyss JM, et al. *Hypertension* 1988;11:55–62.
54. Chen CW, Chen YF, Meng QC, et al. *Brain Res* 1991;5665:135–141.
55. Klangkalya B, Sripairojthikoon W, Oparil S, et al. *Brain Res* 1989;451:77–84.
56. Wyss JM, Yang RH, Jin H, et al. *J Hypertens* 1988;6:805–813.
57. Jin H, Yang R-H, Wyss J, et al. *Hypertension* 1991;18:224–229.
58. Koepke JP, Jones S, DiBona GF. *Hypertension* 1988;11:326–333.
59. DiBona GF, Jones SY. *J Hypertens* 1991;9:543–547.
60. Lawler JE, Barker GF, Hubbard JW, et al. *Psychophysiology* 1980;17:363–370.
61. DiBona GF, Sawin LL. *Am J Physiol* 1978;235:F409–F416.
62. Ricksten S-E, Yao T, DiBona GF, et al. *Acta Physiol Scand* 1981;112:161–167.
63. DiBona GF, Sawin LL. *Proc Soc Exp Biol Med* 1986;182:43–51.
64. Tidgren B, Hjemdahl P. *Am J Physiol* 1989;257:F682–F689.

65. Light KC, Koepke JP, Obrist PA, et al. *Science* 1983;220:429–431.
66. Harshfield GA, Pulliam DA, Alpert BS. *Hypertension* 1991;17:1156–1160.
67. Fauvel JP, Hadj-Aissa A, Laville M, et al. *Am J Hypertens* 1991;4:955–958.
68. Hjemdahl P, Fagius J, Freyschuss U, et al. *Am J Physiol* 1989;257:E654–E664.
69. Anderson EA, Sinkey CA, Mark AL. *Hypertension* 1991;17(suppl III):III43–III49.
70. Herd JA. *Physiol Rev* 1991;71:304–330.
71. Lawton WJ, Sinkey CA, Fitz AE, et al. *Hypertension* 1988;11:529–536.
72. Converse RL, Jacobsen TN, Toto RD, et al. *N Engl J Med* 1992;327:1912–1918.
73. Cowley AC, Roman R. *Am J Nephrol* 1983;3:59–72.
74. Roman RJ, Cowley AW. *Am J Physiol* 1985;248:F190–F198.
75. Ehmke H, Persson PB, Seyfarth M, et al. *Am J Physiol* 1990;259:F466–F473.
76. Brand PH, Coyne KB, Kostrzewski KA, et al. *Am J Physiol* 1991;261:R802–R810.
77. Yoshida M, Satoh S. *Am J Physiol* 1991;260:F81–F85.
78. Roman RJ. *Hypertension* 1987;9(suppl III):III130–III136.
79. Takabatake T, Ushiogi Y. *Am J Physiol* 1990;258:F980–F985.
80. Göthberg G, Folkow B. *Acta Physiol Scand* 1983;117:547–555.
81. Sanchez A, Pettinger WA. *Life Sci* 1981;29:2975–2802.
82. Pettinger WA, Gandler T, Sanchez A, et al. *Clin Exp Hypertens* 1982;A4:819–828.
83. Michel MC, Insel PA, Brodde O-E. *FASEB J* 1989;3:139–144.
84. Akpogomeh BA, Johns EJ. *J Auton Pharmacol* 1990;10:201–212.
85. Akpogomeh BA, Johns EJ. *J Hypertens* 1991;9:373–384.
86. Michel MC, Jäger S, Casto R, et al. *Hypertension* 1992;19:365–370.
87. Jackson CA, Michel MC, Insel PA. *J Cardiovasc Pharmacol* 1992;19:857–862.
88. Meldrum MJ, Singletary N, Dawson R. *Hypertension* 1990;16:49–54.
89. Wilson SK. *J Pharmacol Exp Ther* 1991;256:801–810.
90. Lee MR. *Clin Sci* 1993;84:357–375.
91. Baines AD, Chan W. *Life Sci* 1980;26:253–259.
92. Hayashi M, Yamaji Y, Kitajima W, et al. *Am J Physiol* 1990;258:F28–F33.
93. Ball SG, Lee MR. *Br J Clin Pharmacol* 1977;4:115–119.
94. Goldstein DS, Stull R, Eisenhofer G, et al. *Clin Sci* 1989;76:517–522.
95. Siragy HM, Felder RA, Howell NL, et al. *Am J Physiol* 1989;257:F469–F477.
96. Gesek FA, Schoolwerth AC. *Am J Physiol* 1990;258:F514–F521.
97. Felder CC, Campbell T, Albrecht F, et al. *Am J Physiol* 1990;259:F297–F303.
98. Aperia A, Bertorello A, Seri I. *Am J Physiol* 1987;252:F39–F45.
99. Meister B, Fryckstedt J, Schalling M, et al. *Proc Natl Acad Sci USA* 1989;86:8068–8072.
100. Takemoto F, Satoh T, Cohen HT, et al. *Pflugers Arch* 1991;419:243–248.
101. Bertorello A, Aperia A. *Am J Physiol* 1990;259:F924–F928.
102. Weinman EJ, Shenolikar S, Kahn AM. *Am J Physiol* 1987;252:F19–F25.
103. Bertorello A, Aperia A, Walaas AI, et al. *Proc Natl Acad Sci USA* 1991;88:11359–11362.
104. Bertorello A, Hökfelt T, Goldstein M, et al. *Am J Physiol* 1988;254:F795–F801.
105. Felder RA, Felder CC, Eisner GM, et al. *Am J Physiol* 1989;257:F315–F327.
106. Felder RA, Seikaly MG, Cody P, et al. *Hypertension* 1990;15:560–569.
107. Nishi A, Eklöf A-C, Bertorello AM, et al. *Hypertension* 1993;21:767–771.
108. Felder RA, Kinoshita S, Sidhu A, et al. *Am J Hypertens* 1990;3:96s–99s.
109. Kinoshita S, Sidhu A, Felder Ra. *J Clin Invest* 1989;84:1849–1856.
110. Nishi A, Bertorello AM, Aperia A. *Acta Physiol Scand* 1992;144:263–267.
111. Shikuma R, Yoshimura M, Kambara S, et al. *Life Sci* 1986;38:915–921.
112. Saito I, Takeshita E, Saruta T, et al. *J Hypertens* 1986;4:57–60.
113. Imura O, Shimamoto K. *J Auton Pharmacol* 1990;10(suppl 1):73s–77s.
114. Gill JR, Grossman E, Goldstein DS. *Hypertension* 1991;18:614–621.

Hypertension: Pathophysiology, Diagnosis, and Management, Second Edition, edited by J.H. Laragh and B.M. Brenner, Raven Press, Ltd., New York © 1995.

CHAPTER 82

Control of Renin Release and Glomerular Vascular Tone by the Juxtaglomerular Apparatus

Josephine P. Briggs and Jürgen Schnermann

It is a consistent topographic feature of the mammalian nephron that the distal end of the loop of Henle returns to the vascular pole of its own glomerulus. At the point of contact, specialized epithelial and mesenchymal cells are arranged in a structure called the *juxtaglomerular apparatus* (JGA). Evidence has accumulated to indicate that the JGA has an important function in regulation of body salt-and-water homeostasis. Changes in tubular fluid composition at this site have been shown to produce two effects: an alteration in renin secretion rate and a change in glomerular hemodynamics. This chapter summarizes the available information about the cellular characteristics of the principal cell types of the JGA and reviews the evidence for the functional effects mediated through the JGA. The available information about the

mechanisms by which changes in distal tubular fluid composition produce changes in renin secretion and glomerular filtration rate (GFR) and the evidence that these mechanisms participate in salt conservation in volume-depleted states and are relaxed in volume overload or salt-excess states are summarized, as are studies examining these functions in experimental models of hypertension. Several recent reviews and monographs provide more detailed coverage of these topics (1–4).

HISTORICAL ASPECTS

The existence of a regular connection between the distal nephron and the glomerular vascular pole was first recognized by Golgi (5). In 1889, he concluded on the basis of tubular microdissections that "the ascending limb of the loop of Henle returns with invariable constancy to its respective capsule of origin with which it

J. P. Briggs and J. Schnermann: Departments of Physiology and Internal Medicine, The University of Michigan, Ann Arbor, Michigan 48109.

makes contact at a point where the afferent vessel enters and the efferent exits" (translation). Karl Peter described this relationship in more detail in 1907 (6). By the mid-1930s, the existence of the JGA was well known to several renal anatomists, and the principal structural features were described. Ruyter (7) detected the granular cells in the wall of the afferent arterioles, and Zimmermann (8) drew attention to the specialized plaque of epithelial cells in the wall of the tubule, for which he coined the term *macula densa* (MD). He also observed the cushion (polkissen) of extraglomerular mesangial (EGM) cells that underlie the MD. Goormaghtigh (9), on the basis of many anatomic and pathological observations, was the first to propose a regulatory role for the JGA. In 1937, he suggested that the MD cells may act as "a sensory plaque placed downstream from the most important functional segments of the nephron." Furthermore, he hypothesized, "This creates the possibility of an automatic regulation of the glomerular circulation governed either by the state of emptiness or fullness of the thick ascending limb or by the physicochemical state of the urine flowing there" (translation). He also was the first to speculate that the renal pressor substance (renin) described by Tigerstedt and Bergman (10) might be produced by the granulated cells of the JGA (11).

Tubuloglomerular Feedback

Goormaghtigh's hypothesis for local vascular control resurfaced about 20 years later when in 1957 Harsing and coworkers observed that the administration of a mercurial diuretic or of the glucose transport inhibitor phlorizin caused renal vasoconstriction and a fall in GFR. They speculated that the change in renal vascular tone and filtration rate was initiated by the increases in distal solute concentration that resulted from diuretic or phlorizin-induced proximal transport inhibition. They also clearly recognized that this "tubuloglomerular" adjustment would tend to promote homeostasis by stabilizing the delivery of solute to the distal nephron (12). In the next few years, both Guyton (13) and Thurau (14) expanded on these ideas and particularly emphasized the possible role of distal tubular regulation of vascular tone in autoregulation of blood flow and GFR. In 1965, Thurau and Schnermann (15) reported the first direct evidence in support of this concept: They observed in micropuncture experiments performed in salt-deprived rats that high-NaCl solutions injected into the distal nephron near the MD without control of perfusion pressure and flow produced marked reductions in GFR. The fall of GFR in these studies was inferred from decreases in diameter of the corresponding proximal tubule. Initial attempts to replicate these studies were not successful (16), and the concept of distal tubular control of vascular tone engendered considerable skepticism. With the develop-

ment of improved techniques for assessing single glomerular function and controlling tubular fluid rate and composition, however, many laboratories have demonstrated that increasing distal tubular fluid salt concentration suppresses GFR, and the concept that distal solute concentration is a regulator of glomerular function has become well accepted.

Renin Release

In 1964, based on both anatomic findings and their own physiological observations, Vander and colleagues (17–19) suggested that renin release might be influenced by tubular fluid composition at the MD. They reported that with a variety of manipulations there was an inverse correlation between plasma renin activity (PRA) and sodium excretion but no correlation between renin and mean arterial pressure or renal blood flow (17–19). These data led Vander to suggest that a high-salt delivery to the MD cells might inhibit renin secretion. Studies using micropuncture techniques to manipulate MD NaCl appeared to suggest a different relationship, however. Two groups of investigators (20,21) observed that injection of fluid with a high NaCl concentration into the distal nephron stimulated the activity of renin in the associated glomerulus, which was isolated by microdissection after completion of micropuncture. Because renin secretion was not measured in these studies, these observations were not in direct conflict with those of Vander. Nonetheless, the two data sets were considered discrepant, leading to a vigorous debate as to whether renin secretion was stimulated or inhibited by a high MD NaCl concentration. Whereas the significance of the NaCl effects on local renin activation has not been pursued further, substantial additional evidence from whole animal studies supports an *inverse* relationship between salt concentration and renin release (2,3,17,22). Furthermore, studies in isolated *in vitro* systems have provided direct and quantitative evidence in support of the concept that a high NaCl concentration at the MD inhibits renin secretion (23–25).

CELLULAR ELEMENTS OF THE JGA

To understand the integrated function of the JGA, it is important to consider the anatomy of this structure (Fig. 1) and the characteristics of its cellular components. Information about these cells is accumulating from classic morphologic methods, from application of methods for localization of specific protein and messenger ribonucleic acid (mRNA) species, such as *in situ* hybridization, immunocytochemistry, and histochemistry *in vivo*, and from techniques to isolate and study these cells *in vitro*.

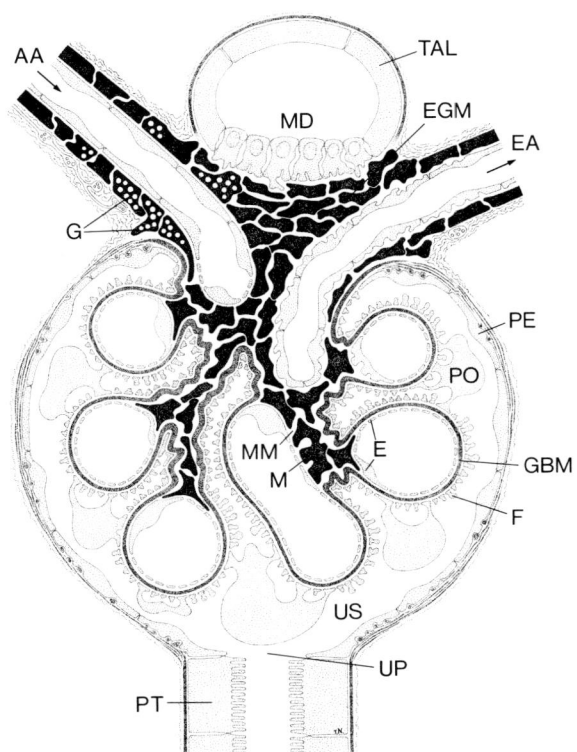

FIG. 1. Juxtaglomerular apparatus. The following structures are illustrated schematically: *MD*, macula densa; *TAL*, thick ascending limb; *EGM*, extraglomerular mesangium; *G*, juxtaglomerular granular cell; *AA*, afferent arteriole; *EA*, efferent arteriole; *M*, mesangium; *MM*, mesangial matrix; *GBM*, glomerular basement membrane; *E*, endothelium; *US*, urinary space; *PT*, proximal tubule; *UP*, urinary pole; *PO*, epithelial podocyte; *F*, foot process; *PE*, parietal epithelium. (Courtesy of Wilhelm Kriz.)

Anatomic Interrelationships in the JGA

The adherent tubule and the afferent and efferent arterioles at the glomerular hilus form a wedge-shaped compartment. The floor of this compartment is the MD, a plaque of distinct epithelial cells in the wall of the distal tubule. The compartment is filled with a cushion of closely packed interstitial cells. These cells are usually referred to as EGM cells, because they are virtually indistinguishable in their fine structure from mesangial cells (26,27) and actually extend into the stalk of the mesangium. The third unique type of cell in the JGA is the renin-containing granular cells, which are located in the media of the arteriolar wall, particularly the afferent arteriole.

The MD is located close to the terminal end of the thick ascending limb (TAL). The position is quite invariant, occurring approximately 100 to 200 μm upstream from the transition from TAL to distal convoluted tubule (27,28) (Fig. 2). Serial reconstructions of the JGA have established that the most extensive and regular con-

tact of the MD cell is with the EGM (29–34). In fact, the MD area usually extends beyond the borders of the EGM (4,31), so that this particular region of the interstitium would appear to be supplied preferentially with absorbate from epithelial transport across the MD. Although contacts between the MD and the afferent and efferent arterioles are not infrequent, they are both less extensive in area and less consistent than the contacts with the EGM (4,31). Contact areas between the TAL in the region before the MD and the efferent arteriole (30) and between the afferent arteriole and the distal connecting tubule (4,32) have also been reported.

Is the MD cell the sensor for JGA-mediated responses? Although the MD is the most consistent point of adherence of the tubule to the vascular pole, the existence of other contacts between vessel and tubule raises the question of other possible signal transmission routes. As reviewed below, there is evidence for functional similarities between the transport properties of the TAL and JGA responses of renin secretion and vascular tone. These observations have raised the question of whether the TAL epithelium that surrounds the MD plaque might actually be the sensor for JGA-mediated responses. Indeed, vascular responses have been observed in amphibian species in which the cells at the tubuloglomerular contact point are not clearly demarcated from their neighbors (35,36), and effects on glomerular vascular tone have been reported with perfusion of the connecting tubule (37). Nevertheless, several arguments suggest that in the mammalian nephron it is probably the MD cell that is the critical sensor of tubule solute composition. Direct electrophysiological and optical studies have established that the MD shares many of the transport properties of the TAL cell (see below). Furthermore, in the past few years, *in vitro* systems for studying

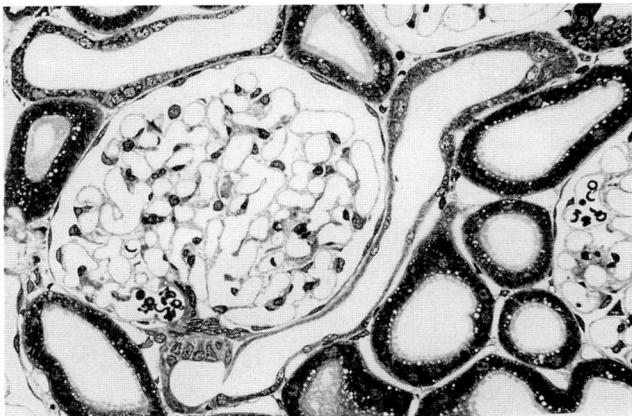

FIG. 2. Photomicrograph of rabbit glomerulus and juxtaglomerular apparatus, showing the macula densa located in the thick ascending limb of the loop of Henle. Note the transition from TAL to distal convoluted tubule is approximately 150 μm upstream from the MD. (Courtesy of B. Kaissling and W. Kriz.)

JGA-mediated responses have been developed in which the tubule and adherent glomerulus are dissected and perfused in isolation (23,38). With microdissection, the contacts between the TAL and the vascular pole are generally disrupted, whereas the adherence point at the MD is very tight and invariably persists *in vitro*. Responses of both renin secretion (23) and vascular tone (38,39) are intact in these preparations, suggesting that the MD is, in fact, the sensor for these effects. Nonetheless, the existence of other interactions between tubular and vascular compartments remains a possibility.

Macula Densa

Morphologic Characteristics

The MD consists of a plaque of 20 to 60 cuboidal epithelial cells per nephron. They differ from their neighbors in having more closely packed nuclei and a higher nuclear-to-cytoplasmic ratio, which gives the cell group the dense appearance. The MD cells have several typical epithelial cell features: They are joined together by tight junctions (4,27) and lie on top of a basement membrane. Specialization of the basement membrane has been noted: It is thinner than surrounding tubular basement membranes and scalloped in appearance, with discontinuities apparent by scanning electron microscopy (40). Mitochondria are abundant in MD cells but are scattered through the cytosol. The intercellular spaces between the cells are prominent and have been observed to become narrower with both mannitol and furosemide diuresis (41).

Biochemical Characteristics

Nitric Oxide Synthase and Glucose-6-Phosphate Dehydrogenase Localization

One of the most striking distinguishing features of the MD cell is a high level of the enzyme nitric oxide synthase (NOS). It has recently been shown by both immunocytochemistry and *in situ* hybridization that the type I or neuronal isoform of NOS is strongly expressed in the MD (42,43) (Fig. 3). Type I NOS is a calcium/calmodulin-dependent enzyme (44–46), raising the possibility that NO production by MD cells is regulated through changes in intracellular calcium. It was shown almost 30 years ago that NADPH-dependent diaphorase is strikingly more intense in the MD than in any other cell type in the kidney (47,48). Recent observations have established that immunocytochemical localization of type I NOS correlates closely with the NADPH diaphorase reaction product even though not all diaphorase activity appears to be caused by the presence of NOS (42).

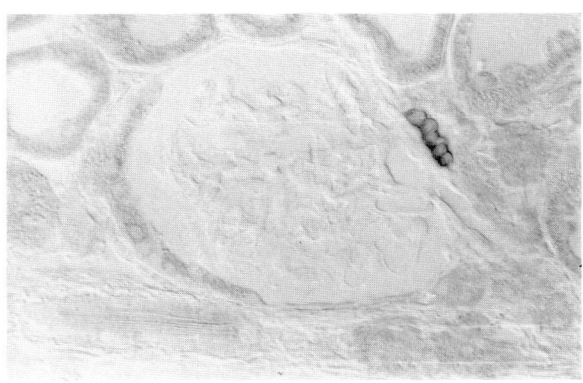

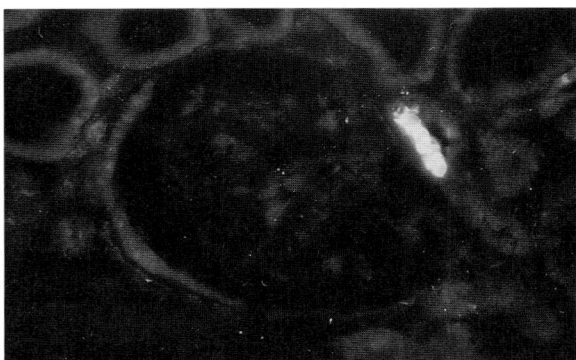

FIG. 3. cNOS localized to the macula densa. **Upper panel** shows reaction product for NADPH diaphorase; **lower panel** shows immunocytochemistry for cerebellar isoform of nitric oxide synthase. (Courtesy of S. Bachmann.)

The MD cell also differs from surrounding tubular cells in that it has higher levels of glucose-6-phosphate dehydrogenase (G6PDH), the enzyme controlling entry of glucose into the pentose shunt pathway (49). Localization of G6PDH to the MD was first observed by histochemical methods (49), and a two- to threefold difference has been confirmed by microenzymatic studies (50). Enzyme activity appears to be regulated; NaCl loading has been shown to reduce G6PDH activity in parallel with renin content (51). Studies in isolated kidneys have shown that 6-amino-nicotinamide, a blocker of the pentose pathway, reduced renin content and virtually abolished its release (52). In general, G6PDH activity is high in cells that use either NADPH or 5-carbon sugars such as ribose. NADPH is a required cofactor for NOS (53); use of NADPH by this enzyme is a possible explanation for the high levels of G6PDH. However, avid uptake of labeled uridine has been shown to occur in MD cells (54), a process inhibited by actinomycin D and therefore probably indicative of high rates of RNA synthesis (54). High uridine incorporation rates suggest an alternate possibility that the high pentose shunt activity might serve to provide ribose-5-phosphate for nucleic acid synthesis. The significance of the high rate of RNA synthesis is unknown.

Other Cell Characteristics

Several other intriguing differences exist between MD cells and surrounding TALs. Luminal membranes of MD cells have a glycoprotein surface coat different from that of TAL cells: Tamm Horsfall protein, a glycoprotein coating luminal and basolateral membranes of TAL cells, is absent in MD cells (55–57), and binding of peanut, soybean, and wheat germ lectin to rat MD luminal membranes can be shown, whereas TAL cells only bind winged pea lectin (58). There is evidence that MD cells possess a relatively high density of benzodiazepine receptors of the peripheral type (59) and possibly of oxytocin receptors (60). Macula densa cells in some species show evidence of a higher carbonic anhydrase activity than TAL cells (61,62). In situ hybridization of preproepidermal growth factor and immunoreactivity of epidermal growth factor, a known product of TAL cells, could not be demonstrated in MD cells (63,64). Recent in situ hybridization studies demonstrate high and specific expression of the recently characterized beta-6-integrin mRNA in the MD of primates (65). This cell surface molecule may function as a fibronectin receptor (66), and high levels of fibronectin expression at the glomerular hilum have been reported (67).

Functional Aspects

With the application of electrophysiological and optical techniques to study of the isolated perfused MD (68–76), substantial progress has been made in delineating its transport characteristics. Using microelectrodes, it was shown that MD cells have a basolateral potential difference of -55 mV, which became more negative in response to furosemide or a reduction in luminal NaCl concentration (69,70). More recently, membrane voltages were measured with patch-clamp electrodes attached to the apical membrane of MD cells. Similar to TAL cells, membrane potentials averaged -72 mV and hyperpolarized in response to furosemide, torasemide, and piretanide but did not change with application of hydrochlorothiazide or muzolimine, agents that do not interact with the Na, K, 2Cl cotransporter (71). Together with the observations that furosemide reduced cytosolic Cl concentrations as well as the volume of MD cells (72–74), these observations indicate that MD cells possess a NaCl uptake mechanism similar to that of TAL cells. Application of the whole-cell patch-clamp approach showed cell membrane depolarizations in response to increases in potassium, or application of barium, indicating the presence of a K^+ conductance, whereas application of a Cl channel blocker to the bath produced hyperpolarization, supporting the presence of basolateral Cl channels (71). Together with the earlier evidence for the presence of luminal K and basolateral Cl conduc-

tances (70,75,76), these results suggest that the mechanisms of NaCl absorption across MD cells are at least qualitatively similar to those of neighboring TAL cells. There is some evidence showing cell alkalinization with increases in luminal NaCl concentration, results consistent with the presence of apical Na/H exchange (69).

Transport rates for the MD cannot be measured directly because of its small size and the inaccessibility of its basolateral surface. Nevertheless, both morphologic features and measurements of Na-K ATPase activity suggest that transport rates are probably less than for the surrounding tubule. Macula densa cells do not have the extensive basal labyrinth and elongated mitochondria found in many transporting epithelia. Basal infoldings are not present, and mitochondria, although numerous, are not in contact with the basal membrane but rather scattered throughout the cytosol (27,33). A low or absent Na,K-ATPase activity in MD cells was suggested by the absence of marked staining with the histochemical reaction product of K-phosphatase (77). Microenzymatic measurement of Na,K-ATPase revealed an enzyme activity of about 0.5 fmol/h/μm^3 of tubular volume (78), which is only about 1/50th of that found in TALs or distal convoluted tubules (79). Low levels of Na,K-ATPase in the basal membranes of MD cells have also been demonstrated by using monoclonal antibodies against the enzyme (80). The low Na,K-ATPase activity correlates well with the low level of Krebs cycle enzymes (81).

Osmotic water permeability of the MD cell plaque has been assessed from the initial cell volume change in response to an osmotic step (73,74). The MD epithelium has been found to be relatively water impermeable, with a hydraulic conductivity similar to that of cortical collecting tubules in the absence of antidiuretic hormone (82). The main restriction to water movement was found to reside in the apical membrane (74). ADH had no effect on MD cells, consistent with the earlier observation that the adenylate cyclase of MD cells is relatively insensitive to vasopressin (83). Wide intercellular spaces are observed between MD cells in isolated perfused specimens and in electron micrographs (43,68). The interspaces resemble those observed between collecting duct cells in the presence of an osmotic gradient and vasopressin (84). Narrowing of these spaces was noted in mannitol and furosemide diuresis (41), suggesting that either blockade of NaCl transport or a reduced transtubular osmotic gradient diminished trans-MD fluid movement. Widening of interspaces during the imposition of an osmotic gradient was directly observed in the perfused MD preparation (68). Because sizable water movement through the epithelial shunt pathway is unlikely, the width of the interspaces may be the result of a high outflow resistance imposed by an interstitium not drained by capillaries. Absence of a correlation between intercellular spaces and water flux has recently been reported in the collecting duct where vasopressin but not cyclic adenosine monophosphate (AMP) caused widening of interspaces even though the increase in osmotic water flux was identical (85). CHIP 28, a likely water channel that is highly expressed in the proximal tubule and descending limb (86), has not been found in MD cells by immunohistochemistry (M. A. Knepper, *personal communication*). The magnitude of the transepithelial water flux is an important determinant of whether there is a buildup of electrolyte concentrations in the JG interstitium. High interstitial solute concentrations have been proposed as a possible intermediate step in the production of vascular responses (87). In Amphiuma, where NaCl transport into the interstitium at the glomerular vascular pole proceeds through the water-impermeable distal epithelium during elevated loop flow rates, substantially hypertonic Cl concentrations were found in this presumably poorly stirred portion of the renal interstitial space (88).

Intracellular Calcium

Two groups of investigators have attempted to determine whether changes in luminal solute concentration result in changes in intracellular Ca concentration in the MD. This question has assumed greater urgency with the recognition, as reviewed above, that a calcium-sensitive NOS is abundant in MD cells. In the first report, a modest and slow increase in cytosolic Ca was observed when the luminal perfusate was changed from a hypotonic perfusate with an osmolarity of 100 mOsm/L to an isotonic solution with an osmolarity 290 mOsm/L (89). However, in a separate and more extensive study, cytosolic Ca was reported to decrease slightly when NaCl concentration was increased whereas changes in osmolarity had no effect (90). Furosemide did not significantly alter intracellular Ca in either TAL or MD cells (91).

Extraglomerular Mesangium

Morphologic Characteristics

Extraglomerular mesangial cells, which have also been called Goormaghtigh or lacis cells, are those cells of the JGA that have the most intimate and regular contact with the MD (37–39). The anatomy and the position of the EGM suggest that they may transmit changes from the MD cells to the glomerular vasculature. They possess long interwoven cytoplasmic processes that, in general, run parallel to the base of the MD cells and that result in expansion of cell membrane surface area (92). Extraglomerular mesangial cells are extensively coupled by gap junctions (93–97), both to each other and to mesangial and granular cells but not to the MD (93). A network of myofilaments are present in EGM cells, suggesting that they, like mesangial cells, may have contractile potential

(97,98). Also, the extracellular matrix contains abundant fibrillar material, the orientation of which suggests a role for the EGM cell region in maintenance of the structural integrity of the glomerular hilum (99).

In striking contrast with the peritubular spaces elsewhere in the cortex is the well-established fact that the basolateral surface of the MD and the interstitial spaces in the EGM cell region are free of capillaries. One of the consequences of this finding may be a retardation of fluid removal from this compartment. In an electron microscopic study, it was found that the interstitial volume density of the EGM cell field increased from 16.9 percent during volume depletion to 29 percent during volume expansion, whereas no changes were noted in the volume density of the peritubular interstitium (100).

In Vivo Studies of Biochemical Characteristics

Most reports localizing expression to the mesangium *in vivo* by methods such as histochemistry or autoradiographic receptor distribution have not distinguished between intraglomerular mesangial and EGM cells. In some cases, localization can be inferred from published material. For example, autoradiographic studies localizing either atrial natriuretic peptide (ANP) or angiotensin II binding suggest labeling over extraglomerular locations (101,102). More recently, *in situ* hybridization studies have shown that angiotensin II type I receptor mRNA is preferentially expressed over the EGM cell field (103). Although EGM cells normally do not synthesize renin, they can be recruited to form renin with chronic stimulation (4,31). Production of renin by intraglomerular mesangial cells would appear to be much more unusual (4).

The thy-1.1 antigen, which is expressed on intraglomerular mesangial cells, appears to be absent or at lower levels in EGM cells (104,105). Decay accelerating factor (DAF), a glycoprotein-limiting complement activation on cell surfaces, is also differentially expressed; in frozen tissue from human kidneys, DAF localization was restricted to EGM with no staining inside the glomerular tuft (106). Cells with phagocytic potential and surface marker expression consistent with bone marrow origin are regularly identified in the mesangium, but these cells appear to be confined to the intraglomerular mesangium and not to occur in the EGM (W. Kriz, *personal communication*). Thus, the available information would suggest that the EGM cell has several features that distinguish it from the intraglomerular mesangial cell.

Functional Aspects

The cultured mesangial cell is one of the most extensively studied cells of renal origin (see excellent reviews in refs. 107 and 108). Review of this work is outside the scope of this chapter, but several observations may be of relevance to understanding the biologic role of the EGM. No method exists, as of yet, to isolate cells of EGM origin separately. Isolated glomeruli, however, the starting material for mesangial cell isolation, include the EGM, and it appears likely that mesangial cells, as cultured with standard techniques, originate from both intra- and extraglomerular locations. Cultured mesangial cells form gap junctions and demonstrate electrical coupling (109). In view of the evidence reviewed below, for anion specificity of JGA-mediated responses, the effects of chloride on mesangial cells are of interest. Studies on mesangial cells indicate the presence of channels that are activated by agonists such as angiotensin II or vasopressin and mediate cell depolarization (110–112). Agonist-induced cell depolarization was found to be inhibited by lowering medium Cl^- concentration, a manipulation that also altered prostaglandin E_2 (PGE_2) production (113).

Granular Cells

Morphologic Characteristics

It is well established that the granular cells in the media of the afferent arteriole are the main renin-producing cells of the kidney. The typical renin-containing cell at the glomerular vascular pole has abundant rough endoplasmic reticulum, a well-developed Golgi apparatus, and a cytoplasm packed with granules (27,98). The renin-containing granules are membrane-bound. Some granules, believed to be the more newly formed, contain mostly prorenin in a crystalline lattice form; others, with an amorphous electron-dense content, are believed to be the more mature form after removal of the prosegment (114,115). Myofibrils may be sparse or even absent in granule-containing cells at the vascular pole. Under control conditions, the bulk of the renin-secreting cells are close to the glomerular vascular pole, but renin is also regularly detected in cells in more proximal locations along the renal microvasculature. These cells often have the typical fusiform or spindle-shaped appearance of a vascular smooth muscle cell and contain abundant myofibrils (4). Stimulation of renin is associated with increased recruitment of renin in these more proximal locations (116,117).

Renin is probably secreted by fusion of the granule membrane with the cell plasma membrane and emptying of granule contents into the interstitium. Electron microscopic evidence is available for a fusion of granules with the plasma membrane (4,115). The classic omega configuration with an open pore to the cell exterior is only rarely encountered, probably reflecting the rare occurrence of the exocytotic event (4). The episodic nature of renin release from isolated afferent arterioles indicates that the frequency of exocytosis may be in the order of only one release episode per JGA per 5 minutes under basal conditions (118).

Functional Aspects

Unfortunately, no method exists for maintaining JG cells in long-term culture without loss of regulated renin synthetic and secretory capacity. Most of the extensive body of experimentation on the regulation of renin secretion (reviewed in detail in ref. 3 and elsewhere in this edition) has used either intact animals or complex in vitro preparations such as cortical renal slices, isolated perfused kidneys, and isolated glomeruli. The granular cell is not directly accessible with these methods, and it is not always possible to infer that the effects of an intervention are the results of a direct effect on the granular cell. The granular cell can be visualized in situ in isolated vessels from mouse kidney, and this preparation is yielding some direct information about its membrane characteristics. Isolated granular cells of reasonably high purity can be obtained by Percoll gradient separation of a cortical cell suspension. After 24 hours in culture, more than 85 percent of cells are renin-immunopositive. The cells can be maintained ex vivo and studied in short-term primary culture (119–121). Renin secretion and renin mRNA levels gradually decline with time in culture (122), but stimulatory and inhibitory effects of a variety of agonists can be demonstrated with this preparation (119–122). The results have been summarized in several reviews (123,124).

Membrane characteristics of in situ JG cells have been studied by using the whole-cell patch-clamp technique (125). Cells possess voltage-dependent K channels with both inward and outward rectifying properties. Blockade of the inward rectifier appears to be a mechanism of cell depolarization by angiotensin II (125). Like mesangial cells, JG cells appear to possess calcium-activated Cl channels (125). It has been proposed that Ca-dependent activation of Cl efflux accompanied by K efflux may cause changes in cell and granule volume that could be responsible for the paradoxical inverse relationship between intracellular Ca concentration and renin secretion (124). Somewhat surprisingly, in view of the well-established action of Ca channel blockers to stimulate renin release (124–127), the granular cells were found to lack voltage-activated Ca channels (125). Renin secretion from isolated granular cell was not stimulated by nifedipine, but in co-culture with mesangial cells, renin secretion was stimulated and voltage-activated Ca channels could be demonstrated on the mesangial cells (128). These data suggest that in vivo Ca channel blockers may stimulate renin secretion by blockade of Ca^{2+} channels on mesangial cells; changes in renin secretion could result either as a consequence of their gap junction coupling with granular cells or via production of a paracrine factor.

INTEGRATED FUNCTION OF THE JGA

Overview

Macula Densa NaCl Concentration

The relationships between the variables controlled through the JGA are indicated schematically in Fig. 4. Important for the regulatory role of the JGA is the fact that NaCl concentration at the MD varies substantially, depending on the rate of flow of fluid into the loop of Henle (Fig. 4A). This characteristic is the consequence of the location of the MD at the distal end of the TAL and is, in fact, rather unique along the nephron. Along the proximal tubule, the concentrations of most solutes deviate only modestly from those in plasma and are not highly dependent on nephron flow rate. In the medullary segments of the loop of Henle, solute concentrations depend on osmotic concentrations prevailing in the interstitium, whereas in more distal nephron segments, solute concentrations depend heavily on the level of certain hormones, particularly ADH and aldosterone. Because of the transport and permeability characteristics of the TAL, the NaCl concentration in the tubule exiting from the loop of Henle is considerably lower than in plasma.

Dilution of salt concentration at the MD cells can reach levels of 20 mEq/L or less during low rates of tubular fluid flow, whereas at high rates of flow, values of 60 to 80 mEq/L are found (129–133). Because loop of Henle flow rate is, in turn, dependent on the rate of delivery from the proximal tubule and therefore on the relative rates of glomerular filtration and proximal tubule reabsorption, alterations in body sodium balance are translated into changes in tubular fluid salt concentration at the MD.

Tubuloglomerular Feedback

The large amount of NaCl filtered into the proximal tubule represents a persistent threat to body NaCl homeostasis by its potential to overwhelm the transport capacity of the nephron. As is reviewed in detail below, the vascular control mechanism, which operates through the JGA, represents one important mechanism to control this risk. Increasing NaCl concentration at the MD, whether a consequence of an increase in filtration rate or decrease in proximal tubular absorption, activates the tubuloglomerular feedback (TGF) control mechanism (Fig. 4B). The resultant reduction in filtration rate limits

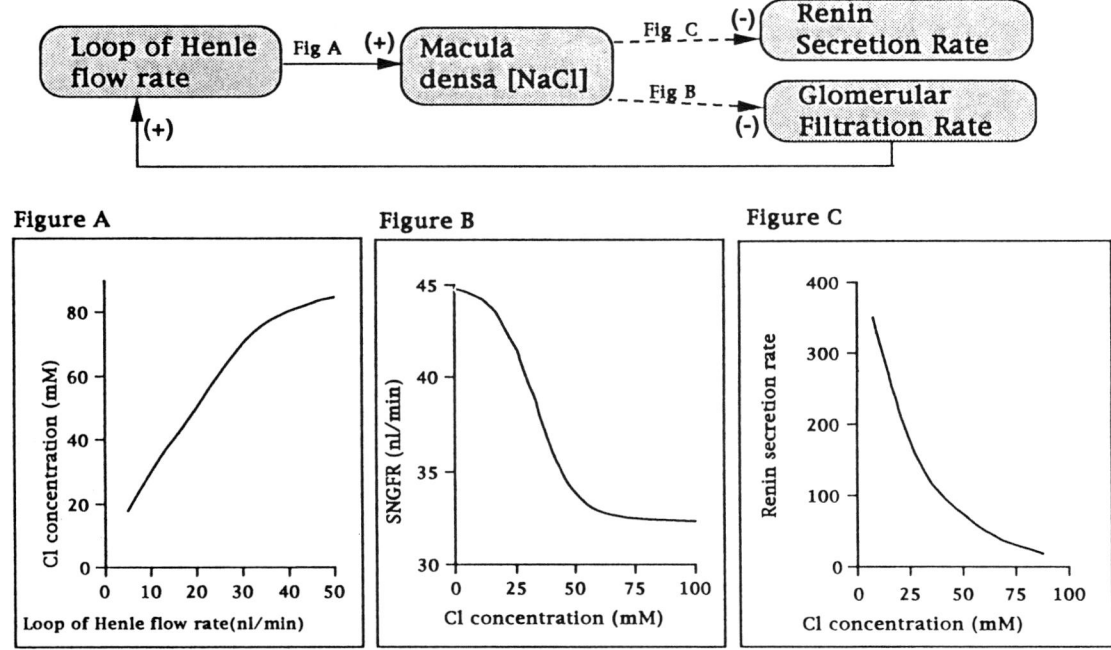

FIG. 4. Functional variables interacting in the juxtaglomerular apparatus. Increasing loop of Henle flow rates results in increasing NaCl concentration at the macula densa. This activates local mechanisms, which result in a decrease in glomerular filtration rate via the tubuloglomerular feedback (*TGF*) mechanism and a decrease in renin secretion rate. The decrease in glomerular filtration rate decreases loop flow rate, thus completing a feedback loop, which stabilizes distal salt delivery. **A:** Relationship between loop of Henle flow rate and Cl concentration at the macula densa, based on data in refs. 130 to 134. **B:** Relationship between Cl concentration and SNGFR is based on data in ref. 135, and previously summarized in ref. 1. **C:** Relationship between Cl concentration and single-nephron renin release rate (nGU/min) is based on data in refs. 22 to 25.

salt delivery into the collecting system, where the capacity to absorb NaCl is low. The magnitude of the filtration rate response to a change in luminal NaCl concentration, the TGF sensitivity, is highly variable: It is high in the volume-depleted state, a condition in which tight control of distal salt delivery is necessary. The functional coupling is relaxed during extracellular volume expansion, permitting an acceleration in the excretion of excess salt.

Renin Secretion

Under normal conditions, renin secretion and synthesis are closely coupled to the salt balance of the organism. The MD sensor for renin release (Fig. 4C) is one of several mechanisms responsible for linking salt balance with activation of the renin-angiotensin system (RAS). It operates synergistically with the other two members of the classic triad of renin release regulators: the baroreceptor and sympathetic nervous system, the redundancy of these control mechanisms probably reflecting the evolutionary importance of salt conservation. A consequence of this redundancy, however, is that in several disease states the system is inappropriately activated, with adverse consequences of excessive salt retention and pathological local effects of the RAS.

Effect of Macula Densa NaCl on Glomerular Filtration Rate

Manipulation and Assessment of Macula Densa NaCl Concentration

A substantial body of information about the JGA has accumulated from studies in which micropuncture methods were used to assess and to manipulate MD tubular fluid composition. However, the MD is not directly accessible by micropuncture, a fact that has resulted in persistent experimental difficulties. The closest accessible site is the early distal tubule, typically 300 to 600 μm downstream. The technique that has been used most widely to change solute composition at the MD is perfusion of the loop of Henle in an orthograde direction from the late proximal tubule (Fig. 5). Because alterations in loop flow are the usual physiological stimulus to change activity of the TGF mechanism, this approach has provided information of value in understanding its regulatory role. Nevertheless, because of the extensive modifications of perfusate in transit through the loop (129–134), this technique has been of limited use in characterizing the tubular signal. A technique has been developed to manipulate MD NaCl concentration by perfusion from the early distal tubule in a retrograde direction (Fig. 5). Although technically more difficult, this approach shortens the distance between perfusion and sensing sites, and at a moderately elevated flow rate, changes in perfusate composition are minimal.

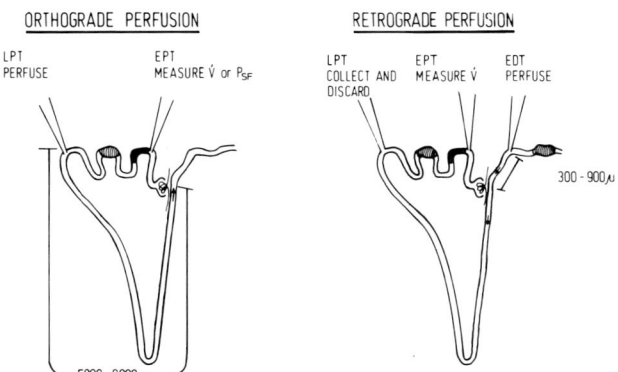

FIG. 5. Micropuncture methods to study tubuloglomerular feedback. **Left panel** illustrates orthograde perfusion of the loop of Henle; **right panel**, retrograde perfusion.

With orthograde perfusion of the loop of Henle, solute concentration, measured in the early distal tubule, depends on perfusion flow rate. Increments in loop of Henle flow rate above normal have been found to be consistently associated with increases in NaCl concentration (129–133). However, early distal NaCl concentration was also observed to increase when loop of Henle flow was reduced below normal (129–133). It is now clear that the biphasic pattern of distal solute concentrations is the result of modifications of tubular fluid between the MD and the surface distal tubule. Computer modeling of loop of Henle transport predicts that NaCl concentration at the MD should be a monotonic function of flow rate, but the relationship is biphasic if a short segment of distal tubule is included (131). When distal tubule fluid conductivity (which correlates with total electrolyte concentration) was measured continuously while stationary fluid from the loop of Henle was abruptly pushed downstream, a transient fall was observed (130), indicating that the minimum NaCl concentration is achieved at a point upstream from the early distal tubule. Other studies examined solute concentrations in nephrons with superficial glomeruli; when fluid collections were made at sites much closer to the MD than usually possible, it was found that Cl concentration almost doubled along the initial distal tubule at the spontaneous low rates of flow (134). These findings provide evidence that the distal tubule epithelium is unable to maintain the degree of dilution achieved by the TAL, and that at normal rates of distal flow, solute concentration at the MD is substantially lower than in the early distal tubule.

Effect of Variation in Loop of Henle Flow Rate on Glomerular Filtration Rate

The maximum response of filtration rate to changes in end proximal flow rate has been measured in many experimental series. As summarized in a previous review, in 26 series in rats, the average decrease in single-nephron GFR (SNGFR) was 13.1 ± 1 nl/min or 40 ± 3 percent in response to increments in loop flow from 0 to 40 or 50 nl/min (1). Responses have also been measured in juxtamedullary nephrons of both rats and hamsters, in which SNGFR fell by approximately 50 percent (136,137), in dogs (138,139), and in a few tubules in isolated human kidneys that were obtained for study because they were not usable for renal transplantation (140). The quantitative relationship between SNGFR and loop of Henle flow rate has been determined by repeat measurements of SNGFR in response to stepwise increments of loop of Henle flow rate. Figure 6 shows results from the most extensive of these studies, in which SNGFR was measured at eight different loop perfusion rates (141). The observed relationship was sigmoidal; three parameters could be estimated, the maximum response, the maximum slope, and the midpoint flow range, $V_{1/2}$ (141) (Fig. 7). One important result to emerge from these studies was that the sensitive flow range corresponded closely to the normal rates of tubular flow. $V_{1/2}$, the flow resulting in the half-maximum response, was 17.5 ± 0.9 nl/min, a value very similar to the normal late proximal flow rate (141). Studies were also undertaken to determine feedback curve parameters for growing rats of different ages. As GFR and kidney weight increased, balanced changes occurred in the feedback response characteristics, with the result that the flow range of maximum sensitivity corresponded in each age group with the normal rate of tubular flow (141). The operating point of the feedback mechanism was thus maintained close to the point of maximum sensitivity. The slope of the curve is a major determinant of the gain of the feedback loop. Gain is a unitless measure of the effectiveness of a feedback system. In the studies in growing rats, gain was observed to increase with age, from 1.7 in young rats to 3.2 in adults. In other studies, gain esti-

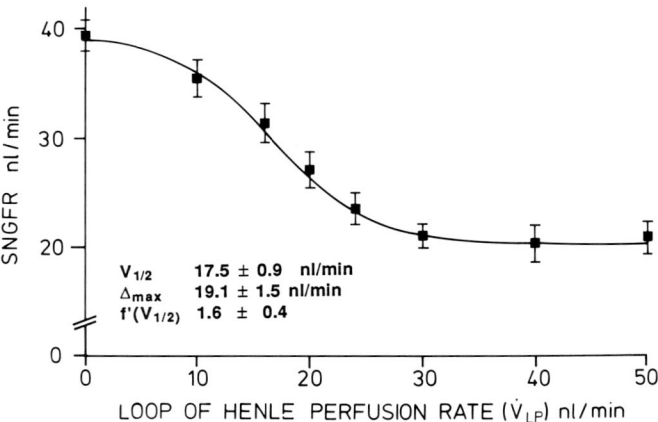

FIG. 6. Tubuloglomerular feedback relationship between loop of Henle flow rate and SNGFR (Data from ref. 141).

mates of between 1.5 and 3.1 have been obtained by measuring the effect on SNGFR of addition or removal of fluid to the late proximal tubule (142–144).

NaCl Dependency of SNGFR

In early studies, it was demonstrated that distal microinjection of isotonic NaCl but not mannitol elicited TGF responses (15), indicating that responses depend on solute characteristics of tubular fluid at the MD and not tubular pressure or flow *per se.* Subsequent retrograde perfusion studies have established the relationship between MD NaCl concentration and SNGFR (135). Single-nephron GFR was found to vary inversely with changes in perfusate NaCl concentration between 15 and 60 mM (or 30 and 120 mOsm), values that extend over the hypotonic range normally occurring at the end of the TAL (130,136). Increments in NaCl concentration

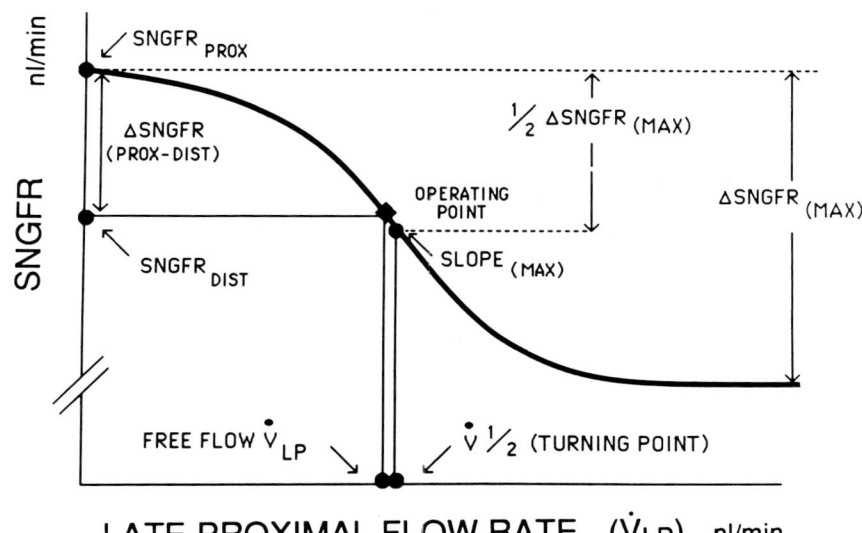

FIG. 7. Feedback relationship. Terms used to describe the relationship between loop of Henle flow and SNGFR. See text.

greater than 60 mM did not further suppress filtration rate. Fitting the equation of a hyperbolic tangent to these results indicates that the half-maximum decrease in SNGFR is caused by a NaCl concentration of 33.5 mEq and that the maximum slope is about 0.5 nl/min/mEq Na^+. No attempt was made in these studies to discriminate between ionic or osmotic effects of the perfusion fluid. Additional evidence, however, indicates that total solute concentration at the MD does not seem to influence measurably the TGF-mediated reductions of SNGFR. In retrograde perfusion experiments in which fluid osmolality and NaCl concentration were varied independently, TGF responses were noted to be exclusively determined by NaCl concentration and not by osmolality (145). Although a correlation between TGF responses and alterations in osmolality has been observed during orthograde perfusion with various solutions (146), the variations in distal osmolality were outside the physiological osmolality range (146). Thus, the cells initiating the vascular TGF response are activated by changes in luminal NaCl concentration, not osmolality. Independence of luminal osmolality is consistent with the relative water impermeability of the MD cell plaque (see above).

TGF Vascular Effector Site

Effect on Glomerular Capillary Pressure

Increasing loop of Henle flow rate has been found to cause a fall in stop flow pressure (P_{SF}) (147), a measure of glomerular capillary pressure applicable to nephrons that do not possess superficial glomeruli (148). In a survey of 23 studies, the average change in P_{SF} was from 39.0 ± 0.8 to 30.3 ± 0.8 mm Hg, a decrease of 22 percent (1). A reduction in P_{SF} was also observed in the dog when loop flow was increased (138,158). Because continuous measurements can be made in a single nephron over relatively extended periods of time, this technique has been widely used as a tool to study TGF-dependent hemodynamic effects (147,149–158). The nonlinear relationship between loop of Henle flow and P_{SF} was apparent long before a similar feedback function for SNGFR was defined (147). Because multiple determinations of P_{SF} can be made in the same nephron with small perfusion flow increments, the technique facilitates characterization of feedback curves. In 15 experimental series, the maximum P_{SF} decrease averaged 7.9 ± 0.6 mm Hg, with a mean $V_{1/2}$ of 20.1 ± 1.1 nl/min (1). The maximum slope varied substantially between studies but typically fell 1 and 2 mm Hg for each nanoliter per minute increase in flow (1). In both hydropenic and euvolemic rats of the Munich-Wistar strain, P_{SF}-derived values for glomerular capillary pressure have been compared with direct measurements and have usually been found to be essentially identical (159). Furthermore, although one contrary report exists (160), several laboratories have reported that the TGF-induced change in P_{SF} is virtually identical to the TGF-induced change in directly measured glomerular pressure (161,162).

Afferent versus Efferent Effector Site

A fall in glomerular pressure could theoretically result from either an increase in preglomerular resistance or a decrease in postglomerular resistance. Distinguishing these two alternatives required assessment of glomerular plasma flow. The micropuncture approach relied on measurements of SNGFR and of single nephron filtration fraction, determined from efferent collections. Increasing loop perfusion rate has been found to reduce plasma flow entering the glomerulus by about 20 percent, consistent with a 30 to 40 percent increase of preglomerular resistance (160,163). Several more direct methods have provided confirmation that the vascular response to increasing MD NaCl is vasoconstrictive and that the afferent arteriole is the dominant site. A TGF-induced reduction in glomerular plasma flow was observed videometrically in capillaries of superficial glomeruli; the rate of arrival of fluorescent particles fell by approximately 25 percent when loop flow was elevated (1). A 30 percent reduction in afferent arteriolar blood flow was also seen in Amphiuma and Necturus kidneys when distal flow rate was increased (88,164). When pre- and postglomerular arteriolar diameter were examined in sections of kidneys snap-frozen during high loop flow, perfusion afferent arteriolar diameter of perfused nephrons was consistently smaller than those belonging to nonperfused nephrons or to nephrons perfused with furosemide-containing solutions (165).

In Vitro Confirmation of a TGF Effect on Afferent Arterioles

More recently, two preparations have been developed that permit TGF activation and direct visualization of the glomerular vasculature. Using a system for in situ blood perfusion of juxtamedullary nephron that permits direct observation of the glomerular vascular pole, it has been observed that increased loop flow induced changes in afferent arteriolar diameter but not in efferent diameter (166,167). Ito and coworkers (38,39) have recently shown that TGF-induced decreases in afferent arteriolar diameter can be demonstrated in vitro using the isolated perfused tubule technique. In technically demanding studies in which both afferent arteriole and the MD tubular segment were perfused, it was shown that increases in MD NaCl concentration produce a local afferent constrictive response (38,39).

Interestingly, the resistance change calculated from

the directly observed diameter changes has generally been greater than the micropuncture estimates. One source of error in the micropuncture determinations is that preglomerular resistance, which is calculated from the artery to glomerulus pressure difference, overestimates true afferent arteriolar resistance, because a portion of the preglomerular resistance resides in the cortical radial arteries (168,169). The relative change caused by the TGF mechanism is thus underestimated, probably by about 15 percent. It is also possible that in the small preglomerular arterioles, resistance may deviate from Poiseuille law. For example, a reduction in blood viscosity caused by the small tube effect (Fahraeus-Lindquist effect) may cause overestimation of resistance based on Poiseuille flow.

The absence of immunoreactive myosin from the renin-containing distal part of the afferent arterioles has been taken as evidence that this vascular segment is noncontractile (115). However, studies in isolated perfused afferent arterioles (170) and in the hydronephrotic kidney (171) have shown that the glomerular entrance segment of the afferent arteriole is contractile, and the *in vitro* preparations have established that it is the main TGF effector site (38,166). Spreading of smooth muscle excitation to proximal portions of the arteriole may occur through electrotonic coupling or through a myogenic response (172).

Other Vascular Effects

In one micropuncture series, increasing loop flow was observed to increase efferent resistance as well as afferent resistance (160). Several studies have shown that in the subnormal flow range (from 0 to 10 nl/min) increasing loop flow is associated with a fall of SNGFR but virtually no change in glomerular pressure, suggesting balanced afferent and efferent vasoconstriction (147,173). During simultaneous inhibition of PG synthetase and converting enzyme, an increase in loop flow was shown to reduce GFR without changing glomerular pressure (162), a result also consistent with the notion of a postglomerular resistance increase. There is also some experimental evidence in support of the possibility that a reduction in the filtration coefficient may also contribute to the TGF-induced reduction of GFR (160), but there has been as of yet no *in vitro* confirmation.

Effect of Macula Densa NaCl on Renin Secretion

Whole Animal Studies of MD Renin Secretion

In the first studies designed to investigate the effect of the MD on renin release, Vander and Miller (19) observed an inverse correlation between venous renin activity and sodium excretion but no correlation between renin and mean arterial pressure, renal plasma flow, fil-

tration fraction, or plasma sodium concentration. These data led them to suggest that a low-salt delivery or concentration at the MD cells might stimulate renin secretion. Shade and coworkers (174) devised an approach to try to separate the MD mechanism from other influences on renin secretion, using dogs with thoracic caval obstruction. They found that intravenous infusion of hypertonic NaCl or KCl was able to substantially inhibit renin secretion in control caval dogs but had no effect in similar animals in which kidneys had been made nonfiltering by ureteral occlusion. In these studies, the hypertonic solutions did not alter renal plasma flow, and the authors concluded that failure to effect renin in the nonfiltering kidney was attributable to the absence of a functioning MD.

Efforts were made to determine whether MD-dependent renin secretion depends only on luminal NaCl concentration or whether it depends on fluid flow rate or NaCl delivery. During ureteral occlusion and superimposed mannitol diuresis, renin secretion was more closely related to changes in Na delivery than concentration (18,175). Additional support for this "sodium load" hypothesis was provided by micropuncture studies (176). Induction of an osmotic diuresis with mannitol was observed to increase Na load but decrease Na concentration in the early distal tubule. In contrast, saline-induced diuresis caused an increase in both concentration and delivery. Because renin secretion was inhibited with both types of diuresis, it was concluded that the initiating signal was a change in Na delivery and not simply concentration. Vander and Carlson (177) demonstrated that furosemide increased renin secretion even when Na-and-water balance were maintained; because furosemide was known to increase salt delivery to the MD, they surmised that furosemide must stimulate renin release via a transport effect. Most early studies assumed Na dependence of renin secretion. However, with administration of a wide variety of Na and Cl salts, Kotchen and coworkers demonstrated that Na without Cl was unable to inhibit renin secretion, whereas Cl without Na retained the inhibitory ability of NaCl (178,179). For example, chronic or acute loading with either NaCl or KCl suppressed renin secretion, whereas loading with $NaHCO_3$ or $KHCO_3$ had no effect. It was therefore proposed on the basis of whole animal studies that renin secretion is inversely related to the rate or magnitude of Cl transport by the MD cells (180).

In Vitro *Methods To Study MD-Mediated Renin Secretion*

Many of the conclusions from these whole animal studies have subsequently been confirmed by more direct approaches. Nonetheless, one review author wrote in 1986, "The existence of a macula densa mechanism for renin secretion remains to be demonstrated" (181).

A variety of obstacles were difficult to overcome in intact animal experiments and limited the general acceptance of the results emerging from these studies (181,182). These included (a) the complexity of the whole animal manipulations; (b) uncertainty about NaCl concentration at the MD; (c) inability to determine renin released from a single JGA quantitatively; and (d) difficulty in isolating the MD signal from the other mechanisms that also influence renin secretion. These difficulties provided the motivation to develop *in vitro* approaches. Juxtaglomerular apparatus specimens consisting of a portion of the TAL, including MD, a portion of the distal tubule, the adherent glomerulus, and fragments of the afferent and efferent arteriole have been dissected from rabbit kidneys and the tubule cannulated and perfused so that fluid at the MD can be varied (23–25). With this technique, it has been demonstrated that high NaCl concentrations at the MD are associated with suppressed levels of renin secretion and that a reduction of NaCl concentration stimulates renin secretion. Macula densa-dependent renin secretion was characterized by prompt (within less than 4 minutes) onset and offset after step changes in NaCl concentration and by essentially complete reversibility (23,24). The sensitive concentration range was similar to that observed with TGF, about 20 to 80 mM (25). Stimulation of renin secretion by a reduction in luminal NaCl at the MD was also seen when perfusate osmolality was kept constant by the addition of mannitol (24). Studies with this technique indicate that renin secretion responds more substantially to a reduction in MD NaCl concentration than NaCl delivery (24), in contrast with the micropuncture data reviewed above (176). The discrepancy probably arises in part from the inaccuracies in estimating MD NaCl concentration from early distal measurements (134). Also, in the earlier studies, systemic administration of mannitol may have produced direct osmotic effects on renin release (175,176).

The *in vitro* studies have yielded a quantitative estimate of the effect of MD NaCl concentration on renin secretion. Assuming a linear correlation between the changes in NaCl concentration and renin release, the *in vitro* results predict that single JGA renin secretion increases by about 0.5 nGU/min/mEq decrement of NaCl concentration (24,25). Using this sensitivity approximation, one can estimate that PRA would increase approximately fivefold if NaCl concentration at the MD fell by 10 mM.

Characterization of the MD Sensing Mechanism for Renin Secretion and TGF

Transport Inhibitor Studies

Inhibition of NaCl transport by application of furosemide or other blockers of Na,K,2 Cl cotransport has been known for some time to be associated with blockade of the TGF mechanism (183). Because distal NaCl concentration increases with application of furosemide, this result indicates that responses do not simply depend on luminal NaCl concentration and suggests that a change in NaCl transport is necessary for the vascular response. Tubuloglomerular feedback blockade has been reported in the presence of loop diuretics such as furosemide (182,183), bumetanide (184), piretanide (184,185), ethacrynic acid (183), triflocin (183), and l-ozolinone (187). Drug concentrations causing transport and feedback inhibition appear similar (about 5×10^{-5} M for furosemide and about 10^{-6} M for bumetanide (182,184). Furthermore, transport inhibition caused by metabolic inhibitors such as cyanide, antimycin A, or uncouplers of oxidative phosphorylation has likewise been found to reduce TGF responsiveness (183,186,188). However, muzolamine, acetazolamide, and amiloride, agents with actions outside the loop of Henle, do not share this effect (183,184,187). Recent studies using *in vitro* perfused JGAs establish that renin secretory responses are also abolished by luminal application of furosemide (25). The electrophysiological and optical evidence for effects of furosemide on MD cells have been reviewed above.

Ion Substitution Studies

That transport via the Na,K,2Cl cotransporter is the initial step in the feedback transmission pathway is further supported by parallelism in the ionic requirements. Although TGF responses can be elicited with a great number of both Na^+ and Cl^- free solutions and even sometimes with nonelectrolyte solutions as well as with orthograde perfusion of the loop of Henle (189), when the loop of Henle is perfused in a retrograde fashion, a clear pattern of ionic specificity emerges (135). Tubuloglomerular feedback responses were not seen during perfusion with isotonic or hypotonic solutions of Na^+ salts such as $NaHCO_3$, $NaNO_3$, NaI, NaSCN, Na acetate, Na gluconate, or Na isethionate (135). In contrast, isotonic solutions of Cl^- salts accompanied by small monovalent cations such as K^+, Rb^+, Cs^+, or NH_4^+ elicited full TGF responses, as did the Br^- salts of Na^+ and K^+ (135). Some of these small cations have been found to be substrates for either the Na^+ or the K^+ site on the cotransporter (190). Similarly, when isolated perfused MD specimens were perfused with salt solutions in which Na^+ was substituted with either choline or Rb^+, renin secretion was inhibited to a comparable degree as observed with NaCl. However, when the Cl^- was substituted with either isethionate or acetate, no inhibitory response to Na^+ could be detected (25). The effect of ion substitutions on responses, the dependency of response magnitude on Cl^- concentration, and the apparent independence of Na^+ concentration are similar to TAL transport (191). In the TAL, half-maximum transport rates require a Cl^- concentration of about 40 to 50 mM but a Na^+ or K^+ concentration of less than 3 mM (191), reflecting a large difference in affinity of the transporter for Cl^- and the cations (191). Even though some discrepancies remain (192), there is now solid experimental support for the concept that NaCl transport initiated by NaCl uptake through the furosemide-sensitive Na,K,2Cl cotransporter is the critical first step in JGA signal transmission.

Stimulus-Response Coupling Mechanisms

Changes in MD NaCl transport initiate complex interactions between the different cell types that make up the JGA. These cell-to-cell signaling steps are only partially understood, but there is evidence to suggest that signal transmission relies on some diffusible extracellular messenger system. As reviewed above, MD cells do not directly contact the renin-secreting granular cells or the afferent arteriole. Their most consistent contact is with the EGM cells, suggesting that signal transmission includes the participation of the EGM interstitial compartment.

Adenosine

Adenosine was initially proposed as a local mediator of metabolic regulation of glomerular blood flow and renin secretion because it was recognized as a metabolic product whose formation rate may depend on solute transport rate (193–195). Substantial evidence, recently reviewed (196), supports this hypothesis. The glomerular entrance segment, the TGF effector site, possesses a high density of vasoconstrictive adenosine$_1$ receptors (197) and is exquisitely sensitive to exogenous adenosine (197). An increase in the interstitial level of adenosine by EHNA, an inhibitor of adenosine deaminase, or by dipyridamole, an inhibitor of cellular adenosine uptake, was associated with an increase in the TGF response magnitude (194,198). Conversely, acceleration of adenosine degradation by adenosine deaminase reduced feedback responses (198). Tubuloglomerular feedback responses could be inhibited by intravenous and MD application of theophylline or other methylxanthines such as IBMX at concentrations at which they may specifically inhibit adenosine receptors (199–202). Finally, a selective antagonist of adenosine$_1$ receptors, 8-cyclopentyl-1,3-dipropylxanthine (CPX), inhibited TGF responses in a concentration of 10 μmol/L, a value close to the concentrations typically required to block adenosine$_1$ receptors (203).

In addition to their vasoconstrictive effect, adenosine$_1$ receptors are known to mediate inhibition of renin release, so adenosine is a possible mediator of the MD-induced changes in renin secretion. Using the isolated perfused JGA technique, it was shown that administra-

tion of the adenosine$_1$-receptor agonist cyclohexyladenosine mimicked the inhibitory effect on renin secretion of a high MD NaCl and that this effect was blocked by the antagonist CPX. Furthermore, administration of CPX was found to blunt the inhibitory effect of high NaCl perfusion itself (204). However, unlike TGF responses, which can be fully blocked by CPX (203), the response of renin to NaCl was only partially inhibited by the antagonist (204). Furthermore, application of the native compound adenosine produced only modest inhibitory effects on renin release, and only at doses at least two logs above the physiological range or in the presence of the adenosine deaminase inhibitor pentostatin (205). These results suggest that, although adenosine may participate in mediating MD-dependent renin secretion, it is unlikely to be the sole determinant of this response.

Solute Concentrations in the Extraglomerular Mesangium

An alteration in MD transport may also affect the vascular elements at the glomerular pole by changing solute concentration or osmolarity in the interstitium of the EGM cell field (87). By using ion-selective microelectrodes, it has been shown that Cl concentrations in the tubuloglomerular contact region of the Amphiuma kidney increase with increasing flow rates to values much higher than plasma (88). There is no direct evidence in mammalian species for or against the occurrence of similar interstitial Cl concentration changes. As reviewed above, reductions in Cl concentration in the medium of cultured mesangial cells have been shown to inhibit the contractile response to angiotensin II, to reduce the accompanying increase in cytosolic Ca and IP$_3$ (110–112), and to stimulate PGE$_2$ formation (113); furthermore exogenous PGE$_2$ mimics the effects of low Cl concentration on agonist-induced increments in cell Ca (113). On the basis of these studies in cultured mesangial cells, it has been inferred that extracellular Cl may act on the EGM to modulate the cellular responses to agonists such as angiotensin II (110). Because EGM and the effector cells of the TGF and renin secretory pathway are coupled by gap junctions, it is conceivable that the intracellular ionic alterations caused by low extracellular Cl may extend to afferent arteriolar smooth muscle and granular cells.

Changes in intracellular Ca of granular cells may also affect renin secretion by an effect on cell volume. Application of the whole-cell patch-clamp technique has shown that granular cells, like mesangial cells, appear to possess Ca-activated Cl channels (125). Thus, an increment in cytosolic Ca may enhance Cl efflux and the accompanying K and water efflux may then cause a reduction of cell volume. In isolated superfused rat glomeruli, Skøtt (206) demonstrated that renin secretion is exquisitely sensitive to changes in extracellular osmolality, with a 16-fold stimulation of renin release caused by a decrease in osmolality of only 25 to 30 percent. Although the evidence for direct osmotic effects on renin secretion is strong, most of the granular cells are located in the wall of the afferent arteriole, outside the EGM field. If MD transport alters local interstitial osmolarity or solute concentration, it is questionable whether this effect extends to the bulk of the renin-secreting cells. Calcium-mediated changes in cell volume, however, may not be limited to the immediate JG region because ionic signals can travel through the many gap junctions existing between mesangial and arteriolar cells.

Arachidonic Acid Metabolites

There is substantial evidence supporting a role for cyclo-oxygenase products in JGA cell-to-cell signaling (207). The effect of PG synthesis inhibition on the renin secretory response to changing MD NaCl concentration has been examined in the isolated perfused JGA preparation (208). Inhibition of cyclo-oxygenase activity with flurbiprofen or flufenamic acid either blunted or completely abolished the stimulation of renin secretion produced by a reduction in luminal NaCl concentration, indicating that MD-mediated stimulation of renin secretion requires an intact cyclo-oxygenase pathway. Immunohistochemical studies have reported localization of cyclo-oxygenase activity in mesangial cells, in epithelial cells of Bowman's capsule, and in endothelial cells of renal arterioles (209) but not in MD cells themselves. The close proximity of the EGM cells to both the MD and the JG cells suggests that inhibition of PG formation by EGM cells may explain these results, possibly as discussed above, via a fall in Cl concentration in the JG interstitium (207).

Other products of arachidonic acid metabolism may influence renin release as well. In anesthetized rats, PRA was suppressed by administration of a thromboxane mimetic and stimulated by blockade of thromboxane synthesis (210). Furthermore, metabolites derived from both lipoxygenase (211) and cytochrome P450 (212) pathways of arachidonate metabolism have been found to inhibit renin release in renal cortical slices. A specific role of these nonprostanoid products in MD-activated renin secretion remains possible but untested. It has been reported that mesangial cells contain both lipoxygenase (107) and P450 monooxygenase (213) activity, in addition to their ability to synthesize PGs and thromboxanes (Tx) (107). This affirms the plausibility that mesangial cells may mediate or at least modulate renin secretion via production of one or more of these agents.

The possibility of a participation of arachidonic acid-derived metabolites in TGF control of vascular tone has been examined by several laboratories. Maximum TGF responses have been shown to be inhibited by the intra-

venous application of cyclo-oxygenase inhibitors, but relatively high doses were required. For example, a dose of 5 mg/kg indomethacin was required to obtain more than 50 percent inhibition of either the SNGFR or the P_{SF} response (214) despite the fact that maximum inhibition of PG synthesis as judged from urinary excretion of PGE_2 or PGF_2 was achieved with a lower dose of indomethacin. Similarly, inhibition of TGF responses by luminal administration of indomethacin required concentrations in the millimolar range (214,215). Intravenous administration of indomethacin did not reduce the maximum TGF response of SNGFR in animals kept on a low-salt diet even though PG synthesis was inhibited to a similar extent (214). Normal TGF responsiveness returned 80 minutes after the intravenous administration of either indomethacin or carprofen, whereas PG production continued to be depressed (214). Similarly, the inhibition of the TGF response achieved by retrograde administration of indomethacin was acutely reversible (214,215) even though inhibition of cyclo-oxygenase is usually long-lasting. With high doses of indomethacin applied by retrograde perfusion, a marked increase in SNGFR rather than the normal decrease was observed (214), indicating that indomethacin in this study acted by producing active vasodilation rather than by blocking the generation of a PG mediator with direct or indirect vasoconstrictor properties. Thus, there is reason to suspect that the attenuation of TGF responses by inhibitors of PG synthesis may not be exclusively related to cyclo-oxygenase inhibition.

A specific role of the vasoconstrictor PG Tx in TGF mediation has been suggested on the basis of the finding that the intravenous administration of Tx-receptor blockers or of Tx-synthesis inhibitors reduced the magnitude of the TGF-induced vasoconstrictor response (216). In other studies, blockade of Tx effects was not found to affect TGF responses measurably, however, so a specific role of Tx in the TGF mechanism remains uncertain (215,217).

Nitric Oxide

With the recent recognition that MD cells possess high levels of the Ca-calmodulin regulated NOS (42,43), the role of NO in MD-mediated vascular and secretory responses has become a topic of active interest. As of yet, there is little information on the factors that regulate NO formation by the MD cell. As reviewed above, the available data on the effects of MD NaCl on intracellular Ca are contradictory, and inferences about the effect of the MD signal on local NO formation through alterations in Ca-calmodulin are therefore speculative.

Inhibition of NO synthesis has been observed to increase TGF responses both *in vivo* (43,218) and *in vitro* (219). A role of NO in modulating TGF responses in high-salt states has been suggested (43,219), although evidence that a high-salt diet stimulates MD NO formation is not yet available. Both stimulatory and inhibitory effects of NO on renin release have been reported. Because NO is known to act via complementary guanosine monophosphate (cGMP) and increases in cGMP are generally believed to inhibit renin release (124), an inhibitory effect might be expected. In fact, studies in renal cortical slices have suggested an inhibitory effect (220), as do studies in anesthetized rats in which renal perfusion pressure and beta-adrenergic activity were held constant (221). Conversely, studies in isolated perfused rat kidneys suggest a potent stimulatory effect of NO on renin secretion (222). In isolated granular cells, the immediate direct effect is inhibition, but with prolonged exposure, stimulation has been observed (223,224). Experiments performed on isolated perfused JGA preparations exhibited a dual effect of NO, depending on which cell types were directly exposed to NOS manipulations. Although agents that increase NO applied to the bathing solutions inhibited renin release, when drugs were administered via the lumen directly to the MD, renin release was stimulated (225). Some of these apparent contradictions may arise because several cell types in the JGA appear to be capable of both NO synthesis and cGMP responses, the renal microvascular endothelium being the prime example. There is evidence for both cytokine-activated and calcium-calmodulin–activated NO synthesis in mesangial cells (226) and high levels of soluble quanylyl cyclase in the EGM region (227). It is possible that NO generated by MD cells may have different effects than NO generated by endothelium, because different concentrations are achieved at potential target cells. Substantial further study is needed to untangle the role of NO in the JGA.

REGULATORY ROLE OF THE TUBULOGLOMERULAR FEEDBACK LOOP

Overview

The JGA control system is constructed as a negative homeostatic feedback loop that will tend to maintain the MD concentration of NaCl within narrow boundaries and to regulate the escape of NaCl into the low-capacity transport system of the distal nephron. The characteristics of this regulatory system, as determined from single-nephron perturbation studies (i.e., refs. 141 to 144), allow the prediction that TGF-induced changes in vascular tone will occur when NaCl concentration at the MD cells deviates from a set value. Long-term recordings of blood pressure in conscious dogs have shown marked fluctuations throughout the day and with changing body activities (228). In the absence of tight control of vascular resistance, glomerular capillary pressure and GFR would

be expected to fluctuate in parallel with blood pressure, causing changes in Na excretion unrelated to the NaCl status of the organism. Because, however, changes in GFR initiate direct changes in distal NaCl concentration, the TGF system will initiate corrective vascular responses that will dampen the amplitude of the predicted GFR changes. Similar rapid hemodynamic adjustments will occur with other perturbations of MD NaCl concentration resulting from variations in cardiac output, renal blood flow, or proximal tubular transport. The role of TGF in chronic alterations in vascular tone is less certain. It is now well established that this system resets its sensitivity when perturbations of MD NaCl concentration are sustained for extended periods of time. It is thus probable that TGF responds primarily to acutely changing signals and may be more important for minute-to-minute adjustments of vascular tone than for its chronic regulation.

One consequence of its nature as a fast and tonic regulator of distal NaCl concentration is that the participation of TGF in the actual setting of vascular tone is not always easy to demonstrate experimentally. It requires the imposition of perturbations and an evaluation of the vascular response to these perturbations in the absence and presence of the TGF system.

Evidence TGF Regulates Distal Salt Concentration

Tonic Nature of the TGF System

For the proposed homeostatic role of the TGF mechanism, it is critical to demonstrate that the resting vascular tone in an animal in normal NaCl balance does include a TGF-dependent component. Several different approaches have shown that GFR does, in fact, change when NaCl concentration is altered in an upward or downward direction. Support for a tonic suppressive action of the TGF system came initially from the observation that GFR in a given nephron is usually higher when measured in a proximal segment than when measurements are performed in the distal tubule (229). As summarized recently, in 39 experimental series, proximal SNGFR exceeded distal SNGFR by an average of 6 nl/min or about 16 percent (1). The interpretation of this result is that the acute withdrawal of fluid necessary to determine GFR of a single nephron will acutely reduce MD NaCl concentration when collections are made in the proximal tubule but will leave MD NaCl unaltered during distal collections (see Fig. 7). Thus, an acute reduction of NaCl from normal to minimum values causes a measurable rise of GFR, indicating that the normal ambient flow exerts control over vascular tone.

Application of closed-loop feedback analysis has confirmed this notion (142–144). Small volumes of fluid were added or withdrawn from the proximal tubule while changes in proximal flow rate were continuously measured by videometric flow velocimetry. Fractional compensation of a flow perturbation was about 60 to 75 percent, indicating that the homeostatic efficiency of the TGF loop is quite high. Furthermore, the maximum compensation in hydropenic animals was found to reside around a zero flow change, indicating that both small increases and small decreases in flow are equally and maximally effective in altering GFR. These observations are in full agreement with the evidence discussed above, that the operating point is positioned at the midpoint of the open-loop feedback function. The midpoint, $V_{1/2}$, corresponds to the point of maximum sensitivity or the point of maximum compensation.

Finally, there is convincing evidence that the basal operation of the TGF loop can result in regular periodic oscillations of vascular tone (230–235). The first evidence for this notion came from the observation that proximal tubule pressure of halothane-anesthetized rats oscillated with a frequency of two to three cycles per minute. These oscillations occurred either spontaneously or, more frequently, could be elicited by small increases in tubule flow (231). Pressure oscillations could be abolished by loop diuretics, suggesting that they were, in fact, generated by the TGF system (232). In more recent studies, distal tubule flow rate and distal Cl concentration have been observed to oscillate with the same frequency but with a fixed-phase shift (233). Thus, the TGF system does appear to have temporal characteristics that can cause stable oscillations of GFR. Mathematical modeling of the TGF system has shown that the generation of TGF-dependent oscillations is consistent with properties of the response. Furthermore, oscillations develop only when the operating point is located in the most sensitive portion of the feedback curve (235,236). Interestingly, as reviewed below, the oscillations are disturbed in hypertensive animals (230,237) (Fig. 8).

Perturbation by Transport Alterations

When the rate of fluid absorption proximal to the MD is decreased, loop flow and MD NaCl concentration are predicted to increase, thereby shifting steady-state GFR to a lower value. This adjustment emphasizes the priority of stabilization of distal salt delivery over GFR constancy.

Hypertonic NaCl Infusion

An example demonstrating this sequence of events is the response of the renal vasculature to the administration of hypertonic NaCl. In most vascular beds, hypertonic NaCl results in vasodilation, but in the renal vas-

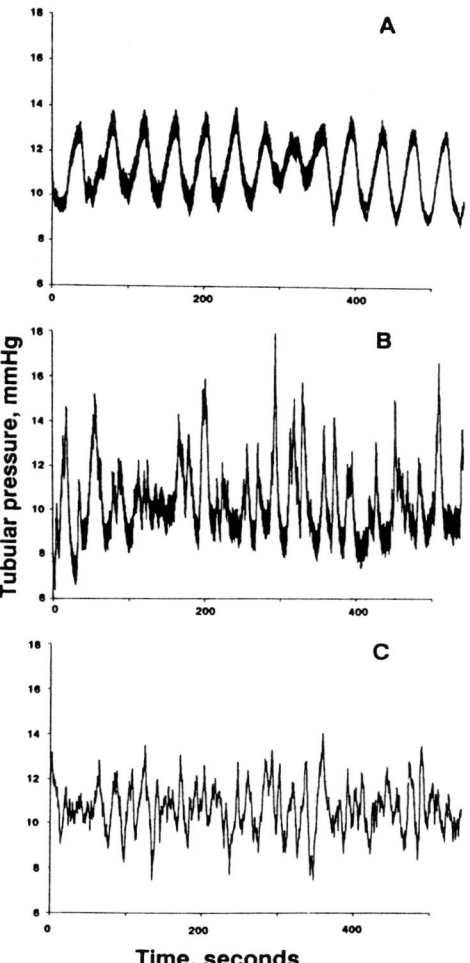

FIG. 8. Oscillations in proximal tubule pressure. **A:** Normal Sprague-Dawley rat. **B:** SHR. **C:** Goldblatt hypertensive rat. (From ref. 315, with permission.)

culature, an anomalous vasoconstriction is produced. There is evidence that this response may be the whole-kidney equivalent of TGF (238,239). Both responses are enhanced by salt depletion (239,240) and inhibited by furosemide, theophylline, or chronic treatment with DOCA-salt (119,240–243). Furthermore, infusion of non–chloride-containing solutions usually does not produce vasoconstriction (238,239). A micropuncture study has directly confirmed that the decrease in GFR is TGF-initiated (238). Hypertonic NaCl has been found to inhibit proximal NaCl absorption and to increase late proximal flow rate from 13.7 to 17 nl/min. As a consequence of this increase in flow, SNGFR fell from 31.4 nl/min to 27.9 nl/min. When the increase in flow was prevented from reaching the MD by a tubular oil block, SNGFR rose instead of falling. In these studies, an increase in tubular flow of 3.3 nl/min resulted in a decrease in GFR of 3.5 nl/min, a gain similar in magnitude to that seen with changes of loop perfusion rate (238).

Protein Feeding

Recent studies in conscious dogs have shown that the acute increase in GFR after a meat meal can be blocked by prior administration of furosemide or ethacrynic acid (244,245). To the extent that the diuretics blocked the TGF mechanism, these results support the concept that the increase in GFR caused by protein feeding is at least in part TGF-dependent. It has been speculated that the acute rise in filtered amino acids causes an increase in proximal Na and fluid absorption and a decrease in MD salt delivery.

There is also evidence that the TGF mechanism may contribute to the increase in GFR with chronic high protein feeding. The difference between proximal and distal SNGFR has been shown to decrease, indicating a shift in the operating point from the midpoint to the shoulder of the feedback curve (246,247). Furthermore, during orthograde perfusion of the loop of Henle, the response curve was shifted to the right, but responses were found to be unaltered when perfusion was retrograde from the distal tubule (248), suggesting a normal JGA transmission mechanism. These results are consistent with the notion that the change in GFR was probably caused by altered transport along the loop of Henle. In fact, NaCl concentration in the distal tubule was found to be 30 percent lower in rats on a high-protein diet than in low-protein–fed animals (248). The augmented NaCl transport may result from structural changes (249).

Proximally Acting Diuretics

Selective inhibition of proximal tubule NaCl transport causes an increase of loop of Henle flow and of MD NaCl concentration. As a result of TGF activation, GFR would be predicted to decrease. In fact, administration of acetazolamide, a carbonic anhydrase inhibitor, caused SNGFR measured in the distal tubule (with the TGF loop intact) to decrease more than proximal SNGFR (with TGF loop interrupted) (250). Similarly, interruption of loop flow prevented benzolamide-induced reductions in filtration rate (251). A recent careful investigation of the effects of acetazolamide on GFR formation has suggested that a substantial part of the decrease in GFR may be due to the increase in proximal tubule pressure (252). Furthermore, from the finding that furosemide did not prevent the acetazolamide-induced decrease in GFR, it was concluded that TGF may not be the most important mechanism responsible for this vascular adjustment (253). These observations may not be surprising in view of the fact that carbonic anhydrase inhibition results in an increase in distal $NaHCO_3$ but not NaCl concentration (250).

TGF Resetting

The importance of TGF control for the maintenance of body Na is underscored by the observation that the functional coupling between MD NaCl concentration and vascular tone varies with salt balance and extracellular fluid volume. This plasticity in the degree of tightness of GFR control by the MD is an appropriate property of a mechanism participating in the control of body Na content, because rigid obligatory coupling would retard the excretion of Na in conditions of excess extracellular Na. Conversely, in states of volume depletion, increased sensitivity of the TGF system will enhance the NaCl conserving effect of this regulatory mechanism.

In fact, infusion of isotonic saline at rates ranging between 4 and 10 percent of body weight reduced response magnitude and slope of the feedback function and increased $V_{1/2}$ in both superficial (254–258) and deep nephrons (259). A similar right shift was observed with plasma expansion (153,260,261). Chronic administration of DOCA in combination with isotonic saline as drinking fluid for more than 1 week has been shown to virtually abolish TGF responses (241,262,263). This reduced sensitivity of the TGF system to luminal NaCl explains why the elevation of distal NaCl that is consistently found in states of volume expansion does not cause afferent constriction and a fall in GFR. The effects of an acute decrease of extracellular volume (ECV) have been studied in rats after acute hypotensive hemorrhage (142,264,265), in dehydrated rats (266), and in rats after furosemide diuresis (267). In general, all these interventions are accompanied by an increase in TGF reactivity. Hypotensive hemorrhage induced a shift of the feedback curve to the left (142,264,265). Because proximal absorption increased at the same time, the operating point tended to move to the shoulder of the reset feedback function (264). The TGF function in rat kidneys after 24 hours of dehydration was similarly altered, although the increase in transport was less pronounced (266); as a consequence, SNGFR and kidney GFR fell significantly. Finally, acute volume depletion of DOCA-salt–treated rats by administration of furosemide completely restored TGF responsiveness (263).

Activity of the RAS

The local activity of the RAS appears to be a main determinant of TGF sensitivity, particularly during changes in body fluid volume. First, in several experimental models, response magnitude correlated with renal renin content. For example, responses were reduced in DOCA-salt–loaded rats (241) and in the nonclipped kidney of Goldblatt hypertensive rats (157) and enhanced in the clipped kidney (157,268). Second, blockade of the RAS has been consistently found to diminish TGF sensitivity. For example, administration of converting enzyme inhibitors reduced the maximum TGF responses of both SNGFR and P_{SF} to about half normal (269–271). A similar effect was seen during angiotensin receptor blockade with angiotensin analogues (271,272). Third, angiotensin infusion partly restored feedback responsiveness during captopril-induced TGF inhibition (273) and greatly enhanced responses in untreated control rats even when a change in arterial pressure was prevented (173). An augmentation of TGF responses was also seen during peritubular infusion of angiotensin at a concentration that in itself did not alter glomerular hemodynamics (274). The effect of angiotensin II on TGF sensitivity does not appear to be a nonspecific consequence of increased vascular tone, because vasopressin or norepinephrine did not affect TGF responses if arterial pressure was held constant (275). Finally, infusion of low nonpressor doses of angiotensin II into volume-expanded animals has been observed to restore feedback responses, producing both a shift of the curve to the right and an increase in the maximum response (276). Restoration was observed at an infusion rate that raised plasma concentration into the range normally found in hydropenic animals (276). Taken together, these observations provide good evidence that angiotensin II plays a specific role in modulating TGF sensitivity. Angiotensin II has been shown to interact with adenosine in constricting afferent arterioles (277). As discussed above, adenosine may be generated by MD cells in a NaCl-dependent manner. Thus, it is possible that angiotensin II acts by its synergistic interaction with the TGF mediator.

The effect of angiotensin II levels on TGF sensitivity gains special importance because changes in NaCl concentration in the tubular fluid in the region of the MD exert two effects on cells of the afferent arteriole. They not only induce direct changes of the tone of contractile smooth muscle cells (the TGF response), but they also inversely affect renin secretion from granular cells. This dual effect has the potential of automatically adjusting TGF sensitivity to the NaCl status of the organism. An increase in NaCl at the MD will lead to an increase in afferent tone, which will tend to lower distal NaCl through its effect on GFR and proximal absorption. This compensation may be incomplete, however, and the persistent error signal will cause a simultaneous decrease in renin secretion. The resulting change in plasma angiotensin II concentration will decrease the sensitivity of the vascular response to NaCl and attenuate the dependency of GFR on the MD signal. These changes will relax control of NaCl at the MD and permit salt excretion to rise. The opposite sequence of events will occur when MD NaCl decreases. Sensitivity regulation by angiotensin II probably contributes to the adjustments in TGF respon-

siveness that are seen during alterations in ECV. Any persistent increase in MD NaCl, for example, with volume expansion, is predicted to uncouple GFR from MD control, because the simultaneous inhibition of renin secretion will gradually reduce TGF sensitivity. Because the resulting increase in GFR will further inhibit renin secretion, a positive feedback cycle is initiated that will allow distal salt delivery to become independent of MD control. However, the fall in angiotensin levels will induce an increasing release of renin secretion from the inhibiting effects of angiotensin. Thus, a new steady state in salt excretion and renin secretion will occur, resulting from a balance of these interconnected feedback loops.

Angiotensin II–dependent resetting also appears to be the reason for the response of the renal vasculature to a pressure change after prolonged reductions of renal artery pressure to subautoregulatory value (278). Clamping of the renal artery to 75 mm Hg for 60 minutes caused a fall in SNGFR that was maintained at the low level for 20 minutes after the clamp had been released. This reduction of SNGFR was TGF-dependent since proximal SNGFR (TGF loop interrupted) promptly returned to normal after release of the clamp. Recent data have shown that the administration of enalapril fully prevented the delay in the return of renal blood flow to normal (276), suggesting that the sustained constrictor influence resulted from an angiotensin II–induced increase in TGF sensitivity.

Interstitial Pressure

A substantial body of experimentation by Persson and coworkers suggests that renal interstitial pressure may also be a factor in determining TGF sensitivity (279–286). This group of investigators observed an inverse correlation between sensitivity and interstitial pressure (the difference between interstitial hydrostatic pressure and oncotic pressure). Responses were observed to increase during peritubular capillary perfusion with a hyperoncotic solution (280). An increase in interstitial pressure was observed during acute NaCl infusion (254,255,281,282), during short-term ureteral obstruction (283), and after contralateral nephrectomy (284,285). In all these conditions, $V_{1/2}$ increased and response magnitude decreased. Conversely, interstitial pressure was reduced after 24 hours of dehydration (266,286) and after release of 24-hour unilateral ureteral occlusion (287), and TGF sensitivity was increased in these conditions.

Marked increases in interstitial volume, restricted to the EGM cell field, have been noted during acute ECV expansion (288). Changes in interstitial volume may underlie the effect of changing interstitial pressure. There are several possible mechanisms by which increases in interstitial volume might impede cell-to-cell transmission in the JGA. Diffusion distances could increase, and cell contact areas could change. Furthermore, the concentrations of humoral or ionic mediators or of modulators such as angiotensin II could be reduced as a result of increases in compartment size.

Other Vasoactive Factors

It has recently been suggested that the baseline vascular tone, defined as the sum of the non-TGF vasomotor inputs, may determine the vascular responsiveness to the TGF signal (289). Tubuloglomerular feedback reactivity is often reduced when the renal vasculature is dilated. Vasodilators that have been shown to reduce responses include ANF (290,291), bradykinin (292), Ca channel blockers (293), dopamine (290,294), and the NO donor sodium nitroprusside (218,289). Furthermore, TGF reactivity is reduced by an acute reduction of arterial blood pressure (295), perhaps as a consequence of non–TGF-mediated autoregulatory vasodilation. The adjustment in TGF sensitivity produced by vasodilators would appear to be a nonspecific consequence of a change in vasomotor tone rather than an intrinsic change in JGA function. The change in response pattern may be a reflection of a dependency of vascular resistance changes on the initial wall thickness/radius ratio (296). Because the predominant effector of the TGF response is the afferent arteriole, this site is the likely candidate for modulation of TGF sensitivity.

Effect of Acute Changes in Arterial Pressure on the TGF System

Participation of TGF in Autoregulation

Acute changes in mean arterial pressure over a wide range are followed by adjustments in renal vascular resistance that effectively prevent sizable alterations of renal blood flow and GFR. It has been postulated that this adjustment in vascular tone is a TGF-mediated event (297,298). A change in arterial pressure is predicted to alter GFR initially and thereby alter the TGF signal. The resulting change of renal vascular resistance would then return GFR to its initial value. This proposal has been tested by comparing the change in SNGFR or P_{SF} when the TGF loop was interrupted with the changes when flow to the MD is intact. In several studies, interruption of the feedback loop has been observed to increase the pressure dependency of filtration rate and glomerular pressure (262,268,299–301), although contrary results have been reported (302,303).

Nonetheless, several lines of evidence suggest that the renal vasculature is capable of autoregulatory adjustments without participation of TGF. Glomerular arterioles in kidney tissue transplanted to the cheek pouch of the hamster showed autoregulatory adjustments despite the lack of a JGA (304), as do renal vessels in a hydronephrotic kidney model that lacks an operating TGF mechanism (305). Several different methods have been used to assess the relative contributions of TGF and other mechanisms to autoregulation. In the blood perfused JG preparation, in which the glomerular vasculature can be directly observed, blockade of TGF by furosemide or mechanical loop blockade only partially blocked autoregulatory resistance changes (306). Changes in arterial pressure had smaller effects on proximal SNGFR (TGF loop interrupted) than predicted from the passive pressure-SNGFR relationship (262,299,300). The passive slope was estimated from either model predictions (262) or by using the pressure dependency of SNGFR in the subautoregulatory range (299). The deviation from the expected slope indicated residual autoregulatory capacity in the absence of TGF, with a relative contribution of about half the autoregulatory changes (262,299).

Frequency domain analysis has also been applied to assess the contribution of TGF to autoregulation in a series of elegant studies combining experimental determinations of blood flow and pressure fluctuations with mathematical data evaluation (307–310). The approach uses Fourier or other signal processing methods to dissect the effect of amplitude fluctuations in arterial blood pressure on the fluctuations in renal blood flow. Mathematical modeling of the TGF mechanism has been used to predict the time delays of TGF-mediated responses of vascular resistance (310). With frequency domain analysis, a rapid response, too fast to be TGF-mediated and generally attributed to an intrinsic myogenic capacity (with a frequency response of ≈ 0.1 Hz), and a slower response with frequency response characteristics (frequency ≈ 0.01 Hz) consistent with TGF mediation, are observed. Interruption of the TGF mechanism by ureteral obstruction or infusion of captopril was observed to eliminate the slower category of vascular autoregulatory adjustments (308,309).

This new body of work has contributed to recognition of the redundancy of renal blood flow regulation. Although in several circumstances a clear and substantial component of autoregulatory resistance changes can be shown to be TGF-mediated, nonetheless other mechanisms can produce relative constancy of renal blood flow. The relative contributions of TGF-dependent and TGF-independent components of autoregulation depends on the time frame of observation, the experimental or physiological condition, and the blood pressure range.

TGF Mechanism in Experimental Hypertension

Spontaneously Hypertensive Rats

Marked abnormalities in glomerular hemodynamics and in the TGF circuit have been demonstrated in young spontaneously hypertensive rats (SHR) in the stage of developing hypertension. Spontaneously hypertensive rats at 6 weeks of age have a markedly reduced renal plasma flow and GFR even though arterial pressure was about 20 mm Hg higher than in age-matched Wistar-Kyoto control rats (311). Blocking the loop of Henle and thereby acutely eliminating the influence of TGF on vascular tone did not normalize the reduced SNGFR in SHRs. Loop perfusion studies in young SHRs showed a shift of the responsive range to lower flows and an increase in the maximum response of both SNGFR and P_{SF}, suggesting that the TGF-induced vasoconstriction might contribute to the reduced blood flow (311). Whether a change in loop transport or in the JGA transmission mechanism is causal in the resetting of TGF sensitivity in SHRs is not known. Furthermore, it is not clear why loop blockade has only modest effects on steady-state SNGFR. It is possible that single-nephron perturbations do not fully reflect the *in situ* situation in which alterations in MD composition affect all nephrons simultaneously. If, as seems likely, afferent arterioles originating from the same interlobular artery can be affected by alterations in MD NaCl concentration in the neighboring nephron (312), vascular tone may be increased through the TGF mechanism even though the loop of Henle is acutely blocked.

In contrast to young SHRs, at 12 weeks of age when hypertension is established, TGF characteristics returned to close to normal (313). Similarly, GFR and renal blood flow remained in the normal range. Thus, in the hypertensive SHR, the increased renal vascular tone appears to be unrelated to TGF activation. Chronic salt loading blunted TGF responses in SHRs to a similar extent as in control rats (314). However, this reduction in TGF sensitivity was not sufficient to prevent a salt-dependent exacerbation of hypertension. Under other experimental conditions, the TGF system of SHRs did not show the blunting of TGF activity seen in normal rats. For example, high-protein diet has no effect on the feedback function in SHRs in contrast to the right shift observed in control rats (1). Furthermore, lowering arterial pressure from hypertensive to normotensive values did not reduce response magnitude even though maximum responses in normal animals are highly pressure-dependent (313).

Recent studies of the dynamic behavior of the TGF system in SHRs have shown that hypertensive animals do not show the pattern of stable oscillations that can be found in normal rats. Rather, oscillations of tubular pressure in SHRs as well as in rats with renal hypertension (2K1C) display irregular fluctuations that can be characterized as deterministic chaos (230,315). The importance of this interesting finding for the development of hypertension is unknown, but it points to a fundamental and highly dramatic difference in the control of afferent arteriolar tone between hypertensive and normotensive animals.

Milan Hypertensive Rats

A different pattern of abnormalities is apparent in another animal model of genetic hypertension, the Milan hypertensive rat. In the prehypertensive phase, at 5 weeks of age, these rats have a higher GFR than age-matched controls and the responses of P_{SF} to changing loop flow rate are greatly diminished (255). During the development of hypertension, at 5 to 7 weeks, GFR did not differ significantly from that of hydropenic control rats, and TGF responses were similar in magnitude and sensitive flow range. However, in this phase, the response to volume expansion and acute unilateral ureteral occlusion differed markedly between normotensive and hypertensive strains (255). In the normotensive animals, volume expansion by administration of Ringer solution at 5 percent of body weight produced a reduction of TGF sensitivity and a 30 percent increase in GFR. In contrast, volume expansion and ureteral occlusion did not blunt TGF responses in the hypertensive rats and only slightly shifted the responsive range, a TGF pattern consistent with the absence of significant increments of GFR in the volume-expanded hypertensive rats. It is conceivable that this alteration in the response to volume expansion causes a delay in the excretion of excess salt and may therefore be a contributory factor to hypertension.

Goldblatt Hypertensive Rats

Clipped and nonclipped kidneys of rats with unilateral renal artery constriction have been found to show profound differences in regard to TGF characteristics. In the clipped kidney, an increased TGF response amplitude and an increase in maximum slope has been reported (157). It is interesting that steady-state GFR and glomerular capillary pressure do not deviate considerably from normal despite the sensitization of the TGF system. In most studies, TGF sensitivity in the nonclipped kidney was found to be reduced, as reflected in a decrease in the response amplitude and a right shift of $V_{1/2}$ (157,158, 268,316). Again, this change in TGF characteristics was not associated with the predicted decrease in vascular tone. Single-nephron GFR and GFR when corrected for body weight were not different from values seen in normotensive control rats, suggesting that the dilatory influence of the TGF system was ineffective in determining vascular resistance in these kidneys. Thus, baseline renal vascular tone in the chronic setting of Goldblatt hypertension does not appear to be determined to a major extent by the TGF system, an observation supporting the notion that TGF is not primarily designed to generate chronic alterations in vascular tone. It is to be predicted, however, that clipped and nonclipped kidneys will respond differently to acute perturbations of MD NaCl concentration. Tubuloglomerular feedback responses in one-clip one-kidney hypertensive rats were found to be comparable with those seen in uninephrectomized control rats (317) even though arterial pressure was increased. Again, renal vascular resistance in this model of hypertension is unlikely to be increased as a consequence of TGF activation.

REFERENCES

1. Schnermann J, Briggs JP. In: Seldin DW, Giebisch G, eds. *The kidney: physiology and pathophysiology.* 2nd ed. New York: Raven Press; 1992:1249–1289.
2. Hackenthal E, Paul M, Ganten D, Taugner R. *Physiol Rev* 1990;70:1067–1116.
3. Lorenz JN, Greenberg SG, Briggs JP. *Semin Nephrol* 1993;13: 531–542.
4. Taugner R, Hackenthal E. *The juxtaglomerular apparatus.* Berlin: Springer-Verlag; 1989.
5. Golgi C. *Atti della Reale Accademia dei Lincei* 1889;5:334–342.
6. Peter K. *Anat Anz* 1907;30:114–124.
7. Ruyter JC. *Z Zellforsch Mikrosk Anat* 1925;2:242–248.
8. Zimmermann KW. *Z Mikrosk Anat Forsch* 1933;32:176–278.
9. Goormaghtigh N. *C R Soc Biol (Paris)* 1937;124:293–296.
10. Tigerstedt R, Bergman PG. *Scand Arch Physiol* 1898;8:223–271.
11. Goormaghtigh N. *Bruxelles Med* 1937;124:293–296.
12. Harsing L, Fonyodi S, Kabat M, Koever G. *Acta Physiol Acad Sci Hung* 1957;12:363–371.
13. Guyton AC. *Physiologist* 1963;6:194.
14. Thurau K. *Proc Int Congress Nephrol* 1963;2:51–61.
15. Thurau L, Schnermann J. *Klin Wochenschr* 1965;43:410–413.
16. Gottschalk CW, Leyssac PP. *Acta Physiol Scand* 1968;74:453–464.
17. Vander AJ. *Physiol Rev* 1967;47:359–382.
18. Vander AJ. *Proc Soc Exp Biol Med* 1968;128:518–520.
19. Vander AJ, Miller R. *Am J Physiol* 1964;207:537–546.
20. Gillies A, Morgan T. *Pflügers Arch* 1978;375:105–110.
21. Thurau K, Gruener A, Mason J, Dahlheim H. *Kidney Int* 1982;22(Suppl 12):S55–S62.
22. Laragh JH, Sealey JE. In: Orloff J, Berliner RW, eds. *Handbook of physiology-renal physiology.* Bethesda, Maryland: American Physiological Society; 1973:831–908.
23. Skøtt O, Briggs JP. *Science* 1987;237:1618–1620.
24. Lorenz JN, Weihprecht H, Schnermann J, Skøtt O, Briggs JP. *Am J Physiol* 1990;259:F186–F193.
25. Lorenz JN, Weihprecht H, Schnermann J, Skøtt O, Briggs JP. *Am J Physiol* 1991;F486–F493.
26. Bucher O, Reale E. *Z Zellforsch* 1961;54:167–181.
27. Kaissling B, Kriz W. *Adv Anat Embryol Cell Biol* 1979;56:1–123.
28. Kaissling B, Peter S, Kriz W. *Cell Tissue Res* 1977;182:111–118.
29. Barajas L. *J Ultrastruct Res* 1970;15:116–147.
30. Barajas L, Latta H. *Lab Invest* 1963;12:257–269.
31. Christensen JA, Meyer DS, Bohle A. *Virchows Arch* 1975;367: 83–92.
32. Christensen JA, Bohle A. *Virchows Arch* 1978;379:143–150.
33. Faarup P. *Acta Anat (Basel)* 1965;60:20–38.
34. Faraj AH, Lindop GBM, Morley AR, Coleman S. *APMIS* 1992;100:29–38.
35. Persson BE, Persson AEG. *Pflügers Arch* 1981;391:129–134.
36. Persson BE, Marsh DJ. *Am J Physiol* 1987;253:F263–F268.
37. Morsing P, Velazquez H, Ellison D, Wright FS. *Acta Physiol Scand* 1993;148:63–68.
38. Ito S, Carretero OA. *Kidney Int* 1990;38:1206–1210.
39. Ito S, Carretero OA. *Kidney Int* 1991;532:583–585.
40. Bonsib SM. *J Ultrastruct Mol Struct Res* 1986;97:103–108.
41. Kaissling B, Kriz W. *Kidney Int* 1982;22(Suppl 12):S9–S17.
42. Mundel P, Bachmann S, Bader M, et al. *Kidney Int* 1992;42: 1017–1019.
43. Wilcox CS, Welch WJ, Murad F, et al. *Proc Natl Acad Sci* 1992;89:11993–11997.
44. Bredt DS, Hwang PM, Glat CE, Lowenstein C, Reed RR, Snyder SH. *Nature* 351:714–718.
45. Moncada S, Palmer RMJ, Higgs EA. *Pharmacol Rev* 1991;43(2): 109–142.
46. Forstermann U, Pollock JS, Schmidt HHW, Heller M, Murad F. *Proc Natl Acad Sci* 1991;88:1788–1792.
47. Wachstein M, Meisel E. *Am J Pathol* 1959;35:1189–1205.
48. Brown JJ, Davies DL, Lever AF, Parker RA, Robertson JIS. *Clin Sci* 1966;30:223–235.
49. Hess R, Gross F. *Am J Physiol* 1959;197:869–872.
50. Norgaard T. *Histochemistry* 1979;63:103–113.
51. Norgaard T. *Histochemistry* 1980;69:49–59.
52. Rostand SG, Work J, Luke RG. *Am J Physiol* 1985;249:F213–F219.
53. Marletta M. *J Biol Chem* 1993;268:12231–12234.
54. Vandewalle A, Cluzeaud F, Chavance M, Bonvalet JP. *Am J Physiol* 1985;248:F552–F564.
55. Bachmann S, Koeppen-Hagemann I, Kriz W. *Histochemistry* 1985;83:531–538.
56. Hoyer JR, Sisson SP, Vernier RL. *Lab Invest* 1979;41:168–172.
57. Sikri KL, Foster CL, MacHugh N, Marshall RD. *J Anat* 1980;132:597–605.
58. Le Hir M, Dubach UC. *Histochemistry* 1982;74:521–530.
59. Beaumont H, Healy DP, Fanestil DD. *Am J Physiol* 1984;247: F718–F724.
60. Stowe NT, Schnermann J, Hermle M. *Kidney Int* 1979;15:473–486.
61. Dobyan D, Magill L, Friedman P, Hebert S, Bulger R. *Anat Rec* 1982;204:185–197.
62. Loennerholm G, Wistrand PJ. *Kidney Int* 1984;25:886–898.
63. Atkin BM, Franklin WA, Bell GI, Toback FG. *Nephron* 1990;54: 313–317.
64. Salido EC, Yen PH, Shapiro LJ, Fisher DA, Barajas L. *Am J Physiol* 1989;256:F632–F638.
65. Breuss JM, Gillett L, Lu L, Sheppard D, Pytela R. *J Histochem Cytochem* 1993;41:1521–1527.
66. Albelda SM, Buck CA. *FASEB J* 1990;4:2868–2880.
67. Blanc-Brunat N, Mutin M, Peyrol S. *Cell Mol Biol* 1989;35:469–484.
68. Kirk KL, Bell PD, Barfuss D, Ribadeneira M. *Am J Physiol* 1985;248:F890–F894.
69. Bell PD, LaPointe JY, Cardinal J, Chang YS. *Kidney Int* 1991;32: S59–S64.
70. Schlatter E, Salomonsson M, Persson AEG, Greger R. *Pflügers Arch* 1989;414:286–290.
71. Schlatter E. *Pflügers Arch* 1993;423:74–77.
72. Salamonsson M, Gonzalez E, Westerlung P, Perrson HEG. *Kidney Int* 1991;39:551–554.
73. Gonzales E, Salomonsson M, Muller-Suur R, Persson AEG. *Acta Physiol Scand* 1988;133:149–157.
74. Gonzales E, Salomonsson M, Muller-Suur R, Persson AEG. *Acta Physiol Scand* 1988;133:159–166.
75. Lapointe JY, Bell PD, Cardinal J. *Am J Physiol* 1990;258:F1466–F1469.
76. Lapointe JY, Bell PD, Hurst AM, Cardinal J. *Am J Physiol* 1991;260:F856–F860.
77. Beeuwkes R III, Rosen S. In: Boulpaep EL, ed. *Current topics in membranes and transport, Vol. 13: Cellular mechanisms of renal tubular ion transport.* New York: Academic Press; 1980:343–345.
78. Schnermann J, Marver D. *Pflügers Arch* 1977;369:39–48.
79. Garg L, Knepper M, Burg M. *Am J Physiol* 1981;240:F536–F544.
80. Kashgarian M, Biemesderfer D, Caplan M, Forbush B. *Kidney Int* 1985;28:899–913.
81. Krompecher-Kiss E, Bucher O. *Histochemistry* 1977;53:265–269.
82. Strange K, Spring KR. *J Memb Biol* 1987;96:27–43.
83. Morel F, Chaardes D, Imbert M. *Kidney Int* 1976;9:264–277.
84. Woodhall PB, Tisher C. *J Clin Invest* 1973;52:3095–3108.
85. Nielsen S, Muller J, Knepper MA. *Am J Physiol* 1993;265:F225–F238.
86. Agre P, Preston GM, Smith BL, et al. *Am J Physiol* 1993;265: F463–F476.
87. Schnermann J, Briggs JP. *Kidney Int* 1982; (Suppl 12):S82–S89.
88. Persson BE, Sakai T, Ekblom M, Marsh DJ. *Am J Physiol* 1988;254:F445–F449.

89. Bell PD, France-Guevara M, Abrahamson DR, Lapointe JY, Cardinal J. In: Persson AEG, Boberg U, eds. *The juxtaglomerular apparatus*. Amsterdam: Elsevier Science Publishers; 1988:63–77.
90. Salomonsson ME, Gonzalez P, Westerlund P, Persson AEG. *Acta Physiol Scand* 1991;142:283–290.
91. Gonzalez D, Salomonsson ME, Westerlund P, Persson AEG. *Kidney Int* 1990;39:555–557.
92. Spanidis A, Wunsch H, Kaissling B, Kriz W. *Anat Embryol* 1982;165:239–252.
93. Taugner R, Schiller A, Kaissling B, Kriz W. *Cell Tissue Res* 1978;186:279–285.
94. Pricam C, Humbert F, Perrelet A, Orci L. *J Cell Biol* 1974;63: F627–F635.
95. Boll HU, Forssman WG, Taugner R. *Cell Tissue Res* 1975;161: 459–469.
96. Forssmann WG, Taugner R. *Cell Tissue Res* 1977;177:291–305.
97. Biava CG, West M. *Am J Physiol* 1966;49:679–708.
98. Latta H, Maunsbach A. *J Ultrastruct Res* 1962;6:547–561.
99. Kriz W, Sakai T. *Anat Embryol* 1987;176:373–386.
100. Schnabel E, Kriz W. *Anat Embryol* 1984;170:217–222.
101. Osborne MJ, Droz B, Meyer P, Morel F. *Kidney Int* 1975;8:245–254.
102. Bacay AC, Mantyh CR, Cohen AH, Mantyh PW, Fine LG. *Am J Kidney Dis* 1989;14(5):386–395.
103. Kakinuma Y, Fogo A, Inagami T, Ichikawa I. *Kidney Int* 1993;43:1229–1235.
104. Mendrick DL, Rennke HG. *J Immunol* 1986;137(5):1517–1526.
105. Paul LC, Rennke HG, Milford EL, Carpenter CB. *Kidney Int* 1984;25(5):771–777.
106. Cosio FG, Sedmar DD, Mahan JD, Nahman NS. *Kidney Int* 1989;36:100–107.
107. Mené P, Simonson MS, Dunn MJ. *Physiol Rev* 1989;69:1347–1424.
108. Kasgarian M, Sterzel RB. The pathobiology of the mesangium. *Kidney Int* 1992;41:524–529.
109. Iijima K, Moore LC, Goligorsky MS. *Am J Physiol* 1991;260: F848–F855.
110. Kurokawa K. *Renal Physiol Biochem* 1993;16:15–20.
111. Okuda T, Yamashita N, Kurokawa K. *J Clin Invest* 1986;78: 1443–1448.
112. Kremer S, Breuer W, Skoreki K. *Kidney Int* 1988;33:162.
113. Okuda K, Kojima I, Ogata E, et al. *J Clin Invest* 1989;84:1866–1872.
114. Barajas L. *J Ultrastruct Res* 1966;15:400–413.
115. Taugner R, Rosivall L, Buhrle CP, Groeschel-Stewart U. *Cell Tissue Res* 1987;248:579–588.
116. Casellas D, Dupont M, Kaskel FJ, Inagami T, Moore LC. *Am J Physiol* 1993;265:F151–F156.
117. Gomez RA, Chevalier RL, Everett AD, et al. *Am J Physiol* 1990;259:F660–F665.
118. Skøtt O. *Pflügers Arch* 1986;407:41–45.
119. Bruna RD, Pinet F, Covol P, Kurtz A. *Am J Physiol* (Renal Fluid Electrolyte Physiol) 1992;31:F397–F402.
120. Kurtz A, Muff R, Born W, et al. *J Clin Invest* 1988;82:538–543.
121. Kurtz A, Pfeilschifter J, Hutter A, et al. *Am J Physiol* 250 (Cell Physiol 19) 1986;C563–C571.
122. Chen M, Schnermann J, Smart A, Brosius F, Killen P, Briggs JP. *J Biol Chem* 1993;268(32):24138–24144.
123. Kurtz A. *Klin Wochenschr* 1986;64:838–846.
124. Kurtz A. *Rev Physiol Biochem Pharmacol* 1989;113:2–40.
125. Kurtz A, Penner R. *Proc Natl Acad Sci* 1989;86:3423–3427.
126. Carmines PK, Navar LG. *Am J Physiol* 1989;256:F1015–F1020.
127. Hess R, Gross F. *Am J Physiol* 1959;197:869–872.
128. Greenberg SG, Yule DI, He X-R, Briggs JP, Schnermann J. *Nieren-und Hochdruckkrankheit* 1993;22:486.
129. Cortney MA, Nagel W, Thurau K. *Pflügers Arch* 1966;287:286–295.
130. Gutsche H-U, Mueller-Suur R, Hegel U, Hierholzer K. *Pflügers Arch* 1980;383:113–122.
131. Baines AD, Basmadjian D, Wang BC. *Biophys J* 1979;27:21–38.
132. Landwehr DM, Schnermann J, Klose RM, Giebisch G. *Am J Physiol* 1968;215:687–695.
133. Wright FS, Schnermann J. *J Clin Invest* 1974;53:1695–1708.
134. Schnermann J, Schubert G, Briggs JP. *Am J Physiol* 1982;243: F160–F166.
135. Schnermann J, Ploth DW, Hermle M. *Pflügers Arch* 1976;362: 229–240.
136. Moore LC. *Fed Proc* 1982;41:A5763.
137. Mueller-Suur R, Ulfendahl HR, Persson AEG. *Am J Physiol* 1983;244:F425–F431.
138. Bell PD, Thomas C, Williams RH, Navar LG. *Am J Physiol* 1978;234:F154–F165.
139. Burke TJ, Navar LG, Clapp JR, Robinson RR. *Kidney Int* 1974;6:230–240.
140. Schnermann J, Stowe NT, Yarimizu S, Magnusson M. *Pflügers Arch* 1977;368(Suppl):R14.
141. Briggs JP, Schubert G, Schnermann J. *Am J Physiol* 1984;247: F808–F815.
142. Moore LC, Mason J. *Am J Physiol* 1983;245:F554–F563.
143. Holstein-Rathlou NH, Marsh DJ. *Am J Physiol* 256 (Renal Fluid Electrolyte Physiol 25):F1007–F1014.
144. Thomson SC, Blantz RC. *Am J Physiol* 264 (Renal Fluid Electrolyte Physiol 33):F930–F936.
145. Briggs JP, Schnermann J, Wright FS. *Am J Physiol* 1980;239: F427–F432.
146. Bell PD, McLean C, Navar LG. *Am J Physiol* 1981;240:F111–F119.
147. Schnermann J, Persson AEG, Agerup B. *J Clin Invest* 1973;52: 862–869.
148. Gertz KH, Mangos JA, Braun G, Pagel HD. *Pflügers Arch* 1966;288:369–374.
149. Bell PD, Navar LG, Ploth DW, McLean CB. *Kidney Int* 1980;18: 460–471.
150. Ploth DW, Rudulph J, Lagrange R, Navar LG. *J Clin Invest* 1979;64:1325–1335.
151. Wunderlich P, Brunner FP, Davis JM, Haeberle D, Thoelen H, Thiel G. *Kidney Int* 1980;17:497–506.
152. Galla JH, Bonduris DN, Sanders PW, Luke RG. *J Clin Invest* 1984;74:2002–2008.
153. Ploth DW, Rudulph J, Thomas C, Navar LG. *Am J Physiol* 1978;235:F156–F162.
154. Bell PD, McLean C, Navar LG. *Am J Physiol* 1981;240:F111–F119.
155. Mueller-Suur R, Gutsche H-U. *Acta Physiol Scand* 1978;103: 353–362.
156. Osswald H, Hermes H. *Kidney Int* 1981;19:251.
157. Mueller-Suur R, Gutsche H-U, Samwer KF, Oelkers W, Hierholzer K. *Pflügers Arch* 1975;359:33–56.
158. Mason J, Kain H, Shiigai T, Welsh J. *Pflügers Arch* 1979;380: 233–243.
159. Arendshorst WJ, Gottschalk CW. *Am J Physiol* 1985;248:F163–F174.
160. Ichikawa I. *Am J Physiol* 1982;243:F447–F455.
161. Briggs JP. *Kidney Int* 1982;22(Suppl 12):S143–S150.
162. Persson AEG, Gushwa LG, Blantz RC. *Am J Physiol* 1984;247: F925–F931.
163. Briggs JP, Wright FS. *Am J Physiol* 1979;236:F40–F47.
164. Persson B-E, Sakai T, Ekblom M, Marsh DJ. *Acta Physiol Scand* 1989;137:93–99.
165. Schnermann J, Briggs JP, Kriz W, Moore L, Wright FS. In: Leaf A, Giebisch G, Bolis L, Gorini S, eds. *Renal pathophysiology*. New York: Raven Press, 1980:165–182.
166. Casellas D, Moore LC. *Am J Physiol* 1990;258:F660–F669.
167. Casellas D, Moore LC. *Am J Physiol* 1993;264:F315–F321.
168. Boknam L, Ericson EC, Aberg B, Ulfendahl HR. *Acta Physiol Scand* 1981;111:159–164.
169. Heyeraas Tonder KJ, Aukland K. *Renal Physiol* 1979/80;2:214–221.
170. Weihprecht H, Lorenz JN, Briggs JP, Schnermann J. *Am J Physiol* 1992;263:F1026–F1033.
171. Steinhausen M, Blum M, Fleming JT, Holz FG, Parekh N, Weigman DL. *Kidney Int* 1989;35:1151–1160.
172. Moore LC, Rich A. *Kidney Int* 1988;33:412.
173. Schnermann J, Briggs JP. *Miner Electrolyte Metab* 1989;15:103–107.
174. Shade RE, Davis JO, Johnson JA, et al. *Circ Res* 1972;31:719–727.

175. DiBona GF. *Am J Physiol* 1971;221:511–514.
176. Churchill PC, Churchill MC, McDonald FD. *Circ Res* 1979;45:786–792.
177. Vander AJ, Carlson J. *Circ Res* 1969;25:145–151.
178. Kotchen TA, Galla JH, Luke RG. *Am J Physiol* 1976;231:1050–1056.
179. Kirchner KA, Kotchen TA, Galla JH, et al. *Am J Physiol* 1978;235:F444–F450.
180. Lorenz JA, Kotchen TA, Ott CE. *Am J Physiol* 1990;258:F1328–F1335.
181. Hackenthal E. *Ann Endocrinol* 1986;47:145–155.
182. Wright FS, Schnermann J. *J Clin Invest* 1974;53:1695–1708.
183. Leyssac PP, Holstein-Rathlou N-H. *Pflügers Arch* 1986;407:285–291.
184. Brunkhorst R, Mueller-Ott KL, Gutsche H-U, Niedermeyer W. *Proc Eur Dial Transplant Assoc* 1978;15:613–616.
185. Odlind B, Beermann B, Selen G, Persson AEG. *J Pharmacol Exp Ther* 1983;225:742–746.
186. Osswald H, Hermes H. *Kidney Int* 1981;19:251.
187. Johnston Pa, Kau ST. *Methods Find Exp Clin Pharmacol* 1992;14:523–529.
188. Briggs JP, Schnermann J. *Pflügers Arch* 1981;389(Suppl):R40.
189. Bell PD, Navar LG, Ploth DW, McLean CB. *Kidney Int* 1980;18:460–471.
190. Kinne R, Kinne-Saffran E, Schutz H, Scholermann B. *J Membr Biol* 1986;94:279–284.
191. Greger R. *Physiol Rev* 1985;65:760–797.
192. Bell PD, Navar LG. *Kidney Int* 1982;22:234–239.
193. Tagawa H, Vander AJ. *Circ Res* 1970;26:327–338.
194. Osswald H, Nabakowski G, Hermle H. *Int J Biochem* 1980;12:263–267.
195. Spielman WS, Thompson CI. *Am J Physiol* 1982;242:F423–F435.
196. Schnermann J, Briggs JP. *Semin Nephrol* 1993;13:236–245.
197. Weihprecht H, Lorenz JN, Briggs JP, Schnermann J. *Am J Physiol* 1991;261:F273–F282.
198. Osswald H, Hermes H, Nabakowski G. *Kidney Int* 1982;22 (Suppl 12):S136–S142.
199. Schnermann J, Osswald H, Hermle M. *Pflügers Arch* 1977;369:39–48.
200. Schnermann J. *Am J Physiol* 1988;255:F33–F42.
201. Bell PD, Navar LG. *Kidney Int* 1985;28:728–732.
202. Franco M, Bell PD, Navar LG. *Am J Physiol* 1990;257:F231–F236.
203. Schnermann J, Weihprecht H, Briggs J. *Am J Physiol* 1989;258:F553–F561.
204. Weihprecht H, Lorenz JN, Schnermann J, Skøtt O, Briggs J. *Am J Physiol* 1990;259:F186–F193.
205. Lorenz JN, Weihprecht H, He XR, Skøtt O, Briggs JP, Schnermann J. *Am J Physiol* 1993;265:F187–F194.
206. Skøtt O. *Am J Physiol* 1988;255:F1–F10.
207. Lorenz JN, Greenberg SG, Briggs JP. *Semin Nephrol* 1993;13:531–542.
208. Greenberg SG, Lorenz JN, He XR, Schnermann J, Briggs JP. *Am J Physiol* 1993;265:F578–F583.
209. Smith WL, Bell TG. *Am J Physiol* 1978;235:F451–F457.
210. Welch WJ, Wilcox CS, Dunbar KR. *Am J Physiol* 1989;257:F554–F560.
211. Antonipillai I. *Proc Soc Exper Biol Med* 1990;194:224–230.
212. Henrich WL, Falck JR, Campbell WB. *Am J Physiol* 1990;258:E269–E274.
213. Sellmayer A, Uedelhoven WM, Weber PC, et al. *J Biol Chem* 1991;266(6):3800–3807.
214. Schnermann J, Schubert G, Hermle M, et al. *Pflügers Arch* 1979;379:269–286.
215. Franco M, Bell PD, Navar LG. *Am J Physiol* 1988;254:F642–F649.
216. Welch WJ, Wilcox CS. *J Clin Invest* 1988;81:1843–1849.
217. Morsing P, Stenberg A, Persson AE. *Kidney Int* 1989;36:447–452.
218. Thorup C, Sundler F, Ekblad E, Persson AE. *Acta Physiol Scand* 1993;148(3):359–360.
219. Ito S, Ren Y. *J Clin Invest* 1993;92:1093–1098.
220. Beierwaltes WH, Carretero OA. *Hypertension* 1992;19(Suppl 11):S68–S73.
221. Sigmon DH, Carretero OA, Beierwaltes WH. *Am J Physiol* 1992;263:F256–F261.
222. Gardes J, Poux JM, Gonzales MF, Alhenc-Gelas F, Menard J. *Life Sci* 1992;50:987–993.
223. Schricker K, Kurtz A. *Am J Physiol* 1993;265:F180–F186.
224. Greenberg SG, He X-R, Briggs JP, Schnermann J. *J Am Soc Nephrol* 1992;3:544.
225. He X-R, Greenberg SG, Schnermann JB, Briggs JP. *FASEB J* 1993;7:A221.
226. Marsden PA, Ballermann BJ. *J Exp Med* 1990;172:1843–1852.
227. Chevalier RL, Fern RJ, Garmey M, El-Dahr SS, Gomez RA, De Vente J. *Am J Physiol* 1992;262:F417–F424.
228. Marsh DJ, Osborne JL, Cowley AW. *Am J Physiol* 1990;258:F1394–1400.
229. Schnermann J, Davis JM, Wunderlich P, Levine DZ, Horster M. *Pflügers Arch* 1971;329:307–320.
230. Holstein-Rathlou NH, Leyssac PP. *Acta Physiol Scand* 1986;126:333–339.
231. Leyssac PP, Baumbach L. *Acta Physiol Scand* 1983;117:415–419.
232. Leyssac PP, Holstein-Rathlou N-H. *Pflügers Arch* 1986;407:285–291.
233. Holstein-Rathlou N-H, Marsh DJ. *Am J Physiol* 1989;256:F1007–F1014.
234. Holstein-Rathlou N-H, Leyssac PP. *Am J Physiol* 1987;252:F560–F572.
235. Holstein-Rathlou N-H, Marsh DJ. *Am J Physiol* 1990;258:F1488–F1459.
236. Pitman EB, Layton HE. *Commun Pure Appl Math* 1989;42:759–787.
237. Yip KP, Holstein-Rathlou N-H, Marsh DJ. *Am J Physiol* 1991;261:F400–F408.
238. Schnermann J, Briggs JP, Wright FS. *Kidney Int* 1981;20:462–468.
239. Wilcox CS. *Clin Invest* 1983;71:726–735.
240. Dev B, Drescher C, Schnermann J. *Pflügers Arch* 1974;346:262–277.
241. Schnermann J, Hermle M, Schmidmeier F, Dahlheim H. *Pflügers Arch* 1975;358:325–338.
242. Gerber JG, Branch RA, Nies AS, Hollifield JW, Gerkens JF. *Am J Physiol* 1979;237:F441–F446.
243. Gerkens JF, Heidemann HT, Jackson EK, Branch RA. *J Pharmacol Exp Ther* 1983;225:611–615.
244. Woods LL, De Young DR, Smith BE. *Am J Physiol* 1991;261:F815–F823.
245. Woods LL. *Am J Physiol* 1993;264:R601–R609.
246. Seney FD, Wright FS. *J Clin Invest* 1985;75:558–568.
247. Schnermann J, Briggs JP. *Renal Physiol* 1984;7:258–259.
248. Seney FD, Persson AEG, Wright FS. *Am J Physiol* 1987;252:F83–F90.
249. Bouby N, Trinh-Trang-Tan M-M, Kriz W, Bankit L. *Kidney Int* 1987;32(Suppl):S57–S61.
250. Persson AEG, Wright FS. *Acta Physiol Scand* 1982;114:1–7.
251. Tucker BJ, Steiner RW, Gushwa LC, Blantz RC. *J Clin Invest* 1978;62:993–1004.
252. Leyssac PP, Karlsen FM, Skøtt O. *Am J Physiol* 1991;261:F169–F178.
253. Yeyati NL, Altenberg GA, Androgue HJ. *Renal Physiol Biochem* 1992;15:105.
254. Boberg U, Persson AEG. *Am J Physiol* 1985;249:F524–F531.
255. Boberg U, Persson AEG. *Am J Physiol* 1986;250:F967–F974.
256. Persson AEG, Schnermann J, Wright FS. *Pflügers Arch* 1979;381:99–106.
257. Persson AEG, Mueller-Suur R, Selen G. *Am J Physiol* 1979;236:F97–F102.
258. Persson AEG, Bianchi G, Boberg U. *Acta Physiol Scand* 1985;123:139–146.
259. Mueller-Suur R, Persson AEG. *Acta Physiol Scand* 1986;126:139–146.
260. Davis JM, Takabatake T, Kawata T, Haeberle DA. *Pflügers Arch* 1988;411:322–327.

261. Davis JM, Haeberle DA, Kawata T, Schmitt E, Takabatake T, Wohlfeil S. *J Physiol* 1988;395:553–576.
262. Moore LC, Schnermann J, Yarimizu S. *Am J Physiol* 1979;237:F63–F74.
263. Moore LC, Yarimizu S, Schubert G, Weber PC, Schnermann J. *Pflügers Arch* 1980;387:39–45.
264. Moore LC, Mason J. *Am J Physiol* 1986;250:F1024–F1032.
265. Kaufman JS, Hamburger RJ, Flamenbaum W. *Renal Physiol* 1982;5:173–181.
266. Selen G, Mueller-Suur R, Persson AEG. *Acta Physiol Scand* 1983;117:83–89.
267. Tucker BJ, Blantz RC. *Kidney Int* 1984;26:112–121.
268. Ploth DW, Schnermann J, Dahlheim H, Hermle M, Schmid-meier F. *Kidney Int.* 1977;12:253–267.
269. Ploth DW, Rudulph J, Lagrange R, Navar LG. *J Clin Invest* 1979;64:1325–1335.
270. Schnermann J, Briggs JP, Schubert G, Marin-Grez M. *Am J Physiol* 1984;247:F912–F918.
271. Stowe NT, Schnermann J, Hermle M. *Kidney Int* 1979;15:473–486.
272. Huang WC, Bell PD, Harvey D, Mitchell KD, Navar LG. *Kidney Int* 1988;34:631–637.
273. Ploth DW, Roy RN. *Kidney Int* 1982;22:S114–S121.
274. Mitchell KD, Navar LG. *Am J Physiol* 1988;258:F537–F544.
275. Schnermann J, Briggs JP. *Kidney Int* 1990;38(Suppl 30):S77–S80.
276. Schnermann J, Briggs JP. *Am J Physiol* 1990;259:F565–F572.
277. Weihprecht H, Lorenz JN, Briggs JP, Schnermann J. *Am J Physiol* 1994;266:F227–F239.
278. Selen G, Persson AEG. *Am J Physiol* 1983;244:F342–F348.
279. Holm L, Morsing P, Casellas D, Persson AEG. *Acta Physiol Scand* 1990;138:395–401.
280. Persson AEG, Muller-Suur R, Selen G. *Am J Physiol* 1979;236:F97–F102.
281. Persson AEG, Bianchi G, Boberg U. *Acta Physiol Scand* 1985;123:139–146.
282. Persson AEG, Hahne B, Selen G. *Can J Physiol Pharmacol* 1982;61:1317–1323.
283. Wahlberg J, Stenberg A, Wilson D, Persson AEG. *Kidney Int* 1984;26:294–302.
284. Mueller-Suur R, Norlen BJ, Persson AEG. *Kidney Int* 1980;18:48–57.
285. Hahne B, Persson AEG. *Kidney Int* 1984;25:42–46.
286. Selen G, Persson AEG. *Acta Physiol Scand* 1983;117:75–81.
287. Persson AEG, Wahlberg J, Safirstein R, Wright FS. *Acta Physiol Scand* 1984;122:35–43.
288. Schnabel E, Kriz W. *Anat Embryol* 1984;170:217–222.
289. Schnermann J. In: Persson AEG, Boberg U, eds. *The juxtaglomerular apparatus.* Amsterdam: Elsevier; 1988:167–176.
290. Huang CL, Cogan MG. *Am J Physiol* 1982;243:F447–F455.
291. Briggs JP, Steipe B, Schubert G, Schnermann J. *Pflügers Arch* 1982;395:271–276.
292. Morsing P, Persson AEG. *Am J Physiol* 1991;260:F868–F873.
293. Mitchell KD, Navar LG. *Am J Physiol* 1990;258:F537–F544.
294. Schnermann J, Todd KM, Briggs JP. *Am J Physiol* 1990;258:F790–F798.
295. Schnermann J, Briggs JP. *Am J Physiol* 1989;256:F421–F429.
296. Folkow B. *Physiol Rev* 1982;62:347–504.
297. Guyton AC, Langston JB, Navar LG. *Circ Res* 1964;14/15(SI):187–196.
298. Thurau K. *Am J Med* 1964;36:698–714.
299. Schnermann J, Briggs JP, Weber PC. *Kidney Int* 1984;25:53–64.
300. Moore LC. *Am J Physiol* 1984;287:F267–F276.
301. Navar LG, Chomdej B, Bell PD. *Am J Physiol* 1975;2229:1596–1603.
302. Knox FG, Ott C, Cuche JL, Gasser J, Haas J. *Circ Res* 1974;34:836–842.
303. Maddox DA, Troy JL, Brenner BM. *Am J Physiol* 1974;227:123–231.
304. Gilmore JP, Cornish KG, Rogers SD, Joyner WL. *Circ Res* 1980;47:226–230.
305. Steinhausen M, Blum M, Fleming JT, Holz FG, Parekh N, Wiegman DL. *Kidney Int* 1989;35:1151–1160.
306. Moore LC, Casellas D. *Kidney Int* 1990;37:1402–1408.
307. Sakai T, Hallman E, Marsh DJ. *Am J Physiol* 1986;250:F364–F373.
308. Daniels FH, Arendshorst WJ, Roberds RG. *Am J Physiol* 1990;258:F1479–F1489.
309. He J, Marsh DJ. *Am J Physiol* 1993;264:F37–F44.
310. Young DK, Marsh DJ. *Am J Physiol* 1981;240:F446–F458.
311. Dilley JR, Stier CT, Arendshorst WJ. *Am J Physiol* 1984;246:F12–F20.
312. Holstein-Rathlou NH. *Pflügers Arch* 1987;408:438–443.
313. Dilley JR, Arendshorst WJ. *Am J Physiol* 1984;247:F672–F679.
314. Ushiogi Y, Takabatake T, Haeberle DA. *Kidney Int* 1991;39:1184–1192.
315. Yip K-P, Holstein-Rathlou N-H, Marsh DJ. *Am J Physiol* 1991;261:F400–F408.
316. Schnermann J, Gokel M, Weber PC, Schubert G, Briggs JP. *Kidney Int* 1986;29:520–529.
317. Ploth DW, McKenzie HS. *Kidney Int* 1991;32:S115–S118.

Hypertension: Pathophysiology, Diagnosis,
and Management, Second Edition,
edited by J.H. Laragh and B.M. Brenner,
Raven Press, Ltd., New York © 1995.

CHAPTER 83

Role of Nitric Oxide on the Intrarenal Regulation of Nephron Function and Its Relevance to Hypertension

Juan Carlos Romero, Vicente Lahera, and Luis Ruilope

In 1980, Furchgott and Zawadzki (1) reported that the vasodilator effects of acetylcholine were mediated by the release of a smooth muscle-relaxing factor from the endothelial cells, which was called endothelium-derived relaxing factor (EDRF). In the years that followed this discovery, significant advances were made on the chemical characterization of EDRF, which was identified as nitric oxide (NO) (2–4), its synthesis precursors (2,4), the pharmacologic and physiological alterations that stimulate the release of NO (2,5), and the mechanism of NO vasodilation (3,5). Furthermore, attempts have also been

made to characterize the pathophysiological consequences derived from a deficient production of NO in endothelial cells. Such a condition, which has been experimentally achieved by the systemic administration of potent inhibitors of NO synthesis, has invariably resulted in a significant increase in mean arterial pressure (6). This NO-dependent hypertension resembles most of the characteristics seen during the development of essential hypertension in humans in the sense that it starts with an increase in intrarenal vascular resistance and a displacement to a lower sensitivity range of pressure-induced natriuresis, which leads to sodium retention (7–9). All these changes are followed by increments in mean arterial pressure, which brings sodium excretion back to normal. In this sequence, the most important event appears to be the resetting of pressure natriuresis, which is a consequence of NO synthesis inhibition.

In this chapter, we examine the importance of NO and prostaglandins (PG) in coupling the intrarenal hemody-

J. C. Romero: Department of Physiology and Biophysics, Mayo Clinic and Mayo School of Medicine, Rochester, Minnesota 55905.
V. Lahera: Department of Physiology, Universidad Complutense, Madrid, Spain.
L. Ruilope: Division of Hypertension, Hospital de Octubre, Universidad Complutense, Madrid, Spain.

namic changes to changes in sodium excretion and the manner in which a deficient synthesis of these two substances could lead to a specific form of sodium retention that has an effect on the maintenance of blood pressure.

GENERAL PRINCIPLES OF THE SYNTHESIS OF NO

Endothelium-derived relaxing factor appears to be mainly represented by NO (Fig. 1), which is synthesized in endothelial cells from a nitrogen atom contained in the guanidino group of the amino acid L-arginine (2,4). Such a reaction does not appear to consist of a simple process of deamination with the formation of NH_3 because exogenous NH_3 cannot be used as a precursor of NO in macrophages (10). The most plausible pathway, as indicated by Marletta (11), involves first a monooxygenase type of hydroxylation-generating N^G-hydroxy-L-arginine, which is subsequently converted to N^G-oxo-L-arginine by the oxidation of the hydroxylamine group. The amino acid radical generated in this last step is so unstable that it fragments to yield NO and a stable compound, N-[(2-amino)-valeryl]-carbodi-imide (11). This amino acid will react with H_2O, yielding citrulline. In support of this pathway of NO formation are the findings that N^G-hydroxy-L-arginine serves as a precursor for NO_2 and NO_3 (12) and that endothelial cells convert L-arginine to citrulline in a reduced nicotinamide adenine dinucleotide (NADH)-dependent fashion (13). Endothelial cells can also metabolize citrulline to L-arginine (13). These findings have raised the notion of the so-called L-arginine salvage pathway, by which citrulline can be recycled to generate L-arginine (14).

Two distinctive NO monooxygenases (NO synthetases), a constitutive form (15) and an inducible form (10,16), have been isolated. The constitutive form is activated by the increase in Ca^{2+} in the cytosol and the resultant binding of this cation to calmodulin. The reaction is NADPH-dependent (13,17–20). The constitutive form of the enzyme is found mostly in endothelial cells (1,2), although it has been shown to exist in other tissues such as the central nervous system (12,21,22) and the tubular epithelium (23).

The inducible form of the enzyme was first discovered in macrophages (10,16) in which its activity was found to be induced by endotoxin, tumor necrosis factor, cytokines, and so forth (24). This enzyme, which is not calcium-dependent, can also be induced in vascular smooth muscle and in endothelial cells (25), particularly by the administration of cytokine (26–28). These observations suggest that the inducible form may be responsible for the hypotension observed during endotoxic shock (29). The inducible enzyme is also activated in cultured mesangial cells by lipopolysaccharides (30), but the significance of these findings remains unknown. It has also been shown that the induction of NO synthetase can be markedly reduced by the administration of steroids (31). This observation has raised the question of the extent to which corticosteroids also inhibit the activity of the constitutive form. This issue is important because it may largely account for the increase in total peripheral resistance and the hypertension that occurs during the continuous administration of mineralocorticoids (32).

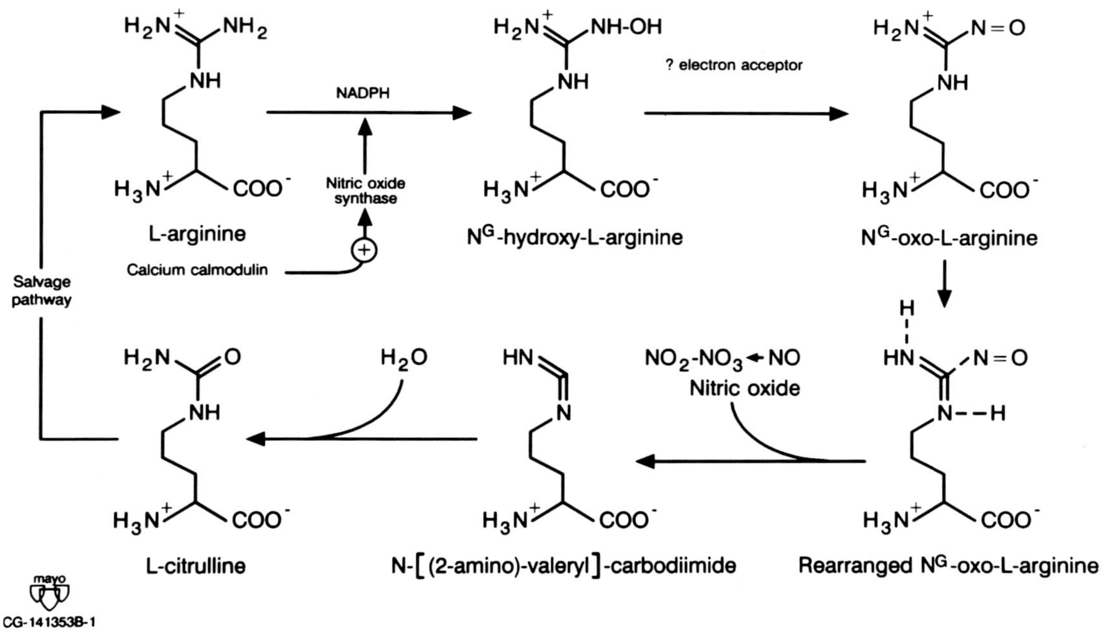

FIG. 1. Possible synthesis pathway of NO from a single amino acid precursor, L-arginine. (Modified from ref. 159.)

Nitrous oxide can also be synthesized from L-homoarginine, methyl and ethyl ester analogues of L-arginine, and certain dipeptide analogues of L-arginine such as L-arginine-L-alanine (5). All these analogues have been shown to be very active in inducing the relaxation of L-arginine–depleted arterial rings. In contrast, substitution of one or both of the two basic amino nitrogen atoms in the guanidino group (N^G) of L-arginine (Fig. 1) results in analogues that competitively antagonize endothelium-dependent relaxation (18). This substitution of N^G atoms with allyl, ethyl, succinyl, or nitro groups confers pronounced inhibitory activity (5). Of all these compounds, the most commonly used have been N^G-monomethyl-L-arginine (L-NMMA) and N^G-nitro-L-arginine methylester (L-NAME). The most likely mechanism of action of these N^G-substituted analogues of L-arginine is competitive inhibition of the conversion of L-arginine or an arginine-containing substance to NO (18). In support of this concept is the demonstration that the inhibitory effect is reversed by increasing the concentration of the precursor L-arginine but not that of the enantiomer D-arginine (18).

A recent, very interesting finding was that an inhibitor of NO synthesis appeared to be synthesized by the organism. Such an inhibitor, which consists of two methyl groups bound to the nitrogen atom of the guanidino group of L-arginine and is known as N^G-D-methyl-arginine or asymmetric dimethylarginine (33), has been isolated from human plasma. More than 10 mg of this substance is excreted in urine over 24 hours. However, in patients with end-stage chronic renal failure who have little or no urine output, the elimination of the inhibitor is impaired and circulating concentrations presumably rise sufficiently to inhibit NO synthesis. Accumulation of endogenous asymmetric dimethylarginine may thus contribute to the development of hypertension and immune system dysfunction associated with chronic renal failure. More studies are needed to determine the mechanism of action of the inhibitor (e.g., whether it regulates the activity of NO synthetase).

Another mechanism of regulation on the biologic activity of NO is by the production of substances that could protect NO from rapid degradation. For example, it is known that NO is rapidly transformed to NO_2 and NO_3 (11). However, the half-life of NO may be prolonged by the presence of "protector molecules," or adductors. Among the chemical species thought to be of potential importance as NO adductors are S-nitrosothiol adducts of the sulfhydryl groups of amino acids, peptides, and proteins. It has recently been shown that NO reacts with free thiol groups of proteins *in vitro* to form S-nitroso-protein-NO adducts, with bioactivities comparable with that of endothelium-derived vasodilating factor but with half-lives on the order of hours (34). Analytic methods that allow the determination of free NO plasma levels and S-nitrosothiols have shown that the concentration of S-nitrosothiols is three to four orders of magnitude greater than that of free NO in mammalian plasma and is mostly composed of the S-nitrosothiol adduct of serum albumin (35). Interestingly, it was also observed that the inhibition of NO synthesis by L-NMMA in rabbits causes a significant decrease in the circulating level of S-nitrosothiol-serum albumin to 60 percent of the initial values by 1 hour after the administration of L-NMMA. Within that time, blood pressure was significantly increased by approximately 25 mm Hg (35). The study suggests that changes in the rate of NO synthesis may be reflected in the plasma levels of S-nitrosothiols. The biologic activity of endogenous NO may also be enhanced by the administration of pharmacologic agents that are thiol donors. Lahera et al. (36) demonstrated that N-acetyl cysteine or N-thiol salicylic acid produced a 20 to 40 percent potentiation of the hypotensive response to acetylcholine.

Under the physiological condition of neutral pH, NO is not very reactive, but its paramagnetic properties (odd number of electrons) account for the remarkable binding affinity for the heme iron (4) and thereby for the inactivation produced by hemoglobin or many other hemoproteins (5). This affinity is closely related to the mechanism of guanylate cyclase activation, because NO binds the heme group of this enzyme. The requirement of reduced iron (Fe^{2+}) in the form of heme for the activation of cytosolic guanylate cyclase (37) has been regarded by Ignarro "as a novel and widespread signal transduction mechanism" that links endothelial signals to the effects of cyclic guanosine monophosphate (GMP) generated in neighboring cells (5). Such a relationship could play a major role in coupling the renal hemodynamic events to changes in the tubular reabsorption of sodium.

SYNTHESIS OF NO AND PGs IN THE KIDNEY: SPECIFIC EFFECTS PRODUCED BY THE STIMULATION OF THESE SUBSTANCES

In the kidney, the administration of endothelium-dependent vasodilators such as bradykinin (38) or acetylcholine (39) produce vasodilation and natriuresis, which are mediated by PGs and NO. The inhibition of NO synthesis alone by L-NMMA does not alter the vasodilation induced by acetylcholine (40). Similarly, inhibiting only PG synthesis leaves all the renal responses to acetylcholine unaltered (40). That is, effective blockade of the intrarenal actions of acetylcholine are obtained only when both NO and PG synthesis are simultaneously blocked (40). Furthermore, increases in total renal blood flow (RBF) are not systematically followed by natriuresis. For example, substances such as secretin (41) and synthetic PGE_2 analogues (42) that produce vasodilation of a magnitude comparable with that produced by bradykinin (38) have minimal effects on urinary sodium ex-

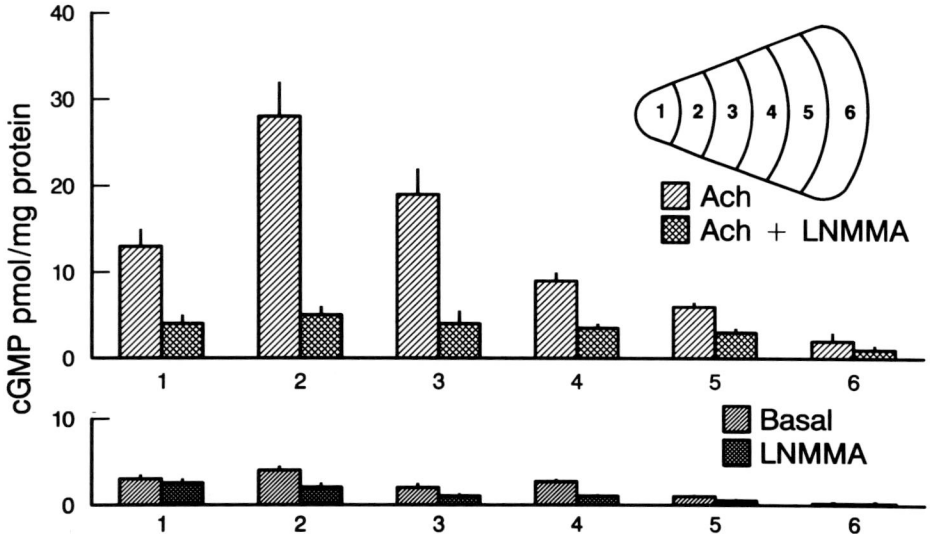

FIG. 2. Distribution of cyclic GMP formation in the most inner (*1*), middle (*2*), and outer (*3*) zones of the renal inner medulla and also the outer medulla (*4*) and inner (*5*) and superficial (*6*) zones of the renal cortex under basal conditions (*lower figure, open columns*), basal condition plus L-NMMA (*lower figure, hatched columns*) during stimulation with acetylcholine (*upper figure, open columns*), or during stimulation with acetylcholine plus L-NMMA (*upper figure, hatched columns*).

cretion (UNaV). It has been suggested (43) that the ability of a renal vasodilator to increase UNaV is intimately linked to its ability to redistribute the total RBF and, specifically, to increase renal medullary blood flow (44) and renal interstitial hydrostatic pressure (44,45). These effects are produced by bradykinin (44,45). In contrast, secretin may not increase medullary blood flow (45) nor alter renal interstitial pressure (41). Evidence from sev-

eral studies suggests that the mechanism coupling changes in medullary blood flow and interstitial pressure to natriuresis may involve NO. Biondi et al. (46) showed that 85 to 90 percent of NO-dependent formation of cyclic GMP takes place in the inner renal medulla (Fig. 2). Stoos et al. (47) demonstrated that NO released from cultured endothelial cells decreased sodium transport (as measured by short-circuit currents) through isolated col-

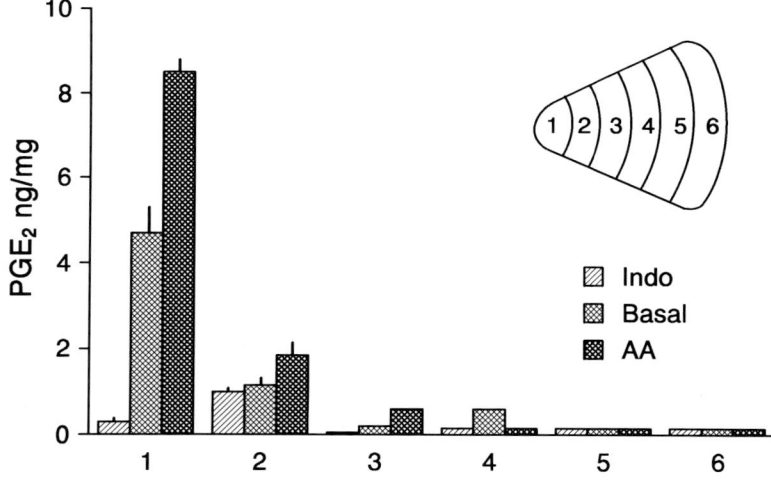

FIG. 3. Distribution of PGE$_2$ synthesis in the inner (*zones 1, 2, and 3*) and outer (*4*) medulla and in the inner (*5*) and outer (*6*) cortex under basal conditions (*cross-hatched columns*) during incubation with indomethacin (*hatched columns*) or arachidonic acid (*open columns*).

lecting ducts. Increases in medullary blood flow could conceivably increase shear stress on medullary vascular endothelial cells (a signal for NO synthesis and release). The NO may then couple the changes in medullary hemodynamics to alterations in sodium excretion. This effect appears to be very critical in volume-induced natriuresis (43).

All these considerations about the possible role of NO on sodium excretion raises the inevitable questions of similar effects exerted by intrarenal PGs. Refoyo et al. (48) have determined the synthesis profile of PGI$_2$ and E$_2$ in the renal medulla and found that these PGs have the distribution very similar to that found for the NO-dependent stimulation of cyclic GMP. In fact, 95 percent of the basal and arachidonic acid–stimulated synthesis of PGE$_2$ takes place in the papilla and the very inner portion of the inner medulla (Fig. 3). Because of this distribution, we ascribed an important role to PGs in mediating the natriuretic activity that is produced when renal medullary blood flow is increased. We thought that changes in interstitial pressure in the renal medulla would stimulate medullary interstitial cells to release PGE$_2$, which will diminish sodium reabsorption in the thick ascending loop of Henle (43). This idea came from the demonstration that PGs mediate the vasodilator action of acetylcholine (40) and bradykinin (38) and that rich binding receptor activity for PGE$_2$ was found in epithelial cells of this tubular segment by Eriksen (49) and by Limas and Limas (50).

ROLE OF NO AND PGs IN MEDIATING PRESSURE-INDUCED NATRIURESIS AND REGULATION OF BLOOD PRESSURE

Increasing renal perfusion pressure (RPP) results in proportional increases in medullary blood flow and interstitial pressure that precede natriuresis (6,51–53).

These changes may be mediated by decreased interstitial levels of renin and angiotensin (43). Under these conditions, blood flow to the renal cortex remains unchanged because of an efficient autoregulatory response (43). The increases in interstitial pressure, however, are quite often very modest, being only 2 to 3 mm Hg (51,53), and are conceivably too small to signal a decrease in renal tubular reabsorption. For these reasons, it has been suggested (6,43) that the effect of changes in interstitial pressure may be significantly amplified by the release of intrarenal natriuretic factors such as PGE$_2$ or NO. This concept is based on evidence showing that blockade of PG synthesis with nonsteroidal anti-inflammatory drugs decreases pressure-induced natriuresis (54,55) (Fig. 4). The natriuresis is restored by infusions of small amounts of synthetic PGE$_2$ analogues that do not produce any hemodynamic effects (55). Intrarenal infusions of comparable amounts of PGI$_2$ do not restore the response (55). Similarly, the blockade of NO also decreases pressure-induced natriuresis, and the response is restored by the administration of L-arginine, the NO synthesis precursor (56). However, blockade of NO does not appear to be as strong as the blockade of PGs in decreasing sodium excretion.

These results are paradoxic because it is very difficult to explain why there are two vasodilator substances, PGE$_2$ and NO, involved in pressure natriuresis. To a large extent, the importance of pressure natriuresis justifies the existence of a redundant system that ensures the elimination of volume that will counteract the elevation of blood pressure. However, this is seldom achieved by producing two substances that exert very similar effects. We examine experimental evidence in the following sections suggesting that NO may be predominantly mediating volume-induced natriuresis whereas PGs could be mostly subserving pressure natriuresis, and both these responses complement each other to preserve volume equilibrium.

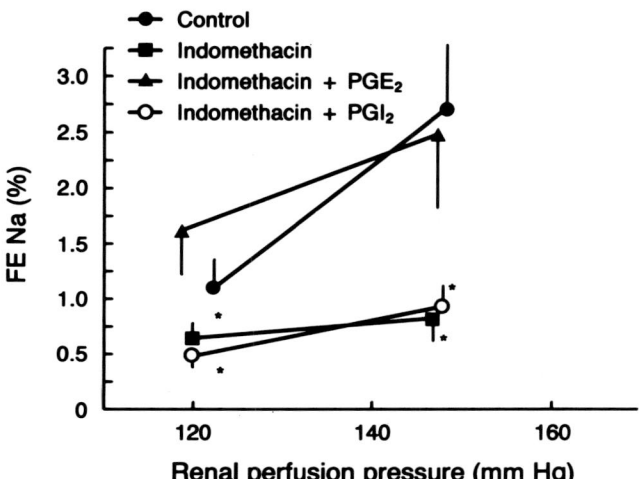

FIG. 4. Changes in pressure-induced natriuresis under control conditions or after the administration of indomethacin alone or with PGE$_2$ or PGI$_2$.

EFFECTS OF NO SYNTHESIS INHIBITION ON THE REGULATION OF SODIUM EXCRETION AND BLOOD PRESSURE

The significance of NO as a mediator of pressure-induced natriuresis was explored by Lahera et al. (57), who systemically induced a progressively greater inhibition of NO synthesis in rats. The earliest and most sensitive alterations produced by small doses of L-NAME (0.1 to 1.0 μg/kg/min) occurred 60 minutes after the start of the infusion and were observed to be decreases in water and sodium excretion. By 120 minutes after beginning the infusion, intrarenal vascular resistance was found to be increased. All these changes took place without any alteration in systemic blood pressure (Table 1). Inhibition of NO synthesis with a higher dose of L-NAME (10 μg/kg/min) was needed to produce increases in systemic blood pressure and in UNaV rates, which overcame the initial antinatriuretic effect of NO synthesis inhibition. This hypertension can then be regarded as an important compensatory mechanism that brings sodium excretion back to normal. Such an effect is illustrated in Fig. 5, which shows the pressure-natriuresis relationship that exists in animals before and after being treated for 2 hours with an infusion of L-NAME, an inhibitor of NO synthesis. In this figure, each point represents one animal in whom mean arterial pressure (represented in the horizontal axis) and sodium excretion rates (represented in the vertical axis) were recorded for 1 hour after 120 minutes of the administration of the L-NAME infusion. It can be seen that before L-NAME treatment mean arterial pressure ranged from 109 to 120 mm Hg and the corresponding values for sodium excretory rates ranged from 13 to 17 mEq/min. After 2 hours of L-NAME infusion,

sodium excretion was significantly decreased by approximately 30 percent in most of the animals in whom mean arterial pressure ranged from 120 to 130 mm Hg. However, in the remaining animals in whom mean arterial pressure increased to 130 to 140 mm Hg, sodium excretion was restored within a range similar to that seen before the treatment. An additional important concept suggested by these studies is that inhibition of NO synthesis could render blood pressure susceptible to be affected by changes in sodium intake. This concept was, in fact, supported by the findings of Salazar et al. (58), who demonstrated that the administration of 0.1 mg/kg/min of L-NAME during 5 consecutive days to normal dogs decreased UNaV without increasing blood pressure (Fig. 6). Blood pressure was markedly increased, however, when the sodium intake in these L-NAME–treated animals was increased from 80 to 300 mEq/day. These observations, which are summarized in Fig. 6, have very important clinical implications because they show that the blockade of the synthesis of a single endogenous vasodilator can render blood pressure volume-dependent. The importance of NO in regulating sodium excretion was further supported by studies (59,60) that showed that blockade of NO synthesis impaired natriuresis induced by volume expansion.

An important issue regarding the effects produced by NO inhibition on renal function and systemic circulation is the extent to which such effects are produced by the activity of pressor systems that are left unbalanced. This issue has been investigated with regard to the renin angiotensin system. Ito et al. (61) and DeNicola et al. (62) presented data suggesting that at least part of the systemic and renal effects produced by the inhibition of NO synthesis are not due to the cessation of the actions

TABLE 1. *Effects of 0.1 and 1.0 μg/kg/min of L-NAME on mean arterial pressure and renal function*[a]

| Dose | Parameters | Control | Time | | |
			60 min	120 min	180 min
Time control	MAP	117 ± 9	113 ± 7	109 ± 6	109 ± 7
	RPF	3.4 ± 0.2	3.3 ± 0.2	3.8 ± 0.4	3.1 ± 0.2
	GFR	1.20 ± 0.06	1.23 ± 0.09	1.30 ± 0.13	1.22 ± 0.13
	UV	93.9 ± 9.6	92.3 ± 15.1	85.6 ± 9.9	79.0 ± 8.7
	UNaV	15.5 ± 1.0	15.0 ± 1.7	13.9 ± 1.7	12.9 ± 1.4
L-NAME	MAP	121 ± 2	120 ± 4	115 ± 4	116 ± 4
(0.1 μg/kg/min)	RPF	3.5 ± 0.4	2.9 ± 0.2	3.4 ± 0.5	3.2 ± 0.2
	GFR	1.2 ± 0.1	1.0 ± 0.1	1.3 ± 0.1	1.2 ± 0.2
	UV	128.4 ± 18.6	93.4 ± 8.5	68.2 ± 6.7*	63.0 ± 13.1*
	UNaV	17.1 ± 2.9	14.5 ± 1.4	13.7 ± 1.8	11.1 ± 2.8
L-NAME	MAP	120 ± 5	122 ± 5	121 ± 5	120 ± 5
(1 μg/kg/min)	RPF	5.4 ± 0.5	3.7 ± 0.7	2.9 ± 0.4*	3.2 ± 0.4*
	GFR	1.4 ± 0.1	1.3 ± 0.2	1.3 ± 0.1	1.2 ± 0.1*
	UV	106.5 ± 9.5	62.5 ± 8.7*	55.0 ± 9.3*	59.5 ± 9.9*
	UNaV	15.9 ± 0.5	11.3 ± 1.0*	10.5 ± 1.4*	9.9 ± 1.4*

Mean arterial pressure (MAP, mm Hg); renal plasma flow (RPF, ml/min); glomerular filtration rate (GFR, ml/min); urine volume (UV/ μl/min); and urine sodium excretion (UNaV, μEq/min) during the control period and at 60, 120, and 180 minutes of the infusion of N^G-nitro-L-arginine methylester (L-NAME). * Indicates P < 0.05 with respect to control period.

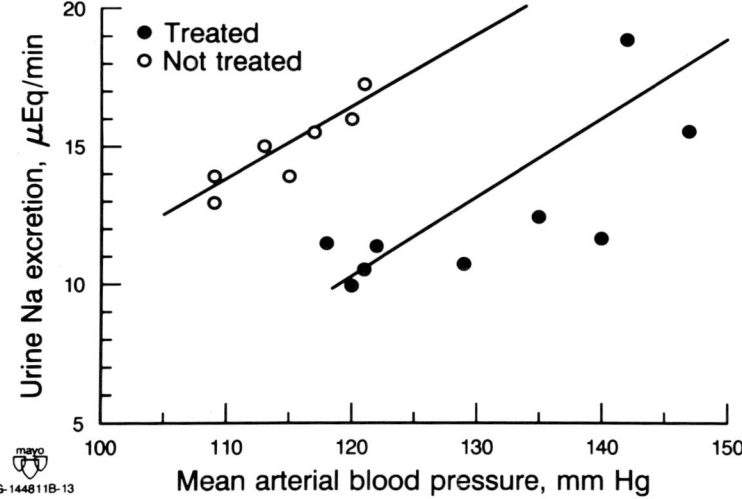

CG-144811B-13

FIG. 5. Pressure-natriuresis relationship in rats before and after being treated 2 hours with and infusion of L-NMMA. (For explanation, see text.)

of NO but are the result of the biologic activity of angiotensin II that becomes manifested after NO tissue concentrations are lowered. In fact, Sigmon et al. (63) showed that the antinatriuresis seen during NO synthesis inhibition with L-NAME was significantly decreased by the prior administration of an angiotensin II receptor antagonist, whereas the increase in systemic blood pressure remained unaltered. However, this issue should be more thoroughly investigated because very recently Pollack et al. (64) have shown that the administration of a specific angiotensin AII receptor antagonist also minimizes the hypertension that develops after the inhibition of NO. The idea that the maintenance of renal function and blood pressure is determined by an equilibrium between the synthesis of NO and PGs on one side and angiotensin on the other is important because the consequences de-

rived from increasing the formation of angiotensin II should be comparable with those obtained by decreasing the synthesis of NO. These two conditions acting together or independently could impair sodium excretion, promoting volume expansion, which in the presence of the reduced cardiovascular compliance would induce hypertension. Furthermore, it is conceivable that the disequilibrium between the synthesis of NO and angiotensin constitute part of a general adaptation to changes in cardiovascular volume. For example, volume expansion promotes a decrease in the formation of angiotensin II (6,43,65) and a concomitant elevation of NO synthesis (6) because of the increases in shear stress produced by the elevation of cardiac output (66). These changes are compatible with the observed vasodilation in renal and systemic circulation and the increase in both cardiovas-

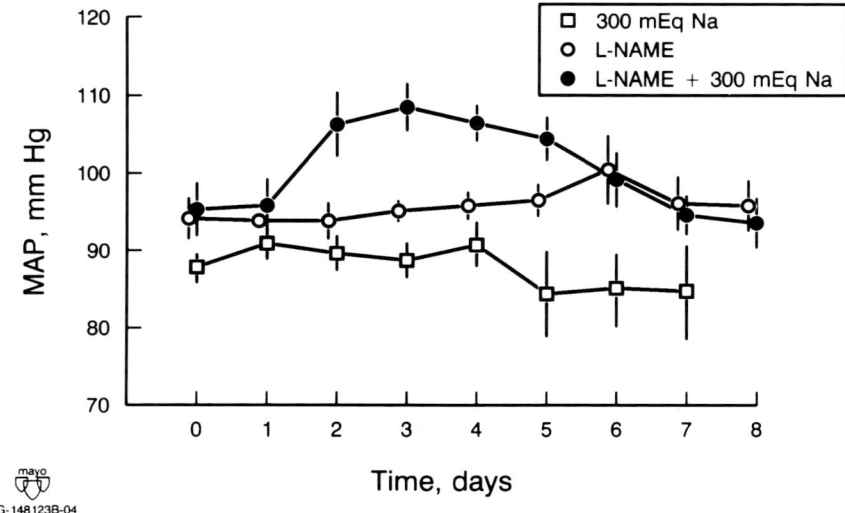

CG-148123B-04

FIG. 6. Changes in mean arterial pressure induced by a daily sodium intake of 300 mmol (□) or by the intravenous infusion of L-NAME (○) at 0.1 μg/kg/min or by L-NAME (0.1 μg/kg/min) + sodium at 300 mmol/day (●).

cular compliance and sodium excretion. The role of NO in promoting natriuresis during volume expansion was demonstrated by the studies of Alberola et al. (59) in mongrel dogs in whom sodium load equivalent was 10 percent of body weight and was performed by infusing 1 L saline solution while the left kidney was being perfused with L-NAME, a potent inhibitor of NO synthesis. The right kidney was used as a control. It was found that the excretion rate of sodium by the left kidney infused with L-NAME was 15 to 20 percent below the excretion rate of the right kidney. This fact is important because it has been found long ago that blockade of PG's synthesis does not alter volume-induced natriuresis. The significance of PGs and NO in the maintenance of volume equilibrium is discussed later.

EFFECTS OF PGs SYNTHESIS INHIBITION ON THE REGULATION OF SODIUM EXCRETION AND BLOOD PRESSURE

The acute blockade of PGs synthesis results in no significant renal hemodynamic alterations and in slight changes in glomerular filtration rate (GFR) in normovolemic experimental animals or humans (67–71). Furthermore, the lack of significant changes in either mean arterial pressure or salt-and-water equilibrium in patients treated for a long term with indomethacin have fostered the idea that PGs do not have any major participation in maintenance of blood pressure or salt-and-water equilibrium. In fact, there is only one study in which measurements of blood pressure, renal hemodynamics, and humoral factors involved in salt-and-water equilibrium were performed in humans treated with large doses of indomethacin for 6 weeks (72). This regime, which produced an 80 percent significant reduction in the urinary excretion of PGE_2, failed to alter mean arterial pressure in a significant manner. It was argued that this lack of effect was most probably caused by the concomitant inhibition of the renin-angiotensin-aldosterone axis, which hampered sodium retention and thereby caused a possible increase in blood pressure. Along this line, it was proved that the most conspicuous alteration produced by the chronic administration of indomethacin was a failure of the renin-aldosterone system to increase during sodium dietary restriction. This study clearly demonstrated that inhibition of PGs synthesis does not produce hypertension.

SPECIFIC EFFECTS EXERTED BY NO AND PGs ON RBF AT DIFFERENT LEVELS OF RPP

There is a general agreement that the basic mechanism responsible for autoregulation is the autonomic contraction of the smooth muscle triggered by the stretch of arterial walls during increments in RPP (43). However, the manner in which the arterial contraction is adjusted to maintain RBF constant remains controversial (73). It has been proposed (73) that NO is not involved in triggering the set of responses that account for the myogenic response of autoregulation; however, during the elevation of RPP, the decrease in arterial diameter results in an elevation of blood flow velocity (because total RBF remains constant) and thereby a proportional increase in shear stress stimulating the release of NO (73) from endothelial cells. This could modulate the myogenic contractility during autoregulation, preventing an excessive fall of RBF (73).

These assumptions are supported by the studies of Salom et al. (74), who found that inhibition of NO by the intravenous infusion of L-NAME in group of euvolemic rats whose kidneys were being perfused at 150 mm Hg

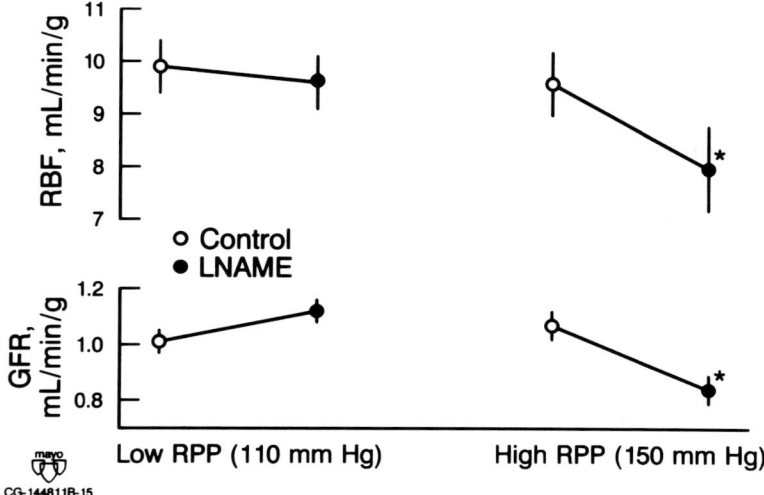

CG-144811B-15

FIG. 7. Effects of NO synthesis inhibition on renal blood flow (*upper figure*) and on GFR (*lower figure*) in rats whose kidneys were being submitted to a high and low RPP.

was followed by a 30 percent reduction in RBF. In contrast, no effects were seen in RBF when L-NAME was given to rats whose RPP was 110 mm Hg (Fig. 7).

In an attempt to determine which are the actual segments that are mainly affected during autoregulation and by NO inhibition, Imig and Roman (75) used a juxtamedullary microvascular preparation in which they first determine the diameter of the arcuate (438 ± 26 μm), interlobular (64 ± 4 μm), and proximal- (30 ± 0.6 μm) and distal-afferent arteriole (20 ± 0.8 μm) at a perfusion pressure of 80 mm Hg. They also observed that the subsequent increase of RPP to 160 mm Hg was followed by an increase in the diameters of arcuate and interlobular arteries of 14 ± 2 and 7 ± 2 percent, respectively, while the diameters of proximal- and distal-afferent arterioles decreased by 3 ± 1 and 7 ± 2 percent, respectively. The administration of L-NAME did not alter the basal diameter of arcuate arteries, but it potentiated the development of active wall tension in interlobular and afferent-proximal and afferent-distal arterioles. These evidences clearly indicate that the arterial segments that are mostly affected by the development of active contraction and thereby by shear stress are the most distal portion of preglomerular circulation. Consequently, one of the main physiological functions of EDRF could be to modulate myogenic contractile response of autoregulation, preventing an excessive fall in RBF and in GFR at high levels of RPP. Such a concept was advanced by us in 1989 (73).

In the dog, the effects of NO synthesis during pressure-induced autoregulation has not yet been well established. However, it would appear from evidence obtained in this animal that the dose of inhibitors of NO synthesis required to alter vascular tone 5 to 10 μg of L-NAME is much higher than the dose needed to alter natriuresis 0.5 to 1 μg/kg/min. Salom et al. (56) has shown that the administration of 1 μg/kg/min failed to modify either the basal renovascular resistance at a perfusion pressure of 100 mm Hg or the efficiency of the autoregulatory response when RPP was elevated to 165 mm Hg. However, no attempts were made to test autoregulatory behavior at higher doses of L-NAME.

All the aforementioned studies in rats and dogs were performed in the absence of PG synthesis inhibition. However, PGs do not appear to have a profound effect on autoregulatory response (55,76,77), although they may contribute to maintained GFR when RPP is driven down to the limit or below the range of autoregulation (78). The evidence indicates the existence of a peculiar interrelationship between NO and PG synthesis in the sense that NO may exert an important modulatory role of RBF at high levels of perfusion pressure (74,75) whereas the inhibition of PG synthesis produces little or no effect. In contrast, an increased synthesis of PGs could exert an important compensatory effect against excessive

decrements of RBF at very low levels of RPP (78,79), whereas the inhibition of NO synthesis appears to have no effect (74,75).

ROLE OF NO AND PGs ON THE RELEASE OF RENIN AS EVOKED BY CHANGES IN RPP

In previous publications, we (43,73) and others (80,81) examined in detail the vascular mechanisms that render renin release dependent on the myogenic response to changes in RPP. This dependency, which is primarily determined by the concentration cytosolic Ca^{2+} in smooth muscle cells and renin secretory cells in the wall of afferent arterioles, could be modulated by PGI_2 and NO. The evidences supporting this assumption are the following.

It has been suggested that the release of NO at high levels of RPP may not only be modulating the smooth muscle contractility triggered by autoregulation but also the arterial pressure-induced decreases of renin release (6). Studies conducted in vitro have supported this notion because incubation of cultured endothelial cells with renal cortical slices for 30 minutes in the presence of indomethacin decreased renin release when the production of NO was stimulated with bradykinin (acetylcholine is a poor stimulator of NO by cultured endothelial cells) (82). These effects were not seen when bradykinin was added to the cortical slices in the absence of endothelial cells or when bradykinin was added to endothelial cells in the presence of oxyhemoglobin, an inactivator of NO.

The inhibitory effects of EDRF on renin were confirmed in additional studies performed by Vidal et al. (83), in which the rate of the secretion of renin from renal cortical slices was significantly decreased in the perfusate exiting from an acetylcholine-stimulated carotid artery (a rich source of NO) (Fig. 8). This inhibitory effect was unaffected when carotid arteries were treated with indomethacin, but it was abolished by hemoglobin or when carotid arteries without endothelial cells were exposed to acetylcholine (83). More recently, Henrich et al. (84) provided strong experimental evidence indicating that the inhibitory effect of NO on renin release is mediated by the formation of cyclic GMP. For example, other agents that increase cyclic GMP accumulation, such as atriopeptins, sodium nitroprusside, and 8-bromo-cyclic GMP, also inhibit the release of renin. Furthermore, inhibition of guanylate cyclase with methylene blue blocks the inhibition of renin release and the increase in cyclic GMP by atriopeptins and sodium nitroprusside.

Consistent with the described effects of NO on renin release, Beierwaltes and Carretero (85) found that incubation of rat kidney slices with L-NMMA (10^{-4} M) en-

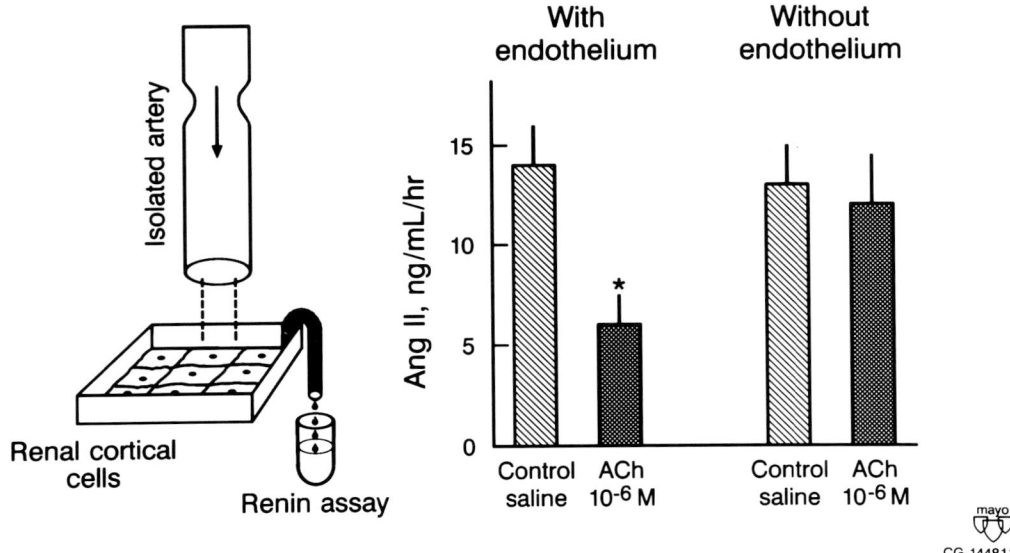

FIG. 8. Inhibitory effects of EDRF on the release of renin from renal cortical cells that were being bathed by a perfusate exiting an isolated carotid artery (*left figure*). The basal release of renin was decreased when EDRF was stimulated with acetylcholine. The effect was not observed when endothelial cells were removed.

hanced renin release by more than 50 percent of control, most probably by removing the inhibitory action of NO. Inhibition of PG synthesis with meclofenamate (1.6×10^{-5} M) did not alter the stimulatory effect of L-NMMA on renin release. Furthermore, the stimulation of renin release produced by a beta-adrenergic agonist (isoproterenol) was not potentiated by L-NMMA, but it was blocked by incubation with the NO precursor L-arginine.

In agreement with this demonstration are the studies of Kurtz et al. (86), which showed that the release of renin under basal conditions, or when stimulated by forskolin or isoproterenol, is markedly attenuated in the presence of endothelial cells (86).

All these *in vitro* demonstrations showing that NO inhibits renin release are to a certain extent correlated by *in vivo* studies. Sigmon et al. (87) proved in rats that the NO synthesis inhibition produces a significant elevation of plasma renin activity. More recently, Lahera et al. (88) have shown that in anesthetized rats, the blockade of NO inhibition produces an increase in blood pressure that is not accompanied by any decrease in renin release.

However, these findings have not been confirmed by other investigators. Johnson and Freeman (89,90) observed that inhibition of NO synthesis with L-NAME in rats is followed by a decrease of renin release, which is observed even when RPP is maintained constant (90). Studies conducted in rat isolated perfused kidney (91,92) are also congruent with a notion that NO produces a strong stimulation of renin release. At present, we cannot offer any logical explanation for these contradictory results.

ROLE OF PGs ON RENIN RELEASE

There is much experimental evidence showing that PGI_2 exerts a potent stimulatory effect on renin release (93–95) and that such an action is very specific (95–99). It is also that PGI_2 stimulates other adenylate cyclase activity (100), inducing the formation of cyclic adenosine monophosphate (AMP) in renal cortical slices, which is associated with the release of renin (100–102). Inhibition of adenylate cyclase blocks the stimulatory action of PGI_2 on renin release.

All these observations on the effects of NO and PGs on renin release, through stimulation of guanylate or adenylate cyclase, respectively, are congruent with the above proposed modulatory role for these substances on RBF. For example, during the increments of RPP, the stimulation of NO is likely to modulate the renal autoregulatory vasoconstriction while decreasing renin release. Conversely, decrements in RPP stimulate the synthesis of PGs, which will compensate for the excessive fall in RBF and will favor the release of renin (73).

GENERAL ADAPTATION TO SODIUM LOAD THROUGH VOLUME AND PRESSURE NATRIURESIS

The studies we have commented about on the role of NO and PGs on the regulation of renal function and blood pressure have significantly changed our concepts about the cardiovascular adaptation to volume expansion in the sense that the activation of these endothelium-derived vasodilators play a role as important as the withdrawal of the vasopressor system (61–64). Such an idea is illustrated in Fig. 9, showing that the reciprocal adaptation of pressor and depressor systems during volume expansion restores sodium balance by increasing UNaV (volume natriuresis) without any significant alteration of blood pressure.

In contrast, an insufficient adaptation of these systems will be translated in a decreased volume natriuretic response with sodium retention and thereby an increase in cardiovascular volume, which will be inappropriate for the existing cardiovascular tone (6,56). Hence, as it is shown in Fig. 9, blood pressure will go up. An insufficient cardiovascular adaptation to volume expansion produced by the lack of modulation of the renin-angiotensin-aldosterone axis was suggested by Shoback et al. (103) and by Hollenberg et al. (104) many years ago. We proposed more recently that a similar situation can be produced by deficient synthesis of NO or PGs in the sense that volume expansion will be poorly modulated because of a significantly decreased volume-induced natriuresis (105).

In any of these cases, the increase in pressure will activate a new set of responses within the kidney, which will produce pressure-induced natriuresis (Fig. 9) that will override the defect responsible for hampering sodium excretion in response to volume expansion, thus restoring sodium balance (57). According to this scheme, the increase in blood pressure should be regarded as a compensatory reaction that is mobilized by the organism to overcome an impairment in the regulation of volume homeostasis (6,105). This sequence of events illustrates how important it is to identify the specific alterations in the kidney that are required to induce natriuresis during volume expansion or during the increments of perfusion

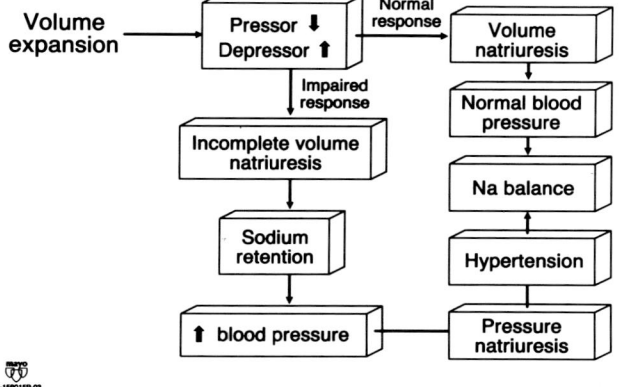

FIG. 9. Volume expansion caused by sodium overload is compensated through volume-induced natriuresis without significant changes in blood pressure. Impairment of this response leads to hypertension, which restored sodium balance through pressure-induced natriuresis.

pressure. These considerations are presented in the following section.

HOMEOSTATIC CONTROL OF NEPHRON FUNCTION DURING CHANGES IN SODIUM EXCRETION

It is well known that the enormous ability of the kidney to eliminate filterable substances from circulation is caused by a large volume of GFR that reaches 180 L in 24 hours. This characteristic poses two basic problems. The first is that an equally large amount of filtered fluid should be reabsorbed by the renal tubules (approximately 99 percent of what was filtered) to prevent volume depletion. The second problem is that fluctuations of blood pressure cannot be reflected in proportional changes in GFR and distal fluid delivery because it will require large compensatory changes that cannot be performed by the distal nephron. To prevent this from happening, the kidney has powerful regulatory mechanisms that constrain the fluctuations of proximal tubule sodium load and proximal reabsorption to very narrow limits. There are indeed three mechanisms involved in such a homeostatic process. The first consists in not allowing the variations of mean arterial pressure to be transmitted to the glomerular capillaries. Such a response is called RBF autoregulation (43). The second mechanism, called glomerular-tubular balance (G-T balance), is a process by which changes in GFR are precisely matched by similar directional changes in proximal tubular fluid reabsorption (106). This minimizes excessive fluctuations of fluid delivered to the loop of Henle.

As it is apparent, the common objective of RBF autoregulation and G-T balance is to control the large amount of plasma being filtered within the reabsorptive ability of the proximal nephron.

Furthermore, the control of the proportionality that must exist between proximal tubular load and fluid delivery to the distal nephrons is so important that a third homeostatic mechanism has evolved within the kidney that couples the autoregulatory vascular response to the distal delivery of tubular fluid. By this mechanism, called tubular-glomerular feedback (T-G feedback), an excessive increase of fluid coming out of the loop of Henle is sensed by the macula densa, which constricts afferent glomerular arterioles until glomerular capillary pressure and thereby GFR are reduced sufficiently to bring distal delivery of fluid back to normal (107). As it is apparent, any maneuver that will increase the excretion rate of sodium in the urine, such as volume expansion or elevation of perfusion pressure, will have to alter these three mechanisms. The functional interrelationship of these mechanisms and the manner in which they are altered during sodium excretion are discussed in the following section.

RBF Autoregulation

This process, which has already been considered in previous sections, consists of minimizing the transmission of changes in aortic blood pressure to the glomeruli by changing intrarenal resistance in a proportional manner. The mechanism responsible for the increase in renal vascular resistance is the rapid entry of calcium into the smooth muscle produced by the stimulation of the stretch-activated calcium channels (43). This process is observed in isolated arteries where the electrical (action potential) and mechanical (vasoconstriction) responses produced by the increase of intraarterial pressure are abolished after the administration of calcium entry blocker such as verapamil (43,108). In general, the stimulation of pressor systems such as an increase of sympathetic tone or plasma renin activity increases vascular tone in the kidney, reducing basal RBF and GFR without modifying the overall autoregulatory response (109). The opposite occurs when the activity of the pressor systems is withdrawn as it happened during volume expansion. In this case, RBF and GFR can be significantly increased above normal. Thus, changes in extracellular fluid volume could alter RBF and GFR in a proportional manner by changing preglomerular vascular tone. As mentioned above, this change in preglomerular vascular tone can also be mediated by the activation of EDRF (74). Consequently, a disregulation in any of these adaptative responses could hamper sodium excretion by resetting GFR at a very low level. This possibility is discussed later in detail.

G-T Balance

As defined above, G-T balance is the ability of proximal tubular reabsorption to change in proportion to GFR. However, the amount of fluid reabsorbed in peritubular capillaries is largely determined by the characteristics of glomerular dynamics. Hence, a previous analysis of the physical forces that determine GFR in proximal tubular reabsorption is required to understand G-T balance.

Glomerular Dynamics

The first step in the formation of urine is the production of an ultrafiltrate of the plasma at the glomerulus (110). Ultrafiltration is driven by Starling forces. These forces acting across the glomerular capillaries are similar to the forces that promote filtration across other capillary beds (Fig. 10).

Both the hydrostatic pressure in the glomerular capillary (Pc) and the oncotic pressure in Bowman's space (πb) promote the movement of fluid from the glomerular capillary into Bowman's space, whereas the hydrostatic

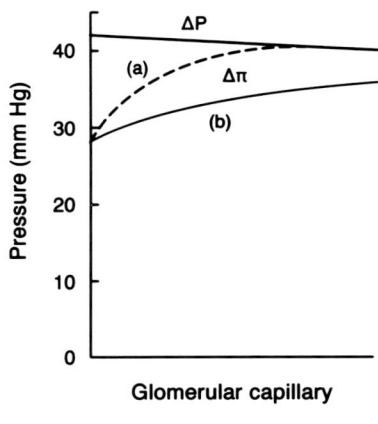

FIG. 10. Changes in hydrostatic (P) and colloidosmotic (π) pressures along the glomerular capillary under filtration equilibrium (*curve a*) and disequilibrium (*curve b*).

pressure in Bowman's space (Pb) and the oncotic pressure in the glomerular capillary (πc) oppose filtration. Consequently, the net ultrafiltration pressure (Puf) can be expressed by the following equation:

$$Puf \text{ or } GFR = (Pc - Pb) - (\pi b - \pi c)$$

As shown in Fig. 10, the mean transglomerular hydrostatic pressure difference (*P*) declines only slightly along the glomerulus (1 or 2 mm Hg) because glomerular capillaries are arranged in parallel, not in series, offering little resistance to circulation (110). In contrast, the corresponding oncotic pressure almost doubles (it raises from 28 mm Hg in the distal end of the afferent arteriole to 36 mm Hg at the distal end of the glomerular capillaries).

By the efferent end of the glomerulus, the oncotic pressure has risen to a value equal (and opposite) to the mean hydrostatic pressure, so that no filtration pressure remains unbalanced (see line *a*, Fig. 10). At this filtration pressure equilibrium, GFR is highly plasma flow–dependent, and exchange across the glomerular capillaries is flow-limited rather than diffusion-limited (110). These characteristics are observed mainly in rats. In dogs and humans, however, the glomerular dynamics are characterized by filtration pressure disequilibrium, which consist in that hydrostatic pressure exceeds oncotic pressure at the end of the glomerulus (see line *b*, Fig. 4). Under these conditions, the dependence of GFR on flow is weaker (110).

Proximal Tubular Reabsorption

Once filtration takes place, solute and fluid go through into the proximal tubule, which reabsorbs approximately 60 percent of the filtered water, sodium, chloride, potassium, and other solutes. Also, all the glucose and amino acids are reabsorbed. As shown in Fig. 11, sodium passes from the tubular lumen to the epithelial cell by virtue of an electrochemical gradient because sodium is positive and the interior of the epithelial cell is negative.

The key element in proximal tubule reabsorption on the basolateral side of the cell is the Na-K ATPase, which is responsible for pumping sodium to the renal interstitium. The accumulation of sodium and the other solutes increases the osmolality of the lateral intercellular space, and water reabsorption follows solute transport. Once the solute and fluid have reached the interstitial space, the reabsorbate may either leak back into the tubular lumen (Fig. 11) or be absorbed into the peritubular capillaries and hence into the blood (111–113).

The variables that determine the net reabsorptive pressure (Pr) acting across the wall of the peritubular capillary are shown in the following equation:

$$Pr = (\pi c - \pi i) - (Pc - Pi)$$

Thus, the oncotic pressure within the peritubular capillary (πc) will favor the uptake of the reabsorbate from the interstitium, whereas the intracapillary hydrostatic pressure (Pc) will oppose this uptake. In contrast, an increase in the hydrostatic pressure in the interstitium (Pi) will largely favor capillary uptake of reabsorbate (and backleak), whereas the interstitial oncotic pressure (πi) will oppose it.

This implies that the forces responsible for the reabsorption of solute and fluid in the proximal tubule are the same as those involved in glomerular filtration, except that the net resulting force favors passage of fluids into the capillaries.

The changes in hydrostatic and colloidosmotic pressure that occurs after the glomeruli are illustrated in Fig. 12. It can be seen that on the efferent end of glomerular capillaries, there is a net hydraulic ultrafiltration force of 40 mm Hg whereas the net colloidosmotic pressure has reached 36 mm Hg. During the passage of blood through the efferent arteriole, there are not alterations in colloidosmotic pressure because no interchange of fluids occurs in this artery. However, hydraulic pressure falls from 40 to 20 mm Hg because of the efferent vascular resistance. In the peritubular capillaries, hydrostatic pressure decreases in proportion to capillary resistance, being 15 mm Hg lower than the existing colloidosmotic pressure. Similarly, the oncotic pressure in the peritubular capillary decreases progressively from 32 to 20 mm Hg as the fluid being reabsorbed produces a progressive dilution of the plasma proteins.

All these considerations lead to the important conclusion that the oncotic pressure gradient across the peritubular capillary (II) is largely determined by the initial peritubular protein concentration at the efferent end of the glomerulus. Similarly, as the interstitial pressure is low (3 to 6 mm Hg), the main hydrostatic pressure opposing the reabsorptive gradient is the peritubular capillary hydrostatic pressure (P), which is mainly determined by the efferent arteriolar vascular resistance. However, the mean hydrostatic pressure gradient across the peritubular capillary (P) is significantly lower than

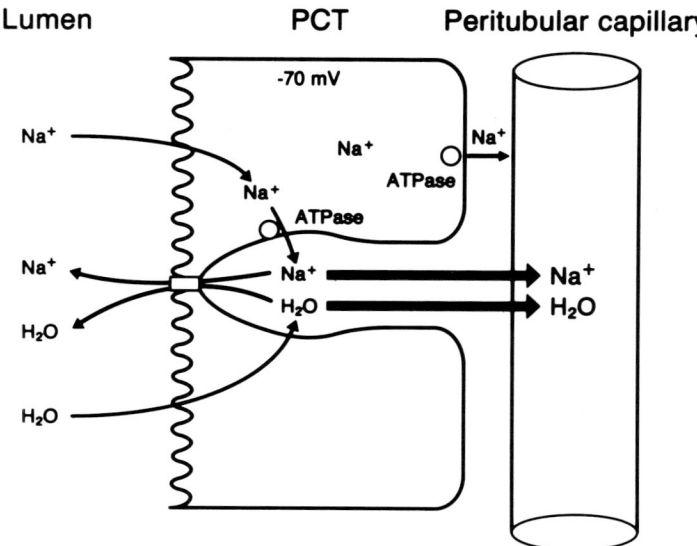

CA-156793B-09

FIG. 11. Schematic representation of proximal tubular sodium reabsorption and backleak in an epithelial cell.

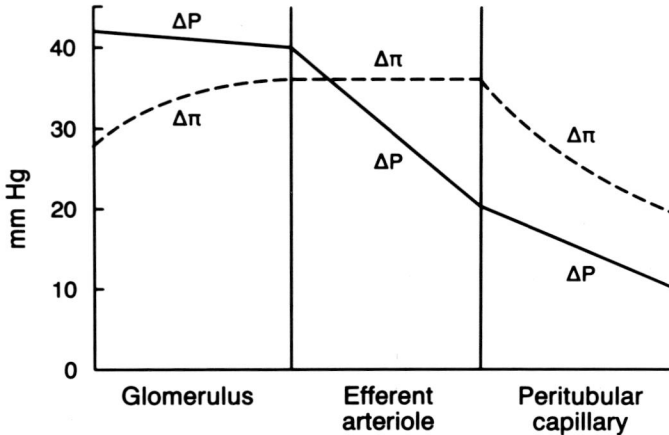

FIG. 12. Interrelated changes in hydrostatic (*P*) and colloidosmotic pressure (π) in the glomerulus, efferent arterioles, and peritubular capillaries during normal (euvolemic) conditions.

peritubular transcapillary oncotic pressure gradient (II). This allows a net positive reabsorptive pressure of 15 mm Hg (Fig. 12). *Consequently, much of the variation that occurs in the reabsorptive forces of peritubular capillaries are the consequence of the alterations in the forces that govern glomerular dynamics. This interplay is what determines the dynamic of G-T balance.* In fact, G-T balance describes the property of the kidney whereby tubular reabsorption is adjusted in proportion to glomerular filtration and by which the percentage (approximately 60 percent) of fluid reabsorption (rather than the amount of reabsorption) remains constant.

It can be derived from Fig. 12 that if more ultrafiltrate is formed from a constant amount of plasma, then the plasma proteins become more concentrated, thus raising the peritubular capillary oncotic pressure. As the peritubular oncotic pressure is directly related to the filtration fraction (FF) (FF = GFR/RPF), a rise in the FF increases the peritubular capillary's oncotic pressure and enhances the uptake of sodium and water. The opposite effect occurs when FF falls because peritubular capillary oncotic pressure will decrease, reducing the tubular uptake of fluid. Under these conditions, some of the fluid and solute that accumulates in the lateral intercellular space returns to the tubular lumen by passive backleak across the tight junctions (see Fig. 11).

As we have examined before, changes in GFR greatly alter the filtered load of sodium. Unless such changes are rapidly accompanied by adjustments in sodium reabsorption, UNaV would fluctuate and disturb whole-body sodium balance. In practice, changes in filtered load are never expressed in full as equivalent changes in UNaV because an important degree of tubular compensation always exists.

In experiments performed in dogs by Landwehr et al. (114), GFR was increased up to 85 percent by protein feeding, dexamethasone administration, infusion of vasodilating drugs, and cross-circulation. They found only

small and inconsistent increments in UNaV. Thus, the total amount reabsorbed rises when the GFR rises and falls when GFR falls. This proportionality is very well illustrated in Fig. 13, in which Giebish et al. (115) showed that changes in GFR from 10 to 70 percent are accompanied by an almost linear increase in proximal tubular reabsorption.

Most of the studies have shown that increments of sodium concentration in the proximal tubule (obtained by inducing hypernatremia) does not alter tubular reabsorption (116–121). In contrast, excellent G-T balance is seen when the filtered load of sodium is changed by varying the GFR (118,120,122,123).

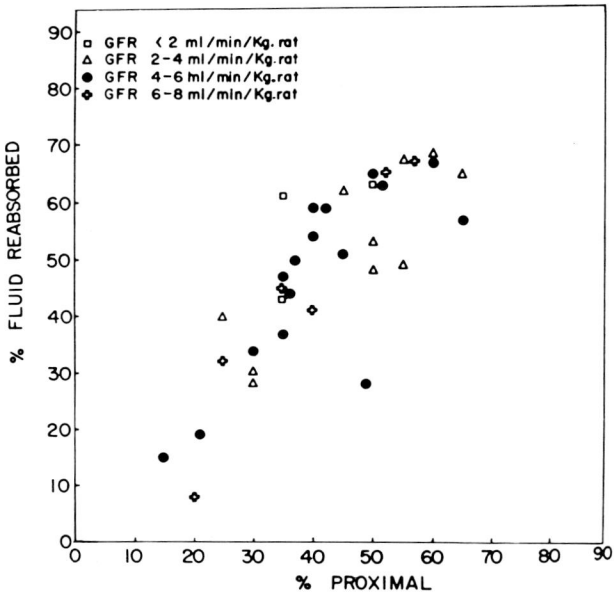

FIG. 13. Influence of spontaneous variations in GFR on the rate of proximal tubular fluid reabsorption. (From ref. 115, with permission.)

G-T Balance During Volume Expansion
Produced by Saline Load

In previous sections, we have emphasized that G-T balance can be regarded as a homeostatic mechanism that prevents excessive delivery of sodium and fluids to the distal nephron. However, this in itself poses a problem under circumstances in which the excretion of sodium needs to be increased significantly such as occurs during excessive sodium intake. Under this condition, there is a gradual displacement of the G-T balance curve toward a decreased proximal reabsorption (124,125). Although the mechanism responsible for such an effect has not been defined completely, it is known that the decrease of plasma colloidosmotic pressure (126–128) is of critical importance. In agreement with this concept, it has been found that the volume of fluid reabsorbed in the proximal tubule is directly correlated with the efferent arterial oncotic pressure (129–131). For example, the perfusion of efferent arterioles in rats that has been submitted to volume expansion with a solution having a colloidosmotic pressure similar to that which existed in the efferent arteriole before the volume expansion restores absolute proximal reabsorption (129). However, absolute proximal reabsorption remained decreased when the arteries were perfused with a concentration of proteins equivalent to that which existed during volume expansion.

The expansion of extracellular fluid volume produces other alterations that affect proximal reabsorption. For example, the fall in plasma renin activity produces a significant decrease of efferent arteriole, which allows that transmission of pressure downstream from the glomeruli. These increments in efferent arteriolar hydrostatic pressure along with the dilution of the efferent arterial plasma protein would reduce the net force for fluid uptake into peritubular capillaries (124,132–135).

Also, saline expansion dilutes interstitial proteins and expands the interstitium, increasing the interstitial hydrostatic pressure. The hydrostatic pressure in the interstitium (Pi) should regulate fluid removal from the interstitial compartment either by promoting fluid uptake into the peritubular capillaries or by promoting paracellular backleak into the tubule. Most of the experimental evidence supports the backleak route, in which increased junctional permeability has been found with volume expansion (136). In *in vivo* studies in Necturus, Boulpaep (113) and Sakin and Boulpaep (137) demonstrated that increased back flux of sodium contributes to reduced net proximal sodium reabsorption during plasma volume expansion and suggested that this was due to increased Pi. This finding agrees with the other reports in which an increase in Pi increases UNaV (138,139) and reduces proximal reabsorption (140,141).

One issue that has been totally neglected in the past is that the permeability of tubular capillaries or the perme-ability of the tight junction may be affected by humoral factors. For example, the release of NO and PGs with a decrease in angiotensin II that occurs during volume expansion may elevate the permeability of a tight junction, favoring the return of fluid toward the tubular lumen. Some observations that have been hitherto difficult to explain may be accounted for by the participation of humoral factors. For example, it has been observed that the marked natriuresis associated with a decrease in proximal tubular reabsorption produced by saline loading can be virtually abolished when the increments induced by volume expansion in RBF and GFR and in interstitial and capillary hydrostatic pressure were prevented by aortic constriction (142–144). However, this preventive effect does not occur if the clamp was placed after the natriuretic response has taken place during volume expansion (142,143,145). In a study conducted by Ichikawa and Brenner (146) to elucidate this issue, it was found that the main difference between the early and late aortic clamp is that with the late clamp, peritubular capillary hydrostatic pressure is not actually decreased, whereas colloidosmotic pressure is diluted to the same extent than with the early clamp. Hence, the natriuresis continues unabated. The difficulties in decreasing capillary hydrostatic pressure with the late clamp could be caused by the difficulties in reversing the elevation in PG and NO production, which must be already triggered during the early phases of volume expansion. This issue should be further explored.

T-G Feedback

The characteristics of the T-G response have been routinely investigated by perfusing the distal tubules (at the level of the macula densa) with fluid of various electrolyte composition. The readers interested in all the details about the T-G response can consult the excellent review written by Schnermann and Briggs (107). Here we will mainly concentrate on the changes that occur in the T-G response during volume expansion. It has been found using distal tubule perfusion technique that in euvolemic animals, fluid perfusion rate of 25 nl/min induces a constriction of the afferent arteriole of 23 percent. However, after volume expansion, higher perfusion rates (35 nl/min) are required to evoke a very mild afferent arteriolar vasoconstriction, which do not exceed 4 percent, a diameter reduction. Recently, Wilcox et al. (106) demonstrated that when the T-G response is stimulated by increasing fluid delivery to the macula densa, the vasoconstriction of afferent arterioles is significantly diminished by the release of NO. This suggests that an enhanced formation of NO in the glomerular pole could be responsible for resetting the T-G response during volume expansion. Furthermore, although extensive review has been written on the nature of T-G response, its physiological meaning has never been clearly defined. We have thought that the T-G response can be regarded as a mechanism that supersedes the autoregulatory responses that control blood flow and glomerular tubular balance. Because these two interdependent responses are autoregulated, they cannot, by definition, reset themselves to a different level. It is then conceivable that volume expansion may decrease the constriction of the afferent arterioles at a lower level, resetting the vascular autoregulatory response to allow a higher GFR. Similarly, under conditions of volume expansion, proximal tubular reabsorption will not offset the increase in filtration because of the resetting of T-G balance by humoral mechanism. This latter effect is not completely understood, but Haberle et al. (147,148) have shown that the activation of feedback response by high perfusion rate of distal nephrons could release from the glomeruli vasoactive principles, which could affect proximal reabsorption and thereby T-G balance. More studies should be conducted to understand this phenomenon fully.

INTEGRATED REVIEW OF THE INTRARENAL MECHANISMS THAT PARTICIPATE IN THE REGULATION OF SODIUM EXCRETION AND BLOOD PRESSURE

Figure 14 intends to summarize the interrelationship that exists among the regulatory mechanisms that control the interchange of fluid and electrolytes along the nephron. From a finalistic standpoint, the large amount of glomerular filtration and proximal tubular reabsorption needs to be protected from wide fluctuations in blood pressure, which may result in unmanageable large deliveries of fluid to the distal nephron. This protection is provided by two important mechanisms: (a) the vascular autoregulatory response because it ensures the constancy of GFR and (b) by the G-T balance, which prevents excessive delivery of fluid to the distal nephron. During

volume expansion, these two processes could be reset by increments in the synthesis of NO produced by the increase of shear stress in endothelial cells. This will induce a marked vasodilation, resetting the autoregulatory response in preglomerular vasculature with the elevation of GFR. This change will not be offset by an equivalent increment in proximal tubular sodium reabsorption because G-T balance will be displaced toward a higher level of sodium rejection by (a) a decrease in colloidosmotic pressure caused by the dilution of plasma and (b) a fall in the intrarenal concentration of pressor antinatriuretic substances, particularly angiotensin II. It should be remembered that the increased synthesis of NO in afferent arterioles may contribute to the decrease of renin release and the corresponding fall of intrarenal concentrations of angiotensin II. All these changes will produce a marked elevation of fluid delivery to the macula densa, which under normal conditions will trigger through a T-G feedback response a vasoconstriction of the afferent arteriole, bringing GFR down to normal. This change will compromise the increased delivery to the distal nephrons. However, during volume expansion, this feedback response may not be effective because the increase in NO synthesis in the glomerular pole will significantly ameliorate the afferent arteriole vasoconstriction. Furthermore, the increase in the distal delivery of fluid will result in an increased volume of urine and sodium excretion because the mechanisms that control sodium reabsorption in the distal nephrons (e.g., aldosterone, vasopressin) are obviously decreased.

All these mechanisms will allow to increase sodium excretion very effectively without increasing mean arterial pressure in a significant manner. However, a deficient synthesis of NO can impair this homeostatic regulation, producing sodium retention with an elevation of mean arterial pressure (Fig. 13). Such an elevation of pressure will then force natriuresis through a mechanism that does not affect renal cortical circulation but it enhances blood flow to the renal medulla (see upper part of Fig. 13). This medullary vasodilation will increase renal

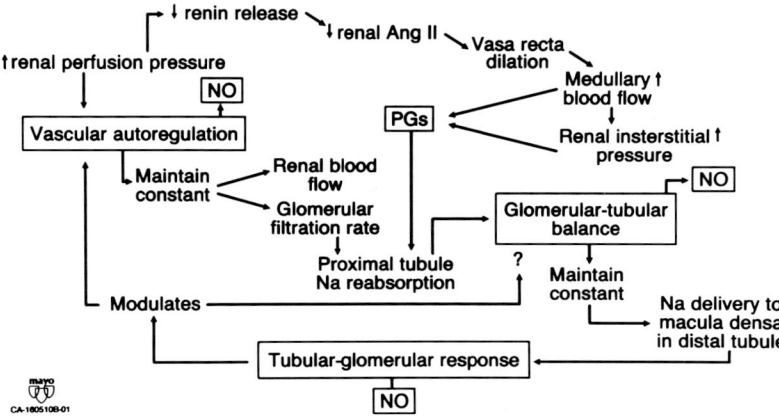

FIG. 14. Interrelationship among vascular autoregulation, G-T balance, and T-G response and modulatory effects of NO and PGs. (For explanation, see text.)

interstitial pressure inhibiting tubular sodium reabsorption per se and/or a concomitant stimulation in the release of PGE_2. The important role of PGs in mediating pressure natriuresis is supported by several experimental evidences. Pawlowska et al. (149) implanted a permeable microcapsule into the renal parenchyma through which the intrarenal interstitial pressure was increased by expanding renal interstitial fluid with microinjections of artificial lymph. These increments in interstitial pressure were immediately followed by a proportional natriuresis that was abolished by the administration of indomethacin, a PG synthesis blocker. The other evidence supporting an important participation of PGs on pressure natriuresis is that the administration of indomethacin abolished the increase in sodium excretion produced by elevation of RPP (54,55). As mentioned above, this blockade of pressure natriuresis is restored by the intrarenal infusion of PGE_2 but not by the administration of PGI_2 (55). The nephron segments where PGE_2 could exert the natriuretic activity have not yet been identified, but recent communications indicate that PGE_2 could greatly increase the permeability of tight junction, promoting backleak in the proximal tubules (150). This finding is in agreement with other experimental demonstrations showing that during pressure natriuresis, most of the fall in tubular reabsorption of sodium occurs at the level of the proximal tubules (138,140,141,152–155).

The importance of the regulatory mechanism that operates on the proximal side of the nephron to control sodium excretion and blood pressure is underscored during the renal escape from the sodium-retaining effects of mineralocorticoids (156). In these circumstances, the continuous administration of aldosterone increases distal tubular reabsorption, producing a 10 to 15 percent body weight expansion of extracellular fluid volume. This will reset the proximal autoregulatory mechanism, increasing sodium delivery to the distal tubules in such a significant amount that it will override the reabsorptive effect of aldosterone in this nephron segment (156,157). This natriuretic effect occurs with small increments of mean arterial pressure that range from 3 to 5 mm Hg (53). However, despite such a mild increase, there is a marked elevation of renal blood flow and renal interstitial pressure because of the withdrawal of the pressor systems that occurs concomitantly with the activation of the vasodilator systems. The importance of allowing the transmission of pressure inside the kidney to induce natriuresis during volume expansion is well illustrated by the experiment of Hall et al. (158). These investigators prevented any significant change in RPP during the continuous administration of aldosterone by placing a servo-controlled automatic cuff in the aorta of dogs. Under these conditions, the volume expansion induced by aldosterone produced a correlative and proportional elevation of mean arterial pressure (from 100 to 130 mm Hg), which was sustained until the aortic constrictive

cuff was released. This maneuver was followed by a massive natriuresis, bringing volume expansion down to normal with a concomitant decrease of blood pressure.

In summary, the results of the studies examined in this chapter show that alterations in the intrarenal concentration of angiotensin II, NO, and PGs are responsible for coupling the changes in renal hemodynamics to sodium handling by the renal tubules. The alteration of this mechanism produces a syndrome that is similar to that observed during the development of a salt-sensitive form of essential hypertension.

REFERENCES

1. Furchgott RF, Zawadzki JV. The obligatory role of endothelial cells in the relaxation of arterial smooth muscle by acetylcholine. *Nature* 1980;299:373–376.
2. Moncada S, Palmer RMJ, Higgs EA. The discovery of nitric oxide as the endogenous nitrovasodilator. *Hypertension* 1988;12:365–372.
3. Furchgott RF, Vanhoutte PM. Endothelium-derived relaxing and contracting factors. *FASEB J* 1989;3:2007–2018.
4. Ignarro LJ. Biosynthesis and metabolism of endothelium-derived nitric oxide. *Annu Rev Pharmacol Toxicol* 1990;30:535–560.
5. Ignarro LJ. Nitric oxide: a novel signal transduction mechanism for transcellular communication. *Hypertension* 1990;16:477–483.
6. Romero JC, Lahera V, Salom MG, Biondi ML. Role of the endothelium-dependent relaxing factor nitric oxide on renal function. *J Am Soc Nephrol* 1992;2:1371–1387.
7. Tolins JP, Palmer RM, Moncada S, Raij L. Role of endothelium-derived relaxing factor in regulation of renal hemodynamic responses. *Am J Physiol* 1990;258:H655–662.
8. Langston JB, Guyton AC, Douglas BH, Dorsett PE. Effect of changes in salt intake on arterial pressure and renal function in nephrectomized dogs. *Circ Res* 1963;12:508–513.
9. Coleman TG, Guyton AC. Hypertension caused by salt loading in the dog. III. Onset transients of cardiac output and other circulatory variables. *Circ Res* 1969;25:152–160.
10. Hibbs JC, Taintor RR, Vavrin Z. Macrophage cytotoxicity: role for L-arginine deiminase and imino nitrogen oxidation to nitrite. *Science* 1987;235:473–476.
11. Marletta MA. Nitric oxide: biosynthesis and biological significance. *Trends Pharmacol Sci* 1989;14:488–492.
12. Garthwaite J, Charles SL, Chess-Williams R. Endothelium-derived relaxing factor release on activation of NMDA receptors suggests role as intercellular messenger in the brain. *Nature* 1988;336:385–388.
13. Palmer RMJ, Moncada S. A novel citrulline-forming enzyme implicated in the formation of nitric oxide by vascular endothelial cells. *Biochem Biophys Res Commun* 1989;158:348–352.
14. Hecker M, Mitchell JA, Harris HJ, Katsura M, Thiemermann C, Vane JR. Endothelial cells metabolize N^G-monomethyl-L-arginine to L-citrulline and subsequently to L-arginine. *Biochem Biophys Res Commun* 1990;167:1037–1043.
15. Leone AM, Palmer RM, Knowles RG, Francis PL, Ashton DS, Moncada S. Constitutive and inducible nitric oxide synthases incorporate molecular oxygen into both nitric oxide and citrulline. *J Biol Chem* 1991;266:23790–23795.
16. Iyengar R, Stuehr DJ, Marletta MA. Macrophage synthesis of nitrite, nitrate, and N-nitrosamines: precursors and role of the respiratory burst. *Proc Natl Acad Sci* 1987;84:6369–6373.
17. Lopez-Jaramillo P, Gonzalez MC, Palmer RM, Moncada S. The crucial role of physiological Ca^{2+} concentrations in the production of endothelial nitric oxide and the control of vascular tone. *Br J Pharmacol* 1990;101:489–493.
18. Palmer RM, Rees DD, Ashton DS, Moncada S. L-arginine is the physiological precursor for the formation of nitric oxide in endothelium-dependent relaxation. *Biochem Biophys Res Commun* 1988;153:1251–1256.

19. Moore PK, al-Swayeh OA, Chong NS, Evans R, Gibson A. L-N^G-nitro arginine (L-NOARG), a novel, L-arginine-reversible inhibitor of endothelium-dependent vasodilatation *in vitro*. *Br J Pharmacol* 1990;99:408–412.

20. Ishii K, Chang B, Kerwin JF, Huang Z-J, Murad F. N^w-nitro-L-arginine: a potent inhibitor of endothelium-derived relaxing factor formation. *Eur J Pharmacol* 1990;176:219–223.

21. Knowles GK, Palacios M, Palmer RM, Moncada S. Formation of nitric oxide from L-arginine in the central nervous system: a transduction mechanism for stimulation of the soluble guanylate cyclase. *Proc Natl Acad Sci* 1989;86:5159–5162.

22. Bredt DS, Snyder SH. Nitric oxide mediates glutamate-linked enhancement of cGMP levels in the cerebellum. *Proc Natl Acad Sci* 1989;86:9030–9033.

23. Ishii K, Chang B, Kerwin JF Jr, Wagenaar FL, Huang ZJ, Murad F. Formation of endothelium-derived relaxing factor in porcine kidney epithelial LLC-PK1 cells: an intra- and intercellular messenger for activation of soluble guanylate cyclase. *J Pharmacol Exp Ther* 1991;256(1):38–43.

24. Nathan CF, Hibbs JB Jr. Role of nitric oxide synthesis in macrophage antimicrobial activity. *Curr Opin Immunol* 1991;3:65–70.

25. Moncada S, Palmer RMJ, Higgs EA. Nitric oxide physiology, pathophysiology, and pharmacology. *Pharmacol Rev* 1991;43:109–142.

26. Busse R, Mulsch A. Induction of nitric oxide synthase by cytokines in vascular smooth muscle cells. *FEBS Lett* 1990;275:87–90.

27. Lamas S, Michel T, Brenner BM, Marsden PA. Nitric oxide synthesis in endothelial cells: evidence for a pathway inducible by TNF-a. *Am J Physiol* 1991;C634–641.

28. Beasley D, Schwartz JH, Brenner BM. Interleukin 1 induces prolonged L-arginine-dependent cyclic guanosine monophosphate and nitrite production in rat vascular smooth muscle cells. *J Clin Invest* 1991;87:602–608.

29. Baker CH, Sutton ET. Arteriolar endothelium-dependent vasodilation occurs during endotoxin shock. *Am J Physiol* 1993;264:1118–1123.

30. Shultz PJ, Tayeh MA, Marletta MA, Raij L. Synthesis and action of nitric oxide in rat glomerular mesangial cells. *Am J Physiol* 1991;261:F600–F606.

31. Radomski MW, Palmer RM, Moncada S. Glucocorticoids inhibit the expression of an inducible, but not the constitutive, nitric oxide synthase in vascular endothelial cells. *Proc Natl Acad Sci* 1990;87:10043–10047.

32. Dananberg J, Sider RS, Grekin RJ. Deoxycorticosterone suppresses the pressor response to nitroarginine [abstract]. *Clin Res* 1992;40:172A.

33. Vallance P, Leone A, Calver A, Collier J, Moncada S. Accumulation of an endogenous inhibitor of nitric oxide synthesis in chronic renal failure. *Lancet* 1992;339:572–575.

34. Stamler JS, Simon DI, Osborne JA, et al. S-nitrosylation of proteins with nitric oxide: synthesis and characterization of biologically active compounds. *Proc Natl Acad Sci USA* 1992;89:444–448.

35. Stamler JS, Jaraki O, Osborne J, et al. Nitric oxide circulates in mammalian plasma primarily as an S-nitroso adduct of serum albumin. *Proc Natl Acad Sci USA* 1992;89:7674–7677.

36. Lahera V, Khraibi AA, Romero JC. Sulfhydryl group donors potentiate the hypotensive effect of acetylcholine in rats. *Hypertension* 1993;22:156–160.

37. Craven PA, DeRubertis FR. Restoration of the responsiveness of purified guanylate cyclase to nitrosoguanidine, nitric oxide, and related activators by heme and heme proteins: evidence of the involvement of the paramagnetic nitrosylheme complex in enzyme activation. *J Biol Chem* 1978;253:8433–8443.

38. Lahera V, Salom MG, Fiksen-Olsen MJ, Romero JC. Mediatory role of endothelium-derived nitric oxide in renal vasodilatory and excretory effects of bradykinin. *Am J Hypertens* 1991;4:260–262.

39. Lahera V, Salom MG, Fiksen-Olsen MJ, Raij L, Romero JC. Effects of N^G-monomethyl-L-arginine and L-arginine on acetylcholine renal response. *Hypertension* 1990;15:659–663.

40. Salom MG, Lahera V, Romero JC. Role of prostaglandins and endothelium-derived relaxing factor on the renal response to acetylcholine. *Am J Physiol* 1991;260:F145–F149.

41. Marchand GR, Ott CE, Lang FC, Greger RF, Knox FG. Effect

42. Haas JA, Hammond TG, Granger JP, Blaine EH, Knox FG. Mechanism of natriuresis during intrarenal infusion of prostaglandins. *Am J Physiol* 1984;247:F475–F479.

43. Romero JC, Knox FG. Mechanisms underlying pressure-related natriuresis: the role of the renin-angiotensin and prostaglandin systems: state of the art lecture. *Hypertension* 1988;11:724–738.

44. Lameire N, Vanholder R, Ringoir S, Leusen I. Role of medullary hemodynamics in the natriuresis of drug-induced renal vasodilation in the rat. *Circ Res* 1980;47:839–844.

45. Fadem SZ, Hernandez-Llamas G, Patak RV, Rosenblatt SG, Lifschitz MD, Stein JH. Studies on the mechanism of sodium excretion during drug-induced vasodilatation in the dog. *J Clin Invest* 1982;69:604–610.

46. Biondi ML, Bolterman RJ, Romero JC. Zonal changes of guanidine 3',5'-cyclic monophosphate related to endothelium-derived relaxing factor in dog renal medulla. *Renal Physiol Biochem* 1992;15:1–7.

47. Stoos BA, Carretero OA, Farhy RD, Scicli G, Garvin JL. Endothelium-derived relaxing factor inhibits transport and increases cGMP content in cultured mouse cortical collecting duct cells. *J Clin Invest* 1992;89(3):761–765.

48. Refoyo A, Bolterman RJ, Bentley MD, Fiksen-Olsen MJ, Sandberg SM, Romero JC. Distribution of prostaglandins E_2 and 6-keto-PGF_{1a} production in the canine kidney. *Hypertension* 1990;15:I-107–I-111.

49. Eriksen EF, Richelson B, Gesser BP, Jacobsen NO, Steengard-Pedersen K. Prostaglandin E_2 receptors in the rat kidney: biochemical characterization and localization. *Kidney Int* 1987;32:181–186.

50. Limas C, Limas CJ. Prostaglandin receptors in the rat kidney. *Arch Biochem Biophys* 1984;233:32–42.

51. Roman RJ, Cowley AW, Garcia-Estañ J, Lombard JH. Pressure-diuresis in volume-expanded rats: cortical and medullary hemodynamics. *Hypertension* 1988;12:168–176.

52. Garcia-Estañ J, Roman RJ. Role of renal interstitial hydrostatic pressure in the pressure diuresis response. *Am J Physiol* 1989;256:F63–F70.

53. Khraibi AA, Haas JA, Knox FG. Effect of renal perfusion pressure on renal interstitial hydrostatic pressure in rats. *Am J Physiol* 1989;256:F165–F170.

54. Carmines PK, Bell PD, Roman RJ, Work J, Navar LG. Prostaglandins in the sodium excretory response to altered renal arterial pressure in dogs. *Am J Physiol* 1985;248:F8–F14.

55. Gonzales-Campoy JM, Long C, Roberts D, Berndt TJ, Romero JC, Knox FG. Renal interstitial hydrostatic pressure and PGE_2 in pressure natriuresis. *Am J Physiol* 1991;260:F643–F649.

56. Salom MG, Lahera V, Guardiola F, Romero JC. Blockade of pressure natriuresis induced by the inhibition of renal synthesis of nitric oxide in dogs. *Am J Physiol* 1992;262:F718–F722.

57. Lahera V, Salom MG, Miranda-Guardiola F, Moncada S, Romero JC. Effects of N^G-nitro-L-arginine methylester on renal function and blood pressure. *Am J Physiol* 1991;261:F1033–F1037.

58. Salazar FJ, Pinilla JM, Alberola A, Romero JC, Quesada T. Salt-induced increase in blood pressure during chronic inhibition of EDRF synthesis [abstract]. *Hypertension* 1991;18:387.

59. Alberola A, Pinilla JM, Quesada T, Romero JC, Salom FJ, Salazar FJ. Role of nitric oxide in mediating renal response to volume expansion. *Hypertension* 1992;19:780–784.

60. Atucha NM, Ramirez A, Quesada T, Garcia-Estañ J. Effects of nitric oxide inhibition on rat renal papillary blood flow response to volume expansion. *Clin Sci (in press)*.

61. Ito S, Johnson CS, Carretero OA. Modulation of angiotensin II-induced vasoconstriction by endothelium-derived relaxing factor in the isolated microperfused rabbit afferent arteriole. *J Clin Invest* 1991;87(5):1656–1663.

62. DeNicola L, Blantz RC, Gabbai FB. Nitric oxide and angiotensin II. Glomerular and tubular interaction in the rat. *J Clin Invest* 1992;89(4):1248–1256.

63. Sigmon DH, Carretero OA, Beierwaltes WH. Angiotensin-dependence of endothelium-mediated renal hemodynamics. *Hypertension (in press)*.

64. Pollack DM, Polakowski JS, Divish BJ, Opgenorth UJ. Angio-

tensin blockade reverses hypertension during long term nitric oxide synthetase inhibition. *Hypertension* 1993;21:660–666.

65. Hall JE. Renal function in one-kidney, one-clip hypertension and low renin essential hypertension. *Am J Hypertens* 1991;4:523S–533S.

66. Olesen S-P, Clapham DE, Davies PF. Haemodynamic shear stress activates a K^+ current in vascular endothelial cells. *Nature (Lond)* 1988;331:168–170.

67. Baer PG. The contribution of prostaglandins to renal blood flow maintenance is determined by the level of activity of the renin-angiotensin system. *Life Sci* 1981;28:587–593.

68. Blasingham MC, Nasjletti A. Differential renal effects of cyclooxygenase inhibition in sodium-replete and sodium-deprived dog. *Am J Physiol* 1980;239:F360–F365.

69. DeForrest JM, Davis JO, Freeman RH, et al. Effects of indomethacin and meclofenamate on renin release and renal hemodynamic function during chronic sodium depletion in conscious dogs. *Circ Res* 1980;47:99–107.

70. Donker AJM, Arisz L, Brentjens JRH, van der Hem GK, Hollemans HJG. The effect of indomethacin on kidney function and plasma renin activity in man. *Nephron* 1976;17:288–296.

71. Campbell WB, Gomez-Sanchez CE, Adams BV, Schmitz JM, Itskovitz HD. Attenuation of angiotensin II- and III-induced aldosterone release by prostaglandin synthesis inhibitors. *J Clin Invest* 1979;64:1552–1557.

72. Ruilope LM, Robles RG, Paya C, et al. Effects of long-term treatment with indomethacin on renal function. *Hypertension* 1986;8:677–684.

73. Romero JC, Bentley MD, Vanhoutte PM, Knox FG. Intrarenal mechanisms that regulate sodium excretion in relationship to changes in blood pressure. *Mayo Clin Proc* 1989;64:1406–1424.

74. Salom MG, Lahera V, Fenoy FJ, Roman R, Romero JC. Role of endothelium-derived relaxing factor (EDRF) in the renal response to changes in renal perfusion pressure [abstract]. *J Am Soc Nephrol* 1990;1:670.

75. Imig JD, Roman RJ. Nitric oxide modulates vascular tone in preglomerular arterioles. *Hypertension* 1992;19:770–774.

76. Blackshear JL, Spielman WS, Knox FG, Romero JC. Dissociation of renin release and renal vasodilation by prostaglandin synthesis inhibitors. *Am J Physiol* 1979;237:F20–F24.

77. Carmines PK, Bell PD, Roman RJ, Work J, Navar LG. Prostaglandins in the sodium excretory response to altered renal arterial pressure in dogs. *Am J Physiol* 1985;248:F8–F14.

78. Schnermann J, Briggs JP. Participation of renal cortical prostaglandins in the regulation of glomerular filtration rate. *Kidney Int* 1981;19:802–805.

79. Dunn MJ, Sambraski EJ. Renal effects of drugs that inhibit prostaglandin synthesis. *Kidney Int* 1980;18:609–622.

80. Fray JCS, Lush DJ, Park CS. Interrelationship of blood flow, juxtaglomerular cells, and hypertension: role of physical equilibrium and Ca. *Am J Physiol* 1986;251:R643–R662.

81. Cohen AJ, Fray JCS. Calcium dependence of myogenic renal plasma flow autoregulation: evidence from the isolated perfused rat kidney. *J Physiol (Lond)* 1982;330:449–460.

82. Boulanger C, Vidal-Ragout M, Fiksen-Olsen M, Romero JC, Vanhoutte PM. Cultured endothelial cells release a non-prostanoid inhibitor of renin release [abstract]. *Clin Res* 1988;36:539A.

83. Vidal MJ, Romero JC, Vanhoutte PM. Endothelium-derived relaxing factor inhibits renin release. *Eur J Pharmacol* 1988;149:401–402.

84. Henrich WL, McAllister EA, Smith PB, Campbell WB. Guanosine 3′-5′-cyclic monophosphate as a mediator of inhibition of renin release. *Am J Physiol* 1988;255:F474–F478.

85. Beierwaltes WH, Carretero OA. Nonprostanoid endothelium-derived factors inhibit renin release. *Hypertension* 1992;19 (Suppl 2):II68–II73.

86. Kurtz A, Kaissling B, Busse R, Baier W. Endothelial cells modulate renin secretion from isolated mouse juxtaglomerular cells. *J Clin Invest* 1991;88:1147–1154.

87. Sigmon DH, Carretero OA, Beierwaltes WH. Endothelium-derived relaxing factor regulates release *in vivo. Am J Physiol* 1992;263:F256–F261.

88. Lahera V, Khraibi AA, Romero JC. Potentiation of the hypotensive effect of acetylcholine by sulfhydryl (SH) group donors [abstract]. *Kidney Int* (submitted).

89. Johnson RA, Freeman RH. Pressure natriuresis in rats during blockade of the L-arginine/nitric oxide pathway. *Hypertension* 1992;19:333–338.

90. Johnson RA, Freeman RH. Sustained hypertension in the rat induced by chronic blockade of nitric oxide production. *Am J Hypertens* 1992;5:919–922.

91. Gardes J, Poux J-M, Gonzalez M-F, Alhenc-Gelas F, Menard J. Decreased renin release and constant kallikrein secretion after injection of L-NAME in isolated perfused rat kidney. *Life Sci* 1992;50:987–993.

92. Münter K, Hackenthal E. The participation of the endothelium in the control of renin release. *J Hypertens* 1991;9(Suppl 6): S236–S237.

93. Bolger PM, Eisner GM, Ramwell PW, Slotkoff LM, Corey EJ. Renal actions of prostacyclin. *Nature (Lond)* 1978;271:467–469.

94. Gerber JG, Branch RA, Nies AS, Gerkins JF, Hollifield JW. Prostaglandins and renin release. II. Assessment of renin secretion following infusion of PGI_2, E_2, and D_2 into the renal artery of anesthetized dogs. *Prostaglandins* 1978;15:81–88.

95. Seymour AA, Davis JO, Freeman RH, DeForrest JM, Rowe BP, Williams GM. Renin release from filtering and nonfiltering kidneys stimulated by PGI_2, and PGD_2. *Am J Physiol* 1982;243: F276–F283.

96. Weber PC, Larsson C, Anggard E, et al. Stimulation of renin release from rabbit renal cortex by arachidonic acid and prostaglandin endoperoxides. *Circ Res* 1976;39:868–874.

97. Whorton AR, Misono K, Hollifield J, Frolich JC, Inagami T, Oates JA. Prostaglandins and renin release. I. Stimulation of renin release from rabbit renal cortical slices by PGI_2. *Prostaglandins* 1977;14:1095–1104.

98. Beierwaltes WH, Schryver S, Sanders E, Strand J, Romero JC. Renin release selectively stimulated by prostaglandin I_2 in isolated rat glomeruli. *Am J Physiol* 1982;243:F276–F283.

99. Schryver S, Sanders E, Beierwaltes WH, Romero JC. Cortical distribution of prostaglandin and renin in isolated dog glomeruli. *Kidney Int* 1984;25:512–518.

100. Herman CA, Zenser TV, Davis BB. Comparison of the effects of prostaglandin I_2 and prostaglandin E_2 stimulation of rat kidney adenylate cyclase-cyclic AMP system. *Biochim Biophys Acta* 1979;582:496–503.

101. Henrich WL, Campbell WB. Relationship between PG and β-adrenergic pathways to renin release in rate renal cortical slices. *Am J Physiol* 1984;247:E343–E348.

102. Henrich WL, Campbell WB. Importance of calcium in renal renin release. *Am J Physiol* 1986;251:E98–E103.

103. Shoback DM, Williams GH, Moore TJ, Dluhy RG, Podolsky S, Hollenberg NK. Defect in the sodium-modulated tissue responsiveness to angiotensin II in essential hypertension. *J Clin Invest* 1983;72:2115–2124.

104. Hollenberg NK, Moore T, Shoback D, Redgrave J, Rabinowe S, Williams GH. Abnormal renal sodium handling in essential hypertension: relation to failure of renal and adrenal modulation of responses to angiotensin II. *Am J Med* 1986;8:412–418.

105. Lahera V, Salazar J, Salom MG, Romero JC. Deficient production of nitric oxide induces volume-dependent hypertension. *J Hypertens* 1992;10:S173–S177.

106. Wilcox CS, Welch WJ, Murad F, et al. Nitric oxide synthase in macula densa regulates glomerular capillary pressure. *Proc Natl Acad Sci* 1992;7:743–749.

107. Schnermann J, Briggs JP. Function of the juxtaglomerular apparatus: control of glomerular hemodynamics and renian secretion. In: Seldin DW, Giebisch G, eds. *The kidney.* New York: Raven Press; 1992:1249–1289.

108. Harder DR, Gilbert R, Lombard JH. Vascular muscle cell depolarization and activation in renal arteries on elevation of transmural pressure. *Am J Physiol* 1987;253:F778–F781.

109. Cowley AW. Long-term control of arterial blood pressure. *Physiol Rev* 1992;72:231–278.

110. Baylis C, Brenner BM. The physiologic determinant of glmerular ultrafiltration. *Rev Physiol Biochem Pharmacol* 1978;80:1–46.

111. Blantz RC, Tucker BJ. Determinants of peritubular capillary fluid uptake in hydropenia and saline and plasma expansion. *Am J Physiol* 1975;228:1927–1935.

112. Deen WM, Robertson CR, Brenner BM. A model of peritubular

capillary control of isotonic fluid reabsorption by the renal proximal tubule. *Biophys J* 1973;3:340–358.

113. Boulpaep EL. Permeability changes of the proximal tubule of necturus during saline loading. *Am J Physiol* 1972;222:517–531.

114. Landwehr DM, Schnermann J, Klose RM, Giebisch G. Effect of reduction in filtration rate on ranal tubular sodium and water reabsorption. *Am J Physiol* 1968;215:687–695.

115. Giebish G, Klose RM, Windhager EE. Micropuncture study of hypertonic sodium chloride loading in the rat. *Am J Physiol* 1964;206:687–693.

116. Blythe WB, Welt LG. Dissociation between filtered load of sodium and its rate of excretion in the urine. *J Clin Invest* 1963;42:1491–1496.

117. Kamm DR, Levinsky NG. Inhibition of renal tubular sodium reabsorption by hypernatremia. *J Clin Invest* 1965;44:1144–1150.

118. Nashat FS, Tappin JW, Wilcox CS. Plasm sodium concentration and sodium excretion in the anesthetized dog. *J Physiol (Lond)* 1976;254:183–202.

119. Puschett JB, Goldstein S, Godshall S, Staum BB, Goldberg M. Effects of filtration rate and plasma sodium concentration on proximal sodium transport. *Am J Physiol* 1971;221:788–794.

120. Toussaint VA, Verestraeten V. Renal tubular trosport in the dog. *Experientia* 1960;16:309–311.

121. Wesson LG, Anslow WP. Relationship of changes in glomerular filtration, plasma chloride and bicarbonate concentration and urinary osmotic load to renal excretion of chloride. *Am J Physiol* 1955;180:237–248.

122. Bresler EH, Nielson DT, Miller MC, Stroud MR. Renal tubular resbsorptive response to hypernatremia. *Am J Physiol* 1976;231:642–649.

123. Kady NN, Nashat FS, Tappin JW, Wilcox CS. Glomerulotubular balance in the whole kidney of the anesthetized doge during infusion of hypertonic saline. *J Physiol (Lond)* 1974;242:114–116P.

124. Schultz I, Ullrich KJ, Fromter E, Holzgreve H, Frick A, Hegel U. Mikropunktion und elektrische Potentialmessung an Schweissdrusen des Menschen. *Pfluger Arch* 1965;284:360–372.

125. Stein RM, Bercovitch DD, Levitt MF. Dual effects of saline loading on renal tubular sodium reabsorption in the dog. *Am J Physiol* 1964;207:826–834.

126. Brenner MD, Troy JL, Daugherty TM. On the mechanism of inhibition in fluid reabsorption by the renal proximal tubule of the volume expanded rate. *J Clin Invest* 1971;50:1596–1602.

127. Daugharty TM, Ueki IF, Nicholas DP, Brenner BM. Renal response to chronic intravenous salt loading in the rat. *J Clin Invest* 1973;52:21–31.

128. Daughtery TM, Ueki IF, Nicholas DP, Brenner BM. Comparative renal effects of isoonocotic and colloid-free volume expansion in the rat. *Am J Physiol* 1972;222:225–235.

129. Brenner BM, Troy JL. Postglomerular vascular protein concentration: evidence for a causal role in governing fluid reabsorption and glomerulotubular balance by the renal porxiam tubule. *J Clin Invest* 1971;40:336–349.

130. Green R, Windhager EE, Giebisch G. Protein oncotic pressure effects on proximal tubular fluid movement in the rat. *Am J Physiol* 1974;226:265–276.

131. Spitzer A, Windhager EE. Effect of peritubular oncotic pressure changes on proximal tubular fluid reabsorption. *Am J Physiol* 1970;218:118–119.

132. Blantz RC, Tucker BJ. Determinants of peritubular capillary fluid uptake in hydropenia and saline and plasma expansion. *Am J Physiol* 1976;228:1927–1935.

133. Ott CE. Effect of saline expansion on peritubular capillary pressures and reabsorption. *Am J Physiol* 1981;240:F106–F110.

134. Quinn MD, Marsh DJ. Peritubular capillary control of proximal tubular reabsorption in the rat. *Am J Physiol* 1979;236:F478–F487.

135. Tucker BJ, Blantz RC. Determinants of proximal tubular reabsorption as mechanisms of glomerulotubular balance. *Am J Physiol* 1978;325:F142–F150.

136. Windhager EE. Sodium chloride transport in membrane transport. In: Giebisch G, ed. *Biology.* Vol IV. *Transport organ.* Berlin: Springer-Verlag; 1979:145–214.

137. Sakin H, Boulpaep EL. Models for coupling of salt and water transport and proximal tubular reabsorption in nectrues kidney. *J Gen Physiol* 1979;66:671–733.

138. Granger JP. Regulation of sodium excretion by renal interstitial hydrostatic pressure. *Fed Proc* 1986;45:1892–1896.

139. Wilcox CS, Sterzel B, Bunckel PT, Mohrmann M, Perfetto M. Renal interstitial pressure and sodium excretion during hilar lymphatic ligation. *Am J Physiol* 1984;247:F344–F351.

140. Granger JP, Haas JA, Pawlowska D, Knox FG. Effect of diuretic increases in renal interstitial hydrostatic pressure on sodium excretion. *Am J Physiol* 1988;254:F527–F532.

141. Haas JA, Granger JP, Knox FG. Effect of direct increase in renal interstitial hydrostaic pressure on superficial and deep proximal sodium reabsorption. *Fed Proc* 1987;46(a).

142. Fitzgibbons JP, Gennari HB, Garfinkel HB, Cortell S. Dependence of saline-induced natriuresis upon exposure of the kidney to the physical effects of extracellular fluid volume expansion. *J Clin Invest* 1974;54:1428–1436.

143. Gennari JJ, Lefavour GS, Caflisch CR, Spevak S, Cotrell S. Identification of two components in the natriuretic response to saline loading in the rat. *Am J Physiol* 1978;235:F126–F130.

144. Osgood RW, Lameire NH, Sorkin MI, Stein JH. Effect of aortic clamping on proximal reabsorption and sodium excretion in the rat. *Am J Physiol* 1977;232:F92–F96.

145. DeWardener HW, Mills IH, Clapham WF, Hayter CJ. Studies on the efferent mechanism of the sodium diuresis which follows the administration of intravenous saline in the dog. *Clin Sci* 1961;21:249–258.

146. Ichikawa I, Brenner BM. Mechanism of inhibition of proximal tubule fluid reabsorption after exposure of the rat kidney to the physical effects of expansion of extracellular fluid volume. *J Clin Invest* 1980;64:1466–1464.

147. Haberle DA, Shiigai T. Flow-dependent volume reabsorption in the proximal convolution of the rat kidney. The role of glomerular-borne tubular fluid for the maintenance of glomerulotubular blance. In: Vogel HG, Ullrich KJ, eds. *New aspects of renal function.* Amsterdam: Excerpta Medica; 1978:198–202.

148. Haberle DA, Muller U, Nagel W. Glomerular tubular balance: mediation by luminal hypotonicity. *Miner Electrolyte Meta* 1989;15:108–113.

149. Pawlowska D, Haas JA, Granger JP, Romero JC, Knox FG. Prostaglandin blockade blunts the natriuresis of elevated renal interstitial pressure. *Am J Physiol* 1988;254:F507–F511.

150. Long CR, Berndt TJ, Haas JA, Knox FG. Effect of saline volume expansion (VE) on the paracellular backflux of ions in the mammalian proximal tubule (PT) [abstract]. *FASEB J* 1993;7:A13.

151. Chou CL, Marsh DU. Role of proximal csonvoluted tubule in pressure diuresis in the rat. *Am J Physiol* 1986;251:F283–F289.

152. Chou CL, Marsh DU. Time course of proximal tubule response to acute arterial hypertension in the rat. *Am J Physiol* 1988;254:F601–F607.

153. Haas JA, Granger JP, Knox FG. Effect of renal perfusion pressure on sodium reabsorption from proximal tubules of superficial and deep nephrons. *Am J Physiol* 1986;250:F425–F429.

154. Kiil R. Principles of sodium and water reabsorption in the proximal convoluted tubules of the kidney. *Scand J Clin Lab Invest* 1988;38:1–6.

155. Roman RJ. Pressure-diuresis in volume-expanded rats. Tubular reabsorption in superficial and deep nephrons. *Hypertension* 1988;12:177–183.

156. Gonzalez-Campoy JM, Kachelski J, Burnett JC Jr, Romero JC, Granger JP, Knox FG. Proximal tubule response in aldosterone escape. *Am J Physiol* 1989;256:R86–R90.

157. Gonzalez-Campoy JM, Romero JC, Knox FG. Escape from the sodium-retaining effects of mineralocorticoids: role of ANF and intrarenal hormone systems. *Kidney Int* 1989;35:767–777.

158. Hall JE, Granger JP, Smith MJ, Preman AS. Role of renal hemodynamics and arterial pressure in aldosterone escape. *Hypertension* 1984;6:I183–I192.

159. Pearson PJ. *Mechanism of coronary vasospasm following reperfusion injury: role of vasoactive factors produced by the endothelium* [Thesis]. Rochester, Minnesota: Mayo Graduate School of Medicine, 1991.

Hypertension: Pathophysiology, Diagnosis, and Management, Second Edition,
edited by J.H. Laragh and B.M. Brenner,
Raven Press, Ltd., New York © 1995.

CHAPTER 84

Nephron Heterogeneity with Unsuppressible Renin Secretion: A Cause of Essential Hypertension[1]

Jean E. Sealey, Jon D. Blumenfeld, Gordon M. Bell, Mark S. Pecker, Sheldon C. Sommers, and John H. Laragh

The kidney plays a central role in blood pressure regulation in two general ways (1–3). Its excretory function determines body sodium content. At the same time, via an interrelated endocrine function, the kidney determines the rate of renin secretion into the circulation. To regulate this latter process, the kidney continuously perceives the amount of sodium chloride delivered to the macula

densa region of the distal tubule of each individual nephron, while renal arteriolar baroreceptors from the same nephron sense and respond to changes in arteriolar perfusion pressure (4,5). These two signals are fundamental determinants of the rate of renin secretion.

Renal afferent arteriolar vasoconstriction is the pathophysiological change that is the hallmark of essential hypertension (2,3,6–8). However, the contribution of this lesion to the pathogenesis of essential hypertension is not well defined. In this chapter we present a new perception of the pathogenesis of essential hypertension and of the renal basis for it, which has evolved from our research and longstanding interest in this problem. We propose that, in essential hypertension, there is a subpopulation of nephrons that is ischemic from either afferent arteriolar vasoconstriction or from an intrinsic narrowing of

---

J. E. Sealey, J. D. Blumenfeld, G. M. Bell, M. S. Pecker, S. C. Sommers, and J. H. Laragh: Cardiovascular Center, New York Hospital–Cornell Medical Center, New York, New York 10021.

[1] Updated from *Journal of Hypertension* 1988;6(10):763–777, with permission. Presented in part as the Presidential Address. International Society of Hypertension, Kyoto, May 1988.

the lumen. Renin secretion from this subgroup of nephrons is tonically elevated. This increased renin secretion then interferes with the compensatory capacity of intermingled normal nephrons to adaptively excrete sodium and, consequently, perturbs overall blood pressure homeostasis.

This new analytical model is based on observations that:

1. all active plasma renin originates from the kidneys (9–11),
2. each individual nephron secretes renin at a rate primarily determined by its own macula densa and baroreceptor detectors (12,13), and
3. the level of renin in the blood is the integrated sum of the secretion of renin from all the individual nephrons (14).

HYPOTHESIS: NEPHRON HETEROGENEITY IN ESSENTIAL HYPERTENSION

We hypothesize that there is nephron heterogeneity in essential hypertension in which two different populations of nephrons are intermingled (Table 1).

There is one population of ischemic nephrons with reduced perfusion pressure, reduced blood flow, and reduced glomerular filtration rate (GFR). These nephrons have tonically elevated renin release for two reasons. First, baroreceptors in the afferent arteriole, downstream from the arteriolar constriction, are underperfused and do not appropriately perceive the systemic hypertension. Second, their filtered load and distal delivery of NaCl are decreased as a result of a reduction in GFR and reduced peritubular capillary hydrostatic pressure. In response to this unchecked renin release and impaired sodium excretion by the dysfunctioning nephrons, arterial pressure rises. The second population, consisting of normal nephrons, then undergoes an adaptive response to the increased systemic arterial perfusion pressure, which results in increased glomerular and postglomerular hydraulic pressures and increased delivery of NaCl to the macula densa (and to the final urine). These several effects result in chronic suppression of renin secretion from the previously normal nephrons. The consequence is that both of these populations of nephrons are exposed to inappropriate levels of angiotensin II. This impairs sodium excretion for several reasons (see Table 1). Because the final plasma renin level is diluted downward by noncontribution from the large population of adapting nephrons, the ischemic nephrons actually receive amounts of renin and angiotensin II that are inadequate to fully maintain GFR by efferent constriction. At the same time, the circulating renin-angiotensin level is inappropriately high for the normal nephrons, and it interferes with their adaptive hypernatriuresis. Angiotensin II acts on these nephrons to:

1. enhance tubular sodium reabsorption, and
2. promote tubuloglomerular feedback (TGF)-mediated afferent vasoconstriction.

Hyperfiltering nephrons have increased proximal tubular sodium reabsorption as a result of the relative excess of renin and angiotensin. In addition, the hyperfiltering nephrons are not exposed to the full force of the arterial pressure; this is because of inappropriate augmentation of TGF by angiotensin II (afferent constriction), as discussed below.

Most patients with essential hypertension do not have overtly reduced renal function. Therefore, it is likely that most of their nephrons are not ischemic and that their nephron number is not unduly reduced, so that they may participate in the adaptive hypernatriuretic response mode. However, a reduction in nephron number related to either age (15) or ischemia could amplify the impaired sodium excretion and promote hypertension (see also Chapter 72).

TABLE 1. *Hypothesis: there is nephron heterogeneity in essential hypertension*

1. There are ischemic nephrons with impaired sodium excretion intermingled with adapting hyperfiltering hypernatriuretic nephrons.
2. Renin secretion is high from ischemic nephrons and very low from hyperfiltering nephrons.
3. The inappropriate circulating renin-angiotensin level impairs sodium excretion because:
   a. In the adapting hypernatriuretic nephrons:
      i. it increases tubular sodium reabsorption and
      ii. it enhances TGF-mediated afferent constriction.
   b. As the circulating renin level is diluted by nonparticipation of adapting nephrons, it becomes inadequate to support efferent tone in hypoperfused nephrons
4. A loss of nephron number with age and from ischemia further impairs sodium excretion.

STRUCTURAL EVIDENCE FOR NEPHRON HETEROGENEITY IN ESSENTIAL HYPERTENSION

In their classic studies (6–8), Sommers and his associates identified afferent arteriolar narrowing as the hallmark renal vascular lesion of uncomplicated essential hypertension (Fig. 1). For their analysis of approximately 1,800 renal biopsy specimens from patients with essential hypertension, a grading system was designed according to the degree of arteriolar thickening or sclerosis, with higher grades representing more luminal narrowing. Focal spasm of afferent arterioles, with an abnormal concentric overlapping of otherwise apparently normal smooth muscle cells, was found in all but one specimen in the lowest grade group. This lesion was not present

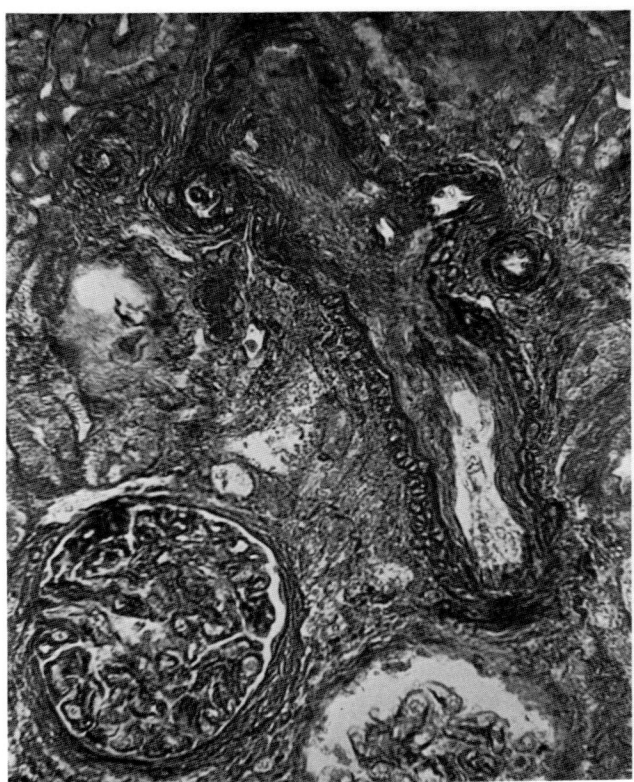

FIG. 1. Variation in the degree of local thickening of larger renal arterioles, with localized collagen deposits, shown as gray fibrillar material. Grade III renal arteriosclerosis. Masson stain ×87. (From ref. 6.)

in a control series of renal biopsies from normotensive subjects. With increasing grades, afferent arteriolar lesions that were observed included endothelial edema, with bulging into a narrowed lumen; vascular smooth cell hypertrophy and widening of the internal elastic lamina, with deposition of PAS-positive material; and degenerative changes and hyalinization, with irregular and focal luminal narrowing.

In typical human Goldblatt-type hypertension, nephrons in the stenotic kidney have diminished blood flow and are exposed to reduced perfusion pressure. As a consequence, the juxtaglomerular cells that produce renin become hyperplastic and heavily granulated (8). These morphological changes in the Goldblatt kidney are correlated with elevated plasma renin activity and with the characteristic renin-dependent hypertension. The contralateral kidney, which is unclipped and therefore exposed to elevated perfusion pressure, does not exhibit hyperplastic changes of juxtaglomerular cells. In addition, renin secretion by that kidney is markedly suppressed.

It follows that if the focal renal afferent arteriolar lesion characteristic of essential hypertension produces ischemia and enhanced renin secretion by some nephrons, while other normal nephrons have augmented re-

nal blood flow and suppressed renin secretion, then a situation analogous to Goldblatt hypertension would occur. This conclusion is supported by the observation of Turgeon and Sommers (8) that, in kidneys of patients with essential hypertension, juxtaglomerular cells are significantly hyperplastic. This was most marked when significant arteriolar thickening was present. Furthermore, only 8 percent of glomeruli were obsolescent in patients with uncomplicated essential hypertension, supporting the clinical observation that significant nephron loss and overt renal insufficiency are not major contributing factors in the pathogenesis of the disease. Thus, we propose that essential hypertension is a consequence of a particular heterogeneity in individual nephron function.

ABNORMAL PATTERNS OF RENIN SECRETION IN ESSENTIAL HYPERTENSION AND THEIR RELEVANCE TO PATHOGENESIS

Plasma renin activity varies inversely in relation to dietary sodium intake. This relationship is determined by changes in macula densa sodium chloride load that stimulate or suppress renin secretion. In Fig. 2 (16), the dashed lines define the normal relationship of renin activity to 24-hrs sodium excretion, the latter being used as an index of sodium intake. In normotensive people, plasma renin activity is very low when salt intake is high. Conversely, when salt is in short supply, renin activity rises sharply. These changes in renin, in normal subjects, offset any effects of accompanying volume expansion or contraction so that blood pressure does not change significantly during wide variations in salt intake. Thus, at high levels of sodium intake, renin is not required for blood pressure maintenance. However, as sodium becomes less available, plasma renin plays a correspondingly important role in sustaining normal levels of blood pressure. In normal subjects the baroreceptor effect on renin release is possibly unimportant because macula densa–mediated changes in renin release operate to maintain normal blood pressure.

Essential hypertensive patients exhibit an abnormally wide splay of renin activity in relation to the state of urinary sodium excretion (16) (Fig. 2). Among patients with hypertension, approximately 30 percent have renin levels that are lower than expected, 50 percent fall within the normal range, and about 20 percent have high plasma renin activity. The questions we would like to address are:

1. Why do hypertensive patients exhibit such a wide range of renin levels?
2. Can our understanding of the mechanisms that determine renin release give us an insight into the underlying pathophysiological mechanisms at work in essential hypertension?

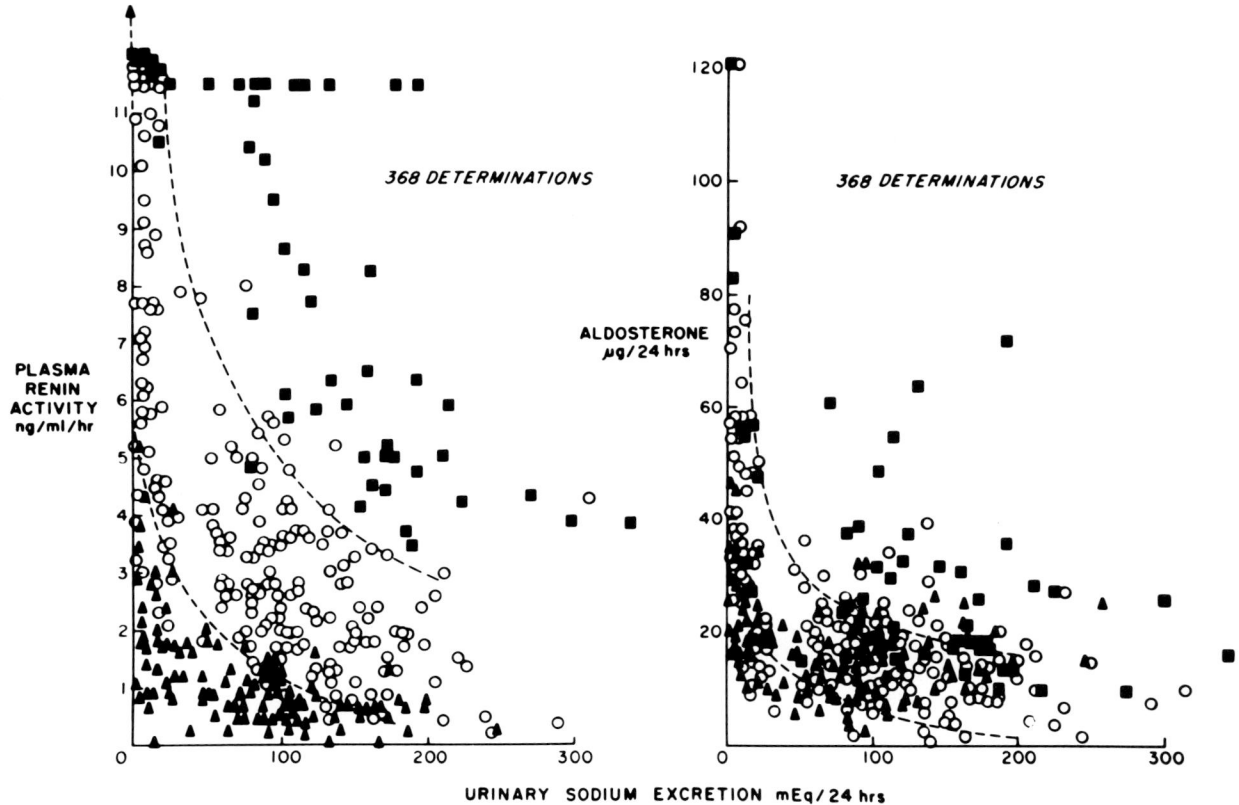

FIG. 2. Relation of the noon ambulatory plasma renin activity (**A**) and of the corresponding daily urinary aldosterone excretion (**B**) to the concurrent daily rate of urinary sodium excretion. The dashed lines define the normal channel derived from the study of normotensive people. A total of 219 patients with untreated essential hypertension were studied, some on several occasions at different levels of sodium intake. ▲, low-renin essential hypertension; ○, normal-renin essential hypertension; ■, high-renin essential hypertension. Three major subgroups are defined by the appropriateness or normality of the plasma renin activity in relation to the rate of sodium excretion, which is used as an index of dietary intake and of sodium balance. Additional abnormal subgroups are defined when aldosterone is included in the analysis. (From ref. 16.) Plasma renin activity results are expressed as nanograms: Angiotension l/ml/hr. Multiply PRA values shown in the figure by 0.64 to conform to the National Bureau of Standards Angiotension I reference standard. (This also applies to Fig. 3 and Fig. 5.)

From the relationship of renin activity and sodium intake and excretion described above for normal subjects, it can be presumed that the low-renin subgroup of hypertensive patients has chronically suppressed renin secretion as a result of an elevated blood pressure, which, in turn, is related to an increased total body sodium. Other support for this conclusion comes from observations that low-renin patients with essential hypertension often become normotensive after dietary or diuretic-induced salt depletion (17). Moreover, the relative lack of renin dependency of this form of hypertension is illustrated by its generally poor response to therapies that block the renin system, such as converting-enzyme inhibitors (18).

In contrast, patients with high-renin hypertension, and even those with "normal"-renin hypertension, have a marked antihypertensive response to converting-enzyme inhibition (18–21). Figure 3 illustrates the re-

sponse of blood pressure in patients with essential hypertension 1 hr after administration of a converting-enzyme inhibitor, either intravenous teprotide (20) (89 patients) or oral captopril (18) (166 patients). It is apparent that when preexisting renin levels are very high, renin blockade produces a commensurate drop in blood pressure, but what is often not appreciated is that when plasma renin activity is within the *normal* range (1–10 ng/ml/ hr), converting-enzyme inhibition often has a considerable beneficial effect on blood pressure. These observations indicate that, in hypertension, even a *normal* level of renin is inappropriate, and they lead to the question of why the baroreceptor signal for renin release does not function appropriately in essential hypertension. As will be discussed below, a normal kidney exposed to high arterial hypertension will promptly turn off its renin secretion.

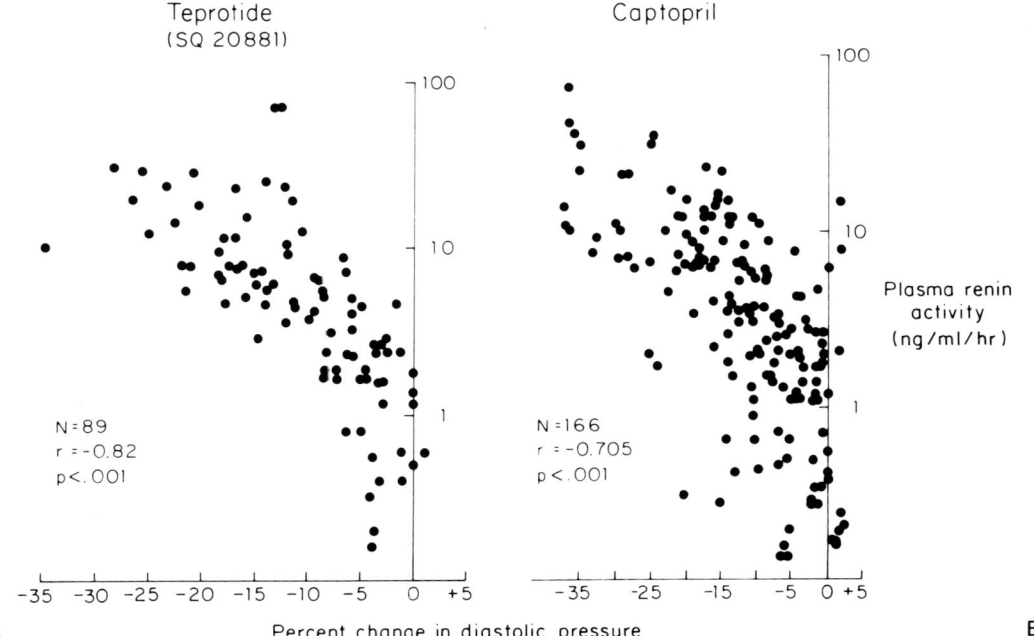

FIG. 3. The acute effects (at 90 min) of intravenous converting-enzyme inhibitors on diastolic blood pressure (DBP). With both drugs, the percentage fall in blood pressure is closely related to the pretreatment levels of plasma renin activity in quietly seated, untreated hypertensive patients. **A:** The effects of administering the nonapeptide isolated from snake venom, teprotide (SW 20881), intravenously to 89 patients; data are re-plotted from refs. 19 and 20. **B:** Changes in seated DBP 90 min after a single oral dose of captopril (25 mg) in 166 patients; data are re-plotted from refs. 18 and 21. Setting aside the errors in cuff pressure measurements, the data reveal remarkable and extremely similar correlations between the level of pretreatment plasma renin and the degree of the induced decrease in blood pressure. Note that patients with plasma renin values < 1.0 ng/ml/hr usually exhibited no change in pressure. The data in both panels also provide strong indirect evidence that the plasma renin value closely reflects the active role of renin in supporting arterial pressure in hypertensive individuals.

FUNCTIONAL EVIDENCE FOR NEPHRON HETEROGENEITY IN ESSENTIAL HYPERTENSION

The Renin-Secretory Response to Sodium Administration or Deprivation: Evidence for the Presence of a Subpopulation of Ischemic Nephrons

Functional evidence for nephron heterogeneity in essential hypertension derives from data demonstrating that the responses of renin secretion to changes in dietary sodium intake, to diuretic therapy, and to saline infusions in hypertensive patients can differ markedly from those observed in normal subjects. Our explanation for these variations is that ischemic nephrons perceive and respond to these interventions differently from the normal, adapting nephrons. Since the number and functional capacity of ischemic nephrons may differ among hypertensive patients, this leads to a heterogeneity in the renin response to a given signal among these patients that is not seen in normotensive subjects.

The Response to Changes in Dietary Sodium

In Fig. 4 (left panel) the plasma renin response to changes in the salt intake of normotensive subjects is compared to that of patients with essential hypertension, in studies performed in our Hypertension Center. The reference value of 100 percent represents the renin value for normal or hypertensive subjects with either low, medium, or high renin levels, at a medium level of salt intake. The values for normal subjects are shown by the open circles with the dashed lines. It is apparent that in normal subjects, plasma renin activity is suppressed by an average of 50 percent during a high-salt diet and increased by nearly 250 percent on a low-salt diet.

In contrast, patients with essential hypertension respond differently to both dietary sodium loading and deprivation. Patients in all three renin subgroups of essential hypertension show a blunted renin response to salt administration, so that even on very high salt intakes they do not suppress their renin secretion as much as normal subjects. On the other hand, during salt depriva-

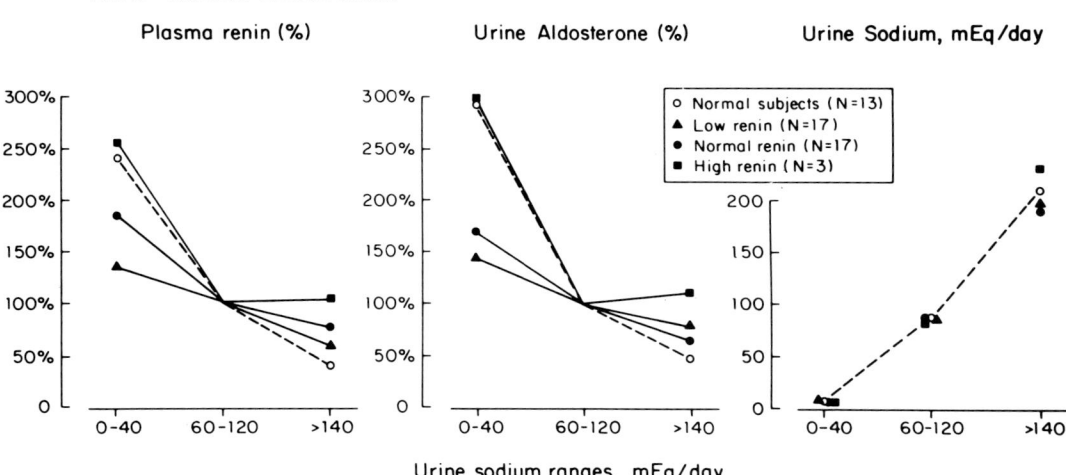

100% = medium sodium intake

FIG. 4. Effect of 5 days of low (10 mmol/liter), medium (100 mmol/liter), or high (200 mmol/liter) constant sodium intake on renin and aldosterone responsiveness and urinary sodium excretion under balanced ward conditions. The reference value of 100 percent represents the renin value for normal subjects (O, $n = 13$), as well as for hypertensive subjects with either low (▲, $n = 17$), normal (●, $n = 17$), or high (■, $n = 3$) renin levels, at a medium level of salt intake.

tion, both low- and medium-renin hypertensive patients exhibit attenuated plasma renin increases, and only the high-renin group appears to exhibit a normal increase in plasma renin activity. Changes in the 24-hr urinary aldosterone secretion parallel the plasma renin changes described above and, thus, verify these abnormal relationships (22). Accordingly, patients with essential hypertension exhibit failure to suppress aldosterone secretion on a high-salt diet and exhibit submaximal stimulation of aldosterone secretion on low-salt diets.

The Response to Diuretic-Induced Sodium Depletion

The plasma renin response to diuretic therapy in hypertensive patients also expresses heterogeneity of responsiveness. Figure 5 illustrates data from a study (23) in which hypertensive patients were treated with chlorthalidone. In this analysis the subjects were grouped as blood pressure responders (left side) or as nonresponders (right side). The responders showed a blunted plasma-renin-secretory response to sodium depletion, and this was associated with an attenuated aldosterone response. In fact, in this group of patients there was virtually no increase in aldosterone upon sodium depletion, very similar to the low-renin group (Fig. 4), who showed very little increase upon sodium deprivation. Conversely, those patients whose blood pressure did not respond to diuretic therapy were quite different. They exhibited striking aldosterone and renin responses, more like those of the high-renin hypertensives and the normal subjects on a low-sodium diet, as illustrated in Fig. 4. It can be deduced from such a study that it is the high renin and

high aldosterone levels that offset the sodium depletion associated with the diuretic, thereby preventing blood pressure from falling by converting an initially salt-supported blood pressure level to one supported by reactive renin secretion. This concept has been verified as follows (24): Hypertensive patients failing to reduce their blood pressure during drastic sodium depletion develop very high renin and aldosterone levels. This reactive renin sustains the hypertension because when a renin-system–blocking drug is given, blood pressure is promptly reduced to normal (24). Altogether, these data provide evidence for the heterogeneity of renin-secretory responsiveness in essential hypertension and its companion relevance to their blood pressure support.

Failure to Suppress Renin Secretion Normally During Acute Saline Infusion in Essential Hypertension

Recently, we have re-examined the relationship between renin secretion and sodium excretion in response to saline infusion in essential hypertension in ongoing studies conducted by Pecker et al. (25). The changes in plasma renin activity in normal subjects were compared to those of patients with essential hypertension after intravenous saline infusion (1 liter over a period of 30 min). The sensitivity of the renin-secretory mechanism to sodium excretion is illustrated in Fig. 6. Normal subjects exhibited a much greater drop in plasma renin activity per mmol/liter salt excreted than did either the low- or normal-renin essential hypertensive patients or those with renovascular hypertension. Thus, in patients with essential hypertension, renin secretion is not nor-

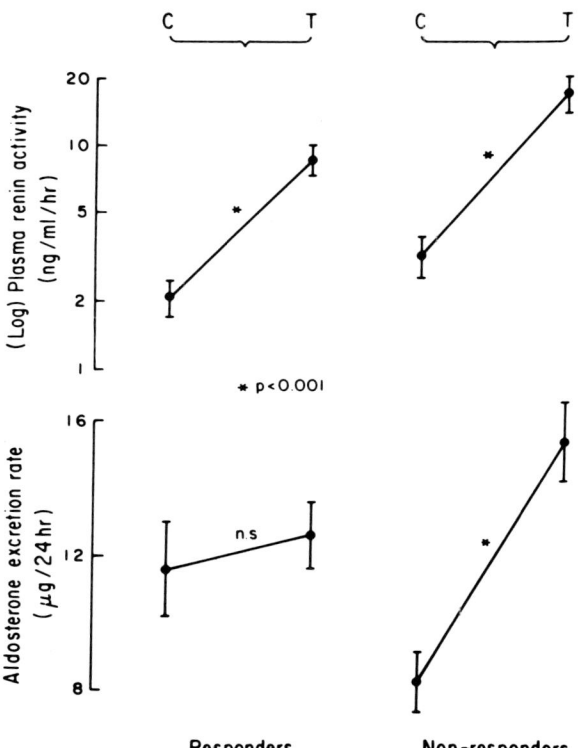

FIG. 5. Comparison of changes in aldosterone excretion and plasma renin activity in the responder and nonresponder groups during treatment. C, control; T, thiazide. (From ref. 23.)

mally suppressed in response to this provocative stimulus, just as it is not normally suppressed when dietary salt intake is increased.

The Pressor Role of the Plasma Angiotensinogen Level When Renin Secretion is Unsuppressible

Renal renin secretion is the only component of the renin system that is directly regulated by the factors that the renin system controls, i.e., blood pressure, renal perfusion pressure, and sodium excretion. However, renin substrate (angiotensinogen) circulates at concentrations that allow renin to generate angiotensin I (Ang I) at only half maximum velocity (26). It follows that, ceteris paribus, changes in the concentration of Aogn will directly affect the rate of Ang I formation (plasma renin activity). Nonetheless, *in vivo,* changes in plasma angiotensinogen do not normally alter PRA levels because renin secretion dynamically adjusts itself to maintain an appropriate rate of Ang II formation for the physiological setting. For example, when plasma angiotensinogen is increased as much as 5-fold by estrogen administration the concentration of renin in plasma falls commensurately, leaving plasma renin activity unchanged (26–28). Also, when plasma angiotensinogen levels are lowered in normal rats by anti-angiotensinogen antibodies blood pressure

falls only transiently (29), most likely because renin secretion increases commensurately to compensate.

In this context, plasma angiotensinogen levels can become the determinant of angiotensin II formation whenever renin secretion cannot suppress appropriately when angiotensinogen increases (30). That explains why some women develop hypertension when angiotensinogen rises during oral contraceptive or estrogen therapy (26,31). It may also be the reason for the increased blood pressure (BP) of people who have a genetic elevation in plasma angiotensinogen levels (32) and for the positive relationship between plasma angiotensinogen levels and BP in hypertensive blacks (33). To study this question we recently investigated if BP is positively related to plasma angiotensinogen in stroke prone spontaneously hypertensive (SHRsp) and Dahl S rats when their renin secretion becomes unsuppressible after 6 weeks of treatment with very high salt diets (34). These rats show no relationship between BP and angiotensinogen under conditions in which renin is normally regulated, i.e., during the first 4 weeks of very high salt diets. However, blood pressure does correlate with angiotensinogen levels in both SHRsp after 6 weeks of high salt diets, i.e., during the time when renin secretion is unsuppressed.

Altogether, the data suggest that angiotensinogen becomes rate limiting for angiotensin II formation whenever renin secretion is unsuppressible as occurs in the presence of nephron heterogeneity.

Hypernatriuresis and Abnormal Renin Responsiveness of Hypertensive Patients: Relation to the Concept of Nephron Heterogeneity and to Pathogenesis

Patients with essential hypertension respond to intravenous saline infusion with a natriuresis that is much

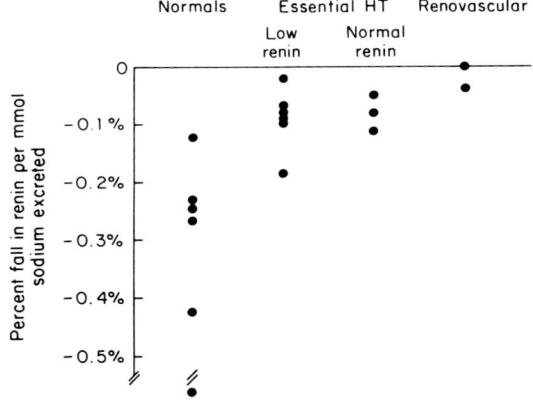

FIG. 6. Suppressibility of plasma renin level by isotonic saline infusion (1 liter in 30 min). The percent fall in the 60-min renin value is related to the absolute rate of sodium excretion between 30 and 60 min. Essential HT, essential hypertension.

more immediate and of much greater magnitude than that observed in normotensive subjects. This cardinal feature of essential hypertension was first recognized by Farnsworth (35), who demonstrated an enhanced chloriuretic response to saline infusion in hypertensive people. This phenomenon has since been verified repeatedly (36–41). However, the pathophysiological basis for this response has not been satisfactorily explained. It is clear that a high arterial pressure is a fundamental prerequisite, since the exaggerated natriuresis disappears with correction of the high blood pressure (42,43). The phenomenon can only partially be reproduced in normal subjects after massive prehydration (44).

The intrarenal changes accompanying the hypernatriuresis have been investigated. Using clearance techniques, Buckalew et al. (45) and Cannon (46) identified a defect in sodium transport in the loop of Henle in hypertensives that was apparent during extracellular fluid expansion. Buckalew et al. (45) found that in hypertensives infused with saline, both $T^c_{H_2O}$ and C_{H_2O} were blunted, indicating that sodium reabsorption in the loop of Henle was decreased at any given rate of distal delivery of sodium. These changes were similar to those described by Cannon (46), who found that C_{H_2O} was decreased at any rate of urine flow in hypertensive patients infused with dextrose rather than saline. An additional set of studies by Buckalew et al. (45) demonstrated that when distal sodium delivery was increased by treatment with acetazolamide without concurrent volume expansion, free water clearance did not differ between the hypertensive and normotensive subjects. Therefore, it was suggested that the abnormality in sodium transport in the loop represented some effect of acute extracellular volume expansion per se, rather than an intrinsic tubular defect of sodium reabsorption. These observations suggest that, during volume expansion in the hypertensive patient, arterial perfusion pressure may be transmitted to the postglomerular circulation, including the vasa recta. Such an increase in postglomerular hydraulic pressures would depress tubular sodium reabsorption throughout the nephron.

Other studies have suggested that additional factors may modulate the natriuretic response to saline infusion in hypertensives. In experimental animals, the wedged renal vein pressure (WRVP) has been shown to closely approximate postglomerular capillary pressures (47,48). Using this technique, Lowenstein et al. (49) investigated the renal hemodynamic basis for the exaggerated natriuresis in hypertensive patients. Prior to saline infusion, they found that WRVP was higher in patients with essential hypertension than in normotensive controls. Surprisingly, there was only a weak correlation between WRVP and mean arterial pressure, demonstrating a heterogeneity in the degree to which arterial pressure is transmitted into the peritubular capillaries in patients with essential hypertension. Interestingly, Lowenstein et

al. (49) were able to relate the degree of hypernatriuresis in hypertensive and normal subjects during saline infusion to the magnitude to which WRVP was increased. These workers proposed that the hypernatriuretic response to saline is induced by afferent arteriolar dilation, with resultant transmission of higher glomerular and postglomerular pressures. Those hypertensive patients not exhibiting such renal hemodynamic changes did not exhibit equivalent hypernatriuresis.

Other studies demonstrated that the heterogeneity of the response to saline infusion is a function of the renin status of the patient. In studying this problem, Krakoff et al. (50) first established that in some hypertensive patients, plasma renin levels were elevated in acute response to a furosemide-induced natriuresis, whereas in others they were not. As a group, the renin nonresponders exhibited lower basal plasma renin levels. Interestingly, the natriuretic response to volume expansion with isotonic saline in these two groups was quite different. The peak rates of sodium excretion and urine flow were more than twofold higher in those patients in whom renin failed to rise after furosemide. In the group that exhibited the lesser natriuresis, higher plasma renin levels were sustained during saline infusion. Altogether, these data suggest that in hypertensive patients, the plasma renin level, or a function related to it, tends to blunt full expression of the typical hypernatriuresis. Krakoff et al. (50) suggested that renin depletion of superficial cortical nephrons might permit hyperperfusion by those cortical glomeruli via redistribution of renal blood flow. In our current analysis we would suggest that in the renin nonresponders, the lack of renin response to furosemide and the hypernatriuretic response to saline infusion would be the result of a preponderance of hyperfiltering hypernatriuretic nephrons, in association with a very few ischemic nephrons and a minimal amount of renin to impair the natriuretic response.

Luft et al. (51) confirmed and extended the observation that the natriuretic response to saline infusion was related to renin status and showed that it was inversely related to the baseline plasma renin in both hypertensive and normal subjects. Participants were categorized according to their renin profile as normal, low, or high. In addition, patients with secondary hypertension (renovascular, primary hyperaldosteronism) were studied. These investigators noted a consistent inverse relationship between the degree of suppression of plasma renin activity and fractional excretion of sodium during saline infusion in patients with essential hypertension and renovascular hypertension and in normal subjects (38). The evidence links two central features of essential hypertension: (a) hypernatriuresis and (b) impaired renin suppressibility.

One other piece of evidence suggests that the presence of renin in some way blunts the natriuretic response to saline infusion. Patients with primary aldosteronism show a complete suppression of renin secretion (52), presumably with a normal preexisting nephron function and number. Saline infusion in these patients results in the very highest rate of sodium excretion (>4,000 mmol/liter/min) and fractional excretion of sodium (>3 percent) observed in any group of hypertensive subjects (52). These patients do not have ischemic nephrons or circulating renin. Therefore, there is no restriction of the degree to which the increased hydrostatic pressure can be transmitted into the peritubular capillaries. Therefore, in primary hyperaldosteronism, hypernatriuresis is most maximal in pace and magnitude.

Taken together, the evidence reviewed demonstrates that in hypertensive subjects receiving acute saline infusions, hypernatriuresis is associated with no change in arterial pressure, with renal vascular dilation, and with an unusual transmittal of hydrostatic pressure into the peritubular capillaries. The degree to which this occurs is related to the renin status. In our hypothesis, the blunting effect of renin on the hypernatriuresis is presumed to be due to unsuppressible renin secretion (and angiotensin formation) from an ischemic population of nephrons. These nephrons show afferent arteriolar narrowing (6–8). This lesion may be structurally fixed, or it may be reversible and due to vasospasm (54,55). Either of these cases would lead to attenuated transmission of the high hydrostatic pressure to the peritubular capillaries in these nephrons and a blunting of sodium excretion. Whatever the case, the fact that a considerable hypernatriuresis does occur in the large majority of hypertensive patients suggests, per se, that a sizeable number of nephrons are capable of adapting to the increased salt load. This supports our postulation of a second, probably relatively large group of adapting hypernatriuretic nephrons.

NORMAL MECHANISMS FOR RENAL RENIN RELEASE

These abnormal responses of renal sodium excretion and of renal renin secretion in essential hypertension to either long-term dietary salt loading or depletion and to acute saline infusion give rise to the following key questions:

1. What are the primary mechanisms for renal renin release?
2. How might their dysfunction explain the differences that occur in sodium excretion and renin secretion in patients with essential hypertension?

The two major intrarenal signals that elicit or suppress renal renin secretion (Table 2) are: (a) the distal tubular sodium chloride supply (5) and (b) the renal arterial perfusion pressure (4). These signals are perceived, respectively, in each nephron by a macula densa detector of

TABLE 2. *Major mechanisms of renin release*

Individual nephron signals:
Macula densa sodium chloride
Afferent anteriolar pressure
Whole-kidney modulating signals:
Angiotensin II feedback
β-receptor
Each individual nephron decides by itself how much renin to secrete, but all nephrons are then exposed to the same circulating renin level.

distal sodium chloride supply or transport and by a baroreceptor in its afferent arteriole. These two primary detectors then modify renin release via activation of local effectors in each nephron.

In addition, numerous signals to the whole kidney can modulate renin-secretory responses (1,56–58). The two most important are (a) the level of circulating plasma angiotensin II that feeds back (5) to suppress renin secretion and (b) β-adrenergic receptor activity, transmitted via the sympathetic nervous system, that enhances renin-secretory activity (5). Either withdrawal of sympathetic tone or β-receptor blockade will reduce total kidney renin secretion. This latter modulator does not play a primary role in the current theory.

We recognize herein a key feature of this control system—that the amount of renin secreted by individual nephrons is determined by two sensors located in each nephron rather than by the kidney as a whole. However, *all* nephrons are then collectively exposed via the renal artery to the *same* circulating renin and angiotensin II levels, generated from the sum total of renin secreted into the renal veins. This angiotensin II, generated in the circulation from plasma renin, then enters the renal artery and all nephrons become exposed equally to it.

THE MACULA DENSA MECHANISM

The macula densa detector–effector mechanism plays a central role in the regulation of renin secretion of each individual nephron and is, to a large degree, responsible for the modulation of renin secretion that occurs in response to changes in dietary sodium intake. The operation of this mechanism is illustrated by a study by Skott and Briggs (12). These investigators utilized a preparation in which they were able to perfuse a single isolated macula densa region, still connected to its juxtaglomerular apparatus. Renin secretion remained constant during continuous perfusion of the distal tubule with isotonic saline. However, upon switching the perfusate to a low-sodium solution, there was a dramatic increase in renin secretion from the attached juxtaglomerular apparatus. Hence, this mechanism for control of renin release occurs individually for each nephron (12). Each nephron detects the signal and then responds to it with a change in its renin release.

THE RENAL BARORECEPTOR MECHANISM

Fray and Lush (13) have directly demonstrated the function of the isolated renal arteriolar baroreceptor. Juxtaglomerular cells in culture were layered on a latex grid with a collagen base. When the latex bed was stretched by approximately 12 percent, renin secretion by those cells fell; renin secretion increased again when the stretch stimulus was removed. Accordingly, individual juxtaglomerular cells can, by themselves, respond to stretch by changing their rate of renin secretion.

How might this individual nephron regulation of renin secretion by the macula densa and baroreceptor mechanisms cause a disruption of blood pressure control if different individual nephrons behaved discordantly?

MODELING RENIN SECRETION PER INDIVIDUAL NEPHRONS

To address the above question we have developed a model to analyze the various normal and abnormal observed patterns of renin secretion in terms of the heterogeneity of individual nephron behavior. Figure 7 illustrates the model in which we depict a kidney as comprising four large nephrons. These four nephrons, two from each kidney, accomplish all of the sodium excretion and all of the renin secretion. Figure 7 shows the predicted responses of these nephrons in a normal person in a steady state, while ingesting 100 mmol/liter ($\sim$5 g) sodium per day. Each of the four nephrons excretes 25

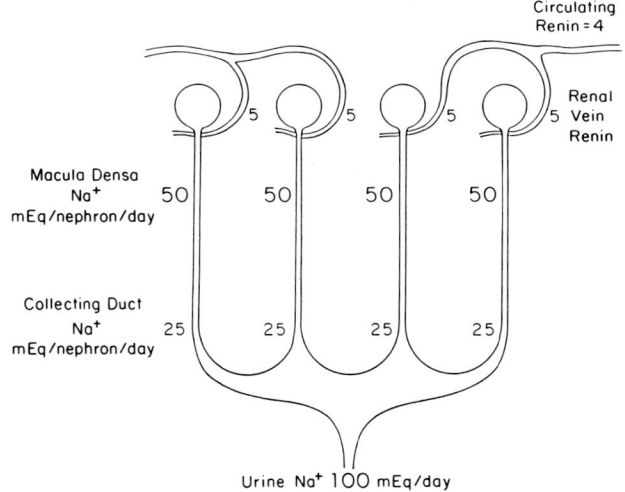

FIG. 7. Relationship between macula densa sodium chloride supply and renin secretion for four big hypothetical normal nephrons, two representing each kidney. Each big nephron thus represents about 500,000 nephrons. Model shown for a normal subject in balance while ingesting 100 mmol/liter Na⁺ and 50 mmol/liter K⁺ per day and assuming no insensible or alimentary losses.

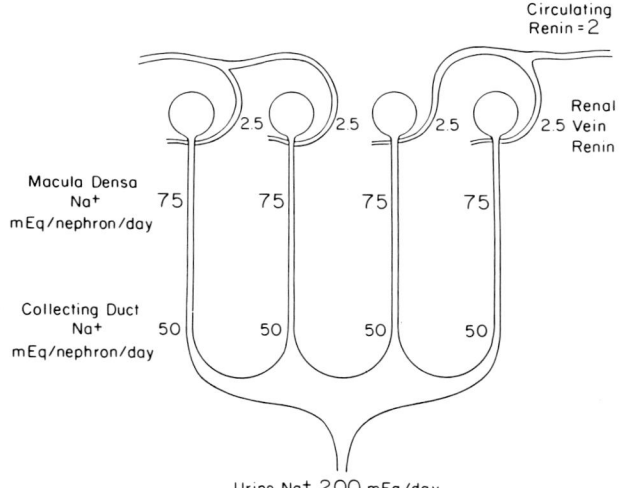

FIG. 8. Relationship between macula densa sodium chloride supply and renin secretion for four big hypothetical normal nephrons, two representing each kidney. Each big nephron thus represents about 500,000 nephrons. Model shown for normal subject in balance while ingesting 200 mmol/liter Na⁺ and 50 mmol/liter K⁺ per day and assuming no insensible or alimentary losses.

mmol/liter sodium per day to account for the total of 100 mmol/liter per day when in balance. The minimum amount of sodium that must arrive at the macula densa of each nephron per day can be estimated from the formula at the bottom of Fig. 7. This is the amount of sodium per nephron excreted in the final urine (25 mmol/liter) plus twice the amount of potassium in the urine, since potassium balance is achieved by tubular secretion in exchange for sodium (2:1) (60). Assuming a K⁺ intake of 50 mmol/liter/day, each nephron would secrete K⁺ at a rate of 12.5 mmol/liter/day in exchange for 25 mmol/liter sodium. Therefore, the minimum amount of sodium delivered to each macula densa should be 50 mmol/liter per nephron per day. At excretion rates of 100 mmol/liter sodium per day, circulating plasma renin averages 4 ng/ml/hr. Our studies have shown that this will result from a renin concentration in the renal vein of 5 ng/ml/hr, or 25 percent higher (61). This steady-state condition is achieved by a commensurate hepatic removal rate (61). Thus, a sodium concentration at the macula densa of 50 mmol/liter per nephron results in a renal vein renin level of 5 ng/ml/hr and a peripheral renin level of 4 ng/ml/hr.

Doubling the salt intake of the model (Fig. 8) to 200 mmol/liter, or $\sim$10 g/day, will result in an increase in urinary sodium to 200 mmol/liter/day. Now each of the four nephrons excretes 50 mmol/liter to make up the total of 200 mmol/liter. Using the same calculation, there are now 75 mmol/liter sodium per nephron reaching each of the four macula densa regions. This signal suppresses renin secretion to 2.0 ng/ml/hr, half of what it was when 100 mmol/liter was being ingested and when the concentration of sodium in the macula densa was 50 mmol/liter per nephron per day. Renal venous renin is again 25 percent higher (2.5 ng/ml/hr).

The hypothetical relationship between macula densa sodium and renin secretion over a wide range of sodium intakes is illustrated in Fig. 9. Renal vein renin concentration per nephron is shown on the ordinate, and the macula densa delivery of sodium per nephron is shown on the abscissa. The line on the right was developed from the model data just described and illustrated in Figs. 7 and 8, and also from similarly modeling a low-sodium diet (20 mmol/liter/day). According to the predictions of these model data, in a normotensive subject, unattainable amounts of sodium chloride would need to be delivered to each distal tubule to make renin secretion approach zero. It would be very difficult to achieve near-zero levels in normal people; in fact, it is rare for renin levels to approach zero in young normotensive subjects. On the other hand, patients with hypertension may have very low plasma renin values, and some older normal subjects exhibit moderately low renin levels.

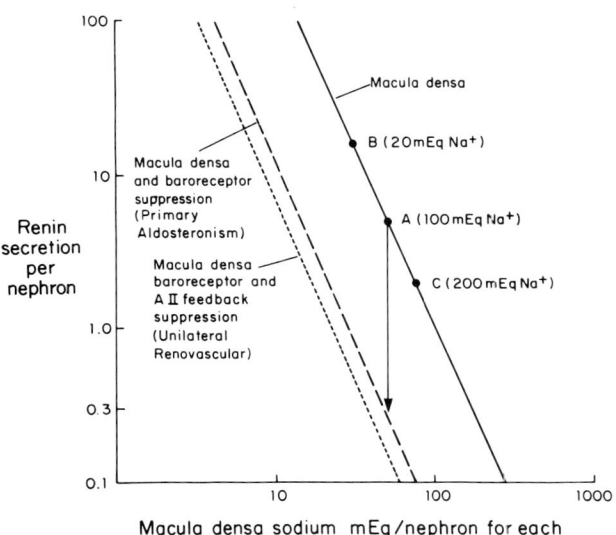

FIG. 9. Data from Fig. 6 (point A here) and Fig. 7 (point C here) are plotted, along with similarly derived data from a normal subject, ingesting 20 mmol/liter/day (point B here). The solid line on the right illustrates the relationship between renin secretion/nephron and macula densa sodium supply for each of the four big hypothetical nephrons in normal subjects. This relationship is shifted to the left in typical primary aldosteronism (— — —) and even more so in the contralateral normal kidney of the patient with unilateral renovascular hypertension (- - -). This shift to the left is due to concurrent suppression of renin secretion from the increased arterial pressure exerted on the afferent arteriolar baroreceptor. The additional suppressing effect in the renovascular model (- - -) is due to angiotensin II feedback suppression, which does not occur in primary aldosteronism where renin secretion is fully turned off (see text).

Thus, the model data suggest that physiologically conceivable increases in the distal sodium supply to the macula densa mechanism cannot, in themselves, explain the suppression of renin secretion seen in these patients. That is to say, operation of the macula densa mechanism by itself cannot explain the renal renin secretion values observed in certain hypertensive patients. Although distal sodium delivery is an important stimulus for the regulation of renin release, the model suggests that invoking this mechanism alone cannot fully explain what is observed. The next obvious question, then, is, To what extent does the baroreceptor mechanism contribute to the observed suppression of renin secretion?

INFLUENCE OF ARTERIAL HYPERTENSION AND THE BARORECEPTOR SIGNAL ON THE RENIN-SECRETORY RESPONSE

When the model kidney is perfused at a high systemic arterial pressure, things change dramatically. The two dashed lines plotted on the left of Fig. 9 were developed from an analysis of the responses of a typical patient with primary aldosteronism and from the contralateral kidney of classic Goldblatt hypertension, respectively. Apart from the fact that they are exposed to arterial hypertension, the kidneys in these two disorders are presumably quite normal.

In the contralateral normal kidney of Goldblatt disease and in primary aldosteronism, renin secretion from this normal contralateral kidney is suppressed completely at a sodium intake of 100 mmol/liter. In contrast, the kidney of a normotensive subject exposed to 100 mmol/liter continues to secrete considerable amounts of renin. (See Fig. 9; solid line on right represents the normotensive reference.) Accordingly, in the presence of high arterial pressure, the normal relationship is shifted to the left, indicating that superimposition of a baroreceptor stretch signal onto the macula densa signal greatly adds to the suppression of renin induced by sodium delivery to the macula densa. In this way, the baroreceptor signal amplifies the macula densa signal by further dampening net renin secretion. In other words, when a nephron is exposed to higher pressures at its afferent arteriole, renin secretion will then be much lower for a given macula densa sodium load. Renin secretion can be suppressed in the contralateral Goldblatt kidney even more so than in primary aldosteronism because of the added renin-suppressing effect of angiotensin II from the ischemic kidney. These model data are especially relevant to our hypothesis on the renal basis of essential hypertension because they illustrate that *any renal renin secretion is abnormal in the presence of arterial hypertension and a normal salt intake.* The response of the normal kidney is to completely turn off renin secretion.

Figure 10 illustrates the classic two-kidney, one-clip

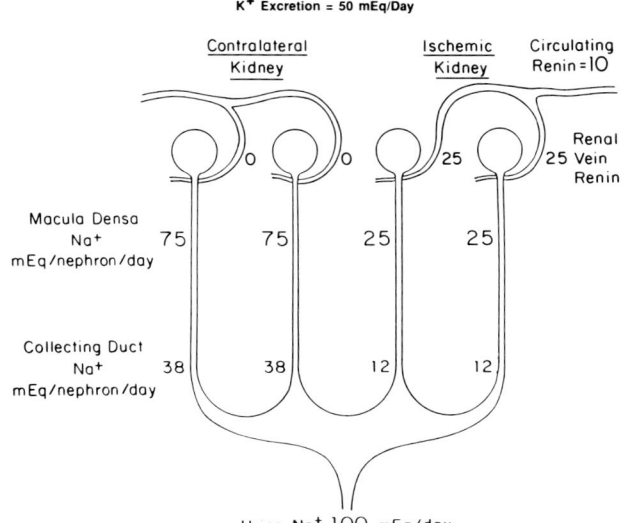

FIG. 10. Typical unilateral renovascular hypertension. The model developed in Fig. 6 is used to illustrate the abnormal patterns of renin secretion, macula densa sodium supply, and renin secretion while in balance, ingesting 100 mmol/liter Na per day (see text). Na$^+$ excretion = 100 mmol/liter/day; K$^+$ excretion = 50 mmol/liter/day.

Goldblatt hypertension using the four-nephron model described in Figs. 7 and 8. In this type of hypertension, 50 percent of the nephrons are ischemic: These are represented by the two nephrons on the right; the other two nephrons on the left represent the normal contralateral kidney (62). This latter kidney is exposed to systemic hypertension and does not make any renin. As in Fig. 7 the sodium intake and output is 100 mmol/liter/day. The difference is that most of the dietary salt is excreted by the unclipped kidney; Na excretion is 38 mmol/liter/day per nephron, as opposed to 12 mmol/liter/day per nephron from the two ischemic nephrons representing the clipped Goldblatt kidney.

Several important points can be made from this model of Goldblatt hypertension. The ischemic kidney secretes large amounts of renin, resulting in a concentration of 25 ng/ml/hr in the ipsilateral renal vein. However, the plasma level is only 10 ng/ml/hr, instead of 20 ng/ml/hr as it would be if both kidneys were supporting the plasma level equally (61). This discrepancy occurs because the unclipped kidney does not contribute any renin to the peripheral circulation so that the renin secreted by the ischemic kidney is diluted by half. Consequently, the ischemic kidney is not exposed to as much angiotensin II as would be expected from the renin it has secreted. That is to say, the reacting level of renin-angiotensin generation, which normally works to support GFR by efferent constriction (63–65), is cut by 50 percent because of the failure of the opposite kidney to contribute any renin

to the circulating pool. Thus, the ischemic kidney, which requires considerable efferent constriction to maintain GFR and enable salt excretion, does not receive sufficient renin and angiotensin II to compensate for the reduced blood flow induced by the afferent arteriolar constriction. Therefore, sodium excretion cannot be maintained adequately by this kidney.

At the same time, the contralateral normal kidney excretes most of the systemic dietary sodium via a pressure natriuresis related to the arterial hypertension; but here again, this adaptive natriuresis is blunted by inappropriate renin activity. The high levels of circulating renin-angiotensin from the ischemic nephrons contribute to sodium retention and to the pathogenesis of hypertension in two ways:

1. The increased plasma angiotensin II increases proximal sodium reabsorption (66,67), thereby blunting the capacity for natriuresis of the good kidney and causing unwanted sodium retention.
2. The high plasma angiotensin II levels induce renal afferent arteriolar constriction in the unclipped kidney by amplifying activity of the intrarenal TGF control mechanism (68).

The latter relationship of the renin-angiotensin system to the TGF mechanism is nicely demonstrated in studies by Mitchell and Navar (69,70). They perfused a distal nephron with isotonic fluid. In the control study, as the luminal perfusion rate to the distal nephron was increased, progressive constriction of its afferent arteriole occurred via the TGF mechanism, an intrarenal feedback control system that modulates GFR in response to changes in distal sodium supply. As a consequence of this mechanism, high distal delivery causes prompt afferent constriction with decreased GFR and vice versa. This mechanism does not depend on the renin system to function, but it is modified by the activity of the renin-angiotensin system in a predictable manner. Thus, when enalaprilat was given to inhibit the generation of angiotensin II, the TGF afferent constrictor response to increased distal perfusion was virtually abolished (70). When angiotensin II was added to the perfusate to correct for the converting-enzyme blockade, full restoration of TGF-mediated constriction occurred. Thus, angiotensin II can induce afferent arteriolar vasoconstriction by amplifying the TGF response to distal sodium delivery.

We propose that, in essential hypertension, an inappropriate amount of circulating renin impairs renal function in both the ischemic nephrons and in the normal hyperfiltering nephrons, but it does so in very different ways. To maintain GFR and an adequate excretion of sodium, the ischemic nephrons require a higher rate of renin secretion than they are actually receiving; this is because at low perfusion pressures, maximal angiotensin II–induced efferent arteriolar constriction is needed to maintain GFR. On the other hand, the compensating hypernatriuretic nephrons become unable to fully excrete dietary sodium because they are unexpectedly exposed to an unwanted, inappropriately high angiotensin II level coming from the ischemic nephrons. As has just been discussed, this angiotensin II impairs sodium excretion by unaffected adapting nephrons by promoting proximal sodium reabsorption and by inducing afferent constriction. The net result is that *all* nephrons are exposed to angiotensin II levels that are inappropriate to their needs. This leads to an impaired ability of both populations of nephrons to excrete sodium, causing sodium retention in the presence of abnormal renin secretion and perpetuation of hypertension.

USING THE MODEL TO EXPLAIN RENAL SODIUM EXCRETION AND RENIN SECRETION IN CLINICAL HYPERTENSION

Let us now examine the spectrum of patients with hypertension and consider how this model, implicating two discordant populations of nephrons, can account for the abnormal relationship between renal renin secretion and renal salt excretion in the pathogenesis of elevated blood pressure. Figure 11 illustrates the interactions of these variables in clinical hypertension. On the ordinate (second line from the top), various possible proportions of ischemic and of hyperfiltering nephrons are depicted as they might occur in various forms of clinical hypertension. The degree of renin secretion from the ischemic subgroup of nephrons is represented by the degree of shading.

Three situations are illustrated for normal people, depicted on the left: young, medium, and old age. In keeping with clinical data, the young have the highest nephron number, the highest renin secretion, and the lowest blood pressure levels. It is well known that, with advancing age, renin secretion falls and blood pressure tends to rise (71). In our view, this is because as the number of functioning nephrons decreases, each surviving nephron adapts by excreting a greater proportion of the dietary sodium load. Thus, an increase in distal sodium supply per nephron is an inevitable consequence of the loss of nephrons from the aging process. Consequently, with more distal sodium delivery per nephron, plasma renin levels fall. In the normotensive subject, as the nephron number falls, sodium excretion per nephron rises, renin secretion falls, salt balance is maintained, and blood pressure stays close to normal.

How is the process modified in hypertension? Two-kidney, one-clip (unilateral) renovascular hypertension is a model (Fig. 10) and a clinical entity with a normal nephron number. In this disorder, 50 percent of the nephrons are ischemic and secrete increased amounts of renin. In contrast, nephrons from the contralateral unclipped kidney are exposed to increased perfusion pressure and have a high distal sodium delivery. Accordingly, they totally suppress their renin secretion to zero. The overall result is a high circulating plasma renin level, a

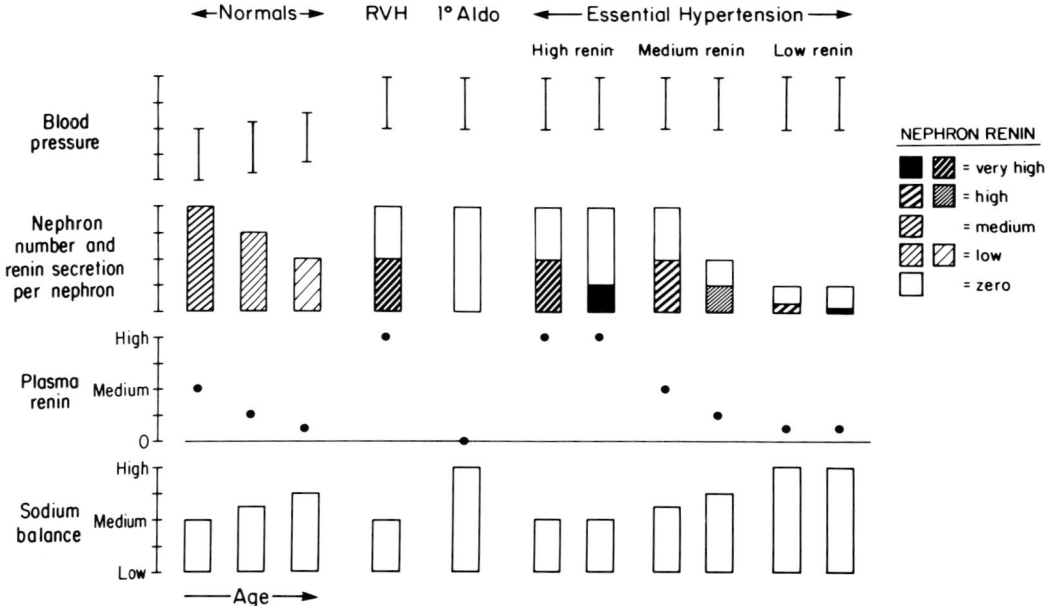

FIG. 11. Renin secretion, plasma renin, sodium balance, and proportions of ischemic and hyperfiltering nephrons and nephron number in normal subjects with age, in unilateral renovascular hypertension, in primary aldosteronism, and in the three renin subgroups of essential hypertension. Relative values shown are derived from data and the hypothetical model reviewed in the text.

normal total nephron number, a neutral or slightly positive sodium balance, and systemic hypertension related to vasoconstriction mediated by excess renin, inappropriate for the state of sodium balance. In this model, inappropriate and unwanted renin secretion from the ischemic nephrons impairs sodium excretion in the uninvolved kidney, while, at the same time, by systemic dilution it becomes insufficient to fully support GFR and renal function in the ischemic nephrons by the mechanisms discussed above.

An exactly opposite form of hypertension occurs in a second basic model of clinical hypertension, namely, primary aldosteronism. This model is also characterized by a normal total nephron number, but in primary aldosteronism, in contrast to the Goldblatt model, renin secretion is suppressed completely in both kidneys. Renal sodium retention occurs in response to aldosterone excess. There is massive sodium-volume expansion, and there is also a huge distal sodium supply that, when combined with renal baroreceptor-mediated inhibition of renin release, reduces renin secretion to zero. Renin secretion is not involved; instead, a sodium-volume-mediated arteriolar vasoconstriction (3) sustains this hypertension.

These two models represent opposite ends of the sodium-renin spectrum of hypertensive diseases: primary aldosteronism is a sodium-volume-mediated, low-renin form of hypertension; the renovascular model is a renin-mediated form of hypertension. These two models express the two long-term, reciprocating mechanisms for arteriolar vasoconstriction (2,3): One is caused by renin-angiotensin; the other is not related to renin but involves, instead, a vasoconstriction state induced by renal sodium retention.

We believe that the spectrum of essential hypertension embodies varying proportions of a disturbance in the delicate interaction between renin secretion and sodium balance. In high-renin patients, two models are possible. One is analogous to the Goldblatt model in which half of the nephrons are ischemic, and the other half are adaptively hyperfiltering—with the defect, instead, being intermingled in both kidneys. The result is an inappropriately high plasma renin activity and a near-normal sodium balance. However, a situation could also exist (Fig. 11) in which there is a high plasma renin level, generated from a smaller fractional population of ischemic nephrons causing the same general effect. Any loss of nephrons would further impair adaptive sodium excretion and would be likely to amplify the hypertension (15).

Further support for this paradigm is provided in studies reported by Hollenberg and Williams (72). These investigators have classified patients with essential hypertension as either nonmodulators or modulators according to their renal hemodynamic responses to saline and angiotensin II infusions. Nonmodulators have impaired plasma renin suppression, renal blood flow, and natriuresis during saline infusion. The latter responses are corrected by converting-enzyme–inhibition therapy, suggesting that inappropriate renin secretion, perhaps from an ischemic subpopulation of nephrons, is an important contributing factor in these patients. In contrast, the modulator group of hypertensive patients responds to saline infusion with an exaggerated natriuresis, and converting-enzyme inhibition does not alter the associated renal hemodynamic responses.

In "normal"-renin hypertension, the circulating plasma renin values are within the normal range in the face of arterial hypertension. Figure 11 depicts two recognized variants: one in which renin secretion is higher than normal, and another in which renin secretion is lower than normal. In each case, renin secretion is increased from the subpopulation of ischemic nephrons and is suppressed in the hypernatriuresing adaptive nephrons. Sodium balance tends to be slightly positive, because, even if the number of nephrons is normal, the adverse effects of inappropriate renin secretion from ischemic nephrons on the hyperfiltering normal nephrons cause a positive sodium balance. Again, a sustained discord between renin activity and sodium excretory capacity leads to hypertension.

In the low-renin form of essential hypertension, total renin secretion is low, but typically it is not suppressed completely. This renin secretion, too, is inappropriate because *any* renin secretion in the presence of arterial hypertension is abnormal, and it works in the same way to impair salt excretion and raise arterial pressure. We suspect that the total nephron number could well be decreased in this form of hypertension; this loss of nephrons further impairs the excretion of sodium. However, in this situation, too, the adverse effect of even small amounts of renin secreted from ischemic nephrons on the adaptive hypernatriuresis of surviving nephrons can support or amplify the hypertension. Pure "renoprival" hypertension due to a loss of nephron number would thus be characterized by:

1. little or no inappropriate renin secretion and by marked to maximal suppression of renin in the surviving normal nephrons because of the high arterial hypertension, and
2. a marked increase in distal sodium supply per nephron; in this situation, the loss of nephrons, rather than the inappropriate renin secretion, would become the predominant factor in pathogenesis.

SUMMARY

We propose herein that there are two functionally abnormal nephron populations in essential hypertension:

1. A group of ischemic nephrons with impaired sodium excretion that chronically hypersecrete renin. Nu-

merically, these ischemic nephrons comprise a minor subgroup, because most patients with essential hypertension exhibit no overt evidence of renal insufficiency.

2. In reaction to this, a more numerous group of normal nephrons appears in adaptive hypernatriuresis. They have an increased distal sodium supply and, consequently, a chronically suppressed renin secretion. One difference between patients with renovascular hypertension and those with essential hypertension is the intermingling of these two populations of nephrons.

In our hypothesis, the adapting hyperfiltering normal nephrons accomplish the hypernatriuresis, in response to saline infusion, that is characteristic of all essential hypertension. However, the unsuppressed secretion of renin that arises from the ischemic nephron population attenuates this compensatory natriuresis in the following ways:

1. It inappropriately acts on the hyperfiltering nephrons to enhance proximal tubular sodium reabsorption.
2. It activates TGF-mediated afferent constriction in these nephrons.
3. Simultaneously, the reactive secretion of renin from ischemic nephrons is diluted by nonparticipation of the adapting hypernatriuretic nephrons so that plasma renin settles at a level that is insufficient to fully compensate GFR in the ischemic nephrons.

These adaptive responses provide a basis for the observation that the inhibition of renin activity with converting-enzyme inhibitors in essential hypertension increases renal blood flow and sodium excretion. They also explain why converting-enzyme inhibitors can effectively reduce blood pressure, even when renin levels are not absolutely elevated, because *any* circulating renin imposed upon the adapting hypernatriuretic nephrons inappropriately impairs their sodium excretion. In addition, the theory explains why basal renin secretion is either not suppressed or inadequately suppressed in patients with essential hypertension. As a result, whole-kidney homeostatic function is compromised because individual nephrons are responding to their individual stimuli to fulfill their individual need, rather than acting in concert with other nephrons. The net effect of this uncoordinated response is to shift total renal function so that systemic arterial hypertension is sustained by abnormal sodium retention for the inappropriately high plasma renin level, or vice versa (1–3).

These concepts are also in keeping with the hallmark multifocal afferent arteriolar narrowing of essential hypertension (6–8) and its characteristic renal hemodynamic pattern of vasoconstriction with reduced renal blood flow and a maintained GFR (73–76). Thus, whereas *total* GFR may be normal, instead of a normal distributional pattern, the GFR is the sum of hypo- and hyperfiltering nephrons. In this pathology, the hallmark

hypernatriuretic response to saline infusion may be (a) directly related in degree to the number of hyperfiltering nephrons and (b) inversely related to total renin secretion. Assessment of this functional nephron discordance in essential hypertension promises to improve its analysis and treatment. This analytical framework could also enable approaches to causation that could reveal fundamental, genetic, neural, or hormonal defects.

REFERENCES

1. Laragh JH, Sealey JE. The renin-angiotensin-aldosterone hormonal system and regulation of sodium, potassium, and blood pressure homeostasis. In: Orloff J, Berliner RW, eds. *Handbook of physiology—renal physiology.* Bethesda: American Physiological Society, 1973;831–908.
2. Laragh JH, Sealey JE, Niarchos AP, Pickering TG. The vasoconstriction-volume spectrum in normotension and pathogenesis of hypertension. *Fed Proc* 1982;41:2415–2423.
3. Laragh JH, Resnick LM. Recognizing and treating two types of long-term vasoconstriction in hypertension. *Kidney Int* 1988; 34(Suppl 25):S162–S174.
4. Tobian L. Interrelationships of electrolytes, juxtaglomerular cells and hypertension. *Physiol Rev* 1960;40:280–312.
5. Vander AJ. Control of renin release. *Physiol Rev* 1967;47:359–382.
6. Sommers SC, Relman AS, Smithwick RH. Histologic studies of kidney biopsy specimens from patients with hypertension. *Am J Pathol* 1958;34:685–715.
7. Sommers SC. Hypertension and kidney disease. *Prog Cardiovasc Dis* 1965;8:210–234.
8. Turgeon C, Sommers SC. Juxtaglomerular cell counts and human hypertension. *Am J Pathol* 1961;38:227–241.
9. Sealey JE, Moon C, Laragh JH, Atlas SA. Plasma prorenin in normal, hypertensive and anephric subjects and its effect on renin measurements. *Circ Res* 1977;40(Suppl 1):41–45.
10. Sealey JE, White RP, Laragh JH, Case DB, Rubin AL. Studies of plasma aldosterone in anephric people: evidence for the fundamental role of the renin system in maintaining aldosterone secretion. *J Clin Endocrinol Metab* 1978;47:42–60.
11. Sealey JE, Atlas SA, Laragh JH. Prorenin and other large molecular weight forms of renin. *Endocr Rev* 1980;1:365–391.
12. Skott O, Briggs JP. Direct demonstration of macula densa-mediated renin secretion. *Science* 1987;237:1618–1620.
13. Fray JCS, Lush DJ. Stretch receptor hypothesis for renin secretion: the role of calcium. *J Hypertens* 1984;2(Suppl 1):19–23.
14. Laragh JH. The meaning of plasma renin measurements: renin and sodium-volume-mediated (low renin) forms of vasoconstriction in experimental and human hypertension and in the oedematous states of nephrosis and heart failure. *J Hypertens* 1984;2(Suppl 1):141–150.
15. Brenner BM, Garcia DL, Anderson S. Glomeruli and blood pressure: less of one, more the other? *Am J Hypertens* 1988;1:335–347.
16. Brunner HR, Laragh JH, Baer L, Newton MA, Goodwin FT, Krakoff LR, Bard RH, Bühler FR. Essential hypertension: renin and aldosterone, heart attack and stroke. *N Engl J Med* 1972;286:441–449.
17. Laragh JH. Vasoconstriction-volume analysis for understanding and treating hypertension: the use of renin and aldosterone profiles. *Am J Med* 1973;55:261–274.
18. Case DB, Atlas SA, Laragh JH, Sealey JE, Sullivan PA, McKinstry DN. Clinical experience with blockade of the renin-angiotensin-aldosterone system by an oral converting-enzyme inhibitor (SQ 14,225, Captopril) in hypertensive patients. *Prog Cardiovasc Dis* 1978;31:195–206.
19. Case DB, Wallace JM, Keim HJ, Weber MA, Sealey JE, Laragh JH. Possible role of renin in hypertension as suggested by renin-sodium profiling and inhibition of converting enzyme. *N Engl J Med* 1977;296:641–646.
20. Case DB, Wallace JM, Keim HJ, Weber MA, Drayer JIM, White

RP, Sealey JE, Laragh JH. Estimating renin participation in hypertension. Superiority of converting enzyme inhibitor over Saralasin. *Am J Med* 1976;61:790–796.

21. Case DB, Atlas SA, Laragh JH. Physiologic effects and diagnostic relevance of acute converting enzyme blockade. In: Laragh JH, Bühler FR, Seldin DW, eds. *Frontiers in hypertension research.* New York: Springer-Verlag, 1981;541–550.

22. Collins RD, Weinberger MJ, Dowdy AJ, Nokes GW, Gonzales CM, Luetscher JA. Abnormally sustained aldosterone secretion during salt loading in patients with various forms of benign hypertension; relation to plasma renin activity. *J Clin Invest* 1970;49:1415–1526.

23. Weber MA, Drayer JIM, Rev A, Laragh JH. Disparate patterns of aldosterone response during diuretic treatment of hypertension. *Ann Intern Med* 1977;87:558–563.

24. Gavras H, Brunner HR, Laragh JH, Sealey JE, Gavras I, Vukovitch RA. An angiotensin converting enzyme inhibitor to identify and treat vasoconstrictor and volume factors in hypertensive patients. *N Engl J Med* 1974;291:817–821.

25. Pecker MS, Cody RJ, Laragh JH, Sala C, Atlas SA. Effect of saline infusion on plasma ANF in normal and hypertensive subjects. *Program and Abstracts, Second World Congress on Biologically Active Atrial Peptides,* 1987;228 (abstract No. B. 179).

26. Newton MA, Sealey JE, Ledingham JGG, Laragh JH. High blood pressure and oral contraceptives. Changes in plasma renin and renin substrate and in aldosterone excretion. *Am J Obstet Gynecol* 1968;101:1037–1045.

27. Derkx FHM, Stuenkel C, Schalekamp MPA, Visser W, Huisveld IH, Schalekamp MADH. Immunoreactive renin, prorenin, and enzymatically active renin in plasma during pregnancy and in women taking oral contraceptives. *J Clin Endocrinol Metab* 1986;63:1008–1015.

28. Krakoff LR. Measurement of plasma renin substrate by radioimmunoassay of angiotensin I: concentration in syndromes associated with steroid excess. *J Clin Endocrinol Metab* 1973;37:110–117.

29. Gardes J, Bouhnik J, Clauser E, Corvol P, Ménard J. Role of angiotensinogen in blood pressure homeostasis. *Hypertension* 1982;4:185–189.

30. Menard J, El Amrani AIK, Savoie F, Bouhnik J. Angiotensinogen: an attractive and underrated participant in hypertension and inflammation. *Hypertension* 1991;18:705–706.

31. Saruta T, Saade GA, Kaplan NM. A possible mechanism for hypertension induced by oral contraceptives. Diminished feedback suppression of renin release. *Arch Intern Med* 1970;126:621–626.

32. Jeunemaitre X, Soubrier F, Kotelevtsev YV, Lifton RP, Williams CS, Charru A, Hunt SC, Hopkins PN, Williams RR, Lalouel J-M, Corvol P. Molecular basis of human hypertension: role of angiotensinogen. *Cell* 1992;71:169–180.

33. Walker WG, Whelton PK, Saito H, Patterson Russell R, Hermann J. Relationship between blood pressure and renin, renin substrate, angiotensin II, aldosterone and urinary sodium and potassium in 574 ambulatory subjects. *Hypertension* 1979;1:287–291.

34. Gahnem F, von Lutterotti N, Camargo MJF, Laragh JH, Sealey JE. Ang II dependent relationship between plasma angiotensinogen and BP in salt-fed Dahl S and SHRsp rats with paradoxically high PRC. *Hypertension* 1993;22:442 (Abstract).

35. Farnsworth EB. Renal reabsorption of chloride and phosphate in normal subjects and in patients with essential arterial hypertension. *J Clin Invest* 1946;25:897–905.

36. Grim CE, Luft FC, Fineberg NS, Weinberger MH. Responses to volume expansion and contraction in categorized hypertensive and normotensive man. *Hypertension* 1979;1:476–485.

37. Cottier PT, Weller JM, Hoobler SW. Effect of an intravenous sodium chloride load on renal hemodynamics and electrolyte excretion in essential hypertension. *Circulation* 1958;17:750–760.

38. Luft F, Weinberg MH. Determinants of exaggerated natriuresis in arterial hypertension. In: Messerli FH, ed. *Kidney in essential hypertension.* Boston: Martinus Nijhoff, 1984;105–123.

39. Hollander W, Judson WE. Electrolyte and water excretion in arterial hypertension. I. Studies in non-medically treated subjects with essential hypertension. *J Clin Invest* 1957;36:1460–1469.

40. Papper S, Belsky JL, Bleifer KH. The response to the administration of an isotonic sodium chloride-actate solution in patients with essential hypertension. *J Clin Invest* 1960;39:876–884.

41. Smith HW. Salt and water volume receptors: an exercise in physiologic apologetics. *Am J Med* 1957;23:623–652.

42. Hollander W, Judson WE. Electrolyte and water excretion in arterial hypertension. II. Studies in subjects with essential hypertension after antihypertensive drug treatment. *Circulation* 1958;17:576–582.

43. Green DM, Ellis EJ. Sodium output-blood pressure relationships and their modification by treatment. *Circulation* 1954;10:536–543.

44. Luft FC, Rankin LI, Bloch R, Weyman AE, Willis LR, Murray RH, Grim CE, Weinberger MH. Cardiovascular and humoral responses to extremes of sodium intake in normal black and white men. *Circulation* 1979;60:697–706.

45. Buckalew VM, Puschett JB, Kintzel JE, Goldberg M. Mechanism of exaggerated natriuresis in hypertensive man: impaired sodium transport in the loop of Henle. *J Clin Invest* 1969;48:1007–1016.

46. Cannon PJ. Effects of five per cent dextrose-water infusions in normal and hypertensive man. Evidence for increased proximal and distal tubular sodium rejection by hypertensive patients and its relation to renal hemodynamics. *Circulation* 1968;37:832–846.

47. Gottschalk GW, Mylle M. Micropuncture study of pressures in proximal tubules and peritubular capillaries of the rat kidney and their relation to ureteral and renal venous pressures. *Am J Physiol* 1956;185:430–439.

48. Wirz H. Druckmessung in Kapillaren und Tubuli der Niere durch Mikropunktion. *Helv Physiol Pharmacol Acta* 1955;13:42–49.

49. Lowenstein J, Beranbaum ER, Chassis H, Baldwin DS. Intrarenal pressure and exaggerated natriuresis in essential hypertension. *Clin Sci* 1970;38:359–374.

50. Krakoff LR, Goodwin FJ, Baer L, Torres M, Laragh JH. The role of renin in the exaggerated natriuresis of hypertension. *Circulation* 1970;42:335–345.

51. Luft FC, Grim CE, Willis LR, Higgins JT, Weinberger MH. Natriuretic response to saline infusion in normotensive and hypertensive man. The role of renin suppression in exaggerated natriuresis. *Circulation* 1977;55:779–784.

52. Laragh JH, Cannon PJ, Ames RP. Aldosterone secretion and various forms of hypertensive vascular disease. *Ann Intern Med* 1963;59:117–120.

53. Biglieri EG, Forsham PH. Studies on the expanded extracellular fluid and the responses to various stimuli in primary aldosteronism. *Am J Med* 1961;30:564–575.

54. Bradley SE, Chasis H, Goldring W, Smith HW. Hemodynamic alterations in normotensive and hypertensive subjects during the pyrogenic reaction. *J Clin Invest* 1945;24:749–758.

55. Hollenberg NE, Borucki LS, Adams DF. The renal vascular lesion in early essential hypertension: evidence for a pathogenetic role. *Medicine* 1978;57:167–178.

56. Keeton TK, Campbell WB. The pharmacologic alteration of renin release. *Pharmacol Rev* 1981;31:81–227.

57. Churchill PC. Calcium channel antagonists and renin release. *Am J Nephrol* 1987;7(Suppl 1):32–88.

58. Hall JE, Guyton AC, Smith MJ, Coleman TG. Blood pressure and renal function during chronic changes in sodium intake: role of angiotensin. *Am J Physiol* 1980;239:F271–F280.

59. Bühler FR, Laragh JH, Baer L, Vaughan ED Jr, Brunner HR. Propranolol inhibition of renin secretion. A specific approach to diagnosis and treatment of renin-dependent hypertensive diseases. *N Engl J Med* 1972;287:1209–1214.

60. Malnic G, Klose RM, Giebisch G. Microperfusion study of distal tubular potassium and sodium transfer in rat kidney. *Am J Physiol* 1966;211:548–559.

61. Sealey JE, Bühler FR, Laragh JH, Vaughn ED Jr. The physiology of renin secretion in essential hypertension: estimation of renin secretion rate and renal plasma flow from peripheral and renal vein renin levels. *Am J Med* 1973;55:391–401.

62. Laragh JH. Renovascular hypertension. A paradigm for all hypertension. *J Hypertens* 1986;5(Suppl 4):S79–S88.

63. Hall JE, Guyton AC, Jackson TE, Coleman TG, Lohmeier TE, Trippodo NC. Control of glomerular filtration rate by renin-angiotensin system. *Am J Physiol* 1977;233:F366–F372.

64. Ichikawa I, Brenner BM. Importance of efferent arteriolar vascular tone in regulation of proximal tubule fluid reabsorption and glomerulotubular balance in the rat. *J Clin Invest* 1980;654:1192–1201.
65. Hall JE, Granger JP. Renal hemodynamic actions of angiotensin II: interaction with tubuloglomerular feedback. *Am J Physiol* 1983;245:R166–R173.
66. Harris PJ, Navar LG. Tubular transport responses to angiotensin. *Am J Physiol* 1985;248:F621–F630.
67. Schuster VL. Angiotensin effects on proximal tubular reabsorption. *Fed Proc* 1986;45:1444–1447.
68. Schnerman J, Haeberle DA, Davis JM, Thurau K. Tubuloglomerular feedback control of renal vascular resistance. In: Windhager EE, ed. *Handbook of physiology—renal physiology,* 2nd edition. Oxford University Press, New York, 1990;in press.
69. Mitchell KD, Navar LG. Amplifications of tubuloglomerular feedback responses during peritubular capillary infusions of angiotensins I and II. *Am J Physiol* 1988;225:F383–F390.
70. Navar LG, Carmines PK, Huang WC, Mitchell KD. The tubular effects of angiotensin II. *Kidney Int* 1987;31(Suppl 20):S81–S88.
71. James GD, Sealey JE, Müller FB, Alderman M, Madhavan S, Laragh JH. Renin relationship to sex, race and age in a normotensive population. *J Hypertens* 1986;4(Suppl 5):S387–S389.
72. Hollenberg NK, Williams GH. Abnormal renal function, sodium-volume homeostasis, and renin system behavior in normal-renin essential hypertension. Chapter in this volume.
73. Bradley SE. Physiology of essential hypertension. *Am J Med* 1948;4:398–415.
74. Chasis H, Goldring W, Breed E, Bolomey A, Smith HW. Effects of salt and protein restriction on blood pressure and renal hemodynamics in hypertensive patients. *J Clin Invest* 1949;28:775 (Abstract).
75. Goldring W, Chasis H, Ranges HA, Smith HW. Effective renal blood flow in subjects with essential hypertension. *J Clin Invest* 1941;20:637–653.
76. Bradley SE, Curry JJ, Bradley GP. Renal extraction of P-amino-hippurate in normal subjects and essential hypertension and chronic diffuse glomerulonephritis. *Fed Proc* 1947;6:79–80 (Abstract).

Hypertension: Pathophysiology, Diagnosis, and Management, Second Edition,
edited by J.H. Laragh and B.M. Brenner,
Raven Press, Ltd., New York © 1995.

CHAPTER 85

Angiotensin II Administration as an Experimental Model of Hypertension

Geza Simon and Gyorgy Abraham

Angiotensin II (ANG II)–induced hypertension has fascinated investigators ever since the agonist became available in pure form. There are several reasons for this fascination. Plasma renin activity, a surrogate measure of plasma ANG II concentration, is increased in renovascular hypertension and in about 16 percent of patients with essential hypertension (1). In other patients with essential hypertension, basal renin secretion and, therefore, plasma ANG II levels may be inadequately suppressed due to a subpopulation of ischemic nephrons that are hypersecreting renin (2). ANG II differs from other vasoconstrictor agents in that its pressor effect is self-potentiating and cumulative (3). The infusion of initially subpressor doses of ANG II will ultimately lead to hypertension (4,5). The mechanisms responsible for the progressive nature of ANG II–induced hypertension are complex and incompletely understood. ANG II has been also shown to stimulate vascular growth (6), and it has been postulated that this trophic effect of the agonist may play an important role in the development of ANG II–induced hypertension (7).

Until recently, methodological problems have limited the use of chronic administration of ANG II as an experimental model of hypertension. There was no reliable measure of plasma ANG II concentration (8). The short half-life of the agonist in biological tissue necessitated intravenous or intraarterial administration, which for the long term is technically difficult to maintain. The long-term administration of ANG II to large animals, such as sheep and dogs, is expensive. Interest in the chronic administration of ANG II as an experimental model of hypertension has been stimulated by the availability of miniaturized, osmotically driven minipumps that can accurately deliver the agonist, dissolved in saline, for several months.

From the beginning, it was apparent that the administration of large doses of renin or ANG II was injurious to small and large arteries (9). The damage was out of proportion to the degree of hypertension, suggesting a direct "toxic" effect of ANG II (see below). When ANG II infusion is used as an experimental model of hypertension, dosing becomes an important issue. The hypertension produced by high doses of ANG II may differ both

  G. Simon: Hypertension Clinic, Veterans Administration Medical Center, Minneapolis, Minnesota 55417.
  G. Abraham: 1st Department of Medicine, Albert Szent-Gyorgyi Medical University, Szeged, Hungary H-6701.

TABLE 1. *Plasma concentrations[a] and threshold pressor doses of ANG II in different species*

	Human	Dog	Rabbit	Rat
Plasma ANG II (pg/ml)				
Normal	2–8	15–20	52 (mean)[b]	8–30
Essential HT	8–30	–	–	–
Renovascular HT	45 (mean)	–	–	55–75
Threshold pressor dose (ng/kg/min)	0.5–1.5 iv	0.5–1.5 iv	6–8 iv	100–200 ip
Plasma ANG II (pg/ml)	~20	20–30	–	~37

[a] Measurements were done by high-pressure liquid chromatography followed by radioimmunoassay.
[b] Radioimmunoassay only.
HT, hypertension.

quantitatively and qualitatively from hypertension produced by small doses of the agonist. Our task in this chapter is to examine the mechanisms of hypertension brought about by varying doses of ANG II, and to decide which model, if any, mimics the development of high-renin (ANG II) human hypertension.

PLASMA ANGIOTENSIN II CONCENTRATION IN HYPERTENSION

Reliable measure of ANG II in plasma became available only recently (8). By separating the different angiotensins by high-pressure liquid chromatography before radioimmunoassay, it has become possible to measure plasma ANG II (1–8 octapeptide) with a limit of detection of about 1 fg/mL and an overall recovery rate of 80 percent or more. The measurements are cumbersome and labor intensive. Systemic plasma ANG II concentrations are in the range of 2–8, 15–20, and 8–30 pg/ml in normal man (8,10), dog (11,12), and rat (13–15), respectively (Table 1). In rabbits, only plasma ANG II measurements performed by immunoassay are available (16). There are few reports of plasma ANG II measurements in human hypertension, using high-pressure liquid chromatography followed by radioimmunoassay. In

patients with unilateral renovascular hypertension, plasma ANG II concentration may rise four- to sixfold, to about 45 pg/ml (Bauer JH, *personal communication*); in essential hypertension, a range of 8 to 30 pg/ml was reported (Table 1) (8). In rats with moderate salt depletion, plasma ANG II concentration increases by about 50 percent (14), and rats with two-kidney, one-clip hypertension of 2 to 3 weeks' duration have ANG II levels in the 55 to 75 pg/ml range (14,17). The pathophysiological range of plasma ANG II concentration does not appear to exceed a five- to sixfold increase, but admittedly reported values are few. By "pathophysiological" we mean concentrations that are reached in nonterminal disease states. In essential hypertension, the increase in plasma ANG II concentration may be considerably less (8).

The threshold dose for an acute pressor effect of ANG II in human subjects and dogs is about 1 ng/kg/min iv (Table 1) (18–23). Interestingly, the estimated normal rate of ANG II production in the circulation of dogs is about the same (1.5 ng/kg/min) (22). Combining the endogenous production of ANG II with the administration of a threshold pressor dose should acutely double the steady-state plasma ANG II concentration. Actual measurements by radioimmunoassay alone bear out these as-

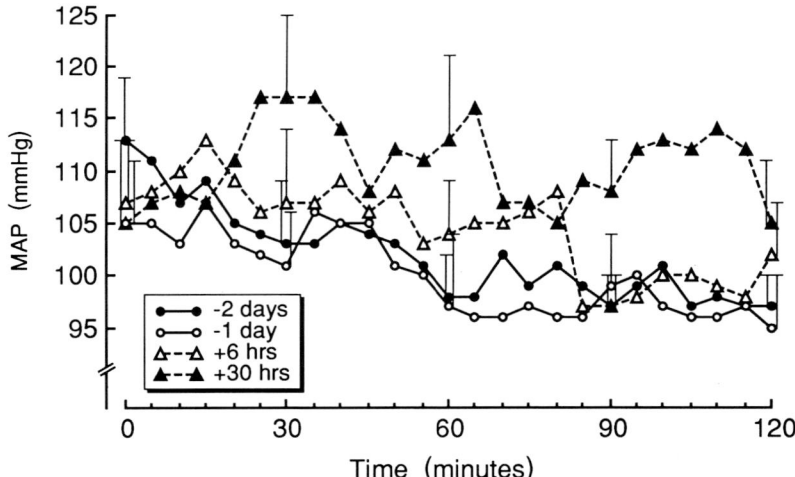

FIG. 1. Two-hour monitoring of mean arterial blood pressure (MAP) (means ± SEM) in seven free-moving, conscious rats, with indwelling aortic catheter, 1 and 2 days before and 6 and 30 h after the start of ANG II treatment (200 ng/kg/min ip), respectively. $p < .05$ for comparison of MAPs 1 day before and 30 h after the start of treatment (repeated measures ANOVA).

sumptions (Table 1) (18–23). In the rabbit, the threshold pressor dose of ANG II is much higher than in human subjects and dogs (Table 1) (4,5). In rats, ANG II is usually delivered either subcutaneously (sc) or intraperitoneally (ip) by osmotic minipump. By subcutaneous delivery, the absorbed ANG II bypasses the liver during its first passage before it enters the systemic circulation; therefore, a lesser dose is required to reach a pressor effect than with the intraperitoneal delivery of the agonist. A dose of 170 to 200 ng/kg/min ANG II sc has an immediate pressor effect in rats (24). The same dose of ANG II delivered ip has either no effect or only a minimal effect on blood pressure during the first 30 hours (Fig. 1) (25–27).

There are indications that the pathogenesis of hypertension brought about by chronic administration of pressor or initially subpressor doses of ANG II may differ substantially. As already mentioned, large doses of ANG II may be "toxic" to the vasculature. Acute elevation of blood pressure may trigger compensatory mechanisms, such as natriuresis and the local production of prostaglandins (see below), that have little to do with the more gradual development of human hypertension. Experiments using pressor and subpressor doses of ANG II will, therefore, be discussed separately.

ADMINISTRATION OF PRESSOR DOSES OF ANGIOTENSIN II

Initially, the focus of attention in human subjects and experimental animals was stimulation of aldosterone secretion by ANG II. The doses used ranged from 15 to 2,500 ng/kg/min iv and were clearly pressor (28). They produced transient sodium retention during the first day or two, followed by a natriuretic effect (20,28–31). In normotensive human subjects receiving ANG II infusion for several days, the interesting observation was made that in order to maintain the arterial pressure rise in the mild-to-moderate hypertensive range the rate of infusion had to be gradually tapered (30). This was in sharp contrast to continuous infusion of equipotent pressor doses of norepinephrine (NE), which resulted in negative sodium balance, and necessitated a gradual increase in the infusion rate in order to maintain the hypertension.

ANG II infusion as an experimental model of hypertension in dogs has been extensively investigated by the Guyton school of physiologists (21–23,32). The doses used ranged from 5 to 20 ng/kg/min iv, resulting in estimated plasma ANG II concentrations of 100 and 400 pg/ml, respectively (12). With the 5 ng/kg/min iv dose, the mean arterial pressure (MAP) of dogs rose by 23 mm Hg on day 1 and by 32 mm Hg on day 2. (A 23 mm Hg rise in MAP corresponds to a blood pressure rise from 130/85 to 160/105) (33). Cumulative sodium balance

was +58 mmol by day 1, +80 mmol by day 3, and +28 mmol by day 8. The maximum sodium retention amounted to sodium contained in about 0.5 L of normal saline. This was borne out by measurements of sodium iothalamate space (extracellular fluid volume, ECFV), which exceeded control values by 646 mL on day 1, although the increase was not statistically significant. By day 8, sodium iothalamate space exceeded control values by only 397 ml (ns). Hall and coworkers (22,32,33), in a series of ingenious and careful studies, have convincingly shown that during ANG II excess the steady-state relationship between MAP and urinary sodium excretion is shifted in the direction of higher pressures. In other words, hypertension is required to maintain sodium balance.

There are, therefore, two remarkable features of ANG II–induced hypertension. One is its progressive nature despite steady doses of the agonist. The other is the shift in the renal pressure–natriuresis relationship that reverses the initial retention of sodium and water. Sodium and water retention does not seem to be sufficient for the progression or the maintenance of the hypertension. Other mechanisms must be operative. To understand these, the experimental model has to be examined in greater detail.

Systemic Hemodynamics

There are no detailed studies of the systemic hemodynamics of ANG II–induced hypertension. In a small number of dogs, using dye-dilution techniques, Olmsted and Page (34) observed a gradual elevation of cardiac output as the infused dose of ANG II was progressively increased from 15 to 150 ng/kg/min iv. Using similar techniques, Cowley and DeClue (21) measured the cardiac output of dogs infused with 5 ng/kg/min ANG II iv for 2 weeks. The cardiac output of dogs was reduced 14 percent during the first 48 hours and, thereafter, rose gradually to 38 percent above control levels on days 4 and 5. An unspecified number of dogs in the study were on a high-sodium diet (120 mmol/day). The increases in cardiac output were observed in the absence of detectable rise in body weight and without evidence for water retention. In dogs infused with ANG II iv, the same group of investigators has observed a small rise in mean circulating pressure, suggesting reduced venous compliance. ANG II, 200 to 1,000 ng/kg/min iv, also increases the mean circulatory pressure of conscious rats in a dose-dependent manner (35). Reduced venous compliance with minor, sometimes statistically insignificant, increases in extracellular fluid volumes constitutes a plausible explanation for the rise of cardiac output in ANG II–infused dogs. If maintained, increased cardiac output may be contributing to chronic ANG II–induced hypertension.

Role of Baroreceptors

Compared to baroreceptor-denervated dogs, the rise of arterial pressure was dampened in intact dogs during the first 24 hours of ANG II administration at 5 ng/kg/min iv (21). Thereafter, arterial pressure rose at the same rate in intact and baroreceptor-denervated dogs, indicating that the baroreceptors no longer influenced the development of hypertension. The plateau of blood pressure reached after 14 days of continuous ANG II infusion was the same in the two groups of dogs. After day 5, in the intact dogs, oscillations in the arterial pressure were increased. This observation was first made by McCubbin and coworkers (36) in conscious dogs infused with 7 ng/kg min ANG II iv (see below). Our own measurements suggest greater oscillations of arterial pressure in rats after the start of ANG II infusion (Fig. 1). These findings may represent baroreceptor dysfunction or bursts of sympathetic activity or both.

Cox and Bishop (37), based on experiments conducted in rabbits, attached greater importance to the role of baroreceptors in ANG II–induced hypertension than Cowley and DeClue (21) did. Rabbits were administered ANG II iv at 50 ng/kg/min for up to 10 days. This dose of ANG II resulted in elevation of MAP by 22 mm Hg on day 1, which was sustained throughout the infusion period. On day 1 there was an acute reduction in plasma NE level and renal nerve sympathetic activity, indicating a dampening effect of baroreceptors on sympathetic outflow. Thereafter, sympathetic activity rose to an intermediate level. The partial return of sympathetic activity toward baseline was prevented, and the chronic phase of ANG II–induced hypertension was attenuated in rabbits with area postrema removal. The interpretation was that resetting of baroreceptors was an important aspect of ANG II–induced hypertension because it allowed sympathetic activity to continue at a level that was inappropriate for the prevailing arterial pressure, and that resetting of baroreceptors occurred through the area postrema. Baroreceptor activity, however, was not tested in these experiments. Much of the interpretation was based on findings in rabbits with the area postrema removed. The chronic hemodynamic response to area postrema ablation may be complex as it is discussed in Neural Mechanisms, below.

Renal Effects

There have been numerous studies of the renal effects of ANG II in human subjects and experimental animals, but there are few that used small, pathophysiological doses of the agonist (20,22,23,29–33,38). With pharmacological doses of ANG II, there has been massive urinary sodium retention, followed by the rapid development of severe hypertension and natriuresis (30,31).

With small doses of ANG II, the fluctuations in sodium balance have been minor; after transient retention, sodium balance was achieved rapidly (23,33). In one study (see below), an initially subpressor dose of ANG II led to mild hypertension without detectable sodium retention initially or long-term (23).

In conscious dogs, the infusion of ANG II, 10 ng/kg/min iv, for 14 days resulted in 15 percent reduction of effective renal plasma flow (ERPF), which was maintained throughout the infusion period (39). The glomerular filtration rate (GFR) of dogs was reduced 5 percent to 6 percent during the first few days, then returned to baseline. Calculated filtration fraction was elevated. These changes were accompanied by a rise of MAP (+38 mm Hg on day 4), marked sodium and water retention, and doubling of ECFV space (sodium iothalamate). When ANG II, 1 ng/kg/min, was infused directly into the renal artery of the remaining kidney of uninephrectomized dogs for 14 days, the same changes in ERPF, GFR, and filtration fraction were observed as with the iv infusion of the agonist (23). After transient sodium retention (+50 mmol) on day 1, sodium balance was achieved starting on day 2, when MAP rose by 9 mm Hg. A small additional increase in MAP (+6 mm Hg) occurred during the rest of the infusion period. By comparison, the infusion of 0.5 ng/kg/min of ANG II iv had no effect on either the blood pressure or sodium balance of dogs during the first 48 hours of infusion. Thereafter, MAP rose by 7 mm Hg without detectable sodium retention. The 0.5 ng/kg/min iv dose was considered to be equipotent with the 1 ng/kg/min dose delivered into the renal artery because of existing evidence that about 50 percent of intraarterially infused ANG II is degraded in the kidney. Histological examinations were not performed to rule out renal damage after 14 days of direct intraarterial infusion of ANG II.

Taken together, the findings indicate that GFR is well preserved during chronic administration of ANG II either iv or into the renal artery. With pharmacological doses of the agonist (10 ng/kg/min iv), there is massive sodium and water retention, which may be contributing to the hypertension (39). With pathophysiological doses of ANG II (1 ng/kg/min ia or 0.5 ng/kg/min iv), the cause-and-effect relationship between sodium and water balance and the hypertension is less clear (23).

Identical observations were made in human subjects. During a 2-hours infusion of 1.5 ng/kg/min of ANG II iv, there was a marked and sustained fall in ERPF and only a minor reduction in GFR (20,38). MAP rose by 5 mm Hg during the first hour and by an additional 3 mm Hg during the second hour. ANG II caused an immediate reduction in urine flow and urinary sodium retention that continued throughout the infusion period. Proximal tubular reabsorption of sodium, estimated by the lithium clearance method, was increased by ANG II. Plasma ANG II concentration was increased threefold during the first 30 min of infusion. Whether these small doses of ANG II, if administered long-term, would lead to chronic, progressive hypertension or not is an important question, but such experiments are not feasible in human subjects.

The antinatriuretic action of ANG II is complex. The topic has been previously reviewed (32,40). ANG II raises efferent arteriolar resistance to a greater extent than afferent arteriolar resistance. Greater receptor density and smaller caliber of efferent vessels account for the difference. GFR and filtered sodium load are preserved because of reduction in the pre- to postglomerular resistance ratio. Because of vasoconstriction, cortical renal blood flow and peritubular capillary hydrostatic pressure are reduced. Filtration fraction and consequently colloid osmotic pressure in peritubular capillaries are increased. The reabsorption of sodium in the proximal renal tubules is facilitated by reduced hydrostatic pressure and increased colloid osmotic pressure in the peritubular capillary network. Further downstream, vasa recta constriction reduces medullary blood flow and increases medullary interstitial fluid osmolarity. Urinary concentrating ability of the medulla is increased, favoring passive reabsorption of sodium. In addition to these hemodynamic effects, ANG II may cause sodium and water retention by direct action on proximal tubular reabsorption. The relative importance of these multiple actions of ANG II in preserving sodium has not been quantitated. While the acute antinatriuretic action of ANG II is fairly well understood, the mechanisms whereby the renal pressure–natriuresis relationship is shifted toward higher pressures during prolonged infusion of the agonist (see above) remains to be investigated.

Neural Mechanisms

There is extensive evidence that infused ANG II stimulates sympathetic outflow from the central nervous system and facilitates sympathetic neurotransmission in the periphery (41,42). The debate is about the relative importance of these effects in the pathogenesis of ANG II–induced hypertension.

Infusion of small doses of ANG II into both vertebral or carotid arteries of conscious dogs raises arterial blood pressure, whereas the intravenous infusion of the same doses does not (43,44). The threshold dose is about 1 ng/kg/min/artery, resulting in estimated increases in the concentration of ANG II in the cerebral circulation of 60 to 100 pg/mL, the upper limit of the "pathophysiological" range (44). The systemic hypertension produced is due primarily to a rise in systemic vascular resistance and can be abolished by the administration of bretylium or by cervical section of the spinal cord (41,43). Nerve recordings showed an uneven distribution of sympathetic discharge: increased preganglionic splanchnic nerve dis-

charge, unchanged cardiac nerve activity, and reduced renal nerve discharge (41). The site of action of ANG II appears to be the area postrema in the medulla oblongata where fenestration of the blood-brain barrier allows direct access to the central nervous system. Unexplained is the finding that ANG II infusion into the carotid artery of dogs produces arterial pressure elevations that are comparable to those produced by intravertebral artery infusion; the carotid arteries do not perfuse the medulla oblongata or other hindbrain regions (44). In the rat, large doses of ANG II (40–160 ng/kg/min) infused into the carotid artery raise arterial pressure more than comparable infusions into the vertebral artery (45). In all the experiments so far cited, infusions of ANG II lasted 5 to 10 minutes. Infusion of 0.7 ng/kg/min ANG II into the right vertebral artery of dogs, the left vertebral artery having been ligated, for 7 days resulted in a 12 mm Hg rise of MAP on the average (46). The same dose of ANG II delivered iv for 7 days caused a small (5 mm Hg), transient rise of MAP on days 2 and 3 of the infusion. This study confirms the findings of the short-term experiments regarding the threshold dose of ANG II needed to raise MAP. The hypertensive response elicited is sustained during the infusion but there is no evidence for progression of the hypertension, which is characteristic of the systemic administration of ANG II.

Another approach to the evaluation of the role of the central nervous system in the pathogenesis of ANG II–induced hypertension has been ablation of the area postrema prior to ANG II administration (37,47). It has been shown that in rabbits and rats surgical ablation of the area postrema attenuates the slow pressor action of ANG II. The approach is, however, complicated by confounding influences. A prolonged recovery period is required between surgical ablation of the area postrema and the start of ANG II infusion. During this waiting period, the ablated animals may become sodium depleted because of renal denervation (48). The rise in plasma renin activity (PRA) with area postrema ablation supports this possibility. During prolonged denervation of the systemic circulation there may be trophic changes in the vasculature, in this case atrophy, especially in still growing experimental animals. These changes may attenuate the arterial pressor response to ANG II independently from direct central nervous system influences.

During chronic ANG II administration sympathetic activity in the renal circulation appears to be reduced and in the mesenteric circulation appears to be increased (12,49). These differences mimic the findings of Ferrario et al. (41), who found increased sympathetic nerve discharge to the mesentery and reduced sympathetic nerve discharge to the kidney during infusion of ANG II into the vertebral circulation of dogs (see above). Carroll and coworkers (12) found reduced renal NE spillover, a measure of sympathetic activity, in dogs infused with 20 ng/kg/min ANG II iv for 6 days. By direct recording, splanchnic sympathetic nerve activity was increased in rats treated with 375 ng/kg/min ANG II sc for 14 days (49). This subcutaneous dose of ANG II corresponds to about 450 ng/kg/min ANG II delivered ip. In both studies, the doses of ANG II used were large, and the pressor response severe.

ANG II infusion also enhances vasoconstrictor responses to peripheral adrenergic nerve stimulation (42). The principal mechanism of action appears to be facilitation of NE release from preganglionic nerve endings. Whether this is a pharmacological action of ANG II or also occurs in certain pathophysiological states of activated renin-angiotensin system is still being debated. The threshold dose of ANG II eliciting the interaction in the canine kidney is highly variable, ranging from 60 to 2,900 pg/ml of perfusing blood (50). In the canine paw, the threshold dose is reproducibly about 60 pg/ml (50). Investigations in human subjects had to rely on plasma NE kinetic measurements during ANG II infusion. ANG II infused iv at 0.5 to 4 ng/kg/min had no effect on either plasma NE concentration or NE spillover to plasma despite a small pressor effect at 2 ng/kg/min dose (18).

Notwithstanding the demonstrated interaction between the sympathetic and the renin-angiotensin system, an intact sympathetic nervous system is not a requirement for the maintenance and progression of ANG II–induced hypertension. The evidence is extensive and varied. Intrarenal and iv infusion of ANG II in doses that are insufficient to have a central nervous system effect can lead to sustained and progressive hypertension (see above). In uninephrectomized rats, denervation of the remaining kidney delays but does not prevent the development of progressive hypertension (51). In dogs infused with 5 ng/kg/min ANG II iv for 10 days, the concomitant administration of guanethidine did not prevent the gradual development of hypertension (52). Sympathectomy with 6-hydroxy dopamine in Wistar-Kyoto rats did not prevent the slow pressor response to infused ANG II (53).

Role of Aldosterone

ANG II is a primary regulator of aldosterone secretion, and one of the main actions of aldosterone is salt and water retention (28,32). In human subjects, stimulation of aldosterone secretion by ANG II is maintained as long as the circulating levels of the agonist are elevated. Because of these findings, it has been assumed that stimulation of aldosterone secretion plays an important role in the maintenance and progression of ANG II–induced hypertension. Experimental findings do not bear out the assumption.

Unlike in human subjects, ANG II–induced stimulation of aldosterone secretion in sheep and dogs is tran-

sient, yet the blood pressure response to ANG II of these species is similar to that of man (28). A fall in plasma potassium concentration and an increase in urinary potassium excretion are prominent features of aldosterone excess, but these changes are either absent or only minimal in ANG II–induced hypertension. In intact dogs, chronic infusion of aldosterone in doses that raise plasma levels two- to fourfold had little or no effect on arterial pressure (54). The same observation was made in dogs infused with ANG II, that is, raising aldosterone levels by infusion in these dogs had no additive effect on the level of blood pressure (55). Finally, adrenelectomy in rabbits does not prevent the gradual development of ANG II–induced hypertension (5).

Humoral Mechanisms

In the central nervous system, large doses of ANG II result in the release of vasopressin into the circulation (44). Only infusion of ANG II into the carotid artery, but not into the vertebral artery, was found to be effective. The estimated increase in plasma ANG II concentration during infusion was about 700 pg/mL, well beyond the pathophysiological range.

Pharmacological doses of ANG II are also needed to stimulate the release of atrial natriuretic factor (26). In the rat, the dose required is about 800 ng/kg/min ip. At this dose, atrial natriuretic factor release is mediated by elevation of left ventricular end-diastolic pressure rather than by a direct effect of ANG II.

ANG II has been shown to stimulate the release of vasodilator and vasoconstrictor prostaglandins from a large variety of tissue, including the kidney, heart, and blood vessels (25,56). Prostaglandins may, therefore, attenuate or amplify the hemodynamic action of ANG II. There are relatively few studies investigating the role of prostaglandins in ANG II–induced hypertension. In general, pressor doses, and in some cases pharmacological doses, of ANG II were required to stimulate prostaglandin production (25,57,58). Pressor doses of ANG II (c. 500 ng/kg/min ip) administered to rats for 12 days increased plasma concentration and urinary excretion of prostaglandin (PGI_2) (25). PGI_2 release was also increased from incubated aortic rings and renal medulla. Smaller doses of ANG II (250–300 ng/kg/min ip) that produced either no hypertension or only minimal rise in blood pressure had no such effects. ANG II administered to rats in large doses, especially in combination with saline administration, also increased urinary excretion of thromboxanes (57). Inhibition of thromboxane synthetase blunted the renal hemodynamic effects of ANG II and attenuated the hypertension (57,58). Because of the large doses used and the severe hypertension produced, it is difficult to determine whether renal and arterial prostaglandin production is intrinsic to the pathogenesis of ANG II–induced hypertension, or whether it is secondary to ANG II–induced vascular damage.

"Toxic" Vascular Effects

In the evaluation of the hemodynamic effects of ANG II, the possibility of vascular "toxicity" has to be ruled out. This has been seldom done. By vascular toxicity is meant histologically demonstrable tissue damage. This is of particular concern when ANG II is infused intraarterially for prolonged periods of time. Under these circumstances, because of laminar flow, segmental vascular beds downstream from the infusion point may be intermittently exposed to large concentrations of the agonist. That ANG II in large concentrations is toxic to arteries has been demonstrated repeatedly (9). In the majority of studies, such large concentrations of ANG II were used that the relevance of the findings to human disease remains in doubt (16,59–64). Lesions included fibrinoid necrosis of small arteries, polyarteritis-like changes of large arteries, renal tubular necrosis, and widespread focal myocardial infarction. Some of these same changes can be found in patients dying from complications of malignant hypertension (16).

An unusual feature of the immediate vascular effects of large concentrations of ANG II has been contraction of endothelial cells. This was demonstrated by electromicroscopy in the iliac artery of rats after injection of ANG II (66,000,000 pg/mL saline!) into the lumen (60). Injections of epinephrine, dopamine, and tyramine had no such effect. Robertson and Khairallah (62) used smaller but still large concentrations of ANG II (500 pg/ml) to demonstrate the phenomenon in the aorta of rabbits. After the administration of ANG II, Evans Blue dye penetrated the arterial wall, staining it blue. Based on these findings, it has been proposed that ANG II–induced endothelial cell contraction increases vascular permeability, allowing the penetration of plasma proteins and platelets into the vessel wall, which form deposits and cause necrosis (fibrinoid necrosis).

Because of the large concentrations of ANG II used, it appeared that these experiments have little bearing on the gradual development of hypertension during chronic administration of small doses of ANG II. However, the issue of vascular toxicity was revived by a recent report of ANG II–induced hypertension in rats (65). Rats were treated with 450 ng/kg/min of ANG II sc for 14 days. Systolic blood pressure of rats rose 48 mm Hg during week 1 and 64 mm Hg during week 2. At the end of the infusion period, small renal arteries showed focal injury with fibrinoid necrosis and medial hyperplasia. There was in addition focal tubulointerstitial injury with tubular atrophy, cast formation, interstitial monocytic infiltrate, and mild interstitial fibrosis. These findings raise disturbing questions about pressor doses of ANG II as

an experimental model of high-renin (ANG II) human hypertension. If similar changes also occur in dogs infused with pressor doses of ANG II either iv or into the renal artery, then renal injury in itself may explain the progressive nature of the hypertension that is produced. In future investigations, it will be necessary to define the dose of ANG II that leads to the gradual development of hypertension without causing renal injury.

There is indirect evidence that high circulating levels of ANG II may be also toxic in human hypertension. During a 5-year period, Brunner and coworkers (1) observed 11 and 14 percent incidence of heart attacks and strokes among patients with high- and normal-renin essential hypertension, respectively. During a similar period of observation, none of 59 patients with low-renin essential hypertension suffered a complication. This study was criticized for being retrospective. In a recent prospective investigation (66), the incidence of myocardial infarction was 14.7, 5.6, and 2.8/1,000 person-years among patients with high-, normal-, and low-renin essential hypertension, respectively. The average follow-up was 8.3 years. There was no difference in the incidence of strokes among the three groups. This being an epidemiological study, a cause-and-effect relationship between ANG II and vascular disease was not established. High circulating levels of ANG II may predispose hypertensive patients to arteriosclerosis.

ADMINISTRATION OF SUBPRESSOR DOSES OF ANGIOTENSIN II

There are two unique features of ANG II–induced hypertension that become apparent when the agonist is administered to experimental animals for prolonged periods of time in initially subpressor doses: autopotentiation and stimulation of vascular growth (3,6). Autopotentiation is the phenomenon whereby the agonist moves its own pressure-dose relationship toward higher pressures during chronic administration. This is contrary to expectations because during long-term administration of vasoconstrictor agents one expects down-regulation rather than up-regulation of responses. The possibility that high circulating levels of ANG II may stimulate vascular growth was raised almost 30 years ago, based on indirect clinical observations (67). More recent tissue culture studies have firmly established the observation that at least *in vitro* ANG II is a potent trophic factor of vascular muscle (6).

Autopotentiation

The observation that the continuous administration of initially subpressor doses of ANG II leads to hypertension was first reported by Dickinson and Lawrence (4,5).

The authors administered small doses of ANG II by iv infusion to rabbits for 3 days and measured changes in MAP at 3 hours and 3 days. Over the 3-day period, the blood pressure–dose relationship shifted toward higher pressures, indicating that potentiation of the hypertensinogenic effect of ANG II has occurred. Some of the doses (6–8 ng/kg/min iv) were subpressor at 3 hours but were mildly pressor by 3 days of continuous administration. This finding raised the possibility that administered long enough acutely ineffective doses of ANG II may be hypertensinogenic in the long run. Comparably increasing sensitivity to small doses of ANG II has been reported in man (3,30), dogs (3,23,28,36,68), and rats (59,69,70), but few of these studies utilized initially subpressor doses of ANG II. One exception was already mentioned— Lohmeier and Cowley (23) infused 0.5 ng/kg/min ANG II iv into dogs for 14 days as control experiments for infusion of the agonist directly into the renal artery of dogs (see above). During the first 48 hours of infusion MAP did not change. Thereafter, MAP rose by 7 mm Hg and remained elevated for the rest of the infusion period. Lachance and Garcia (26) and Diz et al. (25) gave subpressor infusions of ANG II (200–300 ng/kg/min ip) to rats as control experiments for larger doses of ANG II and found no significant increase in systolic blood pressure (BP) over a 7- to 12-day infusion period. However, closer scrutiny of the data reveals a 12 mm Hg rise in systolic BP on days 2 and 3 in both studies. We have administered 200 ng/kg/min ANG II ip to rats and measured MAP continuously for 2 hours daily before and after the start of the infusion. After 6 hours of infusion, there were no significant elevations of systolic BP, but by 30 hours systolic BP was elevated slightly (Fig. 1).

We have investigated the systemic and some of the regional hemodynamic actions of ANG II administered to rats in initially subpressor doses (71,72). Administered for 24 hours, ANG II, 200 ng/kg/min ip, had no effect on either the BP or pressor responses of rats. After 7 to 10 days of continuous ANG II administration, systolic BP rose slightly, and pressor responses were selectively potentiated to ANG II itself but not to NE or serotonin (Fig. 2). Similar observations were made by Bean et al. (68) in dogs and by Basso (70) in rats. In our study, potentiation of pressor responses to ANG II appeared to be due to potentiation of vascular responses because pressure responses to ANG II but not to NE or vasopressin were also increased in the mesenteric circulation of rats, pump-perfused with the rats' own blood (Fig. 3). Interestingly, we did not find autopotentiation of renal vasoconstrictor responses in ANG II–treated rats (*unpublished observations*). There were no detectable changes in baroreceptor sensitivity or intravascular volumes (^{125}I-albumin space) of rats at this stage of ANG II administration (*unpublished observations*). After 5 to 6 weeks of continuous ANG II administration in the same dose as above, systolic BP rose by 12 mm Hg, and pressor responses were increased not only to ANG II but also to NE. Measured after systemic vasodilation with papaverine iv, the wall-to-lumen ratio of small and large mesenteric arteries were unchanged after 7 to 10 days (*unpublished observations*) and increased after 5 to 6 weeks of ANG II administration (Fig. 4). ANG II–specific pressor hyperresponsiveness appears to be a unique feature of the developmental stage of ANG II– induced hypertension and may play an important role in the development of structural vascular changes. In this regard, experimental ANG II–induced hypertension resembles the early stages of human hypertension where, too, pressor hyperresponsiveness was postulated to play an important role in the development of structural vascular changes and of chronic hypertension (73,74).

The mechanisms responsible for the autopotentiation of vasoconstrictor responses by ANG II are unknown. Possibilities include ANG II–specific changes in vascular smooth muscle function and local interaction between ANG II and sympathetic nerve endings. ANG II–specific

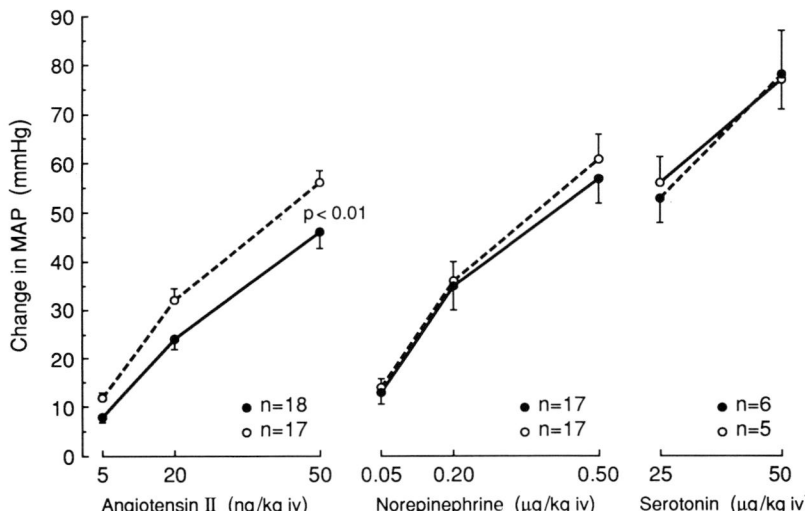

FIG. 2. Mean arterial pressure–dose-response curves (means ± SEM) of rats after 7 to 10 days of ANG II (200 ng/kg/min ip) (*open symbols*) or sham treatment (*solid circles*). Measurements were obtained in chloralose-anesthetized rats after neurohumoral blockade with chlorisondamine, methscopolamine, and vasopressin antagonist. $p < .01$ by repeated measures ANOVA.

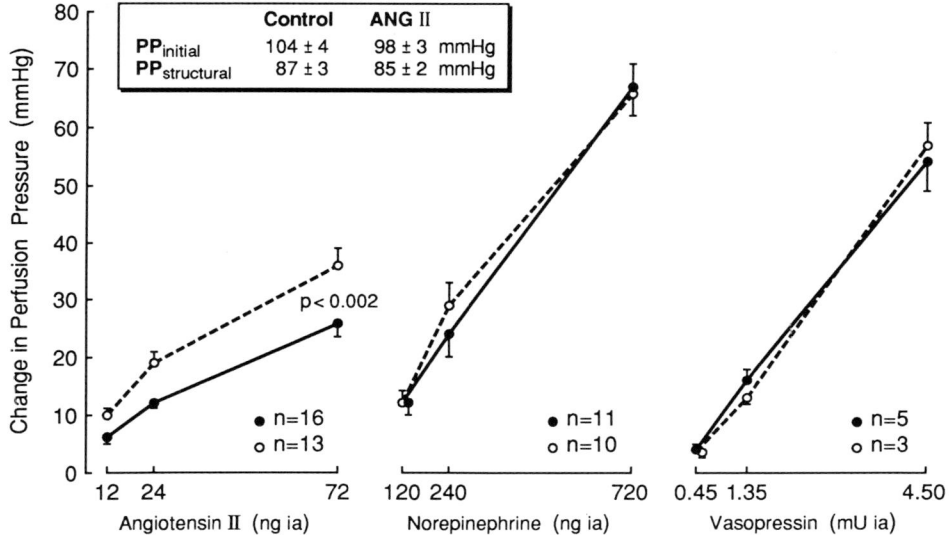

FIG. 3. Mesenteric vascular pressure–dose relationships (means ± SEM) of rats after 7 to 10 days of ANG II (200 ng/kg/min ip) (*open symbols*) or sham treatment (*solid symbols*). PP initial and PP structural indicate perfusion pressure at constant flow at the start of measurements and after maximal vasodilatation (papaverine and sodium-nitroprusside), respectively. *p* < .002 by repeated measures ANOVA.

changes in smooth muscle function may involve up-regulation of receptors or postreceptor mechanisms. Small doses of ANG II administered to rats have been shown to up-regulate glomerular mesangial and adrenal glomerulosa ANG II receptors (75,76). Up-regulation of glomerular mesangial receptors was accompanied by enhanced mesangial cell contractibility. Similar changes may have occurred in the mesenteric circulation of our rats (see above). Possible postreceptor mechanisms include activation of ANG II–specific G protein–transduced pathways (77). It has been shown recently that infusion of ANG II in subpressor doses increases the levels of the G isoforms αi-2 and αi-3 in glomerular and

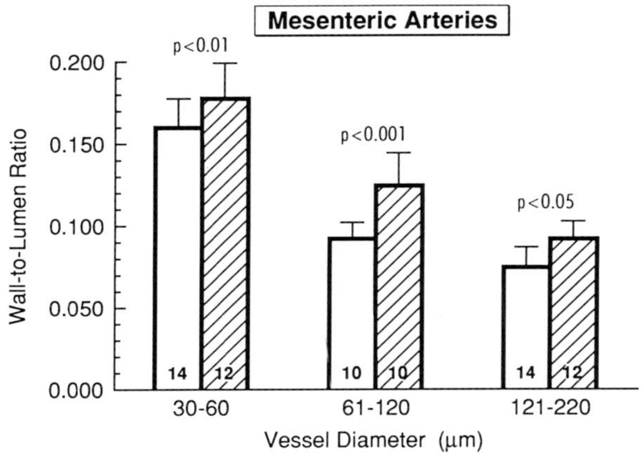

mesenteric vascular membranes of rats. Although an intact sympathetic nervous system may not be a requirement for the onset of ANG II–induced hypertension (see above), a potentiating role of sympathetic innervation in the development of ANG II–induced structural vascular changes cannot be ruled out. Finally, we have advanced our own theory of the mechanisms that underlie the autopotentiation of vasoconstrictor responses by ANG II. It is based on the trophic vascular effects of ANG II (see below).

Lack of Salt and Water Retention

With the administration of pressor doses of ANG II, salt and water retention is invariably present. It has been proposed that some of the early rise in blood pressure is due to a positive sodium balance (22,23,32). In contrast, when ANG II is administered in small or initially subpressor doses, it is difficult to demonstrate sodium and water retention. We have identified experimental data from nine sources, none of which demonstrated significant sodium retention (5,23,25,26,47,51,68,69,78). Some of these studies were detailed and well done. The one by Lohmeier and Cowley (23) was already discussed (see above). The administration of ANG II in initially subpressor doses (0.5 ng/kg/min iv) to dogs for 14 days raised MAP by 7 mm Hg by day 4 without a detectable change in sodium or water balance. Several studies conducted in rats also did not detect sodium or water retention. It can be argued, however, that small changes in sodium balance are difficult to detect in growing rats, which are commonly used for this type of experiment,

FIG. 4. Wall-to-lumen ratio (means ± SD) of mesenteric arteries of rats receiving 200 ng/kg/min ANG II ip for 6 weeks and of vehicle-infused control rats (hatched bars). Arteries were fixed *in situ* after maximal vasodilatation (papaverine). Statistical comparisons were made by two-factor ANOVA. Numbers of observations are shown within bars.

considering that their daily sodium intake is only about 3 mmol, up to 5 percent of which is normally retained daily (79). In one rat study, using pressor doses of ANG II, the progressive development of hypertension was associated with a negative rather than a positive sodium balance (78). In another rat study, pressor doses of ANG II (500 ng/kg/min ip) for 12 days did not result in expansion of ECFV ($^{35}SO_4$-space) (15). There are additional studies conducted in rabbits and dogs that also failed to show sodium retention with the long-term administration of small doses of ANG II (5,68). One has to conclude that sodium and water retention is not a requirement for the slow pressor action of ANG II.

Vascular Trophic Effects of Angiotensin II

There is a burgeoning body of evidence that ANG II in concentrations as low as 100 pg/mL is a trophic factor of vascular smooth muscle cells in tissue culture (6,80). In part, this trophic effect of ANG II is mediated through interaction with autocrine factors, such as transforming growth factor-β (81). The *in vitro* trophic effects of ANG II, including the role of second and third messengers, have been reviewed previously and will not be repeated here (6,82).

In vivo evidence for the trophic vascular effect of ANG II is less extensive than the *in vitro* evidence. As early as 1966 (67), angiopathy resembling hypertensive changes was reported in children with familial chronic diarrhea. Because of chronic dehydration, electrolyte imbalance, and weight loss, these children were normotensive despite chronically elevated plasma renin activity and, presumably, high circulating ANG II levels. It was suggested, therefore, that ANG II may be responsible for arterial wall hypertrophy or hyperplasia or both in this condition. Bartter's syndrome is another condition in which high circulating levels of ANG II are accompanied by normotension and trophic changes of arteries (83). There is also experimental evidence that infusion of ANG II in dogs promotes the growth of collateral vessels independently of pressure stimuli (84). Pressor doses of ANG II in rats produce cardiomegaly and medial hypertrophy of resistance arteries. Coadministration of ANG II and hydralazine prevents the rise in arterial pressure and the development of cardiomegaly but does not inhibit the structural vascular changes, suggesting that nonpressor mechanisms, in this case a direct effect of ANG II, may be contributing to vascular growth (24). When pressor doses of ANG II are administered to rats, and the blood pressure is allowed to rise, it is impossible to separate pressure-related from ANG II–induced changes in vascular growth (85).

We have conducted studies to detect trophic changes of arteries in rats treated with initially subpressor doses of ANG II, before the onset of hypertension (27,86,87).

In some of these studies, trophic changes were also sought in veins in an attempt to dissociate the trophic effects of ANG II from its pressor action. In rats treated with 80 to 260 ng/kg/min ANG II ip for 24 hours, a dose-dependent increase in Na-K pump activity of the aorta was found (27). Increased membrane-bound Na-K pump activity is a requirement for growth (88,89). In rats treated with 200 ng/kg/min ANG II ip, we have detected a bifunctional effect of the agonist on vascular muscle growth; protein (^{35}S-methionine) synthesis of aortic media was stimulated, and DNA (^3H-thymidine) synthesis of aortic media was inhibited (86). Protein synthesis was also increased in the portal vein and bladder wall, but not in the diaphragm, of rats. However, the most pronounced trophic effect of ANG II that we have detected so far is stimulation of vascular proteoglycan synthesis (^{35}S-sulfate). Whereas the increase in protein synthesis of the aorta of ANG II–treated rats amounted to 14 percent, the increase in proteoglycan synthesis at the same dose was 52 percent. Stimulation of proteoglycan synthesis of the aorta was also detected with 100 (instead of 200) ng/kg/min ANG II ip for 48 hours, a clearly subpressor dose. The above measurements were performed *ex vivo*. We have recently extended these investigations by measuring proteoglycan synthesis of vascular and nonvascular tissue of ANG II–treated and control rats *in vivo*, after iv injection of ^{35}S-sulfate. Stimulation of proteoglycan synthesis of the aorta of rats treated with 200 ng/kg/min ANG II ip for 48 hours reached 92 percent (Fig. 5). Proteoglycan synthesis was also increased in mesenteric arteries, right ventricle, and vena cava of ANG II–treated rats, but not in their diaphragm, kidney, or bladder wall. That ANG II may have a pressure-independent effect on myocardial fibrous tissue synthesis has been suggested previously (90). ANG II–induced stimulation of proteoglycan synthesis *in vivo* appears to be cardiovascular tissue–specific.

The early occurrence, magnitude, and cardiovascular tissue–specificity of ANG II–stimulated proteoglycan synthesis suggest that restructuring of extracellular matrix may have a role in the slow pressor action of ANG II. Previously, we have proposed that by binding and attracting sodium ions, the paracellular accumulation of proteoglycans may increase the transmembrane sodium gradient and thereby potentiate the vasoconstrictor action of agonists whose mode of action involves the rapid influx of sodium (27,91,92). ANG II is one such agonist (93). The proposed mechanism may in part account for the autopotentiation of vasoconstrictor responses by ANG II (see above).

Recent interest in trophic factors has prompted a modification of Folkow's original theory of the pathogenesis of human essential hypertension (73). According to Folkow et al. (73), the cause of essential hypertension is the stress-induced intermittent elevation of blood pressure that causes hypertrophy of resistance arteries,

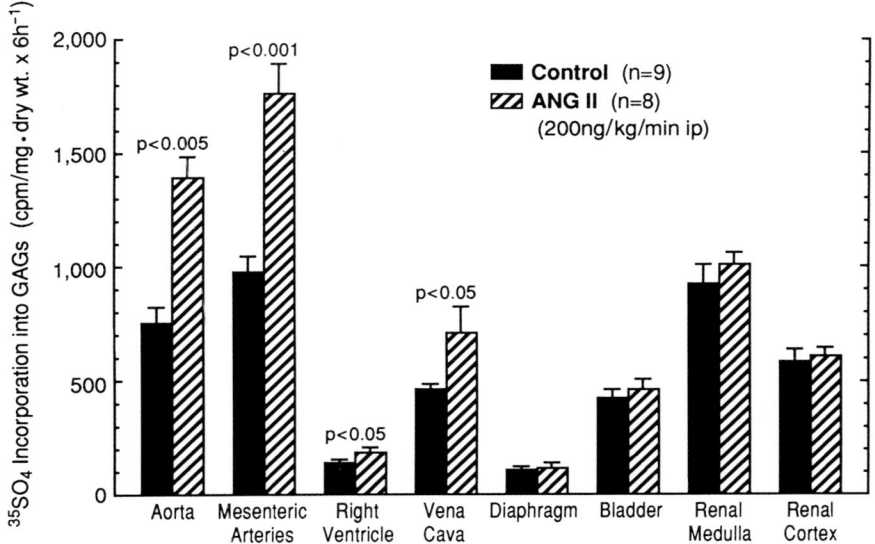

FIG. 5. *In vivo* incorporation of $^{35}SO_4$ into tissue glycosaminoglycans (GAG) (means ± SEM) of rats receiving ANG II (200 ng/kg/min ip) for 48 h and of vehicle-infused control rats. $^{35}SO_4$, 1 µCi/gm body weight, was injected iv 6 h before removal of tissues. Statistical comparisons were made by Student's *t* test for unpaired replicates.

thereby potentiating pressor responses and initiating a vicious cycle that, ultimately, leads to chronic elevation of blood pressure. Lever (7) modified this prescription for hypertension by suggesting that the initiating cause of hypertension may not be the intermittent, stress-related rise in blood pressure but rather medial hypertrophy or hyperplasia of resistance arteries induced by endogenous growth factors. Because of its vascular tissue–specific trophic effects, ANG II is prominent among the candidate growth factors. Subtle, intermittent, inappropriate elevations in plasma ANG II concentrations over several years may be sufficient to promote vascular hypertrophy and initiate the vicious cycle that, ultimately, will lead to chronic elevation of blood pressure.

SUMMARY

It is as if we were confronted with two experimental models of hypertension, one brought about by chronic administration of pressor doses of ANG II, the other by chronic administration of initially subpressor doses of the agonist. The common feature of both is the progressive nature of the hypertension that cannot be explained by the immediate vasoconstrictor action of ANG II. Otherwise, there are important differences between the two models that go beyond the emphasis of the investigators using these models. The hypertension brought about by pressor doses of ANG II is characterized by an acute rise of blood pressure and sodium and water retention that trigger some important compensatory reactions. A further rise in blood pressure reestablishes sodium and water balance (rightward shift of renal pressure natriuresis curve). Other compensatory mechanisms include resetting of baroreceptors, stimulation of tissue prostaglandin synthesis, and secretion of atrial natriuretic factor. The

presence of vascular injury during administration of pressor doses of ANG II is a distinct possibility, in some cases documented, and complicates the interpretation of findings.

By design, when ANG II is administered in initially subpressor doses, the rise of blood pressure is gradual and modest. Sodium and water retention does not play an important role in the slow pressor action of ANG II. The amount of sodium and water retention that may occur but be missed by available techniques is not likely to be hemodynamically significant. Whether there is a rightward shift of the renal pressure–natriuresis relationship is not known. Compensatory mechanisms that play a prominent role in the development of hypertension induced by pressor doses of ANG II do not seem to be activated by small doses of the agonist. Autopotentiation of pressor and vasoconstrictor responses by ANG II is the characteristic feature of the early stages of hypertension induced by small doses of ANG II. Trophic stimulation of vascular tissue, in particular restructuring of extracellular matrix, precedes and may, therefore, be the mechanism responsible for the hemodynamic changes.

CONCLUSIONS

By now, our bias must be clear. The long-term administration of initially subpressor doses of ANG II mimics the development of human hypertension to a greater extent than the administration of pressor doses. The model gives support to the theory that in some forms of hypertension trophic vascular changes may initiate the hypertensive process. Transient autopotentiation of pressor responses by ANG II may function as an amplifier in the vicious cycle that leads to the development of structural vascular changes and, ultimately, of hypertension.

According to Guyton et al.'s (94) view, chronic hypertension is unimaginable without a renal defect, namely, a rightward shift of the renal pressure–natriuresis curve. A corollary to this statement is that systemic vasoconstriction, passive or active, without similar changes in the kidney, does not lead to chronic hypertension (95). The question that has not been asked is whether renal vasoconstriction by itself, without similar changes in the extrarenal circulation, will lead to the type of hypertension that is encountered in clinical practice. Reduction in renal function has to be extreme to cause hypertension without concomitant changes in the rest of the circulation, as in bilateral constriction of the renal arteries and the remnant kidney model of hypertension. This kind of hypertension is characterized by salt and water retention, edema, and renal insufficiency. These are not the features of uncomplicated human essential hypertension. The pressor and subpressor models of ANG II–induced hypertension draw attention to the relative importance of renal and extrarenal mechanisms in the pathogenesis of hypertension. The model of hypertension using pressor doses of ANG II illustrates the importance of renal mechanisms. The model using subpressor doses of ANG II illustrates the importance of changes that take place in the systemic circulation. We submit that in human essential hypertension, as in hypertension induced with small doses of ANG II, renal and nonrenal mechanisms operating together lead to the gradual rise of blood pressure.

The year 1998 will mark the 100th anniversary of the discovery of the pressor properties of renal cortical extracts (96) and the beginning of the era of hypertension research. Almost 100 years of intense research have produced a large body of new information but little progress toward the discovery of the cause of essential hypertension. One cannot help but suspect that there was a basic flaw in our approach. We have tried to discover the cause of a disease that develops over a period of several years by investigating experimental models in which hypertension is produced overnight. Logic would dictate that this cannot be done. The study of the two models of ANG II–induced hypertension, one using pressor, the other initially subpressor, doses, illustrates the point that an entirely different pathophysiological picture emerges when hypertension is induced acutely or gradually by the same agent. To find the cause of human essential hypertension we may have to reorient ourselves toward the investigation of experimental models that lead to hypertension over a prolonged period of time.

ACKNOWLEDGMENTS

This work was supported by a Merit Review Research Grant from the Department of Veterans Affairs and by a Grant-In-Aid Research Grant from the Minnesota Affiliate of the American Heart Association.

REFERENCES

1. Brunner HR, Laragh JH, Baer L, et al. *N Engl J Med* 1972;286: 441–449.
2. Sealey JE, Blumenfeld JD, Bell GM, Pecker MS, Somers SC, Laragh JH. In: Laragh JH, Brenner BM, eds. *Hypertension: pathophysiology, diagnosis and management.* New York: Raven Press, 1990;1089–1103.
3. Robertson JIS, Morton JJ, Tillman DM, Lever AF. *J Hypertens* 1986;4(suppl 4):S95–S103.
4. Dickinson CJ, Lawrence JR. *Lancet* 1963;1:1354–1356.
5. Dickinson CJ, Yu R. *Circ Res* 1967;20–21(suppl II):II-157–II-163.
6. Schelling P, Fischer H, Ganten D. *J Hypertens* 1991;9:3–15.
7. Lever AF. *J Hypertens* 1986;4:515–524.
8. Nussberger J, Waeber B, Brunner HR. *Am J Hypertens* 1989;2: 286–293.
9. Giese J. *Am J Med* 1973;55:315–332.
10. Reams GP, Souther M, Parisi M, VanStone JC, Bauer JH. *J Lab Clin Med* 1989;113:749–752.
11. Villareal D, Wu Z, Baur JH. *Am J Hypertens* 1991;4:84A.
12. Carroll RG, Lohmeier TE, Brown A. *Hypertension* 1984;6:675–681.
13. Seikaly MG, Arant BS, Seney FD. *J Clin Invest* 1990;86:1352–1357.
14. Nussberger J, Fluckiger JP, Hui KY, Evequoz D, Waeber B, Brunner HR. *J Hypertens* 1991;9(suppl 6):S230–S231.
15. Sato Y, Ogata E, Fujita T. *Hypertension* 1991;18:622–629.
16. Gavras H, Kremer D, Brown JJ, et al. *Am Heart J* 1975;89:321–332.
17. Von Thun AM, Hymel AA, Navar LG. *Clin Res* 1991;39:807A.
18. Goldsmith SR, Hasking GJ. *Am J Physiol* 1990;258:H179–H182.
19. Montwani JG, Struthers AD. *Clin Sci* 1992;82:397–405.
20. Eiskjaer H, Sorensen SS, Danielsen M, Pedersen EP. *J Hypertens* 1992;10:1033–1040.
21. Cowley AW, DeClue JW. *Circ Res* 1976;39:779–787.
22. DeClue JW, Guyton AC, Cowley AW, Coleman TG, Norman RA, McCaa RE. *Circ Res* 1978;43:503–512.
23. Lohmeier TE, Cowley AW. *Circ Res* 1979;44:154–160.
24. Griffin SA, Brown WCB, MacPherson F, et al. *Hypertension* 1991;17:626–635.
25. Diz DI, Baer PG, Nasjletti A. *J Clin Invest* 1983;74:466–477.
26. Lachance D, Garcia R. *Hypertension* 1988;11:502–508.
27. Simon G. *Proc Soc Exp Biol Med* 1992;199:424–431.
28. Brown JJ, Casals-Stenzel J, Alison MM, et al. *Hypertension* 1979;1:159–179.
29. Urquhart J, Davis JO, Higgins JT. *Am J Physiol* 1963;205:1241–1246.
30. Ames RP, Borkowski AJ, Sicinski AM, Laragh JH. *J Clin Invest* 1965;44:1171–1186.
31. Louis WJ, Doyle AE. *Clin Sci* 1965;29:489–504.
32. Hall JE. *Am J Physiol* 1986;250:R960–R972.
33. Hall JE, Granger JP, Hester RL, Coleman TG, Smith MJ, Cross RB. *Am J Physiol* 1984;246:F627–F634.
34. Olmsted F, Page IH. *Circ Res* 1965;16:140–149.
35. Tabrizchi R, King KA, Pang CY. *Eur J Pharmacol* 1992;219:141–145.
36. McCubbin JW, DeMoura RS, Page IH, Olmsted F. *Science* 1965;149:1394–1395.
37. Cox BF, Bishop VS. *Am J Physiol* 1991;261:H1284–H1291.
38. Dusing R, Moritz J, Glanzer K, Kramer HJ. *Br J Clin Pharmacol* 1985;19:29–35.
39. Hall JE, Guyton AC, Salgado HC, McCaa RE, Balfe JW. *Am J Physiol* 1978;235:F174–F179.
40. Ichikawa I, Harris RC. *Kidney Int* 1991;40:583–596.
41. Ferrario CM, Gildenberg PL, McCubbin JW. *Circ Res* 1972;30: 257–262.
42. Zimmerman BG, Sybertz E, Wong PC. *J Hypertens* 1984;2:581–587.
43. Ferrario CM, Dickinson CJ, McCubbin JW. *Clin Sci* 1970;39: 239–245.
44. Reid IA, Brooks VL, Rudolph CD, Keil LC. *Am J Physiol* 1982;243:R82–R91.
45. Lappe RW, Brody MJ. *Am J Physiol* 1984;246:R56–R62.
46. Fukiyama K, McCubbin JW, Page IH. *Clin Sci* 1971;40:283–291.
47. Fink GD, Bruner CA, Mangiapane ML. *Hypertension* 1987;9: 355–361.

48. Hyde TM, Miselis RR. *Am J Physiol* 1984;247:R173–R182.
49. Luft FC, Wilcox CS, Unger T, et al. *Hypertension* 1989;14:396–403.
50. Zimmerman BG, Gomer SK, Liao JC. *Fed Proc* 1972;31:1344–1350.
51. Vari RC, Zinn S, Verburg KM, Freeman RH. *Hypertension* 1987;9:345–349.
52. Hall JE, Granger JP. *Fed Proc* 1983;42:589.
53. Li P, Jackson EK. *J Pharmacol Exp Ther* 1989;251:909–921.
54. Young DB, Guyton AC. *Circ Res* 1977;40:138–142.
55. Cowley AW, McCaa RE. *Circ Res* 1976;39:788–797.
56. McGiff JC. *Clin Sci* 1980;59:105s–116s.
57. Mistry M, Nasjletti A. *J Pharmacol Exp Ther* 1990;253:90–94.
58. Wilcox CS, Welch WJ, Snellen H. *Kidney Int* 1991;40:1090–1097.
59. Koletsky S, Rivera-Velez JM, Pritchard WH. *Arch Pathol* 1966;82:99–106.
60. Constantinides P, Robinson M. *Arch Pathol* 1969;88:106–112.
61. Gavras H, Brown JJ, Lever AF, MacAdam RF, Robertson JIS. *Lancet* 1971;2:19–22.
62. Robertson AL, Khairallah PA. *Circ Res* 1972;31:923–931.
63. Wiener J, Giacomelli F. *Am J Pathol* 1973;72:221–240.
64. Giacomelli F, Anversa P, Wiener J. *Am J Pathol* 1976;84:111–138.
65. Johnson RJ, Alpers CE, Yoshimura A, et al. *Hypertension* 1992;19:464–474.
66. Alderman MH, Madhavan S, Ooi WL, et al. *N Engl J Med* 1991;324:1098–1104.
67. Pasternak A, Perheentupa J. *Lancet* 1966;2:1047–1049.
68. Bean BL, Brown JJ, Casals-Stenzel J, et al. *Circ Res* 1979;44:452–458.
69. Brown JJ, Casals-Stenzel J, Gofford S, Lever AF, Morton JJ. *Am J Physiol* 1981;241:H381–H388.
70. Basso N. *Arch Int Pharmacodyn* 1975;215:266–275.
71. Simon G, Abraham G. *Am J Hypertens* 1993;6:24A.
72. Abraham G, Simon G. *Am J Hypertens* 1994;7:269–275.
73. Folkow B, Hallback M, Lundgren Y, Sivertsson R, Weiss SI. *Circ Res* 1972;32(suppl 1):2–16.
74. Pickering TG. *Hypertension* 1990;16:487–500.
75. Aguilera G, Shirar A, Baukal A, Catt KJ. *Circ Res* 1980;46(suppl 1):118–127.
76. Douglas JG. *Hypertension* 1987;9(suppl 3):49–56.
77. Sims C, Ashby K, Douglas JG. *Hypertension* 1992;19:146–152.
78. Textor SC, Brunner HR, Gavras H. *Hypertension* 1981;3:269–276.
79. Mohring J, Mohring B. *J Appl Physiol* 1972;33:688–692.
80. Jackson CL, Schwartz SM. *Hypertension* 1992;20:713–736.
81. Itoh H, Mukoyama M, Pratt RE, Gibbons GH, Dzau VJ. *J Clin Invest* 1993;91:2268–2274.
82. Marsden PA, Brenner BM, Ballermann BJ. In: Laragh JH, Brenner BM, eds. *Hypertension: pathophysiology, diagnosis, and management.* New York: Raven Press, 1990;1247–1272.
83. Fujita T, Sakaguchi H, Sibagaki M, Fukui T, Nomura M, Sekiguchi S. *Am J Med* 1977;63:467–474.
84. Fernandez LA, Caride VJ, Twickler J, Galardy RE. *Am J Physiol* 1982;243:H869–H875.
85. Daemen MJAP, Lombardi DM, Bosman FT, Schwartz SM. *Circ Res* 1991;68:450–456.
86. Simon G, Altman S. *J Hypertens* 1992;10:1165–1171.
87. Simon G, Abraham G, Altman S. *Hypertension* 1994;23(suppl I):I148–I151.
88. Kaplan JG. *Annu Rev Physiol* 1978;40:19–41.
89. Rozengurt E, Mendoza SA. *Curr Top Membr Transport* 1986;27:163–191.
90. Weber KT, Brilla CG. *Circulation* 1991;83:1849–1865.
91. Berczi V, Simon G. *Am J Physiol* 1988;255:H860–H865.
92. Simon G. *Clin Sci* 1990;78:533–540.
93. Smith JB, Brock TA. *J Cell Physiol* 1983;114:284–290.
94. Guyton AC, Cowley AW, Young DB, Coleman TG, Hall JE, DeClue JW. In: Guyton AC, Cowley AW, eds. *Cardiovascular physiology II.* Baltimore: University Park, 1976;341–385.
95. Guyton AC, Coleman TG, Cowley AW, Scheel KW, Manning RD, Norman RA. *Am J Med* 1972;52:584–594.
96. Tigerstedt RAA, Bergman PG. *Scand Arch Physiol* 1898;8:223–271.

Hypertension: Pathophysiology, Diagnosis, and Management, Second Edition,
edited by J.H. Laragh and B.M. Brenner,
Raven Press, Ltd., New York © 1995.

CHAPTER **86**

Intrarenal Actions of Angiotensin II in the Pathogenesis of Experimental Hypertension

Kenneth D. Mitchell and L. Gabriel Navar

The long-standing concept that a cardinal characteristic of the pathophysiology of hypertension involves a renal derangement whereby the kidneys are unable to achieve appropriate salt excretion at normotensive arterial pressures has withstood many challenges and has continued to gain credibility during recent years (1–12). Advocates of this concept have maintained that, without such a derangement, renal compensatory mechanisms are normally so effective that hypertensinogenic processes of nonrenal origin would be appropriately countered by modifications of salt and water balance, extracellular fluid volume, and plasma volume, which would lead to corrections in systemic arterial pressure. With the continued analysis of this premise, it has become apparent that various complex interacting mechanisms can influence the kidney's capability to maintain an appropriate level of salt excretion. Powerful paracrine systems may influence the renal microvasculature and tubular network in a synergistic manner to achieve an intrarenal environment conducive to the development and maintenance of hypertension. The renin-angiotensin system stands at the forefront of the various hypertensinogenic

mechanisms, and its many intricate influences continue to stimulate intensive investigation.

It is well recognized that the renin-angiotensin system serves an essential homeostatic need of the organism to respond to a salt-deficient environment and protect against life-threatening loss of salt and extracellular fluid volume. Unfortunately, the efficiency and power of the renin-angiotensin system also makes it a prime contributor to the pathophysiology of hypertension. This chapter specifically focuses on the interactions among the various intrarenal actions of angiotensin II (ANG II) and the hypertensinogenic processes that develop when this system is inappropriately activated.

ACTIONS OF ANGIOTENSIN II ON TUBULAR TRANSPORT PROCESSES

In addition to its indirect effects mediated in the distal nephron segment by the mineralocorticoid aldosterone, ANG II directly influences tubular sodium reabsorptive mechanisms (13–17). The mechanisms responsible for these direct effects have remained controversial because both natriuretic and antinatriuretic responses to the hormone have been observed (13,14,16). Early studies reported that administration of renal extracts, renin, or ANG II could elicit marked increases in urine flow and

K. D. Mitchell and L. G. Navar: Department of Physiology, Tulane University School of Medicine, New Orleans, Louisiana 70112.

sodium excretion despite decreasing renal blood flow (18–21). However, it became apparent that the direct renal effects of lower (subpressor) doses of ANG II were primarily antidiuretic and antinatriuretic whereas larger doses could cause natriuresis either by a direct effect or as a consequence of the associated increase in arterial blood pressure (13,14,16). Although the antinatriuretic effects of the lower doses were often associated with reductions in both glomerular filtration rate (GFR) and renal blood flow (RBF) (13,14,16), several studies have demonstrated that ANG II can elicit antinatriuretic effects even in the absence of changes in GFR (22–24). These findings indicate that ANG II, at low doses, exerts a direct stimulatory effect on tubular sodium and fluid reabsorption.

Evidence for a direct stimulatory action of ANG II on tubular sodium reabsorption has also been obtained from studies performed with pharmacological inhibitors or antagonists of the renin-angiotensin system. It has been demonstrated that when the associated decreases in arterial pressure are slight, blockade of the renin-angiotensin system results in increases in both absolute and fractional sodium excretion (14–17). In addition, pharmacological blockade of the renin-angiotensin system has been shown to result in a marked augmentation of the slope of the pressure-natriuresis relationship, especially under conditions in which the endogenous activity of the renin-angiotensin system is enhanced (25–27). The potency of the effect of blockade of the renin-angiotensin system to decrease tubular sodium reabsorption was particularly demonstrated in a study in which the kidneys were subjected to a combination of a renin inhibitor, an angiotensin-converting enzyme (ACE) inhibitor, and an ANG II receptor antagonist infused directly into the renal artery of dogs (28). Infusion of these three agents combined, at doses that did not spill over into the systemic circulation to produce systemic hypotension, elicited approximately a tenfold increase in sodium excretion. Although GFR was also increased, the increases in sodium excretion were due primarily to reductions in fractional sodium reabsorption (28). Similarly, infusion of ACE inhibitors to two-kidney, one-clip (2K1C) Goldblatt hypertensive rats can elicit a substantial natriuresis and a decrease in fractional sodium reabsorption in the nonclipped kidney when the associated decreases in arterial pressure are not excessive (29–31). These and other studies performed at the whole kidney level have clearly established that the increased sodium excretion following blockade of the renin-angiotensin system is due in large part to the removal of the stimulatory action of endogenous ANG II on tubular sodium reabsorption.

More direct studies using *in vivo* micropuncture methodology and isolated perfused tubules have indicated that the primary tubular site of action of ANG II is the proximal tubule. In accord with the overall renal re-

sponses, ANG II has been shown to exert a dose-dependent biphasic effect on proximal tubular sodium reabsorption. Experiments utilizing the stationary split-droplet microperfusion technique and isolated perfused tubules have demonstrated that peritubular concentrations of 10^{-12} to 10^{-10} M of ANG II enhance proximal tubular reabsorption rate whereas higher concentrations (greater than 10^{-7} M) inhibit proximal tubular reabsorption rate (32,33). These findings, together with the demonstration that ANG II receptors are present on both the basolateral and luminal membranes of proximal tubule cells (34), have provided compelling evidence that a major tubular site of action of ANG II is the proximal nephron.

Although it is also possible that ANG II may directly influence distal tubular reabsorptive function, there is at present little information regarding the possible direct effects of ANG II on more distal nephron segments. Indeed, the few micropuncture studies that have been performed to evaluate this issue have indicated that ANG II either inhibits or does not affect the reabsorptive function of nephron segments distal to the proximal tubule (35,36). However, most of these experiments evaluated only the effects of high doses of ANG II. In view of the subsequent findings that physiological concentrations of ANG II stimulate proximal tubular reabsorption rate and that ANG II receptors are present on distal tubule cells, albeit in lower numbers than on proximal tubule cells (37), additional studies are required to evaluate more fully the dose-response relationship between ANG II and distal tubular reabsorptive function. Thus, the currently available evidence indicates that the distal nephron sodium-conserving influence of the renin-angiotensin system is mediated primarily by the actions of the mineralocorticoid aldosterone (38).

The stimulatory action of ANG II on proximal tubular reabsorptive function has also been shown by the numerous studies using ANG II receptor antagonists or ACE inhibitors to unmask the preexisting influence being exerted by ANG II. In studies performed on chronically sodium-depleted rats, it was demonstrated that both absolute and fractional proximal tubule reabsorption rates were reduced following blockade of ANG II receptors with saralasin (39). Similarly, ACE inhibition has been shown to result in marked reductions in both absolute and fractional proximal tubule reabsorption rates in the nonclipped kidney of Goldblatt hypertensive rats (30,40). More recently, it was demonstrated that systemic administration of either an ACE inhibitor (captopril) or a nonpeptide AT_1 ANG II receptor antagonist (losartan) to normal rats inhibits proximal tubular solute and fluid reabsorption (41). To the extent that pharmacological blockade of the renin-angiotensin system unmasks the preexisting influence being exerted by ANG II, the results obtained using pharmacological blockers of the renin-angiotensin system indicate that endogenous

ANG II exerts a direct stimulatory influence on proximal tubular reabsorptive function.

Studies utilizing a variety of experimental techniques have provided insight into the mechanisms by which ANG II directly affects proximal tubular transport function. Systemic infusion of a low subpressor dose of ANG II to anesthetized rats markedly stimulates bicarbonate absorption by the early (S_1) segment of the proximal tubule (42). Furthermore, the stimulatory influence of ANG II on proximal bicarbonate reabsorption is inhibited by the luminal application of amiloride, indicating that ANG II enhances proximal tubular reabsorptive function by stimulating the luminal membrane Na^+-H^+ exchanger (43). Experiments using isolated intact proximal tubule cells from rabbits have provided direct evidence in support of this hypothesis (44). In the presence of a transmembrane pH gradient (pH_{in} less than pH_{out}), ANG II, at doses of 10^{-11} to 10^{-9} M, stimulated the initial rate of $^{22}Na^+$ uptake into sodium-depleted, ouabain-treated proximal tubule cells. Similarly, ANG II (10^{-10} M) enhanced the initial rate of intracellular pH recovery of acid-loaded proximal tubule cells (44). Both these stimulatory actions were blocked by amiloride, indicating that the Na^+-H^+ exchanger was the major transport system being stimulated by ANG II. Studies performed using isolated rabbit proximal tubules (45) and membrane vesicles isolated from rabbit renal cortex (46,47) have verified the stimulatory action of ANG II on the luminal membrane Na^+-H^+ exchanger. These studies have provided evidence that ANG II also exerts a direct stimulatory effect on the basolateral membrane Na^+-HCO_3^- cotransport mechanism (45,47). Thus, ANG II directly enhances proximal tubular reabsorptive function by independently stimulating both the luminal membrane Na^+-H^+ exchanger and the basolateral membrane Na^+-HCO_3^- cotransporter.

The stimulatory effect of ANG II on the luminal membrane Na^+-H^+ exchanger appears to be mediated, at least in large part, via an inhibitory G protein (G_i)–induced decrease in intracellular adenosine 3',5'-cyclic monophosphate (cAMP) levels (34,48,49). It has been demonstrated that cAMP inhibits Na^+-H^+ exchange activity in renal proximal tubule brush border membrane vesicles (50), and that ANG II inhibits cAMP production by proximal tubule cells both *in vitro* and *in vivo* (34,48,49). In addition, *in vivo* micropuncture experiments have shown that pertussis toxin pretreatment (which prevents hormone-mediated decreases in cAMP levels) and luminal perfusion with dibutyryl cAMP inhibits ANG II–mediated increases in proximal tubular reabsorption rate (48). In contrast to the growing information on the signal transduction pathway mediating the stimulatory effect of ANG II on the luminal membrane Na^+-H^+ exchanger, the signaling pathway by which ANG II independently stimulates the basolateral membrane Na^+-HCO_3^- cotransporter remains to be elucidated.

Although it is generally accepted that ANG II can effect alterations in proximal tubule cell transport via the activation of specific receptors located on the basolateral membrane, it should be recognized that this is not the only way in which the hormone can directly influence proximal tubule cell transport function. Indeed, as shown in Fig. 1, specific receptors for ANG II are located on both the luminal and basolateral membranes of proximal tubule cells (34), and *in vivo* micropuncture studies have demonstrated that intraluminal application of ANG II can enhance proximal tubule sodium and bicarbonate reabsorption (32,43). Recent micropuncture studies have also demonstrated remarkably high concentrations of ANG II in the proximal tubular fluid (51,52) and the accumulating evidence strongly suggests that the proximal tubule can secrete ANG II or a precursor directly into the tubular lumen (52). Furthermore, ANG II has been shown to stimulate amiloride-sensitive $^{22}Na^+$ uptake by isolated rabbit brush border membrane vesicles (46,47). These data indicate that ANG II can stimulate the luminal membrane Na^+-H^+ exchanger through activation of receptors located on the luminal membrane. As the overall reabsorptive status of the proximal tubule appears to be critically influenced by the prevailing ANG II levels (14,16,17), and in view of the recent findings that proximal tubular fluid contains very high concentrations (nanomolar range) of ANG II (51,52), it is likely that the overall influence of ANG II on proximal tubular reabsorption rate results from the combined influence of luminal and basolateral ANG II receptor activation by ANG II present in both the luminal and interstitial environments. It is also possible that the signaling mechanisms responsible for activating the proximal tubular transport systems may be different for the luminal and basolateral activation pathways (34,46,48,49). Indeed, studies performed using isolated rabbit brush bor-

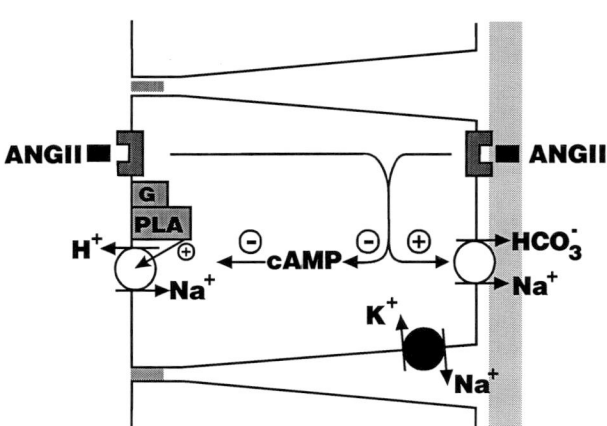

FIG. 1. Schematic representation of the signaling mechanisms by which ANG II directly stimulates proximal tubule cell transport. Based on several studies cited in text.

der membrane vesicles indicate activation of luminal membrane ANG II receptors stimulates Na^+-H^+ exchange activity via a pertussis toxin–sensitive G protein–induced increase in phospholipase A_2 activity (46). The proposed signaling pathways responsible for mediating the direct stimulatory effect of ANG II on proximal tubule cell transport are summarized in Fig. 1. Further

studies are required in order to determine the relative contributions of the luminal and basolateral activation mechanisms to the overall regulation of proximal tubule cell transport by ANG II.

It is worth mentioning that the effects of ANG II on the activities of the luminal membrane Na^+-H^+ exchanger and the basolateral membrane Na^+-HCO_3^- co-

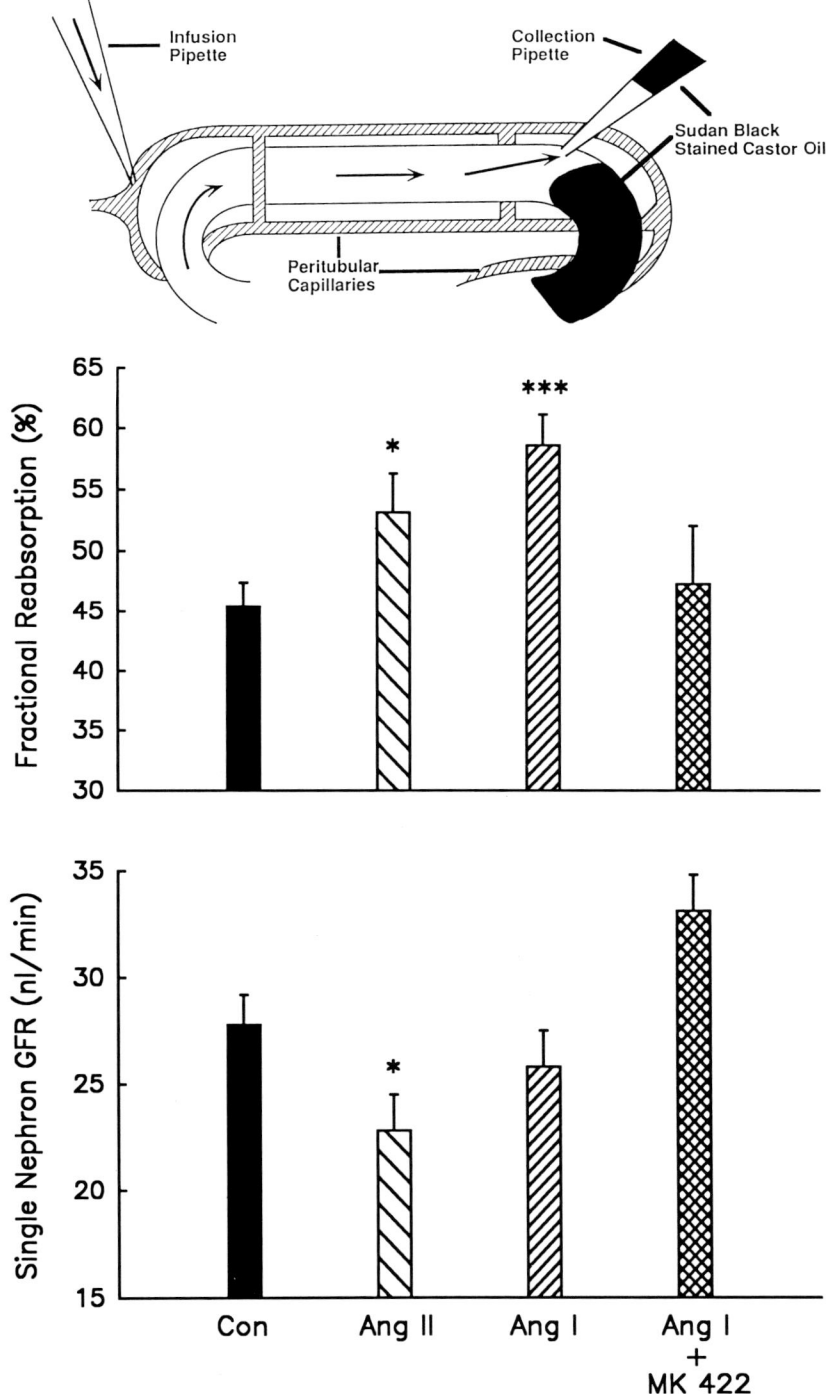

FIG. 2. Effects of peritubular capillary infusion, at a rate of 20 nL/min, of 10^{-7} M angiotensin II (ANG II), 10^{-5} M angiotensin I (ANG I), and 10^{-5} M ANG I together with the ACE inhibitor enalaprilat (MK 422, 10^{-3} M) on proximal tubular fractional fluid reabsorption and single nephron GFR. The schematic figure (**top**) shows the position of the micropipettes used to evaluate the proximal tubular fractional reabsorption rate and single nephron GFR responses to peritubular capillary infusion of ANG II, ANG I, and ANG I + MK 422. $*p < .05$, $**p < .01$, $***p < .001$ compared with the control (Con) value. (Data from ref. 56.)

transporter will result not only in alterations in proximal tubule sodium bicarbonate reabsorption, but also in alterations in proximal tubule sodium chloride reabsorption (53). Transcellular electroneutral sodium chloride reabsorption is effected by the Na^+-H^+ exchanger operating in parallel with Cl^--base$^-$ exchange (54,55). In addition, predominant sodium bicarbonate reabsorption (mediated by the luminal membrane Na^+-H^+ exchanger and the basolateral membrane Na^+-HCO_3^- cotransporter) in the early segment of the proximal tubule provides the driving force for passive paracellular sodium chloride reabsorption in the late proximal tubule by reducing the luminal bicarbonate concentration and increasing the luminal chloride concentration (54,55). Consequently, an ANG II–mediated stimulation of both the luminal membrane Na^+-H^+ exchanger and the basolateral membrane Na^+-HCO_3^{-1} cotransporter will result in an increase in proximal tubule sodium chloride reabsorption (53). This will be reflected as a decrease in the delivery of sodium chloride and water to the distal nephron segments and ultimately as a decrease in urinary salt and water excretion.

Although it is now established that ANG II exerts a substantial influence on proximal tubular reabsorptive function, an issue that has remained unclear is whether increases above the normal endogenous levels in the local intrarenal ANG II concentration result in stimulation or inhibition of proximal tubular reabsorption rate. Indeed, given the dose-response relationship between ANG II and proximal tubular reabsorption rate (32,33), increases in the local intrarenal interstitial ANG II concentration above some critical level of approximately 10^{-9} M might actually inhibit proximal tubular reabsorption. This issue was addressed in a series of *in vivo* micropuncture experiments in which we evaluated the effects of peritubular capillary infusion of ANG II on proximal tubular reabsorption rate (56). By infusing ANG II directly into the peritubular capillaries at a relatively low rate that does not obstruct normal peritubular blood flow, it is possible to selectively increase the local postglomerular capillary and interstitial ANG II concentrations without altering either the circulating ANG II level or arterial blood pressure. With this approach it is possible to mimic the effects elicited by selective increases above the normal endogenous levels in the intrarenal interstitial ANG II concentration.

In these experiments, we also determined if peritubular capillary infusion of ANG I could lead to sufficient *de novo* generation of ANG II in the postglomerular capillary or interstitial environment to elicit effects on proximal tubular reabsorption rate (56). As shown in Fig. 2, peritubular capillary infusion of either ANG I or ANG II, at doses that did not markedly alter the single nephron glomerular filtration rate (SNGFR), elicited significant increases in proximal fractional fluid reabsorption. The stimulatory effect of ANG I on proximal tubule frac-

tional fluid reabsorption was inhibited when the ACE inhibitor, enalaprilat, was infused together with ANG I (Fig. 2). These data, obtained under *in vivo* conditions, indicate that increases above the normal endogenous levels in the local postglomerular interstitial ANG II concentration will primarily cause stimulation of proximal tubular reabsorption rate (56). The stimulatory effect observed with ANG I is of particular interest because it indicates that ANG I can be converted to ANG II in the postglomerular capillary and/or interstitial environment, and that increases in intrarenally generated ANG II, in the absence of changes in circulating levels, will lead to an augmentation of proximal tubular reabsorption rate. It is also worth emphasizing that no evidence for an inhibitory effect of either ANG I or ANG II was observed in the intact nephron setting because higher ANG I and ANG II infusion rates caused SNGFR to fall markedly. These findings indicate that the inhibitory effects of higher intrarenal interstitial ANG II levels on proximal reabsorption rate may not occur because of the concomitant depressive influence of such ANG II concentrations on nephron filtration rate.

INTERACTION BETWEEN ANGIOTENSIN II AND THE TUBULOGLOMERULAR FEEDBACK MECHANISM

The tubuloglomerular feedback mechanism operates at the single nephron level to maintain a balance between the reabsorptive function of each nephron and the amount of solute and fluid filtered at its glomerulus (57–60). The macula densa cells of the thick ascending limb of the loop of Henle detect changes in the composition of the tubular fluid entering the terminal portion of the thick ascending limb of the loop of Henle and transmit signals that alter glomerular vascular resistance, glomerular capillary pressure, and thereby SNGFR. Specifically, increases in the sodium chloride or total solute concentration of the tubular fluid flowing past the macula densa cells in response to increases in fluid flow into the ascending limb of the loop of Henle lead to increases in glomerular vascular resistance and decreases in SNGFR (57–60).

It was formerly postulated that changes in the local ANG II concentrations specifically mediated tubuloglomerular feedback–associated reductions in SNGFR (61). This hypothesis proposed that flow-related increases in the sodium chloride concentration at the macula densa segment would stimulate renin release from the adjacent juxtaglomerular cells and thereby increase the local formation of ANG II, which in turn would constrict the glomerular vasculature and thereby reduce SNGFR. It was recognized, however, that this proposal is at variance with the numerous observations that conditions associated with enhanced renin secretion (i.e., sodium depletion, hemorrhage, increases in sympathetic nervous system activity) result in reductions in sodium chloride delivery to the macula densa and a decreased or unchanged sodium chloride concentration of the tubular fluid at this segment of the nephron (62–64). In addition, the evidence obtained from studies using the isolated perfused and superfused juxtaglomerular apparatus preparation has clearly demonstrated that there is an inverse relationship between the sodium chloride concen-

tration at the macula densa and renin release (65,66). Collectively, these data are incompatible with the concept that ANG II directly mediates tubuloglomerular feedback–induced decreases in SNGFR.

Although the available evidence indicates that ANG II does not directly mediate tubuloglomerular feedback responses, it is clear that the prevailing ANG II levels do exert an important modulatory influence on the overall sensitivity of this mechanism (16,17,60,67,68). Several

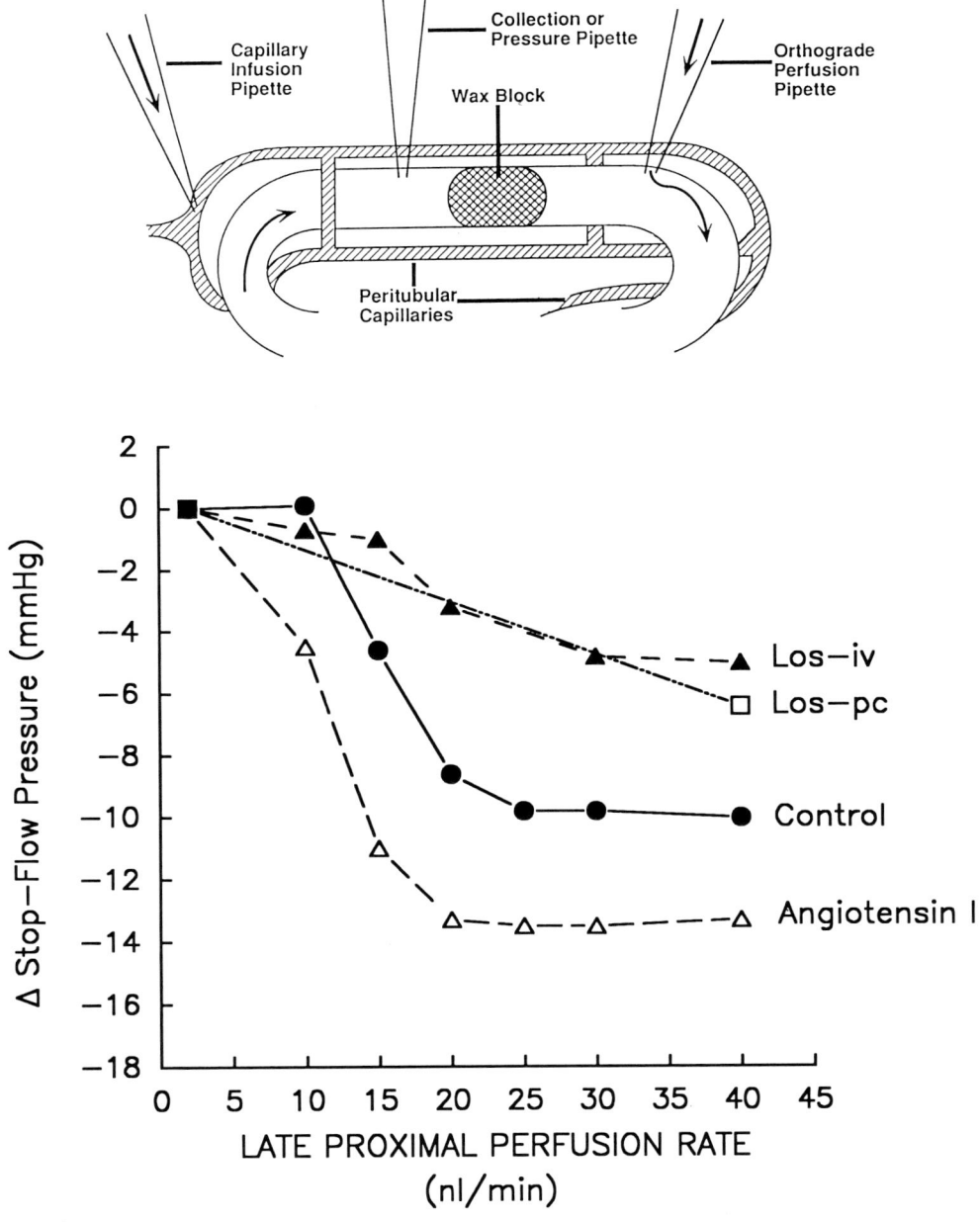

FIG. 3. Representative examples of stop-flow pressure tubuloglomerular feedback responses to increases in late proximal perfusion rate during control conditions, during peritubular capillary infusion of 10^{-5} M angiotensin I (ANG I), during peritubular capillary infusion of the nonpeptide AT_1 receptor antagonist losartan (Los-pc, 10^{-2} M), and following intravenous administration of losartan (Los-iv). **Top panel:** Diagrammatic representation of the micropuncture procedures used to evaluate tubuloglomerular feedback responses. (Data from refs. 73 and 75.)

studies have shown that systemic administration of peptide ANG II receptor antagonists, such as saralasin, or ACE inhibitors, markedly attenuates feedback responsiveness as assessed from stop-flow pressure (SFP) feedback responses to increases in distal nephron perfusion rate (31,69–71). In addition, infusion of exogenous ANG II during conditions of converting enzyme blockade results in partial restoration of feedback responsiveness (31). Furthermore, feedback responsiveness in normal rats is enhanced during systemic infusion of exogenous ANG II (68,72). Collectively, these findings indicate that ANG II acts to enhance the sensitivity of the vascular elements that mediate tubuloglomerular feedback-induced alterations in single nephron hemodynamic function (16,60,67,68). The recent observation that SFP tubuloglomerular feedback responses are attenuated following both systemic and peritubular capillary administration of the nonpeptide ANG II receptor antagonist, losartan, indicates that ANG II exerts its modulatory influence on tubuloglomerular feedback responsiveness via activation of AT_1 receptors (73).

More recent studies have allowed assessment of whether tubuloglomerular feedback responsiveness is modulated by alterations in intrarenal ANG II levels independent of changes in circulating levels. This issue is particularly timely in view of the recent studies demonstrating that intrarenal ANG II levels are generally greater than can be explained on the basis of circulating ANG II levels and are subject to differential regulation (51,52,74). Thus, the role of intrarenally formed ANG II in modulating the sensitivity of the tubuloglomerular feedback mechanism is particularly significant. *In vivo* micropuncture experiments performed to address this specific issue evaluated the effects of peritubular capillary infusions of either ANG I or ANG II on the magnitude of tubuloglomerular feedback–mediated decreases in SFP (75). In these experiments, SFP feedback responses to step increases in orthograde perfusion from a late proximal tubule site were assessed in the same nephrons during control conditions and during simultaneous peritubular capillary infusion of either ANG I or ANG II. Peritubular infusions of both ANG I and ANG II, at rates that did not alter baseline SFP, increased the magnitude of the SFP feedback responses at low proximal perfusion rates of 10 nL/min and at the high proximal perfusion rates (>30 nL/min) that elicited maximal feedback responses (75). The effects of ANG I were blocked by the ANG II receptor antagonist saralasin, indicating that the ANG I–mediated enhancement of feedback sensitivity was due to interaction of intrarenally generated ANG II with ANG II receptors (75). These results provide additional evidence that ANG I can be converted to ANG II in the postglomerular capillary and/or interstitial environment and indicate that increases in the postglomerular interstitial ANG II concentration, independent of changes in the circulating ANG II concentration, can enhance the sensitivity of the tubuloglomerular feedback mechanism. The modulatory effects of changes in, and effectiveness of, the prevailing ANG II levels on tubuloglomerular feedback responsiveness are depicted in Fig. 3.

DIRECT ACTIONS OF ANGIOTENSIN II ON RENAL VASCULATURE AND GLOMERULAR FILTRATION RATE

In addition to its modulatory influence on the tubuloglomerular feedback mechanism, ANG II exerts pronounced direct effects on the renal vasculature. Whole kidney clearance studies have demonstrated that ANG II elicits dose-dependent decreases in RBF, smaller decreases in GFR, and therefore increases in filtration fraction (13,15–17,67,76). The observation that ANG II consistently increases filtration fraction has frequently been cited as evidence indicating that ANG II preferentially constricts the efferent arterioles (15,76). It should be emphasized, however, that this interpretation fails to take into account that increases in filtration fraction can occur as a consequence of parallel increases in both afferent and efferent arteriolar resistances (77). Indeed, *in vivo* micropuncture studies have clearly demonstrated that ANG II elicits reductions in SNGFR and glomerular plasma flow, and increases in both afferent and efferent resistances (78–82).

The decreases in both whole kidney and single nephron filtration rates observed in many experimental studies are also attributable to the effects of ANG II to reduce the glomerular filtration coefficient (K_f) (79,81,83). This effect on K_f has commonly been thought to reflect the actions of the hormone on the contractility of the glomerular mesangial cells; however, the exact mechanism by which mesangial cell contraction reduces K_f remains unclear, and the ANG II concentrations needed to reduce K_f may be higher than the levels normally achieved in physiological states. During systemic infusions of ANG II, afferent arteriolar resistance may increase partially as a consequence of activation of autoregulatory mechanisms secondary to ANG II–induced increases in arterial blood pressure. However, it has been demonstrated that ANG II elicits increases in both afferent and efferent arteriolar resistances when infused directly into the renal artery at doses that do not alter arterial blood pressure (82). Furthermore, studies performed using the *in vitro* blood perfused juxtamedullary nephron preparation have demonstrated that intravascular injections of ANG II elicits decreases in glomerular capillary pressure that are not mimicked by increases in perfusion pressure per se (84), and studies utilizing the peritubular capillary infusion technique have demonstrated that SFP is reduced during peritubular infusion of either ANG I or ANG II (56,75). These studies demonstrate that, *in vivo*,

ANG II increases preglomerular vascular resistance. In addition, ANG II has been shown to constrict both the afferent and efferent arterioles of renal tissue transplanted into hamster cheek pouch (85), and to constrict all preglomerular vessels as well as the efferent arterioles of *in vitro* blood perfused juxtamedullary nephrons (86) and hydronephrotic rat kidneys (87). More recent experiments utilizing isolated perfused arterioles have demonstrated that ANG II constricts both the afferent and efferent arterioles (88,89).

Collectively, these findings indicate that, rather than preferentially constricting the efferent arteriole, ANG II elicits vasoconstrictor actions on both pre- and postglomerular resistance vessels within the kidney. The microvasculature of juxtamedullary nephrons in particular appears to be extremely sensitive to the vasoconstrictor actions of ANG II (86,90,91). This high sensitivity may explain the finding that ANG II, at doses that do not alter whole kidney blood flow or filtration rate, substantially reduces medullary and papillary blood flow (90,91). Such an effect of ANG II to reduce medullary blood flow and thereby increase medullary interstitial fluid osmolality could contribute to the decreased sodium excretion observed during conditions in which the activity of the renin-angiotensin system is enhanced (90,91).

The results obtained during administration of ANG I and ANG II are consistent with those obtained from studies in which pharmacological inhibitors or antagonists of the renin-angiotensin system have been used to unmask the renal hemodynamic effects of endogenous ANG II. Although RBF is generally increased, the GFR response to inhibition of the renin-angiotensin system is more variable. Indeed, GFR has been reported to be either increased (25,28,69,71,92,93), unchanged (94,95), or decreased (96) following pharmacological inhibition of the renin-angiotensin system. The GFR response to inhibition of the renin-angiotensin system is, in large part, dependent upon the magnitude of the associated decrease in arterial blood pressure. When the overall systemic actions of the renin-angiotensin system are high, inhibition of the renin-angiotensin system then results in pronounced hypotension leading to reductions in GFR (67). However, when the associated decreases in arterial blood pressure are more modest, GFR either remains unchanged or even increases slightly. Because the increases in RBF are generally larger in magnitude and more consistent than the changes in GFR, inhibition of the renin-angiotensin system consistently decreases filtration fraction.

The whole kidney hemodynamic responses to blockade of the renin-angiotensin system are consistent with those observed at the single nephron level. *In vivo* micropuncture studies have demonstrated that pharmacological blockade of the renin-angiotensin system in both normal kidneys (25,39,67) and the nonclipped kidneys of 2K1C Goldblatt hypertensive rats (97) results in decreases in both afferent and efferent arteriolar resistances. When arterial pressure is not markedly reduced, ANG II blockade may increase SNGFR as well as single nephron plasma flow (25,30,39,40,69). Thus, the data obtained from micropuncture studies utilizing pharmacological antagonists of the renin-angiotensin system indicate that when the prevailing endogenous ANG II levels are elevated they exert approximately equivalent vasoconstrictor effects on both the pre- and postglomerular resistance vessels.

SYNERGISTIC INTERACTIONS BETWEEN TUBULAR AND VASCULAR EFFECTS OF ANGIOTENSIN II

The data obtained from the numerous studies described above indicate that ANG II exerts a stimulatory influence on proximal tubular reabsorption rate, and that increases in intrarenal interstitial ANG II levels and increased intrarenal ANG II generation further stimulate proximal tubular reabsorption rate. Such an effect of ANG II to stimulate proximal tubular reabsorption rate has been shown to elicit a reduction in end proximal fluid flow (56), which, given the reabsorptive characteristics of the loop of Henle, would result in a decrease in fluid delivery to the macula densa segment. However, a decrease in fluid delivery to the macula densa segment would of itself be expected to elicit a tubuloglomerular feedback–mediated decrease in preglomerular vascular resistance and an increase in SNGFR of sufficient magnitude to offset or counteract the ANG II–mediated increase in proximal tubular reabsorption rate. Consequently, it can be appreciated that, by itself, an ANG II–mediated increase in proximal tubular reabsorption rate would be unable to elicit sustained decreases in distal nephron fluid delivery and sodium excretion because of the compensatory action of the tubuloglomerular feedback mechanism to restore distal nephron volume delivery back toward control levels. However, such a compensatory action of the tubuloglomerular feedback mechanism does not occur in response to an ANG II–mediated decrease in distal nephron volume delivery because of the concomitant modulatory influence of ANG II on tubuloglomerular feedback responsiveness that has just been described.

As shown in Fig. 4, the effect of ANG II to enhance tubuloglomerular feedback responsiveness shifts the operating point of the system and thus allows SNGFR to be maintained at the lower distal nephron volume delivery. Thus, it can be appreciated that during conditions of elevated intrarenal ANG II levels, the modulatory influence of ANG II on tubuloglomerular feedback responsiveness is of pivotal importance in allowing the ANG II–mediated stimulation of proximal tubular reabsorption and the consequent decrease in distal nephron vol-

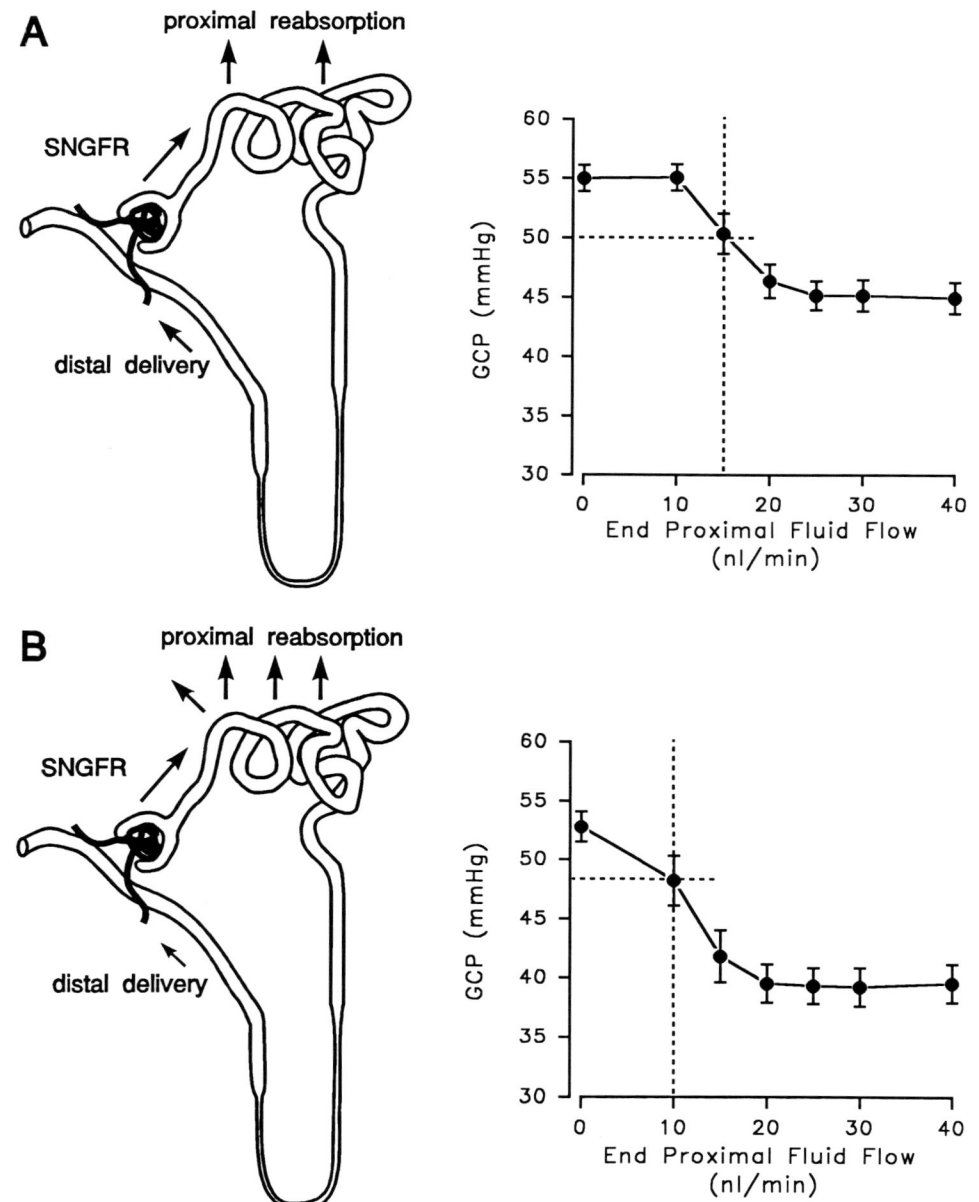

FIG. 4. Representation of the relation between end proximal tubule fluid flow and glomerular capillary pressure (GCP) during control conditions (**A**) and conditions of elevated intrarenal angiotensin II (ANG II) levels (**B**). The effects of elevated intrarenal ANG II levels to augment feedback responsiveness enable GCP, and thus single nephron glomerular filtration rate (SNGFR), to be maintained at reduced distal volume delivery rate that would occur as a consequence of ANG II–mediated stimulation of proximal tubular reabsorption rate. (Data from ref. 75; from ref. 17, with permission.)

ume delivery to be maintained. In this manner, the interactive effects of ANG II to enhance both proximal tubular reabsorption rate and the sensitivity of the tubuloglomerular feedback mechanism enable increases in intrarenal ANG II levels to elicit sustained decreases in distal nephron volume delivery.

These synergistic actions of ANG II on proximal tubular reabsorption rate and tubuloglomerular feedback responsiveness appear to occur at intrarenal concentra-

tions that do not markedly alter baseline vascular resistance or SNGFR (56,75), and thus are probably the most physiologically relevant actions of intrarenal ANG II. However, further increases in intrarenal ANG II levels result in constriction of the glomerular vascular resistance vessels, thereby reducing glomerular capillary pressure, plasma flow, the glomerular ultrafiltration coefficient (K_f), and thus GFR. These direct vasoconstrictor effects of ANG II would act to further reduce distal nephron volume delivery and thus urinary sodium excretion. Although even higher intrarenal ANG II concentrations might elicit direct inhibitory effects on proximal tubular reabsorption rate, such effects would be counteracted by the parallel effects of such concentrations to reduce GFR. Combined with the well-documented stimulatory effects of aldosterone on distal nephron sodium reabsorption (24,38), the direct effects of ANG II on proximal tubular reabsorptive function and glomerular function provide a cascading mechanism by which the renin-angiotensin system can elicit substantial and sustained decreases in urinary sodium and water excretion.

HYPERTENSINOGENIC MECHANISMS MEDIATED BY SYNERGISTIC ACTIONS OF ANGIOTENSIN II ON RENAL TUBULAR AND VASCULAR FUNCTION

It is now clear that activation of the renin-angiotensin system is a pivotal component of the homeostatic responses that maximize sodium conservation and maintain extracellular fluid and blood volume and thus preserve cardiovascular integrity during conditions of reduced sodium chloride intake or volume depletion. It can also be appreciated that inappropriate activation of this system may lead to an excessive retention of salt and water and thereby contribute directly to the development and/or maintenance of hypertension. In this regard, studies performed using two-kidney, one-clip (2K1C) Goldblatt hypertensive rats have indicated that the hypertension in this experimental model is initiated and mediated primarily by an elevated activity of the renin-angiotensin system (2,5,29–31,40,97–99). In response to unilateral renal arterial stenosis, there is an increase in renin secretion from and an increase in renin content of the stenotic or clipped kidney, and both plasma renin activity and circulating ANG II concentrations are elevated (2,5,29,74,100–103).

In addition to the direct vasoconstrictor effects of the elevated circulating ANG II levels, there appear to be pronounced renal effects of the hormone that prevent the nonclipped kidney from responding appropriately to the elevated arterial blood pressure. Although the nonclipped kidney is renin-depleted (2,5,29,100,103–105), it has been reported that the ANG II content of the nonclipped kidney is either normal (100) or even elevated (5,74). Such inappropriately maintained or elevated intrarenal ANG II levels together with the elevated circulating ANG II levels may exert a substantial depressive influence on the excretory function of the nonclipped kidney. Indeed, it has been shown that administration of ANG II receptor antagonists or ACE inhibitors results in renal vasodilation, increased GFR, and increased sodium excretion of the nonclipped kidney (2,5,29–31,40,98,99,106,107). In addition, ACE inhibition elicits

increases in SNGFR and decreases in both proximal reabsorption rate and tubuloglomerular feedback responsiveness in the nonclipped kidney (2,5,30,31,40). Collectively, these findings indicate that the effects of elevated ANG II levels on renal hemodynamics and tubular reabsorptive function act to impair the ability of the nonclipped kidney to achieve a normal level of sodium excretion at normotensive pressures and thus attenuate the magnitude of the natriuretic response of the nonclipped kidney to progressive increases in arterial blood pressure.

On the basis of previous observations that peritubular capillary infusion of ANG II, which mimics the effects of increases in the intrarenal interstitial ANG II levels, increases proximal tubular reabsorption rate and enhances the sensitivity of the tubuloglomerular feedback mechanism (56,75), one would predict that tubuloglomerular feedback responsiveness in the nonclipped kidney would actually be enhanced as a consequence of the inappropriately elevated intrarenal and circulating ANG II levels that occur in this setting. Although previous studies have reported that tubuloglomerular feedback responsiveness in the nonclipped kidney of hypertensive rats is either attenuated (104) or normal (31,105), more recent studies (108) have demonstrated that tubuloglomerular feedback responsiveness in the nonclipped kidney of 2K1C Goldblatt hypertensive rats may even be slightly enhanced as compared with normotensive animals. In these studies, the ANG II–dependency of tubuloglomerular feedback responsiveness in the nonclipped kidney was evaluated using the nonpeptide AT_1 receptor antagonist losartan. Systemic administration of losartan markedly attenuated the magnitude of the SFP tubuloglomerular feedback responses in the nonclipped kidney (108). These recent findings therefore indicate that ANG II, acting via AT_1 receptors, acts to enhance the sensitivity of the tubuloglomerular feedback mechanism in the nonclipped kidney of 2K1C Goldblatt hypertensive rats. Such augmented tubuloglomerular feedback responsiveness, combined with the stimulatory action of ANG II on proximal tubular reabsorptive rate, provides a powerful synergistic mechanism whereby the elevated ANG II levels impair the excretory function of the nonclipped kidney. In this manner, the direct renal vascular and tubular effects of ANG II play an important role in the development and maintenance of hypertension in this setting.

Evidence obtained from a variety of studies indicates that the renal actions of ANG II may also play a role in the development and maintenance of essential hypertension. Although the hypertension in spontaneously hypertensive rats, a model for essential hypertension, is generally considered a normal- or low-renin form of hypertension, experiments performed in spontaneously hypertensive rats have demonstrated that basal renin release, plasma renin activity, and the sensitivity of the renal vasculature to ANG II are increased during the developmental phase of hypertension (109–112). In addition, compared to age-matched Wistar-Kyoto rats, young spontaneously hypertensive rats exhibit reduced RBF and GFR, and increased renal vascular resistance and tubuloglomerular feedback responsiveness (109,113,114). Furthermore, chronic administration of an ACE inhibitor has been shown both to prevent the development of hypertension and to reverse the hypertension in spontaneously hypertensive rats (115–118). These findings, together with the observations that spontaneously hypertensive rats respond to administration of an ACE inhibitor with increases in RBF and GFR (109,110), suggest that the renal actions of ANG II contribute to derangements in renal excretory function in this form of genetic hypertension.

A recently developed animal model of genetic hypertension that promises to provide unique insights into the hypertensinogenic mechanisms mediated by the renal actions of the renin-angiotensin system is the hypertensive transgenic rat [TGR; strain name TGR(mRen2)27] harboring the mouse ren-2 renin gene (119). This transgenic rat line was constructed by inserting the mouse ren-2 renin gene, including approximately 5 kilobases of 5′-flanking sequences and 9 kilobases of 3′-flanking sequences, into the rat genome (119,120). Transgenic rats harboring the ren-2 gene, which is a duplicated form of the renin structural gene and is present in mouse strains expressing high levels of submandibular gland renin, develop fulminant hypertension (119–123). This recently developed model is therefore of considerable interest because, unlike other experimental models of hypertension, it provides an opportunity to evaluate the mechanisms responsible for the derangements in renal excretory function that contribute to the development and maintenance of hypertension that results from a clearly defined genetic alteration. Furthermore, as the genetic alteration results in the overexpression of the ren-2 renin gene, this model also provides the unique opportunity to evaluate the specific renal mechanisms whereby inappropriate activation of the renin-angiotensin system leads to the development and maintenance of hypertension.

The hypertension that occurs as a consequence of overexpression of the ren-2 transgene is associated with suppression of plasma and kidney renin contents (119). In addition, transgenic rats exhibit markedly decreased renin mRNA expression at the juxtaglomerular apparatus, and suppressed renin and ANG II immunoreactivity at the afferent arteriole (121). Although these findings have been taken to indicate that the hypertension in ren-2 transgenic rats is a low-renin form of hypertension (119–123), it should be recognized that circulating ANG II levels are not significantly reduced in ren-2 transgenic rats that have established hypertension (119). In addition, chronic administration of the ACE inhibitor captopril has been shown both to prevent the development of hypertension in young ren-2 transgenic rats and to nor-

malize the blood pressure in transgenic rats that have established hypertension (119,122), indicating that the hypertension in this model is strongly ANG II–dependent. It should be recognized, that just as in the renin-depleted contralateral kidney of the Goldblatt hypertensive rat, renal renin depletion does not mean that renal ANG II levels are depressed. Recent studies in both Goldblatt hypertension (74) and hypertension induced by low-dose ANG II infusions (124) indicate that slight increases in circulating ANG II levels may stimulate the kidneys to increase intrarenal production of ANG II through pathways that do not require elevated renin activity. The mechanism by which this renin-independent augmentation of intrarenal ANG II content occurs has not been determined, but this key finding explains why the presence of a normal kidney does not prevent the development of hypertension in the 2K1C Goldblatt model (124). It remains to be established whether ren-2 transgenic rats also have enhanced intrarenal ANG II levels.

These considerations suggest that the maintained circulating ANG II levels (which can be considered inappropriately high for the level of arterial blood pressure) observed in ren-2 transgenic rats may exert a pronounced influence on renal hemodynamic and tubular reabsorptive function, thereby preventing the kidneys from maintaining normal rates of sodium excretion at normotensive pressure and impairing the natriuretic response to the ANG II–mediated elevation in arterial blood pressure. Studies addressing this issue (125) have recently evaluated the effects on tubuloglomerular feedback responsiveness of the nonpeptide AT_1 receptor antagonist L-158,809 (126). In these experiments, performed on pentobarbital-anesthetized ren-2 transgenic rats aged 7 to 9 weeks (during the development phase of the hypertension), the effects of AT_1 receptor blockade on SFP tubuloglomerular feedback responses to step increases in late proximal perfusion rate were assessed (125). During control conditions, increases in late proximal perfusion rate elicited flow-dependent decreases in SFP. The magnitude of the maximal tubuloglomerular feedback–mediated reduction in SFP averaged approximately 16 mm Hg, a value higher than that normally observed in normotensive rats (75). Administration of the AT_1 receptor blocker decreased mean arterial blood pressure by more than 50 mm Hg and markedly attenuated the magnitude of the SFP tubuloglomerular feedback responses to increases in late proximal perfusion rate (125). These results demonstrate that activation of AT_1 receptors by ANG II is largely responsible for the hypertension in these transgenic rats, and indicate that ANG II, acting via AT_1 receptors, exerts a pronounced stimulatory influence on the sensitivity of the tubuloglomerular feedback mechanism in ren-2 transgenic rats. Such ANG II–induced enhancement of tubuloglomerular feedback responsiveness likely contributes importantly to an impaired renal excretory function and thereby plays an important role in the development and maintenance of hypertension that occurs in ren-2 transgenic rats.

SUMMARY

There is growing awareness that the direct intrarenal actions of ANG II serve as a powerful component of the sodium-conserving influence of the renin-angiotensin system. Low concentrations of ANG II directly stimulate proximal tubular reabsorption rate. Recent studies indicate that this direct stimulatory action is due to an enhanced activity of both the luminal membrane Na^+-H^+ exchanger and the basolateral membrane Na^+-HCO_3^- cotransporter. In addition, increases in intrarenal interstitial ANG II levels, effected either through increased delivery of ANG II from the circulation or as a consequence of conversion of ANG I generated locally, can enhance proximal tubular reabsorption rate. One consequence of enhanced proximal tubular reabsorption rate is reduced distal nephron volume delivery, which would be expected to elicit a tubuloglomerular feedback–mediated afferent arteriolar vasodilation and an increase in SNGFR. It has been demonstrated, however, that peritubular capillary infusions of either ANG I or ANG II, at doses that do not directly alter glomerular dynamics, can increase the sensitivity of the tubuloglomerular feedback mechanism. This enhanced tubuloglomerular feedback responsiveness serves to minimize or prevent tubuloglomerular feedback–mediated increases in SNGFR in the face of reduced distal delivery. With even greater increases in interstitial ANG II concentrations, reductions in glomerular pressure and SNGFR have been observed, demonstrating a powerful action of the hormone on the preglomerular arterioles as well as on the efferent arterioles. At these higher doses, the direct hemodynamic effects of ANG II, combined with the effects on the glomerular ultrafiltration coefficient, will directly reduce filtered sodium load. Through these synergistic actions on both tubular reabsorptive and hemodynamic function and in concert with the indirect effects mediated through the actions of aldosterone on the distal nephron segment, ANG II can elicit a sustained influence over distal nephron volume delivery and urinary sodium excretion.

Although it is clear that the renal tubular and vascular actions of ANG II contribute importantly to the normal homeostatic mechanisms of sodium balance, it can be appreciated that during conditions in which the activity of the renin-angiotensin system is inappropriately activated, the synergistic effects of ANG II to enhance proximal tubular reabsorptive function and reduce hemodynamic function form a potent hypertensinogenic mechanism. In essence, the synergistic effects of inappropriately elevated or maintained ANG II levels on renal tubular and vascular function act to impair the ability of the kidney to achieve normal rates of sodium excretion at normotensive pressures and impair the natriuretic response to sustained elevations in systemic arterial blood pressure. In this manner, the interactive effects of ANG II on renal tubular and vascular function contribute importantly to the development and maintenance of hypertension.

ACKNOWLEDGMENTS

Research studies conducted by the authors have been supported by grants from NHLBI (HL-18426 and HL-26731) and American Heart Association–Louisiana, Inc. (LA-91-G-24 and LA-92-G-31). We thank Dr. Branko Braam, Department of Nephrology and Hypertension, University Hospital Utrecht, The Netherlands, for help with Fig. 4.

REFERENCES

1. Cowley AW, Roman RJ Jr. *Am J Nephrol* 1983;3:59–72.
2. Ploth DW. *Am J Physiol* 1983;245:F131–F141.
3. Guyton AC, Manning RA, Norman RA, Montani JP, Lohmeier TE, Hall JE. *J Hypertens* 1986;4(suppl 4):S49–S56.
4. Zimmerman BG, Arendshorst WJ, DiBona GF, Hostetter TH, Ploth DW, Raij L. *Fed Proc* 1986;45(12):2661–2664.
5. Navar LG, Huang WC, Mitchell KD, Jackson CA, Ploth DW. In: Pholpramol C, Sudsuang R, eds. *Proceedings of the First Congress of Asian and Oceanian Physiological Societies.* Thailand: Physiological Society, 1987;253–261.
6. Williams GH, Moore TJ, Hollenberg NK. *Am J Kidney Dis* 1987;(suppl 1):39–44.
7. Sealey JE, Blumenfeld JD, Bell SM, Pecker MS, Sommers SC, Laragh JH. *J Hypertens* 1988;6:763–777.
8. Rettig R, Folberth CG, Stauss H, et al. *Hypertension* 1990;15:429–435.
9. Hall JE. *Clin Cardiol* 1991;14(suppl IV):IV-6–IV-21.
10. Guyton AC. *Hypertension* 1992;19(suppl I):I-2–I-8.
11. Luke RG. *Hypertension* 1993;21:380–390.
12. Rettig R, Schmitt B, Pelzl B, Speck T. *J Hypertens* 1993;11:883–891.
13. Navar LG, Langford HG. In: Page IH, Bumpus FM, eds. *Angiotensin, Handbuch der experimentellen Pharmakologie,* vol 37. Berlin: Springer-Verlag, 1974;455–474.
14. Harris PJ, Navar LG. *Am J Physiol* 1985;248:F621–F630.
15. Hall JE. *Am J Physiol* 1986;250:R960–R972.
16. Navar LG, Carmines PK, Huang WC, Mitchell KD. *Kidney Int* 1987;31(suppl 20):S581–S588.
17. Mitchell KD, Braam B, Navar LG. *Hypertension* 1992;19(suppl I):I18–I27.
18. Merrill A, Williams RH, Harrison TR. *Am J Med Sci* 1938;196:204–246.
19. Pickering GW, Printmetal M. *J Physiol* 1940;98:314–335.
20. Langford HG, Pickering GW. *J Physiol* 1965;177:161–173.
21. Bonjour JP, Malvin RL. *Proc Soc Exp Biol* 1969;131:469–472.
22. Barraclough MA, Jones NF, Marsden CD. *Am J Physiol* 1967;212:1153–1157.
23. Johnson MD, Malvin RL. *Am J Physiol* 1977;232:F298–F306.
24. Mitchell KD, Navar LG. In: Baylis PH. ed. *Bailliere's clinical endocrinology and metabolism: water and salt homeostasis in health and disease,* vol 3, no 2. London: Bailliere Tindall, 1989;393–430.

25. Navar LG, Jirakulsomchok D, Bell PD, Thomas CE, Huang WC. *Hypertension* 1982;4:58–68.
26. Navar LG, Paul RV, Carmines PK, Chou C-L, Marsh DJ. *Fed Proc* 1986;45:2885–2891.
27. Rosivall L, Youngblood P, Navar LG. *Renal Physiol* 1986;9:18–28.
28. Siragy HM, Howell NL, Peach MJ, Carey RM. *Am J Physiol* 1990;258:F522–F529.
29. Huang W-C, Ploth DW, Bell PD, Work J, Navar LG. *Hypertension* 1981;3:285–293.
30. Huang W-C, Ploth DW, Navar LG. *Am J Physiol* 1982;243:F553–F560.
31. Huang W-C, Bell PD, Harvey D, Mitchell KD, Navar LG. *Kidney Int* 1988;34:631–637.
32. Harris PJ, Young JA. *Pflugers Arch* 1977;367:295–297.
33. Schuster VL, Kokko JP, Jacobson HR. *J Clin Invest* 1984;73:507–515.
34. Douglas JG. *Am J Physiol* 1987;253:F1–F7.
35. Horster M, Nagel W, Schnermann, Thurau K. *Pflugers Arch* 1966;292:118–128.
36. Lowitz HD, Stumpe KO, Ochwadt B. *Nephron* 1969;6:173–187.
37. Mujais SK, Kauffman S, Katz AI. *J Clin Invest* 1986;77:315–318.
38. Laragh JH, Sealey JE. In: Windhager EE, ed. *Handbook of physiology: renal physiology,* section 8, vol II. New York: Oxford University Press, 1992;1409–1541.
39. Steiner RW, Tucker BJ, Blantz RC. *J Clin Invest* 1979;64:503–512.
40. Huang W-C, Jackson CA, Navar LG. *Kidney Int* 1985;28:124–134.
41. Xie M-H, Liu F-Y, Wong PC, Timmermans PBMWM, Cogan MG. *Kidney Int* 1990;38:473–479.
42. Liu F-Y, Cogan MG. *J Clin Invest* 1987;80:272–275.
43. Liu F-Y, Cogan MG. *J Clin Invest* 1988;82:601–607.
44. Saccomani G, Mitchell KD, Navar LG. *Am J Physiol* 1990;258:F1188–F1195.
45. Geibel J, Giebisch G, Boron WF. *Proc Natl Acad Sci USA* 1990;87:7917–7920.
46. Yanagawa N. *Kidney Int* 1991;(suppl 32):S33–S36.
47. Eiam-Ong S, Hilden SA, Johns CA, Madias NE. *Am J Physiol* 1993;265:F195–F203.
48. Liu F-Y, Cogan MG. *J Clin Invest* 1989;84:83–91.
49. Romero MF, Hopfer U, Madhun ZT, Zhou W, Douglas JG. *Renal Physiol Biochem* 1991;14:199–207.
50. Weinman EJ, Shenolikar S, Kahn AM. *Am J Physiol* 1987;252:F19–F25.
51. Seikaly MG, Arant BS, Seney FD. *J Clin Invest* 1990;86:1352–1357.
52. Braam B, Mitchell KD, Fox J, Navar LG. *Am J Physiol* 1993;264:F891–F989.
53. Liu F-Y, Cogan MG. *Am J Physiol* 1990;259:F72–F79.
54. Rector FC Jr. *Am J Physiol* 1983;244:F461–F471.
55. Berry CA, Rector FC Jr. *Kidney Int* 1989;36:403–411.
56. Mitchell KD, Navar LG. *Am J Physiol* 1987;252:F818–F824.
57. Wright FS, Briggs JP. *Physiol Rev* 1979;59:958–1006.
58. Bell PD, Navar LG. *Semin Nephrol* 1982;2:289–301.
59. Navar LG, Bell PD, Burke TJ. *Kidney Int* 1982;22(suppl 12):S157–S164.
60. Schnermann J, Briggs J. In: Seldin DW, Giebisch G, eds. *The kidney: physiology and pathophysiology,* 2nd ed. New York: Raven Press, 1992;1249–1289.
61. Thurau K. In: Page IH, Bumpus FM, eds. *Angiotensin, Handbuch der experimentellen Pharmakologie,* vol 37. Berlin: Springer-Verlag, 1974;475–489.
62. Vander AJ. *Physiol Rev* 1967;47:359–382.
63. Davis JO, Freeman RH. *Physiol Rev* 1976;56:1–56.
64. Churchill PC, Churchill MC, McDonald FD. *Am J Physiol* 1978;235:F611–F616.
65. Skott O, Briggs JP. *Science* 1987;237:1618–1620.
66. Lorenz JN, Weihprecht H, Schnermann J, Briggs JP. *Am J Physiol* 1991;260:F486–F493.
67. Navar LG, Rosivall L. *Kidney Int* 1984;25:857–868.
68. Schnermann J, Briggs J. *Fed Proc* 1986;45:1426–1430.
69. Ploth DW, Rudolph J, LaGrange R, Navar LG. *J Clin Invest* 1979;64:1325–1335.
70. Stowe N, Schnermann J, Hermle M. *Kidney Int* 1979;15:473–486.
71. Ploth DW, Roy RN. *Am J Physiol* 1982;242:F149–F157.
72. Schnermann J, Briggs JP. *Miner Electrolyte Metab* 1989;15:103–107.
73. Mitchell KD, Braam B, Navar LG. *J Am Soc Nephrol* 1991;2(3):524.
74. Guan S, Fox J, Mitchell KD, Navar LG. *Hypertension* 1992;20:763–767.
75. Mitchell KD, Navar LG. *Am J Physiol* 1988;255:F383–F390.
76. Hall JE. *Fed Proc* 1986;45:1431–1437.
77. Carmines PK, Perry MD, Hazelrig JB, Navar LG. *Kidney Int* 1987;31(suppl 20):S229–S232.
78. Myers BD, Deen WM, Brenner BM. *Circ Res* 1975;37:101–110.
79. Blantz RC, Konnen KS, Tucker BJ. *J Clin Invest* 1976;57:419–434.
80. Baylis C, Brenner BM. *Circ Res* 1978;43:889–898.
81. Schor N, Ichikawa I, Brenner BM. *Am J Physiol* 1980;238:F428–F436.
82. Rosivall L, Navar LG. *Am J Physiol* 1983;245:F181–F187.
83. Rosivall L, Carmines PK, Navar LG. *Kidney Int* 1984;26:263–268.
84. Casellas D, Carmines PK, Navar LG. *Kidney Int* 1985;28:752–759.
85. Click RL, Joyner WL, Gilmore JP. *Kidney Int* 1979;15:109–115.
86. Carmines PK, Morrison TK, Navar LG. *Am J Physiol* 1986;251:F610–F618.
87. Steinhausen M, Sterzel RB, Fleming JT, Kuhn R, Weis S. *Kidney Int* 1987;(suppl 20):S64–S73.
88. Yuan BD, Robinette JB, Conger JD. *Am J Physiol* 1990;258:F741–F750.
89. Ito S, Johnson CS, Carretero. *J Clin Invest* 1991;87:1656–1663.
90. Chou SY, Faubert PF, Porush JG. *Fed Proc* 1986;45:1438–1443.
91. Faubert PF, Chou SY, Porush JG. *Kidney Int* 1987;32:472–478.
92. Kimbrough HM Jr, Vaughan ED Jr, Carey RM, Ayers RC. *Circ Res* 1977;40:174–178.
93. Carmines PK, Rosivall L, Till MF, Navar LG. *Renal Physiol* 1983;6:281–287.
94. Fagard RH, Amery AK, Lijnen PJ. *Pflugers Arch* 1978;374:199–204.
95. Clappison BH, Anderson WP, Johnston CI. *Kidney Int* 1981;20:615–620.
96. Hall JE, Guyton AC, Smith MJ Jr, Coleman TG. *Am J Physiol* 1979;237:F424–F432.
97. Ichikawa I, Ferrone RA, Duchin KL, Manning M, Dzau VJ, Brenner BM. *Circ Res* 1983;53:592–602.
98. Masaki Z, Ferrario CM, Bumpus FM. *Hypertension* 1980;2:649–656.
99. Zimmerman BG, Arendshorst WJ, DiBona GF, Hostetter TH, Ploth DW. *Fed Proc* 1986;45:2661–2664.
100. Mendelsohn FAO. *Kidney Int* 1982;22(suppl 12):S78–S81.
101. Brunner H, Desoulles PA, Regoli D, Gross F. *Am J Physiol* 1962;202:795–799.
102. Ten Berg R, DeJong W. *Hypertension* 1980;2:4–13.
103. Jackson CA, Navar LG. *J Hypertens* 1986;4:215–221.
104. Ploth DW, Schnermann J, Dahlheim H, Hermle M, Schmidmeier E. *Kidney Int* 1977;12:253–267.
105. Muller-Suur R, Gutsche HE, Samwer KF, Oelkers W, Hierholzer K. *Pflugers Arch* 1975;359:33–56.
106. Kramer P, Ochwadt B. *Nephron* 1974;12:464–474.
107. Swales JD. *Pharmacol Ther* 1979;7:173–201.
108. Braam B, Mitchell KD, Navar LG. *FASEB J* 1993;7(4):A546.
109. Harrap SB, Doyle AE. *J Hypertens* 1986;4(suppl 3):S249–S252.
110. Arendshorst WA, Chatziantoniou C, Daniels FH. *Kidney Int* 1990;38(suppl 30):S92–S96.
111. Chatziantoniou C, Daniels FH, Arendshorst WA. *Am J Physiol* 1990;259:F372–F382.
112. Henrich WL, Levi M. *Am J Physiol* 1991;260:F530–F535.
113. Dilley JR, Arendshorst WJ. *Am J Physiol* 1984;247:F672–F679.
114. Dilley JR, Stier CT Jr, Arendshorst WJ. *Am J Physiol* 1984;246:F12–F20.
115. Ferrone RA, Antonaccio MJ. *Eur J Pharmacol* 1979;60:131–137.
116. Assad MM, Antonaccio MJ. *Hypertension* 1982;4:487–493.

117. Richer C, Doussau MP, Giudicelli JF. *Hypertension* 1983;5:312–320.
118. Harrap SB, Nicolaci JA, Doyle AE. *Clin Exp Pharmacol Physiol* 1986;13:753–765.
119. Mullins JJ, Peters J, Ganten D. *Nature* 1990;344:541–544.
120. Ganten D, Lindpaintner K, Ganten U, et al. *Hypertension* 1991;17:843–855.
121. Bachmann S, Peters J, Engler E, Ganten D, Mullins J. *Kidney Int* 1992;41:24–36.
122. Barrett GL, Mullins JJ. *Kidney Int* 1992;41(suppl 37):S125–S128.
123. Hilgers KF, Peters J, Veelken R, et al. *Hypertension* 1992;19:687–691.
124. Von Thun AM, Vari RC, El-Dahr SS, Navar LG. *Am J Physiol* 1994;266:F120–F128.
125. Mitchell KD, Mullins JJ. *J Am Soc Nephrol* 1993;4(3):583.
126. Siegl PKS, Chang RSL, Mantlo NB, et al. *J Pharmacol Exp Ther* 1992;262:139–144.

Hypertension: Pathophysiology, Diagnosis, and Management, Second Edition, edited by J.H. Laragh and B.M. Brenner, Raven Press, Ltd., New York © 1995.

CHAPTER 87

Control of Sodium Excretion and Arterial Pressure by Intrarenal Mechanisms and the Renin-Angiotensin System

John E. Hall, Arthur C. Guyton, and Michael W. Brands

The renin-angiotensin system (RAS) is one of the body's most powerful regulators of arterial pressure and body fluid volumes (1–3). This control is exerted through multiple actions of angiotensin II (ANGII) that influence the circulation directly and indirectly via the kidneys and other hormonal systems (1–3). Control of body fluid volume by ANGII includes extrarenal effects, such as stimulation of thirst and aldosterone secretion, and direct intrarenal actions that regulate renal hemodynamics and tubular reabsorption (3–7). Each of these actions contributes to volume regulation, but this chapter concentrates mainly on the intrarenal functions of ANGII because these appear to be especially important in long-term control of renal excretion and, ultimately, fluid balance and arterial pressure.

J. E. Hall, A. C. Guyton, and M. W. Brands: Department of Physiology and Biophysics, University of Mississippi Medical Center, Jackson, Mississippi 39216.

PHYSIOLOGICAL EFFECTS OF ANGII MAY DIFFER FROM PHARMACOLOGICAL EFFECTS

One reason for the rapid growth in our understanding of the RAS has been the development of specific pharmacological blockers of the system, including ANGII antagonists, angiotensin-converting enzyme (ACE) inhibitors, and renin inhibitors (8–10). With these blockers, the physiological effects of endogenous ANGII can be quantitated. Some of these blockers, especially the ACE inhibitors, may have additional effects besides blockade of the RAS. Therefore, it is sometimes useful to determine whether the effects of blocking ANGII formation with ACE inhibitors can be reversed by ANGII infusion at physiological rates.

In examining the actions of exogenous ANGII, it is important to distinguish between physiological and pharmacological effects. Very high levels of ANGII can sometimes elicit effects that are quantitatively and qualitatively different from the physiological actions of ANGII on the kidneys and the circulation. For example, ANGII normally exerts a potent antinatriuretic effect, whereas pharmacological concentrations may cause natriuresis and diuresis (11). Figure 1 shows the quantitative relationships between ANGII infusion rates and plasma ANGII concentrations measured in different conditions. It is apparent that ANGII infusion rates above 40 to 50 ng/kg/min i.v. produce plasma concentrations in excess of those measured even in extreme conditions such as malignant hypertension. Therefore, to mimic the physiological effects of circulating ANGII, infusion rates less than 40 to 50 ng/kg/min must be employed, or plasma concentrations of ANGII must be less than 5 to 6×10^{-10} M. Some of the controversy concerning the mechanisms by which ANGII regulates renal function and blood pressure is undoubtedly the result of failure to take into account the fact that pharmacological levels of ANGII may cause effects that are qualitatively different from those observed at physiological concentrations. In this chapter, we discuss mainly the physiological functions of the RAS as a basis for understanding its role in health and disease.

ANGII IS A POTENT RENAL VASOCONSTRICTOR

ANGII is one of the body's most potent renal vasoconstrictors, and its importance in controlling renal hemodynamics in various physiological and pathophysiological conditions is well established (6,12,13). Infusion of ANGII at low rates, well within the levels that occur under many physiological conditions, causes renal vasoconstriction, especially in the medullary circulation (6,14,15). When the RAS is activated by sodium deprivation, renal artery stenosis, heart failure, or other conditions associated with circulatory depression or volume depletion, blockade of the RAS markedly reduces renal vascular resistance (6,12,13,15). With the availability of effective ACE inhibitors and ANGII antagonists that lack agonistic activity, it has become apparent that blockade of even normal levels of ANGII increases renal

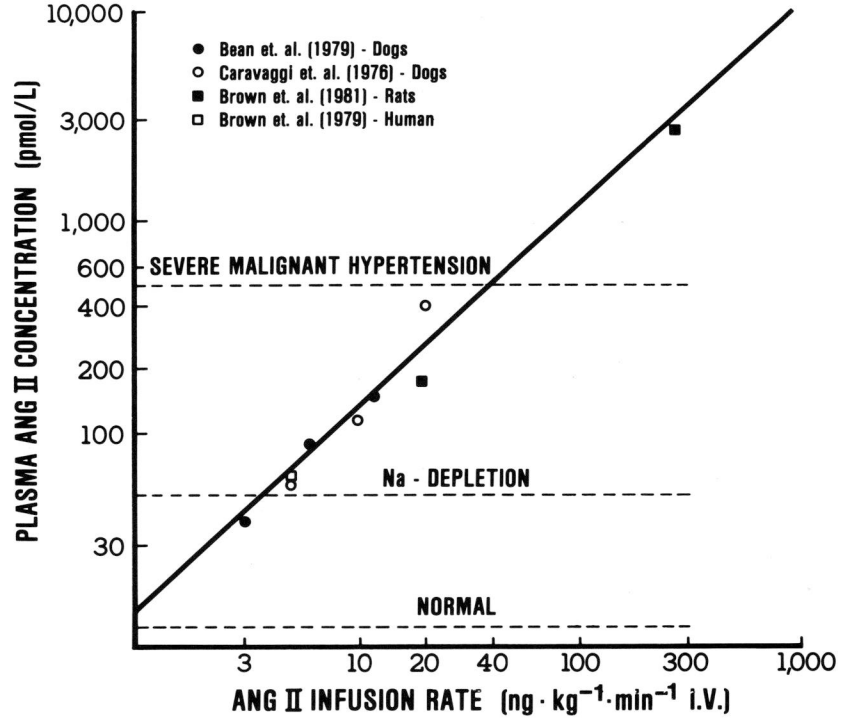

FIG. 1. Relationship between ANGII infusion rate and plasma ANGII concentration. *Dashed lines* show approximate values for plasma ANGII concentrations measured under normal conditions, during sodium depletion, and in malignant hypertension. (From ref. 11, with permission.)

blood flow, indicating that ANGII normally exerts a tonic vasoconstrictor effect on the kidney (6,12,16).

ANGII Preferentially Constricts Efferent Arterioles in Physiological Conditions

Although the importance of ANGII as a renal vasoconstrictor is widely accepted, there is still some controversy concerning the principal site at which ANGII increases renal vascular resistance and its role in glomerular filtration rate (GFR) regulation (5,6,13). ANGII has been suggested to act at almost all sites of the renal vasculature, including preglomerular vessels, the glomerulus, efferent arterioles, and vasa recta (13–18).

The question of where ANGII acts on the renal vasculature is not trivial because vasoconstriction may have quantitatively and qualitatively different effects on some of the major kidney functions, such as excretion of metabolic waste products and sodium, depending on its primary site of action; for example, two actions of ANGII, constriction of efferent arterioles and increased blood pressure, could serve as negative feedback mechanisms to help prevent reductions in GFR and to stabilize excretion of metabolic waste products (19–21) (Fig. 2). However, two other actions of ANGII that have been postulated, constriction of afferent arterioles and contraction of glomerular mesangial cells thus causing decreased glomerular capillary filtration coefficient (K_f), would tend to reduce GFR. If these effects were very powerful, they could initiate a vicious cycle whereby initial decreases in GFR would stimulate renin release (via a macula densa mechanism) and ANGII formation, which would further constrict afferent arterioles and reduce K_f, causing even greater decreases in GFR. Fortunately, this positive feedback does not occur under physiological conditions because the primary renal hemodynamic effect of ANGII seems to be constriction of efferent arterioles, rather than preglomerular vessels (6,16). The primary reason for this is that there are several intrarenal mechanisms that selectively protect preglomerular vessels from ANGII-mediated constriction under normal conditions. In addition, activation of the RAS is often associated with reductions in renal perfusion pressure, due to circulatory depression or volume depletion, which activates other autoregulatory mechanisms that tend to cause dilation rather than constriction of preglomerular vessels.

The conclusion that ANGII normally has a preferential constrictor action on efferent arterioles seems to be contradicted by the observation that ANGII infusion in normal animals usually increases both preglomerular and efferent arteriolar resistances, estimated with micropuncture methods or clearance techniques (13,17). Likewise, blockade of ANGII formation usually decreases afferent and efferent arteriolar resistance, particularly when the RAS is activated (22–25). However, a major part of the preglomerular resistance response to ANGII appears to be secondary to changes in renal perfusion pressure, since this response is attenuated or abolished during intrarenal ANGII infusion or when renal perfusion pressure is held constant (6,26–28).

Part of the vasoconstriction of preglomerular vessels that accompanies ANGII infusion in normal animals may also be caused by enhanced tubuloglomerular feedback (TGF), as discussed in more detail below. To quantify the direct renal vascular actions of ANGII, independent of other autoregulatory mechanisms, we studied the effects of ANGII infusion in dogs in which TGF and pressure-induced changes in renal vascular resistances were blocked (21). When TGF was intact, ANGII infu-

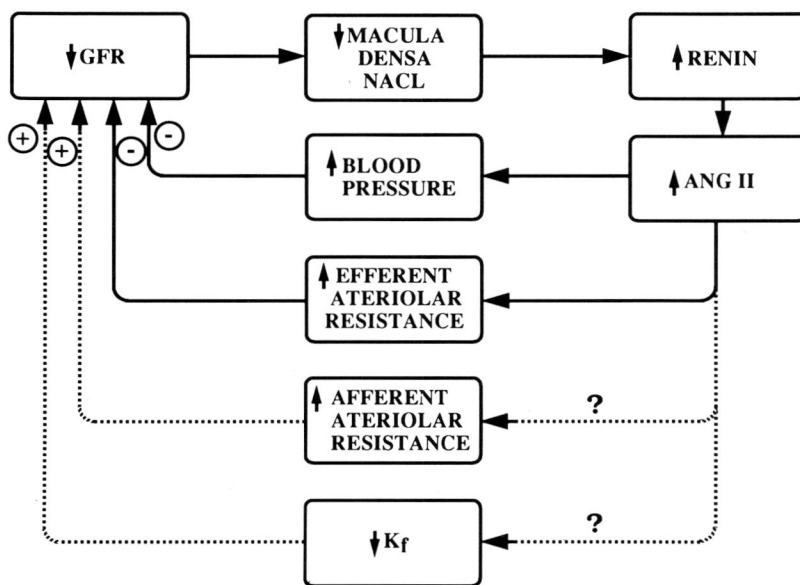

FIG. 2. Postulated actions of ANGII that could influence glomerular filtration rate (GFR) regulation. Two actions, constriction of efferent arterioles and increased blood pressure, serve as negative feedback mechanisms to prevent decreases in GFR, whereas the postulated constriction of afferent arterioles and reduced glomerular capillary filtration coefficient could lead to further decreases in GFR and a positive feedback if the effects were potent.

sion raised preglomerular and efferent arteriolar resistances. In contrast, after TGF blockade and servocontrol of renal artery pressure, ANGII infusion at rates as high as 40 ng/kg/min had no significant effect on preglomerular resistance but markedly increased postglomerular resistance (21). Similarly, ANGII, over a wide range of concentrations, has little or no sustained effect on the diameter of isolated preglomerular vessels, including the afferent arterioles and intralobular arteries, even though it has a potent effect on isolated efferent arterioles (29). Thus, the direct actions of ANGII, at physiological concentrations, appear to be confined mainly to the efferent arterioles, except in special circumstances associated with impaired vascular production of prostaglandins or endothelial-derived relaxing factor (EDRF), or when tissue levels of adenosine are elevated, as discussed below.

Prostaglandins and EDRF Protect Preglomerular Vessels from ANGII-Mediated Constriction

Protection against ANGII-mediated constriction of afferent arterioles by prostaglandins and other autacoid mechanisms may be important in preventing the development of a vicious cycle and acute renal failure in circumstances in which the RAS is activated, such as renal artery stenosis or volume depletion. After infusion of the prostaglandin synthetase inhibitor meclofenamate, ANGII markedly constricted preglomerular vessels (30) (Fig. 3). Because the vasoconstriction was observed even when renal perfusion pressure was servocontrolled and when TGF was blocked, this effect appeared to be a direct action of ANGII on preglomerular vessels, which occurred only after blockade of prostaglandin synthesis. Meclofenamate did not, however, alter the postglomerular resistance response to ANGII. To the extent that the effects of meclofenamate can be attributed to blockade of prostaglandin synthesis, these studies suggest that prostaglandins selectively protect preglomerular vessels from ANGII-mediated constriction without interfering with efferent arteriolar constriction. Similar results have also been reported in other studies using micropuncture or clearance methods (31,32).

Other vasodilators released from the afferent arterioles may also protect them from the constrictor action of

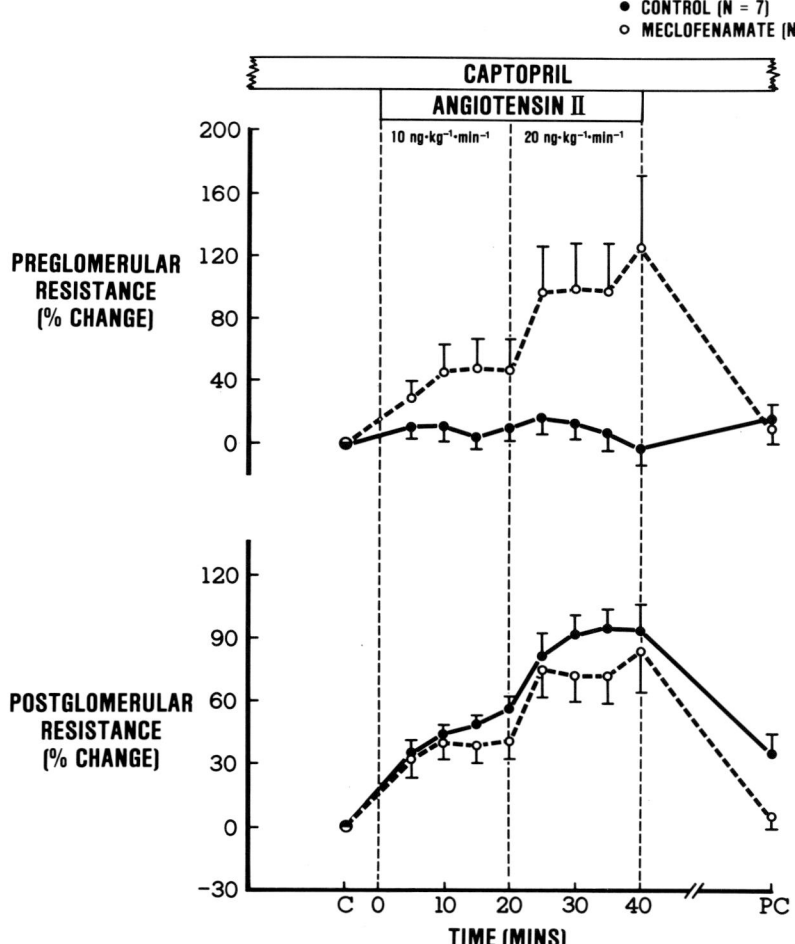

FIG. 3. Effect of ANGII infusion on renal segmental vascular resistance in nonfiltering kidneys during control conditions and after blockade of prostaglandin synthesis with meclofenamate. Endogenous ANGII formation was blocked by infusion of the ACE inhibitor captopril throughout the experiment and the kidneys were made nonfiltering to block changes in tubuloglomerular feedback. (Modified from ref. 30.)

ANGII. Ito et al. (33) found, in completely isolated afferent arterioles, that ANGII normally induced only a transient vasoconstriction that waned in less than a minute. However, after pretreatment of these vessels with N^W-nitro-L-arginine (L-NAME) to inhibit synthesis of nitric oxide, ANGII caused sustained constriction of these vessels. These observations suggest that EDRF, as well as prostaglandins, may selectively protect preglomerular vessels from the constrictor effects of ANGII. The physiological significance of this protection is not completely clear, but studies in intact animals suggest that even low levels of ANGII may markedly reduce GFR, in parallel with reduced renal blood flow, when synthesis of prostaglandins and/or EDRF is impaired (34). It is possible that in pathophysiological conditions associated with widespread renal vascular injury, such as malignant hypertension, high ANGII levels in conjunction with endothelial injury and the inability of the vasculature to produce prostaglandins and/or EDRF may result in a vicious cycle, leading to progressive decreases in GFR.

Adenosine Interacts with ANGII to Constrict Preglomerular Vessels

The presence of increased intrarenal adenosine levels also greatly enhances the effect of ANGII on preglomerular vessels (35) (Fig. 4). This interaction appears to be multiplicative, since neither ANGII nor adenosine alone significantly constricts preglomerular vessels (35). However, when both substances are present in high concentrations, there is a marked increase in preglomerular vascular resistance and parallel decreases in renal blood flow and GFR (35).

The physiological significance of ANGII-adenosine interactions is still uncertain, because tissue adenosine levels are not markedly elevated in most physiological circumstances associated with increased ANGII formation, such as during sodium depletion or moderate reductions in renal perfusion pressure. However, in certain pathophysiological conditions associated with renal ischemia, such as severe renal artery stenosis or with renal vascular lesions in malignant hypertension, it seems

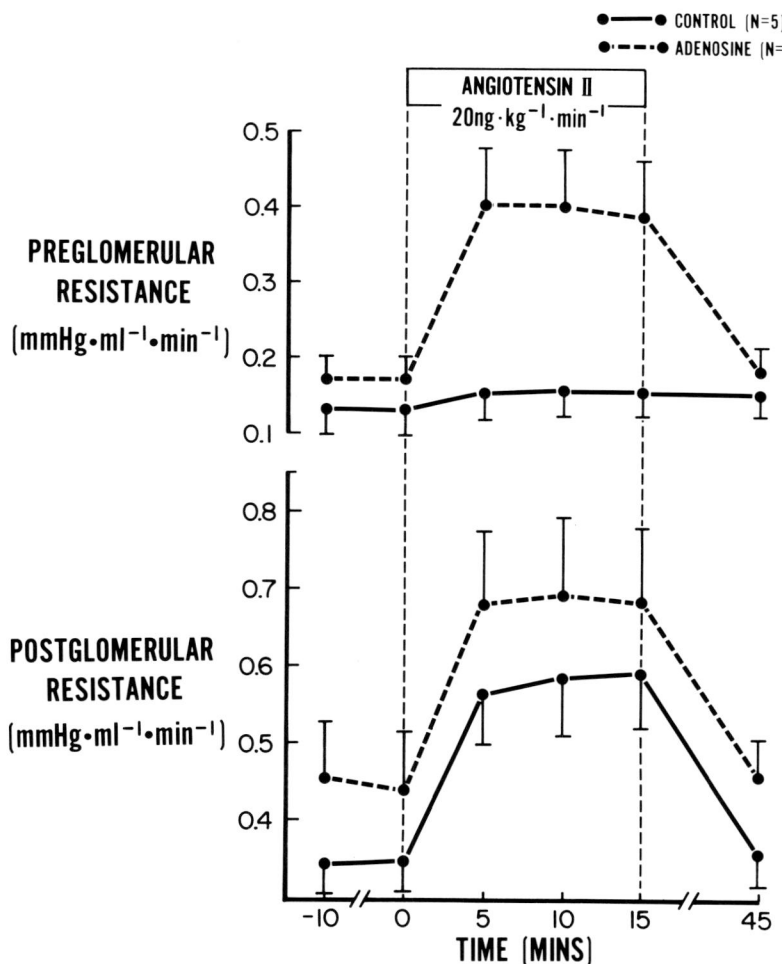

FIG. 4. Effect of ANGII infusion under control conditions and after renal arterial infusions of adenosine (1 μM/min) on renal segmental vascular resistances. Nonfiltering kidneys were used to block changes in tubuloglomerular feedback activity and renal perfusion pressure was held constant to prevent pressure-dependent changes in renal vascular resistances.

more likely that intrarenal levels of adenosine could increase sufficiently to cause preglomerular vasoconstriction. Under these circumstances, simultaneous increases in ANGII and adenosine could conceivably initiate a positive feedback in which decreases in renal blood flow and hypoxia would cause increases in ANGII and adenosine, further vasoconstriction, and eventually renal failure. Additional studies are needed, however, to determine whether such an interaction actually contributes to decreased GFR in these conditions.

Does ANGII Act Directly on the Glomerulus to Decrease K_f

Glomerular mesangial cells are capable of contracting in response to various agonists, including ANGII (36,37). However, the physiological importance of these effects in regulating GFR and renal blood flow is still unclear. In many cases, contraction of mesangial cells has been observed only with pharmacological levels of ANGII, and several investigators have been unable to document responses to ANGII at physiological concentrations using methods that allow direct visualization of the glomeruli (27,38,39). These observations appear to conflict with micropuncture studies that suggest that K_f is reduced when ANGII is infused or stimulated endogenously by chronic sodium depletion (40). However, calculation of K_f using micropuncture methods is indirect and can only be made in superficial nephrons, which may not accurately represent the entire kidney. Thus, the significance of reported effects of ANGII on glomerular contraction and K_f is difficult to assess.

One theoretical consideration that speaks against a major action of ANGII to reduce K_f is the possibility that such an effect could lead to a vicious cycle. If ANGII reduced K_f, this would tend to cause further decreases in GFR, additional stimulation of ANGII formation (via a macula densa mechanism), and still greater decreases in GFR. An experimental observation that also argues against a major effect of ANGII to reduce K_f is the fact that ANGII infusion, at physiological rates, rarely reduces GFR even when there are substantial decreases in renal plasma flow (1,6,16). In fact, ANGII often helps to prevent decreases in GFR when the RAS is activated in circumstances such as renal artery stenosis or congestive heart failure.

ANGII Decreases Vasa Recta Blood Flow

There has been considerable interest in the possibility that the renal medullary circulation may be even more sensitive to the constrictor effects of ANGII than the rest of the kidney (14,41,42). As discussed below, a potent effect of ANGII to reduce medullary blood flow could contribute to the sodium retention, independent of overall effects on renal blood flow and GFR.

There is a high density of ANGII receptors in rat vasa recta bundles and ANGII, at physiological concentrations, decreases renal medullary blood flow (41–43). In fact, ANGII infusion at rates too low to measurably alter total renal blood flow or GFR reduced renal papillary plasma flow (14). Blockade of ANGII formation also increases renal medullary blood flow when the RAS is activated (41,44). These observations suggest that ANGII may have physiological effects on the renal medullary circulation. However, it is not clear whether these effects occur secondarily to increased efferent arteriolar resistance or whether ANGII-mediated changes in medullary blood flow are due to a direct action on the contractile elements of the vasa recta.

ANGII Helps to Prevent Decreased GFR in Hypoperfused Nephrons

Blockade of intrarenal or circulating ANGII, by infusion of either ANGII antagonists or ACE inhibitors, or by renin depletion, often impairs GFR when renal perfusion pressure is reduced (19,20,45). Moreover, this impairment occurs even though renal blood flow autoregulation is well preserved (19,20,45) (Fig. 5). The decreased GFR observed after ANGII blockade appears to be related to inhibition of the constrictor effects of ANGII on efferent arterioles, an effect that is exacerbated by superimposition of other disturbances such as chronic sodium depletion (19,20). Thus, in patients with bilateral renal artery stenosis or stenosis of a solitary kidney, ACE inhibition may cause severe decreases in GFR (46–49). The reduction of GFR in these individuals cannot be attributed solely to low renal perfusion pressure because comparable decreases in blood pressure with other vasodilators, such as nitroprusside, do not reduce GFR (46). It is important to emphasize, however, that in many patients with mild renal artery stenosis and in most essential hypertensives, ANGII blockade does not impair GFR. The primary reason for this is that there are other autoregulatory mechanisms that can reduce afferent arteriolar resistance sufficiently to compensate for efferent arteriolar vasodilation and maintain GFR near normal.

Experimental studies suggest that GFR autoregulation in underperfused nephrons normally involves at least two parallel control systems (Fig. 6). One system, which can operate independently of ANGII, causes dilation of afferent and efferent arterioles when renal perfusion pressure is impaired, probably because of TGF as well as myogenic activity (6,16,50–52). However, as discussed below, ANGII can influence TGF sensitivity. A second mechanism for GFR control is mediated by ANGII, which prevents reductions in efferent arteriolar resis-

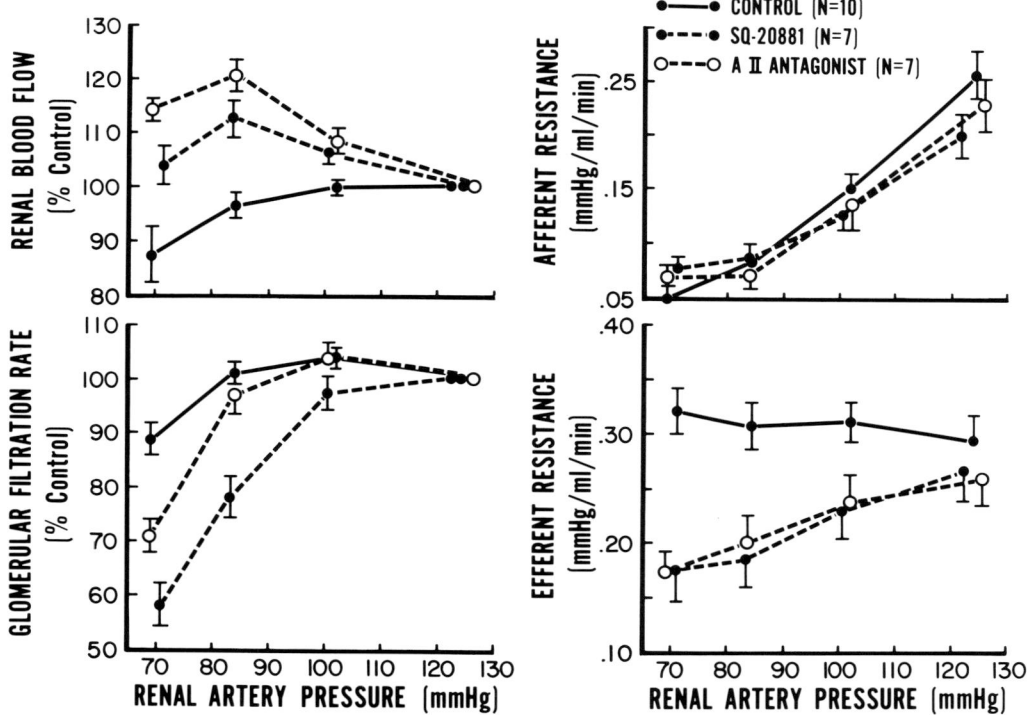

FIG. 5. Effect of decrease in renal artery pressure on renal hemodynamics in normal control dogs and in normal dogs after infusion of the ACE inhibitor, SQ 20881 (teprotide) or the ANGII antagonist (Sar[1]Ile[8]) ANGII. (Modified from refs. 19 and 20.)

tance, thereby stabilizing glomerular hydrostatic pressure and GFR during reduced renal perfusion pressure. The RAS seems to be most important when renal perfusion pressure is reduced to very low levels, near the limits of autoregulation, or when other disturbances such as sodium depletion are superimposed on low renal perfusion pressure (6,16).

In addition to the clinical situation of renal artery stenosis, the renal vasoconstrictor effect of ANGII on efferent arterioles also helps to prevent decreased GFR in circumstances such as sodium deprivation, increased renal venous pressure, renal sympathetic nerve stimulation, congestive heart failure, Bartter's syndrome, or when plasma protein concentration is reduced because of hepatic cirrhosis or hypoalbuminemia (6,12,53–56).

ANGII-Mediated Efferent Arteriolar Constriction Provides Differential Control of Excretion of Sodium and Metabolic Waste Products

The preferential constrictor action of ANGII on efferent arterioles is important not only in regulating GFR but also in causing sodium and water retention (6). Thus, activation of the RAS, which usually occurs in response to circulatory depression or a deficit of sodium and water, decreases sodium excretion while maintaining a rel-

atively constant excretion of metabolic waste products. The reason for this is that excretion of most metabolic waste products, such as urea and creatinine, is usually proportional to the rate of glomerular filtration. Clearance of sodium, however, is determined by the balance between GFR and tubular reabsorption, both of which can vary in different circumstances. By constricting efferent arterioles in hypotensive states, ANGII causes several changes in peritubular capillary dynamics that increase tubular reabsorption of sodium and water, as discussed below. However, efferent arteriolar constriction also raises glomerular hydrostatic pressure, which helps to prevent excessive reductions in GFR and therefore retention of metabolic waste products in hypotensive states. In this way, ANGII provides a mechanism for regulating excretion of metabolic waste products and sodium independently.

Are There Different Roles for Circulating and Intrarenally Formed ANGII in GFR Regulation?

Considerable evidence indicates that significant amounts of ANGII can be formed locally in the kidney as well as in the systemic circulation (13,57–59). Although there has been speculation that intrarenally formed and circulating ANGII may have qualitatively,

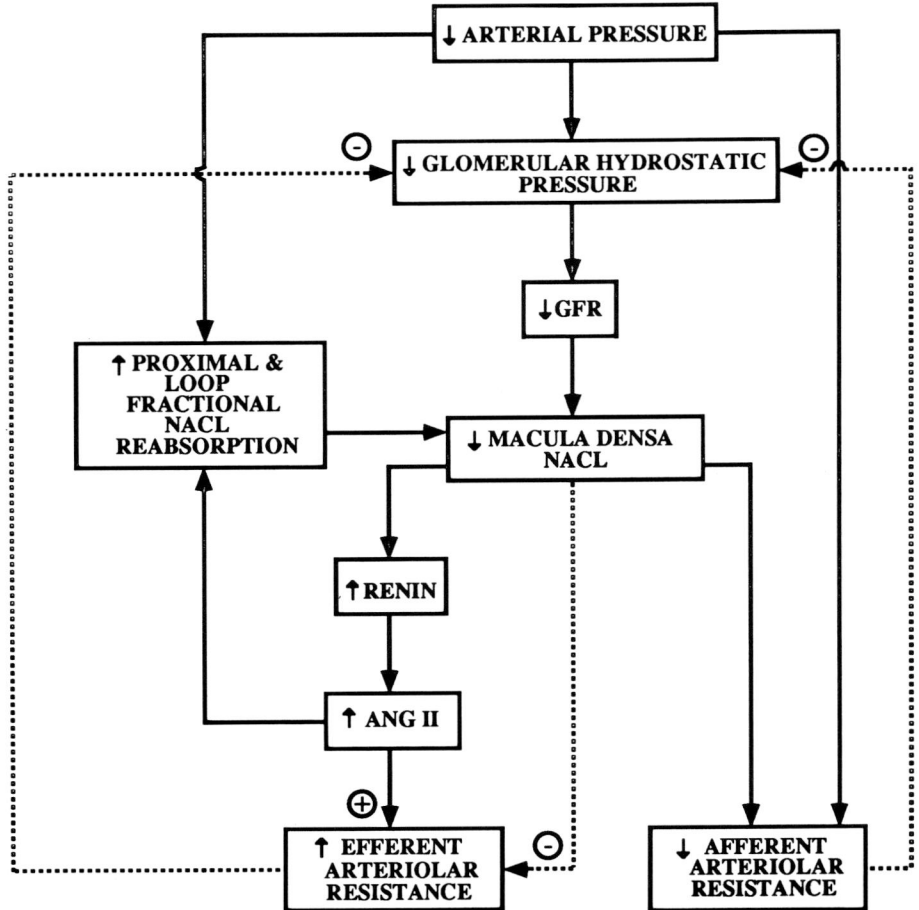

FIG. 6. Interaction of ANGII, macula densa feedback, and pressure-dependent changes in renal vascular resistances on autoregulation of glomerular filtration rate during decreased arterial pressure.

as well as quantitatively, different actions on the renal vasculature, there is little evidence to support this notion. Several studies suggest that both intrarenally formed and circulating ANGII help to preserve GFR by constricting efferent arterioles when renal perfusion is threatened (6,60,61). Although selective inhibition of either intrarenally formed or circulating ANGII does not severely impair GFR, blockade of both mechanisms causes substantial reductions in efferent arteriolar resistance and GFR when renal perfusion is reduced (6,16,60,61). Apparently, both circulating and intrarenally formed ANGII act on the same site of the renal vasculature, mainly the efferent arterioles, with minimal effects on preglomerular vessels.

Although the concentrations of circulating and intrarenally formed ANGII often parallel each other, there may be special circumstances in which they are dissociated. For example, patchy ischemia of the kidney or damage to individual nephrons may result in hypoperfusion and increased renin release in a few nephrons without causing major changes in circulating ANGII (62). Under these conditions, it is conceivable that locally formed ANGII could play an important role in regulating GFR independently of changes in circulating ANGII. However, this hypothesis has been difficult to test experimentally and the role of circulating versus intrarenally formed ANGII in regulating the renal hemodynamics under different physiological and pathophysiological conditions has not been fully elucidated.

ANGII Blockade May Protect Overperfused Nephrons

Although blockade of the constrictor action of ANGII on efferent arterioles often causes a further decline in glomerular hydrostatic pressure and GFR in underperfused nephrons, blocking the constrictor action of ANGII on efferent arterioles may prove to be beneficial in limiting glomerular injury associated with glomerular hyperfiltration in overperfused nephrons.

Experimental studies suggest that ACE inhibition may attenuate the development of proteinuria and glomerular sclerosis in conditions associated with glomerular hyperfiltration and increased hydrostatic pressure; for example, after reducing kidney mass, increased glomerular hydrostatic pressure in the remnant kidney is associated with progressive proteinuria and glomerular capillary damage (63–65). Chronic treatment with ACE inhibitors, by removing the vasoconstrictor action of ANGII on efferent arterioles, reduces glomerular hydrostatic pressure and ameliorates these pathological changes. In contrast, other antihypertensive drugs that reduce systemic arterial pressure to a similar degree, but do not lower glomerular hydrostatic pressure because they dilate preglomerular vessels, do not appear to slow the progression of glomerular damage (63). However, it is possible that there are also nonhemodynamic actions of ACE inhibition that ameliorate glomerular injury.

Thus, the beneficial effects of ACE inhibition in arresting chronic glomerular failure may be due, in part, to decreased glomerular hydrostatic pressure caused by blocking the constrictor action of ANGII on efferent arterioles. If ANGII blockade does indeed prove to be beneficial in preventing glomerular damage in humans through this mechanism, it should be possible not only to ameliorate chronic renal failure but also to block glomerular membrane damage in the early stages of certain diseases associated with glomerular hyperfiltration; for example, there is an increased GFR and glomerular hypertension in diabetes mellitus in the early stages, before diabetic nephropathy and systemic hypertension occur. At that point, it may be useful to reduce systemic arterial pressure and glomerular hydrostatic pressure with ACE inhibitors even before systemic hypertension is present. Although a certain degree of systemic hypotension would be expected after ACE inhibition, the potential for preventing glomerular injury may outweigh this problem.

ANGII Increases Tubuloglomerular Feedback Sensitivity

The existence of a feedback system linking renal tubular function with renal vascular control and renin release is well documented, although there are still uncertainties regarding the exact mechanism by which this feedback system operates (50,51,66,67). When distal tubules of single nephrons are perfused at higher than normal rates, there is a reduction in glomerular hydrostatic pressure and in single nephron GFR (SNGFR), whereas cessation of distal perfusion increases SNGFR. Most of the available evidence suggests that some function of sodium chloride transport by the macula densa cells may be the signal sensed (66,67). There is considerable uncertainty about the mechanism by which macula densa cell transport is ultimately transduced to changes in renal vascular resistance, although several mediators have been postulated (51,67).

The signal sensed by the macula densa is probably not tubular fluid sodium chloride concentration per se, because inhibition of sodium chloride reabsorption in the loop of Henle with furosemide, for example, dissociates distal tubular sodium chloride concentration and TGF (66). Apparently, changes in sodium chloride transport by the macula densa initiate changes in SNGFR via TGF. Under many conditions, sodium chloride transport by the macula densa is directly proportional to the delivery and concentration of sodium chloride in the tubular fluid. In general, an increase in sodium chloride delivery stimulates transport by the macula densa and elicits vasoconstriction of afferent arterioles, thereby reducing SNGFR and returning sodium chloride delivery toward normal. Decreased sodium chloride delivery to the macula densa produces the opposite changes.

Because of the close anatomic association of the juxtaglomerular cells of the afferent arterioles, the primary site of renin secretion, and the macula densa cells, ANGII was postulated to serve as the mediator of TGF (68,69). However, there is considerable evidence that ANGII is not a direct mediator of TGF (6,70), although ANGII may modify the sensitivity of TGF. Infusions of ANGII antagonists or ACE inhibitors blunt TGF, whereas disturbances that stimulate ANGII formation, such as sodium depletion, amplify TGF (70).

The mechanisms by which ANGII modulates TGF are not known. Although ANGII has been suggested to influence TGF by altering baseline afferent arteriolar tone (71), this seems unlikely because ANGII appears to have little or no direct effect on afferent arteriolar resistance, independent of TGF. Moreover, other vasoconstrictors, such as norepinephrine, which are known to have direct effects on afferent arteriolar tone, do not mimic the effect of ANGII on TGF. It seems more likely that ANGII may modify TGF by altering the sensor or mediator step, rather than by directly altering afferent arteriolar resistance.

One mechanism by which ANGII could alter feedback responsiveness is by stimulating macula densa sodium chloride transport. The normal relationship between distal delivery and transported sodium chloride and the postulated effect of ANGII to stimulate sodium transport by these cells are shown in Fig. 7. If ANGII stimulated sodium chloride transport by the macula densa cells, as it does in many other epithelial cells, this would shift the relationship between distal delivery and macula densa transport, thereby increasing the sensitivity of TGF; for any given rate of sodium chloride delivery, a higher rate of transport and greater afferent arteriolar constriction would occur in the presence of elevated ANGII. Conversely, blockade of ANGII formation would reduce sodium chloride transport, thereby decreasing TGF sensitivity.

An effect of ANGII to increase macula densa sodium chloride transport and TGF sensitivity could explain several experimental observations in which simultaneous changes in distal sodium chloride delivery and ac-

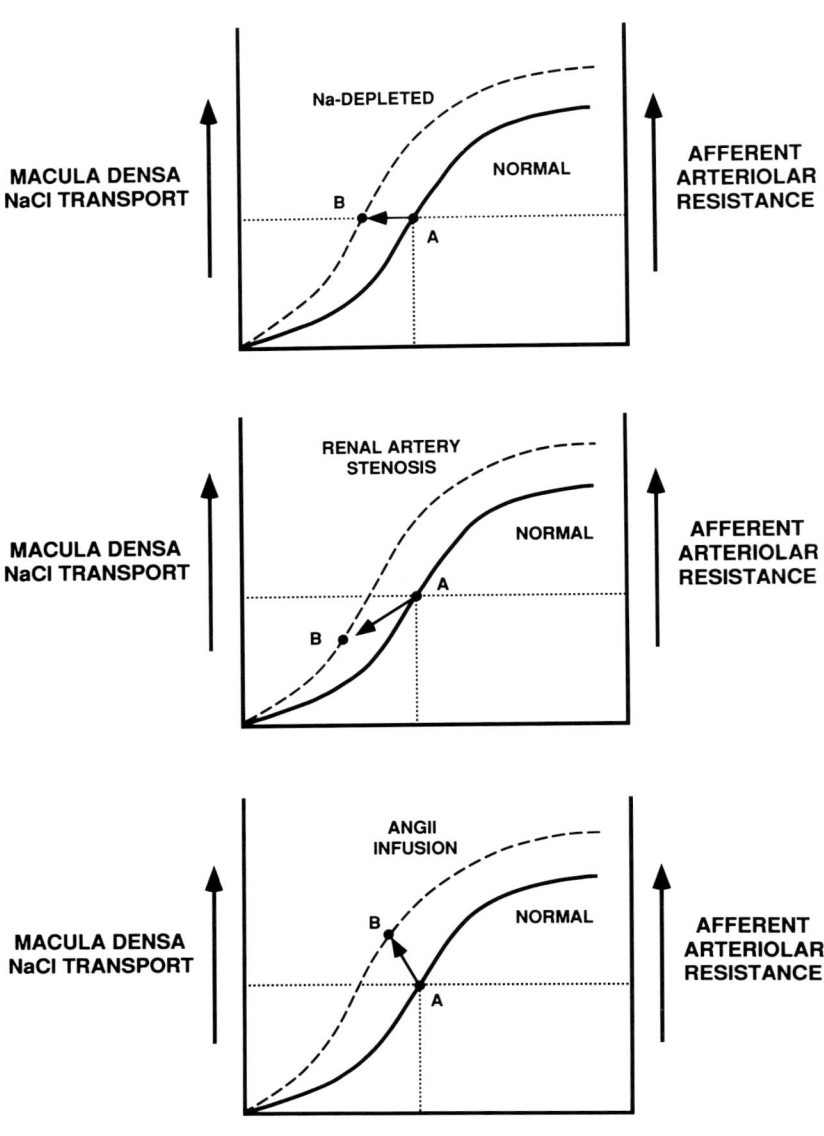

FIG. 7. Postulated relationship between distal sodium chloride delivery and macula densa sodium chloride transport, and effect of ANGII on macula densa sodium chloride transport. Increasing sodium chloride transport at the macula densa is postulated to increase afferent arteriolar resistance via tubuloglomerular feedback. Point A represents normal values for distal sodium chloride delivery, macula densa sodium chloride transport, and afferent arteriolar resistance. Point B represents postulated steady-state values after sodium depletion, renal artery stenosis, or ANGII infusion. (Modified from ref. 16.)

tivity of the RAS occur. For example, with chronic sodium depletion, there is very little change in afferent resistance, although efferent resistance increases markedly (40). Decreased distal tubular sodium chloride delivery, due to small decreases in GFR and increased proximal tubular reabsorption, would tend to decrease distal sodium chloride delivery and cause afferent arteriolar vasodilation during sodium depletion. However, with increased ANGII levels and enhanced TGF sensitivity, there would be little overall change in afferent resistance.

Another example is the response to decreased renal perfusion pressure. With marked decreases in distal sodium chloride delivery after renal artery stenosis, affer-

ent arteriolar vasodilation would occur in the presence of ANGII levels if distal sodium chloride delivery were reduced sufficiently to override increased TGF sensitivity caused by high ANGII. A third example is the renal hemodynamic responses to ANGII infusion. In normal animals, infusion of exogenous ANGII increases afferent and efferent arteriolar resistance, especially if renal perfusion pressure increases and TGF is intact (17,26). When TGF is blocked and renal perfusion pressure is held constant, however, ANGII infusion causes no significant increase in afferent arteriolar resistance (21). Although ANGII infusion may decrease distal sodium chloride delivery, because of enhanced proximal absorption, the reduction in distal delivery may not be sufficient to offset ANGII-mediated increases in TGF sensitivity so that there is a net increase in afferent arteriolar resistance.

Although it is still somewhat speculative, the hypothesis shown in Fig. 7 explains many experimental observations in which there are simultaneous changes in distal sodium chloride delivery and ANGII concentrations. Incorporation of this concept into a mathematical model of the kidney has allowed accurate computer simulations of many of these conditions (72). Although the direct actions of ANGII on macula densa sodium chloride transport have not been examined experimentally, there is evidence that ANGII enhances sodium chloride transport in many other epithelial membranes considered to be analogous to the renal distal tubules (6,7). However, further studies are needed to test this hypothesis experimentally.

Such an effect of ANGII on TGF would be highly beneficial for cardiovascular homeostasis. An increase in TGF sensitivity by ANGII would allow decreases in sodium chloride delivery to occur in circumstances such as sodium depletion without a compensatory TGF-mediated afferent arteriolar vasodilation. The maintained reduction of distal sodium chloride delivery, due to increased proximal tubule reabsorption, could then contribute to decreases in urinary sodium excretion along with other antinatriuretic actions of ANGII that increase sodium reabsorption in more distal parts of the renal tubules, such as stimulation of aldosterone secretion.

ANGII IS A POWERFUL CONTROLLER OF SODIUM EXCRETION

Because ANGII normally acts to prevent reductions in GFR, its antinatriuretic effect is due mainly to increased tubular reabsorption (1,16,73). However, in some pathophysiological circumstances, such as in malignant hypertension, ANGII may contribute to decreases in GFR and reductions in filtered load of sodium.

Stimulation of sodium reabsorption by ANGII occurs via multiple intrarenal and extrarenal effects that influence tubular transport and renal hemodynamics (1,16). The most important extrarenal action of ANGII in regulating sodium reabsorption is stimulation of aldosterone secretion. Although ANGII has also been suggested to enhance sympathetic nerve activity (74–77), considerable evidence indicates that the renal sympathetic nerves do not play a major role in mediating the chronic effects of ANGII on sodium excretion (78–83). The direct intrarenal actions of ANGII are complex and involve hemodynamic effects, such as constriction of efferent arterioles, which alters peritubular capillary dynamics and medullary blood flow, as well as direct actions on tubular

epithelial cell transport. The combined intrarenal and extrarenal actions of ANGII provide the body with one of its most important regulators of sodium excretion.

ANGII Regulates Aldosterone Secretion

ANGII is recognized to be an important regulator of aldosterone secretion (84,85). Since aldosterone is known to stimulate sodium reabsorption, it is often assumed that the primary mechanism by which ANGII controls sodium reabsorption is through aldosterone. Experimental support for this belief, however, is sparse. Although wide extremes in plasma aldosterone concentration are known to have important effects on sodium balance and blood pressure regulation, there is considerable evidence that during many physiological disturbances, such as changes in sodium intake, the effects of aldosterone on sodium excretion and blood pressure regulation may be quantitatively less important than the intrarenal actions of ANGII (1,6,16).

Direct intrarenal infusions of ANGII blockers cause marked increases in sodium excretion independently of changes in plasma aldosterone secretion. In studies from our laboratory (20,86,87), direct intrarenal infusion of either ANGII antagonists or an ACE inhibitor in sodium-depleted dogs increased urinary sodium excretion and decreased fractional sodium reabsorption markedly so that these variables returned to almost normal levels even without changes in plasma aldosterone concentration. Similar results with other blockers of the RAS have been found in other laboratories (88). Also, adrenalectomized dogs on fixed mineralocorticoid replacement during sodium deprivation demonstrated marked natriuresis after intrarenal infusion of an ANGII antagonist, indicating that the changes in sodium excretion cannot be due to alterations in aldosterone secretion (87).

Studies have also shown that chronic blockade of ANGII formation reduces blood pressure and increases renal sodium excretory capability independently of changes in plasma aldosterone concentration (89). In sodium-depleted dogs, the effects of chronic ACE inhibition on blood pressure and renal function could not be reversed by restoring plasma aldosterone concentration to the levels that existed before blockade of ANGII formation (89). In contrast, restoration of circulating ANGII by i.v. infusion almost completely reversed the effects of ACE inhibition on blood pressure and renal function. These observations suggest that the chronic effects of ACE inhibition are caused mainly by ANGII blockade and that decreased plasma aldosterone concentration does not play a major role in mediating these effects.

Studies in adrenalectomized dogs given fixed replacement of mineralocorticoids also support the view that changes in aldosterone secretion may not play a critical role in controlling sodium balance or blood pressure during changes in sodium intake (90). When plasma aldosterone concentration was maintained at a level similar to that measured during normal sodium intake, dogs that were subjected to sodium depletion were able to conserve sodium and maintain arterial pressure as well as dogs with a functional aldosterone system (90). However, adrenalectomized dogs on fixed mineralocorticoid replacement were unable to effectively regulate plasma potassium concentration when challenged with varying sodium and potassium intakes, indicating the importance of aldosterone in regulating potassium balance (91). Patients with adrenal insufficiency who are provided constant aldosterone replacement are also capable of regulating sodium balance effectively even though they are unable to control plasma potassium concentration as well as normal individuals (92).

These observations suggest that changes in aldosterone secretion are normally not essential in maintaining sodium balance or arterial pressure during fluctuations in sodium intake. However, a minimal amount of aldosterone is necessary to prevent excessive sodium loss, and very high levels of aldosterone, such as occurs in patients with aldosterone-secreting tumors (Conn's syndrome), can cause marked sodium retention and increased blood pressure independent of ANGII. Furthermore, blockade of the effects of aldosterone may add to the effects of ACE inhibition in ameliorating sodium retention in patients with congestive heart failure (93). However, in most physiological conditions, variations in plasma aldosterone appear to be much more important in regulating potassium balance than in day-to-day control of sodium balance (91). Apparently, other actions of ANGII, besides stimulation of aldosterone secretion, are primarily responsible for long-term control of sodium excretion and blood pressure by the RAS.

ANGII Controls Sodium Excretion Through Intrarenal Actions

Considerable evidence indicates that powerful antinatriuretic effects of ANGII can occur in the absence of significant decreases in GFR or extrarenal effects such as stimulation of aldosterone, indicating important intrarenal actions of ANGII that stimulate sodium reabsorption (1,2,16). These direct intrarenal actions are, however, complex and involve changes in peritubular capillary dynamics and medullary blood flow as well as direct actions on tubular epithelial cell transport. The quantitative importance of each of these actions in mediating the acute and chronic effects of ANGII on sodium reabsorption is not completely understood, but progress has been made in understanding the fundamental mechanisms by which they operate to conserve sodium.

Insight into the quantitative importance of the different mechanisms by which ANGII influences sodium reabsorption is provided by an analysis of the dose-response relationships between ANGII and its intrarenal and extrarenal actions (Fig. 8). At very low concentrations (10^{-13}–10^{-12} M), ANGII increases sodium and water reabsorption in completely isolated proximal tubules (94,95), an effect that also occurs in other epithelial membrane systems (96–98). Adrenal glomerulosa cells are less sensitive to ANGII (99,100), although enhanced sensitivity occurs during sodium depletion (101,102). Vascular smooth muscle in most parts of the circulation is even less sensitive to ANGII, requiring concentrations of 10^{-10} to 10^{-9} M to cause vasoconstriction and to increase blood pressure during acute infusions (103,104). One exception is the renal efferent arterioles, which constrict with ANGII concentrations as low as 10^{-12} M (29,104). Other vascular segments of the kidney, including the afferent arterioles, interlobar arteries, and interlobular arteries, are much less sensitive to ANGII and in some cases fail to respond to concentrations as high as 10^{-5} M (29,105,106).

Thus, two intrarenal actions of ANGII that occur at very low concentrations and that could increase sodium reabsorption include constriction of efferent arterioles and direct stimulation of tubular sodium transport.

ANGII Increases Sodium Reabsorption by Altering Peritubular Capillary Dynamics

One of the most potent intrarenal effects of ANGII is vasoconstriction of efferent arterioles, an action that not only helps to increase glomerular hydrostatic pressure and to stabilize GFR, but also reduces renal blood flow and causes changes in peritubular capillary dynamics that increase tubular reabsorption (Fig. 9). Efferent arteriolar constriction reduces peritubular capillary hydrostatic pressure and increases peritubular capillary colloid osmotic pressure as a result of decreased renal blood flow and increased filtration fraction. Both of these changes tend to lower renal interstitial fluid hydrostatic pressure and raise interstitial fluid colloid osmotic pressure, thereby increasing the driving force for fluid reabsorption across the tubular epithelium (107–109).

ANGII-mediated changes in interstitial fluid hydrostatic and colloid osmotic pressures could also indirectly increase tubular reabsorption by altering sodium permeability in the tight junctions on the luminal side of the proximal tubular epithelium; this would diminish backleak of sodium actively transported into the intercellular spaces, causing a net increase in reabsorption (109,110). Increased peritubular capillary hydrostatic pressure has been shown to increase electrical conductance of the tubular epithelium and transepithelial flux of polysaccharides that normally do not penetrate the tu-

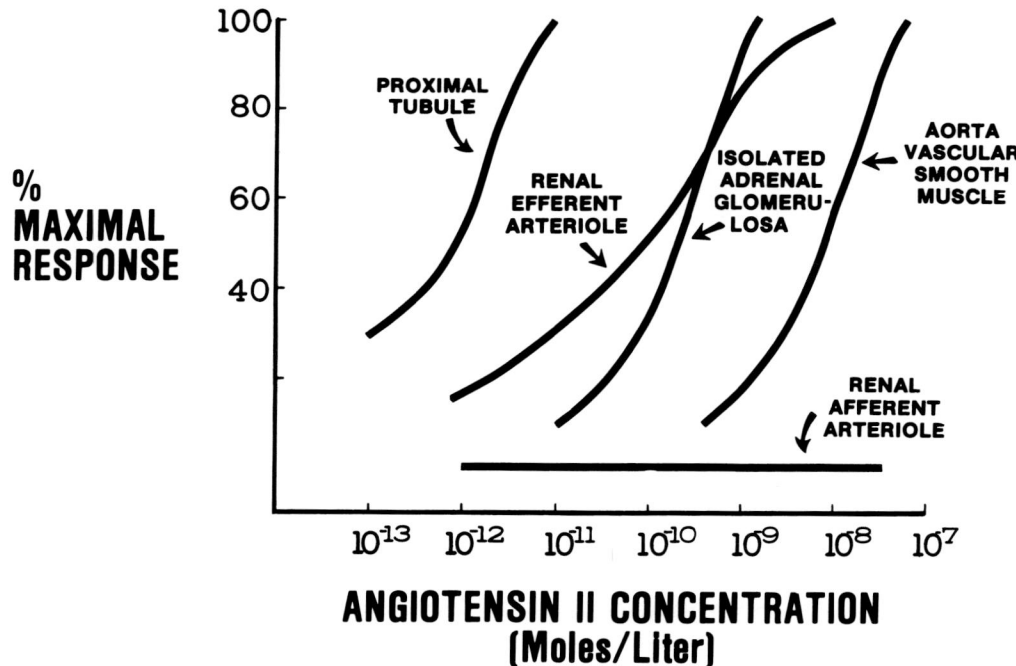

FIG. 8. Approximate dose-response relationships between ANGII concentration and proximal tubular fluid transport, constriction of isolated renal efferent and afferent arterioles, stimulation of aldosterone secretion by isolated adrenal glomerulosa cells or isolated adrenal glands, and contraction of aortic vascular smooth muscle. (Modified from ref. 1.)

bule (111); presumably, ANGII-mediated reductions in peritubular interstitial fluid hydrostatic pressure would cause the opposite effect. Another consequence of reduced interstitial fluid hydrostatic pressure and increased proximal reabsorption is that this would tend to reduce flow rate in the tubular segments of the renal medulla, thereby raising medullary osmolality and passive sodium chloride reabsorption in the thin ascending loops of Henle as well as increasing water reabsorption in the descending loops of Henle and collecting ducts.

Changes in peritubular capillary physical forces have

often been assumed to influence only proximal tubular reabsorption. Interstitial physical forces, however, may also alter reabsorption in more distal parts of the tubule as a result of changes in tubular flow rate and composition of the surrounding interstitium, especially the renal medulla. For example, an increase in proximal reabsorption would reduce flow rate in the tubular segments of the renal medulla, which could raise medullary osmolality and passive sodium chloride reabsorption in the ascending loops of Henle as well as increase water reabsorption in the descending loops of Henle and collecting

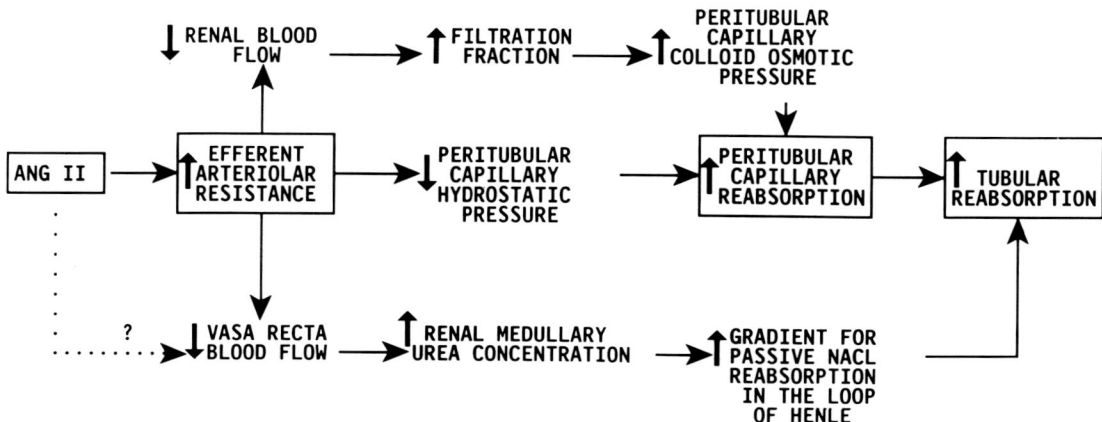

FIG. 9. Possible effects of ANGII on sodium reabsorption through changes in peritubular capillary dynamics.

ducts. Likewise, the effects of ANGII to reduce medullary blood flow would tend to raise renal medullary interstitial osmolality because of the accumulation of urea; increased urea concentration would raise urinary concentrating ability and enhance passive sodium chloride reabsorption in the thin ascending loop of Henle.

Thus, there are several potential mechanisms by which subtle changes in renal hemodynamics, with little or no change in GFR and filtered sodium load, could enhance sodium reabsorption. Micropuncture studies and whole kidney studies have shown that ANGII has important effects on the determinants of peritubular capillary reabsorption (107,112,113), but the contribution of each of the separate hemodynamic effects has been difficult to quantify. Since peritubular capillary uptake is in series with the surrounding interstitium and tubular epithelium, changes in peritubular capillary forces mediated by ANGII must influence tubular reabsorption to some extent. Further studies are needed to quantitate the contribution of changes in interstitial fluid dynamics and medullary tonicity on sodium chloride transport.

ANGII Directly Stimulates Renal Epithelial Cell Sodium Transport

Multiple studies suggest that an important component of the antinatriuretic action of ANGII is related to direct stimulation of tubular transport, independent of changes in renal hemodynamics (1,94,95,114). At high pharmacological concentrations, however, ANGII may directly inhibit tubular reabsorption (94,95), but the inhibitory effect of ANGII probably has very little physiological significance because blockade of the effects of endogenous ANGII has not been shown to directly enhance tubular reabsorption. Instead, inhibition of ANGII formation almost invariably reduces fractional sodium reabsorption in many different physiological and pathophysiological conditions, indicating the importance of the stimulatory effect of ANGII on sodium reabsorption. This stimulation of tubular reabsorption by ANGII appears to occur in proximal tubules and in more distal nephron segments.

ANGII Stimulates Proximal Tubular Reabsorption

Micropuncture and whole kidney studies indicate that ANGII increases proximal tubular sodium reabsorption (1,16,107,115). The direct effects of ANGII on proximal reabsorption have been difficult to quantify because of changes in blood pressure that may also influence sodium reabsorption during ANGII infusion or blockade of ANGII formation; for example, increased arterial pressure during ANGII infusion causes a pressure-mediated reduction in sodium reabsorption that can offset a stimulatory effect of ANGII.

Figure 10 shows the effects of ANGII infusion at various rates ranging from physiological to pharmacological. Note that physiological levels of ANGII caused marked increases in proximal fractional sodium reabsorption and smaller increases in distal fractional reabsorption, estimated with the lithium clearance technique. When renal perfusion pressure was allowed to increase, high rates of ANGII caused natriuresis and diuresis because of decreased proximal and distal tubule sodium reabsorption. This natriuretic and diuretic effect of high doses of ANGII was completely abolished by servocontrolling renal perfusion pressure. These observations indicate that the transition from antinatriuresis to natriuresis with high rates of ANGII infusion was caused by

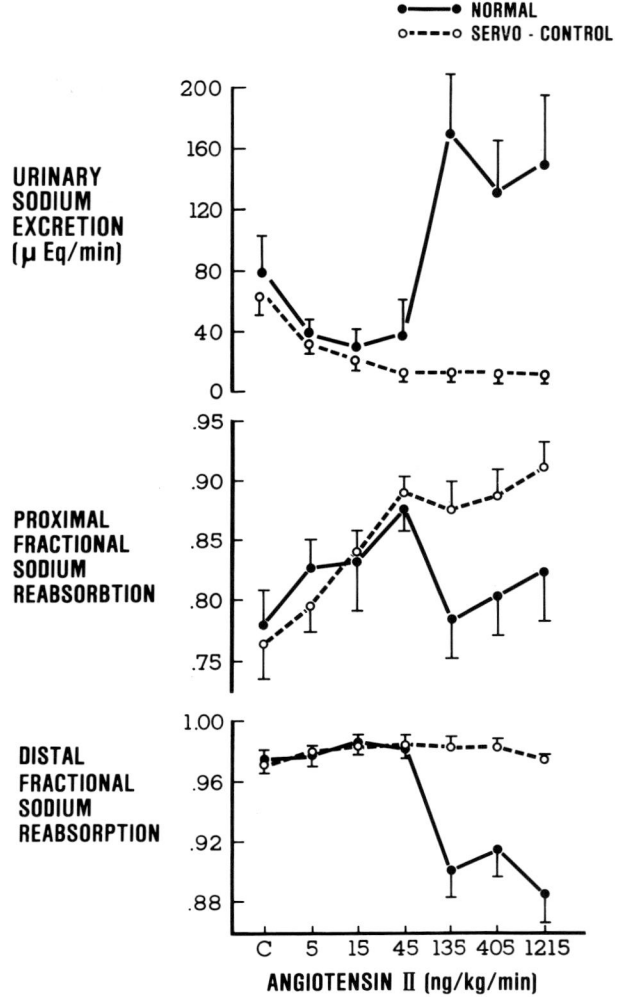

FIG. 10. Changes in urinary sodium excretion, proximal fractional sodium reabsorption (estimated from fractional lithium reabsorption), and distal fractional sodium reabsorption with increasing rates of ANGII infusion, and renal artery pressure either maintained at the control level (servocontrolled) or permitted to increase (normal). "Distal" refers to all parts of the renal tubule beyond the proximal tubule. (Modified from data in ref. 11.)

increased renal perfusion pressure, rather than by a direct inhibitory effect of ANGII on tubular transport. Thus, the net effect of different levels of ANGII on sodium and water excretion depends critically on the balance between the direct antinatriuretic actions of ANGII and the effect of increased renal perfusion pressure, which tends to cause natriuresis.

Micropuncture studies have also demonstrated marked decreases in proximal sodium reabsorption after blockade of ANGII formation. In the untouched kidneys of two-kidney, one-clip Goldblatt hypertensive rats, ACE inhibition decreased absolute and fractional proximal sodium reabsorption (116). Infusion of ANGII antagonists also reduces proximal sodium reabsorption in sodium-depleted rats (113). In all of these studies, however, subtle changes in renal hemodynamics, causing changes in peritubular capillary physical forces or renal medullary blood flow, may have contributed to changes in sodium reabsorption in addition to direct effects of ANGII on tubular sodium transport.

Using a more direct approach to assess renal tubular effects on ANGII, Harris and Young (94) added ANGII to peritubular capillaries while microperfusing rat proximal tubules. Using the steady-state sodium concentration gradient as a measure of proximal reabsorption, they demonstrated that physiological concentrations of

ANGII (10^{-13}–10^{-10} M) increased proximal reabsorption whereas higher concentrations (10^{-9} M) inhibited reabsorption. Similar results were reported by Spinelli and Walther (117). An even more direct demonstration of the stimulatory effect of ANGII on proximal reabsorption comes from the results of Schuster et al. (114), who found that ANGII concentrations of 10^{-11} to 10^{-10} M increased fluid reabsorption in isolated perfused rabbit proximal tubules. A stimulatory effect of ANGII on sodium transport has also been shown in bovine proximal tubule cells grown in primary culture (118) and in kidney cortex slices (119). Thus, there is compelling evidence from a variety of techniques, employing whole kidneys, micropuncture methods, isolated perfused tubules, and individual cells, that ANGII has a direct stimulatory effect on proximal tubule sodium transport.

The specific cellular mechanisms by which ANGII enhances sodium transport have not been completely elucidated, although several studies suggest multiple actions of ANGII on the luminal and basolateral membranes (Fig. 11). The use of nonpeptide ANGII receptor antagonists and radioligand binding studies have led to the identification of two major types of ANGII receptors termed AT_1 and AT_2 (see ref. 120 for review). Most of the available evidence indicates that the physiologically important renal hemodynamic and tubular effects of

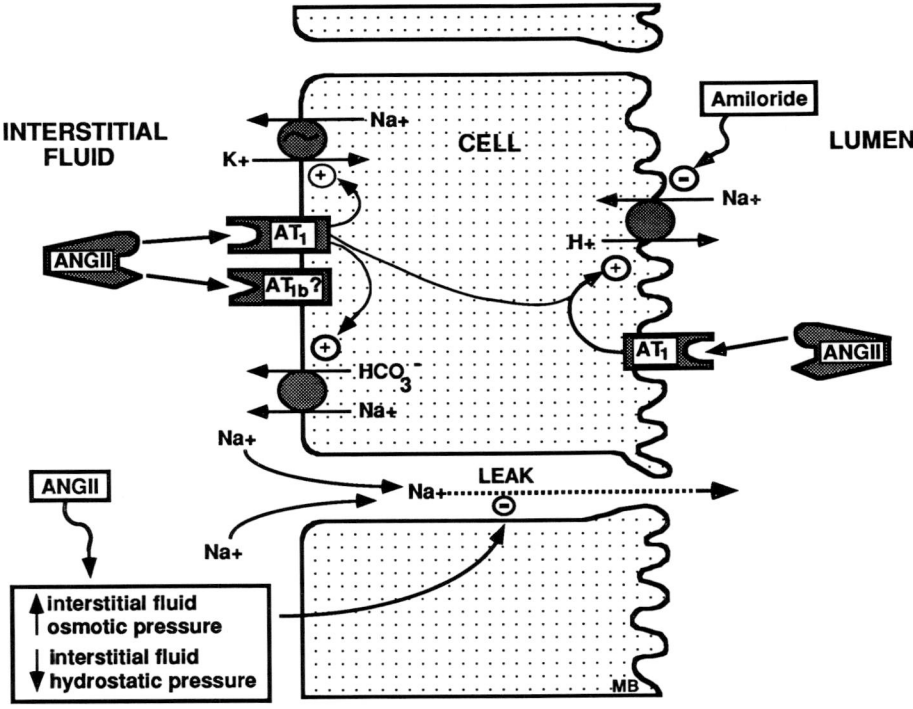

FIG. 11. ANGII increases proximal sodium reabsorption by binding to basolateral or luminal receptors. ANGII binding increases activity of the luminal Na^+/H^+ antiporter and the basolateral Na^+/HCO_3^- cotransporter independently. ANGII also increases activity of the basolateral Na^+, K^+-ATPase pump directly, or indirectly by activating the Na^+-H^+ exchanger. The effects of ANGII on interstitial fluid colloid osmotic and hydrostatic pressures can also affect sodium reabsorption by altering sodium backleak in the proximal tubule.

ANGII are mediated by AT_1 receptors, whereas the functional role of AT_2 receptors remains to be determined (120). Because binding of ANGII to the AT_1 receptor is decreased in the presence of guanine nucleotides, it appears that the AT_1 receptor is coupled to one or more G-proteins. There may be subtypes of AT_1 receptors, based on differences in receptor affinity for ANGII, ligand specificity, amino acid sequence, and signal transduction mechanisms (121–123), but the receptor subtypes that bind ANGII in the renal tubules have not been fully described. Specific binding for ANGII has been demonstrated in luminal and basolateral membranes of the proximal tubule (124–127) and some investigators find that the basolateral membrane has a higher affinity for ANGII (126), consistent with the possibility that there may be different subtypes of the AT_1 receptor in these two membrane systems. However, the functional significance of these differences in regulating tubular transport is still unclear.

Recent studies indicate that ANGII may have multiple actions to stimulate sodium transport in proximal tubules. ANGII stimulates hydrogen ion secretion and sodium bicarbonate reabsorption in the early (S_1) portion of the proximal convoluted tubule (77,128,129). However, the mechanisms by which ANGII increases sodium bicarbonate reabsorption are not certain and could involve a decrease in membrane permeability and subsequent reductions in bicarbonate backleak, increased luminal acidification involving the sodium-hydrogen antiporter, and increased luminal proton pumping. Liu and Cogan (77) found that ANGII decreased bicarbonate permeability, but it seems unlikely that this effect markedly alters bicarbonate reabsorption because luminal membrane bicarbonate permeability is normally very low and baseline backleak of bicarbonate is minimal.

Garvin (130) found that ANGII increased bicarbonate and fluid reabsorption in isolated proximal tubules without altering bicarbonate permeability. This effect was blunted by amiloride, suggesting that ANGII may stimulate the sodium-hydrogen antiporter (77). Amiloride can, however, affect other signal transduction mechanisms and other sodium-dependent transport processes (131). ANGII did not appear to increase the maximum rate of bicarbonate transport in these studies, suggesting that the total number (V_{max}) of hydrogen ion transporters was not altered by ANGII (77). Instead, ANGII may increase the substrate affinity (K_m) of the hydrogen ion transporter, a response that may be analogous to the observation that in vascular smooth muscle ANGII alters K_m but not V_{max} of the sodium-hydrogen exchanger (132). This conclusion is consistent with the finding that ANGII did not alter the maximum transport rate in proximal straight tubules (130).

ANGII may also have effects on the basolateral membrane in addition to its actions on luminal membrane sodium-hydrogen exchange. Specific binding of ANGII in luminal and basolateral membranes has been reported (124–127) and application of ANGII to the luminal surface produces a relatively modest stimulation of sodium transport, compared with administration via the peritubular capillaries and basolateral membranes (94,95). Thus, there is functional evidence that ANGII may have an even greater effect on basolateral than on luminal membrane sodium transport. In support of this possibility, Garvin (130) reported that ANGII stimulated sodium-potassium–adenosine triphosphatase (ATPase) activity in the proximal nephron. Theoretically, stimulation of sodium-potassium–ATPase activity could occur through a second messenger of ANGII or indirectly through changes in intracellular sodium. At least part of the effect of ANGII appears to be a direct action on the sodium-potassium pump, since increased ATPase activity was observed in tubules rendered permeable, which should have prevented major changes in intracellular sodium. There is also evidence that ANGII may stimulate sodium-bicarbonate cotransport in the basolateral membrane. This effect has been found in microperfused superficial S_1 segments of the rabbit proximal tubule as well as in basolateral membrane vesicles from rabbit renal cortex (133,134). Assuming that results from receptor-binding studies and in vitro experiments reflect the physiological actions of ANGII on proximal tubular function, it seems likely that ANGII may increase reabsorption by more than one mechanism, including an effect on sodium entry into the epithelial cells as well as sodium extrusion.

The signal transduction mechanisms by which ANGII stimulates sodium transport in luminal and basolateral membranes are not fully understood. Although the predominant pathway accounting for the stimulatory effect of ANGII on sodium-hydrogen exchange in the luminal membrane appears to be a G-protein–mediated inhibition of adenylcyclase (120), there may also be other pathways. Morduchowicz et al. (135) reported that ANGII activates phospholipase A_2 and directly stimulates sodium uptake in rabbit brush border membrane vesicles via a pertussis toxin–sensitive pathway. Other investigators have found that the stimulatory effects of ANGII on proximal reabsorption could be mimicked by stimulation of protein kinase C with phorbol esters, although this pathway was estimated to account for only about a third of the stimulatory effect of ANGII (136,137). Recently, ANGII has also been shown to stimulate phosphoinositide hydrolysis and inhibit adenylcyclase in rat proximal tubules (138). Further studies will be necessary to characterize more fully the signaling pathways that mediate the stimulatory effect of ANGII on basolateral and luminal transport mechanisms.

ANGII May Stimulate Distal Tubule Reabsorption

Most experimental studies have focused on the proximal tubular actions of ANGII and there is currently very little information on the possible direct effects of physiological levels of ANGII on distal tubular function. Early experiments, using micropuncture methods or whole kidney methods, suggested that ANGII either had no effect or inhibited distal tubular reabsorption (139,140). However, very high pharmacological concentrations were used in those experiments. More recent micropuncture studies have suggested that inhibition of endogenous ANGII formation with ACE inhibitors may reduce sodium reabsorption at a site between the proximal and distal convoluted tubules (141). However, changes in renal hemodynamics in these studies make it difficult to determine whether the effects of ANGII on distal reabsorption were mediated directly or indirectly through changes in intrarenal physical forces.

Several lines of evidence support the possibility that ANGII, at physiological concentrations, may directly increase reabsorption in distal parts of the nephron. Specific binding of ANGII has been demonstrated at almost all sites along the distal nephron, including the thick ascending loop of Henle, the distal convoluted tubule, and the cortical and medullary collecting tubule (142). Autoradiographic studies also suggest a very high level of ANGII binding in the medulla of rat and dog kidneys (43), consistent with a possible action of ANGII on medullary segments of the renal tubule. Moreover, ANGII directly stimulates sodium transport in several epithelial membrane systems considered to be analogous to the distal parts of the renal tubule, suggesting that the stimulatory effect of ANGII on epithelial transport may not be specific to the proximal tubule (1,96–98).

Evidence from whole kidney studies also suggests that physiological concentrations of ANGII increase "distal" fractional sodium reabsorption, estimated with the lithium clearance technique (11). Studies in normal man also indicate that blockade of endogenous ANGII formation reduces fractional sodium reabsorption in the distal nephron, estimated with the lithium clearance technique (143). Since the distal tubule with the lithium clearance method refers to all parts of the nephron beyond the proximal tubule, it was not possible in these studies to determine the specific part of the distal nephron at which ANGII increased reabsorption. To the extent that lithium is reabsorbed in distal parts of the nephron during ANGII infusion, the lithium clearance technique would underestimate the effects of ANGII in stimulating distal tubular sodium reabsorption.

Because ANGII is such a powerful sodium-retaining hormone, capable of reducing sodium excretion to very low levels without significant changes in GFR, one might expect an effect on sodium transport at more than one place, including the distal parts of the nephron where final processing of the urine takes place. One site that may be particularly important in determining final urinary excretion is the macula densa. If ANGII increased macula densa sodium chloride transport, as discussed above, this would explain some of the reported effects of ANGII

on TGF sensitivity as well as the powerful effects on sodium excretion. If ANGII did not have an effect on TGF, ANGII-mediated decreases in urine output of sodium via increased proximal reabsorption would be blunted because a decrease in sodium chloride delivery to the macula densa would elicit a feedback-mediated vasodilation of preglomerular vessels that would tend to increase GFR and return distal delivery toward normal (66,67,144). A stimulatory effect of ANGII on macula densa sodium chloride transport and TGF sensitivity would allow distal sodium chloride delivery to remain reduced without a compensatory increase in GFR, thereby increasing the effectiveness of ANGII as a sodium-conserving hormone. Thus, a stimulating effect of ANGII on TGF sensitivity would act synergistically with the proximal tubular actions to make ANGII more effective in conserving sodium.

Although the importance of ANGII as a physiological regulator of sodium reabsorption is clearly established, its role in the more distal nephron segments is still unclear. In addition, the quantitative importance of direct actions on tubular transport, compared with indirect effects mediated by changes in renal hemodynamics, in causing sodium retention is difficult to ascertain. It seems likely that the contribution of direct tubular and hemodynamic actions of ANGII may vary in different physiological circumstances, depending on the degree of activation of the RAS. As discussed above, the tubular actions of ANGII occur at lower concentrations than are required to produce hemodynamic changes. The combined intrarenal actions of ANGII, including effects on renal hemodynamics and direct stimulation of tubular transport, account for a major part of the antinatriuresis observed with activation of the RAS.

Intrarenally Formed and Circulating ANGII Regulate Sodium Excretion

The importance of circulating ANGII in controlling sodium excretion and renal hemodynamics is well established. ANGII infusion at rates calculated to raise plasma concentrations by only 10 to 15 pg/ml markedly reduces sodium excretion (145). Furthermore, blockade of endogenous ANGII formation in the two-kidney, one-clip Goldblatt hypertension model increases sodium excretion in the contralateral untouched kidney (116), which has suppressed intrarenal ANGII formation but receives blood with normal or elevated circulating ANGII as a result of renin released by the clipped kidney. These and other observations clearly indicate that circulating ANGII plays a major role in the physiological control of sodium excretion.

The contribution of intrarenally formed ANGII in regulating sodium excretion has been more difficult to quantify. Since all of the components of the RAS are found in the kidney and ANGII can be formed locally

(58), there has been considerable interest in the possibility that intrarenally formed ANGII may be even more important than circulating ANGII in controlling sodium excretion. Studies from our laboratory (19,20,86) and others (88) have also shown that intrarenal infusion of ANGII antagonists or ACE inhibitors, at rates that cause no changes in plasma aldosterone concentration or systemic hemodynamics, increase sodium excretion. However, there have been no studies, to our knowledge, that have directly quantified the relative importance of circulating and intrarenally formed ANGII in controlling sodium excretion in various physiological and pathophysiological conditions.

There has also been little information concerning the possibility that circulating and intrarenally formed ANGII may act on different sites of the renal tubules to influence sodium excretion. Since renal renin content decreases from superficial to deep regions of the cortex, it is possible that ANGII generated within the kidney may act primarily on tubular segments of the cortex, whereas circulating ANGII delivered to the tubules by glomerular filtration and by diffusion across the peritubular capillaries may increase reabsorption in medullary as well as cortical nephron segments. However, because there are conditions, such as sodium depletion or renal artery stenosis, in which renin content of juxtamedullary nephrons increases markedly (146,147), the quantitative effects of intrarenally formed and circulating ANGII on tubular reabsorption may be variable.

Recently, ANGII has been suggested to be produced within the renal tubular cells. Angiotensinogen and renin mRNAs have been localized in the proximal and collecting tubular cells (148,149). The presence of mRNA for renin and angiotensinogen in tubular cells, while suggesting the potential for local ANGII production, does not provide direct evidence that physiologically relevant amounts of ANGII are produced in the renal tubular epithelium.

Yanagawa et al. (150) reported evidence of *de novo* synthesis of angiotensinogen and renin in cultured rabbit proximal tubular cells. These observations raised the possibility that ANGII formed in proximal tubular cells could exert local effects independent of circulating ANGII or ANGII formed from other intrarenal sources such as the juxtaglomerular cells. Further evidence that ANGII may be formed in epithelial cells comes from the observation that proximal tubular fluid ANGII concentrations may be considerably higher than found in plasma (151,152). However, the possibility of *in vitro* generation of ANGII, during prolonged collection of tubular fluid in micropipettes, cannot be ruled out and further studies are needed to confirm these findings. In addition, the physiological significance of these findings is still unclear because there is little evidence that blockade of endogenous ANGII formation in isolated tubules or cultured tubular cells has a major effect on epithelial transport.

INTRARENAL ACTIONS OF ANGII CONTRIBUTE TO LONG-TERM BLOOD PRESSURE REGULATION

The importance of the RAS in regulating arterial pressure in various physiological and pathophysiological conditions is well documented. Blockade of ANGII formation lowers arterial pressure during sodium depletion and in pathophysiological conditions such as congestive heart failure, cirrhosis, and renal vascular hypertension (2,3,153–155). With the development and clinical use of orally active ACE inhibitors as an effective treatment for hypertension, the powerful role of the RAS in long-term control of blood pressure has become increasingly apparent.

The mechanisms by which the RAS controls blood pressure chronically are not as well understood as those involved in short-term blood pressure regulation. Although much emphasis has been placed on the vasoconstrictor actions of ANGII, considerable evidence indicates that the chronic blood pressure effects of ANGII are closely intertwined with volume homeostasis, particularly the intrarenal actions that mediate antinatriuresis (1,2,154). Many of the extrarenal actions of ANGII that cause peripheral vasoconstriction are important mainly in short-term blood pressure regulation during acute volume depletion or circulatory depression.

The Renal–Body Fluid Feedback Links Sodium Excretion and Long-Term Blood Pressure

Volume homeostasis and chronic regulation of blood pressure by ANGII are linked through the renal–body fluid feedback mechanism (154). The renal actions of ANGII are particularly important for the effective operation of this feedback and help to prevent excessive decreases in blood pressure during physiological disturbances such as sodium depletion or during conditions associated with circulatory depression, such as congestive heart failure. However, abnormalities of the RAS that result in excessive ANGII levels can also cause hypertension through this same feedback mechanism.

A key component of the renal–body fluid feedback is the effect of blood pressure on sodium excretion, the phenomenon known as pressure natriuresis (154,156–159). Normally, pressure natriuresis provides a powerful means of stabilizing blood pressure; when blood pressure increases above normal, sodium excretion also increases, via pressure natriuresis, and as long as excretion exceeds intake, extracellular fluid volume continues to decrease, thereby reducing venous return and cardiac output until blood pressure returns to normal and fluid intake and output are balanced once again. Conversely, when blood pressure decreases, the kidneys retain salt and water until blood pressure returns to normal.

An important aspect of pressure natriuresis is that various neurohumoral systems, especially the RAS, can amplify or blunt the basic effect of blood pressure on sodium excretion, as discussed below. Another important feature of pressure natriuresis is that it continues to operate until blood pressure is restored to the original set-point, which is determined by renal sodium excretory capability (154). As long as the renal set-point is unaltered, pressure natriuresis provides an "infinite gain" control system to prevent chronic hypertension (see Guyton et al., "The Dominent Role of the Kidneys in Long-Term Arterial Pressure Regulation in Normal and Hypertensive States" in this volume, for further discussion). For hypertension to occur, there must be a change in the renal set-point (i.e., altered pressure natriuresis). It is for this reason that the extrarenal actions of ANGII cannot cause chronic changes in blood pressure unless they also alter the kidneys' capability to excrete sodium and water. This

principle is illustrated in Fig. 12. In this theoretical example, total peripheral resistance is elevated with no change in the renal set-point for pressure natriuresis. Note that blood pressure is transiently elevated, but this increase cannot be maintained because it also raises sodium and water excretion above intake, thereby reducing extracellular fluid volume as long as blood pressure is above normal. If pressure natriuresis is unaltered, the only point at which sodium excretion and intake are in balance is at the normal blood pressure. Thus, sodium balance can be maintained with elevated blood pressure only if there is a concomitant shift of pressure natriuresis.

ANGII Modulates Long-Term Pressure Natriuresis

ANGII has powerful effects on the long-term pressure natriuresis relationship, as shown in Fig. 13. In normal animals and humans, the long-term relationship between blood pressure and sodium excretion is extremely steep, so that minimal changes in blood pressure are needed to maintain sodium balance over a wide range of sodium intakes (154,160). A major reason for the steepness of the normal pressure natriuresis curve is that ANGII levels can be suppressed when sodium intake is raised. When ANGII was infused at low rates so that circulating ANGII could not be suppressed as sodium intake was raised, renal-pressure natriuresis was shifted to higher blood pressures and much larger increases in blood pressure were required to maintain sodium balance (160). Thus, the inability to suppress ANGII formation greatly attenuates the effectiveness of pressure natriuresis and causes blood pressure to be very sensitive to sodium intake.

Blockade of ANGII formation increases renal excretory capability so that sodium balance can be maintained at lower blood pressures (Fig. 13). However, blockade of ANGII formation also causes blood pressure to be sodium-sensitive so that at very high sodium intakes there is little difference between blood pressure in normal and ANGII-blocked subjects. Thus, changes in activity of the RAS have a very important influence on pressure natriuresis and this action is a major factor in long-term blood pressure regulation. As long as the RAS is functioning normally, large variations of sodium intake can be accommodated with minimal changes in blood pressure. With impaired function of the RAS, however, blood pressure becomes much more salt-sensitive.

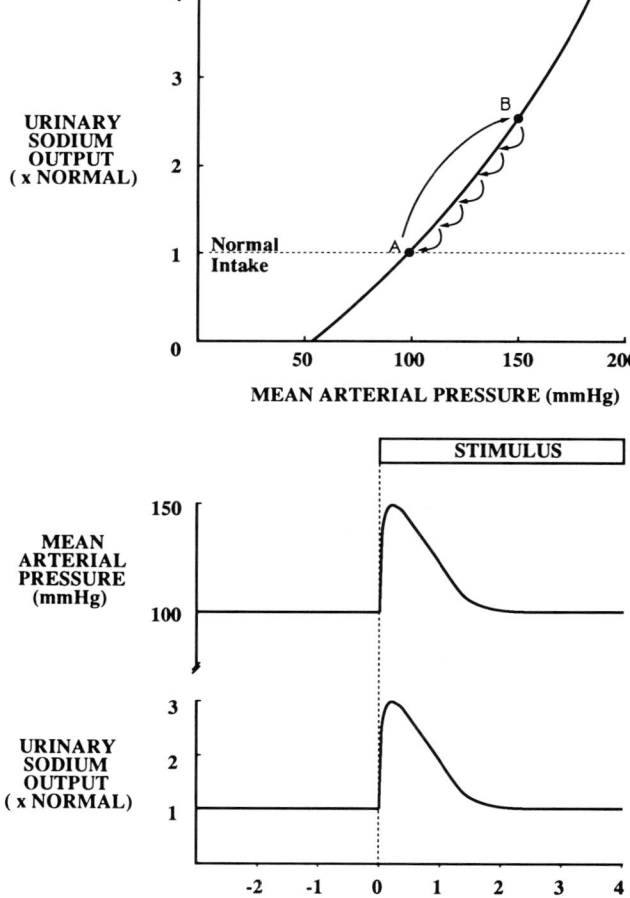

FIG. 12. Predicted long-term effects of a hypertensive stimulus, caused by increased total peripheral resistance or increased cardiac output, with no change in renal-pressure natriuresis. Blood pressure is initially elevated from point A to point B, but cannot be sustained because urinary sodium excretion exceeds intake, thereby reducing extracellular fluid volume until blood pressure returns to normal (point A) and intake and output of sodium are in balance. (Modified from ref. 169.)

Pressure Natriuresis Plays a Dominant Role in "Escape" from ANGII Antinatriuresis

The extreme importance of the interrelationships between blood pressure, renal sodium excretion, and ANGII is illustrated by an experiment designed to examine the chronic effects of ANGII when renal-pressure natriuresis was prevented from operating (161). Excessive

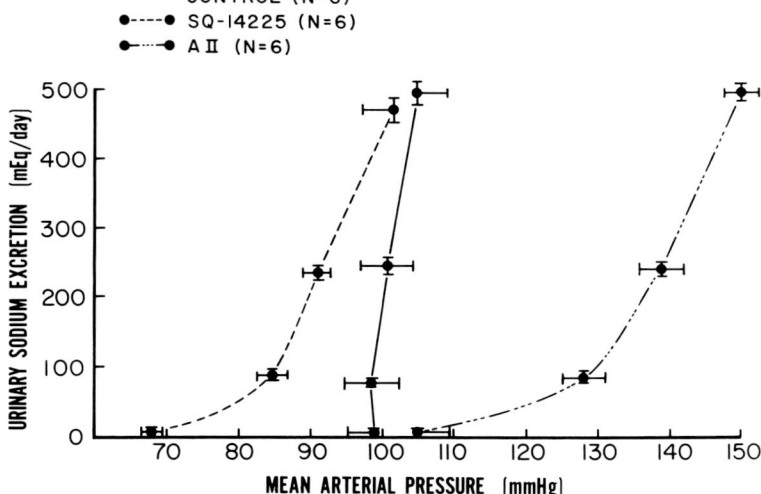

FIG. 13. Steady-state relationships between arterial pressure and sodium excretion in control dogs and in dogs infused with the ACE inhibitor captopril, or ANGII (5 ng/kg/min). (Modified from data in ref. 160.)

formation of ANGII or infusion of physiological amounts of ANGII normally causes a transient decrease in sodium excretion lasting for 1 to 2 days, followed by a gradual return of excretion to normal, similar to the "escape" from sodium retention associated with mineralocorticoid excess (161,162). Several explanations for the renal escape have been postulated, including increased formation of natriuretic factors or decreased sympathetic nerve stimulation. However, as shown in Fig. 14, renal-pressure natriuresis appears to be a primary factor for escape from sodium retention during chronic ANGII infusion. When renal perfusion pressure was held constant with an electronic servocontrol device, escape from sodium retention did not occur during ANGII infusion, and cumulative sodium balance and systemic arterial pressure continued to increase until symptoms of pulmonary edema developed after only a few days. Although the time necessary for the development of severe circulatory disturbances was somewhat variable in these experiments, there was invariably severe fluid retention, extreme hypertension, and symptoms of congestive heart failure and pulmonary edema when renal perfusion pressure was servocontrolled during chronic ANGII infusion. When the servocontroller was stopped and renal artery pressure was allowed to increase to hypertensive levels while ANGII infusion was continued, sodium excretion increased markedly and sodium balance was quickly restored.

We have found similar results in several other models of hypertension caused by chronic infusion of antinatriuretic or antidiuretic hormones such as aldosterone, vasopressin, norepinephrine, and adrenocorticotropic hormone (ACTH) (163–169). In each case, renal-pressure natriuresis appears to play a dominant role in maintaining sodium and water balance when excretory function of the kidney is impaired by excessive levels of antinatriuretic hormones.

The critical role of pressure natriuresis in maintaining fluid balance is somewhat surprising in view of the large number of natriuretic hormones that have been postulated to regulate sodium excretion (170–173). Many of these are believed to be secreted in response to expanded extracellular fluid volume, which rose drastically when renal perfusion pressure was servocontrolled in these models of hypertension. Apparently, if these natriuretic factors are released during volume expansion they are not powerful enough to restore sodium and water balance in the absence of increased renal arterial pressure. Chronic hypertension therefore appears to be an essential trade-off that permits fluid balance to be maintained without severe volume expansion when the kidneys' capability to excrete sodium is reduced markedly by disease or excessive activation of antinatriuretic and antidiuretic mechanisms, such as the RAS (154,168,169).

When high endogenous levels of ANGII occur as a result of diseases that are caused by circulatory depression, such as heart failure and cirrhosis, and are unopposed by pressure natriuresis, sodium retention continues unabated even though other factors associated with volume expansion, such as increased formation of natriuretic hormones, would tend to oppose the antinatriuretic actions of ANGII. The inability to raise blood pressure and to suppress ANGII formation as fluid is retained may explain why escape from sodium retention does not readily occur in these conditions, thereby eventually leading to severe edema.

Increased Blood Pressure Sensitivity to Chronic Increases in ANGII

Unlike many blood pressure control systems, the RAS becomes more effective when it is activated chronically. Infusions of ANGII at rates too low to have an initial

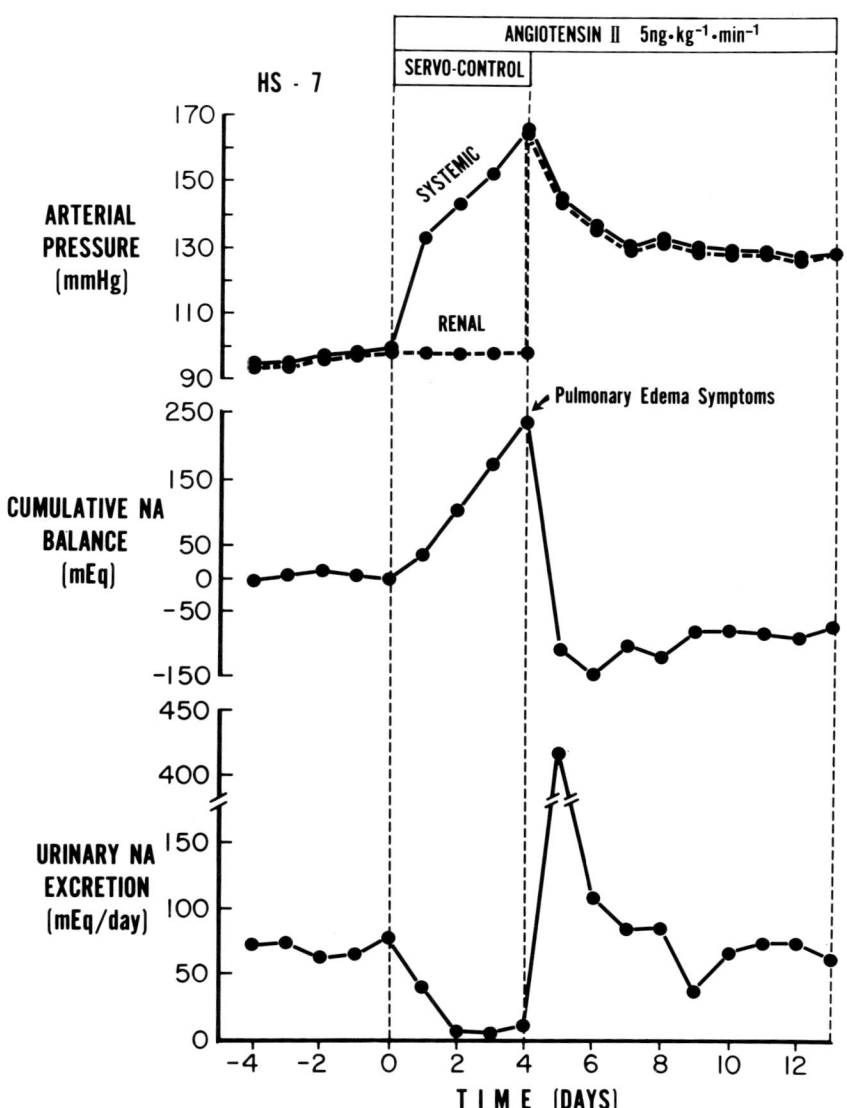

FIG. 14. Effects of ANGII infusion in a dog in which renal perfusion pressure was servocontrolled at the normal level. After 4 days, severe hypertension and sodium and water retention resulted in pulmonary edema. (Modified from ref. 161.)

pressor effect cause a gradual increase in blood pressure over several days (174–176). Ames et al. (174), investigating the effects of prolonged ANGII infusion in normal humans, found that after several days the amount of ANGII needed to maintain a constant level of hypertension was much less than the original rate infused. Thus, blood pressure became more sensitive to ANGII, rather than less sensitive as was observed with norepinephrine infusion (174). Moreover, this increased pressor sensitivity of ANGII was not due to enhanced aldosterone secretion, since plasma aldosterone concentration decreased to normal as the rate of ANGII infusion was reduced.

Several mechanisms have been postulated to explain the development of increased blood pressure sensitivity, including a gradual activation of the sympathetic nervous system (175), "amplification" of blood pressure by vascular hypertrophy (177), and increased cumulative sodium balance, which multiplies the effectiveness of

ANGII in raising blood pressure (154,178). Currently, there is little evidence that the chronic blood pressure or renal actions of ANGII are mediated by the sympathetic nervous system (2,16). The mechanism that has received the most attention in recent years is the possibility that the vascular hypertrophy could "amplify" the blood pressure responses to ANGII. Vascular hypertrophy could be secondary to increased blood pressure or due to the postulated growth promoting effects of ANGII on vascular smooth muscle. Regardless of the cause of vascular hypertrophy associated with high ANGII levels, it seems unlikely that this could act as an amplifier of blood pressure unless the hypertrophy occurred in the renal vasculature and contributed to a shift of pressure natriuresis, as discussed above. Although it is clear that hypertrophy occurs in renal vessels as well as other systemic blood vessels during hypertension, its role as a *cause* of the rise in blood pressure, rather than occurring secondarily to the hypertension, is unclear. Thus far, there is no direct evidence that vascular hypertrophy contributes to increased sensitivity of blood pressure during sustained high levels of ANGII. There is considerable evidence, however, that vascular hypertrophy occurs secondarily to increased blood pressure.

One theoretical objection to the concept that vascular hypertrophy acts as an amplifier of blood pressure is that if this occurred in the renal arterioles it could lead to a vicious cycle (179). An increase in blood pressure would elevate renal vascular resistance, shifting pressure natriuresis to higher levels, causing further increases in blood pressure and further increases in renal vascular resistance, until eventually blood pressure would rise to the point that heart failure developed. Although the sequence may occur in malignant renovascular hypertension, caused by severe renal artery stenosis or diffuse arteriolar lesions that severely impair renal perfusion, it is unlikely that this occurs in most stable forms of hypertension. With chronic ANGII infusion, there is increasing pressor sensitivity, but this increased sensitivity stabilizes within a few days. Also, the fact that increased pressor sensitivity to ANGII occurs over 2 to 4 days makes it unlikely that it is due to vascular hypertrophy, which probably requires a much greater time for development. The vascular hypertrophy hypothesis would also not explain why the blood pressure effects of ANGII gradually increase in contrast to other pressor substances, such as norepinephrine and vasopressin, which have equally potent acute effects on peripheral vascular resistance and blood pressure, but over several days their blood pressure effects begin to wane instead of being amplified (174).

A more likely explanation for the time-dependent increase in blood pressure associated with prolonged elevation of ANGII levels is that a rise in cumulative sodium balance amplifies the blood pressure effects of ANGII. Previous studies have shown that ANGII hypertension closely parallels cumulative sodium balance when pressure natriuresis is impaired (161). Direct intrarenal infusion of ANGII, at rates too low to have systemic effects, causes a gradual rise in blood pressure as sodium and water are retained (180). Also, systemic infusion of ANGII at very low rates may cause marked hypertension when sodium intake is high or when renal excretory function is reduced because of decreased kidney mass (154,181). Very high rates of ANGII infusion chronically do not raise blood pressure much more than low rates of infusion, although high doses initially cause much greater peripheral vasoconstriction and more severe acute hypertension. The inability of high rates of ANGII infusion to raise the chronic level of blood pressure further may be due to the fact that the maximal effects of ANGII on tubular reabsorption occur at relatively low concentrations (10^{-10}–10^{-11} M), whereas the maximal vasoconstrictor actions of ANGII occur at much higher concentrations. The development of hypertension with low doses of ANGII requires a much longer period of time because it depends on cumulative sodium retention.

There is also evidence that the renal tubules may gradually become more sensitive to the effects of ANGII, thereby shifting pressure natriuresis to higher blood pressures during chronic ANGII hypertension. The renal tubular receptors appear to "up-regulate" in response to sustained increases in ANGII levels, at least in vitro (127). If these in vitro observations can be applied to the intact animal, they would indicate that long-term increases in ANGII levels would gradually reduce renal sodium excretory capability, thereby shifting pressure natriuresis and gradually increasing blood pressure.

The gradual increase in blood pressure sensitivity to ANGII explains why blockade of ANGII formation is such a powerful tool for eliciting long-term reductions in blood pressure in hypertensive patients. Although acute ANGII blockade often does not reduce blood pressure markedly in many patients, especially those with normal or slightly reduced plasma renin activity, with chronic ANGII blockade renal sodium excretory capability increases and sodium balance can be maintained at lower blood pressures. After an initial loss of sodium during ANGII blockade, blood pressure becomes increasingly dependent on the RAS. Thus, with long-term ACE inhibition, patients with an initially normal plasma renin activity may, after several days, behave as though they are somewhat sodium depleted. In addition, if renal tubular receptors become less sensitive to ANGII during chronic ACE inhibition, then further increases in renal excretory capability could occur and pressure natriuresis would be shifted to lower blood pressures than observed with acute ACE inhibition.

SUMMARY

The intrarenal actions of ANGII play a powerful role in long-term control of arterial pressure and volume homeostasis. Locally formed and circulating ANGII contribute to this regulation through changes in renal hemodynamics and tubular reabsorption. Although ANGII has multiple extrarenal effects, such as stimulation of aldosterone secretion and peripheral vasoconstriction, evidence indicates that the direct intrarenal actions may play a dominant role in long-term blood pressure control and volume homeostasis.

Two of the most important intrarenal actions of ANGII include constriction of efferent arterioles and direct stimulation of tubular sodium transport. Efferent arteriolar constriction helps to stabilize GFR and excretion of metabolic waste products when renal perfusion is impaired in circumstances such as renal artery stenosis or congestive heart failure. Constriction of efferent arterioles also provides a means of increasing tubular reabsorption by altering peritubular capillary physical forces and by reducing vasa recta blood flow. ANGII also directly increases sodium reabsorption in proximal tubules and perhaps in more distal tubular segments as well, including the macula densa. ANGII-mediated increases in macula densa sensitivity contribute to the effectiveness of ANGII as an antinatriuretic hormone by preventing compensatory changes in renal vascular resistance via TGF during decreased distal tubular sodium chloride delivery.

The intrarenal actions of ANGII contribute to long-term blood pressure regulation mainly by influencing renal-pressure natriuresis. Disturbances that tend to lower blood pressure, such as heart failure and cirrhosis, cause sodium and water retention until blood pressure returns to normal, because of the combined actions of ANGII and reduced blood pressure. Physiologically, the ability to alter ANGII formation also plays a major role in amplifying the effectiveness of pressure natriuresis. For example, with high sodium intake, suppression of ANGII allows sodium balance to be achieved with minimal increases in blood pressure and body fluid volumes. However, when the RAS is inappropriately activated, the sodium-retaining effects of ANGII necessitate increased blood pressure to maintain sodium balance via pressure natriuresis. Because the RAS is so powerful in controlling blood pressure and sodium balance, blockade of this system offers an effective therapeutic tool in diseases such as hypertension and congestive heart failure.

ACKNOWLEDGMENTS

We thank Ivadelle Heidke and Susie Araysi for expert secretarial assistance. The authors research was supported by National Institutes of Health grants HL51971, HL23502, and HL39399.

REFERENCES

1. Hall JE. *Am J Physiol* 1986;250:R960–R972.
2. Hall JE, Mizelle HL, Woods LL. *J Hypertens* 1986;4:387–397.
3. Laragh JH, Sealey JE. In: Orloff J, Berliner RW, eds. *Handbook of physiology, section 8, renal physiology.* Washington DC: American Physiological Society, 1973;831–908.
4. Hall JE, Brands MW. In: Robertson JIS, Nichols MG, eds. *The renin-angiotension system.* London: Gower, 1993; Vol I, 1–48.
5. Hall JE. In: Brenner BM, Stein JH, eds. *Body fluid homeostasis: contemporary issues in nephrology,* vol 16. New York: Churchill Livingstone, 1987;69–100.
6. Hall JE. *Fed Proc* 1986;45:1431–1437.
7. Hall JE, Brands MW. In: Robertson JIS, Nichols MG eds. *The renin-angiotensin system.* London: Gower, 1993;1–43.
8. Haber E, Hui KY. In: Laragh JH, Brenner HR eds. *Hypertension: pathophysiology, diagnosis and management.* New York: Raven Press, 1990;2343–2500.
9. Waeber B, Nussberger J, Brunner HR. In: Laragh BM, Brenner BM eds. *Hypertension: Pathophysiology, diagnosis and management.* New York: Raven Press, 1990;2209–2232.
10. Timmermans PBWM, Carini DJ, Chin AT, et al. In: Laragh BM, Brenner BM eds. *Hypertension: pathophysiology, diagnosis and management.* New York: Raven Press, 1990;2351–2360.
11. Olsen ME, Hall JE, Montani JP, Guyton AC, Langford HG, Cornell JE. *Am J Physiol* 1985;249:F299–F307.
12. Hall JE. In: Guyton AC, Hall JE, eds. *Cardiovascular physiology VI,* vol 26. Baltimore: University Park Press, 1982;243–322.
13. Navar LG, Rosivall L. *Kidney Int* 1984;25:857–868.
14. Chou SY, Faubert PF, Porush JG. *Fed Proc* 1986;45:1438–1443.
15. Robertson JIS, Richards AM. *Kidney Int* 1987;31(suppl 20):s216–s219.
16. Hall JE, Brands MW. In: Seldin DW, Giebish G, eds. *The kidney, physiology and pathophysiology,* 2nd ed. New York: Raven Press, 1992;1455–1504.
17. Blantz RC, Konnen KS, Tucker BT. *J Clin Invest* 1976;57:419–434.
18. Dworkin LD, Ichikawa I, Brenner BM. *Am J Physiol* 1983;244:F95–F104.
19. Hall JE, Guyton AC, Jackson TE, Coleman TG, Lohmeier TE. *Am J Physiol* 1977;233:F366–F372.
20. Hall JE, Coleman TG, Guyton AC, Balfe JW, Salgado HC. *Am J Physiol* 1979;236:F252–F259.
21. Hall JE, Granger JP. *Am J Physiol* 1983;245:R166–R173.
22. Navar LG, LaGrange RA, Bell PD, Thomas CE, Ploth DW. *Hypertension* 1979;1:371–377.
23. Steinhausen M, Kurcherer H, Parrekh N, Weis S, Wiegman D, Weilhelm K-R. *Kidney Int* 1986;30:56–61.
24. Tucker BJ, Blantz RC. *Am J Physiol* 1983;244:F11–F18.
25. Ichikawa I, Pfeffer JM, Pfeffer MA, Hostetter TH, Brenner BM. *Circ Res* 1984;55:669–675.
26. Myers BD, Deen WM, Brenner BM. *Circ Res* 1975;37:101–110.
27. Steinhausen M, Endlich K, Wiegman DL. *Kidney Int* 1990;38:769–784.
28. Ichikawa I, Miele JF, Brenner BM. *Kidney Int* 1979;16:137–147.
29. Edwards RM. *Am J Physiol* 1983;244:F526–F534.
30. Olsen ME, Hall JE, Montani JP, Cornell JC. *Clin Sci* 1986;72:429–436.
31. Baylis C, Brenner BM. *Circ Res* 1978;43:889–898.
32. Heller J, Horacek V. *Renal Physiol* 1986;9:357–365.
33. Ito S, Johnson CS, Carrertero OA. *J Clin Invest* 1991;87:1656–1663.
34. Granger JP, Salazar FJ, Alberola A, Nakamura T. *J Hypertens* 1992;10(4):581.
35. Hall JE, Granger JP. *Am J Physiol* 1986;250:F917–F923.
36. Andrews DM. *Kidney Int* 1981;20:549–562.
37. Marsden PA, Brenner BM, Ballermann BJ. In: Laragh JH, Brenner BM. eds. *Hypertension: pathophysiology, diagnosis and management.* New York: Raven Press, 1990;1247–1272.
38. Zimmerhackl B, Parekh N, Kucherer H, Steinhausen M. *Kidney Int* 1985;27:17–24.
39. Anderson W, Alcorn PD, Gilchrist AI, Whiting JM, Ryan GB. *Am J Physiol* 1989;256:F1021–F1026.
40. Schor N, Ichikawa I, Brenner BM. *Am J Physiol* 1980;238:F428–F436.
41. Faubert PF, Chou SY, Porush JG. *Kidney Int* 1987;32:472–478.
42. Chou S-Y, Porush JG, Faubert PF. *Kidney Int* 1990;37:1–13.
43. Mendelsohn FAO, Dunbar M, Allen A, Chou ST, Millan MA, Aquilera G, Catt KJ. *Fed Proc* 1986;45:1420–1425.
44. Cupples WA, Sakai T, Marsh DJ. *Am J Physiol* 1988;254:F417–F424.
45. Hall JE, Guyton AC, Cowley AW Jr. *Am J Physiol* 1977;232:F215–F221.
46. Textor SC, Tarazi RC, Novick AC, Bravo EL, Fouad FM. *Am J Med* 1984;76:29–37.
47. Hricik DE. *Ann Intern Med* 1985;103:222–223.
48. Hrick DE, Browning PJ, Kopelman R, Goorno WE, Madias NE, Dzau VJ. *N Engl J Med* 1983;308:373–376.
49. Bender W, LaFrance N, Walker WG. *Hypertension* 1984;6(suppl I):I193–I197.
50. Schnermann J, Briggs JP, Weber PC. *Kidney Int* 1984;25:53–64.
51. Navar LG. *Am J Physiol* 1978;234:F357–F370.
52. Aukland K, Qien AK. *Am J Physiol* 1987;252:F768–F783.
53. Williams GM, Davis JO, Freeman RH, DeForrest JM, Seymour AA, Rowe BP. *Am J Physiol* 1979;236:F541–F545.

54. Klaus D, Witzgall H, Zhner J. *Dtsch Med Werbenschr* 1976;101: 1357–1359.
55. Klaus D, Rossler R. *Klin Wochenschr* 1973;51:969.
56. Johns EJ. *J Hypertens* 1989;7:695–701.
57. Hackenthal E, Metz R, Buhrle CP, Taugner R. *Kidney Int* 1987;31(suppl 20):s4–s17.
58. Inagami T, Kawamura M, Naruse K, Okamura T. *Fed Proc* 1986;45:1414–1419.
59. Kriz W. *Kidney Int* 1987;31(suppl 20):s51–s56.
60. Kastner PR, Hall JE, Guyton AC. *Am J Physiol* 1984;246:F897–F906.
61. Hall JE, Coleman TG, Guyton AC, Kastner PR, Granger JP. *Am J Physiol* 1981;241:R190–R197.
62. Sealey JE, Blumenfeld JD, Bell GM, Pecker MS, Sommers SC, Laragh JH. *J Hypertens* 1988;6:763–777.
63. Anderson S, Meyer TW, Rennke HG, Brenner BM. *J Clin Invest* 1985;76:612–619.
64. Anderson S, Rennke HG, Brenner BM. *J Clin Invest* 1986;77: 1993–2000.
65. Brenner BM. *Am J Physiol* 1985;249:F324–F337.
66. Briggs J, Schnermann J. In: Laragh JH, Brenner BM, eds. *Hypertension: pathophysiology, diagnosis and management.* New York: Raven Press, 1990;1067–1087.
67. Schnermann J, Briggs J. In: Seldin DW, Giebisch G. eds. *The kidney: physiology and pathophysiology,* 2nd ed. New York: Raven Press, 1992;1249–1290.
68. Thurau K, Mason J. In: Thurau K. ed. *International review of science: kidney and urinary tract physiology,* vol 6. Baltimore: University Park Press, 1974;357–390.
69. Thurau K. *Am J Med* 1964;36:698–719.
70. Schnermann J, Briggs J. *Fed Proc* 1986;45:1426–1430.
71. Ploth DW, Paul RV. In: Person AEG, Boberg U, eds. *The juxtaglomerular apparatus.* Amsterdam: Elsevier, 1988;257–269.
72. Coleman T, Hall JE. In: Iyengar S, ed. *Computer modelling of complex biological systems,* vol 2. Boca Raton: CRC Press, 1992;89–124.
73. Hall JE, Guyton AC, Smith MJ Jr, Coleman TG. *Clin Sci* 1980;59(suppl):87–90.
74. Ferrario CM, Gildenberg PL, McCubbin JWE. *Circ Res* 1972;30: 257–262.
75. Zimmerman BG, Sybertz EJ, Wong PC. *J Hypertens* 1984;2: 581–588.
76. Levens NR. *Am J Physiol* 1985;249:G3–G15.
77. Liu F-Y, Cogan MG. *J Clin Invest* 1988;82:601–607.
78. Pelayo JG, Blantz RC. *Am J Physiol* 1984;246:F87–F95.
79. Hall JE, Granger JP. *Fed Proc* 1983;42:589.
80. Carroll RG, Lohmeier TE, Brown AJ. *Hypertension* 1984;6:675–681.
81. Mizelle HL, Hall JE, Woods LL, Montani JP, Dzielak DJ, Pan YJ. *Am J Physiol* 1987;252:F291–F298.
82. Mizelle HL, Hall JE, Montani JP, Woods LL. *Am J Physiol* 1988;255:F823–F827.
83. Mizelle HL, Hall JE, Montani JP. *Am J Physiol* 1989;256: F1084–F1093.
84. Sealey J, Laragh JH. In: Laragh JH, Brenner BM, eds. *Hypertension: pathophysiology, diagnosis, and management.* New York: Raven Press, 1990;1287–1317.
85. Davis JO. In: Blascko G, Sayers G, Smith AD, eds. *Handbook of physiology: adrenal physiology.* Washington DC: American Physiological Society, 1975;77–106.
86. Hall JE, Guyton AC, Trippodo NC, Lohmeier TE, McCaa RE, Cowley AW Jr. *Am J Physiol* 1977;232:F538–F544.
87. Lohmeier TE, Cowley AW Jr, Trippodo NC, Hall JE, Guyton AC. *Circ Res* 1977;233:F388–F395.
88. Kimbrough HM Jr, Vaughan ED Jr, Carey RM, Ayers CR. *Circ Res* 1977;40:174–178.
89. Hall JE, Guyton AC, Smith MJ, Coleman GA. *Am J Physiol* 1979;237:F424–F444.
90. Lohmeier TE, Kastner PR, Smith MJ Jr, Guyton AC. *Hypertension* 1980;2:497–505.
91. Young DB. *Endocr Rev* 1985;6:24–44.
92. Rosenbaum JD, Papper S, Ashley MM. *J Clin Endocrinol Metab* 1955;15:1459.
93. Weber KT, Villarreal D. *Am J Cardiol* 1993;71:3A–11A.
94. Harris PJ, Young JA. *Pflugers Arch* 1977;367:295–297.
95. Schuster VL. *Fed Proc* 1986;45:1444–1447.
96. Coviello A, Braukmann ES. *Acta Physiol Lat Am* 1973;23:18–23.
97. Coviello A. *Acta Physiol Lat Am* 1972;22:218–226.
98. Levens NR, Peach MJ, Carey RM. *Circ Res* 1981;48:157–167.
99. Blair-West JR, Coghlan JP, Denton DA, Goding JE, Wintour M, Wright RD. *Rec Prog Horm Res* 1963;19:311–383.
100. Fredlind P, Saltman S, Catt KJ. *Endocrinology* 1975;97:1577–1586.
101. Oelkers W, Brown JJ, Fraser R, Lever AF, Morton JJ, Robertson JIS. *Circ Res* 1974;34:69–77.
102. Brown JJ, Casals-Stenzel J, Cumming AMM, et al. *Hypertension* 1979;1:159–179.
103. Hall MM, Khosla MC, Khairallah PA. *J Pharmacol Exp Ther* 1974;188:222–228.
104. Reid IA. *Am J Physiol* 1984;246:F533–F543.
105. Yuan B, Robinette JB, Conger JD. *Am J Physiol* 1990;258:F741–F750.
106. Strandhoy JW, Cronnelly R, Long JP, Williamson HE. *Proc Soc Exp Biol Med* 1972;141:336–339.
107. Ichikawa I, Harris R. *Kidney Int* 1991;40:583–596.
108. Earley LE, Schrier RW. In: Orlorf J, Berliner RW, eds. *Handbook of physiology: renal physiology.* Washington DC: American Physiological Society, 1973;721–762.
109. Knox FG, Haas JA. *Rev Physiol Biochem Pharmacol* 1982;92: 75–113.
110. Schnermann J. In: Thurau K, ed. *Kidney and urinary tract physiology: international review of physiology,* vol 6. Baltimore: University Park Press, 1974;157–198.
111. Burg M. In: Brenner BM, Rector FC, eds. *The kidney.* Philadelphia: WB Saunders, 1986;145–175.
112. Ichikawa I, Brenner BM. *J Clin Invest* 1980;65:1192–1201.
113. Steiner RW, Tucker BJ, Blantz RC. *J Clin Invest* 1979;64:503–512.
114. Schuster VL, Kokko JP, Jacobson HR. *J Clin Invest* 1984;73: 507–515.
115. Cogan MG. *Hypertension* 1990;15:451–458.
116. Huang WC, Ploth DW, Navar LG. *Am J Physiol* 1982;243:F553–F560.
117. Spinelli F, Walther A. *Colloques Institut National de la Sante et de la Recherches Medicales Colloques et Seminaires* 1978;85: 273–278.
118. Simpson RU, Goodfriend TL. *J Lab Clin Med* 1984;103:255–271.
119. Munday KA, Parsons BJ, Poat JA. *J Physiol* 1971;215:269–282.
120. Edwards RM, Aiyar N. *J Am Soc Nephrol* 1993;3:1643–1652.
121. Douglas JG. *Am J Physiol* 1987;253:F1–F7.
122. Ye MQ, Healy DP. *Biochem Biophys Res Commun* 1992;185: 204–210.
123. Iwai N, Inagami T. *FEBS Lett* 1992;298:257–260.
124. Brown GP, Douglas JG. *Endocrinology* 1982;111:1830–1836.
125. Brown GP, Douglas JG. *Endocrinology* 1983;112:2007–2014.
126. Freedlander AE, Kirschbaum BB, Ris H, Oken DE, Candelora PD. *Clin Res* 1980;28:59a.
127. Douglas JG. *Am J Physiol* 1987;253:F1–F7.
128. Liu FY, Cogan MG. *J Clin Invest* 1987;80:272–275.
129. Liu FY, Cogan MG. *J Clin Invest* 1989;84:83–91.
130. Garvin J. *J Am Soc Nephrol* 1990;1:272–277.
131. Howard MJ, Pullen MD, Insel PA. *Am J Physiol* 1982;253:F21–F25.
132. Beck BC, Aronow MS, Brock TA, Cragoe E JR, Gimbrone MA Jr, Alexander RW. *J Biol Chem* 1987;262:5057–5064.
133. Geibel J, Giebisch G, Boron WF. *Proc Natl Acad Sci USA* 1990;87:7917–7920.
134. Eiam-Ong S, Hilden SA, Johns CA, Madias NE. *Am J Physiol* 1993;265:F195–F203.
135. Morduchowicz GA, Sheilch-Hamad D, Dwyer BE, Stern N, Jo OD, Yanagawa N. *J Membr Biol* 1991;122:43–53.
136. Liu F-Y, Cogan MG. *Am J Physiol* 1990;258:F927–F933.
137. Wang T, Chan YL. *J Pharmacol Exp Ther* 1991;256:309–317.
138. Poggioli J, Lazar G, Houillier P, et al. *Am J Physiol* 1992;263: C750–C758.
139. Vander AJ. *Am J Physiol* 1963;205:133–138.
140. Horster M, Nagel W, Schnermann J, Thurau K. *Pflugers Arch* 1966;292:118–126.

141. Ploth DW, Navar LG. *Fed Proc* 1979;38:2280–2285.
142. Myais SK, Kauffman S, Katz AI. *J Clin Invest* 1986;77:315–318.
143. Hannedouch T, Delgado A, Gnionsahe A, Lacour B, Grunfeld JP. *J Cardiovasc Pharmacol* 1989;13:84–89.
144. Wright FS. *J Hypertens* 1984;2:105–113.
145. Fagard RH, Cowley AW Jr, Navar LG, Langford HG, Guyton AC. *Clin Exp Pharmacol Physiol* 1976;3:539–544.
146. Brown JJ, Davies DL, Lever AF, Parker RA, Robertson JIS. *Clin Sci* 1966;30:223–235.
147. Gavras H, Brown JJ, Lever AF, Robertson JIS. *Clin Sci* 1970;38:409–414.
148. Ingelfinger JR, Zuo WM, Fon EA, Ellison KE, Dzau VJ. *J Clin Invest* 1990;85:417–423.
149. Rajaraman S, Graves K, Kunapuli S. *Kidney Int* 1988;33:169.
150. Yanagawa N, Capparelli AW, Jo OD, Friedal A, Barrett JD, Eggena P. *Kidney Int* 1991;39:938–941.
151. Braam B, Mitchell KD, Fox J, Navar LG. *Am J Physiol* 1993;264:F891–F898.
152. Seikaly MG, Arant BS, Seney FD. *J Clin Invest* 1990;86:1352–1357.
153. Gavras H, Brunner HR, Thurston H, Laragh JH. *Science* 1975;188:1316–1317.
154. Guyton AC. *Arterial pressure and hypertension. Circulatory physiology II*. Philadelphia: WB Saunders, 1980.
155. Sealey JE, Laragh JH. In: Laragh JH, Brenner BM eds. *Hypertension: pathophysiology, diagnosis and management*. New York: Raven Press, 1990;1287–1318.
156. Selkurt EE, Hall PW, Spencer MP. *Am J Physiol* 1949;159:369–384.
157. Thompsen DD, Pitts RF. *Am J Physiol* 1952;168:490–499.
158. Hall JE, Guyton AC, Coleman TG, Mizelle HL, Woods LL. *Fed Proc* 1986;45:2897–2903.
159. Hall JE, Granger JP, Hester HL, Montani JP. *J Hypertens* 1986;4(suppl 4):S57–S65.
160. Hall JE, Guyton AC, Smith MJ Jr, Coleman TG. *Am J Physiol* 1980;239:F271–F280.
161. Hall JE, Granger JP, Hester RL, Coleman TG, Smith MJ Jr, Cross RB. *Am J Physiol* 1984;246:F627–F634.
162. Hall JE, Guyton AC, Salgado HC, McCaa RE, Balfe JW. *Am J Physiol* 1978;235:F174–F179.
163. Hall JE, Montani JP. In: Mantero G, Biglieri J, Funder JW, Scoggins BA, eds. *The adrenal gland and hypertension*. New York: Raven Press, 1985;185–208.
164. Hall JE, Granger JP, Smith MJ Jr, Premen AJ. *Hypertension* 1984;6(suppl I):I183–I192.
165. Hall JE, Montani JP, Woods LL, Mizelle HL. *Am J Physiol* 1986;250:F907–F916.
166. Hall JE, Mizelle HL, Woods LL, Montani JP. *J Hypertens* 1988;6:723–732.
167. Woods LL, Mizelle HL, Hall JE. *Am J Physiol* 1988;255:R894–R900.
168. Hall JE, Guyton AC, Coleman TG, Woods LL, Mizelle HL. In: Kaplan NM, Brenner BM, Laragh JH, eds. *The kidney and hypertension, perspectives in hypertension*, vol 1. New York: Raven Press, 1987;1–20.
169. Hall JE, Mizelle HL, Hildebrandt DA, Brands MW. *Hypertension* 1990;15:547–559.
170. Buckalew VM. *Clin Sci* 1972;42:69–78.
171. Knox FG, Burnett JC Jr, Kohran DE, Spielman WS, Strand JC. *Kidney Int* 1980;17:263–276.
172. Haddy FJ, Pamnani M, Clough D, Huot S. *Life Sci* 1982;30:571–575.
173. De Wardener HE, Graham AM. *Kidney Int* 1980;18:1–9.
174. Ames RP, Borkowski AJ, Sicinski AM, Laragh JH. *J Clin Invest* 1965;44:1171–1186.
175. Dickinson CJ, Yu R. *J Physiol* 1967;190:91–99.
176. Brown AJ. *Am J Physiol* 1981;241:H381–H388.
177. Lever AF. *J Hypertens* 1986;4:515–524.
178. Laragh JH, Sealey JE, Niarchos AP, Pickering TG. *Fed Proc* 1982;41:2415–2423.
179. Guyton AC, Hall JE, Coleman TG, Manning RD Jr. In: Laragh JH, Brenner BM, eds. *Hypertension: pathophysiology, diagnosis and management*. New York: Raven Press, 1990;1029–1052.
180. Lohmeier TE, Cowley AW Jr. *Circ Res* 1979;44:154–160.
181. Hall JE, Mizelle HL, Brands MW, Hildebrandt DA. *Am J Physiol* 1992;262:R61–R71.

Hypertension: Pathophysiology, Diagnosis, and Management, Second Edition, edited by J.H. Laragh and B.M. Brenner, Raven Press, Ltd., New York © 1995.

CHAPTER **88**

Intrarenal Blockade of Angiotensin II in Experimental Genetic Hypertension

Jeanette M. Wood and Nigel R. Levens

The proposal that the kidney is the organ primarily responsible for the initiation and maintenance of essential hypertension dates back many decades (1–3). Convincing evidence for this hypothesis has been provided by transplantation studies in genetically hypertensive rats and in man. However, the mechanisms leading from a primary renal deficit to the development and maintenance of high blood pressure are still not well understood. One of the factors linking the kidney with genetic hypertension may be the renin-angiotensin system (RAS). Angiotensin II has multiple effects upon the kidney, and blockade of the formation of this octapeptide in man and in genetically hypertensive animals leads both to changes in renal function and to a fall in blood pressure. In the following review we have explored the hypothesis that angiotensin II acting within the kidney plays a role in the maintenance of high blood pressure in the spontaneously hypertensive rat and in patients with essential hypertension.

J. M. Wood and N. R. Levens: Cardiovascular Research, CIBA-GEIGY Ltd, Basle, CH-4002, Switzerland.

EXPERIMENTAL GENETIC HYPERTENSION

Inbred rats with genetic hypertension provide the opportunity to gain insight into the mechanisms involved in the pathogenesis of essential hypertension in humans. These strains of rat, having naturally occurring hypertensive disease, were developed by successive brother-to-sister mating of rats selected for the highest blood pressure values. The Okamoto-Aoki strain of spontaneously hypertensive rat (SHR), derived from Wistar-Kyoto (WKY) rats, is the most widely used model of genetic hypertension in cardiovascular research (4). In this strain, arterial pressure progressively increases with age at a much faster rate and to a much higher maximum level than in the control WKY rats, without the need of any surgical or dietary intervention. The SHR shares many common characteristics with patients with essential hypertension and is therefore used as a model of the human disease (4). The hypertension in SHR, as in essential hypertension in man, is associated with an increased total peripheral resistance and a normal cardiac output, extracellular fluid volume, and plasma sodium concentration. Renal vascular resistance is clearly elevated in both forms of hypertension, whereas renal blood flow and glomerular filtration rate are normal or slightly reduced. Although the plasma renin-angiotensin system is not elevated in SHR or in patients with essential hypertension, blockers of the renin-angiotensin system lower blood pressure.

PRIMACY OF THE KIDNEY IN GENETIC HYPERTENSION

Several lines of experimental evidence indicate that the kidney plays a primary role in the etiology of hypertension in SHR. The most compelling evidence for this hypothesis comes from renal transplantation experiments. Hypertension can be consistently transferred with the kidney from genetically hypertensive donors to syngenic normotensive recipients, not only in SHR but also in three other strains of genetically hypertensive rat (5). Conversely, many studies have shown that blood pressure is decreased or the development of hypertension prevented by transplantation of kidneys from genetically normotensive donors to syngenic hypertensive recipients (5). Transplantation of a kidney from a normotensive donor is more effective at reducing blood pressure in SHR at an early stage rather than in a later stage of hypertension. This observation may be related to the structural changes that occur within both blood vessels and the heart with the development of hypertension. Thus, in animals with established hypertension, structural changes may assume a more important role than the kidney in the maintenance of high blood pressure. Hypertension leads to glomerular membrane damage and to the development of nephrosclerosis. It is possible, therefore, that the increase in blood pressure that follows transplantation of kidneys from hypertensive to normotensive animals may be secondary to hypertension-induced renal damage. However, when renal damage in SHR is prevented by chronically lowering blood pressure with antihypertensive drugs, renal transplantation still leads to blood pressure elevation in normotensive recipient animals (5). Furthermore, transplantation of kidneys from prehypertensive SHR to normotensive donors also leads to the development of hypertension (5). These observations would suggest that renal damage is not an explanation for the transfer of hypertension and that the kidney of hypertensive animals contains a primary defect that leads to both the development and maintenance of high blood pressure.

More limited data from human studies also support the hypothesis that essential hypertension in man may have a primary renal component. Although kidneys from hypertensive patients are not usually transplanted into normotensive recipients because the kidneys may be damaged, there are many observations demonstrating that transplantation of a kidney from a normotensive donor to a bilaterally nephrectomized hypertensive recipient with previous end-stage renal disease leads to a fall in blood pressure (6,7). The fall in blood pressure in the hypertensive patients after transplantation is long-lasting and is associated with the maintenance of normal renal function. In contrast, in patients with diabetic nephropathy, renal damage and hypertension rapidly reoccur after removal of the diseased kidneys and transplantation of a healthy kidney, since renal transplantation does not correct the metabolic abnormalities of the disease that are primarily extrarenal.

RENAL FUNCTION IN SHR AND ESSENTIAL HYPERTENSIVES

Guyton and coworkers (8) have suggested that hypertension cannot occur in the absence of a defect in renal function. According to this hypothesis, an increase in blood pressure in the presence of normal renal function would be accompanied by an increase in sodium and water excretion, restoring blood pressure to normotensive levels. Conversely, these investigators have suggested that the kidney in hypertensive individuals has a defect such that a higher than normal blood pressure is needed to maintain extracellular fluid volume balance (Fig. 1).

Spontaneously hypertensive rats have been shown to have an altered pressure-natriuresis relationship from a young age (9). In comparison to the normotensive WKY control strain, young SHR (4–6 weeks) have a reduced glomerular filtration rate and renal blood flow and an increased renal vascular resistance (10,11). At this stage they are only moderately hypertensive. An exaggerated salt and water retention has also been detected in young SHR (10) that may be partly due to an increase in sodium reabsorption from the proximal tubule (12,13). As hypertension develops, glomerular filtration rate and renal blood flow return to normal levels (after 12–14 weeks of age) (10,11). Normal renal blood flow in the face of increased blood pressure indicates an increased renal vascular resistance in SHR with established hypertension.

Cross-breeding studies with SHR and WKY have shown that the reduction in renal blood flow and glomerular filtration rate in young SHR cosegregates with high blood pressure (14). Interestingly, sodium retention did not appear to be important in the genetic determination of blood pressure (15). Thus, the initial defect leading to hypertension may be excessive renal vasoconstriction. The consequent reduction in renal blood flow and glomerular filtration rate may be a stimulus for blood pressure to increase in order to restore renal perfusion. Renal function is returned to normal, but at the expense of an elevated blood pressure (11). The mechanism whereby blood pressure is increased is not clear.

Renal vascular resistance is also clearly increased in patients with essential hypertension (3,4). Renal blood

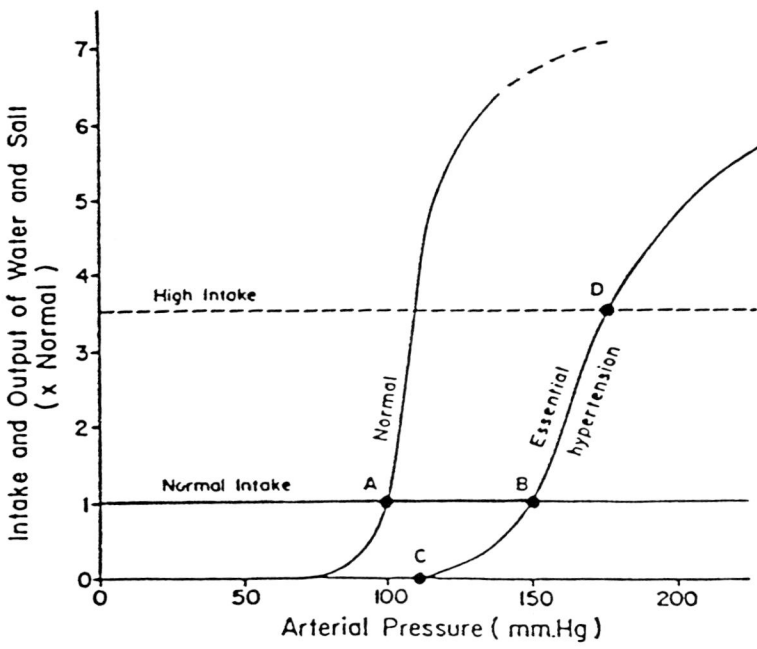

FIG. 1. Plot of the Guyton concept of elevated arterial pressure in essential hypertension (8). Normal steady state with balance between intake and output at normal pressure (A). In normotensives with normal renal function, balance is maintained as salt intake increases without the need for blood pressure to increase. In contrast, with essential hypertension, increasingly higher blood pressures are needed to maintain balance (C, B, and D) as salt intake increases.

flow and glomerular filtration rate are normal or slightly reduced and filtration fraction increased. Renal vasoconstriction may also be present in the prehypertensive stage (3). Normotensive children with both parents having essential hypertension are reported to have a reduced renal blood flow in comparison to children with matched normotensive parents (16).

ROLE OF THE RENIN-ANGIOTENSIN SYSTEM IN SHR AND ESSENTIAL HYPERTENSIVES

Spontaneously hypertensive rats, like most patients with essential hypertension, have a normal-to-low plasma renin activity (17,18) and are not generally considered to be a renin-dependent model of hypertension (4). Renal renin content in SHR generally parallels plasma renin activity and decreases with age and the establishment of hypertension. Some earlier studies have indicated that renal renin content may be elevated in young SHR compared to age-matched WKY. However, there is no difference in the renal renin content between SHR with established hypertension and age-matched WKY.

Although the plasma renin-angiotensin system is not elevated, the antihypertensive efficacy of renin inhibitors (19), angiotensin-converting enzyme inhibitors (19–21), and angiotensin II receptor antagonists (18,22) in SHR and in patients with essential hypertension implicates an involvement of the renin-angiotensin system in the development or maintenance of the hypertension. The observation that the antihypertensive response induced in

SHR by these various blockers of the renin-angiotensin system is abolished after bilateral nephrectomy (18, 20,23) supports the hypothesis that blockade of the effects of angiotensin II on the kidney is central to the mechanism of action of these agents. This conclusion is also supported by the observations that after withdrawal of angiotensin-converting enzyme inhibitor treatment in SHR, the antihypertensive effect persists and is accompanied by a corresponding persistent inhibition of renal angiotensin-converting enzyme activity (24,25) and a reduction in renal vascular resistance (21). In contrast, plasma angiotensin-converting enzyme activity recovers rapidly. Thus, inhibition of the renal effects of intrarenally generated angiotensin II may be important for the mechanism of action of converting enzyme inhibitors.

EFFECTS OF EXOGENOUS ANGIOTENSIN II ON RENAL FUNCTION

Angiotensin II has many effects upon the kidney (26,27). It is one of the most potent endogenous renal vasoconstrictor substances known. The renal vasculature is more sensitive than other vascular beds to the vasoconstrictor effects of angiotensin (28). Lower doses of angiotensin II are required to increase renal vascular resistance than to increase blood pressure (29). The renal vasoconstrictor effect of angiotensin II is predominantly on the efferent arterioles (26,27). Efferent arteriolar constriction lowers the glomerular filtration rate proportionally more than renal blood flow, leading to an increase in the filtration fraction. An increase in filtration fraction leads to an increase in the osmolality of the blood perfusing the peritubular capillaries, thus providing an impetus for ion and water movement from the tubular lumen to the blood. Angiotensin II has been shown to constrict glomerular mesangial cells, leading to a fall in the glomerular filtration coefficient (K_f) and thus contributing to the fall in glomerular filtration rate. Early studies demonstrated that low subpressor infusions of angiotensin II either intravenously or directly into the renal artery produced both antinatriuresis and antidiuresis in the absence of changes in either systemic or renal hemodynamics or the intrarenal distribution of renal blood flow, factors known to affect tubular sodium and water absorption. These indirect observations suggested that angiotensin II exerts a direct effect upon renal tubular transport. More recent studies have confirmed this hypothesis and have demonstrated that direct application of angiotensin II to the basolateral membranes of the isolated proximal convoluted tubule alters sodium absorption in a dose-dependent manner. Angiotensin II stimulates sodium absorption at low "physiological" doses and inhibits absorption at higher doses.

As well as its direct vasoconstrictor effects and direct effects on sodium transport, angiotensin II has growth-promoting effects on vascular smooth muscle and mesangial and tubular cells (30–33). Hypertrophy or proliferation of these cells may also contribute to changes in renal function and blood pressure.

ANGIOTENSIN II AND THE KIDNEY IN SHR

Treatment of young or adult SHR with an angiotensin-converting enzyme inhibitor reduces renal vascular resistance and increases glomerular filtration rate and renal blood flow (21,34). Inhibition of angiotensin-converting enzyme prevents the development of hypertension in young SHR and lowers blood pressure in adult SHR (21). These observations suggest that angiotensin II plays a role in both the renal hemodynamic abnormalities and the development of hypertension in SHR. However, the exact mechanism involved is not clear. There is no consistent evidence that components of the renin-angiotensin system are elevated in the kidney of SHR with established hypertension. One possibility may be that SHR are more sensitive to the renal vasoconstrictor effects of angiotensin II. Differences in sensitivity to vasoconstrictors between SHR and WKY may be due to differences in baseline blood pressure or hypertension-induced changes in blood vessel structure. To overcome this problem, a series of studies was performed in SHR and WKY after blood pressure had been maintained at similar levels by treatment with a converting enzyme inhibitor from 4 weeks of age until the time of study (9–11 weeks) (35). In both SHR and WKY, norepinephrine and angiotensin II induced a slow increase in blood pressure when given by continuous intravenous infusion in a low dose that did not affect blood pressure after acute administration (35). The SHR were more sensitive to the "slow-pressor" effects of angiotensin II than WKY, whereas both strains had a similar sensitivity to the slow-pressor effects of norepinephrine (35). There was no evidence that the enhanced slow-pressor response to angiotensin II in SHR was due to nonrenal actions of this peptide, such as potentiation of sympathetic neurotransmission, increased contraction of nonrenal vascular smooth muscle, or release of aldosterone (35). However, a slow-pressor response was also observed after intrarenal infusion of an even lower dose of angiotensin II that was not effective after intravenous administration (Fig. 2). The increase in blood pressure in these studies was associated with a significant decrease in renal blood flow,

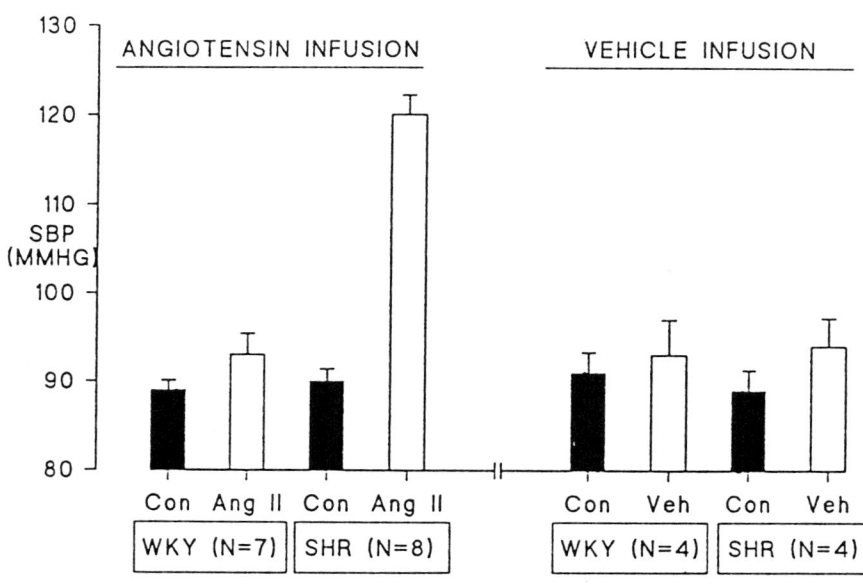

FIG. 2. Slow-pressor response (*left panel*) induced after infusion of a low dose (1 ng/min) of angiotensin II intrarenally over 1 week in 11-week-old spontaneously hypertensive rat (SHR). This dose of angiotensin II had no effects after intravenous administration in SHR or after intrarenal administration in Wistar-Kyoto rats (WKY). Both SHR and WKY had been treated from 4 weeks of age with captopril (100 mg/kg/day) to equalize the blood pressures in the two strains. The infusion of vehicle (*right panel*) had no effect on blood pressure. The values for systolic blood pressure (SBP) are mean ± SEM. (From ref. 35, with permission.)

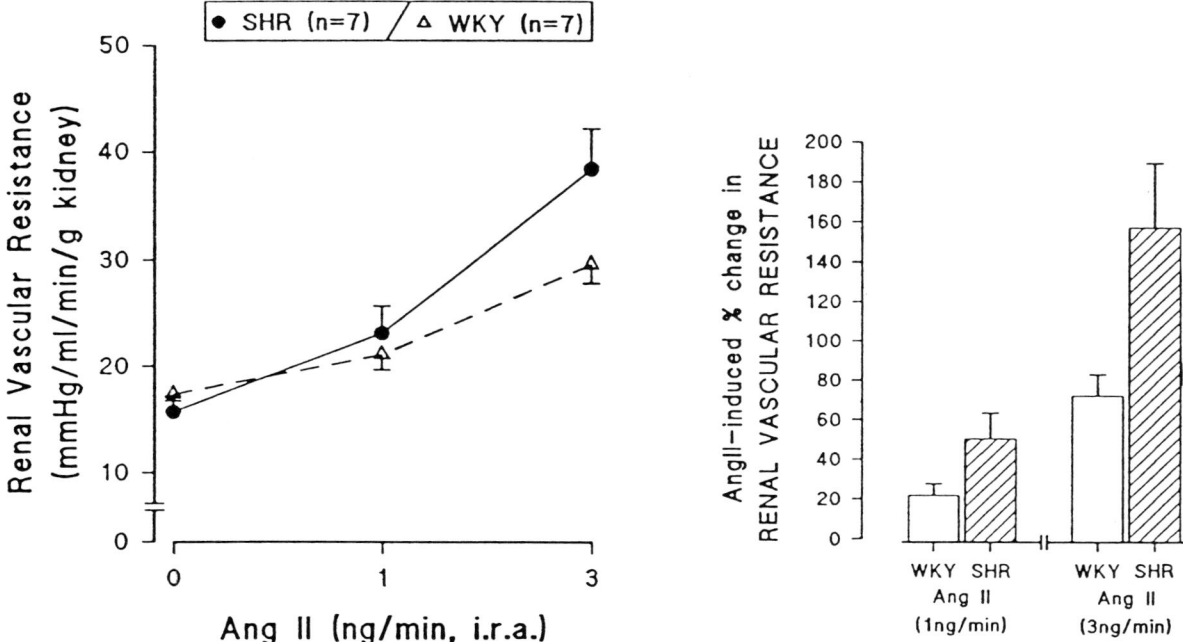

FIG. 3. Effects of intrarenal infusion of angiotensin II on renal vascular resistance in SHR and WKY treated with captopril (100 mg/kg/day) from 4 weeks of age to equalize blood pressure in the two strains. The rats were 9–11 weeks of age at the time of the experiment. Absolute values (*left panel*); percentages of change (*right panel*). Values are mean ± SEM. Angiotensin II induced a significant and dose-dependent increase in renal vascular resistance in both SHR and WKY. The response was significantly enhanced in SHR compared to WKY. (From ref. 36, with permission.)

glomerular filtration rate, and sodium excretion. The same intrarenal dose of angiotensin II did not induce an increase blood pressure in WKY. This suggests that the kidneys mediate the enhanced slow-pressor response to angiotensin II in SHR. A subsequent study demonstrated that SHR are more sensitive to the renal vasoconstrictor effects of angiotensin II than WKY (36) (Fig. 3). This effect appears to be specific to angiotensin II because the response to periarterial nerve stimulation is not enhanced in SHR. The enhanced responsiveness to angiotensin II in SHR appears to be mediated via the AT_1 receptor subtype.

These results suggest that enhanced responsiveness to angiotensin II in SHR may contribute to the development of hypertension. Increased sensitivity to angiotensin II may also explain why this peptide has important renal effects even though its plasma levels are not elevated compared to control animals.

ANGIOTENSIN II RECEPTORS IN THE KIDNEY

Angiotensin II receptors are abundant and widely distributed throughout the kidney (37). Receptor mapping by binding and radioautographic techniques in rat kidney have revealed high concentrations of receptor in the glomerulus, the arterioles, the proximal tubular cells, the

vasa recta bundles, the mesangial cells, and the interstitial medullary cells. Recent studies have shown that there are at least two subtypes of the angiotensin II receptor, designated AT_1 and AT_2 (38). Approximately 90 percent of the receptors found in the rat kidney are of the AT_1 subtype and appear to mediate all of the renal effects of angiotensin II (39). A role for the AT_2 receptor in the modulation of renal function in the rat has not been convincingly demonstrated.

Receptor binding studies have revealed a similar number of angiotensin II receptors in glomeruli from SHR and WKY up to 10 weeks of age, but a higher number in SHR at later stages (40). Receptor affinity was also similar in young SHR, but was increased in old SHR with established hypertension. Since there was no correlation between receptor density or affinity and the development of hypertension in SHR (40), this is probably not the mechanism of the increased sensitivity to the vasoconstrictor effects of angiotensin II. A change in postreceptor signalling pathways may be involved but as yet there are no experimental data to support this proposition.

ANGIOTENSIN II AT_1 RECEPTOR ANTAGONISTS

The first angiotensin II receptor antagonists such as saralasin were modified peptide analogues of the parent peptide. These antagonists are rapidly cleaved *in vivo* and are not orally active. Moreover, the majority, if not all, of the peptide antagonists of angiotensin II are partial agonists, exhibiting agonist properties when the circulating concentrations of angiotensin II are low. They lower blood pressure when circulating concentrations of renin are high as, for example, in experimental renal hypertension in animals or in hypertensive patients with renal arterial stenosis. However, they do not generally lower blood pressure in SHR or in patients with essential hypertension.

More recently, small nonpeptide molecules have been identified that are orally active antagonists of angiotensin II at the AT_1 receptor (41,42). These novel compounds, in contrast to the large peptide analogues, are very selective for the AT_1 receptor subtype, are generally devoid of agonist properties, and lower blood pressure in SHR and in patients with essential hypertension. The peptide analogues are probably ineffective in lowering blood pressure in SHR because of their partial agonist activity. The selective AT_1 antagonists have a similar antihypertensive efficacy to angiotensin-converting enzyme inhibitors in SHR (18,22) and in patients with essential hypertension (43,44).

EFFECTS OF INTRARENAL ANGIOTENSIN II AT_1 RECEPTOR ANTAGONISM IN SHR

Although previous observations suggest that the actions of angiotensin II on the kidney are involved in the development and maintenance of high blood pressure in SHR and that the kidney is an important site of action for blockers of the renin-angiotensin system, they are not direct evidence. Most evidence comes from studies on the effects of exogenous angiotensin II. We therefore performed a series of experiments designed to obtain more direct evidence in support of a role of endogenous angiotensin II. The aim of the experiments was to determine whether blood pressure could be lowered in SHR after infusion of an AT_1 receptor antagonist into the kidney in a dose that selectively blocked the intrarenal actions of angiotensin II. These experiments are described in detail elsewhere (45) and the results are reviewed here. The potent, selective, and competitive AT_1 receptor antagonist valsartan ((s)-N-Valeryl-N-{[2′-(1H-tetrazol-5-yl)biphenyl-4-yl]-methyl}-valine) was used (46). The SHR used in these experiments were between 12 and 14 weeks of age. Under our laboratory conditions, hypertension becomes fully developed in SHR after about 15 weeks.

Effects of Intravenous Valsartan on Blood Pressure

Initial experiments were designed to determine the effective dose range for lowering blood pressure after continuous intravenous infusion of valsartan over 48

hours. Mean arterial blood pressure and heart rate were measured continuously in conscious freely moving SHR via an abdominal aortic catheter. The threshold dose for blood pressure lowering after intravenous infusion was approximately 1 mg/kg/day (Fig. 4). With doses of 1 mg/kg/day and above, the antihypertensive effect developed slowly over 24 hours to reach a maximum after 24 to 48 hours. The maximum lowering of blood pressure in response to intravenous infusion of valsartan was obtained with doses between 3 and 10 mg/kg/day.

Effects of Intrarenal Valsartan on Blood Pressure

To determine the contribution of angiotensin II acting on the kidney to the antihypertensive actions of valsartan, the AT_1 antagonist was infused intrarenally at a dose that was subthreshold for lowering blood pressure when given intravenously (0.3 mg/kg/day). Valsartan was delivered intrarenally via a catheter implanted into the right suprarenal artery. The contralateral kidney (left) was removed to enable the entire renal mass to be perfused with one catheter. When infused intrarenally, this dose of valsartan induced a fall in blood pressure of approximately 25 mm Hg (Fig. 5). The onset of the fall in blood pressure was slow, and the maximum effect was reached after about 48 hours. The fall in blood pressure produced by the intrarenal infusion of valsartan at a dose of 0.3 mg/kg/day approached the maximum antihypertensive response that could be induced after intravenous administration of higher doses (3 mg/kg/day and above) (see Figs. 5 and 6).

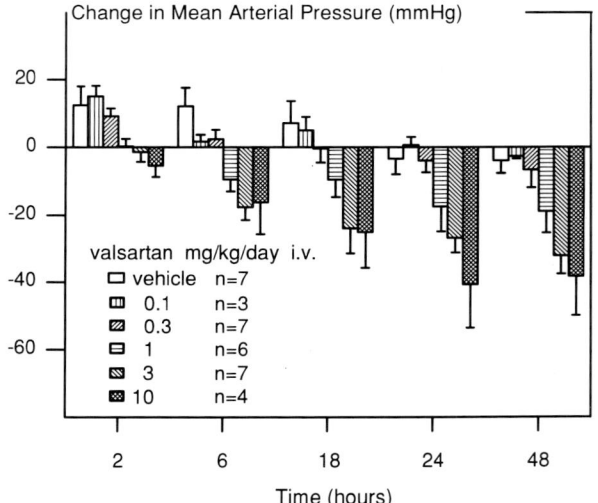

FIG. 4. Dose range of valsartan, a selective angiotensin II AT_1 receptor antagonist required to lower mean arterial blood pressure after intravenous (i.v.) infusion over 48 hours to conscious, freely moving SHR (12–14 weeks). A dose of 0.3 mg/kg/day is subthreshold for blood pressure lowering after i.v. infusion. Values are mean ± SEM. (From ref. 45, with permission.)

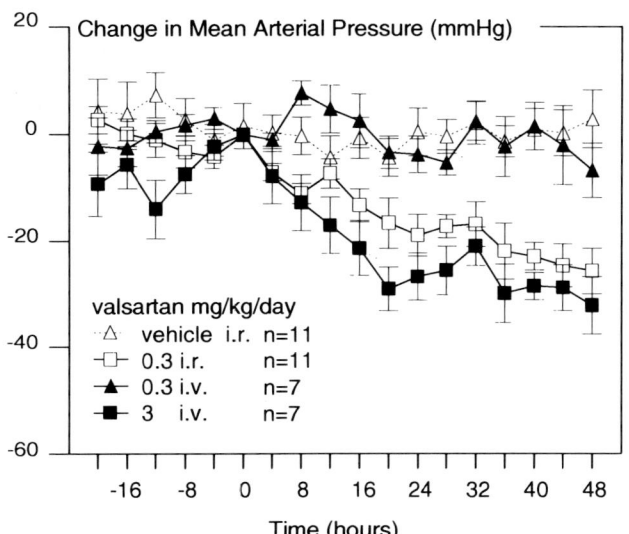

FIG. 5. Decrease in mean arterial blood pressure in conscious, freely moving SHR induced by valsartan, a selective angiotensin II AT$_1$ receptor antagonist, after intrarenal (i.r.) infusion of a dose (0.3 mg/kg/day) that is ineffective after intravenous (i.v.) administration. A tenfold higher dose of valsartan was effective in lowering blood pressure after i.v. administration. Intrarenal delivery of the vehicle had no effect on blood pressure. Values are mean ± SEM. (From ref. 45, with permission.)

Evidence for a Selective Effect of Valsartan on the Kidney After Intrarenal Infusion

The AT$_1$ antagonist valsartan has a long biological half-life in the rat and therefore it could be expected that with time, some compound might spill from the renal into the peripheral circulation. However, although antihypertensive when delivered to the kidney, the same dose did not lower blood pressure when given intravenously. This observation supports a selective intrarenal effect. Further evidence in support of this is provided by the observations that plasma concentrations of valsartan were undetectable after both the intrarenal and intravenous dose of 0.3 mg/kg/day, whereas they were approximately 0.5 μM after the 3 mg/kg/day dose given intravenously. As an additional test for the renal selectivity of the drug delivery, the degree of peripheral blockade of angiotensin II receptors was assessed by measuring the increase in blood pressure induced by a challenge dose of angiotensin II (300 ng/kg) given by bolus intravenous injection. The response in rats receiving the angiotensin II antagonist was compared to that in control rats receiving vehicle. There was some inhibition of the pressor response to angiotensin II after intravenous administration of 0.3 mg/kg/day of valsartan (38 percent), even though this dose was not sufficient to influence baseline blood pressure (Fig. 7). The inhibition of the angiotensin II pressor response was even smaller (20 percent) after in-

trarenal delivery of this dose (see Fig. 7). The small amount of inhibition was probably due to blockade of the constrictor effects of angiotensin II on the renal vascular bed. The renal vasculature is one of the most sensitive vascular beds to the constrictor effects of angiotensin II, and it could be expected that the solitary kidney would have contributed significantly to total peripheral resistance. The tenfold higher dose of valsartan (3 mg/kg/day), delivered intravenously, resulted in almost complete blockade of the angiotensin II pressor response and an antihypertensive response of a magnitude similar to that of the intrarenally delivered dose. Thus, intrarenally administered valsartan appeared to have lowered blood pressure primarily by an interaction with intrarenal AT$_1$ receptors.

EFFECT OF INTRARENAL AT$_1$ BLOCKADE ON PLASMA RENIN CONCENTRATION

Surprisingly, intrarenal infusion of the AT$_1$ receptor antagonist had little effect on plasma renin concentration (see Fig. 8). Other studies have shown that plasma concentrations of renin and angiotensin II are significantly increased after intravenous or oral administration of angiotensin-converting enzyme inhibitors or AT$_1$ receptor antagonists (18,19,47). Indeed, in the present study, a significant increase in plasma renin concentration was observed after an intravenous dose of valsartan

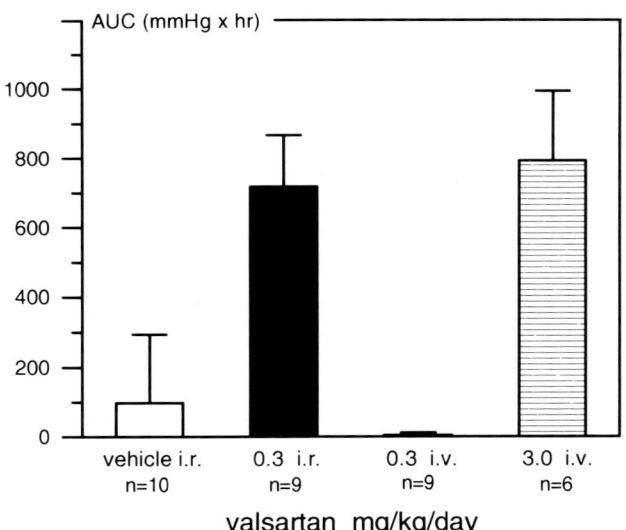

FIG. 6. Total area under the blood pressure curve (AUC) after intrarenal (i.r.) or intravenous (i.v.) infusion of valsartan, a selective angiotensin II AT$_1$ receptor antagonist, to conscious, freely moving SHR. A dose of 0.3 mg/kg/day was ineffective after i.v. administration but lowered blood pressure after i.r. administration. The response to the 0.3-mg/kg/day dose given i.r. was similar to that of a tenfold higher dose (3 mg/kg/day) given i.v. Values are mean ± SEM.

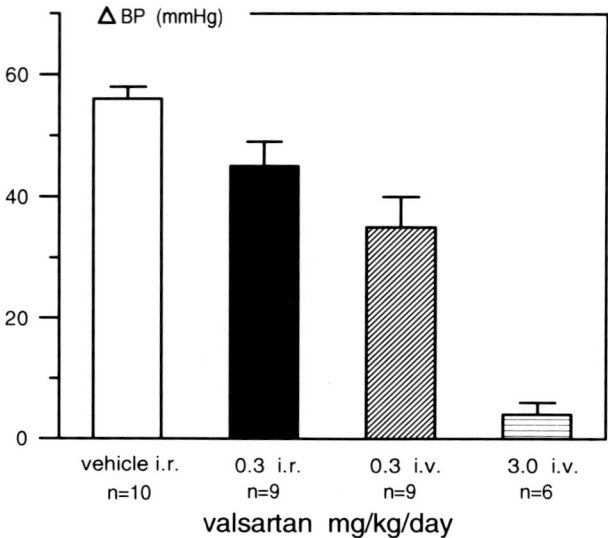

FIG. 7. Blockade of the pressor response induced after intravenous (i.v.) bolus injection of angiotensin II (300 ng/kg) by valsartan, a selective angiotensin II AT_1 receptor antagonist, in conscious, freely moving SHR. Compared to the control response in vehicle-treated rats, the 0.3-mg/kg/day dose of valsartan blocked the pressor response to angiotensin II by 20 percent after intrarenal (i.r.) administration and by 38 percent after i.v. administration. A tenfold higher dose of valsartan given i.v. blocked the response by more than 90 percent. Values are mean ± SEM.

that lowered blood pressure to a similar extent to the intrarenal dose of valsartan (Fig. 8). Release of renin from the kidneys is under the control of several factors, including changes in blood pressure and the negative feedback of angiotensin II on the juxtaglomerular cells. Since in the present study the fall in blood pressure was similar with the intrarenal and a tenfold higher intravenous dose, blood pressure cannot explain the difference in effect on plasma renin concentration. Intrarenal infusion of valsartan may have affected other mechanisms of renin release that were not disrupted during intravenous infusion.

The increase in plasma renin after the intravenous dose was only transient. The peak that was reached after 6 hours may have been due to release of all of the stored renin. The levels may have decreased thereafter because all of the stored renin was depleted and only newly synthesized renin was being released. It may require a longer time period for renin synthesis to be increased.

CONCLUSIONS

Recently AT_1 antagonists coupled to gamma glutamate have been developed (48). The AT_1 antagonists are released from gamma glutamate by the enzyme gamma glutamate transferase. Since this enzyme is located mainly in the kidney, it has been hypothesized that AT_1 antagonists should reach high concentrations selectively within the renal mass after this pro-drug approach of drug delivery. When administered to SHR, gamma-glutamate–derivatized AT_1 antagonists lower blood pressure by 30 mm Hg, without affecting the systemic pressor responses to angiotensin II. These findings appear to support the present observations, indicating that endogenous angiotensin II acting on the kidney is involved in the development and maintenance of high blood pressure in SHR.

All components of the renin-angiotensin system are present within the kidney and the intrarenal formation of angiotensin II does occur (27). Several studies have provided strong evidence for an important physiological role of intrarenally generated angiotensin II in the control of renal function (26,49). Intrarenal infusion of valsartan would be expected to inhibit both the effects of angiotensin II delivered to the kidney from the peripheral circulation and that generated locally within the renal mass. However, the relative contributions of locally versus systemically produced angiotensin II to the response observed in our experiments is not clear.

Although the results of our study demonstrate that selective inhibition of the actions of angiotensin II within the kidney lead to a maximal lowering of blood pressure, the mechanism by which this occurs has not been investigated. There are, however, a number of means by which inhibition of the intrarenal actions of angiotensin II could lead to lower blood pressure.

Adult SHR have a disordered pressure-diuresis/natriuresis relationship, and the primary deficit has been pro-

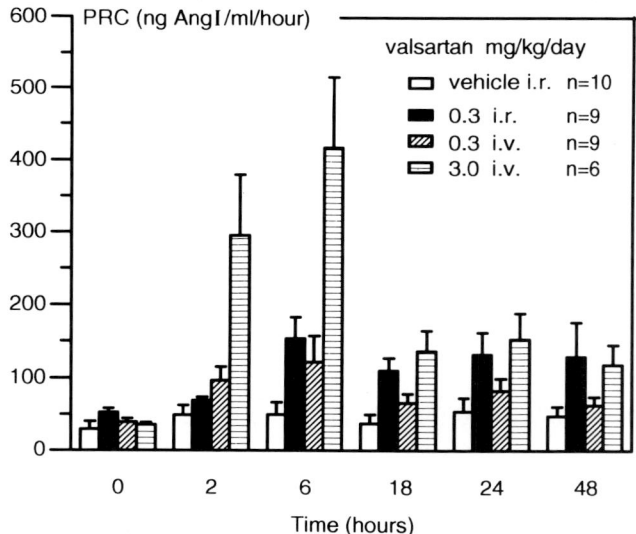

FIG. 8. Plasma renin concentrations (PRC) during intrarenal (i.r.) or intravenous (i.v.) infusion of valsartan or vehicle for 48 hours in conscious, freely moving SHR; PRC was significantly elevated only after the 3.0-mg/kg/day dose given i.v. Values are mean ± SEM. (From ref. 45, with permission.)

TABLE 1. Effects[a] of valsartan, an angiotensin II AT_1 receptor antagonist, on hematocrit, plasma osmolality, plasma sodium, and potassium concentration in spontaneously hypertensive rats[b] before and after 6 and 48 hours of treatment

Treatment	n	Hematocrit (%)			Osmolality (mosmol/L)			Sodium (mEq/L)			Potassium (mEq/L)		
		0	6	48 h	0	6	48 h	0	6	48 h	0	6	48 h
Vehicle i.r.	10	42.0 ± 0.8	39.6 ± 0.9	36.5 ± 0.6	295 ± 3	297 ± 2	296 ± 2	145 ± 2	140 ± 4	148 ± 4	4.5 ± 0.1	4.5 ± 0.2	4.6 ± 0.1
Valsartan (mg/kg/day)													
0.3 i.r.	9	43.6 ± 0.5	40.7 ± 0.6	36.7 ± 0.3	304 ± 2	302 ± 2	296 ± 1	144 ± 1	145 ± 1	140 ± 6	4.4 ± 0.2	4.2 ± 0.1	4.0 ± 0.2
0.3 i.v.	9	42.0 ± 0.5	41.2 ± 0.4	36.7 ± 0.7	302 ± 6	295 ± 3	299 ± 2	145 ± 1	144 ± 1	146 ± 1	4.4 ± 0.1	4.3 ± 0.1	4.4 ± 0.1
3.0 i.v.	9	42.2 ± 0.8	42.3 ± 1.0	36.5 ± 0.6	298 ± 2	295 ± 2	294 ± 1	143 ± 3	143 ± 3	148 ± 5	4.3 ± 0.4	4.3 ± 0.1	4.5 ± 0.1

[a] Values are mean ± SEM.
[b] The rats were 11–14 weeks of age.
Valsartan was delivered by continuous intravenous infusion intrarenally (i.r.) or intravenously (i.v.); n, number of animals.

posed to be an increase in renal vasoconstriction (10,21,35,36). Our study and the other experimental evidence discussed above indicate that angiotensin II is involved. Although renal function was not measured in our study, valsartan most probably lowered blood pressure by inducing vasodilatation in the kidney and may have also decreased sodium reabsortion. After acute systemic administration of blockers of the renin-angiotensin system to SHR, an increase in renal blood flow and in sodium and volume excretion has been observed (21,50). However, the observation that sodium balance remains unchanged when blood pressure is lowered by treatment with an angiotensin-converting enzyme inhibitor, and also as blood pressure recovers after treatment is stopped (21), indicates that changes in sodium balance may not be involved in the antihypertensive response. Moreover, in our own study no changes in hematocrit, plasma osmolality, or the plasma concentrations of sodium and potassium were observed during intrarenal AT_1 blockade (Table 1). However, changes in hematocrit and plasma ions are only crude estimates of volume balance, and studies of renal function obviously need to be performed to determine whether intrarenal infusion of valsartan exerts its antihypertensive effect by promoting renal sodium excretion.

The increased renal vasoconstriction in SHR may be due to an imbalance between an endogenous renal vasoconstrictor such as angiotensin II, and endogenous renal vasodilator systems (10). The antihypertensive effects of intrarenal valsartan could be due to increased release of (or unmasking of) the effects of endogenous vasodilator substances such as prostaglandins (51), nitric oxide (52), or renal medullary lipids (53).

The mechanism whereby blood pressure increases to compensate for the increase in renal vascular constriction is not known. It has been proposed that the derangement in kidney function stimulates the synthesis and release of an endogenous oubainlike factor from the hypothalamus (1,2). It is released primarily to overcome the tendency of the kidney to retain sodium, but as a side effect increases the contractility of peripheral tissues leading to an increase in blood pressure. This factor could be the link between the renal vasoconstrictor effects of angiotensin II and the high blood pressure. However, as yet there is no experimental evidence to support this proposition, and the exact mechanisms involved remain to be elucidated.

Based on the results of our studies (45) and those with the gamma-glutamate–derivatized angiotensin II antagonists (48), the kidney would seem an attractive site for the targeting of blockers of the renin-angiotensin system. By selective delivery to the kidney of a compound with a short half-life in the peripheral circulation, blood pressure could be lowered without peripheral effects of the drug. Such a drug might have a lower incidence of side effects than one that is distributed throughout the body. However, angiotensin-converting enzyme inhibitors have relatively few side effects, and the AT_1 angiotensin II receptor antagonists may have even less. Since angiotensin II may contribute to vascular and cardiac hypertrophy and the development of vascular lesions (54–56), it may be highly desirable to block these effects with a compound that distributes throughout the cardiovascular system. The currently available AT_1 angiotensin II receptor antagonists such as valsartan appear to distribute to the kidney and the vessel wall after systemic administration. Therefore, there is no apparent advantage to target them to the kidney.

Several lines of evidence indicate that the kidney and the renin-angiotensin system play a key role in the development of hypertension in the SHR. We have demonstrated that blood pressure is lowered in SHR after selective intrarenal delivery of an AT_1 antagonist to the kidney in a dose that is inactive after intravenous administration. Our results support the hypothesis that the intrarenal actions of angiotensin II contribute to the elevated blood pressure of SHR and that the kidney is an important target for the antihypertensive action of AT_1 receptor antagonists. These findings may also explain, at least in part, why blockers of the renin-angiotensin system lower blood pressure in SHR although plasma angiotensin II concentrations are not elevated. Further investigation is needed to elucidate the mechanisms involved in mediating the fall in blood pressure after selective intrarenal blockade of intrarenal AT_1 receptors.

REFERENCES

1. de Wardener HE. *Clin Sci* 1990;79:193–200.
2. de Wardener HE. *Clin Sci* 1990;79:289–297.
3. Luke RG. *Hypertension* 1993;21:380–390.
4. Trippodo NC, Frohlich ED. *Circ Res* 1981;48:309–319.
5. Rettig R, Unger T. *TIPS* 1991;12:243–245.
6. Curtis JJ, Luke RG, Dustan HP, et al. *N Engl J Med* 1983;309:1009–1015.
7. Guidi E, Bianchi G, Rivolta E, et al. *Nephron* 1985;41:14–21.
8. Guyton AC, Coleman TG, Cowley AW Jr, et al. *J Med* 1972;52:584–594.
9. Roman RJ. *Hypertension* 1987;9:III-130–III-136.
10. Arendshorst WJ, Chatziantoniou C, Daniels FH. *Kidney Int Suppl* 1990;30:92–S96.
11. Harrap SB, Doyle AE. *J Hypertens* 1986;4[Suppl 3]:S249–S252.
12. Morduchowicz GA, Sheik-Hamad D, Ok DJ, et al. *Kidney Int* 1989;36:576–581.
13. Garg LC, Narang N, McArdle S. *Am J Physiol* 1985;249:F863–F869.
14. Harrap SB, Doyle AE. *Clin Sci* 1988;74:63–69.
15. Harrap SB. *Hypertension* 1986;8:572–582.
16. van Hooft IM, Grabbee DE, Derkx FHM, et al. *N Engl J Med* 1991;324:1305–1311.
17. Sinaiko A, Mirkin BL. *Circ Res* 1974;34:693–696.
18. Bunkenburg B, Schnell C, Baum HP, et al. *Hypertension* 1991;18:278–288.
19. Wood JM. In: MacGregor GA, Severs PS, eds. *Current advances in ACE inhibition 2;* London: Churchill Livingstone, 1991;110–117.

20. Antonaccio MJ, High JP, Rubin B, et al. *Clin Sci* 1979;57:127s–130s.
21. Harrap SB, Nicolaci JA, Doyle AE. *Clin Exp Pharmacol Physiol* 1986;13:753–765.
22. Wong PC, Price WA Jr, Chiu AT, et al. *Hypertension* 1990;15:459–468.
23. Inagami T, Murakami T, Higuchi K, et al. *Am J Hypertens* 1991;4:15S–22S.
24. Unger T, Ganten D, Lang RE, et al. *J Cardiovasc Pharmacol* 1985;7:36–41.
25. Cohen ML, Kurz KD. *J Pharmacol Exp Ther* 1982;220:63–69.
26. Levens NR, Freedlender AE, Peach MJ, et al. *Endocrinology* 1983;112:43–49.
27. Johnston CI, Fabris B, Jandeleit K. *Kidney Int* 1993;44:S59–S63.
28. Hofbauer KG, Criscione L, Neisius D, et al. In: Owman C, Arneklo-Nobin B, eds. *Neuronal messengers in vascular function.* Amsterdam: Elsevier, 1987;271–291.
29. Hollenberg NK. *J Cardiovasc Pharmacol* 1984;6:S176–S183.
30. Ray PE, Aguilera G, Kopp JB, et al. *Kidney Int* 1991;40:764–771.
31. Anderson PW, Do YS, Hsueh WA. *Hypertension* 1993;21:29–35.
32. Norman H, Badie-Dezfooly B, Nord EP, et al. *Am J Physiol* 1987;253:F299–F309.
33. Wolf G, Neilson EG. *J Am Soc Nephrol* 1993;3:1531–1540.
34. Harrap SB. *Am J Hypertens* 1991;4:212S–216S.
35. Li P, Jackson EK. *J Pharmacol Exp Ther* 1989;251:909–921.
36. Kost CK, Jackson EK. *Hypertension* 1993;21:420–431.
37. Mendelsohn FAO, Dunbar M, Allen A, et al. *J Fed Proc* 1986;45:1420–1425.
38. Whitebread S, Mele M, Kamber B, et al. *Biochem Biophys Res Commun* 1989;163:284–291.
39. Edwards RM, Aiyar N. *J Am Soc Nephrol* 1993;3:1643–1652.
40. Messenger EA, Stonier C, Aber GM. *Clin Sci* 1989;76:619–623.
41. Timmermans PBMWM, Carini DJ, Chiu AT, et al. *Blood Vessels* 1990;27:295–300.
42. Timmermans PBMWM, Wong PC, Chiu AT, et al. *Pharmacol Rev* 1993;45:205–251.
43. Smith RD, Chiu AT, Wong PC, et al. *Annu Rev Pharmacol Toxicol* 1992;32:135–165.
44. Tsunoda K, Abe K, Hagino T, et al. *Am J Hypertens* 1993;6:28–32.
45. Wood JM, Schnell CR, Levens NR. *Hypertension* 1993;21:1056–1061.
46. Criscione L, de Gasparo M, Buhlmayer P, et al. *Br J Pharmacol* 1993;110:761–771.
47. Pals DT, Couch SJ. *Clin Exp Hypertension* 1993;15:1–13.
48. Reitz DB, Manning RE. International patent WO 92/04335, 1992
49. Siragy HM, Lamb NE, Rose CE Jr, et al. *Am J Physiol* 1988;255:F749–F754.
50. Fenoy FJ, Milicic I, Smith RD, et al. *Am J Hypertens* 1991;4:321S–326S.
51. Chatziantoniou C, Arendshorst WJ. *Am J Physiol* 1992;263:F573–F580.
52. Pollock DM, Polakowski JS, Divish BJ, et al. *Hypertension* 1993;2:660–666.
53. Muirhead EE, Brooks B, Byers LW, et al. *Hypertension* 1991;18:S158–S163.
54. Baker KM, Booz GW, Dostal DE. *Annu Rev Physiol* 1992;54:227–241.
55. Jackson CL, Schwartz SM. *Hypertension* 1992;20:713–736.
56. Owens GK. *Drug Dev Res* 1993;29:83–87.

Hypertension: Pathophysiology, Diagnosis, and Management, Second Edition,
edited by J.H. Laragh and B.M. Brenner,
Raven Press, Ltd., New York © 1995.

CHAPTER **89**

Biochemistry and Physiology of Multiple Renin Forms

Stephen A. Katz and John A. Opsahl

The renin-angiotensin system (RAS) is a major regulator of blood pressure and sodium balance. Secretion of renin by juxtaglomerular (JG) cells is the rate-limiting step in the control of the activity of the classic (circulating) RAS. Active renin is actually composed of multiple forms that can be readily separated on the basis of charge (isoelectric focusing) or carbohydrate structure (lectin affinity chromatography). This chapter examines the biochemistry and physiological consequences of the heterogeneity of active renin.

During the past 30 years, investigators have reported the presence of multiple forms of active renin in a variety of species (1–3). Early on, the possibility that the multiple forms of renin were artifacts of the separation and purification procedures used in their demonstration could not be excluded. Moreover, the biochemical mechanisms responsible for the heterogeneity of renin

were unknown. However, within the past 12 years, the existence of multiple forms of active renin has been repeatedly verified and demonstrated across a wide evolutionary scale, including fish, amphibians, birds, and mammals (2). Currently, it appears that the heterogeneity of active renin is largely caused by variable glycosylation, although other variations in renin structure or posttranslational attachments may also contribute.

Renin heterogeneity appears to have several important physiological consequences because it affects JG-cell trafficking of renin, acute stimulation of renin secretion, and the hepatic degradation of renin. Plasma renin activity (PRA) is actually the sum of the activities of multiple circulating renin glycoforms. Acute stimulation of renin secretion results in preferential JG-cell release of renin glycoforms, which are rapidly cleared by the liver. Therefore, acute renin secretion results in an increase in PRA with a shorter plasma residence time (shorter half-life). This allows for a more rapid return to basal PRA and potentially limits the physiological effects of acute stimulation of renin secretion, resulting in a fine control mechanism for PRA. Intravenous infusion of purified renin forms leads to variable diuretic and natriuretic responses, indicating the possible involvement of renin heterogeneity in salt-and-water homeostasis. Also, in

   S. A. Katz: Department of Physiology, University of Minnesota, Minneapolis, Minnesota 55455; and Division of Nephrology, Hennepin County Medical Center, Minneapolis, Minnesota 55415.
   J. A. Opsahl: School of Medicine, University of Minnesota, Minneapolis, Minnesota 55455; and Division of Nephrology, Hennepin County Medical Center, Minneapolis, Minnesota 55415.

certain experimental models of hypertension, the proportion of some renin forms in plasma is strongly correlated with blood pressure, suggesting a potential role for renin heterogeneity in the pathophysiology of some forms of hypertension. Finally, vascular wall renin and adrenal renin have been shown to be equal to the sum of the individual activities of multiple renin forms recovered from those tissues. Because renin forms have different net charges at physiological pH, differential access of specific renin forms into various tissue compartments is possible and could be important in determining the target-organ effects of the RAS. The participation of heterogeneous renin forms in salt-and-water balance, hypertension, and tissue RASs are areas of current investigation.

HISTORY

Early reports of the presence of multiple forms of active renin were difficult to interpret because renin heterogeneity was observed with respect to molecular weight, enzymatic activity, isoelectric point, and ligand-binding affinity. Initial studies often used extensive and laborious separation and purification procedures that raised the question of artifactual results. It is now generally accepted that early observations of renin molecular weight heterogeneity were due primarily to molecular weight differences between preprorenin, prorenin, renin, and possibly the cleavage of renin into two polypeptide chains. Most early reports of renin enzymatic heterogeneity can be attributed to inadvertent confusion of active and inactive renin (prorenin), because many initial methods of renin purification included an acidification step that could have reversibly activated inactive renin. However, using isoelectric focusing or affinity chromatography, some investigators were able to distinguish multiple forms of active renin that had approximately the same molecular weight (about 40,000) and the same enzymatic specific activity.

In 1967, Skeggs et al. (4) demonstrated four forms of active hog renin using DEAE-cellulose chromatography. The renin forms eluted off the column at pH values of 5.2, 4.7, 4.5, and 4.25. In 1972, Rubin (5) also partially purified four distinct hog renin fractions with isoelectric points [pH(I)] of 5.1, 5.0, 4.9, and 4.75. All four renin fractions had molecular weights of approximately 40,000. Lauritzen et al. (6) found three renin isozymes in the rat with pH(I) of 5.4, 5.2, and 5.0 in 1976. The molecular weights were between 39,000 and 42,000, and each isozyme had a similar Michaelis constant with rat renin substrate. The immunogenicity of the isozymes also appeared to be the same. Similar findings were also reported in the hog. Importantly, refocusing of renin isoelectric forms did not result in a shift to other isoelectric points. Subsequent attempts to investigate the renin isozymes were unsuccessful because of loss of enzymatic ac-

tivity on further purification. Printz and Dworschack (7) reported isoelectric heterogeneity of rabbit renin and also demonstrated that rabbit renin was a glycoprotein because it bound to concanavalin A (Con A). In 1978, Matoba et al. (8) attempted to purify rat renin and observed three main renin isozymes after the final purification step on CM-cellulose chromatography. The renin isozymes were found to have similar amino acid composition, molecular weight, and specific activity. They possessed pH(I) of 5.22, 5.15, and 5.05 and were also judged to be glycoproteins by their affinity for Con A. Galen et al. (9) found five forms of active human renin in a JG-cell tumor. The pH(I) of the forms ranged from 5.70 to 4.95, and all were glycoproteins. The three main fractions had molecular weights of approximately 40,000 and very similar specific activities. The five forms also appeared to share identical immunogenicity. Conio et al. (10) also isolated multiple forms of active renin from bull kidney with pH(I) of 5.6 to 5.1. In 1981, Druilhet and Overturf (11) separated five to six active multiple renin forms by isoelectric focusing from human, rabbit, hog, and baboon kidney tissue and showed that the isoelectric heterogeneity for each species was somewhat different, but all pH(I)'s ranged from 5.7 to 4.7. Also in 1981, Chang and coworkers (12) found multiple forms of human active renin in both kidney and plasma, with an isoelectric point range of 5.7 to 5.1. Perhaps more importantly, these workers also demonstrated multiple isoelectric points for inactive renin. The isoelectric points were higher for inactive renin (range, 6.4 to 5.3) than for renin and fell on activation with trypsin. Simultaneously, Eggena et al. (13) demonstrated isoelectric heterogeneity of active and inactive renin in human plasma. Again, the isoelectric points of inactive renin were found to be higher than those of active renin. Active renin heterogeneity was also reported in kidney and arterial tissue.

At this point (1981), it was reasonable to conclude that for all species tested, active renin existed as a family of heterogeneous forms or isozymes, with similar molecular weights, specific activities, and common antigenic determinants. The multiple active renin forms had variable affinities for certain ligands and different isoelectric points, which were somewhat species-dependent, but usually in the range of 5.7 to 4.7. Inactive renin was also heterogeneous with respect to isoelectric point. The cause of renin heterogeneity and its physiological significance remained unknown.

Using a pulse-chase strategy with tritiated leucine in dog renal cortical slices, Katz and Malvin (14) found that a portion of secreted renin contained the tritium label. They proposed that some secreted active renin was newly synthesized. However, isoelectric focusing revealed that the newly synthesized secreted renin containing the tritium label focused only at more acidic isoelectric points (greater net negative charge), whereas the less acidic renin activity was devoid of the tritium label. This observation forced the hypothesis that the renal cortical slices were secreting at least two forms of active renin: newly synthesized with relatively high net negative charge, and previously synthesized renin with relatively less net negative charge. Only the renin with less acidic pH(I) (less negative charge) showed an increase in secretion in response to the beta-adrenergic agonist isoproterenol. In another study using rat renal cortical slices, the same workers found six isoelectric forms of secreted rat renin with pH(I) of 5.70, 5.55, 5.30, 5.15, 4.90, and 4.8, representing 1, 62, 18, 9, 8, and 3 percent, respectively, of basal renin secretion (1). Isoproterenol stimulation of renin release from the rat renal cortical slices increased only the secretion of renin with less acidic isoelectric points. From these two studies, it appeared that active renin heterogeneity was somehow involved in JG-cell sorting of active renin into both an isoproterenol responsive storage pool (less acidic isoelectric points) and an immediate secretory path apparently composed of newly synthesized renin (relatively acidic isoelectric points). In other words, the first physiological significance attributable to active renin heterogeneity involved JG-cell trafficking of active renin into storage versus immediate secretory pathways. As discussed below, later work would demonstrate a physiological role for renin heterogeneity not only in JG-cell sorting of renin but also in renin secretion after acute stimulation, the setting of PRA, hepatic clearance of renin, salt-and-water balance, and hypertension.

Further study of active renin heterogeneity revealed that it did not result from measurement artifact or nonspecific interactions because diverse purification and separation protocols from different laboratories yielded the same general results, independent of both the purity of the enzyme and sample pretreatment. Refocusing of individual renin peaks resulted in the same individual

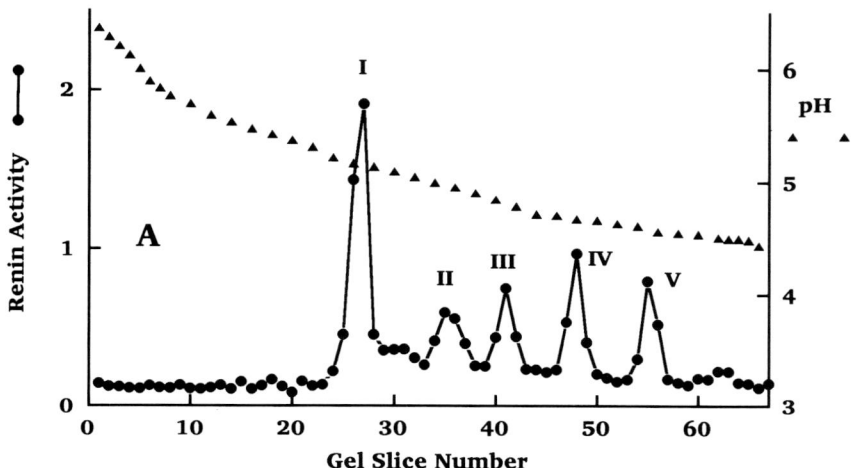

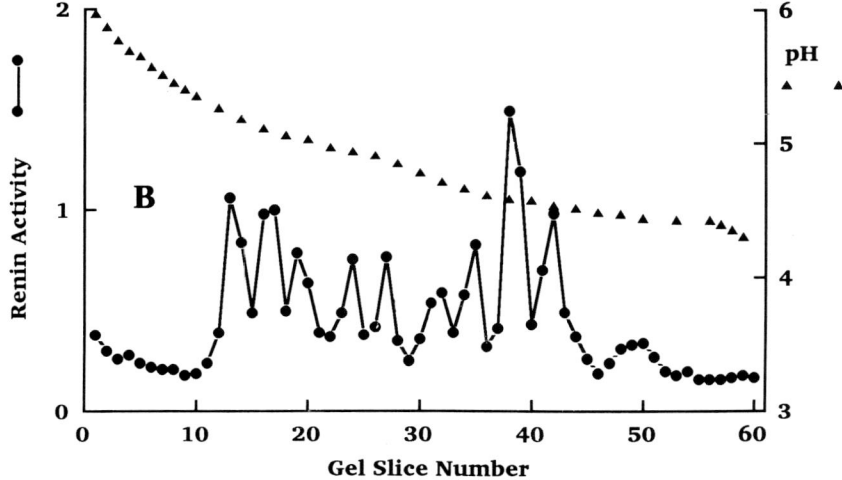

FIG. 1. Representative isoelectric focusing profile of active renin from rabbit plasma using a pH gradient of 0.12 pH units/cm gel (**A**); and a more shallow pH gradient of 0.09 pH units/cm gel (**B**). Renin activity (*left axis*) is expressed as ng AI/ml gel elution/h. The corresponding pH profile (*right axis*) is also shown for each focusing gel. **A:** Five major active renin forms with average isoelectric focusing points of 5.20, 5.00, 4.82, 4.70, and 4.55 are labeled I through V, respectively. (From ref. 17, with permission.)

peak focusing at the same isoelectric point without the appearance of other renin forms (1,6). Complete purification of human kidney renin still resulted in at least five isoelectric forms of renin with similar molecular weights (15). This isoelectric heterogeneity has been shown to exist in all animals studied, across a wide evolutionary scale including fish, amphibians, birds, and mammals, including humans (2). At the present time, seven forms of active human renin can be separated and measured using isoelectric focusing with pH(I) of 5.71, 5.57, 5.49, 5.22, 5.08, 4.93, and 4.82 (16). In the rabbit, up to 10 separate active renin forms can be separated by isoelectric focusing using very shallow pH gradients (17). The number of renin forms separated by isoelectric focusing increases as the pH gradient becomes more shallow (3,17). This is illustrated in Fig. 1 for rabbit plasma renin. Failure to observe renin isoelectric heterogeneity is most often associated with a steep pH gradient, which does not allow resolution of separate renin forms. Neither isoelectric focusing nor affinity chromatography are probably capable of resolving all the different renin forms.

Shallow gradient isoelectric focusing has been commonly used to separate multiple renin forms. However, Con A affinity chromatography has also been used with great success. Kim et al. (18–20) demonstrated three active renin forms with differing affinities for Con A. The renin forms with the greatest affinity for Con A have been shown to be preferentially stored in the kidney, preferentially released in response to acute renin stimulation, present in high concentration in plasma, and preferentially degraded by the liver (18,19,21–24). Inactive renin heterogeneity has also been observed using Con A meth-

odology (20). As will be discussed in the following section, it is our contention that renin form separation by Con A affinity and isoelectric focusing is closely related. Figure 2 shows a representative separation of rat renal renin into three separate active renin forms using Con A affinity chromatography.

BIOCHEMISTRY OF RENIN HETEROGENEITY

Renin is an aspartyl protease glycoprotein that displays isoelectric and ligand-binding heterogeneity. From the previous brief history, one can conclude that the part(s) of the active renin molecule responsible for renin heterogeneity must result in multiple active renin forms with similar molecular weights, specific activities, and common antigenic determinants, as well as variable isoelectric points in the range of 5.7 to 4.7 and dissimilar affinities for certain ligands such as Con A. The molecular moiety responsible for active renin heterogeneity should also result in inactive renin heterogeneity. At this time, the most favored hypothesis explaining renin heterogeneity is that multiple forms of active and inactive renin are the direct result of variable oligosaccharide structures attached to the renin polypeptide chain. Alternative hypotheses are also possible and not necessarily mutually exclusive. Therefore, variable carbohydrate attachment to renin will first be considered as the molecular determinant of renin heterogeneity, followed by discussion of other mechanisms that could also contribute to renin heterogeneity.

Renin Glycoforms

Glycoproteins, including renin, share a common structural theme. In general, the individual polypeptide chain(s) of glycoproteins are post-translationally modified by attachment of heterogeneous oligosaccharide (carbohydrate) structures at specific glycosylation sites. Heterogeneous glycoproteins resulting from differential oligosaccharide attachment are known as glycoforms. In general, polypeptide chain glycosylation creates many separate glycoforms, each with a different oligosaccharide structure, or combination of oligosaccharide structures, attached to the same amino acid sequence (25).

Most proteins synthesized on the rough endoplasmic reticulum are glycosylated at asparagine residues that are one amino acid removed from a serine or threonine. This yields an asparagine-linked (N-linked) glycoprotein. Multiple glycosylation sites on the same glycoprotein are common. Initial glycosylation results from the covalent attachment of a common 14-sugar-residue oligosaccharide-branched chain and occurs as the new polypeptide chain is synthesized and the glycosylation site appears in the endoplasmic reticulum. The initial 14-sugar oligosaccharide chain is then extensively modified

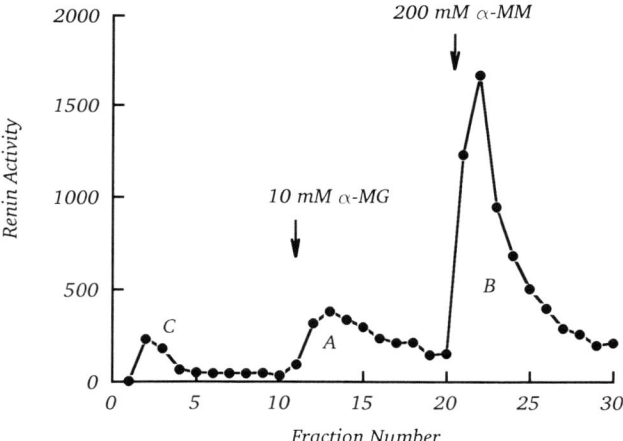

FIG. 2. Concanavalin A (Con A) affinity chromatography of rat renal renin. Renin activity can be resolved into three forms: renin C, unbound renin; renin A, loosely bound renin, eluted with 10 mM alpha-methylglucoside (α-MG); and renin B, tightly bound renin, eluted with 200 mM alpha-methylmannoside (α-MM). Renin activity units are ngAI/ml column fraction/h assay incubation. (Terminology and general methods are from ref. 18.)

while the glycoprotein is still in the endoplasmic reticulum, and further modifications occur in the Golgi apparatus. The modifications to the oligosaccharide chain are the result of enzymatic removal and addition of sugars to the original oligosaccharide chain (26). This process results in heterogeneous oligosaccharide attachments to identical polypeptide chains (25). The glycoforms of a secretory glycoprotein then move from the Golgi apparatus to various transport and storage vesicles.

Renin has two glycosylation sites available for asparagine-linked (N-linked) glycosylation (27,91). Therefore, active renin can be expected to be composed of a family of glycoforms with variable carbohydrate attachment to a single-amino-acid sequence (7,19,24,28,29). About 7 percent of the mass of active renin is carbohydrate. Because initial glycosylation occurs during polypeptide chain elongation, the biosynthetic precursors of renin, especially prorenin (inactive renin), are also glycosylated. Asparagine-linked glycoproteins generally have three types of oligosaccharide attachments; complex, high-mannose, and complex–high-mannose hybrids. Complex oligosaccharide chains tend to terminate with N-acetylneuraminic acid (sialic acid), whereas high mannose oligosaccharides tend to terminate with mannose. All three oligosaccharide types have been observed attached to prorenin secreted from Chinese hamster ovary cells transfected with human prorenin cDNA (28). Figure 3 illustrates a complex oligosaccharide chain compared with a high-mannose oligosaccharide chain.

It seems likely that the isoelectric heterogeneity of renin is caused by variable oligosaccharide attachment because glycosylation of a protein results in attachment of different oligosaccharide structures that may or may not terminate with sialic acid (25,28,30). The nature of N-linked oligosaccharide addition is such that each carbo-

hydrate attachment commonly splits into two to four branches, and each branch may or may not terminate with sialic acid (see Fig. 3). Oligosaccharide termination with sialic acid can explain isoelectric heterogeneity, because sialic acid is the only sugar residue of glycoproteins that bears a net negative charge at physiological pH. Renin bears a variable net negative charge as evidenced by multiple isoelectric forms with acidic isoelectric points. The lower the isoelectric point, the greater the net negative charge.

Approximately nine different N-linked oligosaccharide structures have been found attached to recombinant renin, not counting the highly variable sialic acid attachments, which would greatly increase the number of separate oligosaccharide chains attached to renin (28). Further heterogeneity of renin occurs because it contains two separate N-linked glycosylation sites, which can result in many combinations of paired oligosaccharide attachments.

If sialic acid is responsible for renin isoelectric heterogeneity, then enzymatic removal of sialic acid with neuraminidase (sialidase), removal of oligosaccharide chains with endoglycosidase F, or production of recombinant renin without glycosylation sites should result in decreased isoelectric heterogeneity and a shift of the isoelectric point to a more basic renin species. In fact, three reports have indicated that this is the case (29,31,32), although two other reports failed to observe an isoelectric shift (19,22).

Tunicamycin (TM) blocks the initial step in the eventual addition of oligosaccharides to asparagine (N-linked glycosylation). Addition of TM to the incubation media of rat renal cortical slices significantly altered the secretion profile of active renin isoelectric forms, suggesting that isoelectric heterogeneity is indeed the result of glycosylation (32). The renin profile of cortical slice homogenate (stored renin) was not altered, presumably because TM could not affect the large storage pool of renin synthesized before addition of TM.

Con A affinity chromatography typically resolves active renin into three forms with differing affinities for Con A (18,19). Con A is a leguminous lectin and is part of a class of proteins that can bind specifically and reversibly to certain sugars. Con A has a specific affinity for mannose (33). Human renin Con A glycoforms also display differing affinities toward other plant lectins (22). Therefore, Con A affinity chromatography confirms that renin is heterogeneous with respect to glycosylation.

Because Con A affinity chromatography typically resolves only three glycoforms in the rat and human (17,18,22), compared with the six or more renin forms demonstrated by isoelectric focusing (1,16,34,35), a simple one-to-one correspondence between results derived from Con A and isoelectric focusing would not be expected. Con A has a specific high affinity for mannose (33). Thus, the renin form(s) with the highest Con A

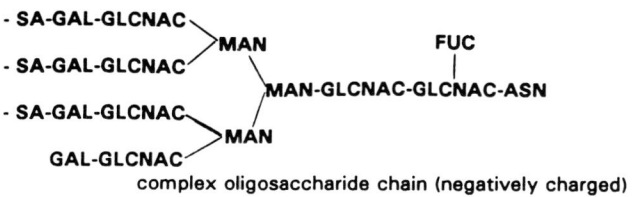

complex oligosaccharide chain (negatively charged)

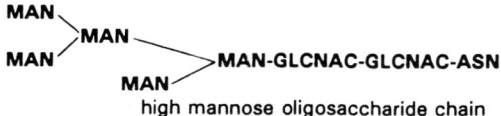

high mannose oligosaccharide chain

FIG. 3. Example of a complex and a high-mannose oligosaccharide structure. Examples were modified from ref. 28. —SA, Sialic acid (negatively charged); GAL, galactose; GLCNAC, N-acetylglucosamine; MAN, mannose; FUC, fucose; ASN, asparagine; from the renin amino acid chain. Note the terminal negatively charged sialic acid attachments on the complex oligosaccharide structure.

affinity should be of the high-mannose glycoform type, whereas the renin form(s) with intermediate affinity should most likely contain hybrid-type oligosaccharide chains, and the renin form(s) with the lowest Con A affinity (zero affinity) should represent complex-type glycoforms with little available mannose. As previously stated, complex-type oligosaccharides tend to terminate in sialic acid and therefore would be expected to possess lower or more acidic isoelectric points because of their greater net negative charge. Thus, it is easy to predict that renin glycoforms with no Con A affinity should have relatively more acidic isoelectric points, whereas high-affinity Con A glycoforms should have relatively less acidic isoelectric points. Preliminary data indicate that this is the case (36,36a). The rat renin fraction with no Con A affinity was composed of more than 63 percent of renin isoelectric forms with very acidic isoelectric points, compared with the renin fraction with the highest Con A affinity, which contained only 10 percent of isoelectric forms focusing with acidic isoelectric points.

Two reports have concluded that glycosylation probably does not contribute to isoelectric-focusing heterogeneity. However, in one, the renin activity studied was unstable, making isoelectric studies of the Con A glycoforms technically impossible (18). In the other, Kim et al. (19) were able to demonstrate isoelectric heterogeneity of each Con A renin glycoform using purified stable rat renal renin. The report concluded that glycosylation probably did not contribute to charge heterogeneity, in part because the isoelectric focusing pattern was similar for all three renin glycoforms. The amount or proportions of the separate isoelectric forms in each renin glycoform were not measured. In newer data (36,36a), six renin isoelectric forms were found to be present in each rat renin glycoform, essentially in agreement with ref. 19. However, careful quantitation of the proportions of the isoelectric forms in each renin glycoform revealed a significantly different isoelectric profile in each of the glycoforms. As stated above, the different isoelectric proportions were sufficient to account for the relationship expected between Con A affinity, sialic acid presence, and isoelectric focusing. Therefore, previous reports of isoelectric heterogeneity and Con A glycoform heterogeneity are actually in agreement.

As explained in greater detail below, renin isoelectric forms with low or very acidic isoelectric points have been previously shown to be constitutively secreted (14,37), whereas the less negatively charged forms are preferentially stored in the kidney (1,16,17), preferentially released in response to acute secretory stimuli (1,14,17), are present in the highest concentration in rat plasma (35), and have the greatest hepatic extraction ratios (35,38,39). Because the less negatively charged renin forms are characterized by high Con A affinity, complementary Con A data should indicate that renin glycoforms with high Con A affinity are preferentially stored

in the kidney, preferentially released in response to acute secretory stimuli, present in highest concentration in rat plasma, and preferentially degraded by the liver. Each of these points has been demonstrated (18,21–23). Therefore, renin isoelectric heterogeneity and renin heterogeneity demonstrated by Con A affinity chromatography must be closely related.

In conclusion, renin is a glycoprotein and thus would be expected to display oligosaccharide-chain heterogeneity. At least nine oligosaccharide chains with variable sialic acid termination have been demonstrated on prorenin secreted from Chinese hamster ovary cells transfected with human prorenin cDNA (28). Because sialic acid bears a net negative charge at physiological pH, variable sialic acid termination of oligosaccharide chains can account for renin isoelectric heterogeneity. Also, removal of sialic acid or oligosaccharide chains, or prevention of oligosaccharide chain attachment, usually results in predictable isoelectric point shifts. Renin is, in fact, heterogeneous with respect to lectin binding, and the Con A binding data are consistent with renin heterogeneity as demonstrated by isoelectric focusing. Finally, the physiological characteristics of renin forms demonstrated by isoelectric focusing and Con A affinity chromatography are in complete agreement. Variable carbohydrate attachment to renin is probably the molecular determinant of renin heterogeneity as measured either by shallow gradient isoelectric focusing or Con A affinity chromatography.

Other Renin Heterogeneity Hypotheses

Several other mechanisms could also contribute to the molecular heterogeneity of renin and result in multiple renin forms with similar molecular weights and specific activities. Such mechanisms are not necessarily exclusive of glycosylation-induced heterogeneity. For example, renin gene polymorphism has been demonstrated in the Dahl rat (40) and in humans (41). Thus, different alleles could cause renin heterogeneity in heterozygote individuals. Variable transcriptional start sites have been reported in some mouse renin genes (42) and could result in renin heterogeneity from the production of more than one type of renin transcript. The attachment of mannose 6-phosphate groups to N-linked oligosaccharides is the marker that allows cells to accumulate certain glycoprotein enzymes in lysosomes. Although renin is not a lysosomal enzyme, it is 46 percent homologous with the lysosomal enzyme cathepsin D (43) and may be partially targeted to the lysosome for proteolytic cleavage. Acquisition of mannose 6-phosphate groups on some renin oligosaccharide chains has been reported for renin expressed in some non–JG-cell culture systems (28,43) and could contribute to renin heterogeneity. Other modifications to oligosaccharide branches are also possible, including sulfated N-acetylgalactosamine attachment (44). Also, alternative forms of active renin with at least the carboxy-terminal one third of the prosegment still attached have been reported (45). Finally, newly synthesized renin may be able to fold spontaneously into multiple stable configurations, which could also contribute to renin heterogeneity (46,47), especially as measured by isoelectric focusing (5). The simplest hypothesis at this time is that most, if not all, of the heterogeneity of active renin measured by isoelectric focusing and Con A chromatography is caused by heterogeneous glycosylation resulting in multiple glycoforms.

PHYSIOLOGY OF RENIN HETEROGENEITY

The presence of oligosaccharide attachments on renin is important for JG-cell processing and secretion, as well as hepatic degradation of renin. The sum of the activities of the circulating renin glycoforms is equal to the PRA. Circulating renin glycoforms are not constant with respect to their individual plasma concentrations or their proportional contribution to PRA. The potential contribution of particular renin forms to salt-and-water balance and certain experimental models of hypertension is not yet fully elucidated but remains intriguing.

JG-Cell Sorting of Renin

Renin heterogeneity is important in JG-cell sorting and processing of renin. Active renin forms with acidic isoelectric points were first shown to be constitutively secreted (immediate nonstimulable release) in dog renal cortical slices (14). A storage pool of previously synthesized renin focusing with less acidic isoelectric points was also shown to be responsive to secretory stimulation (1). This work was later confirmed in rat renal cortical slices (37). These studies showed that the beta-adrenergic agonist isoproterenol could significantly increase active renin release from renal cortical slices but had no effect on the secretion of the newly synthesized active renin, which exhibited elevated net negative charge (relatively acidic isoelectric points). More recently, Opsahl et al. (17,48) demonstrated that the blood perfused *in situ* rabbit kidney contained a large storage pool of renin, only 4 percent of which focused with relatively acidic isoelectric points (17). Acute stimulation of renin secretion (reduction of perfusion pressure and administration of enalapril) caused a 7.3-fold increase in renin secretory rate resulting from the increased secretion of only the less negatively charged renin forms. Renin forms with the greatest net negative charge, focusing at relatively acidic isoelectric points, did not show a significant increase in secretion rate after acute stimulation, yet these same forms accounted for approximately one third of basal renin secretion and PRA (17). Figure 4 compares the iso-

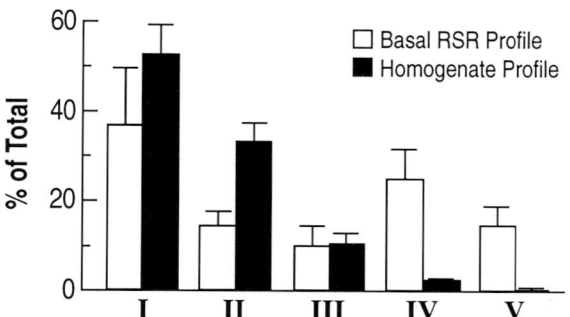

FIG. 4. Proportions of the five isoelectric forms of renin secreted by the rabbit kidney (*open bars*) compared with the same renin forms in renal cortical homogenates (*filled bars*) under basal conditions. The proportion of total active renin composed of forms I and II was significantly greater, and that composed of forms IV and V was significantly less, in the cortical homogenate compared with secreted renin. (From ref. 17, with permission.)

electric focusing profile of renin secreted from the *in situ* perfused rabbit kidney under basal conditions to the corresponding renal cortical homogenate profile. Basal renin secretion and renal renin content were resolved into five separate active renin forms (I to V). Renin forms with the greatest net negative charge (forms IV and V) accounted for more than one third of basal renin secretion and only 4 percent of the renal renin content. Thus, forms IV and V appear to be constitutively secreted.

The segregation of renin into constitutive and regulated pathways in the JG cell is important for renin secretion. *In vivo*, the hourly renin secretory rate (RSR) under basal conditions is approximately 1 percent of renal renin content (17,48–50). Thus, even in the absence of renin synthesis, enough renin is stored to maintain the basal RSR for approximately 100 hours. Release of this large storage pool is responsible for acute increases in RSR (via the regulated pathway), because acute stimulation can result in up to a 5- to 15-fold increase in RSR within a few minutes. Such an increase can be maintained for many hours (17,48,51,52) without corresponding changes in renin mRNA (53). In fact, an acute increase in RSR can occur even when renin synthesis is blocked (54). Constitutive secretion of newly synthesized active renin provides steady basal addition of renin to the plasma compartment. Regulated renin secretion allows for the sudden addition of renin to the plasma compartment in response to acute stimuli for renin release.

The sorting signal directing JG-cell renin into constitutive or regulated secretory pathways is probably differential glycosylation. As previously explained (see *Renin Glycoforms*), constitutively secreted renin appears to be composed primarily of forms that have relatively acidic isoelectric points as a result of attachment of complex-type oligosaccharides with terminal sialic acid residues. Such renin forms are also characterized by low Con

A affinity, and, consistent with the data available regarding the more negatively charged isoelectric forms, renin glycoforms with low Con A affinity are not stored within the kidney and are not preferentially released in response to acute secretory stimuli (18,21–23). Furthermore, TM, which interferes with normal N-linked glycosylation, alters the proportion of secreted renin forms (32). (Tunicamycin does not universally alter secretion of glycoproteins. This has led many investigators to conclude that glycosylation does not generally aid glycoprotein secretion, except for transport to lysosomes via the mannose 6-phosphate signal. However, glycosylation does seem a likely candidate as a signal for at least some glycoprotein sorting in the cell [55].)

In an independent assessment of the role of renin glycosylation in renin secretion, mutated prorenin or renin coding vectors were prepared in which one or both of the asparagine glycosylation sites were altered to prevent glycosylation. Two separate groups of investigators found large alterations in renin and prorenin secretion after introduction of these constructs into cultured cells and concluded that glycosylation was necessary for proper sorting and secretion (27,91). Therefore, secretion of active renin appears to result from two pathways. In the first pathway, newly synthesized renin with attached oligosaccharide chains terminating in sialic acid is immediately secreted and not responsive to secretory stimulation (constitutive pathway). In the second regulated pathway, renin storage granules containing renin with high-mannose–type oligosaccharide attachments are available to release renin in response to acute secretory stimulation. The sorting process appears to be dependent on glycosylation, although not all secreted glycoproteins depend on oligosaccharide attachment to aid in cell sorting. The dual pathway of constitutive and regulated secretory routes is common to many polypeptide endocrine systems (56–58) and, as discussed below, is vital for control of the RAS.

The overall functional significance of these observations is that the specific carbohydrate configurations of the renin oligosaccharide chains, which contribute to isoelectric and Con A heterogeneity, are the intracellular sorting signals for constitutive and regulated secretion and allow the kidney to increase the plasma renin concentration rapidly without relying on synthesis-dependent mechanisms. Acute stimulation of renin secretion results in the immediate release of less negatively charged high Con A affinity renin forms. Thus, the increase in PRA observed after acute stimulation of RSR is caused by an increased plasma concentration and proportion of the less negatively charged renin forms possessing high Con A affinity. This observation has been documented in the rat (35), dog (39), rabbit (17), and in humans, using both isoelectric focusing (59) and Con A affinity chromatography (21). As discussed in the next section, the less negatively charged high Con A affinity renin forms are also preferentially cleared by the liver and kidney.

Hepatic Clearance of Renin

The plasma concentration of renin is set by the RSR as well as the clearance rate from the circulation. The main route of elimination for plasma renin appears to be through the liver, although renal degradation may also play a role (60–63). Reduced hepatic clearance of renin contributes to increased PRA in models of sodium depletion (64,65), heart failure (66), and human hepatic cirrhosis (67–69).

Perhaps the most important physiological consequence of the presence of multiple active renin forms is that the different forms are cleared by the liver at different rates. Canine active renin forms focusing above an arbitrarily selected pH(I) of 5.0 exhibited a combined single-pass hepatic extraction of approximately 40 percent. The combined extraction percentage for renin forms focusing below a pH(I) of 5.0 was significantly less and approximately equal to 20 percent (39). This work has been confirmed and extended in the rat. After nephrectomy, the decay of six isoelectric forms of active rat renin were followed for 100 minutes, and each was fitted to separate double-exponential decay curves. A progressive decrease in the hepatic removal of renin was found as the pH(I) became more acidic (35). This is shown in Fig. 5. In another study of hypertensive humans, active plasma renin was resolved into five main renin forms focusing at pH(I)'s of 5.7, 5.6, 5.5, 5.2, and 5.1, with respective single-pass hepatic extraction percentages of 33, 30, 18, 9, and 11. The combined single-pass hepatic extraction percentage for all active plasma renin was found to be 17.3 (38). In each of the three studies above, renin focusing at less acidic isoelectric points (less net negative charge) was cleared from the circulation between three and five times faster than renin forms focusing with more acidic isoelectric points.

The data available regarding the role of renin glycosylation in hepatic removal of multiple renin forms both complement and extend the isoelectric focusing work reviewed above. Mouse submaxillary renin, which does not possess N-linked oligosaccharide chains, is primarily cleared by the kidney (70), whereas glycosylated renin of renal origin is predominantly cleared by the liver (61,62). Deglycosylation of renin results in reduced hepatic and increased renal uptake (24). Therefore, glycosylation appears necessary for hepatic removal of renin. Kim et al. (18) found that hepatic extraction of rat renin was a direct function of Con A binding. Three active renin glycoforms separated by Con A affinity chromatography showed significant differences in hepatic clearance such

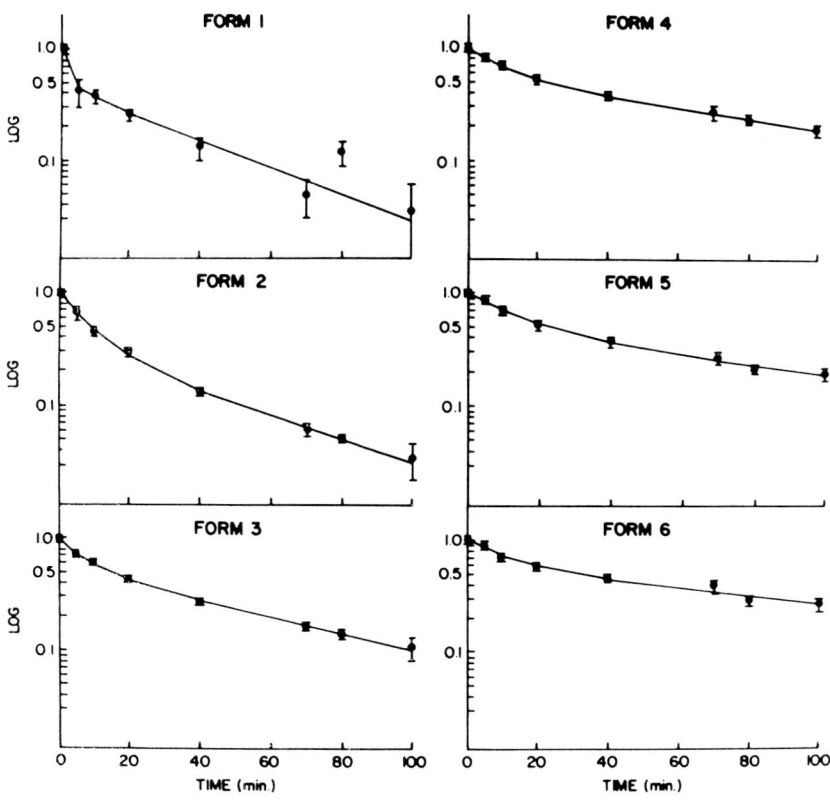

FIG. 5. Plasma decay rates of six isoelectric forms of active renin in the rat after bilateral nephrectomy. Corresponding isoelectric points for forms 1 to 6 were 5.9, 5.7, 5.4, 5.2, 5.0, and 4.8. The continuous curves through the mean data are the result of a weighted least-squares fit of the data by a two-compartment model. Greater net negative charge (more acidic or lower isoelectric point) results in slower hepatic clearance. (From ref. 35, with permission.)

that the higher the Con A affinity, the faster the hepatic clearance. This was confirmed by Marks et al. (23). Because Con A exhibits a specific high affinity for mannose (33), it seems likely that the liver possesses a binding site for some part of the oligosaccharide chains of renin that have sterically available mannose groups. Marks et al. demonstrated such lectin binding for renin on hepatic nonparenchymal cells. The receptor was a mannose-type receptor because hepatic uptake of renin was blocked by mannosylated bovine serum albumin and mannan (23), although at least one other hepatic uptake mechanism was also found for renin. Vertebrate hepatic membrane mannose/N-acetylglucosamine lectins have been previously described (71). Presumably, renin binds to a hepatic mannose/N-acetylglucosamine or similar receptor, initiating receptor-mediated endocytosis and destruction of renin in the lysosomal compartment (23,62).

Thus, the less the net negative charge associated with renin (resulting in higher or less acidic isoelectric points) or the greater the available mannose on the oligosaccharide chains of renin (resulting in high Con A binding), the greater the hepatic extraction of active renin forms. This fits together well because renin forms with less net negative charge tend to be high-mannose–type glycoproteins with corresponding high Con A affinity, whereas renin forms possessing greater net negative charge tend to be complex-type glycoproteins with correspondingly

low affinity for Con A (see *Renin Glycoforms*). In general, heterogeneity of plasma protein glycosylation ensures a range of short-lived and long-lived circulating forms of the glycoprotein (44).

Active renin clearance occurs to a lesser extent in the kidney than the liver (60–63). The most likely route for the renal extraction of renin is via glomerular filtration, followed by reabsorption and subsequent catabolism in proximal tubule cells, although a small fraction of filtered renin appears in the urine (72). Glomerular filtration of proteins as large as renin is a function of net charge. Renal glomerular capillaries are less permeable to negatively charged protein than to equal-sized cationic proteins because of a negatively charged glomerular endothelial surface (73). Therefore, the kidney would be expected to preferentially remove renin forms with less net negative charge, just as observed with the liver. However, preferential hepatic clearance of renin forms is caused by binding of specific high-mannose–type oligosaccharide structures, whereas preferential renal clearance most likely involves the degree of net negative charge. The end result is that preferential clearance of the same renin forms by both the liver and the kidney should occur, although preferential renal clearance has not yet been directly demonstrated.

The different hepatic (and renal) removal rates of multiple active renin forms potentially explain some of the great variability in reported renin half-lives and metabolic clearance rates. Renin half-life has previously been resolved into one or two components with values ranging from 10 to 450 minutes (63). Part of the reason for these disparate results is that active renin can be resolved into a profile of multiple renin forms, each of which exhibits a distinct two-exponential plasma decay curve (35). Moreover, because acute stimulation alters the circulating renin form profile, the half-life of plasma renin after acute stimulation will be shorter than that under steady-state conditions. Similarly, the half-life of renin purified from renal cortical homogenate would be very short because the less negatively charged renin forms with short plasma half-lives predominate in stored renin granules within the JG cells (17).

Physiological Significance of Preferential Renal Secretion and Hepatic Clearance of Active Renin Forms

Acute stimulation of renin secretion results in increased plasma concentrations of less negatively charged high-mannose–type renin forms that are preferentially cleared by the liver and probably the kidney. Acute stimulation results in preferential renal secretion of renin with a short plasma half-life, allowing PRA to return rapidly to prestimulation levels unless the secretory stimulus is sustained (3,17,35,38,39,59). If necessary, an acute increase in RSR can be sustained because of the large storage pool of previously synthesized renin present in the JG cells (17). Chronic stimulation of RSR, as seen with a low-salt diet, is accompanied by an almost proportional increase in the size of the JG-cell renin storage pool (49,74,75), so that acute stimulation of RSR during a high renin state is probably analogous to acute stimulation during a normal renin state. Thus, regulated secre-

tion of active renin provides a variable source of short-lived renin to the plasma compartment, whereas constitutive secretion of newly synthesized renin provides a constant (basal) source of long-lived renin to the plasma compartment. This results in a fine control mechanism for setting PRA and is very consistent with our knowledge of circulating glycoproteins (44). In conclusion, the specific structure of the renin oligosaccharide chains determine JG-cell sorting of renin and hepatic (and renal) degradation of renin. High-mannose oligosaccharide attachments to renin (resulting in less negatively charged renin with high Con A affinity) causes preferential JG-cell storage, preferential release after acute stimulation, and preferential clearance from the circulation. Although it may seem paradoxical that the total clearance of active renin increases at a time when the acute secretory rate is elevated, this situation probably serves to buffer acute increases in PRA when a transient stimulus is not maintained. A diagram of this relationship is shown in Fig. 6.

Multiple Active Renin Forms and Enzymatic Activity

The multiple forms of active renin appear to possess approximately the same specific enzymatic activity (6,8,9,29), and deglycosylation of renin does not appear to affect enzymatic activity (76). Also, mouse submaxillary renin is not glycosylated (70), yet is active enzymatically. These studies indicate that glycosylation is not needed for renin activity. Specific renin inhibitors appear to inhibit each of the main human renin isoelectric forms with the same dose-response characteristics, again indicating that heterogeneity or differential glycosylation of renin does not directly affect enzymatic action (32). Therefore, it is not surprising that the preferential renal

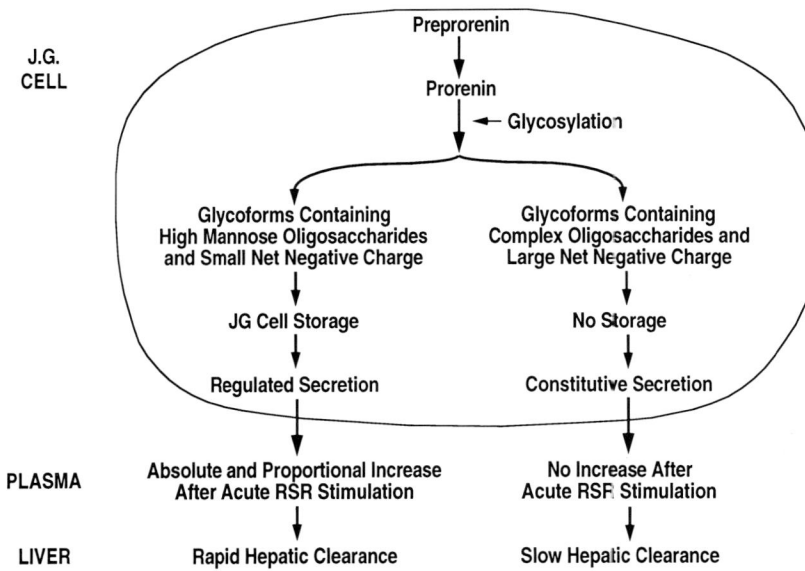

FIG. 6. Schematic overview of multiple active renin forms and their structure-function relationship. Heterogeneity is assumed to result only from variable glycosylation resulting in multiple active renin forms or glycoforms. For simplicity, active renin heterogeneity is represented by only two possible pathways. Also, the conversion of prorenin to active renin and the secretion of prorenin have been omitted. Glycosylation of renin occurs in the endoplasmic reticulum and Golgi apparatus. *RSR,* Renin secretory rate.

secretion and hepatic clearance of multiple renin forms, as discussed above, occurs by mechanisms that are independent of variation in enzymatic-specific activity. However, although glycosylation does not alter renin enzymatic activity, it may provide stability to renin (77), possibly by increasing the water solubility of the enzyme.

Effect of Multiple Active Renin Forms on Salt-and-Water Balance

Because the multiple forms of active renin possess approximately the same specific activity, it would seem unlikely that different forms of the enzyme could be functionally distinct with respect to salt-and-water balance. However, renin forms do differ with respect to charge and animal lectin-binding affinities, both of which could lead to variable tissue access or tissue binding and therefore impart distinctive biologic activities.

One way to assess the biologic effects of renin forms would be to observe the effects of separate purified forms on relevant physiological systems. Kim et al. (78) semipurified and then separated six forms of active rat renin with isoelectric focusing. Equipressor doses of the forms were then injected either intravenously or intraventricularly into anesthetized rats. As expected, the greater the net negative charge of the renin form, the longer the duration of the blood pressure response, reflecting differences in plasma half-life. Unexpectedly, intravenous injection of active renin form IV [fourth most acidic isoelectric point, $pH(I) = 5.2$] caused significant increases in urine flow, excretion of sodium and potassium, and urine osmolality. Other active renin forms were without effect. The renal effects of form IV were abolished by converting enzyme inhibition and were not caused by pressure-induced natriuresis or diuresis, because all six renin forms were given at equipressor doses, and the duration of the blood pressure increase was greater for renin forms V and VI. Further work revealed that plasma aldosterone concentrations were similar after separate renin form infusions and that nonrenin renal proteins copurified with the renin forms were not responsible for the differing effects on renal function (79). Intraventricular infusions of individual renin forms did not raise arterial pressure, yet form VI induced a significant natriuresis that was abolished by converting enzyme inhibition (78). One possible explanation for these results is that certain renin forms have preferential access into particular tissue compartments where the local generation of angiotensin I and II mediates changes in salt-and-water balance.

Similar findings were demonstrated by McKenzie et al. (80) using trypsin-activated prorenin obtained from human ovarian follicular fluid. These investigators injected activated renin forms with $pH(I)$'s of 5.8, 5.6, 5.4, 5.2, 5.1, and 4.9 into anesthetized rats and found large increases in urine volume and sodium excretion for the middle renin forms but no effect for the renin forms focusing at $pH(I)$'s of 5.8 or 4.9. The diuresis and natriuresis were prevented by pretreatment with captopril and not associated with differences in creatinine clearance. Nonactivated prorenin also displayed isoelectric heterogeneity and produced effects similar to the injection of the corresponding activated prorenin forms (80).

Taken together, these studies suggest that multiple renin forms may have functionally significant and different physiological roles. Differential tissue access of circulating renin forms, or direct tissue synthesis of specific renin forms, is a possible mechanism for the differential action of multiple renin forms. This concept has been examined for several tissue systems involved in salt-and-water balance. For instance, both isoelectric and Con A renin heterogeneity have been demonstrated in human pituitary tissue (81), and human prorenin isoelectric focusing patterns were found to be different for amniotic fluid compared with maternal plasma and ovarian tissue (82). In a preliminary report, vascular renin was also shown to focus in different proportions than plasma renin (83). Differences in renin form proportions between tissues and plasma suggest that some renin forms may have preferential access to, or be synthesized by, the tissue.

In addition to the renal and vascular effects already discussed, renin heterogeneity may be important to physiological function in the adrenal gland. Endogenous production of renin by the adrenal gland has been implicated in the regulation of aldosterone production in adrenal glomerulosa cells (84–86). Both isoelectric and Con A heterogeneity of adrenal renin have been demonstrated (84,85). However, the proportions of renin forms in the adrenal gland did not match those in corresponding plasma samples. Also, alterations in salt intake affected the renin form isoelectric profile in the adrenal gland and plasma differently (84). These results reinforce the hypothesis that certain tissues can either preferentially admit specific renin forms from the circulation or produce specific renin forms. Therefore, preferential access of circulating renin forms or tissue synthesis of specific renin forms may be involved in the control of salt-and-water balance. If so, the mechanism(s) responsible for these effects is not yet understood.

Multiple Active Renin Forms and Hypertension

Because of the variability of PRA in various types of hypertension (including essential hypertension), renin heterogeneity would not be expected to play a constant role in its pathogenesis. However, the participation of active renin heterogeneity in several types of experimental hypertension has been examined. The main finding has been a strong positive correlation between the proportions of renin forms focusing at acidic pH and blood pressure.

Sessler and Malvin (87) studied renin heterogeneity in the two-kidney one-clip Goldblatt hypertensive rat (GHR) at 13 to 45 and 90 days postclip. During the first 2 weeks, systolic blood pressure increased from an average of 119 mm Hg to 183 mm Hg. Renin from the incubation medium of renal cortical slices, renal cortical homogenates, and plasma consistently focused into six isoelectric peaks. The proportion of negatively charged renin forms (forms focusing at more acidic pH) was significantly increased in cortical slice incubation medium and renal homogenates derived from the clipped kidney, as well as the plasma of GHR rats compared with controls. The effect tended to be more pronounced at 90 days. The modification of the renin profile in GHR was correlated with time, blood pressure, and renin concentration, although the correlation may have been indirect and not causative. It is possible that the chronic renal artery stenosis caused the increased secretion of acidic renin forms and that the acidic renin forms mediated the increased blood pressure, perhaps by preferential vascular wall access and subsequent local vascular generation of angiotensin I and II.

The isoelectric heterogeneity of active renin has also been examined in spontaneously hypertensive stroke-prone (SHRSP) and normotensive Wistar-Kyoto (WKY) rats. The proportion of each of six renin isoelectric forms secreted by renal cortical slices was different between SHRSP and WKY rats (88). The SHRSP again showed an increase in the proportion of the more negatively charged acidic renin forms, and crossing SHRSP with WKY led to intermediate blood pressures and acidic renin form proportions in F1 progeny. These observations led to the hypothesis that the blood pressure increase in SHRSP was related to the more negatively charged active renin forms and that these traits were under common genetic control. In a second study, there was a remarkable correlation between systolic blood pressure and the fraction of renal renin content that consisted of the three most negatively charged rat renin forms (forms 4 + 5 + 6) in SHRSP, WKY, and their genetic F1 crosses (89). This correlation, which is shown in Fig. 7, did not appear to be secondary to hypertension *per se,* because DOCA hypertensive rats (low renin model of hypertension) did not exhibit the correlation despite increased blood pressure. It was concluded that renin-dependent hypertension may be caused not only by an increased PRA but by the type of renin secreted. The correlation between acidic renin forms and hypertension in some animal models may indicate a causal relationship, but that relationship requires further study.

Prorenin

The physiological significance of prorenin (inactive renin) is not well understood. Prorenin is glycosylated and

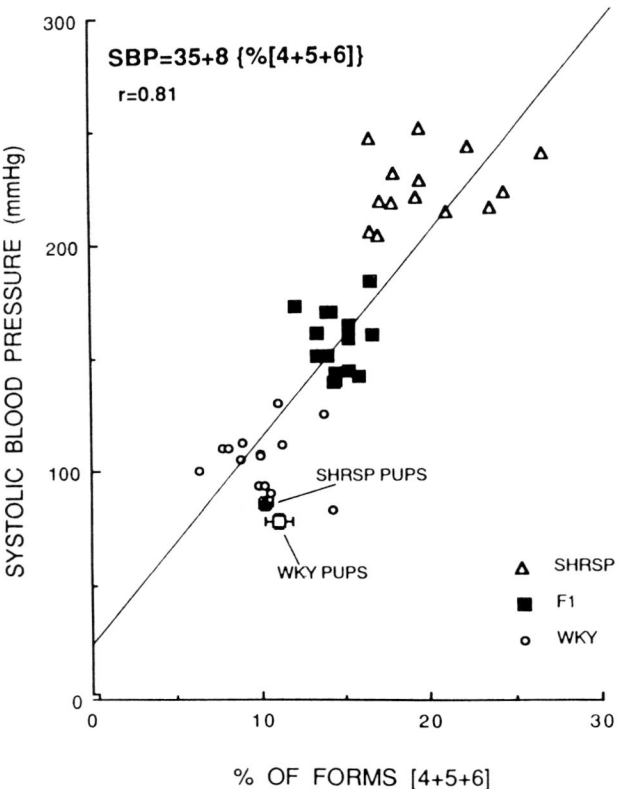

FIG. 7. Relationship between the percentage of the more negatively charged renin forms (4 + 5 + 6) in renal cortical homogenates and systolic blood pressure (*SBP*) in spontaneously hypertensive stroke-prone (*SHRSP*) rats, Wistar-Kyoto (*WKY*) rats, and their genetic crosses (*F1*). (From ref. 89, with permission.)

heterogeneous. Recombinant prorenin contains many heterogeneous oligosaccharide structures (28). As previously mentioned, the heterogeneity of prorenin has been demonstrated by Con A affinity chromatography and isoelectric focusing (12,13,20,31,80,82,84). The reported isoelectric points are generally higher for inactive renin than for renin and fall on activation with trypsin.

In JG cells, prorenin is either converted to renin by a cathepsin B–like enzyme that may be present in immature secretory granules, or secreted into the plasma compartment via a constitutive pathway (90). Glycosylation of prorenin occurs before conversion of prorenin to active renin and before constitutive prorenin secretion.

In one report, only certain isoelectric peaks of inactive prorenin produced a marked diuresis and natriuresis when injected into rats, indicating a possible physiological role for prorenin heterogeneity (80). The possibility that the specific oligosaccharide structures attached to renin can determine JG-cell sorting of prorenin has also been shown (27). The significance of prorenin heterogeneity may not be revealed until the physiological role of prorenin is elucidated.

CONCLUSIONS

Active renin heterogeneity has been shown to exist in all animals studied, across a wide evolutionary scale encompassing fish, amphibians, birds, and mammals, including humans. Both Con A affinity chromatography and shallow gradient isoelectric focusing can resolve active renin into multiple forms. Variable carbohydrate composition of the oligosaccharide structures attached at the two N-linked glycosylation sites on renin are probably responsible for active renin heterogeneity. Heterogeneous glycosylation results in active renin glycoforms, with differing oligosaccharide structures containing varying amounts of mannose and terminating with variable numbers of negatively charged sialic acid residues. Multiple renin glycoforms can therefore be detected by Con A affinity chromatography based on the available mannose and by isoelectric focusing based on the charge heterogeneity imparted by sialic acid. The presence of renin glycoform heterogeneity appears to have several important physiological consequences. First, glycosylation is probably the sorting signal directing JG-cell renin into a constitutive or regulated secretory pathway. Active renin forms with high net negative charge resulting from complex oligosaccharide attachment are constitutively secreted. Renin forms exhibiting high-mannose–type oligosaccharide chains with relatively little net negative charge are stored in the JG cell and released in response to acute stimulation. Second, the high-mannose renin forms with relatively little net negative charge are preferentially cleared by the liver, allowing for fine control of PRA. Finally, renin glycoforms may have functionally significant and different physiological roles despite their apparently equal enzymatic-specific activities. Preferential tissue access of specific circulating renin forms, or tissue synthesis of specific renin forms, may be involved in the control of salt-and-water balance and the setting of blood pressure and may play a pathogenetic role in some forms of hypertension.

REFERENCES

1. Katz SA, Malvin RL. *Endocrinology* 1982;111:814–819.
2. Malvin RL, Katz SA, Kim SH. *Chin J Physiol* 1991;34(1):81–91.
3. Katz SA, Malvin RL. In: Robertson JIS, Nicholls MG, eds. *The renin-angiotensin system*. London: Grover Medical Publishers; 1993:24.1–24.13.
4. Skeggs LT, Lentz KE, Kahn JR, Hochstrasser H. *Circ Res* 1967;(Suppl II)21:II-91–II-100.
5. Rubin I. *Scand J Clin Lab Invest* 1972;29:51–58.
6. Lauritzen M, Damsgaard JJ, Rubin I, Lauritzen E. *Biochem J* 1976;155:317–323.
7. Printz MP, Dworschack RT. *Biochim Biophys Acta* 1977;494:162–171.
8. Matoba T, Murakami K, Inagami T. *Biochim Biophys Acta* 1978;526:560–571.
9. Galen FX, Devaux C, Guyenre T, Menard J, Corvol P. *J Biol Chem* 1979;254:4848–4855.
10. Conio G, Ghiani P, Patrone E, Trefiletti V, Uva B, Vallarino M. *Biochim Biophys Acta* 1980;623:317–328.
11. Druilhet RE, Overturf ML. In: Sambhi MP, ed. *Heterogeneity of renin and renin substrate*. Elsevier North Holland, 1981:89–99.
12. Chang JJ, Kisaragi M, Okamoto H, Inagami T. *Hypertension* 1981;3:509–515.
13. Eggena P, Barrett JD, Wiedman CE, et al. In: Sambhi MP, ed. *Heterogeneity of renin and renin-substrate*. Elsevier North Holland, 1981:215–225.
14. Katz SA, Malvin RL. *Endocrinology* 1982;111:201–207.
15. Do Y-S, Shinagawa T, Tam H, Inagami T, Hsueh WA. *J Biol Chem* 1987;262(3):1037–1043.
16. Katz SA, Abraham PA, Opsahl JA. *Renal Physiol Biochem* 1992;15:240–248.
17. Opsahl JA, Abraham PA, Katz SA. *J Am Soc Nephrol* 1993;4:1054–1063.
18. Kim S, Hosoi M, Hiruma M, Ikemoto F, Yamamoto K. *Am J Physiol* 1989;256(Endocrinol Metab 19):E798–E804.
19. Kim S, Hosoi M, Kikuchi N, Yamamoto K. *J Biol Chem* 1991;266:7044–7050.
20. Kim S, Hoisoi M, Hiruma M, Ikemoto F, Yamamoto K. *Clin Exp Hypertens* [A] 1988;A10(6):1203–1211.
21. Hosoi M, Kim S, Ikemoto F, Yamamoto K. *Life Sci* 1990;47:1903–1913.
22. Hosoi M, Kim S, Yamamoto K. *Clin Sci* 1991;81:393–399.
23. Marks DL, Kost LJ, Kuntz SM, Romero JC, LaRusso NF. *Am J Physiol* 1991;261(Gastrointest Liver Physiol 24):G349–G358.
24. Kim S, Hiruma M, Ikemoto F, Yamamoto K. *Am J Physiol* 1988;255:E642–E651.
25. Rademacher TW, Parekh RB, Dwek RA. *Annu Rev Biochem* 1988;57:786–838.
26. Kornfeld R, Kornfeld S. *Annu Rev Biochem* 1985;54:631–664.
27. Rothwell V, Kosowski S, Hadjilambris O, Baska R, Norman J. *DNA Cell Biol* 1993;4:291–298.
28. Aeed PA, Guido DM, Mathews WR, Elhammer AP. *Biochemistry* 1992;31:6951–6961.
29. Su Y, Reudelhuber TL. *J Hypertens* 1993;11:141–146.
30. Beeley JG. In: Burdon RH, van Knippenberg PH, eds. *Laboratory techniques in biochemistry and molecular biology*. Vol. 16. Amsterdam: Elsevier; 1985:88–90.
31. Egan DA, Grzegorczyk V, Tricarico K, Rueter A, Holleman W, Marcotte P. *Biochim Biophys Acta* 1988;965:68–75.
32. Katz SA, Malvin RL, Lee J, et al. *Proc Soc Exp Bio Med* 1991;197:387–392.
33. Sharon N, Lis H. *FASEB J* 1990;4:3198–3208.
34. Katz SA, Malvin RL. *Renal Physiol* 1984;Basel 7:275–282.
35. Sessler FM, Jacquez JA, Malvin RL. *Am J Physiol* 1986;250(Endocrinol Metab 13):E551–E557.
36. Katz SA, Opsahl JA, Abraham PA. *FASEB J* 1992;6(5):A1810.
36a.Katz SD, Opsahl JA, Abraham PA, Gardner MJ. *Am J Physiol* 1994;(Regulators Integrative Comp. Physiol):in press.
37. Kawamura M, Parmentier M, Inagami T. *Am J Physiol* 1988;255:F100–F107.
38. Abraham PA, Katz SA, Opsahl JA, Miller RP, Stanchfield WR Jr, Andersen RC. *Hypertension* 1990;16:669–676.
39. Shier DN, Malvin RL. *Am J Physiol* 1985;249:79–R84.
40. Rapp JP, Wang S-M, Dene H. *Science* 1989;243:542–544.
41. Soubrier F, Jeunemaitre X, Rigat B, Houot A-M, Cambien F, Corvol P. *Hypertension* 1990;16:712–717.
42. Paul M, Burt DW, Krieger JE, Nakamura N, Dzau VJ. *Am J Physiol* 1992;262(Endocrinol Metab 25):E644–E650.
43. Faust PL, Chirgwin JM, Kornfeld S. *J Cell Biol* 1987;105:1947–1955.
44. Drickamer K. *Cell* 1991;67:1029–1032.
45. Shinagawa T, Do YS, Baxter J, Hsueh WA. *Biochemistry* 1992;31:2758–2764.
46. Englander SW. *Science* 1993;262:848–849.
47. Rahuel J, Priestle JP, Grutter MG. *J Structural Biol* 1991;107:227–236.
48. Opsahl JA, Abraham PA, Katz SA. *Kidney Int* 1990;38:440–446.
49. Park CS, Malvin RL, Murray RD, Cho KW. *Am J Physiol* 1978;234(6):F506–F509.
50. Ludwig G, Ganten D, Murakami K, Fasching U, Hackenthal E. *Mol Cell Endocrinol* 1987;50:223–229.
51. Mangelsen EL, Malvin RL. *Renal Physiol* 1978;1:247–253.
52. Finke R, Gross R, Hackenthal E, Huber J, Kirchheim HR. *Pflugers Arch* 1983;399:102–110.

53. Nakamura N, Soubrier F, Menard J, Pantheir JJ, Rougeon F, Corvol P. *Hypertension* 1985;7:855–859.
54. Katz SA, Malvin RL. *Am J Physiol* 1982;243(Renal Fluid Elect Physiol 12):F434–F439.
55. Olden K, Bernard BA, Humphries MJ, et al. *TIBS* 1985;10:78–82.
56. Kelly RB. *Science* 1985;230:25–32.
57. Chung K-N, Walter P, Aponte GW, Moore H-P. *Science* 1989;243:192–197.
58. Burgess TL, Kelly RB. *Annu Rev Cell Biol* 1987;3:243–293.
59. Opsahl JA, Abraham PA, Katz SA. *Am J Hypertens* 1991;4:126–130.
60. Keiser JA, Romero JC, Kost LJ, LaRusso NF. *Hepatology* 1987;7:1254–1261.
61. Kim S, Iwao H, Nakamura N, Ikemoto F, Yamamoto K. *Am J Physiol* 1987;252:E136–E146.
62. Kim S, Iwao H, Nakamura N, et al. *Am J Physiol* 1987;253:E621–E628.
63. Campbell DJ. In: Robertson JIS, Nicholls MG, eds. *The renin-angiotensin system.* London: Grover Medical Publishers; 1993:23.1–23.23.
64. Johnson JA, Davis JO, Baumber JS, Schneider EG: *Am J Physiol* 1971;220:1677–1682.
65. Echtenkamp SF, Davis JO, Freeman RM, Dietz JR, Villarreal D. *Am J Physiol* 1983;245:H573–H579.
66. Schneider EG, Davis JO, Robb CA, Baumber JS. *Circ Res* 1969;24:213–219.
67. Mitch WE, Whelton PK, Cooke CR, Walker WG, Maddrey WC. *Am J Med* 1979;66:804–810.
68. Barnardo DE, Strong CG, Baldus WP. *J Lab Clin Med* 1969;74:495–506.
69. Wernze H, Rupp W, Tittor W, Schmitt A. In: Langer M, Chiandussi L, Chopra IJ, Martini L, eds. *The endocrines and the liver.* London: Academic Press; 1982:445–448.
70. Nakamura N, Iwao H, Ikemoto F, Yamamoto K. *J Hypertens* 1984;2:241–248.
71. Baroneds SH. In: Liener IE, Sharon N, Goldstein IJ, eds. *The lectins—properties, functions, and applications in biology and medicine.* London: Academic Press; 1986:437–466.
72. Stella A, Zanchetti A. In: Robertson JIS, Nicholls MG, eds. *The renin-angiotensin system.* London: Grover Medical Publishers; 1993:22.1–22.8.
73. Valtin H. Glomerular filtration. In: *Renal function.* 2nd ed. Boston: Little Brown & Co.; 1983:43–63.
74. Naftilan AS, Oparil S. *Am J Physiol* 1981;240(Renal Fluid Electrolyte Physiol 9):F501–F507.
75. Fray JCS. *Am J Physiol* 1978;234:F376–F380.
76. Carilli CT, Vigne J-L, Wallace LC, et al. *Hypertension* 1988;11:713–716.
77. Hori H, Yoshino T, Ishizuka Y, Yamauchi T, Murakami K. *FEBS Lett* 1988;232:391–394.
78. Kim SH, Lloyd MC, Sessler FM, Feng J, Malvin RL. *Am J Physiol* 1988;254:F432–F439.
79. Malvin RL, Chen M, Lloyd MC. *Am J Hypertens* 1989;2:414–418.
80. McKenzie JK, Jones DR, McKenzie IM, Smyth DD. *Am J Physiol* 1991;261:F975–F981.
81. Mizuno K, Ojima M, Hashimoto S, et al. *Life Sci* 1985;37:2297–2304.
82. Khalidi N, McKenzie I, McKenzie JK. *Am J Hypertens* 1991;4:56–59.
83. Katz SA, Zupfer GH, Ayenew W, Opsahl JA. *J Am Soc Nephrol* 1993;4:514.
84. Kim SH, Sessler FM, Malvin RL. *Am J Physiol* 1988;255(Endocrinol Metab 18):E531–E536.
85. Mizuno K, Ojima M, Hashimoto S, et al. *Clin Sci* 1987;72:699–704.
86. Yamaguchi T, Naito Z, Stoner G, Franco-Saenz R, Mulrow P. *Hypertension* 1990;16:635–641.
87. Sessler FM, Malvin RL. *Am J Physiol* 1985;248:E694–E698.
88. Sessler RM, Jokelainen PT, Sing CF, Strack AM, Malvin RL. *Am J Physiol* 1986;251(Endocrinol Metab 14):E367–E372.
89. Lee J, Malvin RL, Jokelainen PT. *Am J Physiol* 1989;257:F275–F279.
90. Hsueh WA, Baxter JD. *Hypertension* 1991;17:469–479.
91. Baxter JD, James MNG, Chu WN, et al. *Yale J Biol Med* 1989;62:493–501.

Hypertension: Pathophysiology, Diagnosis, and Management, Second Edition,
edited by J.H. Laragh and B.M. Brenner,
Raven Press, Ltd., New York © 1995.

CHAPTER 90

Control, Cardiovascular, and Renal Effects of Potassium

David B. Young

A relationship between high dietary potassium intake and prevention of cardiovascular disease is supported by a large, diverse but controversial body of evidence. The support has come from anthropology, epidemiology, population-based research, clinical intervention, trials, and animal experimentation. The first entry on the subject in the modern scientific literature was that by Ambard and Beauchard (1), who reported in 1904 that they had succeeded in lowering the blood pressure in five of eight patients by raising the amount of potassium intake and decreasing the amount of sodium intake. Since then, evidence supporting a protective effect of potassium has accumulated and now represents a convincing argument. Some of the more persuasive and intriguing aspects of the evidence are:

1. Although approximately one-third of the population of industrialized cultures, whose diet is low in potassium and high in sodium, develop hypertension, less than 1 percent of primitive populations who consume a high potassium, low sodium intake develop hypertension (2–5).

2. A diet high in potassium is associated with reduced incidence of stroke in man (6) and animals (7), even in the absence of an effect on blood pressure.

3. Analyses of subgroups of populations from diverse origins demonstrate a consistent increase in blood pressure when a subgroup relocates from its initial condition in which the diet is high in potassium and low in sodium to a new condition in which dietary sodium is high and potassium is low (8,9).

4. In experimental animals, high dietary potassium protects against stroke (7), hypertension (10), cardiac hypertrophy (11), renal glomerular lesions (10), and medial hypertrophy of the arterioles of the kidneys (10) and reduces blood cholesterol and deposition of cholesterol in the aorta (11).

The information supporting potassium's protective effect has been reviewed in detail in the chapter by Tobian, to which the reader is referred for detailed discussion of the data.

The controversy associated with the proposal that potassium has a cardiovascular protective effect is primarily related to three factors: First, raising potassium intake in animals or in man does not always reduce blood pressure or provide a measurable protective effect, and frequently very large increases in potassium intake have

D. B. Young: Department of Physiology and Biophysics, University of Mississippi Medical Center, Jackson, Mississippi 39216-4505.

been reported to be associated with only modest blood pressure reductions. Second, under some conditions large increases in potassium intake are not associated with statistically significant increases in plasma potassium concentration. Finally, there are few established hypotheses capable of accounting for potassium's cardiovascular protection. The first two areas may be related to failure to consider during the design and analysis of the experiments the nature of the system that controls potassium. The control system is complex and contains multiple components, some of which are also involved in regulation of blood pressure and sodium balance. Inadequate appreciation of the nature of the control system could well lead to experimental designs that are not capable of testing hypotheses concerning a relationship between potassium intake and blood pressure regulation. The third source of controversy, absence of accepted hypotheses to explain potassium's protective effects, has stimulated productive investigations in several laboratories that may have provided a framework for analyzing potassium's mechanisms of protection.

The goal of this chapter is to provide information helpful in analyzing potassium's potential role in protection against cardiovascular disease. The chapter will not contain descriptions of studies in which potassium's intake was changed while arterial pressure was measured, for such studies have yielded conflicting results for more than half a century. Nor will the literature concerning the relationship between potassium and blood pressure derived from epidemiological studies be presented here; this subject is covered in depth in the chapter by Tobian. Instead, emphasis will be placed on two subjects: (a) analyses of the physiological regulation of potassium; and (b) the physiological effects of changes in potassium concentration on cardiovascular functions responsible for diseases such as hypertension, heart failure, stroke, and atherosclerosis. From this presentation it is hoped the reader will have an improved perspective of the controversies concerning potassium's protective role against cardiovascular disease.

REGULATION OF POTASSIUM

Approximately 2 percent of the total body potassium is in the extracellular fluid, about 70 mEq for a 70-kg man. During the course of a day, as much as two to three times this amount of potassium may be absorbed from the gut into the extracellular fluid and then be excreted by the kidneys. However, even during the absorptive period plasma potassium concentration must be maintained close to its set-point in order to maintain normal function of neuromuscular tissue. In fact, under normal conditions plasma potassium concentration does not vary more than 15 percent from its desired level throughout the course of a day. The daily rate of intake may

range from one-quarter of the normal level to more than five times normal on a given day or over periods of weeks and months. Even under these conditions plasma potassium concentration must be held within normal limits close to the set-point if normal physiological function is to be maintained.

A highly effective control system operates to maintain plasma potassium concentration and potassium balance within normal limits. The system can operate only by affecting the movement of potassium into and out of the extracellular fluid. Movement of potassium between the intra- and extracellular spaces is an important component of regulation of extracellular fluid potassium concentration, although the mechanisms that control the transmembrane flux act only as short-term buffers of changes. Potassium intake in the diet is not regulated, and absorption from and excretion into the gut are not subject to quantitatively important active regulation. Therefore, long-term regulation of potassium is mediated solely by controlling the rate of renal excretion, which can vary from less than 10 mEq/day to well over 400 mEq/day. The rate of excretion is affected by inherent alterations in nephron function in response to changes in plasma potassium concentration and by changes in the concentration of aldosterone and other hormones reaching the kidney in the blood. The distribution of potassium between the intra- and extracellular spaces can be altered in long-term conditions and is also regulated in part by aldosterone.

A number of factors are capable of affecting potassium distribution and excretion but are not part of the negative feedback control system, which controls the concentration of the ion. For example, insulin and epinephrine both stimulate transfer of potassium from the extra- to the intracellular space. However, these hormones are not part of the control system, for changes in potassium concentration within the physiological range do not affect the rates of secretion of the hormones (see 12 for review). Therefore, changes in the concentrations of epinephrine and insulin represent problems for the control system and are not part of the solution. These hormones are key elements in negative feedback control systems that operate to maintain control of other variables in the body, and when, for example, insulin levels are strongly elevated in the postprandial period, its effect on potassium distribution can cause a sharp fall in potassium concentration. Similarly, during periods of cardiovascular stress such as following myocardial infarction due to coronary artery thrombosis, the extremely high levels of epinephrine present in the circulation can reduce plasma potassium concentration to very low levels. Clearly, these hormones are not acting to control potassium concentration, but rather are creating short-term disturbances in the regulation of potassium.

Analysis of potassium regulation can be confounded by the effects of insulin and epinephrine because insulin concentration may change more than tenfold following a meal. Since changes in concentration of the hormone of this magnitude have the capability of acutely reducing plasma potassium concentration by 15 to 20 percent, measurement of potassium concentration in blood samples drawn in the postprandial period may be considerably lower than during most of the day. To obtain consistent and representative measurements of potassium concentration in the plasma, samples must be taken during a fasting period. Because increases in epinephrine concentration can cause very rapid reductions in potassium concentration in the plasma of 20 percent or more, samples for measurement of the ion's concentration must be obtained from unstressed subjects. This is always difficult in experimental animals and in man, particularly so because the stress that results in elevated epinephrine concentrations may be cold (a very powerful stimulant of epinephrine secretion in small animals), anesthesia, and exercise, as well as anxiety. The artifactual effects of elevated concentrations of these hormones are capable of masking changes in steady-state concentration of potassium that may have developed during the course of an experiment.

In this section, information concerning the operation of the control system will be presented. Because long-term changes in potassium concentration are believed to be required to affect the development of cardiovascular disease, the presentation will be limited to information regarding elements of the long-term control system.

The Nephron

Potassium is freely filtered across the glomerular membrane although the amount entering the nephron from the glomerulus has little influence on the rate of potassium excretion. Approximately 80 percent of the filtered potassium is reabsorbed in the proximal convoluted tubule, and an additional 10 percent is transported out of the tubule along the thick ascending limb of Henle's loop. Further potassium reabsorption can take place along the distal tubule and collecting ducts when potassium conservation is required. However, under normal conditions potassium secretion occurs across the epithelium of the distal nephron and collecting ducts, especially in the most distal sections of the distal tubule (cortical connecting tubule) and the cortical portion of the collecting tubule. Cells in these tubular segments respond to physiological signals by changing their rate of potassium secretion over a wide range. Control of potassium excretion is mediated primarily by modulating function of these cells.

Two cell types are found in the cortical connecting tubule and the cortical collecting tubule, the principal cell and the intercalated cell. Evidence has been presented by Stanton and Giebisch (13) indicating that the principal cells secrete potassium and that the intercalated cells are responsible for potassium reabsorption from the lumen. The potassium absorptive mechanisms are of limited quantitative importance in man, as evidenced by the poor capability to resist potassium depletion during extended periods of low potassium intake. Furthermore, the mechanisms of potassium reabsorption are poorly understood and have not been completely described at this time. On the other hand, the potassium secretory functions of the principal cells are extremely powerful and have been well characterized. Recently, Giebisch (14) reviewed the function of the principal cells and has described five characteristics of their transport mechanisms.

1. *Sodium-potassium adenosine triphosphatase (ATPase) is the main transport element located in the basolateral membrane.* This enzyme system is responsible for uptake of potassium from, and extrusion of sodium into, the peritubular fluid. The sodium-potassium ATPase operates in an electrogenic mode and responds to changes in extracellular potassium concentration, changes in extracellular pH, and variations in mineralocorticoid hormone concentration. In response to increases in aldosterone concentration, activation of the electrogenic sodium-potassium exchange results in hyperpolarization of these cells. Stanton and Giebisch (15) analyzed the direct effect of changes in extracellular potassium concentration on the rate of potassium secretion into the distal nephron. They found that small increases in concentration dramatically raised the rate of secretion (Fig. 1). We designed a series of experiments to quantitatively assess the direct effect of potassium on renal potassium excretion over periods of days and weeks (16). Adrenalectomized dogs were maintained on continuous replacement of aldosterone at the normal level, 50 μg/day given as a continuous intravenous infusion together with a basal level of glucocorticoid supplementation. Sodium intake was held at the normal level throughout the course of the experiment. The dogs received a diet containing 10 mEq/day of potassium. The daily potassium intake was changed in steps of 7 to 10 days' duration by infusing additional amounts so that the total daily intake was increased from 10 to 30, then to 100, and finally to 200 mEq/day. At the conclusion of each level of intake, plasma K and renal excretion, as well as other variables known to influence potassium excretion, were measured. There were minimal changes in arterial pH, mean arterial pressure, extracellular fluid volume, or glomerular filtration rate (GFR) at any of the levels of K intake. Therefore, the change in renal K excretion was related primarily to the change in plasma K, which occurred as a result of alteration of K intake. The two variables were plotted in Fig. 2, with plasma K being the independent variable. The magnitude of the slope of the relationship, 260 mEq/day per mEq/liter increase in concentration

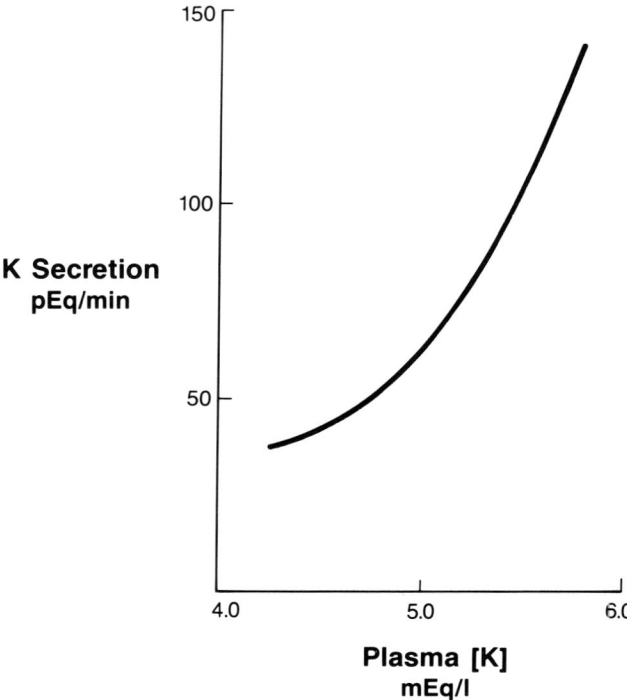

FIG. 1. Potassium secretion rate into the distal tubule as a function of plasma potassium concentration. The distal tubule was perfused at a constant rate throughout the experiment. These results show the magnitude of the direct stimulatory effect of elevating plasma potassium concentration on potassium secretion. (Modified from ref. 15.)

above 4.2 mEq/liter, suggests that this relationship may be the most prominent controller of K excretion above the normal plasma concentration. However, below the normal intake level the slope of the plasma K urinary excretion relationship is much less impressive, 11 mEq/day per mEq/liter.

2. *The basolateral membrane has a conductive pathway for potassium that generates a diffusion potential for potassium ions from cell to peritubular space.* The pathway plays a role in the increased rate of potassium secretion in response to stimulation by mineralocorticoid hormones. With mineralocorticoid treatment, the potassium conductance of the basolateral membrane increases. When the membrane is hyperpolarized as a result of the effect of the hormone on the sodium-potassium ATPase, the electrogenic stimulation of the pump raises the membrane potential above the potassium equilibrium value, causing potassium ions to be driven from the peritubular fluid into the cell. This is in contrast to the situation when the pump is unstimulated and the membrane potential is below the potassium equilibrium value.

3. *In the apical cell membrane, potassium-selective channels are present that provide a route for potassium secretion from cell to lumen.* Potassium enters the tubule lumen, driven by a forcible electrochemical potential gradient. Increasing the potassium concentration difference between cellular fluid and lumen, either by lowering tubular potassium concentration or by increasing cytoplasmic potassium activity, increases the rate of secretion. Similarly, increasing the negativity of the tubular lumen stimulates secretion of the potassium ion. The permeability of the luminal membrane for potassium is subject to regulation and plays an important part in the overall control of the rate of secretion. It is increased by mineralocorticoid administration and is reduced by acidification of the lumen as well as by administration of barium. Exposure to a high-potassium diet increases apical potassium conductance, whereas a diet low in potassium reduces luminal potassium conductance. Analysis of the behavior of single potassium channels in apical membranes of isolated rabbit cortical and collecting tubules has demonstrated that the potassium channels are stimulated by calcium ions and that they are voltage-sensitive. Luminal membrane depolarization results in increased opening of the potassium channels. The voltage sensitivity may explain the increase in potassium conductance of the apical membrane following mineralocorticoid stimulation; the mineralocorticoid stimulation results in a reduction in the apical membrane po-

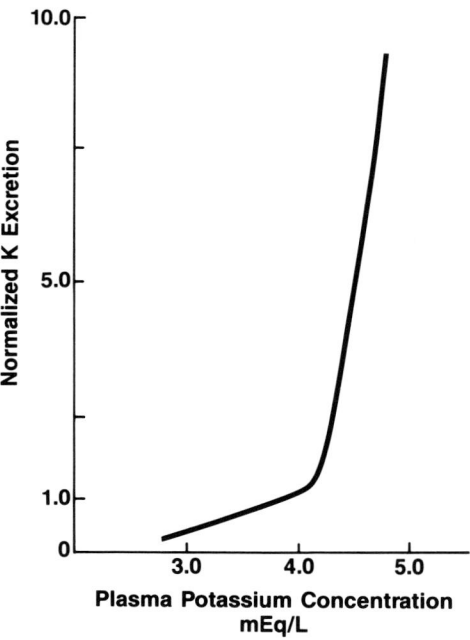

FIG. 2. The relationship between long-term changes and plasma potassium concentration and the rate of renal potassium excretion. Above the normal level of potassium concentration, 4.2 mEq/L, potassium excretion rate increases 26 mEq/day for each 0.1-mEq/L increase in steady-state plasma concentration. The normal rate of excretion from these animals was 22 mEq/day. (Modified from ref. 16.)

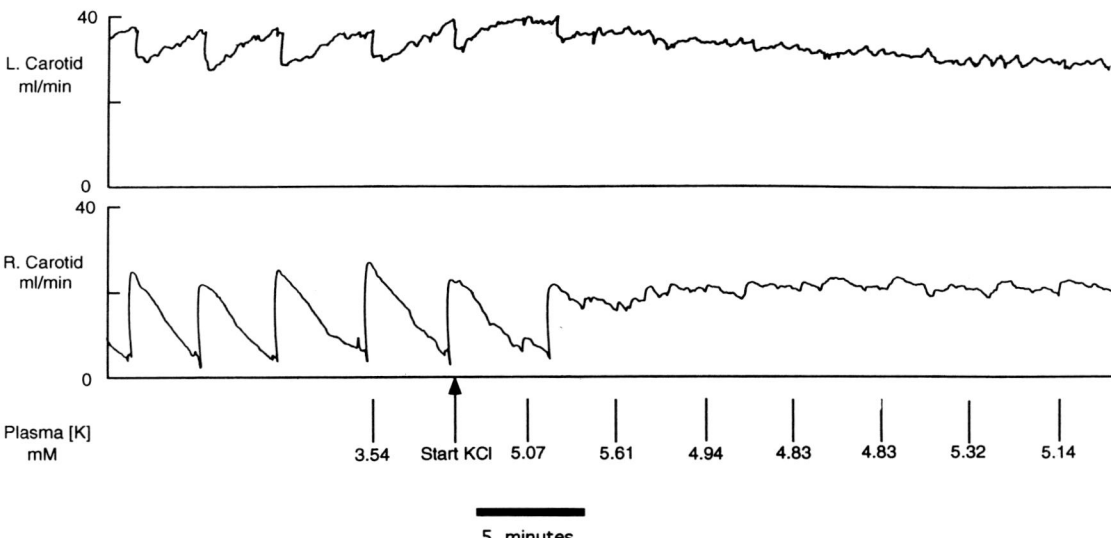

FIG. 12. Left and right carotid artery blood flows of an anesthetized rabbit. The right artery was prepared with damaged endothelium and a constrictor to produce a pattern of thrombus formation resulting in cyclical blood flow reduction. When flow approached zero in the artery the constrictor was temporarily removed, allowing the thrombus to dislodge and disaggregate and blood flow to return to the initial level. At that point the constrictor was replaced and the new thrombus began to form. This consistent pattern of cyclical blood flow reductions due to thrombus formation was interrupted by intravenous KCl infusion resulting in elevation of potassium concentration from 3.54 mEq/L to approximately 5 mEq/L. The concentrations of potassium are given (*bottom*).

incidence of stroke in a study of approximately 1,000 residents of Rancho Bernardo, California. They found that in women there was a statistically significant decrease in stroke associated with a 10-mEq/day increase in potassium intake. Interestingly, Lee and coworkers (58) found in a study of 7,591 Japanese men in Honolulu that increased potassium intake was associated with reduced incidence of thromboembolic strokes but was not associated with a changed incidence of hemorrhagic cerebral vascular incidents. The direct effect of small increases in potassium concentration to inhibit thrombus formation demonstrated in our recent experiments provide a possible mechanism relating increases in potassium intake to protection against stroke in experimental animals and man.

CONCLUSIONS

The control system that maintains potassium homeostasis is extremely effective in preventing changes in potassium concentration when potassium intake is greater than normal. However, this system is relatively inadequate in preventing reductions in potassium concentration below the normal level when potassium intake is reduced to less than the normal daily intake rate. Furthermore, the decrease in plasma potassium concentration as potassium intake falls below normal is accentuated by high levels of sodium intake. These are critical considerations for understanding the relationship between potassium intake and the cardiovascular effects of the ion. Any relationship between change in potassium intake and change in cardiovascular function would be expected to be more pronounced in the range of potassium intake below normal, particularly so if below-normal potassium intake were coupled with greater-than-normal sodium intake. Increasing potassium intake from normal to a value greater than normal may not produce a measurable change in plasma potassium concentration or in the function of the cardiovascular system. However, if potassium intake were increased from well below normal to the normal rate, potassium concentration would be expected to rise measurably and cardiovascular function would be more likely to be affected.

In considering relationships between potassium intake and cardiovascular disease, the importance of time or the duration of the observation period may be important. Changes in potassium intake result in rapid responses of the potassium control system, which bring the rate of potassium excretion toward the rate of intake. However, excretion may not reach the point of balance with the rate of intake for many days; therefore, the plasma potassium concentration may change slowly but measurably over a week or more. This is particularly significant when potassium intake is reduced from a high to a low level, or when sodium intake is raised.

Changes in potassium concentration affect a number

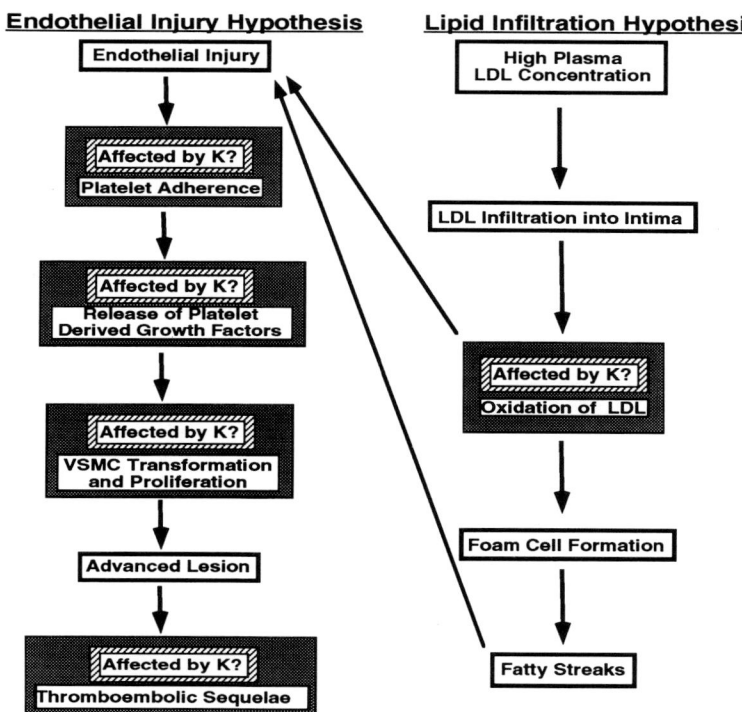

Endothelial Injury Hypothesis

Endothelial Injury

Affected by K?
Platelet Adherence

Affected by K?
Release of Platelet
Derived Growth Factors

Affected by K?
VSMC Transformation
and Proliferation

Advanced Lesion

Affected by K?
Thromboembolic Sequelae

Lipid Infiltration Hypothesis

High Plasma
LDL Concentration

LDL Infiltration into Intima

Affected by K?
Oxidation of LDL

Foam Cell Formation

Fatty Streaks

FIG. 13. Combined endothelial injury–lipid infiltration hypothesis for atherosclerotic lesion formation and points at which increases in potassium concentration may impede lesion development. (Modified from ref. 59.)

of the central components of blood pressure and sodium balance control systems. These include functions that regulate nephron sodium reabsorption, renal blood flow, and GFR. Although the effects of these components have been studied primarily in short-term experiments, some analyses of longer duration have been undertaken and demonstrate a sustained effect of changes in potassium on these systems. Therefore, this interaction between increases in potassium concentration with the central elements of the "pressure natriuresis/body fluid volume/blood pressure control system" may be responsible for the protective effects of high dietary potassium intake against the development of hypertension.

Any proposed relationship between dietary potassium intake and development of vascular lesions will be more complex than the proposed relationship to blood pressure regulation. However, the developing hypothesis concerning the mechanisms involved in formation of atherosclerotic lesions in general will undoubtedly be useful in understanding potassium's potential role. The general hypothesis is illustrated in Fig. 13 (59). One of the earliest events is believed to be the oxidation of LDLs in the subintima of the arteries by reactive oxygen species produced by monocytes, macrophages, and possibly endothelial cells and smooth muscle cells. This is one point at which elevation of potassium concentration may be effective in inhibiting the path toward lesion development. Vascular smooth muscle proliferation in the subendothelium is a process involved in the maturation of the lesion and is also a point at which elevation of potassium concentration may be effective in slowing the prog-

ress of the development. In addition, adherence of platelets to the damaged endothelium overlying the developing lesion may be inhibited by elevations in potassium concentration. Potassium's ability to inhibit the thromboembolic consequences of advanced atherosclerotic lesions is supported by evidence from several sources. Therefore, this aspect of potassium's potential protective effect does have a base of support from experimental and clinical data. However, at this time the quantitative importance of potassium's potential effects and the temporal relationship between changes in potassium intake and vascular protection remain to be determined.

Whether or not potassium is related to blood pressure control and development of cardiovascular disease, as well as its potential for use therapeutically in treatment and prevention of disease, remain to be determined. In view of the potential importance of these questions to the cardiovascular health of the population of the industrialized nations, potassium's potential cardiovascular protective effects demand continued intensive study.

ACKNOWLEDGMENTS

This work was supported by Grants from USPHS HL21435 and 11678. The author expresses his gratitude for the assistance of Drs. Huabao Lin, Richard D. McCabe, Douglas E. Fitzovich, and Yi Jen Pan for their assistance in conducting the research presented from this laboratory.

REFERENCES

1. Ambard L, Beauchard C. *Arch Gen Med* (Paris) 1904;81:520–533.
2. Trowell H, Burkett DP. *Western diseases: their emergence and prevention.* London: Edward Arnold, 1981.
3. Lowenstein FW. *Lancet* 1961;1:389–392.
4. Truswell AS, Kennelly BM, Ansen JD, Lee RD. *Am Heart J* 1972;84:5–12.
5. Cerqueira MT, McMurry M, Fry W, Connor WE. *Am J Clin Nutr* 1979;32:905–915.
6. Khaw KT, Barrett-Connor E. *N Engl J Med* 1987;316:235–240.
7. Tobian L, Lange J, Ulm K, et al. *Hypertension* 1985;7[Suppl 2]:110–114.
8. Page LB, Damon A, Moellering RC Jr. *Circulation* 1974;49:1132–1146.
9. Poulter N, Khaw KT, Hopwood BEC, Mugambi M, Peart WS, Sever PS. *J Cardiovasc Pharmacol* 1984;6:S197–S203.
10. Tobian L, McNeill D, Johnson MA, et al. *Hypertension* 1984;6[Suppl I]:170–176.
11. Tobian L, Jahner TM, Johnson MA. *Am J Hypertens* 1990;3:133–135.
12. DeFronzo RA, Bia M. In: Seldin DW, Giebisch G, eds. *The kidney: normal and abnormal function.* New York: Raven Press, 1985;1179–1206.
13. Stanton BA, Giebisch G. In: Corradino RA, ed. *Functional regulation at the cellular and molecular levels.* Amsterdam: Elsevier, 1982;259–283.
14. Giebisch GM. In: Giebisch G, ed. *Potassium transport: physiology and pathophysiology. Current topics in membrane transport,* vol 28. San Diego: Academic Press, 1987;133–183.
15. Stanton BA, Giebisch GM. *Am J Physiol* 1982;243:F487–F493.
16. Young DB. *Am J Physiol* 1982;242:F599–F604.
17. Berliner RW, Kennedy TJ Jr, Hilton JG. *Am J Physiol* 1950;162:348–367.
18. Stanton BA, Biemesderfer D, Wade JB, Giebisch G. *Kidney Int* 1981;19:36–48.
19. Young DB, Smith MJ Jr, Tipayamontri U, Read RH. *Physiologist* 1982;25:299.
20. Pan YJ, Young DB. *Hypertension* 1982;4:279–287.
21. Young DB, Jackson TE. *Am J Physiol* 1982;243:R526–R530.
22. Young DB, Smith MJ Jr, Jackson TE, Scott RC. *Am J Physiol* 1984;247:E328–E335.
23. Young DB. *Endocr Rev* 1985;6:24–44.
24. Young DB. In: Giebisch G, ed. *Potassium transport: physiology and pathophysiology. Current topics in membrane transport,* vol 28. San Diego: Academic Press, 1987;269–295.
25. Watson RL, Langford HG, Abernethy J, Barnes TY, Watson ML. *Hypertension* 1980;2:I93–I98.
26. Langford HG, Watson RL. In: Paul O, ed. *Epidemiology and control of hypertension.* Miami: Miami Symposium Specialists, 1975;119–128.
27. Berenson GS, Voors AW, Dalferes ER, Webber LS, Shuler SE. *J Lab Clin Med* 1979;93:533–547.
28. Grim CE, Luft FC, Miller JZ, Christian JC, Wienberger MH. *J Chron Dis* 1980;33:87–94.
29. Clausen T, Kjeldsen K. In: G. Giebisch, ed. *Potassium transport: physiology and pathophysiology. Current topics in membrane transport,* vol 28. San Diego: Academic Press, 1987;403–419.
30. Hayslett JP, Mykerey N, Binder HJ, Aronson PS. *Am J Physiol* 1980;239:F378–F382.
31. Baustein MP. *Physiologist* 1976;19:525–540.
32. Brandis M, Keyes J, Windlager EE. *Am J Physiol* 1972;222:421–427.
33. Stokes JB. *Am J Physiol* 1981;241:F395–F402.
34. Sufit CR, Jamison RL. *Am J Physiol* 1983;245:F569–F576.
35. Kirchner KA. *Am J Physiol* 1983;244:F599–F605.
36. Young DB, McCaa RE, Pan YJ, Guyton AC. *Am J Physiol* 1976;231:945–953.
37. Young DB, McCaa RE, Pan YJ, Guyton AC. *Circ Res* 1976;38:II84–II89.
38. Corvol P, Oblin ME, Degoulet P, Fressinaud PH, Menard J. *Endocrinology* 1977;100:1008–1013.
39. Vander AJ. *Am J Physiol* 1970;219:455–459.
40. Sealey JE, Clark I, Bull MB, Laragh JH. *J Clin Invest* 1970;49:2127.
41. Shade RE, Davis JO, Johnson JA, Witty RT. *Circ Res* 1972;31:719–727.
42. Lin H, Young DB, Smith MJ Jr. *Am J Physiol* 1991;260:F170–F176.
43. Lin H, Young DB. *Am J Physiol* 1988;254:F704–F710.
44. Wilkerson PR. *Cardiovasc Med* 1978;3:181–183.
45. Materson BJ, Cushman WC, Goldstein G, et al. *Hypertension* 1990;15:348–360.
46. Harrison CE Jr, Novak LP, Connolly DC, Brown AL Jr. *J Lab Clin Med* 1970;75:185–196.
47. Gunning JF, Harrison CE Jr, Coleman HN III. *J Mol Cell Cardiol* 1972;4:139–153.
48. Brace RA, Anderson DK, Chen W-T, Scott JB, Haddy FJ. *Am J Physiol* 1974;227:590–597.
49. Fitzovich DE, Hamaguchi M, Tull WB, Young DB. *J Am Coll Cardiol* 1991;18:1105–1111.
50. McCabe RD, Young DB, Srivastava K. *FASEB J* 1993;7:A316.
51. McCabe RD, Young DB. *Am J Hypertens* 1994;7:(in press).
52. Srivastava K, McCabe RD, Young DB. *FASEB J* 1993;7:A105.
53. Srivastava K, McCabe RD, Young DB. (*submitted*).
54. Young DB, McCabe RD. *FASEB J* 1992;6:A1698.
55. Lin H, Young DB. *FASEB J* 1993;7:A116.
56. Lin H, Young DB. *Circulation* 1994;89:331–338.
57. Folts JD, Crowell EB, Rowe GG. *Circulation* 1976;54:365–370.
58. Lee CN, Reed DM, MacLean CJ, Yano K. *N Engl J Med* 1988;318:995.
59. Steinberg D, Parthasarathy S, Carew TE, Khoo JC, Witztum JL. *Free Radic Biol Med* 1990;9:155–168.
60. Young DB. *Am J Physiol* 1988;255:F811–F822.

Hypertension: Pathophysiology, Diagnosis, and Management, Second Edition,
edited by J.H. Laragh and B.M. Brenner,
Raven Press, Ltd., New York © 1995.

CHAPTER 91

Lipid-Lowering Agents, Renal Function, and Hypertensive Disease in Experimental Models

Michael P. O'Donnell and William F. Keane

Renal disease, particularly of a chronic nature, is frequently associated with lipid abnormalities and hypertension. It has been appreciated for some time that elevated systemic blood pressure can aggravate the course of renal disease. Indeed, many studies over the past decade have demonstrated a beneficial effect of antihypertensive therapy in slowing the decline in renal function in chronic renal disease. Perhaps less well appreciated is the mounting experimental evidence that lipid abnormalities may contribute to the progression of renal disease. Experiments in several animal models of renal disease and hyperlipidemia, both hypertensive and normotensive models, have suggested that hyperlipidemia may directly injure the glomerulus and contribute to progressive glomerular injury. Many of these experiments have investigated the effects of lipid-lowering agents on the course of experimental renal disease. The first focus of this chapter, therefore, is to summarize the experimental data in the literature that suggest a role for lipids in progressive renal disease. Second, the possible mechanisms by which lipids might injure the glomerulus will be discussed. These include direct effects of lipoproteins on glomerular mesangial cells as well as possible hemodynamic consequences of hyperlipidemia. Last, this chapter will address altered vascular reactivity that may result secondarily from hyperlipidemia in renal disease and how such altered vascular function could contribute to the development of hypertension.

EXPERIMENTAL MODELS OF RENAL DISEASE AND HYPERLIPIDEMIA

The Dahl Salt-Sensitive Rat

The Dahl salt-sensitive (DS) rat has been studied as one experimental model of human essential hypertension. Dahl salt-sensitive rats fed a diet high in sodium

M. P. O'Donnell: Regional Kidney Disease Program, Minneapolis, Minnesota 55404.
W. F. Keane: Division of Nephrology, Department of Medicine, Hennepin County Medical Center, Minneapolis, Minnesota 55415.

chloride (4–8 percent by weight) develop marked systemic hypertension (1,2). The magnitude of the blood pressure increase as well as the rate of development of hypertension are dependent on the level of dietary sodium. By contrast, control Dahl salt-resistant (DR) rats remain normotensive despite a high salt intake (1,2).

Dahl salt-sensitive rats also develop chronic, progressive glomerular disease. Indeed, glomerular abnormalities have been described in DS rats prior to the development of hypertension. Sterzel et al. (3) demonstrated "microalbuminuria" in 6-week-old, prehypertensive DS rats, and this was associated with segmental loss of podocyte foot processes. After initiation of a high salt diet, systemic hypertension and marked albuminuria typically develop in DS rats, and this is associated with progressive glomerular histologic injury characterized by mesangial matrix expansion and focal glomerulosclerosis (3–5).

The mechanisms responsible for initiation and progression of glomerular injury in DS rats are unclear. Recent micropuncture studies (3–6) have demonstrated that glomerular pressures are not elevated in prehypertensive or mildly hypertensive DS rats, suggesting that other factors are responsible for initiation of glomerular injury in this model. Elevated glomerular capillary pressure, however, may occur in older DS rats with more severe hypertension (7) and may be an important determinant of progression of glomerular injury in this model.

Several studies have demonstrated abnormal lipid metabolism in DS rats. O'Donnell et al. (4) found an approximately 30-percent increase in fasting serum triglycerides in 6-week-old, prehypertensive DS rats compared with levels in age-matched control DR rats. Development of hypertension in DS rats fed 4 percent NaCl was associated with progressive increases in both serum triglycerides and serum cholesterol. At 24 weeks of age, triglycerides and cholesterol in hypertensive DS rats were each about twice the respective serum levels in age-matched DR rats (4). Subsequent studies by Reaven et al. (8) and Mondon et al. (9) have confirmed hypertriglyceridemia in male DS rats. These authors did not, however, report whether serum cholesterol levels were increased in DS rats. Mondon et al. also reported that the mechanism of hypertriglyceridemia in DS rats likely involves a combination of increased hepatic triglyceride secretion and decreased triglyceride removal from plasma (9).

One recent study has demonstrated that lipid abnormalities in DS rats, particularly hypercholesterolemia, may be important in the pathogenesis of glomerulosclerosis in this model (5). O'Donnell et al. treated DS rats fed 4 percent NaCl with the HMG-CoA reductase inhibitor lovastatin (Mevacor) for a period of 22 weeks. Lovastatin treatment prevented the rise in serum cholesterol that occurred in untreated DS rats (Fig. 1). Interestingly, lovastatin-treated DS rats also had lower blood pressures

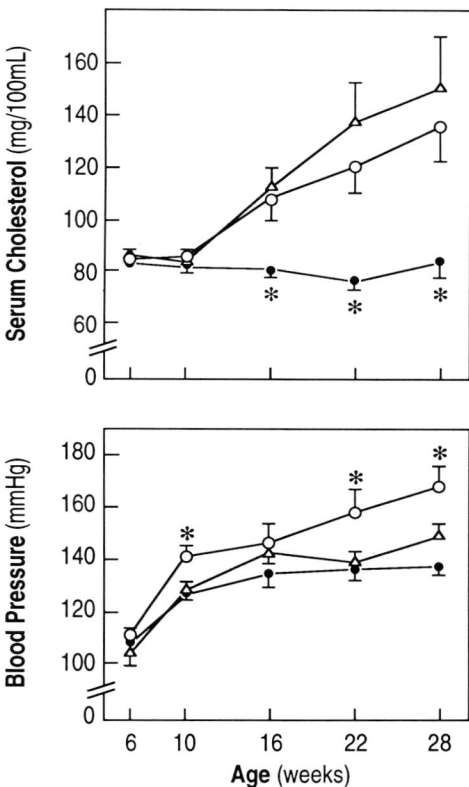

FIG. 1. Fasting serum cholesterol (**top panel**) and awake, systolic blood pressure (**bottom panel**) in vehicle-treated (*open circles*), lovastatin-treated (*closed circles*), and enalapril-treated (*triangles*) Dahl salt-sensitive rats. *$p < .05$ vs other two groups. (Adapted with permission from: O'Donnell MP, Kasiske BL, Katz SA, Schmitz PG, Keane WF. Lovastatin but not enalapril reduces glomerular injury in Dahl salt-sensitive rats. Hypertension 1992;20:651–658. Copyright 1992 American Heart Association.)

than untreated DS rats (see Fig. 1). Throughout the treatment period, lovastatin-treated DS rats had significantly lower urine albumin excretion compared with untreated DS rats (Fig. 2). Moreover, at 28 weeks of age, the percent of glomeruli with glomerulosclerosis was less than 3 percent in lovastatin-treated DS rats, compared with 16 percent in untreated DS rats (see Fig. 2). These results suggested, therefore, that lipids might be important in the development of glomerular injury in DS rats.

In the same study (5), a separate group of salt-fed DS rats was treated with the angiotensin-converting enzyme (ACE) inhibitor enalapril. Although enalapril was effective in lowering blood pressure in DS rats (see Fig. 1), there was no significant effect of enalapril on either urine albumin excretion or glomerulosclerosis (see Fig. 2). This contrasted with beneficial effects of ACE inhibitors to reduce albuminuria and glomerular structural injury in several other experimental models of chronic, progressive renal disease (10–13). The DS rat may be somewhat unique, however, in that this strain, particu-

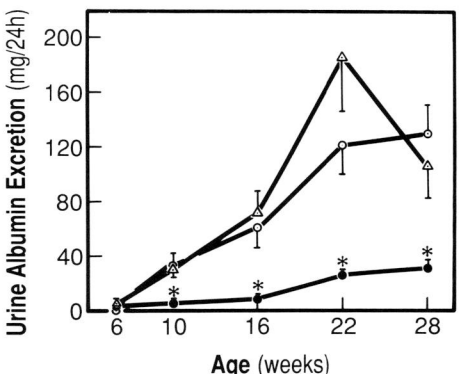

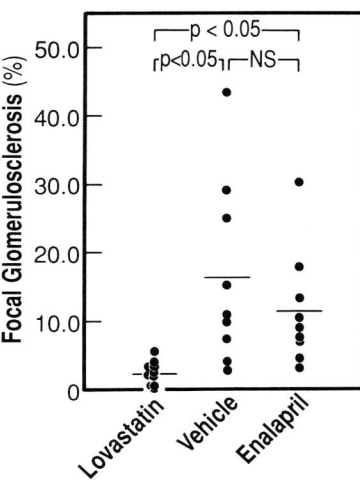

FIG. 2. Top: Albuminuria in vehicle-treated (*open circles*), lovastatin-treated (*closed circles*), and enalapril-treated (*triangles*) Dahl salt-sensitive rats. *$p < .05$ vs other two groups. **Bottom:** Percentage of glomeruli with any focal glomerulosclerosis in each of the three groups of Dahl S rats at 28 weeks of age. The mean percentage in each group is represented (*horizontal bars*). (Adapted with permission from: O'Donnell MP, Kasiske BL, Katz SA, Schmitz PG, Keane WF. Lovastatin but not enalapril reduces glomerular injury in Dahl salt-sensitive rats. Hypertension 1992;20:651–658. Copyright 1992 American Heart Association.)

action was suggested to involve normalization of P450 ω-hydroxylation of renal outer medullary fatty acids and correction of defective loop chloride transport. Whether lovastatin might lower blood pressure in DS rats by a similar mechanism has not been examined.

Remnant Kidney Model of Progressive Renal Disease

Subtotal nephrectomy has been widely used as an experimental maneuver to investigate mechanisms responsible for chronic, progressive glomerular injury. Most studies have been performed in rats, and in most cases, 3/4–5/6 nephrectomy was performed by the combination of unilateral nephrectomy and infarction of portions of the remaining kidney. This "remnant kidney" model is characterized by rapid development of systemic and glomerular hypertension and progressive glomerular disease (17–20). The chronology of glomerular structural changes in 5/6-nephrectomized rats has been described in detail by Floege et al. (21). Increased glomerular cell proliferation was observed from day 5 after renal ablation, peaking at week 2. Glomerular monocyte/macrophages were elevated at week 2 and increased progressively to week 10 when the experiment was terminated. There is much interest in the potential role of glomerular macrophages in mediating both acute and chronic glo-

larly with high salt feeding, demonstrates very low plasma renin activity (14,15). It was suggested, therefore, that in a setting of high salt intake and low renin activity, ACE inhibitors may not be effective in reducing glomerular injury (5).

The mechanism by which lovastatin attenuated the rise in blood pressure in salt-fed DS rats is not known, although this finding suggests that lipids might somehow be involved in the development of hypertension in DS rats. A recent study by Roman et al. (16) also supports this possibility. In their study, DS rats fed 8 percent NaCl and treated with the lipid-lowering agent clofibrate had markedly lower blood pressures compared with untreated DS rats (Fig. 3). The mechanism of the clofibrate

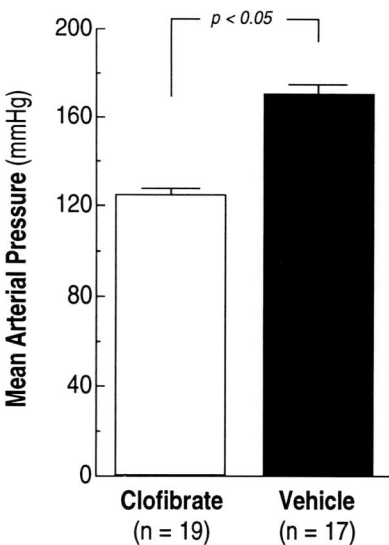

FIG. 3. Effect of clofibrate (80 mg/day) on mean arterial blood pressure in Dahl salt-sensitive rats fed 8.0-percent NaCl diet for 4 weeks. Blood pressures were recorded for 3-hour periods on 4 consecutive days in conscious animals in their home cages. For each rat, a mean value for the entire recording period was determined. (Adapted with permission from: Roman RJ, Ma Y-H, Frohlich B, Markham B. Clofibrate prevents the development of hypertension in Dahl salt-sensitive rats. Hypertension 1993;21:951–958. Copyright 1993 American Heart Association.)

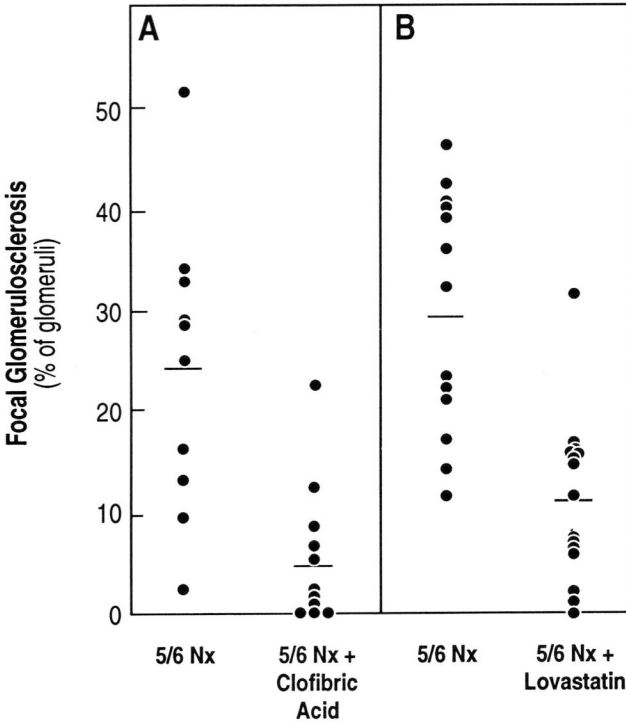

FIG. 4. A: Percentage of glomeruli with focal glomerulosclerosis in control and clofibric acid-treated 5/6-nephrectomy rats at 10 weeks after nephrectomy. The mean percentage in each group is represented (*horizontal bars*). Difference between the means was statistically significant ($p < .05$). **B:** In a separate study, percentage of glomeruli with focal glomerulosclerosis in control and lovastatin-treated 5/6-nephrectomy rats at 10 weeks after nephrectomy. The mean percentage in each group is represented (*horizontal bars*). Difference between the means was statistically significant ($p < .05$). (Adapted with permission from: Kasiske BL, O'Donnell MP, Garvis WJ, Keane WF. Pharmacologic treatment of hyperlipidemia reduces glomerular injury in rat 5/6 nephrectomy model of chronic renal failure. Circulation Research 1988;62: 367–374. Copyright 1988 American Heart Association.)

merular injury. As will be discussed in the next section, macrophages may be important in lipid-mediated glomerular injury. Increased glomerular messenger ribonucleic acid (mRNA) for type I collagen, type IV collagen, and laminin B_2 was also observed 2 weeks after 5/6

nephrectomy and was followed by accumulation of mesangial extracellular matrix material (assessed by periodic acid-Schiff [PAS] staining), increased glomerular tuft area, and the appearance of focal glomerulosclerosis by week 3 after ablation (21).

Rats with subtotal nephrectomy demonstrate elevated serum lipid levels, and there is evidence that lipid abnormalities may be important in the pathogenesis of glomerular disease in remnant nephrons. Fasting serum cholesterol was found to be significantly elevated 2 weeks after ablation in 3/4-nephrectomized rats, and the serum cholesterol level increased progressively to 16 weeks (22). Corresponding to the rise in serum cholesterol, glomerular lipid deposits in remnant glomeruli were detected at 2 weeks after ablation and increased thereafter (22). Moreover, by multiple linear regression analysis, fasting serum cholesterol was found to be a significant predictor of mesangial matrix expansion, suggesting a pathogenetic role for cholesterol in the development of glomerular injury in the remnant kidney (22).

Pharmacological studies have provided more compelling evidence that lipids might participate in glomerular injury in this model. Kasiske et al. (23) demonstrated that two structurally unrelated lipid-lowering drugs, clofibrate and lovastatin (formerly mevinolin), administered daily from the time of renal ablation, each reduced glomerular structural injury in 5/6-nephrectomized rats (Fig. 4). The agents also lowered serum cholesterol levels and albuminuria, but had no effect on elevated systemic and glomerular capillary blood pressures (23) (Tables 1 and 2). The results of this study suggested, therefore, that lipids may be important at least in the initiation of glomerular injury in the remnant kidney model. The importance of hyperlipidemia in the progression of glomerular structural injury in remnant nephrons has not been systematically evaluated. However, a recent preliminary study has demonstrated that lovastatin treatment beginning 8 weeks after 5/6 nephrectomy in rats prevented further progression of albuminuria and reduced the extent of glomerulosclerosis at 16 weeks compared with untreated 5/6-nephrectomized rats (24). Thus, these data suggest that lipids may also play a role in the progression of glomerular injury in the remnant kidney.

TABLE 1. *Effects of clofibric acid on 5/6-nephrectomy rats*

Effects measured	5/6 nephrectomy	5/6 nephrectomy + clofibric acid	Two-kidney controls
Serum cholesterol (mg/dL)*	94 ± 7[a]	53 ± 6[b]	43 ± 3[b]
Albuminuria (mg/24 h)*	62.5 ± 10.0[a]	11.0 ± 4.0[b]	0.6 ± 0.1[c]
Awake systolic blood pressure (mm Hg)**	197 ± 10[a]	183 ± 7[a]	142 ± 2[b]
Glomerular capillary pressure (mm Hg)**	57.8 ± 0.8[a]	56.6 ± 1.5[a]	51.6 ± 1.0[b]

Adapted from ref. 23, with permission.
* Measured 7–10 weeks after nephrectomy.
** Measured 4–6 weeks after nephrectomy.
Results expressed as means ± SEM. Different superscripts indicate $p < 0.05$.

TABLE 2. *Effects of lovastatin on 5/6-nephrectomy rats*

Effects measured	5/6 nephrectomy	5/6 nephrectomy + lovastatin	Two-kidney controls
Serum cholesterol (mg/dL)*	138 $\pm 8^a$	92 $\pm 8^b$	56 $\pm 11^c$
Albuminuria (mg/24 h)*	83.8 $\pm 8.6^a$	43.6 $\pm 7.0^b$	0.8 $\pm$ 0.6^c
Awake systolic blood pressure (mm Hg)**	185 $\pm 5^a$	169 $\pm 7^a$	114 $\pm$ 6^b

* Measured 7–10 weeks after nephrectomy.
** Measured 4–6 weeks after nephrectomy. Adapted from ref. 23, with permission.
Results expressed as mean $\pm$ SEM. Different superscripts indicate $p < 0.05$.

Experimental Nephrotic Syndrome

Administration of puromycin aminonucleoside (PAN) to rats has been frequently used to produce a model of human minimal change nephrotic syndrome. After a single intravenous injection of PAN, overt nephrosis occurs within 1 week and is characterized by marked albuminuria, glomerular macrophage influx, hyperlipidemia, and renal insufficiency (25–30). Reduction in glomerular polyanions, podocyte foot process fusion, and detachment of podocytes from the glomerular basement membrane (GBM) occur within a few days after PAN injection (27). Moreover, the appearance of albuminuria was found to correlate with podocyte detachment (27). Glomerular mRNA levels for the alpha-1 chain of type IV collagen as well as for laminin A, B1, and B2 chains were increased 8 days after PAN, whereas mRNA levels for heparan sulfate proteoglycan, the principal GBM polyanion, were decreased (29).

Within 4 weeks after a single PAN injection the nephrotic syndrome typically resolves, with urine albumin excretion, serum lipids, serum albumin, and renal function returning to normal levels (25,26,28). However, albuminuria resumes about 8 weeks after the PAN injection and increases progressively in association with the development of glomerulosclerosis. Anderson et al. (26) have demonstrated increased glomerular capillary pressure in PAN rats during the resolution phase and have suggested that this is responsible for the subsequent development of progressive glomerular injury. Indeed, administration of the ACE inhibitor enalapril to PAN rats in the resolution phase normalized glomerular pressures and largely prevented subsequent glomerular injury (26).

There is evidence that hyperlipidemia associated with nephrosis in PAN rats may also be important in the ultimate development of glomerulosclerosis. Diamond et al. (28) fed PAN rats a diet supplemented with 5 percent cholestyramine resin. The diet was initiated immediately after PAN injection. Cholestyramine (Cholybar, Questran) significantly attenuated the rise in both urine protein excretion and fasting serum cholesterol 1 week after PAN injection (Fig. 5). Subsequently, the serum cholesterol level was not different between cholestyramine-treated and untreated PAN rats. Cholestyramine administration also attenuated the later rise in urine albumin

excretion (see Fig. 5), and the percent of glomeruli with sclerosis at 24 weeks in cholestyramine-treated nephrotic rats was only one-third that in untreated nephrotic rats. The authors suggested that the lipid-lowering action of cholestyramine in the early nephrotic phase may have been important in the beneficial action of the resin to reduce later glomerular injury.

Chronic nephrotic syndrome has been produced in rats by repetitive subcutaneous injections of low-dose PAN (31–33). In this model, urine albumin excretion in-

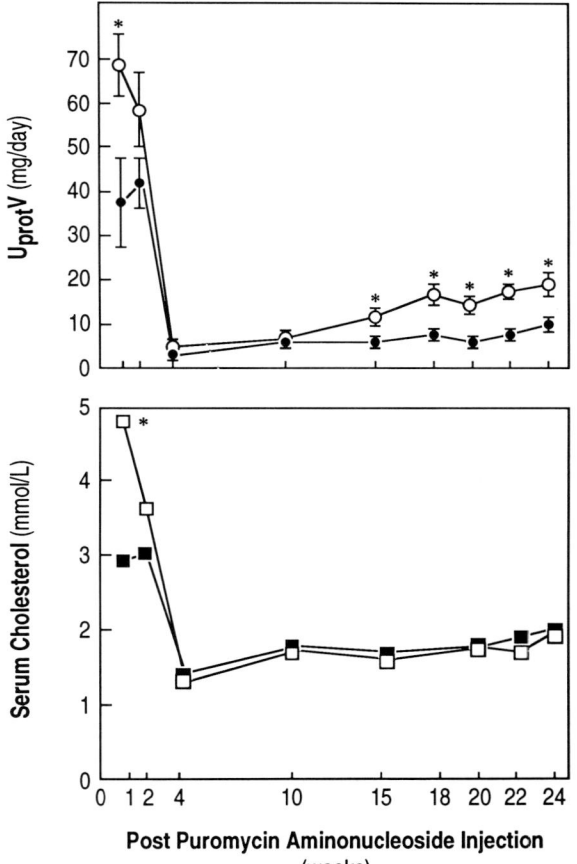

FIG. 5. Urine protein excretion (**top panel**) and fasting serum cholesterol (**bottom panel**) in control (*open symbols*) and cholestyramine-treated (*closed symbols*) nephrotic rats at different time intervals during aminonucleoside nephrosis. *$p < 0.05$. (Adapted from ref. 28, with permission.)

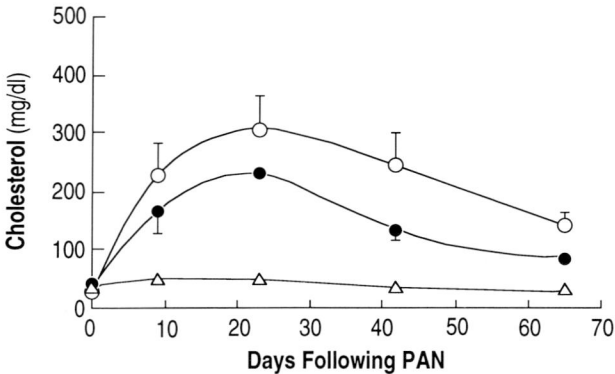

FIG. 6. Effect of lovastatin on plasma cholesterol in uninephrectomized rats administered puromycin aminonucleoside (PAN). Nephrotic rats were given vehicle (*open circles*) or lovastatin (*closed circles*); non-nephrotic control rats were given vehicle (*triangles*). (From ref. 33, with permission.)

creases gradually over several weeks to a maximum and is sustained. Hyperlipidemia and mesangial lipid deposition occur in chronic PAN rats, and Grond et al. (31) have demonstrated focal sclerotic lesions associated with segmental deposition of IgM, fibrinogen, and C3 after 12 weeks of nephrosis. Harris and coworkers (33) demonstrated that lipids may be important in the development of glomerular structural injury in chronic PAN rats. In their study, uninephrectomized rats received repetitive subcutaneous injections of PAN over a period of 40 days. One group of PAN-treated rats also received lovastatin from the time of initiation of PAN injections. Clearance studies and histology were performed at 60 days. Lovastatin reduced serum cholesterol in the nephrotic rats, although cholesterol levels remained substantially higher than those in non-nephrotic rats (Fig. 6). Lovastatin did not significantly affect urine protein excretion in the nephrotic rats but did reduce the severity of glomerular structural injury and preserve renal function. Indeed, inulin clearance in the lovastatin-treated nephrotic rats was about twice that in the untreated nephrotic rats (Fig. 7). The authors concluded that endogenous hyperlipidemia associated with the nephrotic syndrome may play a

role in progressive glomerular damage leading to sclerosis and renal insufficiency.

The mechanism by which hyperlipidemia might contribute to progressive glomerular disease in experimental nephrosis has not been determined. As will be discussed in detail in the next section, evidence has accumulated that oxidized lipoproteins may be injurious to the glomerulus (34,35). Moreover, mesangial cells may be able to oxidize lipoproteins deposited locally in the mesangium (34). Interestingly, two recent studies have implicated reactive oxygen molecules in the development of glomerulosclerosis in PAN rats. In one study, PAN rats fed a diet deficient in selenium had reduced tissue activity of selenium-dependent glutathione peroxidase and significantly greater proteinuria after 4 days compared with selenium-replete PAN rats (36). In another study, PAN rats given the antioxidant taurine in the drinking water had less albuminuria and glomerulosclerosis and higher inulin clearance than PAN rats not given taurine (37). These studies have suggested a role of reactive oxygen species in the development of glomerulosclerosis in nephrotic rats, and it is tempting to speculate that reactive oxygen molecules might be injurious in this model, at least in part, through oxidation of increased levels of lipoproteins associated with the nephrotic state.

Nephrotic rats prepared by either a single intravenous PAN injection or multiple subcutaneous PAN injections, as described above, are typically normotensive. One study, however, has examined the effects of systemic hypertension superimposed on the experimental nephrotic state. Saito and coworkers (38) induced chronic PAN nephrosis in spontaneously hypertensive rats (SHR) and control Wistar-Kyoto (WKY) rats by repetitive PAN injections. At day 80, SHR-PAN rats had higher urine protein excretion and serum creatinine levels than WKY-PAN rats. Serum cholesterol levels were similar in the two groups. Moreover, histologic injury was more severe in the SHR-PAN rats and included advanced focal glomerulosclerosis, interstitial fibrosis, and thickening and fibrinoid necrosis of the intima of small arteries and arterioles. Thus, hypertension superimposed

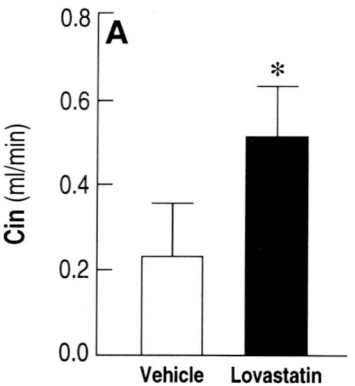

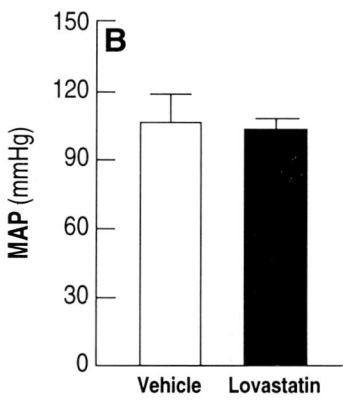

FIG. 7. Values for (**A**) inulin clearance (Cin) and (**B**) mean arterial blood pressure (MAP) at 60 days after the induction of nephrotic syndrome. Nephrotic rats were given vehicle (*open bars*) or lovastatin (*closed bars*). *$p < .05$ vs Cin of vehicle-treated group. (From ref. 33, with permission.)

TABLE 3. *The effects of lipid-lowering agents[1] in obese Zucker rats*

Effects measured	Untreated	Clofibric acid	Lovastatin
Serum cholesterol (mg/dL)[2]	146 ± 10[a]	83 ± 7[b]	91 ± 6[b]
Serum triglycerides (mg/dL)[2]	405 ± 19[a]	397 ± 17[a]	277 ± 41[b]
Urine albumin excretion (mg/24 h)[3]	46.6 ± 6.3[a]	24.1 ± 8.6[b]	9.8 ± 3.0[c]
Systolic blood pressure (mm Hg)[3]	129 ± 5[a]	128 ± 7[a]	114 ± 6[a]
Glomerular capillary pressure (mm Hg)[4]	57.5 ± 1.9[a]	56.1 ± 1.6[a]	55.0 ± 2.0[a]

From ref. 54, with permission.
[1] Injections begun at 8 weeks of age.
[2] Measured at 40 weeks of age.
[3] Measured at 32 weeks of age.
[4] Measured at 14 weeks of age.
Results expressed as mean ± SEM. Different superscripts indicate $p < 0.05$.

on the nephrotic state significantly worsened renal injury independent of effects on serum lipids.

The Obese Zucker Rat

The obese Zucker (OZ) rat has been extensively studied as a model of non–insulin-dependent diabetes mellitus. Obesity in this model is an autosomal recessive trait and the fa/fa genotype is characterized by obesity, peripheral insulin resistance, hyperinsulinemia, and hyperlipidemia (39–43). Obese Zucker rats demonstrate severe hypertriglyceridemia as well as elevations of circulating cholesterol. Glucose intolerance is present in young OZ rats, and fasting hyperglycemia ultimately occurs. Chronic, progressive renal disease develops in OZ rats, and this model has been used to study mechanisms of diabetic nephropathy (44–47). Microalbuminuria and modest mesangial matrix expansion are evident in 12-week-old OZ rats, and glomerular injury increases progressively thereafter (45,47). Marked albuminuria and mesangial expansion as well as focal glomerulosclerosis (FGS) are evident at 28 weeks of age (45,47). Recent studies have reported the percent of glomeruli with sclerosis in 38- to 44-week-old OZ rats to be more than 40 percent (48,49).

Some authors have described hypertension in young OZ rats and have utilized this model to study interrelationships between obesity, insulin resistance, and blood pressure (50,51). Other investigators, including our laboratory, have found that OZ rats are normotensive until renal disease becomes extensive, when modest elevations in systolic blood pressure become evident (13,48,52,53). Glomerular capillary pressure is not altered in young OZ rats (46), but is elevated at 22 to 26 weeks of age when glomerular injury is accelerating (13).

Experimental evidence suggests that lipids may be important in the development of glomerulopathy in OZ rats. Kasiske et al. (54) treated OZ rats for 32 weeks with either clofibrate or lovastatin beginning at 8 weeks of age (54). Both drugs lowered fasting serum cholesterol and lovastatin also reduced fasting serum triglycerides (Table 3). Obese Zucker rats treated with either agent had less albuminuria throughout the treatment period than untreated OZ rats (see Table 3). Moreover, OZ rats treated with the lipid-lowering agents had less mesangial cellularity and matrix expansion and substantially fewer sclerotic glomeruli at the termination of the experiment (Fig. 8). The lipid-lowering drugs had no effect on either systemic blood pressure or glomerular pressures. The results of this study suggested that lipids might play an important role in at least the initiation of chronic, progressive glomerular disease in OZ rats.

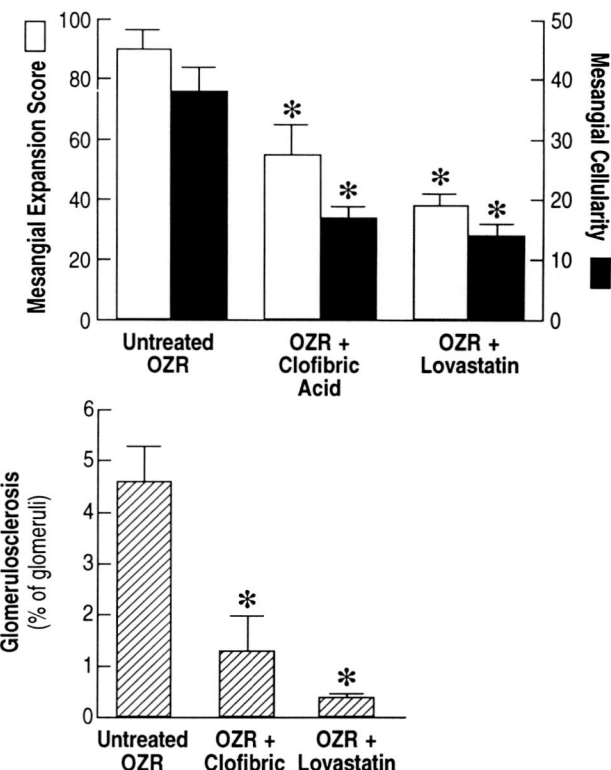

FIG. 8. Top: Mesangial expansion scores and mesangial cellularity scores in obese Zucker rats (OZR) at 40 weeks of age. *$p < 0.05$ vs respective score in untreated OZR. **Bottom:** Percentage of glomeruli with any focal glomerulosclerosis in OZR at 40 weeks of age. *$p < 0.05$ vs. untreated OZR. (Adapted from ref. 54, with permission.)

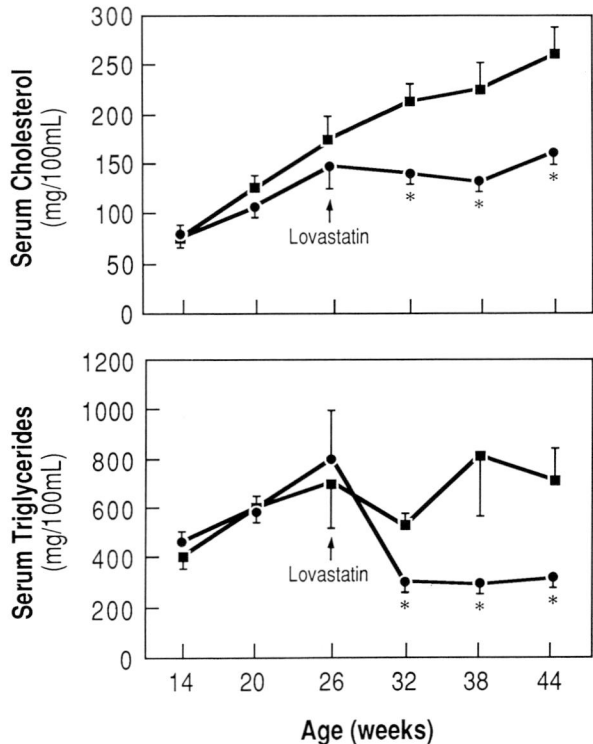

FIG. 9. Top: Fasting serum cholesterol. **Bottom:** triglycerides in vehicle-treated (*squares*) and lovastatin-treated (*circles*) OZ rats. Treatments were initiated at 26 weeks of age. *$p < .05$. (From ref. 48, with permission.)

A more recent study by O'Donnell et al. (48) examined the potential importance of lipids in the progression of glomerular disease in OZ rats. In this study 26-week-old, hyperlipidemic OZ rats with established glomerular disease were treated with daily subcutaneous injections of lovastatin for a period of 18 weeks. Lovastatin lowered serum triglycerides and prevented a further rise in serum cholesterol in the treated OZ rats (Fig. 9). Interestingly, over the first 12 weeks of treatment, lovastatin attenuated the rise in systolic blood pressure that occurred in untreated OZ rats (Fig. 10). Lovastatin also prevented a further rise in urine albumin excretion over the first 12 weeks of treatment (Fig. 11). Indeed, urine albumin excretion declined in the lovastatin-treated rats between 26 and 38 weeks of age. At 44 weeks of age, the percent of glomeruli with sclerosis in the lovastatin-treated rats was one-half that in untreated OZ rats (see Fig. 11). Thus, these data suggested that lipids might be important, not only for initiation but also for progression of glomerular disease in OZ rats.

Other Models

Feeding rats a diet rich in cholesterol has been studied as an experimental model of lipid-induced renal injury

(55,56). In a study by Kasiske et al. (56), rats fed normal chow supplemented with 4 percent cholesterol for 19 weeks developed marked hypercholesterolemia and modest increases in albuminuria, mesangial matrix expansion, and glomerulosclerosis. Blood pressure in the cholesterol-fed rats remained normal. Recently, Kasiske et al. (57) also examined the effects of hypertension in this model. Rats fed normal chow or cholesterol-supplemented chow were subjected to two-kidney, one-clip hypertension by placement of a clip on the left renal artery. Systolic blood pressures in the cholesterol-fed and normal chow rats were similar throughout the study, increasing progressively from 14 to 26 weeks of age and exceeding 190 mm Hg at the end of the study. Hypertension alone in the normal chow rats increased urine albumin excretion and the percent of sclerotic glomeruli in the unclipped kidney. The combination of hypertension and hypercholesterolemia, however, produced even greater increments in urine albumin excretion and sclerotic glomeruli in the cholesterol-fed rats. These results suggested that hypertension and hypercholesterolemia could interact synergistically in the pathogenesis of glomerular injury. Moreover, it was suggested that glomer-

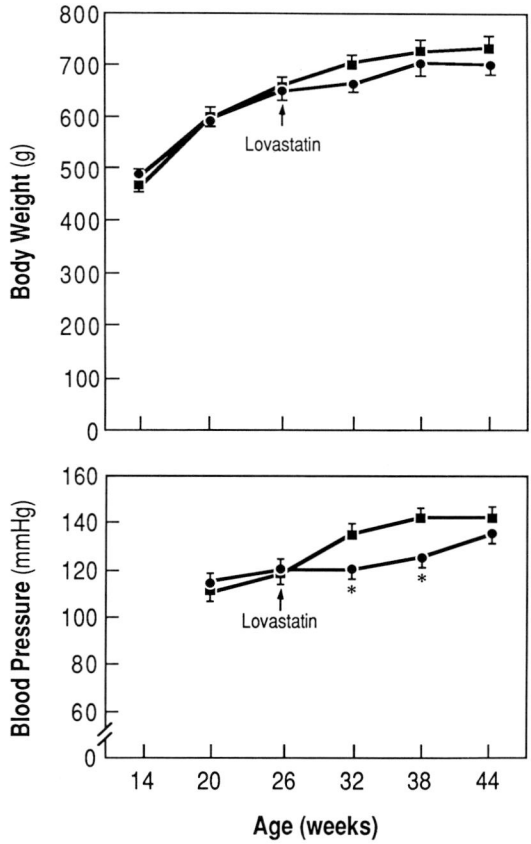

FIG. 10. Top: Body weights. **Bottom:** awake, systolic blood pressures in vehicle-treated (*squares*) and lovastatin-treated (*circles*) OZ rats. Treatments were initiated at 26 weeks of age. *$p < .05$. (From ref. 48, with permission.)

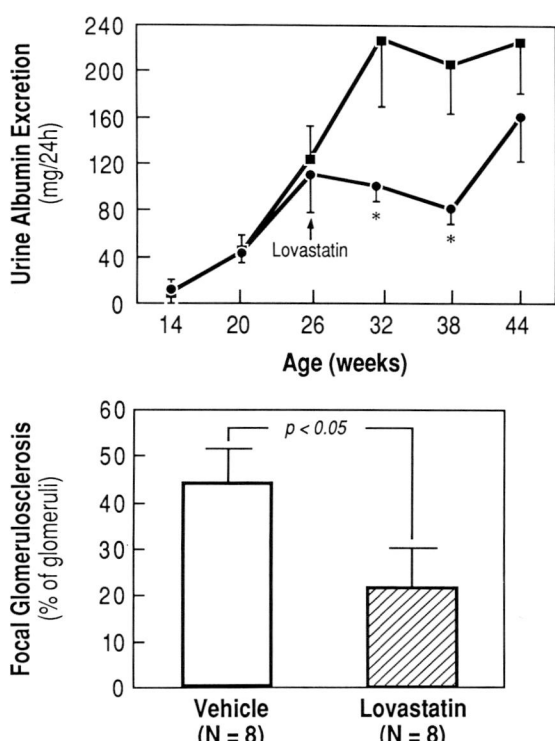

FIG. 11. Top: Albuminuria in vehicle-treated (*squares*) and lovastatin-treated (*circles*) OZ rats. Treatments were initiated at 26 weeks of age. **p < .05.* **Bottom:** Percentage of glomeruli with any focal glomerulosclerosis at 44 weeks of age (18 weeks of treatment) in vehicle-treated and lovastatin-treated OZ rats. (From ref. 48, with permission.)

ular hypertension, resulting from transmission of elevated systemic blood pressure through relatively vasodilated afferent arterioles in the unclipped kidneys, was important in this synergistic interaction (57).

Interaction between hypercholesterolemia and hypertension in the initiation of glomerular injury was also investigated by Tolins and coworkers (58). In their study, DS and DR rats were fed high salt diets containing normal or high cholesterol. Hypercholesterolemia due to high cholesterol intake exaggerated proteinuria and glomerulosclerosis in hypertensive DS rats but not in normotensive DR rats.

Spontaneously hypertensive rats have been frequently studied as a model of human essential hypertension. SHR also develop progressive glomerular injury, albeit at a slower rate than occurs in DS rats or hypertensive rats with a remnant kidney (59,60). One explanation for the relatively slow rate of development of glomerular injury in SHR may be that afferent vasoconstriction in SHR prevents the transmission of elevated systemic blood pressure to the glomerulus so that glomerular pressures remain normal (61). Recently, Reaven and Chang (62) have reported that SHR are insulin resistant, hyperinsulinemic, and hypertriglyceridemic compared with control WKY rats. Whether lipid abnormalities in SHR

contribute to the development of glomerular injury in this model is not known. To date no studies have examined the effects of lipid-lowering agents on glomerular disease in SHR.

MECHANISMS BY WHICH LIPIDS MODULATE EXPERIMENTAL RENAL DISEASE

The preceding section has summarized experimental evidence that suggests an important role for lipids in the pathogenesis of glomerulosclerosis. If lipids do, indeed, contribute to progressive glomerular injury, then one must ultimately define the cellular and biochemical mechanisms by which this occurs. Glomerulosclerosis likely evolves from pathogenic events that begin in the mesangium. Mesangial cell proliferation or increased mesangial cell turnover, together with accumulation of extracellular matrix material, may be fundamental events responsible for mesangial expansion, ultimately causing collapse of glomerular capillaries and development of sclerosis (63–65). Experimental studies over the past few years have begun to examine how lipids might directly alter mesangial cell function and influence these events.

Effects of Native and Oxidized Lipoproteins on Mesangial Cell Proliferation and Accumulation of Extracellular Matrix Proteins

The glomerular mesangium is separated from the glomerular capillary plasma by only a fenestrated endothelium. Thus, circulating lipoproteins, although large particles, can gain access to the mesangium and potentially affect mesangial cell function. Mesangial deposition of apolipoproteins has been documented in both human and rat glomeruli (66–70). Several recent studies have begun to investigate direct effects of lipoproteins on cultured mesangial cells. Mesangial cells can bind and internalize both native low-density lipoprotein (LDL) and oxidized LDL (71–74). *In vitro*, LDL appears to exert a biphasic effect on mesangial cell proliferation (34,75). Lower concentrations stimulate mesangial cell proliferation, whereas high concentrations of LDL inhibit mesangial cell proliferation and may cause cytotoxicity (Fig. 12). The cytotoxic effects of high LDL concentrations may be due to local oxidation of LDL (34). Interestingly, in two human studies, mesangial deposition of apolipoproteins B and E correlated with the degree of mesangial cell proliferation (67,68).

Low-density lipoproteins may also interact synergistically with peptide mitogens such as platelet-derived growth factor (PDGF) (74) and insulin-like growth factor-1 (IGF-1) (76) to stimulate mesangial cell proliferation (Fig. 13). Moreover, PDGF was found to increase

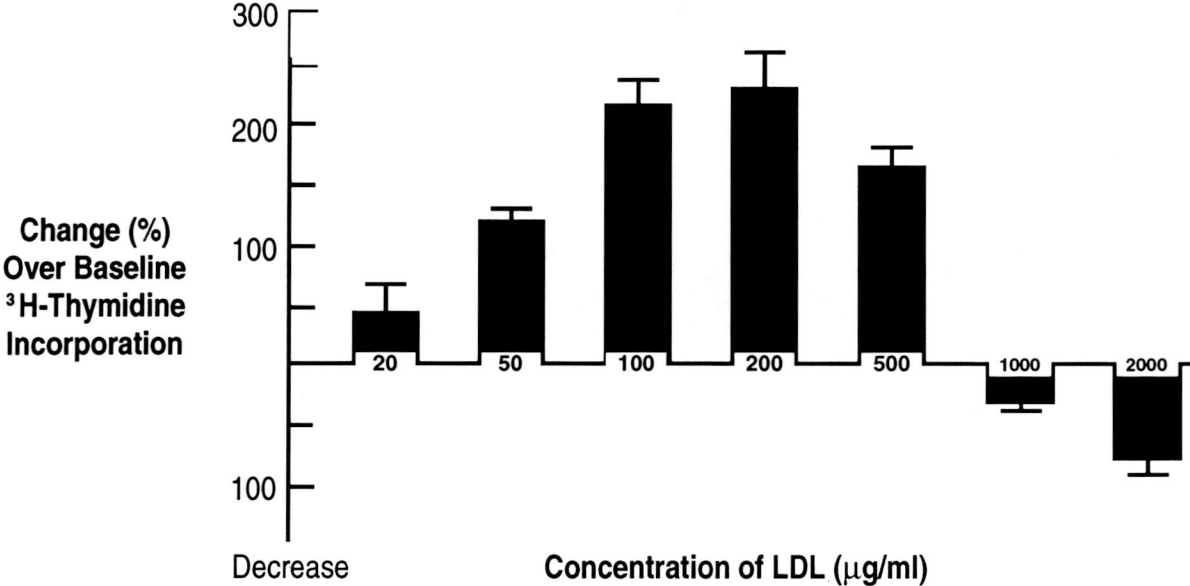

FIG. 12. The effects of adding increasing concentrations of low-density lipoprotein (LDL) to quiescent human mesangial cells. DNA synthesis, as assessed by [³H]thymidine incorporation, was maximal at LDL concentrations between 100 and 200 µg/mL. LDL concentrations of 1,000–2,000 µg/mL demonstrated evidence of cytotoxicity. (From ref. 34, with permission.)

mesangial cell LDL receptors, perhaps providing one mechanism for a synergistic interaction (74). An interaction between lipoproteins and peptide growth factors to stimulate mesangial cell proliferation may be an important mechanism of progressive glomerular disease. Lipoprotein levels are frequently elevated in renal disease, and much evidence indicates that the activities of growth-promoting peptides such as PDGF, IGF-1, and endothelin are often increased in both experimental and clinical renal disease (77–79). Thus, one mechanism by which lipoproteins such as LDL might modulate mesangial expansion and the ultimate development of sclerosis is via stimulatory effects on mesangial cell proliferation.

Local oxidation of lipoproteins may also provide a mechanism of glomerular injury. Keane et al. (34) have recently demonstrated that mesangial cells themselves can oxidize LDL via production of superoxide anion Moreover, infiltrating macrophages may release reactive oxygen species that can cause local oxidation of LDL. Oxidized lipoproteins have been detected in the glomerulus (80), and Coritsides and coworkers (72) have recently shown that mesangial cells preferentially bind oxidized LDL via a scavenger receptor. Oxidized LDL may promote glomerular injury in several ways. First, as discussed above, oxidized LDL may exert direct mesangial cell cytotoxicity (34). Second, oxidized LDL may stimulate accumulation of mesangial extracellular matrix. Mesangial cells produce transforming growth factor-β1 (TGF-β1), a cytokine that has been proposed to be of key importance in processes characterized by accumulation

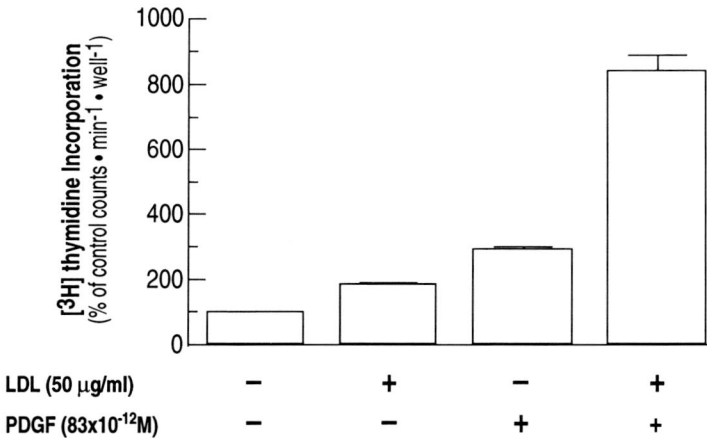

FIG. 13. Effects of low-density lipoprotein (LDL) and platelet-derived growth factor (PDGF), alone and in combination, on DNA synthesis ([³H]thymidine incorporation) in human mesangial cells. Note LDL and PDGF interacted synergistically to cause a marked increase in DNA synthesis. (Adapted with permission from: Gröne EF, Abboud HE, Höhne M, et al. Actions of lipoproteins in cultured human mesangial cells: modulation by mitogenic vasoconstrictors. American Journal of Physiology 1992;263: F686–F696. Copyright 1992 American Physiological Society.)

of extracellular matrix such as wound repair, atherosclerosis, and glomerulosclerosis (81). *In vitro*, oxidized LDL has been found to up-regulate mesangial cell expression of TGF-β1 mRNA (O'Donnell and Keane, *unpublished data*, 1993). Also, mesangial cells exposed to LDL produced increased amounts of fibronectin (82), a matrix protein that accumulates in progressive glomerular injury. *In vivo*, glomerular TGF-β1 and fibronectin mRNA were increased in nephrotic rats fed a high cholesterol diet (83). Although more definitive evidence is needed, these findings suggest that oxidized LDL may promote the accumulation of mesangial matrix.

Last, oxidized lipoproteins may stimulate glomerular monocyte/macrophage recruitment either directly or indirectly via stimulation of synthesis of chemoattractant substances such as monocyte chemoattractant peptide-1 (MCP-1) (82,84). Accumulating evidence indicates that macrophages may be important in glomerulopathies of various etiologies (85). Moreover, lipoprotein-macrophage interactions may lead to glomerulosclerosis via mechanisms similar to those thought to be important in atherosclerosis (86,87). Macrophages produce reactive oxygen molecules that can oxidize LDL. The possible pathogenic actions of oxidized LDL in the mesangium have been discussed. Macrophages can take up oxidized LDL via scavenger receptors and become foam cells (88). Both macrophages and foam cells can release growth factors such as PDGF, which may stimulate mesangial cell proliferation (85). One study has found a correlation between the number of glomerular macrophages and the degree of mesangial cell proliferation (89). Thus, in several ways, lipoprotein-macrophage interactions may be important for lipid modulation of glomerular injury.

Recent preliminary studies have suggested that lovastatin may inhibit glomerular macrophage infiltration, and may do so by directly suppressing mesangial cell production of MCP-1. Rats fed high-cholesterol chow for 2 weeks demonstrated increased glomerular macrophages, and this was prevented by simultaneous daily administration of lovastatin (O'Donnell and Keane, *unpublished data*). *In vitro* experiments demonstrated impaired MCP-1 production by cultured human mesangial cells exposed to lovastatin (90). Moreover, lovastatin markedly suppressed mesangial cell expression of MCP-1 mRNA (90). Thus, these results suggest additional possible mechanisms by which lovastatin may attenuate glomerular injury.

Hyperlipidemia and Glomerular Hypertension

Elevated levels of circulating lipoproteins may also contribute to progressive glomerular injury by elevating glomerular capillary pressure. Micropuncture studies have demonstrated glomerular hypertension in two models of hyperlipidemia and progressive renal disease, i.e., the OZ rat and the cholesterol-supplemented rat.

In OZ rats, glomerular pressures were found to be normal at 10 to 12 weeks of age when only minimal albuminuria and mesangial expansion were evident (46). However, in 22- to 26-week-old OZ rats, glomerular hypertension was present in association with severe hyperlipidemia and accelerating glomerular structural injury (13). Increased glomerular capillary pressure in OZ rats was not dependent on increased systemic blood pressure, but did show a significant correlation with plasma colloid osmotic pressure, which was also increased, possibly as a result of the marked hyperlipoproteinemia.

Two studies have demonstrated glomerular hypertension in rats fed a high cholesterol diet. Kasiske et al. (56) reported that rats fed 4 percent cholesterol for 8 to 10 weeks had marked hypercholesterolemia and elevated glomerular capillary pressures (56). Moreover, as found in OZ rats (13), the elevation in glomerular capillary pressure in the hypercholesterolemic rats correlated with increased colloid osmotic pressure. There was a trend for elevated efferent arteriolar resistance in the cholesterol-fed rats that did not achieve statistical significance. It was suggested that altered glomerular blood rheology associated with hypercholesterolemia may have been responsible, at least in part, for the elevated glomerular pressures (56).

Kaplan et al. (91) also demonstrated glomerular hypertension in cholesterol-fed rats. In their study, rats were fed 4 percent cholesterol chow for 3 weeks. Compared with rats fed standard chow, the cholesterol-supplemented rats had reduced single nephron GFR and increased glomerular pressures. Afferent arteriolar resistance and single nephron filtration fraction were also elevated. Interestingly, treating cholesterol-fed rats with the antioxidant probucol over the 3-week period, or acutely infusing a thromboxane A_2 receptor antagonist on the day of micropuncture, each reversed the hemodynamic alterations. The authors hypothesized that oxidized LDL *in vivo* might cause renal vasoconstriction and elevation of glomerular pressures via stimulation of thromboxane production. Indeed, the cholesterol-fed rats had elevated urine thromboxane excretion that was prevented by probucol treatment (91).

How Does HMG-CoA Reductase Inhibition Reduce Experimental Glomerular Injury?

As has been discussed, several studies have shown that the HMG-CoA reductase inhibitor lovastatin can reduce albuminuria, mesangial expansion, and glomerulosclerosis in experimental models of renal disease (5,23,33, 48,54). The precise mechanism of the beneficial effects of HMG-CoA reductase inhibition has not been elucidated. Reduction in circulating lipoproteins caused by lovastatin might, in itself, attenuate the potential mechanisms of lipid-modulated injury previously discussed, i.e., mesangial lipoprotein deposition, stimulatory and/or cyto-

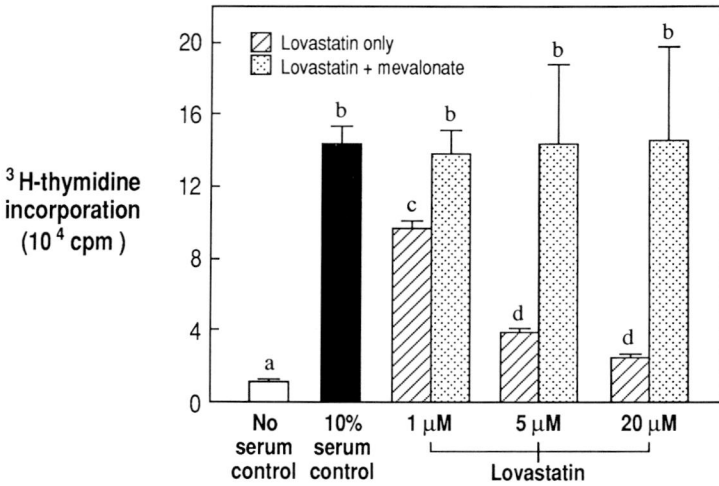

FIG. 14. DNA synthesis ([³H]thymidine incorporation) in confluent rat mesangial cells stimulated by 10-percent fetal bovine serum. Mevalonate concentration was 100 μM. Different letters indicate $p < .05$. (From Journal of Clinical Investigation 1993;91:83–87, by copyright permission of the American Society for Clinical Investigation.)

toxic actions of lipoproteins on mesangial cells, interactions of lipoproteins with macrophages, and stimulation of mesangial matrix accumulation.

One recent study has indicated that lovastatin might also reduce glomerular injury via direct actions on mesangial cells (92). O'Donnell et al. demonstrated that lovastatin directly inhibited serum-stimulated mesangial cell proliferation (Fig. 14). The inhibitory effect of lovastatin was overridden by simultaneous exposure of cells to mevalonate (see Fig. 14), but not to exogenous LDL cholesterol (Fig. 15). These results suggested that one or more nonsterol products of mevalonate metabolism were essential for mesangial cell proliferation. Subsequent experiments demonstrated that lovastatin inhibition of mesangial cell proliferation could be largely prevented by simultaneous exposure of the cells to the isoprenoid farnesol (Fig. 16).

In mammalian cells, farnesol is present as farnesyl pyrophosphate, a critical intermediate in the mevalonate pathway (Fig. 17). Farnesyl can be used to synthesize cholesterol, dolichol, and ubiquinones, all of which are necessary for cell viability and cell proliferation (93). In addition, farnesyl can serve as a substrate for covalent modification, or isoprenylation, of certain intracellular proteins (94–96). The *ras* protein family is one that undergoes such isoprenylation. The proto-oncogene product p21*ras* is a low molecular mass, guanosinetriphosphate (GTP)-binding protein that is thought to be important in mitogenic signaling stimulated by certain growth factors including PDGF (97–99). The proto-oncogene product p21*ras* undergoes covalent modification by farnesyl, which allows the protein to anchor to the inner cell membrane where it may function in signal transduction (96). Treatment of cells with HMG-CoA

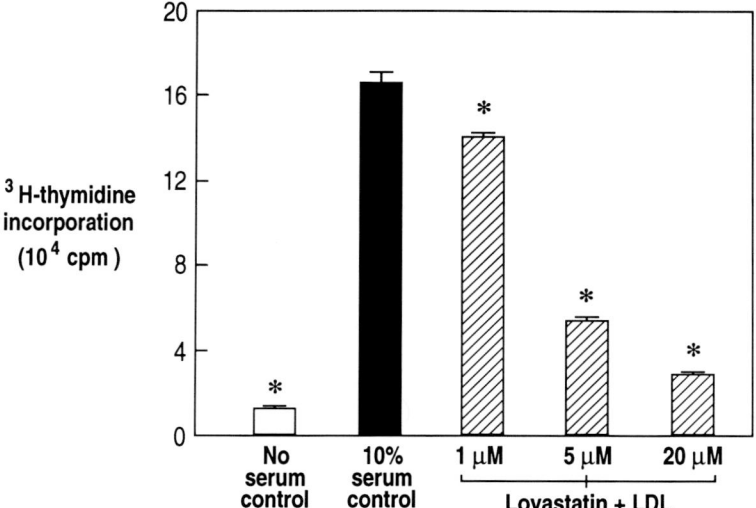

FIG. 15. DNA synthesis ([³H]thymidine incorporation) in confluent rat mesangial cells stimulated by 10-percent fetal bovine serum. Lovastatin was used at the indicated concentrations of 1, 5, and 20 μM. Low-density lipoprotein (LDL) was present at a concentration of 100 μg/mL. *$p < .05$ vs 10 percent serum control. (From Journal of Clinical Investigation 1993;91:83–87, by copyright permission of the American Society for Clinical Investigation.)

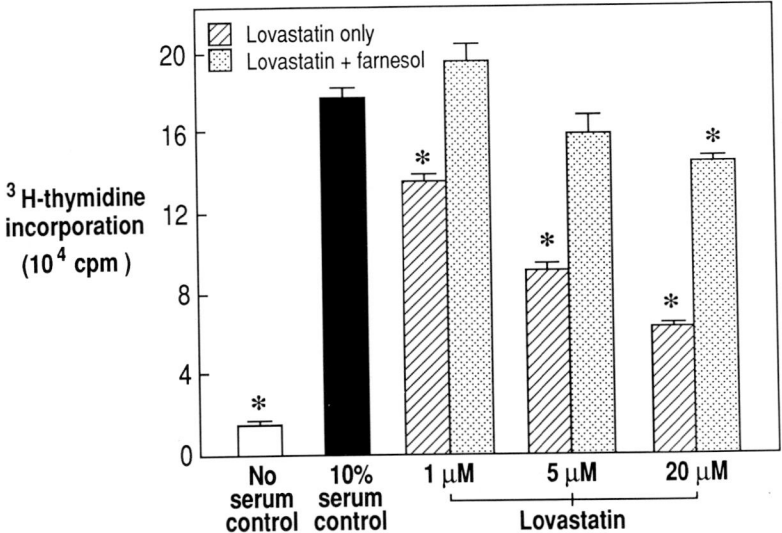

FIG. 16. DNA synthesis ([³H]thymidine incorporation) in confluent rat mesangial cells stimulated by 10-percent fetal bovine serum. Farnesol was used at a concentration of 5 μM. *$p < .05$ vs 10 percent serum control. (From the Journal of Clinical Investigation 1993;91:83–87, by copyright permission of the American Society for Clinical Investigation.)

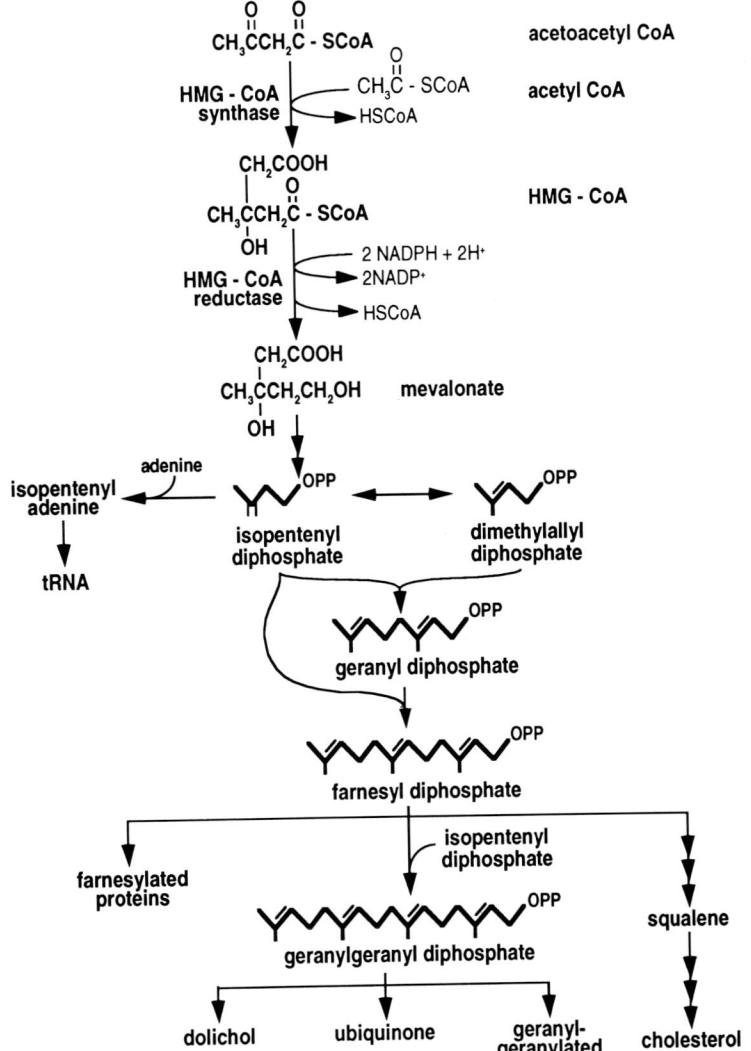

FIG. 17. The mevalonate pathway. Mevalonate is synthesized intracellularly from 3-hydroxy-3-methylglutaryl coenzyme A (HMG-CoA), and this process is catalyzed by the enzyme HMG-CoA reductase. Mevalonate is metabolized to a series of isoprenoid intermediates, of which farnesyl diphosphate (pyrophosphate) is of particular importance. Farnesyl diphosphate can be routed to several end-products necessary for cell viability and cell proliferation. (From ref. 126, with permission.)

reductase inhibitors such as lovastatin or compactin interrupts mevalonate and farnesyl production and has been shown to inhibit proliferation of several cell types, including mesangial cells (92,100–103). Thus, in the experimental studies in which lovastatin reduced glomerular injury, it is conceivable that this may have resulted, at least in part, from a direct effect of lovastatin to inhibit mesangial cell proliferation in response to local release of mitogens that mediate their proliferative effects through p21ras. Whether lovastatin directly affects mesangial cell production of extracellular matrix proteins has not been systematically evaluated. One preliminary study, however, has demonstrated that lovastatin did not affect mesangial cell expression of mRNA for either the alpha-1 chain of type IV collagen or TGF-β1 (104).

HYPERLIPIDEMIA AND VASCULAR REACTIVITY IN EXPERIMENTAL MODELS

Epidemiological studies have demonstrated an increased frequency of lipid abnormalities in patients with essential hypertension. Hypercholesterolemia, hypertriglyceridemia, and reduced HDL cholesterol have been documented in hypertensive men and women, and a direct correlation between blood pressure and the level of serum cholesterol has been reported (105,106). Moreover, it has been suggested that lipoprotein alterations per se may contribute to the development of hypertension (57). In a setting of chronic renal disease associated with hyperlipidemia, therefore, lipids might contribute not only to the progression of renal injury, but also to elevated blood pressure that frequently accompanies renal disease.

There are several potential mechanisms by which lipid alterations might alter vascular reactivity and contribute to the development of hypertension. Recent studies have suggested that hypercholesterolemia may interfere with endothelium-derived relaxing factor/nitric oxide (EDRF/NO). Impaired endothelium-dependent relaxation was found in arteries of cholesterol-fed rabbits (107,108), and this was reversed by treatment with either lovastatin (108) or L-arginine, the precursor of NO (109). In vitro, native LDL and modified LDL have been found to directly inhibit EDRF activity (110,111).

Altered vascular reactivity has been described in experimental models of hyperlipidemia and hypertension, including DS rats and SHR. Simchon and coworkers (112) recently reported decreased renal vasodilatation to nitroprusside and increased renal responsiveness to vasoconstrictors in prehypertensive DS rats (112). Lüscher et al. (113,114) reported impaired endothelium-dependent relaxation in aortic rings of hypertensive DS rats, which was corrected by antihypertensive therapy. Boegehold (115) found decreased basal release of EDRF in skeletal muscle microvasculature of DS rats, although the responsiveness of arteriolar smooth muscle to EDRF was not impaired (115). Interestingly, Chen and Sanders (116) recently reported that treatment of DS rats with L-arginine prevented the development of hypertension. Collectively, these studies suggest that deficiency of EDRF in DS rats contributes to the development of hypertension in this model. The mechanism of impaired endothelial relaxation in DS rats is unknown. It is conceivable, given the evidence that lipids may interfere with EDRF activity (107–111), that lipid abnormalities present in DS rats (4,8,9) may contribute in part to the development of hypertension in this model. In this regard, lovastatin lowered both serum lipids and blood pressure in DS rats (5). Whether this resulted from an action of lovastatin to normalize EDRF activity, however, has not been examined.

Altered vascular reactivity has also been demonstrated in SHR. Lee and Webb (117) have presented evidence that metabolism and/or mobilization of L-arginine in stroke-prone SHR is abnormal, causing altered production of NO. Spontaneously hypertensive rats demonstrate increased renal vascular resistance, and Chatziantoniou and coworkers have found exaggerated renal vascular reactivity to angiotensin II in young SHR. Moreover, it was suggested that this might be due to a deficiency of vasodilator prostaglandin activity in the renal vasculature (118,119). It has been shown that SHR demonstrate hypertriglyceridemia (62), but whether lipid abnormalities in SHR play a role in abnormal vascular reactivity and the development of hypertension is unknown. No studies have investigated whether lipid-lowering agents such as clofibrate or lovastatin can attenuate the rise in blood pressure in this model.

Impaired vascular reactivity has also been noted in rats fed a high cholesterol diet, although these animals typically do not develop hypertension. Kaplan et al. (91) demonstrated altered renal vascular resistance in cholesterol-fed rats, and a subsequent study by the same group showed impaired renal vasodilatation to acetylcholine infusion in cholesterol-fed rats (120). Kasiske and coworkers (121) reported elevated renal vascular resistance in isolated, perfused kidneys obtained from cholesterol-fed rats.

Another experimental model in which the relationship between hyperlipidemia and vascular reactivity has been examined is the OZ rat. As discussed, OZ rats demonstrate severe hypertriglyceridemia as well as substantial increases in serum cholesterol (48,54). Moreover, the serum cholesterol level increases progressively in older OZ rats in association with worsening renal disease (48,54). Blood pressure also rises in older OZ rats (13,48,53). Whether this results in part from lipid-mediated alterations in vascular reactivity has not been investigated. One study has shown, however, that lovastatin attenuated the rise in blood pressure in older OZ rats (48). Limited data are available regarding vascular reactivity in OZ rats. In one study, Harker et al. (122) reported that contractile responses to norepinephrine were not altered in aortic rings isolated from OZ rats. However, aortic rings from older OZ rats had significantly less contractile response to angiotensin II. Thus, the vasculature of OZ rats may not be hyperresponsive to vasoconstrictor agents. Whether endothelium-dependent relaxation is altered in OZ rats has not been investigated and would seem to be an important area of future research in this model.

CONCLUSIONS

There is substantial experimental evidence that lipid alterations can modulate the course of renal disease. Diet-induced hypercholesterolemia has been shown to exaggerate experimental renal disease. In several different models of chronic, progressive renal disease, lipid-lowering agents, particularly the HMG-CoA reductase inhibitor lovastatin, have reduced albuminuria and glomerular structural injury, and improved renal function. The mechanisms by which lipids cause or contribute to glomerular injury, however, are still in question. From experimental studies, it seems possible that lipids may directly influence mesangial cell function and contribute in this way to mesangial matrix expansion and ultimately the development of glomerulosclerosis. Lipid deposition in the glomerulus may also cause macrophage recruitment and foam cell formation. These events might also be important in lipid-mediated renal injury.

The relative importance of lipids in the development and progression of clinical renal disease is not clear. As recently reviewed (123), there are clinical correlations between certain lipid abnormalities and renal disease. On the other hand, however, there does not appear to be an increased prevalence of spontaneous glomerular disease in patients with primary hyperlipidemia (123). Prospective studies involving sufficient patient numbers are needed to define whether specific lipoprotein alterations are independent risk factors for progression of clinical renal disease.

Lipid disturbances frequently accompany human renal disease, and it is conceivable that these disturbances might influence disease progression. Indeed, there are many reports of glomerular lipid deposition in different renal diseases (123). Reports from uncontrolled clinical studies have demonstrated beneficial effects of HMG-CoA reductase inhibitors to reduce proteinuria in patients with renal disease (124,125). To date, however, no long-term, large, controlled clinical trials have been performed to examine the effects of lipid-lowering agents on renal structure and function in patients with progressive renal disease.

Last, it is conceivable that lipid disturbances associated with renal injury may be important in the development of systemic hypertension that frequently accompanies renal disease. There is considerable evidence that elevated cholesterol levels and oxidized lipoproteins can interfere with endothelial-derived relaxation. Altered vascular reactivity has been demonstrated in experimental models in which hypertension and hyperlipidemia coexist. Lovastatin has been shown to lower blood pressure in certain experimental models. Thus, lipid abnormalities may play a role not only in the progression of renal injury but also in disturbances of blood pressure that often accompany renal disease.

ACKNOWLEDGMENTS

The authors thank Ellen Davis and Deanna Gunderson for preparation of the chapter.

REFERENCES

1. Dahl LK, Heine M, Tassinari L. *J Exp Med* 1962;115:1173–1190.
2. Rapp JP. *Hypertension* 1982;4:753–763.
3. Sterzel RB, Luft FC, Gao Y, et al. *Kidney Int* 1988;33:1119–1129.
4. O'Donnell MP, Kasiske BL, Keane WF. *Am J Hypertens* 1989;2:9–13.
5. O'Donnell MP, Kasiske BL, Katz SA, Schmitz PG, Keane WF. *Hypertension* 1992;20:651–658.
6. Roman RJ. *Am J Physiol* 1986;251:F57–F65.
7. Azar S, Limas C, Iwai J, Weller D. *Jap Heart J* 1979;20[Suppl 19]:138–140.
8. Reaven GM, Twersky J, Ho H, Chang H. *Horm Metab Res* 1991;23:44–45.
9. Mondon CE, Plato PA, Dall'Aglio E, Sztalryd C, Reaven G. *Hypertension* 1993;21:373–379.
10. Anderson S, Rennke HG, Brenner BM. *J Clin Invest* 1986;77:1993–2000.
11. Meyer TW, Anderson S, Rennke HG, Brenner BM. *Kidney Int* 1987;31:752–759.
12. Zatz R, Dunn BR, Meyer TW, Anderson S, Rennke HG, Brenner BM. *J Clin Invest* 1986;77:1925–1930.
13. Schmitz PG, O'Donnell MP, Kasiske BL, Katz SA, Keane WF. *Am J Physiol* 1992;263:F496–F502.
14. Iwai J, Dahl LK, Knudsen KD. *Circ Res* 1973;32:678–684.
15. Rodriguez-Sargent C, Cangiano JL, Opava-Stitzer S, Martinez-Moldonado M. *Hypertension* 1981;3[Suppl II]:II-86–II-91.
16. Roman RJ, Ma Y-H, Frohlich B, Markham B. *Hypertension* 1993;21:985–988.
17. Shimamura T, Morrison AB. *Am J Pathol* 1975;79:95–106.
18. Purkerson ML, Hoffsten PE, Klahr S. *Kidney Int* 1976;9:407–417.
19. Hostetter TH, Olson JL, Rennke HG, Venkatachalam MA, Brenner BM. *Am J Physiol* 1981;241:F85–F93.
20. Anderson S, Meyer TW, Rennke HG, Brenner BM. *J Clin Invest* 1985;76:612–619.
21. Floege J, Alpers CE, Burns MW, et al. *Lab Invest* 1992;66:485–497.
22. van Goor H, Fidler V, Weening JJ, Grond J. *Lab Invest* 1991;64:754–765.
23. Kasiske BL, O'Donnell MP, Garvis WJ, Keane WF. *Circ Res* 1988;62:367–374.
24. Lee SK, Lee HB. *Nephrol Dial Transplant* 1992;7:712 [Abstract].
25. Diamond JR, Karnovsky MJ. *Am J Pathol* 1986;122:481–487.
26. Anderson S, Diamond JR, Karnovsky MJ, Brenner BM. *J Clin Invest* 1988;82:1757–1768.
27. Whiteside C, Prutis K, Cameron R, Thompson J. *Lab Invest* 1989;61:650–660.

28. Diamond JR, Hanchak NA, McCarter MD, Karnovsky MJ. *Am J Clin Nutr* 1990;51:606–611.
29. Nakamura T, Ebihara I, Shirato I, Tomino Y, Koide H. *Lab Invest* 1991;64:640–647.
30. Diamond JR, Pesek-Diamond I. *Am J Physiol* 1991;260:F779–F786.
31. Grond J, Weening JJ, Elema JD. *Lab Invest* 1984;51:277–285.
32. Grond J, Muller EW, van Goor H, Weening JJ, Elema JD. *Kidney Int* 1988;33:524–529.
33. Harris KPG, Purkerson ML, Yates J, Klahr S. *Am J Kidney Dis* 1990;15:16–23.
34. Keane WF, O'Donnell MP, Kasiske BL, Kim Y. *J Am Soc Nephrol* 1993;4:187–194.
35. Keane WF, Kasiske BL, O'Donnell MP, Kim Y. *J Am Soc Nephrol* 1992;3:635 [Abstract].
36. Baliga R, Baliga M, Shah SV. *Am J Physiol* 1992;263:F56–F61.
37. Trachtman H, Del Pizzo R, Futterweit S, et al. *Am J Physiol* 1992;262:F117–F123.
38. Saito T, Sato H, Obara K, et al. *J Lab Clin Med* 1990;115:165–173.
39. Schonfeld G, Felski C, Howald MA. *J Lipid Res* 1974;15:457–464.
40. Bray GA. *Fed Proc* 1977;36:148–153.
41. Schirardin H, Bach A, Schaeffer A, Bauer M, Weryha A. *Arch Int Physiol Biochim* 1979;87:275–289.
42. Witztum JL, Schonfeld G. *Diabetes* 1979;28:509–516.
43. Boulange A, Planche E, de Gasquet P. *Metabolism* 1981;30:1045–1052.
44. Shimamura T. *Kidney Int* 1983;24[Suppl 16]:S-259–S-262.
45. Kasiske BL, Cleary MP, O'Donnell MP, Keane WF. *J Lab Clin Med* 1985;106:598–604.
46. O'Donnell MP, Kasiske BL, Cleary MP, Keane WF. *J Lab Clin Med* 1985;106:605–610.
47. Kasiske BL, O'Donnell MP, Keane WF. *J Diabetic Complications* 1987;1:26–29.
48. O'Donnell MP, Kasiske BL, Schmitz PG, Keane WF. *Am J Kidney Dis* 1993;22:83–89.
49. O'Donnell MP. *FASEB J* 1993;7:A454 [Abstract].
50. Kurtz TW, Morris RC, Pershadsingh HA. *Hypertension* 1989;13:896–901.
51. Zemel MB, Peuler JD, Sowers JR, Simpson L. *Am J Physiol* 1992;262:E368–E371.
52. Pawloski CM, Kabagt NL, Mortensen LH, Fink GD. *Hypertension* 1992;19:I-90–I-95.
53. Kasiske BL, O'Donnell MP, Keane WF. *Clin Res* 1991;39:247A [Abstract].
54. Kasiske BL, O'Donnell MP, Cleary MP, Keane WF. *Kidney Int* 1988;33:667–672.
55. Gröne HJ, Walli A, Gröne E, et al. *Lab Invest* 1989;60:433–446.
56. Kasiske BL, O'Donnell MP, Schmitz PG, Kim Y, Keane WF. *Kidney Int* 1990;37:880–891.
57. Kasiske BL, O'Donnell MP, Cowardin W, Keane WF. *Hypertension* 1990;15:443–450.
58. Tolins JP, Stone BG, Raij L. *Kidney Int* 1992;41:1254–1261.
59. Feld LG, Van Liew JB, Galaske RG, Boylan JW. *Kidney Int* 1977;12:332–343.
60. Raij L, Azar S, Keane WF. *Hypertension* 1985;7:398–404.
61. Azar S, Johnson MA, Scheinman J, Bruno L, Tobian L. *Clin Sci* 1979;56:203–209.
62. Reaven GM, Chang H. *Am J Hypertens* 1991;4:34–38.
63. Klahr S, Schreiner G, Ichikawa I. *N Engl J Med* 1988;318:1657–1666.
64. Schultz PJ, Raij L. *Am J Kidney Dis* 1991;17:8–14.
65. Striker LJ, Peten EP, Elliot SJ, Doi T, Striker GE. *Lab Invest* 1991;64:446–456.
66. Sato H, Suzuki S, Kobayashi H, Ogino S, Inomata A, Arakawa M. *Clin Nephrol* 1991;36:127–133.
67. Sato H, Suzuki S, Ueno M, et al. *Kidney Int* 1993;43:430–435.
68. Takemura T, Yoshioka K, Aya N, et al. *Kidney Int* 1993;43:918–927.
69. Joles JA, van Goor H, Grond J, et al. *J Am Soc Nephrol* 1992;3:741 [Abstract].
70. van Goor H, van der Horst MLC, Admosoerodjo J, Joles JA, van Tol A, Grond J. *J Am Soc Nephrol* 1992;3:753 [Abstract].
71. Wasserman J, Santiago A, Rifici V, et al. *Kidney Int* 1989;35:1168–1174.
72. Coritsidis G, Rifici V, Gupta S, et al. *Kidney Int* 1991;39:858–866.
73. Wheeler DC, Fernando RL, Gillett MPT, et al. *Nephrol Dial Transplant* 1991;6:701–708.
74. Gröne EF, Abboud HE, Höhne M, et al. *Am J Physiol* 1992;263:F686–F696.
75. Wheeler DC, Persaud JW, Fernando R, Sweny P, Varghese Z, Moorhead JF. *Nephrol Dial Transplant* 1990;5:185–191.
76. O'Donnell MP, Kasiske BL, Atluru D, Kim Y, Keane WF. *J Am Soc Nephrol* 1992;3:476 [Abstract].
77. Abboud HE. *Kidney Int* 1993;43:252–267.
78. Fine LG, Hammerman MR, Abboud HE. *J Am Soc Nephrol* 1992;2:1163–1170.
79. Orisio S, Benigni A, Bruzzi I, et al. *Kidney Int* 1993;43:354–358.
80. Magil AB, Frohlich JJ, Innis SM, Steinbrecher UP. *Kidney Int* 1993;43:1243–1250.
81. Border WA, Ruoslahti E. *J Clin Invest* 1992;90:1–7.
82. Rovin BH, Tan LC. *Kidney Int* 1993;43:218–225.
83. Ding GH, Pesek-Diamond I, Diamond JR. *Am J Physiol* 1993;264:F577–F584.
84. Quinn MT, Parthasarathy S, Fong LG, Steinberg D. *Proc Natl Acad Sci USA* 1987;84:2995–2998.
85. Schreiner GF. *Semin Nephrol* 1991;11:268–275.
86. Diamond JR, Karnovsky MJ. *Annu Rev Med* 1992;43:83–92.
87. Kamanna VS, Roh DD, Kirschenbaum MA. *Am J Nephrol* 1993;13:1–5.
88. Schonholzer KW, Waldron M, Magil AB. *Nephron* 1992;62:130–136.
89. Diamond JR, Ding G, Frye J, Diamond IP. *Am J Pathol* 1992;141:887–894.
90. Kim SY, Kim Y, Kasiske BL, O'Donnell MP, Keane WF. *J Am Soc Nephrol* 1993;3:599 [Abstract].
91. Kaplan R, Aynedjian HS, Schlondorff D, Bank N. *J Clin Invest* 1990;86:1707–1714.
92. O'Donnell MP, Kasiske BL, Kim Y, Atluru D, Keane WF. *J Clin Invest* 1993;91:83–87.
93. Goldstein JL, Brown MS. *Nature* 1990;343:425–430.
94. Maltese WA. *FASEB J* 1990;4:3319–3328.
95. Casey PJ. *J Lipid Res* 1992;33:1731–1740.
96. Casey PJ, Solski PA, Der CJ, Buss JE. *Proc Natl Acad Sci USA* 1989;86:8323–8327.
97. Santos E, Nebreda AR. *FASEB J* 1989;3:2151–2163.
98. Satoh T, Endo M, Nakafuku M, Nakamura S, Kaziro Y. *Proc Natl Acad Sci USA* 1990;87:5993–5997.
99. Satoh T, Nakafuku M, Kaziro Y. *J Biol Chem* 1992;267:24149–24152.
100. Fairbanks KP, Witte LD, Goodman DS. *J Biol Chem* 1984;259:1546–1551.
101. Habenicht AJR, Glomset JA, Ross R. *J Biol Chem* 1980;255:5134–5140.
102. Perkins SL, Ledin SF, Stubbs JD. *Biochim Biophys Acta* 1982;711:83–89.
103. Quesney-Huneeus V, Galick HA, Siperstein MD, Erickson SK, Spencer TA, Nelson JA. *J Biol Chem* 1983;258:378–385.
104. Guijarro C, O'Donnell MP, Kasiske BL, Kim Y, Atluru D, Keane WF. *J Am Soc Nephrol* 1993 [Abstract].
105. Bnaa KH, Thelle DS. *Circulation* 1991;83:1305–1314.
106. Julius S, Jamerson K, Mejia A, Krause L, Schork N, Jones K. *JAMA* 1990;264:354–358.
107. Osborne JA, Siegman MJ, Sedar AW, Mooers SU, Lefer AM. *Am J Physiol* 1989;256:C591–C597.
108. Osborne JA, Lento PH, Siegfried MR, Stahl GL, Fusman B, Lefer AM. *J Clin Invest* 1989;83:465–473.
109. Cooke JP, Singer AH, Tsao P, Zera P, Rowan RA, Billingham ME. *J Clin Invest* 1992;90:1168–1172.
110. Andrews HE, Bruckdorfer KR, Dunn RC, Jacobs M. *Nature* 1987;327:237–239.
111. Kugiyama K, Kerns SA, Morrisett JD, Roberts R, Henry PD. *Nature* 1990;344:160–162.
112. Simchon S, Manger MW, Shi G-S, Brensilver J. *Hypertension* 1992;20:524–532.

113. Lüscher TF, Raij L, Vanhoutte PM. *Hypertension* 1987;9:157–163.
114. Lüscher TF, Vanhoutte PM, Raij L. *Hypertension* 1987;9[Suppl III]:III-193–III-197.
115. Boegehold M. *Hypertension* 1992;19:290–295.
116. Chen PY, Sanders PW. *J Clin Invest* 1991;88:1559–1567.
117. Lee L, Webb RC. *Hypertension* 1992;19:435–441.
118. Chatziantoniou C, Daniels FH, Arendshorst WJ. *Am J Physiol* 1990;259:F372–F382.
119. Chatziantoniou C, Arendshorst WJ. *Am J Physiol* 1992;263:F573–F580.
120. Bank N, Aynedjian HS. *J Clin Invest* 1992;89:1636–1642.
121. Kasiske BL, O'Donnell MP, Keane WF. *Clin Res* 1987;35:444A [Abstract].
122. Harker CT, O'Donnell MP, Kasiske BL, Keane WF, Katz SA. *J Am Soc Nephrol* 1993;4:1354–1361.
123. Kasiske BL, O'Donnell MP, Kim Y, Keane WF. *Curr Opin Nephrol Hypertens* 1993;2:602–608.
124. Rabelink AJ, Hené RJ, Erkelens DW, Joles JA, Koomans HA. *Lancet* 1988;2:1335–1338.
125. Sasaki T, Kurata H, Nomura K, Utzunomiya K, Ikeda Y. *Jpn J Med* 1990;29:156–163.
126. O'Donnell MP, Kasiske BL, Kim Y, Athiru D, Keane WF. *Mineral Electrolyte Metab* 1993;19:173–179.

Hypertension: Pathophysiology, Diagnosis,
and Management, Second Edition,
edited by J.H. Laragh and B.M. Brenner,
Raven Press, Ltd., New York © 1995.

CHAPTER 92

The Renal Abnormality in Hypertension: A Proposed Defect in Glomerular Filtration Surface Area

Harald S. Mackenzie, Diego L. Garcia, Sharon Anderson, and Barry M. Brenner

That the kidney is invariably implicated in the pathogenesis and maintenance of systemic hypertension was first predicted by Sir Richard Bright (1) in 1863, a notion that has subsequently been supported by many observations, including renal cross-transplantation experiments (2–4). Among the many factors that have been postulated to participate in the pathogenesis of hypertension (5) are alterations in systemic hemodynamics (6), e.g., due to hyperactivity of vasoconstrictors, for example, the renin-angiotensin system (7) or sympathetic nerves (8); or to hypoactivity of vasodilators, e.g., the kallikrein-kinin system (9), or endothelial derived nitric oxide (10). Dietary (11–13) and genetic factors (14), including racial differences (15), have also been implicated.

Abnormalities in renal sodium (Na) handling, especially, have been linked to the pathogenesis of hypertension, the latter often viewed as a cybernetic adaptation to impaired renal Na excretion. In 1963, Ledingham and

Cohen (16) proposed that hypertension was initiated by expansion of extracellular fluid and plasma volume, which in turn causes a rise in central venous pressure and right heart pressures, an increase in cardiac output due to the Starling effect, and finally a rise in blood pressure (BP). Transmission of the elevated perfusion pressure to the renal arteries leads to natriuresis and diuresis by the pressure-natriuresis effect, preventing further expansion of the extracellular fluid volume. Thereafter, in the chronic phase, total peripheral resistance rises and cardiac output returns to normal, inducing a transition from high cardiac output–mediated hypertension to a high peripheral resistance form of chronic hypertension. Similar reasoning led Borst and Borst-de Geus (17) to postulate that certain individuals have an unknown renal defect that requires a higher local perfusion pressure to excrete the increased load of salt and water, thus rendering these individuals susceptible to hypertension. These authors suggested that the treatment of hypertension must involve an increase in the "willingness" of the kidneys to excrete Na.

Guyton et al. (18) have further suggested that hypertension is characterized by abnormalities in the pressure-natriuresis relationship. In the face of an elevated Na intake, increased arterial pressure augments renal Na ex-

H. S. Mackenzie, D. L. Garcia, and B. M. Brenner: Renal Division, Department of Medicine, Brigham and Women's Hospital, Harvard Medical Center, Boston, Massachusetts 02115.

S. Anderson: Division of Nephrology and Hypertension PP262, Oregon Health Sciences University, Portland, Oregon 97201.

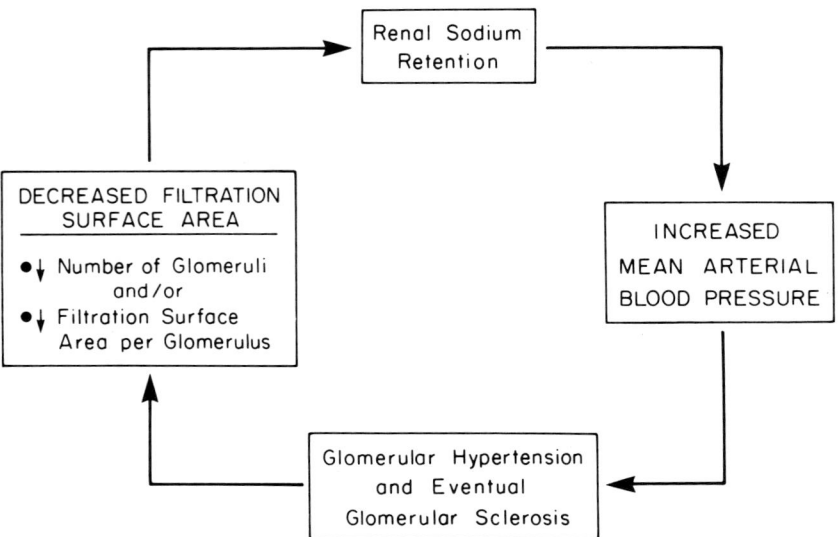

FIG. 1. Relationship between decreased filtration surface area (FSA) and mean arterial pressure. Decreased FSA, due to decreased nephron number and/or FSA per glomerulus, leads to renal sodium retention and thereby leads to increased mean arterial pressure. Systemic hypertension, in turn, promotes glomerular hypertension and eventual sclerosis, thereby further decreasing the functioning filtration surface area.

cretion by increasing filtered Na load and decreasing tubule reabsorption, thereby restoring Na balance. This feedback mechanism thus serves to limit further extracellular fluid volume expansion. Arterial hypertension is the biological price, however, insofar as the kidneys require a supranormal perfusion pressure to restore external sodium balance and maintain near-normal extracellular fluid volume homeostasis.

Whereas dietary Na intake may contribute to hypertension, the association is by no means universal. Individuals (19) as well as populations (20) vary widely in both renal and blood pressure responses to dietary Na intake, suggesting that other factors must be involved in the pathogenesis of hypertension.

We postulate that a major renal abnormality that initiates and contributes to essential hypertension is a decreased filtration surface area (FSA), due to a reduced number of glomeruli and/or a decrease in FSA per glomerulus. Just as alterations in renal hemodynamics, reduced ability to excrete Na, and raised BP characterize the adaptive responses to an acquired decrease in the number of functioning nephrons, so may inborn deficiencies of nephron number enhance susceptibility to essential hypertension. As schematized in Fig. 1, this hypothesis suggests that an initial shortfall in FSA may contribute to renal Na retention, and thus to systemic hypertension. Systemic hypertension then leads to glomerular capillary hypertension and eventual glomerular sclerosis, which in turn further decreases FSA, perpetuating a vicious cycle. In addition, inherited deficiencies in FSA may also explain the highly variable rates of progression of human renal disease, in that the greater hemodynamic burden (i.e., glomerular and systemic hypertension) may render affected individuals less able to

sustain renal function after initial injury than those endowed at birth with a greater number of nephrons.

NEPHRON NUMBER AND HYPERTENSION IN HUMANS

Clinically, major inborn deficits in nephron number are associated with the development of hypertension, as seen in patients with oligomeganephronia (21–23) or a congenital solitary kidney (24–26). Hypertension also often supervenes when a comparable reduction in nephron number occurs later in life as a consequence of ablative surgery. Long-term studies of human subjects who have donated a kidney for transplantation are now becoming available and indicate that although renal function is well maintained in the majority of donors for up to two decades, loss of one kidney may enhance the risk of hypertension and proteinuria when compared to age- and sex-matched controls (27–29). Hypertension is extremely common in renal transplant recipients (30), and for reasons discussed below, this group may represent a population in which the hemodynamic consequences of reduced FSA are especially prominent because functioning nephron numbers in the allograft recipient may be reduced well below 50 percent. Thus, a 50 percent or greater reduction in nephron number, though initially insufficient to induce overt renal insufficiency, clearly enhances the susceptibility to systemic hypertension.

Each human kidney has traditionally been estimated to contain an average of approximately 800,000 to 1,000,000 nephrons (31–34). More recent estimates of glomerular number in humans, however, based on unbiased stereological techniques, give mean values of around 600,000 (35), a figure considerably lower than the "million" commonly stated in textbooks. Moreover, as illustrated in Fig. 2, which depicts nephron numbers in kidneys from individuals under the age of 30 (32), the nephron population ranges widely, from as low as 300,000 to as high as 1,100,000. By these estimates, at least half the population lies between 800,000 and 1,100,000; fewer than 10 percent lie above this range, whereas as many as 40 percent fall below 800,000 per kidney. Few examples of other normal anthropometric characteristics display such extensive variation. No new nephrons are formed after birth, and the number of intact glomeruli tends to decrease after age 40, a consequence of normal aging (36,37).

Are those individuals born with nephron numbers in the low end of the distribution range at higher risk for the development of essential hypertension? Direct studies of nephron number and blood pressure in otherwise normal human subjects are scarce. Hayman et al. (38), in a study of patients with and without renal disease, found systolic BP to be above 150 mm Hg in individuals with fewer than 700,000 glomeruli per kidney, leading these authors to conclude that when nephron number is reduced to this level (about 30 percent below the median in these studies), there is "some change associated with the presence of elevated blood pressure." We suggest that this "change" may be the low nephron number per se. It is tempting to speculate that those individuals whose congenital endowment of nephron numbers falls in the lower range constitute the well-described populations or population subsets that exhibit enhanced susceptibility

to the development of essential hypertension. In addition to the observation that low-birth-weight babies develop increased incidence of essential hypertension in adult life (39) (see chapter 6 by Chertow, *this volume*), it has also been reported that such infants have reduced nephron numbers (40). Does a reduced nephron complement acquired *in utero* account for the relationship between low birth weight and adult essential hypertension? Figure 2 integrates the postulated relationship between nephron number and mean arterial pressure. Those individuals with more than 110 percent of the median number of nephrons may represent the population subset at the lower end of the normal blood pressure range. As nephron numbers fall below the median, blood pressure values rise; those individuals with a critical decrease in nephron number (perhaps below 600,000/kidney) exhibit overt, albeit mild, systemic hypertension. At the extreme low end of the nephron number distribution, blood pressures are greatly elevated.

Alternatively, increased susceptibility to hypertension may result from a decrease in FSA when nephron number is normal, but the filtration surface area per glomerulus is reduced. Glomerular diameter, an indirect measure of FSA, varies as much as threefold in infancy and follows a normal distribution pattern in adult kidneys (41). Glomerular capillary basement membrane surface area, a more direct reflection of net FSA, also varies as much as threefold in normal kidneys (33). Thus, decreased FSA per glomerulus may contribute to hypertension even in the presence of a normal nephron number,

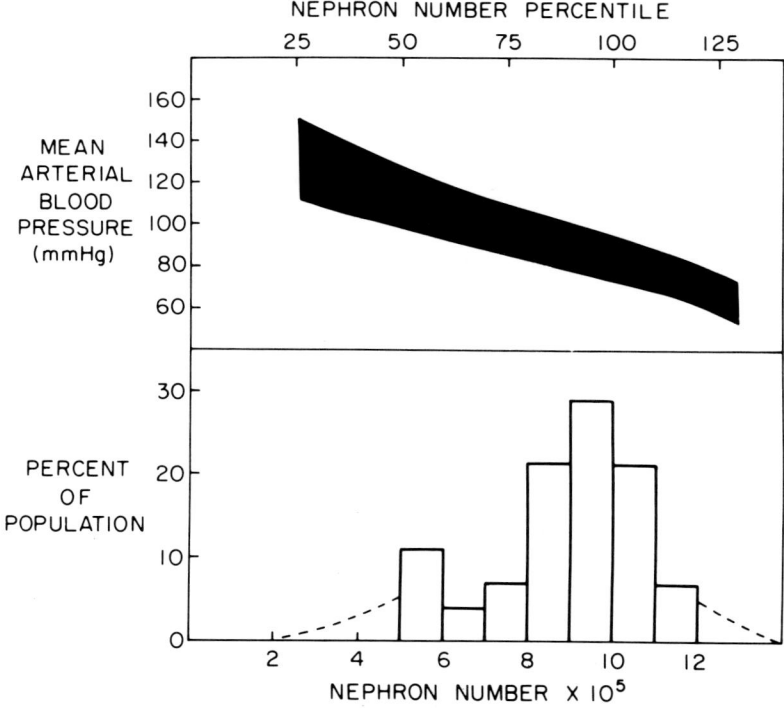

FIG. 2. Nephron number and mean arterial blood pressure. As shown in the *bottom panel*, more than half of the human subjects under 30 years of age possess nephron numbers ranging between 800,000 and 1,100,000 (32)—with approximately 10% exceeding this range, and the remainder falling below. As schematized in the *upper panel*, mean arterial blood pressure (AP) is considered to be within the normal range in those with "normal" nephron numbers, slightly below normal in those with over 1,100,000 nephrons, but elevated in those with reduced nephron numbers. Elevation of AP becomes progressively more marked and variable as nephron number diminishes. Similar patterns would be expected if filtration surface area per glomerulus, rather than number of glomeruli, varied with the same frequency distribution shown here.

TABLE 1. *Nephron number, hypertension, and progressive renal disease*

Abnormal strain	Control strain	Percent of "normal" nephron number	Comments	References
Dahl-sensitive	Dahl resistant	85	High Na intake required to elevate BP; glomerular hypertension and accelerated FGS also develop	49–54
Munich-Wistar-Frömter	Han-Wistar	–	Glomerular density lower; higher BP and accelerated FGS also develop	55–57
Milan hypertensive strain	Milan normotensive strain	83	High BP; absence of severe glomerular hypertension may protect against FGS despite high systemic BP	58–60
Fawn hooded rat		–	Nephron numbers not different, but not quantitated in subset with highest BP and FGS	61
PVG/c		122	Lower BP and resistance to FGS	62

BP, blood pressure; FGS, focal glomerular sclerosis; Na, sodium; –, not measured.

because either or both would serve to reduce total surface area available for filtration.

NEPHRON NUMBER AND HYPERTENSION: EXPERIMENTAL EVIDENCE

Alterations in nephron number could conceivably influence systemic arterial pressure by several mechanisms. For example, it is possible that reducing nephron number may limit renal production of a vasodepressor substance or stimulate secretion of a vasoconstrictive agent. In addition, alterations in nephron number may alter renal sodium handling. When filtration surface area is diminished and sodium intake is not reduced, particularly when proximal tubule sodium reabsorptive mechanisms remain unimpaired, sodium retention may be enhanced.

Experimentally, there are clear associations between nephron number, dietary Na intake, and the incidence of hypertension. In the extreme case, removal of 70 percent or more of the functioning renal mass in the rat leads to systemic and glomerular hypertension, with increased plasma volumes (42) and low plasma renin levels (43,44). Indeed, with such extensive renal ablation, hypertension may be observed even in the absence of a high Na intake (44,45). When the reduction in nephron number is less marked, however, as in the case of uninephrectomy, hypertension usually does not develop in rats on standard diet (46,47), but may be provoked by Na supplementation (47). Koletsky and Goodsitt (48) found that by increasing dietary Na content, hypertension could be induced in 100 percent of rats with 75 percent nephrectomy after 2 weeks, in 94 percent of uninephrectomized rats after 4 months, and in 66 percent of aging rats with intact kidneys after 8 months.

Even in the absence of an acquired reduction in nephron number (i.e., FSA), increasing Na intake enhances susceptibility to hypertension in certain "salt-sensitive"

hypertensive rat strains (49–54). As summarized in Table 1, these animals exhibit a genetic susceptibility to hypertension, the expression of which is greatly enhanced in the presence of a high dietary Na intake. Of note, these salt-sensitive strains are associated with a 15 percent congenital reduction in glomerular number (51,52), suggesting that decreased nephron numbers per se may predispose to an enhanced susceptibility to salt-sensitive hypertension. Indeed, inborn reductions in nephron number may also lead to systemic hypertension in the absence of high Na intake, as shown in other rat strains (55–62) summarized in Table 1. In the spontaneously hypertensive rat (SHR), glomerular numbers are minimally but not significantly lower than in normotensive Wistar-Kyoto (WKY) rats (63), implying that other renal excretory defects may combine with this more subtle reduction in nephron number to predispose to systemic hypertension. However, prehypertensive SHRs exhibit values for the glomerular capillary coefficient that are lower than those in WKY rats, suggesting that FSA and/or the hydraulic permeability properties of the filtering capillaries are also lower in the SHR (64). Although congenital deficiencies in nephron numbers can be induced in rats by exposure to aminoglycoside (65) or low protein diet *in utero* (66), giving rise to eventual glomerular sclerosis (67), it is as yet unknown whether the long-term effect of such manipulations produces hypertension in mature rats (see chapter 6 by Chertow, *this volume*).

SODIUM AND HYPERTENSION

Epidemiologic studies indicate that dietary Na excess is associated with an increased incidence of essential hypertension (20,68–71). Approximately half of essential hypertensives exhibit BP sensitivity to alterations in Na intake (69,70), an effect that may be detected as early as the first few months of life (72). Sodium sensitivity (a decrease in BP after volume depletion, or an increase in

BP after saline loading) follows a gaussian distribution in both hypertensive and normotensive individuals (73).

Clearly, susceptibility to development of essential hypertension is a heritable trait. The risk of hypertension increases dramatically when both parents are hypertensive (14), with a stronger correlation between identical twins than between fraternal twins or siblings (74) and a lack of correlation between parents and their adopted children (75). A compelling familial resemblance has been noted in baseline BP values (76), and also in sodium sensitivity of BP, between parents and their offspring (19). Normotensive first-degree relatives of individuals with essential hypertension exhibit higher basal blood pressures and reduced ability to excrete a Na load, as contrasted with subjects lacking a family history of hypertension (77). Moreover, normotensive teenagers are more likely to exhibit a rise in BP when subjected to a high Na intake, if a parent is hypertensive (78). These observations argue strongly for an inherited renal abnormality in the pathogenesis of essential hypertension.

There may also be a genetic component to the development of hypertension in humans with a solitary kidney. Renal transplant recipients of a kidney from a normotensive donor with a family history of hypertension exhibit higher levels of blood pressure and require more antihypertensive therapy than do recipients of grafts from donors with no family history of hypertension (79). Moreover, these recipients tend to show significant increases in BP during acute rejection episodes (80). Thus, susceptibility to hypertension may be acquired when the kidney comes from a hypertensive donor, but also with a kidney from a normotensive donor with a family history of hypertension. Do such kidneys contain less total FSA (i.e., fewer glomeruli) than those from donors with no such family history?

Because only a minority of the general population is hypertensive, Na intake appears to contribute to the development of hypertension only in individuals with a born susceptibility to the development of hypertension (5). An inherited decrease in nephron number (or FSA), leading to a diminished capacity to excrete a normal Na load, could constitute an important underlying pathogenetic determinant of salt-sensitive essential hypertension in these subjects. As illustrated in Fig. 3, variability in nephron number, with subsequent heterogeneity in BP responses to increased Na intake, may explain the observed variability of arterial pressures at varying levels of Na intake. We postulate that those individuals whose nephron number approximates 100 percent of "normal" exhibit relative insensitivity of BP to changes in Na intake, so that a BP increment is seen only with extreme dietary excess, if at all. However, those individuals whose nephron number falls below the median exhibit progressive increments in BP as Na intake increases. At the low end of the spectrum, as in patients with advanced renal disease, extreme reduction in nephron number greatly

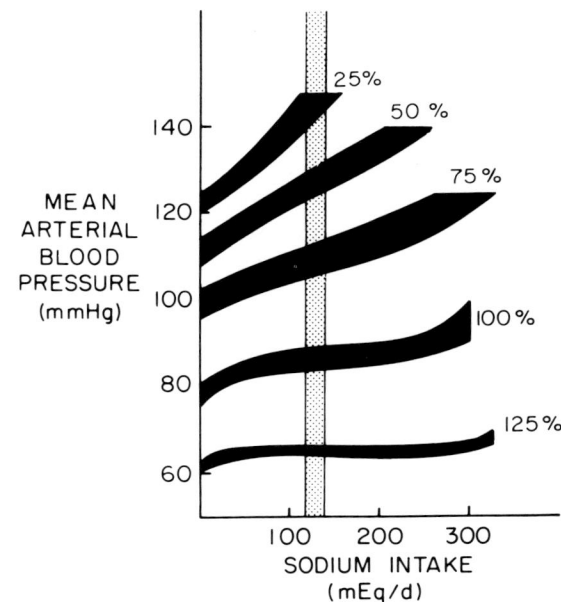

FIG. 3. Filtration surface area (FSA), Na intake, and mean arterial pressure ($\overline{AP}$). "Average" Na intake is depicted by the vertical (*stippled*) band; black bands represent $\overline{AP}$ ranges at indicated FSA percentiles. Individuals whose FSA is in the middle of the normal distribution (i.e., 100% of "normal") are hypothesized to exhibit relative $\overline{AP}$ insensitivity to changes in Na intake. Those with FSA above the median (125% of normal) are likely to exhibit even lower values for $\overline{AP}$ at all levels of Na intake. When FSA is deficient, however, the curve is displaced upward, requiring lesser increases in Na intake to raise $\overline{AP}$. At the extreme low end of the FSA scale, the curve is also steepened, so that greater increases in $\overline{AP}$ are required to maintain external Na balance even at relatively moderate dietary Na intake.

limits capacity to modulate Na excretion, so that greater increases in BP are required to maintain external Na balance, even at relatively moderate dietary Na intake.

Though still largely unexplored, inborn deficits in nephron number could contribute to the observed differences in susceptibility to hypertension (irrespective of dietary factors), which characterize different genetic populations. For example, Japanese subjects exhibit a high incidence of hypertension (81), and autopsy studies demonstrate that this population has smaller kidneys than Caucasians (82). Do these smaller kidneys contain fewer glomerui and/or reduced FSA? Studies among individuals of the same race show that kidney weight correlates highly with nephron number (35), but interracial differences in nephron number have yet to be studied in depth.

Hypertension is both more common and more severe in Americans of African descent (83). In a study of normotensive adults, Luft et al. (84) demonstrated that as compared to Caucasians, black subjects had higher blood pressures with oral Na loading, together with a decreased ability to excrete an intravenous Na load. Helmer (85) proposed that the sensitivity of American black subjects to Na may be related to their African origins, with the tendency to retain Na the consequence of the adaptation of 40,000 or more generations to existence in tropical or subtropical conditions and the resulting stress on Na homeostasis. Greater facility for Na conservation and a lesser capacity to excrete any perceived excess could be a legacy of this geogenetic heritage (86). Although appropriate for a tropical climate, this propensity to retain Na would prove maladaptive in the more temparate climate of North America, thereby contributing to the high incidence of hypertension in Afro-Americans. Helmer further suggested that this tendency toward Na conservation might explain the predilection to low plasma renin activities in black hypertensives, a phenomenon that he was first to identify (85). Black hypertensives exhibit enhanced renal vascular resistance (87), increased plasma volume (88), and a form of hypertension that tends to respond to diuretic therapy (89). A reduction in the glomerular capillary ultrafiltration coefficient has been postulated to contribute to this Na retention in blacks (90) and fewer nephron numbers have also been observed in the black population. Could these and other forms of low renin hypertension result from a diminished capacity of a reduced number of glomeruli (or, alternatively, to a deficient FSA in a normal number of glomeruli) to excrete salt? This latter possibility may be suggested by analogy with *Psammomys obesus,* the desert sand rat. In this mammal, values for glomerular number are higher than those in nondesert rodents, but glomerular diameters, FSA, and single nephron glomerular filtration rates are greatly reduced (91).

Gender may also play a role in the relationship between inherited nephron number and susceptibility to hypertension. Epidemiologic studies in diverse populations indicate that females exhibit greater age-related increases in BP than do males (20,68) and that blood pressures in black women are higher than those in black men (92). Indeed, studies of both race and gender indicate that of all hypertensive groups, black females show the largest decrements in BP following Na and volume depletion (93). Females tend to have smaller kidneys than do males (31), and 10 percent fewer glomeruli (94). Could fewer nephrons account for these smaller kidneys and thereby contribute to enhanced susceptibility to hypertension in females?

Finally, the age-related increase in incidence of hypertension (95) correlates temporally with the decrease in functioning nephron number (36,37) that occurs during normal aging. This gradual but substantial nephron loss may explain the observation that older individuals are less able to excrete an administered or ingested Na load than younger subjects (90), thereby producing hypertension by a mechanism analogous to that postulated in younger subjects with congenitally reduced nephron numbers. As depicted in Fig. 4, both incidence and mag-

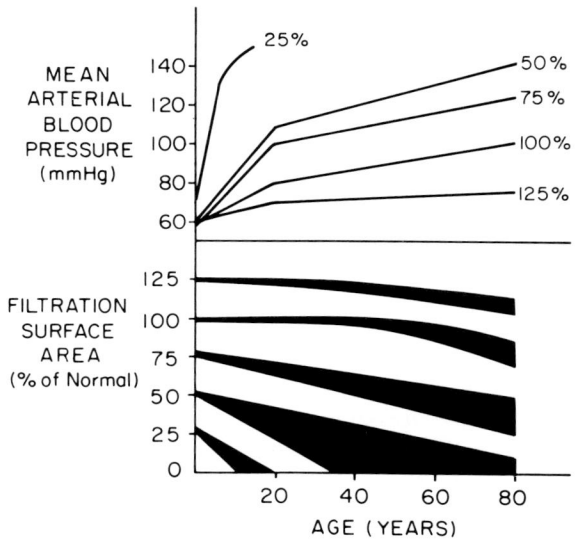

FIG. 4. Age-related increases in mean arterial blood pressure (AP) and loss of filtration surface area (FSA): relationship to initial FSA. As shown in the *top panel,* individuals with 100% of the normal FSA show a slight increase in AP with advancing age. Those with higher nephron numbers, or higher FSA per glomerulus, exhibit little such increase, even in older age, whereas those with lower FSA exhibit hypertension at earlier ages as well as steeper AP increases over time. As shown in the *bottom panel,* age-related loss of functioning glomeruli is minimal in those endowed with higher FSA at birth, moderate in those with normal values, and accelerated when congenital nephron number and/or FSA is substantially below the mean (i.e., designated 100%).

nitude of age-related hypertension and nephron dropout may relate to the congenital endowment of glomerular FSA. Those individuals with supranormal glomerular FSA at birth are envisaged to enjoy normal or low blood pressures throughout life, with relatively little loss of functioning nephron number, or total renal function, even as octogenarians. For those with "normal" FSA, we hypothesize a slight but definable increase in BP as a consequence of the mild nephron loss occurring with advanced age, but neither BP nor renal function is significantly abnormal even in old age. However, those with inborn reductions in FSA are considered to lose nephrons more rapidly and to develop hypertension earlier, perhaps as early as the third or fourth decade of life, the peak age of onset of essential hypertension (96). With severe inborn reductions in FSA, hypertension and nephron loss sufficient to severely compromise renal function are thought to occur at even earlier ages, including childhood and young adulthood.

SODIUM AND RENAL HEMODYNAMICS IN HYPERTENSION

Studies of experimental animals indicate that in chronic hypertension the pressure–natriuresis relationship is abnormal, since Na balance is achieved at the expense of a higher BP. In these models, resetting of the pressure–natriuresis curve serves as a compensatory mechanism maintaining volume homeostasis in the setting of the primary abnormality, a reduced capacity to excrete Na (97). Clinical and experimental studies have yielded considerable information as to the renal hemodynamic mechanisms that serve to initiate and maintain these compensatory adaptations. In 1979, Bianchi et al. (98) studied young normotensive offspring of hypertensive parents and noted a significant increase in renal plasma flow, as well as a numerical increase in glomerular filtration rate, in these "prehypertensive" subjects. As discussed above, these individuals exhibit reduced capacity to excrete a Na load. Recent studies indicate that saline loading induces greater increases in plasma atrial natriuretic peptide (ANP) levels in these subjects than in normals (99), suggesting that this hormone, which augments renal blood flow and glomerular filtration rates as well as renal Na excretion (100,101), may be involved in the renal hemodynamic adaptation to a reduced ability to excrete Na. Conceivably, then, this prehypertensive state is characterized by renal Na retention, which leads to plasma volume expansion and alterations in volume-regulatory hormones that, in turn, contribute to intrarenal hemodynamic adaptations.

An experimental analogue to this condition is found in the prehypertensive Dahl salt-sensitive rat, a hypertensive strain with a congenital reduction in nephron number (54). Of note, the Dahl salt-sensitive rat is also characterized by a reduced glomerular capillary ultrafiltration coefficient (54), a hemodynamic abnormality that may be present even in the prehypertensive stage (102). Dahl salt-sensitive rats have been reported to exhibit a decrease in FSA that correlates with the development of hypertension (103), as well as an impaired glomerular functional response (i.e., rise in GFR) after amino acid infusion in the prehypertensive stage (104). In this model, autoregulation studies indicate that renal blood flow and glomerular filtration rates fall to lower levels with graded decrements in perfusion pressure than in salt-resistant rats (102). Thus, the Dahl salt-sensitive strain exhibits blunting of both the autoregulatory and pressure–natriuresis curves in the prehypertensive stage, thereby suggesting a mechanism to explain similar hemodynamic findings in prehypertensive human subjects (see chapter 94 by Kimura and Brenner, *this volume*). These findings are also reminiscent of "nonmodulators," a subset of essential hypertensives characterized by reduced ability to excrete Na load (105), accompanied by failure of (a) Na loading to enhance basal renal blood flow (106,107), (b) adrenal responsiveness to angiotensin II (106), or (c) the renal vascular response to angiotensin

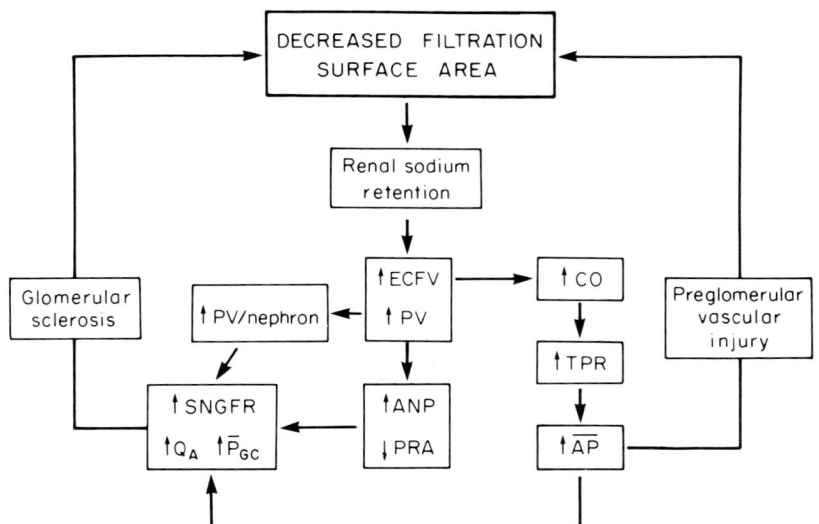

FIG. 5. Postulated mechanism whereby decreased filtration surface area (FSA) leads to alterations in Na balance, renal hemodynamics, and arterial pressure. Decreased FSA, whether congenital or acquired, limits the capacity to excrete Na ($U_{Na}V$), leading to expansion of extracellular fluid volume (ECFV) and plasma volume (PV). This expanded PV leads sequentially to increases in cardiac output (CO), total peripheral resistance (TPR), and mean arterial blood pressure ($\overline{AP}$), the latter serving to restore $U_{Na}V$ (pressure-natriuresis). PV expansion also results in increased plasma atrial natriuretic peptide (ANP) levels and decreased plasma renin activity (PRA); in conjunction with other factors, these humoral alterations lead to increases in the glomerular plasma flow rate (Q_A), mean glomerular capillary hydraulic pressure ($\overline{P}_{GC}$), and single-nephron glomerular filtration rate (SNGFR). Systemic hypertension in itself also contributes to the increase in $\overline{P}_{GC}$, as well as to preglomerular vascular injury. However, systemic hypertension and altered glomerular hemodynamics eventually exert deleterious effects on glomerular structure, resulting in a further loss of FSA and perpetuation of a vicious cycle.

II (106,107). "Nonmodulators" also exhibit (a) delayed suppression of renin release after acute Na loading (105), and (b) correction of most or all of the abnormalities cited with administration of an angiotensin I–converting enzyme inhibitor (107,108). Of note, impaired ability to excrete a Na load (102) and failure to increase renal blood flow after Na loading (109) have been documented in the hypertensive Dahl salt-sensitive rat, suggesting that this strain may share a common underlying renal hemodynamic abnormality with human "nonmodulators." Indeed, a rightward shift of the pressure–natriuresis curve similarly characterizes most, if not all, experimental models of hypertension studied to date (110).

We therefore suggest that congenitally low nephron number may, in part, explain the altered pressure–natriuresis and renal function curves in essential hypertension and may further explain the observed differences in arterial pressure responses to increased Na intake. An integrated scheme whereby congenital or acquired reduction in nephron number (i.e., FSA) leads to alterations in Na balance, renal function, and BP is presented in Fig. 5. Reduction in FSA, in the setting of a normal Na intake, leads to renal Na retention, along with consequent expansion of extracellular fluid and plasma volumes. The latter serves to increase cardiac output, then total peripheral resistance, and finally BP, which enhances urinary Na excretion (pressure–natriuresis). The expanded plasma volume also results in increased plasma ANP levels and decreased plasma renin activity; each of these, in conjunction with other factors that sense the increased plasma volume load per nephron, leads to increases in glomerular capillary plasma flow, hydraulic pressure, and filtration rate. Systemic hypertension in itself contributes to preglomerular vascular disease (111), as well as to elevation of glomerular capillary hydraulic pressure (44,50). Both systemic hypertension and altered glomerular hemodynamics exert deleterious effects on glomerular structure, resulting in a further decrease in functioning nephron number (or acceleration of age-related nephron loss). Thus, the adaptive increases in renal microvascular pressures and flows that serve to enhance urinary Na excretion and to restore external Na balance eventually prove maladaptive and contribute to a further reduction in functioning nephron number, thus perpetuating the cycle.

NEPHRON NUMBER, HYPERTENSION, AND PROGRESSION OF RENAL DISEASE

Whereas a modest congenital deficiency in FSA may contribute to essential hypertension (112,113), it is quite clear that a more extensive reduction, as in acquired renal disease, is often associated with systemic hypertension. We hypothesize that congenital nephron endowment may also be an important determinant of the rate of progression of acquired renal disease. In the extreme case of extensive experimental renal ablation, removal of a critical portion of renal mass results in a syndrome of systemic hypertension, progressive azotemia, proteinuria, and eventual glomerulosclerosis (44,45). Furthermore, the pace of progression accelerates with increasing degrees of ablation and correlates with the compensatory hemodynamic adaptations that occur (114–116). Of note, hemodynamic adaptations eventuate in glomerular destruction not only when nephron number is reduced surgically but also in variant rat strains born with more moderate reductions in nephron number. As summarized in Table 1, modest reductions in congenital nephron number are associated not only with enhanced susceptibility to essential hypertension but also with accelerated age-related proteinuria and glomerular sclerosis (50–52).

Clinical progression to end-stage renal failure is highly variable, in that rates of progression vary widely within the same disease (117,118). We postulate that those individuals born with nephron numbers in the low end of the distribution curve may be the same patients who demonstrate accelerated declines in renal function following initial renal injury. For example, a deficient congenital complement of nephrons could explain the later development of renal insufficiency in those patients who exhibit (a) incomplete initial recovery after acute renal failure (119,120), (b) bilateral renal cortical necrosis (121), and (c) acute post-streptococcal glomerulonephritis (122). Conceivably, the process of repair and compensatory hyperfiltration in surviving glomeruli could serve to preserve renal function at near-normal levels for a period of time, but the excessive hemodynamic burden imposed on a congenitally reduced FSA renders this subset of patients at higher risk for eventual loss of renal function. By analogy to rat strains that exhibit decreased numbers of glomeruli, the reduced number of nephrons in such patients would bear an even greater hemodynamic burden following partial glomerular destruction by disease, exhibit even higher compensatory glomerular capillary flows and pressures, and follow an accelerated course to end-stage renal failure.

Studies in experimental animals lend support to the hypothesis that inborn nephron number may contribute to the rate of progression after renal injury. Whereas chronic renal failure is the major cause of noninfectious death in laboratory rats (123), strains vary greatly in the rapidity of development of age-related renal disease (124–126). Though not directly studied, different rat strains appear to exhibit marked variability in rates of progression to glomerular sclerosis after (a) 5/6 nephrectomy (45,127) or (b) puromycin aminonucleoside nephrosis (128,129).

Conceivably, similar variability in congenital nephron number (i.e., FSA) contributes to the rate of decline in renal function (92,130) and to the development of glomerular sclerosis (36,37) seen in "normal" human aging, as discussed above (see also Fig. 4). Studies of the effects of age, race, and heredity on renal function indicate that glomerular filtration rate (GFR) is partially under the influence of genetic variance (92) and it seems likely that those individuals with fewer nephrons early in life are less able to maintain renal function because nephron dropout engenders hemodynamic maladaptations in remaining glomeruli. Of note, age-related loss of renal function is accelerated in North American blacks as compared to Caucasians (94), perhaps because of a lesser number of nephrons.

NEPHRON NUMBER AND DIABETIC GLOMERULOPATHY

Inborn differences in nephron number may also contribute to susceptibility or resistance to development of renal disease in patients with diabetes mellitus. In both type I (131) and type II (132) diabetics, up to 60 percent of patients eventually develop diabetic glomerulopathy (133), whereas the remainder seem to be spared this complication. Those patients endowed with a reduced FSA might represent the subset of diabetic patients who exhibit (a) persistent hyperfiltration early in the course of the disease and (b) later progression to overt diabetic nephropathy; whereas in those endowed with greater FSA, the risk of overt glomerulopathy might be less. Increased whole-kidney GFR in the face of a reduced nephron number may be explained by marked single nephron hyperfiltration. A 50 percent reduction in nephron number (uninephrectomy) leads to a 40 percent increase in calculated single nephron GFR; therefore, lesser single-nephron hyperfiltration would be required to produce a supranormal whole-kidney GFR in the face of a milder (i.e., 25–30 percent) reduction in congenital nephron number.

Of note, elevated blood pressure typically precedes the appearance of diabetic nephropathy. Patients with type I diabetes exhibit statistical elevations of BP, albeit within the normal range, when urinary albumin levels are not yet elevated (134,135). During the stage of incipient nephropathy, when microalbuminuria is present but before the development of persistent proteinuria, BP values are usually higher than those in normal subjects (134,135). Once glomerulopathy becomes clinically overt, systemic hypertension occurs in the majority of diabetic patients (131) and the severity of hypertension correlates inversely with the level of renal function.

A further correlation between BP and diabetes comes from the important observation that those diabetics who develop renal complications are more likely to have parents with essential hypertension (136,137). Could a congenital nephron deficiency contribute to hypertension in the parents as well as to susceptibility to hypertension in the diabetic offspring?

Several other features of diabetic nephropathy are consistent with such a concept. When diabetic glomerulopathy develops after a renal transplantation (in the setting of one kidney), it does so considerably more rapidly than it did originally in the setting of two native kidneys (138); this enhanced susceptibility in the same patient may relate to the fact that the recipient has only around 50 percent or less of a full nephron complement. Second, the relative risk of end-stage renal disease secondary to diabetic glomerulopathy is almost fourfold higher in blacks than in Caucasians (139), perhaps again reflecting a lesser number of nephrons. Moreover, black women exhibit a relative risk for diabetic glomerulopathy that is even higher than in black males (139). Conceivably, both race and gender contribute to reduction in congenital nephron number and to an enhanced risk for diabetic glomerulopathy.

The theoretical risk of essential hypertension, diabetic glomerulopathy, or end-stage renal failure after acquired renal disease is related to FSA and Na intake in Fig. 6. Those patients with a relative surfeit of nephron number or FSA are considered likely to exhibit (a) relatively low BP and (b) little risk of diabetic glomerulopathy or end-stage renal failure after acquired renal injury. As FSA decreases, relative risk increases, particularly in the setting of enhanced Na intake. At all nephron numbers, reduc-

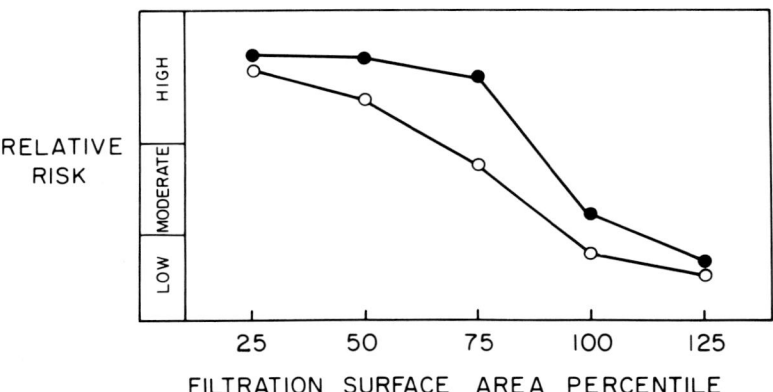

FIG. 6. Theoretical risk of essential hypertension, diabetic glomerulopathy, or end-stage renal failure after acquired renal disease: relationship to filtration surface area (FSA) and Na intake. Those individuals with supranormal nephron numbers or FSA exhibit relatively low blood pressures on high (●) or low (○) Na intake; they also exhibit little risk of diabetic glomerulopathy or of end-stage renal failure after acquired renal disease. In the normal FSA range, relative risk remains low but may be amplified slightly by dietary Na excess. Both relative risk and enhancement of risk with high Na intake increase greatly with FSA below the normal range.

tion of Na intake may reduce, and increased Na intake may enhance, relative risk, though dietary manipulations are insufficient to normalize BP or significantly ameliorate risk when FSA is reduced.

NEPHRON NUMBER AND LATE RENAL ALLOGRAFT FAILURE

Recently it has been suggested that the renal allograft recipient is particularly vulnerable to hypertension by virtue of limited FSA or numbers of functioning nephrons, thus placing the allograft on a programmed course of hemodynamically mediated progressive renal injury from the outset (140). Especially in the setting of cadaveric renal transplantation, nephron numbers are likely to be more extensively reduced than in the case of simple uninephrectomy. Although a single renal allograft could, in theory, provide about 50 percent of the total nephron complement for an individual of similar size to the donor, because of further permanent losses of nephrons through the combined injurious effects of ischemia and reperfusion injury, acute rejection, and cyclosporine nephrotoxicity, the complement of functioning nephrons soon decreases below the original number contained in the graft. Thus, a parallel between the allograft and renal mass ablation models of progressive renal failure is suggested. Given the similarities in the histologic appearances of "chronic rejection" and the kidney with hypertensive nephropathy or other examples of chronic hemodynamically mediated renal injury, this viewpoint has prompted the question: Is the late failure of renal allografts a phenomenon more associated with reduced nephron numbers and the responses to inadequate FSA than one of chronic, alloantigen-directed, immune-mediated injury? Several lines of evidence support this notion. Even before the advent of cyclosporine, the incidence of hypertension in renal allograft recipients approached 50 percent. Furthermore, despite the advances in immunosuppression in recent years, largely responsible for greatly improved 1-year graft survival rates, the long-term attrition rate of renal allografts has remained unchanged over the same period. Are the poorer long-term clinical outcomes encountered after longer cold-ischemia times (141) or more frequent episodes of acute rejection (142,143) the consequence of fewer and fewer nephrons surviving these early events? Body and kidney size discrepancies between donor and recipient may further exacerbate the shortfall between the supply of nephrons and the demands placed upon them (144). Demographic data have been used to infer renal-to-body weight ratios on a population basis (144). As noted above, subtle but consistent shortfalls in total renal mass and nephron numbers have been observed between males and females (94), between the U.S. population of African descent and Caucasians (92,145), and in the el-

derly (35–37). Pediatric kidneys, while having a full complement of nephrons, nevertheless have considerably less FSA when compared with that of the adult organ.

When outcome statistics are analyzed, there is a clear trend for kidneys of black donors to fare worse, irrespective of recipient race, than kidneys from Caucasian donors (146,147). Moreover, kidneys from female donors fare worse in male recipients than male donor kidneys in female recipients (148,149) and the outcome of transplanting kidneys from donors at the extremes of age is worse than for donors of intermediate ages (150–152); however, transplantation of both kidneys from pediatric donors may, in some instances at least, abolish this difference (153). Although kidney weights are not routinely recorded at the time of transplantation, a preliminary report has suggested that donor-to-recipient body surface area ratios of less than 0.8 are associated with poorer early and late graft function (154).

The consistency of these trends, observed across diverse histocompatibility settings, lends support to the concept that the allograft-to-recipient body weight ratio, and hence the number of nephrons or FSA supplied per unit body mass of the recipient, is an independent factor influencing the outcome of cadaveric renal transplantation. The incidence of hypertension under these circumstances is almost certainly increased, as part of the syndrome of the failing allograft, but this dimension has yet to be studied specifically.

Can the development of systemic hypertension and progressive chronic renal allograft failure in the transplant recipient be reduced by matching nephron numbers supplied at transplantation to the recipient's metabolic requirements? Such nephron "dosing" could be based on the donor–kidney weight to recipient–body weight ratio, or donor-to-recipient surface area ratio. Do measures known to reverse the hemodynamic changes resulting from renal mass ablation, e.g., dietary protein restriction, as suggested in some small clinical studies (155–157), or administration of angiotensin-converting enzyme (ACE) inhibitors, ameliorate progression of chronic renal allograft failure? Renal transplantation may well supply the setting in which such fundamental questions about the significance of nephron numbers may be most amenable to study.

SUMMARY AND IMPLICATIONS

Taken together, these observations suggest that a congenital deficiency of glomerular FSA contributes to two processes: (a) limited capacity to excrete a sodium load, leading to a propensity to "essential" hypertension, and (b) susceptibility to accelerated renal failure when FSA is further reduced by surgical ablation or acquired renal injury. Reduction of nephron number, whether congenital or acquired, leads to volume-dependent systemic hypertension and to abnormalities of neurohumoral modulators of renal excretory function including (a) alterations in the renin-angiotensin and adrenergic nervous systems and (b) increased cardiac secretion of ANP. Once systemic hypertension is established, factors such as increased systemic vascular resistance and structural alterations in the renal and extrarenal vasculature tend to perpetuate the process, leading to fixed arterial hypertension. Both systemic hypertension (44,50–53,110) and increased ANP levels (101,158) contribute to glomerular capillary hypertension, which eventuates in glomerular sclerosis. As sclerosis obliterates more and more of the glomerular filtration bed, glomerular destruction further aggravates systemic hypertension. Whereas no therapy is available to directly increase inborn glomerular number or augment the growth of new glomerular capillaries, adequacy of nephron supply at transplantation is a factor that could be addressed by avoiding grossly unfavorable donor–recipient size mismatches. Furthermore, interventions that control systemic and glomerular capillary hypertension (44,110,127,159,160) could interrupt the cycle of progressive injury and minimize risk in those patients most susceptible to hypertension and glomerular injury.

In summary, susceptibility to systemic hypertension, with its underlying abnormalities in renal hemodynamics and Na excretion, may be explained by an inborn deficit in FSA. Deficient filtration capacity may also explain observed increases in BP with normal aging, as well as contribute to the risk of progressive renal disease in diabetics, late allograft failure, and in those with other forms of renal injury. Congenital variability in FSA may explain why only some, but not all, patients exposed to potentially injurious renal stimuli eventually manifest chronic nephropathy, and it may also account for the susceptibility of subsets of type I and type II diabetics to develop overt glomerulopathy. Clinical confirmation of this hypothesis must necessarily await studies correlating glomerular FSA—estimated from nephrectomy or autopsy specimens using reliable glomerular counting methods and morphological measurements of FSA—with systemic arterial pressure. Experimental verification of this heretofore neglected potential risk factor would constitute a major breakthrough in the conceptual and practical approaches to patients with hypertension and progressive renal disease.

REFERENCES

1. Bright R. Tabular view of morbid appearances in 100 cases connected with albuminous urine. *Guy's Hosp Rep* 1863;1:380–410.
2. Dahl LK, Heine M, Thompson K. Genetic influence on the kidneys of blood pressure. Evidence from chronic renal homografts in rats with opposite predispositions to hypertension. *Circ Res* 1973;34:94–101.
3. Bianchi G, Fox U, DiFrancesco DF, et al. Blood pressure changes produced by kidney cross-transplantation between spontaneously hypertensive rats and normotensive rats. *Clin Sci Mol Med* 1974;47:435–438.
4. Curtis JJ, Luke RG, Dustan HP, et al. Remission of essential hypertension after renal transplantation. *N Engl J Med* 1983;309:1009–1015.
5. Genest J, Kuchel O, Hamet P, Cantin M, eds. *Hypertension: pathophysiology and treatment.* 2nd ed. New York: McGraw-Hill; 1983.
6. Lund-Johansen P. Haemodynamics in essential hypertension. State of the art review. *Clin Sci* 1980;59:343s–354s.
7. Laragh JH, Baer L, Brunner HR, et al. Renin, angiotensin and aldosterone in pathogenesis and management of hypertensive vascular disease. *Am J Med* 1972;52:633–652.
8. Oparil S. The sympathetic nervous system in clinical and experimental hypertension. *Kidney Int* 1986;30:437–452.
9. Margolius HS, Geller R, Pisano JJ, Sjoerdsma A. Altered urinary kallikrein in human hypertension. *Lancet* 1971;ii:1063–1065.
10. Panza JA, Quyyumi AA, Brush JE Jr, Epstein SE. Abnormal endothelium-dependent vascular relaxation in patients with essential hypertension. *N Engl J Med* 1990;323:22–27.
11. Freis ED. Salt, volume and prevention of hypertension. *Circulation* 1976;53:589–595.
12. McCarron DA. Is calcium more important than sodium in the pathogenesis of essential hypertension. *Hypertension* 1985;7:607–627.
13. McGregor GA, Smith SJ, Markandu ND, et al. Moderate potassium supplementation in essential hypertension. *Hypertension* 1985;2:567–570.
14. Deutscher S, Epstein FH, Kjelsberg MO. Familial aggregation of factors associated with coronary heart disease. *Circulation* 1966;33:911–924.
15. Gillum RF. Pathophysiology of hypertension in blacks and whites. A review of the racial blood pressure differences. *Hypertension* 1979;1:468–475.
16. Ledingham JM, Cohen RD. The role of the heart in the pathogenesis of renal hypertension. *Lancet* 1963;2:979–981.
17. Borst JGG, Borst-de Geus A. Hypertension explained by Starling's theory of circulatory hemodynamics. *Lancet* 1963;1:677–682.
18. Guyton AC, Coleman PJ, Cowley AW Jr, et al. A systems analysis approach to understanding long range arterial blood pressure control and hypertension. *Circ Res* 1974;35:159–176.
19. Luft FC, Miller JZ, Weinberger MH, et al. Influence of genetic variance on the sodium sensitivity of blood pressure. *Klin Wochenschr* 1987;65:101–109.
20. Denton D. Salt intake and high blood pressure in man. In: Denton D, ed. *The hunger for salt. An anthropological, physiological and medical analysis.* New York: Springer-Verlag; 1982:542–629.
21. Fetterman GH, Habib R. Congenital bilateral oligonephronic renal hypoplasia with hypertrophy of nephrons (oligomeganephronie). *Am J Clin Pathol* 1969;52:199–207.
22. McGraw M, Poucell S, Sweet J, Baumal R. The significance of focal segmental glomerulosclerosis in oligomeganephronia. *Int J Pediatr Nephrol* 1984;5:67–72.
23. Lieberman E. Essential hypertension in children and youth: a pediatric perspective. *J Pediatr* 1974;85:1–11.
24. Kiprov DD, Colvin RB, McCluskey RT. Focal and segmental glomerulosclerosis and proteinuria associated with unilateral renal agenesis. *Lab Invest* 1982;46:275–281.
25. Rugiu C, Oldrizzi L, Lupo A, et al. Clinical features of patients with solitary kidneys. *Nephron* 1986;43:10–15.
26. Thorner PS, Arbus GS, Celemajer DS, Baumal R. Focal and segmental glomerulosclerosis and progressive renal failure associated with a unilateral kidney. *Pediatrics* 1984;73:806–810.
27. Hakim R, Goldszer RC, Brenner BM. Hypertension and proteinuria: long-term sequellae of uninephrectomy in humans. *Kidney Int* 1984;25:930–936.
28. Talsteth T, Fauchald P, Skrede S, et al. Long-term blood pressure and renal function in kidney donors. *Kidney Int* 1986;29:1072–1076.
29. Torres VE, Offord KP, Anderson CF. Blood pressure determinants in living-related allograft donors and their recipients. *Kidney Int* 1987;31:1383–1390.

30. Kirkman RL, Strom TB, Weir MR, Tilney NL. Late mortality and morbidity in recipients of long-term renal allografts. *Transplantation* 1982;34:347–351.
31. Tisher CC, Madsden KM. Anatomy of the kidney. In: Brenner BM, Rector FC Jr., eds. *The kidney.* 3rd ed. Philadelphia: WB Saunders; 1986:3–60.
32. Moore RA. The total number of glomeruli in the normal human kidney. *Anat Rec* 1931;48:153–168.
33. Dunnill MS, Halley W. Some observations on the quantitive anatomy of the kidney. *J Pathol* 1973;110:113–121.
34. Roullier C. General anatomy and histology of the kidney. In: Roullier C, Muller AF, eds. *The kidney: morphology, biochemistry, physiology.* vol 1. New York: Academic Press; 1969:61–156.
35. Nyengaard JR, Bendtsen TF. Glomerular number and size in relation to age, kidney weight, and body surface area in normal man. *Anat Rec* 1992;232:194–201.
36. Kaplan C, Pasternack B, Shah H, Gallo G. Age-related incidence of sclerotic glomeruli in human kidneys. *Am J Pathol* 1975;80:227–234.
37. Kappel B, Olsen S. Cortical interstitial tissue and sclerosed glomeruli in the normal human kidney, related to age and sex. *Virchows Arch* Abt A 1980;387:271–277.
38. Hayman JM Jr, Martin JM, Miller M. Renal function and the number of glomeruli in the human kidney. *Arch Intern Med* 1939;64:69–83.
39. Barker DJP, Osmond C, Golding J, et al. Growth *in utero,* blood pressure in childhood and adult life, and mortality from cardiovascular disease. *Br Med J* 1989;298:564–567.
40. Highcliff SA, Lynch MRJ, Sargent PH, et al. The effect of intrauterine growth retardation in the development of renal nephrons. *Br J Obstet Gynaecol* 1992;99:296–301.
41. Fetterman GH, Schuplock NA, Philipp FJ, Gregg HS. The growth and maturation of human glomeruli and proximal convolutions from term to adulthood. Studies by microdissection. *Pediatrics* 1965;35:601–619.
42. Kaysen GA, Watson JB. Mechanism of hypoalbuminemia in the 7/8-nephrectomized rat with chronic renal failure. *Am J Physiol* 1982;343:F372–F378.
43. Ylitalo P, Hepp R, Oster P, et al. Effects of varying sodium intake on blood pressure and renin-angiotensin system in subtotally nephrectomized rats. *J Lab Clin Med* 1976;88:807–816.
44. Anderson S, Meyer TW, Rennke HG, Brenner BM. Control of glomerular hypertension limits glomerular injury in rats with reduced renal mass. *J Clin Invest* 1985;76:612–619.
45. Purkerson ML, Hoffsten PE, Klahr S. Pathogenesis of the glomerulopathy associated with renal infarction in rats. *Kidney Int* 1976;9:407–417.
46. Hostetter TH, Meyer TW, Rennke HG, Brenner BM. Chronic effects of dietary protein in the rat with intact and reduced renal mass. *Kidney Int* 1986;30:509–517.
47. Koletsky S. Role of salt and renal mass in experimental hypertension. *Arch Pathol* 1959;68:21–32.
48. Koletsky S, Goodsitt AM. Natural history and pathogenesis of renal ablation hypertension. *Arch Pathol* 1960;69:654–662.
49. Dahl LK, Schackow E. Effects of chronic excess salt ingestion: experimental hypertension in the rat. *Can Med Assoc J* 1964;90:155–160.
50. Azar S, Weller D, Bruno L, et al. Single nephron dynamics in the normal Dahl rat on high sodium intake. *Clin Res* 1977;25:504A(abst).
51. Azar S, Limas C, Iwai J, Weller D. Single nephron dynamics during high sodium intake and early hypertension in Dahl rats. *Jap Heart J* 1979;20(Suppl 1):38–40.
52. Azar S, Johnson MA, Hertel B, Tobian L. Single-nephron pressures, flows and resistances in hypertensive kidneys with nephrosclerosis. *Kidney Int* 1977;12:28–40.
53. Azar S, Iwai J, Weller D. Hypertension increases the reduced glomerular filtration coefficient due to high Na load in Dahl rats. *Kidney Int* 1978;14:691A(abst).
54. Raij L, Azar S, Keane WF. Role of hypertension in progressive immune injury. *Hypertension* 1985;7:398–404.
55. Hackbarth H, Buttner D, Jarck D, et al. Distribution of glomeruli in the renal cortex of Munich Wistar Frömter (MWF) rats. *Renal Physiol* 1983;6:63–71.
56. Brunkhorst R, Halbach G, Frei U, et al. Increased glomerular albumin permeability and hyperfiltration in a newly selected rat strain. *Renal Physiol* 1986;9:88–89.
57. Rovira-Halbach G, Alt JM, Brunkhorst R, et al. Single nephron hyperfiltration and proteinuria in a newly selected rat strain with superficial glomeruli. *Renal Physiol* 1986;9:317–325.
58. Baer BG, Bianchi G. Renal micropuncture study of normotensive and Milan hypertensive rats before and after the development of hypertension. *Kidney Int* 1978;13:452–466.
59. Brandis A, Bianchi G, Reale E, et al. Age-dependent glomerulosclerosis and proteinuria occurring in rats of the Milan normotensive strain and not of the Milan hypertensive strain. *Lab Invest* 1986;55:234–243.
60. Boberg U, Persson A. Increased tubuloglomerular feedback activity in Milan hypertensive rats. *Am J Physiol* 1986;250:F967–F974.
61. De Keijzer, Provoost AP. Hyperfiltration and proteinuria in male Fawn Hooded rats with two intact kidneys developing spontaneous hypertension. *Kidney Int* 1987;32:772(abst).
62. Grond J, Beukers JJB, Schilthuis MS, et al. Analysis of renal structural and functional features in two rat strains with a different susceptibility to glomerulosclerosis. *Lab Invest* 1986;54:77–83.
63. Azar S, Johnson MA, Scheinman J, et al. Regulation of glomerular capillary pressure and filtration rate in young Kyoto hypertensive rats. *Clin Sci* 1979;56:203–209.
64. Arendshorst WJ, Beierwaltes WH. Renal and nephron hemodynamics in spontaneously hypertensive rats. *Am J Physiol* 1979;236:F246–F251.
65. Gilbert T, Lelievre-Pegorier M, Merlet-Benichou C. Immediate and long-term renal effects of fetal exposure to gentamicin. *Pediatr Nephrol* 1990;4:445–450.
66. Zeman FJ. Effects of maternal protein restriction on the kidney of the newborn young of rats. *J Nutr* 1968;94:111–116.
67. Gilbert T, Lelievre-Pegorier M, Merlet-Benichou C. Long-term effects of mild oligonephronia induced *in utero* by gentamicin in the rat. *Pediatr Res* 1991;30:450–456.
68. Page LB, Danion A, Moellering RC Jr. Antecedents of cardiovascular disease in six Solomon Islands societies. *Circulation* 1974;49:1132–1146.
69. Dahl LK. Possible role of salt intake in the development of essential hypertension. In: Bock KD, Cottier PT, eds. *Essential hypertension.* Berlin: Springer-Verlag; 1960:53–65.
70. Fujita T, Henry WL, Bartter RC, et al. Factors influencing blood pressure in salt-sensitive patients with hypertension. *Am J Med* 1980;69:334–344.
71. Sinnett PF, Whyte HM. Epidemiologic studies in a total highland population: Tukisenta, New Guinea. Cardiovascular disease and relevant clinical electrocardiographic, radiologic and biochemical findings. *J Chron Dis* 1973;26:265–290.
72. Hofman A, Hazebroek A, Valkenburg HA. A randomized trial of sodium intake and blood pressure in newborn infants. *JAMA* 1983;250:370–373.
73. Weinberger MH. Dietary sodium and blood pressure. *Hosp Pract* 1986;21(Aug):55–64.
74. Havlik RJ, Feinleib M. Dietary sodium and blood pressure. *Hypertension* 1982;4(Suppl III):III121–III127.
75. Biron P, Mongeau J, Bertrand D. Familial aggregation of blood pressure in 558 adopted children. *Can Med Assoc J* 1976;15:773–774.
76. Miller JZ, Daugherty SA, Weinberger MH, et al. Blood pressure response to dietary sodium restriction in normotensive adults. *Hypertension* 1983;5:790–795.
77. Grim CE, McDonough JR, Miller JZ, et al. Effects of sodium loading and depletion in normotensive first-degree relatives of essential hypertensives. *J Lab Clin Med* 1979;94:764–771.
78. Falkener B, Onesti G, Hayes P. The role of sodium in essential hypertension in genetically hypertensive adolescents. In: Onesti G, Kim KE, eds. *Hypertension in the young and the old.* New York: Grune and Stratton; 1981:29.
79. Guidi E, Bianchi G, Rivolta E, et al. Hypertension in man with a kidney transplant: role of familial versus other factors. *Nephron* 1985;41:14–21.
80. Guidi E, Rivolta E, Bianchi G. Blood pressure in recipients of a

"hypertensive" kidney. Effect of acute rejections. *Proc Xth Int Congr Nephrol* 1987;280(abst).

81. Takahashi E, Sasaki N, Takeda J, Ito H. The geographic distribution of cerebral hemorrhage and hypertension in Japan. *Hum Biol* 1957;29:139–166.

82. Tauchi H, Tsuboi K, Okutomi J. Age changes in the human kidney of different races. *Gerontologia* 1971;17:87–97.

83. Final Report of the Subcommittee on Definition and Prevalence of the 1984 Joint National Committee. Hypertension prevalence and the state of awareness, treatment and control in the United States. *Hypertension* 1985;7:457–468.

84. Luft FC, Rankin LI, Bloch R, et al. Cardiovascular and humoral responses to extremes of sodium intake in normal black and white men. *Circulation* 1979;60:697–706.

85. Helmer OM. Hormonal and biochemical factors controlling blood pressure. In: *Les concepts de Claude Bernard sur le milieu interieur,* Paris: Librairies de l'Academie de Medecine; 1967:115–128.

86. Grim CE, Drew CR. On slavery, salt and the greater prevalence of hypertension in black Americans. *Am J Hypertens* 1988;1:57A(abst).

87. Frohlich ED, Messerli FH, Dunn FG, et al. Greater renal vascular involvement in the black patient with essential hypertension. *Miner Electrolyte Metab* 1984;10:173–177.

88. Lilley JJ, Hsu L, Stone RA. Racial disparity of plasma volume in hypertensive man. *Ann Intern Med* 1976;84:707–711.

89. Veterans Administration Cooperative study on Antihypertensive Agents. Comparison of propranolol and hydrochlorothiazide for the initial treatment of hypertension. II. Results of long-term therapy. *JAMA* 1982;72:726–736.

90. Luft FC, Weinberger MH, Grim CE. Sodium sensitivity and resistance in normotensive humans. *Am J Med* 1982;72:726–736.

91. Baines AD, de Rouffignac C. Functional heterogeneity of nephrons. II. Filtration rates, intraluminal flow velocities and fractional water reabsorption. *Pflueg Arch* 1969:260–276.

92. Boyle E. Biological patterns in hypertension by race, sex, body weight and skin color. *JAMA* 1970;213:1637–1643.

93. Luft FC, Fineberg NS, Miller JZ, et al. The effects of age, race and heredity on glomerular filtration rate following volume expansion and contraction in normal man. *Am J Med Sci* 1980;279:15–24.

94. McLachlan MSF, Guthrie JC, Anderson CK, Fuller MJ. Vascular and glomerular changes in the aging kidney. *J Pathol* 1977;121:65–78.

95. Lindeman RD, Tobin JD, Shock NW. Association between blood pressure and rate of decline in renal function with age. *Kidney Int* 1984;26:861–868.

96. Platt R. Heredity in hypertension. *Lancet* 1963;1:899–904.

97. Guyton AC. *Arterial pressure and hypertension.* Philadelphia: WB Saunders; 1980.

98. Bianchi G, Gatti M, Ferrari P, et al. A renal abnormality as a possible cause of "essential" hypertension. *Lancet* 1979;1:173–177.

99. Uchiyama M, Satokata I, Sakai K: Abnormal response of plasma atrial natriuretic factor and sodium to saline infusion in Japanese children with a family history of essential hypertension. *Proc Xth Int Congr Nephrol* 1987;307(abst).

100. Ballermann BJ, Brenner BM. Biologically active atrial peptides. *J Clin Invest* 1985;76:2041–2048.

101. Dunn BR, Ichikawa I, Pfeffer JM, et al. Renal and systemic hemodynamic effects of synthetic atrial natriuretic peptide in the anesthetized rat. *Circ Res* 1986;59:237–246.

102. Roman RJ. Abnormal renal hemodynamics and pressure-natriuresis relationship in Dahl salt-sensitive rats. *Am J Physiol* 1986;251:F57–F65.

103. Azar S, Kabat V, Vernier R. Is the glomerulus the main culprit in the development of Dahl hypertension? *Am J Hypertens* 1988;1:76A(abst).

104. Tobian L, Johnson MA, Hanlon S, Bartemes K. Prehypertensive Dahl S rats show no rise in GFR after amino acid infusion. *Am J Hypertens* 1988;1:71A(abst).

105. Tuck ML, Williams GH, Dluhy RG, et al. A delayed suppression of the renin-aldosterone axis following saline infusion in human hypertension. *Circ Res* 1976;39:711–716.

106. Shoback DM, Williams GH, Moore TJ, et al. Defect in the sodium-modulated tissue responsiveness to angiotensin II in essential hypertension. *J Clin Invest* 1983;72:2115–2124.

107. Redgrave J, Rabinowe S, Hollenberg NK, Williams GH. Correction of abnormal renal blood flow response to angiotensin II by converting enzyme inhibition in essential hypertension. *J Clin Invest* 1985;75:1285–1290.

108. Taylor T, Moore TJ, Hollenberg NK, Williams GH. Converting enzyme inhibition corrects the altered adrenal response to angiotensin II in essential hypertension. *Hypertension* 1984;6:92–99.

109. Fink GD, Takeshita A, Mark AL, Brody MJ. Determinants of renal vascular resistance in the Dahl strain of genetically hypertensive rat. *Hypertension* 1980;2:274–280.

110. Guyton AC. Renal function curve—a key to understanding the pathogenesis of hypertension. *Hypertension* 1987;10:1–6.

111. Baldwin DS, Neugarten J. Hypertension and renal diseases. *Am J Kidney Dis* 1987;10:186–191.

112. Hakim RM, Lazarus JM. Medical aspects of hemodialysis. In: Brenner BM, Rector FC Jr, eds. *The kidney.* 3rd ed. Philadelphia: WB Saunders; 1986:1791–1845.

113. Lazarus J, Hampers CL, Merrill JP. Hypertension and chronic renal failure. Treatment with hemodialysis and nephrectomy. *Arch Intern Med* 1974;133:1059–1066.

114. Hostetter TH, Olson JL, Rennke HG, et al. Hyperfiltration in remnant nephrons: a potentially adverse response to renal ablation. *Am J Physiol* 1981;241:F85–F93.

115. Brenner BM, Meyer TW, Hostetter TH. Dietary protein intake and the progressive nature of kidney disease. *N Engl J Med* 1982;307:652–660.

116. Striker GE, Nagle RB, Kohnen PW, Smuckler EA. Response to unilateral nephrectomy in old rats. *Arch Pathol* 1969;87:439–442.

117. Mitch WE, Walser M, Buffington GA, Lehman J Jr. A simple method for estimating progression of chronic renal failure. *Lancet* 1976;2:1326–1328.

118. Rutherford WE, Blondin J, Miller JP, et al. Chronic progressive renal disease: rate of change of serum creatinine concentration. *Kidney Int* 1977;11:62–70.

119. Finn WF. Recovery from acute renal failure. In: Brenner BM, Rector FC Jr, eds. *The kidney.* 3rd ed. Philadelphia: WB Saunders; 1983:753–774.

120. Hall JW, Johnson WJ, Maher FT, Hunt JC. Immediate and long-term prognosis in acute renal failure. *Ann Intern Med* 1970;73:515–521.

121. Kleinknecht C, Grünfeld JP, Gomez PC. Diagnostic procedures and long-term prognosis in bilateral renal cortical necrosis. *Kidney Int* 1973;4:390–400.

122. Baldwin DS. Chronic glomerulonephritis: nonimmunologic mechanisms of progressive glomerular damage. *Kidney Int* 1982:109–120.

123. Saxton JA Jr, Kimball GC. Relation of nephrosis and other diseases of albino rats to age and to modifications of diet. *Arch Pathol* 1941;32:951–965.

124. Gray JE, van Zwieten MJ, Hollander CF. Early light microscopic changes of chronic progressive nephritis in several strains of aging laboratory rats. *J Gerontol* 1982;37:142–150.

125. Weaver RN, Gray JE, Schulz JR. Urinary proteins in Sprague-Dawley rats with chronic progressive nephrosis. *Lab Anim Sci* 1975;25:705–710.

126. Alt JM, Maess B, Hackbarth H. Species and strain differences in urinary protein excretion. *Renal Physiol* 1985;8:301–309.

127. Meyer TW, Anderson S, Rennke HG, Brenner BM. Reversing glomerular hypertension stabilizes established glomerular injury. *Kidney Int* 1987;31:752–759.

128. Diamond JR, Karnovsky MJ. Focal and segmental glomerulosclerosis following a single intravenous injection of puromycin aminonucleoside. *Am J Pathol* 1986;122:481–487.

129. Anderson S, Diamond JR, Karnovsky MJ, Brenner BM. Mechanisms underlying transition from acute glomerular injury to glomerulosclerosis in a rat model of nephrotic syndrome. *J Clin Invest* 1988;82:1757–1768.

130. Davies DF, Shock NW. Age changes in glomerular filtration rate, effective renal plasma flow, and tubular excretory capacity in adult males. *J Clin Invest* 1950;29:496–507.

131. Hasslacher C, Ritz E, Terpstra J. Natural history of nephropathy

in Type I diabetes. Relationship to metabolic control and blood pressure. *Hypertension* 1985;7(Suppl II):II18–II20.

132. Hasslacher C, Wahl P, Ritz E. Similar risks of nephropathy in Type I and Type II diabetes. *Kidney Int* 1988;11:193(abst).

133. Mogensen CE, Christensen CK. Predicting diabetic nephropathy in insulin-dependent patients. *N Engl J Med* 1984;311:98–93.

134. Feldt-Rasmussen B, Borch-Johansen K, Mathiesen ER. Hypertension in diabetes as related to nephropathy. Early blood pressure changes. *Hypertension* 1985;7(Suppl II):II18–II20.

135. Mogensen CE, Christensen CK. Blood pressure changes and renal function in incipient and overt diabetic nephropathy. *Hypertension* 1985;7(Suppl II):II64–II73.

136. Krolewski AS, Canessa M, Warram JH. Predisposition to hypertension and susceptibility to renal disease in insulin-dependent diabetes mellitus. *N Engl J Med* 1988;318:140–145.

137. Viberti GC, Keen H, Wiseman MJ. Raised arterial pressure in parents of diabetic children. *Br Med J* 1987;295:515–517.

138. Mauer SM, Steffes MW, Connett J, et al. The development of lesions in the glomerular basement membrane and mesangium after transplantation of normal kidneys to diabetic patients. *Diabetes* 1983;32:948–952.

139. Kappel DF, VanTuinen M. Trends in the incidence of treated end-stage renal disease secondary to diabetic nephropathy. *Am J Kidney Dis* 1986;8:234–238.

140. Brenner BM, Milford EL. Nephron underdosing: a programmed cause of chronic renal allograft failure. *Am J Kidney Dis* 1993;21:66–72.

141. Foster MC, Rowe PA, Dennis MJS, et al. Characteristics of cadaveric renal allograft recipients developing chronic rejection. *Ann Roy Coll Surg Engl* 1990;72:23–26.

142. Almond PS, Matas A, Gillingham K, et al. Risk factors for chronic rejection in renal allograft recipients. *Transplantation* 1993;55:752–757.

143. Basadonna GP, Matas AJ, Gillingham KJ, et al. Early versus late acute renal allograft rejection: impact on chronic rejection. *Transplantation* 1993;55:993–995.

144. Brenner BM, Cohen RA, Milford EL. renal transplantation one size may not fit all. *J Am Soc Nephrol* 1992;3:162–169.

145. Oliver J. *Nephrons and kidneys: a quantitative study of development and evolutionary mammalian architectonics.* New York: Harper & Row; 1968.

146. Zhou YC, Terasaki PI, Cecka JM. Race effects on the outcome of

kidney transplants. In: Terasaki P, ed. *Clinical transplants, 1990.* Los Angeles: UCLA Tissue Typing Lab; 1990:447–459.

147. Opelz G. Influence of recipient and donor age on pediatric transplantation. *Transpl Int* 1988;1:95–98.

148. Mickey R, Cho YW, Carnahan E. Long-term graft survival. In: Terasaki P, ed. *Clinical transplants, 1990.* Los Angeles: UCLA Tissue Typing Lab; 1990:385–396.

149. Terasaki PI, Cecka JM, Takemoto S, Yuge J. Overview. In: Terasaki P, ed. *Clinical transplants, 1988.* Los Angeles: UCLA Tissue Typing Lab; 1988:428–430.

150. Alexander JW, Vaughn WK. The use of "marginal" donors for organ transplantation. The influence of donor age on outcome. *Transplantation* 1991;51:135–141.

151. Harmon WE, Jabs K. Special issues in pediatric renal transplantation. *Semin Nephrol* 1992;12:353–363.

152. Hayes JM, Steinmuller DR, Novick SBSC. The development of proteinuria and focal segmental glomerulosclerosis in recipients of pediatric donor kidneys. *Transplantation* 1991;52:813–817.

153. Sutherland DER, Gruessner RWG, Matas AJ, et al. Transplantation of single and double kidneys from pediatric donors. In: Abouna GM, Kumar MSA, White AG, eds. *Organ transplantation 1990.* Dordrecht: Kluwer Academic Publications; 1991:11.

154. Kupin W, Venkat KK, Mozes M, Johnson C. Predictive value of the donor surface area ratio (DSA/RSA) for the outcome of adult primary cadaveric renal transplantation (abst). In: *Proc XII Int Congr Nephrol.* Jerusalem 1993:190.

155. Feehally J, Harris KPG, Bennett SE, Walls J. Is chronic rejection a nonimmunological phenomenon. *Lancet* 1986;2:486–488.

156. Kootte A, 'T Hart-Edermans M, Paul LC. Dietary protein manipulation or cyclosporin therapy in chronic renal allograft therapy. *Clin Transpl* 1988;2:152–159.

157. Salahudeen AK, Hostetter TH, Raatz SK, Rosenberg ME. Effects of dietary protein in patients with chronic renal transplant rejection. *Kidney Int* 1992;41:183–190.

158. Smith S, Anderson S, Ballermann BJ, Brenner BM. Role of atrial natriuretic peptide in adaptation of sodium excretion with reduced renal mass. *J Clin Invest* 1986;77:1395–1398.

159. Zatz R, Meyer TW, Rennke HG, Brenner BM. Predominance of hemodynamic rather than metabolic factors in the pathogenesis of diabetic glomerulopathy. *Proc Natl Acad Sci USA* 1985;82:5963–5967.

160. Zatz R, Dunn BR, Meyer TW, et al. Prevention of diabetic glomerulopathy by pharmacological amelioration of glomerular capillary hypertension. *J Clin Invest* 1986;77:1925–1930.

Hypertension: Pathophysiology, Diagnosis, and Management, Second Edition, edited by J.H. Laragh and B.M. Brenner, Raven Press, Ltd., New York © 1995.

CHAPTER 93

The Role of Nephron Mass and of Intraglomerular Pressure in Initiation and Progression of Experimental Hypertensive-Renal Disorders

Sharon Anderson and Barry M. Brenner

PROGRESSIVE NATURE OF CLINICAL RENAL DISEASE

Once chronic renal insufficiency begins, deterioration of renal function often continues, eventually leading to end-stage renal disease (ESRD). Progressive loss of function occurs after initial injury from several causes, including vesicoureteral reflux (even with surgical repair) (1,2); bilateral renal cortical necrosis (even after a period of relative functional recovery) (3); analgesic nephropathy (whether or not medications are discontinued) (4); after initial recovery from acute poststreptococcal glomerulonephritis (5) or acute renal failure (6,7); and with a congenital reduction in nephron number, as in the case

of oligomeganephronia (8) or a congenital solitary kidney (9). In addition to the extent and severity of the primary renal disease, other factors influence the rate of progression to ESRD. Well-recognized contributing factors include poorly controlled hypertension, urinary tract infection, obstruction, administration of nephrotoxic drugs, and intrarenal deposition of calcium and urate salts. Frequently, however, renal insufficiency progresses despite spontaneous resolution or therapeutic control of the initial disease and attention to the risk factors for disease progression cited above.

In experimental animals, surgical or disease-induced reduction in functioning nephron number leads to a syndrome of systemic hypertension, proteinuria, glomerular sclerosis, and progressive renal insufficiency. After surgical extirpation of renal mass, whole kidney filtration function initially is maintained by structural hypertrophy and by adaptive increases in the capillary pressures and flows in the remaining glomeruli (10). However, when functioning renal mass is reduced extensively,

   S. Anderson: Division of Nephrology and Hypertension, Oregon Health Sciences University, Portland, Oregon 97201.
   B. M. Brenner: Renal Division and Department of Medicine, Brigham and Women's Hospital and Harvard Medical School, Boston, Massachusetts 02115.

these adaptations eventually prove inadequate, and the kidney fails. These observations suggest that, after a certain point, reduction in functioning nephron number leads to failure of the remaining units (10,11). In the hope of interrupting this process, much investigation has centered on the mechanisms that perpetuate injury in the remaining functional nephrons. Studies in animal models, as well as in novel *in vitro* systems, have provided insight into the influence of systemic and intraglomerular hemodynamic adaptations on progression of glomerular injury.

SYSTEMIC HYPERTENSION AND THE PROGRESSION OF RENAL DISEASE

An important risk factor contributing to acceleration of renal disease is systemic hypertension, which may be both cause and consequence of chronic renal disease (12–14). Patients with chronic renal failure (15), including diabetic nephropathy (16), exhibit not only higher blood pressure (BP), but also loss of the usual nocturnal BP decline, so that the mechanisms of hypertensive injury are more continuously operable in these patients at risk. Once present, hypertension is associated with faster loss of renal function in patients with acquired renal disease, as well as acceleration of the more moderate loss of renal function associated with normal aging (17,18).

Hypertension may also initiate renal disease. The incidence of hypertensive nephropathy is difficult to quantify, as the presence of hypertension and absence of a renal biopsy often leads to a presumptive rather than definitive diagnosis of hypertensive nephropathy. Nonetheless, the incidence of ESRD presumably secondary to essential hypertension is considerable and is particularly high in black patients (19).

Studies in experimental hypertensive renal disease have helped to delineate mechanisms of hypertensive injury. Classically, systemic hypertension was believed to cause glomerular obsolescence due to ischemia, with renal vascular disease limiting renal perfusion (20). It is now clear that glomerular sclerosis may occur in the absence of atherosclerotic disease and that it is, in fact, glomerular capillary hyperperfusion and especially hypertension, rather than ischemia, that initiate glomerular structural injury in many cases.

EXPERIMENTAL MODELS OF PROGRESSIVE RENAL DISEASE

An ever-increasing number of models have been developed to represent the variety of human clinical renal diseases. Although certain recurring hemodynamic patterns are found in these models, specific patterns are related in large part to changes in the arterial perfusion pressure and the accompanying patterns of glomerular arteriolar resistances.

Arterial Pressure and Glomerular Arteriolar Resistances: Regulation of Glomerular Capillary Pressure

The normal kidney maintains relative constancy of blood flow despite wide variations in arterial BP. In intact animals, there is near-constancy of the glomerular capillary pressure (P_{GC}) over a wide range of systemic arterial perfusion pressures. The normal kidney's autoregulatory response to increased BP includes an increase in afferent arteriolar resistance (R_A), so that the increased pressure is not fully transmitted into the glomerular capillary network (21) (Fig. 1). However, in some cases, afferent arteriolar vasodilation (or inability to constrict) impairs the ability to counteract the increased systemic BP; the increased perfusion pressure is therefore freely transmitted into the glomerulus, resulting in glomerular capillary hypertension. Thus, defective autoregulation may cause imbalances between systemic and glomerular capillary pressures. As is detailed below, this hemodynamic maladaptation characterizes a variety of experimental renal diseases and, most likely, the patient with loss of functioning nephrons.

Functional Adaptations to Renal Injury

Reduction of functioning renal mass leads to structural and functional hypertrophy of the remaining nephrons (22,23). In clinical (24) and experimental (25) uninephrectomy, glomerular filtration rate (GFR) and renal plasma flow rate (RPF) in the remaining kidney increase by about 40 percent, so that the one-kidney GFR value rises to about 70 percent of the prenephrectomy (two-kidney) value within a few weeks. After uninephrectomy in the rat, increased renal ribonucleic acid and protein synthesis are seen in the contralateral kidney within hours (26), and kidney weight increases within 1 to 2 days (27). Indeed, increased levels of c-*jun* and c-*fos* mRNAs are found as early as 1 hour after uninephrectomy, and messenger ribonucleic acid (mRNA) levels for basement membrane components including the α_1 chain of type IV collagen, laminin B_1 and B_2 chains, and heparan sulfate proteoglycan core protein rise within 12 hours, though glomerular mRNA levels of growth-

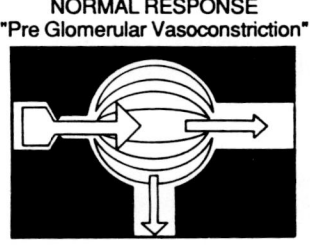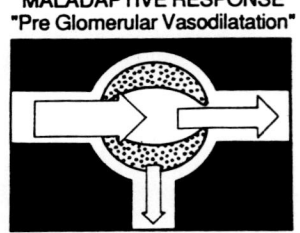

NORMAL RESPONSE "Pre Glomerular Vasoconstriction"   MALADAPTIVE RESPONSE "Pre Glomerular Vasodilatation"

FIG. 1. Preglomerular adaptations to increased systemic blood pressure. (From ref. 21, with permission.)

related proteins do not increase during the first week (28). This structural hypertrophy is accompanied by an increase in the single-nephron GFR (SNGFR) (25). Hemodynamic adaptations are more profound when more renal mass is removed. Micropuncture studies in rats with extensive surgical renal ablation indicate that vascular resistance is reduced in the afferent and efferent arterioles, allowing an increase in the glomerular capillary plasma flow rate (Q_A). Because the decrease in R_A is proportionately greater than that of efferent arteriolar resistance (R_E), P_{GC} rises (10,25). Together, these increases in Q_A and P_{GC} account for the increase in the SNGFR in the remaining nephrons.

Experimentally, the pace of remnant glomerular injury, like the magnitude of remnant hemodynamic change, is correlated with the amount of renal mass excised (29). These observations suggest that the adaptive increases in glomerular capillary pressures and flows, although serving to maintain whole kidney function in the short term, in themselves contribute to the development of glomerular morphologic injury. To examine this hypothesis, Hostetter and coworkers (10) subjected rats to 85 to 90 percent nephrectomy. Glomerular hemodynamic adaptations were apparent as early as 1 week after ablation. Untreated rats exhibited elevations in the SNGFR, due to elevations in both P_{GC} and Q_A (Fig. 2). These hemodynamic adaptations were subsequently shown to be associated with proteinuria and extensive focal and segmental glomerular sclerosis (FSGS) (30). Dietary protein restriction was used to blunt the adaptive hyperfiltration after renal ablation. In animals fed a low-protein diet, values for SNGFR, Q_A, and P_{GC} were nearly normalized, despite equally extensive ablation (Fig. 2). Limitation of Q_A and P_{GC} with dietary protein restriction is associated with slowing of the development of proteinuria and FSGS in this (29,30) and in several other (31,32) experimental models of renal disease.

Of the glomerular hemodynamic determinants of adaptive hyperfiltration, glomerular capillary hypertension appears to be the crucial cause of eventual structural injury. In various models, angiotensin I (Ang I) converting enzyme (ACE) inhibitor (CEI) therapy results in selective control of glomerular capillary hypertension, without affecting the supranormal single-nephron filtration and perfusion rates, and this selective reduction of P_{GC} prevents development of proteinuria and FSGS (13,21,33–36). Conversely, antihypertensive therapy that lowers systemic but not intraglomerular pressure may not protect the kidney at risk. Accordingly, as is detailed below, the relative roles of systemic and glomerular capillary hypertension may be clearly dissociated in studies of experimental renal disease.

Glomerular Hemodynamic Patterns and Structural Injury

Models of hypertensive renal disease may be usefully subdivided into categories based on the presence or absence of systemic and/or glomerular hypertension (10,25,31,34–54) (Table 1). These models will not be detailed here but will be used to illustrate key points in the ensuing text.

Systemic hypertension is accompanied by glomerular capillary hypertension in a variety of experimental renal diseases (Table 1) and probably characterizes the later stages of clinical renal disease as well. In each of these experimental models, systemic and glomerular hypertension are associated with progressive FSGS. That glomerular rather than systemic hypertension is the critical determinant of injury has been shown by demonstrating that therapeutic interventions may affect these pressures independently.

Systemic hypertension need not lead to glomerular hy-

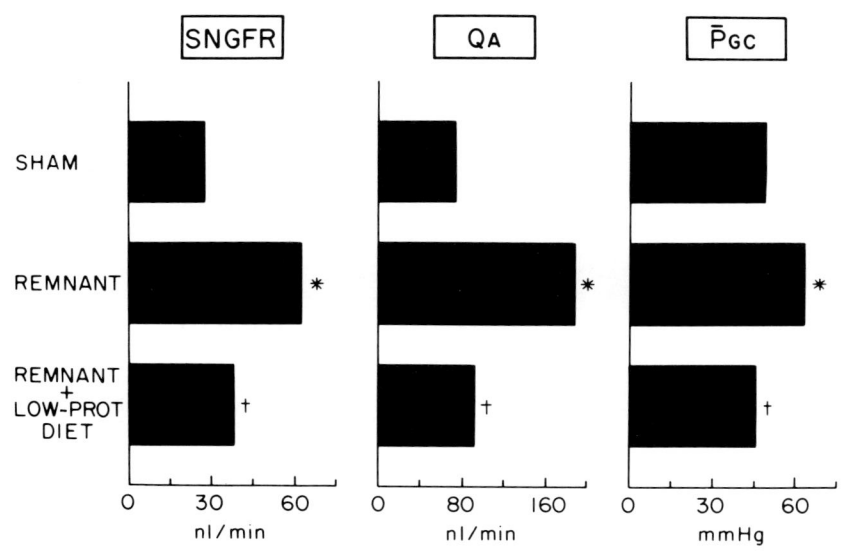

FIG. 2. Effects of renal ablation and of dietary protein restriction on glomerular hemodynamics. As compared with sham-operated animals, rats with a remnant kidney exhibited elevation of the single-nephron glomerular filtration rate (*SNGFR*) caused by elevation of both the glomerular capillary plasma flow rate (*Q_A*) and the glomerular capillary pressure (*P_{GC}*), whereas feeding a low-protein (*LOW PROT*) diet normalized each of these parameters. *$p < .05$ vs. sham, †$p < .05$ vs. remnant. (Adapted from ref. 10.)

TABLE 1. *Systemic and glomerular hypertension: experimental models[a]*

Systemic and glomerular hypertension
    Renal ablation (10,34,35)
    Mineralocorticoid-salt hypertension (37)
    Goldblatt hypertension (38,39)
    Salt-sensitive hypertension (40)
    Spontaneously hypertensive rat with uninephrectomy (41)
    Fawn-hooded rat (42)
    Nephrotoxic serum nephritis/saline (43)
    Chronic blockade of endothelial-derived relaxing
       factor (44)
    Chronic allograft rejection (45,46)
    Adriamycin nephrosis (47)
    Obese Zucker rat (48)
    Cholesterol supplementation (49)
Glomerular hypertension without systemic hypertension
    Uninephrectomy (25)
    Diabetes mellitus (31,36,50)
    Normal aging (51,52)
    Puromycin nephrosis (late stages) (53)
Systemic hypertension without glomerular hypertension
    Spontaneously hypertensive rat (41)
    MWF/Ztm Munich-Wistar substrain (54)

[a] Representative models of systemic and glomerular hypertension. Selected references are given in parentheses.

However, removal of one kidney in the SHR results in lowering of R_A in the remaining kidney, allowing transmission of systemic hypertension and elevation of P_{GC}. This hemodynamic alteration is associated with a sharp increase in $U_{prot}V$ (Fig. 3) and acceleration of FSGS. When the uninephrectomized SHR is fed a low-protein diet, the protective afferent arteriolar vasoconstriction is restored, P_{GC} is maintained at normal levels, and proteinuria and FSGS are prevented (41). Thus, maintenance of normal P_{GC} appears to be an essential element in protection against glomerular injury in experimental hypertension. Restoration of normal afferent arteriolar constriction also reduces P_{GC} and injury in the remnant kidney model (10) (Fig. 4). After partial renal ablation in the untreated rat, high systemic pressure, together with reduced afferent arteriolar resistance, leads to elevation of P_{GC}. Administration of a low-protein diet normalizes R_A, thereby controlling glomerular hypertension and affording protection (10).

Glomerular hypertension may occur in the absence of systemic hypertension. Uninephrectomy in the rat does not result in systemic hypertension (25,29,37); nevertheless, the moderate increases in Q_A and P_{GC} are associated with acceleration of the age-related FSGS in the aging rat (29). Similarly, glomerular hypertension and injury are eventuated in the normotensive kidneys of rats with passive Heymann nephritis (56) and after recovery from acute puromycin nephrosis (53). As is the case with hypertensive renal diseases, dietary or pharmacological therapies that normalize P_{GC} effectively prevent FSGS in normotensive models as well (29,31,36,53).

An extremely important example of this relationship is found in experimental diabetes mellitus. In the insulin-treated diabetic rat, systemic BP is normal, but elevations of Q_A and P_{GC} result in single-nephron hyperfiltration (31,36,50). In this model as well, intraglomerular hyperperfusion and hypertension lead to glomerulosclerosis. As in hypertensive models, therapeutic interventions such as dietary protein restriction, which limit the adaptive increases in SNGFR, P_{GC}, and Q_A, retard the development of albuminuria and glomerular structural injury (31). The critical role of glomerular capillary hy-

pertension, as is demonstrated in the young spontaneously hypertensive rat (SHR), a model of human essential hypertension. In this model, the glomerulus is protected from high systemic BP by relative afferent arteriolar vasoconstriction (41,55). Despite severe systemic hypertension, the superficial nephrons of the young SHR exhibit relatively low values for Q_A, and normal values for P_{GC} and SNGFR, with relative resistance to FSGS. The relatively high values for R_A and normal values for P_{GC} may explain the absence of severe progressive renal disease in this animal model.

The importance of afferent arteriolar vasoconstriction in conferring protection against FSGS in this model is clearly demonstrated when it is diminished or abolished by uninephrectomy. Values for proteinuria ($U_{prot}V$) in the intact SHR are not much higher than those in the normotensive Wistar-Kyoto rat (WKY) (41) (Fig. 3).

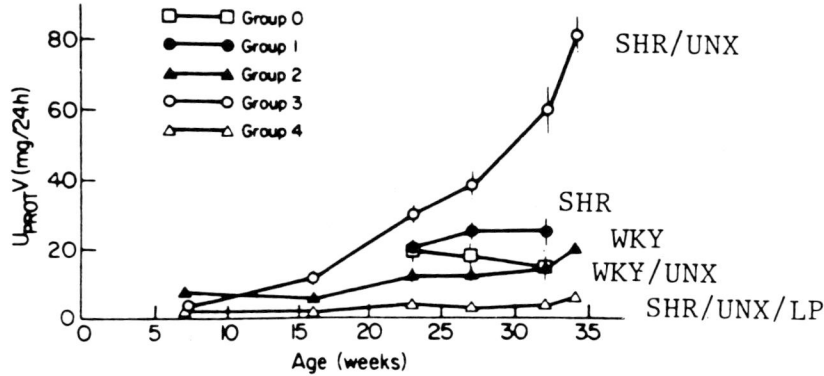

FIG. 3. Effects of systemic hypertension, uninephrectomy (*UNX*), and low-protein (*LP*) diet on urinary protein excretion ($U_{PROT}V$) in the spontaneously hypertensive rat (*SHR*) and the Wistar-Kyoto rat (*WKY*). Intact SHR rats show $U_{PROT}V$ values only slightly higher than those in the intact WKY. UNX dramatically increases $U_{PROT}V$ in the SHR, whereas feeding a low-protein diet abolishes the damaging effect of UNX. (Adapted from ref. 41.)

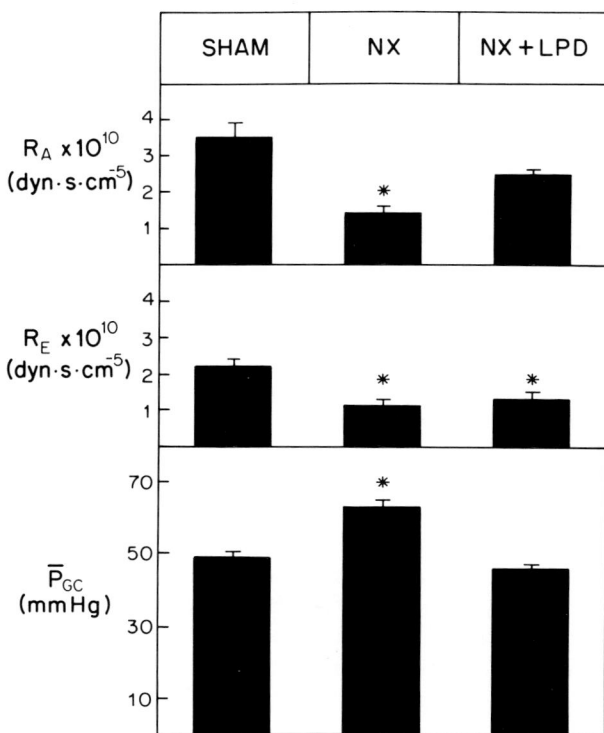

FIG. 4. Effects of renal ablation (*NX*) and a low-protein diet (*LPD*) on afferent (R_A) and efferent (R_E) arteriolar resistances and glomerular capillary pressure (P_{GC}). As compared with sham-operated rats, remnant kidneys exhibited reduced values for arteriolar resistances; the disproportionate reduction in R_A led to elevation of P_{GC}. LPD restored R_A toward normal, thereby normalizing P_{GC}. (Adapted from data in ref. 10.)

Mechanisms of Glomerular Hypertensive Injury

Although glomerular capillary hypertension is an important cause of FSGS, little is yet known of the exact mechanism(s) by which enhanced hydraulic pressure in the glomerular capillary network is translated into morphologic structural injury. Recently, innovative new techniques have been developed to begin to address this question, using a variety of *in vitro* systems. In general, these studies have addressed the hypothesis that increased glomerular capillary pressures and/or plasma flow rates alter the growth and activity of glomerular component cells, inducing the elaboration or expression of cytokines and other mediators, which then stimulate mesangial matrix production and promote structural injury. Hemodynamic physical forces, such as shear stress or changes in blood flow, are well recognized to influence activity of endothelial cells in extrarenal systems (63), and it seems likely that such forces exert cellular actions in the glomerulus as well. For instance, increased shear stress enhances endothelin expression in cultured endothelial cells (64,65), as well as nitric oxide release from cultured endothelial cells (66,67). Recently, it has been shown that growing glomerular capillary endothelial cells under conditions of increased shear stress modulates levels and/or activity of platelet-derived growth factor (PDGF) mRNA (68). Altered hemodynamics may also influence activity of mesangial cells. In support of this notion, it has been postulated that expansion of the glomerular capillaries and stretching of the mesangium in response to hypertension might be a force that translates high P_{GC} into increased mesangial matrix formation (69). Evidence for this mechanism comes from observations in microperfused rat glomeruli, in which increased hydraulic pressure was associated with increased glomerular volume; and in cultured mesangial cells, in which cyclic stretching resulted in enhanced synthesis of protein, total collagen, collagen IV, collagen I, laminin, fibronectin, and transforming growth factor-β (TGF-β) (69,70). Also, growing mesangial cells under pulsatile conditions has been reported to stimulate protein kinase C, calcium influx, and proto-oncogene expression (71), whereas shear stress activates latent forms of TGF-β in mesangial cells (72). Given these new techniques, the mechanisms by which glomerular hypertension leads to structural injury are likely to be elucidated in the coming years.

PHARMACOLOGICAL THERAPY OF SYSTEMIC AND GLOMERULAR HYPERTENSION

Despite the importance of hypertension in accelerating injury, antihypertensive therapy has not proven universally successful in slowing experimental renal disease, as was demonstrated by several studies in the late 1970s

pertension specifically in the pathogenesis of diabetic glomerulopathy has been shown in studies of CEI therapy. A modest reduction of systemic BP within the normal range is associated with selective normalization of P_{GC} and with protection against progression of injury, without affecting the supranormal values for SNGFR and Q_A, or metabolic control (36).

Finally, maneuvers that augment glomerular capillary pressures and flows may hasten glomerular injury even in the absence of increases in BP. The adaptive increases in P_{GC} and Q_A induced by uninephrectomy accelerate FSGS in such diverse forms of experimental renal disease as nephrotoxic serum nephritis, diabetes mellitus, nephrotic syndrome, and lupus-like nephropathy (57–59). Similarly, increasing P_{GC} by such dissimilar maneuvers as high-protein diets (29,31), vasodilatory glucocorticoids (60), elevation of hematocrit (61), or nitric oxide synthase inhibition (62) leads to acceleration of experimental FSGS. Presumably, each of these maneuvers adds to the hemodynamic burden of glomerular capillaries previously subjected to various injurious stresses, thereby accelerating glomerular destruction.

and early 1980s. For example, in the SHR, administration of reserpine, hydralazine, and hydrochlorothiazide ("triple therapy") was found only to delay, rather than prevent, FSGS (73). In the partially nephrectomized rat, this regimen produced only a modest reduction in FSGS, despite excellent control of systemic hypertension (74). Subsequent studies helped to explain the contrasting observations in earlier reports of antihypertensive therapy; studies with various classes of antihypertensive drugs are discussed below.

Ang CEIs and Ang II Receptor Antagonists

Angiotensin CEIs have received intensive attention as potentially protective of the kidney at risk for progressive loss of function. Many studies have established their efficacy in controlling BP, limiting $U_{prot}V$, and slowing development of FSGS in experimental models (13,33–36,46,51,53,60,62). Indeed, of the regimens tested thus far, this class of agents has proven by far the most consistently successful in slowing progression of experimental renal disease (33) (Table 2).

The systemic and intraglomerular hemodynamic consequences of angiotensin CEI have been well described. In the partial nephrectomy model, CEI therapy normalizes both systemic and glomerular capillary pressures (34,35,75–77). The mechanism by which P_{GC} falls relates to effects not only on systemic BP but also on the glomerular arteriolar resistances. CEIs lower R_A, probably representing an autoregulatory response to the decreased renal perfusion pressure. However, CEIs usually induce a greater concurrent fall in R_E, thereby allowing a reduction in P_{GC} with maintenance of Q_A. Also, they are regularly associated with an increase in K_f, the glomerular capillary ultrafiltration coefficient. Thus, maintenance

of Q_A and elevation of K_f allow maintenance of SNGFR at baseline levels, despite the fall in P_{GC}. Studies with CEIs were among the first to establish that of the adaptive changes that characterize renal disease, glomerular capillary hypertension is the crucial determinant of injury (34–36).

These hemodynamic effects are found in virtually all hypertensive models. Exceptions are rare, although not surprisingly, ACE inhibition does not normalize P_{GC} or limit injury in rats with mineralocorticoid-salt hypertension, in which renin levels are virtually undetectable (78). Another important exception is the clipped kidney in Goldblatt (two-kidney, one clip) hypertension, which is critically dependent on Ang II action. In this setting, although CEIs preserve structure and function in the unclipped kidney, they also accelerate loss of function and structure in the clipped kidney (79). In most other models, particularly when CEI therapy is started early in the course of injury, normalization of P_{GC} is associated with slowing of the rate of progression of $U_{prot}V$, and limitation of FSGS. This is a class effect, as such protection has been found with every CEI yet studied. The beneficial effects of CEIs are not limited to hypertensive models. In various normotensive models with glomerular capillary hypertension, as in early diabetes, modestly reducing BP with CEIs results in salutary intraglomerular consequences (i.e., reduction of R_E and P_{GC}) and limitation of $U_{prot}V$ and FSGS (36,51,53).

ACE Inhibition: Mechanisms of Protection

Angiotensin II potently influences many physiological processes, and thus it is no surprise that several different mechanisms have been postulated as contributing to the protective effect of blockade of Ang II production with CEI therapy. As discussed above, control of glomerular hypertension is an important mechanism of action, as correction of this hemodynamic abnormality always affords structural protection. The intraglomerular effects of CEI—specifically, reduction in R_E—most likely relate, in large part, to limitation of Ang II formation and action. Exogenous Ang II increases R_E and P_{GC} and lowers K_f (80); thus, the hemodynamic consequences of CEIs are consistent with those of eradication of Ang II action. In further support for the role of Ang II, recent micropuncture studies with the specific nonpeptide Ang II receptor AT_1 antagonist, losartan (Cozaar; DuP 753, MK 954) confirm that Ang II receptor blockade also reproduces these hemodynamic effects (77,81,82). Although not yet extensively studied, Ang II receptor antagonists have been reported to reduce $U_{prot}V$ and FSGS in several models, including rats with renal ablation (77,83,84) and diabetic rats (85). Thus, preliminary evidence suggests that at least in some models, the beneficial

TABLE 2. *Effects of antihypertensive drugs in experimental renal disease*

	BP	P_{GC}	V_G	FSGS
Angiotensin converting enzyme inhibitors	↓	↓	±	↓
Angiotensin II receptor antagonists	↓	↓	↓	↓
Triple therapy	↓	±	↓	±
Dihydropyridine calcium antagonists	↓	±	↓	±
Diltiazem and related compounds[a]	↓	±	↓	↓
Verapamil	↓	±	±	±
Diuretics[a]	↓	↔	↔	↔
Beta-blockers[a]	↓	↔	?	↔

[a] Data are very limited.
BP, blood pressure; P_{GC}, glomerular capillary pressure; V_G, glomerular volume; ↓, usually reduced; ±, partial or inconsistent effect; ↔, no protective effect; ?, unknown.

effects of CEIs are reproduced with specific Ang II–receptor antagonism. However, these data are as yet preliminary, and exceptions to the rule have already been noted (86,87); further studies are needed to clarify this issue.

In addition to the beneficial hemodynamic effects, other actions of CEIs appear to contribute to their protective effect. Reduction in P_{GC} limits the amount of macromolecules entering the mesangium. Angiotensin II increases mesangial macromolecule uptake in nephrotic rats, whereas infusion of the Ang II–receptor antagonist saralasin blocks this effect (88,89); inhibition of Ang II formation with CEIs may operate in a similar manner. Macromolecular traffic is also reduced into the urinary space; it has been postulated that prolonged proteinuria contributes to the tubulointerstitial injury that usually accompanies glomerular disease (90). In this regard, chronic CEI therapy ameliorates not only FSGS (53) but also chronic tubulointerstitial injury (91) in a model of puromycin nephrosis in the rat. Limitation of proximal tubule procollagen α_1 mRNA levels by CEI therapy in remnant kidney rats (92) lends further support to this potential mechanism of protection.

Angiotensin CEIs reduce proteinuria by multiple mechanisms. One obvious mechanism is reduction of P_{GC}; in many circumstances, the two are directly related. Also, CEIs have been reported to exert a direct effect on glomerular permselectivity, independent of hemodynamic actions (93). Structurally, CEIs have been noted to reverse broadening of epithelial cell foot processes in rats with reduced renal mass (94), a mechanism that might contribute to their antiproteinuric effect.

Somewhat more controversial is the ability of CEIs to reduce glomerular size (95,96). An increase in glomerular size (particularly of uninjured glomeruli) characterizes many forms of progressive renal disease. Studies in a number of experimental models have noted a strong association between increased glomerular size and development of proteinuria and FSGS (37,79,97–100). Enlargement of various intraglomerular components has been noted and linked to postulated mechanisms of injury. In the diabetic kidney, expansion of the mesangial area is prominent. In other models, including mineralocorticoid-salt hypertension (37,101) and partial nephrectomy (100), adaptation to injury includes dilatation of the glomerular capillary lumen and thus an increase in the capillary radius. Indeed, an increase in the glomerular capillary radius is the earliest morphologic finding after uninephrectomy (102,103). The combination of increases in both glomerular capillary intraluminal pressure and capillary radius are postulated to exert increased tension on the glomerular capillary wall (following the Laplace law), thus contributing to disruption of capillary wall integrity and FSGS. The potential additive deleterious effects of glomerular capillary hypertension and glomerular enlargement have also prompted speculation that injury may be mediated by detrimental effects on the glomerular visceral epithelial cells (97,103,104). Still another hypothesis regarding mechanisms of injury related to glomerular enlargement has centered on the concept that glomerular growth promoters, released locally or circulating in response to an injurious stimulus, may possess a capacity not only to enlarge the glomerular tuft but also to augment mesangial matrix formation and/or suppress matrix degradation processes (95,105).

Recognition that some protective interventions are associated with reduction in glomerular size led to the hypothesis that limitation of glomerular enlargement may be a mechanism of protection. However, despite the nearly ubiquitous protective action of CEIs, the influence on glomerular size has not been consistent. Some studies have found that CEIs modestly limit glomerular enlargement, although glomeruli remain significantly enlarged as compared with normal rats (35,106–108). How-ever, in most other studies, CEIs have markedly limited $U_{prot}V$ and FSGS without affecting glomerular size (35,76,94,109–111), suggesting that limiting glomerular size is not necessary for protection (particularly if P_{GC} is reduced). Nevertheless, the combination of increased P_{GC} and increased glomerular size has been associated with more severe injury than either one alone, suggesting a possible synergistic action of these two adverse adaptations. In some circumstances, limitation of glomerular enlargement could be a useful action of CEIs.

Less extensively studied but intriguing are several other potential protective mechanisms of CEIs. Reduction in hematocrit (112), alterations in platelet aggregation (113), and changes in hemorrheology have all been reported with CEI therapy; further information is needed to define the role of these factors. Metabolic mechanisms may contribute as well. These drugs may ameliorate insulin resistance (114), a metabolic abnormality associated with systemic hypertension. Limiting proteinuria with CEIs in nephrotic patients is associated with amelioration of hyperlipidemia (115), a metabolic abnormality recently linked to progressive renal disease. The CEI captopril has been reported to scavenge free radicals directly (116), an effect that could theoretically benefit the glomerulus in certain disease states.

Recognition of beneficial effects on vascular integrity represents an exciting new avenue of investigation with these drugs. For example, the ability of these drugs to preserve or increase serum potassium levels and thereby protect the endothelium (117,118) and to limit experimentally induced atherogenesis (119) could prove to be additional protective mechanisms, limiting the vascular injury component of the preglomerular and possibly glomerular microvessels. Converting enzyme inhibitors have also been noted to prevent functional and morphologic alterations in endothelium (120), possibly by increasing the release or action of endothelium-derived relaxing factor (EDRF) (121), to modulate endothelium-dependent relaxation properties (122), and to reduce aortic and microvascular growth (123) in hypertensive rats, further suggesting a salutary vascular effect.

Finally, the complex interactions among the RAS and interrelated vasoactive hormonal systems preclude exclusion of indirect effects, via altered activity of other vasoactive mediators, as has been suggested for the kallikrein-kinin system (124) and atrial natriuretic peptide (125), to name just two.

Diuretics

Surprisingly, monotherapy with diuretics has received relatively little experimental attention in terms of preventing progressive renal disease. In a study comparing chronic hydrochlorothiazide therapy to sodium restriction in the uninephrectomized SHR, neither regimen lowered BP; sodium restriction, but not diuretic therapy, limited development of proteinuria and FSGS (126). Given the ubiquitous use of diuretics in patients with advanced renal disease, further examination of the potential role of diuretics in renal disease progression certainly seems warranted. Use of diuretics in combination regimens is discussed below.

Calcium Antagonists

The potential ability of calcium antagonists to protect the kidney is of great clinical interest. However, results of calcium channel blockade have been inconsistent in animal models of renal disease. Nifedipine has been reported to ameliorate FSGS in rats with partial nephrectomy, mineralocorticoid-salt hypertension, and uninephrectomized SHR (76,78,127). Other studies have noted a protective effect of verapamil, in nonhypotensive doses, in partially nephrectomized rats (128) and of nicardipine in subtotally nephrectomized SHR (129). Diltiazem has also been reported to limit albuminuria in diabetic rats (130), and the 1,5-benzothiazepine calcium antagonist TA 3090 limits development of albuminuria in diabetic dogs (131). A preliminary report in the partially nephrectomized rat noted equivalent ability of the calcium antagonists diltiazem and TA 3090 and the ACE inhibitors enalapril and captopril to reduce glomerular injury (132).

Other studies, however, have found calcium antagonists to be ineffective. In uninephrectomized diabetic rats, nifedipine fails to reduce P_{GC}, albuminuria, or FSGS, despite excellent reduction of systemic BP (111). In partially nephrectomized rats, neither verapamil in hypotensive doses (106) nor felodipine (133) prevent FSGS. Diltiazem does not ameliorate FSGS in rats with

adriamycin nephrosis (134), and nitrendipine has been reported to accelerate glomerular injury in Goldblatt hypertensive rats (110). In a study comparing the effects of the ACE inhibitor to those of TA 3090 in Dahl salt-sensitive rats, it was noted although while captopril reduced BP, proteinuria, and FSGS (although not glomerular size), equihypotensive doses of TA 3090 were ineffective in limiting development of proteinuria or FSGS, despite limitation of early glomerular enlargement (109). Explanations for these widely diverse findings are lacking, and further studies regarding potential differences in host response of the different models and/or variable efficacy of the structurally diverse calcium antagonists are needed.

Because glomerular hemodynamics were not evaluated in many of these studies, the precise relationship between P_{GC} and injury cannot be inferred. Few studies of the glomerular hemodynamic effects of calcium antagonists in experimental hypertensive renal disease are available. In the partially nephrectomized rat, acute normalization of BP with intravenous verapamil (135,136) or diltiazem (136) results in normalization of both P_{GC} and K_f. In contrast, it has been reported that acute intravenous doses of verapamil (137) and diltiazem (138), which do not entirely normalize BP, are not particularly effective in normalizing P_{GC}. Chronic normalization of BP with nifedipine results in control of glomerular hypertension in the uninephrectomized SHR (127) but not in diabetic rats (111), rats with mineralocorticoid-salt hypertension (78), or partially nephrectomized rats (76). Although protective when started early, nifedipine is ineffective when therapy is delayed in the remnant kidney rat (139). As recently reviewed, renal actions of the calcium antagonists vary greatly with the specific agent used, the experimental model, and the route of administration (140,141).

Vasodilator/Diuretic Combinations

Several studies have evaluated the efficacy of older combination regimens, usually containing a diuretic, a vasodilator, and/or a centrally acting agent. The combination of reserpine, hydralazine, and hydrochlorothiazide ("triple therapy") has been extensively studied, because of its excellent control of BP and its availability long before newer classes of drugs were developed. In some models, this regimen has provided benefit. For example, in rats with salt-sensitive hypertensive glomerulonephritis (43), the uninephrectomized SHR (142), or rats with chronic transplant rejection (46), this regimen normalizes both BP and P_{GC} and ameliorates renal injury; although P_{GC} was not measured, it is also effective in a severely hyperglycemic diabetic rat model (143). However, this regimen is not uniformly protective. Some time ago, administration of triple therapy to the SHR was found only to delay, rather than prevent, glomerular injury (73). In the partially nephrectomized rat, Purkerson and coworkers (74) found only a modest reduction in FSGS, despite excellent control of systemic hypertension, with this regimen. A hemodynamic explanation for the failure of triple therapy to prevent FSGS has been provided by micropuncture studies (35,77). In a study comparing the effects of triple therapy to those of the CEI enalapril in rats subjected to 5/6 nephrectomies, the two regimens were equally effective in controlling systemic hypertension (36). In contrast, however, although CEI markedly limited glomerular injury, triple therapy afforded no protection. Effects of the drugs on BP, P_{GC}, and glomerular size are depicted in Fig. 5. Enalapril re-

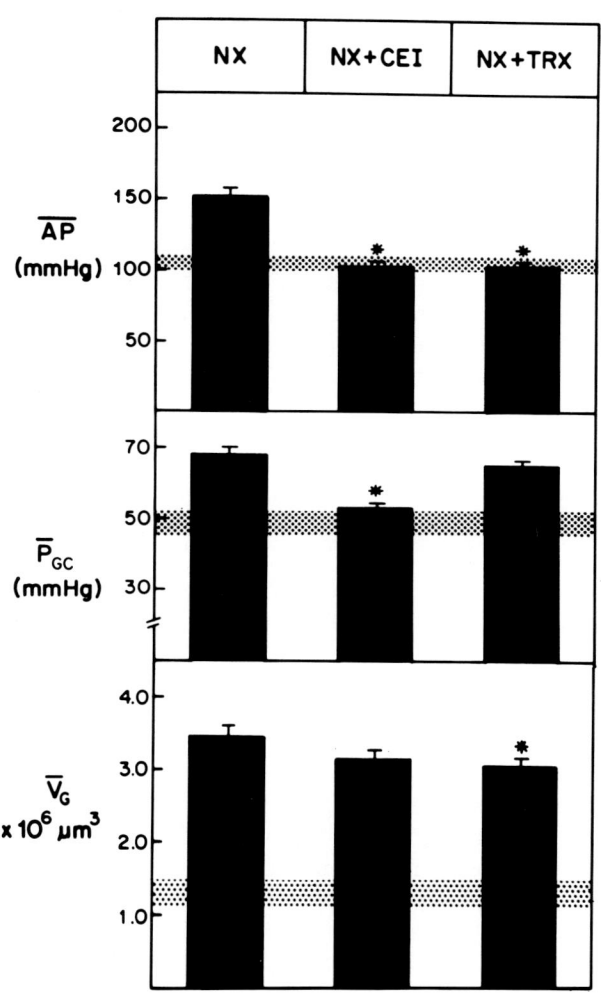

FIG. 5. Effects of converting enzyme inhibitor (*CEI*) therapy and triple therapy (*TRX*) on mean arterial pressure (*AP*), glomerular capillary pressure (P_{GC}), and mean glomerular volume (V_G) in rats with 5/6 nephrectomy (*NX*). In untreated NX rats, all three parameters far exceeded the normal range (*horizontal bands*). CEI normalized both AP and P_{GC} but had no effect on the supranormal glomerular size. TRX normalized AP and slightly but significantly lowered V_G but had no effect on P_{GC}. (Adapted from ref. 35.)

duced systemic and glomerular pressures to the normal range (36), although it did not limit compensatory glomerular enlargement (96). Triple therapy normalized BP and modestly (but significantly) limited glomerular enlargement but had no effect on P_{GC} in this model. Most studies have found this regimen to be ineffective in this model (36,77,83). Failure of triple therapy to protect against FSGS has also been found in mineralocorticoid-salt hypertension (144), in the uninephrectomized SHR with glomerulonephritis (145), in the SHR with renal ablation (146), and in rats with clip hypertension (147). Hydralazine alone fails to lower P_{GC} and offers no protection in diabetic rats (148).

The hemodynamic consequences of this regimen are consistent with the known effects of these drugs on the renin-angiotensin system (RAS). Both the vasodilator and the diuretic stimulate the RAS, and plasma renin concentration levels increase substantially with this regimen (36). Because Ang II increases R_E, it is likely that enhanced Ang II effect contributed to the maintenance of high values for P_{GC}. However, whereas this regimen regularly reduces R_A (probably as an autoregulatory response to the reduced perfusion pressure), its effects on R_E, and thus P_{GC}, differ widely among experimental models (Fig. 6). The disparate effects of this regimen in different experimental models are as yet unexplained, although they may relate, at least in part, to the baseline vascular and hormonal status.

This combination regimen has been somewhat more successful in diabetic rat models. In a relatively short-term study of SHR with untreated diabetes, triple therapy reduced P_{GC} and limited mesangial expansion, but the study was terminated before the development of substantial albuminuria or FSGS (149). A longer study of diabetic SHR found comparable reductions in albuminuria with the CEI perindopril and triple therapy, although morphologic studies were not performed (150). In normotensive diabetic rats, a long-term study comparing triple therapy to CEI therapy found intermediate results; BP reduction with triple therapy significantly limited development of albuminuria and FSGS, as compared with rats not receiving BP therapy. However, the degree of protection afforded with triple therapy was significantly less than that conferred by an equihypotensive dose of the CEI (108). Thus, all three studies suggest that triple therapy is of some benefit in diabetic rats, but the sole long-term morphologic study suggests that it is inferior to CEI therapy in conferring protection.

Beta-Blockers

Beta-blockers as monotherapy have not received intensive study in experimental models; the few available studies are not very promising. Studies examining the hemodynamic effects of the nonselective β-blocker terta-

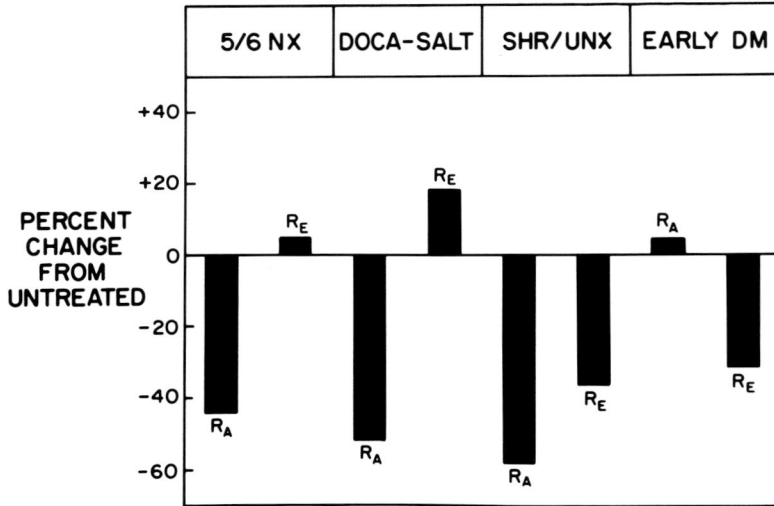

FIG. 6. Effects of combination triple antihypertensive therapy on afferent (R_A) and efferent (R_E) in 5/6 nephrectomized rats (*5/6 NX*), desoxycorticosterone (*DOCA*) salt hypertensive rats, uninephrectomized spontaneously hypertensive rats (*SHR/UNX*), and early diabetes (*DM*). All values are depicted as percentage change from those in the corresponding untreated rats. Values for R_A fell in all three hypertensive models, possibly as an autoregulatory response to the decreased renal perfusion pressure. Values for R_E were variable on this regimen, being reduced by TRX in some models and not in others. (Adapted from data in refs. 35, 108, 142, and 144.)

tolol have established that this agent given acutely raises SNGFR and Q_A without affecting P_{GC} or K_f in normal rats (151). In partially nephrectomized rats, acute infusion of tertatolol but not propranolol increases urine flow rate, GFR, and RPF (152). However, despite effective normalization of systemic BP, chronic tertatolol administration to partially nephrectomized rats fails to influence GFR, RPF, or progressive proteinuria (153).

Finally, although several other antihypertensive regimens have been reported to reduce injury, the absence of intraglomerular hemodynamic study and of confirmation in replicate models currently precludes a thorough analysis of their potential protective effect.

Other Pharmacological Therapies

Anticoagulant Therapy

The observation that fibrinoid material is found within the injured glomerulus prompted speculation that endothelial cell dysfunction (possibly resulting from enhanced shear stress) leads to intracapillary thrombosis and contributes to FSGS (74,154). Indeed, heparin therapy has been found to be protective in limiting FSGS in rats with renal ablation (74,154). The many physiological effects of heparin have precluded any definitive conclusion as to the mechanism(s) of this protective effect. However, hemodynamic factors may play a role, because heparin lowers BP in rats with spontaneous hypertension (155,156) and renal ablation (74), although a micropuncture study of rats in which heparin was briefly withdrawn before study found no significant effect on intraglomerular hemodynamics in the remnant kidney (157). More recently, heparin has been reported to stimulate nitric oxide production (158), which might favorably affect both systemic and intrarenal hemodynamic function.

Antiplatelet Agents and Thromboxane Synthetase Inhibitors

Administration of antiplatelet agents has received attention in recent years, as recently reviewed (159,160). Evidence for a role of platelet aggregation in the pathogenesis of FSGS comes from light, electron, and immunofluorescence microscopy studies of remnant kidneys, which reveal extensive glomerular deposition of platelets and fibrin, as well as coagulated proteins in Bowman's space, and thrombosis of glomerular capillaries (74). Glomerular capillary endothelial damage (caused by hemodynamic stresses or in response to locally released substances) may activate platelets; these activated platelets could then release substances such as platelet-activating factor (PAF), PDGF, TGF-β, and thromboxanes, each of which has been implicated as injurious (159,160). Recent studies have served to clarify the interrelated mechanisms by which antiplatelet agents exert their beneficial effects. For example, studies in partially nephrectomized rats indicate that a selective inhibitor of thromboxane A_2 (TxA_2) serves to inhibit TxA_2-dependent platelet aggregation, lower BP and proteinuria, and limit FSGS (161). More recently, combined TxA_2 synthesis inhibition and increased renal prostaglandin I_2 (PGI$_2$) production has been shown to afford protection (162), as has ticlodipine (which interferes with platelet and platelet-endothelial interactions) (153). Interference with thromboxane formation or action is likely to exert hemodynamic effects, but micropuncture studies have thus far not been performed with these agents.

Prostaglandin Synthesis Inhibitors

Inhibition of vasodilatory PG reduces proteinuria in nephrotic patients (163); studies of glomerular permselectivity indicate that this antiproteinuric effect is caused by a reduction in GFR and also by an improvement of the size-selective characteristics of the glomerular barrier (164). However, chronic PG inhibition may not be beneficial in the nonimmunologic forms of progressive renal disease. In experimental chronic renal failure, indomethacin results in a major decline in GFR, due to reductions in both the Q_A and K_f (165); this compromise in renal flow and filtration may be intolerable to the kidney at risk. Conversely, enhancing PG production by feeding diets rich in PG precursors may favorably affect renal outcome in experimental models (166). More recently, a beneficial effect of the prostacyclin analogue cicaprost in dogs with chronic renal failure has been noted (167). Again, glomerular hemodynamic studies are lacking in such studies and, therefore, effects on P_{GC} are as yet unknown.

Hormonal and Other Interventions

Observations of parallel increases in renal function and size accompanying both normal maturation and altered metabolic states led to the suggestion that endocrine hormones might mediate renal growth, as well as adaptation to reduction in functioning nephron number. As discussed above, the RAS appears to participate in this process. Manipulations of other endogenous hormonal factors may also affect glomerular hemodynamics, growth, and progression of renal disease. Both thyroidectomy (168,169) and hypophysectomy (170) have been reported to limit glomerular hypertension and FSGS in rats with reduced renal mass, without affecting systemic BP. Recent studies have also implicated excessive activity of parathyroid hormone (171), growth hormone (172,173), and insulin-like growth factor-1 (IGF-1). Hemodynamic effects of these hormones are as yet unclear in experimental models. Administration of an antibody to IGF-1 has been shown to decrease SNGFR without affecting P_{GC} in normal rats (174), but effects in disease models are not yet defined.

Although widely used in clinical nephrology, glucocorticoids do not appear particularly useful in the setting of nonimmunologic disease. In animal models, glucocorticoids have little effect on experimental glomerulonephritis, although associated tubulointerstitial processes may be ameliorated (175). However, the hemodynamic consequences of steroid administration may be detrimental to the injured kidney. In addition to their well-known aggravation of systemic hypertension, steroids increase renal blood flow and GFR (176). The glomerular hemodynamic consequences of steroids have been examined in remnant kidney rats. High-dose methylprednisolone therapy accentuated both systemic and glomerular capillary hypertension, in association with marked acceleration of proteinuria and FSGS. As in many other models, concurrent CEI therapy vitiated the hemodynamic sequelae of glucocorticoid therapy (60). Thus, steroids appear to offer little benefit in the setting of nonimmunologic disease, at least in experimental models.

Manipulation of hematocrit also exerts profound influences on systemic and glomerular capillary pressures and FSGS. In rats with renal ablation, accentuating anemia with a low-iron diet ameliorates systemic and glomerular hypertension and affords protection; preventing the anemia that usually accompanies renal disease with exogenous erythropoietin therapy aggravates hemodynamic and structural injury (61). Similar effects have been subsequently reported in other models, including rats with mineralocorticoid-salt hypertension (177) and the male MWF/Ztm model (178). Although the mechanisms are still unknown, changes in blood viscosity, in the RAS (179), and in endothelin levels (180) may play a role.

Endothelial cell–derived vasoactive mediators (including endothelin and EDRF) have recently been implicated in hypertensive renal injury (181,182). Administration of the potent vasoconstrictor endothelin to normal rats induces severe systemic hypertension, constriction of the efferent arteriole, and elevation of P_{GC} (183). A role for endothelin in experimental hypertensive injury is indicated by observations of up-regulation of renal endothelin-1 gene expression in the remnant kidney (184) and of renal protection with administration of a specific endothelin subtype A receptor antagonist (185). Although glomerular hemodynamics have not yet been studied, the mechanism of protection with the endothelin receptor antagonist is likely to be, at least in part, hemodynamic, via reduction in P_{GC}.

Endothelium-derived relaxing factor is an endogenous vasodilator, and blockade of EDRF formation with nitric oxide synthase inhibitor compounds leads to development of systemic and glomerular hypertension, in association with proteinuria and glomerular injury, in normal rats (44,186,187), and acceleration of disease in various experimental models (62). Although hemodynamics have not yet been examined, the protective effect of administering EDRF precursors such as L-arginine (188) is likely to result in part from hemodynamic mechanisms as well.

Another endogenous vasodilator, atrial natriuretic peptide (ANP), has also been implicated in the pathogenesis of FSGS. Administration of ANP to normal rats leads to reduction in R_A and elevation of P_{GC} (189). Although intraglomerular hemodynamics have not yet been studied, administration of an antibody to ANP to diabetic rats (190) or of a specific receptor antagonist to normal rats (191), mineralocorticoid-salt hypertensive rats (192), remnant kidney rats (193), or diabetic rats (194) leads to a reduction in GFR, quite possibly mediated in part by a reduction in P_{GC}.

DIETARY THERAPY OF SYSTEMIC AND GLOMERULAR HYPERTENSION

Dietary interventions may affect systemic and glomerular pressures and disease progression. Although the intraglomerular hemodynamic consequences of such interventions have not been extensively studied, effects on systemic BP and disease progression have received attention (32). Each of the main dietary nutrient groups may affect these parameters. Dietary protein restriction, which reduces P_{GC} and limits injury in many experimental models, usually does not lower BP (10,31,32,41,75). Clinically, there is no consistent relationship between protein intake and systemic BP, although an occasional reduction in BP is noted (195). Although the intrarenal hemodynamic consequences are unknown, progression of experimental renal disease appears to be retarded by restriction of total caloric intake (196,197) and by carbohydrate restriction (198), as well as by enhancing fluid (water) intake (199).

Modulation of lipid intake affects renal disease, at least in part, by hemodynamic mechanisms. Although reduction of cholesterol does not necessarily reduce P_{GC} (200), feeding a high-cholesterol diet aggravates glomerular capillary hypertension and injury (49), perhaps in part by interfering with endothelium-dependent vascular relaxation. Thus it seems likely that as in atherosclerosis, elevated capillary hydraulic pressure and hypercholesterolemia act in synergy as risk factors, with elevated pressure enhancing the deleterious effects of lipid moieties on the vascular wall. Reduction of P_{GC} or reduction in serum cholesterol in the presence of unchanged hydraulic pressure will reduce vascular injury, and presumably reduction of both parameters would prove even more effective.

Other dietary constituents have been less well studied. Phosphate restriction, which retards FSGS in several experimental models (201,202), does not affect systemic BP but limits P_{GC} and injury in uninephrectomized diabetic rats (203). The role of dietary sodium in the progression of hypertensive renal disease has been the subject of recent experimental interest. Severe dietary sodium restriction does not lower BP or P_{GC} in rats with renal injury, but nonetheless appears to ameliorate FSGS in association with limitation of glomerular hypertrophy (100,126,204).

HYPERTENSION AND THE PROGRESSION OF CLINICAL RENAL DISEASE

Although uncontrolled hypertension hastens the decline in GFR that accompanies both normal aging and chronic renal disease, long-term controlled studies of the effect of antihypertensive therapy in slowing the progression of renal disease are only recently being reported. The available clinical studies provide encouraging evidence that these experimental findings may obtain in clinical renal disease. In diabetic renal disease, metanalyses (205,206) and controlled clinical trials (207) indicate that, as in the experimental models, ACE inhibitors are the most consistent in their ability to reduce proteinuria and possibly to prevent progression of renal disease. Data are less abundant in nondiabetic renal disease, but many studies report a beneficial effect of ACE inhibitors (208–210), and no other class of drugs has been reported to be superior to CEI therapy. Thus, agents that control both systemic and glomerular capillary hypertension appear to be most effective in clinical, as well as experimental, renal insufficiency.

SUMMARY AND IMPLICATIONS

The foregoing studies suggest that the progression of renal injury associated with systemic hypertension is mediated by the resultant adaptive increase in P_{GC}, which then contributes to structural injury. The central role of glomerular capillary hypertension in the initiation and progression of FSGS is simply schematized in Fig. 7. Renal ablation or primary renal parenchymal disease leads to systemic hypertension and to glomerular capillary hypertension. Other factors, including normal aging, diabetes, and dietary factors (particularly protein and cholesterol excess), also contribute to elevation of P_{GC}, even when systemic BP is normal. Once present, glomerular hypertension exerts deleterious effects on all glomerular cell constituents. In analogy with atherosclerosis, increased glomerular hydrostatic pressure enhances endothelial cell release of vasoactive substances (e.g., thromboxanes, endothelin), lipid deposition, and intracapillary thrombosis. Injury to the mesangial area includes increased accumulation of injurious macromolecules, which enhances both cell proliferation and matrix production. Glomerular component cells are also induced to elaborate increased levels of PDGF, TGF-β, and other presumed mediators of the eventual sclerotic process. Epithelial cell injury augments glomerular basement membrane permeability and proteinuria. Together, damage to these cellular elements results in FSGS. Progressive nephron destruction in turn contributes to systemic and glomerular hypertension, thus perpetuating the cycle.

Protection is afforded when both systemic and glomerular hypertension are controlled, as is demonstrated in studies using CEI therapy. Reducing P_{GC} limits glomerular injury even in the presence of systemic hypertension, as with dietary protein restriction, whereas control of systemic hypertension with some antihypertensive regimens does not reduce either P_{GC} or injury. Control

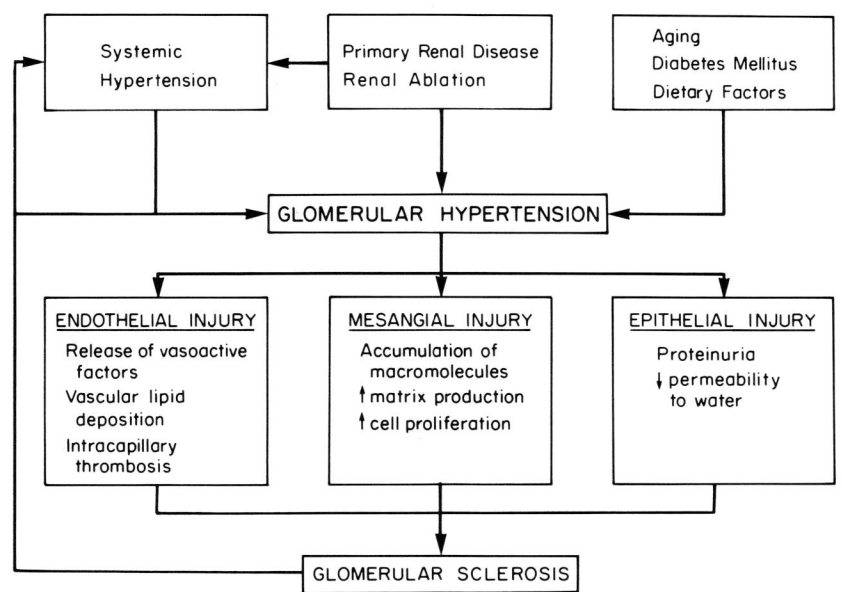

FIG. 7. Central role of glomerular hypertension in the initiation and progression of glomerular injury. See text for discussion.

of glomerular hypertension may afford protection even in normotensive disease, including diabetes. Finally, some interventions that interrupt the process distal to the development of glomerular hypertension, such as heparin, platelet inhibition, and reduction of serum cholesterol, may afford some protection independently when the primary pathogenetic mechanism (glomerular hypertension) is unaffected. However, it is likely that these interventions would prove even more effective if combined with therapy designed to reduce P_{GC} as well. Indeed, it has recently been reported that the combination of a low serum cholesterol level plus CEI therapy more effectively delays the progression of diabetic nephropathy than does either one alone (211). Further studies of the glomerular hemodynamic and functional consequences of other interventions, as well as of the interactions of various risk factors, should allow us to optimize therapies useful in preventing the otherwise predictable loss of renal function in patients at risk for progressive renal injury.

REFERENCES

1. Torres VE, Velosa JA, Holley KE, Kelalis PP, Stickler GB, Kurtz SB. *Ann Intern Med* 1980;92:776–784.
2. Cotran R. *Kidney Int* 1982;21:528–534.
3. Kleinknecht D, Grunfeld JP, Gomez PC, Moreau JF, Garcia-Torres R. *Kidney Int* 1973;4:390–400.
4. Kincaid-Smith P. *Kidney Int* 1980;17:250–260.
5. Baldwin DS. *Kidney Int* 1982;21:109–120.
6. Finn WF. In: Brenner BM, Lazarus JM, eds. *Acute renal failure.* 2nd ed. New York: Churchill Livingstone; 1988:875–918.
7. Georgaki-Angelaki HN, Steed DB, Chantler C, Haycock GB. *Kidney Int* 1989;35:84–89.
8. Royer P, Habib R, Leclerc F. In: Schreiner GE, ed. *Proceedings of the 3rd Intl Congr Nephrol,* vol 2. Basel: Karger; 1967:251–275.
9. Kiprov DD, Colvin RB, McCluskey RT. *Lab Invest* 1982;46:275–281.
10. Hostetter TH, Olson JL, Rennke HG, Venkatachalam MA, Brenner BM. *Am J Physiol* 1981;241:F85–F93.
11. Brenner BM, Meyer TW, Hostetter TH. *N Engl J Med* 1982;307:652–660.
12. Baldwin DS, Neugarten J. In: Mitch WE, Brenner BM, Stein JH, eds. *The progressive nature of renal disease.* New York: Churchill Livingstone; 1986:81–110.
13. Neuringer JR, Anderson S, Brenner BM. In: Mitch WE, Stein JH, eds. *The progressive nature of renal disease.* New York: Churchill Livingstone; 1992:1–22.
14. Weisstuch JM, Dworkin LD. *Kidney Int* 1992; 41(Suppl 36):S-33–S-37.
15. Portaluppi F, Montanari L, Massari M, Di Chiara V, Capanna M. *Am J Hypertens* 1991;4:20–26.
16. Nielsen FS, Rossing P, Gall M-A, Parving H-H. *J Am Soc Nephrol* 1992;3:337 (abstr).
17. Brazy PC, Stead WW, Fitzwilliam JF. *Kidney Int* 1989;35:670–674.
18. Lindeman RD, Tobin JD, Shock NW. *Kidney Int* 1984;26:861–868.
19. U.S. Renal Data System. *USRDS 1992 annual data report.* Bethesda, Maryland: The National Institutes of Health, National Institute of Diabetes and Digestive and Kidney Diseases; August 1992.
20. McManus JFA, Lupton CH Jr. *Lab Invest* 1960;9:413–434.
21. Keane WF, Anderson S, Aurell M, de Zeeuw D, Narins RG, Povar G. *Ann Intern Med* 1989;111:503–516.
22. Hayslett JP. *Physiol Rev* 1979;59:137–164.
23. Rennke HG, Anderson S, Brenner BM. In: Tisher CC, Brenner BM, eds. *Renal pathology.* 2nd ed. Philadelphia: JB Lippincott; 1994:116–142.
24. Pabico RC, McKenna BA, Freeman RB. *Kidney Int* 1975;8:166–175.
25. Deen WM, Maddox DA, Robertson CR, Brenner BM. *Am J Physiol* 1974;227:556–562.
26. Johnson HA, Vera Roman JM. *Am J Pathol* 1966;49:1–13.
27. Phillips TL, Leong GF. *Cancer Res* 1967;27:286–292.
28. Nakamura T, Ebihara I, Tomino Y, Koide H, Kikuchi K, Koiso K. *Am J Physiol* 1992;262:F389–F396.
29. Hostetter TH, Meyer TW, Rennke HG, Brenner BM. *Kidney Int* 1986;30:509–517.
30. Olson JL, Hostetter TH, Rennke HG, Brenner BM, Venkatachalam MA. *Kidney Int* 1982;22:112–126.

31. Zatz R, Meyer TW, Rennke HG, Brenner BM. *Proc Natl Acad Sci (USA)* 1985;82:5963–5967.
32. Modi KS, O'Donnell MP, Keane WF. In: El Nahas AM, Mallick NP, Anderson S, eds. *Prevention of chronic renal failure.* Oxford: Oxford Univ. Press; 1993:117–172.
33. Anderson S. In: El Nahas AM, Mallick NP, Anderson S, eds. *Prevention of chronic renal failure.* Oxford: Oxford Univ. Press; 1993: 173–209.
34. Anderson S, Meyer TW, Rennke HG, Brenner BM. *J Clin Invest* 1985;76:612–619.
35. Anderson S, Rennke HG, Brenner BM. *J Clin Invest* 1986;77: 1993–2000.
36. Zatz R, Dunn BR, Meyer TW, Anderson S, Rennke HG, Brenner BM. *J Clin Invest* 1986;77:1925–1930.
37. Dworkin LD, Hostetter TH, Rennke HG, Brenner BM. *J Clin Invest* 1984;73:1448–1461.
38. Schnermann J, Gokel M, Weber PC, Schubert G, Briggs JP. *Kidney Int* 1986;29:520–529.
39. Steiner RW, Tucker BJ, Gushwa LC, Gifford J, Wilson CB, Blantz RC. *Hypertension* 1982;4:51–57.
40. Azar S, Johnson MA, Hertel B, Tobian L. *Kidney Int* 1977;12: 28–40.
41. Dworkin LD, Feiner HD. *J Clin Invest* 1986;77:797–809.
42. Simons JL, Provoost AP, Anderson S, et al. *J Am Soc Nephrol* 1993;3:1775–1782.
43. Neugarten J, Kaminetsky B, Feiner H, Schacht RG, Liu DT, Baldwin DS. *Kidney Int* 1985;28:135–139.
44. Baylis C, Mitruka B, Deng A. *J Clin Invest* 1992;90:278–281.
45. Junaid A, Kren SM, Rosenberg ME, Nath KA, Hostetter TH. *J Am Soc Nephrol* 1993;4:912 (abstr).
46. Paul LC, Chea R, Davidoff A, Benediktsson H. *J Am Soc Nephrol* 1993;4:917 (abstr).
47. Scholey JW, Miller PL, Rennke HG, Meyer TW. *Kidney Int* 1989;36:816–822.
48. Schmitz PG, O'Donnell MP, Kasiske BL, Katz SA, Keane WF. *Am J Physiol* 1992;263:F496–F502.
49. Kasiske BL, O'Donnell MP, Schmitz PG, Kim Y, Keane WF. *Kidney Int* 1990;37:880–891.
50. Hostetter TH, Troy JL, Brenner BM. *Kidney Int* 1981;19:410–415.
51. Anderson S, Rennke HG, Zatz R. *Am J Physiol* 1994; (in press).
52. Fujihara CK, Limongi DMZP, de Oliveira HCF, Zatz R. *Am J Physiol* 1992;262:R947–R954.
53. Anderson S, Diamond JR, Karnovsky MJ, Brenner BM. *J Clin Invest* 1988;82:1757–1768.
54. Remuzzi A, Puntorieri S, Mazzoleni A, Remuzzi G. *Kidney Int* 1988;34:481–486.
55. Azar S, Johnson MA, Scheinman J, Bruno L, Tobian L. *Clin Sci* 1979;56:203–209.
56. Gabbai FB, Gushwa LC, Wilson CB, Blantz RC. *Kidney Int* 1987;31:1267–1278.
57. Beyer MM, Steinberg AD, Nicastri AD, Friedman EA. *Science* 1977;198:511–513.
58. Velosa JA, Glasser RJ, Nevins TE, Michael AF. *Lab Invest* 1977;36:527–534.
59. Teodoru CV, Saifer A, Frankel H. *Am J Physiol* 1959;196:457–460.
60. Garcia DL, Rennke HG, Brenner BM, Anderson S. *J Clin Invest* 1987;80:867–874.
61. Garcia DL, Anderson S, Rennke HG, Brenner BM. *Proc Natl Acad Sci (USA)* 1988;85:6142–6146.
62. Simons JL, Provoost AP, Anderson S, Rennke HG, Troy JL, Brenner BM. *J Am Soc Nephrol* 1993;4:783 (abstr).
63. Marsden PA, Goligorsky MS, Brenner BM. *J Am Soc Nephrol* 1991;1:931–948.
64. Yoshizumi M, Kurihara H, Fuminaro T, et al. *Circ Res* 1988;78: II-182 (abstr).
65. Kuchan MJ, Frangos JA. *Am J Physiol* 1993;264:H150–H156.
66. Buga GM, Gold ME, Fukuto JM, Ignarro LJ. *Hypertension* 1991;17:187–193.
67. Noris M, Morigi M, Zoja C, et al. *J Am Soc Nephrol* 1993;4:562 (abstr).
68. Ott MJ, Ballermann BJ. *J Am Soc Nephrol* 1992;3:476 (abstr).
69. Riser BL, Cortes P, Zhao X, Bernstein J, Dumler F, Narins RG. *J Clin Invest* 1992;90:1932–1943.
70. Riser BL, Cortes P, Zhao X, Sastry KSS, Hassett CI, Narins RG. *J Am Soc Nephrol* 1992;3:642 (abstr).
71. Homma T, Akai Y, Burns KD, Harris RC. *J Biol Chem* 1992;267:23129–23135.
72. Kaname S, Miyajima Y, Kurokawa K, Ogata E, Uchida S. *J Am Soc Nephrol* 1991;2:439 (abstr).
73. Feld LG, Van Liew JB, Brentjens JR, Boyland JW. *Kidney Int* 1981;20:606–614.
74. Purkerson ML, Hoffsten PE, Klahr S. *Kidney Int* 1976;9:407–417.
75. Meyer TW, Anderson S, Rennke HG, Brenner BM. *Kidney Int* 1987;31:752–759.
76. Dworkin LD, Parker M, Feiner HD. *Kidney Int* 1989;35:427 (abstr).
77. Lafayette RA, Mayer G, Park SK, Meyer TW. *J Clin Invest* 1992;90:766–771.
78. Dworkin LD, Levin RI, Benstein JA, et al. *Am J Physiol* 1990;259:F598–F604.
79. Jackson B, Franze L, Sumithran E, Johnston CI. *J Lab Clin Invest* 1990;115:21–27.
80. Blantz RC, Konnen KS, Tucker BJ. *J Clin Invest* 1976;57:419–434.
81. Anderson S, Jung FF, Ingelfinger JR. *Am J Physiol* 1993;265: F477–F486.
82. Mayer G, Lafayette RA, Oliver J, Deen WM, Myers BD, Meyer TW. *Kidney Int* 1993;43:346–353.
83. Kakinuma Y, Kawamura T, Bills T, Yoshioka T, Ichikawa I, Fogo A. *Kidney Int* 1992;42:46–55.
84. Mackenzie HS, Troy JL, Li Y, et al. *J Am Soc Nephrol* 1993;4: 775 (abstr).
85. Remuzzi A, Perico N, Amuchastegui CS, et al. *J Am Soc Nephrol* 1993;40–49.
86. Hutchison FN, Webster SK. *Am J Physiol* 1992;263:F311–F318.
87. Peten EP, Fogo A, Pesce CM, et al. *J Am Soc Nephrol* 1993;4:780 (abstr).
88. Keane WF, Raij L. *Lab Invest* 1985;52:599–604.
89. Raij L, Keane WF. *Am J Med* 1985;79:24–36.
90. Remuzzi G, Bertani T. *Kidney Int* 1990;38:384–394.
91. Diamond JR, Anderson S. *Am J Pathol* 1990;137:1323–1332.
92. Lee G, Ihm C, Anderson P, et al. *Kidney Int* 1990;37:511 (abstr).
93. Remuzzi A, Puntorieri S, Battaglia C, et al. *J Clin Invest* 1990;85: 541–549.
94. Scholey JW, Miller PL, Rennke HG, Meyer TW. *Kidney Int* 1989;35:437 (abstr).
95. Fogo A, Ichikawa I. *Semin Nephrol* 1989;9:329–342.
96. Lafferty HM, Brenner BM. *Semin Nephrol* 1990;10:294–304.
97. Fries JWU, Sandstrom DJ, Meyer TW, Rennke HG. *Lab Invest* 1989;60:205–218.
98. Yoshida Y, Fogo A, Ichikawa I. *Kidney Int* 1989;35:654–660.
99. Miller PL, Rennke HG, Meyer TW. *Am J Physiol* 1991;261: F459–F465.
100. Daniels BS, Hostetter TH. *Am J Physiol* 1990;258:F1409–F1416.
101. Rennke HG. In: Mitch WE, Brenner BM, Stein JH (eds). *The progressive nature of renal disease.* New York: Churchill Livingstone; 1986:111–131.
102. Nagata M, Schärer K, Kriz W. *Kidney Int* 1992;42:136–147.
103. Nagata M, Kriz W. *Kidney Int* 1992;42:148–160.
104. Miller PL, Scholey JW, Rennke HG, Meyer TW. *J Clin Invest* 1990;85:1119–1126.
105. Motojima M, Nishijima F, Ikoma M, et al. *Kidney Int* 1991;40: 461–469.
106. Brunner FP, Thiel G, Hermle M, Bock HA, Mihatsch M. *Kidney Int* 1989;36:969–977.
107. Yoshida Y, Kawamura T, Ikoma M, Fogo A, Ichikawa I. *Kidney Int* 1989;36:626–635.
108. Anderson S, Rennke HG, Garcia DL, Brenner BM. *Kidney Int* 1989;36:526–536.
109. Tolins JP, Raij L. *Hypertension* 1990;16:452–461.
110. Wenzel UO, Troschau G, Schoeppe W, Helmchen U, Schwietzer G. *Hypertension* 1992;20:233–241.

111. Anderson S, Rennke HG, Brenner BM. *Kidney Int* 1992;41:891–897.
112. Gaston RS, Julian BA, Diethelm AG, Curtis JJ. *Ann Intern Med* 1991;115:954–955.
113. Someya N, Morotomi Y, Kodama K, et al. *J Cardiovasc Pharmacol* 1984;6:840–844.
114. Pollare T, Lithell H, Berne C. *N Engl J Med* 1989;321:868–873.
115. Keilani T, Schlueter MA, Leven ML, Batlle DC. *Ann Intern Med* 1993;118:246–254.
116. Bagchi D, Prasad R, Das DK. *Biochem Biophys Res Commun* 1989;158:52–57.
117. Raij L, Luscher TF, Vanhoutte PM. *Hypertension* 1988;12:562–567.
118. Raij L, Schultz PJ, Tolins JP. *J Hypertension* 1989;7(Suppl 7):S33–S37.
119. Chobanian AV, Haudenschild CC, Nickerson C, Drago R. *Hypertension* 1990;15:327–331.
120. Clozel M, Kuhn H, Hefti F. *Hypertension* 1990;16:532–540.
121. Clozel M. *Hypertension* 1991;18(Suppl II):II-37–II-42.
122. Mombouli J-V, Nephtali M, Vanhoutte PM. *Hypertension* 1991;18(Suppl II):II-22–II-29.
123. Wang D-F, Prewitt RL. *Hypertension* 1990;15:68–77.
124. Kon V, Fogo A, Ichikawa I. *Kidney Int* 1993;44:545–550.
125. Geiger H, Bahner U, Kraus I, et al. *Kidney Int* 1993;44:24–29.
126. Benstein JA, Feiner HD, Parker M, Dworkin LD. *Am J Physiol* 1990;258:F1675–F1681.
127. Dworkin LD, Feiner HD, Parker M, Tolbert E. *Kidney Int* 1991;39:1112–1117.
128. Harris DCH, Hammond WS, Burke TJ, Schrier RW. *Kidney Int* 1987;31:41–46.
129. Katsumata H, Suzuki H, Ohishi A, Nakamoto H, Saruta T, Sakaguchi H. *Lab Invest* 1990;62:474–481.
130. Jyothirmayi GN, Reddi AS. *Hypertension* 1993;21:795–802.
131. Brown SA, Walton CL, Crawford P, Bakris GL. *Kidney Int* 1993;43:1210–1218.
132. Heifets M, Elfenbein IB. *J Am Soc Nephrol* 1990;1:631 (abstr).
133. Jackson B, Debrevi L, Cubela R, Whitty M, Johnston CI. *Clin Exp Pharmacol Physiol* 1986;13:319–323.
134. Podjarny E, Rathaus M, Shapira J, et al. *Nephron* 1990;55:196–202.
135. Yoshioka T, Shiraga H, Yoshida Y, et al. *J Clin Invest* 1988;82:1614–1623.
136. Anderson S. *Hypertension* 1991;17:288–295.
137. Brunner FP, Hermle M, Thiel G. *Proc Xth Intl Congr Nephrol* 1987;497 (abstr).
138. Frei U, Schindler R, Matties V, Koch KM. *J Pharmacol Exp Ther* 1992;263:938–942.
139. Benstein JA, Feiner HD, Ohsumi F, Tolbert E, Dworkin LD. *J Am Soc Nephrol* 1992;3:734 (abstr).
140. Bakris GL. *Am J Hypertens* 1991;4:487S–493S.
141. Dworkin LD, Benstein JA. *Am J Hyperten* 1989;2:162S–172S.
142. Dworkin LD, Grosser M, Feiner HD, Ullian M, Parker M. *Kidney Int* 1989;35:790–798.
143. O'Brien RC, Cooper ME, Jerums G, Doyle AE. *Diabetes* 1993;42:604–609.
144. Dworkin LD, Feiner HD, Randazzo J. *Kidney Int* 1987;31:718–724.
145. Azar S, Keane W, Raij L. *Kidney Int* 1985;27:187 (abstr).
146. Raij L, Chiou X, Owens R, Wrigley B. *Am J Med* 1985;79(Suppl 3C):37–41.
147. Michel J-B, Dussaule J-C, Choudat L, et al. *Kidney Int* 1986;29:1011–1020.
148. Fujihara CK, Padilha RM, Zatz R. *Diabetes* 1992;41:286–293.
149. Bank N, Klose R, Aynedjian HS, Nguyen D, Sablay LB. *Kidney Int* 1987;31:898–905.
150. Cooper ME, Rumble JR, Allen TJ, O'Brien RC, Jerums G, Doyle AE. *Kidney Int* 1992;41:898–903.
151. Gabbai FB, Peterson OW, Prost J-P, Blantz RC. *Am J Hypertens* 1989;2:213S–218S.
152. Delaini F, Perico N, Tagliaferri M, et al. *J Pharmacol Exp Ther* 1988;246:287–293.
153. Zoja C, Perico N, Bergamelli A, et al. *Kidney Int* 1990;37:934–942.
154. Olson JL. *Kidney Int* 1984;25:376–382.
155. Wilson SK, Solez K, Boitnott JK, Heptinstall RH. *Am J Pathol* 1981;102:62–71.
156. Susic D, Mandal AK, Kentera D. *Hypertension* 1982;4:681–685.
157. Ichikawa I, Yoshida Y, Fogo A, Purkerson ML, Klahr S. *Kidney Int* 1988;34:638–644.
158. Yokokawa K, Mandal AK, Kohno M, Takeda T. *J Am Soc Nephrol* 1993;4:527 (abstr).
159. Zoja C, Benigni A, Remuzzi G. In: Mitch WE, Stein JH, eds. *The progressive nature of renal disease.* New York: Churchill Livingstone; 1992:77–98.
160. Remuzzi G, FitzGerald GA, Patrono C. *Kidney Int* 1992;41:1483–1493.
161. Purkerson ML, Joist JH, Yates J, Valdes A, Morrison A, Klahr S. *Proc Natl Acad Sci USA* 1985;82:193–197.
162. Zoja C, Perico N, Corna D, et al. *J Am Soc Nephrol* 1990;1:799–807.
163. Vriesendorp R, Donker AJM, de Zeeuw D, et al. *Am J Med* 1986;81(Suppl 2B):84–94.
164. Neugarten J, Kozin A, Cook K. *Kidney Int* 1989;36:51–56.
165. Nath KA, Chmielewski DH, Hostetter TH. *Am J Physiol* 1987;252:F829–F837.
166. Barcelli UO, Pollak VE. In: Mitch WE, Brenner BM, Stein JH, eds. *The progressive nature of renal disease.* New York: Churchill Livingstone; 1986:65–80.
167. Villa E, Martinez J, Ruilope LM, Mampaso F, Sancho JM, Robles RG. *Am J Hyperten* 1993;6:253–257.
168. Conger JD, Falk SA, Gillum DM. *Am J Kidney Dis* 1989;13:217–225.
169. Falk SA, Buric V, Hammond WS, Conger JD. *Am J Kidney Dis* 1991;17:218–227.
170. Meyer TW, Troy JL, Rennke HG, Brenner BM. *Proc IXth Int Cong Nephrol* 1984;355(abstr).
171. Shigematsu T, Caverzasio J, Bonjour J-P. *Kidney Int* 1993;44:173–181.
172. Doi T, Striker LJ, Quaife C, et al. *Am J Pathol* 1988;131:398–403.
173. El Nahas AM, Bassett AH, Cope GH, Le Carpentier JE. *Kidney Int* 1991;40:29–34.
174. Hirschberg R, Kopple JD. *J Am Soc Nephrol* 1992;2:1417–1422.
175. Saito T, Atkins RC. *Kidney Int* 1990;37:1076–1083.
176. Baylis C, Brenner BM. *Am J Physiol* 1978;234:F166–F170.
177. Lafferty HM, Garcia DL, Rennke HG, Troy HL, Anderson S, Brenner BM. *J Am Soc Nephrol* 1991;1:1180–1185.
178. Remuzzi A, Puntorieri S, Brugnetti B, Bertani T, Remuzzi G. *Kidney Int* 1991;39:647–652.
179. Jamgotchian N, Eggena P, Hu MS, et al. *J Am Soc Nephrol* 1990;1:493 (abstr).
180. Carlini RG, Dusso AS, Obialo CI, Alvarez UM, Rothstein M. *Kidney Int* 1993;43:1010–1014.
181. King AJ, Brenner BM. *Am J Physiol* 1991;260:R653–R662.
182. Raij L, Schultz PJ. *J Am Soc Nephrol* 1993;3:1435–1441.
183. King AJ, Brenner BM, Anderson S. *Am J Physiol* 1989;256:F1051–F1058.
184. Orisio S, Benigni A, Bruzzi I, et al. *Kidney Int* 1993;43:354–358.
185. Benigni A, Zoja C, Corna D, et al. *Kidney Int* 1993;44:440–444.
186. Zatz R, de Nucci G. *Am J Physiol* 1991;261:F360–F363.
187. Ribeiro MO, Antunes E, de Nucci G, Lovisolo SM, Zatz R. *Hypertension* 1992;20:298–303.
188. Reyes AA, Purkerson ML, Karl I, Klahr S. *Am J Kidney Dis* 1992;20:168–176.
189. Dunn BR, Ichikawa I, Pfeffer JM, Troy JL, Brenner BM. *Circ Res* 1986;59:237–246.
190. Ortola FV, Ballermann BJ, Anderson S, Mendez RE, Brenner BM. *J Clin Invest* 1987;80:670–674.
191. Angeli P, Arroyo V, Claria J, et al. *J Am Soc Nephrol* 1993;4:435 (abstr).
192. Zhang PL, Mackenzie HS, Troy JL, Zayas MA, Brenner BM. *J Am Soc Nephrol* 1993;4:527 (abstr).
193. Zhang PL, Mackenzie HS, Troy JL, Li Y, Brenner BM. *J Am Soc Nephrol* 1993;4:591(abstr).

194. Zhang PL, Mackenzie HS, Troy JL, Brenner BM. *J Am Soc Nephrol* 1994;4:1564–1570.
195. Meyer TW, Anderson S, Brenner BM. *Ann Intern Med* 1983;98(Part 2):832–838.
196. Tapp DC, Wortham WG, Addison JF, Hammonds DN, Barnes JL, Venkatachalam MA. *Lab Invest* 1989;60:184–195.
197. Reisin E, Azar S, DeBoisblanc BP, Guzman MA, Lohmann T. *Hypertension* 1993;21:971–974.
198. Kleinknecht C, Laouri D, Hinglais N, et al. *Kidney Int* 1986;30:687–693.
199. Bouby N, Bachmann S, Bichet D, Bankir L. *Am J Physiol* 1990;258:F973–F979.
200. Kasiske BL, O'Donnell MP, Garvis WJ, Keane WF. *Circ Res* 1988;862:367–374.
201. Lumlertgul D, Burke TJ, Gillum DM, et al. *Kidney Int* 1986;29:658–666.
202. Loghman-Adham M. *J Lab Clin Med* 1993;122:15–25.
203. Harris DCH, Falk SA, Conger JD, Hammond WS, Schrier RW. *Am J Kidney Dis* 1988;11:489–498.
204. Lax DS, Benstein JA, Tolbert E, Dworkin LD. *Kidney Int* 1992;42:1527–1534.
205. Kasiske BL, Kalil RSN, Ma JZ, Liao M, Keane WF. *Ann Intern Med* 1993;118:129–138.
206. Wiedmann P, Boehlen L, de Courten M, Shaw SG. *J Am Soc Nephrol* 1992;3:339(abstr).
207. Lewis EJ, Hunsicker LG, Bain RP, Rohde RD. The Collaborative Study Group. *New Engl J Med* 1993;329:1456–1462.
208. Mann JFE, Reisch C, Ritz E. *Nephron* 1990;55(Suppl 1):38–42.
209. Kamper A-L, Strandgaard S, Leyssac PP. *Am J Hypertens* 1992;5:423–430.
210. Zucchelli P, Zuccala A, Borghi M, et al. *Kidney Int* 1992;42:452–458.
211. Björck S, Mulec H, Johnsen SA, Noroen C, Aurell M. *Br Med J* 1992;304:339–343.

Hypertension: Pathophysiology, Diagnosis, and Management, Second Edition,
edited by J.H. Laragh and B.M. Brenner,
Raven Press, Ltd., New York © 1995.

CHAPTER **94**

The Renal Basis for Salt Sensitivity in Hypertension

Genjiro Kimura and Barry M. Brenner

Dahl (1) developed by selective inbreeding two strains of rats: one, a salt-sensitive "S" strain, exhibited hypertension with salt feeding; the other, a salt-resistant "R" strain, remained normotensive despite a high salt intake. Furthermore, replacing the kidneys of "R" rats with the kidneys from "S" rats led to hypertension when these "R" rats were fed a high-salt diet, whereas transplantation of kidneys of "R" into "S" rats prevented the development of hypertension (2). These experiments afforded strong evidence that salt can indeed induce hypertension and that a genetic defect of hypertension in "S" rats is

expressed in the kidneys. This defect, thought to be involved in influencing renal sodium excretory capability, was soon confirmed by Tobian et al. (3), who showed a less steep pressure-natriuresis relationship in perfused kidneys isolated from Dahl S rats.

Bartter and colleagues (4,5) showed for the first time that even in human essential hypertension the blood pressure response to high salt intake was of two types, not unlike that in Dahl rats. They gave a low-sodium diet containing 9 mmol of sodium per day for 7 days, and then switched to a high-sodium diet containing 249 mmol/day for 7 days. Although the change in mean arterial pressures (MAPs) induced by the sodium load seemed to show a regular and continuous distribution from small to large without a clear-cut point of separa-

  G. Kimura and B. M. Brenner: Renal Division, Department of Medicine, Brigham and Women's Hospital and Harvard Medical School, Boston, Massachusetts 02115.

tion, they arbitrarily divided the response into two types: patients were considered "sodium-sensitive" when mean arterial pressure was elevated more than 10 percent, whereas lesser responders were viewed as "non-sodium-sensitive." Some authors followed Bartter's protocol and arbitrary definitions, whereas others modified the amount (6–9) and duration (7–9) of each sodium intake period and also took 5 percent (8) or 10 mm Hg (7,9,10) instead of 10 percent elevation in blood pressure as evidence for a "sodium-sensitive" response.

These inconsistencies made it clear that salt sensitivity should be considered two-dimensionally based on blood pressure elevation as well as the magnitude of sodium load (11–16), since blood pressure elevation can be greater when sodium intake is greater. Also, it became clear that the magnitude of sodium load should be evaluated in each patient as the difference in urinary sodium excretion rate in the steady state of sodium balance at each level of sodium intake. This gave rise to the *sodium sensitivity index,* defined as the ratio of the change in mean arterial pressure (mm Hg) over the change in urinary sodium excretion (mmol/day) (12). As will become evident below, this sodium sensitivity index exactly equals the reciprocal of the slope of the pressure-natriuresis relationship. Since blood pressure and urinary sodium excretion rate are measured in the steady state during sodium balance at each level of sodium intake, this index can readily be compared for results obtained at different levels of sodium intake. In some studies, sodium sensitivity has been examined by observing the blood pressure fall in response to reducing sodium intake (13,14,17). Since, as discussed below, the relationship between urinary sodium excretion rate and systemic mean arterial pressure is approximately linear, the sodium sensitivity index provides insights into true sodium sensitivity, irrespective of whether sodium intake is increased (sodium loaded) or reduced (sodium depleted) (18–20). Even with this more rigorous index for sodium sensitivity, the cut point of separation between salt-sensitive and non–salt-sensitive remains arbitrary. In general, when this index is greater than 10 mm Hg/(200 mmol/day), i.e., 0.05 mm Hg/(mmol/day), blood pressure is usually defined as sodium-sensitive.

IMPORTANCE OF KIDNEY IN LONG-TERM BLOOD PRESSURE CONTROL

When sodium intake is increased, extracellular fluid volume and plasma volume both tend to increase in parallel (except under edematous conditions). This increase in plasma volume in turn induces an elevation in central filling pressures, which increases cardiac output. Eventually, however, whole-body autoregulation results in an increase in total peripheral resistance, thereby returning cardiac output toward normal. Whereas the increase in cardiac output may be minimal, the increase in total peripheral resistance may be substantial. Thus, hypertension becomes of high total peripheral resistance type, instead of high cardiac output type (21). In fact, the concept that blood pressure is determined by total peripheral resistance and cardiac output is valid in the regulation of the steady-state blood pressure only when kidneys are removed (22,23). Normal kidneys minimize salt-induced increases in extracellular fluid and cardiac output and increases in blood pressure; it is the kidneys, therefore, that determine the long-term blood pressure response.

Pressure-Natriuresis Feedback System

The primacy of the kidneys in the regulation of sodium excretion and extracellular fluid volume is well recognized but their importance in blood pressure regulation is less understood. Since sodium is the principal substance maintaining effective osmolality in extracellular fluid, and since extracellular sodium concentration is tightly controlled by the thirst-antidiuretic hormone-renal collecting duct axis, it is the absolute amount of sodium in the extracellular compartment that determines the volume of extracellular fluid. Therefore, although renal sodium excretion determines the extracellular fluid volume, the latter does not serve as a primary regulator of renal sodium excretion. This is because there are no good sensing mechanisms to detect the extracellular fluid volume compartment as a whole. In contrast, changes in blood pressure and intravascular volume can be detected relatively precisely, for example, by carotid baroreceptors, baroreceptors in juxtaglomerular cells, and the degree of distention (stretch) on receptors in right and left atria. In other words, renal sodium excretion–extracellular fluid volume regulation does not constitute a closed 1:1 feedback system. Presumably, this is why edematous disorders can coexist with normally functioning kidneys. Instead, renal sodium excretion is regulated by systemic arterial pressure (i.e., renal perfusion pressure) so that renal sodium excretion–arterial blood pressure regulation constitutes a closed negative feedback system (21,24–27), as illustrated by the pressure-natriuresis relationship (see Fig. 2). In fact, renal perfusion pressure plays a central role in the regulation of urinary sodium excretion by influencing glomerular capillary pressure, renin-angiotensin-aldosterone axis, renal interstitial pressure, medullary blood flow, and so on (28) (Fig. 1). Thus, it may be considered that the regulation of renal sodium excretion is intended to maintain arterial blood pressure rather than extracellular fluid volume (28). Essentially, all regulatory mechanisms of renal sodium excretion that have generally been pro-

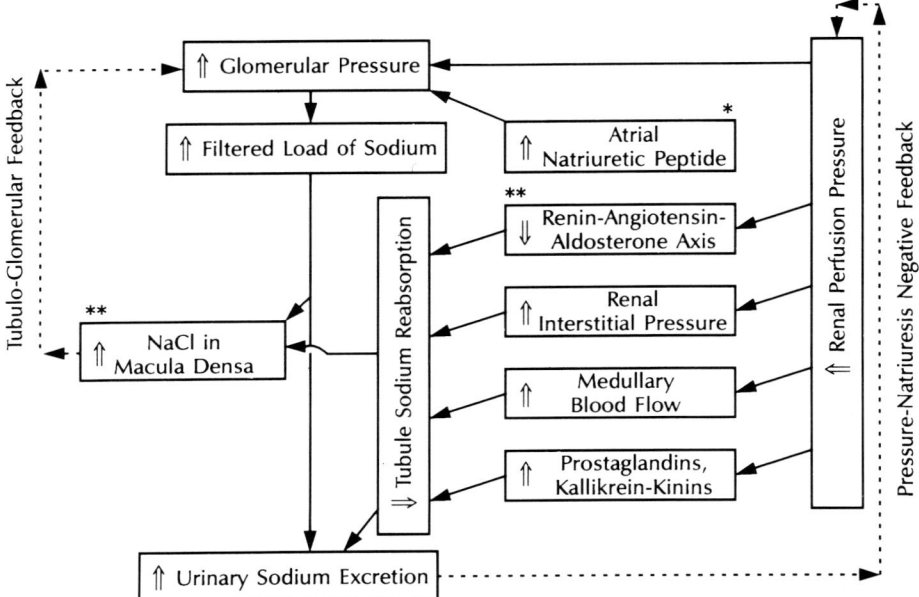

FIG. 1. Regulatory mechanisms of renal sodium excretion and pressure-natriuresis negative feedback system. Essentially all regulatory mechanisms proposed for the regulation of extracellular fluid vol-ume are working for blood pressure (systemic mean and renal perfusion) regulation, and renal sodium excretion-arterial blood pressure regulation constitutes a closed negative feedback system. Stimulation (*continuous arrows*) and inhibition (*broken arrows*) are indicated.

    * Please note that when sodium retention causes the elevation in renal perfusion pressure, the secretion of atrial natriuretic peptide is usually stimulated by atrial distention at the same time.

    ** When the amount of NaCl delivered to macula densa located at the end of thick ascending limb of Henle's loop is increased, the tubuloglomerular feedback mechanism is activated. This results inboth afferent arteriolar vasoconstriction and suppression of renin secretion from juxtaglomerular cells,which inactivates the renin-angiotensin-aldosterone axis, and therefore lowers the glomerular capillary pressure. (From ref. 28, with permission.)

posed for the regulation of extracellular fluid volume are seen here as mainly involved in the regulation of steady-state blood pressure (28).

Implications of Pressure-Natriuresis Relationship

An approximately linear relationship exists (20,21, 24–27,29–33) between the rate of urinary sodium excretion ($U_{Na}V$) and systemic MAP (Fig. 2). This tight pressure-natriuresis relationship constitutes a negative feedback system (see Fig. 1). When the amount of dietary sodium intake is plotted on the $U_{Na}V$ axis of the pressure-natriuresis relationship, the blood pressure value of the crossing point of the above two lines is the equilibrium pressure (21,24,25), indicating that $U_{Na}V$ is equal to the amount of sodium intake only at this equilibrium blood pressure. Unless the pressure-natriuresis relationship is affected, the systemic blood pressure reaches this value in the steady state (as long as sodium intake remains the same). For example, when blood

pressure is elevated beyond the equilibrium pressure by any mechanism, the pressure-natriuresis relationship shows that $U_{Na}V$ exceeds sodium intake. Therefore, sodium balance becomes negative, resulting in a fall in blood pressure such that blood pressure returns to the equilibrium pressure and $U_{Na}V$ becomes equal to sodium intake. Conversely, when blood pressure is lowered below the equilibrium pressure, the pressure-natriuresis relationship shows that $U_{Na}V$ is now less than sodium intake, and sodium balance becomes positive. Therefore, blood pressure rises gradually until an equilibrium pressure is again achieved. Based on the above discussion, Guyton and colleagues (21,24–26) have proposed that the pressure-natriuresis relationship must be affected in the genesis of hypertension regardless of the factors initiating hypertension. When sodium intake is increased, the pressure-natriuresis relationship shows that blood pressure will rise to a new equilibrium pressure. The difference between equilibrium pressures for high and normal sodium intakes gives the actual blood pressure elevation induced by high sodium intake.

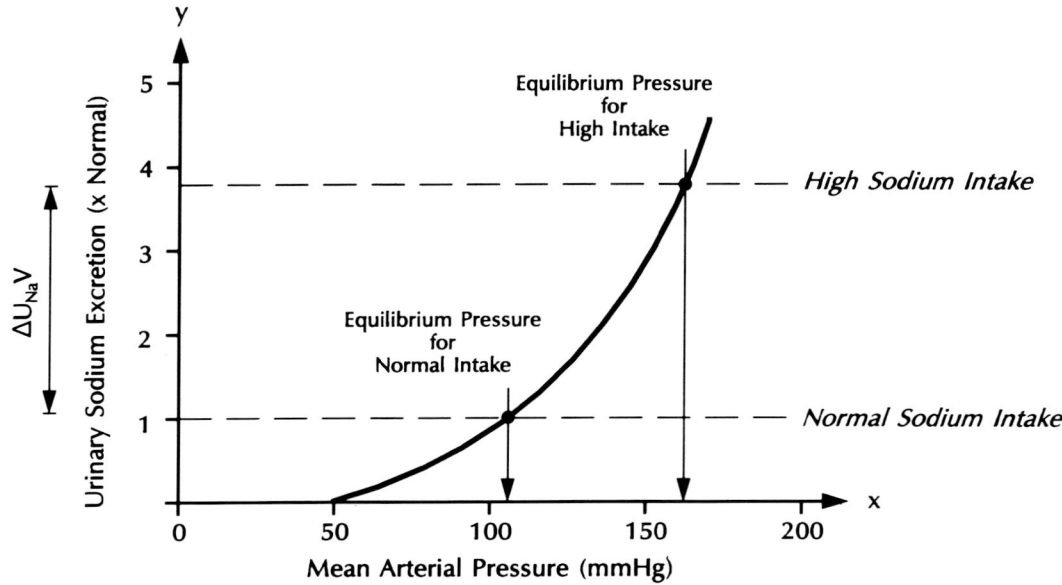

FIG. 2. Pressure-natriuresis relationship. Between the systemic mean arterial pressure (MAP) on the abscissa and urinary sodium excretion rate (U$_{Na}$V) on the ordinate, there exists an approximately linear relationship (pressure-natriuresis relationship). When the two levels of sodium intake are plotted on the ordinate over this relationship, the pressure values of each intercept of the two lines are the equilibrium pressure at which the amount of sodium excreted in urine becomes equal to sodium intake, resulting in zero net sodium balance. Please note that the *sodium sensitivity index,* defined as the ratio of the change in MAP over the change in U$_{Na}$V (ΔMAP/ΔU$_{Na}$V), exactly equals the reciprocal of the slope of this pressure-natriuresis relationship. (From ref. 28, with permission.)

Characterization of Pressure-Natriuresis Relationship

In clinical situations, the pressure-natriuresis relationship has been considered to be linear (11,13–16,20,27,29,30,33,34). Assuming a linear relationship between MAP and U$_{Na}$V, the pressure-natriuresis relationship is drawn by linking two data points obtained in the steady state under two different amounts of sodium intake, low and high, in each subject, where MAP (mm Hg) and U$_{Na}$V (mmol/day) are plotted on the x- and y-axes, respectively (Fig. 3). Using the extrapolated x-intercept (A) and the slope (B), the urinary sodium excretion rate can now be characterized as a first order function of MAP as (35–39):

$$U_{Na}V = B \times (MAP - A) \qquad [1]$$

The x-intercept (A) of the pressure-natriuresis relationship represents the critical level of blood pressure, below which the urinary sodium excretion is halted. The slope (B) represents the reciprocal of the sodium sensitivity of blood pressure (12). When the slope is less steep as shown, blood pressure response to the change in sodium intake is stronger, and the sodium sensitivity becomes higher.

Pressure-Natriuresis Relationship in Hypertension

The pressure-natriuresis relationship in patients with the two most common forms of curable hypertension, unilateral renovascular hypertension and primary aldosteronism, was compared before and after correction procedure (13) (Fig. 4). After correction, the pressure-natriuresis relationship was found normalized in both forms of hypertension. Before correction, however, it was shifted in parallel along the blood pressure axis toward a higher pressure level without significantly affecting the slope in renovascular hypertension, whereas it shifted with the slope depressed in primary aldosteronism. These findings show that the pressure-natriuresis relationship is indeed affected in hypertension, and that renovascular hypertension is of non–sodium-sensitive type, whereas primary aldosteronism is sodium sensitive (13). In patients with essential hypertension, the pressure-natriuresis relationship has also been shown to be shifted in parallel toward a higher blood pressure level without affecting the slope (non–sodium-sensitive type) at an early stage, and shifted further to the higher level with the slope more depressed (sodium-sensitive type) gradually with the progression of essential hypertension (11,14,34).

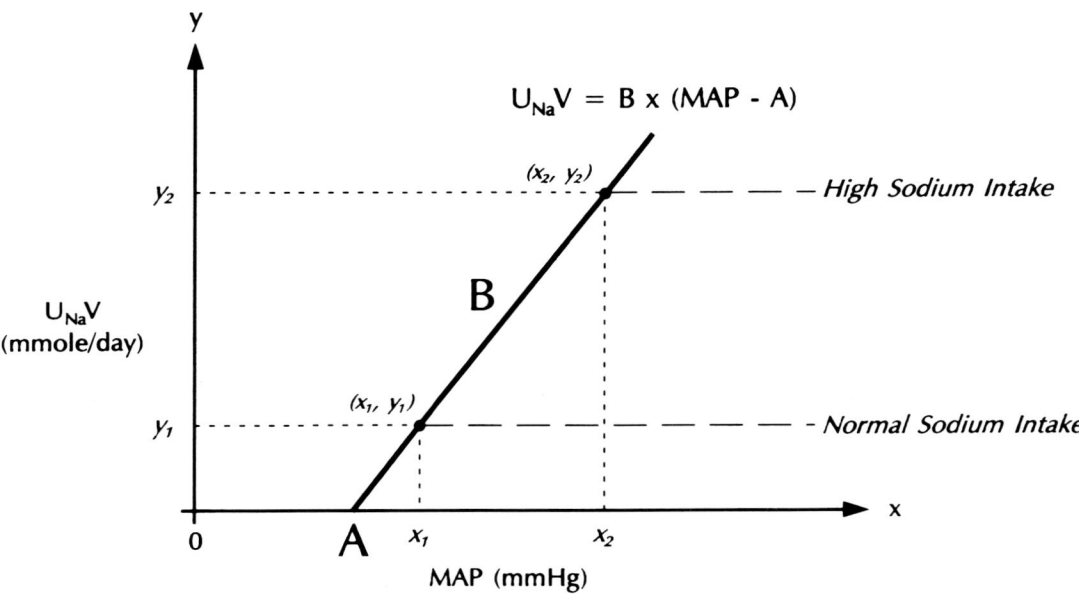

FIG. 3. Characterization of pressure-natriuresis relationship. Assuming a linear relationship between systemic mean arterial pressure (MAP) and daily urinary sodium excretion ($U_{Na}V$), the pressure-natriuresis relationship is drawn by linking two data points, (x_1, y_1), (x_2, y_2), obtained in the steady state under two different amounts of sodium intake, low and high, in each subject, where MAP and $U_{Na}V$ are plotted on the x- and y-axes, respectively. Using the extrapolated x-intercept (A) and the slope (B) of this line, $U_{Na}V$ can now be represented as a first order function of MAP: $U_{Na}V = B \times (MAP - A)$. (From ref. 39, with permission.)

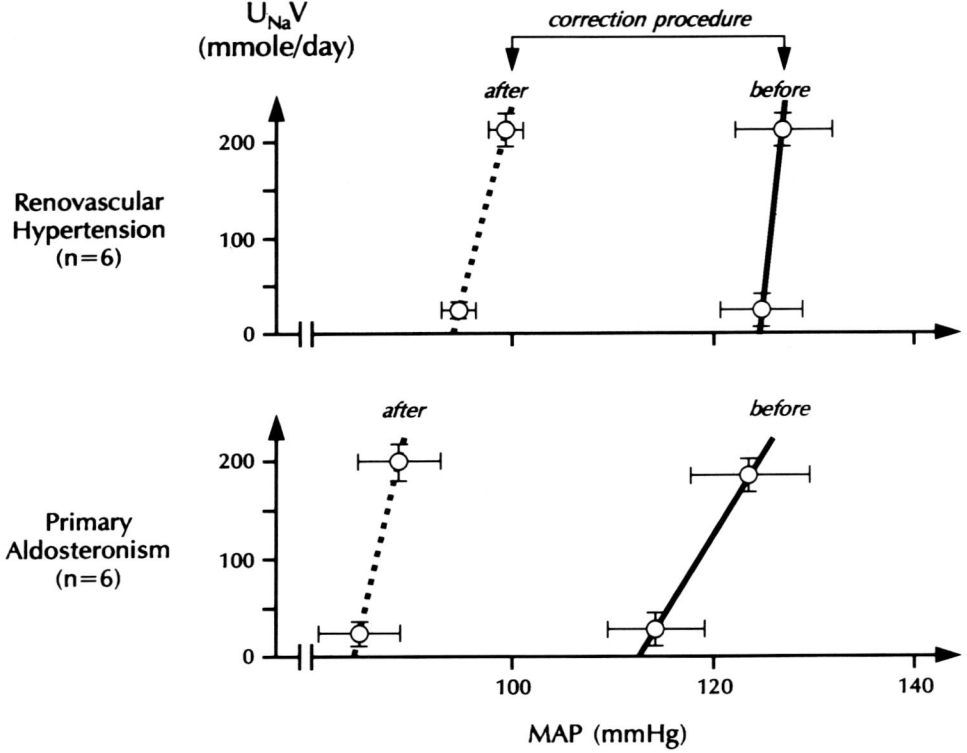

FIG. 4. Pressure-natriuresis relationship in secondary hypertension. Pressure-natriuresis relationship in patients with unilateral renovascular hypertension (n = 6) and primary aldosteronism (n = 6) was compared before and after correction procedure. After correction, the pressure-natriuresis relationship was found normalized in both forms of hypertension. Before correction, however, it was shifted in parallel along the blood pressure axis toward a higher pressure level without significantly affecting the slope in renovascular hypertension, while it shifted with the slope depressed in primary aldosteronism. These findings show that the pressure-natriuresis relationship is indeed affected in hypertension and that renovascular hypertension is of non–sodium-sensitive type, whereas primary aldosteronism is of sodium-sensitive type. (Adapted from ref. 13.)

PHYSICAL PROXY FOR THE PRESSURE-NATRIURESIS RELATIONSHIP BY WATER TANK MODEL

Guyton's theory has made it possible to understand the relationship between blood pressure and sodium metabolism, but did not clarify the renal mechanisms involved. Kimura and colleagues extended Guyton's approach to clarify these renal mechanisms based on the water tank model (35–37,39) (Fig. 5, right). In this model, a water tank with a base area corresponding to the reciprocal of the total peripheral vascular resistance (TPR) is assumed. If an outlet (faucet) is attached to this tank and water is poured into it at a rate corresponding to the amount of sodium intake (Q_{Na}), then an equilibrium will be achieved at a certain water level, tank volume, and outflow volume. The water level represents MAP, the water volume represents cardiac output (CO), and the water output represents $U_{Na}V$. If the base area of the water tank, the height and diameter of the outlet, and the rate of water poured in are known, the changes in water level, volume, and output over time are automatically determined.

Water Tank Model and Pressure-Natriuresis Relationship

As shown on the left side panel of Fig. 5, if MAP is plotted on the x-axis from the bottom to the top, and $U_{Na}V$ on the y-axis from right to left, it can be seen that the x-intercept (A) of the pressure-natriuresis relationship corresponds to the height of the outlet from the tank bottom, and the difference between MAP and A represents the effective pressure on the outlet. Thus, in the water tank model, when MAP is lower than the outlet height (A), no water output occurs, i.e., urinary sodium excretion stops. The slope (B) of the pressure-natriuresis relationship corresponds to the diameter of the outlet in the water tank model, easily explaining why urinary sodium output can be expressed as B times (MAP minus A), that is, the product of the outlet diameter and the effective pressure on the outlet (35,39).

When the pressure-natriuresis relationship is shifted in parallel along the blood pressure axis toward a higher blood pressure level, this corresponds in the water tank model to increasing outlet height from the tank bottom. Therefore, the effective pressure is decreased, resulting in a reduction in $U_{Na}V$ until MAP becomes high enough to keep the effective pressure on the outlet normal. Once a steady state is achieved, the responses to changes in the amount of sodium intake are the same as those in normal control. The net effect of the parallel shift of the pressure-natriuresis relationship is the shift of MAP to higher levels, with hypertension being of non–salt-sensitive type (35,37,39).

On the other hand, when the slope of the pressure-natriuresis relationship is depressed, this corresponds in the water tank model to reducing the diameter of the outlet. Gradual elevation in the effective pressure on the outlet can restore water output from the outlet toward normal. Since the outlet diameter is small, MAP is markedly elevated when Q_{Na} is increased. The resulting hypertension is therefore of salt-sensitive type (35,37,39).

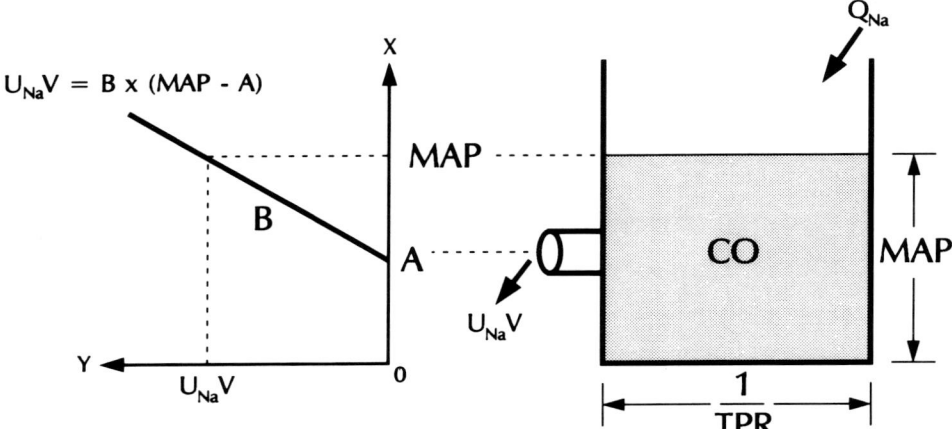

FIG. 5. Water tank model and pressure-natriuresis relationship. A simple model on body fluid volume and blood pressure regulation (*right*) was devised by incorporating the concept of the pressure-natriuresis relationship (*left*). In the assumed water tank, mean arterial pressure (MAP) is equivalent to the water level, cardiac output (CO) to the water volume, and total peripheral resistance (TPR) to the reciprocal of the base area of the water tank. The x-intercept (A) of the pressure-natriuresis relationship corresponds to the height of outlet (faucet), and (MAP minus A) to the effective pressure on the outlet. The slope (B) corresponds to the diameter of the outlet, and the output, i.e., urinary sodium excretion rate ($U_{Na}V$), can be calculated by the formula B × (MAP − A). (From ref. 35, with permission.)

Effective Pressure on the Outlet as Effective Filtration Pressure

The water tank model shows that (MAP minus A) represents the effective pressure on the outlet. This effective pressure is elevated only when blood pressure becomes sodium-sensitive, and the outlet diameter is reduced. Furthermore, the elevation in effective pressure is augmented when sodium intake is high. If water output from the outlet reflects the glomerular filtration rate, the effective pressure (MAP minus A) on the outlet corresponds to the effective filtration pressure across the glomerular capillary walls, and the x-intercept (A) of the pressure-natriuresis relationship corresponds to the sum of the pressure drop from heart to glomeruli plus the opposing pressures against glomerular filtration (39). Thus, interpretation of the pressure-natriuresis relationship based on the water tank model enables us to derive insights regarding glomerular hemodynamics.

When both the pressure-natriuresis relationship and autoregulation curves for glomerular filtration rate (GFR) and renal blood flow rate (RBF) are plotted as functions of systemic mean arterial pressure, GFR becomes zero at the blood pressure level around the x-intercept of the pressure-natriuresis relationship where urinary sodium excretion stops, whereas RBF remains relatively well autoregulated (21,27,29,40) (Fig. 6). Therefore, it may be assumed that GFR is autoregulated when MAP is higher than the x-intercept (A) of the pressure-natriuresis relationship, but falls to zero when MAP reaches A. Furthermore, this phenomenon is assumed to be based on the corresponding change in net effective filtration pressure ($\overline{\Delta P_F}$) across the glomerular capillary walls. In general, $\overline{\Delta P_F}$ is represented as the difference between the mean glomerular capillary hydraulic pressure ($\overline{P}_{GC}$) and the sum of the opposing pressures against filtration at the glomerulus, i.e., hydraulic pressure in Bowman's space (P_T) plus the mean oncotic pressure in glomerular capillaries ($\overline{\Pi}_G$) (41,42):

$$\overline{\Delta P_F} = \overline{P}_{GC} - (P_T + \overline{\Pi}_G) \qquad [2]$$

In turn, $\overline{P}_{GC}$ is represented as the difference between MAP minus the pressure drop from heart to glomeruli, which is the product of the preglomerular vascular resistance (R_A) from heart to glomeruli (mainly in afferent arterioles) and RBF. Thus, $\overline{\Delta P_F}$ can be represented as:

$$\overline{\Delta P_F} = MAP - (R_A \times RBF) - (P_T + \overline{\Pi}_G) \qquad [3]$$

As discussed above, $\overline{\Delta P_F}$ is assumed to be constant when MAP is higher than the x-intercept (A) of the pressure-natriuresis relationship, while assumed to be zero when MAP falls to A. Therefore, in equation [3], $\overline{\Delta P_F}$ becomes 0 when MAP equals A:

$$0 = A - (R_A \times RBF) - (P_T + \overline{\Pi}_G) \qquad [4]$$

Solving this equation [4], A can be represented as the sum of the pressure drop from heart to glomeruli (mainly along the afferent arteriole) plus the opposing pressures

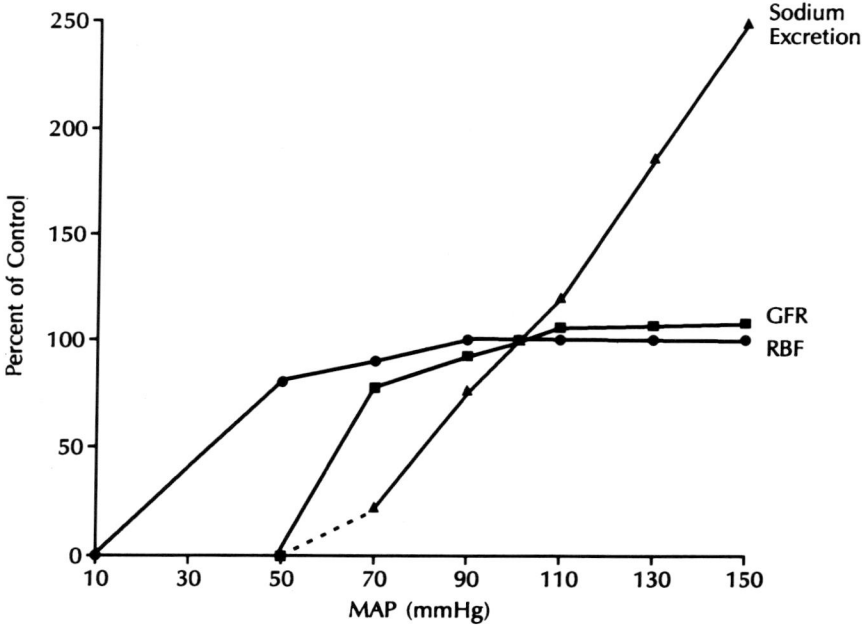

FIG. 6. Pressure-natriuresis relationship and kidney autoregulation. Urinary sodium excretion rate and autoregulation curves for GFR and RBF are plotted as functions of renal perfusion pressure (mean arterial pressure) on the same graph by expressing the ordinate as percent of control values. Around the blood pressure level where urinary sodium excretion stops, GFR also becomes zero whereas RBF remains relatively well autoregulated. (From refs. 27 and 29, with permission.)

against glomerular filtration (38,39,43), as expected from the water tank model:

$$A = (R_A \times RBF) + (P_T + \bar{\Pi}_G) \qquad [5]$$

The left-hand side of equation [5], that is, the x-intercept (A) of the pressure-natriuresis relationship, was plotted as a function of the right-hand side of the equation, i.e., $(R_A \times RBF) + (P_T + \bar{\Pi}_G)$ calculated assuming a normal whole-kidney ultrafiltration coefficient by Gomez's equations (9,44–51). The slope of this regression line was not significantly different from 1, nor was its y-intercept different from 0 mm Hg (38). Although A was obtained independently of values for R_A and RBF, there was a strong 1:1 relationship between these two parameters ($r = 0.72$, $p < .001$), suggesting the validity of the above assumption that the effective filtration pressure becomes zero when MAP equals A (38).

Inserting this relationship [5] into equation [3], $\overline{\Delta P_F}$ can be represented as MAP minus A:

$$\overline{\Delta P_F} = MAP - A \qquad [6]$$

It thus becomes evident that the effective pressure (MAP minus A) on the outlet in the water tank model corresponds to the net effective filtration pressure across the glomerular capillary walls.

Once the effective filtration pressure is obtained, other glomerular hemodynamic parameters such as glomerular capillary pressure and whole-kidney ultrafiltration coefficient can also be calculated consequently. Thus, the above approach gives a clinical way to evaluate glomerular hemodynamics. The detailed discussed appeared elsewhere (39).

CONTROL MECHANISMS OF SALT SENSITIVITY

From the foregoing, it is evident that the steady-state blood pressure as well as its sodium sensitivity are determined by the pressure-natriuresis relationship. Therefore, if specific renal determinants of the pressure-natriuresis relationship are known, then renal mechanisms of sodium sensitivity are clarified necessarily.

Renal Determinants of Pressure-Natriuresis Relationship

The x-intercept (A) of the pressure-natriuresis relationship is shown to be mainly determined by the preglomerular vascular resistance (R_A), mainly in afferent arterioles, as shown by equation [5]. Let us next consider the determinants of the slope (B) of the pressure-natriuresis relationship. First, the pressure-natriuresis relationship is assumed to be linear, as discussed above. Therefore, urinary sodium excretion rate is expressed as a first-order function of MAP using x-intercept A and the slope B, as shown by equation [1]. On the other hand, $U_{Na}V$ is the difference between the filtered load of sodium ($S_{Na} \times GFR$) and simultaneous rate of tubule sodium reabsorption (t_{Na}):

$$B \times (MAP - A) = S_{Na} \times GFR - t_{Na} \qquad [7]$$

Here, S_{Na} is the serum sodium concentration. Since GFR is the product of the whole kidney ultrafiltration coefficient (KF) and effective filtration pressure (MAP minus A), B can be represented as the difference between glomerular and tubule components, an expression of glomerulotubular balance for sodium (39):

$$B = \frac{S_{Na} \times GFR - t_{Na}}{MAP - A} \qquad [8]$$

$$= S_{Na} \times KF - \frac{t_{Na}}{MAP - A} \qquad [9]$$

$$= S_{Na} \times KF \times (1 - FR_{Na}) \qquad [10]$$

Here, FR_{Na} is the fractional sodium reabsorption [$= t_{Na}/(S_{Na} \times GFR)$].

The resulting insights are as follows (Table 1): The x-intercept, i.e., the degree of the shift along the blood pressure axis, is determined by the sum of the pressure drop from heart to glomeruli plus the opposing pressures at glomeruli (38,39,43). The main factor seems to be the preglomerular vascular resistance from heart to glomeruli, mainly due to the afferent arteriolar resistance. The slope is determined by the difference between glomerular (mainly due to the whole kidney ultrafiltration coefficient) and tubule (rate of sodium reabsorption) factors (39).

TABLE 1. *Theoretical determinants of pressure-natriuresis relationship*

Pressure-natriuresis relationship	Determinants	Main factor
x-intercept (A): shift along the blood pressure axis	$(R_A \times RBF) + (P_T + \bar{\Pi}_G)$	Preglomerular resistance
slope (B): reciprocal of sodium sensitivity	$S_{Na} \times KF \times (1 - FR_{Na})$	Glomerulotubular balance

R_A, preglomerular vascular resistance from heart to glomeruli, mainly in afferent arterioles; RBF, renal blood flow rate; P_T, hydraulic pressure in Bowman's space; $\bar{\Pi}_G$, mean oncotic pressure within glomerular capillaries; S_{Na}, serum sodium concentration; KF, whole-kidney ultrafiltration coefficient (filtration surface area per glomerulus × hydraulic permeability of glomerular filtration barrier × the number of glomeruli); FR_{Na}, fractional reabsorption of sodium.

Classification of Hypertension Based on Renal Mechanisms

Let us now attempt to classify various forms of hypertension based on renal mechanisms (Table 2). Theoretically, the pressure-natriuresis relationship can be affected in two different ways to cause hypertension (21,24–26,36,37,39): either a parallel shift toward a higher blood pressure level along the blood pressure axis or a depression in the slope (see Fig. 4). As discussed already, the parallel shift of the pressure-natriuresis relationship induces non–sodium-sensitive hypertension whereas the depressed slope induces sodium-sensitive hypertension. Since the x-intercept of the pressure-natriuresis relationship is determined by the preglomerular vascular resistance from heart to glomeruli (38), as shown by equation [5], the parallel shift should be due to the increased preglomerular vascular resistance. Examples for this mechanism are Goldblatt hypertension in animal models (58,59) and renovascular hypertension in humans (13,50,51). It is well known that these forms of hypertension are based on an increase in vascular resistance due to renal artery stenosis.

There is ample evidence to suggest that spontaneously hypertensive rats of Kyoto strain (SHR) and human essential hypertension result from increased afferent arteriolar resistance (21,38,43,50,60,61). In patients with essential hypertension, the afferent arteriolar resistance was prominently increased, whereas the efferent arteriolar resistance and the mean glomerular hydraulic pressure remained normal. The whole kidney ultrafiltration coefficient was also estimated to be normal (38,43). These findings are consistent with those directly measured in SHR (60,61). The pressure-natriuresis relationship is known to be shifted in parallel along the blood pressure axis toward a higher blood pressure level even at an early stage of essential hypertension and shifted fur-

ther to the higher level with increasing severity and duration of hypertension (11,14,34). There is a strong positive correlation between the systemic mean arterial pressure and afferent arteriolar resistance, which is the main determinant of the shift of the pressure-natriuresis relationship along the blood pressure axis (38). Furthermore, afferent arteriolar resistance is elevated even when blood pressure remains relatively normal (38,50). These results cannot be explained by a simple autoregulatory mechanism in which the afferent arteriolar resistance is increased with elevated systemic arterial pressure in order to maintain constancy of RBF and GFR. Instead, the increase in afferent arteriolar resistance seems to be related to the cause of hypertension itself by shifting the pressure-natriuresis relationship in parallel toward the higher blood pressure level. In this regard, total renal vascular resistance is increased even in mild essential hypertension. Furthermore, the ratio of total renal over total peripheral vascular resistance is increased in essential hypertension, indicating the important role of renal vascular resistance (21).

On the other hand, as we have seen, the depressed slope of the pressure-natriuresis relationship induces sodium-sensitive hypertension. The slope is determined by the difference between the whole kidney ultrafiltration coefficient (KF) and tubule sodium reabsorption, as shown by equation [10]. Therefore, a depressed slope results from a decrease in KF, an increase in tubule sodium reabsorption, or both. KF is the product of the single glomerulus ultrafiltration coefficient (Kf) per glomerulus and the number of glomeruli (41,42). In Dahl salt-sensitive rats and in the early phase of glomerulonephritis, the reduced Kf per glomerulus may contribute to a decreased value of KF (52,53), although there are also data suggesting reduced nephron number (54) and increased tubule sodium reabsorption (55) in Dahl rats. Examples of decreased KF due to the reduced number of glomeruli are Milan hypertensive rats (56), oligo-

TABLE 2. *Classification of hypertension based on renal mechanisms*

Pressure-natriuresis relationship	Glomerular hemodynamics	Experimental model examples	Human hypertension examples
Parallel shift (non-sodium-sensitive)	(Preglomerular) Afferent arteriolar vasoconstriction	Goldblatt SHR	Renovascular hypertension Essential hypertension
Depressed slope (sodium-sensitive)	Decrease in whole kidney ultrafiltration coefficient[a] Increase in tubule sodium reabsorption	Dahl-S rat Milan hypertensive rat DOCA-salt	Glomerulonephritis Hypertension in blacks Primary aldosteronism diabetes mellitus

From ref. 39, with permission. Data from refs. 52–57.
[a] Whole kidney ultrafiltration coefficient can be expressed as the product of the glomerular filtration surface area per glomerulus, the hydraulic conductivity of glomerular capillary walls, and the number of glomeruli. In Dahl rat, a report suggests there is a defect in the glomerular ultrafiltration barrier, whereas there are also data suggesting reduced nephron number (54) and increased tubule sodium reabsorption. In Milan rat and in black people (57), the number of glomeruli seems to be reduced.

meganephronia (62–64), congenital solitary kidney (65–69), extensive renal ablation in humans (70–73), and hypertension in blacks (57). It should be stressed again that the slope of the pressure-natriuresis relationship is determined by glomerulotubular balance, instead by the K_F itself. When the number of glomeruli and nephrons is reduced, both K_F and the rate of tubule sodium reabsorption will be reduced, with little affecting this balance. Thus, the reduced number of nephrons seems to have less impact on the sodium sensitivity than the reduced K_f per glomerulus (21,26).

Enhanced tubule sodium reabsorption clearly contributes to the genesis of hypertension in deoxycorticosterone acetate (DOCA) DOCA-salt hypertension and primary aldosteronism (13). Likewise, in the early phases of diabetes mellitus, increases in tubule sodium reabsorption due to enhanced Na-glucose cotransport may be the principal mechanism for hypertension (74–76).

In brief, hypertension can be ascribed to one of three major renal mechanisms (39): (a) increased preglomerular vascular resistance from heart to glomeruli, mainly due to afferent arteriolar resistance; (b) decrease in whole kidney ultrafiltration coefficient, due to the decrease in filtration surface area per glomerulus, decrease in hydraulic permeability of glomerular filtration barrier, and/or decrease in the number of glomeruli; or (c) increase in the rate of tubule sodium reabsorption. The first produces non–sodium-sensitive hypertension, whereas the latter two produce sodium-sensitive hypertension.

Renal Mechanisms of Salt Sensitivity

Under normal conditions in which renal sodium excretory capability functions fully, the slope is very steep (30–32,77), making blood pressure typically non–sodium-sensitive. When the slope is depressed, however, the pressure-natriuresis relationship indicates that in order to excrete a greater amount of sodium, a much higher level of blood pressure is required. Thus, in response to a high sodium intake, blood pressure must be elevated to a greater extent, resulting in sodium-sensitive hypertension. As noted earlier, the reciprocal of the slope reflects the sodium sensitivity of blood pressure, and in fact exactly equals the sodium sensitivity index (12).

Since the slope is determined mainly by the difference between the whole kidney ultrafiltration coefficient and rate of tubule sodium reabsorption (39), a decrease in the whole kidney ultrafiltration coefficient (K_F) and/or an increase in the rate of tubule sodium reabsorption depress the slope, making blood pressure sodium-sensitive. The impact of changes in GFR on renal sodium excretion is often very large. Under normal conditions, with GFR of ~130 mL/min and serum sodium concentration of 140 mmol/L, some 26,210 mmol/day of sodium are filtered across glomeruli, while 26,080 mmol/day

(99.5 percent of filtered load) of sodium are reabsorbed by the renal tubules, resulting in excretion of only 130 mmol/day of sodium, the average daily level of intake. A change in GFR by 1 mL/min (change by less than 1 percent) affects the filtered load by 200 mmol/day, thus influencing urinary sodium excretion by more than 150 percent if the rate of tubule sodium reabsorption remains constant. Thus, when GFR is reduced, renal sodium excretion and blood pressure must become sodium-sensitive. In fact, it is well known clinically that as GFR declines, blood pressure becomes more sodium-sensitive (12,78). Glomerular filtration rate is the product of K_F and net effective filtration pressure across the glomerular capillary walls. The latter component is a function of glomerular capillary hydraulic pressure (41,42), in turn affected by systemic blood pressure. Therefore, when the effect on blood pressure is considered, K_F, instead of GFR, becomes the independent variable. Reduced K_F decreases the filtered load of sodium created for each mm Hg of glomerular capillary pressure and therefore reduces urinary sodium excretion for any given level of systemic arterial pressure, causing blood pressure to become highly sodium-sensitive (21,26). Furthermore, K_F seems to have greater impact on the blood pressure response to the change in sodium intake than GFR. For example, even when K_F is reduced, GFR can be maintained at normal level by elevating blood pressure and effective filtration pressure. Thus, K_F predicts the elevation in blood pressure, whereas GFR does not. In fact, in many forms of renal disease, blood pressure becomes sodium-sensitive even when GFR remains normal (16) (Kimura and Brenner: *unpublished observations*).

When the rate of tubule sodium reabsorption is enhanced, blood pressure also becomes sodium-sensitive (21,24–26,39). Under normal conditions, the rate of tubule sodium reabsorption is regulated in response to the amount of sodium intake. Enhanced tubule sodium reabsorption makes sodium balance positively dependent on sodium intake, resulting in sodium-sensitive hypertension. In these conditions, GFR is usually increased because of an elevation in glomerular capillary pressure (79), and an increased filtration rate of sodium makes it possible to overcome the enhanced tubule sodium reabsorption (13), resulting in a new sodium balance.

On the other hand, non–sodium-sensitive hypertension is induced by the parallel shift of the pressure-natriuresis relationship along the blood pressure axis, based on an increase in preglomerular resistance anywhere from heart to glomeruli (21,24–26,36,37,39). Systemic arterial pressure must be elevated by exactly the same magnitude as the increase in the pressure drop from heart to glomeruli along the preglomerular vessels in order to keep glomerular capillary hydraulic pressure, and therefore renal sodium excretion, normal (21,26, 39). Once glomerular capillary pressure is restored, the relationship between the elevation in blood pressure and change in sodium intake remains normal, making blood pressure non–sodium-sensitive. Although the systemic arterial pressure-natriuresis relationship is shifted to a higher blood pressure level in parallel, the glomerular capillary pressure-natriuresis relationship, and therefore sodium sensitivity, all remain normal in this type of hypertension (28).

INTERRELATIONSHIPS AMONG SALT SENSITIVITY, SYSTEMIC AND GLOMERULAR HYPERTENSION

As discussed above, in sodium-sensitive states, whether KF is reduced or tubule sodium reabsorption is enhanced, the glomerular capillary hydraulic pressure rises to compensate for the impairments in sodium excretory capability. In other words, it may be considered that both sodium sensitivity and glomerular hypertension reflect adaptations necessary to overcome a defect in the capacity of the kidneys to excrete sodium (28). Elevation in glomerular capillary pressure leads to a syndrome of glomerular hyperfiltration/hypertension characterized by progressive proteinuria, systemic hypertension, eventual glomerular sclerosis, and eventual renal

failure (80–82). If the linkage between sodium sensitivity of blood pressure and glomerular hypertension is as proposed, renal failure may be expected to be more common in sodium-sensitive types of hypertension than in non–sodium-sensitive types (Fig. 7). Indeed, animal models characterized by increased sodium sensitivity of blood pressure with glomerular hypertension show more profound renal injury (9,53,54,57,79,83–88).

A Theoretical Linkage Between Salt Sensitivity and Glomerular Hypertension

In this way, in sodium-sensitive states, whether KF is reduced or tubule sodium reabsorption is enhanced, the glomerular capillary hydraulic pressure seems elevated necessarily to compensate for the impairments in sodium excretory capability. The water tank model (35–37,39) illustrates that when blood pressure becomes sodium-sensitive, and the diameter of the outlet becomes smaller, the effective pressure on the outlet, and therefore the glomerular capillary pressure, are both elevated (39). This linkage can be recognized mathematically as follows. The sodium sensitivity index (SI) exactly equals the reciprocal of the slope (B) of the pressure-natriuresis relationship.

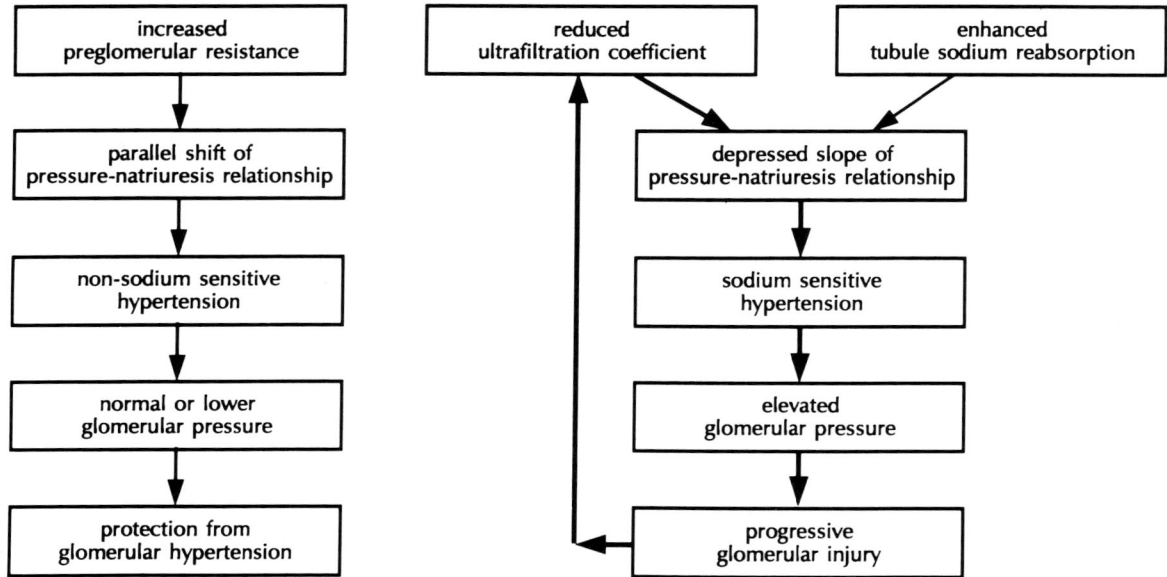

FIG. 7. Sodium sensitivity and glomerular hypertension. The increased preglomerular resistance anywhere from heart to glomeruli causes parallel shift of the pressure-natriuresis relationship toward a higher blood pressure level, and induces non–sodium-sensitive hypertension. In this case, glomeruli are protected from glomerular hypertension. On the other hand, the reduced ultrafiltration coefficient or enhanced tubular sodium reabsorption depresses the slope of the pressure-natriuresis relationship and induces sodium-sensitive hypertension. In this case, glomerular capillary pressure is elevated, and progressive glomerular injury occurs, resulting in further reduction in ultrafiltration coefficient and further depression in the slope of the pressure-natriuresis relationship. Thus, in sodium-sensitive hypertension, a vicious cycle is formed (*thick lines*), leading to eventual glomerulosclerosis. (From ref. 39, with permission.)

$$SI = \frac{1}{B} \qquad [11]$$

Assuming the linearity of the pressure-natriuresis relationship, as shown in equation [1], 1/B can be represented as:

$$\frac{1}{B} = \frac{MAP - A}{U_{Na}V} \qquad [12]$$

Since already we discussed that (MAP minus A) corresponds to the net effective filtration pressure ($\overline{\Delta P_F}$) across the glomerular capillary walls, finally SI can be represented as:

$$SI = \frac{\overline{\Delta P_F}}{U_{Na}V} \qquad [13]$$

Therefore, the net effective filtration pressure is related proportionally to the sodium sensitivity:

$$\overline{\Delta P_F} = SI \times U_{Na}V \qquad [14]$$

This relationship suggests that in patients who have high sodium sensitivity (high SI), the effective filtration pressure and therefore glomerular capillary pressure are elevated, especially under a high sodium intake (i.e., high $U_{Na}V$). Thus, the existence of the linkage between sodium sensitivity and glomerular capillary hypertension can be suggested theoretically.

Animal Models for High Salt Sensitivity with Glomerular Hypertension

Table 3 summarizes the patterns of salt sensitivity and glomerular hemodynamics in various animal models of hypertension. Although animal models provide glomerular hemodynamic data, there are surprisingly few data available on sodium sensitivity. This is in contrast to human diseases, in which only patterns of sodium sensitivity are known. High sodium sensitivity was established in several animal models including Dahl S rats (1–3), DOCA-salt rats (103), Milan rats (104), uninephrectomy (103), extensive renal ablation (98), and obese Zucker rats (105). Experimental models for diabetes mellitus have not been tested for sodium sensitivity, but human studies suggest high sodium sensitivity (10,106,107). On the other hand, it is known that Goldblatt models (19,108) and spontaneously hypertensive rats (SHR) of Kyoto strain (19,109) are not sodium-sensitive. Table 3 clearly shows that in all animal models categorized as "sodium sensitive," the glomerular capillary pressure is elevated, strongly supporting a linkage between sodium sensitivity and glomerular hypertension. The only exception to this rule is seen in the unclipped kidney of Goldblatt (2K-1C) models. In spite of non–sodium-sensitive type of hypertension, glomerular pressure is elevated in the unclipped kidney (58,59), simply because

TABLE 3. *Glomerular hemodynamics in non–salt-sensitive and salt-sensitive forms of hypertension*

Glomerular hemodynamics	MAP	R_A	$\overline{P}_{GC}$	Kf	SNGFR
Non–sodium-sensitive state					
Normal control					
Normal Munich-Wister rats (89)	~	~	~	~	~
Due to increased preglomerular resistance					
Goldblatt (2K-1C)					
Clipped kidney (58)	↑	↑	↓	~	↓
Unclipped kidney (58,59)	↑	~	↑	↓	↑
SHR (60,61)	↑	↑	~	~	~
Sodium-sensitive state					
Due to reduced whole-kidney KF					
Due to reduced single glomerulus Kf					
Glomerulonephritis (90–92)	~ or ↑	↓	↑	↓	~ or ↓
Dahl-S rats (53)	↑	↓	↑	↓	↑
Due to reduced number of glomeruli					
Milan hypertensive rats (56)	↑	na	↑	na	↑
Uninephrectomy (93)	~	↓	↑	~	↑
Extensive renal ablation (94–98)	↑	↓	↑	~	↑
Due to enhanced rate of tubule sodium reabsorption					
DOCA-salt rats (79)	↑	~	↑	~	↑
Diabetes mellitus (99–102)	~	↓	↑[a]	~	↑[a]
Obese Zucker rats (84)	~	↓[a]	↑[a]	~	↑[a]

From ref. 28, with permission.
MAP, systemic mean blood pressure; R_A, preglomerular (afferent arteriolar) resistance; $\overline{P}_{GC}$, glomerular capillary hydraulic pressure; Kf, single-glomerulus ultrafiltration coefficient; KF, whole-kidney ultrafiltration coefficient (KF = Kf × the number of glomeruli); SNGFR, single-nephron glomerular filtration rate; ~, no change; na, data not available; [a], statistically not significant.

non–sodium-sensitive hypertension is based on the clipped kidney. Please note that in Table 3, Kf is the single glomerulus ultrafiltration coefficient, and the whole kidney ultrafiltration coefficient (KF), mentioned earlier, equals the product of Kf and the number of glomeruli (41,42). From the glomerular hemodynamic patterns, it is not yet possible to distinguish the primary defect in each model. In glomerulonephritis (90–92) and Dahl S rats (52,53), the reduced single glomerulus Kf seems the primary mechanism for sodium sensitivity, although the reduced number of glomeruli may also play a role, especially in the latter (54). In Milan rat (56), uninephrectomy, and extensive renal ablation, the reduced whole kidney KF is due primarily to the reduced number of glomeruli, whereas in DOCA-salt rats (103), diabetes mellitus (74–76), and obese Zucker rats (105), an enhanced rate of tubule sodium reabsorption seems to predominate.

Glomerular Hemodynamics and the Renin-Angiotensin Axis in Salt Sensitive States

Let us briefly examine the mechanisms that might link sodium sensitivity with glomerular hypertension (28). When sodium is loaded into normal subjects, the renin-angiotensin-aldosterone axis is suppressed (31,32). This suppression causes renal vasodilation, especially in efferent arterioles and mesangial cells, thereby minimizing changes in glomerular pressure or filtration rate, despite an increase in renal blood flow and ultrafiltration coefficient, as seen in normal animals (89). In fact, in human studies dealing with healthy and non–sodium-sensitive subjects, chronic sodium loading increases GFR only slightly (31,32,77). Since a slight change in GFR has a strong impact on sodium excretion, however, much of the salt load will be excreted at least partially by virtue of this increased GFR.

On the other hand, as discussed previously, in patients who show high sodium sensitivity (whether hypertensive or not), either the whole kidney ultrafiltration coefficient (KF) is reduced or the rate of tubule sodium reabsorption is enhanced. The reduced KF due to the reduced single glomerulus Kf decreases the single nephron GFR and the amount of sodium delivered to the macula densa segment of each nephron, thus resulting in the inhibition

of a tubuloglomerular feedback mechanism (110,111), which in turn dilates the afferent arterioles and activates the local renin-angiotensin-efferent arteriolar vasoconstriction axis, and therefore elevates the glomerular capillary pressure (see Fig. 1). The elevation in glomerular pressure seems to maintain GFR despite the reduced Kf. This pattern is seen typically in experimental glomerulonephritis (90–92) (see Table 3). In glomerulonephritis, the renin-angiotensin axis is usually inappropriately high (112,113) when GFR remains normal despite a sodium-sensitive state. When KF is reduced due to the reduced number of glomeruli, however, the single nephron GFR and the amount of sodium delivered to the macula densa are both increased (114). Therefore, the tubuloglomerular feedback mechanism is expected to be activated, resulting in afferent arteriolar vasoconstriction as well as suppression of the intrarenal renin-angiotensin-efferent arteriolar axis, both of which act to lower the glomerular capillary pressure. On the other hand, the elevation in systemic arterial pressure and elevated plasma atrial natriuretic peptide, both due to sodium retention, probably contribute to the elevation in glomerular pressure and maintenance of GFR. This glomerular hemodynamic pattern is seen in Milan rats (56), uninephrectomy (93), and extensive renal ablation (94–97). When the rate of tubule sodium reabsorption is enhanced, again the elevation in both systemic arterial pressure and plasma atrial natriuretic peptide may contribute to the elevation in glomerular pressure mainly by dilating the afferent arteriole, as seen in DOCA-salt rats (79), diabetes mellitus (99–102), and obese Zucker rats (84). Single nephron and whole kidney GFR as well as the amount of sodium delivered to the macula densa exceed normal, thereby activating the tubuloglomerular feedback mechanism. Thus, the renin-angiotensin axis is suppressed. In this way, in the sodium-sensitive state, the glomerular capillary pressure always seems elevated (28). Furthermore, it may be possible that the low-renin type of sodium-sensitive hypertension is based on the reduced number of glomeruli or an enhanced rate of tubule sodium reabsorption, whereas the normal or high-renin type is based on the reduced single glomerulus Kf due to either the reduced surface area per glomerulus or reduced hydraulic permeability of the glomerular filtration barrier (28) (Table 4). The suppressed renin-angiotensin-aldosterone

TABLE 4. *Differential diagnosis of salt-sensitive states based on glomerular hemodynamics and plasma renin activity*

	Total GFR	$\bar{P}_{GC}$	SNGFR	PRA
Reduced whole-kidney KF				
Reduced single glomerulus Kf	∼ or ↓	↑	∼ or ↓	↑
Reduced number of glomeruli	∼ or ↓	↑	↑	↑↑
Enhanced tubule sodium reabsorption	↑	↑	↑	↓

GFR, glomerular filtration rate; $\bar{P}_{GC}$, glomerular capillary hydraulic pressure; KF, whole-kidney ultrafiltration coefficient; Kf, single-glomerulus ultrafiltration coefficient (KF = Kf × the number of glomeruli); SNGFR, single-nephron glomerular filtration rate; PRA, plasma renin activity.

axis, seen in most cases with sodium-sensitive hypertension, seems to be the consequence of the sodium-sensitive states created by intrarenal mechanisms, rather than the cause of sodium sensitivity.

CLINICAL SYNDROMES CHARACTERIZED BY HIGH SALT SENSITIVITY

In the following human diseases, characterized by high sodium sensitivity, the proposed mechanisms for sodium sensitivity and their relationship with renal injuries will be discussed (28). Edematous disorders such as heart failure and liver disease are not sodium-sensitive because excess fluid is distributed mainly in the interstitial compartment, and therefore blood pressure is not readily affected by the amount of sodium intake.

Chronic Glomerulonephritis

It is well established in advanced chronic renal failure that blood pressure increases and becomes sodium-sensitive (12,78). In the early stage, however, the exact characteristics are still unclear. In general, hypertension occurs more frequently in glomerulonephritis than in tubulointerstitial diseases (115,116). Hypertension occurs in association with normal GFR and increases in frequency as renal function deteriorates (112,115,117–119). Sodium sensitivity becomes greater as GFR declines (12,78). By the time end-stage renal disease ensues, 80 to 90 percent of patients are hypertensive (120,121). Animal experiments (90–92) in glomerulonephritis suggest that even when total GFR remains normal, the single glomerulus Kf and therefore whole kidney KF are reduced, with glomerular capillary pressure rising in compensation. Since, at least theoretically, the reduced KF produces sodium-sensitive hypertension (21,24–26,39,57,86,88,122), we believe that in the early stage of glomerulonephritis, even when GFR is still normal, blood pressure will prove to be sodium-sensitive. Indeed, preliminary data have already been observed in support of this possibility (Kimura and Brenner: *unpublished observations*).

Chronic glomerulonephritis frequently progresses to end-stage renal failure requiring artificial kidney therapy. Once the number of functioning nephrons is reduced, independently of the original pathogenic mechanisms such as immune reactions, the glomerular hemodynamic abnormalities play an important role in leading to eventual glomerular sclerosis and resulting renal failure (80–82). Animal models of extensively reduced nephron number show that normalization of glomerular capillary pressure by protein restriction or angiotensin-I–converting enzyme inhibitors can prevent this progression (95–97). Yet, no definite clinical data are available to draw this conclusion in human glomerulonephritis (123–127).

Essential Hypertension in Blacks

It has been well recognized in black populations that blood pressure is sodium-sensitive (9,128), even when blood pressure is normal (31). Black hypertensives exhibit increased plasma volume (129), low plasma renin activity (130), and a form of hypertension that tends to respond to diuretic therapy (131). Furthermore, age-related declines in renal function are more profound in blacks than in whites (132), and females exhibit higher sodium sensitivity (132) as well as greater age-related elevation in blood pressure (133) than males. Blood pressure in black women tends to be higher than in black men (134). In general, females have smaller kidneys than males and 10 to 20 percent fewer glomeruli (135), and the number of functioning glomeruli tends to decrease after age 40 years as a consequence of normal aging (136). Taken together, Brenner and colleagues proposed that the reduced whole-kidney ultrafiltration coefficient due to the reduced number of glomeruli and/or reduced filtration surface area plays an important role in the genesis of sodium-sensitive hypertension in blacks (57,86, 88) (Fig. 8). Recently, the glomerular capillary pressure was estimated to be elevated in black sodium-sensitive hypertension (9). Moreover, the reduced whole-kidney ultrafiltration coefficient (taken as an index of the number of glomeruli), as well as elevated glomerular capillary pressure, were observed in sodium-sensitive hypertension among Japanese (Kimura, et al.: *unpublished observations*).

Although nephrosclerosis due to essential hypertension in blacks is one of the most common causes of end-stage renal failure requiring maintenance dialysis therapy (137–140), the exact mechanism for higher susceptibility to renal failure is as yet unclear.

Diabetes Mellitus and Obesity

It is well known in diabetes mellitus that blood pressure is sodium-sensitive (10,106,107) and exchangeable sodium is increased (141,142), even before the development of overt diabetic nephropathy. Systolic blood pressure correlates with exchangeable sodium (143), and diuretics restore both exchangeable sodium and blood pressure toward normal (144). Furthermore, there is a tendency for high GFR (145–150) and elevated plasma atrial natriuretic peptide (151,152), both probably due to sodium retention. This sodium–volume–blood pressure state resembles, at least in part, the profile of primary aldosteronism (153–155), a sodium-sensitive form of hypertension due to an enhanced rate of tubule sodium reabsorption (13). The increased tubule sodium reabsorption in diabetes mellitus exclusively takes place in the proximal tubule, whereas the rate of sodium reabsorption by distal nephron remains normal (156). Since insulin acts to stimulate sodium reabsorption in the distal nephron (157), while the sodium-glucose cotransport oc-

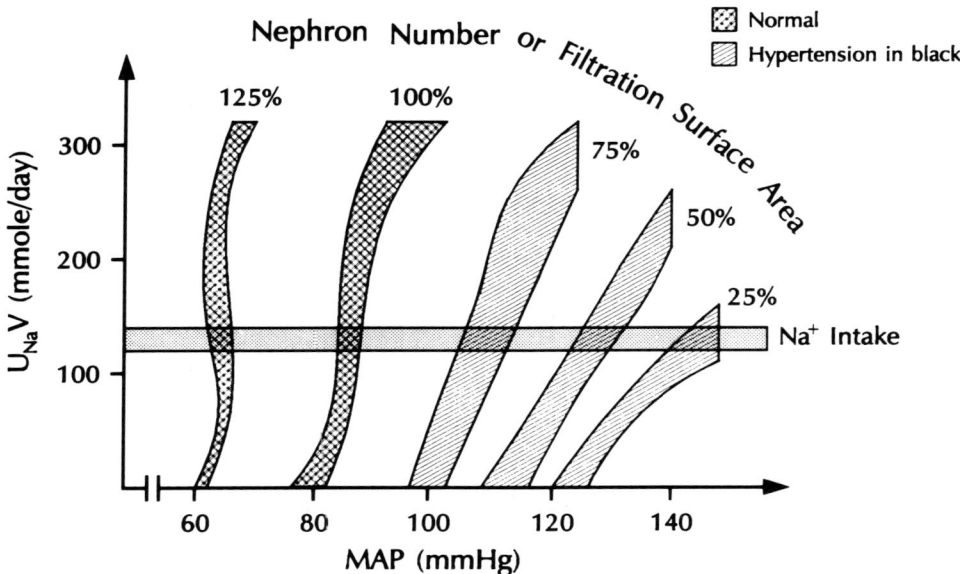

FIG. 8. Proposed mechanism of sodium-sensitive hypertension in blacks. Effect of reduced whole-kidney ultrafiltration coefficient due either to the reduced number of glomeruli or the reduced filtration surface area per glomerulus on the pressure-natriuresis relationship is schematically illustrated. The average daily level of sodium intake is represented (*horizontal shaded area*). In individuals whose ultrafiltration coefficient is in the middle of the normal distribution (i.e., 100 percent of normal), the pressure-natriuresis relationship is steep, and blood pressure remains normal at the average level of sodium intake, being non–sodium-sensitive. Those with ultrafiltration coefficient above the median (125 percent of normal) exhibit even lower blood pressure at all levels of sodium intake. When the ultrafiltration coefficient is reduced, however, the slope is depressed and blood pressure becomes sodium-sensitive. At the extreme low end of the ultrafiltration coefficient, the slope is further depressed, so that a greater elevation in blood pressure is required to maintain sodium balance, even at relatively moderate dietary sodium intake. (Modified from ref. 57.)

curs in the proximal tubule (74–76), the enhanced rate of tubule sodium reabsorption in diabetes is most likely due to the enhanced sodium-glucose cotransport in the proximal tubule (74–76).

Diabetic nephropathy is one of the most common causes of end-stage renal failure leading to dialysis therapy. Animal models of diabetes mellitus show that glomerular capillary hypertension, as shown in Table 3, participates in the progression of renal failure (99–102), and conversely, the normalization of glomerular pressure by protein restriction or angiotensin-I–converting enzyme inhibitors can retard this progression (100–102). Preliminary clinical studies also suggest that protein restriction (125,158–160) and strict antihypertensive therapy (161–165) may slow the deterioration in glomerular filtration rate. Thus, diabetic nephropathy represents a typical syndrome of glomerular hyperfiltration/hypertension characterized by progressive azotemia, proteinuria, and eventual glomerulosclerosis (80–82,166).

In obesity it is known that hypertension is sodium-sensitive and weight loss lowers blood pressure and makes it non–sodium-sensitive (15,167). Extracellular fluid volume (168) and GFR (169) are both increased. Although the mechanisms are unclear, sodium retention seems to participate in the pathogenesis of sodium-sensitive hypertension. Hyperinsulinemia, due to insulin resistance (170,171), which is considered to be a primary cause for obesity, may stimulate sodium reabsorption in the distal nephron (157), where no insulin resistance is assumed. Recently the relationship between obesity and renal disease has been noted. Proteinuria (172), glomerular enlargement (173), focal glomerulosclerosis (174), and nephrotic syndrome (175) are occasionally encountered and, of note, in the hereditary obese Zucker rat with progressive focal glomerulosclerosis (84), the glomerular capillary hydraulic pressure is above normal rodent values.

"Nonmodulating" Essential Hypertension

In the final section of this review, we examine a special form of sodium-sensitive essential hypertension, which Hollenberg and colleagues (176) believe illuminates the pathophysiological basis of sodium sensitivity. Normal "modulating" patients were defined as those in whom angiotensin II infusion at 3 ng/kg/min reduced the renal plasma flow rate (RPF) by more than 125 mL/min/1.73 m^2 on high-sodium diet, whereas in nonmodulators, a lesser change in RPF occurred (7). Modulators were all non–sodium-sensitive (mean arterial pressure elevation less than 10 mm Hg), whereas 12 of 19 nonmodulators were sodium-sensitive (7). In addition to this relatively high frequency of sodium sensitivity, nonmodulators had several characteristics that distinguished them from modulators and normotensives: (a) aldosterone response to angiotensin II was also suppressed (7); (b) basal RPF was relatively low (7,177) and not increased by sodium load (7,178); (c) suppression of plasma renin activity and aldosterone concentration following saline infusion was delayed (177); and (d) following short-term angiotensin-converting enzyme inhibition, basal RPF increased and the response to angiotensin II became normal (178).

Hollenberg and colleagues (176) went on to speculate that the primary defect of nonmodulators is located in the adrenal gland where aldosterone is thought to be hyposecreted in response to angiotensin II. The compensatory hyperactivity of the renin-angiotensin axis is thought to act within the kidneys, especially on the renal vasculature (176), causing sodium retention and sodium-sensitive hypertension (176). However, it is difficult for us to explain the genesis of sodium-sensitive hypertension by this secondary hyperangiotensinism without aldosteronism. Preglomerular vasoconstriction anywhere from heart to glomeruli can cause hypertension (21,24–26,36,37,39), as we already discussed in Goldblatt models and SHR, but this is usually of the non–sodium-sensitive type. Moreover, with renin-secreting tumor or pheochromocytoma (21), hypertension is of the non–sodium-sensitive type, despite the activation of the renin-angiotensin-aldosterone axis. Instead, we believe that the primary defect is probably located in the kidneys, with single glomerulus Kf being reduced (28) (see Table 4). The resulting inhibition of the tubuloglomerular feedback mechanism (111) causes intrarenal activation of the renin-angiotensin-efferent arteriolar vasoconstriction axis as well as afferent arteriolar vasodilatation (110) to maintain single nephron GFR by elevating glomerular capillary pressure. In addition, augmented secretion of atrial natriuretic peptide by sodium retention (179), especially under high sodium intake (180), probably inhibits aldosterone production secondarily (181,182). These assumptions that a primary reduction in single glomerulus Kf and the resulting activation of intrarenal renin-angiotensin axis, as well as secondary suppression of aldosterone, make it possible to easily understand phenomena that otherwise seem complicated. Thus, nonmodulating sodium-sensitive hypertension may differ from other sodium-sensitive forms of hypertension in that the renin-angiotensin axis operates at an inappropriately high level despite high sodium sensitivity.

SUMMARY

The renal basis for sodium sensitivity in hypertension was reviewed. Theoretically, the pressure-natriuresis re-

lationship can be affected in two different ways: either a parallel shift along the blood pressure axis toward a higher blood pressure level or a depression in the slope. The parallel shift of the pressure-natriuresis relationship induces non–sodium-sensitive hypertension, whereas the depressed slope induces sodium-sensitive hypertension. Since the degree of the shift of the pressure-natriuresis relationship is determined by the preglomerular vascular resistance from heart to glomeruli, non–sodium-sensitive hypertension should be based on the increased preglomerular vascular resistance. On the other hand, the slope of the pressure-natriuresis relationship is determined by glomerulotubular balance of sodium, which is mainly controlled by the difference between the whole kidney ultrafiltration coefficient and the rate of tubule sodium reabsorption. Therefore, sodium sensitivity of blood pressure is based on a decrease in the whole-kidney ultrafiltration coefficient (due to a decrease in either filtration surface area per glomerulus, hydraulic permeability of glomerular filtration barrier, or the number of glomeruli) and/or an increase in tubule sodium reabsorption. Thus, sodium sensitivity can be explained based on the renal mechanisms. The suppressed renin-angiotensin-aldosterone axis, seen in most cases with sodium-sensi-tive hypertension, seems to be the consequence of the sodium-sensitive states created by intrarenal mechanisms, rather than the cause of sodium sensitivity. In sodium-sensitive states, whether whole-kidney ultrafiltration coefficient is reduced or tubule sodium reabsorption is enhanced, the glomerular capillary hydraulic pressure rises to compensate for the impairments in sodium excretory capability. In other words, it may be considered that both sodium sensitivity and glomerular hypertension reflect adaptations necessary to overcome a defect in the capacity of the kidneys to excrete sodium. If there is a linkage between sodium sensitivity of blood pressure and glomerular hypertension as proposed, renal failure may be expected to be more common in sodium-sensitive types of hypertension than in non–sodium-sensitive types. Thus, analysis of sodium-sensitive states may provide an important key to understand the pathophysiology of hypertensive diseases as well as the nature of their renal lesions.

REFERENCES

1. Dahl LK. Salt and hypertension. *Am J Clin Nutr* 1972;25:231–244.
2. Dahl LK, Heine M. Primary role of renal homografts in setting chronic blood pressure levels in rats. *Circ Res* 1975;36:692–696.
3. Tobian L, Lange J, Azar S, et al. Reduction of natriuretic capacity and renin release in isolated, blood-perfused kidneys of Dahl hypertensive-prone rats. *Circ Res* 1978;43[Suppl I]:I92–I98.
4. Kawasaki T, Delea CS, Bartter FC, Smith H. The effect of high-sodium and low-sodium intakes on blood pressure and other related variables in human subjects with idiopathic hypertension. *Am J Med* 1978;64:193–198.
5. Fujita T, Henry WL, Bartter FC, Lake CR, Delea CS. Factors influencing blood pressure in salt-sensitive patients with hypertension. *Am J Med* 1980;69:334–344.

6. Takeshita A, Imaizumi T, Ashihara T, Nakamura M. Characteristics of responses to salt loading and deprivation in hypertensive subjects. *Circ Res* 1982;51:457–464.

7. Hollenberg NK, Moore T, Shoback D, Redgrave J, Rabinowe S, Williams GH. Abnormal renal sodium handling in essential hypertension: relation to failure of renal and adrenal modulation of responses to angiotensin II. *Am J Med* 1986;81:412–418.

8. Sullivan JM, Ratts TE. Sodium sensitivity in human subjects. Hemodynamic and hormonal correlates. *Hypertension* 1988;11:717–723.

9. Campese VM, Parise M, Karubian F, Bigazzi R. Abnormal renal hemodynamics in black salt-sensitive patients with hypertension. *Hypertension* 1991;18:805–812.

10. Tuck MT, Corry D, Trujillo A. Salt-sensitive blood pressure and exaggerated vascular reactivity in the hypertension of diabetes mellitus. *Am J Med* 1990;88:210–216.

11. Parfrey PS, Markandu ND, Roulstone JE, Jones BE, Johnes JC, Macgregor GA. Relation between arterial pressure, dietary sodium intake and renin system in essential hypertension. *Br Med J* 1981;283:94–97.

12. Koomans HA, Roos JC, Boer P, Geyskes GG, Dorhout Mees EJ. Salt sensitivity of blood pressure in chronic renal failure: evidence for renal control of body fluid distribution in man. *Hypertension* 1982;4:190–197.

13. Kimura G, Saito F, Kojima S, et al. Renal function curve in patients with secondary forms of hypertension. *Hypertension* 1987;10:11–15.

14. Kimura G, Deguchi F, Kojima S, et al. Antihypertensive drugs and sodium restriction: analysis of their interaction based on pressure-natriuresis relationship. *Am J Hypertens* 1988;1:372–379.

15. Rocchini AP, Key J, Bondie D, et al. The effect of weight loss on the sensitivity of blood pressure to sodium in obese adolescents. *N Engl J Med* 1989;321:580–585.

16. Schmid M, Mann JFE, Stein G, et al. Natriuresis-pressure relationship in polycystic kidney disease. *J Hypertens* 1990;8:277–283.

17. Weinberger MH, Miller JZ, Luft FC, Grim CE, Fineberg NS. Definitions and characteristics of sodium sensitivity and blood pressure resistance. *Hypertension* 1986;8[Suppl II]:II127–II134.

18. DeClue JW, Guyton AC, Cowley AW, Jr, Coleman TG, Norman RA Jr, McCaa RE. Subpressor angiotensin infusion, renal sodium handling, and salt-induced hypertension in the dog. *Circ Res* 1978;43:503–512.

19. Norman RA Jr, Enobakhare JA, DeClue JW, Douglas BH, Guyton AC. Arterial pressure-urinary output relationship in hypertensive rats. *Am J Physiol* 1978;234:R98–R103.

20. Saito F, Kimura G, Shimozaki Y, et al. Hypotensive mechanism of an antihypertensive diuretic, mefruside, based on pressure-natriuresis relationship. *Jap J Nephrol* 1987;29:461–467.

21. Guyton AC. *Arterial pressure and hypertension, circulatory physiology III.* Philadelphia: WB Saunders; 1980.

22. Coleman TG, Bower JD, Langford HG, Guyton AC. Regulation of arterial pressure in the anephric state. *Circulation* 1970;42:509–514.

23. Matsuoka H, Kimura G, Sanai T, et al. Normalization of increased sodium sensitivity by maintenance hemodialysis. *Am J Hypertens* 1990;3:628–631.

24. Guyton AC. Renal function curve—a key to understanding the pathogenesis of hypertension. *Hypertension* 1987;10:1–6.

25. Guyton AC. Dominant role of the kidneys and accessory role of whole-body autoregulation in the pathogenesis of hypertension. *Am J Hypertens* 1989;2:575–585.

26. Hall JE, Mizelle HL, Hildebrandt DA, Brands MW. Abnormal pressure natriuresis: a cause or a consequence of hypertension? *Hypertension* 1990;15:547–559.

27. Knox FG, Granger JP. Control of sodium excretion: an integrative approach. In: Windhager EE, ed. *Handbook of physiology, sect 8.* New York: American Physiology Society; 1992:927–967.

28. Kimura G, Frem GJ, Brenner BM. Renal mechanisms of salt sensitivity in hypertension. *Curr Opin Nephrol Hypertens* 1994;3:1–12.

29. Baer PG, Navar LG, Guyton AC. Renal autoregulation, filtration rate, and electrolyte excretion during vasodilation. *Am J Physiol* 1970;219:619–625.

30. Murray RH, Luft FC, Bloch R, Weyman AE. Blood pressure responses to extremes of sodium intake in normal man. *Proc Soc Exp Biol Med* 1978;159:432–436.

31. Luft FC, Rankin LI, Bloch R, et al. Cardiovascular and humoral responses to extremes of sodium intake in normal black and white men. *Circulation* 1979;60:697–706.

32. Roos JC, Koomans HA, Dorhout Mees EJ, Delawi IMK. Renal sodium handling in normal humans subjected to low, normal, and extremely high sodium supplies. *Am J Physiol* 1985;249:F941–F947.

33. Zoccali C, Mallamaci F, Leonardis D, Gattuso E, Romeo M. A reassessment of the sodium/arterial pressure relationship by accurate estimations of salt intake and BP. *J Am Soc Nephrol* 1992;3:539(abst).

34. Parfrey PS. Salt in essential hypertension. In: Sleight P, Freis ED, eds. *Hypertension.* London: Butterworth, 1982:322–339. (Butterworth's international medical reviews, cardiology 1).

35. Kimura G, Saito F, Deguchi F, et al. Water tank model on body fluid volume versus blood pressure regulation. *J Hypertens* 1986;4[Suppl 5]:S192–S194.

36. Kimura G, Abe H, Ashida T, et al. Hypotensive mechanisms of antihypertensives based on the water tank model. *Am J Hypertens* 1989;2:532–536.

37. Kimura G, Ashida T, Abe H, et al. Sodium sensitive and sodium retaining hypertension. *Am J Hypertens* 1990;3:854–858.

38. Kimura G, Imanishi M, Sanai T, et al. Intrarenal hemodynamics in patients with essential hypertension. *Circ Res* 1991;69:421–428.

39. Kimura G, Brenner BM. A method for distinguishing salt-sensitive from non-salt-sensitive forms of human and experimental hypertension. *Curr Opin Nephrol Hypertens* 1993;2:341–349.

40. Romero JC, Knox FG. Mechanisms underlying pressure natriuresis. *Hypertension* 1988;11:724–738.

41. Maddox DA, Brenner BM. Glomerular ultrafiltration. In: Brenner BM, Rector FC Jr, eds. *The kidney.* Philadelphia: WB Saunders; 1991:205–244.

42. Maddox DA, Deen WM, Brenner BM. Glomerular filtration. In: Windhager EE ed. *Handbook of physiology, sect 8.* New York: American Physiology Society. 1992:545–638.

43. Kimura G, Deguchi F, Kojima S, et al. Effect of a calcium entry blocker, nicardipine, on intrarenal hemodynamics in essential hypertension. *Am J Kidney Dis* 1991;17:47–54.

44. Gomez DM. Evaluation of renal resistances, with special reference to changes in essential hypertension. *J Clin Invest* 1951;30:1143–1155.

45. Smith HW. *The kidney: structure and function in health and disease.* New York: Oxford Press; 1951:575–601.

46. Hall JE, Guyton AC, Cowley AW Jr. Dissociation of renal blood flow and filtration rate autoregulation by renin depletion. *Am J Physiol* 1979;232:F215–F221.

47. Hall JE, Coleman TG, Guyton AC. Control of glomerular filtration rate by circulating angiotensin II. *Am J Physiol* 1981;241:R190–R197.

48. Kobrin I, Pegram BL, Frohlich ED. Acute pressure increase and intrarenal hemodynamics in conscious WKY and SHR rats. *Am J Physiol* 1985;249:H1114–H1118.

49. Isshiki T, Amodeo C, Messerli FH, Pegram BL, Frohlich ED. Diltiazem maintains renal vasodilatation without hyperfiltration in hypertension: studies in essential hypertensive man and the spontaneously hypertensive rat. *Cardiovasc Drugs Ther* 1987;1:359–366.

50. Kimura G, London GM, Safar ME, Kuramochi M, Omae T. Glomerular hypertension in renovascular hypertensive patients. *Kidney Int* 1991;39:966–972.

51. Kimura G, London GM, Safar ME, Kuramochi M, Omae T. Split intrarenal hemodynamics in renovascular hypertension. *Clin Invest Med* 1991;14:559–565.

52. Sterzel RB, Luft FC, Gao Y, et al. Renal diseases and development of hypertension in salt-sensitive Dahl rats. *Kidney Int* 1988;33:1119–1129.

53. Azar S, Weller D, Bruno L, Livingston S, Iwai J. Single nephron dynamics in the normotensive Dahl rat on high salt intake. *Clin Res* 1977;25:504A(abst).

54. Azar S, Johnson MA, Hertel B, Tobian L. Single-nephron pres-

sure, flows and resistance in hypertensive kidneys with nephrosclerosis. *Kidney Int* 1977;12:28–40.

55. Kirchner KA. Greater loop chloride uptake contributes to blunted pressure natriuresis in Dahl salt sensitive rats. *J Am Soc Nephrol* 1990;1:180–186.

56. Baer PG, Bianchi G. Renal micropuncture study of normotensive and Milan hypertensive rats before and after development of hypertension. *Kidney Int* 1978;13:452–466.

57. Brenner BM, Garcia DL, Anderson S. Glomeruli and blood pressure. Less of one, more the other? *Am J Hypertens* 1988;1:335–347.

58. Schwietzer G, Gertz KH. Changes of hemodynamics and glomerular ultrafiltration in renal hypertension of rats. *Kidney Int* 1979;15:134–143.

59. Steiner RW, Tucker BJ, Gushwa LC, Gifford J, Wilson CB, Blanz RC. Glomerular hemodynamics in moderate Goldblatt hypertension in the rat. *Hypertension* 1982;4:51–57.

60. Arendshorst WJ, Beierwaltes WH. Renal and nephron hemodynamics in spontaneously hypertensive rats. *Am J Physiol* 1979;236:F246–F251.

61. Azar S, Johnson MA, Scheiman J, Bruno L, Tobian L. Regulation of glomerular capillary pressure and filtration rate in young Kyoto hypertensive rats. *Clin Sci* 1979;56:203–209.

62. Fetterman GH, Habib R. Congenital bilateral oligonephronic renal hypoplasia with hypertrophy of nephrons (oligomeganephronie). *Am J Clin Pathol* 1969;52:199–207.

63. Lieberman E. Essential hypertension in children and youth: a pediatric perspective. *J Pediatr* 1974;85:1–11.

64. McGraw M, Poucell S, Sweet J, Baumal R. The significance of focal segmental glomerulosclerosis in oligomeganephronia. *Int J Pediatr Nephrol* 1984;5:67–72.

65. Kiprov DD, Colvin RB, McCluskey RT. Focal and segmental glomerulosclerosis and proteinuria associated with unilateral renal agenesis. *Lab Invest* 1982;46:275–281.

66. Thorner PS, Arbus GS, Celermajer DS, Baumal R. Focal segmental glomerulosclerosis and progressive renal failure associated with a unilateral kidney. *Pediatrics* 1984;73:806–810.

67. Bhathena DB, Julian BA, McMorrow RG, Baehler RW. Focal sclerosis of hypertrophied glomeruli in solitary functioning kidneys of humans. *Am J Kidney Dis* 1985;5:226–232.

68. Rugiu C, Oldrizzi L, Lupo A, et al. Clinical features of patients with solitary kidneys. *Nephron* 1986;43:10–15.

69. Gutierrez-Millet V, Nieto J, Praga M, Usera G, Martinez MA, Morales JM. Focal glomerulosclerosis and proteinuria in patients with solitary kidneys. *Arch Intern Med* 1986;146:705–709.

70. Solomon LR, Mallick NP, Lawler W. Progressive renal failure in a remnant kidney. *Br Med J* 1985;291:1610–1611.

71. Stahl RAK, Low I, Schoeppe W. Progressive renal failure in a patient after one and two-thirds nephrectomy. *Klin Wochenschr* 1988;66:508–510.

72. Novick AC, Gephardt G, Guz B, Steinmuller D, Tubbs RR. Long-term follow-up after partial removal of a solitary kidney. *N Engl J Med* 1991;325:1058–1062.

73. Rutsky EA, Dubovsky EV, Kirk KA. Long-term follow-up of a human subject with a remnant kidney. *Am J Kidney Dis* 1991;18:509–513.

74. Carney SL, Wong NLM, Dirks JH. Acute effects of streptozotocin diabetes on rat renal function. *J Lab Clin Med* 1979;93:950–961.

75. Harris RC, Brenner BM, Seifter JL. Sodium-hydrogen exchange and glucose transport in renal microvillus membrane vesicles from rat with diabetes mellitus. *J Clin Invest* 1986;77:724–733.

76. Wald H, Scherzer P, Popovtzer MM. Enhanced renal tubular ouabain-sensitive ATPase in streptozotocin diabetes mellitus. *Am J Physiol* 1986;251:F164–F170.

77. Kirkendall WM, Conner WE, Abboud F, Rastogi SP, Anderson RA, Fry M. The effect of dietary sodium chloride on blood pressure, body fluids, electrolytes, renal function, and serum lipids in normotensive man. *J Lab Clin Med* 1976;87:418–434.

78. Wilkinson R, Luetscher JA, Dowdy AJ, Gonzales C, Nokes GW. Studies on the mechanism of sodium excretion in uremia. *Clin Sci* 1972;42:711–723.

79. Dworkin LD, Hostetter TH, Rennke HG, Brenner BM. Hemodynamic basis for glomerular injury in rats with desoxycorticosterone-salt hypertension. *J Clin Invest* 1984;73:1448–1461.

80. Brenner BM, Meyer TW, Hostetter TH. Dietary protein intake and the progressive nature of kidney disease: the role of hemodynamically mediated glomerular injury in the pathogenesis of progressive glomerular sclerosis in aging, renal ablation, and intrinsic renal disease. *N Engl J Med* 1982;307:652–659.

81. Brenner BM. Hemodynamically mediated glomerular injury and the progressive nature of kidney disease. *Kidney Int* 1983;23:647–655.

82. Brenner BM, Cohen RA, Milford EL. In renal transplantation, one size may not fit all. *J Am Soc Nephrol* 1992;3:162–169.

83. Bianchi G, Cusi D, Guidi E. Renal hemodynamics in human subjects and in animals with genetic hypertension during the prehypertensive stage. *Am J Nephrol* 1983;3:73–79.

84. O'Donnell MP, Kasiske BL, Cleary MP, Keane WF. Effects of genetic obesity on renal structure and function in the Zucker rat. II. Micropuncture studies. *J Lab Clin Med* 1985;106:605–610.

85. Anderson S, Brenner BM. Role of intraglomerular hypertension in the initiation and progression of renal failure. In: Kaplan NM, Brenner BM, Laragh JH, eds. *The kidney in hypertension.* New York: Raven Press; 1987:67–76.

86. Brenner BM, Anderson S. Filtration surface area, salt intake and hypertension. *Contrib Nephrol* 1989;75:45–59.

87. Campese VM, Karubian F. Salt sensitivity in hypertension: implications for the kidney. *J Am Soc Nephrol* 1991;2:S53–S61.

88. Brenner BM, Anderson S. The interrelationship among filtration surface area, blood pressure, and chronic renal disease. *J Cardiovasc Pharmacol* 1992;19[Suppl 6]:S1–S7.

89. Schor N, Ichikawa I, Brenner BM. Glomerular adaptations to chronic dietary salt restriction or excess. *Am J Physiol* 1980;238:F428–F436.

90. Allison MEM, Wilson CB, Gottschalk CW. Pathophysiology of experimental glomerulonephritis in rats. *J Clin Invest* 1974;53:1402–1423.

91. Maddox DA, Bennett CM, Deen WM, et al. Determinants of glomerular filtration in experimental glomerulonephritis in the rat. *J Clin Invest* 1975;55:305–318.

92. Gabbai FB, Gushwa LC, Wilson CB, Blantz RC. An evaluation of the development of experimental membranous nephropathy. *Kidney Int* 1987;31:1267–1278.

93. Deen WM, Maddox DA, Robertson CR, Brenner BM. Dynamics of glomerular ultrafiltration in the rat: VII. response to reduced renal mass. *Am J Physiol* 1974;227:556–562.

94. Hostetter TH, Olson JL, Rennke HG, Venkatachalam MA, Brenner BM. Hyperfiltration in remnant nephrons: a potentially adverse response to renal ablation. *Am J Physiol* 1981;241:F85–F93.

95. Anderson S, Meyer TW, Rennke HG, Brenner BM. Control of glomerular hypertension limits glomerular injury in rats with reduced renal mass. *J Clin Invest* 1985;76:612–619.

96. Anderson S, Rennke HG, Brenner BM. Therapeutic advantage of converting enzyme inhibitors in arresting progressive renal disease associated with systemic hypertension in the rat. *J Clin Invest* 1986;77:1993–2000.

97. Meyer TW, Anderson S, Rennke HG, Brenner BM. Reversing glomerular hypertension stabilizes established glomerular injury. *Kidney Int* 1987;31:752–759.

98. Lax DS, Benstein JA, Tolbert E, Dworkin LD. Effects of salt restriction on renal growth and glomerular injury in rats with remnant kidneys. *Kidney Int* 1992;41:1527–1534.

99. Hostetter TH, Troy JL, Brenner BM. Glomerular hemodynamics in experimental diabetes mellitus. *Kidney Int* 1981;19:410–415.

100. Zatz R, Meyer TW, Rennke HG, Brenner BM. Predominance of hemodynamic rather than metabolic factors in the pathogenesis of diabetic glomerulopathy. *Proc Natl Acad Sci USA* 1985;82:5963–5967.

101. Zatz R, Dunn BR, Meyer TW, Anderson S, Rennke HG, Brenner BM. Prevention of diabetic glomerulopathy by pharmacological amelioration of glomerular capillary hypertension. *J Clin Invest* 1986;77:1925–1930.

102. Anderson S, Rennke HG, Garcia DL, Brenner BM. Short and long term effects of antihypertensive therapy in the diabetic rat. *Kidney Int* 1989;36:526–536.

103. Sugai T, Nakagawa Y, Takeda K, Imai S. Arterial pressure-

urinary output relationship in DOCA-saline hypertensive rats. *Am J Physiol* 1983;245:R633–R636.

104. Bianchi G, Baer PG, Fox U, Zuzzi L, Pagetti D, Giovannetti AM. Changes in renin, water balance, and sodium balance during development of high blood pressure in genetically hypertensive rats. *Circ Res* 1975;36–37[Suppl I]:I153–I161.

105. Zeigler DW, Patel KP. Reduced renal responses to an acute saline load in obese Zucker rats. *Am J Physiol* 1991;261:R712–R718.

106. Roland JM, O'Hare JP, Walters G, Corrall RJ. Sodium retention in response to saline infusion in uncomplicated diabetes mellitus. *Diabetes Res* 1986;3:213–215.

107. O'Hare JP, Roland JM, Walters G, Corrall RJM. Impaired sodium excretion in response to volume expansion induced by water immersion in insulin-dependent diabetes mellitus. *Clin Sci* 1986;71:403–409.

108. Munoz-Ramirez H, Chatelain RE, Bumpus FM, Khairallah PA. Development of two-kidney Goldblatt hypertension in rats under dietary sodium restriction. *Am J Physiol* 1980;238:H889–H894.

109. Kleine RL, Mercer PF. Effect of captopril and hydralazine on arterial pressure-urinary output relationships in spontaneously hypertensive rats. *Hypertension* 1987;10:590–594.

110. Schnermann J, Briggs J. Role of the renin-angiotensin system in tubuloglomerular feedback. *Fed Proc* 1986;45:1426–1430.

111. Briggs JP, Schnermann J. The tubuloglomerular feedback mechanism. In: Laragh JH, Brenner BM, eds. *Hypertension: pathophysiology, diagnosis, and management.* New York: Raven Press; 1990:1067–1087.

112. Brass H, Ochs HG, Armbruster H, Heintz R. Plasma renin activity (PRA) and aldosterone (PA) in patients with chronic glomerulonephritis (GN) and hypertension. *Clin Nephrol* 1976;5:57–60.

113. Shimamoto K, Ishida H, Nakahashi Y, et al. A very sensitive direct radioimmunoassay system for various hypertensive diseases. *Jap Circ J* 1984;48:1228–1235.

114. Bricker NS. Sodium homeostasis in chronic renal disease. *Kidney Int* 1982;21:886–897.

115. Blythe WB. Natural history of hypertension in renal parenchymal disease. *Am J Kidney Dis* 1985;5:A50–A56.

116. Arze RS, Ramos JM, Owen JP, et al. The natural history of chronic pyelonephritis in the adults. *Q J Med* 1982;51:396–410.

117. Danielsen H, Kornerup HJ, Olsen S, Posborg V. Arterial hypertension in chronic glomerulonephritis: an analysis of 310 cases. *Clin Nephrol* 1983;19:284–287.

118. Orofino L, Quereda C, Lamas S, et al. Hypertension in primary chronic glomerulonephritis: analysis of 288 biopsied patients. *Nephron* 1987;45:22–26.

119. Bell PE, Hossack KF, Babow PA, Durr JA, Johnson AM, Schrier RW. Hypertension in autosomal dominant polycystic kidney disease. *Kidney Int* 1988;34:683–690.

120. Stokes GS, Mani MK, Stewart JH. Relevance of salt, water, and renin to hypertension in chronic renal failure. *Br Med J* 1970;3:126–129.

121. Acosta JH. Hypertension in chronic renal disease. *Kidney Int* 1982;22:702–712.

122. Luft FC, Weinberger MH, Grim CE. Sodium sensitivity and resistance in normotensive humans. *Am J Med* 1982;72:726–736.

123. Ihle BU, Becker GJ, Whitworth JA, Charlwood RA, Kincaid-Smith PS. The effect of protein restriction on the progression of renal insufficiency. *N Engl J Med* 1989;321:1773–1777.

124. Rosman JB, Langer K, Brandl M, et al. Protein-restricted diets in chronic renal failure: a four year follow-up shows limited indications. *Kidney Int* 1989;36[Suppl 27]:S96–S102.

125. Mitch WE. Dietary protein restriction in chronic renal failure: nutritional efficacy, compliance, and progression of renal insufficiency. *J Am Soc Nephrol* 1991;2:823–831.

126. Fouque D, Laville M, Boissel JP, Chifflet R, Labeeuw M, Zech PY. Controlled low protein diets in chronic renal insufficiency: meta-analysis. *Br Med J* 1992;304:216–220.

127. Zucchelli P, Zuccala A, Borghi M, et al. Long-term comparison between captopril and nifedipine in the progression of renal insufficiency. *Kidney Int* 1992;42:452–458.

128. Dustan HP, Valdes G, Bravo EL, Tarazi RC. Excessive sodium retention as a characteristic of salt-sensitive hypertension. *Am J Med Sci* 1986;292:67–74.

129. Lilley JJ, Hsu L, Stone RA. Racial disparity of plasma volume in hypertensive man. *Ann Intern Med* 1976;84:707–708.

130. Rowlands DB, DeGiovanni J, McLeay R, Watson RDS, Stallard TJ, Littler WA. Cardiovascular response in black and white hypertensives. *Hypertension* 1982;4:817–820.

131. Veterans Administration Cooperative Study Group on Antihypertensive Agents. Comparison of propranolol and hydrochlorothiazide for the initial treatment of hypertension: II. results of long-term therapy. *JAMA* 1982;248:2004–2011.

132. Luft FC, Fineberg NS, Miller JZ, Rankin LI, Grim CE, Weinberger MH. The effects of age, race and heredity on glomerular filtration rate following volume expansion and contraction in normal man. *Am J Med Sci* 1980;279:15–24.

133. Page LB, Damon A, Moellering RC Jr. Antecedents of cardiovascular disease in six Solomon Islands societies. *Circulation* 1974;49:1132–1146.

134. Boyle E Jr. Biological patterns in hypertension by race, sex, body weight, and skin color. *JAMA* 1970;213:1637–1643.

135. McLachlan MSF, Guthrie JC, Anderson CK, Fulker MJ. Vascular and glomerular changes in the aging kidney. *J Pathol* 1977;121:65–78.

136. Kaplan C, Pasternack B, Shah H, Gallo G. Age-related incidence of sclerotic glomeruli in human kidneys. *Am J Pathol* 1975;80:227–234.

137. Easterling RE. Racial factors in the incidence and causation of end-stage renal disease (ESRD). *Trans Am Soc Artif Intern Organs* 1977;23:28–32.

138. Rostand SG, Kirk KA, Rutsky EA, Pate BA. Racial differences in the incidence of treatment for end-stage renal disease. *N Engl J Med* 1982;306:1276–1279.

139. Dustan HP, Curtis JJ, Luke RG, Rostand SG. Systemic hypertension and the kidney in black patients. *Am J Cardiol* 1987;60[Suppl]:73I–77I.

140. Whelton PK, Klag MJ. Hypertension as a risk for renal disease. Review of clinical and epidemiological evidence. *Hypertension* 1989;13[Suppl I]:I19–I27.

141. O'Hare JA, Ferriss JB, Brady D, Twomey B, O'Sullivan DJ. Exchangeable sodium and renin in hypertensive diabetic patients with and without nephropathy. *Hypertension* 1985;7[Suppl II]:II43–II48.

142. Feldt-Rasmussen B, Mathiesen ER, Deckert T, et al. Central role for sodium in the pathogenesis of blood pressure changes independent of angiotensin, aldosterone and catecholamines in type 1 (insulin-dependent) diabetes mellitus. *Diabetologia* 1987;30:610–617.

143. Weidmann P, Beretta-Piccoli C, Trost BN. Pressor factors and responsiveness in hypertension accompanying diabetes mellitus. *Hypertension* 1985;7[Suppl II]:II33–II42.

144. Weidmann P, Beretta-Piccoli C, Keusch G, et al. Sodium-volume factor, cardiovascular reactivity and hypotensive mechanisms of diuretic therapy in mild hypertension associated with diabetes mellitus. *Am J Med* 1979;67:779–784.

145. Mogensen CE, Andersen MJF. Increased kidney size and glomerular filtration rate in early juvenile diabetes. 1973;22:706–712.

146. Christiansen JS, Gammelgaard J, Frandsen M, Parving H-H. Increased kidney size, glomerular filtration rate and renal plasma flow in short-term insulin-dependent diabetics. *Diabetologia* 1981;20:451–456.

147. Feldt-Rasmussen B, Borch-Johnsen K, Mathiesen ER. Hypertension in diabetes as related to nephropathy: early blood pressure changes. *Hypertension* 1985;7[Suppl II]:II18–II20.

148. Mogensen CE, Christensen CK. Predicting diabetic nephropathy in insulin-dependent patients. *N Engl J Med* 1984;311:89–93.

149. Carr S, Mbanya JC, Thomas T, et al. Increase in glomerular filtration rate in patients with insulin-dependent diabetes and elevated erythrocyte sodium-lithium countertransport. *N Engl J Med* 1990;322:500–505.

150. Rudberg S, Persson B, Dahlquist G. Increased glomerular filtration rate as a predictor of diabetic nephropathy—an 8-year prospective study. *Kidney Int* 1992;41:822–828.

151. Ortola FV, Ballermann BJ, Anderson S, Mendez RE, Brenner BM. Elevated plasma atrial natriuretic peptide levels in diabetic rats. Potential mediator of hyperfiltration. *J Clin Invest* 1987;80:670–674.

152. Sawicki PT, Heinemann L, Rave K, Hohmann A, Berger M. Atrial natriuretic factor in various stages of diabetic nephropathy. *J Diabetic Complications* 1988;2:207–209.

153. Wenting GJ, Man inT Veld AJ, Verhoeven RP, Derkx FHM, Schalekamp MADH. Volume-pressure relationship during development of mineralocorticoid hypertension in man. *Circ Res* 1977;40[Suppl I]:I163–I170.

154. Beretta-Piccoli C, Davis DL, Brown JJ, et al. Relation of blood pressure with body and plasma electrolytes in Conn's syndrome. *J Hypertens* 1983;1:197–205.

155. Weidmann P, Ferrari P. Central role of sodium in hypertension in diabetic subjects. *Diabetes Care* 1991;14:220–232.

156. Ditzel J, Lervang HH, Brochner-Mortensen J. Renal sodium metabolism in relation to hypertension in diabetes. *Diabetes Metab Rev* 1989;15:292–295.

157. DeFronzo RA, Goldberg M, Agus ZS. The effects of glucose and insulin on renal electrolyte transport. *J Clin Invest* 1976;58:83–90.

158. Walker JD, Bending JJ, Dodds RA, et al. Restriction of dietary protein and progression of renal failure in diabetic nephropathy. *Lancet* 1989;ii:1411–1415.

159. Zeller K, Whittaker E, Sullivan L, Raskin P, Jacobson HR. Effect of restricting dietary protein on the progression of renal failure in patients with insulin-dependent diabetes mellitus. *N Engl J Med* 1991;324:78–84.

160. Parving H-H. Protein restriction and renal failure in diabetes mellitus. *N Engl J Med* 1991;324:1743–1744.

161. Mogensen CE. Long-term antihypertensive treatment inhibiting progression of diabetic nephropathy. *Br Med J* 1982;285:685–688.

162. Parving H-H, Andersen AR, Smidt UM, Hommel E, Mathiesen ER, Svendsen PA. Effect of antihypertensive treatment on kidney function in diabetic nephropathy. *Br Med J* 1987;294:1443–1447.

163. Pedersen MM, Christensen CK, Hansen KW, Christiansen JS, Mogensen CE, ACE-inhibition and renoprotection in early diabetic nephropathy. Response to enalapril acutely and in long-term combination with conventional antihypertensive treatment. *Clin Invest Med* 1991;14:642–651.

164. Bjork S, Mulec H, Johnsen SA, Norden G, Aurell M. Renal protective effect of enalapril in diabetic nephropathy. *Br Med J* 1992;304:339–343.

165. Jerums G, Allen TJ, Tsalamandris C, Cooper ME. Angiotensin converting enzyme inhibition and calcium channel blockade in incipient diabetic nephropathy. *Kidney Int* 1992;41:904–911.

166. Anderson S, Brenner BM. Pathogenesis of diabetic glomerulopathy: hemodynamic considerations. *Diabetes Metab Rev* 1988;4:163–177.

167. Tuck ML, Sowers J, Dornfeld L, Kledzik G, Maxwell M. The effect of weight reduction on blood pressure, plasma renin activity, and plasma aldosterone levels in obese patients. *N Engl J Med* 1981;304:930–933.

168. Raison J, Achimastos A, Asmar R, Simon A, Safar M. Extracellular and interstitial fluid volume in obesity with and without associated systemic hypertension. *Am J Cardiol* 1986;57:223–226.

169. Stokholm KH, Brochner-Mortensen J, Hoilund-Carlsen PF. Increased glomerular filtration rate and adrenocortical function in obese women. *Int J Obes* 1980;4:57–63.

170. Sims EAH. Mechanisms of hypertension in the overweight. *Hypertension* 1982;4[Suppl III]:III43–III49.

171. Rutherford PA, Thomas TH, Wilkinson R. Insulin resistance and hypertension-implications for treatment. *Postgrad Med J* 1991;67:869–875.

172. Metcalf P, Baker J, Scott A, Wild C, Scragg R, Dryson E. Albuminuria in people at least 40 years old: effect of obesity, hypertension, and hyperlipidemia. *Clin Chem* 1992;38:1802–1808.

173. Cohen AH. Massive obesity and the kidney. *Am J Pathol* 1975;81:117–127.

174. Kasiske BL, Crosson JT. Renal disease in patients with massive obesity. *Arch Intern Med* 1986;146:1105–1109.

175. Wesson DE, Kurtzman NA, Frommer JP. Massive obesity and nephrotic proteinuria with a normal biopsy. *Nephron* 1985;40:235–237.

176. Hollenberg NK, Williams GH. Abnormal renal function, sodium-volume homeostasis, and renin system behavior in normal-renin essential hypertension. In: Laragh JH, Brenner BM, eds. *Hypertension: pathophysiology, diagnosis, and management.* New York: Raven Press; 1990:1349–1370.

177. Rabinowe SL, Redgrave JE, Shoback DM, Podolsky S, Hollenberg NK, Williams GH. Renin suppression by saline is blunted in nonmodulating essential hypertension. *Hypertension* 1987;10:404–408.

178. Redgrave J, Rabinowe S, Hollenberg NK, Williams GH. Correction of abnormal renal blood flow response to angiotensin II by converting enzyme inhibition in essential hypertensives. *J Clin Invest* 1985;75:1285–1290.

179. Sugawara A, Nakao K, Sakamoto M, et al. Plasma concentration of atrial natriuretic polypeptide in essential hypertension. *Lancet* 1985;2:1426–1427.

180. Matsubara H, Umeda Y, Yamane Y, Nishikawa M, Taniguchi T, Inada M. Role of atrial natriuretic polypeptides for exaggerated natriuresis in essential hypertension. *Am J Cardiol* 1987;60:708–714.

181. Atarashi K, Mulrow PJ, Franco-Saenz R, Snajdar R, Rapp J. Inhibition of aldosterone production by an atrial extract. *Science* 1984;224:992–994.

182. Jonston CI, Hodsman PG, Kohzuki M, Casley DJ, Fabris B, Phillips PA. Interaction between atrial natriuretic peptide and the renin angiotensin aldosterone system. Endogenous antagonists. *Am J Med* 1989;87[Suppl 6B]:24S–28S.

Hypertension: Pathophysiology, Diagnosis, and Management, Second Edition, edited by J.H. Laragh and B.M. Brenner, Raven Press, Ltd., New York © 1995.

CHAPTER 95

The Molecular Biology of Renin Gene Expression

Daniel F. Catanzaro

The renin-angiotensin system (RAS) plays a key role in the long-term regulation of blood pressure and electrolyte homeostasis. Renin released from juxtaglomerular (JG) cells appears to be rate-limiting for the generation of angiotensin II (AII) in the renin-angiotensin-aldosterone cascade (1). Thus, plasma renin levels ultimately determine vascular tone and plasma volume. Moreover, plasma renin levels are related to the incidence of stroke, myocardial infarction, and other vascular injuries (2,3) in hypertensive patients. Because renin release must be accompanied by *de novo* synthesis to replenish depleted JG storage granules, the mechanisms that direct renin

gene expression determine the amount of renin available for release. Therefore, the mechanisms that regulate renin gene expression are likely to play an important role in the pathogenesis and sequelae of hypertension.

Prorenin, the biosynthetic precursor of renin, is also secreted from JG cells and is the final product of renin gene expression at several extrarenal sites (4). Although prorenin normally comprises about 90 percent of the total circulating renin in both humans and rats, it is not converted to active renin in the circulation, suggesting that it may serve some additional function (5,6). Because prorenin is secreted constitutively (7), the rate of renin gene transcription directly affects the rate of prorenin secretion and hence the circulating levels.

Understanding the mechanisms that direct renin gene expression to the renal JG cells as well as to other extra-

D. F. Catanzaro: Cardiovascular Center, Department of Medicine, and Department of Physiology and Biophysics, Cornell University Medical College, New York, New York 10021.

renal sites may reveal genetic and molecular bases for defects in both essential (5,8) and high-renin hypertension (4) and may provide important clues to the function of prorenin. The mechanisms that regulate renin gene expression may also provide targets for new therapies to control hypertension. Because angiotensin-converting enzyme (ACE) inhibitors and angiotensin receptor (AIIR) blockers induce reactive increases in renin secretion that modulate the effects of the drugs, understanding the mechanisms of renin gene expression may also provide better targets for therapies to control hypertension.

The aims of this chapter are to review some of the key studies that have contributed to understanding the molecular mechanisms of renin gene expression and to examine the physiological role these mechanisms may play both in normal physiological homeostasis and in the development of hypertension.

MECHANISMS OF CELL-SPECIFIC GENE EXPRESSION

As a protein-coding gene, the renin gene is transcribed by ribonucleic acid (RNA) polymerase II, a multisubunit enzyme that binds a sequence known as the TATA box situated in the 5'-flanking DNA approximately -30 bp from the startsite of transcription. By convention, the startsite of transcription is labeled $+1$ and the 5'-flanking DNA, which is the sequence upstream of the startsite, is numbered negatively. In addition to the RNA polymerase-binding site, the 5'-flanking DNA contains other sequences called promoter elements, which are usually located within a few hundred base pairs upstream of the TATA box. Promoter elements are sequences 8 to 15 base pairs (bp) long that bind transcription factors. These factors interact with RNA polymerase II to stimulate transcription initiation. The region of 5'-flanking DNA consisting of the TATA box and promoter elements that are sufficient to initiate transcription is referred to as the promoter. Another class of sequences known as enhancers also stimulates transcription but does so from a distance that may be several thousand base pairs away from the transcription startsite. Like promoters, the activity of enhancers is mediated by the transcription factors that they bind. The interplay between promoters and enhancers is thought to determine spatial and temporal patterns of gene expression.

Transcription factors determine both cell specificity and responsiveness to extracellular signals. Transcription factors may be expressed ubiquitously, restricted to a single cell type or to a limited number of cell types. Some transcription factors are, in fact, hormone receptors, such as the steroid/thyroid hormone receptor superfamily, or the final target of second-messenger–mediated signaling pathways. In this way, transcription factors

provide mechanisms to control gene expression in response to extracellular signals. Because transcription factors are themselves generally proteins, a 1:1 correspondence between transcription factors and the genes whose expression they direct would require an infinite number of factors. Therefore, it is generally assumed and supported by experimental findings that cell specificity is accomplished through a combinatorial code that uses different subsets of transcription factors to confer cell specificity. Further discussion of the mechanisms of eukaryotic gene expression may be found in several excellent reviews (9–11).

One of the principal goals of research on the molecular mechanisms of renin gene expression is to identify the promoter and enhancer sequences and their cognate transcription factors that direct renin gene expression. Identification and cloning of transcription factors involved in controlling renin gene expression will provide new probes and targets for genetic analyses of hypertensive patients and possible targets for antihypertensive drugs.

APPROACHES TO STUDYING GENE REGULATORY MECHANISMS

Recombinant DNA technology has made possible both the characterization of naturally occurring mutations that affect gene regulatory elements and the construction of hybrid genes into which specific mutations can be made to test their function. The first of these approaches, the so-called genetic approach (see chapter by Richard Lifton), has revealed mutations that may be involved in the pathogenesis of hypertension. The mutations that have been identified so far are in the regions of genes that encode amino acid sequences. Such mutations may either affect the activity of the molecule in which they occur or may be linked to some other mutation that serves some other structural or regulatory function. However, genetic approaches are limited in that naturally occurring mutations are relatively rare and, even if they do occur, may be deleterious to the cell or organism.

Reverse Genetics and Hybrid Genes

The term *reverse genetics* is sometimes used to describe the approach in which genes, which may be engineered to contain specific mutations, are inserted into a cell to test for function. This approach may be applied to the study of gene regulatory sequences by the use of hybrid genes. The strategy most commonly taken to study gene regulatory mechanisms involves linking the putative promoter and/or enhancer sequences to a heterologous reporter gene to form a hybrid gene, which is then transfected into appropriate cells in culture to test for function. Ideally, the product of such a reporter gene is not normally expressed in mammalian cells, is easily quantified, and is neither toxic nor does it interfere with normal cell function. Although chloramphenicol acetyl transferase (12) has been extensively used as a reporter, more recently luciferase (13), whose activity is more easily quantified over a broad range, has gained in popularity as a reporter.

Once a promoter region is linked to an appropriate reporter, the hybrid gene that is contained in a plasmid may be replicated in bacterial cells, allowing it to be prepared in large quantities. Generally, a set of hybrid gene constructions will contain 5'-flanking DNA sequences fused to the reporter at a fixed position (usually 5 to 50 bp downstream of the transcription startsite) and extending to different positions upstream, depending on the availability of the cloned genomic sequence and the positions of convenient restriction enzyme cleavage sites that are used to piece together the construction. Such a series of 5'-flanking sequences is often referred to as a set of deletions because sequences are usually deleted from the 5' end. Deletional analysis of this type is used to determine the limits of essential regulatory elements. Internal deletions in the 5'-flanking DNA may also be used to identify nonessential sequences that might, for example, separate promoter and enhancer sequences.

To identify key promoter and enhancer elements, two approaches are often used. The first uses systematic mutations through the regulatory sequences to identify functional promoter elements, whereas the second seeks to identify transcription factor binding sites as key regulatory elements.

Scanning Mutagenesis

In the first approach, a scanning mutagenesis (14) of the regulatory sequences is performed. For example, blocks of 5 or 6 bp may be systematically mutagenized throughout the 5'-flanking DNA. Several early studies painstakingly matched deletions from each end of a promoter fragment produced by exonuclease treatment and joined these with a synthetic linker to produce the mutagenized block while maintaining the original spacing of sequences on either side. Although scanning mutagenesis can now be carried out by more rapid methods of site-directed mutagenesis (15,16), these approaches remain time-consuming and costly. Nevertheless, transfection of a set of constructions containing such mutagenized blocks enables the key promoter elements to be systematically identified. The transcription factors interacting with these elements may then be sought. One potential shortcoming of this approach is that if several sites act in concert, mutagenizing a single site may have little effect on promoter activity.

Identification of Transcription Factor Binding Sites

Another approach to characterizing gene regulatory elements is to identify binding sites for transcription factors and then to specifically mutagenize them. Although this narrows down the sequences to be tested for activity, it is limited by the sensitivity of methods to detect DNA binding of transcription factors. The latter is generally accomplished either by footprinting or gel mobility shift assays. Footprinting depends on the ability of a transcription factor to protect the bound DNA sequence from enzymatic digestion. Limited digestion of a DNA fragment labeled at one end with ^{32}P produces a set of nested fragments, the absence of which denotes the footprint. Alternatively, transcription factor binding can be visualized by changes in the mobility of labeled DNA fragments on a nondenaturing acrylamide gel. The principle of this assay is that binding of factors to DNA will produce a complex with reduced electrophoretic mobility in an acrylamide gel, relative to the unbound DNA. Labeling of the DNA fragments with ^{32}P allows the free and complexed DNA to be visualized by autoradiography. The ability of related DNA sequences to compete for binding of common factors can also be assessed by adding an excess of nonradioactive competitor DNA to the binding reaction. Although this method is more sensitive than the footprinting assay, it yields no information about the exact location of the binding site. However, this can be overcome by using short segments of synthetic oligonucleotide DNA (25 to 30 bp). A set of such fragments, designed to overlap by 5 to 10 bp, can be used to identify transcription factor binding sites efficiently in a short segment of DNA ($\sim$100 bp).

In the characterization of most gene regulatory regions, transfection assays and mutagenesis, whether of the scanning type or directed to specific binding sites, together with footprinting and gel mobility shift assays are carried out to determine the sites involved and the transcription factors with which they interact. Also, many studies use transgenic animals to determine whether the sequences identified by transfection experiments are necessary and sufficient for cell-specific, physiologically regulated expression in the context of the intact organism. Extensive reviews of recent advances in the study of renin gene expression in transgenic animals are to be found in several articles by Sigmund and coworkers (17–19).

USE OF CELL CULTURE SYSTEMS IN STUDIES OF RENIN GENE EXPRESSION

To carry out transfection experiments and to isolate transcription factors, it is necessary to have a cell culture system that expresses the gene under investigation and that contains all the factors necessary to direct its expression. Transfection experiments may also be used to identify the elements involved in regulating a gene's expression in response to extracellular signals by testing constructions for responsiveness to these signals and then comparing the effects when various sequences are deleted or mutagenized.

The scarcity of renal JG cells (<0.01 percent) has precluded their isolation and culture for use in studies of renin gene expression. Although Kurtz and coworkers claimed to have produced cultures of rat kidneys containing 50 to 90 percent JG cells (20,21), the supporting evidence provided for this level of enrichment was weak, especially considering that this degree of purification was achieved through a single Percoll gradient centrifugation step followed by differential plating onto plastic. A noteworthy possibility to account for the high-level recovery of renin-expressing cells using the Kurtz protocol is that some aspect of the method may induce the transformation of smooth muscle cells, mimicking the process of recruitment that occurs when renin release is chronically stimulated (see below). In another study (22), similar methods accomplished a modest 10-fold enrichment of JG cells. Even if JG cells could be prepared in high purity, in culture, these cells rapidly lose the ability to express renin. A continuous renal renin-secreting cell line (As4.1) has recently been established using targeted tumorigenesis in transgenic animals (23). The development and applications of this cell line are discussed in later sections. Although As4.1 cells will provide a powerful system with which to study the regulation of renin gene expression, processing, and release, most of our present knowledge on the molecular biology of renin gene expression has been derived from studies using renin-nonexpressing cells or renin-expressing cells of extrarenal origin. Using such cell culture systems, the promoter activity of renin 5'-flanking DNA sequences has been investigated by transfection of hybrid genes containing these sequences linked to various heterologous reporter genes.

Evolutionarily Conserved Sequences in Renin 5'-Flanking DNA

Renin genes from several species including mouse (24), rat (25), and humans (26) have been cloned and sequenced. Alignment of 5'-flanking DNA sequences from rat and human renin genes (Fig. 1) shows that sequences are conserved to approximately 0.5 kb upstream of the transcription startsite. Although interrupted at position −80 by a 476-bp insertion flanked by direct repeats (27), similar sequences are conserved in the 5'-flanking DNA of mouse renin genes (Fig. 2). The conservation of sequence in this 0.5-kb region suggests that it contains important regulatory elements. Within this region, many sequences are very highly conserved (28) (Fig. 2; sites I to XI), whereas several other less highly conserved regions of identity are contained between sites V and VIII. To retain the original numbering system proposed by Burt and coworkers (28), these additional conserved sites are designated as VIa, VIb, etc. Quite often, such highly conserved sequences have been found to function as impor-

HUMAN

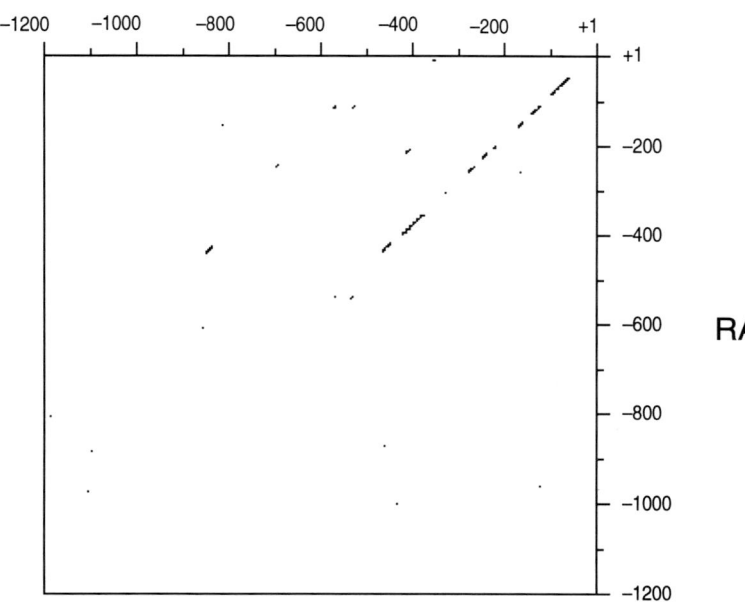

RAT

FIG. 1. Alignment of human and rat renin 5'-flanking DNA sequences. Alignment was carried out using the program DIAGON (113). Sequences were compared using a 25-base window and scored as a match if 75 percent of residues in that window were identical.

```
                                                          I
m  -986    agGTTaCTTTTCCaa.CtAGgcAgcAGcCAaaAg|GAaTCACtcATGaTCa
r  -463    atcTTaCTTTTtcca.CtAGgcAgcAGcCAaaAg|GAqTCACCCATGaTCa
h  -498    ctGTTgCTTTTCCtgcCaAGaaAcaAGtCAtgAa|GAtTCACCCATGtTCt
                                                    II
m  -937    AGATGG.AAgACTaGG|gcaga|GCCTaGGGAGGAGCCAG|....GGgtgAttt
r  -414    gGATGG.AAgACTGGG|.....|GCCTcGGAGGAGCCAG|tcagGGgtAAtaC
h  -448    AGATGGgAAaACTGGG|ctgta|GCCTgGGAGGAGCCAG|tcagGGacAAagC
                    III
m  -892    g|AAgGTTAATATAGA|ttaatagataggttaatatataatattaggttaat
r  -370    a|AAgGTTAATATAGA|................................cg
h  -398    c|AAaGTTAATATAGA|................................ga

m  -842    ATGcAGgtcTCggGGGcATgaGttGGTaGGGtCTGAGtTAGaGgttTG..
r  -353    ATGcAGg.cTCaaGGacATagat.GGTgGGGcCTGAGtTgGaag..TGcA
h  -381    ATGgAGc.tTCcaGGGtATagG..GGTtGGGtCTGAGcTAGgGagcTGgA

m  -794    AAgCcAGGgTcTAtGCTgtgtgtAcccTgacctcatGC.tgaAca.gcaCa
r  -307    AAgCcAGGgTcTAtGCTgtctgtAcccTgacctTatGCttgaAcC.ccaCa
h  -334    AAcCtAGGtTtTAcGCTtgtcccAgttTtgatgTtaGCcctgAgCagtgCt
                    IV                    V
m  -745    GcTcCTCATtAGccTcTG|tCTaag|CtAGaGGTtgCgGGGCCAgGCCA|a..
r  -230    GTTcCTCATCAGCCTCTG|tCgaag|CtAaaGGTtgCAGGGCCAgGCCA|a..
h  -283    GTTtCTCATCAGCCTCTG|cCTgct|CCAGgGGTcaCAGGGCCAaGCCA|gat
                VIa                        VIb
m  -697    AcAGGGactCTAGaGTCAtTGG|gctC.AGc|cacccTTCCCACA.CcccC|a
r  -209    AcAGGGacaCCAGCGTCACTGG|gttCAgcc|aTG.TTTCCCACA.CTc.g|a
h  -233    AgAGGGctqCTAGCGTCACTGG|acacAAGa|tTGcTTTCCCACAgCTgtC|c
                VIc
m  -649    TgCCTgccaCCaCTCTGCTCtgCgacCaGg.t|tCTGctTAtCCTatACCt
r  -162    TTCCTg...CCaCTCTGCTtcgCtTCCGGc.t|CCTGctTAtCCctCACCC
h  -183    TTCCTccagCCcCTCTGCTCccCaTCCGGaaa|CCTGggTAcCCTtCACCC
                VIIa            VIIb            VIII
m  -600    ACCTAaCTtgGTCtCaCAG|gc|TagaATTTAT|.cag|GACTGCCCTGCCAT|g
r  -116    ACCTAGCTtgGcCtCaCgGG|gc|TagATTTAT|.Gag|GgCTGCCCTGCCAT|g
h  -133    ACCTAGCTctGTCcCgCAG|..|TgaGATTTAT|TGct|GACTGCCCTGCCAT|c
                IX
m  -551    gg|CCttgGGG|TAATAAATCAaaGCAG|At...............CCtgTGa
r  -67     gA|CCCtgGGG|TAATAAATCAGaGCAG|gg...............CCtgTG.
h  -85     tA|CCCcaGGG|TAATAAATCAGgGCAG|Agcagaattgcaatcac.CCcaTG.
                X                  XI              +1
m  -40     taCAt|GGtGTGTATAAAAG|....|AaGGCTcAGGG|ggtctqgGCt|A|CA...
r  -33     .....|GGtGTGTATAAAAG|....|AaGGCTcAGGG|..tctggGCt|A|CA...
h  -36     ..CAt|GGaGTGTATAAAAG|ggga|AgGGCTaAGGG|......aGCc|A|CAgaa
```

FIG. 2. Alignment of mouse (m), rat (r), and human (h) 5'-flanking DNA sequences in the conserved region shown in Fig. 1. *Numbered boxes* indicate regions of high-sequence conservation.

tant promoter elements. For example, a sequence contained in the 5'-flanking DNA of growth hormone genes from several species was shown to bind a transcription factor, Zen-15, essential for high-level expression in pituitary somatotrope cells (29). Among the conserved sites shown in Fig. 2, site VIa contains a motif CGTCA that binds the cyclic adenosine monophosphate (AMP) response element binding protein (CREB) (30), and site IX contains an A/T-rich motif that functions as a binding site for the pituitary-specific factor Pit-1 (31) and cell-specific factors expressed in other tissues (see below).

PITUITARY RENIN EXPRESSION

Renin and renin messenger ribonucleic acid (mRNA) have been detected in pituitary cells of several species (32–35). However, the exact cell type in which renin is expressed appears to differ between species. In rats, renin is expressed in gonadotropes, whereas in humans and sheep, renin is expressed in lactotrophs. Although the physiological role(s) of a pituitary RAS is not known, stimulation of AIIR on lactotropes and corticotropes results in increased release of prolactin and adrenocorticotropic hormone (ACTH) (36). Thus, AII produced by rat gonadotropes may play a paracrine role in regulating release of these latter hormones (36).

Our interests in the mechanisms that direct the cell specificity of growth hormone and prolactin genes (37,38) led us to postulate whether a putative binding site for the pituitary-specific transcription factor Pit-1 (39) [also known as GHF-1 (40)] conserved in the 5'-flanking DNAs of rat, human, and mouse renin genes might be involved in the pituitary expression of the renin gene

(31). Pit-1 is a member of the POU family of transcription factors, which are expressed at specific sites in the nervous system and in other organs of the developing embryo (41). As one of the best characterized members of the POU family, Pit-1 has been implicated in the control of proliferation of specific cells in the pituitary, namely, lactotropes, somatotropes, and thyrotropes, and is involved in directing the expression of specific genes that determine the identity of these cells, prolactin, growth hormone, and thyroid-stimulating hormone (TSH).

Pit-1 Binding to a Conserved Sequence in the Human Renin 5′-Flanking DNA

Among the conserved sequences contained in the renin 5′-flanking DNA (see Fig. 1), an A/T-rich region spanning position −70 bears a striking resemblance to the Pit-1–binding site consensus sequence, which has been variously defined as A_T^ATTANCAT (42), $_T^A$TAT$_C^T$CAT (43), and ATATTCA (44).

Gel mobility shift assays demonstrated that the human renin 5′-flanking DNA sequence indeed binds Pit-1 (Fig. 3). The oligonucleotides used for gel mobility shift analysis are shown in Fig. 3A. hRen is the native human renin 5′-flanking DNA sequence (−80/−58), whereas hRenΔ1 and hRenΔ2 contain mutations that alter bases contained in the Pit-1 binding site consensus sequence. The oligonucleotides named Sp1 and AP1 contain binding sites for these two transcription factors that are unrelated either to Pit-1 or each other.

Figure 3B shows the results of mobility shift competition experiments carried out using the native human renin sequence (hRen, −80/−58) as probe. The formation of a predominant group of complexes, which are probably caused by binding of alternatively spliced forms of Pit-1 (45,46), was competed by excess unlabeled hRen sequence or by a strong Pit-1-binding site from the human growth hormone (hGH) gene, but not by the Sp1 or AP1 oligonucleotides. Moreover, mutation of residues in the hRen sequence corresponding to the Pit-1–binding site consensus prevented binding, as evidenced by the inability of oligonucleotides containing these mutations to compete for complex formation on the native sequence.

Proteolytic Clipping Bandshift Assay

The proteolytic clipping bandshift assay (PCBA) (47) permits closer discrimination between factors binding to related sequences by identifying the DNA-binding peptide fragments generated by limited proteolysis. The generation of identical fragments from two different protein-DNA complexes indicates that the same protein is involved in both complexes. Oligonucleotides represent-

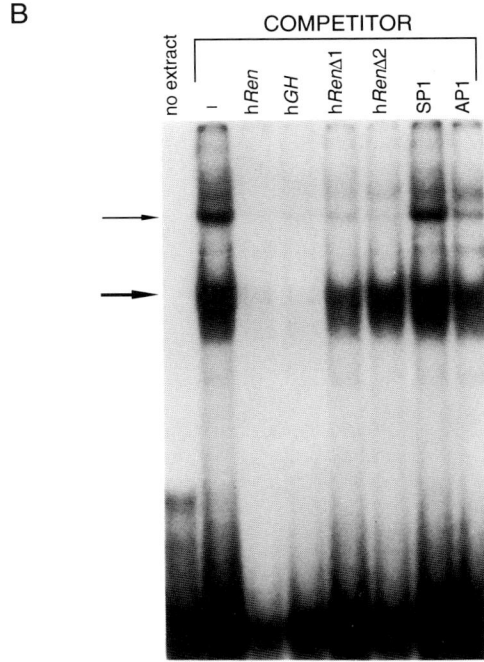

FIG. 3. Gel mobility shift analysis of Pit-1 binding to the human renin 5′-flanking DNA. **A:** Sequences of oligonucleotides used in this analysis. The hRen oligonucleotide, which contains the conserved sequence −80/−58 shown in Fig. 2 (box IX), was used as the probe. Other oligonucleotides are described in the text. **B:** Results of gel mobility shift analysis carried out using GC cell nuclear extract. The *heavy arrow* points to the location of Pit-1 monomer and the *light arrow* to the dimer.

ing Pit-1–binding sites from human renin and growth hormone genes formed quite different complexes, reflecting the predominance of Pit-1 to bind the renin sequence as a monomer and the growth hormone sequence as a dimer (Fig. 4). Titration experiments showed that Pit-1 formed both monomers and dimers on the hRen sequence, as has been previously described for binding to other sites (48), although the higher affinity of the hGH sequence for Pit-1 resulted in greater dimer formation than was observed with the hRen site. Despite these differences, limited proteolysis by staphylococcus V8 protease resulted in a complex of identical mobility between the two different binding sites, suggesting that the same factor binds these two sequences (Fig. 4). Taken

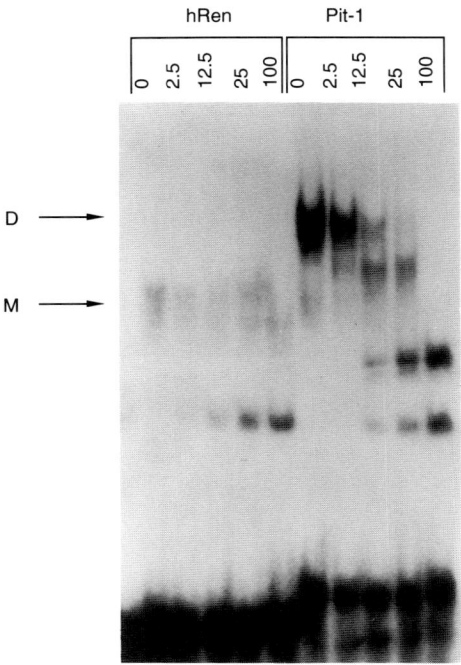

hRen   Pit-1

D →

M →

FIG. 4. Proteolytic clipping bandshift assay of complexes formed on hRen and Pit-1 oligonucleotides. The hRen oligonucleotide is shown in Fig. 3. The Pit-1 oligonucleotide is the same as the sequence labeled hGH in Fig. 3. Numbers above each lane indicate the relative amount of staphylococcus V8 protease added to the extract. Arrows show monomer (M) and dimer (D) formed with each probe. Nuclear extract was from GC cells.

together with the results of gel mobility shift competition experiments, these observations strongly suggested that Pit-1 binds the hRen −80/−58 sequence.

Renin Promoter Activity in GC Pituitary Cells

Because renin is expressed in pituitary cells *in vivo,* the observation that the human renin gene promoter is able to bind Pit-1 prompted studies to examine its activity by transfection of hybrid renin-luciferase genes into a pituitary cell line. GC cells were chosen because they are most closely related to lactosomatotrope precursor cells of the developing pituitary. Although GC cells do not express the endogenous renin gene, this may reflect species-specific differences in the sites of renin gene expression, as rats, from which GC cells are derived, appear to express renin in gonadotrope (33,35). Because the human renin gene is expressed in lactotrope cells (32,34), GC cells might contain the transcription factors necessary and sufficient for lactotrope-specific expression of the human renin gene.

Human renin 5′-flanking DNA sequences from −3,000 to +18 were inserted into the expression vector

pZ*luc,* which consists of a pGEM-based luciferase expression vector containing a polyadenylation cassette trimer upstream of the polylinker region to terminate transcripts originating in the vector (49). This important feature of the luciferase expression vector reduces background to essentially zero, thus permitting low-level promoter activity to be assessed. Figure 5 shows the renin 5′-flanking DNA fragments that were tested and the position within these fragments of the conserved sequences shown in Fig. 2. The most active construct contained hRen sequences −148/+18. The activity of this construction was two to three orders of magnitude above background expression from the promoterless pZ*luc* expression vector.

Deletion of sequences between −3,000 and −148 increased activity up to 20-fold, the greatest change resulting when sequences −3,000/−900 were deleted. Additional increases in activity were observed on deletion of sequences −314/−229 and −229/−148, suggesting that negative control elements are contained in these regions. The low activity of the −323 construct may be caused by deletion of positive control elements in the region −448/−323.

Deletion of sequences downstream of −148 led to sharp reductions in activity. Deletion to −98 reduced activity two- to threefold, suggesting that sequences containing between −148 and −98 contribute to activity. Further deletion to −65, which eliminated the Pit-1–binding site, led to an additional four- to fivefold reduction, the greatest effect on relative activity of any construction. Deletion to −34, which lies immediately upstream of the TATA box, further reduced activity to a level only slightly greater than the promoterless vector pZ*luc.*

Constructions containing mutations that reduced Pit-1 binding (see Fig. 3, Δ1 and Δ2) were also tested to examine the contribution of the Pit-1 site to promoter activity in GC cells. The activities of these constructions (−148Δ1 hRen.luc and −98Δ2 hRen.luc) were reduced approximately fivefold, relative to their counterparts containing the native Pit-1–binding site. These observations suggested that the Pit-1–binding site is the principal determinant of renin promoter activity in GC cells. Further, the finding that the activity of the −148Δ1 hRen.luc was lower than that of the −98 construct suggests that the positive effects of sequences −148/−98 requires the presence of Pit-1.

Coexpression of Pit-1 Activates the Renin Promoter in HeLa Cells

The corollary of the type of experiment described above is to test the activity of hRen.luc hybrid genes in a cell line that does not contain Pit-1, such as HeLa. The effect of Pit-1 can then be assessed by cotransfecting an

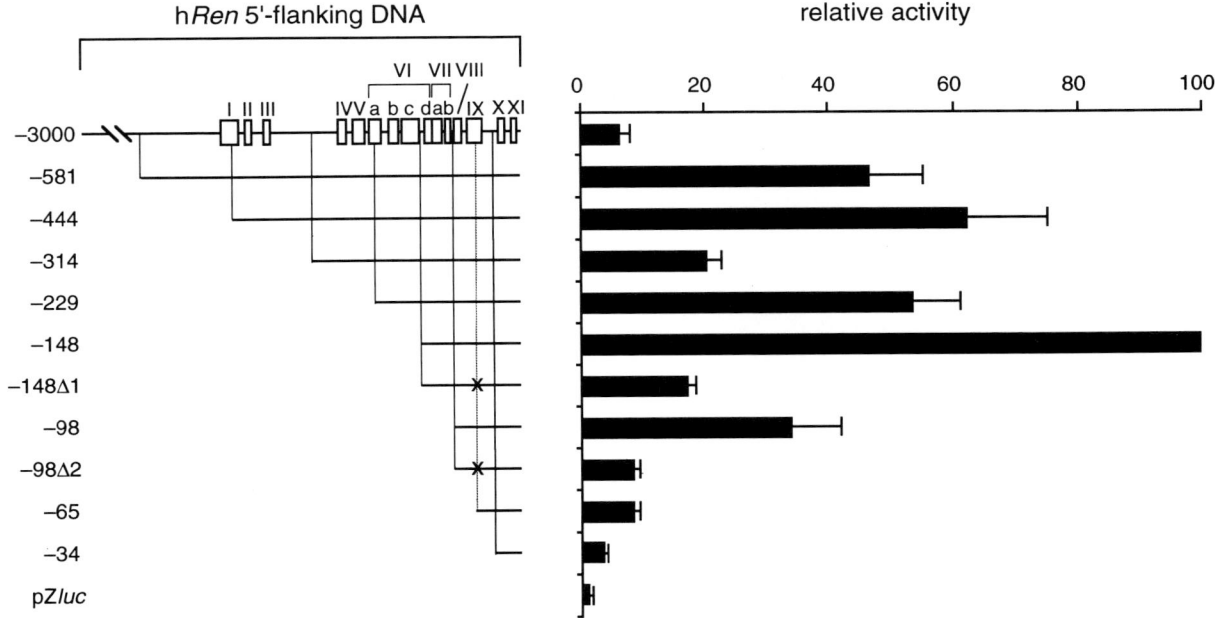

FIG. 5. Activity of hybrid genes containing human renin 5'-flanking DNA sequences linked to luciferase transfected into GC cells. The 5'-end of the human renin 5'-flanking DNA contained in each construction is shown at the *left. Blocks* drawn on the top line indicate the conserved sequences shown in Fig. 2. Transfection was carried out by lipofection (49), and the cells harvested for assay after 48 hours. Results shown are for two separate experiments containing duplicate transfections.

expression vector containing the Pit-1 coding sequences. In the absence of coexpressed Pit-1, the activities of −148 h*Ren.luc* and −148Δ1 h*Ren.luc* were virtually identical, suggesting that the Pit-1 site does not contribute to the low-level expression observed in these cells. However, when Pit-1 was cotransfected, the activity of −148 h*Ren.luc* increased fivefold, whereas the activity of −148Δ1 h*Ren.luc* actually decreased two- to threefold. This reduction in activity was most likely caused by competition for transcription factors by the strong Rous sarcoma virus (RSV) promoter/enhancer. Luciferase activities similar to those obtained with −148 h*Ren.luc* were observed when Pit-1 was coexpressed with a construction containing human chorionic somatomammotropin (h*CS*) sequences −127/+4. Because both h*Ren* and h*CS* (38) constructs contain a single Pit-1 site, these data suggest that Pit-1 binding has a similar effect on the activity of these two promoters. Accordingly, these two constructions yielded similar activities when transfected into GC cells (see Fig. 9 and accompanying text).

POU-Related Transcription Factors and Renin Gene Expression

Taken together, the results of mobility shift assays and transfection experiments strongly suggest that Pit-1 activates the human renin promoter by binding to a specific recognition sequence centered approximately at position −70. Although it is not known whether Pit-1 is involved

in directing pituitary expression of the endogenous renin gene, our findings raise the possibility that other members of the POU family of transcription factors may direct renin gene expression in other tissues.

Among the various sites of renin expression, kidneys and testes express two members of the POU family of transcription factors, Brn-1 and Tst-1, respectively. The POU-specific and POU-homeodomain sequences of Brn-1 and Tst-1, which together with Brn-2 constitute the POU-III group of transcription factors, are highly identical, suggesting that these factors bind similar sequences (50). The binding site consensus sequence for Tst-1, and presumably for these other factors, matches the renin Pit-1–binding site at 7/8 positions. Although expressed predominantly in the central nervous system early in development, expression of these factors in renin-producing tissues occurs at approximately the same time as renin (embryonal day 16 of the mouse) (51). Although Tst-1 and its homologues SCIP and Oct-6 have been shown to act as repressors of Po expression in Schwann cells (41), positive effects on promoters containing the octamer-binding site have also been reported (52). Although members of the POU family of transcription factors such as Brn-1 and Tst-1 may be involved in the regulation of renin expression in kidney and testes, related factors might also be involved. Such distant relationships exist with the homeobox proteins, which are homologous to the POU family in the DNA-binding domain and bind similar AT-rich sites (53). Thus, for example, a JG cell-specific factor might be more closely related to the Hox family than to the POU family of transcription factors. Without resorting to the extensive purification and cloning strategies that were required to identify Pit-1 and some of the other archetypal members of the POU family, a factor that might be found to bind the renin Pit-1 site could be identified using PCBA (described above) to compare the DNA-binding peptide fragments produced from POU and homeodomain proteins produced by recombinant DNA methods.

PLACENTAL RENIN

Renin is present at high concentrations in amniotic fluid (54) and has been detected either enzymatically or immunocytochemically in both chorion laeve (55,56) and amnion (57). Renin has also been found in cultures of chorion laeve (55,58,59) and myometrial tissue (60) but not amnion cells (58). However, a recent study (61) challenged the view that renin is expressed in chorionic tissues, suggesting that contaminating decidua cells are responsible for activity. The principal evidence presented for the lack of renin activity in chorion cells was the absence of renin or renin mRNA in intertwin chorion (which is devoid of decidua) and the secretion of renin from decidua cells placed in culture after removal from sites of ectopic pregnancies. Although the exact cell type that synthesizes placental renin is unknown, the presence of high concentrations of renin mRNA in these tissues (61) and primary cell cultures derived from these tissues (62) demonstrate their ability to synthesize renin actively. These cells appear to express high levels of prorenin through several passages (59). Moreover, placental cell cultures are the only untransformed cell culture systems that express the renin gene.

Duncan et al. (62) made use of primary cultures of decidua to study renin gene expression at the level of endogenous renin mRNA accumulation. They also examined the activity of transfected renin gene promoter constructs. Their studies indicated that placental renin expression and secretion are regulated by forskolin, the effect of which is potentiated by both calcium ionophore and phorbol esters. Sequences contained within 100 bp upstream of the transcription startsite were shown to mediate this pattern of regulation. However, the elements involved were not further delineated. These studies support the results of earlier experiments involving transfection of hybrid promoters containing human renin 5'-flanking sequences linked to the herpes simplex virus thymidine kinase (HSV-TK) promoter into non–renin-producing cells. Cyclic AMP–responsive elements were identified in both mouse and human renin 5'-flanking DNA sequences (63,64) and localized in the human renin gene 5'-flanking DNA sequence to the region −149/+13 (63) (see below). Similar studies on the activity of renin/TK hybrid promoters in choriocarcinoma cells

suggested that negative elements contained in the renin 5'-flanking DNA contribute to the cell specificity of renin gene expression (28,64). However, because the effects were small, the relevance of these findings is unclear. The use of choriocarcinoma cell lines to study renin gene expression is further discussed below.

Renin Promoter Activity in Placental Cell Cultures

Transfection experiments were performed to further characterize renin promoter activity in placental cells (Sun J, Oddoux C, Yan Y, and Catanzaro DF, *unpublished data*). Secondary cultures of both chorion laeve and decidua were transfected with selected renin-luciferase hybrid genes using the calcium phosphate method (65) (Fig. 6). In these experiments, activities were normalized to pRSV.luc transfected in parallel dishes. Although the overall activity differed approximately 10-fold between chorion laeve and decidua cells, the relative activities of h*Ren.luc* constructions were similar between placental cell preparations and resembled the pattern of activities observed in GC cells (31), suggesting that common promoter elements are involved. Accordingly, mutagenesis or deletion of the Pit-1–binding site markedly reduced activity (Fig. 6).

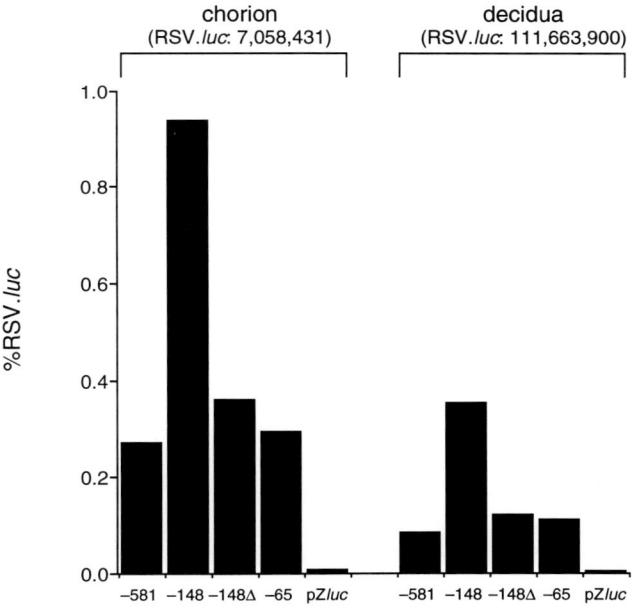

FIG. 6. Activity of hybrid genes containing human renin 5'-flanking DNA sequences linked to luciferase transfected into cultures of chorion laeve and decidua cells. Constructions are as shown in Fig. 5. Transfections were carried out using the calcium phosphate method on 60-mm dishes of each cell preparation at approximately 50 percent confluence. Cells were harvested for assay 48 hours post-transfection. pRSV.luc, which contains the Rous sarcoma virus long terminal repeat, was transfected in parallel, and the data were normalized to the activity of this construct.

Binding of Placental Nuclear Factor(s) to the h*Ren* Pit-1 Site

Nuclear extracts prepared from chorion laeve placental cell cultures were found to contain factors that bind the h*Ren* Pit-1 site. Figure 7 shows the results of mobility shift assays carried out using the h*Ren* Pit-1–binding site as the probe (see Fig. 3) and nuclear extracts from either GC cells, chorion laeve, or decidua cells at various passage numbers. Nuclear extracts from both chorion laeve and decidua cells nuclear resulted in a single band that ran between the monomer and dimer forms of the Pit-1 complex formed with GC cell nuclear extract. This would suggest the presence of a placental cell nuclear factor, different from Pit-1, capable of binding the h*Ren* Pit-1 site. Interestingly, nuclear extracts from later passages, where renin gene expression was reduced (as judged by the rate of prorenin secretion into the media), exhibited proportionally lower formation of this complex. Taken together with the results of transfection experiments described above, these findings suggest that the Pit-1 site and its cognate factor(s) are important in driving renin gene expression in placental cells. However, the cell cultures used in these experiments are relatively heterogeneous. Therefore, it remains to be proved that the factor

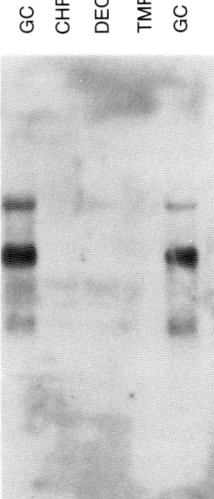

FIG. 8. Northern blot analysis of total cellular RNA from cultures of chorion (*CHR*) and decidua (*DEC*) and from renin-secreting renal tumor cells (*TMR*).

causing the gel shift is actually expressed in renin-expressing cells.

Northern Blot Analysis of POU Gene Expression in Renin-Expressing Tissues

Further studies were carried out to determine whether Pit-1–related sequences are expressed in placental cell cultures; RNA was prepared from chorion laeve and decidua cell primary cultures and subjected to Northern blot analysis using a Pit-1 probe. RNA from GC cells that express the endogenous Pit-1 gene was included as a positive control. Because sequences of the DNA-binding domain of the POU family are highly conserved, this region of the Pit-1 cDNA was used as the probe. Figure 8 shows the results of such a Northern blot analysis carried out at low stringency conditions under which sequences with as little as 50 percent identity to the POU-DNA–binding domain would be expected to bind the probe. Although RNA from GC cells that express high levels of Pit-1 showed a strong band of the expected size, RNA from both chorion laeve and decidua cell cultures showed only very weak hybridization with the probe. Although this might indicate that a POU family factor is expressed at low levels, the intensity of the band observed in gel mobility shift assays with chorion laeve nuclear extracts (described above) suggested that the factor involved is highly abundant. Therefore, it seems more likely that the placental cell factor that binds the h*Ren* Pit-1 site is only distantly related to Pit-1. Because several related factors also bind the Pit-1 site, one of these could account for the observed gel shift and direct renin expression in placental cells.

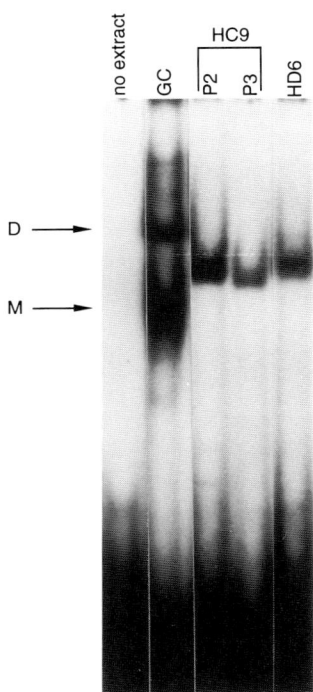

FIG. 7. Gel mobility shift analysis of nuclear factor binding to the human renin Pit-1 site. The h*Ren* oligonucleotide (see Fig. 3) was used as the probe. Nuclear extracts were from GC cells, human chorion (*HC*), and human decidua (*HD*) cell cultures. *P2* and *P3* denote the passage number of the HC culture, whereas HD was secondary culture (*P2*). *M* and *D* indicate monomer and dimer bands.

RENIN EXPRESSION IN HUMAN CHORIOCARCINOMA AND EMBRYONAL KIDNEY CELL LINES

Several studies have suggested that choriocarcinoma cell lines such as JEG-3 may express their endogenous renin genes and be useful in transfection experiments to study renin promoter activity. An early report (63) using hybrid genes containing the native human renin promoter suggested that 892 bp of human renin 5'-flanking DNA directs expression in JEG-3 cells but not in several other non–renin-expressing cell lines. Further studies using hybrid genes containing fragments of renin 5'-flanking DNA sequences linked to the HSV-TK gene were also carried out using JEG-3 cells (64). More recently, the human embryonal kidney cell line 293 has been used in transfection experiments in which the mouse $Ren-1^c$ 5'-flanking DNA sequences were found to be active in directing expression of a linked CAT reporter gene (66). Moreover, the latter study showed that a 293-cell-specific factor bound the Pit-1 site. However, activation by this element was found to be weak unless a sequence contained within the 476-bp insertion specific to mouse renin genes was also present (see Fig. 1).

To determine whether the choriocarcinoma cell lines BeWo, JEG, and JAR might provide a useful system to study renin gene expression, these cells were tested for expression of the endogenous renin gene, and transfection experiments were carried out to determine whether these cells are able to use human renin promoter sequences. Renin activity and prorenin were assayed in culture media from these cells. No renin activity, either before or after trypsin treatment, was detectable in media from these cultures, suggesting that they secrete neither renin nor prorenin. Analysis of choriocarcinoma cell RNA using a highly sensitive ribonuclease protection assay also failed to detect any evidence of renin mRNA. After 1-week autoradiography, which revealed human actin mRNA sequences in as little as 0.01 μg RNA, no renin-specific bands were evident with up to 10 μgRNA (Gilbert MT, Oddoux C, and Catanzaro DF, *unpublished observations*).

Transfection experiments were also conducted to see whether, even in the absence of endogenous renin gene expression, choriocarcinoma or embryonal kidney cells may be able to use renin promoter sequences. Such phenomena are well known, as, for example, in the case of pituitary GC cells that express little endogenous prolactin but efficiently use prolactin promoter and enhancer elements (37). In parallel transfection experiments, the activities of -585 h$Ren.luc$ relative to $RSV.luc$ were 0.06 percent in BeWo cells, 0.3 percent in both JEG-3 and 293 cells, and 2.5 percent in JAR cells. Although relatively high, the activity observed in JAR cells was not affected by deletion of sequences upstream of -38. Although it cannot be ruled out that cell-specific elements

are contained downstream of -38, generally, promoter elements in genes transcribed by RNA polymerase II are found upstream of the TATA box. Moreover, mutations in the Pit-1–binding site had no effect on activity in any of these cell lines. Similar effects were observed for the low expression in 293 cells. Thus, the activity of the mouse $Ren-1^c$ promoter in 293 cells requires sequences that are not found in the hRen 5'-flanking DNA, most likely the 476-bp element inserted at position -80. Therefore, the transcription of hRen hybrid genes observed in these cell cultures reflects basal activity of RNA polymerase, which is only minimally affected by promoter elements outside the TATA box. Taken together with the lack of endogenous renin gene activity, these observations suggest that neither choriocarcinoma nor 293 embryonal kidney cell lines provide useful model systems to study the cell specificity of renin gene expression.

CULTURE SYSTEMS OF RENAL JUXTAGLOMERULAR CELLS

The recent development of a renal renin-expressing cell line (23) has provided a powerful new tool with which to study the molecular biology of renin gene expression. As4.1 cells were produced by targeted tumorigenesis in transgenic mice using mouse renin ($Ren-2$) 5'-flanking DNA sequences linked to the SV 40 T antigen (23). Although their origin has yet to be unequivocally established as JG cells, the renin promoter fragment used to drive expression of T antigen in the transgenic mice directs expression specifically to JG cells. Moreover, these cells constitutively secrete prorenin and process prorenin to renin, which is stored in granules and secreted in response to increases in intracellular cyclic AMP. Because JG cells are the only known site of renin processing, the cell specificity of the $Ren-2$ promoter driving T-antigen expression and the close resemblance of renin synthesis and secretion between As4.1 and renal JG cells suggest that these cells are indeed of JG origin.

Sigmund and coworkers (19) examined the ability of mouse renin 5'-flanking DNA sequences to direct the expression of a linked CAT reporter gene transfected into As4.1 cells. These studies showed that sequences extending to -1.8 kb upstream of the transcription startsite possess only weak promoter activity. However, a segment of $Ren-1^c$ 5'-flanking DNA extending to -4.1 kb stimulated CAT activity approximately 12-fold in As4.1 cells but had no effect in the renin nonproducing L cell line. Further studies showed that $Ren-1^c$ sequences between -4.1 and -2.6 exert cell-specific enhancer activity when linked to more proximal 5'-flanking DNA sequences ($-117/+6$) fused to CAT.

In collaboration with Dr. Gross's group (19), we showed that the human renin 5'-flanking DNA sequences −148/+18 are less active than the corresponding mouse *Ren-1ᶜ* sequences (−117/+6) described above (see Fig. 2) (Gilbert MT, Yan Y, Sun J, and Catanzaro DF, *unpublished observations*). Although the activity of the human renin promoter in these cells was low, mutations in the Pit-1 site that abolished Pit-1 binding reduced activity, suggesting that this site is important for renin promoter activity in JG cells.

ENHANCER ELEMENTS IN THE RENIN GENE

Transfection experiments, using several renin-expressing cell culture systems described above, indicate that the promoter activity of human renin 5′-flanking DNA, encompassing sequences up to 3 kb upstream of the transcription startsite, is relatively weak. In both primary cultures of human placental cells and renin-secreting mouse renal tumor cells, the activity of the most active 5′-flanking DNA fragment was less than 1 percent that of the Rous sarcoma virus long terminal repeat (RSV LTR) (a strong ubiquitously active promoter). Similarly, in GC cells, in which renin promoter activity is dependent on binding of the pituitary-specific factor Pit-1, the activity of the renin promoter was also less than 1 percent that of the RSV LTR.

The weak promoter activity of renin 5′-flanking sequences was also evident in experiments using transgenic mice. Although the mouse *Ren-2* gene containing 2.5 kb of 5′-flanking DNA was sufficient to direct cell-specific renin gene expression in transgenic mice (67), the same 2.5-kb region did not confer cell specificity when linked to a reporter gene (68). However, in agreement with the results of transfection experiments described above, 4.6 kb of *Ren-2* 5′-flanking DNA confers both cell and tissue specificity to the same reporter (17). Studies of human renin gene expression in transgenic animals further showed that as little as 0.9 kb 5′-flanking DNA was required for cell-specific expression when coding and intervening sequences were also present (18,69). These data were interpreted to suggest that sequences that contribute to cell specificity are contained downstream of the transcription startsite, although, at least in the case of the mouse *Ren-2* gene, these may be substituted for by sequences farther upstream in the 5′-flanking DNA (18).

An alternative explanation for the effect of renin-coding sequences on renin gene expression in transgenic mice is that renin mRNA is highly stable and accumulates despite a very weak promoter. Several clinical and experimental observations support this contention. First, prorenin levels change slowly, despite sometimes quite marked changes in plasma renin activity (PRA) (4). Because prorenin is secreted constitutively from renal JG cells, plasma prorenin levels provide a good indication of the rate of renin gene expression. This is consistent with the ongoing translation of a stable mRNA. Second, acute experimental treatments that affect PRA in animal models have often been found to result in much smaller effects on renal renin mRNA levels (27). Third, acute experimental treatments that lead to increased PRA and increased renal renin mRNA content appear to bring about recruitment of afferent arteriolar vascular smooth muscle cells to express renin. For example, treatment with ACE inhibitors resulted in the appearance of renin mRNA in regions of the afferent arteriole more distal to the glomerulus (70), resembling the pattern of renin expression in the fetus in which renin is expressed widely in the renal vasculature (51,70). Although the exact interrelationships between cell number, renin mRNA content, and renin secretion have yet to be determined, this, together with the modest rise in total kidney renin mRNA content, would suggest that chronic stimulation of the RAS results in recruitment of smooth muscle cells rather than increasing the rate at which individual renin genes are transcribed.

Studies have yet to be carried out to determine the effect of renin genomic sequences on cell-specific expression. If renin genomic sequences contain an enhancer activity, then addition of genomic fragments to hybrid genes containing renin 5′-flanking DNA sequences should lead to the cell-specific stimulation of expression. If, however, mechanisms of mRNA stability are involved, it should be possible to replace renin genomic sequences with the corresponding renin cDNA sequences, yet retain cell-specific expression in transgenic mice.

HORMONAL REGULATION OF RENIN RELEASE AND SYNTHESIS

The physiological importance of the renin-angiotensin-aldosterone system has stimulated considerable research into the mechanisms that regulate renin release from JG cells. At the extracellular level, renin secretion is regulated by sodium (or chloride) delivery to the macula densa (71), stretch of the afferent arteriole (72), beta-adrenergic stimulation (73,74), AII (75), and other vasoactive compounds including atrial natriuretic factor (ANF), prostaglandins (20), endothelium-derived relaxing factor (EDRF) (76), and parathyroid hormone (PTH) (77,78). At the intracellular level, renin release is stimulated by cyclic AMP and inhibited by cyclic guanosine monophosphate (GMP) and calcium ion (79–81). Unlike many other proteins whose secretion is stimulated by calcium, the negative effect of calcium appears to be specific to the secretion of renin and PTH (21). Recent studies suggest that this so-called calcium paradox is caused by unusual calcium-activated ion channels on renin- and PTH-secreting cells (21). In the case of JG cells, calcium-activated chloride channels may regulate renin release through changes in cell volume, either directly (21) or through the formation of a myofilament shield that prevents the fusion of secretory granules with the plasma membrane (82). Although these negative effects of calcium ion have not always been observed, a crucial role for calcium has been implicated in many mechanisms of renin release. For example, AII may inhibit renin release by calcium ion and C kinase (83), and PTH may stimulate renin release by preventing calcium influx (77). Similarly, beta-adrenergic stimulation of renin release associated with an increase in intracellular cyclic AMP (84) may be caused by calcium efflux promoted by the rise in cyclic AMP (83). However, cyclic GMP–dependent mechanisms such as those subserving ANF and EDRF appear to be independent of both calcium and cyclic AMP (80).

Although it is not known how a cell determines how much of a stored protein needs to be synthesized, the second messengers, which regulate renin secretion, may also regulate renin gene expression, thus providing a way to replenish cytoplasmic granules depleted by secretion. This would require a mechanism so finely tuned that the second messenger that caused secretion led to the synthesis of exactly the right amount of protein to replace that which was secreted. Alternatively, an intracellular feedback mechanism might sense the amount of protein present in storage granules or released from the cell and direct the activity of the transcriptional machinery accordingly. Such mechanisms might also coexist and operate in concert. Further controls might operate at the level of sorting between the regulated and constitutive pathways (see chapter 97 by Tim Reudelhuber, *this volume*). Also, other hormones could regulate renin gene expression without directly affecting secretion of active renin. Regulation at this level would modulate the rate of prorenin secretion by the constitutive pathway. Defects in any of these regulatory mechanisms could lead to oversecretion and contribute to the development of hypertension.

Studies of Renal Renin Regulation *In Vivo*

Consistent with the mechanisms that are known to regulate renin secretion, most animal studies have found that renal renin mRNA levels increase after feeding a low-sodium diet or treatment with ACE inhibitors and decrease after feeding a high-sodium diet or administration of AII (reviewed in ref. 85). Although changes in renal renin mRNA levels parallel changes in PRA, changes in renal renin mRNA levels are often much smaller than the corresponding changes in PRA (86,87), indicating perhaps that post-transcriptional mechanisms are also involved.

Renin and renin mRNA levels have also been measured in rat models of experimental hypertension. These studies have generally revealed changes consistent with the physiology of the experimental model. In volume-dependent hypertension (DOCA + salt model), PRA is suppressed by the high blood pressure, and renal renin mRNA levels decrease markedly (88). However, in aortic coarction and in the two-kidney, one-clip model (2K1C) of renal hypertension, PRA and renal renin mRNA are usually increased in the ischemic kidney and decreased in the contralateral kidney (89,90). In one of these studies (89), however, the changes in renin mRNA levels reverted to near-normal levels after 14 days. A recent study (91) also reported a transient increase in renin mRNA in the clipped kidney. However, renin mRNA levels in the contralateral kidney exhibited a sustained decrease. This suppression of renin gene expression in the contralateral kidney was found to be independent of compensatory renal growth, blood pressure, AII AT$_1$ receptors, or renal nerves. The authors suggested that an unknown humoral factor might suppress renin gene expression in the contralateral kidney of 2K1C rats.

In spontaneously hypertensive rats (SHR), renin or renin mRNA levels were found not to differ greatly from the normotensive Wistar-Kyoto (WKY) control rats (92). However, in the SHR stroke-prone strain (SHRsp) (93) and Dahl salt-sensitive rats (94), high-salt feeding caused a large paradoxical increase in PRA, which accelerated the development of strokes and other vascular injuries (93).

Studies on the Regulation of Renin Gene Expression in Cell Culture Systems

The lack of renin-expressing cell lines has also hindered studies on the hormonal regulation of renin gene expression. However, GC cells, in which the renin promoter was found to be active, appear to regulate the expression of growth hormone genes in response to several physiological effectors (thyroid hormone, cyclic AMP, and phorbol esters). Therefore, this cell line provides a useful model system in which to study hormonal regulation of renin gene expression. Because studies on renin promoter activity in pituitary, placental, and JG cells suggest that common promoter elements may function in different tissues, GC cells may contain many of the common transcription factors that interact with these sites. These transcription factors are likely to include ones that respond to extracellular signals, either by interacting directly with lipid-soluble hormones or through post-translational modifications mediated by second messengers. Indeed, Pit-1 has been implicated in hormonal regulation of growth hormone gene expression through both protein kinase A– and C–dependent mechanisms (95). At the molecular level, Pit-1 has been shown to be a substrate for phosphorylation by both of these kinases. Thus, as demonstrated for several different transcription factors [e.g., CREB (30)], phosphorylation of Pit-1 could modulate transcriptional regulation of pituitary renin in response to extracellular signals. Pit-1–related factors that have been implicated in the transcriptional regulation of renin gene expression in JG and placental cells might also mediate responsiveness to extracellular signals through similar mechanisms.

Transfection experiments were carried out to investigate the hormonal regulation of renin gene expression in GC cells (Gilbert MT, Sun J, Oddoux C, Lazarus, Yan Y, and Catanzaro DF, *in preparation*). In these experiments, 148 h*Ren.luc,* −148Δ1 h*Ren.luc,* and, as a positively regulated control, −127 h*CS.luc* (38) were transfected into GC cells. The h*CS.luc* construct was selected because it contains a single Pit-1 site and has similar activity to the h*Ren.luc* construct. The activity of the hCS promoter is also positively regulated by both thyroid hormone and cyclic AMP (38,96).

In these experiments (Fig. 9), the highest stimulated activities of h*Ren* and h*CS* constructs were 1 percent and 3 percent of *RSV.luc,* respectively. Whereas triiodothyronine (T_3) had only a small effect on the activity of h*Ren* constructs, T_3 stimulated expression of the h*CS* con-

struct approximately 12-fold. Forskolin, which increases intracellular cyclic AMP levels, stimulated the activity of the native h*Ren* promoter construct sevenfold and had a smaller (fivefold) effect on the h*CS* construct. Although the mutation in the Pit-1 site reduced activity greater than 10-fold, it also reduced the induction by forskolin to about twofold. When T_3 and forskolin were applied together, their effects were additive for the h*CS* construct but antagonistic for the native h*Ren* construct. However, the forskolin-stimulated activity of the mutant h*Ren* promoter construct was not affected by T_3. These findings show that in GC cells h*Ren* promoter activity is regulated by cyclic AMP and is dependent on the Pit-1 site. Moreover, this Pit-1–dependent cyclic AMP regulation appeared to be modulated by thyroid hormone. In the absence of a direct effect of T_3, the negative effect on cyclic AMP–stimulated activity could be caused by some indirect effect such as down-regulation of Pit-1 by thyroid hormone or some post-translational modification that affects either the ability of Pit-1 to bind DNA or its ability to interact with other components of the transcriptional machinery.

Western blot and mobility shift analyses were carried out to determine the effects of hormone treatment on Pit-1 levels and DNA binding. Nuclear extracts from GC cells treated with the various hormones were fractionated by sodium dodecyl sulfate (SDS) polyacrylamide gel electrophoresis and the proteins transferred to a nitrocellulose membrane by electroblotting. Pit-1 levels were determined by immunodetection, using an affinity purified rabbit polyclonal antibody (a generous gift of Dr. Carter Bancroft, Mount Sinai Medical College). Bound antibody was detected by an enzyme-linked chemiluminescence assay and visualized by autoradiography. DNA binding of Pit-1 was determined using a gel mobility shift assay, as described above. Relative levels of Pit-1 and Pit-1 DNA binding were determined by densitometry.

Whereas forskolin had no apparent effect on Pit-1 levels, T_3 lowered Pit-1 levels approximately twofold. Similar results were found when Pit-1 binding was assessed in a gel mobility shift assay, suggesting that differential modification of Pit-1 does not affect its binding to either the h*Ren* or h*CS* sequences. Although these findings do not rule out the possibility that some T_3-mediated post-translational modification of Pit-1 differentially affects its ability to stimulate h*Ren* and h*CS* promoter activities, the effects on Pit-1 levels appear to be sufficient to account for the reduction in h*Ren* promoter activity. The differential effect on h*Ren* and h*CS* promoters may be caused by the higher affinity of the h*CS* sequence for Pit-1 binding. However, Pit-1 may also interact with different factors on the h*Ren* and h*CS* promoters, leading to their different patterns of hormone responsiveness.

Because the Pit-1 site appears to be involved in directing renin gene expression to several different tissues including kidney and placenta, the factors interacting with

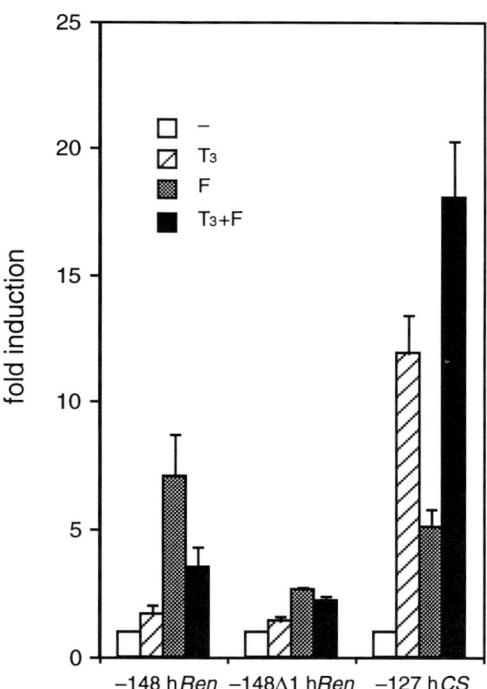

FIG. 9. Regulation of human renin promoter activity in GC cells by thyroid hormone and cyclic AMP. Data are normalized to the activity of the promoterless vector p*Zluc,* which was induced 1.3-, 1.7-, and 1.7-fold by T_3, forskolin, and T_3 + forskolin, respectively. Before transfection, cells were maintained for 48 hours in hormone-depleted medium. After transfection, forskolin and T_3 were added singly or in combination for 48 hours, after which the cells were harvested for assay of luciferase activity or preparation of nuclear proteins for gel shift and Western blot analyses.

this site in these tissues may also be involved in hormonal regulation. Mutations affecting these factors could lead to inappropriate control of renin expression, and thus, the genes encoding these transcription factors represent important candidate genes in the etiology of hypertension.

Although in the experiments described above the effect of T_3 appeared to be indirect, gel mobility shift analyses identified at least five separate thyroid hormone receptor-binding sites between -148 and $+14$. This would suggest either that GC cells lack some factor necessary to transmit the effects of thyroid hormone receptor to RNA polymerase on the h*Ren* promoter or that the receptor-binding sites are not appropriately aligned or distributed to transmit such a positive effect. In mouse renin-expressing renal tumor cells, renin expression increases 9- to 16-fold when serum is withdrawn (19). Because normal fetal bovine serum contains thyroid hormone at concentrations near the K_D for binding to thyroid hormone receptors, withdrawal of serum may derepress transcription through a thyroid hormone–dependent mechanism. It remains to be determined whether this serum responsiveness of the renin gene in As4.1 cells is caused by thyroid hormone and, if so, whether the effect is direct or indirect.

THYROID HORMONE REGULATION OF RENIN GENE EXPRESSION *IN VIVO*

In the hyperthyroid state, increases in cardiac output and blood volume are offset by a decrease in peripheral vascular resistance, and blood pressure falls. Conversely, in the hypothyroid state, despite decreased cardiac output and blood volume, increased peripheral vascular resistance leads to an increase in blood pressure. Although such changes in peripheral resistance could be mediated by the RAS, studies of both humans (97–99) and animals (100–105) have generally found PRA to be positively correlated with thyroid status, the opposite of what would be required for the effects observed. This has led to the conclusion that hypertension associated with hypothyroidism is characterized by low renin levels. A comprehensive discussion of the role of thyroid hormones in hypertension is to be found in the chapter by Irwin Klein.

The molecular findings described above, which suggest that renin gene expression is negatively regulated by thyroid hormones, prompted a review of clinical data to examine the effects of thyroid status on renin biosynthesis. A study of borderline-to-mild hypertensives showed that plasma prorenin levels are inversely related to salt sensitivity (106). Because prorenin is secreted constitutively, plasma prorenin levels provide a better index of renin biosynthesis than measurements of PRA that were examined in previous studies. Among the hypertensive patients whose blood pressure was resistant to changes in dietary salt [salt-resistant (SR)], a statistically significant negative correlation was found between prorenin levels and free thyroxine (T_4) index measured on a medium-salt diet (Pecker MS and Catanzaro DF, *unpublished observations*). Similar trends were also observed in the salt-sensitive (SS) group, although these correlations were not statistically significant.

Although the observations described above suggest that thyroid hormones may indeed suppress renin gene expression, it is necessary to reconcile this negative effect on synthesis with the positive effect thyroid hormones appear to exert on renin release.

One possible mechanism involves beta-adrenergic mechanisms that have frequently been implicated in the control of renin release by thyroid hormones. Thus, hypothyroid patients with low-renin hypertension exhibited decreased sensitivity to catecholamines (107); beta-adrenergic inhibition with propranolol reduced basal levels of AI and PRA, prevented the increase in plasma renin concentration in hyperthyroid rats (104), and returned PRA and serum aldosterone to normal after increases produced by administration of T_3 (101). These interactions between thyroid and adrenergic axes could occur in several ways. Because thyroid hormones increase adrenergic sensitivity by modulating the concentration of beta-adrenergic receptors in several tissues, most notably, in heart and kidney cortex (108,109), renin secretion may be at least transiently stimulated despite decreased synthesis. Propranolol and other membrane-stabilizing beta-blockers that are used to treat thyrotoxicosis are thought to act by inhibiting the peripheral conversion of T_4 to T_3 through a mechanism that appears to be independent of the direct beta-adrenergic antagonist activity of these drugs (110). Thus, drugs such as propranolol could have a twofold action on renin release: first, to block renal beta-adrenergic receptors; and second, to reduce their concentration indirectly through their effects on T_4 conversion. These mechanisms may explain the increase in plasma prorenin levels that are observed after administration of beta-blockers, despite the decreased plasma renin levels. Because T_3 also stimulates angiotensinogen secretion, changes in PRA may also be caused by changes in the levels of renin substrate. In animal studies, this appears to be influenced by the treatment used to induce hypothyroidism; one group (103,105) suggesting that propylthiouracil-induced hypothyroidism has a predominant effect on plasma renin concentration, whereas thyroidectomy exerts a greater effect on angiotensinogen levels. Clearly, the effects of thyroid hormones on renin synthesis and secretion are likely to be complex. Therefore, it will be essential to determine the effects of thyroid hormones on renin gene expression and the interrelationships of these mechanisms with other regulatory systems.

SUMMARY AND CONCLUSIONS

Our understanding of the mechanisms that direct renin gene expression is very much in its infancy. Unlike other genes such as growth hormone and globin for which established cell lines awaited the application of molecular approaches to the study the mechanisms directing their expression, the lack of renin-expressing cell lines has hampered the study of renin gene expression at a molecular level. Nevertheless, some recent progress has been made using pituitary cell lines and placental cell primary cultures. The recent development of a renal renin-expressing cell line through targeted tumorigenesis in transgenic mice has provided the long-awaited cell line, which should facilitate future studies.

Preliminary studies suggest that promoter activity of renin 5′-flanking sequences is very weak. However, common promoter elements appear to drive renin gene expression in pituitary, placental, and renal JG cells, as evidenced by the similar pattern of activities observed with various renin-luciferase hybrid gene constructions in cell culture systems derived from these different tissues. Among these common promoter elements is a site centered at about −70, which binds the pituitary-specific factor Pit-1. Pit-1 is a member of the POU family of transcription factors that belongs to the broader family of homeodomain proteins. Pit-1 binding to this site appears to be the strongest determinant of renin promoter activity in pituitary cells and also appears to be involved in the hormonal regulation of renin gene expression in these cells. Although an abundant factor binding to this site has also been identified in placental cells, Northern blot analysis of mRNA from renin-expressing placental cell cultures and a renin-secreting renal tumor indicates the absence of an abundant Pit-1 factor. This suggests that in renin-expressing placental and JG cells, renin gene expression is driven by more distantly related homeodomain proteins such as the Hox family of transcription factors.

Because the promoter activity of renin 5′-flanking sequences is low, some additional mechanism may account for the efficient expression of renin in JG cells. The level of renin gene expression achieved in renal JG cells may be caused by an enhancer located outside of the renin gene 5′-flanking DNA, possibly within structural or intervening regions of the gene. Alternatively, renin mRNA may be very stable and accumulate despite a weak promoter. However, these hypotheses have yet to be addressed experimentally.

Although inappropriate renin secretion is well known to be associated with hypertension, genetic studies have failed to link mutations in the renin gene with hypertension (111,112). This could be because the lesion is not at the level of the renin structural gene or indeed in the transcriptional regulatory sequences. Instead, the transcription factors that direct renin gene expression may contain structural mutations that affect their activity or regulatory mutations that affect their expression. Identification of the transcription factors that regulate renin gene expression will provide a deeper understanding of the mechanisms involved and provide new candidate genes for genetic studies on the molecular basis of hypertension.

ACKNOWLEDGMENTS

The work described in this chapter was supported by grants from the Mellon, Helmsley, Wallace, and Lounsberry Foundations, the Michael Wolk Heart Fund, a grant-in-aid from the American Heart Association, New York Chapter, and the NIH Hypertension SCOR.

REFERENCES

1. von Lutterotti N, Catanzaro DF, Sealey JE, Laragh JH. *Circulation* 1994;89:458–470.
2. Alderman MH, Madhavan S, OOi WI, Cohen H, Sealey JE, Laragh JH. *N Engl J Med* 1991;324:1098–1104.
3. Brunner HR, Laragh JH, Baer L, Newton MA, Goodwin FT, Krakoff LR. *N Engl J Med* 1972;286:441–449.
4. Sealey JE, Quimby FW, Itskovitz J, Rubattu S. *Frontiers in Neuroendocrinology.* 1990;11:213–237.
5. Sealey JE, von Lutterotti N, Rubattu S, et al. *Am J Hypertens* 1991;4:972–977.
6. Sealey JE, Campbell WG Jr, Ganhem F, Camargo MJF. *JASN* 1993;4:522.
7. Pinet F, Mizrahi J, Laboulandine I, Menard J, Corvol P. *J Clin Invest* 1987;80:724–731.
8. Sealey JE, Rubattu S. *Am J Hypertens* 1989;2:358–366.
9. Dynan WS. *Cell* 1989;58:1–4.
10. Ptashne M. *Nature* 1988;335:683–689.
11. Maniatis T, Goodbourn S, Fischer JA. *Science* 1987;236:1237–1244.
12. Gorman CM, Moffat LF, Howard BH. *Mol Cell Biol* 1982;2:1044–1051.
13. de Wet JR, Wood KV, De Luca M, Helinski DR, Subramani S. *Mol Cell Biol* 1987;7:725–737.
14. McKnight SL, Kingsbury R. *Science* 1982;217:316–324.
15. Ho SN, Hunt HD, Horton RM, Pullen JK, Pease LR. *Gene* 1989;77:51–59.
16. Kunkel TA, Roberts JB, Zakour RA. *Methods Enzymol* 1987;154:367–382.
17. Sigmund CD, Jones CA, Fabian JR, Mullins JJ, Gross KW. *Biochem Biophys Res Commun* 1990;170:344–350.
18. Sigmund CD, Jones CA, Kane CM, Wu C, Lang JA, Gross KW. *Circ Res* 1992;70:1070–1079.
19. Sigmund CD, Fabian JR, Gross KW. *Trends Cardiovasc Med* 1992;2:237–245.
20. Kurtz A, Della Bruna R, Pfeilschifter J, Taugner R, Bauer C. *Proc Natl Acad Sci USA* 1986;83:4769–4773.
21. Kurtz A, Penner R. *Proc Natl Acad Sci USA* 1989;86:3423–3427.
22. Johns DW, Carey RM, Gomez A, et al. *Hypertension* 1987;10:488–496.
23. Sigmund CD, Okuyama K, Ingelfinger J, et al. *J Biol Chem* 1990;265:19916–19922.
24. Mullins JJ, Burt DW, Windass JD, McTurk P, George H, Brammar W. *EMBO J* 1982;1:1461–1466.
25. Burnham CE, Hawelu-Johnson CL, Frank BM, Lynch KR. *Proc Natl Acad Sci USA* 1987;84:5605–5609.
26. Hardman JA, Hort YJ, Catanzaro DF, et al. *DNA* 1984;3:457–468.
27. Sigmund CD, Gross KW. *Hypertension* 1991;18:446–457.
28. Burt DW, Nakamura N, Kelley P, Dzau VJ. *J Biol Chem* 1989;264:7357–7362.
29. Lipkin SM, Naar AM, Kalla KA, Sack RA, Rosenfeld MG. *Genes Dev* 1993;7:1674–1687.

30. Nichols M, Weih F, Schmid W, et al. *EMBO J* 1992;11:3337–3346.
31. Sun J, Oddoux C, Lazarus A, Gilbert MT, Catanzaro DF. *J Biol Chem* 1993;268:1505–1508.
32. Kettani S, Beldent V, Rousselet MC, Ronco P, Verroust P, Saint AJ. *Histochemistry* 1991;95:561–566.
33. Naruse K, Takii Y, Inagami T. *Proc Natl Acad Sci USA* 1981;78:7579–7583.
34. Saint AJ, Rohmer V, Pinet F, Rousselet MC, Bigorgne JC, Corvol P. *Histochemistry* 1989;91:291–297.
35. Deschepper CF, Mellon SH, Cumin F, Baxter JD, Ganong WF. *Proc Natl Acad Sci USA* 1986;83:7552–7556.
36. Ganong WF. *Horm Res* 1989;31:24–31.
37. Jones GJ, Catanzaro DF. *Mol Endocrinol* 1991;5:1836–1844.
38. Tansey WP, Catanzaro DF. *J Biol Chem* 1991;266:9805–9813.
39. Ingraham HA, Chen R, Mangalam HJ, et al. *Cell* 1988;55:519–529.
40. Bodner M, Castrillo J, Theill LE, Deerinck T, Ellisman M, Karin M. *Cell* 1988;55:505–518.
41. Rosenfeld MG. *Genes Dev* 1991;5:897–907.
42. Nelson C, Albert VR, Elsholtz HP, Lu LI, Rosenfeld MG. *Science* 1988;239:1400–1405.
43. Elsholtz HP, Albert VR, Treacy MN, Rosenfeld MG. *Genes Dev* 1990;4:43–51.
44. Sharp ZD, Helsel S, Cao ZD, Barron EA, Sanchez Y. *Nucleic Acids Res* 1989;17:2705–2722.
45. Konzak KE, Moore DD. *Mol Endocrinol* 1992;6:241–247.
46. Morris AE, Kloss B, McChesney RE, Bancroft C, Chasin LA. *Nucleic Acids Res* 1992;20:1355–1361.
47. Schreiber E, Matthias P, Muller MM, Schaffner W. *EMBO J* 1988;7:4221–4229.
48. Ingraham HA, Flynn SE, Voss JW, et al. *Cell* 1990;61:1021–1033.
49. Schadlow VC, Barzilai N, Deutsch PJ. *Mol Biol Cell* 1992;3:941–951.
50. He X, Treacy MN, Simmons DM, Ingraham HA, Swanson LW, Rosenfeld MG. *Nature* 1989;340:35–41.
51. Jones CA, Sigmund CD, McGowan RA, Kane HC, Gross KW. *Mol Endocrinol* 1990;4:375–383.
52. Suzuki N, Rohdewohld H, Neuman T, Gruss P, Scholer HR. *EMBO J* 1990;9:3723–3732.
53. Levine M, Hoey T. *Cell* 1988;55:537–540.
54. Brown JJ, Doak PB, Davies DL, Lever AF, Robertson JIS, Tree M. *Lancet* 1984;2:64.
55. Poisner AM, Wood GW, Poisner R, Inagami T. *Endocrinology* 1981;109:1150–1156.
56. Skinner SL, Lumbers ER, Symonds EM. *Am J Obstet Gynecol* 1968;101:529–533.
57. Poisner AM, Wood GW, Poisner R, Inagami T. *Proc Soc Exp Biol Med* 1982;169:4–6.
58. Acker GM, Galen FX, Devaux C, et al. *J Clin Endocrinol Metab* 1982;55:902–909.
59. Pinet F, Corvol MT, Bourguignon J, Corvol P. *J Clin Endocrinol Metab* 1988;67:1211–1220.
60. Symonds EM, Stanley MA, Skinner SL. *Nature* 1968;217:1152.
61. Shaw KJ, Do YS, Kjos S, et al. *J Clin Invest* 1989;83:2085–2092.
62. Duncan KG, Haidar MA, Baxter JD, Reudelhuber TL. *Proc Natl Acad Sci USA* 1990;87:7588–7592.
63. Burt DW, Nakamura N, Kelley P, Dzau V. *J Hypertens* 1988;6:S429–S431.
64. Nakamura N, Burt DW, Paul M, Dzau VJ. *Proc Natl Acad Sci USA* 1989;86:56–59.
65. Kingston RE. In: Ausubel FM, Brent R, Kingston RE, et al., eds. *Current protocols in molecular biology.* New York: John Wiley and Sons; 1991:9.1.1.
66. Tamura K, Tanimoto K, Murakami K, Fukamizu A. *Nucleic Acids Res* 1992;20:3617–3623.
67. Tronik D, Dreyfus M, Babinet C, Rougeon F. *EMBO J* 1987;6:983–987.
68. Sola C, Tronik D, Dreyfus M, Babinet C, Rougeon F. *Oncogene Res* 1989;5:149–153.
69. Fukamizu A, Hatae T, Kon Y, et al. *Biochem J* 1991;278:601–603.
70. Gomez RA, Chevalier RL, Carey RM, Peach MJ. *Kidney Int* 1990;8(Suppl 30):S18–S23.
71. Kotchen TA, Galla JH, Luke RG. *Kidney Int* 1978;13:201–207.
72. Fray JC. *Am J Physiol* 1976;231:936–944.
73. Ganong WF. *Life Sci* 1974;15:1401–1414.
74. Ganong WF, Reid IA. In: Onesti G, Fernandes M, Kim KE, eds. *Regulation of blood pressure by the central nervous system.* New York: Grune & Stratton, 1976.
75. Johns DW, Peach MJ, Gomez RA, Inagami T, Carey RM. *Am J Physiol* 1990;259:F882–F887.
76. Palmer RM, Ashton DS, Moncada S. *Nature* 1988;333:664–666.
77. Helwig JJ, Musso MJ, Judes C, Nickols GA. *Endocrinology* 1991;129:1233–1242.
78. Nickols GA, Nickols MA, Helwig JJ. *Endocrinology* 1990;126:721–727.
79. Henrich WL, Campbell WB. *Am J Physiol* 1986;251:E98–E103.
80. Henrich WL, McAllister EA, Smith PB, Campbell WB. *Am J Physiol* 1988;255:474–478.
81. Kurtz A, Della BR, Pfeilschifter J, Bauer C. *Kidney Int* 1988;33:798–803.
82. Taugner R, Nobiling R, Metz R, Taugener F, Buhrle C, Hackenthal E. *Cell Tissue Res* 1988;252:687–690.
83. Churchill PC. *Am J Physiol* 1985;248:F175–F184.
84. Matsumura Y, Kawazoe S, Ichihara T, Shinyama H, Kageyama M, Morimoto S. *Am J Physiol* 1988;255:F614–F620.
85. Hackenthal E, Paul M, Ganten D, Taugner R. *Physiol Rev* 1990;70:1067–1116.
86. Nakamura N, Soubrier F, Menard J, Panthier JJ, Rougeon F, Corvol P. *Hypertension* 1985;7:855–859.
87. Catanzaro DF, Mesterovic N, Morris BJ. *Endocrinology* 1985;117:872–878.
88. Makrides SC, Mulinari R, Zannis VI, Gavras H. *Hypertension* 1988;12:404–410.
89. Moffett RB, McGowan RA, Gross KW. *Hypertension* 1986;8:874–882.
90. Samani NJ, Godfrey NP, Major JS, Brammar WJ, Swales JD. *J Hypertens* 1989;7:105–112.
91. Holmer S, Eckardt K-U, Aedtner O, et al. *J Hypertens* 1993;11:1011–1019.
92. Samani NJ, Swales JD, Brammar WJ. *Clin Sci* 1989;77:629–636.
93. Volpe M, Camargo MJF, Mueller FB, et al. *Hypertension* 1990;15:318–326.
94. von Lutterotti N, Camargo MJF, Campbell WJJ, et al. *J Hypertens* 1992;10:949–957.
95. Schaufele F, West BL, Baxter JD. *Mol Endocrinol* 1992;6:656–665.
96. Dana S, Karin M. *Mol Endocrinol* 1989;3:815–821.
97. Richards AM, Nicholls MG, Espiner EA, Ikram H, Turner JG, Brownlie BEW. *Clin Exp Theory Prac* 1985;11:1499–1514.
98. Resnick LM, Laragh JH. *Life Sci* 1982;30:585–586.
99. Elias AN, Kyaw T, Valenta LJ, Meshkinpour H. *Horm Metab Res* 1986;18:349–351.
100. Sernia C, Marchant C, Brown L, Hoey A. *Cardiovasc Res* 1993;27:423–428.
101. Montiel M, Jimenez E, Navaez JA, Morell M. *J Endocrinol Invest* 1984;7:559–562.
102. Montiel M, Jimenez E, Narvaez JA, Ruiz M, Morell M. *Rev Esp Fisiol* 1984;40:431–436.
103. Jimenez E, Montiel M, Narvaez JA, Morell M. *Acta Endocrinol (Copenh)* 1984;105:505–510.
104. Jimenez E, Montiel M, Narvaez JA, Morell M. *Rev Esp Fisiol* 1982;38:35–40.
105. Jimenez E, Montiel M, Narvaez JA, Morell M. *Rev Esp Fisiol* 1982;38:149–154.
106. Pecker MS, James GD, Laragh JH, Sealey JE. *JASN* 1994;4:537.
107. Ruiz M, Montiel M, Jimenez E, Morell M. *J Endocrinol* 1987;115:311–315.
108. Haro JM, Sabio JM, Vargas F. *J Endocrinol Invest* 1992;15:605–608.
109. Pracyk JB, Slotkin TA. *J Dev Physiol* 1991;16:251–261.
110. Eber O, Buchinger W, Lindner W, et al. *Clin Endocrinol (Oxf)* 1990;32:363–372.
111. Soubrier F, Jeunemaitre X, Rigat B, Houot A, Cambien F, Corvol P. *Hypertension* 1990;16:712–717.
112. Jeunemaitre X, Charru A, Rigat B, Houot A, Soubrier F, Corvol P. *Hum Genet* 1992;88:301–306.
113. Staden R. *Nucleic Acids Res* 1982;10:2951–2961.

Hypertension: Pathophysiology, Diagnosis, and Management, Second Edition, edited by J.H. Laragh and B.M. Brenner, Raven Press, Ltd., New York © 1995.

CHAPTER 96

Human Renin: Biochemistry, Crystal Structure, and Opportunities for Development of Specific Inhibitors

Markus G. Grütter and Joseph Rahuel

The renin-angiotensin-aldosterone cascade plays a crucial role in regulating the electrolyte balance of the body (1–3). Imbalance may lead to blood pressure abnormalities such as hypertension or congestive heart failure. Many extensive experimental and clinical studies using inhibitors of the converting enzyme have shown the importance of the renin-angiotensin system (RAS) in blood pressure regulation (4,5). The successful therapeutic application of converting enzyme inhibitors in the treatment of hypertension and congestive heart failure (5–8) has focused interest in compounds that interfere with the cascade at other points in the formation or action of angiotensin II (9–11). For this, renin has been identified as a prime target in recent years.

Renin is the key enzyme of the renin-angiotensin cascade, which regulates the formation of angiotensin II. It is an extremely specific enzyme and its inhibition should provide selective therapy for hypertension (Fig. 1).

In this review, the biochemistry of human renin is briefly summarized, the structural studies on renin alone

and in complex with inhibitors are reviewed, and the implications for structure-based drug design are discussed.

BIOCHEMISTRY

It was initially attempted to isolate and purify renin from several different species (12–17). Because of the scarcity of available material, it was difficult to gain detailed information about renin at the molecular level. The first renin that was completely purified was available in large quantities and had the sequence fully determined from mouse submaxillary gland (18). Several laboratories later described the isolation and sequence analysis of the complementary deoxyribonucleic acid (cDNA) for the mouse renin precursor (18–21) and for the human kidney preprorenin (22–26). The amino acid sequence of the preprorenin deduced from the cDNA sequence is shown in Fig. 2. With these analyses, it became clear that renin is produced with a signal sequence of 23 amino acids. This presequence is cleaved off during secretion to yield the zymogen prorenin. From the primary sequence, it became established for the first time that renin belongs to the well-characterized class of proteolytic enzymes, the aspartic proteases. Members of this family of

M. G. Grütter and J. Rahuel: Biotechnology Research Department, Pharmaceuticals Division, Ciba-Geigy Ltd., CH 4002 Basel, Switzerland.

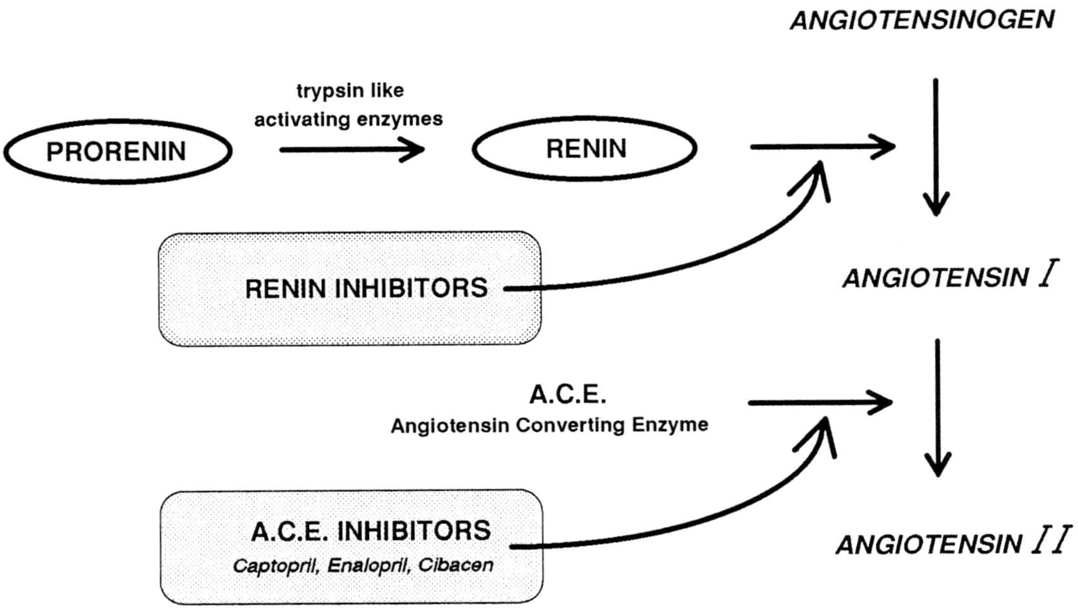

FIG. 1. Renin-angiotensin cascade.

proteases can be characterized by the following features: (a) They consist of two similar N- and C-terminal domains; (b) each domain provides one aspartic acid residue to the active site essential for catalytic activity (27,28); and (c) the enzymes are derived from inactive precursor zymogens with an N-terminal prosequence of roughly 40 amino acids. This prosequence is cleaved off, leading to the active enzyme. The cleaving mechanism is not known in detail.

The three-dimensional structure of several mammalian aspartic proteases has been determined, including porcine pepsin (29), porcine pepsinogen (30), human renin (31–33), and also, those of the fungal enzymes, penicillopepsin (34), rhizopuspepsin (35,36), and endothiapepsin (37,38). These structures reveal that all the enzymes consist of two beta-sheet domains related by an approximate twofold axis. The active site cleft is located between the two domains and extends over eight residues of the corresponding substrate. Each domain provides one of the catalytically essential carboxylates, Asp 32 and Asp 215 (the sequence numbers throughout are based on alignment of the human renin sequence with that of porcine pepsin shown in Fig. 3). These residues are positioned in the center of the substrate binding cleft and are found on two highly conserved and twofold related loops with the sequence Asp-Thr-Gly-Ser/Thr/Ala. More recently, the structures of viral aspartic proteases have become available (39–42). These proteases were assigned as belonging to the aspartic protease family based on active site sequence homology. This subfamily of aspartic proteases, only about one-third the size of the two domain cellular enzymes, is active as homodimers as pre-

dicted by Tang et al. (43). Each monomer provides one of the two conserved aspartic acid residues to the active site, as was shown by the crystal structures of Rous sarcoma virus protease and human immunodeficiency virus 1 (HIV-1) protease (39–42).

One of the most interesting representatives of the cellular enzymes is renin because of its major role in the regulation of blood pressure. In humans, it is an extremely specific enzyme known to cleave only the peptide bond between Leu10 and Val11 of angiotensinogen to form angiotensin I (AI) (see Fig. 1), an inactive decapeptide that is subsequently cleaved by the angiotensin converting enzyme (ACE) to the octapeptide angiotensin II. Angiotensin II is itself a potent vasoconstrictor and also helps regulate blood pressure by triggering the release of aldosterone (9,44).

Prorenin

Expression

Expression of human renin is most successful when the Chinese hamster ovary (CHO) cell line is used as a host. The successful cloning and expression of human prorenin were first reported by Poorman et al. (45) and Fritz et al. (46) in 1986. Sequence analysis (22) of cDNA and genomic DNA analyses (24–26) of human renin and, similarly, amino acid (18) and cDNA sequence analysis of mouse submaxillary gland renin, show or suggest that the enzymes are synthesized as preprorenin with a 23-amino-acid signal sequence and a 43-amino-acid

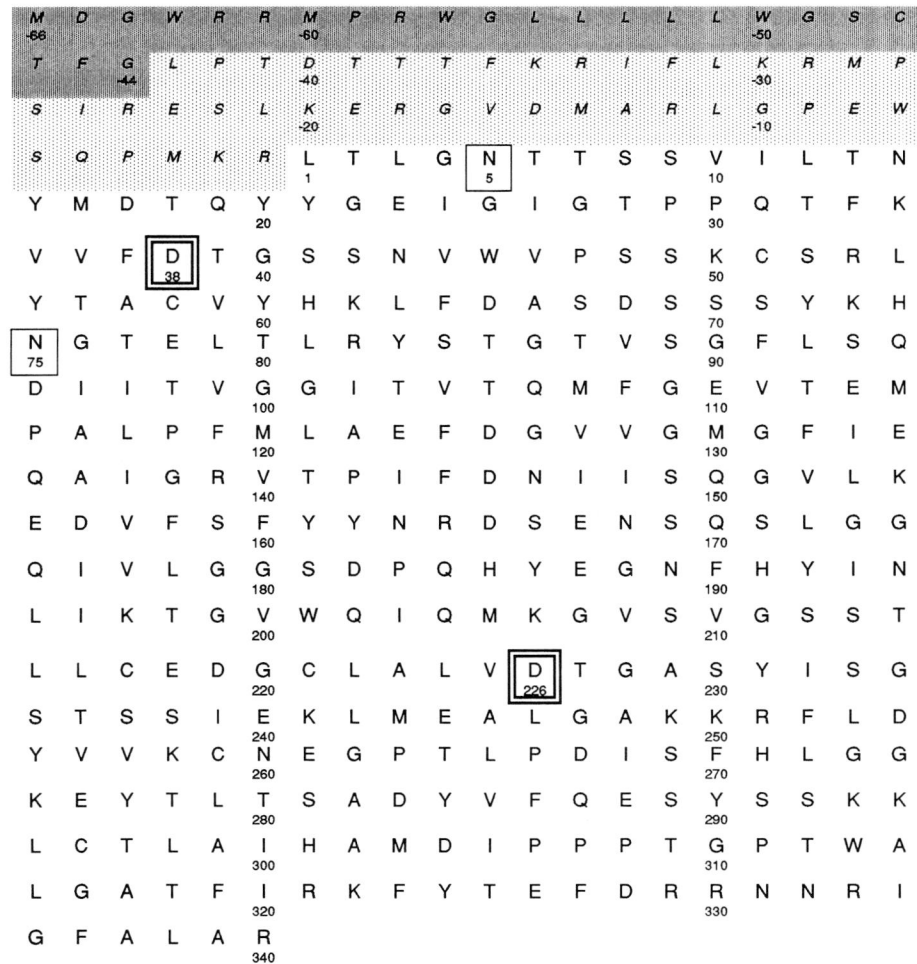

FIG. 2. Complete amino acid sequence of human kidney preprorenin as derived from analysis of the cDNA (22) (renin numbering). Asparaginyl residues in consensus sequences for N-linked glycosylation are boxed, and active site aspartyl residues are doubly boxed. The mature enzyme begins with position 1, the signal sequence is displayed in dark gray, and the pro sequence is in light gray.

pro segment (22) in the case of the human enzyme (see Fig. 2) and an 18-amino-acid amino terminal signal sequence and a 45-amino-acid pro segment in the case of the mouse enzyme (45). The full human renin cDNA (22) was cloned into an eukaryotic expression vector pMTpro containing the regulatory elements and the initiator methionine from the human metallothioneine II gene. Chinese hamster ovary cells transfected with the plasmid designed to express human prorenin secrete the inactive prorenin.

In a similar way, an expression plasmid for human preprorenin was constructed in which the renin genome is driven by the powerful constitutive promoter of the main immediate-early gene of mouse cytomegalovirus and transfected the plasmid into the DHFR-minus CHO cell line DUKXB1 (47). Cell lines that produced the highest amounts of prorenin were selected. To obtain larger quantities of renin for structural analysis as well as

for assay systems, the scale-up of cell culture systems was performed using repeated-batch culture as well as continuous culturing cell techniques. The highest production of renin was achieved with continuous culturing of cells in a chemostat. At steady-state production conditions, about 6 mg of renin (from 10^9 cells) was produced in 2 days, yielding about 1.5 g crude prorenin from a 10 L scale culture (serum free) (47).

Purification and Characterization

Successful purification of large quantities of renin depends on affinity chromatography, which simplifies the purification to essentially a one-step procedure. This was first performed by Poorman et al. (45) and Heinrickson and Poorman (48) who used isosteric peptide inhibitors of renin bound to activated CH-Sepharose according to

```
Renin   LTLGNT  TSSVILTNYM  DTQYYGEIGI  GTPPQTFKVV  FDTGSSNVWV
Pepsin          IGDEPLENYL  DTEYFGTIGI  GTPAQDFTVI  FDTGSSNLWV   40

        PSSKCSRLYT  ACVYHKLFDA  SDSSSYKHNG  TELTLRYSTG  TVSGFLSQDI
41      PSVYCS---SL  ACSDHNQFNP  DDSSTFEATS  QELSITYGTG  SMTGILGYDT   88

        ITVGGITV-T  QMFGEVTEMP  ALPFMLAEFD  GVVGMGFIEQ  AIGRVTPIFD
89      VQVGGISDTN  QIFGLSETEP  GSFLYYAPFD  GILGLAYPSI  SASGATPVFD  138

        NIISQGVLKE  DVFSFYYNRD  SENSQSLGGQ  IVLGGSDPQH  YEGNFHYINL
139     NLWDQGLVSQ  DLFSVYLSSN  DD-----SGSV  VLLGGIDSSY  YTGSLNWVPV  184

        IKTGVWQIQM  KGVSVGSSTL  LCEDGCLALV  DTGASYISGS  TSSIEKLMEA
185     SVEGYWQITL  DSITMSGETI  ACSGGCQAIV  DTGTSLLTGP  TSAIANIQSD  234

        LGAKKRLF-D  YVVKCNEGPT  LPDISFHLGG  KEYTLTSADY  VFQESYSSKK
235     IGAAENSDGE  MVISCSSIDS  LPDIVFTIDG  VQYPLSPSAY  ILQDDD----  281

        LCTLAIHAMD  IPPPTGPTWA  LGATFIRKFY  TEFDRRNNRI  GFALAR
282     SCTSGFEGMD  VPTSSGELWI  LGDVFIRQYY  TVFDRANNKV  GLAPVA     326
```

FIG. 3. Alignment of the sequences of renin and pepsin based on the three-dimensional structures of both proteins. The 127-amino-acid residues are common to renin and pepsin, representing about 40 percent identity. In both enzymes, the proline at position 23 adopts a *cis* conformation. Three additional *cis*-prolines were found in renin, at positions 111, 294, and 297. Renin is glycosylated at the asparaginyl residue 67. The catalytic aspartyl residue numbers are 32 and 215 in renin and in pepsin.

a protocol developed by McIntyre et al. (49). The affinity chromatography step was performed on concentrated crude CHO cell growth media that contains overproduced trypsin-activated renin (up to 100 mg/L). Ninety percent of the renin in the crude growth media was recovered from the affinity column by a decreasing pH gradient (49). The affinity ligand was chosen to optimally mimic the substrate angiotensinogen and has the structure D-His-Pro-Phe-His-Leu-Val-Ile-Tyr with a peptidomimetic part consisting of a reduced peptide bond [—CH(OH)—NH—] between Leu and Val that cannot be cleaved by the protease. Renin isolated and purified by this method was shown to be pure based on sodium dodecyl sulfate-polyacrylamide gel electrophoresis (SDS-PAGE), amino acid composition, and sequence analysis. Carilli et al. (50) have used conventional hydrophobic interaction chromatography and ion exchange chromatography on crude cell growth media containing either prorenin or renin, generated by solid-phase trypsin treatment of the cell growth media.

Different methods have been used to purify recombinant human prorenin from cell cultures. The most efficient ones are based on affinity chromatography. The ligand for affinity chromatography can be either an inhibitor of the enzyme or a monoclonal antibody against human renin.

In our laboratory, purification of renin using immunoaffinity chromatography was chosen. The column used consists of the monoclonal antibody R-3-36-16 (51) coupled with CNBr-activated Sepharose-4B (Pharmacia) at a ratio of 5 mg protein/ml resin. Typically, 1 L crude centrifuged CHO-cell culture medium is applied to a 16-ml column at neutral pH. One fraction containing 6 to 9

mg prorenin in 8 to 12 ml buffer is eluted at pH 3.5. The prorenin obtained in this way is free of contaminants on SDS-PAGE but shows two bands of roughly equal intensity. The prorenin sequence includes two possible sites for *N*-glycosylation and has been reported to contain an average of 1.4 *N*-linked oligosaccharide group per polypeptide chain (52). We therefore suppose the heterogeneity of this material to be caused by glycosylation, although we have not yet performed further investigations to clarify this result.

Renin

Activation of Prorenin

Prorenin can be activated to the mature enzyme by trypsin. Mature, active renin is obtained from the prorenin preparations described above, by incubation at room temperature in the presence of trypsin immobilized on Sepharose. The immobilized enzyme is prepared by reacting tosyl-phenylalanine-chloromethyl-keton–treated trypsin with CNBr-activated Sepharose 4B in the ratio of 5 mg enzyme/ml Sepharose. Approximately 20 mg prorenin can be activated with 50 μl of the immobilized trypsin in a total volume of 10 ml within 1 hour. This activation step has proved to be very efficient and very specific; prorenin disappears in less than 30 minutes, and the mature renin is totally free of additional contaminants as seen by SDS-PAGE (47). Renin also shows at least two bands on SDS-PAGE. Under overloaded conditions, only very minor bands of contaminants are visible. Sequence analysis reveals a single polypeptide chain with the expected sequence Leu-Thr-Leu-Gly at the N terminus. The yield of the process of activation and concentration combined is about 80 percent, the loss being mainly caused by partial precipitation of protein, which is removed by filtration. It was observed that even when the reaction time is lengthened to 24 hours, only negligible traces of undesirable fragments appear. Such polypeptides usually occur when using trypsin in solution as the result of continued proteolysis after the activation of

TABLE 1. *Dihedral angles of CGP 38'560*

Position and residue		Angle (degrees)				
		ϕ	ψ	ω	χ_1	χ_2
P3	'Phe'[a]	−98	146	179	−69	101
P2	His	−140	107	178	−156	93
P1	Cha[b]	−98	56	155	−56	−170
P1'	'Val'[a]	−81	148	175	156	

[a] 'Phe' and 'Val' designate the corresponding amino acid residue in which the main-chain nitrogen is substituted by a carbon.
[b] Cha is for the β-cyclohexyl-L-alanyl residue.

the enzyme. This problem also occurred in early experiments when trying to activate prorenin with a commercial preparation of immobilized trypsin.

With respect to crystallization, the preparation procedure above provides material capable of giving diffraction quality crystals. Therefore, this material was not deglycosylated nor were any attempts to isolate different isoforms of renin made. The deglycosylation of renin is mentioned by Sielecki et al. (31) (30) and Carilli et al. (53) in which the structure determination of renin was first described.

Renin is stable for months when stored in the cold (4°C) at neutral pH. In contrast, we have repeatedly observed that preparations of renin stored at −80°C and then thawed no longer yield diffraction quality crystals but rather many small crystals.

Enzymatic Activity

Enzymatic activity of recombinant human renin was compared with the activity of a World Health Organization (WHO) standard human kidney renin in two different assays (47). In the first, recombinant (0.33 ng/ml) or human kidney renin (0.58 ng/ml) was incubated in buffer containing 10 mg/ml bovine serum albumin and 1 mg/ml neomycin sulfate with a synthetic tetradecapeptide (13.33 μM) corresponding to the 14 amino-terminal amino acids of human angiotensinogen. Alternatively, recombinant renin (0.89 ng/ml) or human kidney renin (0.44 ng/ml) was incubated in 50 percent (v/v) human renin-free plasma in buffer. After 1 hour, the reaction is stopped by adding 1.0 ml ice-cold 100 mM Tris-acetate buffer, pH 7.4, containing 1 mg/ml human serum albumin. The amount of AI generated is determined as prescribed previously (54) and is expressed as nanogram AI generated per hour per nanogram renin. This assay is also used to determine kinetic constants of recombinant human renin.

Renin and prorenin were quantified with an immunoradiometric assay using antibody R1-20-5 and iodinated antibody R3-36-16 (51). This assay was calibrated with renin purified in our laboratory to homogeneity from human kidneys.

The specific activity of recombinant human renin versus human synthetic substrate was 1346 ± 103 ng AI produced per nanogram renin per hour and versus human angiotensinogen was 165 ± 17 ng AI produced per nanogram renin per hour. The values are very similar to those determined for human kidney renin for which versus synthetic substrates 1225 ± 102 ng AI and versus human angiotensinogen 187 ± 24 ng AI were produced. Thus, the specific activities of recombinant and native kidney renin were indistinguishable using either a synthetic tetradecapeptide or human angiotensin as substrate and gave values similar to those previously reported (45,55,56). For this comparative measurement the amount of enzyme was quantified immunologically, because the reference material used was a partially purified preparation of native human kidney renin.

The kinetic parameters of the enzymatic reaction between human recombinant renin and the synthetic substrate are as follows (47): The K_m values measured at pH 7.2 are in agreement with the previously published K_m obtained with human kidney renin acting at this pH on synthetic substrates, 8.4 ± 2.5 μM (57). The catalytic constant K_{cat} is 4.53 times higher than that previously reported for kidney renin acting on the same substrate but at pH 5.7 (58). However, at this low pH a much higher

TABLE 2. *Hydrogen bonds formed between the inhibitor CGP 38'560 and human renin compared with those between CP-69,799 and endothiapepsin*

Inhibitor atom		Renin atom		Distance (Å)	Endothiapepsin atom		Distance (Å)
P3	O	Ser219	N	3.0	Thr219	N	3.05
P3	O	Ser219	O_γ	3.4			
P3	N[a]				Thr219	O_γ	2.68
P2	N	Thr77	O_γ	3.2			
P2	O	Thr77	N	3.2	Asp77	N	3.18
P2	O	Thr77	O_γ	3.4			
P2	O	Ser76	N	3.3	Gly76	N	3.44
P2	$N_{\epsilon2}$	Ser222	O_γ	3.0			
P2	$N_{\delta1}$	Ser76	O_γ	3.2	Thr218	O_γ	2.87
P1	N	Gly217	O	3.4	Gly217	O	3.25
P1	OH	Asp32	$O_{\delta1}$	2.7	Asp32	$O_{\delta1}$	2.70
P1	OH	Asp32	$O_{\delta2}$	3.5	Asp32	$O_{\delta2}$	3.20
P1	OH	Asp215	$O_{\delta1}$	2.4	Asp215	$O_{\delta1}$	2.69
P1	OH	Asp215	$O_{\delta2}$	3.0	Asp215	$O_{\delta2}$	3.06
P1'	O	Ser76	N	3.4	Gly76	N	3.06
P2'	N	Gly34	O	2.8	Gly34	O	3.09

From ref. 32, with permission.
[a] The N_α atom of P3 is substituted by a carbon in CGP 38'560.

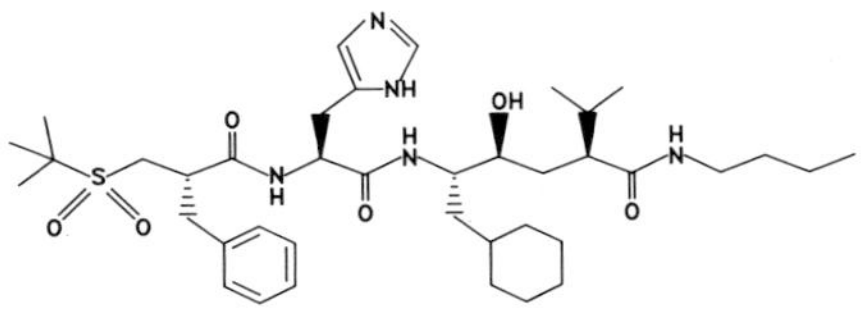

CGP 38'560

FIG. 4. Chemical structure of the renin inhibitor CGP 38'560.

value for K_m was also observed: 20.7 ± 7 μM (58). Higher K_m values have also been reported at higher pH values (e.g., 29 μM at pH 7.5) (59). The pH optimum of renin is highly dependent on the type of substrate used (60), but these data confirm that the optimum pH of the enzymatic reaction between renin and synthetic tetradecapeptides is between pH 6.5 and 7.5 (58).

Crystallization

Using renin purified as described above, two crystal forms of renin have been obtained, both of which were suitable for x-ray structural analysis (32). In one case, renin crystallizes in the presence of the inhibitor CGP 38'560 (Fig. 4). The second type of crystal is obtained with free renin and has also been reported by Lim et al. (61).

Crystals of the complex of renin with CGP 38'560 are obtained from an ammonium sulfate solution and diffract to 2.4 Å resolution. They belong to the tetragonal space group $P4_12_12$ and have unit cell dimensions of $a = b = 90.9$ Å and $c = 109.5$ Å, with one molecule of the complex per asymmetric unit.

Free renin crystallizes in the presence of polyethylene glycol (32,61). These crystals diffract to a maximum of 2.8 Å resolution. They belong to the cubic space group $P2_13$. The cell edges of the unit cell are $a = b = c = 143$ Å, and the asymmetric unit contains two independent molecules. Attempts to crystallize uninhibited renin in the tetragonal crystal form, which diffracts to higher resolution, have failed. Soaking out the inhibitor was also unsuccessful, confirming, as was seen after elucidation of the structure of the complex, that the active site is blocked because of crystal contacts with a symmetry-related molecule. Soaking-in of inhibitors in the cubic crystals is easily accomplished, making them very useful for enzyme-inhibitor complex studies.

STRUCTURES

First Model of Renin

Based on sequence homology with the nonviral aspartic proteases, it was predicted that renin possesses a struc-

ture similar to the other aspartic proteases. The first model of renin based on the structure of the homologous aspartic protease endothia-pepsin was constructed using computer graphics (62). Similar models were constructed later on (63–66). Because of the high-sequence homology with aspartic proteases for which three-dimensional (3-D) structures were available and the fact that there are very few insertions and deletions in the polypeptide sequence of renin, the model of renin has almost all main-chain atoms in identical conformation and a hydrophobic core packing that is similar to the other aspartic proteases. In the absence of an experimentally determined structure, such a model can be regarded as a good representation of the 3-D structure of renin. An analysis of residues forming the active site cleft, and therefore involved in binding substrate, was possible. Aspartic acid residues 32 and 215 in analogy to pepsin were identified as the catalytic residues (see Figs. 2 and 3). The largest differences between renin and the homologous enzymes were observed at the edges of the active site cleft. These differences include a surface loop with residues 237 to 247 and a loop with four proline residues at 293, 294, 295, and 298, partly forming the S4 and the S1/S3 pockets as well as the external surface of the flap that lies across the cleft. With this model, it was possible to investigate the interactions between putative substrates and inhibitors by computer graphics and to design new inhibitor molecules (67). At the same time, crystallization of complexes of renin inhibitors with fungal enzymes (68–73) were used to help design potent renin inhibitors.

Crystal Structure of Deglycosylated Human Renin

The x-ray crystal structure of recombinant deglycosylated human renin was determined at 2.5 Å resolution by Sielecki et al. (31). Secreted human prorenin (46) from transfected CHO cells (45) was converted to active renin by cleavage with immobilized trypsin. The purified renin was treated with endoglycosidase F to remove attached carbohydrates without affecting the specific activity of the enzyme (50). Deglycosylated renin produced in this way was crystallized in the tetragonal space group I4, with unit cell dimensions $a = b = 133.5$ Å and $c = 41.7$ Å, with one renin molecule in the asymmetric unit. The structure was solved by the molecular replacement method (74) using a model based on the known structure of the most homologous aspartic protease, pepsinogen (30).

It was shown for the first time experimentally that renin has the predominantly beta-sheet fold characteristic of the aspartic protease family (Fig. 5). The substrate binding cleft and active site of the enzyme are formed between two structurally similar domains (43). The catalytic residues Asp 32 and 215 are located in the center

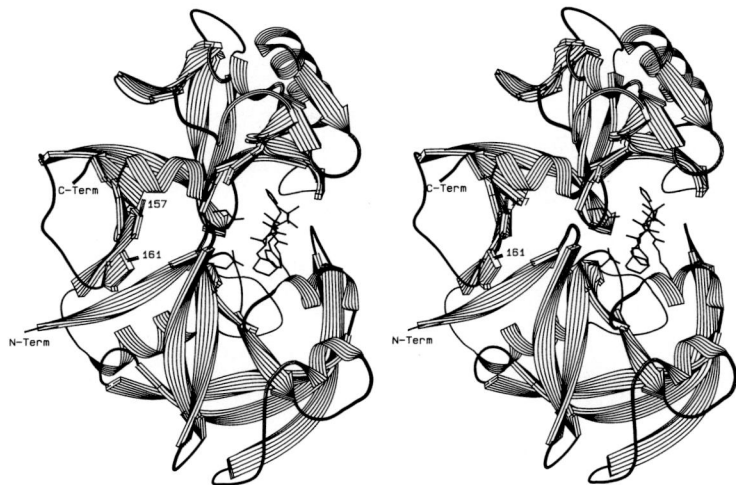

FIG. 5. Stereo ribbon diagram of renin in complex with the inhibitor CGP 38'560. The N-terminal and C-terminal ends and the residues 157 and 161, which delimit a nondefined region of renin, are labeled. The inhibitor CGP 38'560 is shown with the two catalytic aspartic acid residues of renin.

of the cleft (Fig. 5). The carboxylate side chains Asp 32 and 215, which are both followed by type I β turns each with the sequence Asp-Thr-Gly-X (where X is Ser 35 and Ala 218, pepsin numbering), are related by an interdomain twofold axis. This feature was already found in other aspartic protease structures (37). The residues lining the active site in the renin structure, and therefore involved in binding substrate from P4 to P3, were identified and are those predicted in the earlier models (62–65; see also Table 3). Substrate binding residues originating from the central strands of renin have similar conformations to those of the fungal enzymes. Major differences compared with other enzymes of the family are seen in the loops that border the active site.

Structure of Glycosylated Renin

Glycosylated human renin crystallizes in the cubic space group P2₁3 with two independent molecules of renin in the asymmetric unit (61). The structure was solved by the molecular replacement method (74) using the partially refined structure of the renin-inhibitor (CGP

38'560) complex (32) as a search model. The final model, after refinement, has a crystallographic R_{factor} of 22.1 percent for data to a resolution of 2.8 Å (32). Analysis of the structure revealed that the two independent renin molecules in the asymmetric unit of the crystal adapt different conformations. The differences in conformation were analyzed by superimposing the Cα atoms of one domain in each of the two molecules, which indicated a rigid-body domain movement. In one molecule, the C-terminal domain moves toward the N-terminal domain with a small twist. This conformation was called the "closed" form of renin, whereas the other conformation in which the C-terminal domain is farther away from the N-terminal domain was labeled the "open" conformation. The movement can be fairly accurately described as a rigid-body rotation of about 4 degrees around an axis located just behind the active site (Fig. 6). The location of the rotation axis near the active site means that residues in the C-terminal domain contributing to the active site undergo only a relatively small movement (on the average, less than 1 Å). In contrast, residues on the periphery show much larger movements (e.g., the loops 198 to 204 and 236 to 254 shift by about 2.5 Å). The

TABLE 3. *Residues of renin forming the binding pockets with CGP 38'560*

S4 t-Butyl		S3 'Phe'		S2 His		S1 Cha		S1' 'Val'		S2' n-Butyl	
12	Thr	12	Thr	76	Ser	30	Val	76	Ser	34	Gly
219	Ser	13	Gln	77	Thr	32	Asp	213	Leu	35	Ser
220	Tyr	77	Thr	218	Ala	75	Tyr	215	Asp	73	Leu
242	Phe	111	Pro	222	Ser	77	Thr	291	Ile	74	Arg
287	His	112	Phe	287	His	112	Phe	292	Pro	75	Tyr
		114	Leu	289	met	117	Phe	295	Thr	128	Gln
		115	Ala	291	Ile	120	Val	298	Thr	130	Ile
		117	Phe	300	Ala	215	Asp	300	Ala		
		219	Ser			217	Gly				

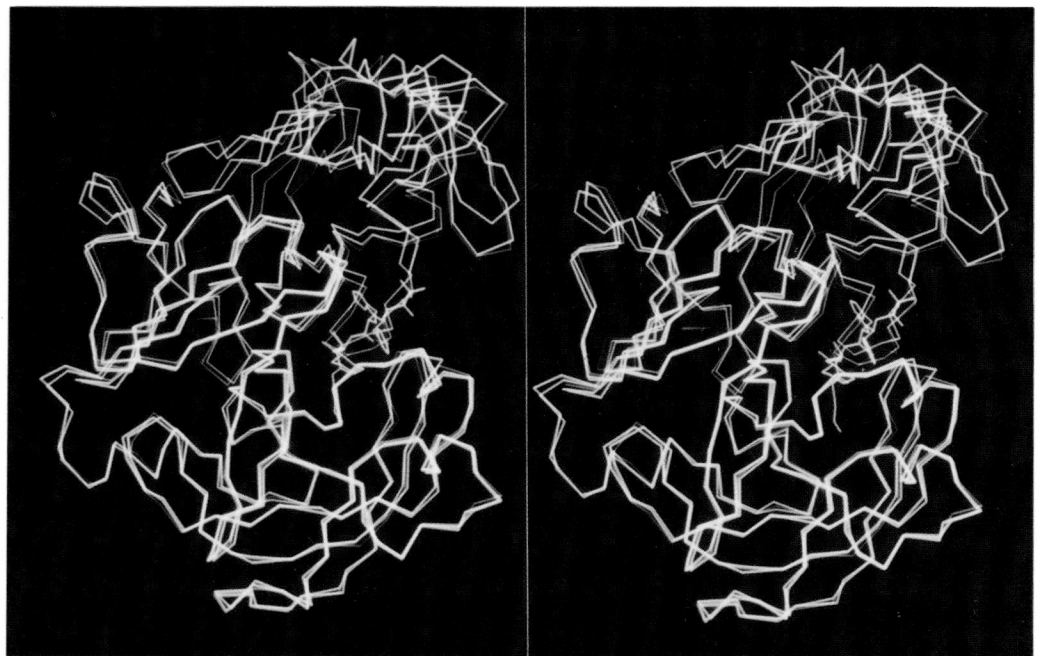

FIG. 6. Cα tracings of inhibited renin from the tetragonal crystals (*red*) with the "open" (*blue*) and "closed" (*yellow*) free renin molecules from the cubic crystals. Superpositioning was carried out using only Cα atoms from the N-terminal domain (*bottom*). The inhibitor CGP 38'560 is shown (*turquoise*). A rotation of 3.8 degrees about the red rotation axis, perpendicular to the plane of the picture, would superimpose the C-terminal domain of the "open" molecule with that of the "closed" molecule. The largest difference (4 Å) between the two forms is found in the loop 237-247 in the C-terminal domain (*top right*), closing down over the active site.

largest movement is that of the C-terminal domain loop over the active site, residues 237 to 247. This loop moves about 4 Å closer to the N-terminal domain, thus closing the active site. The movement of the domains relative to each other is probably induced by crystal packing forces and confirms the flexibility of the domains of renin relative to each other, as has also been seen for other aspartic proteases (73).

Crystal Structure of Renin-Inhibitor Complexes

Many inhibitors have been designed by modifying the Leu10-Val11 scissile bond of N-terminal fragments of the renin substrate according to the transition state inhibition concept (75,76). The inhibitor CGP 38'560 (77) (see Fig. 4) contains the dipeptide isostere (2S,4S,5S)-5-amino-4-hydroxy-2-isopropyl-6-cyclohexyl-hexanoic acid (Cha$\overset{\text{OH}}{-}$Val) at the P1 to P1' position. It mimics the substrate angiotensinogen from residue P3 to P1', according to the Schechter and Berger nomenclature (78). It is a potent specific inhibitor with an IC_{50} of 2 × 10^{-9} M (77).

Structures of aspartic proteases in complex with synthetic inhibitors have already been described [e.g., for penicillopepsin (79), rhizopuspepsin (35), and HIV protease (39,80–82)]. The first human renin-inhibitor complex structure was solved in our laboratory in 1991 (32). The structure of human renin in the tetragonal crystal form was obtained by molecular replacement, starting with a model built from the refined structure of porcine pepsin (83). Refinement of the structure was carried out, leading to a structure with a final crystallographic R_{factor} of 17.6 percent at a resolution of 2.4 Å (32). In 1992, another human renin-inhibitor complex structure with the Pfizer compound CP 85339 was reported by Dhanaraj et al. (33). Similar conclusions as from the study of the human renin CGP 38'560 complex structure can be drawn.

The general folding of renin is shown in Fig. 5. Despite the fact that the overall topology of renin is very similar to that of other human aspartic protease structures (e.g., pepsin), the active site cleft of renin has a more closed conformation. A rigid-body rotation of the C-terminal domain of a few degrees causes a further closing of the active site. In the C-terminal domain, there is a proline-rich loop (Pro 292, Pro 293, Pro 294, Pro 297), which is unique for renin among the aspartic proteases of known structure (Fig. 7). Another loop consisting of residues 241 to 250 is also unique for the renin structure. Human renin contains four *cis*-prolines at positions 23, 111, 294, and 297. The hydrogen bonds involving the threonine

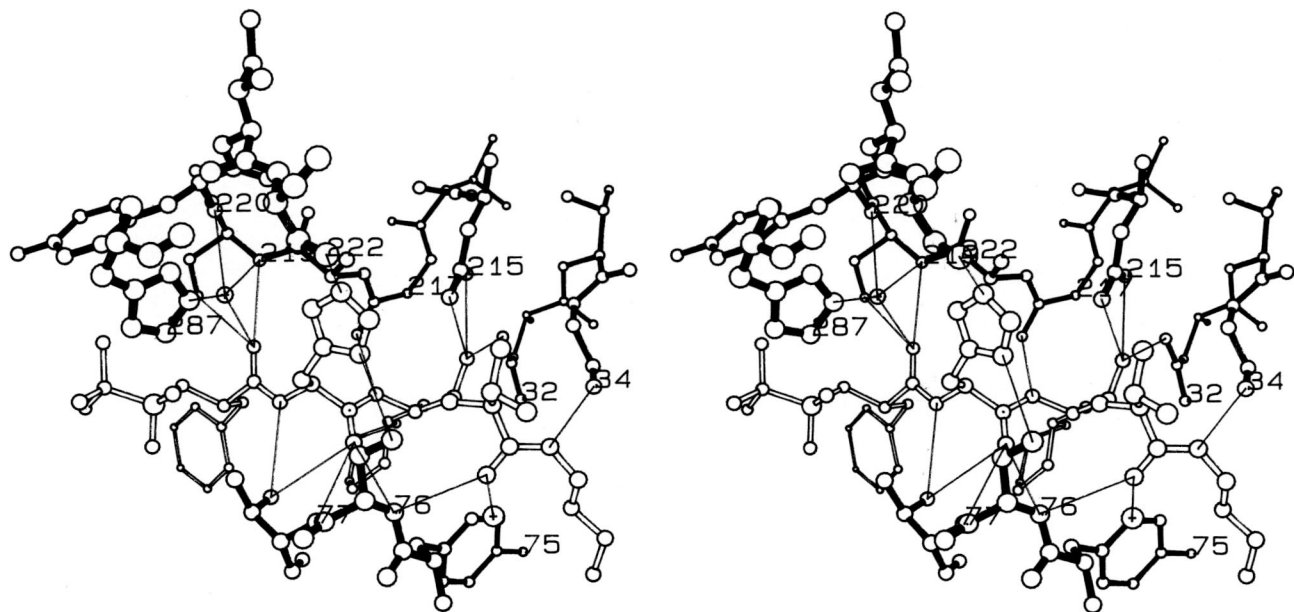

FIG. 7. Hydrogen bonds (Rmin = 3.4 Å) between renin and the inhibitor CGP 38'560 and its environment in the active site of renin. The inhibitor is drawn with open bonds and the enzyme with closed bonds. The hydrogen bonds are presented as *thin lines*. Two water oxygen atom positions are indicated by *crosses*.

residues in the two equivalent beta turns at the catalytic site (Asp-Thr-Gly-Ser/Ala, residues 32 to 35 and 215 to 218), also characteristic for other aspartic proteases, are maintained in the inhibited form: the O_γ of Thr 214 forms hydrogen bonds with the peptide nitrogen of Thr 33 and the carbonyl oxygen of Phe 31.

Inhibitor Binding

The conformation of the inhibitor CGP 38'560 when bound to renin is described in Table 1. The main-chain dihedral angles are similar to those for beta strands in proteins. Whereas the ω dihedral angle for the histidine residue at position P2 in the inhibitor CP 69799 bound to endothiapepsin is significantly different from its ideal value of 180 degrees (73), it is close to ideal in CGP 38'560 when bound to renin. Overall, the inhibitor binds to the enzyme in a conformation that is also energetically favored for the free inhibitor in solution.

The most important interactions between the inhibitor CGP 38'560 and renin, as derived from the tetragonal crystal structure, are presented in Fig. 8. The hydrogen bonding pattern strongly resembles that already described for other aspartic protease/peptidic inhibitor complexes (73,84). In renin, the inhibitor forms 15 hydrogen bonds to the enzyme and 2 to water molecules, themselves hydrogen bonded to the enzyme (see Table 2). The hydroxyl group of the P1 residue of the inhibitor is symmetrically positioned between the two catalytic aspartates of the enzyme. Besides those hydrogen bonds

involving the two catalytic aspartates, seven hydrogen bonds are also found in the complexes of various inhibitors of renin with endothiapepsin. A water molecule that participates in a hydrogen bond with the carbonyl of P3 also forms a hydrogen bond with three residues of renin: to the main-chain nitrogen of Ser 219 and Tyr 220 and to the imidazol ring $N_{\epsilon2}$ of His 287 (see Fig. 7). There are also hydrogen bonds formed between the imidazol nitrogens and the O_γ of Ser 222 and Ser 76.

In clear contrast to what was found in inhibited endothiapepsin (73), the histidine side chain in P2 of CGP 38'560 has a single well-defined conformation in inhibited renin (Fig. 8). The other site found in endothiapepsin is, in the case of renin, occupied by the side chain of His 287 (Fig. 8). The renin residues involved in binding the inhibitor CGP 38'560, and therefore also those interacting with the angiotensinogen substrate from S4 to S2', are listed in Table 3. The substrate-binding residues originating from the central strands forming the back of the active site of renin are similar in conformation to the other aspartic proteases.

Specificity

The residues of the surface loops from the C-terminal domain Arg 240 to Tyr 245 and His 287 to Pro 297 delineate the entrance to the active site binding cleft from one side, whereas the flap residues Leu 71 to Ser 81 close the active site cleft from the N-terminal side (Fig. 8). They include insertion segments in the sequence of renin

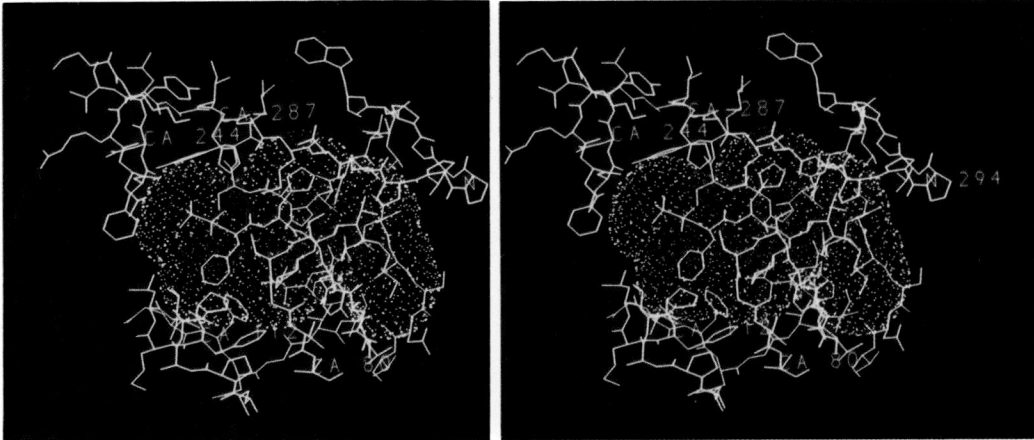

FIG. 8. Van der Waals surface representation (twice Van der Waals radii) of CGP 38'560 in the active site of renin.

when compared with most other aspartic protease sequences (see also ref. 31). The segment Arg 240 to Tyr 245 contributes mainly to the S4-binding pocket, the segment His 287 to Asp 290 contributes to the S2-binding pocket, and the segment Ile 291 and Pro 292 contributes to the S1' and pocket. The loop segment Pro 293 to Pro 297, forming mainly the S1' and S3' pockets, is a feature of the renin structure quite different from other aspartic proteases. These loop segments in renin that differ from the other enzymes provide its specificity and have to be considered important features for the design of potent inhibitors such as CGP 38'560, which, like the substrate angiotensinogen, optimally exploits the active site cleft and its subsites by providing complementary groups to form a maximum number of hydrogen bonds and hydrophobic interactions.

Implications for Rational Drug Design and Development of Specific Inhibitors

Because of renin's important role in the control of blood pressure, the design of renin inhibitors is a field in which many pharmaceutical companies are involved. The number of different compounds synthesized is so large judging from published structures (see reviews in refs. 85 and 86) as well as from structures covered by patent applications that it would be outside the scope of this article to cover all the individual efforts in this area. Instead, only a general description can be given here of the most important features that specific, potent renin inhibitors based on structural knowledge should display.

Based on the knowledge that renin is an aspartic protease and the fact that it is highly specific for angiotensinogen, cleaving the peptide bond between residues Leu 10 and Val 11, peptide fragments and later peptide fragments containing a noncleaveable peptide mimic were

first synthesized to obtain highly specific and tightly binding molecules (see reviews in refs. 48 and 87). Despite the fact that their potency against human renin is in the low nanomolar range and their specificity is extremely high compared with other aspartic proteases such as pepsin and cathepsin D, so far all inhibitors reported have been shown to be rapidly secreted and/or have low oral availability and therefore are only of limited clinical use.

From the structures of the existing renin inhibitor complexes, the specific interactions such as hydrogen bonds, van der Waals contacts, and hydrophobic interactions between enzyme and inhibitor are determined. The space available in the specificity pockets is seen in the structures, as are the surface properties of the particular areas of the enzyme. New molecules exploiting new interactions can be designed, and their binding to the enzyme can be studied. Inhibitors with new nonpeptidic features to optimize properties such as hydrophilicity, size, stability, and oral availability are being designed and synthesized without losing the existing high specificity and tight binding of the previous molecule. The knowledge of the structure of the renin especially in the S2,S1',S3' pockets where it differs from other aspartic protease structures is most valuable. Exploiting these features allows the design of even more specific ligands.

With respect to transition-state isosteres, the inhibitors generally display a hydroxyethylene group, a dihydroxy ethylene group, and in fewer cases, a difluoro-ethylene group, statine and variations on statine. The inhibitors mainly fulfill the requirement for hydrophobic residues in P1', P1, and P3. The P1 pocket (Figs. 8 and 9) can be occupied by a leucyl group or, better, a cyclohexyl group. The P3 moiety of the inhibitors in most cases is a phenylalanine residue, but even larger hydrophobic groups such as napthyl can be accommodated. The variability of the P2 portion among inhibitors can be rather large.

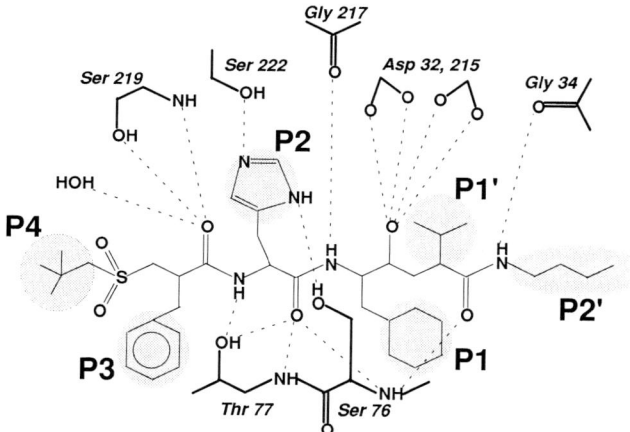

FIG. 9. Schematic diagram representing CGP 38'560 and its interactions with renin. The residues filling the respective enzyme pockets are *shaded;* hydrogen bonds are indicated by *dotted lines.*

Instead of the histidinyl group, a variety of different chemical entities are possible, such as butyl-group, a thiazolidinyl-group, or other hydrophobic groups of similar length (86). Even acidic side chains have been placed in P2 (86). This is possible because of the hydrogen bonding possibility to Ser 222 and Ser 76 of the enzyme. Most of the synthesized molecules show a large variability in the P4 site and on the other side from the P1' site onward.

CONCLUSIONS

The minimum requirement for a potent specific renin inhibitor viewed in the light of the current structural information seems to be the following: (a) a noncleavable peptide mimic, (b) a cyclohexyl or leucyl moiety in P1, and (c) a hydrophobic moiety in P3, preferably Phe or a larger planar group. The P2 site can accommodate a variety of chemical groups such as imidazol, thiazol, butyl, and even acidic groups. In addition to these properties, there is great freedom to add chemical groups to the inhibitors that do not interfere with the spacial requirement of the active site.

Such additional chemical groups as well as the introduction of nonpeptidic features could change the inhibitor's properties with respect to oral availability, stability, solubility, or toxicity. These properties, besides specificity and potency, have to be optimized before a compound can become a useful therapeutic agent. All this is greatly facilitated with the availability of structural information of the target enzymes and their ligands.

ACKNOWLEDGMENTS

We thank J. P. Priestle and S. W. Jacob-Cowan for critical reading of the manuscript and comments.

REFERENCES

1. Reid IA, Morris RJ, Ganong WF. The renin-angiotensin system. *Annu Rev Physiol* 1978;40:377–410.
2. Skeggs LT, Doven FE, Levins M, Lentz K, Kahn JR. The biochemistry of the renin-angiotensin system. In: Johnson JA, Anderson RR, eds. *The renin-angiotensin System.* New York: Plenum Press;1980:1–27.
3. Hofbauer KG, Wood JM. Renin inhibitors as possible antihypertensive agents. *Klin Wochenschr* 1985;66:906–913.
4. Sweet CS, Blaine EH. Angiotensin converting enzyme inhibitors. In: Zanchetti A, Tarazzi RC, eds. *Handbook of hypertension.* Vol 3. Amsterdam: Elsevier;1984:343–363.
5. Johnston CI. Angiotensin converting enzyme inhibitors. In: Zanchetti A, Tarazzi RC, eds. *Handbook of hypertension.* Vol 5. Amsterdam: Elsevier;1984:272–311.
6. Zanchetti A, Tarazzi RC. Symposium on angiotensin-converting enzyme: a developing therapeutic concept. *Am J Cardiol* 1982;49:1381–1579.
7. Hofbauer KG, Hulthén LU, Bülher FR. Antagonists and inhibitors of the renin-angiotensin system for the treatment of hypertension. In: Genest J, Kuchel O, Hamet P, Cantin M, eds. *Hypertension: physiopathology and treatment.* New York: McGraw-Hill; 1983:1225–1238.
8. Brunner NR, Nussberger J, Waeber B. Effects of angiotensin converting enzyme inhibition: a clinical point of view. *J Cardiovasc Pharmacol* 1985;7(Suppl 4):73–81.
9. Ondetti MA, Cushman DW. Enzymes of the renin-angiotensin system and their inhibitors. *Annu Rev Biochem* 1982;51:283–308.
10. Antonaccio MJ. Inhibitors of the renin-angiotensin system as new antihypertensive agents. *Clin Exp Hypertens* 1982;A4:27–46.
11. Hofbauer KG, Wood JM. The renin-angiotensin system: inhibitors and antagonists. In: Zanchetti A, Tarazzi RC, eds. *Handbook of hypertension.* Vol 8. Amsterdam: Elsevier; 1986:466–488.
12. Corvol P, Devaux C, Ito T, Sicard P, Ducloux J, Ménard J. Large scale purification of hog renin. Physiological characterization. *Circ Res* 1977;41:616–622.
13. Inagami T, Murakami K. Pure renin: isolation from hog kidney and characterization. *J Biol Chem* 1977;252:2978–2983.
14. Dzau VJ, Salter EE, Haber E. Complete purification of dog renal renin. *Biochemistry* 1979;18:5224–5228.
15. Yokosawa H, Holladay LA, Inagami T, Haas E, Murakami K. Human renal renin. Complete purification and characterization. *J Biol Chem* 1980;255:3498–3502.
16. Slater EE, Strout V. Pure human renin. Identification and characterization of two major molecular weight forms. *J Biol Chem* 1981;256:8164–8171.
17. Misono KS, Holladay LA, Murakami K, Kuromisu K, Inagami T. Rapid and large-scale purification and characterization of renin from mouse submaxillary gland. *Arch Biochem Biophys* 1982;217:574–581.
18. Misono KS, Chang JJ, Inagami T. Amino acid sequence of mouse submaxillary gland renin. *Proc Natl Acad Sci USA* 1982;79:4858–4862.
19. Rougeon F, Chambraud B, Foote S, Panthier JJ, Nageotte R, Corvol P. Molecular cloning of a mouse submaxillary gland renin cDNA fragment. *Proc Natl Acad Sci USA* 1981;78:6367–6371.
20. Panthier JJ, Foote S, Chambraud B, Stosberg AD, Corvol P, Rougeon F. Complete amino acid sequence and maturation of the mouse submaxillary gland renin precursor. *Nature* 1982;298:90–92.
21. Masuda T, Imai T, Fukushi T, Sudoh M, Hirose S, Murakami K. Molecular cloning of DNA complementary to mouse submandibular gland renin mRNA. *Biomed Res* 1982;3:541–545.
22. Imai T, Miyasaki H, Hirose S, et al. Cloning and sequence analysis of cDNA for human renin precursor. *Proc Natl Acad Sci USA* 1983;80:7405–7409.
23. Soubrier F, Panthier JJ, Corvol P, Rougeon F. Molecular cloning and nucleotide sequence of a human renin cDNA fragment. *Nucleic Acids Res* 1983;11:7181–7190.
24. Hobart PM, Fogliano M, O'Connor BA, Schaefer IM, Chirgwin JM. Human renin gene: structure and sequence analysis. *Proc Natl Acad Sci USA* 1984;81:5026–5030.

25. Hardman J, Hort YJ, Catanzaro DF, et al. Primary structure if the human renin gene. *DNA* 1984;3:457–468.
26. Miyazaki H, Fukamizu A, Hirose S, et al. Structure of the human renin gene. *Proc Natl Acad Sci USA* 1984;81:5999–6003.
27. Chen KCS, Tang J. Amino acid sequence around the epoxide-reactive residues in pepsin. *J Biol Chem* 1972;247:2566–2574.
28. Hartsuck JA, Tang J. The carboxylate ion in the active center of pepsin. *J Biol Chem* 1972;247:2575–2580.
29. Andreeva NS, Zdanov AS, Gutschina AE, Fedorov AA. Structure of ethanol-inhibited porcine pepsin at 2 Å resolution and binding of methyl ester of phenylalanine-diiodotyrosine to the enzyme. *J Biol Chem* 1984;259:11353–11365.
30. James MNG, Sielecki AR. Molecular structure of an aspartic proteinase zymogen, porcine pepsinogen, at 1.8 Å resolution. *Nature* 1986;319:33–38.
31. Sielecki AR, Hayakawa K, Fujinaga M, et al. Structure of recombinant human renin, a target for cardiovascular-active drugs, at 2.5 Å resolution. *Science* 1989;243:1346–1351.
32. Rahuel J, Priestle JP, Grütter MG. The crystal structures of recombinant glycosylated renin alone and in complex with a transition state analog inhibitor. *J Struct Biol* 1991;107:227–236.
33. Dhanaraj V, Dealwis CG, Frazao C, et al. X-ray analyses of peptide-inhibitor complexes define the structural basis of specificity for human and mouse renins. *Nature* 1992;357:466–472.
34. James MNG, Sielecki AR. Structure and refinement of penicillopepsin at 1.8 Å resolution. *J Mol Biol* 1983;163:299–361.
35. Bott R, Subramanian E, Davies DR. Three-dimensional structure of the complex of the *Rhizopus chinensis* carboxyl proteinase and pepstatin at 2.5 Å resolution. *Biochemistry* 1982;21:6956–6962.
36. Suguna K, Bott RR, Padlan EA, et al. Structure and refinement at 1.8 Å resolution of the aspartic proteinase from *Rhizopus chinensis*. *J Mol Biol* 1987;196:877–900.
37. Pearl LH, Blundell TL. The active site of aspartic proteinases. *FEBS Lett* 1984;174:96–101.
38. Blundell TL, Jenkins J, Pearl L, Sewell T, Pedersen V. The high resolution structure of endothiapepsin. In: Kostka V, ed. *Aspartic proteinases and their inhibitors.* Berlin: de Gruyter;1985:151–161.
39. Navia MA, Fitzgerald PMD, McKeever BM, et al. Three-dimensional structure of aspartyl protease from human immunodeficiency virus HIV-1. *Nature* 1989;337:615–620.
40. Lappatto R, Blundell TL, Hemmings A, et al. X-ray analysis if HIV-1 proteinase at 2.7 Å resolution confirms homology among retroviral enzymes. *Nature* 1989;342:299–302.
41. Miller M, Jaskólski M, Rao JKM, Leis J, Wlodawer A. Crystal structure of a retroviral protease proves relationship to aspartic protease family. *Nature* 1989;337:576–579.
42. Wlodawer A, Miller M, Jaskólski M, et al. Conserved folding in retroviral proteases: crystal structure of a synthetic HIV-1 protease. *Science* 1989;245:616–621.
43. Tang J, James MNG, Hsu IN, Jenkins JA, Blundell TL. Structural evidence for gene duplication in the evolution of the acid proteases. *Nature* 1978;271:618–621.
44. Hofbauer KG, Wood JM. Inhibition of renin: recent immunological and pharmacological advances. *Trends Pharmacol Sci* 1985;6:173–177.
45. Poorman RA, Palermo DP, Post LE, et al. Isolation and characterization of native human renin derived from Chinese hamster ovary cells. *Proteins* 1986;1:139–145.
46. Fritz LC, Arfsten AE, Dzau VJ, et al. Characterization of human prorenin expressed in mammalian cells from cloned cDNA. *Proc Natl Acad Sci USA* 1986;83:4114–4118.
47. Asselbergs FAM, Rahuel J, Cumin F, Leist C. Scaled-up production of recombinant human renin in CHO cells for enzymatic and X-ray structure analysis. *J Biotech* 1994;32:191–202.
48. Heinrickson RL, Poorman RA. The biochemistry and molecular biology of recombinant human renin and prorenin. In: Laragh JH, Brenner BM, eds. *Hypertension, pathophysiology, diagnosis, and management.* New York: Raven Press;1990:1179–1196.
49. MacIntyre GD, Leckie B, Hallet A, Szelke M. Purification of human renin by affinity chromatography using a new peptide inhibitor of renin, H.77 (D-His-Pro-Phe-His-Leu—Leu-Val-Tyr). *Biochem J* 1983;211:519–522.
50. Carilli CT, Wallace LC, Smith LM, Wong MA, Lewicki JA. Semi-

51. preparative purification of recombinant human renin and prorenin. *J Chromatogr* 1988;444:203–208.
51. Heusser CH, Bews JPA, Alkan SS, et al. Monoclonal antibodies to human renin: properties and applications. *Clin Exp Hypertens* 1987;A9:1259–1275.
52. Aeed PA, Guido DM, Mathews WR, Elhammer AP. Characterization of the oligosaccharide structures on recombinant human prorenin expressed in Chinese hamster ovary cells. *Biochemistry* 1992;31:6951–6961.
53. Carilli CT, Vigne JL, Wallace LC, et al. Characterization of recombinant human prorenin and renin. *Hypertension* 1988;11:713–716.
54. Hackenthal E, Hackenthal R, Hofbauer KG. No evidence for product inhibition of the renin angiotensin reaction in the rat. *Circ Res* 1977;41(Suppl II):49–54.
55. Vlahos CJ, Walls JD, Berg DT, Grinell BW. The purification and characterization of recombinant human renin expressed in the human kidney cell line 293. *Biochem Biophys Res Commun* 1990;171:375–383.
56. Norman JA, Hadjilambris O, Sharp DY, Kumar R. Stable expression, secretion, and characterization of active human renin in mammalian cells. *Mol Pharmacol* 1992;41:53–59.
57. Poe M, Wu JK, Lin TY, Hoogsten K, Bull HG, Slater E. Renin cleavage of a human kidney renin substrate analogous to human angiotensinogen, H-Asp-Arg-Val-Tyr-Ile-His-Pro-Phe-His-Leu-Val-Ile-His-Ser-OH, that is renin specific and resistant to cathepsin D. *Anal Biochem* 1984;140:459–467.
58. Cumin F, Le-Nguyen D, Castro B, Ménard J, Corvol P. Comparative studies of human renin acting on pure natural or synthetic substrates. *Biochim Biophys Acta* 1987;913:10–19.
59. Burton J, Quinn T. The amino acid residues on the C-terminal side of the cleavage site of angiotensingen influence the species specificity of reaction with renin. *Biochim Biophys Acta* 1988;952:8–12.
60. Holzman TF, Chung CC, Edalji R, et al. Recombinant human renin from CHO cells: expression and purification. *J Protein Chem* 1990;9:663–672.
61. Lim LW, Stegeman RA, Leimgruber NK, Gierse JK, Abdel-Meguid SS. Preliminary crystallographic study of glycosylated recombinant human renin. *J Mol Biol* 1989;210:239–240.
62. Blundell TL, Sibanda BL, Pearl LH. Three-dimensional structure, specificity and catalytic mechanism of renin. *Nature* 1983;304:273–275.
63. Sibanda BL, Blundell T, Hobart PM, et al. Computer graphics modelling of human renin. Specificity, catalytic activity and intron-exon junctions. *FEBS Lett* 1984;174:102–111.
64. Akahane K, Umeyama H, Nakagawa S, et al. Three-dimensional structure of human renin. *Hypertension* (Dallas) 1985;7:3–12.
65. Carlson W, Karplus M, Haber E. Construction of a model for the three-dimensional structure of human renal renin. *Hypertension* (Dallas) 1985;7:13–26.
66. Hemmings AM, Foundling SI, Sibanda BL, Wood SP, Pearl LH, Blundell TL. Energy calculations on aspartic proteinases: human renin, endothiapepsin and its complex with an angiotensinogen fragment analogue. *Biochem Soc Trans* 1985;13:1036–1041.
67. Cohen NC. Molecular mimics and drug design. In: van der Goot H, Domány G, Pallos L, Timmerman H, eds. *Trends in medicinal chemistry 88.* Amsterdam: Elsevier;1989:13–28.
68. Hallett A, Jones DM, Atrash B, et al. Inhibition of aspartic proteinases by transition state substrate analogues. X-ray study of the complex of endothiapepsin with the renin inhibitor H-142. In: Kostka V, ed. *Aspartic proteinases and their inhibitors.* Berlin: de Gruyter;1985:467–478.
69. Foundling SI, Cooper J, Watson FE, et al. High resolution X-ray analyses of renin inhibitor-aspartic proteinase complexes. *Nature* 1987;327:349–352.
70. Blundell TL, Cooper J, Foundling SI, Jones DM, Atrash B, Szelke M. On the rational design of renin inhibitors: X-ray studies of aspartic proteinases complexed with transition-state analogues. *Biochemistry* 1987;26:5585–5590.
71. Cooper JB, Foundling SI, Hemmings A, et al. Inhibitors of aspartic proteinases and their relevance to the design of antihypertensive agents. *Biochem Soc Trans* 1987;15:751–754.
72. Cooper JB, Foundling SI, Hemmings A, et al. The structure of a

synthetic pepsin inhibitor complexed with endothiapepsin. *Eur J Biochem* 1987;169:215–221.

73. Sali A, Veerapandian B, Cooper JB, Foundling SI, Hoover DJ, Blundell TL. High resolution X-ray diffraction study of the complex between endothiapepsin and an oligopeptide inhibitor: the analysis of the inhibitor binding and description of the rigid body shift in the enzyme. *EMBO J* 1989;8:2179–2188.

74. Rossmann MG, ed. *The molecular replacement method. A collection of papers on the use of non-crystallographic symmetry.* New York: Gordon & Breach, 1972.

75. Szelke M, Leckie B, Hallet A, et al. Potent new inhibitors of human renin. *Nature* 1982;299:555–557.

76. Boger J, Lohr NS, Ulm EH, et al. Novel renin inhibitors containing the amino acid statin. *Nature* 1983;303:81–84.

77. Bühlmayer P, Caselli A, Fuhrer W, et al. Synthesis and biological activity of some transition-state inhibitors of human renin. *J Med Chem* 1988;31:1839–1846.

78. Schechter I, Berger A. On the size of the active site of proteases. I. Papain. *Biochem Biophys Res Commun* 1967;27:157–162.

79. James MNG, Sielecki A, Salituro F, Rich DH, Hofman T. Conformational flexibility in the active sites of aspartyl proteinases revealed by a pepstatin fragment binding to penicillopepsin. *Proc Natl Acad Sci USA* 1982;79:6137–6141.

80. Erickson J, Neidhardt DJ, VanDrie J, et al. Design, activity, and 2.8 Å crystal structure of a C_2 inhibitor complexed to HIV-1 protease. *Science* 1990;249:527–533.

81. Fitzgerald PMD, McKeever BM, Van Middleswoth JF, et al. Crystallographic analysis of a complex between human immunodeficiency virus type 1 protease and acetyl-pepstatin at 2 Å resolution. *J Biol Chem* 1990;265:14209–14219.

82. Swain AL, Miller MM, Green J, et al. X-ray crystallographic structure of a complex between a synthetic protease of human immunodeficiency virus 1 and a substrate-based hydroxyethylamine inhibitor. *Proc Natl Acad Sci USA* 1990;87:8805–8809.

83. Sielecki AR, Fedorov AA, Boodhoo A, Andreeva NS, James MNG. Molecular and crystal structures of monoclinic porcine pepsin refined at 1.8 Å resolution. *J Mol Biol* 1990;214:143–170.

84. Blundell TL, Lapatto R, Wilderspin AF, et al. The 3-D structure of HIV-1 proteinase and the design of antiviral agents for the treatment of AIDS. *TIBS* 1990;15:425–430.

85. Greenle WJ. Renin inhibitors. *Med Res Rev* 1990;10:173–236.

86. Greenle WJ, Weber AE. Renin inhibitors. *DN&P* 1991;4:332–339.

87. Wood JM, Stanton JL, Hofbauer KG. Inhibitors of renin as potential therapeutic agents. *J Enzyme Inhib* 1987;1:169–185.

Hypertension: Pathophysiology, Diagnosis, and Management, Second Edition,
edited by J.H. Laragh and B.M. Brenner,
Raven Press, Ltd., New York © 1995.

CHAPTER **97**

Molecular Mechanisms of Processing and Sorting in Renin Secretion

Timothy L. Reudelhuber, Chantal Mercure, Djamel Ramla, Danielle Methot, and Anton Y. Postnov

NATURE AND ORIGIN OF RENIN ACTIVITY IN HUMANS AND OTHER MAMMALS

The renin-angiotensin system (RAS) plays a critical role in the maintenance and modulation of blood pressure in mammals. The RAS has also been implicated, however, in the pathophysiology associated with several diseases including hypertension, cardiac hypertrophy, and myocardial infarction as well as retinopathies and nephropathies (1–4). For this reason, there has been a major effort in the past several years to understand the molecular mechanisms governing the biosynthesis of the components of the RAS so that novel means might be developed to control their activities.

Prorenin and Renin in the Circulation

In the classical view of the RAS (Fig. 1), the glycoprotein angiotensinogen (Aogen) is secreted into the circulation by the liver where it is cleaved by renin, an aspartyl

protease secreted by the kidney, to release the decapeptide angiotensin I (AI). Angiotensin-converting enzyme (ACE), a metalloprotease produced by and anchored to the surface of endothelial cells, then cleaves two amino acids from the carboxy terminus of AI to release the octapeptide angiotensin II (AII). AII exerts its action by binding to specific high-affinity receptors on target cells resulting in vasoconstriction, increased aldosterone secretion from the adrenal gland, feedback regulation on expression of RAS components, and possibly other effects such as stimulating chemotaxis and the proliferation of smooth muscle cells. Aldosterone, in turn, regulates sodium resorption from the proximal tubule and, consequently, fluid and electrolyte balance.

The circulating concentration of Aogen in control human subjects is roughly 1.3 μM (5), which is approximately the K_m (1.15 μM) of purified human renal renin for human angiotensinogen (6). Under these conditions, the rate of generation of AI would be primarily dependent on the concentration of circulating renin. Renin itself is first synthesized as an inactive precursor, or zymogen, called prorenin. Evidence to date suggests that prorenin is analogous to the circulating "big" or "inac-

T. L. Reudelhuber, C. Mercure, D. Ramla, D. Methot, and A. Y. Postnov: Institut de Recherches Cliniques de Montréal, Montreal, Quebec, Canada H2W 1R7.

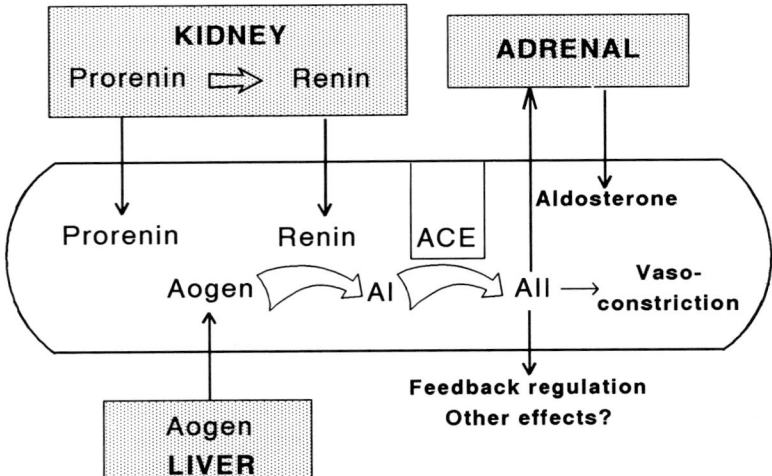

FIG. 1. Schematic representation of the circulating renin-angiotensin system (cRAS). Aogen, angiotensinogen; AI, angiotensin I; ACE, angiotensin-converting enzyme; AII, angiotensin II.

tive" renin and can be present at 3–5 times the level of "active" renin in the circulation of humans (7). Activation of prorenin may occur by a variety of means (Fig. 2). Circulating active renin is generated by the proteolytic removal of a 43 amino acid peptide from the amino terminus of prorenin (6). *In vitro,* acidification (8) or prolonged storage in the cold (9) can result in partial and reversible activation of prorenin in the absence of proteolysis, presumably due to an unfolding of the prosegment and exposure of the active site of the enzyme. It is unlikely that prorenin is activated by any of these means once it is in the circulation, however: Injection of monkeys with large excesses of recombinant human prorenin does not result in a detectable increase in either blood pressure or AII (10,11). Thus, it seems likely that active renin is the major determinant of the activity

of the RAS and that the conversion of prorenin to renin occurs by proteolysis before secretion into the circulation.

Tissue Renin

This view of the so-called circulating RAS (cRAS) has undergone significant evolution in recent years. Protein and/or messenger RNA (mRNA) encoding all of the components of the RAS including angiotensin receptors have been co-localized within several tissues including brain, kidney, adrenal and pituitary glands, heart and vasculature and reproductive tissues (2,12–15), leading to the suggestion that tissue renin-angiotensin systems (tRAS) might function in a locally restricted manner. It should be noted, however, that for a given tRAS to be functionally active, a tissue would presumably need not only to express the renin gene, but to activate the resulting prorenin. In humans, circulating active renin drops to undetectable levels within 2 days after nephrectomy (16). In contrast, while prorenin also drops acutely, it continues to be detected even years after nephrectomy (5,7,17) (Fig. 3A). In rats, the case seems a bit different: Although several extrarenal tissues contain prorenin mRNA and/or protein (18), nephrectomy results in the disappearance of both renin and prorenin from the circulation (19). These results suggest that the kidney releases both prorenin and renin, that the kidney is the predominant (if not exclusive) source of circulating active renin and the nonrenal sources (at least in humans) secrete prorenin.

If the kidney is the sole source of active renin and if renin activity is essential for a functional RAS, one might reasonably ask what happens to angiotensin-generating activity in the absence of the kidney. In anephric patients, circulating AI and AII concentrations fall to less

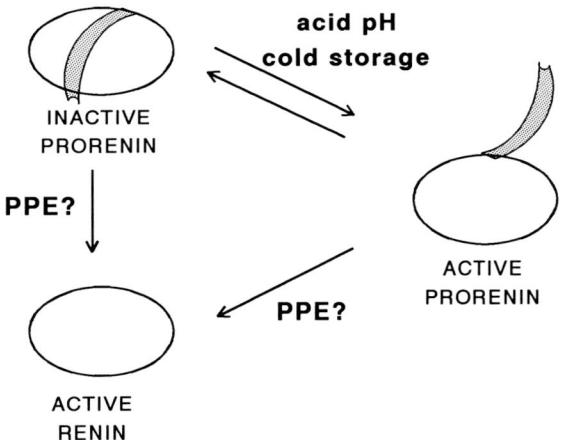

FIG. 2. Schematic representation of the proposed steps in prorenin activation. Stippled area represents the prosegment. PPE, prorenin processing enzyme. It is still unclear whether the proteolytic processing of prorenin to renin *in vivo* requires prior "opening" of the prosegment.

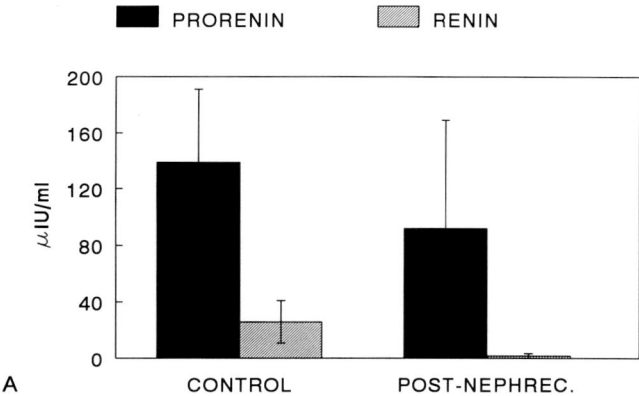

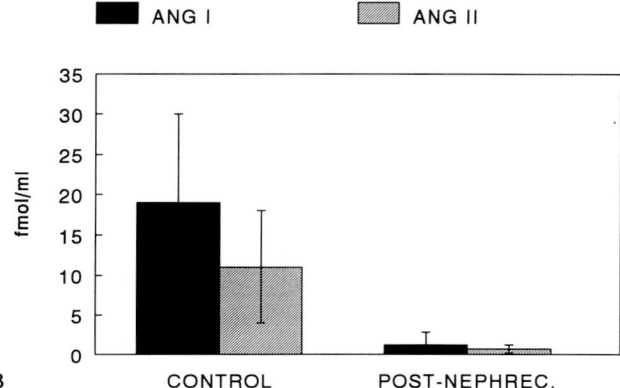

FIG. 3. Effect of chronic nephrectomy on circulating RAS components in humans. Duration of anephric status is between 23 days and 14 years. **A:** Prorenin and renin determined by enzyme kinetic assay are expressed in international units using WHO renin as reference standard. **B:** Plasma concentrations of angiotensin I (ANG I) and angiotensin II (ANG II) as determined by a double HPLC method. (Data are derived from ref. 5.)

Some experiments suggest that the contribution of nonrenal renin to RAS function may not be in direct proportion to its minor role in the generation of *circulating* AII: By microinjecting a mouse renin gene into fertilized rat embryos, Mullins et al. have generated transgenic rats which express both rat and mouse renin (26). Surprisingly, these rats are severely hypertensive even though expression of the mouse transgene is virtually undetectable in the kidney of the transgenic rats. Active mouse renin was also undetectable in the circulation of the transgenic rats although mouse prorenin was present. Notably, the mouse transgene was expressed at high levels in the adrenals of the transgenic rats and was detectable in other tissues such as brain. Could renin be generated within tissues such as the adrenal and act locally to produce AI? In support of this possibility is the finding that explants of normal human adrenal and various adrenal tumors secrete small, but detectable, amounts of active renin when placed in organ culture (27,28).

Thus, although it is difficult from the current findings to be certain about the degree of interaction and the relative contribution of the cRAS and tRAS, it is clear that active renin plays a critical role in cardiovascular physiology and pathophysiology in humans. By contrast, the physiological role of prorenin remains a mystery. The intracellular processes that participate in the generation and secretion of active renin will be the subject of the remainder of this chapter.

BIOSYNTHESIS OF RENIN *IN VIVO*

Transcription, Translation, and Posttranslational Modification

The genes encoding mouse, rat, and human renins have been cloned and characterized (29–33). The genomic organization and deduced amino acid sequence of human renin confirm its close relatedness to other aspartyl proteinases. Human and rat genomes contain only one renin gene (31–34) and while all inbred strains of mice carry the *Ren*-1 structural gene (expressed at high levels in the kidney), some strains contain a second closely linked gene (*Ren*-2) which is expressed at high levels in the submaxillary gland (SMG). In all cases, these genes encode protein precursors of 400–406 amino acids (34–36). A signal peptide encoded at the amino terminus directs the nascent polypeptides to the rough endoplasmic reticulum (RER). Upon insertion into the RER, the signal peptide is removed to generate prorenin and posttranslational modification begins. There are two consensus sequences for N-glycosylation in human renin and three such sites in rat and mouse (Ren-1) renal renin (34,36,37). These sites may be modified to different ex-

than 7 percent of levels in control subjects (5) (Fig. 3B), whereas in rats circulating angiotensins are undetectable within 48 hr after nephrectomy (20). In light of these findings, it might seem surprising that isolated, perfused rat hind limbs are capable of generating angiotensin peptides (21–24). However, peripheral generation of angiotensin peptides is eliminated if the animal is nephrectomized prior to limb isolation and perfusion, suggesting that renin of renal origin can be taken up by peripheral tissues and used to generate angiotensin peptides peripherally (23–25). Taken together, these results suggest that the major mediator of angiotensin biosynthesis in the circulation is active renin secreted by the kidney, but that a small proportion (<10 percent) of the AII found in the circulation may be derived by means other than those involving renal renin.

tents within the RER and Golgi lamellae, resulting in multiple species of renin and prorenin that can be separated by either isoelectric focusing or lectin affinity chromatography (38,39). In human renin, mannose residues on the carbohydrate side chains may also be partially phosphorylated (40), creating a classic lysosomal targeting signal. The importance of the glycosylation of prorenin and renin is most obvious in clearance of the protein from the circulation (41,42), although some evidence has accumulated that glycosylation may also affect intracellular transit time (43), efficiency of intracellular sorting (44), and stability (45) (protease sensitivity?) of prorenin. Rat prorenin can be fractionated into multiple isoelectric species even after enzymatic deglycosylation (46). In contrast, recombinant human prorenin in which the glycosylation sites have been eliminated by protein engineering migrates as a single isoelectric species (47), suggesting that human prorenin does not undergo posttranslational modifications other than N-glycosylation.

Sorting and Processing: Biochemical Studies

Upon their arrival in the terminal lamellae of the trans-Golgi apparatus (the trans-Golgi network or TGN), proteins are segregated to various destinations depending on the posttranslational modifications they have undergone. Proteins in which the carbohydrate side chains have been phosphorylated on mannose residues are targeted to lysosomes (48). Experiments in which recombinant human prorenin has been produced in cultured cells have suggested that a small portion (5–6 percent) of human prorenin may be mannose phosphorylated and transported to lysosomes. The significance of this result is not currently understood, although it may be related to the high degree of similarity between renin and certain lysosomal proteases such as cathepsin D (49).

The bulk of prorenin in the TGN is destined for secretion by one of three pathways (50–54). The first involves direct release from the plasma membrane into the extracellular space. Because there is no evidence of intracellular storage of proteins secreted by this route, it has been called the constitutive secretory pathway. Data suggest that this pathway constitutes the bulk flow or "default" mechanism of protein secretion (50,55) and it is the dominant means of secreting proteins in most eukaryotic cell types. In the constitutive secretory pathway, proteins move from the TGN to the plasma membrane in microtubule-anchored, low-density vesicles (56) with a relatively rapid transit time on the order of minutes to hours (57).

Some specialized endocrine and neuroendocrine cells may also export proteins by the regulated secretory pathway (50,54,58). Proteins secreted in this manner are sorted at the TGN to dense core secretory granules where they are stored until the cell receives a signal which triggers their release. Little is known about the precise molecular signals that target proteins to dense core secretory granules. However, the ability to direct the expression of heterologous proteins in cultured cells of various origins has enabled the definition of certain characteristics of granule targeting signals: Using the model system of mouse pituitary AtT-20 cells, Kelly and co-workers obtained the first evidence that cells from different tissues use a common mechanism to sort proteins to secretory granules (59). AtT-20 cells sort endogenous proopiomelanocortin (POMC) to secretory granules, process POMC to adrenocorticotrophic hormone (ACTH) and other peptides, and release them in response to increases in intracellular cyclic adenosine monophosphate (cAMP). When a recombinant plasmid encoding human proinsulin (an expression vector) is introduced into AtT-20 cells by DNA-mediated gene transfer (transfection), these cells sort and process the encoded prohormone correctly and release human insulin in response to a secretagogue (59). AtT-20 cells have subsequently been shown to correctly sort proteins destined for secretory granules from various species and tissues of origin and to exclude from granules proteins that are known to be secreted in a constitutive manner (60). Further, fusion of a secretory granule–targeted protein with a protein secreted by the constitutive pathway results in secretory granule targeting of the fusion protein (61,62). Taken together, these results suggest that the signals for targeting of proteins to dense core secretory granules are: (a) contained within the targeted protein; (b) universal (i.e., recognized across species and tissue barriers); and (c) dominant (i.e., not by a default mechanism in the absence of a signal). Surprisingly, in spite of this apparent universal nature of the sorting machinery, there exists no extended sequence homology between proteins sorted to granules. There is, in fact, no consensus regarding the actual mechanism of sorting. One hypothesis is that proteins destined for secretory granules interact with a specific secretory granule receptor in much the same way as proteins are sorted to lysosomes. While evidence for the existence of such a "sortase" in dog pancreatic microsomes has been reported (63), there has been no further confirmation of its role as a sorting receptor. Another hypothesis advanced to explain the segregation of granule-targeted proteins in the TGN is selective aggregation (50,64). Many of the proteins that end up in dense core secretory granules show a tendency to aggregate in the presence of calcium and a slightly acidic environment, conditions thought to be present in immature secretory granules (51,64,65). This proposed mechanism is also consistent with microscopic studies demonstrating aggregates in the trans-Golgi network in the process of being encapsulated by membrane (64).

Regardless of the actual mechanism of sorting, the segregated protein is first packaged into a small relatively electron lucid "immature" granule which is often characterized by a clathrin "patch" (51). In some cases, immature granules may fuse with the plasma membrane and release their contents. This pathway, which would result in a seemingly constitutive release of proteins that have been targeted to secretory granules, has been called the "basal" secretory pathway (66). Immature secretory granules not secreted by the basal pathway undergo a maturation process which may involve fusion of multiple immature granules and progressive condensation of their protein content by formation of dense aggregates (51). Mature secretory granules reside at or near the plasma membrane at "docking" sites (50) and fuse with the plasma membrane in response to an extracellular signal. The transit time of proteins in the regulated pathway is longer than that for the constitutive pathway, being in the range of hours to days and depends on the timing of a stimulus for exocytosis (57,67).

The role of the secretory granule in processing prorenin is further supported by biochemical studies: Granule fractions purified from kidney homogenates contain predominantly active renin (68). In addition, renin is secreted more slowly than prorenin from human renal cortical slices and with kinetics that are consistent with its storage in secretory granules (69). Finally, while there must be a mechanism to explain the constant release of both prorenin and renin into the bloodstream, pharmacologic stimuli that cause a release of secretory granules result in an acute and preferential release of active renin into the bloodstream (70). Taken together, these observations suggest a model in which prorenin is secreted constitutively, whereas active renin is generated in maturing secretory granules from which it is released by both the basal and regulated secretory pathways (Fig. 4).

Sorting and Processing: Microscopic Studies

Much of what we understand specifically about the secretion of renin derives from ultrastructural studies on the juxtaglomerular (JG) cells of the kidney, which are the primary site of circulating active renin. JG cells are modified smooth muscle cells which make up approximately 0.1 percent of the cellular mass of the adult kidney (71). While JG cells resemble other neuroendocrine cells in their rich cytoplasmic content of dense core secretory granules (Fig. 5), they are distinguished from these other cell types by two rather striking characteristics: First, rhomboid, paracrystalline structures can sometimes be seen budding off from the TGN and in membrane-bound structures within the cytoplasm (Fig. 6, step 1). These structures are seen most frequently at times of high renin synthesis and may play a role in the

overall mechanism of renin biosynthesis (see below). Second, the secretory granules of JG cells are atypical and display many similarities to lysosomes. At the ultrastructural level, the electron-dense matrix of these granules is sometimes seen to contain multiple vesicular inclusions and membrane fragments (Fig. 6, step 5) and some micrographs suggest that these granules are capable of micropinocytosis and autophagy of other cellular organelles (72,73). In addition, JG cell granules are immunoreactive to antibodies against a number of lysosomal enzymes including acid phosphatase, β-glucuronidase, arylsulfatase, N-acetyl-β-glucosaminidase, and cathepsins B, D, H, and L (73,74). These results, combined with the apparent lack of any recognizable, classic lysosomal structures have led some investigators to suggest that JG cells do not contain the type of secretory granules seen in many endocrine cell types, but rather have adapted lysosomes for the processing, storage, and secretion of prorenin (73).

Using antibodies to various portions of the human prorenin prosegment, Taugner and colleagues have demonstrated that the paracrystalline structures budding off from the TGN of JG cells contain prorenin (75). These structures (Fig. 6, step 1), which have been called protogranules, subsequently fuse together to form a membrane-bound structure containing multiple protogranules, among which small round vesicles can be seen (Fig. 6, step 2). The protogranules eventually lose their individual structures and fuse to form a relatively amorphous, low-density membrane-bound vesicle which has been termed the "immature" or "juvenile" secretory granule (Fig. 6, step 3). In some micrographs these immature granules can be seen to fuse directly with the plasma membrane (73), which would presumably result in the release of prorenin and would correspond, therefore, to the "basal" pathway of protein secretion described above. Immature granules that are not released from the cell become progressively more electron-dense, possibly due to a second stage of aggregation which radiates from a central focal point (Fig. 6, step 4). These structures have been referred to as "intermediate" granules. The most dense granules are referred to as "mature" granules and are frequently seen to contain inclusions which resemble bits of membrane or cellular organelles (Fig. 6, step 5). Evidence suggests that conversion of prorenin to active renin begins in the immature secretory granule. Antibodies specific for the prosegment of human prorenin stain predominantly protogranules and immature granules and show little or no staining of intermediate and mature granules (75). In contrast, an antibody that reacts with both prorenin and renin stains all of these granular structures (75), suggesting that the prosegment is selectively lost at an early stage of granule maturation. These results also suggest that release of immature granules may account for "constitutive-like" or

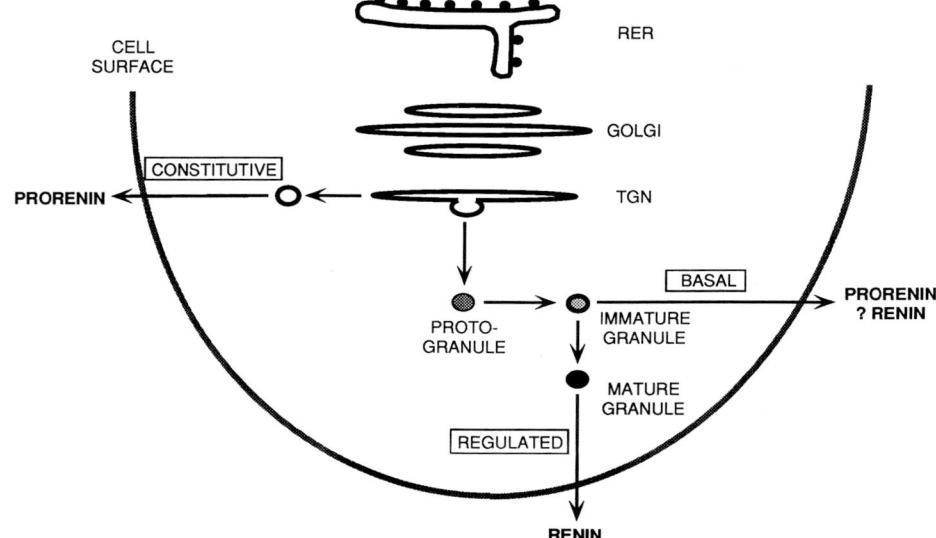

FIG. 4. Schematic representation of potential prorenin and renin secretory pathways in juxtaglomerular cells. RER, rough endoplasmic reticulum; TGN, trans-Golgi network. Boxed labels represent the three potential secretory pathways for prorenin and renin.

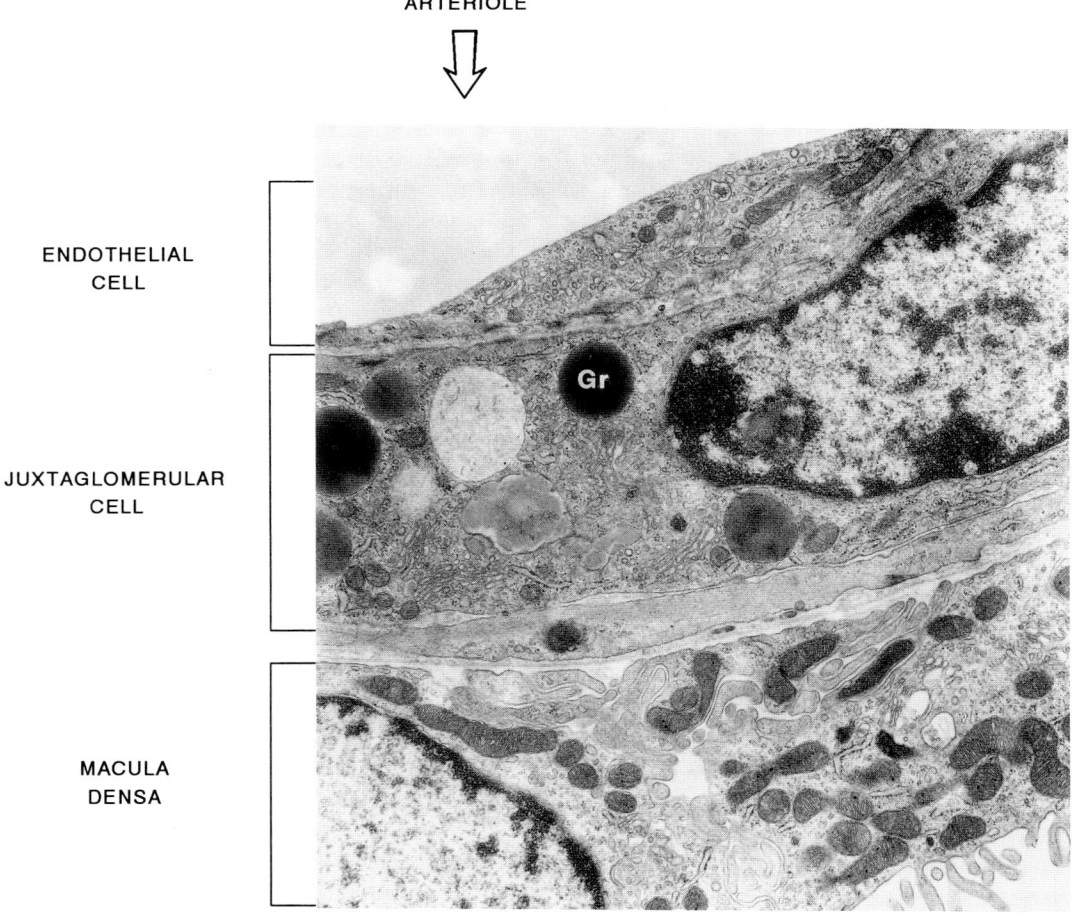

FIG. 5. Electron micrograph of a juxtaglomerular apparatus in a 5-day-old mouse kidney. Gr, dense core secretory granules containing active renin. Original magnification ×15,000.

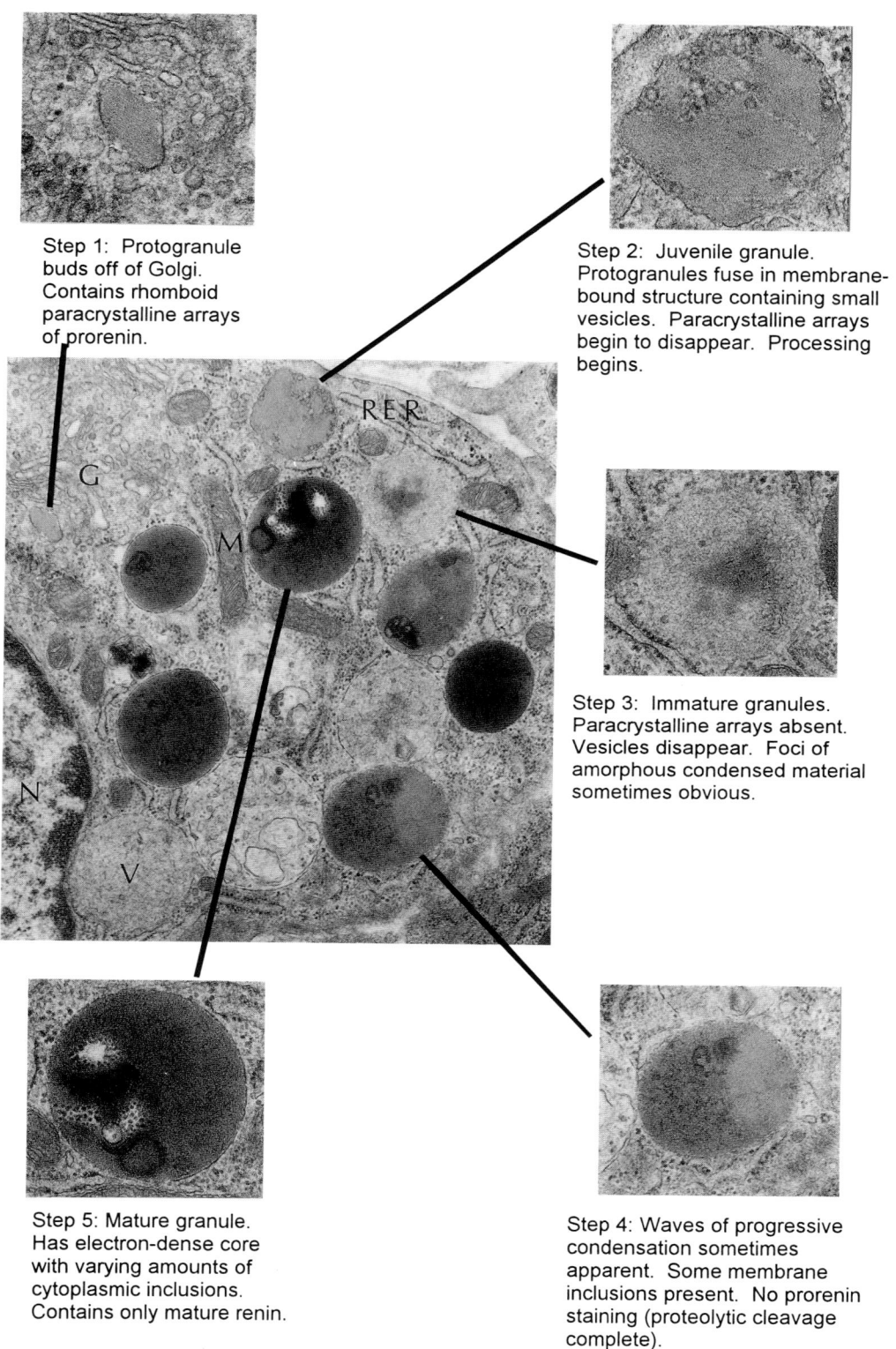

Step 1: Protogranule buds off of Golgi. Contains rhomboid paracrystalline arrays of prorenin.

Step 2: Juvenile granule. Protogranules fuse in membrane-bound structure containing small vesicles. Paracrystalline arrays begin to disappear. Processing begins.

Step 3: Immature granules. Paracrystalline arrays absent. Vesicles disappear. Foci of amorphous condensed material sometimes obvious.

Step 5: Mature granule. Has electron-dense core with varying amounts of cytoplasmic inclusions. Contains only mature renin.

Step 4: Waves of progressive condensation sometimes apparent. Some membrane inclusions present. No prorenin staining (proteolytic cleavage complete).

FIG. 6. Proposed steps in the biosynthesis of renin-containing granules of the 5-day-old mouse juxtaglomerular apparatus. RER, rough endoplasmic reticulum; G, Golgi apparatus; M, mitochondria; N, nucleus; V, vesicular "aneurysms" of the rough endoplasmic reticulum. Original magnification ×22,600.

"basal" release of not only prorenin, but also small amounts of active renin (Fig. 4).

DETERMINANTS OF PRORENIN SORTING

Cell Culture Models

What is the nature of the secretory granule sorting signal on prorenin? Is the seemingly exclusive ability of JG cells to secrete active renin due to the fact that only this particular cell type recognizes secretory granule sorting and processing signals contained on prorenin? This possibility has been directly tested by expressing human, mouse, and rat prorenins in a variety of cell types in tissue culture. Transfection of Chinese hamster ovary (CHO) cells, which contain only a constitutive secretory pathway, with an expression vector encoding human preprorenin leads to secretion of only prorenin (76,77) (Fig. 7). As expected, this prorenin accumulates in a linear fashion in the transfected culture supernatants and secretion is not stimulated acutely by secretagogues. In contrast, transfection of AtT-20 cells, which contain secretory granules and process endogenous POMC, leads to secretion of both prorenin and renin. In addition, whereas prorenin accumulates in culture supernatants constitutively, treatment of the transfected cells with a secretagogue causes a selective and acute release of active renin (76,77) (Fig. 7). This result is characteristic of pro-

teins secreted by the regulated secretory pathway (67) and implies that a portion of the protein is sorted to dense core secretory granules where it is processed and stored for later release. Mouse SMG and renal prorenins (78,79), as well as rat prorenin (79) are also sorted to the regulated secretory pathway in transfected AtT-20 cells. Human prorenin is also sorted to the regulated secretory pathway in PC12 rat pheochromocytoma cells (80) and rat somatomammotrophic GH4 cells (81), although in these two cases prorenin is not activated in granules. These results imply that sorting and activation of prorenin can be seen in cells other than JG cells and that prorenin must contain primary or higher order structural information which directs the cell to carry out these processes.

Molecular Signals

The finding that cells in tissue culture could faithfully direct human prorenin to dense core secretory granules has made it possible to study this intracellular event by modifying the expressed prorenins by site-directed mutagenesis (Fig. 8). Neither the replacement of the native signal peptide of human prorenin with a signal peptide from a constitutively secreted immunoglobulin M (IgM) nor the elimination of the two glycosylation sites on human prorenin prevented its targeting to secretory granules in transfected AtT-20 cells (82) (Fig. 8). The dispens-

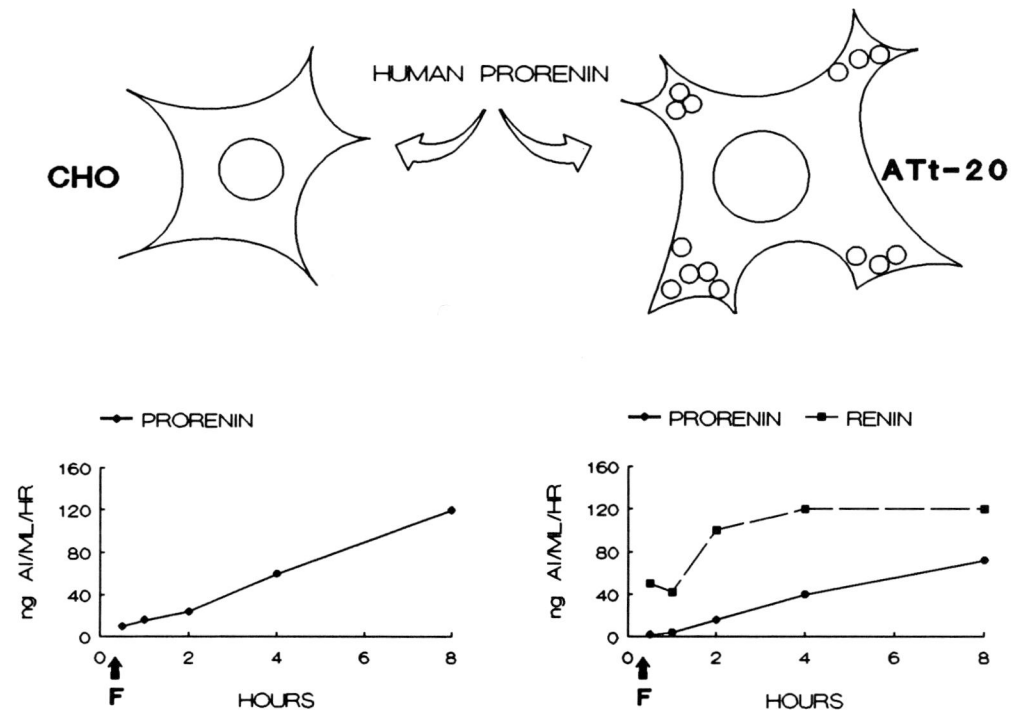

FIG. 7. Cell culture model systems for the study of prorenin sorting, proteolytic cleavage, and secretion. F, point of administration of forskolin, a secretagogue. (Data are derived from ref. 76.)

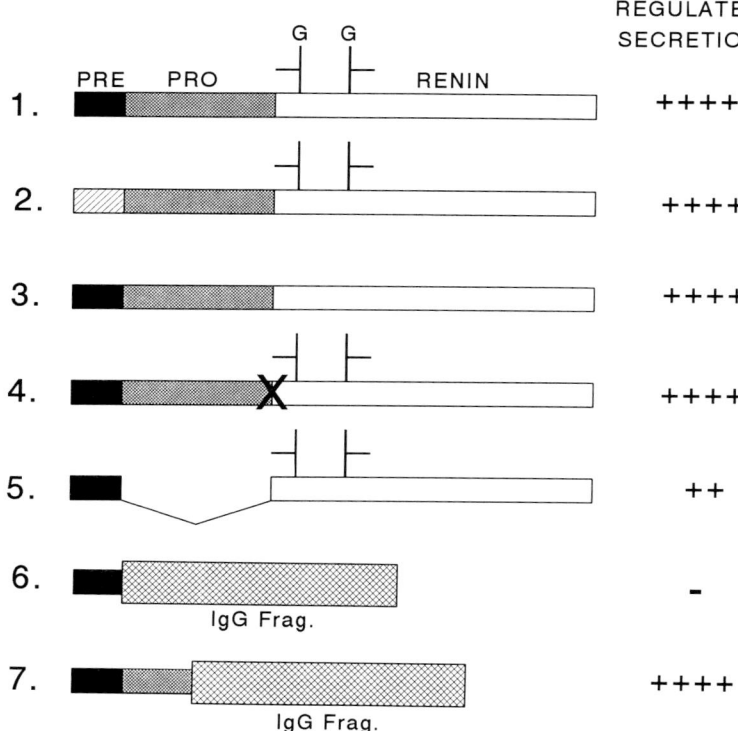

FIG. 8. Summary of mutational effects on secretory granule targeting of human prorenin in transfected AtT-20 cells. G denotes glycosylation sites. 1, native human prorenin; 2, replacement of the signal peptide with that of a mouse IgM; 3, elimination of the glycosylation sites; 4, mutation of the cleavage site to render prorenin noncleavable; 5, elimination of the prosegment; 6, fusion of the prorenin signal peptide to a portion of the mouse IgG heavy chain constant region; 7, fusion of the signal peptide and a portion of the prosegment of human prorenin to the same IgG fragment. (Data are derived from refs. 82–85,95.)

ability of the carbohydrate residues for granule sorting is also evidenced by the fact that mouse SMG prorenin (which is naturally nonglycosylated) is sorted to granules in AtT-20 cells (78). The processing of prorenin to renin also is not required; prorenin molecules containing mutations in the paired basic amino acids at the native processing site can not be activated in AtT-20 cells, but are nevertheless sorted to the regulated pathway and released as prorenin in response to secretagogues (83) (Fig. 8). In addition, regulated secretion of prorenin is seen in transfected PC12 and GH4 cells which contain granules but apparently lack a processing enzyme capable of activating prorenin (80,81). Finally, the prosegment can also be deleted from human prorenin and the resulting "pre-renin" is secreted in a regulated manner in both PC12 and AtT-20 cells (80,82,84) (Fig. 8). By deduction, a sorting signal would appear to be located within the protein domain corresponding to active renin.

To further characterize this sorting sequence, fusion proteins have been constructed which contain a fragment of an immunoglobulin heavy chain constant region (which is constitutively secreted) and fragments of human prorenin. Transfection of AtT-20 cells with the Ig fragment linked to the human prorenin signal peptide alone led to constitutive secretion of the fusion protein (i.e., it was not targeted to secretory granules). However, the addition of a short peptide corresponding to the extreme amino terminus of the human prorenin propeptide led to regulated secretion of the fusion protein in the transfected cells (85) (Fig. 8). The results indicate

that human prorenin contains a peptide within its prosegment that can direct the fusion protein to the regulated secretory pathway. How do these results fit with the finding that the prosegment can be deleted without eliminating secretory granule sorting? The simplest explanation is that more than one domain may be involved in targeting human prorenin to secretory granules; one within its prosegment and another within the active renin portion of the protein.

As previously mentioned, there is no obvious linear homology between the putative sorting peptide in the human prorenin prosegment and peptide sequences contained within other proteins destined for the secretory granule such as POMC, growth hormone, insulin, and atrial natriuretic factor (T. L. Reudelhuber, 1993, *unpublished results*). This result suggests that potential homologies in secretory granule sorting peptides may be in either secondary or tertiary structure rather than the linear amino acid sequence. Alternatively, multiple sorting receptors may exist or a given sorting receptor may have the capacity to interact with a wide spectrum of binding sequences, thereby restricting homologies to subsets of secretory granule sorted proteins. Discrimination between these possibilities will likely have to await the further characterization of minimal sorting peptides in both prorenin and other proteins secreted by the regulated pathway.

In summary, results to date suggest the following regarding the sorting machinery for renin. First, the sorting of prorenin to granules and/or its retention in the maturing granules is not quantitative, either in the JG cells of the kidney or in tissue culture models. In both cases, as much as 80 percent of the prorenin may be secreted in the inactive form by either the constitutive or basal pathway. In this regard, prorenin differs from such proteins as proinsulin which only comprises approximately 15 percent of the total immunoreactive insulin (insulin + proinsulin) in the bloodstream (86). It is unclear at present why this difference exists, but it could presumably be due to differences in the sorting determinants used by the two proteins or in their processing efficiencies once sorted. Second, since the targeting of prorenin to secretory granules can occur in the absence of its proteolytic processing, these two intracellular events appear to be independent. Moreover, since intracellular cleavage of prorenin has not been reported in the absence of targeting to secretory granules, it is likely that targeting precedes processing. This latter conclusion is also supported by immunoelectron microscopic studies of JG cells in which prorenin disappears in the maturing granule and is similar to results reported for insulin in the granules of pancreatic β-cells (87). Third, the signal(s) responsible for directing prorenin to secretory granules appears to be functional in cultured endocrine cells types from a variety of tissues and species. Thus, like the secretory granule sorting determinants on many other granule-targeted proteins, this signal may be universal and thus may not be an ideal target for pharmacologic intervention in the production of renin.

Is the use of an endocrine cell model a reasonable approach to identifying sorting determinants to the lysosome-like granules contained in JG cells? While only 5–6 percent of prorenin expressed in mammalian cells acquires phosphomannosyl residues (40), it is an intriguing possibility that renal prorenins make use of both granular and lysosomal signaling mechanisms to ensure their efficient sorting to the lysosome-like secretory granules in JG cells. Clearly, it will be imperative to test for the function of any potential prorenin sorting peptides in the JG cells of intact animals.

DETERMINANTS OF PRORENIN PROCESSING

Species and Tissue Differences

Amino terminal sequencing of renin isolated from human kidney lysates suggests that activation occurs by the proteolytic removal of a 43 amino acid prosegment from the amino terminus of prorenin (88). This processing site follows a pair of basic amino acids in human renin (Fig. 9). Processing of prorenin in the mouse SMG occurs at the analogous position (89), but processing of rat renal renin seems to occur after a threonine residue which is located 7 amino acids toward the carboxy terminus relative to the analogous position in human renin (46,90)

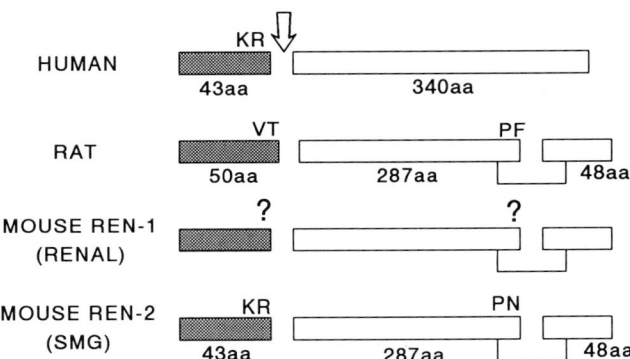

FIG. 9. Proposed cleavage sites for human, rat, and mouse prorenins. Signal peptides are not shown. Numbering is from amino acid 1 of the prosegment. Letters denotes the single letter codes for amino acids. Question marks indicate cleavage sites that have not yet been defined. Drawings are not to scale. (Data are from refs. 6,46,89, and 90.)

(Fig. 9). The processing site for mouse renal renin is currently unknown. Rat renal and mouse SMG renins subsequently undergo an additional internal processing event, converting "one-chain" active renin to a "two-chain" molecule (46,89,90) in which the two halves are held together by a disulfide bridge (Fig. 9). Notably, whereas renal renins appear to be processed within secretory granules, mouse SMG renin may be processed to "one-chain" renin within the Golgi apparatus and only a portion of the protein is further processed in granules to yield the "two-chain" protein (91). Thus, while renins from mice, rats, and humans share many similarities in protein structure and function, differences exist in the way these proteins are modified within the secretory apparatus.

Cleavage Site Selectivity

In the human kidney, cleavage of prorenin is highly specific and occurs at a pair of basic amino acids (Lys-Arg), resulting in removal of a 43 amino acid prosegment from the amino terminus of prorenin (6). There are six additional pairs of basic amino acids in human prorenin (37) including Lys-Lys, Arg-Arg, and Arg-Lys within the body of renin, two Lys-Arg pairs in the prosegment, and the Lys-Lys-Arg triplet in the body of renin, none of which appears to be cleaved in the kidney. Many proteases are capable of activating human renin *in vitro*, including trypsin, plasmin, tissue and plasma kallikreins, and cathepsin B (7,92,93). While some of these enzymes are likely to be physiologically nonrelevant due to their tissue distribution, some nevertheless cleave prorenin with the correct site specificity (94). AtT-20 cells transfected with a human preprorenin expression vector also cleave prorenin at the same site as that reported for renin purified from human kidney lysates (76). What determines this cleavage site selectivity? One hypothesis to explain the cleavage site selectivity displayed by enzymes *in vitro,* AtT-20 cells, and the kidney is that primary and/ or higher order structural determinants on prorenin render the native processing site uniquely sensitive to proteolytic cleavage. This hypothesis was directly tested by introducing single amino acid mutations in human preprorenin surrounding the natural cleavage site and expressing the resultant recombinant proteins to proteolytic activation either by trypsin or by the endogenous processing enzyme in AtT-20 cells (95). The results suggest that amino acids in addition to the pair of basic amino acids surrounding the cleavage site affect the ability of both trypsin and the AtT-20 processing enzyme to cleave prorenin (Fig. 10). Notably, while a proline at position -4 is essential for processing of human prorenin in AtT-20 cells and is correlated with predicted formation of a β-turn at this position, other site-directed mutations suggest that this structural feature in addition to a pair of basic amino acids is not sufficient to lead to proteolytic activation of prorenin (95). In contrast to the case with human prorenin, neither mouse renal prorenin (79) nor rat prorenin (79,96) is processed at the analogous positions in transfected AtT-20 cells. In both cases, mutagenesis of the natural substrates has demonstrated that this is also due to the particular arrangement of amino acids immediately adjacent to the native processing site (76,79,95,97).

Candidate Processing Enzymes

Although many of the enzymes that activate human prorenin *in vitro* may be physiologically irrelevant, there are some notable exceptions. Shinagawa et al. recently characterized an enzyme from human whole kidney lysates which correctly processes human prorenin to active renin (98). Subsequent purification and partial amino acid sequence of this putative prorenin processing enzyme (PPE) revealed that it is cathepsin B (93). While cathepsin B is a lysosomal enzyme which is expressed in a broad variety of cell types (99), it appears to co-localize with renin not only in the lysosome-like granules of JG cells (73,74), but also in the more classic secretory granules of prorenin-containing human pituitary lactotrophs (100). *In vitro,* cathepsin B cleaves human prorenin with the correct specificity and with a substrate constant (K_s) in the nanomolar range (93). For these reasons, cathepsin B has been proposed as the renal PPE. In a similar effort, an enzyme capable of processing mouse SMG prorenin has been isolated from submaxillary glands (101). This enzyme, which has been called prorenin-converting enzyme (PRECE), was subsequently revealed to be identical to the mGK-13 gene product (102) (also known as the epidermal growth factor-binding protein type B), a member of the kallikrein gene family. Although PRECE can activate mouse SMG prorenin to generate "one-chain" renin, it is unable to carry out the second cleavage to yield the "two-chain" form (101). In addition, kidney glandular kallikrein cannot activate mouse SMG prorenin and PRECE is unable to activate mouse renal or human prorenins (101). Recently, a second enzyme capable of converting mouse SMG prorenin to "one-chain" renin has also been isolated from mouse submaxillary gland (103).

As an alternative approach to biochemical purification and *in vitro* testing of candidate PPE, cell culture

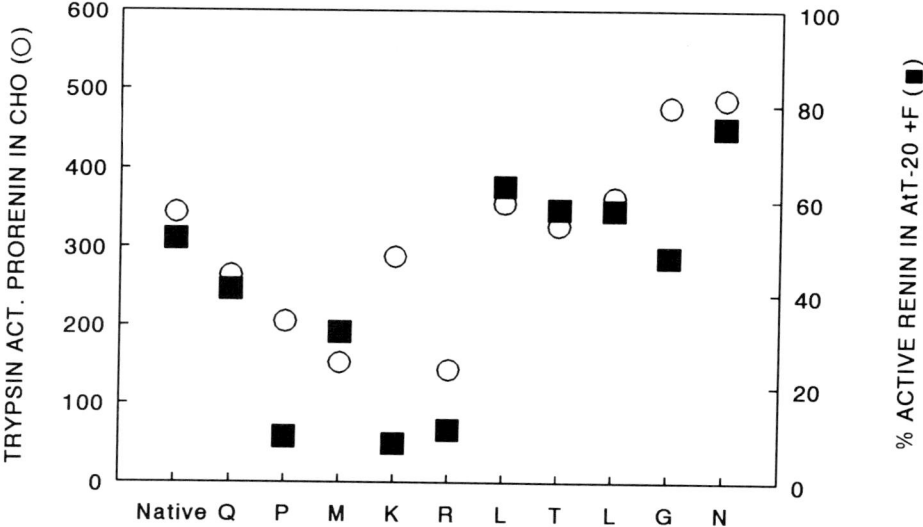

FIG. 10. Effect of site-specific mutations on processing of human prorenin. Single amino acids in the region of the cleavage site of human prorenin were individually converted to alanine. The relative ability of either trypsin (*solid points*) or the endogenous processing enzyme of AtT-20 cells (*open dots*) to activate mutated human prorenins as compared with nonmutated prorenin (native) is shown. Letters under each point represent the single letter code for the amino acid which was replaced. Cleavage normally occurs between R and L. (Data are from ref. 95, with permission.)

transfection assays have been developed to directly test for the ability of candidate processing enzymes to cleave prorenin within the appropriate intracellular environment. Taking into account the reports that prorenin cleavage occurs within the secretory granules of the renal JG cells (see above), we initially identified a cultured cell line which would target human prorenin to granules, but would lack processing enzyme activity. Prorenin expression vectors can then be co-transfected in these cells with expression vectors encoding a variety of processing enzymes, and culture supernatants can be assayed for the presence of active renin (Fig. 11). Transfection of secretory granule–containing GH4 cells with an expression vector encoding human prorenin results in the secretion of prorenin into culture supernatants, confirming the lack of a prorenin processing enzyme in these cells (81) (Fig. 12). When human prorenin is co-transfected into GH4 cells with an expression vector encoding the mouse subtilisin-like endoprotease PC1, the cells are rendered capable of selectively processing prorenin at the identical site as that reported for the human kidney. Interestingly, this processing event does not occur in cells devoid of secretory granules (CHO and BSC-40) and is not due to any apparent differences in processing of PC1 in these cell types (96). When tested in a similar assay, neither furin (81), PC2 (96) nor human cathepsin B (Fig. 12) are able to process human prorenin. Why is cathepsin B unable to process human prorenin within these cells when it is capable of doing so *in vitro?* One possibility is that cathepsin B itself requires activation by enzymes that are lacking in GH4 cells. Another possibility is that the secretory granules in kidney JG cells are sufficiently different in nature from the granules found in GH4 cells that cathepsin B is inactive in the latter. The solution to this problem remains an area of interesting future investigation.

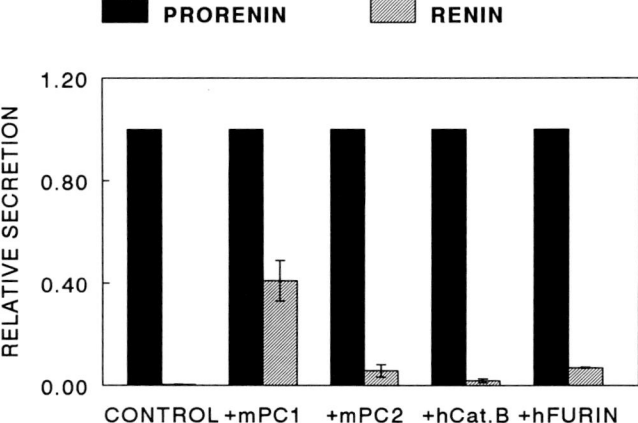

FIG. 12. Effect of candidate PPE on processing human prorenin in GH4 cells. Prorenin (*solid bars*) and renin (*open bars*) detected in culture supernatants 40 hr after co-transfection of cultured cells with expression vectors for human prorenin and corresponding processing enzymes. Active renin is depicted relative to the level of prorenin (set at 100 percent). (Data are derived from ref. 96.)

Is PC1 the enzyme that activates prorenin in mammalian JG cells? Probably not: PC1 is unable to cleave mouse or rat renal prorenins (79,96) and we have obtained no evidence to date for staining of human JG cells with anti-PC1 antibodies (T. L. Reudelhuber, D. Ramla, M. Marcinkiewicz, and N. Seidah, 1993, *unpublished observations*). However, PC1 staining is evident in the human adrenal medulla (T. L. Reudelhuber and D. Ramla, 1994, *unpublished observation*) where the human prorenin gene is also expressed (28). It is possible, therefore, that cathepsin B, PC1, and perhaps other proteases activate human prorenin in a tissue-specific manner.

Transgenic Animals

As mentioned above, rat renal renin does not have the same amino terminus as human renal renin (46,90) and the amino terminus of active mouse renal renin is still unknown. This, combined with the species-specificity of some of the PPE described above, raises the possibility that species-specific differences exist in the processing enzymes that activate prorenins. In contrast to these findings is the experience of expressing prorenins from various species in transgenic animals: Ohkubo et al. have expressed rat renin in ectopic tissues of transgenic mice by placing the prorenin coding sequences under the control of a mouse metallothionein gene promoter (104). Mating of the rat prorenin-expressing mouse strain with another strain which had been rendered transgenic for rat angiotensinogen resulted in a "double transgenic" strain with elevated blood pressure (104). Because only mice containing both of the rat transgenes had elevated pressures, the implication is that the rat prorenin had

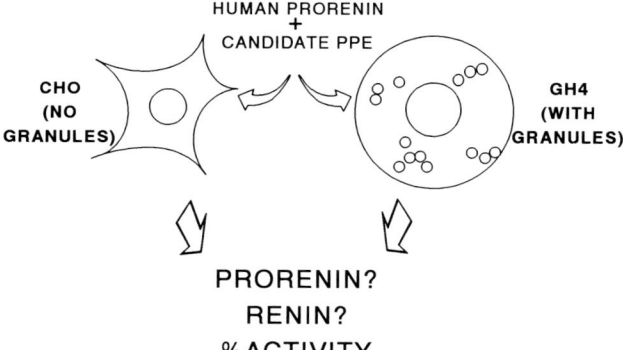

FIG. 11. Schematic representation of a model tissue culture system to test candidate prorenin processing enzymes. Cells either containing (*left*) or lacking (*right*) secretory granules are co-transfected with expression vectors encoding prorenin and various candidate proteases. Culture supernatants are subsequently tested for production of prorenin and active renin.

been activated in the mouse tissues, although the tissue site of activation was not determined. In similar approaches, injection of either mouse (105,106) or rat (107) embryos with the intact human prorenin gene resulted in the generation of transgenic animals with active human renin in their bloodstream. Thus, in spite of the apparent species selectivity of PPE activities reported *in vitro,* the mouse (at the very least) must express an enzyme or enzymes capable of activating prorenins from rats, mice, and humans.

Thus, while it has been possible to purify and characterize candidate PPE by classic biochemical techniques, the occasional promiscuity displayed by processing enzymes *in vitro* and the tendency for cellular colocalization to be misleading regarding function (108,109) has complicated the unequivocal identification of the enzyme responsible for the activation of prorenin in any given tissue. For this reason, it is imperative that these studies be complemented with genetic or other experiments that specifically block the actions of the putative protease *in vivo* before a specific role in prorenin activation can be confirmed.

SUMMARY

Although it has been nearly 100 years since the discovery of renin activity, we continue to gain insight into not only the role of the RAS in physiology and pathophysiology, but also the mechanisms governing the activation and secretion of the rate-limiting component of the RAS, renin. The data available to date not only confirm the critical role of renin of renal origin in the activity of the circulating RAS, but also its possible implication in the activity of tRAS through its uptake from the bloodstream.

Perhaps one of the most perplexing questions that remains regarding the RAS is the role of the prorenin synthesized in various nonrenal tissues. It is possible that this prorenin is activated in a local manner through either proteolytic or other mechanisms, but that the resulting active renin is not released into the bloodstream. There is mounting evidence that such a process occurs in the adrenal gland where prorenin may be activated by an enzyme different from that which produces active renin in the kidney. Other possible explanations for the existence of tRAS must be considered, however. For example, these systems may be vestigial and, as they produce only prorenin, are harmless. This is perhaps the least satisfying explanation due primarily to the rather high conservation in the distribution of components of the tRAS in mammals. Another possibility is that prorenin, in itself, has a biological function in addition to being the precursor to active renin. However, this possibility would fail to explain the presence of the other components of the RAS in many of the tissues expressing pro-

renin. A more appealing possibility is that tRAS plays some important role in gestational development of mammals that is no longer evident in adults. For example, activation of any given tRAS might only require transient expression of a PPE and the generated angiotensin peptides might function not only in regulating local circulation but also perhaps in acting as chemoattractants for cell migration or as angiogenic or generalized growth factors. Such a model might serve to explain the high levels of renin gene expression seen in early gestational sacs in humans (110) and the fluctuating levels of renin gene expression seen in tissues of the developing mouse (111). The ability to selectively "knock-out" specific genes in the mouse genome (112) should enable the testing of such a hypothesis in the near future.

ACKNOWLEDGMENTS

This work was supported by grants from the National Institutes of Health (HL-35706) and the Medical Research Council of Canada (MA-11179 and a Group Grant to the Multidisciplinary Research Group on Hypertension). T. L. Reudelhuber is the recipient of the Merck-Frosst chair in Molecular Pharmacology.

REFERENCES

1. Lindpaintner K, Ganten D. Tissue renin-angiotensin systems and their modulation: the heart as a paradigm for new aspects of converting enzyme inhibition. *Cardiology* 1991;79(Suppl 1):32–44.
2. Griendling KK, Murphy TJ, Alexander RW. Molecular biology of the renin-angiotensin system. *Circulation* 1993;87:1816–1828.
3. Danser AH, van den Dorpel MA, Deinum J, et al. Renin, prorenin, and immunoreactive renin in vitreous fluid from eyes with and without diabetic retinopathy. *J Clin Endocrinol Metab* 1989;68:160–167.
4. Neuringer JR, Brenner BM. Hemodynamic theory of progressive renal disease: a 10-year update in brief review. *Am J Kidney Dis* 1993;22:98–104.
5. Campbell DJ, Kladis A, Skinner SL, Whitworth JA. Characterization of angiotensin peptides in plasma of anephric man. *J Hypertens* 1991;9:265–274.
6. Do YS, Shinegawa T, Tam S, Inagami T, Hsueh WA. Characterization of pure human renal renin: Evidence for a subunit structure. *J Biol Chem* 1987;262:1037–1043.
7. Hsueh WA, Baxter JD. Human prorenin. *Hypertension* 1991;17: 469–479.
8. Derkx FH, Schalekamp MP, Schalekamp MA. Two-step prorenin-renin conversion. Isolation of an intermediary form of activated prorenin. *J Biol Chem* 1987;262:2472–2477.
9. Pitarresi TM, Rubattu S, Heinrikson R, Sealey JE. Reversible cryoactivation of recombinant human prorenin. *J Biol Chem* 1992;267:11753–11759.
10. Lenz T, Sealey JE, Lappe RW, et al. Infusion of recombinant human prorenin into rhesus monkeys. Effects on hemodynamics, renin-angiotensin-aldosterone axis and plasma testosterone. *Am J Hypertens* 1990;3:257–261.
11. Lenz T, Sealey JE, Maack T, et al. Half-life, hemodynamic, renal, and hormonal effects of prorenin in cynomolgus monkeys. *Am J Physiol* 1991;260:R804–R810.
12. Paul M, Wagner J, Dzau VJ. Gene expression of the renin-angiotensin system in human tissues. Quantitative analysis by the polymerase chain reaction. *J Clin Invest* 1993;91:2058–2064.

13. Mulrow PJ. Adrenal renin: a possible local regulator of aldosterone production. *Yale J Biol Med* 1989;62:503–510.
14. Ganong WF, Deschepper CF, Steele MK, Intebi A. Renin-angiotensin system in the anterior pituitary of the rat. *Am J Hypertens* 1989;2:320–322.
15. Ganong WF. Angiotensin II in the brain and pituitary: contrasting roles in the regulation of adenohypophyseal secretion. *Hormone Res* 1989;31:24–31.
16. Sealey JE, Rubattu S. Prorenin and renin as separate mediators of tissue and circulating systems. *Am J Hypertens* 1989;2:358–366.
17. Hosoi M, Kim S, Tabata T, et al. Evidence for the presence of differently glycosylated forms of prorenin in the plasma of anephric man. *J Clin Endocrinol Metab* 1992;74:680–684.
18. Suzuki F, Ludwig G, Hellmann W, et al. Renin gene expression in rat tissues: a new quantitative assay method for rat renin mRNA using synthetic cRNA. *Clin Exp Hypertens* 1988;A10:345–359.
19. Kim S, Hosoi M, Nakajima K, Yamamoto K. Immunological evidence that kidney is primary source of circulating inactive prorenin in rats. *Am J Physiol* 1991;260:E526–E536.
20. Nussberger J, Flückiger J-P, Hui KY, Evéquoz D, Waeber B, Brunner HR. Angiotensin I and II disappear completely from circulating blood within 48 hours after binephrectomy: improved measurement of angiotensins in rat plasma. *J Hypertens* 1991;9(Suppl 6):S230–S231.
21. Campbell DJ, Ziogas J, Kladis A. Metabolism of tetradecapeptide, angiotensinogen and angiotensin I and II by isolated perfused rat hindlimbs. *Clin Exp Pharmacol Physiol* 1990;17:335–350.
22. Kuczera M, Hilgers KF, Lisson C, et al. Local angiotensin formation in hindlimbs of uremic hypertensive and renovascular hypertensive rats. *J Hypertens* 1991;9:41–48.
23. Hilgers KF, Hilgenfeldt U, Veelken R, et al. Angiotensinogen is cleaved to angiotensin in isolated rat blood vessels. *Hypertension* 1993;21:1030–1034.
24. Kato H, Iwai N, Inui H, Kimoto K, Uchiyama Y, Inagami T. Regulation of vascular angiotensin release. *Hypertension* 1993;21:446–454.
25. Danser AHJ, Sassen LMA, Admiraal PJJ, Derkx FHM, Verdouw PD, Schalekamp MADH. Regional production of angiotensins I and II: contribution of vascular kidney-derived renin. *J Hypertens* 1991;9(Suppl 6):S234–S235.
26. Mullins JJ, Peters J, Ganten D. Fulminant hypertension in transgenic rats harbouring the mouse Ren-2 gene. *Nature* 1990;344:541–544.
27. Sarzani R, Fallo F, Dessi-Fulgheri P, et al. Local renin-angiotensin system in human adrenals and aldosteronomas. *Hypertension* 1992;19:702–707.
28. Racz K, Pinet F, Gasc JM, Guyene TT, Corvol P. Coexpression of renin, angiotensinogen, and their messenger ribonucleic acids in adrenal tissues. *J Clin Endocrinol Metab* 1992;75:730–737.
29. Holm I, Ollo R, Panthier J, Rougeon F. Evolution of aspartyl proteases by gene duplication: the mouse renin gene is organized in two homologous clusters of four exons. *EMBO J* 1984;3:557–562.
30. Fukamizu A, Nishi K, Cho T, et al. Structure of the rat renin gene. *J Mol Biol* 1988;201:443–450.
31. Hobart PM, Fogliano M, O'Connor BA, Schaefer IM, Chirgwin JM. Human renin gene: structure and sequence analysis. *Proc Natl Acad Sci (USA)* 1984;81:5026–5030.
32. Miyazaki H, Fukamizu A, Hirose S, et al. Structure of the human renin gene. *Proc Natl Acad Sci (USA)* 1984;81:5999–6003.
33. Hardman JA, Hort YJ, Catanzaro DF, et al. Primary structure of the human renin gene. *DNA* 1984;3:457–468.
34. Burnham CE, Hawelu-Johnson CL, Frank BM, Lynch KR. Molecular cloning of rat renin cDNA and its gene. *Proc Natl Acad Sci (USA)* 1987;84:5605–5609.
35. Murakami K, Hirose S, Miyazaki H, et al. Complementary DNA sequences of renin. State-of-the-art review. *Hypertension* 1984;6:I95–I100.
36. Panthier JJ, Rougeon F. Kidney and submaxillary gland renins are encoded by two non-allelic genes in Swiss mice. *EMBO J* 1983;2:675–678.
37. Imai T, Miyazaki H, Hirose S, et al. Cloning and sequence analysis of cDNA for human renin precursor. *Proc Natl Acad Sci (USA)* 1983;80:7405–7409.
38. Katz SA, Malvin RL, Lee J, et al. Analysis of active renin heterogeneity. *Proc Soc Exp Biol Med* 1991;197:387–392.
39. Hosoi M, Kim S, Yamamoto K. Evidence for heterogeneity of glycosylation of human renin obtained by using lectins. *Clin Sci* 1991;81:393–399.
40. Faust PL, Chirgwin JM, Kornfeld S. Renin, a secretory glycoprotein, acquires phosphomannosyl residues. *J Cell Biol* 1987;105:1947–1955.
41. Shier DN, Malvin RL. Differential secretion and removal of multiple renin forms. *Am J Physiol* 1985;249:R79–R84.
42. Kim S, Hiruma M, Ikemoto F, Yamamoto K. Importance of glycosylation for hepatic clearance of renal renin. *Am J Physiol* 1988;255:E642–E651.
43. Paul M, Nakamura N, Pratt RE, Dzau VJ. Glycosylation influences intracellular transit time and secretion rate of human prorenin in transfected cells. *J Hypertens* 1988;6:S487–S489.
44. Baxter JD, James MN, Chu WN, et al. The molecular biology of human renin and its gene. *Yale J Biol Med* 1989;62:493–501.
45. Hori H, Yoshino T, Ishizuka Y, Yamauchi T, Murakami K. Role of N-linked oligosaccharides attached to human renin expressed in COS cells. *FEBS Lett* 1988;232:391–394.
46. Kim S, Hosoi M, Kikuchi N, Yamamoto K. Amino-terminal amino acid sequence and heterogeneity in glycosylation of rat renal renin. *J Biol Chem* 1991;266:7044–7050.
47. Su Y, Reudelhuber TL. Molecular characterization of human prorenin isoelectric forms. *J Hypertens* 1993;11:141–146.
48. Kornfeld S. Lysosomal enzyme targeting. *Biochem Soc Transac* 1990;18:367–374.
49. Faust PL, Kornfeld S, Chirgwin JM. Cloning and sequence analysis of cDNA for human cathepsin D. *Proc Natl Acad Sci (USA)* 1985;82:4910–4914.
50. Kelly RB. Secretory granule and synaptic vesicle formation. *Curr Opin Cell Biol* 1991;3:654–660.
51. Tooze SA. Biogenesis of secretory granules: implications arising from the immature secretory granule in the regulated pathway of secretion. *FEBS Lett* 1991;285:220–224.
52. Orci L, Ravazzola M, Amherdt M, et al. The trans-most cisternae of the Golgi complex: a compartment for sorting of secretory and plasma membrane proteins. *Cell* 1987;51:1039–1051.
53. Moore HP, Brion C, Chung KN, Lehmicke L, Rivas R, Quinn D. Protein secretion by constitutive and regulated pathways. *Soc Gen Physiol Ser* 1989;44:189–201.
54. Miller SG, Moore H. Regulated secretion. *Curr Opin Cell Biol* 1990;2:642–647.
55. Wieland FT, Gleason ML, Serafini TA, Rothman JE. The rate of bulk flow from the endoplasmic reticulum to the cell surface. *Cell* 1987;50:289–300.
56. Kelly RB. Microtubules, membrane traffic, and cell organization. *Cell* 1990;61:5–7.
57. Moore HP, Kelly RB. Secretory protein targeting in a pituitary cell line: differential transport of foreign secretory proteins to distinct secretory pathways. *J Cell Biol* 1985;101:1773–1781.
58. Rothman JE, Orci L. Molecular dissection of the secretory pathway. *Nature* 1992;355:409–415.
59. Moore HP, Walker MD, Lee F, Kelly RB. Expressing a human proinsulin cDNA in a mouse ACTH-secreting cell. Intracellular storage, proteolytic processing, and secretion on stimulation. *Cell* 1983;35:531–538.
60. Kizer JS, Tropsha A. A motif found in propeptides and prohormones that may target them to secretory vesicles. *Biochem Biophys Res Commun* 1991;174:586–592.
61. Moore HH, Kelly RB. Re-routing of a secretory protein by fusion with human growth hormone sequences. *Nature* 1986;321:443–446.
62. Stoller TJ, Shields D. The propeptide of preprosomatostatin mediates intracellular transport and secretion of alpha-globin from mammalian cells. *J Cell Biol* 1989;108:1647–1655.
63. Chung KN, Walter P, Aponte GW, Moore HP. Molecular sorting in the secretory pathway. *Science* 1989;243:192–197.
64. Reaves BJ, Dannies PS. Is a sorting signal necessary to package

proteins into secretory granules? *Mol Cell Endocrinol* 1991;79: C141–C145.

65. Orci L, Ravazzola M, Anderson RG. The condensing vacuole of exocrine cells is more acidic than the mature secretory vesicle. *Nature* 1987;326:77–79.

66. von Zastrow M, Castle JD. Protein sorting among two distinct export pathways occurs from the content of maturing exocrine storage granules. *J Cell Biol* 1987;105:2675–2684.

67. Burgess TL, Kelly RB. Constitutive and regulated secretion of proteins. *Annu Rev Cell Biol* 1987;3:243–293.

68. Kawamura M, McKenzie JC, Hoffman LH, Tanaka I, Parmentier M, Inagami T. The storage form of renin in renin granules from rat kidney cortex. *Hypertension* 1986;8:706–711.

69. Pratt RE, Carleton JE, Richie JP, Heusser C, Dzau VJ. Human renin biosynthesis and secretion in normal and ischemic kidneys. *Proc Natl Acad Sci (USA)* 1987;84:7837–7840.

70. Toffelmire EB, Slater K, Corvol P, Menard J, Schambelan M. Response of plasma prorenin and active renin to chronic and acute alterations of renin secretion in normal humans. Studies using a direct immunoradiometric assay. *J Clin Invest* 1989;83: 679–687.

71. Taugner R, Bührle CP, Nobiling R. Ultrastructural changes associated with renin secretion from the juxtaglomerular apparatus of mice. *Cell Tissue Res* 1984;237:459–472.

72. Taugner R, Metz R, Rosivall L. Macroautophagic phenomena in renin granules. *Cell Tissue Res* 1988;251:229–231.

73. Taugner R, Hackenthal E. On the character of the secretory granules in juxtaglomerular epithelioid cells. *Int Rev Cytol* 1988;110: 93–131.

74. Matsuba H, Watanabe T, Watanabe M, et al. Immunocytochemical localization of prorenin, renin, and cathepsins B, H, and L in juxtaglomerular cells of rat kidney. *J Histochem Cytochem* 1989;37:1689–1697.

75. Taugner R, Kim SJ, Murakami K, Waldherr R. The fate of prorenin during granulopoiesis in epithelioid cells. Immunocytochemical experiments with antisera against renin and different portions of the renin prosegment. *Histochemis* 1987;86:249–253.

76. Fritz LC, Haidar MA, Arfsten AE, et al. Human renin is correctly processed and targeted to the regulated secretory pathway in mouse pituitary AtT-20 cells. *J Biol Chem* 1987;262:12409–12412.

77. Pratt RE, Flynn JA, Hobart PM, Paul M, Dzau VJ. Different secretory pathways of renin from mouse cells transfected with the human renin gene. *J Biol Chem* 1988;263:3137–3141.

78. Landenheim R, Seidah N, Lutfalla G, Rougeon F. Stable and transient expression of mouse submaxillary gland renin cDNA in AtT20 cells: proteolytic processing and secretory pathways. *FEBS Lett* 1989;245:70–74.

79. Nagahama M, Nakayama K, Murakami K. Sequence requirements for prohormone processing in mouse pituitary AtT-20 cells: analysis of prorenins as model substrates. *Eur J Biochem* 1991;197:135–140.

80. Chidgey MA, Harrison TM. Renin is sorted to the regulated secretory pathway in transfected PC12 cells by a mechanism which does not require expression of the propeptide. *Eur J Biochem* 1990;190:139–144.

81. Hatsuzawa K, Hosaka M, Nakagawa T, et al. Structure and expression of mouse furin, a yeast Kex2-related protease. Lack of processing of coexpressed prorenin in GH4C1 cells. *J Biol Chem* 1990;265:22075–22078.

82. Chu WN, Baxter JD, Reudelhuber TL. A targeting sequence for dense core secretory granules resides in the protein moiety of human prorenin. *Mol Endocrinol* 1990;4:1905–1913.

83. Nakayama K, Nagahama M, Kim WAS, Hatsuzawa K, Murakami K. Prorenin is sorted into the regulated secretory pathway independent of its processing to renin in mouse pituitary AtT-20 cells. *FEBS Lett* 1989;257:89–92.

84. Nagahama M, Nakayama K, Murakami K. Effects of propeptide deletion on human renin secretion from mouse pituitary AtT-20 cells. *FEBS Lett* 1990;264:67–70.

85. Baxter JD, Duncan K, Chu W, et al. Molecular biology of human renin and its gene. *Recent Prog Horm Res* 1991;47:211–257.

86. Gabbay KH, DeLuca K, Fisher JN Jr, Mako ME, Rubenstein

AH. Familial hyperproinsulinemia. An autosomal dominant defect. *New Engl J Med* 1976;294:911–915.

87. Orci L, Ravazzola M, Storch MJ, Anderson RG, Vassalli JD, Perrelet A. Proteolytic maturation of insulin is a post-Golgi event which occurs in acidifying clathrin-coated secretory vesicles. *Cell* 1987;49:865–868.

88. Do YS, Shinagawa T, Tam H, Inagami T, Hsueh WA. Characterization of pure human renal renin. *J Biol Chem* 1987;262:1037–1043.

89. Misono KS, Chang J, Inagami T. Amino acid sequence of mouse submaxillary gland renin. *Proc Natl Acad Sci (USA)* 1982;79: 4858–4862.

90. Campbell DJ, Valentijn AJ, Condron R. Purification and amino-terminal sequence of rat kidney renin: evidence for a two-chain structure. *J Hypertens* 1991;9:29–33.

91. Pratt RE, Ouellette AJ, Dzau VJ. Biosynthesis of renin: multiplicity of active and intermediate forms. *Proc Natl Acad Sci (USA)* 1983;80:6809–6813.

92. Frohlich ED, Iwata T, Sasaki O. Clinical and physiologic significance of local tissue renin-angiotensin systems. *Am J Med* 1990;87(Suppl 6B):19S–23S.

93. Wang PH, Do YS, Macaulay L, et al. Identification of renal cathepsin B as a human prorenin-processing enzyme. *J Biol Chem* 1991;266:12633–12638.

94. Heinrikson RL, Hui J, Zürcher-Neely H, Poorman RA. A structural model to explain the partial catalytic activity of human prorenin. *Am J Hypertens* 1989;2:367–380.

95. Chu WN, Mercure C, Baxter JD, Reudelhuber TL. Molecular determinants of human prorenin processing. *Hypertension* 1992;20:782–787.

96. Benjannet S, Reudelhuber T, Mercure C, Rondeau N, Chrétien M, Seidah NG. Pro-protein conversion is determined by a multiplicity of factors including convertase processing, substrate specificity and intracellular environment. *J Biol Chem* 1992;267: 11417–11423.

97. Hosaka M, Nagahama M, Kim W-S, et al. Arg-X-Lys/Arg-Arg Motif as a signal for precursor cleavage catalyzed by furin within the constitutive secretory pathway. *J Biol Chem* 1991;266: 12127–12130.

98. Shinagawa T, Do YS, Baxter JD, Carilli C, Schilling J, Hsueh WA. Identification of an enzyme in human kidney that correctly processes prorenin. *Proc Natl Acad Sci (USA)* 1990;87:1927–1931.

99. San Segundo B, Chan SJ, Steiner DF. Differences in cathepsin B mRNA levels in rat tissues suggest specialized functions. *FEBS Lett* 1986;201:251–256.

100. Saint-André JP, Rohmer V, Pinet F, Rousselet MC, Bigorgne JC, Corvol P. Renin and cathepsin B in human pituitary lactotroph cells. An ultrastructural study. *Histochemis* 1989;91:291–297.

101. Nakayama K, Kim W-S, Nakagawa T, Nagahama M, Murakami K. Substrate specificity of prorenin converting enzyme of mouse submandibular gland. *J Biol Chem* 1990;265:21027–21031.

102. Kim WS, Nakayama K, Nakagawa T, Kawamura Y, Haraguchi K, Murakami K. Mouse submandibular gland prorenin-converting enzyme is a member of glandular kallikrein family. *J Biol Chem* 1991;266:19283–19287.

103. Kim WS, Nakayama K, Murakami K. The presence of two types of prorenin converting enzymes in the mouse submandibular gland. *FEBS Lett* 1991;293:142–144.

104. Ohkubo H, Kawakami H, Kakehi Y, et al. Generation of transgenic mice with elevated blood pressure by introduction of the rat renin and angiotensinogen genes. *Proc Natl Acad Sci (USA)* 1990;87:5153–5157.

105. Sigmund CD, Jones CA, Kane CM, Wu C, Lang JA, Gross KW. Regulated tissue- and cell-specific expression of the human renin gene in transgenic mice. *Circ Res* 1992;70:1070–1079.

106. Fukamizu A, Sugimura K, Takimoto E, et al. Chimeric renin-angiotensin system demonstrates sustained increase in blood pressure of transgenic mice carrying both human renin and human angiotensinogen genes. *J Biol Chem* 1993;268:11617–11621.

107. Ganten D, Wagner J, Zeh K, et al. Species specificity of renin kinetics in transgenic rats harboring the human renin and angiotensinogen genes. *Proc Natl Acad Sci (USA)* 1992;89:7806–7810.

108. Quinn PS, Judah JD. Calcium-dependent Golgi-vesicle fusion and cathepsin B in the conversion of proalbumin into albumin in rat liver. *Biochem J* 1978;172:301–309.

109. Docherty K, Hutton JC, Steiner DF. Cathepsin B-related proteases in the insulin secretory granule. *J Biol Chem* 1984;259:6041–6044.

110. Itskovitz J, Rubattu S, Levron J, Sealey JE. Highest concentrations of prorenin and human chorionic gonadotropin in gestational sacs during early human pregnancy. *J Clin Endocrinol Metab* 1992;75:906–910.

111. Jones CA, Sigmund CD, McGowan RA, Kane-Haas CM, Gross KW. Expression of murine renin genes during fetal development. *Mol Endocrinol* 1990;4:375–383.

112. Capecchi MR. Altering the genome by homologous recombination. *Science* 1989;244:1288–1292.

Hypertension: Pathophysiology, Diagnosis, and Management, Second Edition, edited by J.H. Laragh and B.M. Brenner, Raven Press, Ltd., New York © 1995.

CHAPTER 98

Expression of the Renin-Angiotensin System in the Kidney

R. Ariel Gomez and James M. Gloor

The renin-angiotensin system (RAS) plays a critical role in the control of blood pressure, fluid and electrolyte homeostasis, and renal hemodynamics. Although first described as a circulating (endocrine) system, it is now recognized that an intrarenal RAS exists that modulates renal function by the paracrine or autocrine action(s) of angiotensin(s). The intrarenal production of angiotensin II (Ang II) requires that the various components of the RAS be accessible and interact with one another. Thus, understanding of the physiology of the intrarenal RAS is enhanced by a better appreciation of the anatomic relationships among the RAS components. The development of molecular biologic and immunocytochemical techniques has permitted the study of the genes of the RAS, their site of expression, and their regulation by physiologic manipulations. This chapter discusses expression of RAS genes in the kidney. The topographic distribution of various components of the RAS is reviewed. Changes in expression of RAS genes and their products in response to physiologic and pathologic stimuli are discussed. When possible, an attempt to elucidate the relation between structure and function is made. Recent investigations of the intrarenal RAS are considered, and areas of controversy in need of further study are identified.

BIOCHEMISTRY AND TOPOGRAPHY OF RAS COMPONENTS IN THE KIDNEY

Renin

Renin is an aspartyl protease that acts on its only known substrate, angiotensinogen (Ao), to generate the decapeptide angiotensin I (Ang I) (1,2). Human renin is highly specific for its homologous substrate. It has poor

R. A. Gomez: Department of Pediatric Nephrology, Child Health Research Center, University of Virginia Health Science Center, Charlottesville, Virginia 22908.

J. M. Gloor: University of Virginia School of Medicine, Charlottesville, Virginia 22908.

affinity for canine or rodent Ao. The human renin gene is approximately 12 kb long and contains ten exons and nine introns (3,4). The 5′ flanking region of the renin gene contains regulatory sequences that confer responsiveness to cyclic adenosine monophosphate (AMP), glucocorticoids, estrogens, and progesterone. The renin gene is expressed in the kidney, adrenal gland, testis, ovary, pituitary gland, and placenta (3). Renin is synthesized as a preprohormone (5). After removal of the leader peptide, the molecule is addressed to the Golgi where it is glycosylated. Glycosylation is partly responsible for the production of renin isoforms with different metabolism and sites of uptake. After leaving the Golgi, prorenin can be secreted constitutively or undergo conversion to renin (presumably in the juxtaglomerular [JG] granule), where on stimulation, renin is released from the cell by degranulation (regulated pathway).

In the adult mammalian kidney, renin is synthesized by the JG cells, a group of myoepithelioid cells located in the afferent arterioles at the entrance to the glomerulus and that comprise part of the JG apparatus (JGA) (6–9). The JGA consists of vascular and tubular components and the extraglomerular mesangium belonging to the same nephron. The vascular portion includes the afferent and efferent arterioles. The tubular portion consists of the macula densa, a segment of the thick ascending loop of Henle located between the afferent and efferent arterioles. The macula densa can be easily recognized by its tall and narrow cells containing nuclei that are closer together than in other parts of the distal tubule. The triangular area bounded by the afferent and efferent arterioles and the macula densa is contiguous with the glomerular mesangium and has been referred to as the extraglomerular mesangium, the lacis, the cells of Goormaghtigh, and the polar cushion (10,11). By virtue of their proximity, intimate contact, and the presence of gap junctions, the various structures of the JGA effectively communicate with one another and transmit signals that regulate renin synthesis and release.

Authentic intracellular renin can be best demonstrated with immunocytochemical techniques using specific antirenin antibodies. Under baseline conditions, in the unstressed adult mammal, immunoreactive renin is restricted to epithelioid cells located in the afferent arteriole as it abuts the glomerulus (classical JG localization) (6,8,12–14) (Figs. 1, 2, 3B, and 4). However, afferent arterioles exhibit considerable heterogeneity in the extent to which they express renin. In fact, there are nephrons in which it is not possible to demonstrate renin immunoreactivity. Interzonal differences in renin expression appear less marked than differences seen in nephrons located in closer proximity to each other (15). Contrary to the pattern of heterogeneity of renin immunoreactivity described above, nephrons from the same population appear to have minimal functional differences whereas significant differences in function are seen between su-

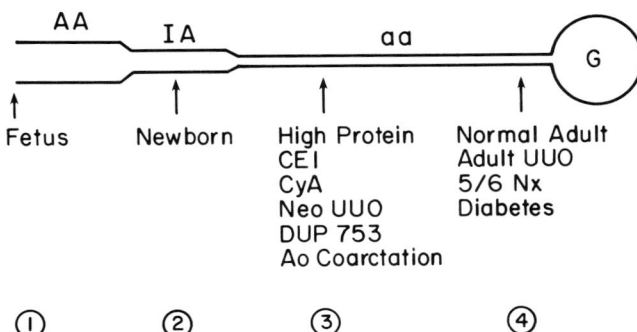

FIG. 1. Schematic representation of changes in the distribution of renin within the renal vasculature in response to various physiologic and pathologic conditions. *Arrows* indicate the approximate boundary of renin immunostaining upstream from the glomerulus along the afferent arteriole (*aa*), whereas manipulations indicated in (*4*) result in renin localization to the juxtaglomerular region, manipulations in (*3*) result in a recruitment of renin-containing cells along the aa. *AA,* Arcuate artery; *IA,* interlobular artery; *G,* glomerulus; *CEI,* converting enzyme inhibition; *CyA,* cyclosporine A; *Neo UUO,* neonatal unilateral ureteral obstruction; *Ao coarctation,* aortic coarctation; *Adult UUO,* adult unilateral ureteral obstruction; *5/6NX,* 5/6 nephrectomy remnant kidney model. (From ref. 106, with permission.)

perficial and juxtamedullary nephrons (16,17). The mechanisms and physiologic significance underlying the heterogeneous expression of renin among different nephrons are not clear and remain to be investigated.

In addition to the afferent arteriole, renin-containing cells have been described in 20 to 40 percent of efferent arterioles in the mouse kidney near the glomerulus (6). As described below, stimuli such as sodium restriction that are known to activate the RAS increase the number of efferent arterioles expressing renin (6). This recruitment of renin-secreting cells in the efferent arteriole may provide a mechanism to increase local Ang II generation, contributing to the observed vasoconstrictive response of this structure to RAS activation (14).

Immunocytochemical techniques combined with electron microscopy have localized renin to a variety of electron-dense granules located within the myoepithelioid cells (9,18,19). Renin occurs in round membrane-bound granules located in the cell periphery, as well as more angular, frequently rhomboidal protogranules located more centrally in areas of protein synthesis. Intermediate forms are also seen, suggesting that protogranules are precursors of the membrane-bound peripheral granules. Also, immunoreactive renin has been demonstrated in the rough endoplasmic reticulum of JG cells (19).

Secretion of renin from granule-containing cells has been proposed to occur by different mechanisms, including exocytosis of mature granules, the formation of cell membrane invaginations that gain access to renin-containing granules deep within the cell, and intracellu-

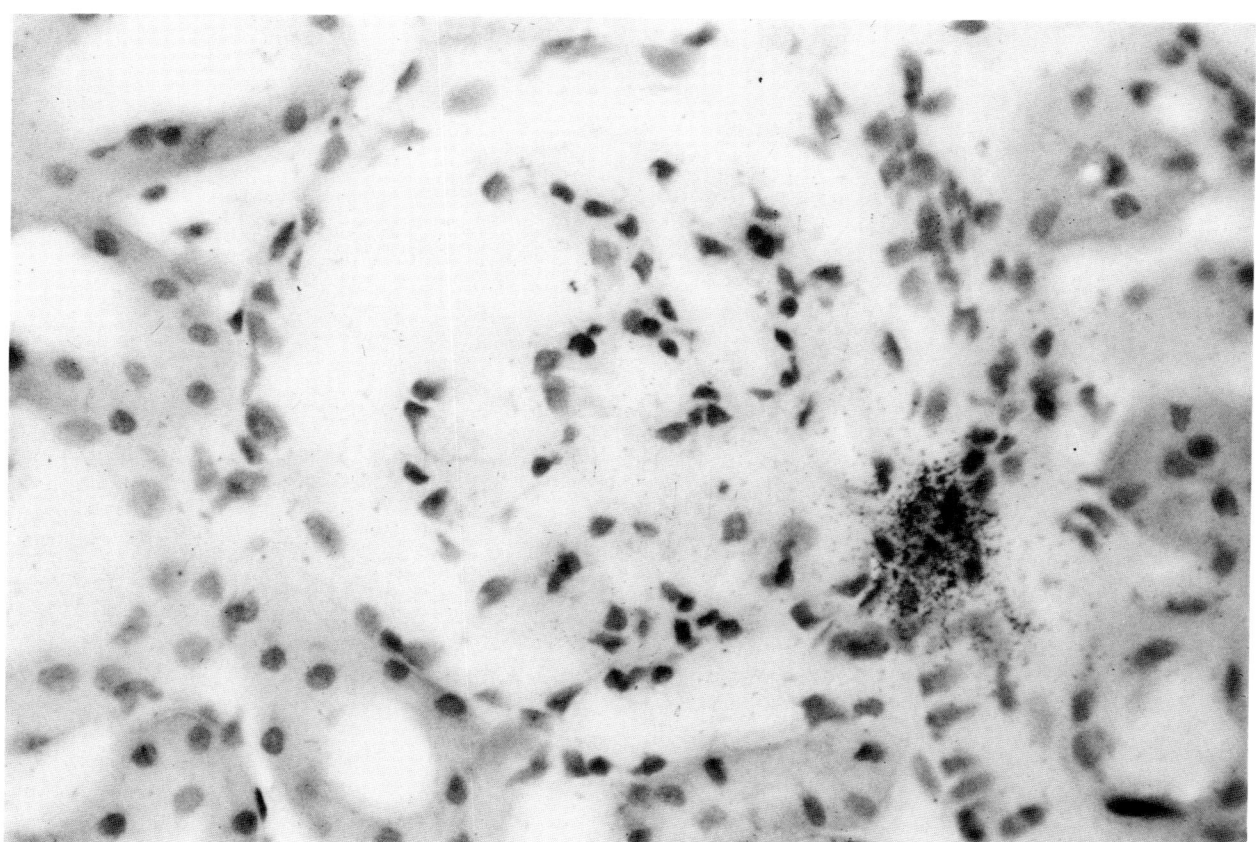

FIG. 2. *In situ* hybridization for renin mRNA. Kidney tissue section from an adult rat showing a mature glomerulus (*center of photograph*). Hybridization signals are restricted to vascular pole of glomerulus. Remainder of afferent arteriole possesses no renin mRNA. Exposure time, 2 days. (From ref. 12, with permission.)

lar solubilization of the stored secretory product (20). Using thin sections and freeze-fracture techniques in mouse kidneys, exocytotic extrusion of electron-dense granules from JG cells has been demonstrated (20).

The presence of immunoreactive renin in granules of epithelioid cells, although illustrating the location of renin storage and secretion, does not necessarily demonstrate the site of synthesis. Cellular uptake of renin syn-

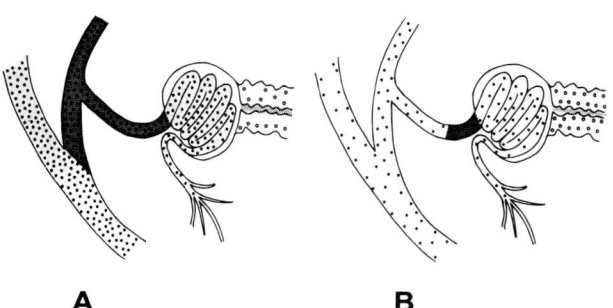

FIG. 3. Intrarenal distribution of Ao (*open circles*), renin (*dark gray*), ACE (*light gray*), and AT1 (*black dots*) mRNAs or their products in newborn (**A**) and adult (**B**) rats. (From ref. 118, with permission.)

thesized elsewhere could potentially give a similar immunohistochemical appearance. *In situ* hybridization studies localizing renin messenger ribonucleic acid (mRNA), however, strongly suggest the site of renin synthesis. Multiple studies using *in situ* hybridization techniques have demonstrated renin mRNA localized to the JGA (21–24) (Fig. 2). The immunocytochemical localization of renin and *in situ* hybridization studies documenting the presence of renin mRNA provide support for the concept that the JGA is the site of renin synthesis, storage, and release.

Renin immunostaining has also been identified in the apical portion of proximal renal tubule cells and in some cells of the connecting and cortical collecting tubules (14). Although low amounts of renin synthesis by epithelial cells is possible, most tubular renin is probably not synthesized in the immunoreactive cells themselves. Rather, filtered renin is taken up by the tubular epithelial cells through a process of pinocytosis (14). This concept is supported by the fact that radioactive-labeled renin injected intraaortically accumulates in the renal cortex, with signal localizing to the apical portion of the proximal tubule epithelial cells (14). Regardless of its source,

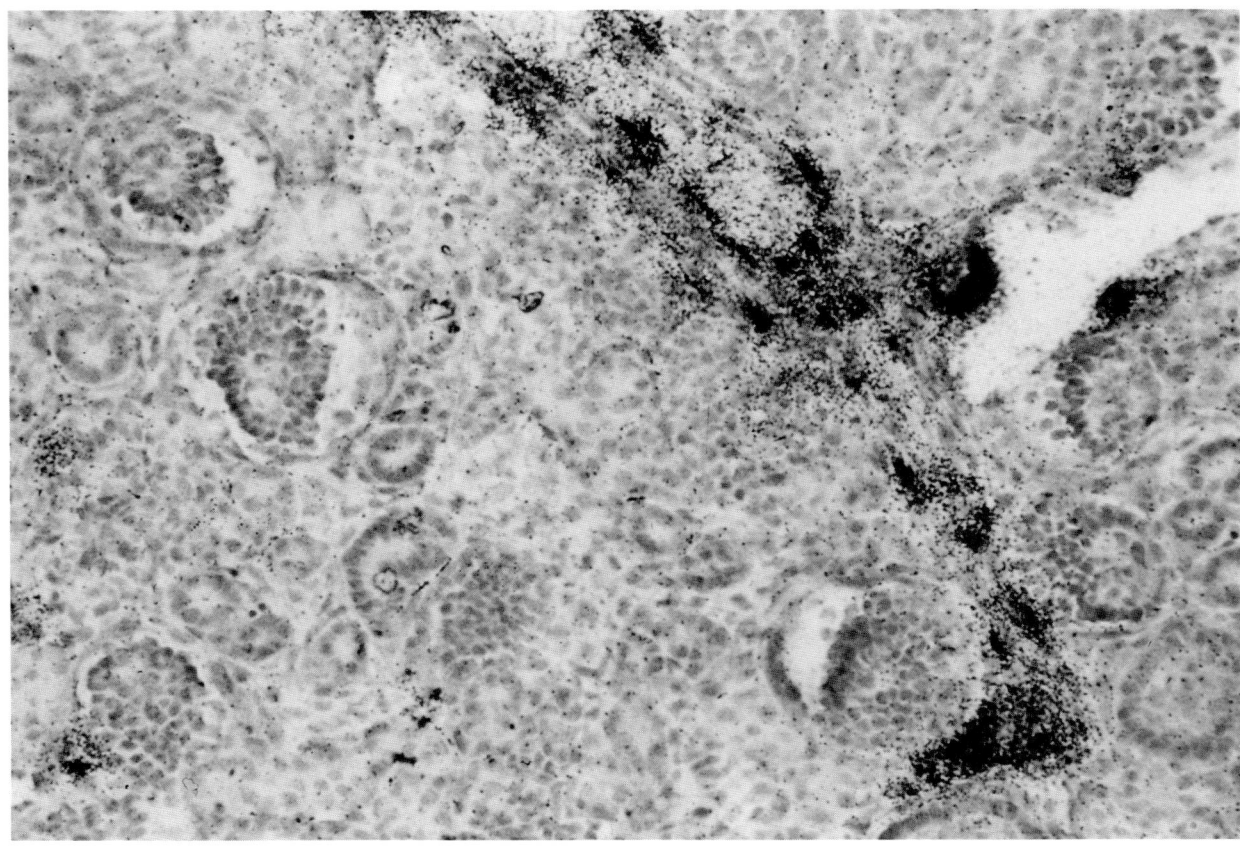

FIG. 4. *In situ* hybridization for renin mRNA. Kidney tissue section from fetal rat at 20 days' gestation. Hybridization signals are located in interlobular and arcuate arteries. Surrounding the arteries are several immature glomeruli in different stages of development. Interstitium and/or glomeruli contain no specific hybridization signals. Magnification ×200. (From ref. 12, with permission.)

the presence of renin in the proximal tubule may result in the cleavage of Ao and the generation of Ang I. Angiotensin-converting enzyme (ACE) is also present in proximal tubular cells. These findings suggest the possibility of a local RAS at the level of the renal tubule. In fact, in euvolemic rats, micropuncture measurements reveal higher Ang II concentration in proximal tubular fluid than in the systemic circulation, suggesting local angiotensin generation (25). Angiotensin II stimulates the sodium-hydrogen exchange and bicarbonate absorption mechanisms in the early proximal tubule (26). Thus, in addition to its effect on the renal circulation, Ang II exerts a direct effect on tubular sodium excretion and bicarbonate reabsorption.

Angiotensinogen

Angiotensinogen or renin substrate is the precursor of angiotensin peptides and the only known substrate for renin. Angiotensinogen is a circulating glycoprotein (55 to 60 kDa) identified in the α_2 globulin fraction of plasma. The Ao gene is encoded by a single copy gene, which in humans has been mapped to chromosome 1 (27). The 5' flanking region of the Ao gene contains several putative regulatory sequences responsive to glucocorticoids, estrogens, and cytokines. The mature Ao mRNA is approximately 1.8 kb, although the length of the molecule varies with the polyadenylation sites used and variations on transcription start site. After removal of its leader peptide, the human protein contains 452 amino acids (27). Post-translational glycosylation results in variable molecular weight and isoelectric point of the circulating protein. It remains to be determined whether elevated high-molecular-weight Ao is responsible for hypertension in pregnant women. Genetic linkage analysis has demonstrated a correlation between high blood pressure and Ao variants (28). The main source of circulating Ao in the adult animal is the liver. Angiotensinogen release by hepatocytes is constitutive. Nevertheless, Ao mRNA has been demonstrated in multiple extrahepatic organs, including the kidney (29–31). In the kidney, Ao mRNA is present in quantities 20 to 30 times less than in the liver (29–31). *In situ* hybridization techniques demonstrate intrarenal Ao mRNA primarily in the proximal renal tubule (Fig. 3) and to a lesser degree in epithelial cells of distal tubular segments and glomerular tufts (32). In support of a proximal tubular site of Ao synthesis, cell cultures obtained from microdissected specimens of rabbit kidney proximal convoluted and straight tubules produce Ao (33). Northern blot analysis of RNA extracted from rat renal microvessels fails to reveal Ao mRNA (34). Immunocytochemical studies using purified Ao antibodies in the rat demonstrate immunoreactive Ao in the apical portion of proximal renal tubular cells (34,35) (Fig. 3).

The ultrastructural localization of Ao has also been studied using electron microscopic immunocytochemistry. Angiotensinogen is distributed evenly throughout the cytoplasm, granules, and other organelles in both proximal tubular cells and JG cells (34). The absence of Ao mRNA in JG cells suggests that immunoreactive Ao peptide is taken up rather than synthesized by the JG cell. Exogenous androgens administered to female rats and to male rats castrated as weanlings result in increased levels of renal Ao mRNA (36). Also, renal Ao mRNA levels fall in adult male rats after castration, suggesting that androgens up-regulate Ao gene expression (36).

In contrast to the effect of androgens on renal Ao gene expression, dexamethasone administered to intact or adrenalectomized rats has no effect on renal Ao mRNA levels, although the expression of the Ao gene in the liver and brain increases (37).

Kidney Ao mRNA levels are lower in spontaneously hypertensive rat (SHR) than in Wistar Kyoto (WKY) rats. Also, the hypertensive rat strain does not seem to respond to a low-salt diet as the WKY strain (38). Studies in opossum renal cells (resembling proximal tubular cells) transfected with the 5′ flanking region of Ao gene linked to a reporter gene demonstrated that thyroxine and cyclic AMP analogues increase promoter expression (39).

The above studies demonstrate the intrarenal synthesis and storage of Ao in the epithelial cells of the proximal tubule. From this site, Ao may be released into the extracellular space, providing a source of substrate for the intrarenal RAS. The colocalization of renin, Ao, and ACE in proximal tubular cells provides a mechanism for the local production of angiotensins.

Angiotensin I Converting Enzyme

Angiotensin I converting enzyme is a zinc-containing dipeptidyl carboxypeptidase that removes carboxyterminal dipeptides from small peptides, including Ang I, from which it generates Ang II (1,40,41). Angiotensin-converting enzyme is identical to kininase II, which degrades bradykinin. Thus, ACE has the dual role of generating a vasoconstrictor and deactivating a vasodilator. Angiotensin-converting enzyme is the product of a single gene that is expressed in multiple tissues, including kidney, lung, endothelium, gut, testis, brain, and lymphocytes (1,40,41). Lung and kidney ACE mRNA are longer than testicular ACE mRNA. The differences in length are caused by differential splicing of the respective transcripts. The protein has a single chain with a molecular weight of 140 to 160 in somatic tissues and 80 in testes (41–43). Angiotensin-converting enzyme is anchored to the cell membrane. Angiotensin-converting enzyme localization on the surface of vascular endothelium makes it ideally suited for the regulation of Ang II generation and systemic vascular tone.

Angiotensin-converting enzyme was initially isolated in blood and later from the microsomal fraction of hog kidney (40,44). The two isolates were later shown to be identical (45). Using immunocytochemical techniques and antibodies directed against rabbit pulmonary ACE, the vascular endothelium of all arteries and arterioles of the kidney can be shown to contain ACE (46,47) (Fig. 3). Immunocytochemical studies also reveal ACE in the endothelial cells of some descending vasa recta as well as portions of the glomerular capillary network, primarily in the region of the glomerular stalk (48). Mesangial cells, peritubular capillaries, and renal veins do not exhibit immunoreactive ACE (48). The intravascular location of ACE permits it to regulate renal hemodynamics through the local production of Ang II. In addition to its vascular location described above, ACE occurs in the proximal tubule (46,47) (Fig. 3). Differential centrifugation studies of homogenates of rat kidney localized the enzyme to the membrane fraction, especially the fraction containing the brush border (47,49–51). Using immunocytochemical techniques, ACE has been demonstrated on the luminal surface of epithelial cells of the proximal convoluted tubules and pars recta in humans, rats, and swine (52–54). Detergent treatment of brush-border membrane fractions solubilize ACE, increasing electrophoretic mobility of the enzyme (51), suggesting that ACE is bound to the epithelial surface by a small hydrophobic anchor (51). Immunoreactive ACE has been less well demonstrated in epithelial cells of the distal tubule (51). Using tritiated ACE substrates, a gradient of increasing ACE activity extending from the glomerulus and epithelial cells of the proximal convoluted tubules to the pars recta of microdissected rabbit nephrons can be demonstrated (55). Angiotensin-converting enzyme activity in brush-border membranes isolated from the inner cortex and outer medulla of the rat kidney is increased tenfold compared with cells of the outer renal cortex, demonstrating interzonal differences in renal ACE activity (56). This is consistent with the structural organization of the kidney, in which the superficial cortex contains a higher proportion of proximal convoluted tubules, whereas in the inner cortex, pars recta predominates. The functional significance of this interzonal difference is unknown.

Using electron microscopic immunocytochemistry,

studies of human kidney proximal tubular cells reveal ACE on the outside of the brush-border plasma membrane and to a lesser extent in vesicular organelles. Angiotensin-converting enzyme also occurs on the basolateral portion of the plasmalemma as well as in the endoplasmic reticulum of proximal tubular cells, consistent with ACE synthesis in the proximal tubular epithelial cell (57). Angiotensin-converting enzyme located in proximal tubular cells is strategically placed to activate Ang I produced by the interaction of tubular renin and Ao. Locally produced Ang II can then interact with its receptors in the proximal tubule to modulate sodium and bicarbonate absorption.

Factors influencing the expression of ACE in the kidney are largely unknown. Renal ACE activity increases in rats made nephrotic by treatment with puromycin (58,59). This may represent a functional adaptation permitting more efficient hydrolysis of filtered protein. Kidney ACE activity also increases with salt depletion. Angiotensin-converting enzyme mRNA levels increase in response to hypoxemia. Increased ACE activity in the aforementioned condition has the potential for increasing local Ang II generation and renal vascular resistance.

Angiotensin II Receptors

Two major receptor subtypes have been identified (60,61). The AT1 receptor has high affinity for Ang II; it is inhibited by DUP753 and is coupled to G proteins and phospholipase C. Activation of these pathways results in phosphoinositide hydrolysis, calcium mobilization, and inhibition of adenylate cyclase. The AT2 receptor binds to PD123177 (nonpeptide) and CGB42112A (peptide) antagonists. All the known actions of Ang II seem to be mediated by the AT1 receptor. The functional role of AT2 receptors is not well defined. It has been suggested that the AT2 receptor mediates a decrease in cyclic guanosine monophosphate (GMP) in neonatal neurons (62,63). It is possible that AT2 may play a role in embryonic development. The AT1 receptor has been cloned (64–66). Analysis of the complementary deoxyribonucleic acid (cDNA) sequence reveals that it encodes 359 amino acids (41 kDa), contains seven transmembrane domains, three glycosylation sites, an N-terminal hydrophobic sequence, a short cytoplasmic loop, and a cysteine residue in each of the four extracellular domains. The latter may be important for ligand binding. Several putative phosphorylation sites (serine, threonine, tyrosine) in the second intracellular loop and in the C-terminal cytoplasmic domain may regulate receptor activity. Two AT1 receptor subtypes exist in rat and mice. AT1A is known as the vascular receptor; AT1B is known as the adrenal receptor. There is 94 percent homology between the two. Two AT1 mRNA transcripts have been identified. A small (2.3 kb) and abundant transcript is present in many tissues, except testes and brain. A larger

(3.5 kb) and less abundant transcript is detected in kidney, liver, adrenal gland, and lung.

The intrarenal localization of ANG II receptors has been studied using autoradiographic ligand-binding techniques. Angiotensin II receptors have been described in high concentration in glomeruli and medullary vascular bundles. Lower concentrations are found in intrarenal pelvis, interstitium, and papillary regions (67–69). Angiotensin II receptor density is down-regulated by treatment with estrogens (70). The AT1 receptor is the predominant subtype seen in the renal vasculature (71). Large preglomerular vessels contain AT2 receptors in adult human kidneys (71). Glomerular AT1 receptors are located on mesangial cells (72). *In situ* hybridization studies of AT1 mRNA have localized AT1 transcripts to glomeruli, the media of arteries of all sizes, and in the vasa recta (73) (Fig. 3B). The intrarenal distribution of Ang II receptors correlates well with the known function of Ang II in the kidney. The demonstration of Ang II receptors on mesangial cells provides an explanation for the observed contractile response of mesangial cells to Ang II, thereby decreasing glomerular ultrafiltration coefficient (K_f) (74). The presence of receptors in the vasa recta provides morphologic evidence for the known Ang II modulation of medullary blood flow and the renal countercurrent concentrating system (68).

Using I^{125}-labeled radioligand binding techniques, Ang II receptors have also been demonstrated in the renal tubular epithelium, although they appear to be present in lower amounts than in glomeruli (67). In microdissected tubules, I^{125}-labeled Ang II binding predominates in the proximal tubular segments (67,75). Angiotensin II binding has been shown to occur in isolated brush-border membranes (76) as well as in isolated basolateral membranes (77). The Ang II receptor located in the renal tubule is not very well characterized. It has a lower affinity for Ang II than the AT1 receptor and, contrary to glomerular receptors, is up-regulated by ANG II and sodium depletion (74,78). It inhibits adenyl cyclase through its interaction with an inhibitory guanosine triphosphate (GTP)-binding protein, resulting in decreased levels of cyclic AMP (78). Radiolabeled Ang II binding to renal tubules is only partially displaced by specific subtype antagonists (78–80). The affinity of the binding sites is much lower than in other sites within the kidney. It is possible that tubular receptors belong to an as-yet-unidentified subtype. However, it has recently been suggested that primary cultures of rabbit proximal tubular cells express the AT1 receptor (81). Because cyclic AMP is known to inhibit proximal tubular sodium/hydrogen exchange, this may represent one mechanism whereby Ang II increases bicarbonate reabsorption. Also, Ang II regulates phospholipase A, releasing arachidonic acid metabolites whose physiologic effect is to attenuate Ang II-induced sodium resorption (81).

Locally produced or taken up, all the components of an angiotensin generating system seem to be present in renal tubules. Concentrations of Ang II in lumens of rat proximal tubules indicate that the peptide must be generated locally, either by release from proximal tubules or intraluminal generation.

Angiotensins

The physiologic actions of the RAS are the result of the interaction of angiotensin(s) with its receptor(s). Cleavage of the decapeptide Ang I by ACE results in the generation of the octapeptide Ang II. Alternative processing of Ang I or Ang II results in the generation of Ang (1–7) and Ang (2–8). The range of activity of these peptides is currently being investigated. It is believed that Ang (1–7) is a counterregulatory vasodilator peptide. Both peptides may have important central actions, acting on unique receptor subtypes. However, most of the well-known actions of the RAS are exerted via Ang II, a potent direct vasoconstrictor. When given intravenously, Ang II rapidly (within 10 to 15 seconds) increases systolic and diastolic blood pressure (1). The response lasts approximately 3 to 5 minutes. In the kidney, Ang II has hemodynamic, tubular, and growth-related effects (74,82). Angiotensin II given intrarenally (without systemic effects) increases renal vascular resistance and decreases renal plasma flow (83). Angiotensin II also participates in the autoregulation of glomerular filtration rate (GFR) (84–88). A decrease in perfusion pressure within the autoregulatory range results in preferential efferent arteriolar constriction, resulting in preservation of GFR. This explains why administration of ACE inhibitors in the setting of bilateral renal artery stenosis could result in a precipitous decline in renal function. Angiotensin II contracts mesangial cells, thus lowering the ultrafiltration coefficient.

Angiotensin II also modulates glomerulo-tubular balance and tubulo-glomerular feedback (74,88). In renal tubules, Ang II increases Na^+-H^+ antiporter activity, ammoniagenesis, and gluconeogenesis. The growth-related effects of angiotensin are dependent on the age of the animals and/or the degree of development of the cells studied. Angiotensin II stimulates proliferation of fetal mesangial cells (89), whereas it stimulates hypertrophy of adult mesangial or tubular cells (81). *In vivo,* Ang II is responsible for nephrovascular development (90). Also, Ang II has a direct negative effect on JG cells (negative feedback loop) on renin release and renin gene expression (91,92).

EXPRESSION OF RAS DURING KIDNEY DEVELOPMENT

Renin

The kidney is the main source of circulating renin in the fetus (93–96). Total kidney renin activity is positively correlated with gestational age. However, renin concentration (corrected for protein content) decreases markedly with fetal age. This is caused by the increase in tubular protein concentration during development. Fetal values (total or corrected) are always higher than adult values. These findings agree with the immunocytochemical and molecular studies described below. Several immunocytochemical studies have shown that the intrarenal distribution of renin changes during kidney development. In the Wistar rat at 15 days' gestation, immunoreactive renin is found in the gonadic arteries (97). Renin-containing cells appear by day 17 in the intrarenal branches of the renal arteries in the Sprague-Dawley rat fetus (98). Subsequently, renin immunostaining progressively extends in a centrifugal distribution to involve the interlobar, arcuate, and interlobular arteries of the developing kidney by day 21 of gestation (8,97,98). After birth, the intrarenal distribution of renin-containing cells gradually decreases, becoming limited to the mature JG distribution by 20 days of postnatal age (8,12,98). Changes in the distribution of renin during maturation are schematically depicted in Figs. 1 and 3.

Using electron microscopic immunocytochemistry, renin immunostaining has been detected in epithelioid cell granules located in both mesonephros and metanephros in the pig (99). In the human, renin immunoreactivity has been detected in the mesonephros as early as 5 to 6 weeks' gestation (100). Metanephric JG epithelioid cells containing renin granules have been shown in an 8-week gestation human fetus (100).

The pattern of changes observed in the distribution of renin with age agrees with analysis of renin mRNA levels. In rats, Northern blot analysis demonstrates a progressive decrease in renin mRNA levels as maturation proceeds (12,96,101). Fetal and newborn mRNA levels have been shown to be 20 and 10 times higher than in adults, respectively (12). The intrarenal distribution of renin mRNA parallels the vascular distribution of renin protein (12). At 20 days' gestation, renin mRNA is seen in larger arteries, involving arcuate, interlobular, and afferent arteries (Fig. 4). During postnatal life, the distribution of renin mRNA expressing cells progressively diminishes to become restricted to the classical JG localization in the adult animal (see Fig. 2). The aforementioned immunocytochemical and molecular findings suggest that the shift in the vascular distribution of renin with maturation is caused by changes in the expression of the renin gene along the developing kidney vasculature. A similar shifting pattern in the distribution of renin has been described in phylogenetic studies and the developing murine kidney (102–105), suggesting a strong evolutionary pressure to conserve the ability to synthesize renin in the large intrarenal vessels of the mammalian fetus.

The changes in renin gene expression noted during development are accompanied by changes in renin secretion. During basal conditions, newborn renal microvessels contain twice as many renin-secreting cells as adult kidney microvessels. In adult animals, Ang II decreases renin release and renin gene expression (106). It was initially speculated that newborn renin-containing cells may be hyporesponsive to Ang II, therefore explaining the high expression and release of renin found in immature animals. However, exposure of newborn and adult cells to Ang II results in a similar percentage decrease in the number of renin-releasing cells. Thus, the physiologic mechanisms regulating the shift in renin gene expression, renin distribution, and renin release remain largely unexplored. The role of paracrine factors, innervation, hormonal milieu, and inductive processes remains to be determined. Similarly, the physiologic signals initiating and/or maintaining the high activity of RAS during early life are not clear. It has been suggested that continuous stimulation of renin release in infants may be necessary for maintaining the positive sodium balance resulting from the avid deposition of sodium in the rapidly growing bone. Supporting this hypothesis, renin mRNA levels are lower in artificially reared pups fed a high-sodium diet than in pups fed normal amounts of sodium (107). However, this hypothesis may not apply to intrauterine life when renin gene expression is at its highest and when the placenta is the main regulator of nutrient exchange. Although speculative, it is possible that the high expression of the renin gene follows a developmentally programmed pattern conserved throughout the phylogenetic scale.

In addition to hemodynamic and tubular actions, the RAS may exert other paracrine effects during ontogeny and phylogeny. Recent evidence indicates that angiotensin may elicit growth responses in a variety of cells and tissues (74,82,89,90). Localization of renin in the developing growing kidney vasculature may provide a mechanism for the local generation of angiotensin, which in turn may act in a paracrine or autocrine fashion to regulate vascular growth. In fact, recent evidence indicates that blockade of AT1 receptors in growing rats impairs nephrovascular development (90).

Angiotensinogen

Unlike the adult animal in which the liver is the primary source of Ao synthesis, there is evidence that in the fetus extrahepatic sources of Ao production may predominate (108). In the rat fetus, Ao has been detected at 11 days' gestational age in embryos and yolk sac placentas (109). Angiotensinogen RNA transcripts are readily detected by Northern blot analysis in kidneys, brown fat, and brain from 20-day-old fetuses (108). The distribution of Ao in the maturing and adult kidney is summarized in Fig. 3A and B. Interestingly, the fetal liver expresses Ao at only a very low level prenatally, although it

is the main site of production in adult life (108). It remains to be determined whether extrahepatic production of Ao contributes to the fetal plasma pool or whether it is used locally, or both. The presence of Ao synthesis in multiple organs in the fetus and of variable regulation of Ao mRNA levels in a tissue-specific manner imply that Ao participates in the local control of the RAS in the fetus.

Angiotensin Converting Enzyme

Renal ACE activity has been shown to increase in an age-dependent manner in the rat (110). The distribution of ACE in the developing kidney has been studied by immunohistochemical techniques (111,112). Angiotensin-converting enzyme occurs in developing proximal tubular epithelial cells on both the basolateral as well the apical surfaces in the human fetus before brush-border differentiation is completed (112). Angiotensin-converting enzyme immunoreactivity is seen in the endothelial cells of developing glomerular capillaries as early as they invade the inferior cleft of the S-shaped body. Angiotensin-converting enzyme is also found in the endothelium of large corticomedullary arteries. As maturation progresses, tubular epithelial cells with more fully developed brush borders exhibit more intense apical immunostaining. Glomerular capillary immunoreactivity progressively becomes less prominent, whereas ACE immunostaining appears in peritubular capillaries (112). No staining is detected in mesangial cells. Changes in the localization of ACE during kidney development are schematically shown in Fig. 3A and B. These changes in distribution of ACE during kidney development suggest that the ACE gene is developmentally regulated. The molecular and physiologic basis for this phenomenon are unresolved. However, both in the developing as well as in the mature kidney, ACE is strategically located to generate Ang II locally and regulate glomerular hemodynamics, tubular function, and perhaps nephrovascular growth and development.

Angiotensin II Receptors

Bioactive Ang II receptors have been detected in the rat fetus as early as 10 days' gestation, and levels increase markedly by 21 days' gestation (34). Study of Ang II receptors in the fetus using the specific antagonists DUP 753 and PD123177 revealed that the AT2 receptor is the predominant subtype in prenatal life (113,114). *In situ* autoradiographic radioligand studies using I^{125}-labeled Ang II reveal Ang II receptors in kidneys from 15-day-old Sprague-Dawley rats (92,113,115). Similar studies in midgestation mouse, monkey, and human fetuses have revealed Ang II receptors as well (116,117). In the fetal rat kidney, radioligand binding is abolished by incubation of the tissue sections with DUP 753, while incubation with PD123177 does not significantly alter signal intensity. These findings suggest that contrary to the predominance of AT2 receptors elsewhere in the fetus, the Ang II receptors in the fetal rat kidney are of the AT1 subtype (113).

The fetal kidney expresses AT1 mRNA as early as 17 days' gestation, and levels increase throughout gestation and early postnatal life to a maximum at 5 days of postnatal age (73). The intrarenal distribution of AT1 receptor mRNA in immature rats differs from the adult as well. In the newborn rat, nephrons at different stages of development are observed, with more mature glomeruli localized to the juxtamedullary cortex. Immature nephrons including S-shaped corpuscles are seen in the subcapsular region. In the juxtamedullary region, AT1 receptor mRNA can be demonstrated by in situ hybridization in glomeruli and arteries in a pattern similar to that seen in the adult animal. AT1 mRNA is also present throughout the nephrogenic cortex. No signal is seen over renal tubular epithelium (73). The pattern of AT1 mRNA expression during maturation parallels the changes in circulating renin, Ang II, and Ang II-binding sites observed in developing animals (73). The localization of AT1 mRNA is schematically summarized in Fig. 3A and B.

The broad distribution of AT1 mRNA in the nephrogenic cortex suggests a role for this receptor in kidney growth and development. In fact, blockade of AT1 receptors with DUP 753 in immature animals results in lower kidney-to-body weight ratio and abnormal nephrovascular development (90,118). Whether the growth effects of angiotensins are direct or mediated through the activation of oncogenes and/or other growth factors (74,82,118–120) remains to be determined.

EXPRESSION OF RAS IN RESPONSE TO PHYSIOLOGIC AND PATHOLOGIC CONDITIONS

Changes in the distribution of renin within the kidney in response to the various conditions discussed below are schematically shown in Fig. 1.

ACE INHIBITION

Angiotensin II inhibits renin gene expression in the kidney (92,121). Angiotensin-converting enzyme inhibition blocks the conversion of Ang I to Ang II, interrupting the negative feedback loop on renin synthesis and release (91,92). Immunocytochemical techniques using specific antirenin antibodies as well as in situ hybridization studies of renin mRNA distribution have been performed to study the effects of ACE inhibition on renin expression (121,122). Angiotensin-converting enzyme

inhibition increases renin mRNA content per JGA and the percentage of JGA expressing renin mRNA and renin protein. Also, afferent arteriolar cells distant from the glomerulus are recruited to express the renin gene (21). Renin mRNA and protein, normally limited to cells in the region of the JGA, extend as far proximally as the interlobular arteries in response to ACE inhibition (15,21,122) (see Fig. 1). These findings explain the increased renin mRNA levels observed in whole kidney homogenate from animals subjected to ACE inhibition (122–125). The increase in renin mRNA levels in ACE-inhibited rats is accompanied by an increase in plasma renin activity (PRA). However, renal renin concentration (RRC) does change significantly (122). Other investigators have found nonproportional changes in PRA and RRC when the RAS is chronically stimulated (126). The discrepancy between increased renin immunoreactivity and the lack of change in RRC suggests that interruption of the Ang II negative feedback results in continuous renin synthesis with accumulation of immature forms of renin maintaining RRC constant while active renin is rapidly secreted into the bloodstream, increasing PRA. Using the reverse hemolytic plaque assay that allows the study of renin release at the single-cell level, it has been demonstrated that the recruitment of renin synthesizing cells is accompanied by an increase in the number of cells secreting renin and in the amount of renin secreted per cell (127). Incubation with Ang II abolishes the increase in the number of renin-secreting cells, although the amount of renin secreted per cell remains unchanged (127).

In summary, Ang II is known to exert a direct negative feedback effect on renin gene expression (92). Interruption of this negative feedback loop by ACE inhibition results in recruitment of more proximal portions of the renal vasculature to express the renin gene. These results suggest that the adult renal vasculature has the capacity to revert to an earlier pattern or renin expression resembling the embryonic pattern. A similar mechanism of cell recruitment has been observed with other cell types (13,122), underscoring its general biologic importance. Overall, these studies demonstrate the plasticity of the kidney vasculature to elicit expression of the renin gene when the physiologic circumstances are appropriate.

SODIUM INTAKE

The state of sodium balance exerts profound effects on the expression of the RAS in the kidney. Renal renin mRNA content analyzed by Northern blot increases in response to dietary sodium restriction, predominantly in the renal cortex (128). In situ hybridization studies demonstrate that sodium depletion increases renin mRNA in the JGA, and the increase in signal intensity is proportional to the duration of depletion (22). This increase in renin mRNA is likely due to increased gene transcription, although changes in renin mRNA stabilization may be a contributing factor (22). Despite an increase in renin mRNA activity in the JGA, no recruitment of renin gene expressing cells from the afferent or efferent arterioles occurs in response to sodium depletion (22).

Renin secretion from isolated kidneys increases in response to sodium depletion, resulting in an increase in PRA (123). This increase in renin secretion occurs due to increases in both the number of renin-secreting cells and the amount of renin secreted per cell (127). Renal renin content does not change, however, suggesting that the newly synthesized renin is rapidly released into the circulation (6,22,123).

Sodium depletion also alters renin immunoreactivity. Although afferent arterioles located in the superficial cortex exhibit slightly increased immunoreactive renin in response to sodium depletion, efferent arterioles of the superficial cortex exhibit a marked increase in renin immunoreactivity (6). This increase in efferent arteriolar renin expression is reflected in the preferential efferent vasoconstrictor tone elicited by Ang II.

The absence of renin mRNA distant from the glomerulus in afferent or efferent arterioles suggests that in sodium depletion recruitment of renin gene expression is limited to the area of the JGA. The presence of renin in afferent and efferent arterioles distant from the site of renin mRNA synthesis is best explained by uptake of circulating renin into the vasculature through a mechanism of endocytosis. This mechanism has been demonstrated in the rat aorta (129). Sodium loading decreases renin and Ang II immunoreactivity in the JGA of the rat (15).

Sodium intake also affects other components of the intrarenal RAS. Dietary sodium restriction increases Ao mRNA levels in both renal cortex and medulla (128). Radioligand-binding studies reveal that glomerular Ang II receptor density increases with sodium loading and decreases with sodium restriction (130). Angiotensin II infusion abolishes the modulating effect of sodium intake on receptor activity in the glomerulus, whereas ACE inhibition reverses the down-regulation of Ang II receptor density induced by sodium restriction (130,131). These studies suggest that the effect of sodium intake on glomerular Ang II receptor density is mediated through its effect on Ang II levels. Contrary to Ang II receptors located in the glomerulus, those present in renal tubules appear to be up-regulated by sodium restriction (74,78). This up-regulation of receptors may function to increase tubular sodium reabsorption in states of sodium depletion.

URETERAL OBSTRUCTION

The activity of the RAS is enhanced during ureteral obstruction contributing to renal vasoconstriction in mature and developing animals. Angiotensin-converting enzyme inhibitors improve renal hemodynamics in chronically obstructed kidneys and single nephrons (132–137). Chronic ureteral obstruction also leads to impaired growth of the obstructed kidney and compensatory hypertrophy of the intact kidney. The compensatory hypertrophy is more pronounced in immature than in adult kidneys (138–141). The effects of ureteral obstruction on renin gene expression differ in neonatal and adult rats (141,142). Complete unilateral ureteral obstruction (UUO) was induced in 2-day-old rats and studied 1 month later. Plasma renin activity and arterial pressure were not different from sham-operated rats. However, marked changes in renin expression were observed. Whereas renin distribution was limited to the classical JG localization in sham rats, recruitment of JGAs and renin-containing cells along the preglomerular vessels was observed not only in the obstructed kidney but also in the intact kidney of UUO animals (see Fig. 1). Interestingly, RRC was increased in the obstructed kidney but decreased in the intact opposite kidney of UUO rats. Renin mRNA remained localized to the JGA in both groups. However, the number of JGA expressing the renin gene was higher in the obstructed kidney than in the contralateral or sham kidneys. These findings illustrate the dissociation between the circulating and intrarenal RAS in the setting of ureteral obstruction. In agreement with these findings, ureteral obstruction in rats and guinea pigs results in increased JG index and RRC, respectively (143,144). The lack of congruence between the broad distribution of renin and the restricted JG localization of its mRNA suggests that the increase renin synthesis results in accumulation of a renin isoform with a longer half-life than its mRNA. Other possibilities include defective renin release, increased translation efficiency, or vascular renin uptake. Regardless of the mechanism(s) involved, the above findings support the notion that the intrarenal RAS plays a role in the vasoconstriction of the obstructed kidney. The increased immunoreactive renin in the intact opposite kidney is more difficult to explain because renal blood flow is increased in these kidneys. However, active renin is decreased in the intact opposite kidney, suggesting that the increased immunoreactivity might be caused by the presence of inactive renin. Recent development of prorenin antibodies (J. Sealey, *personal communication*) may help to solve this important question. Interestingly, chemical or mechanical denervation suppressed the increase in renin gene expression of the neonatal kidney with ipsilateral UUO (145), suggesting that the sympathetic nervous system plays an important role in modulating renin gene expression in the obstructed kidney. It remains to be determined whether increased mechanoreceptor and afferent renal nerve activity during obstruction (145) with its attendant norepinephrine release from nerve endings adjacent to JG cells is responsible for increased renin gene expression during ureteral obstruction. Renal denervation would have decreased renin gene expression by up-regulating Ang II receptors or by inducing hemodynamic changes. In the adult animal, ureteral obstruction of short (24 hour) or 4 weeks' duration did not alter the distribution of renin or its mRNA, although obstruction for 4 weeks resulted in a recruitment of JGAs containing immunoreactive renin (142). Thus, chronic UUO in the adult rat does not alter renin gene expression or the anatomic localization of renin. These findings are in agreement with studies performed in the hydronephrotic mouse kidney (146). The attenuated response of the mature animal obviously suggests an age-dependent response of the intrarenal RAS to UUO. The observed findings in adult animals are difficult to reconcile with the beneficial hemodynamic effects of ACE inhibitors in this condition. Further work assessing intrarenal Ang II concentrations and Ang II receptor expression in the setting of UUO may be needed to answer this question.

CYCLOSPORINE A

Cyclosporine (CyA) treatment is associated with hypertension and alterations in renal function (147–155). The mechanisms responsible for enhanced CyA-mediated vasoconstriction are probably multiple, including enhanced sympathetic activity, increased renal eicosanoid production, increased endothelin activity, and increased renal RAS activity (156–160). Also, CyA induces pathologic and functional changes in the renal microvasculature (161). The renal vascular damage occurs in the distal afferent arteriole. Because this is the same distribution in which renin is located, this raises the possibility of involvement of the RAS. Chronic treatment with CyA increases renal renin content and renin release and alters the distribution of renin in the kidney (161,162). Plasma renin activity is elevated by CyA treatment in rats, although in humans it is decreased or unchanged. The reason for this discrepancy is unclear. Nevertheless, in humans plasma prorenin is increased, resulting in increased total renin concentration, even though active renin is decreased (161). Thus, the conversion of inactive prorenin to active renin may be impaired by treatment with CyA.

In the rat, the percentage of JGA expressing immunoreactive renin and the length of afferent arterioles exhibiting renin immunoreactivity are increased with chronic CyA treatment (see Fig. 1). Renin mRNA levels and intrarenal distribution do not change after chronic CyA administration (162). Increased granule-containing cells are seen along the afferent arteriole during CyA therapy as well (163). In humans, JGA hyperplasia is noted early after starting CyA therapy, but it is not seen in chronic therapy (149,161). The discrepancy between renal renin protein and mRNA levels and distribution with chronic CyA treatment may involve multiple factors. The vasculature is capable of taking up renin from the circulation (129). Uptake of circulating renin into cells of the afferent arterioles, potentially facilitated by CyA-induced endothelial damage, may be involved (153). Alteration in the distribution of expression of various renin isoforms with diminished vascular clearance rates is another possible factor. The presence of an acidic isoform of renin in the kidneys of CyA-treated rats has recently been detected (164), suggesting that CyA may alter intracellular processing and storage of renin. The physiologic mechanisms responsible for CyA-induced changes in RAS expression within the kidneys are not well defined. Because renal denervation only partially reverses vasoconstriction, other stimuli besides the renal nerves may be operative. The renal baroreceptor and macula densa mechanisms are most likely activated during CyA treatment. In fact, renal hypoperfusion by enhanced endothelin and thromboxane activities may play a major role in determining RAS changes within the kidney of CyA-treated individuals.

Chronic CyA treatment suppresses AT1 receptor mRNA levels in the kidney (162), suggesting that increased levels of intrarenal Ang II modulate AT1 gene expression.

Infusion of Ao into isolated pig interlobular arteries provokes an enhanced vasoconstrictive response in the presence of CyA, whereas the response to infusions of Ang I or Ang II is unchanged. Thus, CyA treatment appears to increase the local production of angiotensin. The sensitivity of the vasculature to angiotensin appears to be unchanged. Blockade of the RAS only partially reverses vasoconstriction (154,165). However, alterations in renin and AT1 expression may play a role in the changes in renal vascular reactivity and autoregulation observed in this model (154,165). Down-regulation of AT1 receptors may be responsible for the blunted vascular response to Ang II in this model (165). Further work is necessary to delineate the mechanism(s) and contribution of the RAS to renal arterial disease and hypertension during CyA therapy.

RENAL ABLATION

Reduction of renal mass results in compensatory hypertrophy of the remaining kidney and hyperfiltration leading to glomerulosclerosis, hypertension, and renal failure (166–168). Inhibitors of the RAS improve renal hemodynamics and prevent glomerular alterations. Because PRA does not usually increase in experimental models of renal ablation, activation of the intrarenal RAS has been postulated in the setting of reduced renal mass (169–171). Uninephrectomy does not alter renin mRNA levels or the distribution and concentration of intrarenal renin or PRA. However, severe renal ablation resulting from uninephrectomy and infarction of $\frac{2}{3}$ of the remaining kidney ($\frac{5}{6}$ Nx) results in marked changes in kidney growth and renin expression (23). Four weeks after the procedure, the infarcted area is scarred, and marked hypertrophy develops in the remaining kidney tissue. Recruitment of renin gene-expressing cells is observed only in the infarcted/scarred area (23). However, in the hypertrophic portion (which constitutes the largest portion of the $\frac{5}{6}$ Nx kidney), there is a decrease in renin mRNA levels caused by a decrease in renin mRNA content per JGA and a decrease in the number of JGA expressing the renin gene (23). This is accompanied by a decrease in intrarenal immunoreactive renin (see Fig. 1) and a decrease in PRA. Similar results have been reported by other investigators (172–174). These results are difficult to reconcile with studies suggesting that subtotal nephrectomy results in increased glomerular renin expression and renin enzymatic activity (175). Whereas those studies are not readily comparable, the bulk of the available information suggests that in the hypertrophic portion of the remnant kidney, renin expression is lower than in normal controls. The mechanism(s) mediating the decrease in intrarenal renin expression remains to be elucidated. After renal ablation, GFR increases due to decreased vascular resistance, more pronounced in the afferent than in the efferent glomerular arterioles. The ensuing stretch of JG cells may lead to decreased renin gene expression (176). Similarly, increase in sodium chloride delivery to the distal tubule of remaining nephrons may suppress renin expression by a macula densa mechanism (177). Functional data indicate that Ang II modulates renal hemodynamics in rats subjected to renal ablation (178). Although renin expression is diminished in renal ablation, other components of the RAS may be affected: An increase in angiotensin receptor activity/expression would explain both reduced renin expression and the heightened hemodynamic actions of angiotensin in this condition.

RENAL ISCHEMIA, CHANGES IN CIRCULATING VOLUME, AND PERFUSION PRESSURE

Renal ischemia increases the activity of the RAS and induces hypertension (179,180). Plasma renin activity and circulating Ang II levels increase rapidly after partial constriction of one renal artery or after aortic coarctation (181,182). Changes in circulating renin are accompanied by increased renin secretion, increased kidney renin immunostaining, and enzymatic activity (181,183,184).

In the two-kidney one-clip (2K1C) rat model, Northern blot analysis reveals increased levels of renal renin mRNA in the ischemic kidney at both 4 and 16 to 20 weeks postsurgery. A return to baseline levels of renin mRNA after 2 weeks has also been reported (185–187). Renin mRNA levels are suppressed in the contralateral kidney (185). Although total renin mRNA extracted from combined ischemic and contralateral kidneys is elevated in the 2K1C model of renal hypertension, PRA is increased to a greater degree (187). The nonproportional increase suggests that changes in renin synthesis and alterations in renin processing and release may also play a role in determining PRA, particularly in the early phase of ischemia.

In the 2K1C model, changes in immunoreactive renin appear within 5 days of clipping (181) involving more proximal portions of the renal vasculature, including afferent arterioles and interlobular arteries (15,181). In the contralateral kidney, renin remains confined to the JG region (181). Similar to renin, Ang II immunoreactivity is increased in the ischemic kidney and decreased in the contralateral kidney (15,184). Electron microscopic immunocytochemistry reveals renin as well as Ang II-containing granules in both the ischemic and contralateral kidneys in the 2K1C model (181). The number and size of granules seen in the ischemic kidney appear less than on the contralateral side, the rough endoplasmic reticulum is more abundant, and the Golgi apparatus is larger than in control animals. These ultrastructural changes reflect increased synthetic and secretory activity in the ischemic kidney (181).

In rats subjected to aortic coarctation, interlobular arteries as well as afferent arterioles express both renin protein and renin mRNA (see Fig. 1). Renin protein and mRNA in control rats remain localized to the JGA area (188). These changes appear within 24 hours of coarctation, before the development of hypertension.

In rats, hypervolemia reduces renin activity in isolated JGA from the superficial renal cortex, whereas renin activity from juxtamedullary JGA remains unchanged. Hypovolemia increases JGA renin activity (183).

At low perfusion pressure, renin secretion is predominantly under the control of the baroreceptor mechanism, potentially through the activation of stretch-activated calcium channels (189). It is possible that up-regulation of renin gene expression is mediated through stretch receptors, representing a homeostatic mechanism operating locally to restore renal perfusion. Renin release from isolated perfused kidneys is increased by low perfusion pressure, supporting the stretch receptor hypothesis (190). Also, activation of the macula densa mechanism or increased adrenergic activity could modulate the observed changes in gene expression (191,192). The contribution of each of these mechanisms remains to be determined. However, experiments performed in the nonfiltering denervated kidney demonstrated that the baroreceptor mechanism is the main mechanism stimulating renin secretion under decreased perfusion pressure (192).

In rats subjected to suprarenal aortic coarctation, Northern blot analysis of renal mRNA reveals that the expression of AT1 receptor gene decreases threefold when compared with normal control rats (188). This finding suggests that high Ang II levels (renal and/or systemic) exert a negative feedback on the expression of its own receptor. AT1 receptor down-regulation may also be partially responsible for renin recruitment during decreased perfusion pressure. Down-regulation of glomerular Ang II receptor activity results in decreased renal vascular resistance and increased glomerular K_f, in turn participating in autoregulation of renal function.

DIABETES MELLITUS

Diabetes mellitus is frequently associated with hypertension and renal disease. Altered glomerular hemodynamics, mainly increased glomerular capillary pressure and decreased K_f (193), are partially responsible for glomerular injury and decreased renal function. Treatment with the ACE inhibitor captopril normalizes the glomerular capillary hydrostatic pressure and prevents the development of albuminuria and the pathologic structural changes associated with diabetes (193). Activation of the intrarenal RAS may, therefore, contribute to the functional and morphologic changes observed in diabetes.

In the adult biobreeding (BB) spontaneously diabetic rat, the kidney expresses a high level of renin mRNA during the first 2 to 4 months after the onset of diabetes. Four months after the onset of diabetes, the percentage of JGA exhibiting renin immunoreactivity, the number of renin-containing cells per JGA, and renal renin mRNA content exceed that found in nondiabetic controls. However, by 12 months after the onset of diabetes, these changes decrease to levels lower than in nondiabetic control rats (194) (see Fig. 1).

Streptozocin-induced diabetes increases renal renin content as well as renal renin mRNA compared with nondiabetic controls despite unchanged plasma renin concentration (195). Also, glomerular Ang II receptor density is decreased when compared with treated diabetic controls (195). The mechanisms responsible for changes in renin gene expression during diabetes are not clear. In the diabetic rat, hyperphagia results in increased sodium intake and subsequent plasma volume expansion (193). The elevation of renal renin content in the setting of plasma volume expansion suggests that the control of the intrarenal RAS is disordered in diabetes, with inappropriate expression of the renin gene and possibly enhanced production of Ang II. This possibility is supported by the observed beneficial effects of ACE inhibition in the prevention of diabetes-associated renal complications. Other factors, in addition to volume expansion, such as alterations in atrial natriuretic peptide (ANP) and prostaglandin synthesis, may have contributed to alteration of renin expression in diabetes. Autonomic regulation of renin release is known to be altered in diabetes and may have contributed to the observed findings in renin gene expression within the kidney.

In adult BB spontaneously diabetic rats, Ao mRNA levels appear to be unaltered after the development of diabetes. However, immunoreactive Ao in proximal tubular cells increases after 4 months of diabetes and decreases by 12 months after onset of disease when compared with normal nondiabetic controls (194). The apparent discrepancy between mRNA levels and distribution of immunoreactive Ao may be caused by differences in translational efficiency, transcript degradation, or uptake of circulating Ao by the proximal tubule.

DIETARY PROTEIN INTAKE

High protein intake modulates kidney growth, renal hemodynamics, and the distribution of renin gene-expressing cells in the kidney (196–200). Plasma renin activity is increased by high protein intake (201,202). Blood pressure, however, varies from normal to slightly increased, depending on the experimental setting. Rats fed a high-protein diet from weaning to adulthood exhibit increased intrarenal immunoreactive renin and renin mRNA along afferent arterioles and increased percentage of JG cells expressing renin when compared with normal controls (200) (see Fig. 1). Kidney weight, kidney/body weight ratio, glomerular filtration rate, and renal plasma flow are significantly greater in rats fed a high-protein diet compared with controls (200). DUP 753 blunts these responses, demonstrating that they are mediated through Ang II/AT1 interaction. The mechanism(s) whereby high dietary protein modulates expression of RAS components within the kidney is intriguing. Under normal circumstances, Ang II depresses renin gene expression. However, Ang II actions are increased during a high-protein diet, suggesting that the normal renal negative feedback is altered.

Blunted pressor response to Ang II and normal blood pressure in RAS fed high-protein diets supports this possibility (197,198,201). It is possible that increased local prostaglandin or nitric oxide production mediates Ang II-diminished responsiveness in animals fed high-protein diets (201). Also, up-regulation of both renin and angiotensin may subserve other nonhemodynamic responses. The aforementioned studies suggest a critical role for angiotensin in modulating kidney growth during high-protein feeding.

In rats subjected to $1\frac{2}{3}$ nephrectomy, 2 weeks of a high- (30 percent) versus low- (6 percent) protein diet does not induce a difference in tissue renin content (202). Angiotensin II blockade with Sar 1-Gly 8-Ang II results in decreased single-nephron GFA and glomerular capillary pressure in rats fed high-protein diets. In rats fed a low-protein diet, Ang II blockade does not change renal hemodynamics, demonstrating that in this model the level of RAS activity varies directly with dietary protein intake (202). By decreasing the activity of the RAS, low-protein intake modulates renal vascular resistance and intraglomerular capillary pressure (202). The aforementioned studies at the molecular and physiologic levels provide an explanation for the observation that dietary protein restriction retards the progression of renal insufficiency (196).

AUTOSOMAL-DOMINANT POLYCYSTIC KIDNEY DISEASE

Hypertension is a common finding in patients with autosomal-dominant polycystic kidney disease (ADPKD). Activation of the RAS has been suggested as a cause for the hypertension associated with ADPKD (203). Also, the RAS may function in the process of cyst formation (204).

Immunocytochemistry using antirenin antibodies demonstrates the presence of immunoreactive renin in JGA, in afferent arterioles, and in dilated proximal and distal tubular epithelium from polycystic kidneys (205,206). The percentage of JGA exhibiting immunoreactivity and length of afferent arteriolar immunostaining are unchanged from normal controls. Renin can also be detected in dilated proximal and distal tubules and cysts by Western analysis and enzymatic activity (205). Cyst-derived cell cultures synthesize renin, as demonstrated by detection of renin mRNA by polymerase chain reaction (205). The synthesis of renin by tubular epithelial cells in ADPKD raises the possibility that tubular renin may be involved in the epithelial cell hyperplasia and cyst formation typical of the disease. Thus the RAS, in addition to its role in the pathogenesis of the hypertension associated with ADPKD, may also be responsible for cyst formation.

SUMMARY

Expression of the RAS genes changes markedly during normal kidney development and in response to various physiologic and pathologic conditions. During normal development, high intrarenal expression of RAS genes (renin, AT1) may be responsible for the orderly architectural development of the kidney. In certain physiologic conditions (i.e., salt depletion), enhancement of renin gene expression may have the beneficial effect of increasing renin synthesis and release, with the resultant normalization of blood pressure and circulatory volume. However, in pathologic conditions, alteration of one or more of the components of the RAS may have formidable deleterious effects such as inducing hypertension and contributing to the progression of renal disease. Future developments in cell and molecular biology may allow the specific therapeutic targeting of renal structures expressing RAS components.

ACKNOWLEDGMENTS

This work was supported by the National Institutes of Health, grants P30HD28810 and P50DK45179. The authors thank Ms. Brenda Byers for her administrative assistance.

REFERENCES

1. Peach MJ. *Physiol Rev* 1977;57:313–370.
2. Dzau VJ, Burt DW, Pratt RE. *Am J Physiol* 1988;255:F563–F573.
3. Baxter JD, James MNG, Chu WN. *Yale J Biol Med* 1989;62:493–501.
4. Miyazaki H, Fukamizu A, Shigehisa H, et al. *Proc Natl Acad Sci USA* 1984;81:5999–6003.
5. Hsueh WA, Baxter JD. *Hypertension* 1991;17:469–479.
6. Taugner R, Hackenthal E, Nobiling R, Harlacher M, Reb G. *Histochemistry* 1981;73:75–88.
7. Taugner R, Hackenthal E. *Histochemistry* 1981;72:499–509.
8. Gomez RA, Chevalier RL, Sturgill BC, Johns DW, Peach MJ, Carey RM. *J Hypertens* 1986;4(Suppl 5):S31–S33.
9. Lindop GBM, Lever AF. *Histopathology* 1986;10:335–362.
10. Barajas L, Salido E. *Lab Invest* 1986;54:361–364.
11. Taugner R, Hackenthal E. *The juxtaglomerular apparatus: structure and function.* Heidelberg: Springer-Verlag; 1989:1–306.
12. Gomez RA, Lynch KR, Sturgill BC. *Am J Physiol* 1989;257:F850–F858.
13. Gomez RA, Chevalier RL, Carey RM, Peach MJ. *Kidney Int* 1990;38(Suppl 30):S18–S23.
14. Taugner R, Hackenthal E. *The juxtaglomerular apparatus: structure and function.* Heidelberg: Springer-Verlag; 1989:1–306.
15. Taugner R, Hackenthal E, Helmchen C, et al. *Klin Wochenschr* 1982;60:1218–1222.
16. Minram A, Casellas D. *Kidney Int* 1987;31(Suppl 20):57–63.
17. Oken DE, Wolfert AI, Laveri LA, Choi SC. *Kidney Int* 1985;27:871–878.
18. Lindop GBM, Stewart JA, Downie TT. *Histopathology* 1983;7:421–431.
19. Lindop GBM, Downie TT. *J Hypertens* 1984;2:7–10.
20. Taugner R, Buhrle CP, Nobiling R. *Cell Tissue Res* 1984;237:459–472.
21. Gomez RA, Chevalier RL, Everett AD, et al. *Am J Physiol* 1990;259:F660–F665.
22. Gomez RA, Chevalier RL, Everett AD, Peach MJ, Carey RM. *Kidney Int* 1989;35:300A.
23. Pupilli C, Chevalier RL, Carey RM. *Am J Physiol* 1992;263:F731–F738.
24. Deschepper CF, Mellon SH, Cumin F. *Proc Natl Acad Sci USA* 1986;83:7552–7556.
25. Seikaly MG, Arant BS, Seney FD. *J Clin Invest* 1990;86:1352–1357.
26. Liu FY, Cogan MG. *J Clin Invest* 1988;82:601–607.
27. Lynch KR, Peach MJ. *Hypertension* 1991;17:263–267.
28. Jeunmaitre X, Soubrier F, Kotelevtsev YV, et al. *Cell* 1992;71:169–180.
29. Campbell DJ, Habener JF. *J Clin Invest* 1986;78:31–39.
30. Okhubo H, Nakayama K, Tanaka T, Nakanishi S. *J Biol Chem* 1986;261:319–323.
31. Fried TA, Simpson EA. *Am J Physiol* 1986;250:F347–F377.
32. Ingelfinger JR, Zuo WM, Fon EA. *J Clin Invest* 1990;85:417–423.
33. Yanagawa N, Capparelli AW, Jo OD, Friedal A, Barrett JD, Eggena P. *Kidney Int* 1991;39:938–941.
34. Hunt MK, Ramos SP, Geary KM, et al. *Am J Physiol* 1992;263:F363–F373.
35. Richoux JP, Cordonnier JL, Bouhnik J. *Cell Tissue Res* 1983;233:439–451.
36. Ellison KE, Ingelfinger JR, Pivor M, Dzau VJ. *J Clin Invest* 1989;83:1941–1945.

37. Kalinyak JE, Perlman AJ. *J Biol Chem* 1987;262:460–464.
38. Pratt RE, Zuo WM, Naftilan AJ, Ingelfinger JR, Dzau VJ. *Am J Physiol* 1989;256:F469–F474.
39. Chan JSD, Ming M, Nie Z-R, et al. *J Am Soc Nephrol* 1991;2:396(A).
40. Erdos EG. *Fed Proc* 1977;36:1760–1765.
41. Ehlers MRW, Riordan JF. *Biochemistry* 1989;28:5311–5318.
42. Bernstein KE, Martin BM, Bernstein EA. *J Biol Chem* 1988;263:11021–11024.
43. Soubrier R, Alhenc-Gelas F, Hubert C, et al. *Proc Natl Acad Sci USA* 1988;85:9386–9390.
44. Skeggs LT, Kahn JR, Shumway NP. *J Exp Med* 1956;103:295–209.
45. Yang HYT, Erdos EG, Levin Y. *J Pharmacol Exp Ther* 1971;117:291–300.
46. Caldwell PRB, Seegal BC, Hsu KC. *Science* 1976;191:1050–1051.
47. Ward PE, Gedney CD, Dowben RM, Erdos EG. *Biochem J* 1975;151:755–758.
48. Taugner R, Gauten D. *Histochemistry* 1982;751:191–201.
49. Ward PE, Schultz W, Reynolds RC, Erdos EG. *Lab Invest* 1977;36:599–606.
50. Ward PE, Erdos EG, Gedney CD, Dowben RM, Reynolds RC. *Biochem J* 1976;157:643–650.
51. Ward PE, Sheridan MA. *Biochem Pharmacol* 1983;32:265–274.
52. Defendini R, Zimmerman EA, Weare JA, Alhenc-Gelas F, Erdos EG. *Neuroendocrinology* 1983;37:32–40.
53. Hall ER, Kato J, Erdos EG, Robinson CJG, Oshima G. *Life Sci* 1976;18:1299–1304.
54. Rix E, Ganten D, Schull B, Unger T, Taugner R. *Neurosci Lett* 1981;22:125–130.
55. Marchetti J, Roseau S, Alhenc-Gelas F. *Kidney Int* 1987;31:744–751.
56. Ikemoto F, Song G, Tominaga M, Kanayama Y, Yamamoto K. *Biochem Biophys Res Commun* 1987;144:915–921.
57. Bruneval P, Hinglais N, Alhenc-Gelas F. *Histochemistry* 1986;85:73–80.
58. Ingelfinger JR, Anderson S, Hirsch AT, Dzau VJ, Brenner BM. *Kidney Int* 1990;37:356A.
59. Ingelfinger JR, Anderson S, Hirsch A, Bouyounes B, Brenner BM. *Pediatr Res* 1990;27:330A.
60. Wong PC, Chiu AT, Duncia JV. *Trends Endocrinol Metab* 1992;3:211–217.
61. Bumpus FM, Catt KJ, Chiu AT, et al. *Hypertension* 1991;17:720–721.
62. Bottari SP, King IN, Reichlin S, et al. *Biochem Biophys Res Commun* 1992;183:206–211.
63. Sumners C, Tang W, Zelezna B, et al. *Proc Natl Acad Sci USA* 1991;88:7567–7571.
64. Murphy TJ, Alexander RW, Griendling KK. *Nature* 1991;351:233–236.
65. Iwai N, Yamano Y, Chaki S, et al. *Biochem Biophys Res Commun* 1991;177(1):299–304.
66. Sasaki K, Yamano Y, Bardham S, et al. *Nature* 1991;351:230–233.
67. Mendelsohn FAO, Dunbar M, Allen A. *Fed Proc* 1986;45:1420–1425.
68. Mendelsohn FAO, Millan M, Quirion R, Aguilera G, Sheung-To C, Catt K. *Kidney Int* 1987;20(Suppl):40–44.
69. Gehlert DR, Speth RC, Wamsley JK. *Peptides* 1984;5:1043–1048.
70. Douglas JG. *Am J Physiol* 1987;252:E57–E62.
71. Sechi LA, Grady EF, Griffin CA. *Am J Physiol* 1991;
72. Ernsberger P, Zhou J, Damon TH. *Am J Physiol* 1992;263:F411–F416.
73. Tufro-McReddie A, Harrison JK, Everett AD, Gomez RA. *J Clin Invest* 1993;90:1–9.
74. Ichikawa I, Harris R. *Kidney Int* 1991;40:583–596.
75. Mukais SK, Kauffman S, Katz AI. *J Clin Invest* 1986;77:315–318.
76. Brown GP, Douglas JG. *Endocrinology* 1982;111:1830–1836.
77. Brown GP, Douglas JG. *Endocrinology* 1983;112:2007–2014.
78. Douglas JG. *Am J Physiol* 1987;253:F1–F7.
79. Burns KD, Yamano Y, Inagami T. *J Am Soc Nephrol* 1991;2(A):3395.
80. Douglas JG, Romero M, Hopfer U. *Kidney Int* 1990;38(Suppl 30):S43–S47.
81. Burns KD, Homma T, Harris RC. *Semin Nephrol* 1993;13:13–30.
82. Norman JT. *Renal Physiol Biochem* 1991;14:175–185.
83. Blantz RC, Pelayo JC. *Fed Proc* 1983;42:3071–3074.
84. Hall JE, Guyton AC, Jackson TE. *Am J Physiol* 1977;233:F366.
85. Myers BD, Deen WM, Brenner BM. *Circ Res* 1975;37:101.
86. Navar LG, Rosivall L, Carmines PK, Oparil S. *Fed Proc* 1986;45:1448–1453.
87. Levens NR, Peach MJ, Carey RM. *Circ Res* 1981;48:157–167.
88. Ballerman BJ, Zeidel ML, Gunning ME. Vasoactive peptides in the kidney. In: Brenner BM, Rector FC, eds. *The kidney.* Philadelphia: WB Saunders; 1991:510–583.
89. Ray PE, Aguilera G, Kopp JB, et al. *Kidney Int* 1991;40:764–771.
90. Tufro-McReddie A, Harris JM, Gomez RA. *J Am Soc Nephrol* 1993;4:479A.
91. Keeton TK, Campbell WB. *Pharmacol Rev* 1980;32:81–227.
92. Johns DW, Peach MJ, Gomez RA. *Am J Physiol* 1990;259:F882–F887.
93. Symonds EM, Farler I. *Biol Neonate* 1973;23:133–138.
94. Symonds EM, Craven DJ. *Br J Obstet Gynaecol* 1985;92:618–621.
95. Pelayo JC, Eisner GM, Jose PA. *Clin Perinatol* 1981;8:347–359.
96. Gomez RA. *Pediatr Nephrol* 1990;4:421–423.
97. Richoux JP, Amsaguine S, Grignor G, Bouhnik J, Menard J, Corvol P. *Histochemistry* 1987;88:41–46.
98. Pupilli C, Gomez RA, Tuttle JB. *Pediatr Nephrol* 1991;5:690–695.
99. Egerer G, Taugner R, Tiedemann K. *Histochemistry* 1984;81:385–390.
100. Celio MR, Groscurth P, Inagami I. *Anat Embryol* 1985;173:133–138.
101. Gomez RA, Lynch KR, Chevalier RL, et al. *Am J Physiol* 1988;254:F582–F587.
102. Minuth M, Hackenthal E, Paulsen K, Rix E, Taugner R. *Anat Embryol* 1981;162:173–181.
103. Jones CA, Sigmund CD, McGowan RA, Kane-Haas C, Gross KW. *Mol Endocrinol* 1990;4:375–383.
104. Nishimura H. Comparative endocrinology of renin and angiotensin. Advances in experimental medicine and biology. In: Johnson AJ, Anderson RR, eds. *The renin-angiotensin system.* New York: Plenum Press; 1980:29–77.
105. Nishimura H. *Jpn Heart J* 1978;19:806–822.
106. Gomez RA, Tufro-McReddie A, Everett AD, Pentz ES. *Pediatr Nephrol* 1993;7:635–638.
107. Robillard JE, Kirby RF, Page WV. *Pediatr Res* 1990;27:3378A.
108. Gomez RA, Cassis L, Lynch KR. *Endocrinology* 1988;124(5):2298–2302.
109. Lee EU, Campbell DJ, Habener JF. *Endocrinology* 1987;121:1335–1342.
110. Wallace KB, Bailie MD, Hook JB. *Am J Physiol* 1978;234:R141–R145.
111. Mounier F, Hinglais N, Sich M. *Kidney Int* 1987;32:684–690.
112. Wigger HJ, Stalcup MD. *Lab Invest* 1978;38:581–585.
113. Grady EF, Sechi LA, Griffin CA. *J Clin Invest* 1991;88:921–933.
114. Tsutsumi K, Stromberg C, Viswanathan M, Saavedra JM. *Endocrinology* 1991;129:1075–1082.
115. Millan MA, Carvallo P, Izumi SI. *Science* 1989;244:1340–1342.
116. Zemel S, Millan MA, Aguilera G. *Endocrinology* 1989;124:1774–1780.
117. Zemel S, Millan MA, Feuillan P, Aguilera G. *J Clin Endocrinol Metab* 1990;71:1003–1007.
118. Tufro-McReddie A, Gomez RA. *Semin Nephrol* 1993;13:519–530.
119. Naftilan AJ, Gilliland GK, Eldridge CS, Kraft AS. *Mol Cell Biol* 1990;10:5536–5540.
120. Taubman MB, Berk BC, Izumo S, Tsuda T, Alexander RW, Nadal-Ginard B. *J Biol Chem* 1989;264:526–530.
121. Nakamura A, Iwao H, Fukui K. *Am J Physiol* 1990;258:E1–E6.

122. Gomez RA, Lynch KR, Chevalier RL, et al. *Am J Physiol* 1988;254:F900–F906.
123. Ludwig G, Ganten D, Murakami K, Fashing U, Hackenthal E. *Mol Cell Endocrinol* 1987;50:223–229.
124. Barrett GL, Morgan TO, Smith M, Alcorn D, Aldred P. *Hypertens Dallas* 1989;14:385–395.
125. Catanzaro DF, Mesterovic N, Morris BJ. *Endocrinology* 1985;117:872–878.
126. Nakamara N, Soubrier F, Menard J, Panthier JJ, Rougeon F, Corvol P. *Hypertens Dallas* 1985;7:855–859.
127. Geary KM, Hunt MK, Peach MJ. *Endocrinology* 1992;131:1588–1594.
128. Ingelfinger JR, Pratt RE, Ellison K. *J Clin Invest* 1986;78:1311–1315.
129. Loundon M, Bing RF, Swales JD, Thurston H. *Clin Sci* 1982;63:153–156.
130. Bellucci A, Bilkes BM. *J Clin Invest* 1984;74:1593–1600.
131. Skorecki KL, Ballerman BJ, Rennke HG, Brenner BM. *Fed Proc* 1983;42:3064–3070.
132. Chevalier RL, Peach MJ. *Kidney Int* 1985;28:891–898.
133. Chevalier RL, Jones CE. *J Urol* 1986;136:532–535.
134. Chevalier RL, Gomez RA. *Am J Physiol* 1988;255:F1070–F1077.
135. McDougal WS. *J Urol* 1982;128:418–421.
136. Yarger WE, Schocken DD, Harris RH. *J Clin Invest* 1980;65:400–412.
137. Carmines PK, Tanner GA. *Am J Physiol* 1983;245:F75–F82.
138. Chevalier RL, Sturgill BC, Jones CE, Kaiser DL. *Pediatr Res* 1987;21:338–346.
139. Chevalier RL, Kaiser DL. *Pediatr Res* 1984;18:1266–1271.
140. Zelman SJT, Zenser TV, Davis BB. *Kidney Int* 1983;23:594–598.
141. El-Dahr SS, Gomez RA, Gray MS, Peach MJ, Carey RM. *Am J Physiol* 1990;258:F854–F862.
142. El-Dahr SS, Gomez RA, Khare G, Peach MJ, Carey RM. *Am J Kidney Dis* 1990;15:575–582.
143. Chevalier RL, Gomez RA. *Am J Physiol* 1988;255:F1070–1077.
144. Schubert GER, Standhammer R, Rolle K, Kneissler U. *Urol Res* 1975;3:115–122.
145. El-Dahr SS, Chevalier RL, Gomez RA, Gray MS, Peach MJ, Carey RM. *Kidney Int* 1990;37:354A.
146. Buhrle CP, Hackenthal E, Helmchen U, et al. *Lab Invest* 1986;54:462–471.
147. Mason J. *Pediatr Nephrol* 1990;4:554–574.
148. Bennett WM, Porter GA. *Am J Med* 1988;85:131–133.
149. Myers BD, Sibley R, Newton L, et al. *Kidney Int* 1988;33:590–600.
150. Bantle JP, Paller MS, Boudreau RJ, Olivari MT, Ferris TF. *J Lab Clin Med* 1990;115:233–240.
151. Gillum DM, Truong L, Tasby J, Migliore P, Suki WM. *Transplantation* 1988;46:285–292.
152. Mihatsch MJ, Thiel G, Spickhtin HP, et al. *Transplant Proc* 1983;15(Suppl 1):2821–2835.
153. Yamaguchi Y, Teraoka S, Yagisawa T, Takahashi K, Toma H, Ota K. *Transplant Proc* 1989;21(1):1517–1522.
154. Garr MD, Paller MS. *Am J Physiol* 1990;258:F211–F217.
155. Thomson SC, Tucker BJ, Gabbai F, Blantz RC. *J Clin Invest* 1989;83:960–969.
156. Moss NG, Powell SL, Falk RJ. *Proc Natl Acad Sci* 1985;82:8222–8226.
157. Murray BM, Paller MS. *Clin Nephrol* 1986;25(Suppl 1):S37–S39.
158. Coffman TM, Carr DR, Yarger WE, Klotman PE. *Transplantation* 1987;43(2):282–285.
159. Kon V, Sugiura M, Inagami T, Harvie BR, Ickikawa I, Hoover RL. *Kidney Int* 1990;37:1487–1491.
160. Perico N, Dadan J, Remuzzi G. *J Am Soc Nephrol* 1990;1(1):76–83.
161. Mason J, Muller-Schweinitzer E, Dupont M, et al. *Kidney Int* 1991;39:S28–S32.
162. Kaskel FJ, Devarajan P, Arbeit LA, Moore LC. *Transplant Proc* 1988;20(3):603S–609S.
162. Tufro-McReddie A, Gomez RA, Norling LL, Omar AA, Moore LC, Kaskel FJ. *Kidney Int* 1993;43:615–622.
163. Nittak K, Friedman AI, Nicastri AD, Paik S, Friedman EA. *Transplantation* 1987;44:417–421.
164. Norling LL, Gomez RA, Garmey M, Moore LC, Kaskel FJ. *JASN* 1993;4:757A.
166. Hayslett JP. *Physiol Rev* 1979;59:137–164.
167. Morrison AB. *Methods Achiev Exp Pathol* 1966;1:455–475.
168. Purkerson ML, Hoffsten PE, Klahr S. *Kidney Int* 1976;9:407–417.
169. Anderson S, Meyer TW, Rennke HG, Brenner BM. *J Clin Invest* 1985;76:612–619.
170. Anderson S, Rennke HG, Brenner BM. *J Clin Invest* 1986;77:1993–2000.
171. Jackson B, Hodsman P, Johnston CI. *Am J Hypertens* 1988;1:298–300.
172. El-Dahr SS, Gomez RA, Gray MS, Peach MJ, Carey RM, Chevalier RL. *Am J Physiol* 1990;258:F854–F862.
173. Rosenberg ME, Chmielewski D, Hostetter TH. *J Clin Invest* 1990;85:1144–1149.
174. Terzi F, Beaufils H, Dechaux M, Burtini M, Jouanneau C, Gubler MC. *J Am Soc Nephrol* 1991;2:419A.
175. Rosenberg ME, Correa-Rotter R, Inagami T, Kren SM, Hostetter TH. *Kidney Int* 1991;40:677–683.
176. Fray JCS. *Am J Physiol* 1976;231:936–944.
177. Vander HJ, Miller R. *Am J Physiol* 1964;207:537–546.
178. Pelayo JC, Guan AH, Shanley PF. *Am J Physiol* 1990;258:F414–F422.
179. Goldblatt H. Hypertension due to renal ischemia. *Bull NY Acad Med* 1964;40:745–758.
180. Miller ED, Samuels AI, Haber E, Barger AC. *Science* 1972;177:1108–1109.
181. Cantin M, Gutkowska J, Lacasse J, et al. *Am J Pathol* 1984;115:212–224.
182. Morton JJ, Wallace ECH. *Clin Sci* 1983;64:359–370.
183. Kaufman JS, Hamburger RJ, Flamenbaum W. *Am J Physiol* 1980;238:F488–F490.
184. Taugner R, Marin-Grez M, Keilblach R, Hackenthal E, Nobiling R. *Histochemistry* 1982;76:61–69.
185. Samani NJ, Godfrey NP, Major JS, Brammer WJ, Swales JD. *J Hypertens* 1989;7:105–112.
186. Morishita R, Higaki J, Okunishi H. *J Hypertens* 1991;9:187–192.
187. Moffet RB, McGowan RA, Gross KW. *Hypertension* 1986;8:874–882.
188. Tufro-McReddie A, Chevalier RL, Everett AD, Gomez RA. *Am J Physiol* 1993;264:R696–R702.
189. Lansman JB, Hallam TJ, Rink TJ. *Nature* 1987;325:811–813.
190. Fray JCS. *Am J Physiol* 1976;231:936–944.
191. Briggs JP, Lorenz JN, Weihprecht H, Schnermann J. *Renal Physiol Biochem* 1991;14:164–174.
192. Davis JO, Freeman RH. *Physiol Rev* 1976;56:1–56.
193. Anderson S, Rennke H, Garcia DL, Brenner BM. *Kidney Int* 1989;36:526–536.
194. Everett AD, Scott J, Wilfong N, et al. *Hypertension* 1992;19:70–78.
195. Anderson S, Bouyounes B, Clarey LE, Ingelfinger JR. *J Am Soc Nephrol* 1990;1:621A.
196. Brenner BM, Meyer TW, Hostetter TH. *N Engl J Med* 1982;307:652–659.
197. Hostetter TH, Meyer TW, Rennke HG, Brenner BM. *Kidney Int* 1986;30:509–517.
198. Jakobsson B, Celsi G, Lindbland BS, Aperia A. *Acta Paediatr Scand* 1987;76:293–299.
199. Pullman TM, Alving AS, Dern RJ, Landowne M. *J Lab Clin Med* 1954;44:320–332.
200. Tufro-McReddie A, Arrizurieta EE, Brocca S. *Am J Physiol* 1992;263:F427–F435.
201. Paller MS, Hostetter TH. *Am J Physiol* 1986;251:F34–F39.
202. Rosenberg ME, Chmielewski D, Hostetter TH. *J Clin Invest* 1990;85:1144–1149.
203. Nash DA. *Arch Intern Med* 1977;137:1571–1575.
204. Torres VE, Berndt TJ, Okamura M, et al. *Kidney Int* 1988;33:1130–1139.
205. Torres VE, Donovan KA, Scicli G, et al. *Kidney Int* 1992;42:364–373.
206. Graham PC, Lindop GBM. *Kidney Int* 1988;33:1084–1090.

Hypertension: Pathophysiology, Diagnosis,
and Management, Second Edition,
edited by J.H. Laragh and B.M. Brenner,
Raven Press, Ltd., New York © 1995.

CHAPTER 99

Angiotensinogen: Molecular Biology and Genetics

Xavier Jeunemaitre, Joël Ménard, Eric Clauser, and Pierre Corvol

It has long been known that the pressor factor renin, discovered in the kidney by Tigerstedt and Bergman, is an enzyme that acts on a unique substrate, angiotensinogen (AGT), synthesized mainly by the liver and released into the circulation. Since that time, our knowledge concerning AGT has progressed rapidly thanks to major technologic advances such as radioimmunology, molecular biology, and more recently, molecular genetics. Several recent general reviews have examined various aspects of AGT, mainly its measurement methods (1), biochemistry and purification steps of the protein (2), its molecular structure (3), and hormonal regulation (4). This chapter deals mainly with the recent advances concerning

AGT's expression, regulation, molecular genetics, and putative role in hypertension.

STRUCTURE OF THE ANGIOTENSINOGEN GENE

Structure and Localization of the Human Angiotensinogen Gene

The human AGT complementary deoxyribonucleic acid (cDNA) structure (5) shows the presence of a coding region composed of 1,455 nucleotides, which codes for 485 amino acids. Two possible initiation sites can be predicted from the nucleotide sequence: The first methionine codon is located at position -24 and corresponds to the initiation site of rat pre-AGT messenger ribonucleic acid (mRNA); the second methionine codon is at position -33, closer to the 5' end of the mRNA. The amino acid sequence starts with either of the two initiation sites and with a corresponding signal peptide of 24 or 33 residues. The mature form consists of 452 amino acid resi-

J. Ménard: Centre de Médicine Préventive Cardiovasculaire, Hôpital Broussais, 75014 Paris, France; and INSERM U367, 75005 Paris, France.

X. Jeunemaitre, E. Clauser, and P. Corvol: INSERM U36; Collège d France, 75005 Paris, France; and Service d'Hypertension Artérielle, Hôpital Broussais, 75014 Paris, France.

dues, with the first 10 amino acids corresponding to angiotensin I (Ang I) and the other larger portion to des(ANG I)AGT. The stop codon is followed by a long 3′ untranslated sequence with two different polyadenylation signals, accounting for the existence of two different mRNA species differing in length by 200 nucleotides (5). Rat and human genomic sequences were elucidated shortly after (6–8). The human *AGT* gene encompasses five exons and four introns, spanning 13 kb of genomic sequence (Fig. 1). The first exon is very short (37 nucleotides) and corresponds to the 5′ untranslated sequence of the mRNA. The second exon codes for 59 percent of the protein and contains the nucleotide sequences coding for the signal peptide and Ang I. Exons 3 and 4 code for, respectively, 48 and 62 amino acids of the protein, and the last exon codes for the C-terminal part of the protein and the 3′ untranslated sequence of the mRNA.

A single human *AGT* gene has been localized to chromosome 1q42-3 by *in situ* hybridization (9,10). The renin gene has also been assigned to the long arm of chromosome 1 but in the q32 region. The issue of the genetic proximity of these two genes has been explored using a GT microsatellite repeat at the renin locus (76 percent heterozygosity) (Jeunemaitre and Lifton, *unpublished data*), a GT microsatellite at the *AGT* locus (80 percent heterozygosity) (11), and other markers selected from the consortium map of chromosome 1 (12). Analysis of these markers on pedigrees selected by the Centre d'Etudes du Polymorphisme Humain (CEPH) demonstrated linkage between these two loci (Lod score z =

4.89) for a recombination estimate $\theta = 0.30$ (13). Thus, putative variants of AGT and renin have a 30 percent probability of recombination instead of the 50 percent expected from random recombination events. However, it is interesting to note that the AGT and renin loci do not belong to a syntenic region. In mouse, the *AGT* gene is located on chromosome 8 (14) and the renin 1 and 2 genes are on chromosome 1 (15). In rat, the AGT and renin genes are located on chromosomes 19 and 13, respectively (16,17).

Comparison with Other Serpins

The *AGT* gene belongs to the serpin (*serine protease inhibitor*) superfamily. Angiotensinogen gene structure is similar to those of the human α_1-antitrypsin and α_1-antichymotrypsin genes as far as exon number, size, and splicing sites are concerned (6,18). The main organizational difference between the human *AGT* and α_1-antitrypsin genes resides in exon 2, which is about 200 nucleotides shorter in the latter. Although it has seven exons, the human antithrombin III gene also shares homology with these genes. The percentage of identical amino acids conserved at the same position in human AGT and α_1-antitrypsin is 21 percent and 18 percent for human AGT and antithrombin III. These structural similarities are consistent with the hypothesis that the serine protease inhibitor gene family evolved from a primitive common ancestor some 500 million years ago through

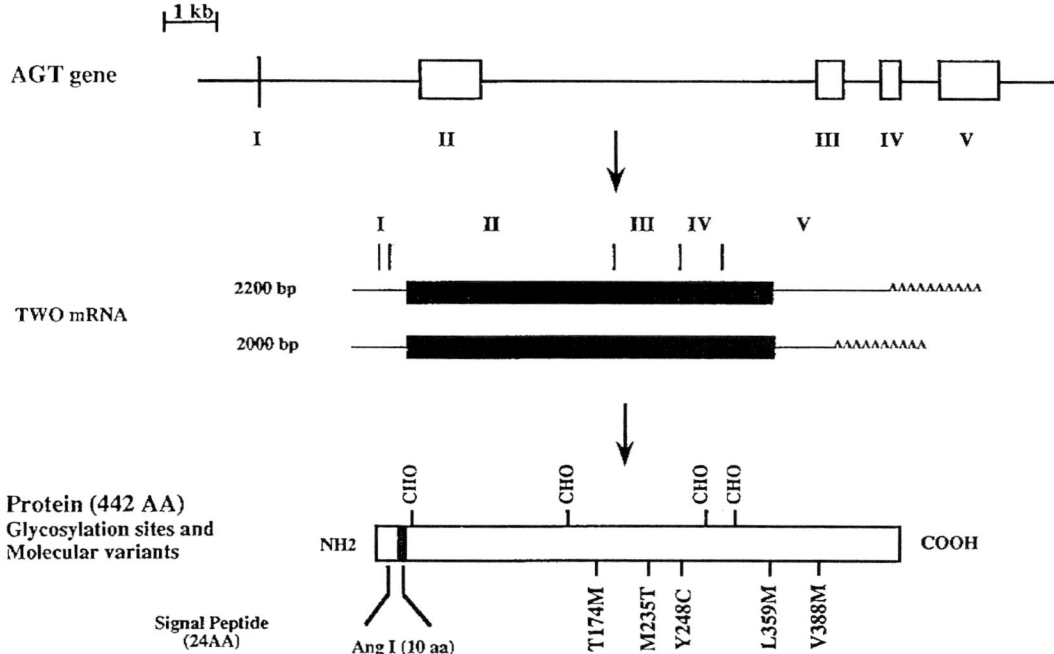

FIG. 1. Human angiotensinogen gene mRNA, protein structure, and molecular variants.

a series of gene duplications, insertions, and deletions (19). The chromosomal localization of the human *AGT* gene (1q42–43) suggests a marked genetic divergence compared with other serpins. Using pulse field gel electrophoresis, Billingsley et al. (20) demonstrated that four different members of the serpin superfamily, namely, α_1-antitrypsin, α_1-antichymotrypsin, corticosteroid-binding globulin, and protein C inhibitor, are all localized to the same chromosomal region (14q32) within a maximum region of 220 kb. This clustering of genes with similar primary sequences and organization strongly suggests that these genes have evolved from a recent ancestor, itself derived from an ancestor gene common to the serpin superfamily.

Thus, AGT is probably one of the more distant serpin superfamily members and has probably lost its serine protease inhibitory activity, as in the case of other serpin superfamily members (e.g., ovalbumin). From a structural point of view, it is difficult to analyze the antiserine protease function of the different serpins because the only three-dimensional structure reported is that of α_1-antitrypsin (21). The primary AGT structure does not suggest any loss of enzymatic property: Exon V, which codes for the antiprotease site, is well conserved between *AGT,* α_1-antitrypsin, and antithrombin III genes. Based on a computer-predicted secondary structure, the distribution of α-helical segments and β-sheet sections is relatively similar in AGT and α_1-antitrypsin (18), and the matched exon–intron junctions between the two genes would also support a possible common biologic function (6). However, experimental evidence has shown that the serpins undergo a striking change in thermal stability after cleavage, with conversion from a stressed to a relaxed form (19). This conformational change has been observed for α_1-antitrypsin, antithrombin, and α_1-antichymotrypsin but not for the noninhibitors ovalbumin and AGT (22). If the stressed conformation is a requirement for the inhibitory function of the serpin's reactive center (21), we could predict that AGT has lost any physiologic serine protease inhibitor activity. Finally, experiments conducted in this laboratory failed to show any AGT antiesterase activity against various serine esterases (Wei, Clauser, and Corvol, *unpublished data*).

CHARACTERIZATION OF THE PROTEIN

Purification and characterization of AGT was a major achievement of biochemistry (23,24), and the different steps of its purification have already been extensively reviewed (2). Human AGT is a globular glycoprotein with a molecular mass varying between 55 and 65 kDa according to its state of glycosylation. It contains four *N*-linked glycosylation sites (Asn-X-Ser/Thr), each of which can bind complex oligosaccharide chains. No

physiologic role of this glycosylation process has yet been demonstrated. Polyclonal and monoclonal antibodies were developed, allowing direct immunoassay of AGT and of its inactive C-terminal part des(Ang I)AGT (25,26). This technique provides precise quantification of AGT in tissues such as the liver, where multiple enzymes capable of metabolizing AGT are present, making the interpretation enzymatic assay results difficult. Comparison of the results of direct AGT quantification by immunoassay with those of its enzymatic assay through exhaustion by an excess of renin revealed that, under circumstances in which renin secretion is high (e.g., in sodium-depleted patients treated with captopril [27] and other conditions of renin stimulation [26]), des(Ang I)AGT accumulates in plasma.

Comparison with Other Species

Angiotensinogen has been purified and partially sequenced from different species including hog (28), sheep (29), dog (30), and rat (31). Based on complete cDNA sequences, human (5) and rat (32) AGTs have been compared on the basis of their respective amino acid sequences and their hydropathy profiles (18). Only 65 percent of the amino acid positions are identical in the two proteins, but an 80 percent similarity is observed for their hydropathy profiles. The more divergent region is located in the 5′ region of the gene following the Ang I sequence. Predicted from the Asn-X-Ser sequence, four and three glycosylation sites are present in the mature human and rat AGTs, respectively. The more important discovery was the explanation of the well-known species specificity of AGT cleavage by renin: Renin cleaves a Leu-Val bond in human AGT and a Leu-Leu bond in rat and other mammalian AGTs (23,33). Although human AGT is cleaved only by human and primate renin, other mammalian AGTs are cleaved by renins originating from most species, including humans. This led to improved understanding of the species specificity of the reaction between renin and its substrate, a key issue for the design and biologic testing of renin inhibitors, because the cleavage of AGT by renin is influenced by the structure of the P'_1 to P'_4 sites (34). This species specificity has been confirmed in transgenic experiments (35).

ANGIOTENSINOGEN AND THE RENIN-ANGIOTENSIN SYSTEM

Role of Angiotensinogen as the Substrate for Renin

The circulating renin-angiotensin system (RAS) has quite particular quantitative aspects. Angiotensin II, the active peptide, has an affinity for its receptor in the nanomolar range but circulates at plasma levels in the picomolar range. These observations suggest the existence of a local Ang II-concentrating process in the vicinity of its receptor and that plasma Ang II levels are not entirely responsible for the effects of the system. The plasma renin concentration is in the picomolar range and varies up to tenfold in usual physiologic circumstances. Angiotensinogen, mainly synthesized in the liver, is the unique substrate for renin, and its plasma concentration is in the micromolar range. Angiotensinogen, distributed both in plasma and extracellular fluid, can be considered as a "reservoir" for the action of renin. Another reservoir is the cerebrospinal fluid (CSF), which has the highest proportion of AGT (per mg of total protein) of all biologic fluids (25,36). Short-term regulation of the RAS does not seem to depend on changes in plasma AGT concentration. For example, rapid adaptation to changes in sodium intake changes is mediated by abrupt modification of renin release by the renal juxtaglomerular (JG) cells, but similar rapid changes in plasma AGT concentration do not occur.

The issue of AGT's limiting role is debated. The K_m of renin for AGT is about 1.25 ± 0.1 μmol/L, more than tenfold lower than that for the homologous synthetic tetradecapeptide substrate (20.7 ± 7 μmol/L) (2,37). Because plasma AGT concentrations in rat and humans are about 1 μmol/L, ten times more AGT than is naturally present would be necessary for reaching a zero-order enzymatic reaction. This is why it is generally accepted that the large amount of AGT present in plasma does not provide an excess of substrate for renin. Direct evidence supporting the limiting role of plasma AGT in Ang I generation comes from (a) the decreased blood pressure and plasma renin activity (PRA) after injection of anti-AGT antibodies (38); this blood pressure fall was dependent on sodium balance and was not present in binephrectomized animals, and (b) the increased blood pressure after injection of pure AGT in salt-depleted rats (39). This has important implications for the quantification of plasma RAS components. A profound decrease of hepatic AGT synthesis can cause an underestimation of renin levels when these are determined by PRA measurements. This has been confirmed by comparison with true levels determined by radioimmunoassay (40).

Assuming that the rate of Ang I formation at the usual plasma AGT concentration is one-half maximal, it appears logical to suspect that the rise in AGT induced by administration of synthetic estrogens or glucocorticoids plays a role in the pathophysiology of some secondary forms of hypertension, such as oral contraceptive-induced hypertension (41) or Cushing's syndrome (42). However, in a physiologic state, the short feedback loop of Ang II on renin release limits the direct effect of plasma AGT changes on blood pressure. An exclusively AGT-dependent hypertension is thus theoretically difficult to imagine, although two exceptional cases of hypertension associated with hepatic cell tumors producing large amounts of AGT have been reported (43,44).

Does Angiotensinogen Play Another Role in the Renin-Angiotensin System?

Angiotensinogen can be considered as the prohormone of Ang I, this transformation occurring extracellularly. This contrasts with the case of renin, which is processed intracellularly from prorenin in the JG cells before being released. It remains surprising that the organism produces a large protein of 452 amino acids to generate a peptide of only 10 amino acid residues. On the basis that the reaction between AGT and renin has a high K_a and a low K_{cat}, which characterize inhibitors, an inhibitory function of des(Ang I)AGT on renin activity or on other proteolytic reactions has been proposed (45) but never documented further.

TISSUE AND CELLULAR LOCALIZATION OF ANGIOTENSINOGEN

The possibility of detecting the presence of AGT and renin mRNA in various tissues has stimulated research on local RASs. These tissue systems differ from the circulating RAS by the local production of the active peptide Ang II, which may have paracrine or autocrine effects. These may well be regulated locally, independently of the circulating system. Biochemical and molecular biology techniques have been used to discover these local RASs. One of the difficulties of localizing AGT by immunohistochemistry is its lack of storage in synthesizing cells. For instance, immunohistochemical studies of the liver could only detect AGT after colchicine treatment causing AGT accumulation in the hepatic cells. *In situ* hybridization detected hepatic AGT (9) more easily because of its relatively high rate of expression. Other pitfalls may arise from the characterization of AGT by its ability to release Ang I, and then Ang II after the action of angiotensin converting enzyme (ACE). Angiotensin II has not always been well characterized, and purification and isolation of "true" Ang II should be demonstrated by high-power liquid chromatography (HPLC) characterization in addition to its immunoassay by specific polyclonal or monoclonal antibodies. Moreover, Ang II can be produced from AGT by enzymes other than renin, and Ang I can be converted to Ang II by enzymes other than ACE. The N-terminal part of AGT (AGT tetradecapeptide) has frequently been used as a substitute for pure AGT to investigate "local" renin. Because it has intrinsic vasoactive properties and is degraded by several metabolic pathways, this tetradecapeptide is not suitable for the study of local renin in various tissues (46).

For these reasons, the method of choice for localizing AGT is probably the detection of its mRNA. The presence of AGT mRNA in tissues has been demonstrated using Northern blot analysis, nuclease S_1 protection assay, and polymerase chain reaction (PCR). Competitive PCR assays after reverse transcription allow quantification of alterations in gene expression of the components of the RAS (47). Because of the possibility of amplification of very few molecules, these techniques raise questions about the physiologic significance of the very low (but still detectable) levels of mRNA. *In situ* hybridization techniques have permitted precise intracellular localization of mRNA in tissues.

Angiotensinogen is a widely expressed glycoprotein (see ref. 48). The liver is the main site of synthesis, and plasma AGT levels mainly reflect this hepatic synthesis (49). Brain, large arteries, kidney, and adipose tissue are other established sites of AGT synthesis (50,51). In brain, *in situ* hybridization and immunohistochemistry have shown that astrocytes are the most likely source of AGT (52–54). Astrocyte cultures derived from human brain tissue express AGT (55). The synthesis of AGT has been shown in two neuroblastoma cell cultures (56,57). Presence of AGT mRNA has only been demonstrated in astroglial cells (53), whereas immunoreactive AGT has been demonstrated in both astrocytes and neurons (58,59). Therefore, it has been hypothesized that glial cells could synthesize the renin substrate that would be taken up by neurons, these cells constituting a paracrine RAS system (60). Brain and CSF AGT is diminished by adrenalectomy (61) and increased by dexamethasone (62) with a lesser extent than liver AGT (63). The exact location of AGT within the vessel wall is still a matter of debate, especially whether it is located in vascular smooth muscle cells or in the adventitia (64–66). Interestingly, Naftilan et al. (66) found an expression in the aortic medial smooth muscle layer that depended on sodium status. More recently, increased expression of AGT mRNA was found in the medial layer of the injured aorta, suggesting a role of AGT in the myointimal proliferation after vascular injury (67). Because the main source of AGT mRNA in the rat aorta seems to be located in the brown adipose tissue (64), the presence of highly vascularized adipose tissue surrounding this vessel raises the possibility of a local RAS in which adipose cells would synthesize AGT and Ang II would be generated through circulating renin and endothelial ACE.

In heart, AGT mRNA is expressed mostly in the atria and less abundantly in the ventricles (50,68). The cardiac presence of mRNA of the different components of the RAS, including Ang II receptors, supports the hypothesis of a physiologic role of the RAS in cardiac function. In addition to hormonal regulation of the cardiac expression of AGT (50), AGT mRNA expression has been found to increase after a low-salt diet (69) and to decrease after treatment with ACE inhibitors (70). Increased ACE activity and AGT expression have also been demonstrated after experimental left ventricular hypertrophy (71), suggesting with other studies that the cardiac RAS may have an important role in modulating growth and hypertrophy of the heart.

Angiotensinogen mRNA is detectable in kidney at much lower levels than in the liver (50,72). Ingelfinger et al. (73) demonstrated that AGT mRNA is present in proximal tubular cells. Proximal convoluted and straight tubular cells obtained from microdissected rabbit proximal tubule and cultured *in vitro* are able to produce AGT (and reninlike activity) (74). However, AGT mRNA is apparently not present in JG cells, where Ang II has been detected by immunohistochemistry (75). Changes in sodium diet are able to regulate kidney AGT expression: A low-salt diet increases AGT mRNA in proximal tubular cells (76), whereas periaortic fat and liver mRNA levels remain unchanged. Alteration of renal hemodynamics caused by experimental heart failure has been shown to induce a renal-specific increase in AGT mRNA, suggesting its contribution to activation of the intrarenal RAS (77). Even though renal AGT level is mainly dependent on circulating AGT (78), it seems to be an important rate-limiting factor for the generation of renal Ang I under converting enzyme inhibitors, suggesting the importance of AGT in determining renal angiotensin peptides and renal vascular resistance (79).

The investigation of local RASs involves the exact cel-

TABLE 1. *Main expression sites of angiotensinogen*

Tissues	Localization	Intensity (% total mRNA compared with liver)	References
Liver	Hepatocytes	100	50,51,65
Brain	Hypothalamus, cerebellum brainstem, spinal cord	20–40	50,51,53,65
Adipose tissue	Brown fat > white fat	5	48,50,67
Kidney	Cortex > medulla	4–20	50,72,76
Adrenals	Cortex > medulla	1–5	50,51,65
Vessels	Adventitia > media	1–2	50,66,123
Heart	Atria > ventricules	5	50,51,80
Ovary	Granulosa	3–4	50,65

lular localization of the four main proteins of this system (AGT, renin, ACE, and Ang II receptors). Because regulation of AGT expression is tissue-specific, local synthesis sites may play biologic roles that are independent of that of circulating AGT. However, the biochemical or molecular evidence for the presence of RAS components (mRNA or protein) should ideally be supported by the demonstration of a biologic effect of their stimulation or their blockade, in isolated organs such as the heart (70,80) or the perfused rat hindquarters (81).

REGULATION

Hormonal Regulation of Angiotensinogen

In contrast with the rapid changes documented in plasma renin (occurring within seconds or minutes), changes in plasma AGT are rather slow (occurring over hours or days). Angiotensinogen is secreted constitutively (i.e., it is not stored within secretory granules). In a great variety of *in vivo* and *in vitro* models, investigators have repeatedly demonstrated that administration of glucocorticoids (especially dexamethasone), estrogens, Ang II, and thyroid hormones is able to stimulate the synthesis and release of AGT (see refs. 1–4). These effects are neutralized by antiglucocorticoids and antiestrogens, and adrenalectomy and thyroidectomy decrease plasma AGT levels. The stimulatory effect of Ang II on AGT synthesis and release is important to consider in parallel with its opposite effect on renin synthesis and release: The fall in plasma AGT during ACE inhibition is probably caused by both its increased consumption due to the rise in plasma renin and decreased synthesis (82).

There is a parallel rise in plasma AGT and estrogens during pregnancy (83). A high-molecular-weight form of AGT (HM$_r$ A) has been found in plasma of pregnant women (accounting for approximately 10 percent of circulating levels) and is the predominant form (60 to 70 percent) of AGT in amniotic fluid (84). This HM$_r$ A, possibly of placental origin, has kinetic properties with renin similar to those of the classical AGT (LM$_r$ A). Based on a multiple-step AGT purification procedure, Tewksbury and Tryon (85) hypothesized that the HM$_r$ A could contain two subunits identical to LM$_r$ A, bound together by disulfide bonds, hydrophobic interactions, and a still unknown protein. The physiologic significance of this HM$_r$ A is still unknown. Angiotensinogen stimulation by estrogens also occurs with administration of oral contraceptive pills, containing ethinyl-estradiol, which induces a dose-dependent rise in plasma AGT (86). This stimulatory effect is not observed with percutaneous estrogen administration (87), likely due to the absence of accumulation of estradiol in the hepatic cells. Angiotensinogen's increased expression is modulated by estrogen receptors levels and is tissue-dependent: Although

estrogen's stimulatory effect on liver is important, no stimulating effect has been observed in adipose tissue; contradictory results have been observed in brain (54). Binephrectomy is another situation in which AGT's hepatic synthesis and plasma concentration are increased, albeit via a mechanism thus far unknown (2,88). Finally, the additive effect of these various stimuli suggests that they trigger AGT synthesis through different transcriptional pathways.

Transcriptional Regulation of Angiotensinogen

Most of the biochemical results previously obtained in the whole organism or in isolated cells have been extended by the study of AGT mRNA levels and, in some instances, by that of AGT's rate of transcription. Glucocorticoids, estrogens, Ang II, and thyroid hormones increase the amount of AGT mRNA in rat liver (50,65,89,90). Binephrectomy increases the liver content of AGT mRNA (91). The hormonal regulation of AGT mRNA has also been studied in both hepatic (92) and nonhepatic cell lines, such as Chinese hamster ovary cells (93), pancreatic cells (94), or adipocytes (95). It is likely that the main part of AGT regulation occurs at the transcriptional level, although a post-transcriptional regulatory process, such as modification of the stability of the mRNA, has been documented in the case of Ang II-increased AGT mRNA levels (96). Cells that synthesize and secrete AGT do not possess secretory granules, and the main characteristic of AGT release is the use of a constitutive pathway. This was well demonstrated by Deschepper and Reudelhuber (97), who compared the pattern of secretion of AGT with that of endogenous adrenocorticotrophic hormone (ACTH), which is secreted by AtT-20 cells through a regulated pathway. In these cells, db-cyclic adenosine monophosphate (AMP) and potassium chloride triggered ACTH secretion, and monensin, which impairs the constitutive secretory pathway, reduced ACTH secretion slightly. In the cells transfected with rat AGT cDNA, neither db-cyclicAMP nor potassium chloride were able to release AGT, whose secretion was greatly decreased by monensin. This observation is important because in the same cells transfected with human renin, renin is secreted by the regulated secretory pathway. Therefore, AGT and active renin, at least in these cells, are not cocompartmentalized in dense core secretory granules. Also, it is likely that AGT and renin are produced by different cells in a given local RAS.

Regulation of Angiotensinogen Gene Expression

The 5' regulatory region of eukaryotic genes is involved in the hormonal regulation of their transcription and in their tissue-specific expression. They contain short nucleotidic stretches (*cis*-regulatory elements) involved in protein–DNA interactions that regulate transcription and that are generally well conserved between species. Based on comparison with corresponding consensus sequences, the presence of several putative hormone responsive elements (HRE) in the 5' region of the human *AGT* gene has been reported (7,8). Three putative glucocorticoid responsive elements (GRE) are located at −126 to −133 bp, −202 to −217 bp and −670 to −675 bp of the human *AGT* gene. Potential estrogen (−324 to −338 bp) and thyroid receptor responsive elements (−370 to −384 bp) are present in the 5' flanking sequence of the human *AGT* gene. Other sequences potentially involved in the transcriptional regulation of the human gene include a cyclicAMP-responsive element (−833 to −839 bp), an acute-phase responsive element (APRE) (−270 to −278 bp), and a heat shock element (−561 to −573 bp).

To investigate the *in vivo* tissue specificity of the putative regulatory regions of the *AGT* gene, transgenic mice were created by using a minigene as the reporter of transcription (98). Sequences necessary and sufficient for mediating induction by glucocorticoids, estrogen, and bacterial endotoxin were contained in a minigene bearing 0.75 kb of DNA upstream of the capsite. This construct was also able to confer tissue specificity in most organs known to produce AGT (liver, brain, kidney, brown adipose tissue, and to a lesser extent, lung and heart).

Based on experiments involving transfection of AGT-CAT reporter plasmids into rat hepatoma cells, Feldmer et al. (99) identified the sequences from −569 to −589 and −460 to −480 as functional GREs of the rat *AGT* gene. The *in vitro* transcriptional regulation of rat AGT expression in liver by glucocorticoids and acute-phase proteins has been extensively studied by the Habener's group (100–103). They performed a series of elegant studies using the H35 rat hepatoma cell line into which they transfected different constructs consisting of various 5' sequences of the *AGT* gene promoter linked to a reporter gene, such as luciferase. The cytokine-induced increase in AGT expression appears only when the cells are cultured in the presence of glucocorticoid, due to a *cis*-acting APRE DNA element (−552 to −537) localized in the 615 bp of the AGT promoter. The cytokine-inducible transcription of AGT is activated through a "hormonally inducible enhancer unit" comprising the APRE with one upstream and one downstream GRE, both of which mediate glucocorticoid-stimulated transcription *in vivo* (103). Point mutations in these two rat AGT GREs abolished binding of the glucocorticoid receptor and the stimulatory effect of interleukin 1. Ron *et al* (102) proposed a model in which competition between an inducible binding protein (BPi) such as NFkB and a constitutively present binding protein (BPc) for the common APRE binding site results in modulation of the activity of the *AGT* gene APRE. The dependence of the response to cytokines on glucocorticoids was further explained by the interactions between glucocorticoids, the BPi and BPc, and the "hormonally inducible enhancer unit." Occupation of this unit by different proteins in different cell types could explain tissue-specific activation of AGT transcription (102). Finally, a differentiation-specific element (DSE), located at −1,000 bp in the 5' flanking region of the rat *AGT* gene, could act as a binding site for a pou-homeodomain class of transcription factors and thus play an important role in the developmental switch for the expression of AGT during the differentiation of fibroblasts to adipocytes (104).

ANGIOTENSINOGEN AND HYPERTENSION

Animal Genetic Studies

Multiple experiments have been performed in animals, usually in rats, to test the importance of the renin substrate in the activation of the RAS and blood pressure regulation. Specific rat AGT antiserum was able to decrease blood pressure in rats, to a greater extent in those on a normal than a low-sodium diet, and was devoid of effect in binephrectomized animals (38). We also demonstrated a 30-mm Hg rise in blood pressure in anesthetized rats after injection of 250 μg pure rat AGT. This pressor effect of AGT was shown when rats were salt-depleted, with a marked reduction in plasma AGT caused by its consumption by the increased renin activation (39). These results confirm the importance of the *in vivo* dependency of AGT concentration on renin activation status.

Transgenic Animals Expressing Angiotensinogen

The mouse is particularly suitable for AGT transgenic experiments because it is known to have low circulating AGT levels (105) and because mouse renin is capable of cleaving rat AGT (106). Kimura et al. (107) generated transgenic mice expressing the entire rat *AGT* gene including 1.6 kb of 5' flanking sequences. These animals developed hypertension, especially in males and when AGT was overexpressed in liver and brain. In this study, specific cerebral expression seemed to be a prerequisite for the hypertensive phenotype. Other transgenic animals have been generated by Ohkubo et al. (35), who introduced in mice either the *rat* renin gene, the *rat AGT* gene, or both, under the control of the mouse metallothionine I promoter. A similar chimeric RAS was constructed through cross-mating separate lines of transgenic mice carrying either the human renin or *AGT* genes (108). In both models, captopril-sensitive hypertension was present only in the transgenic mice carrying both transgenes. These experiments documented *in vivo* the species specificity of the renin-AGT reaction that had already been established *in vitro*. Although these transgenic experiments clearly demonstrated that overexpression of the renin and *AGT* genes led to increased blood pressure, their relevance to the pathogenesis of human hypertension is highly questionable. Incidentally, such transgenic animals offer the possibility of studying the antihypertensive effect of specific human renin inhibitors (108).

Human Genetic Studies

Essential Hypertension

In humans, different studies have indicated a relationship between plasma AGT level and blood pressure. A high correlation between the renin substrate and blood pressure ($r = .39$, $p < .0001$) has been reported in a large study involving 574 subjects (109). Higher levels of plasma renin substrate have been observed in hypertensives and offspring of hypertensive parents compared with normotensives (110). In a study using a four-corners approach to identification of the genetic determinants of blood pressure, increased plasma AGT was associated with increased blood pressure in offspring with contrasted parental predisposition to hypertension (111). More recently, Tiret et al. (*in preparation*) have performed a segregation analysis in healthy nuclear families, showing that plasma AGT level is in part genetically determined, with a high correlation between mother and offspring ($r = .47 \pm 0.07$) and between offsprings ($r = .35 \pm 0.09$). A positive relation was found between plasma AGT levels and diastolic blood pressure, significant in females but not in males. All these studies are concordant, supporting the hypothesis of AGT being a determinant of blood pressure.

Another way of determining the role of AGT in blood pressure regulation is to apply the molecular genetics approach to hypertensive subjects. Multiple markers have recently been characterized at the AGT locus. The only reported diallelic restriction fragment length polymorphism (RFLP) is located in exon 4 of the *AGT* gene, with an amino acid change (Leu to Met) that eliminates a recognition site for the restriction enzyme *Pst* I (112). More recently, a highly polymorphic dinucleotide GT repeat (80 percent heterozygosity) has been described (11), displaying ten alleles and located in the 3' region of the *AGT* gene. Other diallelic polymorphisms, detected by the single-strand conformation technique (113) and located in the 5' regulatory region of the gene and in intronic sequences, have also been described (114).

An extensive study of the potential role of the *AGT* gene in human essential hypertension was recently performed in two large series (Utah and Paris, France) of hypertensive sibships yielding a total of 379 sib pairs (115). Using the highly polymorphic GT microsatellite described above, we obtained evidence of genetic linkage between the *AGT* gene and hypertension. In particular, a strong linkage (17 percent excess of allele sharing) was found in patients characterized by a diastolic blood pressure greater than 100 mm Hg or the prescription of two or more antihypertensive medications. In both the Utah and Paris groups, although significant linkage was obtained in male pairs, none was observed in female comparisons, suggesting the influence of an epistatic hormonal phenomenon. We screened the genomic sequences of the AGT locus by the means of multiple PCR fragments and searched for mutations in nondenaturing conditions (113). Among the 15 observed variants, 5 were missense mutations (3 rare, observed in single families [Fig. 1]). In both Caucasian groups, the M235T variant (Met → Thr in amino acid position 235) was found

TABLE 2. *Relations between angiotensinogen and blood pressure in humans*

Studies	Findings	References
Essential hypertension		
Correlation between plasma angiotensinogen and blood pressure	$r = .39$	109
Increased plasma angiotensinogen	HTN vs NTN	110
Association with molecular variants		
Probands of hypertensive families (Paris and Salt Lake City)	M235T and T174M	114
Unselected hypertensives (Paris)	M235T	116
Unselected hypertensives (Japan)	M235T	117
Positive sib-pair linkage study		
Patients with diastolic blood pressure ≥ 100 mm Hg or treated with ≥ 2 drugs	17% excess	115
Male–male pairs	13% excess	
Pregnancy-induced hypertension		
Association with molecular variants		
Utah and Japanese women	M235T	120
Positive sib-pair linkage study		121
Icelandic and Scottish women		

more frequently in hypertensive probands, especially in the more severe index cases (0.50), than in controls (0.38). More important, plasma AGT levels were found to be significantly increased in patients with the M235T variant, with 10 and 20 percent increases in heterozygotes (MT) and homozygotes (TT), respectively, compared with wild-type homozygotes (MM). These initial results have been confirmed in Caucasian (116) and Japanese (117) hypertensive patients without selection for a family history of hypertension. The corroboration of these studies supports the interpretation that molecular variants of the *AGT* gene, such as M235T or those in linkage disequilibrium with this variant, constitute inherited predispositions to essential hypertension in humans.

Pregnancy-induced Hypertension

The presence of a susceptible allele of the *AGT* gene associated with increased plasma AGT concentration and an increase in blood pressure could be more striking when AGT expression is stimulated, such as in pregnancy or during oral estrogen administration. Clinical studies have documented a familial tendency to develop preeclampsia, and familial studies have suggested both a genetic inheritance and the influence of environmental factors (118,119). A significant plasma HM_r A increase has been observed in women with pregnancy-induced hypertension compared with normotensive pregnant women (84). Two recent reports indicate that the AGT locus could play an important role in the occurrence of pregnancy-induced hypertension. Ward et al. (120) found a significant association between the 235T variant and preeclampsia in both Caucasian and Japanese samples. Using another strategy (analysis of allelic inheritance of the GT microsatellite in 52 sibling pairs of preeclamptic sisters), Arngrimsson et al. (121) were able to demonstrate significant linkage between the AGT locus and preeclampsia in Icelandic and Scottish families. Thus, although the mechanisms proposed for preeclampsia and essential hypertension are different, a frequent variant of the *AGT* gene could predispose to both diseases.

Oral administration of natural or synthetic estrogens stimulates the production of AGT, but no direct relation exists between the increase in plasma AGT and blood pressure level. However, subtle changes in renal blood flow were observed in women whose AGT levels were increased by oral treatment with synthetic estrogens (122). Chronically increased plasma AGT might facilitate hypertension in predisposed individuals who would have in addition an abnormal short feedback loop between Ang II and renin release.

OTHER ROLES

Angiotensinogen, Obesity, and Blood Pressure

Angiotensinogen is expressed in adipocytes from multiple anatomic sites (123). Together with other markers of adipocyte function, AGT production appears at the time of differentiation from fibroblast to preadipocyte cell lines (124). A differentiation-specific element located in the 5′ flanking region of the gene could be implicated in this developmental pattern of expression (see Regulation of Angiotensinogen Gene Expression). Angiotensinogen expression in white adipocytes seems influenced by nutrition, with a 15 to 30 percent reduction during fasting conditions and a twofold increase in refed rats (95). In obesity, plasma AGT levels have been shown to correlate strongly with blood pressure during weight loss (125).

The abundance of AGT in adipose tissue should also be considered. As stated above, local AGT synthesis could be part of a paracrine system influencing the release of Ang II in the vicinity of the vascular smooth muscle cell. Thus, an increase in the number of adipocytes could lead to a parallel increase in AGT production, which would cause vasoconstriction and increased peripheral resistance. The nutritional status could therefore play a role in influencing blood supply to adipose tissue and thus affect vascular resistance and blood pressure in obese individuals. Interestingly, a study of 67 obese Japanese women showed that those who were hypertensive exhibited a higher intraabdominal/subcutaneous area fat index than the normotensives (126). In the same study, a strong and significant correlation was found between this fat index and systolic and diastolic blood pressure (r = .62 and .63, respectively), independently of age and body mass index. The association between intraabdominal fat accumulation and hypertension raises the question of whether the renin substrate is involved in the pathogenesis of hypertension in obese individuals. In the ECTIM (Etude Cas-Témoin de l'Infarctus du Myocarde) population, the M235T AGT variant was only associated with hypertension in individuals who were not overweight (Tiret et al., *submitted*). All these results suggest that AGT expression and regulation in adipose tissue may interact with blood pressure levels.

Angiotensinogen and Inflammation

A completely different aspect of AGT regulation is its stimulation during inflammation and tissue injury. Bing (127) first reported that plasma AGT was elevated in injuries known to increase acute-phase proteins. In patients suffering from various streptococcal infections,

AGT increases by 70 percent, along with similar increases of acute-phase proteins (128). Consumption of this increased AGT is shown by the accumulation of des(Ang I)AGT in patients suffering from bacterial sepsis or the adult respiratory distress syndrome (129).

Kageyama et al. (130) examined the response of AGT mRNA to inflammation in rat liver and brain. During the first 5 hours after *Escherichia coli* lipopolysaccharide (LPS) administration, liver mRNA increased fivefold, but there was no change in brain mRNA levels. Different models of inflammation were tested by Bouhnik et al. (131), who compared the changes in T-kininogen, a major acute-phase protein-inhibiting cysteine proteinase (132), and AGT (133) in various inflammation models. Lipopolysaccharide increased both T-kininogen and AGT, but turpentine increased only T-kininogen. Itoh et al. (133) reported that, in the presence of dexamethasone, Reuber H35 hepatoma cells produced more AGT when the incubation medium contained 50 and 500 U/ml interleukin 6. The identification of APRE in the rat AGT promoter by Ron et al. (101) is consistent with this observed increase in AGT expression in inflammation.

The physiologic significance of the increase in AGT during acute inflammation is still unknown. In these inflammatory states, AGT could be a neutral marker of inflammation devoid of any role or could inhibit a proteolytic enzyme that has not yet been recognized. In the presence of fever-induced vasodilation, activation of the RAS could counteract vasodilation locally and help maintain blood pressure.

CONCLUSIONS

Angiotensinogen remains a promising protein, justifying continued biologic and clinical research. Although AGT's function has long been considered as being limited to providing a plasma reservoir for renin action, new interest has recently been generated from basic experiments demonstrating the diversity of its expression and the tissue specificity of its regulation. In these multiple sites of expression, AGT is mainly present in extracellular fluids. Because local tissular concentrations of the RAS are still unknown, it is difficult to speculate whether local AGT concentrations could be limiting in these local RAS activities. Another focus of interest comes from recent findings of molecular variants of human AGT suggesting that a chronic state of AGT overexpression might predispose to the development of hypertension. The use of precise enzymatic assays and radioimmunoassays to measure plasma AGT concentration and of modern molecular biology tools to identify variations of the *AGT* gene should be important in determining the precise role of AGT in the RAS and in blood pressure homeostasis.

ACKNOWLEDGMENTS

The authors thank N. Braure and C. Loury for preparation of this manuscript.

REFERENCES

1. Robertson JIS. Angiotensinogen measurement. In: Robertson JIS, Nicholls MG, eds. *The renin angiotensin system, biochemistry–physiology.* Gower Medical Publishing; 1993:14.1–14.8.
2. Tewksbury DA. Angiotensinogen: biochemistry and molecular biology. In: Laragh JJ, Brenner BM, eds. *Hypertension, pathophysiology, diagnosis and management.* New York: Raven Press; 1990:1197–1216.
3. Lynch KR, Peach MJ. Molecular biology of angiotensinogen. *Hypertension* 1991;17:263–269.
4. Deschepper CF, Hong-Brown LQ. Hormonal regulation of the angiotensinogen gene in liver and other tissues. In: Raizada MK, Philips MI, Sumners C, eds. *Cellular and molecular biology of the renin angiotensin system.* Boca Raton, FL: CRC Press; 1993:149–166.
5. Kageyama R, Ohkubo H, Nakanishi S. Primary structure of human preangiotensinogen deduced from the cloned cDNA sequence. *Biochemistry* 1984;23:3603–3609.
6. Tanaka T, Ohkubo H, Nakanishi S. Common structural organization of the angiotensinogen and α_1-antitrypsin genes. *J Biol Chem* 1984;259:8063–8065.
7. Gaillard I, Clauser E, Corvol P. Structure of human angiotensinogen gene. *DNA* 1989;8:87–99.
8. Fukamizu A, Takahashi S, Min Seok SEO, et al. Structure and expression of the human angiotensinogen gene. Identification of a unique and highly active promoter. *J Biol Chem* 1990;265:7576–7582.
9. Gaillard-Sanchez I, Bruneval P, Clauser E, et al. Successful detection by in situ cDNA hybridization of three members of the serpin family: angiotensinogen, alpha 1 protease inhibitor, and antithrombin III in human hepatocytes. *Modern Pathol* 1990;3:216–222.
10. Isa MN, Boyd E, Morrison N, Harrap E, Clauser E, Connor JM. Assignment of the human angiotensinogen gene to chromosome 1q42-q43 by nonisotopic *in situ* hybridization. *Genomics* 1990;8:598–600.
11. Kotelevtsev YV, Clauser E, Corvol P, Soubrier F. Dinucleotide repeat polymorphism in the human angiotensinogen gene. *Nucleic Acids Res* 1991;19:6978.
12. Dracopoli NC, O'Connell P, Elsner T, et al. The CEPH consortium linkage map of human chromosome 1. *Genomics* 1991;9:686–700.
13. Jeunemaitre X, Lifton RP. Genes of the renin angiotensin system and the genetics of human hypertension. In: Raizada MK, Phillips MI, Sumners C, eds. *Cellular and molecular biology of the renin angiotensin system.* Boca Raton, FL: CRC Press; 1993:73–94.
14. Clouston WM, Evans BA, Haralambidis J, Richards RI. Molecular cloning of the mouse angiotensinogen gene. *Genomics* 1988;2:240–248.
15. Chirgwin JM, Schaefer IM, Diaz JA, Lalley PA. Mouse kidney renin gene is on chromosome 1. *Somatic Cell Mol Genet* 1984;10:633.
16. Mori M, Ishizaki K, Yamada T, et al. Restriction fragment length polymorphisms of the angiotensinogen gene in inbred rat strains and mapping of the gene on chromosome 19q. *Cytogenet Cell Genet* 1989;50:42–45.
17. Pravenec M, Simonet L, Kren V, et al. The rat renin gene: assignment to chromosome 13 and linkage to the regulation of blood pressure. *Genomics* 1991;9:466–472.
18. Doolittle RF. Angiotensinogen is related to the antitrypsin-antithrombin-ovalbumin family. *Science* 1983;222:417–419.
19. Carrell RW, Boswell DR. Serpins: the superfamily of plasma serine proteinase inhibitors. In: Barrett, Salvesen, eds. *Proteinase inhibitors.* Elsevier Science Publishers BV; 1986:403–420.

20. Billingsley GD, Walter MA, Hammond GL, Cox DW. Physical mapping of four serpin genes: α1 antitrypsin, α1-antichymotrypsin, corticosteroid-binding globulin, and protein C inhibitor, within a 280-kb region on chromosome 14q32.1 *Am J Hum Genet* 1993;52:343–353.

21. Hüber R, Carrell RW. Implications of the three-dimensional structure of a₁-antitrypsin for structure and function of serpins. *Biochemistry* 1989;28:8951–8966.

22. Stein PE, Tewksbury DA, Carrell RW. Ovalbumin and angiotensinogen lack seroin S-R conformational change. *Biochem J* 1989;262:103.

23. Printz MP, Printz JM, Dworschack RT. Human angiotensinogen. Purification, partial characterization and a comparison with animal prohormones. *J Biol Chem* 1977;252:1654–1662.

24. Tewksbury DA, Dart RA, Travis J. The amino terminal aminoacid sequence of human angiotensinogen. *Biochem Biophys Res Commun* 1981;99:1311–1315.

25. Genain C, Bouhnik J, Tewksbury D, Corvol P, M ¦nard J. Characterization of plasma and CSF human angiotensinogen and desangiotensin I angiotensinogen by direct radioimmunoassay *J Clin Endocrinol Metab* 1984;59:478–484.

26. Bouhnik J, Clauser E, Gardes J, Corvol P, Ménard J. Direct radioimmunoassay of rat angiotensinogen and its application to rats in various endocrine states. *Clin Sci* 1982;62:355–360.

27. Rasmussen S, Nielsen M, Giese J. Captopril combined with thiazide lowers renin substrate concentration: implications for methodology in renin assays. *Clin Sci* 1981;60:591–593.

28. Skeggs LT Jr, Lentz KE, Hochstrasser H, Kahn JR. The purification and partial characterization of several forms of hog renin substrate. *J Exp Med* 1963;118:73–98.

29. Fernley RT, John M, Niall HD, Coghlan JP. Purification and characterization of ovine angiotensinogen. *Eur J Biochem* 1986; 154:597–601.

30. Moffett RB. Purification of multiple forms of plasma angiotensinogen: molecular weight and charge heterogeneity. *Biochim Biophys Acta* 1987;912:1–8.

31. Bouhnik J, Clauser E, Strosberg D, Frenoy JP, Ménard J, Corvol P. Rat angiotensinogen and des (angiotensin I) angiotensinogen: purification, characterization and partial sequencing. *Biochemistry* 1981;20:7010–7015.

32. Ohkubo I, Kageyama R, Ujihara M, Hirose T, Inayama S, Nakanishi S. Cloning and sequence analysis of cDNA for rat angiotensinogen. *Proc Natl Acad Sci USA* 1983;20:2196–2200.

33. Quinn T, Burton J. Amino acid sequence of angiotensinogen as a basis for species-specificity of renin. *Chem Abst* 1982;97:276.

34. Haber E, Hui KY. Specific renin inhibitors. The concepts and prospects. In: Laragh JH, Brenner BM, eds. *Hypertension: pathophysiology, diagnosis and management.* New York: Raven Press, 1990; 2343–2350.

35. Ohkubo H, Kawakami H, Kakehi Y, et al. Generation of transgenic mice with elevated blood pressure by introduction of the rat renin and angiotensinogen genes. *Proc Natl Acad Sci* 1990;87:5153–5157.

36. Ito T, Eggena P, Barrett JD, Katz D, Metter J, Sambhi MP. Studies on angiotensinogen of plasma and cerebrospinal fluid in normal and hypertensive human subjects. *Hypertension* 1980;2: 432–436.

37. Cumin F, Le-Nguyen D, Castro B, Ménard J, Corvol P. Comparative enzymatic studies of human renin acting on pure natural or synthetic substrates. *Biochim Biophys Acta* 1987;913:10–19.

38. Gardes J, Bouhnik J, Clauser E, Corvol P, Ménard J. Role of angiotensinogen in blood pressure homeostasis. *Hypertension* 1982; 4:185–189.

39. Ménard J, El-Amrani AIK, Savoie F, Bouhnik J. Angiotensinogen: an attractive and underrated participant in hypertension and inflammation. *Hypertension* 1991;18:705–706.

40. Arnal JF, Cudek P, Plouin PF, Guyene TT, Michel JB, Corvol P. Low angiotensinogen levels are related to the severity and liver dysfunction of congestive heart failure: implications for renin measurements. *Am J Med* 1991;90:17–22.

41. Laragh JH, Sealey JE, Ledingham JGG, Newton MA. Oral contraceptives. Renin, aldosterone and high blood pressure. *JAMA* 1967;201:918–922.

42. Krakoff LR, Einsenfeld AJ. Hormonal control of plasma renin substrate (angiotensinogen). *Circ Res* 1977;41:II-43–II-46.

43. Ueno N, Yoshida K, Hirose S, Yokoyama H, Uehara H, Murakami K. Angiotensinogen-producing hepato-cellular carcinoma. *Hypertension* 1984;6:931–933.

44. Kew MC, Leckie BJ, Greef MC. Arterial hypertension as a paraneoplastic phenomenon in hepato cellular carcinoma. *Arch Intern Med* 1989;149:2111–2113.

45. Poulsen K, Jacobsen J. Is angiotensinogen a renin inhibitor, and not the substrate for renin? *J Hypertens* 1986;4:65–69.

46. Campbell DJ, Ziogas J, Kladis A. Metabolism of tetradecapeptide, angiotensinogen and angiotensin I and II by isolated perfused rat hindlimbs. *Clin Exp Pharmacol Physiol* 1990;17:335–350.

47. Paul M, Wagner J, Dzau VJ. Gene expression of the renin-angiotensin system in human tissues. Quantitative analysis by the polymerase chain reaction. *J Clin Invest* 1993;91:2058–2064.

48. Phillips MI, Speakman EA, Kimura B. Tissue renin-angiotensin systems. In: Raizada MK, Phillips MI, Summers C, eds. *Cellular and molecular biology of the renin angiotensin system.* Boca Raton, FL: CRC Press; 1993:97–130.

49. Clauser E, Bouhnik J, Coezy E, Corvol P, Ménard J. Synthesis and release of immunoreactive angiotensinogen by rat liver slices. *Endocrinology* 1983;114:776–785.

50. Campbell DJ, Habener JF. Angiotensinogen gene is expressed and differentially regulated in multiple tissues of the rat. *J Clin Invest* 1986;78:31–39.

51. Dzau VJ, Ellison KE, Brody T, et al. A comparative study of the distribution of renin and angiotensinogen mRNA in rat and mouse tissues. *Endocrinology* 1987;120:2334–2338.

52. Lynch KR, Simnad VI, Ben-Ari ET, Garrison C. Localization of preangiotensinogen messenger RNA sequences in the rat brain. *Hypertension* 1986;8:540–543.

53. Stornetta RL, Hawelu-Johnson CL, Guyenet PG, Lynch KR. Astrocytes synthesize angiotensinogen in brain. *Science* 1988; 242:1444–1446.

54. Bunnemann B, Fuxe K, Ganten D. The renin angiotensin system in the brain: an update 1993. *Regul Pept* 1993;46:487–509.

55. Milsted A, Barna BP, Ransohoff RM, Brosnihan KB, Ferrario CM. Astrocyte cultures derived from human brain tissue express angiotensinogen mRNA. *Proc Natl Acad Sci USA* 1990;87:5720–5723.

56. Okamura T, Clemens DL, Inagami T. Renin, angiotensins, angiotensin-converting enzyme in neuroblastoma cells: evidence for intracellular formation of angiotensins. *Proc Natl Acad Sci* 1981;78:6940–6943.

57. Petrossian G, Oliver JA. Synthesis of angiotensinogen by renincontaining neuroblastomas. *Am J Physiol* 1989;257:C185–C189.

58. Imboden H, Harding JW, Hilgenfeldt U, Celio MR, Felix D. Localization of angiotensinogen in multiple cell types of rat brain. *Brain Res* 1987;410:74–77.

59. Thomas WG, Greenland KJ, Shinkel TA, Sernia C. Angiotensinogen is secreted by pure rat neuronal cell cultures. *Brain Res* 1992; 588:191–200.

60. Deschepper CF, Bouhnik J, Ganong WF. Colocalization of angiotensinogen and glial fibrillary acidic protein in astrocytes in the rat brain. *Brain Res* 1986;374:195–198.

61. Wallis CJ, Printz MP. Adrenal regulation of regional brain angiotensinogen content. *Endocrinology* 1980;106:337–342.

62. Schelling P, Muller J, Clauser E. Regulation of angiotensinogen in cerebrospinal fluid and plasma in rats. *Am J Physiol* 1983;244: R466–R471.

63. Deschepper CF, Flaxman M. Glucocorticoid regulation of rat diencephalon angiotensinogen production. *Endocrinology* 1990; 126:923–970.

64. Campbell DJ, Habener JF. Cellular localization of angiotensinogen gene expression in brown adipose tissue and mesentery: quantification of messenger ribonucleic acid abundance using hybridization *in situ. Endocrinology* 1987;121:1616–1626.

65. Ohkubo H, Nakayama K, Tanaka T, Nakanishi S. Tissue distribution of rat angiotensinogen mRNA and structural analysis of its heterogeneity. *J Biol Chem* 1986;261:319–323.

66. Naftilan AJ, Zou WM, Ingelfinger JR, Ryan TJ, Pratt RE, Dzau VJ. Localization and differential regulation of angiotensinogen

mRNA expression in the vessel wall. *J Clin Invest* 1991;87:1300–1311.

67. Rakugi H, Jacob HZ, Krieger JE, Ingelfinger JR, Pratt RE. Vascular injury induces angiotensinogen gene expression in the media and neointima. *Circulation* 1993;87:283–290.

68. Lindpaintner K, Jin M, Niedermaier N, Wilhelm MJ, Ganten D. Cardiac angiotensinogen and its local activation in the isolated perfused beating heart. *Circ Res* 1990;67:564–573.

69. Dzau VJ. Circulating versus local renin-angiotensin system in cardiovascular homeostasis. *Circulation* 1988;77[Suppl I]:I-4–I-13.

70. Lindpaintner K, Wilhelm MJ, Jin M, et al. Tissue renin-angiotensin systems: focus on the heart. *Circ Res* 1990;67:564–570.

71. Schunkert H, Dzau VJ, Tang SS, Hirsch AT, Apstein CS, Lorell BH. Increased rat cardiac angiotensin converting enzyme activity and mRNA expression in pressure overload left ventricular hypertrophy. Effects on coronary resistance, contractility and relaxation. *J Clin Invest* 1990;86:1913–1930.

72. Fried TA, Simpson EA. Intrarenal localization of angiotensinogen mRNA by RNA-DNA dot-blot hybridization. *Am J Physiol* 1986;250:F374–F377.

73. Ingelfinger JR, Zuo WM, Fon EA, Ellison KE, Dzau VJ. *In situ* hybridization evidence for angiotensinogen messenger RNA in the rat proximal tubule. *J Clin Invest* 1990;85:417–423.

74. Yanagana N, Capparelli N, Jo OD, Friedal A, Barrett JD, Eggena P. Production of angiotensinogen and renin-like activity by rabbit proximal tubular cells in culture. *Kidney Int* 1991;39:938–941.

75. Inagami T, Mizuno K, Naruse K, Okamura T, Kawamura M. Intracellular formation and release of angiotensins from juxtaglomerular cells. *Kidney Int* 1990;38:S33–S37.

76. Ingelfinger JR, Pratt RE, Ellison K, Dzau VJ. Sodium regulation of angiotensinogen mRNA expression in rat kidney cortex and medulla. *J Clin Invest* 1986;78:1311–1315.

77. Schunkert H, Ingelfinger J, Hirsch AT, et al. Evidence for tissue specific activation of renal angiotensinogen mRNA expression in chronic stable experimental heart failure. *J Clin Invest* 1992;90:1523–1529.

78. Misumi J, Gardes J, Gonzales M-F, Corvol P, Ménard J. Angiotensinogen's role in ANG formation, renin release, and renal hemodynamics in isolated perfused kidney. *Am J Physiol* 1989;256:F719–F727.

79. Campbell DJ, Lawrence AC, Towrie A, Kladis A, Valentijn AJ. Differential regulation of angiotensin peptide levels in plasma and kidney of the rat. *Hypertension* 1991;18:763–773.

80. Kunapuli SP, Kumar A. Molecular cloning of human angiotensinogen cDNA and evidence for the presence of its mRNA in rat heart. *Circ Res* 1987;60(5):786–790.

81. Oliver JA, Sciacca X. Local generation of angiotensin II as a mechanism of regulation of peripheral vascular tone in the rat. *J Clin Invest* 1984;74:1247–1251.

82. Jaramillo H, Sanibhi M, Bouhnik J, Corvol P, Ménard J. Liver angiotensinogen synthesis and release during captopril treatment in sodium-depleted rats. *Endocrinology* 1987;120:1384–1390.

83. Skinner SL, Lumbers ER, Symonds EM. Analysis of changes in the renin angiotensin system during pregnancy. *Clin Sci* 1972;42:479–488.

84. Tewksbury DA, Dart RA. High molecular weight angiotensinogen levels in hypertensive pregnant women. *Hypertension* 1982;4:729–734.

85. Tewksbury DA, Tryon ES. Immunochemical comparison of high molecular weight angiotensinogen from amniotic fluid, plasma of men and plasma of pregnant women. *Am J Hypertens* 1989;2:411–413.

86. Derkx FHM, Stuenkel C, Schalekamp MPA, Visser W, Huisveld IH, Schalekamp MADH. Immunoreactive renin, prorenin and enzymatically active renin in plasma during pregnancy and in women taking oral contraceptives. *J Clin Endocrinol Metab* 1986;63:1008–1015.

87. DeLignieres B, Basdevant A, Thomas G, et al. Biological effects of estradiol-17β in postmenopausal women: oral versus percutaneous administration. *J Clin Endocrinol Metab* 1986;62:536–541.

88. Eggena P, Barrett JD. Regulation and functional consequences of angiotensinogen gene expression. *J Hypertens* 1992;10:1307–1311.

89. Kunapuli SP, Benedict CR, Kumar A. Tissue specific hormonal regulation of the rat angiotensinogen gene expression. *Arch Biochem Biophys* 1987;254:F582–F587.

90. Nakamura A, Iwao H, Fukui K, et al. Regulation of liver angiotensinogen and kidney renin mRNA levels by angiotensin II. *Am J Physiol* 1990;258:E1–E6.

91. Iwao H, Kimura S, Fukui K, et al. Elevated angiotensinogen mRNA levels in rat liver by nephrectomy. *Am J Physiol* 1990;258:E413–417.

92. Chang E, Perlman AJ. Multiple hormones regulate angiotensinogen messenger ribonucleic acid levels in a rat hepatoma cell line. *Endocrinology* 1987;121:513–519.

93. Wei L, Gaillard I, Corvol P, Clauser E. Expression and characterization of recombinant human angiotensinogen in a heterologous eukaryotic cell line. *Biochem Biophys Res Commun* 1988;156:1103–1110.

94. Brasier AR, Philippe J, Campbell DJ, Habener JF. Novel expression of the angiotensinogen gene in a rat pancreatic islet cell line. Transcriptional regulation by glucocorticoids. *J Biol Chem* 1986;261:16148–16154.

95. Frederich RC, Kahn BB, Peach MJ, Flier JS. Tissue-specific nutritional regulation of angiotensinogen in adipose tissue. *Hypertension* 1992;19:339–344.

96. Klett C, Hellmann W, Müller F, et al. Angiotensin II controls angiotensinogen secretion at a pretranslational level. *J Hypertens* 1988;6[Suppl 4]:S442–S445.

97. Deschepper CF, Reudelhuber TL. Rat angiotensinogen is secreted only constitutively when transfected into AtT-20 cells. *Hypertension* 1990;16:147–153.

98. Clouston WM, Lyons IG, Richards RI. Tissue-specific and hormonal regulation of angiotensinogen minigenes in transgenic mice. *EMBO J* 1989;8:3337–3343.

99. Feldmer M, Kaling M, Takahashi S, Mullins JJ, Ganten D. Glucocorticoid and estrogen-responsive elements in the 5′-flanking region of the rat angiotensinogen gene. *J Hypertens* 1991;9:1005–1012.

100. Brasier AR, Tate JE, Ron D, Habener JF. Multiple *cis*-acting DNA regulatory elements mediate hepatic angiotensinogen gene expression. *Mol Endocrinol* 1989;3:1022–1034.

101. Ron D, Brasier AR, Habener JF. Transcriptional regulation of hepatic angiotensinogen gene expression by the acute-phase response. *Mol Cell Endocrinol* 1990;74:C97–C104.

102. Ron D, Brasier AR, Wright KA, Habener JF. The permissive role of glucocorticoids on interleukin-1 stimulation of angiotensinogen gene transcription is mediated by an interaction between inducible enhancers. *Mol Cell Biol* 1990;10:4389–4395.

103. Brasier AR, Ron D, Tate JE, Habener JF. A family of constitutive c/EBP-like DNA binding proteins attenuate the IL-1a induced, NF$_K$B mediated trans-element. *EMBO J* 1990;9:3933–3944.

104. McGehee RE, Ron D, Brasier AR, Habener JF. Differential-specific element: a *cis*-acting developmental switch required for the sustained transcriptional expression of the angiotensinogen gene during hormonal-induced differentiation of 3T3-L1 fibroblasts to adipocytes. *Mol Endocrinol* 1993;7:551–560.

105. Weaver D, Skinner S, Walker L, Sangster M. Phenotypic inhibition of the renin angiotensin system, emergence of the Ren-2 gene, and adaptive radiation in mice. *Gen Comp Endocrinol* 1991;83:306–315.

106. Oliver WJ, Gross F. Unique specificity of the mouse angiotensinogen to homologous renin. *Proc Soc Exp Biol* 1981;122:923–930.

107. Kimura S, Mullins JJ, Bunneman B, et al. High blood pressure in transgenic mice carrying the rat angiotensinogen gene. *EMBO J* 1992;11:821–827.

108. Fukamizu A, Sugimura K, Takimoto E, et al. Chimeric renin angiotensin system demonstrates sustained increase in blood pressure of transgenic mice carrying both human renin and human angiotensinogen genes. *J Biol Chem* 1993;268:11617–11621.

109. Walker WG, Whelton PK, Saito H, Patterson Russel R, Hermann J. Relation between blood pressure and renin, renin substrate, angiotensin II, aldosterone and urinary sodium and potassium in 574 ambulatory subjects. *Hypertension* 1979;1:287–291.

110. Fasola AF, Martz BL, Helmer OM. Plasma renin activity during supine exercise in offspring of hypertensive patients. *J Appl Physiol* 1968;25:410–415.

111. Watt GCM, Harrap SB, Foy CJW, et al. Abnormalities of glucocorticoid metabolism and the renin angiotensin system: a four-corners approach to the identification of genetic determinants of blood pressure. *J Hypertens* 1992;10:473–482.

112. Kunapuli SP, Kumar A. Difference in the nucleotide sequence of human angiotensinogen cDNA. *Nucleic Acids Res* 1986;14:7509.

113. Orita M, Iwahana H, Hayashi K, Sekiaya T. Detection of polymorphisms of human DNA by gel electrophoresis as single-strand conformation polymorphisms. *Proc Natl Acad Sci USA* 1989;86:2766–2770.

114. Jeunemaitre X, Soubrier F, Kotelevtsev Y, et al. Molecular basis of human hypertension. Role of angiotensinogen. *Cell* 1992;71:169–178.

115. Jeunemaitre X, Lifton RP, Hunt SC, Williams RR, Lalouel J-M. Absence of linkage between the angiotensin converting enzyme locus and human essential hypertension. *Nature Genet* 1992;1:72–75.

116. Jeunemaitre X, Charru A, Chatellier G, et al. M235T variant of the human angiotensinogen gene in unselected hypertensive patients. *J Hypertens* 1993;11[Suppl:5]:580–581.

117. Hata A, Namikawa C, Sasaki M, et al. Angiotensinogen as a risk factor for essential hypertension in Japan. *J Clin Invest* 1994;93:1285–1287.

118. Sutherland A, Cooper D, Howie P, Liston W, MacGillivary I. The incidence of severe pre-eclampsia amongst mothers and mothers-in-law of pre-eclamptics and controls. *Br J Obstet Gynaecol* 1981;88:785–789.

119. Chesley LC, Cooper DW. Genetics of hypertension in pregnancy: possible single gene control of pre-eclampsia and eclampsia in the descendants of eclamptic women. *Br J Obstet Gynaecol* 1986;93:898–903.

120. Ward K, Hata A, Jeunemaitre X, et al. A molecular variant of angiotensinogen associated with pre-eclampsia. *Nature Genet* 1993;4:59–61.

121. Arngrimsson R, Purandare S, Connor M, et al. Angiotensinogen: a candidate gene involved in preeclampsia? *Nature Genet* 1993;4:114–115.

122. Hollenberg NK, Williams GH, Burger B, Chenitz W, Hossmand I, Adams DF. Renal blood flow and its response to angiotensin II. An interaction between oral contraceptive agents, sodium intake and the renin-angiotensin system in healthy young women. *Circ Res* 1976;38:35–40.

123. Cassis LA, Saye JA, Peach MJ. Location and regulation of rat angiotensinogen messenger RNA. *Hypertension* 1988;11:591–596.

124. Saye JA, Lynch KR, Peach MJ. Changes in angiotensinogen messenger RNA in differentiating 3T3-F442A adipocytes. *Hypertension* 1990;15:867–871.

125. Eggena P, Sowers J, Maxwell MH, Barrett JD, Golub MS. Hormonal correlates of weight loss associated with blood pressure reduction. *Clin Exp Hypertens* [A] 1991;13:1447–1456.

126. Kanai H, Matsuzawa Y, Kotani K, et al. Close correlation of intra-abdominal fat accumulation to hypertension in obese women. *Hypertension* 1990;16:484–490.

127. Bing J. Relation between renin substrate and acute phase proteins. *Acta Pathol Microbiol Immunol Scand* [A] 1972;80:646–650.

128. Nielsen AHJ, Knudsen F. Angiotensinogen is an acute-phase protein in man. *Scand J Clin Lab Invest* 1987;47:175–178.

129. Hilgenfeldt U, Kellermann W, Kienapfel G, Jochum M. Relationship between angiotensinogen, alpha 1-protease inhibitor elastase complex, antithrombin III and C-reactive protein in septic ARDS. *Eur J Clin Pharmacol* 1990;38:125–131.

130. Kageyama R, Ohkubo H, Nakanishi S. Induction of rat liver angiotensinogen mRNA following acute inflammation. *Biochem Biophys Res Commun* 1985;129:826–832.

131. Bouhnik J, Savoie F, Corvol P. Differential effects of inflammation models on rat T-kininogen and rat-angiotensinogen. *Biochem Pharmacol* 1988;37:1099–1102.

132. Okamoto H, Hatta A, Itoh N, Ohashi Y, Arakawa K, Nakanishi S. Acute phase responses of plasma angiotensinogen and T-kininogen in rat. *Biochem Pharmacol* 1987;36:3069–3073.

133. Itoh N, Matsuda T, Ohtani R, Okamoto H. Angiotensinogen production by rat hepatoma cells is stimulated by B cell stimulatory factor 2/interleukin-6. *FEBS Lett* 1989;244:6–10.

Hypertension: Pathophysiology, Diagnosis, and Management, Second Edition,
edited by J.H. Laragh and B.M. Brenner,
Raven Press, Ltd., New York © 1995.

CHAPTER 100

The Angiotensin-converting Enzyme: Molecular Biology and Implication of the Gene Polymorphism in Cardiovascular Diseases

François Cambien and Florent Soubrier

The angiotensin I-converting enzyme (ACE) plays an important role in vascular homeostasis. ACE exists predominantly as an ectoenzyme of vascular endothelial cells and is a component of the renin-angiotensin and kallikrein-kinin systems, as it activates angiotensin I (AI) into angiotensin II (AII) and inactivates bradykinin (BK). These two peptide hormones have opposite effects on vascular tone and on smooth muscle cell (SMC) proliferation. Inhibition of these effects probably largely explains the beneficial action of ACE inhibitors in hypertension and heart failure. Important progress has been

made in recent years concerning the molecular biology and genetics of ACE and its possible involvement as a risk factor in several cardiovascular disorders. This chapter provides an update of these different aspects.

BIOCHEMISTRY AND MOLECULAR BIOLOGY OF ACE

Biochemistry of ACE

The angiotensin I-converting enzyme (ACE) is an ectoenzyme anchored to the cell membrane, with its catalytic sites exposed at the extracellular surface of the cell. ACE is a zinc metallopeptidase with a wide substrate

F. Cambien and F. Soubrier: INSERM SC7 and INSERM U36, 75005 Paris, France.

specificity, although it was initially described for its catalytic properties on two vasoactive peptides, AI and BK. On these two peptides, ACE acts as a dipeptidyl carboxypeptidase, processing AI into the active octapeptide AII and degrading BK into inactive peptides by two successive cleavages (1). The substrate for which ACE has the lowest Michaelis constant (K_m) is BK (0.2 mmol/L), this K_m being 80-fold lower than for AI (16 mmol/L) (Table 1). ACE is able to hydrolyze a wide range of oligopeptides *in vitro,* such as enkephalins, neurotensins, and the chemotactic peptide FMet-Leu-Phe via its dipeptidyl carboxypeptidase activity (1). However, on some substrates, ACE can also act as an endopeptidase, releasing predominantly C-terminal tripeptides from some substrates such as substance P (2) and des-Arg^9-BK (3) or amidated C-terminal dipeptides from cholecystokinin-8 and various gastrin analogues (4). On luteinizing hormone-releasing hormone (LHRH), ACE releases a tripeptide from the amidated C terminus and in addition an N-terminal tripeptide (5). The K_m for these substrates is usually high, resulting, even with high catalytic rate constant (K_{cat}), in low K_{cat}/K_m ratios, which seem unfavorable for metabolism *in vivo* (6). However, conditions for hydrolysis of these peptides could be fulfilled in some particular tissular environments.

The widely distributed form of ACE, present in endothelial and epithelial cells, is called the somatic form in contrast to the germinal isoform of ACE found in male spermatids. These two forms differ by their primary structures which have been determined in humans by molecular cloning of the two cDNA (7–9) (Fig. 1).

The somatic form has a molecular weight of 170 kDa and has a repetitive structure with two homologous domains. A consensus sequence for zinc metallopeptidases (H-E-X-X-H) is found in each homologous domain. In this sequence, by analogy to the structure of thermolysin, the two histidine residues are coordinated to the zinc atom and the glutamic acid is the base donor. The presence of the zinc-binding consensus sequence in each domain of ACE suggests the presence of two active sites in

each enzyme molecule, and this was further supported by the presence of two zinc atoms per mole of enzyme and the binding of two competitive ACE inhibitor molecules per mole of enzyme (10,11).

Monovalent anions, especially chloride, enhance the activity of ACE toward all known substrates although the presence of chloride is not always essential (12); for example, BK is hydrolyzed in the absence of chloride. This activation is thought to be a consequence of a change in protein conformation occurring on chloride binding to a putative lysine residue located in the region of the active site (13).

Many other residues implicated in catalysis have not yet been identified, for example His 231 of thermolysin, which stabilizes the transition state of the substrate, and Glu 166, which provides the third zinc-coordinating ligand (14). Although we proposed histidine 404 and 1,002, and glutamic acid 389 and 987 as candidate residues for these functions, respectively, their role has not been confirmed. A tyrosine and a lysine residue have also been identified as essential residues in rabbit lung ACE by inactivation of the purified enzyme with 1-fluoro-2,4,-dinitrobenzene (Dnp-F) (15), confirming previous findings (16). By peptide mapping and sequencing, these amino acids have been identified as lysine 694 and tyrosine 776 in the C domain. Similarly, Dnp-F reacts with lysine 122 and tyrosine 204 of rabbit testicular ACE, which correspond to lysine 118 and tyrosine 200 of human testicular ACE (17). A mutant human testicular ACE in which tyrosine 200 was replaced by a phenylalanine, was expressed in Chinese hamster ovary (CHO) cells (18). This mutant ACE exhibited a 15-fold decrease of the K_{cat} for the hydrolysis of the synthetic substrate furanacryloyl-phe-gly-gly and a 7-fold decrease for AI hydrolysis. The K_m values of the mutant enzyme for these substrates were slightly increased, but the specific ACE inhibitor, lisinopril, was 100-fold less tightly bound to the mutant enzyme compared to the wild-type enzyme. However, these results were not confirmed by Sen et al. (19), by site-directed mutagenesis of the rabbit tes-

TABLE 1. *Kinetic parameters for the hydrolysis of BK and AI by wild-type recombinant ACE and ACE mutants, allowing the assessment of the catalytic activity of the C and N domains^a*

ACE	BK			AI		
	K_m mM	K_{cat} s^{-1}	K_{cat}/K_m ($\times 10^{-6}$) M^{-1} s^{-1}	K_m mM	K_{cat} s^{-1}	K_{cat}/K_m ($\times 10^{-6}$) M^{-1} s^{-1}
Wild-type	0.18	11	61	16	40	2.5
C domain^b	0.24	8	33	18	34	1.9
N domain^b	0.54	5	9	15	11	0.7

(Adapted from ref. 50.)
^{a} Initial velocities were measured in 50 mM NaCl, pH 7.5.
^{b} C domain and N domain: mutant ACE bearing a catalytically active carboxy terminal or amino terminal domain, respectively.

BK, bradykinin; AI, angiotensin I; ACE, angiotensin I-converting enzyme; K_{cat}, catalytic rate constant; K_m, Michaelis constant.

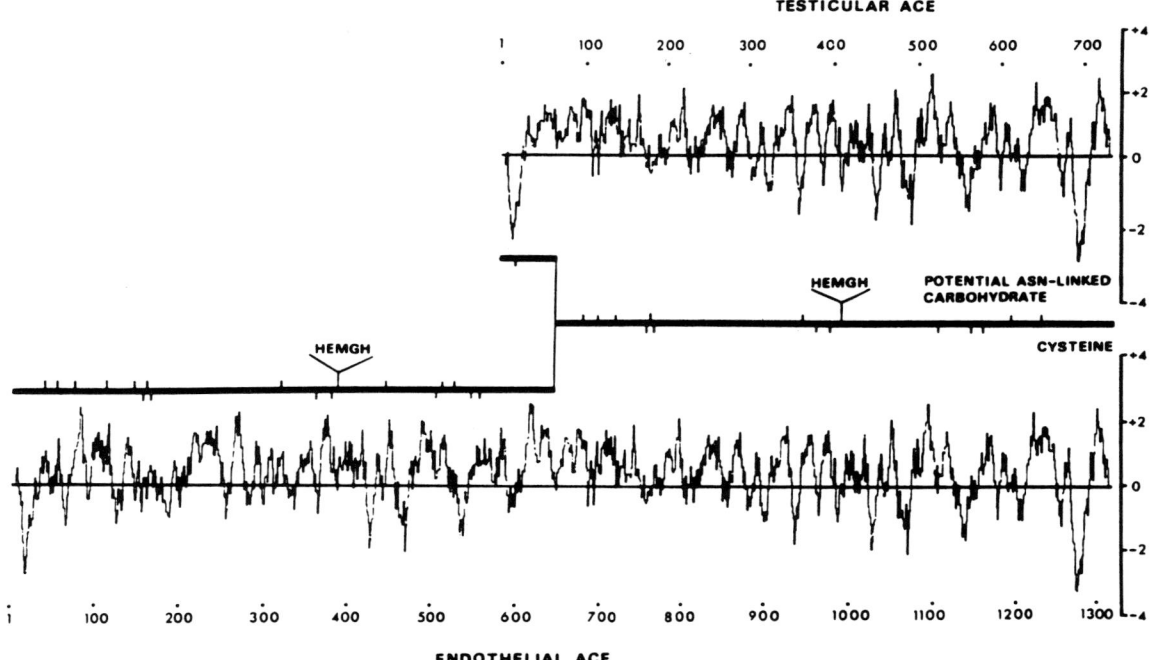

FIG. 1. Schematic representation of the testicular and endothelial ACE enzymes. **Middle:** Diagram showing the cysteine positions, the potential asparagine-linked glycosylation sites, and the positions of the putative residues of the active site of the two enzymes. Beyond the point of divergence, the testicular enzyme is figured on the upper line and the endothelial enzyme on the lower line. **Top and bottom:** Hydropathy plots of the predicted testicular (*top*) and endothelial (*bottom*) amino acid sequences. Amino acid numbering is presented above and under the hydropathy plots. (From ref. 8, with permission.)

ticular ACE. Separate mutagenesis of the Dnp-F reactive Lys or Tyr did not produce any changes in the enzymatic properties. In contrast combined mutagenesis of both residues altered several enzymatic characteristics, which suggests a slight modification of the three-dimensional structure.

The pulmonary enzyme contains 30 percent carbohydrate which includes fucose, mannose, N-acetylglucosamine, galactose, and sialic acid (20). The pulmonary enzyme contains a higher proportion of sialic acid than kidney ACE (21).

The germinal form of ACE has a smaller molecular weight of 90 kDa in humans but was known to possess enzymatic properties similar to the somatic enzyme (22). Its primary structure, deduced from the cDNA sequence, is completely identical to the C-terminal moiety of the somatic enzyme, but it possesses an N-terminal specific sequence of 67 amino acids, which includes the signal peptide and a serine-threonine-rich region, corresponding to potential O-glycosylation sites (8,9). The germinal isoform thus contains only one potential active site, corresponding to the C domain of the somatic isoform. The substrate of germinal ACE is not known and the importance of its physiological role in reproduction has not been determined. The activity of germinal ACE is preserved during chronic oral treatment by ACE inhibitors,

as these molecules usually do not cross the blood-testis barrier (23).

Biosynthesis and Mechanisms of ACE Anchoring and Secretion

ACE is synthesized as a precursor with a signal peptide at its N-terminal extremity which is cleaved during biosynthesis, as this peptide is no longer present in the mature molecule (7). ACE is anchored to the cell membrane by a hydrophobic peptide, 17 amino acids long, which is located at its C terminus (24,25). This mechanism of anchoring was demonstrated by several studies. Immunohistochemistry of ACE with an antiserum raised to the C-terminal part of the molecule beyond the anchoring peptide demonstrated that no cleavage occurred for positioning of ACE on the membrane, when ACE is expressed in CHO cells. On Western blotting, the same antiserum also reacted with ACE solubilized from kidney membranes by detergents (24). Expression of mutant ACE with a deletion of the hydrophobic peptide led to a secreted form of the enzyme (24). The anchored form of ACE is found on endothelial cells and on several epithelia. A secreted form of ACE is also found in biological fluids, such as plasma, cerebrospinal fluid, amniotic fluid (26), and semen (27). The release of ACE from the cell membrane probably results from a proteolytic process which cleaves the C-terminal part of the enzyme as suggested by the fact that plasma ACE is not recognized by an antiserum raised against the C-terminal extremity of the enzyme (24). The proteolytic release of ACE also occurs in CHO cells, transfected with the ACE cDNA, and these cells offer a good model for the *in vitro* study of this process (24,25). The sequence of the carboxy terminus of ACE secreted by CHO cells and of human plasma ACE was determined by caboxyl-terminal microsequencing (28). This sequence corresponds to a cleavage between Arg-1137 and Leu-1138 of human ACE. Site-directed mutagenesis of Arg-1137 into glutamine did not prevent the secretion of ACE in CHO cells, showing that this amino acid does not confer any specificity of the cleavage site by the putative cleaving enzyme. Indeed, a secretase activity from pig kidney microvilli, able to convert the amphipathic membrane-bound enzyme into the soluble form, has been partially characterized (29). The secretase activity is inhibited by the metal chelator EDTA, and is not sensitive to inhibitors of serine-, thiol-, or aspartic proteases and is not affected by reducing agents.

Localization of ACE

Because of the association of ACE with the plasma membrane of vascular endothelial cells, the enzyme displays a ubiquitous tissue distribution. In addition to an endothelial location, high concentrations of ACE are also found in the brush borders of absorptive epithelia, such as the apical microvillosities of the small intestine and the kidney proximal convoluted tubule (30). Other epithelial locations of ACE include the choroid plexus, where the enzyme is found at a high concentration and is probably the source of ACE in the cerebrospinal fluid (31,32), the prostate and epididymis of the male genital tract (33,34), and gastric epithelial cells in rabbits (35). ACE is also found in mononuclear cells, such as monocytes after macrophage differentiation and T-lymphocytes, and in fibroblasts (36–38).

In vitro autoradiography, employing radiolabeled specific ACE inhibitors, and immunohistochemical studies have mapped the locations of ACE in brain, mainly in the rat, the monkey, and in humans. ACE was found primarily in the choroid plexus, ependyma, subfornical organ, basal ganglia (caudate putamen and globus pallidus) but, most notably, the enzyme was localized in the striatonigral neuronal pathway (39–41). Using striatal *N*-methyl-D-aspartate lesions in the rat, a significant decrease of ACE was observed in the caudate putamen, globus pallidus, entopeduncular nucleus, and substantia nigra pars reticulata on the lesioned side (42). This demonstrates that ACE is associated with neurons and

terminals which descend from the caudate putamen and globus pallidus to the substantia nigra. As few AII receptors are present in the basal ganglia (43), these results suggest a role for ACE in the metabolism of a neuropeptide present in the same pathway. Substance P co-localizes with ACE to the same neuronal pathway, however, neutral endopeptidase, also highly abundant in this area, is more likely to be involved in the *in vivo* degradation of substance P (44,45). High levels of ACE were found in rat neurosecretory nuclei, such as paraventricular, and supraoptic nuclei, the median eminence, and posterior pituitary. In these regions, the level of AII is also high (45). High concentrations of ACE are detected in the hippocampus and in the Purkinje cell layer of the cerebellum. In the monkey, high levels are also found throughout the cerebral cortex and in the interpeduncular and suprachiasmatic nuclei (47).

Neuronal ACE is slightly smaller in size compared to the endothelial enzyme and this observation has been attributed to differences in the extent of N-glycosylation (48). However, both forms of the enzyme display the same neuropeptide specificities and inhibition profiles and therefore do not represent distinct isoforms (49).

In the rat heart, ACE was localized by *in vitro* quantitative autoradiography with an iodinated ACE inhibitor (50). High densities of binding sites were found on valve leaflets (aortic, pulmonary, mitral, and tricuspid), but the binding was low on the endocardium. A dense labeling was observed in the coronary arteries, and the labeling was more dense in the right atrium than in the other parts. In the aorta, the labeling was high both in the endothelial and adventitial layers, and low in the media.

The Catalytic Properties of Each Active Site of ACE

Several studies have assessed the activity of each catalytic site present in each homologous domain of ACE. The catalytic properties of the N domain and the C domain were assessed by transfecting, in CHO cells, cDNA constructs of the somatic ACE in which one of the two active sites was either inactivated or deleted (51). These experiments showed that the two active sites have a similar K_m for the two main substrates, AI and BK, but they show striking differences in the K_{cat}. At optimal chloride concentration, the active site of the N domain has a K_{cat} 3 and 10 times lower than the C-domain active site for AI and the specific synthetic substrate Hip-His-Leu, respectively (51). In all these experiments, both domains appeared to function independently since the activity of the wild-type enzyme was equal to the sum of the activities of the N and C domains (51). These studies established that ACE possesses two functional catalytic sites, which were both dependent on a zinc co-factor.

It is well established that chloride has a marked influence on ACE activity (13) and it is interesting to note that the catalytic activity of the two domains was affected differently by chloride (51). For AI hydrolysis, the N active site exhibited low levels of activity in the absence of chloride and optimal activity at a concentration of 10 mM chloride. In contrast, the C active site was essentially inactive in the absence of chloride and required much higher chloride concentrations for optimal activity (30 mM). Bradykinin was hydrolyzed efficiently by both active sites with similar K_{cat} values in the presence of NaCl but again with different chloride activation profiles (52).

The interaction of the two active sites of ACE with competitive ACE inhibitors was also investigated (53). Both the N and the C domains contain a high-affinity binding site for [³H]-trandolaprilat, a potent ACE inhibitor. Chloride stabilizes the enzyme-inhibitor complex and slows the dissociation rate, an effect which is more marked for the C domain than for the N domain.

The binding of different ACE inhibitors was studied, using purified lung and testis rat ACE (10). Binding parameters for the two binding sites of lung ACE were deduced from displacement of the ACE inhibitor, ^{125}I-Ro 31-8472 with either Ro 31-8472 or 351A, a *p*-hydroxybenzamidine analogue of lisinopril. Whereas analogues K_d were found for the two binding sites of lung ACE with Ro 31-8472, contrasted K_d values were found for 351A, the K_d for the N domain being more than a hundred-fold higher than for the C domain. As the main structural difference between these two inhibitors concerns the length of their side chains, it was suggested that the side chain may encounter steric hindrance at a deeply recessed active site in the N terminal domain of ACE. Thus, further studies with various ACE inhibitors may help to elucidate the structure/function of these two active sites and possibly lead to the design of specific inhibitors for each active site.

As the N domain cleaves less efficiently the main substrates of ACE than the C domain, AI and BK, one can hypothesize that the N domain has another substrate specificity. Although no specific substrate was found for the N active site, it was shown that the release of the amino-terminal tripeptide of LHRH was more efficiently performed by the N domain than by the C domain (52).

Structure, Expression, and Evolution of the ACE Gene

By Southern blot experiments and gene cloning, it was demonstrated that the somatic and germinal ACE mRNA are transcribed from a unique gene (54). The complete intron-exon structure of the human ACE gene was determined by restriction mapping of genomic clones and by sequencing of the intron-exon boundaries (54). The human ACE gene contains 26 exons (Fig. 2).

Several studies have demonstrated the presence of two functional promoters in the ACE gene allowing the transcription of the somatic and germinal mRNAs, each having its own regulation and being expressed with its own cell specificity. The somatic ACE mRNA seems to be constitutively expressed in the human kidney; the low level of ACE mRNA contrasts with the high concentration of the enzyme. The somatic promoter is located on the 5' side of the first exon of the gene and leads to the transcription of all exons. In the mature somatic ACE mRNA, exons 1 to 26 are found, except exon 13 which is spliced. Fusions of various size fragments of the somatic ACE promoter to a reporter gene in transfection experiments showed the presence of positive regulatory elements inside the 132 bp region upstream the transcription start site and also suggested the presence of negative regulatory elements between −132 bp and −343 and between position −472 bp and −754 (55). Similarly, a strong negative element was identified in the rabbit ACE promoter between nucleotide position −692 and −610 (56). The negative effect on transcription of this element was shown to be independent of its position, orientation, and to be dose-dependent. The *trans*-acting factor which putatively binds this element has not yet been identified.

The presence of an internal alternative promoter was suggested by the transcription of another mRNA, with a completely different pattern of expression and regulation from the somatic transcript. The germinal transcript of ACE is expressed exclusively by male germ cells with a precise stage-specific pattern, after the meiosis, starting in round spermatids and finishing in spermatozoa (57). In the absence of germ cell maturation, before puberty or after experimental hypophysectomy in the rat, no ACE expression is detected in the testis. Restoration of spermatogenic cell maturation by androgens or pituitary gonadotrophins is able to restore ACE expression (58). The germinal ACE mRNA is not detected out of the testis in the mouse, even after reverse transcription, cDNA amplification, and southern hybridization (59). The germinal mRNA contains exon 13 to exon 26 of the gene.

The location of the germinal promoter on the 5' flanking region of exon 12, the germinal-specific exon, was suggested by several experiments. Primer extension and

TABLE 2. *Familial resemblance of plasma ACE level in the Nancy Study 1[a]*

	Fathers	Mothers	Offspring
n	87	87	169
Age	41.7 (5.0)	39.4 (5.2)	14.2 (2.6)
SBP (mm Hg)	125.9 (13.1)	117.8 (13.7)	112.8 (11.0)
ACE (U/L)	34.1 (10.7)	30.7 (10.4)	43.1 (17.2)*

(Adapted from ref. 84.)
[a] Much higher plasma ACE levels were observed in offspring than in parents.
* $p < 10^{-6}$.
SBP, systolic blood pressure.

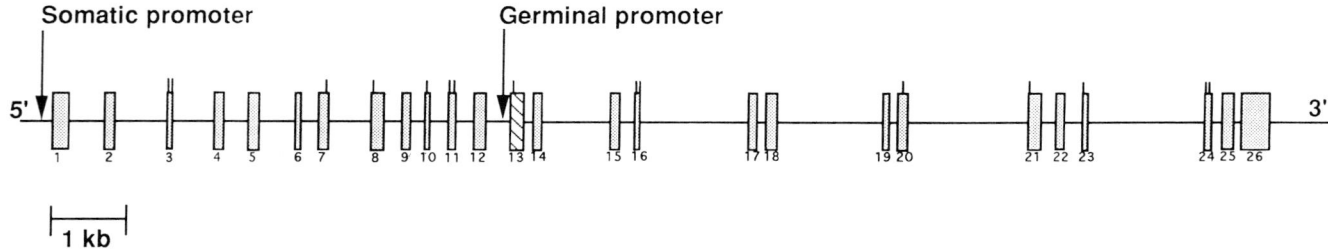

FIG. 2. Organization of the human ACE gene. Location of the 26 numbered exons (*vertical bars*). Exon 13 (*open bar*) is specific to the testicular ACE mRNA. The two promoters are indicated by vertical arrows. Vertical bars above the exon boxes indicate the location of the cysteine residues. (Adapted from ref. 54.)

ribonuclease (RNase) protection assays on testicular RNAs were performed in mice, rabbits, and humans (54,60). In all species investigated, the 5′ extremity of the germinal ACE mRNA corresponded to the 5′ end of exon 13. Therefore, intron 12, corresponding to the genomic sequence flanking the 5′ region of the testicular-specific exon 13, as deduced from the complete analysis of the ACE gene in humans, was proposed as the putative germinal ACE promoter (54).

The promoter function of this sequence was firmly established by using intron 12 to drive the transcription of a reporter gene in a germinal-specific fashion (61). A 689 bp fragment, containing intron 12, exon 13, and a part of intron 12 of the mouse ACE gene fused to the beta-galactosidase coding sequence, was used to construct transgenic mice. A histochemical analysis of the transgenic mice revealed that the beta-galactosidase was only expressed, together with the ACE gene, in elongating spermatozoa. In another series of transgenic mice, a 91 bp fragment of intron 12 of the ACE gene was used as promoter and was able to confer to the transgene a germinal-cell-restricted pattern of transcription (62). Further mapping of elements controlling transcription by deoxyribonuclease (DNAse) footprint experiments and gel mobility shift assays showed that a sequence between position -42 and -62 specifically binds to nuclear factors from testicular extracts and contains a consensus cyclic adenosine monophosphate (cAMP) responsive element (CRE) (62).

To our knowledge, this is the only example of an intragenic, alternative promoter, present inside a duplicated gene and driving transcription of the ancestral nonduplicated form of the gene.

The structure of the human ACE gene provides further support for the duplication of an ancestral ACE gene (Fig. 2). Exons 4–11 and 17–24, encoding the two homologous domains of the ACE molecule are highly similar both in size and in sequence (54). In contrast, intron size separating homologous exons is not conserved. The ACE gene duplication appears to have occurred early in evolution. In all mammalian species where the ACE gene has been cloned, that is, rabbits, mice, and humans, the ACE gene is duplicated. A dipeptidyl carboxypeptidase, affinity-purified from the electric organ of *Torpedo marmorata,* was recognized by a polyclonal antiserum raised against pig kidney ACE and was activated by chloride (63). The molecular weight of *Torpedo* ACE is 190,000, and therefore this enzyme would also appear to be transcribed from a duplicated ACE gene. If this is the case, then the duplication of the ACE gene must have occurred more than 300 million years ago. Conservation in remote species of the two transcription units inside the ACE-duplicated gene reflects their physiological significance, although a local and specific substrate of testicular ACE, which would definitively signify its function, is not yet known.

An ACE-like enzyme has been characterized in the housefly, *Musca domestica* (64). This enzyme is able to cleave the ACE substrate Hip-His-Leu and is inhibited by captopril with an inhibition of protein constant, 50 percent (IC50) of 0.4 mM. A cDNA coding for an enzyme with high sequence similarity to ACE also has been cloned in *Drosophila* (65). The amino-acid identity reaches 65 percent in the region of the zinc-binding motif. Interestingly, the *D. meganoster* ACE-like enzyme gene does not seem to be duplicated as the full length cDNA is 2.1 kb, an observation which is in agreement with the 87 kDa found for the ACE-like enzyme from *Musca domestica.* Therefore, this gene likely represents the ancestral nonduplicated form of the ACE gene.

Regulation of ACE

Pharmacologic Stimulation of ACE Secretion and Expression

Several agents, such as cAMP analogues (66), methylxanthines, calcium ionophore A23187, and sodium ionophore monensin (67) have been shown to induce ACE secretion from cultured bovine endothelial cells. ACE secretion is also increased by glucocorticoid hormones on cultured endothelial cells (68), cultured rabbit alveolar macrophages (69), and human monocytes (36). Glucocorticoid responsive elements are indeed present in the somatic promoter of the ACE gene and an increased ACE gene expression might be responsible for the increased ACE secretion (54). However, studies using the ACE promoter-driving transcription of a reporter gene transfected in various cell types were unable to detect any effect of glucocorticoids on transcription, suggesting that these responsive elements are not functional and that glucocorticoids act through responsive elements located elsewhere or by another mechanism (55). ACE secretion is also increased in cultured endothelial cells by thyroid hormones, a result which is in accordance with the observation that ACE is increased during hyperthyroidism in humans (70).

The most intriguing observation is the increase of serum ACE levels and ACE concentrations in tissues after ACE inhibitor treatment in rats (71,72). The increase of plasma ACE was also observed in patients treated with the ACE inhibitor captopril in humans (73). In cultured human endothelial cells, the ACE inhibitor captopril was able to increase the ACE concentration inside the cell and in the medium (74). In another study on porcine-cultured pulmonary artery endothelial cells, it was shown that ACE mRNA and ACE transcription were increased by captopril treatment of the cells at a comparable level to the increased ACE activity (75). This result was confirmed by *in vivo* experiments which showed an increase of rat lung ACE mRNA after treatment of the animals during 3 days with an ACE inhibitor (76). Interestingly, this work also showed a decrease of ACE mRNA level in the lung of rats receiving AII infusion, which was associated with a moderate change in pulmonary ACE activity and no change in serum and testicular ACE concentrations.

ACE Expression in Experimental Models of Hypertension and Cardiac Failure

The expression of the ACE gene was studied during experimental overload of the heart by aortic stenosis in the rat (77). Both ACE activity and ACE mRNA were increased in the left ventricle wall. In the experimental model of heart failure by left coronary ligature in the rat, the ACE activity was also increased in the right ventricle which was unaffected by experimental myocardial infarction (MI) (78). The aortic ACE mRNA was also studied in the two-kidney, one-clip model of rat hypertension at 4 and 12 weeks after clipping (79). At both stages an increase of ACE mRNA was observed, together with an increase of ACE activity in this tissue. In contrast, no modification of ACE mRNA was observed in other tissues, such as the lung, and the plasma ACE concentration was unchanged. The local expression of ACE is also increased in the scar tissue of MI in the rat (80).

THE GENETICS OF ACE IN HUMANS

Repeated measurement of plasma ACE in adult humans has shown that the concentration of the enzyme is very stable within individuals. Conversely, plasma ACE level differs strongly from person to person and is independent of a large number of environmental, metabolic, and hormonal factors (81). The high circulating level of ACE in sarcoidosis is the consequence of an increased ACE secretion by monocyte-derived cells (82,83). ACE concentrations in middle-aged men and women are very similar, whereas an important temporary increase is observed during adolescence (84,85).

Genetic Control of Plasma ACE Level

A low intraindividual, but high interindividual variability and a lack of association with environmental factors suggested that plasma ACE level was genetically determined. To test this hypothesis, plasma ACE level was measured in a sample of nuclear families composed of healthy individuals, the Nancy Study 1 (Table 2). Statistical analyses were performed to assess the familial correlations of the enzyme and the compatibility of ACE levels with the presence of a major gene segregating in the families (84). Higher plasma ACE levels were observed in offspring than in parents: 43.1 (standard deviation [SD] 17.2), 34.1 (SD 10.7), and 30.7 (10.4) units/L in offspring, fathers, and mothers respectively ($p < 0.001$). The correlations between spouses, fathers and offspring, mothers and offspring, and between offspring were 0.02 (nonsignificant [NS]), 0.17 ($p < 0.05$), 0.33 ($p < 0.001$), and 0.31 ($p < 0.01$) respectively. The results of the segregation analysis testing the presence of a major gene effect are reported in Table 3, for the model best

TABLE 3. *Segregation analysis of plasma ACE in the 87 nuclear families included in the Nancy Study 1*

Parameters estimated in the segregation analysis	Parameter estimates for the best-fitting model
Residual means (U/L)	
Fathers	29.6
Mothers	26.6
Offspring	32.3
Residual familial correlations	(0)[a]
Frequency of alleles S/s	0.24/0.76
Major gene effects in parents	
Heterozygotes/homozygotes	8.1/21.4
Major gene effects in offspring	
Heterozygotes/homozygotes	21.4/48.7
Departure from Mendelian transmission	(1/0.5/0)[a]

(Adapted from ref. 84.)
[a] Not significantly different from the specified value. All other parameter estimates are significantly different from 0 ($p < 0.05$).

fitting the data. A major gene transmission was much better supported than a polygenic or a nongenetic transmission. The frequencies of alleles *S/s* associated with high/low plasma ACE levels were 0.24/0.76. The effect of *S* was codominant and stronger in offspring than in parents. In parents, the level of plasma ACE was approximately 1 SD higher in *Ss* heterozygotes and 2 SD higher in *SS* homozygotes than in *ss* homozygotes. In offspring, the effects were twice as important. No residual familial correlation was present after taking into account the major gene effect. According to the segregation analysis, the postulated polymorphism *S/s* accounted for 29 percent and 75 percent of the variance of plasma ACE in parents and offspring, respectively.

These results strongly suggested that plasma ACE level was largely determined by the effect of a single major gene; however the identity of this gene was unknown.

The ACE Gene and Its Polymorphism

After the ACE cDNA was cloned, it was possible to elucidate the structure of the gene and investigate its polymorphism (7,54). A frequent insertion (*I*)/deletion (*D*) polymorphism (ACE *I/D*), characterized by the presence/absence of a 287 bp fragment and corresponding to an *Alu* sequence in the 16th intron of the gene was identified by hybridization with a cDNA probe (86).

The ACE *I/D* Polymorphism Is Associated with Plasma ACE Level

The relationship between the ACE *I/D* polymorphism and plasma ACE level was studied in a sample of 80 healthy adults (86). The concentration of ACE in plasma, measured by radioimmunoassay (RIA), was strongly associated with the genetic polymorphism. In *II* homozygotes, *ID* heterozygotes, and *DD* homozygotes, the mean levels of ACE were 299, 393, and 494 μg/L respectively ($p < 0.001$). The effect of the gene was

strictly codominant and accounted for 47 percent of the interindividual variability of plasma ACE.

ACE Activity in T-Lymphocytes Is Associated with the ACE *I/D* Polymorphism

Costerousse et al. (37) have recently studied ACE activity in human circulating mononuclear cells. The highest enzyme level was found in T-lymphocytes in which ACE activity was approximately 30 times that found in monocytes. No detectable activity could be found in B-lymphocytes. ACE activity in T-lymphocytes was measured in 35 healthy individuals. As for plasma ACE, the cellular level was very stable within individuals but highly variable between individuals. The correlation between the plasma and T-lymphocyte levels of ACE was 0.42 ($p < 0.01$). The ACE *I/D* polymorphism was also investigated in these subjects. Mean ACE levels in T-lymphocytes of *II*, *ID*, and *DD* individuals were respectively 277 (SD 58), 362 (78), and 487 (101) μU/mg protein ($p < 0.001$).

Thus, not only plasma ACE, but also ACE in T-lymphocytes is largely determined by a polymorphism probably affecting the ACE gene. From these results, it is tempting to extrapolate that the polymorphism could also affect ACE expression in other types of cells; this could have important consequences, in particular in the vessel wall.

The ACE *I/D* Polymorphism Is a Genetic Marker in Strong Linkage Disequilibrium with an Unknown Functional Variant (ACE *S/s*) Located Within or Near the ACE Gene

In the Nancy Study 1 (84), no DNA had been stored; it was thus impossible to determine the genotype of the individuals participating in this study. A new set of 98 nuclear families composed of healthy individuals was recruited (Nancy Study 2), in which the ACE *I/D* polymor-

TABLE 4. *Blood pressure and plasma ACE level (means [SD]) according to the ACE I/D polymorphism in the Nancy Study 2[a]*

	II	ID	DD	p Value
Parents	*n* = 33	*n* = 103	*n* = 60	
SBP (mm Hg)	119.1 (11.0)	121.3 (12.5)	120.0 (11.9)	NS
DBP (mm Hg)	71.9 (6.7)	74.7 (8.9)	73.5 (8.1)	NS
ACE (UI/L)	61.1 (23.0)	83.7 (23.8)	107.5 (24.0)	<0.001
Offspring	*n* = 43	*n* = 94	*n* = 71	
SBP (mm Hg)	113.7 (9.5)	115.5 (8.7)	115.7 (8.5)	NS
DBP (mm Hg)	61.1 (5.6)	61.6 (5.8)	63.0 (5.3)	NS
ACE (UI/L)	81.7 (28.4)	119.9 (38.0)	141.4 (44.7)	<0.001

(Adapted from ref. 85.)

[a] Blood pressure is not associated with the polymorphism. Plasma ACE is strongly and codominantly positively associated with the *D* allele.

ACE *I/D*, insertion (*I*)/deletion (*D*) polymorphism; SBP, systolic blood pressure; DBP, diastolic blood pressure; NS, nonsignificant.

TABLE 5. *Linkage-segregation analysis of plasma ACE and the ACE I/D polymorphism in the Nancy Study 2[a]*

Parameters estimated in the linkage-segregation analysis	Parameter estimates (SE) for the best-fitting model
Frequency of *D/I*	0.57/0.43
Frequency of *S* on *I*	(0)[b]
Frequency of *S* on *D*	0.78
m*ss*	−0.888
m*sS*	0.137
m*SS*	1.07
Residual SD	0.745
Residual h²	(0)[b]

(Adapted from ref. 85.)

[a] ACE levels were adjusted on age and standardized before analysis. As a consequence, the means (m) and residual SD are expressed in term of SD of the crude level of ACE.

[b] Not significantly different from the specified value. All other parameter estimates are significantly different from 0 ($p < 0.05$).

phism was genotyped by the polymerase chain reaction (PCR) technique (87) and plasma ACE activity was measured (85). The aim of this study was to establish whether the *S/s* polymorphism, inferred from segregation analysis in the Nancy Study 1 but not identified at the molecular level, and the ACE *I/D* molecular polymorphism were identical. For that purpose, a statistical technique called linkage-segregation analysis was used. In this study, as in the Nancy Study 1, much higher plasma ACE levels were observed in offspring than in parents (Table 4). The best-fitting model for the linkage-segregation analysis performed on age-adjusted ACE level (Table 5) yielded a frequency of 0.57 for the *D* allele and frequencies of *S* on alleles *I* and *D* of 0 and 0.78, respectively. These results suggested that the postulated *S/s* polymorphism was present within or near the ACE gene (ACE *S/s*) and that the ACE *I/D* polymorphism was a marker of ACE *S/s*. The best-fitting model suggested that allele *S* was always found on allele *D* but the two alleles were not identical since a significant fraction (0.22) of the *D* alleles were carrying *s*. In this study, the *S/s* susceptibility polymorphism and the *I/D* marker polymorphism explained, respectively, 44 percent and 28 percent of the interindividual variance of plasma ACE level.

THE ACE GENE, A CANDIDATE GENE FOR CARDIOVASCULAR DISEASE

The ACE *I/D* Polymorphism Is Not Related to Blood Pressure in Humans

Positional cloning has identified a locus, called BP/1, linked to blood pressure in a cross between stroke-prone spontaneously hypertensive rats (SHRsp) and Wistar-Kyoto (WKY) rats (88,89), especially when the rats were salt loaded. The BP/1 locus is located on chromosome 10 and belongs to a syntheny group with a locus located on chromosome 17q23 in humans which includes the ACE gene. New crosses will be required to map BP/1 more precisely. The implication of the ACE locus has also been demonstrated in Dahl hypertensive rats (90). As a consequence of the role of ACE in the renin-angiotensin system, it was logical to hypothesize that the ACE gene could be a candidate for human hypertension. However in the different studies that we have performed (see, for example, Table 4), the ACE *I/D* polymorphism was never associated with blood pressure. A study in pairs of hypertensive sibs using a highly informative marker located close to the ACE gene on the growth hormone locus has also failed to demonstrate a linkage between the ACE locus and hypertension (91). In another study, the distribution of the ACE *I/D* genotypes did not significantly differ in groups of offspring contrasted for blood pressure and parental history of high blood pressure (92) and a lack of association between the polymorphism and blood pressure has also been reported in a Dutch study (93). In a comparison of hypertensives and normotensives of Japanese origin, the distribution of ACE *I/D* genotypes was also similar in both groups (94). Interestingly, in this study, the frequency of allele *D* (0.40 in controls) was lower than in Caucasian populations where its frequency is generally found between 0.53 and 0.57. We have checked in a sample of 150 healthy individuals from northern China that the *D* allele is effectively less frequent (0.37) in northern Asians than in Caucasians (*unpublished result*). Until now, the only significant association of the ACE *I/D* polymorphism with hypertension was found by Zee et al. (95) in a study involving 80 Caucasian hypertensives and 93 normotensives in Australia. In this study the frequency of the insertion allele (*I*) was 0.56 in hypertensives, whereas it was 0.41 in normotensives ($p < 0.01$). In the analysis of the 188 control subjects age 60 or older included in the ECTIM study (see below), a highly significant association between diastolic blood pressure and the ACE *I/D* polymorphism was found, higher levels being observed in presence of the *I* allele. This association was homogeneous across the four populations studied and after adjustment on population, age, and body mass index, the mean levels of diastolic blood pressure were 77.8 (standard error of the mean [SEM] 1.9), 84.8 (1.4), and 86.3 (2.2) mm Hg in *DD*, *ID*, and *II* individuals, respectively (test for trend: $p < 0.003$). In the younger age group, no association was found. This observation is in agreement with the results of Zee et al. (95) and it may appear paradoxical in view of the positive association between the *D* allele and plasma and cellular ACE. However, given the association between the ACE *D* allele and coronary heart disease (CHD) risk described below, it is possible that the association between blood pressure and the *I* allele may result from selection by death of ACE *DD* hypertensive subjects.

The ACE Gene: A Candidate Gene for CHD

By inducing AII production and BK degradation, an elevated ACE activity could favor chronic vasoconstriction in specific arterial territories or exacerbate the acute response to vasoconstrictor triggers. Furthermore, given the growth-modulating effects of AII and BK, high ACE levels could favor SMC proliferation and remodeling of the exposed arteries. Arrythmias could also be favored by high AII levels. Coronary constriction, proliferation of SMC, and arrythmias are involved in the pathophysiology of CHD and its complications such as MI and sudden death. It is then plausible that the ACE *D* allele as a consequence of its association with high plasma and cellular levels of ACE may predispose to CHD.

The ACE *I/D* Polymorphism and MI in the ECTIM Study

The Etude Cas-Témoin de l'Infarctus du Myocarde (ECTIM) study is a case-control study specially designed to identify genetic variants associated with MI. Four populations covered by CHD registries (WHO/MONICA) were targets for study: three populations in France in the regions of Lille, Strasbourg, and Toulouse and one population in Northern Ireland, in the region of Belfast. France is one of the industrialized countries where the frequency of MI is the lowest, whereas among middle-aged men, this disease is 3 to 4 times more frequent in Northern Ireland than in France. In the ECTIM study, male patients with definite MI aged 35–64 were recruited 3 to 9 mo after the acute episode and during a period of 2.5 years starting at the end of 1988. Random samples of control subjects were recruited during the same period and in the same age range as the cases, using electoral rolls in France and the lists of general practitioners held by the Central Services Agency in Belfast (96). The participants were of Caucasian origin, parents of cases and controls had to be born in the same regions and their four grandparents had to be born in Europe. The ACE *I/D* polymorphism was genotyped by PCR (87) in all the subjects recruited.

Randomly Selected Subjects Who Have a CHD Are More Likely to Have the DD Genotype Than Their Unaffected Counterparts

Among the randomly selected subjects included in the ECTIM study, 18 (9 percent) in Belfast and 25 (4.3 percent) in France had a CHD. Figure 3 shows the distribution of the ACE *I/D* genotypes in these subjects according to the presence or absence of CHD. In this analysis *ID* and *II* individuals were pooled, because the number of *II* homozygotes with CHD was very small. In Belfast

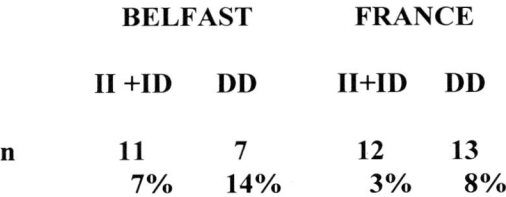

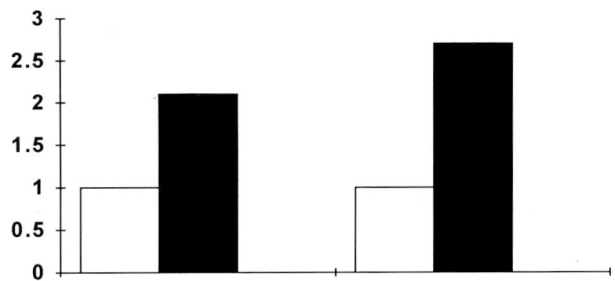

| | BELFAST | | FRANCE | |
	II +ID	DD	II+ID	DD
n	11	7	12	13
	7%	14%	3%	8%

odds ratio

FIG. 3. ECTIM Study: Prevalence of coronary heart disease (CHD) in relation to the ACE polymorphism in the population samples. The prevalence of CHD is increased in *DD* homozygotes; adjusted odds ratio: 2.4 (1.2–4.7), $p < 0.008$.

and France, a larger number of *DD* homozygotes was observed in subjects with CHD; the overall odds ratio (relative risk) of *DD* subjects adjusted on population was 2.4 ($p < 0.008$).

Randomly Selected Subjects Carrying the D Allele Are More Likely to Have Parents Who Died from MI

In the ECTIM study the parental history of MI, including age of occurrence, was recorded by questionnaire. In France, for legal reasons, it was impossible to check the reported history; but in Belfast, the data were validated using records of general practitioners, hospital records, and death certificates. Subjects from Belfast for whom this validation was not possible (15 percent) were excluded from the analysis of parental history. Figure 4 shows the frequency of parental history of fatal MI in Belfast and France, according to the ACE *I/D* polymorphism. As expected, parental history was much more frequent in Belfast than in France (about 4 times). In both countries the frequency of the *D* allele was increased in those having a parental history. Taking the *II* genotype as reference, very similar odds ratios for parental fatal MI associated with the *DD* and *ID* genotypes were observed in Belfast and France; the odds ratio adjusted on population being 2.7 ($p < 0.02$) for *DD* versus *II* and 1.9 ($p = 0.1$) for *ID* versus *II*. Paternal and maternal histories were similarly associated with the presence of the *D* allele in the offspring (97).

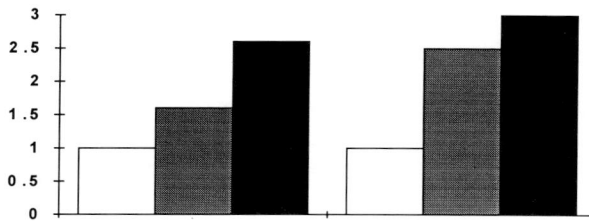

BELFAST   FRANCE

II   ID   DD   II   ID   DD

n   8   23   16   3   22   14
     20% 28% 39%   3%   7%   9%

odds ratio

FIG. 4. ECTIM Study: Parental history of fatal MI in relation to the ACE polymorphism in the population samples. Parental history of fatal MI is more frequent when allele *D* is present; adjusted odds ratio: *DD/II* 2.7 (1.2–6.4), *p* < 0.02; *ID/II* 1.9 (0.9–4.1), *p* = 0.1.

Patients with MI Have a Higher Frequency of the ACE D Allele Than Controls

For the case-control comparisons all the patients with CHD in the control groups and a biased sample of individuals included in the Toulouse center after May 1990 (98) were excluded.

In the whole population, the odds ratio (relative risk) for MI was 1.57 for *DD* versus *II* and 1.26 for *ID* versus *II* (test for trend, *p* < 0.003). This association was not significantly heterogeneous across populations and the frequency of the two alleles was similar in the different control groups (Table 6).

In view of the association between the ACE *I/D* polymorphism and MI, different variables potentially re-

lated to MI were compared between ACE *I/D* genotypes in the control groups. No difference could be detected, for plasma lipid variables, fibrinogen, factor VII, plasminogen-activator inhibitor-1 (PAI-1), body mass index (BMI), cigarette consumption, or blood pressure. Furthermore, the prevalence of hypertension, defined by the presence of a diastolic blood pressure higher than 100 mm Hg or of antihypertensive treatment, was similar in the three genotypes: 22.0 percent, 17.7 percent, and 20.3 percent in genotypes *DD*, *ID*, and *II*, respectively (non-significant difference).

Since the influence of the ACE *I/D* polymorphism on MI appeared independent of the classic risk factors, we hypothesized that it could be particularly important in MI patients considered to be at low risk according to common criteria. Because hyperlipidemia and obesity are important contributors to the CHD epidemic in Western countries, a low-risk group was defined according to plasma apolipoprotein B (ApoB) level and BMI. This low-risk group included subjects with a plasma ApoB level lower than 125 mg/dl (the approximate median of ApoB in controls), not treated with hypolipidemic drugs and with a BMI < 26 kg/m² (the approximate median of BMI in controls). In this group (Fig. 5), the association between the ACE *I/D* polymorphism and MI was highly significant and homogeneous across populations (test for trend, *p* < 0.005); however the increased risk of MI was present only in *DD* individuals, and the overall odds ratio adjusted on population comparing *DD* and *ID* + *II* individuals was 2.7 (*p* < 0.0005). Conversely, in the high-risk group which included all subjects who were not in the low-risk group defined above (Fig. 6), the ACE *I/D* polymorphism was less strongly related to MI, although the test for trend was still significant (*p* < 0.05). In the whole population, adjustment on age, cigarette consumption, plasma ApoAI, plasma Lp(a), blood pressure, and social class did not affect the association observed between the ACE *I/D*

TABLE 6. *ECTIM study: distribution of the ACE (I/D) genotypes in cases and controls—all subjects*

	Belfast		Lille		Strasbourg		Toulouse[a]	
	Cases	Controls	Cases	Controls	Cases	Controls	Cases	Controls
Genotype								
DD	51	44	31	44	68	55	27	28
ID	111	96	27	75	108	98	28	60
II	40	43	7	32	30	41	12	19
Odds ratio[b]								
DD/II	1.25		3.22		1.69		1.53	
ID/II	1.24		1.65		1.51		0.74	

[a] Toulouse subjects recruited after June 1990 were excluded because the genotype distribution after that date in Toulouse controls was in strong Hardy-Weinberg disequilibrium. As a consequence the results slightly differ from those reported in ref. 99, where no exclusion was performed. Although the results are similar, this presentation gives a better account of the codominant association between the polymorphism and MI.

[b] Adjusted odds ratio: *DD/II* 1.57; *ID/II* 1.26; test for trend adjusted on center: *p* < 0.003.

odds ratio

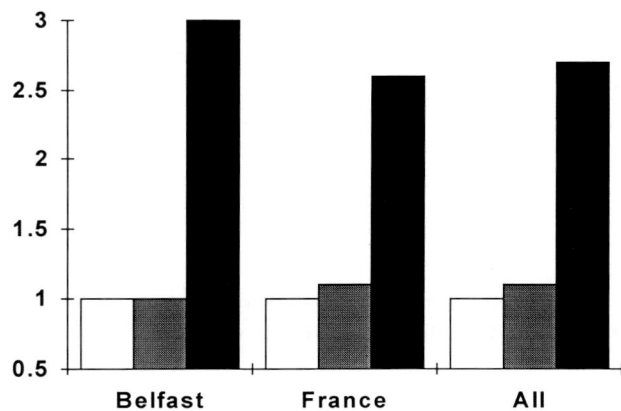

FIG. 5. ECTIM Study: Distribution of the ACE (*I/D*) genotypes in cases and controls—Low-risk subjects. Genotypes: *II*, white bar; *ID*, gray bar; *DD*, black bar. Toulouse subjects included after June 1990 were excluded (see Table 6). In cases with low risk the *DD* genotype is more frequent; adjusted odds ratio: *DD/II* 2.7; *ID/II* 1.1. Test for comparison *DD/II* + *ID* adjusted on population: *p* < 0.0005.

polymorphism and MI. The ACE *I/D* polymorphism was thus an independent risk factor for MI in the ECTIM study.

We defined our low-risk group by reference to plasma ApoB level, hypolipidaemic treatment, and BMI; the results were very similar (but slightly less significant) when total or LDL cholesterol was used instead of ApoB. In contrast, the association between the ACE polymorphism and MI was similar in the groups defined according to the median of cigarette consumption, ApoAI, Lp(a), or fibrinogen. Since a substantial proportion of MI patients received potent drugs likely to affect blood pressure, we were unable to define a normotensive low-risk group.

It is unlikely that population heterogeneity could explain these results; within each population, cases and controls were carefully selected to minimize ethnic heterogeneity. All subjects participating in our study were Caucasians, and in the other samples of general population of Caucasian origin that we have studied, the frequency of the ACE *I/D* polymorphism was fairly similar to that found in the ECTIM study. The fact that the associations were very homogeneous across populations also provides a strong argument against a possible confounding effect of population heterogeneity (99).

Why a Stronger Association in Low-risk Subjects?

It is well known that established risk factors for MI have a cumulative effect on MI risk, i.e., the relative risk associated with a particular risk factor is fairly constant over the range of variations of other risk factors. How-

ever there is no reason to exclude the possibility that other risk factors may act preferentially in particular subgroups of individuals. Such risk factors would be less easy to identify and there is a clear rationale for searching for them in patients devoid of known risk factors.

A weaker association between the ACE *I/D* polymorphism and MI in high-risk than in low-risk subjects could also be the consequence of selection due to a high mortality rate in high-risk *DD* or *ID* patients suffering a coronary event. From the difference in genotype distribution between cases and controls in the ECTIM study, a lower odds ratio for parental history of fatal MI associated with the ACE *I/D* polymorphism would have been predicted. This could be the consequence of an underestimation of the case-control difference due to the selection mentioned above. In the ECTIM study, patients were included 3–9 mo after the acute event. Several sources of evidence suggest that approximately 30 percent of the patients who develop an acute coronary event die before arriving at the hospital and that during the first 3 mo after hospitalization, about 8 percent of the patients die from a complication of their MI. Thus, in our study, 30–40 percent of the patients with acute coronary events died before being eligible for the study. Such a selection could strongly affect an association between a risk factor for death and MI and could lead to an underestimation of the effect of the risk factor.

Cases with Recurrent MI More Frequently Carry the ACE D Allele in Belfast

Not all cases included in the ECTIM study were first MI. Among cases, 22 percent in Belfast and 12.5 percent

odds ratio

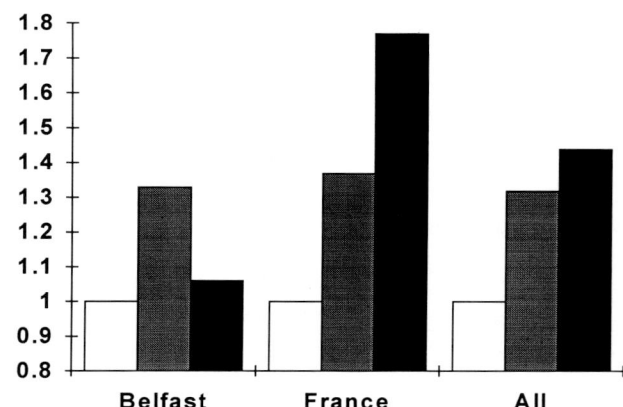

FIG. 6. ECTIM Study: Distribution of the ACE (*I/D*) genotypes in cases and controls—High-risk subjects. Genotypes: *II*, white bar; *ID*, gray bar; *DD*, black bar. Toulouse subjects included after June 1990 were excluded (see Table 6). Adjusted odds ratio: *DD/II* 1.44; *ID/II* 1.32. Test for trend adjusted on center: *p* = 0.036.

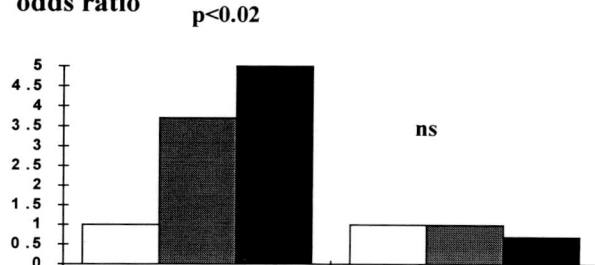

	BELFAST			**FRANCE**		
	II	**ID**	**DD**	**II**	**ID**	**DD**
n	3	26	15	9	28	14
%	7.7	23.6	29.4	13.8	14.3	9.6

FIG. 7. ECTIM Study: Frequency of recurrent MI in relation to the ACE polymorphism in cases. In Belfast, cases with recurrent MI are more frequently *DD* or *ID* than cases with first MI; *p* < 0.02.

in France had a recurrent MI. When compared to patients with first infarct, these patients had a higher frequency of the ACE *D* allele in Belfast (*p* < 0.02) but not in France (Fig. 7). This particular association in the high-risk population of Belfast could be the consequence of an earlier mean age of occurrence of first MI in ACE *D* carriers.

Plasma ACE Activity Is Increased in Young MI Patients Independently of the ACE I/D Polymorphism

Plasma ACE activity was measured in the ECTIM study from frozen plasma samples. There was a strong association between plasma ACE level and MI in the younger patients (aged less than 55, the median age in the study) but not in the older patients. Furthermore, as shown in Fig. 8, plasma ACE was elevated in the younger cases within each ACE *I/D* genotype, indicating that this association was independent of the polymorphism (100). In this analysis it was possible to infer the frequency of the ACE *S* allele in cases and controls and according to age by a commingling analysis of the ACE distribution conditioned on the ACE *I/D* polymorphism. ACE *S* was more frequent in cases before than after age 55: 0.45 and 0.32, respectively (*p* < 0.01). This may be due to a high mortality in MI patients carrying the *D* allele. Interestingly the commingling analysis further indicated that the ACE *S/s* and ACE *I/D* polymorphisms were not in complete linkage disequilibrium since a small proportion of ACE *I* alleles were carrying ACE *S*. The Nancy Study 2 (85) was apparently of insufficient power to detect this incomplete linkage.

Consistency of the Results of the ECTIM Study

The results of the ECTIM study are consistent in showing a positive association between the ACE *D* allele and MI: The prevalence of CHD and the parental history of fatal MI were increased in the presence of the *D* allele in the random samples of populations, and MI patients had a higher frequency of ACE *DD* than controls, in particular in the presence of low risk. Results in patients with recurrent MI also suggested that the first MI occurred earlier in patients carrying the *D* allele. The effect of the *D* allele on risk appears codominant, except in the low-risk group where a recessive effect was observed. Furthermore, MI patients younger than 55 years of age had a higher mean plasma ACE level than controls within each ACE *I/D* genotype. Other studies in different populations should be performed to definitively establish the association. The results of the ECTIM study also suggest that the ACE *D* allele might be associated with an increased risk of death in patients developing a CHD. This is a crucial question and even if the results are only suggestive, the possibility of a genetic trait predisposing to sudden death warrants further studies, in particular, prospective studies and postmortem studies on DNA obtained from tissues of patients who died from a CHD.

Mechanisms Proposed for the Possible Effect of the ACE Gene Polymorphism on MI

In the plasma and on the surface of endothelial cells, ACE converts the inactive decapeptide AI into the highly vasoactive and aldosterone-stimulating octapeptide AII.

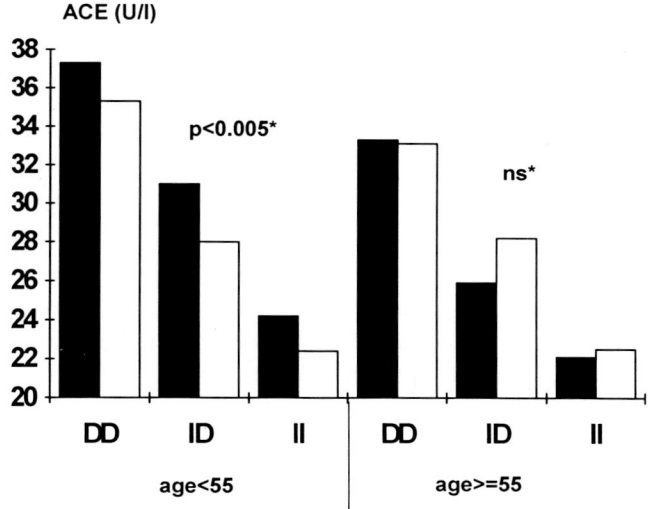

FIG. 8. ECTIM Study: Plasma ACE level in cases and controls, according to the ACE *I/D* polymorphism and age. Cases: black bar; controls: white bar. *Cases-controls difference. In younger subjects, higher levels of plasma ACE are observed in cases within each ACE *I/D* genotype; *p* < 0.005.

AII is a powerful coronary vasoconstrictor (101,102) which may modulate the growth of vascular SMC and induce myointimal hyperplasia after endothelial injury (103). Bradykinin, the other best-known substrate of ACE, is a potent vasodilator and inhibitor of SMC proliferation which by interacting with the BK B2 receptor induces the release of endothelial factors, including nitric oxide and prostacyclin (104–106). Bradykinin is inactivated by ACE; this could account for some of the effects associated with high ACE expression and for part of the beneficial effect of ACE inhibitors (105,107,108).

Since allele ACE *S* is associated with high plasma and cellular levels of ACE, it can be proposed that a chronic increased expression of ACE, by modulating the level of AII and BK in specific sites, affects cardiovascular homeostasis and is responsible for the increased risk of MI. ACE probably acts locally in the coronary arteries and/or in the heart. This is suggested by experimental results (109) and is compatible with a possible beneficial effect of ACE inhibition on CHD complications and cardiac hypertrophy independent of blood pressure reduction. The paracrine and autocrine effects of vascular or cardiac renin-angiotensin (110) and kallikrein-kinin (111,112) systems could explain the local action of ACE and of ACE inhibitors. The variable availability of AII receptors of AT1 and AT2 subtypes in different tissues and cells and in different physiopathological circumstances could also account for local effects attributable to AII (113,114).

Vascular dysfunction and/or injury of endothelium or SMC, followed by monocyte recruitment and macrophage formation, lipid deposition, SMC proliferation, and extracellular matrix synthesis are sequential events involved in the pathogenesis of atherosclerosis (115). During this chronic process, several cells including endothelial cells, macrophages, T-lymphocytes, and SMC play a major role by secreting and responding to growth factors or other mediators (116) including ACE, AII, and BK. An important component in the development of atherosclerosis is the rupture of the plaque, which is a frequent complication of relatively small, lipid-rich plaques, and leads to thrombosis and coronary constriction, and eventually to acute coronary occlusion (115,117). Given the important roles of AII and BK as modulators of cellular growth and of vasomotoricity, their respective deleterious and beneficial implication at different stages of the atherosclerotic process and during the acute events leading to MI or sudden death can be postulated. In patients with coronary artery disease, ACE inhibition attenuates sympathetic coronary vasoconstriction. This may be due to the removal of the facilitating influence of AII on sympathetic modulation of coronary vasomotor tone (118). Furthermore, ACE inhibition has a potent effect to reduce experimental infarct size, probably by increasing collateral flow (119). This may be clinically relevant since viability of the myocardium in patients with MI appears to depend on the presence of collateral blood flow within the infarct bed (120). AII could also interfere with thrombogenesis. *In vitro* studies have shown that AII induces the synthesis of PAI-1 in a dose-dependent fashion in cultured endothelial cells (121) and infusion of AII in humans results in a rapid and dose-dependent increase in circulating PAI-1 (122), thus AII might contribute to the development of a prothrombic state.

It is also possible that high ACE expression in the heart may be able to increase the generation of AII and predisposes to left ventricular hypertrophy. The ACE gene is expressed in the heart and its regulation is under the control of hemodynamic variations. In rats, ACE mRNA is increased in hearts with pressure overload left ventricular hypertrophy (75) and a tissue-specific activation of cardiac ACE has also been observed in a rat model of compensated heart failure due to coronary artery ligature (76). ACE overexpression might be a marker of hypertrophy or might promote hypertrophy. Indeed, AII could have a trophic role in the heart since AII receptors of the AT1 subtype are present (123). ACE is also expressed in the fibrous scar after experimental MI in the rat (78). Moreover, ACE inhibitors are more effective than other antihypertensive drugs to prevent cardiac hypertrophy in pressure overload models in the rat and a direct effect of the drug has been proposed (124). The results of the Framingham study have clearly demonstrated that electrocardiographic or echocardiographic evidence of left ventricular hypertrophy were strong risk factors for clinical events, including death, attributable to cardiovascular disease (125). Hence, if ventricular hypertrophy was the main consequence of ACE overexpression, the ACE polymorphism could be a risk factor for MI and sudden cardiac death independent of atherosclerosis development. In this context, it is worth noting that patients with ischemic or idiopathic dilated myocardiopathy are more frequently ACE *DD* homozygotes than controls (126) and that patients with hypertrophic myocardiopathy have an increased frequency of the ACE *D* allele, in particular in the presence of a family history of sudden cardiac death (127).

The higher plasma ACE in children observed in the two Nancy studies probably reflects the increased expression of the enzyme during growth. This increased expression is apparently modulated by the ACE polymorphism. A genetic factor acts very early in life and it is conceivable that its phenotypic effects observed in adult life may only reflect the influence of the genetic factor during critical periods of development. This is connected with the concept of programming which has been proposed to account for environmental influences operating at sensitive periods of development and resulting in long-term changes in the structure and the function of the organism (128,129). The recently published results of an autopsy study of newborn children in Finland have demonstrated that intimal thickening of coronary arteries in infants was strongly associated with a family history of coronary artery disease (CAD), suggesting that intimal thickening was a morphological manifestation of predisposition to CAD and that this possibly genetic predisposition was operating very early in life (130). Programming may then be the result of an interaction between variable environmental exposition and genetic predisposition.

CONCLUSIONS

Important progress has been made recently in understanding the molecular biology, genetics, and epidemiology of ACE. However several important questions remain:

- Are there important unknown substrates for ACE?
- Is there a specific substrate for the N domain of ACE?
- What are the functions of ACE in the central nervous system and germinal cells?
- If ACE is a risk factor for CHD and myocardial hypertrophy, what are the mechanisms involved and what is the impact of genetically determined high ACE expression on artery and heart physiology?
- Is the ACE polymorphism functionally important in the central nervous system?
- What is the molecular basis of the ACE *S/s* polymorphism?

There is little doubt that these questions will occupy several research groups for the next few years.

REFERENCES

1. Erdös EG. *Hypertension* 1990;16:363–370.
2. Yokosawa H, Endo S, Ogura Y, Ishii S. *Biochem Biophys Res Commun* 1983;116:735–742.
3. Inokuchi JJ, Nagamatsu A. *Biochem Biophys Acta* 1981;662:300–307.
4. Dubreuil P, Fulcrand P, Rodriguez M, et al. *Biochem J* 1989;262:125–130.
5. Skidgel RA, Erdös EG. *Proc Natl Acad Sci (USA)* 1985;82:1025–1029.
6. Skidgel RA, Erdös EG. In: Turner AJ, ed. *Neuropeptides and their peptidases.* UK: Ellis Horwood, Chichester, 1987:165–182.
7. Soubrier F, Alhenc-Gelas F, Hubert C, et al. *Proc Natl Acad Sci (USA)* 1988;85:9386–9390.
8. Lattion AL, Soubrier F, Allegrini J, et al. *FEBS Lett* 1989;252:99–104.
9. Ehlers MRW, Fox EA, Strydom DJ, Riordan JF. *Proc Natl Acad Sci (USA)* 1989;86:7741–7745.
10. Perich RB, Jackson B, Rogerson F, et al. *Mol Pharmacol* 1992;42:286–293.
11. Williams TA, Barnes K, Kenny AJ, et al. *Biochem J* 1992;288:878–881.
12. Bünning P, Riordan JF. *Biochemistry* 1983;22:110–116.
13. Shapiro R, Holmquist B, Riordan JF. *Biochemistry* 1983;22:3850–3857.
14. Kester WR, Matthews BW. *Biochemistry* 1977;16:2506–2516.
15. Bünning P, Kleemann SG, Riordan JF. *Biochemistry* 1990;29:10488–10492.
16. Bünning P, Holmquist B, Riordan JF. *Biochem Biophys Res Commun* 1978;83:1442–1449.
17. Chen YNP, Riordan JF. *Biochemistry* 1990;29:10493–10498.
18. Chen YNP, Ehlers MRW, Riordan JF. *Biochem Biophys Res Commun* 1992;184:306–309.
19. Sen I, Kasturi S, Jabbar MA, Sen GC. *J. Biol Chem* 1993; 268:25748–25754.
20. Das M, Soffer RL. *J Biol Chem* 1975; 250:6762–6768.
21. Weare JA, Gafford JT, Lu HS, Erdös EG. *Anal Biochem* 1982;123:310–319.
22. Lanzillo JJ, Stevens J, Dasarathy Y, et al. *J Biol Chem* 1985;260:14938–14944.
23. Jackson B, Cubela RB, Sakaguchi K, Johnston CI. *Endocrinology* 1988;122:50–55.
24. Wei L, Alhenc-Gelas F, Soubrier F, et al. *J Biol Chem* 1991;266:5540–5546.
25. Ehlers MRW, Riordan JF. *Biochemistry* 1991;30:7118–7126.
26. Yasui T, Alhenc-Gelas F, Corvol P, Ménard J. *J Lab Clin Med* 1984;104:741–751.
27. El-Dorry HA, MacGregor JS, Soffer RL. *Biochem Biophys Res Commun* 1983;115:1096–1100.
28. Beldent V, Michaud A, Wei L, et al. *J Biol Chem* 1993; 268:26428–26433.
29. Oppong SY, Hooper NM. *Biochem J* 1993;292:597–603.
30. Bruneval P, Hinglais N, Alhenc-Gelas F, et al. *Histochemistry* 1986;85:73–80.
31. Arregui A, Iversen LL. *Eur J Pharmacol* 1978;52:147–150.
32. Schweisfurth H, Schioberg-Schiegnitz S. *Enzyme* 1984;32:12–19.
33. Yokoyama M, Takada Y, Iwata H, et al. *J Urol* 1982;127:368–370.
34. Cushman DW, Cheung HS. *Biochim Biophys Acta* 1971;250:261–265.
35. Nonotte I, Laliberté MF, Duperray C, et al. *Mol Cell Endocrinol* 1993;92:167–174.
36. Friedland J, Setton C, Silverstein E. *Biochem Biophys Res Commun* 1978;83:843–849.
37. Costerousse O, Allegrini J, Lopez M, Alhenc-Gelas F. *Biochem J* 1993;290:33–40.
38. Weinberg KS, Douglas WHJ, MacNamee DR, et al. *In Vitro* 1982;18:400–406.
39. Defendini R, Zimmerman EA, Weare JA, et al. *Neuroendocr* 1983;37:32–40.
40. Barnes K, Matsas R, Hooper NM, et al. *Neuroscience* 1988;27:799–817.
41. Chai SY, McKenzie JS, McKinley MJ, Mendelsohn FAO. *J Comp Neurol* 1990;291:179–194.
42. Chai SY, Christie MJ, Beart PM, Mendelsohn FAO. *Neurochem Int* 1987;10:101–107.
43. Mendelsohn FAO, Quirion R, Saavedra JM, et al. *Proc Natl Acad Sci (USA)* 1984;81:1575–1579.
44. Matsas R, Kenny AJ, Turner AJ. *Biochem J* 1984;223:433–440.
45. Oblin A, Danse MJ, Zivkovic B. *Neurosci Lett* 1988;84:91–96.
46. Chai SY, Mendelsohn FAO, Paxinos G. *Neuroscience* 1987;20:615–627.
47. Chai SY, McKinley MJ, Paxinos G, Mendelsohn FAO. *Neuroscience* 1991;42:483–495.
48. Hooper NM, Turner AJ. *Biochem J* 1987;241:625–633.
49. Williams TA, Hooper NM, Turner AJ. *J Neurochem* 1991;57:193–199.
50. Yamada H, Fabris B, Allen AM, et al. *Circ Res* 1991;68:141–149.
51. Wei L, Alhenc-Gelas F, Corvol P, Clauser E. *J Biol Chem* 1991;266:9002–9008.
52. Jaspard E, Wei L, Alhenc-Gelas F. *J Biol Chem* 1993;268:9496–9503.
53. Wei L, Clauser E, Alhenc-Gelas A, Corvol P. *J Biol Chem* 1992;267:13398–13405.
54. Hubert C, Houot AM, Corvol P, Soubrier F. *J Biol Chem* 1991;266:15377–15383.
55. Testut P, Soubrier F, Corvol P, Hubert C. *Biochem J* 1994; in press.
56. Goraya TY, Kessler SP, Kumar RS, et al. *Nucl Acids Res* 1994;22:1194–1201.
57. Sibony M, Gasc JM, Soubrier F, et al. *Hypertension* 1993;21:827–835.

58. Velletri PA, Aquilano DR, Bruckwick E, et al. *Endocrinology* 1985;116:2516–2522.
59. Nadaud S, Houot AM, Hubert C, et al. *Biochem Biophys Res Comm* 1992;189:134–140.
60. Kumar RS, Thekumkara TJ, Sen G. *J Biol Chem* 1991;266: 3854–3862.
61. Langford KG, Shai SY, Howard TE, et al. *J Biol Chem* 1991;266: 15559–15562.
62. Howard T, Balogh R, Overbeek P, Bernstein KE. *Mol Cell Biol* 1993;13:1–27.
63. Turner AJ, Hryszko J, Hooper NM, Dowdall MJ. *J Neurochem* 1987;48:910–916.
64. Lamango N, Isaac RE. *Biochem Soc Trans* 1993;21:245S.
65. Cornell MJ, Coates D, Isaac RE. *Biochem Soc Trans* 1993;21: 243S.
66. Krulewitz AK, Fanburg BL. *J Cell Physiol* 1986;129:147–150.
67. Dasarathy Y, Fanburg BL. *J Cell Physiol* 1991;148:327–335.
68. Krulewitz AH, Baur WE, Fanburg BL. *Am J Physiol* 1984;247: C163–C168.
69. Friedland J, Setton C, Silverstein E. *Science* 1977;197:64–65.
70. Yotsumoto H, Imai Y, Kuzuyu N, et al. *Ann Intern Med* 1982;96: 326–328.
71. Kokubu TE, Ueda E, Ono M, et al. *Eur J Pharmacol* 1980;62: 269–275.
72. Fyhrquist F, Florslund T, Tikkanen I, Gronhagen-Riska C. *Eur J Pharmacol* 1980;67:473–475.
73. Larochelle P, Genest J, Kuchel O, et al. *Can Med Assoc J* 1979;121:309–316.
74. Fyhrquist F, Hortling L, Gronhagen-Riska C. *J Clin Endocrinol Metab* 1982;55:783–786.
75. King SJ, Oparil S. *Am J Physiol* 1992;263:C743–C749.
76. Schunkert H, Ingelfinger JR, Hirsch AT, et al. *Circ Res* 1993;72: 312–318.
77. Schunkert H, Dzau VJ, Tang SS, et al. *J Clin Invest* 1990;86: 1913–1920.
78. Hirsch AT, Talsness CE, Schunkert H, et al. *Circ Res* 1991;69: 475–482.
79. Shiota N, Miyasaki M, Okunishi H. *Hypertension* 1992;20:168– 174.
80. Johnston CI, Mooser V, Sun Y, Fabris B. *Clin Exp Pharmacol Physiol* 1991;18:107–110.
81. Alhenc-Gelas F, Richard J, Courbon D, et al. *J Lab Clin Med* 1991;117:33–39.
82. Lieberman J. *Am J Med* 1974;59:365–372.
83. Okabe TK, Yamagata M, Fujisawa J, et al. *J Clin Invest* 1985;75: 911–914.
84. Cambien F, Alhenc-Gelas F, Herbeth B, et al. *Am J Hum Genet* 1988;43:774–780.
85. Tiret L, Rigat B, Visvikis S, et al. *Am J Hum Genet* 1992;51:197– 205.
86. Rigat B, Hubert C, Alhenc-Gelas F, et al. *J Clin Invest* 1990;86: 1343–1346.
87. Rigat B, Hubert C, Corvol P, Soubrier F. *Nucl Acids Res* 1992;20: 1433.
88. Hilbert P, Lindpaintner K, Beckmann J, et al. *Nature* 1991;353: 521–526.
89. Jacob HJ, Lindpaintner K, Lincoln SE, et al. *Cell* 1991;67:213– 224.
90. Deng Y, Rapp JP. *Nature Genet* 1992;1:267–272.
91. Jeunemaitre X, Lifton RP, Hunt SC, et al. *Nature Genet* 1992;1: 72–75.
92. Harrap SB, Davidson HR, Connor JM, et al. *Hypertension* 1993;21:455–460.
93. Schmidt S, Van Hooft IMS, Grobbee DE, et al. *J Hypertens* 1993;11:345–348.
94. Higashimori K, Zhao Y, Higaki J, et al. *Biochem Biophys Res Commun* 1993;191:399–404.
95. Zee RYL, Lou YK, Griffiths LR, Morris BJ. *Biochem Biophys Res Commun* 1992;184:9–15.
96. Parra HJ, Arveiler D, Evans AE, et al. *Arteriosclerosis and Thrombosis* 1992;12:701–707.
97. Tiret L, Kee F, Poirier O, et al. *Lancet* 1993;341:991–992.
98. Cambien F. *Clin Genet* 1994; (In press).
99. Cambien F, Poirier O, Lecerf L, et al. *Nature* 1992;359:641–644.
100. Cambien F, Costerousse O, Tiret L, et al. *Circulation* 1994; (In press).
101. Whelan RF, Scroop GC, Walsh JA. *Am Heart J* 1969;77:546– 565.
102. Magrini F, Reggiani P, Roberts N, et al. *Am J Med* 1988;84(Suppl 3A):55–60.
103. Powell JS, Clozel JP, Müller RKM, et al. *Science* 1989;245:186– 188.
104. Pelc LR, Gross GJ, Warltier DC. *Circulation* 1991;83:2048– 2056.
105. Farhy R, Khang-loon Ho, Carretero OA, Scicli AG. *Biochem Biophys Res Commun* 1992;182:283–288.
106. Schrör K. *J Cardiovasc Pharmacol* 1992;20(Suppl 9):S68–S73.
107. Linz W, Schölkens BA. *J Cardiovasc Pharmacol* 1992;20(Suppl 9):S83–S90.
108. Wiemer G, Schölkens BA, Becker RHA, Busse R. *Hypertension* 1991;18:558–563.
109. Linz W, Schölkens BA. *J Cardiovasc Pharmacol* 1987;10(Suppl 7):S75–S82.
110. Paul M, Wagner J, Dzau VJ. *J Clin Invest* 1993;91:2058–2064.
111. Saed GM, Carretero OA, MacDonald RJ, Scicli AG. *Circ Res* 1990;67:510–516.
112. Scicli AG, Farhy R, Scicli G, Nolly H. In: Bönner G, Schölkens BA, Scicli AG, eds. *The role of bradykinin in the cardiovascular action of the converting enzyme inhibitor ramipril.* Frankfurt: Hoechst Aktiengesellschaft, 1992; 17–28.
113. Janiak P, Pillon A, Prost JF, Vilaine JP. *Hypertension* 1992;20: 737–745.
114. Sudhir K, MacGregor JS, Gupta M, et al. *Circulation* 1993;87: 931–938.
115. Badimon JJ, Fuster V, Chesebro JH, Badimon L. *Circulation* 1993; 87(Suppl II):II3–II16.
116. Russell Ross. *Nature* 1993;362:801–809.
117. Fuster V, Badimon L, Badimon JJ, Chesebro JH. *New Engl J Med* 1992;326:310–318.
118. Perondi R, Saino A, Tio RA, et al. *Circulation* 1992;85:2004– 2013.
119. Ertl G, Kloner RA, Alexander R, Braunwald E. *Circulation* 1982;65:40–48.
120. Sabia PJ, Powers ER, Ragosta M, et al. *N Engl J Med* 1992;327: 1825–1831.
121. Vaughan DE, Shen C, Lazos SA. *Circulation* 1992;86:(Suppl I):I-557.
122. Ridker PM, Gaboury CL, Conlin PR, et al. *Circulation* 1993;87: 1969–1973.
123. Sechi LA, Griffin CA, Grady EF, et al. *Circ Res* 1992;71:1482– 1489.
124. Baker KM, Chernin MI, Wixson SK, Aceto JF. *Am J Physiol* 1990;259:H324–H332.
125. Kannel WB. *J Hyperten* 1991;9(Suppl 2):s3–s9.
126. Raynolds MV, Bristow MR, Bush EW, et al. *Lancet* 1993;342: 1073–1075.
127. Marian AJ, Yu QT, Workman R, et al. *Lancet* 1993;342:1085– 1086.
128. Lucas A. In: Bock GR, Whelan J, eds. *Ciba Found Symp 156.* Chichester: Wiley; 1991:38–55.
129. Barker DJP, ed. *Fetal and infant origins of adult disease,* 1st ed. London: *Br Med J*; 1992.
130. Kapprio J, Norio R, Pesonen E, Sarna S. *Circulation* 1993;87: 1960–1968.

Hypertension: Pathophysiology, Diagnosis, and Management, Second Edition, edited by J.H. Laragh and B.M. Brenner, Raven Press, Ltd., New York © 1995.

CHAPTER 101

Tissue Distribution of Angiotensin-Converting Enzyme

Siew Yeen Chai and Colin I. Johnston

The renin-angiotensin system plays an important role in the maintenance of blood pressure and fluid and electrolyte homeostasis. Although the effector peptide angiotensin II can be formed via different pathways from the precursor angiotensinogen, the primary enzymes involved are renin (EC 3.4.23.15) and angiotensin-converting enzyme (ACE) (EC 3.4.15.1) (Fig. 1). The renin-angiotensin system was originally regarded as a circulating hormonal system. However, discovery of its different components within tissues suggests more extensive roles in the local maintenance of tissue function. ACE exists (a) in plasma (circulating hormone), (b) in the interstitium (tissue), or (c) intracellularly. However, ACE is predominantly a membrane-bound ectoenzyme and hence, formation of angiotensin II probably occurs extracellularly in the interstitium (Fig. 2).

ENZYME CHARACTERISTICS

Structure of ACE

ACE occurs generally as a membrane-bound dimeric glycoprotein of 146 kDa that contains a large hydrophilic extracellular domain which is anchored in the membrane by its small hydrophobic C-terminal sequence (1) (Fig. 3). The first full-length cDNA sequence of ACE obtained from human endothelial cells consists of 4,024 nucleotides which encode 1,306 amino acids with 17 potential glycosylation sites. The extracellular domain consists of a 29 amino acid leader sequence followed by two regions of high sequence homology, both of which contain active site sequences (2).

The somatic form of the enzyme appears to be the same in all tissues studied except for the testis. The testicular form of the enzyme has only one active site and has an identical sequence to the C-terminus of the endothelial enzyme except for its short N-terminal portion (3) (Fig. 3).

Soluble forms of the enzyme also exist in plasma, ce-

S. Y. Chai and C. I. Johnston: University of Melbourne, Department of Medicine, Austin Hospital, Heidelberg, Victoria 3084, Australia.

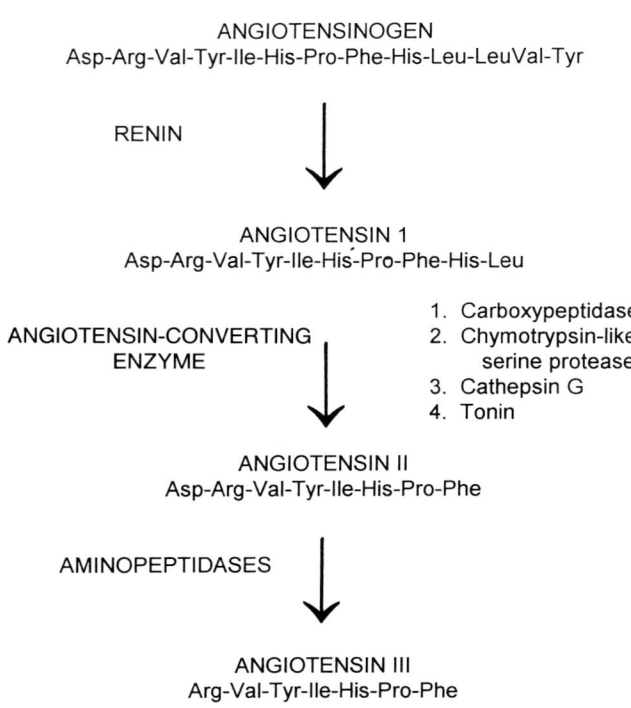

ANGIOTENSINOGEN
Asp-Arg-Val-Tyr-Ile-His-Pro-Phe-His-Leu-LeuVal-Tyr

RENIN

ANGIOTENSIN 1
Asp-Arg-Val-Tyr-Ile-His-Pro-Phe-His-Leu

ANGIOTENSIN-CONVERTING ENZYME

1. Carboxypeptidase
2. Chymotrypsin-like serine protease
3. Cathepsin G
4. Tonin

ANGIOTENSIN II
Asp-Arg-Val-Tyr-Ile-His-Pro-Phe

AMINOPEPTIDASES

ANGIOTENSIN III
Arg-Val-Tyr-Ile-His-Pro-Phe

FIG. 1. Components of the renin-angiotensin system.

rebrospinal fluid, aqueous humor of the eye, and seminal plasma. Characteristics of plasma ACE are virtually identical to somatic forms of the enzyme except for the lack of the transmembrane and intracellular sequence which has been removed presumably by proteolytic cleavage (4). Whether this cleavage is by a specific enzyme or due to cell aging is not known. Also, the relationship between and control of the plasma to the somatic enzyme is unclear.

ACE Gene

The human, mouse, and rabbit gene has been cloned and the enzyme is the product of one gene (2,3,5). The human and mouse genes are made up of 26 exons and 25 introns. Most somatic forms of ACE appear to be transcribed from all exons except exon 13 which encodes the unique N-terminal region of the testicular enzyme. The gene expression for the two forms of the enzyme appears to be under different controls; a glucocorticoid-responsive element is present in the regulatory region of somatic ACE whereas a steroid-responsive element is found in the testicular regulatory region (6). Testicular ACE appears to be the ancestral form of the enzyme since the somatic form of ACE contains two regions of high sequence homology which are coded for by exons of similar sizes suggesting that it is the result of gene duplication (6).

The human ACE gene is localized to the q23 portion of chromosome 17. Polymorphism as a result of a 287 base pair insertion-deletion in intron 16 of the human gene is found to be responsible for the large variability in plasma ACE levels in the population. The genotype with deletion of the 287 base pair results in higher plasma ACE levels (7).

Active Sites and Substrate Specificity

ACE is a zinc-dependent carboxypeptidase which hydrolyzes di- and tripeptides from the C-terminus of peptides. Each active site of the enzyme appears to bind one atom of zinc (8) which is crucial for its catalytic activity. Zinc is thought to participate directly in the catalysis of peptide substrates since replacement with other divalent

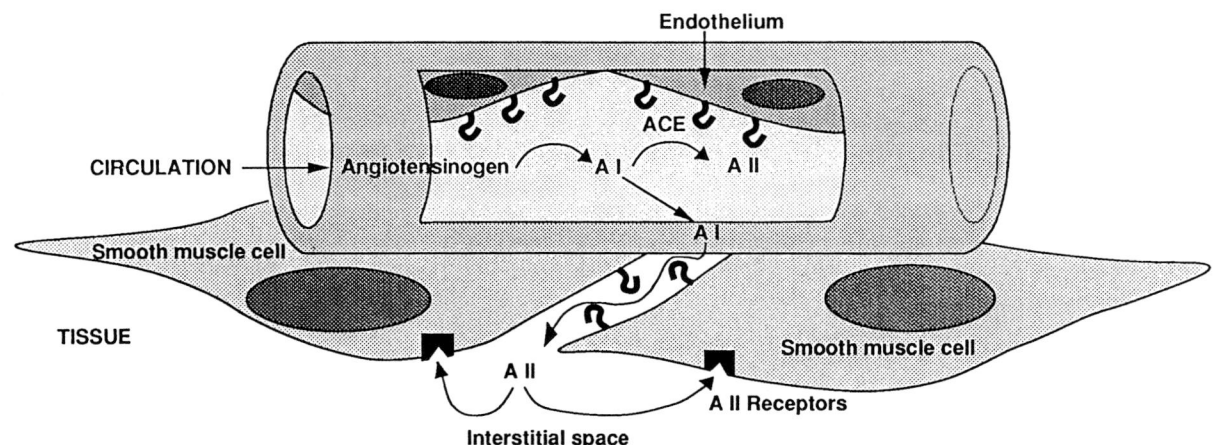

FIG. 2. Sites of conversion of angiotensin II by ACE in the vascular endothelium and in the interstitium of vascular smooth muscle cells.

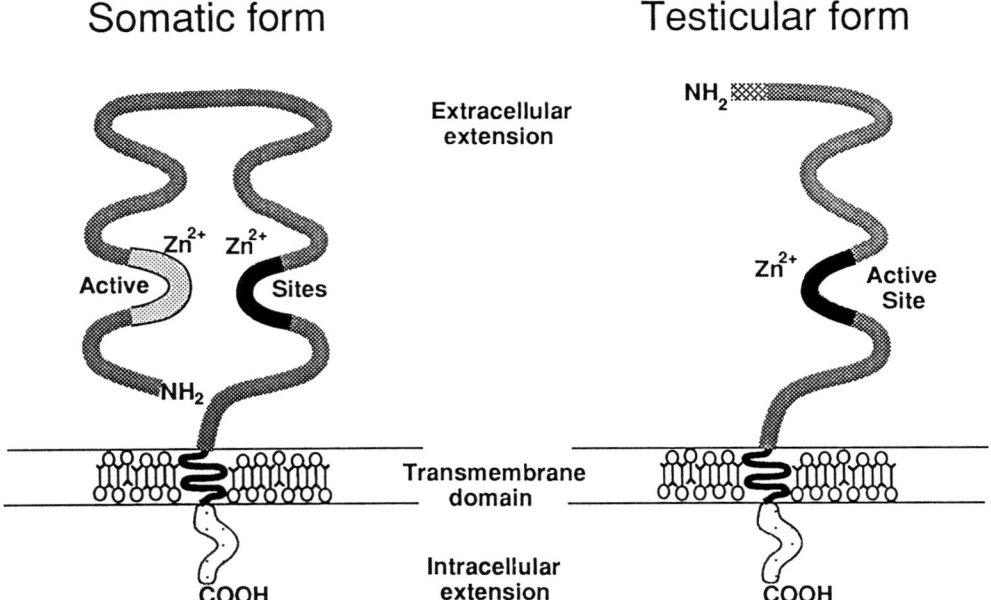

Somatic form

Testicular form

Extracellular extension

Transmembrane domain

Intracellular extension

FIG. 3. Structure and conformation of somatic and testicular ACE as deduced from the amino acid sequences of the enzyme.

cations affects the rate of conversion with little effect on the affinity (9,10). ACE is also activated by monovalent anions, particularly chloride, which is highly dependent on the nature of the substrate. The monovalent anions appear to be important for substrate binding (11).

Although the ACE molecule has two catalytically active sites, only the C-terminal site appears to be responsible for most of the hydrolysis of angiotensin I as demonstrated by site-directed mutagenesis. The affinity of angiotensin I for the two sites is similar but the conversion rate is greater in the C-terminal site (12).

The ability of ACE inhibitors to bind to the active sites appears to depend on their structural configuration. A recent inhibitor binding study with ^{125}I-Ro 31-8472, which has a smaller configuration, detected twice the number of binding sites per mole of somatic ACE compared to the testicular enzyme (13). In contrast, studies with [125]I-351A, a substituted N-carboxymethyl dipeptide with a lysyl-tyrosyl side chain, detected only one active site in both the somatic and testicular enzyme, indicating that it only bound to the C-terminus active site (14). These studies suggest the two active sites of ACE have different conformational requirements and therefore may preferentially cleave different peptide substrates. An important implication of these studies is the design of specific inhibitors for each of these sites to selectively block the formation or degradation of a particular endogenous substrate.

In addition to the classic role of ACE in the conversion of angiotensin I to angiotensin II and the degradation of

bradykinin, the enzyme can also cleave a range of different peptides (Table 1) including substance P, opioid peptides, neurotensin, cholecystokinin, bombesin, and luteinizing hormone-releasing hormone (LHRH) (15). It is not known if ACE has significant roles *in vivo* in the hydrolysis of these other peptides. The conversion rate of the different substrates *in vitro* is dependent on the source of the enzyme and tissue system studied. For ex-

TABLE 1. *Putative substrates of angiotensin-converting enzyme*

Angiotensin
Bradykinin
Lys-bradykinin
des-Arg9-bradykinin
Tachykinins
Substance P
Neurokinin A (?)
Physalaemin
Opioids
Met-enkephalin
Leu-enkephalin
Met-enkephalin-Arg6-Phe7
Met-enkephalin-Arg6-Gly7-Leu8
Dynorphin [1-6]
Dynorphin [1-8]
Beta-neo-endorphin
Neo-kyotorphin
Neurotensin
Cholecystokinin-8
Bombesin
Luteinizing hormone-releasing hormone

ample, ACE purified from rat striatum is reported to hydrolyze neurokinin A whereas rat lung ACE does not (16) and ACE appears to be more important for the metabolism of met- and leu-enkephalin in lung and serum than in the brain (17–19).

Unique among the putative substrates of ACE is LHRH which can be cleaved from both the N- and C-termini, releasing tripeptides from either end (20). The hydrolysis of LHRH is exquisitely chloride-dependent, high chloride concentrations favoring cleavage of the N-terminus and at low chloride levels, hydrolysis occurs at both ends. Moreover, hydrolysis of LHRH is 300 times faster in somatic ACE than in the testicular enzyme, suggesting that the N-terminus active site is more important in the hydrolysis of this peptide (21). Although *in vitro* alternative pathways for the formation of angiotensin II have been suggested particularly by a specific cardiac chymase (22), studies *in vivo* in humans demonstrate that ACE inhibitors block 90 percent of angiotensin II conversion across peripheral vascular beds including the heart (23).

DISTRIBUTION AND MAPPING

ACE is widely distributed throughout the body. It is a membrane component of all endothelial cells as well as many epithelial and neuronal cells (Table 2). More recently, it has been associated with cells of the hemopoietic and reticuloendothelial system.

Cardiovascular System

Although ACE was first isolated from horse plasma (24), it was later detected on the luminal surface of all vascular beds by immunohistochemistry (25). More re-

TABLE 2. *Distribution of angiotensin-converting enzyme in tissues*

Endothelial cells
Epithelial cells
  Gastrointestinal tract
  Renal proximal tubular cells
  Submandibular glands
  Choroid plexus
Reproductive tracts
Cardiovascular structures
  Heart
  Vascular adventitia
  Adrenal cortex
Brain
  Neurons in the basal ganglia
  Cells in the posterior pituitary
  Purkinje cells of the cerebellum

cently, ACE has also been found in high concentration in the vasa vasorum of the adventitia of larger blood vessels as demonstrated by *in vitro* autoradiography (Fig. 4) (26–28). This finding is consistent with earlier isolated organ studies which found that removal of the endothelium had little effect on the formation of angiotensin II which was sensitive to ACE inhibitors (29,30).

ACE concentrations vary markedly in different types of rat vessels, where the highest concentration is found in mesenteric resistance vessels and lower levels in the aorta and cerebral microvessels (31). However, it is not known if this difference in ACE levels is due to a variation in endothelial or adventitial enzyme concentrations.

In the rat heart, high concentrations of ACE occur in the valve leaflets and in coronary arteries. Lower levels are found in the right atrium followed by the left atrium (27). In contrast, in the human heart, ACE is homogenously distributed throughout the heart, with only low levels in the valves (32).

The contributions of ACE in the maintenance of blood pressure and cardiovascular function via the renin-angiotensin system have been well studied and are discussed in the section entitled Functional Role.

Central Nervous System

ACE is widely distributed in the brain, in association with the cerebral vasculature as in all other tissues but also within neurons (33). Extremely high concentrations of the enzyme are detected in the rat choroid plexus (Fig. 4A) where it occurs on the brush border of the epithelial cells (34). The human choroid plexus contains significantly lower levels of the enzyme (35). In most of the species studied, including human, the distribution of ACE could be broadly grouped into the following: (a) The forebrain circumventricular organs which have deficient blood-brain barriers where the high concentrations of ACE occur primarily in association with plasma membranes of astrocytes (33,35,36). These are sites in which ACE could convert circulating angiotensin I to angiotensin II which could then act locally on the high densities of angiotensin II receptors. (b) Moderate to high levels of ACE which are found in sites corresponding to the distribution of angiotensin II immunoreactive cell bodies and fibers and angiotensin II receptors. These include the paraventricular and supraoptic hypothalamic nuclei and the dorsal vagal complex (33,35,37,38). (c) Sites in the brain which are not generally associated with the angiotensin II system like the basal ganglia (Figs. 4A and 5), hippocampus (Fig. 4A), cerebellum (Fig. 4A), inferior olivary nuclei, and the spinal trigeminal nucleus (33,35).

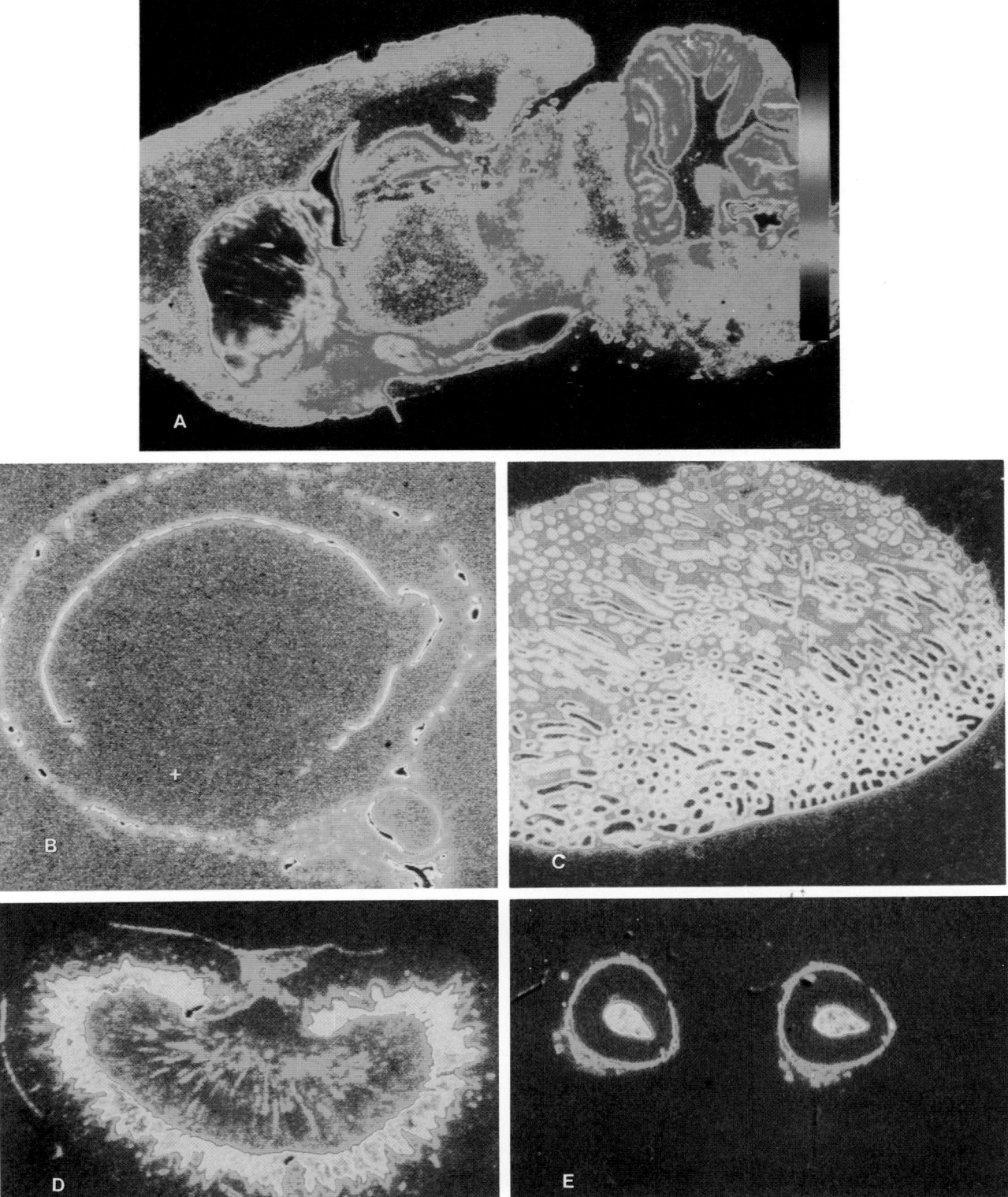

FIG. 4. Computer-generated pseudo-color images of ACE distribution in the rat brain (**A**), dog aorta (**B**), rat testis (**C**), rat kidney (**D**), and rat adrenals (**E**).

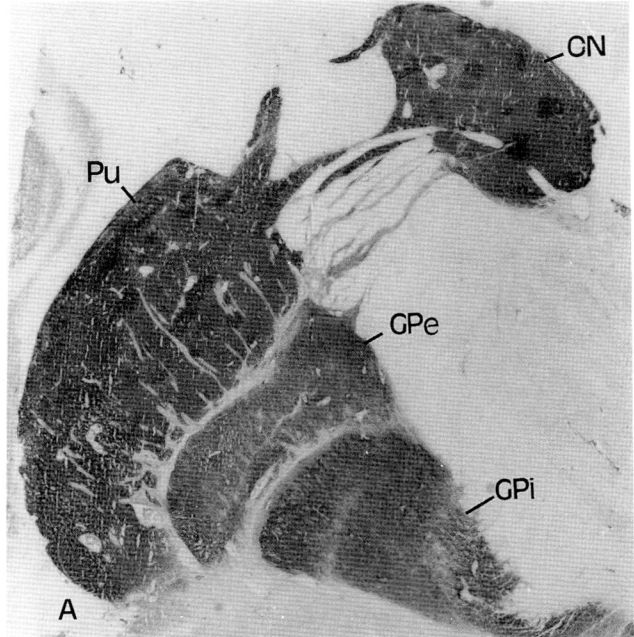

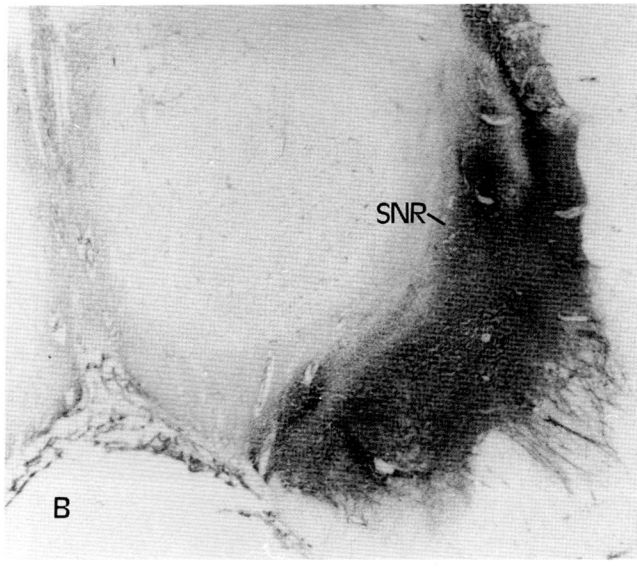

FIG. 5. ACE distribution in the human basal ganglia; striatum (**A**) and substantia nigra (**B**). CN, caudate nucleus; GPe, external globus pallidus; GPi, internal globus pallidus; Pu, putamen; SNR, substantia nigra pars reticulata.

Kidney and Adrenal

The kidney was the first tissue where ACE was demonstrated in nonendothelial cells. ACE occurs in high concentrations in epithelial cells lining the brush border of the proximal tubules (Fig. 4D). In addition to the well-known effects of angiotensin II in the regulation of renal blood flow and glomerular filtration rate, the peptide also exerts a biphasic response on tubular sodium reabsorp-

tion (39). Although circulating angiotensin II is probably the main contributor to the more traditional renal effects of the peptide, there is evidence that intrarenally formed angiotensin II may regulate some renal function (40), particularly in the proximal tubules where high concentrations of angiotensin II have been demonstrated (41). Further support for a physiological role of angiotensin II on sodium reabsorption is the finding that treatment of patients with chronic heart or renal failure with ACE inhibitors results in diuresis and natriuresis.

In the rat and human adrenal, ACE is present throughout the medulla (Fig. 4E). In the rat it is associated with the plasma membrane of chromaffin cells (42,43). In the cortex, ACE is found in the vasculature of the capsule. Hypophysectomy in rats markedly increases ACE in the adrenal medulla, an effect which is not regulated by glucocorticoids (42). Angiotensin II stimulates aldosterone production in many species of mammals, glucocorticoid secretion in some, and adrenal medullary catecholamine release in all species examined (44,45). Receptors for angiotensin II have also been found in the zona glomerulosa and medulla (46). In view of the multiple actions of angiotensin II in the adrenal, ACE may have an important role in the regulation of the local synthesis of the peptide.

Reproductive Systems

In the rat testis, extremely high concentrations of ACE have been demonstrated in mature spermatid heads and in the lumen of seminiferous tubules (Fig. 4C). In the epididymis, ACE occurs in the lumen and on the lumenal surface of epithelial cells (47). The enzymes from the above locations were found to be of the testicular isozyme except for the epithelial ACE which was of the somatic form. High levels of ACE are also present in the seminal fluid (48). The presence of ACE in association with spermatozoa in the seminiferous tubules suggests a role for the enzyme in sperm development. Further support for this is the finding of increased ACE activity following spermatogenesis initiation (49). There is conflicting evidence concerning the effect of ACE on sperm motility (50,51) although the gradient of increasing enzyme levels along the epididymis correlated with increased sperm motility and viability (49).

In the rat ovary, ACE is present in the corpus luteum, granulosa cells in some follicles, and on the germinal epithelium (52,53). The concentration of ACE is increased following maturity of the follicles (53).

Gastrointestinal Tract

In the rat and human small intestines, ACE is present in high concentrations on the epithelial cells lining the brush border (54,55) where it is solely located on the plasmalemmal membrane (56). The function of ACE in this site is not known although the enzyme is able to metabolize small peptides presumably to reduce their sizes to aid absorption (57).

ACE has also been demonstrated in the fundic mucosa of the rabbit stomach where it is found intracellularly in granules in the neck and chief cells in contrast to other sites in which ACE is an ectoenzyme (58).

FUNCTIONAL ROLE

Despite its lack of substrate specificity *in vitro*, the primary function of ACE *in vivo* is the synthesis of angiotensin II and probably a role in bradykinin degradation. Although the contribution of the circulating renin-angiotensin system in the regulation of blood pressure and fluid and electrolyte homeostasis is well studied, the role of endogenous tissue angiotensin systems is not fully understood. Many components of the renin-angiotensin system have been localized in association with ACE in the blood vessels, heart, and brain. However, high concentrations of ACE also occur in the epithelial cells of the gastrointestinal and reproductive tracts and choroid plexus and in fibroblasts and differentiated macrophages, which suggests more extensive physiological roles for ACE than the synthesis of angiotensin II. It is possible that tissue ACE provides an additional mechanism and step controlling the rate of formation of angiotensin II in the interstitial compartment of peripheral tissues.

Cardiovascular System

Various components of the renin-angiotensin system have been demonstrated in blood vessels (Table 3) where angiotensin II has multiple actions. Renin, angiotensinogen, ACE, and angiotensin II receptors have all been

TABLE 3. *Components of the renin-angiotensin system in the blood vessels*

Endothelial cell	Angiotensinogen
	Angiotensinogen mRNA
	Renin (?)
	ACE
	Angiotensin II receptors
Smooth muscle	Angiotensinogen
	Angiotensinogen mRNA
	Renin
	ACE (?)
	Angiotensin II receptors
	Angiotensinogen (perivascular
Adventitia	fat)
	ACE (vasa vasorum)

demonstrated in cultured aortic smooth muscle and endothelial cells (59). More recently, angiotensinogen mRNA has been demonstrated in vascular smooth muscle, endothelium, and perivascular fat (60) although renin mRNA cannot be detected (61). The decline of vascular renin activity after bilateral nephrectomy suggests the uptake of renin from the circulation (62). Despite the absence of renin mRNA, local formation of angiotensin II in the rat hindlimb vasculature which is dependent on circulating renin has been demonstrated (63).

Local formation of angiotensin II in the interstitium of blood vessels controlled by tissue ACE may provide further regulation of regional blood flow.

In addition to its direct action on the vascular smooth muscles, angiotensin II stimulates release of prostaglandin and nitric oxide from the endothelial cells (64). Moreover, angiotensin II may act as a mitogen to stimulate hyperplasia and hypertrophy (65). Further evidence in support of the involvement of the vascular renin-angiotensin system in vascular hypertrophy and neointimal hyperplasia is discussed in the section entitled Hypertrophy and Remodeling.

Angiotensin II is also known to facilitate release of noradrenaline and prevent its reuptake from sympathetic nerve terminals (66). Therefore, another role for the local angiotensin system may be to modulate vascular sympathetic activity.

All the components of the renin-angiotensin system have been demonstrated in the heart. Angiotensinogen mRNA is more abundant in the atria than ventricles (67) as is ACE (68). Angiotensin II receptors are found in high concentrations in the atrioventricular node, in the intracardiac ganglia, and over parasympathetic nerve bundles in the rat heart (69). Angiotensin II has direct inotropic and chronotropic actions in the heart (45) and also facilitates sympathetic nerve activity (70) and decreases vagal tone (71). Similar to the blood vessels, angiotensin II is also postulated to have growth-modulating effects in the heart. The possible role of an intrinsic cardiac renin-angiotensin system in ventricular hypertrophy and remodeling is discussed under Hypertrophy and Remodeling.

Central Nervous System

Angiotensin II has many actions in the brain including stimulation of drinking, regulation of autonomic function, modulation of pituitary hormone release, and possibly facilitation of monoamine release (72). All components of the renin-angiotensin system have been demonstrated in the brain although the presence of renin has been disputed (Table 4).

Angiotensin II-like immunoreactivity (38), angiotensin II receptors (37) and angiotensin converting enzyme

TABLE 4. *Components of the renin-angiotensin system in the brain*

Angiotensinogen	Neurons, glial cells
Angiotensinogen mRNA	Predominantly glial cells
Renin	(?)
ACE	Cerebral vasculature
	Neurons, epithelial cells
Angiotensin II receptors	Neurons, others (?)

(33) exist in many brain regions which are thought to be important for central pressor and dipsogenic effects and modulation of pituitary hormone release. These sites, which include the forebrain circumventricular organs and paraventricular hypothalamic nucleus, are responsive to locally applied angiotensin II (73,74). Similarly, in the hindbrain, various components of the angiotensin system occur in the dorsal vagal complex and in the ventrolateral medulla, sites involved in the baroreflex control of cardiovascular and other autonomic function which are also responsive to angiotensin II (75–77). In these brain structures, the high densities of angiotensin II receptors and moderate to high levels of ACE are conserved across the different species of mammals studied.

Although ACE and angiotensinogen are both present in the rat basal ganglia (33,78,79), angiotensin II receptors cannot be demonstrated. This led to the hypothesis that ACE may be involved in the processing of other neuropeptides. However, in the human basal ganglia, high concentrations of angiotensin II receptors have been detected in association with the dopaminergic projections from the substantia nigra to the striatum (80). Exogenous angiotensin II has been shown to stimulate dopamine release and endogenous angiotensin II to tonically regulate its release from these neurons (81). This strongly suggests a previously unsuspected physiological role for angiotensin II in the basal ganglia. ACE, however, is present in neurons arising from the striatum which projects to the globus pallidus and substantia nigra.

The existence of ACE in brain regions not enriched with angiotensin supports alternative roles for the enzyme in the degradation of other neuropeptides.

REGULATION AND DISEASE STATES

Although renin is considered the rate-limiting enzyme in the cascade, there is little doubt that ACE is an important enzyme in the formation of angiotensin II since the conversion of angiotensin I to angiotensin II can be totally prevented in all peripheral vascular beds by ACE inhibitors. The catalytic properties and the tissue distribution of the enzyme are well studied but not much is understood about the regulation of the enzyme or its gene. Endothelial cell ACE is increased by glucocorticoids (82) and the expression of testicular ACE is under

the control of pituitary hormones and androgens (83). These observations were confirmed by the finding of glucocorticoid and steroid responsive elements in the somatic and testicular regulatory regions respectively of the ACE gene.

Plasma ACE is increased in some inflammatory states particularly sarcoidosis where the elevated enzyme level is due to excessive production of ACE in the activated macrophages (84). Plasma ACE is also induced after treatment with ACE inhibitors although ACE in most other tissues except the lung remains unchanged (85,86). Angiotensin II levels or salt status appears to have little effect on plasma or tissue ACE concentrations.

Hypertension

The renin-angiotensin system plays a very important role in the control of blood pressure. The circulating renin-angiotensin system responds rapidly to changes in fluid balance, blood pressure, and blood flow with angiotensin II acting on peripheral and central receptors to provide immediate hemodynamic stability. In contrast, the tissue renin-angiotensin systems, particularly in the blood vessels and heart, are thought to be more involved in the maintenance of tissue structure and function thereby providing long-term regulation of blood pressure.

Although a defective vascular renin-angiotensin system has been implicated in the development of hypertension, the evidence is far from conclusive due to conflicting reports on the changes in vascular ACE levels in the spontaneously hypertensive rat and in the two-kidney, one-clip Goldblatt hypertensive rat (87–89). In the one-kidney, one-clip Goldblatt hypertensive rat, an experimental model of hypertension with normal renin levels, increases in ACE were consistently found in the mesenteric vessels and in the heart (89) with no change in the plasma enzyme levels. The brain angiotensin system is also thought to be modified in hypertensive states (90). Whether these reported changes are the cause of the hypertension or the consequence of the disease has not been delineated.

The possible association between abnormalities in ACE levels and blood pressure has been demonstrated in spontaneously hypertensive rats. Short-term treatment of these rats during the critical period prior to the development of hypertension with an ACE inhibitor delayed or prevented the rise in blood pressure long after the treatment was discontinued (91). Moreover, it has been reported that the gene for blood pressure cosegregates with the portion of the genome that contains the ACE gene (92,93). Although suggestive, this observation is not conclusive since an unrelated gene in close proximity to the ACE gene could equally well be linked to the hypertensive trait.

Hypertrophy and Remodeling

There is some evidence that local tissue renin-angiotensin systems may be involved in vascular and cardiac hypertrophy. Angiotensin II has been shown to stimulate hyperplasia and hypertrophy in cultured smooth muscle cells and induce release of platelet-derived growth factor. It also has the ability to activate the proto-oncogenes c-fos and c-myc (65).

In the rat carotid artery, the myointimal proliferation that follows denudation of the endothelium could be abolished by treatment with an ACE inhibitor (94). Moreover, denudation of the endothelium results in an initial fall in vascular ACE levels followed by an increase (95). ACE mRNA is also increased in the proliferating tissue (96). However, clinical trials on the prevention of restenosis after coronary angioplasty have failed to demonstrate any benefit.

The association of angiotensin II with cardiac hypertrophy has been reinforced by the observation that ACE mRNA is increased in the hypertrophied ventricle following aortic banding in rats (97). In similar experiments, pretreatment with an ACE inhibitor caused significant regression of the ventricular hypertrophy even at a dose that did not lower blood pressure (98). In contrast, in the spontaneously hypertensive rats, the beneficial effects of ACE inhibitors in preventing ventricular hypertrophy were shown to be related to the blood-pressure-lowering effects of these drugs (99). Increases in cardiac ACE are well correlated with increases in left-ventricular weight in the Goldblatt one-kidney, one-clip experimental model of hypertension (100). A close correlation has also been demonstrated between left ventricular weight and left ventricular angiotensin II levels in spontaneously hypertensive rats (101). However, left ventricular hypertrophy is a more complex process than just an increase in ventricular size or number of cells and may involve restructuring of collagen and supporting elastic fibers (102).

In experimental myocardial infarction in rats obtained by occlusion of the left coronary artery, the remaining cardiac tissue undergoes marked hypertrophy and remodeling which is associated with increases in myocardial ACE (103) and angiotensin II receptors. Treatment with ACE inhibitors suppresses cardiac ACE with resulting regression in cardiac hypertrophy and improved survival (103).

Inflammation

It is well known that serum ACE is elevated in some inflammatory states, particularly in sarcoidosis. This increase is attributed to increased enzyme activity in granulomas (104). ACE is also induced when monocytes are differentiated into macrophages (105) and has been demonstrated on T-lymphocytes. More recently, ACE has been shown to be increased in the necrotic myocardium and in scar tissues following acute myocardial infarction. In addition, ACE is reported to be involved in neointimal hyperplasia after denudation of the endothelium (94). Angiotensinogen is known to be an acute-phase protein. These observations taken together suggest that ACE may play a role in the inflammatory response and be involved in the repair of tissues following damage.

Moreover, substrates of ACE have been shown to be involved in inflammation. Bradykinin which regulates the hyperemic response and increases capillary permeability, substance P which is an important mediator of pain, and a chemotactic peptide N-formyl-Met-Leu-Phe which is involved in inflammation (106) can all be inactivated by ACE.

INHIBITION BY ACE INHIBITORS

ACE inhibitors are important therapeutic agents in the treatment of cardiovascular disease. Although it was initially thought that their antihypertensive actions were due to the blockade of formation of circulating angiotensin II, several lines of evidence suggest that their blood-pressure-lowering effects are also the result of a series of actions at the tissue level. First, there is a lack of association between the time course of plasma ACE inhibition and the ACE inhibitor–induced fall in blood pressure. Moreover, during the chronic stages of the drug administration, the blood pressure reduction is not associated with similar falls in plasma renin or angiotensin II levels. The hypotensive effect of these inhibitors also does not correlate with the renin status of the different forms of hypertension, being effective in renin-dependent and nonrenin-dependent hypertensive states.

As demonstrated in rat studies, most tissue ACE is susceptible to blockade by an oral dose of ACE inhibitor except for the testicular isozyme which appears to be protected by a blood-testis barrier (107–109). The inhibition of brain ACE, on the other hand, is highly dependent on its locality, the dose regime, and the lipophilicity of the drug used. ACE in the circumventricular organs, not within the blood-brain barrier, is readily inhibited whereas the enzyme present in neurons is only blocked by high doses of the more lipophilic drugs (110). The time course of the blood-pressure-lowering effect of the ACE inhibitors more closely parallels that of the inhibition of tissue ACE than of blockade of plasma ACE levels. This provides further support for the hypothesis that inhibition of tissue ACE may account for the chronic blood-pressure-lowering effect of the ACE inhibitors. Apart from the brain and testis, ACE inhibitors appear to inhibit tissue ACE in a dose- and time-dependent manner to similar proportions across tissues. Furthermore, the binding affinity and dissociation rate of the inhibitors from tissue ACE vary and determine their pharmacokinetics and hence dosing frequency.

CONCLUSIONS

ACE is a widely distributed enzyme. In most sites (endothelial and epithelial), it is a membrane-bound ectoenzyme and may therefore control the formation of circulating and interstitial angiotensin II concentration. Its physiological role in many sites (brain, reproductive and gastrointestinal tracts) is not known. In the cardiovascular system, it probably provides a secondary control mechanism for regulating the concentration of angiotensin II in peripheral tissues. Here it could serve a number of important cardiovascular functions, including regulation of peripheral regional blood flow, modulation of local sympathetic activity as well as stimulation of growth and hypertrophy and thus cardiovascular structure. The beneficial effects of ACE inhibitors in cardiovascular disease may be due both to their favorable hemodynamic effects and to their inhibition of local tissue ACE.

ACKNOWLEDGMENTS

Studies by the authors are supported by grants from the National Health and Medical Research Council and National Heart Foundation of Australia. Siew Yeen Chai is a National Health and Medical Research Council Australian Postdoctoral Fellow.

REFERENCES

1. Hooper NM, Keen J, Pappin DJC, Turner AJ. *Biochem J* 1987;247:85–93.
2. Soubrier F, Alhenc-Gelas F, Hubert C, et al. *Proc Natl Acad Sci (USA)* 1988;85:9386–9390.
3. Kumar RS, Kusari J, Roy SN, Soffer RL, Sen GC. *J Biol Chem* 1989;264:16754–16758.
4. Das M, Hartley JL, Soffer RL. *J Biol Chem* 1977;252:1316–1319.
5. Bernstein KE, Martin BM, Edwards AS, Bernstein EA. *J Biol Chem* 1989;264:11945–11951.
6. Hubert C, Houot AM, Corvol P, Soubrier F. *J Biol Chem* 1991;266:15377–15383.
7. Rigat B, Hubert C, Alhenc-Gelas F, Cambien F, Corvol P, Soubrier F. *J Clin Invest* 1990;86:1343–1346.
8. Riordan JF, Chen YNP, Kleeman SG, Bunning P. *Biomed Biochem Acta* 1991;50:809–814.
9. Bunning P, Riordan JF. *J Inorg Biochem* 1985;24:183–198.
10. Schullek JP, Wilson JB. *Arch Biochem Biophys* 1988;265:346–350.
11. Bunning P, Riordan JF. *Biochemistry* 1983;22:110–116.
12. Wei L, Alhenc-Gelas F, Corvol P, Clauser E. *J Biol Chem* 1991;266:9002–9008.
13. Perich RB, Jackson B, Attwood MR, Prior K, Johnston CI. *Pharm Pharmacol Lett* 1991;1:41–43.
14. Perich RB, Jackson B, Rogerson FM, Mendelsohn FAO, Paxton D, Johnston CI. *Mol Pharmacol* 1992;420:280–293.
15. Skidgel RA, Defendini R, Erdos EG. In: Turner AJ, ed. *Neuropeptides and their peptidases.* Chichester, U.K.: Ellis Horwood, 1987;165–182.
16. Strittmatter SM, Thiele EA, Kapiloff MS, Snyder SH. *J Biol Chem* 1985;260:9825–9832.
17. Patey G, De La Baume S, Schwartz JC, et al. *Science* 1981;212:1153–1155.
18. Gillespie MN, Krechniak JW, Crooks PA, Altiere RJ, Olson JW. *J Pharmacol Exp Ther* 1985;232:675–681.
19. Shibanoki S, Weinberger SB, Beniston D, et al. *J Pharmacol Exp Ther* 1991;256:650–655.
20. Skidgel RA, Erdos EG. *Proc Natl Acad Sci (USA)* 1985;82:1025–1029.
21. Ehlers MRW, Riordan JF. *Biochemistry* 1991;30:7118–7126.
22. Urata H, Healy B, Stewart RW, Bumpus M, Husain A. *Circ Res* 1990;66:883–890.
23. Schalekamp MADH. *J Hypertens* 1991;9s6:S10–S17.
24. Skeggs JT, Kahn JR, Shumway NP. *J Exp Med* 1956;103:295–299.
25. Caldwell PRB, Seegal BC, Hsu KC, Das M, Soffer RL. *Science* 1976;191:1050–1051.
26. Wilson SK, Lynch DR, Snyder SH. *J Clin Invest* 1987;80:841–851.
27. Yamada H, Fabris B, Allen AM, Jackson B, Johnston CI, Mendelsohn FAO. *Circ Res* 1991;68:141–149.
28. Rogerson FM, Schlawe I, Chai SY, Murray WK, Marley PD, Mendelsohn FAO. *J Hypertens* 1992;10:615–620.
29. Saye JA, Singer HA, Peach MJ. *Hypertension* 1984;6:216–221.
30. Story DF, Ziogas J. *Br J Pharmacol* 1986;87:249–255.
31. Jandeleit K, Jackson B, Perich R, Paxton D, Johnston CI. *Clin Exp Pharmacol Physiol* 1991;18:353–356.
32. Zhuo J, Allen AM, Yamada H, Sun Y, Mendelsohn FAO. In: Lindpaintner K, Ganten D, eds. *The cardiac renin-angiotensin system.* New York: Futura Medical Publishers (In press).
33. Chai SY, Mendelsohn FAO, Paxinos G. *Neuroscience* 1987;20:615–627.
34. Pickel VM, Chan J, Ganten D. *J Neurosci* 1986;6:2457–2469.
35. Chai SY, McKenzie JS, McKinley MJ, Mendelsohn FAO. *J Comp Neurol* 1990;291:179–194.
36. Mendelsohn FAO, Allen AM, Chai SY, McKinley MJ, Oldfield BJ, Paxinos G. *Trends in Endocrinol Metab* 1990;1:189–198.
37. Mendelsohn FAO, Quirion R, Saavedra JM, Aguilera G, Catt KJ. *Proc Natl Acad Sci (USA)* 1984;81:1575–1579.
38. Lind RW, Swanson LW, Ganten D. *Neuroendocrinol* 1985;40:2–24.
39. Harris PJ, Young JA. *Pflueg Arch* 1977;367:295–297.
40. Levens NR, Peach MJ, Carey RM. *Circ Res* 1981;48:157–167.
41. Braam B, Mitchell KD, Fox J, Navar LG. *Am J Physiol* 1983;33:F891–F898.
42. Strittmatter SM, De Souza EB, Lynch DR, Snyder SH. *Endocrinol* 1986;118:1690–1699.
43. Gonzalez-Garcia C, Keiser HR. *J Hypertens* 1990;8:433–441.
44. Kaplan NM. *J Clin Invest* 1965;44:2029–2039.
45. Peach MJ. *Physiol Rev* 1977;57:313–370.
46. Mendelsohn FAO. *J Hypertens* 1985;3:307–316.
47. Strittmatter SM, Snyder SH. *Endocrinol* 1984;115:2332–2341.
48. El-Dorry HA, MacGregor JS, Soffer RL. *Biochem Biophys Acta* 1983;115:1096–1100.
49. Jaiswal AK, Panda JN, Kumar MV, Singh LN. *Andrologia* 1983;15:347–349.
50. Mizutani T, Schill WB. *Andrologia* 1985;17:150–157.
51. Krassnigg F, Niederhauser H, Placzek R, Frick J, Schill WB. *Adv Exp Med Biol* 1986;198:477–485.
52. Speth RC, Husain A. *Biol Reprod* 1988;38:695–702.
53. Daud AI, Bumpus FM, Husain A. *Endocrinol* 1990;126:2927–2935.
54. Takada Y, Unno M, Hiwada K, Kokubu T. *Clin Sci* 1981;61:253s–256s.
55. Duggan KA, Mendelsohn FAO, Levens NR. *Am J Physiol* 1989;257:G504–G510.
56. Bruneval P, Hinglais N, Alhenc-Gelas F, et al. *Histochemistry* 1986;85:73–80.
57. Yoshioka M, Erickson RH, Woodley JF, Gulli R, Guan D, Kim YS. *Am J Physiol* 1987;253:G781–G786.
58. Laliberte F, Laliberte MF, Nonotte I, Bali JP, Chevillard C. *J Histochem Cytochem* 1991;39:1519–1529.
59. Dzau VJ. *J Hypertens* 1989;7:933–936.

60. Naftilan AJ, Zuo WM, Ingelfinger J, Ryan TJ, Pratt RE, Dzau VJ. *J Clin Invest* 1991;87:1300–1311.
61. Ekker M, Tronik D, Rougeon F. *Proc Natl Acad Sci (USA)* 1989;86:5155–5158.
62. Thurston H, Swales JD, Bing RF, Hurst BC, Marks ES. *Hypertension* 1979;1:643–649.
63. Hilgers KF, Mann JFE. *Arzneim-Forsch* 1993;43:198–201.
64. Mombouli JV, Nephtali M, Vanhoutte PM. *Hypertension* 1991;18:11–22.
65. Schelling P, Fischer H, Ganten D. *J Hypertens* 1991;9:3–15.
66. Ziogas J, Story DF, Rand MJ. *Clin Exp Pharmacol Physiol* 1984;11:314–318.
67. Lindpaintner K, Jin M, Niedermeyer N, Wilhelm MJ, Ganten D. *Circ Res* 1990;67:564–570.
68. Fabris B, Jackson B, Cubela R, Mendelsohn FAO, Johnston CI. *Clin Exp Pharmacol Physiol* 1989;16:309–316.
69. Allen AM, Yamada H, Mendelsohn FAO. *Int J Cardiol* 1990;28:25–33.
70. Ziogas J, Story DF, Rand MJ. *Eur J Pharmacol* 1984;106:11–18.
71. Lumbers ER, McCloskey DI, Potter EK. *J Physiol* 1979;294:69–80.
72. Phillips MI. *Ann Rev Physiol* 1987;49:413–435.
73. Harding JW, Felix D. *Brain Res* 1987;410:130–134.
74. Mangiapane ML, Simpson JB. *Neuroendocrinol* 1980;31:380–384.
75. Casto R, Phillips MI. *Am J Physiol* 1986;250:R193–R198.
76. Allen AM, Dampney RAL, Mendelsohn FAO. *Am J Physiol* 1988;255:H1011–H1017.
77. Allen AM, Mendelsohn FAO, Gieroba ZJ, Blessing WW. *J Neuroendocrinol* 1990;2:867–873.
78. Thomas WG, Sernia C. *Neuroscience* 1988;25:319–341.
79. Bunnemann B, Fuxe K, Ganten D. In: Fuxe K, Agnati L, eds. *Volume transmission in the brain: novel mechanisms for neural transmission.* New York: Raven Press; 1991:131–158.
80. Allen AM, Paxinos G, McKinley MJ, Chai SY, Mendelsohn FAO. *J Comp Neurol* 1991;312:291–298.
81. Mendelsohn FAO, Jenkins T, Berkovic S. *Brain Res* 1994 (In press).
82. Mendelsohn FAO, Lloyd CJ, Kachel C, Funder JW. *Clin Exp Pharmacol Physiol* 1982;7:57–62.
83. Velletri PA, Aquilano DR, Bruckwick E, Tsai-Morris CH, Dufau ML, Lovenberg W. *Endocrinol* 1985;116:2516–2522.
84. Pertzchuk LP, Silverstein E, Friedland J. *Am J Clin Pathol* 1981;75:350–354.
85. Fyhrquist F, Forslund T, Tikkanen I, Gronhagen-Riska C. *Eur J Pharmacol* 1980;67:473–475.
86. Kohzuki M, Johnston CI, Chai SY, et al. *J Hypertension* 1991;9:579–587.
87. Okamura R, Miyazaki M, Inagami T, Toda N. *Hypertension* 1986;8:560–565.
88. Morishita R, Higaki J, Okunishi H, et al. *J Hypertens* 1991;9:187–192.
89. Jandeleit K, Perich R, Jackson B, Johnston CI. *Clin Exp Pharmacol Physiol* 1992;19:348–352.
90. Saavedra JM, Correa FM, Kurihai M, Shigematsu K. *J Hypertens* 1986;4:s27–s30.
91. Giudicelli JF, Freslon JL, Glasson S, Richer C. *Clin Exp Hypertens* 1980;2A:1083–1096.
92. Hilbert P, Lindpaintner K, Beckmann JS, et al. *Nature* 1991;353:521–528.
93. Jacob HE, Lindpaintner K, Beckmann JS, et al. *Cell* 1991;67:213–224.
94. Powell JS, Clozel JP, Muller RKM, et al. *Science* 1989;245:186–188.
95. Johnston CI, Jandeleit K, Mooser V, et al. *J Cardiovasc Pharmacol* 1994 (In press).
96. Dzau VJ, Gibbons GH, Pratt RE. *Hypertension* 1991;18(Suppl II):II100–II105.
97. Schunkert H, Dzau VJ, Tan SS, Hirsch AT, Apstein CS, Lorell BH. *J Clin Invest* 1990;86:1913–1920.
98. Linz W, Scholkens BA, Ganten D. *Clin Exp Hypertens* 1989;A11:1325–1350.
99. Mooser V, Katopothis A, Harrap SB, Johnston CI. In: Sassard J, ed. *Genetic hypertension.* Paris: Colloques Inserm Series 218, Libbey Eurotext; 1992:253–255.
100. Jandeleit K, Johnston CI, Hiettierachichi M, Paxton D, Perich R, Jackson B. In: MacGregor GA, Sever PS, eds. *Current advances in ACE inhibition.* London: Churchill Livingstone; 1991:230–233.
101. Nagano J, Higaki J, Mikami H, et al. *J Hypertens* 1991;9:595–599.
102. Weber KT, Janicki JS. *Br J Clin Pharmacol* 1989;28:141s–150s.
103. Johnston CI, Mooser V, Sun Y, Fabris B. *Clin Exp Pharmacol Physiol* 1990;18:107–110.
104. Weinstock JV. *Sarcoidosis* 1986;3:19–26.
105. Friedland J, Setton C, Silverstein J. *Biochem Biophys Res Commun* 1978;83:843–849.
106. Erdos EG. *Hypertension* 1990;16:363–370.
107. Sakaguchi K, Chai SY, Jackson B, Johnston CI, Mendelsohn FAO. *Neuroendocrinol* 1988;48:223–228.
108. Sakaguchi K, Chai SY, Jackson B, Johnston CI, Mendelsohn FAO. *Hypertension* 1988;11:230–238.
109. Sakaguchi K, Jackson B, Chai SY, Mendelsohn FAO, Johnston CI. *J Cardiovasc Pharmacol* 1988;12:710–727.
110. Chai SY, Perich R, Jackson B, Mendelsohn FAO, Johnston CI. *Clin Exp Pharmacol Physiol* 1992;19(Suppl 19):7–12.

Hypertension: Pathophysiology, Diagnosis, and Management, Second Edition,
edited by J.H. Laragh and B.M. Brenner,
Raven Press, Ltd., New York © 1995.

CHAPTER 102

Characteristics of Angiotensin II Receptors and Their Role in Cell and Organ Physiology

Marc de Gasparo, Serge Bottari, and Nigel R. Levens

THE RENIN-ANGIOTENSIN SYSTEM

The main components of the renin-angiotensin system (RAS) are shown in Fig. 1. Renin is an aspartic proteinase which is synthesized within modified smooth muscle cells of the renal afferent arteriole. The activity of the RAS is regulated mainly through variations in the secretion of renin by the kidney. Once released into the circulation, renin acts upon an $\alpha2$-macroglycoprotein, angiotensinogen, which is continuously synthesized and released from the liver. The first 10 amino acids of angiotensinogen represent angiotensin I (Ang I) which is released by the hydrolytic action of renin. Angiotensin I is converted to the octapeptide Ang II upon circulation through organs and in plasma, by the action of the predominantly endothelium-bound enzyme angiotensin-I-converting enzyme (ACE). Angiotensin II is rapidly hydrolyzed both in tissues and in blood to Ang III and a number of peptide fragments. All components of the RAS are dynamic in their expression, and there are feedback loops to coordinate their activity (1).

Angiotensin II is the main effector of the renin-angiotensin system, but certain peptide fragments particularly

Ang (2-8) (Ang III), and possibly Ang (1-7) and Ang (3-6) have biological activity (2). Localization of all components of the RAS and the demonstration of Ang II formation within tissues has led to the suggestion that Ang II may function not only as an endocrine hormone but also as an autocrine or paracrine factor (3–7).

Angiotensin II constricts vascular smooth muscle and enhances the activity of the sympathetic nervous system by increasing central sympathetic outflow and by enhancing the quantity of norepinephrine released from sympathetic nerve terminals per neural impulse. Angiotensin II also stimulates the release of norepinephrine and epinephrine from the adrenal medulla. Angiotensin II exerts antinatriuretic and antidiuretic effects in the kidney and promotes the release of vasopressin from the pituitary and aldosterone release from the adrenal glomerulosa. By a combination of these actions, the RAS plays a major role in the control of blood pressure and the extracellular fluid volume (see Fig. 1). In addition to effects on cardiovascular homeostasis, Ang II also has a role in the regulation of cerebral function and contributes to the control of cellular growth (8–13).

To produce changes in tissue function, Angiotensin II interacts with specific receptors on the surface of target cells. Ang II receptors are coupled to molecular mechanisms which are responsible for the generation of intracellular signals and which, in turn, produce the ultimate tissue response, i.e., contraction, secretion, or prolifera-

M. de Gasparo and N. R. Levens: Cardiovascular Research, CIBA-GEIGY, Basel CH 4002, Switzerland.

S. Bottari: Centre d'Etudes Nucleaires, INSERM U244, B. P. 85X, F-38041, Grenoble, France.

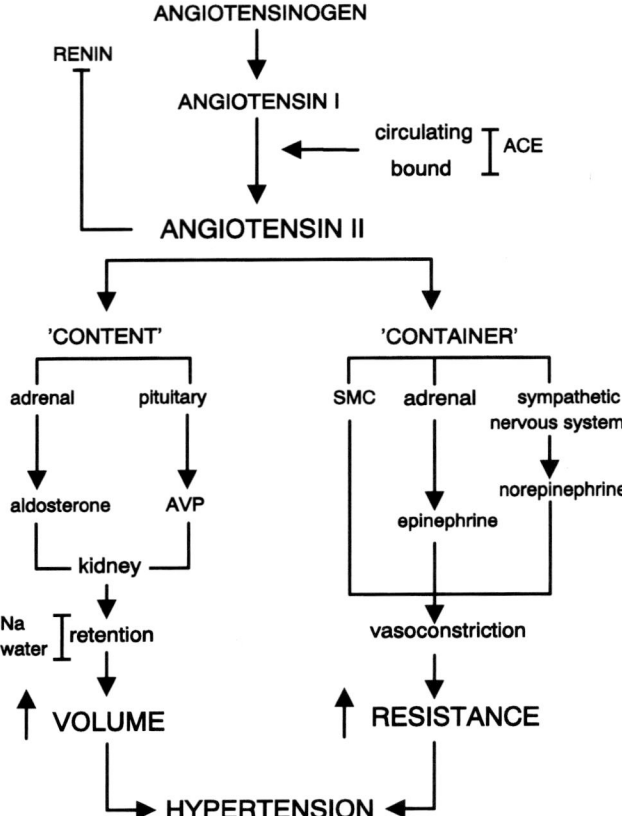

FIG. 1. Angiotensin II (Ang II) is one of the key hormones in the pathogeny of hypertension as it acts directly or indirectly on both the circulating fluid and the vascular tree. Angiotensin II has additional properties as it influences also gene regulation. The multiplicity of endocrine, paracrine, and autocrine effects of Ang II in a variety of tissues has led to the concept of Ang II receptor heterogeneity.

tion. The existence of Ang II receptor subtypes has been suggested by numerous studies conducted over the past 20 years (14,15). This hypothesis was initially based upon observations that the structure-activity relationship of Ang I, II, and III varied between tissues. Additional support for the existence of different receptor subtypes came also from the fact that certain ions, sulfhydryl reducing agents, and guanyl nucleotides exhibited differential effects on Ang II binding in different tissues. However, none of the early proposed classifications of Ang II receptor subtypes could be extended to more than a few tissues or species. The recent availability of new, highly modified peptide and nonpeptide ligands has allowed the characterization of at least two distinct Ang II receptor subtypes, called AT₁ and AT₂. The majority of the actions of Ang II can be described by an interaction of the peptide with either of these two receptor subtypes (16–19). However, it is also highly likely that additional receptor subtypes exist and that there are subclasses within the AT₁ and AT₂ receptor classification.

ANGIOTENSIN II RECEPTOR SUBTYPES

Eleven years after the synthesis of the peptide antagonist saralasin, the first nonpeptide compounds capable of blocking Ang II receptors were synthesized (20), and several new Ang II receptor subtype-specific ligands soon followed (Figs. 2, 3). The classification of Ang II receptors into two distinct subpopulations is based on the binding characteristics of these new ligands (19,21–25). For example, tetrazolbiphenylimidazoles represented by losartan and analogues (see Fig. 2) have a high affinity (5–50 nM) for the Ang II receptor in vascular smooth muscle cells (SMC) and liver membranes. In contrast, other ligands such as the pentapeptide Ang II analogue CGP 42112, and tetrahydroimidazopyridines such as PD 123177 and PD 123319 (see Fig. 3) display a much lower affinity (0.5 μM and >10 μM, respectively) (19,21,26,27). Angiotensin II receptors exhibiting these binding characteristics are referred to as AT₁ (28). In some tissues, such as human myometrium and bovine cerebellum, Ang II receptors bind CGP 42112, PD 123319, and PD 123177 with high affinity (<1 nM and 10–100 nM, respectively); whereas their affinity for losartan and related analogues is low (>1 μM) (19,29,30). Angiotensin II receptors having such binding characteristics are designated AT₂ (28). Examples of competition binding curves for Ang I, Ang II, Ang III and selective AT₁ and AT₂ ligands in vascular SMC and human myometrium are shown in Fig. 4.

The AT₁ Receptor

Angiotensin Peptide Binding

The AT₁ receptor binds the angiotensin family of peptides with the following order of potency: Ang II > Ang III > Ang I. Ang III has five- to tenfold lower affinity and Ang I, 1000-fold lower affinity than Ang II for the AT₁ receptor (31). The peptide breakdown products of Ang II, Ang (1-7) and Ang (3-8) also bind to the AT₁ receptor, but with low affinity. Peptide antagonists such as saralasin bind to the AT₁ receptor with an affinity greater or equal to that of Ang II (24).

Effect of Sulfhydril Reducing Agents

In many early binding studies, dithiothreitol (DTT) was used to prevent the breakdown of Ang II. However, it has recently been shown that DTT and other sulfhydryl-reducing agents inhibit the binding of Ang II to the AT₁ receptor (19,32). The observed decrease in affinity for Ang II after DTT treatment is probably secondary to disruption of the disulfide bridges between the cysteine residues present in each of the four extracellular loops of the receptor (33). Thus, studies where DTT has been

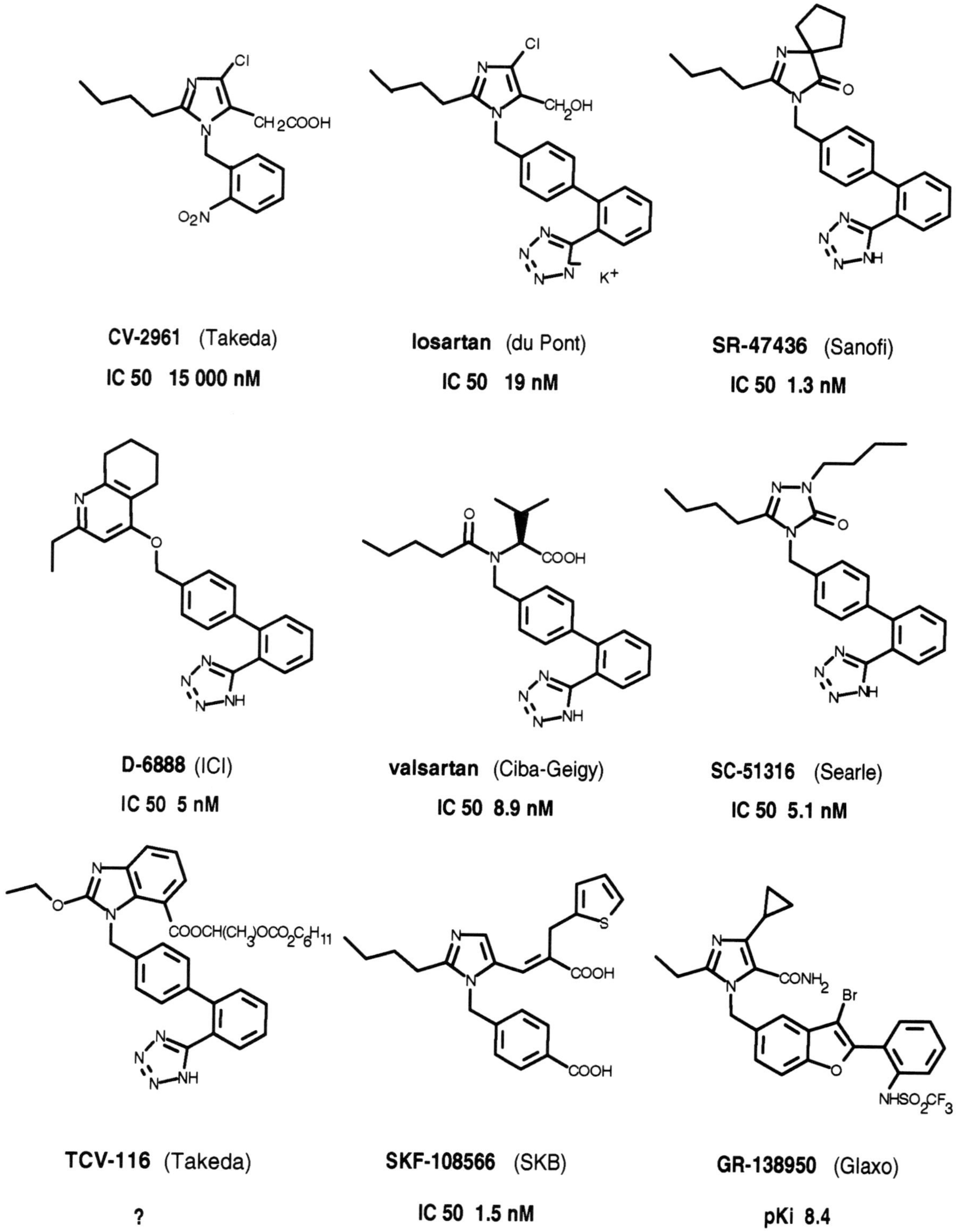

CV-2961 (Takeda)

IC 50 15 000 nM

losartan (du Pont)

IC 50 19 nM

SR-47436 (Sanofi)

IC 50 1.3 nM

D-6888 (ICI)

IC 50 5 nM

valsartan (Ciba-Geigy)

IC 50 8.9 nM

SC-51316 (Searle)

IC 50 5.1 nM

TCV-116 (Takeda)

?

SKF-108566 (SKB)

IC 50 1.5 nM

GR-138950 (Glaxo)

pKi 8.4

FIG. 2. Structure of some best-known nonpeptidic AT_1 antagonists derived from the early benzyl-imidazole-5-acetic acid of Takeda. Variations of all three basic structural features, i.e., imidazole, biphenyl, and acid functions of losartan have been claimed. These compounds are presently evaluated in human subjects. From Furukawa et al. (20), Buehlmayer (275), and Dudley and Hamby (276).

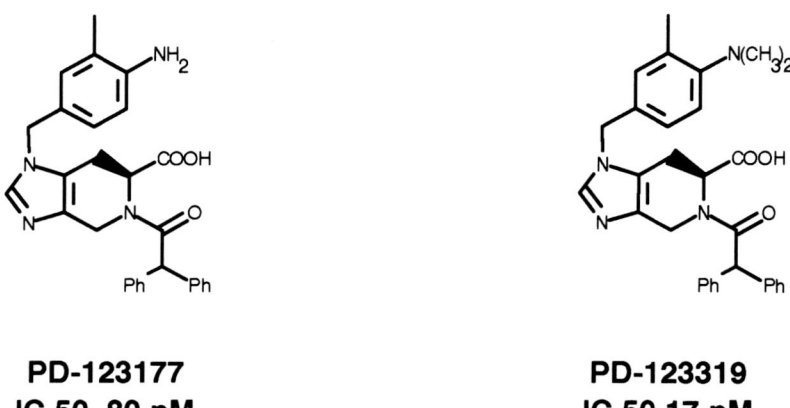

CGP42112
IC 50 0.21 nM

PD-123177
IC 50 80 nM

PD-123319
IC 50 17 nM

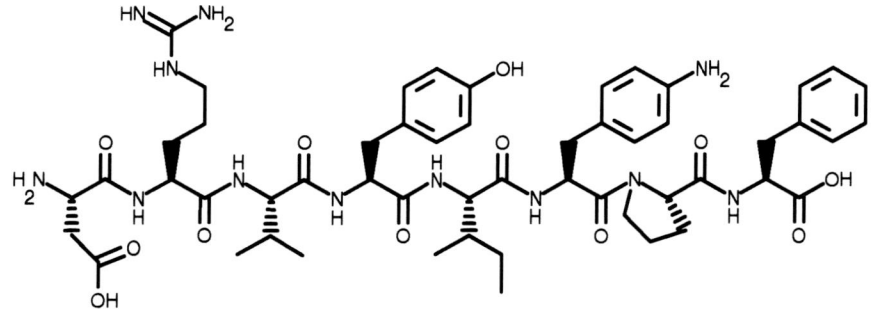

p-aminophenyl Ang II
IC 50 3.6 nM

FIG. 3. Structure of peptidic and nonpeptidic compounds with high affinity for the AT$_2$ receptor.

TABLE 1. *Distinctive properties of the AT_1 and AT_2 receptors*

Item	AT_1	AT_2	
Previous name	Ang II-1	Ang II-2	
	Ang II-α	Ang II-β	
	Ang II-B	Ang II-A	
Specific tissues	smooth muscle	human myometrium	
	liver	bovine cerebellum	
		ovarian follicles	
Potency order	Ang II > Ang III	Ang III $\geq$ Ang II	
Specific ligand	losartan (DuP 753)	CGP 42112	PD123177
pK$_i$ [^{125}I-Ang II]			
SMC	7.8	5.8	<4.3
h.myometrium	<4.3	9.8	7.1
Property	antagonist	agonist	antagonist
Effect of DTT	inhibition	in most cases: stimulation	
Effect of Na$^+$/Ca^{2+}	↑affinity for agonist	none	
Endocytosis	yes	no or doubtful	
Molecular weight (kDa)	40.9,58–79	41.3,49–52	
Isoelectric point	6.8	6.3	
Coupling mechanism	G-protein	phosphotyrosine phosphatase (?)	
Effectors	↑ PLC (Gq)	↓ cGMP	
	↓ CAMP (Gi)	↓ T-type Ca^{2+} current	
	ion channels (Go)	others ?	
Clone	AT_{1a}-AT_{1b}	AT_{2a}-AT_{26}	

SMC, smooth muscle cells; DTT, dithiothreitol; PLC, phospholipase C; cAMP, cyclic adenosine monophosphate; cGMP, cyclic guanosine monophasphate; ?,

used give an incomplete picture of Ang II binding, since the AT_1 receptor must be at least partially inactivated in these experiments. Interestingly, in contrast to Ang II, the binding of radioactive nonpeptidic ligands such as losartan is unaffected by disturbance of the disulfide bridges obtained by mutation of the Cys residues to Gly in the extracellular loop of the receptor (34).

Effects of Ions and pH

Various ions also affect Ang II binding to the AT_1 receptor. For example, sodium, magnesium, and calcium ions increase the affinity of the AT_1 receptor for *agonists* such as Ang II and Ang III, probably through an allosteric interaction with the receptor. In contrast, these ions do not affect the binding affinity of Ang II *antagonists* such as saralasin and losartan for the AT_1 receptor (35–37).

Low pH (6.8) appears to increase and high pH (8.0) to decrease Ang II binding to the AT_1 receptor. However, changes in pH primarily affect receptor number rather than receptor affinity (38).

Physicochemical Properties

The molecular weight of the AT_1 receptor was initially reported to be as high as 126 kDa (39). However, this is probably an overestimation of the true molecular weight, since chemical cross-linking of adjacent proteins to the receptor, or of G-protein subunits together with the hormone-receptor complex appear to have occurred in these experiments. More recently, polyacrylamide gel electrophoresis studies of solubilized AT_1 receptors from various tissues obtained from different species have revealed bands with molecular weights ranging from 58 to 79 kDa (39). The variations in molecular weight produced by the electrophoretic technique appear to be related to different degrees of glycosylation of the receptor, since enzymatic deglycosylation decreases the size of the AT_1 receptor in bovine and rat adrenal to 35 kDa.

The cDNA encoding for the 7-transmembrane domain AT_1 receptor isolated from rat vascular SMC or bovine adrenal encodes a protein of 359 amino-acid residues and a relative molecular mass of 40.9 kDa. This value is close to the molecular weight of the deglycosylated rat liver receptor measured by traditional photoaffinity labeling (40.7 kDa) and electrophoresis (35 kDa) (40,41).

Internalization

In rat aortic SMC, which express only the AT_1 receptor, 65 percent of radioactive Ang II is internalized at 21 degrees C ($t_{1/2}$ = 6 min). This phenomenon is attenuated by a covalent sulfhydryl-modifying agent phenylarsine oxide, and by cooling (42). After internalization, the Ang II receptor is reinserted into the plasma membrane ($t_{1/2}$ = approximately 15 min), thus preventing membrane receptor loss. Similar findings have been obtained using an Ang II-colloidal gold complex (43). The inter-

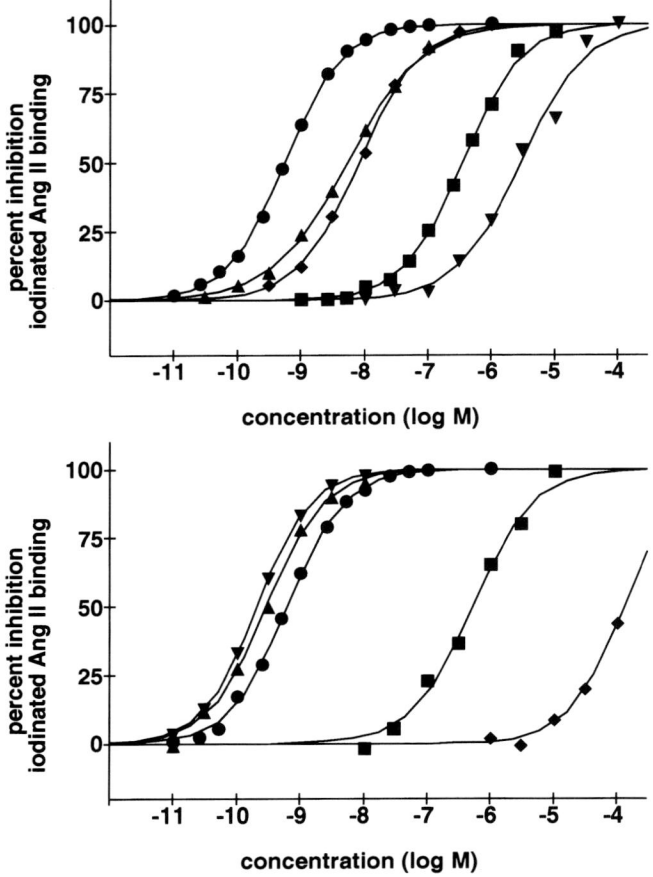

FIG. 4. Competition for [^{125}I]Ang II binding in rat vascular smooth muscle cells (AT$_1$, *upper panel*) and human myometrium (AT$_2$, *lower panel*) membrane particulates by Ang I (■), Ang II (●), Ang III (▲), valsartan (◆), and CGP 42112 (▼). The method has been described in {19}. The concentration of radioiodinated Ang II was 0.15 nM. The binding buffer contained 2 mg/mL bovine serum albumin. Ang I and Ang II do not distinguish the AT$_1$ and AT$_2$ receptors, whereas the affinity of Ang III for AT$_2$ is greater than for the AT$_1$ receptor. Valsartan {17} and CGP 42112 {19} bind preferentially to the AT$_1$ and AT$_2$ receptor, respectively.

nalization process in smooth muscle cells is blocked by losartan, confirming that it is an event mediated by the AT$_1$ receptor (43). Similarly, in neuroblastoma NIE-115 cells, Ang II downregulates 85 percent of the AT$_1$ receptors within 5 min at 37 degrees C. There is a rapid but incomplete recovery within 4 hours which involves receptor recycling and an 80-percent recovery by 18 hours that requires protein synthesis and new receptor formation (44).

Subtypes of AT$_1$ Receptors, Evidence from Binding Studies

There appears to be subtle differences between the binding properties of central and peripheral AT$_1$ receptors. Indeed, AT$_1$ receptors in the brain appear to be less

sensitive to DTT than their corresponding peripheral counterparts, and some reports have indicated a tenfold difference in affinity for Ang II between central and peripheral AT$_1$ receptors (45,46). The AT$_1$ receptor in the kidney has recently been subdivided into two subpopulations termed AT_{1a} and AT_{1b} (47). The AT$_{1a}$ receptor has a high affinity for losartan (K$_i$ 7.9 nM) whereas the AT$_{1b}$ receptor subtype demonstrates 100-fold lower affinity for losartan (K$_i$ 650 nM) but a 10,000-fold higher affinity for PD 123319 (K$_i$ 1.2 nM). The AT$_{1b}$ subtype, despite its high affinity for PD 123319, differs from the typical AT$_2$ subtype in having a low affinity for CGP 42112 (K$_i$ 1.4 μM) and being coupled to a G-protein. Functionally, the AT$_{1a}$ and AT$_{1b}$ receptor subtypes in the kidney are both linked to IP$_3$ generation, calcium mobilization and adenylate cyclase inhibition (48). The AT$_{1a}$ receptors also appear to mediate Ang-II-induced protein synthesis (49).

Subtypes of AT$_1$ Receptors, Evidence from Molecular Biology Techniques

In addition to the binding studies outlined above, molecular biology has provided strong evidence for AT$_1$ receptor heterogeneity in animals. For example, the AT$_1$ receptor expressed by *Xenopus* oocytes after inoculation with rat brain messenger ribonucleic acid (mRNA), discriminates poorly between Ang II and Ang III. This is in contrast to the AT$_1$ receptor expressed in this cell type after liver or pituitary mRNA inoculation which discriminates highly between Ang II and Ang III (50).

In rat adrenal, two clones encoding for different AT$_1$ receptor subtypes have been identified from genomic libraries (51–53). These AT$_1$ receptor clones, also termed AT_{1a} and AT_{1b}, bear little resemblance to the AT$_{1a}$ and AT$_{1b}$ receptor classification proposed from binding studies in rat kidney (47). The two rat adrenal clones, which have a 90-percent identity, differ in their amino-acid sequence, primarily in the last intracellular loop of the receptor. The AT$_{1a}$ gene, located on chromosome 17, is mainly expressed in rat vascular smooth muscle, in the rat kidney, and in rat lung. The AT$_{1b}$ gene, located on chromosome 2, is expressed in rat adrenal glomerulosa, pituitary, and liver (51). An additional cDNA, AT$_{1c}$, which is highly homologous to the AT$_{1a}$ and AT$_{1b}$ genes, has recently been identified in cultured rat vascular smooth muscle cells and in rat mesangium (54). Hybridization experiments using brain cDNA probes have also revealed the existence of additional mRNAs, suggesting differences between central and peripheral Ang II receptors (55). Interestingly, transfected COS-7 cells express both AT$_{1a}$ and AT$_{1b}$ receptors. When these cells are labeled with radioactive Ang II, solubilized, and the supernatant run on isoelectric focusing gels, a single peak of specific radioactivity (pI 6.8) is obtained (56). These results as well as the similar binding signature of the clones

(57) indicate that AT_{1a} and AT_{1b} receptors may actually be isoforms rather than specific subtypes of the AT_1 receptor. In contrast to the rat, only one single gene encoding for the AT_1 receptor has been reported so far in bovine and human tissues. Recently, however, a novel type of human AT has been cloned from placental CDHA library. It has identity with the receptor cloned from human heart CDHA and appears pharmacologically distinct (41,58–60).

The regulation of the expression of both AT_{1a} and AT_{1b} receptors differs. Angiotensin II downregulates AT_{1a} mRNA in vascular SMC but induces the upregulation of AT_{1b} mRNA in rat adrenal (61). Furthermore, bilateral nephrectomy is accompanied by a decreased expression of the AT_{1a} receptor in liver and by an increase of the AT_{1b} receptor in the adrenal (36). Treatment with adrenocorticotropic hormone (ACTH) or Ang II antagonists downregulates AT_{1b} mRNA in adrenal, whereas insulin upregulates it (33). These observations indicate that both receptor subtypes are regulated, but in opposite directions. It has been proposed that at least two pathways downregulate AT_1 mRNA in rat glomerular mesangial cells (62). One pathway is an Ang-II-induced, protein-kinase-C-independent but cycloheximide-sensitive pathway, indicating that it involves protein synthesis. The other is Ang-II-independent, induced by cyclic adenosine monophosphate (cAMP) but is cycloheximide-insensitive.

Are the AT_{1a} and AT_{1b} receptor subtypes pharmacologically and functionally different? Indeed, Ang III appears more potent when acting through the AT_{1b} receptor subtype than through the AT_{1a} receptor subtype. In addition, the dose-response curves for Ang-II-induced calcium mobilization differ between the two receptor subtypes (63). Moreover, the two subtypes seem differentially coupled to inhibition of adenylate cyclase, since ACTH-induced CAMP formation is inhibited by Ang II in adrenocortical tumor cells transfected with the AT_{1a}—but not the AT_{1b} receptors (64). Thus, although there appear to be some pharmacological differences between the two AT_1 receptor subtypes, there is so far no conclusive evidence indicating a difference in their functional roles.

Distribution of the AT_1 Receptor

The anatomical distribution of the AT_1 receptor has received considerable attention and conventional receptor binding methodology, as well as autoradiography, have been used to identify AT_1 receptors in several tissues from various species, including humans. Reports that have identified AT_1 receptors in somatic and brain tissues are summarized in Table 2. Some tissues express a nearly homogeneous population of AT_1 receptors, while others are characterized by a mixture of both the AT_1 and AT_2 receptor subtypes (6,24,65,66). In general, AT_1 receptors predominate in virtually all organs and tissues

involved in fluid-electrolyte balance and blood pressure regulation. Thus, the AT_1 receptor is found primarily in adrenals, vascular smooth muscle, kidney, and heart. AT_1 receptors are also present in specific brain areas such as the circumventricular organs, the hypothalamus, the suprachiasmatic nucleus, the supraoptic nucleus, the paraventricular nucleus, and the nucleus of the solitary tract which are implicated in the dipsogenic actions of Ang II, the release of vasopressin, and the neurogenic control of blood pressure (67,68).

Major differences exist in the distribution of AT_1 receptors between species (6,24). For example, bovine adrenal glomerulosa and human adrenal cortical cells express only AT_1 receptors; whereas rat, rabbit, and dog adrenal cortex exhibit both AT_1 and AT_2 receptors (19,21,69,70). In rat and rabbit kidney, only the AT_1 receptor is expressed, but both receptors are present in the kidney parenchyme of the rhesus monkey (71,72) and in the large cortical vessels of human kidney (73). Similar variations between species have been observed in the distribution of the AT_1 receptor in the brain. For example, human locus coeruleus, cerebellum, and the subthalamic nucleus express the AT_1 subtype, whereas the same brain areas of the rat contain mainly AT_2 receptors (46,74–80).

Similar species differences are found with regard to the relative proportion of AT_1 and AT_2 receptors in tissues where both receptors are expressed (24). Thus, in rabbit aorta, 90 percent of Ang II receptors are of the AT_1 receptor subtype, whereas in rat and monkey aorta, only 60 percent of the Ang II receptors are of the AT_1 subtype. Furthermore, rat heart differs from rabbit, monkey, and human heart in expressing over 90-percent AT_1 receptors (81–83). These observations indicate that a marked species variation exists in both the distribution and the proportion of the Ang II receptor.

The AT_1 Receptor-Signaling Mechanisms

G-proteins

The AT_1 receptor has been recently cloned and is a member of the 7-transmembrane domain, G-protein coupled receptor superfamily (40,41). The AT_1 receptor has been shown to be independently coupled through G-proteins (G_i and G_q) to a variety of signal transduction pathways, including adenylate cyclase, phospholipase C, phospholipase A_2, phospholipase D, and ion channels (39,174–176). These various mechanisms mediate a variety of tissue responses to Ang II which have been extensively reviewed (6,177).

Adenylate Cyclase

Angiotensin II has been found to either inhibit or stimulate adenylate cyclase. In the majority of studies, Ang II inhibits adenylate cyclase. For example, in adrenal and

TABLE 2. *Distribution of the angiotensin II subtypes in various tissues of different species*

System	Species	AT$_1$	AT$_2$	Reference
Cardiovascular				
Heart	Rabbit, pig, monkey	+	+	(81,82,84,85)
	Rat, guinea pig	+	−	(81,86–89)
	Human	+	+	(83)
Aorta	Rabbit, pig, dog	+	−	(81,90)
	Rat, monkey	+	+	(81,91–93)
	Rat fetus	±	+	(94)
Renal artery	Human	+	+	(19)
Pulmonary artery	Rat	+	−	(95)
Anterior cerebral artery	Rat	−	+	(96)
Portal vein	Rat	+	−	(97)
Mesenteric artery	Rat	+	?	(98)
Vascular SMC	Rat, human	+	−	(19,27,99,100)
Neointima	Rat	+	+	(101,102)
		+	−	(103)
Spleen	Rat	+	−	(104)
Platelet	Human	+	−	(105)
Excretory				
Kidney	Rat, rabbit	+	−	(71,73,81,87,106–108)
	Monkey, human	+	+	(71,81,109)
Glomeruli	Rat, human	+	−	(109–113)
Mesangial cells	Rat	+	−	(47)
Proximal tubule	Rat, rabbit	+	−	(114,115)
Tick ascending loop	Rat	+	−	(115)
LLC-PK1 cells	Pig tubular epithelial cell	+	−	(116)
Capsule	Rabbit	−	+	(106)
Preglomerular vessel	Rat	+	−	(117)
	Human	−	−	(118)
Urinary Bladder	Guinea pig	+	−	(119)
Endocrine				
Adrenal				
Cortex	Rat, rabbit, dog, human	+	+	(19,21–23,27,30,69,81,106,108)
	Bovine, monkey	+	−	(69,81)
Fasciculata	Bovine, human	+	−	(70,120)
Medulla	Rat, human	±	+	(19,21,27,30,69,81,108)
	Rabbit	−	−	(106)
	Bovine	+	±	(69,121,122)
Pituitary	Rat	+	−	(123,124)
	Murine anterior pituitary tumor	+	−	(125)
PC12W cells	Rat pheochromocytoma	−	+	(25,127,208)
Digestive system				
Liver	Rat, rabbit	+	−	(25,27,128,129)
	Rat fetus	+	±	(94)
PLC-PRF-5 cells	Hepatoma cell line	+	−	(130)
Clone 9	Rat liver cell line	+	±	(22,131)
Intestine	Guinea pig, rat	+	±	(132–134)
Pancreas	Dog	±	+	(135,136)
Reproductive system				
Uterus	Rat, rabbit	+	+	(19,22,27)
	Monkey, human	−	+	(19,137)
	Ovine during pregnancy	+	−	(138)
	Ovine outside pregnancy	−	+	(138)
Ovary atretic follicle	Rat, bovine	−	+	(139–141)
corpus luteum	Rat	+	−	(139)
Placenta	Rat, human	+	−	(142–144)
	Rabbit (fetal portion)	−	+	(145)
	Guinea pig, rabbit (chorion)	+	−	(145)
Vas Deferens	Rabbit	+	−	(146)
Epididymis	Rat	+	−	(147)
Adipocyte	Rat epididymis	+	−	(148)

TABLE 2. *Continued.*

System	Species	AT₁	AT₂	Reference
Respiratory system				
Lung	Rat	+	−	(142,149)
	Rat fetus	+	+	(94)
Nervous system				
Brain	Rat, monkey	+	+	(46,75,79,81,99,150)
	Rabbit	+	±	(81)
Astrocytes	Rat	+	−	(151)
Choroid plexus	Rat	+	−	(78,152)
Circumventricular organ				
Organum vasculosum laminae terminalis	Rat, rabbit	+	−	(46,76,77,108,153–155)
Area postrema	Rat, human	+	−	(74,76–78)
	Rabbit	−	−	(74,153,157)
Median eminence	Rat, rabbit, human	+	−	(74,77,152,153,158,159)
Septum and hypothalamus				
Hypothalamus	Rat	+	+	(46,75,79,123)
Suprachiasmatic nucleus	Rat	+	−	(46,76,78,123)
	Hamster	−	−	(160)
Supraoptic nucleus	Rat, rabbit	+	−	(46,78,153–155,161)
Thalamus				
Paraventricular nucleus	Rat, rabbit, human	+	−	(46,74,78,79,153,155,156,161,162)
Subthalamic nucleus	Rat	−	+	(76,77)
	Human	+	−	(74)
	Rabbit, hamster	−	−	(153,160)
Mediodorsal thalamic nucleus	Rat	±	−	(76–79,155)
	Rabbit	−	−	(153)
Amygdala				
Medial amygdala	Rat	−	+	(76,78,152)
Dentate gyrus	Rat	−	−	(153)
	Rabbit	+	−	(153)
Midbrain and pons				
Superior colliculus	Rat	+	+	(46,76–79,108,123,157)
Locus ceruleus	Rat	−	+	(76–78,123)
	Rabbit	±	−	(153)
	Human	+	+	(74)
Substantia nigra	Rat	−	−	(153)
	Rabbit	+	−	(153)
	Human	+	±	(74)
Medial geniculate nucleus	Rat	−	+	(108,152,157)
	Human, hamster	+	−	(74,160)
Medulla oblongata				
Nucleus tractus solitarius	Rat, human, rabbit	+	−	(76–79,123,155)
Dorsal motor neuron of vagus	Rat, Human	+	−	(74,76,77,79)
Inferior olive	Rat, human	−	+	(74,76–78)
	Rabbit, hamster	−	−	(153,160)
	Human	+	+	(80)
NG108-15 cells	Mouse neuroblastoma × rat glioma hybrid	−	+	(163)
NIE-115 cells	Murine neuroblastoma	+	+	(44,164)
Glial cells	Rat	+	−	(165,166)
Neuronal cells	Rat	−	+	(165,166)
Miscellaneous				
Fetal/newborn skin	Human, rat, monkey,	±	+	(142,167–172)
Skeletal muscle	Rat fetus	±	+	(94)
Fibroblast	Rat fetal skin	+	+	(171)
R3T3 cells	Line derived from Swiss 3T3 fibroblasts	−	+	(173)

in kidney membrane particulate (177–180). However, in intact adrenal glomerulosa cells, in bovine adrenal fasciculata, in fetal fibroblasts in culture, in freshly isolated and cultured microvessel endothelial cells, as well as in cultured vascular smooth muscle cells, Ang II stimulates cAMP production (171,181–184). The effect of Ang II to stimulate adenylate cyclase activity may not be via a direct interaction of the AT_1 receptor with adenylate cyclase through G_i but may be secondary to 1,4,5-triphosphate (IP_3) stimulation of a calcium-calmodulin-dependent mechanism (183) or may result from the activation of other pathways such as phospholipase A_2, responsible for the generation of prostanoids, which in turn can stimulate adenylate cyclase.

Phospholipase C

Interaction of Ang II with AT_1 receptors results in the activation of phospholipase C, which hydrolyzes phosphatidylinositol bisphosphate (PIP_2) leading to the production of inositol 1,4,5 trisphosphate (IP_3) and 1,2-diacylglycerol (DAG). Each of these two metabolites activates a different pathway. Generation of IP_3 results in the release of calcium from intracellular stores whereas DAG activates protein kinase C (PKC). These two pathways are the most extensively investigated signal transduction pathways of Ang II (180).

IP_3 Generation

The rapid rise in intracellular calcium induced by IP_3 generation initiates a variety of cellular responses, including the synthesis and secretion of aldosterone (180), the secretion of peptide hormones such as prolactin, ACTH, vasopressin and oxytocin (185), vasoconstriction (186), and protein-tyrosine phosphorylation (187). Increased intracellular calcium has also been shown to decrease intracellular cyclic guanosine monophosphate (GMP) levels, secondary to activation of a calcium-calmodulin-dependent phosphodiesterase (188). Interestingly, mutation of Asp[74] in the AT_1 receptor to Asn or Gln decreases tenfold the affinity for losartan, increases 20-fold that of CGP 42112 and the mutants become unable to stimulate IP_3 production and Ca^{2+} mobilization. This indicates that Asp[74] is essential for the signaling mechanism of the AT_1 receptor (189).

DAG Formation

DAG has a dual role: it activates PKC and it stimulates arachidonic acid formation which leads to the formation of eicosanoids. Protein kinase C phosphorylates various cellular proteins including hormone receptors and acts synergistically with cytosolic-free calcium to initiate a wide variety of cellular responses. For example, DAG

formation in response to hormone-receptor binding may feedback to terminate IP_3 generation and calcium mobilization (190). This process is involved in desensitization of the cell to Ang II. Protein kinase C also contributes to the stimulation of prostaglandin (PG) synthesis and smooth muscle cell contraction (186,191,192). Recently it has been suggested that this enzyme also modulates cardiac sodium channels and can stimulate steroidogenesis (193,194). In addition, PKC probably plays an essential role in the growth-promoting effects of Ang II by activating kinases such as MAP kinase and Raf-1 kinase (195) involved in the mitogenic cascade, and by inducing the expression of growth factors such as platelet-derived growth factor (PDGF), insulin-like growth factor (IGF), or transforming growth factor-β (TGF-β) and proto-oncogenes like *fos, myc,* jun and jun-B (9,10,12, 196–199). However, Ang II can also activate protein phosphorylation through PKC-independent mechanisms (195).

Phospholipase A_2 and Phospholipase D

In mesangial cells, Ang II has been shown to stimulate phospholipase A_2 through a pertussis toxin-sensitive G-protein (186) and phospholipase D through a G-protein as yet undetermined (200).

Phospholipase A_2

Phospholipase A_2 (PLA_2) hydrolyses phospholipids to generate PG, prostacyclin, thromboxane A_2, and other eicosanoids. These molecules probably play a role in the regulation of Ang II actions since PG formation by Ang II has been shown to attenuate vasoconstriction induced by the peptide. Furthermore, a PG metabolite, 5,6-epoxyeicosatrienoic acid, has been suggested to inhibit sodium entry in proximal tubules, probably through stimulation of voltage-gated calcium channels. Thus, stimulation of phospholipase A_2 may also contribute to modulation of the renal actions of Ang II on proximal tubular ion transport (177). Interestingly, pertussis toxin that abolishes Ang-II-induced decrement in CAMP production does not inhibit Ang II stimulation of PLA_2 in proximal tubular epithelium (177).

Phospholipase D

Stimulation of phospholipase D in glomerular mesangial cells and vascular SMC results in hydrolysis of phosphatidylcholine and generation of DAG and phosphatidic acid, two metabolites which activate PKC and lead to the synthesis of PGs (200,201). The physiological role of this enzyme has not yet been elucidated, but it may be involved in stimulation of cell growth and contraction.

Regulation of Calcium, Potassium, Sodium, and Chloride Channels

Calcium Channels

In adrenal glomerulosa cells, Ang II acting via the AT_1 receptor stimulates voltage-gated calcium channels and blocks potassium channels [204]. These two mechanisms are responsible for an increase in intracellular calcium concentration which ultimately leads to aldosterone release (180,202–204). The nature of the type of calcium channel activated by Ang II is still controversial and may vary according to the species and tissue. It has been suggested that in bovine glomerulosa the channels involved in Ang II stimulus-secretion coupling are of the T type (205), whereas in proximal tubular epithelium they are of the L type (177).

Potassium Channels

A low-conductance, adenosine-triphosphate (ATP)-sensitive potassium channel has been found to be inhibited by Ang II via the AT_1 receptor in cultured porcine coronary artery smooth muscle cells (206). Blockade of potassium channels in this tissue results in depolarization and sustained calcium influx through voltage-dependent channels as described previously in glomerulosa cells and may be involved in Ang II induced vasoconstriction (204,206).

Sodium Channels

Angiotensin II modulates sodium channels in isolated rat ventricular cardiomyocytes (193). In these cells, which express only AT_1 receptors (81), Ang II increases the frequency of opening of sodium channels and hence the rate of activation of single-channel sodium currents (193). The phorbol ester TPA mimics the effect of Ang II, suggesting the involvement of PKC as the second messenger.

Chloride Channels

Angiotensin II has been reported to increase calcium-activated chloride conductance in mesangial cells (190,207). This effect is thought to be mediated by an increase in the concentration of intracellular calcium secondary to IP_3 generation and to the activation of PKC (207).

The AT_2 Receptor Subtype

The binding characteristics and the distribution of the AT_2 receptor have been well described. In contrast to the AT_1 receptor, however, much less is known about its signaling mechanism and its physiological role.

Binding Properties

The AT_2 receptor binds Ang peptides with the following order of potency: Ang III ≥ Ang II > Ang (3-8) > Ang (1-7) = Ang I. The AT_2 receptor has a 10-times-higher affinity for Ang III (pK_i 9.5) than the AT_1 receptor (24,173,208). As described previously, the AT_2 receptor has a low affinity for losartan ($K_i \geq 10^{-4}$ M) and related compounds but a high affinity for CGP 42112, a peptide analogue of Ang II (K_i | 1 nM) and nonpeptidic, spinacine derivatives, examplified by PD 123319 and analogues ($K_i \sim 10$ nM) (19,21,22). CGP 42112 and PD 123319 have at least a 2000-fold greater affinity for the AT_2 than for the AT_1 receptor (28).

Biochemical Properties

In contrast to their effect on the binding properties of the AT_1 receptor, reducing agents such as DTT either increase or have no effect on the binding of Ang II to the AT_2 receptor (19,22,32,81,94,139,141,209,210). Sodium ions do not affect the binding of Ang II to the AT_2 receptor, except in bovine cerebellum where the affinity is lowered two- to threefold (35).

Physicochemical Properties

The molecular weight of the AT_2 receptor has been characterized by covalent cross-linking and photoaffinity labeling (137,139,173). In R3T3 cells, a mouse fibroblast cell line derived from Swiss 3T3 cells, a specifically labeled protein corresponding to the AT_2 receptor has been detected with a molecular weight of 100 kDa. In ovarian granulosa cells, a molecular weight of 79 kDa has been reported (139). Similar experiments performed using membranes prepared from NG108-15 hybridoma cells and human myometrium indicate that glycosylated AT_2 receptors in these tissues have molecular weights of 92 and 68 kDa, respectively. After deglycosylation, the molecular weight of the AT_2 receptor in NG108-15 cells falls to 56 kDa and to 49 kDa in human uterus [(137); Bonnafous et al., *personal communication*]. The difference in the molecular weights of the AT_2 receptor in different cell lines or tissues, together with the observed differences in glycosylation, raises the possibility that the AT_2 receptor may be a heterogeneous protein. The AT_2 receptor in rat adrenal tissue has an isoelectric point of 6.3 (56,211). Using expression cloning from fetal and pheochromocytoma cell line (PC12W) libraries, two groups of investigators have recently reported the successful isolation of a full-length cDNA encoding the AT_2

receptor based on its identical binding specificities, DTT enhancement of binding, and developmental and tissue-specific expression. Surprisingly, this cloned AT$_2$ receptor has a 7-transmembrane topology, but ligand binding was unaffected by guanosine triphosphate (GTP) analogues. The novel receptor is a protein of 363 aminoacid residues with an estimated molecular weight of 40.9 kDa. It has 32% homology with the AT$_1$ receptor (356–358). This finding will certainly catapult research on the AT$_2$ receptor into a new era.

Internalization

Unlike the AT$_1$ receptor, the AT$_2$ receptor expressed in ovarian atretic follicles and in R3T3 cells does not undergo agonist-induced endocytosis (139,173). Upregulation of the AT$_2$ receptor has been noted in R3T3 cells treated with AT$_2$ ligands (212). In contrast, in neuroblastoma NIE-115 cells, which express both AT$_1$ and AT$_2$ receptors, there is a late downregulation of the AT$_2$ receptor occurring 30 minutes after exposure to Ang II (44). These observations may suggest that AT$_2$ receptors in neural and peripheral tissues are heterogeneous.

Relative Proportion and Distribution

Proportion

The proportion of Ang receptors that are of the AT$_2$ subtype varies between tissues and species (see Table 2). As an example of interspecies variations, nonpregnant sheep, marmosets, and human myometrium express only the AT$_2$ receptor, whereas nonpregnant rabbit and rat myometrium express both receptors (19,137,138). An example of intertissue variations has been reported in the monkey where the relative proportion of the AT$_2$ receptor varies between less than 10 percent to a maximum of 58 percent in adrenal and kidney cortex respectively (81).

Distribution

A number of studies have been published describing the distribution of Ang II receptors in brain (see Table 2). The AT$_2$ receptor is located mainly in areas related to the control and learning of motor activity, as well as in sensory and visual areas and in the limbic system (213). Centers involved in the regulation of blood pressure, drinking, salt appetite, and vasopressin release do not express AT$_2$ receptors. AT$_2$ receptors are particularly abundant in the fetus where they show a transient pattern of expression (142,209,214). They will be described later in relation to their hypothesized role in growth and development.

Signaling Mechanisms

Cells such as atretic follicular cells, NG108-15 cells, R3T3 cells, and PC12W pheochromocytoma cells express only the AT$_2$ receptor and have been extensively utilized to study the intracellular mechanisms linked to this receptor. Despite extensive studies in these cell lines, the exact nature of the intracellular mechanisms coupled to the AT$_2$ receptor have not been clearly determined (139,173,208,215). Thus, the AT$_2$ receptor does not signal through G-proteins and does not affect inositol phosphate production, phosphatidylcholine turnover, intracellular calcium mobilization, or arachidonate metabolism. Neither does Ang II binding to the AT$_2$ receptor affect CAMP or tyrosine kinase activity (25,35,37,127,139,141,173,208).

Working with cultured neurones isolated from neonatal rat brain, which express predominantly AT$_2$ receptors, Sumners et al. (166) recently demonstrated that Ang II decreased intracellular cyclic guanosine monophosphate (cGMP). This effect of Ang II in neuronal cultures was found to be blocked by high doses of PD 123177 and CGP 42112, suggesting the involvement of AT$_2$ receptors. However, this effect appears to be linked to a Ca^{2+}-calmodulin-dependent phosphodiesterase mechanism. Recent studies by Bottari et al. (6,216) indicate that in PC12W cells stimulation of AT$_2$ receptors leads to a 40-percent decrease in both basal and atrial-natriuretic-peptide (ANP)-stimulated cGMP levels regardless of the presence of a phosphodiesterase inhibitor. There is no effect on nitroprusside-stimulated cGMP levels, ruling out interactions between the AT$_2$ receptor and *soluble* guanylate cyclase (217). Particulate guanylate cyclase activity in both membrane particulates as well as in intact PC12W cells maintained in culture was inhibited by Ang II. These effects of Ang II were not affected by losartan but were mimicked by CGP 42112 (6,216,218–220). Using the same experimental model, such an effect was not observed in smooth muscle cells, excluding suggestion that the effects of Ang II in PC 12W cells are AT$_1$-linked. These data suggest that *particulate* guanylate cyclase and especially the ANP-receptor are targets of the AT$_2$ receptor.

Bottari et al. (6,216) have also demonstrated that the effect of Ang II on intracellular cGMP levels in PC12W cells can be abolished by 100-μM sodium orthovanadate, an inhibitor of protein tyrosine phosphatase, but not by okadaic acid which is a serine/threonine phosphatase inhibitor. Immunoblotting experiments using an antiphosphotyrosine monoclonal antibody have shown that Ang II induces a rapid dephosphorylation of tyrosine-phosphorylated proteins in PC12W cells and that this effect is inhibited by orthovanadate. Furthermore (Fig. 5), Ang II dose-dependently stimulates the protein tyrosine phosphatase activity of PC12W cell membranes using paranitrophenyl-phosphate as a sub-

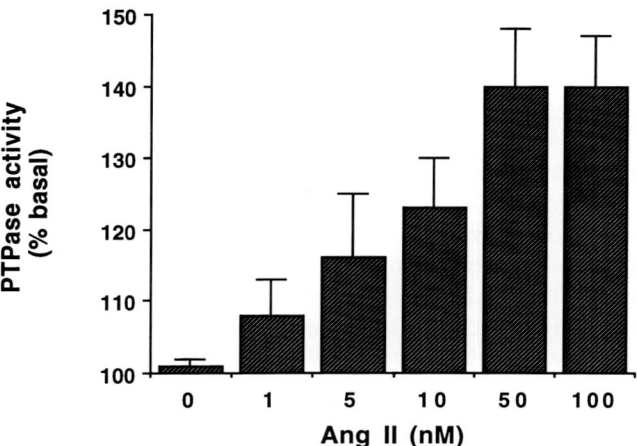

FIG. 5. Effect of Ang II on phosphotyrosine phosphatase (PTPase) activity in PC12W plasma membrane particulate (mean ± SEM; n = 7). Membranes were preincubated for 20 mins at room temperature in the presence of increasing concentrations of Ang II. PTPase activity was determined after 60 min incubation using para-nitrophenylphosphate as a substrate. The results are expressed as the percentage of basal PTPase activity. (Florio et al. [222] and Pan et al. [223]).

strate (221). It is therefore suggested that AT_2 receptors signal by stimulating protein tyrosine phosphatase activity which modulates a series of cellular effector systems. A similar pathway has been recently reported for two members of the 7-transmembrane domain receptor superfamily, somatostatin and dopamine receptors (222,223).

Decreased levels of cyclic GMP in response to Ang II is not a conclusion shared by all investigators who have utilized this cellular system (127,208,356). Moreover, in stably transfected cells, Ang II mediated on inhibition of protein cytosine phosphatase or was devoid of effect (357,358). Thus, the observations of Bottari et al. in PC12W cells need to be confirmed and extended to other tissue systems before this putative signaling system of the AT_2 receptor can be accepted.

Another cellular target for the AT_2 receptor has recently been described in NG108-15 hybridoma cells which express only the AT_2 receptor (163). Using the technique of whole cell patch-clamping, Ang II, as well as CGP 42112, have been shown to inhibit T-type calcium currents at membrane potentials higher than −40 mV and to shift the current voltage curve to lower potentials. These effects are not affected by losartan but are inhibited by orthovanadate. The intracellular mechanisms mediating these effects of Ang II have not yet been determined.

Heterogeneity

Tsutsumi and Saavedra (224) have recently shown the presence of Ang II binding sites in rat brain that have a high affinity for CGP 42112 and PD 123177 but which differ from "classical" AT_2 receptors in their sensitivity to DTT, GTP-γ-S, and pertussis toxin (224,225). These newly discovered binding sites which are found in the ventral thalamic nuclei, the medial geniculate nucleus, and the locus ceruleus have been designated AT_{2a} while the "classic" AT_2 receptor found in the inferior olive is designated as AT_{2b} in this classification. Fluharty et al. (226,227) have also demonstrated the existence of two populations of AT_2 receptors in cells of the NIE-115 neuroblastoma line, both of which exhibit a high affinity for CGP 42112 but no affinity for losartan. They differ in their sensitivity to PD 123319 and to DTT (Fluharty, *personal communication*). Moreover, using a specific anti-PLC-α antiserum, these investigators suggest that one of the CGP-42112-sensitive receptor subpopulations is coupled to PLC-α through a Gq-like protein. Classification of putative subpopulations will be postitive when more receptors will have been cloned.

Angiotensin Binding Sites Other Than AT_1 and AT_2

The Cytosolic Binding Protein

A cytosolic protein with high affinity for Ang II and particularly Ang III has been detected in many tissues including liver, neonatal rat cardiomyocytes, myometrium, and in the brain (228–231). This Ang-II-binding protein of 80.8 kDa which has been isolated, purified, and cloned (230), shares no sequence homology with the AT_1 receptor. Neither losartan nor PD 123177 have any reasonable affinity for this protein (228). CGP 42112, however, shows a low affinity for this binding site (1 μM), similar to its affinity for the AT_1 receptor (24).

The Nuclear Binding Site

Early studies demonstrated that injection of tritiated Ang II into the left ventricle of adult rats resulted in radioactivity appearing in the nucleus of endothelial and smooth muscle cells. These observations, which have since been confirmed in rat liver and spleen, suggest that Ang II or a fragment binds to a nuclear protein and may exert an action on nuclear function (232,233).

The nuclear Ang II receptor binds losartan with high affinity but has a very low affinity for PD 123177 (234,235). Thus, the nuclear receptor appears to have binding properties similar to AT_1 receptors present in the plasma membrane and has a similar molecular weight. Another similarity between the nuclear binding protein and the plasma membrane AT_1 receptor is its coupling to G-proteins in a manner similar to that recently reported for the somatostatin nuclear receptor. The nature of the nuclear second messengers linked to the nuclear-binding-receptor–G-protein complex has not yet been reported, but possible candidates for signal transduction such as PKC, calcium-ATPase, and inositol trisphosphate-sensitive calcium channels are known to be localized in the nucleus (236,237). Slight differences between their binding properties and binding requirement suggest that the nuclear receptor, the cytosolic binding protein, and the plasma membrane AT_1 receptor are independent entities (24).

Binding Sites for the Angiotensin II Fragments Ang (1-7) and Ang (3-8)

Angiotensin II is rapidly degraded both in blood and in tissues (238–240). Among the various metabolites of Ang II, a heptapetide (Ang 1-7) and a hexapeptide (Ang 3-8) have been detected (241).

Ang (1-7)

Ang (1-7) has been shown to stimulate vasopressin release and to decrease blood pressure after injection into the area postrema, the nucleus of the tractus solitarius, or into the ventrolateral medulla (242,243). Ang (1-7) enhances prostaglandin synthesis in endothelial cells, vascular smooth muscle cells, astrocytes, glioma cells, and in perfused rat hearts (244–247). Furthermore, in the rat kidney, Ang (1-7) produces a substantial natriuresis and diuresis and an increase in glomerular filtration rate without affecting renal vascular resistance (248). In contrast to Ang II, Ang (1-7) does not produce peripheral vasoconstriction or dypsogenesis and does not stimulate aldosterone secretion (242).

Since Ang (1-7) has actions different from those of Ang II and has only a weak affinity for either AT_1 and AT_2 receptors (24), it has been proposed that this heptapeptide acts via a separate receptor subtype. However, Ang (1-7) has a high affinity for the AT_{1b} receptor subtype present in proximal tubular epithelium (47). Thus in the kidney, Ang (1-7) may affect renal sodium and water handling by interacting with the AT_{1b} receptor (248).

Ang (3-8)

Although Ang (3-8) has been termed *Ang IV*, a physiological role for this peptide has not yet been precisely defined. It has, however, been proposed that Ang (3-8) may be involved in endothelial cell-dependent vasodilation, renal cortical blood flow, and learning acquisition (249–251). Definite and distinct binding sites for Ang (3-8) have been described in sensitive tissues from a variety of species (250,252,253). Ang (3-8) binding in these tissues is saturable, reversible, and specific. Its affinity for its binding site is high, in the nanomolar range. Neither losartan nor CGP 42112 or PD 123177 are able to compete with radiolabeled Ang (3-8) for binding. Ang (3-8)

itself exhibits very little affinity for either AT_1 or AT_2 receptors (24). The density of this putative Ang (3-8) binding site is generally higher than that of AT_1 and AT_2 receptors. GTP-γ-S has no effect on the binding of Ang II (3-8) in bovine aorta smooth muscle cells, indicating that this receptor is probably not coupled to a G-protein (254). Possible intracellular signaling mechanisms of this "receptor" have not been defined. However, calcium metabolism may be involved, since in rat aorta smooth muscle cells, Ang (3-8) produces a sustained increase in intracellular calcium and inositol trisphosphate, which are not altered by treatment with pertussis toxin (255). It has been proposed to call this receptor AT_4.

Nonmammalian Angiotensin II Receptors

Ang II receptors expressed in amphibian and avian tissues, as well as in mycoplasma, appear to differ from mammalian receptors (24).

Amphibian Receptors

In amphibians, Ang II receptors are functionally similar to the AT_1 subtype since they mediate phosphoinositide hydrolysis and calcium mobilization. However, they bind peptide and nonpeptide ligands with different affinities than either mammalian AT_1 or AT_2 receptors. Thus, amphibian Ang II receptors have virtually no affinity for either losartan or PD 123177. CGP 42112, which selectively binds to the mammalian AT_2 receptor, also has high (nM) affinity for the amphibian Ang II receptor (256,257). Functionally, CGP 42112, in contrast to losartan or PD 123177, inhibits Ang-II-induced increased calcium flux in frog oocytes, a pathway typical of the AT_1 receptor (257,258). Molecular cloning and sequencing of an amphibian Ang II receptor have pointed to a 60-percent amino acid identity and 65-percent nucleotide homology with the coding region of the mammalian AT_1 receptor (258).

Avian Receptors

Losartan and PD 123319 bind poorly to Ang II receptors present in vascular smooth muscle and endothelial cells obtained from chicken tissues, as well as from the chicken egg chorio-allantoic membrane (259). CGP 42112, however, binds with high affinity to the Ang II receptor present in the chorio-allantoic membrane (260) and in this respect resembles the Ang II receptor found in amphibian membranes. In contrast to the mammalian AT_1 receptor, nonhydrolyzable GTP analogues do not alter the dissociation rate of Ang II bound to the avian receptor (261). Functionally, CGP 42112 is able to inhibit Ang-II-induced angiogenesis of pre- and postcapillary vessels, whereas PD 123319 and losartan are ineffective (260). In contrast, the initial blood pressure reduction induced by the natural ligand, Val^5-Ang II, in the anesthetized chicken was attenuated by both losartan and PD 123319 (259). These conflicting reports suggest that the avian receptor may not be identical to mammalian AT_1 or AT_2 receptors. Recently, a receptor has been cloned from turkey adrenocortical cells. It shows 78-percent amino acid identity and 85-percent nucleotide homology with the rat aortic smooth muscle AT_1 receptor (262).

Microorganisms

Microorganisms of the class Mollicutes such as *Mycoplasma* and *Acholeplasma* are common cell culture contaminants which also express an Ang II binding site. This binding site, which differs markedly from mammalian AT_1 and AT_2 receptors (263,264), is characterized by a very low affinity for Ang III and a high affinity for both Ang (1-7) and Ang I. Losartan, PD 123319, and CGP 42112 do not bind to this site. Low concentrations of DTT increase the affinity of Ang II for this binding site by 35–50 percent, whereas bacitracin inhibits binding (IC_{50} 30 μM). It is unknown at the present time whether the Ang II binding site in *Acholeplasma* is coupled to intracellular second messengers or whether Ang II mediates a physiological function through this site. Therefore, it cannot yet be considered a true receptor.

Miscellaneous Angiotensin II Binding Sites

Other poorly characterized Ang II binding sites have been described (24).

Mouse Neuroblastoma (Neuro-2a)

This cell line expresses a binding site that has a high affinity for Ang II but not for Ang III. Ligand binding in neuro-2a cells is not blocked by losartan or PD 123319 and is not affected by GTP analogues. Disulfide bridge integrity does not play an essential role in ligand binding since DTT has only minor effects on receptor affinity. This site has been tentatively named AT_3 since its binding properties differ from the AT_1 and AT_2 receptors that are present in mammalian cells (265). In neuro-2a cells, Ang II at concentrations 1000-fold higher than its K_d for binding, causes a concentration-dependent increase in soluble guanylate cyclase activity which is not blocked by losartan or PD 123319 (266). This stimulatory effect on guanylate cyclase appears to be secondary to an increase in nitric oxide synthesis. Increased calcium influx via an ion channel distinct from the L type or N type may be the initiatory event in this response (267). In terms of receptor binding, the "AT_3 receptor" in neuro-2a cells closely resembles the Ang-II-binding site in *Acholeplasma* and *Mycoplasma*.

Mas-Oncogene

The mas-oncogene has been reported to code for a novel neuronal Ang II receptor. This receptor has been cloned and is reported to possess a molecular weight of 37.5 kDa (268). When transfected into *Xenopus* oocytes, binding sites appear which mediate increased membrane chloride conductance and intracellular calcium mobilization in response to high concentrations ($\geq 10^{-6}$ M) of Ang II and Ang III. These findings suggest that the binding site encoded by the mas-oncogene in *Xenopus* oocytes is coupled to the endogenous inositol lipid/calcium mobilizing pathway in these cells. The changes in intracellular biochemistry produced by Ang II in this cell line are not blocked either by losartan or PD 123177 (269), suggesting that the mas-oncogene does not code for a classical, functional AT_1 or AT_2 receptor (270). Indeed, the recent cloning of AT_1 receptor cDNA has revealed that mas bears only a minor structural resemblance with less than 10 percent overall identity to this receptor. Several groups have cloned mas-related gene [mrg, rat thoracic aorta (RTA)] (271,272). Neither mrg nor RTA have been detected in tissues which display Ang II binding. Thus the 7-transmembrane proteins encoded by the mas gene family are not authentic Ang II receptors. They appear, however, to enhance the expression or signaling sensitivity of endogenous Ang II receptors and their signaling pathways.

Additional Angiotensin II Binding Sites

Additional Ang II binding sites have been described in fetal mesenchyme (142) and after nephrectomy in the adrenal cortex (273). These are not typical AT_1 or AT_2 receptors as they have poor affinity, if any, for losartan, PD 123177, or CGP 42112. More binding sites will be most probably discovered in the near future as our tools become more sophisticated.

The Physiological Role of AT_1 and AT_2 Receptors

Since the development of subtype-specific ligands, it has been possible to determine which tissues express Ang II receptor subtypes. In many tissues the intracellular processes and the ultimate response or responses mediated through the AT_1 receptor have been clearly established. It appears that the majority, if not all, of the known effects of Ang II are mediated through the AT_1 receptor (274). A large number of selective antagonists have been synthesized (see Fig. 3) (275,276) and all studies have demonstrated that, following activation of the renin-angiotensin system, blockade of the AT_1 receptor decreases blood pressure (BP) and aldosterone release, affects drinking behavior, and modulates many of the effects of Ang II on renal function (277). Thus, AT_1 antagonists, like ACE inhibitors, may have utility in the clinical settings of hypertension and congestive heart failure. In addition to effects on BP and fluid balance, Ang II acting through the AT_1 receptor stimulates the growth of various cells in culture and can reverse cardiac hypertrophy and neointima proliferation after experimental balloon angioplasty (278–282). Finally, AT_1 receptor blockade may also influence neural transmission and, at least in rodents, affect general behavior (283,284). In view of the numerous actions of AT_1 antagonists on systems other than hemodynamics and fluid balance, future studies with this class of compounds are anticipated to reveal potential therapeutic indications beyond hyper-

tension and heart failure. A description of the tissue responses linked to the AT_1 receptor has recently been the subject of several excellent journal reviews and are discussed in detail in other chapters of this book (6,66,277,285). The interested reader is therefore referred to these and other sources for further detailed information concerning the physiological processes linked to the AT_1 receptor.

Blockade of the AT_1 receptor in animal and in man is accompanied by a compensatory increase in circulating Ang II (219,275,276,286–292). This may result in Ang II exerting some effects via the unblocked, i.e., non-AT_1 receptors (Fig. 6). The functional importance and clinical relevance of receptors other than AT_1 are not known

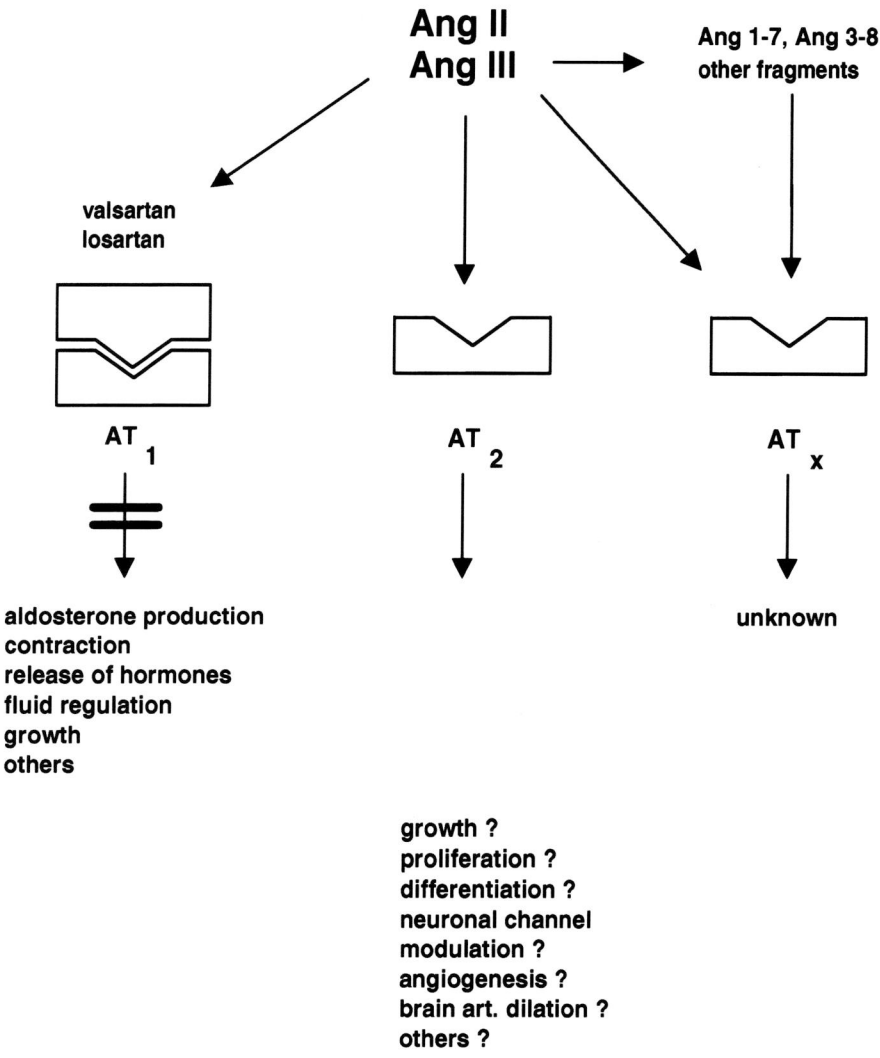

FIG. 6. Blockade of the AT_1 receptor on the juxtaglomerular cells leads to an increase in renin and Ang II plasma levels. The unblocked receptors are accessible to Ang II and its various metabolites. This may lead to additional effects, the clinical relevance of which is still unknown, as the function of the AT_2 receptor and other binding sites is still poorly understood. So far, the tolerance of the AT_1 antagonists is good in both animals and humans.

and further investigation is therefore required to understand the possible therapeutic application of Ang II receptor blockade in cardiovascular and other diseases.

Is There a Physiological Role for the AT_2 Receptor?

In contrast to our knowledge of the AT_1 receptor, the intracellular mechanisms and physiological processes mediated through the AT_2 receptor are still poorly, if at all, understood. Nonetheless, many reports have appeared in the recent literature demonstrating that AT_2 selective ligands have actions in several organ systems. Whether these observations can be considered evidence of functional AT_2-mediated responses is a matter of debate. Part of the confusion concerning the interpretation of studies using AT_2 specific ligands is related to our poor understanding of their mechanism of action. For example, it is often assumed that CGP 42112, PD 123319, and PD 123177 are antagonists of Ang II acting at AT_2 receptors. However, this assumption has not been convincingly demonstrated. Indeed, it appears, at least in two cell lines, that CGP 42112 is a full agonist at AT_2 receptors (163,218); whereas both PD 123319 and PD 123177 display antagonistic properties (218,358). Furthermore, none of the selective ligands available for study are completely specific for the AT_2 receptors (29). Therefore, many studies performed with AT_2 selective ligands are virtually impossible to interpret because of the very high concentrations of these compounds used. Indeed, it has recently been very clearly shown that at high doses CGP 42112 acts as a partial agonist at AT_1 receptors (293) and that PD 123319 may have some agonistic properties (48).

In view of the confusion concerning the use of AT_2-specific ligands and the difficulty in correctly interpreting data from experiments where they have been used in whole animal studies, this section is confined to a critical review of the current literature concerning the functional role of the AT_2 receptor.

Effects of AT_2 Ligands on the Central Actions of Angiotensin II

Ang II exerts many actions within the brain by modulating neuronal function (294). For example, when administered centrally, Ang II enhances sympathetic outflow leading to an increase in blood pressure. Angiotensin II stimulates thirst and salt appetite and leads to the release of several hormones including vasopressin, prolactin, luteinizing hormone, and ACTH. Angiotensin II has also been shown to modify behavior in rodents. In view of this multiplicity of action and the large distribution of both receptors, the brain has been the focus of studies designed to determine the role of AT_2 receptors in mediating the central actions of Ang II.

Angiotensin II-Induced Pressor Response

Selective administration of Ang II into the cerebral ventricles or into certain brain structures, such as the paraventricular nucleus, leads to peripheral vasoconstriction and to an increase in systemic BP. There appears to be almost universal agreement that the pressor response to centrally administered Ang II is mediated by AT_1 receptors (277). Thus, in both conscious and anesthetized rats and in the spontaneous hypertensive rat, intracerebroventricular (ICV) injection of 40–350 ng Ang II directly into the paraventricular nucleus produces an increase in BP which is completely blocked by losartan (0.7–10.0 μg ICV or 3 mg/kg ICV), but is unchanged by PD 123177 or PD 123319 (7.0 μg ICV or 10 mg/kg IV) (295–301). The observations suggesting that the central cardiovascular effects of Ang II are mediated by AT_1 receptors are in agreement with the distribution of this receptor subtype in areas of the brain where Ang II produces its pressor action. In contrast, AT_2 receptors are present only outside areas involved in cardiovascular regulation (76).

Interestingly, ICV injection of PD 123319 (80 μg) has recently been shown to produce a long-lasting antagonism (>48 hours) of the pressor effects of centrally administered Ang II (100 ng) (300). However, in this study PD 123319 was used at a high dose and the possibility exists that the AT_2 antagonist may be blocking the central effects of Ang II at the AT_1 receptor or be exhibiting nonspecific properties (300).

Angiotensin-II-Induced Thirst

Injection of Ang II (40–100 ng) into the brain ventricles causes drinking in animals. This response to Ang II appears to be mediated by AT_1 receptors since it is blocked by <4 μg losartan and not by doses of up to 4 μg PD 123319 or CGP 42112 (296,297,302–307).

Angiotensin-II-Induced Release of Vasopressin, Luteinizing Hormone, and Prolactin

There appears to be controversy in the published literature concerning the subtype of receptor through which Ang II exerts its effects on vasopressin release. Thus, in the explanted rat hypothalamo-neurohypophyseal system, the release of vasopressin in response to 1 and 5 μM Ang II can be blocked by both CGP 42112 (5 μM) and PD 123177 (30 μM) but not by losartan (10 μM) (308). However, the depolarization of supraoptic nuclei by 1–25 μM Ang II is antagonized by 5–20 μM losartan but not by equimolar concentrations of PD 123177 (309). A consistent response to the intraventricular injection of Ang II is the release of vasopressin into the systemic circulation. In the conscious rat, 50-ng Ang II given ICV increases vasopressin release, a response which can be significantly but not completely blocked by up to 0.7–10 μM losartan and up to 7.0 μM PD 123319 (297). In the brain, the release of vasopressin in response to Ang II appears to be mediated in part by AT_1 receptors acting upon alpha-adrenergic terminals (310). Recent studies have shown that AT_2 receptors are present in the hypophyseal arteries supplying the pituitary. Changes in blood flow to the pituitary modulated by AT_2 ligands may therefore contribute to the effect of these compounds on pituitary vasopressin release (158).

In estrogen- and progesterone-treated ovariectomized rats, ICV injection of Ang II (100 ng) stimulates luteinizing hormone (LH) and inhibits prolactin release into the systemic circulation. The changes in LH and prolactin release in response to Ang II appear to be mediated by both the AT_2 and AT_1 receptors since both are blocked by either 1 μg losartan or 1 μg PD 123177 (304).

Behavior

Angiotensin-I-converting enzyme inhibitors have been shown to enhance cognitive performance in animals, suggesting the involvement of Ang II (13). This notion is further supported by the ability of losartan (0.1–1.0 mg/kg PO) to significantly suppress avoidance behavior, habituation, and to overcome the cognitive impairment produced by scopolamine (0.25 mg/kg IP) (283,284). In contrast, PD 123177 (0.01–1.0 mg/kg IP) did not affect aversion but 10 ng/kg ip.bd enhanced performance in a habituation test and improved scopolamine-induced cognitive impairment (311).

Angiotensin-II-Sensitive Neurons

Sympathetic ganglia. Angiotensin II interacts with specific receptors present upon the postganglionic cells of sympathetic ganglia leading to depolarization of the neural membrane and to the generation of an action potential (312). Recent studies have shown that the membrane depolarization in sympathetic ganglia produced by Ang II (10^{-8} M to 10^{-5} M) could be inhibited by losartan (0.03–0.1 μM) but not by PD 123177 (3 μM) (313).

Central neurons. Neurons of the inferior olive express essentially a single population of AT_2 receptors. The spontaneous firing of neurons in this brain region is excited by Ang II and blocked by PD 123177 and CGP 42112, while losartan is ineffective even at high doses (314,315).

Neuronal Cultures

In neuronal cultures prepared from brainstem (medulla oblongata and pons) and hypothalamus, electro-

physiological studies have demonstrated that Ang II (0.1 nM–10 μM) is able to cause either an increase or a decrease in net outward current, depending on the neuron population (315,316). The observed *increase* in net outward current in these studies could be blocked by both 100 nM PD 123177 and PD 123319, but not by losartan (100 nM). In contrast, the *decrease* in outward current could be blocked by losartan (100 nM), but not by 100 nM PD 123177. In nondifferentiated NG 108-15 cells which contain only AT_2 receptors, Ang II (100 nM) inhibits T-type calcium currents. CGP 42112 (100 nM) has the same effects as Ang II (100 nM) (163).

The AT₂ Receptors and the Cardiovascular System

Blood Pressure and Blood Flow

Considerable effort has been directed toward determining whether Ang II, acting through AT_2 receptors, plays a role in the control of cardiovascular hemodynamics. Early studies demonstrated that Ang-II-induced contractions of isolated rabbit aortic rings were antagonized by losartan but were unaffected by the AT_2 antagonist PD 123177 even at doses as high as 10^{-4} M (295). In a similar manner, the pressor effects of intravenously injected Ang II in the anesthetized pithed and conscious rat can be antagonized by losartan but are unaffected by PD 123177 at doses up to 100 mg/kg (295,317,318). The reduction in blood flows to the kidney, intestinal tract, and the hindquarters produced by Ang II in the conscious and anesthetized rat can also be effectively antagonized by the active metabolite of losartan but not by the AT_2 antagonists PD 123319 or by the AT_2 ligand CGP 42112 (10 mg/kg) (319). Furthermore, in the renal hypertensive rat and the anesthetized sodium-depleted rat, models dependent upon the renin-angiotensin system for BP maintenance, both PD 123319 and CGP 42112 have no effect on BP at doses up to 100 mg/kg (293,295). These observations would suggest that the AT_1 but not the AT_2 receptor plays a key role in the control of cardiovascular hemodynamics. While AT_2 ligands do not appear to affect hemodynamics acutely, they appear to do so after chronic administration and at plasma concentrations low enough to bind only to the AT_2 receptor (93). Furthermore, it has been shown that Ang II exerts a biphasic effect on BP after bolus administration with an initial pressor effect and a later depressor response. The initial pressor response can be blocked with losartan while the later depressor effect can be blocked by PD 123319 (320).

Cardiac Function

Angiotensin II has been shown to exert positive inotropic effects on the heart which are antagonized by losartan (10^{-6} M) but not by the AT_2 antagonist PD 121981 (10^{-4} M), (84,321). Both AT_1 and AT_2 receptors are present within the rabbit ventricular myocardium and human atria (82,83). Interestingly, in man, the relative proportion of atrial AT_1 and AT_2 receptors appears to be correlated with left and right atrial pressures as well as with left ventricular ejection fraction (83,219). Thus, the percentage of AT_1 receptors is higher and the percentage of AT_2 receptors lower with increasing left ventricular ejection fraction. Conversely, the percentage of AT_1 receptors is lower and the percentage of AT_2 receptors higher with increasing left and right atrial pressures (83,219). The fact that the number and proportion of AT_2 receptors increases in response to heart failure may suggest that this receptor is in some way involved in this pathological process and is borne out by recent physiological experiments (281,322–324). A "balance" between AT_1 and AT_2 receptors has been suggested (219), and it has been proposed that the AT_2 receptor may counteract the action of the AT_1 receptor (325).

Cerebral Blood Flow Regulation

Cerebral blood flow displays the complex phenomenon of autoregulation which is mediated by changes in tone of the cerebral blood vessels. Angiotensin II has been suggested to contribute to the control of cerebral blood flow (CBF) regulation by dilating large cerebral blood vessels (326,327). Large cerebral blood vessels express only AT_2 receptors (96) and so the hypothesis has been advanced that Ang II, acting through AT_2 receptors, contributes to upper limit of cerebral autoregulation where the tone of the large vessels assumes increasing importance. In this regard, it has recently been shown in rats that PD 123319 can prevent the norepinephrine-induced increase in CBF (328). In another study PD 123319 (10 mg/kg or 0.36 mg/kg/min) and losartan (10 mg/kg) shifted the upper limit of CBF regulation in rats toward higher pressures (329).

The Kidney

There have been many recent reports suggesting that AT_2 ligands affect renal function. For example, the AT_2 receptor ligands PD 123177 and PD 123319 have been shown to antagonize the renal vasoconstrictor response to exogenous Ang II and to induce an increase in urine volume and free water formation in the anesthetized dog (330–332). Furthermore, in the conscious rat, PD 123177 has been shown to increase renal blood flow following experimental myocardial infarction and, in the anesthetized rat, to increase glomerular filtration rate, urine volume, and chloride and bicarbonate excretion (333,334). Since, in the aforementioned studies, PD 123177 and PD 123319 were used at very high doses,

and in the majority of cases produced effects qualitatively similar to AT_1 receptor antagonists, the possibility exists that PD 123177 and PD 123319 influence renal function by interacting with the AT_1 receptor or may exhibit nonspecific properties. Both PD 123177 and PD 123319 are closely related compounds (see Fig. 2), and studies of renal function with other ligands selective for the AT_2 receptor have not yet been performed. Therefore, it is unknown whether the renal actions of PD 123177 and PD 123319 are specific for this class of compounds or are a property of all ligands selective for the AT_2 receptor. Recently, the role of AT_2 receptors in the control of kidney function has been reassessed (293) using the highly selective AT_2 ligand CGP 42112. In these experiments, the renal actions of CGP 42112 in comparison to PD 123319 and losartan were investigated in sodium-depleted anesthetized rats. The results in Fig. 7 illustrate that PD 123319 at infusion rates of 1–1000 µg/kg/min had no effect on renal function, while CGP 42112 affected renal function only at an infusion rate of 1000 µg/kg/min. During these experiments the plasma levels of both compounds were monitored and compared to their known affinities for AT_1 and AT_2 receptors. Assuming the plasma concentrations of CGP 42112 and PD 123319 to be in equilibrium with those at the receptor level, then at infusion rates between 1 and 1000 µg/kg/min, PD 123319 (plasma levels 70 nM and 25 µM, respectively) would be expected to interact essentially with an exclusive population of AT_2 receptors. At doses between 1 and 100 µg/kg/min, CGP 42112 (plasma levels 14 and 700 nM, respectively) would be expected to bind to AT_2 receptors, but at 1000 µg/kg/min (plasma levels 2.2 µM) to bind to 80 percent of the available AT_1 population. The results therefore suggest that when used at doses that were compatible with an AT_2-selective interaction, the AT_2 receptors are not involved in the control of renal function. It remains to be determined whether this is also the case in other animal species.

Ovarian Regulation

Angiotensin II receptors are present on many structures of the ovary, including the follicular granulosa, the thecal cell layers, interstitium, corpora lutea, blood vessels, and surface epithelium. In the rat ovary, follicular granulosa cells appear to express only AT_2 receptors, while all other ovarian cells express the AT_1 receptor (139). In contrast, in bovine ovary AT_2 receptors are expressed only by thecal cells (140). All components of the renin-angiotensin system are found within the ovary, and Ang II levels are higher in this organ than in the surrounding plasma. Therefore, it has been suggested that locally formed Ang II can alter ovarian function (335,336). Within the ovary, Ang II has been shown to stimulate estrogen formation and also appears to control ovulation since saralasin can inhibit ovulation in imma-

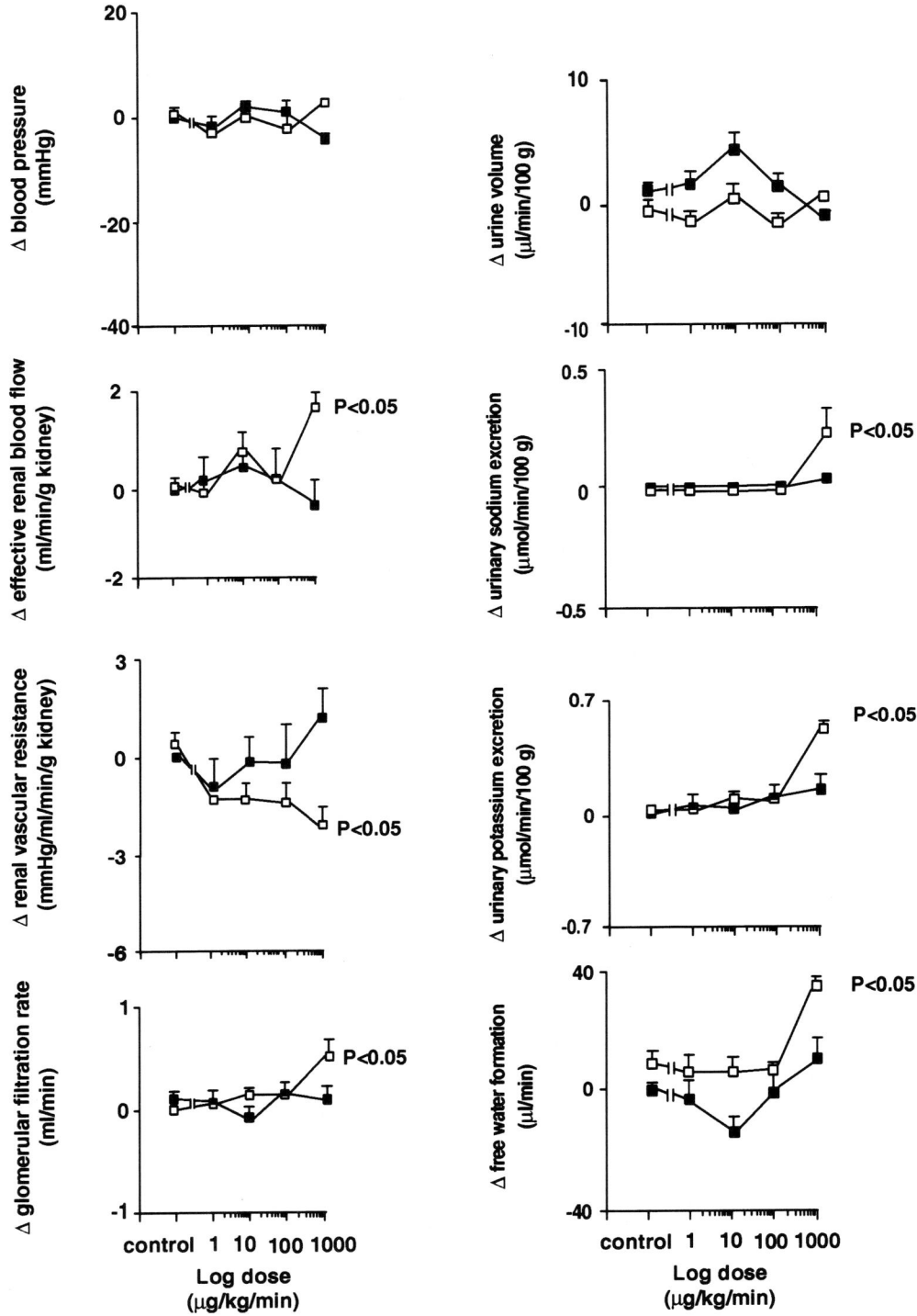

FIG. 7. Effect of AT$_2$ ligands on blood pressure and renal function in the sodium-depleted rat. Results are expressed as mean ± SEM from 5 to 13 rats at each dose. Statistics compare each dose of PD 123319 (●) and CGP 42112 (□) with vehicle controls by ANOVA or unpaired t tests. For additional details of methods see Macari et al. (293).

ture female rats primed with pregnant mare's serum gonadotrophin (337). These observations have led to the suggestion that Ang II, acting via the AT_2 receptor, may control aspects of ovarian function like follicular maturation and atresia.

Growth and Development

Angiotensin II has been shown to stimulate cellular growth both directly and also through the actions or expression of other growth factors such as IGF, EGF, and PDGF (11,12,198). The expression of the AT_2 receptor has been shown to be enhanced in the fetus and following damage to the skin and the interior surface of the aortic wall. These experimental observations have led to the conclusion that Ang II, acting through the AT_2 receptor, may play a role in tissue growth and differentiation.

Fetal Growth

Recent studies have shown the presence of Ang II receptors in the rat fetus as early as day 10 of gestation. Angiotensin II receptors in the developing fetus are predominantly of the AT_2 subtype, are abundant by days 14–18 of gestation, particularly within the mesenchymal tissue and brain, and decline shortly after birth (78,142,213,338). All components of the renin-angiotensin system are present within the developing fetus and formation of Ang II does occur. Therefore, it has been suggested that Ang II, acting through the AT_2 receptor, plays a role in fetal development. The number of AT_2 receptors in cerebral arteries from 2-week-old animals is higher than in adult rats, leading to the suggestion that Ang II, acting via the AT_2 receptor, may also play a role in postnatal development (92,96). However, the lower number of AT_2 receptors in some rapidly dividing cells may suggest on the contrary that the AT_2 receptor has no function in cell replication or growth (212,339). This controversial issue will require additional studies.

Experimental Wound Healing

Skin expresses both AT_1 and AT_2 receptors and, after wounding, the expression of the AT_2 receptor is significantly enhanced, both in the dermis and in the superficial dermis of the skin around the wound. Interestingly, Ang II levels in the skin increase after wounding, which has led to the hypothesis that Ang II, acting via the AT_2 receptor, contributes to skin repair after wounding (172,339–341).

Restenosis

Injury to the blood vessel wall has been shown to result in smooth muscle cell proliferation and migration at the site of damage and to the formation of a neointimal layer. Treatment of animals with ACE inhibitors has been shown to reduce the formation of this neointimal layer, suggesting the involvement of Ang II in the remodeling process (342).

Recent studies that have considered the subtype of receptor mediating these actions of Ang II have shown that either the AT_1- or AT_2-receptor number increases in the aortic wall after injury (103,219,279,282). Blockade of AT_1 receptors can clearly prevent the formation of neointima formation; the involvement of the AT_2 receptor subtypes remains puzzling (279,280,282,343).

AT_2 Blockade Potentiates the Actions of AT_1 Antagonists

There is an increasing number of experimental observations suggesting that, while AT_2 antagonists may be themselves inactive, they can potentiate the action of AT_1 antagonists in a number of organ systems. Thus, for example, the increase in systemic blood pressure and, in some studies, the release of vasopressin in response to Ang II, is not inhibited by PD 123319. However, in these studies PD 123319 potentiated the antagonistic effect of submaximal but not maximal doses of losartan (319,344–346). These interesting observations have been interpreted as secondary to the displacement of losartan from nonspecific binding sites resulting in higher and more effective concentrations of the AT_1 inhibitor or as an unmasked effect of Ang II acting through AT_2 receptors following AT_1 blockade.

Physiology of Angiotensin II at Binding Sites Other Than AT_1 and AT_2 Receptors

The Cytosolic Binding Protein

At present, the role of the cytosolic Ang-II-binding protein is unclear. It may be an intracellular transporter protein conveying internalized Ang II to the nucleus where the hormone may affect the expression of some regulatory elements. Alternatively, the cytosolic protein may carry Ang II from an intracellular site of synthesis to the plasma membrane for release, protecting it from intracellular degradation.

The Nuclear Binding Site

Angiotensin II stimulates angiotensinogen mRNA (347,348), increases RNA synthesis in isolated hepatic nuclei (349), and induces changes in chromatin conformation (350). A direct effect on cell growth and cell proliferation has been observed (11,278,351–353). It may be hypothesized that such a nuclear effect may result from binding of the hormone-receptor complex to specific

DNA sequences, leading to change in the expression of target genes. In this sense, Ang II does not differ from other hormones and growth factors for which nuclear binding sites have already been identified (354). The mechanism, however, of translocation of Ang II from the extracellular space to or near the nucleus remains to be defined, as there was no evidence for nuclear association of Ang-II-gold probe, even 60 minutes after internalization had begun (43).

CONCLUSIONS

The recent discovery of Ang II receptor subtypes has given an impetus to extensive work in the molecular biology, physiology, and pharmacology of Ang II. The cloning and sequencing of Ang II receptors and the availability of new selective Ang II receptor ligands will allow a new level of understanding of the biology of Ang II. Although most, if not all, of the commonly known actions of Ang II can be explained by interaction of the peptide with the AT_1 receptor, the existence of other receptor subtypes, such as the AT_2 receptor and other binding sites, may lead to the discovery of additional target sites and functions for Ang II. The existence, at least in rodents, of isoforms of the AT_1 receptor, if confirmed in humans, may have pharmacological implications in mediating tissue-specific functions, receptor regulation, signal transduction, and desensitization mechanisms (355). It may open the road to a better targeting of new compounds. The potential of the other receptors is poorly understood as the physiological role of the AT_2 and other putative receptors is still largely undetermined. The beneficial effect of blocking nonspecifically all Ang II receptors remains to be demonstrated. Therefore, better knowledge of the molecular structure and the signaling mechanisms of the members of this heterogeneous Ang II receptor family will surely prove exciting and informative. Molecular, biological, and chemical tools and methods are already available which could help us to disclose new therapeutic applications.

REFERENCES

1. Bernstein KE. *Ann Med* 1993;24:113–115.
2. Goodfriend TL. *Hypertension* 1991;17:139–140.
3. Chang RSL, Lotti VJ, Keegan ME. *Biochem Pharmacol* 1982;31:1903–1906.
4. Dzau VJ. *Am J Cardiol* 1992;70:C4–C11.
5. Dzau VJ, Gibbons GH. *Am J Cardiol* 1987;60:991–1031.
6. Bottari SP, de Gasparo M, Steckelings UM, Levens NR. *Front Neuroendocrinol* 1993;14:123–171.
7. Dzau VJ. *Basic Res Cardiol* 1993;88:1–14.
8. Schelling P, Fischer H, Ganten D. *J Hypertens* 1991;9:3–15.
9. Naftilan AJ, Pratt RE, Dzau VJ. *J Clin Invest* 1989;83:1419–1424.
10. Naftilan AJ, Pratt RE, Eldridge CS, Lin HL, Dzau VJ. *Hypertension* 1989;13:706–711.
11. Itoh H, Mukoyama M, Pratt RE, Gibbons GH, Dzau VJ. *J Clin Invest* 1993;91:2268–2274.
12. Delafontaine P, Lou H. *J Biol Chem* 1993;268:16866–16870.
13. Barnes JM, Barnes NM, Costall B, et al. *J Cardiovasc Pharmacol* 1992;19[Suppl 6]:S63–S71.
14. Peach MJ. *Physiol Rev* 1977;57:313–370.
15. Papadimitriou A, Worcel M. *Br J Pharmacol* 1974;50:291–297.
16. Timmermans PBMWM, Carini DJ, Chiu AT et al. In: Laragh JH, Brenner BM, eds. *Hypertension: pathophysiology and management.* New York: Raven Press; 1990;2351–2360.
17. Criscione L, de Gasparo M, Buehlmayer P, Whitebread S, Ramjoue HP, Wood JM. *Br J Pharmacol* 1993;110:761–771.
18. Blankley CJ, Hodges JC, Klutchko SR, et al. *J Med Chem* 1991;34:3248–3260.
19. Whitebread S, Mele M, Kamber B, de Gasparo M. *Biochem Biophys Res Commun* 1989;163:284–291.
20. Furukawa Y, Kisshimoto S, Nishikawa K. *US patent* 1982; 4′340′598: 4′355′040.
21. Chiu AT, Herblin WF, McCall DE, et al. *Biochem Biophys Res Commun* 1989;165:196–203.
22. Dudley DT, Panek RL, Major TC, et al. *Mol Pharmacol* 1990;38:370–377.
23. Chang RS, Lotti VJ. *Mol Pharmacol* 1990;37:347–351.
24. de Gasparo M, Whitebread S, Bottari SP, Levens NR. in: Timmermans PB, Wexler RR, eds. *Medicinal chemistry of the renin angiotensin system.* Amsterdam: Elsevier, 1994; (in press).
25. Speth RC, Kim KH. *Biochem Biophys Res Commun* 1990;169:997–1006.
26. Timmermans PB, Carini DJ, Chiu AT, et al. *Hypertension* 1991;18:III136–III142.
27. de Gasparo M, Whitebread S, Mele M, et al. *J Cardiovasc Pharmacol* 1990;16[Suppl 4]:S31–S35.
28. Bumpus FM, Catt KJ, Chiu AT, et al. *Hypertension* 1991;17:720–721.
29. Smith RD, Timmermans PBMWM. Human angiotensis receptor subtypes. *Curr Opin Nephrol Hypertens* 1994;3:112–122.
30. Wiest SA, Rampersaud A, Zimmerman K, Steinberg MI. *J Cardiovasc Pharmacol* 1991;17:177–184.
31. Pendleton RG, Gessner G, Horner E. *J Pharmacol Exp Ther* 1991;256:614–620.
32. Chiu AT, McCall DE, Nguyen TT, et al. *Eur J Pharmacol* 1989;170:117–118.
33. Inagami T, Iwai N, Sasaki K, et al. *J Hypertension* 1992;10:713–716.
34. Yamano Y, Ohyama K, Chaki S, Guo DF, Inagami T. *Biochem Biophys Res Commun* 1992;187:1426–1431.
35. Bottari SP, Taylor V, King IN, Bogdal Y, Whitebread S, de Gasparo M. *Eur J Pharmacol* 1991;207:157–163.
36. McQueen J, Semple PF. *Mol Pharmacol* 1989;35:809–817.
37. Michel AD, Barnes JC. *Br J Pharmacol* 1991;102:205P.
38. Carroll JE, Landry AS, Elliott ME, Goodfriend TL. *J Lab Clin Med* 1986;108:23–29.
39. Catt KJ, Carson MC, Hausdorff WP, et al. *J Steroid Biochem* 1987;27:915–927.
40. Murphy TJ, Alexander RW, Griendling KK, Runge MS, Bernstein KE. *Nature* 1991;351:233–236.
41. Sasaki K, Yamano Y, Bardhan S, et al. *Nature* 1991;351:230–233.
42. Ullian ME, Linas SL. *J Clin Invest* 1989;84:840–846.
43. Anderson KM, Murahashi T, Dostal DE, Peach MJ. *Am J Physiol* 1993;264:C179–C188.
44. Reagan LP, Ye X, Maretzski CH, Fluharty SJ. *J Neurochem* 1993;60:24–31.
45. Chang RS, Lotti VJ, Chen TB, Faust KA. *Biochem Biophys Res Commun* 1990;171:813–817.
46. Obermuller N, Unger T, Culman J, Gohlke P, de Gasparo M, Bottari SP. *Neurosci Lett* 1991;132:11–15.
47. Ernsberger P, Zhou J, Damon TH, Douglas JG. *Am J Physiol* 1992;263:F411–F416.
48. Zhou J, Ernsberger P, Douglas JG. *Hypertension* 1993;21:1035–1038.
49. Madhun ZT, Ernsberger P, Ke FC, Zhou J, Hopfer U, Douglas JG. *Regul Pept* 1993;44:149–157.
50. Cantau B, Bartolami S, Baskevitch PP, Desarnaud F, Chicot D, Jard S. *Biochem J* 1991;277:729–733.
51. Iwai N, Inagami T. *FEBS Lett* 1992;298:257–260.

52. Elton TS, Stephan CC, Taylor GR, et al. *Biochem Biophys Res Commun* 1992;184:1067–1073.
53. Sasamura H, Hein L, Krieger JE, Pratt RE, Kobilka BK, Dzau VJ. *Biochem Biophys Res Commun* 1992;185:253–259.
54. Hahn AWA, Jonas U, Buehler FR, Resink TJ. *Biochem Biophys Res Commun* 1993;192:1260–1265.
55. Sunar-Akbasak B, Kiss A. *75th Annual Meeting The Endocrine Society* 1993;186–544B.
56. Barker S, Marchant W, Clark AJL, et al. *Biochem Biophys Res Commun* 1993;192:392–398.
57. Chiu AT, Dunscomb JH, McCall DE, Benfield P, Baubonis W, Sauer B. *Regul Pept* 1993;44:141–147.
58. Takayanagi R, Ohnaka K, Sakai Y, et al. *Biochem Biophys Res Commun* 1992;183:910–916.
59. Bergsma DJ, Ellis C, Kumar C, et al. *Biochem Biophys Res Commun* 1992;183:989–995.
60a.Furuta H, Guo DF, Inagami T. *Biochem Biophys Res Commun* 1992;183:8–13.
60b.Konishi H, Kuroda S, Inada Y, Fujisawa Y. Novel subtype of human angiotensin II type 1 receptor-cDNA cloning and expression. *Biochem Biophys Res Commun* 1994;199:467–474.
61. Iwai N, Yamano Y, Chaki S, et al. *Biochem Biophys Res Commun* 1991;177:299–304.
61a.Iwai N, Yamano Y, Chaki S, et al. Rat angiotensin II receptor: cDNA sequence and regulation of the gene expression. *Biochem Biophys Res Commun* 1991;177:299–304.
61b.Iwai N, Inagami T, Ohmichi N, et al. Differential regulation of rat AT1a and AT1b receptor mRNA. *Biochem Biophys Res Commun* 1992;188:298–303.
62. Makita N, Iwai N, Inagami T, Badr KF. *Biochem Biophys Res Commun* 1992;185:142–146.
63. Sandberg K, Ji H, Clark AJ, Shapira H, Catt KJ. *J Biol Chem* 1992;267:9455–9458.
64. Sandberg K, Tian Y, Ji H. *75th Annual Meeting The Endocrine Society* 1993;355–1220B.
65. Hodges JC, Hamby JM, Blankley CJ. *Drugs Future* 1992;17:575–593.
66. Smith RD, Chiu AT, Wong PC, Herblin WF, Timmermans PB. *Annu Rev Pharmacol Toxicol* 1992;32:135–165.
67. Steckelings UM, Obermuller N, Bottari SP, Qadri F, Veltmar A, Unger T. *Pharmacol Toxicol* 1992;70:S23–S27.
68. Bunnemann B, Fuxe K, Ganten D. *Regul Pept* 1993;46:487–509.
69. Balla T, Baukal AJ, Eng S, Catt KJ. *Mol Pharmacol* 1991;40:401–406.
70. Naville D, Lebrethon MC, Kermabon AY, Rouer E, Benarous R, Saez J. *FEBS Lett* 1993;321:184–188.
71. Gibson RE, Thorpe HH, Cartwright ME, et al. *Am J Physiol* 1991;261:F512–F518.
72. Edwards RM, Aiyar N. *J Amer Soc Nephrol* 1993;3:1643–1652.
73. Simon M, Fluegge G, Fuchs E, Groene HJ. *FASEB J* 1991;5:A870–2904.
74. Barnes JM, Steward LJ, Barber PC, Barnes NM. *Eur J Pharmacol* 1993;230:251–258.
75. Leung KH, Smith RD, Timmermans BM, Chiu AT. *Neurosci Lett* 1991;123:95–98.
76. Rowe BP, Grove KL, Saylor DL, Speth RC. *Regul Pept* 1991;33:45–53.
77. Song K, Allen AM, Paxinos G, Mendelsohn FA. *Clin Exp Pharmacol Physiol* 1991;18:93–96.
78. Tsutsumi K, Saavedra JM. *Am J Physiol* 1991;261:R209–R216.
79. Gehlert DR, Gackenheimer SL, Reel JK, Lin HS, Steinberg MI. *Eur J Pharmacol* 1990;187:123–126.
80. Barnes JM, Barber PC, Barnes NM. *Neuroreport* 1991;2:605–608.
81. Chang RS, Lotti VJ. *Life Sci* 1991;49:1485–1490.
82. Rogg H, Schmid A, de Gasparo M. *Biochem Biophys Res Commun* 1990;173:416–422.
83. Rogg H, de Gasparo M, Graedel E, Stulz P, Erne P. *Schweiz Med Wochenschr* 1991;121(11)[Suppl 36]:23.
84. Scott AL, Chang RS, Lotti VJ, Siegl PK. *J Pharmacol Exp Ther* 1992;261:931–935.
85. Schambelan M, Sechi LA, Grady EF, Griffin CA, Kalinyak JE. *FASEB J* 1991;5:A870.
86. Sechi LA, Griffin CA, Grady EF, Kalinyak JE, Schambelan M. *Circ Res* 1992;71:1482–1489.
87. Sechi LA, Grady EF, Griffin CA, Kalinyak JE, Schambelan M. *J Hypertens Suppl* 1991;9:S224–S225.
88. Feolde E, Vigne P, Frelin C. *Eur J Pharmacol* 1993;245:63–66.
89. Megges LG, Coupet J, Huang H, et al. *Circ Res* 1993;72:1149–1162.
90. Leung KH, Roscoe WA, Smith RD, Timmermans PBMWM, Chiu AT. *FASEB J* 1991;5:A1767.
91. Tsutsumi K, Saavedra JM. *J Neurochem* 1991;56:348–351.
92. Viswanathan M, Tsutsumi K, Correa FM, Saavedra JM. *Biochem Biophys Res Commun* 1991;179:1361–1367.
93. Keiser JA, Major TC, Lu GH, Davis LS, Panek RL. *Drug Develop Res* 1993;29:94–99.
94. Feuillan PP, Millan MA, Aguilera G. *Regul Pept* 1993;44:159–169.
95. Chiu AT, Carini DJ, Duncia JV, et al. *Biochem Biophys Res Commun* 1991;177:209–217.
96. Tsutsumi K, Saavedra JM. *Am J Physiol* 1991;261:H667–H670.
97. Zhang JS, Van Meel JC, Pfaffendorf M, van Zwieten PA. *Naunyn Schmiedebergs Arch Pharmacol* 1993;347:220–224.
98. Edwards RM, Aiyar N, Ohlstein EH, et al. *J Pharmacol Exp Ther* 1992;260:175–181.
99. Chiu AT, McCall DE, Ardecky RJ, Duncia JV, Nguyen TT, Timmermans PB. *Receptor* 1990;1:33–40.
100. Itazaki K, Shigeri Y, Fujimoto M. *Eur J Pharmacol* 1993;245:147–156.
101. Pratt RE, Wang D, Hein L, Dzau VJ. *Hypertension* 1992;20:432–P52(abst).
102. Panek R, Kaplan C, Overhiser R, et al. *Circulation* 1992;86:I-168(abst).
103. Viswanathan M, Stromberg C, Seltzer A, Saavedra JM. *J Clin Invest* 1992;90:1707–1712.
104. Tsutsumi K, Stromberg C, Saavedra JM. *Peptides* 1992;13:291–296.
105. Burnier M, Centeno G, Grouzmann E, Walker P, Waeber B, Brunner HR. *Am J Hypertens* 1991;4:438–443.
106. Herblin WF, Diamond SM, Timmermans PB. *Peptides* 1991;12:581–584.
107. Zhuo J, Song K, Harris PJ, Mendelsohn FA. *Renal Physiol Biochem* 1992;15:231–239.
108. Song K, Zhuo J, Allen AM, Paxinos G, Mendelsohn FA. *Cardiology* 1991;79[Suppl 1]:45–54.
109. Grone HJ, Simon M, Fuchs E. *Am J Physiol* 1992;262:F326–F331.
110. Gauquelin G, Garcia R. *Receptor* 1992;2:207–212.
111. Edwards RM, Stack EJ, Weidley EF, et al. *J Pharmacol Exp Ther* 1992;260:933–938.
112. Chansel D, Czekalski S, Pham P, Ardaillou R. *Am J Physiol* 1992;262:F432–F441.
113. Sechi LA, Grady EF, Griffin CA, Kalinyak JE, Schambelan M. *Am J Physiol* 1992;262:F236–F240.
114. Burns KD, Inagami T, Harris RC. *Am J Physiol* 1993;264:F645–F654.
115. Meister B, Lippoldt A, Bunnemann B, Inagami T, Ganten D, Fuxe K. *Kidney Int* 1993;44:331–336.
116. Wolf G, Zahner G, Mondorf U, Schoeppe W, Stahl RA. *Nephrol Dial Transplant* 1993;8:128–133.
117. Deleon H, Garcia R. *Receptor* 1992;2:253–260.
118. Goldfarb DA, Diz DI, Tubbs RR, Ferrario CM, Novick AC. Angiotensin II receptor subtypes in the human renal cortex and renal cell carcinoma. *J Urol* 1994;151:208–213.
119. Leung E, Eglen RM. *FASEB J* 1991;5:A871.
120. Ouali R, Poulette S, Penhoat A, Saez JM. *J Steroid Biochem Mol Biol* 1992;43:271–280.
121. Hedberg A, Cohen RB, Liu ECK, Webb ML, Dickinson KEJ. *FASEB J* 1991;5:2871–2909.
122. Rasmussen-Ortega K, Printz MP. *FASEB J* 1991;5:A869–2900.
123. Rowe BP, Saylor DL, Speth RC. *Neuroendocrinology* 1992;55:563–573.
124. Seltzer A, Pinto JE, Viglione PN, et al. *Neuroendocrinology* 1992;55:460–467.
125. Crawford KW, Frey EA, Cote TE. *Mol Pharmacol* 1992;41:154–162.
127. Leung KH, Roscoe WA, Smith RD, Timmermans PB, Chiu AT. *Eur J Pharmacol* 1992;227:63–70.

128. Bauer PH, Chiu AT, Garrison JC. *Mol Pharmacol* 1991;39:579–585.
129. Gonzalez Espinosa C, Garcia Sainz JA. *Biochim Biophys Acta* 1992;1136:309–314.
130. Wintersgill HP, Warburton P, Bryson SE, Ball SG, Balmforth AJ. *Eur J Pharmacol* 1992;227:283–291.
131. Kozlowski MR, Arcuri M, Zynardi L. *J Recept Res* 1993;13:1031–1040.
132. Eglen RM, Rapp JM, Leung E. *FASEB J* 1991;5:A869–2898.
133. Schinke M, Doods HN, Ganten D, Wienen W, Entzeroth M. *Eur J Pharmacol* 1991;204:165–170.
134. Sechi LA, Valentin JP, Griffin CA, Schambelan M. *Am J Physiol* 1993;265:G21–G27.
135. Chappell MC, Diz DI, Jacobsen DW. *Peptides* 1992;13:313–318.
136. Chappell MC, Millsted A, Diz DI, Brosnihan KB, Ferrario CM. *J HYPERTENS* 1991;9:751–759.
137. Servant G, Boulay G, Bosse R, Escher E, Guillemette G. *Mol Pharmacol* 1993;43:677–683.
138. Cox BE, Ipson MA, Kamm KE, Shaul PW, Horning KM, Rosenfeld CR. *FASEB J* 1992;6:A1578–3718.
139. Pucell AG, Hodges JC, Sen I, Bumpus FM, Husain A. *Endocrinology* 1991;128:1947–1959.
140. Brunswig-Spickenheier B, Mukhopadhyay AK. *Endocrinology* 1992;131:1445–1452.
141. Aiyar N, Griffin E, Edwards R, Weinstock J, Samanen J, Nambi P. *Pharmacology* 1993;46:1–8.
142. Grady EF, Sechi LA, Griffin CA, Schambelan M, Kalinyak JE. *J Clin Invest* 1991;88:921–933.
143. Kalenga MK, de Gasparo M, De Hertogh R, Whitebread S, Vankrieken L, Thomas K. *Reprod Nutr Dev* 1991;31:257–267.
144. Kalenga MK, De Hertogh R, Whitebread S, Vankrieken L, Thomas K, de Gasparo M. *Rev Fr Gynecol Obstet* 1991;86:585–591.
145. Kalenga MK, de Gasparo M, Whitebread S, Vankrieken L, Thomas K, De Hertogh R. *Reprod Nutr Dev* 1992;32:47–54.
146. Hegde SS, Clarke DE. *J Pharmacol Exp Ther* 1993;265:601–608.
147. Grove KL, Speth RC. *Endocrinology* 1989;125:223–230.
148. Crandall DL, Herzlinger HE, Saunders BD, Zolotor RC, Feliciano L, Cervoni P. *Metabolism* 1993;42:511–515.
149. Entzeroth M, Hadamovsky S. *Eur J Pharmacol* 1991;206:237–241.
150. Tsutsumi K, Viswanathan M, Stromberg C, Saavedra JM. *Eur J Pharmacol* 1991;198:89–92.
151. Bottari SP, Obermuller N, Bogdal Y, Zahs KR, Deschepper CF. *Brain Res* 1992;585:372–376.
152. Gehlert DR, Gackenheimer SL, Schober DA. *Neuroscience* 1991;44:501–514.
153. Aldred GP, Chai SY, Song KF, Zhuo JL, MacGregor DP, Mendelsohn FAO. *Regul Pept* 1993;44:119–130.
154. Phillips MI, Shen L, Richards EM, Raizada MK. *Regul Pept* 1993;44:95–107.
155. Wamsley JK, Herblin WF, Alburges ME, Hunt M. *Brain Res Bull* 1990;25:397–400.
156. Bunnemann B, Iwai N, Metzger R, Fuxe K, Inagami T, Ganten D. *Neurosci Lett* 1992;142:155–158.
157. Heemskerk FMJ, Zorad S, Seltzer A, Saavedra JM. *Neuroreport* 1993;4:103–105.
158. Tsutsumi K, Saavedra JM. *Endocrinology* 1991;129:3001–3008.
159. Steckelings UM, Bottari SP, Unger T. *Trends Pharmacol Sci* 1992;13:365–368.
160. Saylor DL, Perez RA, Absher DR, et al. *Brain Res* 1992;595:98–106.
161. Pfister J, Felix D, Imboden H. *Regul Pept* 1993;44:109–117.
162. Foucart S, Murphy TV, Majewski H. *J Auton Nerv Syst* 1990;30:221–232.
163. Buisson B, Bottari SP, de Gasparo M, Gallo-Payet N, Payet M. *FEBS LETT* 1992;309:161–164.
164. Zarahn ED, Ye X, Ades AM, Reagan LP, Fluharty SJ. *J Neurochem* 1992;58:1960–1963.
165. Sumners C, Richards EM, Tang W, Raizada MK. *Regul Pept* 1993;44:181–188.
166. Sumners C, Tang W, Zelezna B, Raizada MK. *Proc Natl Acad Sci USA* 1991;88:7567–7571.
167. Zemel S, Millan MA, Aguilera G. *Endocrinology* 1989;124:1774–1780.
168. Millan MA, Carvallo P, Izumi S, Zemel S, Catt KJ, Aguilera G. *Science* 1989;244:1340–1342.
169. Shanmugan S, Monnot C, Corvol P, Gasc JM. Distribution of type 1 angiotensin II receptor subtype messenger RNAs in the rat fetus. *Hypertension* 1994;23:137–141.
170. Zemel S, Millan MA, Feuillan P, Aguilera G. *J Clin Endocrinol Metab* 1990;71:1003–1007.
171. Johnson MC, Aguilera G. *Endocrinology* 1991;129:1266–1274.
172. Viswanathan M, Saavedra JM. *Peptides* 1992;13:783–786.
173. Dudley DT, Hubbell SE, Summerfelt RM. *Mol Pharmacol* 1991;40:360–367.
174. Ohnishi J, Ishido M, Shibata T, Inagami T, Murakami K, Miyazaki H. *Biochem Biophys Res Commun* 1992;186:1094–1101.
175. Pobiner BF, Northup JK, Bauer PH, Fraser ED, Garrison JC. *Mol Pharmacol* 1991;40:156–167.
176. Sims C, Ashby K, Douglas JG. *Hypertension* 1992;19:146–152.
177. Douglas JG, Romero M, Hopfer U. *Kidney Int Suppl* 1990;30:S43–S47.
178. Jard S, Cantau B, Jackobs KH. *J Biol Chem* 1981;256:2603–2606.
179. Pobiner BF, Hewlett EL, Garrison GC. *J Biol Chem* 1985;260:16200–16209.
180. Catt KJ, Balla T, Baukal AJ, Hausdorff WP, Aguilera G. *Clin Exp Pharmacol Physiol* 1988;15:501–515.
181. Missale C, Memo M, Sigala S, Carruba MO, Spano P. *Regul Pept* 1989;24:167–178.
182. Rainey WE, Byrd EW, Sinnokrot RA, Carr BR. *Mol Cell Endocrinol* 1991;81:33–41.
183. Kubalak SW, Webb JG. *Am J Physiol* 1993;264:H86–H96.
184. Baranczyk-Kuzma A, Audus KL, Guillot FL. *Neurochem Res* 1992;17:209–214.
185. Sumners C, Myers LM, Kalberg CJ, Raizada MK. *Prog Neurobiol* 1990;34:355–385.
186. Pfeilschifter J. *Eur J Clin Invest* 1989;19:347–361.
187. Huckle WR, Dy RC, Earp HS. *Proc Natl Acad Sci USA* 1992;89:8837–8841.
188. Smith JB, Lincoln TM. *Am J Physiol* 1987;253:C147–C150.
189. Bihoreau C, Monnot C, Davies E, et al. *Proc Natl Acad Sci USA* 1993;90:5133–5137.
190. Pfeilschifter J, Fandrey G, Ochsner M, Whitebread S, de Gasparo M. *FEBS Lett* 1990;261:307–311.
191. Smith JB, Smith L, Brown ER, et al. *Proc Natl Acad Sci USA* 1984;81:7812–7816.
192. Tsuda T, Kawahara Y, Ishida Y, Koide M, Shii K, Yokoyama M. *Circ Res* 1992;71:620–630.
193. Moorman JR, Kirsch GE, Lacerda AE, Brown AM. *Circ Res* 1989;65:1804–1809.
194. Nilius B, Tytgat J, Albitz R. *Biochim Biophys Acta* 1989;1014:259–262.
195. Molloy CJ, Taylor DS, Weber H. *J Biol Chem* 1993;268:7338–7345.
196. Stouffer GA, Owens GK. *Circ Res* 1992;70:820–828.
197. Gibbons GH, Pratt RE, Dzau VJ. *J Clin Invest* 1992;90:456–461.
198. Ververis JJ, Ku L, Delafontaine P. *Circ Res* 1993;72:1285–1292.
199. Lyall F, Dornan ES, McQueen J, Boswell F, Kelly M. *J Hypertens* 1992;10:1463–1469.
200. Pfeilschifter J, Huwiler A, Merriweather C, Briner VA. *Eur J Pharmacol* 1992;225:57–62.
201. Lassegue B, Alexander RW, Clark M, Akers M, Griendling KK. *Biochem J* 1993;292:509–517.
202. Capponi AM, Lew PD, Jornot L, Vallotton MB. *J Biol Chem* 1984;259:8863–8869.
203. Capponi AM, Lew PD, Vallotton MB. *Biochem J* 1987;247:335–340.
204. Brauneis U, Vassiev PM, Quinn SJ, Williams GH, Tillotson DL. *Am J Physiol* 1991;260:E772–E779.
205. Cohen CJ, McCarthy RT, Barrett PQ, Rasmussen H. *Proc Natl Acad Sci USA* 1988;85:2412–2416.
206. Miyoshi Y, Nakaya Y. *Biochem Biophys Res Commun* 1991;181:700–706.
207. Kurokawa K, Okuda T. *Kidney Int* 1990;38:S48–S50.
208. Webb ML, Liu EC, Cohen RB, et al. *Peptides* 1992;13:499–508.
209. Tsutsumi K, Saavedra JM. *Cell Mol Neurobiol* 1991;11:295–299.
210. Speth RC, Rowe BP, Grove KL, Carter MR, Saylor D. *Brain Res* 1991;548:1–8.

211. Montiel M, Barker S, Vinson GP, Jimenez E. *J Mol Endocrinol* 1993 [in press].
212. Dudley DT, Summerfelt RM. *Regul Pept* 1993;44:199–206.
213. Tsutsumi K, Stromberg C, Viswanathan M, Saavedra JM. *Endocrinology* 1991;129:1075–1082.
214. Cook VI, Grove KL, McMenamin KM, Carter MR, Harding JW, Speth R. *Brain Res* 1991;560:334–336.
215. Carrithers MD, Ghoneim W, Shelman W, Weyhenmeyer JA. Regulation of tyrosine phosphorylation by angiotensin II in differentiated NG108-15 cells. *Soc Neurosci Abstracts* 1992; 18: 488,2.
216. Bottari SP, King IN, Reichlin S, Dahlstroem I, Lydon N, de Gasparo M. *Biochem Biophys Res Commun* 1992;183:206–211.
217. Brechler V, Reichlin S, Levens NR, de Gasparo M, Bottari SP. *Recept & Channels* 1994 (in press).
218. Brechler V, Jones PW, Levens NR, de Gasparo M, Bottari SP. *Regul Pept* 1993;44:207–213.
219. de Gasparo M, Whitebread S, Levens N, et al. in: Saez JM, Brownie AC, Capponi A, Chambaz EM, Mantero F, eds. *Cellular and molecular biology of the adrenal cortex; vol 222.* London: Colloque INSERM/John Libbey Eurotext; 1992;3–17.
220. de Gasparo M, Levens NR, Kamber B, et al. in: Timmermans PB, Saavedra JM, eds. *Angiotensin receptor.* New York: Plenum; 1994 (in press).
221. Brechler V, de Gasparo M, Bottari SP. *Recept & Channels* 1994 (in press).
222. Florio T, Pan MG, Newman B, Hershberger RE, Civelli O, Stork PJS. *J Biol Chem* 1992;267:24169–24172.
223. Pan MG, Florio T, Stork PJS. *Science* 1992;256:1215–1217.
224. Tsutsumi K, Saavedra JM. *Mol Pharmacol* 1992;41:290–297.
225. Tsutsumi K, Zorad S, Saavedra JM. *Eur J Pharmacol* 1992;226: 169–173.
226. Siemens IR, Adler HJ, Addya K, Mah SJ, Fluharty SJ. *Mol Pharmacol* 1991;40:717–726.
227. Mah SJ, Ades AM, Mir R, Siemens IR, Williamson JR, Fluharty SJ. *Mol Pharmacol* 1992;42:217–226.
228. Kiron MA, Soffer RL. *J Biol Chem* 1989;264:4138–4142.
229. Hagiwara H, Sugiura N, Wakita K, Hirose S. *Eur J Biochem* 1989;185:405–410.
230. Sugiura N, Hagiwara H, Hirose S. *J Biol Chem* 1992;267:18067–18072.
231. Sen I, Rajasekaran AK. *J Mol Cell Cardiol* 1991;23:563–572.
232. Robertson AL, Khairallah PA. *Science* 1971;172:1138–1139.
233. Re RN, MacPhee AA, Fallon JT. *Clin Sci* 1981;61:245S–247S.
234. Tang SS, Rogg H, Schumacher R, Dzau VJ. *Endocrinology* 1992;131:374–380.
235. Booz GW, Conrad KM, Hess AL, Singer HA, Baker KM. *Endocrinology* 1992;130:3641–3649.
236. Smith CD, Wells WW. *J Biol Chem* 1983;258:9368–9373.
237. Nicotera P, Orrenius S, Nilsson T, Berggren PO. *Proc Natl Acad Sci USA* 1990;87:6858–6862.
238. Wagner LA, Andree T, Buckley JP. *Res Commun Chem Pathol Pharmacol* 1978;22:267–275.
239. Abhold RH, Harding JW. *J Pharmacol Exp Ther* 1988;245:171–177.
240. Ferrario CM, Brosnihan KB, Diz DI, et al. *Hypertension* 1991;18[Suppl III]:123–133.
241. Chappell MC, Brosnihan KB, Diz DI, Ferrario CM. *J Biol Chem* 1989;288:16518–16523.
242. Schiavone MT, Khosla MC, Ferrario CM. *J Cardiovasc Pharmacol* 1990;16[Suppl 4]:S19–S24.
243. Silva LCS, Fontes MAP, Campagnolesantos MJ, et al. *Brain Res* 1993;613:321–325.
244. Jaiswal N, Diz DI, Chappell MC, Khosla MC, Ferrario CM. *Hypertension* 1992;19:II49–II55.
245. Jaiswal N, Tallant EA, Diz DI, Khosla MC, Ferrario CM. *Hypertension* 1991;17:1115–1120.
246. Jaiswal N, Diz DI, Tallant EA, Khosla MC, Ferrario CM. *Am J Physiol* 1991;260:R1000–R1006.
247. Jaiswal N, Tallant EA, Jaiswal RK, Diz DI, Ferrario CM. *J Pharmacol Exp Ther* 1993;265:664–673.
248. Dellipizzi AM, Hilchey SD, Quilley CP. *Hypertension* 1994; (in press).
249. Haberl RL, Decker PL, Einhaeupl KM. *Circ Res* 1991;68:1621–1627.
250. Swanson GN, Hanesworth JM, Sardinia MF, et al. *Regul Pept* 1992;40:409–419.
251. Braszko JJ, Kupryszewski G, Witczuk B, Wisniewski K. *Neuroscience* 1988;27:777–783.
252. Jarvis MF, Gessner GW, Ly CQ. *Eur J Pharmacol* 1992;219: 319–322.
253. Harding JW, Cook VI, Millerwing AV, et al. *Brain Res* 1992;583: 340–343.
254. Hall KL, Hanesworth JM, Ball AE, Felgenhauer GP, Hosick HL, Harding JW. *Regul Pept* 1993;44:225–232.
255. Dostal DE, Murahashi T, Peach MJ. *Hypertension* 1990;15:815–822.
256. Sandberg K, Ji H, Millan MA, Catt KJ. *FEBS Lett* 1991;284: 281–284.
257. Ji H, Sandberg K, Catt KJ. *Mol Pharmacol* 1991;39:120–123.
258. Ji H, Sandberg K, Zhang Y, Catt KJ. *Biochem Biophys Res Commun* 1993;194:756–762.
259. Nishimura H, Walker OE, Patton CM. *Hypertension* 1992;20: 435.
260. Lenoble FAC, Schreurs NHJS, vanStraaten HWM, et al. *Am J Physiol* 1993;264:R460–R465.
261. Kawano M, Koshikawa T, Kanzaki T, Morisaki N, Saito Y, Yoshida S. *Eur J Clin Invest* 1993;23:84–90.
262. Carsia RV, Mcilroy PJ, Kowalski KI, Tilly JL. *Biochem Biophys Res Commun* 1993;191:1073–1080.
263. Bergwitz C, Madoff S, Abou Samra AB, Juppner H. *Biochem Biophys Res Commun* 1991;179:1391–1399.
264. Whitebread S, Pfeilschifter J, Ramjoue H, de Gasparo M. *Regul Pept* 1993;44:233–238.
265. Chaki S, Inagami T. *Biochem Biophys Res Commun* 1992;182: 388–394.
266. Chaki S, Inagami T. *Eur J Pharmacol* 1992;225:355–356.
267. Chaki S, Inagami T. *Mol Pharmacol* 1993;43:603–608.
268. Jackson TR, Blair LAC, Marshall J, Goedert M, Hanley MR. *Nature* 1988;335:437–440.
269. Hanley MR. *J Cardiovasc Pharmacol* 1991;18[Suppl 2]:S7–13.
270. Ambroz C, Clark AJ, Catt KJ. *Biochim Biophys Acta* 1991;1133: 107–111.
271. Ross PC, Figler RA, Corjay MH, et al. *Proc Natl Acad Sci USA* 1990;87:3052–3056.
272. Monnot C, Weber V, Stinnakre J, et al. *Mol Endocrinol* 1991;5: 1477–1487.
273. Song K, Shiota N, Okunishi H, Miyazaki M. *Life Sci* 1992;51: PL165–PL170.
274. Timmermans PB, Chiu AT, Herblin WF, Wong PC, Smith RD. *Am J Hypertens* 1992;5:406–410.
275. Buehlmayer P. *Drugs Future* 1992;2:1693–1718.
276. Dudley DT, Hamby JM. *Drugs Future* 1993;3:581–596.
277. Timmermans PB, Benfield P, Chiu AT, Herblin WF, Wong PC, Smith R. *Am J Hypertens* 1992;5:221S–235S.
278. Geisterfer AAT, Peach MJ, Owens GK. *Circ Res* 1988;62:749–756.
279. Prescott MF, Sawyer WK. *Drug Develop Res* 1993;29:88–93.
280. Kauffman RF, Bean JS, Zimmerman KM, Brown RF, Steinberg MI. *Life Sci* 1991;49:223–228.
281. Smits JF, van Krimpen C, Schoemaker RG, Cleutjens JP, Daemen MJ. *J Cardiovasc Pharmacol* 1992;20:772–778.
282. Azuma H, Niimi Y, Hamasaki H. *Br J Pharmacol* 1992;106: 665–671.
283. Barnes NM, Champaneria S, Costall B, Kelly ME, Murphy DA, Naylor RJ. *Neuroreport* 1990;1:239–242.
284. Barnes NM, Costall B, Kelly ME, Murphy DA, Naylor RJ. *Neuroreport* 1990;1:20–21.
285. Timmermans PBMWM, Wong PC, Chiu AT, et al. *Pharmacol Rev* 1993;45:205–251.
286. Bunkenburg B, Schnell C, Baum HP, Cumin F, Wood JM. *Hypertension* 1991;18:278–288.
287. Ohtawa M, Takayama F, Saitoh K, Yoshinaga T, Nakashima M. *Br J Clin Pharmacol* 1993;35:290–297.
288. Goldberg MR, Tanaka W, Barchowsky A, et al. *Hypertension* 1993;21:704–713.
289. Christen Y, Waeber B, Nussberger J, et al. *Circulation* 1991;83: 1333–1342.
290. Mizuno K, Tani M, Hashimoto S, et al. *Life Sci* 1992;51:367–374.

291. Abdelrahman AM, Burrell LM, Johnston CI. *J Hypertension* 1993;11:S23–S26.
292. Mizuno K, Niimura S, Tani M, et al. *Life Sci* 1992;51:PL183–PL187.
293. Macari D, Whitebread S, de Gasparo M, Bottari SP, Levens N. *Eur J Pharmacol* 1993;249:85–93.
294. Moffet RB, Bumpus FM, Husain A. *Life Sci* 1987;41:1867–1879.
295. Wong PC, Hart SD, Zaspel AM, et al. *J Pharmacol Exp Ther* 1990;255:584–592.
296. Kirby RF, Thunhorst RL, Johnson AK. *Brain Res* 1992;576:348–350.
297. Hogarty DC, Speakman EA, Puig V, Phillips MI. *Brain Res* 1992;586:289–294.
298. Bains JS, Potyok A, Ferguson AV. *Brain Res* 1992;599:223–229.
299. Yang RH, Jin HK, Wyss JM, Oparil A. Depressor effect of blocking angiotensis subtype-1 receptor in anterior hypothalamus. *Hypertension* 1992;19:475–481.
300. Widdop RE, Gardiner SM, Kemp PA, Bennett T. *Am J Physiol* 1993;264:H117–H125.
301. Speakman EA, Hogarty D, Puig V, Phillips MI. *FASEB J* 1992;6:5416.
302. Beresford MJ, Fitzsimons JT. *Exp Physiol* 1992;77:761–764.
303. Dourish CT, Duggan JA, Banks RJ. *Eur J Pharmacol* 1992;211:113–116.
304. Stephenson KN, Steele MK. *J Neuroendocrinol* 1992;4:441–447.
305. Blair-West JR, Denton DA, McKinley MJ, Weisinger RS. *Am J Physiol* 1992;262:R204–R210.
306. Fregly MJ, Rowland NE. *Brain Res Bull* 1991;27:97–100.
307. Barbella Y, Cierco M, Israel A. *Proc Soc Exp Biol Med* 1993;202:401–406.
308. Schiavone MT, Brosnihan KB, Khosla MC, Ferrario CM. *Hypertension* 1991;17:425.
309. Yang CR, Phillips MI, Renaud LP. *Am J Physiol* 1992;263:R1333–R1338.
310. Veltmar A, Culman J, Qadri F, Rascher W, Unger T. *J Pharmacol Exp Ther* 1992;263:1253–1260.
311. Barnes NM, Costall B, Kelly ME, Murphy DA, Naylor RJ. *Neuroreport* 1991;2:351–353.
312. Reit E. *Fed Proc* 1972;31:1338–1343.
313. Hawcock AB, Barnes JC, Michel AD. *Br J Pharmacol* 1992;105:686–690.
314. Ambuhl P, Felix D, Imboden H, Khosla MC, Ferrario CM. *Regul Pept* 1992;38:111–120.
315. Ambuhl P, Felix D, Imboden H, Khosla MC, Ferrario CM. *Regul Pept* 1992;41:19–26.
316. Kang J, Sumners C, Posner P. *Brain Res* 1992;580:317–324.
317. Abdelrahman A, Pang CC. *Can J Physiol Pharmacol* 1992;70:716–719.
318. Wong PC, Chiu AT, Duncia JV, Herblin WF, Smith RD, Timmermans PBMWM. *Trends Endocrinol Metab* 1992;3:211–217.
319. Widdop RE, Gardiner SM, Kemp PA, Bennett T. *Br J Pharmacol* 1992;107:873–880.
320. Scheuer DA, Perrone MH. *Am J Physiol* 1993;264:R917–R923.
321. Koch-Weser J. *Circ Res* 1964;14:337–344.
322. Ruzicka M, Yuan B, Harmsen E, Leenen FH. *Circulation* 1993;87:921–930.
323. Sudhir K, MacGregor JS, Gupta M, et al. *Circulation* 1993;87:931–938.
324. Hartman JC, Hullinger TG, Wall TM, Shebuski RJ. *Eur J Pharmacol* 1993;234:229–236.
325. Kambayashi Y, Bardhan S, Inagami T. *Biochem Biophys Res Commun* 1993;194:478–482.
326. Paulson OB, Waldemar G. *Blood Vessels* 1991;28:231–235.
327. Brix J, Haberl RL. *FASEB J* 1992;6:A1264–1896(abst).
328. Stromberg C, Naveri L, Saavedra JM. *Neuroreport* 1992;3:703–704.
329. Stromberg C, Naveri L, Saavedra JM. *J Cereb Blood Flow Metab* 1993;13:298–303.
330. Clark KL, Robertson MJ, Drew GM. *Br J Pharmacol* 1992;106:19.
331. Keiser JA, Bjork FA, Hodges JC, Taylor DG, Jr. *J Pharmacol Exp Ther* 1992;262:1154–1160.
332. Clark KL, Robertson MJ, Drew GM. *Br J Pharmacol* 1993;109:148–156.
333. Cogan MG, Liu FY, Wong PC, Timmermans PB. *J Pharmacol Exp Ther* 1991;259:687–691.
334. Mento PF, Maita ME, Wilkes BM. *Hypertension* 1992;20:426–P66.(abst)
335. Andrade-Gordon P, Zreck T, Apa R, Naftolin F. *Biochem Pharmacol* 1991;42:715–719.
336. Yoshimura Y, Karube M, Koyama N, Shiokawa S, Nanno T, Nakamura Y. *FEBS Lett* 1992;307:305–308.
337. Peterson CM, Zhu C, Mukaida T, Butler TA, Woessner JF Jr., Lemaire WJ. *Am J Obstet Gynecol* 1993;168:242–245.
338. Ferrari Dileo G, Davis EB, Anderson DR. *Invest Ophthalmol Vis Sci* 1991;32:21–26.
339. Grady EF, Kalinyak JE. *Regul Pept* 1993;44:171–180.
340. Phillips MI, Kimura B, Krim AJ, Konicek JR, Fossum GT. *FASEB J* 1991;A904–3103.
341. Gyurko R, Kimura B, Kurian P, Crews FT, Phillips MI. *Biochem Biophys Res Commun* 1992;186:285–292.
342. Powell JS, Clozel JP, Mueller RKM, et al. *Science* 1989;245:186–188.
343. Janiak P, Pillon A, Prost JF, Vilaine JP. *Hypertension* 1992;20:737–745.
344. Toney GM, Porter JP. *Neuropharmacology* 1993;32:581–589.
345. Toney GM, Porter JP. *Brain Res* 1993;603:57–63.
346. Wong PC, Cnrist DD, Timmermans PB. *Eur J Pharmacol* 1992;220:267–270.
347. Nakamura A, Iwao H, Fukui K, et al. *Am J Physiol* 1990;258:E1–E6.
348. Hermann H, Dzau VJ. *Circ Res* 1988;52:328–334.
349. Re RN, Parab M. *Life Sci* 1984;34:647–651.
350. Re RN, LaBiche RA, Bryan SE. *Biochem Biophys Res Commun* 1983;110:61–68.
351. Aceto JF, Baker KM. *Am J Physiol* 1990;258:H806–H813.
352. Wolf G, Neilson EG. *Am J Physiol* 1990;259:F768–F777.
353. Anderson PW, Do YS, Hsueh WA. *Hypertension* 1993;21:29–35.
354. Burwen SJ, Jones AL. *Trends Biochem Sci* 1987;12:159–162.
355. Dzau VJ, Sasamura H, Hein L. *J Hypertens* 1993;11[Suppl 3]:S13–S18.
356. Takahasi K, Bardhan S, Kambayashi Y, Shirai H, Inagami T. Protein tyrosine phosphatase inhibition by angiotensin II in rat pheochromocytoma cells through type 2 receptor, AT2. *Biochem Biophysic Res Commun* 1994;198:60–66.
357. Mukoyama M, Nakajima M, Horiuchi M, Sasamura H, Pratt RE, Dzau VJ. Expression cloning of type 2 angiotensin II receptor reveals a unique class of seven-transmembrane receptors. *J Biol Chem* 1993;268:24539–24542.
358. Kambayashi Y, Bardhan S, Takahashi K, et al. Molecular cloning of a novel angiotensin II receptor isoform involved in phosphotyrosine phosphatase inhibition. *J Biol Chem* 1993;268:24543–24546.
359. Nakajima M, Mukoyama M, Pratt RE, Horiuchi M, Dzau VJ. Cloning of cDNA and analysis of the gene for mouse angiotensin II type 2 receptor. *Biochem Biophys Res Commun* 1993;197:393–399.